ADULT
CHEST SURGERY

David J. Sugarbaker, MD

Director, The Lung Institute
Chief, Division of Thoracic Surgery
The Olga Keith Weiss Chair of Surgery
Baylor College of Medicine
Baylor St. Luke's Medical Center
Houston, Texas

Raphael Bueno, MD

Professor of Surgery
Harvard Medical School
Chief, Division of Thoracic Surgery
Vice Chair of Surgery for Cancer and Translational Research
Brigham and Women's Hospital
Boston, Massachusetts

Yolonda L. Colson, MD

Professor of Surgery
Harvard Medical School
Associate Administrative Chief
Division of Thoracic Surgery
Brigham and Women's Hospital
Boston, Massachusetts

Michael T. Jaklitsch, MD

Associate Professor of Surgery
Harvard Medical School
Brigham and Women's Hospital
Boston, Massachusetts

Mark J. Krasna, MD

Medical Director, Oncology
Meridian Cancer Care
Jersey Shore University Medical Center
Neptune, New Jersey

Steven J. Mentzer, MD

Professor of Surgery
Harvard Medical School
Senior Surgeon, Division of Thoracic Surgery
Brigham and Women's Hospital
Boston, Massachusetts

ADULT CHEST SURGERY

SECOND EDITION

Editors

David J. Sugarbaker
Raphael Bueno
Yolonda L. Colson
Michael T. Jaklitsch
Mark J. Krasna
Steven J. Mentzer

With

Marcia Williams
Ann Adams

Mc Graw Hill Education

New York Chicago San Francisco Athens London Madrid Mexico City
Milan New Delhi Singapore Sydney Toronto

Adult Chest Surgery, Second Edition

1 2 3 4 5 6 7 8 9 0 CTP/CTP 19 18 17 16 15 14

ISBN 978-0-07-178189-3
MHID 0-07-178189-7

NOTICE

Medicine is an ever-changing science. As new research and clinical experience broaden our knowledge, changes in treatment and drug therapy are required. The authors and the publisher of this work have checked with sources believed to be reliable in their efforts to provide information that is complete and generally in accord with the standards accepted at the time of publication. However, in view of the possibility of human error or changes in medical sciences, neither the authors nor the publisher nor any other party who has been involved in the preparation or publication of this work warrants that the information contained herein is in every respect accurate or complete, and they disclaim all responsibility for any errors or omissions or for the results obtained from use of the information contained in this work. Readers are encouraged to confirm the information contained herein with other sources. For example and in particular, readers are advised to check the product information sheet included in the package of each drug they plan to administer to be certain that the information contained in this work is accurate and that changes have not been made in the recommended dose or in the contraindications for administration. This recommendation is of particular importance in connection with new or infrequently used drugs.

This book was set in Warnock Pro by Aptara® Inc.
The editors were Brian Belval and Peter J. Boyle.
The production supervisor was Richard Ruzycka.
Project management was provided by Indu Jawwad, Aptara, Inc.
The designer was Alan Barnett.
China Translation & Printing, Ltd., was the printer and binder.

This book was printed on acid-free paper.

Library of Congress Cataloging-in-Publication Data

Adult chest surgery / editors, David J. Sugarbaker, Raphael Bueno, Yolonda L. Colson, Michael T. Jaklitsch, Mark J. Krasna, Steven J. Mentzer with Marcia Williams, Ann Adams. – Second edition.
p. ; cm.
Includes bibliographical references and index.
ISBN 978-0-07-178189-3 (hardcover : alk. paper) – ISBN 0-07-178189-7 (hardcover : alk. paper)
I. Sugarbaker, David J., editor. II. Bueno, Raphael, editor. III. Colson, Yolonda L., editor. IV. Jaklitsch, Michael T., editor. V. Krasna, Mark, editor. VI. Mentzer, Steven J., editor.
[DNLM: 1. Thoracic Surgical Procedures–methods. 2. Esophageal Diseases–surgery. 3. Lung Diseases–surgery. 4. Mediastinal Diseases–surgery. 5. Pleural Diseases–surgery. WF 980]
RD536
617.5'4059–dc23

2014027058

DEDICATION

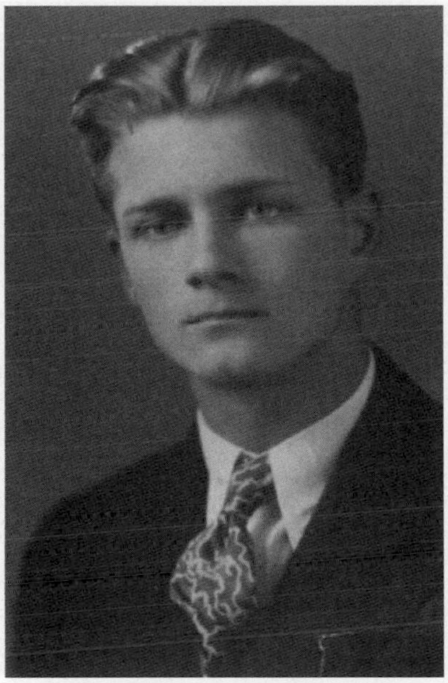

Everett D. Sugarbaker, MD

— 1910 to 2001 —

"Wherever you are, it is 90% you and 10% institution."

Cornell University Medical College, MD, 1935
Memorial Hospital, New York, 1937
Chief of Surgery, National Cancer Institute, Bethesda, Maryland, 1940
Chief of Surgery/Chief of Staff, Ellis Fischel Hospital, Columbia, Missouri, 1942
Sugarbaker Tumor Clinic, Jefferson City, Missouri, 1948 to 1983

To my father, Everett D. Sugarbaker: inventor, author, researcher, mentor, and master surgeon.

IN MEMORIAM

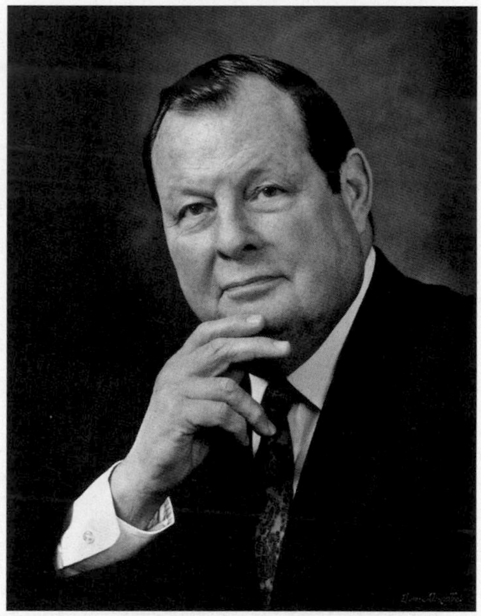

Harold C. Urschel, Jr., MD

1930 to 2013

Professor of Surgery,
Department of Cardiothoracic Surgery,
Baylor University Medical Center, Dallas, Texas

Our colleague, Harold (Hal) C. Urschel, has passed since the first edition of this book was published. He will be greatly missed. Hal was not only a master surgeon, author, and mentor, but also our true friend.

Contents

Contributors

Ann Adams
Sr. Consulting Medical Writer
Department of Surgery
Massachusetts General Hospital
Boston, Massachusetts
Chapter 68, Overview of Anatomy and Pathophysiology of Lung Cancer
Chapter 103, Surgical Treatment of Thoracic Fungal Infections

Hiroshi Akiyama, MD
Emeritus Director of Toranomon Hospital
Tokyo, Japan
Chapter 20, Three-Field Esophagectomy

Naveed Zeb Alam, MD, FRCSC, FRACS
Consultant Thoracic Surgeon
St. Vincent's Hospital Melbourne, Department of Surgery
Senior Lecturer, University of Melbourne
Melbourne, Victoria
Australia
Chapter 121, Pleurectomy and Decortication for Malignant Pleural Diseases

Ali O.M. Al Dameh, MD
Division of Thoracic Surgery
Harvard Medical School
Brigham and Woman Hospital
Boston, Massachusetts
Chapter 9, Techniques for Pleural Drainage and Chest Tube Management

Majed A. Al-Mourgi, FRCS
Department of Surgery
Taif University
Taif, Kingdom of Saudi Arabia
Chapter 44, Techniques for Dilation of Benign Esophageal Stricture

Miguel Alvelo-Rivera, MD
Associate Professor of Surgery
Cardiothoracic Surgery
Harper University Hospital
Wayne State University
Chapter 144, Thoracoscopic First Rib Resection with Dorsal Sympathectomy

Rafael S. Andrade, MD
Section of Thoracic and Foregut Surgery
Department of Surgery
University of Minnesota
Minneapolis, Minnesota
Chapter 151, Plication of the Diaphragm from Below

Luis M. Argote-Greene, MD
Chief, Thoracic Surgery
National Institute of Medical Science and Nutrition "Salvador Zubiran"
National Autonomous University of Mexico (UNAM)
Mexico City, Mexico
Chapter 159, Thoracoscopic Approach to Thymectomy with Advice on Patients with Myasthenia Gravis

Simon K. Ashiku, MD
Northern California Thoracic Group
Permanente Medical Group
Walnut Creek Medical Center
Walnut Creek, California
Chapter 64, Resection of the Carina

Nasser K. Altorki, MD
Professor of Thoracic Surgery
New York Presbyterian-Weill Cornell Medical College
New York, New York
Chapter 19, Radical En Bloc Esophagectomy

Edward D. Auyang, MD, MS
Assistant Professor of Surgery
University of New Mexico
Albuquerque, New Mexico
Chapter 41, Surgery and Endoscopic Interventions for Barrett Esophagus

Lindsey Robert Baden, MD
Associate Professor of Medicine
Harvard Medical School
Department of Medicine—Infectious Disease
Brigham and Women's Hospital
Boston Massachusetts
Chapter 102, Lung Infections and Interstitial Lung Disease: Overview and General Approach to Lung Infections

Elizabeth H. Baldini, MD, MPH
Associate Professor of Radiation Oncology
Harvard Medical School
Department of Radiation Oncology
Lowe Center for Thoracic Oncology
Dana-Farber Cancer Institute/Brigham and Women's Hospital
Boston, Massachusetts
Chapter 87, Neoadjuvant and Adjuvant Radiation Therapy in Lung Cancer
Chapter 118, Radiation Therapy for Mesothelioma

Mark L. Barr, MD
Associate Professor of Surgery
University of Southern California
Keck School of Medicine
Los Angeles, California
Chapter 110, Living Lobar Lung Transplantation

Hasan F. Batirel, MD, PhD
Professor of Thoracic Surgery
Department of Thoracic Surgery
Marmara University Faculty of Medicine
Ministry of Health of Turkey
Marmara University Hospital
Istanbul, Turkey
Chapter 100, Minimally Invasive Methods of Managing Giant Bullae: Monaldi Procedure

Richard A. Baum, MD, MPA, MBA
Director of Interventional Radiology
Associate Professor of Radiology
Harvard Medical School
Brigham and Women's Hospital
Boston, Massachusetts
Chapter 131, Percutaneous Therapy for Traumatic Chylothorax

Rabih Bechara, MD
Chief of Interventional Pulmonology
Pulmonary and Critical Care Medicine
Southeastern Regional Medical Center
Atlanta, Georgia
Chapter 127, Medical Management of Nonmalignant Pleural Effusions

Angeliks Behrens, MD
Department of Internal Medicine II
Teaching Hospital of the University of Mainz
Wiesbaden, Germany
Chapter 173, Endoscopic Resection Techniques

S. Christopher Bellot, MD
Assistant Professor of Surgery
Surgical Director of Cardiovascular Surgery ICU
Surgical Director of ECMO Program
Division of Cardiovascular and Thoracic Surgery
University of Alabama at Birmingham
Birmingham, Alabama
Chapter 154, Acute and Chronic Traumatic Rupture of the Diaphragm

Mark F. Berry, MD
Associate Professor of Cardiothoracic Surgery
Stanford University
Falk Cardiovascular Research Center
Stanford University Medical Center
Stanford, California
Chapter 60, Overview
Chapter 62, Techniques of Tracheal Resection
Chapter 82, Bronchopleural Fistula After Pneumonectomy

Ankit Bharat, MD
Assistant Professor of Surgery
Northwestern University Feinberg School of Medicine
Surgical Director, Lung Transplantation
Northwestern Memorial Hospital
Chicago, Illinois
Chapter 109, Lung Transplantation Technique
Chapter 142, Supraclavicular Approach for Thoracic Outlet Syndrome

Amit Bhargava, MD
Attending Thoracic Surgeon, Montefiore Medical Center
Assistant Professor of Cardiothoracic Surgery, Albert Einstein College of Medicine
New York, New York
Chapter 146, Thoracoscopic Sympathectomy for Hyperhidrosis and Vasomotor Disorders

Thomas J. Birdas, MD
Associate Professor of Clinical Surgery
Indiana University School of Medicine
Indianapolis, Indiana
Chapter 132, Fibrothorax and Decortication

Costas S. Bizekis, MD
Assistant Professor of Cardiothoracic Surgery
Director of Esophageal Surgery Program
Division of Thoracic Surgery
Department of Cardiothoracic Surgery
NYU Langone Medical Center
New York, New York
Chapter 120, Thoracoscopy with Intrapleural Sclerosis for Malignant Pleural Effusion

Justin D. Blasberg, MD
Department of Surgery
University of Wisconsin Hospitals and Clinics
University of Wisconsin School of Medicine and Public Health
Madison, Wisconsin
Chapter 48, Management of Esophageal Perforation

Ayesha S. Bryant, MD
Assistant Professor of Surgery
Division of Thoracic Surgery
University of Alabama
Birmingham, Alabama
Chapter 128, Pneumothorax and Pneumomediastinum

Raphael Bueno, MD
Chief, Division of Thoracic Surgery
Vice Chair of Surgery for Cancer and Translational Research
Brigham and Women's Hospital
Professor of Surgery
Harvard Medical School
Boston, Massachusetts
Chapter 14, Esophagoscopy
Chapter 39, Nissen Fundoplication
Chapter 42, Management of Shortened Esophagus
Chapter 43, Management of the Failed Reflux Operation
Chapter 44, Techniques for Dilation of Benign Esophageal Stricture
Chapter 56, Use of Tracheobronchial Stents

Robert Burakoff, MD, MPH, FACG, FACP, AGAF
Clinical Chief, Division of Gastroenterology
Brigham and Women's Hospital
Associate Professor of Medicine
Harvard Medical School
Boston, Massachusetts
Chapter 33, Overview of Esophageal Motility Disorders

Bryan M. Burt, MD
Assistant Professor of Cardiothoracic Surgery
Stanford University Medical Center
Stanford, California
Chapter 78, Pulmonary Metastasectomy

Charles E. Butler, MD
Professor with Tenure
Director of Graduate Medical Education Programs
Department of Plastic Surgery
University of Texas MD Anderson Cancer Center
Houston, Texas
Chapter 138, Options for Soft Tissue Chest Wall Reconstruction

John G. Byrne, MD, MBA
Lawrence H. Cohn Professor of Surgery
Harvard Medical School
Chief, Division of Cardiac Surgery
Brigham and Women's Hospital
Boston, Massachusetts
Chapter 81, Cardiopulmonary Bypass for Extended Thoracic Resections

Phillip C. Camp, Jr., MD
Director, Transplant Administration
Associate Medical Director, New England Organ Bank
Director, Lung Transplant Program
Administrative Director, ECMO Program
Associate Program Director, CT Residency
Assistant Professor, Harvard Medical School
Division of Thoracic Surgery
Department of Surgery
Brigham and Women's Hospital
Boston, Massachusetts
Chapter 108, Overview of Lung Transplantation with Anatomy and Pathophysiology
Chapter 111, Medical Management of Lung Transplant Patients
Chapter 130, Management of Acute Bronchopleural Fistula

Stephanie Cardarella, MD
Instructor, Harvard Medical School
Dana-Farber Cancer Institute and
Brigham and Women's Hospital
Boston, Massachusetts
Chapter 89, Adjuvant and Neoadjuvant Chemotherapy

Shamus R. Carr, MD
Associate Chief of Thoracic Surgery
Assistant Professor
Division of Thoracic Surgery
University of Maryland School of Medicine
Baltimore, Maryland
Chapter 73, Segmentectomy for Primary Lung Cancer
Chapter 134, Overview of Chest Wall and Sternal Tumors

Giorgio Cavallesco, MD
Associate Professor of Surgery
U.O. di Chirurgia Generale e Toracica
University of Ferrara
Ferrara, Italy
Chapter 90, Overview of Benign Lung Disease: Anatomy and Pathophysiology

Robert James Cerfolio, MD, MBA
Chief of Thoracic Surgery at University of Alabama at Birmingham
James Estes Endowed Chair of Lung Cancer Research
Birmingham, Alabama
Chapter 128, Pneumothorax and Pneumomediastinum

Walter W. Chan, MD, MPH
Director, Center for Gastrointestinal Motility
Brigham and Women's Hospital
Assistant Professor of Medicine
Harvard Medical School
Boston, Massachusetts
Chapter 33, Overview of Esophageal Motility Disorders

Andrew C. Chang, MD
Associate Professor and Head, Section of Thoracic Surgery
John Alexander Distinguished Professor
University of Michigan Medical School
Ann Arbor, Michigan
Chapter 170, Genomics, Molecular Markers, and Targeted Therapies in Esophageal Cancer

Albert S.Y. Chang, MD
Assistant Professor of Surgery
Division of Cardiovascular and Thoracic Surgery
Duke University School of Medicine
Raleigh, North Carolina
Chapter 58, Surgical Repair of Congenital and Acquired Tracheoesophageal Fistulas

Michael Y. Chang, MD, MPH
Department of Surgery
Kaiser Permanente Medical Center
Los Angeles, California
Chapter 156, Cervical Mediastinoscopy and Anterior Mediastinotomy
Chapter 49, Blunt and Penetrating Esophageal Trauma

Lucian R. Chirieac, MD
Associate Professor of Pathology
Harvard Medical School
Pathologist
Brigham and Women's Hospital
Boston, Massachusetts
Chapter 69, Role of the Pathologist and Pathology-Specific Treatment of Lung Cancer

Gary W. Chmielewski, MD
Associate Professor of Surgery
Rush University
Department of Cardiac and Thoracic Surgery
Rush University Medical Center
Chicago, Illinois
Chapter 164, Resection of Patients with Superior Vena Cava Syndrome

Michael H. Cho, MD, MPH
Member, Pulmonary and Critical Care Medicine Division and Channing Division of Network Medicine
Brigham and Women's Hospital
Assistant Professor of Medicine, Harvard Medical School
Boston, Massachusetts
Chapter 97, Overview of Chronic Obstructive Pulmonary Disease

Leigh-Anne Cioffredi, MD, MPH
Resident
University of North Carolina School of Medicine
Chapel Hill, North Carolina
Georgetown University School of Medicine
Washington, District of Columbia
Chapter 117, Systemic Chemotherapy for Mesothelioma

Daniel M. Cohen, MD
Chief of Thoracic Surgery, Veteran's Administration Hospital
Attending Thoracic Surgeon, Brigham and Women's Hospital
Instructor in Surgery, Harvard Medical School
Boston, Massachusetts
Chapter 83, Management of Hemoptysis in Lung Cancer
Chapter 105, Adjuvant Surgery for Tuberculosis
Chapter 141, Surgical Repair of Complex (Recurrent) Pectus Excavatum in Adults

Yolonda L. Colson, MD, PhD
Professor of Surgery
Harvard Medical School
Associate Administrative Chief, Division of Thoracic Surgery
Brigham and Women's Hospital
Boston, Massachusetts
Chapter 54, Tracheostomy
Chapter 104, Role of the Thoracic Surgeon in the Diagnosis of Interstitial Lung Disease
Chapter 155, Overview of Benign and Malignant Mediastinal Disease
Chapter 168, Sentinel Node Mapping in Lung Cancer
Chapter 171, Nanoparticle Therapy in Lung Cancer

Carolyn E. Come, MD, MPH
Pulmonary and Critical Care Medicine
Brigham and Women's Hospital
Boston, Massachusetts
Chapter 101, Endoscopic Approaches for Treatment of Emphysema

William A. Cook, MD
Thoracic and Cardiac Surgeon
North Andover, Massachusetts
Chapter 106, Thoracoplasty for Tuberculosis

Willy Coosemans, MD
University Hospitals Leuven
Department of Thoracic Surgery
Leuven, Belgium
Chapter 18, Ivor Lewis Esophagectomy
Chapter 40, Other Reflux Procedures (Toupet, Dor, and Hill)

Joseph M. Corson, MD
Professor of Pathology
Department of Pathology
Brigham and Women's Hospital
Boston, Massachusetts
Chapter 115, Pathology of Pleural Malignant Mesothelioma

Daniel Geraldo Cuadrado, MD
Surgeon
Madigan Army Medical Center
Tacoma, Washington
Chapter 81, Cardiopulmonary Bypass for Extended Thoracic Resections

Marcelo Cypel, MD, MSc
Canada Research Chair in Lung Transplantation
Assistant Professor of Surgery
University of Toronto
Canada Research Chair in Lung Transplantation (Tier 2)
Thoracic Surgeon, University Health Network
Assistant Professor of Surgery
Division of Thoracic Surgery
University of Toronto
Toronto, Ontario, Canada
Chapter 172, Ex Vivo Lung Perfusion

Harry J. D'Agostino, Jr., MD
Associate Professor, Department of Surgery
Chief, Division of Cardiothoracic Surgery
College of Medicine
University of Florida
Jacksonville, Florida
Chapter 160, Radical Transsternal Thymectomy

Jonathan C. Daniel, MD
Thoracic Surgeon
Providence Cancer Center
Providence Portland Medical Center
Providence St. Vincent Medical Center
Portland, Oregon
Chapter 141, Surgical Repair of Complex (Recurrent) Pectus Excavatum in Adults

Marcelo C. DaSilva, MD
Chief of Thoracic Surgery
Loyola University Medical Center - Chicago
Associate Professor of Thoracic Surgery and General Surgery
Stritch School of Medicine
Chicago, Illinois
Chapter 123, Intracavitary Hyperthermic Chemotherapy for Malignant Mesothelioma
Chapter 137, Chest Wall Stabilization and Novel Closures of the Chest

Paul De Leyn, MD, PhD
Professor of Surgery
KU Leuven University
Thoracic Surgeon
University Hospitals Leuven
Leuven, Belgium
Chapter 73, Segmentectomy for Primary Lung Cancer

Herbert Decaluwé, MD
Thoracic Surgeon
University Hospitals Leuven
Leuven, Belgium
Chapter 73, Segmentectomy for Primary Lung Cancer

Malcolm M. DeCamp, MD
Fowler McCormick Professor of Surgery
Northwestern University Feinberg School of Medicine
Chief, Division of Thoracic Surgery
Northwestern Memorial Hospital
Chicago, Illinois
Chapter 38, Belsey-Mark IV Fundoplication/Collis Gastroplasty
Chapter 64, Resection of the Carina

Steven R. DeMeester, MD
Professor of Cardiothoracic Surgery
University of Southern California School of Medicine
Los Angeles, California
Chapter 30, Resection of Esophageal Diverticula

Todd L. Demmy, MD
Chair, Department of Thoracic Surgery
Roswell Park Cancer Institute
Buffalo, New York
Chapter 86, Management of Superficial Central Airway Lung Cancers

Claude Deschamps, MD
Professor of Surgery
University of Vermont
Burlington, Vermont
Chapter 46, Techniques for Repair of Paraesophageal Hiatal Hernia

Phillip M. Devlin, MD
Chief, Division of Brachytherapy
Institute Physician, Dana Farber Cancer Institute
Associate Professor of Radiation Oncology
Harvard Medical School
Boston, Massachusetts
Chapter 88, Innovative Radiation Techniques: Role of Brachytherapy and Intraoperative Radiotherapy in Treatment of Lung Cancer

Enrique Diaz-Guzman, MD
Assistant Professor of Surgery
Medical Director, Lung Transplant Program
University of Kentucky
Lexington, Kentucky
Chapter 113, Artificial Lung

Miguel J. Divo, MD
Instructor in Medicine, Harvard Medical School
Associate Physician, Brigham and Women's Hospital
Boston, Massachusetts
Chapter 7, Mechanical Ventilation

Christopher T. Ducko, MD
Instructor in Surgery
Harvard Medical School
Thoracic Surgeon
Brigham and Women's Hospital
Boston, Massachusetts
Chapter 76, Radical Lymphadenectomy
Chapter 133, Surgical Management of Chylothorax
Chapter 152, Diaphragm Pacing

André Duranceau, MD
Department of Surgery
Université de Montréal
Division of Thoracic Surgery
Centre Hospitalier de l'Université de Montréal
Montreal, Québec, Canada
Chapter 32, Complications of Esophageal Surgery

Michael I. Ebright, MD
Assistant Professor of Clinical Surgery
Section of Thoracic Surgery
Columbia University Medical Center
New York, New York
Chapter 10, Overview of Esophageal and Proximal Stomach Malignancy
Chapter 24, Esophageal Malignancy: Palliative Options and Procedures

Christian Ell, MD
Chief, Department of Medicine
Professor of Medicine
Sana Klinikum Offenbach
Offenbach am Main, Germany
Chapter 173, Endoscopic Resection Techniques

Armin Ernst, MD
President and Chief Executive Officer
Reliant Medical Group
Worcester, Massachusetts
Chapter 67, Ablative Endoscopic Therapy for Endobronchial Lesions
Chapter 127, Medical Management of Nonmalignant Pleural Effusions

Christopher H. Fanta, MD
Member, Pulmonary and Critical Care Medicine Division, Brigham and Women's Hospital
Director, Partners Asthma Center
Professor of Medicine, Harvard Medical School
Boston, Massachusetts
Chapter 97, Overview of Chronic Obstructive Pulmonary Disease

Alexander S. Farivar, MD
Attending, Division of Thoracic Surgery
Swedish Cancer Institute and Medical Center
Seattle, Washington
Chapter 157, Resection of Substernal Goiter

Mark K. Ferguson, MD
Professor, Department of Surgery and the Cancer Research Center
Head, Thoracic Surgery Service
Director, Residency Program in Cardiothoracic Surgery
University of Chicago Medicine and Biological Sciences
Chicago, Illinois
Chapter 28, Overview: Anatomy and Pathophysiology of Benign Esophageal Disease
Chapter 29, Resection of Benign Tumors of the Esophagus

Hiran C. Fernando, MD
Department of Cardiothoracic Surgery
Boston University School of Medicine
Boston, Massachusetts
Chapter 24, Esophageal Malignancy: Palliative Options and Procedures

Pasquale Ferraro, MD
Department of Surgery
Université de Montréal
Division of Thoracic Surgery
Centre Hospitalier de l'Université de Montréal
Montreal, Québec, Canada
Chapter 32, Complications of Esophageal Surgery

Neil A. Fine, MD
Associate Clinical Professor
Northwestern University Feinberg School of Medicine
Northwestern Specialists in Plastic Surgery
Chicago, Illinois
Chapter 138, Options for Soft Tissue Chest Wall Reconstruction

Raja M. Flores, MD
Ames Professor of Thoracic Surgery
Chairman, Department of Thoracic Surgery
Mount Sinai Health System
New York, New York
Chapter 121, Pleurectomy and Decortication for Malignant Pleural Diseases

Joseph S. Friedberg, MD
Chief of Thoracic Surgery
PENN Presbyterian Medical Center
Division of Thoracic Surgery
University of Pennsylvania
Philadelphia, Pennsylvania
Chapter 60, Overview
Chapter 62, Techniques of Tracheal Resection
Chapter 73, Segmentectomy for Primary Lung Cancer
Chapter 124, Photodynamic Therapy in the Management of Pleural Tumors

Anne L. Fuhlbrigge, MD, MS
Pulmonary and Critical Care Medicine
Brigham and Women's Hospital
Harvard Medical School
Boston, Massachusetts
Chapter 4, Preoperative Evaluation of Thoracic Surgery Patient

Ziv Gamliel, MD
Division of Thoracic Surgery
University of Maryland
St. Joseph Medical Group
Towson, Maryland
Chapter 16, Transhiatal Esophagectomy

Sidhu P. Gangadharan MD
Chief, Division of Thoracic Surgery and Interventional Pulmonology
Beth Israel Deaconess Medical Center
Assistant Professor of Surgery
Harvard Medical School
Boston, Massachusetts
Chapter 38, Belsey-Mark IV Fundoplication/Collis Gastroplasty
Chapter 126, Overview of Benign Pleural Conditions: Anatomy and Physiology of Pleura
Chapter 162, Neurogenic Tumors of the Posterior Mediastinum

Gary A.J. Gelfand, MD, MSc, FRCSC
Clinical Assistant Professor of Surgery
Division of Thoracic Surgery
University of Calgary
Foothills Medical Centre
Calgary, Alberta, Canada
Chapter 147, Surgical Treatment of Chest Wall Infections

Ritu R. Gill, MD, MPH
Assistant Professor of Radiology
Harvard Medical School
Division of Thoracic Radiology
Brigham and Women's Hospital
Boston, Massachusetts

Denis M. Gilmore, MD
Division of Thoracic Surgery
Brigham and Women's Hospital
Boston, Massachusetts
Chapter 168, Sentinel Node Mapping in Lung Cancer

John J. Godleski, MD
Associate Professor of Pathology
Department of Pathology
Brigham and Women's Hospital
Boston, Massachusetts
Chapter 115, Pathology of Pleural Malignant Mesothelioma

Hilary J. Goldberg, MD, MPH
Assistant Professor of Medicine
Harvard Medical School
Associate Physician
Brigham and Women's Hospital
Boston, Massachusetts
Chapter 111, Medical Management of Lung Transplant Patients

David B. Graham, MAJ USAF, MD
Cardiothoracic Surgeon
San Antonio Military Medical Center
Joint Base San Antonio
Fort Sam Houston
San Antonio, Texas
Chapter 166, Robotics: Esophagectomy

Kimberly S. Grant, MD
Department of Surgery
University of Southern California Keck School of Medicine
Los Angeles, California
Chapter 30, Resection of Esophageal Diverticula

Mark W. Grinstaff, PhD
Distinguished Professor of Translational Research
Professor of Biomedical Engineering
Professor of Chemistry
Professor of Materials Science and Engineering
Director, NIH T32 Program in Translational Research in Biomaterials
Director, Center for Nanoscience and Nanobiotechnology
Boston University
Chapter 171, Nanoparticle Therapy in Lung Cancer

Sean C. Grondin, MPH, MD, FRCSC
Clinical Associate Professor of Surgery
Division of Thoracic Surgery
University of Calgary
Foothills Medical Centre
Calgary, Alberta, Canada
Chapter 147, Surgical Treatment of Chest Wall Infections

William Grossi, MD
Thoracic Surgeon
U.O. di Chirurgia Generale e Toracica
University of Ferrara
Ferrara, Italy
Chapter 90, Overview of Benign Lung Disease: Anatomy and Pathophysiology

Timothy M. Haffey, MD
Head and Neck Institute
Cleveland Clinic Foundation
Cleveland, Ohio
Chapter 63, Subglottic Resection of the Airway

Zane T. Hammoud, MD
Associate Professor of Surgery
Division of Cardiothoracic Surgery
Wayne State University School of Medicine
Detroit, Michigan
Chapter 53, Overview of Benign Disorders of the Upper Airways

David H. Harpole, Jr., MD
Professor of Surgery
Division of Thoracic Surgery
Duke University Medical Center
Durham, North Carolina
Chapter 82, Bronchopleural Fistula after Pneumonectomy

Philip M. Hartigan, MD
Assistant Professor of Anaesthesia
Harvard Medical School
Director of Thoracic Anesthesia
Department of Anesthesiology, Perioperative and Pain Medicine
Brigham and Women's Hospital
Boston, Massachusetts
Chapter 5, Anesthesia Management

Jona Hattangadi-Gluth, MD
Assistant Professor of Radiation Oncology
University of California, San Diego
San Diego, California
Chapter 27, Radiation Therapy in the Management of Esophageal Cancer

W. Hardy Hendren III, MD
Honorary Surgeon at Massachusetts General Hospital
Robert E. Gross, Distinguished Professor of Surgery, Harvard Medical School
Chief of Surgery, Emeritus, Childrens Hospital Boston
Boston, Massachustts
Chapter 51, Congenital Disorders of the Esophagus in Infants and Children

Mark W. Hennon, MD
Roswell Park Cancer Institute
Buffalo, New York
Chapter 91, Benign Lung Masses

Roy S. Herbst, MD, PhD
Yale Comprehensive Cancer Center
Smilow Cancer Hospital at Yale-New Haven
Yale School of Medicine
New Haven, Connecticut
Chapter 169, Genomics, Molecular Markers, and Targeted Therapies in Non–Small-Cell Lung Cancer

Marcelo W. Hinojosa, MD
Acting Instructor
Department of Surgery
University of Washington
Seattle, Washington
Chapter 34, Esophagocardiomyotomy for Achalasia (Heller)

Wayne Hofstetter, MD
Associate Professor of Surgery
Department of Thoracic and Cardiovascular Surgery
University of Texas MD Anderson Cancer Center
Houston, Texas
Chapter 23, Options for Esophageal Replacement

Edward Hong, MD
General Surgeon, Thoracic Surgeon
Chicago, Illinois
Chapter 70, Techniques for Staging and Restaging of Lung Cancer

Charles W. Hoopes, MD
Associate Professor of Surgery
Alexander Gill Professor of Thoracic Surgery
Director, Comprehensive Transplant Institute
University of Kentucky
Lexington, Kentucky
Chapter 113, Artificial Lung

Nicholas C. Issa, MD
Instructor in Medicine
Harvard Medical School
Infectious Disease Specialist
Brigham and Women's Hospital
Boston, Massachusetts
Chapter 102, Lung Infections and Interstitial Lung Disease: Overview and General Approach

Yoshimi Iwanuma, MD
Associate Professor
Department of Esophageal and Gastroenterological Surgery
Juntendo University Hospital
Tokyo, Japan
Chapter 20, Three-Field Esophagectomy

David M. Jackman, MD
Assistant Professor of Medicine, Harvard Medical School
Medical Director of Clinical Pathways, Dana-Farber Cancer Institute
Boston, Massachusetts
Chapter 117, Systemic Chemotherapy for Mesothelioma

Francine L. Jacobson, MD, MPH
Assistant Professor of Radiology
Harvard Medical School
Division of Thoracic Radiology
Brigham and Women's Hospital
Boston, Massachusetts
Chapter 3, Chest Imaging: Role of CT, PET/CT, and MRI

Michael T. Jaklitsch, MD
Associate Professor of Surgery
Harvard Medical School
Division of Thoracic Surgery
Brigham and Women's Hospital
Boston, Massachusetts
Chapter 2, Thoracic Incisions
Chapter 76, Radical Lymphadenectomy
Chapter 78, Pulmonary Metastasectomy
Chapter 83, Management of Hemoptysis in Lung Cancer
Chapter 114, Overview and Historical Context of Malignant Pleural Diseases
Chapter 145, Thrombosis of the Subclavian Vein: Paget–Schroetter Syndrome
Chapter 149, Incision, Resection, and Replacement of the Diaphragm
Chapter 150, Plication of the Diaphragm from Above
Chapter 159, Thoracoscopic Approach to Thymectomy with Advice on Patients with Myasthenia Gravis

Bruce E. Johnson, MD
Professor of Medicine
Harvard Medical School
Lowe Center for Thoracic Oncology
Dana-Farber Cancer Institute
Boston, Massachusetts
Chapter 89, Adjuvant and Neoadjuvant Chemotherapy

David R. Jones, MD
Chief, Thoracic Service
Professor, Department of Surgery
Memorial Sloan Kettering Cancer Center
New York, New York
Chapter 132, Fibrothorax and Decortication

Yoshiaki Kajiyama, MD
Professor
Department of Esophageal and Gastroenterological Surgery
Juntendo University Hospital
Tokyo, Japan
Chapter 20, Three-Field Esophagectomy

Robert J. Keenan, MD
Professor of Cardiothoracic Surgery
Temple University
Division Director, Thoracic Surgery
Allegheny Health Network
Pittsburgh, Pennsylvania
Chapter 132, Fibrothorax and Decortication

Steven M. Keller, MD
Director of Thoracic Surgery
Weiler Hospital
Montefiore Medical Center
Professor of Cardiothoracic Surgery
Albert Einstein College of Medicine
New York, New York
Chapter 146, Thoracoscopic Sympathectomy for Hyperhidrosis and Vasomotor Disorders

Kemp H. Kernstine, Sr., MD, PhD
Professor and Chief, Division of Thoracic Surgery
University of Texas Southwestern Medical Center
Dallas, Texas
Chapter 166, Robotics: Esophagectomy

Shaf Keshavjee, MD
Surgeon in Chief, University Health Network
James Wallace McCutcheon Chair in Surgery
Professor, Division of Thoracic Surgery
University of Toronto
Toronto, Ontario, Canada
Chapter 158, Transcervical Thymectomy
Chapter 172, Ex Vivo Lung Perfusion

Mark J. Krasna, MD
Medical Director, Oncology
Meridian Cancer Care
Jersey Shore University Medical Center
Neptune, New Jersey
Chapter 10, Overview of Esophageal and Proximal Stomach Malignancy
Chapter 16, Transhiatal Esophagectomy
Chapter 22, Left Transthoracic Esophagectomy (Ellis)
Chapter 79, Resection of Bronchogenic Carcinoma with Oligometastatic Disease
Chapter 80, Pancoast Syndrome: Extended Resection in Superior Pulmonary Sulcus and Anterior Approach

Eric S. Lambright, MD
Assistant Professor
Department of Thoracic Surgery
Surgical Director, Lung Transplant
Chief of Thoracic Surgery, Veterans Affairs Medical Center, Nashville
Vanderbilt University Medical Center
Nashville, Tennessee
Chapter 81, Cardiopulmonary Bypass for Extended Thoracic Resections

Rodney J. Landreneau, MD
Vice Chairman, Department of Surgery, Clinical Program Development
Chief, General Thoracic Surgery
Medical Director, Ochsner Cancer Institute
Ochsner Medical Center
New Orleans, Louisiana
Chapter 77, Open and VATS Wedge Resection for Lung Cancer
Chapter 107, Surgical Approaches for Chronic Empyema and for Management of Chronic Bronchopleural Fistula
Chapter 144, Thoracoscopic First Rib Resection with Dorsal Sympathectomy

Marzia Leacche, MD
Assistant Professor of Surgery
Harvard Medical School
Staff Surgeon
Brigham and Women's Hospital
Boston, Massachusetts
Chapter 81, Cardiopulmonary Bypass for Extended Thoracic Resections

Abraham Lebenthal, MD
Instructor in Surgery, Harvard Medical School
Division of Thoracic Surgery, Brigham and Women's Hospital
West Roxbury VA Hospital
Boston, Massachusetts
Chapter 9, Techniques for Pleural Drainage and Chest Tube Management
Chapter 15, Minimally Invasive Esophagectomy
Chapter 39, Nissen Fundoplication
Chapter 42, Management of Shortened Esophagus
Chapter 43, Management of the Failed Reflux Operation
Chapter 47, Treating Traumatic Chest Injuries in a Limited Resource Setting

Jay M. Lee, MD
Associate Professor of Surgery
David Geffen School of Medicine/UCLA
Chief, Thoracic Surgery
Ronald Regan UCLA Medical Center
Los Angeles, California
Chapter 122, Extrapleural Pneumonectomy for Pleural Malignancies
Chapter 136, Sternal and Clavicular Chest Wall Resection and Reconstruction

Jacqueline J. Lee, MD
Division of Thoracic Surgery
Geisinger Health System
Scranton, Pennsylvania
Chapter 139, Overview: Benign Disorders of Chest Wall

Paul C. Lee, MD
Professor of Cardiothoracic Surgery
Division of Thoracic Surgery
Weill-Cornell Medical College
New York, New York
Chapter 166, Robotics: Esophagectomy

Toni Lerut, MD, PhD
Emeritus Professor in Surgery and Emeritus Chairman, Department of Thoracic Surgery
The Huub and Imelda Spierings Chair in Thoracic and Esophageal Surgery
University Hospital Gasthuisberg
Leuven, Belgium
Chapter 13, Surgical Approach to Esophagogastric Junction Cancers
Chapter 18, Ivor Lewis Esophagectomy
Chapter 40, Other Reflux Procedures (Toupet, Dor, and Hill)
Chapter 46, Techniques for Repair of Paraesophageal Hiatal Hernia

Zhigang Li, MD
Assistant Professor of Surgery, The Second Military Medical University
Department of Thoracic and Cardiovascular Surgery
Changhai Hospital
Shanghai, China
Chapter 26, Salvage Surgery for Recurrent Esophageal Cancer

Moishe Liberman, MD, PhD
Department of Surgery
Université de Montréal
Division of Thoracic Surgery
Centre Hospitalier de l'Université de Montréal
Montreal, Québec, Canada
Chapter 33, Overview of Esophageal Motility Disorders

Jules Lin, MD
Assistant Professor, Section of Thoracic Surgery
Surgical Director of Lung Transplant
Department of Surgery
University of Michigan Medical School
Ann Arbor, Michigan
Chapter 170, Genomics, Molecular Markers, and Targeted Therapies in Esophageal Cancer

Philip A. Linden, MD
Chief, Division of Thoracic Surgery
Associate Professor of Surgery
Case Western Reserve School of Medicine
Cleveland, Ohio
Chief, Division of Thoracic and Esophageal Surgery
University Hospitals Case Medical Center
Cleveland, Ohio
Chapter 37, Overview: Anatomy and Pathophysiology of Esophageal Reflux Disease
Chapter 133, Surgical Management of Chylothorax

Bradley C. Linden, MD
Department of Surgery
Boston Children's Hospital
Harvard Medical School
Boston, Massachusetts
Chapter 153, Long-Term Outcomes After a Congenital Diaphragmatic Hernia Repair: Implications for Adult Thoracic Surgeons

Michael J. Liptay, MD
The Mary and John Bent Professor and Chairperson
Department of Cardiovascular and Thoracic Surgery
Rush University Medical Center
Chicago, Illinois
Chapter 53, Overview of Benign Disorders of the Upper Airways
Chapter 70, Techniques for Staging and Restaging of Lung Cancer
Chapter 164, Resection of Patients with Superior Vena Cava Syndrome
Chapter 168, Sentinel Node Mapping in Lung Cancer

Gregory M. Loewen, DO
Spokane Respiratory Consultants, Pulmonary Oncologist
Spokane, Washington
Chapter 86, Management of Superficial Central Airway Lung Cancers

Robert R. Lorenz, MD
Staff Physician, Head and Neck Institute
Cleveland Clinic Foundation
Cleveland, Ohio
Chapter 63, Subglottic Resection of the Airway

Brian E. Louie, MD, MHA, MPH, FRCSC
Director, Thoracic Research and Education
Co-Director, Minimally Invasive Thoracic Surgery Program
Asst. Program Director, MIS Thoracic and Esophageal Fellowships
Division of Thoracic Surgery
Swedish Cancer Institute
Seattle, Washington
Chapter 36, Esophagectomy for Primary or Secondary Motility Disorders

Jeanne M. Lukanich, MD
Baystate Thoracic Surgery
Baystate Medical Center
Springfield, Massachusetts
Chapter 50, Surgical Management of Corrosive Injury to the Esophagus

James D. Luketich, MD
Henry T. Bahnson Professor and Chairman Department of Cardiothoracic Surgery
University of Pittsburgh Medical Center
Pittsburgh, Pennsylvania
Chapter 15, Minimally Invasive Esophagectomy
Chapter 107, Surgical Approaches for Chronic Empyema and for Management of Chronic Bronchopleural Fistula

Susan E. Mackinnon, MD, FRCS(C)
Sydney M. Shoenberg, Jr. and Robert H. Shoenberg Professor, Surgery
Chief, Plastic and Reconstructive Surgery
Department of Surgery
Washington University School of Medicine
Barnes-Jewish Hospital
St. Louis, Missouri
Chapter 142, Supraclavicular Approach for Thoracic Outlet Syndrome

Mitchell J. Magee, MD
Cardiopulmonary Research Science and Technology Institute
Medical City Dallas Hospital
Dallas, Texas
Chapter 25, Management of Malignant Esophageal Fistula

Raymond H. Mak, MD
Assistant Professor, Department of Radiation Oncology
Lowe Center for Thoracic Oncology
Brigham and Women's Hospital
Dana-Farber Cancer Institute
Harvard Medical School
Boston, Massachusetts
Chapter 87, Neoadjuvant and Adjuvant Radiation Therapy in Lung Cancer

Harvey Mamon, MD, PhD
Clinical Director, Department of Radiation Oncology
Brigham and Women's Hospital
Dana Farber Cancer Institute
Associate Professor of Radiation Oncology
Harvard Medical School
Boston, Massachusetts
Chapter 27, Radiation Therapy in the Management of Esophageal Cancer

Jeremiah T. Martin, MD, MB BCh
Assistant Professor of Surgery
University of Kentucky
Lexington, Kentucky
Chapter 113, Artificial Lung

David P. Mason, MD
Department of Thoracic Surgery
Baylor University Medical Center
Dallas, Texas
Chapter 58, Surgical Repair of Congenital and Acquired Tracheoesophageal Fistulas
Chapter 75, Sleeve Resection/Bronchoplasty for Lung Cancer

Douglas J. Mathisen, MD
Hermes Grillo Professor of Surgery
Harvard Medical School
Massachusetts General Hospital
Boston, Massachusetts
Chapter 21, Left Thoracoabdominal Approach

David C. Mauchley, MD
Resident, Cardiothoracic Surgery
Division of Cardiothoracic Surgery
University of Colorado
Denver School of Medicine
Aurora, Colorado
Chapter 94, Surgery for Bronchiectasis

Shannon S. McKenna, MD
Medical Director
Thoracic Surgical Intensive Care Unit
Department of Anesthesiology, Perioperative and Pain Medicine
Brigham and Women's Hospital
Boston, Massachusetts
Chapter 6, Critical Care for the Thoracic Surgery Patient

Ciaran J. McNamee, MD
Instructor in Surgery
Harvard Medical School
Attending Thoracic Surgeon, Division of Thoracic Surgery
Brigham and Women's Hospital
Boston, Massachusetts
Chief of Thoracic Surgery
Milford Hospital
Milford, Massachusetts
Chapter 9, Techniques for Pleural Drainage and Chest Tube Management
Chapter 68, Overview of Anatomy and Pathophysiology of Lung Cancer
Chapter 103, Surgical Treatment of Thoracic Fungal Infections
Chapter 105, Adjuvant Surgery for Tuberculosis
Chapter 129, Benign Tumors of the Pleura
Chapter 161, Resection of Benign Anterior and Middle Mediastinal Cysts and Tumors
Chapter 163, Malignant Primary Anterior Mediastinal Tumors

Steven J. Mentzer, MD
Professor of Surgery, Harvard Medical School
Associate Surgeon, Division of Thoracic Surgery
Brigham and Women's Hospital
Boston, Massachusetts
Chapter 8, Postoperative Management
Chapter 59, Tracheobronchial Injuries
Chapter 61, Bronchoscopy, Rigid and Flexible
Chapter 108, Overview of Lung Transplantation with Anatomy and Pathophysiology
Chapter 130, Management of Acute Bronchopleural Fistula
Chapter 156, Cervical Mediastinoscopy and Anterior Mediastinotomy

Carlos M. Mery, MD, MPH
Assistant Professor of Surgery and Pediatrics
Baylor College of Medicine
Associate Surgeon, Congenital Heart Surgery
Texas Children's Hospital
Houston, Texas
Chapter 78, Pulmonary Metastasectomy

Bryan F. Meyers, MD
Patrick and Joy Williamson Professor of Surgery
Washington University School of Medicine
Chief, Division of Cardiothoracic Surgery
Washington University
St. Louis, Missouri
Chapter 99, Lung Volume Reduction Surgery
Chapter 112, Management of Surgical Complications of Lung Transplantation

John D. Mitchell, MD
Professor and Chief, Division of Cardiothoracic Surgery, University of Colorado Denver School of Medicine
Aurora, Colorado
Chapter 94, Surgery for Bronchiectasis

Biren P. Modi, MD
Department of Surgery
Boston Children's Hospital
Boston, Massachusetts
Chapter 52, Minimally Invasive Techniques for Esophageal Repair

J. Ernesto Molina, MD, PhD
Professor of Surgery
University of Minnesota Medical School
Cardiothoracic Surgery
Minneapolis, Minnesota
Chapter 145, Thrombosis of the Subclavian Vein: Paget-Schroetter Syndrome

Daniel Morgensztern, MD
Associate Professor, Division of Medical Oncology
University of Washington School of Medicine
St. Louis, Missouri
Chapter 169, Genomics, Molecular Markers, and Targeted Therapies in Non–Small-Cell Lung Cancer

Christopher R. Morse, MD
Assistant Professor of Surgery
Harvard Medical School
Thoracic Surgery
Massachusetts General Hospital
Boston, Massachusetts
Chapter 21, Left Thoracoabdominal Approach

Aneil A. Mujoomdar, MD, FRCS
Thoracic Surgeon
Moncton Hospital
Moncton, New Brunswick, Canada
Chapter 139, Overview: Benign Disorders of Chest Wall

Sudish C. Murthy, MD, PhD
Surgical Director, Center of Major Airway Disease
Thoracic and Cardiovascular Surgery
Cleveland Clinic
Cleveland, Ohio
Chapter 55, Endoscopic Treatments for Benign Major Upper Airways Disease
Chapter 75, Sleeve Resection/Bronchoplasty for Lung Cancer

Subhakar Mutyala, MD
Radiation Oncology
Scott and White Memorial Hospital
Bronx, New York
Chapter 88, Innovative Radiation Techniques: Role of Brachytherapy and Intraoperative Radiotherapy in Treatment of Lung Cancer

Philippe Nafteux, MD
Clinical Head
Department of Thoracic Surgery
University Hospital Gasthuisberg
Leuven, Belgium
Chapter 13, Surgical Approach to Esophagogastric Junction Cancers
Chapter 18, Ivor Lewis Esophagectomy
Chapter 40, Other Reflux Procedures (Toupet, Dor, and Hill)

Chaitan K. Narsule, MD
Tufts Medical Center
Division of Cardiothoracic Surgery
Boston, Massachusetts
Chapter 24, Esophageal Malignancy: Palliative Options and Procedures

Daniel G. Nicastri, MD
Thoracic Surgeon
LCDR, MC, U.S. Navy
Department of Cardiothoracic Surgery
Walter Reed National Military Medical Center Bethesda, Maryland
Assistant Professor
Department of Surgery
Uniformed Services University of Health Sciences Bethesda, Maryland
Chapter 65, Mediastinal Tracheostomy
Chapter 74, VATS Lobectomy

Michael S. Nussbaum, MD
Professor and Chair
Department of Surgery
University of Florida College of Medicine—*Jacksonville*
Surgeon-in-Chief, Shands Jacksonville
Jacksonville, Florida
Chapter 160, Radical Transsternal Thymectomy

Chumy E. Nwogu, MD
Roswell Park Cancer Institute
Elm and Carlton Streets
Buffalo, New York
Chapter 91, Benign Lung Masses

David D. Odell, MD, MMSc
Assistant Professor of Cardiothoracic Surgery
University of Pittsburgh Medical Center
Pittsburgh, Pennsylvania
Chapter 38, Belsey-Mark IV Fundoplication/Collis Gastroplasty

Robert D. Odze, MD, FRCPc
Chief, Gastrointestinal Pathology
Professor of Pathology
Brigham and Women's Hospital
Harvard Medical School
Boston, Massachusetts
Chapter 11, Pathology of Esophageal Cancer

Brant K. Oelschlager, MD
Byers Endowed Professor of Surgery
University of Washington
Byers Endowed Professor of Esophageal Research
Chief, Gastrointestinal and General Surgery and Center for Videoendoscopic Surgery
Department of Surgery
University of Washington
Seattle, Washington
Chapter 34, Esophagocardiomyotomy for Achalasia (Heller)
Chapter 41, Surgery and Endoscopic Interventions for Barrett's Esophagus

Daniel S. Oh, MD
Assistant Professor of Surgery
Division of Thoracic Surgery
University of Southern California
Los Angeles, California
Chapter 129, Benign Tumors of the Pleura

Kazunori Okabe, MD
Division of Thoracic Surgery
National Hospital Organization
Yamaguchi Ube Medical Center
Ube, Yamaguchi, Japan
Chapter 92, Bronchoplasty for Benign Lung Lesions

Isabelle Opitz, MD
Division of Thoracic Surgery
University Hospital Zurich
Zürich, Switzerland
Chapter 125, Induction Chemotherapy Followed by Surgery for Malignant Pleural Mesothelioma

Dennis P. Orgill, MD, PhD
Vice Chairman for Quality Improvement
Department of Surgery, Brigham and Women's Hospital
Professor of Surgery, Harvard Medical School
Boston, Massachusetts
Chapter 138, Options for Soft Tissue Chest Wall Reconstruction

Bernard J. Park, MD
Deputy Chief of Clinical Affairs, Thoracic Service
Memorial Sloan Kettering Cancer Center
New York, New York
Chapter 164, Resection of Patients with Superior Vena Cava Syndrome
Chapter 165, Robotics: Lobectomy
Chapter 167, Robotics: Thymectomy

Jennifer Paruch, MD
Department of Surgery
University of Chicago
Chicago, Illinois
Chapter 28, Overview: Anatomy and Pathophysiology of Benign Esophageal Disease
Chapter 29, Resection of Benign Tumors of the Esophagus

Ital M. Pashtan, MD
Radiation Oncologist
Dana Farber Cancer Institute and Brigham and Women's Hospital
Boston, Massachusetts
Chapter 88, Innovative Radiation Techniques: Role of Brachytherapy and Intraoperative Radiotherapy in Treatment of Lung Cancer

Harvey I. Pass, MD
Professor and Chief Thoracic Oncology
New York University Medical Center
New York, New York
Chapter 120, Thoracoscopy with Intrapleural Sclerosis for Malignant Pleural Effusion

Amit N. Patel, MD
Associate Professor of Surgery (Tenured)
University of Utah
Salt Lake City, Utah
Chapter 143, Thoracic Outlet Syndromes
Chapter 144, Thoracoscopic First Rib Resection with Dorsal Sympathectomy

G. Alexander Patterson, MD
Joseph C. Bancroft Professor of Surgery
Division of Cardiothoracic
Washington University School of Medicine
St. Louis, MO
Chapter 109, Lung Transplantation Technique
Chapter 142, Supraclavicular Approach for Thoracic Outlet Syndrome

Subroto Paul, MD, MPH
Associate Professor of Cardiothoracic Surgery
Associate Professor of Health Policy and Research in Cardiothoracic Surgery
Department of Cardiothoracic Surgery
Weill Cornell Medical College
New York Presbyterian Hospital
Chapter 31, Techniques and Indications for Esophageal Exclusion
Chapter 49, Blunt and Penetrating Esophageal Trauma
Chapter 54, Tracheostomy
Chapter 104, Role of the Thoracic Surgeon in the Diagnosis of Interstitial Lung Disease
Chapter 119, Nonoperative Treatment of Malignant Pleural Effusions

Olliver Pech, MD
Head of Gastroenterology and Interventional Endoscopy
St. John of God Hospital
Regensburg, Germany
Chapter 173, Endoscopic Resection Techniques

Brian L. Pettiford, MD
Thoracic Surgeon
Good Samaritan Hospital
York, Pennsylvania
Chapter 107, Surgical Approaches for Chronic Empyema and for Management of Chronic Bronchopleural Fistula

Christian G. Peyre, MD
Assistant Professor of Surgery
Division of Thoracic and Foregut Surgery
University of Rochester
New York, New York
Chapter 17, Three-Hole Esophagectomy: The Brigham and Women's Hospital Approach

Victor Pinto-Plata, MD
Director Pulmonary Function Laboratory
Staff Physician-Brigham and Women's Hospital
Lecturer in Medicine, Harvard Medical School
Boston, Massachusetts
Chapter 4, Preoperative Evaluation of Thoracic Surgery Patient

J. Mark Pool, MD
Cardiac and Thoracic Surgeon
Texas Health Presbyterian Hospital
Dallas, Texas
Chapter 143, Thoracic Outlet Syndromes

Siva Rija, MD, PhD
Cleveland Clinic
Cleveland, Ohio
Chapter 55, Endoscopic Treatments for Benign Major Upper Airways Disease
Chapter 58, Surgical Repair of Congenital and Acquired Tracheoesophageal Fistulas
Chapter 75, Sleeve Resection/Bronchoplasty for Lung Cancer

Yael Refaely, MD
Thoracic Surgeon
Head of Thoracic Surgery
Soroka Medical Center
Senior Lecturer at the Ben Gurion University
Beer Sheva
Israel
Chapter 134, Overview of Chest Wall and Sternal Tumors

Thomas W. Rice, MD
The Karen and Daniel Lee Endowed Chair in Thoracic Surgery
Professor of Surgery, Cleveland Clinic Lerner College of Medicine of Case Western Reserve University
Head, Section of General Thoracic Surgery
Department of Thoracic and Cardiovascular Surgery
Heart and Vascular Institute
Cleveland Clinic
Cleveland, Ohio
Chapter 12, Esophageal Cancer Staging
Chapter 26, Salvage Surgery for Recurrent Esophageal Cancer
Chapter 66, Cancers of the Upper Aero-digestive Tract: Cervical Exenteration

William G. Richards, PhD
Assistant Professor, Department of Surgery, Harvard Medical School
Research Associate, Surgery, Brigham and Women's Hospital
Boston, Massachusetts
Chapter 116, Mesothelioma Staging

John R. Roberts, MD, MBA
Tri-Star Thoracic
Sarah Cannon Cancer Center
Nashville, Tennessee
Chapter 71, The Five Lobectomies
Chapter 72, Pneumonectomy

Loring W. Rue, III, MD
Professor and Vice Chair, Clinical Affairs
Director, Division of Trauma, Burns and Surgical Critical Care
John H. Blue Chair in General Surgery
University of Alabama at Birmingham
Senior Vice President, Quality, Patient Safety and Clinical Effectiveness
UAB Health System
Birmingham, Alabama
Chapter 154, Acute and Chronic Traumatic Rupture of the Diaphragm

Mirco Santini, MD
Staff Surgeon
U.O. di Chirurgia Generale e Toracica
Azienda Ospedaliera Universitaria S. Anna
Ferrara, Italy
Chapter 90, Overview of Benign Lung Disease: Anatomy and Pathophysiology

Mandeep Singh Saund, MBBS
Clinical Fellow
Division of Thoracic Surgery
Brigham and Women's Hospital
Boston, Massachusetts
Chapter 156, Cervical Mediastinoscopy and Anterior Mediastinotomy

Matthew P. Schenker, MD
Assistant Professor of Radiology
Harvard Medical School
Brigham and Women's Hospital
Boston, Massachusetts
Chapter 131, Percutaneous Therapy for Traumatic Chylothorax

Matthew J. Schuchert, MD
Department of Cardiothoracic Surgery
University of Pittsburgh Medical Center
Pittsburgh, Pennsylvania
Chapter 77, Open and VATS Wedge Resection for Lung Cancer

Prashant C. Shah, MD
Assistant Professor of Surgery
Thoracic Surgeon Attending
Fox Chase Cancer Center
Philadelphia, Pennsylvania
Chapter 163, Malignant Primary Anterior Mediastinal Tumors

Robert C. Shamberger, MD
Robert E. Gross Professor of Surgery
Harvard Medical School
Chief, Department of Surgery
Boston Children's Hospital
Chapter 96, Pediatric Primary and Secondary Lung Tumors

David J. Sher, MD, MPH
Assistant Professor of Radiation Oncology
Department of Radiation Oncology
Rush University Medical Center
Chicago, Illinois
Chapter 85, Radiotherapy for Inoperable Non–Small-Cell Lung Cancer

Joseph B. Shrager, MD
Professor of Cardiothoracic Surgery
Stanford University School of Medicine
Chief, Division of Thoracic Surgery
Thoracic Oncology Program Leader
Stanford Hospitals and Clinics
Staff Surgeon, Veterans Affairs Palo Alto Healthcare System
Stanford, California
Chapter 148, Overview of Anatomy, Physiology, and Pathophysiology of the Diaphragm

Eero Sihvo, MD
Associate Professor of Surgery
Division of General Thoracic and Esophageal Surgery
Helsinki University Central Hospital
Finland
Chapter 158, Transcervical Thymectomy

Joshua R. Sonett, MD
Professor of Clinical Surgery
Department of Surgery
Columbia University
New York-Presbyterian Hospital
New York, New York
Chapter 25, Management of Malignant Esophageal Fistula
Chapter 98, Resection of Blebs, Bullae, and Giant Bullae

Amitabh Srivastava, MD
Department of Pathology
Brigham and Women's Hospital
Boston, Massachusetts
Chapter 11, Pathology of Esophageal Cancer

Vaughn A. Starnes, MD
Chair, Department of Surgery
Surgeon-in-Chief
Keck Hospital and Norris Cancer Hospital
University of Southern California
Los Angeles, California
Chapter 110, Living Lobar Lung Transplantation

Stacey Su, MD
Assistant Professor of Surgical Oncology
Fox Chase Cancer Center
Philadelphia, Pennsylvania
Chapter 50, Surgical Management of Corrosive Injury to the Esophagus
Chapter 155, Overview of Benign and Malignant Mediastinal Disease

David J. Sugarbaker, MD
Director, The Lung Institute
Chief, Division of Thoracic Surgery
The Olga Kieth Weiss Chair of Surgery
Baylor College of Medicine
Baylor St. Luke's Medical Center
Houston, Texas
Chapter 1, Introduction
Chapter 17, Three-Hole Esophagectomy: The Brigham and Women's Hospital Approach
Chapter 35, Long Esophageal Myotomy: Open, Thoracoscopic, and Peroral Endoscopic Approach
Chapter 68, Overview of Anatomy and Pathophysiology of Lung Cancer
Chapter 122, Extrapleural Pneumonectomy for Pleural Malignancies
Chapter 123, Intracavitary Hyperthermic Chemotherapy for Malignant Mesothelioma
Chapter 159, Thoracoscopic Approach to Thymectomy with Advice on Patients with Myasthenia Gravis

Paul H. Sugarbaker, MD
Washington Cancer Institute
Washington, D.C.
Chapter 123, Intracavitary Hyperthermic Chemotherapy for Malignant Mesothelioma

Scott J. Swanson, MD
Professor of Surgery
Harvard Medical School
Director of Minimally Invasive Thoracic Surgery
Brigham and Women's Hospital
Chief Surgical Officer
Dana Farber Cancer Institute
Boston, Massachusetts
Chapter 65, Mediastinal Tracheostomy
Chapter 74, VATS Lobectomy

Nitika Thawani, MD
Assistant Professor of Radiology
Texas A&M Health Science Center
College of Medicine
Temple, Texas
Chapter 88, Innovative Radiation Techniques: Role of Brachytherapy and Intraoperative Radiotherapy in Treatment of Lung Cancer

Masahiko Tsurumaru, MD
Professor
Department of Esophageal and Gastroenterological Surgery
Juntendo University Hospital
Tokyo, Japan
Chapter 20, Three-Field Esophagectomy

Harushi Udagawa, MD
Chief of Surgery
Department of Surgery
Toranomon Hospital
Tokyo, Japan
Chapter 20, Three-Field Esophagectomy

Harold C. Urschel, Jr., MD
Deceased
Professor of Surgery
Baylor University Medical Center
Dallas, Texas
Chapter 80, Pancoast Syndrome: Extended Resection in Superior Pulmonary Sulcus and Anterior Approach
Chapter 143, Thoracic Outlet Syndromes

Karl Fabian L. Uy, MD
Assistant Professor
Division of Thoracic Surgery
UMass Memorial Medical Center
University of Massachusetts Medical School
Worcester, Massachusetts
Chapter 57, Techniques of Tracheal Resection and Reconstruction

Eric Vallières, MD, FRCSC
Surgical Director of the Lung Cancer Program
Medical Director Division of Thoracic Surgery
Swedish Cancer Institute
Seattle, Washington
Chapter 36, Esophagectomy for Primary or Secondary Motility Disorders
Chapter 157, Resection of Substernal Goiter

Victor van Berkel, MD, PhD
Division of Cardiothoracic Surgery
University of Louisville School of Medicine
Louisville, Kentucky
Chapter 99, Lung Volume Reduction Surgery

Dirk Van Raemdonck, MD, PhD, FEBTS
Professor of Surgery
KU Leuven University
Thoracic Surgeon
University Hospitals Leuven
Leuven, Belgium
Chapter 73, Segmentectomy for Primary Lung Cancer

Jeffrey B. Velotta, MD
Division of Thoracic Surgery
Brigham and Women's Hospital
Boston, Massachusetts
Chapter 136, Sternal and Clavicular Chest Wall Resection and Reconstruction

Urs von Holzen, MD
Associate Professor of Surgery
Department of Surgery
University Hospital Basel
Basel, Switzerland
Chapter 47, Treating Traumatic Chest Injuries in a Limited Resource Setting

Thomas K. Waddell, MD, MSc, PhD
Professor and Chair
Division of Thoracic Surgery
University of Toronto
Toronto, Canada
Chapter 57, Techniques of Tracheal Resection and Reconstruction

Wenping Wang, MD
Department of Surgery
Université de Montréal
Division of Thoracic Surgery
Centre Hospitalier de l'Université de Montréal
Montreal, Québec, Canada
Chapter 32, Complications of Esophageal Surgery

George R. Washko, MD, MMSc
Assistant Professor of Medicine
Harvard Medical School
Staff Pulmonologist, Division of Pulmonary Medicine
Brigham and Women's Hospital
Boston, Massachusetts
Chapter 7, Mechanical Ventilation
Chapter 101, Endoscopic Approaches for Treatment of Emphysema

Walter Weder, MD
Division of Thoracic Surgery
University Hospital Zurich
Zürich, Switzerland
Chapter 125, Induction Chemotherapy followed by Surgery for Malignant Pleural Mesothelioma

Jon O. Wee, MD
Co-Director of Minimally Invasive Thoracic Surgery
Division of Thoracic Surgery
Brigham and Women's Hospital
Boston, Massachusetts
Chapter 15, Minimally Invasive Esophagectomy
Chapter 35, Long Esophageal Myotomy: Open, Thoracoscopic, and Peroral Endoscopic Approach
Chapter 45, Endoscopic Techniques in Antireflux Surgery
Chapter 84, Percutaneous Thoracic Tumor Ablation

Christopher B. Weldon, MD, PhD
Department of Surgery
Boston Children's Hospital
Boston, Massachusetts
Chapter 51, Congenital Disorders of the Esophagus in Infants and Children
Chapter 52, Minimally Invasive Techniques for Esophageal Repair
Chapter 96, Pediatric Primary and Secondary Lung Tumors
Chapter 137, Chest Wall Stabilization and Novel Closures of the Chest

Daniel C. Wiener, MD
Assistant Professor, Department of Surgery
Tufts University School of Medicine
Tufts Medical Center
Boston, Massachusetts
Chapter 149, Incision, Resection, and Replacement of the Diaphragm

Andrea Wolf, MD, MPH
Assistant Professor
Department of Thoracic Surgery
Mount Sinai Medical Center
New York, New York
Chapter 69, Role of the Pathologist and Pathology-Specific Treatment of Lung Cancer

Cameron D. Wright, MD
Professor of Surgery
Harvard Medical School
Division of Thoracic Surgery
Massachusetts General Hospital
Boston, Massachusetts
Chapter 48, Management of Esophageal Perforation

Jane Yanagawa, MD
Division of Cardiothoracic Surgery
Ronald Reagan UCLA Medical Center
Los Angeles, California
Chapter 112, Management of Surgical Complications of Lung Transplantation

Jaime Yun, MD
Director of Minimally Invasive Thoracic Surgery
Lutheran Medical Center
Brooklyn, New York
Director of Minimally Invasive Thoracic Surgery
Wyckoff Heights Hospital
Brooklyn, New York
Chapter 65, Mediastinal Tracheostomy

Jill M. Zalieckas, MD, MPH
Department of Surgery
Boston Children's Hospital
Boston, Massachusetts
Chapter 140, Primary Repair of Pectus Excavatum

Lambros Zellos, MD, MPH
Director of Thoracic Surgery
Henry Dunant Hospital
Athens, Greece
Chapter 31, Techniques and Indications for Esophageal Exclusion
Chapter 93, Pulmonary Sequestration
Chapter 95, Pulmonary Arteriovenous Malformation
Chapter 100, Minimally Invasive Methods of Managing Giant Bullae: Monaldi Procedure
Chapter 119, Nonoperative Treatment of Malignant Pleural Effusions

Michael D. Zervos, MD
New York University Medical Center
New York, New York
Chapter 120, Thoracoscopy with Intrapleural Sclerosis for Malignant Pleural Effusion

Marie Ziesat, MD
Department of Surgery
University of Chicago
Chicago, Illinois
Chapter 28, Overview: Anatomy and Pathophysiology of Benign Esophageal Disease
Chapter 29, Resection of Benign Tumors of the Esophagus

Kimberly A. Zubris, PhD
Departments of Biomedical Engineering and Chemistry
Boston University, Boston, Massachusetts
Chapter 171, Nanoparticle Therapy in Lung Cancer

Joseph B. Zwischenberger, MD
Johnston-Wright Professor and Chairman of Surgery
Professor of Surgery, Pediatrics, Biomedical Engineering, and Diagnostic Radiology
Surgeon-in-Chief, UK Health Care
University of Kentucky
Lexington, Kentucky
Chapter 113, Artificial Lung

Foreword

Adult Chest Surgery is the culmination of a team effort. It would be unfair to single out any surgeon in particular, yet every team needs a vision, a driving force, an individual who is able to articulate that vision, recognize talent, acquire resources, seize opportunity, delegate responsibility, and lead. That is the hidden message of this book. Every surgeon who contributed to this volume is a leader in his or her own right. More than just a compilation of technical procedures, every author is trying to tell you something important, something they learned from the school of hard knocks, something that can make the difference between a successful and unsuccessful operation, and something that may impact your career in thoracic surgery. This impressive list of contributing authors also emphasizes the number of national and international surgeons who have dedicated their careers to the pursuit of general thoracic surgery. These individuals are the product of a focused and dedicated approach to general thoracic surgical training as practiced at multiple institutions worldwide.

As I look back upon my own experience, the unique events leading to the establishment of a separate division and training program for general thoracic surgery at Toronto General Hospital had far-reaching implications, the details of which I will relate herein.

Happenstance and good fortune placed me in the general surgery training program at Toronto General Hospital in the early 1950s when the seeds of our profession were sown. This was the same hospital where my predecessors, Dr. Norman Shenstone and Dr. Robert Janes, pioneered the Shenstone/Janes lung tourniquet in 1932. The purpose of the tourniquet was to control intraoperative hemorrhage, decrease mortality, and reduce the incidence of postoperative fistulae, and thereby ensure the safety of pneumonectomy and lobectomy for the treatment of suppurative lung diseases like tuberculosis. Previous to this, surgeons used to hold their breath during the difficult dissection of the hilum. As a result of this innovation, Toronto quickly became a leading center for general thoracic surgery in North America.

When my surgical career began, four surgeons (still operating within the division of general surgery) were responsible for the care of thoracic patients at Toronto General Hospital, including my mentor, Dr. Fredrick Kergin, as well as Drs. Norman Shenstone, Robert Janes, and Norman Delarue. Dr. Kergin played a key role in my development as well as in the evolution of general thoracic surgery. He was one of three general surgeons practicing thoracic surgery at the time and had an international reputation for his contributions to that specialty. Among his many contributions, he was largely responsible for the creation of a separate division of general thoracic surgery at Toronto General Hospital and for his foresight in bringing endoscopy (esophagoscopy and bronchoscopy) into the practice of general thoracic surgery. Previously, endoscopy had been the exclusive domain of otolaryngologists and ENT surgeons. This was the case not only in Canada but also throughout North America and most of the world.

Dr. Wilfred G. Bigelow, a young general surgeon with training in vascular disease, also played an important role. He introduced me to the more practical aspects of scientific research through a one-year fellowship in his physiology laboratory in 1951 to 1952. In 1953, Dr. Bigelow was named head of one of three hospital divisions of general surgery. Recognizing the need to develop specialized training for cardiac surgeons, he used his persuasion as surgeon-in-chief to create a dedicated division and training program for cardiovascular surgery. This decision influenced later events at Toronto General Hospital, and, eventually, across North America.

In 1958, just preceding a staff appointment to Toronto General Hospital, I benefited from a one-year traveling fellowship to Great Britain and Scandinavia. The McLaughlin Fellowship, as it was called, had been established to give young surgeons exposure to the international community prior to assuming a staff appointment. I spent six months as a senior house officer with the renowned esophageal surgeon, Ronald Belsey, in Bristol, England, and seven months in Sweden and Denmark, where I gained valuable exposure to mediastinoscopy. I was especially fortunate, after a chance meeting in the surgeons lounge while visiting the Karolinska Institute in Stockholm, Sweden, to be invited by Dr. Carlens to assist him in the operating room where I observed mediastinoscopy first hand.

In 1960, after returning to Canada, I joined the surgical staff of the Toronto General Hospital and we began to train a new generation of general thoracic surgeons. In 1966, with Dr. Kergin's blessing, Norman Delarue and I proposed that Toronto General Hospital establish the University's first dedicated thoracic surgical service. By 1968, the Royal College of Physicians and Surgeons of Canada had recognized general thoracic surgery as a distinct subspecialty, and I became chief of the first Division of Thoracic Surgery at Toronto General Hospital. Benefiting from my fellowship in Scandinavia and Great Britain, our division contributed to the development of mediastinoscopy, techniques of modern tracheal surgery, and the treatment of esophageal reflux disease through the introduction of the Collis-Belsey procedure. Subsequently, the "Toronto Program" became known internationally for its pioneering work in lung transplantation, minimally invasive procedures, and basic and clinical research. The training program in general thoracic surgery we had instituted at Toronto General Hospital became a model for training programs worldwide. The rest, as they say, is history.

Eventually, the notion of having independent, dedicated training programs in cardiac and general thoracic surgery expanded into the United States, with the creation of the first division of thoracic surgery at Brigham and Women's Hospital in 1988. Many academic centers followed suit. Indeed, today, the majority of academic thoracic surgery is performed by dedicated thoracic surgeons working in separate divisions or sections. This is a stark change from earlier days when cardiothoracic surgeons did it all.

This brings me full circle to the present. It is worth noting that although I have stressed the importance and value of dedicated thoracic training, thoracic surgeons are not the only professional groups qualified to perform these procedures. As a result of differences in postgraduate programs or constraints sometimes imposed by the custom of practice where care is delivered, thoracic cases may be handled by a cardiothoracic surgeon with training in both cardiac and thoracic procedures or even a general surgeon who is comfortable operating in the chest. This book is intended for all three professional groups. In my opinion, the authors and editors of *Adult Chest Surgery* have prepared a masterful presentation of the thoracic discipline that is well worth your time and attention.

F. Griffith Pearson
Professor of Surgery Emeritus
Toronto, Canada

Preface

Adult Chest Surgery is your guide to the future of thoracic surgery. Now in its second edition, this internationally recognized, authoritative resource builds on the reputation of the first edition, which garnered numerous awards and laudatory reviews for art, production, and science.[1-3] Intended for residents preparing for a case, surgeons seeking management tips, and surgeon specialists preparing for board recertification, the second edition remains steadfast in its mission to provide a comprehensive yet practical guide to the modern practice of general thoracic surgery. Broad in scope and straightforward in style and presentation, the volume is an excellent reference for anyone desiring a comprehensive description of the clinical nature of general thoracic surgery.

By updating the second edition in record time for a volume of this length and complexity, the editors of the second edition have assured that the information is current and applicable to present day practice. The concise description of current techniques and surgical principles for the most common thoracic surgical problems encountered in the clinic and the operating room are the thrust of this text. It expands generously on the content of the first edition with 40 new chapters devoted to a range of topics including new endoscopic techniques for antireflux surgery; percutaneous thoracic tumor ablation; peroral esophageal myotomy; robotic techniques for lobectomy, esophagectomy, and thymectomy; and other new minimally invasive approaches to standard thoracic resections.

More than 250 detailed illustrations of procedures have been added to the text, bringing the total to 850. The volume continues to represent several generations of internationally recognized surgical innovators conversant in a range of innovative techniques and technologies, as well as leading medical experts in thoracic oncology and pulmonary disease. These thought leaders have trained in centers of surgical excellence that have contributed to the discipline of general thoracic surgery. We are indebted to these individuals and especially their mentors, who sustained and nurtured general thoracic surgical education and training from the infancy of the discipline.

The editors wish to acknowledge the continued support of Ann Adams and Marcia Williams, who have brought continuity to the second edition through their excellent and precise editorial and artistic contributions.

We also acknowledge our spouses Linda Sugarbaker, Kate Poverman, Gray Lorig, Bridget Jaklitsch, Diane Krasna, and Barbara Smith for putting up with our hectic schedules; our parents Geneva V. and Everett D. Sugarbaker, Rachel and David Bueno, Thomas and Shirley Colson, Frederick and Evelyn Jaklitsch, Anne and Irwin Krasna, and Loy and James Mentzer, who inspired and supported us in our educational pursuits; our partners, trainees, and colleagues, who carry the field forward; and our patients, who put their trust and hope in our hands.

David J. Sugarbaker
Raphael Bueno
Yolonda L. Colson
Michael T. Jaklitsch
Mark J. Krasna
Steven J. Mentzer

1. Prose Awards American Association of Publishers, 2009
2. Association of Medical Illustrators, 2009
3. British Medical Association, Medical Book Awards, 2010

PART 1

OVERALL CARE

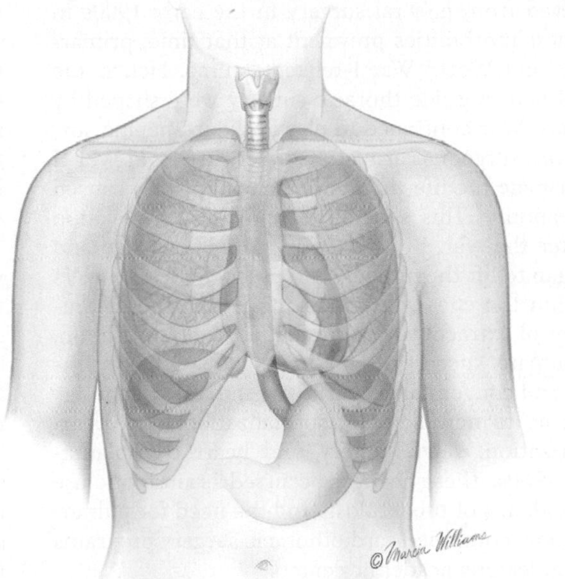

1 Introduction

David J. Sugarbaker

The emergence of general thoracic surgery in North America as a surgical subspecialty distinct from general surgery, congenital heart surgery, and adult cardiac surgery occurred through dramatic and tumultuous changes that once threatened but ultimately strengthened the integrity of the discipline. The discipline evolved from general surgery in the early 1900s in response to chest morbidities prevalent at that time, primarily tuberculosis and World War I-related trauma. Hence, the systems established to guide thoracic surgery were shaped by general surgeons. War continued to play a role in shaping surgery. In the 1940s, surgeons caring for soldiers in World War II struggled to manage the life-threatening chest injuries caused by modern weaponry. This spurred technological innovation during and after the war. By the 1950s, new knowledge and technology began to lift the physical and psychological barriers to surgery within the chest, including the heart. The technical achievement of extracorporeal circulation by John Gibbon, first used in humans successfully in 1953, allowed the extension of cardiac and congenital heart surgery into more complex problems, leading to new fields of specialization in myocardial revascularization, valve surgery, and heart transplantation in the late 1960s. These changes occurred as antibiotic use reduced the incidence of tuberculosis and the need for pulmonary surgery. Soon, combined cardiothoracic surgery programs began to form at leading academic centers.

The union between thoracic and cardiac surgery, however, was not altogether ideal, and thoracic training often played second fiddle to cardiac training. In 1981, Dr. Donald Paulson, President of the American Association for Thoracic Surgery, focused on the inadequacy of training in general thoracic surgery. In his presidential address, he stated: "Failure to correct the imbalance in training of thoracic surgery has resulted in a vacuum, which could lead to disintegration of the specialty."[1] By the 1990s, the realm of general thoracic surgery was so eclipsed by the dramatic developments in cardiovascular disease that funding in combined cardiothoracic programs began to be diverted in favor of cardiac training.

This pattern was played out largely in the United States, United Kingdom, and Europe, and threatened the ability of such programs to attract top-notch general thoracic surgeons. In an editorial published in 1991 in the *Annals of Thoracic Surgery*, the President of the American Association for Thoracic Surgery, Dr. John Waldhausen, addressed the broad concern that American thoracic surgery programs were failing to attract the "brightest candidates." Later that year an educational workshop was convened in Snow Bird, Utah, to define the deficiencies in American thoracic surgery.

Meanwhile, although similarly influenced by the pace of development in cardiac and congenital heart surgery, events transpired somewhat differently in Canada, where dedicated resources were committed to a separate general thoracic service and training program. Dr. F. Griffith Pearson, the first Chief of the first Division of General Thoracic Surgery at Toronto General Hospital, is widely known for his role in establishing thoracic surgery as a bona fide surgical subspecialty in North America. You can read his personal account of the Toronto experience in the Foreword to this book.

Dr. Pearson had tremendous impact in the field of general thoracic surgery[2] and is widely regarded as the father of thoracic surgery in North America. Throughout his tenure as Chief of the thoracic division at Toronto General Hospital (1967–1984) and subsequently as a staff surgeon until he retired in 1999, he oversaw important developments in lung transplantation, thoracic oncology, and clinical and basic research, mentoring many surgical leaders around the globe. American surgeons with an interest in general thoracic surgery were attracted to the Canadian programs. After training, the many successful graduates of these programs brought their experiences and commitment back to the United States, where lack of specific funding for thoracic surgery training had led to a shortage of qualified surgeons as described above.

The inevitable consequence of this pent-up demand fueled the trend of establishing separate programs in cardiac and general thoracic surgery in the United States. Dedicated thoracic surgery programs were better able to compete for funding, and training programs improved. These university centers flourished over the next several decades and have trained countless general thoracic surgeons and have promoted a multitude of group practices in general thoracic surgery.

In the first half of the 20th century, pulmonary tuberculosis was the primary focus for thoracic surgeons. After an effective chemotherapy was developed, thoracoplasty faded away in favor of drug therapy and resection only when necessary. In the second half of the century lung cancer replaced tuberculosis as the primary focus of thoracic surgery. Lung cancer became the leading cause of cancer death worldwide, and this in turn, spurred new knowledge and technological developments in general thoracic surgery.

The role of the general thoracic surgeon is diverse. Practitioners are sometimes diagnosticians, sometimes surgeons, and sometimes scientists. Today, surgical extirpation of lung and other pulmonary cancers dominates general thoracic practice, and surgical complete macroscopic resection remains the foundation of therapy in solid tumors. Over time, thoracic surgeons have made steady progress in the technical conduct of surgery, thereby reducing the morbidity and mortality of surgical resection. The primary challenge that remains for many malignancies is the propensity of these cancers to exhibit locoregional and systemic recurrence. Surgical participation in new strategies to effectively control micrometastatic disease will be required for significant progress to be made. The answers to these conundrums lie, presumably, at the molecular level. The relevance of the thoracic surgeon in this scenario continues to grow as surgeons play an increasing role in the development of translational research strategies. In this regard, the emergence of tissue banks, organized and administered by thoracic surgeons, has promoted progress in collaboration with translational and basic science.

The education and training of general thoracic surgeons has seen much progress. The recent emergence of specialized thoracic surgery training tracks and the reorganization of training programs that will facilitate the training of highly skilled surgeons is one example. The emergence of programs that accept medical students who have decided on a focus in cardiothoracic surgery, as well as programs selecting residents midway through their general thoracic training, is another example. All of these efforts permit greater focus on individual specialties and support the training of competent and innovative surgeons. New fellowship programs are also being developed to refine specific operative skill sets. For example, fellowships in minimally invasive surgery, thoracic oncology, and more recently, robotic surgery seek to refine unique skills in a subset of members of our surgical community.

The ongoing divergence of the two subspecialties of cardiothoracic surgery is attributable to the specialization of skills and knowledge required for the diagnosis and treatment of cardiac versus lung and chest wall disease. While it is has been demonstrated that surgeons who work hard and keep abreast of their personal continuing medical education can be competent in both cardiac and thoracic operations, it is my personal belief that to create new knowledge in either field and to train dedicated cardiac or thoracic residents, a career dedicated to one or the other discipline is prerequisite. It goes without saying, for example, that acquiring sufficient knowledge to teach residents about the multitude of new cardiac valve replacement prostheses necessarily precludes the level of knowledge required to teach residents about the appropriate chemotherapy approaches in the multidisciplinary care of thoracic oncologic processes.

If asked to offer a piece of advice I have found most valuable in my role as surgical educator and mentor, it would be the following. The success of one's career depends not only on accomplished and industrious academic pursuit, but also on the ability to identify and pursue select goals with focus and singularity of purpose. This principle is illustrated in the following parable.

A young surgeon walked up to the granite wall of human disease. The wall was so shiny and black, he could see his face reflected on the surface. Anxious to make his mark, he grabbed a pick axe lying nearby and started swinging at the wall, but the blade bounced off. He tried this repeatedly without raising a speck of dust. Further down the wall, several other young surgeons were having the same problem. Feeling frustrated and discouraged, the young man stopped to rest. Suddenly, he became aware of an old surgeon sitting on a bench nearby quietly surveying the scene. He decided to approach him for advice. The surgeon took the young man's axe, held it in his hands, and looked thoughtfully at the blade, rolling it over several times. He then studied the other young surgeons flailing at the granite wall, unable to make their marks. After what seemed like an eternity, he spoke. "I notice," he said, "that everyone here is using the broad end of the pick." He swung the axe around, pulled a grind stone out of his bag, and honed the fine end of the pick to an extremely sharp point. "Try that," he suggested when he was satisfied with his work. The young surgeon walked to the wall and swung the pick with its narrow focused point. Before too long, dust began to fly, and the young man began to make progress.

The moral of this story is clear. For a surgeon to make real progress in the treatment of human disease, a clarity of purpose and focused attention will be required or the effort will be frustrating and progress slow.

It is difficult to enumerate the challenges that lie ahead for our specialty. Many factors—technological, biological, sociological, political—have the potential to influence our future course. We have the opportunity to build upon the firm base in general thoracic training and education that was established by our mentors in the 1980s. The future of our specialty will be shaped by the quality of our education and the institutions that have been established to keep our practitioners current and informed. The pursuit of excellence in our individual practices will have an untold influence on the collective practice of our specialty. Although this book is a reflection of individuals who have focused their careers in thoracic surgery, it is equally intended for general thoracic surgeons, cardiothoracic surgeons, and general surgeons who operate in the chest. Indeed, the only prerequisite for benefiting from this book is that one practice some form of general thoracic surgery. The pioneers of our profession participated in an exciting, almost unparalleled era in the history of medicine, but the story is not over. I have no doubt that the readers of this book will continue to witness and contribute to major advances in our field across the spectrum of evolving surgical therapies. Above all, this text seeks to promote and support the attainment of individual excellence in the practice of thoracic surgery so that we can continue to provide our patients with the highest quality of surgical care.

References

1. Paulson DL. A time for assessment. *J Thorac Cardiovasc Surg.* 1981;82:163–168.
2. Pearson FG. Adventures in surgery. *J Thorac Cardiovasc Surg.* 1990;100:639–651.

2 Thoracic Incisions

Michael T. Jaklitsch

Keywords: Thoracic incisions, posterolateral thoracotomy, anterolateral thoracotomy, axillary thoracotomy, bilateral thoracosternotomy (clamshell), median sternotomy, partial sternotomy, anterior mediastinoscopy (parasternal Chamberlain), open thoracostomy, Eloesser flap, Clagett window

A surgical incision opens an aperture into the thorax to permit the work of the planned operation to proceed. If placed correctly, the operation proceeds with unimpeded visualization of the important anatomy. If placed incorrectly, it can lead to frustrating delays and difficulty in the operation. Dr. Robert E. Gross' admonition, "If an operation is difficult, you are not doing it properly," applies directly to the incision used.* This chapter is designed for both the novice and those who have already gained some experience with thoracic incisions. The artwork is designed to explain important relationships for the inexperienced. We also have provided subtle pearls that will rekindle an appreciation of different incisions for the more experienced. More important, we have tried to explain the logic behind the incisions.

Each incision is described in terms of its current general use, technical details, advantages, and disadvantages. We also provide details of chest wall anatomy, with particular attention to structures that can be injured while developing the incision. Finally, we provide surface anatomy landmarks that can be used to place the incision properly.

As the thoracic surgeon gains experience, these incisions frequently will be modified to accommodate the primary surgical objective of a given operation. Furthermore, as technology progresses, these standard incisions may begin to change. For instance, in the modern era of video-assisted techniques, even classic open incisions are decreasing in length as surgeons become more comfortable with the concept of centering the incision on the anatomy that is critical for the operation to progress. In this regard, these standardized incisions can be thought of as building blocks, similar to the notes of a musical chord. It is our belief that the more the surgeon understands the strengths, weaknesses, and possibilities of each incision, the quicker he or she will learn to use the full variety of possible incisions tailored to the individual patient.

*Personal communication with W. Hardy Hendren on the origin of Dr. Gross' sign, September 20, 2007: "The sign was made by Dr. Robert E. Gross. He was the William E. Ladd Professor and surgeon-in-chief of Children's Hospital in Boston from 1947 to 1967, when he was succeeded by Dr. Judah Folkman. Dr. Gross was then appointed cardiovascular surgeon-in-chief until he retired in 1972. The sign hung in OR 3, which, sadly, became an anesthesia workroom when the OR suite was enlarged. Dr. Folkman saved the sign, which was an important relic of the past. In 1982, Dr. Folkman elected to spend full time in his burgeoning laboratory. He was succeeded by W. Hardy Hendren, who had been for 22 years head of pediatric surgery at the Massachusetts General Hospital. When Dr. Hendren was appointed chief of surgery at Children's Hospital in 1982, Dr. Folkman presented the sign to him. It hung in OR 7 until the operating suite was once again enlarged, and the room was changed into a nursing administrative office. Alas, planners have no appreciation of historical places. Only the original Ida Smith ward, where the surgical neonates were housed back to the Ladd era, has thus far escaped the wrecker's ball. When Bob Shamberger became chief of surgery, I passed on to him 'The Sign.' It is now in his office. Perhaps it will find its way back to the OR. I hope the above will correct the record on the famous sign. Best regards, Hardy."

POSTEROLATERAL THORACOTOMY

General Use

Posterolateral thoracotomy is the standard workhorse for most thoracic surgeons. It offers excellent direct visualization of the entire thoracic cavity, including the posterior diaphragmatic sulcus and apex of the hemithorax. The incision generally is centered over the fifth intercostal space, which corresponds to the greater fissure of the lung. This provides an unobstructed view of the base of the fissure, the pulmonary artery, and the hilum. The incision generally is used for anatomic lung resections, including pneumonectomy and lobectomy. It offers the easiest access for radical lymphadenectomy. An extended posterolateral thoracotomy is used for Pancoast resection, extrapleural pneumonectomy, and aortic transection.

Technique

The patient is placed in a standard lateral decubitus position, with the ipsilateral arm extended forward. The inferior tip of the scapula is palpated and generally marked. The incision begins approximately 3 cm posterior to the scapula tip and approximately halfway between the scapula and the spinous process. The incision curves around the tip to lie along the top margin of the sixth rib (fifth intercostal space). In general, it extends to the anterior axillary line (Fig. 2-1). The soft tissue and Scarpa's fascia are divided. The latissimus dorsi muscle is divided. The auscultatory triangle, the space bounded by the lower border of the trapezius, the serratus anterior, and the medial margin of the scapula can be identified at this time. The serratus anterior muscle can be spared by freeing it from the soft tissue of the auscultatory triangle and the muscle rotated forward. Preservation of the serratus anterior muscle helps to preserve the motion of the shoulder girdle and quickens recovery time. An intact serratus anterior muscle can limit the spread of the fifth and sixth ribs. This can be overcome by detaching the lower slips of attachment of the muscle from the eighth, seventh, and sixth ribs (Fig. 2-2).

If the ribs are to be preserved, the attachment of the intercostal muscles is divided from the top of the sixth rib. It is important to stay on the top surface of the lower rib to avoid injury to the neurovascular bundle of the upper rib. This is best done by proceeding from posterior to anterior along the line of

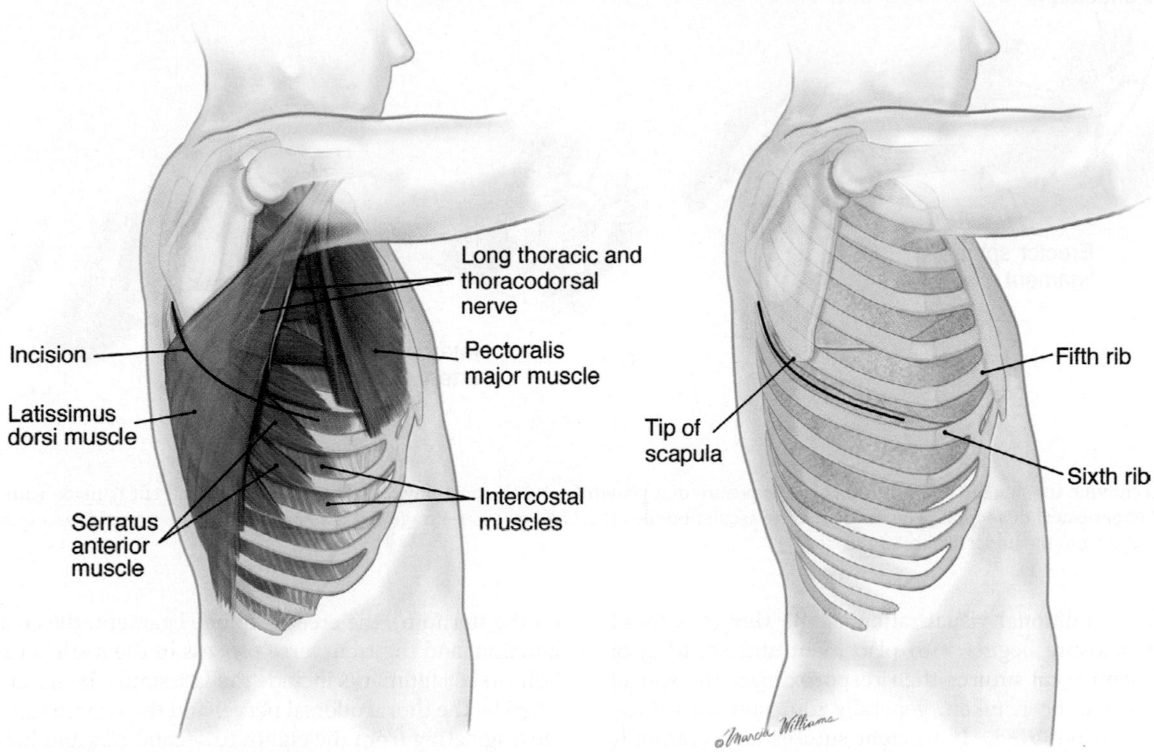

Figure 2-1. Standard posterolateral thoracotomy incision, with extrathoracic musculature and surface landmarks. The incision wraps around the tip of the scapula and parallels the course of the sixth rib.

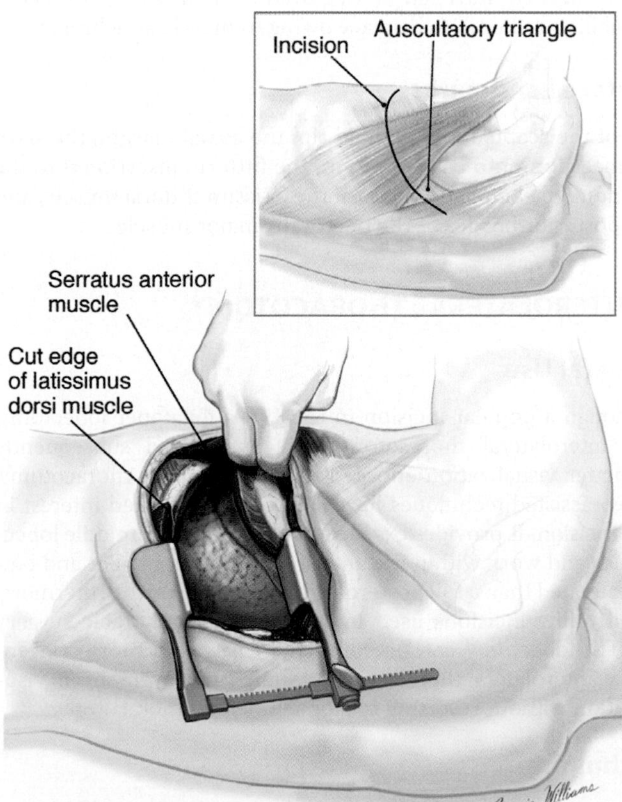

Figure 2-2. Posterolateral thoracotomy divides the latissimus dorsi muscle and rotates the serratus anterior muscle forward. The incision appears centered on the greater fissure of the lung, providing access to the pulmonary artery at the base of the fissure.

the external intercostal fibers. For maximal spread of the ribs, it is important to take down these attachments as far forward as the costochondral junction and as far posterior as the transverse processes of the vertebral body. Both these landmarks can be palpated by a finger passed just superficial to the intercostal muscle layer. In general, there is no need to disrupt the erector spinae ligament, which passes perpendicular to the posterior rib behind the posterior axillary line.

Either removing the rib or "shingling" the posterior rib can achieve additional spread of the ribcage. To remove the rib, the periosteum is raised initially by cautery, and then the plane between the cortical bone and the periosteum is dissected with a periosteal elevator. The neurovascular bundle is pushed out of the inferior groove of the rib with the elevator. The elevator is passed from posterior to anterior above the rib and from anterior to posterior below the rib to take advantage of the angle of the superficial intercostal muscle fibers as they insert into the bone. The direction of these fibers can be remembered simply by thinking of the angle of your arm when you place your hand in your pocket. After the periosteum is raised, the rib is cut, usually with a guillotine rib cutter. This device cuts the bone to one side and thus needs to be turned to remove the entire stripped portion of bone.

"Shingling" a rib involves removal of approximately a centimeter length of rib just anterior to the erector spinae ligament to allow further distraction of the fifth and sixth ribs without a subsequent midshaft fracture of the rib (Fig. 2-3). These small bony defects are much less painful than midshaft fractures. It is important to free the intercostal neurovascular bundle from beneath the inferior groove of the posterior segment of the remaining rib to prevent neuropraxia of the nerve. Increasing the distraction of the ribs can stretch the nerve if it remains fixed to the undersurface of the posterior fragment. Freeing this

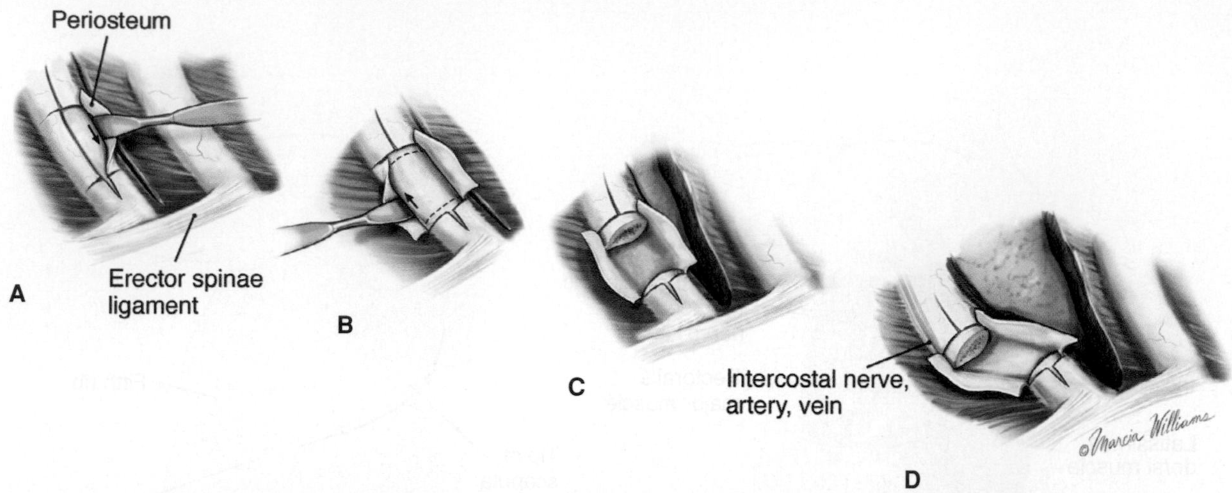

Figure 2-3. Technique to "shingle" the rib to increase exposure of a posterolateral thoracotomy. (*A*) The initial periosteal cut is made with a bovie and elevated. (*B*) Subperiosteal dissection protects the neurovascular bundle. (*C*) The osseous rib fragment is removed. (*D*) The nerve is susceptible to stretch injury unless freed from the undersurface of the rib.

nerve provides additional visualization of the thorax without nerve injury. Closure begins with placement and securing of chest tubes. Paracostal sutures then reapproximate the spread ribs. If no rib has been taken, generally four sutures suffice. If a rib has been removed, six to eight sutures are commonly required to prevent a chest wall hernia. If a midshaft rib fracture has occurred, the paracostal sutures should be placed to prevent movement of the fracture. Fracture ends sometimes are best treated by removing the jagged portion of the rib with a rib cutter, with the end result similar to a "shingle." The ribs should be approximated but not brought tightly in apposition to each other because this frequently causes the bones to fuse subsequently, which can limit surgical choices for redo thoracotomies. The serratus anterior muscle is reapproximated to the soft tissue overlying the auscultatory triangle, and then the latissimus dorsi muscle is sewn back together. Approximation of the latissimus dorsi fascia with minimal bulky muscle will minimize pain and provide a superior cosmetic result. Two additional layers of closure reapproximate Scarpa's fascia and the skin.

Advantage

The posterolateral thoracotomy incision provides the best unobstructed view of the entire hemithorax (Fig. 2-4).

Disadvantages

A generally long incision, the posterolateral thoracotomy is associated with more tissue injury to the extrathoracic musculature and soft tissue. It is also associated with a longer recovery time than almost any other incision (with the exception of the clamshell incision, which is generally slightly more morbid). It takes more time to open and close this incision compared with minimally invasive incisions. Epidural catheters have improved acute postoperative pain control and are especially helpful in the face of impaired lung function.

Chest Wall Anatomy

Key bony landmarks (Fig. 2-1) include the tip of the scapula,[1] the sixth rib (identified as the first rib contributing to the costal margin), the fifth rib (identified as the last rib inserting directly on the sternum), the erector spinae ligament, the costochondral junction, and the transverse process of the sixth vertebral body. Soft tissue landmarks include the latissimus dorsi muscle (innervated by the thoracodorsal nerve) and the serratus anterior muscle originating from the eighth to second ribs and innervated by the long thoracic nerve. A small vascular perforator enters each of the slips of the serratus anterior muscle where they insert on the rib. Both the thoracodorsal nerve and the long thoracic nerve can be injured. Ribs can be fractured if the distraction exceeds the ability of the rib to displace owing to muscle attachments.

Surface Landmarks

Tip of the scapula, the xiphoid tip, the costal margin, the sixth rib insertion onto costal margin, the fifth rib insertion into the sternum, the anterior border of the latissimus dorsi muscle, and the posterior border of the pectoralis major muscle.

ANTEROLATERAL THORACOTOMY

General Use

Although a popular incision in the 1950s for upper lobectomy, the anterolateral thoracotomy was supplanted subsequently by better visualization afforded by posterolateral thoracotomy. Video-assisted techniques have spawned a rekindled interest in this incision. It provides excellent visualization for middle lobectomies and work within the anterior chest. It is smaller and better tolerated than a full posterolateral thoracotomy. Furthermore, small utility incisions used for video-assisted thoracic surgery (VATS) lobectomy can be converted easily to a more conventional anterolateral thoracotomy for quick improvements in visualization without resorting to a posterolateral thoracotomy.

Technique

These incisions generally are placed in the fourth or fifth intercostal space (Fig. 2-5). The fourth interspace (over the top of the fifth rib) provides excellent visualization of the anterior mediastinum and hilum at the level of the superior pulmonary vein. The fifth intercostal space (over the top of the sixth rib) provides

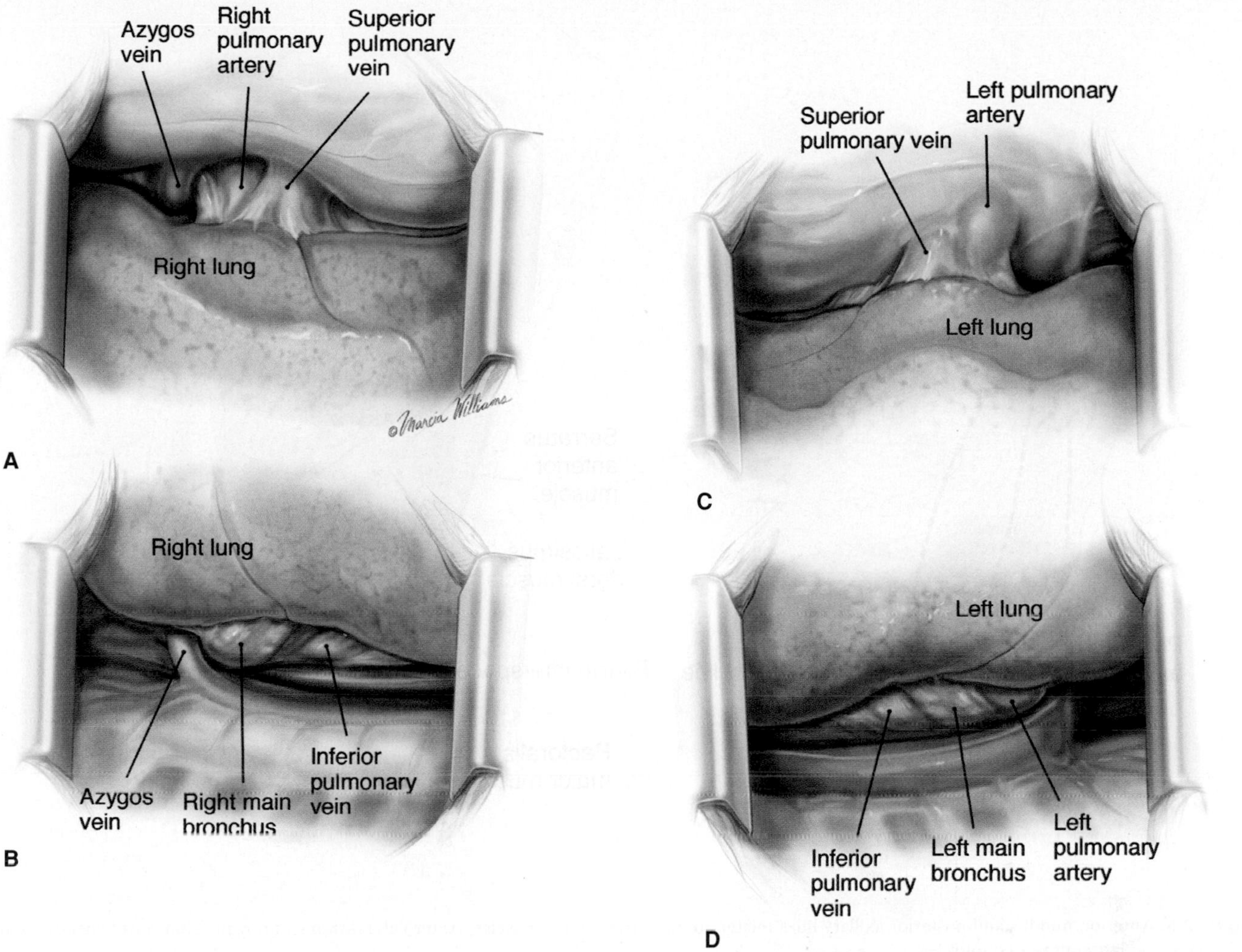

Figure 2-4. Anterior and posterior views of the hilum of the lung from a standard posterolateral thoracotomy. *A.* Anterior view of right lung. *B.* Posterior view of right lung. *C.* Anterior view of left lung. *D.* Posterior view of left lung.

better visualization for a middle lobectomy because it provides visualization of both the lower portion of the superior pulmonary vein and the top portion of the inferior pulmonary vein (Fig. 2-6).

The patient is placed in the same lateral decubitus position as for a posterolateral thoracotomy. The arm is placed in a more classic "swimmer" position with 90-degree abduction of the upper arm to allow easier access to the fourth intercostal space.

The incision starts approximately 1 cm posterior to the pectoralis major muscle and runs along the top of the rib for approximately 10 to 15 cm. The skin and Scarpa's fascia are divided. The posterior border of the pectoralis major muscle is frequently seen but not divided. The latissimus dorsi muscle is not seen. The serratus anterior muscle is divided along the course of its fibers and not rotated. The intercostal muscle is lifted from the top of the inferior rib. The intercostal muscle can be further undercut beneath the more superficial soft tissues by bluntly developing a plane just superficial to the intercostal muscle and then dividing it while not dividing the more superficial soft tissues. It is important to remove the intercostal muscle from the top portion of the lower rib to avoid injury to the neurovascular bundle of the upper rib. Although ribs can be removed or "shingled," this is rarely needed because the intercostal space gets larger as the ribs pass anteriorly. Thus there is a greater natural distraction of ribs at the anterior axillary line compared with the posterior axillary line.

Advantages

The anterolateral incision is smaller and associated with a quicker recovery compared with the posterolateral incision. The latissimus dorsi muscle is not divided, leaving better shoulder function postoperatively and preserving future use of a latissimus dorsi flap if the patient is at risk of developing a bronchopleural fistula.

Disadvantages

Although the incision provides good visualization of the anterior hemithorax, visualization of the posterior hemithorax and inferior portions of the chest are impaired. These disadvantages can be offset by the use of thoracoscopy, hence the frequent use of this incision in VATS procedures. Quick extension of the incision is hampered by the potential of injury to the long thoracic nerve posteriorly and the bulk of the pectoralis major muscle anteriorly.

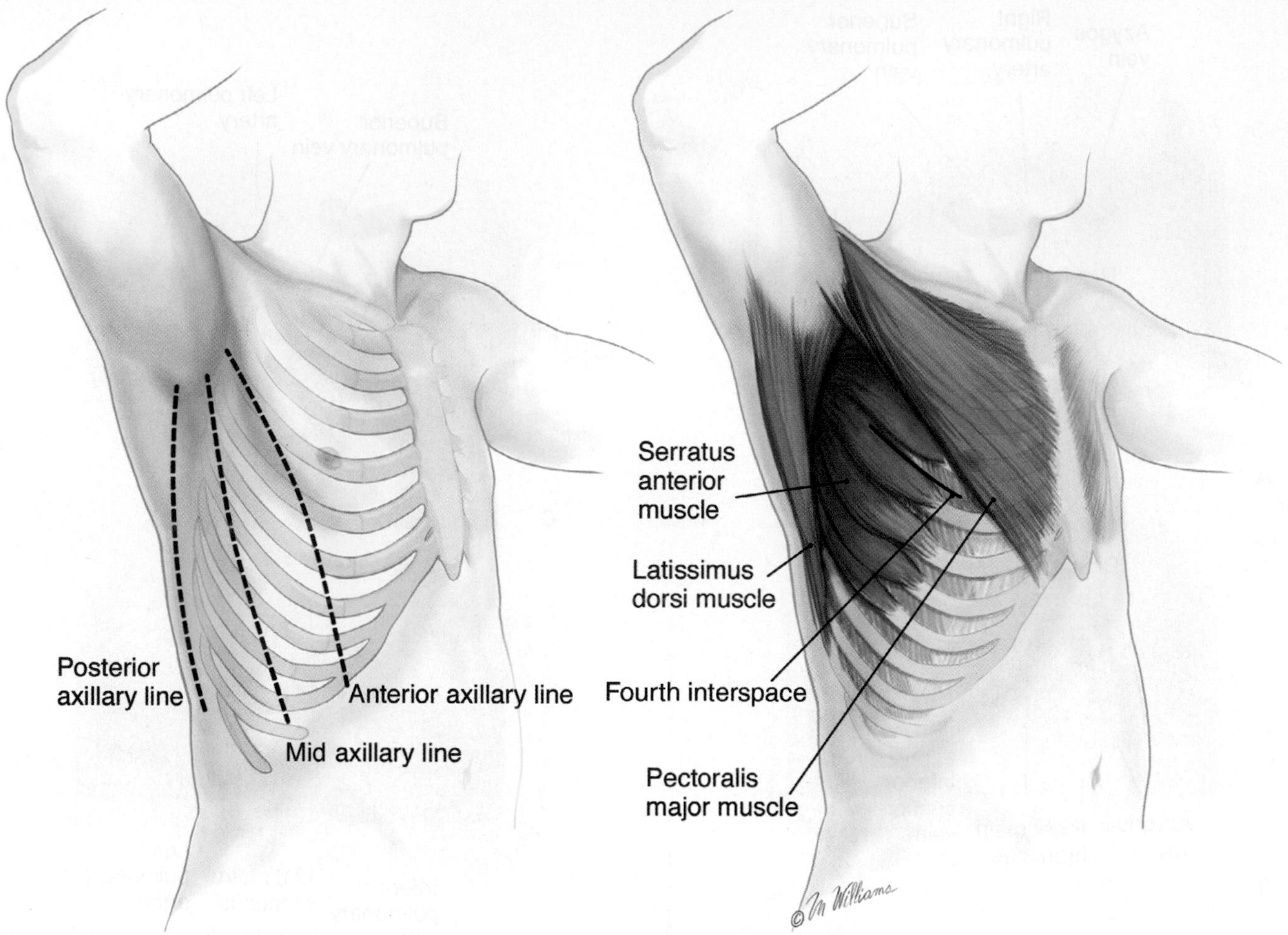

Figure 2-5. Anterior, middle, and posterior axillary lines related to the extrathoracic muscles. Anterolateral thoracotomy incision runs beneath the pectoralis major and latissimus dorsi muscles.

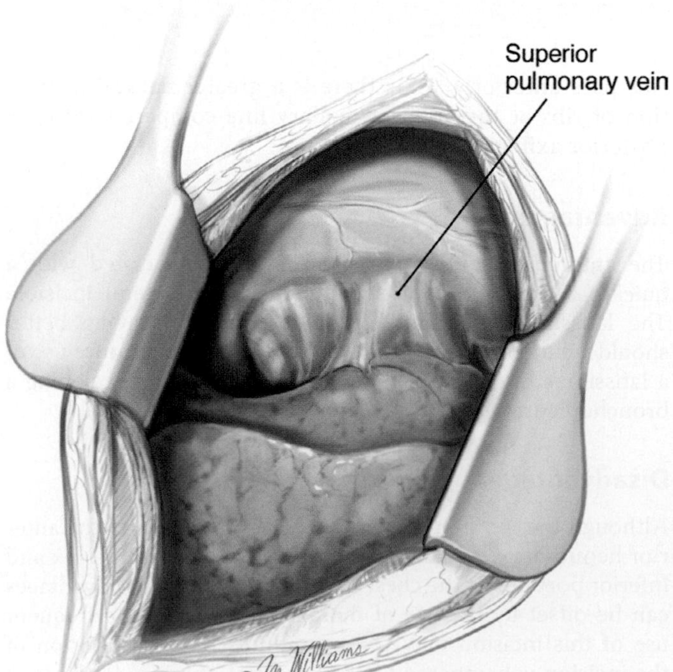

Figure 2-6. View of the right hilum from an anterolateral thoracotomy.

Chest Wall Anatomy

Key bony landmarks include the sixth rib (identified as the first rib contributing to the costal margin), the fifth rib (identified as the last rib inserting directly on the sternum), and the costochondral junction. The most important soft tissue landmark is the long thoracic nerve that innervates the serratus anterior muscle and runs just beneath the anterior border of the latissimus dorsi muscle. Since the serratus anterior muscle is divided along its fibers and not rotated, this nerve can be injured by posterior extension or misplacement of the incision.

Surface Landmarks

Posterior border of the pectoralis major, the sixth rib insertion onto the costal margin, the fifth rib insertion into the sternum, and the anterior border of the latissimus dorsi muscle.

AXILLARY THORACOTOMY

General Use

An axillary thoracotomy can be thought of as an anterolateral thoracotomy incision in the first, second, or third interspace (Fig. 2-7). It provides access to the apex of the hemithorax and is

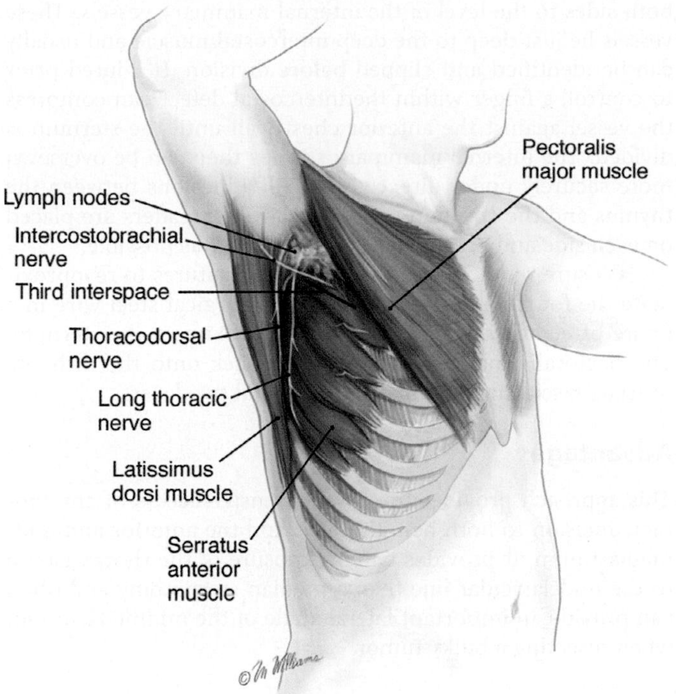

Figure 2-7. Extrathoracic structures at risk for injury with an axillary thoracotomy and proper placement of the incision.

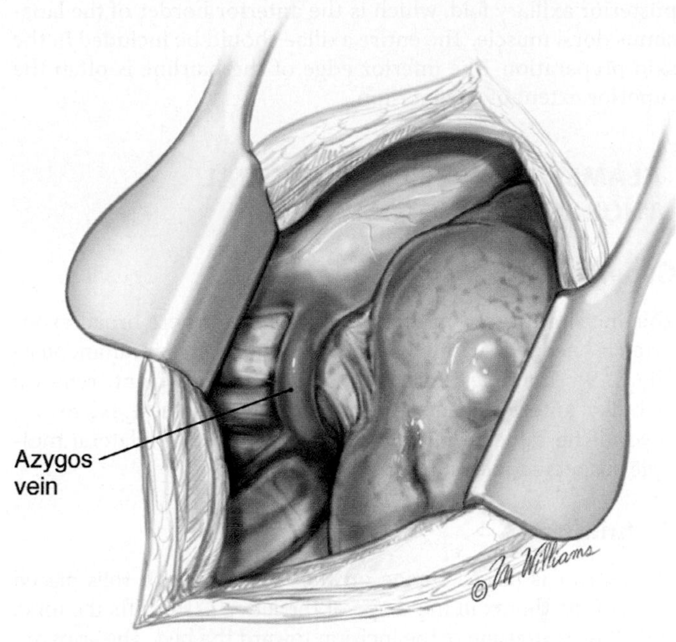

Figure 2-8. View of the right hilum from an axillary thoracotomy.

particularly useful for mobilizing a scarred apical segment from the parietal pleura during thoracoscopic procedures,[2] visualization of the posterior portion of the apex of the lung during bullectomy, and mobilization of the thymus when using a thoracoscopic approach. Because the apex of the lung lacks the bulk of the lower portion, it is easily displaced, and the anterior, middle, and posterior upper mediastinum can be visualized easily. This same incision is used for first rib resection via an axillary approach.

Technique

The ipsilateral arm needs to be put into true swimmer's position, with a 90- to 120-degree angle between the thorax and the humerus. Deep palpation of the axilla should identify the second and third intercostal space and even the first intercostal space in very thin patients. In general, the third intercostal space between the third and fourth ribs is the easiest position for this incision in males and the second intercostal space in females. The incision extends across the base of the axilla, between the anterior border of the latissimus dorsi muscle and the posterior extent of the pectoralis major muscle. This is the auscultatory triangle. It has no underlying muscles. It contains clavipectoral fascia and underlying lymphatics and lymph nodes. It is important to ligate or cauterize these lymphatics to avoid postoperative lymphoceles. Once one enters the thorax, the incision lies to the anterior side of the hilum at the level of the azygos–caval junction (Fig. 2-8). This is one rib interspace above the superior pulmonary vein.

Advantages

This approach provides adequate visualization of the upper mediastinum and posterior portion of the apex of the lung. Recovery time is very quick, and pain is modest. In general, the higher the interspace, the lower is the pain, most likely because there is less excursion of the ribs during respiration. Maximum excursion of the ribcage during forced respiration is at the level of the seventh and eighth ribs.

Disadvantages

The correct interspace for the incision needs to be considered carefully based on the goal of the operation. A second interspace incision will not allow proper visualization of the superior pulmonary vein. Incisions in the upper interspaces also do not allow much extension of the incision, if desired. Thoracoscopy can be used to place the incision, guided by direct inspection of the surface lung landmarks correlated with soundings at the skin level. This thoracoscopic port then can be used for chest tube placement at the conclusion of the procedure.

Chest Wall Anatomy

The major structures in danger of injury are the long thoracic nerve to the serratus anterior muscle, the thoracodorsal nerve to the latissimus dorsi muscle, and the intercostobrachial nerve (Fig. 2-7). The long thoracic nerve can be identified as it passes under the axillary vein at the level of the second rib. It travels inferiorly along the serratus anterior muscle parallel with the lateral thoracic artery. The thoracodorsal nerve can be identified posterior to the long thoracic nerve, just anterior to the border of the latissimus dorsi muscle. The higher the interspace chosen, the shorter is the length of the bordering ribs, and the higher is the probability of injury to these nerves, especially if the incision is extended posteriorly. If the incision is placed in the first intercostal space, the intercostobrachial nerve also can be injured, resulting in numbness to the medial side of the arm.

Surface Landmarks

Surface landmarks include the anterior axillary fold, which is the posterior border of the pectoralis major muscle, and the posterior axillary fold, which is the anterior border of the latissimus dorsi muscle. The entire axillae should be included in the skin preparation. The inferior edge of the hairline is often the superior extent of any incision.

CLAMSHELL INCISION (BILATERAL THORACOSTERNOTOMY)

General Use

This incision is used in rare circumstances where broad exposure is needed within both hemithoraces simultaneously (Fig. 2-9). Examples include double lung transplant, removal of bulky anterior mediastinal masses with lateral extensions beyond the midclavicular lines, and removal of bilateral multiple suspected metastases.[3]

Technique

The patient is placed supine on the OR table with rolls placed beneath the thorax in the shape of the letter *I*. This lifts the torso and allows extension of the incision toward the bed. The arms are extended above the head and suspended with the upper arms distracted from the thorax at approximately a 120-degree angle. The incision runs beneath each inframammary crease and crosses the sternum in the fourth intercostal space. The incision extends into the inferior portion of each axilla. The pectoralis major muscle is lifted off the top of the fifth rib anteriorly. The intrapleural space is entered by dividing the intercostal muscles at the midclavicular line. Dissection then extends medially on both sides to the level of the internal mammary vessels. These vessels lie just deep to the deep intercostal muscle and usually can be identified and clipped before division. If injured prior to control, a finger within the intercostal defect can compress the vessel against the anterior chest wall until the sternum is divided. The internal mammary stumps then can be oversewn more securely under direct vision. All adhesions between the thymus and the sternum are divided. Rib spreaders are placed on each side and often can be opened as far as possible.

Closure requires multiple paracostal sutures to reapproximate the fourth and fifth ribs. A no. 5 surgical steel wire in a figure-of-eight pattern is used to reapproximate the sternum. The pectoralis major muscle is sewn back onto the fifth rib. Scarpa's fascia and skin make up the final two layers.

Advantages

This approach provides the most extensive access of any thoracic incision to both hemithoraces and the anterior and mid-mediastinum. It provides better exposure of the thorax lateral to the midclavicular line than a median sternotomy and often can provide an important lateral angle of the midmediastinum when resecting a bulky tumor.

Disadvantages

Because this incision is associated with extensive disruption of muscle and bone, as well as extended length, recovery from this incision is more difficult than with all other thoracic incisions. Furthermore, the disruption of the intercostal and accessory muscles of respiration at the level of the fourth and fifth

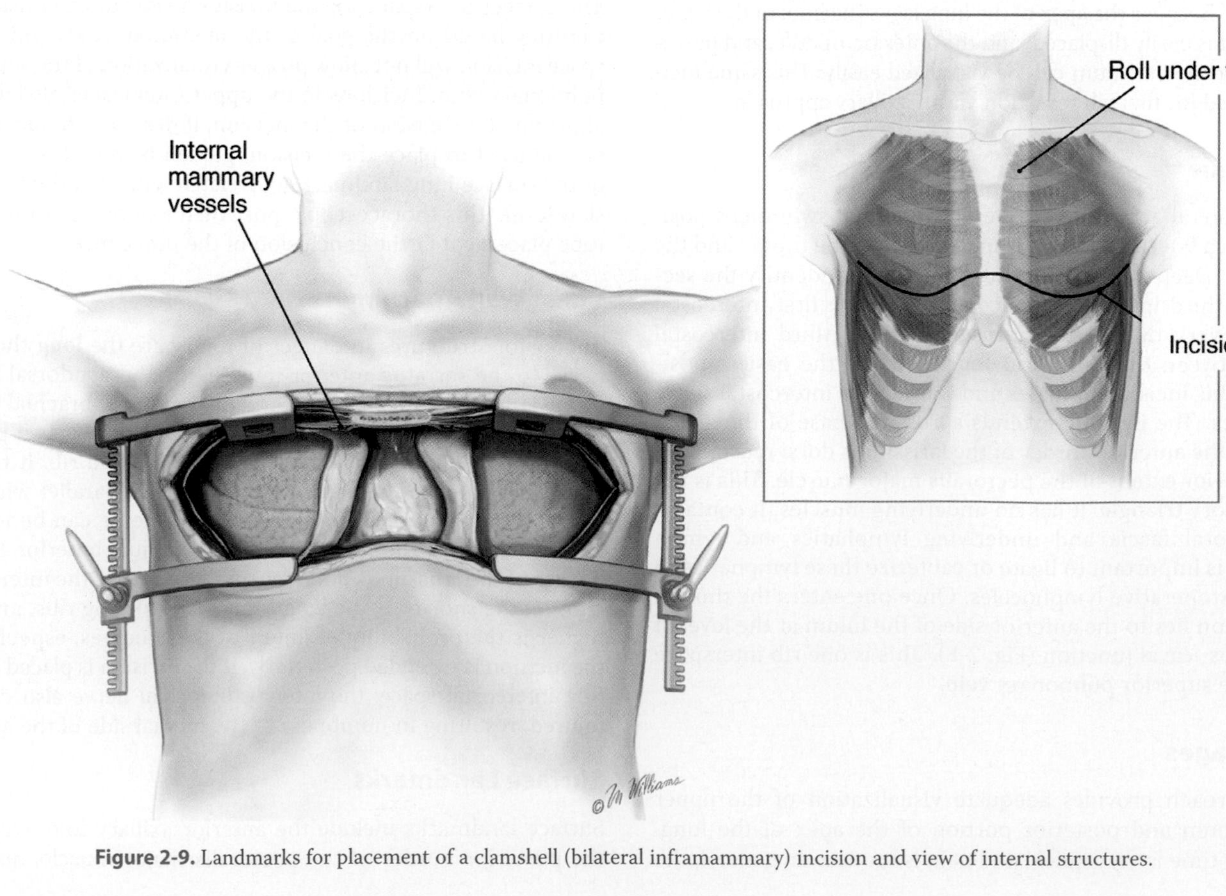

Figure 2-9. Landmarks for placement of a clamshell (bilateral inframammary) incision and view of internal structures.

interspaces has a serious impact on chest wall excursion and breathing mechanics. As a result, this incision should not be considered for frail patients. Both the phrenic nerves are susceptible to injury, especially when mobilizing adhesions close to their insertions in the diaphragm or at the level of the manubrium. In addition, it provides poor exposure of the posterior mediastinum.

Chest Wall Anatomy

Important landmarks include clear identification of the fourth, fifth, and sixth ribs and their insertions into the sternum or costal margin. The sternomanubrial junction, or angle of Louis, denotes the second intercostal space.

Surface Landmarks

The incision runs through the inframammary crease but must cross the sternum at the level of the fourth intercostal space. Once the pectoralis major muscle has been lifted, the fourth intercostal space is easily brought into the base of the wound, but the skin incision should cross the sternum at the level of the planned osteotomy.

MEDIAN STERNOTOMY

General Use

This incision is used widely for cardiac surgery, resection of anterior mediastinal masses, radical thymectomies, and dissections of the upper mediastinum. It also can provide access to both hemithoraces for bilateral pulmonary nodules or lung volume reduction surgery.

Technique

The most important goal of this incision is to be precisely in the vertical midline of the sternum. This begins with positioning on the OR table. The patient must be supine with a transverse roll beneath the most kyphotic portion of the back. The hips must be even. The sternal notch and tip of the xiphoid are marked, and vigorous palpation of the edge of the sternum in each intercostal space is used to mark the midline of the sternum. The skin incision should extend from the sternomanubrial junction to 2 cm below the tip of the xiphoid (Fig. 2-10). Dissection is carried down through Scarpa's fascia between the origins of the two pectoralis major muscles. Dissection is extended above the sternal notch. A transverse venous branch frequently crosses the sternal notch and should be cauterized. The clavicular–clavicular ligament can be palpated just deep to the undersurface of the manubrium and links the two heads of the clavicles. This is divided with cautery. The linea alba is divided for 2 cm caudal to the tip of the xiphoid process. A second transverse venous branch is found at the sternoxiphoid junction and needs to be cauterized. The surgeon passes a finger through the defect in the linea alba deep to the xiphoid to bluntly open the diaphragmatic hiatus directly behind the sternum. Likewise, the surgeon's finger passes deep to the manubrium at the cranial end of the incision to bluntly dissect the tissue away from the back of the bone (Fig. 2-11). The saw footplate is placed deep to the bone and pushed or pulled through the center in a careful, steady fashion.

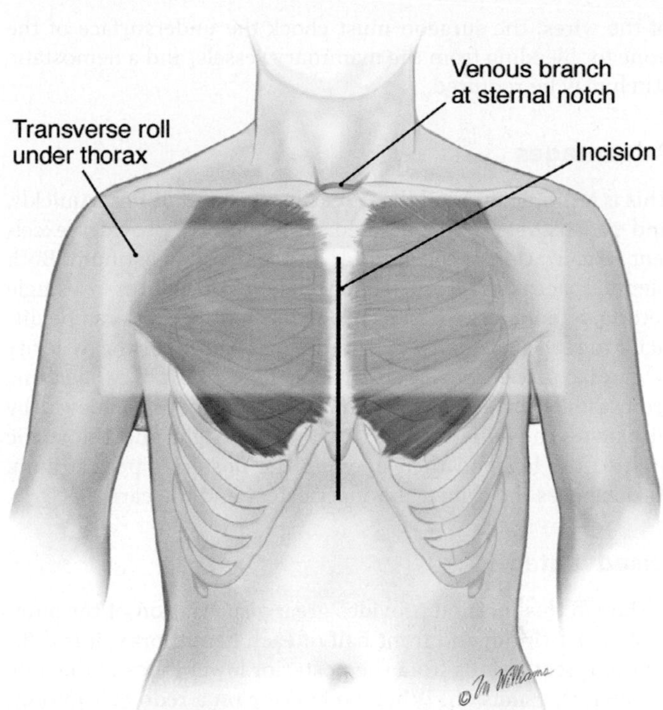

Figure 2-10. Landmarks for placement of skin incision for a median sternotomy.

Hemostasis is achieved by cauterizing the edges of the periosteum and the application of either bone wax or a topical coagulant, such as Gelfoam, soaked in thrombin. A sternal retractor then is placed.

At the conclusion of the procedure, mediastinal drainage tubes are placed through the rectus sheaths with care not to injure abdominal organs. The bone remnants are reapproximated with surgical steel wire. Generally, no. 5 wire is used. Most commonly, two simple wires are placed in the manubrium, and four to five additional wires are placed in the body. Many other sternal fixation devices are currently available. After placement

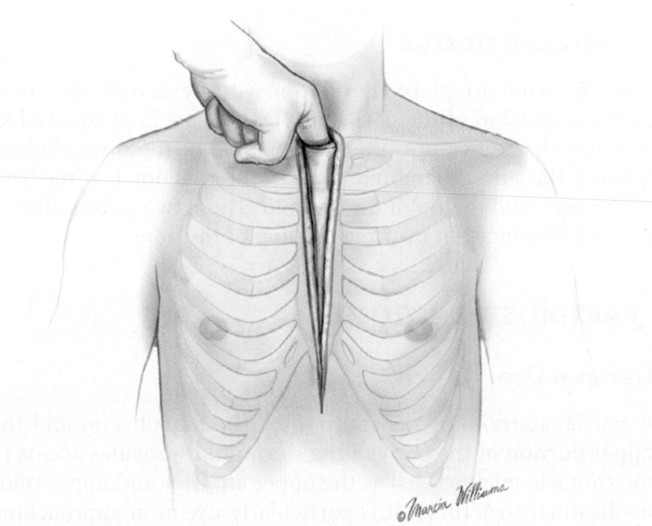

Figure 2-11. Undermining the soft tissues beneath the sternal notch of the manubrium after division of the ligament attaching the two clavicular heads to the sternum.

of the wires, the surgeon must check the undersurface of the bone for bleeding from the mammary vessels, and a hemostatic stitch may be required.

Advantages

This is a simple incision that is easily mastered. It heals quickly, and pain is very well tolerated. This incision provides excellent visualization of the anterior and upper mediastinum. Both pleural spaces can be opened for bilateral procedures in a single setting, although the posterior portions of the chest can be difficult to reach. Median sternotomy can be used for the majority of cardiac procedures. It also can be used to expose the carina from a different angle than thoracotomy. This is achieved by displacing the superior vena cava to the right and the aortic arch to the left and then opening the posterior pericardium. This exposes the right pulmonary artery and the carina.

Disadvantages

Although this incision provides great visualization of the anterior mediastinum and front half of each hemithorax, it is difficult to resect lesions from the posterior lower lobes of the lung through this incision. When embarking on a redo sternotomy, care must be taken to avoid inadvertent entry into the heart, which may be adhered to the underside of the sternum. A lateral radiograph can reveal the degree of adhesion, and preparation for possible emergency cardiopulmonary bypass support can be planned.

Chest Wall Anatomy

The sternum has three component parts: manubrium, body, and xiphoid. The manubrium extends from the sternal notch at the base of the neck to the angle of Louis. The xiphoid is easily palpated. Once the deep fascia is opened over the length of the sternum, the rib insertions into the lateral sternum can be palpated. With a finger pushing into bilateral interspaces at the lateral edge of the body of the sternum, the midpoint of the bone can be marked by electrocautery in the periosteum, facilitating the goal of keeping the saw cut in the midportion of the bone.

Surface Landmarks

Care is taken to place a roll transversely across the most kyphotic portion of the back, and the hips are kept squared so that the chest does not pitch to one side or the other. Subsequently, the surface landmarks are the sternal notch at the base of the neck and the tip of the xiphoid. These two points allow a straight-line incision over the midline of the bone.

PARTIAL STERNOTOMY

General Use

A partial sternotomy generally splits the manubrium and the upper portion of the body of the sternum. It provides access to the thoracic inlet, as well as the upper anterior and upper mid-mediastinal structures. It is particularly useful in approaching the thymus gland and is easily combined with neck incisions to provide proximal and distal control of upper mediastinal arteries and veins.

Technique

The patient is positioned supine with a transverse roll behind the most kyphotic portion of the back. To ensure a vertical midline incision, the hips must be even. A midline incision is made from the angle of Louis inferiorly for about four fingerbreadths. A subcutaneous tunnel is developed superficial to the pectoralis major fascia up to the sternal notch. A transverse venous branch frequently crosses the sternal notch, at the deep level of the manubrium, and should be cauterized. The clavicular–clavicular ligament can be palpated just deep to the undersurface of the manubrium and links the two heads of the clavicles. This is divided with cautery.

This incision can favor the right to displace the right sternal fragment laterally, favor the left to displace the left fragment, or combine with a transverse sternotomy to allow the combined displacement of both fragments (Fig. 2-12). The pectoralis major insertion on the sternum and costal cartilages of the second and third ribs is lifted with electrocautery on the side the incision will favor. A small perforator from the internal mammary vessels can be used to identify the location of the unseen deep artery and both veins. The periosteum of the manubrium is burned in the midline to the angle of Louis. The burn is then extended in a curvilinear manner to the interspace between the second and third or third and fourth ribs. The surgeon's finger passes deep to the manubrium at the sternal notch to bluntly dissect tissue away from the back of the bone. A metal clamp or right angle is used to develop the lateral edge of the bone of the body of the sternum in the rib interspace to insure that the mammary vessels are safely displaced away from the bone. The saw footplate is placed deep to the bone in the sternal notch and pushed or pulled through the center of the manubrium in a careful steady fashion. The saw is gently turned to the rib interspace after the angle of Louis, following the burn in the periosteum. Alternatively, a sternal Lebsche knife can be used to finish the cut into the intercostal space.

Hemostasis is achieved by cauterizing the edges of the periosteum and the application of either bone wax or a topical coagulant, such as Gelfoam soaked in thrombin. A sternal retractor then is placed. The lateral displacement of the fragment is not as much as that occurs with a full sternotomy, but is sufficient to do most dissections in the upper anterior mediastinum.

At the conclusion of the procedure, pleural tubes are placed if the pleurae are open. If the pleurae remain closed, a drainage catheter is frequently not placed since there has been no anticoagulation. The bone fragments are reapproximated with no. 5 surgical steel wires. Most commonly, two simple wires are placed in the manubrium.

Advantages

A partial sternotomy provides nearly the same visualization of the upper anterior mediastinum. Since the angle of Louis corresponds with the carina, any structure in the anterior or middle mediastinal compartment above the level of the carina can be easily approached with this incision. The extension into the neck with a hockey stick incision or a transverse collar incision allows proximal and distal control of the subclavian and carotid arteries, aortic arch, and internal jugular, subclavian, innominate, and brachiocephalic veins. This incision keeps the lower body of the sternum and the costal margins intact. This preserves the respiratory function of the lower ribs for patients with compromised respiratory function. There is less pain and

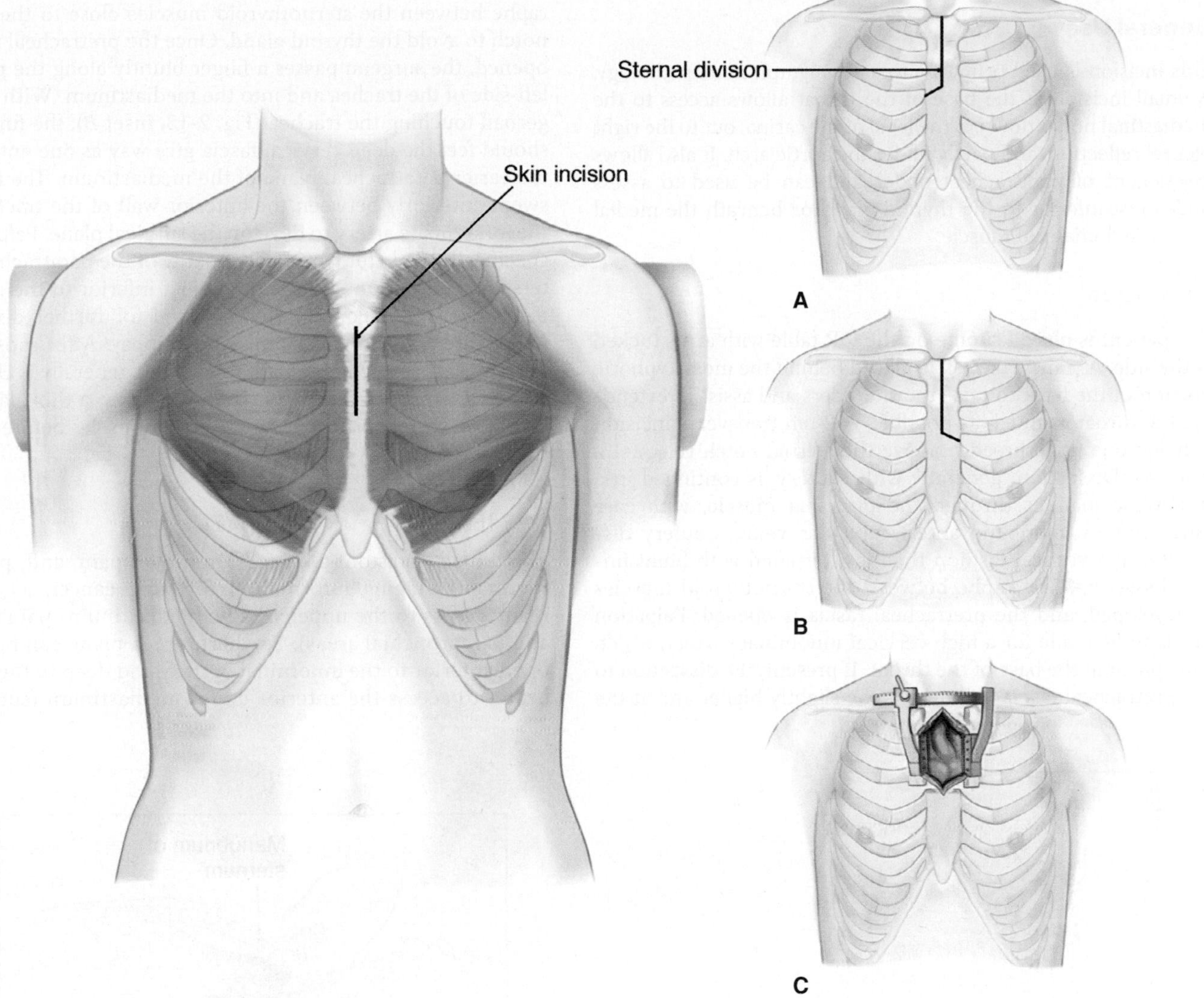

Figure 2-12. Location of incision to favor the right to displace the right sternal fragment laterally (inset *A*). Location of incision to favor the left to displace the left fragment (inset *B*). Location of incision combined with transverse sternotomy to allow the combined displacement of both fragments (inset *C*).

fewer lifting restrictions are required owing to the partial osteotomy. Lifting after partial sternotomy is frequently limited to 20 lbs for 3 weeks, whereas with median sternotomy the lifting restrictions are generally imposed for 8 weeks. Finally, for obese patients, there is less lateral pull to disrupt the partial sternal closure because the lower body of the sternum is intact.

Disadvantage

Since it is only a partial sternotomy, the visualization can be limited at the inferior portion of the osteotomy and laterally at the edges of dissection. If the lateral portion of the osteotomy goes in the interspace between the second and the third rib, the inferior portion of a very large thymus gland may not be seen. If a transverse sternotomy is made, a careful reapproximation of both fragments to the remnant of the body of the sternum must be made. Finally, there is limited visualization into the pleural spaces, and pleural drain placement can be difficult.

Chest Wall Anatomy

The sternum has three component parts: manubrium, body, and xiphoid. The manubrium extends from the sternal notch to the angle of Louis (the cartilage-filled joint between manubrium and upper body of sternum). Once the deep fascia is opened over the planned sternal cut, the rib insertions into the lateral portions of the body of the sternum can be palpated. The rib that inserts into the angle of Louis directly is the second rib.

Surface Landmarks

Care is taken to place a roll transversely across the most kyphotic portion of the back, and the hips are kept squared so that the chest does not pitch to one side or the other. Subsequently, the surface landmarks are the sternal notch at the base of the neck and angle of Louis, where the angle of the manubrium changes from the angle of the body, and the tip of the xiphoid.

CERVICAL MEDIASTINOSCOPY

General Use

This incision is used primarily to assess lymph node pathology. A small incision at the base of the throat allows access to the mediastinal nodes down to the level of the carina, out to the right pleural reflection, and partly under the aortic arch. It also allows assessment of paratracheal nodes and can be used to assess nodes just inferior to the thyroid gland or beneath the medial sternocleidomastoid muscle.

Technique

The patient is placed supine on the OR table with arms tucked at the side. A transverse roll is placed behind the most kyphotic portion of the back to raise the shoulders and assist in extending the throat as much as possible. A 2-cm transverse incision is made one fingerbreadth above the sternal notch (Fig. 2-13, inset *A*). Dissection, generally with cautery, is continued in a transverse manner through the platysma muscle, with care taken not to injure the anterior jugular veins. Cautery dissection in a vertical fashion then is alternated with blunt finger dissection. The raphe between the sternothyroid muscles is developed, and the pretracheal fascia is opened. Palpation needs to be made for a high cervical innominate artery, which can appear at the base of the throat. If present, the dissection to the pretracheal fascia will need to be slightly higher and at the level of the isthmus of the thyroid (one cartilaginous ring below the cricoid cartilage). If not present, we prefer to dissect the raphe between the sternothyroid muscles close to the sternal notch to avoid the thyroid gland. Once the pretracheal fascia is opened, the surgeon passes a finger bluntly along the patient's left side of the trachea and into the mediastinum. With the fingernail touching the trachea (Fig. 2-13, inset *B*), the finger pad should feel the deep cervical fascia give way as one enters into the easier paratracheal plane of the mediastinum. The finger is swept anteriorly between the anterior wall of the trachea and the innominate artery to develop the surgical plane. Palpation is specifically made for lymphadenopathy of the paratracheal gutters and the station 3 lymph node just inferior to the innominate artery. The scope is then inserted for further dissection under direct vision and lymph node biopsy. After satisfactory hemostasis has been obtained, the wound generally is closed in two layers (platysma and skin). Alternatively, a third layer can be placed by reapproximating the strap muscles before closing the platysma.

Advantages

This small incision produces minimal pain and provides invaluable staging information for lung cancer, as well as ready access to the upper middle mediastinum (paratracheal and parabronchial areas). Furthermore, a plane can be developed anterior to the innominate artery and deep to the manubrium to access the anterior upper mediastinum (substernal

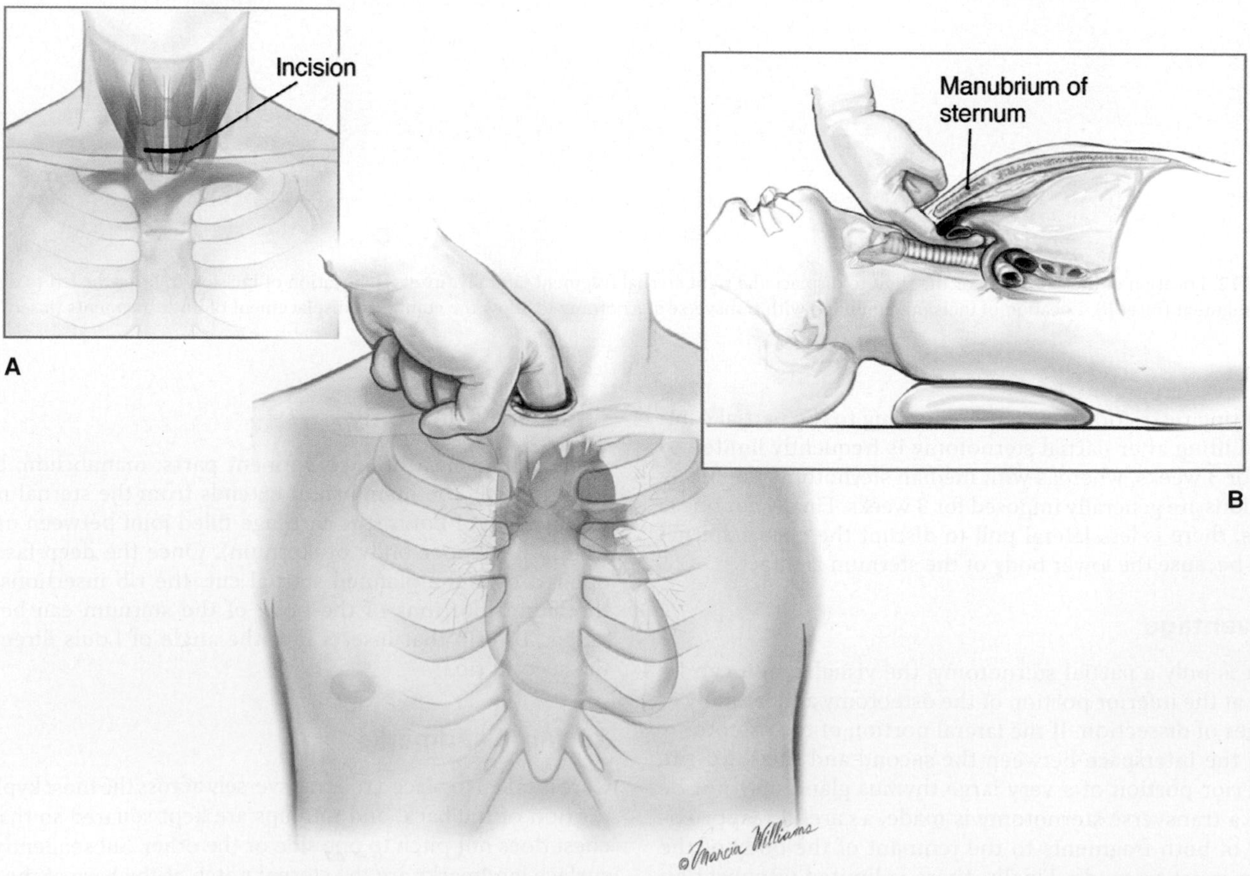

Figure 2-13. Location of incision for cervical mediastinoscopy (inset *A*). The surgeon passes his or her finger bluntly along the anterior border of the trachea into the mediastinum. The tip of the finger feels specifically for adenopathy at station 3 (inset *B*).

mediastinoscopy). The greatest advantage is that this central incision offers bilateral access to lymph nodes in the supraclavicular and paratracheal areas, differentiating IIIA (N2 nodes) from IIIB (N3 nodes) disease in the pathologic staging of lung cancer. The supraclavicular nodes can be accessed by bluntly dissecting laterally beneath the sternocleidomastoid muscle with a finger and then passing the scope onto a firm node, if found.

Disadvantages

Comfort with this incision requires training and experience. Mediastinal vascular structures can be injured, and catastrophic bleeding can occur. Packing the mediastinoscopy wound may be inadequate to control bleeding, and an emergency sternotomy or thoracotomy may be necessary. A sternal saw should be available whenever performing mediastinoscopy.

Chest Wall Anatomy

Cricoid cartilage, sternal notch, heads of the clavicles, sternal heads of the sternocleidomastoid muscles, and the trachea.

Surface Landmarks

The most inferior transverse skin crease of the throat, the sternal notch, the tip of the thyroid cartilage, the anterior curve of the trachea, and the heads of the sternocleidomastoid muscle are used to center the incision.

ANTERIOR MEDIASTINOSCOPY (PARASTERNAL, CHAMBERLAIN)

General Use

This approach is used most commonly to biopsy anterior mediastinal masses that abut the anterior chest wall or biopsy the prevascular (station 6) or aortopulmonary window (station 5) nodes within the left hemithorax. This incision can provide access to all structures medial to the midclavicular lines and anterior to the bronchi, including the internal mammary nodes, the thymus, the pericardium, and the phrenic nerve.

Technique

This incision can be placed in either a right or left parasternal location, within the second to fourth interspace (Fig. 2-14). The most common location is over the top of the third rib in the left parasternal location, which provides access to the aorticopulmonic window nodes. A 2-cm transverse incision is made just to the left of the edge of the sternum (approximately 2 cm lateral to the midpoint of the sternum) and extended over the top of the third rib. Pectoralis major fibers are split along their course, and pectoralis minor fibers generally are more lateral. At the fascia over the external intercostal muscle, a branch of the internal mammary vessels generally can be identified, localizing the hidden vertical course of those vessels. The superficial and deep intercostal muscles are lifted

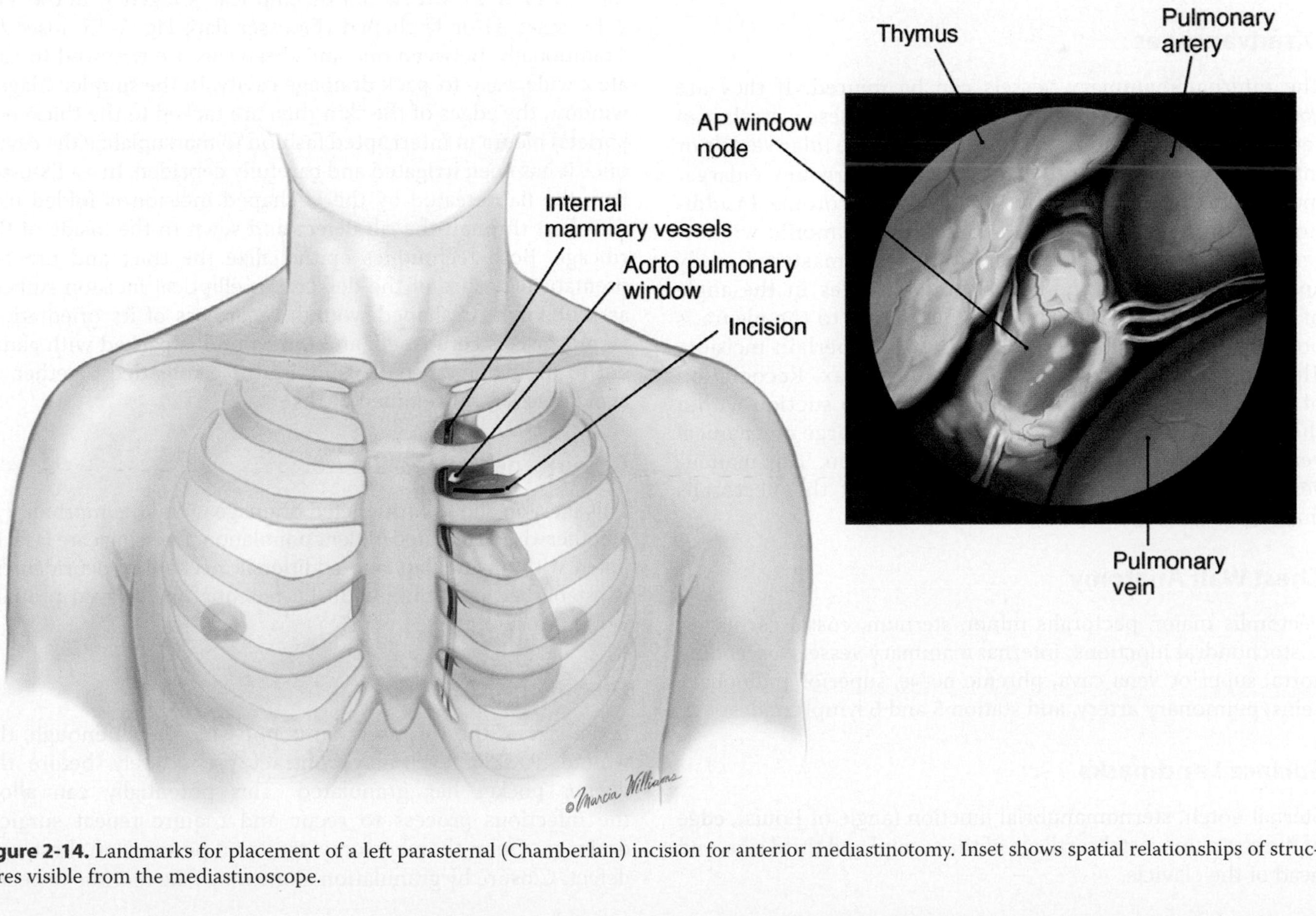

Figure 2-14. Landmarks for placement of a left parasternal (Chamberlain) incision for anterior mediastinotomy. Inset shows spatial relationships of structures visible from the mediastinoscope.

from the top of the third rib down to the level of the intact pleura. The pleura is kept closed and is dissected bluntly from beneath the medial aspect of the incision, separating the pleura from the internal mammary vessels. Blunt dissection is continued beneath the sternum and onto the lateral border of the ascending aorta. At this point, a mediastinoscope is inserted, and dissection is continued with blunt insertion of the scope and a sucker tip to the level of the aorticopulmonic window. Some surgeons prefer a double-lumen endotracheal tube for lung isolation, which may facilitate keeping the pleura closed during the mediastinal dissection. The vacuum within the pleural space pulls the mediastinal pleura laterally during deflation of the ipsilateral lung.

The classic Chamberlain procedure involves a 5- to 6-cm incision over the second costal cartilage, division of the pectoralis major, and resection of the second costal cartilage.[4] The internal mammary artery is divided. The mediastinum then is entered through the posterior perichondrium. This approach is seldom necessary.

Before closure of the anterior mediastinotomy, an aspiration catheter is placed deep into the intercostal muscles. After the first two layers of closure, a Valsalva maneuver is delivered by the ventilator while aspirating the catheter, which then is removed.

Advantages

This small incision provides well-tolerated access to the mediastinal nodes and anterior mediastinal masses. It can be done under local anesthesia with intravenous sedation in patients unable to tolerate general anesthesia.

Disadvantages

The internal mammary vessels can be injured. If they are completely avulsed, the bleeding ends of these vessels can retract beneath the adjacent ribs. Injury to the hilar vessels or internal mammary vessels can force an emergency enlargement of the incision to an anterolateral thoracotomy. In addition, accurate appreciation of the aorticopulmonic window requires experience. This operation is not mastered easily and requires understanding of subtle changes in the angle of the mediastinoscope. Finally, a disruption to the pleura is possible with lateral extension of the Chamberlain incision. This will produce an ipsilateral pneumothorax. Recognition of such a defect in the pleura should lead to suction within the pleura via a red rubber catheter during a large mechanical ventilator breath before closure of the incision. This maneuver generally is performed after closure of the pectoralis major muscle.

Chest Wall Anatomy

Pectoralis major, pectoralis minor, sternum, costal cartilages, costochondral junctions, internal mammary vessels, ascending aorta, superior vena cava, phrenic nerve, superior pulmonary veins, pulmonary artery, and station 5 and 6 lymph nodes.

Surface Landmarks

Sternal notch, sternomanubrial junction (angle of Louis), edge of the sternum, costal cartilage of the second and third ribs, and head of the clavicle.

OPEN THORACOSTOMY (ELOESSER FLAP AND CLAGETT WINDOW)

General Use

The Eloesser flap was used originally in the treatment of tuberculous empyema.[5] Since its description in 1935, the Eloesser procedure has been modified.[6] Dr. Clagett described his simpler technique for treating postpneumonectomy empyema in 1963.[7] Both techniques are used today in the treatment of chronic empyemas related to parapneumonic effusions and bronchopleural fistulas in frail patients after lung resection. Usually an attempt is made to provide drainage and/or decortication of an infected pleural space with thoracoscopy or thoracotomy as first-line therapy. When these maneuvers fail to completely treat a chronic space infection or the patient is too debilitated to withstand these procedures, open thoracostomy can be used to control the septic process. These chronic openings into the chest allow the wound to granulate and close over time with repeated bedside dressing changes. Alternatively, it may act as a bridge to secondary but definitive wound closure with muscle or omental flaps once the acute infection is under control.

Technique

Under most circumstances, the patient is somewhat debilitated. While the previous thoracotomy incision can be used again, a new incision generally is made in the most dependent location of the chest space to facilitate gravity drainage. Computed tomographic (CT) scan is invaluable in locating the best site for this incision, which can be elliptical (Clagett window; Fig. 2-15, inset *A*) or U-shaped (Eloesser flap; Fig. 2-15, inset *B*). Traditionally, between one and three ribs are removed to create a wide, easy-to-pack drainage cavity. In the simpler Clagett window, the edges of the skin then are tacked to the thickened parietal pleura in interrupted fashion to marsupialize the cavity once it has been irrigated and carefully debrided. In an Eloesser flap, the flap created by the U-shaped incision is folded into the chest through the rib defect and sewn to the inside of the ribcage. Both techniques epithelialize the tract and prevent premature closure of the defect. An elliptical incision suffices as much as a U-shaped wound, regardless of its orientation. Hemostasis is confirmed, and the wound is packed with gauze cut to fit as one piece or using multiple rolls tied together, to avoid inadvertent retained packs.

Advantages

This incision allows for targeted drainage with little morbidity in an otherwise debilitated patient population. Dressing care is facilitated with a wide flap, and additional mechanical debridement is established over time with the potential for delayed primary wound closure.

Disadvantages

If the size of the rib resection is not wide or tall enough, the wound at skin level may contract prematurely, before the deeper pocket has granulated. This potentially can allow the infectious process to recur and require repeat surgical drainage. Open thoracostomy creates a permanent chest wall defect. Closure by granulation alone may take months to years.

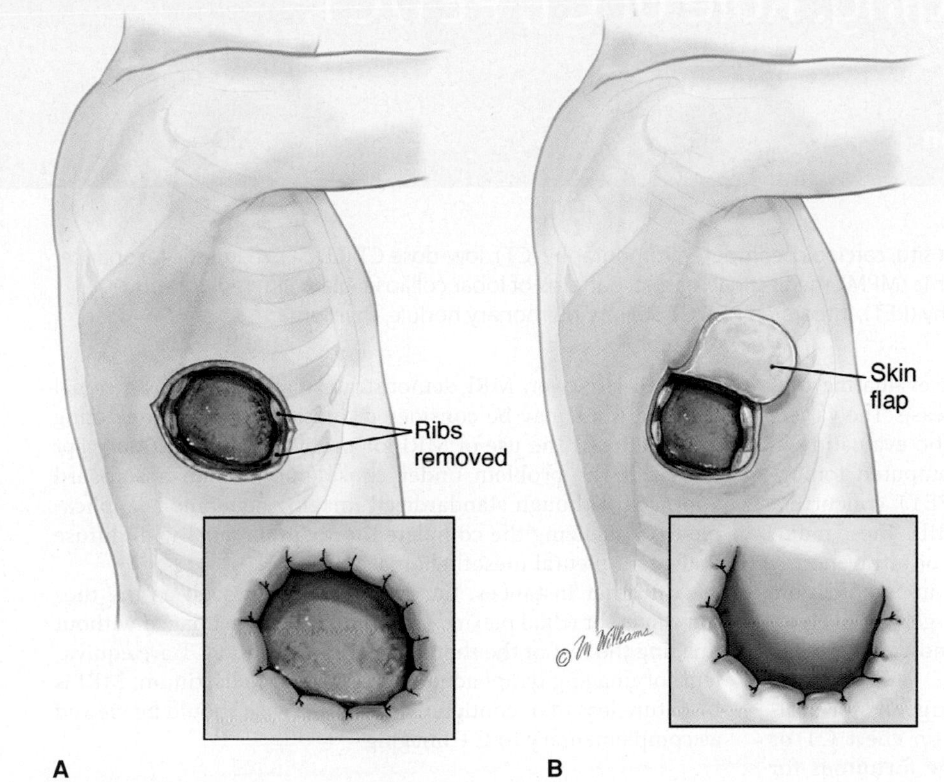

Figure 2-15. Typical appearance of completed surgical thoracostomy with Clagett (inset *A*) window or Eloesser flap (inset *B*) with pleural–cutaneous symphysis. These defects are typically placed at the most dependent part of the thorax.

The process generally is accelerated by closure with muscle flaps once the bed of the thorax is clean.

Chest Wall Anatomy

Correlation with CT scanning is important in accessing the infected space at the correct level. Dependent drainage is the key. It is also important to consider future muscle flap options when placing the incision. Depending on previous incisions, the surgeon should make attempts to spare the latissimus or serratus muscle for later use as flaps.

Surface Landmarks

Surface landmarks include the tip of the scapula, the xiphoid process, the costal margin, the anterior border of the latissimus dorsi muscle, and the posterior border of the serratus anterior muscle. Previous incisions should be noted and marked for use as needed during the drainage procedure. Surface landmarks should be correlated with the CT scan images when targeting the fluid collection in question and choosing the approach.

EDITOR'S COMMENT

The choice of thoracic incision is the key initial part of every chest operation, but details regarding this choice are often omitted from thoracic surgery textbooks. This chapter was written for the novice. It is unique in its approach to explaining the advantages, disadvantages, uses, and limitations of each incision. It also provides important surface landmarks to use in centering the incision in the correct area. This chapter has been heavily thumbed in the first edition of Adult Chest Surgery kept outside the Brigham Thoracic Surgery operating rooms. It has become an important real-time reference for fellows, residents, students, and nurses.

—MTJ

References

1. Salazar JD, Doty JR, Tseng EE, et al. Relationship of the long thoracic nerve to the scapular tip: an aid to prevention of proximal nerve injury. *J Thorac Cardiovasc Surg.* 1998;116:960–964.
2. Frank MW, Backer CL, Mavroudis C, et al. Axillary thoracoscopy. *Ann Thorac Surg.* 1998;66:590–591.
3. Bains MS, Ginsberg RJ, Jones WG 2nd, et al. The clamshell incision: an improved approach to bilateral pulmonary and mediastinal tumor. *Ann Thorac Surg.* 1994;58:30–32.
4. McNeill TM, Chamberlain JM. Diagnostic anterior mediastinotomy. *Ann Thorac Surg.* 1966;2:532–539.
5. Eloesser L. Recollections: of an operation for tuberculous empyema. *Ann Thorac Surg.* 1969;8:355–357.
6. Symbas PN, Nugent JT, Abbott OA, et al. Nontuberculous pleural empyema in adults. The role of a modified Eloesser procedure in its management. *Ann Thorac Surg.* 1971;12:69–78.
7. Clagett OT, Geraci JE. A procedure for the management of postpneumonectomy empyema. *J Thorac Cardiovasc Surg.* 1963;45:141–145.

3 Chest Imaging: Role of CT, PET/CT, and MRI

Francine L. Jacobson

Keywords: Adenocarcinoma, adenocarcinoma in situ, carcinoid, computed tomography (CT), low-dose CT (LDCT), magnetic resonance imaging (MRI), malignant pleural mesothelioma (MPM), mediastinal masses, patterns of lobar collapse, plain film radiography, pleural tumors, positron-emission tomography (PET), integrated PET/CT, solitary pulmonary nodule, thymoma

Chest imaging is a critical diagnostic tool for evaluating thoracic anomalies in anatomic structure and disease. The variety of imaging technologies available for diagnostic evaluation in the chest includes plain-film radiography, computed tomography (CT), positron-emission tomography (PET), concurrent PET/CT, and magnetic resonance imaging (MRI). These radiologic procedures are further enhanced by oral or intravenously administered contrast materials used alone or in combination. The role of radiologic imaging in thoracic surgery is likely to gain even more importance as imaging technologies provide ever more accurate means of visualization.

Patients often are referred to thoracic surgeons for evaluation and treatment of incidental findings on chest CT or radiography. These incidental findings can be fortuitous for the patient, providing the opportunity for treatment before the development of symptoms heralding advanced disease. The thoracic surgeon may choose to further the evaluation with registered PET/CT or to follow indeterminate findings over time with serial CT scans.

CT is the backbone imaging modality for preoperative evaluation. The adrenal glands are always included in routine chest CT images because this is a common site of lung cancer metastases. CT can be supplemented with PET/CT or MRI for special purposes. These modalities are often useful for problem solving. PET/CT has dramatically increased the ability of imaging to contribute to accurate preoperative staging in lung cancer, thereby setting patients on the proper treatment course from the outset. The resulting change in lung cancer staging flows from the ability of PET/CT both to recognize unsuspected distant metastases and to identify coexisting benign disease. For example, before the availability of PET/CT, inflammation in contralateral lymph nodes often was attributed erroneously to a tumor of more advanced stage and patients were not offered potentially curative resection. Adjuvant PET/CT can provide preoperative staging information capable of upstaging (30%) or downstaging (15%) disease in an individual patient.[1] In the setting of heterogeneous disease, PET/CT can be used to select the "best" biopsy site, in turn decreasing the number of biopsy specimens required to definitively classify difficult-to-identify cancers such as diffuse malignant pleural mesothelioma.

MRI is less useful than PET/CT, particularly with the advent of multidetector CT scanners, which permit data to be acquired with voxels of equal dimension in all three planes, thus providing sagittal and coronal images with CT that were previously only possible with MRI. This is not to say that MRI is without advantages. MRI can sensitively differentiate tissues, including blood, by differentiating the various states of hemoglobin. In addition, fascial planes are more sharply delineated by MRI. However, MRI demonstrates calcification as a signal void and thus may be considered inferior to CT for detecting calcifications. The use of MRI for problem solving is more apt to reflect the problem under consideration than a standard approach, although standardized imaging generally is applicable for visualizing the complete thorax in patients with diffuse malignant pleural mesothelioma.

In other instances, the area of interest, such as the thoracic inlet, brachial plexus, or lung apex, will be imaged without imaging the rest of the thorax by MRI. MRI and CT are equivalent for imaging lymphadenopathy in the mediastinum. MRI is by nature less than contiguous and otherwise should be viewed as complementary to CT imaging.

COMPUTED TOMOGRAPHY

CT provides detailed anatomic images of the chest in which a variety of soft tissues can be recognized, along with water, fat, and bones; the resulting basic transaxial images are the in vivo equivalent of transaxial anatomic pictures of a cadaver (Fig. 3-1). State-of-the-art multidetector CT scanners are capable of

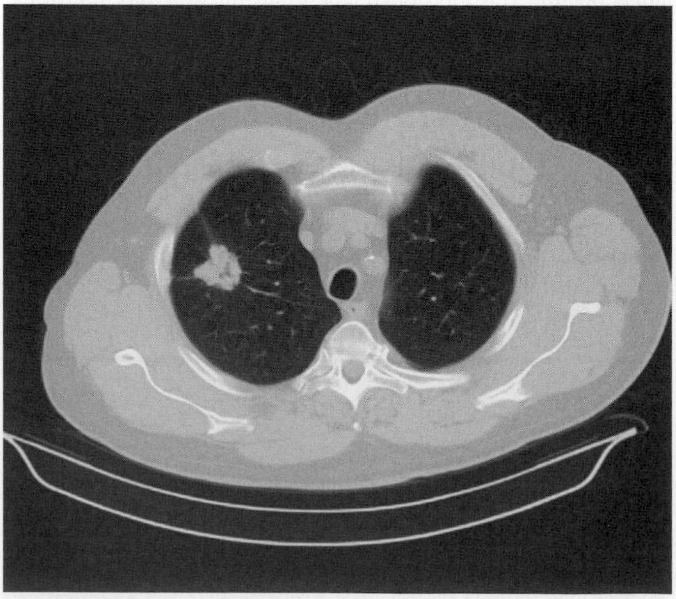

Figure 3-1. Transaxial CT image above level of aortic arch, presented in lung window. Skin, muscles, bones, and mediastinum are all visible. Right and left brachiocephalic veins are seen anterior to the principal branches of the aorta. This patient has adenocarcinoma in the right upper lobe.

acquiring ever-increasing numbers of individual slices of data at one time. Four-detector scanners are capable of scanning the chest in approximately 20 seconds, a practical time for patient breath-holding. Readily available clinical models with the capability of producing 16 to 64 slices at one time can scan the chest in 10 seconds or less. Alternatively, very small structures can be studied using ever-smaller slice thicknesses. Development of this technology is currently focused on providing up to 256 slices at one time. Along with cardiac gating, this technology permits unprecedented in vivo evaluation of ultrastructure in the lungs as well as the heart.

The technical parameters of CT scanning can be altered to improve the visualization of different tissues. CT of the chest is performed with a small focal spot using kilovolts between 100 and 120 and milliamperes between 20 and 200 or more. Reconstructed images include contiguous 5-mm images with soft tissue smoothing for visualization of the heart, great vessels, and mediastinal structures. These are generally referred to as mediastinal images and are displayed with a window level of 25 to 40 Hounsfield units (HU) and a relatively narrow window width, such as 360 HU. In addition, separate images with edge enhancement for optimizing visualization of lung ultrastructure are displayed with a window level of −600 HU and a wide window width of 1500 to 2000 HU.

Hounsfield units derive their name from the developer of the CT scanner, Nobel laureate Sir Godfrey N. Hounsfield. The scale arbitrarily assigns water the attenuation value of 0, air −1000, and bone up to +1000. These numerical values of normalized x-ray attenuation define the gray scale of all CT images. The display windows highlight various structures based on the relationships between the underlying fundamental gray scale and the composition of various tissues in the body.

Intravenous iodinated contrast material is used commonly to provide optimal delineation of vascular structures, particularly when they lie in close proximity to the pathologic entity. Thus lung cancer staging is performed most often with intravenous contrast. NPO conditions should be instituted 4 hours before the examination to minimize nausea and vomiting. In many instances, patients with a history of contrast material allergy may be imaged with MRI instead of CT. When it is mandatory to use CT in a patient who has had a prior contrast material reaction, pretreatment with oral steroids and Benadryl can be considered. Oral contrast material is rarely used because air and fat often provide adequate contrast for identifying gastrointestinal tract structures.

Increasing concern for nephrogenic systemic fibrosis has led to the institution of reduced-dose regimens for patients with impaired renal function. Half the standard dose of contrast material is used for patients with an estimated glomerular filtration rate of between 30 and 60 mL/min/1.73 m^2; intravenous contrast material should not be given to a patient with an estimated glomerular filtration rate less than 30 mL/min/1.73 m^2. In the setting of impaired renal function, as with contrast material allergy, consulting the radiologist before the study will ensure that the best possible study is selected for the given patient. Even with normal renal function, it is advisable to separate examinations that require administration of intravenous contrast material by at least 24 hours.

Varying the section thickness sometimes can improve visualization. The thinnest section that can be obtained is directly related to the size of the focal spot with which the scan was performed, currently providing images as thin as 0.6 mm. Images of 1 to 2 mm reconstructed with an edge-enhancing algorithm are still the most commonly provided thin-section images of lungs. These high-resolution CT (HRCT) images can be derived from the same data acquisition on multidetector scanners. Interspersed HRCT images permit visualization of the lung parenchyma and pleura and are most helpful for evaluating diffuse diseases such as emphysema and bronchiectasis. Contiguous or overlapping thin-section images are used for studying small nodules. These are appropriate for evaluating the features of a given nodule when reconstructed using a lung algorithm and identifying fat and calcification when reconstructed using a soft tissue algorithm.

Edge enhancement produces artifacts that can be mistaken for calcification. Thus, evaluating for the presence of calcifications should be performed using mediastinal soft tissue reconstruction. A second caveat must be offered when looking for calcified pulmonary nodules. Since contrast material may give small vessels a dense appearance very similar to calcification, non–contrast-enhanced CT may be preferable in the setting of prior granulomatous infection. Nodule surveillance guidelines published by the Fleischner Society in November 2005 can help to minimize the number of CT examinations performed, particularly for very small nodules in patients at low risk for lung cancer[2] (Table 3-1). In December 2013, the Fleischner Society issued on update focused on the management of subsolid pulmonary nodules detected on CT to complement the 2005 recommendations for incidentally detected solid pulmonary nodules. Since peripheral adenocarcinomas account for the most common type of lung cancer, and there is evidence of increasing frequency, developing a standardized approach to interpreting and managing subsolid nodules remains an important goal.[3] The American Association for Thoracic Surgery has also published guidelines for the surgical management of pulmonary nodules in lung cancer survivors and other high-risk patients who undergo lung cancer screening with low-dose CT.[4]

Table 3-1

FLEISCHNER SOCIETY 2005 RECOMMENDATIONS FOR CT FOLLOW-UP OF SMALL NODULES

NODULE SIZE (mm)	LOW-RISK PATIENT	HIGH-RISK PATIENT
≤4	No follow-up required	If no change at 12 mo, no further follow-up required.
4–6	If no change at 12 mo, no further follow-up required	Follow-up CT at 6–12 mo. If no change, CT at 18–24 mo.
6–8	Follow-up CT at 6–12 mo. If no change, then CT at 18–24 mo.	Follow-up CT at 3–6 mo. If no change, then CT at 18–24 mo.
>8	CT at 3, 9, and 24 mo or contrast-enhanced CT or PET/CT or biopsy	CT at 3, 9, and 24 mo or contrast-enhanced CT or PET/CT or biopsy

Specialized CT examinations are performed according to disease-specific algorithms. Interstitial lung disease is evaluated on 1- to 2-mm thick images obtained without contrast material. Increasingly, these thin-section HRCT images are obtained from volumetric data acquired from a single breath-hold and reconstructed retrospectively at specified intervals. Radiologists generally will evaluate HRCT images in conjunction with standard renderings of the volumetric CT data set. It is very important to obtain and view HRCT images with the proper field of view. Reducing the size of the image reduces the information available from the images.

CT pulmonary angiography is performed with a higher concentration of iodine, such as 370 g/100 mL, compared with 300 g/100 mL for ordinary chest CT contrast. With the more crucial timing requirement for imaging contrast material in pulmonary arteries, a test bolus or automated bolus tracking software is often used to refine the timing rather than relying on an approximation of the circulation time from the antecubital fossa to the main pulmonary artery at 20 seconds. Rendering of CT pulmonary angiographic images requires thin-section imaging and often uses a variety of special reconstructions and multiplanar images in sagittal and coronal planes. A plane for reconstruction also may be chosen to follow the axis of the pulmonary arteries at the bifurcation. It is important to remember, especially when working with patients who have hypercoagulable states owing to processes such as cancer, that pulmonary emboli may be visualized on standard CT images, such as those performed for staging. Secondary criteria, including atelectasis and pleural effusions, may be absent. In patients who have had a lung resection, particularly pneumonectomy, a common location for the accumulation of thrombus is at the site of lung resection in the terminus of the pulmonary artery stump. Thrombus in such a location may persist for long periods of time.

Three-dimensional reconstruction is performed increasingly for understanding the anatomy in relation to the function and pathology. This strategy is being used to evaluate airways for bronchomalacia and in the fitting of bronchial stents, as well as in patients in whom virtual bronchoscopy can provide visualization of a point beyond the proximal obstruction. Functional information regarding obstruction may be added to such examinations by acquiring a second CT data set at reduced dose, such as 80 mA, during expiration. Acquiring images in frank expiration to eliminate respiratory motion is a useful strategy when the suspected level of obstruction is distal, at a level such as the terminal bronchioles. Pathology in the midmediastinum with a complex relationship to the heart and great vessels may be mapped using three-dimensional reconstruction with color rendering of the images for surgical planning. Cardiac gating can eliminate confusion that may arise from cardiac motion for this purpose. Since the cardiac gating increases the dose required, it should be used for imaging only when it will provide crucial information.

Some centers evaluate nodules with dynamic imaging during and following administration of intravenous contrast material. A nodule is likely benign if enhancement is less than 10 HU. The nodule is likely malignant if enhancement is greater than 20 HU. A nodule that demonstrates enhancement of 15 HU or more is not usually a granuloma. This technique has proved to be user-dependent and therefore may yield disappointing results in centers where it is not performed commonly. It can be used when PET/CT is not available; however, and may be advantageous in regions where there is endemic granulomatous disease such as histoplasmosis.

Perioperative CT scans are performed for a variety of reasons and may or may not include the administration of intravenous contrast material. Infected pleura may enhance with contrast material and better delineate lung from pleural effusion. Evaluations related to pneumothoraces generally do not benefit from intravenous contrast material administration. Oral contrast material may be used for the evaluation of potential leaks after surgery such as esophagectomy. The oral contrast material should be water soluble and administered by a surgeon with clear purpose in choosing both the route of administration and volume of contrast material. Preliminary images performed before the administration of oral contrast material are often the most important images obtained. These images permit the detection of subtle changes such as those caused by the introduction of oral contrast material that leaks into spaces such as the pleural space. The preliminary images eliminate confusion related to a variety of sources of radiopaque materials such as surgical clips and previously administered contrast material. Barium can remain in the lung and in the pleural space permanently.

POSITRON-EMISSION TOMOGRAPHY WITH REGISTERED CT

The PET/CT scanner combines a gamma camera and multidetector CT scanner in the same instrument, allowing the images from both examinations to be displayed together with registration to increase the identification of subtle signs of pathology. The PET scanner records the positron emissions from a radioactive tracer, that is, [^{18}F]fluorodeoxyglucose (^{18}F-FDG), hence the name PET. Both scans generally image from the top of the skull through the pubic symphysis. In the case of melanoma, the lower-extremity imaging is extended. The long range of PET/CT scans provides a total body examination but also permits physiologic motion over time, which creates the potential for discordance between PET and CT images. This can occur as a result of peristalsis in the gastrointestinal tract and, especially, breathing. Although a patient could not be expected to breath-hold through the entire examination, lasting minutes, a separate chest CT can be obtained during a breath-hold to improve the resolution of lung imaging. In some centers, PET/CT is a routine procedure for indications such as solitary pulmonary nodule, lung cancer, and mesothelioma.

Concurrent PET/CT imaging combines the ability to detect subtle metabolic changes through the preferential uptake of ^{18}F-FDG by metabolically active cells responsible for the growth of abnormal cells (PET) with precise anatomic location of disease (CT), tumor, or affected tissue (Fig. 3-2). It is currently a reimbursable procedure when used for diagnosing solitary pulmonary nodules and tumor staging. The patient usually must fast for a minimum of 6 hours before the injection of ^{18}F-FDG. In some centers, the patient may be instructed to have very specific meals at specified times before the examination to reduce cardiac uptake of ^{18}F-FDG through saturation of receptors. The patient rests quietly for approximately 1 hour after intravenous injection of the radioisotope to permit the tracer to disperse throughout the body before imaging. Some institutions also give dilute oral contrast material to improve visualization and identification of abdominal structures. The PET and CT scans

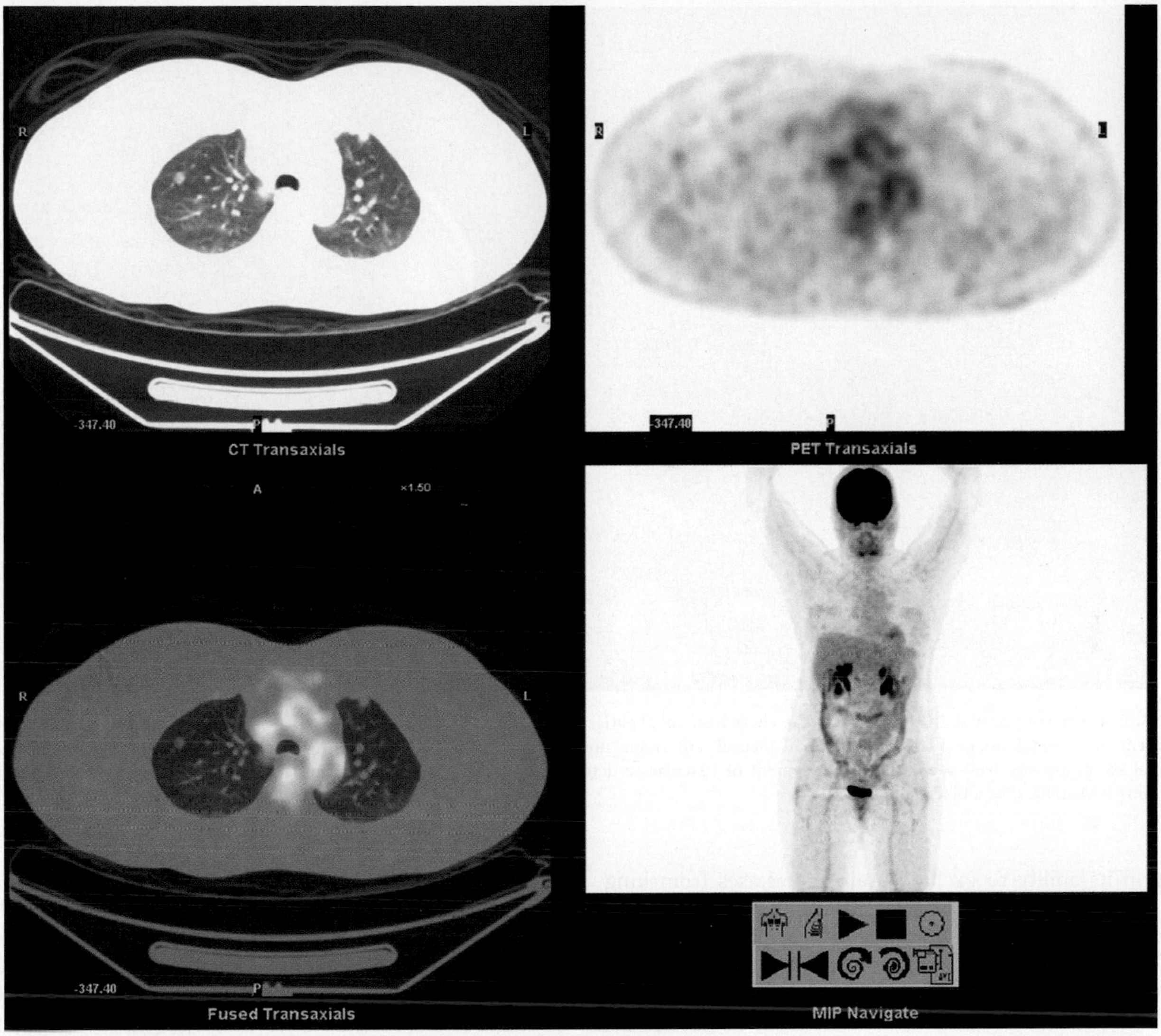

Figure 3-2. Transaxial CT and transaxial PET images presented over a fused transaxial image and projection image, which also can rotate during interpretation. Small nodule in right upper lobe demonstrates no ^{18}F-FDG avidity. This determination is reliable only for nodules larger than 7 mm in diameter.

are both performed on the same scanner without moving the patient. Patients having the examination for the investigation of pathology within the chest also should have a CT of the chest during a breath-hold while in the same position. Although this scan is generally of lower quality than a diagnostic CT, such a scan will improve evaluation of the lungs significantly compared with a standard CT obtained to correct for attenuation. Intravenous contrast material is not yet a standard feature of this examination because conventional iodine contrast agents interfere with the PET scan portion of the examination.

Pulmonary nodules that measure 7 to 8 mm in diameter or greater can be evaluated reliably with PET/CT. Although it is possible for smaller pulmonary nodules and lymph nodes to demonstrate avidity for ^{18}F-FDG, the scan requires very high metabolic activity, leaving uncertainty when a nodule is not apparently avid for ^{18}F-FDG.

PET scans also require calibration for accuracy. The process of quantifying ^{18}F-FDG avidity, or uptake, is complex, with extensive quality control measures. Quantification procedures vary somewhat between institutions, particularly in regard to correction and reporting of the standard uptake value (SUV). The SUV relates the activity concentration in a volume of tissue to the amount of injected dose and the patient's body weight. The maximum SUV indicates the affinity of a pathologic process, such as a tumor, for glucose. This correlates with the aggressiveness of a tumor histologically. There is no correlation between SUV and CT attenuation measured in Hounsfield units.

The pitfalls of PET/CT scanning remain numerous at this time despite its extreme utility for thoracic surgical evaluations. Investigations of intravenous contrast material and more widespread addition of breath-hold images for the lungs, it is hoped, will lead to a diagnostic-level CT scan within a PET/CT investigation and enable radiologists to keep the radiation of patients as low as reasonably achievable. PET/CT provides the best preoperative staging currently possible. The results of the two types of scans combined may be thought of as concordant or discordant based on whether the findings can be correlated. The consistency with pathologic truth is a separate and equally important consideration. PET/CT has not replaced conventional

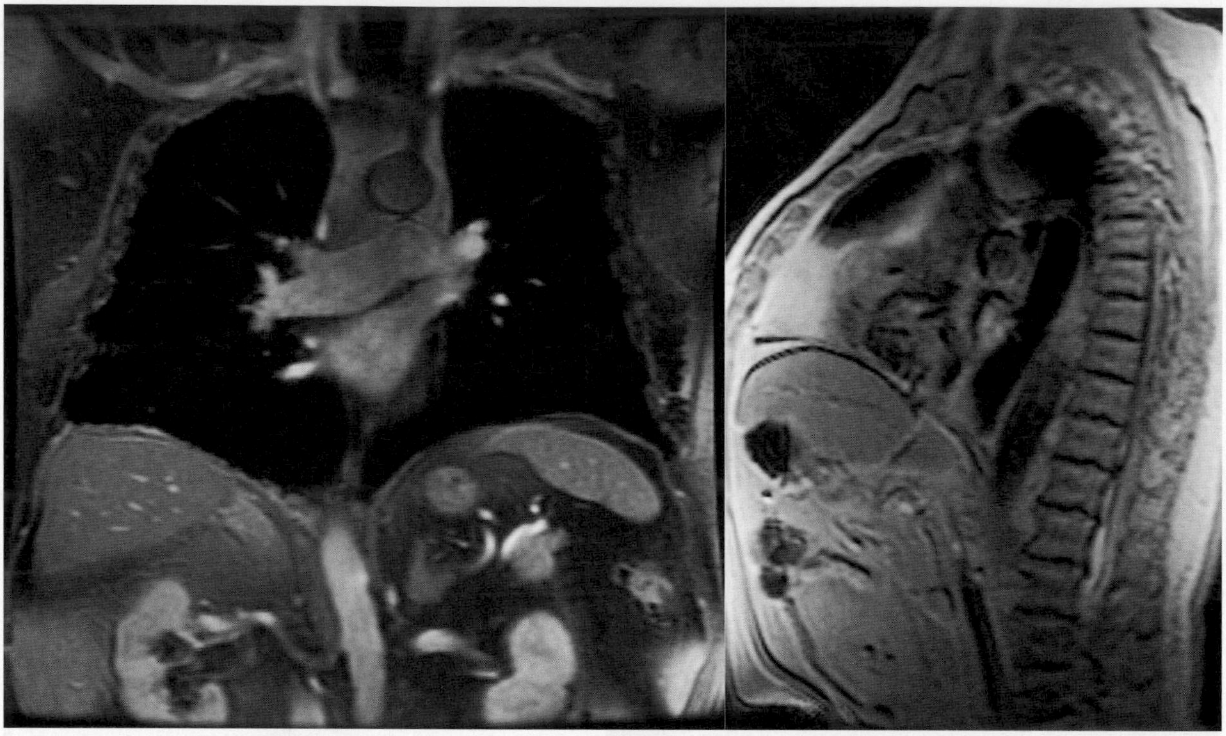

Figure 3-3. Coronal and sagittal MRI images of the chest have less spatial resolution than CT images, whereas contrast resolution is greater. Contrast enhancement on coronal image (left) reveals small pleural soft tissue nodules above the black-appearing fascial plane at the right hemidiaphragm. Mediastinal structures are well seen with enhancement of vascular structures. Sagittal T2-weighted image (right) reveals intact diaphragmatic fascia. Cortical bone is visualized as a black signal void.

imaging in its ability to exclude brain metastases from lung cancer. The accuracy and therefore utility of PET/CT for the brain are limited. Although brain metastasis may be found on PET/CT, the lack of a finding does not exclude metastasis. The pitfalls of PET/CT correlative imaging in bone also have proved to be a significant limitation. Metastases, depending on phase and rate of bone destruction, can be concordant or discordant, leading to a number of confusing situations, some of which would be better resolved with conventional radionuclide bone scanning. In a number of potentially confusing situations, evaluation of SUV in various locations may reconcile PET and CT findings with the pathologic processes present. Inflammation can have a very high SUV but generally will have low-to-moderate values, whereas an avid tumor will have a much higher SUV (e.g., tumor SUV of 10 and inflammatory process SUV of 3). It is also possible for tumors to have little or no avidity for ^{18}F-FDG. Two tumors in the lung are particularly important in this regard, adenocarcinoma in situ and carcinoid. The ^{18}F-FDG uptake of a tuberculoma can be extremely high, with an SUV as high as 20. The decision to operate must consider factors from CT and the clinical evaluation of the patient. Clarity is sometimes increased by serial PET/CT scans to watch lesions over time.

MAGNETIC RESONANCE IMAGING

MRI uses a variety of pulse sequences to identify unique characteristics of soft tissues and fluids that cannot be detected with CT scanning. MRI can sensitively identify blood and determine the length of time it has been present based on the state of hemoglobin as it changes to deoxyhemoglobin and further degradation products. MRI can readily determine the direction of blood flow in a vessel, useful information not provided at the same level by CT and not addressed by PET/CT. The use of MRI in the chest has increased as data acquisition times have diminished, allowing breath-hold imaging of the lungs (Fig. 3-3). MRI examinations are customized to the problem being evaluated. Coils used to perform the examination not only provide improved imaging but also control technical parameters such as field of view. The bore of the available MRI scanner itself may limit the sizes of patients who can have chest MRI. Larger-bore and open scanners have decreased this limitation, but a patient may have to go to a special location to have such an examination. It is helpful to explore patient claustrophobia before ordering the examination. Patients who are concerned about having the examination often benefit from oral premedication that permits normal outpatient scanning. Of course, the standard exclusions for any MRI, such as aneurysm clip, recent surgery, and pacing devices, apply to chest MRI.

The need to visualize blood vessels, nerves, and the variety of substances, including blood, that can be found in the pleural or pericardial space serves as a guide in choosing MRI for a particular patient. As a problem-solving tool, the examination will be customized by the radiologist. In unusual situations, it is best to discuss the problem with the radiologist before ordering the examination. This will ensure adequate scanner time and the best chance that important clinical questions will be answered. Until recently, 20 mL of intravenous gadolinium contrast material was administered routinely both to identify the tissue-enhancement characteristics of many tumors and to perform magnetic resonance angiography. As with iodinated contrast material for CT scans, however, documented cases of nephrogenic systemic fibrosis have led to the restriction of contrast material administration, particularly in the setting of impaired renal function.

MRI is the primary imaging modality for thoracic outlet syndrome. For this type of evaluation, the patient is imaged with the arms up and with the arms down. The vessels and nerves of the thoracic inlet and brachial plexus region are studied using limited field of view and special blood flow techniques.

MRI is also performed routinely for diffuse malignant pleural mesothelioma. This is the most standardized chest MRI examination, and images the complete chest and upper abdomen. Intravenous gadolinium contrast material is administered to detect the enhancement of tumor masses. Of note, recent incorporation of PET/CT into mesothelioma protocols has resulted in more specific identification of sites that will yield a productive tumor biopsy than can be achieved with MRI alone. The MRI itself is more helpful for clarifying the integrity of fascial planes at the diaphragmatic and mediastinal boundaries of the tumor. Operability is determined through this combination of tests to determine unforeseen distant disease and local extension beyond the scope of extrapleural pneumonectomy (see Chapter 122).

Pancoast tumors also are imaged with MRI to best evaluate relationships between the brachial plexus and apex (see Chapter 80). Depending on lesion size and clinical considerations, the examination may be planned as a brachial plexus examination or a full field-of-view examination, as performed for mesotheliomas.

MRI is a primary tool for the noninvasive evaluation of adrenal masses. When an adrenal lesion does not exhibit the low attenuation associated with adrenal adenomas, the MRI may confirm the presence of an adenoma and obviate the need for biopsy.

Cardiac MRI, performed with cardiac gating to eliminate the motion of the heart, is also used increasingly for surgical planning in the removal of large central mediastinal masses and evaluation of structures adjacent to the heart that are not well seen on CT scans.

RADIOLOGIC ANATOMY

Projection radiography results in overlapping of structures with limited differentiation based upon radiographic densities of metal, calcium, water, and air. The fifth radiographic density, fat, is not reliably differentiated from water. Water density thus encompasses the range between fat and most soft tissue, including muscles. CT scanning is able to resolve more subtle differences in tissue attenuation and eliminate overlap between structures that can be confusing. Anatomic differentiation is more similar between CT, PET/CT, and MRI.

The orientation of the radiologist to anatomy is derived from the anatomic position. Projection radiographs therefore are viewed as you would look at the patient, placing the patient's right side at your own left side. Coronal cross-sectional images use the same orientation, generally presented from anterior to posterior. Axial images are viewed from the perspective of standing at the supine patient's feet, again placing the patient's right side at your own left side. Sagittal images generally are presented from the patient's left side to the right side, although this convention is not applicable to all studies, particularly in MRI. It is helpful to reconcile the position of the heart in determining whether sagittal images are on the right or left side of the patient's body. The Visible Human Project and the proliferation of Web-based medical education materials now allow easy access to comparison images for anatomic identification in all three of these planes. Sophisticated image processing of volumetric CT data sets increasingly enables radiologists to provide data for surgery in the perspective of the surgeon. Surgeons also have learned to use conventional axial CT images to determine operability and plan specific surgeries.

The localization of anatomy on PA and lateral chest radiographs requires concordance in localization between views. An anatomic structure must be in the correct location on both views or it has not been correctly identified. This correlation extends also to localization of pathology. The lobes of each lung are covered by a thin linear pleura, visible between aerated lung parenchyma when tangential to the x-ray beam. Identifying the fissures that divide the lungs into lobes is facilitated by focusing on the expected anatomic localization. The right minor fissure has a rather constant location on a PA chest radiograph, laterally extending to the right lateral sixth rib. The major fissures are more consistently seen on the lateral chest radiograph. The left major fissure is generally more vertical. The right major fissure is also frequently identified by the confluence with the right minor fissure. The adult lateral chest radiograph is obtained with the left side up to the film or detector. The x-ray beam diverges according to the inverse square law, leading to a lateral chest radiograph with sharper smaller left hemithorax inside larger less sharp right hemithorax. Lobar localizations need to respect the fissures on both views.

Observations are frequently more apparent on one view than the other. In this case, looking at an expected location increases the confidence in identification on the second view whereby the pathology is localized. Three landmarks are helpful for this type of comparison, the top of the aortic arch, the carina, and the pulmonary venous confluence. In older adults, the aortic arch is well seen on both PA and lateral chest radiographs. The carina can be accurately located on PA view by following the left mainstem bronchus back to the carina. The lateral view is less intuitive although the location is just under the well seen aortic arch that can serve as a surrogate. The pulmonary venous confluence is well seen on the lateral chest radiograph, where it frequently simulates a mass. A corresponding retrocardiac mass representing the right pulmonary venous confluence is uncommonly visualized on the PA chest radiograph. The location on the PA chest radiograph can be learned from studying the course of engorged pulmonary veins on patients with interstitial pulmonary edema. The location is above the dome of the diaphragm. The lateral view best demonstrates the large volume of lung below this landmark that is comparatively hidden by the superior extent of the abdomen. Hidden areas on chest radiographs also benefit from review of abdominal, neck, and shoulder radiographs.

Lung

Lung anatomy most frequently presents three lobes in the right lung and two lobes in the left lung. The right upper lobe consists of three segments: anterior, posterior, and apical. The apical bronchus may be thought of as the chimney of the lung with its vertical orientation. The right middle lobe consists of two segments, medial and lateral. The lateral segment extends more

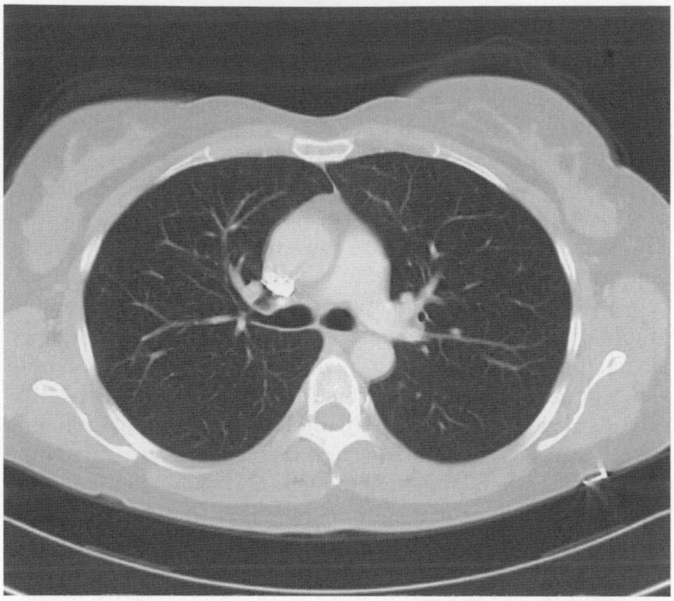

Figure 3-4. Transaxial CT image of the chest rendered for lungs at the level of the carina. Segmental airways to the right upper lobe are well seen. An avascular plane localizing the major fissure is better seen on the left than on the right.

posteriorly, causing it to project behind the right lung on a lateral view of the chest. The right lower lobe also has an apical segment, as well as four basilar segments: medial, anterior, lateral, and posterior. The left upper lobe includes a combined apical-posterior segment, an anterior segment, and superior and inferior lingular divisions. The left lower lobe is similar to the right lower lobe, although the basilar segmental anatomy is somewhat more variable, commonly having only three segments, such as anterior, lateral, and posterior. Segment identification is best confirmed by reconciling both airway and fissure anatomy (Figs. 3-4 to 3-7).

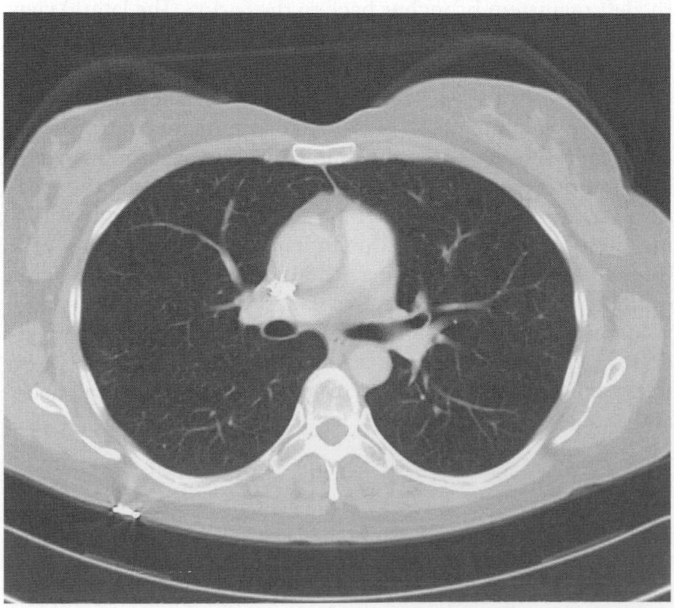

Figure 3-5. Transaxial CT image of the chest rendered for lungs at the level of the right minor fissure. Bronchus intermedius is well seen on the right. Complete left major fissure extends to the left hilum.

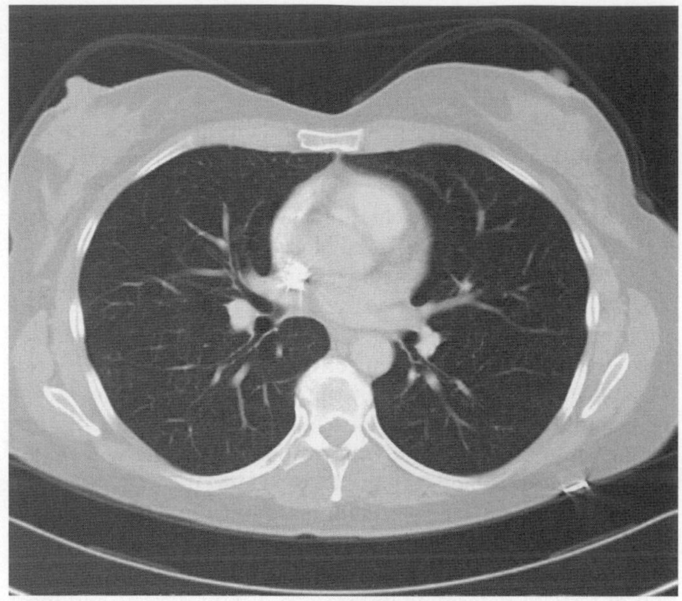

Figure 3-6. Transaxial CT image of the chest rendered for lungs at the level of the lower lobe airway bifurcations. Right middle lobe bronchus gives rise to medial and lateral branches. The medial branch is also seen dividing on this image. Pulmonary veins are entering the left atrium. Lung medial to the vein (V_3B) on the right is in the right upper lobe. Left lower lobe segmental bronchi are demonstrated behind the left major fissure.

It is helpful to be familiar with classic lobar collapse patterns that are specific to the anatomy of each lobe and the differences in airway anatomy between the right and the left lung. The anatomic differences also apply to the distributions of consolidation. The mid-lung division on the right occurs at the bronchus intermedius with right upper lobe collapse of

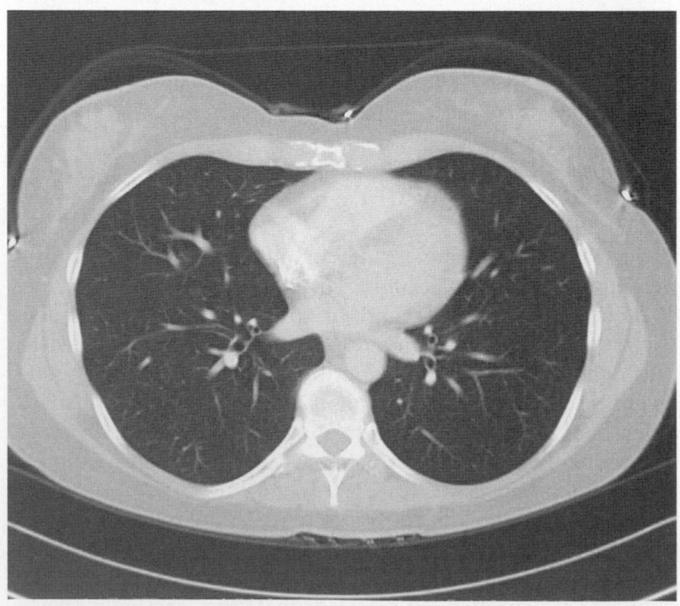

Figure 3-7. Transaxial CT image of the chest rendered for lungs at the level of the pulmonary venous confluence. Major fissures are seen anterior to the pulmonary venous confluence in each lung. Minor thickening of the right major fissure produces a subtle line on this 5-mm image, whereas the left major fissure is visualized only as an avascular plane. HRCT images at this level, along with images at the level of the aortic arch and carina, respectively, are useful for assessing the distribution of diffuse lung diseases in lung parenchyma.

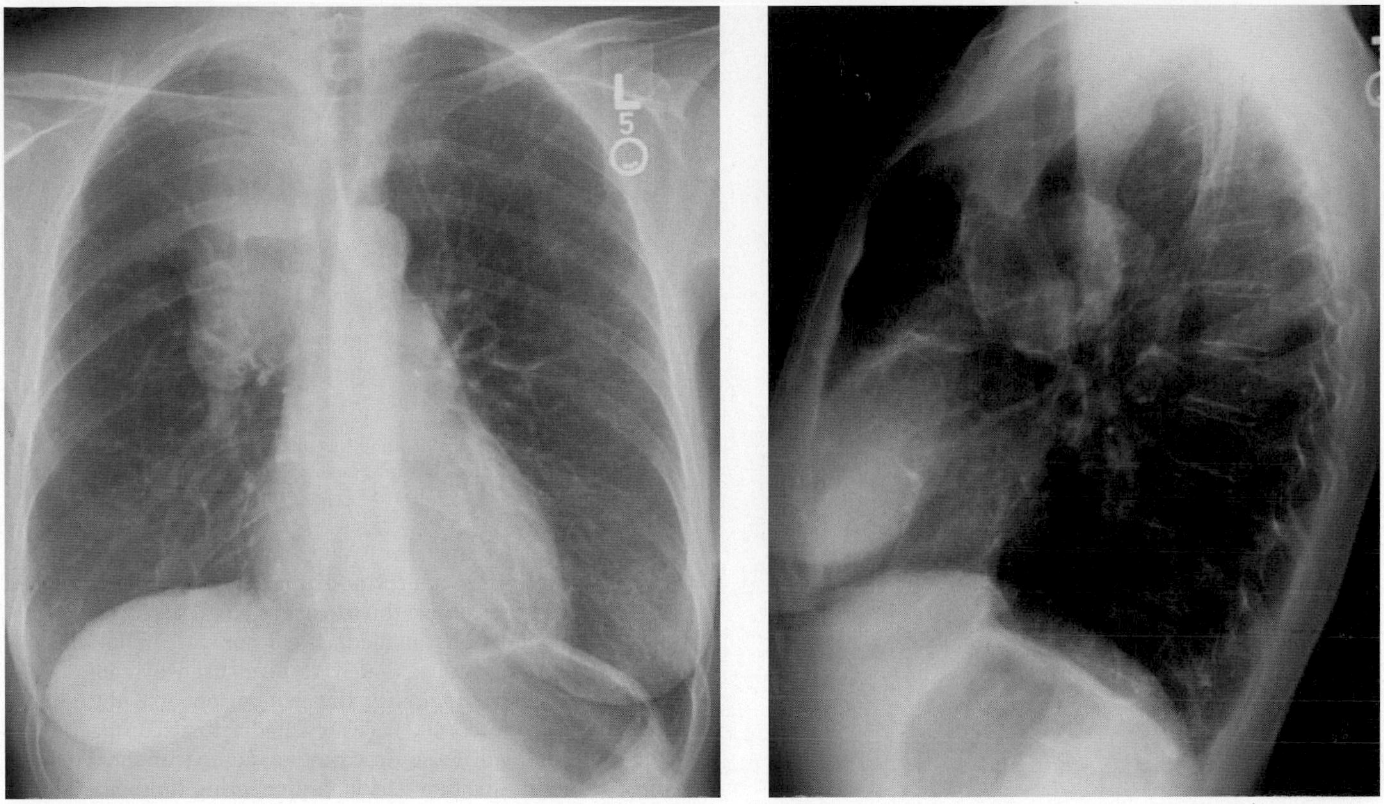

Figure 3-8. Right upper lobe collapse shown in frontal (*A*) and lateral (*B*) views.

three independent segments (Fig. 3-8). The elevated right minor fissure forms the inferior border. When a mass causes postobstructive collapse of the lobe, the curvature is referred to as the reverse S sign of Golden or, more simply, Golden S sign (Fig. 3-9). The right middle lobe and right lower lobe can be individually collapsed (Figs. 3-10 and 3-11) or collapsed together as a unit at the level of the bronchus intermedius (Fig. 3-12). The right middle and right lower lobe collapse patterns are similar to the

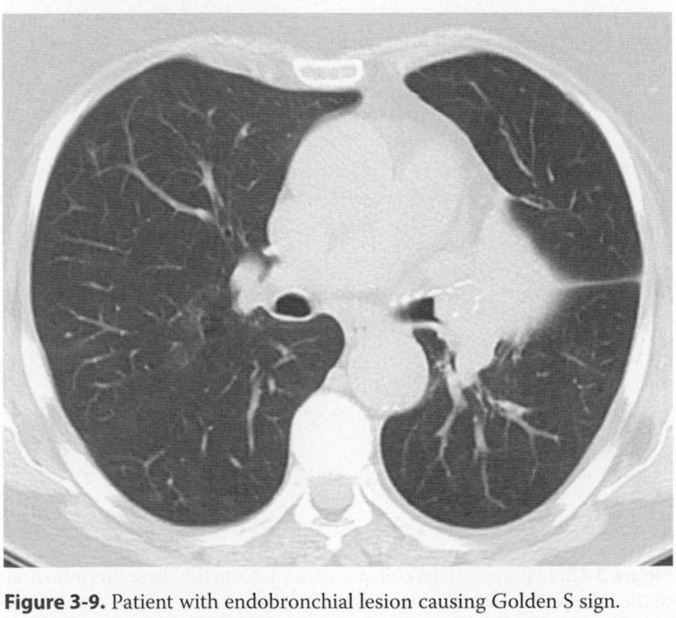

Figure 3-9. Patient with endobronchial lesion causing Golden S sign.

patterns of collapse in the lingula and left lower lobe. Complete lower lobe collapse toward the spine may be quite subtle although the overall volume loss in the affected lung should be obvious. The pattern of collapse in the left upper lobe (Figs. 3-13 and 3-14) is distinctive and differs from the right lung collapse patterns owing to the inclusion of the lingular division in the left upper lobe. The collapse of this lobe moves the left major fissure anteriorly with hyperexpansion of the left lower lobe producing apical lucency. Although infrequent, the lingula can collapse without collapse of the entire lobe (Fig. 3-15). The difference in appearance between the right middle lobe consolidation and lingular consolidation primarily is seen as the presence or absence of the minor fissure on the lateral view. The anatomy of the lungs determines when a single lesion could not produce the effect in both lobes. Although collapse of the right upper and right middle lobe might look like left upper lobe collapse, two separate lesions would be required in the right lung whereas a single lesion would produce this appearance in the left lung.

Pleura

The periphery of the lung is covered in visceral pleura, along the chest wall and each fissure. Fissures are frequently incomplete. Common anatomic variants include the superior and inferior accessory fissures, the azygos fissure (when azygos vein migration is incomplete), and the left minor fissure. Unlike the cobblestone structure of the lung, the pleura is a primary source of linear structure in the lungs. On CT images, fissures are seen as avascular planes on 5-mm images and as

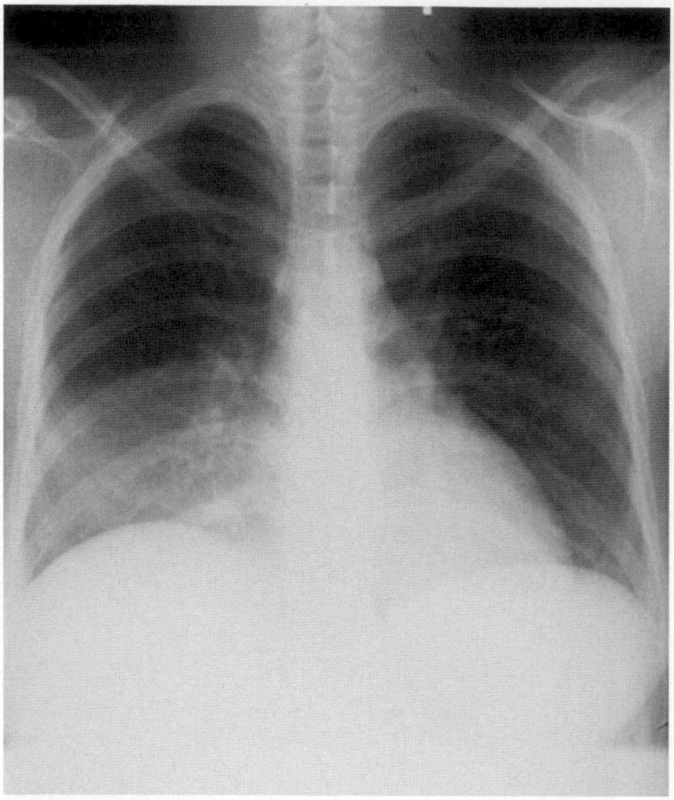

Figure 3-10. Right middle lobe collapse pattern.

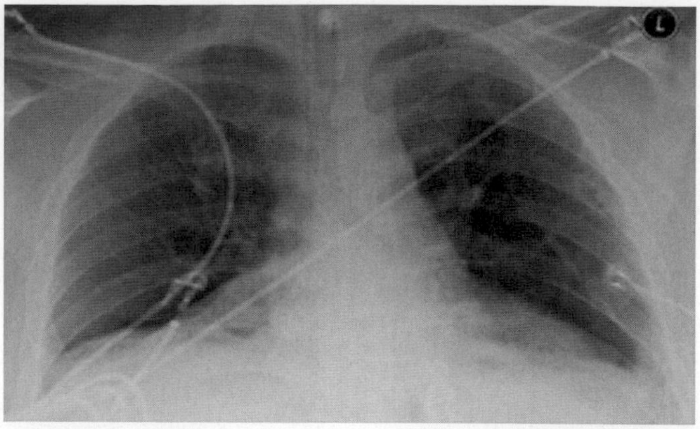

Figure 3-12. Combined RML and RLL collapse pattern in intubated patient with mucus plug in bronchus intermedius.

fine white lines on images up to approximately 2 mm in thickness. Mediastinal pleural surfaces are least well seen by CT and benefit from MRI, whereas fissures are not visualized on many MRI sequences unless they are abnormally thickened (Fig. 3-16).

Mediastinum

The mediastinum is divided into three compartments: anterior mediastinum, middle mediastinum, and posterior mediastinum. The superior mediastinum is not a mediastinal compartment, but it is commonly understood to include lymph nodes and normal structures above the top of the aortic arch. There exist several classifications of mediastinal compartments, besides the anatomic divisions, that have been used by radiologists for many years to simplify the generation of a differential diagnosis (see Table 3-1). Felson mediastinal compartments and the "modified" Felson mediastinal compartments are used most commonly.[5,6] Ben Felson, a pioneering thoracic radiologist, defined projection radiography boundaries for the mediastinum, bringing the anterior mediastinum from the anterior chest wall through the retrosternal clear space to the anterior wall of the trachea. The later modification drew this posterior boundary at the anterior wall of the ascending aorta. In both, the posterior mediastinum begins 1 cm behind the anterior margin of the vertebral bodies, behind the anatomic mediastinum. In this way, differential diagnosis is simplified for the posterior compartment without undue complication of the middle

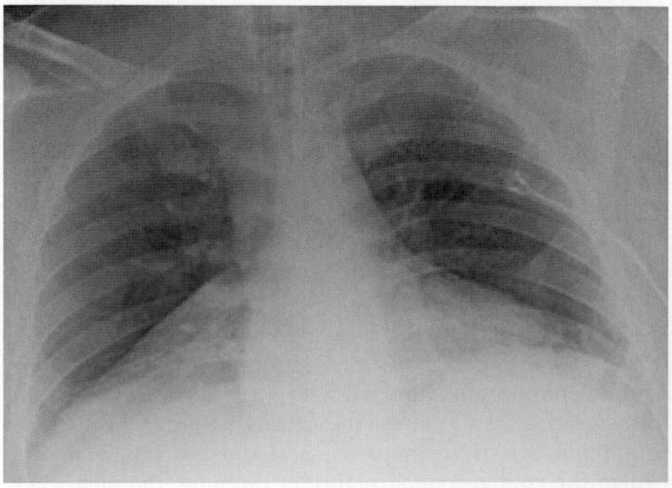

Figure 3-11. Right lower lobe collapse pattern in intubated patient with mucus plug.

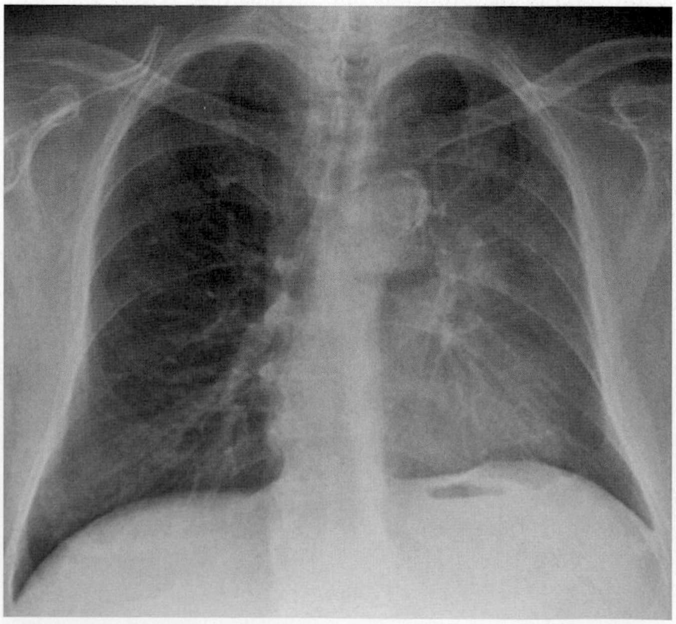

Figure 3-13. Left upper lobe collapse pattern. Note the abrupt termination of the left upper lobe bronchus at its origin.

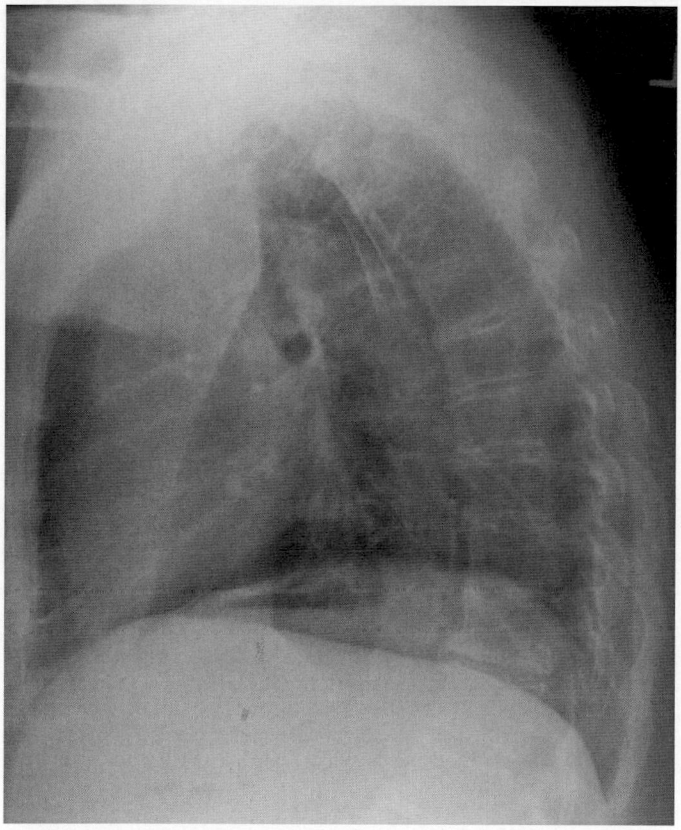

Figure 3-14. Lingula-sparing left upper lobe collapse pattern.

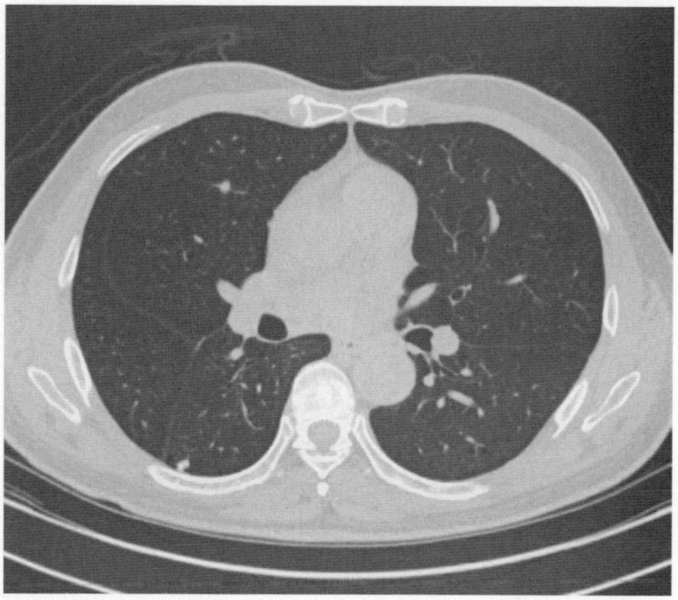

Figure 3-16. Transaxial HRCT image of the chest rendered for pleura reveals detail regarding airways seen here, with minimal dilatation in the right lower lobe lung parenchyma, and precisely defines the location of pleural fissures visualized as thin white lines. The right middle lobe only exists within the circle of pleura defining the minor fissure. Lung parenchyma surrounding the minor fissure is in the right upper lobe. Subpleural nodules are noted in the right lower lobe. HRCT images for lung parenchyma are not appropriate for the detection of calcium, as suggested by this image.

mediastinum. Adding the esophagus to the middle mediastinal compartment can be useful for creating clear differential diagnoses that are directly applicable to clinical practice. The choice between the two versions of Felson mediastinal compartments is best made based on the logic employed by the individual radiologist and mirrors variations within surgical practices as well. Those who want to work with short differential diagnosis lists and can readily remember to look at the potential pathology arising from an adjacent space will be well served by the modified Felson criteria applied to lateral chest radiographs. One further reminder is in order: The internal mammary vessels and any accompanying lymphadenopathy project with, but are not part of, the anterior mediastinum (Figs. 3-17 to 3-20).

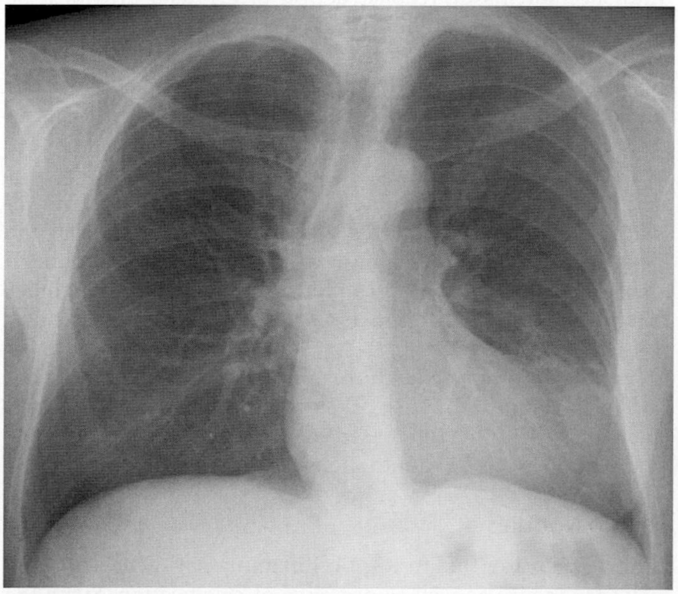

Figure 3-15. Lingular collapse that spares the lung.

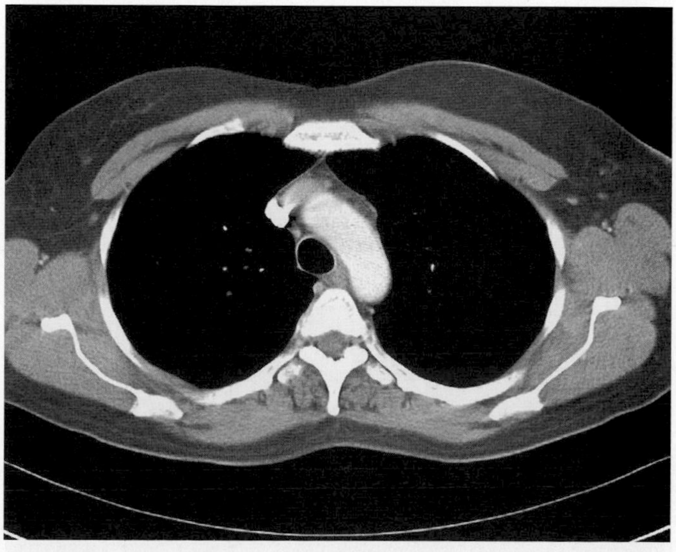

Figure 3-17. Transaxial CT image of the chest rendered for mediastinum at the level of the aortic arch. Brachiocephalic veins are joining to form the superior vena cava. Anterior mediastinal fat has a triangular shape in the thymic bed region of the anterior mediastinum.

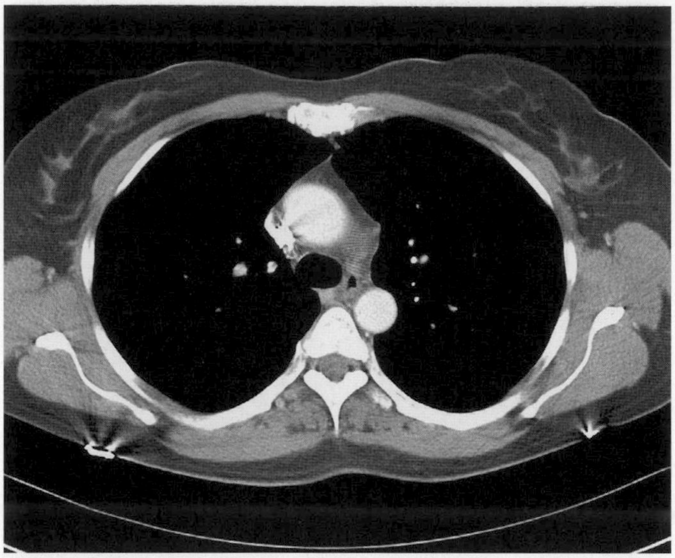

Figure 3-18. Transaxial CT image of the chest rendered for mediastinum at the level of the aorticopulmonic window. Small lymph node adjacent to the left side of the trachea and origin of left main stem bronchus is in station 4R, whereas the small lymph node lateral to the ligamentum arteriosum is in the aorticopulmonic window lymph node station. Anterior mediastinal fat again demonstrates normal thymic fat in a middle-aged adult. Internal mammary vessels are well seen flanking the sternum.

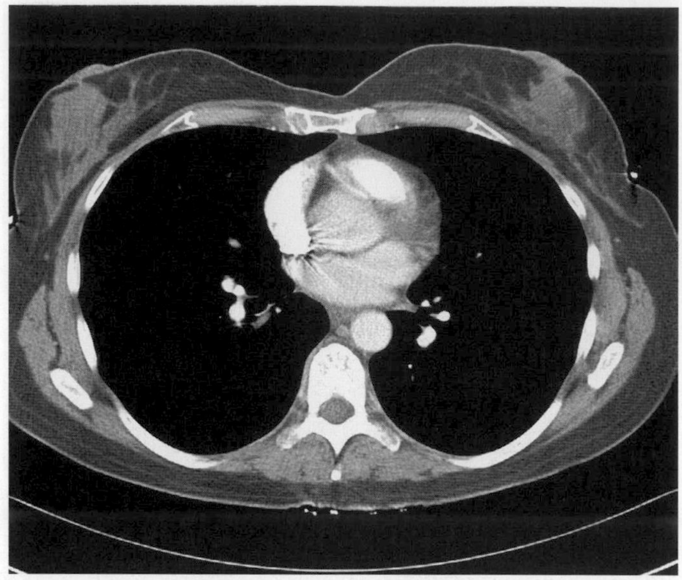

Figure 3-20. Transaxial CT image of the chest rendered for mediastinum at the level of the aortic root. The right atrium is right of aortic root, and the pulmonary outflow tract is left of the aortic root. The left atrium is posterior to the aortic root and anterior to the descending thoracic aorta. The azygos vessels flank the descending thoracic aorta. The esophagus is collapsed between the left atrium, the descending thoracic aorta, and the azygos vein. The posterior mediastinal compartment begins behind the descending thoracic aorta.

PRACTICAL APPROACHES TO SPECIFIC PROBLEMS

Solitary Pulmonary Nodule

A solitary pulmonary nodule found on a plain-chest radiograph should be further analyzed with CT to characterize the nodule, determine whether additional nodules are present, and assess other associated findings, including lymphadenopathy and pleural effusions.[2,4,7–10] The term mass is reserved for large nodules; over time, the definition has decreased progressively from 6 to 4 cm to, most recently, 3 cm. The size of a nodule itself correlates positively with the probability of malignancy, even in the absence of additional features to suggest malignancy. The margins of the nodule, pattern of calcification (if present), and presence or absence of fat help to distinguish benign from malignant lung nodules. Special features such as enlarged feeding and draining vessels also can help to indicate a very specific diagnosis. A nodule containing dense central calcification, whether solid or lamellated, is benign, requiring no further follow-up to determine the nature of a calcified granuloma. Thin-slice soft tissue reconstruction of CT data provides the most accurate assessment in this regard.[11] The common causes of solitary pulmonary nodules are listed in Table 3-2.

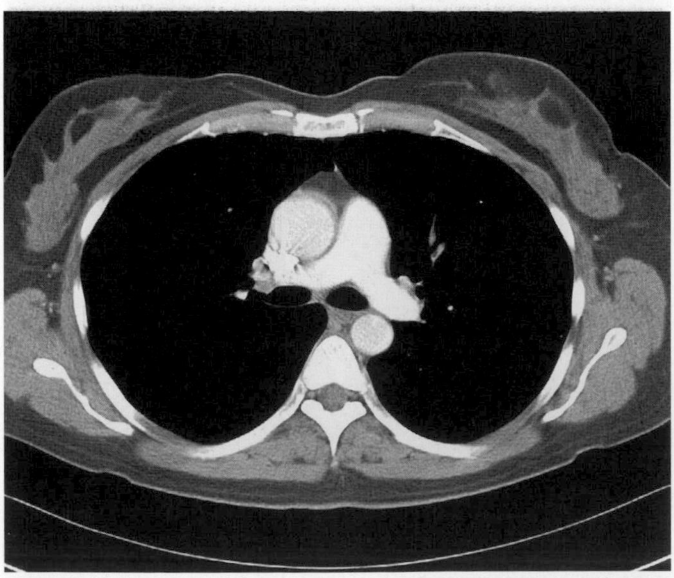

Figure 3-19. Transaxial CT image of the chest rendered for mediastinum at the level of the bifurcation of the carina and pulmonary arteries.

Solitary pulmonary nodules and small solid nodules are studied with serial CT examinations over 2 or more years to determine whether a nodule is benign or malignant. One outcome of screening studies such as the Early Lung Cancer Action Project is recognition of the extremely low incidence of cancer in tiny nodules.[12] This observation contributed to the Fleischner Society Guidelines, which currently recommend only a single follow-up CT scan for solitary pulmonary nodules that measure less than 4 mm in diameter and then only in high-risk patients (Tables 3-1 to 3-3). Clinical practitioners have yet to become comfortable with this "no follow-up" recommendation for patients at low risk of developing lung cancer, but this change has definitely increased patient and practitioner comfort with the 6- to 12-month interval surveillance CT.

Benign Nodules

Granulomas are the result of inflammatory processes and may vary in size as well as presence of calcification. Since the dense, solid, calcified nodule can vary in size, it is important to

Table 3-2

DIFFERENTIAL DIAGNOSIS FOR SOLITARY PULMONARY NODULES

NODULE ETIOLOGY	DISTINGUISHING CHARACTERISTICS
Granuloma	Smooth margins Solid or lamellated calcifications
Carcinoid	Lobulated margins Dystrophic, eccentric calcifications
Hamartoma	Lobulated margins Calcifications appear in rings or arcs Fat
AVM	Lobulated margins Infrequent calcification (vascular) Feeding/draining vessels
Lung cancer	Spiculated, lobulated, or smooth margins Dystrophic calcifications Large lesions with necrosis Cavitation in squamous cell carcinoma and adenocarcinoma
AIS/MIA	≤5 mm of atypical adenomatous hyperplasia Ground-glass opacity Well-demarcated margins Part-solid nodule Cystic spaces Focal extensions to pleura Very slow growth
Solid pulmonary metastasis	Nonspecific, although may have appearance characteristic of primary tumor

AVM, arteriovenous malformation; AIS/MIA, adenocarcinoma in situ/minimally invasive carcinoma.

remember that such nodules are benign calcified granulomas. Granulomas are not necessarily calcified, though. A solitary noncalcified granuloma must be treated as an indeterminate pulmonary nodule. It is helpful to consider the prevalence of granulomatous disease in the patient population, which also will reflect the presence of endemic granulomatous diseases in the community. The size of the nodule is also a factor because tiny nodules, measuring less than 4 mm in diameter, rarely signify early malignancy.

Hamartomas can contain specific calcifications, described as rings and arcs, owing to cartilage that may be present within the hamartoma. Fat also may be seen in the same pulmonary nodule. As with carcinoid tumors, hamartomas also may have a lobulated contour. In the case of a hamartoma, the identification of fat on thin-section images is the most convincing evidence of benignity. Fat also can be seen in nodules or even consolidations if the lesion is caused by the aspiration of mineral oil, commonly referred to as lipoid pneumonia.

Arteriovenous malformations (AVMs) may be single or multiple, as in the case of syndrome such as Osler–Weber–Rendu syndrome of hereditary hemorrhagic telangiectasia (HHT). Enlarging vessels leading to nodules are most helpful for identification. Contrast-enhanced CT scanning with PE protocol for vessel enhancement may identify additional more subtle lesions. Very small lesions may only be detected by echocardiographic bubble study. Although an AVM is not malignant, complications can include bleeding and spread of infection from lung through systemic circulation to seed brain abscesses. Treatment options include interventional radiologic embolization as well as surgery.

Malignant Nodules

The recognition of malignant potential in small nodules has increased through more than a decade of lung cancer screening trials and is now well supported by CT technology allowing volumetric imaging of nodules with slice thicknesses of less than 1 mm. The relationship to mortality risk from these lesions is less clear than the radiopathologic correlation consistently demonstrated. Through such radiopathologic correlations, we have learned that invasive adenocarcinoma is often present in the lesions described previously as BAC owing to lepidic growth characteristics[13,14] (Fig. 3-21). The increased understanding of the significance of specific features of nonsolid and part-solid nodules and the progression of adenocarcinoma in situ to invasive adenocarcinoma has resulted in earlier resection of many such lung cancers. The lepidic growth of tumor along alveolar walls defines both atypical adenomatous hyperplasia (AAH) and adenocarcinoma in situ (AIS, formerly BAC). Only size distinguishes between these two entities, with AAH used to describe ground-glass opacities up to 5 mm in diameter and AIS used to describe lesions larger than 5 mm in diameter. The diagnosis no longer rests on morphology, which has been replaced by emerging biomarkers that allow analysis of transthoracic biopsy specimens chiefly by cytology to provide diagnosis and necessary biomarkers for selecting chemotherapy, obviating the need for many excisional biopsies.

On CT, the presence of lepidic growth can have the appearance of well demarcated but subtle ground-glass opacity, which, by definition, allows visualization of vessels and airways within the nodule. The importance of these subtle opacities, particularly when present with findings suggestive of more advanced lung cancer, has caused them to be reclassified as nonsolid nodules. As the tumor increases, such nodules develop areas

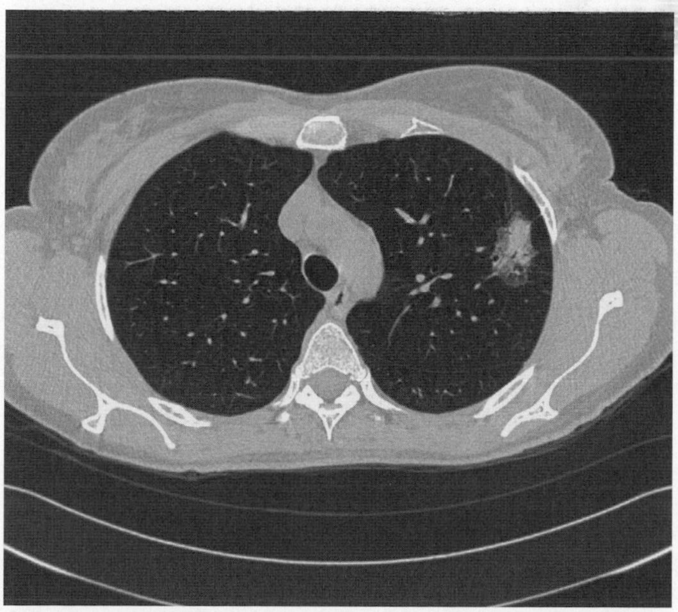

Figure 3-21. Transaxial 1-mm HRCT image of the chest rendered for lungs at the level of the aortic arch reveals adenocarcinoma with AIS features in the periphery of the left upper lobe. It contains a solid component anteriorly, ground-glass opacity medially and posteriorly, along with a small cystic feature centrally and focal radiations extending to the pleural surface anteriorly and laterally.

Table 3-3

DIFFERENTIAL DIAGNOSIS OF MEDIASTINAL MASSES

MASS	DIFFERENTIAL DIAGNOSIS	LOCATION	FEATURES
Anterior mediastinal mass	Thyroid mass	Contiguous with thyroid gland	Deviation of trachea
	Thymoma or thymic cyst	Thymic bed	Smoothly marginated
	Lymphoma and small cell lung cancer	All lymph node stations in superior mediastinum, thymic bed, prevascular space, aorticopulmonic window Extramediastinal location hilar lymph nodes	May be lobulated Mass may involve multiple lymph node groups Hilar lymph node enlargement may be asymmetric Hodgkin disease spreads from thymic bed to middle mediastinum to hilar lymph nodes
	Germ cell tumor	Variable, including prevascular space and thymic bed	Fat, hair, and teeth are diagnostic May be homogeneous with smooth margins
Middle mediastinal mass	Duplication cyst (includes bronchogenic cyst)	Most often located at bifurcation of trachea and central airways May be paraesophageal or intraparenchymal	Smoothly marginated High-attenuation fluid
	Lymphadenopathy	All lymph node stations, including subcarinal space	May appear as separate enlarged nodes or as a multiple lymph node mass May be homogeneous or heterogeneous Low attenuation indicates tuberculosis Single site with enhancement indicates Castleman disease
	Pericardial cyst	Adjacent to heart, especially in cardiophrenic sulcus	Smoothly marginated Water attenuation Can also represent pericardial diverticulum if history of mediastinoscopy
	Thyroid mass (intrathoracic goiter)	Thyroid, extending into thorax 15% of these masses extend behind the trachea	Appearance of thyroid tissue is heterogeneous, can include calcifications and focal fluid
	Tracheal tumor	Within or surrounding trachea	Narrowing of trachea Adenoid cystic carcinoma has more tumor outside the trachea than within it, so-called toothpaste lesion
	Vascular variants and abnormalities	Posterior to trachea Anterior or posterior to esophagus	Diverticulum of Kommerall with aberrant subclavian artery Vascular rings and slings
Posterior mediastinal mass	Esophageal abnormalities and masses	Large esophageal mass can occupy middle and posterior mediastinal compartments	Esophageal cancer Foregut duplication cyst
	Neurogenic tumor	Connected to neural foramen	Smoothly marginated or lobulated May have low attenuation May contain fat
	Extramedullary hematopoiesis	Paraspinal masses	Masses are often paired Smoothly marginated

Note: Radiographic division of middle mediastinum may include esophagus, thyroid, and lymph nodes, leaving neurogenic tumors and extramedullary hematopoiesis as primary considerations in posterior mediastinum.

of more solid opacity that can result in a part-solid nodule. In this context, the development of bars corresponds to invasive adenocarcinoma. Small cysts, some of which may be indistinguishable from bronchi, and focal extensions to pleural surfaces, with and without deflection of the pleural reflection, are also seen. Since these lesions can be unifocal or multifocal and require different treatment strategies, extensive follow-up CT scanning is performed. Comparison of size measurements also has become more complex as tumor evolution has become better demonstrated on CT scans. Tumor progression may be expressed by increase in density of part or all of the well-demarcated ground-glass opacity accompanied by decrease in size of the lesion or a part of the lesion. Thin-section reconstruction in lung kernel provides the most consistent data for comparison. Short-term follow-up reveals resolution of many such opacities, particularly after a course of antibiotic therapy. In the case of persistent ground-glass opacity, more than 2 years of follow-up may be required to prove the lack of growth over time.

Carcinoid

The new WHO classification for lung cancer places carcinoid tumors within the category of lung cancer, regardless of whether typical or atypical, in the spectrum of neuroendocrine malignancies, which also include small cell lung cancer.[15] Carcinoid tumors present as endobronchial lesions with a cherry-like appearance on bronchoscopy, often associated with mucoid impaction of the distal airways. Dystrophic calcification in a lobulated nodule seen obstructing a bronchus, perhaps with mucoid impaction also evident, is a classic description of a carcinoid tumor. Not all carcinoid tumors have every one of these features; however, and the presence or absence of individual imaging features does not correlate with typical versus atypical carcinoid. The most extreme form of neuroendocrine tumor,

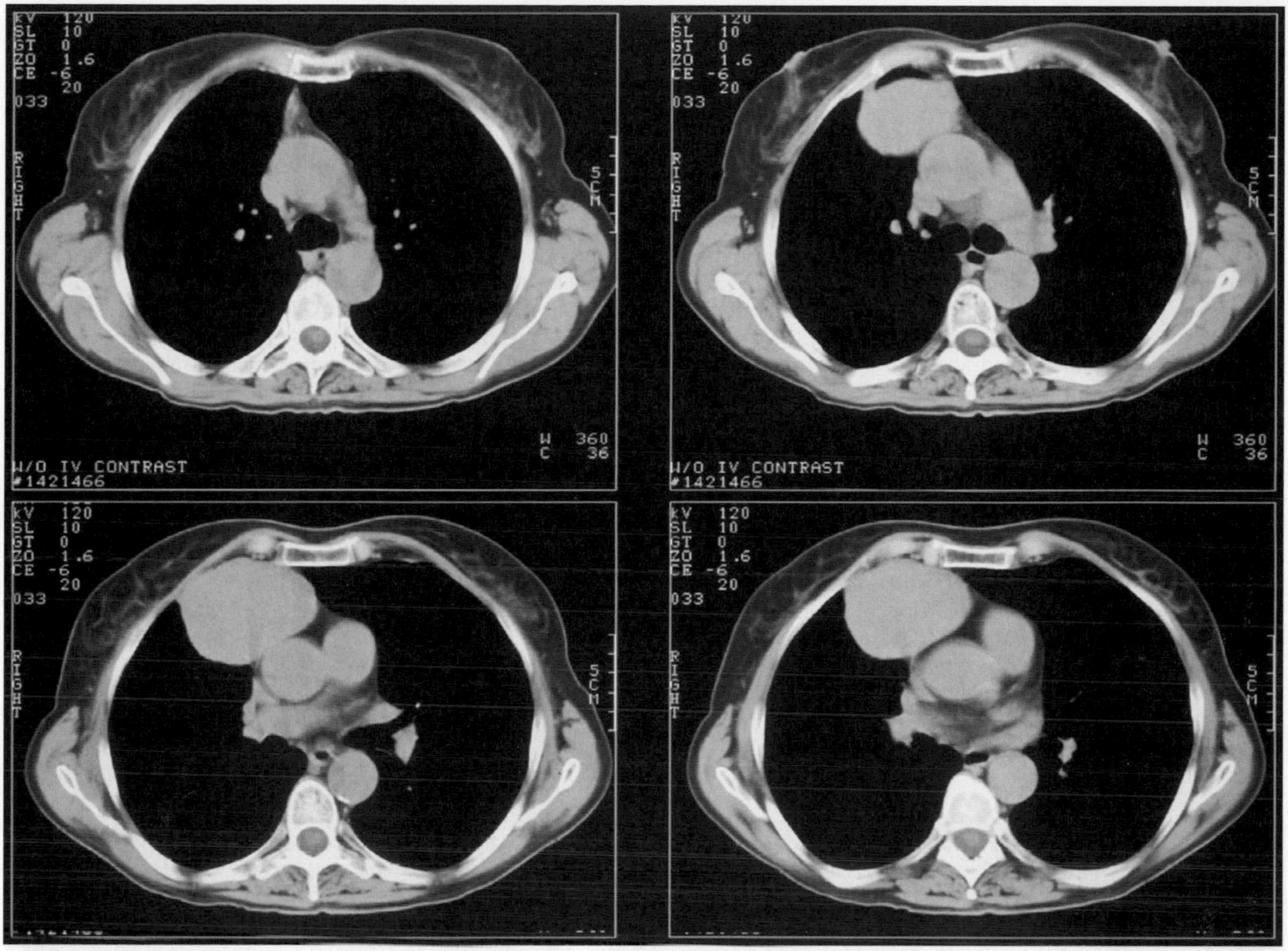

Figure 3-22. Transaxial 5-mm non–contrast-enhanced images of the chest rendered for mediastinum reveal a homogeneous, smoothly marginated mass in the right side of the thymic bed. This appearance is classic for a thymoma, especially when seen in middle age.

small cell lung cancer, may present with no obvious lung nodule but with striking lymph node enlargement.

The presence of tumor elsewhere in the body also may increase concern for metastasis, although the lung nodule may be the initial presentation of an extrathoracic malignancy. Colon cancer, common in the age group of patients who develop lung cancer, is particularly associated with large "cannon ball" and potentially solitary pulmonary metastases.

Mediastinal Mass

Mediastinal masses can be tricky to image with CT. The most difficult decision is regarding the administration of intravenous contrast material. If a patient has a thyroid mass that can be treated with radioactive ^{131}I, the administration of iodine contrast material is contraindicated. The administered iodine contrast material would saturate the iodine receptors to which radioactive ^{131}I also binds, requiring a 3-month delay in treatment to allow the receptors to become available again to ^{131}I. Not giving iodine contrast material, on the other hand, masks the diagnosis of Castleman disease. In the case of Castleman disease, or angiofollicular lymph node hyperplasia, the enhancement of the mass is most apparent by comparing scans before and after the administration of intravenous contrast material. Adopting the strategy of paired CT scans with and without contrast material for all nonthyroid mass examinations unnecessarily increases the radiation exposure for most patients. Thymoma, lymphoma, and teratoma may be imaged with or without contrast material. Contrast material sometimes adds clarity to the examination of mediastinal masses. The age of the patient is generally more helpful than contrast enhancement with these tumors (Fig. 3-22).

Extensive Pleural Disease—Diffuse Malignant Pleural Mesothelioma

The pleural space is not well vascularized and therefore can provide an environment for infection that is not easily treated with antibiotics. Hence extensive pleural disease requires attention from the thoracic surgeon whether it is benign or malignant. Since 800 mL of pleural fluid or a change in pleural fluid volume of this magnitude can be undetectable on a bedside chest radiograph, pleural effusions detected by imaging are often significant. The characterization of small, medium, and large for the size of a pleural effusion is a gross approximation on chest radiographs, although such imaging may be more helpful for quantification than CT and MRI. Differences in patient position during the examination make it difficult to directly compare the sizes of pleural effusions over time using different modalities. The volume of a pleural effusion is often overstated on cross-sectional imaging reports compared with chest radiography. In the absence of quantification, the size of a pleural effusion on axial CT images is often determined by cranial-caudal extent, resulting in overestimation of the size of many significant pleural effusions. The same problem also applies to reporting the size of a pneumothorax. As image processing enters the clinical practice of radiology, more quantification may be provided on a routine basis. The more pressing issue in this regard is in the setting of primary pleural tumor with extensive pleural disease, such as in malignant pleural mesothelioma. Fluid and tumor masses may encase the lung with a thickness that warrants measurement despite the complexities involved. In some instances, the additional findings such as extrathoracic lymph nodes and invasion of vital structures, whether in the mediastinum or the abdomen or by extensive involvement of the chest wall, may be more important than quantification of tumor mass, fluid, or both within the pleural space (Fig. 3-23).

Since the pleural surface is very thin, pleurectomy may not be recognized on postoperative CT. Adjacent hemorrhage is often seen without conveying its postoperative significance. The performance of the extrapleural pneumonectomy (see Chapter 119), most often for malignant pleural mesothelioma but also on occasion appropriate for the more common adenocarcinomatosis of the pleural space and unusual tumor metastases, requires careful consideration of preoperative cross-sectional imaging, generally with CT, MRI, and PET/CT.[16] The use of ultrasound is limited primarily to the localization of small collections of pleural fluid. Imaging modalities generally are complementary, but caution is warranted regarding the limitation of each modality in the assessment of extensive pleural disease.

Contrast-enhanced chest CT is the most basic of these imaging techniques, but it can be the best imaging modality for detection of small extrathoracic lymph nodes, chest wall tumors, and bone destruction. CT is not sensitive to focal invasion of the abdomen and may overestimate invasion of mediastinal structures by contiguous tumor. Secondary signs, such as a pericardial effusion in the setting of pericardial invasion, may be helpful for correct assessment of disease extent by CT. Multiplanar reconstruction has increased the utility of the volumetric CT data conventionally acquired by multidetector CT.

MRI, performed with multiplanar T1- and T2-weighted sequences and intravenous injection of 20 mL of gadolinium contrast agent, provides the best demonstration of fascial

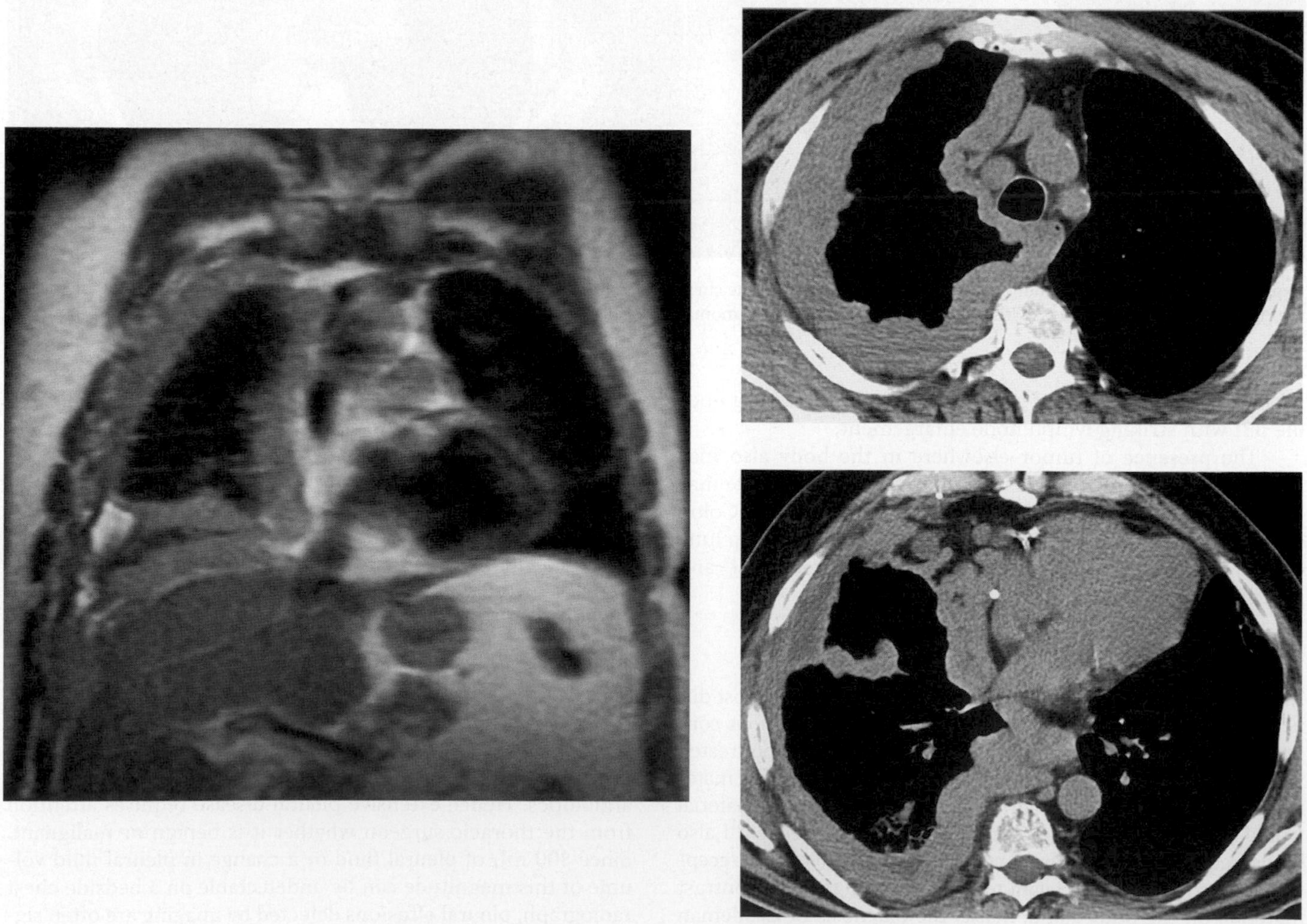

Figure 3-23. Coronal MRI and transaxial CT images demonstrate lobulated pleural thickening with small collections of fluid encasing the right lung. MRI demonstrates the fascial plane between the pleural disease and the chest wall, diaphragm, and mediastinum. Note the extrapleural lymph nodes in the right anterior diaphragmatic region on the bottom CT image.

planes. In particular, sagittal MRI provides the best preoperative evaluation for the integrity of the hemidiaphragm, and all three planes contribute in a similar manner to detection of mediastinal fascial planes. MRI demonstration of tissue characteristics also highlights the distinction between tumor masses and fluid in the pleural space. Diffusion characteristics may allow preoperative determination of epithelial and sarcomatoid tumor subtypes and be useful in selection of biopsy site. MRI provides less spatial resolution and may not image small structures, including tiny lung nodules, even when the structure is within the image. Furthermore, MRI sequences are not volumetric in the manner of CT scans and thus can fail to image small structures.

PET/CT is not always performed; however, it is being used increasingly to select the best possible biopsy target, thereby improving the initial diagnosis of malignant pleural mesothelioma. Multimodality therapy also may be offered on the basis of PET/CT findings, particularly when intense ^{18}F-FDG activity is seen in extrathoracic lymph nodes despite being smaller than can reliably be detected by the radioisotope and smaller than can be reliably identified by contrast-enhanced CT. Volumetric measurement of tumor burden also will be enhanced by functional information from PET scanning. Consequent improvements in the evaluation of treatment for malignant pleural mesothelioma also can lead to the use of PET/CT for evaluation of treatment adequacy in benign processes such as empyema.

Horizons: CT Screening and Tumor Ablation

The use of CT to improve survival of lung cancer patients is no longer controversial as it is widely accepted that CT will find smaller, presumably earlier lesions, whether it is the patient's first lung cancer, a recurrent lung cancer, or independent development of a new lung cancer in a patient who already has had lung cancer. For more than 50 years, screening trials failed to demonstrate decreased lung cancer–specific mortality. In 2011, the National Lung Screening Trial (NLST) succeeded for the first time in demonstrating a lung cancer–specific mortality reduction of 20% through low-dose lung cancer screening CT.[17] In 2012, the American Association for Thoracic Surgery (AATS) published guidelines for the provision of lung cancer screening also to include provision of equivalent low-dose screening CT (LDCT) scan surveillance to long-term lung cancer survivors after the surveillance period for recurrence.[4] Lung cancer screening CT scans should strive to maintain dose equivalent to NLST recommendations (1.5 mSv) and should be undertaken with a multidisciplinary team including board-certified thoracic surgeons to ensure the very lowest morbidity and mortality that is necessary for results comparable to the NLST.

The use of imaging for screening of patients at high risk for developing lung cancer may change significantly over the next few years. In addition to guidelines regarding who should receive CT, at what age, and at what intervals in time, we may well see the introduction of a biomarker screening test for lung cancer. Image-guided therapy and the introduction of new drugs to treat tumors will further hone diagnostic evaluation with imaging and shape the future practice of thoracic surgery.

Pulmonary thermal ablation, initially performed with radiofrequency (RF) electrodes for palliation in nonoperative candidates, is likely to be superseded by microwave ablation that would be a more suitable treatment strategy for early lung cancer.[18,19] The advantage of microwave energy over RF and laser is the larger and faster volume of tissue heating that allows more complete ablation of larger tumors. Microwave energy provides greater control over the size and shape of the ablation zone and is able to reduce the effect on adjacent blood and airflow, thereby reducing complications seen with RF ablation. This therapy ultimately may become part of a multimodality approach to lung cancer, requiring less radical surgery and permitting cure of patients who are presently unsuitable candidates for surgery. Microwave ablation may provide effective therapy, capable of replacing resection for early lung cancers, particularly in the elderly.

SUMMARY

This chapter provides fundamental information regarding the selection of imaging modalities and strategies for correlating images with anatomy and pathology commonly encountered in thoracic surgery. Radiologic imaging plays a central role in the management of thoracic disease. Familiarity with the various imaging modalities can facilitate the relationship between the thoracic radiologist and surgeon and best address clinical problems. Lung cancer diagnosis, surgical planning, and long-term management of patients with thoracic problems benefit from close collaboration between thoracic surgeons and thoracic radiologists.

EDITOR'S COMMENT

Thoracic surgeons are adept at reading plain-chest x-ray films and CT scans. They offer an additional perspective to that of the thoracic radiologist; they can correlate the images with what they see in the operating room. Preoperative radiographic imaging is key to planning the operation in terms of proper incision placement and magnitude of resection required. This chapter has been improved with the addition of several new images highlighting lobar collapse and consolidation. These representative images should be memorized by residents and fellows, so that collapse can be recognized in the postoperative period.

—Michael T. Jaklitsch

References

1. Seltzer MA, Yap CS, Silverman DH, et al. The impact of PET on the management of lung cancer: the referring physician's perspective. *J Nucl Med.* 2002;43(6):752–756.
2. MacMahon H, Austin JH, Gamsu G, et al. Guidelines for management of small pulmonary nodules detected on CT scans: a statement from the Fleischner Society. *Radiology.* 2005;237(2):395–400.
3. Naidich DP, Bankier AA, MacMahon H, et al. Recommendations for the management of subsolid pulmonary nodules detected at CT: a statement from the Fleischner Society. *Radiology.* 2013;266(1):304–317.
4. Jaklitsch MT, Jacobson FL, Austin JH, et al. The American Association for Thoracic Surgery guidelines for lung cancer screening using low-dose computed tomography scans for lung cancer survivors and other high-risk groups. *J Thorac Cardiovasc Surg.* 2012;144(1):33–38.

5. Felson B. Standard terminology in computerized tomography. *Semin Roentgenol.* 1978;13(3):185–186.
6. Whitten CR, Khan S, Munneke GJ, et al. A diagnostic approach to mediastinal abnormalities. *Radiographics.* 2007;27(3):657–671.
7. Colson Y, Sanders J, Nason L, et al. Primary care physicians and the fight against lung cancer. *Primary Care Report.* 2007;13:1–9.
8. Jeong YJ, Yi CA, Lee KS. Solitary pulmonary nodules: detection, characterization, and guidance for further diagnostic workup and treatment. *AJR Am J Roentgenol.* 2007;188(1):57–68.
9. Miller JC, Shepard JA, Lanuti M, et al. Evaluating pulmonary nodules. *J Am Coll Radiol.* 2007;4(6):422–426.
10. Carr S, Pechet T. *Assessment of a Solitary Pulmonary Nodule.* Chicago, IL: WebMD.COM; 2006.
11. Li F, Sone S, Abe H, Macmahon H, et al. Malignant versus benign nodules at CT screening for lung cancer: comparison of thin-section CT findings. *Radiology.* 2004;233(3):793–798.
12. International Early Lung Cancer Action Program Investigators, Henschke CI, Yankelevitz DF, et al. Survival of patients with stage I lung cancer detected on CT screening. *N Engl J Med.* 2006;355(17):1763–1771.
13. Travis WD, Brambilla E, Noguchi M, et al. International association for the study of lung cancer/american thoracic society/european respiratory society international multidisciplinary classification of lung adenocarcinoma. *J Thorac Oncol.* 2011;6(2):244–285.
14. Travis WD, Brambilla E, Noguchi M, et al. Diagnosis of lung cancer in small biopsies and cytology: implications of the 2011 International Association for the Study of Lung Cancer/American Thoracic Society/European Respiratory Society Classification. *Arch Pathol Lab Med.* 2013;137:668–684.
15. Detterbeck FC, Boffa DJ, Tanoue LT. The new lung cancer staging system. *Chest.* 2009;136(1):260–271.
16. Gerbaudo VH, Sugarbaker DJ, Britz-Cunningham S, et al. Assessment of malignant pleural mesothelioma with (18)F-FDG dual-head gamma-camera coincidence imaging: comparison with histopathology. *J Nucl Med.* 2002;43(9):1144–1149.
17. National Lung Screening Trial Research Team, Aberle DR, Adams AM, et al. Reduced lung-cancer mortality with low-dose computed tomographic screening. *N Engl J Med.* 2011;365(5):395–409.
18. Dupuy DE, Zagoria RJ, Akerley W, et al. Percutaneous radiofrequency ablation of malignancies in the lung. *AJR Am J Roentgenol.* 2000;174(1):57–59.
19. Sharma A, Abtin F, Shepard JA. Image-guided ablative therapies for lung cancer. *Radiol Clin North Am.* 2012;50(5):975–999.

4 Preoperative Evaluation of Thoracic Surgery Patient

Victor Pinto-Plata and Anne L. Fuhlbrigge

Keywords: Preoperative evaluation, pulmonary function testing, regional lung function assessment, integrative exercise testing, cardiopulmonary reserve

The decision to proceed with any surgical procedure involves a careful consideration of the anticipated benefits of surgery and an assessment of the risks associated with the operation. An important component of estimating the benefit of surgery is knowledge of the natural history of the condition in question. It is a popular, though inaccurate, conception of the preoperative evaluation that the evaluating physician "clears" the patient for surgery. This implies a binary clinical scenario: Either the patient is at low risk and is "cleared" or the risk is excessive and the patient is "turned down" for surgery. The reality, of course, is more complex and often more gray than black and white. A more accurate view of preoperative evaluation fulfills two goals: first, to accurately define the morbidity and risks of surgery, both short and long term, and second, to identify specific factors or conditions that can be addressed preoperatively to modify the patient's risk of morbidity. The formulation of an approach to accomplish these goals requires knowledge of both the specific characteristics of the patient population and the general effects of thoracic surgery on patients.

PATIENT POPULATION UNDERGOING THORACIC SURGERY

Many patients undergoing a noncardiac thoracic surgical procedure do so as a consequence of known or suspected lung or esophageal cancer. These diseases share the common risk factor of a significant and prolonged exposure to cigarette smoking and commonly include older individuals. The combination of age and prolonged cigarette smoking yields a population with a significant incidence of comorbid factors beyond the primary diagnosis. A major source of comorbidity in the population of patients with lung cancer is the presence of chronic obstructive pulmonary disease (COPD). The diagnosis of COPD is an independent risk factor for the development of lung cancer, after controlling cigarette smoke exposure.[1,2] The combination of these factors, plus the magnitude of the surgical procedures, presents a challenge to the clinicians evaluating such patients. The potential for perioperative morbidity and mortality is substantial, but at the same time, the lack of effective alternative therapy for the patient's malignancy means that the consequence of not being a surgical candidate is almost certain death. This quandary led Gass and Olsen to ask, "What is an acceptable surgical mortality in a disease with 100% mortality?"[3]

The Charlson Comorbidity Index (CCI),[4] which generates a score based on the presence of comorbid conditions, was originally designed as a measure of the risk of 1-year mortality attributable to comorbidity of hospitalized patients. This index has been demonstrated to stratify the risk of postoperative complications in thoracic surgery patients.[4,5] In nonsmall cell lung cancer patients, the CCI is a better predictor of survival than individual comorbid conditions and has been recommended for use in the selection of patients for NSCLC surgery.[6] A recent study, compared the CCI to another comorbidity index, the Kaplan–Feinstein index (KFI), and demonstrated the CCI performed better at predicting perioperative mortality and death from noncancer causes after surgery.[7]

PHYSIOLOGIC EFFECTS OF THORACIC SURGERY

Surgical procedures and the anesthesia administered to permit such procedures have significant impact on respiratory physiology that contributes to the development of postoperative pulmonary complications. Because the incidence of pulmonary complications is directly related to the proximity of the planned procedure to the diaphragms, patients undergoing pulmonary, esophageal, or other thoracic surgical procedures fall into the category of patients at high risk for postoperative respiratory complications.[8]

Intraoperatively, the use of inhaled volatile agents can affect gas exchange by altering diaphragmatic and chest wall function. These changes occur without corresponding alterations in blood flow and give rise to areas of low ventilation/perfusion and cause the gradient for alveolar–arterial oxygen to widen.

In the postoperative period, a number of factors contribute to the development of complications. These include an alteration in breathing pattern to one of rapid shallow breaths with the absence of periodic deep breaths (sighs) and abnormal diaphragmatic function. These breathing derangements are caused by pain and diaphragmatic dysfunction secondary to splanchnic efferent neural impulses arising from the manipulation of abdominal contents. This has the effect of reducing the functional residual capacity (FRC), that is, the resting volume of the respiratory system. The FRC declines by an average of 35% after thoracotomy and lung resection and by approximately 30% after upper abdominal operations.[9] If the FRC declines sufficiently to approach closing volume—the volume at which small airways closure begins to occur—patients may develop atelectasis and are predisposed to impairment in gas exchange and infectious complications.[10] The closing volume is elevated in patients with underlying lung disease, narrowing the distinction between the FRC and the closing volume.

The alterations in lung volume that occur as a result of reduction in both the inspiratory capacity (the maximal inhalation volume attained starting from a given lung volume) and the expiratory reserve volume (the maximal exhalation volume from a given lung volume) contribute to a decline in the effectiveness of cough and cause increased difficulty in clearing pulmonary secretions.

MOST COMMON COMPLICATIONS AFTER THORACIC SURGERY

The complications associated with thoracic procedures are reviewed in Chapter 8 and are discussed with greater specificity in the many surgical technique chapters of this book. In general, however, the most common complications after major thoracic procedures are respiratory and cardiovascular. Although the exact frequency varies from series to series, pneumonia, atelectasis, arrhythmias (particularly atrial fibrillation), and congestive heart failure are the most common. Myocardial infarction, prolonged air leak, empyema, and bronchopleural fistula, although less common, also occur with significant frequency.[11] It follows, therefore, that particular attention to pulmonary and cardiac reserve and risk factors should be a major component of the preoperative evaluation.

GOALS OF PREOPERATIVE EVALUATION

The clinicians evaluating a patient for a major thoracic surgical procedure have several goals for the evaluation process. The foremost objective is to provide an accurate assessment of the short- and long-term risks of morbidity and mortality for a given procedure in a given patient while identifying factors that can be addressed preoperatively to reduce the possibility of adverse events. Less obvious benefits of the comprehensive evaluation include identification of risk factors and other health issues that may facilitate institution of interventions regardless of the plans for surgery.

HISTORY AND PHYSICAL EXAMINATION

History

Although the field of thoracic surgery has been dramatically altered by the development of new technologies, both in imaging and in therapeutics, the history and physical examination remain the most important components of the preoperative evaluation. There is no substitute for a careful history and physical examination when it is performed by an experienced clinician. Table 4-1 highlights the important components of the patient history. Although age is a risk factor for perioperative morbidity and often a factor used by both patient and physician to assess the risk and potential benefit of surgery,[12–15] much of this added risk is a consequence of the accompanying comorbidities. Recent publications suggest age alone is not an independent factor predicting mortality. Chambers et al.[16] showed that 30-day mortality rates, hospital length of stay, and global quality of life (QoL) were not influenced by age (age <70 years vs. age ≥70 years). Similar findings were found by Okami et al.,[17] who reported that octogenarian patients with stage I lung cancer had reasonable long-term outcomes.

Table 4-1

IMPORTANT COMPONENTS OF THE HISTORY IN PREOPERATIVE EVALUATION

- Presenting symptoms and/or circumstances of diagnosis
- Prior diagnosis of pulmonary or cardiac disease
- Comorbid conditions such as diabetes mellitus, liver disease, renal disease
- Prior experiences with general anesthesia and surgery
- Cigarette smoking: never, current, ex-smoker (If ex-smoker, when did the patient stop?)
- Inventory of functional capacity of patient
- Medications/allergies
- Alcohol use, including prior history of withdrawal syndromes

Although many of the elements of the history are self-explanatory, several bear further exposition.

Patients who are current smokers should be advised to quit. Importantly, there is a better chance of achieving smoking cessation in COPD patients after a lung cancer diagnosis (over 50%)[18] compared with smokers without this diagnosis, and better survival has been reported for those who quit after a diagnosis of early-stage lung cancer versus those who continue to smoke.[19] In addition, smokers compared with nonsmokers are at greater risk of postoperative complications including delayed wound healing, pulmonary and cardiovascular complications, and mortality as shown in randomized trials.[20] A meta-analysis found a relative risk reduction of 41% for prevention of postoperative complications with trials of 4 weeks smoking cessation having the largest treatment effect.[20] The ideal time for quitting is still controversial. A small number of observational studies have described a paradoxical increase in the risk of postoperative complications in patients who quit within 2 months of surgery,[21] which may be related to a selection bias (sicker subjects at increased risk of complications were more likely to quit).[20] A large retrospective study of in-hospital outcomes for 7990 primary lung cancer resections found an increased mortality for current smokers with adjusted odd ratio (AOR) 3.5 and confidence intervals (CIs) 1.1 to 11 and for those who quit for less than a month prior to surgery (AOR: 4.6, CI: 1.2–18).[22] However, there was no difference in mortality between current smokers and those who quit within a month. Therefore, it is recommended that patients be advised to quit smoking before surgery regardless of the time and, if possible, allow for a month of smoking abstinence to reduce the risk of postoperative complications to the level of a nonsmoker.[23]

Pharmacotherapy improves the likelihood of successful abstinence. Combining the use of nicotine replacement therapy and counseling has a higher rate of success.[24] Currently available pharmacotherapies include nicotine replacement therapy, bupropion, and nicotine agonist, varenicline.[24]

A critical component of the preoperative evaluation is the assessment of the patient's functional status. It is well established that there is a broad range of symptoms and functional impairments in patients with similar pulmonary function test results.[25] As described below, functional capacity is a major determinant of operative candidacy and an important component of the decision algorithm for both the pulmonary and cardiac elements of the preoperative evaluation. A number of approaches have been taken to determine functional capacity. These include questionnaires, tests of locomotion (e.g., the 6-minute walk or stair climbing tests), and cardiopulmonary exercise testing (CPET) (discussed below).

Physical Examination

Although most patients being evaluated for thoracic surgery have a normal or near-normal physical examination, it is an important component of the evaluation. The examination of the patient should include an assessment of general overall appearance, including signs of wasting. Respiratory rate and the use of accessory muscles of respiration should be noted. Careful observation of the patient as he or she moves around the examining room, climbs onto the examination table, lies down, and sits up can provide important information about functional status. Examination of the head and neck should include assessment of adenopathy and focal neurologic deficits or signs, particularly Horner syndrome in patients with a Pancoast tumor. The pulmonary examination should include an assessment of diaphragmatic motion (by percussion) and note of any paradoxical respiratory pattern in the recumbent position. The presence of rales should raise the possibility of pneumonia, heart failure, or pulmonary fibrosis. The cardiac examination should include assessment of a third heart sound to suggest left ventricular failure, murmurs to suggest valvular lesions, and an accentuated pulmonic component of the second heart sound to suggest pulmonary hypertension. The heart rhythm and the absence or presence of any irregular heartbeats should be noted. The abdominal examination should note liver size, presence or absence of palpable masses or adenopathy, and any tenderness. The examination of the extremities should note any edema, cyanosis, or clubbing. The presence of clubbing should not be attributed to COPD and raises the possibility of intrathoracic malignancy or congenital heart disease. The patient's gait should be observed both as an assessment of neurologic function and to confirm the patient's ability to participate in postoperative mobilization.

Pulmonary rehabilitation improves exercise capacity in patients with moderate and severe COPD. This intervention can improve the exercise performance in patients with severely reduced exercise capacity (<10 mL/kg/min or nonsurgical candidates) to a potentially resectable level (mean improvement 2.8 mL/kg/min).[26] However, the recommended duration of these programs (6–8 weeks) restricts the implementation of this intervention in the great majority of cases. Although there is evidence that the length of hospital stay could be shortened by 3 days with this intervention,[27] there is scarce information of other beneficial effects. Therefore, the use of pulmonary rehabilitation before surgical treatment for lung cancer may have a role limited to those patients with much reduced exercise capacity and early-stage lung cancer.

Laboratory Studies

It is a reasonable practice to check electrolytes, renal function, and clotting parameters and to order a complete blood count as part of the preoperative assessment. In patients with known or suspected malignancy, liver function tests and serum calcium also should be checked. Arterial blood gases may have a role in documenting a patient's baseline for future comparison, but the previously held view that resting hypercarbia (elevated P_{CO_2}) in isolation is a contraindication to thoracic surgery is no longer valid.[28]

Imaging Studies

The options for radiologic imaging are reviewed in Chapter 3 and are covered with specificity in the surgical technique chapters of this text.

Pulmonary Function Testing

The utility of preoperative pulmonary function testing in part depends on the type of operative procedure being planned. Preoperative pulmonary function testing is unlikely to contribute to the preoperative evaluation of patients undergoing mediastinoscopy, drainage of pleural effusions, or pleural biopsy when there is no prior history of lung disease or unexplained dyspnea. For patients who report dyspnea, significant functional limitation, prior pulmonary resection, or a diagnosis of COPD with a recent change in functional capacity; however, pulmonary function testing is an appropriate component of the evaluation.

Preoperative pulmonary function testing is mandatory for patients who are being considered for pulmonary parenchymal resection. Although a number of pulmonary function tests have been examined in this setting, two have emerged with predictive value for postoperative complications. These are the forced expiratory volume in 1 second (FEV_1) measured during spirometry and the diffusing capacity of the lung for carbon monoxide (D_{LCO}). Either of these values can be used to provide an estimate of the risk of operative morbidity and mortality. In addition, they are used to calculate the *predicted postoperative (ppo)* values for FEV_1 and D_{LCO} (ppo-FEV_1 and ppo-D_{LCO}, respectively).[29]

Prediction of Postoperative Lung Function

The ppo lung function has been demonstrated to be an important predictor of operative risk. In general, the available methods for calculating postoperative lung function underestimate actual measured lung function once the patient has recovered from surgery.[29] The two common approaches for calculating postoperative lung function are simple calculation (recommended for lobectomies) and regional assessment of lung function (recommended for pneumonectomy).[30]

Simple calculation is based on the assumption that the patient's lung function is homogeneously distributed. The calculation requires knowledge of the number of segments to be resected and the preoperative value. For FEV_1, the formula is ppo-FEV_1 = preoperative $FEV_1 \times$ (1 − (number of unobstructed segments to be resected/total number of unobstructed segments)). The calculation is similar for D_{LCO}. For most patients, this simple approach to calculation is sufficient and, as mentioned earlier, results in a conservative prediction of pulmonary function after recovery from surgery. Traditionally, a ppo-FEV_1 or D_{LCO} of 40% or lower was used to categorize a patient as a high risk for lung surgery. However, advances in perioperative management and surgical techniques (concomitant lung volume reduction and minimally invasive surgery) have further reduced the lower ppo limit to 30% in selected cases.[29] For patients with ppo-FEV_1 or ppo-D_{LCO} values <40%, the predicted postoperative product (PPP) may be used (where PPP = ppo-$FEV_1 \times$ ppo-D_{LCO}). Patients with PPP<1650 have been shown to have a high risk of operative mortality.[31]

In certain situations, simple calculation does not predict postoperative lung function accurately. The clinical situations for which regional assessment of lung function is indicated are summarized in Table 4-2. A number of approaches have

Table 4-2

INDICATIONS FOR PREOPERATIVE ASSESSMENT OF THE REGIONAL DISTRIBUTION OF LUNG FUNCTION

- Significant airflow obstruction on spirometry (FEV_1 <65% of predicted and FEV_1/FVC <0.70)
- Reduced exercise capacity: 35%–75% or 10–20 mL/kg
- Significant pleural disease
- Known or suspected endobronchial obstruction
- Central lung mass or planned pneumonectomy
- History of prior lung resection
- Presence of lobar collapse or major atelectasis on imaging

FVC, forced vital capacity.

Table 4-3

RISK ASSESSMENT FOR PULMONARY SURGERY

HIGHER RISK	LOWER RISK
Higher extent of resection	FEV_1 >2 L for pneumonectomy; >1 L for lobectomy; >0.6 L for segmentectomy
Poor exercise performance	Predicted postoperative FEV_1 >30%–40% of predicted (pneumonectomy > lobectomy > wedge resection)
Low predicted postoperative FEV_1	Stair climbing >5 flights for pneumonectomy; 3 flights for lobectomy
Low predicted postoperative D_{LCO}	Cycle ergometry >83 W
High PCO_2 or age >70 yrs (controversial)	Predicted postoperative D_{LCO} >40% of predicted
	Maximal oxygen uptake >15–20 mL/kg/min

been used to attempt to assess the regional distribution of lung function, including lateral position testing, bronchospirometry, quantitative radionuclide ventilation/perfusion scanning, and quantitative CT scanning. Although quantitative CT scanning holds promise in this regard, the current standard test is radionuclide scanning. Typically, the data from quantitative radionuclide perfusion scans are reported as the percent function contributed by the six lung regions: upper third, middle third, and lower third of each hemithorax. These data, combined with the preoperative lung function value and the location and planned extent of surgical resection, permit a calculation to be made of the ppo value. Using the quantitative $\dot{V}/\dot{Q}$ data, the ppo-FEV_1 or ppo-D_{LCO} is calculated as ppo value = baseline value × (100 − percent perfusion in the region of planned resection)/100.

Assessment of Functional Capacity

In many ways, assessment of functional capacity is the most critical component of the preoperative assessment in patients considering thoracic surgery. It is a decisive factor for determining whether further cardiac evaluation is needed (as outlined below) and is the major factor for determining the operative suitability of patients with significant impairment of lung function. As outlined at the beginning of this chapter, such patients are "overrepresented" in this population by virtue of the additional independent risk engendered by obstructive lung disease. As outlined in Table 4-3, there are reasonable guidelines for identifying patients at low risk for morbidity and mortality after thoracic surgery. Although lung function and calculation of anticipated postoperative function can fairly reliably identify patients at low risk, these factors do less well at defining which high-risk patients have prohibitive risk. For further refinement of risk in this group, an assessment of functional capacity needs to be obtained.

Although the clinician can derive an assessment of functional capacity based on the initial history and physical examination, for patients whose history suggests significant functional impairment or who have abnormal pulmonary function tests (FEV_1 or D_{LCO} <80% predicted), a test of performance is indicated.

Performance Tests of Functional Capacity

Historically, clinicians have used tests of ambulation as a semiquantitative assessment of functional capacity. Early teaching in the field used stair climbing as a measure of functional reserve, establishing a threshold of performance that connotes acceptable risk. This test has held up remarkably well over time. Patients able to climb three flights of stairs (54 steps) have adequate reserve for lobectomy and approximately five flights for a pneumonectomy.[11,32,33] A recent report of 640 patients who underwent lobectomy or pneumonectomy confirmed the utility of stair climbing in assessing postoperative risk; they observed a significant decrease in the risk of postoperative complications and mortality in the group of patients who climbed 22 m or more (110 steps) compared with those who climbed 12 m (approximately 60 steps in the United States).[34]

More recently, much of the literature has focused on the use of incremental CPET, with expired gas analysis, to quantify cardiopulmonary reserve. Such testing that can be performed with either a treadmill or cycle ergometer (preferred method) allows quantification of maximal exercise capacity, expressed as maximal oxygen uptake rate (MVO_2). This can be expressed as an absolute value in units of milliliters of O_2 per kilogram of body mass per minute or as a percent of predicted. Studies using this approach have established that patients with an MVO_2 of greater than 15 to 20 mL/kg/min have an acceptable risk for pulmonary resection.[29,30] Conversely, patients with an MVO_2 of less than 10 mL/kg/min have a high risk of postoperative complications and perioperative mortality.[29]

Most recently, reports have used the ppo exercise capacity (ppo-MVO_2) as a predictor of postoperative risk. This value is calculated using the results of both the CPET and quantitative lung function testing in a manner analogous to that used to calculate ppo-FEV_1. A ppo-MVO_2 of less than 10 mL/kg or 35% predicted is associated with a high postoperative mortality.[29]

Not surprisingly, in addition to being predictive of mortality, functional capacity is also predictive of perioperative complications and hospital length of stay.[35]

There is no consensus as to the sequence of testing one should follow in evaluating patients for thoracic surgery. The American Thoracic Society (ATS),[36] American College of Chest Physicians (ACCP),[30] and European Respiratory Society/European Society of Thoracic Surgery[29] have published guidelines for preoperative evaluation of patients with COPD that recommend several approaches to this situation. They differ primarily in respect to whether exercise testing or quantitative lung function assessment is the first test performed in patients with abnormal lung function and/or a history suggestive of a low functional capacity. The ATS has published a validated algorithm that incorporate these concepts (Fig. 4-1) and a second more simplified algorithm that includes stair climbing as the measure of functional capacity (Fig. 4-2). We acknowledge that the particular sequence used often depends on local practice and the availability of testing, particularly CPET. A typical sequence of evaluation is the history, physical examination, screening spirometry, and initial blood tests. For patients with airflow obstruction on spirometry and/or reduced diffusion capacity or those who report substantial functional impairment, further evaluation with a CPET is indicated.[29] According to the exercise capacity level, estimation of the ppo lung function by simple calculation or perfusion scintigraphy is indicated. Alternatively, lung function testing and ppo lung function calculation could be estimated first, followed by a CPET when indicated.

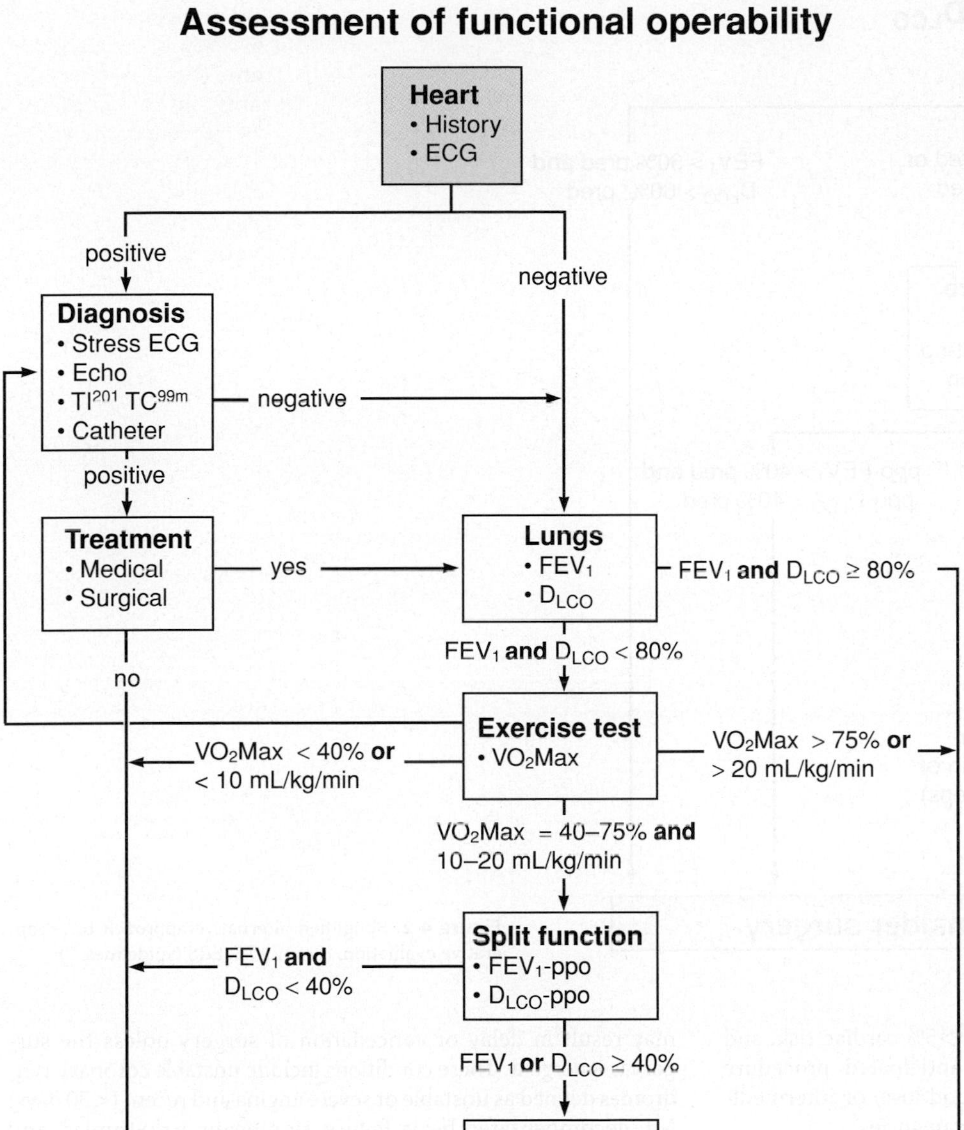

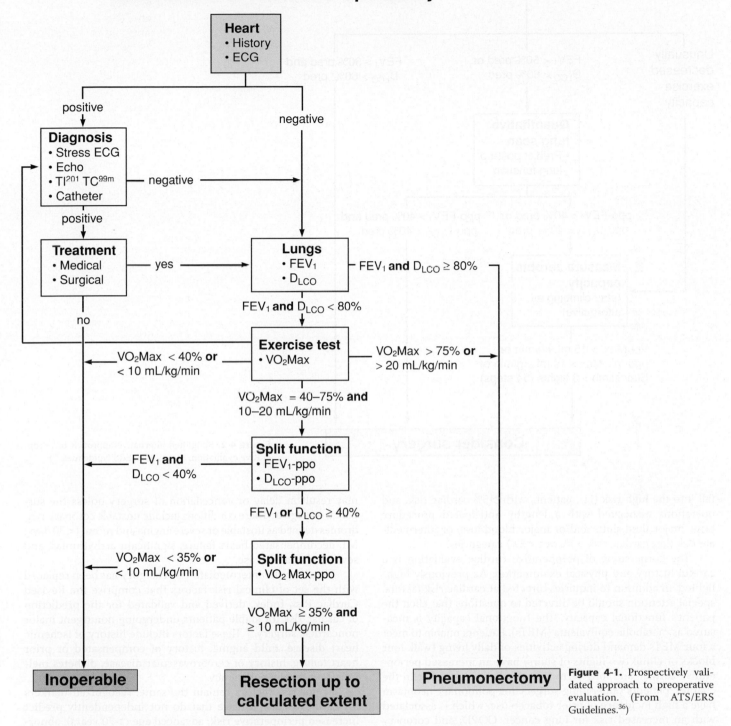

Figure 4-1. Prospectively validated approach to preoperative evaluation. (From ATS/ERS Guidelines.[36])

CARDIAC ASSESSMENT

The basic philosophy of cardiac assessment for surgical procedures has changed in recent years, as reflected in the recent guidelines jointly formulated by the American College of Cardiology and the American Heart Association.[37] The preoperative evaluation is now viewed as an opportunity to perform a general cardiac assessment and to initiate risk-factor modification/management rather than a specific intervention centered on surgery. The practice is to institute medical management as indicated by the patient's condition rather than specific preoperative recommendations. As a consequence, coronary revascularization, either by catheter approach or via bypass grafting, is rarely indicated solely to reduce operative risk in a particular patient.

The preoperative cardiac evaluation incorporates consideration of both the cardiac risks associated with the operation under consideration and the specific risk factors of the patient under consideration. In general, thoracic surgical procedures

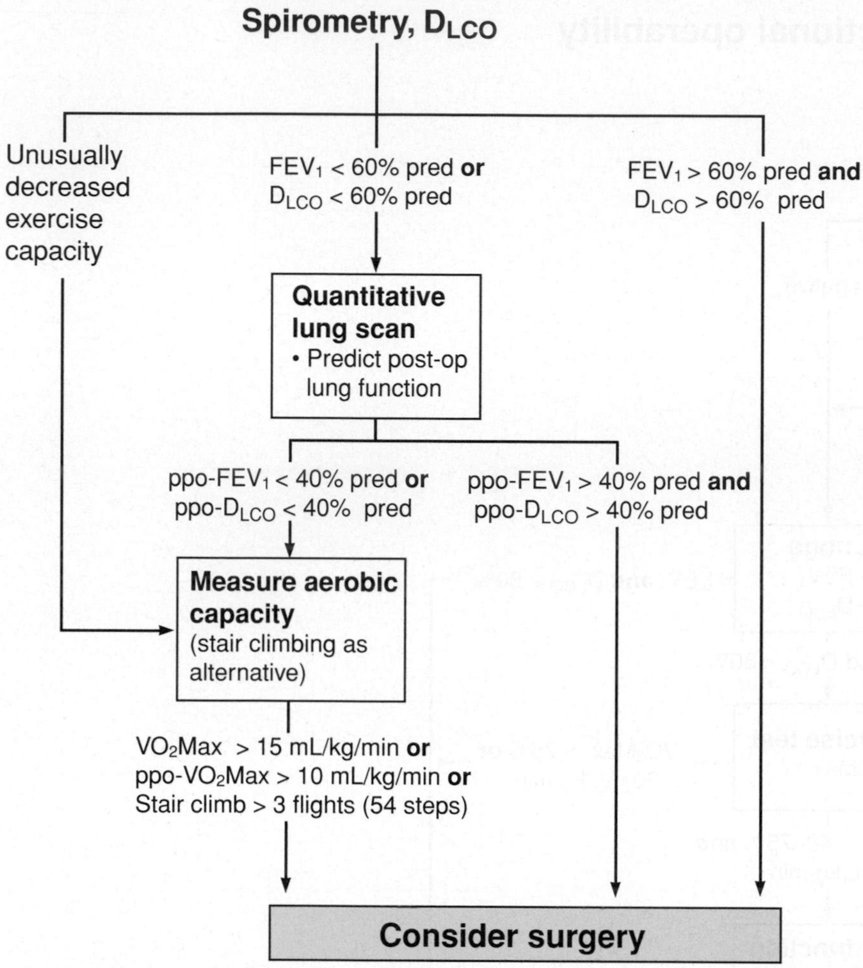

Figure 4-2. Simplified alternative approach to preoperative evaluation. (From ATS/ERS Guidelines.[36])

fall into the high risk (i.e., patients with >5% cardiac risk, and operations associated with a lengthy anticipated procedure time, major fluid shifts and/or major blood loss) or intermediate risk (i.e., cardiac risk >1% but <5%) categories.

The cornerstone of preoperative cardiac evaluation is a careful history and physical examination. As previously highlighted, in addition to inquiries directed at cardiac risk factors, special attention should be directed to questions that elicit the patient's functional capacity. The functional capacity is measured as metabolic equivalents (METs). Patients unable to meet a four METs demand during activities of daily living (walk four blocks or climb two flights of stairs) have an increased perioperative cardiac and long-term risk. As discussed earlier in the chapter, patients undergoing surgery for pulmonary neoplasm have a high incidence of prior tobacco use, which is associated with an increased risk for lung cancer, COPD, and coronary arterial disease (CAD). In addition, assessment of CAD is more difficult among these patients because limitations in exercise tolerance can be due to either CAD, lung disease, or both. It is wise to have a higher index of suspicion of comorbid CAD in patients undergoing intrathoracic surgery.

In the 2002 ACC/AHA guidelines, the committee chose to segregate clinical risk factors into major, intermediate, and minor risk factors. The 2007 guidelines modified this classification.[37] The updated guidelines continue to identify a set of active cardiac conditions, of which, the presence of one or more of these conditions mandates intensive management and may result in delay or cancellation of surgery unless the surgery is emergent. These conditions include unstable coronary syndromes defined as unstable or severe angina and recent (<30 days) MI, decompensated heart failure, significant arrhythmias, and severe valvular disease.

However, the intermediate-risk category has been replaced with the set of clinical risk factors that comprise the Revised Cardiac Risk Index, derived and validated for the prediction of cardiac risk for stable patients undergoing nonurgent major noncardiac surgery.[38] These factors include history of ischemic heart disease, mild angina, history of compensated or prior heart failure, history of cerebrovascular disease, diabetes mellitus, and renal insufficiency.

Minor risk factors remain the same; recognized markers for cardiovascular disease that do not independently predict increased perioperative risk; advanced age (>70 years), abnormal ECG (LV hypertrophy, left bundle branch block, ST-T abnormalities), rhythm other than sinus, and uncontrolled systemic hypertension.

The revised guidelines recommend a stepwise approach to the evaluation after a comprehensive history, physical examination, and review of the electrocardiogram.

For all patients, any long-term issues meriting consideration of risk-factor modification and/or therapy should be addressed in the postoperative period and appropriate therapy should be instituted when the patient is stable enough to tolerate the proposed treatment.

SUMMARY

The cornerstone for evaluating any patient under consideration for a thoracic procedure is a well-performed history and physical examination. For patients considering major thoracic procedures, this often should be supplemented by screening pulmonary function testing. Subsequent evaluation will be dictated by the results of this initial process. For patients with significant functional impairment or abnormal testing, estimation of postoperative function should be performed and consideration should be given to a formal test of functional capacity. Previously held concepts that advanced age and resting hypercarbia are absolute contraindications to surgery are no longer valid. Any patient who is an active smoker at the time of evaluation should be instructed to quit and offered pharmacotherapeutic assistance; ideally, this should be done at least 4 weeks before surgery.

A common clinical scenario begins with review by the evaluating physician of imaging studies, prior test results, screening spirometry, and perhaps a letter from a referring physician. Armed with this information, the clinician then enters the examination room and interviews and examines the patient. In this scenario, clinicians often state that a patient looks "better" or "worse" than expected based on the previously available information. This clinical impression is often supported by the results of functional capacity assessment; patients who "look better" than expected often have a functional capacity that permits major surgery with relatively low postoperative mortality.[28,39]

ACKNOWLEDGMENT

We wish to acknowledge Dr. John J. Reilly for his contribution to prior versions of this chapter.

References

1. Mannino DM, Aguayo SM, Petty TL, et al. Low lung function and incident lung cancer in the United States: data From the First National Health and Nutrition Examination Survey follow-up. *Arch Intern Med.* 2003;163:1475–1480.
2. Tockman MS, Anthonisen NR, Wright EC, et al. Airways obstruction and the risk for lung cancer. *Ann Intern Med.* 1987;106:512–518.
3. Gass GD, Olsen GN. Preoperative pulmonary function testing to predict postoperative morbidity and mortality. *Chest.* 1986;89:127–135.
4. Charlson ME, Pompei P, Ales KL, et al. A new method of classifying prognostic comorbidity in longitudinal studies: development and validation. *J Chronic Dis.* 1987;40:373–383.
5. Ra J, Paulson EC, Kucharczuk J, et al. Postoperative mortality after esophagectomy for cancer: development of a preoperative risk prediction model. *Ann Surg Oncol.* 2008;15:1577–1584.
6. Birim O, Kappetein AP, Bogers AJ. Charlson comorbidity index as a predictor of long-term outcome after surgery for nonsmall cell lung cancer. *Eur J Cardiothorac Surg.* 2005;28:759–762.
7. Wang CY, Lin YS, Tzao C, et al. Comparison of Charlson comorbidity index and Kaplan-Feinstein index in patients with stage I lung cancer after surgical resection. *Eur J Cardiothorac Surg.* 2007;32:877–881.
8. Smetana GW. Preoperative pulmonary evaluation. *N Engl J Med.* 1999; 340:937–944.
9. Meyers JR, Lembeck L, O'Kane H, et al. Changes in functional residual capacity of the lung after operation. *Arch Surg.* 1975;110:576–583.
10. Rothen HU, Sporre B, Engberg G, et al. Airway closure, atelectasis and gas exchange during general anaesthesia. *Br J Anaesth.* 1998;81:681–686.
11. Ploeg AJ, Kappetein AP, van Tongeren RB, et al. Factors associated with perioperative complications and long-term results after pulmonary resection for primary carcinoma of the lung. *Eur J Cardiothorac Surg.* 2003; 23:26–29.
12. Smetana GW. Preoperative pulmonary assessment of the older adult. *Clin Geriatr Med.* 2003;19:35–55.
13. Schuurmans MM, Diacon AH, Bolliger CT. Functional evaluation before lung resection. *Clin Chest Med.* 2002;23:159–172.
14. Jaklitsch MT, Mery CM, Audisio RA. The use of surgery to treat lung cancer in elderly patients. *Lancet Oncol.* 2003;4:463–471.
15. Jaklitsch MT, DeCamp MM Jr, Liptay MJ, et al. Video-assisted thoracic surgery in the elderly. A review of 307 cases. *Chest.* 1996;110:751–758.
16. Chambers A, Routledge T, Pilling J, et al. In elderly patients with lung cancer is resection justified in terms of morbidity, mortality and residual quality of life? *Interact Cardiovasc Thorac Surg.* 2010;10:1015–1021.
17. Okami J, Higashiyama M, Asamura H, et al. Pulmonary resection in patients aged 80 years or over with clinical stage I non-small cell lung cancer: prognostic factors for overall survival and risk factors for postoperative complications. *J Thorac Oncol.* 2009;4:1247–1253.
18. Baser S, Shannon VR, Eapen GA, et al. Smoking cessation after diagnosis of lung cancer is associated with a beneficial effect on performance status. *Chest.* 2006;130:1784–1790.
19. Parsons A, Daley A, Begh R, et al. Influence of smoking cessation after diagnosis of early stage lung cancer on prognosis: systematic review of observational studies with meta-analysis. *BMJ.* 2010;340:b5569.
20. Mills E, Eyawo O, Lockhart I, et al. Smoking cessation reduces postoperative complications: a systematic review and meta-analysis. *Am J Med.* 2011;124:144–154.e8.
21. Nakagawa M, Tanaka H, Tsukuma H, et al. Relationship between the duration of the preoperative smoke-free period and the incidence of postoperative pulmonary complications after pulmonary surgery. *Chest.* 2001;120:705–710.
22. Mason DP, Subramanian S, Nowicki ER, et al. Impact of smoking cessation before resection of lung cancer: a Society of Thoracic Surgeons General Thoracic Surgery Database study. *Ann Thorac Surg.* 2009;88:362–370; discussion 370–371.
23. Raviv S, Hawkins KA, DeCamp MM Jr, et al. Lung cancer in chronic obstructive pulmonary disease: enhancing surgical options and outcomes. *Am J Respir Crit Care Med.* 2011;183:1138–1146.
24. Chandler MA, Rennard SI. Smoking cessation. *Chest.* 2010;137:428–435.
25. Jones PW. Health status measurement in chronic obstructive pulmonary disease. *Thorax.* 2001;56:880–887.
26. Bobbio A, Chetta A, Ampollini L, et al. Preoperative pulmonary rehabilitation in patients undergoing lung resection for non-small cell lung cancer. *Eur J Cardiothorac Surg.* 2008;33:95–98.
27. Benzo R, Wigle D, Novotny P, et al. Preoperative pulmonary rehabilitation before lung cancer resection: results from two randomized studies. *Lung Cancer.* 2011;74:441–445.
28. Kearney DJ, Lee TH, Reilly JJ, et al. Assessment of operative risk in patients undergoing lung resection. Importance of predicted pulmonary function. *Chest.* 1994;105:753–759.
29. Brunelli A, Charloux A, Bolliger CT, et al. ERS/ESTS clinical guidelines on fitness for radical therapy in lung cancer patients (surgery and chemo-radiotherapy). *Eur Respir J.* 2009;34:17–41.
30. Brunelli A, Kim AW, Berger KI, Addrizzo-Harris DJ. Physiologic evaluation of the patient with lung cancer being considered for resectional surgery: diagnosis and management of lung cancer 3rd ed: American college of chest physicians evidence-based clinical practice guidelines. *Chest.* 2013;143(5 Suppl): e166S–e190S.
31. Pierce RJ, Copland JM, Sharpe K, et al. Preoperative risk evaluation for lung cancer resection: predicted postoperative product as a predictor of surgical mortality. *Am J Respir Crit Care Med.* 1994;150:947–955.
32. Pollock M, Roa J, Benditt J, et al. Estimation of ventilatory reserve by stair climbing. A study in patients with chronic airflow obstruction. *Chest.* 1993;104:1378–1383.

33. Brunelli A, Monteverde M, Al Refai M, et al. Stair climbing test as a predictor of cardiopulmonary complications after pulmonary lobectomy in the elderly. *Ann Thorac Surg*. 2004;77:266–270.
34. Brunelli A, Refai M, Xiumé F, et al. Performance at symptom-limited stair-climbing test is associated with increased cardiopulmonary complications, mortality, and costs after major lung resection. *Ann Thorac Surg*. 2008;86:240–247; discussion 247–248.
35. Weinstein H, Bates AT, Spaltro BE, et al. Influence of preoperative exercise capacity on length of stay after thoracic cancer surgery. *Ann Thorac Surg*. 2007;84:197–202.
36. http://www.thoracic.org/clinical/copd-guidelines/resources/copddoc.pdf.
37. Fleisher LA, Beckman JA, Brown KA, et al. ACC/AHA 2007 Guidelines on Perioperative Cardiovascular Evaluation and Care for Noncardiac Surgery: Executive Summary: a report of the American College of Cardiology/American Heart Association Task Force on Practice Guidelines (writing committee to revise the 2002 Guidelines on Perioperative Cardiovascular Evaluation for Noncardiac Surgery): developed in collaboration with the American Society of Echocardiography, American Society of Nuclear Cardiology, Heart Rhythm Society, Society of Cardiovascular Anesthesiologists, Society for Cardiovascular Angiography and Interventions, Society for Vascular Medicine and Biology, and Society for Vascular Surgery. *Circulation*. 2007;116:1971–1996.
38. Lee TH, Marcantonio ER, Mangione CM, et al. Derivation and prospective validation of a simple index for prediction of cardiac risk of major noncardiac surgery. *Circulation*. 1999;100:1043–1049.
39. Linden PA, Bueno R, Colson YL, et al. Lung resection in patients with preoperative FEV1 < 35% predicted. *Chest*. 2005;127:1984–1990.

5 Anesthesia Management

Philip M. Hartigan

Keywords: Thoracic anesthesia management, one-lung ventilation, single-lung ventilation, jet ventilation, double-lumen tube, single-lumen tube, endobronchial intubation, bronchial blocker, thoracic epidural analgesia, pain management

Anesthetic management of the thoracic surgical patient may improve operative conditions, efficiency, and outcome. Overlap exists in the territories of responsibility between thoracic surgeons and anesthesiologists, highlighting the importance of communication and mutual understanding. This chapter provides a brief overview of the general conduct of anesthesia for pulmonary resections, followed by a discussion of selected concepts in thoracic anesthesia of utility to thoracic surgeons.

OVERVIEW: CONDUCT OF THORACIC ANESTHESIA FOR PULMONARY RESECTION

Barring extremes of pathophysiology (e.g., end-stage chronic obstructive pulmonary disease), lesion-related hazards (e.g., compression of vital structures), or important coexisting disease states, the conduct of anesthesia for pulmonary resection is largely dictated by the surgical approach. For thoracotomy, the most common strategy consists of general anesthesia with paralysis, an arterial catheter (and possibly a central venous catheter), double-lumen tube (DLT), thoracic epidural, and immediate postoperative extubation.

Before induction, antibiotics, sedatives, and nebulized bronchodilator treatments are administered as indicated and the epidural is positioned and tested. After induction, diagnostic bronchoscopy may be performed via a large (8–8.5 mm) endotracheal tube or laryngeal mask airway (LMA). Findings that may affect the lung isolation plan should be noted by the anesthesia team at this time. Lung isolation by DLT or bronchial blocker (BB) then is imposed, with confirmation of position by pediatric fiberoptic bronchoscopy. After lateral decubitus positioning, repeat bronchoscopy is recommended. Ventilator parameters must be adjusted with initiation of one-lung ventilation (OLV) to ensure adequate gas exchange and to prevent barotrauma. Surgical entrance of the pleural space permits direct evaluation of the quality of lung isolation. Suctioning of secretions may aid atelectasis. Blood products should be available and checked before hilar dissection. Cross-clamp of the pulmonary artery typically does not cause changes in central venous pressure (CVP) or hemodynamics in patients with adequate cardiopulmonary reserve, and oxygenation should improve (see below). On cross-clamping of the bronchus, unchanged ventilatory compliance should be confirmed. If available, bronchoscopic visualization of the stump is useful before stapling. A "leak test" is commonly used by providing 20 to 30 cm H_2O of positive pressure ventilation to the submerged stump. Recruitment of any remaining lung is accomplished with incremental 5-second periods of 20 to 40 cm H_2O of positive pressure (recruitment maneuvers). After closure and supine repositioning, a final bronchoscopy via a large tube or LMA may necessitate a tube exchange. Rapid emergence and extubation depend on the strategic use of short-acting anesthetic agents; limited narcotic use; full reversal of muscle relaxation; control of secretions, bronchospasm, and pain (thoracic epidural); and return of airway reflexes, sensorium, and adequate respiratory efforts. Respiratory mechanics are greatly aided by raising the head of the bed more than 30 degrees at emergence (see Chapter 8).

Variations on the foregoing and procedure- or lesion-specific issues are presented as "bullet points" at the conclusion of this chapter.

PREOPERATIVE ASSESSMENT

The anesthesiologist should equally invest in assessments of cardiopulmonary reserve and coexisting disease states, as discussed in Chapter 4. Beyond that, the broad goal of the preoperative anesthetic evaluation is to identify issues with an aim toward reducing perioperative risk through preemption or preparation. The history, physical examination, and review of radiographic information should be targeted to anticipate problems with induction, airway management, lung isolation, vascular access, and pain management. Acute processes (e.g., respiratory infections) or the need to optimize treatment of existing conditions occasionally may justify postponement, but the semielective nature of thoracic oncologic surgery often mandates a higher risk tolerance.

Induction risk is increased in patients with threatened major airways, tamponade physiology, difficult airway anatomy, and traumatic or emergency scenarios. Paraneoplastic or associated syndromes (e.g., carcinoid syndrome, myasthenia gravis, Eaton–Lambert syndrome) have specific management implications (see below). Factors predictive of desaturation during OLV may be identified in advance (Table 5-1).

Patient medication regimens, in general, should not be disrupted, with the exception of insulin, oral hypoglycemic agents, and anticoagulants. Guidelines for how long anticoagulants should be held before placing an epidural have been published in a consensus statement by the American Society

Table 5-1

FACTORS ASSOCIATED WITH DESATURATION DURING OLV

- High-percent perfusion or ventilation to operative lung
- Low baseline Pa_{O_2}
- Right-sided surgery
- Normal or restrictive pattern by spirometry
- Supine surgical position

Table 5-2

RECOMMENDED DURATION TO HOLD ANTICOAGULANTS BEFORE EPIDURAL

ANTICOAGULANT	DURATION
Aspirin/nonsteroidal anti-inflammatory drug/COX-2	0
Unfractionated heparin (5000 units subcutaneous)	0
Unfractionated heparin (intravenous, therapeutic)	4 h
Low-molecular-weight heparin	
High dose	24 h
Low dose	12 h
Coumadin	3 d
Selective ADP inhibitors	
Clopidogrel (Plavix)	7 d
Ticlopidine (Ticlid)	14 d
Glycoprotein IIb/IIIa inhibitors	
Tirofiban (Aggrastat)	2 h
Eptifibatide (Integrilin)	4 h
Abciximab (Reopro)	36 h

Adapted from reference.[1]

of Regional Anesthesia[1] (Table 5-2). Patients with ischemic cardiac disease may benefit from thoracic epidural analgesia (TEA) and invasive hemodynamic monitoring despite a minimally invasive surgical approach. In such patients, perioperative beta-adrenergic blockade should not be withheld for fear of bronchospasm. Avoiding inhalational anesthetics and narcotics by use of total intravenous anesthetic (TIVA) techniques, together with TEA, may enable early extubation despite severe obstructive lung disease.

MONITORING

Invasive arterial blood pressure monitoring is indicated for most thoracotomies and many lesser procedures in which there is unstable or severe cardiac disease or the opportunity for catastrophic bleeding. Central venous blood pressure monitoring is significantly distorted by alterations in intrathoracic pressure during thoracic surgery, but such catheters are useful when venous access is problematic or for postoperative volume management. Central lines are best placed on the operative side because a pneumothorax in the nonoperative chest would be problematic during OLV.

Pulse oximetry is a standard, invaluable monitor but possesses limitations that deserve to be understood. Pulse oximetry does not measure oxygen saturation directly. Red (660 nm) and near-infrared (940 nm) light is emitted from diodes and attenuated by the tissue and blood through which it passes. The pulsatile portion of the signal is presumed to be arterial blood. The Spo_2 value is derived from the ratio of pulse-added absorbances at 940 nm (oxygenated hemoglobin) and 660 nm (reduced hemoglobin). Motion, ambient light, and venous pulsations can introduce artifact. Other species of hemoglobin will introduce error. Carboxyhemoglobin falsely elevates SpO_2. High methemoglobin levels lead to an Spo_2 of 85% regardless of Pao_2. Spo_2 readings below 85% should not be considered precise.

Monitoring for myocardial ischemia is compromised during left-sided thoracic surgery by the inability to place electrocardiogram leads in physiologic positions. Even in right-sided surgery, the position of the heart relative to the chest is altered, reducing electrocardiographic sensitivity. Transesophageal echocardiography may prove useful as a monitor of ischemia as well as right-sided heart function in response to pulmonary artery cross-clamping but does not necessarily predict subsequent right-sided heart failure. Transesophageal echocardiography also may help to guide surgical decisions in the evacuation of loculated pericardial effusions or the assessment of pulmonary venous anastomoses after lung transplantation. Pulmonary artery catheters are used infrequently in thoracic surgery because of the potential pitfalls in interpretation,[2] the risk of entrapment in resection staple lines, and the limited need for left-sided filling pressures or cardiac output determinations. Right-sided heart pressures (CVP) are generally of greater value.

Capnography has become a standard monitor and reliably confirms alveolar ventilation and cardiac output. The capnogram shape roughly correlates with the degree of obstructive disease (Fig. 5-1). The gradient between end-tidal CO_2 and $Paco_2$ is affected by the amount of dead space, which can be significant and variable in thoracic surgical patients. Acute changes in capnogram waveforms may signal bronchospasm,

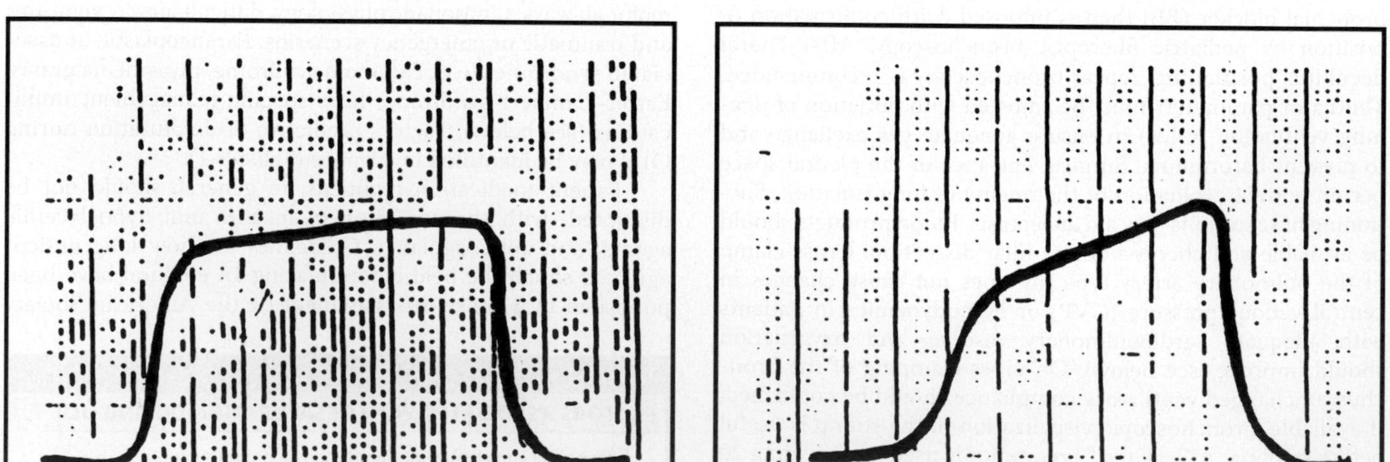

A B

Figure 5-1. Capnograms depicting exhaled CO_2 in a patient with normal (*A*) and severely obstructive pulmonary function (*B*).

tube malposition, circuit disconnection, ventilator valve malfunction, or exhausted CO_2 absorbant. Acute pulmonary embolism results in a sudden decrease in end-tidal CO_2 (increased dead space). High end-tidal CO_2 levels also can be the earliest sign of malignant hyperthermia. Effective chest compressions during cardiac arrest are reflected by the return of a capnogram.

POSITIONING

In the lateral decubitus position, the head and neck should be supported in line with the spine, with attention to protecting the eyes and dependent ear. Lateral neck flexion may cause traction injury of the suprascapular nerve and postoperative shoulder pain. An axillary roll placed caudad to the axilla relieves pressure on the dependent humeral head and axillary nerves and vessels. Excessive abduction of the nondependent arm (>90 degrees to the torso) may cause brachial plexus injury or contribute to shoulder pain. Ulnar nerves at the elbow and the dependent peroneal nerve are vulnerable and should be padded.

INDUCTION

Induction implies loss of consciousness. Inhalation of volatile anesthetics (e.g., sevoflurane or desflurane) can achieve induction with maintenance of spontaneous ventilation. Intravenous inductions (e.g., propofol, thiopental, or etomidate) usually produce apnea. Propofol is used most commonly for its favorable antiemetic and kinetic profile. As a continuous infusion, propofol (with or without narcotic) is a TIVA or a useful sedative in lower doses. Etomidate is a cardiostable induction agent, but is associated with greater nausea and may inhibit adrenal function. Ketamine has sympathomimetic and analgesic activity but may cause tachycardia, increased pulmonary artery pressure, and disturbing hallucinations. Ketamine is most useful for inducing patients with hypovolemia, tamponade, or bronchospasm or as an adjunct.

Physiology of Induction

It is critically important to understand the negative effects of induction on venous return and the caliber of airways. Induction in the supine position causes a 20% reduction in functional residual capacity (FRC), amounting to roughly 500 mL. This reduction in FRC occurs irrespective of the agents used (excepting ketamine), the imposition of paralysis, or the preservation of spontaneous ventilation and it persists for some hours after emergence. Airway calibers and resistance to airflow may be affected correspondingly. Patients with variable obstruction of major airways (e.g., anterior mediastinal mass effect) may convert to life-threatening complete obstruction on induction.

Induction impairs venous return by removal of the thoracic pump effect, imposition of positive-pressure ventilation, and vasodilation from induction agents. Increased intrathoracic pressure from positive end-expiratory pressure (PEEP; from the ventilator or auto-PEEP) will further reduce the gradient for venous return. Dynamic hyperinflation of lungs from auto-PEEP may exert pressure on the heart (with a closed chest), further impairing diastolic filling. Induction thus may unmask tamponade-like effects from large pleural or pericardial effusions or anterior mediastinal masses. Great vessels may be held open by traction during spontaneous ventilation but partially collapse under the weight of a large tumor on induction. The common mechanistic denominator, venous return to the heart, must be considered and defended at the time of induction.

Strategies for High-Risk Inductions

Threatened Major Airway Obstruction

Collapse of threatened major conducting airways may occur as a result of the decrease in FRC, as well as loss of the traction effect of inspiration that accompanies induction. Such "dynamic obstruction" may result from intraluminal masses, tracheomalacia, or large anterior mediastinal masses. Predicting which patients will lose patency with induction remains a judgment based primarily on symptoms and radiographic studies. Generally, patients who are asymptomatic at full expiration while supine will tolerate an intravenous induction. Coughing or dyspnea with this maneuver or tracheal lumens of less than 50% of normal by computed tomographic (CT) scan are treated more conservatively at my institution. Upright and supine flow-volume loops will sensitively illustrate dynamic obstruction but are of limited predictive value for induction. Intermediate concern may prompt a spontaneous-breathing (inhalation) induction, or an awake, topically anesthetized fiberoptic examination before induction. If the latter reveals nonreassuring anatomy, the stenotic region should be stented with an endotracheal tube before induction. Rigid bronchoscopy, patient repositioning, and jet ventilation (JV) are potential rescue maneuvers that should be immediately available. Short-acting agents for induction and muscle relaxation should be used initially in the event that resumption of spontaneous ventilation is required. Distal tracheal/carinal obstruction should prompt a more conservative approach because of the greater difficulty of emergently stenting such lesions with a tube or rigid bronchoscope. It is possible to place a DLT into a bronchus as a stent under local anesthesia. Placement of an LMA with topical anesthesia to the pharynx offers a convenient approach for awake fiberoptic examination of the entire trachea (Fig. 5-2).

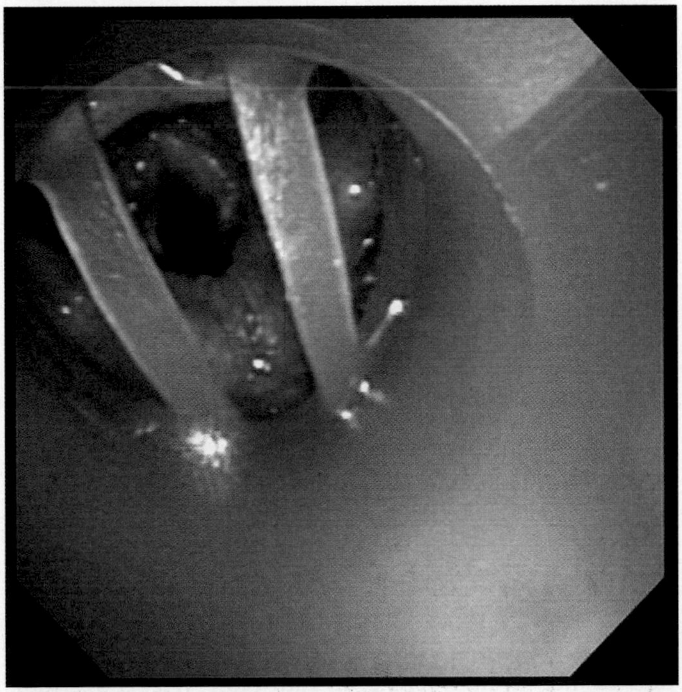

Figure 5-2. Bronchoscopic view of the vocal cords via a laryngeal mask airway (LMA).

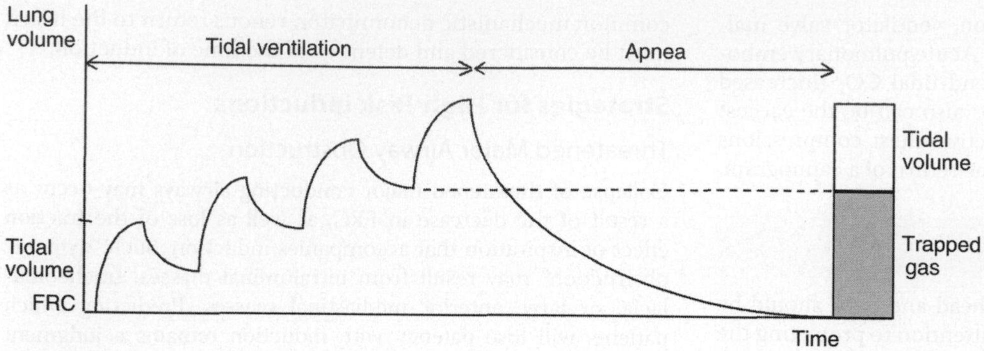

Figure 5-3. Schematic depiction of the development of dynamic pulmonary hyperinflation (auto-PEEP) and its resolution with a period of apnea. (Reproduced with permission from Myles PS, Ryder IG, Weeks AM, et al. *J Cardiothorac Vasc Anesth.* 1997;11:100.)

Local anesthetic delivered through the working port of the bronchoscope then can anesthetize the vocal cords and trachea. Rapid absorption by mucosal surfaces makes it important to be cognizant of the recommended thresholds for local anesthetic toxicity.

Threatened Venous Return

Patients at risk include those with large pleural or pericardial effusions, hypovolemia, severe obstructive lung disease, or large masses compressing the heart or great veins. Preemptive vasoconstrictors, intravascular volume expansion, use of cardiostable induction agents, patient positioning, avoidance of an epidural test dose, and use of graded inspiratory volumes and long expiratory times will preserve venous return in most inductions. When clinical and/or radiographic/echocardiographic evidence suggests higher risk, induction with maintenance of spontaneous ventilation is a more conservative approach. Preinduction drainage of pericardial or pleural fluid under local anesthesia should be considered in symptomatic (dyspneic) patients. Lower-extremity large-bore intravenous access is essential for patients with superior vena cava syndrome. Tension pneumothorax should be considered in patients with bullous emphysema and recalcitrant hypotension after induction. Intra-arterial blood pressure monitoring before induction is indicated for all high-risk patients, as is a plan for resuscitation should cardiovascular collapse occur.

Other Inductions of Increased Risk

Induction risk is also increased for patients with unfavorable airway anatomy, significant symptoms of gastroesophageal reflux, bronchospasm, or unstable coronary or severe valvular heart disease. Not uncommonly, competing priorities mandate compromise of one or the other concern. While aspiration risk argues for a rapid-sequence intravenous induction, this avenue may be contraindicated by difficult airway anatomy. Patients with unfavorable upper airway anatomy predictive of a difficult intubation (e.g., morbid obesity or micrognathia) should have an airway established under local anesthesia (e.g., LMA or awake fiberoptic intubation) before induction unless it is documented or apparent that the patient can be ventilated by mask. Use of short-acting agents (e.g., propofol or succinylcholine) is prudent whenever the airway is in question.

AUTO-PEEP

Failure to fully expire the preceding tidal volume at inspiration results in air trapping or auto-PEEP (Fig. 5-3). Auto-PEEP may lead to hemodynamic instability (including cardiac arrest) and barotrauma from dynamic hyperinflation. During OLV, excessive auto-PEEP in the dependent lung impairs gas exchange by diverting pulmonary blood flow to the nondependent lung. The incidence and severity of auto-PEEP roughly correlate with the severity of obstructive disease (Fig. 5-4) and is further exacerbated by the higher airflow resistance of DLTs and by inappropriate ventilator settings.

LUNG ISOLATION

Options for lung isolation remain threefold: DLTs, BBs, and endobronchial intubation.

Double-Lumen Tubes

The default choice for lung isolation in most cases is a left DLT for its ease of insertion, comfortable margin for error, and capacity to deflate either lung depending on which lumen is clamped. Auscultation may be used to confirm position, but direct visualization by fiberoptic bronchoscopy is increasingly a standard of care (Fig. 5-5). Up to 30% of patients with DLTs positioned by auscultation require repositioning when subsequently examined by fiberoptic bronchoscopy.[3] If the left DLT passes into the right main stem bronchus instead of the left, the

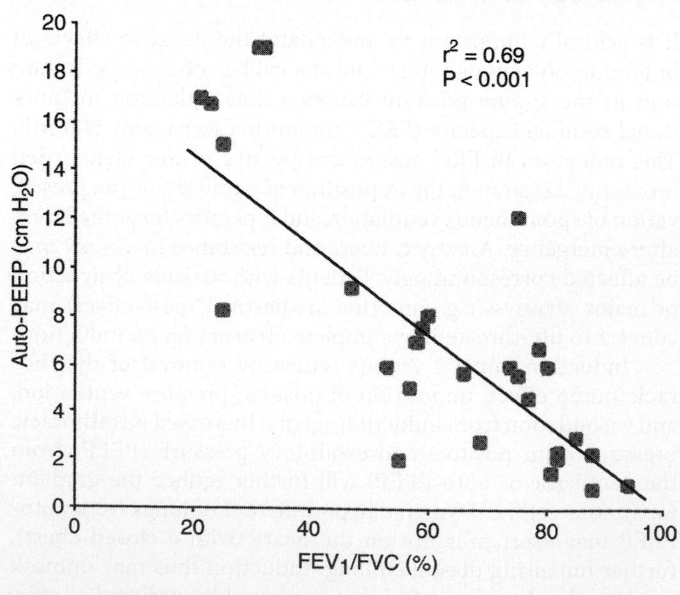

Figure 5-4. Relationship between the degree of airflow obstruction (FEV_1/FVC) and dynamic pulmonary hyperinflation (auto-PEEP). (Reproduced with permission from Ducros L, Moutafis M, Castelain MH, et al. *J Cardiothorac Vasc Anesth.* 1999;13:35.)

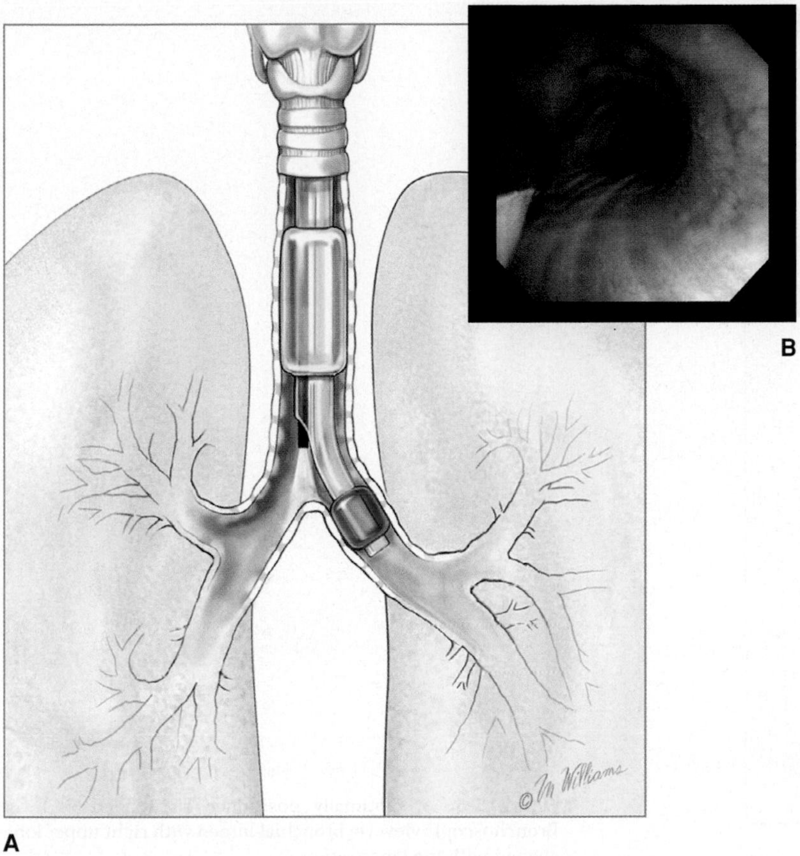

Figure 5-5. *A.* Optimally positioned left-sided DLT. *B.* Bronchoscopic view via tracheal lumen of carina, DLT, and bronchial cuff (blue) correctly positioned.

fiberoptic bronchoscope may be used as a stylette via the bronchial lumen to guide the tube into the left bronchus after withdrawal to the trachea. Reconfirmation of DLT position should be performed after turning the patient to the lateral decubitus position.

Right-sided DLTs have a fenestration in the bronchial lumen for the right upper lobe that must be aligned by fiberoptic bronchoscopy (Fig. 5-6). Common indications include any surgery in which pathology exists or any surgery intended in the left main stem bronchus (e.g., left pneumonectomy, sleeve resection, bronchopleural fistula repair, or left single-lung transplant). The likelihood of displacement is greater for a right-sided DLT than for a left-sided DLT. Because of this, some practitioners prefer to use a left-sided DLT (or a BB) for left pneumonectomy and to withdraw the apparatus before division of the bronchus. Right-sided DLTs cannot accommodate an anomalously short right main stem bronchus.

Current DLTs have D-shaped lumens with favorable airflow resistance characteristics. They are disposable and made of polyvinylchloride with low-pressure, high-volume cuffs. They are stiffer and larger than single-lumen tubes and have the potential to traumatize vocal cords and the distal airway. Compared with BBs, the large lumens of DLTs offer a route for air egress and active suctioning to accelerate collapse of the operative lung.

Bronchial Blockers

BB options now range from simple balloon-tipped Fogarty vascular embolectomy catheters to blocker systems (e.g., Univent [Fuji Systems Corporation, Tokyo, Japan], Arndt [Cook Critical Care, Bloomington, IN, USA], and Cohen [Cook Critical Care, Bloomington, IN, USA]) (Fig. 5-7). Blockers are generally easier to place than DLTs in patients with anatomically difficult airways, and they obviate the need for multiple tube changes. Blockers may also be used to achieve lung isolation via nasotracheal intubations or tracheostomy tubes, to isolate hemoptysis, or to tamponade mucosal bleeding from a bronchial lesion. Modern blocker systems have central lumens that permit air egress and insufflation of oxygen (CPAP). They can even be positioned to selectively deflate individual lobes in patients who would not tolerate complete lung collapse. BBs are more useful for left-sided procedures. When positioned in the short right main stem bronchus, they are easily displaced with repositioning or surgical manipulation of the lung. A sudden inability to ventilate when using a BB likely signifies a blocker that has popped out into the trachea. The appropriate reflex is to announce the situation and deflate the blocker balloon to establish ventilation if time does not permit bronchoscopic examination.

Endobronchial Intubation

Endobronchial intubation may be achieved with traditional single-lumen tubes advanced into main stem bronchi or with specifically designed endobronchial tubes with more favorable (short and distal) cuff designs and a fenestration for the right upper lobe. Indications for endobronchial intubation in adults include carinal resections or patients with prior pneumonectomy and bronchopleural fistula. In emergent massive hemoptysis from the left lung, blind advancement of an endobronchial tube into the right main stem bronchus can be lifesaving. Endobronchial intubation is also useful for pediatric patients in whom currently available DLT sizes fail to fit.

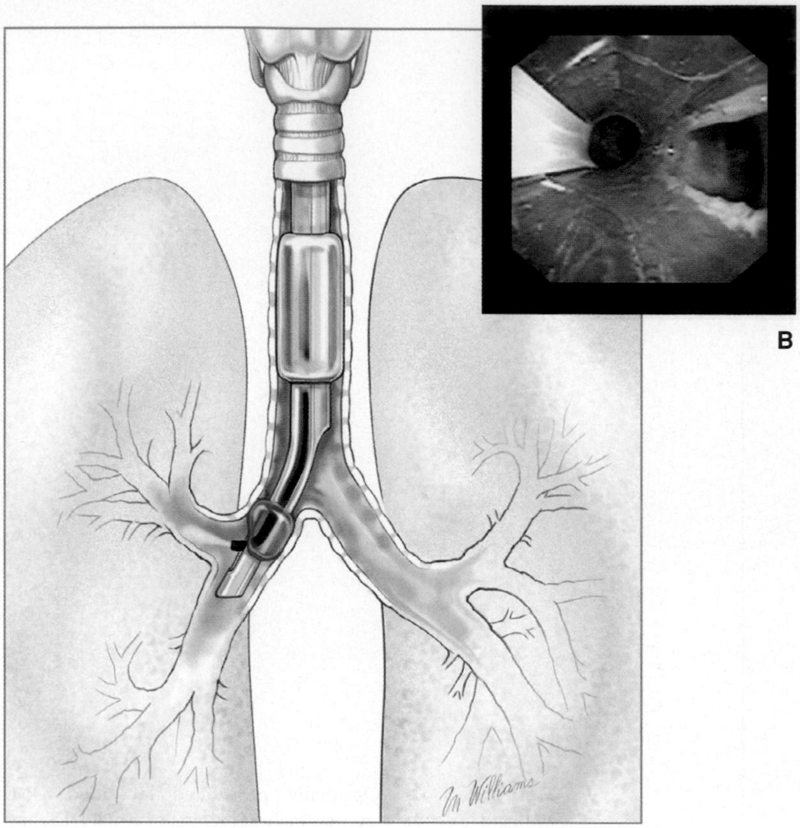

B

A

Figure 5-6. *A.* Optimally positioned right-sided DLT. *B.* Bronchoscopic view via bronchial lumen with right upper lobe aligned with the fenestration.

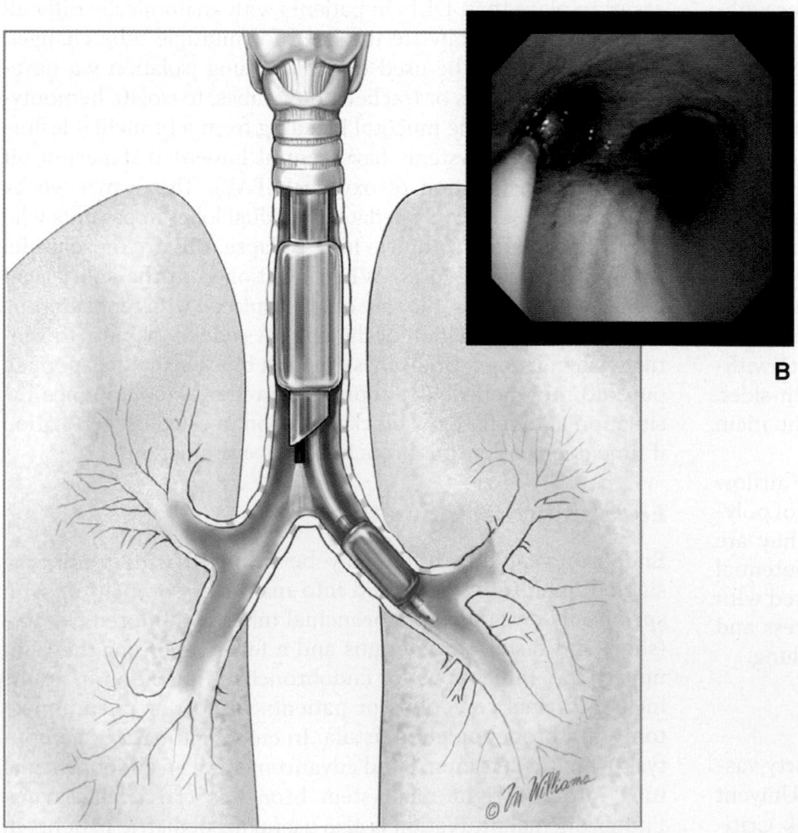

B

A

Figure 5-7. *A.* Arndt wire–guided BB (Cook) passed through a single-lumen tube into the left main stem bronchus. *B.* Bronchoscopic view of the same BB.

Special Lung Isolation Situations

Tracheal deviation or a splayed carina may make intubation of the left main stem bronchus difficult. A right-sided DLT or BB, if appropriate, likely is often easier than a left-sided DLT for such situations. Saber-sheath tracheas may occlude the tracheal lumen of a DLT. An anomalous short right main stem bronchus predicts a poor fit for a right-sided DLT. A left-sided DLT, BB, or endobronchial tube (depending on the planned surgery) should be considered instead. An efficient option for lung isolation for patients with difficult intubation status is to perform a fiberoptic intubation with a single-lumen tube together with a BB or, alternatively, to change to a DLT over an airway-exchange catheter. A BB can be placed in an individual lobe for selective lobar atelectasis if full OLV is not tolerated.

PATHOPHYSIOLOGY OF OLV

Efficient gas exchange depends on tight matching of pulmonary ventilation ($\dot{V}$) and perfusion ($\dot{Q}$). This relationship is severely disrupted by OLV, the lateral decubitus position, positive-pressure ventilation, general anesthesia, and paralysis, as well as by underlying lung disease. This scenario, applicable to most thoracic surgeries, typically results in a reduction of Pa_{O_2} from the 400 mm Hg range (at $F_{IO_2} = 1$) to approximately 150 mm Hg. Generally, the greatest single cause of ($\dot{V}$)/($\dot{Q}$) mismatch is the residual blood flow through the operative, nondependent lung, which constitutes pure shunt. Although individual variations can be substantial, blood flow to that lung is reduced on average from 45% to 55% of cardiac output to approximately 20%, principally by gravity and hypoxic pulmonary vasoconstriction (HPV). Additional shunt is invariably present in the dependent lung as well owing to the circumferential restrictive forces imposed by the weight of the mediastinum, the dependent hemidiaphragm, and the anteroposterior stabilizers. ($\dot{V}$)/($\dot{Q}$) mismatch also may exist to varying degrees within the ventilated dependent lung from parenchymal diseases such as chronic obstructive pulmonary disease, secretions, bronchospasm, or other pathology. Maneuvers to minimize nondependent and dependent lung shunt and dependent lung ($\dot{V}$)/($\dot{Q}$) mismatch are the basis for optimizing oxygenation during OLV.

HYPOXIC PULMONARY VASOCONSTRICTION

HPV is critical both to reduce nondependent lung blood flow and to fine-tune ($\dot{V}$)/($\dot{Q}$) matching in the dependent lung. The detailed mechanism of HPV remains unknown but appears to be mediated by voltage-sensitive potassium channels in response to (primarily) alveolar hypoxia and (secondarily) low mixed venous oxygen saturation. HPV is a rapid local response unique to the pulmonary vasculature and does not depend on intact vascular endothelium or autonomic innervation. Most vasodilators inhibit HPV, including nitrates (e.g., nitroglycerin and nitroprusside), nitric oxide, isoproterenol, terbutaline, adenosine, dobutamine, and to a lesser extent, calcium channel antagonists. Inhaled anesthetic agents (e.g., isoflurane, sevoflurane, desflurane, and halothane) inhibit HPV in a dose-dependent fashion. Within clinically relevant concentrations (<1 minimum alveolar concentration); however, their effect is of minimal significance. Hypercapnia/acidosis enhances and hypocapnia/alkalosis inhibits HPV. The net effect of any variable on oxygenation during OLV depends on the combined effects on HPV (direct and indirect), cardiac output, and mixed venous oxygen tension and often cannot be predicted.

SINGLE-LUNG VENTILATION STRATEGIES

Optimal single-lung ventilatory settings are controversial and often require a compromise between optimal recruitment of the dependent lung (large tidal volumes) and risk of barotrauma. This balance is most delicate in patients with severe obstructive disease who are prone to auto-PEEP. Such patients may benefit from a protective ventilatory strategy (5–7 mL/kg tidal volumes) and transient permissive hypercapnia. There is no firm evidence at this time, however, that "traditional" ventilatory strategies (10 mL/kg) are injurious or that protective ventilatory strategies improve outcome.

HYPOXEMIA DURING OLV

The incidence of hypoxemia during OLV has dropped from more than 20% in the 1970s to less than 1%[4] owing to improved DLT designs, increased use of the fiberoptic bronchoscope, and improved understanding of the physiology of OLV. Treatment options for hypoxemia during OLV are listed in Table 5-3. Which maneuver to employ first depends on the clinical scenario. In rapid, severe desaturation, reinflation should be the first move, coordinated with the surgeon. If time permits, passage of a bronchoscope to confirm tube/blocker position and to rule out secretions, blood, kinks, or other causes of obstruction is prudent.

CPAP and Optimal Peep During OLV

Continuous positive airway pressure (CPAP; 5–10 cm H_2O) delivered to the nondependent lung generally will improve oxygenation but may partially reinflate the lung and interfere with the conduct of surgery. PEEP delivered to the dependent lung may improve oxygenation through recruitment of atelectatic lung units. Each patient has an optimal PEEP level beyond which oxygenation will deteriorate as a consequence of increased nondependent lung shunt. Extreme air trapping may result in hemodynamic instability and barotrauma. The degree of auto-PEEP is not measurable by standard operating

Table 5-3

TREATMENT OPTIONS FOR HYPOXEMIA DURING OLV

- $F_{IO_2} = 1$
- Bronchoscopy to rule out
  - Tube malposition
  - Secretions
  - Other sources of obstruction
- PEEP to the dependent lung
- CPAP to the nondependent lung
- Reinflate nondependent lung
- Cross-clamp nondependent pulmonary artery (if surgically appropriate)

room ventilators but can be detected by briefly disconnecting the circuit and observing for end-expiratory airflow. Patients likely to benefit from dependent lung PEEP are patients predisposed to dependent lung atelectasis (e.g., those with restrictive disease, obesity, and young patients with a normal FEV_1). In contrast, patients with severe obstructive disease likely will have unavoidable levels of auto-PEEP equal to or in excess of their optimal PEEP. Low levels of extrinsic (ventilator imposed) PEEP will not increase total PEEP in patients with significant auto-PEEP. A useful strategy therefore is to begin with less than 5 cm H_2O of extrinsic PEEP and to increase PEEP incrementally with Spo_2 as a guide in patients who are hypoxemic during OLV. PEEP is more effective when preceded by a recruitment maneuver to the dependent lung.

Other Strategies to Improve Oxygenation During OLV

If bronchospasm is suspected, nebulized bronchodilators delivered to the dependent lung may be helpful. When surgical cross-clamping of the pulmonary artery is imminent, marginal saturations can be tolerated with the knowledge that cross-clamping invariably will improve oxygenation by reducing or eliminating (in the case of pneumonectomy) nondependent lung shunt. Minor improvements in oxygenation occasionally can be achieved through intermittent recruitment maneuvers to the dependent lung, or by eliminating drugs that inhibit HPV. Because inhalational anesthetics inhibit HPV and most intravenous agents do not, TIVA has been proposed to improve oxygenation during OLV. Clinical studies are currently inconclusive on this matter, which is complicated by secondary effects on oxygenation through changes in cardiac output and mixed venous oxygen saturation.[5] Similarly, inhaled nitric oxide, which might be expected to reduce nondependent lung shunt and improve dependent lung blood flow, has proved to be ineffective in improving one-lung oxygenation in a number of human studies.[5]

CHOICE OF AGENTS

The priority for early extubation of pulmonary resection patients influences most anesthesiologists to select relatively short-acting agents. For induction, propofol is widely favored for its low incidence of nausea as well as its kinetics. Vecuronium is a convenient muscle relaxant because of its neutral hemodynamic effects as well as its intermediate duration. Of the currently used potent inhalational agents, sevoflurane and desflurane are both rapidly eliminated as a consequence of their low solubility. Desflurane has more airway irritant effects than sevoflurane, but this is not a clinically significant issue when adequate anesthetic depth is present. Both are eliminated more rapidly than isoflurane. Nitrous oxide is often avoided because of the potential to expand in closed spaces (e.g., blebs, pneumothoraces, and endotracheal tube cuffs) and because its use requires a reduction in Fio_2. Unless contraindicated (e.g., history of bleomycin therapy), a high Fio_2 is often necessary to achieve a safe margin of oxygenation during OLV. Narcotics are useful in limited doses as a supplement to anesthetic depth and to blunt airway reflexes. Excessive narcotic effect blunts respiratory drive, clouds the sensorium, induces nausea and constipation, and delays extubation. Therefore, narcotics generally are used judiciously before intubation and sparingly thereafter. The ultra-short–acting narcotic remifentanil is particularly useful to blunt airway reflexes before tube exchanges at the terminus of the case without delaying extubation. TIVA (usually propofol $\pm$ remifentanil) is advantageous for maintenance in patients with severe obstructive disease (delayed elimination of inhaled agents), for patients undergoing rigid bronchoscopy, or for surgeries involving an open airway (e.g., tracheal resection).

INTRAOPERATIVE MANAGEMENT OF THORACIC EPIDURALS

A midthoracic epidural catheter is justified for most thoracotomies, whether full posterolateral or limited muscle-sparing, and is best placed before induction. An awake patient will respond dramatically and early to any needle contact with nerve roots or spinal cord. Epidural needle-induced nerve damage has been reported with thoracic epidurals performed in anesthetized patients. After aspiration, an initial test dose (e.g., 3 mL of 2% lidocaine with epinephrine 1:200,000) should be administered with monitors in place to serve three vital functions. Failure to aspirate clear fluid and absence of dense motor block or exaggerated hypotensive response suggest that the catheter position is not erroneously subarachnoid. Failure to aspirate blood and absence of an epinephrine-induced spike in heart rate suggest that the catheter is not erroneously positioned within a blood vessel. Third, the development of a midthoracic band of analgesia within 10 to 15 minutes strongly suggests an appropriately positioned epidural catheter.

After induction, if significant blood loss or hypotension is probable, it is wise to delay the imposition of a dense thoracic epidural (sympathetic) block. Patients with unstable coronary disease may benefit from early initiation of the block, with care to preserve coronary perfusion (diastolic) pressure. In all other situations, the timing of initiation and intraoperative management of the TEA is largely dictated by the blood pressure. However it is managed, a dense blockade at the terminus of surgery is imperative to achieve extubation after thoracotomy. Claims of a "preemptive analgesic" advantage from early initiation of TEA have not been established.

FLUID MANAGEMENT AND POSTPNEUMONECTOMY PULMONARY EDEMA

Barring unusual blood loss, a target positive fluid balance in the first 24 hours of less than 20 mL/kg with less than 2 L of intraoperative crystalloid has been recommended for pulmonary resection surgery.[5] This relatively restrictive practice, particularly intended for pneumonectomy patients, stems from the finding that postpneumonectomy pulmonary edema (PPE; incidence = 2%–4%) has a high mortality and has been associated with higher fluid balances.[6] Although the etiology of such PPE is unknown, it is characterized by low pulmonary wedge pressures and high protein edema fluid. Thus increased pulmonary capillary permeability is presumed and any intravascular fluid over and above what is essential to hemodynamic stability will redistribute to pulmonary interstitium proportionately. Contributing factors include reduced lymphatic drainage and right-sided surgery (because lymphatic compromise is greater after right pneumonectomy).

Postulated causes of PPE, besides fluid overload, include oxygen toxicity, lung hyperinflation, or ventilator-induced lung injury. The latter possibility has influenced many anesthesiologists to limit OLV tidal volumes to 6 to 7 mL/kg rather than to the traditional 10 mL/kg. Prolonged elevated airway pressures during OLV for thoracic surgery have been identified as the risk factors for PPE.[7] Postoperative management of chest drainage also may influence the degree of hyperinflation of the residual lung. Whether prevention of lung hyperinflation will eliminate PPE remains to be tested. Although fluid restriction alone fails to eliminate PPE,[8] it is sensible to limit the magnitude of pulmonary capillary transudates should endothelial injury occur. The essential caveat is that intravascular volume should not be reduced to the point where the thoracic epidural is not tolerated or to the peril of end-organ perfusion.

ALTERNATIVE FORMS OF VENTILATION

JV systems deliver pulses of oxygen from a high-pressure source (20–50 lb/in^2) via a narrow orifice attachment or catheter placed either within the airway or attached to a rigid bronchoscope. Upper or lower airway surgery may be performed by JV without the interference or fire hazard of an endotracheal tube. The manually triggered Sanders JV system (Fig. 5-8) is the simplest example. By Bernoulli principle, ambient air is entrained at the mouth of the jet, increasing the tidal volume and decreasing the FIO_2 by an unpredictable amount. Because it is an open system, inhalational anesthetics cannot be used, and end-tidal CO_2 cannot be monitored. There is risk of aspiration and barotrauma, but in experienced hands, JV is safe and effective. Most commonly, JV is used for surgery (including laser surgery) of major conducting airways.

High-frequency ventilation is an umbrella term for any of a variety of delivery systems that use small (e.g., 2 mL) tidal volumes at frequencies of 60 to 2400 breaths/min. High-frequency ventilation may be delivered through a standard endotracheal tube or through a small-diameter jet orifice (high-frequency JV). Mechanisms of gas exchange in high-frequency ventilation include mass movement, Taylor dispersion (i.e., enhanced diffusion), coaxial gas flow, and pendelluft movement. Purported advantages include lower mean airway pressures and a motionless operative field. Advantageous applications to patients with large bronchopleural fistulas or tracheobronchial disruptions have been advocated but poorly supported by data. As with JV, the ability to use small-diameter catheters improves surgical conditions and exposure.

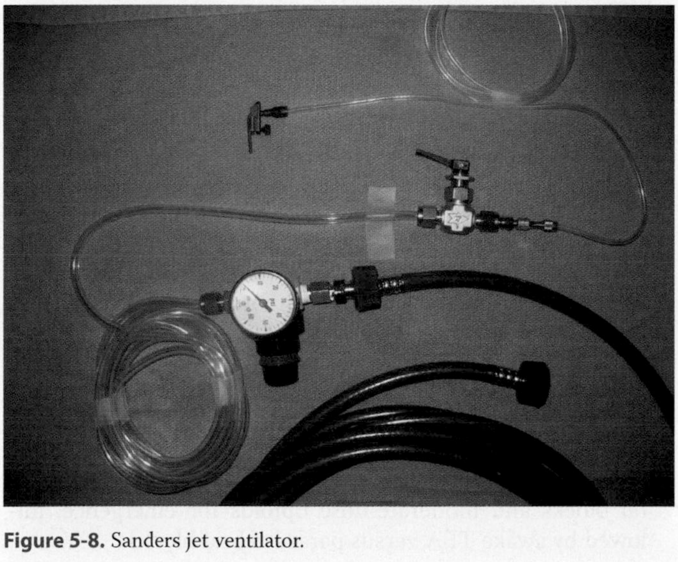

Figure 5-8. Sanders jet ventilator.

High-frequency oscillatory ventilation improves gas exchange by its push–pull effect but results in a shimmering operative field, which may disrupt surgery. Low-flow apneic ventilation (essentially turning the ventilator off and applying CPAP with 100% O_2) can sustain adequate oxygen saturations in many patients for 5 to 10 minutes when there is a surgical need for a motionless field. Acidosis and CO_2 accumulation (which rises by 6 mm Hg in the first minute and then by 3 mm Hg/min thereafter) limit the duration of apneic oxygenation.

PAIN MANAGEMENT

Sources of pain after thoracotomy include soft tissue, ribs, intercostal nerves, pleura, diaphragm, and pulmonary parenchyma. Afferents mediating this pain include intercostal nerves (4–8) and the vagal and phrenic nerves. No single modality ablates all sources of thoracotomy pain.

Ipsilateral shoulder pain is reported by 80% of thoracotomy patients who have functional epidurals. It is likely that the epidural unmasks shoulder pain by covering the dominant incisional pain. Shoulder pain is multifactorial. Postulated causes include referred pain (from the diaphragm, pericardium, pleura, or bronchus) and pain from ligamentous injuries to the shoulder due to positioning or surgical mobilization of the scapula. Phrenic blockade reduces the incidence of shoulder pain by more than 50%,[9] and shoulder blocks have variable efficacy. Systemic nonsteroidal anti-inflammatory drugs are the most consistently effective but carry risk of renal, gastrointestinal, or bleeding complications.

Chronic postthoracotomy pain syndrome (persistent pain along incision site for more than 2 months after thoracotomy, unrelated to recurrence or infection) is reported in over 50% of patients. The pain is neurolytic in nature and presumed to result from trauma to intercostal nerves. Entrapment by sutures, direct trauma, and crush injuries from retractors or instruments (including thoracoscopes) are among the postulated mechanisms. The severity is variable, with fewer than 10% of patients seeking treatment for postthoracotomy pain syndrome.

Thoracic Epidural Analgesia

TEA represents the current standard for acute postthoracotomy pain control. Small-bore multiport catheters inserted via 17-gauge needles into the midthoracic epidural space provide an avenue for intermittent bolus, continuous infusion, or patient-controlled delivery of analgesics. Most use a dilute solution of local anesthetic (e.g., bupivacaine, ropivacaine, or levobupivacaine) and opioid. The combination produces synergism of effect and permits reduced dosages. Fentanyl, meperidine, and hydromorphone are popular opioid choices because they possess intermediate lipophilicity. Highly lipophilic opioids (e.g., sufentanil) are absorbed quickly and produce greater systemic symptoms (i.e., sedation). Morphine is hydrophilic and thus spreads more broadly within the epidural space with

Table 5-4

COMPLICATIONS OF THORACIC EPIDURAL ANALGESIA

- Postdural puncture headache
- Inadvertent subarachnoid (spinal) block
- Local anesthetic toxicity—seizures, heart block, cardiac arrest
- Epidural infection
- Epidural hematoma
- Nerve injury (direct—from needle or catheter)
- Nerve injury (indirect—from compression by epidural hematoma or abscess)
- Horner syndrome
- Hypotension
- Urinary retention
- Sedation
- Respiratory depression
- Pruritus
- Failure to work

risk of higher levels, pruritus, and delayed respiratory depression. The very dilute dose of bupivacaine, enabled by the synergistic effect of the opioid, has the advantage of producing very little motor blockade of respiratory muscles.

The most common side effect from TEA is hypotension from local anesthetic blockade of presynaptic sympathetic nerves. Sympatholysis results in dilation of venous capacitance vessels, venous pooling (especially in the splanchnic bed), and possibly reduced cardiac contractility. Treatment consists of intravascular volume expansion, vasopressors, and inotropes. Other complications of TEA are listed in Table 5-4.

Evolving neurologic deficits in a patient who had a TEA should prompt urgent magnetic resonance imaging to rule out an epidural hematoma or abscess with spinal cord compression. Local anesthetic toxicity generally produces jitteriness progressing to seizures. Bupivacaine toxicity may manifest first with blockade of cardiac conduction. Treatment requires supportive care until the local anesthetic effects wear off. Intralipid infusions may ameliorate toxicity. In extreme bupivacaine toxicity, cardiopulmonary bypass may be required for support. Central nervous system toxicity may not be evident during general anesthesia, highlighting the importance of a test dose preceding induction. Aspiration from the catheter before each injection serves to rule out migration of the catheter into blood vessels.

Contraindications to TEA include coagulopathy, infection at the insertion site, local anesthetic allergy (extremely rare), and patient refusal. Relative contraindications include sepsis, preexisting neurologic deficit, and tumor involvement at the site.

Perioperative outcome is improved by epidural analgesia. Meta-analyses indicate that epidural analgesia is associated with reduced pulmonary (infection, atelectasis)[10] and cardiac (myocardial infarction)[11] complications. Even when compared with equianalgesic systemic narcotic regimens, TEA confers superior "dynamic" analgesia while coughing. The cardiosympatholytic effect protects against myocardial ischemia and reduces postoperative supraventricular arrhythmias. The cardioprotective effects of TEA depend on how it is managed. Significant hypotension may counteract its beneficial anti-ischemic effects. Chronic postthoracotomy pain is reduced in patients with aggressive management of acute postoperative pain with TEA, lending support for a potential preemptive effect.

Pain Management Other Than TEA

Intravenous patient-controlled analgesia with opioids is used most commonly for video-assisted thoracic surgery (VATS) or sternotomy incisions, which, barring significant cardiopulmonary disease, do not warrant TEA. If TEA is used for sternotomy incisions, parenteral narcotics or parasternal blocks are often required to supplement the most cephalad portion. As mentioned previously, dynamic analgesia with patient-controlled analgesia is inferior to TEA. The need for adjuncts, including intercostal or paravertebral blocks, nonsteroidal anti-inflammatory drugs, or ketamine, is not uncommon. Paravertebral blocks rival TEA and only impose a unilateral sympathectomy but have a higher technical failure rate and last only 12 to 18 hours. Intercostal blocks are simple and familiar to surgeons. Rapid vascular uptake of local anesthetics after intercostal blockade limits duration to 4 to 8 hours and raises the risk of toxicity. To include the lateral cutaneous branch, intercostal blocks must be applied posterior to the posterior axillary line. A rule-of-thumb safe limit for intercostal blocks using bupivacaine with epinephrine is 2.5 mg/kg.

Cryotherapy to exposed intercostal nerves before chest closure produces a blockade lasting up to 6 months. Concern that it might cause chronic neuralgia has prevented its widespread acceptance.

Interpleural catheters delivering local anesthetics tend to be unreliable because the agents distribute within the chest by gravity and are lost to chest drainage. Transcutaneous electrical nerve stimulation, acupuncture, and hypnotherapy are used only occasionally as adjuncts in thoracic anesthesia. Lumbar intrathecal morphine (0.2–0.3 mg) provides 24 hours of good analgesia for patients in whom TEA is contraindicated. The high incidence of pruritus and concern over delayed respiratory depression from ascension within the spinal canal have limited its popularity.

SYNOPSIS OF ANESTHETIC ISSUES FOR SPECIFIC PROCEDURES

Cervical Mediastinoscopy

- Intravenous access adequate for potential bleeding
- Right-hand pulse oximeter (or arterial line, if indicated) to detect innominate artery compression
- Limit nitrous oxide usage (pneumothorax potential)

Vats Pulmonary Resection

- TEA and arterial line if poor cardiopulmonary reserve or high probability to convert to open resection.
- Consider TEA when large utility port is anticipated (e.g., VATS lobectomy).
- Early lung isolation and active suctioning of operative lung secretions to promote atelectasis in operative lung.
- Avoid operative lung CPAP if possible.
- Leak test after resection (sustained positive pressure of 20–30 cm H_2O with chest filled with saline).
- Recruitment maneuvers (up to 40 cm H_2O sustained positive pressure) to maximally re-expand remaining lung.
- If converted to thoracotomy without TEA, employ intercostal blocks and moderate-dose opioids for emergence, followed by awake TEA versus paravertebral blocks.

Pneumonectomy

- Ensure absence of anesthesia "hardware" in operative bronchus and pulmonary artery.
- Assess stability at time of pulmonary artery test-clamp (CVP should not change).
- Assess for compliance changes with bronchial cross-clamp before staples are fired.
- Leak test as above.
- Conservative fluid management because of the risk of PPE.
- Be prepared for cardiac herniation when returning patient to supine position (especially right pneumonectomy).
- Mediastinal shift may be cause of moderate instability at end of case.
- Assiduous care to avoid disruption of bronchial stump when exchanging tubes.

Extrapleural Pneumonectomy

- Large intravenous access, arterial line, TEA, CVP on operative side, nasogastric tube.
- Four units of bank blood in operating room.
- Avoid sympathetic (epidural) block until hemostasis is achieved.
- Prevent exacerbation of blood loss by hypertension during dissection phase.
- Be prepared for intermittent hypotension from surgeon-induced impairment of venous return. Temporize with vasopressors, and communicate with surgeons.
- PEEP to dependent lung frequently advantageous (restrictive physiology).
- Leak test after specimen is removed, as per pneumonectomy.
- Benign transient ST-segment elevation on electrocardiogram is frequently seen during "wash phase" (? temperature effect).
- Terminus of case as per pneumonectomy; higher risk of cardiac herniation (especially with right EPP).

Esophagectomy

- TEA, arterial line, large intravenous access, ±CVP (sparing left neck), nasogastric tube.
- Liberalize intravenous fluids to account for deficit and substantial insensible losses.
- Avoid dense sympathetic block until final anastomosis.
- Avoid large doses of alpha-adrenergic agonists because they may affect conduit tone (length).
- Have glucagon (1 mg) available if requested for smooth muscle relaxation (conduit length).
- Assiduous care to avoid esophageal intubation at time of endotracheal tube exchange (consider tube exchange catheter).
- Consider postoperative ventilation if there is significant airway edema.

Anterior Mediastinal Mass

- See "Strategies for High-Risk Inductions."
- Lower-extremity intravenous access if superior vena caval compression.
- Assess risk of tamponade by echocardiogram.
- Consider awake, topically anesthetized fiberoptic assessment of airway in symptomatic patients.
- Rigid bronchoscopy option must be available as a backup.
- Maintain spontaneous ventilation until airway is ensured.
- Assess risk of airway obstruction based on symptoms and CT scan.
- Arterial line for symptomatic patients.

Tracheostomy

- Low FIO_2 during electrocautery with open trachea (fire hazard).

Rigid Bronchoscopy/Core-Out

- Initial bronchoscopy awake or spontaneously breathing if airway is tenuous (as above).
- Ventilate by jet or sideport of rigid scope.
- Total intravenous anesthesia.
- Arterial line to assess $PaCO_2$ (if using jet).
- Consider heliox if severely stenotic.

Laser Core-Out

- Lowest possible FIO_2; avoid N_2O (supports combustion).
- Wavelength-specific eye protection for patient and personnel.
- Fuel sources away from laser path.
- Saline-filled syringe within reach.
- LMA or rigid bronchoscope for distal airway lesions.
- If intubation is required, use "laser safe" tube (with saline in cuff).
- Consider heliox if severely stenotic.
- Induction considerations as per threatened major airways.

Photodynamic Therapy

- Blue goggle eyewear protection for patient and personnel.
- Limit patient's skin exposure to overhead/intense light.
- Rotate pulse oximeter probe to new site every hour.
- General anesthesia is not imperative but is often expedient and allows for motionless target.

Lung Volume Reduction Surgery

- Similar anesthesia whether VATS or sternotomy.
- Arterial line, TEA, ± CVP.
- Support induction with vasopressors/fluid bolus.
- Dynamic hyperinflation is unavoidable.
- Delicate balance between adequate ventilation and barotrauma.
- Err on side of permissive hypercapnia rather than barotrauma to dependent lung during OLV.
- Minimal or no intravenous narcotics or sedatives (except remifentanil).
- Total intravenous anesthesia.
- Arterial blood gases to establish $ETCO_2$–$PaCO_2$ gradient.

Tracheal Resection/Reconstruction

- Be prepared to ventilate distal, divided trachea via jet (with catheter) or sterile tube over the field.
- Alternative technique is use of long, thin endotracheal tube placed orally, advanced beyond lesion, with surgeon working around it.

- A third technique is to jet via an orally placed catheter with tip situated near lesion.
- Induction considerations as per threatened major airways.
- Smooth emergence may be facilitated by use of remifentanil for final bronchoscopy.
- Prevent head extension after anastomosis.

Bronchopleural Fistula

- If small air leak, single-lumen tube for initial bronchoscopy.
- If large, consider awake bronchoscopy, followed by lung (fistula) isolation, before positive-pressure ventilation.
- Ensure patient chest drain before positive-pressure ventilation.
- Attention to prevent further disruption of stump by endotracheal tube.
- If large, consider alternative modes of ventilation (spontaneous, JV, high-frequency JV) and TIVA.
- Protect against cross-contamination with position and lung isolation.

Carcinoid Syndrome

- Arterial line for prompt detection of carcinoid crisis.
- Octreotide (somatostatin analog) pretreatment, infusion, or immediate availability.
- Avoid sympathomimetic drugs.
- Thoracic epidural to blunt sympathetic response to thoracotomy.
- Potential significant bleeding or mediator release from tumor manipulation.
- Evaluate for carcinoid heart disease or associated endocrinopathies.
- Hyperglycemia.
- Cushing syndrome.
- Increased antidiuretic hormone (ADH) and melanocyte-stimulating hormone (MSH).

Myasthenia Gravis

- Associated with thymoma.
- Skeletal muscle weakness owing to autoimmune destruction of acetylcholine receptors at neuromuscular junction.
- Increased sensitivity to nondepolarizing muscle relaxants.
- Resistance to succinylcholine.
- Increased sensitivity to narcotics.
- Symptomatic improvement with preoperative plasmapheresis.
- Maintain preoperative anticholinesterase treatment.
- Eliminate nondepolarizing muscle relaxant use if possible.
- Succinylcholine is usually okay, but duration may be prolonged by plasmapheresis and anticholinesterase usage.
- Monitor for myasthenic versus cholinergic crisis.
- Close observation for postoperative respiratory failure.
- Low threshold for postoperative ventilatory support.

Myasthenic (Eaton–Lambert) Syndrome

- Associated with small cell carcinoma of the lung.
- Proximal limb skeletal muscle weakness.
- Improved strength with activity (posttetanic facilitation) in contrast to myasthenia gravis.
- Autoimmune-mediated reduction in quanta of acetylcholine released from motor neurons.
- Increased sensitivity to both nondepolarizing and depolarizing muscle relaxants.
- Poor response to anticholinesterase drugs.
- Avoid all muscle relaxants if possible.

EDITOR'S COMMENT

A successful thoracic operation requires coordination between members of the anesthesia team and members of the surgical team. The partnership between surgeon and anesthesiologist is clearest in cases of airway management. The effect of induction of anesthesia on respiratory function is an extremely important topic that should be well understood by all thoracic surgeons. The strategies for high-risk inductions are clearly presented in this chapter. Also of tremendous practical value are the strategies of managing hypoxia during OLV. There are several disadvantages to reinflating the operative lung prematurely, including risk of losing the localization of nodules, risk of changing the orientation of the operative approach, and risk of injury to the lung by surgical instruments, as well as added time waiting for lung atelectasis. These strategies can prevent laissez-faire inflation of the lung.

—MTJ

References

1. Horlocker TT, Wedel DJ, Benzon H, et al. Regional anesthesia in the anticoagulated patient: defining the risks (Second ASRA Consensus Conference on Neuraxial Anesthesia and Anticoagulation). *Reg Anesth Pain Med.* 2003;28:172–197.
2. Benumof J. Monitoring (Chapter 7). *Anesthesia for Thoracic Surgery*. 2nd ed. Philadelphia, PA: Saunders; 1995:266–268.
3. Klein U, Karzai W, Bloos F, et al. Role of fiberoptic bronchoscopy in conjunction with the use of double-lumen tubes for thoracic anesthesia: a prospective study. *Anesthesiology*. 1998;88:346–350.
4. Slinger P. Management of one-lung anesthesia: review course lectures. *Anesth Analg.* 2005;100:89.
5. Ramsay JG, Murphy M. Postoperative respiratory failure and treatment (Chapter 18). In: Kaplan J, Slinger P, eds. *Thoracic Anesthesia*. 3rd ed. Philadelphia, PA: Churchill Livingstone; 2003:397–422.
6. Zeldin RA, Normandin D, Landtwing D, et al. Postpneumonectomy pulmonary edema. *J Thorac Cardiovasc Surg.* 1984;87:359–365.
7. Licker M, de Perrot M, Spiliopoulos A, et al. Risk factors for acute lung injury after thoracic surgery for lung cancer. *Anesth Analg.* 2003;97:1558–1565.
8. Turnage WS, Lunn JJ. Postpneumonectomy pulmonary edema: a retrospective analysis of associated variables. *Chest.* 1993;103:1646–1650.
9. Scawn ND, Pennefather SH, Soorae A, et al. Ipsilateral shoulder pain after thoracotomy with epidural analgesia: the influence of phrenic nerve infiltration with lidocaine. *Anesth Analg.* 2001;93:260–264.
10. Ballantyne JC, Carr DB, deFerranti S, et al. The comparative effects of postoperative analgesic therapies on pulmonary outcome: cumulative meta-analyses of randomized, controlled trials. *Anesth Analg.* 1998;86:598–612.
11. Beattie WS, Badner NH, Choi P. Epidural analgesia reduces postoperative myocardial infarction: a meta-analysis. *Anesth Analg.* 2001;93:853–858.

6 Critical Care for the Thoracic Surgery Patient

Shannon S. McKenna

Keywords: acute respiratory distress syndrome (ARDS), goal-directed therapy for sepsis and shock, intensive insulin therapy, fluid management, nosocomial complications, idiopathic acute lung injury, atrial fibrillation

INTRODUCTION

The thoracic surgery patient population can present significant challenges to clinical care. Patients often are older, current, or former smokers, and sicker than other surgical populations. It is not uncommon for these patients to present with underlying chronic lung disease, some form of arteriovascular disease, hypertension, diabetes, and baseline renal insufficiency. They have diminished physiologic reserve and more limited ability to recover from perioperative complications. In particular, they are prone to pulmonary complications, which are very poorly tolerated. As a result, they may require the services of an intensive care unit (ICU) and its highly trained, specialized staff more frequently than other patient populations. This chapter reviews critical care issues specific to thoracic surgery patients, general issues of management related to sepsis and acute respiratory distress syndrome (ARDS), and strategies for avoiding the common nosocomial complications of critical care.

COMMON CRITICAL CARE ISSUES AFTER THORACIC SURGERY

Secretion Retention, Atelectasis, Pneumonia

Thoracic surgery patients are at increased risk of secretion retention and atelectasis. General anesthesia, particularly when accompanied by one lung ventilation (OLV), causes a marked decrease in functional residual capacity (FRC), which promotes atelectasis. Surgical manipulation of the lung can lead to retained blood and secretions, with partial or complete airway obstruction. Gas flow is further hindered by bronchospasm and decreased compliance of the operative lung. Splinting from postoperative pain, or conversely, respiratory depression from opiates or benzodiazepines further limit lung expansion. Patients with preexisting chronic obstructive pulmonary disease (COPD), asthma, bronchitis, or pneumonia will be at greatest risk. Similarly, patients with impaired cough reflexes, including those who have had airway resection with anastomosis (e.g., sleeve resection) would be expected to have greater difficulty clearing secretions. Secretion retention over time results in both hypoxemia and hypercarbia. It also predisposes the patient to pneumonia.

Preventing secretion retention and atelectasis requires a systematic, multidisciplinary approach. Time under general anesthesia should be limited to the minimum required to complete the procedure. Patients should be extubated immediately whenever possible. Fiberoptic bronchoscopy immediately before extubation facilitates the removal of blood and secretions from the proximal airways. Excellent analgesia combined with aggressive early ambulation will promote recruitment of lung volume and clearance of secretions. Chest physiotherapy further aids this process. Any patient with a preoperative pulmonary infection should undergo aggressive, culture-directed, antibiotic therapy during the immediate perioperative period.

Treatment of retained secretions and atelectasis includes aggressive chest physiotherapy and mobilization. Humidified oxygen, nebulized saline, and bronchodilators can help thin secretions and promote gas flow. Patients with copious, thick secretions may benefit from nebulized N-acetylcysteine or dornase (DNAse), with bronchodilator pretreatment to mitigate treatment-induced bronchospasm. Any patient having significant trouble clearing their secretions should be evaluated for the possibility of vocal cord dysfunction, which is a known complication of certain thoracic surgical procedures and results in a markedly impaired cough. A small subset of patients may require more aggressive interventions including repeated awake fiberoptic bronchoscopy, intermittent noninvasive ventilation, use of an Acapella® device or vibratory vest, assisted cough using an inexuflator device, or in the most severe cases, intubation and mechanical ventilation. Patients who require intubation primarily for secretion clearance should be evaluated for early tracheostomy.

Postpneumonectomy Pulmonary Edema

Approximately 2% to 9% of pneumonectomy patients will experience early onset idiopathic acute lung injury (ALI). It is characterized by the development of diffuse infiltrates followed by significant hypoxemia in the first 1 to 3 days postoperatively. In contrast to late onset ALI, no etiology is readily apparent. Pulmonary capillary wedge pressures are normal to low, and the alveolar fluid has high protein content. Studies using radiolabeled albumin have been consistent with a pulmonary capillary leak syndrome.[1] The relative rarity of this event has precluded the possibility of prospective analysis.

Retrospective analyses have identified multiple factors associated with the development of postpneumonectomy pulmonary edema (Table 6-1).[2] The exact etiology remains unknown. It has

Table 6-1

FACTORS ASSOCIATED WITH POSTPNEUMONECTOMY PULMONARY EDEMA

- Right-sided pneumonectomy
- High intraoperative ventilatory pressures
- High intraoperative fluid administration
- Duration of surgery
- Fresh-frozen plasma administration
- Advanced age
- Prior chest irradiation

been postulated that ventilator-induced lung injury, oxygen toxicity, tissue injury with cytokine release, loss of lymphatic drainage, pulmonary hypertension, and shear injury to the capillary endothelium from increased blood flow through the remaining pulmonary artery all contribute to the development of capillary leak and the subsequent accrual of interstitial lung water. Once a capillary leak develops, movement of fluid from the pulmonary vasculature to the interstitium is governed by hydrostatic and colloid osmotic pressures, as described by Starling's law. Few recommendations can be made regarding strategies to prevent postpneumonectomy pulmonary edema, but it would seem prudent to use lung-sparing ventilation with lower tidal volumes and plateau pressures and to limit intravascular fluid to the minimum needed to support end-organ perfusion. Likewise, hypercarbia, hypoxia, and pain should be avoided because of the propensity to increase pulmonary arterial pressures. Once established, postpneumonectomy pulmonary edema is treated the same as any other case of ALI or ARDS, with lung-sparing ventilation and good supportive care.

Atrial Arrhythmias

Atrial fibrillation and atrial flutter are common after thoracic surgery. The incidence can be as high as 44% following extrapleural pneumonectomy.[3] A number of factors have been associated with the occurrence of atrial arrhythmias (Table 6-2). Etiologies may include elevated catecholamines, myocardial ischemia, pulmonary hypertension, atrial enlargement, hypoxemia, electrolyte imbalances, mechanical displacement of the heart, and vagal nerve irritation. Trials in the cardiac surgery population have shown that prophylaxis with beta blockers, calcium channel blockers, sotalol, amiodarone, statins, or corticosteroids may decrease the incidence of atrial fibrillation.[4,5]

The few clinical trials performed in lung resection patients suggest that both calcium channel blockers and beta blockers, given prophylactically, decrease the incidence of atrial tachydysrhythmia by roughly 50%.[6] Hemodynamically stable patients with atrial arrhythmias can be treated with beta blockers or calcium channel blockers to achieve rate control. The ability of calcium channel blockers to reduce pulmonary vascular resistance (PVR) and right ventricular pressures makes this drug class an appealing choice for primary treatment in lung resection patients.

Digoxin may be used as an additional agent to improve rate control but care must be taken to avoid toxicity, particularly in the setting of renal insufficiency. Amiodarone is a useful agent for those patients who maintain a high ventricular response rate despite maximum therapy with other agents or who become hypotensive with first line agents. However, amiodarone can cause primary acute lung toxicity in patients who have undergone thoracic resections, and, therefore should be reserved as a second line therapy.[7]

Table 6-2

FACTORS ASSOCIATED WITH ATRIAL ARRHYTHMIAS

- Underlying cardiac disease
- Advanced age
- Electrolyte abnormalities
- Increased pulmonary vascular resistance
- Volume of lung resected
- Intrapericardial dissection
- Postoperative pulmonary edema

The risk of third-degree heart block must be carefully evaluated if more than one nodal blocking agent is to be used simultaneously. Unstable patients may require electrical cardioversion to restore sinus rhythm. Unfortunately, the factors that led to the atrial arrhythmia are usually still present after surgery, and recurrence of the arrhythmia is common after either electrical or initial chemical cardioversion. Of note, however, the majority of patients with *new onset* atrial arrhythmia after surgery will be back in sinus rhythm within 6 weeks. This makes rate control with anticoagulation, if not otherwise contraindicated, a practical approach in this patient population.

Bronchospasm and Chronic Obstructive Pulmonary Disease Exacerbation

COPD is a common comorbidity in the thoracic surgery patient population. Intubation and airway manipulation can exacerbate a patient's COPD. The increased resistance to airflow increases the work of breathing and may result in frank respiratory distress. Associated "auto-peep" or dynamic hyperinflation, resulting from trapped alveolar gas, further increases the work of breathing, adversely affects gas exchange, and causes hemodynamic instability if venous return is impaired. Patients with COPD should be maintained on their home bronchodilator and inhaled steroid regimen throughout the perioperative period. The rare patient will require systemic steroids to treat an exacerbation of their COPD. Early extubation followed by aggressive mobilization is critical to avoiding the cycle of airway irritability, bronchospasm, dynamic hyperinflation, and respiratory distress.

Hypotension

Postoperative hypotension can be categorized as problems of pump function or venous return. Myocardial ischemia is a cause of acute ventricular dysfunction. Likewise, acute onset or worsening of pulmonary hypertension can lead to right ventricular failure (see Hyperglycemia). Venous return problems limiting effective diastolic filling of the heart are more common. Dehydration or acute hemorrhage leads to absolute hypovolemia. Tension pneumothorax, pericardial tamponade, pulmonary embolism, severe dynamic hyperinflation, mediastinal shift, and cardiac herniation will limit venous return despite normal intravascular volume. Finally, some patients may exhibit hypotension with a normal cardiac output and a low systemic vascular resistance. The increase in venous capacitance creates a state of relative hypovolemia. This low-tone state is typical of sepsis, but may also be seen with sympathectomies that are either pharmacologically induced from local anesthetics given via a thoracic epidural, or mechanically induced from trauma to the sympathetic chain during surgery. Central venous pressure (CVP) monitoring can be very helpful in distinguishing between the various causes of postoperative hypotension. If pulmonary hypertension and right heart failure is suspected, early placement of a pulmonary artery catheter (PAC) is advised.

Pulmonary Hypertension and Right Ventricular Failure

Acute onset of pulmonary hypertension with subsequent right ventricular failure is one of the most dreaded perioperative complications following thoracic surgery. Unless it is immediately recognized and successfully managed it can become rapidly fatal. Preexisting COPD, with its intrinsic loss of pulmonary microvasculature, limits the ability of the remaining lung to compensate for an abrupt increase in pulmonary blood flow following pulmonary resection and predisposes the patient to acute perioperative pulmonary hypertension. Preoperative evaluation, including echocardiography and cardiac catheterization can help to identify those patients with significant preoperative pulmonary hypertension. It should be understood, however, that these tests are done at rest, and sometimes under conscious sedation; therefore, may not accurately predict the pulmonary artery pressures that may occur postoperatively under the conditions of stress and hypermetabolism. Even a reassuring preoperative catheterization with a balloon occlusion trial does not completely rule out the possibility of postoperative right ventricular failure.

Patients with acute right ventricular failure will often present with hypotension and evidence of low cardiac output including oliguria, a high CVP and peripheral edema. Patients also may complain of dyspnea and lightheadedness, particularly with exertion. Unlike patients with biventricular failure, there generally is an absence of pulmonary edema, and left atrial pressures are low. Right ventricular dysfunction can occur in the setting of right ventricular pressure overload, volume overload, or impaired contractility. An electrocardiogram and echocardiogram will help exclude right ventricular ischemia or infarction, which if present, may require urgent therapy to treat an acute coronary syndrome. Likewise, the patient should be assessed for the likelihood of acute pulmonary embolism, as this can cause pulmonary hypertension and right ventricular failure and requires specific therapy.

Initial treatment of right ventricular failure is aimed at correcting reversible causes of pulmonary hypertension including hypoxia, hypercarbia, and acidosis. Pain and fever, because of their associated hypermetabolic state, can also cause pulmonary hypertension and should be rapidly treated. Volume management can be complex. Cardiac output is preload dependent; however, right-sided volume overload can adversely affect left ventricular output through septal shift and intraventricular dependence. The combination of echocardiography and PAC measurements can be helpful in identifying the optimum volume status for each patient. Right ventricular function and systemic blood pressure can be supported with the use of inotropes (dopamine, epinephrine, and norepinephrine) and inodilators (dobutamine, milrinone). A PAC is helpful for titrating therapy. If an inodilator results in an improved cardiac output but worsened systemic hypotension, low-dose vasopressin may be used to maintain systemic blood pressure without increasing pulmonary artery pressures. Unfortunately, the inotropes and inodilators are all arrhythmogenic and also increase myocardial oxygen consumption.

Pulmonary vasodilators reduce PVR and increase the right ventricular cardiac output without causing arrhythmias or increasing myocardial oxygen consumption. Unfortunately, the common vasodilators, including nitroglycerine, sodium nitroprusside, and hydralazine, usually result in significant systemic hypotension. Inhaled nitric oxide can decrease PVR and does not cause systemic hypotension. Recent experience has shown that many patients respond well to inhaled epoprostenol, which is considerably less costly than nitric oxide. Intravenous epoprostenol or enteral sildenafil may also be useful. Patients who develop chronic pulmonary hypertension should be evaluated by specialists with expertise in long-term management of pulmonary hypertension. Options for long-term management include: prostanoids (epoprosentol, treprostinil, and iloprost), endothelin receptor antagonists (bosentan, ambrisentan), and phosphodiesterase-5 inhibitors (sildenafil, tadalafil, vardenafil).[8]

Massive Hemoptysis

Massive hemoptysis defined as more than 600 mL of blood loss in 24 hours, is uncommon but can be rapidly fatal. It is associated with pulmonary infections, bronchiectasis, tumor erosion into a pulmonary or bronchial artery, pulmonary artery rupture during pulmonary artery catheterization, and trauma. Patients with massive hemoptysis are at imminent risk of death from asphyxiation. The patient should be turned bleeding side down to protect the good lung and intubated early rather than late. A bronchial blocker can be used to isolate the site of bleeding. Although double-lumen endotracheal tubes do allow for lung isolation, difficult positioning and very small internal lumens make them difficult to use in this setting. Once the patient is stabilized, focus should shift to determining the source of bleeding. Bronchoscopy, CT scanning, and angiography all may be useful. Further management is dictated by the specific cause of the hemoptysis.

Bronchopleural Fistula

The breakdown of an airway anastomosis or stump can result in the formation of a large proximal bronchopleural fistula (BPF). Alveolar rupture, persistent leak at a resection margin, or traumatic injury to the pulmonary parenchyma will create a more distal air leak. Empyema, tumor recurrence, irradiation, and poor wound healing all contribute to BPF formation. Early aggressive treatment of infection is critical. Maximizing the patient's nutritional status is a priority. Every effort should be made to keep patients ambulatory and breathing without mechanical assistance. If a patient requires mechanical ventilation, volume loss through the BPF can be quantified by comparing the inspiratory and expiratory tidal volumes recorded on the volume versus time loop of the ventilator graphics. Patients with significant volume loss may be easier to ventilate using pressure modes of ventilation. If the patient is awake, pressure support can be used if the ventilator model permits adjustment of the expiratory flow cut-off. Failure to increase the expiratory flow cut-off above the standard 25% may result in a sustained inspiration and subsequent ventilator dyssynchrony. No matter which ventilator mode is used, inspiratory pressure and volume should be minimized to limit the airflow across the BPF. In some cases, lung isolation may be required to permit adequate ventilation. This is particularly true for BPFs that occur after pneumonectomy, especially if the remaining lung is compromised. In this setting, double-lumen endotracheal tubes, endobronchial tubes or specially made tracheotomy tubes that are custom measured to sit below the carina will allow exclusion of the BPF. Unfortunately, it is difficult to maintain any of these tubes in constant position, and the emergent need to reposition these tubes occurs with some frequency.

CARE OF THE PATIENT WITH ARDS

Meticulous supportive care remains the mainstay of treatment for patients with ARDS. It is vitally important to manage the mechanical ventilation with a view toward avoiding ventilator-induced lung injury. The ARMA trial, published in 2000, showed that low tidal volume ventilation (6 mL/kg ideal body weight), with a plateau pressure of 30 cm H_2O or less, resulted in an 8% decrease in absolute mortality.[9] This has now become the standard of care for patients with, or at risk of developing, ARDS. Ideally, the level of positive end-expiratory pressure (PEEP) should be set to prevent cyclic alveolar collapse at end expiration. Unfortunately, at this time there is no clear consensus on how to determine optimum PEEP in routine clinical practice. A pragmatic approach is to titrate the PEEP up until maximum pulmonary compliance and best oxygenation is achieved.

During the late 1970s and early 1980s, a number of trials were undertaken to investigate the use of high-dose corticosteroids in early ARDS.[10] All of these studies were negative, with some actually resulting in increased mortality. The steroid debate reemerged in 1998 with the publication of a very small single center trial of prolonged methylprednisolone for late-stage ARDS.[11] This trial reported a significant decrease in mortality in the treatment group but was plagued by serious methodological problems in the trial design and execution. In 2006, the ARDSNet trials group published the results of a large, multicenter randomized trial of steroids for late ARDS.[12] The treatment group did, in the initial 4 weeks of treatment, have more ventilator-free and shock-free days, as well as improved oxygenation and pulmonary compliance. There was no difference in mortality at 60 or 180 days. Of note, if methylprednisolone was started more than 14 days after the onset of ARDS, there was a significant increase in mortality at both 60 and 180 days. The only subgroup that appeared to benefit from treatment was the group with elevated procollagen III levels in the alveolar fluid at the time of enrollment. *At this time corticosteroids cannot be recommended for routine treatment of ARDS.*

The ARDSNet Trials Group recently completed a complex but well-designed trial comparing a liberal versus restrictive fluid policy for patients with ARDS.[13] The restrictive protocol targeted a CVP of 4 mm Hg or less provided the patient was not in shock and did not display signs of end-organ hypoperfusion. The liberal protocol targeted pressures of 10 to 14 mm Hg. There was no difference in mortality, but the restrictive protocol resulted in earlier liberation for the ventilator and earlier discharge from the ICU without any increase in organ failure. Another arm of the study executed the same fluid interventions but used a PAC rather than a central venous catheter. There was no advantage to PAC use in ARDS. This study reassuringly supports the common clinical practice of moderate fluid restriction.

GOAL-DIRECTED MANAGEMENT OF THE SEPTIC PATIENT

Historically, mortality from septic shock has exceeded 40%. In 2001, Emanuel Rivers published a randomized prospective clinical trial of early goal-directed therapy. He focused on protocol-driven resuscitation within the first 6 hours of presentation.[14] Mortality in this clinical setting was decreased from 46.5% to 30.5%. Bernard et al. published another study in 2001 regarding the results of a randomized, prospective trial of activated protein C (APC). APC led to a 6% absolute reduction in mortality, making APC the first pharmacologic substance to have proven efficacy in sepsis.[15]

In 2004, the Society of Critical Care Medicine, in conjunction with multiple other organizations, launched the Surviving Sepsis Campaign, which underwent substantial revision in 2008.[16] The guidelines integrate findings from all recent high-quality sepsis trials. Care goals are bundled into the first 6 hours and the first 24 hours, reflecting increasing evidence that outcomes from sepsis are dependent on the timeliness of treatment.

Within the first 6 hours the focus should be on obtaining cultures, starting an appropriate broad-spectrum antibiotic regime, and executing rapid and effective fluid resuscitation. Specific recommendations for fluid resuscitation include the early placement of an arterial line and central venous line. Either crystalloids or colloids may be used to reach a CVP target of 8 to 12 mm Hg. If the patient is mechanically ventilated, a higher goal of 12 to 15 mm Hg is appropriate. Mean arterial pressure (MAP) should be maintained at greater than 65 mm Hg. If the target CVP has been reached and the MAP is still low, the patient should be started on vasopressors. Urine output (at least 0.5 mL/kg/h), trends in lactic acid levels, and the central venous oxygen saturation ($SvcO_2$) are followed for evidence of tissue hypoperfusion. If the $SvcO_2$ is less than 70%, the urine output remains low, or lactic acid levels are climbing, the patient may be a candidate for inotropic therapy and/or transfusion to a hematocrit of 30%, with the goal being to increase cardiac output and oxygen delivery.[14] Norepinephrine and dopamine are considered the vasopressors of choice and dobutamine is the inotrope of choice. Source control is vital to the successful treatment of sepsis and any focal area of infection amenable to drainage or debridement should be addressed early.

Mechanically ventilated patients should be treated using the lung protective strategies outlined in the previous section. Appropriate glucose control should be instituted (see Hyperglycemia below). Routine evaluation for adrenal insufficiency is no longer recommended on the basis of the results of the CORTICUS trial.[17] Corticosteroid therapy should be reserved for those septic shock patients who are poorly responsive to both fluid and vasopressors.

PREVENTION OF SECONDARY COMPLICATIONS

In many situations, a critically ill patient may survive their initial illness only to succumb to complications of their care. There are a number of well-recognized nosocomial complications that are common to ICU patients throughout the world. Most are preventable with appropriate attention to detail and protocolized care. The most common and significant nosocomial complications are discussed below.

Thromboembolism

Deep venous thrombosis (DVT) initially is a silent disease, and when accompanied by pulmonary embolism, it can be quite morbid in the thoracic surgery population because of limited pulmonary reserve. Virtually all thoracic surgery patients should receive aggressive prophylaxis for DVT, including mechanical venous compression devices and pharmacologic therapy with either low-dose unfractionated heparin or low-molecular-weight heparin. Even with appropriate prophylaxis, DVT does occur, and it is necessary to maintain a high index of suspicion for thrombotic and thromboembolic events in this population.

Stress Ulcers

Shallow gastric mucosal ulcerations, usually located in the proximal stomach, are common in ICU patients and develop rapidly after the onset of acute illness. In a small percentage, the ulceration will progress to involve the submucosal layers and can result in bleeding or perforation. Histamine-2-receptor antagonists are the mainstay of prophylaxis in the ICU setting. They have been shown to effectively decrease the rate of clinical bleeding from stress ulcers. Proton-pump inhibitors have also been used for this purpose. Unfortunately, both of these classes of drugs result in alkalization of the stomach resulting in overgrowth with gram-negative bacilli. A growing body of evidence shows that stress ulcer prophylaxis with pH-modifying drugs increases the rate of ventilator-associated pneumonia (VAP).[18,19]

Pressure Sores

Pressure sores remain a troublesome issue for ICU patients. Many patients have multiple risk factors including immobility, heavy sedation, poor nutrition, impaired tissue perfusion, and frequent incontinence. Pressure sores are both morbid and costly to treat. Early identification of at-risk patients, combined with aggressive efforts at prevention, is needed. Preventative measures include correcting nutritional deficits, restoring tissue perfusion, minimizing sedation, and emphasizing early return to mobility even for ventilated patients. For patients who are immobile, redistributing body weight over bony prominences at least every 2 hours is mandatory. In addition, the skin must be kept clean and dry, and care must be taken to avoid sheer injury to the skin during turns. High-risk patients may benefit from special low air loss therapy beds.

Malnutrition

Inadequate nutrition is an insidious problem that can ultimately lead to severe consequences. It contributes to wound breakdown and infection, the development of pressure sores, immune suppression, and generalized weakness which in turn limits mobility and impairs weaning from mechanical ventilation. In addition, malnourished patients tend to have lower colloid osmotic pressures and more trouble mobilizing edema fluid. Corticosteroid use, when necessary, will further compound muscle catabolism and amplify the systemic effects of malnutrition. It is vitally important to begin nutritional repletion as soon as possible in all ICU patients. Enteral feeding is strongly preferred. Theoretically, postpyloric feeding should be associated with a lower risk of aspiration and improved ability to reach nutritional goals. Unfortunately, multiple trials have failed to demonstrate this benefit.[20] Decisions about enteral access should be made on an individual patient basis. Those patients who are not candidates for enteral feeding in the short term should be supported with total parenteral nutrition (TPN). Since TPN is associated with significant complications, initiation of TPN should be done concomitantly with reassessment of options to promote enteric function and allow for a rapid transition to enteric feeding. Critically ill patients should be regularly reevaluated to determine if their nutritional needs are being adequately met.

Hyperglycemia

Surgery and critical illness both result in a systemic stress response. Even nondiabetic patients will develop insulin resistance and hyperglycemia. A single center trial showed promising results with tight control targeting blood glucose of 80 to 110 mg/dL in critically ill patients.[21] Unfortunately, subsequent studies, including the NICE-SUGAR trial,[22] which enrolled 6104 patients have not confirmed these results. Currently the consensus recommendations from the American Diabetes Association and the American Association of Clinical Endocrinologists[23] recommend starting an insulin infusion for blood glucose greater than 180 mg/dL and targeting glucose of 140 to 180 mg/dL for critically ill patients. Further research is needed to identify the optimum blood glucose target in different populations and to test closed-loop systems that continuously monitor blood glucose and automatically titrate insulin.

Nosocomial Blood Stream Infection

Catheter-related blood stream infections (CRBSIs) are associated with an increased length of stay, increased cost of care, and significant attributable mortality. Recent research indicates that catheter-related blood stream infections are nearly completely preventable. The Centers for Disease Control and Prevention (CDC) publishes practice-based guidelines with which all clinicians caring for patients with central lines should be familiar.[24] A bundled approach that emphasizes hand hygiene, full body draping during insertion, chlorhexidine skin preparation, avoidance of the femoral site, use of a real-time checklist, and daily assessment for catheter removal has been remarkably effective at decreasing CRBSI rates in multiple institutions.[25]

Ventilator-Associated Pneumonia

Certain thoracic surgical patients will require postoperative mechanical ventilation. Up to 25% of ventilated patients develop VAP. VAP is associated with significant morbidity and mortality and therefore prevention of VAP should be a priority for all ICUs. A number of simple interventions can reduce the incidence of VAP. Patients should be nursed in the semi-recumbent position, with the head of bed elevated at least 30 degrees at all times. Routine oral care, including twice daily chlorhexidine, has been shown to have a significant impact on VAP rates. Each institution should develop a standardized policy for mouth care of intubated patients. All patients should undergo standardized daily assessment for readiness to extubate, which may include the measurement of the rapid shallow breathing index (RISBI) or a spontaneous breathing trial. Any patient on continuous sedation should have a daily sedation holiday, unless contraindicated, with the assessment for readiness to be extubated timed to the sedation holiday. As mentioned previously, some evidence supports the use of sucralfate rather than pH-modifying agents for stress ulcer prophylaxis. Use of specialized endotracheal tubes with subglottic suctioning or silver impregnation may be appropriate for patients likely to be intubated for greater than 72 hours. Finally, the CDC has published guidelines on the care of respiratory equipment, including humidifiers, nebulizers, and tonsil tip suction devices. Institutional practices should be periodically reviewed to verify compliance with these guidelines in an effort to prevent such equipment from serving as a nidus of infection. Institutions that have bundled interventions to prevent VAP with universal training and frequent monitoring and feedback have been able to significantly reduce VAP rates across all patient populations.

Delirium and Over Sedation

For years, physicians and nurses have sedated mechanically ventilated patients to minimize the physiologic stress response and maximize patient comfort. Although these are laudable goals, these practices have resulted in the unexpected complications of increased delirium, delayed ventilator weaning, increased VAP, and severe physical deconditioning. Delirium in turn is associated with increased length of stay and higher mortality. All ICUs should use standardized sedation scores (e.g., RASS) and delirium assessment tools (e.g., CAM-ICU).[26,27] These standardized tools help to prevent over sedation and allow for early diagnosis and intervention for delirium. Writing sedation orders to target a specific sedation score, combined with daily interruption of sedative infusions, is particularly effective at minimizing over sedation and promoting early extubation. Patients who require heavy sedation to tolerate oral intubation should be evaluated for early tracheostomy.

Renal Dysfunction

Acute renal failure is a common complication in critically ill patients. Unfortunately, it is also a highly morbid one, with reported mortality rates greater than 50% in some trials. Prerenal azotemia refers to compromised renal function secondary to impaired renal perfusion but absent any actual damage to the nephron. This occurs in patients who are hypovolemic or have severely decreased cardiac output. It is rapidly reversible provided the underlying condition is recognized and corrected. Persistent renal hypoperfusion, such as that occurs in shock states, can result in cellular damage to the nephron or glomerulus, thus converting prerenal azotemia into intrinsic renal failure. Administration of nephrotoxic agents can amplify the injury or even result in de novo injury to the nephron in the absence of renal ischemia. Finally, the clinician must remember to evaluate every patient with acute renal failure for potential postrenal obstructive processes.

Close attention should be paid to avoiding renal injury in critically ill patients. Nephrotoxic drugs should be avoided whenever possible. Consideration should be given to pretreatment with n-acetylcysteine or sodium bicarbonate before intravenous contrast administration. Hypotension, hypovolemia, and hypoxia must be rapidly corrected. Patients with new onset of acute renal failure should have urine electrolytes and urine sediment evaluated. CVP monitoring may be helpful in detecting hypovolemia. An echocardiogram can provide a rapid assessment of overall cardiac function. If there is any concern for obstructive pathology, an immediate renal ultrasound should be performed. Although positive findings are rare, often they are amenable to intervention. It is important to carefully review the patient's medication list, eliminating all potentially nephrotoxic agents and renally dosing the rest. Should renal replacement therapy be needed, most critically ill patients tolerate a continuously administered replacement best. It is important to appreciate that it may take weeks for renal function to recover and it is impossible to accurately predict renal recovery.

Critical Illness Polyneuropathy and Acute Myopathy

Critical illness polyneuropathy occurs in up to 50% of patients who are septic for more than 2 weeks. The etiology remains unknown. Clinically, it presents as severe muscle weakness (distal worse than proximal), respiratory muscle weakness with difficulty weaning from mechanical ventilation, and decreased deep tendon reflexes. Pathologically, it is a disease of axonal degeneration and denervation. Nerve conduction studies show normal conduction velocities with prominent denervation. Patients who survive their underlying illness will regain muscle strength over a period of weeks to months. Treatment and prevention focus on avoiding compounding factors such as unnecessary use of corticosteroids or nondepolarizing neuromuscular blockers, both of which are thought to cause acute myopathy.[28] If paralytic agents cannot be avoided, every effort should be made to limit the duration of use to less than 48 hours. Beyond 48 hours, the incidence of myopathy becomes quite high. Malnutrition, heavy sedation, and prolonged immobility need to be avoided. At-risk patients should receive daily physical therapy with the goal of early resumption of mobility, even in the setting of prolonged mechanical ventilation. Ventilated patients may be ambulated with the help of a walker and either an Ambu bag or portable mechanical ventilator.

EDITOR'S COMMENT

The management of the critically ill patient requiring thoracic surgery is facilitated by a partnership between a thoracic intensivist and a thoracic surgeon. Furthermore, this patient population frequently requires daily interventions, such as bronchoscopy, invasive monitoring, and nutritional support. This concise chapter provides clear instruction in the management of the most common issues, including secretion retention, arrhythmias, and avoidance of secondary complications. Management of pulmonary hypertension is frequently the focus of therapeutic intervention, and I call the reader's attention to this particular area. Specifics in ventilator management are discussed in Chapter 7.

—MTJ

References

1. Waller DA, Keavey P, Woodfine L, et al. Pulmonary endothelial permeability changes after major lung resection. *Ann Thorac Surg.* 1996;61(5):1435–1440.
2. Grichnik KP, D'Amico TA. Acute lung injury and acute respiratory distress syndrome after pulmonary resection. *Semin Cardiothorac Vasc Anesth.* 2004;8(4):317–334.
3. Sugarbaker DJ, Jaklitsch MT, Bueno R, et al. Prevention, early detection, and management of complications after 328 consecutive extrapleural pneumonectomies. *J Thorac Cardiovasc Surg.* 2004;128(1):138–146.
4. Dunning J, Treasure T, Versteegh M, et al. Guidelines on the prevention and management of de novo atrial fibrillation after cardiac and thoracic surgery. *Eur J Cardiothorac Surg.* 2006;30(6):852–872.

5. Passannante AN. Prevention of atrial fibrillation after cardiac surgery. *Curr Opin Anaesthesiol.* 2011;24(1):58–63.
6. Sedrakyan A, Treasure T, Browne J, et al. Pharmacologic prophylaxis for postoperative atrial tachyarrhythmia in general thoracic surgery: evidence from randomized clinical trials. *J Thorac Cardiovasc Surg.* 2005;129(5):997–1005.
7. Ashrafian H, Davey P. Is amiodarone an underrecognized cause of acute respiratory failure in the ICU? *Chest.* 2001;120(1):275–282.
8. Shah SJ. Pulmonary hypertension. *JAMA.* 2012;308(13):1366–1374.
9. Ventilation with lower tidal volumes as compared with traditional tidal volumes for acute lung injury and the acute respiratory distress syndrome. The Acute Respiratory Distress Syndrome Network. *N Engl J Med.* 2000;342(18):1301–1308.
10. Thompson BT. Glucocorticoids and acute lung injury. *Crit Care Med.* 2003;31(4):S253–S257.
11. Meduri GU, Headley AS, Golden E, et al. Effect of prolonged methylprednisolone therapy in unresolving acute respiratory distress syndrome: a randomized controlled trial. *JAMA.* 1998;280(2):159–165.
12. Steinberg KP, Hudson LD, Goodman RB, et al. Efficacy and safety of corticosteroids for persistent acute respiratory distress syndrome. *N Engl J Med.* 2006;354(16):1671–1684.
13. Wiedemann HP, Wheeler AP, Bernard GR, et al. Comparison of two fluid-management strategies in acute lung injury. *N Engl J Med.* 2006;354(24):2564–2575.
14. Rivers E, Nguyen B, Havstad S, et al. Early goal-directed therapy in the treatment of severe sepsis and septic shock. *N Engl J Med.* 2001;345(19):1368–1377.
15. Bernard GR, Vincent JL, Laterre PF, et al. Efficacy and safety of recombinant human activated protein C for severe sepsis. *N Engl J Med.* 2001;344(10):699–709.
16. Dellinger RP, Levy MM, Carlet JM, et al. Surviving Sepsis Campaign: international guidelines for management of severe sepsis and septic shock: 2008. *Crit Care Med.* 2008;36(1):296–327.
17. Sprung CL, Annane D, Keh D, et al. Hydrocortisone therapy for patients with septic shock. *N Engl J Med.* 2008;358(2):111–124.
18. Laheij R, Sturkenboom M, Hassing R, et al. Risk of community-acquired pneumonia and use of gastric acid-suppressive drugs. *JAMA.* 2004;292(16):1955–1960.
19. Herzig SJ, Howell MD, Ngo LH, et al. Acid-suppressive medication use and the risk for hospital-acquired pneumonia. *JAMA.* 2009;301(20):2120–2128.
20. Davies AR, Morrison SS, Bailey MJ, et al. A multicenter, randomized controlled trial comparing early nasojejunal with nasogastric nutrition in critical illness. *Crit Care Med.* 2012;40(8):2342–2348.
21. van den Berghe G, Wouters P, Weekers F, et al. Intensive insulin therapy in critically ill patients. *N Engl J Med.* 2001;345(19):1359–1367.
22. Finfer S, Chittock DR, Su SY, et al. Intensive versus conventional glucose control in critically ill patients. *N Engl J Med.* 2009;360(13):1283–1297.
23. Moghissi ES, Korytkowski MT, DiNardo M, et al. American Association of Clinical Endocrinologists and American Diabetes Association consensus statement on inpatient glycemic control. *Endocr Pract.* 2009;15(4):353–369.
24. O'Grady NP, Alexander M, Burns LA, et al. Guidelines for the prevention of intravascular catheter-related infections. *Am J Infect Control.* 2011;39(4 Suppl 1):S1–S34.
25. Pronovost P, Needham D, Berenholtz S, et al. An intervention to decrease catheter-related bloodstream infections in the ICU. *N Engl J Med.* 2006;355(26):2725–2732.
26. Ely EW, Truman B, Shintani A, et al. Monitoring sedation status over time in ICU patients: reliability and validity of the Richmond Agitation-Sedation Scale (RASS). *JAMA.* 2003;289(22):2983–2991.
27. Ely EW, Inouye SK, Bernard GR, et al. Delirium in mechanically ventilated patients: validity and reliability of the confusion assessment method for the intensive care unit (CAM-ICU). *JAMA.* 2001;286(21):2703–2710.
28. Schweickert WD, Hall J. ICU-acquired weakness. *Chest.* 2007;131(5):1541–1549.

7 Mechanical Ventilation

Miguel J. Divo and George R. Washko

Keywords: Postoperative management of mechanical ventilation

Ventilator management for most thoracic surgery patients involves two distinct phases: (1) support in the operating room while the patient is *undergoing surgery* and receiving general anesthesia, and (2) support in the postoperative recovery room or intensive care unit (ICU) as the patient is *recovering from surgery.* Issues relating to the intraoperative ventilator management of thoracic surgery patients are largely the responsibility of the anesthesiologist and are discussed in Chapter 5. Issues relating to the postoperative management of mechanical ventilation are the responsibilities of the thoracic surgeon and intensivist.

EFFECTS OF ANESTHESIA AND THORACIC SURGERY ON RESPIRATORY SYSTEM PHYSIOLOGY

In the transition from the operating room to the recovery room or ICU it is important to appreciate that general anesthesia and thoracic surgery adversely affect nearly all aspects of respiratory physiology. These include anesthetic-related alterations in respiratory drive, reductions in lung volume due to loss of chest wall tone, changes in the ventilation perfusion relationship, and increased airway resistance in the setting of diminished lung volumes. Given the postoperative structural changes in the lung as well as its native state of disease, these alterations may have variable effect on overall function and be unpredictable in duration. They certainly must be taken into account during initial ventilatory management.

POSTOPERATIVE VENTILATOR STRATEGIES

The overall approach to mechanical ventilation in the postoperative thoracic surgery patient is similar to that used in the critically ill medical patient. Preexisting lung disease, intraoperative complications, and known physiologic alterations associated with a planned surgery require more innovative approaches.

There are two basic approaches to mechanical ventilation in patients who have undergone thoracic surgery. These are (1) methods used to support postoperative patients who are kept intubated after surgery for a specific indication that is expected to resolve within hours, allowing for rapid discontinuation of ventilator support; and (2) methods used to support patients who develop hypoxic or hypercarbic respiratory failure as a consequence of a primary process that will resolve over a period of days to weeks and may require more gradual weaning.

EXTUBATION OF THE STABLE PATIENT

In most patients, the physiologic alterations caused by anesthesia and thoracic surgery are well tolerated. These patients generally have minimal to mild preexisting pulmonary disease and are either extubated in the operating room or arrive in the postoperative recovery area or ICU ready for extubation with normal PaO_2 and $PaCO_2$ blood gas values on minimal ventilator support. Successful extubation in this group is associated with: (1) intact mental status; (2) reasonable assurance that the patient will have the ability to cough and protect his or her airway; and (3) initiation of an analgesic protocol that optimizes respiratory mechanics without causing undue respiratory depression.

Although mental status is usually simple to assess, often it is not possible to confirm intact recurrent laryngeal nerve (RLN) function before attempting extubation simply by relying on the patient's ability to cough and swallow secretions. The risk of injury to the RLN is increased in the thoracic surgery population because many procedures involve anatomic dissection or traction on structures near the left mainstem bronchus where the RLN branches from the vagus.[1] Postextubation evaluation revealing a weak voice and ineffective cough should prompt direct laryngoscopic evaluation of the hypopharynx and vocal cords, followed by vocal cord medialization if indicated.[2]

Several factors contribute to respiratory muscle dysfunction after thoracic surgery. Pain is a major contributor. Thus, selection of an appropriate analgesic regimen is essential for preventing postoperative respiratory failure.[3] Studies of respiratory muscle function also have demonstrated that diaphragmatic contractility is compromised by somatic reflex inhibition of the phrenic nerve as a consequence of afferent intercostal stimulation.[4] Thus analgesic regimens that address both these factors should provide optimal management. Epidural anesthesia with local anesthetic agents (i.e., bupivacaine) accomplishes this objective and can be administered either alone or in combination with opioids. Patient-controlled anesthesia (PCA) also may be an effective adjunct, but care must be taken in titration to minimize the degree of respiratory depression.[5]

VENTILATOR SUPPORT WITH POSTOPERATIVE RESPIRATORY COMPROMISE

A substantial number of patients undergoing thoracic surgery will require ventilator support postoperatively. A successful ventilator strategy for longer-term management involves the following general principles:

1. Selecting a *mode* of ventilation that prevents high airway pressures and optimizes patient-ventilator synchrony.

2. Early weaning of FIO_2 to prevent adsorption atelectasis and limit possible oxygen toxicity, especially in patients receiving medications that have been associated with free-radical lung injury (e.g., bleomycin).
3. Selecting an appropriate sedation/analgesia regimen to ensure patient comfort while permitting periodic assessments of mental status and respiratory function.
4. Initiating nutritional support and deep venous thrombosis prophylaxis.
5. Closely monitoring the intravascular fluid status to prevent development of pulmonary edema, especially in areas of lung tissue that have been manipulated during surgery.

No guidelines exist for selecting the "single best" mode of ventilation for the postoperative thoracic surgery patient. Anecdotal experience indicates that many surgeons select pressure-controlled modes of ventilation in which the user-specified independent variable is airway pressure rather than tidal volume. This ensures that airway pressures will not exceed a known value, thus limiting stress on newly created staple or suture lines. There are no data to indicate that this approach improves respiratory physiology or ICU outcomes in this patient population.[6] Furthermore, appropriate selection of ventilator parameters using volume-cycled modes can ensure equivalent limiting of airway pressures. Thus, in most instances, user preference and experience will dictate ventilator settings.

ANATOMY OF THE VENTILATOR

Mechanical ventilation has evolved dramatically in the last 100 years, revolutionizing the concept of intensive care. Mechanical ventilation can be provided as either negative pressure ventilation (iron lung, cuirass shell, or rocking bed) or more commonly as positive pressure inflation by using an endotracheal tube or mask (known as noninvasive positive pressure ventilation). Positive pressure ventilation is also classified as manual (hand bag valve mask) or mechanical. The latter is provided by transport, critical care, and neonatal/pediatric ventilators.

There are many models of commercially available ventilators and it is important for the physician to understand the core components of these devices (Fig. 7-1). The most widely used system is positive pressure ventilation, which is administered through an endotracheal tube.[7] Positive pressure ventilation requires the following components: an oxygen source (if O_2 mixture above 21% is needed), a mixing chamber, a compressor, an electronically controlled inspiratory valve, a ventilator circuit (with inhalation, "Y" connector, and exhalation limb), and an exhalation valve to form a closed circuit. The core of the apparatus is a computer, which controls the manner in which the ventilator breaths are triggered, cycled, and limited. These parameters are organized as preset modes. The computer also monitors pressure and flow sensors, providing a feedback and safety system. The array of information generated by the

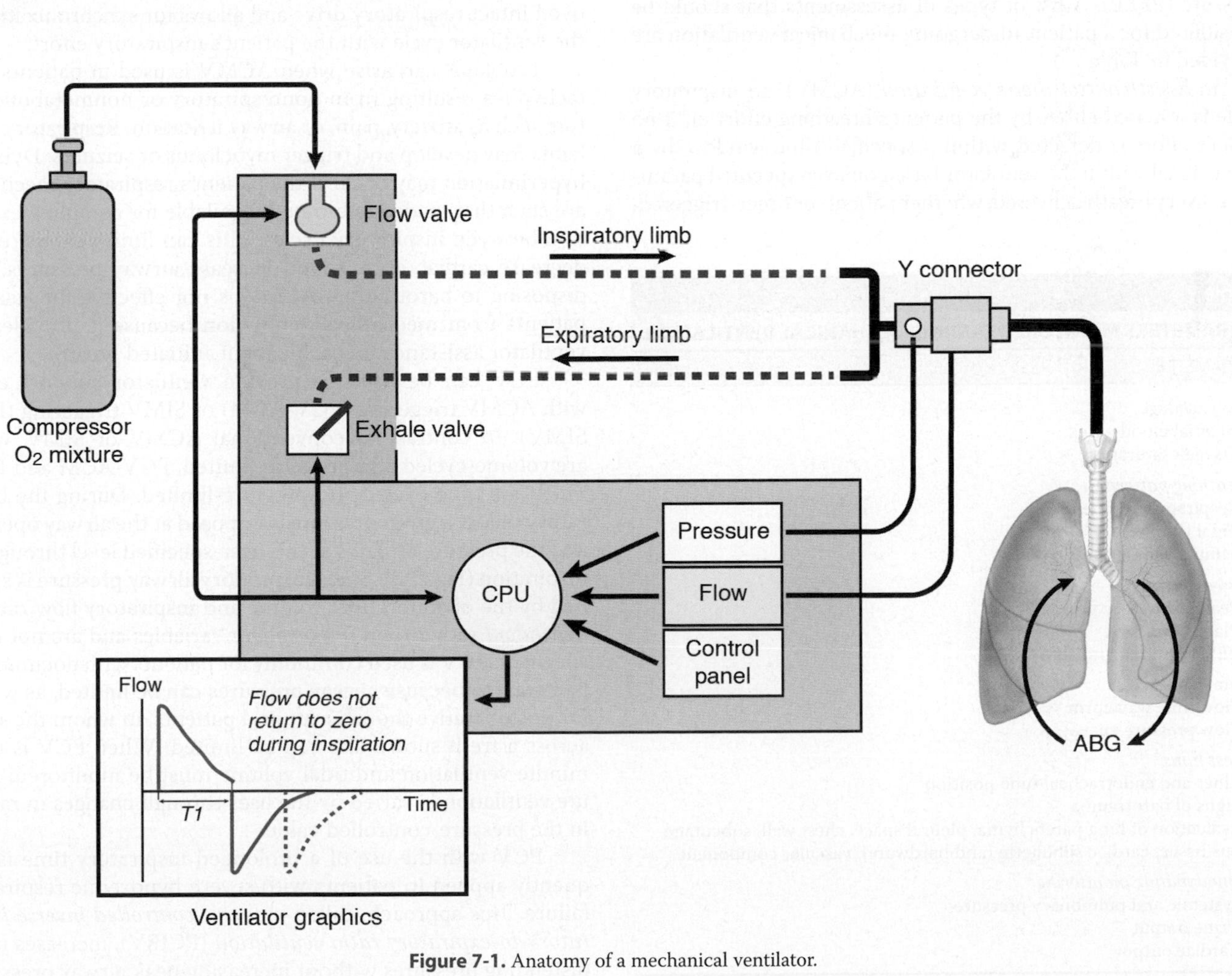

Figure 7-1. Anatomy of a mechanical ventilator.

computer is displayed on a monitor in tabular or graphic format. In this way, the clinician can adjust the patient's ventilatory strategy based on the patient's clinical status while minimizing potential harm.

CONVENTIONAL MODES OF VENTILATION

Commonly used modes available on most commercial ventilators include assist/control, pressure-controlled ventilation (PCV), pressure-support ventilation (PSV), and continuous positive airway pressure (CPAP). The setup and operation of these modes are described below.

When choosing ventilator settings, the *mode refers* specifically to the manner in which ventilator breaths are triggered, cycled, and limited. The *trigger*, either an inspiratory effort or a time-based signal, defines what the ventilator senses to initiate an assisted breath. *Cycle* refers to the factors that determine the end of inspiration. For example, in volume-cycled ventilation, inspiration ends when a specific tidal volume is delivered to the patient. Other types of cycling include pressure cycling, time cycling, and flow cycling. *Limiting factors* are operator-specified values, such as airway pressure, that are monitored by transducers internal to the ventilator circuit throughout the respiratory cycle. If the specified values are exceeded, inspiratory flow is immediately stopped, and the ventilator circuit is vented to atmospheric pressure or the specified positive end-expiratory pressure (PEEP). A list of types of assessments that should be considered for a patient undergoing mechanical ventilation are provided in Table 7-1.

In *assist/control mode ventilation* (ACMV), an inspiratory cycle is initiated either by the patient's breathing effort or, if no patient effort is detected within a specified time window, by a timer signal within the ventilator based on user-specified parameters. Every breath delivered, whether patient- or timer-triggered,

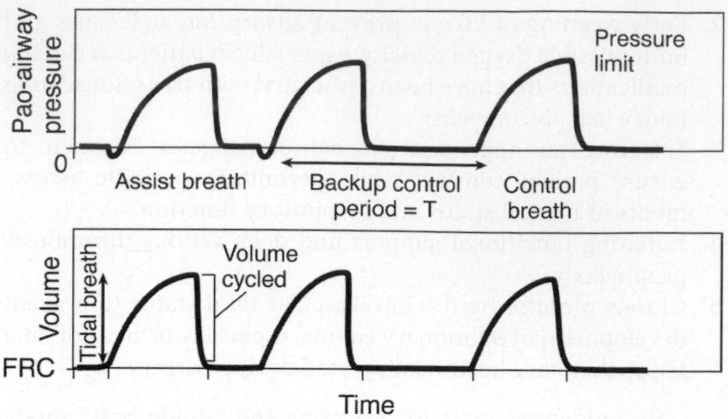

Figure 7-2. Assist/control mode ventilation (ACMV) airway pressure and delivered tidal volume profiles. In ACMV ventilation, two types of breaths can occur. *Assisted breaths* are initiated by the patient and are fully supported by the ventilator, which delivers a user-specified tidal volume. *Ventilator-controlled breaths* are initiated by the ventilator at the backup rate specified by the user and are triggered by the timer system in the ventilator if the patient fails to initiate a breath after a specified period.

consists of the operator-specified tidal volume. Ventilatory rate is determined either by the patient or by the operator-specified backup rate, whichever is of higher frequency (Fig. 7-2). ACMV is used commonly for initiation of mechanical ventilation because it ensures a backup minute ventilation in the absence of an intact respiratory drive and allows for synchronization of the ventilator cycle with the patient's inspiratory effort.

Problems can arise when ACMV is used in patients with tachypnea resulting from nonrespiratory or nonmetabolic factors such as anxiety, pain, or airway irritation. Respiratory alkalemia may develop and trigger myoclonus or seizures. Dynamic hyperinflation may occur if the patient's respiratory mechanics are such that inadequate time is available for complete exhalation between inspiratory cycles. This can limit venous return, decrease cardiac output, and increase airway pressures, predisposing to barotrauma. ACMV is not effective for weaning patients from mechanical ventilation because it provides full ventilator assistance on each patient-initiated breath.

PCV can be used to provide ventilator support either with ACMV triggering (PCV-ACM) or SIMV triggering (PCV-SIMV). In contrast to conventional ACMV or SIMV, which are volume-cycled and pressure-limited, PCV-ACM and PCV-SIMV are time-cycled and pressure-limited. During the inspiratory phase, a given pressure is imposed at the airway opening, and the pressure remains at this user-specified level throughout inspiration (Fig. 7-3). Since inspiratory airway pressure is specified by the operator, tidal volume and inspiratory flow rate are *dependent* rather than *independent* variables and are not user-specified. PCV is used commonly for patients with documented barotrauma because airway pressures can be limited, as well as for postoperative thoracic surgical patients, in whom the stress across a fresh suture line can be limited. When PCV is used, minute ventilation and tidal volume must be monitored; minute ventilation is varied by the user through changes in rate or in the pressure-controlled value.

PCV with the use of a prolonged inspiratory time is frequently applied to patients with severe hypoxemic respiratory failure. This approach, called *pressure-controlled inverse inspiratory-to-expiratory ratio ventilation* (PCIRV), increases mean distending pressures without increasing peak airway pressures.

Table 7-1

PARAMETERS MONITORED DURING MECHANICAL VENTILATION

PARAMETER
Gas exchange
• Arterial blood gases
• Oxygen saturation
Breathing pattern
• Respiratory frequency
• Tidal volume
• Minute ventilation
Airway pressure
• Peak inspiratory pressure
• Plateau pressure
• PEEP, external and auto
Flow
• Flow time waveform
• Flow pressure curve
Chest films
• Lines and endotracheal tube position
• Signs of barotrauma
• Evaluation of lung parenchyma, pleural space, chest wall, subcutaneous tissue, cardiac silhouette (and hardware), vascular component
Hemodynamic monitoring
• Systemic and pulmonary pressure
• Urine output
• Cardiac output

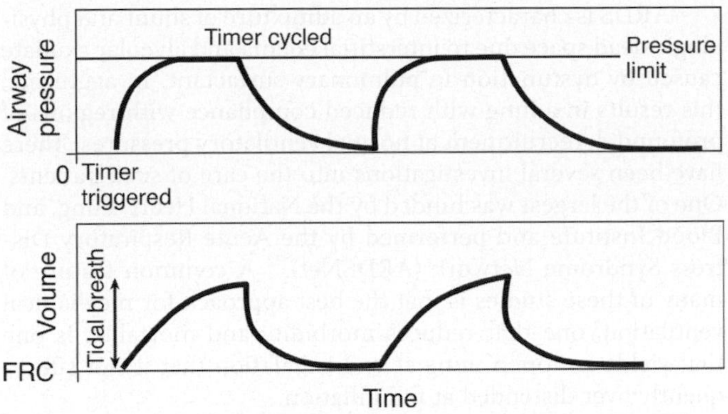

Figure 7-3. Pressure-control ventilation (PVC) delivers airway inflation pressure using time cycling rather than a user-specified tidal volume using volume cycling. In this figure, all breaths are shown as timer-cycled, although PCV can be programmed to trigger according to an assist/control algorithm or synchronized intermittent mandatory algorithm.

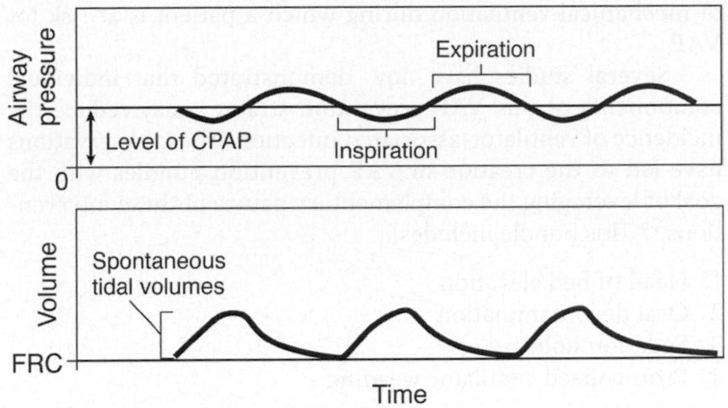

Figure 7-5. Continuous positive airway pressure (CPAP) charges the ventilator circuit to a user-specified continuous airway pressure but provides ventilator assist with respiratory efforts. All ventilation occurs through the spontaneous efforts of the patient.

It is thought to work in conjunction with PEEP to open collapsed alveoli and improve oxygenation. In acute lung injury (ALI), PCIRV may be associated with fewer deleterious effects than conventional volume-cycled ventilation, which requires higher peak airway pressures to achieve an equivalent reduction in shunt fraction, but there are no convincing data to show that PCIRV improves outcomes in ALI or adult respiratory distress syndrome.[8,9]

PSV is a form of ventilation that is patient-triggered, flow-cycled, and pressure-limited; it is designed specifically for use in the weaning process but is also used commonly to ventilate patients with new-onset respiratory failure who are agitated and become asynchronous with other modes of ventilator support. During PSV, the inspiratory phase is terminated when the inspiratory flow rate falls below a certain level; in most ventilators, this flow rate cannot be adjusted by the operator. When PSV is used, patients receive ventilator assist only when the ventilator detects an inspiratory effort (Fig. 7-4). Thus it is mandatory that the patient have an intact respiratory drive to be maintained safely on this mode of ventilation without additional backup ventilator support.

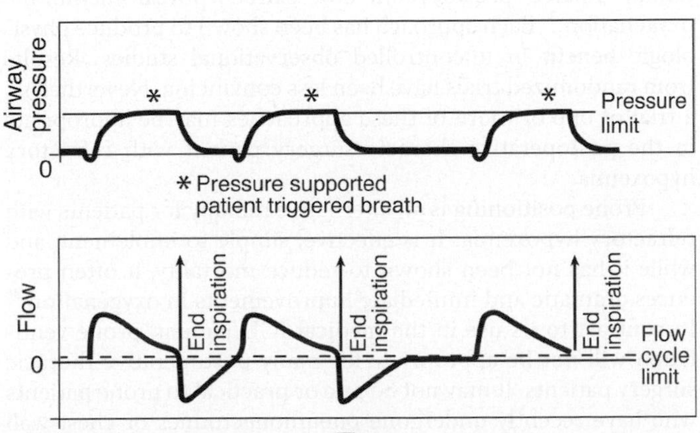

Figure 7-4. Pressure-support ventilation (PSV) requires patient triggering for every breath. The ventilator assists every patient effort by applying a user-specified amount of positive pressure throughout the airway circuit. As the lung fills, inspiratory flow slows. When flow falls below a set value, inspiratory assist ceases, and the expiratory valve opens, allowing for exhalation. The size of each breath is dictated by the patient's inspiratory efforts, which augment ventilator assist. Respiratory rate is determined by the frequency of triggering by the patient.

PSV is well tolerated by most patients who are being weaned. PSV parameters can be set to provide full or nearly full ventilator support that can be withdrawn slowly over a period of days in a systematic fashion to gradually load the respiratory muscles and allow the patient to fully resume spontaneous breathing.

CPAP is not a true support mode of ventilation because ventilation occurs through the patient's spontaneous efforts. The ventilator provides fresh gas to the breathing circuit with each inspiration and charges the circuit to a constant operator-specified pressure that can range from 0 to 20 cm H_2O (Fig. 7-5). CPAP is used to assess extubation potential in patients who have been weaned effectively and are requiring little ventilator support.

COMPLICATIONS OF PROLONGED MECHANICAL VENTILATION

One of the most serious complications associated with mechanical ventilation is ventilator-associated pneumonia (VAP). VAP is defined as a pulmonary parenchymal infection that has developed after at least 48 hours of mechanical support.[10] It is the most common infection acquired in the ICU, accounting for up to 50% of the antibiotics prescribed in this setting, and has an attributable mortality rate between 5.8% and 27%.[11–15] Because of these ominous statistics, there is great interest in disease pathogenesis and prevention.

Several mechanisms have been proposed for the development of VAP. The most common is pathogenic colonization of the aerodigestive tract. From this point, bacteria can enter the lung via the blood and lymphatics or may be introduced into the airways through or around the endotracheal tube (ETT).[10,16–18] Based upon these proposed mechanisms, several preventive strategies have been implemented to reduce infection. These include decontamination of the aerodigestive tract via topical/oral antimicrobial medications, elevation of the head of the bed, sedation holidays, and aggressively implemented weaning protocols.[19–25] The latter two are focused not on interrupting the translocation of bacteria but rather on shortening the duration of mechanical ventilation during which a patient is at risk for VAP.

Several studies have now demonstrated that individual components of this VAP prevention strategy may reduce the incidence of ventilator-associated infection. These observations have led to the creation of VAP prevention bundles with the goal of leveraging the complementary nature of these interventions.[26] This bundle includes:

1. Head of bed elevation
2. Oral decontamination
3. Sedation holidays
4. Protocolized ventilator weaning

Recently, Morris and colleagues reported that following the implementation of such a protocol, the rate of VAP decreased from 32 cases per 1000 ventilator days to 12 cases per 1000 ventilator days ($p < 0.001$).[26] These and other similar investigations strongly support the use of VAP prevention bundles as a routine part of clinical care in the ICU.

As mentioned, one of the proposed mechanisms of bacterial entry into the lung is by the endotracheal tube, more specifically around the endotracheal tube. By design, the endotracheal tube has a low-pressure high-volume inflatable cuff on its distal end that provides tube stability and reduces the leakage of air. Although this cuff facilitates ventilatory strategies such as increased PEEP or driving pressures, it also serves as a local nidus of secretions that have collected above it in the proximal trachea. In attempt to mitigate the potential for the drainage of secretions into the lung from this source, manufacturers offer endotracheal tubes that have continuous suction ports in this space to evacuate pooled secretions. Such devices have demonstrated efficacy in reducing VAP and are increasingly being adopted in the ICU.

Finally, there is increasing evidence that some prophylactic interventions commonly used in the inpatient setting may have unintended consequences. Recently, Herzig et al.[27] demonstrated that in a single-center survey of over 63,000 hospital admissions, medical suppression of gastric acid was associated with a 30% increased odds of hospital-acquired pneumonia. These data and other investigations linking pharmacologic acid suppression to VAP suggest that altering the pH of gastric secretions may facilitate pathologic colonization.[28,29] Further investigation is required to determined how best to weigh the apparent risks of these medications with their obvious benefits.

VENTILATION OF THE POSTOPERATIVE THORACIC SURGERY PATIENT WITH HYPOXEMIC RESPIRATORY FAILURE

A commonly used metric to assess the severity of hypoxemic respiratory failure is the ratio of the partial pressure of oxygen in the arterial blood (PaO_2) divided by the fraction of inspired oxygen (FiO_2: ranging from 0.21 or ambient gas to 1 which corresponds to 100% oxygen). A patient with a PaO_2/FiO_2 ratio less than 300 but more than 200 is categorized as having ALI whereas those with a ratio less than or equal to 200 is categorized as having acute respiratory distress syndrome (ARDS).[30] It is estimated that the mortality associated with ARDS is between 25% and 40%.[31,32] And while it is increasingly clear that one of the greatest risks for the development of this condition is the presence of ALI, there are no specific recommendations pertaining to ventilatory strategies in this cohort.

ARDS is characterized by an admixture of shunt and physiologic dead space due to interstitial edema and alveolar exudate caused by dysfunction in pulmonary surfactant. In aggregate, this results in a lung with reduced compliance with regions of profound derecruitment at normal ventilatory pressures. There have been several investigations into the care of such patients. One of the largest was funded by the National Heart, Lung, and Blood Institute and performed by the Acute Respiratory Distress Syndrome Network (ARDSNet).[32] A common feature of many of these studies is that the best approach for mechanical ventilation, one that reduces morbidity and mortality, is one that yields an "open" lung at end exhalation that is not subsequently over distended at full inflation.

The open lung strategy of ventilation is thought to work by recruiting damaged, collapsed alveoli and improving oxygenation without causing overdistention and ventilator-associated lung injury in less damaged areas of lung.[33] Open lung ventilation is not a distinct mode of ventilation. Rather, it is a strategy for applying either volume-cycled or pressure-controlled ventilation to patients with severe respiratory failure. The level of PEEP is selected to help avoid cyclic opening and closing of alveolar units, thereby allowing the majority of alveoli to remain inflated during tidal ventilation. Achievement of eucapnia and normal blood pH through adjustments in ventilator tidal volume and breathing frequency are of lower priority. Hypercapnia and consequent respiratory acidosis tend to be well tolerated physiologically, except in patients with significant hemodynamic compromise, ventricular dysfunction, cardiac dysrhythmias, or increased intracranial pressure. Furthermore, data suggest that hypercapnia may have direct beneficial anti-inflammatory effects in the inflamed lung.[34] Open lung ventilation has been shown to primarily benefit medical ICU patients with hypoxemic respiratory failure owing to ALI. Although open lung ventilation has not been specifically evaluated in the thoracic surgery patient population, it is reasonable to presume that similar benefits will be observed in thoracic surgery patients with this condition.

Other nonconventional strategies that have been used to manage critically ill patients with hypoxemic respiratory failure include prone-position ventilation, nitric oxide supplementation, inhaled prostacyclin, and extracorporeal membrane oxygenation.[35] Each approach has been shown to produce physiologic benefit in uncontrolled observational studies. Results from randomized trials have been less convincing. Nevertheless, a trial of one or more of these approaches may be appropriate in the postoperative thoracic surgery patient with refractory hypoxemia.

Prone positioning is an alternative therapy for patients with refractory hypoxemia. It is effective, simple to implement, and while it has not been shown to reduce mortality, it often produces dramatic and immediate improvements in oxygenation.[36] In contrast to its use in the medical ICU patient, prone ventilation will not be appropriate for many postoperative thoracic surgery patients. It may not be safe or practical to prone patients who have recently undergone pneumonectomies or chest wall resections or have multiple anterior chest tubes. Nevertheless, in patients in whom proning is safe, a trial should be considered for the severely hypoxic patient. Prone positioning can be used in combination with any mode of ventilator support. Patients are rotated from the supine position to the prone swimmer's position. Pads are required for bony dependent areas such as the forehead, elbows, ankles, and knees, and frequent turning is required to prevent skin breakdown.

The physiologic basis for improvement in gas exchange after proning appears to result from improved $\dot{V}/\dot{Q}$ matching in newly dependent lung zones and recruitment of damaged areas of lung through gravity-assisted redistribution of transpulmonary pressures.[22] Several small nonrandomized trials have demonstrated improvements in oxygenation with proning. Results of a recently completed randomized clinical trial confirmed these observations but failed to demonstrate a mortality benefit from an initial 10-day course of prone ventilation.[37] Nevertheless, prone ventilation still may improve oxygenation in selected postoperative patients for whom it can be instituted safely and thus should be considered as a supplement to conventional ventilation for the patient with refractory hypoxemia.

Inhaled nitric oxide (NO: 2–40 ppm) also has been combined with mechanical ventilation to treat patients with hypoxemic respiratory failure.[38] Benefits in oxygenation and reductions in pulmonary artery pressures have been observed in many patients receiving NO, although physiologic benefit has not been universal, and clinical parameters to identify responders have not yet been identified.[39] Two randomized clinical trials conducted in patients with hypoxemic respiratory failure have failed to show mortality benefits or decreased resource utilization from NO therapy.[40] Although not universally effective, inhaled NO still may be effective in selected patients with postoperative hypoxemic respiratory failure. The primary limitation to its widespread implementation is cost which has led many centers to embrace other inhaled therapies for refractory hypoxemia such as prostacyclin.

Inhaled prostacyclin (PGI_2: 0–50 ng/kg/min) is a pulmonary vasodilator that promotes smooth muscle relaxation by increasing cytoplasmic adenosine monophosphate. Its half-life is less than 5 minutes and it has effects similar to those observed with inhaled NO.[35] Prostacyclin is formulated to be administered intravenously or via inhalation but the former limits its beneficial impact on ventilation perfusion matching and has the disadvantage of causing systemic hypotension. Although there have been no large randomized trials of inhaled prostacyclin, it is simple to use, requires no special monitoring for administration, and is less expensive than NO.

Extracorporeal membrane oxygenation also may be used in the management of the posttransplantation patient with severe hypoxemia secondary to ischemia-reperfusion injury or severe acute rejection. Although randomized trials have failed to demonstrate consistent benefits from use of extracorporeal membrane oxygenation for established ARDS, posttransplantation hypoxemic respiratory failure has been managed successfully using this approach.[41,42]

WEANING FROM MECHANICAL VENTILATION

Mechanical ventilation can successfully support ventilation and gas exchange during surgery, the perioperative period, and during episodes of acute respiratory failure, but it is associated with considerable risks and complications that increase with the duration of intubation.[7,43] Therefore, it is imperative to recognize when sufficient improvement occurs to expeditiously shift attention to liberation from mechanical ventilation. The clinician must carefully weigh the benefits of rapid liberation against the risks of premature trials of spontaneous breathing and extubation. For the majority of patients (~75%), there is no need for a step-by-step prolonged decrease in ventilatory support. Several studies have demonstrated that the process can be carried out safely by performing three simple steps[43–45]: (1) Establish readiness for spontaneous breathing trial (SBT) by recognizing adequate recovery of gas exchange and respiratory muscle function followed by; (2) SBT; and (3) extubation (Fig. 7-6).

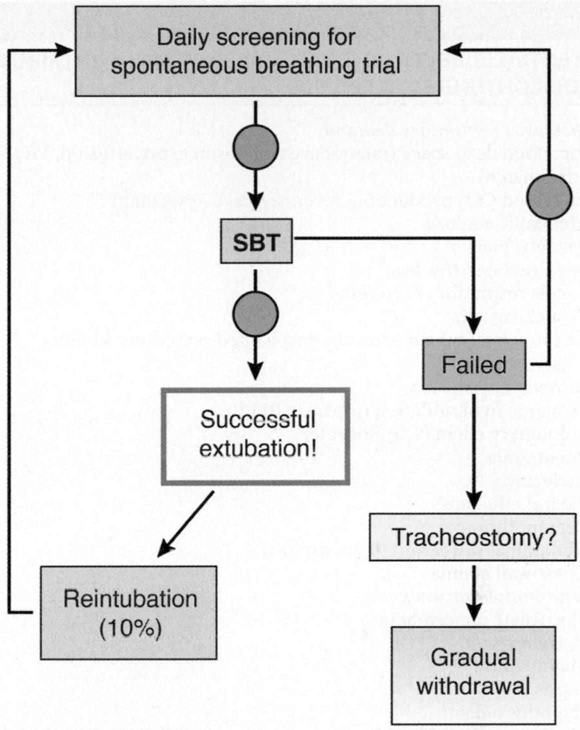

Figure 7-6. Protocolized weaning.

The clinician should consider each step as a test with a minimal threshold that has to be met before proceeding with weaning. The assessment for readiness is conducted on a daily[22] (or twice daily) basis as soon as mechanical ventilation is initiated. The critical step in this process is to recognize when the causes(s) of respiratory failure have reversed (Table 7-2) to a degree that makes spontaneous breathing possible.

PERSISTENT WEANING FAILURE

Up to 20% of mechanically ventilated patients may have several failed SBT attempts, despite efforts to reverse the initial cause(s) of respiratory failure (Table 7-2). In these cases it is reasonable to consider tracheostomy to transition to a more gradual withdrawal of ventilatory support. This should be considered earlier when upper airway obstruction, coma, or irreversible or slowly reversible neuromuscular disease complicates clinical care. Tracheostomy tubes have several benefits including patient comfort which affords a reduction in sedation, better oral care, possible speech restoration, provision of more secure airway, and reductions in the work of breathing.

SPECIAL CONSIDERATIONS IN THE PNEUMONECTOMY PATIENT

The guidelines outlined in the preceding section are satisfactory for weaning most thoracic surgery patients from mechanical

Table 7-2

POTENTIALLY REVERSIBLE FACTORS THAT MAY CONTRIBUTE TO DISCONTINUATION FAILURE

1. *Increased ventilatory demand*
   Increased dead space (pulmonary embolism, hypoperfusion, $\dot{V}/\dot{Q}$ mismatch)
   Increased CO_2 production (fever, sepsis, overfeeding)
   Metabolic acidosis
   Anxiety, pain
2. *Increased resistive load*
   Excess respiratory secretions
   Bronchospasm
   Endotracheal tube narrowing (inspissated secretions, kinking, narrow tube)
3. *Increased elastic load*
   Dynamic hyperinflation (intrinsic PEEP)
   Pulmonary edema (cardiogenic)
   Pneumonia
   Atelectasis
   Pleural effusions
   Pneumothoraces
   Abdominal distention (ileus, ascites)
   Chest wall edema
4. *Neuromuscular weakness*
   Electrolyte abnormalities
   Corticosteroids
   Malnutrition
   Sepsis
   Hypothyroidism
   Medications (NMBs)
5. *Reduced ventilatory drive*
   Oversedation
   Metabolic alkalosis
   CNS process
   Obesity hypoventilation syndrome
6. *Myocardial ischemia*
7. *Psychological factors*

ventilation. Patients who have undergone a pneumonectomy, however, often present special challenges that can slow weaning and complicate postoperative management. Shift of the mediastinum toward the remaining lung owing to rapid accumulation of fluid within the hemithorax can increase pleural pressures and thus decrease transpulmonary distending pressures in the remaining lung. This imposes an added, severe restrictive physiologic load on the respiratory system postoperatively that can precipitate respiratory failure. Destabilization of the mediastinum can have additional adverse consequences on lung physiology. The loss of transpulmonary distending pressures owing to mediastinal shift can lead to collapse of small airways and can produce wheezing on examination. This pseudo-obstruction pattern tends to be refractory to bronchodilators and compromises breathing by increasing the work of breathing. Therapeutic drainage of fluid from the side of the pneumonectomy, restoration of pressure equilibrium between the hemithoraces, and reestablishment of a midline mediastinal position lead to resolution of this problem.

Hemodynamic instability also may occur after pneumonectomy because of several factors that influence right-sided heart function. Loss of a portion of the functioning pulmonary vascular bed may contribute to increased pulmonary pressures in patients with limited preexisting reserve. Lowering the intrathoracic pressure by removing excess air or fluid from the pneumonectomized side can acutely increase right ventricular afterload and contribute to right-sided heart failure. Conversely, increased intrathoracic pressures resulting from rapid accumulation of fluid on the pneumonectomized side can decrease preload and cause hypotension and reduced cardiac output. Reinstituting drainage of the chest cavity to atmospheric pressure via a chest tube connected to a water seal represents effective management.

ACKNOWLEDGMENT

We wish to acknowledge Dr. Edward P. Ingenito for his contribution to prior versions of this chapter.

EDITOR'S COMMENT

This chapter has been specifically geared to the novice, although everyone will find value in its pages. A simple description of the anatomy of the ventilator is a good place to start to understand this complex issue. The authors then explain the conventional modes of ventilation and explain the acronyms that many students find confusing. There is a lot of practical information in this chapter, including positioning of the patient, sedation management, and special considerations for ventilating the pneumonectomy patient. This chapter is written in a clear style that makes it of practical value to anyone working in a thoracic ICU.

–MTJ

References

1. Sugarbaker DJ, Jaklitsch MT, Bueno R, et al. Prevention, early detection, and management of complications after 328 consecutive extrapleural pneumonectomies. *J Thorac Cardiovasc Surg.* 2004;128:138–146.
2. Schneider B, Schickinger-Fischer B, Zumtobel M, et al. Concept for diagnosis and therapy of unilateral recurrent laryngeal nerve paralysis following thoracic surgery. *Thorac Cardiovasc Surg.* 2003;51:327–331.
3. Bromage PR, Camporesi E, Chestnut D. Epidural narcotics for postoperative analgesia. *Anesth Analg.* 1980;59:473–480.
4. Shannon R. Intercostal and abdominal muscle afferent influence on medullary dorsal respiratory group neurons. *Respir Physiol.* 1980;39:73–94.
5. Keats AS, Girgis KZ. Respiratory deression associated with relief of pain by narcotics. *Anesthesiology.* 1968;29:1006–1013.
6. Campbell RS, Davis BR. Pressure-controlled versus volume-controlled ventilation: does it matter? *Respir Care.* 2002;47:416–424; discussion 424–416.
7. Esteban A, Anzueto A, Frutos F, et al. Characteristics and outcomes in adult patients receiving mechanical ventilation: a 28-day international study. *JAMA.* 2002;287:345–355.
8. Shanholtz C, Brower R. Should inverse ratio ventilation be used in adult respiratory distress syndrome? *Am J Respir Crit Care Med.* 1994;149:1354–1358.
9. Mercat A, Titiriga M, Anguel N, et al. Inverse ratio ventilation (I/E = 2/1) in acute respiratory distress syndrome: a six-hour controlled study. *Am J Respir Crit Care Med.* 1997;155:1637–1642.
10. American Thoracic Society; Infectious Diseases Society of America. Guidelines for the management of adults with hospital-acquired, ventilator-associated, and healthcare-associated pneumonia. *Am J Respir Crit Care Med.* 2005;171:388–416.
11. Chastre J, Fagon JY. Ventilator-associated pneumonia. *Am J Respir Crit Care Med.* 2002;165:867–903.

12. Melsen WG, Rovers MM, Bonten MJ. Ventilator-associated pneumonia and mortality: a systematic review of observational studies. *Crit Care Med.* 2009;37:2709–2718.
13. Vincent JL, Bihari DJ, Suter PM, et al. The prevalence of nosocomial infection in intensive care units in Europe. Results of the European Prevalence of Infection in Intensive Care (EPIC) Study. EPIC International Advisory Committee. *JAMA.* 1995;274:639–644.
14. Craven DE. Preventing ventilator-associated pneumonia in adults: sowing seeds of change. *Chest.* 2006;130:251–260.
15. NNIS System. National Nosocomial Infections Surveillance (NNIS) System report, data summary from January 1990–May 1999, issued June 1999. A report from the NNIS System. *Am J Infect Control.* 1999;27:520–532.
16. Tablan OC, Anderson LJ, Besser R, et al. Guidelines for preventing health-care–associated pneumonia, 2003: recommendations of CDC and the Healthcare Infection Control Practices Advisory Committee. *MMWR Recomm Rep.* 2004;53:1–36.
17. Safdar N, Crnich CJ, Maki DG. The pathogenesis of ventilator-associated pneumonia: its relevance to developing effective strategies for prevention. *Respir Care.* 2005;50:725–739; discussion 739–741.
18. Bonten MJ, Kollef MH, Hall JB. Risk factors for ventilator-associated pneumonia: from epidemiology to patient management. *Clin Infect Dis.* 2004;38:1141–1149.
19. van Nieuwenhoven CA, Vandenbroucke-Grauls C, van Tiel FH, et al. Feasibility and effects of the semirecumbent position to prevent ventilator-associated pneumonia: a randomized study. *Crit Care Med.* 2006;34:396–402.
20. Drakulovic MB, Torres A, Bauer TT, et al. Supine body position as a risk factor for nosocomial pneumonia in mechanically ventilated patients: a randomised trial. *Lancet.* 1999;354:1851–1858.
21. Jackson DL, Proudfoot CW, Cann KF, et al. The incidence of sub-optimal sedation in the ICU: a systematic review. *Crit Care.* 2009;13:R204.
22. Ely EW, Baker AM, Dunagan DP, et al. Effect on the duration of mechanical ventilation of identifying patients capable of breathing spontaneously. *N Engl J Med.* 1996;335:1864–1869.
23. Chlebicki MP, Safdar N. Topical chlorhexidine for prevention of ventilator-associated pneumonia: a meta-analysis. *Crit Care Med.* 2007;35:595–602.
24. Labeau SO, Van de Vyver K, Brusselaers N, et al. Prevention of ventilator-associated pneumonia with oral antiseptics: a systematic review and meta-analysis. *Lancet Infect Dis.* 2011;11:845–854.
25. Pileggi C, Bianco A, Flotta D, et al. Prevention of ventilator-associated pneumonia, mortality and all intensive care unit acquired infections by topically applied antimicrobial or antiseptic agents: a meta-analysis of randomized controlled trials in intensive care units. *Crit Care.* 2011;15:R155.
26. Morris AC, Hay AW, Swann DG, et al. Reducing ventilator-associated pneumonia in intensive care: impact of implementing a care bundle. *Crit Care Med.* 39:2218–2224.
27. Herzig SJ, Howell MD, Ngo LH, et al. Acid-suppressive medication use and the risk for hospital-acquired pneumonia. *JAMA.* 2009;301:2120–2128.
28. Prod'hom G, Leuenberger P, Koerfer J, et al. Nosocomial pneumonia in mechanically ventilated patients receiving antacid, ranitidine, or sucralfate as prophylaxis for stress ulcer. A randomized controlled trial. *Ann Intern Med.* 1994;120:653–662.
29. Cook DJ, Reeve BK, Guyatt GH, et al. Stress ulcer prophylaxis in critically ill patients. Resolving discordant meta-analyses. *JAMA.* 1996;275:308–314.
30. Bernard GR, Artigas A, Brigham KL, et al. The American-European Consensus Conference on ARDS. Definitions, mechanisms, relevant outcomes, and clinical trial coordination. *Am J Respir Crit Care Med.* 1994;149: 818–824.
31. Zilberberg MD, Epstein SK. Acute lung injury in the medical ICU: comorbid conditions, age, etiology, and hospital outcome. *Am J Respir Crit Care Med.* 1998;157:1159–1164.
32. Ventilation with lower tidal volumes as compared with traditional tidal volumes for acute lung injury and the acute respiratory distress syndrome. The Acute Respiratory Distress Syndrome Network. *N Engl J Med.* 2000;342:1301–1308.
33. Amato MB, Barbas CS, Medeiros DM, et al. Effect of a protective-ventilation strategy on mortality in the acute respiratory distress syndrome. *N Engl J Med.* 1998;338:347–354.
34. Laffey JG, Tanaka M, Engelberts D, et al. Therapeutic hypercapnia reduces pulmonary and systemic injury following in vivo lung reperfusion. *Am J Respir Crit Care Med.* 2000;162:2287–2294.
35. Cranshaw J, Griffiths MJ, Evans TW. The pulmonary physician in critical care – part 9: non-ventilatory strategies in ARDS. *Thorax.* 2002;57:823–829.
36. Albert RK, Leasa D, Sanderson M, et al. The prone position improves arterial oxygenation and reduces shunt in oleic-acid-induced acute lung injury. *Am Rev Respir Dis.* 1987;135:628–633.
37. Gattinoni L, Tognoni G, Pesenti A, et al. Effect of prone positioning on the survival of patients with acute respiratory failure. *N Engl J Med.* 2001;345:568–573.
38. Rossaint R, Gerlach H, Schmidt-Ruhnke H, et al. Efficacy of inhaled nitric oxide in patients with severe ARDS. *Chest.* 1995;107:1107–1115.
39. Dellinger RP, Zimmerman JL, Taylor RW, et al. Effects of inhaled nitric oxide in patients with acute respiratory distress syndrome: results of a randomized phase II trial. Inhaled Nitric Oxide in ARDS Study Group. *Crit Care Med.* 1998;26:15–23.
40. Taylor RW, Zimmerman JL, Dellinger RP, et al. Low-dose inhaled nitric oxide in patients with acute lung injury: a randomized controlled trial. *JAMA.* 2004;291:1603–1609.
41. Kollef MH. Rescue therapy for the acute respiratory distress syndrome (ARDS). *Chest.* 1997;111:845–846.
42. Anderson H, 3rd, Steimle C, Shapiro M, et al. Extracorporeal life support for adult cardiorespiratory failure. *Surgery.* 1993;114:161–172; discussion 172–163.
43. Brochard L, Rauss A, Benito S, et al. Comparison of three methods of gradual withdrawal from ventilatory support during weaning from mechanical ventilation. *Am J Respir Crit Care Med.* 1994;150:896–903.
44. Esteban A, Alia I, Gordo F, et al. Extubation outcome after spontaneous breathing trials with T-tube or pressure support ventilation. The Spanish Lung Failure Collaborative Group. *Am J Respir Crit Care Med.* 1997; 156:459–465.
45. Frutos-Vivar F, Ferguson ND, Esteban A, et al. Risk factors for extubation failure in patients following a successful spontaneous breathing trial. *Chest.* 2006;130:1664–1671.

8 Postoperative Management

Steven J. Mentzer

Keywords: Postoperative management, thoracic duct injury, vocal cord paralysis, pulmonary edema after lobectomy, pulmonary embolism, deep vein thrombosis, esophageal anastomotic leak, bronchopleural fistula, air leak, fluid management, extubation, pain, aspiration, ventilation, atrial fibrillation

Postoperative care of the thoracic surgery patient requires an active rehabilitative approach. Both the type of surgical procedure and the underlying disease can present a significant challenge to postoperative management. An illustration of this approach is early ambulation after surgery. Early postoperative ambulation confers multiple systemic benefits in any surgical setting but is uniquely valuable to the recovering thoracic surgery patient (Table 8-1). Ambulation promotes airway clearance and decreases the risk of pneumonia. These benefits are amplified in patients who have surgically related or underlying lung dysfunction. Thus the nature and extent of surgical resection in thoracic patients require a well-trained staff and specialized equipment for monitoring patient status, which together can have a significant impact on morbidity and mortality.

PRINCIPLES OF POSTOPERATIVE CARE

Although many principles of postoperative care in the thoracic surgery population are common to other areas of surgery, there are some important differences. For example, fluid management in thoracic patients differs significantly from strategies used in nonthoracic patients. Lung edema and its effect on pulmonary compliance are closely linked to extracellular fluid volume. Many maneuvers made during thoracic surgery result in an increase in lung water. To compensate, it may be appropriate to restrict fluid administration postoperatively. In general, minimizing total body water improves pulmonary compliance and overall lung function.

Mediastinal dissection, whether for mediastinal tumor or esophageal surgery, can be associated with idiopathic pleural and pericardial effusions. Similarly, esophageal surgery, whether for motility disorder, reflux disease, or tumor, is associated with an increased risk for aspiration pneumonia. An additional consequence of esophagectomy is that it entails a complete vagotomy. In the acute setting, the complete vagotomy may result in prolonged dysmotility, enhancing the risk of malnutrition and even aspiration.

Table 8-1

BRAT STAGING PROTOCOL

STAGE	ACTIVITY	ROOM AIR O_2 SATURATION LTP	ROOM AIR O_2 SATURATION NON-LTP
0	Resting	<85	<90
1	Resting	>85	>90
2	Sitting	>85	>90
3	Standing	>85	>90
4	Walking 1–6 minutes	>85	>90
5	Walking >6 minutes	>85	>90

BRAT, Brigham Room Air Tolerance (BRAT) staging protocol. The BRAT assessment was developed to provide a quantifiable measurement of a patient's oxygen saturation level during physical activity. The BRAT stage is determined daily and documented on the patient flow sheet.; LTP, lung transplant patient.

The range of issues that affect the recovery period include extubation, pain, air leak/chest tube management, fluid management, aspiration, ventilation, and the prevention of atrial fibrillation or pulmonary embolism. Specific complications related to a particular thoracic procedure may involve thoracic duct injury, vocal cord paralysis, pulmonary edema after lobectomy, esophageal anastomotic leak, and bronchopleural fistula.

Extubation

Early extubation is the overriding goal of thoracic anesthesia and should be performed immediately after the surgical procedure. Immediate extubation not only improves patient mobilization but also promotes airway clearance. In rare circumstances, it may be beneficial to ventilate the postoperative patient overnight. Indications for postoperative ventilation include (1) bleeding that requires large-volume resuscitation, (2) inadequate pain control requiring high-dose parenteral narcotics, (3) decortication or visceral pleurectomy, and (4) a high-risk airway.

Pain

Postoperative pain control is essential for recovery, particularly in patients undergoing thoracotomy or sternotomy. For patients with severely impaired lung function, a preoperative epidural catheter is often indicated, even for thoracoscopic procedures. Chest wall pain can result in a restrictive chest wall and low lung volumes. Diminished forced vital capacity (FVC) and functional residual capacity (FRC) lead to fatigue and eventual hypoxemia. To prevent this consequence of chest wall pain in high-risk lung surgery patients, epidural catheters or, in selected patients, a paraspinal blockade should be used preemptively. Intravenous analgesics are not an acceptable substitute for epidural analgesia. Intravenous narcotics, whether patient-controlled or controlled by nursing, result in inevitable sedation and potential hypercarbia.

Air Leak/Chest Tube Management

Chest drains are used to evacuate fluid that accumulates in the pleural space after surgery. Blood that collects in the pleural space needs to be evacuated because it may compromise lung function. Similarly, air in the pleural space indicates that the lung is inadequately filling the hemithorax, causing a proportionate impairment in lung function.

The amount of suction applied to the chest tube should be the minimum required to obtain full expansion of the lung. Too much suction may exclude the chest tube if locally compliant tissue occludes the holes of the tube. The chest tube also may be excluded if it is poorly positioned, such as in a fissure or in the lateral pleural space. Owing to the geometry of the thorax and lung, at least one chest tube should be placed in the apical thorax to facilitate optimal cephalad expansion of the lung and maintain control of the apical space. Often a basilar tube is also used to complement the apical tube and prevent the accumulation of subpulmonic air or fluid.

Pleural suction, usually applied using a pleural drainage unit, should also be minimized to limit airflow through the pleural space. Depending on the location of the pleural drain relative to the air leak, increasing the suction simply may increase the leak volume. A large ongoing air leak eventually will result in bacterial contamination as oral flora are entrained through the lung and deposited in the pleural space.

Proper chest tube management requires the recognition of several typical clinical situations:

- *Large swings in the water seal chamber.* Tidal ventilation results in big swings in the chest tube water seal when there is a large residual pleural space. The chest contains relatively compliant structures. Therefore, the larger the space, the bigger is the swing. A large swing in the water seal chamber may reflect significant atelectasis or volume loss in the remaining lung.
- *Chest tube not draining a pneumothorax.* The presence of a "paradoxical" pneumothorax implies one of two easily distinguishable clinical scenarios: (1) the unrecognized loss of pleural suction or (2) an air leak sufficiently large to overwhelm the suction provided by the pleural drainage unit. When there is a sudden loss of suction, it is commonly due to compression of the tube by either the patient or the wheel of the bed. An uncontrolled air leak of approximately 50 L/min usually indicates a systemic disconnection or, more ominously, a central airway communication.
- *Accumulation of pleural air with decreasing vacuum.* When weaning the patient off chest tube suction, one should routinely check for the accumulation of pleural air. This "functional test" occasionally involves increasing the amount of applied vacuum. A rush of air through the drainage system at a higher suction setting implies that the previous setting was inadequate; that is, air was inappropriately accumulating at the lower setting. This test is far more sensitive than chest x-ray to determine the appropriateness of discontinuing suction (so-called water seal).
- *Small or intermittent air leak.* The presence of a very small or intermittent air leak can be difficult to detect. One approach is to reconnect the suction device while the water seal chamber is observed carefully. A rush of air suggests that air was accumulating in the pleural space. A related approach is to clamp the chest tube for a period of time, place the tube back on suction, and then release the clamp while observing the water seal chamber.

A CT scan of the chest may be needed to determine the amount of air in the thoracic cavity and assess the relative advantage of placing additional chest drains (Fig. 8-1).

Fluid Management

Intraoperative fluid management is critical to maintaining lung compliance. Injudicious fluid administration combined with surgical trauma may lead to a loss of pulmonary compliance and impaired postoperative ventilation. Patients with impaired lung function may require ventilatory support, but ventilation should be avoided whenever possible, because mechanical ventilation can cause a separate set of complications.

Postoperative lung edema and pulmonary compliance are closely related to extracellular fluid volume. This is particularly

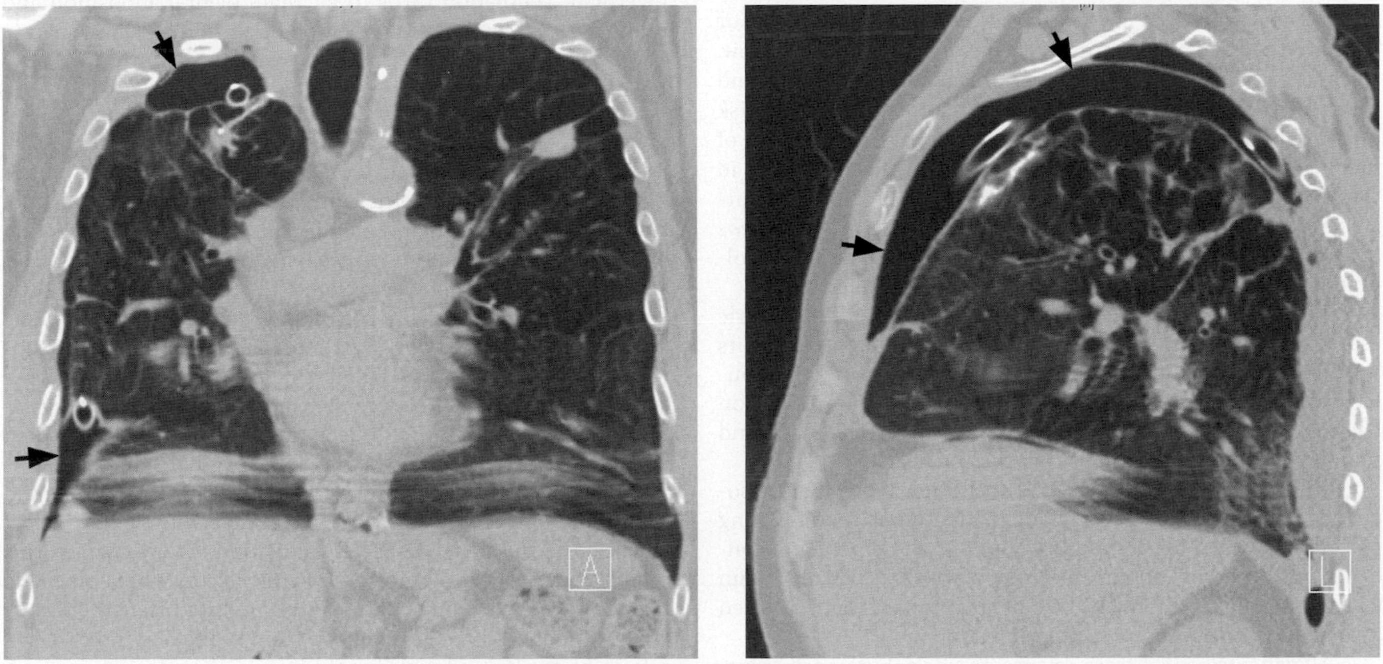

A B

Figure 8-1. Chest CT scans showing the presence of intrathoracic air on coronal (*A*) and sagittal (*B*) views.

so in patients recovering from pulmonary resection, where lung tissues have been insulted from the surgical procedure itself. Fluid volumes must be monitored closely. Generally speaking, anything that can be done to minimize total body water in the recovery period will improve pulmonary compliance and overall lung function. Fluid management also plays a role in the surgical resection of mediastinal tumors because mediastinal dissection can be associated with idiopathic pleural or pericardial effusion.

Aspiration

The risk for aspiration pneumonia is particularly high in individuals undergoing esophageal surgery, whether for a motility disorder, reflux disease, or esophageal tumor. Complete vagotomy performed in conjunction with esophagectomy in the acute setting may result in prolonged dysmotility, which enhances the risk of malnutrition and aspiration.

Aspiration causes the tracheobronchial tree to be contaminated with material from the upper digestive tract. The two primary sources of aspirated substances are the oropharynx and the stomach. Oropharyngeal aspiration commonly results in bacterial contamination by anaerobic organisms, alone or in combination with aerobic and/or microaerophilic organisms. In most intensive care settings, the pathogens are hospital-acquired flora that disseminate via oropharyngeal colonization (e.g., enteric gram-negative bacteria and staphylococci).

The aspiration of gastric contents can result in chemical pneumonitis. The degree of pulmonary parenchymal injury depends on the chemical composition and volume of the aspirated material. Even small volumes of aspirated fluid with a pH less than 2.5 have been associated with severe chemical pneumonitis (Mendelson syndrome).[1]

Oropharyngeal and small-volume gastric aspiration is a common event in healthy individuals. The aspirated material is cleared by airflow (e.g., cough), mucociliary action, and pulmonary phagocytes. A major contributor to airway clearance is sustained airflow. Effective airflow depends on unobstructed airways and adequate lung volumes. Endotracheal tubes or mucus impaction are common reasons for inadequate airflow. Ventilator-associated pneumonias are a well-established and dangerous consequence of prolonged intubation.[2] The risk of pneumonia is likely due to both the relative obstruction of mucociliary clearance and the presence of artificial surfaces in the airway. (Bacterial adherence, the so-called biofilm, is a characteristic of many species of bacteria, including *Pseudomonas aeruginosa* and *Staphylococcus aureus.*) Inadequate lung volumes result from recumbent posture and immobilization.

The treatment for oropharyngeal and small-volume gastric aspiration is mobilization and ambulation. Ambulation recruits lung volumes and improves airflow. Patients can be ambulated while requiring some ventilatory support, but extubation has the additional benefit of improving airway clearance and removing artificial surfaces within the trachea.

Because large-volume gastric aspiration typically is associated with acute respiratory failure, treatment requires long periods of intubation, ventilatory support, and emergent bronchoscopy. Broad-spectrum antibiotic coverage is usually begun at the time of aspiration, because the pulmonary injury is often associated with subsequent superinfection.

All patients benefit from reverse Trendelenburg positioning, which tilts the entire plane of the bed such that the head is elevated with respect to the legs (Fig. 8-2). Merely raising the head end of the bed by 30 degrees is inadequate because it is difficult to maintain the patient in this position and can even increase intraabdominal pressure. Patients who have had a left pneumonectomy are at particular risk for aspiration. The elevated left hemidiaphragm compromises hiatal antireflux mechanisms, and the single remaining lung makes any aspiration life threatening. Other patients at high risk for aspiration are esophagectomy patients. These patients may have prolonged gastrointestinal dysmotility because of acute thoracic vagotomy. To improve drainage of the gastric interposition graft, a pyloroplasty usually is performed,[3] and some type of tube compression is often required for up to a week after surgery.

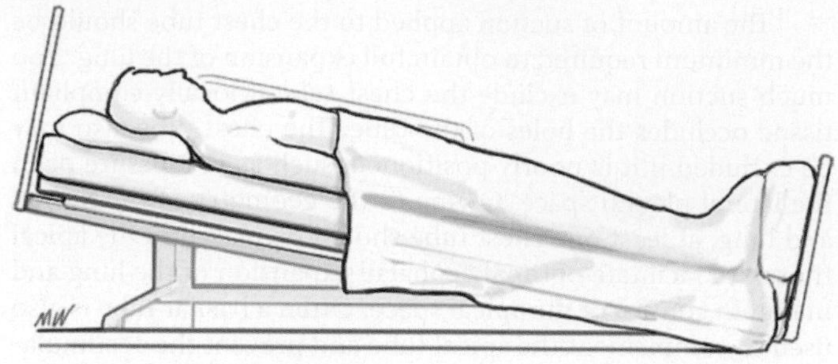

Figure 8-2. Reverse Trendelenburg position.

Ventilation

In rare circumstances, it may be beneficial or necessary to ventilate the postoperative patient overnight. Indications for postoperative ventilation include (1) a high-risk airway, (2) bleeding requiring large-volume replacement, (3) inadequate pain control requiring high-dose parenteral narcotics, and (4) decortication or visceral pleurectomy.

Postoperative ventilation can be beneficial to patients undergoing decortication or visceral pleurectomy. Both procedures result in a loss of lung compliance secondary to surgical trauma to the parenchyma. In addition, these procedures are often associated with a bloody pleural space and several days of air leak. Overnight ventilation helps to facilitate pleural apposition and minimize the accumulation of blood or air in the pleural space.

Atrial Fibrillation

Cardiac myocytes undergo transient depolarization and repolarization that is triggered by external (e.g., nerve depolarization) or intracellular stimulation. The cardiac action potential is distinct from those found in nerve or muscle cells. The cardiac action potential is several hundred times longer (200–400 ms), and calcium plays a role in depolarization (Fig. 8-3).

Atrial fibrillation is a common complication of thoracic surgery. Thirty percent of all patients who undergo major thoracic surgery develop atrial dysrhythmias. Almost all these arrhythmias present between 24 and 96 hours after surgery. The mechanism of atrial fibrillation is unknown, but high endogenous catecholamine levels appear to participate.[4]

Almost all patients undergoing thoracic surgery should receive perioperative prophylactic treatment with a beta blocker, because the frequency of atrial fibrillation is very high in this population. Exclusion criteria for cardioselective beta blockade include severe cardiomyopathy and rare drug insensitivities. A trial of preoperative beta-blocker therapy may be indicated in selected patients to determine the appropriate dosing.

In the acute setting, the initial evaluation of atrial fibrillation should focus on (1) treatment of precipitating factors and (2) rate control.[4] Precipitating factors include electrolyte abnormalities,

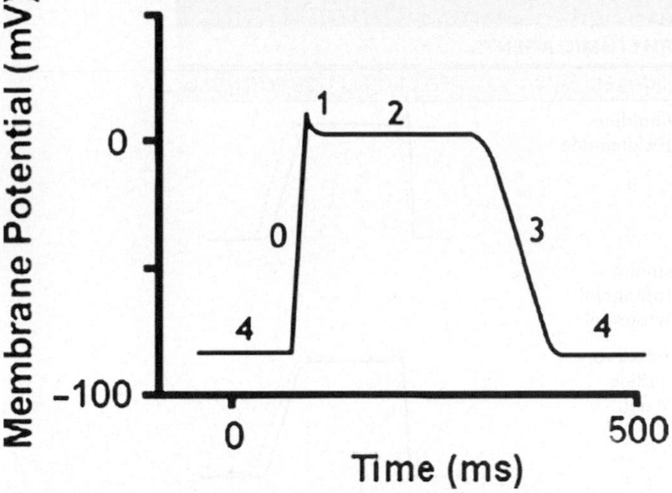

Figure 8-3. The cardiac action potential consists of five phases. Phase 4 is a resting membrane potential. Phase 0 is the rapid depolarization caused by a transient increase in fast Na^+ channel conductance. Phase 1 represents an initial repolarization that is caused by the opening of a special type of K^+ channel. Phase 2 reflects a large increase in calcium conductance. Phase 3 occurs with an increase in K^+ conductance.

high catecholamine states secondary to pain, and the administration of arrhythmogenic agents (e.g., dopamine or epinephrine).

Supported by clinical trials in nonsurgical settings (e.g., AFFIRM[5] and RACE[6]), the treatment of thoracic surgery patients should emphasize rate control over rhythm control. Acute rhythm control is rarely successful in the immediate postoperative period. Potential reasons for the failure of rhythm control include high endogenous catecholamine levels related to volume depletion and pain. Further, local inflammation after intrapericardial dissection may prevent the return to sinus rhythm. Despite problems with rhythm control in the first week, almost all patients revert to stable spontaneous sinus rhythm within 6 weeks of surgery.

Rapid atrial fibrillation can lead to hyperperfusion pulmonary edema, an important reason to emphasize rate control. In some patients, rapid atrial fibrillation is associated with a fall in cardiac output. This may increase central venous pressures and slightly increase lung water but is not a life-threatening emergency. In contrast, other patients have increased cardiac output caused by an increase in intraventricular conduction. If these patients have a limited vascular bed because of a pneumonectomy or other surgical resection, they may rapidly develop pulmonary edema (Fig. 8-4). The clinical spiral believed to be

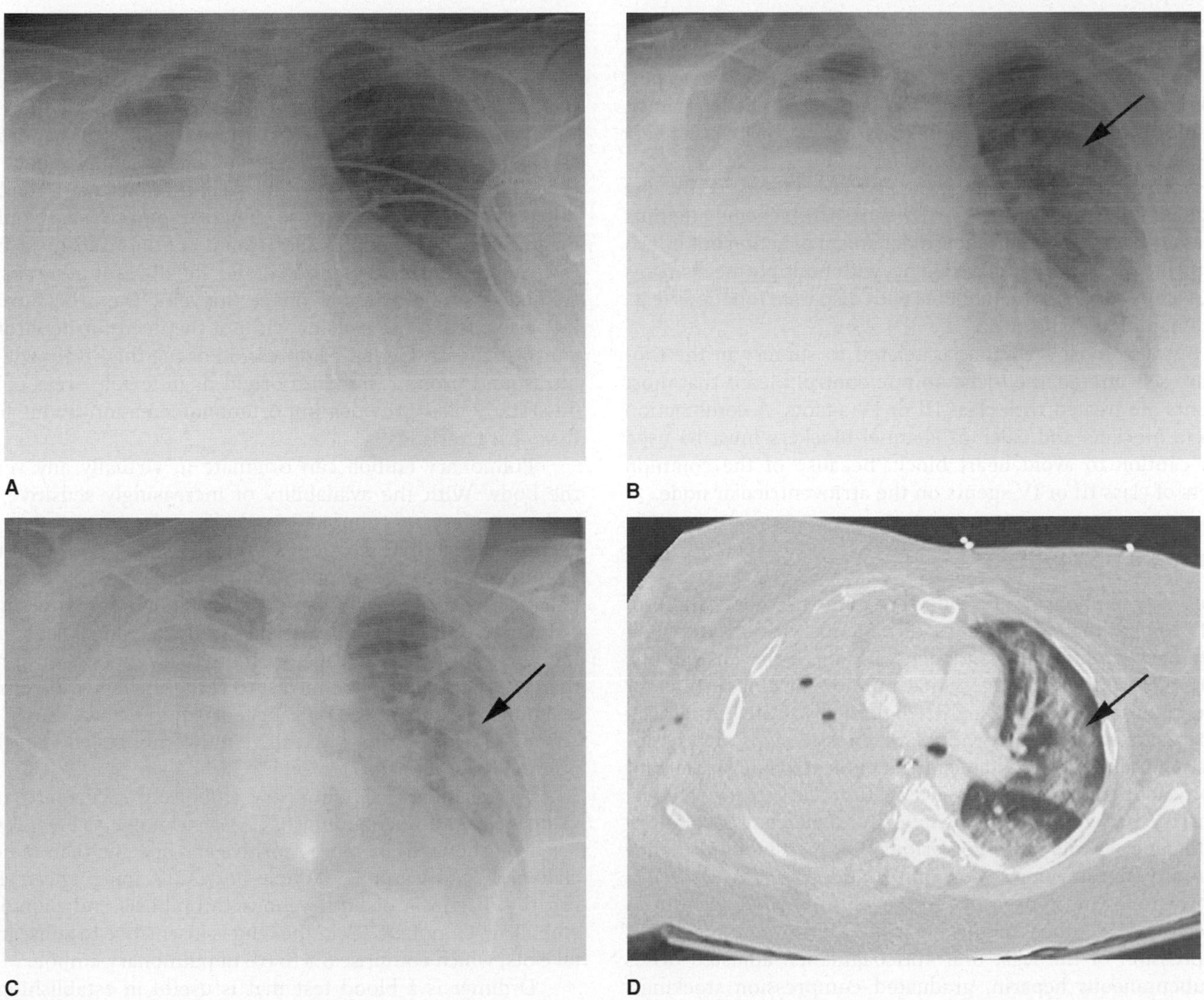

Figure 8-4. This patient developed hyperperfusion pulmonary edema within 4 hours of pneumonectomy and rapid atrial fibrillation within 24 hours. The chest X-rays show the lungs at 1 hour (*A*), 4 hours (*B*) and 8 hours (*C*) after surgery. The CT scan demonstrates the pulmonary edema 12 hours (*D*) after surgery. The patient responded to rate control and diuresis.

Table 8-2

VAUGHAN WILLIAMS CLASSIFICATION OF ANTIARRHYTHMIC AGENTS

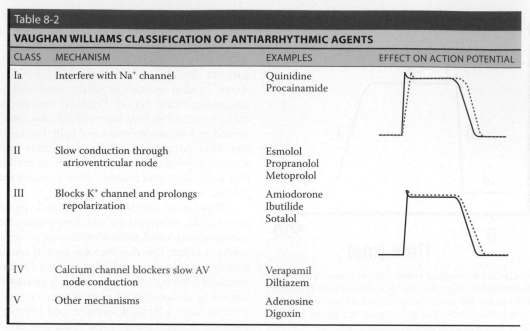

CLASS	MECHANISM	EXAMPLES	EFFECT ON ACTION POTENTIAL
Ia	Interfere with Na^+ channel	Quinidine Procainamide	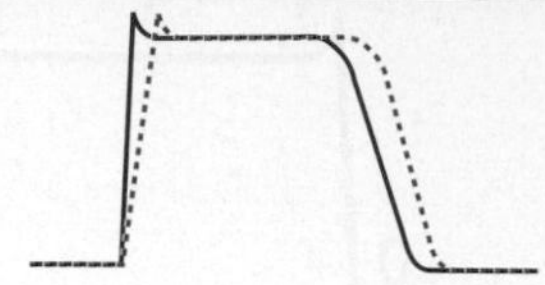
II	Slow conduction through atrioventricular node	Esmolol Propranolol Metoprolol	
III	Blocks K^+ channel and prolongs repolarization	Amiodorone Ibutilide Sotalol	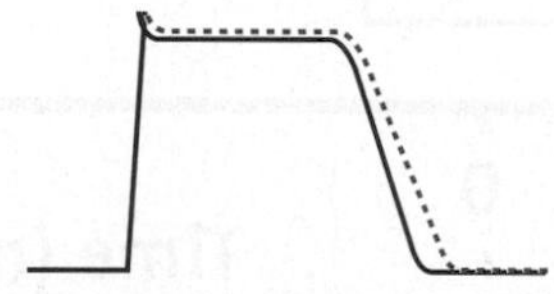
IV	Calcium channel blockers slow AV node conduction	Verapamil Diltiazem	
V	Other mechanisms	Adenosine Digoxin	

Source: From Hagens VE, Ranchor AV, Van Sonderen E, et al. Effect of rate or rhythm control on quality of life in persistent atrial fibrillation. Results from the Rate Control Versus Electrical Cardioversion (RACE) Study. *J Am Coll Cardiol.* 2004;43(2):241–247.

related to plasma ultrafiltration in excess of oncotic reabsorption or lymphatic drainage results in rapidly progressive pulmonary edema. The treatment is rapid control of heart rate. This may even require the administration of a short-acting beta blocker such as esmolol.

Antiarrhythmic agents typically are classified by the Vaughan Williams classification system. This scheme attempts to classify agents based on their mechanism of action but is limited by the need to account for agents with multiple mechanisms (e.g., sotalol) or active metabolites with disparate functions (e.g., procainamide)[7] (Table 8-2).

Because most arrhythmias related to surgery in the thorax are self-limited, the focus on rate control means that most patients are treated with class III or IV agents. A combination of beta blockers and calcium channel blockers must be used with caution to avoid heart block, because of the common effects of class III or IV agents on the atrioventricular node.

Pulmonary Embolism

Pulmonary embolism is a life-threatening complication of DVT. Approximately one-third of patients with an untreated pulmonary embolism eventually will die from an embolic event. Autopsy series suggest that pulmonary embolism is far more common than is recognized clinically. Clot in the deep venous system may not produce diagnostic signs and symptoms. The subtleties of establishing a clinical diagnosis warrant prophylactic treatment for DVT in all thoracic surgery patients. High-risk patients with any clinically significant respiratory insufficiency should undergo periodic noninvasive surveillance by noninvasive imaging.

The following approaches to preventing DVT have proven value: low-dose subcutaneous heparin, intermittent pneumatic compression of the legs, oral anticoagulants, adjusted doses of subcutaneous heparin, graduated compression stockings, and low-molecular-weight heparin. Antiplatelet agents such as aspirin are less effective for preventing DVT. Patients at high risk for DVT include those with any of the following characteristics: age over 60 years, obesity, malignancy, surgery, immobility, pregnancy, and active phlebitis or a history of prior DVT.

Venography cannot be performed repeatedly, and some studies indicate that the radiographic dye actually may promote blood clot formation. These limitations have rendered duplex ultrasound the most effective noninvasive tool for diagnosing DVT.[8] Duplex ultrasound can be used most effectively to diagnosis thigh blood clots. The ultrasound uses high-frequency sound waves to image the vein. The procedure can be performed at the bedside without the need for nephrotoxic contrast agents. Gentle compression of the thigh vein with the ultrasound probe can identify rigid or inflexible areas of clot. This study also provides important information about blood flow characteristics.

Pulmonary emboli can originate in virtually any vein in the body. With the availability of increasingly sensitive procedures to test for pulmonary embolism, the current data suggest that nearly every patient with a large vein thrombosis will have some evidence of pulmonary embolism. Approximately half these patients will have no clinical symptoms to suggest pulmonary embolism. Clot arising in the popliteal segment of the femoral vein is the cause of pulmonary embolism in more than 60% of patients. In contrast to earlier beliefs, calf veins are a significant source of DVT. Recent studies have shown that 33% to 46% of patients with calf vein thromboses will develop a pulmonary embolism.

The diagnosis of pulmonary embolism is currently made using helical CT angiography (CTA), also known as PE-CT. CTA has been shown to be more sensitive and specific than radionuclide perfusion scanning.[9] Whole-body CTA imaging can establish the diagnosis of both venous thrombosis and pulmonary embolism. Of note, CTA in the lung is insensitive to subsegmental clots, which comprise 3% to 6% of pulmonary emboli.

D-dimer is a blood test that is useful in establishing the diagnosis of pulmonary embolism as well as DVT, acute myocardial infarction, and disseminated intravascular coagulation.

D-dimer is formed only when fibrin is cross-linked. Therefore, the release of D-dimer fragments in the blood reflects thrombin and plasmin activity.

PROCEDURE-SPECIFIC COMPLICATIONS

Thoracic Duct Injury

The thoracic duct transports lymph from the intraabdominal triangular dilatation called the *cisterna chyli* to the junction of the left subclavian vein with the left internal jugular vein in the neck. Although there are many anatomic variants, the thoracic duct typically ascends along the right side of the thoracic vertebra, crossing to the left side at the level of the subcarinal space.

Thoracic duct fluid is composed of chyle and lymph plasma. Chyle is composed of the long-chain fatty acids that are absorbed in the intestines and then secreted in chylomicrons into the intestinal lymphatics. Lymph plasma is composed of serum electrolytes, a relatively high concentration of protein (particularly albumin), and lymphocytes.

The chylous portion of the thoracic duct leak may not manifest until the patient begins eating. A test for triglycerides is typically abnormal *if the patient is receiving enteral nutrition,* because triglycerides (glycerol plus fatty acids) are the dominant component of chylomicrons. In the absence of enteral feeding, the triglyceride levels will reflect plasma concentrations.

Patients at increased risk for thoracic duct injury include individuals undergoing esophagectomy or extensive extrapleural or mediastinal dissections. The possibility of a thoracic duct injury should be raised when a patient has (1) chest tube output more than 1 L/day and (2) a recent extrapleural or mediastinal dissection.

The diagnosis of thoracic duct leak can be made after the introduction of enteral feedings. The fluid accumulating in the chest has a milky appearance and elevated triglyceride levels.

Treatment of small accessory duct leaks with relatively low output (~1 L/day) can be managed without intervention if adequate nutrition can be maintained. Placing the chest tube on water seal (20 cm H_2O resistance) avoids the vacuum-assisted "sump" created by the chest tube. Increased resistance to lymph flow is believed to encourage lymph flow through existing vessels and decrease drainage.

Persistent outputs of 3 to 5 L/day, however, must be managed aggressively to avoid hypoproteinemia and malnutrition. Although percutaneous decompression or occlusion of the cisterna chyli can be useful, surgical ligation of the main thoracic duct typically is indicated. The duct has valves and myoepithelial elements. Therefore, the fluid may accumulate under considerable pressure. The ligation is best performed as caudally as possible within the right chest, because of the possibility of collateral leaks or "blowouts" proximal to the ligation. The ligation typically is performed with a pledget to prevent injury to the duct. Sclerosis of the pleural space generally is ineffective because of the pressure generated by the thoracic duct. Attempts at sclerosis either fail completely or result in loculated pleural collections.

More recently, thoracic duct embolization has been used to treat chylothoraces. Thoracic duct embolization involves pedal lymphangiography, transabdominal needle puncture of the thoracic duct, and subsequent embolization. Currently, disadvantages of the procedure include prolonged procedure times and variable success rates. A recent review indicates that approximately two-thirds of patients benefit from the procedure, either because the thoracic duct was successfully embolized or because the cisterna chyli was disrupted and presumably decompressed by the procedure. The morbidity and mortality of this procedure appears to be low (<2%).[10]

Vocal Cord Paralysis

The recurrent laryngeal nerve is a branch of the vagus nerve that supplies the motor component of the intrinsic muscles of the larynx and a portion of the cricopharyngeus. The recurrent laryngeal nerve also provides a sensory component to the laryngeal mucosa below the vocal cords.

The recurrent laryngeal nerve takes a different course in each hemithorax. The left recurrent laryngeal nerve passes under the aortic arch and along the tracheoesophageal groove. The right recurrent laryngeal nerve loops under the right subclavian artery and ascends to the larynx with a more lateral course than the left nerve (Fig. 8-5).

The left recurrent laryngeal nerve is the nerve most commonly injured in thoracic surgical procedures. The left recurrent laryngeal nerve typically is injured during cervical mediastinoscopy or esophagectomy procedures. Nerve injuries during mediastinoscopy are caused by direct trauma to the nerve or the ill-advised use of electrocautery during the dissection of 2 or 4 L lymph nodes. Similarly, recurrent laryngeal nerve injuries during esophagectomy are associated with excessive traction or direct trauma.

The diagnosis of vocal cord paralysis may be delayed because of vocal cord edema in the immediate postoperative period. Usually within 24 hours a patient with vocal cord paralysis will demonstrate a weak voice and unusual effort required with phonation.

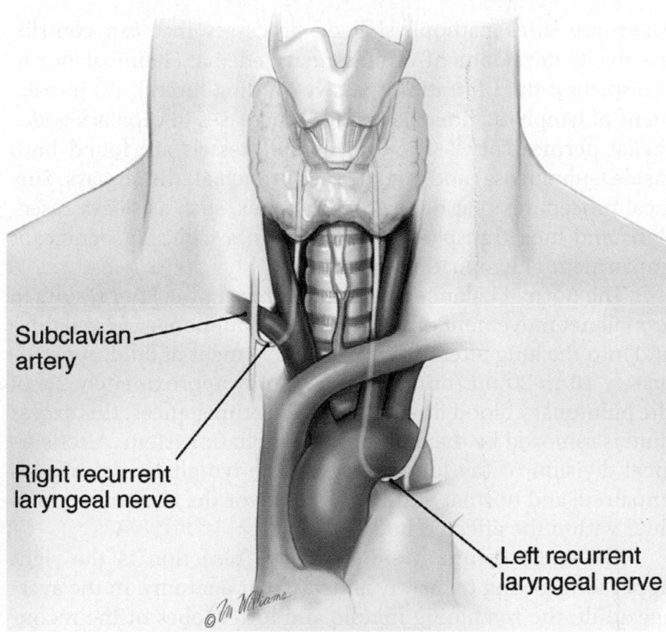

Figure 8-5. The left recurrent laryngeal nerve passes under the aortic arch along the tracheoesophageal groove. The right recurrent laryngeal nerve loops under the right subclavian artery and ascends to the larynx with a more lateral course than the left nerve.

The configuration and mobility of the vocal cords are best evaluated using a fiberoptic laryngoscopy. The vocal cord and arytenoid are immobile on the paralyzed side, resulting in a glottal gap with phonation. Although the paralyzed vocal cord may have a variable position, paralyzed vocal cords typically are abducted 1.5 to 2 mm from the midline. In unusual circumstances, typically those associated with traumatic intubations, vocal cord dysfunction is a consequence of subluxation of the arytenoid.

Spirometry shows abnormalities in the patient's flow-volume loop. Patients with vocal cord paralysis may show blunting or truncation of the inspiratory loop—evidence of extrathoracic airflow obstruction.

In addition to the fatigue associated with ineffectual phonation, vocal cord paralysis is associated with aspiration. In particular, liquids are aspirated during the pharyngeal phase of swallowing. Post-swallow aspiration also may occur when the residual food bolus is retained in the piriform sinus on the paralyzed side. The most telling sign of vocal cord paralysis in the thoracic surgical patient is an ineffective cough.

Fatigue and airway clearance are the primary indications for treatment of vocal cord paralysis in the early postoperative period. There are two main approaches to treating vocal cord paralysis.

- An injection of a temporary or absorbable material is used to stiffen and medialize the vocal cord because some patients may recover nerve function spontaneously. The injection can be performed through a laryngoscope under local anesthesia. Teflon also can be injected, but this procedure should be considered permanent.
- A more definitive solution is a lateral laryngeal implant. This procedure requires an external neck incision, but it can be performed under local anesthesia. The lateral laryngeal implant has a high success rate but is potentially reversible.

Pulmonary Edema After Sleeve Lobectomy

There are three pathophysiologic processes that can contribute to the development of pulmonary edema: (1) imbalance in transpleural fluid filtration (passive Starling forces), (2) impairment of lymphatic drainage, and (3) increases in capillary endothelial permeability.[11] The lung lymph vessels are found both inside (submucosa) and outside (peribronchial) the airways. Surgical procedures that divide the bronchus, such as sleeve resections and lung transplantation, result in a clinically significant impairment of lymphatic drainage.

The normal balance of Starling forces in the lung results in a small net movement of fluid out of the pulmonary vasculature and into the lung interstitium. This movement of fluid, approximately 10 to 20 mL/min, represents only approximately 2% of the pulmonary blood flow. In normal circumstances, this excess fluid is removed by the pulmonary lymphatic system. After surgical division of the lung, however, the lymphatic drainage is impaired, and normal Starling forces favor the accumulation of fluid within the affected lung.

The most common site of sleeve resection is the right upper lobe, owing to airway and vascular anatomy. In the average adult, the remaining middle and lower lobes of the reconstructed right lung will accumulate approximately 500 mL of lung water within the first 2 days after surgery. This progressive pulmonary edema typically results in unexpected hypoxemia 2 to 3 days after sleeve lobectomy. In some patients, hypoxic vasoconstriction of the affected lung results in an apparent "hyperperfusion" pulmonary edema of the contralateral lung.

The treatment of pulmonary edema relies on active reversal of passive Starling forces, namely, a diuresis sufficiently vigorous to cause a net movement of fluid out of the lung interstitium and into the vasculature. Empirical observations after lung transplantation suggest that passive Starling forces will reverse after an acute diuresis equivalent to 20% of the patient's circulating blood volume. In the average 70-kg patient, the total blood volume is 5 L (65 mL/kg for females and 75 mL/kg for males). As a consequence, treatment of pulmonary edema secondary to lymphatic impairment requires a diuresis of approximately 250 mL/h for 4 hours. The clinical complaint of thirst and a serum sodium concentration in the low 140s corroborate the hemoconcentration.

Esophageal Anastomotic Leak

Leaks from a gastroesophageal anastomosis occur most commonly within the first 48 hours or 7 to 10 days after esophagectomy. Early leaks typically reflect technical complications at the time of surgery. Late anastomotic leaks reflect ischemia of the gastric (or colonic) interposition graft. Ischemic complications are more likely to occur in cervical esophageal anastomoses (20%) than in intrathoracic anastomoses (1%).

Early anastomotic failures are characterized by the drainage of bilious material from the chest drain or the rapid accumulation of a pleural effusion. Accompanying these ominous signs are fever, leukocytosis, and the toxicity of acute mediastinitis.

Late anastomotic leaks usually are associated with subtle signs and symptoms. A slight increase in the blood leukocyte count and tenderness in the neck incision may herald an anastomotic leak. Although cervical esophageal anastomoses are more commonly associated with leaks, these can be drained quite easily by opening up the skin of the neck incision. Prompt drainage of the cervical collection can avoid the septic complications of the leak. Anastomotic leaks appear to be associated with a higher incidence of anastomotic stricture, but a cervical leak is usually not life threatening.

Bronchopleural Fistula

Bronchopleural fistulas are communications between the central airways and the pleural space. Although all air leaks technically communicate with the central airways, the term *bronchopleural fistula* usually is reserved for the breakdown of a surgical closure of the lobar or mainstem bronchus.

After pulmonary resection, most surgeons test their bronchial closure by submerging the stump and looking for air bubbles during active ventilation. Consequently, early technical failures of stump closure are rare. A more common complication is the breakdown of a pneumonectomy stump in the weeks to months after surgery. The mechanism of bronchopleural fistula in most cases is believed to be the ischemic breakdown of the stump closure with a secondary infection of the distal pleural space. (Supporting this mechanism is the observation that longer stumps are generally located in the "watershed" region of bronchial artery perfusion.) Patients typically present with increasing dyspnea, a new infiltrate in the remaining lung, and a decrease in the air–fluid level in the pneumonectomy space. On questioning, the patient may report brown or rust-colored sputum.

A related complication, but with a more insidious presentation, is the gradual wasting and cachexia associated with chronic empyema. Patients with a chronic pneumonectomy space infection may be afebrile and have a normal leukocyte count. It is not uncommon for a medical oncologist to assume that the patient has a recurrent cancer.

Bronchopleural fistula is treated initially by draining the pneumonectomy space to prevent massive aspiration. A tube thoracostomy should be placed at or above the level of the pneumonectomy incision to account for the contraction of the pleural space. A useful technique is to direct a right-angled tube into the costophrenic sulcus to optimize drainage of the hemithorax. The procedure should be performed with local anesthesia and spontaneous ventilation.

The suspected fistula should be evaluated by bronchoscopy performed during spontaneous ventilation. Small fistulas may be difficult to see but may be effectively demonstrated by the disappearance of stump fluid during inspection. The space distal to the bronchopleural fistula is, by definition, infected. The use of plugs or glues is rarely helpful because they do not address the primary problem, that is, ischemic breakdown of the airway with secondary space infection. In the setting of a suspected bronchopleural fistula, general anesthesia can be a major risk. General anesthesia and even the positioning of the patient for intubation are associated with increased risk of contamination of the remaining lung. If the pneumonectomy space has been drained, positive-pressure ventilation may be ineffective or result in tension pneumothorax. The loss of effective positive airway pressure in an anesthetized patient will result in a loss of lung volume and progressive hypoxemia. The average length of the right mainstem bronchus is very short (1.3 ± 0.3 cm). Therefore, selective intubation of the mainstem bronchus is only practical with a remaining left lung.

Even when selective intubation is achieved, it is difficult to maintain. The angle and luminal diameter of the left mainstem bronchus result in an intermittent tube obstruction or displacement. In addition, the selective intubation of the left mainstem bronchus requires a 6 F endotracheal tube, which effectively limits bronchoscopic access to the remaining lung.

In the patient with respiratory failure, the management principle is to avoid the circumstance of ongoing soilage of the remaining lung. The problem with tube drainage (with or without irrigation) is that it provides only partial control of the pneumonectomy space. Drainage is limited by the position of the tube or inflammatory loculations within the chest. To ensure adequate drainage and to prevent ongoing contamination of the remaining lung, an open thoracic "window" should be created. A thoracic window or Clagett procedure[12] involves the resection of one or more ribs in the dependent lateral chest wall to facilitate irrigation and packing of the empyema space. In contrast to the Clagett procedure, the Eloesser flap was proposed to facilitate drainage of an empyema in the setting of functioning ipsilateral lung tissue requiring spontaneous ventilation (see Chapter 2).[13]

Positive-pressure ventilation can be maintained in a patient with a large bronchopleural fistula and a thoracic window by tightly packing the chest with rolls of mineral oil-soaked gauze. The chest must be packed tightly. Dressing changes, usually performed once a day, need to be performed expeditiously.

Most surgeons wait 6 weeks to 6 months before closing the window. During that time, nutrition is optimized, and control of the infection is ensured. Ideally, the fistula is healed before closure of the thoracic window. In addition, patients with malignancy should be restaged radiographically. Closure of the chest wall involves rotation of muscle into the chest to facilitate antibiotic delivery and to minimize the residual space.

SUMMARY

Thoracic surgery creates unique physiologic stresses in the immediate postoperative period. Optimal postoperative management relies on multiple pre- and perioperative interventions. Daily preoperative conditioning programs can improve the patient's exercise capacity and facilitate early ambulation after surgery. Early ambulation after surgery promotes airway clearance and decreases the risk of pneumonia. Early mobility also decreases the risk of pulmonary embolus. Careful attention to fluid management can improve pulmonary compliance and gas exchange in the immediate postoperative period. Cardiac rate and rhythm disturbances are a common feature of postoperative management. Other complications can be directly related to the operative thoracic procedure, such as thoracic duct injury, vocal cord paralysis, pulmonary edema after lobectomy, esophageal anastomotic leak, and bronchopleural fistula. Most of these complications are best managed by a well-equipped facility with a highly trained staff.

EDITOR'S COMMENT

This well-written chapter is obligatory reading for everyone involved in the postoperative management of the thoracic surgery patient. In a simple prose style filled with common sense, Dr. Mentzer identifies the most significant risks for patients. The chapter combines scientific knowledge with practical personal experience. The underlying message is clear; aggressively look for early signs of these potential complications and intervene early to prevent tragedy. This philosophy has led an interesting paradox in the modern thoracic surgery literature. Although reported morbidities have increased compared to the literature of 20 years ago, the reported mortalities have dramatically reduced.

—MTJ

References

1. Mendelson CL. The aspiration of stomach contents into the lungs during obstetric anesthesia. *Am J Obstet Gynecol.* 1946;52:191–205.
2. Melsen WG, Rovers MM, Koeman M, et al. Estimating the attributable mortality of ventilator-associated pneumonia from randomized prevention studies. *Crit Care Med.* 2011;39(12):2736–2742.
3. Cheung HC, Siu KF, Wong J. Is pyloroplasty necessary in esophageal replacement by stomach? A prospective, randomized controlled trial. *Surgery.* 1987;102(1):19–24.
4. Dunning J, Treasure T, Versteegh M, et al. Guidelines on the prevention and management of de novo atrial fibrillation after cardiac and thoracic surgery. *Eur J Cardiothorac Surg.* 2006;30(6):852–872.

5. Wyse DG, Waldo AL, DiMarco JP, et al. A comparison of rate control and rhythm control in patients with atrial fibrillation. *N Engl J Med.* 2002; 347(23):1825–1833.
6. Hagens VE, Ranchor AV, Van Sonderen E, et al. Effect of rate or rhythm control on quality of life in persistent atrial fibrillation. Results from the Rate Control Versus Electrical Cardioversion (RACE) Study. *J Am Coll Cardiol.* 2004;43(2):241–247.
7. Vaughan Williams EM. Classification of antiarrhythmic drugs. In: Sandoe E, Flensted-Jansen E, Olesen K, eds. *Symposium on Cardiac Arrhythmias.* Sodertalje, Sweden: AB Astra; 1970:449–472.
8. Duwe KM, Shiau M, Budorick NE, et al. Evaluation of the lower extremity veins in patients with suspected pulmonary embolism: a retrospective comparison of helical CT venography and sonography. 2000 ARRS Executive Council Award I. American Roentgen Ray Society. *AJR Am J Roentgenol.* 2000;175(6):1525–1531.
9. Blachere H, Latrabe V, Montaudon M, et al. Pulmonary embolism revealed on helical CT angiography: comparison with ventilation-perfusion radionuclide lung scanning. *AJR Am J Roentgenol.* 2000;174(4):1041–1047.
10. Marcon F, Irani K, Aquino T, et al. Percutaneous treatment of thoracic duct injuries. *Surg Endosc.* 2011;25(9):2844–2848.
11. Michel RP, Zocchi L, Rossi A, et al. Does interstitial lung edema compress airways and arteries? A morphometric study. *J Appl Physiol.* 1987;62(1):108–115.
12. Clagett OT, Geraci JE. A procedure for the management of postpneumonectomy empyema. *J Thorac Cardiovasc Surg.* 1963;45:141–145.
13. Eloesser L. Of an operation for tuberculous empyema. *Ann Thorac Surg.* 1969;8(4):355–357.

9 Techniques for Pleural Drainage and Chest Tube Management

Ali O.M. Al Dameh, Abraham Lebenthal, and Ciaran J . McNamee

Keywords: Water seal, thoracostomy, pneumothorax, pleural effusion, empyema

The concept of chest tube drainage was first advocated by Hippocrates when he described the treatment of empyema by means of incision, cautery, and insertion of metal tubes.[1] The technique was not widely used until the influenza epidemic of 1917 which saw an increased use of intercostal drainage for postpneumonic empyema.[2] The use of chest tubes was imperative in the management of World War II causalities requiring thoracotomy and was reported in 1922 for post-operative care.[3] The concept of emergency thoracostomy for acute trauma gained wider popularity following the Korean War in 1945.[4] Today the use of chest tubes is part of the day-to-day management of acute trauma and care of thoracic surgery patients.

Chest tubes are indicated for both emergent and elective situations.[4–6] The most common indication for tube thoracostomy is pneumothorax and/or hemothorax. Other indications are summarized in Table 9-1. There are no absolute contraindications to drainage by means of chest tube, especially in the case of life-threatening emergency.[4] Relative contraindications to chest tube insertion include postoperative inflammatory and infective pleural space adhesions, presence of a diaphragmatic hernia, or hepatic hydrothorax with documented coagulopathy.[7]

TECHNIQUE

The essential steps to inserting a pleural drainage tube are summarized in Table 9-2. The technique can also be viewed online.[8] Good insertion technique and appropriate post-insertion care are associated with less morbidity and shorter hospital stays.[9] The most common site of insertion is the "safe triangle," which as the name implies, is the safest entry into the chest.[10,11] The boundaries of this triangle are identified by the anterior border of the latissimus dorsi, the lateral border of the pectoralis major muscle, and a line superior to the horizontal level of the nipple and an apex below the axilla (Fig. 9-1). In this space, the likelihood of damaging vital structures during insertion is considerably low.[12] As the diaphragm can rise to the fifth rib at nipple level during expiration, chest tubes should be placed above this level to avoid inadvertent damage to abdominal structures.

An incision 1.5 to 2 cm in length is made parallel to the rib. A Kelly clamp or an artery forceps is used bluntly to dissect through the subcutaneous layers and intercostal muscles. The path of dissection should aim toward the upper superior intercostal space. A dissection plane is created through the subcutaneous tissue layers and the intercostal muscles on the superior surface of the rib. Adhering to the superior surface will avoid inadvertent injury to the neurovascular bundle located at the inferior surface. The blunt bevel of the dissecting instrument is used to gently puncture through the parietal pleura. Digital penetration (usually with the index finger) is followed to avoid puncturing any adjacent lung tissue. Once entry into the pleura is confirmed, the Kelly clamp is withdrawn and the tube is inserted along the established tract. When thoracostomy is needed to drain an apical pneumothorax, an anticlockwise wrist maneuver will permit the tube to slide away from the fissure and lie in the desired position in the apex of the lung. Mattress or interrupted sutures are used on both sides of the incision to close the ends (Fig. 9-2). The loose ends of the sutures are wrapped around the tube and tied to anchor the tube to the chest wall. The tube is then taped to the side of the patient and wrapped by a petroleum-based gauze dressing. Several pieces of regular sterile gauze and multiple pressure dressings are used to secure the chest tube in place. A chest x-ray is obtained to confirm placement.[13]

Table 9-1 INDICATIONS FOR CHEST TUBE INSERTION
Emergent
Pneumothorax in the setting of:
• Mechanical ventilation
• A large pneumothorax
• Clinically unstable patient
• Tension pneumothorax after emergency decompression
• Chest trauma
• Hemopneumothorax
• Esophageal rupture with evidence of leak into pleural space
Nonemergent
• Malignant pleural effusion
• Treatment with pleurodesis agents
• Pleural effusion
• Parapneumonic effusion or empyema
• Chylothorax
• Postoperative care (e.g., esophagectomy, after coronary bypass, thoracotomy, or lobectomy)

Table 9-2 ESSENTIAL STEPS FOR INSERTING A PLEURAL CHEST TUBE
1. Infiltrate overlying area with local anesthesia
2. Make a 3–4 cm incision through the skin and subcutaneous tissues between the fourth and fifth ribs, parallel to the rib margins
3. Bluntly dissect through the intercostal muscles down to the pleura
4. Insert Kelly clamp through the pleura and spread jaws parallel to the direction of the ribs
5. Introduce forefinger into the thoracic cavity
6. Insert chest tube and secure with nonabsorbable suture

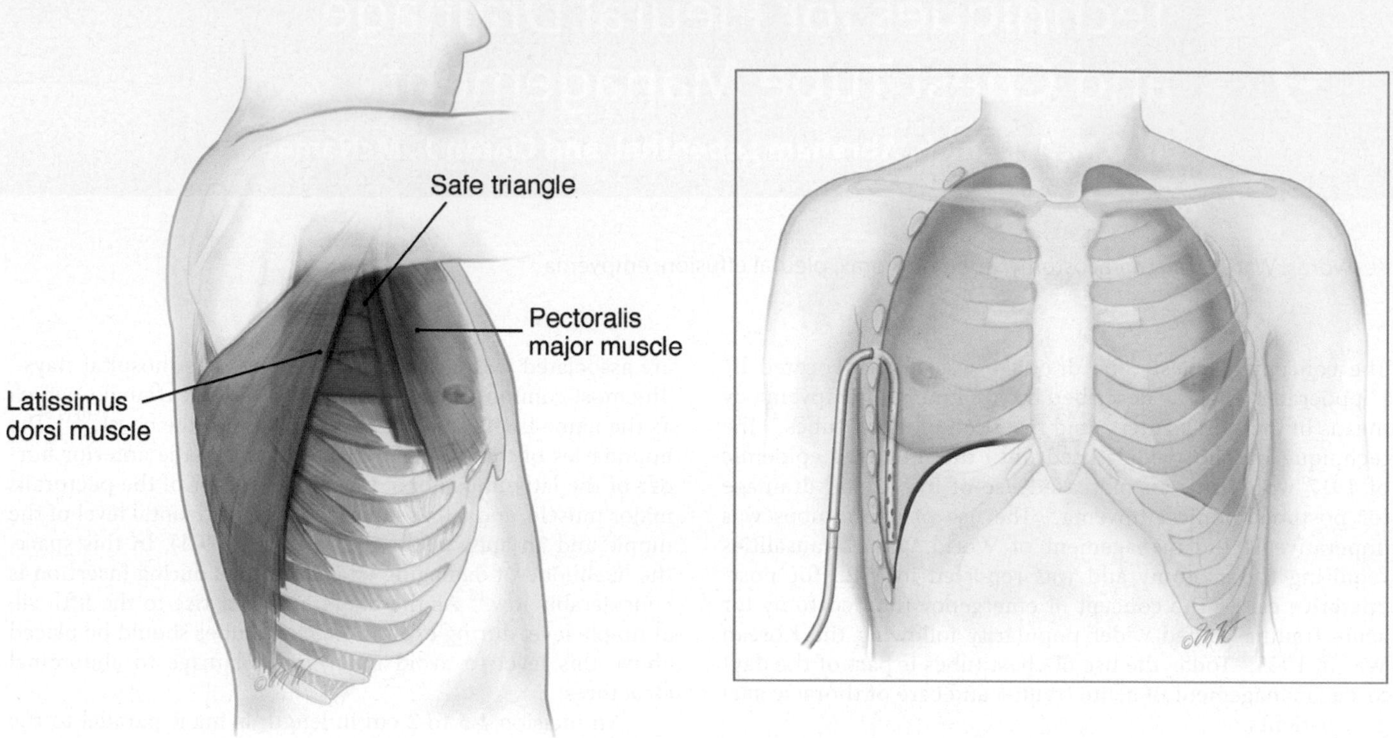

Figure 9-1. The "Safe Triangle" for pleural chest tube insertion.

The tube is then connected to a water seal drainage container. This allows the air and fluid to be evacuated and avoids inadvertent suction into the chest cavity. The water seal container connected to the chest tube also permits one-way movement of air and liquid from the pleural cavity. Traditionally, the underwater seal drainage apparatus comprises a series of up to three reusable glass bottles connected to one another and attached to the chest tube (Fig. 9-3). The water seal drainage container normally is filled with approximately 250 to 350 mL of sterile water to a marked level. The first bottle provides the collection chamber. The second, the water seal valve. It has an afferent tube that is kept below water level. Fluid and air can egress from the tube. The vacuum produced by inhalation draws fluid into the tubing but does not allow air to be re-introduced into the pleural cavity. The intrapleural vacuum can be countered by the application of suction to the third bottle, the suction control. In addition to the afferent and efferent tubes, the suction control bottle has a third tube open to air. The depth at which the tube penetrates below the fluid level determines the degree of suction; hence the familiar measure of surgical suction in centimeters. Currently, commercially available clear plastic disposable containers are used instead. These consist of either a single chamber with an underwater seal (Fig. 9-4) or a three-chamber container with a collection chamber, suction chamber, and water seal chamber in the middle (Fig. 9-5).

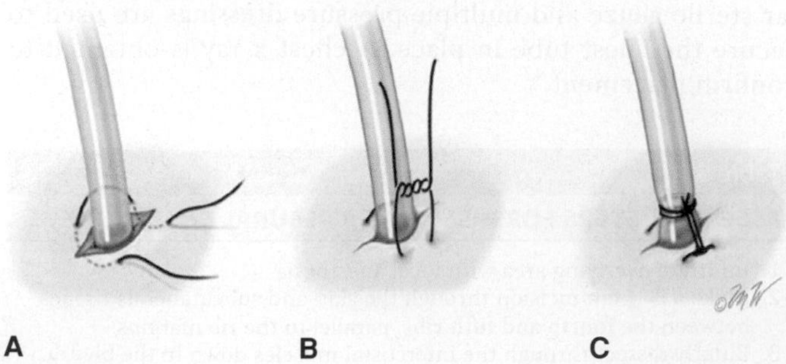

Figure 9-2. Securing the chest drain. The chest tube is secured by placing a stitch around the incision, using heavy suture (0/ or 1/), as shown in (*A*). Mattress or interrupted sutures are used to secure the stitch and both ends of the incision (*B*). The loose ends of the sutures are wrapped around the tube and tied to anchor it to the chest wall (*C*).

COMPLICATIONS

Complications of chest tube insertion are summarized in Table 9-3. The most important complications include bleeding from intercostal artery perforation, perforation of visceral organs (lung, heart, diaphragm, or intra-abdominal organs), and perforation of major vascular structures.[4]

Table 9-3

COMPLICATIONS OF CHEST TUBE INSERTION

1. Intercostal artery perforation
2. Perforation of visceral organs (lung, heart, diaphragm, or intra-abdominal organs)
3. Perforation of major vascular structures (aorta or subclavian vessels)
4. Intercostal neuralgia and trauma of neuromuscular bundles
5. Subcutaneous emphysema
6. Rexpansion pulmonary edema
7. Infection of the drainage site, pneumonia, and empyema
8. Technical problems (intermittent tube blockage with blood clot, pus, or debris, or incorrect positioning of the tube)

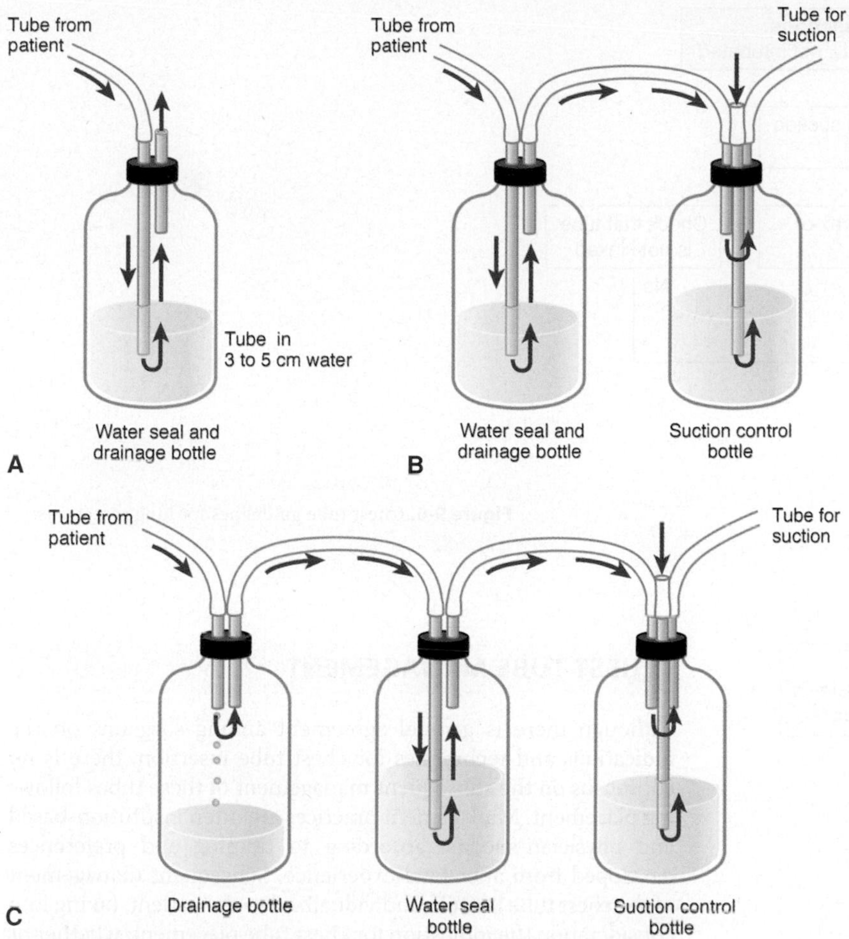

Figure 9-3. A typical water seal drainage system is comprised of up to three reusable glass bottles. In (*A*), a single bottle is used both for collection of the drainage and water seal without suction. In (*B*), a second bottle has been added for suction. In (*C*) three bottles are used, one each for collection, water seal, and suction, respectively.

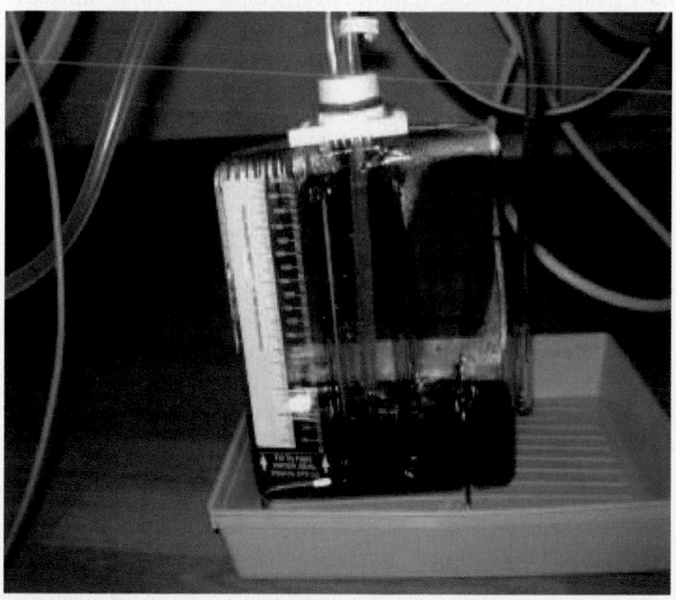

Figure 9-4. A single-chamber chest tube drainage container with markings for a basic underwater seal.

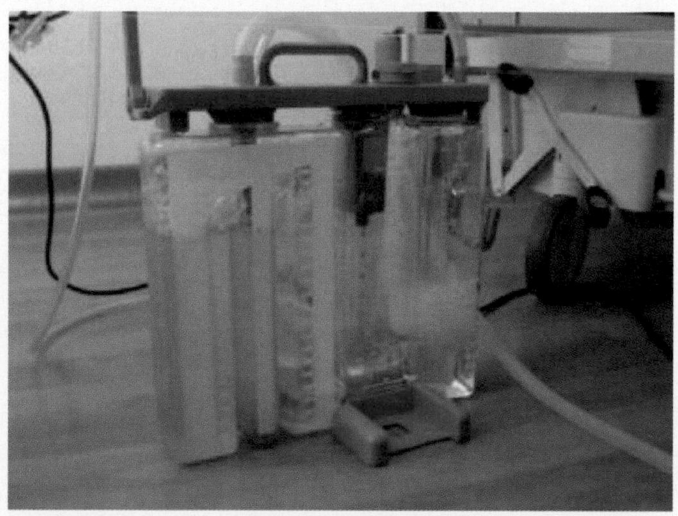

Figure 9-5. A three-chamber chest tube drainage container system.

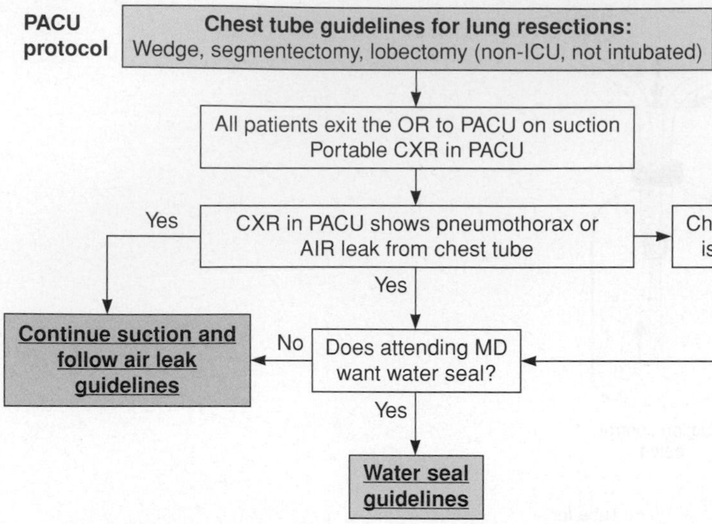

Figure 9-6. Chest tube guidelines for lung resections.

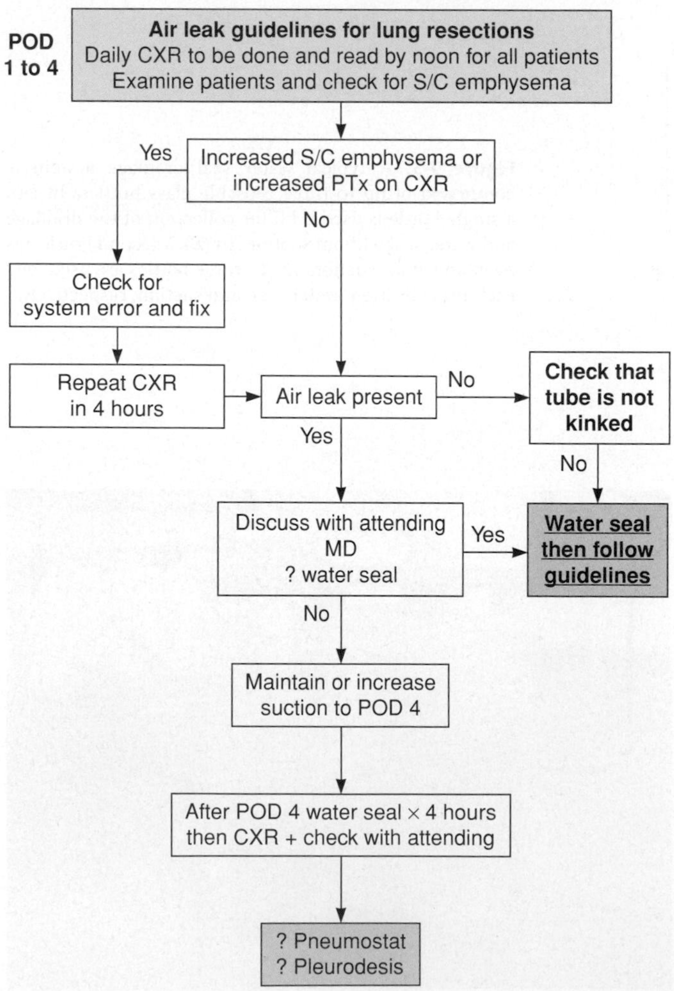

Figure 9-7. Air leak guidelines for lung resections.

CHEST TUBE MANAGEMENT

Although there is general agreement among surgeons on the indications and techniques for chest tube insertion, there is no consensus on the subsequent management of these tubes following placement. Management practices are often institution-based and physician-specific according to training and preferences developed from anecdotal experience. Subsequent management of the chest tube must be individualized to the patient, taking into consideration the indication for chest tube placement, whether or not the patient has had pulmonary resection or is dependent on mechanical ventilation, and if the patient has a bronchopulmonary fistula. Premature removal of the tube, as well as unnecessary delay, leads to increased hospital stays and unjustified costs.

The timing of chest tube removal in regard to drainage volume has been investigated by Younes et al.[14] in a prospective randomized trial. There was no major difference in the rate of fluid accumulation and need for thoracentesis between groups with drainage amounts of ≤100, ≤150, or ≤200 mL/day, respectively. Using a daily threshold of 200 mL could lead to quicker removal of the chest tube, thereby reducing hospitalization time and overall cost. The ideal timing of chest tube removal in regard to the respiratory cycle also has been investigated. A prospective, randomized by Bell and colleagues evaluated whether recurrent pneumothorax was more likely when the chest tube was removed at end-inspiration or end-expiration. This study concluded that the risk of recurrent pneumothorax was similar between both groups and that either method of chest tube removal was safe.[15]

The ideal algorithm has yet to be determined for managing chest tubes. Specifically, wide variation in management practices exist in regard to timing and parameters under which chest tubes should be removed, the best method of removal, and the need for chest x-rays to monitor patients pre- and post-chest tube removal. An algorithm developed for chest tube management at Brigham and Women's is provided in Figures 9-6 to 9-8.

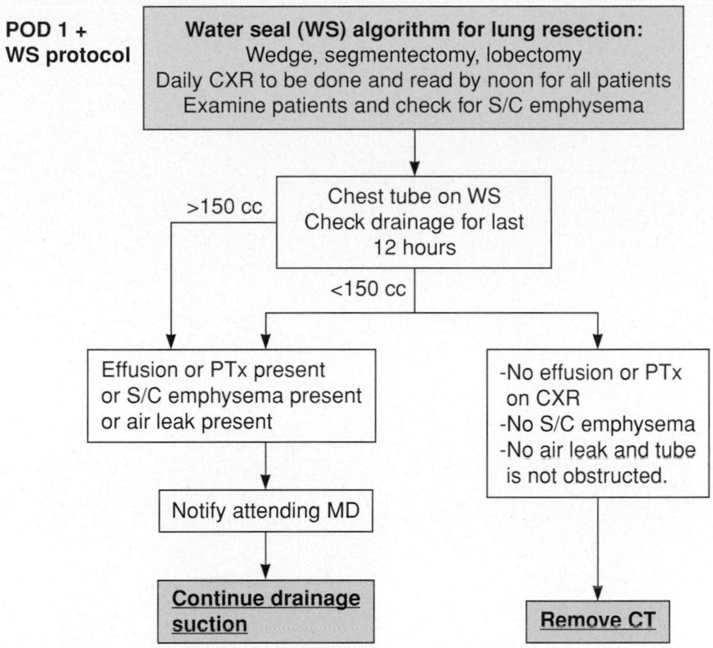

Figure 9-8. Water seal algorithm for lung resections.

EDITOR'S COMMENT

Few aspects of Thoracic Surgery are surrounded with more confusion than chest tube management. Yet, this topic is so important and commonplace we felt justified in adding this chapter to the new edition of the book. We are grateful for the authors for presenting a straightforward and short review to demystify these drains. Chest tubes are actually a surprisingly recent development. The authors explain their history and the physics behind the water seal mechanism. Most importantly, they present (with internet video support) a safe and simple way to place a chest tube. This chapter should be required reading for every resident rotating onto a Thoracic Surgery Service.

—Michael T. Jaklitsch

References

1. Hippocrates. Genuine Works of Hippocrates: Sydenham Society; 1847.
2. Graham E, Bell R. Open pneumothorax: its relation to the treatment of empyema. *Am J Med Sci*. 1918;156:839–871.
3. Lilienthal H. Resection of the lung for supportive infections with a report based on 31 consecutive operative cases in which resection was done or intended. *Ann Surg*. 1922;75:257–320.
4. Miller K, Sahn S. Chest tubes: indications, technique, management and complication. *Chest*. 1987;91:259–264.
5. Tang AT, Velissaris TJ, Weeden DF. An evidence-based approach to drainage of the pleural cavity: evaluation of best practice. *J Eval Clin Pract*. 2002;8:333–340.
6. Laws D, Neville E, Duffy J. BTS guidelines for the insertion of a chest drain. *Thorax*. 2003;58(Suppl 2):ii53–ii59.
7. Runyon B, Greenblatt M, Ming R. Hepatic hydrothorax is a relative contraindication to chest tube insertion. *Am J Gastroenterol*. 1986;81: 566–567.
8. Dev SP, Nascimiento B, Jr., Simone C, et al. Videos in clinical medicine. Chest-tube insertion. *N Engl J Med*. 2007;357:e15.
9. Dordevic I, Stanic V, Nestorovic M, et al. [Failures and complications of thoracic drainage]. *Vojnosanit Pregl*. 2006;63:137–142.
10. Ellis H. The applied anatomy of chest drain insertion. *Br J Hosp Med (Lond)*. 2010;71:M52–M53.
11. Ellis H. The applied anatomy of chest drain insertion. *Br J Hosp Med (Lond)*. 2007;68:M44–M45.
12. Griffiths JR, Roberts N. Do junior doctors know where to insert chest drains safely? *Postgrad Med J*. 2005;81:456–458.
13. Henry M, Arnold T, Harvey J. BTS guidelines for the management of spontaneous pneumothorax. *Thorax*. 2003;58(Suppl 2):ii39–ii52.
14. Younes RN, Gross JL, Aguiar S, et al. When to remove a chest tube? A randomized study with subsequent prospective consecutive validation. *J Am Coll Surg*. 2002;195:658–662.
15. Bell RL, Ovadia P, Abdullah F, et al. Chest tube removal: end-inspiration or end-expiration? *J Trauma*. 2001;50:674–677.

PART 2

ESOPHAGEAL AND PROXIMAL STOMACH MALIGNANCY

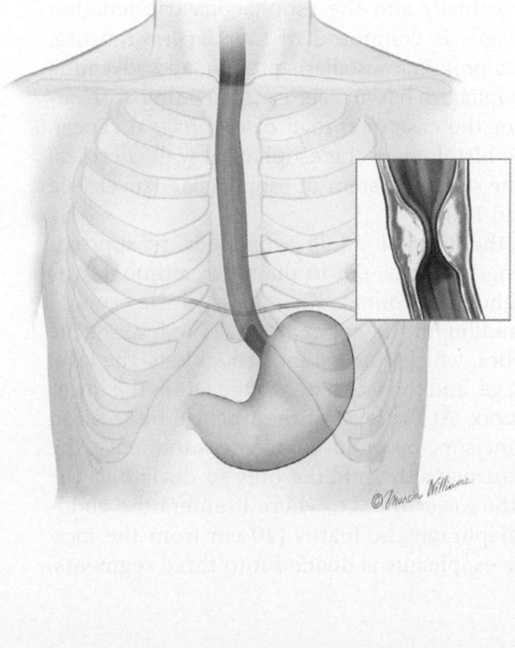

10 Overview of Esophageal and Proximal Stomach Malignancy

Michael I. Ebright and Mark J. Krasna

Keywords: Adenocarcinoma, squamous cell carcinoma, Barrett esophagus, multimodality treatment, esophageal cancer, staging of esophageal cancer

Esophageal cancer is the eighth most frequent cancer worldwide. It is the sixth most common cause of cancer death, accounting for 5.4% of all cancer deaths.[1] Although the annual incidence of esophageal cancer in the United States is 4.5 per 100,000, some of the highest incidences are found in Asia, with roughly 100 per 100,000 individuals affected in the Linxian Province of central China.[2,3] Esophageal cancer remains one of the most lethal of all malignancies, with incidence and mortality rates roughly equal. Once a diagnosis is established, the prognosis is dismal, with a 5-year survival rate of 17%.[4] The results of single-modality treatment have been poor, with the exception of surgery for early esophageal cancer. More recently, neoadjuvant chemotherapy, radiotherapy, and combined chemoradiation therapy have been added as treatment modalities to enhance local control, increase resectability rates, and improve disease-free survival.[5] The initial results of these multimodality treatments have been encouraging. Since management of esophageal cancer and survival of patients is stage dependent, accuracy of clinical staging is vital. An array of technologies such as CT, MRI, and PET of the esophagus, as well as endoscopic ultrasound (EUS) and minimally invasive thoracoscopic/laparoscopic staging (Ts/Ls), offer more reliable preoperative diagnosis and staging of patients with esophageal cancer. This may result in allocation of patients to stage-specific regimens with resulting improved cure rates.

ANATOMY

The boundaries of the esophagus are the inferior cricopharyngeal constrictor proximally and the esophagogastric junction distally. The esophagus is composed of four layers: mucosa, submucosa or lamina propria, muscularis propria, and adventitia (Fig. 10-1). The esophagus has no serosa, providing a teleologic explanation for the ease of spread of esophageal cancer. Familiarity with the histology of the esophageal wall is critical to understanding the staging system of esophageal cancer (see also Chapters 11 and 12).

Anatomically, the normal adult esophagus is approximately 35 cm in length and 2.5 cm in diameter, although it is not uniform throughout its course. The course of the esophagus begins in the midline in the upper neck at the level of the sixth cervical vertebra, which corresponds roughly to the level of the cricoid cartilage, and then deviates to the left in the lower neck and upper thorax. At the level of the tracheal bifurcation (24 cm from the incisors by endoscopic measurement), the esophagus again returns to the midline only to deviate to the left once again in the lower thorax, where it enters the abdomen through the diaphragmatic hiatus (40 cm from the incisors). Clinically, the esophagus is divided into three segments, the cervical, middle, and distal segments. The cervical segment ranges from the cricoid cartilage to the thoracic inlet (10–18 cm from the incisors). The middle esophageal segment ranges from the thoracic inlet to the midpoint between the tracheal bifurcation and the esophagogastric junction (19–34 cm). The distal esophageal segment extends from the midpoint between the tracheal bifurcation and the esophagogastric junction (35–44 cm). Three distinct narrowings are present in the esophagus. The first narrowing is formed by the cricopharyngeus muscle and is the narrowest segment of the gastrointestinal tract, located 12 to 15 cm from the incisors in the adult. The second narrowing is caused by the tracheal bifurcation and aortic arch at approximately 24 to 26 cm from the incisors. The last narrowing is located at the lower esophageal sphincter, approximately 40 to 44 cm from the incisors.[6]

The arterial blood supply of the esophagus is segmental (Fig. 10-2). The upper esophagus is supplied by branches from the inferior thyroid and subclavian arteries. The midesophagus receives blood from the bronchial arteries and direct branches from the thoracic aorta. The lower esophagus is supplied by branches of the inferior phrenic and gastric vessels. Venous drainage of the esophagus is segmental as well. The upper esophagus drains via the inferior thyroid veins. The midesophagus drains into the bronchial and azygos or hemiazygos veins. The lower esophagus drains into the coronary vein. As with the arterial network, the rich plexus of veins in the submucosa makes venous congestion unlikely.

Lymphatic drainage of the esophagus consists of two longitudinal interconnecting networks, the lymph channels and the lymph nodes. The intraesophageal or mucosal network of lymph channels is connected to the submucosa through transverse

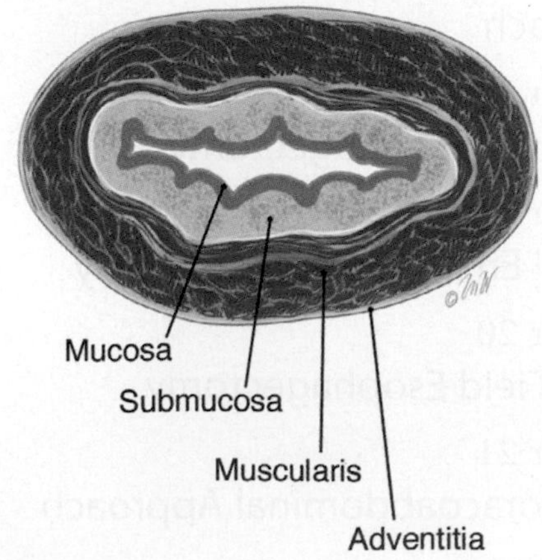

Figure 10-1. The four layers of the esophagus: mucosa, submucosa or lamina propria, muscularis propria, and adventitia.

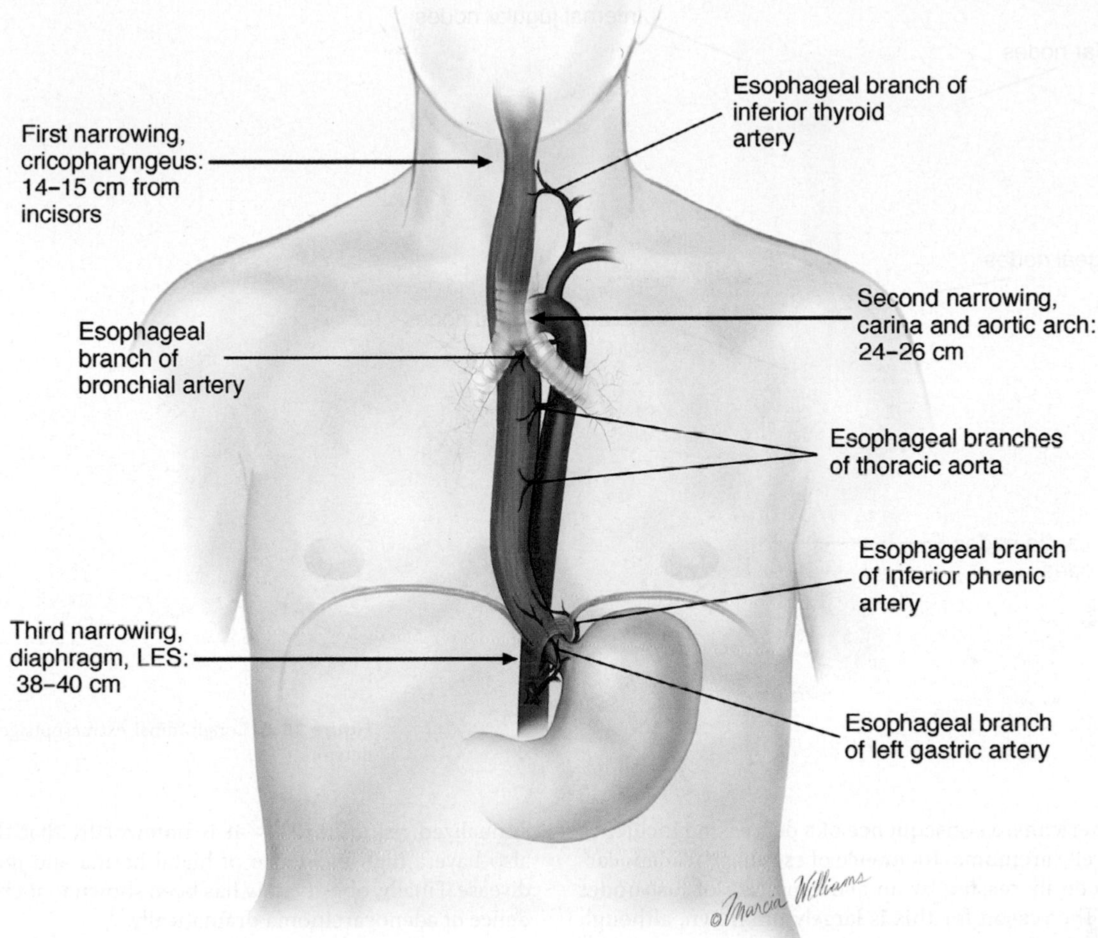

Figure 10-2. Arterial blood supply of the esophagus.

interconnections (Fig. 10-3). These collecting lymph channels merge, forming larger channels that feed into the extraesophageal lymph nodes (Fig. 10-4). It is estimated that the longitudinal flow is significant, which also may explain the frequency of spread of tumor along lymphatics. Flow proceeds in either direction freely and can be influenced by intrathoracic pressure differences and/or obstruction of lymphatic channels. The typical drainage pattern, however, is as follows: Cervical lymphatics drain into the internal jugular and supraclavicular nodes, the midesophagus drains into the paraesophageal and periesophageal nodes in the mediastinum, and the inferior esophagus drains below the diaphragm to the region of the cardia, left gastric vessels, lesser curve of the stomach, and celiac axis.[7,8]

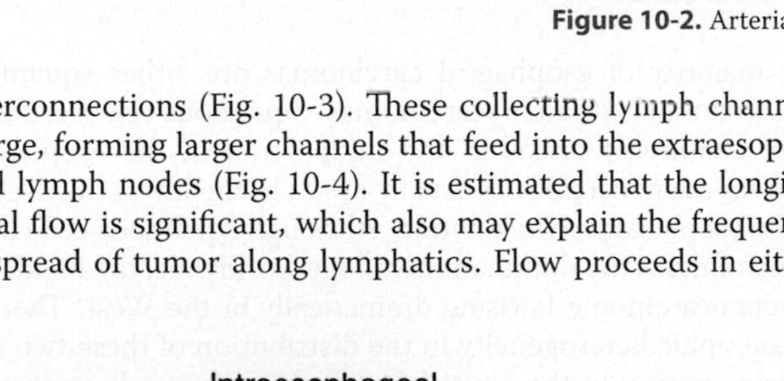

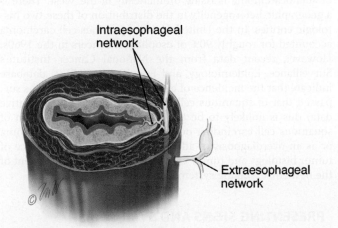

Figure 10-3. Two longitudinal networks of intraesophageal lymph channels traverse the muscularis feeding into the regional extraesophageal lymph node network.

EPIDEMIOLOGY

Esophageal cancer is a disease primarily of men (male:female ratio, 3:1) that occurs in the sixth and seventh decades of life with a median age of 67 years. In the United States, the incidence is 4.5 per 100,000 population, whereas in China it may be as high as 140 per 100,000 population. In addition, Russia, Japan, Scotland, and the Scandinavian countries have a higher incidence than the United States or Western Europe. In the United States, the incidence of adenocarcinoma of the esophagus is increasing dramatically across all socioeconomic boundaries. The incidence of adenocarcinoma in White men is roughly three times that in Black men, whereas the incidence of squamous cell carcinoma of the esophagus is six times higher in Blacks. Esophageal cancer rates have been declining

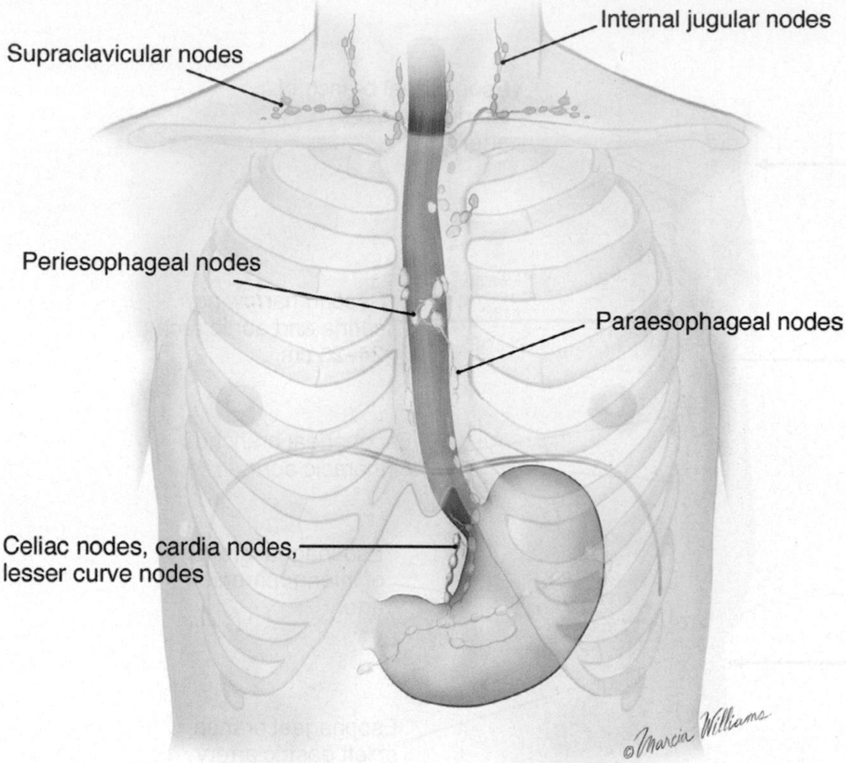

Figure 10-4. Longitudinal extraesophageal lymph node network.

in African Americans, a consequence of a decreasing incidence of squamous cell carcinoma. Incidence of esophageal adenocarcinoma has been increasing by an alarming rate of just under 2% per year.[9] The reason for this is largely unknown, although the worsening obesity epidemic may be partially responsible.[10] Several environmental factors have been implicated in the etiology of this disease, but none has been proved scientifically. Tobacco has been shown to increase the risk of esophageal cancer approximately 10-fold, whereas alcohol abuse increases the risk from 20- to 50-fold. Furthermore, the combination of tobacco and alcohol use may increase the risk 100-fold. Adenocarcinoma has a stronger association with tobacco use, whereas squamous cell carcinoma is more closely linked to alcohol use. In addition, diets high in nitrosamines and foods contaminated with molds (*Fusarium*) and fungus (*Geotrichum candidum*) also have been implicated, as well as diets in which hot liquids are consumed. Nutritional deficiencies also have been implicated. Diets low in beta carotene, vitamins B and C, magnesium, and zinc all have been implicated. Environmental exposure to asbestos, perchloroethylene, and radiation also has been shown to contribute to increased incidence.[11]

PATHOPHYSIOLOGY

Several premalignant conditions have been shown to predispose to esophageal carcinoma. Achalasia causes esophageal irritation and is associated with a 5% to 10% incidence in squamous cell carcinoma over 15 to 25 years. This tumor tends to occur in younger individuals and carries a poor prognosis. Gastroesophageal reflux disease causing distal esophageal metaplasia (Barrett esophagus) appears to be related to the increased incidence of adenocarcinoma in White males. Patients with Barrett esophagus have an 11-fold risk of developing esophageal adenocarcinoma, with an annualized risk of 0.12%.[12] It is noteworthy that these patients also have a high incidence of hiatal hernia and duodenal ulcer disease. Finally, obesity now has been shown to increase the incidence of adenocarcinoma dramatically.[10]

HISTOLOGY

The majority of esophageal carcinomas are either squamous cell carcinomas or adenocarcinomas. Squamous cell carcinoma most commonly arises in the midportion of the esophagus, whereas adenocarcinoma usually arises in the lower third, close to the esophagogastric junction. Although squamous cell carcinoma remains the dominant histology worldwide, the incidence of adenocarcinoma is rising dramatically in the West. There is a geographic heterogeneity in the distribution of these two histologic entities. In the United States, squamous cell carcinoma accounted for roughly 90% of esophageal cancers in the 1960s. However, recent data from the National Cancer Institute's Surveillance, Epidemiology, and End Results (SEER) database indicate that the incidence of adenocarcinoma actually has surpassed that of squamous cell carcinoma. Based on correlative data, this is unlikely to be the result of the reclassification of squamous cell carcinoma or adjacent gastric adenocarcinoma or as an overdiagnosis of adenocarcinoma. The importance of tumor histology and tumor grade is apparent with the advent of the new AJCC staging system (see Chapters 11 and 12).

PRESENTING SIGNS AND SYMPTOMS

Esophageal cancer often presents in an insidious and nonspecific manner, with indigestion, retrosternal discomfort, and transient dysphagia comprising the leading complaints. Often patients may present late because they have been able to compensate subconsciously for symptoms of dysphagia by eating softer foods or chewing their food more thoroughly. Dysphagia is the most commonly presenting symptom of esophageal carcinoma. It can progress to odynophagia and eventually to complete obstruction. Pain may be transient, associated with swallowing, or constant. It may be retrosternal or epigastric in location. Weight loss may be due to dietary changes, starvation, or tumor anorexia. Patients may experience regurgitation of undigested food, that is, food that has not been tainted with acidic gastric secretions. Patients also may develop respiratory sequelae primarily from aspiration but also from other causes such as direct invasion of tumor into the tracheobronchial tree or even a tracheoesophageal fistula, usually involving the left mainstem bronchus. Symptoms may include cough, dyspnea, and pleuritic pain. Hoarseness can result from direct involvement of the recurrent laryngeal nerve, a poor prognostic sign. Also, in advanced cases of near-complete or complete esophageal obstruction, patients may become severely dehydrated, even hypokalemic, because of their inability to swallow potassium-rich saliva.

DIAGNOSTIC TECHNIQUES

The most commonly used diagnostic and staging modalities are the barium swallow study, chest radiography, esophagoscopy, bronchoscopy, CT, MRI, and EUS with fine-needle aspiration (FNA). Additional adjuncts include thoracoscopic and laparoscopic staging, and PET scan. Usually, the first diagnostic method is a barium swallow, followed by endoscopy with biopsy. After a histologic diagnosis of carcinoma is confirmed, a CT scan of the thorax and abdomen should be obtained for the purpose of staging, paying particular attention to tumor extension, lymphadenopathy, and distant metastases. In some countries, abdominal ultrasound is often performed instead of CT to diagnose liver or celiac lymphatic metastasis.

Chest radiography has a minimal role in the modern diagnosis and staging of esophageal cancer, although it can reveal an abnormal finding in almost half of the patients with esophageal cancer. However, in some countries it is still used routinely to identify hilar or mediastinal adenopathy, evidence of pulmonary metastases, secondary pulmonary infiltrates caused by aspiration, elevation of the bronchus by midesophageal tumors and pleural effusion.[13] Bronchoscopy is often necessary to determine involvement of the tracheobronchial tree for patients with middle- and upper-third disease.[14,15] Gallium scanning can be useful for the detection of bony metastases but generally has been replaced by PET scan in the United States. Endoscopy remains the method of choice for the confirmation of esophageal cancer.[16] Its ability to detect early lesions can be improved with the use of staining techniques and, more recently, narrow-band imaging.[17]

Although the role of CT in evaluating esophageal cancer has been studied thoroughly, questions regarding its utility still remain. Although CT is highly effective in the assessment of mediastinal esophageal carcinomas, it is less helpful in the staging of cervical or gastroesophageal junction carcinomas. It plays a key role in assessing initial tumor bulk for radiation therapy planning and is also useful in monitoring tumor response to the cytoreductive therapy. CT is also helpful in depicting extraesophageal tumor spread to contiguous structures and distant metastases. CT evaluation is performed from the thoracic inlet through the liver to include the upper abdominal lymph node groups. Either thin barium or water-soluble oral contrast agents are administered routinely. Adequate distention of the esophagogastric junction is essential to exclude tumor involvement of this anatomic segment. Intravenous contrast material should be administered by the dynamic bolus technique to ensure optimal opacification of the heart, mediastinal vessels, and liver. Measurements of esophageal wall thickness greater than 5 mm are abnormal regardless of the degree of distention. Intraluminal air is seen in 60% of normal patients. CT staging of esophageal cancer includes assessment of (1) the extent of involvement of the esophageal wall by tumor, (2) tumor invasion of the periesophageal fat and adjacent structures, and (3) metastases to regional lymph nodes or distant organs.

The two key prognostic features of esophageal cancer are (1) the depth of tumor infiltration into or through the esophageal wall and (2) the presence or absence of visceral metastasis. Although the thickness of the esophageal wall often can be determined by CT, the individual layers of the esophageal wall cannot.[18] T1 and T2 lesions generally show an esophageal mass thickness between 5 and 15 mm, and T3 lesions show a thickness greater than 15 mm. T4 lesions show invasion of contiguous structures on CT. Specific findings of tracheobronchial invasion include demonstration of a tracheobronchial fistula or extension of tumor into the airway lumen. If an esophageal tumor indents or displaces the adjacent airway, luminal invasion is likely. Thickening of the wall of the tracheobronchial tree also suggests invasion. Generally, direct visualization with bronchoscopy is necessary to rule out airway invasion (usually distal trachea or left mainstem bronchus) for upper- and middle-third tumors. Although CT is useful in determining the extent of local disease, it is not as accurate in the staging of lymph node involvement; it is limited in differentiating between small normal nodes and nodes invaded by tumor but small in size. It has been suggested that mediastinal nodes greater than 10 mm in diameter in the short axis should be classified as pathologic and that subdiaphragmatic nodes greater than 8 mm in diameter should be considered abnormal. The accuracy of CT in predicting lymph node involvement ranges from 83% to 87% for abdominal lymph nodes but only 51% to 70% for mediastinal nodes.

MRI offers an alternative to CT for the evaluation of esophageal cancer. Its application in esophageal carcinoma has received scant attention. Like CT, MRI is highly accurate for detecting distant metastases of esophageal cancer, especially to the liver, and for determining advanced local spread (T4). However, it is less reliable in defining early infiltration (T1–3). MRI appears to be as sensitive as CT in predicting mediastinal invasion. One advantage of MRI is the loss of signal in the vessels and the air-filled trachea and bronchi, which may provide a clear delineation between the tumor and the aorta and the tracheobronchial tree. Like CT, MRI is poor at detecting tumors restricted to mucosa or submucosa and also tends to understage the regional lymph nodes.[19] MRI is not customarily used in the evaluation of esophageal cancer, as alternative modalities are often more reliable for determining local invasion and distant disease.

EUS has now become routine for the staging of esophageal cancer. EUS combines the technologies of flexible endoscopy and ultrasonic imaging. Tio et al.[20] found that the accuracy of EUS for T1a and T1b cancer was 85% versus 12% for CT. Luminal stenosis is a definite limiting factor for EUS, as it is occasionally not possible to traverse the tumor with the endoscope. Lymph nodes at a distance of more than 2 cm from the esophageal lumen cannot be imaged because of the very limited penetration depth of ultrasound. For patients with severe stenosis, a nonoptical, wire-guided echoendoscope can markedly reduce the occurrence of incomplete esophageal cancer staging and improve the detection of metastatic disease. EUS is also of help in the assessment of unresectability. The most important findings of unresectability are tumor invasion into the left atrium (with loss of smooth, flexible movement of the pericardium on real-time EUS), the wall of the descending aorta, the spinal body, the pulmonary vein or artery, or the tracheobronchial system. The latter should be confirmed with bronchoscopy with transbronchial FNA. EUS appears most helpful in predicting the superficial T1 tumors as well as the T3/4 tumors with greater depth of penetration. The positive predictive value of EUS for T2 tumors, however, is only 23%, with most tumors overstaged.[21] Clinically, T1N0 and T2N0 tumors are found to have unanticipated nodal disease 24% and 39% of the time, respectively.[22] Furthermore, for clinically T2 tumors, EUS understages nodal disease roughly two-thirds of the time.[23] It is possible to enhance specificity with ultrasound-guided needle biopsies through the EUS endoscope. The use of EUS-guided FNA was first reported in the diagnosis of esophageal cancer recurrence after distal esophageal resection in 1989.[24] One must use caution to avoid traversing the primary tumor with a needle resulting in a false-positive lymph node biopsy. At this time, EUS, especially when combined with FNA, is the most accurate imaging modality for locoregional staging of esophageal cancer.

Since multimodal neoadjuvant treatment for esophageal cancer has been used with increased frequency, tumor restaging remains fundamental in evaluating the response to therapy and in planning an operation. Many studies have evaluated the role of EUS in this setting. Although EUS is extremely accurate for staging untreated esophageal cancer, its accuracy in staging tumors after neoadjuvant chemoradiotherapy is relatively poor, with most errors caused by overstaging.[25] Although EUS is close to 90% accurate in predicting initial T stage, after neoadjuvant therapy, accuracy ranges from 27% to 82%. N stage is from 38% to 73% accurate after neoadjuvant therapy, whereas FNA can be expected to increase the accuracy further. Errors in posttherapy staging are likely due to the similar echogenic appearance of fibrosis and residual tumor. Residual nodal disease is an ominous finding. EUS, when combined with FNA, is very useful in detecting residual cancer within the lymph nodes. Others have found that ultrasound evidence of tumor regression is predictive of pathologic response to neoadjuvant therapy.

Recent evidence regarding the use of endoscopic mucosal resection (EMR) (see Chapter 173) particularly for early-stage tumors has emphasized the importance of this technology in determining the correct stage and differentiating T1a from T1b tumors when a superficial carcinoma is suspected.[26]

As with many other malignancies, [^{18}F]fluoro-2-deoxy-D-glucose (FDG)-PET is becoming a useful adjunct to conventional radiographic staging. PET improves staging and facilitates selection of patients for operation by detecting distant disease not identified by CT scanning alone. PET and CT are effective in showing the primary tumor and are equally sensitive in the demonstration of periesophageal nodes. The American College of Surgeons Oncology Group embarked on a prospective trial (Z0060) investigating the utility of PET scanning in the initial staging of esophageal cancer.[27] With 189 patients evaluated, roughly 5% of patients had a biopsy-confirmed distant metastasis detected with PET over CT alone. However, an additional 9.5% of patients had unconfirmed PET findings accepted by the treating surgeon as sufficient evidence to preclude resection. This particular study did not utilize PET/CT composite technology, which may have hampered the results. PET/CT is now accepted to have a routine role in esophageal cancer staging, with additional studies reporting the ability to detect distant metastatic disease in a significant number of patients.[28–30] Recent evidence suggests that PET scanning also may be used to measure the biologic activity of a tumor and thereby assess response to neoadjuvant therapy, stratifying survival after resection.[31] Maximal standard uptake values (SUVmax) have been shown to be independent predictors of prognosis.[32] The clinical relevance of this finding is most powerful in those patients with early-stage disease and high SUVmax who may be predicted to benefit from induction therapy.

Brain metastases are very rare in patients presenting with esophageal carcinoma. Autopsy studies reveal the prevalence of brain metastases in patients who died from esophageal cancer to be 0% to 1.8%. They tend to occur in patients with large tumors or aggressive nodal disease. Brain imaging is not generally performed during the evaluation of an esophageal cancer patient in the absence of neurologic symptoms.[33,34]

PATHOLOGY/STAGING

The treatment of esophageal cancer is rigorously stage-driven. Patients with early-stage esophageal cancer may have a 5-year survival of over 75%, yet with more advanced disease, survival drops precipitously. The ability to recommend effective treatment algorithms and predict prognosis relies on the determination of a clinical stage for each patient with current technology.

The sixth edition of the AJCC staging system for esophageal cancer was introduced in 2002, and was not significantly different from an earlier version from 1987 because of lack of convincing survival data. Our cancer staging systems need to evolve as newer diagnostic modalities and treatments emerge, and as knowledge of the disease accumulates. As such, the staging system for esophageal carcinoma was recently revised with the introduction of the 7th edition of the AJCC staging manual (see Chapter 12) (Tables 10-1, 10-2A, and 10-2B).[35] Data used to generate the new staging system were assembled by a worldwide esophageal cancer collaboration, which included over 4600 patients.[36] Although the previous system was logical, straightforward, and simple, modifications were necessary as limitations became apparent (Table 10-3). The most important change pertains to the N descriptor. In the previous edition, the N descriptor was binary—N0 indicated no known nodal metastasis and N1 indicated any metastasis, regardless of tumor burden. The distinction was somewhat arbitrary an N1 node versus a distant M1a nodal metastasis which was not supported by recent data. The N descriptor in the new system now ranks lymph node burden with gradations from N0 through N3.

The staging system for gastric cancer includes groupings within the N descriptor based on number of involved lymph nodes. This has been shown to be relevant to prognostication for esophageal cancer as well.[37–39] The number of involved lymph nodes correlates with survival, irrespective of tumor

Table 10-1

7TH EDITION AJCC/UICC TNM CLASSIFICATIONS

Primary tumor (T)	
TX	Primary tumor cannot be assessed
T0	No evidence of primary tumor
Tis	High-grade dysplasia[a]
T1	Tumor invades lamina propria, muscularis mucosae, or submucosa
	T1a Tumor invades lamina propria or muscularis mucosae
	T1b Tumor invades submucosa
T2	Tumor invades muscularis propria
T3	Tumor invades adventitia
T4	Tumor invades adjacent structures
	T4a Resectable tumor invading pleura, pericardium, or diaphragm
	T4b Unresectable tumor invading other adjacent structures, such as aorta, vertebral body, trachea, etc.
Regional lymph nodes (N)[b]	
NX	Regional lymph nodes cannot be assessed
N0	No regional lymph node metastasis
N1	Regional lymph node metastases involving 1 to 2 nodes
N2	Regional lymph node metastases involving 3 to 6 nodes
N3	Regional lymph node metastases involving 7 or more nodes
Distant metastasis (M)	
M0	No distant metastasis
M1	Distant metastasis
Histopathologic type	
Squamous cell carcinoma	
Adenocarcinoma	
Histologic grade (G)	
GX	Grade cannot be assessed—stage grouping as G1
G1	Well differentiated
G2	Moderately differentiated
G3	Poorly differentiated
G4	Undifferentiated—stage grouping as G3 squamous
Location[c]	
Upper or middle—cancers above lower border of inferior pulmonary vein	
Lower—below inferior pulmonary vein	

[a]Includes all noninvasive neoplastic epithelium that was previously called carcinoma in situ. Cancers stated to be noninvasive or in situ are classified as Tis.
[b]Number must be recorded for total number of regional nodes sampled and total number of reported nodes with metastases.
[c]Location (primary cancer site) is defined by position of upper (proximal) edge of tumor in esophagus.

depth of invasion. The prior subgrouping of M1 as M1a and M1b appears unfounded. The former M1a indicated distant nodal disease, but may have simply been a surrogate for large lymph node burden. This distinction has been eliminated in the new system. The seventh edition of the AJCC cancer staging manual also recommends harvesting a minimum number of lymph nodes based on the T descriptor. Ten nodes must be resected for T1, 20 for T2, and at least 30 for T3 or T4. These numbers are supported by data indicating that survival improves as a greater number of nodes are resected with the specimen.[40] This may be due at least in part to stage migration rather than resection of nodal micrometastases. It has been reported, however, that most resections fail to harvest an adequate number of lymph nodes.[41] The harvest is improved when the surgeon takes the time to individually submit lymph node stations distinct from the resected esophagogastric specimen.

Histologic tumor type also has been shown to be of prognostic significance, with adenocarcinoma having a somewhat better prognosis than squamous cell carcinoma.[42] These two tumor types now have their own stage groupings (see Tables 10-2A and 10-2B). Histologic grade was introduced as an important variable, as well-differentiated (G1) yet higher T-stage tumors have a similar prognosis to less well-differentiated tumors that are of lower T-stage.

Many surgical studies show a significant stratification of survival after resection of esophageal cancer based on accurate pathologic staging. Multimodality treatment of this disease has been introduced; however, it is difficult to compare different

Table 10-2A

STAGE GROUPINGS BY HISTOLOGY FOR ADENOCARCINOMA

STAGE	TUMOR (T)	NODE (N)	METASTASES (M)	GRADE (G)
0	Tis (HGD)	0	0	1
IA	1	0	0	1–2
IB	1	0	0	3
	2	0	0	1–2
IIA	2	0	0	3
IIB	3	0	0	Any
	1–2	1	0	Any
IIIA	1–2	2	0	Any
	3	1	0	Any
	4a	0	0	Any
IIIB	3	2	0	Any
IIIC	4a	1–2	0	Any
	4b	Any	0	Any
	Any	N3	0	Any
IV	Any	Any	1	Any

HGD, High-grade dysplasia.

Table 10-2B

STAGING GROUPINGS BY HISTOLOGY FOR SQUAMOUS CELL CARCINOMA

STAGE	TUMOR (T)	NODE (N)	METASTASES (M)	GRADE (G)	LOCATION
0	Tis (HGD)	0	0	1	Any
IA	1	0	0	1	Any
IB	1	0	0	2–3	Any
	2–3	0	0	1	Lower
IIA	2–3	0	0	1	Upper, middle
	2–3	0	0	2–3	Lower
IIB	2–3	0	0	2–3	Upper, middle
	1–2	1	0	Any	Any
IIIA	1–2	2	0	Any	Any
	3	1	0	Any	Any
	4a	0	0	Any	Any
IIIB	3	2	0	Any	Any
IIIC	4a	1–2	0	Any	Any
	4b	Any	0	Any	Any
	Any	N3	0	Any	Any
IV	Any	Any	1	Any	Any

HGD, High-grade dysplasia.

Table 10-3

SUMMARY OF CHANGES—7TH EDITION AJCC ESOPHAGEAL CANCER TNM STAGING SYSTEM

- Tumors that arise at the esophagogastric (EG) junction or tumors that arise in the stomach and are greater than 5 cm from the EG junction and cross the EG junction are staged according to the TNM system for esophageal adenocarcinoma.
- Tis is redefined and T4 is subclassified.
- Regional lymph nodes are redefined. N is subclassified according to the number of regional lymph nodes containing metastasis.
- M is redefined.
- Separate stage groupings for squamous cell carcinoma and adenocarcinoma.
- Stage groupings are reassigned using T, N, M, and G classifications.

treatment modalities because of the lack of precise preoperative staging. Preoperative minimally invasive surgical staging in esophageal cancer may solve this problem, just as the successful use of mediastinoscopy in preoperative staging has solved this problem for lung cancer. Such staging in esophageal cancer may separate advanced disease from early local disease. Prognostication in patients with esophageal cancer may allow more appropriate allocation of chemotherapy and/or radiation therapy, thus reducing the morbidity and mortality associated with esophageal cancer treatment.

Murray et al.[43] first reported their experience with minimally invasive surgical staging for esophageal cancer in 1977. They used mediastinoscopy and minilaparotomy prospectively in 30 esophageal cancer patients. Seven were found to have positive lymph nodes by mediastinoscopy, and celiac lymph nodes were identified in 16. Dagnini et al.[44] did routine laparoscopy in 369 esophageal cancer patients, and they noted intra-abdominal metastases in 14% and celiac lymph node metastases in 9.7%. All these patients with metastasis avoided unnecessary resection.

Diagnostic laparoscopy with laparoscopic ultrasound revealed previously unknown findings, particularly in patients with locally advanced adenocarcinoma of the distal esophagus or cardia (hepatic metastases in 22% and peritoneal tumor spread or free tumor cells in the abdominal cavity in 25%), whereas the diagnostic gain was low in patients with squamous cell esophageal cancer.[45]

With the advances in thoracoscopic (Ts) and laparoscopic (Ls) techniques, Ts/Ls has been used for staging esophageal cancer in some centers. Recent reports show that Ts/Ls staging can correctly predict nodal metastasis for esophageal cancer, as mediastinoscopy does for lung cancer. Krasna and McLaughlin[46] first described the efficacy of thoracoscopic lymph node staging in esophageal cancer. They further reported their successful experience with combined Ts/Ls for staging disease in the chest and abdomen in a follow-up series from three institutions of the Cancer and Leukemia Group B with an accuracy of over 90%.[47] A more recent report of 65 patients showed 94% accuracy with laparoscopy and 91% accuracy with thoracoscopy in esophageal cancer staging.[48] When compared with EUS, Ts/Ls staging is superior for detecting lymph node metastases. The study also demonstrated that clinical stage evaluation based on noninvasive diagnostic methods including CT, MRI, and EUS may be used to guide surgeons to focus on suspicious areas for the most high-yield biopsy targets when doing Ts/Ls staging.[49] The main advantage of Ts/Ls staging is that it provides greater accuracy in evaluation of regional and celiac lymph nodes. Such information is very important in patient stratification and selection of therapy, especially in the setting of new treatment protocols. Furthermore, the histologic status of mediastinal and abdominal lymph nodes is critical for design of the field for irradiation. It permits one to maximize the dose delivery to areas of known disease while minimizing dose to surrounding sensitive, normal tissue. Minimally invasive surgical techniques in combination with new molecular diagnostic techniques may improve the ability to stage cancer patients. Reverse transcriptase-polymerase chain reaction of carcinoembryonic antigen mRNA has been used to increase the detection of micrometastases in lymph nodes from esophageal cancer patients with minimally invasive staging.[50] Krasna et al.[51] found that immunohistochemistry study of the molecular marker of p53 also can be used for this purpose; immunohistochemistry study of cytokeratin, an antibody to epithelial cells, also can be used to detect occult micrometastasis in Ts/Ls lymph nodes, and patients with positive cytokeratin findings tend to have poor survival.

GUIDELINES FOR DIAGNOSIS AND STAGING

Recently, the task force of the Society of Thoracic Surgeons (STS) conducted an evidence-based evaluation of diagnostic studies for esophageal cancer (Table 10-4).[16] Based on this analysis, a Class I recommendation was made for flexible endoscopy with biopsy (level of evidence *B*).[16] The task force also evaluated the efficacy of diagnostic tools for staging based on the current stage groupings published in the 7th edition of the AJCC staging manual for esophageal cancer (see also Chapter 12). In making these recommendations, esophageal cancer was defined as early-stage (T1a), locoregionalized (T2b-T4, any N, and M0), and distant (M1 disease). A class I recommendation (level of evidence B) was made for the use of computed tomography (CT) of the chest and abdomen as an optional test for staging. CT of the chest and abdomen was recognized as the recommended test for staging of locoregionalized esophageal cancer (Class I recommendation; level of evidence B). A Class IIA recommendation was made for the use of positron emission tomography (PET) as an optional test for early-stage cancer. A class IIA recommendation also was made for endosonography (EUS) in the absence of metastatic disease as a tool for improving the accuracy of clinical staging.

THERAPEUTIC OPTIONS

Esophageal cancer can metastasize to virtually any organ in the body. Widespread distant metastases are almost always present at the time of death. The extensive lymphatic drainage pathways in the esophagus and the long-time interval during which tumors typically remain asymptomatic may contribute to the high incidence of lymph node metastases. For all but the earliest stage tumors, surgical resection alone is inadequate. In fact, as many as 30% of patients with early (T1) lesions may have lymph node metastases. For this reason, multimodality regimens have been designed to achieve better survival in this disease.

Table 10-4

EVIDENCE-BASED GUIDELINES OF THE STS TASKFORCE ON DIAGNOSIS AND STAGING[16]

CLASS/LEVEL OF EVIDENCE	RECOMMENDATION
Class I (evidence level B)	For early-stage esophageal cancer, computed tomography (CT) of the abdomen and chest is an optional test for staging.
Class I (evidence level B)	For locoregionalized esophageal cancer, CT of the chest and abdomen is a recommended test for staging.
Class IIA (evidence level B)	For early-stage esophageal cancer, positron emission tomography (PET) is an optional test for staging.
Class IIA (Evidence level B)	For locoregionalized esophageal cancer, PET is a recommended test for staging.
Class IIA (Evidence level B)	In the absence of metastatic disease, endosonography (EUS) is recommended to improve the accuracy of clinical staging.
Basis for Classification Recommendations:	
Class I (the treatment/procedure SHOULD be performed)	
Class II (the treatment/procedure is REASONABLE to perform but additional focused studies are needed)	
Class III (the procedure is not helpful or there is no proven benefit to the procedure)	
Class IV (Both the treatment and procedure are not helpful and may be harmful)	
Basis for Levels of Evidence:	
Level A: Multiple populations evaluated. Data derived from multiple randomized clinical trials or meta-analyses.	
Level B: Limited populations evaluated. Data derived from a single randomized trial or nonrandomized studies.	
Level C: Very limited populations evaluated. Only consensus opinion of experts, case studies, or standard of care are available.	

Neoadjuvant Radiotherapy

The rationale for using preoperative radiotherapy is to reduce marginally resectable tumors to a more resectable size, to reduce the risk of tumor spread during surgical manipulation, and to treat extension of tumor beyond the surgical specimen. Surgery then removes the central, more radioresistant tumor mass. It does not appear that preoperative radiotherapy has an adverse effect on resectability or surgical morbidity.

Preoperative radiation doses of 30 to 45 Gy have been reported to result in a complete pathologic response rate of 15% to 30%. It is important to note that precise reporting of the rates of tumor sterilization is not possible, because not all patients who are irradiated undergo surgery and not all those operated on are resectable. Some clinical trials have suggested that survival after preoperative radiotherapy is correlated with the extent of tumor destruction seen in the resected specimen. A multicenter randomized controlled trial conducted by the European Organization for Research and Treatment of Cancer involved the administration of 33 Gy in 10 fractions in the treatment arm, followed by esophagectomy within 8 days. There were no significant differences in resectability or operative mortality between the study arms. Locoregional failure was decreased significantly in the radiotherapy arm from 67% to 46%. This was not associated with a survival benefit.[52] Current consensus sees no role for neoadjuvant XRT alone.

Neoadjuvant Chemotherapy

Neoadjuvant chemotherapy in patients with esophageal cancer who appear to have locoregional disease may diminish the incidence of unrecognized systemic metastases. The potential benefits of preoperative chemotherapy include downstaging the disease to facilitate surgical resection, improving local control, and eradicating micrometastatic disease. Surgical resection subsequently provides an opportunity to assess the tumor response to chemotherapy and to evaluate the patient for possible postoperative adjuvant therapy. In patients with localized, resectable tumors, chemotherapy-related toxicity occasionally can result in prolonged delay or even cancellation of planned surgical resection, risking further spread of disease. The resulting need for careful patient selection for participation in clinical trials of preoperative chemotherapy can bias treatment results. An American multi-institutional randomized trial of 440 patients compared surgery alone versus neoadjuvant chemotherapy followed by surgery. Preoperative chemotherapy consisted of three cycles of fluorouracil (5-fluorouracil or 5-FU) and cisplatin. Surgical resection followed 2 to 4 weeks later. Patients received two additional cycles of chemotherapy postoperatively. There was no significant difference in perioperative morbidity and mortality between the two groups. There was no significant difference in 1-year survival (60%), 2 year survival (35%), or local or distant recurrence rates. Survival did not differ between patients with squamous cell carcinoma and adenocarcinoma. Median survival time was 15 to 16 months in both treatment arms.[53] A smaller randomized trial comprising 147 esophageal cancer patients from Hong Kong demonstrated a higher rate of curative resection, yet failed to show a survival benefit with neoadjuvant chemotherapy.[54]

A British randomized controlled trial of 802 patients also studied the use of preoperative 5-fluorouracil and cisplatin. The rate of microscopically complete resection was significantly higher for patients undergoing preoperative chemotherapy than for those undergoing surgery alone (60% vs. 54%). Postoperative complication rates were similar in both groups (41% vs. 42%). Patients undergoing preoperative chemotherapy achieved significantly improved median survival (16.8 vs. 13.3 months) and 2-year survival (43% vs. 34%).[55] Results of this trial were updated in 2009, reporting 5-year survival of 23% for the neoadjuvant chemotherapy group versus 17% for the surgery alone group.[56] The results of this trial, however, are potentially confounded by the fact that clinicians were allowed the option of giving preoperative radiotherapy to their patients irrespective of randomization.

An oft-quoted study is the Medical Research Council Adjuvant Gastric Infusional Chemotherapy (MAGIC) Trial which randomized 503 patients with gastroesophageal cancer to either perioperative chemotherapy or surgery alone.[57] The chemotherapy was comprised of three cycles of epirubicin, cisplatin, and 5-fluorouracil followed by surgery and three additional cycles of the same regimen. It was originally designed to include gastric cancer only, but inclusion criteria were later extended to include cancers of the lower third of the esophagus. There was a survival benefit for perioperative chemotherapy (36% 5-year survival vs. 23%). It should be kept in mind, however, that only a quarter of these patients had tumors of the lower esophagus or gastroesophageal junction; the remainder were gastric cancers. Another more recent multicenter randomized study by Ychou et al.[58] investigated a similar question of perioperative chemotherapy (cisplatin and 5-fluorouracil) versus resection alone for cancers of the esophagogastric junction. Of 224 patients, 11% involved the lower esophagus, 25% the stomach, and the remainder were true gastroesophageal junction tumors. There was again a survival benefit conferred by perioperative chemotherapy. Although some are conflicting, the majority of recent data, suggest a benefit of perioperative chemotherapy over surgery alone for the treatment of esophageal cancer.

Neoadjuvant Chemoradiotherapy

Both chemotherapy and radiotherapy have been reported to improve survival in patients with esophageal cancer when administered preoperatively. The notion of downstaging esophageal cancer before surgical resection is appealing. In an attempt to improve resectability and survival in esophageal cancer, chemotherapy has been combined with radiotherapy in the neoadjuvant setting. Most reports of so-called trimodality therapy for esophageal carcinoma describe concurrent neoadjuvant chemoradiation using combinations of cisplatin and 5-fluorouracil while administering 30 to 45 Gy of radiation. Some studies have used additional postoperative chemotherapy. The results appear comparable at most experienced centers.

In an Irish study of 113 patients who had esophageal adenocarcinoma, patients were randomly allocated to surgery alone versus trimodality therapy with neoadjuvant chemoradiation.[59] Patients randomized to the trimodality arm received two cycles of 5-fluoruracil and cisplatin given concurrently with 40 Gy of radiation, followed by surgery. Neoadjuvant chemoradiation was associated with a pathologic complete response rate of 25%. Trimodality therapy was associated with significantly increased median survival (16 vs. 11 months) and 3-year survival (32% vs. 6%). It should be noted that, at the time of surgery, the incidence of lymph node involvement was significantly higher in the group undergoing surgery alone. Survival with surgery alone was lower than that reported in most other series.

A French randomized trial of 282 patients compared surgery alone with two cycles of cisplatin chemotherapy and concurrent radiotherapy (total 37 Gy) followed 2 to 4 weeks later by surgery.[60] Neoadjuvant chemoradiation was associated with a pathologic complete response rate of 26% but with significantly increased operative mortality (12.3% vs. 3.6%). Despite a significantly increased rate of microscopically complete resection, longer local disease-free survival time, longer overall disease-free survival time, and fewer cancer-related deaths in the trimodality arm, overall survival time was 18.6 months in both treatment arms. A randomized trial from the University of Michigan looked at 100 patients receiving either preoperative chemoradiation (total 45 Gy) or surgery alone.[61] All resections were performed using a transhiatal approach. With a median follow-up of 8 years, there was no difference in survival.

Meta-analyses of randomized trials of trimodality therapy versus surgery alone for esophageal carcinoma have revealed a trend toward increased treatment-related mortality and slightly increased overall survival. Among patients treated with trimodality therapy for esophageal carcinoma, the best predictor of survival appears to be the finding of a pathologic complete response at the time of surgical resection.[62,63]

Cancer and Leukemia Group B 9781 was a prospective, randomized intergroup trial of trimodality therapy versus surgery alone for the treatment of stages I to III esophageal cancer.[64] Patients were randomized to treatment with either surgery alone or cisplatin (100 mg/m^2) and 5-fluorouracil (1000 mg/m^2 per day $\times$ 4 days) during weeks 1 and 5 concurrent with radiation therapy (50.4 Gy at 1.8 Gy/daily fraction over 5.6 weeks) followed by esophagectomy with lymph node dissection. A total of 56 patients were entered into the study between October 1997 and March 2000 when the trial was closed as a consequence of poor accrual. Thirty patients were randomized to trimodality therapy and 26 to surgery alone. An intent-to-treat analysis showed a median survival of 4.5 versus 1.8 years in favor of trimodality therapy (log rank $p = 0.02$). A log-rank test with stratifications by N stage, staging approach, and histology demonstrated a p value of 0.005. The 5-year survival was 39% (95% confidence interval: 21%–57%) versus 16% (95% confidence interval: 5%–33%) in favor of trimodality therapy.

Van der Gaast et al.[65] presented results in 2010 of the largest randomized study to date looking at neoadjuvant chemoradiotherapy compared to surgery alone. The multicenter phase III CROSS trial investigated 363 esophageal cancer patients undergoing neoadjuvant chemoradiation (utilizing a different chemotherapy regimen and a total of 41.4 Gy) versus surgery alone. The R0 resection rate was 92% in the neoadjuvant arm versus 65% in the surgery alone arm. Median survival was 49 months compared to 26 months in favor of trimodality therapy. The benefit was most pronounced in patients with squamous cell histology. The final results have recently been published in manuscript form and confirm these findings.[66]

An Australian randomized phase II trial investigated whether the addition of concurrent radiation to a preoperative chemotherapy regimen is advantageous.[70] Seventy-five patients with esophageal adenocarcinoma received either neoadjuvant chemotherapy or chemoradiotherapy. There was no statistically significant difference in survival. The major pathologic response rate (pCR + <10% viable cells) was significantly improved in the arm receiving radiation (8% vs. 31%; $p = 0.01$). However, the advantage in 5-year survival was not statistically significant, suggesting that the study may have been underpowered.

To date, there is no completely reliable preoperative method for identifying a pathologic complete response after neoadjuvant chemoradiation. There is conflicting evidence regarding whether a restaging PET scan is a reliable predictor of a complete pathologic response prior to resection.[67,68] However, we now know that the survival of patients with microscopic residual disease approaches that of patients with a complete pathologic response, whereas gross residual disease is a poor prognostic factor.[69]

At this point, there is adequate prospective evidence that the addition of radiation to a neoadjuvant chemotherapy regimen improves survival, as well as the rate of a complete pathologic response.[66]

Adjuvant Radiotherapy

Radiotherapy is commonly considered postoperatively to "sterilize" residual microscopic disease and to control gross residual locoregional tumor. As an advantage, reserving radiotherapy for postoperative use avoids the necessity of subjecting all patients with completely resectable disease to the damaging effects of radiation. As a disadvantage, the use of postoperative radiation in patients who have undergone gastric pull-up or colonic interposition exposes large volumes of normal tissue to harm and is a potential cause of late morbidity. A French randomized trial of 221 patients with squamous cell carcinoma arising in the distal two-thirds of the esophagus compared surgical resection alone versus surgery followed by postoperative radiotherapy doses of 45 to 55 Gy in daily fractions of 1.8 Gy. Among patients with negative lymph nodes, local recurrence rates were lower in the group that received postoperative radiotherapy. There was no significant difference in survival between the two groups.[71] A randomized trial from Hong Kong studied 130 patients undergoing either palliative or curative resection for esophageal cancer. Patients randomized to the postoperative radiotherapy arm of the study received doses of 49 to 52.5 Gy in daily fractions of 3.5 Gy. The very high daily radiation dose used in this study was associated with a significantly decreased median survival compared with surgery alone (8.7 vs. 15.2 months). In patients undergoing curative resection, postoperative radiotherapy was not associated with any improvement in local control. Although postoperative radiotherapy was associated with improved local control in patients undergoing palliative resection with gross residual disease, there was no survival benefit.[72] A prospective Chinese study of 495 patients who had undergone surgical resection of esophageal cancer randomized patients to a postoperative radiotherapy group or a control group. A midplane dose of 50 to 60 Gy was administered in daily fractions of 2 Gy. A trend toward improved 5-year survival in patients who received postoperative radiotherapy (41.3% vs. 31.7%) was not statistically significant. This trend was somewhat stronger in patients with positive lymph nodes (29.2% vs. 14.7%, $p = 0.07$). Postoperative radiotherapy was associated with a statistically significant improvement in 5-year survival only among patients with stage III disease (35.1% vs. 13.1%).[73] This is corroborated by a more recent retrospective analysis of the Surveillance, Epidemiology and End Results (SEER) database suggesting a survival benefit for stage III patients with either squamous cell carcinoma or adenocarcinoma who receive postoperative radiation as opposed to resection alone. There was no benefit associated with postoperative radiation among stage II patients.[74]

Adjuvant Chemotherapy

Adjuvant chemotherapy also has been studied. A multi-institutional Japanese randomized controlled trial of 242 patients who had undergone complete surgical resection for esophageal squamous cell carcinoma studied the effects of adjuvant chemotherapy with two cycles of cisplatin and 5-fluorouracil. Adjuvant chemotherapy was associated with significantly improved 5-year disease-free survival in patients with lymph node involvement (52% vs. 38%). Despite improved disease-free survival, there was no significant improvement in overall survival. Among node-negative patients receiving adjuvant chemotherapy, a trend toward improved 5-year disease-free survival (76% vs. 70%) was not statistically significant.[75] To date, there are no published North American data suggesting that postoperative chemotherapy in the absence of documented metastatic disease is associated with prolonged survival.

Definitive Chemoradiotherapy

In light of the relatively high morbidity and mortality rates associated with esophageal resection, definitive chemoradiation has been advocated as a reasonable approach for the treatment of esophageal cancer. Two similar phase III studies compared the efficacy of neoadjuvant chemoradiotherapy and definitive chemoradiotherapy, with concordant results. A French study only randomized chemoradiotherapy nonresponders (of 444 eligible patients, only 259 were randomized). Of the remaining patients who responded clinically to chemoradiation, there was no difference in survival when surgery was added to the treatment regimen. However, the surgical arm had more early deaths yet better local control and palliation of dysphagia.[76] A German study also failed to reveal a survival difference between treatment arms, yet resected patients had better progression-free survival. Clinical response to induction chemotherapy was a good prognostic factor in each group.[77] For elderly patients, however, definitive chemoradiation is associated with significant morbidity and poor survival.[78] It may be reasonable to consider resection alone for elderly patients who are of acceptable surgical risk.

It is clear from patterns-of-care study surveys that a multimodality approach is increasing in popularity across the country.[79] Novel restaging techniques, as well as further study of the risks and benefits of neoadjuvant chemoradiotherapy, are needed.

Although patients with early localized disease benefit from complete surgical resection, there is increasing evidence that multimodality therapy (neoadjuvant chemoradiation followed by surgical resection) has increased survival benefits when compared to surgery alone for more advanced stages.[59]

ROLE OF SURGERY

The success rate for treatment of esophageal cancer with surgery alone is related to the disease stage. If the depth of tumor invasion is limited to the submucosa without regional lymph node involvement or distant metastases (T1N0M0), most patients undergoing complete resection will survive 5 years. In most cases of esophageal cancer presenting with dysphagia, however, management is complicated by the prevalence of locally advanced disease (T3 or T4), involvement of regional lymph nodes (N1–3), or distant (often occult) metastases (M1). Curative treatment of esophageal cancer must address local control of the primary lesion as well as the control and/or prevention of metastases.

There has been a significant variation within the literature with regard to morbidity and mortality rates after esophagectomy. A Veterans Affairs National Surgical Quality Improvement Program database of 1777 patients undergoing esophagectomy revealed morbidity and mortality rates of 50% and 10%, respectively.[80] A more recent study gleaned from 2315 patients entered into the Society of Thoracic Surgeons (STS) General Thoracic Database revealed a much lower mortality rate of 2.7%.[81] This difference may be due, in part, to the fact that participation in the STS database is voluntary and comprised mostly of board-certified thoracic surgeons. Nevertheless, risk factors for poor outcomes were identified to include congestive heart failure, coronary artery disease, peripheral vascular disease, diabetes, hypertension, steroid use, smoking status, and a high American Society of Anesthesiology (ASA) score. Interestingly, induction therapy was found not to be a risk factor for increased morbidity. Several recent studies have documented the importance of institution and surgeon experience as measured by volume of esophagectomies.[82–86]

Although esophagectomy remains the preferred treatment for the earliest stage intramucosal tumors (T1aN0), endoscopic approaches are gaining in popularity. Endoscopic radiofrequency ablation and EMR have been used for metaplasia and dysplasia of the mucosa, and indications are now broadening to include these superficial tumors. Studies have shown successful treatment of T1aN0 tumors using EMR.[87,88] These series are highly selective, comprised of small tumors staged with EUS and excluding poorly differentiated tumors. Patients were followed endoscopically and some required repeated treatments. Although endoscopic treatment of these highly selected lower-risk tumors may be reasonable, there must be a commitment by both patients and their physicians to rigorous long-term surveillance.[89] Endoscopic treatment is certainly a good option for the high-risk surgical patient.

For most patients with localized esophageal cancer, surgical resection affords the best chance for local control and the best means of palliation of dysphagia. In all but the earliest stages of esophageal cancer (T1N0M0 or T2N0M0), however, both local and systemic recurrence of disease is common when surgical resection is performed as the sole treatment modality. With the exception of these early lesions, surgery alone with complete resection of all grossly apparent disease is associated with median survival ranging from 12 to 18 months in most centers and 5-year survival rarely exceeding 20%. Because of the low cure rates associated with the treatment of esophageal cancer by surgery alone, other modalities have been added to the treatment regimen.[90,91]

SUMMARY

Esophageal cancer is the fastest growing malignancy in terms of incidence in the North American and the Western nations. A multimodality approach generally is needed to treat this disease. With newer imaging and minimally invasive staging techniques, careful determination of pathologic TNM staging can be achieved before treatment. Patients can receive stage-specific treatment regimens, including chemotherapy, radiation therapy, and surgery, appropriate to their disease. With further advances in the identification of molecular markers, patients with esophageal cancer will be able to receive treatments based on a specific profile of genome expression, as is currently being done for patients with cancers of the breast and lung.

EDITOR'S COMMENT

The main message from this chapter is that esophageal cancer must be approached in a stage-specific fashion, just as one would approach any other solid-organ malignancy. New diagnostic and staging algorithms, recently endorsed by the STS Taskforce, suggest the use of EGD, PET, and EUS with FNA for all but the most superficial tumors. Using the revised TNM staging system, surgeons should carefully allocate treatment (resection, neoadjuvant and adjuvant therapy) as appropriate for each subgroup based on stage. The results of two recent randomized trials (CALGB 9781 and the CROSS study) have codified neoadjuvant chemoradiation as the approach of choice for locoregional disease. Until a definitive method of restaging patients postchemo/radiation induction therapy is developed, surgery should always be considered as part of the multimodality regimen in nonmetastatic patients.

—Mark J. Krasna

References

1. Ferlay J, Shin HR, Bray F, et al. Estimates of worldwide burden of cancer in 2008: GLOBOCAN 2008. *Int J Cancer*. 2010;127:2893–2917.
2. Howlader N, Noone AM, Krapcho M, et al. *SEER Cancer Statistics Review, 1975–2008*. Bethesda, MD: National Cancer Institute.
3. Ke L. Mortality and incidence trends from esophagus cancer in selected geographic areas of China circa 1970–90. *Int J Cancer*. 2002;102:271–274.
4. Siegel R, Naishadham D, Jemal A. Cancer statistics, 2012. *CA Cancer J Clin*. 2012;62:10–29.
5. Ellis FH, Jr., Heatley GJ, Krasna MJ, et al. Esophagogastrectomy for carcinoma of the esophagus and cardia: a comparison of findings and results after standard resection in three consecutive eight-year intervals with improved staging criteria. *J Thorac Cardiovasc Surg*. 1997;113:836–846; discussion 846–848.
6. Standring S, Borley MR, Collins P, et al. Chapter 55: Mediastinum. In: *Gray's Anatomy: The Anatomical Basis of Clinical Practice*. 40th edition. Elsevier, 2009.
7. Refaely Y, Krasna MJ. Multimodality therapy for esophageal cancer. *Surg Clin North Am*. 2002;82:729–746.
8. Rafaely Y, Krasna M. Lymphaic drainage of the esophagus. In: Shields T, ed. *General Thoracic Surgery*. 6th ed. Philadelphia, PA: Lippincott, Williams & Wilkins; 2005:1894–1902.
9. Cancer Facts & Figures. American Cancer Society, 2012. http://www.cancer.org/research/cancerfactsfigures/cancerfactsfigures/cancer-facts-figures-2012. Accessed February 28, 2013.
10. Lagergren J, Bergstrom R, Nyren O. Association between body mass and adenocarcinoma of the esophagus and gastric cardia. *Ann Int Med*. 1999;130:883–890.
11. Pohl H, Welch HG. The role of overdiagnosis and reclassification in the marked increase of esophageal adenocarcinoma incidence. *J Natl Cancer Inst*. 2005;97:142–146.
12. Hvid-Jensen F, Pedersen L, Drewes AM, et al. Incidence of adenocarcinoma among patients with Barrett's esophagus. *N Engl J Med*. 2011;365:1375–1383.
13. Lindell MM, Jr., Hill CA, Libshitz HI. Esophageal cancer: radiographic chest findings and their prognostic significance. *AJR Am J Roentgenol*. 1979;133:461–465.
14. Choi TK, Siu KF, Lam KH, et al. Bronchoscopy and carcinoma of the esophagus II. Carcinoma of the esophagus with tracheobronchial involvement. *Am J Surg*. 1984;147:760–762.
15. Choi TK, Siu KF, Lam KH, et al. Bronchoscopy and carcinoma of the esophagus I. Findings of bronchoscopy in carcinoma of the esophagus. *Am J Surg*. 1984;147:757–759.
16. Varghese T, Hofstetter W, Risz N, et al. The Society of Thoracic Surgeons Guidelines on the diagnosis and staging of patients with esophageal cancer. *Ann Thorac Surg*. 2013;96(1):346–356.
17. Uedo N, Fujishiro M, Goda K, et al. Role of narrow band imaging for diagnosis of early-stage esophagogastric cancer: current consensus of experienced endoscopists in Asia-Pacific region. *Dig Endosc*. 2011;23(Suppl 1):58–71.

18. Inculet RI, Keller SM, Dwyer A, et al. Evaluation of noninvasive tests for the preoperative staging of carcinoma of the esophagus: a prospective study. *Ann Thorac Surg*. 1985;40:561–565.
19. Furukawa H. [Magnetic resonance (MR) imaging for the detection of the invasion into neighboring structures in esophageal cancers]. *Nihon Geka Gakkai Zasshi*. 1991;92:636–644.
20. Tio TL, Cohen P, Coene PP, et al. Endosonography and computed tomography of esophageal carcinoma. Preoperative classification compared to the new (1987) TNM system. *Gastroenterology*. 1989;96:1478–1486.
21. Rice TW, Blackstone EH, Adelstein DJ, et al. Role of clinically determined depth of tumor invasion in the treatment of esophageal carcinoma. *J Thorac Cardiovasc Surg*. 2003;125:1091–1102.
22. Crabtree TD, Yacoub WN, Puri V, et al. Endoscopic ultrasound for early stage esophageal adenocarcinoma: implications for staging and survival. *Ann Thorac Surg*. 2011;91:1509–1515; discussion 15–16.
23. Stiles BM, Mirza F, Coppolino A, et al. Clinical T2-T3N0M0 esophageal cancer: the risk of node positive disease. *Ann Thorac Surg*. 2011;92:491–496; discussion 6–8.
24. Reed CE, Mishra G, Sahai AV, et al. Esophageal cancer staging: improved accuracy by endoscopic ultrasound of celiac lymph nodes. *Ann Thorac Surg*. 1999;67:319–321; discussion 22.
25. Lightdale CJ, Kulkarni KG. Role of endoscopic ultrasonography in the staging and follow-up of esophageal cancer. *J Clin Oncol*. 2005;23:4483–4489.
26. Young PE, Gentry AB, Acosta RD, et al. Endoscopic ultrasound does not accurately stage early adenocarcinoma or high-grade dysplasia of the esophagus. *Clin Gastroenterol Hepatol*. 2010;8:1037–1041.
27. Meyers BF, Downey RJ, Decker PA, et al. The utility of positron emission tomography in staging of potentially operable carcinoma of the thoracic esophagus: results of the American College of Surgeons Oncology Group Z0060 trial. *J Thorac Cardiovasc Surg*. 2007;133:738–745.
28. Block MI, Patterson GA, Sundaresan RS, et al. Improvement in staging of esophageal cancer with the addition of positron emission tomography. *Ann Thorac Surg*. 1997;64:770–776; discussion 6–7.
29. van Westreenen HL, Westerterp M, Bossuyt PM, et al. Systematic review of the staging performance of 18 F-fluorodeoxyglucose positron emission tomography in esophageal cancer. *J Clin Oncol*. 2004;22:3805–3812.
30. Luketich JD, Schauer PR, Meltzer CC, et al. Role of positron emission tomography in staging esophageal cancer. *Ann Thorac Surg*. 1997;64:765–769.
31. Downey RJ, Akhurst T, Ilson D, et al. Whole body 18FDG-PET and the response of esophageal cancer to induction therapy: results of a prospective trial. *J Clin Oncol*. 2003;21:428–432.
32. Rizk N, Downey RJ, Akhurst T, et al. Preoperative 18[F]-fluorodeoxyglu cose positron emission tomography standardized uptake values predict survival after esophageal adenocarcinoma resection. *Ann Thorac Surg*. 2006;81:1076–1081.
33. Edge S, ed. *American Joint Committee on Cancer*. New York, NY: Springer; 2010.
34. Mao YS, Suntharalingam M, Krasna MJ. Management of late distant metastases after trimodality therapy for esophageal cancer. *Ann Thorac Surg*. 2003;76:1742–1743.
35. Edge SB, American Joint Committee on Cancer. *AJCC Cancer Staging Manual*. 7th ed. New York, NY: Springer; 2010.
36. Rice TW, Rusch VW, Apperson-Hansen C, et al. Worldwide esophageal cancer collaboration. *Dis Esophagus*. 2009;22:1–8.
37. Rizk N, Venkatraman E, Park B, et al. The prognostic importance of the number of involved lymph nodes in esophageal cancer: implications for revisions of the American Joint Committee on Cancer staging system. *J Thorac Cardiovasc Surg*. 2006;132:1374–1381.
38. Kang CH, Kim YT, Jeon SH, et al. Lymphadenectomy extent is closely related to long-term survival in esophageal cancer. *Eur J Cardiothorac Surg*. 2007;31:154–160.
39. Greenstein AJ, Litle VR, Swanson SJ, et al. Effect of the number of lymph nodes sampled on postoperative survival of lymph node-negative esophageal cancer. *Cancer*. 2008;112:1239–1246.
40. Altorki NK, Zhou XK, Stiles B, et al. Total number of resected lymph nodes predicts survival in esophageal cancer. *Ann Surg*. 2008;248:221–226.
41. Veeramachaneni NK, Zoole JB, Decker PA, et al. Lymph node analysis in esophageal resection: American College of Surgeons Oncology Group Z0060 trial. *Ann Thorac Surg*. 2008;86:418–421; discussion 21.
42. Siewert JR, Stein HJ, Feith M, et al. Histologic tumor type is an independent prognostic parameter in esophageal cancer: lessons from more than 1,000 consecutive resections at a single center in the Western world. *Ann Surg*. 2001;234:360–367; discussion 8–9.
43. Murray GF, Wilcox BR, Starek PJ. The assessment of operability of esophageal carcinoma. *Ann Thorac Surg*. 1977;23:393–399.
44. Dagnini G, Caldironi MW, Marin G, et al. Laparoscopy in abdominal staging of esophageal carcinoma. Report of 369 cases. *Gastrointest Endosc*. 1986;32:400–402.
45. Stein HJ, Kraemer SJ, Feussner H, et al. Clinical value of diagnostic laparoscopy with laparoscopic ultrasound in patients with cancer of the esophagus or cardia. *J Gastrointest Surg*. 1997;1:167–172; discussion 72–73.
46. Krasna MJ, McLaughlin JS. Efficacy and safety of thoracoscopy for diagnosis and treatment of intrathoracic disease: the University of Maryland experience. *Surg Laparosc Endosc*. 1994;4:182–188.
47. Krasna MJ, Reed CE, Jaklitsch MT, et al. Thoracoscopic staging of esophageal cancer: a prospective, multiinstitutional trial. Cancer and Leukemia Group B Thoracic Surgeons. *Ann Thorac Surg*. 1995;60:1337–1340.
48. Krasna MJ, Flowers JL, Attar S, et al. Combined thoracoscopic/laparoscopic staging of esophageal cancer. *J Thorac Cardiovasc Surg*. 1996;111:800–806; discussion 6–7.
49. Luketich JD, Nguyen NT, Weigel T, et al. Minimally invasive approach to esophagectomy. *JSLS*. 1998;2:243–247.
50. Luketich JD, Kassis ES, Shriver SP, et al. Detection of micrometastases in histologically negative lymph nodes in esophageal cancer. *Ann Thorac Surg*. 1998;66:1715–1718.
51. Krasna MJ, Mao YS, Sonett JR, et al. P53 gene protein overexpression predicts results of trimodality therapy in esophageal cancer patients. *Ann Thorac Surg*. 1999;68:2021–2024; discussion 4–5.
52. Launois B, Delarue D, Campion JP, et al. Preoperative radiotherapy for carcinoma of the esophagus. *Surg Gynecol Obstet*. 1981;153:690–692.
53. Kelsen DP, Ginsberg R, Pajak TF, et al. Chemotherapy followed by surgery compared with surgery alone for localized esophageal cancer. *N Engl J Med*. 1998;339:1979–1984.
54. Lam KY, Law S, Ma LT, et al. Pre-operative chemotherapy for squamous cell carcinoma of the oesophagus: do histological assessment and p53 overexpression predict chemo-responsiveness? *Eur J Cancer*. 1997;33:1221–1225.
55. MRC. Surgical resection with or without preoperative chemotherapy in oesophageal cancer: a randomised controlled trial: Medical Research Council Oesophageal Cancer Working Group. *Lancet*. 2002;359:1727–1733.
56. Allum WH, Stenning SP, Bancewicz J, et al. Long-term results of a randomized trial of surgery with or without preoperative chemotherapy in esophageal cancer. *J Clin Oncol*. 2009;27:5062–5067.
57. Cunningham D, Allum WH, Stenning SP, et al. Perioperative chemotherapy versus surgery alone for resectable gastroesophageal cancer. *N Engl J Med*. 2006;355:11–20.
58. Ychou M, Boige V, Pignon JP, et al. Perioperative chemotherapy compared with surgery alone for resectable gastroesophageal adenocarcinoma: an FNCLCC and FFCD multicenter phase III trial. *J Clin Oncol*. 2011;29:1715–1721.
59. Walsh TN, Noonan N, Hollywood D, et al. A comparison of multimodal therapy and surgery for esophageal adenocarcinoma. *N Engl J Med*. 1996;335:462–467.
60. Bosset JF, Gignoux M, Triboulet JP, et al. Chemoradiotherapy followed by surgery compared with surgery alone in squamous-cell cancer of the esophagus. *N Engl J Med*. 1997;337:161–167.
61. Urba SG, Orringer MB, Turrisi A, et al. Randomized trial of preoperative chemoradiation versus surgery alone in patients with locoregional esophageal carcinoma. *J Clin Oncol*. 2001;19:305–313.
62. Urschel JD, Vasan H. A meta-analysis of randomized controlled trials that compared neoadjuvant chemoradiation and surgery to surgery alone for resectable esophageal cancer. *Am J Surg*. 2003;185:538–543.
63. Sjoquist KM, Burmeister BH, Smithers BM, et al. Survival after neoadjuvant chemotherapy or chemoradiotherapy for resectable oesophageal carcinoma: an updated meta-analysis. *Lancet Oncol*. 2011;12:681–692.
64. Tepper J, Krasna MJ, Niedzwiecki D, et al. Phase III trial of trimodality therapy with cisplatin, fluorouracil, radiotherapy, and surgery compared with surgery alone for esophageal cancer: CALGB 9781. *J Clin Oncol*. 2008;26:1086–1092.
65. van der Gaast A, van Hagen P, Hulshof M, et al. Effect of preoperative concurrent chemoradiotherapy on survival of patients with resectable esophageal or esophagogastric junction cancer: result from a multi-center randomized phase III study. *J Clin Oncol*. 2010;28:4004.

66. van Heijl M, van Lanschot JJ, Koppert LB, et al. Neoadjuvant chemoradiation followed by surgery versus surgery alone for patients with adenocarcinoma or squamous cell carcinoma of the esophagus (CROSS). *BMC Surg.* 2008;8:21.
67. Port JL, Lee PC, Korst RJ, et al. Positron emission tomographic scanning predicts survival after induction chemotherapy for esophageal carcinoma. *Ann Thorac Surg.* 2007;84:393–400; discussion.
68. Cerfolio RJ, Bryant AS, Talati AA, et al. Change in maximum standardized uptake value on repeat positron emission tomography after chemoradiotherapy in patients with esophageal cancer identifies complete responders. *J Thorac Cardiovasc Surg.* 2009;137:605–609.
69. Koshy M, Greenwald BD, Hausner P, et al. Outcomes after trimodality therapy for esophageal cancer: the impact of histology on failure patterns. *Am J Clin Oncol.* 2011;34:259–264.
70. Burmeister BH, Thomas JM, Burmeister EA, et al. Is concurrent radiation therapy required in patients receiving preoperative chemotherapy for adenocarcinoma of the oesophagus? A randomised phase II trial. *Eur J Cancer.* 2011;47:354–360.
71. Ténière P, Hay JM, Fingerhut A, et al. Postoperative radiation therapy does not increase survival after curative resection for squamous cell carcinoma of the middle and lower esophagus as shown by a multicenter controlled trial. French University Association for Surgical Research. *Surg Gynecol Obstet.* 1991;173:123–130.
72. Fok M, Sham JS, Choy D, et al. Postoperative radiotherapy for carcinoma of the esophagus: a prospective, randomized controlled study. *Surgery.* 1993;113:138–147.
73. Chiu PW, Chan AC, Leung SF, et al. Multicenter prospective randomized trial comparing standard esophagectomy with chemoradiotherapy for treatment of squamous esophageal cancer: early results from the Chinese University Research Group for Esophageal Cancer (CURE). *J Gastrointest Surg.* 2005;9:794–802.
74. Schreiber D, Rineer J, Vongtama D, et al. Impact of postoperative radiation after esophagectomy for esophageal cancer. *J Thorac Oncol.* 2010;5:244–250.
75. Ando N, Iizuka T, Ide H, et al. Surgery plus chemotherapy compared with surgery alone for localized squamous cell carcinoma of the thoracic esophagus: a Japan Clinical Oncology Group Study–JCOG9204. *J Clin Oncol.* 2003;21:4592–4596.
76. Bedenne L, Michel P, Bouche O, et al. Chemoradiation followed by surgery compared with chemoradiation alone in squamous cancer of the esophagus: FFCD 9102. *J Clin Oncol.* 2007;25:1160–1168.
77. Stahl M, Stuschke M, Lehmann N, et al. Chemoradiation with and without surgery in patients with locally advanced squamous cell carcinoma of the esophagus. *J Clin Oncol.* 2005;23:2310–2317.
78. Mak RH, Mamon HJ, Ryan DP, et al. Toxicity and outcomes after chemoradiation for esophageal cancer in patients age 75 or older. *Dis Esophagus.* 2010;23:316–323.
79. Suntharalingam M, Moughan J, Coia LR, et al. Outcome results of the 1996–1999 patterns of care survey of the national practice for patients receiving radiation therapy for carcinoma of the esophagus. *J Clin Oncol.* 2005;23:2325–2331.
80. Bailey SH, Bull DA, Harpole DH, et al. Outcomes after esophagectomy: a ten-year prospective cohort. *Ann Thorac Surg.* 2003;75:217–222; discussion 22.
81. Wright CD, Kucharczuk JC, O'Brien SM, et al. Predictors of major morbidity and mortality after esophagectomy for esophageal cancer: a Society of Thoracic Surgeons General Thoracic Surgery Database risk adjustment model. *J Thorac Cardiovasc Surg.* 2009;137:587–595; discussion 96.
82. Verhoef C, van de Weyer R, Schaapveld M, et al. Better survival in patients with esophageal cancer after surgical treatment in university hospitals: a plea for performance by surgical oncologists. *Ann Surg Oncol.* 2007;14:1678–1687.
83. Padmanabhan RS, Byrnes MC, Helmer SD, et al. Should esophagectomy be performed in a low-volume center? *Am Surg.* 2002;68:348–351; discussion 51–52.
84. Santin B, Kulwicki A, Price P. Mortality rate associated with 56 consecutive esophagectomies performed at a "low-volume" hospital: is procedure volume as important as we are trying to make it? *J Gastrointest Surg.* 2008;12:1346–1350.
85. Santin BJ, Price P. Laparoscopic transhiatal esophagectomy at a low-volume center. *JSLS.* 2011;15:41–46.
86. Birkmeyer JD, Stukel TA, Siewers AE, et al. Surgeon volume and operative mortality in the United States. *N Engl J Med.* 2003;349:2117–2127.
87. Peters FP, Kara MA, Rosmolen WD, et al. Endoscopic treatment of high-grade dysplasia and early stage cancer in Barrett's esophagus. *Gastrointest Endosc.* 2005;61:506–514.
88. Ell C, May A, Pech O, et al. Curative endoscopic resection of early esophageal adenocarcinomas (Barrett's cancer). *Gastrointest Endosc.* 2007;65:3–10.
89. Narsule CK, Montgomery MM, Fernando HC. Evidence-based review of the management of cancers of the gastroesophageal junction. *Thorac Surg Clin.* 2012;22:109–121, vii–viii.
90. Krasna MJ, Mao YS. Making sense of multimodality therapy for esophageal cancer. *Surg Oncol Clin North Am.* 1999;8:259–278.
91. Orringer MB. Transhiatal esophagectomy without thoracotomy for carcinoma of the thoracic esophagus. *Ann Surg.* 1984;200:282–288.

11 Pathology of Esophageal Cancer

Amitabh Srivastava and Robert D. Odze

Keywords: Squamous cell carcinoma (SCC) of esophagus and histologic variants, verrucous SCC, carcinosarcoma (spindle cell carcinoma), basaloid SCC, adenocarcinoma of esophagus and histologic variants, Barrett esophagus, non–Barrett-associated adenocarcinomas, carcinomas with mixed squamous and glandular differentiation, adenoid cystic carcinoma, choriocarcinoma, carcinoid tumors, malignant melanoma, gastrointestinal stromal tumor (GIST)

INTRODUCTION

Esophageal cancer is a gastrointestinal malignancy that encompasses a range of pathologic entities. Squamous cell carcinomas constitute at least 90% of all cancers worldwide.[1] Adenocarcinoma is the second most common type of cancer. Other types, such as small cell carcinoma and malignant melanoma are rare. The incidence of esophageal adenocarcinoma has increased in the United States from 0.5 to 0.9/100,000 in the 1970s to 3.2 to 4.0/100,000 in the 1980s and 1990s. Although esophageal adenocarcinoma accounted for about 16% of all esophageal cancers among White men in the United States in the mid-1970s, by the late 1990s, this number approached 50%. This increase has been seen across all socioeconomic groups[2] but has been most pronounced in affluent populations.[3–7] Over the same period of time, there has been a decline in both esophageal squamous cell carcinomas and adenocarcinomas of the distal stomach.[8,9] Barrett esophagus is a metaplastic condition in which normal squamous mucosa of the distal esophagus is transformed into intestinalized columnar epithelium. Barrett esophagus is the established precursor lesion for nearly all esophageal adenocarcinomas.

SQUAMOUS CELL CARCINOMA AND VARIANTS

Squamous cell carcinoma of the esophagus is relatively infrequent in much of Western Europe and North America, but is a major disease for a large proportion of the world's population. About 80% of cases occur within developing countries.[10] In the United States, squamous cell carcinoma continues to represent the most common type of esophageal cancer in African Americans. The highest rates are found in the Asian esophageal cancer belt region, which extends from Turkey to Iran, Iraq and Kazakhstan to Northern China. Squamous cell carcinoma is the most prevalent type of esophageal cancer in this region. However, even within this region, there are sharp gradients of incidence between regions that lie only a few hundred miles apart. In Europe, where the incidence of squamous cell carcinoma is low, pockets of high incidence occur, such as in Normandy and Brittany.[11]

Etiology and Associations

The etiology of squamous cell carcinoma is most likely multifactorial. Epidemiological studies have provided evidence that causative agents may act synergistically and may differ between geographical regions and between high-risk versus low-risk areas.

Cigarette smoking and alcohol consumption have both been associated with an increased predisposition for esophageal cancer, and the association is stronger with squamous cell carcinoma compared to adenocarcinoma. Smokers are at three to seven times greater risk of developing squamous cell carcinoma compared with the general population.[12–15] There is a statistically higher incidence of esophageal carcinomas among patients who smoke or chew tobacco, and this is equally true for pipe users, cigar, and cigarette smokers.[16] Among combined drinkers and smokers, the risk rises considerably with increased alcohol consumption, compared to increasing tobacco consumption.[15] In the United Kingdom, variations in the rate of esophageal cancer have closely paralleled total alcohol consumption, with only a short lag, suggesting that the effect of alcohol may be on the later stages of carcinogenesis, as a tumor promoter.

Esophageal carcinomas are frequently associated with multiple primary tumors in the mouth, pharynx, stomach, or intestine.[17,18] It has been suggested that this finding may be related to ingestion of nicotine and other carcinogenic substances.[18] In some high-risk populations in South Africa and India, tobacco appears to play a more important role than alcohol.[19,20]

Fungal esophagitis, mostly due to Candida spp., is very common in the Linxian province of China and has been postulated as a possible etiological factor in esophageal carcinogenesis. Recent research has focused on the role of human papillomavirus (HPV) infection in esophageal carcinoma.[21–27] Histological changes in esophageal squamous cell carcinomas similar to condylomatous genital lesions have been observed.[28] The reported prevalence of HPV in squamous cell carcinoma of the esophagus has varied widely from 0% to 71%. The variation may be due to true geographic variation in pathogenesis, variation in techniques used to detect HPV, different thresholds to classify cases as being HPV positive, and, in some instances, it may simply reflect sample contamination. The marked difference in association of esophageal cancer with HPV infection has led the International Agency for Research on Cancer to recently conclude that "there is inadequate evidence in humans for carcinogenicity of HPV in the esophagus."[29]

There is an increased risk of esophageal carcinoma after ingestion of lye (crude sodium hydroxide with sodium carbonate), typically after a time interval of 40 years.[30,31] The evidence for development of cancer in strictures from other causes is less convincing.[32] Esophageal cancer has been reported following therapeutic radiation for neck and spinal diseases,[33] after radiation to the chest for breast carcinoma and, less frequently, for lymphoma.[34] Polycyclic aromatic hydrocarbons may also play a role in the pathogenesis of esophageal cancer.[35,36]

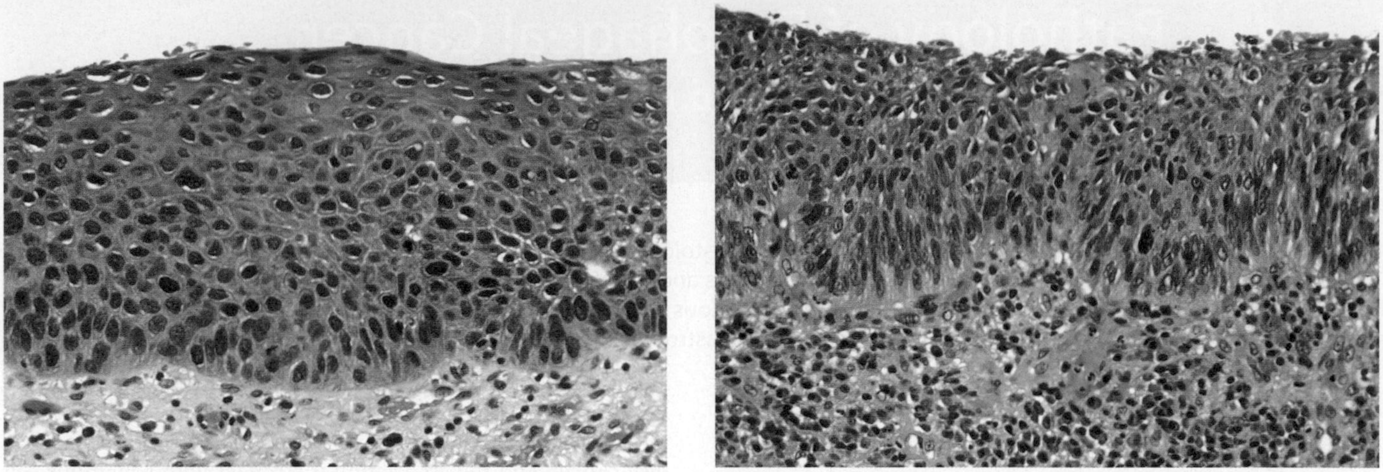

A

B

Figure 11-1. Squamous cell dysplasia is categorized as low grade when the thickness of mucosa involved with basaloid undifferentiated cells is less than 50% (*A*) and as high grade when it exceeds 50% (*B*).

A study from Northern Iraq found a positive family history of esophageal cancer in 47.1% of patients in high-risk regions, compared with only 2% among the low-risk population.[37] Familial esophageal cancer in families associated with keratosis palmaris and plantaris (tylosis), inherited as a dominant trait, have been described.[38–40] The tylosis esophageal cancer (TOC) gene locus was recently mapped to chromosome 17q25.[41] This locus is also commonly deleted in sporadic esophageal squamous cell carcinomas, suggesting the existence of a tumor suppressor gene for esophageal squamous cell carcinoma at this site.[42]

Acetaldehyde, produced during alcohol metabolism, is eliminated from the body by aldehyde dehydrogenase which is a product of the *ALDH2* gene. The *1/*2 heterozygous polymorphism of the *ALDH2* gene has been shown to confer an increased risk of esophageal squamous cell carcinoma.[43,44] In addition, the *2/*2 homozygous genotype of *ALDH2* gene is associated with a lower risk of squamous cell carcinoma.[45] Another example of genetic susceptibility for esophageal cancer involves the C677 T polymorphism in the *MTHFR* (methylenetetrahydrofolate reductase) gene. The TT and TC genotypes of this gene have been shown to confer an increased risk of squamous dysplasia, and cancer, compared to the CC genotype.[46]

Other conditions associated with an increased risk of esophageal cancer include achalasia, diverticulosis,[47,48] Plummer-Vinson syndrome,[49] and celiac disease.[50,51] Esophageal carcinoma is also associated with tumors of the oropharynx and larynx,[52,53] presumably due to shared risk factors such as heavy smoking and high alcohol intake.[54]

Pathology

Precancerous Lesions

Chronic esophagitis is common in populations with a high incidence of esophageal carcinoma, and usually involves the middle and lower thirds of the esophagus. "White" patches are seen at endoscopy, which corresponds to acanthosis and swollen clear squamous cells. Squamous dysplasia is a precursor of esophageal squamous cell carcinoma. Dysplasia may appear endoscopically as areas of friable or erythematous mucosa, erosions, plaques, or nodules. Ill-defined irregularities of the mucosal surface, or white patches, also may be present. In a very small proportion of cases, foci of dysplasia, or cancer, may appear endoscopically normal.[55] The age distribution of dysplasia and carcinoma suggested a continuous progression from mild to severe dysplasia and carcinoma in situ. Further evidence of the role of dysplasia as a precancerous lesion comes from its frequent occurrence in areas adjacent to, or distant from, invasive squamous carcinoma when esophagectomy specimens have been studied in detail.[56–59] Prevalence of dysplasia at the margins of invasive carcinoma is reported to be inversely related to the depth of invasion of the main lesion. This suggests that dysplasia represents a precursor lesion rather than cancerization of overlying benign epithelium by the invasive carcinoma.[60] Multicentric tumors may be present in 15% to 30% of squamous cell carcinomas further supporting the idea of a "field effect" in carcinogenesis.[61,62]

The histological criteria for dysplasia include architectural and cytological abnormalities. Two classifications have been used. The original classification defined dysplasia as mild when <25% of the epithelium was involved, moderate when 25% to 50% of the epithelium was involved, and severe when more than 50% of the mucosa was involved. A two-tiered system, where low-grade dysplasia is defined as <50% and high-grade dysplasia as >50% involvement of the epithelium with neoplastic cells, is preferred (Fig. 11-1A,B). Cytological features of dysplasia include high nuclear-cytoplasmic ratio, nuclear hyperchromasia and pleomorphism, and increased mitotic activity. Dysplasia also may spread in a pagetoid fashion or into underlying esophageal gland ducts.[63,64] In some cases, the presence of koilocytotic change may reflect an underlying HPV infection.[65,66]

In the presence of significant inflammation, a diagnosis of dysplasia should be made with caution because regenerative changes secondary to inflammation, radiation, or chemotherapy may mimic dysplasia. Unlike dysplasia, regenerative epithelium shows surface maturation and does not show significant nuclear crowding and loss of polarity, and atypical mitoses are typically absent. Vesicular chromatin, with prominent nucleoli, is often present in regenerating epithelium. In cases of uncertainty, a diagnosis of "indefinite for dysplasia" should be rendered.

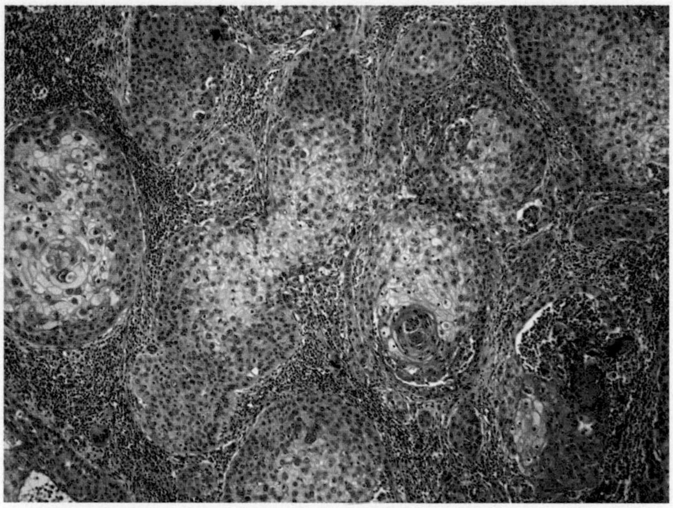

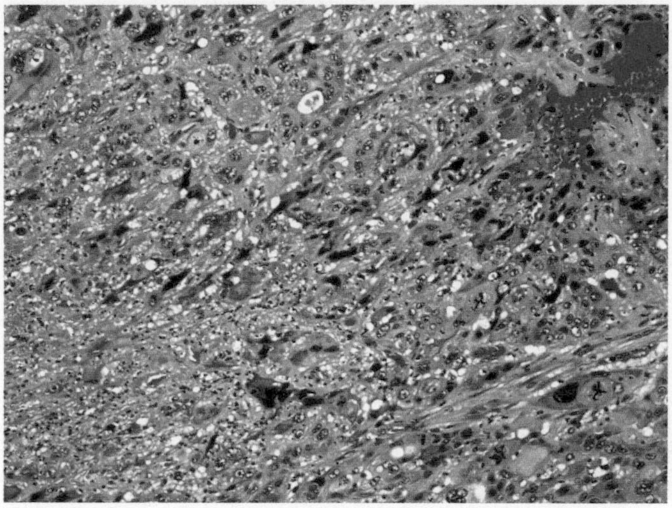

A B

Figure 11-2. The spectrum of invasive squamous cell carcinoma ranges from well-differentiated tumors (*A*) with bland, monomorphic nuclei with minimal cytological atypia to those that are poorly differentiated (*B*) and show marked nuclear hyperchromasia, pleomorphism, and abundant atypical mitoses.

Gross Pathology of Squamous Cell Carcinoma

Squamous cell carcinoma is rare in the upper third of the esophagus, most common in the middle third, and less frequent in the lower third. The distribution in one large series was in the upper third of the esophagus in 11.7%, the middle third in 63.3%, and the lower third in 24.9%.[67] Macroscopically, squamous carcinomas may be exophytic, ulcerating or infiltrating, or show a combination of these features. Irregular, friable and, hemorrhagic strictures may be present. Papillary or verrucous squamous cell carcinomas are uncommon, and occur as large, warty, slowly growing neoplasms.[68] Most have been reported in the upper third.[69–71] Rarely, a diffuse infiltrative pattern, resembling a "leather bottle stomach," may involve the esophagus. Superficial spreading carcinomas, with extensive intramucosal involvement and a propensity to permeate lymphatics and metastasize to lymph nodes, have also been described.[72]

Microscopic Pathology of Squamous Cell Carcinoma

Esophageal squamous cell carcinomas show all grades of differentiation. Well-differentiated lesions are composed of well-defined nests of tumor cells with keratinization while poorly differentiated tumors show sheets of undifferentiated tumor cells without any evidence of keratinization (Fig. 11-2A,B). Some tumors may show a predominance of basaloid tumor cells with peripheral palisading similar to a basal cell carcinoma. In most tumors, keratin pearls or intercellular bridges are present. Variation of cellular differentiation in different parts of the tumor is common. Histochemical, immunohistochemical, and ultrastructural studies have confirmed morphological heterogeneity. Focal adenocarcinomatous differentiation may be present in some tumors.[73–75]

Histologic Variants of Squamous Cell Carcinoma

Verrucous Squamous Cell Carcinoma of the esophagus is extremely rare. These are large, exophytic neoplasms with a papillary or warty appearance and are often associated with stricture formation. The age range of patients is broad, but there is a male predilection. These tumors can arise at any site in the esophagus. But in most cases occur in the upper third.[69] Histologically, verrucous carcinoma consists of papillary projections of well-differentiated squamous cells, with parakeratosis and hyperkeratosis most prominent between papillae (Fig. 11-3). Evidence of invasion is frequently lacking in biopsies. Pathologists may interpret the "bland" features as a benign process if they are unaware of the endoscopic appearance. Invasion is typically in the form of a broad pushing front, and may be difficult to diagnose with certainty even in resection specimens. Despite low-grade morphology, and a low risk of distant metastases,[68] this tumor has a poor prognosis because of its propensity to invade locally, and develop fistulas.[76]

Carcinosarcoma (Spindle Cell Carcinoma) was first described by Virchow in 1865. It is also termed "polypoid

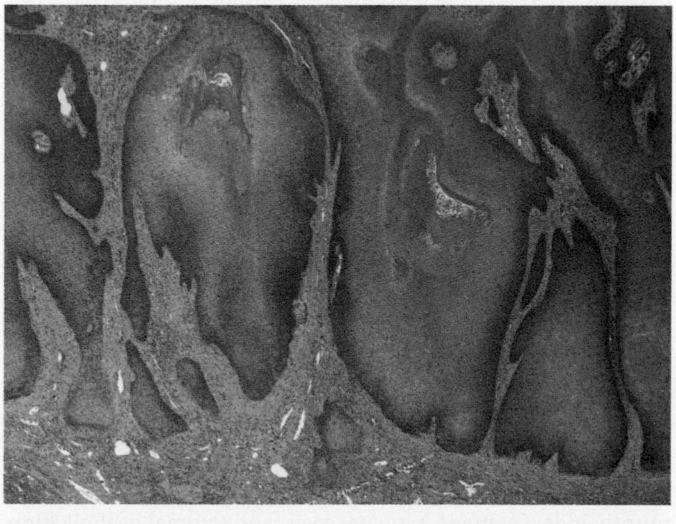

Figure 11-3. Verrucous carcinomas show papillary fronds of extremely well-differentiated squamous cells with marked parakeratosis and hyperkeratosis. Invasion is typically along a broad front with pushing margins and may be difficult to demonstrate even in resection specimens.

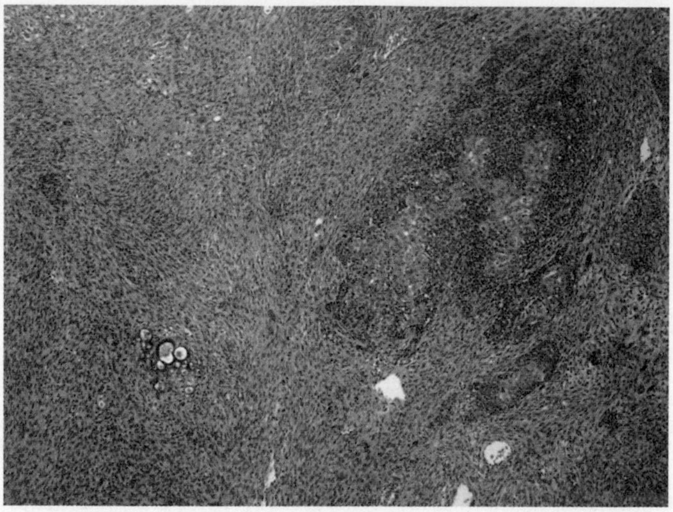

Figure 11-4. Carcinosarcomas are biphasic tumors with epithelial and sarcomatous elements. The latter is usually in the form of intersecting fascicles of spindle-shaped cells but cartilaginous or osseous differentiation may also be present in some cases.

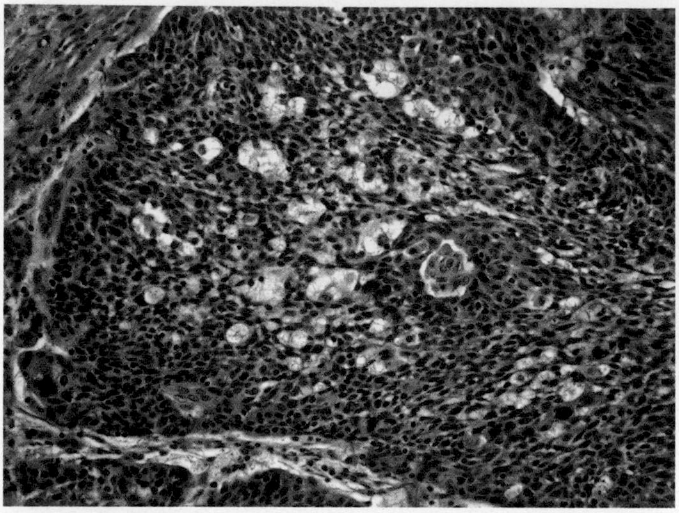

Figure 11-5. Squamous cell carcinomas with basaloid features may demonstrate microcystic spaces that impart a pseudoglandular appearance to the tumor. Basaloid tumors with this morphology have been mistaken for adenoid cystic carcinomas in the past.

carcinoma," "sarcomatoid carcinoma," and "spindle cell carcinoma." These tumors represent about 2% of all esophageal carcinomas. It affects predominantly adult men between 40 and 90 years of age, and presents as a bulky polypoid tumor in the middle or lower esophagus. Microscopically, the tumors show a mixture of "sarcomatous" and epithelial elements, the former showing interlacing bundles of spindle-shaped cells. Osseous and cartilaginous differentiation and bizarre giant cells may occur as well (Fig. 11-4). An epithelial component of squamous or undifferentiated carcinoma is typical, but these foci may be small and difficult to detect. Occasionally, an adenocarcinomatous,[70] adenocystic,[78] neuroendocrine, or glandular component may be present.[79] In most tumors, the sarcomatous pattern predominates, and the squamous cell carcinoma component is inconspicuous and confined to small areas at the base of the pedicle. Areas of transition from typical squamous carcinoma to sarcoma are often present.[78,80] The demonstration of tonofibrils and well-developed desmosomes in the spindle cells[77,81] on ultrastructural examination, suggests that the sarcomatous cells are squamous in origin. Immunohistochemical studies have demonstrated disparate findings. Some authors have shown immunoreactivity to keratin in the spindle cell component[82,83] whereas others have reported negative reactions to keratin and variable positivity for desmin, smooth muscle actin, vimentin, alpha-1-antichymotrypsin, and alpha-1-antitrypsin.[79,84,85] Although hematogenous spread is more common in carcinosarcomas than pure squamous cell carcinoma, the overall 5-year survival rate has been shown to be similar.[77,86]

Basaloid Squamous Cell Carcinomas comprise about 2% to 11% of all squamous cell carcinomas[87,88] and usually occur in elderly males, in the mid or distal esophagus. Presentation at an advanced stage is typical. There is, by definition, a variable amount of undifferentiated basaloid component in the form of solid sheets, anastomosing trabeculae, festoons or microcystic structures, and these areas are associated with a high mitotic index, comedo-type necrosis, and stromal hyalinization (Fig. 11-5). The neoplastic, in situ or invasive squamous component may be inconspicuous. The prognosis of patients with basaloid–squamous carcinoma does not differ significantly from conventional squamous cell carcinoma.[88] The majority of cases in the literature reported as "adenoid cystic carcinomas" of the esophagus probably represent basaloid–squamous cell carcinomas. True esophageal adenoid cystic carcinoma has a less aggressive clinical course (see below).[89,90]

Natural History and Prognosis of Squamous Cell Carcinoma

Squamous cell carcinoma confined only to the mucosa or the submucosa, with or without lymph node metastasis, is referred to as "superficial cancer." However, the prognosis of early esophageal cancer differs from early gastric cancer, with 5-year survival rates for esophagus in the 50% to 60% range for tumors with submucosal infiltration. This is related to the fact that 30% to 40% of esophageal tumors with submucosal invasion also have lymph node metastasis.[91–93] This has led some authors to suggest that the term "early" esophageal cancer should be restricted to cases in which there is carcinoma in situ (intraepithelial dysplasia/neoplasia), or mucosal carcinoma only, in which the prognosis approaches 100%.[93–95] The presence of an elevated component in superficial esophageal cancer may be predictive of submucosal invasion, and a high probability of lymph node involvement.[96] Superficial carcinomas may occupy a large area of the esophagus[64,97,98] in some cases. Endoscopic ultrasonography has been used in cases of superficial esophageal carcinoma to assess depth of invasion and lymph node metastasis.[99] Nonsurgical interventions such as photodynamic therapy[100] and endoscopic mucosal resection[101] are being increasingly used in the treatment of precursor lesions and superficial cancer.

The risk of nodal metastasis increases with depth of invasion and rises dramatically once tumors have penetrated the submucosa. Thus, intramucosal tumors have a $<5\%$ risk of nodal metastasis compared to tumors that invade the submucosa, where the risk approaches 45%.[102,103] Skip metastases may be present in esophageal cancers and distant metastasis to lungs and liver have been reported in up to 50% of all squamous cell carcinomas.[53] Overall, the 5-year survival rate in squamous cell

Table 11-1

TNM STAGING OF ESOPHAGEAL CARCINOMA (7TH EDITION, 2010)

T—Primary tumor
- pT1 Tumor invades lamina propria, muscularis mucosa, or submucosa
  - T1a: invades lamina propria or muscularis mucosa
  - T1b: invades submucosa
- pT2 Tumor invades muscularis propria
- pT3 Tumor invades adventitia
- pT4 Tumor invades adjacent structures
  - T4a: resectable tumor invading pleura, pericardium, or diaphragm
  - T4b: unresectable tumor invading other structures (aorta, vertebra, trachea, etc.)

N—Regional lymph nodes
- pN0 No regional lymph node metastasis
- pN1 Regional lymph node metastasis involving 1–2 nodes
- pN2 3–6 positive lymph nodes
- pN3 7 or more positive lymph nodes

M—Distant metastasis
- M1 Distant metastasis present

carcinoma is about 26%. Tumor stage remains the most significant prognostic factor in patients treated with esophagectomy. The TNM (tumor, node, metastasis) staging system proposed by the American Joint Committee on Cancer (AJCC) has been revised recently and is significantly different from the prior edition (see Chapter 12). The staging criteria in the new proposal are outlined in Table 11-1. The number of lymph nodes examined in esophagectomy specimens has been shown to be an independent prognostic factor in a number of studies.[104–106] Histopathologic examination for extent of residual tumor has also been proposed as a prognostic factor following neoadjuvant therapy for esophageal squamous cell carcinoma.[107]

ADENOCARCINOMA AND VARIANTS

Clinical Features

Barrett esophagus is a metaplastic precancerous lesion involving the distal esophagus that occurs in patients with chronic gastroesophageal reflux disease and is present in the majority of patients with esophageal adenocarcinoma. The distal third of the esophagus is the most common location for esophageal adenocarcinoma. The overall incidence of esophageal adenocarcinoma has increased from 3.6 per million in 1973 to 25.6 per million in 2006.[2,8,108] The incidence of adenocarcinoma has also risen among Black males and women during this period, but the rates have remained at much lower levels. Increasing rates of esophageal adenocarcinoma have also been reported from the United Kingdom, Scandinavia, France, Switzerland, Australia, and New Zealand.[109–114] Interestingly, recent incidence trend analysis for esophageal adenocarcinoma using the SEER database shows that the increase in incidence of esophageal adenocarcinoma may have slowed down and possibly reached a plateau. The rising trend appears to have slowed down from an annual 8.2% increase prior to 1996 to 1.3% in subsequent years. This is largely due to changes in incidence of early stage disease, which has changed from a 10% annual increase prior to 1999, to a 1.6% decline subsequently.[115]

Etiology and Associations

The underlying risk factors for adenocarcinoma of the distal esophagus and the gastroesophageal junction are significantly different from those of esophageal squamous cell carcinoma. Gastroesophageal adenocarcinomas show an association with reflux disease, obesity, dietary factors, smoking, and alcohol consumption, and are inversely associated with gastric colonization by *Helicobacter pylori*. Obesity and overweight have been consistently shown to be associated with esophageal adenocarcinoma, but not to squamous cell carcinoma.[116,117] This may be related to increased abdominal pressure predisposing to gastroesophageal reflux disease and increasing likelihood of developing Barrett esophagus.[118,119] The impact of smoking on risk of esophageal adenocarcinoma is weak compared to squamous cell carcinoma. There is a two- to threefold increased risk in smokers, but unlike squamous cell carcinoma, the risk of esophageal adenocarcinoma does not decrease substantially after cessation of smoking.[120–122] Alcohol consumption has not been consistently related to an increased risk for esophageal adenocarcinoma. The use of aspirin or other nonsteroidal antiinflammatory drugs (NSAIDs) may reduce the risk of esophageal cancer. A 35% decrease in the risk of esophageal cancer among NSAID users compared with nonusers was shown in a recent meta-analysis.[123–127] Single nucleotide polymorphisms (SNPs) involving Caspase-7 and Caspase-9 genes are reported to be significantly associated with an increased risk of esophageal adenocarcinoma. SNP in the *PR* (progesterone receptor) gene among women carrying the variant G allele may exert a protective effect.[128]

Pathologic Features

Gross Pathology of Adenocarcinoma

The majority of esophageal adenocarcinomas involve the distal third of the esophagus and present as ulcerating, infiltrative lesions (40%–50%), frequently associated with stenosis of the esophageal lumen. Others are fungating (20%–25%), flat (10%–15%), or polypoid (5%–10%) in appearance.[129,130] A diffusely infiltrative growth pattern resembling linitis plastica in the stomach is seen in rare instances.[131] Early cancers detected during surveillance of patients with Barrett esophagus may be invisible on endoscopy or appear as small depressed or elevated lesions.[132] Multicentric tumors have also been described.[130,133] Barrett esophagus is often apparent in the background, although in large tumors this may be obliterated completely by the tumor mass. Patients in whom esophagectomy is performed after neoadjuvant chemoradiation therapy may not show any residual lesion upon gross examination. Only a flat ulcerated lesion or an indurated scar may be present at the primary tumor site.[134]

Microscopic Pathology of Adenocarcinoma

Histologically, these tumors show a similar spectrum of changes as adenocarcinomas that develop in the stomach. High-grade dysplasia is commonly seen in adjacent columnar epithelium.[129,135] The majority of tumors show a tubular or papillary growth pattern with variable grades of differentiation. Well-differentiated tumors show >95% gland formation, with columnar to cuboidal cells, hyperchromatic or vesicular nuclei, and a variable amount of eosinophilic or clear cytoplasm. Moderately differentiated tumors show gland formation in 50% to 95% of the tumor and poorly differentiated tumors show <50%

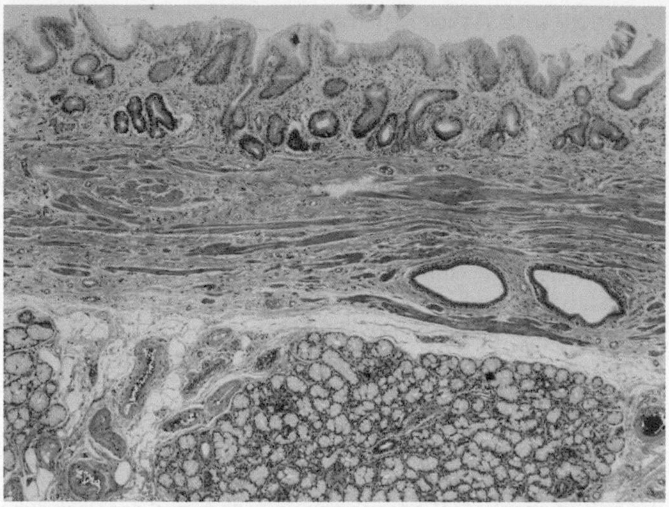

A

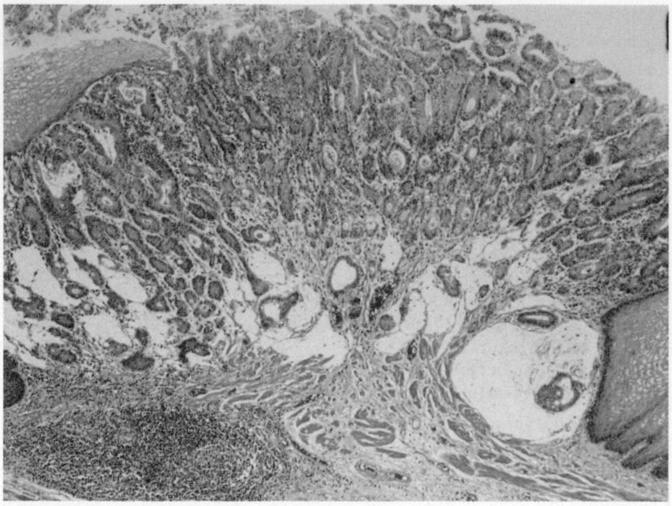

B

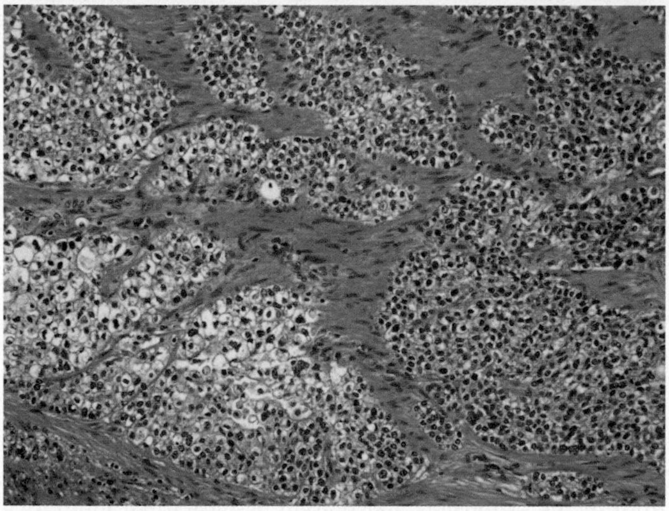

C

Figure 11-6. *A*. The majority of esophageal adenocarcinomas arise in a background of Barrett esophagus (BE) in which esophageal squamous mucosa is replaced by a metaplastic columnar epithelium with goblet cells (top). The esophageal location of the metaplastic epithelium can be confirmed by the presence of esophageal submucosal glands/ducts (bottom). *B*, *C*. Adenocarcinomas are graded on the basis of the degree of gland formation. At one end of the spectrum are well-differentiated adenocarcinomas with more than 95% gland formation (*B*) whereas at the other end are poorly differentiated tumors with a solid architecture barely recognizable as an adenocarcinoma (*C*).

glandular differentiation (Fig. 11-6A,B). The degree of nuclear pleomorphism parallels the grade of differentiation. Large, bizarre pleomorphic nuclei are more commonly seen in poorly differentiated tumors. About 5% to 10% tumors are of the mucinous (colloid) type and show prominent pools of extracellular mucin with floating clusters of tumor cells (Fig. 11-7). Signet ring cell carcinoma is less common (5% of cases) than in the stomach. Foci of squamous, neuroendocrine, and Paneth cell differentiation have been described in esophageal adenocarcinomas and represent multidirectional differentiation in the tumor.[136] Pagetoid spread into overlying squamous epithelium occurs, at times, in poorly differentiated adenocarcinomas.[137] The presence of a double muscularis mucosa in patients with Barrett esophagus may lead to errors in staging of early adenocarcinomas. The deep layer of muscularis mucosae is often thick and may be mistaken for muscularis propria[138–140] in an endoscopic mucosal resection specimen which may lead to over staging of invasive carcinomas in about 7% cases.[139] Carcinomas that invade between the two layers of muscularis mucosae are associated lymphovascular invasion in about 10% of cases.[139,140]

In esophagectomies performed after neoadjuvant therapy, residual tumor is often present in small, isolated clusters in

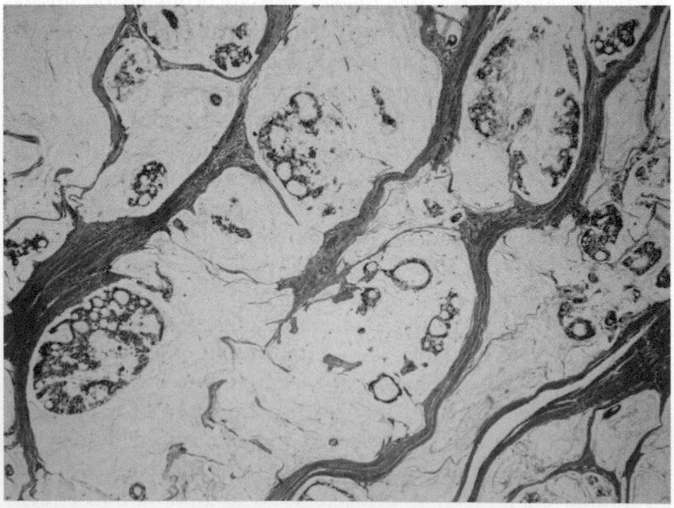

Figure 11-7. Mucinous (colloid) adenocarcinomas of the esophagus are uncommon and show tumor cells in small clusters and aggregates floating in abundant pools of extracellular mucin.

association with dense fibrosis or pools of acellular mucin. Tumor cells may appear more pleomorphic and show neuroendocrine differentiation as a consequence of treatment. Large pools of mucin without any viable tumor cells, with or without calcific deposits, may be present and should not be reported as residual tumor[141] since these are not associated with an increased risk of recurrence or distant metastasis. The amount of residual carcinoma (0%, 1%–50%, and >50%) seen in resections performed after preoperative chemoradiation has been shown to be a reproducible predictor of survival in some studies.[142]

Ancillary Studies

Isolated tumor cells in postneoadjuvant therapy resection specimens may be difficult to distinguish from reactive mesenchymal cells. Immunostains for keratins can be helpful in these cases. Keratin stains may also help determine the deepest extent of tumor invasion for accurate staging when the residual tumor is present predominantly as single cells. In small biopsy specimens, distinction of primary esophageal adenocarcinoma from secondary tumors may be an issue. Esophageal spread from gastric, pulmonary, or breast carcinoma is the most common consideration in the differential diagnosis. Immunoreactivity for TTF-1 and estrogen receptor is useful in distinguishing esophageal tumors from pulmonary and breast primaries, respectively. Distinguishing gastric carcinomas with extension into the esophagus from primary esophageal adenocarcinoma is virtually impossible using immunohistochemical studies. The presence of Barrett esophagus with dysplasia adjacent to the carcinoma is the only truly reliable form of evidence in favor of an esophageal primary.

Molecular Findings

Esophageal adenocarcinoma arises from Barrett esophagus through a progressive, step-wise accumulation of genetic abnormalities. Aneuploidy and tetraploidy, on flow cytometric analysis of mucosal biopsies, are strong predictors of risk of progression to adenocarcinoma in patients with Barrett esophagus. Common alterations in adenocarcinomas include inactivation of p16, p27, and p53 through mutation or transcriptional silencing, and overexpression of cyclin D1.[143–145] Cyclin D1 overexpression has been reported in up to 64% of adenocarcinomas. *TP53* mutations in esophageal adenocarcinoma are predominantly G:C to A:T transitions at CpG dinucleotide sites and loss of heterozygosity of the 17p locus of the gene is associated with increased risk for aneuploidy and tetraploidy, as well as high-grade dysplasia. *CDKN2 A* inactivation occurs through promoter hypermethylation or 9p loss of heterozygosity and may be a critical early event in Barrett esophagus–associated neoplasia. Amplification of EGFR and HER2 also occur in 15% to 30% of cases.[146,147] Upregulation of miR-196a has been shown in esophageal adenocarcinoma and is believed to target annexin-A1 leading to suppression of apoptosis and enhance cell survival.[148]

Adenocarcinoma Variants

Non-Barrett-Associated Adenocarcinomas

Occasional reports have described adenocarcinomas arising in heterotopic gastric mucosa in the cervical esophagus.[149–153] Salivary gland type adenocarcinomas may rarely occur in the middle third of the esophagus, which presumably arise from the submucosal gland/ducts.

Carcinomas with Mixed Squamous and Glandular Differentiation

These are uncommon aggressive tumors in which the tumor shows bidirectional differentiation. They have been termed as adenosquamous or mucoepidermoid carcinoma in literature depending on whether the two components are discrete (adenosquamous) or intimately associated with each other (mucoepidermoid). Adenosquamous carcinomas also show a greater degree of nuclear pleomorphism in the squamous component compared to mucoepidermoid carcinoma. A background of Barrett esophagus is often present.[130,154–156] The prognosis of patients with these tumors remains uncertain due to their rarity.

Adenoid Cystic Carcinoma

True adenoid cystic carcinomas of the esophagus are extremely rare.[89,90,157] They show a biphasic phenotype with predominance of basal/myoepithelial cells and interspersed ductal structures. The growth pattern is solid, cribriform, or tubular and abundant basement membrane like myxohyaline stroma is present. Marked nuclear pleomorphism, brisk mitotic activity, and necrosis are not features of adenoid cystic carcinoma and should alert the pathologist to the possibility of a basaloid squamous cell carcinoma with which these tumors have been confused in the past. The ductal cells stain with keratin and the basal/myoepithelial cells with S100 and actin. Adenoid cystic carcinomas are slow growing tumors that rarely metastasize, and have a much better prognosis than basaloid squamous cell carcinomas.

Choriocarcinoma

Choriocarcinoma of the esophagus is a rare tumor that has been reported in both adult men and women.[158–161] They are large, exophytic, fungating tumors with extensive hemorrhage and necrosis. Foci of typical squamous cell carcinoma or Barrett esophagus–associated adenocarcinoma coexist in many cases. An admixture of syncytiotrophoblast and cytotrophoblast is present on histological examination. Tumors with yolk-sac like differentiation have also been described.[160] The possibility of contiguous spread from a mediastinal germ cell tumor should be excluded. Most patients have widespread metastatic disease at presentation. The overall prognosis is extremely poor.

Natural History and Prognosis of Adenocarcinoma

Tumor stage remains the best prognostic indicator in esophageal adenocarcinoma. Survival rates between 80% and 100% are reported for tumors confined to the mucosa or submucosa but decline significantly to about 10% to 20% for those that invade deep into the muscularis propria.[162–164] Nodal metastasis to periesophageal and perigastric lymph nodes occurs in 50% to 60% of patients and appears to be closely related to the depth of tumor infiltration. Risk of nodal metastasis is <5% for intramucosal cancers and rises to over 30% for tumors with submucosal invasion. The number of positive lymph nodes is also of prognostic value[165–167] and this is reflected in the recently updated TNM classification which is summarized in Table 11-1. Histological type is not considered an independent prognostic factor, but mucinous and signet ring cell carcinomas have been shown to be associated with poor survival on multivariate analysis in some studies.[168] Absence of residual tumor (complete pathologic response) in resections performed after neoadjuvant therapy is associated with a good outcome whereas persistent nodal disease is a strong adverse prognostic indicator.[169–171]

Neuroendocrine Tumors

Carcinoid tumors are now designated as well-differentiated neuroendocrine tumors in the new WHO classification. Initially described in 1969, esophageal carcinoids are the rarest of all GI carcinoid tumors. In a meta-analysis of 8305 carcinoids of various sites, only three were located in the esophagus.[172] The patients show a male predominance (6:1) of variable ages. The majority of tumors occur in the distal third of the esophagus or at the gastroesophageal junction. Carcinoids of the esophagus occur in two clinical scenarios: as solitary, circumscribed, polypoid lesions, or in association with Barrett esophagus. Increased numbers of endocrine cells have been described in some cases of Barrett esophagus[173,174] and this may contribute to the development of esophageal carcinoids. The morphology is similar to carcinoid tumors seen elsewhere in the gastrointestinal tract. The tumors show nested or trabecular architecture and the cells are monomorphic with a characteristic salt and pepper nuclear chromatin pattern (Fig. 11-8). Immunohistochemical markers of neuroendocrine differentiation, such as chromogranin and synaptophysin are invariably positive. Esophageal carcinoids were initially thought to be associated with a poor prognosis. More recent data suggests that cases previously reported as esophageal carcinoids with an adverse outcome may have been examples of small cell carcinoma because there was evidence of high mitotic activity and necrosis in the tumors.[175–177] Hoang et al.[178] described four new cases in 2002 and reviewed the outcome of other reported cases in literature. All 11 patients with primary esophageal carcinoids were alive and disease free after 1 to 23 years of follow-up. This suggests that the prognosis of esophageal carcinoids is favorable. Neuroendocrine tumors of the gastrointestinal tract are now graded on the basis of the mitotic activity and proliferative index on a Ki67 immunostain.[175] The prognostic value of this scheme for esophageal carcinoids remains uncertain given the rarity of these tumors. A brief summary of the current grading scheme is provided in Table 11-2.

Table 11-2

WHO GRADING SCHEME FOR NEUROENDOCRINE TUMORS OF THE GASTROINTESTINAL TRACT

GRADE	MITOTIC COUNT	Ki-67 PROLIFERATIVE INDEX (%)
1 (Low grade)	<2 per 10 high power fields AND	<3
2 (Intermediate grade)	2–20 per 10 high power fields OR	3–20
3 (High grade)	>20 per 10 high power fields OR	>20

Note: Most well-differentiated neuroendocrine (carcinoid) tumors fall under the Grade 1 or 2 category. Grade 3 tumors usually correspond to poorly differentiated (small cell or large cell) neuroendocrine carcinoma.

Small Cell Carcinomas constitute 1% to 2.4% of all esophageal carcinomas.[175,179–182] In the majority of cases, these tumors are large, protuberant, and arise in the middle and lower thirds of the esophagus. On histological examination, small, fusiform, or polygonal-shaped cells with little cytoplasm, hyperchromatic nuclei, and inconspicuous nucleoli are present, arranged in sheets or anastomosing cords and ribbons (Fig. 11-9). Crush artifact of the tumor cells is common, particularly in biopsy material and rosette formation may be present. Squamous differentiation has been described, as well as foci of glandular differentiation, particularly in resection specimens.[183] About a third of cases may shows areas of squamous cell carcinoma in situ.[184] Carcinoid-like areas within an otherwise typical small cell carcinoma have also been reported occasionally.[181] Confirmation that the tumor is a primary small cell carcinoma and not an undifferentiated squamous cell carcinoma depends on demonstration of neuroendocrine differentiation by chromogranin and synaptophysin immunostains or the finding of

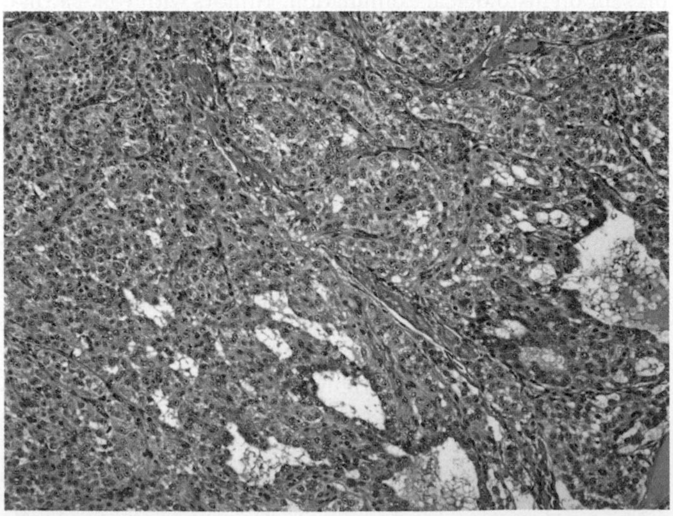

Figure 11-8. Well-differentiated neuroendocrine (carcinoid) tumors show nested or trabecular architecture. The tumor cells are monomorphic with a fine granular nuclear chromatin and show immunoreactivity for markers of neuroendocrine differentiation, such as chromogranin and synaptophysin.

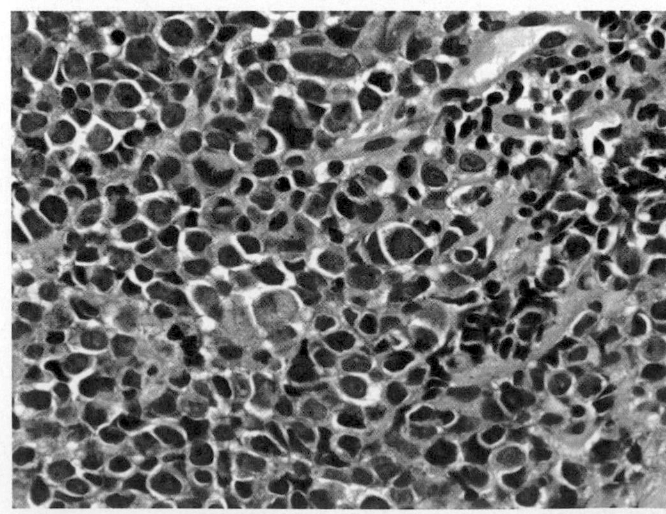

Figure 11-9. Small cell carcinomas show sheets of round to oval cells with a high nuclear-cytoplasmic ratio, marked nuclear hyperchromasia, nuclear molding, "salt and pepper" chromatin pattern and brisk mitotic activity. Necrosis and crush artifact may also be present.

neurosecretory granules on ultrastructural examination. Poorly differentiated squamous cell carcinomas and adenocarcinomas stain positively with p63 and CDX2, respectively, and are helpful in arriving at the correct diagnosis. The prognosis of these tumors is poor with a median survival between 3 and 12 months,[180] although occasional long-term survivors have been reported.[185–187]

Malignant Melanoma

It is now well recognized that melanocytes may be identified in normal esophageal mucosa in about 4% to 8% of normal individuals.[188–191] Benign appearing melanocytosis and atypical junctional lesions, similar to those seen in the skin, have also been described in association with primary esophageal malignant melanomas. Melanocytosis has been reported in about 25% of primary melanomas of the esophagus.[192] Metastatic malignant melanoma involves the esophagus in about 4% of patients with disseminated disease.[193] Therefore, a melanoma presenting in the esophagus is still much more likely to represent a metastasis rather than a primary tumor. In a recent analysis using the SEER database, the age-adjusted rates of cutaneous, anorectal, and esophageal malignant melanoma were 70.1, 0.27, and 0.03 per million, respectively.[194] The diagnostic criteria for primary esophageal melanoma require demonstration of melanocytes in adjacent epithelium with melanocytosis or junctional changes.[195] The majority of primary esophageal melanomas is melanotic and show pigmentation upon gross and microscopic examination, although primary amelanotic melanomas of the esophagus have also been reported.[196] Primary malignant melanomas have been reported mostly in elderly people in the sixth to seventh decade of life. They are twice as common in men and most often involve the middle or lower third of the esophagus. Most lesions appear as large, polypoid, and friable lesions that bulge into the lumen upon endoscopy. Satellite lesions, melanocytosis, or atypical junctional lesions are often present.[197–201] Histologically, spindle and/or epithelioid tumor cells are present which contain melanin pigment (Fig. 11-10) and are positive for S100, Melan-A, and HMB45 immunostains.[202]

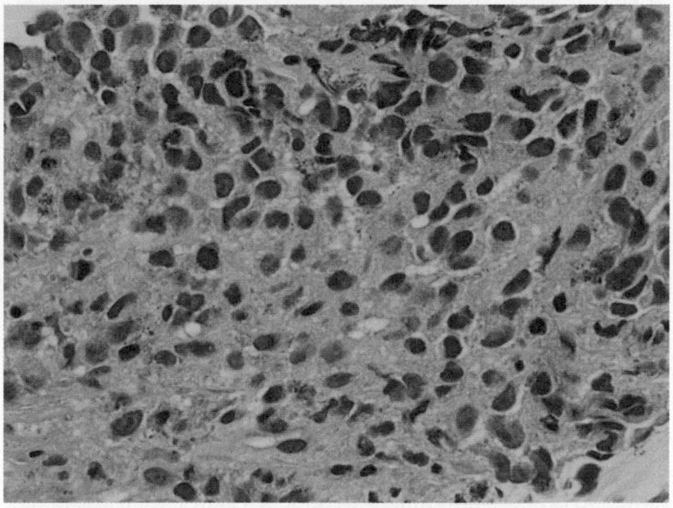

Figure 11-10. Primary malignant melanoma of the esophagus is rare. Large, spindle to ovoid tumor cells with abundant amphophilic cytoplasm and marked nucleolar prominence are seen. Melanin pigment is present in this example but in amelanotic tumors, immunostaining for markers of melanocytic differentiation (S-100, HMB-45, Melan-A) is helpful in confirming the diagnosis.

Both primary and secondary malignant melanomas involving the esophagus have a poor prognosis. The mean survival after diagnosis is only about 13 months.[203]

Gastrointestinal Stromal Tumor

Symptomatic gastrointestinal stromal tumors (GISTs) are uncommon in the esophagus. However, a significant number of esophageal GISTs are detected incidentally during examination of esophagectomies performed for another type of malignancy. In a series of 150 esophagectomies performed for esophageal or gastroesophageal junction adenocarcinomas, incidental GISTs were detected in 10% of cases.[204] Most tumors occur in the lower third of the esophagus.[205] The histological and immunophenotypic features of esophageal GISTs are similar to their counterparts in the stomach (Fig. 11-11). Both spindle

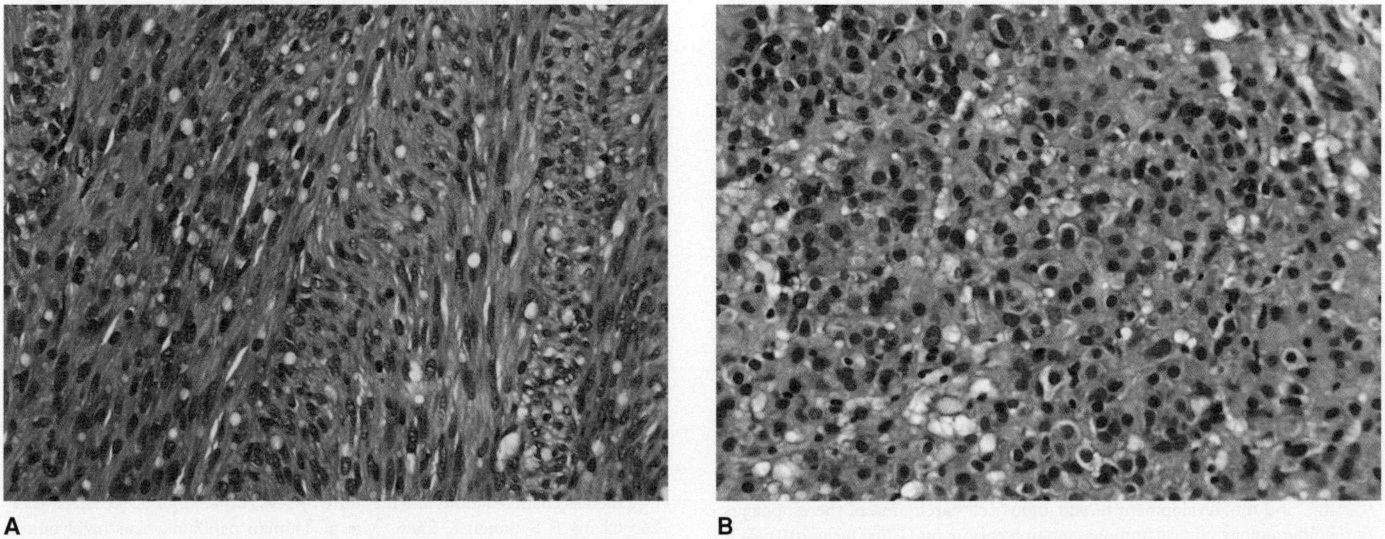

A B

Figure 11-11. Gastrointestinal stromal tumors may show a spindle (*A*) or epithelioid (*B*) morphology. Most tumors are positive for c-kit and/or CD34 and risk stratification is based on tumor size and mitotic activity.

and epithelioid cell types have been described. The tumor cells stain consistently with KIT and CD34.[206,207] KIT positivity is also seen in malignant melanoma and is a potential pitfall in diagnosis because primary or metastatic amelanotic melanoma involving the esophagus may be mistaken for a GIST.[208] Melanocytic markers Melan-A and HMB45 are helpful in arriving at the correct diagnosis. Miettinen et al.[205] reported a series of 17 GISTs in which nine patients died of disease. However, all fatal cases were more than 10 cm in size and one had more than five mitoses per 50 high power fields. The incidentally detected tumors in esophagectomy specimens are invariably associated with an excellent outcome.

Miscellaneous

Primary sarcomas of the esophagus have also been reported.[209–216] It is important to sample a tumor extensively to exclude the possibility of sarcomatous differentiation in a spindle cell carcinoma before a diagnosis of primary esophageal sarcoma can be established with certainty. Secondary tumors in the esophagus are rare but may cause obstruction and mimic a primary tumor. They may be the result of direct spread from adjacent organs, or of spread by lymphatics or bloodstream. Direct spread occurs most commonly from carcinoma of the stomach into the lower end of the esophagus, less commonly from the bronchus or thyroid.[217–218] Immunohistochemical analysis with TTF-1 may be particularly helpful in these latter instances to exclude an esophageal primary. Lymphatic spread has been described from carcinomas of the breast,[217,219,220] and bloodstream metastasis has been reported from primary tumors of the testis, prostate,[221,222] kidney,[223] endometrium,[224] and pancreas.[217]

EDITOR'S COMMENT

With the incidence of esophageal carcinoma increasing worldwide, the importance of differentiating histologic subtypes and staging classifications is paramount. The authors explain the histologic and pathologic differences with an emphasis on light microscopic findings. In addition, the recent identification of genetic variants that encode for specific pathologic changes as well as familial and pathogenic predisposition are reviewed. The importance of understanding the discrete differences between squamous carcinoma and adenocarcinoma, as well as the grade of the tumor, are apparent with the new AJCC staging strategy (7th edition). Likewise, the correlation between the depth of penetration and prevalence of lymph node metastasis is increasingly important as the new staging system includes the number of lymph nodes involved.

—Mark J. Krasna

References

1. Kamangar F, Dores GM, Anderson WF. Patterns of cancer incidence, mortality, and prevalence across five continents: defining priorities to reduce cancer disparities in different geographic regions of the world. *J Clin Oncol*. 2006;24(14):2137–2150.
2. Jemal A, Siegel R, Xu J, et al. Cancer statistics, 2010. *CA Cancer J Clin*. 2010;60(5):277–300.
3. Vizcaino AP, Moreno V, Lambert R, et al. Time trends incidence of both major histologic types of esophageal carcinomas in selected countries, 1973–1995. *Int J Cancer*. 2002;99(6):860–868. Erratum in: *Int J Cancer*. 2002 Oct 20;101(6):599.
4. Botterweck AA, Schouten LJ, Volovics A, et al. Trends in incidence of adenocarcinoma of the esophagus and gastric cardia in ten European countries. *Int J Epidemiol*. 2000;29(4):645–654.
5. Wu X, Chen VW, Andrews PA, et al. Incidence of esophageal and gastric cancers among Hispanics, non-Hispanic whites and non-Hispanic blacks in the United States: subsite and histology differences. *Cancer Causes Control*. 2007;18(6):585–593.
6. Trivers KF, Sabatino SA, Stewart SL. Trends in esophageal cancer incidence by histology, United States, 1998–2003. *Int J Cancer*. 2008;123(6):1422–1428.
7. Baquet CR, Commiskey P, Mack K, et al. Esophageal cancer epidemiology in blacks and whites: racial and gender disparities in incidence, mortality, survival rates and histology. *J Natl Med Assoc*. 2005;97(11):1471–1478.
8. Blot WJ, Devesa SS, Kneller RW, et al. Rising incidence of adenocarcinoma of the esophagus and gastric cardia. *JAMA*. 1991;265:1287.
9. Blot WJ, Devesa SS, Fraumeni JF Jr. Continuing climb in rates of esophageal adenocarcinoma: an update (letter). *JAMA*. 1993;270:1320.
10. Parkin DM, Bray F, Ferlay J, et al. Global cancer statistics, 2002. *CA Cancer J Clin*. 2005;55;74–108.
11. Tuyns AJ, Masse LMF. Mortality from cancer of the esophagus in Brittany. *Int J Epidemiol*. 1973;2:242.
12. Morita M, Kumashiro R, Kubo N, et al. Alcohol drinking, cigarette smoking, and the development of squamous cell carcinoma of the esophagus: epidemiology, clinical findings, and prevention. *Int J Clin Oncol*. 2010;15(2): 126–134.
13. Islami F, Fedirko V, Tramacere I, et al. Alcohol drinking and esophageal squamous cell carcinoma with focus on light-drinkers and never-smokers: a systematic review and meta-analysis. *Int J Cancer*. 2010; 129(10): 2473–2484.
14. Wang JM, Xu B, Rao JY, et al. Diet habits, alcohol drinking, tobacco smoking, green tea drinking, and the risk of esophageal squamous cell carcinoma in the Chinese population. *Eur J Gastroenterol Hepatol*. 2007;19(2):171–176.
15. Pandeya N, Williams G, Green AC, et al. Australian Cancer Study Alcohol consumption and the risks of adenocarcinoma and squamous cell carcinoma of the esophagus. *Gastroenterology*. 2009;136(4):1215–1224.
16. Paymaster JC, Sanghui LD, Gangadharan P. Cancer of the gastrointestinal tract in Western India: epidemiological study. *Cancer*. 1968;21:279.
17. Epstein SS, Payne PM, Shaw HJ. Multiple primary malignant neoplasms in the air and upper food passages. *Cancer*. 1960;13:137.
18. Shanta V, Krishnamurthi S. Further study in aetiology of carcinomas of the upper alimentary tract. *Br J Cancer*. 1963;17:8.
19. Jussawalla DJ, Deshpande VA. Evaluation of cancer risk in tobacco chewers and smokers: an epidemiologic assessment. *Cancer*. 1971;28:244.
20. Bradshaw E, Schonland M. Smoking, drinking and oesophageal cancer in African males of Johannesburg, South Africa. *Br J Cancer*. 1974;30:157.
21. Chen B, Yin H, Dhurandar N. Detection of human papillomavirus DNA in esophageal squamous cell carcinomas by the polymerase chain reaction using general consensus primers. *Hum Pathol*. 1994;25:920.
22. Suzuk L, Noffsinger AE, Hui YZ, et al. Detection of human papillomavirus in esophageal squamous cell carcinoma. *Cancer*. 1996;78:704.
23. Fidalgo PO, Cravo ML, Chaves PP, et al. High prevalence of human papillomavirus in squamous cell carcinoma and matched normal esophageal mucosa. Assessment by polymerase chain reaction. *Cancer*. 1995;76:1522.
24. Turner JR, Shen LH, Crum CP, et al. Low prevalence of human papillomavirus infection in esophageal squamous cell carcinomas from North America: analysis by a highly sensitive and specific polymerase chain reaction-based approach. *Hum Pathol*. 1997;28:174–178.
25. Poljak M, Cerar A, Seme K. Human papillomavirus infection in esophageal carcinomas: a study of 121 lesions using multiple broad-spectrum polymerase chain reactions and literature review. *Hum Pathol*. 1998;29:266–271.
26. Chang F, Syrjanen S, Shen Q, et al. Human papillomavirus involvement in esophageal carcinogenesis in the high-incidence area of China: a study of 700 cases by screening and type-specific in situ hybridization. *Scand J Gastroenterol*. 2000;35:123–130.

27. Farhadi M, Tahmasebi Z, Merat S, et al. Human papillomavirus in squamous cell carcinoma of esophagus in a high-risk population. *World J Gastroenterol.* 2005;11:1200–1203.
28. Syrjänen KJ. Histological changes identical to those of condylomatous lesions found in esophageal squamous cell carcinomas. *Arch Geschwulstforsch.* 1982;52:283.
29. International Agency for Research on Cancer. Human papillomaviruses. *IARC Monogr Eval Carcinog Risks Hum.* 2007;90:1–636.
30. Kiviranta UK. Corrosion carcinoma of the esophagus: 381 cases of corrosion and 9 cases of corrosion carcinoma. *Acta Otolaryngol.* 1953;42:89.
31. Appelqvist P, Salmo M. Lye corrosion carcinoma of the esophagus. A review of 63 cases. *Cancer.* 1980;45:2655.
32. Benedict EB. Carcinoma of the esophagus developing in benign stricture. *N Engl J Med.* 1941;224:408.
33. Chudecki B. Radiation cancer of the thoracic esophagus. *Br J Radiol.* 1972; 45:303.
34. Fekete F, Mosnier H, Belghiti J, et al. Esophageal cancer after mediastinal irradiation. *Dysphagia.* 1994;9:289.
35. Roth MJ, Guo-Qing W, Lewin KJ, et al. Histopathologic changes seen in esophagectomy specimens from the high-risk region of Linxian, China: potential clues to an etiologic exposure? *Hum Pathol.* 1998;29(11):1294–1298.
36. Roth M, QIAO Y, Rothman N, et al. High urine 1-hydroxypyrene glucoronide concentration in Linxian, China, an area of high risk for squamous oesophageal cancer. *Biomarkers.* 2001;6(5):381–386.
37. Ghadirian P. Familial history of esophageal cancer. *Cancer.* 1985;56:2112.
38. Howel-Evans W, McConnell RB, Clarke CA, et al. Carcinoma of the esophagus with keratosis palmaris et plantaris (tylosis): a study of two families. *Q J Med.* 1958;27:413.
39. Ashworth MT, Nash JGR, Ellis A, et al. Abnormalities of differentiation and maturation in the oesophageal squamous epithelium of patients with tylosis: morphological features. *Histopathology.* 1991;19:303.
40. Marger RS, Marger D. Carcinoma of the esophagus and tylosis. A lethal genetic combination. *Cancer.* 1993;72:17.
41. Kelsell DP, Risk JM, Leigh IM, et al. Close mapping of the focal nonepidermolytic palmoplantar keratoderma (PPK) locus associated with oesophageal cancer (TOC). *Hum Mol Genet.* 1996;5:857.
42. Iwaya T, Maesawa C, Ogasawara S, et al. Tylosis esophageal cancer locus on chromosome 17q25.1 is commonly deleted in sporadic human esophageal cancer. *Gastroenterology.* 1998;114:1206.
43. Yokoyama A, Kato H, Yokoyama T, et al. Genetic polymorphisms of alcohol and aldehyde dehydrogenases and glutathione S-transferase M1 and drinking, smoking, and diet in Japanese men with esophageal squamous cell carcinoma. *Carcinogenesis.* 2003;23:1851–1859.
44. Yokoyama A, Muramatsu T, Ohmori T, et al. Alcohol and aldehyde dehydrogenase gene polymorphisms and oropharyngolaryngeal, esophageal and stomach cancers in Japanese alcoholics. *Carcinogenesis.* 2001;22:433–439.
45. Lewis SJ, Smith GD. Alcohol, ALDH2, and esophageal cancer: a meta-analysis which illustrates the potentials and limitations of a Mendelian randomization approach. *Cancer Epidemiol Biomarkers Prev.* 2005;14:1967–1971.
46. Larsson SC, Giovannucci E, Wolk A. Folate intake, MTHFR polymorphisms, and risk of esophageal, gastric, and pancreatic cancer: a meta-analysis. *Gastroenterology.* 2006;131:1271–1283.
47. Shin MS. Primary carcinoma arising in the epiphrenic esophageal diverticulum. *South Med J.* 1971;64:1022.
48. Saldana JG, Cone RO, Hopens TA. Carcinoma arising in an epiphrenic esophageal diverticulum. *Gastrointest Radiol.* 1982;7:15.
49. Wynder EL, Hultberg S, Jacobsson F, et al. Environmental factors in cancer of upper alimentary tract: Swedish study with special reference to Plummer–Vinson (Paterson–Kelly) syndrome. *Cancer.* 1957;10:470.
50. Holmes GKT, Stokes PL, Sorahan TM, et al. Coeliac disease, gluten-free diet, and malignancy. *Gut.* 1976;17:612.
51. Cooper BT, Holmes GKT, Ferguson R, et al. Celiac disease and malignancy. *Medicine.* 1980;59:249.
52. Goodner JT, Watson WL. Cancer of the esophagus: its association with other primary cancers. *Cancer.* 1956;9:1248.
53. Mandard AM, Chasle J, Marnay J, et al. Autopsy findings in 111 cases of esophageal cancer. *Cancer.* 1981;48:329.
54. Morita M, Kuwano H, Ohno S, et al. Multiple recurrence of carcinoma in the upper aerodigestive tract associated with esophageal cancer. Reference to smoking, drinking and family history. *Int J Cancer.* 1994;58:207.
55. Dawsey SM, Wang G-Q, Weinstein WM, et al. Squamous dysplasia and early esophageal cancer in the Linxian region of China: distinctive endoscopic lesions. *Gastroenterology.* 1993;105:1333.
56. Mandard AM, Marnay J, Gignoux M, et al. Cancer of the esophagus and associated lesions: detailed pathologic study of 100 esophagectomy specimens. *Hum Pathol.* 1984;15:660.
57. Kuwano H, Morita M, Matsuda H, et al. Histopathologic findings of minute foci of squamous cell carcinoma in the human esophagus. *Cancer.* 1991;68:2617.
58. Nagamatsu M, Mori M, Kuwano H, et al. Serial histologic investigation of squamous epithelial dysplasia associated with carcinoma of the esophagus. *Cancer.* 1992;69:1094.
59. Morita M, Kuwano H, Yasuda M, et al. The multicentric occurrence of squamous epithelial dysplasia and squamous cell carcinoma in the esophagus. *Cancer.* 1994;74:2889.
60. Kuwano H, Matsuda H, Matsuoka H, et al. Intra-epithelial carcinoma concomitant with esophageal squamous cell carcinoma. *Cancer.* 1987;59:783.
61. Kuwano H, Ohno S, Matsuda H, et al. Serial histologic evaluation of multiple primary squamous cell carcinomas of the esophagus. *Cancer.* 1988;61:1635.
62. Pesko P, Rakic S, Milicevic M, et al. Prevalence and clinicopathologic features of multiple squamous cell carcinoma of the esophagus. *Cancer.* 1994;73:2687.
63. Tajima Y, Nakanishi Y, Tachimori Y, et al. Significance of involvement by squamous cell carcinoma of the ducts of esophageal submucosal glands: analysis of 201 surgically resected superficial squamous cell carcinomas. *Cancer.* 2000;89:248–254.
64. Chu P, Stagias J, West AB, et al. Diffuse pagetoid squamous cell carcinoma in situ of the esophagus: a case report. *Cancer.* 1997;79:1865–1870.
65. Winkler B, Capo V, Reumann W, et al. Human papillomavirus infection of the esophagus. A clinico-pathologic study with demonstration of papillomavirus antigen by the immunoperoxidase technique. *Cancer.* 1985;55:149.
66. Hille JJ, Markowitz S, Margolius KA, et al. Human papillomavirus and carcinoma of the esophagus. *N Engl J Med.* 1985;312:1707.
67. Liu FS. Pathology of the esophageal cancer. *Cancer Res Prev Treat.* 1976; 3:74.
68. Meyerowitz BR, Shea LT. The natural history of squamous verrucose carcinoma of the esophagus. *J Thorac Cardiovasc Surg.* 1971;61:646.
69. Minielly JA, Harrison EG Jr, Fontana RS, et al. Verrucous squamous cell carcinoma of the esophagus. *Cancer.* 1967;20:2078.
70. Parkinson AT, Haidak GL, McInerney RP. Verrucous squamous cell carcinoma of the esophagus following lye stricture. *Chest.* 1970;57:489.
71. Agha FP, Weatherbee L, Sams JS. Verrucous carcinoma of the esophagus. *Am J Gastroenterol.* 1984;79:844.
72. Soga J, Tanaka O, Sasaki K, et al. Superficial spreading carcinoma of the esophagus. *Cancer.* 1982;50:1641.
73. Kuwano H, Ueo H, Sugimachi K, et al. Glandular or mucus-secreting components in squamous cell carcinoma of the esophagus. *Cancer.* 1985;56:514.
74. Takubo K, Sasajima K, Yamashita K, et al. Morphological heterogeneity of esophageal carcinoma. *Acta Pathol Jpn.* 1989;39:180.
75. Newman J, Antonakopoulos GN, Darnton SJ, et al. The ultrastructure of oesophageal carcinomas: multidirectional differentiation. A transmission electron microscopic study of 43 cases. *J Pathol.* 1992;167:193.
76. Biemond P, ten Kate FJ, van Blankenstein M. Esophageal verrucous carcinoma: histologically a low-grade malignancy but a fatal disease. *J Clin Gastroenterol.* 1991;13:102.
77. du Boulay CEH, Isaacson P. Carcinoma of the esophagus with spindle cell features. *Histopathology.* 1981;5:403.
78. Talbert JL, Cantrell JR. Clinical and pathologic characteristics of carcinosarcoma of the esophagus. *J Thorac Cardiovasc Surg.* 1963;45:1.
79. Robertson NJ, Rahamim J, Smith MEF. Carcinosarcoma of the esophagus showing neuroendocrine, squamous and glandular differentiation. *Histopathology.* 1997;31:263.
80. Guarino M, Reale D, Micoli G, et al. Carcinosarcoma of the esophagus with rhabdomyoblastic differentiation. *Histopathology.* 1993;22:493.
81. Osamura RY, Watanabe K, Shimamura K, et al. Polypoid carcinoma of the esophagus. A unifying term for 'carcinosarcoma' and "pseudosarcoma". *Am J Surg Pathol.* 1978;2:201.
82. Kuhajda FP, Sun T-T, Mendelsohn G. Polypoid squamous carcinoma of the esophagus: a case report with immunostaining for keratin. *Am J Surg Pathol.* 1983;7:495.
83. Gal AA, Martin SE, Kernen JA, et al. Esophageal carcinoma with prominent spindle cells. *Cancer.* 1987;60:2244.
84. Linder J, Stein RB, Roggli VL, et al. Polypoid tumor of the esophagus. *Hum Pathol.* 1987;18:692.
85. Kimura N, Tezuka F, Ono I, et al. Myogenic expression in esophageal polypoid tumors. *Arch Pathol Lab Med.* 1989;113:1159.

86. Iyomasa S, Kato H, Tachimori Y, et al. Carcinosarcoma of the esophagus: a twenty case study. *Jpn J Clin Oncol.* 1990;20:99–106.
87. Abe K, Sasano H, Itakura Y, et al. Basaloid-squamous carcinoma of the esophagus. A clinicopathologic, DNA ploidy, and immunohistochemical study of seven cases. *Am J Surg Pathol.* 1996;20:453.
88. Sarbia M, Verreet P, Bittinger F, et al. Basaloid squamous cell carcinoma of the esophagus. Diagnosis and prognosis. *Cancer.* 1997;79:1871.
89. Kabuto T, Taniguchi K, Iwanaga T, et al. Primary adenoid cystic carcinoma of the esophagus: report of a case. *Cancer.* 1979;43:2452.
90. Bell-Thomson J, Haggitt RC, Ellis FH. Mucoepidermoid and adenoid cystic carcinoma of the esophagus. *J Thorac Cardiovasc Surg.* 1980;79:438.
91. Bogomoletz WV, Molas G, Gayet B, et al. Superficial squamous cell carcinoma of the esophagus. A report of 76 cases and review of the literature. *Am J Surg Pathol.* 1989;13:535.
92. Tajima Y, Nakanishi Y, Ochiai A, et al. Histopathologic findings predicting lymph node metastasis and prognosis of patients with superficial esophageal carcinoma: analysis of 240 surgically resected tumors. *Cancer* 2000;88:1285–1293.
93. Goseki N, Koike M, Yoshida M. Histopathologic characteristics of early stage esophageal cancer. A comparative study with gastric carcinoma. *Cancer.* 1992;69:1088.
94. Kitamura K, Ikebe M, Morita M, et al. The evaluation of submucosal carcinoma of the esophagus as a more advanced carcinoma. *Hepatogastroenterology.* 1993;40:236.
95. Kumagai Y, Makuuchi H, Mitomi T, et al. A new classification system for early carcinomas of the esophagus. *Dig Endosc.* 1993;5:139.
96. Sugimachi K, Ohno S, Matsuda H, et al. Lugol-combined endoscopic detection of minute malignant lesions of the thoracic esophagus. *Ann Surg.* 1988;208:179.
97. Tsutsui S, Kuwano H, Yasuda M, et al. Extensive spreading carcinoma of the esophagus with invasion restricted to the submucosa. *Am J Gastroenterol.* 1995;90:1858.
98. Aouad K, Aubertin J-M, Bouillot J-L, et al. Extensive spread of squamous cell carcinoma in situ of the esophagus: an unusual case. *Am J Gastroenterol.* 1996;91:2421.
99. Yoshikane H, Tsukamoto Y, Niwa Y, et al. Superficial esophageal carcinoma: evaluation by endoscopic ultrasonography. *Am J Gastroenterol.* 1994; 89:702.
100. Sibille A, Lambert R, Souquet J-C, et al. Long-term survival after photodynamic therapy for esophageal cancer. *Gastroenterology.* 1995;108:337.
101. Kitamura K, Kuwano H, Yasuda M, et al. What is the earliest malignant lesion in the esophagus? *Cancer.* 1996;77:1614.
102. Ando N, Ozawa S, Kitagawa Y, et al. Improvement in the results of surgical treatment of advanced squamous esophageal carcinoma during 15 consecutive years. *Ann Surg.* 2000;232:225–232.
103. Eguchi T, Nakanishi Y, Shimoda T, et al. Histopathological criteria for additional treatment after endoscopic mucosal resection for esophageal cancer: analysis of 464 surgically resected cases. *Mod Pathol.* 2006;19:475–480.
104. Twine CP, Lewis WG, Morgan MA, et al. The assessment of prognosis of surgically resected oesophageal cancer is dependent on the number of lymph nodes examined pathologically. *Histopathology.* 2009;55(1):46–52.
105. Kelty CJ, Kennedy CW, Falk GL. Ratio of metastatic lymph nodes to total number of nodes resected is prognostic for survival in esophageal carcinoma. *J Thorac Oncol.* 2010;5(9):1467–1471.
106. Hu Y, Hu C, Zhang H, et al. How does the number of resected lymph nodes influence TNM staging and prognosis for esophageal carcinoma? *Ann Surg Oncol.* 2010;17(3):784–790.
107. Brucher BL, Becker K, Lordick F, et al. The clinical impact of histopathologic response assessment by residual tumor cell quantification in esophageal squamous cell carcinomas. *Cancer.* 2006;106:2119–2127.
108. Brown LM, Devesa SS, Chow WH. Incidence of adenocarcinoma of the esophagus among white men by sex, stage and age. *J Natl Cancer Inst.* 2008;100:1184–1187.
109. Powell J, McConkey CC. The rising trend in esophageal adenocarcinoma and gastric cardia. *Eur J Cancer Prev.* 1992;1:265.
110. Tuyns AJ. Oesophageal cancer in France and Switzerland: recent time trends. *Eur J Cancer Prev.* 1992;1:275.
111. McKinney PA, Sharp L, MacFarlane GJ, et al. Oesophageal and gastric cancer in Scotland 1960–90. *Br J Cancer.* 1995;71:411.
112. Armstrong RW, Borman B. Trends in incidence rates of adenocarcinoma of the esophagus and gastric cardia in New Zealand 1978–92. *Int J Epidemiol.* 1996;25:941.
113. Thomas RJ, Lade S, Giles GG, et al. Incidence trends in oesophageal and proximal gastric carcinoma in Victoria. *Aust N Z J Surg.* 1996;66:271.
114. Hansen S, Wiig JN, Giercksky KE, et al. Esophageal and gastric carcinoma in Norway 1958–92: incidence time trend variability according to morphological subtypes and organ subsites. *Int J Cancer.* 1997;71:340.
115. Pohl H, Sirovich B, Welch HG. Esophageal adenocarcinoma incidence: are we reaching the peak? *Cancer Epidemiol Biomarkers Prev.* 2010; 19(6):1468–1470.
116. Hampel H, Abraham NS, El-Serag HB. Meta-analysis: obesity and the risk for gastroesophageal reflux disease and its complications. *Ann Intern Med.* 2005;143(3):199–211.
117. Kubo A, Corley DA. Body mass index and adenocarcinomas of the esophagus or gastric cardia: a systematic review and meta-analysis. *Cancer Epidemiol Biomarkers Prev.* 2006;15(5):872–878.
118. Brown LM, Swanson CA, Gridley G. Adenocarcinoma of the esophagus: role of obesity and diet. *J Natl Cancer Inst.* 1995;87:104.
119. Chow WH, Blot WJ, Vaughan TL, et al. Body mass index and risk of adenocarcinomas of the esophagus and gastric cardia. *J Natl Cancer Inst.* 1998;90:150.
120. Kabat GC, Ng SKC, Wynder EL. Tobacco, alcohol intake, and diet in relation to adenocarcinoma of the esophagus and gastric cardia. *Cancer Causes Control.* 1993;4:123.
121. Brown LM, Silverman DT, Pottern LM, et al. Adenocarcinoma of the esophagus and esophagogastric junction in white men in the United States: alcohol, tobacco, and socioeconomic factors. *Cancer Causes Control.* 1994; 5:333.
122. Gammon MD, Schoenberg JB, Ahsan H, et al. Tobacco, alcohol, and socioeconomic status and adenocarcinomas of the esophagus and gastric cardia. *J Natl Cancer Inst.* 1997;89:1277.
123. Corley DA, Kerlikowske K, Verma R, et al. Protective association of aspirin/NSAIDs and esophageal cancer: a systematic review and meta-analysis. *Gastroenterology.* 2003;124(1):47–56.
124. Lindblad M, Lagergren J, Garcia Rodriguez LA. Nonsteroidal anti-inflammatory drugs and risk of esophageal and gastric cancer. *Cancer Epidemiol Biomarkers Prev.* 2005;14(2):444–450.
125. Anderson LA, Johnston BT, Watson RG, et al. Nonsteroidal anti-inflammatory drugs and the esophageal inflammation-metaplasia-adenocarcinoma sequence. *Cancer Res.* 2006;66(9):4975–4982.
126. Ranka S, Gee JM, Johnson IT, et al. Non-steroidal anti-inflammatory drugs, lower oesophageal sphincter-relaxing drugs and oesophageal cancer. A case-control study. *Digestion.* 2006;74(2):109–115.
127. Fortuny J, Johnson CC, Bohlke K, et al. Use of anti-inflammatory drugs and lower esophageal sphincter-relaxing drugs and risk of esophageal and gastric cancers. *Clin Gastroenterol Hepatol.* 2007;5(10):1154–1159.
128. Liu C, Wu MC, Chen F, et al. A large scale genetic association study of esophageal adenocarcinoma risk. *Carcinogenesis.* 2010;31:1259–1263.
129. Thompson JJ, Zinsser KR, Enterline HT. Barrett's metaplasia in adenocarcinoma of the esophagus and gastroesophageal junction. *Hum Pathol.* 1983;14:42.
130. Smith RRL, Hamilton SR, Boitnott JK, et al. The spectrum of carcinoma arising in Barrett's epithelium: a clinicopathologic study of 26 patients. *Am J Surg Pathol.* 1984;8:563.
131. Chejfec G, Jablokow VR, Gould VE. Linitis plastica carcinoma of the esophagus. *Cancer.* 1981;51:2139.
132. Reid BJ, Weinstein WM, Lewin KJ, et al. Endoscopic biopsy can detect high-grade dysplasia or early adenocarcinoma in Barrett's esophagus without grossly recognizable neoplastic lesions. *Gastroenterology.* 1988;94(1):81–90.
133. Witt TR, Bains MS, Zaman MB, et al. Adenocarcinoma in Barrett's esophagus. *J Thorac Cardiovasc Surg.* 1983;85:337.
134. Dunne B, Reynolds JV, Mulligan E, et al. A pathological study of tumour regression in oesophageal adenocarcinoma treated with preoperative chemoradiotherapy. *J Clin Pathol.* 2001;54:841–845.
135. Hamilton SR, Smith RRL. The relationship between columnar epithelial dysplasia and invasive adenocarcinoma arising in Barrett's esophagus. *Am J Clin Pathol.* 1987;87:301.
136. Banner BF, Memoli VA, Warren WH, et al. Carcinoma with multi-directional differentiation arising in Barrett's esophagus. *Ultrastruct Pathol.* 1983;4:205.
137. Abraham SC, Wang H, Wang KK, et al. Paget cells in the esophagus: assessment of their histologic features and near universal association with underlying esophageal adenocarcinoma. *Am J Surg Pathol.* 2008;32:1068–1074.
138. Takubo K, Sasajima K, Yamashita K, et al. Double muscularis mucosae in Barrett's esophagus. *Hum Pathol.* 1991;22(11):1158–1161.

139. Lewis JT, Wang KK, Abraham SC. Muscularis mucosae duplication and the musculo-fibrous anomaly in endoscopic mucosal resections for barrett esophagus: implications for staging of adenocarcinoma. *Am J Surg Pathol.* 2008;32(4):566–571.
140. Abraham SC, Krasinskas AM, Correa AM, et al. Duplication of the muscularis mucosae in Barrett esophagus: an underrecognized feature and its implication for staging of adenocarcinoma. *Am J Surg Pathol.* 2007;31(11):1719–1725.
141. Hornick JL, Farraye FA, Odze RD. Prevalence and significance of prominent mucin pools in the esophagus post neoadjuvant chemoradiotherapy for Barrett's-associated adenocarcinoma. *Am J Surg Pathol.* 2006;30(1):28–35.
142. Wu TT, Chirieac LR, Abraham SC, et al. Excellent interobserver agreement on grading the extent of residual carcinoma after preoperative chemoradiation in esophageal and esophagogastric junction carcinoma: a reliable predictor for patient outcome. *Am J Surg Pathol.* 2007;31(1):58–64.
143. Wongsurawat VJ, Finley JC, Galipeau PC, et al. Genetic mechanisms of p53 LOH in Barrett's esophagus: implications for biomarker validation. *Cancer Epidemiol Biomarkers Prev.* 2006;15:509–516.
144. Lai LA, Paulson TG, Li X, et al. Increasing genomic instability during premalignant neoplastic progression revealed through high resolution array-CGH. *Genes Chromosomes Cancer.* 2007;46:532–542.
145. Wong DJ, Paulson TG, Prevo LJ, et al. P16INK4 a lesions are common, early abnormalities that undergo clonal expansion in Barrett's metaplastic epithelium. *Cancer Res.* 2001;61:8284–8289.
146. Thompson SK, Sullivan TR, Davies R, et al. HER-2/neu gene amplification in esophageal adenocarcinoma and its influence on survival. *Ann Surg Oncol.* 2011;18(7):2010–2017.
147. Cronin J, McAdam E, Danikas A, et al. Epidermal growth factor receptor (EGFR) is overexpressed in high-grade dysplasia and adenocarcinoma of the esophagus and may represent a biomarker of histological progression in Barrett's esophagus (BE). *Am J Gastroenterol.* 2011;106(1):46–56.
148. Kan T, Meltzer SJ. MicroRNAs in Barrett's esophagus and esophageal adenocarcinoma. *Curr Opin Pharmacol.* 2009;9:727–732.
149. Christensen WN, Sternberg SS. Adenocarcinoma of the upper esophagus arising in ectopic gastric mucosa;two case reports and review of the literature. *Am J Surg Pathol.* 1987;11:397.
150. Ishii K, Ota H, Nakayama J, et al. Adenocarcinoma of the cervical esophagus arising from ectopic gastric mucosa. The histochemical determination of its origin. *Virchows Arch A Pathol Anat.* 1991;419:159.
151. Takagi A, Ema Y, Horii S, et al. Early adenocarcinoma arising from ectopic gastric mucosa in the cervical esophagus. *Gastrointest Endosc.* 1995;41:167–170.
152. Lauwers GY, Scott GV, Vauthey GN. Adenocarcinoma of the upper esophagus arising in cervical ectopic gastric mucosa: rare evidence of malignant potential of so-called "inlet patch". *Dig Dis Sci.* 1998;43:901–907.
153. Alrawi SJ, Winston J, Tan D, et al. Primary adenocarcinoma of cervical esophagus. *J Exp Clin Cancer Res.* 2005;24:325–330.
154. Bosch A, Frias Z, Caldwell WL. Adenocarcinoma of the esophagus. *Cancer.* 1979;43:1557.
155. Ter RB, Govil YK, Leite L, et al. Adenosquamous carcinoma in Barrett's esophagus presenting as pseudoachalasia. *Am J Gastroenterol.* 1999;94:268–270.
156. Lam KY, Dickens P, Loke SL, et al. Squamous cell carcinoma of the esophagus with mucin-secreting component (mucoepidermoid carcinoma and adenosquamous carcinoma): a clinicopathologic study and a review of literature. *Eur J Surg Oncol.* 1994;20:25–31.
157. Morisaki Y, Yoshizumi Y, Hiroyasu S, et al. Adenoid cystic carcinoma of the esophagus: report of a case and review of the Japanese literature. *Surg Today.* 1996;26:1006–1009.
158. Sasano N, Abe S, Satake O. Choriocarcinoma mimickry of an esophageal carcinoma with urinary gonadotropic activities. *Tohoku J Exp Med.* 1970;100:153.
159. Kikuchi Y, Tsuneta Y, Kawai T, et al. Choriocarcinoma of the esophagus producing chorionic gonadotropin. *Acta Pathol Jpn.* 1988;38:489.
160. Wasan HS, Schofield JB, Krausz T, et al. Combined choriocarcinoma and yolk sac tumor arising in Barrett's esophagus. *Cancer.* 1994;73:514.
161. Merimsky O, Jossiphov J, Asna N, et al. Choriocarcinoma arising in a squamous cell carcinoma of the esophagus. *Am J Clin Oncol.* 2000;23:203–206.
162. Paraf F, Flejou JF, Pignon JP, et al. Surgical pathology of adenocarcinoma arising in Barrett's esophagus: analysis of 67 cases. *Am J Surg Pathol.* 1995;19:183–191.
163. Torres C, Turner JR, Wang HH, et al. Pathologic prognostic factors in Barrett's associated adenocarcinoma: a follow-up study of 96 patients. *Cancer.* 1999;85:520–528.
164. van Sandick JW, van Lanschot JJ, ten Kate FJ, et al. Pathology of early invasive adenocarcinoma of the esophagus or esophagogastric junction: implications for therapeutic decision making. *Cancer.* 2000;88:2429–2437.
165. Rice TW, Blackstone EH, Rybicki LA, et al. Refining esophageal cancer staging. *J Thorac Cardiovasc Surg.* 2003;125(5):1103–1113.
166. Wijnhoven BP, Tran KT, Esterman A, et al. An evaluation of prognostic factors and tumor staging of resected carcinoma of the esophagus. *Ann Surg.* 2007;245(5):717–725.
167. Thompson SK, Ruszkiewicz AR, Jamieson GG, et al. Improving the accuracy of TNM staging in esophageal cancer: a pathological review of resected specimens. *Ann Surg Oncol.* 2008;15:3447–3458.
168. Chirieac LR, Swisher SG, Correa AM, et al. Signet-ring cell or mucinous histology after preoperative chemoradiation and survival in patients with esophageal or esophagogastric junction adenocarcinoma. *Clin Cancer Res.* 2005;11:2229–2236.
169. Chirieac LR, Swisher SG, Ajani JA, et al. Posttherapy pathologic stage predicts survival in patients with esophageal carcinoma receiving preoperative chemoradiation. *Cancer.* 2005;103:1347–1355.
170. Rohatgi P, Swisher SG, Correa AM, et al. Characterization of pathologic complete response after preoperative chemoradiotherapy in carcinoma of the esophagus and outcome after pathologic complete response. *Cancer.* 2005;104:2365–2372.
171. Gu Y, Swisher SG, Ajani AJ, et al. The number of lymph nodes with metastasis predicts survival in patients with esophageal or esophagogastric junction adenocarcinoma who receive preoperative chemoradiation. *Cancer.* 2006;106:1017–1025.
172. Modlin IM, Sandor A. An analysis of 8305 cases of carcinoid tumors. *Cancer.* 1997;79:813–829.
173. Buchanan AMJ, Grant S, Freeman HJ. Regulatory peptides in Barrett's esophagus. *J Pathol.* 1985;146:227–234.
174. Griffin M, Sweeney EC. The relationship of endocrine cells, dysplasia and carcinoembryonic antigen in Barrett's mucosa to adenocarcinoma of the esophagus. *Histopathology.* 1987;11:53–62.
175. Arnold R, Capella C, Klimstra DS, et al. Neuroendocrine neoplasms of the oesophagus. In: Bosman FT, Carneiro F, Hruban RH, Theise ND, eds. *World Health Organization Classification of Tumors of the Digestive System.* Lyon, France: IARC Press; 2010:32–34.
176. Oz MC, Ashley PF, Oz M. Atypical gastroesophageal carcinoid: a case report and review of the literature. *Del Med J.* 1897;12:785–788.
177. Ready AR, Soul JO, Newman J, et al. Malignant carcinoid tumor of the esophagus. *Thorax.* 1989;44:594–596.
178. Hoang MP, Hobbs CM, Sobin LH, et al. Carcinoid tumors of the esophagus. A clinicopathologic study of four cases. *Am J Surg Pathol.* 2002;26:517–522.
179. McKeown F. Oat-cell carcinoma of the esophagus. *J Pathol Bacteriol.* 1952; 64:889.
180. Casas F, Ferrer F, Farrús B, et al. Primary small cell carcinoma of the esophagus. A review of the literature with emphasis on therapy and prognosis. *Cancer.* 1997;80:1366.
181. Briggs JC, Ibrahim NBN. Oat cell carcinoma of the esophagus: a clinicopathological study of 23 cases. *Histopathology.* 1983;7:261.
182. Law SY-K, Fok M, Lam K-Y, et al. Small cell carcinoma of the esophagus. *Cancer.* 1994;73:2894.
183. Mori M, Matsukuma A, Adachi Y, et al. Small cell carcinoma of the esophagus. *Cancer.* 1989;63:564.
184. Takubo K, Nakamura K, Sawabe M, et al. Primary undifferentiated small cell carcinoma of the esophagus. *Hum Pathol.* 1999;30:216–221.
185. Nichols GL, Kelsen DP. Small cell carcinoma of the esophagus: the Memorial Hospital experience 1970–87. *Cancer.* 1989;54:1531.
186. Hussein AM, Feun LG, Sridhar KS, et al. Combination chemotherapy and radiotherapy for small-cell carcinoma of the esophagus. A case report of long-term survival and review of the literature. *Am J Clin Oncol.* 1990;13: 369.
187. McCullen M, Vyas SK, Winwood PJ, et al. Long-term survival associated with metastatic small cell carcinoma of the esophagus treated by chemotherapy, autologous bone marrow transplantation, and adjuvant radiation therapy. *Cancer.* 1994;73:1.
188. De la Pava S, Nigogosyan G, Pickren JW, et al. Melanosis of the esophagus. *Cancer.* 1963;16:48–50.
189. Ohashi K, Kato Y, Kanno J, et al. Melanocytes and melanosis of the esophagus in Japanese subjects: analysis of factors effecting their increase. *Virchows Arch A Pathol Anat Histopathol.* 1990;417:137–143.

190. Sharma SS, Venkateswaran S, Chacko A, et al. Melanosis of the esophagus: an endoscopic, histochemical, and ultrastructural study. *Gastroenterology.* 1991;100:13–16.
191. Bogomoletz WV, Lecat M, Amoros F. Melanosis of the esophagus in a Western patient. *Histopathology.* 1997;30:498–499.
192. DiCostanzo DP, Urmacher C. Primary malignant melanoma of the esophagus. *Am J Surg Pathol.* 1987;11:46–52.
193. Wysocki W, Komorowski A, Daradz Z. Gastrointestinal metastases from malignant melanoma: report of a case. *Surg Today.* 2004;34:542–546.
194. Cote TR, Sobin LH. Primary melanomas of the esophagus and anorectum: epidemiologic comparison with melanoma of the skin. *Melanoma Res.* 2009; 19:58–60.
195. Raven RW, Dawson I. Malignant melanoma of the esophagus. *Br J Surg.* 1964;51:551.
196. Stringa O, Valdez R, Beguerie JR, et al. Primary amelanotic melanoma of the esophagus. *Int J Dermatol.* 2006;45:1207–1210.
197. Sakornpant P, Barlow D, Bevan CM. Two cases of primary malignant melanoma of the esophagus. *Br J Surg.* 1964;51:386.
198. Piccone VA, Klopstock R, Leveen HH, et al. Primary malignant melanoma of the esophagus associated with melanosis of the entire esophagus. First case report. *J Thorac Cardiovasc Surg.* 1970;59:864.
199. Muto M, Saito Y, Koike T, et al. Primary malignant melanoma of the esophagus with diffuse pigmentation resembling superficial spreading melanoma. *Am J Gastroenterol.* 1997;92:1936.
200. Musher DR, Lindner AE. Primary melanoma of the esophagus. *Dig Dis Sci.* 1974;19:855.
201. Sabanathan S, Eng J, Pradhan GN. Primary malignant melanoma of the esophagus. *Am J Gastroenterol.* 1989;84:1475–1481.
202. Gown AM, Vogel AM, Hoak D, et al. Monoclonal antibodies specific for melanocytic tumors distinguish subpopulations of melanocytes. *Am J Pathol.* 1986;123:195.
203. Chalkiadakis G, Wihlm JM, Morand G, et al. Primary malignant melanoma of the esophagus. *Ann Thorac Surg.* 1985;39:472–475.
204. Abraham SC, Krasinskas AM, Hofstetter WL, et al. "Seedling" mesenchymal tumors (gastrointestinal stromal tumors and leiomyomas) are common incidental tumors of the esophagogastric junction. *Am J Surg Pathol.* 2007;31:1629–1635.
205. Miettinen M, Sarlomo-Rikala M, Sobin LH, et al. Esophageal stromal tumors: a clinicopathologic, immunohistochemical, and molecular genetic study of 17 cases with comparison with esophageal leiomyomas and leiomyosarcomas. *Am J Surg Pathol.* 2000;24:211.
206. Miettinen M, Virolainen M, Rikala MS. Gastrointestinal stromal tumors. Value of CD34 antigen in their identification from true leiomyomas and schwannomas. *Am J Surg Pathol.* 1995;19:207.
207. Sarlomo-Rikala M, Kovatich A, Barusevicius A, et al. CD117: a sensitive marker for gastrointestinal stromal tumors that is more specific than CD34. *Mod Pathol.* 1998;11:728.
208. Wang S, Thamboo TP, Nga M, et al. C-kit positive amelanotic melanoma of the esophagus: a potential diagnostic pitfall. *Pathology.* 2008;40: 527–530.
209. Bloch MJ, Iozzo RV, Edmunds LH Jr, et al. Polypoid synovial sarcoma of the esophagus. *Gastroenterology.* 1987;92:229.
210. Anton-Pacheco J, Cano I, Cuadros J, et al. Synovial sarcoma of the esophagus. *J Pediatr Surg.* 1996;31:1703.
211. Aagaard MT, Kristensen IB, Lund O, et al. Primary malignant non-epithelial tumours of the thoracic esophagus and cardia in a 25-year surgical material. *Scand J Gastroenterol.* 1990;25:876.
212. Willen R, Lillo-Gil R, Willen H, et al. Embryonal rhabdomyosarcoma of the esophagus: case report. *Acta Chir Scand.* 1989;155:59.
213. Vartio T, Nickels J, Hockerstedt K, et al. Rhabdomyosarcoma of the esophagus. *Virchows Arch Pathol Anat.* 1980;386:357.
214. Friedman SL, Wright TL, Altman DF. Gastrointestinal Kaposi's sarcoma in patients with acquired immunodeficiency syndrome. Endoscopic and autopsy findings. *Gastroenterology.* 1985;89:102.
215. Mansour KA, Fritz RC, Jacobs DM, et al. Pedunculated liposarcoma of the esophagus: a first case report. *J Thorac Cardiovasc Surg.* 1983;86: 447.
216. McIntyre M, Webb JN, Browning GCP. Osteosarcoma of the esophagus. *Hum Pathol.* 1982;13:680.
217. Toreson WE. Secondary carcinoma of the esophagus as a cause of dysphagia. *Arch Pathol.* 1944;38:82.
218. Hale RJ, Merchant W, Hasleton PS. Polypoidal intra-oesophageal thyroid carcinoma: a rare cause of dysphagia. *Histopathology.* 1990;17:475.
219. Polk HC Jr, Camp FA, Walker AW. Dysphagia and oesophageal stenosis: manifestations of metastatic mammary cancer. *Cancer.* 1967;20: 2002.
220. Varanasi RV, Saltzman JR, Krims P, et al. Breast carcinoma metastatic to the esophagus: clinicopathological and management features of four cases, and literature review. *Am J Gastroenterol.* 1995;90:1495.
221. Gross P, Freedman LJ. Obstructing secondary carcinoma of the esophagus. *Arch Pathol.* 1942;33:361.
222. Gore RM, Sparberg M. Metastatic carcinoma of the prostate to the esophagus. *Am J Gastroenterol.* 1982;77:358.
223. Nussbaum M, Grossman M. Metastases to the esophagus causing gastrointestinal bleeding. *Am J Gastroenterol.* 1976;66:467.
224. Zarian LP, Berliner L, Redmond P. Metastatic endometrial carcinoma to the esophagus. *Am J Gastroenterol.* 1983;78:9.

12 Esophageal Cancer Staging

Thomas W. Rice

Keywords: TNM classification for esophageal cancer, Stage groupings for esophageal cancer, AJCC/UICC Cancer Staging Manual, 7th edition

Cancer staging is an evolutionary process. The Tumor-Node-Metastasis (TNM) esophageal cancer staging, first introduced in 1968, rapidly developed, but unfortunately then stagnated for decades. T classifications had not changed since 1988, N classifications for thoracic esophageal cancer since 1977, and M classifications since 1997. The principal hindrance to evolution was the long held concept of stage groupings of esophageal cancer which was incorrectly based on a simple, orderly arrangement of increasing anatomic T, then N, then M classifications. This assumption was consistent with neither cancer biology nor survival data. Worldwide collaboration[1] has provided data for a unique, modern machine-learning analysis[2] that has produced data-driven staging for cancer of the esophagus and esophagogastric junction (EGJ).[3] This new system is the basis for the 7th editions of the AJCC and UICC Cancer Staging Manuals.[4,5] It is more representative of and consistent with the survival following esophagectomy of patients with esophageal cancer. The changes address problems of empiric stage grouping and prior disharmony with stomach cancer staging. In addition, TNM classifications have been reviewed and revised where data analysis and consensus demonstrated a need for change. For the first time, nonanatomic cancer characteristics, primary cancer site (location), histologic grade (grade), and histopathologic type (cell type) are incorporated in esophageal cancer staging.

THE DATA

At the request of the AJCC, the Worldwide Esophageal Cancer Collaboration was inaugurated in 2006. Thirteen institutions from five countries and three continents (Asia, Europe, and North America) submitted de-identified data by July 2007. A database of 4627 esophagectomy patients who had no induction or adjuvant therapy was created.[1]

THE ANALYSIS

Multiple previously proposed revisions of esophageal cancer staging have examined goodness of fit or *p* values to test for a statistically significant effect of stage on survival. Instead, staging for the 7th edition used Random Forest (RF) analysis, a machine-learning technique that focuses on predictability for future patients.[2] RF analysis makes no *a priori* assumptions about patient survival, is able to identify complex interactions among variables, and accounts for nonlinear effects. RF may be viewed as a "backward" analysis which determines the anatomic classifications (TNM) and nonanatomic cancer characteristics that are associated with specific survival groups.

RF analysis first isolated cancer characteristics of interest from other factors influencing survival by generating risk-adjusted survival curves for each patient. Unlike previous approaches that began by placing cancer characteristics into proposed groups, RF analysis produced distinct groups with monotonically decreasing risk-adjusted survival without regard to cancer characteristics. Then, anatomic and nonanatomic cancer characteristics important for stage group composition were identified within these groups. Finally, homogeneity within groups guided both amalgamation and segmentation of cancer characteristics between adjacent groups to arrive at the final stage groups.[3–5]

7TH EDITION TNM CLASSIFICATIONS: CHANGES AND ADDITIONS

Primary tumor (T) classification has been changed only for Tis and T4 cancers (Fig. 12-1, Table 12-1). Tis is now defined as high-grade dysplasia and includes all noninvasive neoplastic epithelium that was previously called carcinoma in situ. T4, tumors invading local structures, has been subclassified as T4a and T4b. T4a tumors are resectable cancers invading adjacent structures such as pleura, pericardium, or diaphragm. T4b are unresectable cancers invading other adjacent structures, such as aorta, vertebral body, or trachea. Otherwise, T classifications are unchanged.

A regional lymph node has been redefined to include any paraesophageal lymph node extending from cervical nodes to celiac nodes. This revolutionary change in esophageal cancer classification requires a refocusing in staging mentality. Regional lymph node classification has been radically changed. Data analyses support convenient coarse groupings of number of cancer-positive nodes.[2–4] Regional lymph node (N) classification comprises N0 (no cancer-positive nodes), N1 (1 or 2), N2 (3–6), and N3 (7 or more). N classifications for cancers of the esophagus and EGJ are identical to stomach cancer N classifications.

The subclassifications M1a and M1b have been eliminated, as has MX. Distant metastases are simply designated M0, no distant metastasis, and M1, distant metastasis.

7TH EDITION: NONANATOMIC CANCER CHARACTERISTICS

Nonanatomic classifications identified as important for stage grouping are histopathologic cell type, histologic grade, and tumor location (Fig. 12-2). The difference in survival between adenocarcinoma and squamous cell carcinoma is best managed by separate stage groupings for stages I and II. Increasing

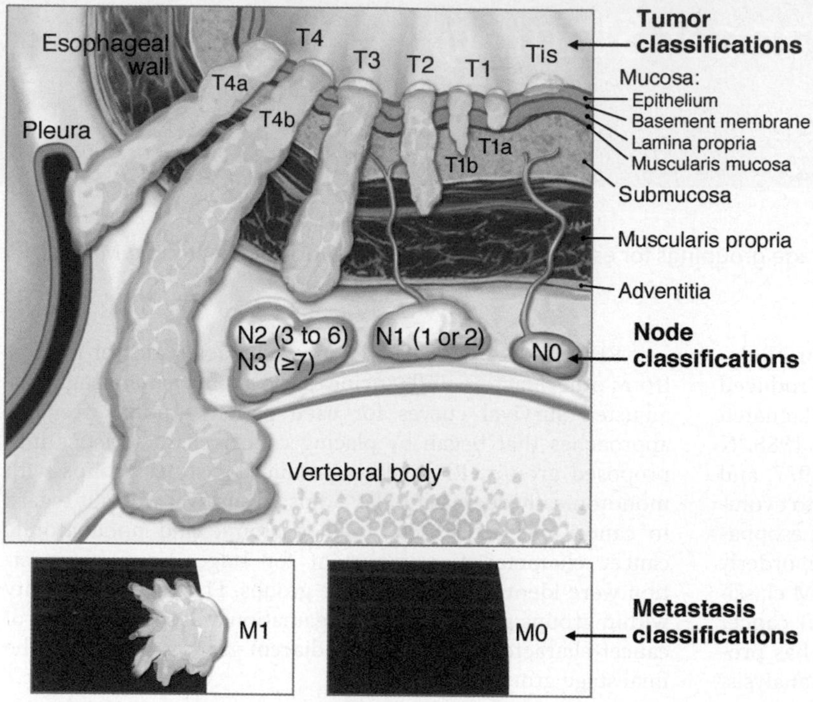

Figure 12-1. 7th edition TNM classifications. T is classified as Tis: high-grade dysplasia; T1: cancer invades lamina propria, muscularis mucosae, or submucosa; T2: cancer invades muscularis propria; T3: cancer invades adventitia; T4a: resectable cancer invades adjacent structures such as pleura, pericardium, or diaphragm; and T4b; unresectable cancer invades other adjacent structures, such as aorta, vertebral body, or trachea. N is classified as N0: no regional lymph node metastasis; N1: regional lymph node metastases involving 1 to 2 nodes; N2: regional lymph node metastases involving 3 to 6 nodes; and N3: regional lymph node metastases involving 7 or more nodes. M is classified as M0: no distant metastasis; and M1: distant metastasis.

Table 12-1

7TH EDITION AJCC/UICC TNM CLASSIFICATIONS

Primary tumor (T)	
TX	Primary tumor cannot be assessed
T0	No evidence of primary tumor
Tis	High-grade dysplasia[a]
T1	Tumor invades lamina propria, muscularis mucosae, or submucosa
T1a	Tumor invades lamina propria or muscularis mucosae
T1b	Tumor invades submucosa
T2	Tumor invades muscularis propria
T3	Tumor invades adventitia
T4	Tumor invades adjacent structures
T4a	Resectable tumor invading pleura, pericardium, or diaphragm
T4b	Unresectable tumor invading other adjacent structures, such as aorta, vertebral body, trachea, etc.
Regional lymph nodes (N)[b]	
NX	Regional lymph nodes cannot be assessed
N0	No regional lymph node metastasis
N1	Regional lymph node metastases involving 1–2 nodes
N2	Regional lymph node metastases involving 3–6 nodes
N3	Regional lymph node metastases involving 7 or more nodes
Distant metastasis (M)	
M0	No distant metastasis
M1	Distant metastasis
Histopathologic type	
Squamous cell carcinoma	
Adenocarcinoma	
Histologic grade (G)	
GX	Grade cannot be assessed—stage grouping as G1
G1	Well differentiated
G2	Moderately differentiated
G3	Poorly differentiated
G4	Undifferentiated—stage grouping as G3 squamous
Location[c]	
Upper or middle—cancers above lower border of inferior pulmonary vein	
Lower—below inferior pulmonary vein	

[a]Includes all noninvasive neoplastic epithelium that was previously called carcinoma in situ. Cancers stated to be noninvasive or in situ are classified as Tis.

[b]Number must be recorded for total number of regional nodes sampled and total number of reported nodes with metastases.

[c]Location (primary cancer site) is defined by position of upper (proximal) edge of tumor in esophagus.

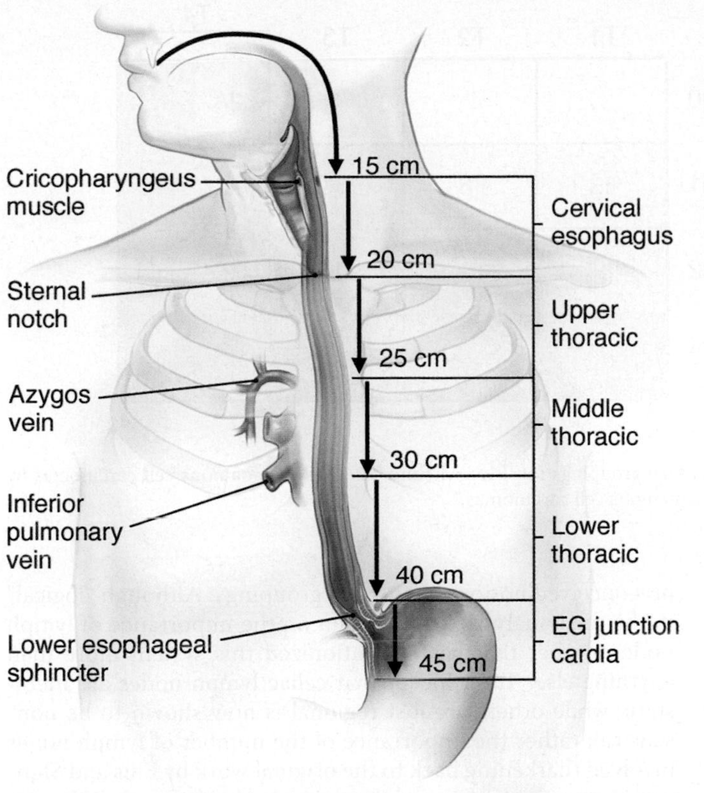

Figure 12-2. Cancer location. Cervical esophagus, bounded superiorly by the cricopharyngeus and inferiorly by the sternal notch, is typically 15 to 20 cm from the incisors at esophagoscopy. Upper thoracic esophagus, bounded superiorly by the sternal notch and inferiorly by the azygos arch, is typically >20 to 25 cm from the incisors at esophagoscopy. Middle thoracic esophagus, bounded superiorly by the azygos arch and inferiorly by the inferior pulmonary vein, is typically >25 to 30 cm from the incisors at esophagoscopy. Lower thoracic esophagus, bounded superiorly by the inferior pulmonary vein and inferiorly by the lower esophageal sphincter, is typically >30 to 40 cm from the incisors at esophagoscopy; it includes cancers whose epicenter is within the proximal 5 cm of the stomach that extend into the EGJ or lower thoracic esophagus.

histologic grade is associated with incrementally decreasing survival for early-stage cancers. For adenocarcinoma, distinguishing G1 and G2 (well and moderately differentiated) from G3 (poorly differentiated) is important for stage I and IIA cancers. For squamous cell carcinoma, distinguishing G1 from G2 and G3 is important for stage I and II cancers. Tumor location (upper and middle thoracic versus lower thoracic) is important for grouping T2-3N0M0 squamous cell cancers.

7TH EDITION STAGE GROUPINGS

Stages 0 and IV are by definition (not data driven) TisN0M0 and T any N any M1, respectively. Strict adherences to these definitions, as required by the AJCC for the 7th edition, unfortunately hindered the production of true homogeneous groupings at the extremes of stage groupings. Hopefully these definitions will be loosened, liberalized, or abandoned for the 8th edition.

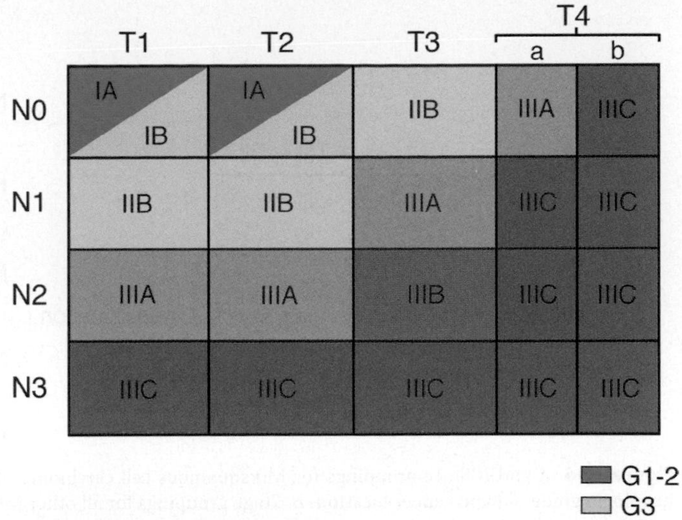

Figure 12-3. Stage groupings for M0 adenocarcinoma by T and N classification and histologic grade (G).

Stage groupings for M0 adenocarcinoma are shown in Figure 12-3. For T1N0M0 and T2N0M0 adenocarcinoma, subgrouping is by histologic grade: not G3 (G1 and G2) versus G3.

Stage groupings for M0 squamous cell carcinoma are shown in Figure 12-4. For T1N0M0 squamous cell carcinoma, subgrouping is by histologic grade: G1 versus not G1 (G2 and G3) (Fig. 12-4A). For T2N0M0 and T3N0M0 squamous cell carcinomas, stage grouping is by histologic grade and location. The four combinations range from G1 lower thoracic squamous cell carcinoma (stage IB), which has the best survival, to G2-G4 upper and middle thoracic squamous cell carcinomas (stage IIB), which have the worst. G2-G4 lower thoracic squamous cell carcinomas and G1 upper and middle thoracic squamous cell carcinomas are grouped together (stage IIA), with intermediate survival.

Stage 0, III, and IV adenocarcinoma and squamous cell carcinoma (Fig. 12-4B) are identically stage grouped. Adenosquamous carcinomas are staged as squamous cell carcinoma.

ESOPHAGOGASTRIC JUNCTION CANCERS

The arbitrary 10-cm segment encompassing the distal 5 cm of the esophagus and proximal 5 cm of the stomach (cardia), with the EGJ in the middle, has been an area of contention. Besides being data driven, the 7th edition of the Cancer Staging Manual harmonizes staging of cancer across the EGJ. Previous staging editions produced different stages for these cancers depending on use of either esophageal or stomach stage groupings. The 7th edition staging is for cancers of the esophagus and EGJ and includes cancer within the first 5 cm of the stomach that invade the EGJ. All other cancers with an epicenter in the stomach greater than 5 cm distal to the EGJ, or those within 5 cm of the EGJ but not extending into the EGJ or esophagus, are staged grouped using the gastric (non-EGJ) cancer staging system.

CONCLUSIONS

7th edition staging of cancer of the esophagus and EGJ is data driven and harmonized with stomach cancer staging. This

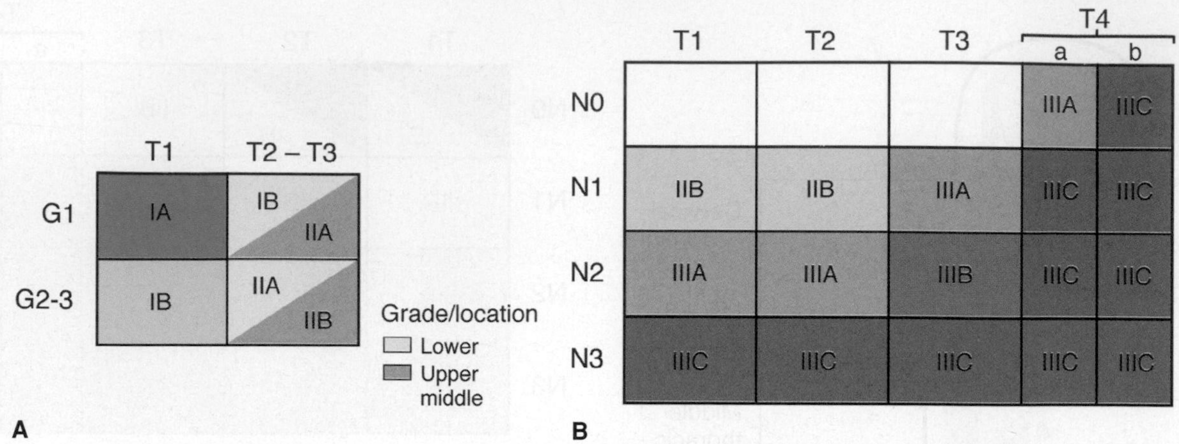

Figure 12-4. *A* and *B* Stage groupings for M0 squamous cell carcinoma. *A*. Stage groupings for T1N0M0 and T2-3N0M0 squamous cell carcinomas by histologic grade (G) and cancer location. *B*. Stage groupings for all other M0 squamous cell carcinomas.

required changes in TNM definitions and addition of nonanatomic cancer characteristics. For cancers of the esophagus and EGJ, stages 0, III, and IV are identical for both adenocarcinoma and squamous cell carcinoma. However, stage groupings differ for stage I and II cancers based on histopathologic cell type, histologic grade, and cancer location.

The new era of data-driven staging of esophageal cancer promises a bright future for staging of all cancers.[6] However, for further evolution, the 8th edition requires more extensive worldwide collaboration to refine TNM classifications and identify cancer and patient characteristics that influence esophageal cancer stage and impact survival.

EDITOR'S COMMENT

This new chapter in the esophagus section of Adult Chest Surgery highlights one of the momentous changes and improvements in managing esophageal cancer. The new AJCC 7th edition staging system is finally a data-driven system without preconceived notions as to stage groupings. Although "logical" in the final analysis, it is the data on the importance of lymph node number that has revolutionized this system more than anything else. The concept that celiac lymph nodes are metastatic while others are just regional is now shown to be nonsensical; rather the importance of the number of lymph nodes involved (harkening back to the original work by Ellis and Skinner in the 1980s) is now the primary determinant. Likewise the ability to use a uniform system for esophageal, EGJ, and gastric cancers in terms of lymph node groupings will make the comparison of data from the United States, Europe, and Asia possible. Finally, recognizing the differences in early-stage squamous versus adenocarcinoma with the weight of tumor grade represented appropriately in each, is a huge step forward. Dr. Rice and his collaborators have tried to lobby for many of these data-driven changes for over two decades and this new system has vindicated many of the esophageal surgeons who have published on the failings of the prior system.[7,8]

—Mark J. Krasna

References

1. Rice TW, Rusch VW, Apperson-Hansen C, et al. Worldwide esophageal cancer collaboration. *Dis Esoph.* 2009;22:1–8.
2. Ishwaran H, Blackstone EH, Apperson-Hansen C, et al. A novel approach to cancer staging: application to esophageal cancer. *Biostatistics.* 2009;10:603–620.
3. Rice TW, Rusch VW, Ishwaran H, et al. Cancer of the esophagus and esophagogastric junction: data-driven staging for the 7th edition of the AJCC cancer staging manual. *Cancer.* 2010;116:3763–3773.
4. American Joint Committee on Cancer. *AJCC Cancer Staging Manual.* 7th ed. New York: Springer; 2010.
5. International Union Against Cancer. *TNM Classification of Malignant Tumors.* 7th ed. Oxford, UK: Wiley-Blackwell; 2009.
6. Rusch VW, Rice TW, Crowley J, et al. The seventh edition of the American Joint Committee on Cancer/International Union Against Cancer Staging Manuals: the new era of data-driven revisions. *J Thorac Cardiovasc Surg.* 2010;139:819–821.
7. Skinner DB, Little AG, Ferguson MK, et al. Selection of operation for esophageal cancer based on staging. *Ann Surg.* 1986;204(4):391–401.
8. Ellis FH Jr, Watkins E Jr, Krasna MJ, et al. Staging of carcinoma of the esophagus and cardia: a comparison of different staging criteria. *J Surg Oncol.* 1993;52(4):231–235.

13 Surgical Approach to Esophagogastric Junction Cancers

Toni Lerut and Philippe Nafteux

Keywords: Esophagogastric junction (EGJ) tumors, Siewert classification of adenocarcinoma of the esophagogastric junction (AEG), esophageal resection operations

INTRODUCTION

Esophageal cancer is ranked among the top 10 most common cancers in the world, with more than 480,000 new cases diagnosed annually.[1] The proportion of cases involving the two most common histopathological entities, adenocarcinoma and squamous cell carcinoma, is changing. While adenocarcinoma of the esophagus is rising rapidly in Western countries; squamous cell carcinoma remains unchanged.[2] The true incidence of adenocarcinoma is difficult to determine because cancer of the esophagogastric junction (EGJ) is classified by some as a gastric cancer while by others as an esophageal cancer (see Chapter 12). This explains, in part, the ongoing controversy over which strategy to follow when it comes to surgical approach and technique.

In an effort to rationalize what had been a rather indiscriminate approach to EGJ tumors and to provide clearer guidelines, in 1998, Siewert and Stein[3] published a classification for adenocarcinoma of the esophagogastric junction (AEG). Tumors of the AEG were defined as tumors with an epicenter equal to or less than 5 cm proximal and distal to the anatomic EGJ (anatomic cardia).

Three entities were distinguished:

1. Adenocarcinoma of the distal esophagus, usually arising in Barrett intestinal metaplasia,
2. True carcinoma of the EGJ, which may arise from the cardiac epithelium or from Barrett intestinal metaplasia, and
3. Subcardial adenocarcinoma arising from the gastric fundus.

Using this classification and drawing on their own data, Siewert and Stein proposed guidelines on which surgical strategy to use according to each of the above-described subtypes. This classification is based entirely on identifying the "anatomical" cardia and measuring the center of the tumor in relation to this anatomical cardia on the resected specimen (i.e., pathological staging). However, measuring the center of the tumor turns out to be impractical if not impossible for the purposes of clinical staging. It is important to have accurate clinical staging because it ensures the appropriateness of the therapeutic decision (e.g., in the presence of a hiatal hernia). Not surprisingly, Omloo et al.[4] recently reported a substantial discrepancy between the clinical and pathological staging when using the Siewert classification.

The 7th edition of the TNM classification system,[5] which is based on evidence derived from a large international multinational database, also addressed this issue. It classifies and stages tumors that have their epicenter in the EGJ, or within the proximal 5 cm of the stomach and extending into the EGJ or esophagus, similarly to an adenocarcinoma of the esophagus. Tumors centered in the stomach that are located more than 5 cm from the EGJ, or tumors within 5 cm of the EGJ but without extension into the esophagus, are classified and staged as gastric tumors.[6]

As a result, the strategies related to surgical approaches and techniques are, in general, similar to those intended for cancers of the esophagus. These strategies in particular are related to the patterns of lymphatic spread observed with esophageal cancer.

Lymphatic dissemination is an early event and has a negative influence on survival. Lymph node metastases are found in less than 5% of intramucosal tumors, but in as many as 30% to 40% of submucosal tumors, that is, when the tumor spreads beyond the mucosa. The esophageal wall is characterized by an extensive submucosal lymphatic plexus, which not only supplies a drainage route for early dissemination, but also gives rise to jump metastases (i.e., lymph nodes adjacent to the primary tumor are not affected, but more distantly located lymph nodes contain metastases).[7]

The pattern of lymphatic dissemination therefore is difficult to predict. Nevertheless, carcinomas of the proximal and middle thirds of the esophagus tend to metastasize to the cervical region, whereas more distal-lying tumors and tumors of the EGJ more commonly metastasize to the lymph nodes around the celiac trunk. This is also the case for adenocarcinoma of the EGJ. These tumors typically drain by an extraperitoneal route into the retropancreatic area and into the left renal hilum.[8] Adenocarcinoma of the EGJ also has a tendency to spread to the thoracic lymph nodes including subcarinal, paratracheal, and aortopulmonary window nodes. Lagarde et al.[9] evaluated a group of 50 patients with a EGJ tumor that underwent extensive lymphadenectomy through a transthoracic approach and found that 22% of them had lymph node involvement of the more proximal nodes. These findings need to be taken into consideration when determining surgical strategies.

PRINCIPLES OF SURGERY

For decades surgeons have been combining transthoracic and abdominal esophagectomy to remove the esophagus and cardia, together with the primary tumor and adjacent lymph nodes, under direct vision.[10] It has been suggested that long-term survival might benefit from a more radical resection and a more extensive lymphadenectomy in the thorax and abdomen.[11]

The Radical En Bloc Resection

The radical en bloc resection extends the standard treatment to encompass a wide local resection of the primary tumor with a radical lymph node dissection of the middle and distal thirds of the posterior mediastinum.[12] The concept of extensive en bloc resection was first reported in 1963, but the associated mortality of more than 20% discouraged its general acceptance.

Skinner and Akiyama reintroduced this method in the 1980s. Ultimately, they were able to reduce operative mortality to 5%, with 5-year survival rates of 18% and 42% respectively.[13,14] Over time the results steadily improved worldwide. Today, mortality rates are well below 5%, and 5-year survival figures routinely reach 40% at experienced centers.

The Two-Field Lymph Node Dissection

Early lymphatic dissemination, characterized by longitudinal spread of tumor along the esophagus via the submucosal plexus to the upper mediastinum and abdomen, was the rationale for advancing to a two-field lymphadenectomy.[7] This approach, which originated in Japan, adds the following elements to a wide local excision of the primary tumor: lymphadenectomy of the entire posterior mediastinum, the lymph nodes along the celiac trunk, common hepatic and splenic arteries, as well as the lymph nodes along the lesser gastric curvature and in the lesser omentum.

Transhiatal Resection

Despite some indication that surgical techniques with extensive lymph node dissections tend to improve long-term survival, a less radical transhiatal approach was developed to decrease early postoperative risk by eliminating the need for thoracotomy. This approach has been popularized in the Western world by Orringer.[15]

Attempting to close the ongoing debate between advocates of radical esophagectomy via the transthoracic approach versus advocates of the less radical esophagectomy via the transhiatal approach, Hulscher et al.[16] of The Netherlands instituted a multi-institutional randomized clinical trial. This trial compared limited transhiatal resection to transthoracic resection with extended en bloc lymph node dissection for adenocarcinoma of the esophagus and EGJ. The results revealed no statistically significant overall difference between the two surgeries, but there was a clear long-term trend in favor of the more extensive approach which yielded a 39% 5-year survival compared with a 29% 5-year survival for the more limited resection. Particularly for adenocarcinoma of the distal esophagus, a subsequent analysis revealed a 17% survival benefit in favor of the more extensive transthoracic approach.[17] This trial remains the only randomized study to compare these two approaches, but several other studies have supported the overall findings that long-term survival may benefit from a more radical esophagectomy combined with extensive two-field lymphadenectomy. Indeed, data from many centers seem to endorse a better overall 5-year outcome, often exceeding 40% after two-field lymphadenectomy, as compared with the less radical lymphadenectomy with 5-year survival figures in the range of 20% to 25%.[18]

Concerning the recommended number of lymph nodes to be dissected, there is no general agreement. Historically, 15 nodes have been considered the minimum. However, a recent multivariate analysis by Peyre et al.[19] in a large patient population found that the absolute number of lymph nodes removed during esophagectomy was a strong independent predictor of survival. They reported an optimal survival benefit required resection of at least 23 lymph nodes, and this finding was not the result of stage migration. Within every tumor stage (I–III), patients with more than 23 resected lymph nodes had better survival than patients with less than 23 resected nodes, thus strongly emphasizing the importance of performing an adequate lymph node dissection.

Within the compartments of a two-field dissection (thoracic and superior abdominal compartment), in addition to the nodes along the lesser curvature and left gastric artery, the celiac, hepatic, and splenic artery nodes also should be routinely removed during the abdominal stage of any en bloc resection. Since 1994 lymph node dissection in the chest has been defined as standard (lower periesophageal and subcarinal nodes), extended (including some upper mediastinal nodes, i.e., right paratracheal nodes), and total thoracic lymph node dissection (including the uppermost mediastinal nodes, i.e., left and right paratracheal and aortopulmonary window nodes).[20] In a classic two-field lymphadenectomy at least the periesophageal and subcarinal nodes should be removed and preferably also the node at the aortopulmonary window and the right paratracheal nodes.

As to safe margins, a wide peritumoral or en bloc resection should be attempted whenever possible to obtain an R0 status (clear circumferential, proximal, and distal margins on pathological examination). At the side of the esophagus a proximal gross length of at least 5 cm or even more to achieve a microscopically negative proximal margin is advocated. This is particularly true for the more advanced T3 and T4 cancers as shown recently by Ito et al.[21]

The extent of stomach resection will depend on the location and the length of the tumor. For adenocarcinoma of the distal esophagus and EGJ, a resection margin of 5 cm below the distal pole of the tumor will suffice. This permits use of the stomach for reconstruction after resection of the lesser curvature and its lymph nodes to create a gastric tube with an anastomosis high in the chest or the neck. If the tumor extends more than 5 cm over the fundus or lesser curve, a total gastrectomy with Roux-en-Y jejunal reconstruction is mandatory.

Currently, there are several approaches to the surgical treatment of adenocarcinoma of the distal esophagus and EGJ. These include the right-sided abdominotransthoracic approach with anastomosis high in the chest (Ivor Lewis) or in the neck (McKeown, also called 3-hole resection), a left-sided abdominotransthoracic approach with anastomosis in the chest (Sweet) or in the neck (Belsey), a transhiatal resection with anastomosis in the neck (Orringer), and the minimally invasive esophagectomy (MIE).

It is generally accepted that in patients who are medically fit for surgery, a radical esophagectomy with at least a two-field lymphadenectomy is the preferred intervention. The transhiatal resection is reserved for older patients and/or patients who are medically unfit for a radical resection.

The Ivor Lewis, McKeon, or 3-hole esophagectomy, and MIE are described in Chapters 15, 17, and 18 of this book. In this chapter we describe our approach to the transhiatal and the left-sided transthoracic technique for resection of EGJ tumors (also see Chapters 16, 21, and 22).

Transhiatal Esophagectomy

The transhiatal esophagectomy without thoracotomy has a number of practical advantages, that is, a short operative duration, probably lower incidence of pulmonary complications, and the avoidance of postthoracotomy pain. The method is particularly applicable to tumors of the distal esophagus and EGJ, where the lower mediastinum can be approached through a surgically widened hiatus. The stomach is preferred for reconstruction and is anastamosed to the remaining cervical esophagus. This can be achieved via the esophageal bed (the so-called prevertebral route) or via the retrosternal route. The latter is preferable if macroscopic locoregional tumor residue is left behind in the posterior mediastinum.

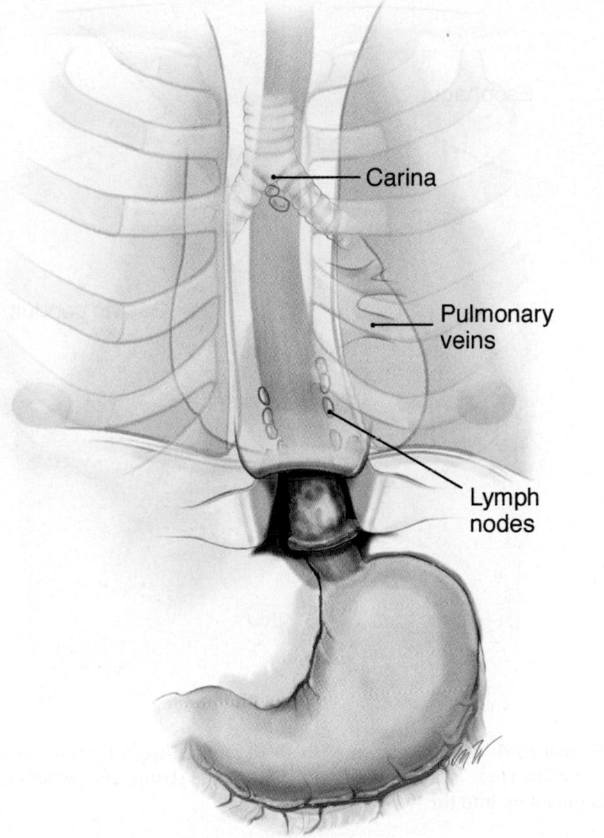

Figure 13-1. The esophagus is freed in the hiatus, along with a surrounding cuff of diaphragm if necessary.

Operative Technique

The operation begins with a median laparotomy, the incision extending from the xiphoid process to just below the umbilicus. The abdominal cavity is inspected and palpated in search of distant metastases, as this would be a contraindication for proceeding to resection. After mobilizing the left lobe of the liver, the esophageal hiatus can be inspected and tumors of the EGJ can be assessed for invasion of adjacent organs. Subsequently, the stomach is mobilized. The esophagus is freed in the hiatus, and if necessary, a surrounding cuff of diaphragm can be included in the resection specimen (Fig. 13-1). Next, the central tendon of the right hemi-diaphragm is incised, thus opening the lower mediastinum (Fig. 13-2A).

The periesophageal fatty tissues, the left and right parietal pleura, and if needed the pericardium are included in the surgical specimen. This procedure can be advanced at least as far as the inferior pulmonary veins. The more proximal and unmobilized part of the (normal) esophagus is bluntly mobilized or stripped, using a vein stripper through a neck incision (Fig. 13-2B).

After the intra-abdominal dissection is complete, the lesser curvature is resected and a neoesophagus is created, by fashioning a narrow 3 to 4 cm wide gastric tube from the remainder of the stomach (Fig. 13-3).

In this manner the lymph nodes along the right and left gastric artery are also removed. The gastric tube is then pulled/pushed (Fig. 13-4) to the neck via the prevertebral route, where an esophagogastrostomy is created (Fig. 13-5A,B).

When the retrosternal route is used, a tunnel is created by blunt retrosternal dissection from the xiphoid process up to the jugular notch. This retrosternal tunnel must be spacious enough that it does not compromise the perfusion of the interposed

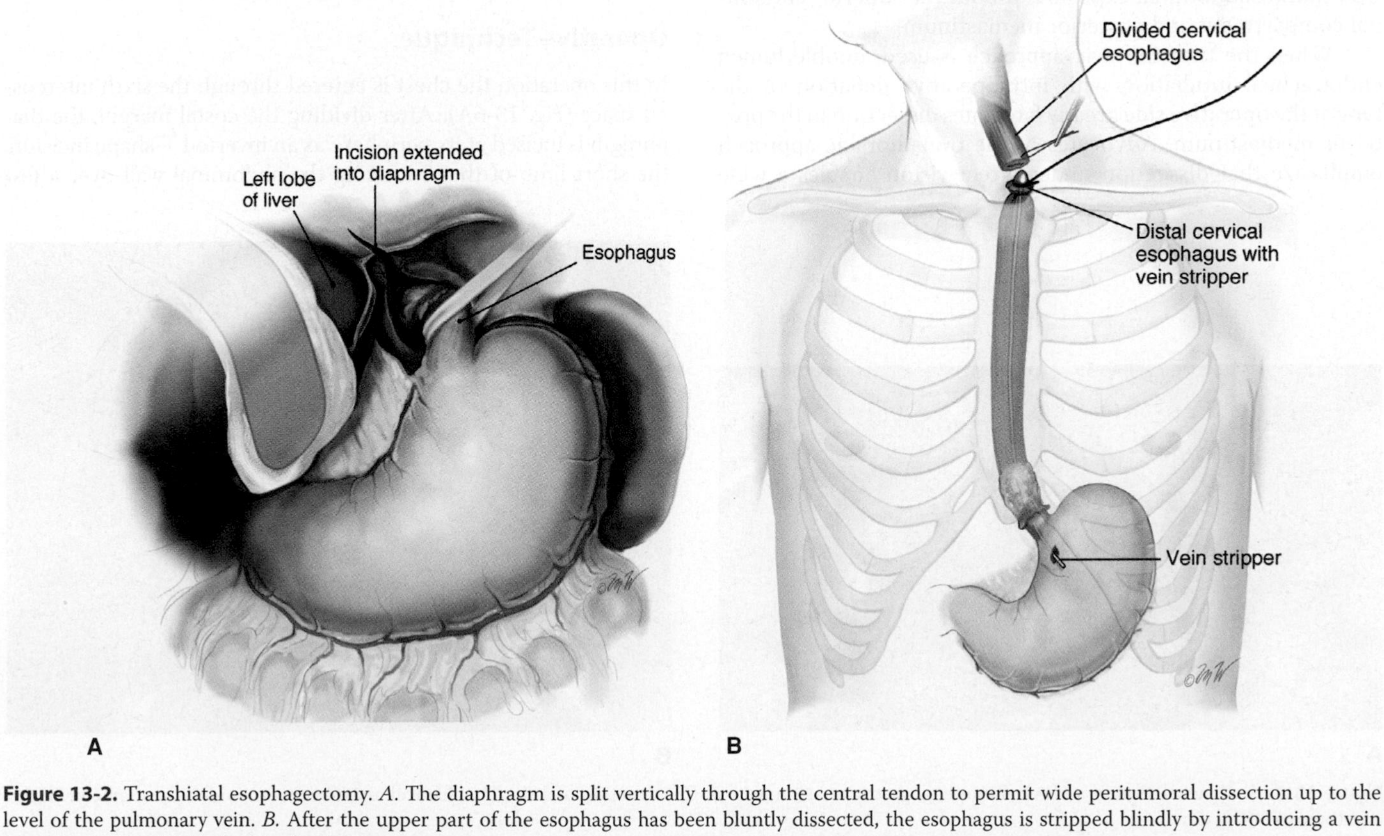

Figure 13-2. Transhiatal esophagectomy. *A*. The diaphragm is split vertically through the central tendon to permit wide peritumoral dissection up to the level of the pulmonary vein. *B*. After the upper part of the esophagus has been bluntly dissected, the esophagus is stripped blindly by introducing a vein stripper. A string is attached to the stripper.

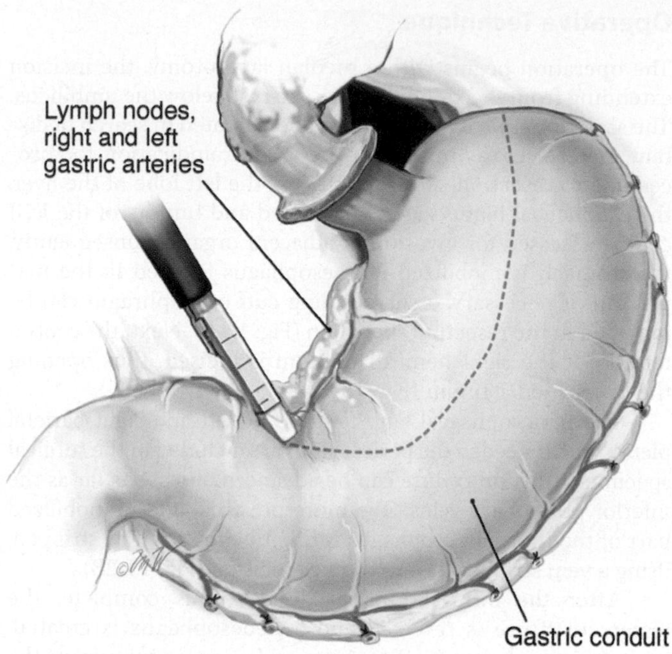

Figure 13-3. The lesser curvature of the stomach is resected.

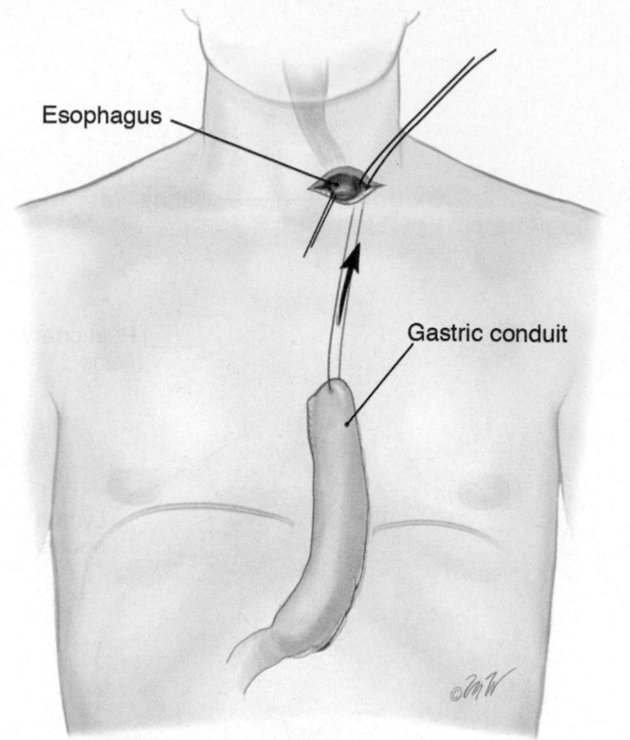

Figure 13-4. After resection of the lesser curvature, a narrow gastric tube is constructed. The top end is attached to the string, after which the tube is pulled up into the neck.

conduit by undue compression. This may in some cases require resection of the sternoclavicular joint.

Transthoracic Esophagectomy

The left thoracic approach is considered by many surgeons to be the standard approach for carcinoma of the lower esophagus and cardia. This operation was popularized by Sweet.[22] The left posterolateral approach may be extended anteriorly across the costal margin as advocated by Belsey.[23] The latter provides a true thoracoabdominal exposure of both the superior abdominal compartment and posterior mediastinum.

When the transthoracic approach is used, double lumen endotracheal intubation with intraoperative deflation of the lung at the operative side greatly facilitates dissection in the posterior mediastinum. Advocates of the transthoracic approach emphasize that dissection under direct vision enables a wide peritumoral en bloc esophagectomy as well as meticulous intrathoracic lymph node dissection. The chief disadvantage is the probably higher incidence of pulmonary complications.

Operative Technique

In this operation the chest is entered through the sixth intercostal space (Fig. 13-6A). After dividing the costal margin, the diaphragm is incised at its periphery as an inverted T-shape incision, the short limb of the T incising the abdominal wall over a few

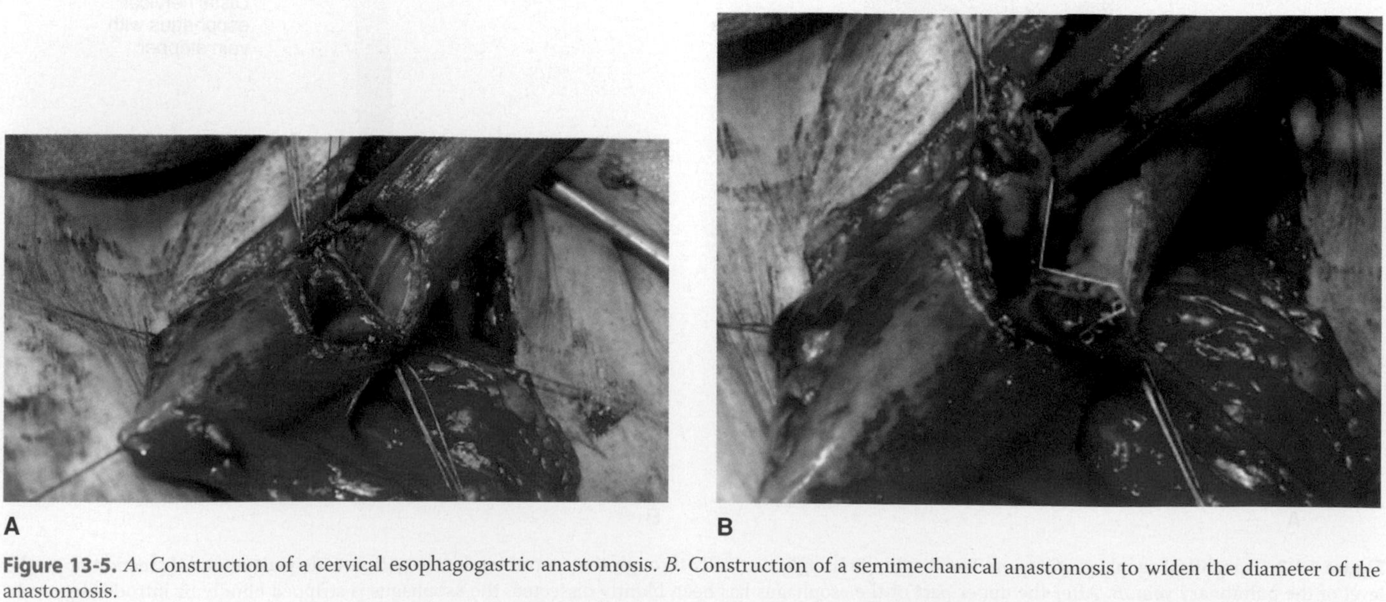

A B

Figure 13-5. *A.* Construction of a cervical esophagogastric anastomosis. *B.* Construction of a semimechanical anastomosis to widen the diameter of the anastomosis.

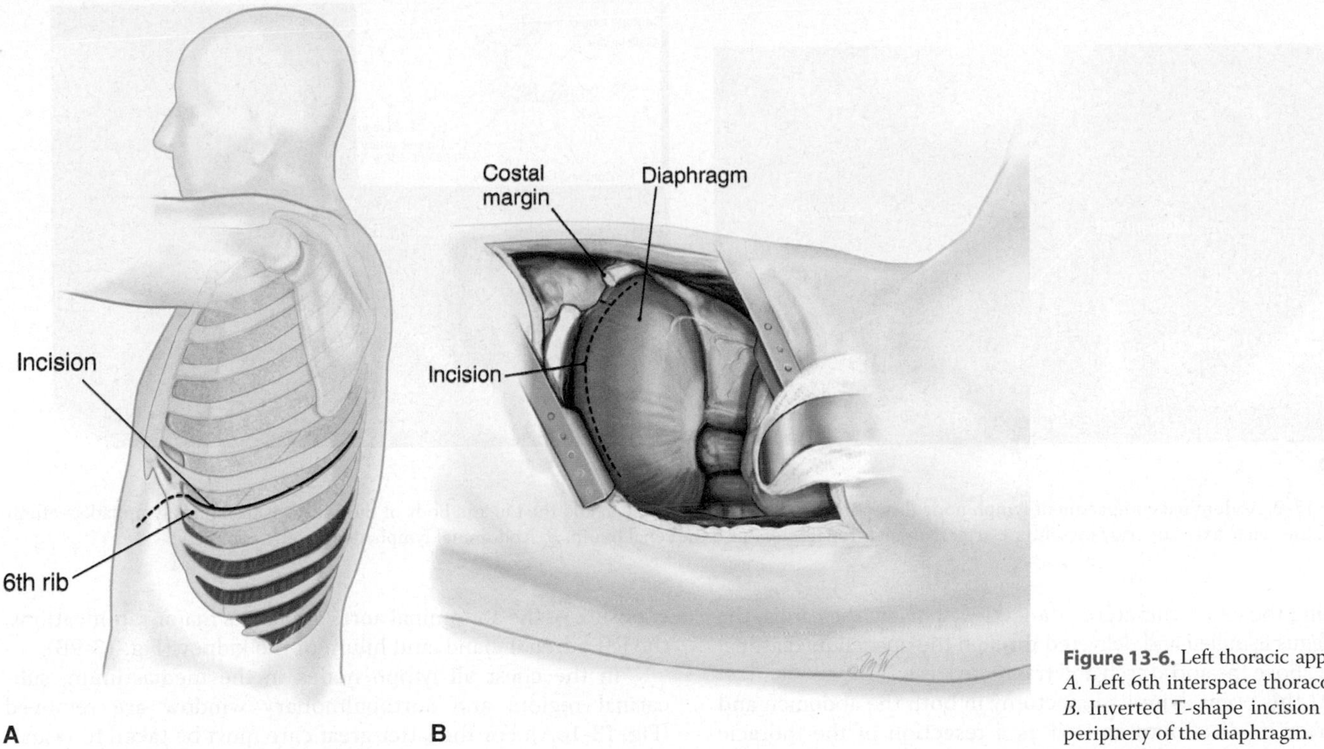

Figure 13-6. Left thoracic approach; *A.* Left 6th interspace thoracotomy. *B.* Inverted T-shape incision at the periphery of the diaphragm.

centimeters. By incising the diaphragm at its periphery, innervation and consequently function are well preserved (Fig. 13-6B).

This approach permits optimal direct vision of both the abdomen and chest cavity through one single incision. As a result, some claim that by using this incision, maximum radicality can be achieved. The entire thoracic esophagus can be dissected through the left-sided approach. In case of a EGJ tumor it may be necessary to resect a cuff of the diaphragmatic muscle surrounding the tumor (Fig. 13-7).

Dissecting the esophagus from beneath the aortic arch, requires ligation and transection of the bronchial arteries just below the arch (Fig. 13-8). The mobilization is then continued by blunt finger dissection behind the aortic arch and up into the apex of the chest. The mediastinal pleura above the aortic arch is opened. After

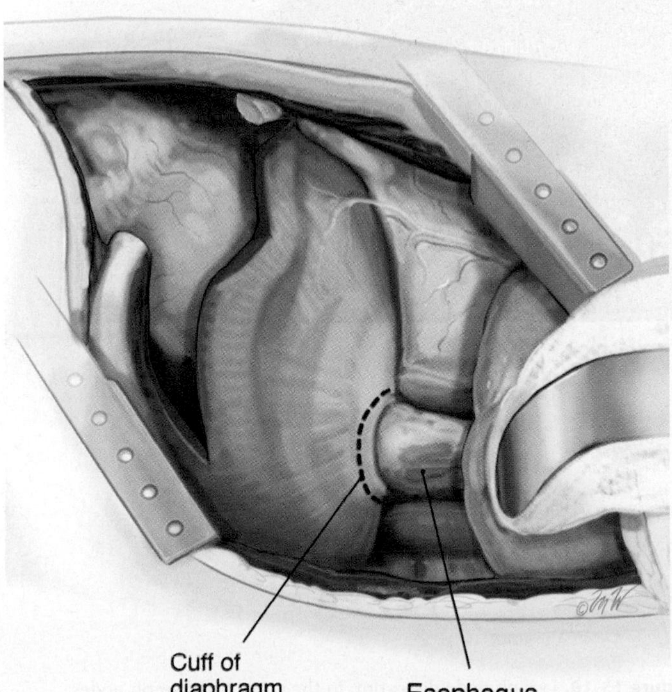

Figure 13-7. It may be necessary to resect a cuff of the diaphragm muscle surrounding the tumor when mobilizing and dissecting a EGJ tumor.

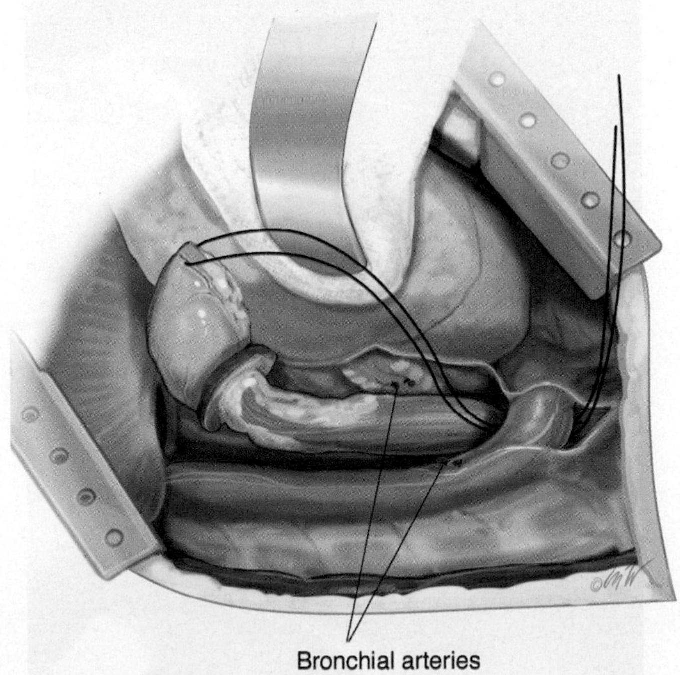

Figure 13-8. After ligating the aortic branches to the esophagus and bronchus, the esophagus is mobilized bluntly underneath the aortic arch. The mediastinal pleura above the aortic arch is opened allowing the esophagus to be pulled through.

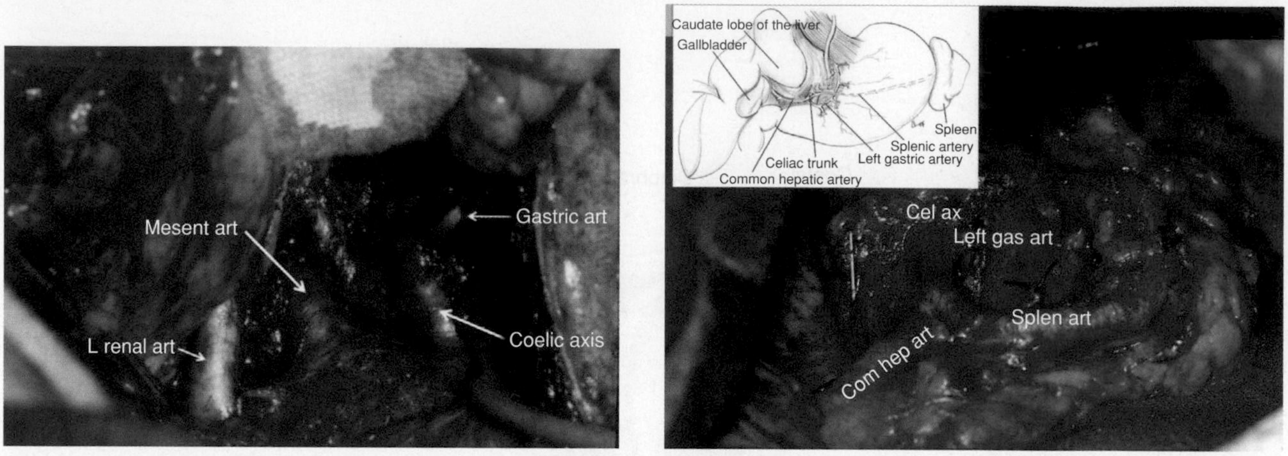

Figure 13-9. Abdominal compartment lymph node dissection. *A*. Mobilizing the spleen and the tail and body of the pancreas facilitates lymphadenectomy around the celiac axis, superior mesenteric artery, and left renal artery into the renal hilum. *B*. Abdominal lymphadenectomy completed.

resecting the lesser curvature at a level well below the cardia, the esophagus is pulled and delivered through the opened mediastinal pleura above the aortic arch and transected as well.

At this point, lymphadenectomy in both the abdomen and posterior mediastinum as well as a resection of the thoracic duct is performed. Mobilizing the spleen and the tail-body of the pancreas can be performed by incising the peritoneal reflection dorsally behind the spleen (Fig. 13-9A). The spleen and pancreas are flipped over to the right side yielding a perfect exposure of the abdominal aorta and all its major ramifications, the left adrenal gland, and hilum of the kidney (Fig. 13-9B).

In the chest all lymph nodes in the mediastinum, subcarinal region, and aortopulmonary window are removed (Fig. 13-10A). For the latter great care must be taken to visualize and preserve the left recurrent nerve.

Transecting the fibrotic remnant of the ductus arteriosus opens the left paratracheal space for further lymph node clearance (Fig. 13-10B).

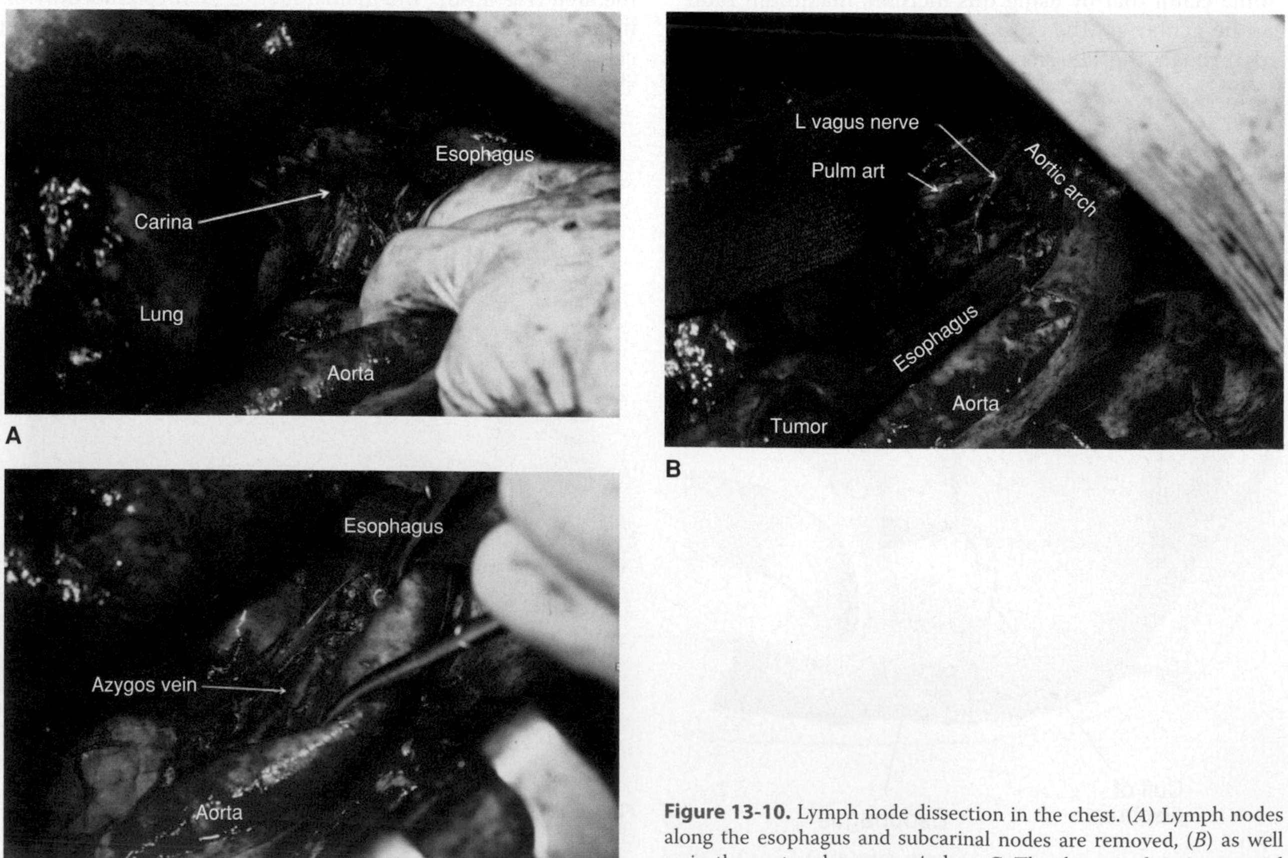

Figure 13-10. Lymph node dissection in the chest. (*A*) Lymph nodes along the esophagus and subcarinal nodes are removed, (*B*) as well as in the aortopulmonary window. *C*. The thoracic duct is resected and ligated.

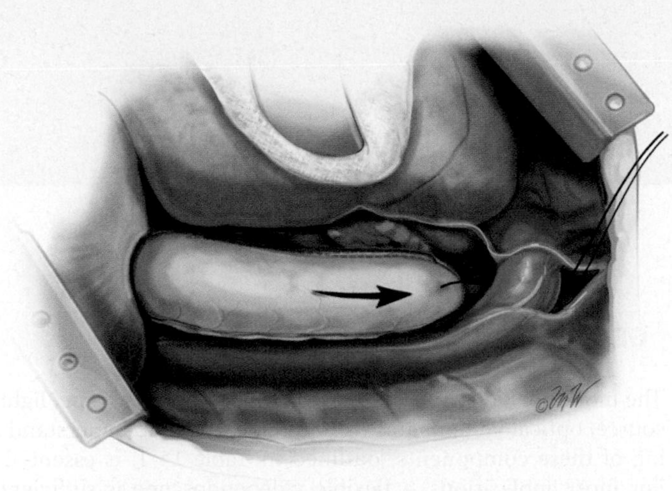

Figure 13-11. The gastric tube is brought up through the esophageal hiatus, underneath the aortic arch, and temporarily fixed to the proximal stump of the transected esophagus in the top of the chest.

Finally, resection and ligation of the thoracic duct also is the best way to prevent a chyle leak postsurgery (Fig. 13-10C).

A narrow gastric tube is constructed and brought upward through the hiatus and behind the aortic arch and temporarily fixed to the esophageal stump in the apex of the chest (Fig. 13-11).

The incision is then closed and the patient is turned to supine position. Through a left cervicotomy the esophageal stump with the attached gastric tube is exteriorized into the operative field and a cervical esophagogastrostomy is performed. According to the use of vascular pedicle, several modes of creating a gastric tube have been described. Whether or not it is a good idea to perform a gastric drainage procedure (pyloroplasty, pyloromyotomy, or more recently by injecting the pylorus with Botox) remains controversial. There is, however, a tendency to leave the pylorus intact at the time of surgery. If a gastric outlet problem occurs after surgery, it is in general well managed with prokinetic drugs and/or by performing balloon dilatation of the pylorus.[24]

In cases where the EGJ tumor extends greater than 5 cm onto the stomach, a total gastrectomy followed by a Roux-en-Y jejunal reconstruction with an intrathoracic infra-aortic esophagojejunostomy becomes mandatory.

EDITOR'S COMMENT

Siewert classification was originally described to allow surgeons to approach each section of the distal esophagus and proximal stomach logically. With the advent of the 7th edition of the AJCC staging system, the location of the tumor is an innate and critical part of the system. Arbitrary pathological description of the location of the epicenter, less relevant for a therapeutic approach, has been abandoned in exchange for a clinically relevant description which needs only to clarify whether or not the EGJ tumor extends more than 5 cm distally into the stomach. The authors have described their preferred surgical approaches to these tumors. Other modifications of this approach, as described in Chapters 21 and 22, are also recommended.

—Mark J. Krasna

References

1. Ferlay J, Shin HR, Bray F, et al. Estimates of worldwide burden of cancer in 2008: GLOBOCAN 2008. *Int J Cancer*. 2010;127(12):2893–2917 .
2. Devesa SS, Blot WJ, Fraumeni JF, Jr. Changing patterns in the incidence of esophageal and gastric carcinoma in the United States. *Cancer*. 1998;83(10): 2049–2053.
3. Siewert JR, Stein HJ. Classification of adenocarcinoma of the oesophagogastric junction. *Br J Surg*. 1998;85(11):1457–1459.
4. Omloo JM, Lagarde SM, Hulscher JB, et al. Extended transthoracic resection compared with limited transhiatal resection for adenocarcinoma of the mid/distal esophagus: five-year survival of a randomized clinical trial. *Ann Surg*. 2007;246(6):992–1000; discussion 1000–1001.
5. UICC. In: Sobin L, Gospodarowicz M, Wittekind C, eds. *TNM Classification of Malignant Tumors*. 7th ed. Oxford, UK: Wiley-Blackwell; 2009.
6. Rice TW, Blackstone EH, Rusch VW. 7th edition of the AJCC Cancer Staging Manual: esophagus and esophagogastric junction. *Ann Surg Oncol*. 2010;17(7):1721–1724.
7. Akiyama H, Tsurumaru M, Kawamura T, et al. Principles of surgical treatment for carcinoma of the esophagus: analysis of lymph node involvement. *Ann Surg*. 1981;194(4):438–446.
8. Dresner SM, Lamb PJ, Bennett MK, et al. The pattern of metastatic lymph node dissemination from adenocarcinoma of the esophagogastric junction. *Surgery*. 2001;129(1):103–109.
9. Lagarde SM, Cense HA, Hulscher JB, et al. Prospective analysis of patients with adenocarcinoma of the gastric cardia and lymph node metastasis in the proximal field of the chest. *Br J Surg*. 2005;92(11):1404–1408.
10. Schattenkerk ME, Obertop H, Mud HJ, et al. Survival after resection for carcinoma of the oesophagus. *Br J Surg*. 1987;74(3):165–168.
11. Skinner DB, Dowlatshahi KD, DeMeester TR. Potentially curable cancer of the esophagus. *Cancer*. 1982;50(11 Suppl):2571–2575.
12. DeMeester TR, Zaninotto G, Johansson KE. Selective therapeutic approach to cancer of the lower esophagus and cardia. *J Thorac Cardiovasc Surg*. 1988;95(1):42–54.
13. Skinner DB. En bloc resection for neoplasms of the esophagus and cardia. *J Thorac Cardiovasc Surg*. 1983;85(1):59–71.
14. Akiyama H, Tsurumaru M, Udagawa H, et al. Radical lymph node dissection for cancer of the thoracic esophagus. *Ann Surg*. 1994;220(3):364–372; discussion 72–73.
15. Orringer MB. Transhiatal esophagectomy without thoracotomy for carcinoma of the thoracic esophagus. *Ann Surg*. 1984;200(3):282–288.
16. Hulscher JB, van Sandick JW, de Boer AG, et al. Extended transthoracic resection compared with limited transhiatal resection for adenocarcinoma of the esophagus. *N Engl J Med*. 2002;347(21):1662–1669.
17. Hulscher JB, van Lanschot JJ. Individualised surgical treatment of patients with an adenocarcinoma of the distal oesophagus or gastro-oesophageal junction. *Dig Surg*. 2005;22(3):130–134.
18. Lerut T, Decker G, Coosemans W, et al. Quality indicators of surgery for adenocarcinoma of the esophagus and gastroesophageal junction. *Recent Results Cancer Res*. 2010;182:127–142.
19. Peyre CG, Hagen JA, DeMeester SR, et al. The number of lymph nodes removed predicts survival in esophageal cancer: an international study on the impact of extent of surgical resection. *Ann Surg*. 2008;248(4): 549–556.
20. Fumagalli U. Resective surgery for cancer of the thoracic esophagus: results of a consensus conference. *Dis Esoph*. 1996;9(suppl):30–38.
21. Ito H, Clancy TE, Osteen RT, et al. Adenocarcinoma of the gastric cardia: what is the optimal surgical approach? *J Am Coll Surg*. 2004;199(6): 880–886.
22. Sweet R. Surgical management of carcinoma of the midthoracic esophagus. Preliminary report. *N Engl J Med*. 1945;233:1–7.
23. Belsey R. Surgical exposure of the esophagus. In: Skinner D, Belsey R, eds. *Management of Esophageal Disorders*. Philadelphia, London, Toronto, Montreal, Sydney, Tokyo: WB Saunders Company; 1988:192–201.
24. Lerut TE, van Lanschot JJ. Chronic symptoms after subtotal or partial oesophagectomy: diagnosis and treatment. *Best Pract Res Clin Gastroenterol*. 2004;18(5):901–915.

14 Esophagoscopy

Abraham Lebenthal and Raphael Bueno

Keywords: Esophagogastroduodenoscopy, foregut endoscopy

Esophagoscopy is an endoscopic procedure that permits visualization of the internal lumen of the esophagus. It is usually accomplished as a part of a more extended procedure called *esophagogastroduodenoscopy* (EGD), which includes the stomach and duodenum. This visual examination is performed by using a specially designed endoscope (flexible or rigid). Since its invention by Philip Bozzini in 1806, the endoscope, which at that time consisted of a rigid tube, external light source, and a viewer, has evolved to become smaller, flexible, and more versatile. Currently, flexible endoscopes are equipped with video imaging systems that generate magnified, clear images that can be viewed by the entire operating room staff. Although flexible esophagoscopy can be performed with topical anesthesia, conscious sedation, or general anesthesia, rigid esophagoscopy is usually performed with the patient under general anesthesia.

Esophagoscopy is the primary diagnostic tool for any disease suspected to involve the esophagus. It also can be used for many different therapeutic applications, including delivery of ablative energy (cautery and photodynamic or laser therapy) for tumors, banding of varices, cauterization or injection for bleeding, deployment of stents, removal of foreign objects, and other surgical manipulations. Expertise in esophagoscopy is a requisite for all esophageal and general thoracic surgeons, and guidelines for skill attainment have been established and published by a number of surgical societies.[1–5]

Table 14-1

COMPONENTS OF AN ENDOSCOPIC SYSTEM

The scope
- Rigid tube containing a lens and a light source.
- Flexible tube containing a flexible light and optic fibers. Flexible scopes have a control panel that enables steering in two or four directions.

The light source
- Usually located outside the body, the light source transmits light waves through an optical fiber system to the distal end of the scope, thereby illuminating the organ or object under inspection.

The optical system
- A lens system that transmits the image to the viewer from the fiberscope, or video chip, at the end of the scope.
- Newer systems relay a video image to a television monitor and may have recording capabilities.

The working port
- The channel used for diagnostic and therapeutic modalities. The working port facilitates the administration of drugs, irrigation, and suction, as well as implementation of energy-delivery systems, including cautery, photodynamic therapy, or laser. Through this port, endoscopic instrumentation is also introduced, including guidewires, forceps, scissors, brushes, snares, and baskets, all of which are used to enable tissue biopsy, removal of foreign bodies, dilation, and focal surgical procedures such as polypectomy.

GENERAL PRINCIPLES

The modern endoscopic system consists of an endoscope, light source, optical system, and working port. A basic understanding of these components, outlined in Table 14-1, is essential. For most applications, a flexible videoendoscope is sufficient and preferred. Flexible endoscopes come in many sizes. The larger sizes allow for wider suction and working ports while providing excellent images. The smaller sizes are more comfortable for the patient and allow sufficient room for additional devices to be placed through the lumen of the esophagus at the same time. Rigid esophagoscopes are large, inflexible metal cylinders that come in different widths and lengths. These are used only for work that requires a very wide lumen, such as removing a foreign object or repositioning a stent.

EGD is indicated when there is a clinical suspicion of pathology of the upper gastrointestinal tract, before surgery of the esophagus or stomach, and for specific therapy of known disorders. This procedure enables the surgeon to visualize the endoluminal anatomy in great detail, as well as structural anomalies, disorders, and defects of the gastrointestinal tract. In addition, endoscopy is an excellent way to obtain tissue biopsy for histologic diagnosis or to examine the mediastinum or the rest of the layers of the esophagus with ultrasound.

Endoscopy should be performed in a controlled, well-equipped setting staffed and monitored by experienced personnel. Such locations usually include freestanding endoscopy suites and operating rooms. In emergent cases, the equipment and personnel can be moved to the bedside in the ICU or emergency ward, obviating the need to move a critically ill patient. As for any other procedure, the endoscopist should be well trained and have proper credentials to perform the procedure. Clear indications and expectations for any procedure should be discussed with the patient before endoscopy. It is also important for the surgeon to be familiar with the potential complications of endoscopy and to take proactive measures to reduce overall morbidity (Table 14-2). Several good practices are (1) to avoid applying undue force when maneuvering the instrument through the patient's oropharynx or esophagus because this may lead to perforation or unsafe instrumentation, (2) to

Table 14-2

COMMON PITFALLS

- Failure to establish a clear indication for procedure
- Failure to recognize or evaluate the patient's premorbid state
- Coagulopathy (primary or secondary to medication)
- Patient compliance with NPO status preprocedure
- Endoscopist attempting procedure beyond limits of training
- Equipment failure
- Undue force used in working with instrumentation during procedure
- Performing endoscopy when there are additional tubes in place

remove all tubes that are in place (e.g., nasogastric tube) before starting the procedure, and (3) to not compromise patient care by lack of the equipment required to perform the proposed procedure, a particular concern in the office setting.

PATIENT SELECTION AND PREPROCEDURAL ASSESSMENT

The risk of endoscopy arises from the patient's medical condition, anesthetic management, and, the actual procedure. A careful and thorough preprocedural assessment of the patient, including evaluation, selection, and preparation, is the first step for any surgical procedure. Particular attention should be focused on history of coagulopathy (primary or secondary to medication) because this can increase the procedural risk significantly. Patients deemed high risk secondary to other comorbid disease or procedures that may require technology not readily available in the outpatient setting should be treated in a hospital setting. All patients are assessed for their relative risk of undergoing anesthesia using standard American Society of Anesthesiologists' (ASA) guidelines.[6] Anesthesia-related risks include aspiration, intravenous conscious sedation or general anesthesia, and anaphylaxis. Patients with an ASA score of 4, defined as a "patient with severe systemic disease that is a constant threat to life," should not undergo endoscopy in the office setting. Patients with an ASA score of 3 (a "patient with severe systemic disease") should undergo additional preoperative assessment to determine the appropriateness of office endoscopy. Before the endoscopic procedure, patients must be given clear instructions that stress the importance of fasting for at least 6 to 8 hours before the procedure. Aspiration can be a catastrophic complication. Procedural complications are reduced in the hands of an experienced endoscopist.

TECHNIQUE

Preoperative Setup

Before performing esophagoscopy, all equipment (endoscopic, monitoring, and resuscitative) must be assembled and examined for proper function (Table 14-3). The endoscope should be examined for sterility and external integrity (e.g., the plastic coating must be completely intact without visible fractures). All knobs and buttons should be fit snugly in place and should be tested for proper function, including axial motion, air insufflation, water instillation, and suction. The video monitor should be turned on, the patient data should be entered in the electronic record, and the scope should be balanced for image clarity. The monitor should be placed directly in front of the endoscopist, and the room lights should be dimmed to maximize the quality of the image on the video monitor.

Anesthesia

The patient's status with respect to oral intake is confirmed (NPO for at least 6 hours). Anesthesia has already been selected on the basis of surgeon preference and the goals of the procedure. Standard procedures for anesthesia or conscious sedation are instituted. For general anesthesia, the patient is placed in the supine position on the operating table, induced, and intubated. The conscious patient is placed in left lateral decubitus position, and a mouth guard is placed both to enable passage of the scope into the mouth and to prevent the patient from biting the scope.

Table 14-3

MONITORING AND SEDATION FOR OFFICE-BASED ENDOSCOPY

- Confirm patient's NPO status.
- Place intravenous line before administering sedatives, and maintain intravenous line until patient has recovered sufficiently to permit safe discharge.
- Monitoring baseline pulse, respiratory rate, oxygen saturation, and blood pressure, recorded before administration of any sedatives. Pulse oximetry, cardiac monitoring, automated blood pressure recording, and supplemental oxygen should be employed routinely.
- Endoscopy suite must have emergency medications and equipment used for cardiopulmonary resuscitation (including oral suction, defibrillator, ambu bag, laryngoscope, and an emergency airway tray). This equipment must be readily available and checked on a daily basis.
- Staff must be appropriately trained in resuscitation. An advanced cardiac life support (ACLS)-certified provider must accompany all sedated patients throughout their stay.
- An assistant trained at least in basic cardiac life support (BCLS) should be present during all procedures to monitor the patient.
- A registered nurse should monitor the patient in the recovery area.
- A formal transport agreement with an acute care facility capable of managing endoscopic complications must be in place and easily executed when necessary.

Equipment

Two types of flexible endoscopes are available: videoscopic and those that utilize eye pieces. The standard endoscope is 140 cm long. It has a diameter of 5 to 11 mm and a working port that is 2.8 mm wide. Adult endoscopes typically have two dials that enable four directional control (left and right as well as up and down), whereas pediatric endoscopes have only one dial. In anesthetized adults we typically use a 9- to 12-mm scope, while 5-mm endoscopes are reserved for awake patients and those with tight strictures. All equipment should be examined for proper function prior to the procedure. This includes checking for maneuverability, light, insufflation, suction, and irrigation. Flexible endoscopic equipment is expensive. Proper maintenance (cleaning and storage) of the endoscope, including all its detachable parts, must be maintained to assure long-term function.

Esophagoscopy

After the patient has been inducted with general anesthesia, the endoscope is placed into the oropharynx and esophagus by extending the lower jaw anteriorly and placing the endoscope behind the endotracheal tube (Fig. 14-1). Alternatively, endoscopy can be performed under intravenous conscious sedation or with the patient fully awake. A bite blocker is placed between the teeth to prevent damage to the scope. The conscious patient is positioned on his or her side, usually the left. Monitored sedation is then administered using short-acting intravenous medications, after which the endoscope is carefully introduced. Alternatively, in a cooperative patient, awake endoscopy can be performed with a small scope inserted via the nose or regular endoscope after aerosolized analgesia of the oropharynx. The awake patient can aid the endoscopist by active "swallowing."

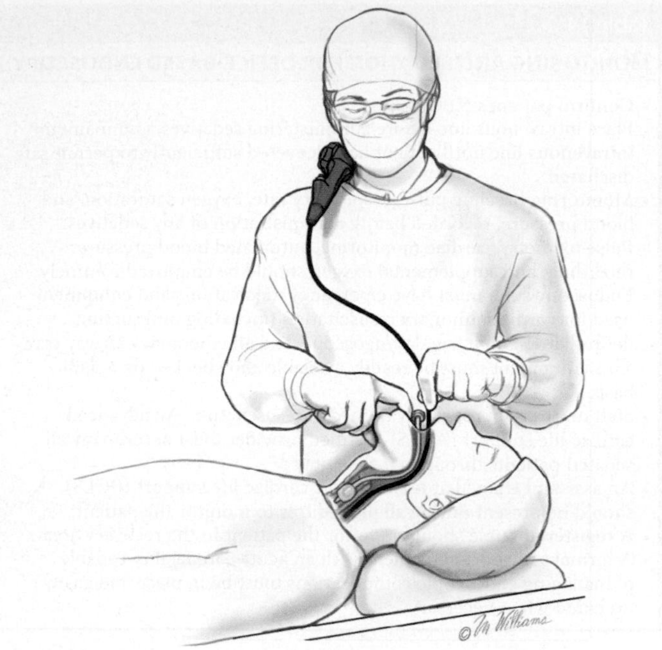

Figure 14-1. Inserting the endoscope for esophagoscopy.

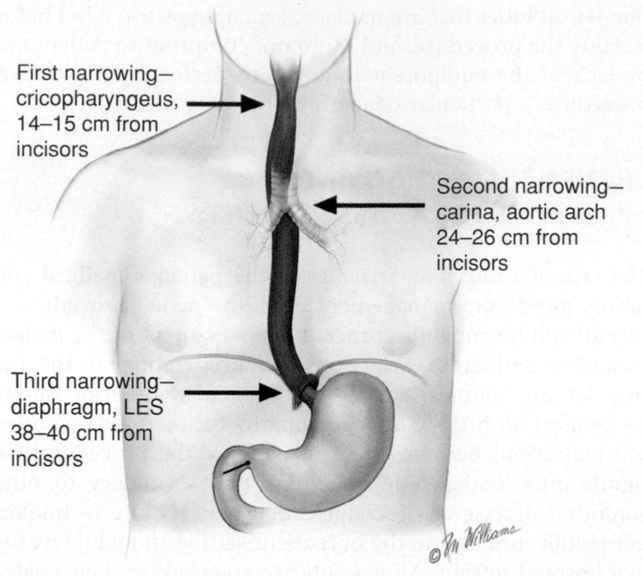

Figure 14-2. Anatomic regions of esophageal and proximal foregut narrowing. Cricopharyngeus (14 cm in females, 15 cm in males). Carina and aortic arch (24–26 cm). Diaphragmatic constriction in the area of the lower esophageal sphincter (LES; 36–38 cm in females, 38–40 cm in males). Pylorus (small arrow).

The endoscope is maneuvered by rotation in the hands of the operator, who at all times should be attempting to center the lumen on the video monitor, which decreases the chance of perforation, and by using insufflation as needed before advancing the endoscope farther along. The scope should be in the unlocked position. The scope should be advanced with minimal force. During endoscopy, the majority of the maneuvering is done by the dominant hand on the scope while the fine tuning is done by the nondominant hand on the dials. Typically, in the anesthetized patient, the scope can be passed directly into the mid-esophagus with the nondominant hand. The mouth and chin are elevated and the scope is gently advanced. If resistance is encountered, the endoscopist should draw back 1 to 2 cm, center the scope, and only then gently advance. After the scope is beyond the first narrowing of the upper esophageal sphincter at the cricopharyngeus, the esophagus is insufflated with air and the mucosa examined as the scope is advanced (Fig. 14-2).

A second narrowing occurs in the area of the aortic arch and carina, approximately 24 to 25 cm from the incisors. The final anatomic narrowing occurs at the lower esophageal sphincter (LES), which is about 40 cm from the incisors. The esophageal, gastric, and duodenal mucosae are examined visually for lesions, strictures, webs, ulcers, dilatations, diverticula, and other pathology (Fig. 14-3). The Z-line is identified, and the length is measured (incisors to Z-line) and documented.

The stomach is entered, insufflated, and examined in its entirety. Retroflexion is performed by advancing the scope into the greater curvature and then angling it to achieve maximal retroflexion. The scope is pulled back toward the gastroesophageal junction and turned 360 degrees, providing good visualization of the esophagogastric junction and its relation to the hiatus from within the stomach. The greater and lesser curvatures of the stomach, as well as the antrum and pylorus, are insufflated and examined. The scope is then passed into the second part of the duodenum to exclude the presence of additional pathology and determine how tight the pylorus may be. In our practice, endoscopy routinely includes visualization up to and including the second part of the duodenum. Before withdrawing the scope from the duodenum, air is removed by suction.

Depending on the indication for esophagoscopy, after visual examination, diagnostic procedures such as biopsy using flexible biopsy forceps or therapeutic procedures can be performed. Visual examination of the mucosa is typically performed using white light. Attention is paid to the regularity of the mucosa, in addition to color and presence of nodularity, ulceration, or masses. Newer scopes may have customized features such as a narrow band imaging (NBI) mode that accentuates the microvasculature and can help the endoscopist identify subtle changes. Additional diagnostic endoscopic modalities include life-scope and confocal technologies. Currently, these are not widely used. Biopsy should be performed when suspected pathology is encountered. This can be accomplished with regular or jumbo forceps. Endoscopic mucosal resection (EMR) may provide diagnostic as well as therapeutic benefit (see Chapter 173). In the event of stricture, a guidewire may be inserted to cross the stricture before (if the stricture is very tight) or after the scope has traversed it. The scope is withdrawn, and serial dilations are carried out using Savary dilators. Alternatively, a pneumatic dilator can be placed over the guidewire and the stricture dilated using preset pressure and diameter. Completion endoscopy is then carried out to evaluate the results of the dilation and to rule out procedure-related injury. In cases where stenting is indicated a guidewire can be placed beyond the target lesion, and a stent placed under direct endoscopic vision or using fluoroscopy.

PROCEDURE-SPECIFIC COMPLICATIONS

Prevention is key to avoiding the complications of endoscopy, namely, oversedation, aspiration, bleeding, perforation, systemic

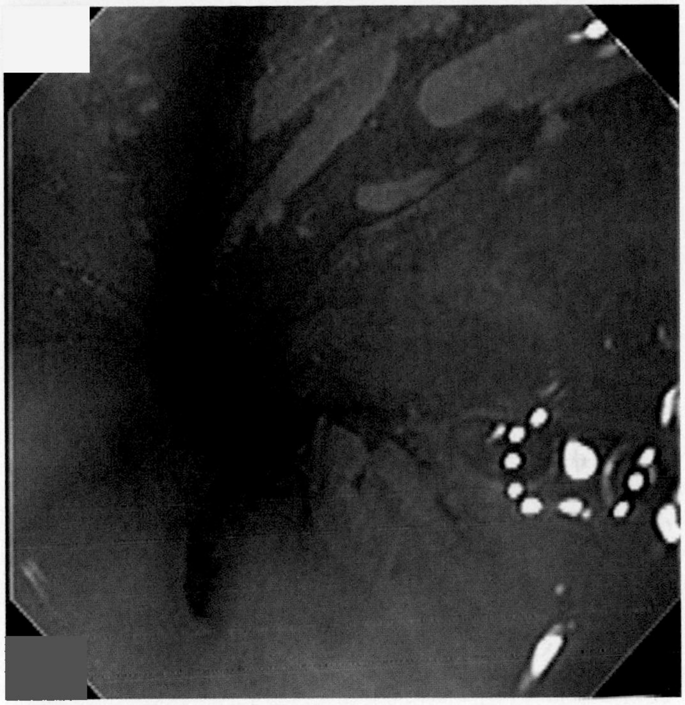

A

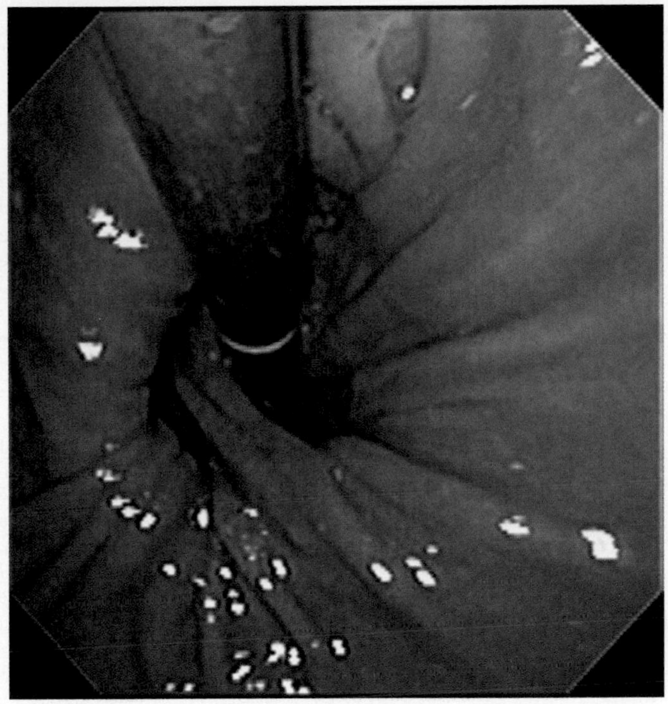

B

Figure 14-3. Representative pathology. *A.* Barrett's distal esophagus. *B.* Retroflex view showing slipped Nissen fundoplication.

processes, and injury incidental to recovery (Table 14-4). Oversedation can be avoided by judicious use of sedatives, but when it occurs, it is best managed by postprocedural monitoring or intubation and monitoring in an intensive care unit setting. The major risks of oversedation are central respiratory suppression and loss of gag reflex. The risk of aspiration is minimized with proper patient preparation (i.e., NPO for at least 6 hours), by avoiding excessive insufflation, and through judicious use of sedation and monitoring. Bleeding can be minimized by gentle maneuvering of the endoscope, cessation of anticoagulant medication preoperatively, and if encountered, cauterization of bleeding sites as soon as they are identified. Parenthetically, some of the flexible biopsy forceps also have the capability of functioning as electrocautery. Perforation can be avoided largely by careful maneuvering of the endoscope without forcing it through tight spots. Perforations usually occur at the site of one of the three narrow points described earlier or next to the diseased portion. It is important to recognize perforation early because immediate therapy reduces mortality. A high index of suspicion is important. Patients with perforation usually complain of pain and may have tachycardia and/or subcutaneous emphysema. A chest x-ray may demonstrate a pneumothorax or air tracking in the mediastinum. A contrast study such as an upper gastrointestinal series or CT scan may be helpful to identify a perforation before the repair.

Table 14-4

COMPLICATIONS

- Oversedation
- Aspiration
- Bleeding
- Perforation
- Systemic

Finally, systemic complications are extremely rare except in critically ill patients. These can be secondary to medications (i.e., hypotension, arrhythmias, and rarely, anaphylaxis). Instrumentation insufflation can lead to a vasovagal reflex, and rarely, translocation of bacteria has been reported to precipitate sepsis, as has the use of instruments not sterilized properly.

SUMMARY AND FUTURE DIRECTIONS

Esophagoscopy is an evolving and important diagnostic and therapeutic operation. Hybrid procedures are emerging that combine the advantages of multiple therapeutic and technologically advanced platforms. Reports of initial experiences with long-distance endoscopy are encouraging and in future could facilitate improved medical care to remote and underserved regions. The experimental field of natural orifice transluminal endoscopic surgery (NOTES) one day may expand the indications for use of this important technology.[7] Endoscopes with sewing ports are currently used for plication of the gastroesophageal junction. The longevity and efficacy of these procedures, however, have yet to be proved. In addition, early reports of using natural orifices for organ removal, with intentional internal perforation of the stomach for cholecystectomy and appendectomy, are unproved in terms of safety and long-term benefit. Intriguing emerging technologies that one day may replace diagnostic endoscopy, thus reducing the procedural risks associated with sedation and instrumentation, are also being developed. Examples include the wireless capsule endoscopy and virtual endoscopy with three-dimensional computed tomographic reconstruction. Despite the aforementioned advances, acquiring the skills for conventional endoscopy is paramount to the surgeon interested in foregut practice and will be needed for some time to come.

EDITOR'S COMMENT

This concise and clearly written chapter describes the indications for and the technique of endoscopy of the esophagus. Taking great care with patient preparation and having appropriate backup monitoring as well as OR capability are key to performing this procedure safely. Although not all esophageal surgeons do their own esophagoscopy, there is a trend for more surgeons to do this at the time of resection. EGD with biopsy is the first confirmatory diagnostic test to prove the presence of esophageal cancer. Safe dilation in skilled hands can allow EUS to be performed to further assess the depth of wall invasion as well as judge the presence of regional lymph nodes. It also permits a palliative therapy, such as stent or laser procedures, to be undertaken at the same time, allowing neoadjuvant or definitive chemoradiation to be undertaken without the loss of GI alimentation.

—Mark J. Krasna

References

1. *Guidelines for Endoscopic Surgery.* Society of American Gastrointestinal and Endoscopic Surgeons, 2007; http://www.sages.org/sagespublication.php?doc+09. Accessed July 20, 2014.
2. Cass O, Freeman M, ACES Study Group, et al. Acquisition of competency in endoscopic skills (ACES) during training: a multicenter study (abstract). *Gastrointest Endosc.* 1993;43:308.
3. Cass OW, Freeman ML, Peine CJ, et al. Objective evaluation of endoscopic skills during training. *Ann Intern Med.* 1993;118:40–44.
4. Cosgrove JM, Cohen JR, Wait RB, et al. Endoscopy training during general surgery residency. *Surg Laparosc Endosc.* 1995;5:393–395.
5. Galandiuk S. A surgical subspecialist enhances general surgical operative experience. *Arch Surg.* 1995;130:1136–1138.
6. American Society of Anesthesiology Physical Status Score. http://www.asahq.org/clinical/physicalstatus.htm. Accessed July 20, 2014.
7. Giday SA, Kantsevoy SV, Kalloo AN. Principle and history of Natural Orifice Translumenal Endoscopic Surgery (NOTES). *Minim Invasive Ther Allied Technol.* 2006;15:373–377.

15 Minimally Invasive Esophagectomy

Jon O. Wee and James D. Luketich

Keywords: Minimally invasive esophagectomy, thoracoscopy, laparoscopy, Barrett esophagus

INTRODUCTION

First described in AD 160 by Galen, the esophagus has proved to be a challenging organ to understand and manipulate. Its complex physiology and treacherous location in the posterior mediastinum precluded surgical manipulation until the 20th century. The first thoracic esophageal resection was described by Torek in 1915.[1] He illustrated a resection of the midesophagus with an extra-anatomic reconstruction. Although he described only one survivor, this event heralded the beginning of esophageal surgery. For the remainder of this century and into the next, surgeons have endeavored to improve the technique and outcomes of this thoracic specialty.

Orringer and Sloan[2] popularized a transhiatal approach to esophageal resection and a gastric tube reconstruction. McKeown[3] described a three-field approach requiring a thoracotomy to perform the majority of the esophageal dissection, followed by a laparotomy for the gastric mobilization, and finally, a cervical incision for anastomosis. Variations in approaches and reconstructions have provided today's surgeons with a large armament of techniques and fodder for debate over the ideal approach.

Open surgical procedures remain the standard of care for esophageal resections in most medical centers. However, the morbidity and mortality associated with open procedures and the diseases for which they are required still reveal the need for further improvement. A 10-year review of the esophagectomy experience within the Veterans' Affairs hospital system revealed a morbidity of 50% and a mortality of 10%.[4] Birkmeyer et al.,[5] in a recent analysis of a national Medicare database, revealed that the mortality rates from esophagectomy in the United States ranged from 8% in high-volume centers to 23% in low-volume centers.

BEGINNINGS OF MIE

The advent of laparoscopy and thoracoscopy in the 1980s opened the door to the possibility of a minimally invasive approach to esophageal surgery. Initial experience with laparoscopic Nissen fundoplications formed the basis of the early surgical experience, followed by the use of laparoscopic and thoracoscopic staging of lymph nodes. Collard et al.[6] were the first to describe a thoracoscopic technique for esophageal dissection. Although multiple reports of laparoscopic-assisted esophagectomies followed, it was not until DePaula et al. published their initial experience in 1996 that a totally laparoscopic esophagectomy was documented.[7] Although this report detailed a laparoscopic transhiatal approach,[8–10] our center and others have used primarily a combined thoracoscopic and laparoscopic approach.[11–14] The thoracoscopic approach affords better visualization of the periesophageal structures, especially near the main airways and subcarinal areas. It is also less affected by patient height and body habitus and, in our experience, improves nodal dissection and overall visualization compared with the totally laparoscopic method. In 2000, Nguyen et al.[15] compared the minimally invasive approach with open transthoracic and transhiatal esophagectomy. The minimally invasive approach documented shorter operative times, less blood loss, and shorter stays in the intensive care unit with no increase in morbidity compared with the open approach.

Indications

Indications for the minimally invasive approach for esophagectomy include Barrett esophagus with high-grade dysplasia, end-stage achalasia, esophageal strictures, and esophageal cancer.[16–20] While most T4 esophageal cancers generally are not amenable to any surgical approach, all other T stages should be amenable to minimally invasive esophagectomy (MIE) in experienced hands. Downstaged cancer with neoadjuvant chemoradiation is also resectable by a minimally invasive approach. Previous thoracic and abdominal surgery is not necessarily a contraindication depending on the extent of the previous surgery and the experience of the surgeon performing the esophagectomy.

Operative approaches to MIE have varied from a 3-hole modified McKeown to the Ivor Lewis approach. While our initial experience was largely the 3-hole approach with the initial dissection starting in the chest, over the past several years we have favored the Ivor Lewis approach.[21] A high thoracic anastomosis can be performed thoracoscopically approaching the same level as a neck dissection. In addition, avoidance of a neck dissection minimizes recurrent nerve injury, dysphagia, and aspiration. Furthermore, the anastomosis is generally performed at a level on the gastric conduit that is better perfused by blood and hence is less likely to be damaged by ischemia. Below we describe the minimally invasive Ivor Lewis approach but modifications for the 3-hole approach are also discussed.

Technique

Positioning

Esophagogastroscopy is performed in all patients to confirm the location of the tumor and the suitability of the stomach for tubularization. For midesophageal tumors, a bronchoscopy is also indicated. The patient is intubated with a double-lumen endotracheal tube at the start of the case. Both lungs are ventilated during the abdominal dissection. The right lung is isolated during the thoracic dissection to provide adequate visualization and mobilization of the esophagus.

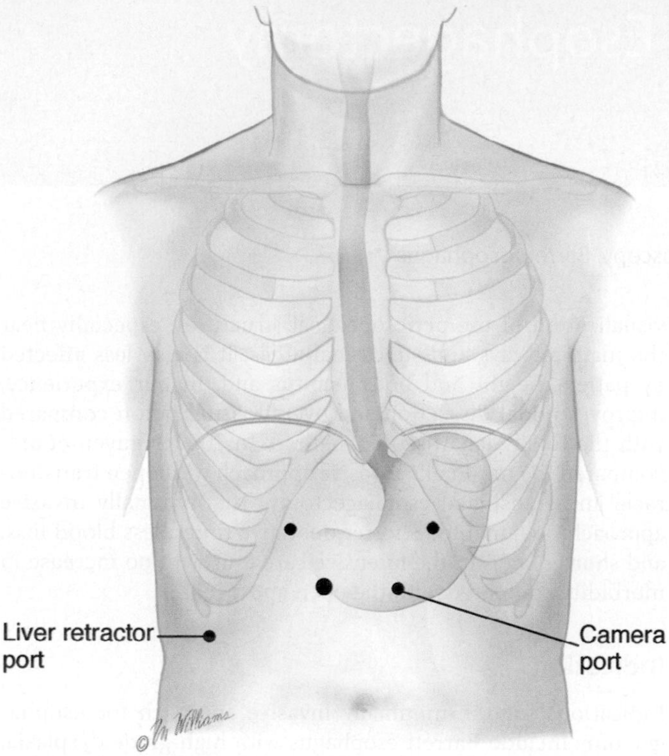

Figure 15-1. Abdominal port placement.

Laparoscopy

The patient is placed supine. Five ports are used for the gastric mobilization (Fig. 15-1). A 10-mm port is placed right of midline in the epigastrium, slightly below the midpoint between the xiphoid process and the umbilicus. The port is inserted under direct vision. The patient is placed in a steep reverse Trendelenburg position. A 5-mm port is placed to the left of midline at the same level as the original port. A 5-mm, 30-degree camera is placed through this port. Additional 5-mm ports are placed at the left subcostal margin and the right subcostal margin. A 5-mm port is placed in the right flank to support a liver retractor. A self-retaining retractor is used to elevate the left lobe of the liver and expose the hiatus (Fig. 15-2). The gastrohepatic ligament is divided to expose the right crus. The esophagogastric junction is freed from the hiatus by dissection up the right crus. The phrenoesophageal ligament is taken down, and the dissection is extended to the left crus. The right gastroepiploic arcade is identified, and the gastrocolic ligament is divided lateral to this arcade. Dissection is carried up along the greater curvature of the stomach, taking down the short gastric arteries. Once dissection is carried up toward the left crus, the posterior attachments of the gastroesophageal junction can be divided. The stomach is retracted superiorly and to the right to expose the celiac vessels. Celiac and gastric nodal tissue is dissected free and left with the specimen. The left gastric artery then is isolated and divided at the base using an Endo-GIA vascular stapler (Covidien, Norwalk, CT). The stomach itself must be handled with care at all times to minimize traumatic injuries to the tissue.

A Kocher maneuver is performed, and the retrogastric and duodenal attachments are carefully dissected to achieve adequate mobilization of the gastric tube. Adequate mobilization should permit the pylorus to reach the right crus with ease. This should be reassessed at several time points during the mobilization to inform the surgeon of the degree of dissection required. If there is any difficulty with this maneuver, further pyloroantral mobilization generally is required.

The gastric tube construction is now initiated by firing the Endo-GIA stapler across the lesser-curve vessels and fat at an angle pointing toward the incisura. For the first firing, we generally use a vascular load (white) with a staple height of 2.5 mm to minimize small-vessel oozing along the lesser curve (Fig. 15-3A). The right gastric vessels are preserved. The angle of the first few staple firings will determine the gastric tube diameter, and the staples should be placed accordingly. We prefer to create a gastric tube that is approximately 4 to 5 cm wide. In addition, we apply slight caudal and simultaneous

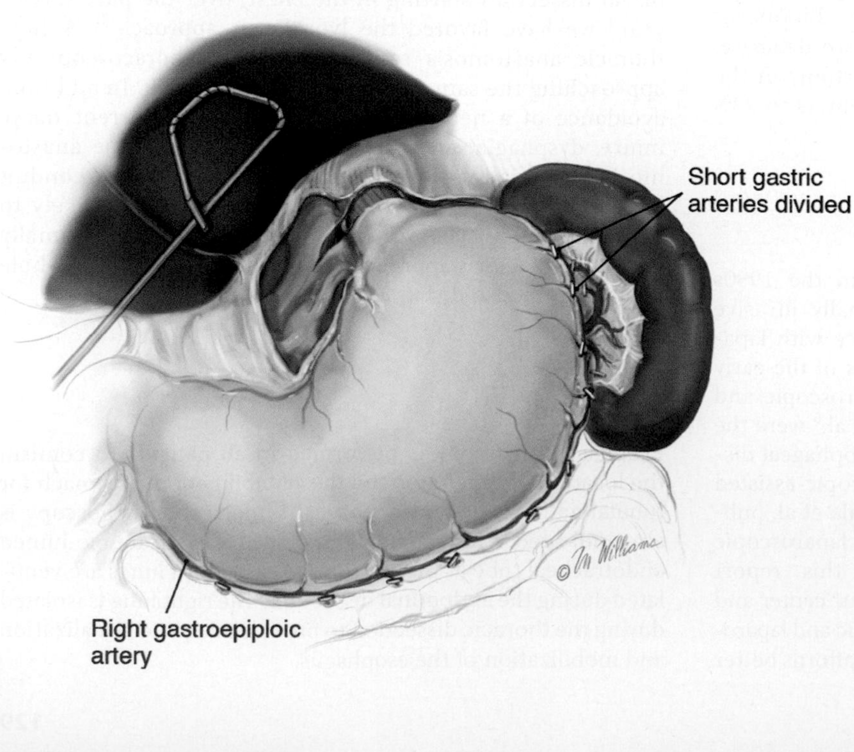

Figure 15-2. Gastric mobilization.

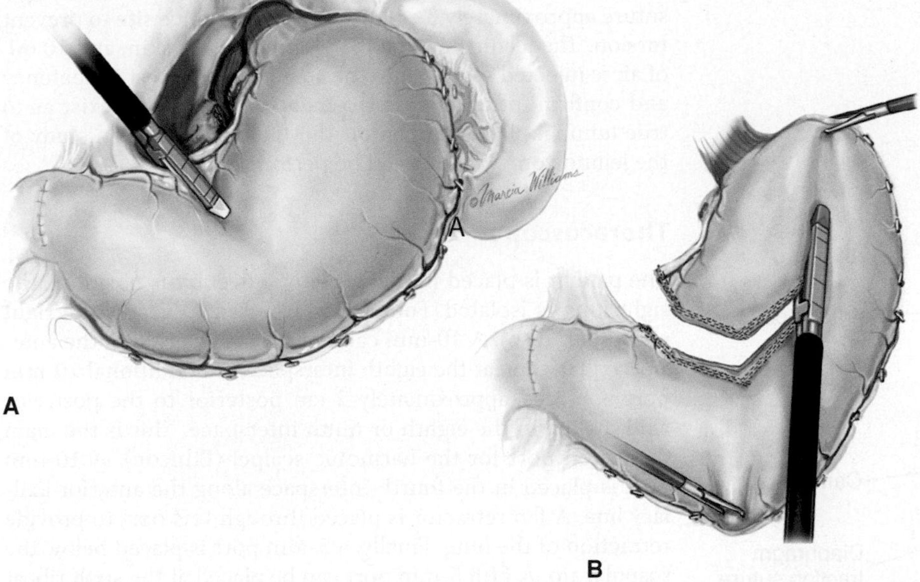

Figure 15-3. *A.* The Endo-GIA staper is fixed across the lesser curvature vessels at an angle pointing toward the incisura. *B.* A gastric tube is created approximately 4 to 5 cm wide. The stapler should be in line with the greater curvature to avoid twisting.

cephalad traction during application of the stapler to keep the gastric tube on slight stretch (Fig. 15-3B). This will afford better length of the final tube. Subsequent firings of the stapler should be maintained in a line parallel to the greater-curvature arcade to create a consistent tube width and avoid spiraling of the tubularized gastric conduit. The staple load used along the thick gastric antrum may require the green stapling cartridge (4.8-mm height). As the stapling continues toward the fundus, we generally use the blue loads (3.5-mm height). The staple line is inspected for hemostasis. The conduit is observed while the pyloroplasty is completed. A pyloroplasty is performed in Heinecke-Mikulicz fashion (see Chapter 17). An Endo Stitch (Covidien, Norwalk, CT USA) is placed superiorly and inferiorly on the pylorus to provide retraction. Ultrasonic shears are used to incise the pylorus, and the opening is closed transversely using 2-0 interrupted endosutures. The resected specimen is attached to the gastric tube with two endosutures (Fig. 15-4). These sutures should be placed from the tip of the fundic portion of the tube to the lesser-curve portion of the resected specimen. This technique tends to minimize the bulk as the specimen and gastric tube are passed through the hiatus (Fig. 15-5).

FEEDING JEJUNOSTOMY

An additional 10-mm port is placed in the right lower quadrant to facilitate jejunostomy tube placement. The transverse colon is retracted cephalad using a grasper applied to the adjacent fatty

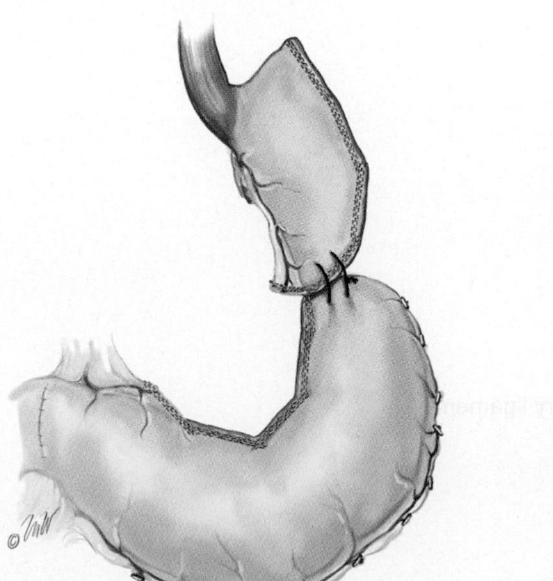

Figure 15-4. Attachment of specimen to gastric conduit.

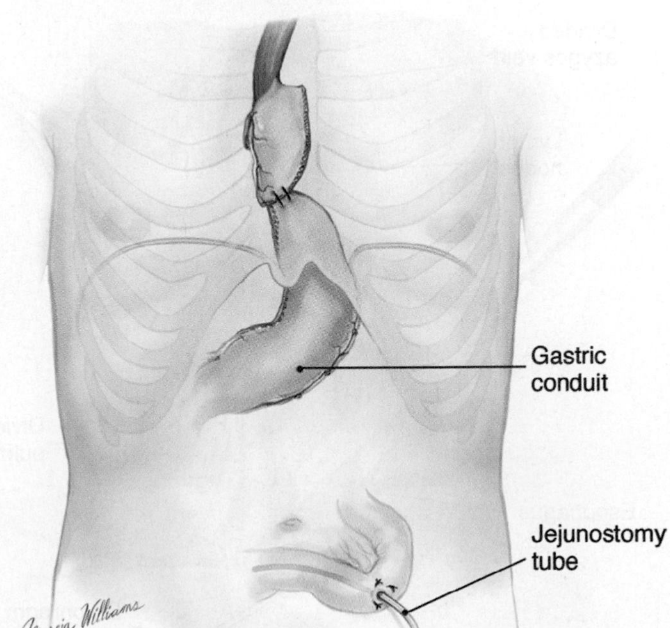

Figure 15-5. Gastric pull-up.

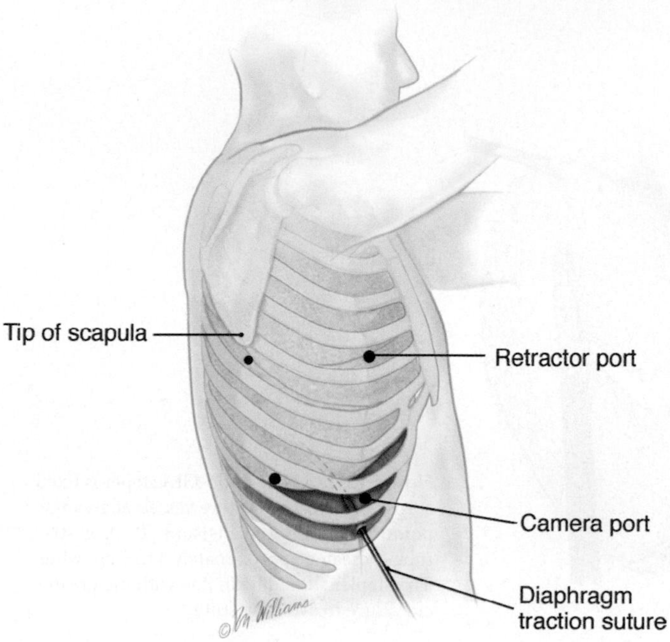

Figure 15-6. Thoracic port placement.

epiploicae, and the ligament of Treitz is identified. Approximately 40 cm from the ligament of Treitz, a loop of jejunum is attached to the anterior abdominal wall in the left lower quadrant using an Endo Stitch. A 10-Fr laparoscopic feeding jejunostomy tube is inserted into the jejunum percutaneously using the Seldinger technique. The guidewire is threaded into the small bowel, followed by the catheter, to a distance of approximately 20 cm. The jejunum is further tacked to the anterior abdominal wall using three additional endosutures as well as a single suture approximately 3 cm distal to the entrance site to prevent torsion. The feeding catheter is secured on the skin, and 10 mL of air is injected rapidly into the small bowel to test for patency and confirm intraluminal placement. If any doubts exist as to true luminal placement, an on-the-table Gastrografin study of the jejunostomy tube should be performed.

Thoracoscopy

The patient is placed in the left lateral decubitus position. The right lung is isolated. Four ports are used to access the right chest (Fig. 15-6). A 10-mm camera port is inserted in the anterior axillary line at the eighth interspace. An additional 10-mm port is placed approximately 2 cm posterior to the posterior axillary line in the eighth or ninth interspace. This is the main dissection port for the harmonic scalpel (Ethicon). A 10-mm port is placed in the fourth interspace along the anterior axillary line. A fan retractor is placed through this port to provide retraction of the lung. Finally, a 5-mm port is placed below the scapular tip. A fifth 5-mm port can be placed at the sixth rib, at the anterior axillary line, for suction by the assistant. The addition of insufflation can depress the diaphragm to give better visualization of the hiatus. Alternatively, an Endo Stitch can be placed in the central tendon of the right diaphragm and brought out percutaneously through the lower chest wall near the costal margin using the Endo-Close device (Covidien, Norwalk, CT). Downward traction on this stitch pulls the diaphragm inferiorly and allows better visualization of the lower esophagus and hiatus.

Dissection is begun by taking down the inferior pulmonary ligament (Fig. 15-7). The mediastinal pleura is dissected

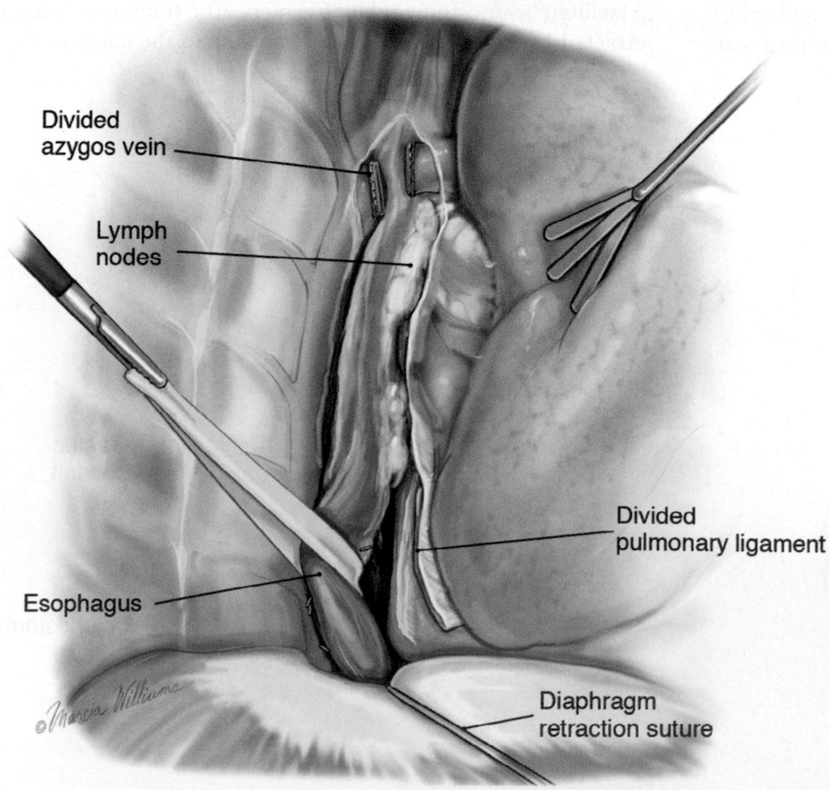

Figure 15-7. Esophageal mobilization.

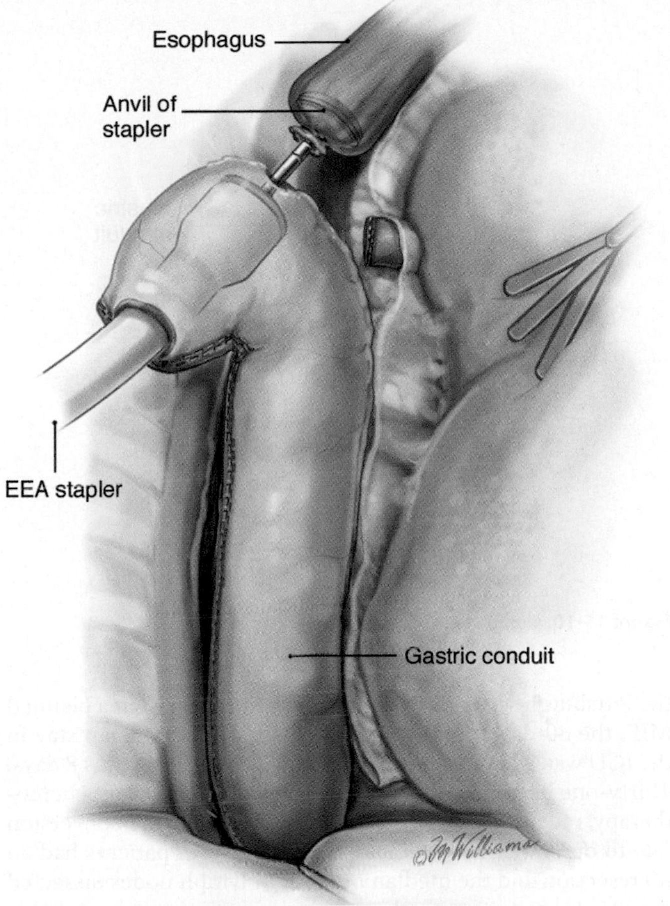

Figure 15-8. Creation of the esophagogastric anastomosis.

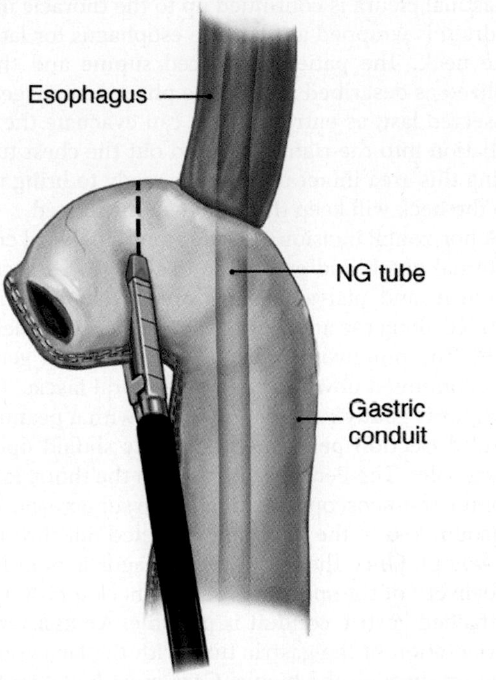

Figure 15-9. The gastrotomy is closed with an Endo-GIA stapler.

anteriorly along the plane between the edge of the lung and the esophagus and is resected with the specimen up to the azygos vein. The subcarinal lymph nodes are taken en bloc with the esophagus. Care is exercised to avoid injury to the posterior membrane of the right mainstem bronchus, carina, and trachea. Dissection is carried up to the azygos vein, and the vein is divided with an Endo-GIA stapler (Covidien, Norwalk, CT).

The mediastinal pleura is also divided inferiorly near the hiatus (Fig. 15-7) Tributaries from the thoracic duct to the esophagus are at risk for subsequent leak. Liberal use of endoclips here will minimize the chances of a postoperative chylous leak. Aortoesophageal attachments are also isolated, clipped, and divided. All surrounding soft tissue is taken with the esophagus, including the lymph node packets. Once the dissection is carried up to the divided azygos vein, the vagus nerve is divided, and the dissection is now performed close to the esophagus. By dissecting the surrounding tissue away from the esophagus, traction on the vagus nerve is minimized, and the risk of recurrent nerve injury is decreased. Care is taken to preserve the mediastinal pleura above the azygos vein. This precaution is an aid to maintaining the gastric tube in the mediastinum and seals the surrounding tissue to minimize leakage of any cervical drainage into the chest.

Periesophageal dissection can be taken all the way up to the thoracic inlet. Once the esophagus is mobilized, the specimen and the gastric conduit are brought into the field with gentle retraction of the esophagus. The suture is divided separating the specimen and gastric conduit. Once the esophagus is fully mobilized up to the upper chest cavity, the esophagus is sharply divided with endoshears, dividing the proximal esophagus and separating the specimen. The posterior inferior dissection port is increased by 2 cm and fitted with a wound protector (Alexis, Applied Medical). The specimen is removed through the wound.

The open esophagus is gently dilated with a balloon and the anvil of an end-to-end anastomosis (EEA) stapler is placed within the lumen. The edges of the esophagus are then suture closed with two rows of purse-string suture. Use of an endosuture (Covidien) or free-hand suture is generally required to form a snug fit around the anvil. The gastric conduit is brought up into the field, and the proximal end is divided to open the conduit. The handle of the EEA stapler is placed through the posterior incision and into the open end of the conduit. The spike is brought out along the greater curvature at a site that is distal to the opening and well perfused (Fig. 15-8). This spike is attached to the anvil, reapproximated, and fired to form the anastomosis. The EEA stapler is gently removed. Once an NG tube is placed, the open end of the gastric conduit can be resected flush, in line with the body of the conduit with the Endo-GIA stapler, closing the opening and leaving generally an in-line conduit in the esophageal bed (Fig. 15-9). If adequate omentum has been brought up to the chest, it can be used to buttress the anastomosis and staple lines. The chest is washed with multiple liters of saline. Chest tubes are placed, including a Blake drain near the conduit. The chest is closed, completing the reconstruction.

Three-Hole Approach and Cervical Anastomosis

For a 3-hole modified McKeown approach, the dissection is started in the right chest with the patient in the left lateral decubitus position. Full mobilization is performed using similar port placement as described for the thoracoscopic phase of the Ivor Lewis MIE. In this case, however, the dissection of the mediastinal pleura is continued up to the thoracic inlet. A Penrose drain is wrapped around the esophagus for later retrieval in the neck. The patient is placed supine and the stomach mobilized as described above. The phrenoesophageal ligament is dissected last, as entrance here can evacuate the abdominal insufflation into the right chest and out the chest tube. Hence, keeping this area intact until one is ready to bring the conduit up to the neck will keep the abdomen insufflated.

A horizontal incision is made along a cervical crease above the sternal notch and extending to the left. Dissection is carried down, and platysmal flaps are developed. Dissection is continued along the anterior border of the sternocleidomastoid muscle. The omohyoid muscle is divided, and gentle dissection is continued down to the prevertebral fascia. The cervical esophagus is gently retracted medially with a peanut dissector. Careful dissection performed inferiorly should open into the thoracic inlet. The Penrose drain left in the thoracic inlet at the end of the thoracoscopic portion of the surgery should be readily encountered in the neck and retracted out through the cervical wound. Once the cervical esophagus is bluntly dissected free, delivery of the specimen out the neck incision along with the attached gastric conduit is possible. An assistant observes the orientation of the gastric tube with the laparoscope as it is guided up through the hiatus. Care must be taken to preserve proper orientation and prevent spiraling or tension at the hiatus. Once the gastric tube is delivered into the neck, the two endosutures are divided. The proximal gastric tube is assessed for viability. The proximal cervical esophagus is mobilized. An auto–purse-string device (Covidien, Norwalk, CT) is applied 2 to 3 cm distal to the cricopharyngeus, and the esophagus is divided. A 25-mm EEA stapler is used to perform the anastomosis. The anvil is placed in the cervical esophagus, and the purse string is tied. The proximal gastric tube tip is opened, and the EEA stapler is inserted and directed posteriorly between the staple line and the line of the short gastric arteries. Usually, the gastric tube is sufficiently long to permit the anvil to exit the gastric tube 6 to 8 cm distally. Once the anastomosis is complete, a nasogastric tube is guided under direct vision. The gastrotomy opening is closed by stapling off the distal 5 to 6 cm of the proximal gastric tube with an Endo-GIA stapler.

Attention is directed back into the abdomen. Graspers are applied to the antral area, and gentle downward traction is applied until the cervical anastomosis dips into the neck incision. This maneuver ensures the absence of redundant gastric tube above the hiatus that may have been pulled up during creation of the neck anastomosis. The gastric tube is tacked to the hiatus to prevent future herniation (Fig. 15-10). Care must be taken to avoid injury to the vascular supply. We generally apply three sutures, one from the greater-curve side to the left crus, one from the lesser-curve side to the right crus, and one on the anterior gastric tube to the central edge of the diaphragmatic hiatus. The cervical anastomosis is irrigated, and the skin is only loosely approximated with one or two staples. In our experience, multilayer suture closure of the cervical incision may lead to downward tracking of an anastomotic leak, should one occur.

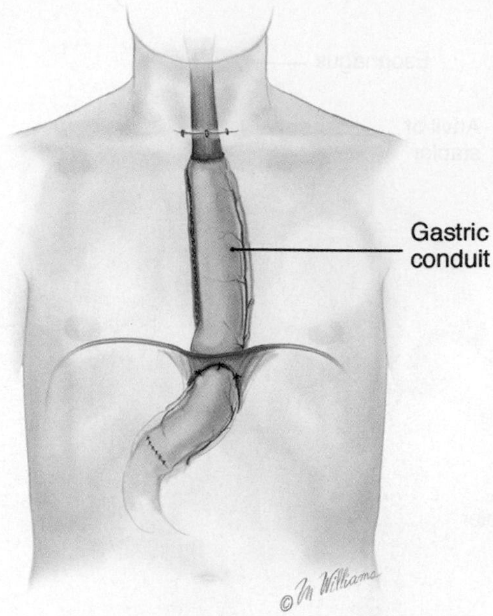

Figure 15-10. Completed reconstruction.

RESULTS

The largest reported experience with MIE to date highlights some of the potential advantages and pitfalls of this approach. In the Pittsburgh series of 1011 patients who underwent a planned MIE, the 30-day operative mortality was 1.7%. Median stay in the ICU was 2 days, and total hospital length of stay was 8 days. Thirty-one percent of all patients received neoadjuvant chemotherapy, radiation therapy, or both before MIE. The conversion rate to open was 4.5%. Ninety-eight percent of patients had an R0 resection and the median number of lymph nodes dissected was 21. Stage-for-stage, the survival curves were comparable with those of open esophagectomy.[22]

Nguyen et al.,[23] in a smaller series of 46 patients undergoing MIE, reported a mean operative time of 350 minutes, blood loss of 270 mL, and an overall mortality of 4.3%. The minimally invasive approach yielded comparable, if not better, outcomes than open approaches, as reported in the literature, in terms of length of stay (16.6 days), operating room time (336 minutes), and mortality (5.5%).[24] In another analysis of MIE in patients over the age of 75 years, there were no operative deaths in 41 patients, and overall survival in 36 patients with esophageal cancer was 81% at 20 months.[25] These findings suggest that MIE can be performed in high-risk patients who otherwise might not be considered for surgery. A meta-analysis of open versus minimally invasive studies demonstrated equivalent survival between open esophagectomy and MIE.[26]

COMPLICATIONS

Morbidity associated with open esophagectomy can be significant, ranging from 35% to 50% in reported studies. An analysis of minimally invasive series reveals that the absolute rate of complications is similar, but the degree of the insult to the patient appears to be less in terms of impact on mortality and length of hospital stay. Comparing some of the largest series of MIEs, transhiatal esophagectomies, and transthoracic esophagectomies with a 10-year review of all esophagectomies performed at the Veterans' Affairs hospital system illustrates a favorable outcome in mortality, length of stay, and several major complication criteria (Table 15-1).

Table 15-1

COMPLICATIONS

	LUKETICH et al.[13,22] (*n* = 1011) MIE	ORRINGER et al.[28,37] (*n* = 2007) THE	SWANSON et al.[38] (*n* = 250) TTE	BAILEY et al.[4] (*n* = 1777) MIXED
Anastomotic leak	4.8%[a]	12%	8%	N/A
Vocal cord paresis/paralysis	4.2%	4.5%	14%	N/A
Cervical anastomosis	7.7%			
Thoracic anastomosis	0.9%			
Chylothorax	3.2%[b]	1.2%	9%	N/A
Tracheal tear	0.9%[b]	0.4%	1%	N/A
Gastric tube necrosis	2.4%	0.7%	0.8%	N/A
Myocardial infarction	2.0%	N/A	N/A	1.2%
Pneumonia	7.7%[b]	2%	5%	21.4%
Pulmonary embolism	1.4%[b]	N/A	1%	0.7%
Mortality	1.7%	3%	3.6%	9.8%
Length of stay	8 d	8 d[c]	13 d	N/A

MIE, minimally invasive esophagectomy; THE, transhiatal esphagectomy; TTE, transthoracic esophagectomy; N/A, result not available.

[a]Anastomotic leak requiring surgery.

[b]In 222 patients who underwent modified McKeown MIE.

[c]In 718 patients since July 1998.

Operative Complications

Thorax

Bleeding and transfusion requirements are less with the minimally invasive approach,[27] but it is important to note that even small amounts of bleeding can obscure the operative field and may require conversion to an open procedure. Hence, the aortoesophageal branches must be identified and clipped. Bleeding from the azygos vein and peribronchial arteries also must be avoided. Injury to the posterior membranes of the bronchus and trachea must be carefully avoided, especially during lymph node dissection. Cautery and harmonic scalpel use in close proximity to the posterior membranous trachea or mainstem bronchus can lead to tissue damage resulting in an air leak, local ischemia, herniation of the gastric conduit, and subsequent development of a tracheogastric conduit fistula.

The thoracic duct is at risk for subtle injuries leading to the development of chylothorax. Early in our initial series of 77 patients undergoing MIE, we noted 3 patients with delayed chylothorax. This complication led us to be more cautious in this area and to use metal clips on all branches from the thoracic duct. Vocal cord paralysis resulting from injury to the recurrent laryngeal nerve is minimized by dividing the vagus nerve just above the azygos vein and dissecting it away from the esophagus. We generally do not dissect lymph nodes above this level because of the risk of injury to the recurrent laryngeal nerves and the lack of definitive evidence that lymph node clearance is essential in this location for esophagogastric junction tumors.

Abdomen

Disruption of the epiploic arcade can be devastating to the viability of the gastric tube. Likewise, one must make sure that there is adequate room at the hiatus for the conduit to lie without strangulation. In our series, the incidence of gastric tip necrosis was 2.4%.[22] Although this is slightly higher than the rate reported by Orringer or Swanson, it was mostly associated with use of a narrow 3-cm gastric tube, which has since been abandoned for a more generous 4- to 5-cm tube.[12] Furthermore, the overall mortality in over 1000 patients was 1.7%, which is significantly lower than many open series.[22]

Delayed hiatal herniation of abdominal viscera also can occur if the gastric conduit is not properly tacked to the hiatus. We have observed four delayed hiatal hernias in our 222 patient series.[13] All were repaired successfully. Orringer's series identified a 2% rate of splenectomy in 2007 open transhiatal esophagectomies.[28] In our series of 1011 MIEs, splenectomy was only required in 0.2%.[22]

Orringer's open series also reported a 3% incidence of wound infection and dehiscence.[28] The national Veterans' Affairs study revealed a 10.9% rate of wound infection with a 3.7% rate of wound dehiscence after open esophagectomy.[4] When open transhiatal and transthoracic procedures were evaluated prospectively, the transhiatal approach was associated with a 5% incidence of wound dehiscence, and the transthoracic approach was associated with only 2% wound dehiscence.[29] Delayed incisional hernias are seldom reported but are estimated to occur in 5% to 10% of long-term survivors. In our minimally invasive series of 222 patients who underwent MIE using a modified McKeown approach, only a 0.9% incidence of minor wound infection was seen with one early port hernia, and no wound dehiscences were observed.[13]

Postoperative Complications

The postoperative complications observed after MIE generally are comparable with those of an open procedure. In our series of 222 patients who underwent MIE using the modified McKeown approach, our overall cervical anastomotic leak rate was 11%. Of note, the anastomotic leak rate increased to 26% in a subset of 56 patients in whom a very narrow diameter (3-cm) gastric tube was constructed. However, in the other 166 patients, we constructed a 5-cm gastric conduit and observed a leak rate of only 6%.[30] In our recent series of 1011 patients who underwent a planned MIE, the rate of anastomotic leaks requiring surgery dropped to 5%.[22] The reported leak rate for open procedures is approximately 9.1%.[23]

The most common cardiopulmonary complications encountered in our series[13] included atrial fibrillation (11.7%), pleural effusion (6.3%), and pneumonia (7.7%). Delayed gastric emptying was seen in only 1.8% of patients, and only 4% of patients complained of recalcitrant long-term postoperative reflux symptoms.[13] Moderate strictures at the gastroesophageal cervical anastomosis are common and generally can be managed with one or two outpatient dilations.

Alternative Approaches

MIE encompasses an array of thoracoscopic and laparoscopic techniques that all seek to reduce the morbidity of an open procedure. We favor the thoracoscopic/laparoscopic approach with an intrathoracic anastomosis. Several other groups have reported variations in technique that may provide insight in this emerging field. Bonavina and colleagues described the use of a laparoscopic transhiatal approach with a video mediastinoscope from the cervical incision to assist their mediastinal dissection. They reported 10 of 12 successful operations with a mean operative time of 270 minutes.[31] Mean hospital stay was 10 days with no ICU stays. Jobe et al.[32] used a nasogastric tube to invert the esophagus to assist the laparoscopic transhiatal dissection. Costi et al.[33] describe an alternative approach with an intrathoracic anastomosis. Jarral et al.[34] reviewed the prone approach for esophagectomy. Several groups[35,36] described the use of robotics to assist in transhiatal esophagectomy. Horgan's group published a single case report on one patient who underwent a robotic dissection of the esophagus with a laparoscopic gastric mobilization and an open cervical anastomosis.

CONCLUSION

MIE is a technically challenging operation. Recent reports clearly demonstrate comparable, if not improved, mortality and morbidity following MIE in centers with significant experience in open and minimally invasive techniques. Currently, an intergroup trial (ECOG 2202) is under way to assess the outcomes of MIE in a multicenter trial setting. The preliminary results of this study suggest that MIE is safe and feasible with low perioperative morbidity and mortality and good oncologic results.

EDITOR'S COMMENT

The authors, leaders in the field of MIE, have described the metamorphosis of their MIE technique over the last decade and a half. Although initially, a routine 3-hole total esophagectomy was used, they currently recommend a thoracoscopic/laparoscopic "Ivor Lewis" type approach. With the use of automated stitching devices and the future expansion of robotic suture techniques, this operation should continue to receive broader acceptance, especially by the next generation of thoracic surgeons already facile in minimally invasive techniques. One final key message is that the operation should not "skimp" on any standard steps especially when done for cancer. If dissection of the mediastinal pleura or routine dissection of the upper paratracheal lymph nodes is usually done, the surgeon should strive to achieve the same approach laparoscopically. Likewise, if the accepted routine neoadjuvant therapy for locally advanced esophageal cancer is chemoradiation, then that should be applied even to patients who are to undergo an MIE in the future. Rather than deny a patient routine neoadjuvant chemoradiation, we should develop the technique further to assure that this operation can be applied safely to these patients.

—Mark J. Krasna

References

1. Torek F. The operative treatment of carcinoma of the esophagus. *Ann Surg.* 1915;61:385–405.
2. Orringer MB, Sloan H. Esophagectomy without thoracotomy. *J Thorac Cardiovasc Surg.* 1978;76:643–654.
3. McKeown KC. Total three-stage oesophagectomy for cancer of the oesophagus. *Br J Surg.* 1976;63:259–262.
4. Bailey SH, Bull DA, Harpole DH, et al. Outcomes after esophagectomy: a ten-year prospective cohort. *Ann Thorac Surg.* 2003;75:217–222; discussion 22.
5. Birkmeyer JD, Stukel TA, Siewers AE, et al. Surgeon volume and operative mortality in the United States. *N Engl J Med.* 2003;349:2117–2127.
6. Collard JM, Lengele B, Otte JB, et al. En bloc and standard esophagectomies by thoracoscopy. *Ann Thorac Surg.* 1993;56:675–679.
7. DePaula AL, Hashiba K, Ferreira EA, et al. Laparoscopic transhiatal esophagectomy with esophagogastroplasty. *Surg Laparosc Endosc.* 1995;5(1):1–5.
8. Swanstrom LL. Minimally invasive surgical approaches to esophageal cancer. *J Gastrointest Surg.* 2002;6:522–526.
9. Law S, Wong J. Use of minimally invasive oesophagectomy for cancer of the oesophagus. *Lancet Oncol.* 2002;3:215–222.
10. Luketich JD, Nguyen NT, Schauer PR. Laparoscopic transhiatal esophagectomy for Barrett's esophagus with high grade dysplasia. *JSLS.* 1998;2:75–77.
11. Fernando HC, Christie NA, Luketich JD. Thoracoscopic and laparoscopic esophagectomy. *Semin Thorac Cardiovasc Surg.* 2000;12:195–200.
12. Litle VR, Buenaventura PO, Luketich JD. Minimally invasive resection for esophageal cancer. *Surg Clin North Am.* 2002;82:711–728.
13. Luketich JD, Alvelo-Rivera M, Buenaventura PO, et al. Minimally invasive esophagectomy: outcomes in 222 patients. *Ann Surg.* 2003;238:486–494; discussion 494–495.
14. Nguyen NT, Schauer PR, Luketich JD. Combined laparoscopic and thoracoscopic approach to esophagectomy. *J Am Coll Surg.* 1999;188:328–332.
15. Nguyen NT, Follette DM, Wolfe BM, et al. Comparison of minimally invasive esophagectomy with transthoracic and transhiatal esophagectomy. *Arch Surg.* 2000;135:920–925.
16. Pierre AF, Luketich JD. Technique and role of minimally invasive esophagectomy for premalignant and malignant diseases of the esophagus. *Surg Oncol Clin N Am.* 2002;11:337–350.
17. Nguyen NT, Schauer P, Luketich JD. Minimally invasive esophagectomy for Barrett's esophagus with high-grade dysplasia. *Surgery.* 2000;127:284–290.
18. Luketich JD, Nguyen NT, Weigel T, et al. Minimally invasive approach to esophagectomy. *JSLS.* 1998;2:243–247.
19. Luketich JD, Schauer PR, Christie NA, et al. Minimally invasive esophagectomy. *Ann Thorac Surg.* 2000;70:906–911; discussion 11–12.

20. Fernando HC, Luketich JD, Buenaventura PO, et al. Outcomes of minimally invasive esophagectomy (MIE) for high-grade dysplasia of the esophagus. *Eur J Cardiothorac Surg*. 2002;22:1–6.
21. Wee JO, Morse CR. The 2011 Minimally invasive thoracic surgery summit. Section VI - Malignant Esophagus: Minimally invasive Ivor Lewis esophagectomy. *J Thorac Cardiovasc Surg*. 2012;144(3):S60–S62.
22. Luketich JD, Pennathur A, Awais O, et al. Outcomes after minimally invasive esophagectomy: review of over 1000 patients. *Ann Surg*. 2012;256(1): 95–103.
23. Nguyen NT, Roberts P, Follette DM, et al. Thoracoscopic and laparoscopic esophagectomy for benign and malignant disease: lessons learned from 46 consecutive procedures. *J Am Coll Surg*. 2003;197:902–913.
24. Traverso LW, Shinchi H, Low DE. Useful benchmarks to evaluate outcomes after esophagectomy and pancreaticoduodenectomy. *Am J Surg*. 2004;187: 604–608.
25. Perry Y, Fernando HC, Buenaventura PO, et al. Minimally invasive esophagectomy in the elderly. JSLS. 2002;6:299–304.
26. Dantoc MM, Cox MR, Eslick GD. Does minimally invasive esophagectomy (MIE) provide for comparable oncologic outcomes to open techniques? A systematic review. *J Gastrointest Surg*. 2012;16(3):486–494.
27. Makay O, van den Broek WT, Yuan JZ, et al. Anesthesiological hazards during laparoscopic transhiatal esophageal resection: a case control study of the laparoscopic-assisted vs the conventional approach. *Surg Endosc*. 2004;18:1263–1267.
28. Orringer MB, Marshall B, Chang AC, et al. Two thousand transhiatal esophagectomies: changing trends, lessons learned. *Ann Surg*. 2007;246(3):363–374.
29. Rentz J, Bull D, Harpole D, et al. Transthoracic versus transhiatal esophagectomy: a prospective study of 945 patients. *J Thorac Cardiovasc Surg*. 2003;125:1114–1120.
30. Schuchert MJ, Luketich JD, Fernando HC. Complications of minimally invasive esophagectomy. *Semin Thorac Cardiovasc Surg*. 2004;16:133–141.
31. Bonavina L, Incarbone R, Bona D, et al. Esophagectomy via laparoscopy and transmediastinal endodissection. *J Laparoendosc Adv Surg Tech A*. 2004; 14:13–16.
32. Jobe BA, Reavis KM, Davis JJ, et al. Laparoscopic inversion esophagectomy: simplifying a daunting operation. *Dis Esophagus*. 2004;17:95–97.
33. Costi R, Himpens J, Bruyns J, et al. Totally laparoscopic transhiatal esophagogastrectomy without thoracic or cervical access: the least invasive surgery for adenocarcinoma of the cardia? *Surg Endosc*. 2004;18:629–632.
34. Jarral OA, Purkayastha S, Athanasiou T, et al. Thoracoscopic esophagectomy in the prone position. *Surg Endosc*. 2012;26(8):2095–2103.
35. Horgan S, Berger RA, Elli EF, et al. Robotic-assisted minimally invasive transhiatal esophagectomy. *Am Surg*. 2003;69:624–626.
36. Dunn DH, Johnson EM, Morphew JA, et al. Robot-assisted transhiatal esophagectomy: a 3-year single-center experience. *Dis Esophagus*. 2012;26:159–266.
37. Orringer MB, Marshall B, Iannettoni MD. Transhiatal esophagectomy for treatment of benign and malignant esophageal disease. *World J Surg*. 2001; 25:196–203.
38. Swanson SJ, Batirel HF, Bueno R, et al. Transthoracic esophagectomy with radical mediastinal and abdominal lymph node dissection and cervical esophagogastrostomy for esophageal carcinoma. *Ann Thorac Surg*. 2001;72:1918–1924; discussion 24–25.

16 Transhiatal Esophagectomy

Ziv Gamliel and Mark J. Krasna

Keywords: Transhiatal esophagectomy, esophageal cancer, upper midline laparotomy, left cervical incision

Transhiatal esophagectomy was popularized by Orringer in the late 1970s as a less invasive approach to esophagectomy.[1,2] This approach avoids thoracotomy and has been endorsed primarily by nonthoracic general surgeons who perform esophagectomy. For trained thoracic surgeons, the main drawbacks of this approach are the inability to perform an extensive lymph node dissection and the risk of injury to the great vessels and main airways with tumors of grade T3 or greater.[3,4] We describe herein our current technique for transhiatal esophagectomy, which includes minor modifications to the original Orringer technique.

Comparisons of transhiatal versus transthoracic esophagectomy published in the last decade have included retrospective studies,[5,6] prospective studies,[7] randomized controlled studies,[8] and meta-analyses.[9] The published evidence suggests that transhiatal esophagectomy is associated with a reduced risk of pulmonary complications and in-hospital mortality as well as a shortened length of hospital stay, but an increased risk of anastomotic leakage and postoperative vocal cord paralysis. Although there is no clear difference in overall long-term survival, there is an apparent trend toward improved 5-year survival with transthoracic esophagectomy in patients with a limited number of involved lymph nodes.[10] Published data comparing transhiatal esophagectomy with totally minimally invasive esophagectomy is rather limited.[11,12]

TECHNICAL PRINCIPLES

Transhiatal esophagectomy is performed via an upper midline laparotomy incision and a left neck incision. Unlike the left transthoracic approach, the transhiatal approach offers excellent exposure of the abdominal cavity.[13–15] A generous Kocher maneuver can be performed, allowing the pylorus to extend almost to the hiatus. This helps to provide the length needed to pull the stomach into the neck. A pyloromyotomy or pyloroplasty can be performed easily, helping to decrease symptomatic gastric stasis postoperatively. There is ample exposure to allow a feeding jejunostomy to be created, aiding in postoperative nutrition.

The lack of a thoracotomy incision in transhiatal esophagectomy has potential advantages. The incisional pain associated with thoracotomy is avoided. The need for one-lung anesthesia is obviated. A chest tube is usually not required. These factors may be of particular importance in patients with severe chronic obstructive pulmonary disease, poor pulmonary function, or both. On the other hand, the lack of exposure of the mediastinum limits the surgeon's ability to fully assess that portion of the surgical field and to perform radical resection.[4] Moreover, the surgeon's hand dissects bluntly behind the heart for a significant length of time during the procedure, making this approach more risky intraoperatively in patients with compromised cardiac function.[16]

The left neck incision used in transhiatal esophagectomy affords excellent exposure of the cervical esophagus. The esophageal resection can be extended fairly high in the neck, encompassing even high esophageal lesions adequately. The length of gastric conduit required to reach the neck results in higher leak and stricture rates compared with intrathoracic anastomoses. In the event of a cervical esophagogastric anastomotic leak, however, satisfactory drainage is easily obtained by reopening the neck wound, making the clinical consequences less severe than those of an intrathoracic anastomotic leak. Although methods have been described for performing a stapled cervical esophagogastric anastomosis, the lack of an ideally suited stapling device makes these techniques somewhat awkward. The anastomosis is usually hand sewn and may take no more time to complete than a stapled anastomosis.

The left recurrent laryngeal nerve is at risk in transhiatal esophagectomy, and left vocal cord palsy is a well-recognized complication. In addition to increasing the risk of aspiration owing to incoordination of swallowing, vocal cord palsy may reduce the effectiveness of coughing and compromise tracheobronchial toilet. Peristalsis in the proximal esophageal remnant may help to decrease clinically significant gastroesophageal reflux postoperatively. The relatively short length of remaining cervical esophagus after transhiatal esophagectomy may represent less of a barrier to inevitable postoperative gastroesophageal reflux than the longer esophageal remnant found with intrathoracic anastomoses.

ONCOLOGIC PRINCIPLES

The upper midline abdominal incision used in transhiatal esophagectomy affords excellent exposure of the entire abdomen. Unlike the left transthoracic approach, this exposure permits the surgeon to search thoroughly for abdominal metastatic disease before undertaking any resection. Metastases typically may be found in the omentum, mesentery, or liver and may be biopsied readily. In the absence of distant metastatic disease, the exposure afforded by the upper midline incision used in transhiatal esophagectomy allows for complete resection of the left gastric and celiac axis lymph nodes en bloc with the esophagogastrectomy specimen.

The lack of a thoracotomy incision results in virtually no exposure of thoracic or mediastinal structures. To a large extent, dissection of the esophagus is performed blindly and bluntly. Segmental arteries are avulsed close to the esophageal wall, and an adequate radial resection margin is not easily achievable.[17] There is no reliable way to remove lymph node—bearing periesophageal fat en bloc with the specimen.[18] Furthermore, with the transhiatal approach, there is no effective way to examine the lung for metastases. These factors underscore the need to ascertain early-stage disease preoperatively before committing to the transhiatal approach.

IDEAL PATIENT CHARACTERISTICS AND PREOPERATIVE ASSESSMENT

The patient's ability to withstand the procedure and its possible complications should be carefully evaluated preoperatively. Pulmonary and cardiac function should be assessed. Significant carotid artery stenosis and coronary artery disease should be ruled out. As a result of the high incidence of deep vein thrombosis in patients with esophageal cancer, preoperative lower-extremity venous duplex scanning should be considered.

Transhiatal esophagectomy affords little or no exposure of the upper and middle thirds of the thoracic esophagus for the surgeon. To avoid intraoperative airway injury or vascular injury, any possibility of adherence or direct invasion of the tumor into adjacent structures such as the trachea, aorta, or azygos vein should be excluded before undertaking this approach. For tumors arising above the distal third of the thoracic esophagus in particular, a high-quality CT scan with intravenous and oral contrast material is important. More detailed evaluation for tumor invasion into surrounding structures can be achieved with endoscopic ultrasound (EUS). Currently available clinical (preoperative) staging methods may often fail to identify nodal metastases.[19] Unlike approaches that involve a thoracotomy incision, the technique of transhiatal esophagectomy does not permit en bloc mediastinal lymphadenectomy. The transhiatal approach does not afford exposure of any but the most inferiorly located mediastinal nodes.[20] Every effort should be made to exclude metastatic tumor involving lymph nodes above the esophageal hiatus, which would result in an unrecognized incomplete resection. The use of CT and PET scans may be helpful.

TECHNIQUE

Patient Preparation

An epidural catheter may be placed before induction of anesthesia to facilitate postoperative pain management. Pneumatic intermittent calf compression boots are applied. With the patient in the supine position under general single-lumen tube endotracheal anesthesia, a Foley catheter and a radial arterial line are placed. Central venous access may be obtained via the right side of the neck.

To confirm the location of the tumor and/or extent of Barrett epithelium, as well as to rule out gastric/duodenal pathology, upper endoscopy may be performed using minimal air insufflation. After removing the endoscope, an 18F Salem sump nasogastric tube is placed, and the stomach is decompressed. A transverse roll is placed beneath the shoulders, and the head is placed on a gel donut and turned to the right. The entire abdomen and left neck are prepared and draped in continuity (Fig. 16-1). An intravenous antibiotic is administered before making the skin incision, and additional doses are given periodically as appropriate throughout the procedure for wound prophylaxis.

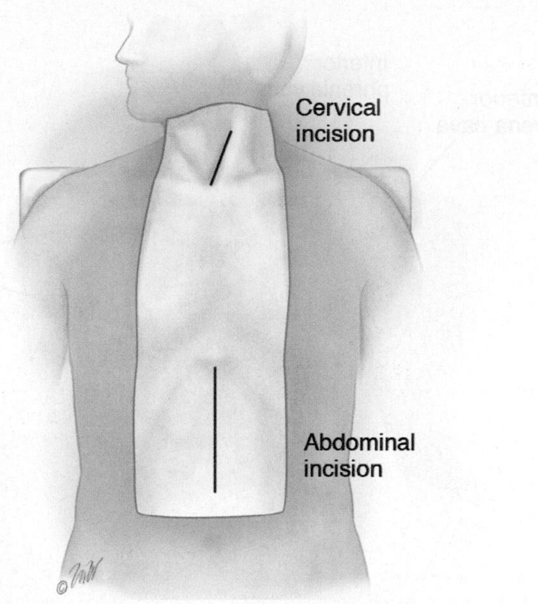

Figure 16-1. Patient setup for transhiatal esophagectomy.

Preparation of the Stomach

An upper midline laparotomy incision is made. The peritoneal cavity and abdominal viscera are examined for evidence of metastatic disease or other pathology. The xiphoid process is excised with electrocautery. A Buchwalter retractor is placed. A bladder blade is used to retract the lower sternum cephalad, and Richardson blades are used to retract the rectus muscles laterally (Fig. 16-2). The left triangular hepatic ligament is divided

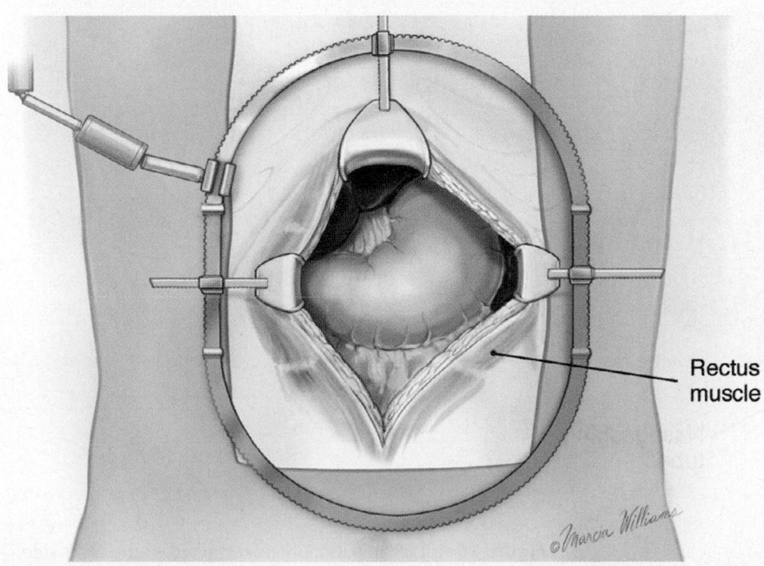

Figure 16-2. Buchwalter retractor in place.

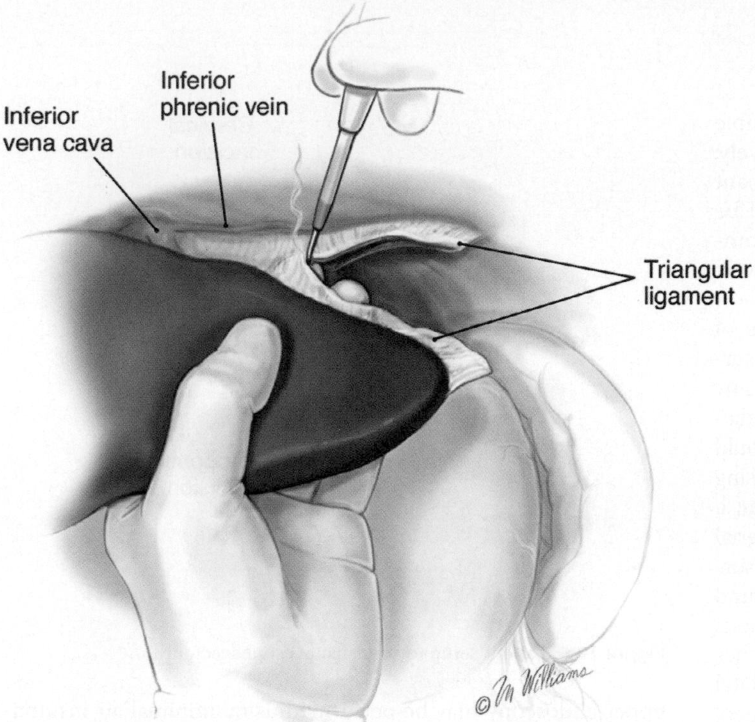

Figure 16-3. Division of left triangular hepatic ligament.

with electrocautery (Fig. 16-3). The mobilized left hepatic lobe is retracted rightward with a wide Deaver blade covered with a laparotomy sponge (Fig. 16-4).

The nasogastric tube is positioned along the greater curvature of the stomach with its tip near the pylorus and is used as a handhold on the stomach. The abdominal esophagus is dissected from its crural attachments with electrocautery, encircled, and elevated on a Penrose drain. Alternatively, for lesions that are possibly directly invading the area of the esophagogastric junction (EGJ), a cuff of diaphragm can be resected with cautery under direct vision. The greater curvature of the stomach is mobilized using a harmonic scalpel, taking great care to avoid injury to the gastroepiploic arcade (Fig. 16-5).

The gastric fundus is mobilized using a harmonic scalpel to divide the short gastric vessels. Divided branches may be reinforced with ligatures or clips. The posterior gastric vessel, a penultimate branch usually well visualized off the splenic artery, is carefully divided and ligated. The left gastric vessels

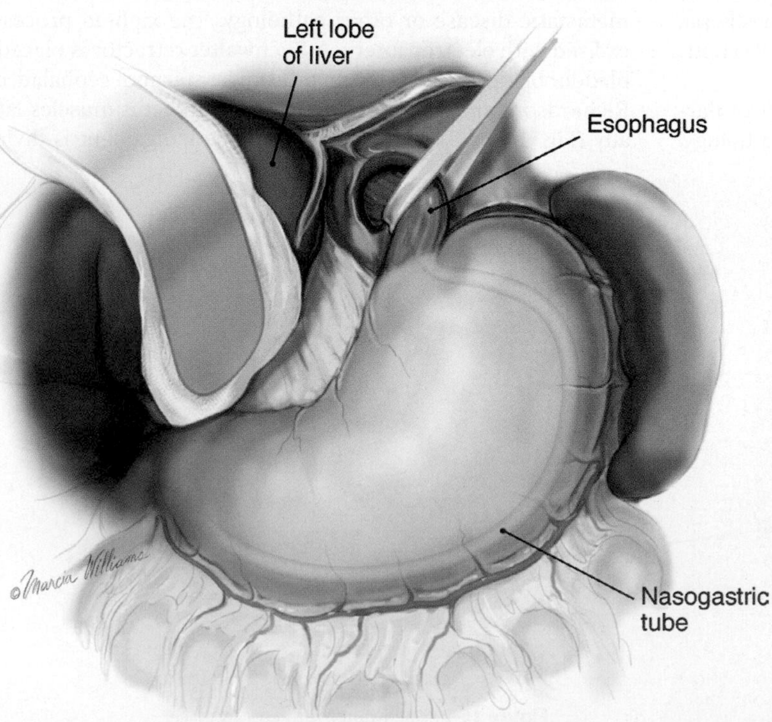

Figure 16-4. Left hepatic lobe is retracted to the right side.

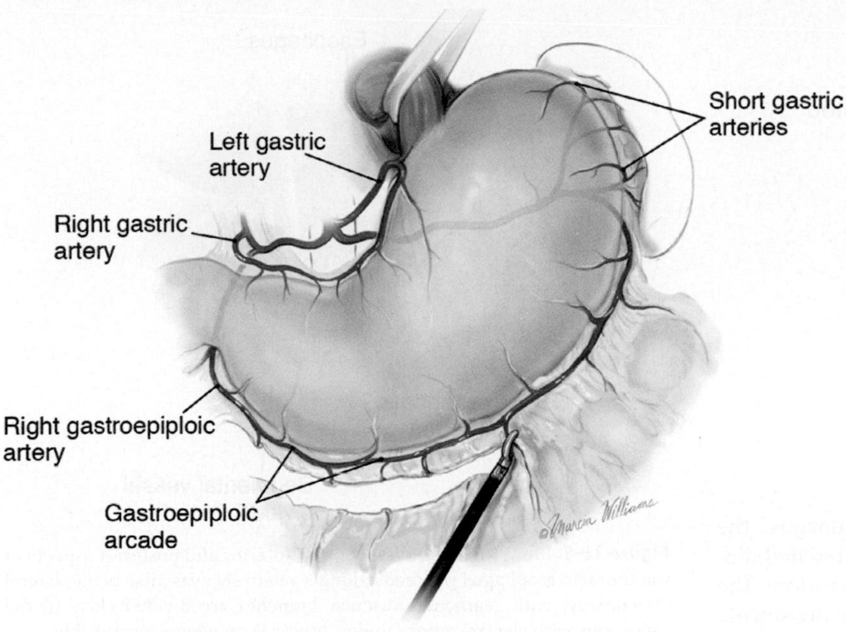

Figure 16-5. Division of gastrocolic ligament with a harmonic scalpel.

are dissected, reflecting the left gastric lymph nodes toward the stomach. The left gastric vessels are divided using a roticulating vascular stapler (Fig. 16-6).

A generous Kocher maneuver is performed. The serosa overlying the anterior wall of the pylorus is incised with electrocautery, avoiding the great pyloric vein of Mayo. A complete pyloromyotomy is performed using straight Mayo scissors or a #15 blade. Alternatively, a formal Heineke-Mikulicz pyloroplasty may be performed (see Chapter 17).

Mobilization of the Abdominal, Thoracic, and Cervical Esophagus

Attention is turned to the diaphragmatic hiatus, where the peritoneal reflection and phrenoesophageal ligament are taken with electrocautery dissection, completely mobilizing the esophagus in the hiatus. Transhiatal exposure is achieved by manual retraction using the hooked handles of two narrow Deaver retractors (Fig. 16-7).

Mobilization of the intrathoracic esophagus proceeds cephalad while maintaining downward traction on the stomach. Blunt manual dissection is performed along the anterior and posterior aspects of the thoracic esophagus in a relatively avascular plane. Lateral attachments containing segmental vascular branches are divided close to the esophagus using electrocautery under direct vision whenever possible (Fig. 16-8). Divided lymphatics are meticulously ligated with surgical clips. Care is taken to avoid injury to the inferior pulmonary veins.

As mobilization of the esophagus proceeds cephalad, direct visualization becomes impossible. Blunt "blind" manual dissection is undertaken anteriorly and posteriorly using the palpable nasogastric tube within the esophageal lumen as a guide. Care is taken to avoid injury to the membranous wall of the trachea anteriorly and to the aorta and azygos vein posteriorly (Fig. 16-9). Lateral attachments containing segmental vessels are hooked on the surgeon's finger and gently avulsed close to the esophagus using a downward motion using hemaclips and cautery when possible.

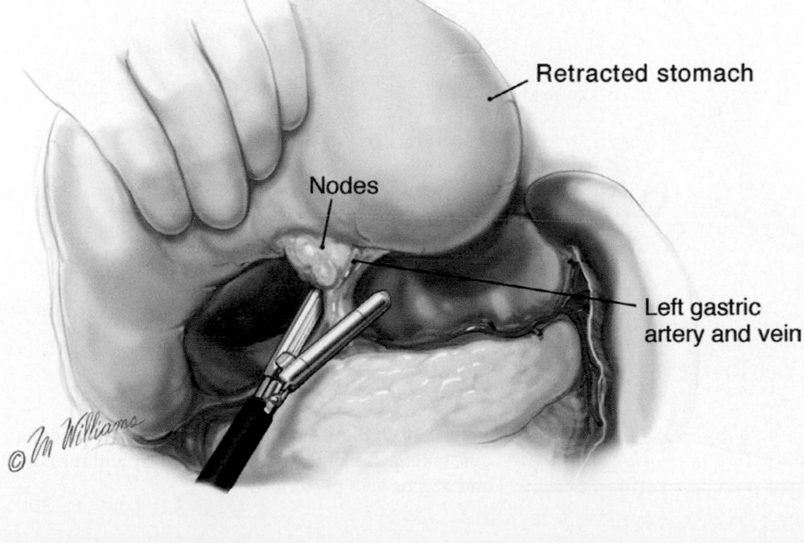

Figure 16-6. Stapling across the left gastric artery and vein.

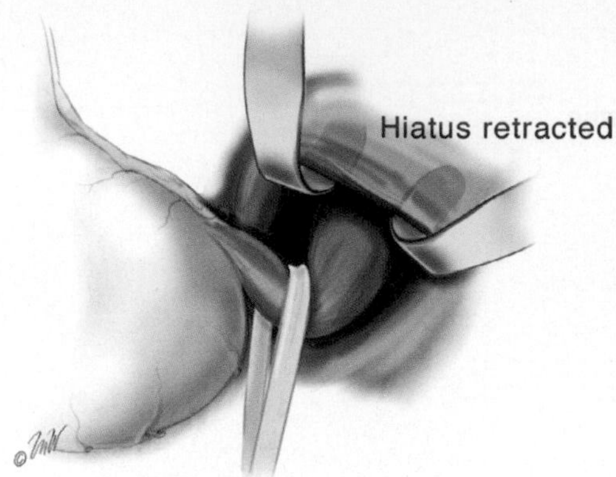

Figure 16-7. Exposure of the hiatus.

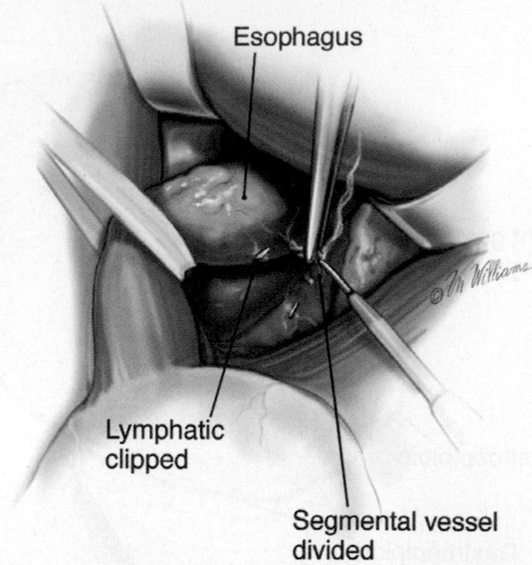

Figure 16-8. Blunt (manual) dissection of anterior and posterior aspects of the thoracic esophagus proceeds along a relatively avascular plane; lateral attachments with segmental vascular branches are divided close to the esophagus with electrocautery under direct vision whenever possible.

While mobilizing the superior thoracic esophagus, the surgeon's entire hand will be passed through the stretched diaphragmatic hiatus, working into a retrocardiac position. The surgeon must closely monitor the arterial line tracing during this portion of the procedure. If hypotension develops, it may be necessary for the surgeon to remove his or her hand from the chest intermittently to permit the blood pressure to recover. Major vascular injury must be recognized promptly; although repair may be possible through the dilated hiatus, emergency anterolateral thoracotomy is sometimes required.[21] The thoracic esophagus is mobilized in this fashion to the level of the thoracic inlet.

After the entire thoracic esophagus has been completely mobilized, attention is turned to the left neck, where an incision is made along the anterior border of the sternocleidomastoid muscle and deepened through the platysma. This step can often be facilitated by a second surgeon starting on the neck just as the surgeon is starting the periesophageal dissection from below; this can shorten the overall time and make good use of the two surgeons working from opposite ends through the completion of the anastomosis. The omohyoid muscle is divided with electrocautery. The contents of the carotid sheath are reflected posteriorly with the sternocleidomastoid muscle. The middle thyroid vein is divided between surgical ties. Dissection is continued through an areolar plane to the vertebral bodies, reflecting the thyroid, trachea, and esophagus anteromedially. Blunt digital dissection is carried out along the vertebral bodies in a caudal direction until the thoracic inlet is entered. The surgeon's fingers from above and below should be able to touch without difficulty while again observing the blood pressure monitor. The esophagus is encircled in the thoracic inlet using blunt digital dissection. A Penrose drain is passed around the distal cervical esophagus and is used to elevate it into the incision (Fig. 16-10).

The esophagus is separated from the membranous wall of the cervical trachea with careful blunt dissection aided by

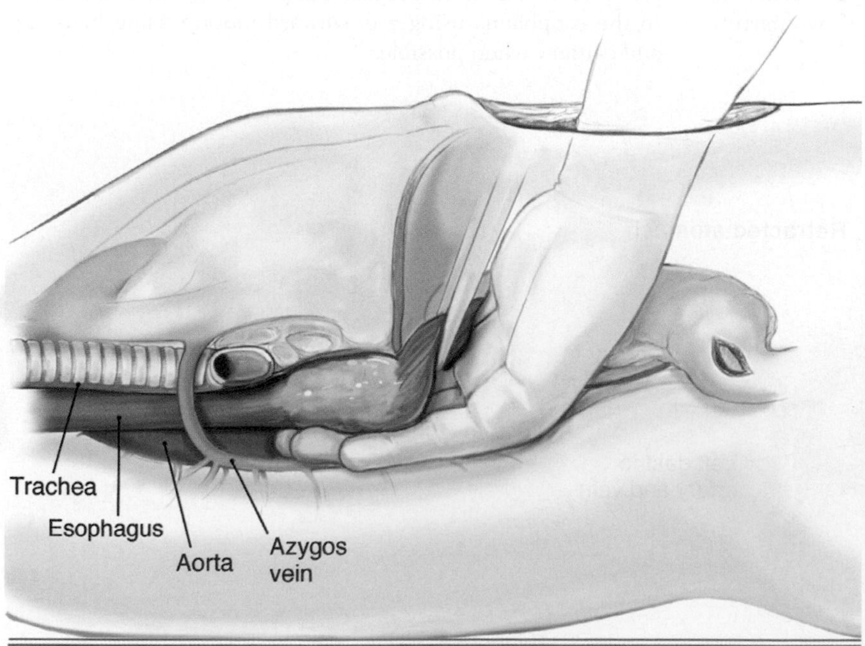

Figure 16-9. Blunt (manual) dissection of the esophagus, taking care of the trachea anteriorly and the aorta and azygos vein posteriorly.

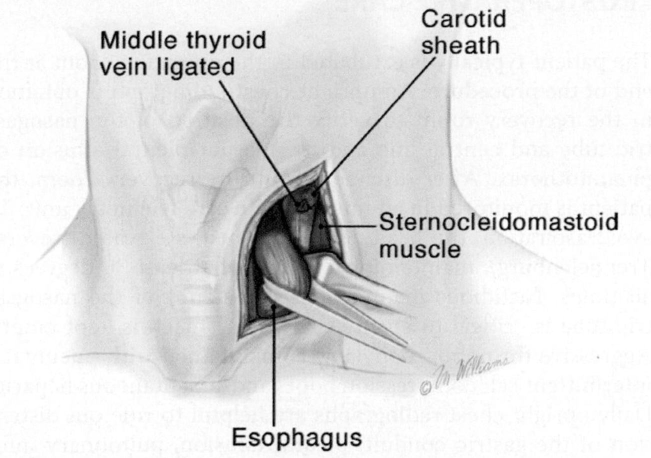

Figure 16-10. Mobilization of the cervical esophagus.

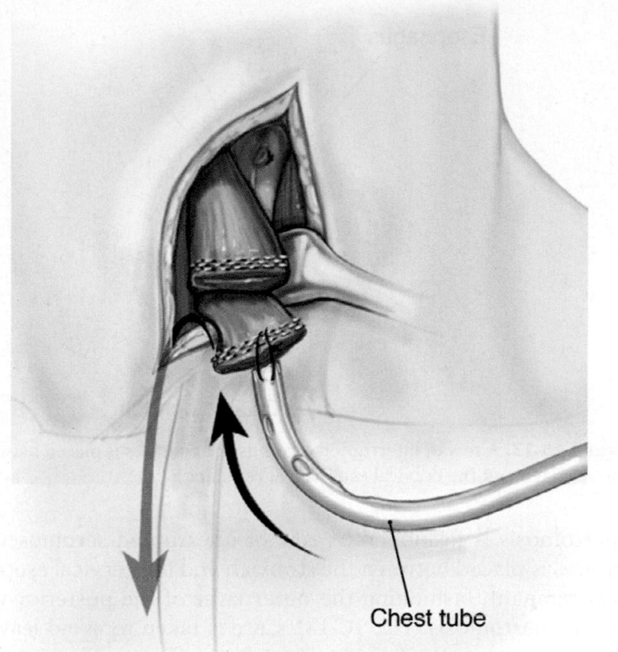

Figure 16-11. The fenestrated end of a large chest tube is sutured to the distal end of the divided cervical esophagus. Using downward traction on the mobilized stomach, the mobilized esophagus, and the attached chest.

electrocautery. Special care is taken to avoid injury to the recurrent laryngeal nerves.

Resection of the Specimen and Delivery of the Stomach to the Neck

The tip of the nasogastric tube is pulled back to the top of the cervical esophagus, which is divided well above the thoracic inlet using a GIA stapler. The fenestrated end of a large chest tube is sutured to the distal end of the divided cervical esophagus (Fig. 16-11). With downward traction on the mobilized stomach, the mobilized esophagus and the attached chest tube are pulled inferiorly through the posterior mediastinum until the fenestrated end of the chest tube appears through the diaphragmatic hiatus in the abdomen. The greater curvature of the stomach is fashioned into a long tube using sequential firings of the GIA stapler, taking care to obtain an adequate margin around the lesser curvature of the stomach. The detached esophagogastrectomy specimen is delivered from the operative field.

The long gastric staple line is oversewn with imbricating seromuscular suture. The newly fashioned gastric tube is placed in a sterile plastic endoscopic camera sleeve. The endoscopic camera sleeve is sutured to the fenestrated (abdominal) end of the chest tube that was passed through the posterior mediastinum (Fig. 16-12). Sheathed in the sterile plastic camera sleeve, the gastric tube is delivered cephalad via the diaphragmatic hiatus into the posterior mediastinum in the surgeon's hand. Simultaneous traction on the cervical end of the posterior mediastinal chest tube is used to pull the sterile plastic camera sleeve upward, delivering the gastric tube atraumatically through the thoracic inlet into the cervical incision.

Creation of the Anastomosis and Feeding Jejunostomy

A suitable point on the stomach, away from the long gastric staple line, is selected for the anastomosis. A hand-sewn two-layer

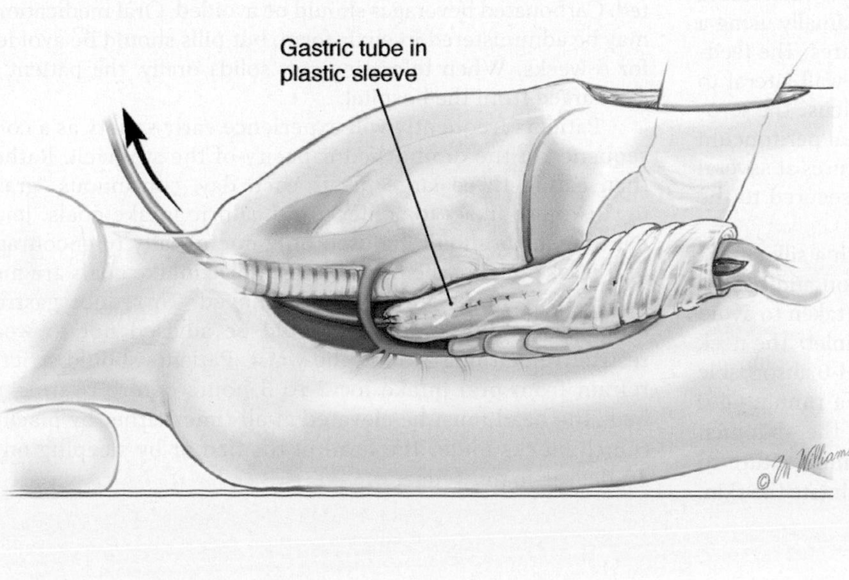

Figure 16-12. Delivery of the gastric conduit to the neck.

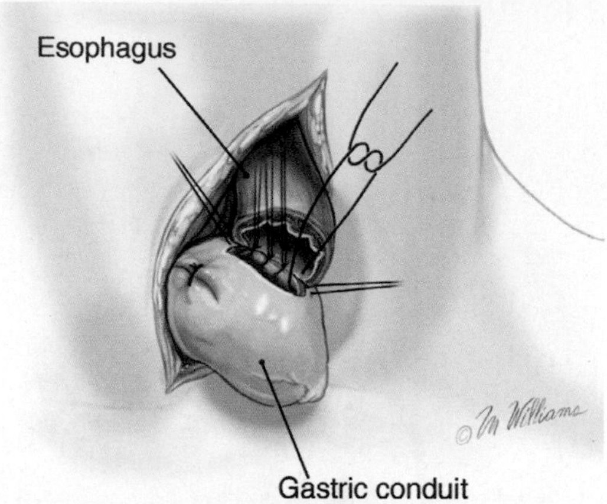

Figure 16-13. A row of interrupted seromuscular sutures is placed between the stomach and the cervical esophageal remnant.

anastomosis is fashioned. A row of interrupted seromuscular sutures is placed between the stomach and the cervical esophageal remnant, fashioning the outer layer of the posterior wall of the anastomosis (Fig. 16-13). Care is taken to avoid leaving an excessive length of cervical esophagus. Every effort is made to ensure that the anastomosis remains both tension free and above the level of the thoracic inlet. The esophageal staple line is grasped in a Kocher clamp and excised using a scalpel blade. The stomach is entered with electrocautery and suctioned. The inner layer of the posterior wall of the anastomosis is fashioned with interrupted absorbable suture.

The nasogastric tube is advanced beyond the anastomosis into the stomach and positioned with its tip at the level of the diaphragmatic hiatus. It is then placed on suction and secured to the skin of the nasal septum with a heavy nonabsorbable monofilament suture. The inner layer of the anterior wall of the anastomosis is completed with running or interrupted absorbable suture. The outer layer of the anterior wall of the anastomosis is completed with a row of interrupted seromuscular sutures. Alternatively, a modified "Orringer" posterior wall stapled anastomosis using an EndoGIA stapler can be performed, then closing the anterior wall in two layers.

A feeding jejunostomy is created. The tip of an 18F red rubber catheter is trimmed and passed through two concentric seromuscular purse-string sutures of absorbable material placed in the antimesenteric wall of the jejunum 40 cm beyond the ligament of Treitz. The red rubber catheter is imbricated into the antimesenteric wall of the jejunum proximally using a row of interrupted seromuscular absorbable sutures. The feeding tube is brought out through the abdominal wall lateral to the rectus muscle sheath at the level of the umbilicus. The serosal surface of the jejunum is sutured to the parietal peritoneum at the jejunostomy tube site using absorbable sutures at several points to prevent volvulus. The feeding tube is secured to the skin with a heavy silk suture.

A short 1-inch Penrose drain is secured with a silk suture to the skin at the inferior end of the neck incision and passed behind the esophagogastric anastomosis. Care is taken to avoid passage of the Penrose drain below the thoracic inlet. The neck incision is closed in two layers using a running 3-0 absorbable suture to reconstitute the platysma muscle and a running 4-0 subcuticular suture to reapproximate the skin. The abdomen is closed in two layers using #1 absorbable running suture to reconstitute the linea alba and staples to reapproximate the skin.

POSTOPERATIVE CARE

The patient typically is extubated in the operating room at the end of the procedure. An upright chest radiograph is obtained in the recovery room to verify the position of the nasogastric tube and central line and to rule out pleural effusion or pneumothorax. After discharge from the recovery room, the patient is monitored in an intermediate care telemetry unit. To avoid aspiration, the head end of the bed is elevated (reverse Trendelenburg), maintaining an angle of at least 30 degrees at all times. Fastidious maintenance of patency of the nasogastric tube is critical to ensure that the stomach is kept empty. Aggressive thromboprophylaxis is maintained with pneumatic intermittent calf compression boots and subcutaneous heparin. Daily upright chest radiographs are helpful to rule out distention of the gastric conduit, pleural effusion, pulmonary infiltrates, and ileus. Patient-controlled analgesia, chest physical therapy, and incentive spirometry are used to prevent atelectasis. Early ambulation is encouraged.

The Penrose drain is removed from the neck on the first postoperative day, after bile leak and hemorrhage have been excluded. No oral intake of any kind is permitted initially. Tube feedings may be started via the jejunostomy when appropriate and are increased gradually to the goal rate. A bowel regimen is helpful for avoiding constipation. Plasma electrolyte levels are monitored daily, and potassium and magnesium level determinations are repleted aggressively.

Throat discomfort related to the nasogastric tube may be alleviated with topical anesthetic spray. After 6 days without any oral intake, ice chips are permitted sparingly. Seven days postoperatively, a fluoroscopic swallow study is performed with the nasogastric tube in place. Small amounts of contrast material are frequently aspirated during this examination. Because of its propensity to cause chemical pneumonitis when aspirated, water-soluble contrast medium should be avoided completely and barium used instead. There are no known adverse consequences of barium extravasation in the chest. In the absence of a leak, the nasogastric tube is removed, and the patient is allowed to continue taking ice chips orally.

If there are no signs or symptoms of leak or infection, the patient's diet is advanced to clear fluids on the first morning after a normal barium swallow. Full fluids are permitted the next day. When appropriate, a mechanical soft diet is permitted. Carbonated beverages should be avoided. Oral medications may be administered in elixir form, but pills should be avoided for 6 weeks. When tolerating soft solids orally, the patient is discharged from the hospital.

Patients frequently will experience early satiety as a consequence of the diminished capacity of the stomach. Rather than eating three large meals each day, continuous "grazing" is more likely to achieve oral caloric intake goals. Jejunal tube feeds should be used only nocturnally to encourage oral intake during the day. When caloric intake goals are met orally, the jejunostomy tube is removed. To reduce gastroesophageal reflux, patients should be advised not to wear restrictive clothing around the waist. Patients should strictly refrain from oral intake for 2 to 3 hours before retiring to bed. The head must be elevated at all times either by placing 6-inch blocks under the head of the bed or by sleeping on a 30-degree foam wedge.

PROCEDURE-SPECIFIC COMPLICATIONS

Early Complications

During the course of esophageal mobilization in the neck, the recurrent laryngeal nerves (especially on the left side) may be injured, resulting in vocal cord paresis or paralysis. This reduces the effectiveness of coughing and impairs the patient's ability to expectorate tracheobronchial secretions. Furthermore, vocal cord weakness increases the patient's vulnerability to aspiration. The result is an increased risk of postoperative pneumonia. Patients with postoperative vocal cord dysfunction must receive especially close attention to tracheobronchial toilet and nasogastric tube patency. In some cases, medialization of the impaired vocal cord may be warranted.

During the course of blunt dissection of the thoracic esophagus, the mediastinal pleura may be breached on either side. This sometimes can lead to delayed accumulation of unilateral or even bilateral pleural effusion. If a divided lymphatic vessel is not ligated properly, a chylothorax may result. To avoid respiratory embarrassment, postoperative pleural effusions should be drained immediately and completely with a pigtail catheter or chest tube. In the event of a chylous leak, tube feeds should be stopped immediately and parenteral nutrition instituted. Early surgical intervention is warranted for large lymph leaks that persist despite a withdrawal of enteral nutrition.

Respiratory problems are among the most common postoperative complications associated with esophagectomy, even when performed via the transhiatal approach. Aspiration of gastric contents is frequently the cause. Aspiration is often due to occlusion of the nasogastric tube with resulting gastric distention, excessive oral intake, or failure to maintain head elevation at all times. Many patients undergoing esophagectomy have a history of excessive alcohol consumption and are prone to delirium and other symptoms. Careful attention should be paid to a history of excess alcohol consumption, and appropriate prophylaxis with short-acting benzodiazepines should be instituted. Care should be taken to avoid inadvertent removal of the nasogastric tube by delirious patients.

Anastomotic Leak

An early anastomotic leak is attributable to technical error and should be readily appreciated when saliva and/or bile is seen draining from the Penrose drain in the neck on the first or second postoperative day. Leaks are more commonly due to a failure of anastomotic healing and usually occur on the sixth or seventh postoperative day, long after the Penrose drain has been removed. Signs of a delayed cervical anastomotic leak include erythema, fluctuance, and crepitus in the neck, as well as drainage of saliva and/or bile from the cervical incision. Early reopening and drainage of the inferior aspect of the cervical wound are imperative to prevent tracking of infection into the mediastinum. This usually can be accomplished satisfactorily at the bedside. The neck should be explored at the bedside with a gloved finger introduced via the reopened wound to ensure that any collection in the neck has been drained adequately. A large Penrose drain should be reintroduced via the lower end of the neck wound with its tip positioned behind the anastomosis. The drain may be sutured to the skin at the lower end of the neck wound. Its external end should be trimmed to a length of 2 to 3 cm and secured with a large safety pin to prevent it from becoming lost inside the wound. In the absence of fever and leukocytosis, a barium contrast swallow study is performed. If there is no extravasation of contrast material into the mediastinum, oral fluid intake is permitted, and the patient's diet is gradually advanced to soft solids. The patient should be instructed to push gently on the neck wound dressing when swallowing to decrease the leakage of food and drink. The anastomotic leak typically resolves in 2 to 3 weeks.

The development of mediastinal emphysema, pleural effusion, fever, hypoxia, hypotension, oliguria, acidosis, or a decline in mental status should lead the clinician to suspect mediastinitis. Although anastomotic leaks usually are drained effectively by reopening the neck wound, leaked secretions occasionally may track below the thoracic inlet into the mediastinum and/or pleural cavity. In this event, early and aggressive resuscitation of the patient along with institution of intravenous antibiotics is mandatory. Intubation and mechanical ventilation may be required. When the patient's condition has been stabilized, CT imaging is essential to rule out intrathoracic collections requiring drainage. Early and complete chest tube drainage or CT-guided percutaneous drainage of all collections is essential.

Occasionally, despite early intervention for a cervical anastomotic leak, the patient may remain septic. Under such circumstances, ischemia or gangrene of the proximal aspect of the gastric tip should be suspected. The characteristic odor of gangrenous tissue may be detectable from the cervical wound or the mouth. Very gentle flexible endoscopy may be performed—using minimal air insufflation—to assess mucosal viability. Full-thickness ischemia of the proximal gastric tip can be identified by more aggressive exploration of the neck incision in the operating room. When necrosis of the gastric tip has resulted in a leak that tracks below the thoracic inlet, the anastomosis should be taken down. The proximal esophageal end should be sutured to the skin in the neck as an end-esophagostomy. The stomach should be brought back down into the abdomen, and the gangrenous portion should be resected. The proximal end of the gastric remnant then can be secured to the parietal peritoneum in the left upper quadrant as an end-gastrostomy. Four to six months later, when the patient is doing well at home on jejunostomy feedings, continuity of the upper gastrointestinal tract can be restored electively. The gastric remnant is often long enough to permit an extra-anatomic (typically substernal) gastric pull-up with primary reanastomosis in the neck.

Stricture

Healing of the cervical esophagogastric anastomosis may be complicated by stricture, resulting in dysphagia to solids. The incidence of anastomotic stricture is increased if an anastomotic leak occurs postoperatively.[22] Anastomotic strictures usually respond to repeated dilatation. Dilatation may be instituted as early as 4 weeks postoperatively, even if there is ongoing residual anastomotic drainage from the cervical wound. Initially, Savary bougies are used in the operating room under brief general anesthesia. Patients are encouraged to resume eating a mechanical soft diet immediately after undergoing dilatation to inhibit immediate recurrence of the anastomotic stricture. Dilatations are performed every 2 to 3 weeks until the dysphagia subsides. In the rare instance that requires numerous dilatations for complete resolution of the stricture, patients may be taught to dilate themselves at home every 4 to 7 days in an upright seated position using a Maloney bougie.[23]

SUMMARY

At our institution, we perform most esophagectomies with an open thoracotomy approach (i.e., left transthoracic [see Chapter 21], Ivor Lewis [see Chapter 17], or McKeown/three-hole [see Chapter 16] technique). In certain circumstances we do use the transhiatal technique as described earlier. These include primarily high-risk patients with poor pulmonary function who have early-stage localized tumors as well as patients with long-segment Barrett dysplasia.

CASE HISTORY

A 77-year-old White man with long-segment Barrett esophagus presented with high-grade dysplasia near the esophagogastric junction. The patient had a history of coronary artery disease and mild chronic obstructive pulmonary disease. He underwent a transhiatal esophagectomy after an extensive workup showed no revascularizable lesions in the coronary arteries and no evidence of carcinoma on multiple biopsies. His postoperative course was unremarkable, and he underwent a barium swallow on postoperative day 7 that was read as normal. One day later, after eating a mint lozenge, he noticed a swelling over his left neck incision. On examination, he had fluctuant swelling over the anastomotic site with minimal redness and no fever or leukocytosis. His incision was opened and explored at the bedside. No obvious leak was noted, and no gangrene was found. The wound was irrigated and packed with wet-to-dry gauze dressings for 2 weeks. He was discharged home on postoperative day 10 in good condition tolerating a soft mechanical diet. He presented 6 weeks later with dysphagia and on esophagogastroduodenoscopy was found to have an anastomotic stricture. He required balloon and later Savary bougie dilations every 1 to 2 months for almost a year, after which his stricture resolved.

EDITOR'S COMMENT

Although rarely used by most thoracic esophageal surgeons for esophageal cancer, transhiatal esophagectomy still has many proponents. In addition to general surgeons who prefer this technique as it can be done without a thoracotomy, in certain situations this operation can be helpful. For example, this operation can be performed in patients who are found to have Barrett esophagus with moderate-to-severe dysplasia or patients with a T1a or T1b distal esophageal cancer, since the risk of lymph node metastasis is below 10%. In addition, patients who have severe pulmonary dysfunction may benefit from this approach, which avoids thoracotomy. Despite the potential advantages inherent with this approach, careful attention to technical details is paramount.

—Mark J. Krasna

References

1. Orringer MB, Sloan H. Esophagectomy without thoracotomy. *J Thorac Cardiovasc Surg*. 1978;76(5):643–654.
2. Orringer MB, Marshall B, Iannettoni MD. Transhiatal esophagectomy for treatment of benign and malignant esophageal disease. *World J Surg*. 2001;25(2):196–203.
3. Gandhi SK, Naunheim KS. Complications of transhiatal esophagectomy. *Chest Surg Clin N Am*. 1997;7(3):601–610; discussion 611–612.
4. Herbella FA, Del Grande JC, Colleoni R. Efficacy of mediastinal lymphadenectomy in transhiatal esophagectomy with and without diaphragm opening: a cadaveric study. *Dis Esophagus*. 2002;15(2):160–162.
5. Chang AC, Ji H, Birkmeyer NJ, et al. Outcomes after transhiatal and transthoracic esophagectomy for cancer. *Ann Thorac Surg*. 2008;85(2):424–429.
6. Connors RC, Reuben BC, Neumayer LA, et al. Comparing outcomes after transthoracic and transhiatal esophagectomy: a 5-year prospective cohort of 17,395 patients. *J Am Coll Surg*. 2007;205(6):735–740.
7. Rentz J, Bull D, Harpole D, et al. Transthoracic versus transhiatal esophagectomy: a prospective study of 945 patients. *J Thorac Cardiovasc Surg*. 2003;125(5):1114–1120.
8. Omloo JM, Lagarde SM, Hulscher JB, et al. Extended transthoracic resection compared with limited transhiatal resection for adenocarcinoma of the mid/distal esophagus: five-year survival of a randomized clinical trial. *Ann Surg*. 2007;246(6):992–1000; discussion 1000–1001.
9. Boshier PR, Anderson O, Hanna GB. Transthoracic versus transhiatal esophagectomy for the treatment of esophagogastric cancer: a meta-analysis. *Ann Surg*. 2011;254(6):894–906.
10. Colvin H, Dunning J, Khan OA. Transthoracic versus transhiatal esophagectomy for distal esophageal cancer: which is superior? *Interact Cardiovasc Thorac Surg*. 2011;12(2):265–269.
11. Biere SS, Cuesta MA, van der Peet DL. Minimally invasive versus open esophagectomy for cancer: a systematic review and meta-analysis. *Minerva Chir*. 2009;64(2):121–133.
12. Bakhos CT, Fabian T, Oyasiji TO, et al. Impact of the surgical technique on pulmonary morbidity after esophagectomy. *Ann Thorac Surg*. 2012;93(1):221–226; discussion 6–7.
13. Bolton JS, Teng S. Transthoracic or transhiatal esophagectomy for cancer of the esophagus-does it matter? *Surg Oncol Clin N Am*. 2002;11(2): 365–375.
14. Hulscher JB, Tijssen JG, Obertop H, et al. Transthoracic versus transhiatal resection for carcinoma of the esophagus: a meta-analysis. *Ann Thorac Surg*. 2001;72(1):306–313.
15. Hulscher JB, van Sandick JW, de Boer AG, et al. Extended transthoracic resection compared with limited transhiatal resection for adenocarcinoma of the esophagus. *N Engl J Med*. 2002;347(21):1662–1669.
16. Kuppusamy MK, Felisky CD, Helman JD, et al. Assessment of intraoperative haemodynamic changes associated with transhiatal and transthoracic oesophagectomy. *Eur J Cardiothorac Surg*. 2010;38(6): 665–668.
17. Rizzetto C, DeMeester SR, Hagen JA, et al. En bloc esophagectomy reduces local recurrence and improves survival compared with transhiatal resection after neoadjuvant therapy for esophageal adenocarcinoma. *J Thorac Cardiovasc Surg*. 2008;135(6):1228–1236.
18. Veeramachaneni NK, Zoole JB, Decker PA, et al. Lymph node analysis in esophageal resection: American College of Surgeons Oncology Group Z0060 trial. *Ann Thorac Surg*. 2008;86(2):418–421; discussion 21.
19. Stiles BM, Mirza F, Coppolino A, et al. Clinical T2-T3N0M0 esophageal cancer: the risk of node positive disease. *Ann Thorac Surg*. 2011;92(2):491–496; discussion 6–8.
20. Wolff CS, Castillo SF, Larson DR, et al. Ivor Lewis approach is superior to transhiatal approach in retrieval of lymph nodes at esophagectomy. *Dis Esophagus*. 2008;21(4):328–333.
21. Javed A, Pal S, Chaubal GN, et al. Management and outcome of intrathoracic bleeding due to vascular injury during transhiatal esophagectomy. *J Gastrointest Surg*. 2011;15(2):262–266.
22. Schuchert MJ, Abbas G, Nason KS, et al. Impact of anastomotic leak on outcomes after transhiatal esophagectomy. *Surgery*. 2010;148(4):831–838; discussion 8–40.
23. Davis SJ, Zhao L, Chang AC, et al. Refractory cervical esophagogastric anastomotic strictures: management and outcomes. *J Thorac Cardiovasc Surg*. 2011;141(2):444–448.

17 Three-Hole Esophagectomy: The Brigham and Women's Hospital Approach

Christian G. Peyre and David J. Sugarbaker

Keywords: Three-hole esophagectomy, esophageal malignancy, esophageal resection

The management of esophageal cancer has evolved tremendously over the past decade. Increasingly, patients are treated with an aggressive multimodal approach including neoadjuvant chemoradiotherapy followed by surgical resection.[1] Despite these changing trends in the treatment paradigm for esophageal cancer, esophagectomy remains the crucial component to long-term survival.

The key to success in managing patients with esophageal cancer is surgeon experience.[2] There are numerous approaches to esophageal resection and replacement, both open and minimally invasive, but all have the potential for a high rate of morbidity and mortality. Each esophageal surgeon must develop and refine a technique of resection that is safe and expeditious to minimize morbidity while aggressively pursuing standard oncologic principles including adequate resection margins and complete lymphadenectomy to help assure long-term survival.

The selection of operative approach is based on numerous factors: type and location of the lesion, extent of invasion, stage of disease, need for lymphadenectomy, history of previous surgeries, and type of conduit chosen for esophageal replacement (i.e., stomach, colon, or jejunum). Surgeon preference and experience plays an important role in the selection of the operation. Popular methods of esophageal resection in the United States are based on methods developed by Ivor Lewis and McKeown, among others.[3–5] They differ by the approach, number of incisions, and location of the anastomosis (intrathoracic or cervical) (Table 17-1). The three-hole esophagectomy

Table 17-1

POPULAR METHODS OF ESOPHAGEAL RESECTION AND REPLACEMENT IN THE UNITED STATES

TECHNIQUE	INCISION(S)	ADVANTAGES	DISADVANTAGES	LESIONS
LTE	Left thoracoabdominal Good exposure for GEJ tumors	Single incision High risk of postoperative reflux	Proximal margin limited by aorta	GEJ
Transhiatal[a]	Upper midline laparotomy Left cervical	No thoracotomy	Limited lower mediastinal lymphadenectomy Blind midthoracic dissection	Benign disease, high-grade dysplasia, GEJ and lower esophageal tumors
Ivor Lewis[b]	Right thoracotomy Laparotomy	Direct-vision thoracic dissection Lymphadenectomy	Thoracotomy Limited proximal margin Intrathoracic anastomosis/leak Increased risk of postoperative bile reflux	Middle and lower thirds
Modified McKeown[c]	Right thoracotomy Midline laparotomy Right cervical	Good proximal margin Direct-vision thoracic dissection Lymphadenectomy Cervical anastomosis	Thoracotomy Three incisions Exposure to right RLN during dissection Increased incidence of postoperative reflux	Middle third
Brigham THE[d]	Muscle-sparing right thoracotomy Simultaneous abdominal and left cervical	Unlimited proximal margin Direct-vision esophageal dissection Cervical anastomosis avoids morbidity of an intrathoracic leak and anastomosis located out of potential radiation field Reduced risk of postoperative reflux RLN avoided from left approach Serratus muscle-sparing thoracotomy Expeditious two-stage procedure Complete lymphadenectomy	Thoracotomy Three incisions	Middle third Upper and middle thirds if neoadjuvant therapy is given
MIE	Right thoracoscopy Laparoscopy +/− left cervical	No thoracotomy Reduced postoperative pain More rapid recovery	Technically challenging	

LTE, left thoracoabdominal esophagectomy; RLN, recurrent laryngeal nerve; GEJ, gastroesophageal junction; THE three-hole esophagectomy; MIE, minimally invasive esophagectomy.

[a]Orringer MB, Sloan H. Esophagectomy without thoracotomy. *J Thorac Cardiovasc Surg.* 1978;76:643.

[b]Lewis I. The surgical treatment of carcinoma of the esophagus with special reference to a new operation for growths of the middle third. *Br J Surg.* 1946;34:18.

[c]Modified McKeown K: Trends in oesophageal resection for carcinoma. McKeown first described the operation with a right thoracotomy and a left paramedian abdominal incision. The Modified McKeown is the right thoracotomy with a midline laparotomy. *Ann R Coll Surg Engl.* 1972;51:213.

[d]Swanson SJ, Batirel HF, Bueno R, et al. Transthoracic esophagectomy with radical mediastinal and abdominal lymph node dissection and cervical esophagogastrostomy for esophageal carcinoma. *Ann Thorac Surg.* 2001;72:1918.

at the Brigham and Women's hospital has evolved over time and is designed specifically to limit morbidity by assimilating the best elements of each of the predecessor surgeries in a safe and expeditious procedure.[6–9] This chapter will delineate the conduct of the operation and establish principles that can be applied to any approach for esophagectomy whether open or minimally invasive.

GENERAL PRINCIPLES

Even for experienced centers, esophagectomy is a difficult procedure to perform and is associated with a considerable risk of morbidity and mortality (Table 17-2). Careful preoperative assessment, as well as the prevention, detection, and early treatment of procedure-specific complications, is essential to an excellent outcome. The Brigham three-hole esophagectomy is conducted in two stages. First, the thoracic dissection is conducted under direct vision by means of a limited right muscle-sparing posterolateral thoracotomy. The patient then is moved from the left lateral decubitus position to the supine position for the second stage of the procedure, beginning with simultaneous upper midline and left cervical incisions.

The operation allows direct visualization of the entire esophagus for resection with ample longitudinal margins and the ability to perform a complete lymphadenectomy in both the chest and abdomen. The specimen and surrounding lymph tissues are removed en bloc before the conduit is fashioned and placed. We prefer to use a gastric conduit whenever feasible, but other conduits may be used (i.e., colon or jejunum). The operation is completed with a cervical anastomosis, which is easy to care for in the event of postoperative leak and associated with a lower incidence of recurrent gastric reflux than operations requiring an intrathoracic anastomosis.

The three-hole esophagectomy is ideal for patients with upper, middle, or lower third esophageal lesions. It is also suitable for patients with bulky tumors or with dense adhesions secondary to radiation therapy or caustic injuries, since the dissection is enhanced by the direct vision afforded by thoracotomy. Patients with a history of preoperative neoadjuvant radiation, in whom there is an increased expectation of inflammation and fibrosis of the mediastinal structures, likewise do well with this surgery. The procedure is preferred for malignant disease because it ensures excellent circumferential visualization and dissection.

PREOPERATIVE ASSESSMENT AND PERIOPERATIVE CARE

Before the patient is considered for resection, diagnostic studies include esophagogastroduodenoscopy to evaluate the extent of proximal and distal disease along with endoscopic ultrasound and a PET/CT scan to complete clinical staging and rule out distant metastases. The majority of patients with stage II or III disease are considered for neoadjuvant therapy. It is important to restage patients following neoadjuvant treatment with CT scan or PET/CT to identify those patients who may have progressed on therapy.

All patients are screened carefully for cardiopulmonary reserve. Patients identified as high risk on the basis of cardiopulmonary screening may undergo additional optimization procedures such as cardiac revascularization, valve repair or replacement, smoking cessation, or cardiopulmonary rehabilitation.

Table 17-2

PROCEDURE-SPECIFIC COMPLICATIONS

- Pulmonary
- Anastomotic leak
- Conduit necrosis
- Anastomotic stricture
- Recurrent gastric acid reflux
- Tracheoesophageal fistula
- Injury to recurrent laryngeal nerve

Our preference is to use the stomach for reconstruction for its ease of use, need for only one anastomosis, and reliable blood supply. For patients who have had previous abdominal surgery, specifically gastric resections that might compromise the vascular supply of potential conduits, we routinely obtain preoperative angiograms to evaluate the vascular anatomy.

Forty-eight hours before surgery, all patients receive a course of oral antibiotics and mechanical bowel cleanout. An epidural catheter is placed for postoperative analgesia to reduce pulmonary complications secondary to pain. Preinduction intravenous antibiotics are administered prophylactically.

SURGICAL TECHNIQUE

Stage I: Thoracic Dissection

The patient is induced with general anesthesia and intubated with a double-lumen tube to allow for single left lung ventilation. (For a detailed description of anesthetic technique, see Chapter 5.) For those patients with upper or middle third tumors, we first perform a bronchoscopy through a single-lumen endotracheal tube to assess the posterior membranous wall of the airway for tumor invasion.

The patient is turned to the left lateral decubitus position. A limited right posterolateral thoracotomy incision is made in the fifth interspace, sparing the serratus anterior muscle (Fig. 17-1).

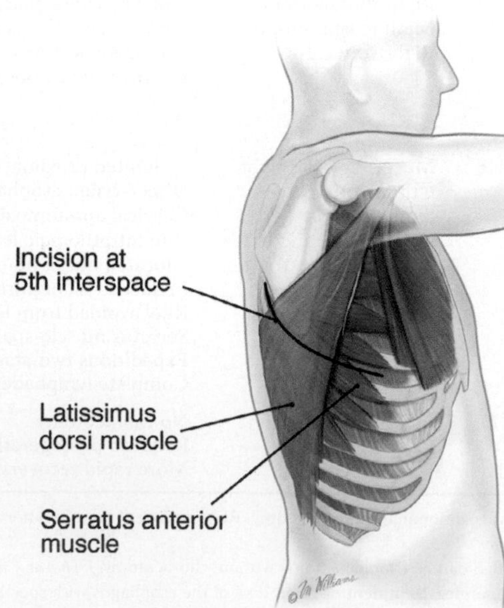

Figure 17-1. A muscle-sparing right posterolateral thoracotomy incision is made at the fifth interspace.

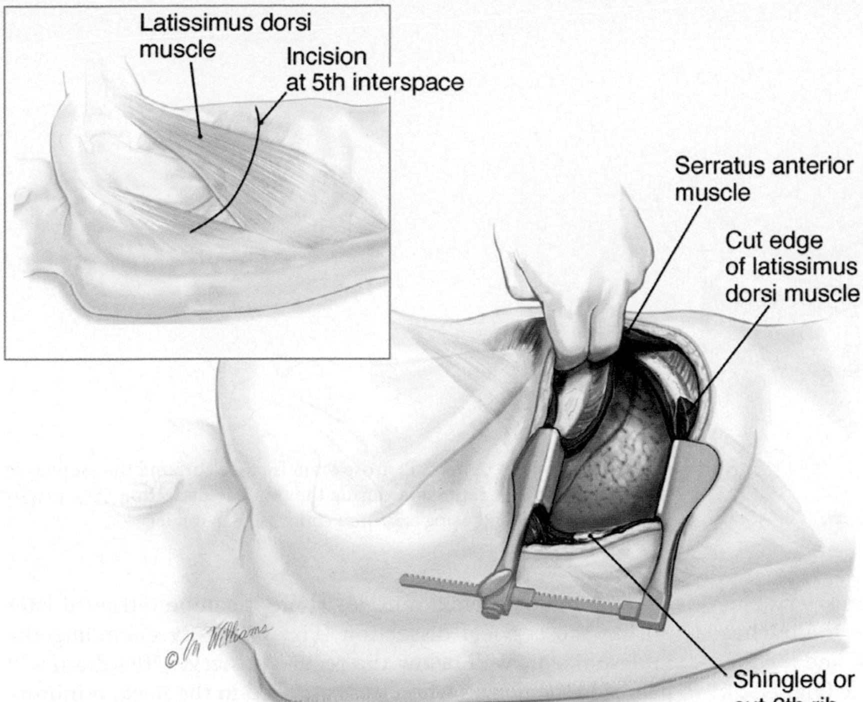

Figure 17-2. The fifth interspace is opened, the sixth rib is removed or "shingled," and the ribs are gently retracted.

The fifth interspace is opened, and the sixth rib is shingled to permit better access to the thoracic cavity (Fig. 17-2). The ribs were spread using gentle retraction.

The lung is retracted anteriorly and the inferior pulmonary ligament is divided. The posterior mediastinal pleura is opened from the apex of the chest to the diaphragm at the level of the vertebral bodies thereby exposing the esophagus (Fig. 17-3). The esophagus is then mobilized in a region above the tumor. A 1-cm Penrose drain is passed around the esophagus and used for gentle retraction during the remainder of the thoracic dissection. Retracting the esophagus in this manner permits evaluation of the tumor for resectability from its surrounding structures. The azygos vein is usually divided using a 30-mm endovascular stapler to improve access to the upper thoracic esophagus (Fig. 17-4). If the tumor is deemed to be resectable, the surgeon proceeds with near-total esophagectomy, carrying the dissection cephalad along the esophagus toward the apex of the chest using a combination of electrocautery and blunt dissection with constant traction from the Penrose drain, and countertraction provided by the first assistant's sponge stick. For mid- and distal esophageal tumors, the dissection of the upper thoracic esophagus proceeds close to the esophagus to avoid injury to the right

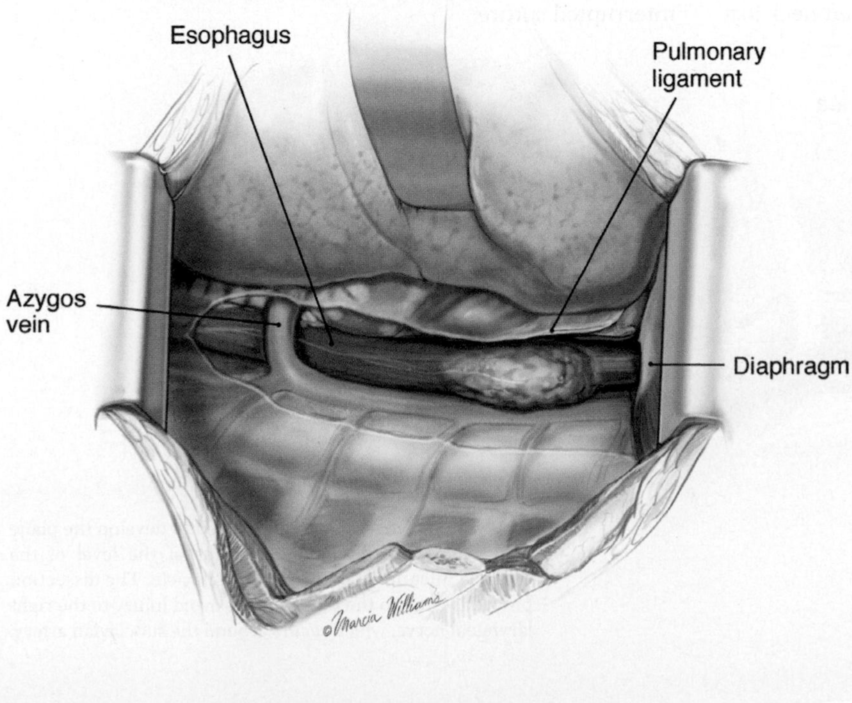

Figure 17-3. The posterior mediastinal pleura is opened over the esophagus from the apex of the chest to the diaphragm.

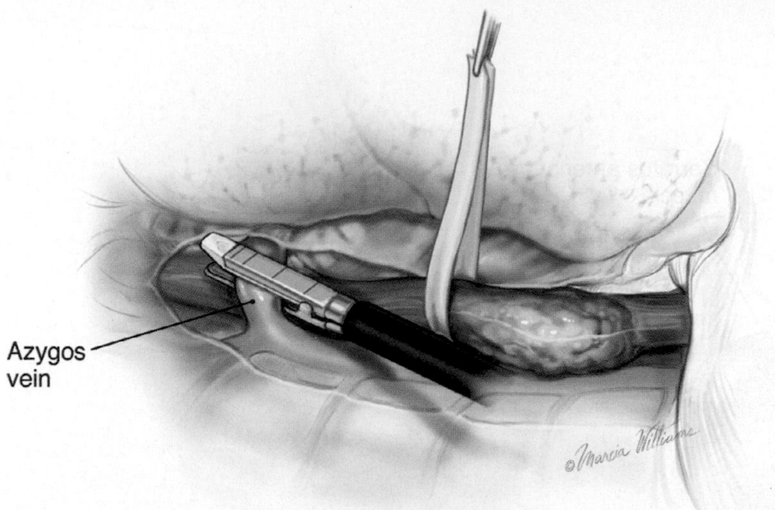

Figure 17-4. A 1-cm Penrose drain is passed around the esophagus and used for retraction during the thoracic dissection. The azygos vein is divided using a 30-mm endovascular stapler.

laryngeal nerve, which recurs around the subclavian artery. Finger dissection is used to define the plane between the trachea and the esophagus at the level of the thoracic inlet, and the finger dissection is carried up to the level of the clavicle (Fig. 17-5).

After packing the apex of the chest with a laparotomy sponge to minimize bleeding, the dissection proceeds caudad between the aorta and esophagus, where the arterial branches are divided. A second Penrose drain can be placed around the lower esophagus, distal to the tumor if possible, to provide countertraction for the posterior dissection. Any pericardium that adheres to the tumor is removed as well as adherent pleura along both sides of the mediastinum. A small rim of diaphragm is incised circumferentially around the esophageal hiatus. The peritoneal cavity is entered posteriorly, and the posterior wall of the stomach is palpated by the surgeon's finger. In particular, when the lesion is at the carina and densely adherent, using the two Penrose drains above and below the lesion allows safe access to the most densely adherent level where the tumor abuts the posterior wall of the airway and anterior wall of the aorta.

At this point, the first upper Penrose drain is loosely knotted around the esophagus and pushed up into the left neck just beneath the omohyoid muscle, where it can be retrieved later during the cervical dissection (Fig. 17-6). By encircling the midesophagus well below the recurrent nerves, the drain will be inside the nerves when it is retrieved in the neck, minimizing traction or direct injury to the recurrent nerve. The second Penrose drain is loosely knotted around the lower esophagus and passed into the peritoneal cavity to be retrieved at the time of the laparotomy to facilitate dissection of the gastroesophageal junction (Fig. 17-7). Although the goal is to resect the nodal tissue en bloc with the esophagus, any nodal tissue that has not been dissected with the specimen is resected separately and labeled appropriately. The region of the thoracic duct is identified near the aortic hiatus and ligated with a 0 silk suture to prevent chyle leak. If the duct cannot be visualized easily, a mass ligature is placed around all of the tissue between the spine and the aorta at the level of the diaphragm. Hemostasis is achieved, and a straight 28 French chest tube is placed in the posterior chest to the apex and brought out through a separate inferior stab incision. The thoracotomy is closed in layers in typical fashion after reapproximating the ribs with interrupted suture.

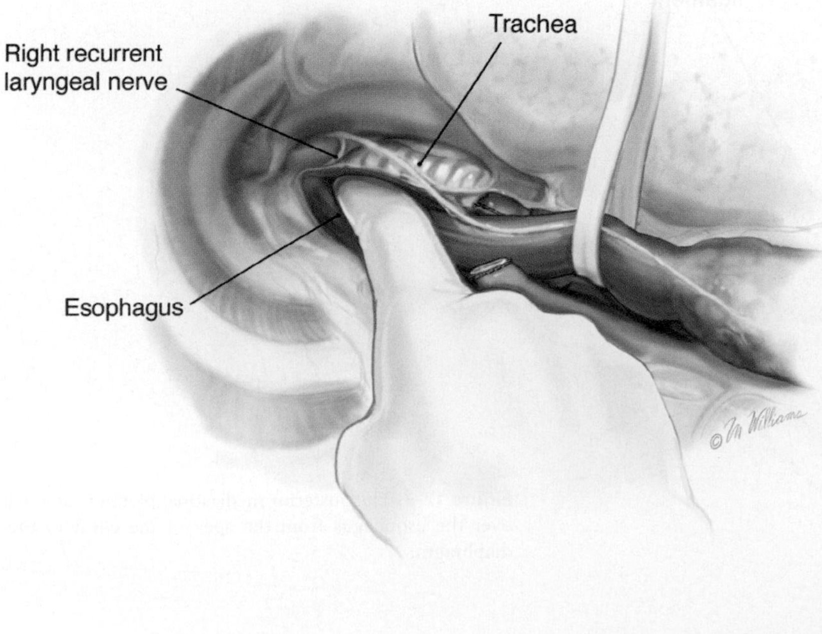

Figure 17-5. Finger dissection is used to develop the plane between the trachea and esophagus at the level of the thoracic inlet up to the level of the clavicle. The dissection proceeds close to the esophagus to avoid injury to the right laryngeal nerve, which recurs around the subclavian artery.

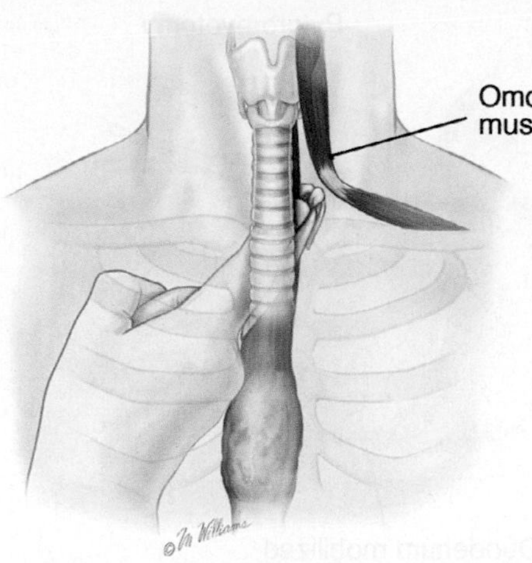

Figure 17-6. After the esophagus has been dissected to the level of the clavicle, the end of the Penrose drain is knotted and pushed behind the esophagus up through the thoracic inlet for use later in the cervical dissection.

Stage II: Abdominal and Cervical Dissections

The patient is repositioned supine for the abdominal and left cervical dissections. At this juncture, the double-lumen tube is replaced with a single-lumen tube to avoid the need to replace the endotracheal tube after the conclusion of the case once the cervical anastomosis has been created and airway edema is at its worst. If dissection around the trachea or carina was difficult due to radiation fibrosis or tumor, a bronchoscopy can be performed at this junction to ensure no injury to the airway has occurred. The patient's head is rotated 45 degrees to the right, and a shoulder roll is placed. The patient is prepped from the jaw to the pubic symphysis. An upper midline laparotomy and left cervical incisions can be performed simultaneously (Fig. 17-8).

Abdominal Dissection

The abdomen is explored for resectability. With the availability of improved CT and PET/CT technology for preoperative surgical staging, it is unlikely at this stage to find any evidence of metastatic disease. In the event that metastatic disease is identified, the patient can be safely closed after removing the Penrose drains and inserting a feeding tube. The esophagus has a rich longitudinal submucosal blood supply and will continue to survive. As patients with stage IV esophageal cancer have a short median survival, palliative esophagectomy may not be the best choice for a quick recovery and discharge from the hospital. Palliation of dysphagia from an obstructing tumor can often be achieved endoscopically at a later date if necessary.

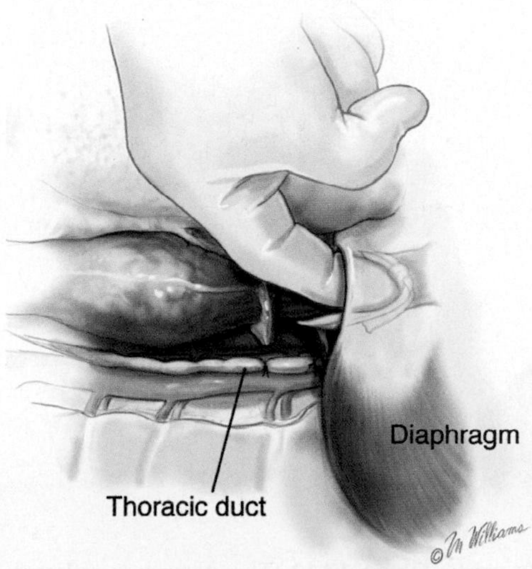

Figure 17-7. A second Penrose drain is knotted around the lower esophagus and pushed into the peritoneal cavity for use later in the laparotomy and dissection of the gastroesophageal junction.

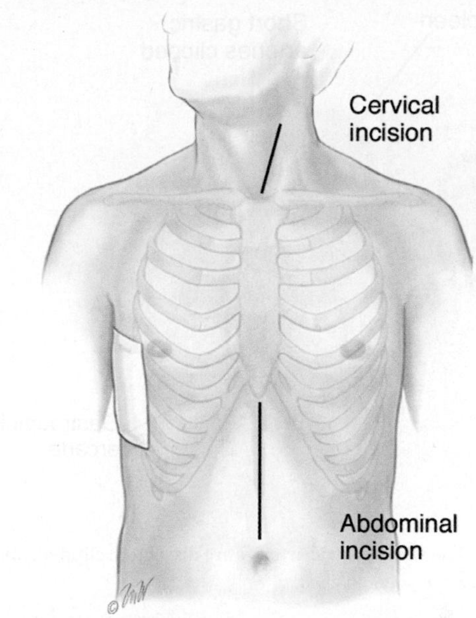

Figure 17-8. After the thoracic dissection is complete, the patient is placed in the supine position, and different surgical teams working simultaneously make two incisions, a midline abdominal incision and a left cervical incision.

If no evidence of metastatic disease is found, the triangular ligament to the left lobe of the liver is divided and the left lobe is folded down and retracted to the right with a moist laparotomy pad and a deep self-retaining retractor. We use upper-hand and Balfour retractors to provide exposure after taking down the triangular ligament. The Penrose drain placed during thoracotomy is identified and used for retracting the esophagus at the level of the gastroesophageal junction (Fig. 17-9). Adequate

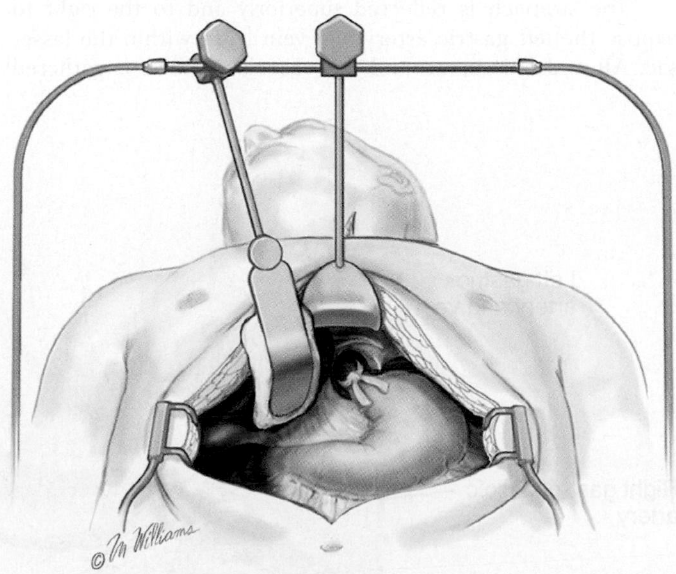

Figure 17-9. The abdomen is explored for resectability through the midline incision. Upper-hand and Balfour retractors are placed to provide exposure after taking down the triangular hepatic ligament. The second Penrose drain that was placed during thoracotomy is identified.

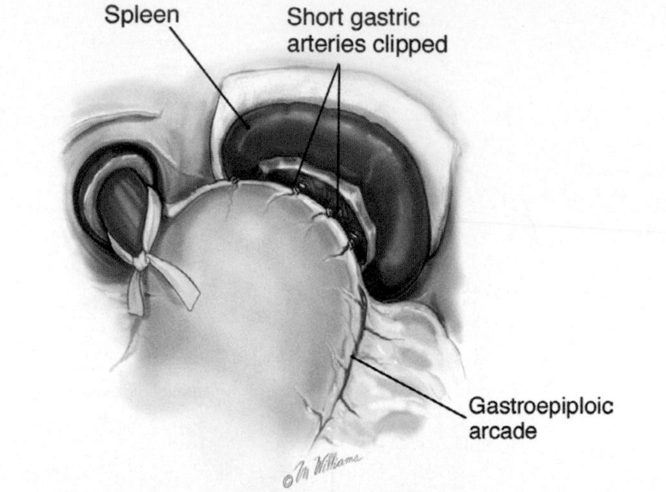

Figure 17-10. The short gastric arteries are dissected, clipped, and divided.

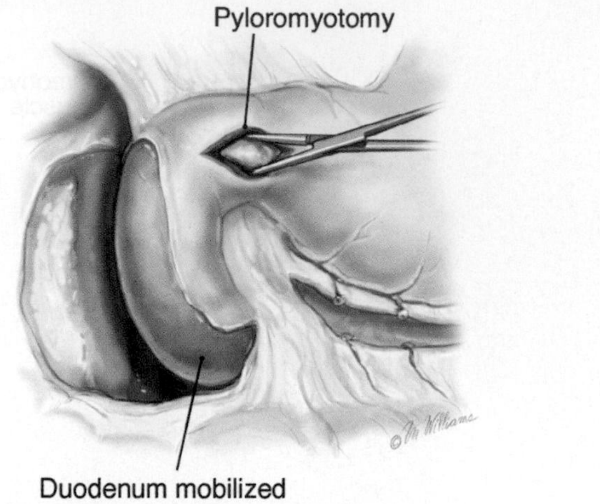

Figure 17-11. The duodenum is mobilized using a Kocher maneuver. A pyloromyotomy or Heineke-Mikulicz type of pyloroplasty using single layer of 3-0 silk is done to create the egress from the conduit.

pulse is confirmed in the right gastroepiploic artery, after which the surgeon proceeds to locate and divide the short gastric vessels. If the spleen is located deep in the left upper quadrant such that it limits visualization of the gastric vessels, a laparotomy pad can be placed behind the spleen to bring the short gastric vessels into view. Once the short gastric vessels are identified, they can be transected with ties and clips, harmonic scalpel, or endovascular linear staplers (Fig. 17-10). With the short gastric arteries divided to the level of the hiatus, dissection is carried along the greater curvature toward the pylorus, dividing the omentum from the stomach, taking care to avoid injury to the gastroepiploic arcade and pedicle. The lesser sac is entered and the posterior attachments of the stomach to the pancreas are sharply divided. A generous Kocher maneuver is carried out to mobilize the duodenum to the midline. A pyloromyotomy or Heineke-Mikulicz type of pyloroplasty using a single layer of 3-0 silk is created to provide adequate drainage of the conduit (Fig. 17-11).

The stomach is reflected superiorly and to the right to expose the left gastric artery and vein from within the lesser sac. All nodal tissue around this vascular pedicle is gathered up onto the specimen. The left gastric pedicle is palpated at its takeoff from the celiac axis and ligated with a single firing of the endovascular 30-mm linear stapler. Before firing the stapler, it is important to recheck the pulse of the right gastroepiploic pedicle to be sure that the celiac axis itself has not been clamped (Fig. 17-12). The lesser omentum is divided and the gastric conduit is now ready to be divided.

Left Cervical Dissection

A left cervical incision can be performed simultaneously with the upper midline laparotomy by a separate surgical team. A left neck incision is preferred as the path of the left recurrent nerve is more predictable and less likely to be injured during dissection. A short left neck incision is created along the anterior border of the sternocleidomastoid muscle (Fig. 17-13). The sternocleidomastoid muscle is mobilized laterally along with the carotid sheath. Dissection is deepened lateral to the thyroid gland. The middle thyroid vein may need to be divided. Care is taken not to impinge the left recurrent nerve with retractors. The use of self-retaining metal retractors should be avoided to prevent recurrent laryngeal nerve injury and carotid artery

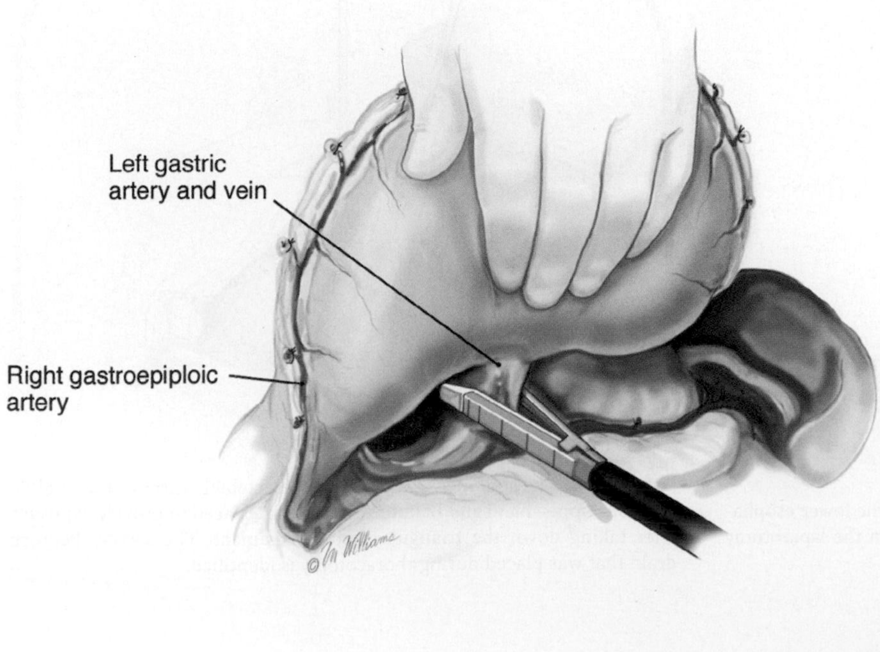

Figure 17-12. The stomach is reflected superiorly and to the right, exposing the left gastric vein and artery, which are ligated using an endostapler near their origin in the celiac axis.

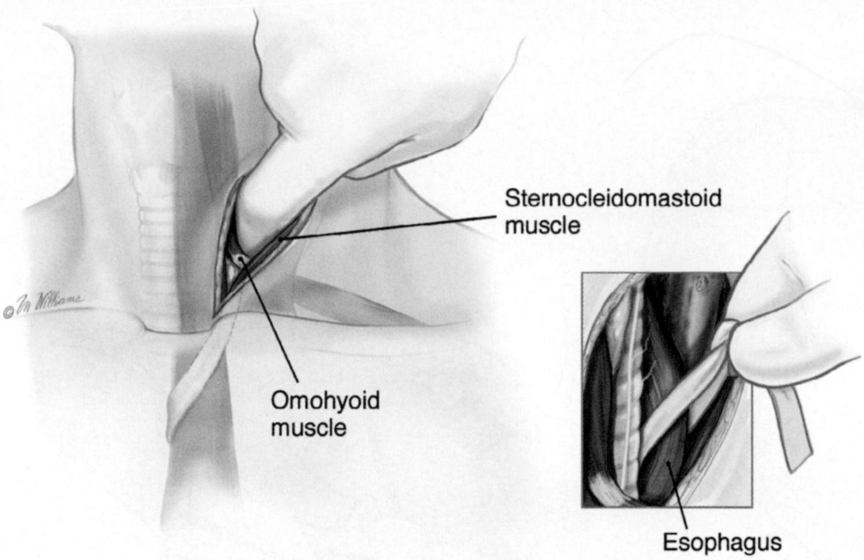

Figure 17-13. While the first team mobilizes the esophagus below the diaphragm, the second team creates a short left cervical incision along the anterior border of the sternocleidomastoid muscle and locates the first Penrose drain.

lesions, particularly if carotid plaques are suspected. The omohyoid and sternohyoid muscles may be divided with electrocautery for improved esophageal exposure. Using gentle blunt finger dissection, the surgeon proceeds posterior to the cervical esophagus and anterior to the vertebral bodies where the upper Penrose drain placed during the thoracic dissection can be found. The drain is brought into the wound and traction from the Penrose drain permits further blunt mobilization of the cervical esophagus. The entirety of the esophagus should now be mobile.

The cervical esophagus is divided with a linear 75 mm stapler (Fig. 17-14). A long #1 silk suture is placed in the distal esophageal staple line, and the specimen is retrieved from the abdomen. In this manner, the silk tie, which is pulled down into the mediastinum with the specimen, can later be used to guide the gastric conduit up through the posterior mediastinum into the neck (Fig. 17-15).

PREPARATION OF THE CONDUIT AND ALIMENTARY RECONSTRUCTION

With the specimen delivered into the abdomen, a linear cutter 75-mm stapler is used to divide the stomach to ensure an adequate distal margin from the tumor and to fashion a narrow tube-shaped conduit. The outline for the conduit begins along the greater curvature of the stomach, high on the fundus, and is drawn toward the lesser curvature just above the crow's foot (Fig. 17-16). The staple line along the gastric conduit can be reinforced with invaginating "Lembert" seromuscular sutures. Maintaining a narrow conduit is important physiologically to ensure adequate emptying of the neoesophagus. The hiatus is dilated manually to permit four fingers to be placed through it.

A sterile arthroscopic camera bag is attached to the proximal end of a 30-mL Foley catheter secured to the distal end of the silk tie (Fig. 17-17). The gastric conduit is placed inside the bag and the bag is unfolded. A small aliquot of saline is added inside the bag and suction is applied to the distal end of the Foley drain to maintain traction on the conduit. The Foley catheter, camera bag, and gastric conduit are gently pushed

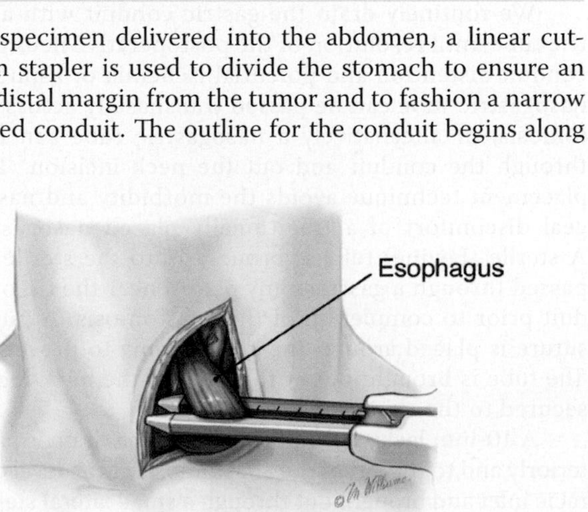

Figure 17-14. The cervical esophagus is divided with a linear cutter, 75-mm (GIA) stapler.

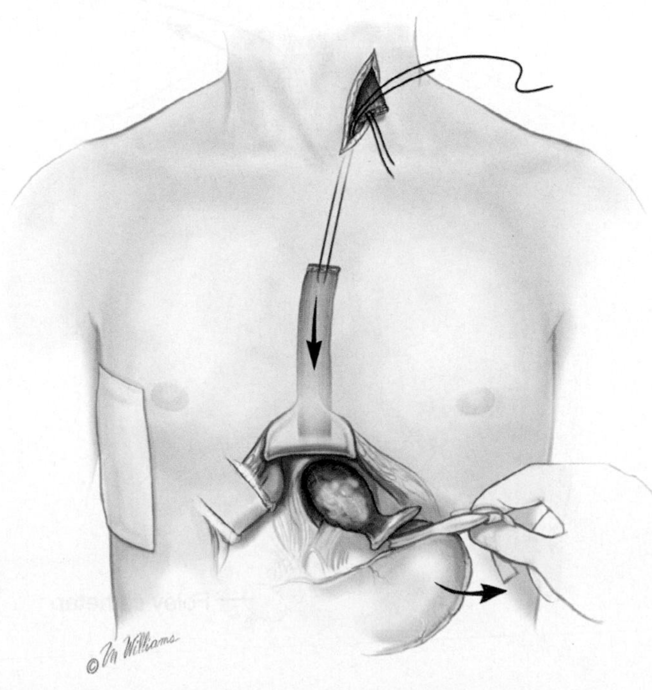

Figure 17-15. A long, heavy silk suture is attached to the cervical end, and the specimen is brought down through the abdominal incision and removed.

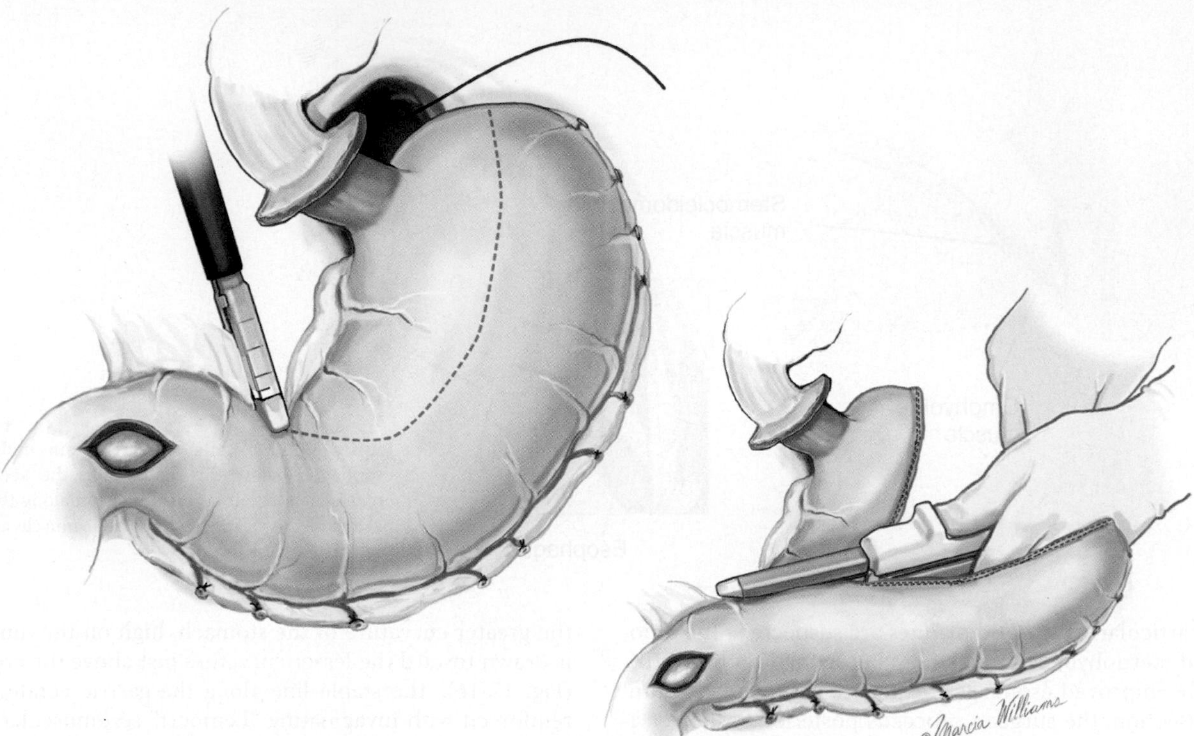

Figure 17-16. A linear cutting stapler is used to create the gastric conduit. The conduit is fashioned by creating a semicircular line along the greater curvature of the stomach beginning high on the fundus and ending at a point along the lesser curvature just above the crow's foot.

into the mediastinum and out the left cervical incision taking care to prevent twisting of the conduit (Fig. 17-18). The conduit should be gently pushed or fed up the mediastinum rather than pulled up to prevent injury to the walls of the conduit or

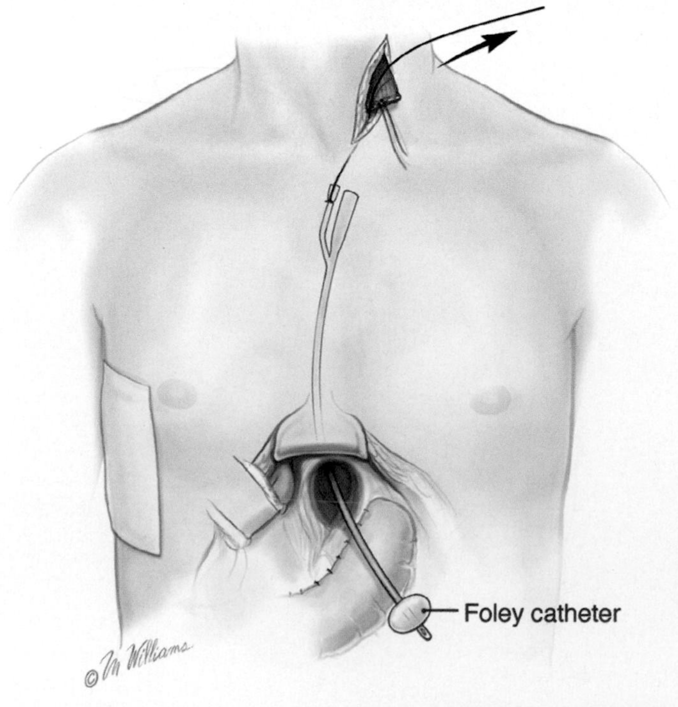

Figure 17-17. The silk tie is attached to the port of a 30-mL Foley balloon catheter, and the catheter is pulled up until it is partway through the neck incision.

the vascular pedicle. When oriented properly, the gastric staple line lies on the right side of the neck incision from the patient's perspective, and the pylorus rests at the hiatus (Fig. 17-19). The esophagogastric anastomosis can be performed in one of two ways: hand sewn or stapled. For a hand-sewn anastomosis, the proximal esophageal staple line is cut off and a gastrotomy is made 3 cm below the tip of the conduit. A single layer of interrupted 3-0 silk sutures is used to create the anastomosis (Fig. 17-20). For a stapled anastomosis, a functional end-to-end anatomic side-to-side anastomosis is created using a linear cutting stapler and a thoracoabdominal-30 (TA-30) stapler to close the enterotomies (Fig. 17-21).

We routinely drain the gastric conduit with a nasogastric tube until resolution of the postoperative ileus to prevent conduit distention and potential ischemia or aspiration. The nasogastric tube can be passed transnasally across the anastomosis, or alternatively a nasogastric tube can be passed through the conduit and out the neck incision. This latter placement technique avoids the morbidity and nasopharyngeal discomfort of a traditionally placed nasogastric tube. A sterile (Levine) tube is brought onto the sterile field and passed through a gastrostomy placed near the tip of the conduit prior to completion of the anastomosis. A purse-string suture is placed around the gastrostomy to prevent leakage. The tube is brought out at the apex of the neck incision and secured to the skin.

A 10-mm Jackson-Pratt closed suction drain is passed posteriorly and to the left of the anastomosis at the level of the thoracic inlet and brought out through a small lateral stab incision. This tube prevents seroma and provides an outlet for drainage in the event of an early leak in the anastomosis. A jejunal feeding tube is inserted routinely for postoperative feeding and to

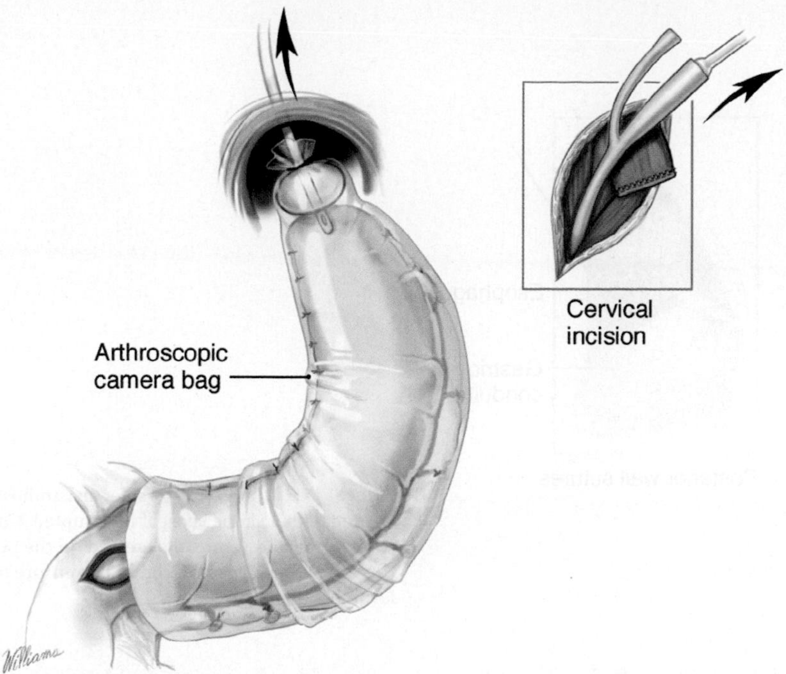

Figure 17-18. The other end of the Foley catheter is attached to an arthroscopic camera bag. The neoesophagus is placed into the folded bag, being careful to ensure proper axial orientation (i.e., the neoesophagus is oriented with the staple line on the patient's right side). A Yankauer suction device is attached to collapse the bag around the neoesophagus.

provide access for enteral nutrition if problems with oral feeding occur postoperatively.

Procedure-Specific Morbidity

Morbidity following esophagectomy is common, most frequently from cardiopulmonary and anastomotic complications (Table 17-3). Thorough knowledge of the common sources of morbidity and mortality following esophagectomy can facilitate prevention, early detection, and rapid treatment of complications, which is essential for satisfactory outcome.

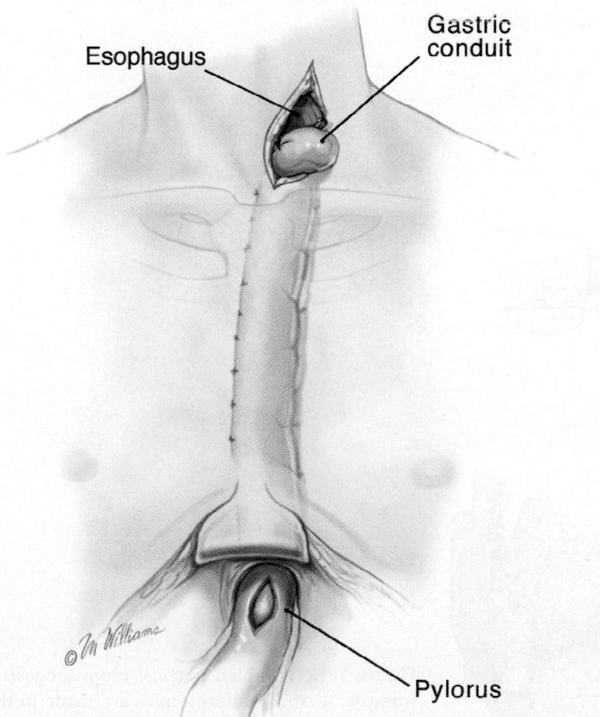

Figure 17-19. The gastric conduit is pulled through the posterior mediastinum into the cervical wound.

Cardiopulmonary Complications

Many esophagectomy patients are ultimately, often malnourished individuals and frequently have a history of smoking and alcohol use. Often, they have comorbid conditions that compromise their cardiovascular and pulmonary status, prolong recovery, and complicate the postoperative management. Pulmonary complications including pneumonia, aspiration, and respiratory failure requiring prolonged intubation are common after esophagectomy and occur at a rate of 20% to 30% at high-volume centers.[10] A preoperative epidural catheter for pain control is critical to improve postoperative pulmonary toilet. Conversely, the incidence of cardiovascular complications is relatively low, occurring in 5% to 10% of patients in most large series. Atrial fibrillation is most common but myocardial infarction, arrhythmias, congestive heart failure, deep venous thrombosis, and pulmonary embolism can occur as well.[10]

Anastomotic Leak

Anastomotic leak remains the Achilles heal of esophageal surgery. Most leaks manifest within 10 days of surgery. General factors that influence the development of anastomotic leak include tension on the anastomosis, quality of the arterial and venous blood supplies, location of the anastomosis, manner in which it was performed, and surgeon experience. Anastomotic leaks that are not quickly identified and treated remain a major source of operative mortality. We prefer a cervical as opposed to intrathoracic anastomosis, as in our experience it is easier to treat a leak in the neck than one in the chest. Early initiation of antimicrobial therapy, opening of the neck wound, and making the patient NPO is usually all that is necessary to resolve the leak and prevent severe sepsis. Soilage into the mediastinum is uncommon. Conversely, intrathoracic leaks may necessitate reoperation to adequately drain the source of the mediastinal

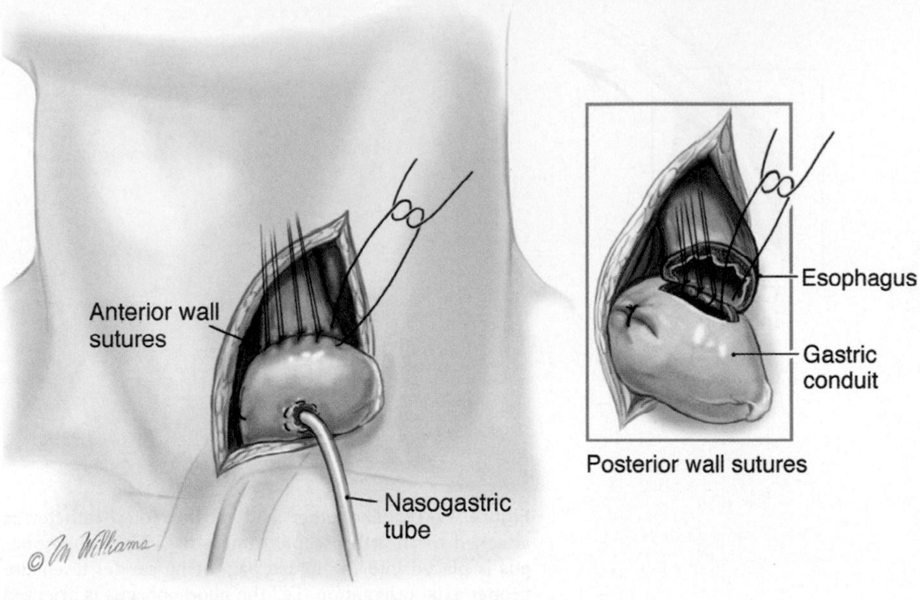

Figure 17-20. An end-to-side anastomosis is created with a single layer of interrupted 3-0 silk suture. The anastomosis is created on the posterior aspect of the gastric conduit to ensure more favorable drainage.

sepsis. Recently, some have advocated the use of endoluminal stents to seal leaks.

Hemorrhage

There are many potential sources for hemorrhage after esophagectomy, including unrecognized or poorly controlled injury to the spleen, azygos vein, intercostal vessels, omentum, right gastric artery, and lung parenchyma. Traction injuries of the heart and pericardium can lead to cardiac tamponade. Injury to the phrenic veins during mobilization of the left lateral segment of the liver extending to the vena cava also can give rise to internal bleeding. Patients with unsuspected cirrhosis can have bleeding of the esophageal varices intraoperatively. Prevention of intraoperative bleeding requires close attention to technique and vigilant examination of all potential bleeding sites before closure. Postoperative hemorrhage requires urgent reexploration and occurs with an incidence of 3% to 5%. Diagnosis of postoperative bleeding is usually delayed by 12 to 24 hours. Unexpected tachycardia and decreased urine output are early signs of a developing problem. Since esophagectomy patients have sizable fields of dissection, where the blood can hide, they generally require large-volume blood replacement. After patients are resuscitated with blood products to correct coagulopathies, they are reexplored. This source of bleeding usually can be prevented with meticulous surgical technique.

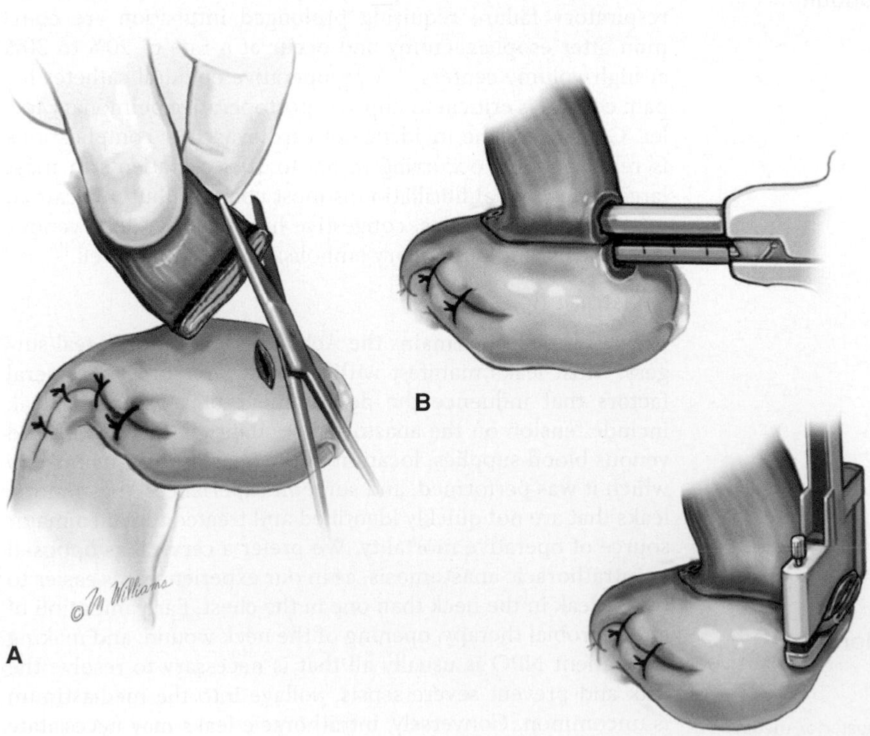

Figure 17-21. Stapled cervical esophagogastric anastomosis. *A.* small enterotomies are made in the distal esophagus and posterior wall of the gastric conduit. *B.* Using a linear GIA stapler, the posterior wall of the esophagus and gastric conduit are joined. *C.* The remaining enterotomy is closed with a TA stapler.

Table 17-3

MAJOR COMPLICATIONS OF THREE-HOLE ESOPHAGECTOMY (*N* = 250)

COMPLICATION	FREQUENCY (%)	*N*
Recurrent laryngeal nerve injury	14	35
Chylothorax	9	22
Anastomotic leak	8	19
Pneumonia	5	13
Postoperative bleeding	2	5
Tracheoesophageal fistula	1	2
Adult respiratory distress syndrome	1	2
Empyema	1	2
Sepsis	0.4	1
Mediastinitis	0.4	1

Reprinted with permission from Sugarbaker D, DeCamp M, Liptay M. *Surgical procedures to resect and replace the esophagus.* In: Zinner MJ, Schwartz SI, Ellis H, eds. Maingot's Abdominal Operations. 10th ed. Stamford, CT: Appleton & Lange; 1997.

Chylothorax

The thoracic duct follows a similar course to the esophagus, comes in close proximity to the aorta and vertebral bodies, and is at risk of being injured during esophagectomy. Chylothorax occurs with an incidence of 1% to 5%. Diagnosis is made on demonstration of a pleural effusion consisting of a milky white fluid with high triglyceride and lymphocyte counts. It should be suspected with the development of a new right pleural effusion on chest radiographs following early removal of the chest drains or if the chest tube output remains elevated beyond postoperative day 4. The fluid may be clear and have a low triglyceride level if the patient has been NPO for a few days and may not turn milky until enteral feeds have been initiated. Although chylothorax can be managed conservatively in some patients with parenteral nutrition and restriction of enteral intake, the course is frequently prolonged and may lead to significant protein loss. We favor an aggressive reoperative approach with mass suture ligation of the thoracic duct via right thoracotomy if high chest tube outputs persist beyond the seventh postoperative day. To avoid this complication, we routinely ligate the thoracic duct at time of esophagectomy.

Pleural Effusion and Pneumothoraces

Other possible complications of esophagectomy include pleural effusion and pneumothorax. These conditions can be managed conservatively with percutaneous drainage or thoracostomy after other causes have been eliminated, including hemorrhage, chylothorax, conduit leak, metastatic disease, and airway injury. Dissection through the left pleura may result in fluid or air originating in the right hemithorax communicating with the left pleural space.

Recurrent Laryngeal Nerve Injury

A serious complication of esophagectomy is recurrent laryngeal nerve palsy. This injury affects the vocal cords and phonation but more importantly impacts the ability of the patient to detect and protect their airways against life-threatening aspirations. It occurs with an incidence of 10% to 20% in patients receiving a cervical anastomosis.[7] Care must be taken in patients receiving oral nutrition with a recurrent nerve palsy to avoid aspiration. We frequently pursue early medialization of the vocal cord if a recurrent nerve palsy is identified.

Airway Injuries

Rarely, a tracheobronchial injury arises intraoperatively. If undetected at surgery, it can result in a postoperative tracheogastric fistula with persistent pulmonary soiling and recurrent pneumonias. We routinely perform bronchoscopy after the thoracic dissection to look for airway injuries. The risk of injury to the membranous wall of the trachea is minimized when the dissection is carried out under direct vision during the thoracic dissection, which is not possible during a transhiatal approach. If an airway injury does occur, it can be repaired primarily and buttressed with pericardium, omentum, and/or transposed muscle.

Delayed Gastric Emptying

Up to 10% of patients undergoing esophagectomy experience delayed gastric emptying in the postoperative period. We routinely perform a pyloromyotomy for all patients undergoing a three-hole esophagectomy to avoid this disabling complication. If a gastric drainage procedure is not added, delayed gastric emptying can often be managed with endoscopic balloon dilatation but the surgeon must be vigilant toward the early detection of retained gastric juices and oral intake to avoid life-threatening aspiration.

Late Sequelae

It is important for the surgeon to educate the patient and family to recognize some of the late complications that can occur following esophagectomy that may warrant intervention. These include anastomotic stricture, paraesophageal hernia, intestinal motility problems (e.g., dumping syndrome), bile reflux, and post-thoracotomy pain syndrome.

Esophageal Anastomotic Stricture

Tension and inadequate blood supply can lead to esophageal stricture weeks to months after surgery. Patients who develop an anastomotic leak are at high risk for later development of a stricture. Dysphagia is the first sign of an esophageal stricture, and patients should be evaluated with an upper endoscopy and/or barium swallow. We have a low threshold for early endoscopy and dilatation. Anastomotic stricture is a frequent problem for a cervical anastomosis although serial dilatation is very effective and typically resolves the problem without the need for reoperation.

SUMMARY

The mortality rate for esophagectomy is proportional to experience. Mortality ranges from a high of 10% at low-volume centers to a low of 2% to 3% at high-volume centers. Attention to all aspects of the procedure includes careful patient selection, meticulous surgical technique, and diligent perioperative care.[9,10] A high suspicion for procedure-specific complications yields a safe procedure with acceptable morbidity and mortality when the surgery is performed by an experienced surgical team (Table 17-4). Highlights of the most important technical aspects of this approach include use of a muscle-sparing right posterolateral thoracotomy, direct vision for the thoracic dissection, complete thoracic lymphadenectomy (which yields the best chance for cure and guidance for adjuvant treatment regimens), and clear margins. Placing the anastomosis in the left neck provides easy postoperative maintenance, reduces the morbidity of anastomotic leaks in comparison with an intrathoracic

Table 17-4

STRATEGIES FOR PREVENTION OF COMPLICATIONS

Preoperative strategies

Preoperative cardiopulmonary screening to identify risk factors
- Surgical and medical optimization for selected patients, e.g., coronary artery bypass graft surgery, smoking cessation

Previous surgery
- Preoperative angiogram to assess condition and availability of conduits

Preoperative measures 48 h in advance of surgery
- Mechanical bowel cleanout
- Oral antibiotics

Day of Surgery
- Preinduction intravenous prophylactic antibiotic administration
- Epidural catheter placement for postoperative pain control to reduce pulmonary complications

Intraoperative strategies
- Meticulous hemostasis
- Pyloroplasty or pyloromyotomy to ensure appropriate gastric emptying and potentially minimize postoperative aspiration
- Jejunostomy feeding tube for postoperative enteral feeding
- Prophylactic ligation of the thoracic duct
- Appropriate drainage of right pleural space and cervical anastomosis

anastomosis, and is associated with a lower incidence of postoperative bile reflux. Survival data have not revealed a clear benefit of one surgery over another in a comparison of the transhiatal and transthoracic techniques. The technical complications are fewer when thoracic esophageal dissection is performed under direct vision rather than with blunt dissection. This is especially the case after caustic injuries and neoadjuvant radiation therapy. However, several recent randomized studies have demonstrated a trend toward improved survival with the transthoracic approach.[11]

EDITOR'S COMMENT

The technical details of the "three-hole approach" are clearly described in this chapter. Although this is the favored route of the "Brigham group" it has been abandoned by those performing MIE and others in favor of the standard Ivor Lewis approach. There is no doubt that the three-hole approach allows the best access to all of the lymph node fields one might consider removing. Likewise, if one were to do the three-field approach, the technique described above is well thought out and meticulous in attention to detail and will yield excellent results. The key unanswered issue remains whether there is any benefit to the residual esophagus after esophagectomy. If there is a perceived benefit to having a longer, functional remnant, an Ivor Lewis should be preferred for most lesions of the distal esophagus and esophagogastric junction. On the other hand, this modification is my operation of choice for patients with squamous cell carcinoma as these are generally of the mid-esophagus and total esophagectomy with neck anastomosis is the preferred option.

—Mark J. Krasna

ACKNOWLEDGMENT

The authors wish to acknowledge Luis Argote-Greene, MD, for his contributions to this chapter in the first edition.

References

1. van Hagen P, Hulshof MC, van Lanschot JJ, et al. Preoperative chemoradiotherapy for esophageal or junctional cancer. *N Engl J Med.* 2012;366(22):2074–2084.
2. Birkmeyer JD, Stukel TA, Siewers AE, et al. Surgeon volume and operative mortality in the United States. *N Engl J Med.* 2003;349(22):2117–2127.
3. Lewis I. The surgical treatment of carcinoma of the oesophagus; with special reference to a new operation for growths of the middle third. *Br J Surg.* 1946;34:18–31.
4. Orringer MB, Marshall B, Iannettoni MD. Transhiatal esophagectomy: clinical experience and refinements. *Ann Surg.* 1999;230(3):392–400; discussion 400–403.
5. McKeown KC. Trends in oesophageal resection for carcinoma with special reference to total oesophagectomy. *Ann R Coll Surg Engl.* 1972;51(4):213–239.
6. Sugarbaker D, DeCamp M, Liptay M. *Surgical procedures to resect and replace the esophagus.* In: Zinner MJ, Schwartz SI, Ellis H, eds. Maingot's Abdominal Operations. 10th ed. Stamford, CT: Appleton & Lange; 1997.
7. Swanson SJ, Batirel HF, Bueno R, et al. Transthoracic esophagectomy with radical mediastinal and abdominal lymph node dissection and cervical esophagogastrostomy for esophageal carcinoma. *Ann Thorac Surg.* 2001;72(6):1918–1924; discussion 24–25.
8. Swanson SJ, Sugarbaker DJ. The three-hole esophagectomy. The Brigham and Women's Hospital approach (modified McKeown technique). *Chest Surg Clin N Am.* 2000;10(3):531–552.
9. Wee J, Sugarbaker D. Surgical procedures to resect and replace the esophagus. In: Zinner M, Ashley S, eds. *Maingot's Abdominal Operations.* 12th ed. New York, NY: McGraw-Hill; 2006.
10. Kuo EY, Chang Y, Wright CD. Impact of hospital volume on clinical and economic outcomes for esophagectomy. *Ann Thorac Surg.* 2001;72(4):1118–1124.
11. Hulscher JB, van Sandick JW, de Boer AG, et al. Extended transthoracic resection compared with limited transhiatal resection for adenocarcinoma of the esophagus. *N Engl J Med.* 2002;347(21):1662–1669.

18 Ivor Lewis Esophagectomy

Phillippe Nafteux, Willy Coosemans, and Toni Lerut

Keywords: Ivor Lewis esophagectomy, esophageal malignancy, adenocarcinoma, squamous cell carcinoma, esophageal resection

For surgeons familiar with the unique and extraordinary challenges presented by surgery of esophageal malignancy, the words of Ivor Lewis appear as valid today as they were when first written over 50 years ago: "There is little doubt that the successful outcome of radical curative surgery for esophageal carcinoma remains one of the great challenges of surgical practice."[1] A satisfactory result necessitates optimization of the patient's physical state and tumor staging, a high degree of surgical skill and experience, and teamwork involving close coordination of the surgical, anesthetic, physiotherapeutic, and nursing modalities of treatment.

GENERAL PRINCIPLES AND PATIENT SELECTION

The procedure first described in 1946 by Ivor Lewis now represents the middle road between "minimal" transhiatal esophagectomy without radical lymph node dissection, as described by Orringer et al.,[2] and extensive radical resection combined with three-field lymphadenectomy, as described by Akiyama et al.[3] The operation combines an extended resection of the esophagus with either standard or extensive thoracic and abdominal lymph node dissection under direct vision through a combined abdominal and thoracic approach. For this reason, the Ivor Lewis esophagectomy is a preferred approach in many centers for patients with resectable tumor of the middle to lower third of the esophagus and gastroesophageal junction.

The procedure has several drawbacks that, in our view, confine its use to a select group of patients. The operation may limit the proximal extent of the esophageal resection, which can be a major concern in the case of skip lesions or tumors that spread through the submucosa. By terminating the dissection at the apex of the chest, one may not appreciate the presence of positive lymph nodes in the neck or reap the potential benefits of a third-field lymphadenectomy. Indeed from our own experience in a series of 174 patients with three-field lymphadenectomy,[4] we observed that 23% of patients with adenocarcinoma (distal third or gastroesophageal junction) and 25% with squamous cell carcinoma presented with positive cervical lymph nodes. Unforeseen changes in the TNM classification because of such lymph node involvement were observed in 12% of patients. Five-year survival in patients with middle-third esophageal squamous cell carcinoma was 27.7%, and 4- and 5-year survival in patients with distal-third adenocarcinoma was 35.7% and 11.9%, respectively. Finally, the intrathoracic anastomosis, as compared with the cervical anastomosis, is thought to be associated with a higher risk of life-threatening sepsis in the event of leak. For these reasons, we reserve the Ivor Lewis technique for patients with resectable tumors in whom a neck anastomosis is contraindicated. This category includes patients with a past history of cervical malignancy that has been treated by either radical radiotherapy or major surgery and patients with other contraindications to surgery in the cervical region.

PREOPERATIVE ASSESSMENT

The preoperative evaluation should establish the histologic diagnosis and extent of local and distant disease, as well as the patient's physiologic status, which should be improved preoperatively if necessary. Esophagoscopy should be performed to obtain tissue diagnosis and to document the precise location of the tumor and the presence of associated findings (e.g., Barrett esophagus). A bronchoscopy is mandatory in all proximal- and middle-third tumors to evaluate airway invasion or a synchronous second primary. Endoscopic ultrasound has been established as key to evaluating the depth of tumor penetration and involvement of regional lymph nodes. Endoscopic ultrasound also offers the possibility of fine-needle aspiration biopsy for suspicious lymph nodes, especially nodes of the celiac trunk.

Barium swallow is used to document the location and extent of the lesion. CT scan of the chest and abdomen is also obtained routinely, although CT is not as effective as endoscopic ultrasound for determining the extent of intra- and transmural penetration or nodal involvement. CT is more valuable for assessing tumor extension into adjacent structures, such as the aorta, and for the detection of visceral and occult metastasis, especially in combination with a PET scan.

The role of thoracoscopy and laparoscopy in the evaluation of tumor resectability, staging of local and distant lymph nodes, identification of peritoneal implants, and detection of liver or lung metastasis is less clear mainly because of the expense, technical difficulty, and time associated with these procedures.

Careful preoperative assessment of pulmonary and cardiovascular function is mandatory. Routine investigations also include a full blood count, urea and electrolytes, liver function tests, and tumor markers. Physiotherapy is instituted to improve the patient's mobility and pulmonary function, as well as to enhance the patient's general condition. Adequate levels of nutrition and hydration also must be ensured. If necessary, the patient should be begun on nutritional supplements or total parenteral nutrition.

TECHNIQUE

Anesthesia

The anesthetic technique must be of the highest standard. All patients undergoing the Ivor Lewis procedure should have an epidural catheter placed whenever possible to obtain satisfactory levels of analgesia postoperatively, thereby facilitating physiotherapy and respiratory function. A double-lumen endotracheal tube permits single-lung ventilation, which is required to obtain proper visualization and radical resection of the area concerned. Arterial and central venous pressure lines are inserted. Urinary output should be monitored with a Foley catheter. A gastric tube is placed to ensure adequate drainage during the procedure. The patient is positioned with the aid of a vacuum beanbag during thoracotomy. Twenty-four-hour antibiotic prophylaxis is instituted before incision.

Surgical Management

The Ivor Lewis esophagectomy is a two-stage procedure consisting of laparotomy for gastric mobilization and tubularization, followed by a right thoracotomy for esophageal resection and reconstruction. A radical lymphadenectomy is performed in the upper abdomen and chest. During the procedure, careful dissection is mandatory to avoid bleeding, limit the need for transfusion, and minimize manipulation of the heart.

Abdominal Dissection

The patient is positioned in a supine manner for laparotomy, and an upper midline incision is performed. Full abdominal exploration ensues with special attention to evidence of tumor dissemination in the form of unforeseen peritoneal or serosal implants, liver metastasis, or both. An abdominal self-retaining retractor is useful. The left lobe of the liver can be retracted cephalad and to the right after dividing the triangular ligament.

The dissection of the stomach starts by entering the lesser sac at a point well away from the gastroepiploic artery. The greater omentum is divided along the greater curvature by ligating and transecting the branches of the gastroepiploic arteries to the epiploon. During this maneuver, great care is taken to protect the gastroepiploic vessels needed for future vascularization of the stomach. The short gastric vessels are ligated sequentially and divided as close to the spleen as possible to avoid interrupting the epiploic arcade, thus preserving the circulation to the gastric fundus. Injury to the fundus of the stomach is assiduously avoided because this will serve as the site of the future anastomosis. While dissecting the gastrocolic omentum toward the duodenum, the stomach is lifted upward to allow the various adhesions between the stomach and pancreas down to the posterior surface of the first part of the duodenum to be transected. At this point in the operation the right gastroepiploic artery origin or venous communicating branch to the mesocolon is most vulnerable to injury. The duodenum is mobilized generously with a Kocher maneuver, and any loose adhesions between the duodenum and gallbladder fundus are divided.

Attention is turned to the lesser omentum, which is divided close to the undersurface of the left liver lobe up to the esophageal hiatus. The vagal branches to the liver are transected, and if a left liver lobe artery is found, care is taken to preserve this artery if at all possible. The right gastric vessels are identified, dissected, ligated sequentially, and divided approximately 1 inch proximal to the pylorus. The stomach is lifted up by the assistant, bringing into the surgeon's view a bundle of tissue connecting the lesser curvature to the posterior abdominal wall (i.e., the celiac trunk). Palpation confirms pulsation of the left gastric artery within this tissue. Careful dissection permits the artery and vein to be visualized individually and tied off. The surrounding fat and lymph nodes are also removed during this maneuver. The left gastric artery is divided and ligated close to its origin from the celiac axis. The remaining loose adherent tissue, which contains a few small vessels, is divided, bringing the crura of the diaphragm into view. Gentle posterior pressure between the two pillars permits access to the posterior mediastinum, where loose areolar tissue can be broken down with gentle dissection. The phrenoesophageal ligament is transected around the esophagus to complete the mobilization. During this procedure, a cuff of diaphragmatic muscle can be resected if diaphragmatic invasion is suspected. After opening the diaphragmatic hiatus, access is gained to the fibrofatty and lymphatic tissue that separates the esophagus from the pericardium. This fibrofatty and lymphatic tissue is reflected away from the surrounding structures. In this way, much of the dissection of the lower esophagus can be achieved through the abdomen under direct vision. The gastric tubularization is performed using several linear staplers, starting from the gastric fundus down to the place on the small curvature where the right gastric artery has been ligated. The staple line is placed such that it leaves a gastric tube of 4 to 5 cm in width (Fig. 18-1). The staple line is

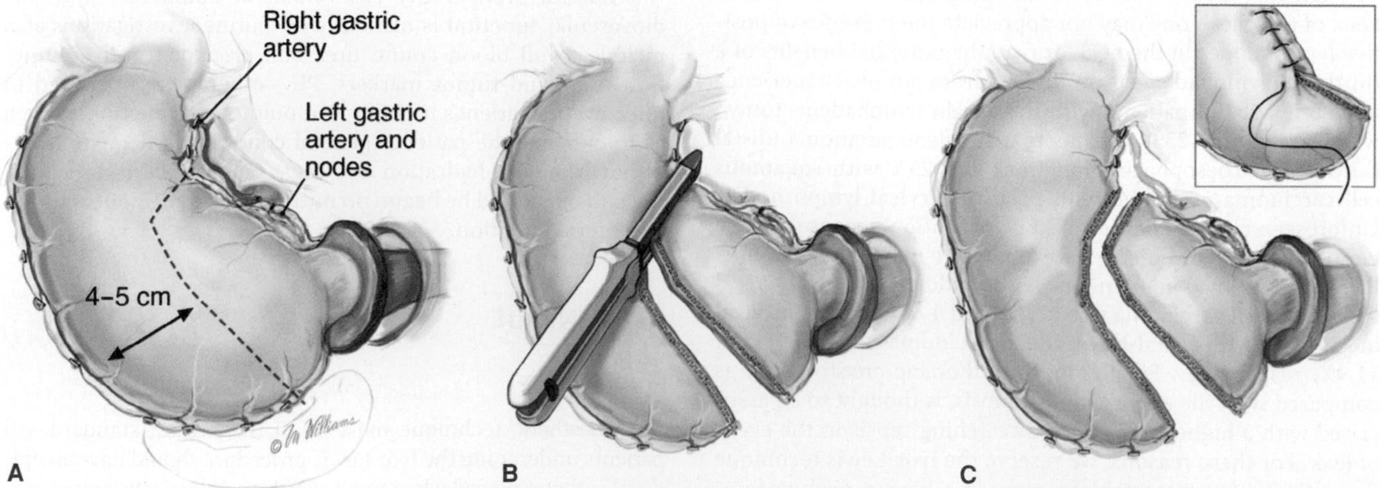

Figure 18-1. Gastric tube performed with staplers.

oversewn in a running fashion, although some surgeons prefer to use interrupted sutures. Thus, by resecting the lesser curvature, all lymphatic tissue in this area is removed. A lymph node dissection along the splenic artery, common hepatic artery, and celiac axis is performed. This also can be done en bloc with the dissection of the left gastric artery. The gastric tube is fixed to this separated lesser curvature by using two stay sutures.

At the end of the first stage of the procedure, it should be possible to place the pylorus at the hiatus, ensuring sufficient length for the reconstruction. Pyloroplasty is not carried out, but digitoclasy of the pylorus may be useful. The abdomen is closed.

Thoracic Dissection

A lateral thoracotomy (which can be extended anteriorly or posteriorly depending on the surgeon's preference) is performed through the fifth interspace. The serratus muscle is spared if possible.

The right lung is selectively deflated and retracted anteriorly. First, the azygos vein is dissected, ligated, and transected, as well as the underlying intercostobronchial artery. The mediastinal pleura anterior to the esophagus is opened widely from the azygos vein to the top of the chest. The proximal esophagus is dissected circumferentially and looped with an umbilical tape. The dissection is carried cephalad toward the apex of the chest, separating the esophagus from its tracheal and prevertebral attachments using the tape for traction and countertraction. Great care is taken to avoid injury to the membranous part of the trachea.

Similar dissection of the esophagus is achieved by encircling it with a tape distally from the distal pole of the tumor. During this dissection, it is important to remove the esophagus en bloc along with the surrounding tissues, including the thoracic duct and azygos vein, to achieve radical resection, especially if transmural extension is suspected. Dissection of the esophagus proceeds inferiorly, encompassing all tissue between the aorta and pericardium, including all periesophageal and subcarinal nodes. Both vagal nerves are transected.

A further lymph node dissection is performed along the left and right paratracheal spaces, along the aortopulmonary window, and along the right recurrent nerve at the level of the brachiocephalic trunk. To facilitate exposure of the right recurrent nerve, slight traction is exerted on the right vagus nerve, slightly stretching the recurrent nerve. Avoiding electrocautery is mandatory in this region to avoid injury to the nerve. Similarly, the left recurrent nerve is identified, and careful lymph node clearance is performed.

At this point, the gastric tube can be pulled up into the chest cavity, being careful to avoid axial rotation of the tube during this process (Fig. 18-2). A suitable point at least 5 cm above the tumor is chosen for transecting the esophagus. After transection, a frozen section must be obtained of the proximal resection margin to confirm the absence of tumor extension in the suture line.

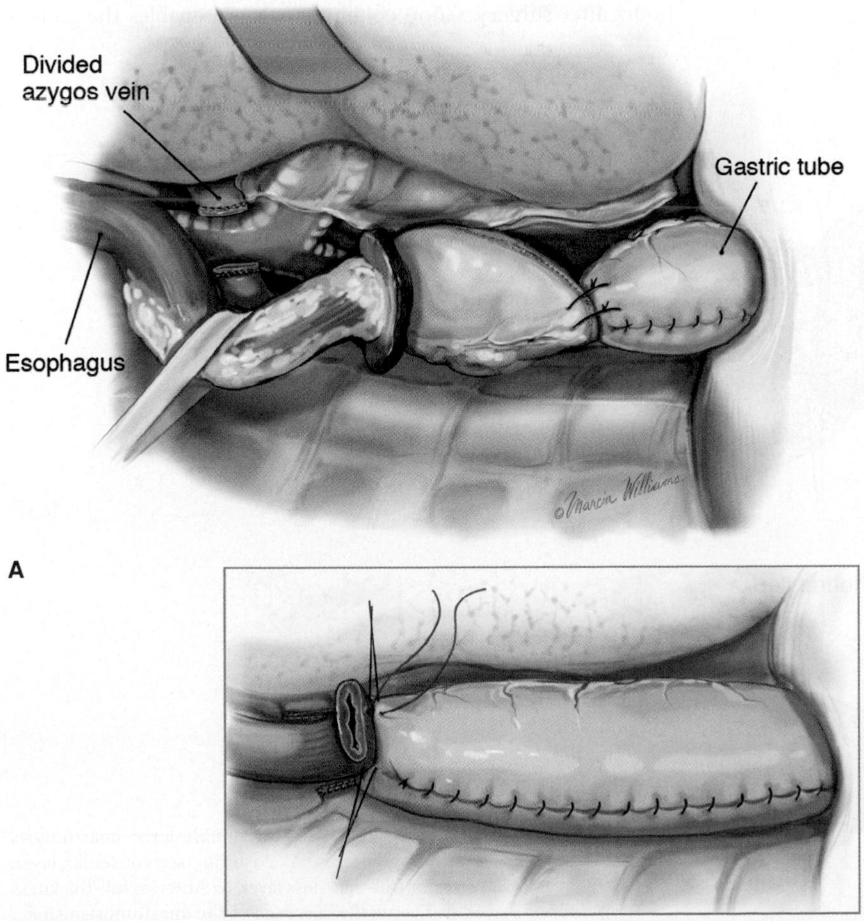

A

B

Figure 18-2. Hand-sewn anastomosis at the level of the azygos vein.

Anastomosis

A number of techniques have been described for esophagogastrostomy, including use of a circular stapler or hand-sewn anastomosis.

Stapled Anastomosis

For a mechanical anastomosis, the esophagus is transected, and a purse-string suture with, for example, Prolene 4-0 running suture, is placed through the mucosa and muscular layer. The anvil head of the circular stapler (size at least 25) is placed into the esophagus, and the purse-string suture is tied snugly around the shaft of the anvil head. An incision is made at the top of the gastric tube to insert the gun of the circular stapler. The site where the gun will perforate the gastric wall is chosen carefully on the posterior aspect of the gastric tube, away from previous staple lines and the greater curvature vessels. One also must verify that once the anastomosis is performed, it will not be under tension because this can lead to postoperative complications. After penetrating the gastric wall, the pointed shaft of the gun is detached, and the gun is connected to the anvil head. The gun then is fired in the customary manner, and the doughnuts are inspected to ensure the integrity and completeness of the anastomosis. Several nonabsorbable stitches can be placed between the muscular layer of the esophagus and the seromuscular lining of the stomach to strengthen and protect the anastomosis. The nasogastric tube then is advanced through the anastomosis into the gastric tube. The redundant part of the gastric tube including the opening used to insert the gun is then transected with a linear stapler, and the staple line is inverted with a running suture.

Hand-Sewn Anastomosis

For a hand-crafted anastomosis (Fig. 18-3), the posterior seromuscular aspect of the anastomosis is performed using separated nonabsorbable suture, for example, Ticron 3-0 stitches. The esophagus and gastric tubes then are incised along this suture line using electrocautery. The posterior layer comprising the full thickness of both the esophagus and gastric wall then is performed with separated absorbable suture, for example, Maxon 3-0 stitches. The gastric tube is advanced across the anastomosis. The anterior part of the esophageal wall is transected. The anastomosis is finalized using separated absorbable suture, for example, Maxon 3-0 for the anterior layer, and separated nonabsorbable suture, for example, Ticron 3-0 for the outer seromuscular layer. Some authors use a running suture, whereas others prefer a single-layer anastomosis.

In most cases we use a pleural flap to cover the anastomosis to protect the chest cavity from anastomotic leakage. The thoracic cavity is usually drained using a 36F chest drain placed in the paraspinous position. The chest wall is closed in layers.

POSTOPERATIVE MANAGEMENT

To optimize the results of surgery, this procedure should be performed at an appropriately equipped high-volume center with meticulous management of the postoperative course by an experienced staff. A chest radiograph is obtained in the OR to confirm complete lung expansion and appropriate placement of chest drains. Most patients can be extubated immediately or a few hours after surgery. Good epidural analgesia enables the patient

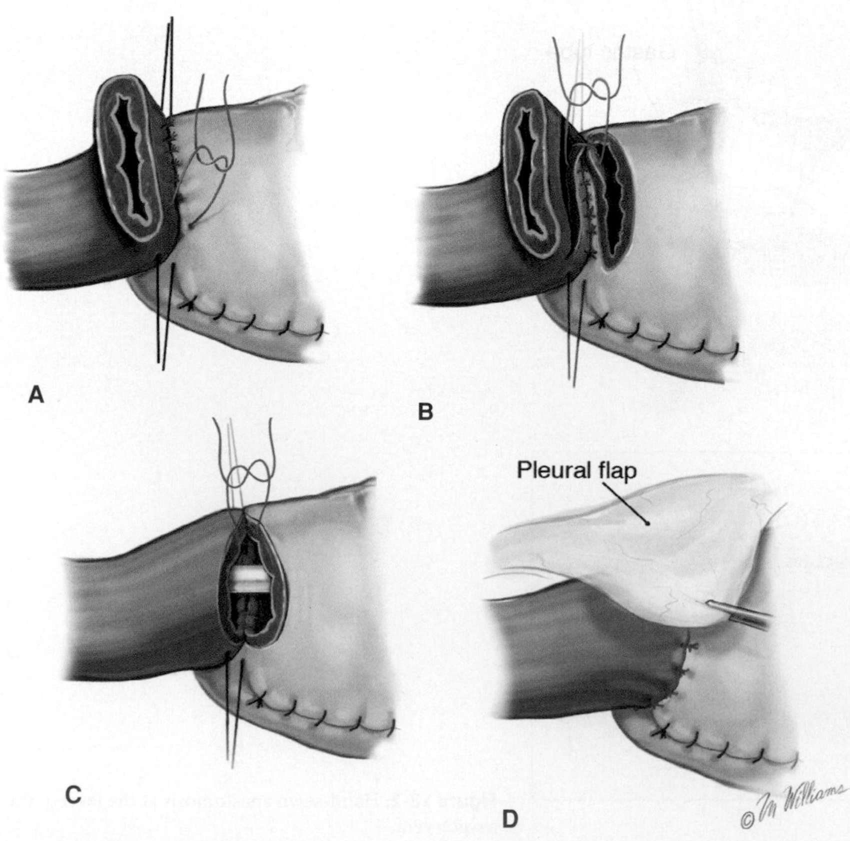

Figure 18-3. Technique of double-layer anastomosis with running sutures. *A.* Posterior seromuscular layer. *B.* Posterior full-thickness layer. *C.* Anterior full-thickness layer. *D.* Eventually coverage of the anastomosis using a pleural flap.

to sit upright in bed, breathe deeply, and cooperate fully with physiotherapy. If necessary, bronchoscopy or eventually a mini-tracheostomy either at the time of surgery or sometime thereafter to ensure enhanced bronchial cleaning can be performed.

Fluid balance and oxygen saturation should be closely monitored, and oxygen supplementation is mandatory. Fluid restriction is used to avoid cardiac and respiratory complications, especially in patients having neoadjuvant therapy. It is also vital to maintain adequate and balanced nutrition during the early postoperative period because many of these patients have suffered significant weight loss and are malnourished. Total parenteral nutrition is preferred.

Thrombosis prophylaxis is continued by subcutaneous low–molecular-weight heparin injections and prophylactic antibiotics given for 2 days.

Since it is essential to avoid intragastric stasis in the stomach tube, the nasogastric tube is kept in place to prevent respiratory complications secondary to aspiration.

On day 5, a contrast study is performed to evaluate the integrity of the anastomosis. If no leak is visualized, oral feeding is started. On the same day, the epidural catheter is removed, and the patient is encouraged to mobilize fully. Oral pain therapy can be started. The chest drain will be removed when the effluent amounts to less than 200 mL of fluid.

Patients are discharged when they are able to tolerate a soft diet and the pain is sufficiently controlled to permit normal mobilization. The patient is seen in the outpatient clinic 1 month after discharge, and based on the patient's general condition, further follow-up is arranged. After 1 year, the follow-up interval is every 6 months, and a clinical examination is routinely completed with CT chest abdomen and biochemistry.

COMPLICATIONS

Atelectasis and Respiratory Complications

Atelectasis and other respiratory problems are very common after transthoracic esophagectomy. Good analgesia, physiotherapy, adequate hydration (i.e., avoiding overhydration of the lungs), and early mobilization are key to minimizing these respiratory complications.

Anastomotic Leak

Anastomotic leaks may occur in the early postoperative period (2–3 days) owing to a technical failure. Leaks also can occur later (3–7 days) and are thought to be due to ischemic changes in the stomach, usually at the suture line and occasionally as a result of necrosis of the proximal end of the gastric tube. A subclinical leak detected on a contrast study usually heals without specific treatment. In case of minor leaks conservative treatment (i.e., nil by mouth, antibiotics, total parenteral nutrition, jejunostomy feeding, proton pump inhibitors, nasogastric tube, and possibly octreotide) will suffice. Early endoscopy is useful for determining the viability of the gastric tube and for evaluating a leak. Early dilation, if needed, is mandatory to allow free passage of saliva. Larger leaks in the chest that remain contained are treated the same way but will require adequate drainage of all collections through a pigtail catheter or chest tube, preferably placed under CT guidance for optimal positioning. Reintervention is necessary occasionally to control sepsis, in particular in the presence of diffuse intrathoracic collections. In the event of endoscopically documented gastric tube necrosis, immediate reintervention with resection of the necrotic stomach and diverting esophagostomy is the safest option. Placement of a jejunostomy tube for feeding is mandatory, if not already performed at the time of the esophagectomy. Reconstruction will be planned after 3 to 6 months, usually with a retrosternal colon.

Anastomotic Stricture

In many reports, at least a third of patients develop a stricture at the anastomosis. Dilation of the stricture can be accomplished by several means. The preferred method is endoscopic dilation with Savary dilators. The success rate, eventually, after several dilations, is high (>80%). When dealing with a more resistant stricture, balloon dilation and local steroid injection usually resolve the problem. The need for reintervention is extremely rare.

Delayed Gastric Emptying

Causes of delayed gastric emptying include lack of a pyloric drainage procedure when the whole stomach or wide gastric tubes are used, obstruction at a severely narrowed passage through the hiatus, and a redundant intrathoracic stomach resulting in kinking, axial twisting, or both. This infrequent but sometimes very bothersome complication is best tackled by endoscopic balloon dilation of the pylorus along with prokinetic agents (e.g., metoclopramide or erythromycin). If conservative management fails, reoperation with an adequate drainage procedure or repositioning of the gastric tube may become necessary.

Reflux

Reflux is a common problem after gastric pull-up, especially with an intrathoracic anastomosis. The level of severity seems to vary with the location of the anastomosis, with those above the azygos vein having a lower incidence than those below this level.[5] Small, frequent feedings, avoidance of liquids with meals, avoidance of the supine position after meals, and elevation of the patient's head while lying in bed are helpful in remediating these symptoms. Acid reflux is best treated with proton pump inhibitors to avoid the higher risk of anastomotic stricture formation through the caustic effect of the acid on the anastomosis. Intestinal metaplasia may develop in the remaining proximal esophagus as a result of mixed acid and biliary reflux. Therefore, regular endoscopic surveillance during follow-up is mandatory.

RESULTS

Modern-day results of the Ivor Lewis procedure have shown that the technique can be performed safely with a low morbidity and mortality (Table 18-1). Survival after Ivor Lewis esophagectomy for cancer of the esophagus has been described in several studies.[6–10] Visbal et al.[7] in their series of 220 consecutive patients had an overall 5-year survival of 25.2% (squamous cell and adenocarcinoma). In a series of 264 Ivor Lewis resections for squamous cell carcinoma of the esophagus, Lozac'h et al.[11] reported an overall survival of 33.3%. Survival was stage-dependent in both the series. Stage I was 94.4% and

Table 18-1

RECENTLY PUBLISHED OUTCOMES AFTER IVOR LEWIS ESOPHAGOGASTRECTOMY

SOURCE	TIME PERIOD (YEARS)	NUMBER OF PATIENTS	POSTOPERATIVE MORBIDITY	ANASTOMOTIC LEAKS	MORTALITY	MEDIAN LENGTH OF STAY (DAYS)
Lozac'h et al., 1998[11]	—	264	16% pulmonary	7%	4.5%	—
Gluch et al. 1999[8]	10	33	60.6%	9.1%	6.1%	26 overall 2.9 ICU
Karl et al., 2000 [6]	10	143	29%	3.5%	2.1%	13.5 overall 3.3 ICU
Visbal et al., 2001[7]	3	220	37.7%	0.9%	1.4%	11 overall ICU NA
Griffin et al., 2002[9]	10	228	45% overall 10% major	2%	4%	13 overall 1 ICU
Cerfolio et al., 2004[10]	4	90	26.6% overall 17.7% major	0%	4.4%	7 overall 0 ICU

53.2%, respectively; stage IIa was 36.0% and 38.8%, respectively; stage IIb in the first series was 14.3%, and stage III was 10% and 13.4%, respectively. In these two studies, the comparison between positive and negative lymph nodes after pathologic examination showed a significant improvement in 5-year survival for N0 (56.5% and 44.8%, respectively) versus N+ tumors (9.6% and 15.2%, respectively).

SUMMARY

The Ivor Lewis esophagectomy is a safe surgical approach with low morbidity and mortality in experienced hands. It allows for a radical resection under direct vision of most of the lymph node stations at risk. Because of the possibility of developing an intrathoracic leak at the anastomosis site and the absence of a third-field lymph node dissection, which is especially pertinent in cases of middle-third esophageal cancer, we prefer a three-hole (McKeown) approach. Nevertheless, for selected patients with previous neck surgery or cervical malignancy, for whom neck dissection and anastomosis are contraindicated, we still find the Ivor Lewis a suitable and preferred option. Recent advances in minimally invasive esophagectomy (MIE) focus on applying the Ivor Lewis approach by performing an intrathoracic anastomosis by means of video-assisted thoracic surgery (VATS).

CASE HISTORY

A 56-year-old man presented with dysphagia for solid food and weight loss of approximately 10 kg during the last month. His past medical history was positive for a hypopharyngeal carcinoma 4 years earlier that was treated with chemoradiation and surgery. The clinical examination was unremarkable except for induration of the neck region owing to fibrosis secondary to radiotherapy and surgery. At endoscopy, a tumor was noted in the middle third of the esophagus that proved on pathologic examination to be a moderately differentiated squamous cell carcinoma. Endoscopic ultrasound revealed invasion of the esophageal muscular layer and possibly localized invasion of the surrounding fat without lymph node involvement (uT3N0). Bronchoscopy appeared to be normal. CT scan of the chest and abdomen confirmed the presence of the lesion in the esophagus without enlarged lymph nodes and without liver or lung metastases. A control CT scan of the neck revealed no evidence of local recurrence of the previous hypopharyngeal carcinoma or enlarged lymph nodes. The PET scan showed enhanced uptake only on the primary tumor, without evidence of metastatic spread of the disease. Electrocardiogram, pulmonary function tests, and blood examination were normal. As a result, this patient was judged to be a good candidate for curative surgery. Furthermore, because of the extensive neck changes from previous radiotherapy and surgery, we opted to perform the Ivor Lewis operation, with anastomosis high in the chest.

The operation was performed as described earlier. No metastatic deposits were found in the liver, lung, or elsewhere. Esophagectomy was combined with a two-field lymph node dissection, resulting in a complete resection. The esophagogastrostomy was created using a mechanical anastomosis, as described earlier.

The pathologic examination of the specimen showed a 3-cm-long tumor of the middle third of the esophagus with invasion of the muscular wall (muscularis propria) of the esophagus but no breakthrough and with negative section planes. All 32 resected lymph nodes were free of tumor (pT2N0M0-R0).

The patient was extubated quickly and discharged to the thoracic surgery ward the day after surgery. On the second postoperative day, he developed atrial fibrillation, treated with IV amiodarone with conversion to normal sinus rhythm. On the fifth postoperative day, a routine contrast barium swallow showed absence of leak and good emptying of the gastric tube (Fig. 18-4). The nasogastric tube was removed, and oral feeding was started. The patient was discharged on day 10. At the first outpatient clinic appointment 1 month after surgery the patient presented with no dysphagia, slight pain at the thoracotomy level, and a slight degree of shortness of breath. The chest x-ray was unremarkable. Four years after surgery, this patient remains disease-free but is experiencing some degree of acid reflux, which has been treated successfully with proton pump inhibitors.

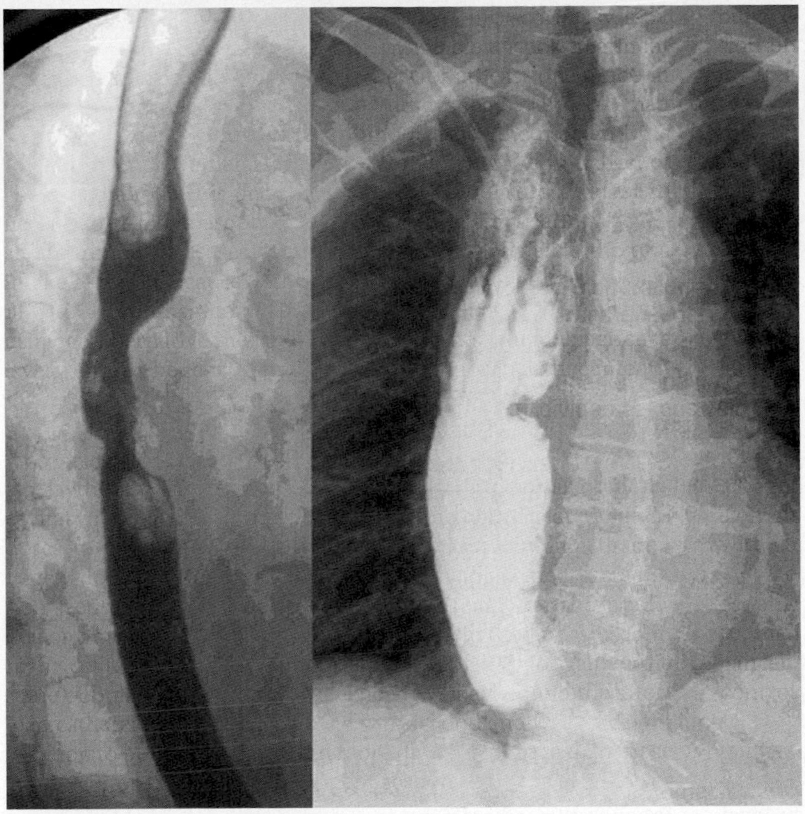

A B

Figure 18-4. Contrast swallow showing a middle-third esophageal neoplasm *(A)* and the contrast swallow 5 days after an Ivor Lewis esophagectomy *(B)*.

EDITOR'S COMMENT

In my opinion, this operation remains the mainstay for all esophageal cancer surgery. Especially in patients who have had neoadjuvant chemoradiation therapy or those with prior thoracic disease, this approach, whether done open or by laparoscopy/thoracoscopy, offers the best exposure to the esophagus and regional lymph nodes, as well as adjacent structures, aiding their resection and avoiding inadvertent injury. Although it does not permit three-field lymph node dissection, the need for this approach in distal GEJ tumors is as yet unproven. There are several minor technical differences in my own approach to this operation. I generally transect the stomach in the abdomen and then fashion the gastric tube before closing the belly. A routine feeding jejunostomy is performed at the initial laparotomy. At the time of the thoracotomy and anastomosis, more or less stomach can be pulled up into the chest as desired. This minimizes the amount of "redundant" gastric tube left lying in the chest, thereby avoiding the subsequent sequelae of reflux and dysphagia. Finally, when operating after chemoradiation, I routinely harvest an intercostal muscle flap when I enter the chest and use it to wrap the completed anastomosis and cover the gastric suture line.

—Mark J. Krasna

References

1. Lewis I. The surgical treatment of carcinoma of the esophagus with special reference to a new operation for growths of the middle third. *Br J Surg.* 1946;34:18–31.
2. Orringer MB, Marshall B, Stirling MC. Transhiatal esophagectomy for benign and malignant disease. *J Thorac Cardiovasc Surg.* 1993;105:265–276; discussion 76–77.
3. Akiyama H, Tsurumaru M, Udagawa H. Systematic lymph node dissection for esophageal cancer: effective or not? *Dis Esoph.* 1994;7:2–13.
4. Lerut T, Nafteux P, Moons J, et al. Three-field lymphadenectomy for carcinoma of the esophagus and gastroesophageal junction in 174 R_0 resections: impact on staging, disease-free survival, and outcome. A plea for adaptation of TNM classification in upper-half esophageal carcinoma. *Ann Surg.* 2004;240:962–972; discussion 72–74.
5. De Leyn P, Coosemans W, Lerut T. Early and late functional results in patients with intrathoracic gastric replacement after oesophagectomy for carcinoma. *Eur J Cardiothorac Surg.* 1992;6:79–84; discussion 85.
6. Karl RC, Schreiber R, Boulware D, et al. Factors affecting morbidity, mortality, and survival in patients undergoing Ivor Lewis esophagogastrectomy. *Ann Surg.* 2000;231:635–643.
7. Visbal AL, Allen MS, Miller DL, et al. Ivor Lewis esophagogastrectomy for esophageal cancer. *Ann Thorac Surg.* 2001;71:1803–1808.
8. Gluch L, Smith RC, Bambach CP, et al. Comparison of outcomes following transhiatal or Ivor Lewis esophagectomy for esophageal carcinoma. *World J Surg.* 1999;23:271–275; discussion 5–6.
9. Griffin SM, Shaw IH, Dresner SM. Early complications after Ivor Lewis subtotal esophagectomy with two-field lymphadenectomy: risk factors and management. *J Am Coll Surg.* 2002;194:285–297.
10. Cerfolio RJ, Bryant AS, Bass CS, et al. Fast tracking after Ivor Lewis esophagogastrectomy. *Chest.* 2004;126:1187–1194.
11. Lozac'h P, Topart P, Perramant M. Ivor Lewis procedure for epidermoid carcinoma of the esophagus: a series of 264 patients. *Semin Surg Oncol.* 1997;13:238.

19 Radical En Bloc Esophagectomy

Paul C. Lee and Nasser K. Altorki

Keywords: Esophageal cancer, radical en bloc esophagectomy, two- or three-field esophagectomy, staging, extended lymphadenectomy

Despite improvements in perioperative care, surgical techniques, and neoadjuvant therapy over the last decade, the prognosis of esophageal cancer remains poor. More than 95% of new cases diagnosed annually in the United States succumb to disease. Among the subset of patients resected with curative intent (R0 resection), the 5-year survival after transthoracic esophagectomy or transhiatal esophagectomy rarely exceeds 30% based on reports from large surgical series.[1–4] The principal justification for these poor results is the finding that most patients develop metastatic disease and already may have disseminated disease at the time of diagnosis. A careful analysis of the patterns of failure after surgical resection also implicates inadequate locoregional control. The locoregional failure rates are unacceptably high after conventional surgical resection, ranging from 30% to 60%.[5–8] The addition of preoperative therapy of any kind does not meaningfully reduce the high rate of local failure.[6–8] Thus a meaningful improvement in the survival of patients with esophageal cancer is unlikely without adequate locoregional control.

En bloc resection for tumor of the lower esophagus and cardia was first described by Logan in 1963.[9] The reported 5-year survival was unparalleled at the time but was achieved at the cost of high operative mortality. In 1979, Skinner revisited the en bloc approach and extended its use to tumors of the middle and proximal esophagus, publishing his first report in 1983.[10] A few years earlier, Orringer and Sloan[11] published their first report on the transhiatal approach for esophagectomy without thoracotomy. The controversy continues to the present concerning the efficacy of radical en bloc esophagectomy, and most surgeons favor conventional techniques of esophageal resection through either a transthoracic or a transhiatal approach. However, we and others continue to advocate radical en bloc esophageal resection as the optimal procedure for maximizing locoregional control and improving long-term survival in patients with esophageal cancer.[12] The basic concept of en bloc esophagectomy is resection of the tumor-bearing esophagus with a wide margin of surrounding tissues. Thus, for tumors of the middle or lower thoracic esophagus, the en bloc specimen includes the tumor-bearing esophagus, the pericardium anteriorly, both pleural surfaces laterally, and the thoracic duct and all other lymphoareolar tissue wedged posteriorly between the esophagus and the spine. The associated lymphadenectomy includes en bloc resection of all nodal groups in the middle and lower mediastinum as well as the upper abdomen.

For a selected group of patients, the lymphadenectomy is extended to include the superior mediastinal and cervical lymph nodes (three-field lymph node dissection). The three-field concept was first introduced by Japanese surgeons, prompted by their observation that up to 40% of patients resected by radical two-field esophagectomy developed isolated recurrences in the cervical nodes.[13] In 1991, Isono et al.[14] reported nationwide results of three-field lymph node dissection and found that occult cervical node metastases occurred in one-third of patients. Even for lower-third tumors, up to 20% of patients harbored cervical metastases. Most Western surgeons have been reluctant to adopt the three-field dissection technique for two principal reasons: skepticism that long-term survival can be achieved once nodal disease is present and the reported high morbidity associated with the operation. In particular, injury to one or both recurrent laryngeal nerves has been described in as many as 50% of patients with a consequent high risk for tracheostomy.[15,16]

PREOPERATIVE ASSESSMENT

Preoperative assessment is directed toward establishing, as accurately as possible, the clinical stage of the disease, as well as assessing the patient's ability to tolerate the planned operation. Our standard diagnostic and staging workup includes an upper endoscopy with biopsy and CT scan of the chest and upper abdomen in all patients. In addition, patients currently undergo endoscopic ultrasonography as well as positron emission tomography. The former is useful in selecting patients for clinical trials of preoperative induction therapy, whereas the latter is a more sensitive test for detecting distant visceral and skeletal metastases. Generally, patients are considered for primary surgical resection if the preoperative evaluation reveals no evidence of distant visceral metastases or clear evidence of direct neoplastic invasion of the airway or major vascular structures. The presence of extensive nodal disease is not considered a contraindication to resection unless it clearly extends beyond the proposed fields of dissection. Finally, all patients are evaluated for pulmonary and cardiac function to determine their ability to withstand the planned procedure.

OPERATIVE TECHNIQUE

The basic principle underlying en bloc esophagectomy is resection of the tumor-bearing esophagus within a wide envelope of periesophageal tissue, which includes both pleural surfaces laterally, a patch of pericardium anteriorly, and the thoracic duct posteriorly, along with the mediastinal lymph nodes from the tracheal bifurcation to the hiatus (Fig. 19-1).

An upper abdominal lymphadenectomy is also performed, including the celiac, common hepatic, left gastric, parahiatal, lesser curvature, and retroperitoneal lymph nodes. A "third field" nodal dissection can be incorporated by extending the lymphadenectomy to include the superior mediastinal and

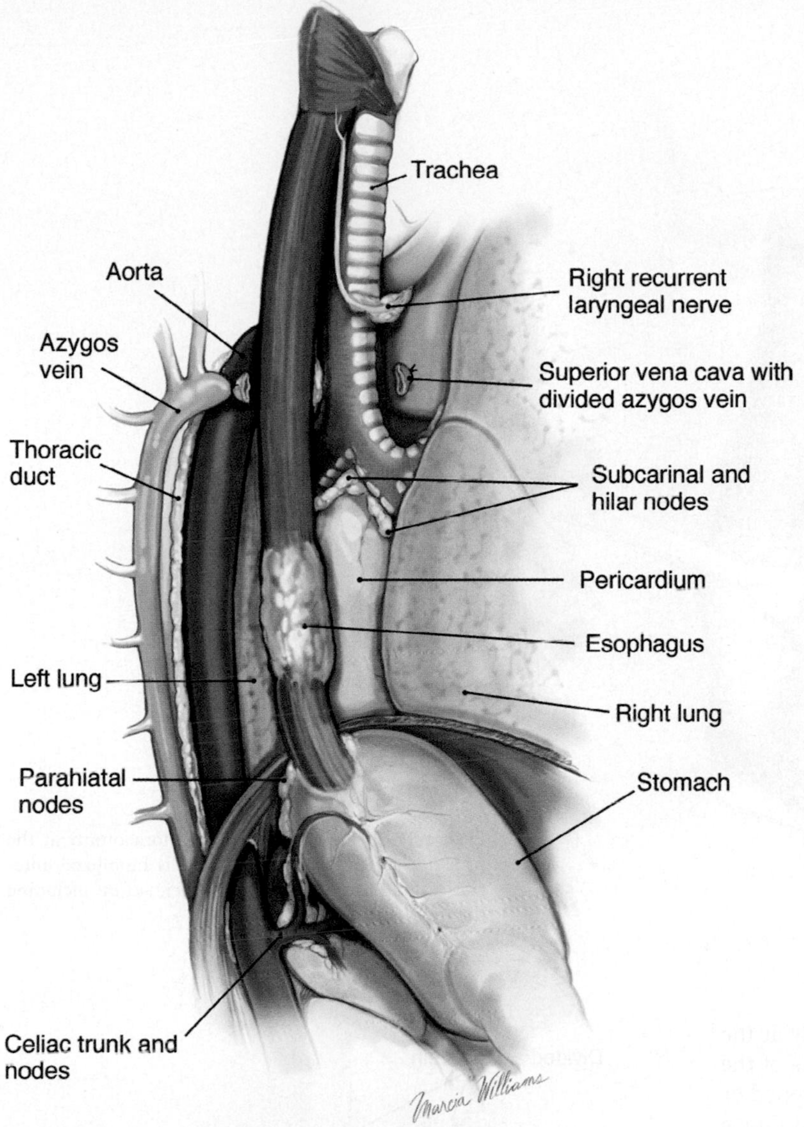

Figure 19-1. Radical en bloc esophagectomy entails resection of the tumor-bearing esophagus within a wide envelope of periesophageal tissue from the tracheal bifurcation to the hiatus.

cervical lymph nodes (Fig. 19-2). The procedure is almost always carried out through three incisions: a right thoracotomy, followed by a laparotomy and collar neck incision. More recently, the thoracic and abdominal portions of the dissection are accomplished by a minimally invasive approach.

The Thorax

A right fifth interspace thoracotomy is performed regardless of the location of the tumor within the esophagus (Fig. 19-3, inset). The "first field" comprises the middle and lower mediastinum and is bound superiorly by the tracheal bifurcation, inferiorly by the esophageal hiatus, anteriorly by the hilum of the lung and pericardium, and posteriorly by the descending thoracic aorta and the spine. Dissection of the middle and lower mediastinum begins by incising the mediastinal pleura over the anterior aspect of the azygos vein from the level of the azygos arch superiorly to the aortic hiatus inferiorly. The dissection proceeds leftward anterior to the aorta and across the mediastinum to the opposite pleura, which is entered along the entire length of the incision. The thoracic duct thus is mobilized

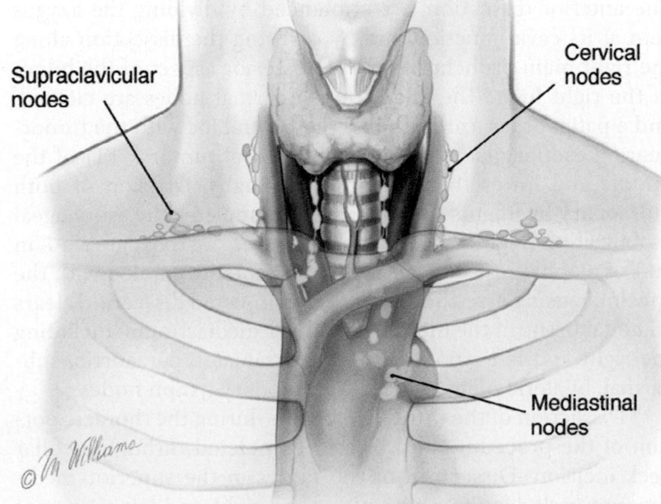

Figure 19-2. A "third field" nodal dissection is performed by extending the lymphadenectomy to include the superior mediastinal and cervical lymph nodes.

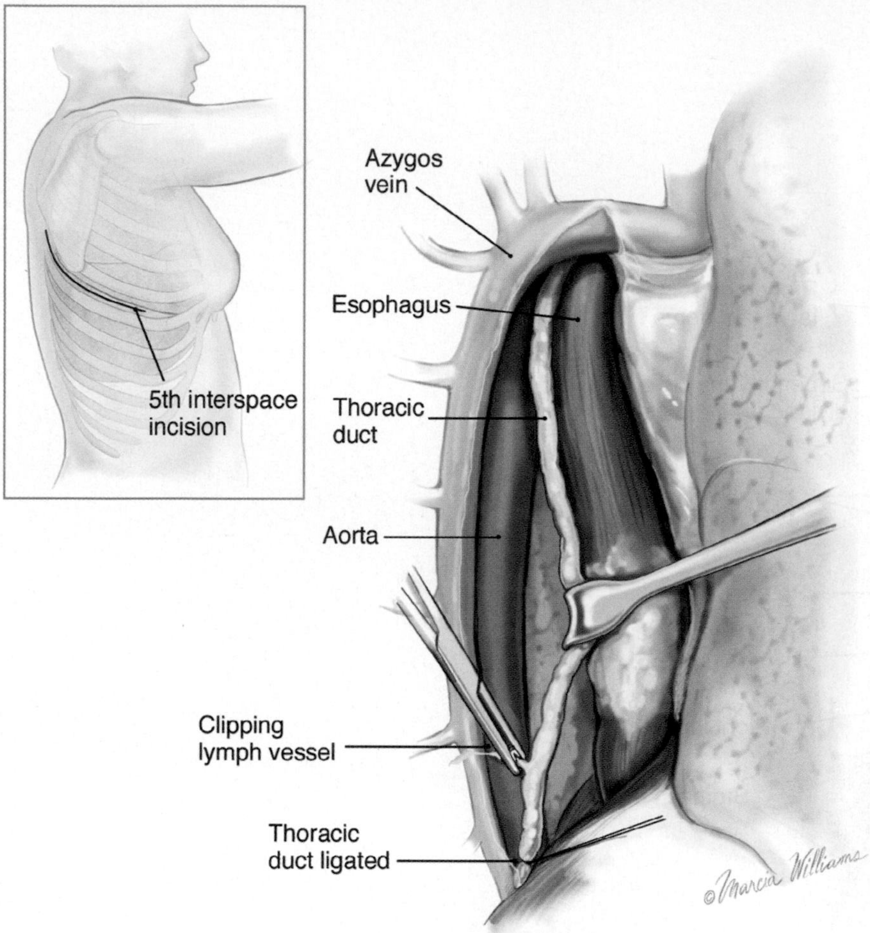

Figure 19-3. View from a right thoracotomy at the fifth interspace (inset). Specimen is mobilized anteriorly along the descending thoracic aorta, including the thoracic duct.

anteriorly toward the specimen and is ligated inferiorly at the aortic hiatus and superiorly as it crosses to the left side of the mediastinum (Fig. 19-3). All lymphatic channels are clipped or ligated between the thoracic duct and the spine to minimize the probability of a chylothorax. The arch of the azygos vein, but not its main trunk, is resected en bloc with the specimen. The anterior dissection is commenced by dividing the azygos vein at its caval junction and by carrying the dissection along the right main bronchus and the posterior aspect of the hilum of the right lung. The hilar and subcarinal nodes are cleared, and a patch of pericardium is resected en bloc with the tumor-bearing esophagus for all but submucosal tumors (T1) of the middle and lower thirds of the esophagus. Division of both pulmonary ligaments (left and right) completes the esophageal mobilization (Fig. 19-4). For tumors traversing the hiatus, a 1-in cuff of diaphragm is excised circumferentially en bloc with the specimen using electrocautery. The completed dissection clears all nodal tissue in the middle and lower mediastinum, including the right and left paraesophageal, parahiatal, paraaortic, subcarinal, bilateral hilar, and aortopulmonary lymph nodes.

Dissection of the third field begins during the thoracic portion of the procedure and is later completed through a collar neck incision. Dissection of the nodes in the superior mediastinum includes the nodes along the right and left recurrent laryngeal nerves throughout their mediastinal course. The paratracheal retrocaval compartment is not disturbed. The left recurrent nerve is dissected using a "no touch" technique, and

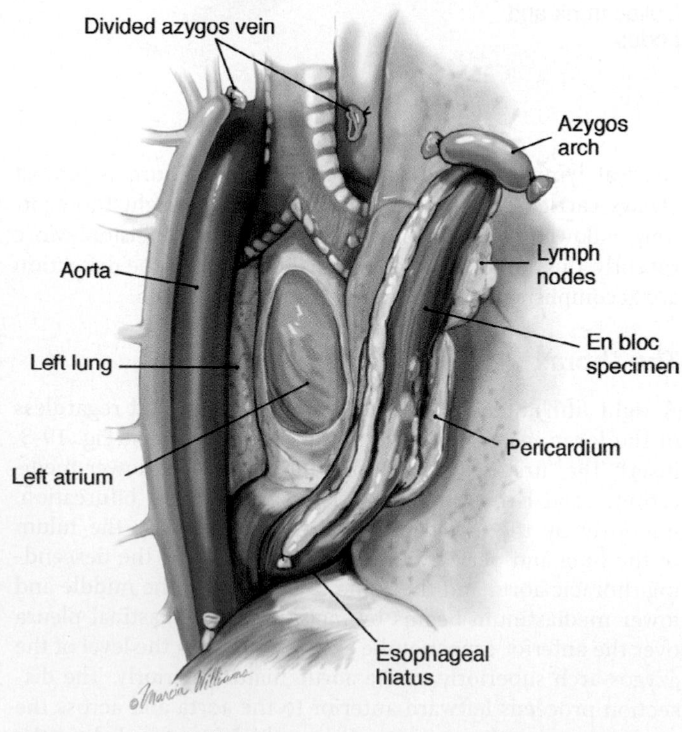

Figure 19-4. The en bloc specimen is completely mobilized, revealing the left lung, the tracheal bifurcation, and the pericardium.

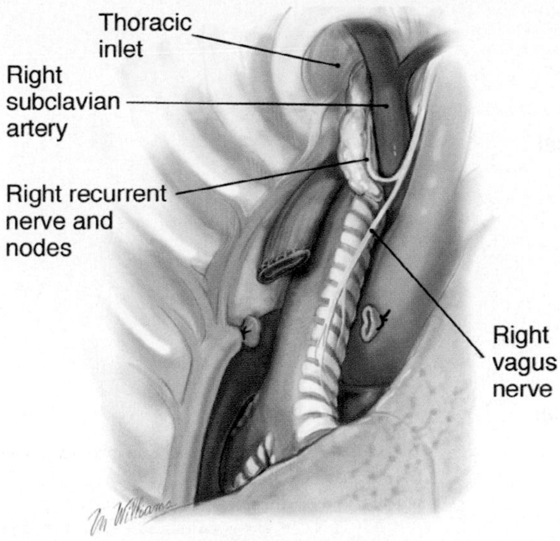

Figure 19-5. The right recurrent nerve is carefully exposed near its origin at the base of the right subclavian artery. The right vagus nerve serves as a guide to locate the right recurrent nerve. The right recurrent nodal chain begins at that level and forms a continuous package that extends through the thoracic inlet to the neck.

nodes along its anterior aspect are carefully excised. Notably, there is a paucity of nodal tissue along the left nerve in nearly all Caucasians. The right recurrent nerve is carefully exposed near its origin at the base of the right subclavian artery (Fig. 19-5). The right vagus nerve serves as a good guide to locate the right recurrent nerve. The right recurrent nodal chain begins at that level and forms a continuous package that extends through the thoracic inlet to the neck. Again, the nerve is dissected using a strict no touch technique. Through the cervical incision, the remainders of the recurrent nodes are dissected, as are the lower deep cervical nodes located posterior and lateral to the carotid sheath. Thus the third field includes a continuous anatomically inseparable chain of nodes that extends from the superior mediastinum to the lower neck. These nodes should be appropriately labeled cervicothoracic nodes rather than cervical nodes.

The Abdomen

The abdomen is entered through a midline incision (Fig. 19-6, inset). The omentum is separated from the colon in the avascular plane, and the lesser sac is entered. After dividing the short gastric vessels, the retroperitoneum is incised along the superior border of the pancreas (Fig. 19-6). The retroperitoneal lymphatic and areolar tissues are swept superiorly toward the esophageal hiatus and medially along the splenic artery to the celiac trifurcation. The left gastric artery is divided flush with its celiac origin, and the nodes along the common hepatic artery are dissected toward the specimen. This retroperitoneal dissection is bound by the dissected esophageal hiatus superiorly, the hilum of the spleen laterally, and the common hepatic artery and inferior vena cava medially. Finally, the lesser curvature and left gastric nodes are included with the specimen as the gastric tube is prepared. The omentum is resected as a separate specimen at least 1 in outside the gastroepiploic arcade.

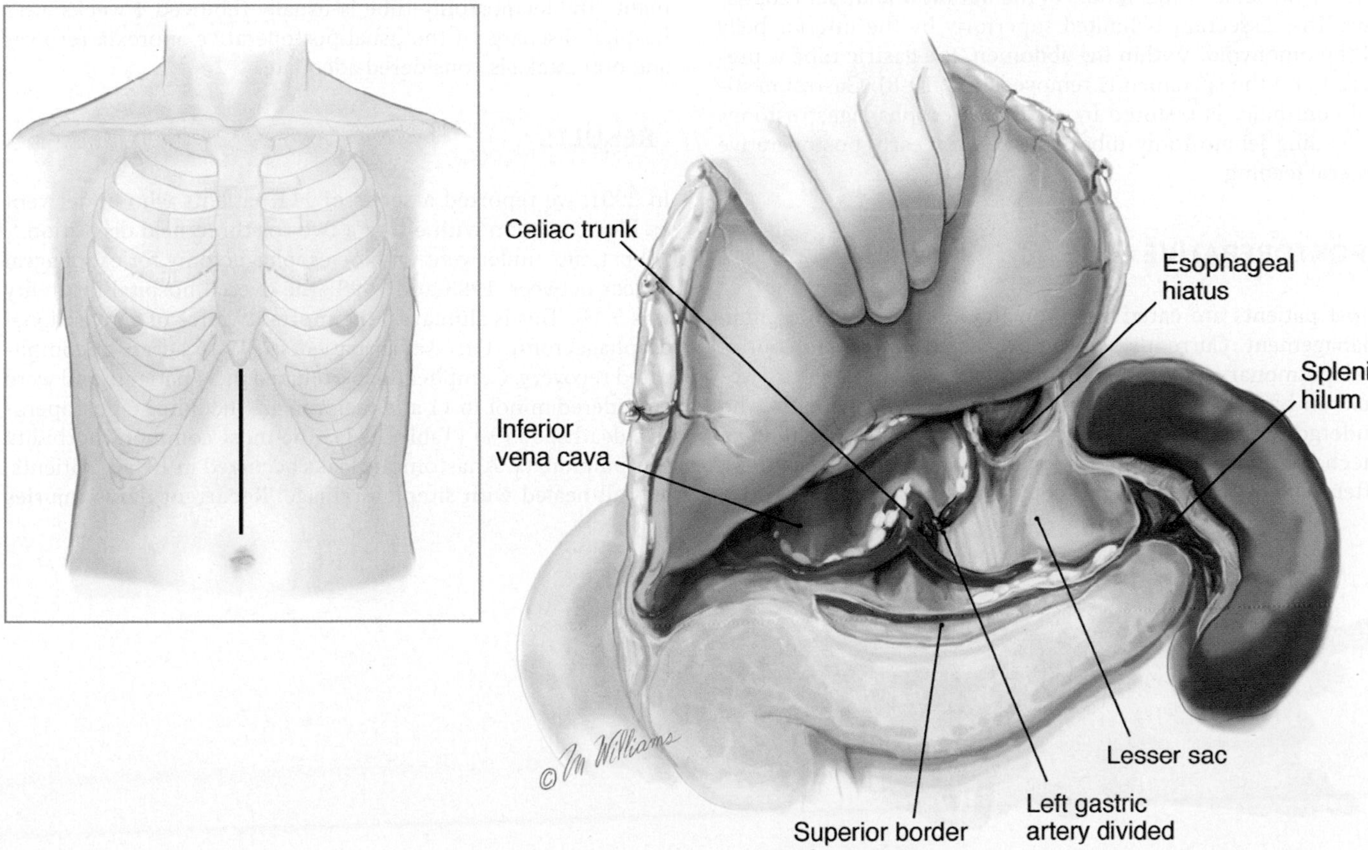

Figure 19-6. Illustration of abdominal en bloc dissection.

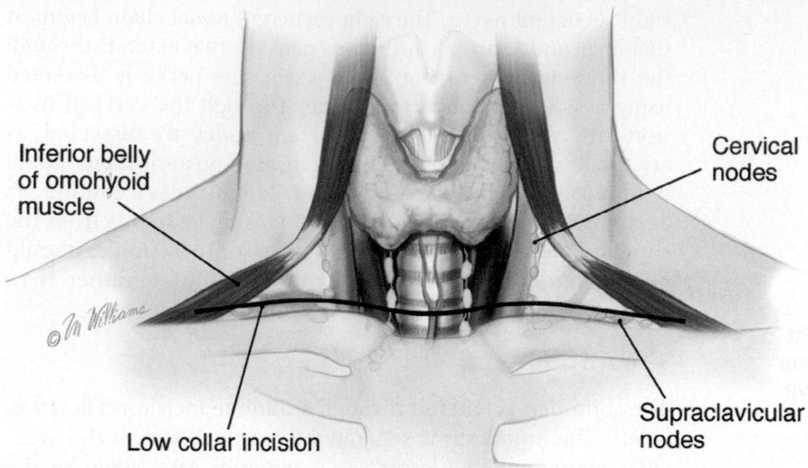

Figure 19-7. Low collar incision provides access for dividing the esophagus.

The Neck

A generous low collar incision is performed, and subplatysmal flaps are raised inferiorly and superiorly (Fig. 19-7). The strap muscles and the medial heads of the sternocleidomastoid are divided. The esophagus (previously fully mobilized from the thorax) is retrieved from the prevertebral space. The esophagus is divided distally, and the specimen is retrieved in the abdomen. The previously dissected recurrent nerves are easy to visualize (especially the right recurrent nerve), and any residual nodal tissue is excised. Next, the nodes posterior and lateral to the carotid sheath are removed, along with the supraclavicular nodes, particularly for tumors of the middle and upper esophagus. The dissection is limited superiorly by the inferior belly of the omohyoid. Within the abdomen, the gastric tube is prepared and the specimen is removed (Fig. 19-8). Gastrointestinal continuity is restored by a cervical esophagogastrostomy. A feeding jejunostomy tube is placed for early postoperative enteral feeding.

POSTOPERATIVE CARE

Most patients are cared for in an ICU for 24 hours for fluid management. Currently, with improved epidural pain control and pulmonary physiotherapy, patients who undergo a two-field en bloc resection are extubated in the OR. Patients who undergo a three-field en bloc resection often require 24 hours of mechanical ventilation. Intense pulmonary hygiene is required, often with repeated bronchoscopy for the first 48 hours after extubation, because most patients have bronchorrhea, which generally resolves on the third or fourth postoperative day. Patients often demonstrate significant fluid sequestration postoperatively, with spontaneous diuresis by the third postoperative day. Aggressive physical therapy is essential for getting patients out of bed and ambulating. Enteral jejunostomy feeding is started by the fourth or fifth postoperative day. Chest tubes are removed when drainage is less than 250 mL/day. Oral intake is begun once anastomotic integrity is confirmed by a contrast study on the sixth or seventh postoperative day. Patients are discharged by the tenth postoperative day on a regular diet but often require supplemental jejunostomy feeding at night. The jejunostomy tube is usually removed 4 weeks after hospital discharge if the usual postoperative anorexia resolves and oral intake is considered adequate.

RESULTS

In 2001, we reported a series of 111 patients who underwent en bloc resection with either a two- or three-field dissection.[17] All patients underwent en bloc esophagectomy for esophageal cancer between 1988 and 1998. The overall hospital mortality was 5.4%. This is similar to the mortality rates of conventional esophagectomy. Fifty-seven patients (51%) had an uncomplicated recovery. Complications occurred in 54 patients and were considered minor in 11 and major in 43 (including 6 postoperative deaths; 38.7%) (Table 19-1). The most common morbidity was pulmonary. Anastomotic leaks occurred in 13% of patients, and all healed with simple drainage. Recurrent nerve injuries

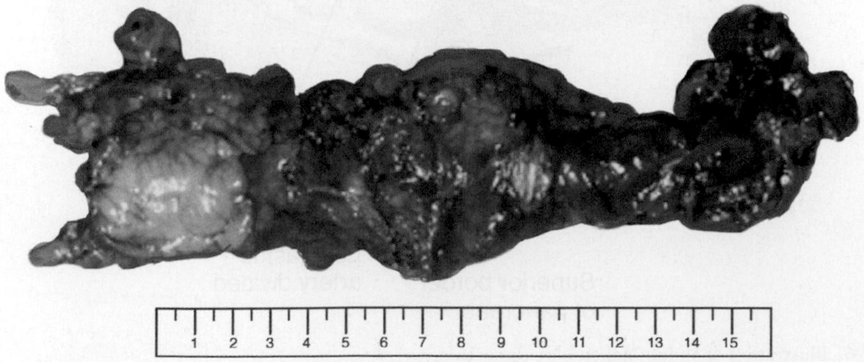

Figure 19-8. The surgical specimen is removed through the abdomen.

Table 19-1

SURGICAL COMPLICATIONS

Leak	15 (13.5%)
Anastomotic	10 (9%)
Gastric tip necrosis	5 (4.5%)
Pulmonary	30 (27%)
Reintubation	17
Tracheostomy	10
Lobar collapse	9
Pneumonia	8
Cardiac	11 (11.7%)
Myocardial infarction	1
Supraventricular arrhythmia	10
Pericarditis	2
Infectious complications	11 (10%)
Wound	2
Abscess	1
Urinary tract infection	1
Empyema	8[a]
Chylothorax	2
Recurrent nerve injury (unilateral)	4
Other	11 (10%)
Splenectomy	1
Renal failure	1
Stroke	1
Pulmonary embolism	2
Delirium tremens	5
Peritonitis	1

[a]Including six patients with anastomotic leaks. From Altorki N, Skinner D. Should en bloc esophagectomy be the standard of care for esophageal carcinoma? *Ann Surg*. 2001;234:581–587., with permission.

occurred in only four patients and were unilateral in all. No patients required tracheostomy as a result of recurrent nerve injury.

Overall 5-year survival for all patients was 40%, with a median survival of 38 months (Fig. 19-9). Node-negative patients had a significantly improved 5-year survival of 75% compared with 26% in node-positive patients. More impressively, the 5-year survival for stage III patients was 39% compared with 11% after conventional transthoracic esophagectomy, as reported previously.[18] This is especially important because most of the patients presenting with esophageal cancer

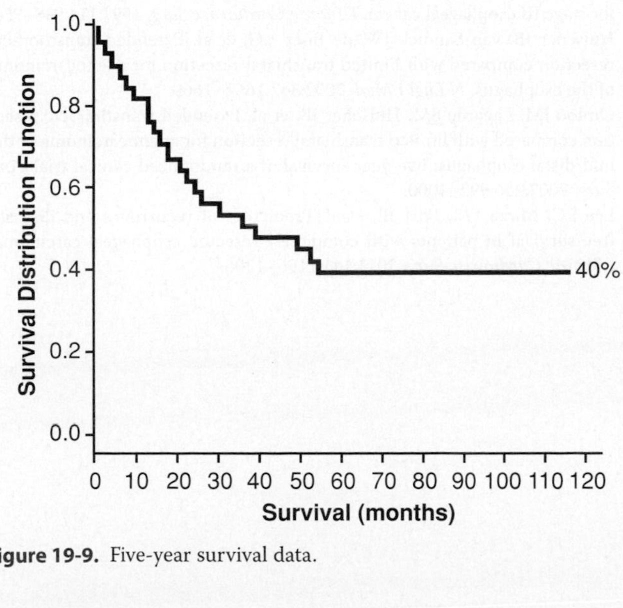

Figure 19-9. Five-year survival data.

have stage III disease. It is interesting to observe that for stage IV patients, 5-year survival was 27%. Survival also was significantly better for patients with locoregional N1 nodal metastases compared with distant M1a nodal metastases (31% vs. 21%, $p = 0.03$). Nonetheless, even for patients with distant nodal metastases (celiac or recurrent laryngeal nodes), there were long-term survivors. These data suggest that these patients should be classified as a subgroup of stage III rather than stage IV. Overall local recurrence rate was 8%, comparing favorably with the 31% to 45% incidence of local recurrence reported after conventional esophagectomy.

In 2004, Lerut published the results of a cohort of 174 R0 resections in patients with esophageal cancer using en bloc esophagectomy with three-field lymphadenectomy.[12] Hospital mortality was 1.2%, and morbidity was 58%. Overall 3-and 5-year survivals were 51% and 41.9%, respectively, with disease-free survival of 51.4% and 46.3%, respectively. The locoregional lymph node recurrence was impressively low at 5.2%. The 5-year survival for node-negative patients was 80.2% compared with 24.5% for node-positive patients. The prevalence of metastatic disease to the cervical nodes was high: 23% in patients with adenocarcinoma and 25% in patients with squamous cell carcinoma. The 5-year survival in patients with positive cervical nodes in middle-third carcinomas was 27.2%, leading the author to suggest that these nodes should be considered as regional (N1) rather than distant metastasis (M1b) in middle-third carcinomas.

A randomized trial comparing transthoracic en bloc esophagectomy with transhiatal resection was published by Hulscher in 2002.[19] Although the difference in survival between the two groups was not statistically significant, there was a trend toward a survival benefit with en bloc resection at 5 years. Five-year overall and disease-free survival rates in the en bloc group were 39% and 39%, respectively, compared with 29% and 27% in the transhiatal group. Transthoracic en bloc esophagectomy was associated with higher morbidity than transhiatal esophagectomy, consistent with the wider extent of dissection and complexity of the resection. The authors subsequently published a subgroup analysis showing that in patients with Siewert type I tumors, en bloc resection was associated with an absolute survival advantage of 14% compared to transhiatal resection (51% vs. 37%).[20] Further analysis suggested that the benefit may be limited to patients with 1 to 8 positive nodes rather than those with higher nodal burden or those without nodal metastases.

Recently, we reported our series of 465 patients who had a R0 resection for esophageal cancer.[21] A total of 328 patients (71%) had an en bloc resection (two-field lymphadenectomy in 129, three-field in 199). The remaining 137 patients (29%) had a conventional esophagectomy. Multivariate regression analysis was used to identify independent predictors of freedom from recurrence and disease-free survival. Other than good performance status and early pathologic stage, en bloc resection was a significant independent predictor of improved freedom from recurrence and disease-free survival.

SUMMARY

Radical en bloc esophagectomy can be performed with low mortality and similar morbidity to conventional transthoracic or transhiatal esophagectomy. It provides the most thorough staging information. Locoregional recurrence rates are substantially reduced, with improved disease-free survival. En bloc resection appears to have a favorable impact on survival, especially in patients with limited nodal metastases.

CASE HISTORY

Surveillance endoscopy on a 72-year-old man with a long history of Barrett esophagus showed an ulcerated lesion of the distal esophagus. Biopsy results showed squamous cell carcinoma. CT of the chest and upper abdomen showed no obvious esophageal mass or nodal metastases. Endoscopic ultrasonography demonstrated a T2N0 esophageal carcinoma. Preoperative cardiopulmonary evaluation indicated that the patient was a good candidate for surgical resection, and he underwent en bloc esophagectomy with three-field lymphadenectomy. The patient was extubated on postoperative day 1 and had an episode of atrial fibrillation on postoperative day 3 that was successfully treated pharmacologically. Barium study on postoperative day 6 revealed no evidence of a leak, and oral diet was commenced. The patient was discharged home on postoperative day 8 on supplemental jejunostomy feeding. Final pathology revealed a T1N1M0 (stage IIB) squamous cell carcinoma of the distal esophagus with a single nodal metastasis in the right recurrent laryngeal nodal chain. The patient received no adjuvant therapy. After 5 years of follow-up, the patient remains disease-free.

EDITOR'S COMMENT

Clearly, this technique has not "caught on" yet among the majority of esophageal surgeons. The Cornell group is to be commended, however, as their careful reporting of the data also has resulted in their recent adaptation of this technique to minimally invasive esophagectomy. As yet, no convincing data comparing radical versus nonradical or two-field versus three-field esophagectomies have emerged to show a survival advantage stage by stage. It will be interesting to see whether there are differences going forward, especially given the changes in N that appear in the new AJCC staging system (7th edition). Other than the major risk of tracheostomy postoperatively, the procedure can be done with similar results by experienced surgeons.

—Mark J. Krasna

References

1. Orringer MB, Marshall B, Iannettoni MD. Transhiatal esophagectomy: clinical experience and refinements. *Ann Surg.* 1999;230:392–400.
2. Ellis FH Jr, Heatley GJ, Krasna MJ, et al. Esophagogastrectomy for carcinoma of the esophagus and cardia: a comparison of findings and results after standard resection in three consecutive eight-year intervals with improved staging criteria. *J Thorac Cardiovasc Surg.* 1997;113:836–846.
3. Lieberman MD, Shriver CD, Bleckner S, et al. Carcinoma of the esophagus: prognostic significance of histologic type. *J Thorac Cardiovasc Surg.* 1995;109:130–138.
4. Putnam JB Jr, Suell DM, McMurtrey MJ, et al. Comparison of three techniques of esophagectomy within a residency training program. *Ann Thorac Surg.* 1994;57:319–325.
5. Altorki NK. The rationale for radical resection. *Surg Oncol Clin North Am.* 1999;8:295–305.
6. Herskovic A, Martz K, Al-Sarraf M, et al. Combined chemotherapy and radiotherapy compared with radiotherapy alone in patients with cancer of the esophagus. *N Engl J Med.* 1992;326:1593–1598.
7. Kelsen DP, Ginsberg R, Pajak TF, et al. Chemotherapy followed by surgery compared with surgery alone for localized esophageal cancer. *N Engl J Med.* 1998;339:1979–1984.
8. Law S, Fok M, Chow S, et al. Preoperative chemotherapy versus surgical therapy alone for squamous cell carcinoma of the esophagus: a prospective, randomized trial. *J Thorac Cardiovasc Surg.* 1997;114:210–217.
9. Logan A. The surgical treatment of carcinoma of the esophagus and cardia. *J Thorac Cardiovasc Surg.* 1963;46:150–161.
10. Skinner DB. En bloc resection for neoplasms of the esophagus and cardia. *J Thorac Cardiovasc Surg.* 1983;85:59–71.
11. Orringer MB, Sloan H. Esophagectomy without thoracotomy. *J Thorac Cardiovasc Surg.* 1978;76:643–654.
12. Lerut T, Nafteux P, Moons J, et al. Three-field lymphadenectomy for carcinoma of the esophagus and gastroesophageal junction in 174 R_0 resections: impact on staging, disease-free survival, and outcome. A plea for adaptation of TNM classification in upper-half esophageal carcinoma. *Ann Surg.* 2004;240:962–972.
13. Isono K, Onoda S, Okuyama K, et al. Recurrence of intrathoracic esophageal cancer. *Jpn J Clin Oncol.* 1985;15:49–60.
14. Isono K, Sato H, Nakayama K. Results of a nationwide study on the three-field lymph node dissection of esophageal cancer. *Oncology.* 1991;48:411–420.
15. Fujita H, Kakegawa T, Yamana H, et al. Mortality and morbidity rates, postoperative course, quality of life, and prognosis after extended radical lymphadenectomy for esophageal cancer: comparison of three-field lymphadenectomy with two-field lymphadenectomy. *Ann Surg.* 1995;222:654–662.
16. Nishihira T, Hirayama K, Mori S. A prospective, randomized trial of extended cervical and superior mediastinal lymphadenectomy for carcinoma of the thoracic esophagus. *Am J Surg.* 1998;175:47–51.
17. Altorki N, Skinner D. Should en bloc esophagectomy be the standard of care for esophageal carcinoma? *Ann Surg.* 2001;234:581–587.
18. Altorki NK, Girardi L, Skinner DB. En bloc esophagectomy improves survival for stage III esophageal cancer. *J Thorac Cardiovasc Surg.* 1997;114:948–956.
19. Hulscher JB, van Sandick JW, de Boer AG, et al. Extended transthoracic resection compared with limited transhiatal resection for adenocarcinoma of the esophagus. *N Engl J Med.* 2002;347:1662–1669.
20. Omloo JM, Lagarde SM, Hulscher JB, et al. Extended transthoracic resection compared with limited transhiatal resection for adenocarcinoma of the mid/distal esophagus: five-year survival of a randomized clinical trial. *Ann Surg.* 2007;246:992–1000.
21. Lee PC, Mirza FM, Port JL, et al. Predictors of recurrence and disease-free survival in patients with completely resected esophageal carcinoma. *J Thorac Cardiovasc Surg.* 2011;141:1196–1206.

20 Three-Field Esophagectomy

Masahiko Tsurumaru, Yoshiaki Kajiyama, Yoshimi Iwanuma, Harushi Udagawa, and Hiroshi Akiyama

Keywords: Radical resection, three-field lymphadenectomy, esophageal cancer, squamous cell carcinoma

The esophagus traverses the neck, mediastinum, and abdomen. Cancer of the thoracic esophagus can metastasize to lymph nodes and locate in any or all of these compartments.[1] The rate of lymph node involvement is very high. Approximately 50% of tumors that invade the submucosa develop lymph node metastases, and the rate increases with increasing depth of invasion. Radical surgery for esophageal cancer therefore requires three-field lymphadenectomy. Our group has been performing three-field lymph node dissections since 1984 for all thoracoesophageal cancers. In this chapter we lay down the principles, describe the procedure, and discuss the outcome of this mode of treatment based on our experience.

The overall 5-year survival rate for squamous cell carcinoma of the esophagus has improved from 20% to 60%. We believe this improvement in survival can be directly related to extensive and meticulous lymphadenectomy.[2] This view has been corroborated by multivariate analysis. The key to three-field lymphadenectomy therefore is meticulous dissection of the upper mediastinum and cervical nodes that lie along the course of both recurrent laryngeal nerves. Preserving the right bronchial artery and pulmonary branches of the vagus nerve decreases the rate of pulmonary complications. Using this comprehensive approach, we have achieved a postoperative mortality rate of less than 2%.

LYMPH NODE METASTASES

Esophageal cancer is biologically more aggressive than other gastrointestinal malignancies and has a higher incidence of lymph node metastasis.[3] Lymph node metastasis is an important and independent factor for predicting the prognosis of esophageal cancer. The number of metastatic lymph nodes is thought to reflect the aggressiveness of the cancer.[4] Accurate documentation of the extent of lymph node involvement therefore is essential to determining the appropriate treatment strategy for esophageal cancer.

Histopathologic assessment remains the gold standard for accurate lymph node staging. Proper assessment also requires that an adequate number of lymph nodes be presented to the pathologist. Since 1984, all tumors determined to have invasion of the submucosa or beyond undergo three-field dissection at our institution. *Three-field dissection* is defined as an extended en-bloc lymph node dissection throughout the cervical, thoracic, and abdominal fields.[5]

CUMULATIVE EXPERIENCE AT JUNTENDO UNIVERSITY

A total of 1123 patients underwent transthoracic esophagectomy with extended en-bloc cervicothoracoabdominal (three-field) lymphadenectomy between January 1998 and December 2011 at Juntendo University in Japan for carcinoma of the esophagus. A total of 120,722 lymph nodes were dissected, and the average number of dissected lymph nodes per patient was 108. The lymph nodes removed en bloc with the specimen were dissected and classified into respective lymph node groups immediately after the operation by the surgeons who performed the esophagectomy, as outlined in the Japanese *Guidelines for Clinical and Pathologic Studies on Classification of Esophageal Cancer*[6] (Fig. 20-1). This provides a more detailed lymph node classification than the *AJCC Cancer Staging Manual*.[7] The pattern of lymphatic spread was investigated in detail, and the final pathologic diagnosis of lymph node metastasis was compared with the preoperative clinical evaluation to assess the accuracy of preoperative diagnosis for each lymph node station and each field.

LYMPHATIC SPREAD

Rate of Lymph Node Metastasis

Three hundred forty-eight patients did not have any lymph node metastases, whereas 775 patients had one or more metastatic lymph nodes, yielding a metastatic rate of 69.1%. The rate of lymph node metastasis increased with the depth of tumor invasion and was 54.7% for pT1b, 66.4% for pT2, and 81.0% for pT3 or pT4 disease (Fig. 20-2). The TNM classification divides pT1 tumors into two subclasses, pT1a and pT1b. A pT1a tumor invades only mucosa, including muscularis mucosae (mucosal cancer), and pT1b tumor invades the submucosal layer (submucosal cancer). In the normal esophagus, many lymphatic vessels are found in the lamina propria mucosa.[8] Therefore, lymphatic invasion can develop in comparatively early-stage cancer.

As shown in Figure 20-2, the rate of lymph node metastasis in esophageal cancer is three times higher than that of gastric cancer even for submucosal invasion (pT1b). The mean number of dissected lymph nodes was 41 in the neck, 35 in the mediastinum, and 31 in the abdomen. The mean number of metastatic lymph nodes was 0.7 in the neck, 1.8 in the mediastinum, and 1.6 in the abdomen.

The frequency and distribution of lymph node metastases differ according to the location of the tumor. The rate of lymph node metastasis was 65.6% in the upper thoracic esophagus ($n = 163$), 69.1% in the middle thoracic esophagus ($n = 651$), and 70.6% in the lower thoracic esophagus ($n = 309$) (Fig. 20-3). Upper esophageal tumors had a greater frequency of metastases to cervical lymph nodes than tumors of the middle and lower esophagus. The frequency of metastasis to abdominal nodes was higher with lower esophageal cancer than with tumors of the middle and upper esophagus. However, we did sometimes find abdominal lymph node metastasis in upper esophageal cancer and cervical node metastasis in lower esophageal cancer. Midesophageal tumors frequently metastasized to lymph nodes

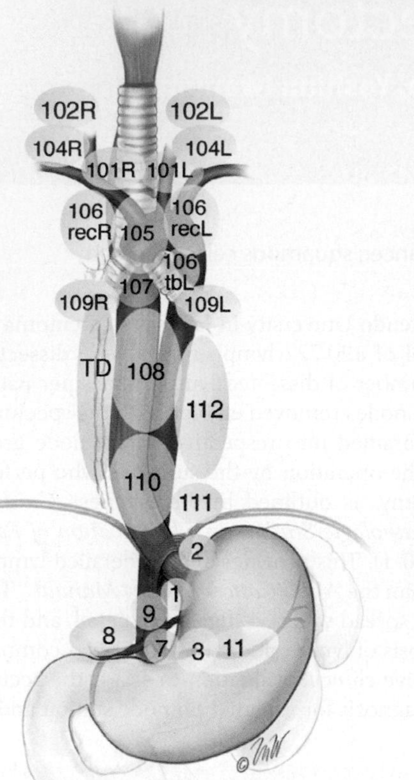

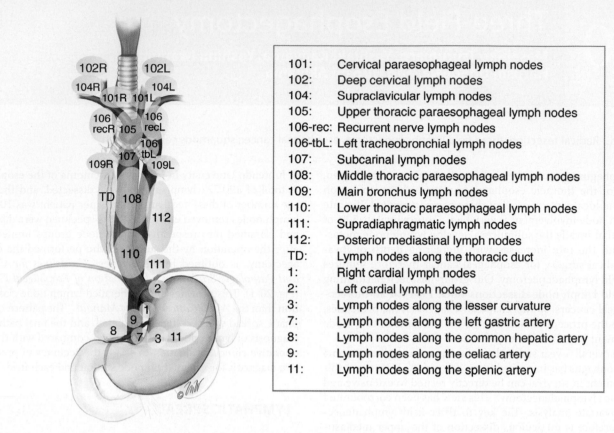

101:	Cervical paraesophageal lymph nodes
102:	Deep cervical lymph nodes
104:	Supraclavicular lymph nodes
105:	Upper thoracic paraesophageal lymph nodes
106-rec:	Recurrent nerve lymph nodes
106-tbL:	Left tracheobronchial lymph nodes
107:	Subcarinal lymph nodes
108:	Middle thoracic paraesophageal lymph nodes
109:	Main bronchus lymph nodes
110:	Lower thoracic paraesophageal lymph nodes
111:	Supradiaphragmatic lymph nodes
112:	Posterior mediastinal lymph nodes
TD:	Lymph nodes along the thoracic duct
1:	Right cardial lymph nodes
2:	Left cardial lymph nodes
3:	Lymph nodes along the lesser curvature
7:	Lymph nodes along the left gastric artery
8:	Lymph nodes along the common hepatic artery
9:	Lymph nodes along the celiac artery
11:	Lymph nodes along the splenic artery

Figure 20-1. Precise classification and station numbers of regional lymph nodes according to the Japanese Classification of Esophageal Cancer. (Illustration adapted from an original sketch provided by author.)

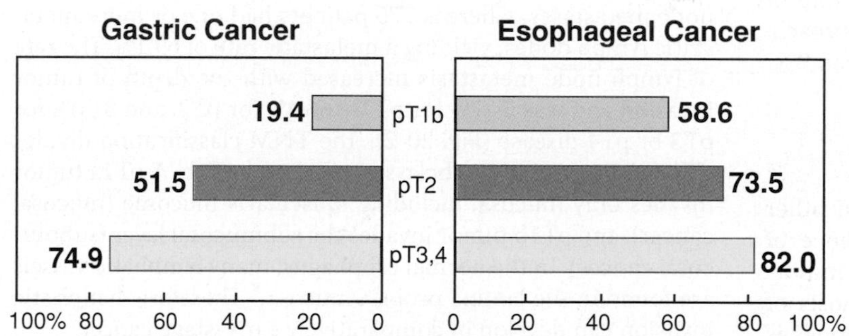

Figure 20-2. Rate of lymph node metastasis according to tumor invasion. Comparison between esophageal cancer and gastric cancer.

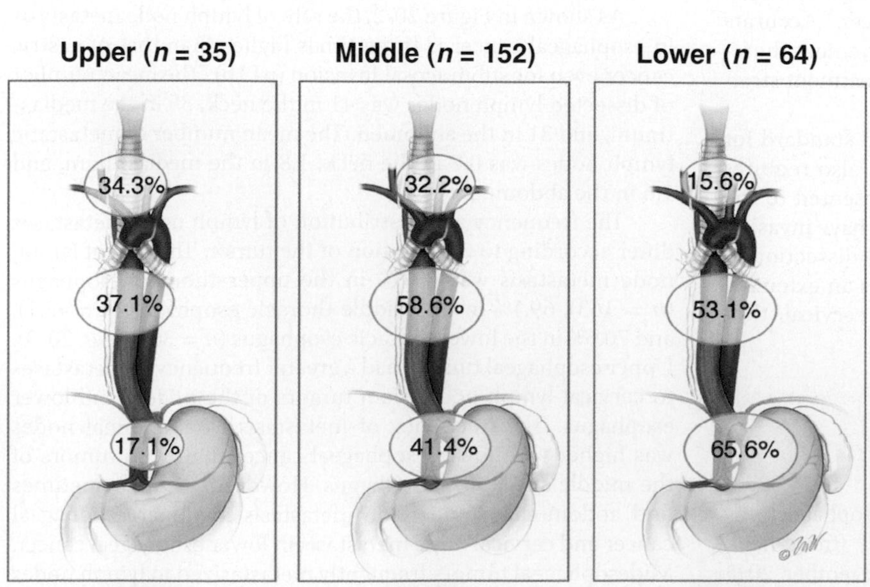

Figure 20-3. Frequency and distribution of lymphatic spread according to location of esophageal cancer. (Illustration adapted from an original sketch provided by author.)

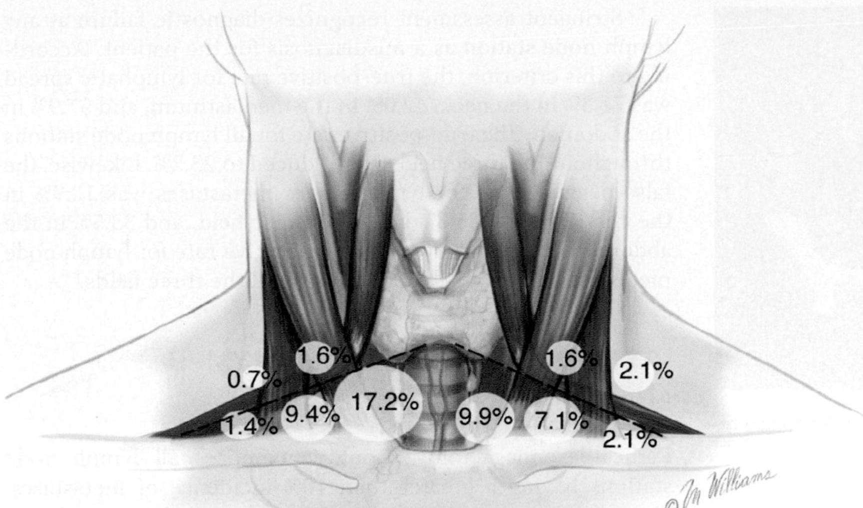

Figure 20-4. Lymph node metastasis in the neck. Among 140 patients with cervical metastatic nodes, 122 patients (87.1%) had positive nodes caudal to the omohyoid muscle. (Illustration adapted from an original sketch provided by author.)

in the neck and abdomen. Approximately 90% of cervical node metastases were caudal to the superior belly of the omohyoid muscle (Fig. 20-4).

Which Are the Frequently Involved Lymph Node Groups?

Analysis of lymphatic spread revealed that the sites with a metastatic rate of more than 20% (main metastatic sites) were located along the right recurrent laryngeal nerve in the upper mediastinum (106-recR: 23.8%) and along the lesser curvature of the proximal stomach (3: 21.6%) (Fig. 20-5). The sites with a metastatic rate ranging from 10% to 20% (common metastatic sites) were the right supraclavicular area (104: 14.4%), right cervical paraesophageal area along the recurrent laryngeal nerve (101R: 10.1%), along the left recurrent laryngeal nerve in the upper mediastinum (106-recL: 18.8%), the subcarinal area (107: 10.0%), the middle thoracic paraesophageal area (108: 13.0%), the lower thoracic paraesophageal area (110: 11.6%), the posterior mediastinal area (112: 17.0%), along the thoracic duct (TD: 10.0%), the right (1: 14.5%) and left (2: 16.6%) pericardial area, and along the left gastric artery (7: 18.0%). The nodes involved less often by metastases (metastatic rate <5%) were the middle deep cervical nodes (102R: 1.3%, 102L: 2.9%), the diaphragmatic nodes (111: 1.2%), the nodes along the common hepatic artery (8: 4.0%), and the nodes along the splenic artery (11: 4.4%).

As noted earlier, this detailed analysis of the lymphatic spread of esophageal cancer based on pathologic findings revealed two main metastatic sites: one along the recurrent laryngeal nerve in the upper mediastinum, which Haagensen called the *recurrent nerve*,[9] and the other along the lesser curvature of the proximal stomach. Unlike other gastrointestinal malignancies, frequent metastases to distant nodes are a distinctive feature of esophageal cancer.

PREOPERATIVE ASSESSMENT

The preoperative diagnostic workup for lymph node metastasis consists of endoscopic ultrasonography, conventional ultrasonography of the neck and abdomen, and CT scan from the neck to the lower abdomen. A PET scan is done as indicated.

Criteria for Preoperative Diagnosis

Mediastinal and abdominal lymph nodes were considered to be metastatic when the largest diameter was greater than 10 mm, the node was almost round, the internal CT density or ultrasound echogenicity was low, and the margin of the node was

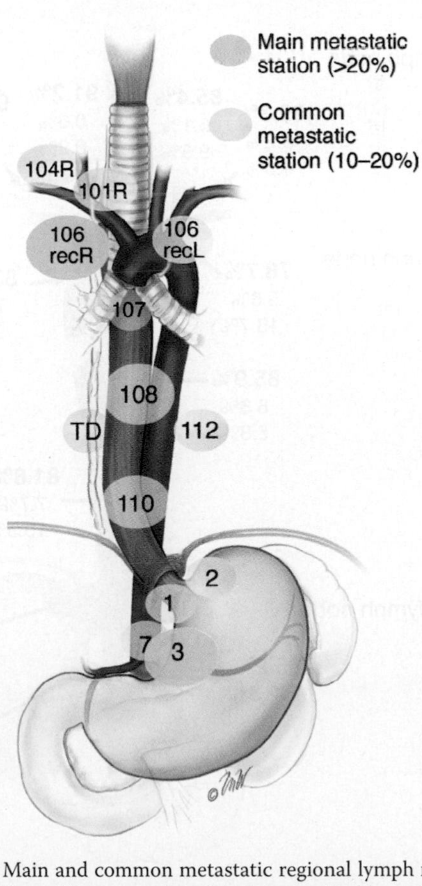

Figure 20-5. Main and common metastatic regional lymph node stations. (Illustration adapted from an original sketch provided by author.)

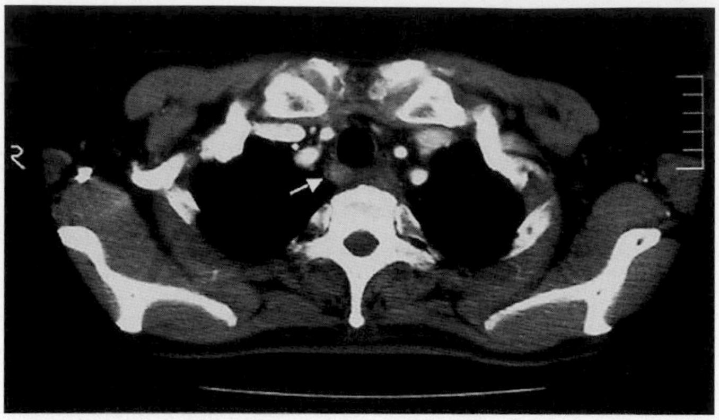

Figure 20-6. The *arrow* shows a metastatic node along the right recurrent laryngeal nerve (106-recR).

clear. For cervical lymph nodes, the same criteria were applied, except that the diameter was set at greater than 5 mm. Figure 20-6 shows a metastatic lymph node along the right recurrent nerve in the superior mediastinum at the root of the right subclavian artery.

Accuracy of Preoperative Diagnosis

Figure 20-7 depicts the accuracy of preoperative diagnosis of lymph node metastases compared with the subsequent pathologic examination. For each lymph node station, the true-positive rate was 85% to 94% in the neck, 79% to 86% in the thorax, and 78% to 86% in the abdomen. The false-negative and false-positive rates for metastatic lymph nodes are also shown in the figure.

Stringent assessment recognizes diagnostic failure at any lymph node station as a misdiagnosis for the patient. According to this criterion, the true-positive rate for lymphatic spread was 71.3% in the neck, 42.0% in the mediastinum, and 57.9% in the abdomen. The true-positive rate for all lymph node stations throughout the three fields was reduced to 23.2%. Likewise, the false-negative rate for lymph nodes metastases was 13.9% in the cervical field, 35.6% in the thoracic field, and 33.5% in the abdominal field. The overall false-negative rate for lymph node metastases increases to 53.7% across all the three fields.

TECHNIQUE OF THREE-FIELD LYMPH NODE DISSECTION

Radical esophagectomy should encompass all lymph node stations having a greater than 10% incidence of metastases. Nevertheless, lymphatic metastasis cannot be diagnosed precisely either by ultrasonography or CT imaging before surgery. Therefore, radical surgery for cancer of the thoracic esophagus requires complete three-field lymph node dissection.

The first step of the operation is an anterolateral thoracotomy through the fourth intercostal space. The thoracic duct, azygos vein, pleura, and periesophageal tissues including lymph nodes and lymphatic channels in the mediastinum are dissected en bloc. The right and left recurrent laryngeal nerves are identified, and the upper mediastinal lymph nodes (including the node group of the recurrent laryngeal nerve chain) are cleared (Fig. 20-8). After this procedure, paratracheal lymph nodes on both sides (Fig. 20-9), subcarinal, right and left hilar lymph nodes, posterior mediastinal lymph nodes adjacent to the descending aorta and left pleura, and diaphragmatic lymph

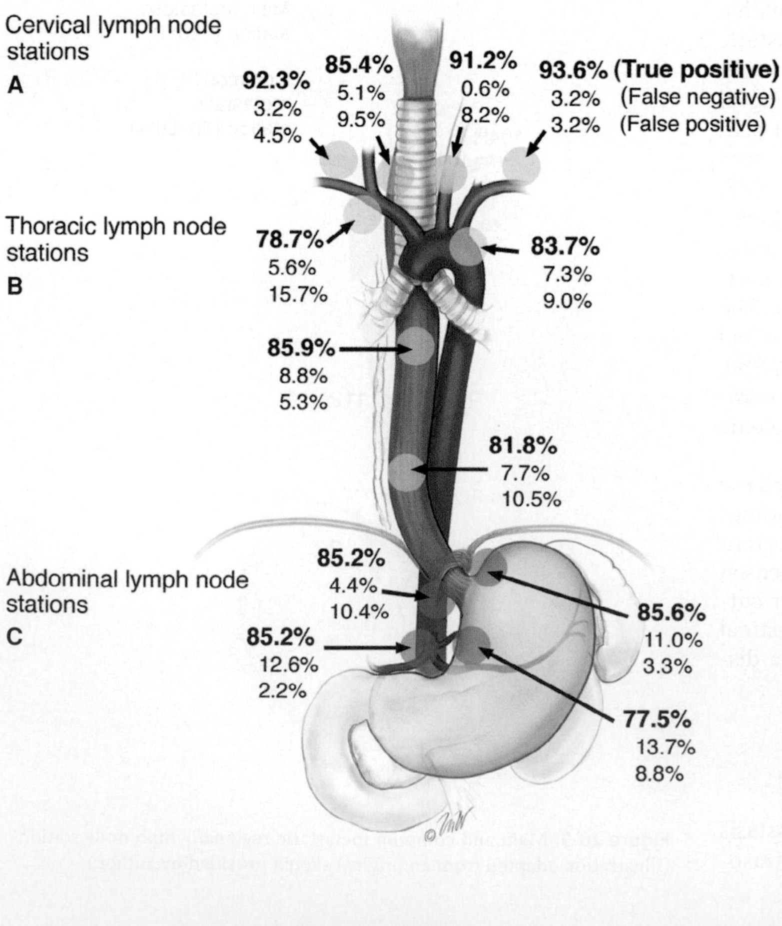

Figure 20-7. True-positive, false-negative, and false-positive clinical diagnostic rates for lymph nodes metastases at each regional lymph node station. *A*. Cervical field. *B*. Thoracic field. *C*. Abdominal field. (Illustration adapted from an original sketch provided by author.)

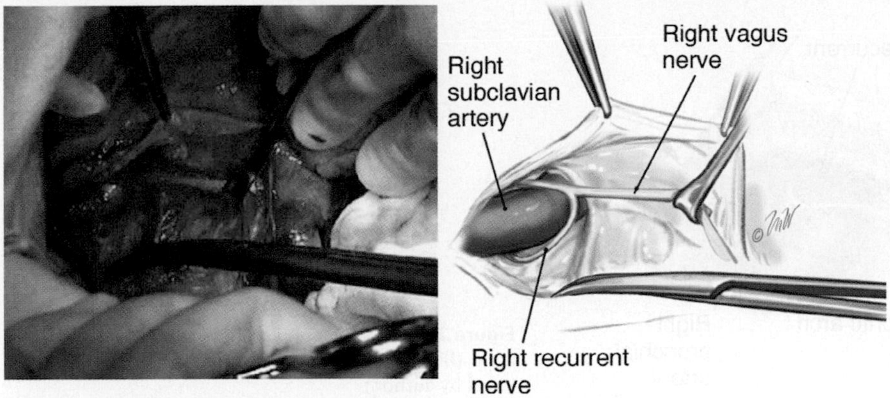

Figure 20-8. Lymph node dissection is started with identification of the right recurrent laryngeal nerve in the utmost upper mediastinum. (Illustration adapted from an original sketch provided by author.)

nodes are dissected en bloc (Fig. 20-1). The lymph nodes inside the aortic arch (left tracheobronchial) are dissected separately (Fig. 20-10). To avoid ventilatory impairment, the right or left bronchial artery and the pulmonary branches of the vagus nerve should be preserved (Fig. 20-11).

For the abdominal procedure, after an upper midline laparotomy, en-bloc dissection of lymph nodes is carried out along the cardia, lesser curvature, left gastric artery, celiac axis, common hepatic artery, and splenic artery (Fig. 20-12). The left gastric artery is cut at its origin. Along with all these dissected lymph nodes, the proximal stomach is cut between the junction of the right and left gastric arteries to the farthest point in the fundus using a linear stapler (Fig. 20-13). The gastric remnant, based on the right gastroepiploic artery and right gastric artery, is used for esophageal reconstruction. We do not perform pyloroplasty. The extent of abdominal lymph node dissection is very similar to that of D_2 lymph node dissection for gastric cancer surgery.

In the neck, a collar incision is made as in thyroidectomy. The middle deep cervical and supraclavicular lymph nodes (102 and 104 in Fig. 20-1), which are located lateral to the common carotid artery, ventral to the anterior scalene muscle and phrenic nerve, and inferior to the superior belly of the omohyoid muscle, are removed. Then the lymph nodes along the cervical recurrent laryngeal nerve are excised (Fig. 20-14). These lymph nodes are between the common carotid artery and trachea (101 in Fig. 20-1), and they should be removed meticulously and carefully so as not to traumatize the recurrent laryngeal nerve.

Postoperative Morbidity

The patient is usually extubated in the operating theater when the PaO_2 level (torrs) exceeds three times the FIO_2 (%). The patient is transferred to the surgical ICU and is monitored there for a period of approximately 1 week.

The surgeon should be aware of four main complications in the postoperative course of esophagectomy with three-field lymph node dissection (Fig. 20-15). They consist of pulmonary complications, cardiac complications, anastomotic leakage, and recurrent nerve paralysis. Among these, pulmonary complications are by far the most common and of grave concern. Pulmonary compromise may be caused by the wide dissection around the trachea and bronchi, which leads to various degrees of ischemia of the respiratory tract and a decreased cough reflex.

Pulmonary Complications

Hypoxemia requires inhalation of a high concentration of oxygen and was seen in 25.4% of the study group (Fig. 20-16). It

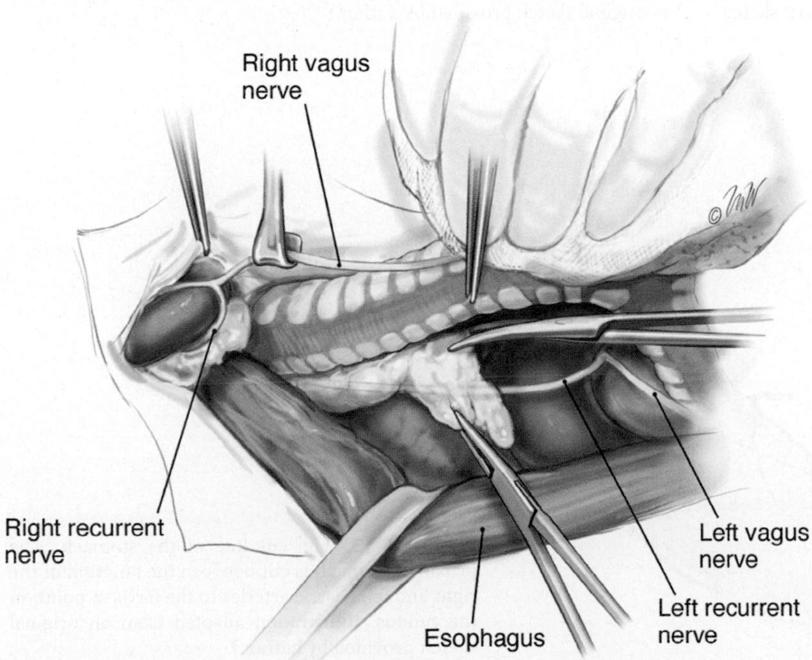

Figure 20-9. Upper mediastinal dissection. The right and left recurrent nerves are separated, and tissues are cleared around the nerves. (Illustration adapted from an original sketch provided by author.)

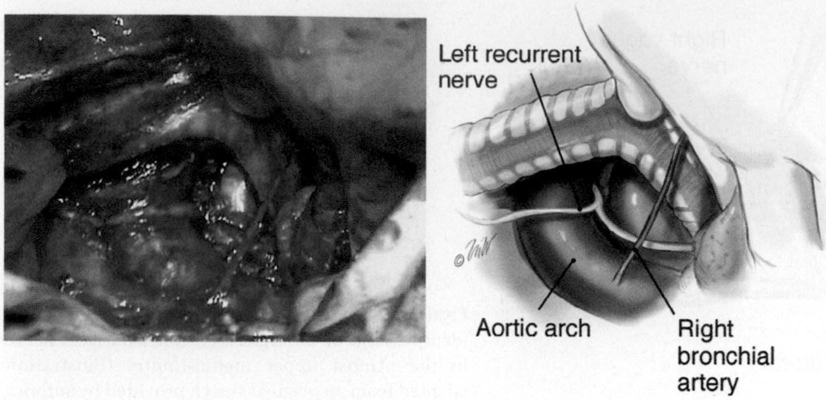

Figure 20-10. Completion of dissection inside the aortic arch. (Illustration adapted from an original sketch provided by author.)

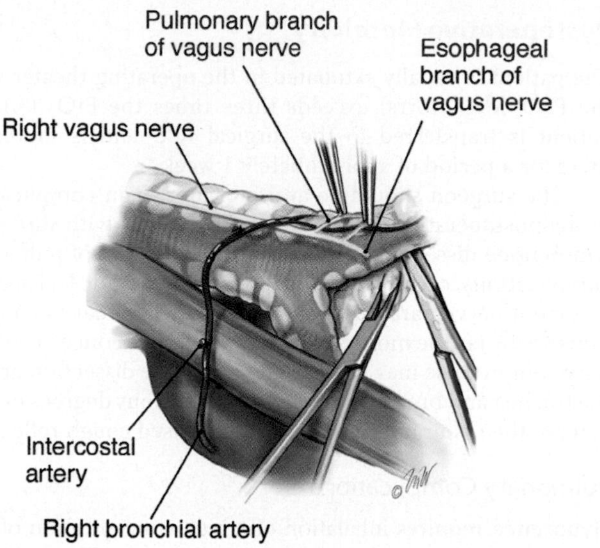

Figure 20-11. Preservation of the right bronchial artery and pulmonary branches of the vagus nerve. (Illustration adapted from an original sketch provided by author.)

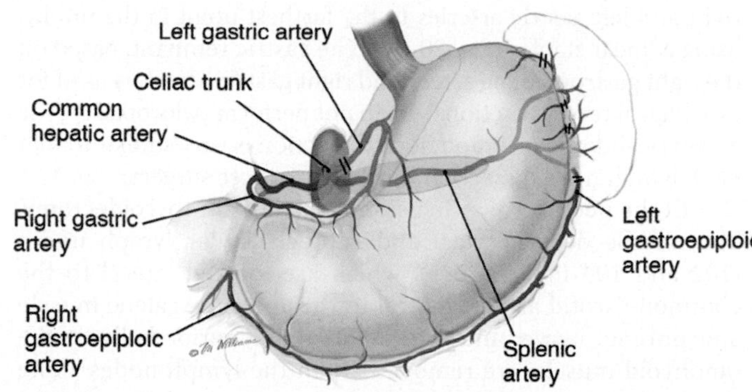

Figure 20-12. Dissection areas in the abdomen. (Illustration adapted from an original sketch provided by author.)

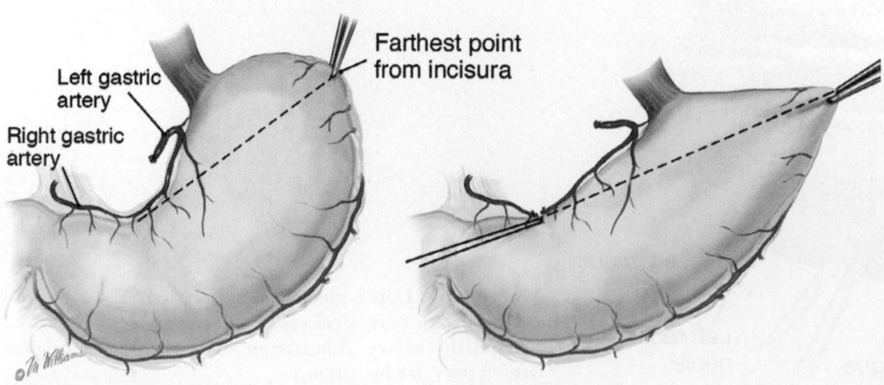

Figure 20-13. The cut line of the stomach. The proximal stomach is cut between the junction of the right and left gastric arteries to the farthest point on the fundus. (Illustration adapted from an original sketch provided by author.)

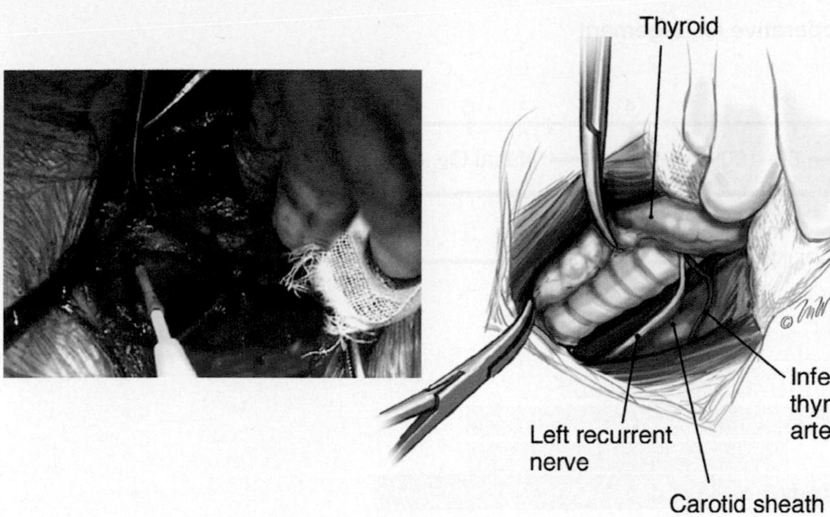

Figure 20-14. Dissection along the cervical recurrent laryngeal nerve on the left side. (Illustration adapted from an original sketch provided by author.)

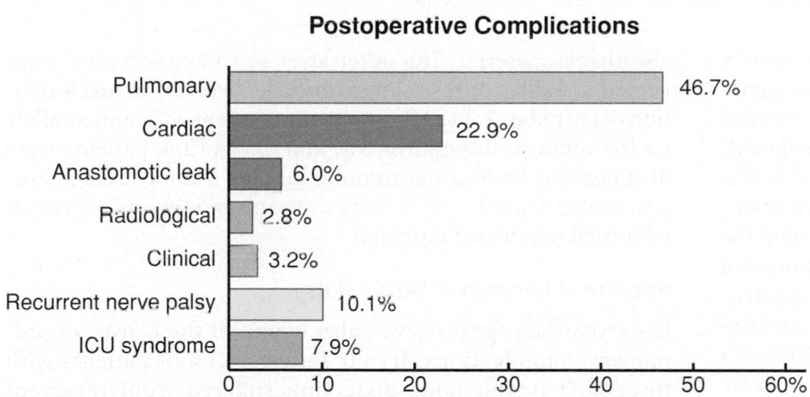

Figure 20-15. Postoperative complications after three-field dissection. Anastomotic leakage includes radiologic minor leakage (2.8%) and clinical fistula formation (3.2%).

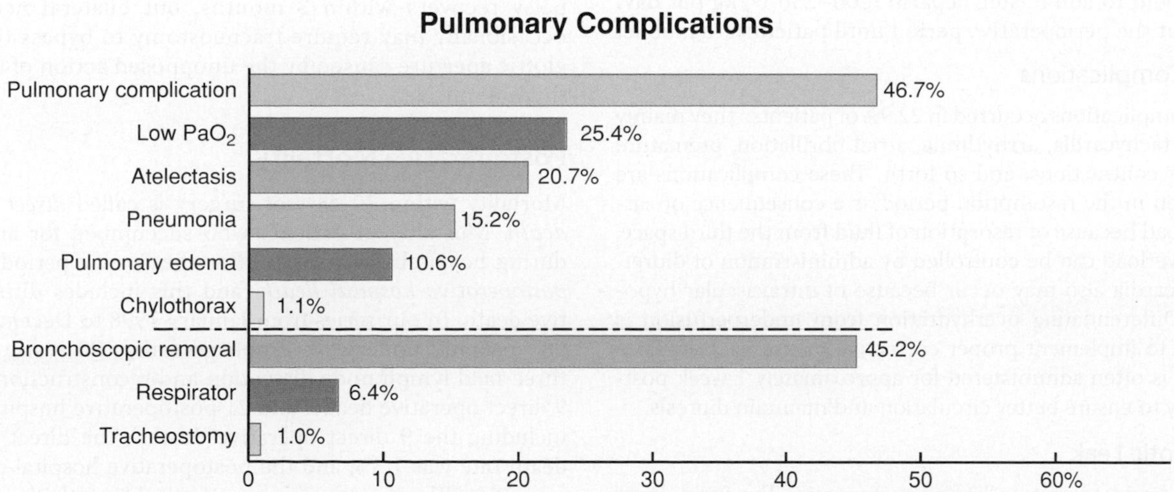

Figure 20-16. Pulmonary complications after three-field dissection.

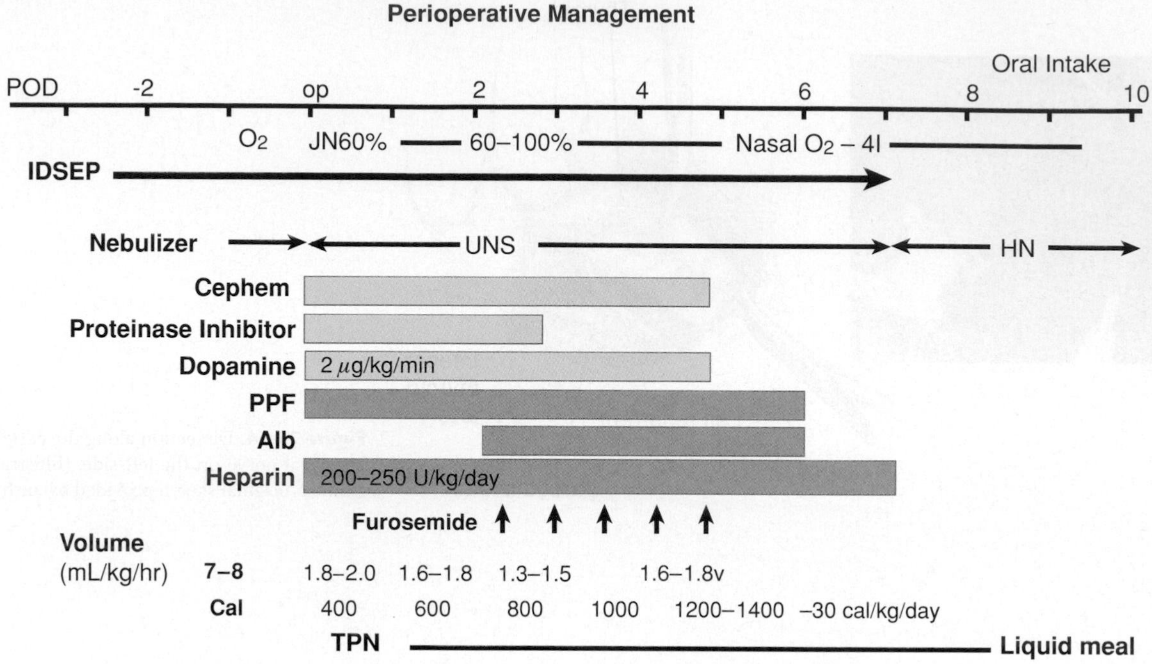

Figure 20-17. Perioperative management of three-field dissection.

is caused mainly by pneumonia, atelectasis, and pulmonary edema. Pulmonary edema or potential pulmonary edema sometimes develops in radical esophagectomy patients after removal of the thoracic duct, which causes lymphatic retention in the retroperitoneum, hypoproteinemia, and depletion of intravascular volume. The rate of fluid infusion during the procedure is maintained at approximately 7 to 8 mL/kg/h, taking into account the blood loss and urine output (Fig. 20-17). Consequently, potential pulmonary edema can occur in the resorption period approximately 48 hours postoperatively. It can be controlled successfully by administration of dopamine, albumin, and diuretics (e.g., furosemide). It should be borne in mind that intraoperative restriction of fluid transfusion to keep the lungs "dry" can result in tachycardia with serious hypotension postoperatively.

Pulmonary embolism is a less common complication, but one should maintain a high degree of suspicion in patients with no obvious cause of hypoxemia. Its prevention is very important. It is advisable to use pneumatic pressure garments on both legs and to administer heparin (200–250 U/kg per day) throughout the perioperative period until patients are mobile.

Cardiac Complications

Cardiac complications occurred in 22.9% of patients. They mainly consist of tachycardia, arrhythmia, atrial fibrillation, premature ventricular contractions, and so forth. These complications are usually seen in the resumption period as a consequence of cardiac overload because of resorption of fluid from the third space. Cardiac overload can be controlled by administration of diuretics. Tachycardia also may occur because of intravascular hypovolemia. Differentiating overhydration from underperfusion is important to implement proper corrective measures. Low-dose dopamine is often administered for approximately 1 week postoperatively to ensure better circulation and maintain diuresis.

Anastomotic Leak

We use a hand-sewn two-layer anastomosis. The inner-layer suture is continuous and consists of a 5-0 monofilament absorbable material. The outer layer is completed with interrupted fine silk sutures. Clinical leakage involving fistula formation occurred in 3.2%. All patients underwent a barium swallow on the ninth postoperative day, and 6.0% of the patients were diagnosed as having anastomotic leakage. Minor leakage usually healed within 1 to 2 weeks of conservative management with total parenteral nutrition.

Recurrent Laryngeal Nerve Palsy

Recurrent laryngeal nerve palsy is one of the causes of pulmonary complications. In our series, 10.1% of patients with three-field lymph node dissection suffered from recurrent laryngeal nerve palsy, and 95% of them had impairment of the left recurrent nerve. This may cause silent aspiration of saliva, which contains bacteria from the oral cavity. Inadequate glottic closure also impairs the cough reflex and expulsion of retained secretions by preventing buildup of adequate intratracheal pressure. Hoarseness owing to unilateral nerve palsy recovers within 3 months, but bilateral nerve palsy occasionally may require tracheostomy to bypass the closed glottic aperture caused by the unopposed action of the cricothyroid muscle.

Postoperative Mortality

Mortality within 30 days of surgery is called *direct operative death.* Mortality of patients who succumbed for any reason during hospitalization even after the 30-day period is called *postoperative hospital death,* and this includes direct operative death. In our series from January 1998 to December 2011, 687 patients underwent esophagectomy (R0 resection) with three-field lymph node dissection and reconstruction. We had 9 direct operative deaths and 21 postoperative hospital deaths, including the 9 direct operative deaths. The direct operative death rate was 1.3%, and the postoperative hospital death rate was 3.1%. These rates compare favorably with the mortality rates reported in other large series.

Table 20-1

INDEPENDENT PROGNOSTIC FACTORS EXAMINED BY COX REGRESSION MODEL

COVARIATES	SIGNIFICANCE	RISK RATIO
Age	<0.0001	1.0308
Number of positive node	<0.0001	1.0539
Cell differentiation	0.0056	
MQ:PQ	0.0051	1.4999
MQ:WQ	0.1615	0.7935
Gender (f: m)	<0.0001	2.3296
Residual tumor	0.0466	
R0:R1	0.9444	0.9795
R0:R2	0.0175	0.7265
2-F/3-F	<0.0001	0.5501
TNM pM	0.0008	
pMO:pM1 (HEP)	0.0089	14.7106
pMO:pMl (LYM)	0.0042	1.5600
TNM pT	<0.0001	
pTl:pT2	0.0004	1.9575
pTl:pT3	<0.0001	2.3917
pTl:pT4	<0.0001	3.1654
pTl:pTis	0.7062	0.7969

LONG-TERM PROGNOSIS

The long-term survival rate was calculated according to the Kaplan–Meier method, and the statistical difference was considered to be significant at a p value of less than 0.05.

Statistical Analysis

The survival curve of the three-field dissection group was compared with the survival curve of the historical group (limited two-field dissection) before 1984. The overall 5-year survival rate for the three-field group was 62.5%, whereas in the limited two-field group it was 37.1% ($p < 0.001$). The effect of extensive lymph node dissection on long-term survival also was examined using multivariate analysis (Cox regression model). Ten factors such as age, gender, tumor location, number of metastatic nodes, extent of lymph node dissection (three vs. two fields), cellular differentiation, curativity, pT category, pN category, and clinical M category were entered into the model as covariates. Consequently, the extent of lymph node dissection was selected as one of the independent prognostic factors with a risk ratio of 0.5501 (Table 20-1). This means that systematic lymph node dissection contributes to improved long-term survival for squamous cell carcinoma of the thoracic esophagus.

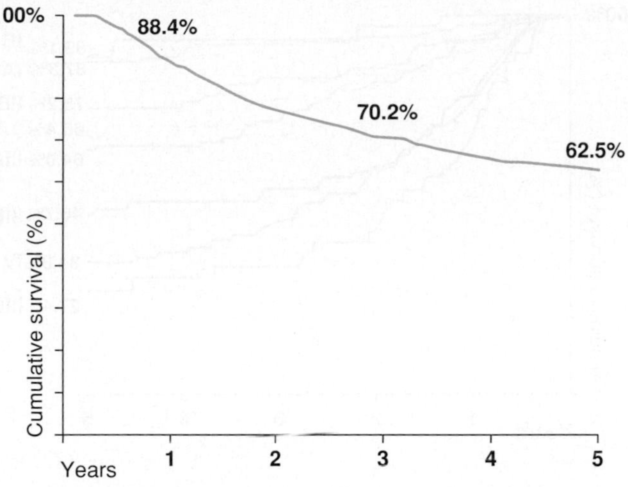

Figure 20-18. Overall survival for all cases. (Kaplan–Meier method).

Relationship Between the Pattern of Lymph Node Metastasis and Prognosis

The long-term survival rate of our series is shown in Figure 20-18. The 5-year survival rate was 62.5%. The survival rate decreased as the number of metastatic lymph nodes increased irrespective of the site of metastasis. The prognosis of 687 patients who underwent three-field lymph node dissection was analyzed to correlate lymph node metastasis pattern with prognosis.

The number of positive nodes has a close relationship with prognosis. According to the version 7 TNM classification, the cases were categorized into four groups. N0 for no LN metastasis, N1 for metastasis in 1 to 2 regional lymph nodes, N2 metastasis in 3 to 6 regional lymph nodes, N3 for metastasis in 7 or more regional lymph nodes. Therefore, the number of lymph node metastases is an independent predictor of prognosis. The 5-year survival rates for patients of the N0, N1, N2, and N3 groups were 81.0%, 69.3%, 44.9%, and 19.1%, respectively (Fig. 20-19). Figure 20-20 shows survival rates of the patients

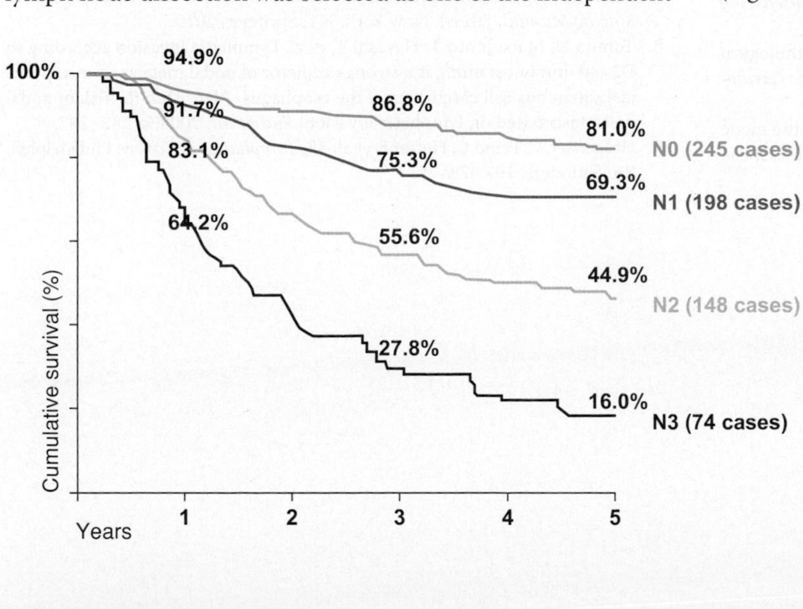

Figure 20-19. Survival curves according to N category.

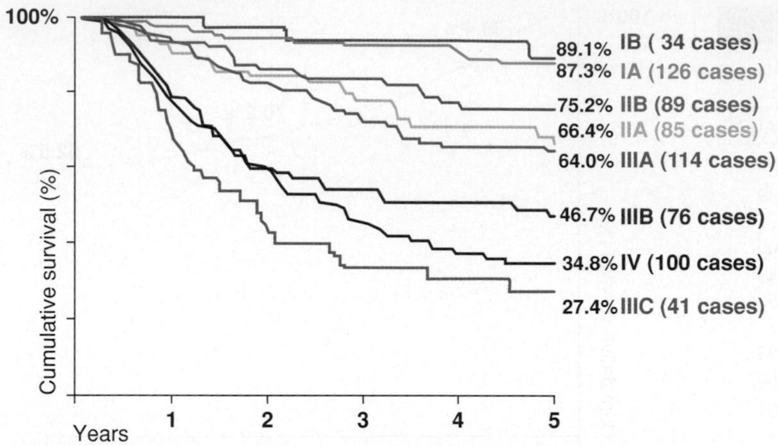

Figure 20-20. Survival curves according to stage groupings.

grouped by TNM stage. The 5-year survival rates decreased according to stage for stages I to III. However, stage IV cases, which include M1, survived 5 years at a rate of 34.8%. In our series, the 5-year survival rate of stage IV exceeded that of stage IIIC, but it was not statistically significant. The reason of this phenomena was not clear, but thought to be derived from overestimation of M1 category which includes lymph node metastasis in the neck. This clearly demonstrates that extensive lymph node dissection in the neck, mediastinum, and abdomen can contribute to long-term survival in esophageal cancer.

SUMMARY

In Japan, three-field lymph node dissection is used routinely for the surgical treatment of squamous cell carcinoma of the thoracic esophagus. However, this procedure has not been universally accepted. Doubts continue to persist regarding the need for such extensive dissection and the subsequent benefits conferred.[10] We analyzed the extent and frequency of lymph node metastasis of squamous cell carcinoma of the esophagus and its impact on long-term survival. We found that the lymph node stations involved depend on the site of the primary tumor. Positive nodes were found in all three fields irrespective of the location of the tumor. It was thought previously that metastases to neck nodes were distant metastases, and they were considered to indicate incurability. In our experience, however, some patients with metastatic neck nodes can have prolonged survival with radical three-field dissection. Extended lymph node dissection of the neck, mediastinum, and abdomen should be considered mandatory for complete eradication of carcinoma of the thoracic esophagus.

References

1. Akiyama H. Squamous cell carcinoma of the thoracic esophagus. In: Akiyama H, ed. *Surgery for Cancer of the Esophagus*. Baltimore, MD: Williams & Wilkins; 1990.
2. Udagawa H, Tsutsumi K, Kinoshita Y. Surgical treatment of squamous cell cancer of the esophagus. In: Pinotti HW, ed. *Recent Advances in Diseases of the Esophagus*. Bologna: Monduzzi Editore; 2001:585–588.
3. Kuwano H, Nakajima M, Miyazaki T, et al. Distinctive clinicopathological characteristics in esophageal squamous cell carcinoma. *Ann Thorac Cardiovasc Surg*. 2003;9:6–13.
4. Hosch SB, Stoecklein NH, Pichlmeier U, et al. Esophageal cancer: the mode of lymphatic tumor cell spread and its prognostic significance. *J Clin Oncol*. 2001;19:1970–1975.
5. Akiyama H, Tsurumaru M, Udagawa H, et al. Radical lymph node dissection for cancer of the thoracic esophagus. *Ann Surg*. 1994;220:364–372; discussion 72–73.
6. *Japanese Society for Esophageal Diseases: Japanese Classification of Esophageal Cancer.* Tokyo: Kanehara; 2008.
7. Edge SB, Byrd DR, Compton CC, et al. *American Joint Committee on Cancer Staging Manual*. 7th ed. New York, NY: Springer; 2010.
8. Tomita N, Matsumoto T, Hayashi T, et al. Lymphatic invasion according to D2-40 immunostaining is a strong predictor of nodal metastasis in superficial squamous cell carcinoma of the esophagus. Algorithm for risk of nodal metastasis based on lymphatic invasion. *Pathol Int*. 2008;58:282–287.
9. Haagensen C, Feind C, Herter F, et al. *The Lymphatics in Cancer.* Philadelphia, PA: Saunders; 1972:78–79.

21 Left Thoracoabdominal Approach

Christopher R. Morse and Douglas J. Mathisen

Keywords: Thoracoabdominal esophagectomy, distal esophageal cancer, adenocarcinoma, esophageal cancer

A thoracoabdominal approach to resection of the esophagus is most useful with tumors of the distal esophagus that lie inferior to the aortic arch as well as lesions of the gastric cardia. Eggers first reported the use of a left thoracoabdominal incision for a partial resection of the esophagus in 1931.[1] Eventual resection of the distal esophagus and replacement with mobilized stomach was described by Adams and Phemister in 1938.[2] Finally, Sweet[3] described the technique of anastomosis on the basis of the principles of meticulous technique and attention to detail. The thoracoabdominal incision provides excellent access to the abdomen. With extension of the incision through the costal arch, left rectus muscle, and diaphragm, the esophagus can be mobilized and replaced with stomach, colon, or jejunum depending on the situation. In addition, with an upward paravertebral extension of the incision and Sweet's double-rib resection, one can reach almost any lesion of the intrathoracic esophagus.[3]

PREOPERATIVE ASSESSMENT

Because of the magnitude of a thoracoabdominal esophagectomy or any esophagectomy, it is important to engage in a rigorous selection and staging work-up before proceeding with surgical intervention. Although patients with widely disseminated disease and extreme comorbid illnesses are easily eliminated from surgical consideration, most patients undergo a systematic evaluation of resectability and a review of risk factors.

The initial evaluation of patients with esophageal carcinoma should include a contrast esophagogram and upper gastrointestinal endoscopy. Esophagoscopy with biopsy of the lesion is essential to obtain a tissue diagnosis, to confirm that there is not a second synchronous esophageal carcinoma, and to obtain a more accurate assessment of the extent of the tumor both grossly and microscopically by mucosal biopsy. Endoscopy also Barrett's esophagus and evaluation of potential gastric involvement.

Further evaluation by CT imaging of the thorax and abdomen provides information regarding invasion of adjacent structures (e.g., pericardium and diaphragm), tracheobronchial invasion, and mediastinal lymph node involvement. However, recent reports have noted the accuracy of CT imaging for the presence of locoregional disease to be as low as 50%.[4,5] CT imaging of the abdomen with contrast material also assists in the detection of hepatic metastasis.

Endoscopic ultrasound (EUS) is used commonly in the local staging of esophageal cancer. It provides valuable data regarding the depth of tumor invasion, potential nodal involvement, and the opportunity for fine-needle aspiration of adjacent lymph nodes. Accuracy in predicting T status with EUS in esophageal cancer is greater than 80%, and accuracy in predicting N status ranges around 70%.[6] EUS is clearly superior to CT in T staging, and appears more accurate in predicting T_4 disease.[7]

PET imaging is becoming a more valuable tool in the evaluation of distant metastatic disease. PET scans have almost no role in the determination of T status, but in regard to metastatic disease, the results are encouraging, with reports of greater than 90% accuracy.[8] (PET imaging may have a further application in monitoring for disease recurrence.)

An evaluation of preoperative risk factors includes an assessment of pulmonary and cardiovascular function. Pulmonary function testing should be obtained if there are any questions as to the patient's respiratory status. Smoking should be stopped well in advance of surgery. A cardiovascular assessment also should be performed with a history and physical examination, as well as an ECG and, if deemed necessary, a stress test or cardiac catheterization.

TECHNIQUE

It is suggested that all esophageal procedures, including thoracoabdominal esophagectomy, begin with endoscopy in the operating room. Repeat endoscopy provides confirmation of the location of the tumor and evaluation of the esophagus for a second lesion or extension into the stomach. With tumors of the middle and upper thirds of the esophagus, bronchoscopy also should be performed. A double-lumen endotracheal tube is placed, permitting deflation of the left lung during the thoracic dissection, and broad-spectrum antibiotics are given before surgical incision and may need redosing during the procedure. We encourage the liberal use of an epidural catheter in the management of postoperative pain, given the extend of the incision.

The patient is positioned in the right lateral decubitus position, which permits access to both the left side of the chest and the upper abdomen. The initial step is an exploration of the abdomen through the medial portion of the incision. A valuable landmark in planning the abdominal portion of the incision is to aim the medial aspect at a point halfway between the xiphoid and umbilicus. The abdominal portion of the incision permits inspection of the liver, palpation of the celiac nodes, and further evaluation of the stomach. With no metastatic disease identified, the incision is carried into the chest over the seventh or eighth rib (Fig. 21-1). The higher the interspace, the easier it is to perform the anastomosis. As the diaphragm is divided, it should be clearly marked with stitches to allow reapproximation at the conclusion of the case.

Thoracic Dissection

Thoracic exploration begins with an inspection of the left lung, diaphragm, pericardium, and pleural space. Opening of the mediastinal pleura permits further inspection of the extent of the tumor, evaluation of possible invasion of the aorta or lung,

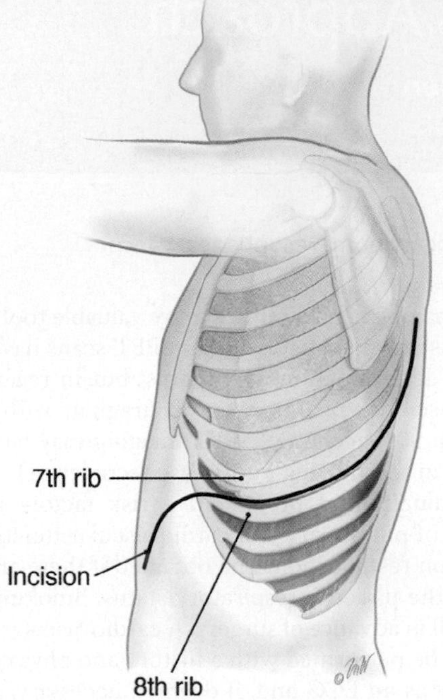

Figure 21-1. The incision is carried into the chest over the seventh rib. The higher the interspace, the easier it is to perform the anastomosis. As the diaphragm is divided, it should be clearly marked with stitches to allow reapproximation at the close of the procedure.

and determination of metastases to the paraesophageal and paraaortic lymph nodes.

Dissection begins in the chest, freeing the esophagus and harvesting all adjacent lymph nodes. The descending aorta is completely bared by division of the aortoesophageal branches. Aortic involvement precludes resection. The esophagus is encircled after the dissection is carried medially along the posterior aspect of the mediastinum up to the level of the left main stem bronchus, away from the proximal tumor margin. Gentle traction on the esophagus facilitates dissection of the paraesophageal nodes and fat. The thoracic duct is rarely seen with the left thoracoabdominal approach and is not routinely ligated.

It may be necessary to mobilize the esophagus superior to the level of the aortic arch. Division of aortic intercostal vessels is necessary to gain adequate mobilization of the arch. With mobilization of the arch, the left recurrent nerve must be carefully preserved. In addition, it is at this point that the thoracic duct is most vulnerable to injury, and the left main stem bronchus also must be examined for injury to the membranous wall.

Abdominal Dissection

Mobilization of the stomach begins with the division of the greater omentum. This is performed outside the gastroepiploic arcade formed by the left gastroepiploic artery arising from the splenic artery and the right gastroepiploic artery arising from the gastroduodenal artery at the pylorus. Use of the stomach to replace the esophagus hinges on the patency of the right gastroepiploic artery and to a lesser degree, the right gastric artery. The transverse colon is placed on stretch, and the lesser sac is entered at the thinnest portion of the omentum. The dissection is carried toward the pylorus, dividing the small omental branches of the epiploic artery. Cautery coagulation is used sparingly for fear of damaging the gastroepiploic arcade. Dissection then is carried toward the spleen, where the left gastroepiploic artery is ligated at the upper end of the arcade as it arises from the splenic artery. Management of the short gastric arteries deserves special attention, and it must be ensured that the ties on the stomach are secure because they can slip with distention of the stomach within the thorax. Alternative methods for controlling the short gastric vessels include use of the Harmonic Scalpel (Ethicon-Endosurgery, Inc.) or the LDS (US Surgical, Norwalk, CT) stapling device.

At the level of the esophagogastric junction, the reflection of the peritoneum is divided, and the esophagus is encircled. Passage of a Penrose drain allows for upward traction on the abdominal esophagus and dissection of the lesser curve. The thin avascular gastrohepatic ligament is divided, and placement of a second thin Penrose drain around the stomach at the level of the incisura can further assist with dissection of the lesser curve. The gastrohepatic ligament should be inspected for an accessory branch of the left hepatic artery. If one is identified, it should be occluded temporarily with a bulldog clamp and the liver assessed for viability. If concern exists about the vascular supply of the liver, the accessory branch must be preserved. This can be done by skeletonizing the accessory branch to its origin from the left gastric artery and preserving these vessels.

Management of the left gastric artery is best accomplished by exposing it with the greater curve rotated to the right, often with the assistance of the Penrose drains. The filmy retrogastric adhesions can be taken down sharply to the level of the pylorus, and the celiac axis can be identified by palpation. With further dissection, the left gastric artery is exposed, doubly tied, and suture ligated at its origin with 2-0 silk suture. The left gastric vein is also suture ligated and divided. At this point in the operation, the stomach is free except for the pylorus/duodenum and right gastroepiploic artery arising from the gastroduodenal artery.

Transection of the Stomach

For a distal esophagectomy performed for cancer, the celiac axis nodes and the nodes along the left gastric artery should have been swept up with the specimen. The stomach should be transected from a point on the greater curvature opposite the emergence of the left gastroepiploic artery to a point on the lesser curvature below the lowest branch of the left gastric artery. The fundus should be preserved to maximize the length of the gastric tube, and it is important not to assume adequate gastric length and amputate the conduit prematurely (Fig. 21-2). After the stapler is fired and the stomach is divided, the staple line is turned in with 4-0 silk Lembert stitches (Fig. 21-3).

If required, further mobilization of the stomach is performed via a Kocher maneuver starting at the pylorus and extending around the curve of the duodenum. Care must be taken to avoid the right gastric artery and the common bile duct during the dissection. The duodenum and pancreas then are swept off the inferior vena cava by blunt dissection. The Kocher maneuver can mobilize the stomach sufficiently to reach to the thoracic inlet, which is rarely needed for the thoracoabdominal approach.

Drainage of the stomach remains controversial. In our opinion, a gastric drainage procedure makes sense from a physiologic perspective; that is, after vagotomy, there is clinical

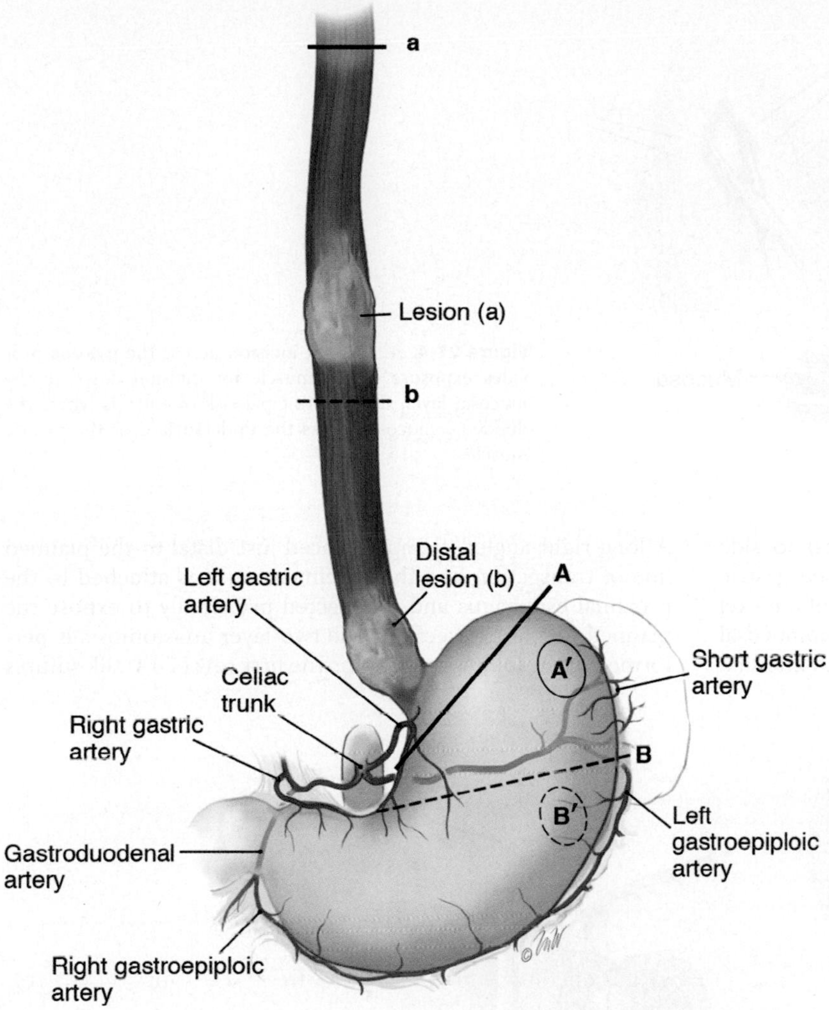

Figure 21-2. The fundus should be preserved (*A, solid line*) to maximize gastric length, which permits extension of the gastric tube to the neck (*a, solid line*) if necessary. For a distal lesion where only a portion of the esophagus needs to be resected (*b, dashed line*), more of the gastric fundus may be taken in creating the gastric conduit (*B, dashed line*). It is important not to assume adequate gastric length and amputate the conduit prematurely. The *circles* marked *A′* and *B′* indicate the proposed esophagogastric site.

experience to suggest that obstructive symptoms are encountered without a drainage procedure. A pyloromyotomy is preferred because it does not distract from the length of the stomach. The pyloric muscle may retain some of its barrier capacity against bile reflux into the esophagus (Fig. 21-4). Initially, traction sutures are placed on either side of the pyloric vein to facilitate exposure. Once the submucosal plane is reached, the incision is carried onto the first portion of the duodenum and distal stomach. The myotomy is usually limited to 2 cm. If the mucosa is inadvertently violated, the safest course of action is to convert the procedure to a Heineke-Mikulicz pyloroplasty with coverage of the pyloroplasty with omentum.

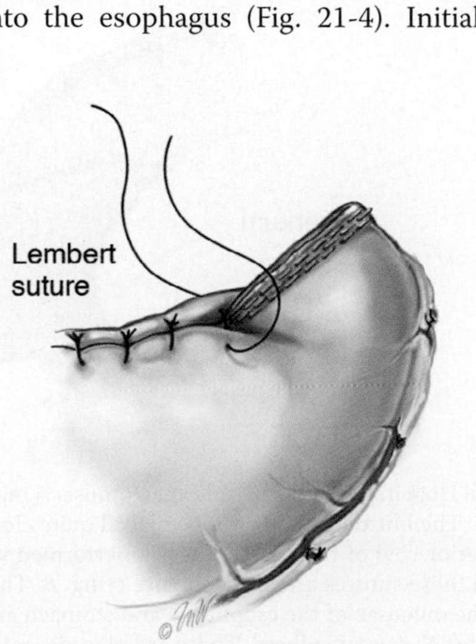

Figure 21-3. The staple line of the gastric conduit is turned in with interrupted Lembert sutures before completing the anastomosis.

Anastomosis

There are multiple options for performing the gastroesophageal anastomosis. Many advocate for a stapled approach which can be done in a number of different ways. However, we prefer a two-layer hand-sewn technique with interrupted 4-0 silk sutures (Fig. 21-5). Basic principles of performing the anastomosis are (1) to avoid placing crushing clamps on tissue to be included in the anastomosis and (2) to transect the esophagus with a fresh knife blade rather than cautery. No matter how preformed, there must be no tension on the anastomosis. The interrupted fashion of the anastomosis does not allow for purse-stringing and permits blood vessels to reach the anastomotic edge. If the anastomosis is sufficiently secure after these basic principles are followed, there should be no concern about placing the anastomosis in the mediastinum.

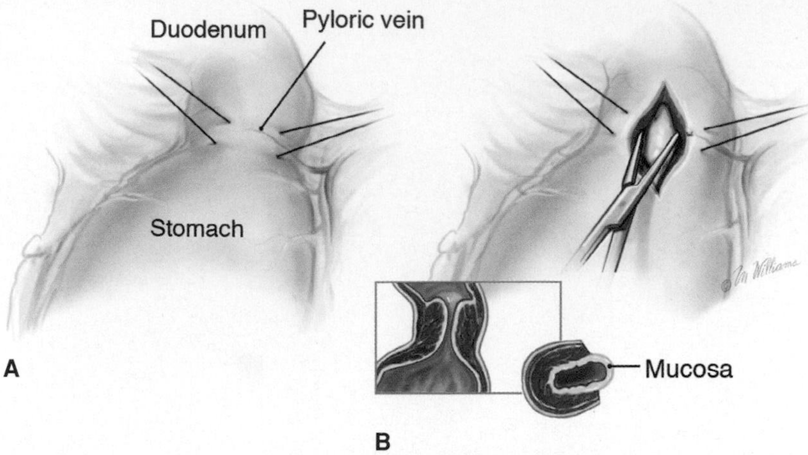

Figure 21-4. *A.* A 2-cm incision across the pylorus provides exposure of the muscle for division down to the mucosal layer. *B.* The principal risk of entry is where the duodenal mucosa covers the undersurface of the pyloric muscle.

The anastomosis is performed end (esophagus) to side (gastric tube). A point approximately 2 cm from the gastric suture line is selected, and a small circle of the size of a nickel is scored in the serosa with a knife blade. The small submucosal vessels exposed by this maneuver then are ligated with fine silk. A long right-angled clamp is placed just distal to the planned line of transection and the specimen remains attached to the proximal esophagus and is reflected proximally to expose the planned line of transection. The two-layer anastomosis is performed in the following fashion: The first row of 4-0 silk sutures

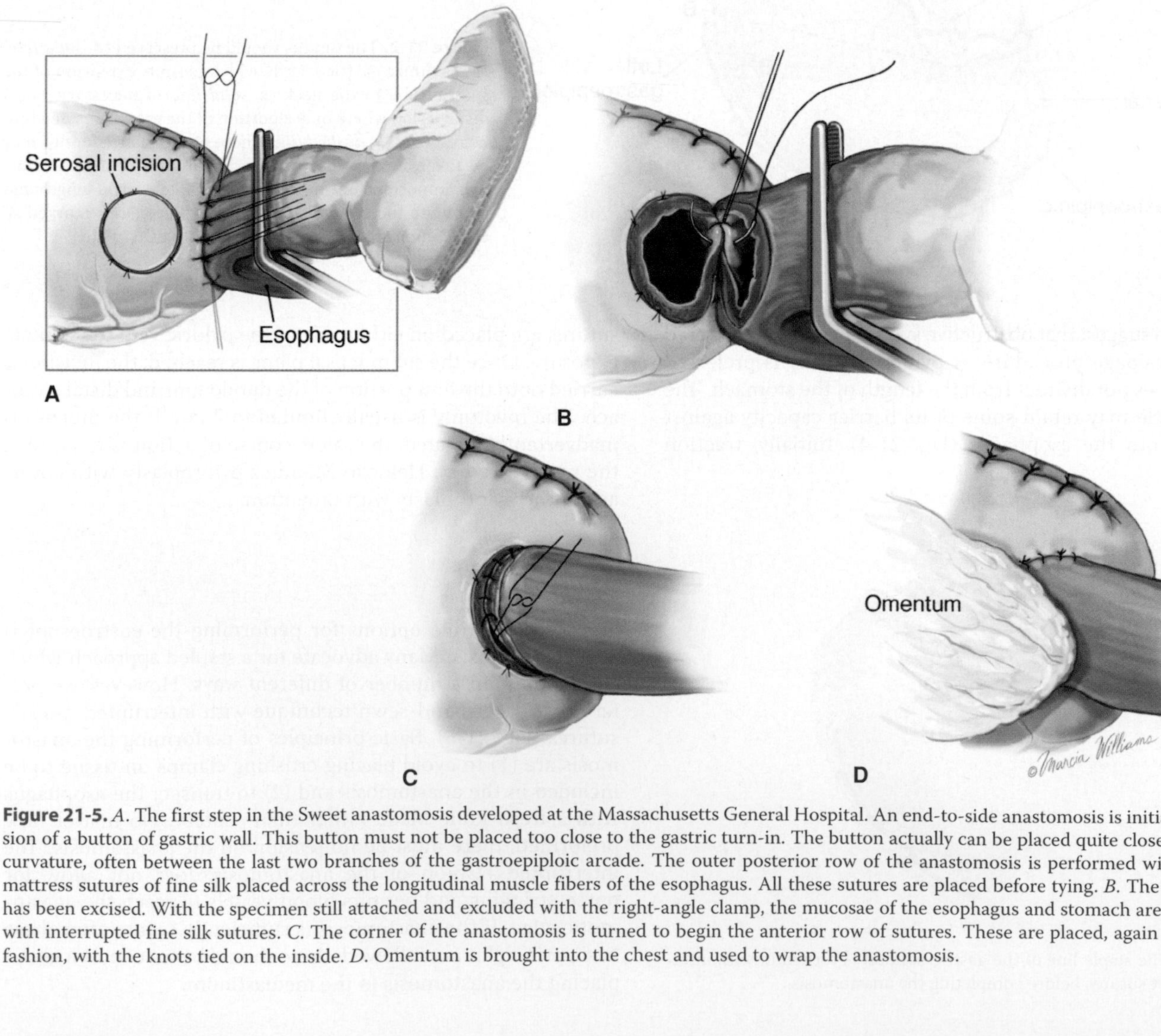

Figure 21-5. *A.* The first step in the Sweet anastomosis developed at the Massachusetts General Hospital. An end-to-side anastomosis is initiated with excision of a button of gastric wall. This button must not be placed too close to the gastric turn-in. The button actually can be placed quite close to the greater curvature, often between the last two branches of the gastroepiploic arcade. The outer posterior row of the anastomosis is performed with interrupted mattress sutures of fine silk placed across the longitudinal muscle fibers of the esophagus. All these sutures are placed before tying. *B.* The gastric button has been excised. With the specimen still attached and excluded with the right-angle clamp, the mucosae of the esophagus and stomach are approximated with interrupted fine silk sutures. *C.* The corner of the anastomosis is turned to begin the anterior row of sutures. These are placed, again in interrupted fashion, with the knots tied on the inside. *D.* Omentum is brought into the chest and used to wrap the anastomosis.

is placed in a horizontal mattress fashion between the muscularis of the esophagus and the serosa–muscular layer of the stomach. A total of four to six sutures are placed posteriorly and tied while the stomach is brought up to the esophagus (because the esophagus is a fixed structure). This outer posterior layer should cover only one-third of the circumference, which provides exposure for placement of an inner layer.

The esophagus then is opened sharply 4 to 5 mm distal to the initial row of sutures, and the incision is extended to each corner. The mucosal button of the stomach then is opened, and the inner back row of oiled 4-0 silk sutures is placed. Each stitch is placed approximately 5 mm back from the cut edge. The sutures should include the full thickness of the stomach and submucosa and mucosa of the esophagus. Attempts should be made not to manipulate the mucosa. Elevating the previous stitch guides placement of the next. Once the posterior row is complete, the esophagus can be transected. The nasogastric tube is advanced through the anastomosis to the level of the gastric antrum. The anterior inner row is completed in a similar fashion such that the knots are always within the lumen with complete inversion of the mucosa. The outer layer of horizontal mattress sutures is completed over the remaining two-thirds of the circumference. The stomach is suspended by a series of nonabsorbable sutures to the fascia overlying the thoracic spine. Omentum is brought into the chest and used to wrap the anastomosis.

A jejunostomy tube is placed at the conclusion of the case for feeding purposes to speed recovery, to improve nutrition, and to promote healing. Patients are usually discharged on tube feeding and limited oral intake. The jejunostomy tube is usually removed at the first postoperative visit.

POSTOPERATIVE MANAGEMENT

Patients spend the first night in an ICU. With a significant amount of dissection and mobilization of stomach and esophagus, it is important to maintain an adequate volume status and not engage in the use of pressors for the management of blood pressure. This avoids spasm of the right gastroepiploic artery and compromise of the anastomosis.

The nasogastric tube remains in place for several days, and a barium swallow evaluation is performed approximately 1 week after surgery. During the course of the first week, patients are often started on enteral feeds via the jejunostomy tube, and these feedings are increased over the course of several days.

The epidural catheter is typically left in place for 3 to 4 days following the procedure. Occasionally, if patient comorbidities allow, we will add ketorolac as a supplement to the epidural if needed. As the patient is transitioned to enteral feeding pain medication, typically narcotics, they can be delivered via the feeding tube and the epidural discontinued. Once oral intake is established, patients usually convert to oral narcotics until the pain resolves.

The left chest tube is left in place until drainage slows, which often takes several days. We prefer to start tube feeding and advance to goal prior to removal to ensure there is not a chyle leak. It is not necessary to leave the chest tube in place until the barium swallow is performed, and it is often discontinued between postoperative days 4 and 6.

PROCEDURE-SPECIFIC COMPLICATIONS

Many potential complications exist after a thoracoabdominal esophagectomy, the most dreaded being an anastomotic leak. Smaller anastomotic leaks that appear to drain back into the esophagus can be followed in a conservative manner and should heal. A leak developing after 2 to 4 weeks may only give rise to a localized empyema, which may be managed initially with percutaneous drains but may need a more definitive procedure. A large intrathoracic leak during the early postoperative period can cause an acute pyopneumothorax, fever, dyspnea, and shock. These patients need to be emergently explored and potentially diverted.

Other potential complications include gastric conduit necrosis, aortoanastomotic fistula, delayed gastric emptying, and anastomotic stricture. Approximately 5% to 10% of patients develop an anastomotic stricture, and most respond to a single dilation.

Reflux is also a common complaint after esophagectomy and gastric pull-up. It has been demonstrated that the severity of the reflux depends on the height of the anastomosis, with lower anastomoses leading to more reflux. Often conservative measures are sufficient to control reflux, including smaller, more frequent meals, elevation of the head of the bed, and acid suppression.

SUMMARY

Thoracoabdominal esophagectomy is one of several surgical approaches to carcinoma of the esophagus. In a series from the Massachusetts General Hospital, we reported a 2.9% mortality with no anastomotic leaks in 101 patients, thus demonstrating excellent results with a low mortality and morbidity.[9] Before proceeding to surgery, a standard and logical staging evaluation should be completed and clearance obtained from a cardiac and pulmonary perspective. Postoperative care is similar to that for other techniques of esophageal resection, with careful attention paid to pulmonary physiotherapy and early mobilization. Potential complications include anastomotic stricture, anastomotic leak, and reflux.

CASE HISTORY

A 76-year-old man presented with worsening dysphagia and moderate weight loss. His past medical history was significant for coronary artery disease status, postcoronary artery bypass grafting, and diabetes mellitus. Physical examination was unremarkable. An initial barium swallow demonstrated a mass lesion in the distal esophagus. Endoscopy revealed a tumor at 37 cm from the incisors with thickening of the gastroesophageal junction on retroflexed view. Biopsies were read as adenocarcinoma. Further work-up included EUS, which staged the tumor as uT2N0, as well as PET/CT imaging of the chest and abdomen that were without enlarged lymph nodes and metastases. Other preoperative testing included an ECG, a stress test, pulmonary function tests, and a full laboratory evaluation, which were within normal limits. With the tumor located in the distal third of the esophagus, we proceeded with a thoracoabdominal esophagectomy. No metastatic disease was found at the time of surgery, and the patient underwent a complete lymph node dissection. A hand-sewn esophagogastric anastomosis was performed. Pathology returned a T_2 tumor with no evidence of metastatic disease in 28 lymph nodes sampled.

The patient was extubated in the OR and transferred to the surgical ICU after the procedure. He was transferred to the general thoracic surgical floor on postoperative day 1. Physical therapy began immediately to mobilize the patient. With the return of bowel function, tube feeds were started and advanced slowly. A nasogastric tube remained in place. On postoperative day 7, a barium swallow demonstrated no anastomotic leak and adequate gastric emptying. The patient started oral feeding and was discharged on postoperative day 9. At clinical follow-up, he complained of mild reflux symptoms that were controlled adequately with proton-pump inhibitors. Follow-up imaging has been negative for recurrence, and the patient has not required subsequent dilations.

EDITOR'S COMMENT

This approach used by the MGH group was popularized by Sweet after being described by Adams and Phemister. It has been used successfully for several decades. Although it is similar to the Ellis left transthoracic esophagectomy (see chapter 22), in terms of exposure of the esophagogastric junction, it does afford better access to the abdomen and therefore the possibility of doing a pyloroplasty and feeding jejunostomy. Both versions of the left transthoracic approach can be modified and extended to allow for a high supraaortic anastomosis as is popular in China and Russia. On the other hand, the transcostal is the most painful incision in thoracic surgery and should be avoided if at all possible.

—Mark J. Krasna

References

1. Eggers C. Resection of the thoracic portion of the esophagus for carcinoma. *Surg Gynecol Obstet*. 1931;52:739.
2. Adams W, Phemister D. Carcinoma of the lower thoracic esophagus: report of a successful resection and esophagogastrectomy. *J Thorac Surg*. 1938;7:621.
3. Sweet R. Surgical management of carcinoma of the mid-thoracic esophagus: preliminary report. *N Engl J Med*. 1945;223:1.
4. Wu LF, Wang BZ, Feng JL, et al. Preoperative TN staging of esophageal cancer: comparison of miniprobe ultrasonography, spiral CT and MRI. *World J Gastroenterol*. 2003;9:219–224.
5. Chandawarkar RY, Kakegawa T, Fujita H, et al. Comparative analysis of imaging modalities in the preoperative assessment of nodal metastasis in esophageal cancer. *J Surg Oncol*. 1996;61:214–217.
6. Lightdate C. Staging of esophageal cancer: endoscopic ultrasonography. *Semin Oncol*. 1994;21:438–446.
7. Riedel M, Stein HJ, Mounyam L, et al. Predictors of tracheobronchial invasion of suprabifurcal oesophageal cancer. *Respiration*. 2000;67:630–637.
8. Meltzer CC, Luketich JD, Friedman D, et al. Whole-body FDG positron emission tomographic imaging for staging esophageal cancer comparison with computed tomography. *Clin Nucl Med*. 2000; 25(11):882–887.
9. Mathisen DJ, Grillo HC, Wilkins EW Jr, et al. Transthoracic esophagectomy: a safe approach to carcinoma of the esophagus. *Ann Thorac Surg*. 1988;45:137–143.

22 Left Transthoracic Esophagectomy (Ellis)

Mark J. Krasna

Keywords: Esophagectomy, esophageal adenocarcinoma, esophageal resection and reconstruction, left transthoracic approach, Ellis esophagectomy, gastric conduit

The worldwide estimate for new cases of esophageal cancer was 482,300 in 2008.[1] In 2012 over 17,500 new cases of esophageal cancer were diagnosed in the United States alone, with over 15,000 deaths. Despite advances in chemotherapeutic agents and radiation therapy, surgery remains the core component of treatment of this disease. Especially in early-stage disease, surgery is still offered as definitive therapy. The incidence of esophageal adenocarcinoma has been increasing steadily in the United States.[2,3] Adenocarcinoma of the esophagus develops predominantly in a segment of intestinal metaplasia, and thus the increased incidence of esophageal adenocarcinoma translates into an increasingly prevalent disease in the distal third of the esophagus.[4] Given the anatomic configuration of the esophagus within the thoracic cavity, no one surgical incision provides uniform access to the entire esophagus. The surgical approach therefore must be tailored to the individual patient, permitting adequate exposure to the diseased region of the esophagus with the least amount of invasiveness.

Although resection of the distal esophagus via a left transthoracic incision was first described in the 1930s, the increasing prevalence of distal esophageal cancer has renewed interest in this surgical approach.

Likewise, for Barrett esophagus and high-grade dysplasia, the left transthoracic approach can be optimal allowing a safe complete resection through a single incision with much shorter operating times (about 2 hours).[5]

PARTICULARITIES WITH THIS APPROACH

The advantage of left transthoracic esophagectomy is readily apparent in that it affords a surgical resection with a single incision. In addition to the obvious advantage of decreasing the patient's discomfort, the left transthoracic esophagectomy also can be performed in much less time than the Ivor Lewis or McKeown esophagectomy, with operative time averaging 2 to 3 hours.[6] The left transthoracic approach does have a number of disadvantages that should be noted. First, although the division of the diaphragm provides excellent visualization of the left upper quadrant of the abdomen via the left chest, the remainder of the abdomen cannot be accessed using this approach. As a result of the limited abdominal exposure, adequate dissection of the pylorus cannot be achieved to perform pyloromyotomy. Many surgeons profess that gastric drainage is an essential component of esophageal reconstruction with gastric conduit placement after esophagectomy and identify the inability to perform a drainage procedure as a significant limitation of the left transthoracic approach. Evidence for the vital role of gastric drainage, however, is lacking. A meta-analysis of randomized controlled trials revealed that although pyloric drainage decreased the incidence of early gastric drainage dysfunction, the incidence of gastric drainage dysfunction in patients not receiving pyloric drainage was only 10%.[7] Results from this study that suggest a trend toward increased bile reflux in patients treated with pyloric drainage have led some surgeons to question, in general, the value of pyloric drainage in esophageal reconstruction.

A further limitation of the left transthoracic approach is the lack of adequate exposure to perform a feeding jejunostomy. Early enteral nutrition has been demonstrated in some studies to be associated with improved outcome after esophagectomy in comparison with parenteral nutrition.[8] Although jejunostomy is not easily accomplished via the left chest approach, enteral nutrition still may be possible using a nasojejunal feeding tube. To prevent inadvertent anastomotic injury from a blind tube insertion, the nasojejunal tube may be placed at the time of surgery using direct visualization to guide the tube through the anastomosis and endoscopic guidance to position the tube within the jejunum. The position of the nasal feeding tube within the jejunum may be secured using an endoscopic clip to fix the tube to the bowel wall. Alternatively, enteral access may be achieved laparoscopically using a jejunostomy tube or a percutaneous jejunal feeding tube placed under radiologic guidance.

A more subtle limitation of the left transthoracic approach is the technical challenge of performing the esophageal anastomosis within the left chest. Considering the relationship of the distal esophagus to the heart and great vessels within the left thorax, right-handed surgeons may experience some increased technical difficulty when performing the hand-sewn anastomosis from this exposure. The initial technical challenge of performing an esophagogastric anastomosis within the left chest arises from the unfamiliar angle of approach to the operative field for most right-hand dominant surgeons. This can be overcome with experience in this approach. The exposure and approach are identical with the left chest approach for Heller myotomy and Belsey repair. Finally, if a resection requires more extensive dissection, and a left neck anastomosis is thought to be the best approach, the mobilization can be completed under the aortic arch and the conduit prepared for a separate new approach by repositioning the patient.

In fact, in Asia, most surgeons perform total esophagectomies for squamous cell cancer through a sole left thoracotomy approach. Recently, there has been adoption of the standard Ivor Lewis approach in China, as a way of accomplishing a more extensive lymph node dissection. Still, many Asian surgeons perform the resection through the classical Ellis approach.

PREOPERATIVE ASSESSMENT

The limited exposure of the abdomen and thorax resulting from the left thoracotomy approach increases the importance of thorough preoperative staging to rule out metastatic disease.

CT scanning, PET scanning, and endoscopic ultrasound (EUS) are essential components of preoperative staging. Any evidence of metastatic disease identified by CT, PET, or EUS is further investigated using EUS-guided fine-needle aspiration if accessible. At our institution, we continue to pursue an aggressive approach to surgical staging of all patients with esophageal cancer using laparoscopic and thoracoscopic staging for any patient evidencing a suggestion of advanced disease on CT, PET, or EUS. With the advent of more successful EUS-FNA of thoracic lymph nodes, the number of node-negative patients subjected to surgical staging has dropped to about 25%. In patients requiring laparoscopic staging because of suspicion of advanced disease, a jejunal feeding tube may be placed laparoscopically at the time of staging to facilitate perioperative alimentation.

In addition to oncologic staging and standard preoperative testing, preoperative cardiac stress testing and pulmonary function testing should be obtained to confirm the patient's ability to tolerate single-lung ventilation. The patient is placed on a full liquid diet 48 hours before surgery, advancing to a clear liquid diet 24 hours before surgery. Some surgeons still use an antibiotic bowel preparation with oral neomycin and erythromycin base the day before surgery.

TECHNICAL PRINCIPLES

After placing a dual-lumen endotracheal tube in the correct position, as confirmed by bronchoscopy, an 18F nasogastric tube is placed. The patient is placed in the right lateral decubitus position with the arm positioned such that it is flexed 45 to 90 degrees at the shoulder and elbow. The bed is then flexed at the patient's hips to widen the intercostal spaces. The surgeon stands to the patient's left side with the assistant to the patient's right side (Fig. 22-1).

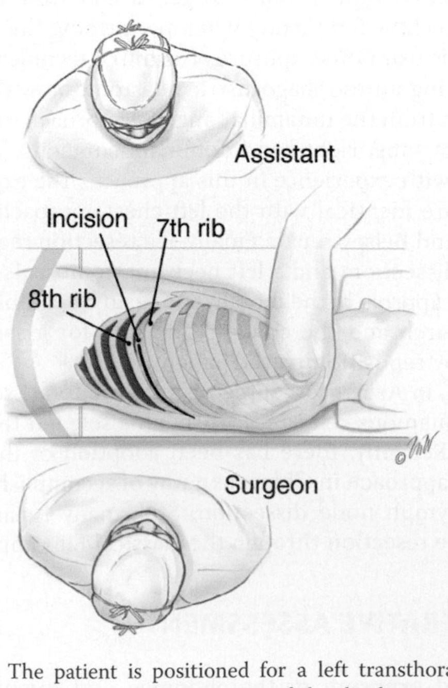

Figure 22-1. The patient is positioned for a left transthoracic esophagectomy. Skin incision provides exposure of the diaphragm and thoracic esophagus. The surgeon stands on the left side of the patient, and the first assistant stands on the right side of the patient.

The patient's skin is prepared and draped widely to the right of the midline in the event that a laparotomy or thoracoabdominal incision is required. The eighth rib is identified by counting the ribs from caudad to cephalad by palpation. The skin is incised over the seventh intercostal space from 4 cm lateral to the costal margin to the posterior axillary line. The latissimus dorsi muscle is divided, but care is taken to preserve the serratus anterior muscle by freeing the inferior attachment of the muscle and thus allowing the muscle to be retracted superiorly. The ribs are again counted to confirm the position of the eighth rib. The seventh intercostal space is entered along the superior edge of the eighth rib. For patients who receive preoperative chemotherapy and radiation, the seventh intercostal muscle bundle is harvested during entry into the thorax to buttress the esophageal anastomosis.

The rib is cut posteriorly just at the junction of the paraspinous muscles, and a small portion of the rib is resected. A rib spreader is used to permit exposure of the left chest. A systematic exploration of the left hemithorax is performed, and mediastinal lymph nodes are sampled for staging. The inferior pulmonary ligament is divided to permit cephalad retraction of the left lung, and the inferior pulmonary ligament lymph nodes (level 9) are removed for pathologic staging. The lung may be palpated for evidence of metastasis.

The mediastinal pleura overlying the esophagus is incised anteromedially in a plane along the pericardiopleural reflection and posterolaterally along the medial aspect of the aorta (Fig. 22-2A). Dissection is continued for several centimeters superiorly and inferiorly to permit sufficient mobilization of the esophagus to identify and palpate the tumor. The nasogastric tube is used as a guide to identify the plane of dissection, and the esophagus is mobilized circumferentially using blunt finger dissection and then encircled with a Penrose drain (Fig. 22-2B). Esophageal mobilization is continued proximally to a point 5 cm above the superior edge of the tumor and distally until the surgeon's fingers can pass easily into the abdomen.

After the esophagus is fully mobilized, the diaphragm is incised in a semilunar fashion approximately 2 to 4 cm from the costal margin. Given the direction of travel of the phrenic nerve fibers, radial incisions should be avoided on the diaphragm to prevent postoperative diaphragmatic paresis. As the diaphragm is being divided, marking sutures are placed on both sides of the divided diaphragm approximately every 5 cm along the incision line to assist with proper orientation of the diaphragm during closure. Care must be taken not to injure the underlying spleen or left colon.

After dividing the diaphragm, the surgeon next explores the abdomen, paying particular attention to the celiac axis and liver. The peritoneum overlying the gastroesophageal junction is incised, and the gastroesophageal junction is freed by blunt finger dissection. The gastroesophageal junction then is encircled with a second Penrose drain (Fig. 22-3). A Harrington retractor is used to retract the left lateral lobe of the liver medially to provide exposure of the hiatus. Gentle retraction with a laparotomy pad or "sponge stick" over the spleen completes the exposure.

The peritoneal reflection is incised to the left of the hiatus close to the gastric serosa. The peritoneum overlying the short gastric vessels is divided, and the vessels themselves are divided using a Harmonic Scalpel (Ethicon-Endosurgery, Inc.), taking care to divide the short gastric vessels well away from the gastroepiploic artery to maximally preserve the right gastroepiploic

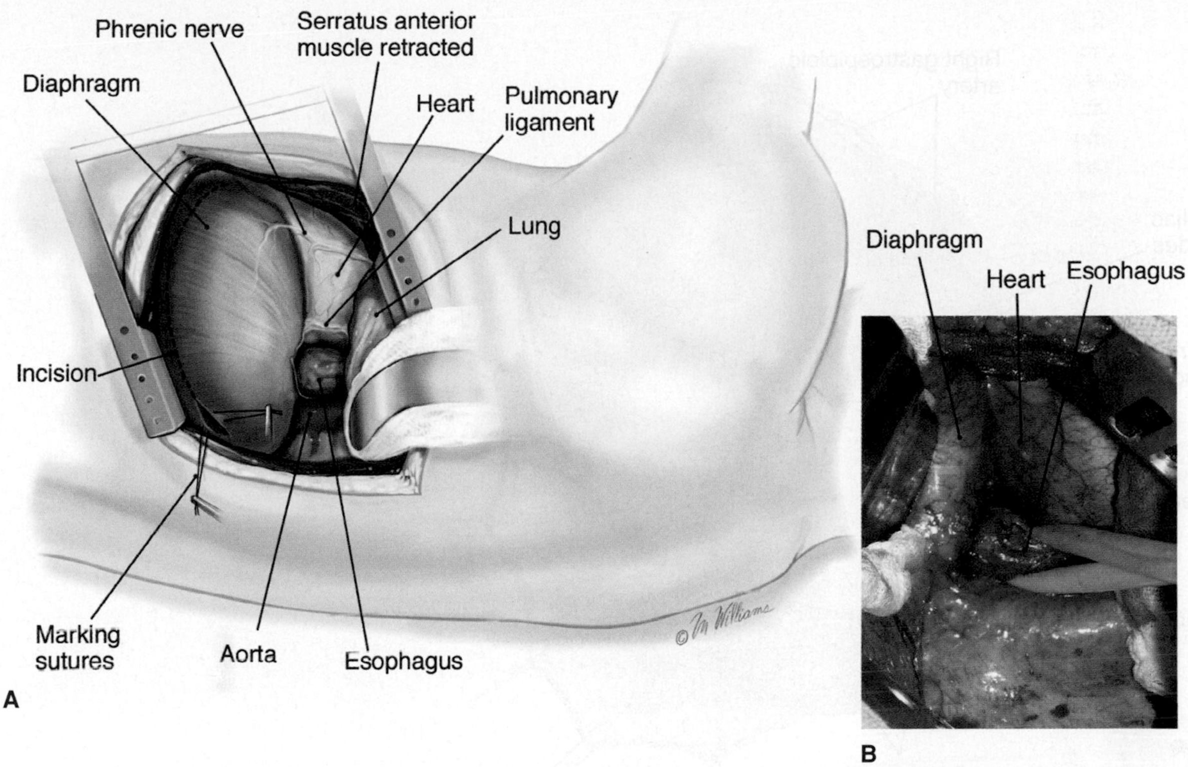

Figure 22-2. *A.* Exposure of the distal esophagus and planned diaphragm incision. *B.* Intraoperative photograph of the same exposure.

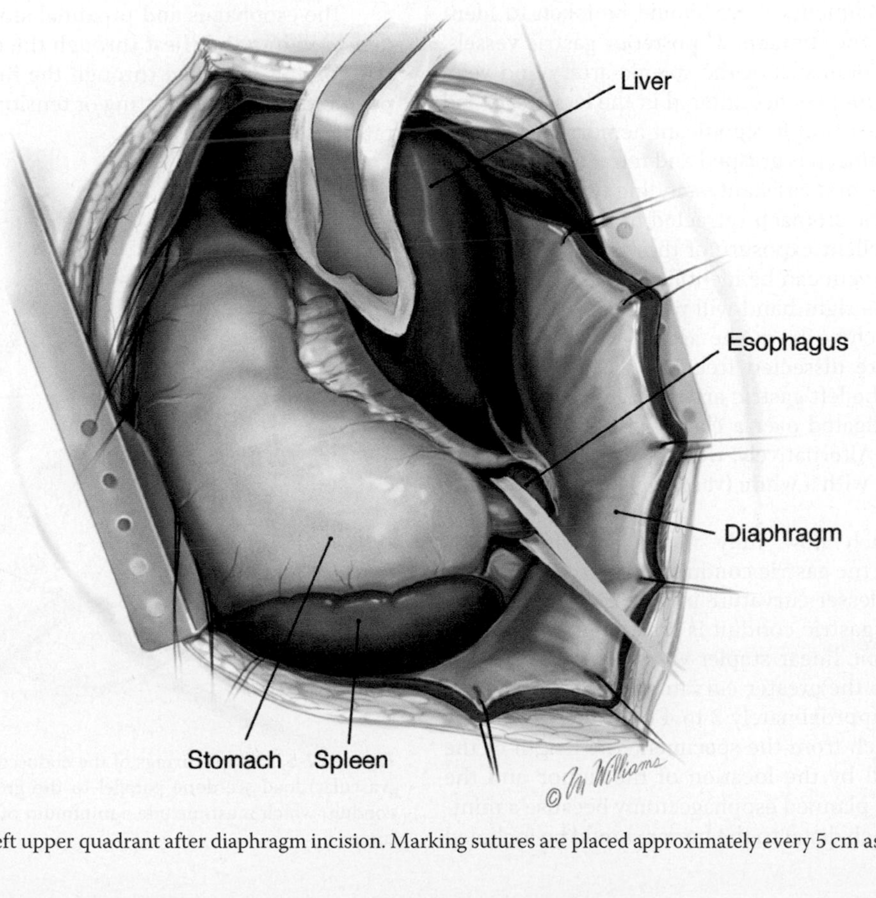

Figure 22-3. Exposure of the left upper quadrant after diaphragm incision. Marking sutures are placed approximately every 5 cm as the diaphragm is incised.

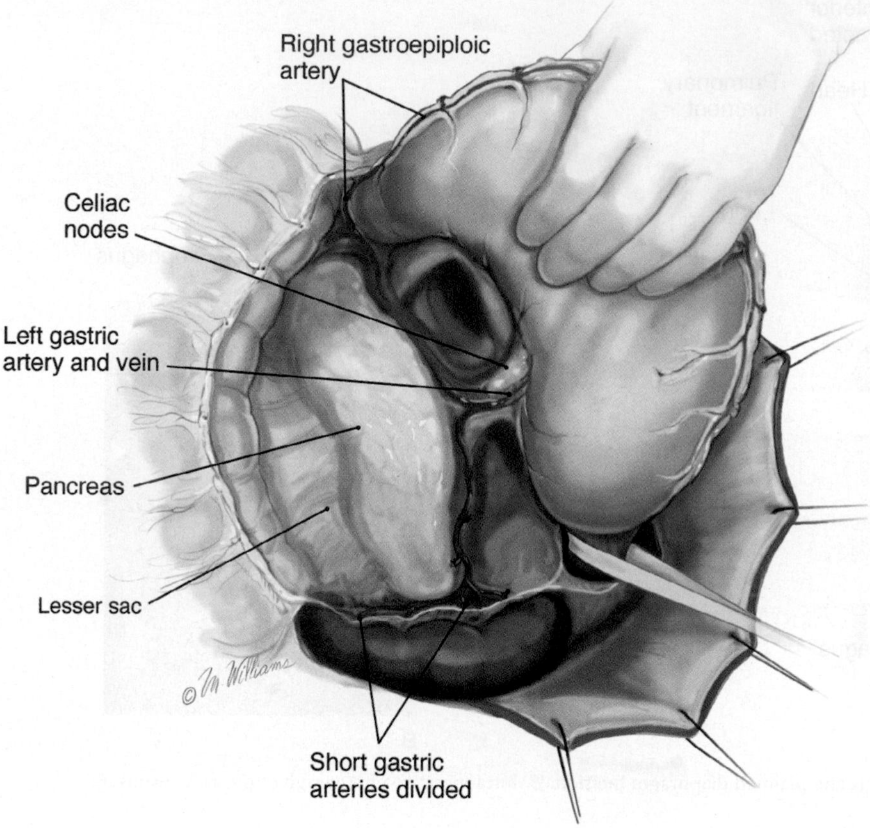

Figure 22-4. After division of the gastrocolic omentum, the stomach is retracted cranially to expose the left gastric artery and vein.

artery. If involved with tumor, the spleen may easily be included with the specimen. The stomach is further mobilized by dividing the posterior attachments. Care should be taken to identify, ligate, and divide the "unnamed" posterior gastric vessels, which arise as direct branches of the splenic artery and vein. These vessels are commonly encountered in the lesser sac, and inadvertent injury may result in significant hemorrhage.

The mobilized stomach is grasped and retracted superiorly and to the right by the first assistant, standing to the right side of the patient. With the stomach retracted in this manner, the surgeon achieves excellent exposure of the lesser sac, and the left gastric artery and vein can be identified (Fig. 22-4). Palpation with the surgeon's right hand will permit identification of the celiac trunk branching from the aorta. Any celiac lymph nodes encountered are dissected free and are included with the specimen. Next, the left gastric artery and vein are sharply dissected, separately ligated over a clamp with 2-0 silk suture ligature, and divided. Alternatively, we now use an endoscopic linear vascular stapler with a white (vascular) load to divide the left gastric artery.

With the stomach now fully mobilized, attention is directed to fashioning the gastric conduit. The nasogastric tube is pushed toward the lesser curvature in preparation for dividing the stomach. The gastric conduit is created using multiple firings of an endoscopic linear stapler with a large green load along a line parallel to the greater curvature of the stomach to create a gastric tube approximately 3 to 4 cm wide, eventually transecting the stomach from the specimen. The length of the conduit is determined by the location of the tumor and the proximal extent of the planned esophagectomy because a minimum of 5 cm of stomach distal to the tumor should be included with the conduit (Fig. 22-5). The staple line is reinforced using 3-0 silk interrupted Lembert sutures.

The esophagus and proximal stomach specimens then are delivered into the chest through the diaphragm. Next, the gastric conduit is passed through the hiatus into the chest and is positioned without twisting or tension along the aorta in preparation for anastomosis.

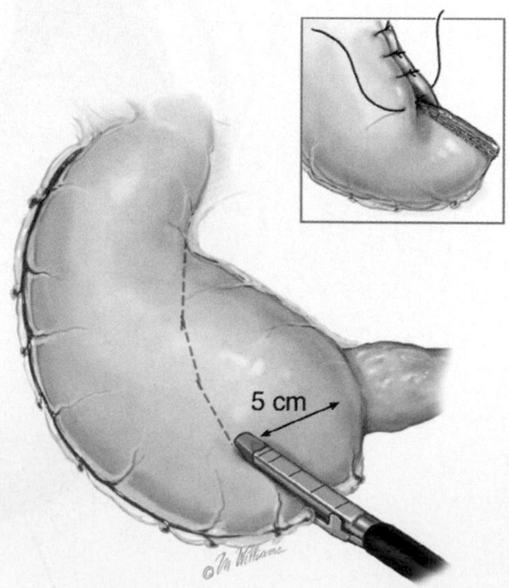

Figure 22-5. Multiple firings of the endoscopic linear stapler with a green (vascular) load are done parallel to the greater curvature to fashion the conduit, which must include a minimum of 5 cm of stomach distal to the tumor.

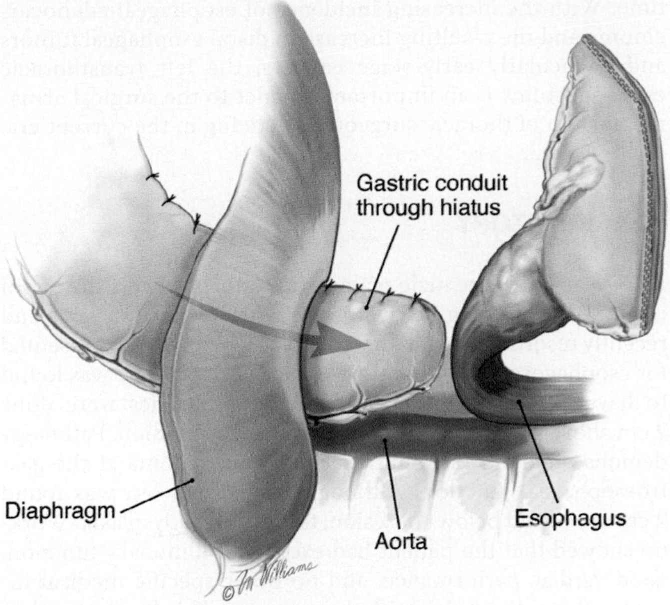

Figure 22-6. The gastric tube (with staple line oversewn) is brought up into the left posterior mediastinum through the hiatus.

The esophagogastrostomy is performed as a two-layer anastomosis. The posterior wall anastomosis is performed before the esophagus is divided and the specimen is removed, because by retracting the intact specimen superiorly, the posterior esophagus is exposed to facilitate suturing (Fig. 22-6). The posterior wall outer-layer anastomosis is performed using interrupted 3-0 silk horizontal mattress sutures (Fig. 22-7A). After the posterior row of sutures is placed, the posterior esophagus is opened using an angled knife blade. The anterior half of the esophagus is not yet divided, again to permit traction on the specimen to expose the anastomotic site. Any large arterial vessels that are bleeding are point cauterized, but care is taken to minimize electrocautery along the anastomotic line.

The gastrotomy is performed next, also using sharp incision through the gastric serosa and then mucosa. The inner layer of the anastomosis is performed using 4-0 interrupted absorbable sutures taking full-thickness bites of the esophagus and large seromuscular and small mucosal bites on the stomach (Fig. 22-7B). When the posterior half of the inner row of sutures is completed, the sutures are placed on clamps and retracted laterally, and the remainder of the esophagus is transected along a bevel to create a slightly longer esophageal length anteriorly than posteriorly (Fig. 22-7C). Before completing the anastomosis, the nasogastric tube is advanced under direct vision through the anastomosis and into the stomach (Fig. 22-7D). The anterior inner full-thickness anastomosis is then completed such that the knots are within the lumen at the completion of the inner layer. Finally, the anterior outer layer of interrupted 3-0 silk horizontal mattress suture is placed to complete the anastomosis.

At this point, the anastomosis may be further buttressed by using an intercostal muscle bundle harvested during initial thoracotomy. The intercostal bundle is secured over the anastomosis with interrupted 3-0 absorbable sutures. Alternatively,

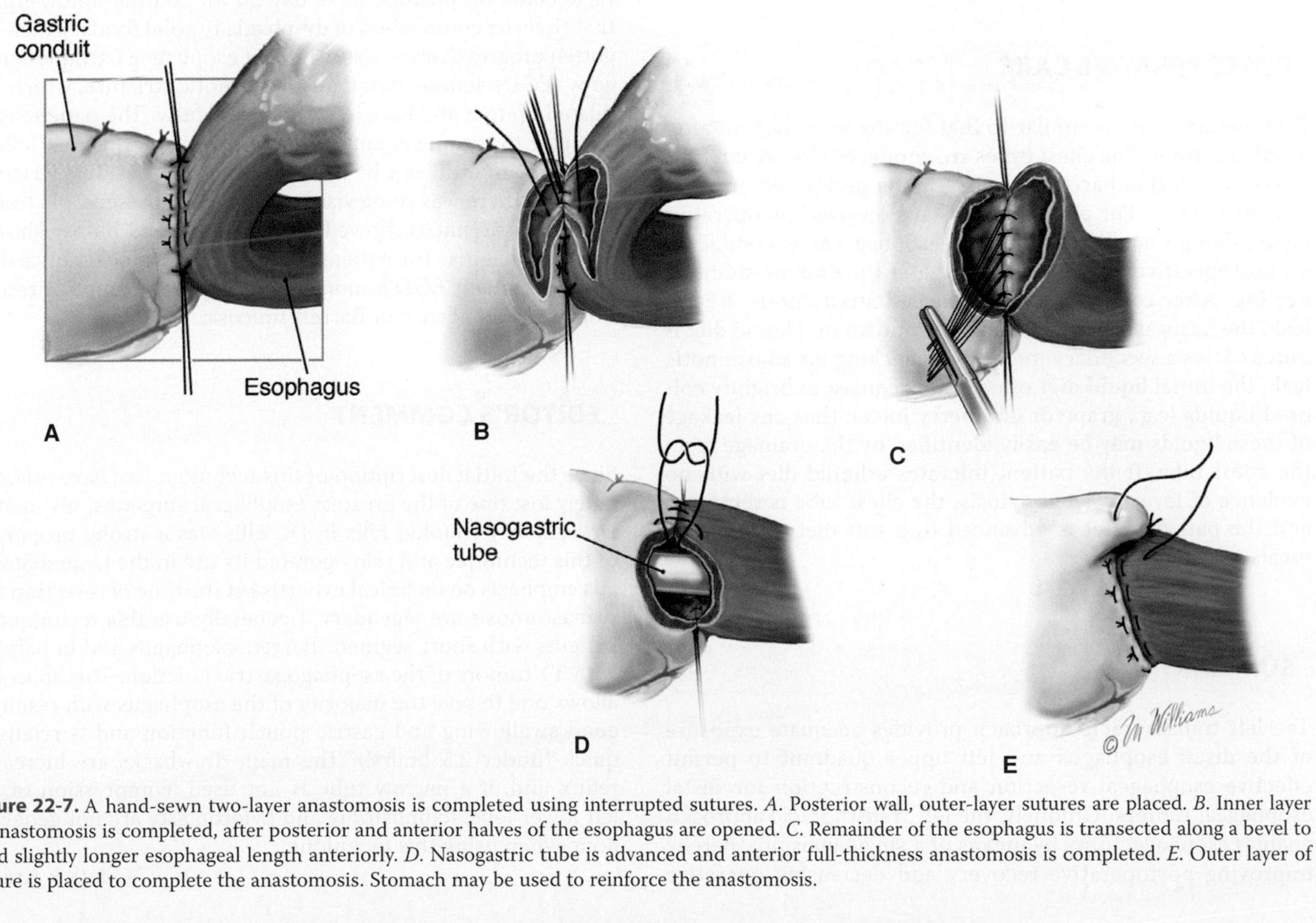

Figure 22-7. A hand-sewn two-layer anastomosis is completed using interrupted sutures. *A.* Posterior wall, outer-layer sutures are placed. *B.* Inner layer of anastomosis is completed, after posterior and anterior halves of the esophagus are opened. *C.* Remainder of the esophagus is transected along a bevel to yield slightly longer esophageal length anteriorly. *D.* Nasogastric tube is advanced and anterior full-thickness anastomosis is completed. *E.* Outer layer of suture is placed to complete the anastomosis. Stomach may be used to reinforce the anastomosis.

the stomach may be used to reinforce the anastomosis (Fig. 22-7E). By taking a second row of Lembert sutures over the anterior suture line, the stomach serves to bury the entire anterior suture line, creating a so-called "ink well." Some surgeons prefer a stapled anastomosis for this approach as well, in which case a circular load is probably easier than a linear load. After this, any redundant stomach is returned to the abdomen to avoid future technical issues related to torsion or sacculation of the gastric conduit.

After ensuring adequate hemostasis, attention is directed to closing the diaphragmatic defect. The previously placed sutures within the diaphragm are used as markers for orientation, and the diaphragm is reapproximated using interrupted figure-of-eight absorbable monofilament sutures. To prevent herniation into the abdomen and subsequent traction on the anastomosis, the gastric tube may be secured to the mediastinal pleura and/or diaphragm with a number of interrupted 3-0 silk sutures. The chest is drained with a single 36F chest tube placed inferiorly and posteriorly to provide dependent drainage. After thorough reexpansion of the lung, the chest is closed using #1 absorbable PDS suture for the paracostal sutures, as well as #1 absorbable running suture to reapproximate the muscle layers. The subcutaneous tissues are closed using a 2-0 absorbable suture in a running fashion, and the skin is reapproximated with a running 3-0 subcuticular suture.

Before the patient emerges from anesthesia, the nasogastric tube is secured in position using a bridle technique by passing an umbilical tape around the choana or suturing the tube to the septum with a large nylon suture. The patient is extubated in the OR after gaining consciousness.

POSTOPERATIVE CARE

Postoperative care is similar to that for any other patient after esophagectomy. The chest tubes are connected to −20 cm H_2O of suction. A thin barium esophagram is performed on postoperative day 7. For patients who have received preoperative chemotherapy and radiation, the esophagram is conducted on postoperative day 10 to allow greater time for anastomotic healing. After confirming a well-healed anastomosis, free of leak, the nasogastric tube is removed and an oral liquid diet is initiated. As a secondary method of checking for anastomotic leak, the initial liquid diet offered may consist of brightly colored liquids (e.g., grape or cranberry juice); thus any leakage of these liquids may be easily identified by the drainage from the chest tube. If the patient tolerates a liquid diet with no evidence of fever or leukocytosis, the chest tube is removed, and the patient's diet is advanced to a soft diet of six small meals a day.

SUMMARY

The left transthoracic approach provides adequate exposure of the distal esophagus and left upper quadrant to permit effective esophageal resection and reconstruction for distal esophageal tumors. Uniquely, the left transthoracic approach enables esophagectomy by means of a single incision, thereby improving postoperative recovery and decreasing operative time. With the increasing incidence of esophageal adenocarcinoma and the resulting increase in distal esophageal tumors and particularly early-stage cancers, the left transthoracic esophagectomy is an important adjunct to the surgical armamentarium of thoracic surgeons practicing in the current era.

CASE HISTORY

A 55-year-old white male malpractice attorney had a history of reflux. After treating his symptoms with Rolaids for years and recently resorting to over-the-counter H_2 blockers, he presented for esophagoscopy. At the time of his endoscopy, he was found to have Barrett mucosa. Four quadrant biopsies were done 2 cm above and below the gastroesophageal junction. Pathology demonstrated a T1a noninvasive adenocarcinoma at the gastroesophageal junction. Although Barrett mucosa was found 2 cm above and below the lesion, there was no dysplasia. Workup showed that the patient had excellent pulmonary function, good cardiac performance, and no other specific medical illnesses. After discussion with the patient and his family, the thoracic surgeon decided that a left transthoracic esophagectomy would allow the best swallowing in the postoperative period, although the patient still may experience some symptoms of reflux. The patient concurred, and a left transthoracic esophagectomy with anastomosis at the level of the inferior pulmonary vein was done using a two-layer hand-sewn anastomosis. The patient had a normal swallow study on postoperative day 7 and was discharged from the hospital on postoperative day 10 able to eat six small meals per day. He presented back to the thoracic clinic on postoperative day 30 for routine follow-up. At that time, he complained of dysphagia to solid foods, which had gotten progressively worse. A repeat esophagogastroduodenoscopy (EGD) demonstrated an anastomotic stricture, which was dilated up to a 40F bougie without difficulty. The patient again was able to resume eating six small meals a day, and at follow-up EGD 1 month later he had no evidence of residual stricture, although there was some visible esophagitis present. pH testing of the gastric juices showed a normal pH, and biopsy showed mild esophagitis. The patient resumed his H_2 blocker once daily and subsequent EGD 6 months later showed complete resolution and no evidence of Barrett mucosa.

EDITOR'S COMMENT

Since the initial description of this technique, we have unfortunately lost one of the greatest esophageal surgeons, my mentor Dr. F. Henry (Bunky) Ellis Jr. Dr. Ellis was a strong proponent of this technique and reinvigorated its use in the United States. His emphasis on technical expertise at the time of resection and reanastomosis are legendary. I generally use this technique in patients with short-segment Barrett esophagus and in patients with T1 tumors of the esophagogastric junction. This approach allows one to save the majority of the esophagus with resultant good swallowing and gastric pouch function and is relatively quick (under 2.5 hours!). The main drawbacks are increased reflux and, if a narrow tube is not used, compression of the left lower lobe. Jejunostomy and pyloroplasty are not generally done when using this technique.

—Mark J. Krasna

References

1. American Cancer Society. Global Facts and Figures 2008. http://www.cancer.org/acs/groups/content/@epidemiologysurveilance/documents/document/acspc-027766.pdf. Accessed December 28, 2012.
2. American Cancer Society. Facts and Figures 2012. http://www.cancer.org/acs/groups/content/@epidemiologysurveilance/documents/document/acspc-031941.pdf. Accessed June 11, 2014.
3. Bollschweiler E, Wolfgarten E, Gutschow C, et al. Demographic variations in the rising incidence of esophageal adenocarcinoma in white males. *Cancer.* 2001;92:549–555.
4. Theisen J. Preferred location for the development of esophageal adenocarcinoma within a segment of intestinal metaplasia. *Surg Endosc.* 2006;20:235–358.
5. Adams W, Phemister D. Carcinoma of the lower thoracic esophagus: report of a successful resection and esophagogastrostomy. *J Thorac Surg.* 1938;7:62.
6. Krasna M. Left transthoracic esophagectomy. *Chest Surg Clin North Am.* 1995;5:543–554.
7. Urschel JD, Blewett CJ, Young JE, et al. Pyloric drainage (pyloroplasty) or no drainage in gastric reconstruction after esophagectomy: a meta-analysis of randomized, controlled trials. *Dig Surg.* 2002;19:160–164.
8. Gabor S, Renner H, Matz V, et al. Early enteral feeding compared with parenteral nutrition after oesophageal or oesophagogastric resection and reconstruction. *Br J Nutr.* 2005;93:509–513.

23 Options for Esophageal Replacement

Wayne Hofstetter, MD

Keywords: Esophagectomy, esophageal reconstruction, conduit, jejunum, colon, stomach

INTRODUCTION

Reestablishing gastrointestinal continuity after esophagectomy can be challenging for patient and surgeon alike. There are no perfect substitutes, since every reconstructive alternative is inferior to the native, normal esophagus. Ultimately, the goals for reconstruction include the maintenance of continuity, ability to swallow followed by adequate transit of food through the replacement conduit, provision of some barrier to reflux and aspiration, and independence from nutritional sources other than a normal oral diet. Simultaneously, every surgeon has the obligation to minimize morbidity, mortality, and long-term alterations in quality of life to the greatest extent possible. At odds to these objectives are the indications for removing the native organ and the extent to which it must be sacrificed. Clearly, situations that require complete removal of the esophagus up to the base of the tongue necessitate different reconstructive efforts compared to junctional tumors where a portion of the thoracic esophagus can remain intact. Esophageal surgeons must be adept and versatile at many different replacement options. This chapter focuses on the description of reconstructive options, emphasizing conduits other than stomach as described in foregoing chapters (Fig. 23-1). To the greatest extent possible, an attempt is made to compare our experiences with the various conduit options with the caveat that there is no level 1 data pertaining to such comparison.

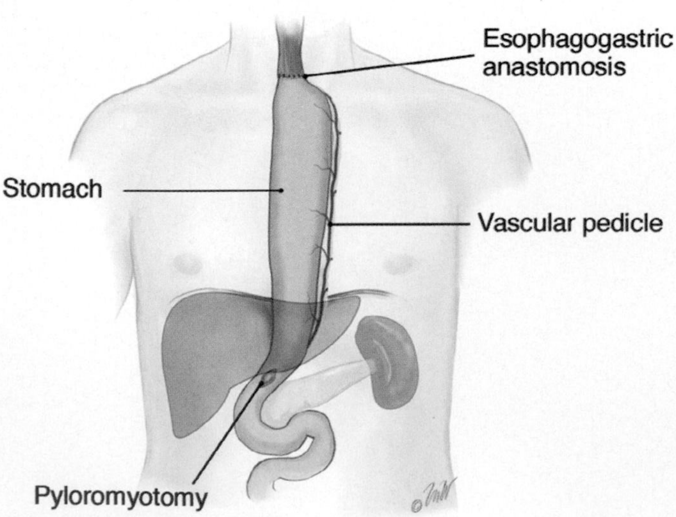

Figure 23-1. Stomach is the preferred graft for malignant esophageal replacement. Several configurations have been devised. Depicted here is a conduit in which the whole stomach is used.

ORGAN ALTERNATIVES

Whenever a reconstruction alternative other than stomach is used, the complexity of the procedure significantly increases. Rather than a single esophagogastric anastomosis, alternative reconstructive efforts will require two to three anastomoses to reestablish continuity. Establishing adequate blood supply to the transposed reconstruction also may be more challenging in contrast to using a well-vascularized gastric conduit. For these reasons, modified whole stomach options are generally considered the first alternative to the native esophagus, despite the relative disadvantages generated by transposing the gastric reservoir into the chest, such as life-long reflux and aspiration risk (Fig. 23-2).

When the stomach is not available, however, alternative conduits for esophageal replacement become necessary. The decision to choose one option over another depends on patient and surgeon factors. The more common preferences include the colon or jejunum in variations of length and vascular supply. Prior abdominal operations or preexisting pathology may limit the use of either organ, and a thorough history is an essential part of planning for reconstruction.

JEJUNUM

The jejunum is an option for either partial or total esophageal replacement (Fig. 23-3). There are several advantages to consider with small bowel reconstruction. It generally remains free of intrinsic disease throughout a patient's life span and does not undergo senescent lengthening. Compared to the native esophagus, the size-match is excellent. There is a relative abundance of the organ, which permits reconstruction of the whole esophagus with adequate length to maintain nutritional demands. The jejunum also has a reliable blood supply with fairly consistent anatomy that does not routinely require preoperative evaluation. In the past, there were limitations on the length of esophagus that could be reconstructed with the jejunum, but this issue largely has been overcome with microvascular augmentation techniques that can accommodate grafts spanning from the base of the neck to the abdomen.

Indications

Jejunal interpositions can be tailored to any length necessary to replace the resected esophagus. We have found jejunal interpositions to be especially useful for secondary reconstruction attempts after a gastric conduit loss that has resulted in esophageal diversion. Conduit position is also determined in part by the indication requiring reconstruction. Most often placed in the retrosternal position, a supercharged jejunal conduit also

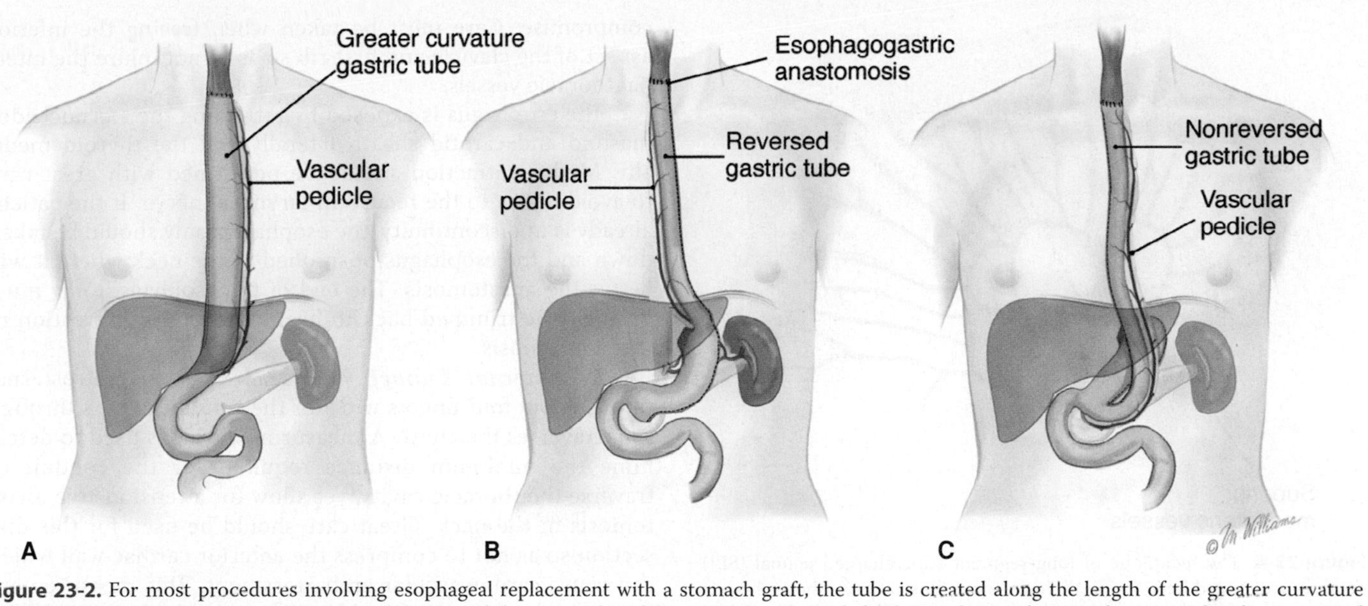

Figure 23-2. For most procedures involving esophageal replacement with a stomach graft, the tube is created along the length of the greater curvature (between the gastric antrum and the splenic hilum), and the remainder of the stomach is discarded (*A*). *B* and *C*. Techniques for reversed and nonreserved gastric tubes, respectively.

may be placed in the posterior mediastinum or less often subcutaneously on the anterior chest. We believe the microvascular anastomosis and subsequent lie of the conduit are best when the conduit is in the substernal position. If local recurrence in the posterior mediastinum is a factor, or the need for radiation exists, the conduit should be placed away from this field.

Surgical Technique

Long Segment Supercharged Jejunal Conduit

Preoperative Evaluation Routine preoperative evaluation is necessary when planning a supercharged jejunal conduit for esophageal replacement. A complete history and physical examination should be performed, and it is important to take note of any previous abdominal, thoracic, or sternal incisions as they may alter the surgical plan and position of the conduit. In the setting of esophageal cancer, complete staging should be performed, including esophagogastroduodenoscopy/endoscopic ultrasound (EGD/EUS) and PET/CT. A CT chest/abdomen with contrast will help rule out metastatic disease, along with abnormalities of the small bowel or major abdominal vessels. Consultation with a plastic surgeon in addition to the thoracic surgeon is necessary when planning a supercharged jejunal conduit. Thorough preoperative patient education and counseling focusing on postoperative expectations, including dietary and lifestyle modifications that will be necessary following the

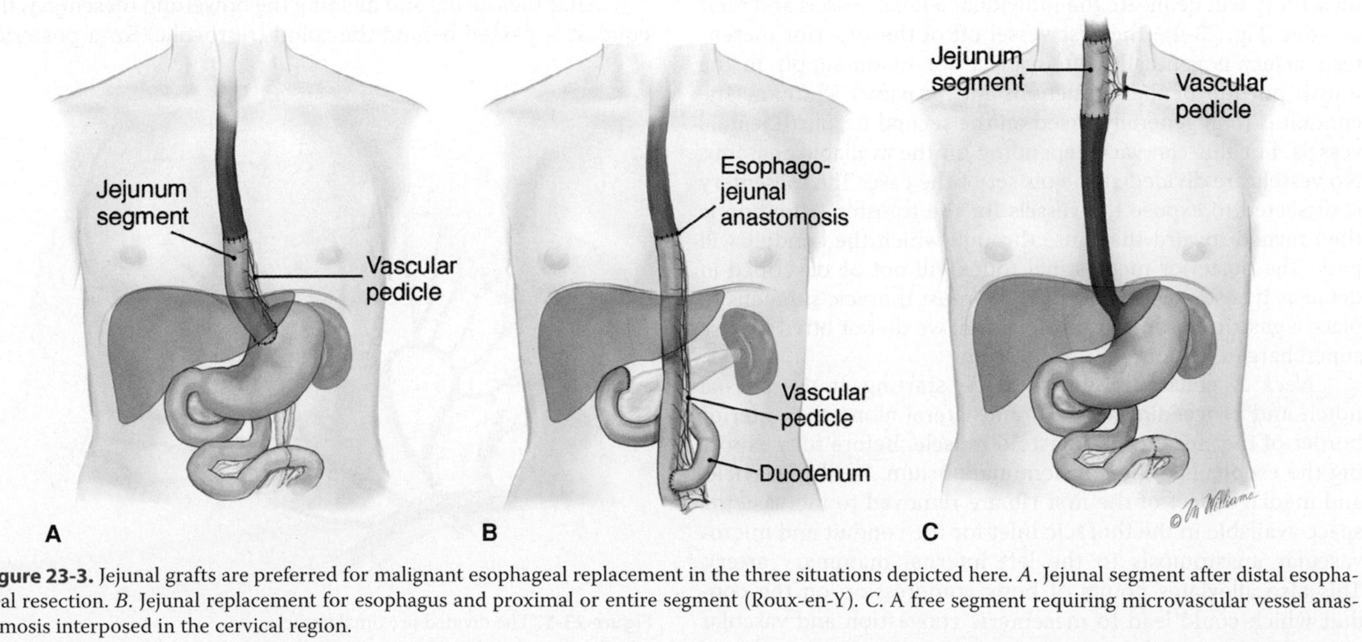

Figure 23-3. Jejunal grafts are preferred for malignant esophageal replacement in the three situations depicted here. *A*. Jejunal segment after distal esophageal resection. *B*. Jejunal replacement for esophagus and proximal or entire segment (Roux-en-Y). *C*. A free segment requiring microvascular vessel anastomosis interposed in the cervical region.

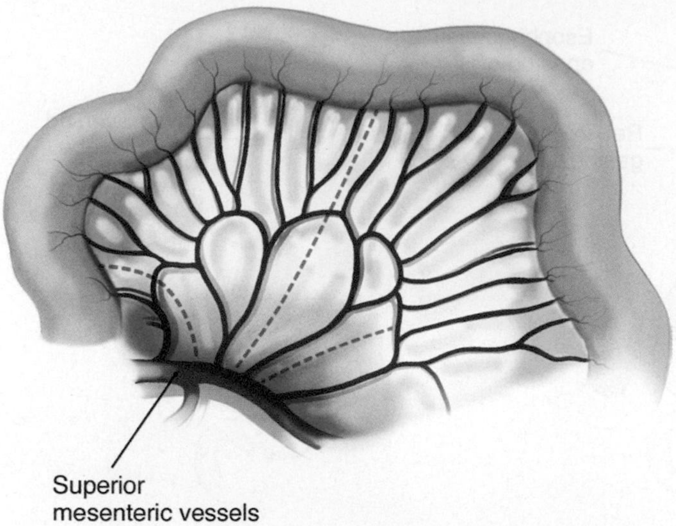

Figure 23-4. The technique of long-segment supercharged jejunal (SPJ) conduit is depicted here and in the next three illustrations. Shown here is the vascular anatomy of the proximal jejunum.

procedure should be provided. In contrast to a colon interposition, there is no need for presurgical preparation of the bowel. Naturally, if one is concerned about the viability of the small bowel as a useable conduit, it is not a bad idea to have the colon prepared as another alternative.

Surgical Procedure The patient is positioned supine with a shoulder roll in place and the head turned slightly to the right. The left neck, chest, and abdomen are prepped into the field. The legs may be prepped into the field at the discretion of the plastic surgeon for possible harvest of a saphenous vein graft.

Abdomen An upper midline incision is made and the ligament of Treitz identified along with the proximal jejunum. A complete lysis of adhesions should be performed and any prior feeding jejunostomy or gastrostomy should be taken down and the bowel repaired. Transillumination of the proximal jejunal mesentery will delineate the individual jejunal vessels and their arcades (Fig. 23-4). The first vessel off of the superior mesenteric artery is generally left in place for blood supply to the fourth portion of the duodenum and proximal jejunum. The conduit is then generally based on the second to fourth jejunal vessels, but this can vary depending on the available anatomy. No vessels are divided at the outset of the case. The mesentery is dissected to expose the vessels for the transfer. Attention is then turned toward the route through which the conduit will pass. The posterior mediastinal route will not be described in detail as it is standard procedure for most thoracic surgeons to place a gastric conduit in this location; we do not often place a supercharged jejunum in this location.

Neck A collar incision is made starting at the sternal notch and proceeding upward and lateral along the anterior border of the sternocleidomastoid muscle. Before fully exposing the esophagus, the left hemimanubrium, head of clavicle, and medial aspect of the first rib are removed to increase the space available in the thoracic inlet for the conduit and microvascular anastomosis to the left internal mammary artery. This also alleviates points of bony compression on the conduit which could lead to mesenteric congestion and vascular compromise. Care must be taken when freeing the inferior aspect of the clavicle and first rib so as to not injure the internal thoracic vessels.

The esophagus is exposed by retracting the sternocleidomastoid and carotid sheath laterally and the thyroid medially. Medial retraction should be performed with great care to avoid injury to the recurrent laryngeal nerve. If the patient already is in discontinuity, the esophagostomy should be taken down and the esophagus positioned in the neck where it will lie for the anastomosis. The end of the esophagostomy must generally be trimmed back to healthy mucosa for creation of the anastomosis.

Retrosternal Tunnel We usually create a retrosternal tunnel about four fingers wide for the conduit to pass through as it traverses the chest. A measuring device is used to determine the minimum distance required for the conduit to traverse the thoracic cavity, yet allow for a tension-free anastomosis in the neck. Great care should be used for this dissection so as not to compress the anterior cardiac wall which can cause cardiovascular embarrassment. This measurement is critical because it is used to determine the location of the distal aspect of the conduit. As much as is practically possible, the conduit should lie in a straight line with no redundancy or large mesenteric loops in the bowel. The position of the conduit is critical to forming a straight, well-functioning jejunal interposition.

Conduit Creation and Passage The proximal pedicle of the jejunum, usually the second jejunal vessel, is divided close to its origin from the superior mesenteric artery (Fig. 23-5). The bowel is divided a few centimeters proximal to this point. The next jejunal vascular pedicle, usually the third, is also divided close to its origin. The mesentery that lies between these two vessels is divided toward the mesenteric border of the bowel to allow the jejunum to unfurl and straighten (Fig. 23-6). This step is key to establish a straight course through the mediastinum and a more accurate estimate of the length needed.

For a jejunogastric anastomosis, the length is measured to the posterior wall of the stomach, and the distal aspect of the jejunum is divided at the appropriate length. For a Roux limb, the distal jejunum does not require division.

After measuring and dividing the bowel and mesentery, the conduit is passed behind the colon (retrocolic) for a posterior

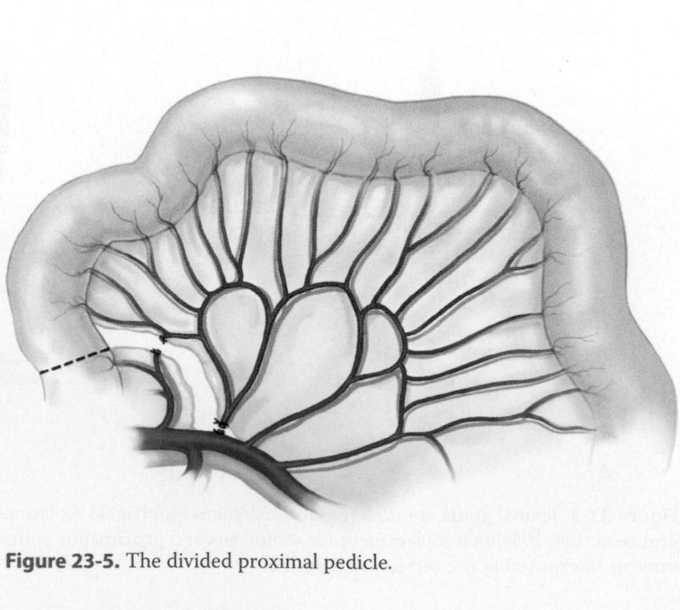

Figure 23-5. The divided proximal pedicle.

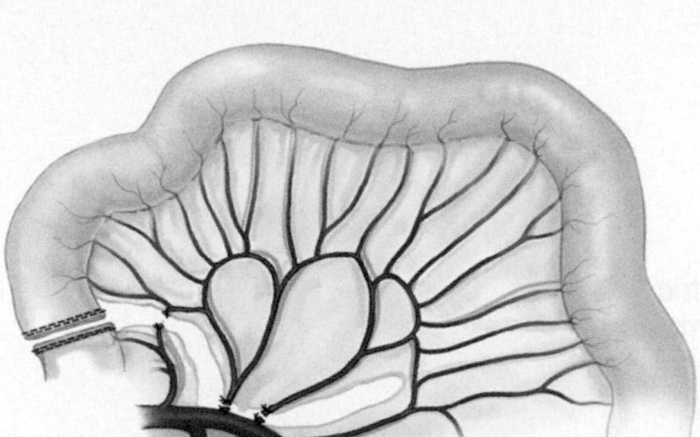

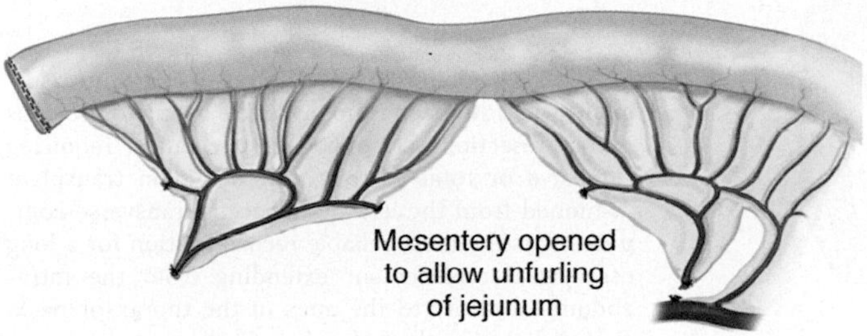

Figure 23-6. Opening the mesentery.

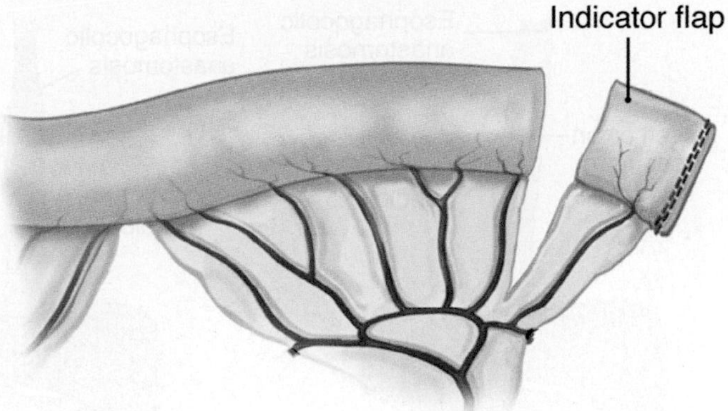

Figure 23-7. Indicator flap.

mediastinal reconstruction, or in front of the colon (antecolic) for a retrosternal reconstruction. The conduit is placed inside a plastic bag to allow safe passage through the mediastinum. The plastic bag provides protection for small vessels as the conduit is pulled through the chosen mediastinal route. One must ensure that no twisting of the conduit occurs as it is pulled through the mediastinum. Care also must be taken to avoid excess traction on the conduit as this can lead to tearing of the mesentery and result in ischemic areas. Once positioned in the neck, the recipient vessels are prepared and the vascular augmentation is performed. The venous anastomosis is typically performed to the internal jugular vein. Saphenous vein grafts can be used if there is a length discrepancy. The arterial anastomosis is then performed under the operating microscope. Usually the artery can be connected directly to the carotid; if there is a length issue it can be anastomosed to a branch vessel or a short Gore-tex graft can be used.

An "indicator flap" can be created with the distal most 2 or 3 cm of jejunum. The distal 2 to 3 cm of the jejunum and its intact mesentery is separated from the main conduit and set aside to be externalized at the completion of the procedure as an indicator flap (Fig. 23-7).

Reconstruction The esophagojejunal anastomosis is performed via a hand-sewn or stapled technique. A stapled functional end-to-end anastomosis may be performed with a posterior linear staple line between the esophagus and jejunal conduit followed by hand-sewn or TA closure of the "hood" (modified Collard or Orringer technique). Alternatively the circular EEA device may be used, but care must be taken to avoid a blind pouch that will lead to a pseudo-Zenker's phenomenon.

The abdominal reconstruction is performed either by creating a "Roux" limb and distal jejunojejunal anastomosis or via a jejunogastric anastomosis low on the posterior wall of the stomach. We generally create a Roux limb as more often there is no remaining stomach for reconstruction. If stomach is chosen we advocate a prior 2/3 gastrectomy to avoid gastric stasis issues created by a vagotomized stomach. A feeding jejunostomy is then performed. If there is remaining stomach that is not in continuity with the conduit (i.e., a Roux limb was created), a drainage procedure at the pylorus should be performed.

When closing the neck incision the indicator flap should be positioned at the inferior aspect of the wound in a straight course so as not to compromise the blood supply. Once a drain is placed and the wound closed, one or both ends of the indicator segment should be opened to allow for drainage of secretions. This flap is left externalized as a monitor for the perfusion of the proximal bowel segment until just prior to discharge. At that point, it can be amputated at the bedside.

Complications

Most of the complications seen after a supercharged jejunal conduit are similar to those seen after esophagectomy. Bowel ischemia resulting in conduit loss is infrequent. Thrombosis or diminished flow through the vascular anastomosis may occur and if perfusion is compromised, the vascular augmentation should be revised to avoid graft loss. The indicator flap serves as a guide to the viability of the conduit and should be monitored frequently. Suspicion of conduit ischemia should prompt evaluation.

Other complications such as bleeding, aspiration pneumonia, recurrent laryngeal nerve damage, redundant bowel loop, and stricture formation are managed using standard techniques.

Results

Recently presented data update the 10-year experience from MD Anderson Cancer Center. Sixty patients received a supercharged jejunal conduit, largely for reconstruction related to esophageal cancer. Postoperative complications included 18 (30%) patients with pneumonia, 19 (31.7%) patients with an anastomotic leak (9 required major intervention, others were managed conservatively), and 4 (6.7%) patients with graft loss. The majority of patients (88%) were able to return to a regular diet after jejunal reconstruction. Thirty-day mortality, including in-hospital mortality, was 5% with a 90-day mortality of 10%. Median survival was 28 months, and the 5-year overall survival in this series is 30%. These results represent a group of high-risk patients, 42% of which were undergoing reversal of discontinuity. Given these results, we prefer a supercharged

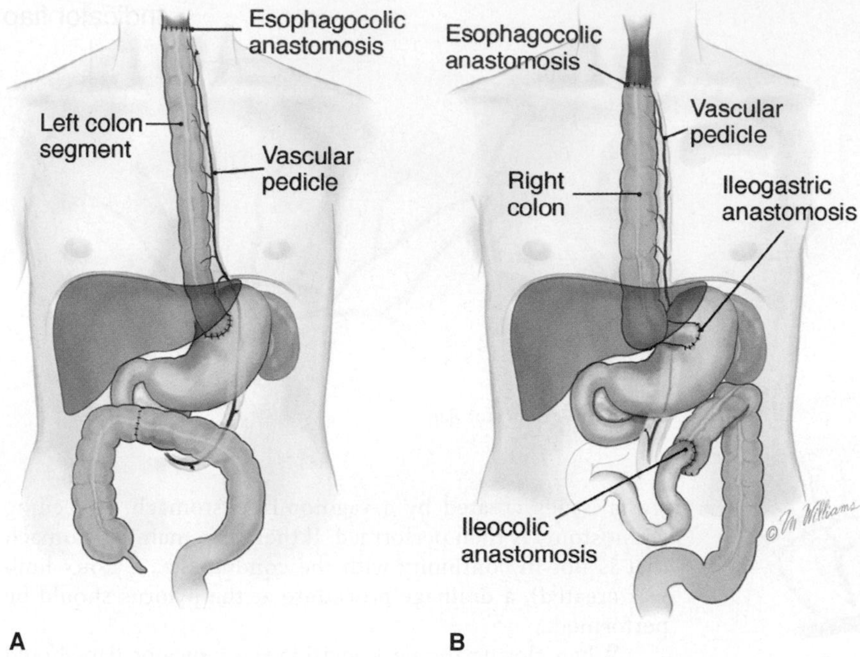

Figure 23-8. Colon interposition is used by most surgeons when stomach is not available owing to previous gastric resection or esophagogastric cancer requiring extensive or total gastrectomy. *A.* Colon transplant fashioned from the left and adjacent transverse components is the most reliable reconstruction for a long esophageal replacement extending from the intra-abdominal cavity to the apex of the thorax or neck. *B.* Pedicled transplant of right colon.

jejunal conduit for esophageal reconstruction only when the stomach is not available.

COLON INTERPOSITION

When the stomach is not available, the colon is another viable option for esophageal reconstruction (Fig. 23-8). Either the right or the left colon may be used for reconstruction and each can provide adequate length to reach the pharynx. The transverse colon is an integral part of the conduit whether it is based on vessels from the right or left colon. A left colon graft is based on the ascending branch of the left colic artery, whereas the middle colic vessels are the primary blood supply for a right colon graft. We prefer to use an isoperistaltic left colon conduit, as opposed to a right colon conduit, because it has a better size-match to the native esophagus and thicker wall. Some believe the colon is the best choice for reconstruction if the patient has an extended life expectancy because it is resistant to peptic strictures and provides a barrier to reflux into the proximal esophagus.

Preoperative Evaluation

The preoperative evaluation is similar to that for a jejunal conduit, which pays special attention to the colonic vessels. A CT angiogram should be obtained to identify and delineate the vascular supply to both right and left colon, including marginal arteries that connect the left and middle colic arcades. Bear in mind that the marginal artery around the splenic flexure may be inadequate or absent in approximately 5% of patients.

Previous abdominal operations or bowel resections also may limit the use of colon if the vessels already have been sacrificed or if the mesentery is scarred and foreshortened. In addition to a CT scan, a colonoscopy or double-contrast barium enema should be obtained to rule out any primary colonic lesions, diverticular disease, or vascular malformations. Patients should be placed on a liquid diet and given a mechanical bowel preparation 24 to 48 hours prior to the operation to remove bulky stool from the conduit.

Surgical Procedure

Here, we describe esophageal replacement with a left colon conduit. Begin by mobilizing the left colon completely and removing the omentum from the transverse colon (Fig. 23-9). Preserve the mesenteric vessels at all times during mobilization and identify the ascending branch of the left colic artery, as this will serve as the vascular pedicle for the conduit. Transillumination of the mesentery facilitates vessel identification. The middle colic artery also needs to be identified in the transverse colon mesentery.

An umbilical tape may be used to approximate the length needed for reconstruction. Measure the distance from a point

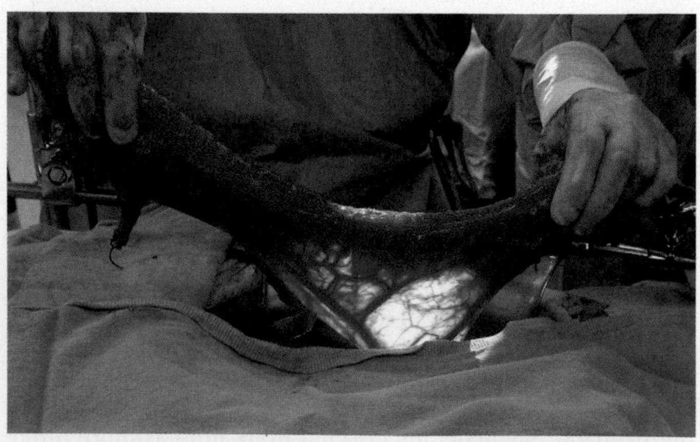

Figure 23-9. Left colon interposition. First the colon is completely mobilized and the omentum is removed from the transverse colon.

5 cm below the xiphoid to the ear lobe. After determining the length needed for transposition, begin vascular isolation of the pedicle. Open the transverse mesocolon on the right side of the middle colic vessels. The mesentery should be opened on both sides of the left colic artery as well. Place small bulldog clamps on the vessels that will be ligated, leaving them in place for 5 to 10 minutes to confirm graft viability. Begin ligating the vessels if the graft appears healthy after vascular isolation. Ligate the left branch of the middle colic at its origin from the middle colic, and ligate the marginal artery beyond the branches supplied by the left colic going distal in the left colon. Confirm the length needed and then transect the colon to the appropriate length. If there is a question about the viability of the segment, either intraoperative Doppler flow or fluorescein dye can be used to assure segmental viability.

The conduit should be placed retrogastric and can be passed through the posterior mediastinum, retrosternal, or via subcutaneous route to its final position in the neck. A plastic bag should again be used when passing the conduit to protect the mesentery and ensure a straight and untwisted course through the mediastinum. If using the retrosternal route, the ipsilateral hemimanubrium, clavicular head, and medial aspect of the first rib should be removed as described above for a jejunal conduit. The anastomosis is done similar to the jejunal anastomosis described above.

Complications

Some of the early complications associated with colonic conduits are secondary to vascular or anastomotic problems. There is generally no indicator flap with a colonic conduit. Therefore, one must monitor the patient carefully for any signs of conduit ischemia. Three colonic anastomoses are used with this method of reconstruction and a leak may occur from any one or more of these anastomoses if ischemia or tension is present. Leaks in the neck are generally managed by opening the neck incision and allowing for wide drainage. Managing intra-abdominal leaks may require more aggressive measures ranging from percutaneous drainage to possible reexploration if less invasive means of controlling the leak are unsuccessful. Late complications are unfortunately not uncommon secondary to senescent lengthening and dilation of the colon interpolate.

Results

The literature on colon interposition for esophageal reconstruction demonstrates good short- and long-term results. Rates of anastomotic leak, graft loss, and perioperative mortality are not significantly different than those associated with gastric pull-up procedures when reported by experienced centers. There are some disadvantages to a colon interposition. Although this is classified as an isoperistaltic graft, the peristalsis is unlikely to be functionally effective and colon interposition really represents a passive conduit. It is also somewhat difficult to avoid creating a colon interposition without introducing some degree of redundancy and angulation. Late reoperation for conduit dilation, stasis, and regurgitation has been described and is used as necessary in up to 30% of patients.

COMPARISON

Limited functional data exist comparing swallowing function with colon compared to jejunal grafts but it is thought that jejunal conduits maintain intrinsic peristalsis after transposition that may actually assist in functional outcomes. The intrinsic peristalsis of the jejunal interposition is also a potential downside; the peristalsis is not coordinated to swallowing in any fashion. Therefore, patients will often complain of some dysphagia during meals early in the transition to peroral intake. This is part of a learning curve, and once patients recognize the symptom they are able to reprogram their swallowing to effectively "wait" until the jejunum is receptive to a bolus swallow. The high incidence of cervical anastomotic leaks in the jejunal series is also of concern.

SUMMARY

Both the colon and augmented jejunum are acceptable options for long-segment esophageal reconstruction when the stomach is not available. There are technical aspects unique and critical to the success of each operation and surgeons will often prefer one technique over others given past experiences. Neither has been definitively proved to be superior in the literature in terms of immediate postoperative outcomes or long-term functional results. Knowledge and adeptness in both techniques are important for the frequent esophageal surgeon.

EDITOR'S COMMENT

This chapter by one of the champions of the "supercharged" jejunal graft is a key component to a successful esophageal surgery practice. Knowledge of all the alternatives is crucial, in the event that either oncologic findings or technical limitations challenge the esophageal surgeon from being able to use a gastric conduit. The availability of jejunum and the ability to use the graft without a preoperative bowel preparation make this an attractive option. When possible, preoperative assessment of vascular compatibility for both jejunal and colonic conduits is preferred. Although the choice of conduit should generally depend on the location of the tumor and the level of the planned anastomosis, occasionally an alternate should be expected up front such as when there has been prior partial gastric resection or numerous prior laparotomies. The authors also mention an important technical trick, not mentioned in any of the other esophagectomy chapters. Before the esophagus is fully exposed, they recommend removing the left hemimanubrium, head of clavicle, and medial aspect of the first rib to increase the space available in the thoracic inlet for the conduit and microvascular anastomosis to the left internal mammary artery. As the authors describe, this also alleviates points of bony compression on the conduit which could lead to mesenteric congestion and vascular compromise. This trick is helpful for any type of esophagectomy where a neck anastomosis must be performed in difficult situations, such as very obese or very thin individuals.

—Mark J. Krasna

Recommended Readings

Ascioti A, Hofstetter W, Miller M, et al. Long-segment, supercharged, pedicled jejunal flap for total esophageal reconstruction. *J Thorac Cardiovasc Surg.* 2005;130(5):1391–1398.

Chen H, Rampazzo A, Gharb B, et al. Motility differences in free colon and free jejunum flaps for reconstruction of the cervical esophagus. *Plast Reconstr Surg.* 2008;122(5):1410–1416.

Doki Y, Okada K, Miyata H, et al. Long-term and short-term evaluation of esophageal reconstruction using the colon or the jejunum in esophageal cancer patients after gastrectomy. *Dis Esophagus.* 2008;21(2):132–138.

Isolauri J, Reinikainen P, Markkula H. Functional evaluation of interposed colon in esophagus. Manometric and 24-hour pH observations. *Acta Chir Scand.* 1987;153(1):21–24.

Klink CD, Binnebösel M, Schneider M, et al. Operative outcome of colon interposition in the treatment of esophageal cancer: a 20-year experience. *Surgery.* 2010;147(4):491–496.

Motoyama S, Kitamura M, Saito R, et al. Surgical outcome of colon interposition by the posterior mediastinal route for thoracic esophageal cancer. *Ann Thorac Surg.* 2007;83:1273–1278.

Swisher S, Hofstetter W, Miller M. The supercharged microvascular jejunal interposition. *Semin Thorac Cardiovasc Surg.* 2007;19(1):56–65.

24 Esophageal Malignancy: Palliative Options and Procedures

Chaitan K. Narsule, Michael I. Ebright, and Hiran C. Fernando

Keywords: Esophageal stents, photodynamic therapy (PDT), cryoablation, Nd:YAG laser, chemoradiation, brachytherapy

INTRODUCTION

Esophageal cancer has an incidence that varies between 12,000 and 18,000 new cases. Unfortunately, the overall survival for esophageal cancer is dismal because patients usually present when symptomatic with dysphagia and/or weight loss, by which time the tumor has metastasized. The symptoms from an obstructing esophageal tumor can have a significant impact on quality of life. Fortunately, palliative treatment options of limited risk are available which can improve swallowing, allow for continued oral intake, and help prevent aspiration.

Options for palliating the patient with dysphagia from advanced, unresectable esophageal cancer include stenting, photodynamic therapy (PDT), cryoablation, laser ablation, and chemoradiation. Of these, the therapies that are most widely used in the United States are esophageal stenting and PDT. Cryoablation is a newer modality that is gaining in popularity. These three therapies are the focus of this discussion. Generally they deliver rapid relief and provide patients with the ability to consume an oral diet with some modifications.

TECHNICAL PRINCIPLES

Stents

Historically, stenting to relieve malignant strictures of the esophagus involved the use of plastic stents. Typically, these stents had a 10-mm internal diameter with proximal and distal flanges and were placed using an open traction or pulsion technique. With the traction technique, the patient underwent a laparotomy and a gastrotomy. A bougie was advanced orally and retrieved through the gastrotomy. The stent was attached to the bougie and pulled into place. With the pulsion technique, which could be performed under sedation, a guidewire was placed, the obstructing stricture was dilated, and the stent was advanced into position using an introducer device. Complications associated with plastic stents included stent displacement, food impaction, and intractable reflux for stents positioned across the gastroesophageal junction. In one report of 409 patients, this approach improved symptoms of dysphagia in 80% of patients but was associated with a 3% mortality rate.[1] In another report comparing traction and pulsion techniques, mortality and length of stay were lower for patients treated using the pulsion technique (14% and 8.4 days, respectively) than those treated using the traction technique (23% and 18.6 days, respectively).[2]

Fortunately, the advent of self-expanding metal stents (SEMSs) has simplified palliation. The SEMS can be placed under endoscopic and fluoroscopic guidance. This approach does not require general anesthesia (though this may be preferable) or aggressive dilation of the malignant stricture. The stent itself is embedded within the tumor. Consequently, the likelihood of migration is small. The benefits of SEMSs over the earlier plastic stents have been demonstrated in a clinical trial, which showed similar improvement in dysphagia scores using both the techniques, but absence of early complications among patients treated with metal stents as compared to 20% early morbidity and 16% mortality among patients treated with plastic stents.[3]

In general, over 85% of patients are palliated immediately from their dysphagia symptoms when an SEMS approach is used. In cases where stenting is not able to relieve dysphagia, technical issues, such as poor stent expansion or malposition, are generally to blame and may be remedied by removing the stent and replacing it with a more appropriately sized device. In addition, an alternate treatment—such as cryoablation or PDT—may be used concurrently.

The newer generation SEMSs are constructed from various materials that include cobalt alloys (Wallstent, Schneider, Minneapolis, MN), stainless steel (Z-stent, Cook, Bloomington, IN), and a nickel—titanium alloy called nitinol (Esophacoil, Medtronic, Minneapolis, MN; Ultraflex, Boston Scientific, Natick, MA). These materials are resistant to corrosion and biologically inert.

The wire stents may be woven (Wallstent), knitted (Ultraflex), or bent into a zigzag (Z-stent) or coil (Esophacoil) configuration. Some stents also have windsock-type valves that serve as antireflux mechanisms (Dua Z-stent, Cook; FerX-ELLA, ELLA-CS, Czech Republic). The stent design influences its retraction properties. Retraction percentage is higher with the coil than with the zigzag configuration. The shape—memory characteristics of these metals and alloys permit the stent to reexpand to its original tubular shape even after it has been compressed into a delivery system.

The SEMS systems vary in deployment mechanisms. Some may be deployed with the removal of a suture (Ultraflex) whereas others are released using a sheath and pusher-rod mechanism. Also, the available systems include stents that can be deployed from the proximal end, the center, or the distal end. Proximal deployment (where the stent expands from a proximal-to-distal direction) is better suited for proximal strictures close to the cricopharyngeus muscle, whereas distal deployment (where the stent expands from a distal-to-proximal direction) is more suitable for obstructions located close to the gastroesophageal junction.

The SEMS is also available as a covered or uncovered device. Covered designs help to reduce tumor ingrowth but also increase the risk of migration. Because most stents are uncovered at the proximal and distal ends, the tendency for migration may be limited albeit at the expense of potential tumor ingrowth. In cases of excessive ingrowth, the tumor may be ablated using cryotherapy, PDT, or laser therapy, and additional stents may be deployed. If laser ablation is considered for treating tumor ingrowth, it should only be used with uncovered stents because of the risk of fire with covered stents. Covered stents also have properties especially suited for the management of tracheoesophageal fistulas,[4] and can play a role in the management of anastomotic leaks and perforations.[5] Examples of covered SEMS include the Ultraflex stent and the Alveolus stent (Merit Medical Endotek, South Jordan, UT). The wide range of available diameters and lengths permits the use of the SEMS for most esophageal lesions.

A recent innovation in stent technology is the self-expanding plastic stent (Polyflex Esophageal Stent, Boston Scientific, Natick, MA). As with the SEMS, these stents can be placed without the need for aggressive predilation. However, the self-expanding plastic stent also can be removed because there is no tissue ingrowth, and, for this reason, it is preferred for benign strictures. The self-expanding plastic stents have a high migration rate reported from 25–46%.[6–8]

Photodynamic Therapy

PDT is a nonthermal, light-activated ablative treatment option. In this approach, a patient is given an intravenous administration of a photosensitive substance that accumulates in the esophageal tumor. This photosensitizing agent, when activated by a light source of a specific wavelength, causes selective tissue destruction with the goal of restoring esophageal patency. Currently, Photofrin (porfimer sodium; Pinnacle Biologics, Inc, Bannockburn, IL) is the only photosensitizer approved by the Food and Drug Administration for esophageal cancer and high-grade dysplasia of the esophagus, and its optimal wavelength of light absorption is 630 nm.

Photosensitizing agents accumulate in all cells of the body. However, after 1 to 4 days following administration, higher concentrations are found within the substance of the tumor. This phenomenon is thought to be either due to altered lymphatic drainage, neovascularization associated with the tumor, or increased cellular proliferation. Light of a specific wavelength that is delivered to the esophageal tumor—with a concentrated amount of the photosensitizer—triggers a series of processes that catalyze the formation of oxygen radical species that promote cell destruction. The targets of the oxygen radical species are cellular components—phospholipid membranes, amino acids, nucleosides, etc. Typically, the depth of penetration and tumor necrosis with this approach is 5 mm. Because of this limited degree of ablation, the risk of perforation is lower with PDT than when a thermal laser is used. However, PDT may be inadequate in the presence of large and bulky tumors, or if there is significant extrinsic compression, for instance, from nodal disease outside the lumen of the esophagus.

Cryoablation

Cryoablation using endoscopic spray cryotherapy (CryoSpray Ablation System; CSA Medical, Baltimore, MD) is a relatively newer treatment modality. In this approach, low-pressure liquid nitrogen is sprayed onto the esophageal tumor under endoscopic visualization. Clinical use of this technology was first reported by Johnston et al.[9] in treating Barrett's metaplasia in 2005. A follow-up case report by the same group[10]—describing the efficacy of this approach in treating a medically inoperable 73-year-old man with malignant dysphagia—demonstrated the potential utility of spray cryotherapy in the palliation of esophageal cancer.

Spray cryotherapy with low-pressure liquid nitrogen is designed to deliver a high rate of thermal energy transfer through a 7-Fr catheter—placed through the working channel of an endoscope—without making direct contact to the esophageal mucosa or tumor. This approach delivers approximately 25 W of energy to the targeted area, and is similar to the energy transfer of a laser and even several factors greater than the energy transfer of cryotherapy using a standard cryotherapy probe. The use of liquid nitrogen in rapidly delivering thermal energy at −196°C effectively flash-freezes the tissue and results in immediate cell death. Spray cryotherapy maintains the underlying tissue architecture and fosters a favorable wound healing response with minimal scarring. We have successfully used spray cryotherapy to treat bleeding related to esophageal tumors, as well as areas of tumor ingrowth/overgrowth around stents. We find it less useful for palliation of dysphagia in patients with obstructing tumors, since it is necessary to place a decompression tube into the stomach alongside the gastroscope. This tube is necessary to prevent overexpansion of the stomach as the liquid nitrogen vaporizes into gas with warming.

Laser Ablation

Laser ablation for malignant esophageal strictures initially involved the use of either an argon or neodymium:yttrium-aluminum-garnet (Nd:YAG) laser. Over time, the Nd:YAG laser gained in popularity due to its efficacy, although it is also associated with a perforation rate of 7% to 10%. It is an especially useful treatment option in the patient with advanced esophageal cancer with bleeding from the tumor. Treatment with Nd:YAG laser therapy usually involves the delivery of up to 90 W of energy in pulses of up to 1 second, at a wavelength of 1064 nm. While it is more useful for tumors of the airway, which tend to be only a few centimeters in length, we use it occasionally to treat small endoluminal tumors of the esophagus in patients with tumor overgrowth close to an uncovered stent or at the site of a previous esophagogastrostomy.

Generally, under fluoroscopic guidance, a guidewire is advanced beyond the malignant stricture, which is widened with a Savary dilator. Thereafter, a laser probe is advanced through an endoscope which is brought into approximation with the tumor. The luminal surface of the obstructing or bleeding tumor is treated with the laser in a point-by-point fashion. This process has the potential to be time-consuming for larger tumors. Also, because this approach may be of limited benefit within patients with bulky tumors causing extraluminal compression, and on account of the increased rate of perforation associated with both the laser treatment and the simultaneous dilation procedure that is often needed, patients are often better palliated with stents, PDT, or cryoablation.

Chemoradiation

Chemoradiation therapy can also be used to palliate patients with dysphagia from esophageal cancer, although the effects of this approach are not immediate and in many cases there is initial worsening of symptoms before improvement is achieved. In a report by Harvey et al.[11], 106 patients with malignant dysphagia from esophageal cancer were evaluated and treated by chemoradiation therapy for palliative intent. Dysphagia was measured using a modified DeMeester (4-point) scoring system. In this series, 78% of the 102 patients available for posttreatment dysphagia scoring had an improvement of at least one grade in their dysphagia, 49% of patients had no dysphagia, and 14% had no improvement with treatment. Importantly, the median time to clinical improvement was 6 weeks following the initiation of chemoradiation. This delay in treatment response is thought to be due to reactive esophagitis that results from treatment even as the tumor decreases in size, which adversely affects the oral intake of food. Because of this, patients with an expected survival of 3 to 4 months should preferably be evaluated for palliation using an alternative method, as these patients would experience a very limited benefit from chemoradiation for palliative intent.

Brachytherapy

Brachytherapy refers to the placement of interstitial or intracavitary radioactive sources to facilitate the delivery of radiation doses to tumors, with relative sparing of surrounding tissues. High—dose-rate brachytherapy involves the placement of radiation seeds via blind-ended afterloading catheters for short periods of time. Although high—dose-rate brachytherapy is used in many centers for airway tumors, this therapy has not gained the same popularity for esophageal cancer. We have found the afterload catheters currently approved by the Food and Drug Administration to be cumbersome and more difficult to place than those approved for the airway. Treatment response time is also slower than that seen with PDT. A recent randomized study from Sweden comparing stent insertion and brachytherapy demonstrated a more rapid relief of dysphagia in stent patients, with improved dysphagia scores at 1 month.[12] Median survival was similar for both groups (132 vs. 109 days, stent vs. brachytherapy).

IDEAL PATIENT CHARACTERISTICS

All patients with malignant dysphagia from esophageal cancer for whom there are no plans for esophagectomy should be considered for palliation (Table 24-1).

For the immediate relief of dysphagia, SEMSs have minimal risk, immediate effect, and are useful when tumors are either predominantly endoluminal or extraluminal. Tumor location, however, is a very important consideration in using stents. In the case of proximal esophageal tumors, placement of stents near the cricopharyngeus muscle may impart a persistent foreign-body sensation and may be intolerable. Also, for bulky cervical tumors, stent deployment may lead to compression of the airway, which may require a separate airway stent for treatment. With distal tumors, stents that are placed close to (or along) the gastroesophageal junction can cause significant reflux. Early on, the development of antireflux stents was thought to be able to mitigate these symptoms. However, in spite of the promising results of an early series, subsequent reports of antireflux stents have been mixed.[13–16] Therefore, PDT or cryoablation may be preferable for palliating cancers in the proximal or distal esophagus.

For midesophageal tumors, stenting, PDT, or cryoablation are all potentially effective. An advantage of stenting or cryoablation is that there is no period of sun sensitivity that patients experience with PDT, which requires strict avoidance of direct sunlight. Alternatively, if definitive chemoradiation is selected for the patient, the use of PDT or cryoablation to manage these malignant strictures may avoid the complications of stent erosion and esophageal perforation that is sometimes associated with chemotherapy.[17]

Covered stents may be useful for the treatment of tracheoesophageal fistulas. Another group of patients who are difficult to manage are those with advanced, perforated esophageal cancer. In these cases, a covered stent may achieve adequate control of sepsis.[4,5,18]

PREOPERATIVE ASSESSMENT

All patients with esophageal cancer are evaluated first for esophagectomy. In the process of staging, all patients will have a computed tomographic (CT) scan of the chest and abdomen. Barium esophagram and endoscopy are useful in determining the location and length of the tumor, as well as the degree of the obstruction. Also, risk stratification can be carried out based on the patient's preexisting medical comorbidities.

If PDT is planned, preoperative patient education is essential to minimize complications related to photosensitivity. Patients will remain sensitive to light for a period of approximately 4 weeks after treatment. Direct sunlight exposure must be avoided during this period. After 4 weeks, patients are gradually reexposed to sunlight. When outdoors during the period of photosensitivity, patients must cover their skin by wearing hats, sunglasses, long-sleeve shirts, gloves, and long pants. Even indoors, it is necessary to avoid sitting next to windows and to keep blinds or curtains closed. Education of hospital staff is also important, and the use of labels to identify a

Table 24-1
COMPARISON OF PALLIATIVE TREATMENT OPTIONS FOR ESOPHAGEAL CANCER

	SEMS	PDT	CRYOABLATION	LASER	CHEMORADIATION
Onset of relief of dysphagia	Immediate	Days	Days	Immediate	Weeks
Intraluminal tumors	Effective	Effective	Effective	Effective	Effective
Tumors causing extrinsic compression	Effective	Not effective	Not effective	Not effective	Effective
Bleeding	Not effective	Effective	Effective	Effective but rarely used	Not immediately effective
Palliation of gastroesophageal junction tumors	Limited by reflux, data on antireflux SEMS unavailable	Preferred	Preferred	Effective but rarely used	Preferred, but not for patients with limited life expectancy
Photosensitivity	No	Yes	No	No	No

photosensitive patient may minimize untoward light exposure during transfers for imaging studies or other procedures.

TECHNIQUE

Self-Expanding Metal Stents

SEMS placement can be carried out under sedation or general anesthesia. Esophageal stents are available in a range of lengths (6–15 cm), although most have a similar maximal internal diameter (17–23 mm). If the opening of the malignant stricture is not wide enough to accept the endoscope, it may need to be dilated or partially fulgurated with a laser before measurements can be made accurately. Once the tumor is identified endoscopically, fluoroscopy is used to mark the proximal and distal extents of the obstruction. Several radiopaque markers—typically in the form of unbent paper clips—are taped to the chest wall at the areas corresponding to the proximal and distal aspects of the tumor. Sometimes, depending on the location of the tumor, it is helpful to mark the position of the gastroesophageal junction or the upper esophageal sphincter complex to avoid incorporating these areas during stent deployment.

Once the length of the tumor is determined, an appropriately sized stent is selected. In general, a stent is chosen of a length that is a few centimeters longer than the stricture to avoid crimping and infolding of the proximal and distal ends. A guidewire is passed through the obstruction, and the endoscope is withdrawn. Under fluoroscopic guidance, the stent delivery system is advanced over the guidewire through the obstruction and is positioned with the assistance of the radiopaque markers. The stent is deployed under real-time imaging and expands within the esophagus. Positioning and deployment is then confirmed endoscopically. In rare cases where the stent deploys in an area distal to the target lesion, minor adjustments can be made by grasping the proximal end of the stent, or the stent retraction suture, with endoscopic forceps and pulling the stent proximally. Once deployed, however, it is not possible to advance the stent distally. Some stents, such as the Polyflex stent, can be removed and reinserted if not positioned appropriately.

In cases where the tumor is bulky and located in the cervical esophagus, bronchoscopy should also be performed. Since the diameter of most esophageal stents are in the range of 18 to 23 mm, a balloon dilator or bougie of corresponding size can be placed through the malignant stricture while a bronchoscopy is performed, which will allow for assessment of the airway and help to determine the need of a tracheal or bronchial stent.

Photodynamic Therapy

This treatment begins with the intravenous administration of porfimer sodium (1.5–2 mg/kg), which is done in the outpatient clinic. The patient is scheduled for endoscopy and delivery of the light therapy 24 to 48 hours later. At the time of endoscopy, patients are either sedated or placed under general anesthesia. A cylindrical diffuser fiber is advanced through the scope and used to deliver light therapy to the tumor. These fibers are available in three sizes (1, 2.5, and 5 cm), with the larger sizes used typically for treating esophageal tumors. The fiber is positioned alongside the tumor, and depending on the length of the tumor relative to the length of the probe, multiple light illumination cycles are administered for a total energy transfer of 300 to 400 J/cm to the tumor. Care is taken to avoid exposure of the normal regions of the esophagus to the light therapy as this could result in the formation of strictures and scarring. In fact, because of the tendency of the light therapy to activate and cause damage to normal esophageal mucosa, a lower dosimetry is used when patients are treated for high-grade dysplasia using PDT.

Forty-eight hours later, a repeat endoscopy is performed—and occasionally a third endoscopy is performed 48 hours beyond that—remove necrotic debris using a combination of irrigation, suction, and forceps techniques. In addition, a dilated balloon can be useful in dislodging necrotic tumor and exposing underlying viable tumor. Depending on the extent of the tumor burden that remains, additional light treatments can be administered. For palliating dysphagia, an effect is usually achieved in 5 to 7 days.

Cryoablation

With this approach, patients first undergo upper endoscopy to identify the malignant stricture. Thereafter, a guidewire is advanced through the stricture and into the stomach, and the endoscope is withdrawn. A modified 16-Fr orogastric tube—which serves as a gastric decompression tube—is advanced over the guidewire through the mouth and into the stomach. This decompression tube contains ports along the distal 12 in to allow for venting of the nitrogen gas from the stomach and esophagus during treatment, and is connected to a suction system throughout the cryoablation procedure. The venting of the nitrogen gas is an important safety consideration, as the liquid-to-gas expansion ratio of nitrogen (1:694 at 20°C) can translate into immense pressure exerted onto the alimentary tract, putting patients at risk of perforation. (In our practice experience, no perforations have occurred to date.)

Next, a 7-Fr cryotherapy catheter is connected to the cryospray machine and primed with liquid nitrogen. The catheter is then advanced through the working channel of the endoscope, and a suction cap—which helps prevent ice formation over the lens, preserving the endoscopic view—is placed on the end of the scope. The endoscope is then advanced alongside the decompression tube through the mouth, to a point about 1 to 2 cm proximal to the upper margin of the tumor. The cryospray machine is activated, and once the liquid nitrogen is seen spraying out of the open end of the catheter, the stream is directed about the surface of the tumor, freezing it and forming a white frost, in a cycle that lasts 20 seconds. The frost is then allowed to completely thaw, in a period that takes up to 45 seconds. This "freeze-thaw" treatment cycle is repeated twice more, for a total of three 20-second freezing cycles.

POSTOPERATIVE CARE

All patients treated with either SEMS, cryoablation, PDT, or laser ablation should have a postoperative chest x-ray in the postanesthesia care unit to confirm the absence of pneumomediastinum or pneumothorax, and to document stent location in cases of stent placement. A barium esophagram is also very useful for assessing patency at the site of the treated malignant stricture and can rule out an iatrogenic perforation whenever it is suspected. When ablative therapies are used, delaying a barium esophagram to assess patency provides time for tissue edema to decrease. Also, as mentioned previously, patients who undergo PDT must avoid exposure to sunlight. In all of these patients, proton pump inhibitors are recommended to minimize problems with esophagitis after the ablative therapies are used, or bleeding and reflux after stent placement.

PROCEDURE-SPECIFIC COMPLICATIONS

Patients who undergo palliative treatment for esophageal cancer are often considered to be medically high risk and cannot tolerate an esophagectomy. In spite of this, the rates of complications are very low with these treatment options. The SEMS is associated with extremely low rates of major complications (0% death, 1%–3% perforation, <1% airway compression) and minor complications (0%–10% migration, 8% food impaction, 0%–6% bleeding, 11% reflux, <2% chest pain, and 4%–33% tumor ingrowth or overgrowth).[17,19] Other early complications include inadequate deployment (3.1%) and pain requiring stent removal (1.6%). In one report,[17] the most severe complication was erosion of the stent through the esophagus leading to sepsis, which occurred in three patients (two of whom received chemotherapy).

PDT likewise has a favorable safety profile when used for palliation. A series of 215 patients from the University of Pittsburgh[20] demonstrated a mortality rate of 1.8%, esophageal perforation rate of 2%, and a stricture rate of 2%, which is far less than the stricture rate (~30%) that is commonly seen when PDT is used for high-grade dysplasia. Similarly, the safety profile of spray cryotherapy has been evaluated in the setting of treatment for high-grade dysplasia and esophageal cancer. Among two recent series, complication rates include 1.3% for perforation, 3% to 4% for stricture, and up to 2% for severe chest pain requiring treatment with oral narcotic medications.[21,22] With Nd:YAG laser therapy, the esophageal perforation can be as high as 7%, as demonstrated in one randomized trial comparing this intervention with PDT[23]; interestingly, in the eight perforations that occurred with laser therapy in this series, four occurred in association with dilation of the malignant stricture and the remainder with laser therapy alone. Also, another study has demonstrated a stricture rate as high as 10% with Nd:YAG laser therapy.[24]

Occasionally, patients may require repeat intervention during follow-up. For instance, in cases where patients are palliated with SEMS, tumor ingrowth can lead to recurrent dysphagia. Treatment with PDT, cryotherapy, or Nd:YAG laser therapy can restore luminal patency. As mentioned previously, laser ablation is of limited use in cases where covered stents have been deployed due to a risk of fire. Also, secondary intervention after PDT or cryoablation may include another course of PDT, cryoablation, or stent placement depending on the reasons for the underlying recurrent dysphagia.

SUMMARY

Although patients with advanced esophageal cancer have a poor survival, palliative therapies such as stent placement, PDT, and cryoablation can significantly improve their quality of life. These therapies fulfill the principal goals of the palliative treatment of esophageal cancer: resumption of oral intake, ease of treatment, and limited hospital stay. They are very effective and have a safety profile that is generally associated with low morbidity and mortality. The surgeon should be familiar with each of these methods of intervention, and should tailor therapy in accordance with the tumor's characteristics and patient's wishes. In many cases, these therapies are complementary, and one approach is not mutually exclusive of the others.

CASE PRESENTATION

An 80-year-old man with a history of hypertension, diabetes, congestive heart failure, coronary artery disease, end-stage renal disease requiring dialysis, and stroke presented on an outpatient basis with weight loss and dysphagia to solids and liquids. An esophagogastroduodenoscopy (EGD) revealed a large fungating mass in the middle third of the esophagus. Biopsies identified the tumor as a squamous cell carcinoma, and endoscopic ultrasonography allowed for clinical staging as T3N0 Mx. Also, PET imaging revealed localized disease (Fig. 24-1).

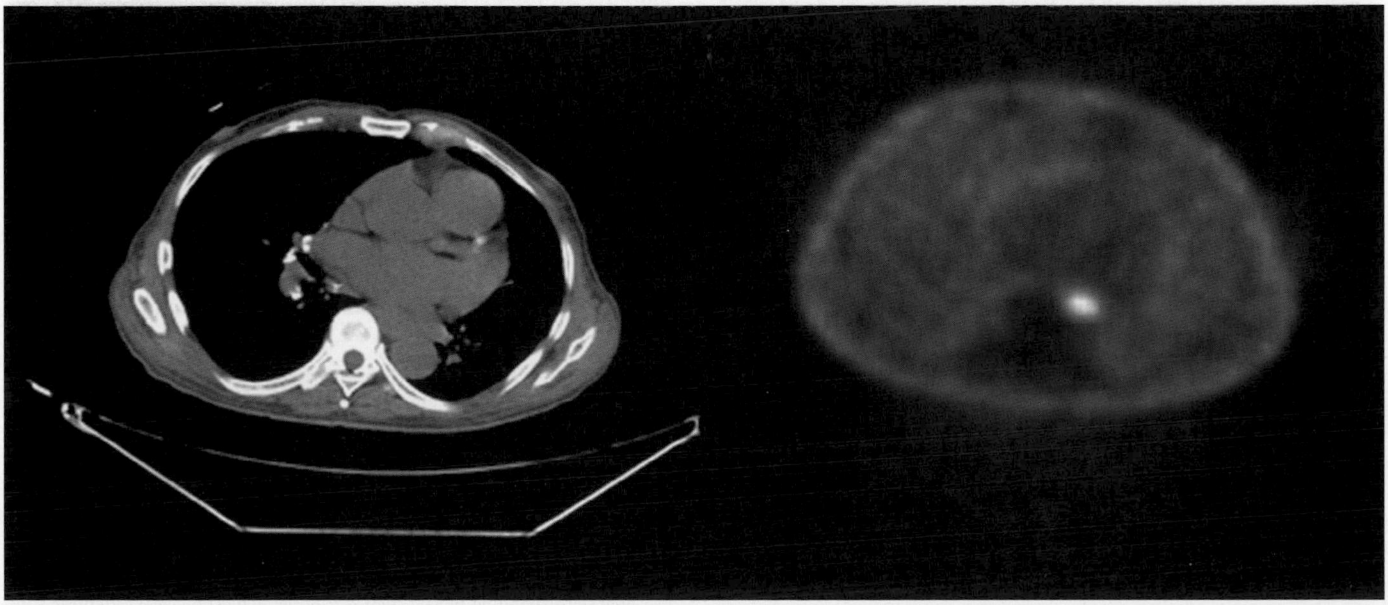

Figure 24-1. PET/CT imaging revealing FDG-avidity of the esophageal cancer. (Left: CT axial image. Right: PET axial image at the same level.)

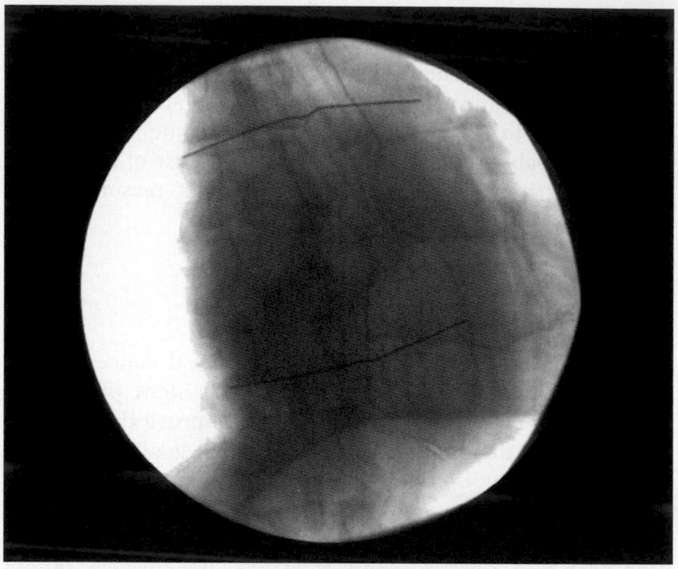

Figure 24-2. Fluoroscopic stent image of deployed esophageal stent. Note the radiopaque markers (which denote the proximal and distal margin of the tumor).

On account of the patient's preexisting comorbidities, he was deemed to be high risk for esophagectomy and chemotherapy. His dysphagia was so severe, endoscopic palliation was necessary. The location of the tumor, lent itself to an approach involving stent placement. Both cryotherapy and PDT were not considered good options because the stricture was extremely tight and there was only a small component of endoluminal disease. Under general anesthesia, we performed our own endoscopy, which revealed that the tumor was located 30 cm from the incisors. Although it was initially difficult to advance the scope beyond the tumor, this was ultimately achieved with careful maneuvering. The length of the tumor was approximately 4 cm, and the proximal and distal extents of the tumor were marked under fluoroscopic visualization with unbent paper clips taped to the patient's chest wall (Fig. 24-2). Thereafter, a guidewire was placed, and a covered stent was advanced over the guidewire into the esophagus. Once the stent was positioned to achieve ample overlap beyond the proximal and distal margins, it was deployed (Fig. 24-2).

The patient was extubated successfully. A postoperative chest x-ray confirmed the absence of pneumomediastinum and pneumothorax. A barium esophagram performed a few days later demonstrated a patent esophagus (Fig. 24-3). Subsequently, the patient resumed a modified diet and was able to drink liquids.

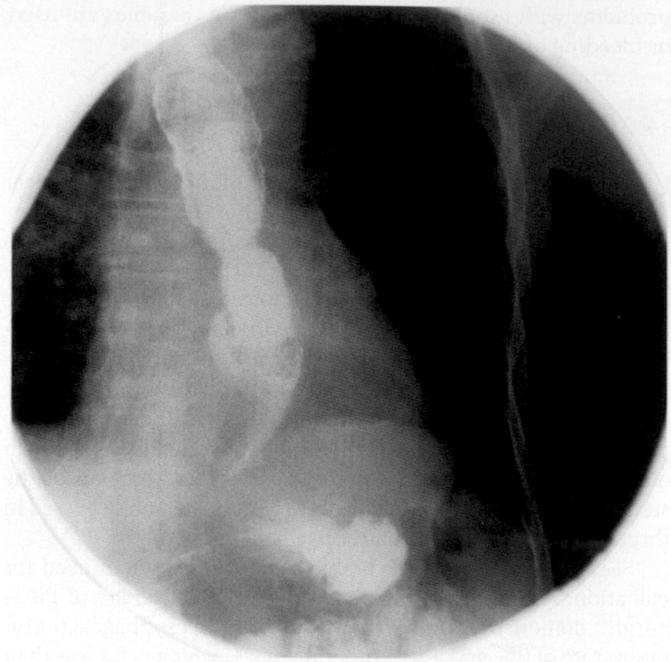

Figure 24-3. Barium esophagram following placement of the esophageal stent. Note a "waist" that appears at the midportion of the stent, corresponding to the location of the malignant stricture.

EDITOR'S COMMENT

Palliation of dysphagia is one of the aims of treating esophageal cancer. In patients for whom a curative resection cannot be undertaken because of the presence of metastases or comorbidities, early palliation should still be done even before any cytotoxic therapy is given. The concept that one should wait 2 to 8 weeks to see if there is shrinkage of the tumor from chemoradiation is to be deplored. Likewise, even when considering definitive curative therapy with or without surgical resection, early palliation of dysphagia should be considered for most patients. In the past, we would remove the esophagus with the stent in place; currently we advocate using a plastic removable stent, which is then removed prior to esophagectomy or once the patient's dysphagia has resolved after successful chemoradiation. Finally, it should be noted that all these techniques can be used together to improve swallowing function, that is, a stent may give rapid improvement but later ablation and even brachytherapy are always possible if symptoms worsen or recur.

—Mark J. Krasna

References

1. Cusumano A, Ruol A, Segalin A, et al. Push-through intubation: effective palliation in 409 patients with cancer of the esophagus and cardia. *Ann Thorac Surg*. 1992;53:1010–1014.
2. Unhurt HW, Pagliero KM. Pulsion intubation versus traction intubation for obstructing carcinomas of the esophagus. *Ann Thorac Surg*. 1985;40:337–342.
3. De Palma GD, di Matteo E, Romano G, et al. Plastic prosthesis versus expandable metal stents for palliation of inoperable esophageal thoracic carcinoma: a controlled prospective study. *Gastrointest Endosc*. 1996;43:478–482.
4. van den Bongard HJ, Boot H, Baas P, et al. The role of parallel stent insertion in patients with esophagorespiratory fistulas. *Gastrointest Endosc*. 2002;55:110–115.
5. D'Cunha J, Rueth NM, Groth SS, et al. Esophageal stents for anastomotic leaks and perforations. *J Thorac Cardiovasc Surg*. 2011;142(1):39–46.
6. Adler DG, Fang J, Wong R, et al. Placement of Polyflex stents in patients with locally advanced esophageal cancer is safe and improves dysphagia during neoadjuvant therapy. *Gastrointest Endosc*. 2009;70(4):614–619.
7. Costamagna G, Shah SK, Tringali A, et al. Prospective evaluation of a new self-expanding plastic stent for inoperable esophageal strictures. *Surg Endosc*. 2003;17:891–895.

8. Oh YS, Kochman, ML, Ahmad NA, et al. Clinical outcomes after self-expanding plastic stent placement for refractory benign esophageal strictures. *Dig Dis Sci.* 2010;55(5):1344–1348.
9. Johnston MH, Eastone JA, Horwat JD, et al. Cryoablation of Barrett's esophagus: a pilot study. *Gastrointest Endosc.* 2005;62:842–848.
10. Cash BD, Johnston LR, Johnston MH. Cryospray ablation (CSA) in the palliative treatment of squamous cell carcinoma of the esophagus. *World J Surg Oncol.* 2007;5:34.
11. Harvey JA, Bessell JR, Beller E, et al. Chemoradiation therapy is effective for the palliative treatment of malignant dysphagia. *Dis Esophagus.* 2004;17:260–265.
12. Bergquist H, Wenger U, Johnsson E, et al. Stent insertion or endoluminal brachytherapy as palliation of patients with advanced cancer of the esophagus and gastroesophageal junction: results of a randomized, controlled clinical trial. *Dis Esophagus.* 2005;18:131–139.
13. Laasch HU, Marriott A, Wilbraham L, et al. Effectiveness of open versus antireflux stents for palliation of distal esophageal carcinoma and prevention of symptomatic gastroesophageal reflux. *Radiology.* 2002;225:359–365.
14. Homs MY, Wahab PJ, Kuipers EJ, et al. Esophageal stents with antireflux valve for tumors of the distal esophagus and gastric cardia: a randomized trial. *Gastrointest Endosc.* 2004;60(5):695–702.
15. Shim CS, Jung IS, Cheon YK, et al. Management of malignant stricture of the esophagogastric junction with a newly designed self-expanding metal stent with an antireflux mechanism. *Endoscopy.* 2005;37(4):335–339.
16. Wegner U, Johnsson E, Arnelo U, et al. An antireflux stent versus conventional stents for palliation of distal esophageal or cardia cancer: a randomized clinical study. *Surg Endosc.* 2006;20(11):1675–1680.
17. Christie NA, Buenaventura PO, Fernando HC, et al. Results of expandable metal stents for malignant esophageal obstruction in 100 patients: short-term and long-term follow-up. *Ann Throac Surg.* 2001;71:1797–1801.
18. White RE, Mungatana C, Topazian M. Expandable stents for iatrogenic perforation of esophageal malignancies. *J Gastrointest Surg.* 2003;7:715–719.
19. Therasse E, Oliva VL, Lafontaine E, et al. Balloon dilation and stent placement for esophageal lesions: indications, methods, and results. *Radiographics.* 2003;23:89–105.
20. Litle VR, Luketich JD, Christie NA, et al. Photodynamic therapy as palliation for esophageal cancer: experience in 215 patients. *Ann Throac Surg.* 2003;76:1687–1692.
21. Greenwald BD, Dumot JA, Horwat JD, et al. Safety, tolerability, and efficacy of endoscopic low-pressure liquid nitrogen spray cryotherapy in the esophagus. *Dis Esophagus.* 2010;23(1):13–29.
22. Shaheen NJ, Greenwald BD, Peery AF, et al. Safety and efficacy of endoscopic spray cryotherapy for Barrett's esophagus with high-grade dysplasia. *Gastrointest Endosc.* 2010;71:680–685.
23. Lightdale CJ, Heier SK, Marcon NE, et al. Photodynamic therapy with porfimer sodium versus thermal ablation therapy with Nd:YAG laser for palliation of esophageal cancer: a multicenter randomized trial. *Gastrointest Endosc.* 1995;42:507–512.
24. Heier SK, Rothman KA, Heier LM, et al. Photodynamic therapy for obstructing esophageal cancer: light dosimetry and randomized comparison with Nd:YAG laser therapy. *Gastroenterology.* 1995;109:63–72.

25 Management of Malignant Esophageal Fistula

Mitchell J. Magee and Joshua R. Sonett

Keywords: Self-expanding metal stents (SEMSs), palliative treatment for esophageal malignant esophageal fistulae

INTRODUCTION

Malignant esophageal fistula occurs infrequently, yet remains one of the most challenging complications encountered in thoracic oncology. It may occur in the setting of complicated esophageal cancer, presenting at an advanced stage of disease, or as a complication of treatment. The fundamental tenets of successful management of any fistula, such as relief of distal obstruction, treatment of infection, nutrition, and treatment of underlying malignancy, should be kept in mind but unfortunately are inherent to the disease process and usually overwhelming for patient and clinician. Improvements in completely covered self-expanding metallic stents (SEMSs) and associated delivery systems have dramatically changed the approach to managing esophageal fistulae, particularly involving the tracheobronchial tree. Palliation and not cure is the objective in the majority of patients afflicted with this uniformly fatal complication, which most often occurs in the setting of advanced stage disease. A multidisciplinary approach to accurate and precise diagnosis and treatment is essential.

GENERAL PRINCIPLES: PATIENT EVALUATION AND DIAGNOSIS

Malignant esophageal fistula usually presents with clinical symptoms of recurrent aspiration or less commonly hemoptysis or hematemesis. An esophageal fistula may also be suspected on the basis of transmission of oral flora through the fistula tract and the development of associated infection of the body cavity or organ in communication with the esophagus, such as recurrent pneumonia, empyema, and abscess. The majority of patients will present with known locally advanced or metastatic tumor and will frequently already be undergoing treatment with chemotherapy and radiation. The diagnosis is confirmed with fluoroscopy during administration of dilute barium oral contrast followed by thin-cut computed tomography (CT), which will usually define the precise location and extent of the fistula. A small fistula may be missed on radiographic evaluation and aspiration of swallowed barium can be confused with a fistula to the respiratory tract, particularly with proximal third esophageal lesions. Flexible esophagoscopy and bronchoscopy often are required for confirmation and anatomic assessment of the suspected fistula and provide additional information needed for treatment planning in addition to the therapeutic benefit of clearing the contaminated airway.

A tracheobronchial–esophageal fistula is often visualized more easily with bronchoscopy rather than esophagoscopy, as the esophageal mucosal folds and tumor sometimes obscure the origin of the fistula. It is also important to visualize any luminal compromise of the airway from tumor compression, as this may be exacerbated with esophageal stenting.

Once the diagnosis is established, broad-spectrum antibiotics should be instituted to include coverage for gram-positive bacteria, anaerobes, and yeast. Oral intake should be withheld and alternative forms of nutrition established. The ensuing treatment plan should then be directed toward:

1. Limiting or eliminating ongoing contamination of the respiratory tract or other body cavities.
2. Draining contained foci of infection such as the pleural, peritoneal, and pericardial spaces.
3. Maintaining adequate nutrition for healing.
4. Minimizing distal obstruction.
5. Treating the cancer if feasible.

Traditionally, contamination was controlled by surgical exclusion or diversion with a cervical esophagostomy and possible placement of a gastrostomy to limit reflux contamination, along with a jejunal feeding tube. Any contaminated fluid collections identified in the mediastinum, pleural space, peritoneal cavity, or pericardium should be adequately drained percutaneously or surgically.

Partially or fully covered SEMSs are now the primary treatment option for most fistulae, and offer an attractive alternative to some of the described surgical options. It is important to remember that contaminated fluid collections still require drainage. Primary thoracoscopic debridement and decortication may prevent the need for thoracotomy. Advantages of SEMSs in the management of esophageal fistulae related to esophageal cancer include ease and expediency of deployment with essentially immediate control of ongoing contamination from both antegrade and retrograde secretions. Tumor or treatment-related stricture and associated obstruction distal to the fistula are effectively managed simultaneously with stent placement across the fistula and through the stricture or obstructed lumen of the esophagus. Oral enteral nutrition can be resumed promptly without the need for a surgically placed feeding tube. The most common clinically significant complication of SEMSs is stent migration, which is more common in the absence of stricture or partial obstruction by tumor. It is important, particularly in the absence of stricture, to maximize the diameter and length of the stent both to increase the purchase of the stent and decrease migration. As well, it is important to ensure that the length of the covered portion of the stent extends 2 to 4 cm proximal and distal to the fistula. The stent should be long enough to include any stricture, both to facilitate oral intake and minimize stent migration. More than one stent occasionally may be required. SEMSs successfully control the fistula in essentially all patients with a very low complication rate.[1]

PREOPERATIVE ASSESSMENT AND PATIENT SELECTION

Once the diagnosis is confirmed, it is important to determine the location (proximal, middle, or distal third of the esophagus) of the fistula, its size, communication with other organs or body cavities, presence or absence of abscess cavities or effusions, and whether it is wholly contained within the mediastinum. Broad-spectrum antimicrobial coverage already should have been instituted, often even before the diagnosis is established, and the patient should be resuscitated, stabilized, and the airway secured with endotracheal intubation if necessary. Each of these components are integral to making an adequate assessment of the fistula, along with CT and endoscopy as described above, and are essential to formulating a treatment plan.

Once clinically stabilized, patients then are selected for conservative nonoperative management or surgical intervention, based on the size and location of the fistula and other associated pathology. A combined approach that is commonly employed in the operating room with anesthesia may include endoscopy with SEMS placement under fluoroscopic guidance, a surgical drainage procedure and decortication, and placement of a gastrostomy or jejunostomy tube for drainage or enteral access.

SURGICAL APPROACH AND TECHNIQUE

Perforations or fistulae involving the proximal third of the esophagus may be contained within the mediastinum or communicate with the airway via the membranous trachea. Fistulae that are contained within the mediastinum, depending on size, can be managed nonoperatively or by placing a closed drain in the mediastinum via a left neck incision. Caution should be exercised in placing SEMSs in the esophagus that extend proximally toward the hypopharynx as proximal migration can occur resulting in airway compromise and even asphyxiation. Proximal lesions involving the airway are better managed with a tracheal stent and a cervical drain.

Esophageal fistulae of the middle or distal third of the esophagus may involve the airway, one or both pleural spaces, the pericardium, the peritoneum, or the aorta (Fig. 25-1). These are best managed in the operating room with anesthesia and with supplies and equipment available, including flexible esophagogastroscope, flexible bronchoscope, thoracoscope, fluoroscopy, and a variety of sizes of completely covered SEMSs for the esophagus and airway. The presence of an esophageal–aortic fistula is usually a premorbid event; however, endoluminal aortic stenting may be considered to salvage these patients. In patients awaiting planned surgical resection following neoadjuvant chemoradiation, occasionally a heroic attempt at resection may allow urgent palliation if combined with an endograft or open aortic replacement. This should only be contemplated if the patient is in excellent condition; in the era of endografting, this would be the preferred primary approach.

SEMSs are available in the United States from several different manufacturers and may be uncovered, partially covered, or fully covered. Fully covered stents are most appropriate in the management of malignant esophageal fistulae as they more effectively prevent ongoing leak from the esophagus and disrupt communication through the fistula tract. Fully covered SEMSs, as opposed to partially covered stents, are less prone to tissue ingrowth and thereby more easily removed or repositioned, but consequently also more prone to migration. Flexible esophagoscopy (Fig. 25-2A,B) should be performed in the

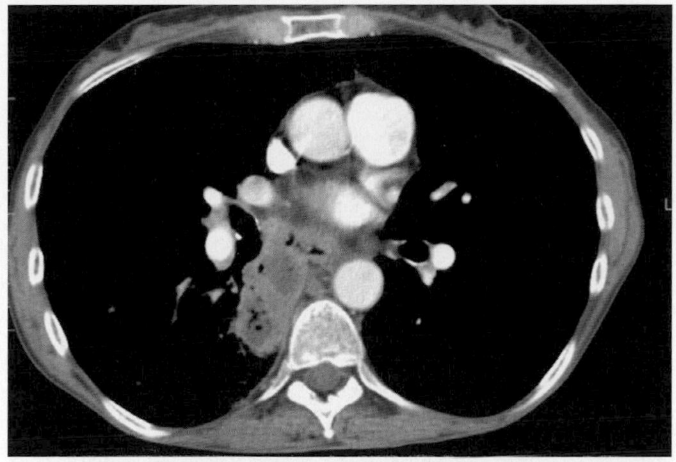

Figure 25-1. Mid-esophageal perforation, contaminating the mediastinum and contained right pleural collection.

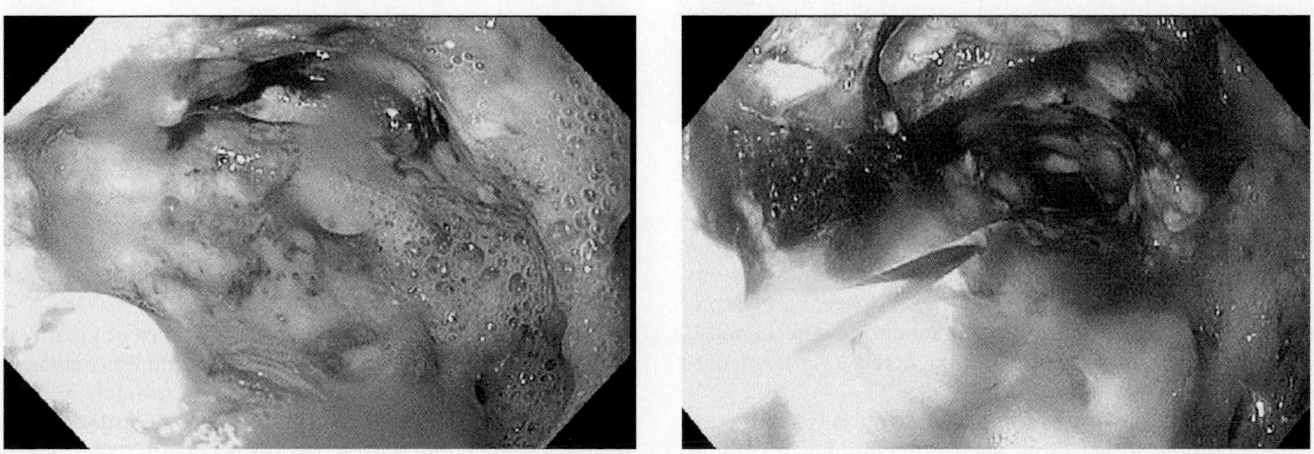

A B

Figure 25-2. *A.* Endoscopy of esophageal perforation identified on CT scan. The communicating perforation can be visualized. *B.* True lumen is identified and guidewire is passed under direct vision and fluoroscopy guidance.

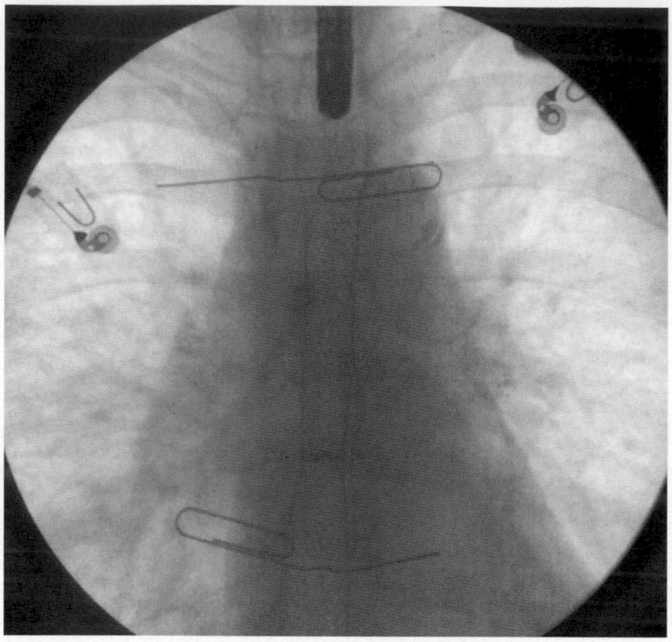

Figure 25-3. Placement of stent is seen as visualized by fluoroscopy as well as direct proximal visualization.

operating room with fluoroscopy and a variety of lengths of large diameter SEMSs available. The fistula is visualized endoscopically and the proximal and distal extent marked with internal or external surface radiopaque marker under fluoroscopic guidance. The stent should be at least 4 cm longer than the desired area to be covered, which should include the entire length of the fistula and any tumor or stricture associated with, or distal to, the fistula (Fig. 25-3). If an obstructing tumor or stricture is present, it must be dilated to an internal diameter of 6 to 10 mm to permit passage of the predeployed stent delivery system. It is important to avoid overdilating the stricture as this may exacerbate the fistula as well as facilitate stent migration. It is important to attempt to limit the extent of the stent distally that resides across the lower esophageal sphincter and in the stomach, as this can promote reflux and aspiration and potentially lead to obstruction or ulceration through contact with the opposing gastric wall. If the CT scan suggests the presence of bulky tumor adjacent to the trachea posing a potential risk for external tracheal compression, then consideration should be given to placing a tracheal stent before placing an esophageal stent.

Decortication of the contaminated pleural space, including unroofing of any mediastinal abscess protruding into the pleural space (but contained by mediastinal pleura) and drainage of contaminated pleural or pericardial effusions, can usually be accomplished with video-assisted thoracoscopy. Routine drains should be placed as with any infected closed space. Rarely, consideration for an end esophagostomy should be entertained if the patient is becoming septic, although the long-term outcome from these situations is dismal.

If prolonged delay in resuming oral nutrition is anticipated because of complicating factors, such as pneumonia or respiratory compromise requiring mechanical ventilation, then a surgically placed feeding tube should be considered before leaving the operating room.

POSTOPERATIVE MANAGEMENT

Not less than 24 hours following placement of the stent or as soon as the patient is capable of swallowing oral contrast, an esophagram is obtained to confirm proper seating of the stent and seal of the fistula as evidenced by absence of contrast leak. If no contrast leak is detected, oral liquids are resumed and the patient is advanced to a mechanical soft diet. Leaks due to migration or improper seating of the stent due to enfolding of the proximal stent may be corrected by endoscopic repositioning or occasionally require removal and replacement of the stent. Potential stent migration can be easily monitored with routine chest radiographs. After sufficient time for healing has passed, usually 4 to 6 weeks, the stent is removed in the operating room under general anesthesia and healing confirmed by endoscopy. If incomplete healing is suspected, the stent is replaced and managed accordingly. If the fistula is closed, then a confirmatory contrast esophagram is obtained within 48 hours and if negative for leak the patient is discharged home on a mechanical soft diet.[2]

RESULTS

Experience and expected outcomes in the management of malignant esophageal fistulae are mostly anecdotal, as no large series exist. Attempting to extrapolate results from the management of iatrogenic perforations or other etiologies of perforation or fistula formation provides little insight into expected results with this uncommon complication of esophageal cancer and its treatment. Confounding factors include malnutrition and compromised immunity, both of which affect healing and infection control, and the presence of luminal obstruction. All of these factors would be expected to impact a complicated open surgical repair or diversion and drainage procedure with its attendant morbidity and mortality to the same or greater degree as the contemporary recommendation described in this chapter. In this regard, improvements in completely covered SEMSs and associate delivery systems have dramatically changed the approach to managing esophageal fistulae. Older series report a median survival of 2 to 6 months following development of malignant esophageal fistula, regardless of treatment. Utilizing SEMS for fistula management to (1) rapidly and effectively control the leak and associated contamination, (2) provide rapid return of enteral nutrition, and (3) manage infection with antimicrobial agents and a minimally invasive approach to drainage, appears to provide the least morbid and most effective palliation for this uniformly fatal complication, and in most instances, is a better alternative to direct surgical intervention.

EDITOR'S COMMENT

As noted above, these cases represent an almost uniformly fatal scenario. Older series, where this complication was managed by routine exclusion and diversion, describe extremely high perioperative morbidity and mortality. The current options utilizing SEMSs are much more attractive as they do not have the procedure-related complications experienced with prior approaches (including "palliative esophagectomy"). In this author's experience, the only time an open procedure with possible resection and reconstruction should be considered is when the patient has completed neoadjuvant therapy, is doing well clinically, and suddenly presents acutely with either a perforation or airway or vascular fistula. Despite this possible scenario, a recognition that these "heroic" approaches have an extremely high morbidity and mortality should always lead the surgeon to be less than sanguine toward an open direct surgical approach.

—Mark J. Krasna

References

1. Raijman I, Siddique I, Ajani J, et al. Palliation of malignant dysphagia and fistulae with coated expandable metal stents: experience with 101 patients. *Gastrointest Endosc*. 1998;48(2):172–179.
2. Freeman RK, Ascioti AJ, Giannini T, et al. Analysis of unsuccessful esophageal stent placements for esophageal perforation, fistula, or anastomotic leak. *Ann Thorac Surg*. 2012;94:959–965.

26 Salvage Surgery for Recurrent Esophageal Cancer

Zhigang Li and Thomas W. Rice

Keywords: Salvage esophagectomy, failed esophagectomy, R0 versus R1, R2 resections, definitive chemoradiotherapy, neoadjuvant chemoradiotherapy

INTRODUCTION

Recurrent (after a disease-free period) or persistent esophageal cancer following definitive therapy, particularly for locally advanced cancer, is common. Treatment failure following definitive chemoradiotherapy in RTOG-8501 was 46% at a minimum of 5 years follow-up.[1] Twenty percent of patients had recurrence after clinical complete response and 26% persistent cancer. In RTOG-8911 following R0 esophagectomy, at a median follow-up of 8.8 years, cancer recurrence was reported in 52% of patients receiving induction chemotherapy and 56% of patients with esophagectomy alone.[2]

Treatment of recurrent or persistent esophageal cancer after primary therapy is typically palliative and most commonly nonsurgical. However, in rare situations, salvage esophagectomy has been reported to be useful in highly selected patients in a final attempt to cure. To determine indications for salvage esophagectomy, the literature must be carefully assessed.

LITERATURE REVIEW

Failed Definitive Chemoradiotherapy

In 2007, Gardner-Thorpe et al.[3] reviewed nine single institution series of salvage esophagectomy following definitive chemoradiotherapy. A total of 105 patients, predominantly with squamous cell carcinoma, were included in this simple evaluation. Salvage esophagectomy was an uncommon operation. With centers performing one to two salvage esophagectomies a year, this represented 1.7% to 4.2% of their esophagectomy volume. Morbidity was significant and three centers reported it was more than following neoadjuvant chemoradiotherapy. Anastomotic leak was reported in 18% of patients and conduit complications (necrosis and fistula) in 5%. Complications accounted for 42% of the 11% in-hospital mortality. Median survival ranged from 7 to 32 months. Almost all deaths after discharge were due to cancer. R0 resection was associated with improved survival in four series. In three series, no patient with R1 or R2 resection survived more than 13 months. There was some evidence that patients with recurrent cancer after chemoradiotherapy did better than those with persistent cancer.

Nishimura et al.[4] reported results of salvage esophagectomy in 46 patients treated 1 to 7 months following definitive chemoradiotherapy. This group comprised 16% of patients with persistent or recurrent cancer after chemoradiotherapy. Operative mortality was 15%. Complications were frequent; the most common was anastomotic leak in 22% of patients. Median survival was 22 months, and 3-year survival was 17%. There were no clear predictors of survival; however, the three long-term survivors were ypN0 at salvage esophagectomy.

Piessen et al.[5] reported salvage esophagectomy in 98 (20%) of 472 patients treated with definitive chemoradiotherapy. Sixty-two percent had R0 resection which was associated with improved median survival, 19 months in R0 patients versus 9 months in R1 and R2 patients ($p < 0.001$). In-hospital mortality was 3.1% and morbidity 33%. There were no R1 or R2 survivors after 26 months. Predictors of R0 resection were cancer length ≤5 cm on barium esophagram ($p = 0.05$) and contact between the primary cancer and aorta ≤90° on CT ($p = 0.04$).

D'Journo et al.[6] reported their 10-year salvage esophagectomy experience in 24 patients (9% of esophagectomies). In this series, 88% had R0 resection and 30- and 90-day mortality was high at 21% and 25%, respectively. Forty-five percent of patients had a complication. Radiation dose greater than 55 Gray (Gy, unit of absorbed radiation dose) was associated with increased mortality, morbidity, length of stay, and blood transfusions. Five-year disease-free survival was 21%. R0 resection was associated with best 5-year survival (36% for R0 vs. 0% for R1 and R2), but this small experience did not reach statistical significance ($p = 0.7$).

Four studies have compared salvage esophagectomy to esophagectomy alone or esophagectomy as a component of neoadjuvant chemoradiotherapy.[7–10] Smithers et al.[7] reported the results of salvage esophagectomy in 14 patients (4% of patients treated with definitive chemoradiotherapy) and compared them to 53 patients treated with neoadjuvant chemoradiotherapy. No statistical assessments of the comparisons were made. Median time from chemoradiotherapy to esophagectomy was 28 weeks in salvage patients versus 4 weeks in neoadjuvant patients. Salvage esophagectomy patients had more respiratory complications and longer ICU and hospital stays. Anastomotic leaks, transfusion requirements, and operative mortality were greater in salvage patients. Survival at 3 years was 24% for salvage patients and 53% for neoadjuvant patients. Survival following salvage esophagectomy was better for patients with recurrent cancer (25 months) than for those with persistent cancer (13 months).

Chao et al. reported 84 patients treated definitively with chemoradiotherapy.[8] Forty-seven had persistent or recurrent cancer, of which 27 had salvage esophagectomy. Compared to patients receiving definitive chemoradiotherapy alone, salvage esophagectomy patients had a significantly better survival, 0% 5-year survival for definitive chemoradiotherapy versus 25% for salvage esophagectomy ($p = 0.003$). Compared to patients receiving neoadjuvant therapy, salvage esophagectomy patients were significantly older ($p = 0.04$), had more cervical and upper third thoracic cancers ($p = 0.05$), had fewer R0 resections ($p = 0.001$), more pulmonary complications ($p = 0.006$), more anastomotic leaks ($p = 0.002$), and higher operative mortality. However, survival was similar. In salvage esophagectomy patients, multivariable analysis identified low preoperative albumin level ($p = 0.07$) and anastomotic leak ($p = 0.02$)

as predictors of hospital mortality and R1 and R2 resections ($p = 0.04$) as the predictor of disease-specific mortality.

Morita et al.[9] reported 27 salvage esophagectomy patients and compared them to both patients who received neoadjuvant therapy and patients who received esophagectomy alone. Complications were associated with the use of chemoradiotherapy and were most common in salvage patients (25% esophagectomy alone, 40% neoadjuvant therapy, and 59% salvage esophagectomy, $p < 0.001$). Salvage patients were four times more likely to experience a pulmonary complication than those receiving esophagectomy alone. Preoperative therapy and retrosternal or subcutaneous routes of reconstruction were associated with increased risk of anastomotic leak. Operative mortality was increased in salvage patients but not statistically significant (2.4% vs. 2.0% vs. 7.4%, respectively). Compared to patients who had salvage esophagectomy for recurrent cancer, patients who had salvage esophagectomy for persistent cancer were less likely to have an R0 resection ($p = 0.07$) and had a worse 5-year survival (15% vs. 70%, respectively, $p = 0.008$).

Tachimori et al.[10] treated 59 patients who had failed definitive chemoradiotherapy (radiation dose >60 Gy) with salvage esophagectomy and compared them to 553 patients who had esophagectomy alone. Salvage esophagectomy patients had significantly more respiratory complications (32% vs. 20%, respectively, $p = 0.05$), anastomotic leaks (31% vs. 25%, $p = 0.003$), wound infections (27% vs. 15%, $p = 0.02$), and hospital mortality (8% vs. 2%, $p = 0.01$), compared to patients who had esophagectomy alone. Tracheobronchial and gastric conduit necroses were highly lethal complications of salvage esophagectomy. Three-year survival following salvage esophagectomy was 38% compared to 58% following esophagectomy alone, T4 cancer and R1 and R2 resections were confounded in the analysis, thus leading the authors to conclude that only R0 resection was associated with improved survival in salvage esophagectomy patients.

Failed Esophagectomy

The literature is scarce for salvage esophagectomy following esophagectomy and typically anecdotal. In this setting, salvage esophagectomy is primarily used to treat anastomotic recurrence. Schipper et al.[11] reported a 30-year experience in which 27 patients were considered for salvage esophagectomy, 23 (85%) for anastomotic recurrence, and 4 for cancer recurrence (3 esophageal remnant and 1 gastric conduit). Salvage surgery was possible in 19 (70%), 10 completion esophagogastrectomies and 9 anastomotic resections. Eight patients had exploration only. Operative mortality was 7% and 59% of patients had postoperative complications. Five-year survival was 35% in salvage patients, no patient undergoing exploration only survived 3 years. Predictors of survival were disease-free interval between esophagectomy and salvage surgery greater than 2 years ($p < 0.05$) and R0 resection ($p < 0.02$).

GENERAL PRINCIPLES

Although the quality of evidence is poor, the overwhelming message from the literature is *R0 resection is a prerequisite if salvage esophagectomy is to offer a survival benefit.*

Preoperative identification of an R0 patient is problematic. The published salvage esophagectomy experience represents only a miniscule fraction of the 1% of patients with failed therapy for esophageal cancer. Thus these patients represent a highly selected group. Even in these patients, R0 resection was not assured. It is evident that only the rare patient with failed therapy is presently considered for or will benefit from salvage surgery. Although not absolute, an R0 resection may be more likely in the setting of recurrence after definitive chemoradiotherapy and less likely with persistent cancer following definitive chemoradiotherapy or failed esophagectomy. In these patients, a longer disease-free interval is more favorable. Salvage esophagectomy of smaller cancers and cancers without clinical evidence of invasion of adjacent structures (T4) are more likely to produce R0 resection. A surrogate for R0 resection may be a ypN0/rpN0 cancer.

PREOPERATIVE ASSESSMENT AND PATIENT SELECTION

The Recurrence: Cancer Restaging

Patients with M1, T4, and most N+ (N1 relative contraindication and N2 or N3 absolute contraindication) cancers are not candidates for salvage esophagectomy. First, M1 cancers must be excluded. CT/PET scanning is the essential restaging imaging modality. Any distant hypermetabolic focus must be sampled to confirm its nature. MRI of the brain is indicated for clinical signs or symptoms. However, its performance as a last step in restaging (all other restaging excludes nonbrain M1, T4, and N+) of all potential candidates for salvage esophagectomy can be argued because of a 13% prevalence of brain metastases following definitive chemoradiotherapy for esophageal cancer.[12] Additional imaging will be dictated by the findings of these principal restaging tools.

Esophagogastroduodenoscopy (EGD) with biopsy and endoscopic ultrasound (EUS) is the next step in restaging. However, repeat esophagoscopy and rebiopsy may not identify residual mucosal cancer after aggressive therapy. Residual cancer at biopsy after chemoradiotherapy had sensitivity and negative predictive value of 23% and specificity and positive predictive value of 92% for cancer in the esophagectomy specimen.[13] Biopsy positive patients were more likely to have residual positive regional lymph nodes compared to biopsy negative patients.

EUS is inaccurate in determining T classification following chemoradiotherapy, with reported accuracies ranging from 27% to 47%. The most common error is overstaging because EUS is unable to distinguish cancer from inflammation and fibrosis produced by chemoradiotherapy. EUS accuracy for N classification after chemoradiotherapy is poor and ranges from 49% to 71%. The primary reasons for this inaccuracy are alterations in the ultrasound appearance of lymph nodes after chemoradiotherapy, such that established EUS criteria do not apply, and residual foci of cancer within the nodes that are too small for detection by any modality other than pathologic analysis.

EUS-directed fine-needle aspiration is necessary for restaging. Any hypermetabolic focus detected by PET and any EUS abnormality must be sampled to differentiate recurrent or persistent cancer from reactive and inflammatory changes. This includes all suspicious mural findings, regional lymph nodes, and periesophageal M1 sites.

Use of ancillary staging modalities will be dictated by the classification to be defined (T4, N+, M1), tissue to be sampled, site of recurrence, and prior therapy. These procedures include laryngoscopy, bronchoscopy, mediastinoscopy, thoracoscopy, laparoscopy, surface ultrasonography, and simple incisional or excisional biopsy. At least aspiration and cytologic review is necessary, but biopsy and histopathologic review is preferred.

The Patient: Present State of Health

Critical inpatient assessment is a comparison of the patient's present state of health to that prior to original therapy. Any deterioration in health or poor tolerance or complications of original therapy may preclude salvage esophagectomy. The present performance status should be normal (Zubrod 0, Karnofsky 100-90). Cardiopulmonary status, a major determinate of early postoperative course, should be optimized and not impaired. ASA status should be 1 (normal) and no less than 2 (mild systemic impairment). The patient should have normal protein and albumin levels and not be anemic.

The Prior Therapies: Bridges Burned

A plan for resection and reconstruction must be formulated before salvage esophagectomy is undertaken. It may be discovered that prior therapies have burned bridges necessary for successful salvage esophagectomy. For re-resection and re-reconstruction, explanations for failed esophagectomy and a strategy to avoid repeating these mistakes are needed.

Any plan must include alternatives for both extent of resection and organs and routes of reconstruction. The impact of the prior "curative" therapy on salvage esophagectomy must be considered. For patients who have undergone definitive chemoradiotherapy, the dose and fields of treatment must be evaluated and their impact on salvage esophagectomy, both resection and reconstruction, must be assessed. Salvage esophagectomy for recurrence after R0 esophagectomy requires assessment of the impact of the prior esophagectomy on re-resection of the recurrence and answers to the questions: What adjacent structures are in jeopardy? Will resection of these be possible? What organ will be available for reconstruction? What route of reconstruction is most available?

The patient should be aware of and prepared for exploratory surgery without salvage esophagectomy and resection without reconstruction. Although reconstruction may be staged (planned or unplanned), it may not be possible.

OPERATIVE TECHNIQUE AND POSTOPERATIVE CARE

The literature provides little direction in techniques of salvage esophagectomy. However, principles followed for esophagectomy in the neoadjuvant setting are applicable. It is imperative that salvage esophagectomy provide an R0 resection including the radial margin. An adequate lymphadenectomy is crucial for restaging and in directing further adjuvant therapy, thus optimizing survival. However, there is no literature guidance for extent of lymphadenectomy. Organ and route of reconstruction will depend upon the prior therapy and findings at salvage esophagectomy. Anastomotic technique should be optimal to prevent leakage and conduit necrosis. A staged reconstruction is preferable to a failed reconstruction.

Similarly, the literature provides little direction in postoperative care following salvage esophagectomy. Principles of postoperative care following esophagectomy in the neoadjuvant setting are applicable.

PROCEDURE-SPECIFIC COMPLICATIONS

Compared to esophagectomy in other clinical settings, complications are much increased in patients undergoing salvage esophagectomy, and perhaps are the highest seen. Complications are typically those following esophagectomy and are most frequently pulmonary and anastomotic. Conduit and airway necroses following salvage esophagectomy are frequently lethal. Prior high-dose radiation therapy and patient debility (reflected by low serum albumin) have been reported to be predictive of postoperative morbidity and mortality. Complications are associated with postoperative mortality following salvage esophagectomy.

RESULTS

The infrequent, supremely selected patient, who is a candidate for salvage esophagectomy following definitive therapy, can at best expect a median survival of 12 to 36 months, a 5-year survival of 25% to 35%, and a disease-free survival of 10% to 20% if R0 resection is possible. Death is frequently due to persistent or recurrent cancer. In patients undergoing R1 or R2 resections, it is rare to survive 2 years following salvage esophagectomy.

SUMMARY

Salvage esophagectomy is a rare treatment option in patients that fail definitive treatment of esophageal cancer. The ideal patient has recurrent cancer with a long disease-free interval. R0 resection is necessary if long-term survival is to be realized. Patients with small recurrent cancers without M1, T4, or N+ disease are most likely to benefit from salvage esophagectomy. Complications are frequent and are typically pulmonary or anastomotic. Mortality is significant. Survival is 25% to 35% at most following R0 resection. Most deaths are secondary to cancer or salvage esophagectomy. R1 and R2 resections are to be avoided.

AN ILLUSTRATED CASE HISTORY

A 56-year-old white man presented with sudden onset of solid dysphagia and weight loss 2 years prior. He was found to have a cG2T3N1M0 adenocarcinoma of the esophagogastric junction. He received neoadjuvant therapy with three courses of platinum-based chemotherapy and radiation to 54 Gy. He underwent an Ivor Lewis esophagectomy, with anastomosis at 24 cm from the incisors. Pathologic review revealed this to be ypGT3N0M0 adenocarcinoma. The inked radial margin was involved by cancer.[14] A stormy postoperative course prevented any postoperative adjuvant therapy.

Fifteen months after diagnosis, esophagoscopy revealed recurrent adenocarcinoma at the anastomosis and distally for 2 cm into the stomach. This was staged as rG3T3N0M0 adenocarcinoma. The patient's performance status was excellent (Zubrod 0). However, he was anemic with otherwise normal laboratory studies. His young age and belief that R0 resection was possible led his surgeon to offer thoracic esophagectomy and completion gastrectomy. Colon interposition was used for reconstruction. Review of the resection specimen revealed rG3T4bN1M0 adenocarcinoma with positive radial margin at the carina (R1) and metastases to three of six regional lymph nodes resected.

His postoperative course was complicated by pneumonia and anastomotic leak. The esophagocolic anastomotic leak was treated with local measures and tracheostomy was avoided. Unfortunately, ongoing conduit necrosis eventually involved the proximal 2 cm of the colon. The neck wound was converted to an ostomy, nutrition was provided via his jejunostomy tube. He was kept npo and palliative care was administered for the next 3 months until his death in hospice.

EDITOR'S COMMMENT

The authors present a challenging scenario: what to do with the patient who is now being considered for resection after the so-called "definitive chemoradiation" or the rare patient who has an infield (visceral or anastomotic) recurrence. Given that the recurrence rate after chemoradiation alone approaches 50%, the most important challenge for the thoracic esophageal surgeon is to be involved in a prospective multidisciplinary discussion before any "definitive" treatment is begun. Otherwise, all other options involve a less than optimal scenario where a patient who would have been a good candidate is now frail; or where the wrong combination therapy was given for a particular patient. Especially since there is no advantage to a radiation dose exceeding 54 Gy, patients should be discussed *a priori* by a multidisciplinary team and a course agreed upon up front. Naturally, there are rare situations where a decision to operate late may occur as the result of severe symptoms, but if the surgeon were involved up front, the patient could be selected appropriately. A recent series from MD Anderson has shown similar excellent results with the so-called salvage esophagectomy, but again with higher morbidity and mortality.[15–19]

—Mark J. Krasna

References

1. Cooper JS, Guo MD, Herskovic A, et al. Chemoradiotherapy of locally advanced esophageal cancer: long-term follow-up of a prospective randomized trial (RTOG 85–01). Radiation Therapy Oncology Group. *JAMA.* 1999;281:1623–1627.
2. Kelsen DP, Winter KA, Gunderson LL, et al. Long-term results of RTOG trial 8911 (USA Intergroup 113): a random assignment trial comparison of chemotherapy followed by surgery compared with surgery alone for esophageal cancer. *J Clin Oncol.* 2007;25:3719–3725.
3. Gardner-Thorpe J, Hardwick RH, Dwerryhouse SJ. Salvage esophagectomy after local failure of definitive chemoradiotherapy. *Br J Surg.* 2007;94:1059–1066.
4. Nishimura M, Daiko H, Yoshida J, et al. Salvage esophagectomy following definitive chemoradiotherapy. *Gen Thorac Cardiovasc Surg.* 2007;55:461–465.
5. Piessen G, Briez N, Triboulet JP, et al. Patients with locally advanced esophageal carcinoma nonresponder to radiochemotherapy: who will benefit from surgery. *Ann Surg Oncol.* 2007;14:2036–2044.
6. D'Journo XB, Michelet P, Doddoli C, et al. Indications and outcome of salvage esophagectomy for oesophageal cancer. *Eur J Cardiothorac Surg.* 2008;33:1117–1123.
7. Smithers BM, Cullinan M, Thomas JM, et al. Outcomes of salvage esophagectomy post definitive chemoradiotherapy compared with resection following preoperative neoadjuvant chemoradiotherapy. *Dis Esophagus.* 2007;20:471–477.
8. Chao YK, Chan SC, Chang HK, et al. Salvage surgery after failed chemoradiotherapy in squamous cell carcinoma of the esophagus. *Eur J Surg Oncol.* 2009;35:289–294.
9. Morita M, Kumashiro R, Hisamatsu Y, et al. Clinical significance of salvage esophagectomy for remnant or recurrent cancer following definitive chemoradiotherapy. *J Gastroenterol.* 2011;46:1284–1291.
10. Tachimori Y, Kanamori N, Uemura N, et al. Salvage esophagectomy after high-dose chemoradiotherapy for esophageal squamous cell carcinoma. *J Thorac Cardiovasc Surg.* 2009;137:49–54.
11. Schipper PH, Cassivi SD, Deschamps C, et al. Locally recurrent esophageal carcinoma: when is re-resection indicated? *Ann Thorac Surg.* 2005;80:1001–1006.
12. Smith RS, Miller RC. Incidence of brain metastasis in patients with esophageal carcinoma. *World J Gastroenterol.* 2011;17:2407–2410.
13. Yang Q, Cleary KR, Yao JC, et al. Significance of post-chemoradiation biopsy in predicting residual esophageal carcinoma in the surgical specimen. *Dis Esophagus.* 2004;17:38–43.
14. Verhage RJJ, Zandvoort HJA, ten Kate FJW, et al. How to define a positive circumferential resection margin in T3 adenocarcinoma of the esophagus. *Am J Surg Pathol.* 2011;35:919–926.
15. Taketa T, Correa AM, Suzuki A, et al. Outcome of trimodality-eligible esophagogastric cancer patients who declined surgery after preoperative chemoradiation. *Oncology.* 2012;83(5):300–304.
16. Sepesi B, Swisher SG, Walsh GL, et al. Omental reinforcement of the thoracic esophagogastric anastomosis: an analysis of leak and reintervention rates in patients undergoing planned and salvage esophagectomy. *J Thorac Cardiovasc Surg.* 2012;144(5):1146–1150.
17. Marks JL, Hofstetter W, Correa AM, et al. Salvage esophagectomy after failed definitive chemoradiation for esophageal adenocarcinoma. *Ann Thorac Surg.* 2012;94(4):1126–1132; discussion 1132–1133.
18. Kim JY, Correa AM, Vaporciyan AA, et al. Does the timing of esophagectomy after chemoradiation affect outcome? *Ann Thorac Surg.* 2012;93(1):207–212; discussion 212–213.
19. Minsky BD, Pajak TF, Ginsberg RJ, et al. INT 0123 (Radiation Therapy Oncology Group 94–05) phase III trial of combined-modality therapy for esophageal cancer: high-dose versus standard-dose radiation therapy. *J Clin Oncol.* 2002;20(5):1167–1174.

27 Radiation Therapy in the Management of Esophageal Cancer

Jona Hattangadi and Harvey Mamon

Keywords: Multimodality treatment of esophageal cancer

Radiation therapy plays an important role in the multimodality treatment of esophageal cancer. Only 30% to 40% of patients with esophageal cancer have potentially resectable disease at presentation. In combination with chemotherapy in the neoadjuvant setting, radiation has been shown to improve survival over surgery alone. Radiation also can be very effective in the palliative setting. In this chapter, we discuss the general background and data on the use of radiation in the management of esophageal cancer.

RADIATION ALONE

There are few studies of radiation alone for esophageal cancer, and these have generally had poor outcomes. Historically, radiation was used for patients with extensive disease or those unfit for surgery. In a review of 49 early series of patients treated with radiation alone for esophageal squamous cell carcinoma, the overall survival rate at 5 years was 6%.[1] In a British study of 101 patients with clinically localized esophageal cancer, who received definitive radiation doses of 45 to 53 Gray (Gy, unit of absorbed radiation dose), the 5-year survival rate was 21%.[2] In a randomized trial (Radiation Therapy Oncology Group [RTOG] 85-01) of combined chemoradiation versus radiation alone to 64 Gy for 121 patients with mostly esophageal squamous cell carcinoma, 5-year overall survival in the radiation alone arm was 0.[3,4] For this reason, radiation alone for esophageal cancer is generally considered palliative rather than curative in intent. However, there are some studies exploring whether early-stage (stage I) esophageal cancer could be effectively treated with radiation alone.[5]

DEFINITIVE CHEMORADIATION

Definitive concurrent chemotherapy and radiation therapy have been studied as an alternative to operative management for esophageal cancer, particularly for patients who are not good surgical candidates. RTOG 85-01 was a prospective, randomized phase III trial of patients with nondisseminated adenocarcinoma or squamous cell carcinoma of the thoracic esophagus.[3,4,6] Patients were randomized between radiation alone (64 Gy in 32 fractions over 6.5 weeks) versus concurrent chemoradiation (2 cycles of infusional 5-FU plus cisplatin and radiation [50 Gy in 25 fractions over 5 weeks]). The trial closed early because a planned interim analysis showed a significant survival advantage for chemoradiation (5-year survival 27% vs. 0%) as well as a reduction in locoregional and distant failures. However, 46% of patients in the chemoradiation arm had persistent or locally recurrent disease in the esophagus at 12 months. Severe acute but not late toxicity was significantly higher in the chemoradiation arm.

The follow-up trial to RTOG 85-01 asked the question whether radiation dose escalation may improve local control rates. In the Intergroup 0123 study (RTOG 94-05), 236 patients with nonmetastatic squamous cell carcinoma or adenocarcinoma of the thoracic esophagus received concurrent cisplatin and 5-FU, and the patients were randomized between two different radiation doses: 50.4 Gy in 28 fractions or 64.8 Gy in 36 fractions.[7] Radiation treatment was given daily, five fractions per week. There was no significant difference in median survival (13 vs. 18 months) or locoregional failure and persistence of disease (56% vs. 52%) between the high-dose and standard-dose arms, respectively. There was also a significantly higher rate of deaths in the high-dose arm (nine vs. two events). However, of the nine treatment-related deaths in the high-dose arm, six occurred before reaching 5040 cGy, suggesting that the deaths were not related to the higher radiation dose. Nevertheless, higher radiation dose does not appear to provide a survival or local control benefit, so 5040 cGy remains the standard of care in the United States at this time.

Patients of advanced age or those with significant comorbidities may not be good candidates for surgical management of esophageal cancer. Older patients have higher rates of postoperative morbidity and mortality after esophagectomy.[8] Studies suggest that definitive chemoradiation may be well tolerated in elderly patients, with outcomes comparable to those in younger patients.[8,9]

ADDITION OF SURGERY OVER DEFINITIVE CHEMORADIATION

As definitive chemoradiation in contemporary series have shown near equivalent long-term survival as surgical series, the question becomes whether patients undergoing chemoradiation for esophageal cancer benefit from surgery. The results of the 8501 study demonstrated a locoregional recurrence rate of over 45%. Although there is no clear survival benefit, studies suggest that resection leads to improved locoregional control, predominantly in squamous cell carcinoma.

In a French trial, patients with operable T2N0–1 thoracic esophageal cancer received induction chemoradiation with either protracted (46 Gy in 4.5 weeks) or split course (15 Gy, days 1–5 and 22–26) radiation concurrent with 5-FU/cisplatin. Patients with at least a partial response ($n = 259$) were randomly assigned to surgery or continued chemoradiation. At a median follow-up of 47 months, survival was not significantly different between the two groups (median survival 18 vs. 19 months), but the surgical arm had lower locoregional recurrence (34% vs. 43%, $p = 0.001$) and need for palliative stents.[10] Quality of life was similar between the arms at 2 years.[11] A German trial randomized 172 patients with locally advanced esophageal squamous cell carcinoma to induction chemotherapy and chemoradiation (40 Gy) followed by surgery or the same induction regimen followed by chemoradiation (65 Gy or greater) without surgery.[12] At 5 years, overall survival was equivalent between the arms, but local progression-free survival was better in the surgery group (64% vs. 53%, $p = 0.003$). However, treatment-related mortality was also higher in the surgery group (12.8% vs. 3.5%, $p = 0.03$).

Two studies have compared definitive chemoradiation (with surgical salvage) and surgery alone for resectable thoracic esophageal squamous cell carcinoma. In a Chinese prospective randomized trial where 80 such patients received 50 to 60 Gy with concurrent 5-FU/cisplatin or esophagectomy alone, there was no difference in survival.[13] In a similar but nonrandomized study comparing those receiving 60 Gy concurrent with 5-FU/cisplatin or surgery alone, survival rates were similar, but the surgery alone arm had a higher rate of metastases.[14]

NEOADJUVANT THERAPY FOR ESOPHAGEAL CANCER

The rationale for preoperative (neoadjuvant) therapy for esophageal cancer is three-fold: to decrease micrometastases and control systemic disease, to improve resectability by tumor shrinkage, and to assess in vivo tumor response to therapy.

Preoperative Chemoradiation

The use of chemotherapy concurrent with radiation preoperatively is based on the notion of radiosensitization, namely, that the chemotherapy makes radiation more effective. This treatment paradigm is also called trimodality treatment: chemotherapy and radiation preoperatively, followed by surgical resection. There are seven major randomized trials of surgery with or without preoperative chemoradiation for patients with potentially resectable esophageal cancer, three of which showed a statistically significant survival benefit for chemoradiation.

In the Irish trial by Walsh and colleagues, 113 patients with esophageal or gastroesophageal (GE) junction adenocarcinoma were randomized to surgery alone or cisplatin/5-FU–based chemoradiation before surgery.[15] Chemoradiation improved survival (32% vs. 6% at 3 years), although the surgery alone arm had a lower than expected survival. CALGB 9781 randomized 56 patients with squamous cell carcinoma or adenocarcinoma of the thoracic esophagus to trimodality therapy or surgery alone. With median follow-up of 6 years, median survival was significantly improved with preoperative chemoradiation (4.5 vs. 1.8 years, $p = 0.002$).[16] In the Dutch CROSS trial, 366 patients with potentially resectable esophageal or GE junction cancer (mostly adenocarcinoma) were randomized to preoperative chemoradiation (chemotherapy was paclitaxel and carboplatin, radiation was given to 41.4 Gy over 5 weeks) versus surgery alone. The study showed a significant overall survival benefit with preoperative chemoradiation (median survival 49 months vs. 24 months), and this 29% of patients in this arm achieved a pathologic complete response.[17] There was also a higher complete (R0) resection rate in the chemoradiation-surgery group (92% vs. 69%, $p < 0.001$).

Three other randomized trials of surgery alone versus preoperative chemoradiation followed by surgery did not show a statistically significant survival benefit to trimodality treatment.[18–20] Adequate statistical power may have been an issue. As well, three studies comparing sequentially delivered chemotherapy and radiation preoperatively to surgery alone also failed to show any survival benefit to trimodality therapy.[21–23]

Preoperative Chemotherapy

Multiple randomized phase III trials have evaluated the benefit of preoperative chemotherapy followed by surgery compared with surgery alone (no radiation in either arm). Results are mixed, with four negative trials[24–27] and three showing a survival benefit to preoperative chemotherapy.[28–30]

Comparing Preoperative Regimens

A German study published in 2009 randomized 119 patients with locally advanced adenocarcinoma of the lower esophagus or gastric cardia to (A) induction chemotherapy (5-FU, leucovorin, cisplatin, 15 weeks) followed by surgery or (B) chemotherapy (12 weeks) followed by chemoradiation (30 Gy in 15 fractions over 3 weeks with concurrent cisplatin/etoposide) followed by surgery.[31] The study closed early on account of low accrual. At a median follow-up of 46 months, the chemoradiation arm had a higher rate of pathologic complete response (16% vs. 2%, $p = 0.03$) and node negative disease at surgery (64% vs. 38%, $p = 0.01$). Three-year overall survival was 47% in the chemoradiation arm compared with 28% in the chemotherapy arm, but this did not reach statistical significance ($p = 0.07$). This may have been due to insufficient power.

Meta-Analyses

With conflicting results from different randomized trials, we can look to meta-analyses with their increased statistical power to determine whether preoperative treatment provides a survival benefit in esophageal cancer. Sjoquist et al.[32] looked at 12 trials of neoadjuvant chemoradiation versus surgery alone ($n = 1854$), 9 trials of neoadjuvant chemotherapy versus surgery alone ($n = 1981$), and 2 trials comparing neoadjuvant chemoradiation and neoadjuvant chemotherapy ($n = 194$), all in patients with resectable esophageal cancer. Overall, neoadjuvant chemoradiation improved survival by 22% over surgery alone. This survival benefit was seen in both adenocarcinoma (17% survival benefit) and squamous cell carcinoma (20% survival benefit). Neoadjuvant chemotherapy without radiation, compared with surgery alone, provided a 13% survival improvement. This benefit was seen in adenocarcinoma patients (17% survival benefit), but there was no significant survival benefit of neoadjuvant chemotherapy over surgery alone for squamous cell carcinoma. When chemoradiation and chemotherapy were indirectly compared, there was weak evidence favoring chemoradiation, although this was not statistically significant.

Another recently published meta-analysis found similar results.[33] The authors report that neoadjuvant chemoradiation provides a 19% overall survival benefit over surgery alone, and neoadjuvant chemotherapy a 7% survival benefit. They did not find a significant increase in morbidity rates after neoadjuvant chemoradiation, and reported that the likelihood of a complete (R0) resection was 15% higher after neoadjuvant treatment. They found no significant survival difference between definitive chemoradiation and neoadjuvant treatment followed by surgery or surgery alone, although treatment-related mortality rates were over seven-fold lower.

These meta-analyses provide strong evidence for a survival benefit of neoadjuvant chemoradiation or chemotherapy over surgery alone in esophageal cancer. Although there appears to be no clear advantage of neoadjuvant chemoradiation over neoadjuvant chemotherapy, the data do suggest that chemoradiation may have a marginally greater survival benefit and higher pathologic response rate.

Measuring Response to Neoadjuvant Therapy: Implications for Individualized Treatment

Although neoadjuvant therapy followed by surgery has emerged as the standard of care for locally advanced esophageal cancer, there is variability in response to neoadjuvant treatment. Some patients may have a complete response but will go on to resection and be exposed to the risks of surgery. Similarly, for patients who do not respond to neoadjuvant chemotherapy, their prognosis after this treatment might be worse than that of a primary surgical approach, especially if there was local disease progression.

A German phase II trial (MUNICON) used FDG-positron emission tomography (PET) imaging to identify early responders to neoadjuvant chemotherapy.[34] Patients ($n = 119$) with locally advanced adenocarcinoma of the distal esophagus or gastric cardia had a baseline PET scan, then went on to receive 2 weeks of 5-FU/platinum-based induction chemotherapy. Those with a decrease of 35% or more in tumor glucose standard uptake value (SUV) on repeat PET were defined as metabolic responders and went on to receive 12 more weeks of chemotherapy and then surgery. Patients who did not have a sufficient response on PET to the 2 weeks of induction chemotherapy were considered nonresponders and went straight to surgical resection. Median event-free survival was higher among PET responders (30 months vs. 15 months, $p = 0.002$), and these patients were also more likely to have an R0 resection and complete pathologic response at surgery.

A follow-up study, MUNICON II, treated nonresponders to induction chemotherapy with salvage neoadjuvant chemoradiation before surgery.[35] With this salvage treatment, nonresponders had an improved histopathologic response rate when compared with the MUNICON I results. A recent retrospective study showed that PET complete response predicted improved survival after definitive chemoradiation, but not after trimodality therapy for esophageal cancer (neoadjuvant chemoradiation + surgery).[36] These preliminary data suggest that FDG-PET may help to identify patients in whom surgery might be avoided, but would need to be tested in a prospective study. The goal of identifying responders to neoadjuvant treatment is to potentially tailor therapies based on tumor biology and response.

POSTOPERATIVE RADIATION

In patients who undergo surgery for esophageal cancer, there is limited data on postoperative radiation. There are only three older randomized trials which address this issue. A trial from Hong Kong randomized 130 patients after curative or palliative esophageal resection to postoperative radiation (49 Gy in 14 fractions) or no additional treatment.[37] Among patients who had palliative resections, postoperative radiation decreased local recurrence (20% vs. 46%), but there was no significant effect on local control in patients who had curative resection. In fact, there was a detriment to overall median survival with postoperative radiation (9 months vs. 15 months) and a higher rate of complications (37% vs. 6%), with 17 cases of gastric ulceration and 5 deaths from bleeding. These data are from 1986 to 1989 using older radiation planning and delivery techniques. A French study, from 1979 to 1985, randomized 221 patients with esophageal squamous cell carcinoma to surgery alone or surgery followed by postoperative radiation (45–55 Gy).[38] Although local recurrence was lower in the radiation arm (15% vs. 30%), there was no difference in survival (median 18 months both arms). A Chinese study randomized 485 patients with esophageal squamous cell cancer from 1986 to 1997 to surgery versus surgery followed by radiation (50–60 Gy).[39] The addition of radiation in this group of patients did not improve overall survival.

To assess whether the addition of concurrent chemotherapy improves outcomes with adjuvant radiation in esophageal patients, we can extrapolate from the Intergroup 0116 trial.[40] In this study 556 patients with adenocarcinoma of the stomach or GE junction were randomized to resection alone or resection plus postoperative treatment. Approximately 20% of the patients had tumors located in the GE junction. The adjuvant treatment arm consisted of one cycle of postoperative chemotherapy (5-FU/leucovorin), then concurrent chemoradiation (45 Gy and 5-FU/leucovorin), followed by two more cycles of chemotherapy. Adjuvant chemoradiation improved overall survival (median 36 months vs. 27 months) and relapse-free survival (median 30 months vs. 19%). Based on these data, adjuvant chemoradiation is generally recommended for patients with GE junction cancers who undergo surgery as initial management.

We do not routinely use postoperative radiation therapy in esophageal cancer above the GE junction, since modern studies exhibit improved outcomes with neoadjuvant treatment. In addition, postoperative radiation fields are generally much larger to treat the anastomotic site (Fig. 27-1). Larger fields that extend high into the thorax and neck can involve normal tissues that are sensitive to the effects of radiation, particularly the lung and heart. Neoadjuvant chemoradiation is thus preferable to postoperative treatment for locally advanced esophageal cancer. Although the results of INT-0116 support the use of postoperative treatment for GE junction tumors, the rationale for neoadjuvant therapy applies to tumors of the cardia and GE junction, and neoadjuvant chemoradiation is therefore our preferred treatment strategy for locally advanced tumors of the esophagus, GE junction, and cardia.

BRACHYTHERAPY

Brachytherapy, which involves the temporary or permanent insertion of radioactive sources into the tumor or peritumoral tissues, is the most conformal radiation treatment modality available. It allows for focal dose escalation to the tumor, with sparing of surrounding normal tissue.[41] RTOG 9207 was a prospective phase I/II study of 49 patients with inoperable esophageal cancer who received concurrent chemoradiation (50 Gy with 5-FU/cisplatin) followed by esophageal brachytherapy (15–20 Gy).[42] Unfortunately, life-threatening treatment-related toxicity was 24% and treatment-related deaths were 10%. Six patients developed esophageal fistulas, resulting in three deaths, and median survival was only 11 months.

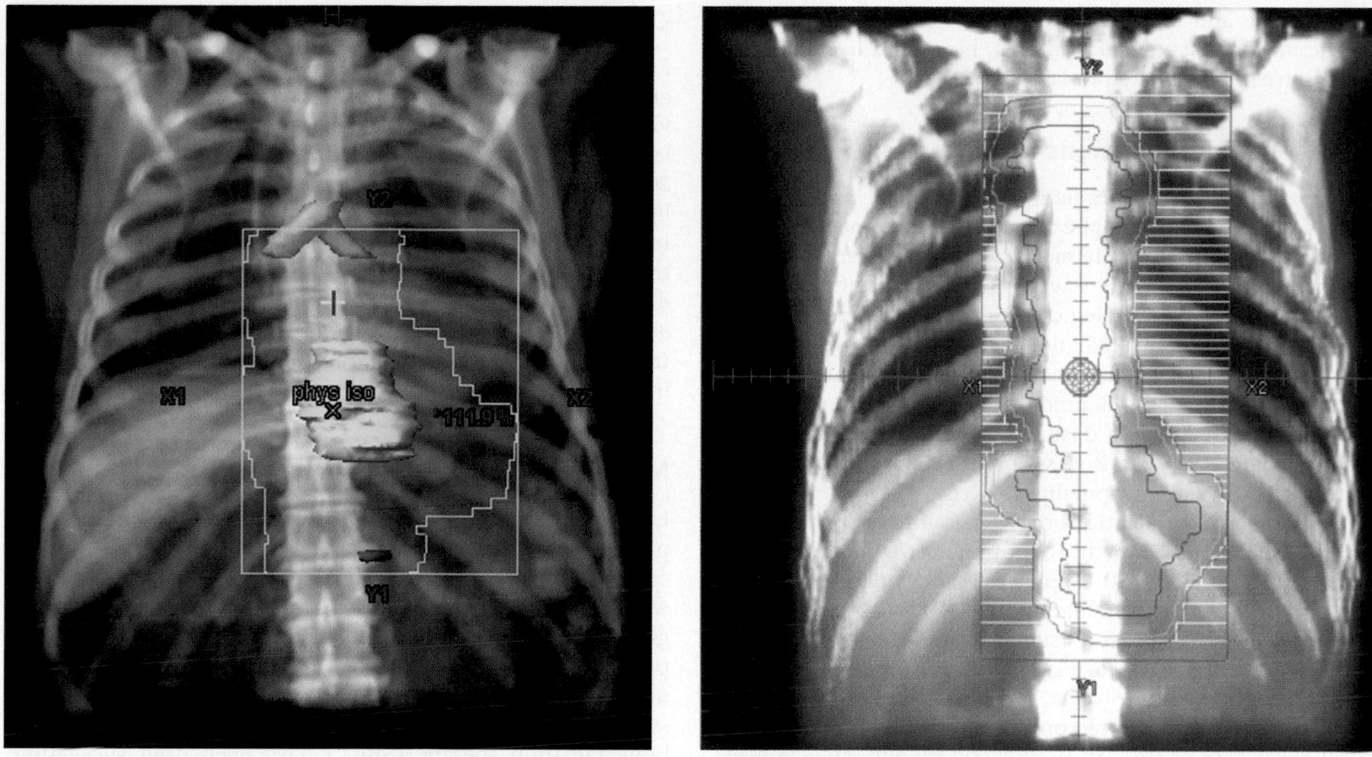

A B

Figure 27-1. *A.* Anterior-posterior (AP) field for preoperative treatment of a GE junction tumor. *B.* AP field for postoperative treatment of a GE junction tumor. Note that the field extends much farther superiorly, to the level of the clavicles rather than the level of the carina. The larger field results in the treatment of significantly more normal tissue, particularly heart and lung.

Intraluminal brachytherapy was used alone or as additional dose following external beam radiation therapy for patients with T1N0 esophageal cancer in a retrospective Japanese series.[43] The authors reported good overall outcomes (75% local control and 84% overall survival at 5 years) but 7% grade 3 to 4 toxicity including grade 4 and 5 esophageal ulcers. Another recent Japanese series reviewed 97 cases of stage I esophageal cancer treated with radiation (external beam with or without brachytherapy) and chemotherapy.[44] The addition of brachytherapy showed no survival or local control benefit, but the rate of serious adverse effects including lethal esophageal ulcers was significantly higher. Thus, for curative esophageal cancer, the addition of brachytherapy to external beam radiation has yet to demonstrate a local control or survival advantage. However, treatment-related toxicities, including esophageal ulcers and fistulas, can be significant.

The use of intraluminal brachytherapy for palliation of obstructive symptoms in locally advanced esophageal cancer is much more promising. A multicenter Danish phase III trial randomized 209 patients with dysphagia from inoperable esophageal or GE junction cancer to esophageal stent placement or single-dose brachytherapy (12 Gy).[45] Dysphagia improved more rapidly after stent placement, but long-term relief was more sustained after brachytherapy. Quality of life scores were better with brachytherapy. A Polish series of 91 patients with unresectable locally advanced esophageal cancer demonstrated a significant improvement in dysphagia with palliative high-dose-rate brachytherapy (22.5 Gy in 3 fractions per week).[46] Whether the addition of external beam radiation to brachytherapy can improve palliation has been addressed in two prospective phase III randomized trials. A Canadian multicenter trial randomized 60 patients with inoperable esophageal cancer to intraluminal brachytherapy (16 Gy in 2 fractions over 3 days) with or without additional external beam radiation (30 Gy in 10 fractions over 2 weeks).[47] At 6 months follow-up, the authors found no significant benefit of external beam radiation for symptom relief or overall survival. A study by the International Atomic Energy Agency randomized 219 patients with obstructive squamous cell esophageal cancer to high-dose–rate brachytherapy (2 fractions of 8 Gy each, within 1 week) with or without additional external beam radiation therapy (30 Gy in 10 fractions).[48] Combined modality treatment (brachytherapy + external beam) improved symptoms of dysphagia, odynophagia, regurgitation, and chest pain compared with brachytherapy alone, although there was no difference in survival outcomes.

Besides brachytherapy, other esophageal recanalization methods, with the aim of debulking the tumor, include laser therapy,[49] photodynamic therapy (PDT),[50] and argon plasma coagulation (APC).[51] These methods were compared directly in a randomized trial of 93 patients with obstructive dysphagia from esophageal cancer: APC + brachytherapy, APC + PDT, or APC alone. Palliative combination treatment with APC and brachytherapy or PDT was more effective than APC alone. APC with brachytherapy was associated with the best quality of life and the least treatment-related complications.

TREATMENT-RELATED TOXICITY

Radiation treatment for esophageal cancer can be challenging because of the advanced presentation of esophageal tumors, and the large fields that are often needed to adequately cover gross disease and submucosal spread. These large fields can include normal tissues, such as lung, heart, and liver, and can result in treatment-related toxicity.

Pulmonary Complications

Patients receiving chemoradiation for esophageal cancer are at risk for pulmonary complications. Radiation pneumonitis is a subacute complication characterized by persistent cough or shortness or breath arising 6 weeks to 6 months after therapy. There is often also a radiologic correlation seen on CT within the photon beam path. Radiation oncologists try to minimize complications based on dose metrics to normal tissue. There is evidence that the risk of pneumonitis correlates with mean lung dose and data points on a dose–volume histogram (Fig. 27-2), although there is no definitive set of dose parameters that correlates perfectly with low pneumonitis risk.[52]

Pulmonary complications that occur after esophagectomy can contribute substantially to postoperative morbidity and mortality. A study of 110 esophageal cancer patients treated with preoperative chemoradiation followed by esophagectomy found that dosimetric factors such as higher mean lung doses and worse lung sparing correlated with postoperative pulmonary complications.[53] However, a recent German study comparing patients who received preoperative chemoradiation followed by surgery or surgery alone found no difference in perioperative pulmonary toxicity.[54]

Cardiac Toxicity

Long-term cardiac morbidity from esophageal radiation is generally unknown because of the small number of long-term survivors of locally advanced esophageal cancer and the fact that late cardiac toxicity from radiation does not occur until 10 to 20 years after treatment. Extrapolating from the breast cancer literature, however, shows that there are excess cardiac deaths in patients who received high doses of radiation to the left ventricle.[52] Thus, as cure rates for esophageal cancer improve, cardiac late effects may become more important. Techniques such as three-dimensional (3D) CT planning, intensity-modulated radiation therapy, and high resolution imaging may help to improve dose distributions to the heart and lung.

Metastatic Disease

Unfortunately, 50% to 60% of patients with esophageal cancer present with unresectable locally advanced or metastatic disease. The most common sites of distant metastases in patients with esophageal cancer are the liver, lungs, bone, and adrenal glands. Metastases can progress quickly and cause significant pain and discomfort, impacting quality of life. Palliative external beam radiation can be very effective in improving pain from symptomatic bone metastases.[55] New advances in stereotactic body radiation therapy (SBRT) have been used successfully for palliation of spinal[56] and liver metastases.[57] Thus radiation

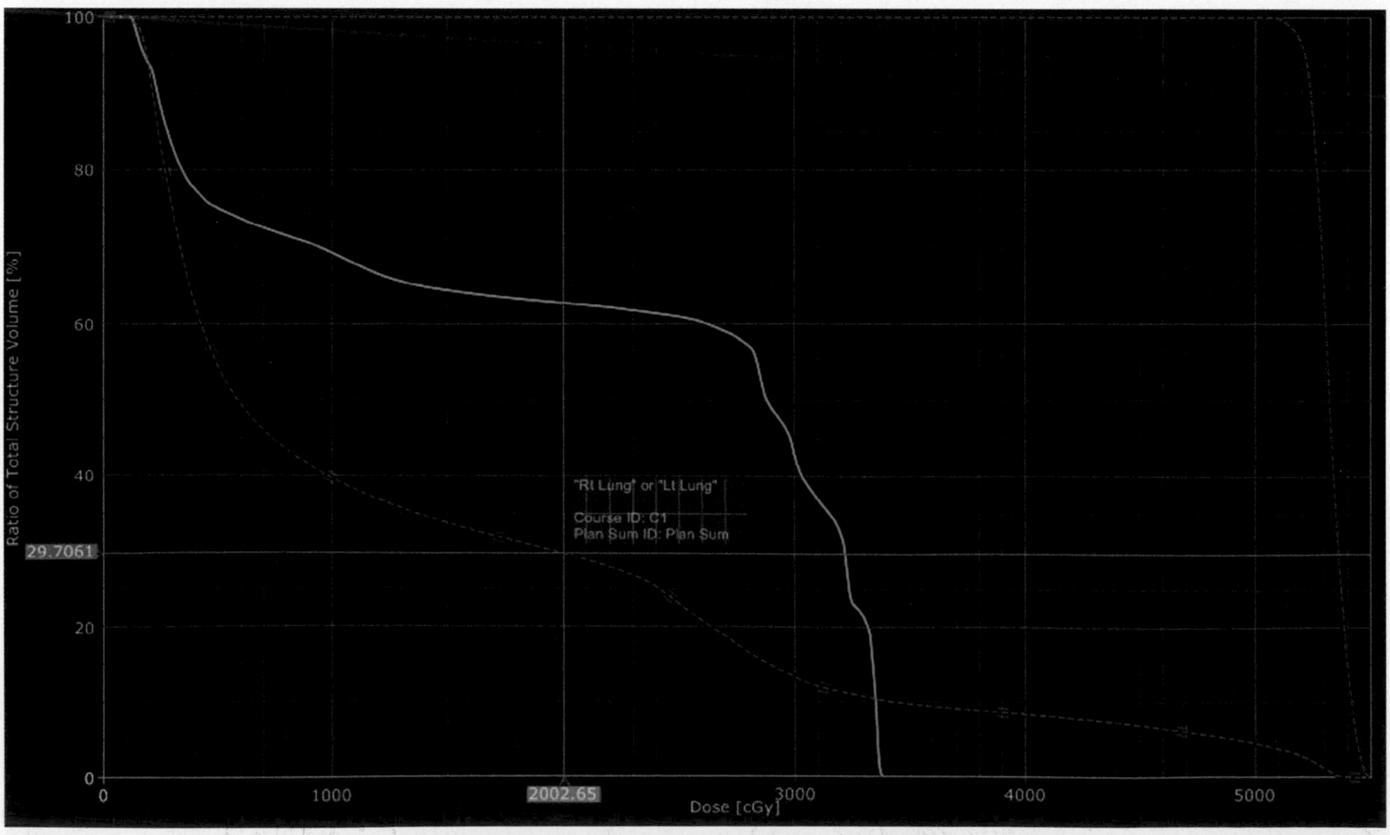

Figure 27-2. Dose–volume histogram (DVH) of a patient receiving radiation therapy for esophageal cancer. The red dotted line represents the esophageal tumor, all of which receives the prescribed dose of 5040 cGy. The green solid line represents the spinal cord, which receives a maximal dose of 3400 cGy, well below the tolerance of 4500 cGy. The blue dashed line represents the combined lung volume, with 30% of this volume receiving a dose of 2000 cGy, which is associated with a low risk of clinically significant pneumonitis.

therapy is frequently part of the overall palliative management of patients with metastatic esophageal cancer.

EDITOR'S COMMENT

This chapter reviews the data supporting the use of radiation therapy (XRT) as an adjunct in treating patients with esophageal cancer. Whether as definitive therapy, used in conjunction with chemotherapy, or as a form of palliation (with external beam or brachytherapy), XRT has an important role and should be considered early in the decision-making process. One of the most important factors currently under evaluation is the ability to minimize toxicity from XRT, not only to adjacent organs such as the heart, lungs and spine, but also to minimize XRT dose to the future gastric conduit. Several techniques are available that should be pursued prospectively in these patients. First, a determination of the degree of lymph node involvement should be made. This can generally be done at the time of EUS with FNA. If these lymph nodes are negative or not evaluable, thoracoscopy/laparoscopy lymph node staging can be performed. These techniques will allow the radiooncologist to limit the dose, using 3D conformal and IMRT dose planning, to a smaller field if lymph nodes are not involved as opposed to a large field (conceivably more than 5 cm beyond the proximal and distant extent of the primary tumor). Another potential technique is to treat patients with a full stomach (using a liquid "meal") at each treatment. This has been shown to act as a weight and pull the greater curvature of the stomach (the future conduit) laterally into the left upper quadrant. This allows full dose XRT to be delivered to the celiac axis without directly damaging the conduit or its vascular branches.

—Mark J. Krasna

References

1. Earlam R, Cunha-Melo JR. Oesophogeal squamous cell carcinomas: II. A critical view of radiotherapy. *Br J Surg.* 1980;67:457–461.
2. Sykes AJ, Burt PA, Slevin NJ, et al. Radical radiotherapy for carcinoma of the oesophagus: an effective alternative to surgery. *Radiother Oncol.* 1998;48:15–21.
3. Al-Sarraf M, Martz K, Herskovic A, et al. Progress report of combined chemoradiotherapy versus radiotherapy alone in patients with esophageal cancer: an intergroup study. *J Clin Oncol.* 1997;15:277–284.
4. Herskovic A, Martz K, al-Sarraf M, et al. Combined chemotherapy and radiotherapy compared with radiotherapy alone in patients with cancer of the esophagus. *N Engl J Med.* 1992,326:1593–1598.
5. Sasaki T, Nakamura K, Shioyama Y, et al. Treatment outcomes of radiotherapy for patients with stage I esophageal cancer: a single institute experience. *Am J Clin Oncol.* 2007;30:514–519.
6. Cooper JS, Guo MD, Herskovic A, et al. Chemoradiotherapy of locally advanced esophageal cancer: long-term follow-up of a prospective randomized trial (RTOG 85-01). Radiation Therapy Oncology Group. *JAMA.* 1999;281:1623–1627.
7. Minsky BD, Pajak TF, Ginsberg RJ, et al. INT 0123 (Radiation Therapy Oncology Group 94-05) phase III trial of combined-modality therapy for esophageal cancer: high-dose versus standard-dose radiation therapy. *J Clin Oncol.* 2002;20:1167–1174.
8. Davies L, Lewis WG, Arnold DT, et al. Prognostic significance of age in the radical treatment of oesophageal cancer with surgery or chemoradiotherapy: a prospective observational cohort study. *Clin Oncol (R Coll Radiol).* 2010;22:578–585.
9. Tougeron D, Di Fiore F, Thureau S, et al. Safety and outcome of definitive chemoradiotherapy in elderly patients with oesophageal cancer. *Br J Cancer.* 2008;99:1586–1592.
10. Bedenne L, Michel P, Bouche O, et al. Chemoradiation followed by surgery compared with chemoradiation alone in squamous cancer of the esophagus: FFCD 9102. *J Clin Oncol.* 2007;25:1160–1168.
11. Bonnetain F, Bouche O, Michel P, et al. A comparative longitudinal quality of life study using the Spitzer quality of life index in a randomized multicenter phase III trial (FFCD 9102): chemoradiation followed by surgery compared with chemoradiation alone in locally advanced squamous resectable thoracic esophageal cancer. *Ann Oncol.* 2006;17:827–834.
12. Stahl M, Stuschke M, Lehmann N, et al. Chemoradiation with and without surgery in patients with locally advanced squamous cell carcinoma of the esophagus. *J Clin Oncol.* 2005;23:2310–2317.
13. Chiu PW, Chan AC, Leung SF, et al. Multicenter prospective randomized trial comparing standard esophagectomy with chemoradiotherapy for treatment of squamous esophageal cancer: early results from the Chinese University Research Group for Esophageal Cancer (CURE). *J Gastrointest Surg.* 2005;9:794–802.
14. Ariga H, Nemoto K, Miyazaki S, et al. Prospective comparison of surgery alone and chemoradiotherapy with selective surgery in resectable squamous cell carcinoma of the esophagus. *Int J Radiat Oncol Biol Phys.* 2009;75:348–356.
15. Walsh TN, Noonan N, Hollywood D, et al. A comparison of multimodal therapy and surgery for esophageal adenocarcinoma. *N Engl J Med.* 1996;335:462–467.
16. Tepper J, Krasna MJ, Niedzwiecki D, et al. Phase III trial of trimodality therapy with cisplatin, fluorouracil, radiotherapy, and surgery compared with surgery alone for esophageal cancer: CALGB 9781. *J Clin Oncol.* 2008;26:1086–1092.
17. van Hagen P, Hulshof MC, van Lanschot JJ, et al. Preoperative chemoradiotherapy for esophageal or junctional cancer. *N Engl J Med.* 2012;366(22):2074–2084.
18. Burmeister BH, Smithers BM, Gebski V, et al. Surgery alone versus chemoradiotherapy followed by surgery for resectable cancer of the oesophagus: a randomised controlled phase III trial. *Lancet Oncol.* 2005;6:659–668.
19. Urba SG, Orringer MB, Turrisi A, et al. Randomized trial of preoperative chemoradiation versus surgery alone in patients with locoregional esophageal carcinoma. *J Clin Oncol.* 2001;19:305–313.
20. Mariette C, Seitz JF, Maillard E, et al. Surgery alone versus chemoradiotherapy followed by surgery for localized esophageal cancer: analysis of a randomized controlled phase III trial FFCD 9901 (abstract 4005). *J Clin Oncol.* 2010;28:302s.
21. Bosset JF, Gignoux M, Triboulet JP, et al. Chemoradiotherapy followed by surgery compared with surgery alone in squamous-cell cancer of the esophagus. *N Engl J Med.* 1997;337:161–167.
22. Le Prise E, Etienne PL, Meunier B, et al. A randomized study of chemotherapy, radiation therapy, and surgery versus surgery for localized squamous cell carcinoma of the esophagus. *Cancer.* 1994;73:1779–1784.
23. Nygaard K, Hagen S, Hansen HS, et al. Pre-operative radiotherapy prolongs survival in operable esophageal carcinoma: a randomized, multicenter study of pre-operative radiotherapy and chemotherapy. The second Scandinavian trial in esophageal cancer. *World J Surg.* 1992;16:1104–1109.
24. Ancona E, Ruol A, Santi S, et al. Only pathologic complete response to neoadjuvant chemotherapy improves significantly the long term survival of patients with resectable esophageal squamous cell carcinoma: final report of a randomized, controlled trial of preoperative chemotherapy versus surgery alone. *Cancer.* 2001;91:2165–2174.
25. Kelsen DP, Ginsberg R, Pajak TF, et al. Chemotherapy followed by surgery compared with surgery alone for localized esophageal cancer. *N Engl J Med.* 1998;339:1979–1984.
26. Roth JA, Pass HI, Flanagan MM, et al. Randomized clinical trial of preoperative and postoperative adjuvant chemotherapy with cisplatin, vindesine, and bleomycin for carcinoma of the esophagus. *J Thorac Cardiovasc Surg.* 1988;96:242–248.

27. Schuhmacher C, Schlag P, Lordick F, et al. Neoadjuvant chemotherapy versus surgery alone for locally advanced adenocarcinoma of the stomach and cardia: randomized EORTC phase III trial (Abstract #4510). *J Clin Oncol.* 2009;27:204s.
28. Medical Research Council Oesophageal Cancer Working Group. Surgical resection with or without preoperative chemotherapy in oesophageal cancer: a randomised controlled trial. *Lancet.* 2002;359:1727–1733.
29. Boige V, Pignon J, Saint-Aubert B, et al. Final results of a randomized trial comparing preoperative 5-fluorouracil/cisplatin to surgery alone in adenocarcinoma of stomach and lower esophagus (ASLE): FNLCC ACCORD07-FFCD 9703 trial (abstract). *J Clin Oncol.* 2007;25:200s.
30. Cunningham D, Allum WH, Stenning SP, et al. Perioperative chemotherapy versus surgery alone for resectable gastroesophageal cancer. *N Engl J Med.* 2006;355:11–20.
31. Stahl M, Walz MK, Stuschke M, et al. Phase III comparison of preoperative chemotherapy compared with chemoradiotherapy in patients with locally advanced adenocarcinoma of the esophagogastric junction. *J Clin Oncol.* 2009;27:851–856.
32. Sjoquist KM, Burmeister BH, Smithers BM, et al. Survival after neoadjuvant chemotherapy or chemoradiotherapy for resectable oesophageal carcinoma: an updated meta-analysis. *Lancet Oncol.* 2001;12:681–692.
33. Kranzfelder M, Schuster T, Geinitz H, et al. Meta-analysis of neoadjuvant treatment modalities and definitive non-surgical therapy for oesophageal squamous cell cancer. *Br J Surg.* 2011;98:768–783.
34. Lordick F, Ott K, Krause BJ, et al. PET to assess early metabolic response and to guide treatment of adenocarcinoma of the oesophagogastric junction: the MUNICON phase II trial. *Lancet Oncol.* 2007;8:797–805.
35. Meyer Zum Buschenfelde C, Herrmann K, Schuster T, et al. 18 F-FDG PET-guided salvage neoadjuvant radiochemotherapy of adenocarcinoma of the esophagogastric junction: the MUNICON II trial. *J Nucl Med.* 2011;52:1189–1196.
36. Monjazeb AM, Riedlinger G, Aklilu M, et al. Outcomes of patients with esophageal cancer staged with [(1)F]fluorodeoxyglucose positron emission tomography (FDG-PET): can postchemoradiotherapy FDG-PET predict the utility of resection? *J Clin Oncol.* 2010;28:4714–4721.
37. Fok M, Sham JS, Choy D, et al. Postoperative radiotherapy for carcinoma of the esophagus: a prospective, randomized controlled study. *Surgery.* 1993;113:138–147.
38. Teniere P, Hay JM, Fingerhut A, et al. Postoperative radiation therapy does not increase survival after curative resection for squamous cell carcinoma of the middle and lower esophagus as shown by a multicenter controlled trial. French University Association for Surgical Research. *Surg Gynecol Obstet.* 1991;173:123–130.
39. Xiao ZF, Yang ZY, Liang J, et al. Value of radiotherapy after radical surgery for esophageal carcinoma: a report of 495 patients. *Ann Thorac Surg.* 2003;75:331–336.
40. Macdonald JS, Smalley SR, Benedetti J, et al. Chemoradiotherapy after surgery compared with surgery alone for adenocarcinoma of the stomach or gastroesophageal junction. *N Engl J Med.* 2001;345:725–730.
41. Czito BG, Siddiqi NH, Mamon HJ. Gastrointestinal brachytherapy. In: Devlin PM, ed. *Brachytherapy: Applications and Techniques.* Philadelphia, PA: Lippincott Williams & Wilkins; 2006.
42. Gaspar LE, Winter K, Kocha WI, et al. A phase I/II study of external beam radiation, brachytherapy, and concurrent chemotherapy for patients with localized carcinoma of the esophagus (Radiation Therapy Oncology Group Study 9207): final report. *Cancer.* 2000;88:988–995.
43. Murakami Y, Nagata Y, Nishibuchi I, et al. Long-term outcomes of intraluminal brachytherapy in combination with external beam radiotherapy for superficial esophageal cancer. *Int J Clin Oncol.* 2012; 17(3):263–271.
44. Kodaira T, Fuwa N, Tachibana H, et al. Retrospective analysis of definitive radiotherapy for patients with superficial esophageal carcinoma: consideration of the optimal treatment method with a focus on late morbidity. *Radiother Oncol.* 2010;95:234–239.
45. Homs MY, Steyerberg EW, Eijkenboom WM, et al. Single-dose brachytherapy versus metal stent placement for the palliation of dysphagia from oesophageal cancer: multicentre randomised trial. *Lancet.* 2004;364:1497–1504.
46. Skowronek J, Piotrowski T, Zwierzchowski G. Palliative treatment by high-dose-rate intraluminal brachytherapy in patients with advanced esophageal cancer. *Brachytherapy.* 2004;3:87–94.
47. Sur R, Donde B, Falkson C, et al. Randomized prospective study comparing high-dose-rate intraluminal brachytherapy (HDRILBT) alone with HDRILBT and external beam radiotherapy in the palliation of advanced esophageal cancer. *Brachytherapy.* 2004;3:191–195.
48. Rosenblatt E, Jones G, Sur RK, et al. Adding external beam to intra-luminal brachytherapy improves palliation in obstructive squamous cell oesophageal cancer: a prospective multi-centre randomized trial of the International Atomic Energy Agency. *Radiother Oncol.* 2010;97:488–494.
49. Swain CP, Bown SG, Edwards DA, et al. Laser recanalization of obstructing foregut cancer. *Br J Surg.* 1984;71:112–115.
50. Kashtan H, Konikoff F, Haddad R, et al. Photodynamic therapy of cancer of the esophagus using systemic aminolevulinic acid and a non laser light source: a phase I/II study. *Gastrointest Endosc.* 1999;49:760–764.
51. Akhtar K, Byrne JP, Bancewicz J, et al. Argon beam plasma coagulation in the management of cancers of the esophagus and stomach. *Surg Endosc.* 2000;14:1127–1130.
52. Hong TS, Crowley EM, Killoran J, et al. Considerations in treatment planning for esophageal cancer. *Semin Radiat Oncol.* 2007;17:53–61.
53. Wang SL, Liao Z, Vaporciyan AA, et al. Investigation of clinical and dosimetric factors associated with postoperative pulmonary complications in esophageal cancer patients treated with concurrent chemoradiotherapy followed by surgery. *Int J Radiat Oncol Biol Phys.* 2006;64:692–699.
54. Dahn D, Martell J, Vorwerk H, et al. Influence of irradiated lung volumes on perioperative morbidity and mortality in patients after neoadjuvant radiochemotherapy for esophageal cancer. *Int J Radiat Oncol Biol Phys.* 2011;77:44–52.
55. Nguyen J, Chow E, Zeng L, et al. Palliative response and functional interference outcomes using the brief pain inventory for spinal bony metastases treated with conventional radiotherapy. *Clin Oncol (R Coll Radiol).* 2011;23:485–491.
56. Chang EL, Shiu AS, Mendel E, et al. Phase I/II study of stereotactic body radiotherapy for spinal metastasis and its pattern of failure. *J Neurosurg Spine.* 2007;7:151–160.
57. Rusthoven KE, Kavanagh BD, Cardenes H, et al. Multi-institutional phase I/II trial of stereotactic body radiation therapy for liver metastases. *J Clin Oncol.* 2009;27:1572–1578.

PART 3

RESECTION TECHNIQUES FOR BENIGN ESOPHAGEAL DISEASE

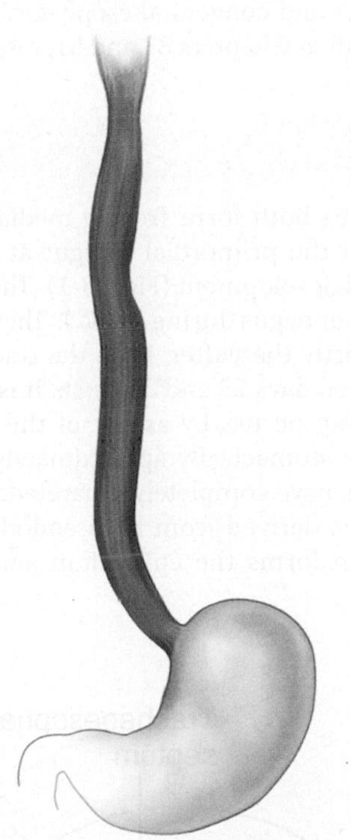

28 Overview: Anatomy and Pathophysiology of Benign Esophageal Disease

Marie Ziesat, Jennifer Paruch, and Mark K. Ferguson

Keywords: esophageal anatomy, esophageal pathophysiology leiomyoma, esophageal cyst, esophageal benign neoplasm, esophageal diverticulum, esophageal web, esophageal ring

The term "esophagus" derives from the Greek root "oisein" (to carry) and "phagos" (to eat). The esophagus' intricate components perform in symphony to provide a muscular conduit between the pharynx and stomach. Even small deviations in structure can lead to dysfunction. Benign esophageal lesions can obstruct the esophageal lumen and produce symptoms. This chapter discusses esophageal development and anatomy as well as the pathophysiology of benign esophageal diseases. Chapter 29 details the surgical and endoscopic approaches to these diseases. Motility disorders and congenital esophageal diseases are discussed in more detail in Chapters 33 and 51, respectively.

EMBRYOLOGY

The esophagus and trachea both form from a medial ventral diverticulum arising from the primordial foregut at approximately day 22 or 23 of fetal development (Fig. 28-1). The foregut divides into trachea and esophagus during week 4. The stomach bud forms posteriorly shortly thereafter. Both the trachea and esophagus elongate between days 23 and 34 or 36. It is thought that esophageal lengthening occurs by ascent of the pharynx rather than descent of the stomach. By approximately day 36, the trachea and esophagus have completely separated.[1]

The esophageal wall is derived from both endoderm and mesoderm. The endoderm forms the epithelium and glands, whereas the mesoderm eventually forms the muscular layers, connective tissue, and angioblasts. During the seventh and eighth weeks of development, the esophageal epithelium proliferates to fill the lumen, leaving only small irregular channels open. These channels grow to form vacuoles, which then coalesce to create one lumen by the 10th week of gestation (Fig. 28-2). Ciliated epithelium initially lines the embryological esophagus, but it is replaced by the fourth month of gestation by stratified squamous epithelium. By the sixth week, the mesenchymal circular muscular coat forms, and the splanchnic mesenchyme surrounds the esophagus and trachea. The splanchnic mesenchyme enables the formation of the smooth muscle of the lower esophagus. The longitudinal musculature forms during weeks 9 through 12, and the muscularis mucosa forms by week 16. Blood vessels start to enter the esophageal wall in week 28, but the lymphatic capillaries do not form until the third to fourth month of gestation.[1]

Congenital anomalies of the esophagus occur in 1 in 3500 births and typically are the result of a genetic defect or maternal event. They are more common in premature infants, and 60% are associated with other congenital anomalies, including VACTERL syndrome (associated vertebral, anal, cardiac, tracheal, esophageal, renal, and limb congenital anomalies).[2] For further information regarding congenital anomalies of the esophagus, including atresia, stenosis, clefts, and tracheoesophageal fistula, see Chapter 51.

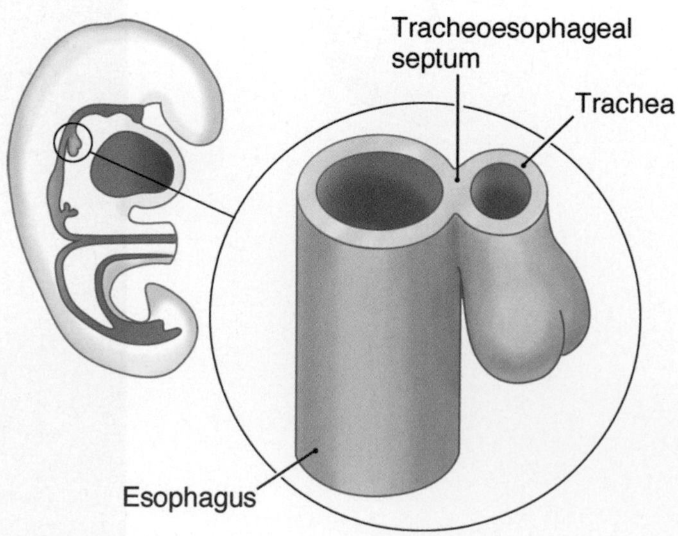

Figure 28-1. The embryonic tracheoesophageal septum forms to separate the esophagus and trachea. The lungs then bud off ventrally from the trachea.

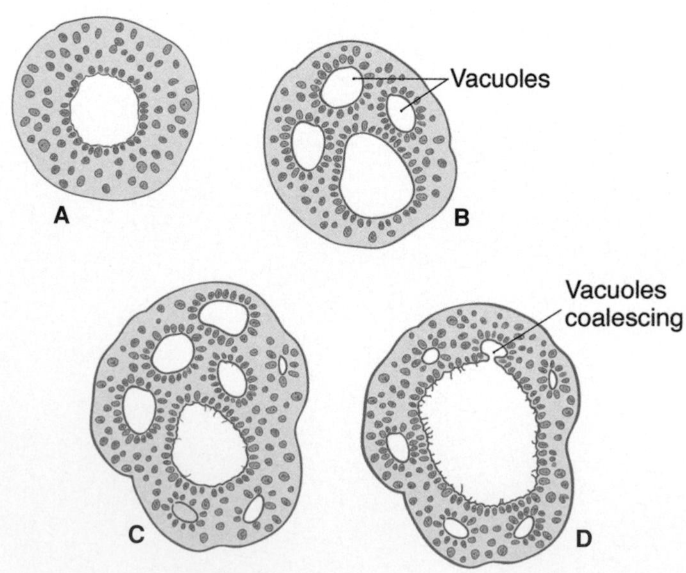

Figure 28-2. *A*. Epithelial cells initially fill the obliterated esophagus, then isolated vacuoles form (*B*) and eventually coalesce (*C*) to form a patent lumen (*D*).

ANATOMY

Esophageal terminology can be classified by function, anatomy, or surgical divisions. Anatomically, the esophagus is divided into cervical, thoracic, and abdominal portions. Surgeons further classify esophageal anatomy based on therapeutic approach and adjacent structures as cervical, proximal, middle, distal thoracic, and abdominal.

The esophagus ranges from 21 to 34 cm in length from the cricopharyngeus to the lower esophageal sphincter (LES), with an average length of 23 cm in females and 28 cm in males. The cervical esophagus ranges from 3 to 5 cm in length, the thoracic portion 18 to 22 cm, and the abdominal portion 3 to 5 cm. The distance from the incisors to the cricoid cartilage is 13 cm.[3]

Nonkeratinizing, stratified squamous epithelium lines most of the esophageal lumen. This mucosa contains only alveolar serous glands, which are small, tubular mucus glands originating from the submucosa. In the terminal esophagus, cardiac glands, much like those found in the stomach, project through the epithelium to form papillae. Endoscopically, the transition between the esophageal squamous mucosa and the columnar gastric mucosa starts as four-to-six pink tongues projecting up through the paler distal esophagus at what is known as the "Z-line" just proximal to the esophagogastric junction. Replacement of the distal esophageal squamous mucosa by columnar epithelium is diagnostic of Barrett esophagus, a premalignant condition.[3] For further information on Barrett esophagus, see Chapter 41.

The lamina propria mucosa lies deep to the mucosa and consists of an areolar, elastic, and collagenous network of fibers that contains small blood vessels, follicles, and mucus glands. The muscularis mucosa is a thin layer of smooth muscular bundles. The submucosa consists of loose areolar connective tissue and elastic and collagen fibers with numerous blood vessels, lymphatics, nerves (including Meissner plexus), and deep mucus glands (Fig. 28-3).

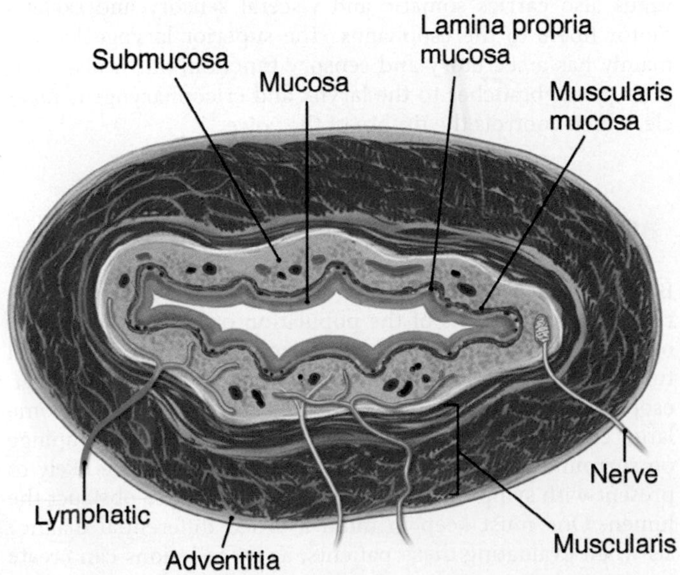

Figure 28-3. The esophagus is lined with stratified squamous epithelium. The mucosa of the esophagus is comprised of epithelium, lamina propria, and muscularis mucosa. The submucosa is deep to this, then the inner circular muscular layer and the outer longitudinal muscular layer.

The pharyngeal and esophageal muscles coordinate to form coordinated contractions to make swallowing and speech possible. Pharyngeal muscle is striated, whereas the esophagus transitions to more smooth muscle as it descends past the level of the carina and the lower two-thirds of the esophagus. The tunica muscularis is composed of oblique muscle fibers in a single layer in the pharynx, but two layers throughout the esophagus: a longitudinal outer layer and circular inner layer. The circular layer is an extension of the cricopharyngeus muscle.[3]

The upper esophageal sphincter (UES) acts as the gatekeeper for entry of a food bolus from the pharynx to the esophagus during swallowing. The posterior cricoid cartilage forms the anterior wall of the UES, and a muscular sling of the lower inferior pharyngeal constrictor forms the posterior UES. This sphincter functions to prevent esophageal distension during respiration and to prevent reflux, as it remains in a tonic state of contraction with 30 to 142 mm Hg of pressure between episodes of swallowing.

The LES does not have anatomy as discrete as the UES. The LES is composed in part from a thickening of the circular esophageal fibers that superimpose on each other approximately 3 cm from the gastroesophageal junction. It is not macroscopically or grossly detectable. The LES, in conjunction with the diaphragmatic crura, angle of His, and intra-abdominal length of esophagus, provides a tonic pressure of 14.5 to 34 mm Hg to prevent reflux.[3] Liebermann-Meffert[4] described short transverse clasp fibers and oblique sling fibers in cadavers that curve around the greater curve that aid in the sphincter effect and help account for the asymmetric anatomy of the LES. For more information regarding the pathophysiology of the esophageal sphincters, see Chapter 33.

Only loose adventitia adheres the esophagus to its surrounding mediastinum, as it has no serosa or mesentery. These loose attachments allow for considerable cephalocaudal movement during respiration.

Arterial Supply

The esophagus receives arterial blood from multiple sources as it courses through the neck, chest, and abdomen.

The superior thyroid artery gives off smaller arteries that supply the UES and pharynx. The inferior thyroid arteries supply the cervical esophagus. They give off 2 to 3 cm branches called tracheoesophageal arteries that travel inferiorly and medially on each side. The tracheoesophageal arteries subdivide into tracheal and esophageal branches, which in turn subdivide several more times before they eventually enter the esophageal wall.[3]

The thoracic esophagus derives its blood supply from the superior and inferior thyroid arteries superiorly and the aorta inferiorly. Both the tracheobronchial arteries and the bronchoesophageal artery originate from the aortic arch and further subdivide to provide branches to the trachea. The proper aortic esophageal arteries are unpaired and arise from the descending aorta.[3]

The abdominal esophagus is supplied by the left gastric artery, ascending branches from the left phrenic artery, and the splenic artery. The splenic artery delivers arterial blood to the posterior and left lateral distal esophagus. Branches from both extend beyond the diaphragmatic hiatus. The repetitive branching of the arterial supply eventually forms

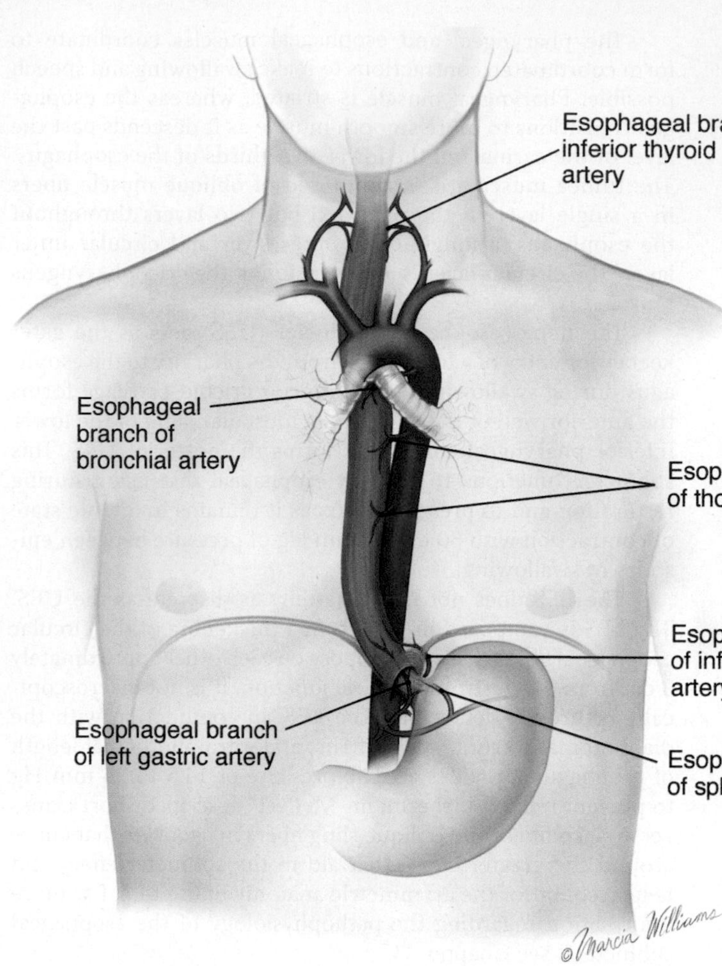

Figure 28-4. Arterial blood supply to the esophagus. The cervical esophagus is supplied by the inferior thyroid arteries. The thoracic esophagus is mainly supplied by direct branches off the aorta, and the abdominal esophagus is supplied by the left gastric and inferior phrenic arteries.

a rich submucosal arterial plexus that allows for ligation of extramural vessels without compromising the underlying esophagus (Fig. 28-4).

Venous Drainage

A submucosal venous plexus drains blood from the subepithelial venous network. This plexus then empties into communicating veins that traverse the muscular wall along with the perforating arteries. The superior esophagus drains into the internal jugular veins or the azygos or hemiazygos veins. The inferior veins drain into the left gastric and splenic veins. There are no valves in the esophageal venous system.[3]

Lymphatic Drainage

The lymphatic system of the esophagus is poorly described. Lymph from the thoracic esophagus likely drains to paratracheal, tracheobronchial bifurcation, juxtaesophageal, and intra-aorticoesophageal nodes. The abdominal esophagus likely drains to superior gastric, pericardiac, and inferior diaphragmatic nodes. All areas of the esophageal lymph system eventually empty into the thoracic duct. Lymphatic channels are more abundant as longitudinal submucosal channels than in the muscular layers.[3]

Innervation

The visceral autonomic nervous system innervates the esophagus, pharynx, and larynx. The sympathetic efferent pathways cause vasoconstriction, sphincter contraction, and relaxation of the muscular wall via the cervical and thoracic sympathetic chains. The parasympathetic nervous system increases glandular and peristaltic activity via the vagus (cranial nerve X). The vagus also carries somatic and visceral sensory and skeletal motor fibers to the esophagus. The superior laryngeal nerve mainly has a secretory and sensory function, but it also supplies motor branches to the larynx and cricopharyngeus muscle, which controls the timbre of the voice.[3]

BENIGN ESOPHAGEAL NEOPLASMS

Benign esophageal neoplasms are rare lesions, most occurring in less than 0.5% of the population on autopsy. A review of 20,000 autopsies in 1962 found only 90 benign esophageal tumors, or a prevalence of 0.45%.[5] The majority of benign esophageal tumors do not cause symptoms unless they become large enough to obstruct the esophageal lumen or impinge on surrounding structures. Mucosal lesions are more likely to present with symptoms, as they are more likely to obstruct the lumen. One must keep in mind a broad differential diagnosis when evaluating these patients, as these lesions can create mechanical obstruction and symptoms common to many other esophageal diseases (Table 28-1). Adult patients with cancer, gastroesophageal reflux, motility disorders, esophagitis, or

Table 28-1

BENIGN ESOPHAGEAL LESIONS AND ENDOSCOPIC AND MICROSCOPIC APPEARANCE

ORIGIN	LESION	HISTOPATHOLOGY	ENDOSCOPIC APPEARANCE
Mucosal	Papilloma	Finger-like projections of squamous epithelium	Exophytic, wart-like
	Adenoma	Glandular mucosa	Polypoid mucosa
	Web/Membranous ring	Squamous mucosa	Shelf of mucosa projecting into lumen
Submucosal	Granular cell tumor	Large cells with eosinophilic granules, neural	Pale, yellow, firm
	Fibrovascular polyp	Fibrous/vascular/adipose cells	Rubbery polyp, +/− feeding vessel
	Lymphangiomas		Yellow, translucent
	Hemangiomas		Reddish-blue, blanching
Muscular	Leiomyoma	Spindle cells with fibrous core	Fleshy compressible lesion
	Muscular ring	Hypertrophied muscular ring with normal overlying mucosa	Circumferential projection of rings into lumen
Heterotopic	Inlet patch	Gastric mucosa	Pink patch, distal esophagus
Extraluminal	Duplication cyst	Fluid-filled cyst under muscular layer	No communication with lumen
	Tubular duplication	Normal esophageal wall	Communicates with true lumen

even psychiatric illness can have similar presentations to these benign lesions.

These lesions are typically found incidentally on imaging or on endoscopy and typically do not warrant resection unless they mechanically compress mediastinal structures. Generally, removal is recommended for patients with symptoms or larger lesions.

LESIONS OF THE MUCOSAL LAYER

Papillomas

Esophageal papillomas are small (typically subcentimeter) benign sessile lesions arising from the lamina propria in the distal esophagus.[6] Histologically, they have finger-like projections of squamous-lined epithelium over a core of connective tissue. Endoscopically, they appear as pale exophytic, wart-like lesions that can be mistaken for verrucous squamous cell carcinoma, granulation tissue, or papillary leukoplakia. They occur most often in the fifth decade of life.[7] They rarely cause symptoms, but large lesions can cause dysphagia.

Differing theories exist regarding the origin of esophageal papillomas. A theory of local inflammation giving rise to papillomas is supported by an association with reflux, esophagitis, and mucosal irritants as well as the distal location of papillomas.[8] Animal studies have shown a causative relationship between chemical mucosal irritation and the development of esophageal papillomas.[9] Some evidence points to a role of the human papilloma virus (HPV) in the development of esophageal papillomas based on varying reports on the prevalence of HPV in patients with esophageal papillomas. Although HPV has been linked to laryngeal and cervical cancers, there is no conclusive evidence for a relationship between HPV and esophageal malignancy (Fig. 28-5).

Adenomas

Esophageal adenomas are hyperplastic epithelial cells in a polypoid configuration, similar to adenomas elsewhere in the gastrointestinal tract. Esophageal adenomas arise almost exclusively in the setting of Barrett esophagus and are more likely a polypoid dysplastic tissue than purely adenomatous tissue. Isolated esophageal adenomas are exceedingly rare, with only a handful of cases reported in the literature. An association of these lesions with concomitant adenocarcinoma further supports their relationship to Barrett esophagus. Given this association to cancer, these lesions should be treated as premalignant and should be removed.[10] They appear as polypoid mucosal lesions and should be removed endoscopically. If found in the setting of normal esophageal mucosa, multiple biopsy specimens of the surrounding tissue should be taken to evaluate for evidence of metaplasia. For further detail regarding the management of Barrett esophagus and the pathology of esophageal cancer, see Chapters 41 and 10, respectively.

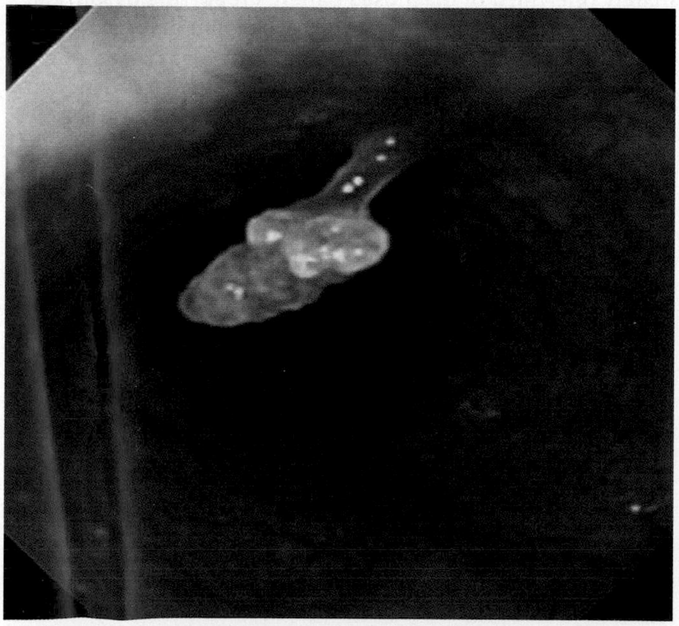

Figure 28-5. Esophageal papilloma appears as an isolated, wart-like exophytic projection on endoscopy. (Reproduced with permission from Feldman M, Friedman L, Brandt L. *Sleisenger and Fordtran's Gastrointestinal and Liver Disease*. 9th ed. Philadelphia, PA: Saunders; 2010, Figure 48-16).

Inflammatory Polyps

Inflammatory polyps are edematous folds of gastric mucosa occurring at the gastroesophageal junction. These benign lesions are the result of gastroesophageal reflux. Microscopically, they appear as inflamed gastric mucosa with plasma cells, eosinophils, fibroblasts, and multinucleated giant cells surrounding the epithelium. They typically resolve with treatment of reflux and do not need to be resected.[11]

LESIONS OF THE SUBMUCOSAL LAYERS

Fibrovascular Polyps

Fibrovascular polyps represent a group of fibrous benign lesions consisting of fibrous, vascular, and adipose tissues covered by normal gastrointestinal submucosa. They are extremely rare and represent only 0.5% to 1% of all benign esophageal lesions.[12] The group includes lipomas, myomas, fibromas, and fibrolipomas. They occur more in the proximal esophagus, where large lesions (as large as 20 cm) have been reported to cause dysphagia, cough, nausea, vomiting, and even asphyxiation.[13] An endoscopic ultrasound can diagnose a polyp with a large feeding vessel, which, if present, would preclude endoscopic resection. An endoscopist can successfully remove symptomatic lesions if they have a visible stalk and do not have a large feeding vessel.[14]

Granular Cell Tumors

Granular cell tumors can arise from skin, breast, tongue, and gastrointestinal tract. They are rare tumors—only 10% occur in the gastrointestinal tract and 65% of those occur in the esophagus. They occur most commonly in men ages 45 to 60 years old. They are usually asymptomatic, with approximately one-third of diagnosed patients reporting dysphagia.[15] Granular cell tumors are neural in origin and likely arise from Schwann cells. Microscopically, they appear as nests of cells with pyknotic nuclei, abundant eosinophilic granular cytoplasm, and strong S-100 positivity.[6] They appear pale or yellow on endoscopy and feel firm or rubbery when palpated with forceps (Fig. 28-6).

Unlike most other benign lesions discussed in this chapter, granular cell tumors have malignant potential. In a series of 183 patients with granular cell tumors, 4% were malignant. All of the malignant lesions found were larger than 4 cm.[15] Despite their malignant potential, recurrence after endoscopic resection has not been described. These lesions are generally treated with endoscopic resection with biopsy forceps or endoscopic mucosal resection for lesions larger than 1 cm.

Lymphangiomas

Lymphangiomas are the result of congenitally malformed lymphatic tissue. Lymphangiomas are found most commonly in the skin, and they are extremely rare benign lesions in the esophagus. Fewer than 15 cases of esophageal lymphangiomas have been reported, all found in children younger than the age of 2 years. They appear as a translucent, yellow mass on endoscopy, and are generally managed conservatively, as most lesions are less than 5 mm. If they grow to a size of 4 to 5 cm and the patient becomes symptomatic, treatment such as band-assisted mucosectomy may be appropriate.[16]

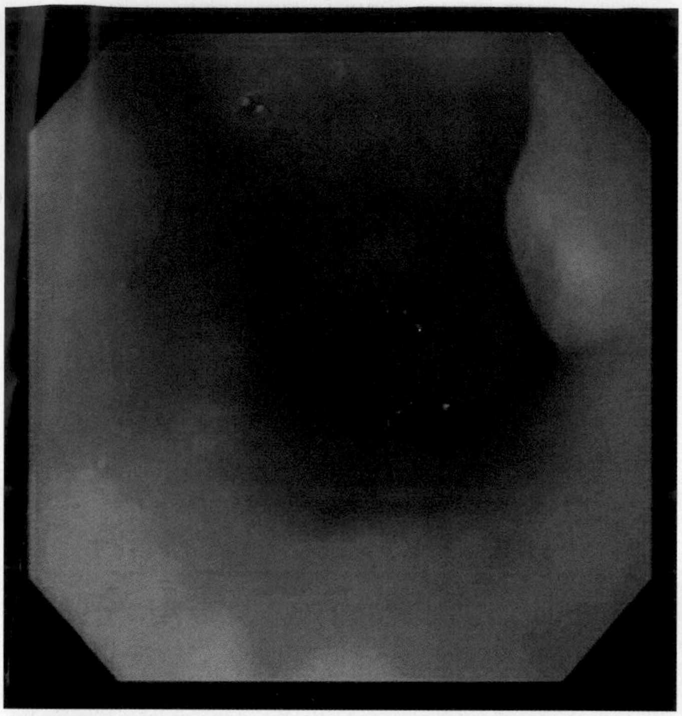

Figure 28-6. Endoscopic view of esophageal granular cell tumor. (Reprinted with permission from *J Pediatr Gastroenterol Nutr.* 2004;38(1):97–101).

Hemangiomas

Hemangiomas are also extremely rare diseases in the esophagus and are typically found incidentally. On endoscopy, they appear as nodular, soft, blanching bluish-red lesions that can be mistaken for Kaposi sarcoma. If symptoms exist, they usually consist of bleeding or dysphagia. Surgical or endoscopic resection has been used to treat symptomatic patients.[17]

LESIONS OF THE MUSCULAR LAYERS

Leiomyoma

Leiomyomas are the most common benign neoplasms found in the esophagus. They are smooth muscle lesions that arise from the muscularis propria and on occasion from the muscularis mucosa. They appear as spindle-shaped muscle fibers in a cascade or whirl-like pattern surrounded by a fibrous capsule on histology. One should suspect malignancy if increased cellularity, atypia, or mitotic figures are identified histologically.

Leiomyomas very seldom cause symptoms, but dysphagia, chest pain, bleeding (if ulcerated), reflux (if distal), and obstruction (if larger than 5 cm) all have been described. On esophogram, these lesions appear as rounded filling defects; on endoscopy, they appear as firm nodules with normal overlying mucosa (Fig. 28-7). Because the mucosa is normal, forceps biopsy is rarely helpful (unless the lesion happens to arise from the muscularis mucosa). On endoscopic ultrasound, they are

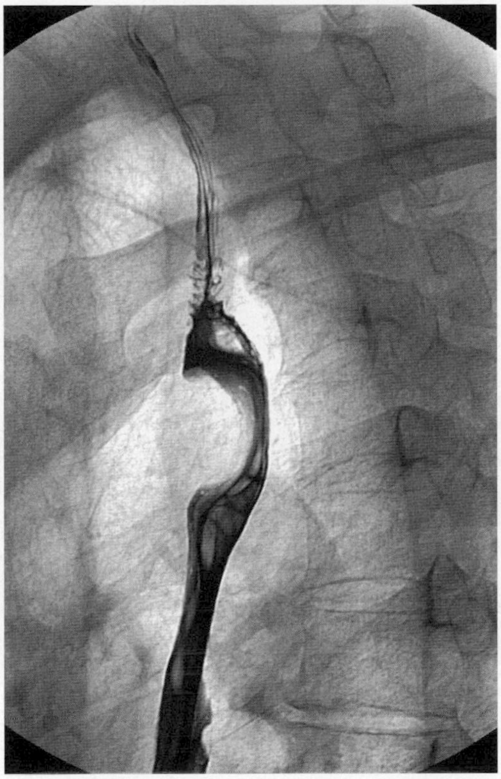

Figure 28-7. Smooth filling defect on barium esophogram of an esophageal leiomyoma.

hypoechoic and arise from the muscular layer of the esophagus, whereas computed tomography is not always useful in determining the layer of origin (Fig. 28-8A,B). These lesions are slow growing, and if encountered incidentally, smaller asymptomatic lesions can be treated conservatively. As with most muscle-derived tumors, such as sarcomas and gastrointestinal stromal tumors, lesions larger than 4 cm have an increased risk of malignancy and should be treated with resection.[6] Unlike other parts of the gastrointestinal tract, however, leiomyomas are far more common in the esophagus than their malignant counterparts. Given the difficulty of clear diagnosis with endoscopic biopsy or fine-needle aspiration, resection is recommended to confirm the diagnosis of benign disease. Lesions that are greater than 2 cm or that are symptomatic should be surgically resected.

HETEROTROPIC MUCOSA (INLET PATCH)

An inlet patch is an area of heterotopic gastric mucosa found just distal to the UES in up to 10% of thorough endoscopies (Fig. 28-9A). They are generally thought to be congenital in origin and result from incomplete replacement of columnar gastric epithelium with esophageal squamous epithelium.[18] The patches appear as red velvety patches from 0.5 to 2 cm in diameter and can be composed of either antral- or fundic-type gastric mucosa. Fundic mucosa contains chief and parietal cells that have the capability of producing acid (Fig. 28-9B). Inlet patches are usually asymptomatic, but there has been a suggested association with globus sensation, which resolves with ablation.[19] There have also been reports of association with helicobacter pylori infection and esophageal webs, rings, or strictures.[20] Only 24 reports of associated gastric adenocarcinoma have been published.[18]

EXTRALUMINAL ESOPHAGEAL MASSES

Inclusion Cysts

Esophageal cysts are the second most common benign esophageal tumor. Inclusion cysts are intramural and typically occur near the tracheal bifurcation. They are filled with a brownish mucoid fluid and are lined with either ciliated columnar or stratified squamous epithelium.[11]

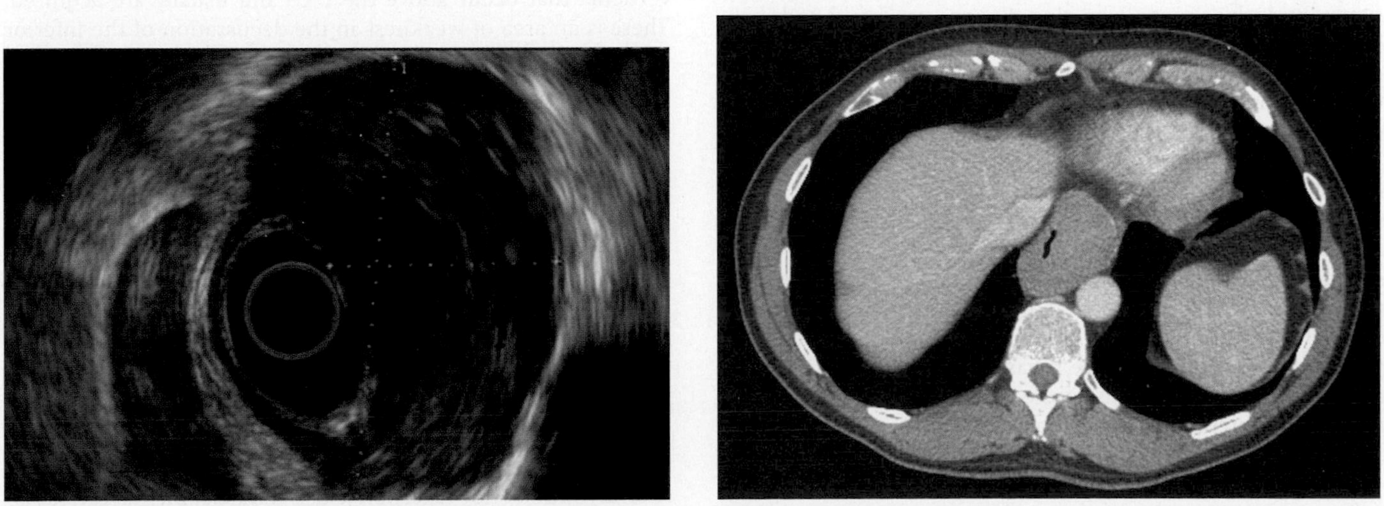

A B

Figure 28-8. *A.* Endoscopic ultrasound of a hypoechoic homogeneous mass originating from the muscularis propria found to be a giant leiomyoma on pathology. (Image provided by Dr. Irving Waxman and Dr. Mariano Gonzalez-Haba Ruiz, University of Chicago, Department of Gastroenterology.) *B.* Computed tomogram demonstrating a large leiomyoma of the distal esophagus.

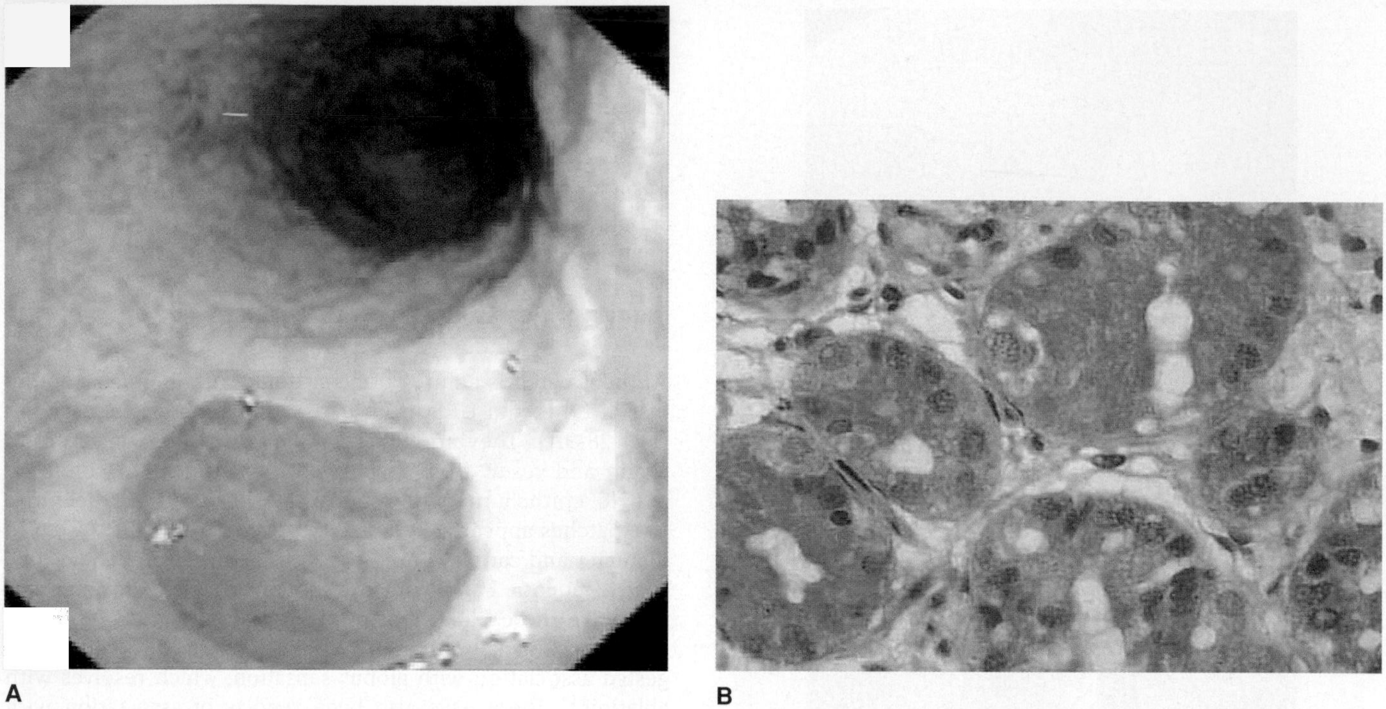

Figure 28-9. Heterotopic gastric mucosa on endoscopy *(A)* and microscopy *(B)*. (Reprinted with permission from *Gastrointest Endosc.* 2001;53(7):717–721).

Duplication Cysts

It is important to distinguish esophageal tubular duplications from duplication cysts. True intestinal duplications are rare parallel channels that communicate with the alimentary tract; whereas duplication cysts do not communicate with the alimentary tract. The esophagus is the most common location for foregut duplication. Congenital tubular (or enteral) duplications are discussed in Chapter 51 (Fig. 28-10).

Esophageal duplication cysts are fluid-filled structures that typically occur in the posterior mediastinum, have a mucosal epithelial lining, and are located within the muscular wall of the esophagus.[1] Duplication cysts can produce a variety of respiratory and gastrointestinal symptoms as a result of extrinsic compression. Respiratory symptoms include cough, wheezing, dyspnea, aspiration, and pneumonia; and gastrointestinal symptoms include regurgitation, dysphagia, regurgitation, epigastric pain, and anorexia.[21] More rarely, they are associated with hemorrhage, perforation, chest pain, cardiac arrhythmias, spinal cord symptoms, and malignancy.[1]

Duplication cysts may be seen on esophogram as a compression on the esophageal lumen, or on endoscopy, as a submucosal mass (Fig. 28-11). These lesions are visible on CT or MRI and manifest as anechoic lesions on endoscopic ultrasound. An endoscopic fine-needle aspiration of the cyst fluid can help to find neoplastic cells in masses that are found incidentally, although only surgical excision truly rules out neoplasm.[21] Surgical excision is the favored treatment because it has low morbidity.[22] Occasionally, emergency endoscopic needle decompression is needed to treat life-threatening airway complications of duplication cysts.

ESOPHAGEAL DIVERTICULA

An esophageal diverticulum is an outpouching of the esophageal wall. These abnormalities can include the entire wall (a true diverticulum) or just a part of the wall (a pseudodiverticulum involving protrusion of either the mucosa or possibly submucosa through the muscularis propria). They also may be categorized as pulsion versus traction. Pulsion diverticula occur as a result of propulsive forces from a bolus of food that causes herniation of part of the esophageal wall through a weakness in the muscular fibers. A traction diverticulum is a rare true diverticulum that results most commonly from chronically inflamed mediastinal lymph nodes that attach to and pull on the esophagus, eventually causing a protrusion of the entire esophageal wall.[6]

Esophageal diverticula also may be classified by their location. Proximal, more specifically pharyngoesophageal (Zenker's), diverticula are the most common. These are pseudodiverticula that occur above the UES and usually are acquired. There is an area of weakness in the decussation of the inferior pharyngeal constrictors called Killian triangle, where the circular muscular layer of the esophagus does not exist. Mucosa and submucosa typically protrude through this defect just above the cricopharyngeus.[3] They occur more commonly in women and approximately 50% occur in patients in their seventh or eighth decade. They are thought to account for less than 5% of reported cases of dysphagia[6] (Fig. 28-12).

Zenker diverticula are usually asymptomatic and are found incidentally on esophagoscopy or endoscopy as a posterior hypopharyngeal protrusion. A barium swallow is diagnostic. If symptoms do occur, patients report a vague sticking or globus sensation. Larger diverticuli can cause gurgling or even regurgitation. Some patients have reportedly learned maneuvers to empty the pouch.[6] Asymptomatic patients do not need treatment. If troubling symptoms exist, however, several options for excision exist: endoscopic diverticulostomy, diverticulopexy, or diverticulectomy. A cricopharyngeal myotomy is included as part of the procedure to eliminate the distal functional obstruction that contributed to the formation of the pseudodiverticulum. For details regarding resection of diverticula, see Chapter 30.

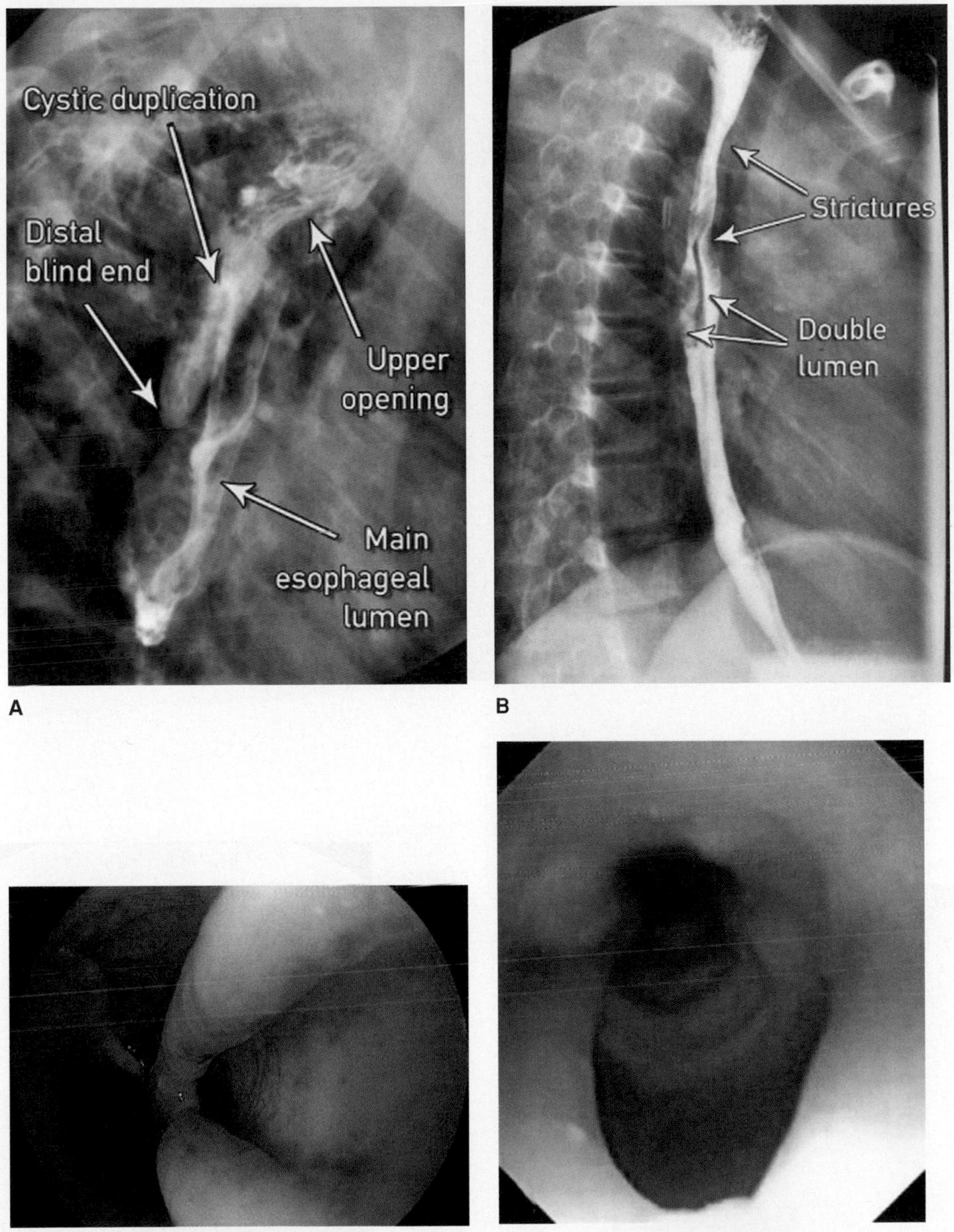

Figure 28-10. Barium swallow (*A, B*) and endoscopic views (*C, D*) of a tubular esophageal duplication. (Reprinted with permission from *Gastrointest Endosc.* 2010;71(4):827–830).

Midesophageal diverticula can be traction or pulsion diverticula. Patients with chronic inflammatory thoracic disease such as tuberculosis or fungal infections can have inflammatory lymph nodes that scar and pull on the esophagus to cause traction diverticula. Motor dysfunction causing abnormal forces on the esophageal wall in patients with achalasia, LES dysfunction, spasm, or nonspecific motility disorders have been reported to cause pulsion midesophagus diverticula in some patients.[23]

Distal or epiphrenic diverticula are the second most common type of diverticulum in Western society and can occur at all ages. These diverticula are usually the result of motor dysfunction, such as discoordination between the distal esophagus and the LES, achalasia, or diffuse esophageal spasm. Patients are usually asymptomatic, but the severity of the symptoms depends on the motor abnormality, the size of the diverticulum, and the size of the mouth of the diverticulum. A small diverticular mouth may limit spontaneous emptying of the diverticulum and contribute to symptoms of regurgitation. Symptoms described include chest pain and, less commonly, regurgitation. These lesions are typically diagnosed on barium swallow[6] (Fig. 28-13). Symptomatic lesions

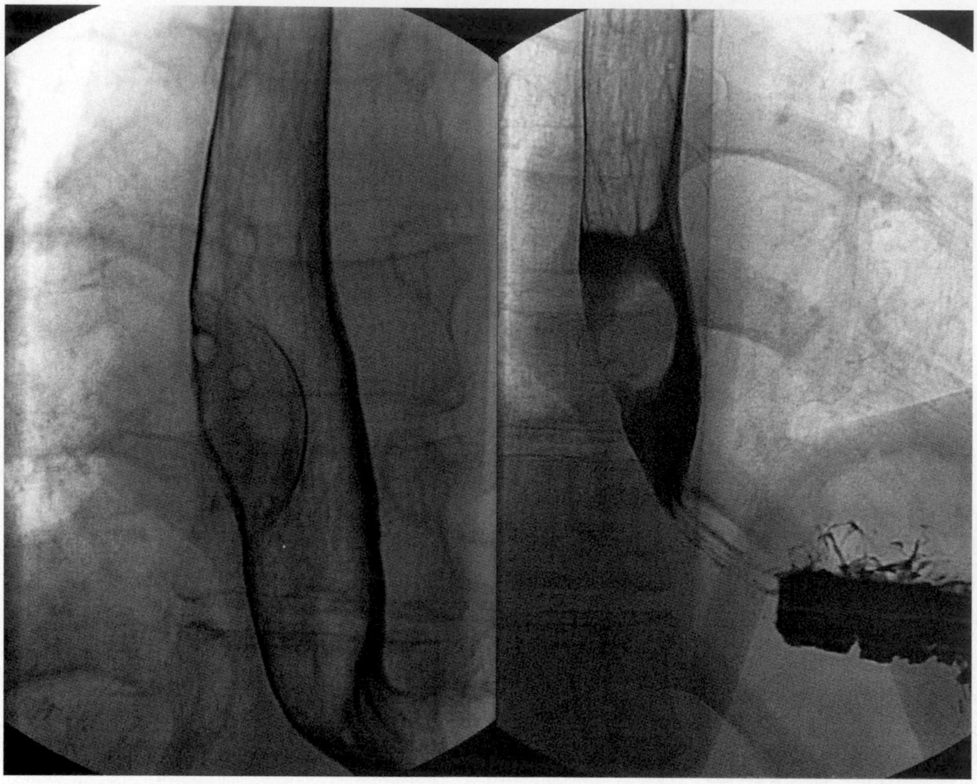

Figure 28-11. Barium swallow demonstrating an esophageal duplication cyst. (Image provided by The Human Imaging Research Office at The University of Chicago).

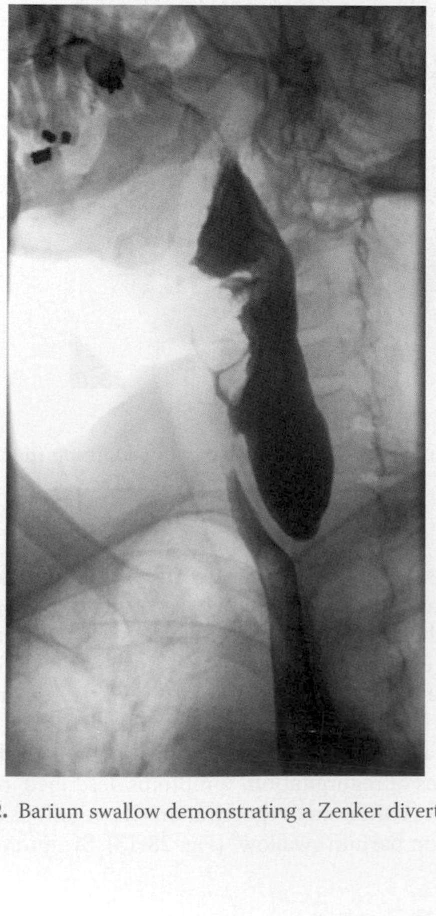

Figure 28-12. Barium swallow demonstrating a Zenker diverticulum.

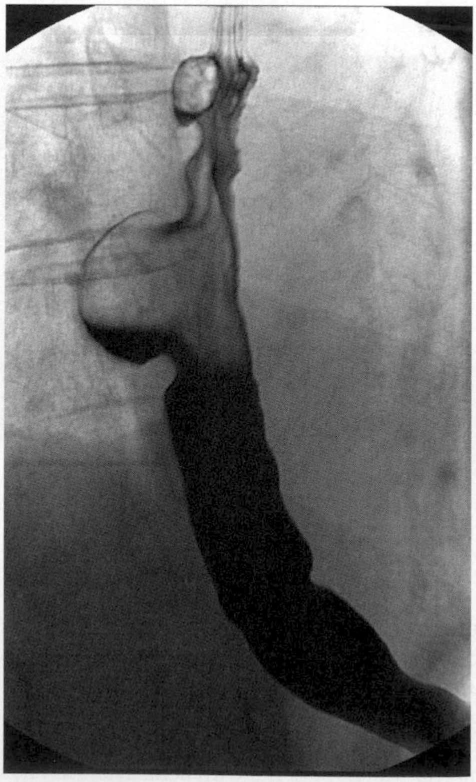

Figure 28-13. Pulsion diverticula evident on barium swallow. (Image provided by The Human Imaging Research Office at The University of Chicago).

are treated with either laparoscopic or thoracoscopic diverticulectomy and possibly fundoplication. Consideration also should be given to concurrent esophageal myotomy distal to the diverticulum. For details of the surgical approach to epiphrenic diverticula, see Chapter 30.

ESOPHAGEAL WEBS

Esophageal webs are membranous diaphragms composed of stratified squamous epithelium, typically located in the cervical or midesophageal region. They usually are acquired and rarely are congenital. They may occur in an otherwise normal esophagus or may be associated with congenital anomalies such as tracheoesophageal fistula. Webs are found in 5% to 15% of patients undergoing radiologic or endoscopic evaluation for dysphagia.[24] Esophageal webs are similar to webs found in the small intestine and typically are composed of mucosa only.

Plummer—Vinson syndrome is described as an association between iron deficiency anemia and esophageal webs, although one report showed no correlation between the two.[25] Acquired esophageal webs can be the result of chronic ingestion of substances such as quinidine, aspirin, phenytoin, tetracycline, potassium chloride, and vitamin C[1]. Esophageal webs are seen on esophogram as a shelf, best seen on a lateral view (Fig. 28-14). Most are asymptomatic, but they can cause dysphagia to solids. Webs are delicate tissue that can be treated easily with either passage of the endoscope at the initial diagnostic endoscopy or with more formal dilation.[26]

Congenital webs are extremely rare, with only 30 reported cases. Congenital webs occur by incomplete coalescence of the vacuoles in the epithelial cells that fill the esophagus at approximately week 10 of gestation. If the diaphragm completely occludes the lumen, the treatment is surgical excision of the membrane shortly after birth.[1] More commonly, however, these diaphragms are incomplete and behave clinically as any other type of esophageal stenosis. Unlike esophageal rings (see below), they rarely encircle the entire esophagus, and typically project from the anterior or lateral esophagus.

ESOPHAGEAL RINGS

There are two types of esophageal rings: mucosal rings (also termed "Schatzki ring") and the rarer muscular ring. These rings partially occlude the lumen and can cause dysphagia. Muscular rings occur congenitally and are formed by a band of hypertrophied muscle covered by squamous epithelium approximately 2 cm proximal to the squamocolumnar junction. If symptomatic, these lesions can be treated either with dilation or with botulinum toxin.[27,28]

Schatzki first described the "Schatzki ring" in 1944. It is a shelf-like membranous esophageal diaphragm of squamous mucosa located at the junction of the esophageal vestibule and the gastric cardia. These rings generally are asymptomatic but have been reported to cause dysphagia, most commonly in middle-aged men, when they narrow the lumen (<13 mm) enough that a food bolus cannot pass.[29] They are fairly common, with an incidence between 6% and 14% on esophogram.[30] They appear as a radiographic shelf in the mid-to-distal esophagus on esophogram[1] (Fig. 28-15). It is important to dilate the distal esophagus sufficiently to be able to see the ring on endoscopy. Most rings can be treated successfully with large bougie or balloon dilation with a recurrence rate of 13% in one series.[31]

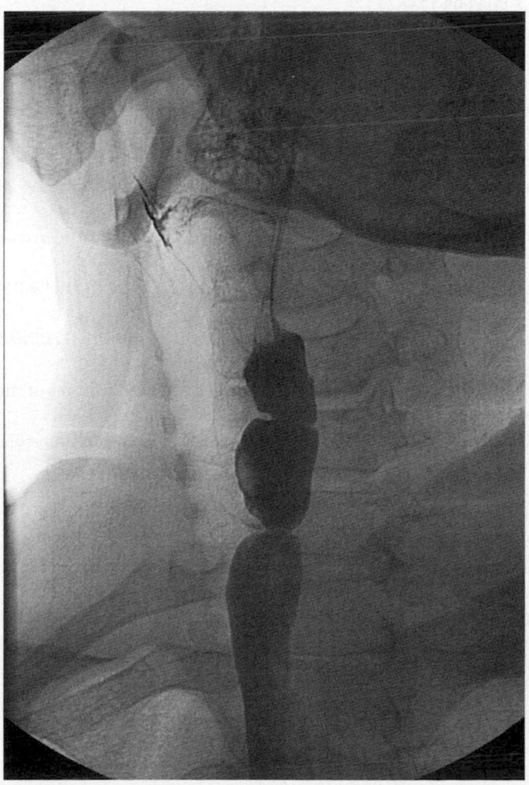

Figure 28-14. Barium swallow of an esophageal web. (Image provided by The Human Imaging Research Office at The University of Chicago).

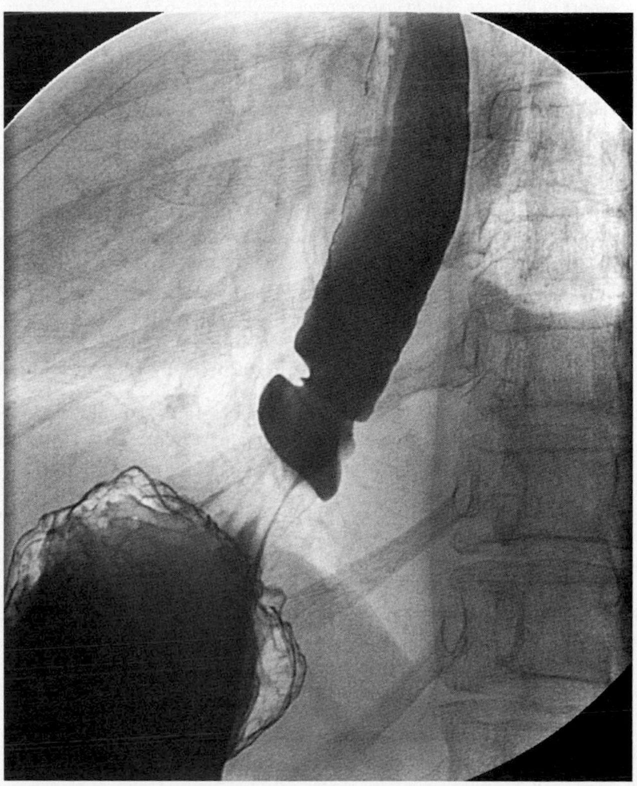

Figure 28-15. Barium swallow of an esophageal ring. (Image provided by The Human Imaging Research Office at The University of Chicago).

Disruption of the ring with electrocautery has also been shown to be effective.[26]

The benign esophageal diseases discussed in this chapter are limited to benign neoplasms and several structural abnormalities. Management of these lesions is discussed in the Chapters 29 and 30. For details regarding congenital esophageal disease, consult Chapters 50 and 51. See Chapters 32 to 35 for a detailed discussion of motility disorders. For more information regarding the pathophysiology and surgical treatment of esophageal malignancy, see Chapters 10 through 25.

EDITOR'S COMMENT

The anatomy and histological anatomy of the esophagus are critical to the understanding of esophageal disease, staging of esophageal cancer, and therapeutic interventions. For example, the depth of invasion of early esophageal cancer needs to be determined precisely before deciding whether mucosal resection or esophagectomy is best for the patient, and new depth measurements (mucosal: m1–3, submucosal: sm1–3) have been proposed.

For leiomyoma, it is clear that large tumors (>4 cm) and symptomatic tumors need to be removed, preferably by minimally invasive enucleation. The dilemma is how to treat intermediate, asymptomatic tumors (>2 and <4 cm). One option is to follow up the patient every 6 months, and ultimately annually, with EUS or MRI to monitor the progression or stability of the lesion. Another option is to perform EUS-guided biopsies to determine the status of the biomarker, tyrosine-protein kinase (Kit or cKIT), and then only aggressively treat tumors that are cKIT positive. The one limitation to this approach is that the biopsy can cause local inflammation and increase the risk of a postoperative esophageal leak. We currently favor minimally invasive enucleation, particularly in cKIT-negative lesions, as opposed to esophagectomy.

—Raphael Bueno

References

1. Skandalakis JE, Gray SW. *Embryology for Surgeons*. 2nd ed. Baltimore, MD: Williams & Wilkins; 1994.
2. Keckler SJ, Peter SD, Valusek PA, et al. VACTERL anomalies in patients with esophageal atresia: an updated delineation of the spectrum and review of the literature. *Pediatr Surg Int.* 2007;23:309–313.
3. Skandalakis JE. *Surgical Anatomy: Embryologic and Anatomic Basis of Esophageal Surgery*. Baltimore, MD: Williams & Wilkins; 2004.
4. Liebermann-Meffert D, Allgöwer M, Schmid P, et al. Muscular equivalent of the lower esophageal sphincter. *Gastroenterology.* 1979;76:31–38.
5. Plachta A. Benign tumors of the esophagus. Review of the literature and report of 99 cases. *Am J Gastroenterol.* 1962;38:639–652.
6. Castell, DO, Richter, JE. *The Esophagus*. 4th ed. Philadelphia, PA: Lippincott Williams and Wilkins; 2004.
7. Odze R, Antonioli D, Shocket D, et al. Esophageal squamous papillomas. A clinicopathologic study of 38 lesions and analysis for human papillomavirus by the polymerase chain reaction. *Am J Surg Pathol.* 1993;17:803–812.
8. Godey SK, Diggory RT. Inflammatory fibroid polyp of the oesophagus. *World J Surg Oncol.* 2005;3:30.
9. Nakamura T, Matsuyama M, Kishimoto H. Tumors of the esophagus and duodenum induced in mice by oral administration of N-ethyl-N'-nitro-N-nitrosoguanidine. *J Natl Cancer Inst.* 1974;52:519–522.
10. Lee RG. Adenomas arising in Barrett's esophagus. *Am J Clin Pathol.* 1986;85:629–632.
11. Choong CK, Meyers BF. Benign esophageal tumors: introduction, incidence, classification, and clinical features. *Semin Thorac Cardiovasc Surg.* 2003;15:3–8.
12. Palanivelu C, Rangarajan M, John SJ, et al. A rare cause of intermittent dysphagia: giant fibrovascular polyp of the proximal esophagus. *J Coll Physicians Surg Pak.* 2007;17:51–52.
13. Owens JJ, Donovan DT, Alford EL, et al. Life-threatening presentations of fibrovascular esophageal and hypopharyngeal polyps. *Ann Otol Rhinol Laryngol.* 1994;103:838–842.
14. Avezzano EA, Fleischer DE, Merida MA, et al. Giant fibrovascular polyps of the esophagus. *Am J Gastroenterol.* 1990;85:299–302.
15. Orlowska J, Pachlewski J, Gugulski A, et al. A conservative approach to granular cell tumors of the esophagus: four case reports and literature review. *Am J Gastroenterol.* 1993;88:311–315.
16. Saers T, Parusel M, Brockmann M, et al. Lymphangioma of the esophagus. *Gastrointest Endosc.* 2005;62:181–184.
17. Sogabe M, Taniki T, Fukui Y, et al. A patient with esophageal hemangioma treated by endoscopic mucosal resection: a case report and review of the literature. *Med Invest.* 2006;53:177–182.
18. Von Rahden BHA, Stein HJ, Becker K, et al. Heterotopic gastric mucosa of the esophagus: literature-review and proposal of a clinicopathologic classification. *Am J Gastroenterol.* 2004;99:543–551.
19. Meining A, Bajbouj M, Preeg M, et al. Argon plasma ablation of gastric inlet patches in the cervical esophagus may alleviate globus sensation: a pilot trial. *Endoscopy.* 2006;38:566–570.
20. Gutierrez O, Akamatsu T, Cardona H, et al. *Helicobacter pylori* and heterotopic gastric mucosa in the upper esophagus (the inlet patch). *Am J Gastroenterol.* 2003;98:1266–1270.
21. Berrocal T, Torres I, Gutierrez J, et al. Congenital anomalies of the upper gastrointestinal tract. *Radiographics.* 1999;19:855–872.
22. Cioffi U, Bonavina L, De Simone M, et al. Presentation and surgical management of bronchogenic and esophageal duplication cysts in adults. *Chest.* 1998;113:1492–1496.
23. D'Ugo D, Cardillo G, Granone P, et al. Esophageal diverticula. Physiopathological basis for surgical management. *Eur J Cardiothorac Surg.* 1992;6:330–334.
24. Tobin RW. Esophageal rings, webs, and diverticula. *J Clin Gastroenterol.* 1998;27:285–295.
25. Elwood PC, Jacobs A, Pitman RG, et al. Epidemiology of the Kelly Patterson Syndrome. *Lancet.* 1964;2:716–720.
26. Feldman M, Friedman L, Brandt L. *Sleisenger and Fordtran's Gastrointestinal and Liver Disease*. 9th ed. Philadelphia, PA: Saunders; 2010.
27. Hirano I, Gilliam J, Goyal RK. Clinical and manometric features of the lower esophageal muscular ring. *Am J Gastroenterol.* 2000;95:43–49.
28. Varadarajulu S, Noone T. Symptomatic lower esophageal muscular ring: response to Botox. *Dig Dis Sci.* 2003;48:2132–3134.
29. Schatzki R. The lower esophageal ring. Long term follow-up of symptomatic and asymptomatic patients. *Am J Roentgenol Radium Ther Nucl Med.* 1963;90:805–810.
30. Jalil S, Castell DO. Schatzki's ring. A benign cause of dysphagia in adults. *J Clin Gastroenterol.* 2002;35:295–298.
31. Scolapio JS, Pasha TM, Gostout CJ, et al. A randomized prospective study comparing rigid to balloon dilators for benign esophageal strictures and rings. *Gastrointest Endosc.* 1999;50(1):13–17.

29 Resection of Benign Tumors of the Esophagus

Jennifer Paruch, Marie Ziesat, and Mark K. Ferguson

Keywords: esophagus, tumor, benign, leiomyoma polyp, esophagus, cyst, papilloma, granular cell tumor

INTRODUCTION

Benign tumors of the esophagus are rare cases encountered by a variety of specialists including gastroenterologists, general surgeons, and thoracic surgeons. The clinical presentation of these lesions may vary from asymptomatic, incidentally discovered tumors (most common) to large lesions resulting in important dysphagia or airway compromise. The development of minimally invasive approaches to esophageal pathology over the last decade has expanded the diagnostic and treatment options for these lesions.

Benign tumors represent less than 1% of all esophageal tumors, and less than 10% of all surgically resected esophageal lesions.[1,2] They may be classified based on either histology or location within the esophageal wall (mucosal, submucosal, or extraluminal) (Tables 29-1 and 29-2). The most common lesions include leiomyomas, esophageal cysts, fibrovascular polyps, and granular cell tumors. The development of endoscopic ultrasound (EUS) has improved the preoperative diagnosis of these lesions and is a helpful adjunct for clinical decision-making. Many of these lesions have a characteristic radiological appearance that eliminates the need for biopsy in many cases. Fine-needle aspiration (FNA) is often not required for diagnosis and may not be diagnostic in all lesions (e.g., in differentiating leiomyoma from leiomyosarcoma). Forceps biopsy is appropriate for mucosal lesions, but usually is unhelpful for submucosal or deeper lesions.

Table 29-1

CLASSIFICATION OF BENIGN ESOPHAGEAL LESIONS BY CELL TYPE

Epithelial	Squamous cell papilloma Fibrovascular polyp Adenoma Inflammatory pseudotumor/polyp
Nonepithelial	Leiomyoma Hemangioma Fibroma Neurofibroma Schwannoma Rhabdomyoma Lipoma Lymphangioma Hamartoma
Heterotopic	Granular cell tumor Chondroma Osteochondroma Giant cell Amyloid Eosinophilic granuloma

GENERAL PRINCIPLES

Benign tumors are generally asymptomatic and are discovered incidentally on imaging studies. Dysphagia is the most common presenting symptom and is more common with intraluminal tumors. Other presenting symptoms vary depending on the lesion, as described below, but may include vomiting, weight loss, gastrointestinal (GI) bleeding, substernal discomfort, cough, or regurgitation of pedunculated cervical lesions. Examples of intraluminal tumors include squamous cell papillomas, fibrovascular polyps, inflammatory pseudopolyps, and fibroneuroid tumors. Fibrovascular polyps are the most common, arise from the cervical esophagus, and generally are seen in men in the sixth or seventh decade of life. Squamous cell papillomas are small, sessile lesions found in the distal esophagus, most commonly seen in elderly patients.

Submucosal and intramural lesions are more commonly asymptomatic until they have grown to >5 cm in transverse diameter. Large tumors can cause obstructive symptoms such as dysphagia and emesis. Examples of these tumors include leiomyomas, granular cell tumors, lipomas, hamartomas, and neurofibromas. These tumors are difficult to differentiate on endoscopy, and EUS is helpful for making a diagnosis. Mucosal biopsy is not helpful for these lesions, and should be avoided in such cases because mucosal disruption may compromise subsequent enucleation of the lesions. FNA may be used in situations in which a diagnosis cannot be made by EUS alone, and does not threaten mucosal integrity.

PREOPERATIVE ASSESSMENT

All patients undergoing resection for a benign tumor should undergo a standard preoperative work-up and risk stratification as described in Chapter 4. The majority of benign tumors are asymptomatic, and other potential esophageal pathology should

Table 29-2

CLASSIFICATION OF ESOPHAGEAL LESIONS BY LOCATION

TUMOR TYPE	ANATOMIC LOCATION	EUS LAYER
Leiomyoma	Muscularis propria	4
Esophageal cyst	Extramural	4–5
Fibrovascular polyp	Mucosa	1–2
Squamous cell papilloma	Mucosa	1–2
Granular cell tumor	Mucosa/submucosal	1–3
Hemangioma	Submucosa	2–3
Lipoma	Submucosa	3

Note: Endoscopic ultrasound (EUS) layers correspond as follows: superficial mucosa (1, hyperechoic), deep mucosa (2, hypoechoic), submucosa (3, hyperechoic), muscularis propria (4, hypoechoic), paraesophageal tissue (5).

be evaluated carefully with a history, physical examination, and diagnostic studies to avoid an inappropriate operation. Evaluating for other esophageal pathology such as gastroesophageal acid reflux disease (GERD), achalasia, hiatal hernia, or a diverticulum also may help with assessing the need for additional procedures during resection of a benign tumor.

Diagnostic imaging for individual lesions is discussed in detail below, but often will involve a combination of barium swallow, endoscopy, and endoscopic ultrasound. Barium studies may help identify small lesions, especially those that are covered with normal mucosa and may easily be missed on endoscopy. Barium studies also will reveal other pathology including hiatal hernia, reflux, and diverticula that may need to be addressed at the time of surgery and may prompt additional preoperative testing. Endoscopy provides valuable information regarding the location of the tumor, whether there are multiple lesions, the continuity of the mucosa overlying the lesion, and other potential pathology. Endoscopic ultrasonography is invaluable in characterizing the size, layer of origin, and internal characteristics of lesions. EUS-directed FNA is frequently feasible as an aid to diagnosis. Intraoperative endoscopy also may be of assistance as described below.

INTRALUMINAL AND MUCOSAL LESIONS

Fibrovascular Polyp

Clinical Presentation and Diagnosis

Fibrovascular polyps commonly cause obstructive symptoms such as dysphagia, regurgitation, vomiting, and weight loss. These tumors originate near the thoracic inlet, adjacent to the cricopharyngeus muscle at C6, and grow on a pedunculated stalk. Symptoms may range from episodic regurgitation of the mass to laryngeal impaction and asphyxiation.[3,4] Large tumors are prone to ulceration at the tip and may be a source of GI bleeding.

On barium esophagram, these characteristically appear as smooth, lobulated, elongated filling defects starting at the level of the cervical esophagus (Fig. 29-1A,B). Computed tomography (CT) or magnetic resonance imaging (MRI) will show a dilated esophagus with a homogeneous, intraluminal soft tissue mass without invasion of surrounding structures. These studies can also identify the level of origin of the stalk. Endoscopy may be useful for identifying the site of origin and size of the lesion (Fig. 29-1C). However, small lesions may be missed because they are typically lined with normal-appearing mucosa. EUS is useful for identifying feeding vessels and predicting risk of significant bleeding during excision.

Management

Fibrovascular polyps are benign and may be treated with endoscopic excision; those with thin pedicles may be endoscopically ligated or cauterized.[3] Factors that preclude safe endoscopic removal include vascular stalks that need to be ligated or cauterized, or tumors too large to be delivered through the upper esophageal sphincter. These lesions may require cervical esophagotomy for excision.[4,5] Lesions with features concerning for malignancy or those too large to be removed through a cervical esophagotomy may require a formal esophagectomy (see Chapters 15–22). Resection is recommended for all large fibrovascular polyps because of the risk of regurgitation and asphyxiation.

For fibrovascular polyps that are treated surgically, the location of the tumor stalk or pedicle should be evaluated preoperatively as described above. It is helpful to have endoscopy available for intraoperative localization. Consideration likewise should be given to performing a gastrotomy if necessary to facilitate removal of large lesions that extend into the stomach. The patient should be positioned and draped appropriately with these considerations in mind. The esophagus is approached through a longitudinal neck incision anterior to the sternocleidomastoid muscle on the side opposite to the tumor. Fibrovascular polyps generally originate just inferior to the cricopharyngeus muscle. A longitudinal esophagotomy is made at the level of the stalk origin. The incision must be long enough to deliver the tumor through the incision while the stalk is intact. The incision can then be extended distally to expose the entire stalk, allowing for submucosal resection of the tumor with the stalk (Fig. 29-2). The base of the stalk is then ligated, taking care to control any vessels supplying the tumor through the stalk. Complete excision of the pedicle is necessary to prevent recurrence. The esophagus is closed in two layers. Drains are not routinely placed.

Postoperative Care and Complications

Reported complications from this procedure are rare. A nasogastric tube is not routinely used. The patient can typically begin taking clear liquids on the first postoperative day. No routine postoperative imaging is required. Recurrence of fibrovascular polyps is rare but has been reported and appears to occur more commonly after endoscopic polyp resection.[6]

Squamous Cell Papillomas

Squamous cell papillomas are rare tumors typically found in the lower third of the esophagus. They are thought to be etiologically linked to human papillomavirus (HPV) and GERD. They are small in diameter (usually <1.5 cm), pink or white in color, soft, and have a smooth or slightly rough surface. They may appear similar to superficial squamous cell carcinomas, but can easily be differentiated histologically. There is no evidence that they progress to malignancy, and thus do not need to be removed unless they are symptomatic.[2,7] Their small size and superficial location make these lesions good candidates for endoscopic resection. The recurrence rate is low for lesions that have been completely excised.

SUBMUCOSAL AND INTRAMURAL LESIONS

Leiomyoma

Clinical Presentation and Diagnosis

Leiomyomas are the most common benign tumors of the esophagus, accounting for more than half of all benign tumors in some reports.[8,9] They typically present between the ages of 20 and 69 years, and the peak incidence is between the third and fifth decades. As with other benign tumors, they often are asymptomatic. Patients with symptoms may describe dysphagia, weight loss, chest pain, or early satiety. The lesions grow slowly, arise from smooth muscle cells, and are predominantly found in the lower two-thirds of the esophagus. Leiomyomas rarely ulcerate or bleed. There is some controversy regarding the malignant potential of these lesions.[9]

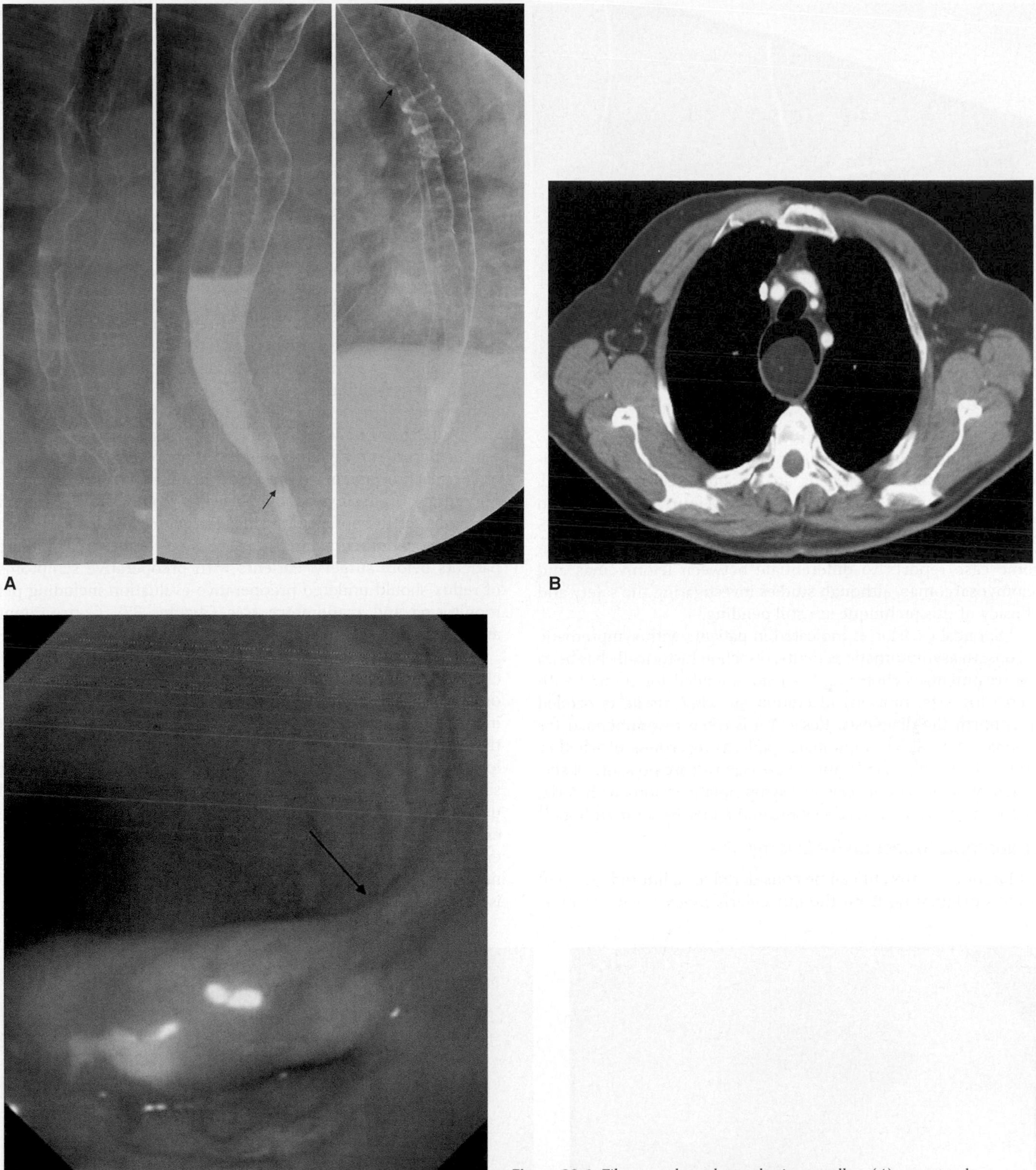

Figure 29-1. Fibrovascular polyp on barium swallow (*A*), computed tomography (*B*), and gross specimen (*C*).

Leiomyomas have a typical appearance on barium swallow as rounded, smoothly marginated intraluminal filling defects. Large tumors show an acute angle with the wall of the esophagus and the tumor edge. A contrast swallow is useful for identifying the level and laterality of the lesion for surgical planning. Endoscopy may be useful in identifying the location of the tumor. Endoscopic characteristics of leiomyomas include normal-appearing overlying mucosa, mobile lesions, and projection into the lumen (Fig. 29-3A). Endoscopic forceps biopsy is contraindicated in patients with leiomyomas since it has not been shown to assist in obtaining a definitive diagnosis and puts patients at increased risk for complications such as

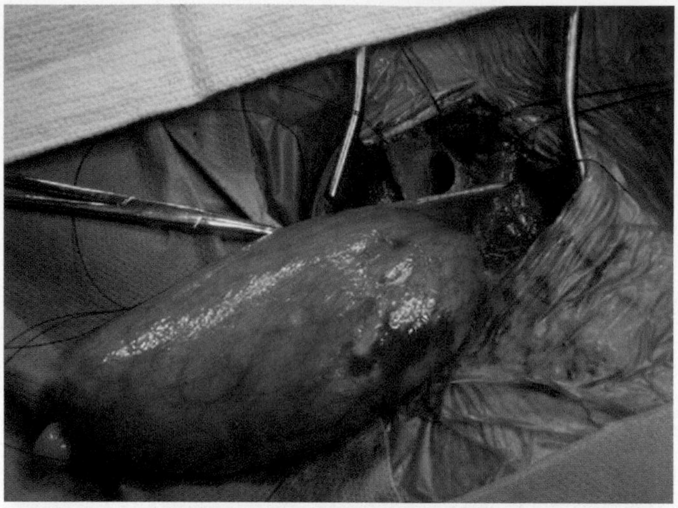

Figure 29-2. Cervical esophagotomy for fibrovascular polyp.

bleeding, infection, and perforation at the time of enucleation. On EUS, these lesions are smooth, well-circumscribed, hypoechoic tumors originating from the fourth layer with an intact and uninvolved overlying mucosa[10] (Fig. 29-3B). EUS provides the opportunity for FNA, which has been used in some case reports to differentiate between leiomyomas and leiomyosarcomas, although studies investigating the safety and efficacy of this technique are still pending.

Surgical excision is indicated in patients with symptomatic lesions. In asymptomatic patients, resection historically has been the treatment of choice and is recommended for tumors with increasing size, mucosal ulceration, or when tissue is needed to confirm the diagnosis. Resection is often recommended for lesions >4 cm in asymptomatic patients regardless of whether other abnormalities indicating increased risk are present. Observation of small, characteristic, asymptomatic lesions with serial EUS every 1 to 2 years has been recommended by some authors.[11]

Endoscopic Resection for Leiomyoma

Endoscopic treatment can be considered for a limited group of lesions originating from the muscularis mucosa with intraluminal growth or polypoid growth patterns.[12] Tumors smaller than 2 cm that are pedunculated may be resected via endoscopic lumpectomy, while larger lesions may be treated with ethanol injection followed by lumpectomy. Lumpectomy is performed with a snare wire and suction cylinder after dissecting the tumor free from the submucosa using hypertonic saline injection. For larger lesions, multiple ethanol injections are administered over several weeks. Use of both of these techniques is more prevalent in Japan and is not yet common in Western countries. Reports have shown complete resolution of symptoms, negligible mortality, and low rates of recurrence.[12]

Surgical Enucleation for Leiomyoma

The location of the tumor should be evaluated preoperatively with endoscopy to facilitate surgical planning. Endoscopy should be available in the operating room for localization, transillumination, and leak identification during resection. The patient is positioned to facilitate either a right or left approach according to the level of the lesion (see below). Double-lumen endotracheal intubation is used to improve intraoperative exposure if a transthoracic approach is selected. Laparoscopy or an upper midline laparotomy may be used for distal esophageal lesions.

Tumors in the lower esophagus may require mobilization of the cardia and disruption of the hiatal structures. Performance of a simultaneous antireflux procedure should be discussed with these patients before surgery. Patients with preoperative symptoms of reflux should undergo preoperative evaluation including pH monitoring and manometry (see Chapter 37). Concomitant antireflux procedures are also recommended in these patients.

Transthoracic enucleation has been the procedure of choice for removal of most leiomyomas.[11,13] Open thoracotomy or video assisted thoracic surgery (VATS) may be used according to surgeon preference. Tumors in the upper two-thirds of the esophagus are usually accessed from the right side, while lower third lesions are removed from either the left or the right side. After the esophagus is exposed, the lesion is identified using palpation and/or transillumination with endoscopy. The esophagus is mobilized sufficiently to identify the circumferential extent of the tumor. The azygos vein may be divided as necessary to gain adequate exposure. A longitudinal myotomy is then made overlying the tumor; this incision can be smaller

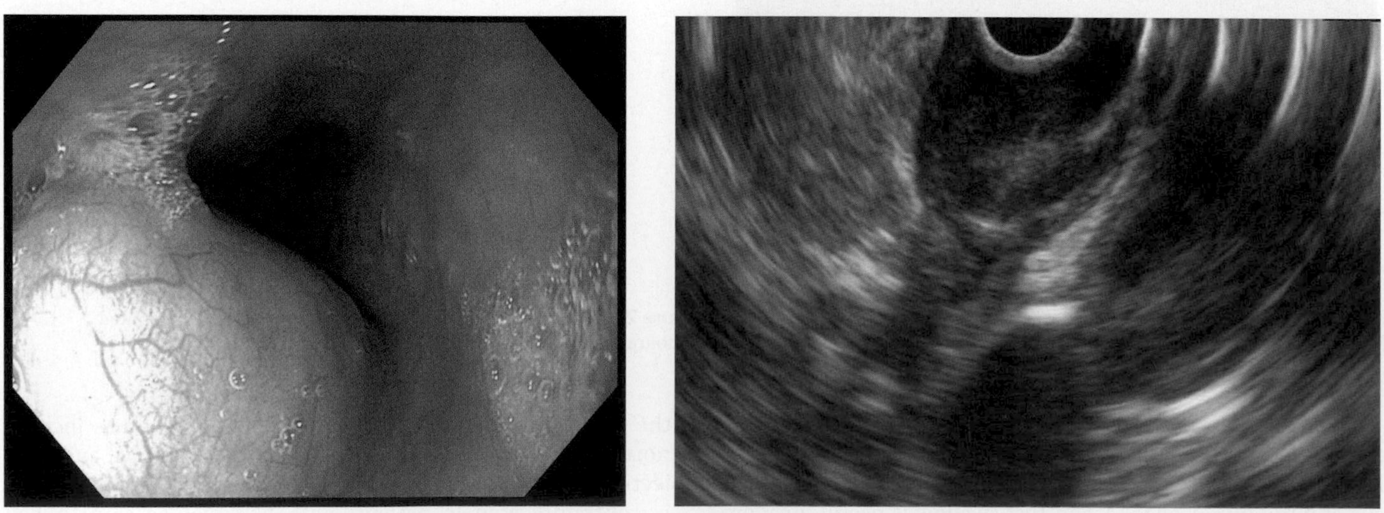

A B

Figure 29-3. Leiomyoma on flexible esophagoscopy (*A*) and endoscopic ultrasonography (*B*).

than the length of the tumor. The leiomyoma will appear as a smooth, avascular, gray-white mass. Blunt dissection, hook cautery, and scissors are used to mobilize the tumor from the muscle layer and underlying submucosa. A traction suture may be placed in the tumor to assist in freeing it from the underlying tissue. Endoscopic visualization can be used during dissection to identify any mucosal damage.

After the tumor is removed, the endoscope is used for insufflation, possibly using distal occlusion of the esophagus. The esophagus is submerged in saline to observe for any air leak, which is an indication of a mucosal leak. Preoperative endoscopic biopsy predisposes to scar tissue formation that makes the tumor more adherent to the mucosa and increases the risk of intraoperative mucosal damage. Mucosal damage identified during surgery is repaired in two layers with absorbable sutures. In this case, delay of oral feedings for several days should be considered. After mucosal integrity is confirmed, the muscular layer is approximated without tension. Some authors suggest not closing the muscular layer if there is evidence of significant trauma after resection. A flap of pleura, pericardium, diaphragm, omentum, or pedicled intercostal muscle may be used as a buttress for the closure, but this is rarely necessary if the muscle layer is preserved in good condition and the closure of the muscle layer is secure. Failure to close the muscle layer or otherwise reinforce the area of myotomy may predispose to the development of a pseudodiverticulum (Fig. 29-4).

Postoperative Care and Complications

Nasogastric tubes are used according to surgeon preference, but likely provide little benefit. Patients without mucosal damage or evidence for a leak may be started on a clear liquid diet on the day of surgery, while feeding should be deferred for at least 1 day in patients who require mucosal repair. The diet is advanced to pureed and then mechanical soft foods over 7 to 10 days. Routine postoperative imaging of the esophagus is not required.

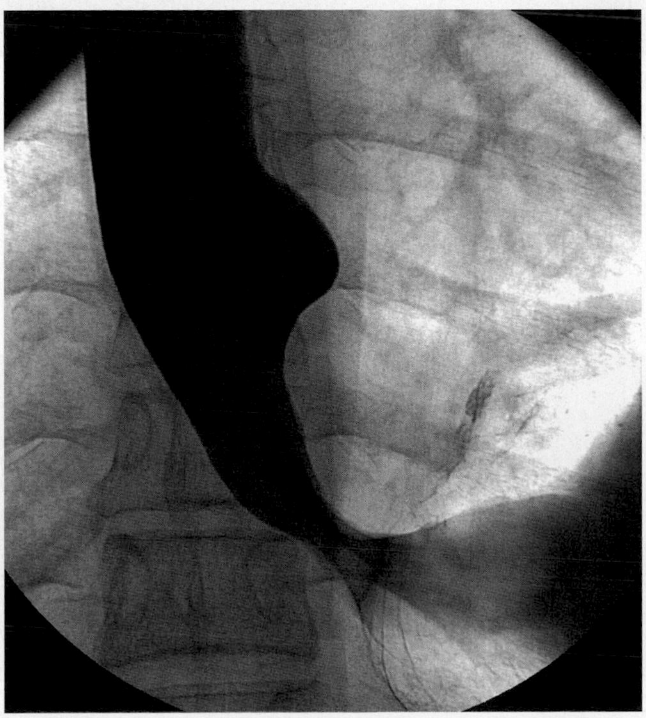

Figure 29-4. Pseudodiverticulum after enucleation for leiomyoma.

Enucleation of leiomyomas gives excellent results, with 89% to 95% of patients free of symptoms at 5 years.[11,13] Mortality rates range from 0% to 1.3%. Postoperative complications include acid reflux, esophagitis, fistula, stenosis, and diverticulum formation. Some of these may result from impairment in esophageal propulsion and inability to clear acid after resection of large tumors when the muscle layer is not adequately reapproximated.

Segmental Resection

Segmental esophageal resection should be considered for large tumors (>8 cm), circumferential tumors, those with significant distortion of the musculature, or those with high suspicion for leiomyosarcoma based on imaging or FNA. It should also be considered in patients undergoing enucleation when there is extensive damage to the esophageal mucosa predisposing the patient to a high risk of postoperative leak. Preoperative planning in all of these patients should include consideration of conduit reconstruction. Reconstructive options include gastric pull-up or colonic or jejunal interposition. Preoperative preparation and positioning are similar to those for enucleation procedures. Techniques and postoperative care for segmental esophageal resection are discussed in Chapters 15–22.

OTHER INTRAMURAL TUMORS

Lipomas and granular cell tumors have typical appearances on EUS and can be diagnosed without biopsy. Granular cell tumors are yellow, firm nodules located in the distal esophagus that arise from the first or second layer as seen on EUS. They have a 1% to 3% malignancy rate, and resection should be considered for lesions >1 cm in diameter or those that are symptomatic. Endoscopic mucosal resection (EMR) has been described for these lesions with good outcomes.[12] Those that are not resected should be followed with endoscopy and EUS to rule out malignancy.

Lipomas are soft, yellow lesions covered with normal mucosa. They appear as homogeneous, hyperechoic lesions confined to the submucosal layer on EUS. They do not progress to malignant lesions, and resection is generally indicated only for symptomatic lesions. Asymptomatic lipomas do not require any specific follow-up.

Hemangiomas are typically located in the middle and lower esophagus. They may present with bleeding or dysphagia and sometimes are mistaken for varices. On EUS, they are hypoechoic, have sharp borders, and arise from the second or third layer. Biopsy is not recommended as this has been associated with significant hemorrhage. Treatment options include sclerotherapy, fulgurization, radiotherapy, EMR, tumor enucleation, and formal esophagectomy, depending on the size of the lesion and the patient's clinical presentation.[12] Reports of treatment with EMR and other endoscopic techniques are largely anecdotal, with successful immediate outcomes but limited long-term follow-up.[14]

EXTRAMURAL LESIONS

Esophageal Cysts

Esophageal cysts are the second most common benign esophageal tumor. They are typically extramural, with epithelial and muscular components that are continuous with the muscularis propria. They are commonly located near the tracheal bifurcation. They are evident as cystic lesions on CT and endoscopic ultrasound, but sometimes may appear dense because of thickened contents or previous hemorrhage. Cysts can lead to a host of complications including ulceration, hemorrhage, perforation, airway obstruction, dysphagia, and repeated pulmonary infections.[2] Resection is recommended for all esophageal cysts. They are discussed in more detail in Chapter 28.

CASE REPORT

A 59-year-old male presented to surgery clinic after an annual whole-body CT scan revealed an intramural mass just proximal to the gastroesophageal (GE) junction (Fig. 29-5A). He denied any symptoms from the lesion, including dysphagia, pain, weight loss, or reflux. He had no other significant past medical or surgical history. His physical examination was unremarkable. His preoperative laboratory results revealed a normal hematocrit (45.5%). An upper endoscopy and EUS were performed and revealed a tortuous, intramural, noncircumferential lesion extending from the distal thoracic esophagus to the GE junction (38–42 cm from the incisors) (Fig. 29-5B). It originated from the fourth layer on EUS, and had well-circumscribed borders (Fig. 29-5C). It was 6 cm in diameter (Fig. 29-5D). The remainder of the esophagus was normal. An FNA was performed, and cytology confirmed the diagnosis of leiomyoma; immunohistochemistry was negative for S100, CD117, and DOG1. Resection was performed via a laparoscopic approach. The distal 10 cm of the esophagus was exposed, and the mass was readily apparent anteriorly. The esophagus was mobilized circumferentially in the mediastinum to bring the cephalad aspect of the mass to the level of the hiatus. Intraoperative endoscopy was used to confirm the proximal and distal margins of the mass. The muscular layers on the anterior surface of the esophagus were incised to expose the mass, and a combination of blunt dissection, hook monopolar cautery, and LigaSure™ (Covidien, Mansfield, MA) were used to mobilize the mass from the submucosa.

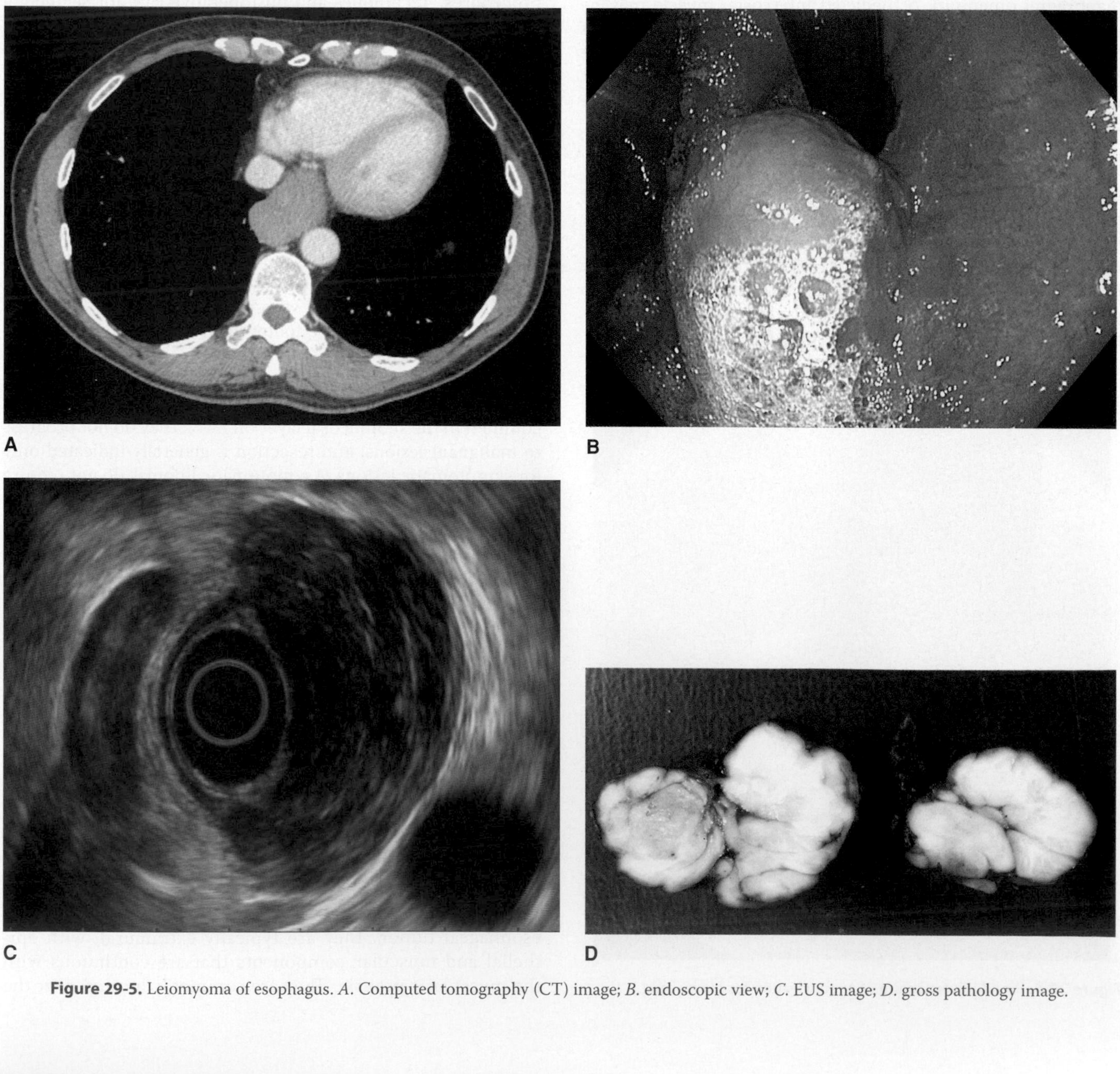

A B C D

Figure 29-5. Leiomyoma of esophagus. *A.* Computed tomography (CT) image; *B.* endoscopic view; *C.* EUS image; *D.* gross pathology image.

The mass was removed and endoscopic insufflation was used to confirm that the submucosa remained intact. The posterior crural pillars were reapproximated and a partial anterior (Dor) fundoplication was performed. No drains were left. The patient was given clear liquids by mouth on the first postoperative day, and then was advanced to a soft mechanical diet the next day. He was discharged home on day 3, and was seen 2 weeks postoperatively, at which time he was tolerating a regular diet without symptoms of reflux or dysphagia. The final pathology revealed a 6.5-cm leiomyoma.

SUMMARY

Benign esophageal tumors are rare, frequently are asymptomatic, and usually are discovered incidentally on CT, barium esophagram, or endoscopy. They are classified according to histology or esophageal layer of origin. Accurate diagnosis of these tumors is usually possible through imaging using barium esophagram, endoscopy, EUS, and CT scan. Biopsy is generally not required to establish a diagnosis, and is usually contraindicated for intramural tumors that may require enucleation. Many of these tumors require no treatment or may be safely resected using endoscopic techniques. Surgery is reserved for fibrovascular polyps, very large tumors of other histologic types, and those for which imaging is not able to rule out malignancy. Outcomes for surgical resection of these lesions are excellent and will continue to improve with the increased use of minimally invasive approaches.

EDITOR'S COMMENT

Benign esophageal lesions generally can be resected by means of minimally invasive surgery and/or endoscopic surgery. Preoperative evaluation, diagnosis, and staging are paramount to exclude cancer and define the surgical objectives. The distal esophagus and GE junction can be easily accessed via a laparoscopic approach, which permits enucleation of even large and circumferential leiomyomas provided that adequate pre- and frozen-section evaluation excludes the presence of an aggressive tumor. Such extensive resection often requires complete mobilization of the GE junction followed by a complete or at least partial fundoplication, both to protect the mucosa and to reestablish the lower esophageal sphincter.

—Raphael Bueno

References

1. Skinner DB, Belsey RHR. *Management of Esophageal Disease*. Philadelphia, PA: W.B. Saunders Company; 1988.
2. Choong CK, Meyers BF. Benign esophageal tumors: introduction, incidence, classification, and clinical features. *Semin Thorac Cardiovasc Surg.* 2003;15(1):3–8.
3. Caceres M, Steeb G, Wilks SM, et al. Large pedunculated polyps originating in the esophagus and hypopharynx. *Ann Thorac Surg.* 2006;81(1):393–396.
4. Peltz M, Estrera AS. Resection of a giant fibrovascular polyp. *Ann Thorac Surg.* 2010;90:1017–1019.
5. Goenka AH, Sharma S, Ramachandran V, et al. Giant fibrovascular polyp of the esophagus: report of a case. *Surg Today.* 2011;41:120–124.
6. Drenth JPH, Wobbes T, Bonenkamp JJ, et al. Recurrent esophageal fibrovascular polyps: case history and review of the literature. *Dig Dis Sci.* 2002;47(11):2598–2604.
7. Mosca S, Manes G, Monaco R, et al. Squamous papilloma of the esophagus: long-term follow up. *J Gastroenterol Hepatol.* 2001;16(8):857–861.
8. Seremetis MG, Lyons WS, deGuzman VC, et al. Leiomyomata of the esophagus. An analysis of 838 cases. *Cancer.* 1976;38:2166–2177.
9. Hatch GF 3rd, Wertheimer-Hatch L, Hatch KF, et al. Tumors of the esophagus. *World J Surg.* 2000;24(4):401–411.
10. Rice TW. Benign Esophageal tumors: esophagoscopy and endoscopic esophageal ultrasound. *Semin Thorac Cardiovasc Surg.* 2003;15:20–26.
11. Lee LS, Singhal S, Brinster CJ, et al. Current management of esophageal leiomyoma. *J Am Coll Surg.* 2004;198(1):136–146.
12. Kinney T, Waxman I. Treatment of benign esophageal tumors by endoscopic techniques. *Semin Thorac Cardiovasc Surg.* 2003;15(1):27–34.
13. Sampire J, Nafteux P, Luketich J. Minimally invasive techniques for resection of benign esophageal tumors. *Semin Thorac Cardiovasc Surg.* 2003; 15(1):34–43.
14. Sogabe M, Taniki T, Fukui Y, et al. A patient with esophageal hemangioma treated by endoscopic mucosal resection: a case report and review of the literature. *J Med Invest.* 2006;53(1–2):177–182.

30 Resection of Esophageal Diverticula

Kimberly S. Grant, Steven R. DeMeester

Keywords: Esophageal diverticulum, Zenker diverticulum, myotomy, stapled diverticulotomy

Esophageal diverticula are unusual but interesting abnormalities that can develop in any part of the esophagus. The most common esophageal diverticulum occurs in the cervical region and is known as a Zenker diverticulum. An esophageal diverticulum may also occur in the midesophagus near the pulmonary hilum or as an epiphrenic diverticulum near the gastroesophageal junction. There are two categories of esophageal diverticula—pulsion and traction. Each has a distinct etiology. Pulsion diverticula are the most common type in the United States, and develop as a consequence of a motility abnormality in the esophagus distal to the site of the diverticulum.[1] They are false diverticula since they are not composed of the entire wall of the esophagus, but instead the mucosa herniates or protrudes through the muscle layers (Fig. 30-1).

The other type, traction diverticula, develop secondary to inflamed mediastinal lymph nodes, and represent a true diverticulum since all layers of the esophageal wall are involved. The prevalence of all types of diverticula increases with age.

Pulsion diverticula are the most common type of diverticula, and the most common pulsion diverticulum is a Zenker diverticulum. These develop in the cervical region secondary to repetitive pharyngeal pressure on boluses of food that are held up by a dysfunctional cricopharyngeus muscle.[2] Over time, this pressure causes a posterior herniation of the esophageal mucosa through *Killian dehiscence*, a weak point at the junction of the inferior constrictor and cricopharyngeus muscles. Epiphrenic diverticula are also pulsion diverticula. These develop secondary to a motility disorder in the distal esophagus, most commonly at the gastroesophageal junction and most commonly achalasia.[3] Radiographically, pulsion diverticula typically have a wide neck, rounded contour, and retain contrast material on a barium swallow (Fig. 30-2). Symptoms associated with pulsion diverticula are often initially related to the underlying motility abnormality, but as the size of the diverticulum increases the symptoms may become more attributable to the pouch itself. Thus, while dysphagia is often the primary initial symptom, as the pouch enlarges, regurgitation may become more prominent. It is not unusual for these symptoms to lead to a misdiagnosis of gastroesophageal reflux disease before the diverticulum itself is identified (Fig. 30-3). However, careful questioning will usually elicit the key information that the regurgitated material tastes bland, not bitter, since the regurgitated food or fluid was trapped in the pouch and never made it to the stomach. Other symptoms attributable to a diverticulum are halitosis, cough, and aspiration of debris retained within the pouch. The larger and more proximal the pouch, the more troublesome these symptoms may be for patients.

Traction diverticula are caused by granulomatous inflammation of mediastinal lymph nodes, and occur most commonly in areas where tuberculosis or histoplasmosis is endemic. The inflamed nodes attach to the esophagus, and as the acute inflammation subsides, the nodes contract, pull on the esophagus, and create a conical outpouching. Traction diverticula are true diverticula, since the entire wall of the esophagus is involved. In contrast to pulsion diverticula, traction diverticula tend to have a pointed tip on radiographs and empty well on barium swallow (Fig. 30-4). Symptoms generally are less significant compared to patients with a pulsion diverticulum, and are

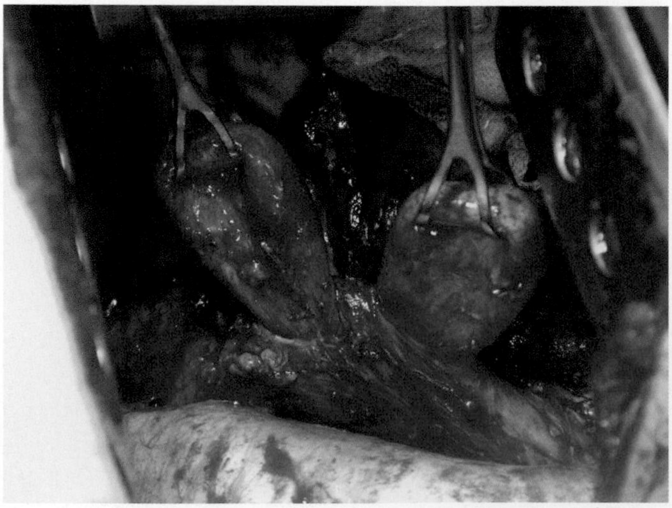

A

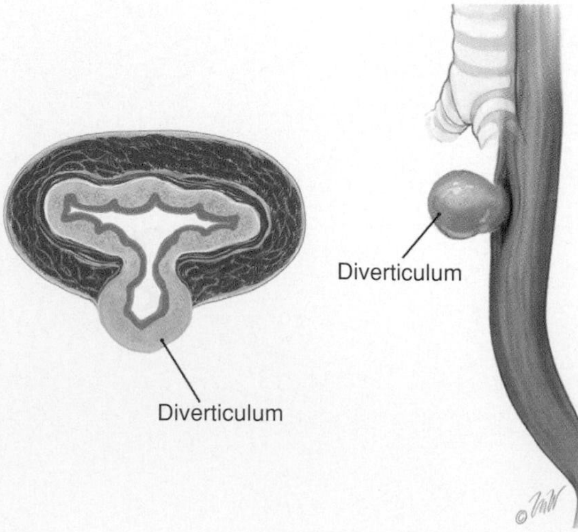

B

Figure 30-1. *A*. The epiphrenic esophageal diverticulum depicted in the intraoperative photograph is of the pulsion variety. Pulsion diverticula (*B*) are not covered by the muscle layers of the esophageal wall and thus are considered false diverticula.

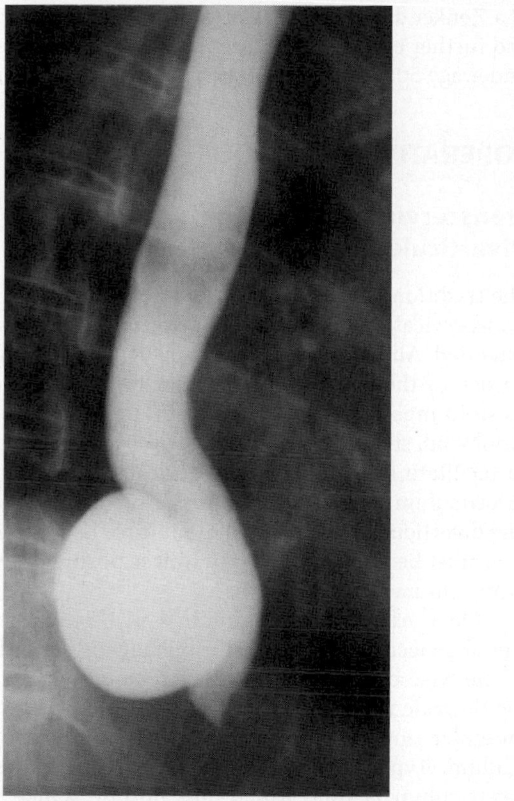

Figure 30-2. Barium swallow of a patient with a large epiphrenic diverticulum.

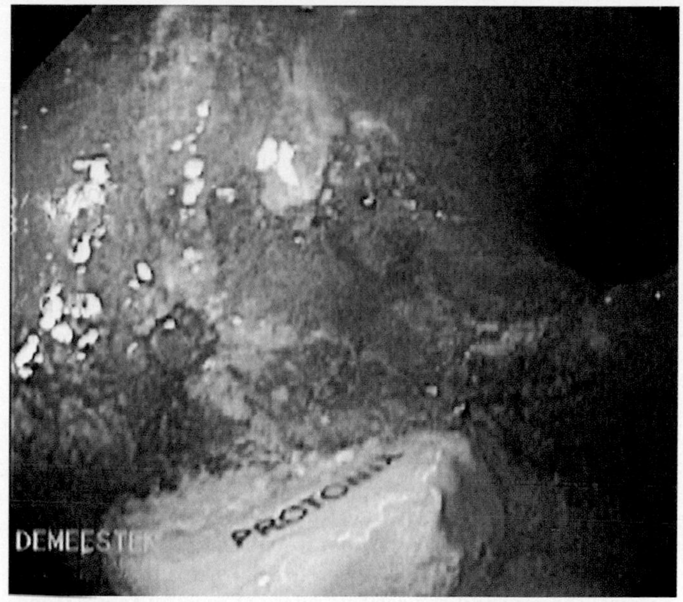

Figure 30-3. Regurgitation symptoms are common in patients with a large diverticulum, and often they are assumed to have reflux and are placed on a proton pump inhibitor. A key distinction is that the material regurgitated in a patient with a diverticulum is bland, not bitter or acidic.

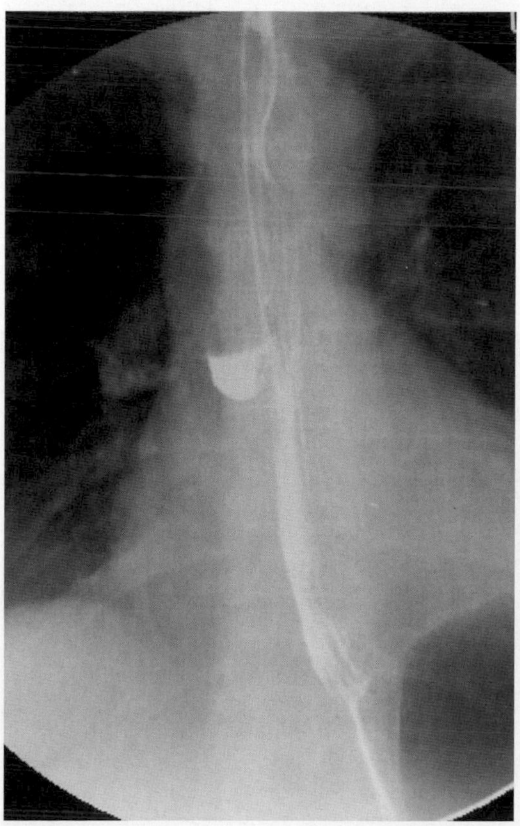

A

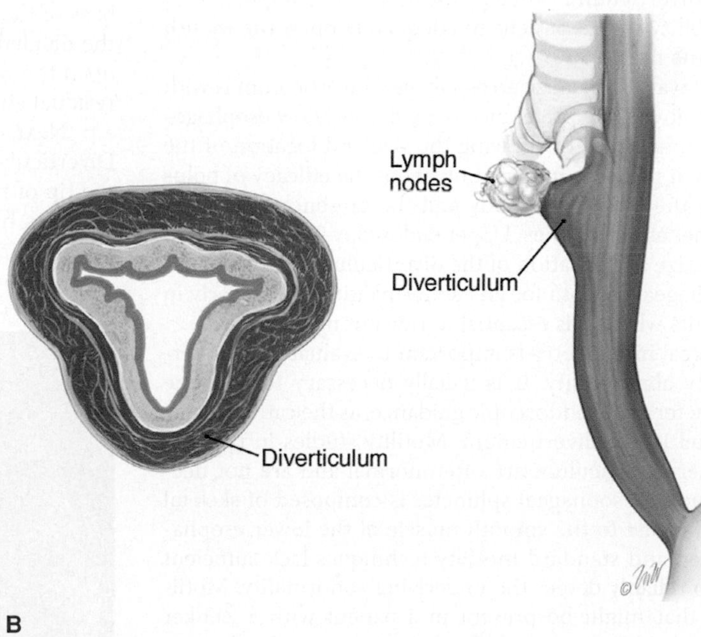

B

Figure 30-4. *A*. Barium swallow of a patient with a midesophageal traction diverticulum. Note the calcified nodes in hilum. *B*. Illustration of a true diverticulum showing involvement of the complete esophageal wall.

related to the diverticulum or mediastinal inflammation since there is no underlying motility abnormality.

Surgery is the only effective therapy for esophageal diverticula. Dilation of the cricopharyngeus muscle has been attempted in patients with Zenker diverticulum with limited success. Even if the dilation is helpful, it only addresses the dysphagia component of the patient's symptoms. The surgical plan for patients with a pulsion diverticulum includes myotomy of the dysfunctional esophageal muscle adjacent and distal to the diverticulum and either excision or suspension of the diverticulum based on its size and location. Failure to divide the dysfunctional muscle leads to a high rate of recurrence and increases the risk of a leak from the suture or staple line if the diverticulum has been excised.[4] For patients with a symptomatic traction diverticulum, only excision of the diverticulum is necessary, but the fibrotic nodes that caused the diverticulum can make the dissection tedious. Approaches to both pulsion and traction diverticula include the traditional open techniques and more recent transoral, laparoscopic, and thoracoscopic minimally invasive options. Given the absence of effective nonsurgical therapy and the relative safety of most of these procedures, symptomatic patients with an esophageal diverticulum should be considered for surgical therapy regardless of age.

PREOPERATIVE ASSESSMENT

The physical examination of patients with an esophageal diverticulum generally is unrevealing, even when a large Zenker diverticulum. However, if a transoral approach for correction of a Zenker diverticulum is being considered, it is important to assess the ability of the patient to adequately open the mouth and extend the neck.[5]

The best way to visualize an esophageal diverticulum is with a barium swallow.[4] Our preference is a video swallow esophagogram, since in addition to showing the size and location of the diverticulum, it provides information about the efficacy of bolus transport by the esophageal body and the presence of a hiatal hernia or other abnormalities. Upper endoscopy is useful both to measure the size and location of the diverticulum, and to evaluate the esophageal mucosa for any abnormalities, particularly in elderly patients where it is essential to rule out malignancy.

Esophageal manometry is important to evaluate the underlying motility abnormality. It is usually necessary to pass the motility catheter using endoscopic guidance, as the catheter may otherwise coil in the diverticulum. Motility studies in patients with a Zenker diverticulum are often normal and are not necessary. The upper esophageal sphincter is composed of skeletal muscle, in contrast to the smooth muscle of the lower esophageal sphincter, and standard motility techniques lack sufficient sensitivity to reliably detect the underlying abnormality. Motility findings that might be present in a patient with a Zenker diverticulum include an increased bolus pressure in the pharyngeal contraction wave (evidence of outflow obstruction distally) and mistimed or incomplete relaxation of the cricopharyngeus with a swallow.[2] Most patients with a Zenker diverticulum are elderly, and the cause of the cricopharyngeal dysfunction is usually related to prior neck injury, radiation, or neurologic abnormalities such as a stroke. Young patients (<50 years old) with a Zenker diverticulum often have no predisposing factors, but frequently have symptoms of gastroesophageal reflux disease. This raises the possibility that proximal reflux can induce dysfunction of the cricopharyngeus muscle and lead to the development of a Zenker diverticulum. Certainly, reflux should be considered and further evaluated if present in an otherwise healthy patient under age 50 who presents with a Zenker diverticulum.

OPERATIVE TECHNIQUE

Transcervical Cricopharyngeal Myotomy and Diverticulectomy or Suspension

The traditional approach for repair of a Zenker diverticulum is transcervical, with the patient positioned supine and the neck extended. An incision is made in the left neck along the anterior border of the sternocleidomastoid muscle. The sternocleidomastoid muscle and carotid sheath are retracted laterally. The omohyoid, sternothyroid, and sternohyoid muscles are divided to facilitate exposure of the cervical esophagus. The Zenker diverticulum will be located posterior to the cricoid cartilage. The diverticulum is sheathed in multiple layers of fibrous tissue that must be teased apart to permit exposure of the base of the diverticulum (Fig. 30-5).

Once exposed, a longitudinal myotomy on the posterolateral aspect of the cervical esophagus is started just inferior to the base of the diverticulum. It should extend inferiorly to the thoracic inlet, and then it is carried superiorly through the muscular ring of the cricopharyngeus at the base of the diverticulum. Typically, the muscle in the area of the base of the diverticulum is quite thick and fibrotic. Once released, the diverticulum should be clearly visualized. To ensure that all the dysfunctional fibers are divided, we also incise the lower fibers of the inferior pharyngeal constrictor superiorly from the base of the diverticulum for 1 to 2 cm. In addition, the edges of the divided muscle should be bluntly dissected to widely splay open the mucosa and permit identification and division of any residual circular muscle fibers.

Next, the diverticulum is either suspended or excised. Diverticula 2 cm or less in size are easily suspended by tacking the tip of the diverticulum with 3-0 Prolene to the precervical fascia as high up in the neck as necessary to fully upend the pouch. Larger pouches are difficult to fully upend and are best

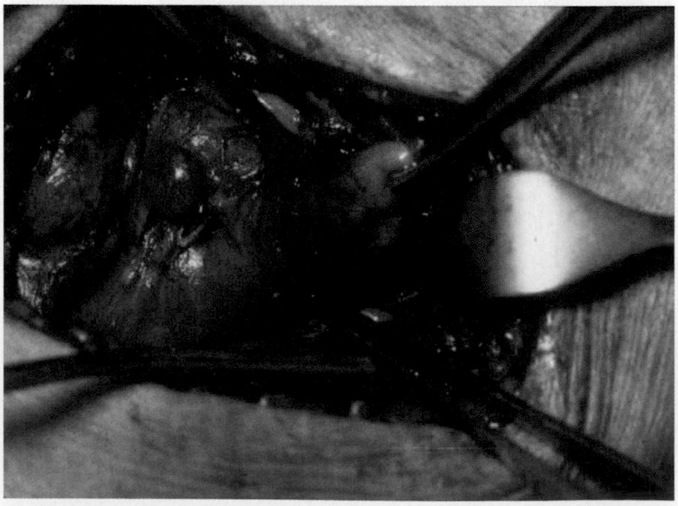

Figure 30-5. Open repair of Zenker diverticulum. The Zenker diverticulum will be located posterior to the cricoid cartilage. The diverticulum is sheathed in multiple layers of fibrous tissue that must be teased apart to permit exposure of the base of the diverticulum.

excised using a TA stapler with a 52F bougie in the esophagus to prevent narrowing of the esophageal lumen. The staple line and/or myotomy can be checked for leaks by passing a nasogastric tube into the area and insufflating air to distend the mucosa while the neck incision is filled with saline. This also provides an opportunity to ensure the mucosa distends fully with no residual bands in the area of the myotomy. Before neck closure, it is critical to ensure perfect hemostasis, because a hematoma requiring reexploration can develop from even small vessels secondary to coughing or straining as the patient awakens from anesthesia. We leave a small closed suction drain in place and approximate the platysma and skin to complete the operation.

Transoral Endoscopic-Stapled Diverticulotomy

A transoral endoscopic approach is another option for treating a Zenker diverticulum. This approach is attractive largely because it eliminates the neck incision, but limited because the pouch must be at least 3 cm in length and the patient must be able to extend the neck and open the mouth widely. Inability to extend the neck and open the mouth makes placement of the Storz rigid diverticuloscope difficult or impossible. If the diverticulum is less than 3 cm in length, it may not be possible to completely divide the dysfunctional cricopharyngeus muscle, leading to persistent or recurrent symptoms. Patients with evidence of malignancy inside the pouch are also not candidates for transoral stapling technique and instead require excision of the pouch.[6] Although the procedure is quick and well tolerated, and in suitable patients produces excellent relief of dysphagia and regurgitation symptoms, patients must be warned of the possibility of chipped teeth secondary to the rigid scope insertion. In addition, most patients have considerable tongue swelling for a day or two after the procedure.

Before the procedure commences, a 30-mm GIA laparoscopic stapler is modified by cutting off the tip of the stapler with an orthopedic circular saw such that the knife blade and the staple line reach the end of the modified tip. The tip should be smoothed with a rasp or file. The patient is placed under general anesthesia and positioned supine with the neck extended, and the Storz diverticuloscope is inserted under

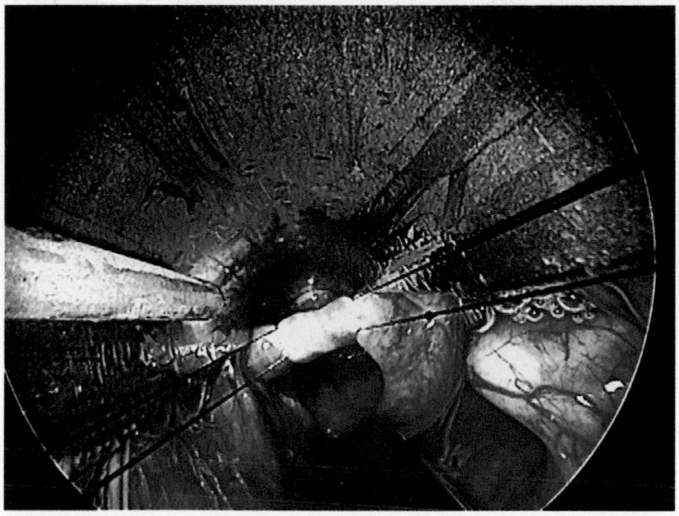

Figure 30-7. Traction sutures in place in preparation for the stapling.

direct visualization and advanced into the esophagus. It is helpful to have a pediatric flexible esophagoscope to facilitate placement of the rigid scope. The goal is to advance the longer anterior blade into the true lumen of the esophagus whereas the shorter posterior blade is advanced into the diverticulum. Once positioned, the blades of the scope are separated to permit clear visualization of the cricopharyngeus muscle band (Fig. 30-6). Using a laparoscopic needle holder, 3-0 Prolene traction sutures are placed on each side of the cricopharyngeus muscle (Fig. 30-7). With gentle traction on these stitches, the bar is held in position as the modified GIA stapler is inserted and fired (Fig. 30-8). Several applications of the stapler are typically necessary to divide the muscle bridge all the way to the tip of the diverticulum (Fig. 30-9). In this fashion, the cricopharyngeus muscle is divided, and the pouch is incorporated into the esophagus to create a single common cavity. If the diverticulum is less than 3 cm in length, the cricopharyngeus muscle will not be adequately divided, leading to a high rate of symptomatic failure and a significant risk for the development

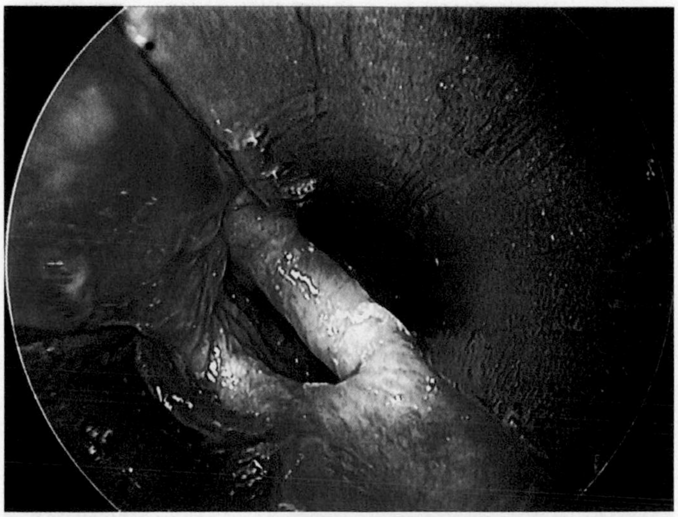

Figure 30-6. Diverticuloscope positioned with the longer upper blade in the true lumen of the esophagus and the shorter blade in the diverticulum (lower left of picture). The cricopharyngeus muscle band is clearly seen between the blades.

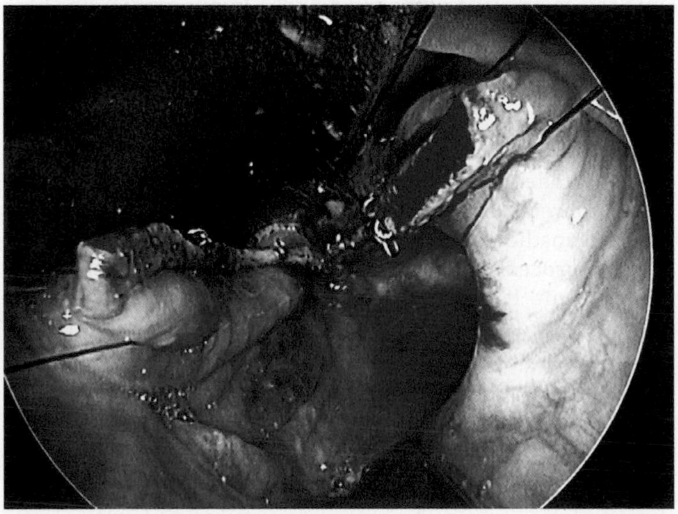

Figure 30-8. Complete transection of the cricopharyngeus achieved with multiple loads of a 30-mm GIA stapler. A common chamber now has been created between the true esophageal lumen and the diverticulum, and the dysfunctional cricopharyngeus muscle has been completely divided.

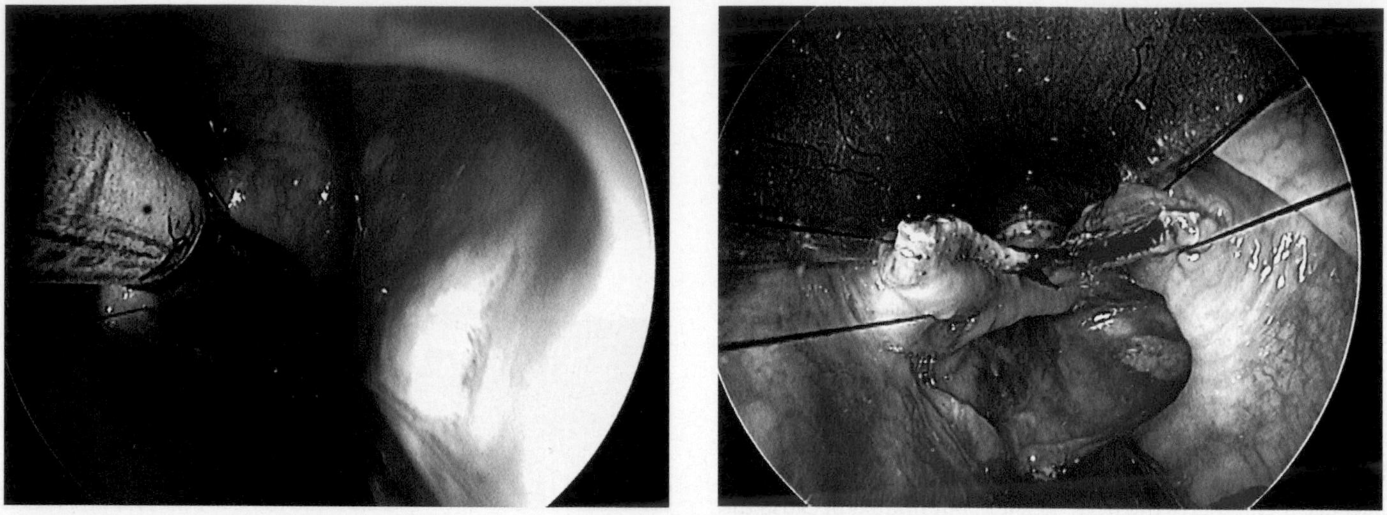

A B

Figure 30-9. *A.* Modified 30-mm GIA stapler inserted and ready. *B.* Partial transection of the cricopharyngeus after use of a single 30-mm GIA stapler. Note the residual pouch.

of a recurrent diverticulum. It is important to modify the stapler to minimize the amount of residual pouch with the transoral approach, since even a 1-cm remnant can lead to persistent symptoms. Although it is nearly impossible to completely eliminate the pouch, in our experience, patients with less than 4 to 5 mm of residual pouch remain asymptomatic.

Laparoscopic, Transabdominal, or Transthoracic Esophageal Myotomy; Diverticulectomy; and Partial Fundoplication (Triple Treat)

The objectives of the procedure for an epiphrenic diverticulum are identical regardless of the approach, and include division of the dysfunctional esophageal muscle distal and adjacent to the diverticulum, excision of the diverticulum, and partial fundoplication to protect the esophagus from gastroesophageal reflux.[1,7] A myotomy that ends at the gastroesophageal junction is associated with a higher incidence of persistent or recurrent dysphagia compared to a myotomy that extends 2 to 3 cm onto the gastric side of the junction.[1,7,8] In our opinion the best location for the myotomy is along the left lateral aspect of the esophagus with continuation down across the angle of His on the greater curvature side of the stomach. Further, it is clear that the addition of a partial fundoplication reduces esophageal acid exposure after myotomy,[9] and therefore a partial fundoplication is added to the myotomy in all patients.

Epiphrenic diverticula can be treated via a transabdominal or transthoracic approach, and as an open or minimally invasive procedure depending on the size and location of the diverticulum. If the diverticulum is located near the hiatus, a laparoscopic diverticulectomy with esophageal myotomy and partial fundoplication is readily accomplished, but it is important to recognize that many diverticula are more proximal than they appear radiographically, and only those very close to the gastroesophageal junction are amenable to a transabdominal or laparoscopic approach (Fig. 30-10). Some epiphrenic diverticula are located 5 to 10 cm proximal to the gastroesophageal junction, and for these patients, a transthoracic approach is optimal. The approach is via left thoracotomy in the eighth intercostal space. After incision of the mediastinal pleura and identification of the esophagus, the diverticulum can be dissected. Once the diverticulum is dissected it can be excised using a TA stapler with a 52F or larger bougie in the esophagus to avoid narrowing the lumen. Subsequently, the muscle is reapproximated over the staple line with interrupted 3-0 silk sutures (Fig. 30-11), and a myotomy is performed on the opposite side of the esophagus and carried down for several centimeters on the greater curvature side of the stomach (Fig. 30-12). Typically, a Dor partial fundoplication is performed (Fig. 30-13), but if there is a hiatal hernia, then crural closure with a Belsey partial fundoplication is preferred. Diverticula underneath the aortic arch are difficult to excise from the left chest and are better visualized from the right. In this setting, a two-stage approach offers some advantages. The first stage is a laparoscopic myotomy and partial fundoplication, and then 6 weeks later the patient can be brought back for a thoracoscopic diverticulectomy and long esophageal myotomy through the right chest.

Traction diverticula occur secondary to mediastinal adenopathy, and a myotomy is unnecessary. Treatment entails

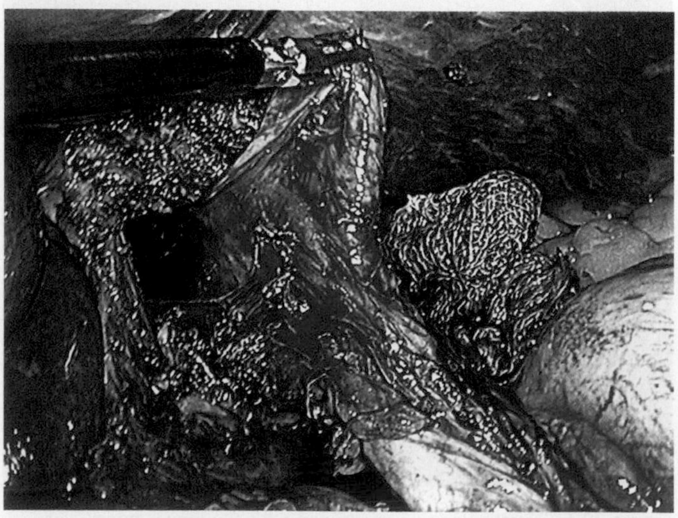

Figure 30-10. Epiphrenic diverticulum dissected by a laparoscopic approach.

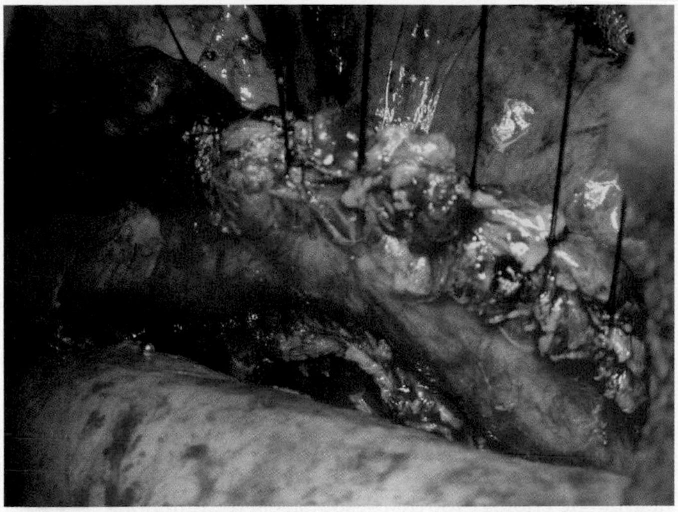

Figure 30-11. Muscle approximated in interrupted fashion over the staple line after diverticulectomy over a 52F bougie. The myotomy is visible below the reapproximated muscle layers.

separating the esophagus from the culprit nodes (often difficult secondary to intense inflammation, fibrosis, and/or calcification) and excising the diverticulum. This is best accomplished in most patients via the right chest either as an open or thoracoscopic procedure. It is recommended that pleura or intercostal muscle is placed between the esophageal repair and any residual mediastinal nodes to prevent leakage or recurrence.

POSTOPERATIVE CARE

Patients are kept NPO after the procedure until the following day, or 24 to 48 hours longer when the diverticulum has been excised. We typically obtain a Gastrografin esophagogram before starting oral feeds, both to document the integrity of the myotomy ± diverticulectomy staple line and to verify that the patient is able to swallow without aspiration, particularly in a patient who has undergone surgery for a Zenker diverticulum.

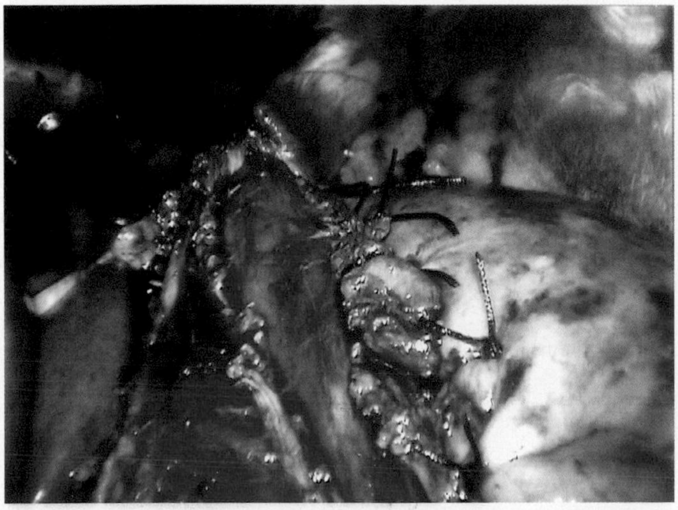

Figure 30-12. Laparoscopic myotomy along the anterolateral aspect of the esophagus exposing the mucosa across the gastroesophageal junction.

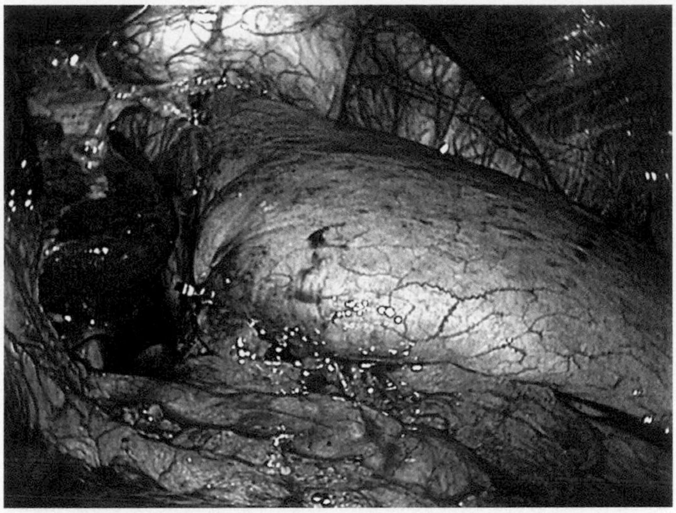

Figure 30-13. Completed Dor partial fundoplication.

COMPLICATIONS AND RESULTS

Major morbidity is uncommon, but potential complications include a leak from the myotomy or suture line if the diverticulum was excised, mediastinitis, fistula formation, hoarseness from vocal cord paralysis, incomplete myotomy, luminal stenosis, and wound infection. Long-term complications include recurrence of the diverticulum, particularly if no or an inadequate myotomy is done in patients with a pulsion-type diverticulum, and development of gastroesophageal reflux when the myotomy is carried across the gastroesophageal junction. Most procedures are well tolerated, have minimal morbidity, and provide excellent symptomatic relief for patients.

SUMMARY

Esophageal diverticula are uncommon but interesting esophageal abnormalities. The pulsion-type diverticulum develops as a consequence of an underlying esophageal motility disorder, and occurs most commonly in the cervical region as a Zenker diverticulum. These are false diverticula, and treatment entails a myotomy through the dysfunctional muscle distal to the diverticulum with suspension or resection of the diverticulum. For epiphrenic diverticula a partial fundoplication is added to complete the so-called "triple treat." The other type of diverticulum is called a traction diverticulum. These develop secondary to inflamed mediastinal lymph nodes and are true diverticula that involve the entire esophageal wall. Treatment for symptomatic patients entails excision of the diverticulum.

Surgical therapy should be considered in all symptomatic patients since there is no effective medical therapy for the regurgitation and aspiration problems associated with a diverticulum. In addition to the traditional open approaches, new minimally invasive or transoral approaches are applicable in some patients and may reduce procedure-related morbidity and hasten recovery. Careful patient evaluation and technical precision during the procedure will ensure excellent results.

CASE HISTORY

An 85-year-old woman was referred with a 5-year history of dysphagia, primarily for solid food and pills, but occasionally for liquids if she drank too quickly. She also noticed a frequent gurgling sensation in the neck and experienced regurgitation of undigested food particles, particularly at night when lying down. She endured severe heartburn symptoms for 20 years that she self-treated with over-the-counter medications, but recently was placed on Prilosec with excellent relief.

On physical examination, her neck was supple with good extension, and she was able to open her mouth widely. She had a barium swallow study that revealed a several-centimeter Zenker diverticulum and a sliding hiatal hernia. She underwent an upper endoscopy, which demonstrated an approximately 3-cm Zenker pouch, a sliding hiatal hernia, and a columnar-lined distal esophagus with intestinal metaplasia on biopsy. She was offered surgical therapy for her Zenker diverticulum. The option of open versus transoral endoscopic approach was discussed, and it was thought that she would be a good candidate for the transoral technique.

Under general anesthesia, she was positioned with the neck extended. A Storz diverticuloscope was introduced transorally and advanced into the esophagus. The pouch was exposed but was determined to be of insufficient size to permit complete division of the cricopharyngeus muscle. Therefore, the diverticuloscope was withdrawn, and the patient had an open cricopharyngeal myotomy with suspension of the diverticulum. She had an uncomplicated postoperative hospital course and reported significant improvement in her swallowing. A barium swallow study showed a widely patent cricopharyngeal region with no filling of the suspended Zenker pouch.

EDITOR'S COMMENT

When suspending a Zenker diverticulum, one must be cautious not to directly suture it to the prevertebral fascia, as this can result in osteomyelitis. A better place to suture is the cricopharyngeal muscle proximally. Furthermore, many patients presenting with symptoms consistent with Zenker diverticulum are elderly and frail and must be carefully monitored postoperatively. One must also exclude from surgery those who have neurologic etiology for their esophageal dysfunction.

Occasionally, a relatively small epiphrenic diverticulum can be treated by laparoscopic Heller myotomy and Dor fundoplication without diverticulectomy, particularly when the symptoms are mostly obstructive. Finally, there are those patients with severe long-standing reflux who develop strictures that result in small diverticulum. These patients require careful preoperative assessment to identify and will likely require a full wrap to effectively treat their reflux.

—Raphael Bueno

References

1. Nehra D, Lord RV, DeMeester TR, et al. Physiologic basis for the treatment of epiphrenic diverticulum. *Ann Surg*. 2002;235:346–354.
2. Bremner CG, DeMeester TR. Endoscopic treatment of Zenker's diverticulum. *Gastrointest Endosc*. 1999;49:126–128.
3. Aly A, Devitt PG, Jamieson GG. Evolution of surgical treatment for pharyngeal pouch. *Br J Surg*. 2004;91:657–664.
4. Salerno C, Mitchell JD, Whyte RI. Congenital and acquired esophageal diverticula. In: Yang SC, Cameron DE, eds. *Current Therapy in Thoracic and Cardiovascular Surgery*. St Louis, MO: Mosby; 2004:432–435.
5. Balaji NS, Peters JH. Minimally invasive surgery for esophageal motility disorders. *Surg Clin North Am*. 2002;82:763–782.
6. Sen P, Bhattacharyya AK. Endoscopic stapling of pharyngeal pouch. *J Laryngol Otol*. 2004;118:601–606.
7. Rosati R, Fumagalli U, Bona S, et al. Diverticulectomy, myotomy, and fundoplication through laparoscopy: A new option to treat epiphrenic esophageal diverticula? *Ann Surg*. 1998;227:174–178.
8. Del Genio A, Rosetti G, Maffetton V, et al. Laparoscopic approach in the treatment of epiphrenic diverticula: long-term results. *Surg Endosc*. 2004;18:741–745.
9. Richards WO, Torquati A, Holzman MD, et al. Heller myotomy versus Heller myotomy with Dor fundoplication for achalasia: a prospective, randomized, double-blind clinical trial. *Ann Surg*. 2004;240(3):405–412; discussion 412–415.

31 Techniques and Indications for Esophageal Exclusion

Subroto Paul and Lambros Zellos

Keywords: Esophageal exclusion and diversion, penetrating trauma, Boerhaave syndrome, iatrogenic injury

The four main causes of esophageal perforation are spontaneous perforation associated with protracted vomiting, also known as Boerhaave syndrome, iatrogenic injury from instrumentation, breakdown of esophageal reconstructions after esophagectomy, and penetrating trauma.[1–4] Regardless of the etiology, mediastinal contamination from salivary, gastric, and biliary secretions, with the associated bacteria, leads to both local and systemic inflammatory responses. If the perforation is not controlled promptly, it will give rise to sepsis, which if left untreated, nearly 100% of the time, will result in mortality within 1 week.[1,4,5] Despite advances in surgical technique and critical care over the past decades, esophageal perforation remains a challenging clinical problem. Early diagnosis and prompt surgical treatment are the hallmarks of successful outcome after spontaneous (i.e., Boerhaave syndrome) and iatrogenic esophageal perforation. Advocates for stenting, primary esophageal repair, drainage with a T-tube, esophageal exclusion, esophageal diversion, and esophagectomy with upfront reconstruction for perforations can be found. This chapter describes the techniques and indications for esophageal exclusion.

CLINICAL PRESENTATION

The extent of the inflammatory response depends on the location of the injury and the length of time from the injury, both of which correlate with extent of mediastinal contamination. Cervical perforations often are limited to the neck, resulting in minimal to absent mediastinal contamination. Such perforations are best managed by local drainage techniques.[1,6] However, intrathoracic and intra-abdominal perforations generally cannot be managed successfully by drainage alone and require either repair with diversion or exclusion in addition to drainage procedures. The choice whether to proceed with primary repair or with esophageal exclusion rests on multiple factors.

IDEAL PATIENT CHARACTERISTICS AND PREOPERATIVE ASSESSMENT

Numerous studies have shown that the length of time from injury to diagnosis is an important determinant of outcome. Cases diagnosed more than 24 hours after injury are associated with increased mortality.[1,2] The length of time from injury to diagnosis is proportional to the degree of mediastinal or abdominal contamination, the severity of inflammation and tissue edema, and ultimately, the need for esophageal diversion. Rather than focusing on absolute lengths of time, however, when formulating a plan for treatment, it is better to evaluate the patient as a whole, considering the extent of injury, the overall physiologic status of the patient, the quality of the tissues on exploration, and the underlying esophageal pathophysiologic process. Otherwise healthy patients who sustain iatrogenic perforation to the intrathoracic or intra-abdominal esophagus and are diagnosed immediately are ideal candidates for primary repair with drainage. Elderly, malnourished, septic patients on vasopressors who go undiagnosed for several days after perforation and on exploration are found to have "woody," edematous, and inflamed tissues remain poor candidates for primary repair and are best served by diversion and drainage procedures.

Primary esophageal resection for perforation has been touted by some to produce superior mortality results to primary repair or diversion.[1,2,7] For the most part, however, these opinions emanate from older nonrandomized, retrospective studies that often do not adequately account for patient comorbidity. Clearly, resection remains an option for patients with extensive tissue destruction who require resection for control of sepsis. All too often, the primary objective of treating esophageal perforation—to have a patient who is alive at the end of the day—is forgotten.

For patients with an underlying primary esophageal malignancy, esophageal resection with or without reconstruction is a viable option depending on the physiologic status of the patient, the degree of obstruction, and the stage of the malignancy. Younger patients with early-stage disease, minimal mediastinal contamination, and good-quality tissues are best served by resection with immediate reconstruction. Older patients or those with poor physiologic reserve should be resected without immediate reconstruction. Patients with involvement of the esophagus and the airway are more appropriately managed with exclusion and diversion techniques or esophageal stenting (see Chapter 56).

TECHNIQUES

Esophageal Exclusion

Midthoracic esophageal perforations generally are explored via right thoracotomy through the fifth intercostal space (Fig. 31-1). One should consider harvesting an intercostal muscle flap on entry because it may be beneficial to buttress the repair with intercostal muscle.

Distal thoracic or intra-abdominal esophageal perforations can be approached via left thoracotomy incision through the seventh intercostal space with takedown of the diaphragm as needed (Fig. 31-1). After entry, the chest is thoroughly explored with full visualization of the extent of esophageal injury, often requiring sharp dissection of the overlying esophageal muscle to reveal the full extent of mucosal injury (Fig. 31-2). The degree of contamination and the nature of the esophageal injury and surrounding tissues are noted.

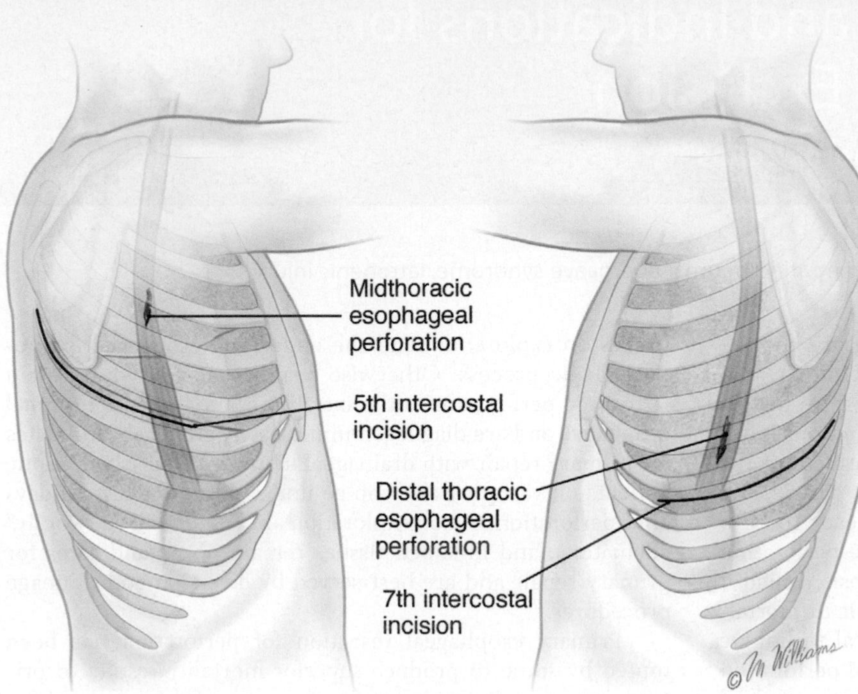

Figure 31-1. Exploration of midthoracic esophageal perforation via right thoracotomy through the fifth intercostal space (*left*). Distal thoracic or intra-abdominal esophageal perforations via left thoracotomy incision through the seventh intercostal space (*right*).

Debate persists as to whether both proximal and distal exclusions are needed. Some surgeons find that a gastric tube is sufficient for distal drainage of bile, whereas others prefer a distal exclusion. If the decision is made to proceed to esophageal exclusion, the mediastinal pleura is incised, and the esophagus proximal and distal to the perforation is mobilized as needed to facilitate exposure. If the plan is to close the perforation before exclusion and diversion, the esophageal musculature is dissected to define the extent of mucosal injury. The perforation then is repaired with interrupted sutures, and the repair may be buttressed by using a pleural flap or intercostal muscle pedicle. After the perforation has been repaired, the esophagus proximal and distal to the perforation is isolated and ligated either with a heavy absorbable tie or, more commonly, with a stapling device (Ethicon TA-30 stapler; Johnson & Johnson, Somerville, NJ) without division of the esophagus (Fig. 31-3).[6] It is important to use the same stapling device for both the proximal and distal ligations because recanalization of the esophagus occurs at different rates for different staple thicknesses. This can lead to potential problems if the perforation has not healed prior to recanalization, with bile reflux of salivary and gastric or biliary secretions through recanalized segments. After the distal esophagus has been ligated, the thoracic cavity is well drained and irrigated, and the chest is closed. A nasogastric tube is left in the proximal esophagus for drainage.

Cervical Esophageal Diversion

Exclusion may not be possible in patients in whom the tissue is too edematous and inflamed to hold sutures or staples. In this case, the perforation can be left alone, with reliance on diversion and drainage to heal the tear. Alternatively, for large perforations, an esophagocutaneous fistula can be formed by placing a T-tube through the perforation, which is

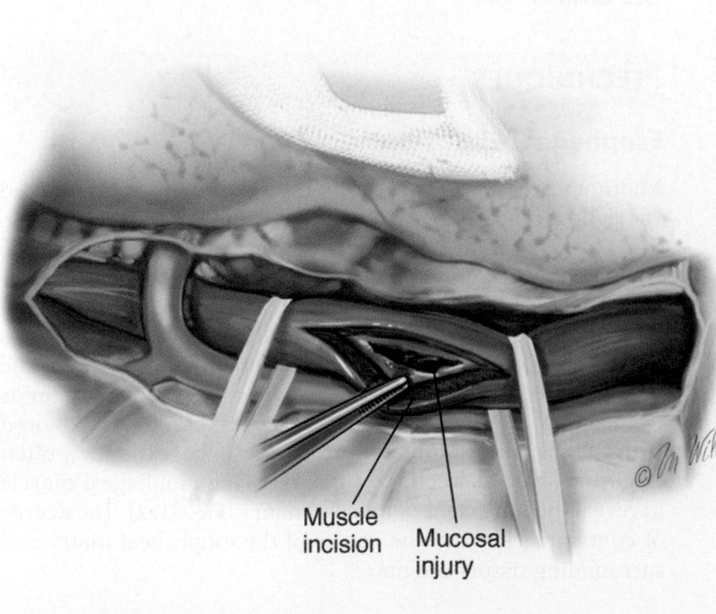

Figure 31-2. Sharp dissection of the overlying esophageal muscle at the site of visible perforation is often required to reveal the full extent of the underlying mucosal injury.

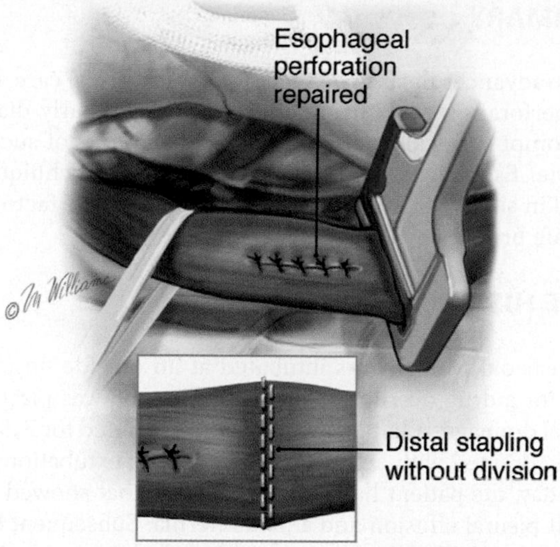

Figure 31-3. Isolation and ligation of the esophagus are performed proximally or distally or both proximally and distally at the surgeon's discretion using a heavy absorbable tie or a stapling device *without division.*

then tunneled outside the chest (Fig. 31-4).[1,2] With adequate proximal and distal exclusion or diversion, the creation of an esophagocutaneous fistula is not necessary, and debate persists as to whether a T-tube either for primary repair or in the setting of exclusion or diversion is ever needed.

The patient is then turned supine with neck extension that is facilitated by placement of a towel roll under the patient's shoulders with the head turned to the right to expose the left neck. Both the neck and abdomen are widely prepped. The proximal esophagus is exposed through the left neck with an incision along the anterior sternocleidomastoid muscle (Fig. 31-5). The sternocleidomastoid muscle is retracted laterally. The strap muscles along with the middle thyroid vein are divided if needed. The carotid sheath then is identified and retracted laterally. The esophagus is palpated along the cervical spine and carefully encircled with a Penrose drain, with attention being paid to the recurrent laryngeal nerve to avoid injury.[1,6] The esophagus then is mobilized proximally to the level of the cricopharyngeus muscle and distally to the thoracic inlet. The proximal esophagus then can be brought out through the bottom of the incision, with a transverse incision being made in the proximal esophagus that later will be matured as a loop esophagostomy. Before this is matured, the distal end of the cervical esophagus is isolated and ligated using either sutures or a stapling device (Fig. 31-6). After the distal cervical esophagus is ligated, the remaining cervical esophagus proximal to the ligated esophagus is brought out through the wound, a transverse or longitudinal incision is made in the esophagus, and the loop esophagostomy is matured using interrupted absorbable sutures (Fig. 31-7). Alternatively, the distal cervical esophagus can be ligated and divided, and an end esophagostomy can be matured. Although this eliminates the possibility of any proximal source of soilage, end esophagostomy requires a more extensive procedure when reestablishing esophageal continuity.

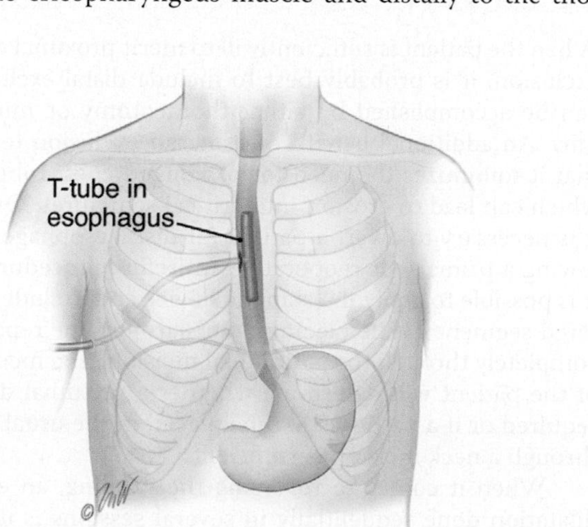

Figure 31-4. An esophagocutaneous fistula can be formed by placing a T-tube through the perforation, which is then tunneled outside the chest.

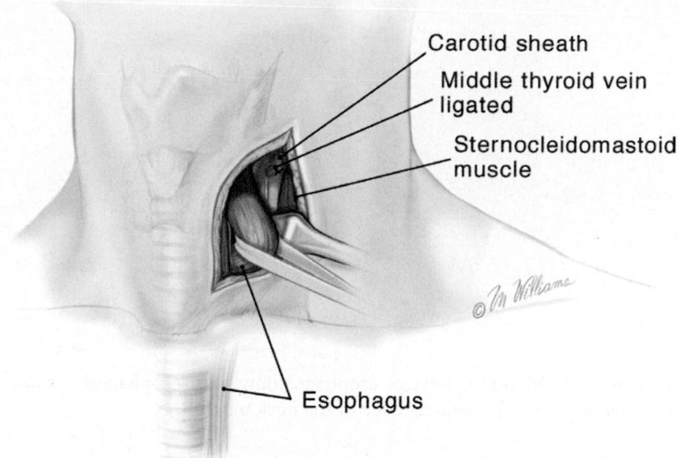

Figure 31-5. The cervical esophageal diversion is performed through the left neck with an incision along the anterior sternocleidomastoid muscle.

Feeding Tubes

The abdomen is explored through the midline if a right thoracotomy was used initially to explore the chest. It is important to explore the abdomen to ensure that the intra-abdominal esophagus has not been injured. If the intra-abdominal esophagus

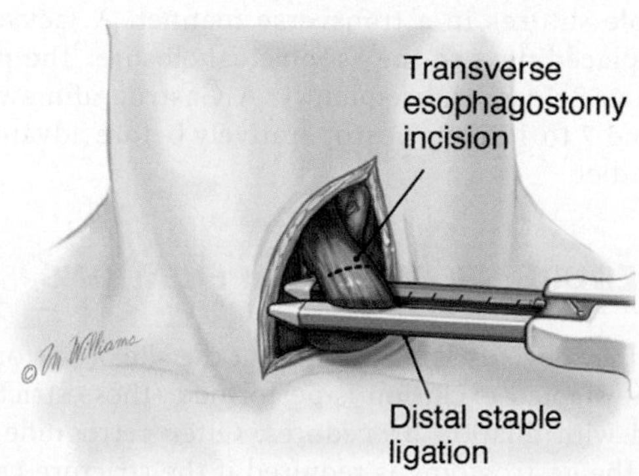

Figure 31-6. In preparation for the matured loop esophagostomy, the distal end of the cervical esophagus is isolated and ligated using either sutures or a stapling device.

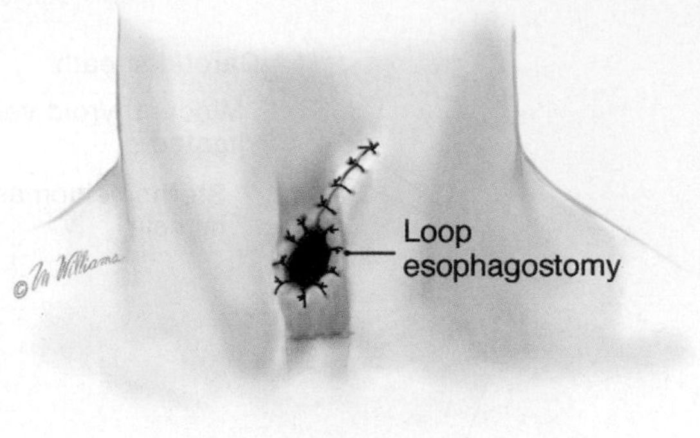

Figure 31-7. Matured cervical esophagostomy with esophageal ostomy incorporated into the inferior edge of the neck incision.

is injured, a gastrostomy is performed in addition to a feeding jejunostomy. The abdomen is then closed after irrigation, with placement of drains near the intra-abdominal esophageal perforation. Without any evidence of injury to the intra-abdominal esophagus, the gastrostomy may be omitted and only a feeding jejunostomy placed before the abdominal closure. However, typically, both a gastrostomy and jejunostomy are placed. Placement of a gastrostomy permits retrograde dilation of the esophagus if any stricture forms postoperatively.

POSTOPERATIVE CARE

The patient is supported throughout the postoperative period. The historical survival rate for exclusion and diversion procedures in a meta-analysis was 24%.[1] Although this survival rate is higher than that reported for primary repair and resective procedures, none of the studies is prospective, nor do they stratify patient comorbidities as discussed earlier. It is likely that those who underwent exclusion and diversion procedures had more comorbidities and were more likely to be septic with flora.

Once the patient has made adequate recovery, the loop cervical esophagostomy is closed at the minimum of 6 to 8 weeks postoperatively. If the esophagus has not been divided completely, the loop cervical esophagostomy can close spontaneously. However, more typically, the patient is taken to the operating room for closure. In these cases, the skin around the esophagostomy is incised, and the esophagus is mobilized. The esophagostomy then is closed with interrupted absorbable sutures in a transverse manner. A Jackson-Pratt drain is placed next to the esophageal closure. The platysma and skin are closed subsequently. A Gastrografin swallow is performed 7 to 10 days postoperatively before advancing the patient's diet.

PROCEDURE-SPECIFIC COMPLICATIONS

Patients may develop late strictures at the site of perforation or where the stapled exclusion is performed. These strictures are managed with dilation procedures. Often retrograde dilation through the gastrostomy is required if the stricture cannot be passed antegrade, as has been described.[8] Late strictures frequently require esophageal resection with reconstruction using either stomach or colon as a conduit.[6]

SUMMARY

Despite advances in surgical technique and critical care, esophageal perforation remains a clinical challenge. Early diagnosis and prompt surgical treatment are the hallmarks of successful outcome. Esophageal exclusion and diversion techniques are needed in situations where patient and local tissue factors prohibit safe primary esophageal repair and drainage.

CASE HISTORY

A 52-year-old woman was intubated at an outside hospital for 8 days for a drug overdose. A nasogastric tube was placed with minimal drainage. A left pleural effusion was noted for 7 days and partially drained with a pigtail catheter. After extubation on the eighth day, the patient had a chest CT scan that showed persistent left pleural effusion and a hiatal hernia. Subsequent barium swallow revealed a distal esophageal perforation with contrast material flowing freely into the left chest. The patient was transferred to our hospital for further management. On presentation, she appeared sick and had chest pain and an elevated white blood cell count. She was taken to the OR, and esophagogastroduodenoscopy was performed. The defect was identified in the distal esophagus. The patient underwent left thoracotomy. Two liters of bilious material was drained, and areas of necrotic parietal pleura were resected. The esophagus was noted to be edematous and inflamed. The esophagus could not be mobilized to fully identify the medial defect. Hence the esophagus was excluded proximal and distal to the perforation using TA and Endo-GIA knifeless staplers. Several chest tubes were placed to drain the chest. A gastrostomy and feeding jejunostomy were performed. The patient did well for 2 weeks but then developed renewed clinical signs of esophageal leakage. Chest CT scan revealed a persistent esophageal leak. At esophagogastroduodenoscopy, it was discovered that the proximal staple line had recanalized. A cervical esophagostomy was performed with resolution of the patient's sepsis. Several months later, the esophagostomy was taken down, and the esophagus was dilated at the stapled line of distal esophageal exclusion. The esophagus had healed completely.

EDITOR'S COMMENT

When the patient is sufficiently ill to merit proximal esophageal exclusion, it is probably best to include distal exclusion. This can be accomplished by either thoracotomy or mini-laparotomy. An additional benefit of using an exclusion technique is that it minimizes the need for prolonged chest tube drainage, which can lead to erosion into critical structures. On occasion it is necessary to divert a patient for distal esophageal leak following a primary or reoperative antireflux procedure. Usually, it is possible to apply the stapling device and exclude the perforated segment (while placing drains around the repaired hole) completely through the abdominal incision. The medical status of the patient will determine whether a proximal diversion is required or if a nasogastric tube placed in the usual fashion or through a neck incision is sufficient.

When it comes to reversing the stapling, an endoscopic dilatation done sequentially in several sessions is usually sufficient. Additional perspective on this situation is also offered in chapter 32 by André Duranceau.

—Raphael Bueno

References

1. Brinster CJ, Singhal S, Lee L, et al. Evolving options in the management of esophageal perforation. *Ann Thorac Surg.* 2004;77:1475–1483.
2. Kim-Deobald J, Kozarek RA. Esophageal perforation: an 8-year review of a multispecialty clinic's experience. *Am J Gastroenterol.* 1992;87:1112–1119.
3. Salo JA, Isolauri JO, Heikkila LJ, et al. Management of delayed esophageal perforation with mediastinal sepsis: esophagectomy or primary repair? *J Thorac Cardiovasc Surg.* 1993;106:1088–1091.
4. Vial CM, Whyte RI. Boerhaave's syndrome: diagnosis and treatment. *Surg Clin North Am.* 2005;85:515–524.
5. Newton E, Mandavia S. Surgical complications of selected gastrointestinal emergencies: pitfalls in management of the acute abdomen. *Emerg Med Clin North Am.* 2003;21:873–907.
6. Koniaris LG, Spector SA, Staveley-O'Carroll KF. Complete esophageal diversion: a simplified, easily reversible technique. *J Am Coll Surg.* 2004;199:991–993.
7. Jones WG 2nd, Ginsberg RJ. Esophageal perforation: a continuing challenge. *Ann Thorac Surg.* 1992;53:534–543.
8. Bueno R, Swanson SJ, Jaklitsch MT, et al. Combined antegrade and retrograde dilation: a new endoscopic technique in the management of complex esophageal obstruction. *Gastrointest Endosc.* 2001;54:368–372.

32 Complications of Esophageal Surgery

André Duranceau, Wenping Wang, Pasquale Ferraro, and Moishe Liberman

Keywords: Antireflux surgery, minimally invasive surgery, gastroesophageal reflux disease (GERD), iatrogenic injury, vagal nerve injury, organ perforation, gastroesophageal leak

COMPLICATIONS OF OPERATIONS FOR HIATAL HERNIAS AND REFLUX DISEASE

There has been a huge increase in antireflux operations over the last two decades. The emergence of minimally invasive surgery has led to a widening of surgical indications for the operation. Reflux disease remains a functional disorder and it must still be assessed with objectivity if unequivocal evidence of mucosal damage within the esophagus is to be documented before indicating a medical treatment or a surgical approach. As hiatal hernias and reflux esophagitis have been closely associated over the last half century, complications in their surgical management will be treated together.

Preoperative Complications

Gastroesophageal reflux disease (GERD) is a pathologic reflux disorder that causes mucosal damage. The presence of symptoms suggestive of reflux without any mucosal alteration is considered a functional reflux disorder.[1] As all humans have physiologic episodes of reflux, the diagnosis, to be clear, must be based on objective criteria if a wrong diagnosis with its unhappy results is to be avoided. Operations should not be planned on the basis of symptoms, alone, as they bear little relationship to the degree of damage present in the esophagus. At a minimum, radiologic and endoscopic documentation of the disease must be obtained. Classification of damage using the MUSE (**M**etaplasia, **U**lcerations, **S**tricturing, and **E**rosions) classification or the Los Angeles classification are considered objective as they only consider mucosal breaks in the esophagus to be evidence of damage (Table 32-1).

Complications during the Operation

Most of the antireflux operations completed today are by laparoscopic approach. The reported morbidity varies from 4% to 7% with a 0.1% mortality.[2] Morbidity, however, even if these new approaches have modified its prevalence, must be looked at independently of open abdominal, thoracic, or minimally invasive incisions. Open repairs, especially those utilizing laparotomy, are thought to produce more splenic trauma, primarily during mobilization of the gastric fundus for fundoplication or by simple traction on the omentum causing avulsion of adhesions on the splenic capsule. The open approach is also associated with a greater number of incisional hernias. However, the transition from open surgery to minimally invasive operations has not resulted in morbidity becoming part of the past. Looking at medical liability issues in Canada in 109 closed liability files allowed us to document that while 37% of these files before the era of minimally invasive surgery were related to antireflux operations, that proportion increased to 76% during the 15-year period following the appearance of the new approach. Central issues for complaint were mostly iatrogenic injuries incurred during the operation. Organ perforations (esophagus, stomach, small and large bowel) were the most frequent complications. Vagal nerve injuries were responsible for 7% of these files, whereas major vessel (vena cava, left hepatic vein, aorta, inferior pulmonary vein) injuries accounted for 8%. Splenic injury also remained a major source of intraoperative complications. These lesions emphasize the need for conversion readiness whenever immediate control of bleeding is needed. Although a 1% to 3% prevalence of splenic injury is reported during open repairs[3,4] in a much larger cohort of patients treated laparoscopically, the overall frequency of splenic injury was only 0.2%.[5]

Esophageal perforation results from blind dissection of the posterior intra-abdominal esophagus. Urschel[6] reported it in 2% of operated patients. Zaninotto et al.[7] reported the complication in 1% of patients with a minimally invasive approach. Dissection under direct vision with palpation when open, or careful visual mobilization during laparoscopy, should prevent the problem. When present, the traumatized organ must be repaired primarily, observing all the principles of esophageal perforation repair. Healthy tissue coverage over the repair

Table 32-1

THE MUSE (*METAPLASIA, ULCERATION, STRICTURE, EROSION*) CLASSIFICATION

	METAPLASIA	ULCERATION	STRICTURE	EROSION
Grade 0	M0 absent	U0 absent	S0 absent	E0 absent
Grade 1	M1 one	U1 one	S1 >9 mm	E1 one
Grade 2	M2 circumferential	U2 ≥ 2	S2 ≤9	E2 circumferential

The Los Angeles Classification

Grade A	≥1 Mucosal break <5 mm long that dose not extend between the tops of 2 mucosal folds
Grade B	≥1 Mucosal break >5 mm long that dose not extend between the tops of 2 mucosal folds
Grade C	≥1 Mucosal break that extends between the tops of ≥2 mucosal folds involving <75% of the esophageal circumference
Grade D	≥1 Mucosal break that involves ≥75% of the esophageal circumference

is essential. Inadvertent gastrotomy or enterotomy usually results from inappropriate manipulation or from the excessive use of the cautery. In Urschel's report, gastroesophageal leaks occurred in 2% of open antireflux surgery and this increased to 8% if previous hiatal surgery had been completed.

Nerve injury to both vagal trunks can occur during the esophageal dissection or when constructing the fundic wrap around the esophagus. Reoperations are always seen as a major risk for vagal injury, especially those with a thoracic approach. When this occurs, delayed gastric emptying with gastric outlet obstruction can be expected. Pyloric dilatation or an eventual pyloromyotomy or pyloroplasty can be planned after a reasonable attempt at conservative management. Pneumothorax may occur when an abdominal or a minimally invasive approach is used, or when using a left thoracic incision, and consequently is part of the repair. Entry into the right chest through the middle mediastinum behind the heart is considered an important part of the operation for repair of the hiatus for both antireflux and massive paraesophageal hernia repairs. This ensures proper identification of the right diaphragmatic crus for proper suture positioning on both cruses behind the esophagus. The additional use of mesh is not indicated with this technique.

Postoperative Complications

Immediate: Intra-abdominal Infections

Complications resulting in fistula formation are rare but may result from unrecognized injuries during the dissection or from poorly repaired injuries during the operation. Thick stitches on the wall of the esophagogastric junction can produce similar results when transmural necrosis occurs at their level. Prolonged ileus and progressive abdominal or mediastinal sepsis must be managed aggressively by reoperation to obtain control of the contamination site. Emergency esophagectomy or gastrectomy may even be indicated to control the septic condition.

Bleeding, although rare, may result from direct injury to the liver or spleen or from poor hemostasis on the gastrosplenic vessels.

Early

Dysphagia following antireflux operations usually results from unmeasured tension exerted by the fundic wrap on the esophageal wall. Although dysphagia may be transient when influenced by postoperative inflammation and with the repair, it may persist over time if the tension exerted affects the integrity of the esophageal lumen. This is usually prevented by using a 48F or 50F bougie within the esophageal lumen during the repair. Severe dysphagia can also result from tight crural sutures behind the esophagus. This is rarely seen when the index finger passes easily between the newly repaired hiatus and the esophageal wall at the end of the repair. A total fundoplication made too long will result in the same obstructive effects. Reoperation becomes indicated if complete obstruction is present or if significant obstruction persists over time. Acute early herniation of the fundoplication or even major portions of the stomach may occur after complete dissection of the hiatus with division of the phrenoesophageal attachments. Tenuous suture repair of the hiatus with significant intra-abdominal pressure may simply push the stomach above the hiatus. This is seen mostly in obese patients or in patients who produce sudden pressure increases immediately after the operation. The presence of shortened esophagus, as seen with stricture or in patients with massive hernias or with a circumferential Barrett esophagus, is usually the result of a repair under tension if a standard antireflux operation has been used: early migration in the mediastinum is frequently seen in these patients.

Late

Failure of the antireflux repair over time may be secondary to wrap disruption or malposition of the wrap around the gastric smaller curvature. A slipped fundoplication from a periesophageal position to a perigastric position creates an hourglass stomach with reflux symptoms and dysphagia. Pressure of the fundoplication on a tightly closed hiatus may produce this complication, especially if the wrap has not been fixed to the esophageal wall and if the esophagus is shortened. Complete transhiatal herniation of the wrap usually results from a deficient hiatal repair or from an esophagus shortened by disease. If a partial fundoplication has been completed, reflux disease will result with the fundoplication in the chest. If a total fundoplication has been used, it may still offer good reflux control even if in the mediastinum. Proper gastric drainage is important in that situation and the hiatus must be widely open to allow easy emptying of the herniated stomach.

Complications Related to Massive Hernia Repair

Massive paraesophageal hernias show a failure rate of 10% to 18% when an open abdominal approach is used. Maziak and Pearson[8,9] when using an elongation gastroplasty reported a recurrence rate of 4%. Laparoscopic repair of paraesophageal hernias shows an early recurrence rate of 15% to 66%. The three significant aspects of massive hernia repairs that are still open to discussion in the surgical literature are: first, the notion of esophageal shortening, second, the prevalence of reflux disease and its evolution and third, the large hiatal defect. These three factors are probably influential in the early failure rate of the operations selected to treat them.

COMPLICATIONS OF OPERATIONS FOR MOTOR DISORDERS

Primary esophageal dysfunction is seen at the pharyngoesophageal junction or on the esophageal body and at the esophagogastric junction. Cricopharyngeal myotomy is the preferred treatment offered to patients with oropharyngeal dysphagia of various causes. Esophageal body myotomy and the modified Heller myotomy aim at controlling symptoms resulting from primary esophageal motor disorders. These operations, even if successful in the majority of patients, can be responsible for significant morbidity and even mortality.

Operations on the Pharyngoesophageal Sphincter

Idiopathic Oropharyngeal Dysphagia

This form of idiopathic dysphagia affects the cricopharyngeus but has no neurologic or muscular condition to explain it. It is seen as an obstructive upper esophageal sphincter by itself or accompanied by its complication, the pharyngoesophageal or Zenker diverticulum. The cause for the muscle abnormality resulting in this constrictive and obstructive condition remains unknown. In the previous era, when no antibiotics were available, it was considered a treacherous problem where inflammation, perforation, mediastinitis, tracheoesophageal fistulas, and carcinoma formation could be expected when untreated. These complications are rarely seen today. Still, 61% of patients treated today complain of dysphagia and 17% mention aspiration episodes and pulmonary symptoms.[10] Complications at operation for Zenker diverticulum may first be related to poor exposure. We prefer an incision along the anterior border of the sternocleidomastoid muscle, which allows wide exposure of the pharyngoesophageal junction. Small oblique incisions along the skin lines are limiting. These incisions were used in all the patients presenting with an incomplete myotomy that had failed to improve the oropharyngeal dysphagia.[11] Sacrifice of the superficial branch of the cervical cutaneous nerve results in hypoesthesia and paresthesia of the ipsilateral submandibular area. This may subside over time.

The diverticulum, if large, is usually visualized under the buccopharyngeal fascia, the fibroareolar tissue covering the posterior pharyngoesophageal junction. As the majority of the diverticula seen today are smaller than 3 cm, they can be easily missed if this fascia is not opened, allowing protrusion of the diverticulum. Once exposed, its tip is seized with a small Duval clamp and lifted to allow the safe insertion of an intraesophageal bougie. This bougie serves as a stent to support the myotomy, while also protecting the esophageal lumen integrity. As diverticulectomy alone for a Zenker has been reported to result in a high recurrence rate over time, a myotomy or myectomy of the pharyngoesophageal junction is considered the essential part of the treatment whereas diverticulectomy or diverticulum suspension is seen as treatment for the complication of the dysfunction.

Mucosal perforation during the myotomy is usually recognized and repaired using small resorbable sutures. When the diverticulum is resected, the endoluminal bougie is there to prevent narrowing of the esophageal lumen during the resection. The resection line is usually made transverse. When the diverticulum is suspended, its tip is usually tied to the transected muscle margin of the hypopharynx. Fixation to the prevertebral fascia has been seen to cause fasciitis and osteomyelitis as the sutures made through the tip of the diverticulum are considered contaminated. To be complete, a cricopharyngeal myotomy must include the fibers of the inferior constrictor of the pharynx, the cricopharyngeus, itself, and a small portion of the cervical esophagus musculature. The cut margins of the myotomy must allow outpouching of the mucosa over 50% of the circumference to avoid reclosure of the myotomy.

Postoperative complications may be significant. This is not only related to the technique, but also to age as a majority of those patients are elderly and frail. Wound infection and fistula formation are the most frequent complications seen. For a one-stage diverticulectomy, the reported infection rate was 3%, with half of these patients showing a fistula. In our own experience, with close to 100 patients, infection was the most frequent complication. The fistula rate was 1.5%. The Mayo Clinic experience suggests a recurrent nerve palsy in 3% of their 888 patients.[12] When reoperated, however, patients can expect the morbidity to increase to as high as 20%, explained by a more difficult mobilization of structures. When a fistula occurs, wide drainage of the wound is preferred as a first step. If there is no spontaneous early closure, a pedicled muscle flap of the sternocleidomastoid muscle is used to repair the fistula.

Recurrences were seen in 7% of Payne's experience with 164 patients followed 5 to 14 years. Nicholson[13] in a radiologic follow-up of 20 patients showed that 13 had a recurrent pouch. Hansen et al.[14] saw recurrences in 3 of 19 patients, Bertelsen and Aasted[15] in 14 of 68 cases, and Einarsson and Hallen[16] in 17 of 20 patients. Pouch formation probably develops over a significant period of time. This emphasizes that long-term radiologic documentation is necessary if objective results are to be obtained. When only cricopharyngeal myotomy is offered to treat the diverticulum, less than satisfactory results are found in patients in whom a small but dependent pouch persists.

Endoscopic esophagodiverticulostomy had initially been popularized by Dohlman using coagulation and, later, using laser to create a single lumen between the diverticulum and the cervical esophagus.[17] The use of surgical linear staplers has gained popularity in recent years. Initially proposed for high-risk patients, it has now been used in large reported series. Although clinical results seem less satisfactory, the complication rate is low. Decreased operating time and avoidance of recurrent nerve injury are often proposed as advantages. Chang et al.[18] report a 2% complication rate without mortality. These include dental complications (7%), fever (4%), aspiration pneumonia (0.7%), and esophageal perforation (0.7%). Transient cord paralysis was seen in one patient. Case and Baron[19] reported minor bleeding in 23%, perforation in 27%, and neck abscesses in 4.5% of treated patients.

Neurologic, Myogenic, and Idiopathic Dysphagia

Table 32-2 describes the morbidity and mortality resulting from cricopharyngeal myotomy for indications other than Zenker's diverticulum. With proper selection, significant improvement in oropharyngeal dysphagia can be obtained.

Although in neurologic patients the dysphagia is usually related to poor coordination between swallowing, pharyngeal contraction, and upper sphincter relaxation, patients with muscular dysphagia have symptoms resulting from poor pharyngeal contraction and propulsion with incomplete sphincter opening. Adequate symptom documentation and quantification with videoradiologic assessment are essential for appropriate patient selection. Complications related to the myotomy in these patients are less frequent than in Zenker's patients. Mucosal penetration, although frequent, is rarely followed by infection or fistula formation. Campbell et al.,[20] however, report pharyngeal leaks in 8% of their patients. In our experience, primary repair with resorbable sutures or a pedicled muscle flap is usually satisfactory to prevent this complication. Persistent aspiration with pulmonary complications may have to be approached by a permanent tracheostomy with laryngeal diversion or resection.

Table 32-2

CRICOPHARYNGEAL MYOTOMY MORBIDITY AND MORTALITY

	NEUROLOGIC 28 PATIENTS	MYOGENIC 153 PATIENTS	IDIOPATHIC 129 PATIENTS
Technical Complications			
Mucosal tear	1	9	0
Fistula	0	0	2
Infection	1	3	12
Systemic Complications			
Pulmonary	6	10	6
Cardiac	3	8	7
Urinary	3	3	9
Metabolic	2	3	3
Mortality	0	4	0

Mortality was seen mostly in the muscular dysphagia group (4%) and is always secondary to severe lung infection.

Operations on the Esophageal Body and the Lower Esophageal Sphincter

Achalasia

Achalasia is the most frequent and best described esophageal motor dysfunction. The diagnostic criteria are well established and recently three types of the same abnormalities were proposed to classify these dysfunctions.[21] A wrong diagnosis remains a possibility as a number of medical conditions can mimic this primary disorder clinically, radiologically, and manometrically. Pseudoachalasia by an obstructive subcardial lesion must especially be ruled out before reaching the diagnosis. A comprehensive approach to investigation is essential to allow an objective diagnosis in all patients and prevent misdirected therapy.

Preoperative Complications They are related primarily to the consequences of esophageal retention/obstruction. Aspiration pneumonia was reported in 10% of patients by Ellis and Olsen[22] and Clouse and Lustman,[23] whereas Effler et al.[24] observed nocturnal aspiration in 24% of their patients and Black et al.[25] in 46%. Olsen[26] reported a 10% incidence of pulmonary infection in their series, including a chronic form of mycobacterial infection suspected to be caused by the fatty supernatant found frequently in the achalasic esophagus. Acute airway obstruction may require rapid intubation. This is seen mostly with end-stage achalasia. One of the dreaded complications is massive aspiration during the induction of anesthesia. Allen and Clagett reported that one of the two deaths in their series resulted from that complication.[27] Whenever an esophagus is dilated with documented retention, a safe approach remains a liquid diet for the days preceding the operation, emptying and lavage of the esophagus the morning of the operation, and awake intubation by the anesthetist before the induction of anesthesia.

Intraoperative Complications These are related to the technique and to the type of approach selected. Even to this day there is no consensus on what an ideal myotomy for achalasia should be. The modified Heller myotomy in use today varies significantly in length on the esophagus and in its extension on the gastric wall. Independent of the surgical approach selected, the principles for treatment should be identical: remove the obstructive effect of the lower esophageal sphincter. The overall mortality reported varies between 0.7% and 2.8% with smaller series showing a higher mortality.[28] Mucosal perforations during the myotomy are usually inadvertent and immediately repaired using resorbable sutures. Andreollo and Earlam[29] documented mucosal penetration in 1.1% of their review of over 5000 myotomies. This led to a fistula and empyema in 0.4% of all patients. Moreno González et al.[30] found a similar prevalence in their European study. In most large series, the morbidity is related to mucosal penetration. Ellis[31] reported it in 25 of their 262 patients whereas Okike et al.[32] observed leaks and sepsis in 1% of their 468 patients. Repeat myotomies are at higher risk of mucosal damage.[33–35] Little et al.[36] proposed a posterior myotomy in this situation to improve the safety of the operation. Mortality in surgery for achalasia is usually the immediate consequence of fistula formation and sepsis. In view of the severity of this technical mishap, added protection after the repair is indicated with the use of a partial fundoplication, or pleural or muscular flap, depending on the level of the mucosal damage in the myotomized area.

Persistent dysphagia immediately after the operation usually results from an incomplete myotomy.[37] Reoperation gives satisfactory results in 75% of the group.

Paraesophageal hernias are usually the result of a disrupted hiatus after the operation. This complication has been reported frequently in open surgery series.[38–41] Immediate reoperation is indicated to prevent complications on the herniated stomach or on the mucosa denuded of its muscularis. Anatomic restoration of the hiatus with a partial Belsey-type fundoplication should allow a proper seal of the abdominal cavity from the chest.

Late Complications Complications can result from altering the function of the lower esophageal sphincter;[38–41] or when esophageal body dysfunction is not modified by the operation and aperistalsis persists; an insufficient myotomy fails to relieve dysphagia; or adequate sphincter division exposes to the possibility of reflux disease.

When dysphagia recurs 6 months to 1 year after the operation, this usually suggests healing of the myotomy.[31,42] The absence of esophagitis at endoscopy with a competent lower esophageal sphincter on manometry and at endoscopy suggests either rehealing or an incomplete myotomy. Difficulty in identifying the myotomy zone at the operation usually confirms that impression. Periesophageal sclerosis with hyalinization also has been reported by Fekete and Lortat-Jacob[37] and Peracchia et al.[43] Recurrent dysphagia is also seen with late-stage achalasia. Esophageal cancer must be ruled out.

Reflux esophagitis and stricture are the most frequent complications of the modified Heller myotomy. Extension of the myotomy on the gastric wall is considered important but if the myotomy extends more than 2 cm on the stomach, reflux disease will result in all patients.[44,45] Reflux disease increases with the passage of time: 24% at 1 year, 48% at 10 years, and stabilization at 52% after 13 years. At that time, 19% of patients present with a stricture. The more objective the evaluation, the higher the prevalence of reflux complications on the esophageal mucosa. Failed myotomies are predominantly caused by peptic esophagitis. Long-term reflux exposure may induce the appearance of columnar-lined metaplasia with its related morbidity. Ulcerations, fistulas, strictures, perforations, and malignant transformation may ensue if the condition goes untreated.

Diverticulization of the myotomized esophagus is another potential problem. The longer the myotomy on the esophageal body, the higher the chances of observing progressive diverticulization of the mucosa through the myotomized area. This has been observed in over 60% of patients with a long myotomy. It happened in patients with a total fundoplication at the end of their myotomy but also in those who had a partial fundoplication of the Belsey type.[46,47] We have now reduced the length of the myotomy to 4 cm, when the lower esophageal sphincter alone is divided. Extension on the stomach is 2 cm. The myotomy zone is then completely covered by the partial fundoplication. Dysphagia is well controlled, the denuded mucosa is protected, but reflux control remains imperfect.

The advent of minimally invasive operations has significantly influenced the management of achalasia patients. This approach, however, must respect the same principles for treatment. The same objective reassessment must take place to rule out the complications that have been documented in open surgery series. Achalasia patients are at increased risk of developing a cancer.

This risk is about 140-fold than that of the general population.[48] This has not been modified by cardiomyotomy. When achalasia is untreated for more than 20 years, the esophageal mucosa irritation by the stagnant and putrescent food is seen as increasing the risk for transformation significantly.[49] Once treated by myotomy, 1.5% to 2.2% of the patients can be expected to develop an esophageal cancer.[50,51]

Spastic Disorders

Spastic or hyperdynamic esophageal disorders include diffuse esophageal spasm, hyperperistalsis, and the hypertensive lower esophageal sphincter. The importance of obtaining an objective and reliable diagnosis cannot be overemphasized. A wrong diagnosis and a wrong orientation in treatment are bound to produce poor results.[52]

The high strung personality in these patients requires special care and evaluation. Following psychological evaluation and treatment with calcium channel blocking agents and anxiety medication, endoscopic botulinum injection can be considered.[53] Surgery is never a first approach in treatment. When an epiphrenic diverticulum is present, most patients are found to have an associated spastic disorder. Treatment in that condition must be similar to that of achalasia. Division of the lower esophageal sphincter must accompany the esophageal body myotomy to the upper level of the diverticulum as the lower sphincter shows intermittent abnormal relaxation. Failure to extend the myotomy on the stomach wall may result in significant morbidity and even mortality, especially if a diverticulectomy has created a suture line on the esophageal body.[54] The complications of myotomy for spastic disorders are similar to those seen and reported for achalasia.

COMPLICATIONS OF ESOPHAGEAL INJURY

Injury to the esophageal wall may result from multiple causes. Those have been summarized by Bladergroen et al.[55] in their series: 55% are iatrogenic, 15% are spontaneous or postemetic (barotrauma), 14% are secondary to foreign-body impaction and/or transgression, and 10% are seen after a trauma. Five to seven percent of esophageal perforations are associated with the evolution of an esophageal pathology. Trends in survival have improved over the last 50 years, mainly the result of earlier diagnosis and treatment as well as improvement in intensive care management. However, the overall mortality remains high at 22% and is still significantly influenced by the delay in diagnosis.[56] Thoracic esophageal perforations result in a 20% to 30% mortality if the repair is completed within the first 24 hours after the rupture. The mortality exceeds 60% when more than 24 hours have passed since the perforation. Extensive mediastinal contamination by the buccopharyngeal flora is usually responsible for the rapid progression of pain, sepsis, and shock. For these reasons, procrastination in the investigation and management of these patients can only lead to uncontrollable sepsis and mortality. Treatment of mediastinitis requires correction or removal of the cause. Surgery is urgent, especially if best supportive care does not result in stabilization and improvement. For these reasons, in patients remaining septic after a delay in diagnosis of more than 72 hours, resection of the perforated esophagus with creation of a long parasternal esophagostome with gastric decompression and feeding jejunostomy has been shown by Gouge et al.[57] to be a safe and life-saving approach. Esophageal replacement is best delayed for when the patient is well recuperated from these events.

Complications after Primary Surgical Repair

Esophageal perforations require thorough cleaning and debridement of contaminants and necrotic tissue in the mediastinum. With the pleural contamination and empyema resulting from complete decortication one must permit full reexpansion of the pulmonary parenchyma. Once the esophagus is freed from its mediastinal attachments, the perforated area is inspected and debrided of all damaged esophageal muscle. The muscular layer must be myotomized to clarify the length of the mucosal laceration underneath. Once all layers of the esophageal wall are clearly identified, a single-layer repair of the esophageal wall is preferred using large resorbable sutures positioned with a distance of 0.5 cm from each other. As this repair is completed in a contaminated field, coverage protection with a muscular flap, thickened pleura, or healthy gastric fundic tissue is indicated. Gouge[57], in his review, documented that persistent sepsis and fistula formation occurred in 39% of all patients when the repair was completed without any buttressing. The mortality resulting was then 25%. If the same repair without coverage is made in patients with a late repair, persistent leaks and sepsis will be seen in 50% of treated patients. When the added protection of a well-vascularized muscle flap or fundic tissue is added, the documented fistula formation is reduced to 13% and the mortality to 6%. Richardson[58] reports persistent leaks in 17% and a mortality of 1.5% when the primary repair is covered with the added protection of a pleural or muscle flap. In those patients with a delayed diagnosis or a perforation related to esophageal disease, 13 of 14 patients undergoing an esophagectomy had excellent results. Vogel et al.[59] reported treating 47 patients with aggressive drainage of collections and frequent radiographic studies using gastrografin and computerized tomography documentation of the evolution. Two of 37 patients with thoracic perforations died but 34 patients were considered healed at discharge without operative treatment. Wright et al.[60] reported on 28 patients receiving either early or late treatment. All had reinforced primary closure. None of the patients treated early died and two showed a contained leak. Among those 13 receiving late treatment, 7 leaks occurred and 4 deaths resulted.

Alternative methods of treatment result in high morbidity and mortality: pleural drainage 43% to 66%, esophageal exclusion 35% to 42%, T-tube directed fistula with drainage 36% to 50%. Esophageal exclusion entails a complex reconstruction. More recently Linden et al.[61] treated esophageal perforations in 43 patients with the use of T-tube drainage. Their observed morbidity was 47% with a mortality of 7%. If the condition was treated early, the mortality was 5%. If the diagnosis was delayed, it was 8.7%. If treatment was offered in less than 24 hours, the morbidity was less than 20%. This increased to 42% when the diagnosis was obtained between 24 and 72 hours, and to 82% if later than 72 hours.

A number of reports on endoscopic management of esophageal perforations have appeared in the literature with the appearance and popularity of self-expanding stents as an additional tool to help palliation and treatment of esophageal disease.[62] Most published series, however, where stents are used to treat perforations are either for instrumental perforations or for postoperative fistula formation. Metallic stents must be fully covered to allow removal once healing is complete. Uncovered stents lead to progressive esophageal wall encrustation and they cannot be removed later. In a contaminated cavity, metallic stents also have been reported to erode into major vessels. The potential advantages of covered stents remain the reduction or elimination of the contamination, the possibility of better nutrition if the damaged area is well sealed, and the return to a normal healed structure after removal of the stent.[63]

External trauma to the esophagus may be difficult to document on account of the presence of associated conditions. Delays that usually result might explain the overall complication rate of 47% to 53% and 7% to 19% mortality reported from major trauma centers.[64]

Caustic Injury

Whether accidental or self-induced, ingestion of caustic agents may result in significant damage to the esophageal wall. Type and concentration of the agent and duration of the exposure will influence the extent of damage.

Alkali Agents

Sodium hydroxide causes liquefaction necrosis of the esophageal mucosa with rapid diffusion through the esophageal wall within 30 seconds of the exposure. Cell destruction with inflammation and vascular thrombosis follows. Secondary bacterial invasion supervenes. Necrotic tissue sloughing results in granulation deposition and chronic fibrotic strictures. The constant deposition of fibrous tissue is responsible for lifelong strictures.

Acid Agents

Strong acids (sulfuric, sulfanic, nitric) when exposed to the esophageal mucosa cause rapid coagulation of tissues on contact. Prolongation of the exposure results in deeper damage that may progress to transmural inflammation, necrosis, and perforation. With the ingestion of strong acids, as the longer exposure is frequently in the stomach, distal gastric wall damage is often documented as the end result of the exposure.

The ingestion of solid or liquid lye results in the greatest morbidity. Progressive and recurrent esophageal strictures with malnutrition and chronic aspirations are seen frequently. Normal esophageal function is lost.[24] Ten to twenty-five percent of patients present with chronic strictures requiring treatment. The liquid form of lye causes the worst damage. Anderson et al.[65] documented that no benefit can be expected from the use of corticosteroids to prevent damage. When initial assessment reveals mucosal necrosis and ulcerations, acute mediastinitis will be present in 20% and up to 15% of esophageal perforation will occur. The mortality approximates 5% and is usually related to extensive necrosis requiring total esophagectomy and total gastrectomy. Esophageal cancer may develop 30 to 40 years after the insult: its incidence is 1000 times greater in lye stricture patients when compared to the general population.[66,67] The severity of the stricture will usually be the indication for an esophageal resection with reconstruction using either the stomach or the colon.

Foreign Bodies

Food impaction is the most frequent cause for obstruction by a foreign body seen in adults. Some materials may be pointed or sharp and perforate the esophageal wall. Usually the impaction and subsequent damage will result from pressure and progressive erosion and ulceration through the esophageal wall. The fragility of the wall with the inflammation and relative ischemia may explain the ease of instrumental perforation when attempting to extract these impacted boluses.

When a foreign body remains impacted in the esophagus or progresses into the stomach cavity after impaction, 40% of patients will show an esophageal injury. With persistent impaction, superficial lacerations are seen in 28%, deeper wounds in 9%, and perforations in 4%.When the impacted bolus has progressed into the stomach, lacerations are still seen frequently but perforations are rarely documented. When bones are part of the impacted bolus, more injuries occur (76%) and perforations are seen more often (8%). Pure food impaction is considered as less threatening.

Endoscopic extraction is usually followed by radiologic control of the esophageal wall integrity. Wide-spectrum antibiotics are administered if there is any doubt of mediastinal contamination. Rapid initiation of treatment, with or without stent installation, is mandatory as soon as a perforation is documented. Close monitoring may dictate a surgical approach with a reinforced repair of the damaged area if the contamination area is not controlled and results in sepsis progression.

COMPLICATIONS OF ESOPHAGECTOMY

Esophagectomy is the most extensive operation performed in thoracic surgery. The risks related to the operation parallel its importance. Complications related to the underlying condition will not be considered here. Difficulties, morbidity, and mortality resulting from the operation itself are to be considered.

Preoperative Complications

Besides the natural evolution of conditions indicating an esophagectomy, especially when a malignancy is present, a number of key points should be considered if morbidity and mortality are to be anticipated and prevented.

Patient Selection

A good general condition with an adequate cardiopulmonary reserve is essential. Patients who have lost more than 10% of their body weight rapidly are at risk of morbidity, especially if already debilitated. Patients in their eighth decade, even if well in appearance, have a limited capacity to react to any form of trauma or complication. Heavy smokers should help themselves by complete abstinence from tobacco before the operation. Complications in these patients are not limited to the high risk of lung infection. Risks to the vascular supply of the interposed organ to be used as replacement must be part of the informed consent given to the patients. Catastrophic necrosis of the proximal stomach is seen mostly in this category of patients. In our multi- and univariate analysis of complications following esophagectomy, tobacco smoking remained the most significant risk factor resulting in pulmonary and vascular complications to the interposed stomach. A number of studies looking at risk factors and risk factor scores in patients undergoing esophagectomy have been published.[68–72]

Hospital Volume

This is considered an important aspect to be considered by those interested in the management of esophageal diseases. Esophagectomy is a complex operation that should not be completed by a surgeon who can realize it only occasionally. Begg et al.[73] reported that whenever esophagectomies are completed by a surgeon who does fewer than five per year, the hospital mortality approximates 17%. This mortality decreases to 3.4% in high-volume hospitals.[74] These facts have led to regionalized care in many countries.

Operative Complications

Esophagectomy can be completed through a number of approaches (see Chapters 12–22). Complications during the operation can occur in the abdomen, in both chest cavities, or in the neck. In the abdomen, splenic injury may occur by either simple traction on the greater omentum during exploration or during the mobilization of the gastrosplenic vessels for the preparation of the gastric interposition. Conservative measures are used first for splenic conservation, as the bleeding lesion is usually limited to the capsule. If significant bleeding persists at the completion of the operation, a splenectomy is preferred. Mobilization of the stomach and duodenum may result in injury of the head of the pancreas. And if extensive node dissection is carried along the celiac axis, on the superior border of the pancreas, injury can occur as well, resulting in postoperative pancreatitis. If any damage is suspected, peripancreatic drainage is advisable. An extramucosal pyloromyotomy is usually completed to favor better gastric emptying. Once the mucosa is freed, the horizontal muscular layer is reapproximated vertically to insure pyloric enlargement. Mucosal penetration is rare but usually occurs on the anterior recess of the duodenal mucosa. If this is seen, the myotomy is transformed into a formal pyloroplasty closed by a single layer of separate sutures then covered by an epiploplasty.

A feeding jejunostomy is added in all esophagectomy patients as insurance against either potential complications or to prevent any malnutrition especially during the readaptation period after esophagectomy. The jejunostomy is created with a no. 18 t-tube installed on the antimesenteric border of the first jejunal loop. It is exteriorized and secured in a left paramedial position. Feeding is usually started on the third or fourth day after the operation when active peristalsis is heard. Resection of the diaphragmatic hiatus is considered part of the esophageal resection. The left pleura is frequently opened during this part of the procedure. Drainage of the left chest cavity is performed as insurance against the development of pneumothorax and for the prevention of pleural effusion which is frequent after resection. Complications during the thoracic part of the operation require attention to the azygos and hemiazygos veins especially if a modified radical resection is preferred where all intercostal veins are dissected and ligated to remove the vein "en bloc" with the thoracic duct and the adventitia of the aorta. Other risk areas for operative complications are injuries to the membranous trachea and bronchi, for example, the left recurrent laryngeal nerve lying deep in the mediastinum while the retrotracheal esophagus is dissected and the thoracic duct emerging behind the right crus of the diaphragm with some branches lying occasionally on the adjacent vertebral bodies. Most of the life-threatening vascular injuries (1.4%) have been reported during transhiatal esophagectomy (see Chapter 16).[75] Dissection in the left neck is frequently completed with resection of the left clavicular head in continuity with the manubrium and first rib. Once the deep cervical fascia is opened, the esophageal remnant is easily accessible if mobilization of the esophagus has been completed in the right chest. Safe and careful dissection of the left recurrent laryngeal nerve is usually completed under direct vision.

Postoperative Complications

Early Complications

Cardiac Complications These are mostly supraventricular arrhythmias and myocardial infarctions. This is recorded in over 35% of operated patients. Patients with ischemia on preoperative evaluation must be treated before proceeding to esophagectomy.

Pulmonary Complications These are mostly infectious and related to atelectasis and pneumonia. The respiratory distress syndrome with respiratory insufficiency is seen mostly in patients who have received neoadjuvant chemoradiotherapy. Prevention of atelectasis by early mobilization, physiotherapy, and aggressive tracheobronchial toilet is essential. This has been helped significantly by offering epidural analgesia for the postoperative period until the chest tubes are removed. Gastric tube decompression is insured to prevent tracheobronchial aspiration as gastric interposition is recognized as a free duodenogastroesophageal reflux model. Absent gastric retention and active peristalsis signal removal of gastric drainage. If significant restriction of pulmonary function has been documented, the transhiatal approach is preferred to limit the after effects of thoracotomy.[76,77]

Anastomotic Complications Leakage at the anastomosis is always feared after esophagectomy. An intact repair depends on a good vascular supply to the esophageal remnant and to the stomach. Faulty anastomosis, when not technical, is usually the result of poor vascular supply to the proximal part of the stomach. The absence of tension on the reconstruction and healthy transection margins are the other conditions essential to good healing of the anastomosis. When this complication occurs, it causes mediastinitis, pleural contamination, and empyema. The leak rate in the chest seems less frequent than when the anastomosis is in the neck.[78–80] Orringer et al.[81] report a less than 3% leak rate for cervical anastomosis. Although leakage in the neck usually requires wide drainage, leakage in the chest may require a more aggressive approach, especially if it is documented within 48 hours of the operation. This usually means necrosis and dehiscence of the anastomosis which then must be reconstructed immediately if mobilization and transplant quality are there. Sepsis and pneumothorax during the initial postoperative week also suggest disruption of the reconstruction or a vascular complication of the transplant. Reexploration to correct the situation is essential. Repositioning of the stomach in the abdomen and an esophagostome may be necessary. If the leak at the anastomosis is small and contained, a positive evolution can be expected. If, however, significant ischemia and necrosis are present on the proximal stomach, meticulous assessment of the available viable tissue is necessary before deciding if repair must be attempted, usually with a pedicled muscle transplant, or, if a more complex reconstruction must be planned at a later date. For smaller leaks, the use of self-expandable completely covered stents may help in sealing the leak and allowing more rapid healing of the defect.[82,62]

Chylothorax

The prevalence of thoracic duct injury during esophagectomy is approximately 2%. It is reported as more frequent if esophagectomy is completed without thoracotomy.[83,84] Centers recognized for a high esophagectomy volume and experienced with this approach do not confirm this. Early management of large chylous fluid drainage may require temporary intravenous hyperalimentation. Nutritional and immunologic depletions are the disturbing consequences of prolonged conservative management. In their review of the problem, Wemyss-Holden et al.[85] report a mortality rate of 50% to 82% when a conservative approach is maintained. A more aggressive management is suggested by Lagarde et al.[86] If a high daily output persists despite 2 days of optimal conservative therapy, mass ligation of the thoracic duct is advised. We proceed with rethoracotomy over the ninth rib if chest drainage of more than 1000 mL per day persists for more than 5 days.

Recurrent Nerve Palsy

Injury to the left recurrent nerve may occur during exposure of the cervical esophagus in the left neck or during dissection of the esophagus in the chest.[87] In the neck, undue traction or compression results in left vocal cord paralysis. The immediate consequences are significant difficulties in obtaining a successful tracheobronchial toilet. The nonapposition of the cords reduces the efficacy of coughing and increases the risks of pulmonary infection. Oropharyngeal dysphagia may occur later with secondary aspirations. Adaptation, however, will usually result in improvement of the symptoms.

Late Complications

Technically, reconstruction with an end-to-side circular stapler has been shown to cause more strictures, possibly because of the mucosal gap present between the esophageal squamous epithelium and the gastric mucosa after the anastomosis. Strictures are seen mostly if there has been a leak or an infection at the anastomosis level. These strictures may also result from infection around the anastomosis, even if no fistula has become manifest. Early endoscopy with guided dilatation is a safe approach and offers good control of early dysphagia. Over time, narrowing of the anastomosis may also be the result of gastroesophageal reflux affecting the esophageal remnant. This is usually diagnosed by endoscopy as the symptoms are not as typical as in patients with idiopathic reflux disease.[88]

Delayed gastric emptying results from gastric denervation. The pylorus is usually widened by pyloroplasty or pyloromyotomy. If no drainage procedure has been offered gastric retention may be increased, leading to more regurgitations and aspirations.

This can be managed by balloon dilatation, or if persistent in time, by pyloroplasty. The use of proton pump inhibitors (PPIs) with prokinetics (erythromycin, domperidone) has helped with gastric emptying. Duodenogastroesophageal reflux is a mixed refluxate, and the most damaging to the mucosal integrity of the esophageal remnant. Dumping may occur. Diarrhea may be debilitating but it usually decreases within the first 3 to 6 months after the reconstruction.

Hiatal Herniation of Abdominal Content

Resection and widening of the diaphragmatic hiatus may allow some space to persist between the wall of the stomach used for reconstruction and the resected hiatus. Although herniation through that space may be seen acutely immediately after the operation, it is usually seen and documented as a late complication, sometimes many years after the operation. Even if asymptomatic, these hernias must be repaired with closure of the opening that allows herniation.

Complications of the Interposed Stomach or of the Excluded Esophagus

The use of gastric interposition, even if bilateral vagotomy and pyloroplasty is part of the esophageal resection, shows normal acid secretion within a year after reconstruction of the esophagus.[89] The mixed refluxate in the gastric cavity may cause significant damage not only to the esophageal remnant but also to the gastric wall: gastric ulcers can bleed, perforate, or create a gastrobronchial communication. If, in a long-term survivor, damaging reflux disease is documented in the esophageal remnant, antral resection with a Roux-en-Y reconstruction has been shown to offer good results to protect the esophageal remnant.[90] For tracheogastric or bronchogastric fistulas, resection and repair of the affected tracheobronchial tree with resection of the stomach ulcer may control this difficult situation. A well-vascularized muscle transposition may help protect the repaired stomach and the reconstructed tracheobronchial tree.

In the rare situation where the esophagus must be excluded in the mediastinum, it must be decompressed since normal peristaltic activity persists with every swallow. Blowouts of the proximal or distal ends of the excluded esophagus could happen as in any closed loop obstruction. A Foley catheter installed distally as a directed fistula is usually sufficient to prevent these complications.[91] The other complication that can be seen in that situation is a large mediastinal mucocele.

EDITOR'S COMMENT

Complications after any type of esophageal surgery usually have significant impact because of the central role of the esophagus in alimentation and its location, which traverses the neck, thorax, and abdomen. Ensuring that the operation to be done is indicated and that the patient is prepared to undergo the surgery safely is paramount. Precise and careful anatomic dissection is mandatory with particular attention to avoiding esophageal injury and can help improve outcome. In surgery for reflux, for example, appropriate mobilization of the distal intrathoracic esophagus can reduce complications associated with "shortened esophagus." Careful attention to postoperative progress with an almost expectant attitude regarding complications will lead to early identification, prevention, and treatment with lower ultimate mortality and earlier return to normal function. Any suspicious symptom must be aggressively pursued to ensure early diagnosis and treatment of potential esophageal perforation, leak, or necrosis. In this way, mortality can be reduced to less than 1%. The particular solution to a complication must be tailored to fit the specific complication, patient, and institutional expertise.

—Raphael Bueno

References

1. Jameson GG, Duranceau AC. Gastroesophageal reflux. Philadelphia, PA: W.B. Saunders; 1988.
2. Rantanen TK, Salo JA, Sipponen JT. Fatal and life-threatening complications in antireflux surgery: analysis of 5,502 operations. *Br J Surg.* 1999;86(12):1573–1577.
3. Donahue PE, Samelson S, Nyhus LM, et al. The floppy Nissen fundoplication. Effective long-term control of pathologic reflux. *Arch Surg.* 1985;120(6):663–668.
4. DeMeester TR, Bonavina L, Albertucci M. Nissen fundoplication for gastroesophageal reflux disease. Evaluation of primary repair in 100 consecutive patients. *Ann Surg.* 1986;204(1):9–20.
5. Carlson MA, Frantzides CT. Complications and results of primary minimally invasive antireflux procedures: a review of 10,735 reported cases. *J Am Coll Surg.* 2001;193(4):428–439.
6. Urschel JD. Complications of antireflux surgery. *Am J Surg.* 1993;166(1):68–70.
7. Zaninotto G, Molena D, Ancona E. A prospective multicenter study on laparoscopic treatment of gastroesophageal reflux disease in Italy: type of surgery, conversions, complications, and early results. Study Group for the Laparoscopic Treatment of Gastroesophageal Reflux Disease of the Italian Society of Endoscopic Surgery (SICE). *Surg Endosc.* 2000;14(3):282–288.
8. Maziak DE, Todd TR, Pearson FG. Massive hiatus hernia: evaluation and surgical management. *J Thorac Cardiovasc Surg.* 1998;115(1):53–60; discussion 1–2.
9. Pearson FG. Hiatus hernia and gastroesophageal reflux: indications for surgery and selection of operation. *Semin Thorac Cardiovasc Surg.* 1997;9(2):163–168.
10. Duranceau A, Ferraro P. Pharyngeal and cricopharyngeal disorders. In: Patterson GA, Cooper JD, Deslauriers J, Lerut AEMR, Luketich JD, Rice TW, eds. *Pearson's Thoracic and Esophageal Surgery.* Philadelphia, PA: Churchill Livingstone/Elsevier; 2008.
11. Brigand C, Ferraro P, Martin J, et al. Risk factors in patients undergoing cricopharyngeal myotomy. *Br J Surg.* 2007;94(8):978–983.
12. Payne WS, King RM. Pharyngoesophageal (Zenker's) diverticulum. *Surg Clin North Am.* 1983;63(4):815–824.
13. Nicholson WF. The late results of operations for pharyngeal pouch. *Br J Surg.* 1962;49:548–552.
14. Hansen JB, Jagt T, Gundtoft P, et al. Pharyngo-oesophageal diverticula. A clinical and cineradiographic follow-up study of 23 cases treated by diverticulectomy. *Scand J Thorac Cardiovasc Surg.* 1973;7(1):81–86.
15. Bertelsen S, Aasted A. Results of operative treatment of hypopharyngeal diverticulum. *Thorax.* 1976;31(5):544–547.
16. Einarsson S, Hallen O. On the treatment of esophageal diverticula. *Acta Otolaryngol.* 1967;64(1):30–36.
17. Dohlman G, Mattsson O. The endoscopic operation for hypopharyngeal diverticula: a roentgencinematographic study. *AMA Arch Otolaryngol.* 1960;71:744–752.
18. Chang CY, Payyapilli RJ, Scher RL. Endoscopic staple diverticulostomy for Zenker's diverticulum: review of literature and experience in 159 consecutive cases. *Laryngoscope.* 2003;113(6):957–965.
19. Case DJ, Baron TH. Flexible endoscopic management of Zenker diverticulum: the Mayo Clinic experience. *Mayo Clin Proc.* 2010;85(8):719–722.
20. Campbell BH, Tuominen TC, Toohill RJ. The risk and complications of aspiration following cricopharyngeal myotomy. *Am J Med.* 1997;103(5A):61S–63S.
21. Kahrilas PJ. Esophageal motor disorders in terms of high-resolution esophageal pressure topography: what has changed? *Am J Gastroenterol.* 2010;105(5):981–987.
22. Ellis FH Jr., Olsen AM. Achalasia of the esophagus. *Major Probl Clin Surg.* 1969;9:1–221.
23. Clouse RE, Lustman PJ. Psychiatric illness and contraction abnormalities of the esophagus. *N Engl J Med.* 1983;309(22):1337–1342.
24. Effler DB, Loop FD, Groves LK, et al. Primary surgical treatment for esophageal achalasia. *Surg Gynecol Obstet.* 1971;132(6):1057–1063.
25. Black J, Vorbach AN, Collis JL. Results of Heller's operation for achalasia of the oesophagus. The importance of hiatal repair. *Br J Surg.* 1976;63(12):949–953.
26. Olsen AM. The spectrum of aspiration pneumonitis. *Ann Otol Rhinol Laryngol.* 1970;79(5):875–888.
27. Allen TH, Clagett OT. Changing concepts in the surgical treatment of pulsion diverticula of the lower esophagus. *J Thorac Cardiovasc Surg.* 1965;50(4):455–462.
28. Hollender LF, Meyer C, Jamart J, et al. Heller's operation in the treatment of idiopathic mega-esophagus. Reflections on 22 cases. *Med Chir Dig.* 1977;6(2):89–94.
29. Andreollo NA, Earlam RJ. Heller's myotomy for achalasia: is an added antireflux procedure necessary? *Br J Surg.* 1987;74(9):765–769.
30. Moreno González E, Garcia Alvarez A, Landa Garcia I, et al. Results of surgical treatment of esophageal achalasia. Multicenter retrospective study of 1,856 cases. GEEMO (Groupe Europeen Etude Maladies Oesophageennes) Multicentric Retrospective Study. *Int Surg.* 1988;73(2):69–77.
31. Ellis FH Jr. Esophagomyotomy for esophageal achalasia. *Surg Clin North Am.* 1973;53(2):319–325.
32. Okike N, Payne WS, Neufeld DM, et al. Esophagomyotomy versus forceful dilation for achalasia of the esophagus: results in 899 patients. *Ann Thorac Surg.* 1979;28(2):119–125.
33. Fekete F, Breil P, Tossen JC. Reoperation after Heller's operation for achalasia and other motility disorders of the esophagus: a study of eighty-one reoperations. *Int Surg.* 1982;67(2):103–110.
34. Ellis FH Jr., Crozier RE, Watkins E, Jr. Operation for esophageal achalasia. Results of esophagomyotomy without an antireflux operation. *J Thorac Cardiovasc Surg.* 1984;88(3):344–351.
35. Adebo OA, Grillo IA, Osinowo O, et al. Oesophagomyotomy for achalasia of the oesophagus: experience at the University College Hospital, Ibadan. *East Afr Med J.* 1980;57(6):390–398.
36. Little AG, Soriano A, Ferguson MK, et al. Surgical treatment of achalasia: results with esophagomyotomy and Belsey repair. *Ann Thorac Surg.* 1988;45(5):489–494.
37. Fekete F, Lortat-Jacob JL. [Failures and suggested failures of Heller's operation for idiopathic megaoesophagus. Study of 55 reoperated cases (author's transl)]. *Ann Chir.* 1977;31(6):515–524.
38. Frobese AS, Stein GN, Hawthorne HR. Hiatal hernia as a complication of the Heller operation. *Surgery.* 1961;49:599–605.
39. Yon J, Christensen J. An uncontrolled comparison of treatments for achalasia. *Ann Surg.* 1975;182(6):672–676.
40. Vallieres E, Waters PF. Incarcerated parahiatal hernia with gastric necrosis. *Ann Thorac Surg.* 1987;44(1):82–93.
41. Fletcher PR. Acute hiatal hernia with oesophageal perforation following Heller's operation. *Br J Surg.* 1978;65(7):486–488.
42. Bremner CG. Benign strictures of the esophagus. *Curr Probl Surg.* 1982;19(8):401–489.
43. Peracchia A, Nosadini A, Tremolada C, et al. [Reoperation after Heller's operation for megaesophagus]. *Chirurgie.* 1986;112(1):50–55.
44. Jara FM, Toledo-Pereyra LH, Lewis JW, et al. Long-term results of esophagomyotomy for achalasia of esophagus. *Arch Surg.* 1979;114(8):935–936.
45. McVey JL, Schlegel JF, Ellis FH Jr. Gastroesophageal sphincteric function after the Heller myotomy and its modifications. An experimental study. *Bull Soc Int Chir.* 1963;22:419–423.
46. Chen LQ, Chughtai T, Sideris L, et al. Long-term effects of myotomy and partial fundoplication for esophageal achalasia. *Dis Esophagus.* 2002;15(2):171–179.
47. Almarhabi Y, D'Journo XB, Chen LQ, et al. A short 4-cm oesophageal myotomy relieves the obstructive symptoms of achalasia. *Eur J Cardiothorac Surg.* 2009;36(5):894–900.
48. Brucher BL, Stein HJ, Bartels H, et al. Achalasia and esophageal cancer: incidence, prevalence, and prognosis. *World J Surg.* 2001;25(6):745–749.
49. Loviscek LF, Cenoz MC, Badaloni AE, et al. Early cancer in achalasia. *Dis Esophagus.* 1998;11(4):239–247.
50. Liu JF, Zhang J, Tian ZQ, et al. Long-term outcome of esophageal myotomy for achalasia. *World J Gastroenterol.* 2004;10(2):287–291.
51. Zaninotto G, Rizzetto C, Zambon P, et al. Long-term outcome and risk of oesophageal cancer after surgery for achalasia. *Br J Surg.* 2008;95(12):1488–1494.
52. Bombeck CT, Battle WS, Nyhuss LM. Spasm in the differential diagnosis of gastroesophageal reflux. *Arch Surg.* 1972;104(4):477–483.
53. Bashashati M, Andrews C, Ghosh S, et al. Botulinum toxin in the treatment of diffuse esophageal spasm. *Dis Esophagus.* 2010;23(7):554–560.

54. D'Journo XB, Ferraro P, Martin J, et al. Lower oesophageal sphincter dysfunction is part of the functional abnormality in epiphrenic diverticulum. *Br J Surg*. 2009;96(8):892–900.
55. Bladergroen MR, Lowe JE, Postlethwait RW. Diagnosis and recommended management of esophageal perforation and rupture. *Ann Thorac Surg*. 1986;42(3):235–239.
56. Jones WG 2nd, Ginsberg RJ. Esophageal perforation: a continuing challenge. *Ann Thorac Surg*. 1992;53(3):534–543.
57. Gouge TH, Depan HJ, Spencer FC. Experience with the Grillo pleural wrap procedure in 18 patients with perforation of the thoracic esophagus. *Ann Surg*. 1989;209(5):612–617; discussion 7–9.
58. Richardson JD. Management of esophageal perforations: the value of aggressive surgical treatment. *Am J Surg*. 2005;190(2):161–165.
59. Vogel SB, Rout WR, Martin TD, et al. Esophageal perforation in adults: aggressive, conservative treatment lowers morbidity and mortality. *Ann Surg*. 2005;241(6):1016–1021; discussion 21–23.
60. Wright CD, Mathisen DJ, Wain JC, et al. Reinforced primary repair of thoracic esophageal perforation. *Ann Thorac Surg*. 1995;60(2):245–248; discussion 8–9.
61. Linden PA, Bueno R, Mentzer SJ, et al. Modified T-tube repair of delayed esophageal perforation results in a low mortality rate similar to that seen with acute perforations. *Ann Thorac Surg*. 2007;83(3):1129–1133.
62. Swinnen J, Eisendrath P, Rigaux J, et al. Self-expandable metal stents for the treatment of benign upper GI leaks and perforations. *Gastrointest Endosc*. 2011;73(5):890–899.
63. Dantas RO, Mamede RC. Esophageal motility in patients with esophageal caustic injury. *Am J Gastroenterol*. 1996;91(6):1157–1161.
64. Asensio JA, Chahwan S, Forno W, et al. Penetrating esophageal injuries: multicenter study of the American Association for the Surgery of Trauma. *J Trauma*. 2001;50(2):289–296.
65. Anderson KD, Rouse TM, Randolph JG. A controlled trial of corticosteroids in children with corrosive injury of the esophagus. *N Engl J Med*. 1990;323(10):637–640.
66. Moore WR. Caustic ingestions. Pathophysiology, diagnosis, and treatment. *Clin Pediatr (Phila)*. 1986;25(4):192–196.
67. Ramasamy K, Gumaste VV. Corrosive ingestion in adults. *J Clin Gastroenterol*. 2003;37(2):119–124.
68. Lagarde SM, Reitsma JB, Maris AK, et al. Preoperative prediction of the occurrence and severity of complications after esophagectomy for cancer with use of a nomogram. *Ann Thorac Surg*. 2008;85(6):1938–1945.
69. Steyerberg EW, Neville BA, Koppert LB, et al. Surgical mortality in patients with esophageal cancer: development and validation of a simple risk score. *J Clin Oncol*. 2006;24(26):4277–4284.
70. Nagamatsu Y, Shima I, Yamana H, et al. Preoperative evaluation of cardiopulmonary reserve with the use of expired gas analysis during exercise testing in patients with squamous cell carcinoma of the thoracic esophagus. *J Thorac Cardiovasc Surg*. 2001;121(6):1064–1068.
71. Forshaw MJ, Strauss DC, Davies AR, et al. Is cardiopulmonary exercise testing a useful test before esophagectomy? *Ann Thorac Surg*. 2008;85(1):294–299.
72. Ferguson MK, Durkin AE. Preoperative prediction of the risk of pulmonary complications after esophagectomy for cancer. *J Thorac Cardiovasc Surg*. 2002;123(4):661–669.
73. Begg CB, Cramer LD, Hoskins WJ, et al. Impact of hospital volume on operative mortality for major cancer surgery. *JAMA*. 1998;280(20):1747–1751.
74. Metzger R, Bollschweiler E, Vallbohmer D, et al. High volume centers for esophagectomy: what is the number needed to achieve low postoperative mortality? *Dis Esophagus*. 2004;17(4):310–314.
75. Javed A, Pal S, Chaubal GN, et al. Management and outcome of intrathoracic bleeding due to vascular injury during transhiatal esophagectomy. *J Gastrointest Surg*. 2011;15(2):262–266.
76. Donohoe CL, O'Farrell NJ, Ravi N, et al. Evidence-based selective application of transhiatal esophagectomy in a high-volume esophageal center. *World J Surg*. 2012;36(1):98–103.
77. Hulscher JB, van Sandick JW, de Boer AG, et al. Extended transthoracic resection compared with limited transhiatal resection for adenocarcinoma of the esophagus. *N Engl J Med*. 2002;347(21):1662–1669.
78. Biere SS, Maas KW, Cuesta MA, et al. Cervical or thoracic anastomosis after esophagectomy for cancer: a systematic review and meta-analysis. *Dig Surg*. 2011;28(1):29–35.
79. Hulscher JB, Tijssen JG, Obertop H, et al. Transthoracic versus transhiatal resection for carcinoma of the esophagus: a meta-analysis. *Ann Thorac Surg*. 2001;72(1):306–313.
80. Iannettoni MD, Whyte RI, Orringer MB. Catastrophic complications of the cervical esophagogastric anastomosis. *J Thorac Cardiovasc Surg*. 1995;110(5):1493–500; discussion 500–501.
81. Orringer MB, Marshall B, Iannettoni MD. Eliminating the cervical esophagogastric anastomotic leak with a side-to-side stapled anastomosis. *J Thorac Cardiovasc Surg*. 2000;119(2):277–288.
82. van Boeckel PG, Sijbring A, Vleggaar FP, et al. Systematic review: temporary stent placement for benign rupture or anastomotic leak of the oesophagus. *Aliment Pharmacol Ther*. 2011;33(12):1292–1301.
83. Bolger C, Walsh TN, Tanner WA, et al. Chylothorax after oesophagectomy. *Br J Surg*. 1991;78(5):587–588.
84. Merigliano S, Molena D, Ruol A, et al. Chylothorax complicating esophagectomy for cancer: a plea for early thoracic duct ligation. *J Thorac Cardiovasc Surg*. 2000;119(3):453–457.
85. Wemyss-Holden SA, Launois B, Maddern GJ. Management of thoracic duct injuries after oesophagectomy. *Br J Surg*. 2001;88(11):1442–1448.
86. Lagarde SM, Omloo JM, de Jong K, et al. Incidence and management of chyle leakage after esophagectomy. *Ann Thorac Surg*. 2005;80(2):449–454.
87. Hulscher JB, van Sandick JW, Devriese PP, et al. Vocal cord paralysis after subtotal oesophagectomy. *Br J Surg*. 1999;86(12):1583–1587.
88. D'Journo XB, Martin J, Ferraro P, et al. The esophageal remnant after gastric interposition. *Dis Esophagus*. 2008;21(5):377–388.
89. Gutschow C, Collard JM, Romagnoli R, et al. Denervated stomach as an esophageal substitute recovers intraluminal acidity with time. *Ann Surg*. 2001;233(4):509–514.
90. D'Journo XB, Martin J, Gaboury L, et al. Roux-en-Y diversion for intractable reflux after esophagectomy. *Ann Thorac Surg*. 2008;86(5):1646–1652.
91. Duranceau AC, Lafontaine ER, Archambault SC, et al. Motor function in the excluded esophagus and its implications in the management of patients with unresectable carcinoma of the esophagus. *Ann Surg*. 1987;206(6):787–790.

PART 4

ACHALASIA AND ESOPHAGEAL MOTILITY DISORDERS

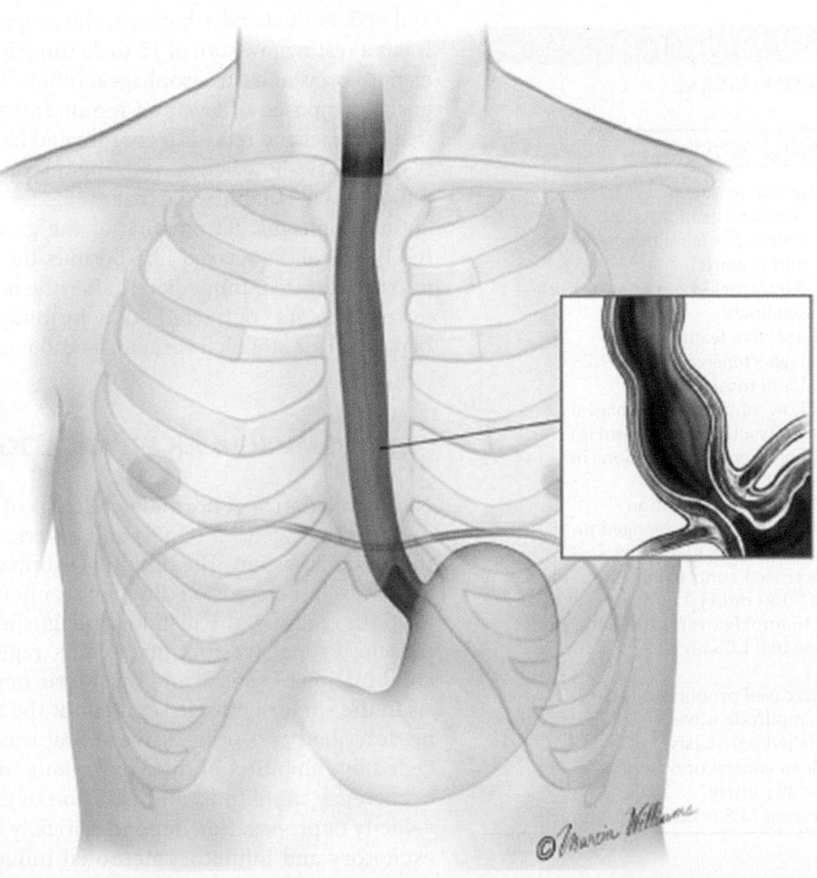

33 Overview of Esophageal Motility Disorders

Robert Burakoff and Walter W. Chan

Keywords: Achalasia, diffuse esophageal spasm, nutcracker esophagus, hypercontracting esophagus, hypertensive lower esophageal sphincter, primary esophageal motility disorders

Primary esophageal motility disorders are characterized by abnormalities of esophageal peristalsis or contractions that interfere with swallowing and transit of food through the esophagus, producing symptoms of dysphagia and chest pain. The disorder is considered primary (idiopathic) when the cause of the patient's symptoms and altered motility cannot be attributed to other systemic diseases (e.g., diabetes mellitus, scleroderma, amyloidosis, or neuromuscular disorders that affect striated muscle). The classic presentation is achalasia, a disorder characterized by failure of the lower esophageal sphincter (LES) to relax. There are several nonspecific esophageal motility disorders, including diffuse esophageal spasm (DES), nutcracker esophagus, ineffective esophageal motility (IEM), and other abnormalities of the LES. Whether these represent true disorders, a continuum of disease or merely abnormal motility patterns that are associated with but not the physiologic causes of symptoms remains a controversy (Table 33-1). Lack of a meaningful classification system adds to this confusion. Current systems classify the disorder based on aberrant esophageal motility patterns documented on manometric studies in the context of dysphagia and pain that cannot be explained by other thoracic or cardiac disease. These systems fall short because the cause of most motility abnormalities is unknown. Patients can have abnormal manometric tracings and be perfectly healthy. Conversely, therapies may correct the abnormal tracing, but symptoms do not improve. Strategies for managing esophageal dysmotility disorders include conservative management, treatment with drugs and other agents, and surgery. In the sections that follow we review current knowledge about the pathophysiology of the primary esophageal motility disorders and recent advances in diagnosis and treatment.

Table 33-1

CLASSIFICATION OF PRIMARY ESOPHAGEAL MOTILITY ABNORMALITIES

DIAGNOSIS	MOTILITY FINDINGS
Achalasia	Essential features: – Aperistalsis in distal 2/3 of esophagus (simultaneous onset and isobaric) – Abnormal LES relaxation with swallows Supportive features: – Hypertensive baseline LES (>45 mmHg) – Low amplitude esophageal contractions (<30 mmHg)
Diffuse esophageal spasm (DES)	Simultaneous contractions in ≥20% wet swallows Normal LES relaxation Other features: prolonged pressure waves, repetitive peaks (≥3)
Hypercontracting esophagus	Increased contraction amplitude (>180 mmHg) or duration (>7.5 sec)
Hypertensive peristalsis (Nutcracker esophagus)	
Hypertensive LES	>45 mmHg over intragastric pressure
Incomplete LES relaxation	Residual LES pressure >8 mmHg
Hypocontracting esophagus	Increased proportion (≥30%) of low amplitude waves (<30 mmHg) or failed peristalsis
Ineffective esophageal motility (IEM)	Mean contraction amplitude <30 mmHg
Hypotensive LES	Resting LES pressure <10 mmHg

LES, lower esophageal sphincter.

PATHOPHYSIOLOGY

Normal Esophagus

The normal human esophagus uses two sphincters to control the passage of food and prevent the reflux of stomach contents: the upper esophageal sphincter (UES) and the LES. The LES is often adversely affected in primary esophageal motility disorders. The normal LES is located in the most distal portion of the esophagus and acts as the barrier between the esophagus and the stomach. It has a resting pressure of 15 to 25 mm Hg, which is usually sufficient to prevent gastroesophageal reflux. The body of the esophagus is composed of layers of motor, mixed, and smooth muscle that contract and relax in a coordinated fashion during peristalsis. A normal swallow begins with the relaxation of the LES and initiation of a peristaltic wave that moves the food bolus through the entire esophagus, terminating at the gastroesophageal junction (GEJ), where the relaxed LES permits the food bolus to progress into the stomach. Immediately after the bolus passes, the sphincter resumes its contracted state, forming a barrier between the highly caustic stomach contents and the esophageal lumen.

NEUROMUSCULAR PHYSIOLOGY

Neuronal control of normal peristalsis of the human esophagus involves both central (CNS) and enteric (ENS) components of the nervous system. The proximal esophagus, composed of striated muscle, depends on direct motor neuron sequencing by the CNS. In contrast, the distal esophagus is composed of smooth muscle. Propulsive motility in this region is controlled by a combination of central and myenteric neural circuitry. Peristalsis in the smooth muscle segment of the healthy esophagus can be described as a progressive aboral wave of contraction, preceded by inhibition of distal segments, including the LES. The occurrence, amplitude, and duration of the contraction and the velocity of propagation depend critically on the coordination of excitatory and inhibitory neuronal influences.[1] The excitatory innervation is mediated predominantly by acetylcholine, which acts on the muscarinic receptors, whereas inhibitory innervation involves mostly nitric oxide (NO) synthesis.[2]

The inhibitory function of NO is ubiquitous in the gastrointestinal tract.[3] Its synthesis from l-arginine results from the activation of neuronal nitric oxide synthase (nNOS). NO mediates smooth muscle relaxation via an enzymatic cascade involving activation of soluble guanylate cyclase, production of guanosine 3,5-monophosphate (cGMP), and stimulation of cGMP-dependent protein kinase. Nerves and fibers immunoreactive for nNOS in the esophagus are localized to circular muscle in the distal segment.[2] The normal peristaltic contraction likely depends on a balance between a cholinergic excitatory tone and an inhibition that is progressively more profound in distal segments.[2] NO also plays a critical role in relaxation of the LES,[4] although inhibitory neuropeptides, particularly vasoactive intestinal peptide, also have been implicated in LES relaxation.[5]

NEUROPATHY IN PRIMARY MOTOR DISORDERS

It has been proposed that nutcracker esophagus, DES, and achalasia may represent a continuum of disease resulting from a progressive neuropathy primarily involving inhibitory innervation in the distal esophagus and LES.[6] The nature of the pathology underlying the loss of inhibitory innervation is not clear, although an autoimmune interpretation is supported by the finding that sera obtained from a subset of achalasia patients bind to myenteric neuronal elements, including apparently nNOS-containing neurons.[7] This model offers an appealingly cogent interpretation of these esophageal disorders. At early stages, such a pathologic process would be expected to alter the balance in favor of excitation, leading to the high amplitude but still peristaltic contractions characteristic of nutcracker esophagus. Further compromise of inhibitory influence would lead to loss of coordinated propagation, as observed in diffuse spasm, and finally, aperistalsis, loss of LES relaxation, and the sequelae of obstruction that is characteristic of achalasia (Fig. 33-1).

This interpretation is supported by case reports of apparent clinical transition from nutcracker esophagus to diffuse spasm[8,9] and from diffuse spasm to achalasia.[6,10] It is also in agreement with a variety of clinical and pathologic experimental evidence. In patients with diffuse spasm, achalasia, or intermediate disease, the degree of swallow-induced receptive inhibition measured manometrically correlates inversely with peristaltic velocity.[11] IV glyceryl trinitrate, an NO donor, produces dose-dependent increases in latency and propagation velocity, decreases the duration of swallow-induced contractions, and alleviates the symptoms in patients with DES.[12] In achalasia patients, distal relaxation in response to esophageal distention is impaired, but proximal contractile responses are preserved.[13] In vitro circular smooth muscle strips from the LES of normal control individuals exhibit spontaneous tone and relaxation during electrical field stimulation, whereas similar strips from patients with achalasia exhibit a contraction mediated by muscarinic receptors.[14]

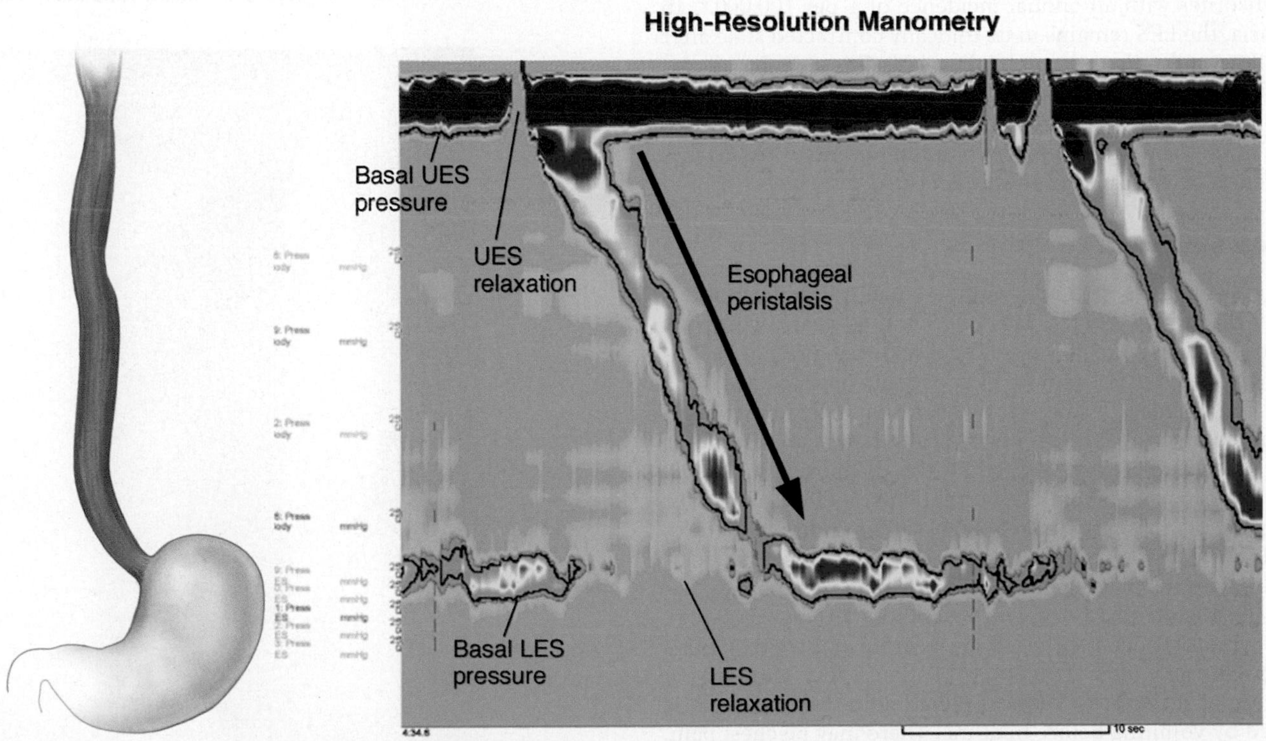

Figure 33-1. The normal human esophagus uses two sphincters to control the passage of food and prevent the reflux of stomach contents: the upper esophageal sphincter (UES) and the LES. The LES is often adversely affected in primary esophageal motility disorders as shown on high-resolution manometry. **Normal Swallow:** After swallow, food bolus is transmitted through the esophagus by waves of peristaltic contractions; the LES undergoes a brief period of relaxation just after the swallow to allow the bolus to pass into stomach before returning to normal resting pressure (15–25 mm Hg). **Nutcracker Esophagus:** Increased distal peristaltic amplitude (mean value >180 mm Hg), increased distal peristaltic duration (mean value >6 seconds), normal LES. **Diffuse esophageal spasm (DES):** Simultaneous contractions, repetitive contractions (>3 peaks), prolonged duration of contractions (6 seconds), intermittent peristalsis, and prolonged LES relaxation. **Achalasia:** Loss of peristaltic activity in the distal esophagus with decreased simultaneous contractions, incomplete LES relaxation (residual pressure >8 mm Hg), elevated resting LES pressure (>45 mm Hg), increased baseline esophageal pressure.

Histologic quantitation of NADPH-diaphorase–positive (nNOS containing) neurons in LES and gastric fundus muscles of achalasia patients indicates a significant reduction of such neurons relative to cancer control individuals.[15] Similarly, immunohistochemical staining demonstrates an absence of nNOS in the LES of achalasia patients.[16] Normal esophageal smooth muscle is innervated by fibers immunoreactive for vasoactive intestinal peptide and neuropeptide Y, whereas few such fibers are evident in smooth muscles obtained from patients with achalasia.[17]

Knowledge of this pathophysiology has suggested several strategies for medical treatment. Sildenafil blocks enzymatic degradation of cGMP and thus enhances relaxation of smooth muscle. In normal volunteers, sildenafil reduces contraction amplitude in the esophageal body and LES tone, and this drug shows apparent benefit for a subset of patients with nutcracker esophagus.[18] Botulinum toxin acts by inhibiting autonomic acetylcholine release and has been shown to be an effective treatment for achalasia by reducing LES pressure.[19] Though less effective, it provides a less risky alternative to more invasive treatments such as dilation or myotomy.

ACHALASIA

Etiology

The term achalasia originates from Greek, meaning "does not relax." The etiology of achalasia is unknown. It is a rather uncommon disorder with an annual incidence of 1 per 100,000.[20] In achalasia, the LES remains in its tonically contracted state after a swallow and fails to completely relax. This may be associated with the loss of peristalsis in the body of the esophagus, predominantly in the smooth muscle segment, or lower two-thirds of the esophagus. The loss of inhibitory neuronal drive is believed to be the cause of these effects.

Clinical Spectrum

The disease affects men and women equally. The diagnosis is usually made between the ages of 25 and 60 years, with peak diagnosis at ages 30 to 40 years. The disease can present in children (see Chapter 51) as well as in patients over the age of 65 years. The hallmark features at presentation include dysphagia for liquids and solids. Patients typically have had symptoms for at least 2 to 3 years preceding the diagnosis. Dysphagia for solids occurs in about 90% of patients, and dysphagia for liquids occurs in approximately 85%. Other common features include difficulty belching, regurgitation (often undigested food is noted on one's pillow on awakening from a recumbent position), chest pain, heartburn, and weight loss (average 5–10 kg). These symptoms occur either singly or in various combinations in approximately 50% of patients.[21] Patients very often have a sensation of retrosternal fullness radiating to the throat that is relieved by vomiting before bedtime. There may be chest pain, especially in younger patients, but attempts to differentiate these symptoms by manometric characteristics have not been forthcoming.[22] Heartburn is usually associated with decreased LES pressures and resultant reflux. In patients with achalasia, heartburn may occur due to inflammatory changes in the esophageal mucosa secondary to candidiasis or irritation from pills, various ingested foods, and exposure to lactate from the bacterial formation of carbohydrates. Additional symptoms reported by patients include hiccups, possibly secondary to obstruction of the distal esophagus, and a globus sensation from esophageal distention caused by retained food. Children with achalasia may present with deficient tear production or alacrima and adrenal glucocorticoid deficiency (Allgrove syndrome). In one published report from the adult literature, 4 of 20 patients (20%) with achalasia had alacrima.

In addition to clinical symptoms, patients with achalasia carry a significant risk of developing squamous cell carcinoma of the esophagus. In a Scandinavian study, the calculated risk of developing esophageal cancer over several years was 16 times higher in achalasia patients compared to controls. In one study of over 200 patients in the United States, a similar risk was noted. Despite these findings, the cost-effectiveness of routine endoscopic screening for cancer among achalasia patients has not been established.

Diagnosis

The diagnosis of achalasia is based initially on clinical symptoms and confirmed by radiographic, endoscopic, and manometric evaluation and criteria. Many patients are treated initially for gastroesophageal reflux disease or misdiagnosed as a result of the very often slow progression of clinical symptoms. In one study, the average duration of symptoms before diagnosis was 4 to 5 years.[22] Therefore, patients occasionally don't get diagnosed until later stages of the disease. In these cases, signs of achalasia can sometimes even be seen on plain chest films that demonstrate a widened mediastinum secondary to

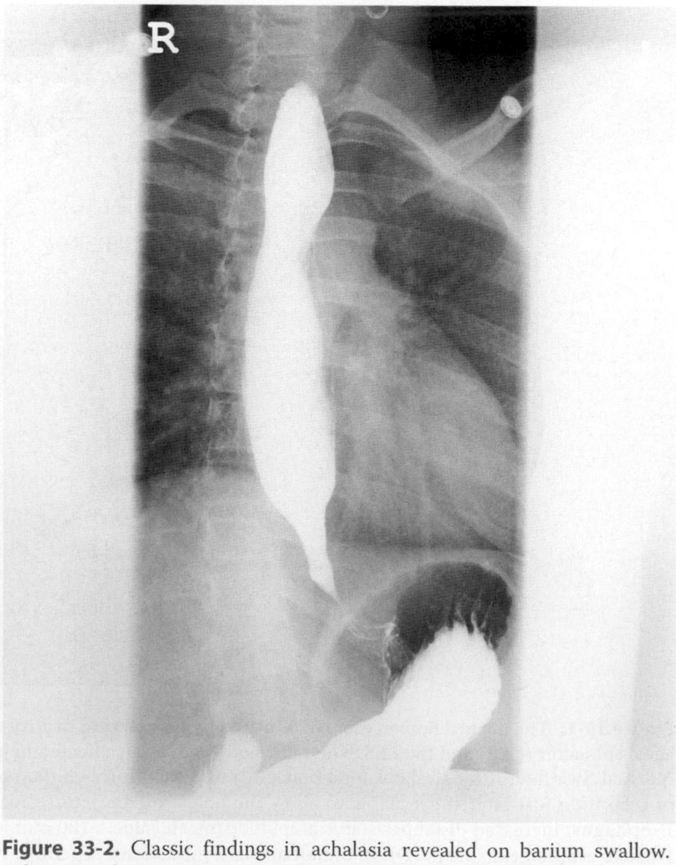

Figure 33-2. Classic findings in achalasia revealed on barium swallow. Dilatation of the esophagus and "bird's beak" at the GEJ. (Courtesy of John M. Braver, MD)

a dilated esophagus. In addition, a gastric air bubble is often absent because of incomplete relaxation of the LES.

Barium swallow is the initial radiographic examination of choice for patients with suspected achalasia. The classic finding is a dilated esophagus with a beak-like narrowing at the GEJ. This finding is over 90% accurate for the diagnosis of achalasia[23] (Fig. 33-2). The beak-like narrowing is caused by the persistent contraction of the LES, which fails to relax completely, thus decreasing the passage of contrast through the area. With primary achalasia, the narrowing at the GEJ is symmetric. One must suspect a secondary cause of achalasia (e.g., invasion of the GEJ by a tumor) if the narrowing is asymmetric. On fluoroscopy, loss of peristalsis can be noted in the smooth muscle, or lower two-thirds, segment of the esophagus. Occasionally, high-amplitude nonperistaltic contractions termed vigorous achalasia are noted.

ESOPHAGEAL MOTILITY STUDY (MANOMETRY)

Esophageal manometry performed with nonperfused catheter systems can confirm the initial presumptive diagnosis of achalasia made from clinical symptoms and radiographic findings.[24] The classic features of achalasia on conventional esophageal manometry include: (1) aperistalsis in the smooth muscle segment of the esophagus, usually accompanied by low-amplitude contractions secondary to a dilated esophagus, (2) elevation of the LES resting pressure, and (3) incomplete relaxation of the sphincter after a wet swallow (Fig. 33-3). Often, the esophageal body resting pressure may be higher than the gastric pressure, as the elevated LES pressure prevents the intraluminal pressure from relaxing to the gastric baseline. Achalasia is classified as vigorous when the amplitude of the simultaneous contractions in the esophageal body is greater than the lower limit of normal (>30 mm Hg). The vigorous form may represent an earlier presentation of achalasia when some of the intramural ganglion cells are still present, and some prior studies suggested that the response to therapy may be better in this subgroup.[25]

High-resolution manometry (HRM) utilizes a larger number of pressure sensors spaced throughout the catheter than conventional manometry, providing enhanced details in the characterization of each swallow. Data from high-resolution esophageal manometry can be interpreted and displayed in

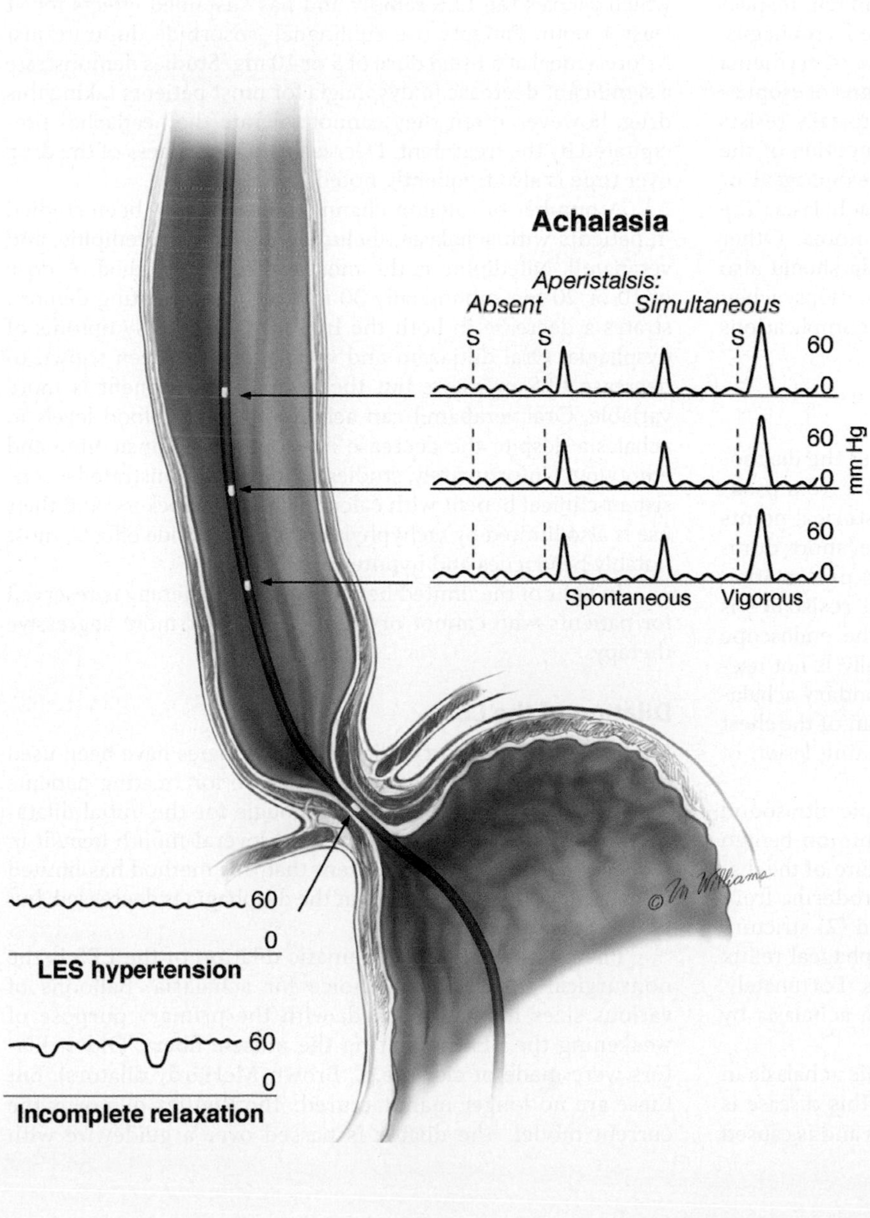

Figure 33-3. Classic features of achalasia revealed on esophageal manometry (LES, lower esophageal sphincter; S, swallow).

color-coded plots called esophageal pressure tomography or Clouse Plot.[26] With HRM, esophageal motility disorders can be categorized according to the Chicago Classification using several calculated parameters. Under this system, achalasia is defined by impaired GEJ deglutitive relaxation (normal: eSleeve 3-second nadir <15 mm Hg) and aperistalsis. It can be further classified into three subtypes (I, II, and III), distinguished by the esophageal body intraluminal pressure response with each swallow. Type I achalasia shows no change in esophageal body pressurization with swallowing, whereas type II achalasia results in panesophageal simultaneous pressurization (>30 mm Hg). Type III (spastic) achalasia is characterized by simultaneous, abnormal, lumen-obliterating contractions or spasm.[27] Among the three subtypes, type II has been shown to be most responsive to therapy regardless of modality, and is an independent predictor of treatment success. On the other hand, type III achalasia has been associated with the lowest treatment response rate and is a negative predictor of treatment response.[27]

Endoscopy

Endoscopy should be included in the evaluation of patients with a presumptive diagnosis of achalasia to examine the esophageal mucosa, GEJ, and cardia and fundus of the stomach. Inspection of the esophagus may demonstrate a dilated esophagus, whereas the esophageal mucosa may reveal signs of erythema and/or ulcerations secondary to stasis of food. Signs of esophageal candidiasis may also be present. The GEJ usually resists passage of the endoscope into the stomach. Inspection of the GEJ may reveal a tumor invading from either esophageal or gastric mucosa, indicating secondary or pseudoachalasia. The most common neoplasm is gastric adenocarcinoma. Other obstructive lesions leading to secondary achalasia should also be ruled out. Endoscopy also permits appropriate biopsy when necessary to rule out inflammatory or infectious complications or neoplasm.

Differential Diagnosis

The most important consideration in establishing the diagnosis of achalasia is differentiating primary achalasia from pseudoachalasia or secondary achalasia. The key historical points that raise suspicion for a malignant cause are short duration of symptoms (<6 months), advanced age at presentation (>60 years), and usually weight loss. Significant resistance is usually encountered when attempting to pass the endoscope through the GEJ. Esophageal manometry generally is not useful for distinguishing between primary and secondary achalasia. We recommend that patients undergo CT scan of the chest and abdomen to determine if there is an infiltrating lesion of the mediastinum or gastric cardia or fundus.

If endoscopic biopsy is unrevealing, endoscopic ultrasound with fine-needle aspiration may be helpful. Common benign conditions that mimic achalasia include (1) stricture of the distal esophagus with esophageal dilatation in scleroderma from collagen infiltration of the submucosal layers and (2) stricture of the distal esophagus from chronic gastroesophageal reflux disease resulting in dilatation of the esophagus. Fortunately, these disease entities can be differentiated from achalasia by manometry and endoscopic evaluation.

Chagas disease presents similarly to idiopathic achalasia in terms of manometric and endoscopic findings. This disease is endemic in regions of Central and South America and is caused by the parasite *Trypanosoma cruzi*. Evidence to raise suspicion for this diagnosis can be elicited from the history.

Treatment

The pathogenesis of achalasia involves the degeneration of ganglion cells in the myenteric plexus of the esophagus with a predilection for the abnormality to be present in the region of the LES. Treatment is targeted toward decreasing LES pressure to ease the passage of food into the stomach. There is no treatment that can restore peristalsis in the body of the esophagus. Therapy for achalasia includes medical treatment, pneumatic dilation, botulinum toxin injection, and surgery[28] (see Table 33-1; see also Chapters 33–35).

Medical Therapy

The goal of medical therapy is to promote relaxation of the LES through the use of appropriate pharmacologic agents. Unfortunately, none of the medications currently available provide sustained relief of symptoms. Calcium channel blockers and nitrates can relax the smooth muscles of the LES. The best results have been achieved with sublingual isosorbide dinitrate, which relaxes the LES rapidly and has sustained effects for at least 1 hour. Patients use sublingual isosorbide dinitrate just before a meal at a usual dose of 5 or 10 mg. Studies demonstrate a significant decrease in dysphagia for most patients taking this drug; however, often they cannot tolerate the headaches precipitated by the treatment. Decreasing effectiveness of the drug over time is also frequently noted.

A number of calcium channel blockers have been studied in patients with achalasia, including diltiazem, nifedipine, and verapamil. Nifedipine is the most extensively studied. A dose of 10 or 20 mg sublingually 30 minutes before eating demonstrates a decrease in both the LES pressure and symptoms of dysphagia. Oral diltiazem and verapamil have been shown to decrease LES pressure, but the symptomatic benefit is more variable. Oral verapamil can achieve adequate blood levels in achalasia despite the decrease in esophageal transit time and emptying. Unfortunately, studies have not demonstrated a consistent clinical benefit with calcium channel blockers, and their use is also limited by tachyphylaxis and other side effects, most notably headaches and hypotension.[29]

In light of the limited benefits, medical therapy is reserved for patients who cannot or will not consider more aggressive therapy.

Dilation of the LES

Rubber bougie: Mercury-filled rubber bougies have been used to dilate the LES as a temporal measure for treating patients with achalasia, using a 50 to 60F bougie for the initial dilatation. Despite some data purporting a several-month benefit in reducing dysphagia, it is apparent that this method has limited value. Many patients report that the dysphagia is decreased, but the effect is very short-lived.

Pneumatic dilation: Pneumatic dilation of the LES is the nonsurgical treatment of choice for achalasia. Balloons of various sizes have been used, with the primary purpose of weakening the LES by tearing the muscle fibers. Older dilators were made of cloth (e.g., Brown-McHardy dilators), but these are no longer manufactured. The Rigiflex dilator is the current model. The dilator is passed over a guidewire with fluoroscopic guidance, and a Witzel balloon is passed through the endoscope and inflated under direct visualization.[30] Many methods have been developed for balloon dilation, with variables including balloon size (diameter range 2.5–5.0 cm), number of inflations, and amount of time the balloon remains deployed. Regardless of technique, the results are similar. A good-to-excellent result lies in the range of 60% to 85% dilation depending on the study cited. Approximately two-thirds of patients have good-to-excellent results after one or more dilations for a median follow-up of 11 years. Most prospective studies suggest that approximately 50% of patients will require a second dilation within 5 years.[31] In direct comparison between pneumatic dilation and surgical myotomy, the success rates between the two treatment modalities appear to be similar.

Prior studies have suggested young age, postdilation LES pressure greater than 20 mm Hg, and the use of smaller balloons to be negative predictors for sustained treatment response from pneumatic dilation. On the other hand, the emptying time of barium from the esophagus after dilation appears to be the best indicator for a sustained benefit.[32] If barium emptying time is prompt on examination 3 months after pneumatic dilation, most patients will experience a sustained benefit over the next several years. If pneumatic dilation is repeated for a second time and prompt emptying of barium from the esophagus is not observed, surgical correction with myotomy would be recommended (described in Chapters 34 and 35).

Although it is the current nonsurgical procedure of choice, pneumatic dilation is not performed without risk. The rate of perforation associated with this procedure ranges from 2% to 6%. Most of the perforations occur on the left side. Therefore, a modified barium swallow with Gastrografin is recommended routinely after dilation to rule out perforation. Fortunately, mortality associated with perforation is rare (<0.2%). When an obvious perforation is diagnosed, immediate surgical repair is undertaken. If Gastrografin swallow or CT scan fails to reveal an obvious perforation but the patient continues to have chest pain and fever, he or she should be kept at nothing by mouth and given a course of antibiotics, with repeat barium swallow (with or without a CT scan) to confirm resolution.

Given its success rate and less invasive nature, endoscopic pneumatic dilation has been compared to surgical myotomy for treatment outcome. The most recent prospective trial in Europe randomizing 201 achalasia patients to pneumatic dilation versus laparoscopic Hellar myotomy found no significant difference between the two groups with regard to all parameters of treatment response, including symptoms, LES pressure, esophageal emptying, quality of life, and esophageal acid exposure.[33] As patients in this study were only followed for a mean of 43 months, further studies are needed to compare the longer-term outcomes between the two therapies.

Botulinum (Botox) Injection

Botulinum toxin inhibits release of acetylcholine from neurons. It has been theorized that endoscopic injection of botulinum toxin in the anatomic area of the LES would inhibit the release of acetylcholine in neurons that play a role in LES smooth muscle tone, thereby decreasing LES pressure. Several small studies have demonstrated the benefit of endoscopic botulinum toxin injection. Unfortunately, although these initial studies demonstrated up to 90% immediate symptomatic relief, the benefit was relatively short-lived. Subsequent studies showed the median duration of benefit to be only about 6 months. Approximately two-thirds of patients were asymptomatic at 6 months, with the remission rate further decreasing to 45% at 1 year. Botulinum toxin injection has also been found to be significantly more effective in patients over age 50 (80% vs. 40%).[25] Even if a sustained result is not achieved, no data have demonstrated that toxin injection results in increased morbidity or worse outcomes if pneumatic dilation or surgery should follow. The drawback to using toxin injection is the high cost (approximately $300 for a vial of botulinum toxin). The advantage is its excellent safety profile. Fewer than 25% of patients receiving botulinum toxin injection experience transient mild chest pain, and fewer than 5% experience reflux symptoms.

Various treatments are available for achalasia. Medical therapy with nitrate and calcium channel blockers has a short-term, limited role. The effect of botulinum toxin injection, although safe, is relatively short-lived and may be most useful for older patients (age 50 and older), in whom the risk of pneumatic dilation or surgery is escalated. Pneumatic dilation for most patients is the first-line nonsurgical therapy, capable of yielding a sustainable benefit in 70% of patients. When dilation fails, surgical myotomy is the treatment of choice.

NONSPECIFIC ESOPHAGEAL MOTILITY DISORDERS

Diffuse Esophageal Spasm

DES was first described by William Osler in 1892 in a hypochondriacal patient with chest pain. Today, DES is considered part of the spectrum of esophageal motility disorders, and it is diagnosed by esophageal manometry in patients who present with symptoms of dysphagia, chest pain, or both.

Historically, there are three requirements to make the diagnosis of DES: (1) dysphagia and/or chest pain, (2) radiographic study demonstrating tertiary or spontaneous contractions resulting in the classic radiographic finding of the "corkscrew esophagus" or "rosary bead esophagus" (Fig. 33-4), and (3) esophageal manometry study demonstrating spontaneous, repetitive, and prolonged-duration contractions (Fig. 33-5). However, more recent esophageal manometry studies in patients with DES have identified additional distinguishing criteria.[34] Patients who present with dysphagia as the predominant symptom tend to have lower-amplitude contractions than those who present with chest pain. Despite the increased contraction amplitude, DES patients with chest pain rarely have sustained pressure greater than 180 mm Hg. The diagnostic criteria on esophageal manometry include simultaneous contractions of at least 30 mm Hg for more than 20% of measured wet swallows. In addition, approximately 30% to 40% of patients have abnormalities of the LES that consist of either high resting pressure or incomplete relaxation after a wet swallow. Radiographic studies also may be entirely normal in patients who have dysphagia as their predominant symptom. In fact, measurement of bolus transit using electrical impedance as a part of the manometry catheter has demonstrated abnormal bolus transit even with normal radiographic examination. Patients with chest pain and higher-amplitude spontaneous contractions usually have normal bolus transit time. The pathophysiology of this disorder is still not fully elucidated, but there is evidence for a defect in the synthesis of NO (see above). On HRM, DES patients are found to have

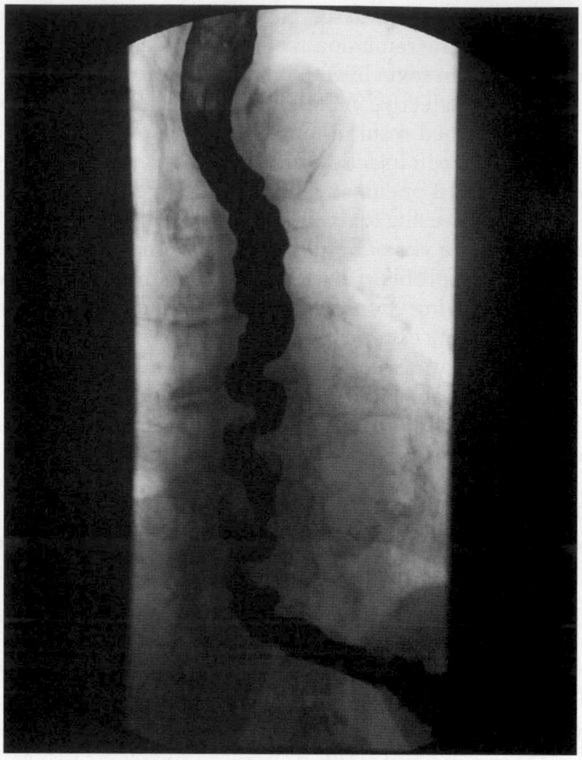

Figure 33-4. On barium swallow, spontaneous and tertiary contractions yield a "corkscrew esophagus" appearance in diffuse esophageal spasm. (Courtesy of John M. Braver, MD)

simultaneous contractions and pressurization of the distal esophagus with usually normal relaxation of the LES. They usually have a rapidly propagated pressurization of the esophagus, with a contractile front velocity >8 cm/s in at least 20% of swallows per Chicago Classification.

Nutcracker Esophagus

Nutcracker esophagus is the term ascribed to a state of high-amplitude (>180 mm Hg) peristaltic contractions in the distal esophagus associated with dysphagia and/or chest pain (Fig. 33-6). It is seen most commonly in women and carries a higher prevalence than DES in the general population. It is often part of the spectrum of irritable bowel syndrome and is associated with increased visceral sensitivity. Patterns of DES or nutcracker esophagus have been observed during periods of chest pain in patients undergoing prolonged esophageal manometric monitoring. A radiographic study obtained is frequently normal, and because contractions are peristaltic, impedance studies also demonstrate normal bolus transit. In the Chicago Classification for HRM, nutcracker esophagus or hypertensive peristalsis is defined by a contractile front velocity <8 cm/s in more than 90% of swallows and a mean distal contractile integral (a parameter integrating the length, contraction amplitude, and duration of a contraction) of >5000 mm Hg-s-cm.

Nutcracker esophagus may also be associated with a hypertensive or poorly relaxing LES. The pathophysiology is still not well clarified, but, similar to other hypercontractile disorders of

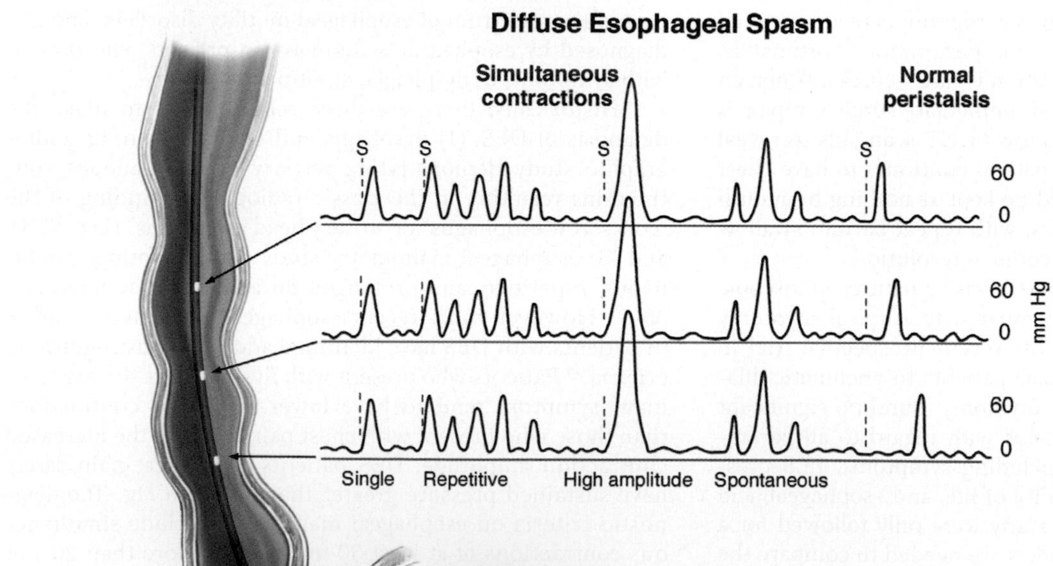

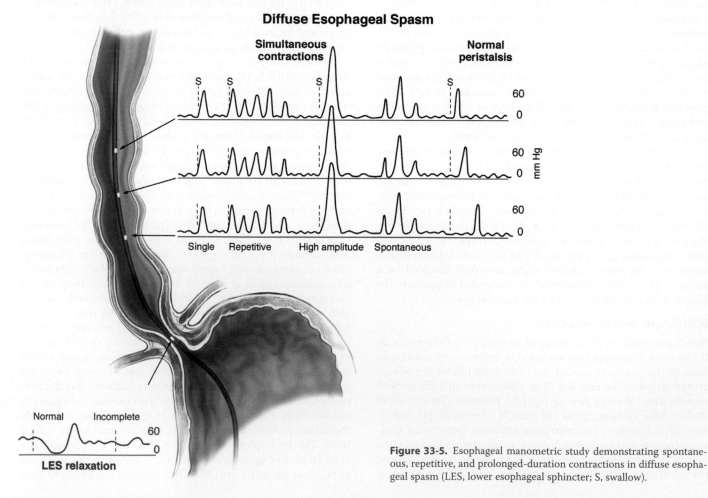

Figure 33-5. Esophageal manometric study demonstrating spontaneous, repetitive, and prolonged-duration contractions in diffuse esophageal spasm (LES, lower esophageal sphincter; S, swallow).

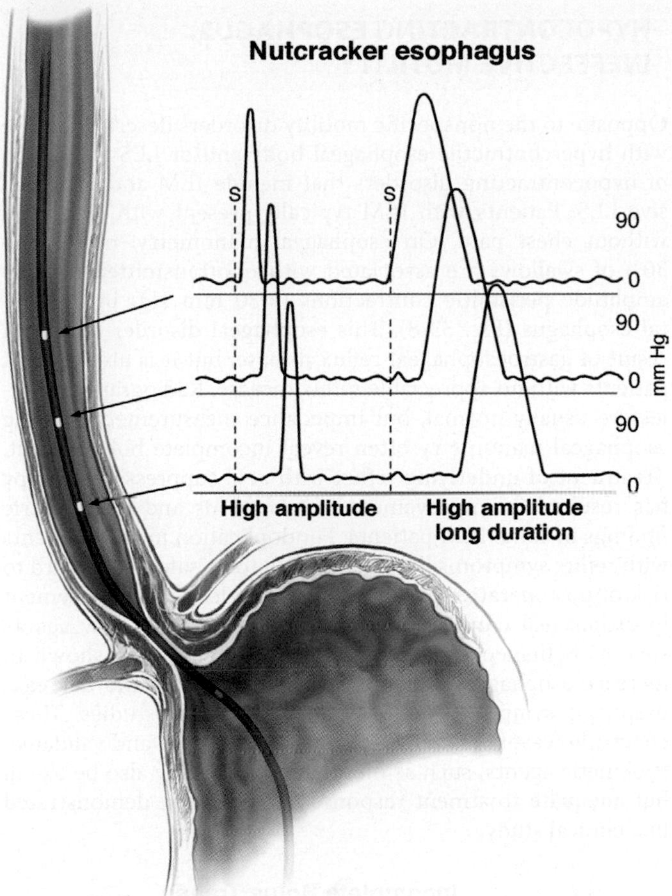

Figure 33-6. Nutcracker esophagus yields a state of high-amplitude (>180 mm Hg) peristaltic contractions in the distal half of the esophagus (LES, lower esophageal sphincter; S, swallow).

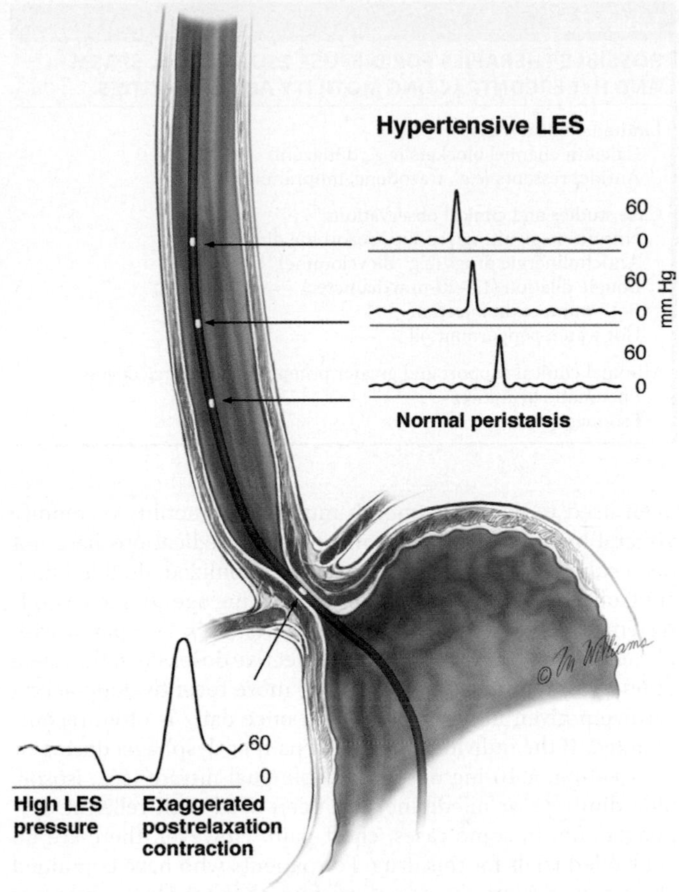

Figure 33-7. Hypertensive LES, defined as a basal LES pressure of more than 45 mm Hg, is found often in patients who present with dysphagia.

the esophagus, changes in NO synthesis and degradation may be involved (see above).

Hypertensive LES

Hypertensive LES, defined as a basal LES pressure of greater than 45 mm Hg, is found often in patients who present with dysphagia. It is associated with high-amplitude peristaltic contractions in the distal esophagus in approximately 50% of the patients who present with chest pain (Fig. 33-7). Hypertensive LES also may be associated with incomplete relaxation of the LES after a wet swallow, which may be present in DES as well as in high-amplitude contraction abnormalities. As one can surmise from this discussion, there is an entire spectrum of abnormal motility patterns with various combinations that may include one, a few, or all the abnormalities described earlier in patients presenting with chest pain and or dysphagia (Table 33-2).

MEDICAL MANAGEMENT OF NONSPECIFIC ESOPHAGEAL DYSMOTILITY DISORDERS

Since the pathophysiology of the nonspecific disorders described earlier is poorly understood, there is significant treatment overlap for DES, nutcracker esophagus, and hypertensive sphincter disorders (Table 33-3). Numerous medications have

Table 33-2

MANAGEMENT OF ACHALASIA

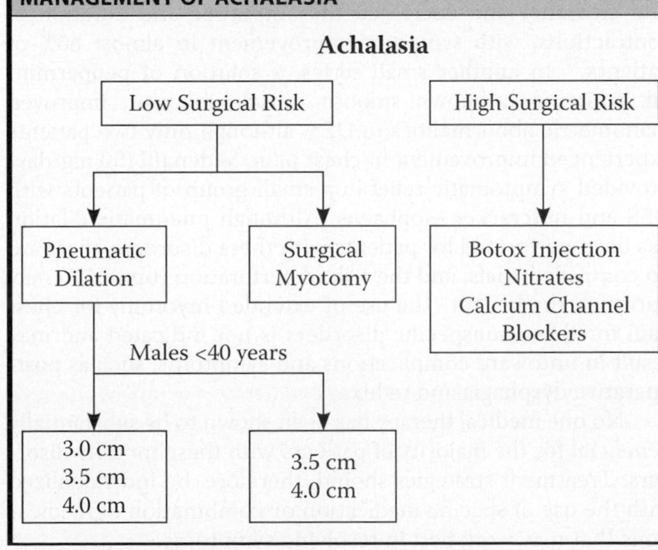

Table 33-3

POSSIBLE THERAPIES FOR DIFFUSE ESOPHAGEAL SPASM AND HYPERCONTRACTING MOTILITY ABNORMALITIES

Limited clinical trials
Calcium channel blockers (e.g., diltiazem)
Antidepressants (e.g., trazodone, imipramine)
Case studies and clinical observations
Nitrates (e.g., nitroglycerine, isosorbide dinitrate)
Anticholinergic drugs (e.g., dicyclomine)
Bougie dilation (17–20-mm diameter)
Botulinum toxin injection
Hot water, peppermint oil
Minimal clinical support and greater potential for adverse effects
Pneumatic dilatation
Esophagomyotomy

been used to decrease smooth muscle contractility or modify visceral hypersensitivity, but most of the medications have not been subjected to large prospective, randomized, double-blind, controlled trials. Calcium channel blocking agents such as diltiazem have been shown to relieve chest pain compared with placebo in nutcracker esophagus. Effective doses lie in the range of 60 to 90 mg four times daily, but more recently, long-acting cardizem given in doses of 240 mg once daily is often recommended. If the individual has chest pain or dysphagia during or after eating, a 10-mg dose of a sublingual nitrate (e.g., isosorbide dinitrate or nifedipine) has been used with relief of dysphagia and, in some cases, chest pain. However, there are no controlled trials for this drug. For patients who have continued chest pain despite the use of calcium channel blocking agents or nitrates, some have benefited from tricyclic antidepressants (e.g., trazodone in a dose range of 75–150 mg/day and imipramine at 50 mg/day), which modify visceral hypersensitivity rather than alter esophageal dysmotility. More recently, several uncontrolled trials have demonstrated a good effect with botulinum toxin injections (100 units injected circumferentially at the GEJ) in reducing chest pain in patients with nonspecific esophageal motility disorders.[35,36] Improvement was observed in 70% of patients, with approximately 50% of patients having complete relief of chest pain and a sustained benefit of up to 7 months.

Other treatments with reported benefit in single studies include hot water taken with meals, which improved esophageal clearance and decreased the amplitude and duration of contractions, with symptom improvement in almost 60% of patients.[37] In another small series, a solution of peppermint oil, which is a known smooth muscle relaxant, improved manometric abnormalities in DES, although only two patients experienced improvement in chest pain. Sildenafil (50 mg/day) provided symptomatic relief in a small group of patients with DES and nutcracker esophagus. Although pneumatic dilation has been performed for patients with these disorders, there are no controlled trials, and the risk of perforation (up to 5%) may outweigh the benefit. The use of extended myotomy for chest pain for these nonspecific disorders is not indicated and may result in untoward complications and symptoms, such as postoperative dysphagia and reflux.

No one medical therapy has been shown to be substantially beneficial for the majority of patients with these motility disorders. Treatment strategies should, therefore, be individualized with the use of specific medication or combination of medications that may work best in resolving symptoms.

HYPOCONTRACTING ESOPHAGUS: INEFFECTIVE MOTILITY

Opposite to the nonspecific motility disorders described above with hypercontractile esophageal body and/or LES is a group of hypocontracting disorders that include IEM and hypotensive LES. Patients with IEM typically present with dysphagia without chest pain. On esophageal manometry, more than 30% of swallows are associated with nontransmitted or low-amplitude peristaltic contractions (<30 mm Hg) in the distal esophagus (Fig. 33-8). This esophageal disorder may be a result of gastroesophageal reflux disease, but it is also present patients with no appreciable reflux disease. Radiographic studies are usually normal, but impedance measurements during esophageal manometry often reveal incomplete bolus transit. Treatment of underlying reflux with acid suppression therapy has resulted in improvement in symptoms and manometric findings in some IEM patients. Fundoplication in IEM patients with reflux symptoms has been shown to be safe with regard to risk of postoperative dysphagia and may lead to improvement in esophageal contractions on manometry.[38,39] A few agents such as bethanechol and buspirone have also been shown to increase esophageal body and LES contractions and decrease dysphagia symptoms in IEM patients in small studies. These effects, however, need to be further investigated and validated. Prokinetic agents, such as metoclopramide, may also be useful but adequate treatment response has not been demonstrated in a clinical study.

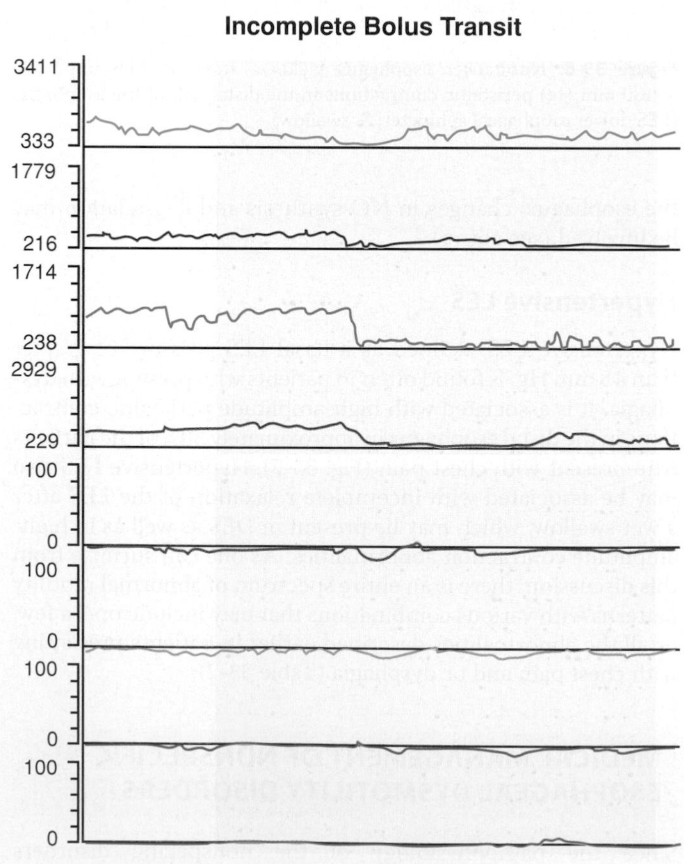

Figure 33-8. Impedance determinations during esophageal manometry reveal incomplete bolus transit in patients with hypocontracting esophagus.

SUMMARY

Primary esophageal motility disorders may result from esophageal body and LES hypocontraction, hypercontraction, or mixed response. Depending on the underlying pathophysiology and esophageal function, options for treatment may include conservative management, pharmacologic treatment, endoscopic therapy, and surgery (see Chapters 34–36). Further development of more specific medical therapies in the future will depend on a more profound understanding of the pathogenesis of these disorders.

EDITOR'S COMMENT

The spectrum of esophageal motility disorders includes those that are surgically manageable and those for which there are no current surgical solutions. A comprehensive multidisciplinary approach to evaluation is required prior to surgical manipulation, despite the insistence of some patients that a surgical "cure" be attempted. Frankly, the differential diagnoses described eloquently in this chapter should prompt every surgeon to insist on manometric evaluation of every patient before undertaking any surgery for benign motility disorders or reflux.

—Raphael Bueno

References

1. Richards WG, Grondin SC, Sugarbaker DJ. *Physiology of Esophageal Peristalsis*. Philadelphia, PA: Harcourt Health Sciences; 2002.
2. Richards WG, Sugarbaker DJ. Neuronal control of esophageal function. *Chest Surg Clin North Am*. 1995;5:157–171.
3. Takahashi T. Pathophysiological significance of neuronal nitric oxide synthase in the gastrointestinal tract. *J Gastroenterol*. 2003;38:421–430.
4. Tlottrup A, Forman A, Funch-Jensen P, et al. Effects of postganglionic nerve stimulation in oesophageal achalasia: an in vitro study. *Gut*. 1990;31:17–20.
5. Ny L, Alm P, Larsson B, et al. Nitric oxide pathway in cat esophagus: localization of nitric oxide synthase and functional effects. *Am J Physiol*. 1995;268:G59–G70.
6. Vantrappen G, Janssens J, Hellemans J, et al. Achalasia, diffuse esophageal spasm, and related motility disorders. *Gastroenterology*. 1979;76:450–457.
7. Verne GN, Sallustio JE, Eaker EY. Anti-myenteric neuronal antibodies in patients with achalasia. A prospective study. *Dig Dis Sci*. 1997;42:307–313.
8. Traube M, Aaronson RM, McCallum RW. Transition from peristaltic esophageal contractions to diffuse esophageal spasm. *Arch Intern Med*. 1986;146:1844–1846.
9. Narducci F, Bassotti G, Gaburri M, et al. Transition from nutcracker esophagus to diffuse esophageal spasm. *Am J Gastroenterol*. 1985;80:242–244.
10. Longstreth GF, Foroozan P. Evolution of symptomatic diffuse esophageal spasm to achalasia. *South Med J*. 1982;75:217–220.
11. Sifrim D, Janssens J, Vantrappen G. Failing deglutitive inhibition in primary esophageal motility disorders. *Gastroenterology*. 1994;106:875–882.
12. Konturek JW, Gillessen A, Domschke W. Diffuse esophageal spasm: a malfunction that involves nitric oxide? *Scand J Gastroenterol*. 1995;30:1041–1045.
13. Paterson WG. Esophageal and lower esophageal sphincter response to balloon distention in patients with achalasia. *Dig Dis Sci*. 1997;42:106–112.
14. Tottrup A, Svane D, Forman A. Nitric oxide mediating NANC inhibition in opossum lower esophageal sphincter. *Am J Physiol*. 1991;260:G385–G389.
15. De Giorgio R, Di Simone MP, Stanghellini V, et al. Esophageal and gastric nitric oxide synthesizing innervation in primary achalasia. *Am J Gastroenterol*. 1999;94:2357–2362.
16. Mearin F, Mourelle M, Guarner F, et al. Patients with achalasia lack nitric oxide synthase in the gastro-oesophageal junction. *Eur J Clin Invest*. 1993;23:724–728.
17. Wattchow DA, Costa M. Distribution of peptide-containing nerve fibres in achalasia of the oesophagus. *J Gastroenterol Hepatol*. 1996;11:478–485.
18. Eherer AJ, Schwetz I, Hammer HF, et al. Effect of sildenafil on oesophageal motor function in healthy subjects and patients with oesophageal motor disorders. *Gut*. 2002;50:758–764.
19. Brisinda G, Bentivoglio AR, Maria G, et al. Treatment with botulinum neurotoxin of gastrointestinal smooth muscles and sphincters spasms. *Mov Disord*. 2004;19 Suppl 8:S146–S156.
20. Howard PJ, Maher L, Pryde A, et al. Five year prospective study of the incidence, clinical features, and diagnosis of achalasia in Edinburgh. *Gut*. 1992;33:1011–1015.
21. Eckardt VF, Stauf B, Bernhard G. Chest pain in achalasia: patient characteristics and clinical course. *Gastroenterology*. 1999;116:1300–1304.
22. Eckardt VF, Kohne U, Junginger T, et al. Risk factors for diagnostic delay in achalasia. *Dig Dis Sci*. 1997;42:580–585.
23. Ott DJ, Richter JE, Chen YM, et al. Esophageal radiography and manometry: correlation in 172 patients with dysphagia. *AJR Am J Roentgenol*. 1987;149:307–311.
24. Hirano I, Tatum RP, Shi G, et al. Manometric heterogeneity in patients with idiopathic achalasia. *Gastroenterology*. 2001;120:789–798.
25. Pasricha PJ, Rai R, Ravich WJ, et al. Botulinum toxin for achalasia: long-term outcome and predictors of response. *Gastroenterology*. 1996;110:1410–1415.
26. Pandolfino JE, Ghosh SK, Rice J, et al. Classifying esophageal motility by pressure topography characteristics: a study of 400 patients and 75 controls. *Am J Gastroenterol*. 2008;103:27–37.
27. Pandolfino JE, Kwiatek MA, Nealis T, et al. Achalasia: a new clinically relevant classification by high-resolution manometry. *Gastroenterology*. 2008;135:1526–1533.
28. Spiess AE, Kahrilas PJ. Treating achalasia: from whalebone to laparoscope. *JAMA*. 1998;280:638–642.
29. Gelfond M, Rozen P, Gilat T. Isosorbide dinitrate and nifedipine treatment of achalasia: a clinical, manometric and radionuclide evaluation. *Gastroenterology*. 1982;83:963–969.
30. West RL, Hirsch DP, Bartelsman JF, et al. Long term results of pneumatic dilation in achalasia followed for more than 5 years. *Am J Gastroenterol*. 2002;97:1346–1351.
31. Ghoshal UC, Kumar S, Saraswat VA, et al. Long-term follow-up after pneumatic dilation for achalasia cardia: factors associated with treatment failure and recurrence. *Am J Gastroenterol*. 2004;99:2304–2310.
32. Farhoomand K, Connor JT, Richter JE, et al. Predictors of outcome of pneumatic dilation in achalasia. *Clin Gastroenterol Hepatol*. 2004;2:389–394.
33. Boeckxstaens GE, Annese V, des Varannes SB, et al. Pneumatic dilation versus laparoscopic Heller's myotomy for idiopathic achalasia. *N Engl J Med*. 2011;364:1807–1816.
34. Sperandio M, Tutuian R, Gideon RM, et al. Diffuse esophageal spasm: not diffuse but distal esophageal spasm (DES). *Dig Dis Sci*. 2003;48:1380–1384.
35. Storr M, Allescher HD, Rosch T, et al. Treatment of symptomatic diffuse esophageal spasm by endoscopic injection of botulinum toxin: a prospective study with long term follow-up. *Gastrointest Endosc*. 2001;54:18A.
36. Miller LS, Pullela SV, Parkman HP, et al. Treatment of chest pain in patients with noncardiac, nonreflux, nonachalasia spastic esophageal motor disorders using botulinum toxin injection into the gastroesophageal junction. *Am J Gastroenterol*. 2002;97:1640–1646.
37. Triadafilopoulos G, Tsang HP, Segall GM. Hot water swallows improve symptoms and accelerate esophageal clearance in esophageal motility disorders. *J Clin Gastroenterol*. 1998;26:239–244.
38. Tsereteli Z, Sporn E, Astudillo JA, et al. Laparoscopic Nissen fundoplication is a good option in patients with abnormal esophageal motility. *Surg Endosc*. 2009;23:2292–2295.
39. Ravi N, Al-Sarraf N, Moran T, et al. Acid normalization and improved esophageal motility after Nissen fundoplication: equivalent outcomes in patients with normal and ineffective esophageal motility. *Am J Surg*. 2005;190:445–450.

34 Esophagocardiomyotomy for Achalasia (Heller)

Marcelo W. Hinojosa and Brant K. Oelschlager

Keywords: Cardiomyotomy, minimally invasive esophagocardiomyotomy, achalasi

INTRODUCTION

In 1914, Ernest Heller described the first cardiomyotomy for the treatment of achalasia.[1] He described an anterior and posterior myotomy along the gastroesophageal junction (GEJ) using a thoracoabdominal incision. The operation was subsequently modified by Groenveldt and Zaaijer to include only the anterior myotomy. Owing to the morbidity of the open approach, this operation was performed primarily in patients who failed medical management. It was not until the early 1990s with the advent of minimally invasive techniques that minimally invasive esophagocardiomyotomy became a viable first-line therapy. This operation has yielded excellent results, with 90% to 95% of patients receiving durable relief of dysphagia.[2–5] At the University of Washington, we converted from a thoracoscopic approach to a laparoscopic Heller myotomy in 1994, and along with most centers, we now consider laparoscopic esophageal myotomy to be an excellent first-line therapy because of the low morbidity, durability, and the high levels of success after minimally invasive esophagocardiomyotomy.[3,6–9]

GENERAL PRINCIPLES

Clinical Characteristics of Achalasia

Achalasia is characterized by aperistalsis of the mid-to-distal esophageal body combined with lack of LES relaxation. Although it is the most common primary esophageal motility disorder, it is rare. The reported incidence in North America is 0.5 to 1 per 100,000 people. Achalasia was first described as cardiospasm in the 17th century by Sir Thomas Willis. The name achalasia, *meaning* "failure to relax," was coined by Lendrum in 1937.[10]

Achalasia manifests most commonly with progressive dysphagia, starting with solids and progressing to liquids. The diagnosis usually is made between the ages of 20 and 50 years without a gender predilection. Ineffective relaxation of the LES and loss of esophageal peristalsis lead to impaired emptying and gradual esophageal dilatation, resulting in severe dysphagia. Patients may use various maneuvers to attempt to clear the esophagus, including drinking liquids, standing after swallowing, walking around during meals, raising hands over head, and extending or flexing the neck. Patients also may complain of regurgitation of undigested food, cough, aspiration, wheezing, and choking. These symptoms often are made worse in the recumbent position, when esophageal contents flow back into the airway, and in some can lead to recurrent aspiration pneumonia.

Chest pain is commonly reported, and it is postulated to be a result of esophageal overdistention and uncoordinated peristalsis. Stress or cold liquids can also exacerbate these symptoms in some. A subset of patients with simultaneous contractions of normal or near-normal amplitude on manometry, are considered to have a variation of Achalasia termed *vigorous achalasia*.[11] In reality, achalasia may be a heterogeneous collection of disorders or subtypes as has been recently described by Pandolfino et al.[12] As with other hypercontractile esophageal motility disorders, simultaneous contractions are postulated as one cause of chest pain, but this seems unlikely for most patients with achalasia who demonstrate little even simultaneous contractile activity. Heartburn may occur but is usually the result of fermentation of unevacuated food in the esophagus and not gastroesophageal reflux disease (GERD). Misdiagnosis with GERD or the presence of aspiration pneumonia can lead to a delay in treatment.

Mild weight loss is occasionally a manifestation of the disease. Rapid or significant drop in weight of more than 10 lb (4 kg) along with advanced age (>60 years) or rapid onset of symptoms (<6 months) should alert clinicians to the possibility of an esophageal malignancy that has caused obstruction (and with it all the other manifestations of achalasia). This entity is often referred to as pseudoachalasia. If any diagnostic doubt exists, CT should be considered. Alternatively, if available, esophagogastroscopy combined with endoscopic ultrasound is a highly specific and sensitive method of confirming or excluding tumors and can be used to simultaneously biopsy suspicious masses or lymph nodes.

Surgical Treatment With Laparoscopic (Heller) Myotomy

Until the early 1990s surgical myotomy was accomplished via open transthoracic or transabdominal approach, both of which were associated with the morbidity and mortality of a major open operation. Since the introduction of minimally invasive surgery for the treatment of achalasia the use of Heller myotomy has expanded, and it has become an attractive first option as a result of its improved overall risk-benefit ratio.

The laparoscopic approach has been demonstrated to be superior to both open and thoracoscopic procedures with respect to complications, morbidity, mortality, relief from dysphagia, prevention of postoperative reflux, operative times, and hospital stay.[11,13] Additional advantages of the laparoscopic approach include improved visualization of the esophageal muscle layers, better access to perform a longer gastric myotomy owing to improved esophageal and gastric access, substantial reduction in postoperative pain, and ease of performing an antireflux procedure.

As previously mentioned, the laparoscopic approach to Heller myotomy has been our preferred method since 1994. We found that the limited gastric myotomy (0.5–1.0 cm) afforded by the thoracoscopic approach did not protect patients from gastroesophageal reflux, and in fact, pH monitoring revealed that 80% of patients had pathologic reflux. In our experience with the thoracoscopic approach we also found that 17% of patients returned with recurrent dysphagia, half of which required a laparoscopic revision of the myotomy with extension onto the stomach. The laparoscopic approach permitted a long esophageal myotomy that could be extended onto the stomach.

In our initial experience with the laparoscopic approach we performed a traditional 1 to 2 cm gastric myotomy, and the majority of patients showed excellent improvement in their dysphagia. Still, there were some with recurrent dysphagia that needed an operative revision, and we noted that extending the gastric portion of the myotomy improved their symptoms.[6] Therefore, in 1998, we began extending the myotomy to a full 3 cm on the gastric side and also began performing a Toupet rather than a Dor fundoplication.[14] We reasoned that an anterior fundoplication would be more difficult with a 3-cm cardiomyotomy and suspected that the posterior Toupet would provide better control of reflux.

Subsequently, Di Martino et al.[15] found similar results using an animal model. They performed a 6-cm myotomy with a 3-cm gastric extension which thus disrupted the sling fibers of the stomach and led to a more effective ablation of the LES on manometry. We have found that dysphagia was both less frequent (once a month vs. once a week on average) and less severe (3.2 vs. 5.3 on a 10-point visual analog scale) in the extended myotomy with Toupet fundoplication group. Perhaps most importantly, no patient has required surgical intervention for recurrent dysphagia in the last 13 years in our center. The need for endoscopic treatment was also rare.[14] We also found that completely obliterating the LES did not result in more reflux long-term because the mean distal esophageal acid exposure was equivalent between the two groups (extended myotomy with Toupet fundoplication 6.3% vs. shorter myotomy with Dor fundoplication 3.5%).

Antireflux Procedure

Whether to perform an antireflux procedure is no longer controversial and is accepted by most surgeons. It is also uniformly accepted as good practice, and has been validated by a randomized trial, that a partial fundoplication provides better control of reflux without adversely affecting the relief of dysphagia.[16] In their study, Richards and colleagues enrolled 43 patients to either undergo Heller myotomy with Dor fundoplication versus Heller myotomy alone and found pathologic gastroesophageal reflux in 9.1% versus 47.6% of patients respectively. They also noted that there was no negative effect on relief of dysphagia.

Which antireflux procedure to perform does remain a matter of debate. Reported results of postoperative reflux after esophageal myotomy with Dor fundoplication range from 4% to 25%.[16,17] Several studies support use of the Toupet fundoplication, reporting similarly successful results.[18,19] A recent multicenter randomized trial comparing laparoscopic Dor versus Toupet fundoplication following Heller myotomy showed that there was no difference in esophageal symptoms between the two groups.[19] There was a trend toward higher percentage of abnormal 24-hour pH-test results in the Dor group (41.7% vs. 21.0%); however, this was not statistically significant.

Most surgeons find that performing an antireflux procedure whether it be Dor or Toupet fundoplication in conjunction with laparoscopic myotomy does not add significant time or morbidity to the operation and is not associated with increased postoperative dysphagia. We find that the Toupet fundoplication provides an effective barrier to reflux as well as possibly preventing scarring and reapproximation of the divided muscle edges. However, the proponents of the Dor like the fact that it covers the mucosa of the myotomy and might be protective if there is an injury. Also, a Dor does not require posterior esophageal mobilization or division of the short gastric vessels. A total fundoplication for the most part is not used as it results in a high incidence of recurrent dysphagia when compared to a partial fundoplication.[20]

Surgical Treatment With Robotic (Heller) Myotomy

Recently, robotic assisted Heller myotomy has emerged as a safe alternative to the laparoscopic approach. Some believe that robotics improves visualization, degree of instrument freedom, and tremor control. Three retrospective studies exist comparing robotic versus laparoscopic Heller myotomy.[21–23] All of these studies show no intraoperative perforations with the robotic approach, an 8% to 16% perforation rate with the laparoscopic approach, and no differences in postoperative dysphagia. The information that can be extrapolated from these studies is limited, however, since they were not randomized, the groups were heterogeneous, and the operations were performed at different times within each group's operative experience, and in some cases in different groups altogether.

In our experience using both the laparoscopic and robotic approaches, we have found that the laparoscopic approach yields excellent outcomes with low intraoperative perforation rates. The robotic approach does provide the "feeling" of more precision, and may indeed be beneficial for surgeons with less experience. Whether this is worth the added cost and time associated with the robotic approach is open for debate.

Endoscopic Treatments

Before the development of laparoscopic techniques in the early 1990s, the first-line therapy for achalasia was endoscopic dilation. The concept of dilating the LES to provide relief for patients with achalasia was first performed in the 17th century by Sir Thomas Willis when he used a whalebone to perform a dilation. Today, endoscopic techniques such as pneumatic dilation and endoscopic administration of botulinum toxin are still used by some as first-line treatments before surgery. However, the low morbidity and long durability of laparoscopic esophageal myotomy is making laparoscopic Heller myotomy a more attractive first-line therapy.

More recent advances in therapeutic endoscopy have led some surgeons to begin performing endoscopic esophageal myotomy. These procedures are termed peroral esophageal myotomy (POEM).[24,25] Using an endoscope, an 8-cm esophagogastric myotomy of the circular muscle fibers is performed via a submucosal tunnel after an incision is made in the mucosa of the midesophagus. The longitudinal muscle fibers are left intact and the mucosa is closed on the way out. Initial reports with regard to dysphagia have been promising; however, further longer-term studies are needed to better elucidate the efficacy and complication profile of this procedure. Specifically, it is unclear whether relief of dysphagia is equivalent when only the circular muscle fibers are divided, and we do not know if gastroesophageal reflux is more frequent since a fundoplication cannot be performed. The adaptation of this technique for long myotomies is discussed in Chapter 35.

PREOPERATIVE ASSESSMENT

Manometry

Esophageal manometry is the standard for diagnosing achalasia. Classically described findings for achalasia are aperistalsis of the distal two-thirds of the esophageal body and incomplete relaxation of the LES (Figs. 34-1–34-4). The body of the esophagus typically demonstrates nonpropagated or undulating isobaric simultaneous waves due to the transmission of pharyngeal and upper esophageal contractions down the fluid-filled esophagus. Vigorous achalasia has simultaneous normal or high-amplitude waves without normal progression (Fig. 34-5). Although hypertension of the LES is often found, the LESP is usually in the normal range and a hypertensive LES is not required for the diagnosis. The use of high-resolution manometry allows for detailed topographical visualization of the UES, LES, and esophageal body simultaneously and is adding to our knowledge of achalasia and the variations in manometric presentations (Figs. 34-2 and 34-4).

Upper Gastrointestinal Series

Findings on upper gastrointestinal studies usually include esophageal dilation, tapering of the GEJ "bird's beak" appearance, and slow passage of contrast typically with a barium fluid column (Fig. 34-5). As the esophageal dilatation worsens, it may become sigmoid-shaped. An air–fluid level in the esophagus is seen commonly, arising from slow clearance of the contrast material bolus. Particulate food matter may be seen in the contrast material, even though patients fast for several hours before study.

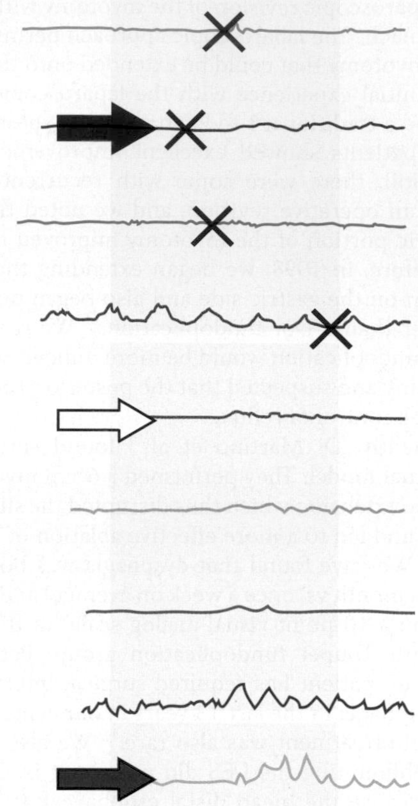

Figure 34-1. Manometry tracing showing aperistalsis of the esophageal body (*white arrow*) and incomplete LES relaxation (*red arrow*). Top four impedance tracings showing no drop in impedance and lack of bolus transit (*black arrow*).

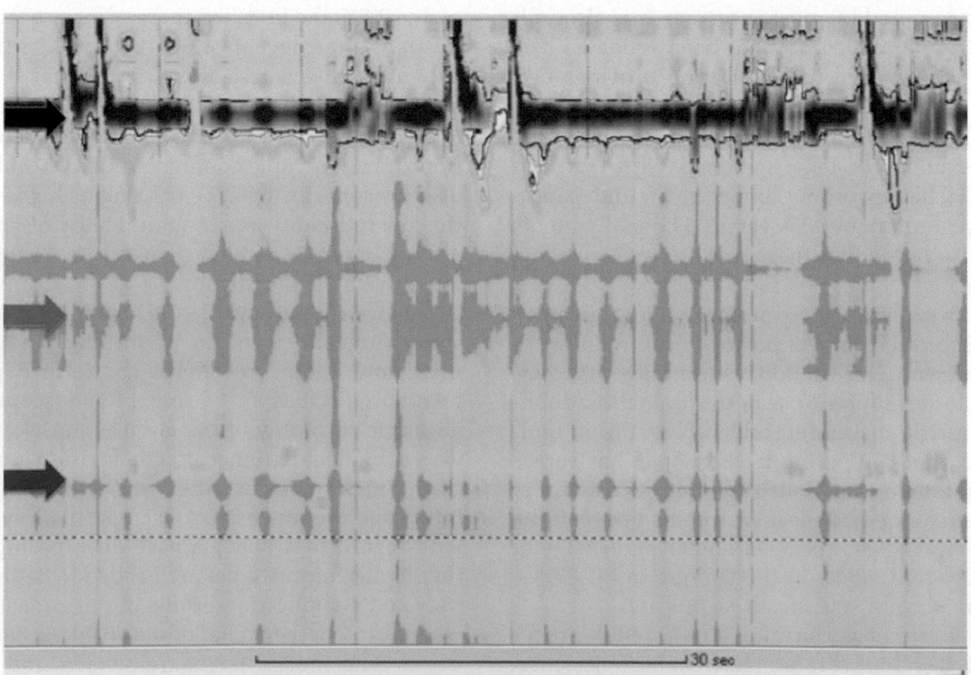

Figure 34-2. High-resolution manometry showing the upper esophageal sphincter (*black arrow*), aperistalsis of the esophageal body (*green arrow*) and the LES (*red arrow*).

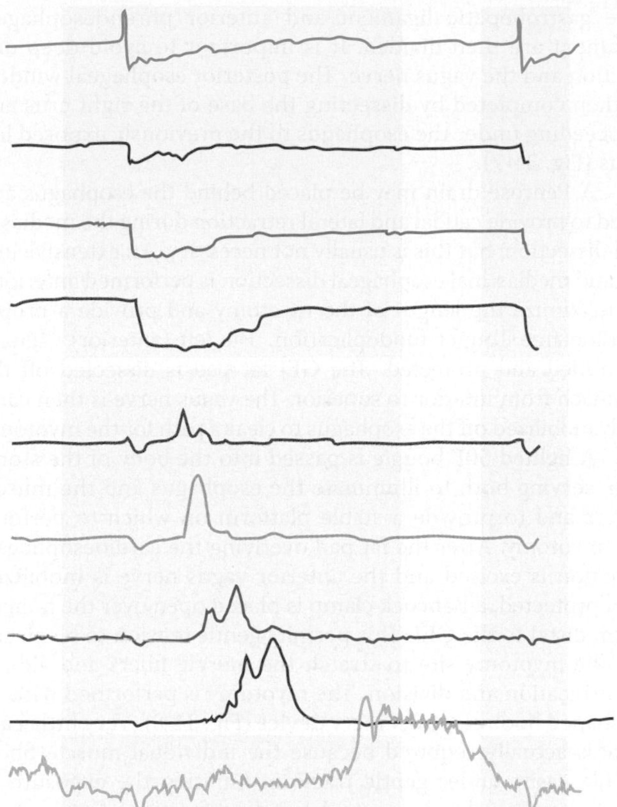

Figure 34-3. Normal esophageal manometry with progression of peristaltic wave and LES relaxation. Top four tracings show normal progressive drop in impedance followed by recovery after bolus transit.

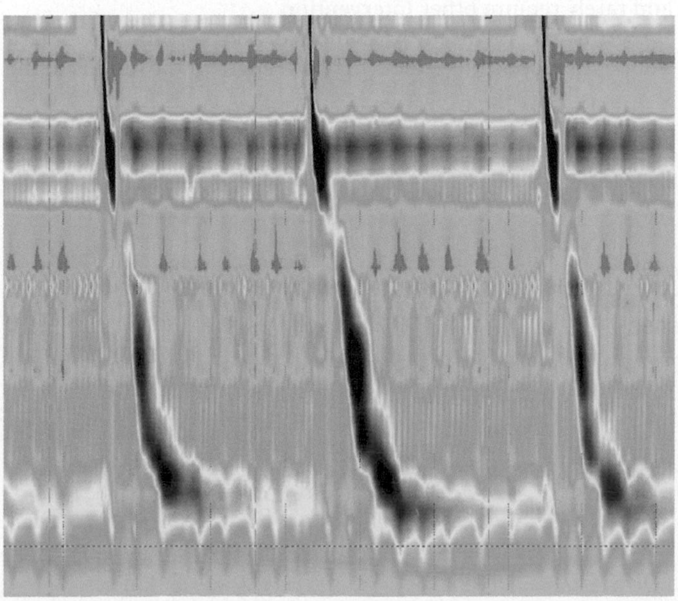

Figure 34-4. Normal high-resolution esophageal manometry with progression of peristaltic wave and LES relaxation.

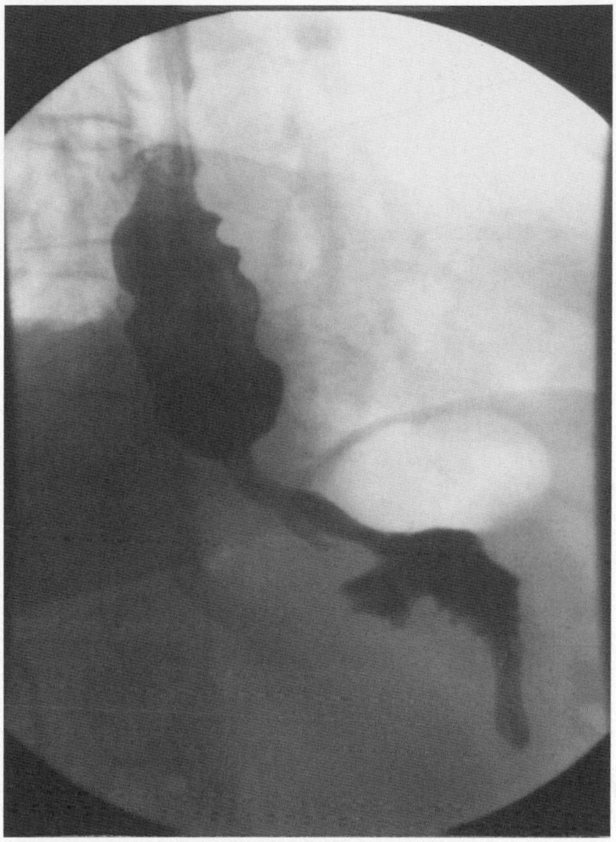

Figure 34-5. Upper gastrointestinal esophagram showing a dilated esophagus and incomplete relaxation of the LES, allowing minimal fluid passage.

Esophagogastroscopy

Endoscopic findings include normal mucosa, usually without stigmata of reflux or esophagitis. Patients with long-standing achalasia may have thicker, abnormal mucosa. Retained food or fluid is often found. Passage of the endoscope through the LES has been described as a "pop" or "sudden release." The esophagogastroscopy, apart from the findings of achalasia, is often completely normal but is required to rule out pseudoachalasia. Any abnormal findings or variations in the presentation necessitate the performance of EUS or CT scan.

Laparoscopic Operative Technique

Preoperatively, the patient is made NPO at midnight prior to the operation. The patient is placed on a liquid diet for 4 to 5 days prior to the operation to allow for adequate emptying of esophageal contents. Immediately preoperatively the patient is given chemical deep venous thrombosis prophylaxis. Prior to the incision a first-generation cephalosporin is given as antibiotic prophylaxis.

In the operating room, the patient is placed in a modified lithotomy position with a beanbag allowing steep reverse Trendelenburg position. Four standard ports and a Nathanson liver retractor are placed (Fig. 34-6). We begin with the left upper quadrant port, placed just lateral to the midclavicular line at the costal margin. Pneumoperitoneum is obtained using a Veress needle followed by placement of a 10-mm optical trocar. The 10-mm camera port is positioned at 10 to 12 cm from the costal margin and 2 cm left of the umbilicus. A 10-mm left lateral port

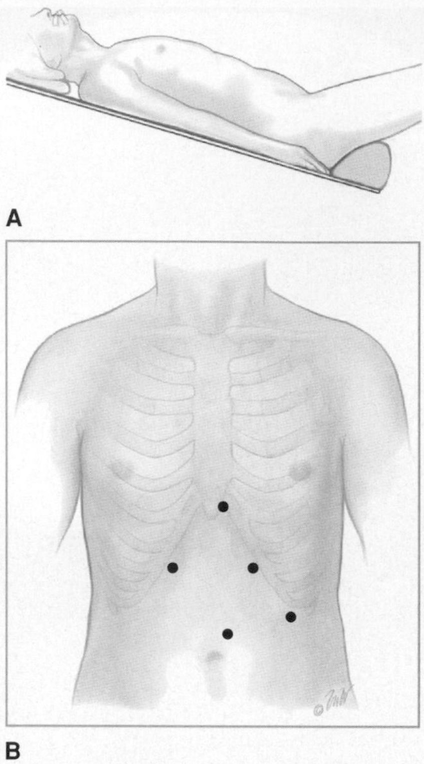

Figure 34-6. Positioning (*A*) and port placement (*B*) allow access to the hiatus, with care to avoid pressure points and to maintain joint neutrality.

along the anterior axillary line at the level of the camera port is then placed, followed by placement of a right 5-mm subcostal port. Finally, a Nathanson liver retractor is placed just to the left of midline high in the epigastrum. If the liver is large, the Nathanson retractor can be substituted with a paddle retractor from a right lateral position.

We begin by first dividing the left phrenogastric ligament to expose the posterior left crus. This facilitates division of the superior-most short gastric vessels and releases the spleen. We mobilize the gastric fundus, dividing the proximal short gastric vessels and posterior attachments of the proximal stomach to minimize tension on the subsequent fundoplication. The gastrohepatic ligament and anterior phrenoesophageal ligament are then divided. It is important to avoid deep dissection and the vagus nerve. The posterior esophageal window is then completed by dissecting the base of the right crus and proceeding under the esophagus to the previously exposed left crus (Fig. 34-7).

A Penrose drain may be placed behind the esophagus and used to provide caudal and lateral retraction during the mediastinal dissection, but this is usually not necessary. An extensive hiatal and mediastinal esophageal dissection is performed anteriorly to maximize the length of the myotomy and provide a proper tension-free Toupet fundoplication. The left (anterior) vagus is identified and protected. The GEJ fat pad is dissected off the stomach from inferior to superior. The vagus nerve is then carefully mobilized off the esophagus to clear a path for the myotomy.

A lighted 50F bougie is passed into the body of the stomach, serving both to illuminate the esophagus and the muscle layers and to provide a stable platform on which to perform the myotomy. After the fat pad overlying the cardioesophageal junction is excised and the anterior vagus nerve is mobilized and protected, a Babcock clamp is placed open over the bougie, 3 cm distal to the GEJ. This permits gentle tension to be placed on the myotomy site to stretch the muscle fibers and aids in identification and division. The myotomy is performed with an L-shaped hook electrocautery device (Fig. 34-8). Very little cautery is actually required because the individual muscle fibers divide easily under gentle traction. Limiting the exposure to electrocautery also prevents delayed perforations from unrecognized thermal mucosal injury. The longitudinal muscle fibers are divided first, exposing the inner circular muscle, which is divided next, leaving the submucosa intact (Fig. 34-9). Controlling submucosal or muscle bleeding with gentle pressure and time prevents mucosal injury, and further intervention is rarely required. The distal dissection is most difficult because of poor differentiation of the muscular layers and a thinner mucosa, especially at the GEJ. Performing a longer myotomy, at least 3 cm onto the gastric cardia and dividing all tangential sling fibers, aids in avoiding recurrent dysphagia. Mucosal perforations should be repaired with fine (4-0 or 5-0) absorbable suture and rarely require other intervention.

After the myotomy is complete, we perform a standard Toupet fundoplication, securing both edges of the fundus to the

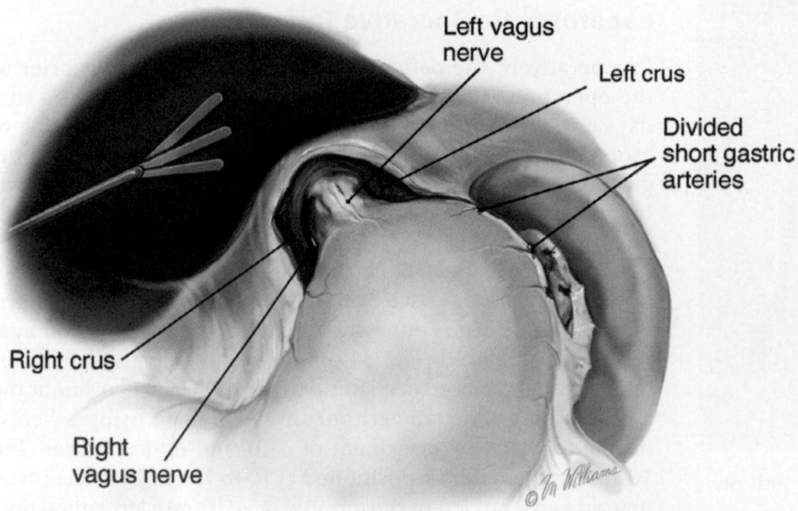

Figure 34-7. Dissection and mobilization of the esophagus.

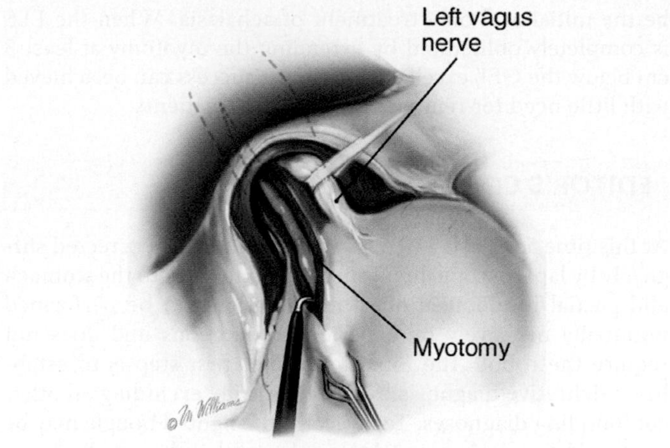

Figure 34-8. The myotomy is carried as far proximally as possible (usually 6–8 cm) and at least 3 cm onto the stomach.

muscle edges of the myotomy and to the diaphragm (Fig. 34-10). The hiatus is not closed except in the rare case of encountering a very large hiatal hernia. Should mucosal lacerations occur, a prudent choice is to perform a Dor anterior fundoplication to buttress the repaired mucosa to avoid esophageal leak or fistula. We then routinely perform intraoperative endoscopy to assure that the GEJ is open and not angulated by the fundoplication, as well as assuring no injury to the mucosa.

Postoperative Management

Patients generally start liquids the night of their procedure and are advanced to a soft diet on postoperative day 1. A trained nutritionist evaluates each patient postoperatively and provides dietary guidance. Average hospital stay is 1 to 2 days, and resumption of normal diet and activities occurs within 3 to 4 weeks. The patient is followed up at 1 to 3 weeks, and thereafter, follow-up is tailored to patient needs, including continued nutritionist input. We perform manometry and 24-hour pH studies on our patients 6 months after surgery to evaluate acid exposure, correlate symptoms with pH results, and assess outcomes. Patients with abnormal pH monitoring are placed on proton pump inhibitors to reduce their risk of chronic injury to the distal esophageal mucosa.

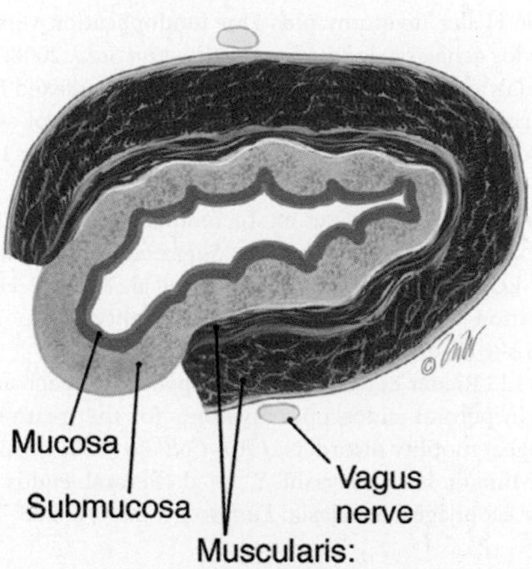

Figure 34-9. The muscle fibers are divided to the plane between the circular muscularis and the submucosa.

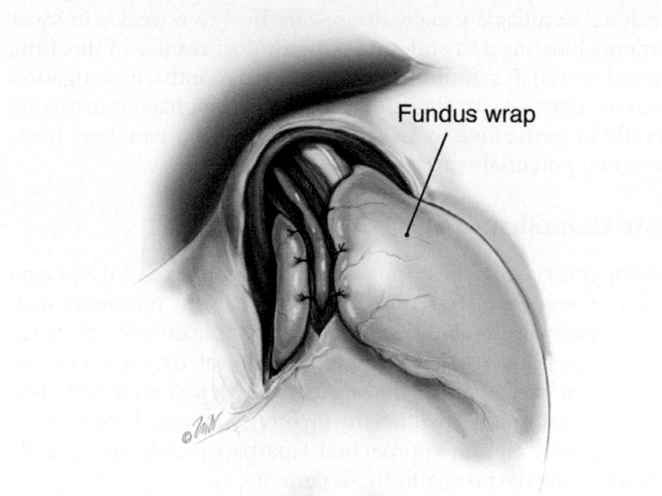

Figure 34-10. A standard Toupet fundoplication is performed after the myotomy by first securing superior edges of the fundus to each side of the myotomy and to the diaphragm. The two inferior stiches are then placed from the myotomy to the fundus.

Contraindications

The inability to undergo surgery or general endotracheal anesthesia is an absolute contraindication. Previous hiatal or esophageal surgery may be a relative barrier to laparoscopic or open surgery, but subject to surgeon comfort and experience. Prior esophageal perforations or thoracic operations may make mediastinal dissection and myotomy technically difficult. Knowledge of laparoscopic and open abdominal and thoracic approaches provides alternatives for those with prior operations or perforation.

Some believe that megaesophagus or grade IV dilatation (>8 cm) is a contraindication to myotomy because of poor dysphagia relief and technical difficulty. By using minimally invasive techniques, however, little is lost or risked in attempting a myotomy while reserving esophagectomy for failures. Most patients with severe or even sigmoid-shaped esophagi are relieved of dysphagia and subsequently avoid esophagectomy and its higher associated morbidity and mortality (2%–8%).[4]

We do usually avoid a fundoplication in patients with a sigmoid esophagus tortuosity at the GEJ, as it can provide further angulation that can negate any benefits from the myotomy.

COMPLICATIONS

Early Complications

Perforations occur in 1% to 5% of patients in most series, and most are recognized and repaired, adding little morbidity to or deleterious effect on successful relief of dysphagia. Pneumothorax, bleeding, intra-abdominal abscess, and wound infection occur in approximately 3% of patients. Pneumothorax rarely requires treatment because the carbon dioxide used for insufflation is readily absorbed. Other complications, such as vagal injuries, unrecognized mucosal perforations, or splenic injuries, are reported but rare.

Bloating and the inability to belch occasionally bother patients after Nissen fundoplication. Patients rarely complain of similar symptoms after esophagomyotomy and fundoplication.

Residual dysphagia usually disappears by 4 to 6 weeks. In most patients bloating and abdominal discomfort resolve in this time period as well. If symptoms remain after 3 months, investigation with an upper gastrointestinal study and esophagogastroscopy should be performed to assess fundoplication orientation, position, and potential scarring of the myotomy.

Late Complications

Postoperative complications related to recurrent dysphagia and reflux account for most clinically relevant problems with esophagomyotomy and fundoplication. Occasionally, diarrhea occurs, possibly owing to increased bowel osmotic load or changes in gastric emptying. In many patients, recurrent dysphagia is caused by insufficient myotomy length. Lengthening the myotomy can be approached laparoscopically and usually alleviates the dysphagia in these patients.

SUMMARY

Laparoscopic eosphagocardiomyotomy with partial fundoplication for patients with an acceptable operative risk should be the initial and only treatment of achalasia. When the LES is completely obliterated by extending the myotomy at least 3 cm below the GEJ, excellent long-term success can be achieved with little need for reintervention in most patients.

EDITOR'S COMMENT

At this time achalasia is a disease that should be corrected surgically by laparoscopic myotomy with extension to the stomach and partial fundoplication. The operation can be performed minimally invasively by experienced surgeons and does not require the robot. The most important first step is to establish a definitive diagnosis by systematically excluding all other confounding diagnoses. Technically, the lighted bougie may be replaced by an endoscope that can be used at the conclusion of the myotomy both to confirm the success of the procedure and to rule out perforation. Reoperation for the failed myotomy also may be performed laparoscopically. To reduce the risk of perforation, we usually place the new myotomy more to the patient's left on the esophagus and stomach (at the line of the greater curvature).

—Raphael Bueno

References

1. Heller E. Extramukose kardioplastik beim chronischen kardiospasmus it dilatation des oesophagus. *Mitt Grenzgeb Med Chir.* 1914;27:141–149.
2. Pellegrini CA. Impact and evolution of minimally invasive techniques in the treatment of achalasia. *Surg Endosc.* 1997;11:1–2.
3. Oelschlager B, Pellegrini CA. Surgical management of achalasia. *MedGenMed.* 2003;5(4):31.
4. Patti MG, Fisichella PM, Perretta S, et al. Impact of minimally invasive surgery on the treatment of esophageal achalasia: a decade of change. *J Am Coll Surg.* 2003;196:698–703; discussion 703–705.
5. Chapman JR, Joehl RJ, Murayama KM, et al. Achalasia treatment: improved outcome of laparoscopic myotomy with operative manometry. *Arch Surg.* 2004;139(5):508–513; discussion 513.
6. Oelschlager BK, Chang L, Pellegrini CA. Improved outcome after extended gastric myotomy for achalasia. *Arch Surg.* 2003;138:490–495; discussion 5–7.
7. Zaninotto G, Costantini M, Rizzetto C, et al. Four hundred laparoscopic myotomies for esophageal achalasia: a single centre experience. *Ann Surg.* 2008;248:986–993.
8. Zaninotto G, Annese V, Costantini M, et al. Randomized controlled trial of botulinum toxin versus laparoscopic heller myotomy for esophageal achalasia. *Ann Surg.* 2004;239:364–370.
9. Woltman TA, Oelschlager BK, Pellegrini CA. Surgical management of esophageal motility disorders. *J Surg Res.* 2004;117:34–43.
10. Lendrum F. Anatomic features of the cardiac orifice of the stomach with special reference to cardioaspasm. *Arch Intern Med.* 1937;59:474–511.
11. Ramacciato G, Mercantini P, Amodio PM, et al. The laparoscopic approach with antireflux surgery is superior to the thoracoscopic approach for the treatment of esophageal achalasia. Experience of a single surgical unit. *Surg Endosc.* 2002;16:1431–1437.
12. Pandolfino JE, Kwiatek MA, Nealis T, et al. Achalasia: a new clinically relevant classification by high-resolution manometry. *Gastroenterology.* 2008;135:1526–1533.
13. Luketich JD, Fernando HC, Christie NA, et al. Outcomes after minimally invasive esophagomyotomy. *Ann Thorac Surg.* 2001;72:1909–1912; discussion 12–13.
14. Wright AS, Williams CW, Pellegrini CA, et al. Long-term outcomes confirm the superior efficacy of extended Heller myotomy with Toupet fundoplication for achalasia. *Surg Endosc.* 2007;21:713–738.
15. Di Martino N, Monaco L, Izzo G, et al. The effect of esophageal myotomy and myectomy on the lower esophageal sphincter pressure profile: intraoperative computerized manometry study. *Dis Esophagus.* 2005;18:160–165.
16. Richards WO, Torquati A, Holzman MD, et al. Heller myotomy versus Heller myotomy with Dor fundoplication for achalasia: a prospective randomized double-blind clinical trial. *Ann Surg.* 2004;240:405–412; discussion 12–15.
17. Donahue PE, Horgan S, Liu KJ, et al. Floppy Dor fundoplication after esophagocardiomyotomy for achalasia. *Surgery.* 2002;132:716–722; discussion 22–23.
18. Hunter JG, Trus TL, Branum GD, et al. Laparoscopic Heller myotomy and fundoplication for achalasia. *Ann Surg.* 1997;225:655–664; discussion 64–65.
19. Rawlings A, Soper NJ, Oelschlager B, et al. Laparoscopic Dor versus Toupet fundoplication following Heller myotomy for achalasia: results of a multicenter, prospective, randomized-controlled trial. *Surg Endosc.* 2012;26:18–26.
20. Rebecchi F, Giaccone C, Farinella E, et al. Randomized controlled trial of laparoscopic Heller myotomy plus Dor fundoplication versus Nissen fundoplication for achalasia: long-term results. *Ann Surg.* 2008;248:1023–1030.
21. Horgan S, Galvani C, Gorodner MV, et al. Robotic-assisted Heller myotomy versus laparoscopic Heller myotomy for the treatment of esophageal achalasia: multicenter study. *J Gastrointest Surg.* 2005;9:1020–1029; discussion 9–30.
22. Iqbal A, Haider M, Desai K, et al. Technique and follow-up of minimally invasive Heller myotomy for achalasia. *Surg Endosc.* 2006;20:394–401.
23. Huffmanm LC, Pandalai PK, Boulton BJ, et al. Robotic Heller myotomy: a safe operation with higher postoperative quality-of-life indices. *Surgery.* 2007;142:613–618; discussion 8–20.
24. Swanstrom LL, Rieder E, Dunst CM. A stepwise approach and early clinical experience in peroral endoscopic myotomy for the treatment of achalasia and esophageal motility disorders. *J Am Coll Surg.* 2011;213:751–756.
25. Inoue H, Minami H, Kobayashi Y, et al. Peroral endoscopic myotomy (POEM) for esophageal achalasia. *Endoscopy.* 2010;42:265–271.

35 Long Esophageal Myotomy: Open, Thoracoscopic, and Peroral Endoscopic Approach

Jon O. Wee and David J. Sugarbaker

Keywords: Surgical treatment of diffuse esophageal spasm, open esophageal myotomy, minimally invasive thoracoscopic myotomy, peroral endoscopic myotomy

Diffuse esophageal spasm (DES) is one of several nonspecific smooth muscle esophageal motility disorders associated with intermittent debilitating dysphagia and chest pain. The efficacy of long esophageal myotomy for the surgical treatment of DES has not been as favorable as myotomy has been for achalasia (see Chapter 33). Surgical treatment in this patient group therefore remains controversial. Long esophageal myotomy was first described for the treatment of DES in 1950 by Professor Lortat-Jacob of Paris, France.[1] Although the surgical principles remain the same, a few modifications have been made in the approach to diagnosis and treatment.

GENERAL PRINCIPLES AND PATIENT SELECTION

The pathophysiology of DES is still poorly understood. It is thought to be a neuropathy involving the smooth muscle layer of the esophageal wall that causes an inhibitory effect in the distal esophagus and hypotension of the lower esophageal sphincter (LES), giving rise to incomplete LES relaxation after a wet swallow. Gastroesophageal reflux disease (GERD) also has been implicated in the etiology of DES.[2] Dysphagia to solids and liquids, sometimes exacerbated by very cold or very hot foods, and intermittent chest pain are the predominant symptoms. The dysmotility, which is characterized by the presence of incoordinated nonperistaltic esophageal contractions of high, medium, or low amplitude, may progress or, in rare cases, has been observed to normalize. Progression of DES to achalasia is uncommon but has been reported in a prospective cohort study. No manometric or demographic predictors of progression have been identified.[3]

The condition continues to represent a therapeutic challenge. For some patients, medical therapy with smooth muscle relaxants (e.g., long-acting nitrates), calcium channel antagonists, and/or psychotropic drugs has proved beneficial.[4,5] Anticholinergics, pneumatic dilation, and botulinum toxin (Botox) injections produce brief and partial symptomatic relief.

Surgery is offered when symptoms are refractory to medical treatment or when complications arise. In general, surgical therapy can control symptoms in approximately 80% of patients. Patients with spastic disorder in addition to a pulsion diverticulum will benefit more from surgery than patients with spastic disorder only.[6] Long myotomy is often combined with an antireflux operation.

A successful outcome for surgical treatment of DES requires the elimination or reduction of episodes of dysphagia and/or chest pain and prevention of postoperative GERD. Some consider long esophageal myotomy for DES to be a palliative procedure because swallowing is never perfectly restored.

PREOPERATIVE ASSESSMENT

Since esophageal motility dysfunction is thought to represent a continuum of disease, establishing the correct diagnosis is important to selecting the most appropriate treatment, reducing the incidence of postoperative complications, and achieving the best therapeutic outcome. The standard diagnostic work-up for DES includes barium swallow, esophageal manometry, esophagogastroduodenoscopy (EGD), and endoscopic ultrasound (EUS). pH studies can confirm the presence or absence of gastroesophageal reflux and may guide therapeutic maneuvers.

Radiologic examination with barium swallow reveals the characteristic corkscrew appearance of the esophagus first described by Moersch and Camp (Fig. 35-1).[7] The contractions are relatively constant in their location and usually confined to the lower half of the intrathoracic esophagus. On esophageal manometry, DES is characterized by the presence of intermittent simultaneous contractions (30–100 mm Hg) intermixed with normal peristalsis (Fig. 35-2). The disorder is variously defined as the presence of 10% to 30% or more simultaneous contractions after 10 wet swallows.[8,9] The greater the percentage of simultaneous contractions, the more certain is the diagnosis. The mean simultaneous contraction amplitude in DES should exceed 30 mm Hg. Other manometric findings may include spontaneous contractions and repetitive contractions (multiple-peaked contractions).[8,10]

EGD is indicated to exclude organic pathology such as an obstructing lesion, benign stricture, or cancer. Endoscopic observation of DES also has revealed that the tighter muscular rings tend to be fixed in location and that the less constricting spastic muscle causes the mucosa to have a corrugated appearance (Fig. 35-3).[11,12]

EUS can be quite useful for assessing the extent of the spastic segment when used in combination with barium esophagram and manometric analysis. The spastic segment is revealed by a thickened muscle layer in the esophageal wall (Fig. 35-4).[13] The esophageal wall muscle is thicker at rest (baseline) in patients with DES than in normal subjects, and there is a significant correlation between baseline muscle thickening and peak pressure.[11,14]

SURGICAL TECHNIQUE

Anesthesia and Positioning

Long esophageal myotomy is usually performed via thoracotomy or minimally invasive thoracoscopy. Whenever a thoracotomy is planned, an epidural catheter should be placed. With

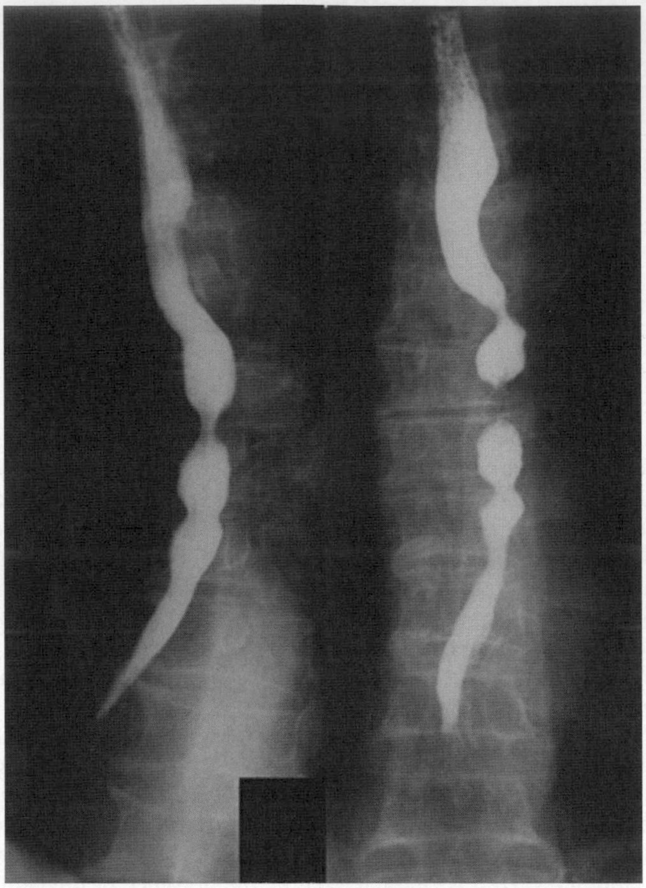

Figure 35-1. Barium swallow from a patient with DES showing poorly sequenced peristaltic waves that produce the classic corkscrew appearance of the esophagus below the infra-aortic arch. (Reproduced with permission from Maruyama K, Motoyama S, Okuyama M, et al. Successful surgical treatment for diffuse esophageal spasm. *Jpn J Thorac Cardiovasc Surg*. 2005;53:169–172.)

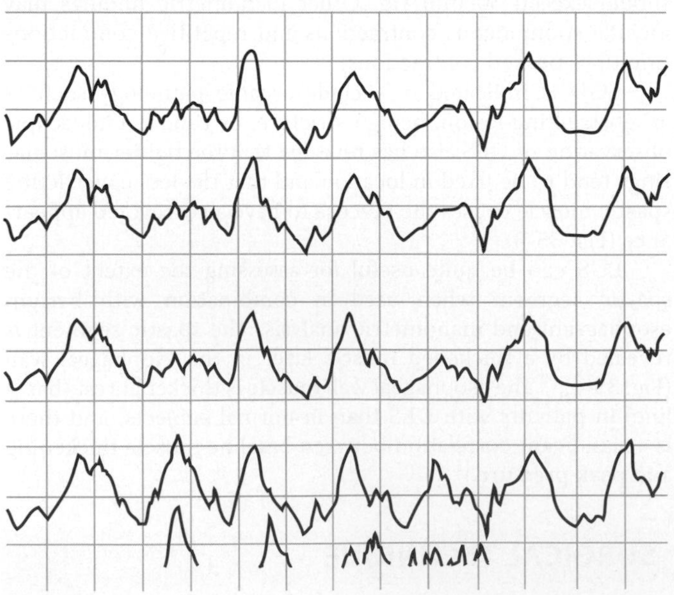

Figure 35-2. Esophageal manometry showing intermittent simultaneous contractions (30–100 mm Hg) and the presence of these contractions after 50% of wet swallows. (Reproduced with permission from Maruyama K, Motoyama S, Okuyama M, et al. Successful surgical treatment for diffuse esophageal spasm. *Jpn J Thorac Cardiovasc Surg*. 2005;53:169–172.)

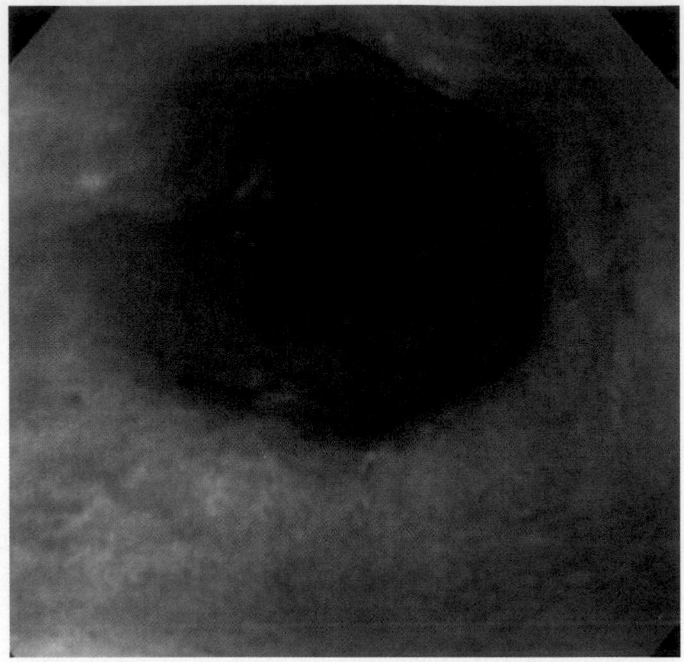

Figure 35-3. Esophagoscopy revealing tight muscular rings and corrugated appearance of the esophageal mucosa. (Reproduced with permission from Maruyama K, Motoyama S, Okuyama M, et al. Successful surgical treatment for diffuse esophageal spasm. *Jpn J Thorac Cardiovasc Surg*. 2005;53:169–172.)

the minimally invasive approach, depending on the surgeon's experience and confidence that the procedure can be completed without conversion to open technique, the epidural may not be necessary.[15] A double-lumen endotracheal tube permitting lung isolation is necessary, regardless of approach. A nasogastric tube is inserted, and the patient is placed in right lateral

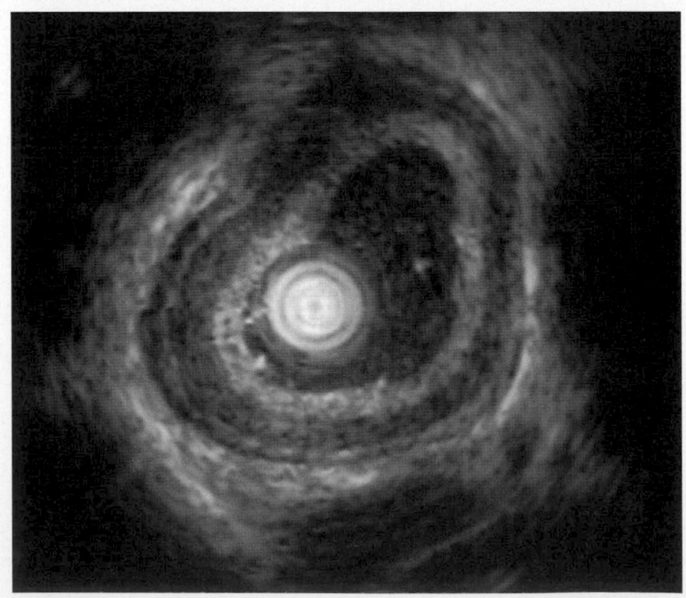

Figure 35-4. Endoscopic ultrasonography showing the thickness of the muscle layer at rest in the spastic region of the esophagus located 23 cm from the incisors. (Reproduced with permission from Maruyama K, Motoyama S, Okuyama M, et al. Successful surgical treatment for diffuse esophageal spasm. *Jpn J Thorac Cardiovasc Surg*. 2005;53:169–172.)

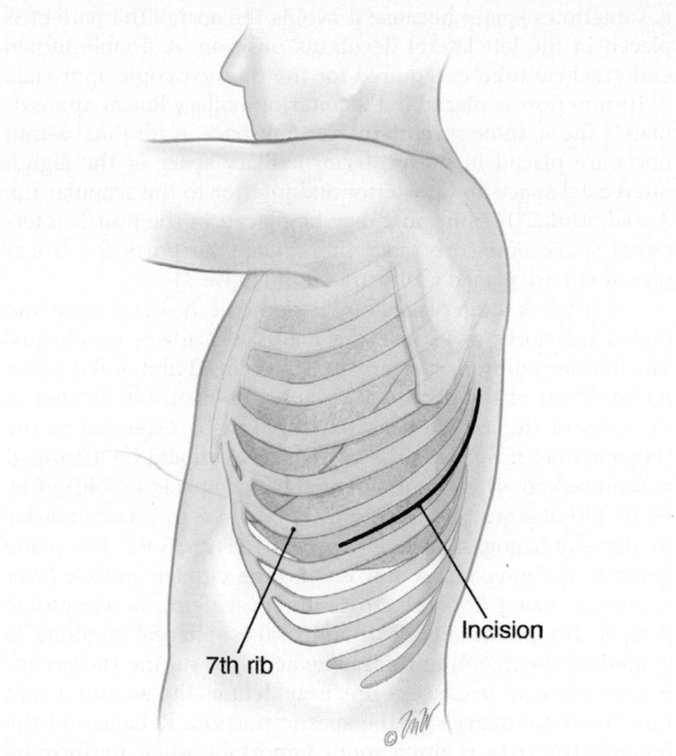

Figure 35-5. Incision for left open thoracotomy approach.

decubitus position. The position of the endotracheal tube is reconfirmed before draping.

Open Thoracotomy Approach

A left posterolateral thoracotomy is preferred because it is easier to perform an antireflux procedure if needed through the left chest. The left lung is isolated. The sixth or preferably seventh intercostal space is entered (Fig. 35-5). The inferior pulmonary ligament is mobilized up to the inferior pulmonary vein. The lung is retracted medially and cephalad, and the mediastinal pleura is incised over the esophagus. A Penrose drain is placed around the esophagus to assist with mobilization. Care should be taken to identify and preserve both vagal nerve trunks. A complete longitudinal extramucosal myotomy in the spastic segment of the esophagus is made using scissors, knife, diathermy, LigaSure (Valleylab, Boulder, CO), or Harmonic Scalpel (Ethicon Endosurgery, Inc.). The segment of spastic smooth muscle usually is located in the middle and lower esophageal wall in patients with DES. The myotomy thus is usually performed inferior to the level of the aortic arch.

The surgical technique described by Henderson et al.[16] involved a total thoracic myotomy that extended to the thoracic inlet. Ellis[17] found later that a total intrathoracic myotomy was rarely indicated. In most patients with DES, the LES is normal, and therefore, a myotomy extending superiorly to the aortic arch level is sufficient (Fig. 35-6). If the preoperative work-up reveals an abnormal LES, the myotomy should be extended inferiorly onto the gastric cardia. This, however, increases the risk of postoperative gastroesophageal reflux, and a fundoplication or fundic patch procedure ranging from 2 to 3 cm in length may be required.[18]

The reasons for performing a fundic patch procedure are to preserve the separation of each myotomized edge, to reinforce the wall of the surface of the myotomized mucosa, and to avoid postoperative leak complications. Some surgeons claim that the patch procedure also prevents adhesion and contraction of the myotomy wound and the possible development of postoperative segmental diverticular dilatation at the myotomy site. The number of patients who have been reported to undergo this technique, however, is limited, and there is no long-term follow-up.[13]

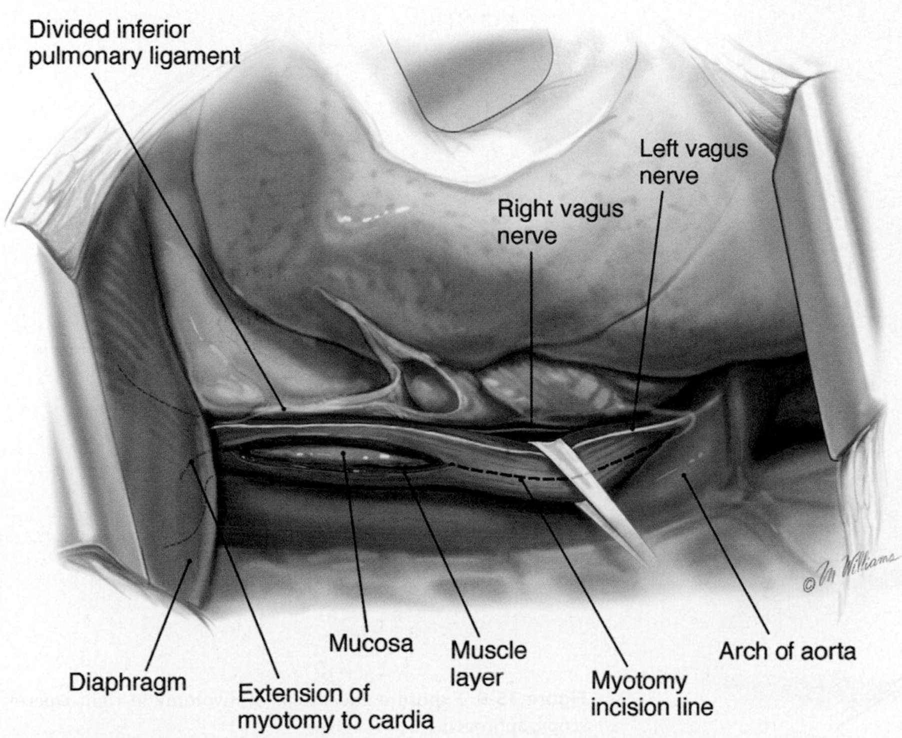

Figure 35-6. Long myotomy with the spastic segment commencing above the LES, with myotomy carried superiorly to the level of the aortic arch. Dashed lines indicate extension onto the gastric cardia when there is LES involvement.

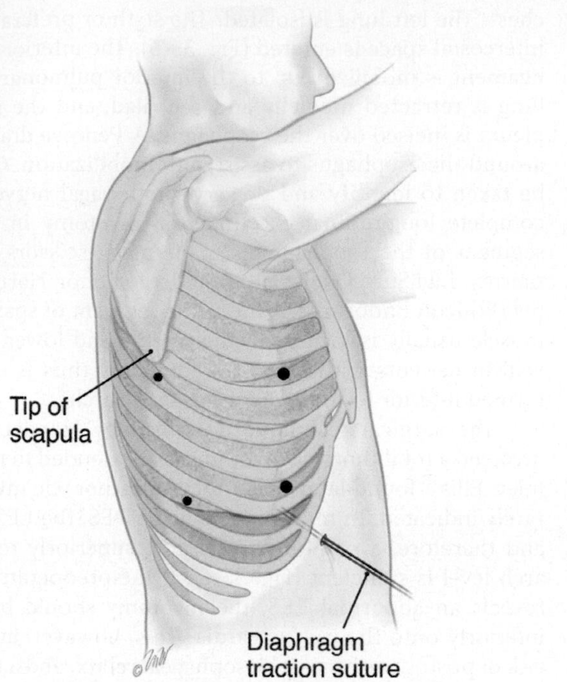

Figure 35-7. Port placement for minimally invasive long myotomy.

Thoracoscopic Approach

Thoracoscopic esophageal myotomy has been performed in several centers with early satisfactory results.[19–21] Although in the open approach the esophagus is exposed through the left chest, in a minimally invasive approach, a right-sided approach is sometimes easier because it avoids the aorta. The patient is placed in the left lateral decubitus position. A double-lumen endotracheal tube is required for the thoracoscopic approach. A 10-mm port is placed in the anterior axillary line at approximately the sixth or seventh intercostal space. Additional 5-mm ports are placed in the posterior axillary space at the eighth intercostal space and posterior and inferior to the scapular tip. An additional 10-mm port may be placed in the fourth intercostal space anteriorly near the axilla. The ports for trocar placement are placed as illustrated in Figure 35-7.

A stitch is often placed on the dome of the diaphragm and pulled inferiorly to expose the hiatus and lower esophagus. The inferior pulmonary ligament is mobilized first, followed by mobilization of the distal esophagus. The pleura is divided to the level of the azygos vein, but this can be extended to the thoracic inlet if needed. The vagus nerves should be identified and preserved. The circumferential esophagus is mobilized by 90 to 120 degrees. The myotomy is begun 6 to 7 cm superior to the esophagogastric junction (EGJ) (Fig. 35-8). The plane between the muscularis mucosa and the circular muscle layer is entered using hook electrocautery, LigaSure, or Harmonic Scalpel. The extent of the extramucosal esophageal myotomy is guided by the manometric tracing acquired during the preoperative work-up because it precisely defines the anatomic and functional boundaries of the spastic portion. Reliance on the manometric data is often more important when performing redo surgery after an incomplete myotomy has failed.

The mucosa should be inspected closely to identify mucosal perforations irrespective of the approach to surgery. Filling the pleural space with saline and gently insufflating air into the esophagus is a useful technique in this regard, but it is far from 100% accurate. Before closure, the pleural space is drained with a single 28F chest tube.

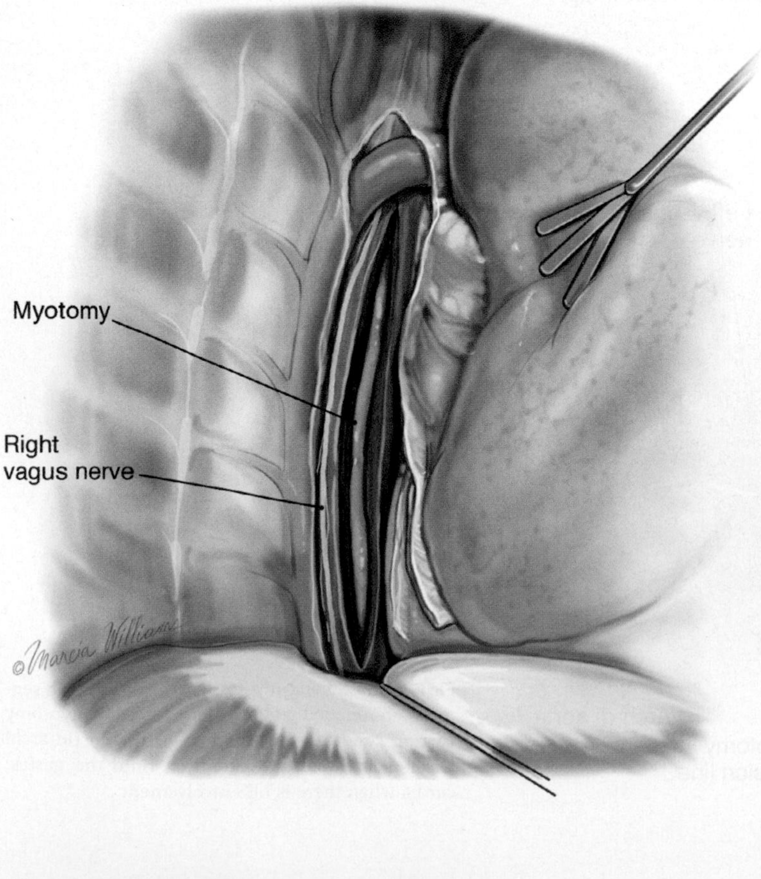

Figure 35-8. Exposure and extent of myotomy in right laparoscopic approach.

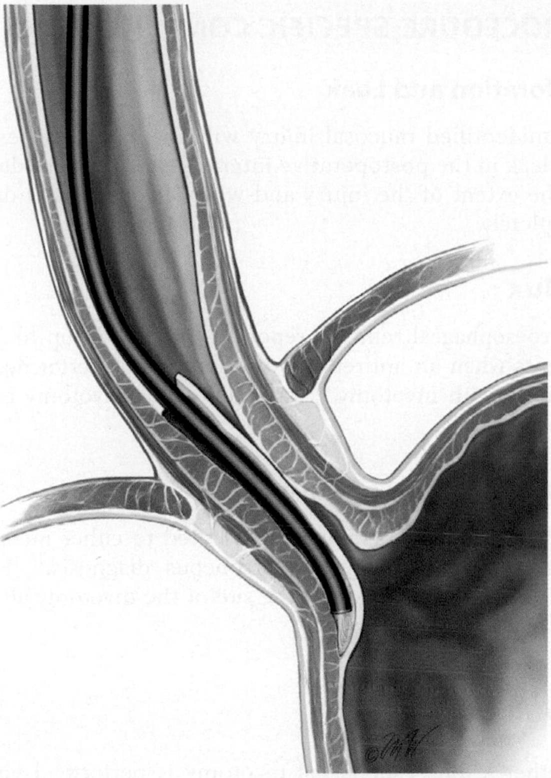

Figure 35-9. Peroral endoscopic myotomy (POEM). The endoscope is placed in the submucosal space and a tunnel is created by insufflating with CO_2 and saline infusion.

Peroral Endoscopic Myotomy

Peroral endoscopic myotomy (POEM) has emerged as a possible alternative approach to the traditional myotomy. As an advent of natural orifice transluminal endoscopic surgery (NOTES), this technique has been described for the treatment of achalasia,[22,23] but the technique also can be adapted for longer myotomies. In general, a mucostomy is performed with the endoscope. The endoscope is placed in the submucosal space and an endoscopic tunnel is created using gentle CO_2 insufflation and saline infusion (Fig. 35-9). An endoscopic triangular-shaped needle knife (TT-knife, Olympus) is used to divide the inner circular muscular layer (Fig. 35-10). The longitudinal muscles remain intact. The scope is then withdrawn and the mucosal lining is closed with endoscopic hemoclips (Fig. 35-11).

Swanström et al.[23] described five patients who underwent POEM for achalasia with no complications and initial favorable outcomes. Von Renteln et al.[22] report a prospective trial in Europe of 16 patients with achalasia. At 3 months follow-up, patients had decreased LES pressures with improvement in 94% of patients. Hence, this may be a method that can be adapted for long myotomies, although current data are lacking for this indication.

POSTOPERATIVE CARE

Postoperative care after long myotomy for DES follows the same principles of care for any noncardiac surgery of the chest. Unique to surgery of the esophagus, however, is a high index

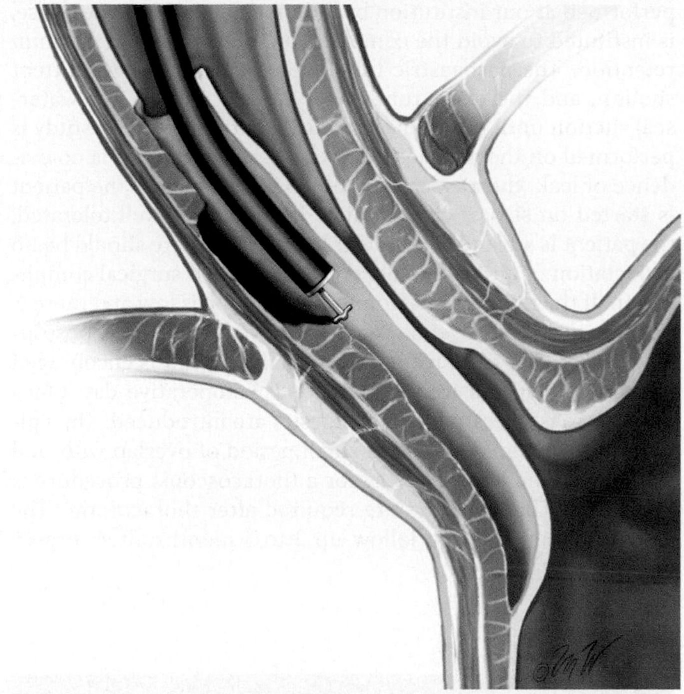

Figure 35-10. A triangular-shaped endoscopic needle knife (TT-knife; Olympus) is used to divide the inner circular muscular layer, leaving the longitudinal muscles intact.

of suspicion for unidentified esophageal leak, for this can be a catastrophic complication. Patients are extubated preferably in the OR or postanesthesia recovery room. At our institution, patients are admitted to a step-down thoracic ICU. Attention to pulmonary toilet is essential, and chest physiotherapy,

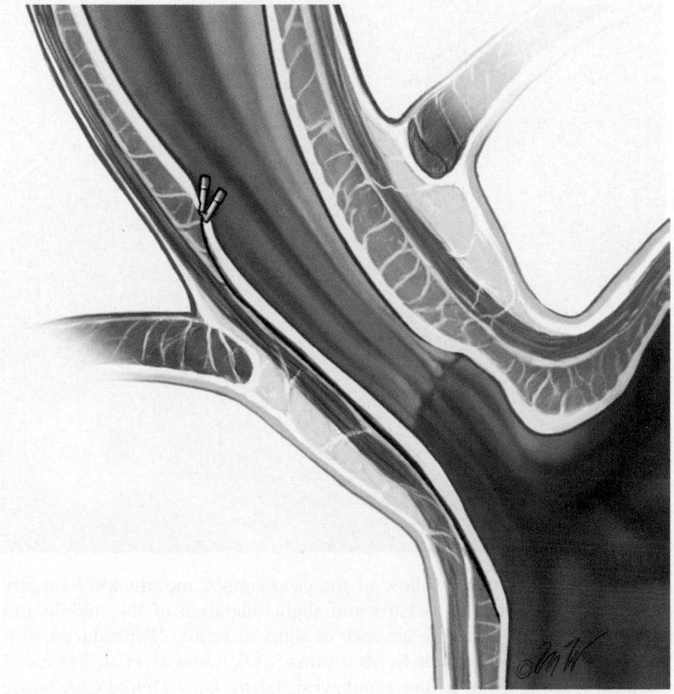

Figure 35-11. The scope is withdrawn and the mucosal lining is closed with endoscopic hemoclips.

performed at our institution by a thoracic intensive care nurse, is instituted to avoid the complication of atelectasis or sputum retention. The nasogastric tube is placed on low intermittent suction, and the chest tube is set at −20 cm H_2O of water-seal suction until the next morning. A barium swallow study is performed on the first postoperative day, and if there is no evidence of leak, the nasogastric tube is removed, and the patient is started on sips of clear liquids. If liquids are well tolerated, the patient is advanced to a clear liquid diet. There should be no expectation of air leak unless there is a known surgical complication. If the fluid output from the chest tube is low and there is no air leak, the chest tube can be removed on the first postoperative day after the barium swallow. The patient is encouraged to ambulate aggressively on the first postoperative day. Once oral intake is tolerated, oral analgesics are introduced. The epidural is later removed after a small period of overlap with oral analgesics. The length of stay for a thoracoscopic procedure is 1 to 3 days. Longer stays are required after thoracotomy. The patient is seen again in follow-up 2 to 3 months after surgery (Fig. 35-12).

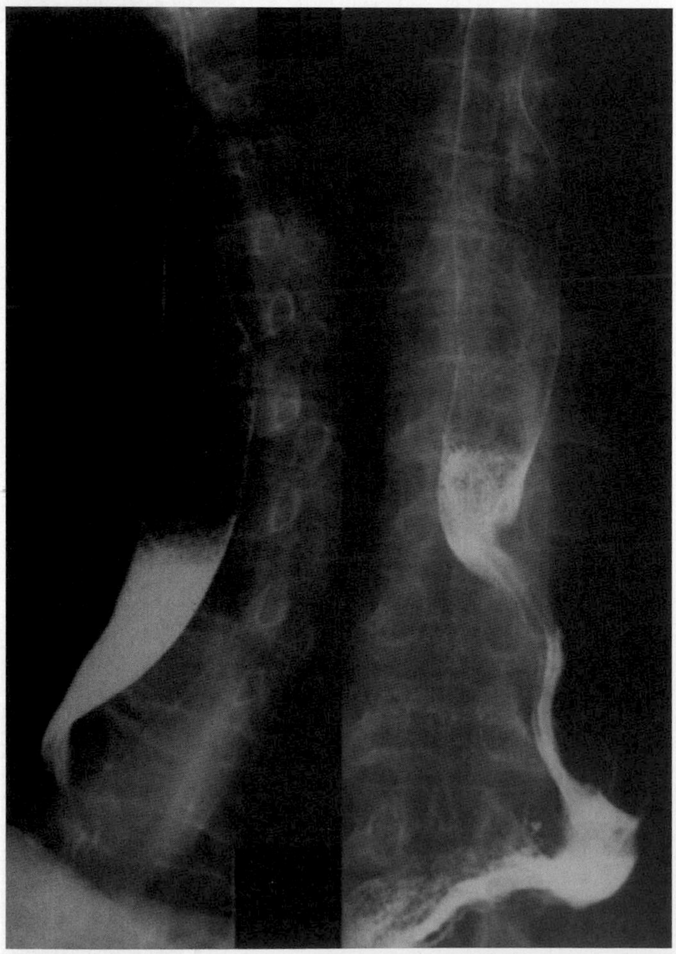

Figure 35-12. Barium swallow of the esophagus 2 months after surgery showing the absence of spasms and slight dilatation of the middle and lower esophagus. Note the absence of signs of reflux. (Reproduced with permission from Maruyama K, Motoyama S, Okuyama M, et al. Successful surgical treatment for diffuse esophageal spasm. *Jpn J Thorac Cardiovasc Surg.* 2005;53:169–172.)

PROCEDURE-SPECIFIC COMPLICATIONS

Perforation and Leak

An unidentified mucosal injury will give rise to an esophageal leak in the postoperative interval. Management depends on the extent of the injury and whether or not it is drained completely.

Reflux

Gastroesophageal reflux is reported to occur in up to 50% of patients when an antireflux procedure is not performed concomitant with myotomy,[24] especially if the myotomy extends onto the cardia.

Dysphagia and Failure

Surgical failures generally are attributed to either incomplete myotomy or incomplete or erroneous diagnosis.[16] Fibrous adhesions or contraction at the site of the myotomy also may result in failure.

SUMMARY

Whether a long esophageal myotomy is performed via posterolateral thoracotomy or minimally invasive thoracoscopy, one should ensure that the correct diagnosis has been made and that all the preoperative investigations are reviewed thoroughly. Extending the myotomy superiorly to the level of the aortic arch will ensure that the spastic segment is completely excluded. The vagus trunks should be identified and preserved, and all the extramucosal layers should be divided. A debate still exists as to whether an antireflux procedure should be included in the operative plan. In our practice, we base this decision on the following factors: Whenever the spastic segment extends onto the gastric cardia or if the patient has pre-existing symptoms of reflux that have been confirmed with pH studies, we always include an antireflux operation. In this case, we generally perform a Dor or Belsey wrap. The procedure can be performed through the left chest or abdomen. If there is minimal or limited distal involvement of the cardia with no reflux symptoms, we opt for a sphincter-sparing myotomy with good long-term outcome.

EDITOR'S COMMENT

It may be technically advantageous to place a gastroscope into the stomach instead of a nasogastric tube during the conduct of the operation. The gastroscope distends the esophagus, but not too much, and facilitates the performance of the myotomy. It also allows the surgeon to immediately verify, endoscopically, the sufficient extent of the myotomy and absence of leak. As noted above, the number of patients who are truly candidates for long myotomy is small. We advise multi-modality care for these patients and a team decision before offering them surgery since many such patients may not be much better after surgery.

—Raphael Bueno

References

1. Lortat-Jacob JL. La myomatosa nodulaire diffuse de l'oesophage. Les Acquisitions Medicales Recentes. *Ed Med Flammarion.* 1950;195:103–111.
2. Robson K, Rosenberg S, Lembo T. GERD progressing to diffuse esophageal spasm and then to achalasia. *Dig Dis Sci.* 2000;45:110–113.
3. Khatami SS, Khandwala F, Shay SS, et al. Does diffuse esophageal spasm progress to achalasia? A prospective cohort study. *Dig Dis Sci.* 2005;50:1605–1610.
4. Swamy N. Esophageal spasm: clinical and manometric response to nitroglycerine and long acting nitrites. *Gastroenterology.* 1977;72:23–27.
5. Richter JE, Dalton CB, Buice RG, et al. Nifedipine: a potent inhibitor of contractions in the body of the human esophagus: studies in healthy volunteers and patients with the nutcracker esophagus. *Gastroenterology.* 1985;89:549–554.
6. Nastos D, Chen LQ, Ferraro P, et al. Long myotomy with antireflux repair for esophageal spastic disorders. *J Gastrointest Surg.* 2002;6:713–722.
7. Moersch H, Camp J. Diffuse spasm of the lower part of the esophagus. *Ann Otol Rhinol Laryngol.* 1934;43:1165–1173.
8. Richter JE. Oesophageal motility disorders. *Lancet.* 2001;358:823–828.
9. Clouse R, Hallett J. What degree of impaired peristalsis is important for the diagnosis of diffuse esophageal spasm. *Am J Gastroenterol.* 1992;87:1246A.
10. Spechler SJ, Castell DO. Classification of oesophageal motility abnormalities. *Gut.* 2001;49:145–151.
11. Maruyama K, Motoyama S, Okuyama M, et al. Successful surgical treatment for diffuse esophageal spasm. *Jpn J Thorac Cardiovasc Surg.* 2005;53:169–172.
12. Skinner D, Belsey R. *Management of Esophageal Disease.* Philadelphia, PA: Saunders; 1988:431–440.
13. Kuwano H, Miyazaki T, Masuda N, et al. Long myotomy of the esophagus and gastric cardia with a complete fundic patch procedure for diffuse esophageal spasm. *Hepatogastroenterology.* 2004;51:1729–1731.
14. Pehlivanov N, Liu J, Kassab GS, et al. Relationship between esophageal muscle thickness and intraluminal pressure in patients with esophageal spasm. *Am J Physiol Gastrointest Liver Physiol.* 2002;282:G1016–G1023.
15. Patti MG, Pellegrini CA, Arcerito M, et al. Comparison of medical and minimally invasive surgical therapy for primary esophageal motility disorders. *Arch Surg.* 1995;130:609–615; discussion 15–16.
16. Henderson RD, Ryder D, Marryatt G. Extended esophageal myotomy and short total fundoplication hernia repair in diffuse esophageal spasm: five-year review in 34 patients. *Ann Thorac Surg.* 1987;43:25–31.
17. Ellis FH Jr. Long esophagomyotomy for diffuse esophageal spasm and related disorders: an historical review. *Dis Esophagus.* 1998;11:210–214.
18. Eypasch EP, DeMeester TR, Klingman RR, et al. Physiologic assessment and surgical management of diffuse esophageal spasm. *J Thorac Cardiovasc Surg.* 1992;104:859–868; discussion 68–69.
19. Filipi CJ, Hinder RA. Thoracoscopic esophageal myotomy—a surgical technique for achalasia diffuse esophageal spasm and "nutcracker esophagus". *Surg Endosc.* 1994;8:921–925; discussion 925–926.
20. Pellegrini C, Wetter LA, Patti M, et al. Thoracoscopic esophagomyotomy. Initial experience with a new approach for the treatment of achalasia. *Ann Surg.* 1992;216:291–296; discussion 296–299.
21. Shimi SM, Nathanson LK, Cuschieri A. Thoracoscopic long oesophageal myotomy for nutcracker oesophagus: initial experience of a new surgical approach. *Br J Surg.* 1992;79:533–536.
22. von Renteln D, Inoue H, Minami H, et al. Peroral endoscopic myotomy for the treatment of achalasia: a prospective single center study. *Am J Gastroenterol.* 2012;107:411–417.
23. Swanström LL, Rieder E, Dunst CM. A stepwise approach and early clinical experience in peroral endoscopic myotomy for the treatment of achalasia and esophageal motility disorders. *J Am Coll Surg.* 2011;213(6):751–756.
24. Pellegrini CA. Impact and evolution of minimally invasive techniques in the treatment of achalasia. *Surg Endosc.* 1997;11:1–2.

36 Esophagectomy for Primary or Secondary Motility Disorders

Brian E. Louie and Eric Vallières

Keywords: Motility disorders, esophagectomy, achalasia, outcomes, surgery

INTRODUCTION

Esophageal resection and reconstruction in patients with primary or secondary motility disorders of the esophagus are very uncommon. Often, consideration of esophagectomy is the final decision in a long and difficult plan of care by both the gastroenterologist and esophageal surgeon. Fortunately, the majority of motility disorder patients are seen in expert centers, where they usually undergo extensive evaluation and are treated appropriately with reasonable palliation of their symptoms. Patients who are not well palliated usually present with disabling symptoms associated with obstruction or pseudo-obstruction, uncontrollable pain with eating, and/or refractory gastroesophageal reflux disease. In addition, these patients may have undergone not one but several prior esophageal and/or gastroesophageal surgeries.

Esophagectomy in these situations is viewed as a "Hail Mary" and may not be given enough credit owing to the significant risk of mortality and morbidity that have been attributed to this operation. However, recent technical improvements have lessened these risks and perhaps esophagectomy should be considered earlier in the treatment course rather than after repeated attempts at repair. In skilled hands, the improvement in quality of life (QOL) and swallowing function after esophagectomy may outweigh the risks of the operation for many of these patients.

This chapter briefly reviews the features, initial treatment(s), complications of treatment, and long-term outcomes of the most common primary and secondary motility disorders. It outlines the indications for esophagectomy, discusses current controversies in management, describes the technique of vagal-sparing esophagectomy (VSE) for reconstruction in these settings, and finally, summarizes the outcomes of esophagectomy in patients with benign disease.

PRIMARY AND SECONDARY MOTILITY DISORDERS

Detailed review of the primary and secondary motility disorders is beyond the scope of this chapter. For meaningful discussion of the role of esophagectomy, however, it is helpful to have some idea of the salient features of the most common primary and secondary motility disorders, as well as the recommended diagnostic evaluation, manometric findings, appropriate primary surgical therapy, and long-term complications. This information is summarized in Table 36-1.

Aside from collagen vascular disorders such as scleroderma, progressive systemic sclerosis, and systemic lupus erythematosus, the other causes of secondary motility disorders such as diabetes mellitus, alcohol, amyloidosis, myxedema, and psychiatric diseases are exceptionally rare and few if any reports exist that outline the role of esophagectomy let alone primary surgical therapy in these situations. As a principle, treatment is directed at the underlying cause of the motility disorder followed by careful evaluation with upper endoscopy, manometry, and pH testing to ensure the appropriate course of treatment may be undertaken. Secondary motility disorders are commonly associated with GERD and often complicate antireflux surgery. Whether these disorders result from, cause, or exacerbate GERD is unclear. The management of recurrent GERD and failed antireflux surgery is discussed in Chapter 43.

CLINICAL MANIFESTATIONS AND INDICATIONS FOR SURGERY

Patients with esophageal motility disorders who contemplate esophagectomy present with a wide variety of symptoms. In one large series, the most common symptoms include dysphagia (90%), regurgitation (57%), heartburn (52%), weight loss (32%), and chest pain (25%).[3] In some instances, the symptoms will be germane to the original disease process such as chest pain in nutcracker esophagus or dysphagia in achalasia. Symptoms such as regurgitation, aspiration, and dysphagia may be derived from the previous medical and surgical therapies. Rarely, patients present acutely with hemorrhage, ulceration, perforation, or fistulization. In most instances, these symptoms will be the reason to consider additional surgery, but it is important to recognize that some of these symptoms may indicate a more significant underlying process such as a benign reflux stricture that is refractory to dilation or a cancer of the esophagus. Indications for surgery that may be secondary to the motility disorder or the previous surgical therapy are listed in Table 36-2.

PREOPERATIVE EVALUATION AND DECISION MAKING

The preoperative evaluation in some ways is more thorough and complex than a similar evaluation would be for a patient with esophageal cancer considering esophagectomy. This is largely because of the number of surgical options for benign disease. Although staging investigations are not required, the patient must undergo a complete physiologic esophageal and gastric evaluation. The primary goal of this evaluation is to determine whether the patient's symptoms may be palliated with esophagectomy or if a lesser intervention, surgical or not, will suffice.

Table 36-1

FEATURES, TREATMENT, AND LONG-TERM COMPLICATIONS IN NAMED MOTILITY DISORDERS[1]

	FEATURES	PRIMARY SURGICAL TREATMENT	LONG-TERM COMPLICATIONS
Achalasia	• Dysphagia, regurgitation and heartburn • EGD, barium swallow, manometry • Aperistalsis, absent or incomplete LES relaxation or Type I classic with minimal pressure, Type II compression, or Type III spastic	• Laparoscopic modified Heller myotomy and partial fundoplication • Relief of symptoms in >90% at 5 years • Relief of symptoms in 73% at 16 years	• GERD and GERD strictures • Recurrent dysphagia and obstruction • Barrett metaplasia • Squamous cancer
Diffuse or Segmental Esophageal Spasm	• Dysphagia and/or chest pain • EGD, barium swallow, manometry, pH, cardiac studies • Normal peristalsis interrupted by simultaneous contractions in >20%, hypertensive LES (50%), abnormal LES relaxation (70%)	• Myotomy with partial fundoplication • Length of myotomy based on manometry ◦ Laparoscopic ± VATS • Relief of symptoms in 70%–95% >5 years of follow-up	• Recurrent dysphagia and/or obstruction • GERD and GERD strictures • Regurgitation • Diverticula formation
Nutcracker Esophagus	• Chest pain but may also have dysphagia • EGD, manometry, pH, cardiac studies • Normal peristalsis with high amplitude (>180 mm Hg CM or >216 HRM) contractions and/or prolonged duration	• Myotomy based on manometry ± fundoplication ◦ If dysphagia primary and LES pressure increased • Relief of dysphagia in >80% • Relief of chest pain in <50%	• Recurrence of chest pain in 75% • Recurrent dysphagia
Hypertensive LES	• Chest pain and/or dysphagia • EGD, manometry and pH (to rule out GERD as secondary cause) • LES basal pressure >3 SD above upper limit of normal (45 mm Hg CM or 41 mm Hg HRM), normal peristalsis, incomplete relaxation, increased intrabolus pressure	• pH– : Laparoscopic myotomy and partial fundoplication • Relief of symptoms in >90% • pH+: Laparoscopic Nissen fundoplication	• See Achalasia • Recurrent chest pain
Collagen Vascular Disease[2] (Scleroderma, systemic lupus erythematosus systemic sclerosis)	• GERD and dysphagia • EGD, barium swallow, pH, manometry • Dysmotility to aperistalsis with absent LES basal pressures • Short esophagus	• Laparoscopic partial or Nissen fundoplication ± Collis gastroplasty • Laparoscopic modified RYGBP more recently • Dysphagia in 31%–70% • Failure with time ultimately	• Persistent dysphagia • Persistent GERD/erosive esophagitis • Long segment strictures • Barrett metaplasia ± dysplasia • Regurgitation

SD, standard deviation; LES, lower esophageal sphincter; CM, conventional manometry; HRM, high-resolution manometry; +, positive; –, negative; EGD, esophagogastroduodenoscopy; RYGP, Roux-en-Y gastric bypass.

Esophageal Function Testing

A comprehensive history by an experienced esophageal surgeon is likely to reveal a significant amount of information about the indications for esophagectomy before the objective evaluation begins. Obvious lines of questioning relate to aspiration events, food bolus impaction, severe dysphagia and odynophagia, and weight loss. It is often enlightening to ask the patient about their daily routines since they may have modified or adapted to their disorder in significant ways which seem normal to them but will strike outsiders as being somewhat unusual. Some examples include eating while standing up to make the food pass easier, keeping a bucket by the bedside for nighttime regurgitation, or eating the last meal of the day at 3 PM to avoid evening and nighttime symptoms of GERD.

Table 36-2

INDICATIONS FOR ESOPHAGECTOMY IN PATIENTS WITH MOTILITY DISORDERS

Advanced motility disorder with refractory symptoms (chest pain, dysphagia)
End-stage gastroesophageal reflux
Recurrent aspiration due to regurgitation
Malnutrition
Esophageal obstruction
Nondilatable stricture
Cancer
Barrett metaplasia with dysplasia

On the basis of the history, objective tests are ordered to confirm our initial suspicions. These may include some or all of the following tests.

A contrast radiologic upper gastrointestinal evaluation (UGI) can be highly instructive if completed by an experience radiologist and performed with the surgeon in attendance or recorded for playback. The use of liquid barium and solids such as hamburger coated in barium replicate most eating scenarios. Often liquids produce minimal to no symptoms, but the addition of hamburger or egg salad sandwich can elicit pain when the bolus of food does not pass through the gastroesophageal (GE) junction and the patient reports severe pain (Fig. 36-1) or regurgitates from the stomach back up the proximal esophagus. Alternatively, the food bolus may pass relatively easily while the patient may be experiencing a variety of symptoms. Other pathologies such as the development of a diverticulum post long myotomy for diffuse esophageal spasm (DES) or achalasia (Fig. 36-2) may be documented. Peristalsis in the esophagus and

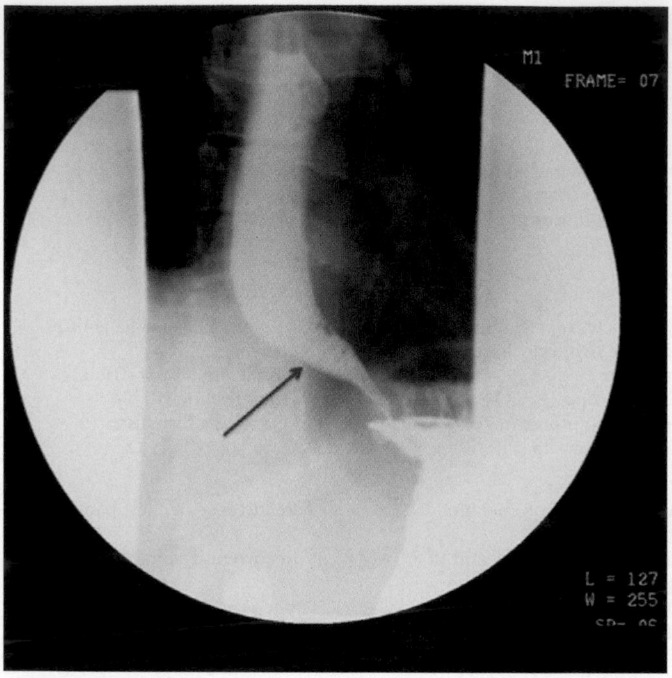

Figure 36-1. Food-coated barium swallow. Barium swallow demonstrating hold up of the hamburger-coated barium (noted by arrow) at the gastroesophageal junction in a patient with achalasia and a reflux stricture.

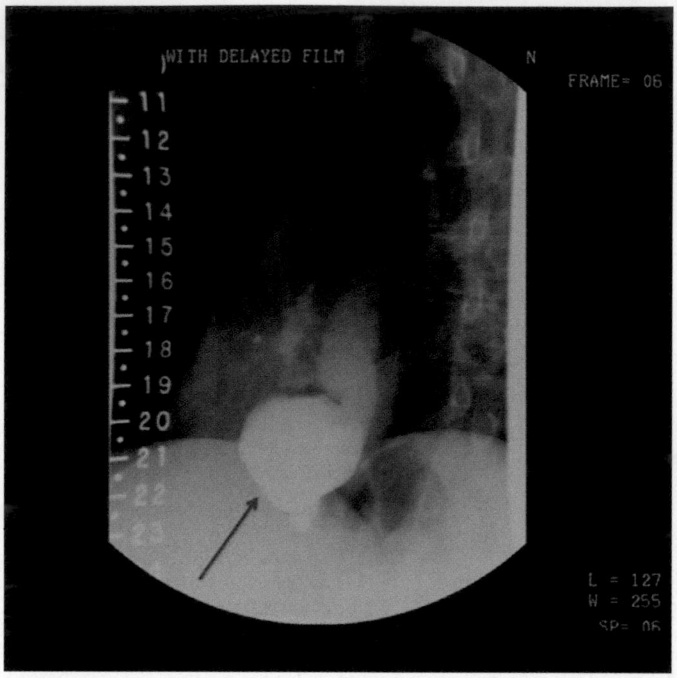

Figure 36-2. Myotomy complicated by diverticulum. Barium swallow demonstrating an epiphrenic diverticulum 6 years after myotomy for achalasia now with recurrent episodes of aspiration.

particularly in the gastric antrum along with pyloric relaxation should be noted as a surrogate measure of intact vagal function.

A modification of the UGI is the timed barium swallow where patients are instructed to drink 250 mL of barium within 30 to 45 seconds.[4] Spot films are taken under fluoroscopy at 1, 2, and 5 minutes with the height and width of the barium column along with the changes over time (emptying or stasis). This has been particularly useful in making decisions about esophagectomy in postmyotomy achalasia patients with symptoms of dysphagia and/or chest pain. In addition to showing end-stage esophageal function, it also can be used to correlate and educate patients about their symptoms and eating. Some patients may experience symptoms despite the complete passage of barium in normal time limits, whereas others have profound chest pain with transient hold up of barium and esophageal distension. The latter patient is more likely to benefit from reoperative surgery.

High-resolution manometry (HRM) should be repeated during preoperative evaluation to determine and confirm the current status of the motility disorder. This study is critical since it may demonstrate a recent change in the motility disorder. The spastic disorders (DES and nutcracker) can progress into achalasia, which would dictate a different surgical approach. In addition, postmyotomy dysphagia and partial fundoplication for achalasia may be due to a tight wrap, postsurgical scarring, herniation of a prior repair, or malpositioning of the repair (Fig. 36-3). More subtle findings such as bolus pressurization indicating outflow obstruction, a nonrelaxing LES, and absent body peristalsis not only may indicate the etiology of the symptoms, but also provide clues to severe esophageal dysfunction that is beyond repair. For patients with spastic disorders, it may be helpful to have patients with dysphagia ingest 5 × 1 cm cubes of bread in addition to the standard water swallows, and if necessary, a standard meal of rice and ground beef (125 mL) to replicate their symptoms and define the length of hypercontractile esophagus.

pH testing via 24-hour nasal catheter, 48-hour wireless catheter, or 24-hour impedance-pH catheter is helpful since such testing can provide correlation between symptoms and acid and/or nonacid reflux in the case of impedance. In the case of GERD-positive symptoms, treatment should be directed at addressing the GERD with optimized medical therapy or with a surgical option other than esophagectomy since the motility disorder may be secondary to pathologic reflux.

Upper endoscopy with biopsy prior to surgery can also reveal more insights into the function of the esophagus and stomach. The presence of retained food, cobble-stoning of the esophagus, stricture, Barrett esophagus, and even cancer are possible findings. The former three findings suggest poor esophageal function due to delayed emptying and esophageal stasis, and this information may aid the decision to proceed with esophagectomy.

Other objective tests such as computed tomography, nuclear medicine gastric-emptying scans, and endoscopic ultrasound are ordered as appropriate. Colonoscopy is standard if a colon interposition is being considered. The role of mesenteric angiography is controversial in standard colon interposition, but in the setting of multiple previous surgeries and uncertainty regarding reconstruction options, we favor complete assessment of the celiac and both mesenteric systems.

Cardiopulmonary Evaluation

Given the surgical physiologic impact of esophagectomies and often of the redo nature of surgeries in these settings, we believe every potential candidate should undergo full cardiac evaluation prior to esophagectomy. Pulmonary function tests including diffusing capacity should also be obtained.

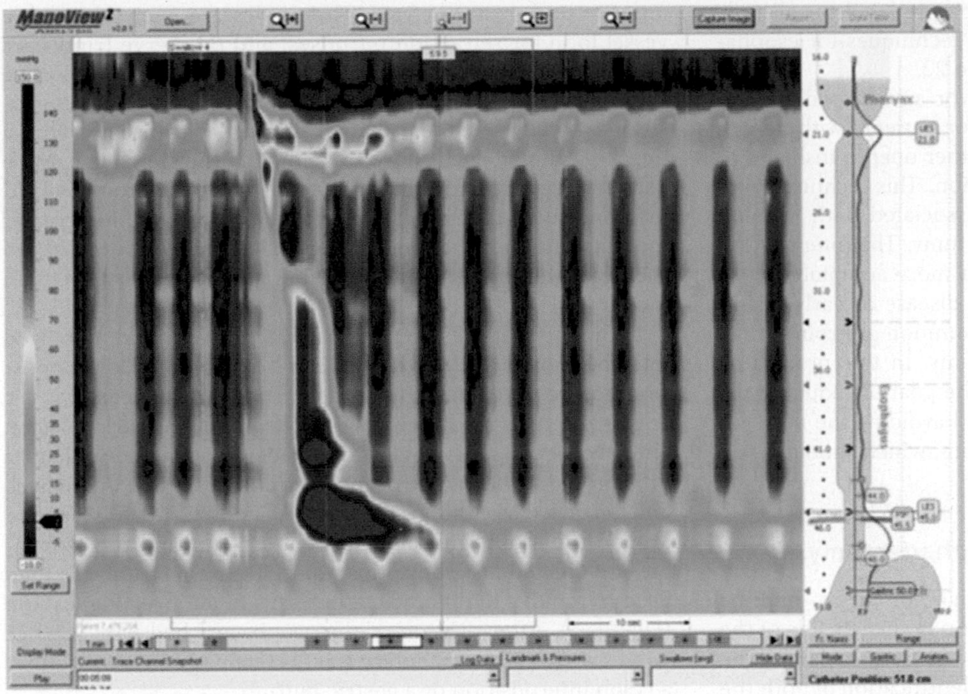

Figure 36-3. High-resolution manometry for postmyotomy achalasia. High-resolution manometry demonstrating an aperistaltic esophagus with distal pressurization and a high-pressure zone at the gastroesophageal junction in a previously myotomized patient with overly tight wrap.

CONSIDERATIONS AFTER FAILURE OF INITIAL THERAPY

When initial medical and then surgical therapy fail, the esophageal surgeon is confronted with one of the most challenging situations: to attempt a revision or modification of the original surgery or to recommend a larger, extirpative resection followed by reconstruction. More often than not, the instinct of the surgeon, referring physician, and patient is to proceed with the former hoping to avoid or delay esophagectomy even when esophagectomy may be more appropriate in palliating the patient's symptoms.

If a decision is made to revise or modify the original surgery, the surgeon must be aware that the second or third attempts are prone to aggravate local tissue destruction, ischemia, distortion of the native anatomy and potential for vagal injury. As a result, redo surgery not only may lead to worsened dysphagia, pain, regurgitation, and weight loss, but also may complicate eventual esophagectomy or potentially eliminate the option of a minimally invasive and/or VSE.

In evaluating these patients for potential intervention, one must first consider the severity of symptoms. In some cases, the patient's symptoms are minor, intermittent, and often related to what or how the patient eats. These may be easily managed by diet modification: avoidance of foods provoking symptoms, changing the patient's eating habits such as adding fluids, chewing longer, and eating slowly. The addition of medications may also help alleviate or lessen the severity of symptoms. However, in more advanced cases, the patient may be experiencing repeated food bolus impactions or dysphagia, gross regurgitation, symptoms of aspiration or pneumonia, profound weight loss, and unremitting GERD, which may be better palliated by esophagectomy.

The second consideration is the necessity of removing the esophagus. Obviously, if the pathology or symptoms are derived from the esophagus, resection is reasonable. However, when GERD (heartburn or reflux) is the predominant symptom, one alternative to esophagectomy is a modified Roux-en-Y gastric bypass. This approach has several benefits over esophagectomy including a lower operative mortality, for obese patients the opportunity to lose weight, derive improvement in comorbid conditions, and very good GERD control.[5]

Lastly one must consider the various options for reconstruction after esophagectomy. The obvious and most well-known options are tubularized stomach and colon interposition. The techniques for reconstruction, including its advantages and disadvantages are covered in Chapter 23. Our preference depends on the patient's symptoms and whether or not the majority of the esophagus requires removal. When symptoms are due to a nonfunctional esophagus such as with end-stage achalasia with sigmoid esophagus, we favor stomach for reconstruction. Comparatively, the patient with a nondilatable stricture due to GERD and multiple GE junction surgeries, may be better suited to undergo left thoracoabdominal resection and reconstruction with a short colon interposition or esophago-jejunostomy to reestablish GI continuity while simultaneously achieving GERD control.

TECHNIQUES OF ESOPHAGECTOMY FOR BENIGN DISEASE

Every known combination of incisions to access the esophagus has been described with none more common than the other. Both prior operation(s) and methods of reconstruction will be key drivers in the choice of access. Fortunately, the majority of initial operations for motility disorders are now performed laparoscopically or thoracoscopically. However, many patients with achalasia and DES operated long ago were approached through a thoracotomy. Thus, in the setting of benign disease that requires esophagectomy, previous surgeries may dictate the approach, and the surgeon must be prepared for all possibilities. A description of the various techniques for esophagectomy can be found in Chapters 13 to 22.

When technically possible, we favor a VSE as described by DeMeester.[6] VSE is ideally suited for patients with benign disease and can be accomplished by either open transhiatal or laparoscopic approach with neck incision. This technique was developed to avoid the morbidities associated with division of the vagi during standard esophagectomy. The intent of the operation is to make esophagectomy a more acceptable therapy to patients with end-stage benign disease or early malignant disease by avoiding some of the common gastrointestinal side effects of a standard esophagectomy. In this procedure, the vagus nerves are preserved with the goal of reducing the frequency of dumping and diarrhea and avoiding the need for gastric resection or a drainage procedure, which should result in improved alimentary function.

Technique of Vagal-Sparing Esophagectomy

VSE can be performed either through an upper midline abdominal incision and a second incision in the left side of the neck or laparoscopically with a left-sided neck incision. The abdominal operation begins with the identification of both the anterior and posterior vagi. The nerves are encircled with a vessel loop for retraction purposes, and the nerve trunks are mobilized from the GE junction by a limited highly selective vagotomy along the lesser curve (Fig. 36-4). If a colon interposition is to be used, the proximal stomach is transected with a linear stapling device above this point. If the stomach is to be used for reconstruction, the highly selective vagotomy is simply continued distally on the stomach to provide for greater mobility and the creation of the gastric tube without injury to the vagus nerves. This allows the left gastric vessels to remain intact.

The esophagus is then exposed in the neck and mobilized into the thoracic inlet where it can be divided as low as possible to preserve length for construction of the anastomoses. A gastrotomy is made proximal to the point of gastric division and a vein stripper is passed antegrade through an esophagotomy made just below the proposed transection line in the neck and retrieved via the gastrotomy. A stout ligature is applied around the esophagus, and the vein stripper and the esophagus are divided just above this point. The vein stripper is then used to remove the thoracic esophagus in an inverting fashion (Fig. 36-5). After dilation of the esophageal bed with a 90-cc Foley catheter, the alimentary tract is reconstructed with either a colon interposition or a gastric pull-up.

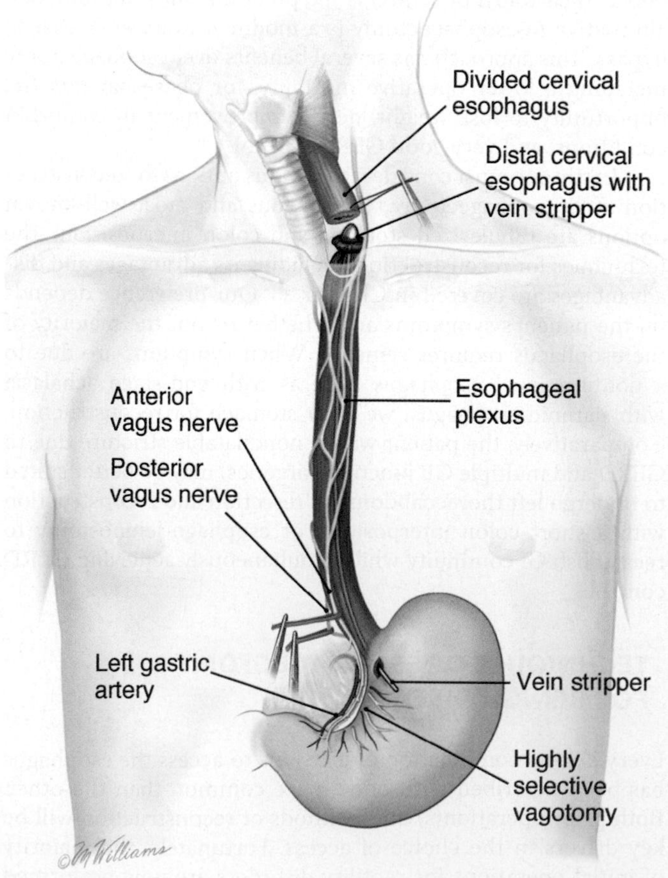

Figure 36-4. Technique of vagal-sparing esophagectomy. This figure highlights the identification of both vagal nerves that are encircled and the area of highly selective vagotomy. The neck incision has been opened and the proximal esophagus already divided.

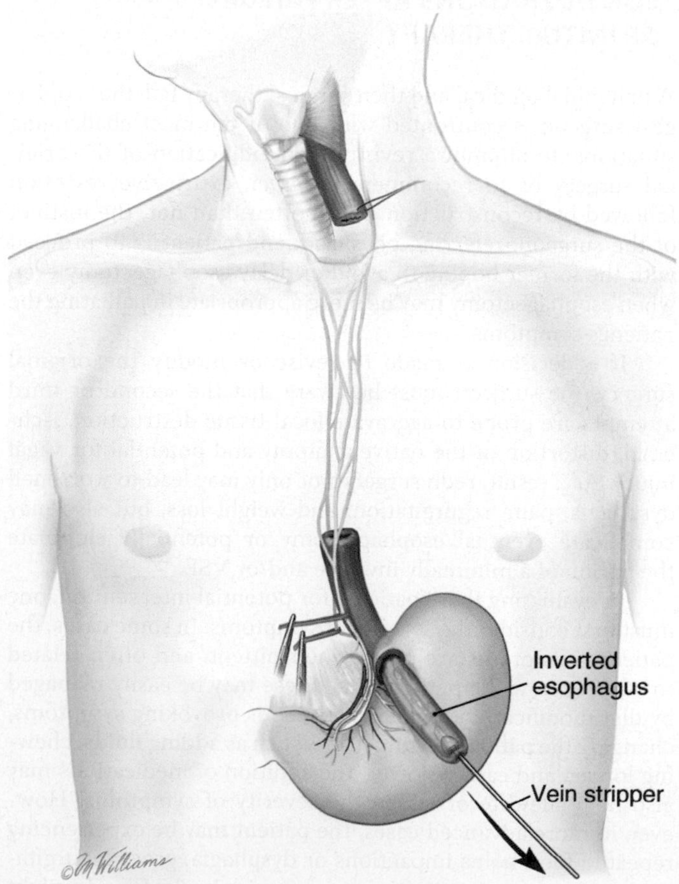

Figure 36-5. Technique of vagal-sparing esophagectomy. This figure shows the stripping of the esophagus by the inversion technique using the vein stripper.

CLINICAL OUTCOMES AND QUALITY OF LIFE

The measures of whether esophagectomy for benign motility disorders is successful include operative mortality and morbidity, but more important are the functional outcomes such as the ability to eat and the absence of symptoms and ultimately, the patient's interpreted QOL.

Mortality from esophagectomy in this situation ranges from 1.9% to 5.1% in the more recently published series.[3,7,8] This is similar to mortality rates reported for esophagectomy for locally advanced carcinoma with or without induction therapy in high-volume centers. But, when compared to the mortality for esophagectomy for high-grade dysplasia, which ranges from 0% to 4% or averages 1.2% (2/168) for esophagectomies in 11 of the most recent series, it is perhaps slightly higher. One possible explanation for this difference is the fact that most patients undergoing esophagectomy for a benign motility disorder have had at least one prior operation on their esophagus, with a median of two prior surgeries.[7] Nevertheless, the mortality for esophagectomy in benign disease is low in high-volume centers.

Operative complications remain a significant source of morbidity and are similar to those of cancer esophagectomies. Overall rates of morbidity range from 35% to 60% with pulmonary issues and arrhythmias accounting for the majority of complications. Once outside the perioperative period, anastomotic stricture after a leak is a common problem and many patients will require subsequent anastomotic dilation (10%–15%). However, recently described improvements in the anastomotic technique using a functional side-to-side stapled esophagogastrostomy suggest that this problem may be less common now than in the past.[9]

The functional results after esophagectomy are also quite varied. There is unfortunately little detail in most reports about whether the symptoms leading to esophagectomy were palliated or not. One has to remember that the most common symptoms preoperatively are dysphagia, regurgitation, and heartburn, which are all likely to be present to some degree after esophagectomy. Despite the presence of these symptoms, in one series, nearly 75% of patients reported improvement in their symptoms and 25% felt their preoperative symptoms were cured by esophagectomy.[3] In a different report, the Mayo group[7] reported that 32% of patients reported an excellent result postesophagectomy for benign disease with no symptoms, although when reflux and dysphagia (35%) were present, only a "fair" result was obtained. Last, this series also reported that when followed over time 25% to 30% of patients will require a reoperation for complications related to the esophagectomy.[7] This pattern of outcome is redemonstrated in a more recent series with 50.6% of patients reporting good-to-excellent outcomes and 12% of patients requiring reoperation after intestinal continuity was established.[8] This important observation is very relevant to any discussion one should have with a potential candidate for "benign" esophagectomy, since unlike esophageal cancer patients, patients with benign disease have a longer life expectancy.

The QOL in these patients has been difficult to interpret since no reported series has captured and compared pre- and postesophagectomy QOL scores of their patients. Most series have compared the postoperative QOL to that of existing standard populations and not unexpectedly they are lower than population normals particularly on long-term follow-up.[10] As a possible hint to this important aspect of the expected results, Moraca et al.[2] found similar perceptions of general, mental, and physical health on the SF-36 QOL questionnaire when evaluating patients before and after esophagectomy for high grade dysplasia and early esophageal cancer. Some differences were seen in bodily pain and overall physical health, which was slightly worse post surgery.

The addition of VSE into the surgical armamentarium for benign and early esophageal cancers in 2002 has resulted in an improved functional outcome. When compared with the results of a standard transhiatal esophagectomy with gastric pull-up and to esophagectomy with colon interposition, vagal secretory function was better preserved after the VSE as was vagal motor function. Gastric reservoir function was also more normal and there was a significantly lower frequency of dumping and diarrhea after the VSE.[11] Further evaluation of VSE demonstrated a shortened length of stay, substantial reduction in postoperative complications, less anastomotic stricturing and minimal postvagotomy side effects such as dumping and weight maintenance. However, symptoms of regurgitation, and aspiration were unchanged.[6] Obviously, long-term results and follow-up of VSE after 10 years are not yet available.

SUMMARY

Primary and secondary motility disorders produce a number of symptoms where dysphagia and chest pain predominate. Although primary surgical treatments are reasonably effective, a number of patients will progress onward with taxing long-term complications that necessitate additional interventions. In this situation, the challenge facing the esophageal surgeon is whether to attempt revision of the prior operation in hopes of ameliorating the symptoms or if it is better to consider a larger extirpative surgery in esophagectomy. Careful objective evaluation to determine the origin of symptoms is key in choosing the appropriate candidate for esophagectomy. Esophagectomies of all types can be performed with low mortality in experienced centers, but it remains a formidable operation as evidenced by the postoperative morbidity. When feasible a VSE is an attractive option with its apparent reduced morbidity and improved functional outcomes on short-term follow-up. Roux-en-Y gastric bypass is an alternative to esophagectomy particularly in patients with GERD-predominant symptoms.

EDITOR'S COMMENT

Surgery for benign esophageal disease should be rare and carefully considered. Reoperative surgery (at least once and sometimes twice) can be effective in expert hands. Even with low mortality and morbidity the results of esophagectomy are not ideal and the patient should be made aware of this in advance of surgery. We usually use a multimodality team of gastroenterologists and psychologists to discover whether other options are possible. Psychological consultation is often helpful to discover those patients with unrealistic expectations.

—Raphael Bueno

References

1. Herbella FA, Tineli AC, Wilson JL, et al. Surgical treatment of primary esophageal motility disorders. *J Gastrointest Surg.* 2008;12:604–608.
2. Moraca RJ, Low DE. Outcomes and health-related quality of life after esophagectomy for high-grade dysplasia and intramucosal cancer. *Arch Surg.* 2006;141(6):545–549; discussion 549–551.
3. Watson TJ, DeMeester TR, Kauer WK, et al. Esophageal replacement for end stage benign esophageal disease. *J Thorac Cardiovasc Surg.* 1998;115(6):1241–1249.
4. Kostic SV, Rice TW, Baker ME, et al. Timed Barium Esophagogram: a simple physiologic assessment for achalasia. *J Thorac Cardiovasc Surg.* 2000;120:935–946.
5. Awais O, Luketich JD, Tam J, et al. Roux-en-Y near esophagojejunostomy for intractable gastroesophageal reflux after anti-reflux surgery. *Ann Thorac Surg.* 2008;85:1954–1961.
6. Peyre CG, DeMeester SR, Rizzetto C, et al. Vagal-sparing esophagectomy: the ideal operation for intramucosal adenocarcinoma and barrett with high-grade dysplasia. *Ann Surg.* 2007;246(4):665–671; discussion 671–674.
7. Young MM, Deschamps C, Trastek VF, et al. Esophageal reconstruction for benign disease: early morbidity, mortality, and functional results. *Ann Thorac Surg.* 2000;70(5):1651–1655.
8. Chang AC, Lee JS, Sawicki KT, et al. Outcomes after esophagectomy in patients with prior antireflux or hiatal hernia surgery. *Ann Thorac Surg.* 2010;89:1015–1023.
9. Orringer MB, Marshall B, Iannettoni, MD. Eliminating the cervical esophagogastric anastomotic leak with a side-to-side stapled anastomosis. *J Thorac Cardiovasc Surg.* 2000;119:277–288.
10. Young M, Deschamps C, Allen M. Esophageal reconstruction for benign disease: self-assessment of functional outcome and quality of life. *Ann Thorac Surg.* 2000;70:1799–1802.
11. Banki F, Mason RJ, DeMeester SR, et al. Vagal-sparing esophagectomy: a more physiologic alternative. *Ann Surg.* 2002;236(3):324–335; discussion 335–336.

PART 5

ESOPHAGEAL REFLUX DISORDERS

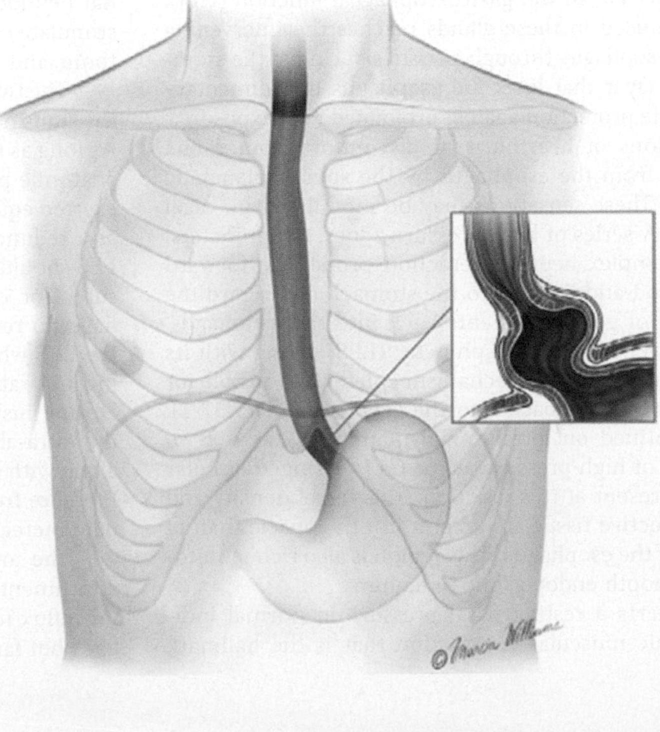

37 Overview: Anatomy and Pathophysiology of Esophageal Reflux Disease

Philip A. Linden

Keywords: Gastroesophageal reflux disease (GERD), heartburn, lower esophageal sphincter (LES), hiatal hernia, peptic stricture, Barrett metaplasia

EPIDEMIOLOGY

Gastroesophageal reflux disease (GERD) is one of the most common disorders seen in the general population. Approximately 10% of all people experience heartburn daily, 15% in any given week, and about half the population in any given year.[1] The spectrum of disease ranges from occasional postprandial substernal discomfort to the development of peptic stricture or even carcinoma in the setting of Barrett esophagus. It is important for physicians to identify and select appropriate treatments for patients at risk of developing complications. This chapter reviews the etiology, diagnosis, complications, and treatment of GERD.

NORMAL ANATOMY AND PHYSIOLOGY

The esophagus is lined with a stratified nonkeratinizing squamous epithelium consisting of three layers: superficial, intermediate, and basal. The basal cell layer comprises 15% of the total epithelial thickness and is the only layer that normally contains mitotic figures. The lamina propria, which lies deep to the squamous epithelium, contains glandular structures similar to those found in the gastric cardia. The epithelium is covered by a protective layer of mucin and surface bicarbonates that are produced by salivary glands located in the proximal esophagus and in the region adjacent to the gastroesophageal junction (GEJ). The mucus produced in these glands reaches the intervening sections of the esophagus through peristalsis. Unlike the stomach, the mucus layer that lines the esophagus is rudimentary and provides little protection against prolonged acid exposure.

The sensations of heartburn or discomfort from reflux are transmitted from the esophagus by the spinal splanchnic afferent nerves. These sensations may be modulated by vagal afferent nerves. A series of high-pressure zones, or sphincters, and zones of complex neural interaction propel the forward movement of food and liquid into the stomach and retard the return or reflux of gastric contents back into the esophagus. The intrinsic lower esophageal sphincter (LES), along with its extrinsic components, is the mechanism chiefly responsible for preventing gastric reflux back into the esophagus (Fig. 37-1). The LES is identified on intraluminal manometry as a 2- to 4-cm-long zone of high pressure at the GEJ. A ringed circular muscle is also present at this junction. The vessel density and amount of connective tissue are greater in LES muscle than in the remainder of the esophagus. This region is also rich in mitochondria and smooth endoplasmic reticulum.

The LES exerts a resting basal pressure in normal individuals. The tonic muscular contraction that is the hallmark of the LES contributes to the resting tone, distinguishing this region from the esophageal body. Inhibition of LES contraction is mediated largely through nitric oxide, whereas excitation is mediated through acetylcholine. Even with ablation of all neural input, the LES maintains its intrinsic basal smooth muscle tone. This muscular tone is distributed unevenly throughout the sphincter. The pressure is greatest in the lowest 2 cm of the LES and on the left side, where the left crus and sling fibers of the stomach exert force on the LES. The basal pressure also varies according to the respiratory cycle. During inspiration, the pressure in the upper half of the LES decreases, whereas the pressure in the lower half increases. This finding may be related to the respiratory contractions of the diaphragmatic crural fibers or relative intrathoracic and intra-abdominal pressures. A small shift in the position of the LES can have dramatic effects on these pressure gradients.

Relaxation of the LES occurs naturally during deglutition, about 2 seconds after the initiation of swallowing. At this time, the pressure in the LES decreases to a level approximating the intragastric pressure. This period of decreased pressure may last as long as 8 to 10 seconds. Distention of the esophagus produces a reflex relaxation of the LES that is distinct from the relaxation elicited during initiation of swallowing, such as that produced from tactile pharyngeal stimulation. A number of hormones and neurotransmitters also can produce LES relaxation. These include gastric inhibitory peptide, glucagon, cholecystokinin, nitric oxide, progesterone, vasoactive intestinal peptide, and prostaglandin E. Conversely, hormones that stimulate contraction include gastrin, bombesin, motilin, serotonin, and somatostatin (Table 37-1).

The two components of the *extrinsic* portion of the LES are the transmitted intra-abdominal pressure and the crural fibers. As long as the LES is situated below the diaphragm (the normal anatomic position), increases in intra-abdominal pressure are exerted equally on the LES and stomach. The crural fibers serve as a redundant means of maintaining LES pressure. A normal LES should be able to resist most increases in intragastric pressure. For this reason, many individuals with a hiatal hernia have no reflux. The crural fibers exert increased pressure on the LES when the tendency toward reflux is greatest (i.e., during inspiration and with increases in intra-abdominal pressure). During inspiration, the intrathoracic pressure decreases, and the intra-abdominal pressure increases. Crural fibers contract along with the diaphragm, causing an increase in LES pressure. Pressure from the crural fibers also increases during independent increases in intra-abdominal pressure.

The anatomy of the proximal stomach and its angle of attachment to the LES (angle of His) counteract the tendency for reflux to occur. The esophagus joins the stomach not at its apex but farther down along the lesser curvature. It is believed

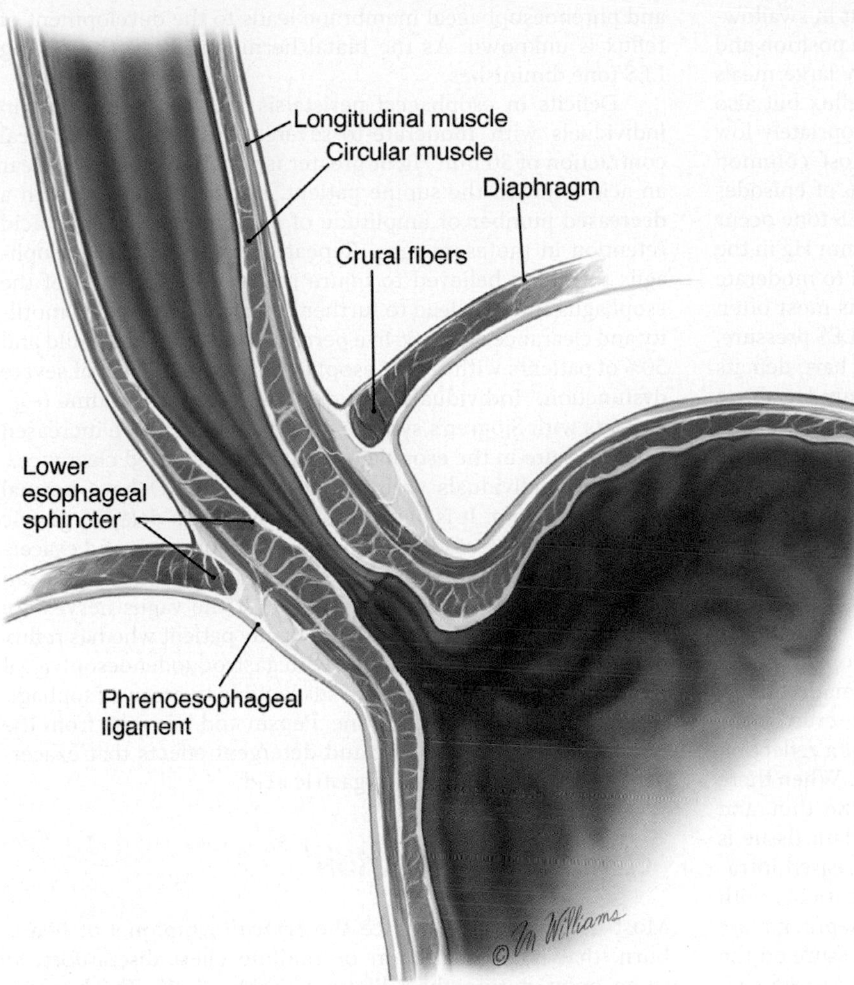

Figure 37-1. Normal anatomy of the lower esophageal sphincter (LES).

that the lateral fold of the gastric mucosa acts as a flap valve, helping to close the entrance to the LES during episodes of raised intra-abdominal and intragastric pressure. The fundus and cardia of the stomach act as a reservoir to minimize the increase in intragastric pressure associated with meals. The anatomic significance of the angle of His and its relationship to the fundic reservoir is apparent in studies showing a larger degree of reflux when individuals lie on the right side as opposed to the left.

Table 37-1

AGENTS AFFECTING LES TONE

Increased tone	
	Gastrin
	Bombesin
	Motilin
	Serotonin
	Somatostatin
Decreased tone	
	Gastric inhibitory peptide
	Glucagon
	Cholecystokinin
	Nitric oxide
	Progesterone
	Vasoactive intestinal peptide
	Prostaglandin E

Normal esophageal motility and clearance are important to minimizing the effects of gastric refluxate. Reflux into the esophagus is normally followed by waves of secondary peristalsis that move the contents back into the stomach. This secondary wave of peristalsis also brings bicarbonate-rich saliva into the esophagus to neutralize the remaining gastric acid. Although impaired esophageal motility occasionally may result from severe reflux esophagitis, it also may contribute to it, such as occurs in patients with scleroderma.

PATHOPHYSIOLOGY OF GASTROESOPHAGEAL REFLUX

Factors that affect the degree of gastroesophageal reflux include esophageal motility, the amount and composition of the saliva and other protective esophageal factors, the intrinsic LES, alterations in the transthoracic—transabdominal pressure gradient, the extrinsic LES (including the crural muscles), the integrity of the angle of His, gastric emptying, and the nature of the refluxate.

The LES is the most important component of the antireflux apparatus. Decreased resting LES tone and transiently decreased LES tone both may contribute to reflux. Transient relaxation is induced by gastric distention and pharyngeal stimulation. The former condition allows eructation with relief of gastric pressure, whereas the latter is important in swallowing. Transient relaxation is inhibited in the supine position and during sleep. The consumption of inappropriately large meals not only provides a pressure gradient favoring reflux but also induces transient relaxation of LES tone. Inappropriately low transient LES pressure is believed to be the most common cause of reflux and may account for 60% to 70% of episodes of heartburn. Pathologic transient decreases in LES tone occur when the LES pressure decreases by more than 5 mm Hg in the absence of a swallow. Reflux in patients with mild to moderate disease and no endoscopic evidence of esophagitis most often occurs as a consequence of transient decreases in LES pressure, whereas patients with severe reflux typically also have deficits in resting LES tone. Normal LES tone is 10 to 30 mm Hg above gastric pressure. Less than 2.5% of the population has a resting LES pressure of less than 6 mm Hg. Most patients with mild reflux have normal LES tone. Patients with erosive esophagitis usually have a low resting LES tone, and the degree of esophagitis typically correlates with the lack of LES tone. There is evidence in animals that repeated exposure of the LES to acid via transient relaxation may damage the sphincter, leading to a lower resting LES tone.

A *hiatal hernia* is defined as the separation and cranial displacement of the GEJ from the diaphragmatic hiatus. In normal individuals, the GEJ is anchored to the crus by the phrenoesophageal ligament, which is composed of a reflection of peritoneum fused with fibrous tissue (Fig. 37-2). When there is a hiatal hernia, the crura are often stretched and thin, and the phrenoesophageal ligament is lax. The redundant tissue is termed the *hernia sac*. In normal individuals, increased intra-abdominal pressure does not lead to reflux. In patients with hiatal hernia, however, the contribution of the diaphragmatic crura and effects of increased intra-abdominal pressure on the intra-abdominal esophagus are lost, leading to increased susceptibility to strain-induced reflux. Whether prolonged reflux leads to fibrosis and shortening of the esophagus with development of a hiatal hernia, or if the primary laxity in the crura and phrenoesophageal membrane leads to the development of reflux is unknown. As the hiatal hernia enlarges, the resting LES tone diminishes.

Deficits in esophageal peristalsis are seen commonly in individuals with moderate-to-severe GERD. An esophageal contraction of 30 mm Hg or greater is usually adequate to clear an acid bolus in the supine patient. Poor contractility, with a decreased number or amplitude of contractions, leads to acid retention in the esophagus. Repeated exposure of the esophagus to acid is believed to injure the intrinsic muscles of the esophagus and may lead to further deficits in esophageal motility and clearance. Twenty-five percent of patients with mild and 50% of patients with severe esophagitis have evidence of severe dysfunction.[2] Individuals with decreased salivary volume (e.g., patients with Sjögren's syndrome and smokers) have increased acid exposure in the esophagus owing to decreased clearance.

Most individuals with symptomatic GERD have normal gastric emptying. It is evident, however, that a delay in gastric emptying will increase gastric volume and pressure and exacerbate GERD in patients predisposed to the condition. This can be seen after any surgery on the GEJ if the vagus nerves are injured, and it must be considered in any patient who has reflux despite fundoplication. Patients with gastroduodenoesophageal reflux *and* GERD may be more susceptible to erosive esophagitis than those with GERD alone. Pepsin and bile salts from the duodenum have proteolytic and detergent effects that exacerbate the damaging effects of gastric acid.

CLINICAL PRESENTATION

Most individuals experience the *typical* symptoms of heartburn, that is, regurgitation or midline chest discomfort, at some point during their lifetime (Table 37-2). The burning pain or pressure associated with heartburn is caused by reflux of acid into the esophagus. Frequently, symptoms are more prevalent after meals or in the supine position. Certain foods

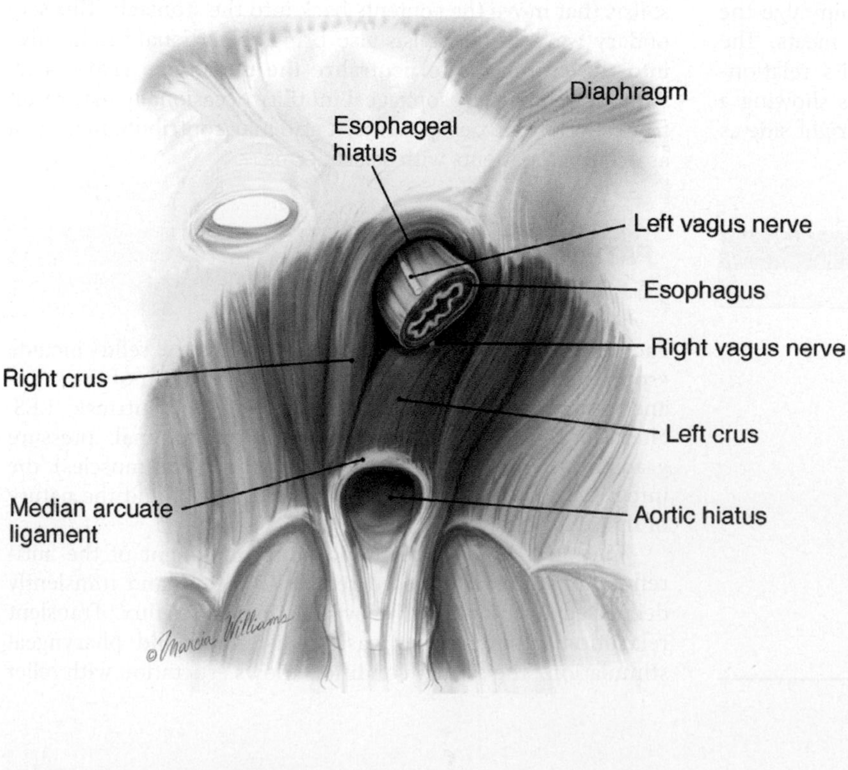

Figure 37-2. Normal anatomy of the esophageal hiatus.

Table 37-2

SYMPTOMS OF GERD

Typical
- Heartburn
- Sour-tasting regurgitation

Atypical
- Cough
- Pneumonia
- Asthma
- Hoarseness
- Noncardiac chest pain (tightness)

Symptoms of complicated GERD
- Dysphagia
- Odynophagia
- Hematemesis/Melena

associated with decreased LES tone, such as high-fat meals, caffeine, chocolate, peppermint, and alcohol, may exacerbate these symptoms. In general, individuals who experience heartburn only after certain foods tend to have higher resting LES pressures than those who experience heartburn with almost all types of foods. Patients with daily symptoms are more likely to have resting LES pressures of less than 10 mm Hg.[1] Relief of symptoms immediately after ingestion of water or antacids supports the diagnosis of GERD. Substernal pressure may be related to esophageal spasm caused by esophagitis or exposure to acid. If the pain is related to exertion and stops on cessation of activity, cardiac ischemia should be considered, although a significant number of these patients also may have reflux. The severity and frequency of symptoms do not necessarily reflect the severity of the underlying esophagitis. One-quarter of all patients with severe reflux and Barrett esophagus have no symptoms at all.[3] Likewise, a significant number of patients with frequent and severe complaints are not found to have esophagitis by endoscopy.

Respiratory symptoms such as hoarseness, cough, asthma, and recurrent pneumonia are referred to as *atypical* symptoms (Table 37-2). Although a significant number of patients with chronic asthma or cough also may have GERD, these symptoms are less specific than typical symptoms, and surgical fundoplication is, in general, less effective for symptom control. A randomized controlled trial by Larrain et al.[4] treated 94 intrinsic asthma patients with reflux documented by either barium swallow or pH probe analysis. The patients were randomized to placebo, cimetidine, or surgery. The surgery and cimetidine groups had roughly 75% improvement in wheezing and respiratory function versus only 34% in the control group. Long-term follow-up showed that 50% of the surgical group was asthma-free compared with only 5% of the control group. Individuals with respiratory symptoms who may be more likely to respond to GERD treatment are those with nonallergic asthma, nocturnal symptoms, abnormal proximal esophageal acid exposure, and those who had reflux symptoms before developing asthma.

Patients with odynophagia (i.e., pain on swallowing) or dysphagia (i.e., difficulty swallowing) are more likely to have severe esophagitis, abnormal motility, or structural abnormalities of the esophagus. Odynophagia may be associated with severe esophagitis or esophageal spasm. Dysphagia may be related to motor diseases (typically, dysphagia to both solids and liquids) or to a narrowing caused by a peptic stricture, ring, or tumor (dysphagia more with solids than with liquids).

DIAGNOSTIC TECHNIQUES

Diagnostic techniques focus on three aspects of GERD: objective documentation and quantification of reflux (usually by pH probe), definition of the pathophysiology (usually by manometry), and assessment of mucosal complications of reflux such as stricture, metaplasia, ulcers, or neoplasia (by barium swallow or endoscopy) (Table 37-3).

Barium Swallow

Barium swallow is a noninvasive means of obtaining valuable information about the esophagus. The fundamental techniques employed with barium swallow include (1) full-column examination, in which the esophagus is filled with barium and inspected for hiatal hernia, contour deformity, rings, and strictures; (2) analysis of mucosal patterns, in which the empty esophagus is coated with barium and inspected for irregular, thickened folds or varices; (3) fluoroscopic observation and motion recordings employing real-time observation of contractions and reflux; and (4) double-contrast examination, in which the esophagus is coated with barium and then distended with air to reveal fine mucosal abnormalities. The barium swallow is overall a relatively insensitive tool for diagnosing GERD. Mild esophagitis may not be visible on barium swallow, although air-contrast techniques increase the sensitivity. Moreover, reflux of barium from the stomach into the esophagus can be seen in a significant number (20%–25%) of patients with no reflux symptoms and infrequently in patients with severe symptoms. Barium swallow is most effective for detecting the following conditions: moderate-to-severe esophagitis, presence of a hiatal hernia, and any associated stricture or mass lesion. The

Table 37-3

WORKUP OF THE GERD BEFORE FUNDOPLICATION

Typical symptoms
- Step 1: Lifestyle and diet modification: avoidance of caffeine, tobacco, alcohol, or inciting foods; weight loss; smaller meals; low-fat meals; avoidance of eating 3 h before recumbence. If continued symptoms, then
- Step 2: PPI therapy, 8 wk. If continued symptoms and age <50, then (if age >50, proceed to EGD)
- Step 3: May consider double-dose PPI therapy for 3 mo. If continued symptoms or recurrent symptoms, then
- Step 4: EGD, 24-h pH probe, and manometry
- Step 5: If pH probe test is positive: 360-degree fundoplication if normal motility, partial wrap if motility impaired

Atypical symptoms (e.g., chronic cough, recurrent aspiration pneumonia, hoarseness, adult-onset or recumbent asthma)
- Step 1: 24-h pH probe study; if positive, then
- Step 2: PPI therapy or directly to fundoplication after EGD and manometry

presence of a hiatal hernia containing gastric mucosal folds and the presence of a stricture above these folds are fairly specific for peptic stricture in the setting of Barrett esophagus.

Radionuclide Scintigraphy

Radionuclide scintigraphy was proposed initially as a means of documenting reflux and assessing reflux severity. A radioisotope (technetium-99 m sulfur colloid) is swallowed and followed for reflux. Manual compression of the abdomen or straining maneuvers can be used to elicit reflux. The sensitivity and specificity of this test have been questioned, and it is not employed commonly in the workup of GERD. Radionuclide scintigraphy is sensitive and specific for detecting delayed gastric emptying and can be employed if this disorder is suspected. It should be part of the routine workup of recurrent or persistent reflux after fundoplication or for patients in whom gastric emptying dysfunction is suspected based on symptoms, associated disorders (diabetes mellitus), or in patients taking medications that may slow gastric emptying.

Endoscopy

Endoscopy is the first and preferred diagnostic procedure when reflux fails medical treatment, if symptoms recur after a course of medical treatment, or when patients have significant odynophagia or dysphagia. Endoscopy permits direct visualization and biopsy. Metaplasia, ulcers, strictures, and erosions seen during endoscopy can be graded to standardize reflux severity. Patients with reflux and mild esophagitis may have an endoscopically normal-appearing esophagus. Random mucosal biopsy should be taken 5 cm above the LES because even normal individuals may exhibit some metaplastic change in the most distal esophagus. Microscopic changes that are apparent with esophagitis include a basal epithelial layer exceeding 15% of the total epithelial thickness and the presence of lamina propria papillae that extend more than two-thirds deep into the epithelial layer. Neutrophils and eosinophils in the lamina propria are considered to be better indicators of reflux esophagitis, as are erosion, ulceration, stricture, and a columnar-lined mucosa. The presence of retained food in the stomach during endoscopy should also alert the physician to the possibility of gastric emptying dysfunction.

pH Probe Analysis

pH probe analysis is the most sensitive and specific means for quantifying acid reflux in the esophagus. In patients with typical symptoms of reflux and esophagitis documented by endoscopy, pH probe analysis adds little to the overall management. This technique is applicable to (1) patients with typical reflux symptoms in the absence of esophagitis, (2) patients with atypical symptoms with or without esophagitis, (3) before consideration of antireflux surgery, or (4) for the evaluation of unsuccessful antireflux treatment. Proton pump inhibitors (PPIs) must be stopped 7 days before study, and H_2-receptor antagonists should be stopped 48 hours before study.

The electrode, made of either glass or antimony, is positioned 5 cm above the LES (as defined by manometry). Dual-probe catheters are available that simultaneously measure acid in the upper esophagus and lower pharynx. The catheter is left in place for 24 hours, and the patient is asked to record the duration of meals, time spent in the supine position, and the occurrence of any reflux symptoms. Studies have shown that the variable *percentage of time with pH <4* is the most reproducible measurement (85% reproducibility). This measurement is termed the *reflux time or acid exposure time* and correlates better with esophagitis grade than the variable *number of episodes with pH <4*. Normal patients typically have acid exposure times of less than 7%. Patients with values in the 7% to 12% range may have some degree of mild inflammation, whereas acid exposure times of greater than 12% are usually found with more severe forms of esophagitis. For example, patients with columnar-lined esophagitis have an average exposure time of 26%.

DeMeester and Johnson developed a composite score based on six variables of acid exposure: total time with pH <4, upright time with pH <4, supine time with pH <4, total number of episodes with pH <4, number of episodes >5 minutes with pH <4, and duration of longest episode of pH <4. It is not clear that this composite score characterizes the severity of reflux any better than the simple variable *number of episodes of pH <4*.[5]

Some patients are bothered by placement of a 24-hour transnasal pH probe catheter that is worn externally. A Bravo capsule, consisting of a wireless transmitter and pH electrodes in a 25 mm by 6 mm capsule, can monitor acid reflux in the esophagus and transmit information wirelessly. This capsule sends data to an external receiver and recorder, which is worn by the patient. The capsule is typically placed at the time of endoscopy and is secured on the wall of the esophagus via small pins into the mucosa. Twenty-four-hour collection is typically performed, and the capsule usually sloughs off and is passed within 5 to 7 days.

Approximately 10% to 20% of patients who have endoscopy and biopsy-proved esophagitis demonstrate negative 24-hour pH studies. A percentage of these patients may have significant reflux of duodenal contents into the esophagus. In theory, patients with bilious reflux should have an esophageal pH greater than 7, but duodenogastroesophageal reflux typically occurs with gastroesophageal reflux, and the esophageal pH is rarely, if ever, greater than 7. Reflux of bile and duodenal enzymes has been proposed as factors contributing to the development of esophagitis and Barrett esophagus. Bilirubin-sensitive probes are available for measuring bile reflux. These probes rely on detecting significant light absorption near 450 nm, the characteristic absorption peak of bilirubin. A fiberoptic probe is used to calculate the difference in light absorption at 470 nm (bilirubin peak) and 565 nm (reference) at the tip of the probe. There is a reasonably good correlation between these readings and direct aspiration and measurement of bilirubin levels. Manometry, often used to evaluate esophageal function before fundoplication, is discussed in Chapter 33.

Impedance

Impedance is the ratio of voltage to current and is inversely proportional to conductivity. Using a catheter placed in the esophagus one can make sum measurements of the impedance of the esophagus and its contents. Impedance electrodes are typically placed at 2-cm intervals along a transnasal catheter that traverses the length of the esophagus. By measuring bolus transit, conclusions regarding functional peristalsis can be made, although it is not clear yet whether impedance transit measurements offer anything additional to high-resolution manometry.

Impedance measurements do, however, add to our knowledge of the chemical composition of refluxate in the esophagus. Multichannel intraluminal catheters which combine impedance and pH measurements are more sensitive to the detection of combined acidic and nonacidic reflux events. Typically, the catheter is placed for 24 hours, and patients are asked to keep a log of symptoms. Using impedance, for example, it is now known that many patients on PPIs do not have less reflux, but only have fewer episodes of low pH reflux. Patients with continued symptoms on PPI may be more appropriately offered antireflux surgery if it can be documented that continued nonacidic reflux events persist. In theory, a single multichannel impedance pH catheter could give complete information regarding esophageal peristalsis, reflux episodes, and reflux composition.

MANAGEMENT OF GERD

Lifestyle Modifications

The first phase of therapy for symptomatic GERD involves lifestyle modifications aimed at factors that have been shown to increase symptoms and acid exposure in the esophagus (Table 37-3). Elevating the head by 6 inches in the supine position has been shown to decrease esophageal clearance time and esophageal acid exposure in reflux patients. Certain foods have been shown to increase acid exposure in the esophagus by causing increased acid production, decreased LES tone, decreased gastric emptying, decreased esophageal clearance, or a variety of these factors. Chocolate, peppermint, alcohol, high-fat meals, and smoking all have been shown to decrease LES pressure. Fatty foods also significantly delay gastric emptying. The effect of caffeine on LES pressure is less clear, but it is believed to increase acid production and acid exposure in the esophagus. There is a correlation between obesity, low LES pressure, and GERD. Alterations in diet and lifestyle with antacid therapy may provide significant relief to individuals with occasional heartburn or mild GERD, but studies in patients with reflux esophagitis show a good or excellent response in only approximately 20% (vs. a 75% response rate in surgical patients).[6]

Motility Agents

Motility agents should, in theory, increase acid clearance, and if gastric emptying and LES pressure are increased, they should decrease acid exposure of the esophagus. Metoclopramide increases LES tone, improves esophageal contraction, and increases gastric emptying. When used for prolonged periods, however, there is a significant incidence of side effects such as restlessness and agitation. Even in combination with H_2-receptor antagonists, it does not seem to be as effective as the better-tolerated PPIs. Cisapride, another promotility agent, is similar in efficacy to metoclopramide but is no longer available for use in the US owing to its proarrhythmic effects.

H_2-Receptor Antagonists

Although antacids are effective in raising the esophageal pH above 4 (the threshold for esophageal healing), they are short-acting and give only transient relief. H_2-receptor antagonists such as cimetidine (300 mg qid), ranitidine (150 mg bid), famotidine (20 mg bid), and nizatidine (150 mg bid) were used initially for 6- to 12-week durations to treat reflux that did not respond to conservative measures. These dosages are effective in 50% to 70% of patients, with higher doses needed to reliably heal moderate-to-severe cases of esophagitis.

Proton Pump Inhibitors

PPIs provide more rapid relief of symptoms and promote healing of erosive esophagitis far more effectively. They are used today in preference to H_2-receptor antagonists. PPIs omeprazole (40 mg per day), lansoprazole (30 mg per day), pantoprazole (40 mg per day), and rabeprazole (20 mg per day) are approximately 90% effective in healing erosive esophagitis after 8 weeks. Patients who do not heal with once-daily dosing should be put on a twice-daily regimen for better 24-hour control of gastric acid production. Most patients with erosive esophagitis treated with PPIs heal, but they have recurrent symptoms within 6 to 9 months. An additional 10% have recurrent esophagitis without symptoms. PPIs have few known side effects. However, the complete suppression of acid secretions is known to stimulate goblet cells, resulting in hypergastrinemia, although the development of carcinoid tumors or gastrinomas has not been seen in humans. The appearance of significant numbers of metaplastic cells in the esophageal mucosa with PPI treatment is also theoretically of concern in relation to Barrett esophagus. Although PPIs stop acid production, limit acid exposure in the esophagus, and decrease the quantity of refluxate, they do not stop the act of reflux. The possibility of bile salts and digestive enzymes contributing to the progression of Barrett esophagus and the development of dysplasia, cancer, or both also has been raised. Despite these concerns, there is no clear-cut relationship between the use of PPIs and an increased risk of Barrett metaplasia.

Role of Surgery

For the uncomplicated patient with GERD, surgical therapy cannot be recommended over PPI therapy. There appears to be no difference in response of esophagitis, symptoms, patient satisfaction, or death from cancer between the two modes of treatment. After fundoplication, the need for PPIs decreases, but a significant percentage of patients continue to take these medications (in one study 37%).[7] In a patient with complicated GERD (Barrett and/or stricture), surgery may very well be more effective than PPI therapy (see Chapter 41).

Laparoscopic fundoplication is indicated for patients who do not respond to or cannot tolerate high-dose PPI therapy, as well as for those who require long-term therapy but do not wish to take PPIs long term (see Chapters 38–40). A thorough evaluation before fundoplication includes a 24-hour pH probe analysis, esophageal manometry, and an esophagogastroduodenoscopy (EGD). Patients must meet two criteria before being offered the option of fundoplication. They must have symptoms of acid reflux into the esophagus (i.e., esophagitis or sequelae of esophagitis, pain, or atypical symptoms) and documentation of abnormal acid exposure. Alternatively, patients should manifest complications clearly caused by GERD, such as peptic strictures, Barrett esophagitis, or ulcers. Patients are stratified as those with typical or atypical symptoms and those without esophagitis, with esophagitis, or with complicated esophagitis. Patients with typical symptoms and evidence of esophagitis are good candidates for fundoplication. (Some surgeons would argue that pH and manometry in these patients adds little to overall management.[8]) Those with typical symptoms but without esophagitis also may be candidates for surgical therapy if PPIs are not effective or not tolerated, provided that the acid reflux has been documented by pH/manometry testing. Patients with atypical symptoms, such as frequent pneumonia, chronic cough, adult-onset asthma, and esophagitis, also should undergo pH/manometry testing. Overall, laparoscopic Nissen fundoplication is more successful in relieving typical symptoms (93% successful) than atypical symptoms[9] (56% successful) (see Chapter 39). Patients with atypical symptoms without evidence of esophagitis must be studied carefully before being considered for fundoplication. The absence of mucosal damage does not mean that reflux is absent. These patients still may be suffering from reflux and aspiration but have the ability to quickly clear residual fluid from the esophagus. PPIs stop acid production, decrease the amount of gastric secretions, and decrease the amount of gastric contents refluxed, but the upper airway still may be exposed to damage from bile acids and enzymes. Nonetheless, patients with atypical symptoms without esophagitis who respond to PPIs have a better response to fundoplication than those who do not.[10] This is attributable in large part to the diagnostic capability of PPI therapy to select atypical patients with symptoms secondary to reflux.

Patients who have recurrent symptoms after surgical fundoplication should undergo EGD to document the presence of esophagitis and recurrent hernia. Repeat pH and manometry testing provides objective evidence of recurrent reflux or motor disorders. Gastric emptying also must be assessed. If vagal nerves were injured at the time of the original fundoplication, delayed gastric emptying may be contributing to reflux despite the presence of an adequate fundoplication. Treatment for this condition would be a promotility agent, such as metoclopramide, followed by either pyloromyotomy or pyloroplasty if symptoms continue.

HIATAL HERNIA

A *hiatal hernia* is a type of paraesophageal hernia defined as a loosening of the phrenoesophageal membrane resulting in displacement of the LES away from its attachments to the diaphragm. There are four types of paraesophageal hernias (Fig. 37-3). All four types are associated with symptomatic and asymptomatic GERD. Type I, also termed a *sliding hiatal hernia,* is a simple herniation of the LES into the chest, often associated with esophageal shortening. The hernia itself is not harmful and requires no surgical correction. A large number of people have an asymptomatic hiatal hernia. Any surgical treatment offered for a type I hernia is dictated by the need to treat the associated GERD. Adequate surgical correction of a significant type I hernia often requires esophageal lengthening (see Chapter 42).

The LES in type II hiatal hernia, also termed *paraesophageal,* remains fixed in position at the level of the hiatus, but a portion of the stomach herniates along with the LES into the chest through a small defect in the phrenoesophageal membrane. Type II hiatal hernias are quite rare, but because they involve only a partial defect of the phrenoesophageal membrane, the incidence of incarceration and strangulation is high. Surgical repair is indicated to prevent strangulation or further herniation of the involved portion of the stomach.

Type III hernias have both sliding and paraesophageal components. As a sliding hernia progresses, the mobile greater curvature of the stomach is drawn into the chest and it begins to rotate until it eventually resides in the right chest. This condition is termed *organoaxial rotation.* Several complications can occur from large type III hernias. Vascular insufficiency may arise from arterial obstruction or venous congestion. There also may be ulceration, bleeding, or frank necrosis and perforation. Chronic iron-deficiency anemia is common in patients with type III hernias and is thought to be due to the slow, chronic loss of blood from the stomach. Partial or complete obstruction may occur either from organoaxial rotation or from compression of the conduit which often occur as a result of a meal.

Type IV hernias are simply type III hernias that involve displacement of additional structures and organs into the chest, such as the omentum, spleen, or colon.

COMPLICATIONS OF GASTROESOPHAGEAL REFLUX

Peptic Stricture

Approximately 10% of patients seeking treatment for GERD suffer from peptic stricture. Like other patients suffering from complicated GERD, these patients tend to have a lower resting

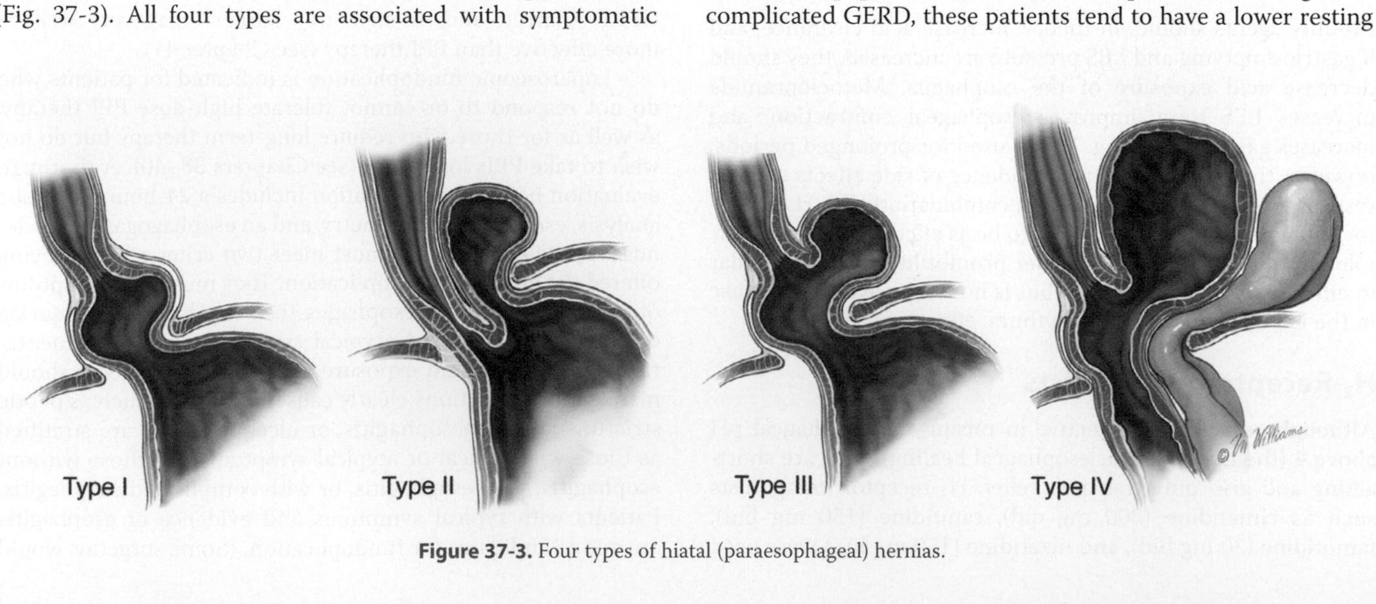

Figure 37-3. Four types of hiatal (paraesophageal) hernias.

LES pressure. One study noted that 64% of patients with stricture suffered from motility disorders versus 32% of patients without stricture, suggesting that impaired clearance of acid may be a causative factor in GERD.[11]

Strictures usually form in the lower esophagus as a result of severe esophagitis. When esophagitis extends to the full thickness of the esophageal wall, healing may result in stricture. Schatzki rings are short, web-like stenoses associated with GERD. They may be the result of mucosal and submucosal inflammation and subsequent fibrosis. The ring does not involve the muscular portion of the esophagus. Peptic strictures typically present at the squamocolumnar junction. (In patients with Barrett esophagitis, the squamocolumnar junction lies above the GEJ.) These strictures usually measure 1 cm in length or less and are rarely longer than 3 cm. Other factors predisposing to stricture formation include Zollinger—Ellison syndrome, prolonged nasogastric tube placement, and scleroderma.

Dysphagia is the most common presenting symptom of peptic stricture. Many strictures form gradually. Patients tend to adapt their diet to prevent the physical discomfort, and therefore, complaints regarding the severity of dysphagia correlate very loosely with severity of the stricture. Because the stricture is a mechanical obstruction, the dysphagia typically is more pronounced with solid foods than with liquids. Most patients have a prior history of GERD, along with an associated hiatal hernia. Weight loss is uncommon with peptic stricture in contrast to malignant strictures, which typically occur in patients over 50 years of age, develop more suddenly, may not be accompanied by a hiatal hernia, and are almost always associated with weight loss.

Strictures typically are diagnosed by barium swallow. As noted earlier, benign strictures are located at the squamocolumnar junction; associated with a hiatal hernia; and typically have smooth, tapered proximal and distal segments. Associated esophagitis may be present. In contrast, malignant strictures may not be associated with a hiatal hernia and have irregular narrowing with abrupt or "shouldered" proximal or distal edges. EGD should be performed. Associated esophagitis is seen often. Biopsy should be performed proximally throughout the stricture and beyond, if possible. Use of a thinner pediatric endoscope may facilitate passage. Coexisting Barrett metaplasia may be found. Dilation of the stricture with serial Maloney dilators may permit passage of the endoscope and yield a more detailed examination.

Initial management of peptic stricture involves dilation (see Chapter 44) and PPI therapy. Use of PPIs rather than H_2-receptor antagonists results in a lower incidence of stricture recurrence. Three different types of esophageal dilators may be used. The soft, flexible, mercury-filled Maloney dilator is used more commonly for benign strictures. These tapered dilators come in various sizes up to 60F (20 mm). They are designed with flexible tips to follow the course of the esophageal lumen. These dilators are preferred for their ease of use, provided that the stricture is not extremely tight or tortuous. Savary dilators are similar in shape to the Maloney dilators, but they are stiffer, have a central channel, and are designed to be passed over a flexible guidewire. These dilators are used for more tortuous or tight strictures, where there is a greater concern for perforation, or if there may be difficulty engaging the stricture. The wire is passed through the stricture under direct vision and is verified with fluoroscopy to end in the stomach. A series of dilators then may be passed using Seldinger technique. These dilators range in size from 15 to 60 F (5–20 mm). Through-the-scope balloon dilators are also available, although they are disposable and more expensive.

The typical peptic stricture may be dilated safely with Maloney dilators without the use of fluoroscopy. The risk of perforation should be <1%. One-third to one-half of patients require long-term repeat dilations. After two or more dilations, additional dilations are required in nearly all patients. Surgery is indicated in patients who cannot be dilated, as well as in patients who have recurrent strictures while on PPI therapy. The preferred treatment in patients who can be dilated is a laparoscopic fundoplication. Any patient who has concomitant esophageal shortening also should undergo an esophageal lengthening procedure. If the patient cannot be dilated, then esophagectomy is usually needed; however, this is extremely rare, and a thorough effort should be made to exclude unusual malignancies. In a patient with an otherwise healthy esophagus, distal esophagectomy is an acceptable procedure. Colon or jejunum interposition typically is used because a high incidence of recurrent reflux and stricture has been described with the gastric pull-up procedure after distal esophagectomy. Distal esophagectomy is also reasonable in patients suffering from perforation after dilation, especially if they have required several dilations. In these patients, repair of the perforation is associated with a very high incidence of recurrent, difficult-to-dilate strictures. Repair of the stricture and perforation using a Thal patch of stomach to widen the esophagus has been described. This technique is prone to leakage and often leaves the patient with wide-open reflux. For this reason, distal esophagectomy usually is preferred.

Barrett Metaplasia

Barrett metaplasia is defined as the presence of a "specialized" columnar epithelium in the distal esophagus. The term *specialized* is used because the epithelium is different from that found in the gastric cardia, with features of gastric, small intestinal, and colonic mucosa, including goblet cells. It is most similar to intestinal epithelial cells. Before Barrett metaplasia can be diagnosed, first it must be identified by the endoscopist. The GEJ is defined endoscopically as the point where the gastric folds are first apparent in the minimally distended esophagus. The squamocolumnar junction, or Z-line, typically coincides with the GEJ. Barrett metaplasia exists when the usual pale pink stratified squamous epithelium of the distal esophagus is replaced by a beefy red columnar intestinal mucosa. The exact location of the GEJ may be difficult to discern, especially in patients with a hiatal hernia. Varying distances have been proposed for the length of columnar mucosa that must be identified before the diagnosis of Barrett esophagus can be made. Patients with less than 3 cm of Barrett metaplasia have short-segment Barrett. Those with more than 3 cm of metaplasia have long-segment Barrett. This distinction is important because patients with short-segment Barrett may not have the same risk of dysplasia.

Barrett metaplasia is caused by frequent, repeated, and prolonged exposure of the esophagus to the gastroduodenal contents. Patients with Barrett metaplasia have been shown to have more severe reflux than patients with esophagitis. Average LES pressure in Barrett patients is about half that of patients with uncomplicated reflux esophagitis (5 vs. 9 mm).[12] Most Barrett patients have a hiatal hernia of significant size

(76% vs. 50% with uncomplicated esophagitis).[13] Exposure to acid and bile is higher in Barrett patients than in patients with non-Barrett esophagitis. The origin of the specialized metaplastic cells is unclear. A number of hypotheses have been proposed. For example, these specialized cells may result from migration of gastric cardia cells to the distal esophagus, they may represent metaplasia of esophageal squamous cells, or they may develop from esophageal glandular cells. Experimental and clinical evidence exists for each of these hypotheses without clear consensus.

Approximately 10% of patients with esophagitis eventually will develop Barrett metaplasia. The disease is twice as prevalent in men as in women. Barrett patients have a 30- to 125-fold chance of developing esophageal adenocarcinoma compared with the general population. The rate of cancer development is 1 in 200 patient-years for those with metaplasia. Not all Barrett patients are at equal risk of developing adenocarcinoma. Risk factors for the development of adenocarcinoma in these patients include male gender, smoking, greater length of Barrett esophagus, Barrett ulcer, peptic stricture, white race, and older age. Most Barrett patients have symptoms that are indistinguishable from those of uncomplicated esophagitis. Barrett patients tend to have more complications from esophagitis (e.g., bleeding and stricture). The development of a stricture at the squamocolumnar junction well above the GEJ in a patient with a hiatal hernia is nearly pathognomonic for Barrett esophagus.

Barrett carcinoma is believed to progress in the following sequence: metaplasia < low-grade dysplasia < high-grade dysplasia < adenocarcinoma. Progression from low-to-high—grade dysplasia may take many years, whereas progression from high-grade dysplasia to adenocarcinoma occurs on average in 14 months.[14] The annual incidence of the development of cancer in a patient with Barrett esophagus has been estimated to be from 0.2% to 1.9%.[15] Dysplasia indicates the development of neoplastic changes that consist of alterations in the cellular and glandular architecture. Cell nuclei may be hyperchromatic and enlarged, with increased mitotic figures. The nuclei may show loss of polarity and, instead of appearing uniformly at the base of cells, may migrate toward the luminal surface. In high-grade dysplasia, nuclei extend toward the luminal one-third of the cell. The differentiation between low- and high-grade dysplasia is often difficult.

The treatment of Barrett esophagus with low-grade and high-grade dysplasia is controversial and continues to evolve. The natural history and progression of low-grade dysplasia to high-grade dysplasia to intramucosal carcinoma and eventually to cancer with metastatic potential has yet to be well defined. The surveillance and treatment of Barrett Esophagus is discussed in detail in Chapter 41.

EDITOR'S COMMENT

GERD is both common and heterogeneous. It is related but not limited to obesity and modern Western lifestyle. Careful elucidation of all symptoms, as well as thorough clinical evaluation including endoscopy, pH study, and a manometric evaluation, are recommended prior to surgical therapy or any other interventions. Whenever suspected because of medical history or symptoms, gastric emptying should be assessed to avoid operating on patients with poor gastric motility. This disorder is often treated by multiple specialists including gastroenterologists, general surgeons, thoracic surgeons, otolaryngologists, and pulmonologists. Behavior modification can improve the symptoms of many but not all patients. It is important to remember to design individualized treatments that are best for each patient rather than fit the patient to a specialized treatment strategy.

—Raphael Bueno

References

1. Nebel OT, Fornes MF, Castell DO. Symptomatic gastroesophageal reflux: incidence and precipitating factors. *Am J Dig Dis.* 1976;21:953–956.
2. Kahrilas PJ, Dodds WJ, Hogan WJ. Effect of peristaltic dysfunction on esophageal volume clearance. *Gastroenterology.* 1988;94:73–80.
3. Galmiche J, Bruley S. Symptoms and disease severity in gastroesophageal reflux disease. *Scand J Gastroenterol.* 1994;29:62–68.
4. Larrain A, Carrasco E, Galleguillos F, et al. Medical and surgical treatment of nonallergic asthma associated with gastroesophageal reflux. *Chest.* 1991;99:1330–1335.
5. Schindlbeck NE, Heinrich C, Konig A, et al. Optimal thresholds, sensitivity, and specificity of long-term pH-metry for the detection of gastroesophageal reflux disease. *Gastroenterology.* 1987;93:85–90.
6. Behar J, Sheahan DG, Biancani P, et al. Medical and surgical management of reflux esophagitis: a 38-month report of a prospective clinical trial. *N Engl J Med.* 1975;293:263–268.
7. Spechler SJ, Lee E, Ahnen D, et al. Long-term outcome of medical and surgical therapies for gastroesophageal reflux disease: follow-up of a randomized, controlled trial. *JAMA.* 2001;285:2331–2338.
8. Frantzides CT, Carlson MA, Madan AK, et al. Selective use of esophageal manometry and 24-hour pH monitoring before laparoscopic fundoplication. *J Am Coll Surg.* 2003;197:358–363; discussion 63–64.
9. So JB, Zeitels SM, Rattner DW. Outcomes of atypical symptoms attributed to gastroesophageal reflux treated by laparoscopic fundoplication. *Surgery.* 1998;124:28–32.
10. Hinder RA. Surgical therapy for GERD: selection of procedures, short- and long-term results. *J Clin Gastroenterol.* 2000;30:S48–50.
11. Ahtaridis G, Snape WJ Jr, Cohen S. Clinical and manometric findings in benign peptic strictures of the esophagus. *Dig Dis Sci.* 1979;24:858–861.
12. Iascone C, DeMeester TR, Little AG, et al. Barrett's esophagus: functional assessment, proposed pathogenesis, and surgical therapy. *Arch Surg.* 1983;118:543–549.
13. Cameron AJ. Barrett's esophagus: prevalence and size of hiatal hernia. *Am J Gastroenterol.* 1999;94:2054–2059.
14. Reid BJ, Blount PL, Rubin CE, et al. Flow-cytometric and histological progression to malignancy in Barrett's esophagus: prospective endoscopic surveillance of a cohort. *Gastroenterology.* 1992;102:1212–1219.
15. Drewitz DJ, Sampliner RE, Garewal HS. The incidence of adenocarcinoma in Barrett's esophagus: a prospective study of 170 patients followed 4.8 years. *Am J Gastroenterol.* 1997;92:212–215.

38 Belsey–Mark IV Fundoplication/Collis Gastroplasty

David D. Odell, Sidhu P. Gangadharan, and Malcolm M. DeCamp

Keywords: Gastro-esophageal reflux disease (GERD), hiatal hernia, para-esophageal hernia, short esophagus, peptic esophageal stricture, partial fundoplication, high resolution manometry

INTRODUCTION

The management of gastroesophageal reflux disease and hiatus hernia has continually evolved in both general and thoracic surgery over the last century. Although the introduction of improved medical management in the form of H_2 blockers and proton pump inhibitors (PPIs) has reduced the number of patients presenting to the surgeon for management of this disease, a well-defined role for surgical treatment remains in the circumstances of medical failure or medication intolerance as well as for a fixed anatomical abnormality. Beginning in the late 1950s with the work of Belsey, Nissen, Hill, and Collis and extending through the present day, there has been great debate as to the optimal surgical approach to reflux disease and repair of paraesophageal hernia. Most recently, minimally invasive approaches have gained favor. However, the traditional techniques of open hiatal hernia repair and fundoplication are required in select patient groups. This chapter will discuss the current application of the transthoracic Collis–Belsey approach to hiatal hernia repair with a focus on appropriate patient selection and evaluation.

GENERAL PRINCIPLES

The operation now attributed to Belsey is the culmination of several rounds of clinical experimentation spanning over a decade's worth of experience. Dr. Belsey's original intent was to create a general approach to the management of reflux disease, and several iterations were needed to arrive at the Mark IV version, which is most commonly used today.[1] In parallel to Belsey's work, Collis also sought to develop a surgical solution for gastroesophageal reflux, focusing on the importance of obtaining an adequate length of intra-abdominal esophagus to allow for a tension-free acute angle of esophageal entry into the stomach. Looking for ways to achieve this, he published the first description of the tubularization of a section of the lesser curvature of the stomach for use as a distal esophageal equivalent in 1957.[2] In 1971, Pearson et al.[3] published a series of 24 patients with peptic stricture of the distal esophagus treated with a combination gastroplasty and Belsey hiatal hernia repair. They reported excellent results with either resolution or improvement in the symptoms of dysphagia in all patients.

The "Collis–Belsey" operation, as described by Pearson, gained a great amount of support as an approach to hiatal hernia repair and a viable antireflux procedure. In recent years, however, the advent of efficacious minimally invasive approaches to the surgical treatment of GERD has limited application of the Collis–Belsey procedure to a relatively specific subset of patients with esophageal stricture and foreshortened esophagus. The operation also has a defined role as an option in the repair of hiatal hernia in the obese patient in whom the bulk and pressure from the abdominal viscera and omentum limit visualization with an abdominal or laparoscopic approach.

A transthoracic approach to paraesophageal hernia may also be preferred in the reoperative setting in patients who have had a prior abdominal repair. In addition, patients with impaired esophageal motility identified preoperatively may benefit from the improved esophageal clearance provided by the partial fundoplication of the Belsey procedure as compared with the "tighter" circumferential wrap described by Nissen. In the setting of incarcerated paraesophageal hernia with gastric volvulus, when an urgent operation is indicated to prevent gastric necrosis or bleeding, it may not be known whether the patient has normal motility or a foreshortened esophagus. A Collis–Belsey approach will address both concerns in this setting.

PREOPERATIVE ASSESSMENT

A thorough assessment of the patient is of paramount importance in determining the appropriate surgical approach. A detailed history of symptoms and prior interventions can give an accurate impression of the severity of the disease process. All patients should undergo esophagogastroduodenoscopy (EGD) both to assess the anatomic relationship of the esophagogastric junction (EGJ) to the diaphragm as well as the degree of esophagitis and the presence of stricture. EGD also can define the size and degree of organoaxial volvulus of a paraesophageal hernia. A barium esophagram may be helpful to further assess esophageal length and the anatomy of the paraesophageal hernia. A foreshortened esophagus will produce tension on the hiatal repair or fundoplication and these patients benefit greatly from an esophageal lengthening procedure. Peptic stricture of the distal esophagus is indicative of a transmural inflammatory process which, as it heals, causes a cicatricial scar which binds the esophageal mucosa and submucosa to the muscularis. Fibrosis involving the inner circular muscle layer produces luminal stricture, whereas involvement extending to the outer longitudinal muscle layer leads to esophageal shortening.

An assessment of esophageal motility with a manometric pressure catheter is essential. This instrument affords appropriate characterization of the intrinsic esophageal function, which, if abnormal, may mandate partial fundoplication to avoid significant dysphagia postoperatively. A complete evaluation will include quantification of the extent of reflux with 24-hour pH monitoring and correlation of symptoms with periods of decreased distal esophageal pH.

The recent introduction of accurate high-resolution manometric (HRM) studies has paved the way for even more accurate characterization of both motility within the esophageal body and function of the lower esophageal sphincter. The technique uses a manometry catheter with multiple, closely spaced sensors to gather accurate manometric data throughout the entire length of the esophagus rather than from a limited number of isolated positions. These data may be independently evaluated as a pressure tracing. More recently, a technique known as esophageal pressure topography (EPT) plotting[4] has provided even more detailed analysis of HRM studies. This process uses an interpolated average of data between sensors to create a seamless isobaric color plot, which permits the function of the entire esophagus to be presented in a single visual display. The improved data have rendered this approach the new gold standard for the diagnosis of esophageal motility disorders.[5] Distinct HRM patterns are identifiable for each pathologic condition,[6] allowing the surgeon to make accurate preoperative assessments of the extent of dysmotility and to develop the appropriate operative plan. This is especially important with respect to the choice of fundoplication.

Occasionally, a hiatal hernia may be detected incidentally on plain chest radiographs (Fig. 38-1). It may manifest as a retrocardiac air-fluid level. If a paraesophageal hernia is causing symptoms of postprandial pain, retching, or early satiety, an abdominal CT scan may reveal the abnormally positioned intrathoracic stomach (Fig. 38-2).

Once the patient is deemed an appropriate surgical candidate, a careful evaluation of their pulmonary function and cardiac health should be undertaken both by the surgeon and the anesthesiologist. We routinely recommend preoperative anesthesia consultation both to achieve this goal and to discuss thoracic epidural placement and other strategies for postoperative pain control.

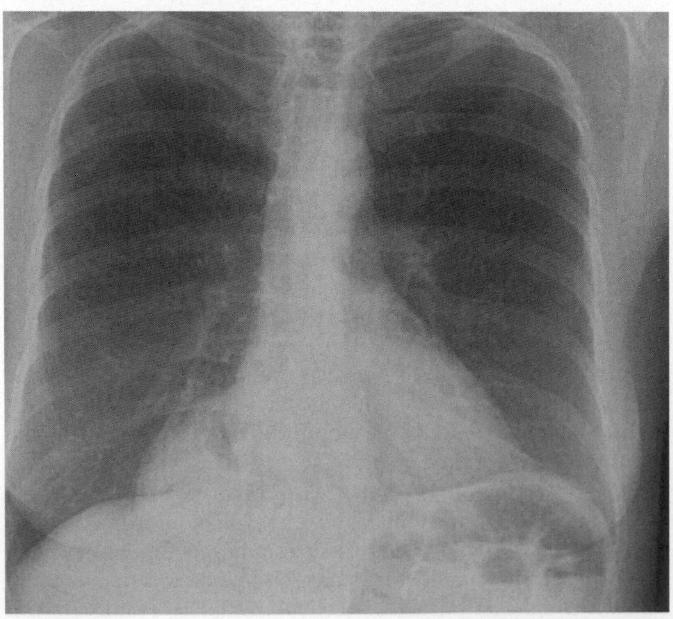

Figure 38-1. Standard plain film shows a soft tissue density at the retrocardiac and the right heart border. This density represents a large paraesophageal hernia.

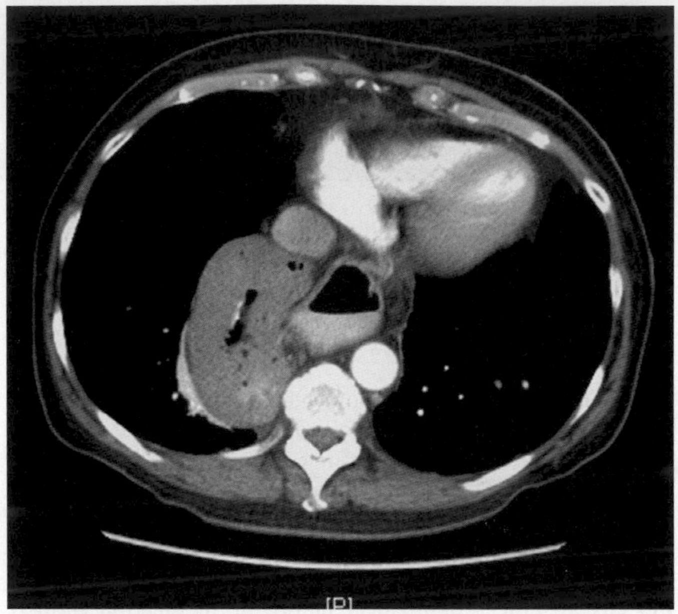

Figure 38-2. Abdominal CT scan done for epigastric and substernal pain reveals an incarcerated stomach with organoaxial volvulus.

TECHNIQUE

We are indebted to Pearson's excellent description of the Collis–Belsey procedure in the chapter on open gastroplasty in his textbook of *Esophageal Surgery*.[7]

Anesthesia

A thoracic epidural catheter and arterial line are placed in the preoperative holding area. After induction of general anesthesia, a double lumen endotracheal tube is placed to provide optimal lung isolation and maximal exposure. The anesthesiologist will also assist with placement of the esophageal Bougie to aid proper sizing of the gastroplasty.

Positioning and Incision

An upper endoscopy may be performed at the outset of the procedure to assess for the presence of stricture or other pathology before commencing the fundoplication and gastroplasty. This would not be obligatory in the setting of an elective repair, when all the obligatory data have been obtained. However, when gastric volvulus and the threat of gastric necrosis necessitate an urgent trip to the operating room, it is prudent to inspect endoscopically before making an incision. Upper endoscopy is performed most easily when the patient is still in the supine position.

When the operative procedure begins, the patient should be in the left thoracotomy position, with pressure points padded appropriately. After properly securing the patient, the operating table should be flexed to open the left interspaces for maximal exposure. A generous sixth or seventh interspace posterolateral thoracotomy is created, dividing the muscle of the latissimus dorsi but sparing the serratus anterior. Occasionally, a rib will need to be "shingled" posteriorly to achieve better exposure, but this is not common if the interspace is opened slowly and widely to allow gentle rib spreading.

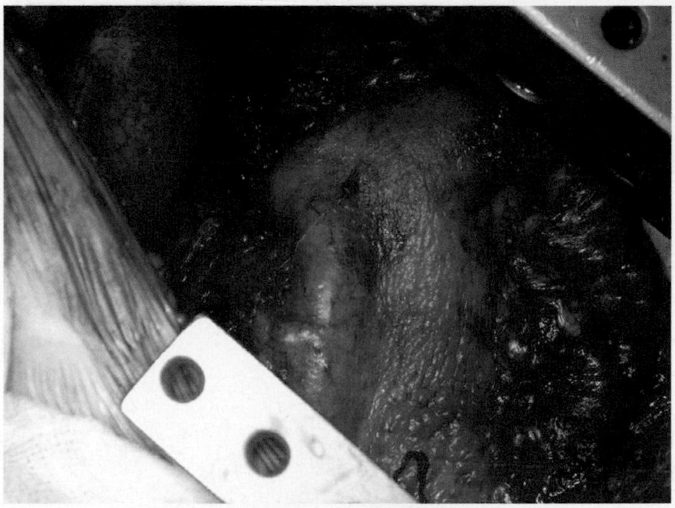

Figure 38-3. View of the incarcerated stomach from left thoracotomy after dissection of hiatal hernia sac.

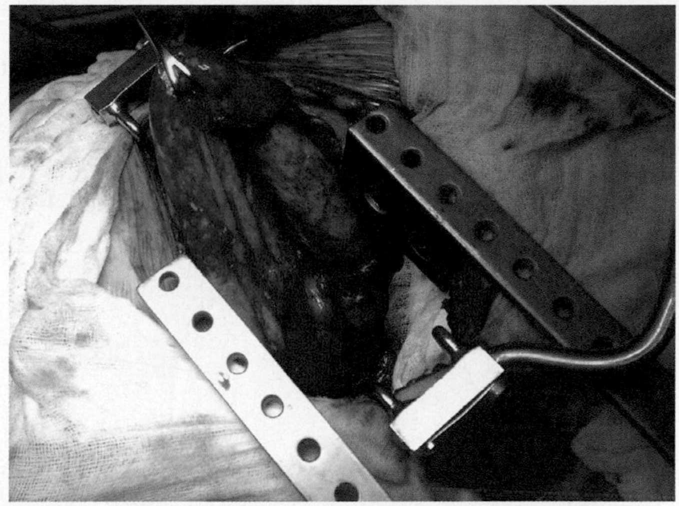

Figure 38-4. The fundus is shown retracted by a Babcock clamp.

Dissection of the Esophagus and Stomach

The inferior pulmonary ligament is divided with electrocautery to permit the lung to retract into the upper hemithorax and expose the esophagus, which lies anterior to the descending aorta and posterior to the pericardium. There may be a large hernia sac above the hiatus. Whether this is present or not, the initial circumferential dissection of the esophagus should be at the level of the inferior pulmonary vein to permit identification of both vagus nerves. Beginning the dissection at this level allows one to mobilize a sufficient length of esophagus to facilitate the gastroplasty and a tension-free return to the abdomen. A Penrose drain is passed around the esophagus and used for gentle retraction.

Attention is then turned to the hiatus. The hiatal hernia sac (which consists of parietal pleura), phrenoesophageal membrane, and peritoneum should be dissected from the hiatus circumferentially. By dividing the hernia sac, the serosa of the stomach is exposed, and the abdomen may be entered safely (Fig. 38-3). The crura should be dissected free during this stage. To freely deliver the stomach into the chest, the gastrohepatic omentum, which tethers the cardia below the diaphragm, is divided at this point. To more fully mobilize the fundus, the highest 2 to 3 short gastric vessels may be ligated and divided (Fig. 38-4). These maneuvers are especially helpful in situations of intrathoracic gastric volvulus to ensure that proper orientation of the stomach is maintained once it is reduced to the abdomen. Three to five crural closure sutures (0 braided polyester) are placed but left untied.

The gastroesophageal junction (GEJ) is identified with its overlying fat pad. Dissection of the fat pad, elevating it off the GEJ, commences at its posterolateral aspect, just to the left of the posterior (right) vagus nerve. As the fat pad is dissected anteriorly, the anterior (left) vagus nerve is mobilized along with the fat pad and retracted to the right and away from the EGJ. Small vessels coursing between the fat pad and the gastric wall may need to be controlled individually with electrocautery, vascular clips, or direct ligation.

Creation of the Gastric Tube (Esophageal Lengthening)

A gastric tube is created from the cardia of the stomach (Fig. 38-5A). A 48 to 50F Bougie is passed into the stomach along the lesser curvature by the anesthesiologist and guided by the surgeon to avoid malpositioning or perforation during placement. The fundus is retracted and a thick tissue stapler is placed alongside the Bougie and fired to add 4 to 5 cm of extra length to the esophagus (Fig. 38-5B). This permits the *neo*-GEJ to lie without tension below the diaphragm. However, since this neoesophagus (gastric tube) will not retain normal esophageal motility, segments longer than 4 to 5 cm are not advised. We oversew the gastroplasty staple line with 3-0 polypropylene suture, taking care not to narrow the gastric tube.

Fundoplication and Return to the Abdomen

The fundoplication is a partial wrap of 270 degrees created with three rows of horizontal mattressed, double-armed 2-0 or 3-0 braided polyester or silk sutures. The sutures should be placed partial thickness (seromuscular), but must be deep enough to permit apposition of the fundus to the esophagus without tearing out. The middle suture of each *row* should straddle the staple line used to create the gastric tube (Fig. 38-6A). The other sutures of each row are therefore 135 degrees left and right of the middle suture. The next row is spaced 1.5 cm from the fold created by tying down the sutures in the previous row (Fig. 38-6B). The last row of sutures is not tied down after placement; rather, the needles are passed into the abdomen via the hiatus and then back up through the diaphragm to anchor the reconstruction (Fig. 38-6C). A malleable retractor or sterile spoon can be used to protect the abdominal viscera during this maneuver. The transdiaphragmatic sutures should continue the 270-degree spacing of the fundoplication. The GEJ, with its fundoplication in place, is then returned to the abdomen and the transdiaphragmatic sutures are tied down to anchor the wrap to the underside of the diaphragm anteriorly (Figs. 38-7 and 38-8). The crural sutures are then tied down, establishing an adequate length of the posterior aspect of the hiatus. When tied, the reconstructed hiatus should remain lax enough to admit a finger alongside the esophagus. A completion flexible endoscopy may be of assistance in ensuring both the fundoplication and crural repair are appropriate.

A nasogastric tube is placed with guidance by the surgeon at the field. The chest is irrigated, and a flexible or standard chest drain is placed. The chest is closed in standard fashion

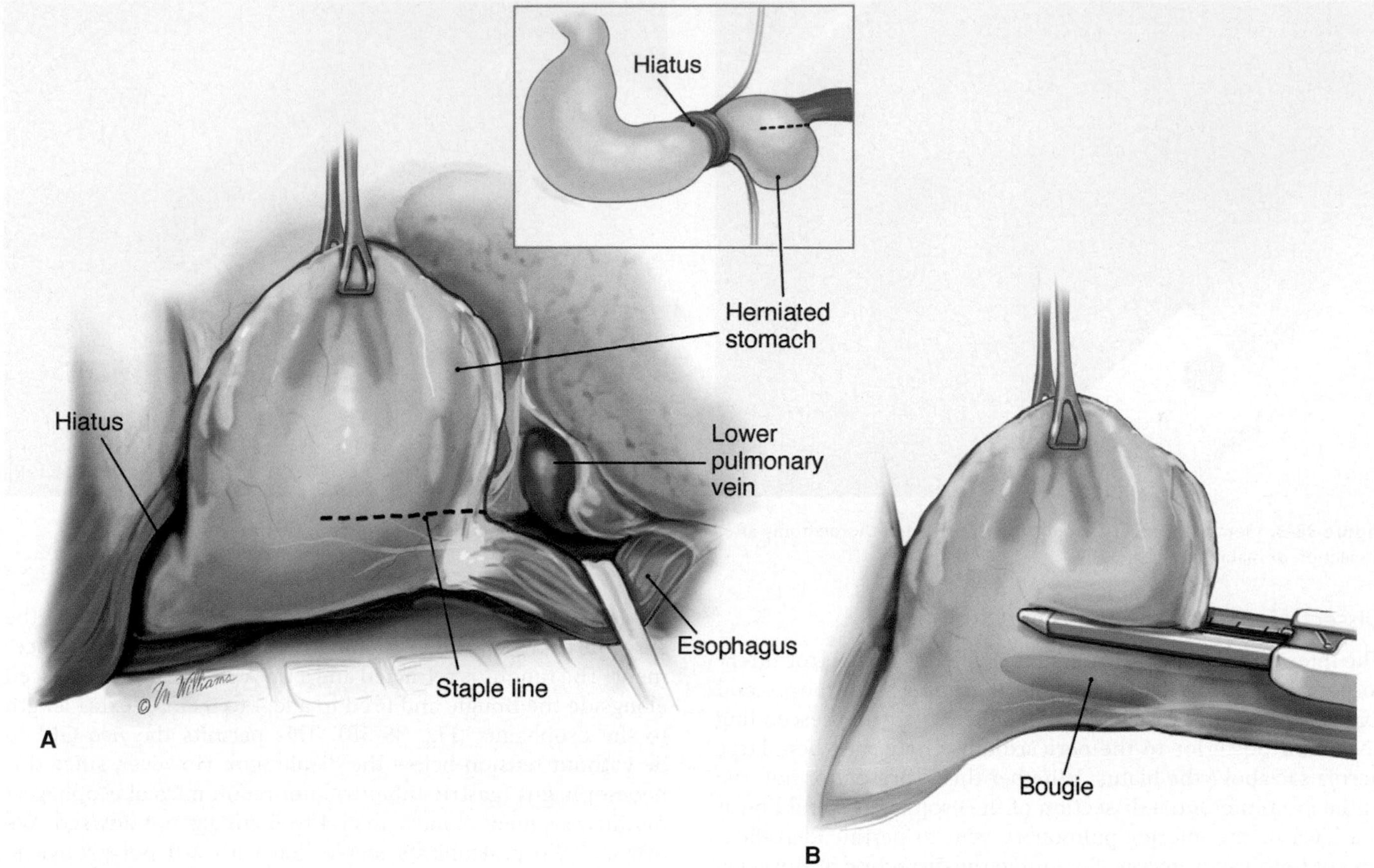

Figure 38-5. Collis gastroplasty for esophageal lengthening. *A.* The fundus is retracted with a Babcock clamp. *B.* A thick tissue stapler is placed at the angle of His alongside a 48 to 50F esophageal bougie. A 4- to 5-cm staple line is created (Inset). The staple line is subsequently oversewn with 3-0 polypropylene suture (not shown).

after ensuring good lung reexpansion. Every effort is made to extubate the patient in the operating room at the completion of the case.

POSTOPERATIVE MANAGEMENT

In the recovery room, the patient is assessed for adequacy of analgesia. A chest radiograph is obtained to assess lung reexpansion and confirm the placement of the chest and nasogastric drains. The patient should be positioned in the bed with 20 to 30 degrees of head elevation. Maintenance IV fluid is provided at a minimal hourly rate and care is taken to avoid fluid overload to both prevent pulmonary dysfunction and minimize bowel edema which might contribute to both ileus and early difficulty with passage of esophageal contents beyond the fundoplication. By postoperative day 1, ambulation and significant time out of bed should be a mandatory goal for all patients.

Perioperative antibiotics are continued for 24 hours. Prophylactic subcutaneous heparin or enoxaparin and lower extremity pneumatic compression boots are used.

The chest tube is typically able to be removed by postoperative day 2, provided the daily output is less than 200 to 300 cc. The nasogastric tube is discontinued either postoperative day 1 or 2 with adequate recovery of bowel function. After the nasogastric tube is removed, a barium swallow may be performed both to ensure that edema at the level of the fundoplication does not cause temporary dysphagia and to check for occult leak at the gastroplasty staple line or at the sites of the esophageal or gastric sutures. If the swallow is unremarkable, the patient is allowed sips of clear liquids and, once tolerated, advanced to clear liquids ad lib. The next day, soft solid food may be introduced. The patient is typically discharged on this diet as well. Pills may be taken orally when required; but if possible, liquid formulations (i.e., oral liquid narcotic analgesics) or crushed pills should be used to avoid the possibility of medication impaction at the level of the fundoplication. The hospital length of stay is typically 4 to 5 days. At the postoperative follow-up visit, more substantial food may be reintroduced provided the patient has no significant complaints of dysphagia.

COMPLICATIONS

Dysphagia

Dysphagia represents the most common both immediate and delayed complication of the procedure. In almost all cases, this is related to stricture of the distal esophagus, usually present at the time of the operation. Treatment should be approached endoscopically with Bougie dilation. In many cases, postoperative esophageal edema may be the etiology of dysphagia, though repeated dilation may be necessary over an interval of time in some patients.

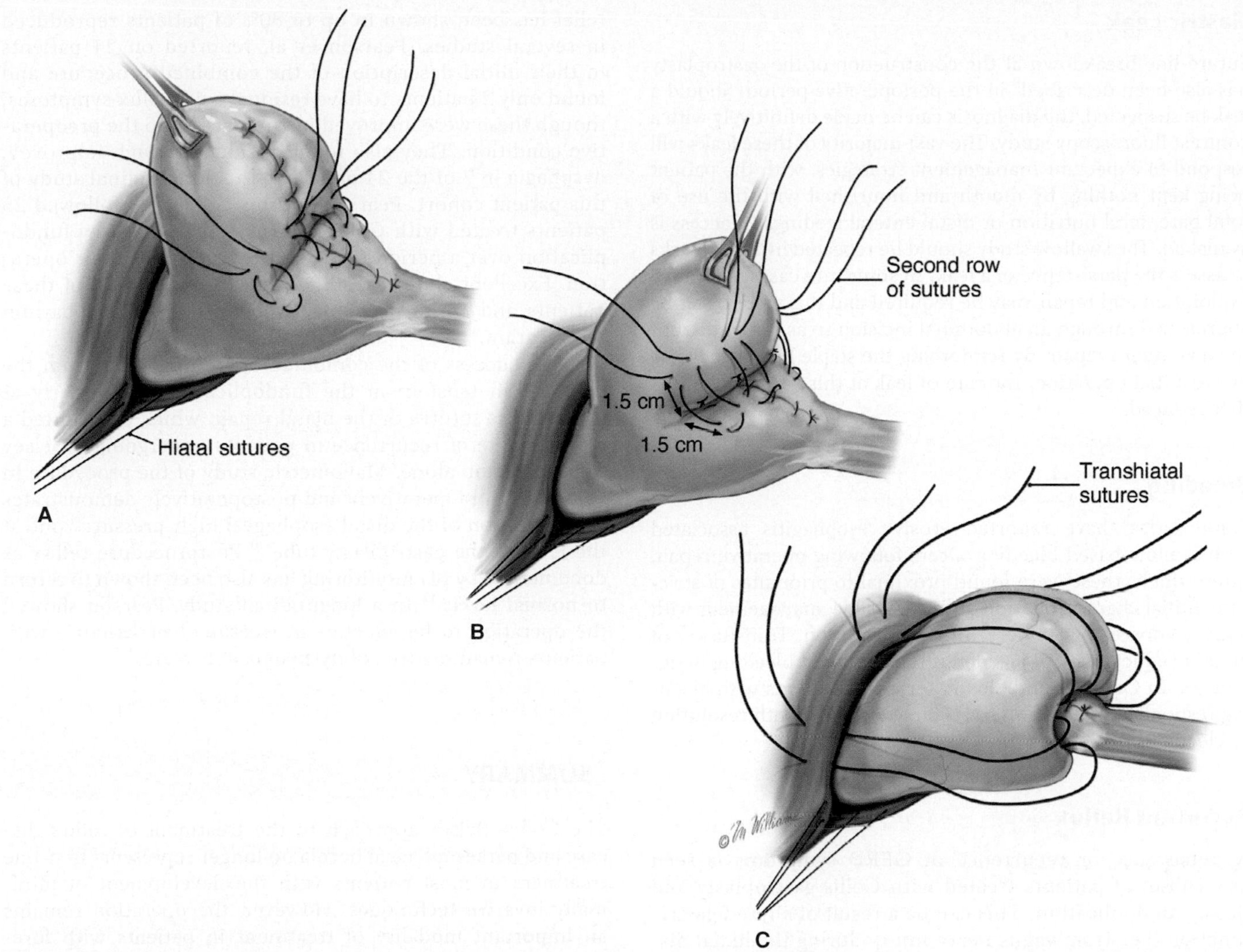

Figure 38-6. Fundoplication. *A.* Initial middle suture is placed in mattress fashion on either side of oversewn gastroplasty staple line to begin fundoplication. Left and right mattress sutures then are placed 135 degrees to either side of this initial middle suture for this row. *B.* The first-row sutures have been tied down, the middle row of the next suture is placed and the next row's middle suture is placed, again straddling the staple line. Note that the sutures are placed 1.5 cm away from the fold created by the first row of sutures. Again, sutures will be placed to the left and right of this middle suture to continue to create the 270-degree fundoplication. *C.* Finally, the last row is placed in similar fashion but not tied down until the needles are passed through the diaphragm, and the gastroesophageal junction and fundoplication are returned to the abdomen.

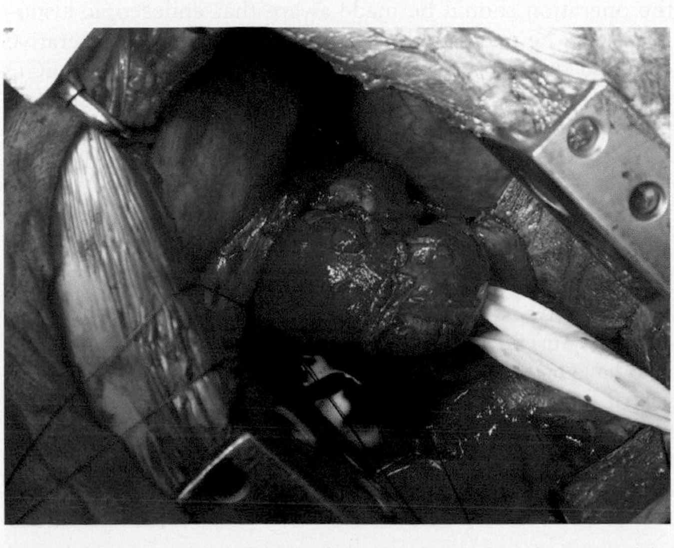

Figure 38-7. Appearance of the fundoplication just before placement of the third and final row of sutures. Note the presence of the untied crural sutures.

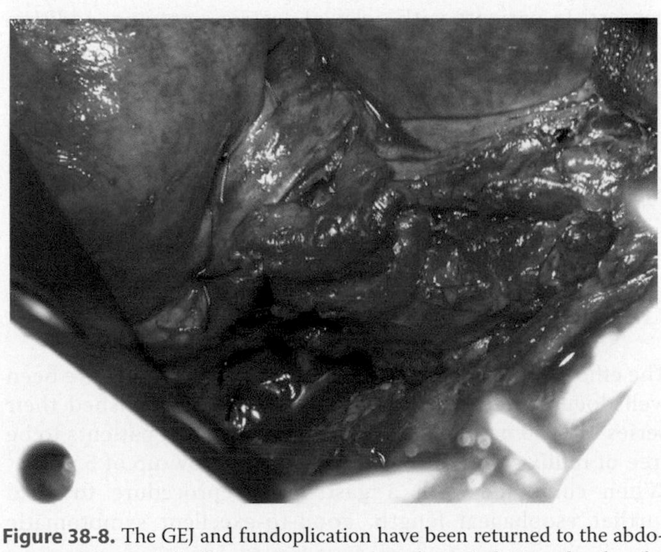

Figure 38-8. The GEJ and fundoplication have been returned to the abdomen, and the transdiaphragmatic sutures have been tied. Note also that the crural sutures also have been tied at this stage.

Gastric Leak

Suture-line breakdown at the construction of the gastroplasty has also been described[8] in the perioperative period. Should a leak be suspected, the diagnosis can be made definitively with a contrast fluoroscopy study. The vast majority of these leaks will respond to expectant management strategies, with the patient being kept nothing by mouth and nourished with the use of total parenteral nutrition or distal enteral feedings (if access is available). The swallow study should be repeated in 2 to 3 weeks to assess the persistence of a leak. In some rare cases, operative exploration and repair may be required and this would best be approached through an abdominal incision so as not to disrupt the diaphragm repair. By reinforcing the staple line at the time of the initial operation, the rate of leak at this site may be further reduced.

Bleeding

Some series[8] have reported erosive esophagitis associated with shallow-based bleeding ulcers following operative repair. Interestingly, these were found proximal to prior sites of stricture. Initial characterization and, if possible, management with upper endoscopy is preferred in this situation. Transfusion of blood products may be needed if the degree of bleeding is significant. In Orringer and Sloan's series, all patients with bleeding responded to addition of H_2 blocker or PPI with resolution of bleeding.

Recurrent Reflux

A persistence or recurrence of GERD symptoms is seen in a subset of patients treated with Collis gastroplasty and Belsey fundoplication. This can be a result of altered gastric function (i.e., from vagus nerve injury during the hiatal dissection) or may demonstrate a failure of the reconstructed esophagogastric junction to act as a physiologic barrier. A gastric emptying study using technetium-labeled food products can be beneficial in determining the contribution of relative gastroparesis to the reflux symptom complex. In fact, this is a part of the routine preoperative evaluation in some centers. In patients with delayed gastric emptying, addition of a promotility agent (metoclopromide, erythromycin, etc.) often result in amelioration of symptoms. Long-term use may not be required. In the patient group with normal gastric motility, reflux symptoms can usually be well controlled with the addition of PPIs to the postoperative medication regimen.

RESULTS

The efficacy and safety of the Belsey fundoplication have been well documented since Skinner and Belsey published their series of 1030 patients in 1967 showing 85% of patients to be free of reflux symptoms at a minimum follow-up of 5 years.[1] When combined with a gastroplasty procedure to yield further esophageal length, good-to-excellent symptomatic relief has been shown in up to 80% of patients reproduced in several studies. Pearson et al. reported on 24 patients in their initial description of the combined procedure and found only 2 patients to have residual acid reflux symptoms, though these were improved in comparison to the preoperative condition. They also found residual, though improved, dysphagia in 7 of the 24 patients.[3] In a longitudinal study of this patient cohort, Pearson and his colleagues followed 25 patients treated with Collis gastroplasty and Belsey fundoplication over a period of at least 5 years from their operation. Excellent clinical results were achieved in 24 of these patients and confirmed objectively with EGD and barium esophagram.[9]

The success of the combined operation stems from the decrease in tension on the fundoplication; particularly at the buttress sutures of the hiatal repair, which constituted a common site of recurrence in patients undergoing a Belsey fundoplication alone. Manometric study of the procedure in vivo both intraoperatively and postoperatively demonstrates reconstitution of the distal esophageal high-pressure zone at the level of the gastroplasty tube.[10] Postprocedure reflux as documented by pH monitoring has also been shown to return to normal levels.[11] In a longitudinal study, Pearson showed the operation to be effective in treatment of stricture with patients remaining free of dysphagia at 5 years.[9]

SUMMARY

The Collis–Belsey approach to the treatment of reflux disease and paraesophageal hernia no longer represents first-line treatment in most patients with the development of minimally invasive techniques. However, the operation remains an important modality of treatment in patients with foreshortened esophagus and distal esophageal stricture. In this difficult patient subset, an excellent long-term result may be achieved. A thorough preoperative evaluation is essential in the selection of appropriate operative candidates with careful attention being paid to the anatomy of the distal esophagus and the motility of the esophageal body. Patients undergoing the operation should be made aware that endoscopic evaluation may be necessary in the course of their postoperative care and the surgeon should be aggressive in pursuing EGD in patients with persistent symptoms of reflux or dysphagia postoperatively.

EDITOR'S COMMENT

The open transthoracic surgical approach to reflux can be extremely useful in reoperative cases, particularly in patients who have had multiple upper abdominal procedures including gastric bypass surgery. Less stomach is required than for a complete wrap, making definitive therapy possible. This approach may also be applicable to patients who require urgent surgery for a perforation of a peptic stricture.

—Raphael Bueno

References

1. Skinner DB, Belsey RH. Surgical management of esophageal reflux and hiatus hernia. Long-term results with 1030 patients. *J Thorac Cardiovasc Surg.* 1967;53(1):33–54.
2. Collis JL. An operation for hiatus hernia with short esophagus. *J Thorac Surg.* 1957;34:768–788.
3. Pearson FG, Langer B, Henderson RD. Gastroplasty and Belsey hiatus hernia repair. An operation for the management of peptic stricture with acquired short esophagus. *J Thorac Cardiovasc Surg.* 1971;61(1):50–63.
4. Clouse RE, Staiano A. Topography of the esophageal peristaltic pressure wave. *Am J Physiol.* 1991;261(4 Pt 1):G677–G684.
5. Bansal A, Kahrilas PJ. Has high-resolution manometry changed the approach to esophageal motility disorders? *Curr Opin Gastroenterol.* 2010;26(4):344–351.
6. Pandolfino JE, Roman S. High-resolution manometry: an atlas of esophageal motility disorders and findings of GERD using esophageal pressure topography. *Thorac Surg Clin.* 21(4):465–475.
7. Pearson F. Gastroplasty/Open Gastroplasty. In: Pearson F, ed. *Esophageal Surgery*. Philadelphia, PA: Churchill-Livingston; 2002.
8. Orringer MB, Sloan H. Complications and failings of the combined Collis-Belsey operation. *J Thorac Cardiovasc Surg.* 1977;74(5):726–735.
9. Pearson FG, Henderson RD. Long-term follow-up of peptic strictures managed by dilatation, modified Collis gastroplasty, and Belsey hiatus hernia repair. *Surgery*. 1976;80(3):396–404.
10. Cooper JD, Gill SS, Nelems JM, Pearson FG. Intraoperative and postoperative esophageal manometric findings with Collis gastroplasty and Belsey hiatal hernia repair for gastroesophageal reflux. *J Thorac Cardiovasc Surg.* 1977;74(5):744–751.
11. Orringer MB, Sloan H. Collis-Belsey reconstruction of the esophagogastric junction. Indications, physiology, and technical considerations. *J Thorac Cardiovasc Surg.* 1976;71(2):295–303.

39 Nissen Fundoplication

Abraham Lebenthal and Raphael Bueno

Keywords: Esophageal reflux disorders, gastroesophageal reflux disease (GERD), high-resolution manometry, laparoscopic and open surgical techniques

Gastroesophageal reflux disease (GERD) is caused by the chronic reflux of gastric acid from the stomach to the esophagus. This may be the result of an incompetent lower esophageal sphincter (LES) or poor gastric emptying. GERD is an anatomic and physiologic problem that may lead to surgical consultation for treatment of either the symptoms or sequelae of reflux. It was first recognized as a clinical entity in the 1930s. Today, it is the most prevalent upper gastrointestinal disorder in the Western world.[1]

GERD gives rise to a spectrum of symptoms that range in intensity from mild to severe. Up to 80% of patients present with so-called typical symptoms of GERD. These include heartburn, regurgitation, sour taste, and intermittent dysphagia but no evidence of esophageal inflammation or injury. Approximately 20% of patients present with atypical symptoms, namely, chest pain, hoarseness, nocturnal choking, chronic cough, asthma, shortness of breath, and pneumonia. For some, GERD causes severe medical disabilities, such as recurrent aspiration, ulceration, end-stage lung disease, or recurrent esophageal stricture. Left untreated, these complications may lead to disability and rarely mortality. For most, however, GERD is a non-life-threatening condition and patients suffering from this disease seek treatment mainly to improve their quality of life.

The treatment options for GERD range from lifestyle change and medical therapy to antireflux surgery based on the severity of the patient's symptoms or presence of complications. Long-term treatment with proton pump inhibitor (PPI) therapy is highly effective in terms of symptoms but may require indefinite duration because 82% of patients have recurrent symptoms within 6 months of discontinuation. When conservative treatment fails, several interventions are possible. Herein, we describe both the open Nissen fundoplication and the laparoscopic adaptation, the current surgical standard for the treatment of GERD. These operations were designed to fix the anatomic and physiologic problems that give rise to GERD.

GENERAL PRINCIPLES AND PATIENT SELECTION

The Nissen fundoplication consists of hiatal closure and a 360-degree wrap of stomach posteriorly around the distal esophagus to augment and restore the function of the LES. The laparoscopic adaptation is associated with reduced morbidity compared with the open approach; however, a history of previous abdominal operation with dense scar and adhesion still poses a significant challenge. Since its conception,[2] the Nissen fundoplication has been a successful operation with excellent long-term outcomes. The morbidity associated with the upper midline incision of the open approach; however, limited its application to patients with symptoms refractory to medical therapy and severe complications of GERD.

The laparoscopic adaptation, first reported in 1991,[3] revitalized interest in the surgical treatment of GERD. Factors underlying this increased interest included the rising incidence of GERD in Western countries, the decreased morbidity and mortality of the minimally invasive approach, poor compliance or dissatisfaction with long-term medical treatment, recognition of an association between GERD and esophageal cancer, and curative potential of the surgery. Patient demand for a permanent treatment led many surgeons to acquire expertise in the minimally invasive approach. The learning curve for laparoscopic fundoplication is relatively short, reaching a plateau at 20 cases for the individual surgeon[4,5] and 50 cases for an institution.[6] A two-surgeon collaborative approach can further reduce the learning curve.[7] The long-term results of open and laparoscopic fundoplication appear to be equivalent, with larger series showing a sustained benefit in 95% of patients at 5 years and approximately 90% at 10 years.[1]

A recent survey of 2261 consecutive cases over a 20-year period cites a conversion rate of 3.2%, a 5% rate of reoperation within 1 year, 9.6% within 10 years, and 1.4% beyond 10 years. The latter figure may not carry much value since less than one-third of the patients were followed beyond 10 years.[8] Patient selection is critical. Those that benefit most from medical therapy have the best long-term results.

General indications for antireflux surgery include esophageal ulceration, severe esophagitis, Barrett esophagitis, severe pulmonary symptoms, recurrent stricture, dysplasia, and failure or inability to comply with medical therapy. To be considered for this surgery, the patient must have normal esophageal motility and a normal-length esophagus. Patients with foreshortened esophagus likely will require a Collis extension coupled with this procedure.

It is essential to conduct an adequate preoperative evaluation to confirm the diagnosis because the symptoms of GERD overlap substantially with the primary esophageal motility disorders, which require different therapies for treatment (see Part 4). Experience with the open technique is a prerequisite because rapid conversion to the open procedure may be required if the laparoscopic approach fails or in the event of a serious complication. Depending on specific anatomic considerations, other procedures described in this section also may be necessary (e.g., a Nissen–Collis procedure or partial fundoplication). Obesity is associated with GERD; however, for patients with a body mass index greater than 40, bypass or other weight-loss procedures have superior results.[9]

Table 39-1

STANDARD STUDIES FOR THE EVALUATION OF ANTIREFLUX

pH studies	Positive for reflux if the composite reflux score is more than 14.7 (Table 39-2)
Esophagoduodenogastroscopy	To assess esophageal length, webs and strictures, mucosal anomalies, the coexistence of a hiatal hernia or other pathology
Esophagram	Detects structural changes and evaluates surgical anatomy; sensitive in the detection of achalasia and diffuse esophageal spasm, both of which contraindicate Nissen fundoplication
Manometry	To rule out esophageal motility disorders, which would call for a different operative approach

PREOPERATIVE ASSESSMENT

Patients referred for surgical treatment of GERD often have long-standing symptoms and have pursued at least medical and often lifestyle changes without success or satisfaction. Lifestyle changes include dietary modifications that reduce the consumption of fatty foods, peppermint, and alcohol, cessation of tobacco smoking, and weight loss.

The evaluation for antireflux procedures is best accomplished by studies designed to exclude related disorders of the esophagus [10] (Table 39-1). These are the barium or cine esophagram (upper gastrointestinal series), endoscopy (esophagogastroduodenoscopy [EGD]), esophageal manometry, and esophageal pH probe analysis. If the findings are inconclusive, esophageal and gastric-emptying studies, and even provocative testing may be useful.

NONINVASIVE DIAGNOSTIC PROCEDURES

Barium Esophagram

The barium swallow or esophagram is the diagnostic modality of choice for the evaluation of dysphagia and chest pain likely to be related to the esophagus. It is a sensitive diagnostic modality for achalasia and diffuse esophageal spasm but not for nutcracker esophagus or scleroderma, the latter representing secondary esophageal motility disorders. Only 40% of patients with classic GERD symptoms have a positive esophagram. Spontaneous regurgitation or moderate-to-severe reflux of contrast material to the esophagus confirms GERD.

Cine Esophagram

The cine esophagram is a dynamic video contrast study that records the transfer of contrast material from the oral cavity to the pharynx, showing the coordinated motion of the tongue, palate, epiglottis, laryngeal and pharyngeal walls, inferior constrictors, and upper esophageal sphincter. This study is indicated for patients with atypical chest pain and normal findings on barium esophagram.

INVASIVE DIAGNOSTIC PROCEDURES

Esophagogastroduodenoscopy

Fiberoptic EGD is the most important tool for the diagnosis and management of esophageal disease. It is usually performed with topical anesthesia and IV conscious sedation in an outpatient setting (see Chapter 14). We routinely perform EGD before surgery for GERD to assess esophageal length, define and treat any strictures, exclude other pathology such as cancer, evaluate Barrett esophagitis, and determine the presence of a hiatal hernia (esophageal or paraesophageal).

Esophageal Manometry

Esophageal manometry provides information about the motor function of the esophagus and its sphincters (upper and lower) at rest and during swallowing. Conventional manometry is performed using a water-perfused catheter which has pressure sensors located at several points along the length of the catheter. These catheters produce limited data, however, because of the large gaps between the sensors. A new generation of catheters has been developed for high-resolution manometry (HRM). The HRM catheters are equipped with intraluminal pressure transducers. They enable the clinician to simultaneously measure the entire esophagus (from hypopharynx to stomach). This not only increases the accuracy of the test but also provides more information. The data generated from these catheters is visualized on a spatiotemporal color plot, called a Clouse plot, which is more intuitive and easier for clinicians to interpret.[11]

Patients who undergo Nissen fundoplication must have a relatively normally functioning esophagus. Impaired motility increases the risk for obstructive symptoms postoperatively. One exception is the entity known as esophageal stunning that is caused by prolonged acid exposure and reflected in decreased motility of the distal esophagus. This entity occasionally may be confused with diffuse esophageal spasm. At rest, the normal LES is a 3- to 4-cm high-pressure zone in the distal esophagus. It relaxes with a food bolus, permitting food to pass into the stomach. The LES has three components: resting pressure at midrespiration, overall length, and abdominal length (the lower limits of normal are 6 mm Hg, 2 cm, and 1 cm, respectively). If just one of these values is low, the LES will not function properly. Esophageal manometry is most useful for identifying nonobstructive causes of dysphagia because it is sensitive to pressure changes and does not provide information about the passage of food. It provides a definitive diagnosis of achalasia, diffuse esophageal spasm, nutcracker esophagus, hypertensive LES, and scleroderma, all of which are contraindications to Nissen fundoplication.

Esophageal pH Probe Monitoring

Ambulatory esophageal pH monitoring was introduced in 1985 for the diagnosis of GERD. The patient must cease H_2-blocker therapy 48 hours before monitoring and PPI therapy 2 weeks in advance of study. The basic instrument consists of a tube with

Table 39-2

COMPOSITE REFLUX (DEMEESTER) SCORE[12]

Components	
Percent of total time pH <4	
Percent of upright time pH <4	
Percent of supine time pH <4	
Total number of episodes pH <4	
Number of episodes pH <4 lasting >5 min	
Number of minutes of longest episode pH <4	
Score	
<14.7 indicates absence of reflux (95% confidence interval)	

a number of pH channels. This tube is placed in the esophagus for 24 hours. The tube is positioned such that the first probe is located 5 cm above the LES (determined by manometry). The second is connected to the skin, and both are connected to a portable data recorder. The pH is sampled and recorded every second. In general, the patient is asked to eat a regular diet and carry out normal daily activities. A diary is used to document meals, symptoms, and sleep time. A composite reflux score is calculated, and a value above 14.7 represents pathologic exposure to acid. Ninety-five percent of individuals score under 14.7. The composite reflux score has a sensitivity of 90% and specificity of 85% for GERD. It is especially useful in diagnosing reflux with atypical pulmonary symptoms such as chronic cough, wheezing, asthma, and recurrent pneumonia. It can be used to assess the efficacy of medical therapy or the success of surgical therapy. It should be used to confirm GERD in all patients before antireflux procedures. This test does not detect "alkaline reflux," that is, reflux owing to bile with a pH >7. It is considered the single most useful objective test for evaluating GERD[12] (Table 39-2).

Newer devices have been developed that cause less discomfort to the patient. The wireless Bravo capsule (Bravo, pH Monitoring System, Medtronic, Inc., Minneapolis, MN), for example, is clipped to the esophageal wall during endoscopy and is capable of transmitting pH data to a small external recorder for up to 48 hours. A new generation of commercially available catheters has been developed that measure pH and impedance simultaneously at multiple sites in the esophagus via a single multichannel intraluminal device, whereas other catheters measure HRM and impedance. These contribute to the understanding of the relationship between GERD and motility.

ADDITIONAL NONINVASIVE PROCEDURES

On occasion, findings on the aforementioned studies are inconclusive. Nuclear scintigraphy (esophageal and gastric emptying studies) uses food (e.g., cereal, eggs, or juice) labeled with radioactive technetium-99m or indium-111 to record the transit of food over time through the body. Abnormal studies demonstrate rapid or delayed emptying. Normal transit time through the esophagus is 10 to 17 seconds, and 50% of gastric emptying occurs within 15 to 90 minutes for liquids and 45 to 100 minutes for solids.

Provocative testing was developed because many patients, particularly those with atypical symptoms, may be asymptomatic at the time of testing. These studies reproduce the type of pain characteristic of GERD but do not provide insight into the underlying pathology. Of historical interest is the Bernstein acid perfusion test that was developed in 1958 to distinguish esophageal from other causes of chest pain. A tube is placed in the distal esophagus, and 0.1N hydrochloric acid is infused continuously at a rate of 5 to 10 mL/min for 10 to 30 minutes. The test is positive if the patient experiences pain when acid is introduced, and the pain abates with saline.

SURGICAL TECHNIQUE

Laparoscopic Nissen Fundoplication

The critical steps of this operation are (1) placing the ports, (2) dividing the short gastric arteries, (3) hiatal dissection, (4) mobilization of the fat pad and assessment of esophageal length, (5) hiatal closure, and (6) fashioning and securing the wrap. The procedure is performed under general anesthesia. EGD should be performed by the surgeon at the time of the operation to confirm the anatomic findings, in particular, esophageal length. The bladder is decompressed, antibiotics are given, and prophylactic measures to prevent pulmonary embolus are instituted. The procedure can be performed in the supine or lithotomy position, with both arms tucked in at the sides.

OR Setup and Trocar Placement

Our preference is to perform the operation with the patient in the lithotomy position. The surgeon stands between the patient's legs, and the first assistant is positioned to the left of the surgeon (Fig. 39-1).

Typically, we create an 11-mm incision in the periumbilical region for the camera port using a modified Hassan technique to minimize inadvertent injury to the abdominal viscera. Although it adds a few additional minutes in overall time, to date, we have not experienced a single laparoscopic port catastrophe when using this technique. We then create a pneumoperitoneum by insufflating the abdomen with carbon dioxide to a maximal pressure of 15 to 19 mm Hg. At our institution, we use a CO_2 insufflator (Lexion Medical, Inc., St. Paul, MN), which humidifies and heats the peritoneum, improves visualization, and decreases hypothermia during surgery. Thereafter, we insert a fully adjustable 10-mm laparoscope with a deflectable tip to permit multiple planes of visualization; others use a 30-degree laparoscope. The table is positioned in a steep reverse Trendelenburg position for the duration of the procedure. Laparoscopy is performed to assess for the presence of adhesions. The remaining ports are placed sequentially under direct visualization in areas devoid of adhesions and are used, if needed, to perform further adhesiolysis until all five standard ports have been placed (Fig. 39-1). All ports should be placed such that the instruments point naturally in the direction of the dissection (i.e., toward the gastroesophageal junction [GEJ]).

Dividing the Short Gastric Arteries to Mobilize the Fundus and Prevent Splenic Injury

The assistant raises the left lobe of the liver using a self-retaining liver retractor. A grasper is placed high on the greater curvature, retracting the greater curve caudally, anteriorly, and medially, whereas a second grasper elevates the gastrosplenic ligament laterally (Fig. 39-2). An avascular plane is identified along the greater curvature at the midlevel of the short gastric arteries. Using a 5-mm LigaSure (Valleylab, Boulder, CO) device, the

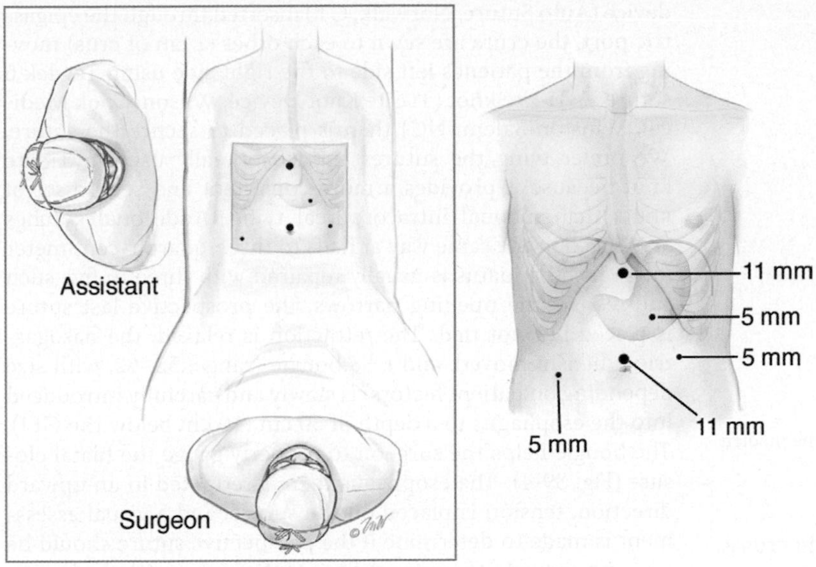

Figure 39-1. With the patient in the lithotomy position, the surgeon stands between the patient's legs, and the first assistant is positioned to the left of the surgeon.

gastrosplenic ligament is gradually divided all the way to the left crus. The two leaves should be divided separately. All lateral attachments to the upper portion of the greater curve of the stomach are completely divided to mobilize the stomach. It is important to completely mobilize the fundus to later enable a tension-free wrap of the esophagus.

Hiatal Dissection

After reaching the left crus, the left gastrophrenic ligament is opened, exposing the left crus down to its confluence with the right crus. Care must be taken to avoid injury to the anterior vagus, which courses between 3 o'clock and 12 o'clock. If a hiatal hernia is identified, as is extremely common in patients with GERD, its contents are reduced into the abdomen, and the peritoneal sac is amputated. Most often the hernia is of the sliding type (see Chapter 46), and the sac is very small. If the hernia is larger than 4 cm, special attention should be given to ensuring adequate esophageal length. Attention to detail during crural dissection is critical. It is important to preserve the peritoneal covering over the crural fibers. The fibers are not covered by fascia and we believe that the future integrity of closure is improved when the peritoneum is left intact.

With the stomach retracted laterally, the lesser curvature is opened in an avascular region near the liver, exposing the caudate lobe, until the right crus of the hiatus is seen. Care is required to avoid the left gastric artery, a possible replaced hepatic artery, and vagal branches. Occasionally, a small branch from the left gastric artery to the left hepatic artery is divided

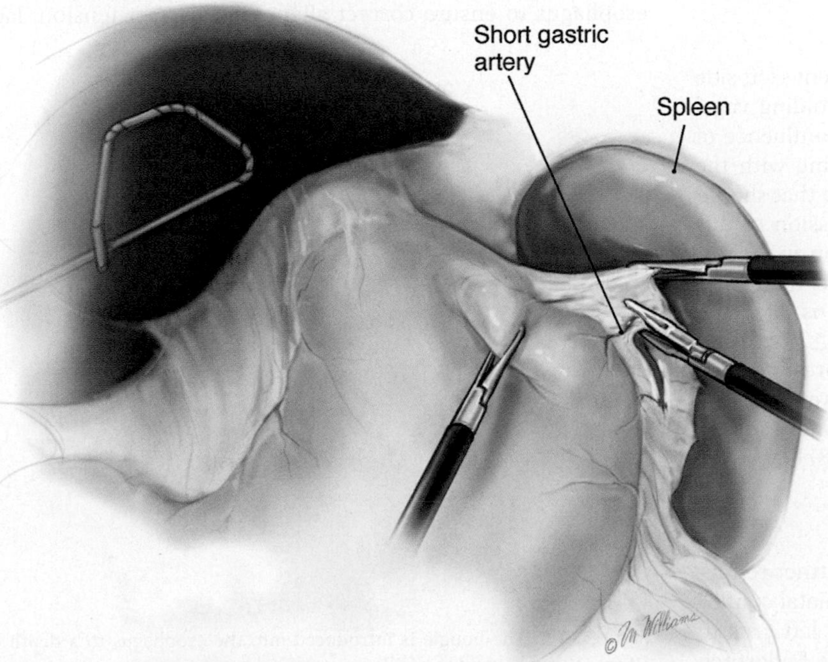

Figure 39-2. The first grasper is placed high on the greater curvature, retracting the greater curve caudally, anteriorly, and medially, and a second grasper elevates the gastrosplenic ligament laterally.

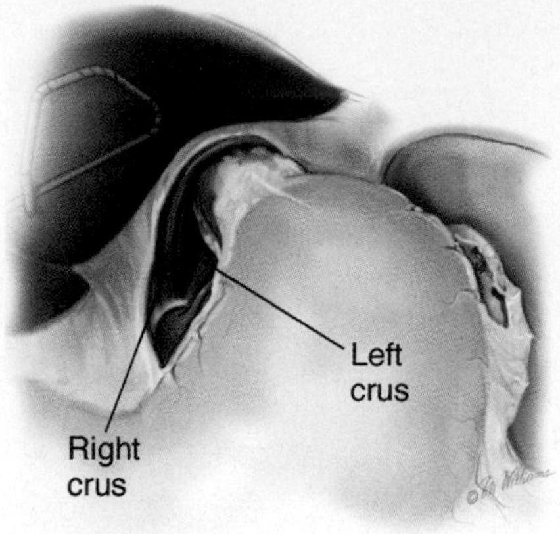

Figure 39-3. The right crus is dissected from its confluence to the median arcuate ligament, where it joins the left crus.

without consequence to improve the exposure. The right crus is identified, and the overlying peritoneum is opened, exposing its edge. *The risk of esophageal perforation is sufficiently high that we do not attempt to directly identify the esophagus before opening the crus.* The right crus is dissected from its confluence to the median arcuate ligament, where it joins the left crus (Fig. 39-3). This dissection is done meticulously taking only a thin layer of peritoneum, and the esophagus is revealed by its orientation, longitudinal muscle fibers, and position of the posterior vagus nerve, which courses between 9 o'clock and 6 o'clock. Using blunt dissection with traction and countertraction, the peritoneum and phrenoesophageal ligaments are divided, proceeding in a plane perpendicular to the esophagus. We divide the esophagophrenic attachments and peritoneum in a semicircular fashion down to the median arcuate ligament, with all due caution to avoid injury to the anteroposterior branches of the vagus. Great care is taken to avoid perforating the esophagus or stomach when mobilizing the GEJ. The esophagus is retracted upward, and a window is bluntly opened and widened to reveal the left side of the abdomen.

Mobilization of the Fat Pad and Assessment of Esophageal Length

The fat pad is medialized proceeding from the patient's left side to center, thereby exposing the true GEJ and avoiding vagal injury. The GEJ is identified by recognizing the confluence of the longitudinal muscles of the esophagus merging with the sling muscles of the stomach. This is a critical step that should not be omitted. In Dr. Pearson's experience, omission of this step will lead to misjudgment of the GEJ location in 30% of the patients. Of note: the GEJ is not perpendicular but rather oblique. In approximately 90% of patients, there is adequate tension-free length of the abdominal esophagus (≥2 cm), and a lengthening procedure is not required. If a foreshortened esophagus is encountered (i.e., if the esophagus retracts into the mediastinum and there is <1 cm of abdominal esophagus), we perform a Collis extension (see Chapter 38) before the hiatus is closed.

Closing the Hiatus

The esophagus is retracted using an endoscopic Kittner retractor (Ethicon Endo-Surgery, Cincinnati, OH). The hiatal confluence then is visualized and closed by sewing the left crus to the right crus beginning at the confluence. Using the Endostitch device (Auto Suture, Norwalk, CT) inserted through the epigastric port, the crura are sewn to each other (1 cm of crus) moving from the patient's left side to the right side using Tevdek 0 suture. A Ti-rite knot (Ti-rite Knot Device, Wilson-Cook Medical, Winston-Salem, NC) then is placed to secure the suture. We prefer tying the sutures extracorporeally using a Ti-rite knot because it provides a more consistent and secure set of knots than manual intracorporeal tying. Additional stitches are placed in the same way at half- to three-quarter-centimeter intervals. The hiatus is usually repaired with three to five such sutures. As the opening narrows, the prospective last suture is placed but not tied. The retraction is relaxed, the nasogastric tube is removed, and a 58 bougie (range: 52–60, with size depending on patient factors) is slowly and carefully introduced into the esophagus to a depth of 50 cm (10 cm below the GEJ). The bougie helps the surgeon to properly gauge the hiatal closure (Fig. 39-4). The esophagus then is retracted in an upward direction, tension is placed on the suture, and a visual assessment is made to determine if the prospective suture should be tied or removed. When the caliber of the hiatus with the bougie in the esophagus is deemed snug but not constricted, the bougie is retracted to 25 cm. If the hiatus is still lax, the bougie is withdrawn, and an extra suture is placed.

Creating the Wrap

The GEJ is elevated, and a reticulating grasper is brought under the esophagus to pull the apical tip of the greater curvature to the right of the right side. The inverted stomach is grabbed with an endoscopic grasper. The surgeon aids by pushing the gastric fundus behind the esophagus, enabling the surgeon to assess the configuration of the wrap. After bringing the gastric fundus behind the esophagus, we choose the most apical point along the line of the greater curvature (the line of the short gastric vessels). *Choosing the correct region of the stomach to wrap is essential for the success of the fundoplication.*

Babcock clamps are applied to both sides of the stomach that now encircles the esophagus, and the 58 bougie is carefully readvanced into the stomach. Using the Babcock clamps, the stomach is "shoeshined" at both ends around the distal esophagus to ensure correct alignment, correct tension, lack

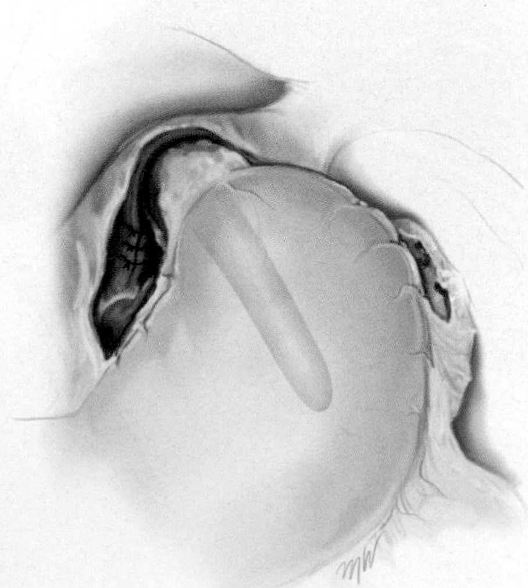

Figure 39-4. The bougie is introduced into the esophagus to a depth of 50 cm (10 cm beyond the GEJ).

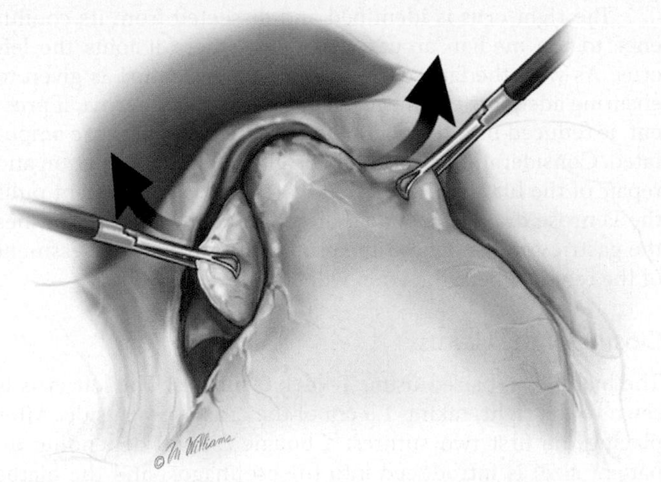

Figure 39-5. The wrap is "shoeshined" at both ends around the distal esophagus to ensure proper placement.

of excess redundancy, and correct placement of the wrap (Fig. 39-5). The fat pad is now pulled caudad from the greater curvature in the area of the GEJ to enable better adhesion of the stomach to the esophagus.

Securing the Nissen Fundoplication

Using the Endostitch device, sutures are passed from the left side of the wrap to the esophagus and then to the right side of the wrap, taking 1 cm of stomach on each side, and the sutures are tied with a Ti-rite knot (Fig. 39-6). Additional stitches are placed in the same way at 5-mm intervals. The length of the fundoplication is 2 to 2.5 cm and typically consists of four nonabsorbable Tevdek 2-0 stitches. The first three stitches are taken through all three layers: stomach–esophagus–stomach. The last stitch is made from stomach to stomach. It is important to take small bites of serosa and muscularis without mucosa because the latter can lead to necrosis and leak if tied too tightly. After removing the bougie, an 18F nasogastric tube is placed by the anesthesiologist, and its entrance into the stomach and positioning are confirmed visually. The repair then is examined visually to ensure that the wrap is configured correctly. Hemostasis is ensured and the fasciae underneath the large ports are closed, as is the skin.

Open Nissen Fundoplication

At one time, the open Nissen fundoplication, developed by Rudolph Nissen in the 1950s,[2] was the "gold standard" of antireflux surgery. It was simple, easy to learn, yielded excellent outcome with an overall 10-year success rate of better than 90%, and was technically less challenging than other operations for reflux. However, after Dallemagne et al.[3] adapted the technique laparoscopically in 1991, high patient demand for the minimally invasive procedure quickly followed. As a consequence, the open approach is now indicated only in the diminishing circumstances where a laparoscopic approach is not possible. In experienced hands, these circumstances are rare. Frankly, the laparoscopic approach is easier to perform and safer because of its better visualization and access. In our practice, we try to accomplish the wrap first laparoscopically, even when we plan to open the abdomen subsequently for another reason. We recommend that the equipment required for conversion be readily available and a system set up for rapid conversion. It is important for the staff to periodically discuss and simulate the conversion sequence.

The open procedure is performed with the patient in the supine position with the right arm extended or tucked and the left arm tucked in at the side. The bed is placed in a shallow reverse Trendelenburg position. A nasogastric tube is inserted for drainage and decompression of the stomach.

Incision and Exposure

The abdomen is explored through an upper midline incision (Fig. 39-7). (If needed, the incision can be extended below the umbilicus.) Lysis of adhesions can be carried out in the left upper quadrant as needed. The falciform suspensory ligament

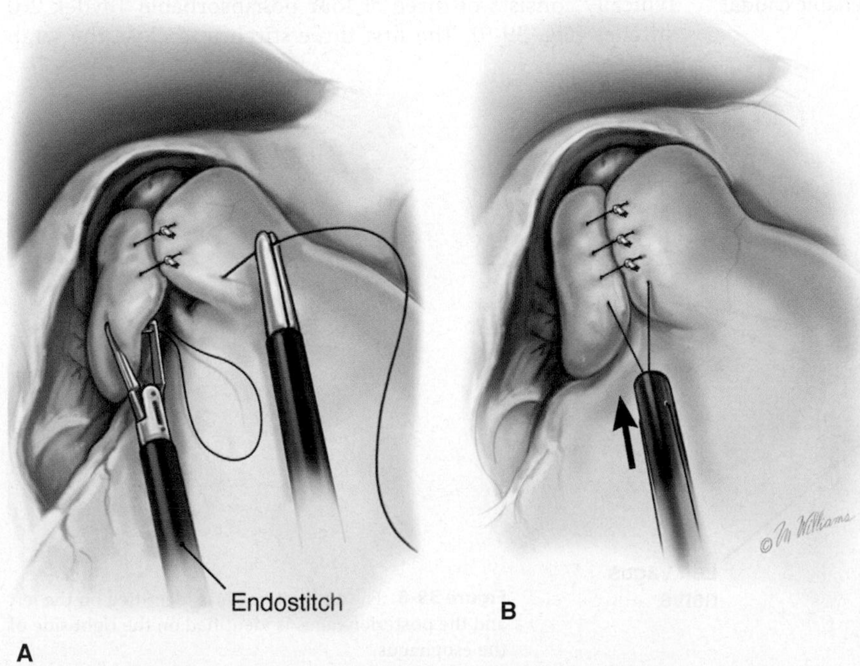

Figure 39-6. The Endostitch device is used to secure the wrap. *A.* Sutures are passed from the left side of the wrap to the esophagus and then to the right side of wrap and tied with a Ti-rite knot. *B.* Additional stitches are placed at 5-mm intervals.

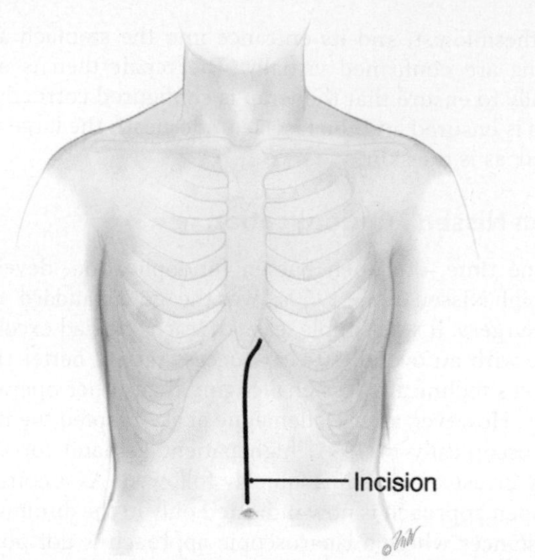

Figure 39-7. Midline incision for open technique.

is divided, and the triangular ligament (hepatophrenic ligament) is excised. An upper-hand retractor is placed to elevate the costochondral portion of the chest. A moist laparotomy pad is placed behind the spleen, and a liver retractor is positioned to retract the left lobe, exposing the esophageal hiatus.

Mobilization of the Distal Esophagus and Proximal Stomach

As with the laparoscopic approach, three or four short gastric arteries are ligated either with clamps or with the LigaSure device (Valleylab, Boulder, CO) to avoid splenic injury. The phrenoesophageal ligament is opened using Metzenbaum scissors to make a semicircular incision. The anterior vagus is identified on the left and the posterior vagus is identified on the right side of the esophagus (Fig. 39-8). The gastrohepatic ligament is opened close to the liver, with vigilance to avoid injury to the left gastric artery, a replaced hepatic artery, or branches of the vagus. A finger is placed behind the esophagus, and then a Penrose drain is passed behind the esophagus to enable caudal retraction.

The right crus is identified and dissected from its confluence to the median arcuate ligament, where it joins the left crus. As with the laparoscopic approach, attention is given to ensuring adequate esophageal length, and hiatal hernia, if present, is reduced into the abdomen and the peritoneal sac amputated. Consideration also should be given to reconstruction and repair of the hiatus with mesh if warranted. The assistant pulls the Penrose drain in a caudal direction as the surgeon pushes the gastric fundus behind the esophagus, enabling assessment of the region where the wrap will lie.

Closure of the Hiatus

The hiatus is repaired using Tevdek 0 sutures. The left crus is sewn to the right, taking 1.5 cm of the crus on each side. After placing the first two sutures, a bougie (58–60 depending on patient size) is introduced into the esophagus, and the hiatus is closed with a few additional sutures to correctly gauge the closure. Note that insertion of the bougie is a critical step. If performed incorrectly, this maneuver can lead to esophageal or gastric perforation. It must be done under direct vision in a controlled manner to minimize potential complications.

Nissen Fundoplication

After the gastric fundus has been brought behind the esophagus, the apical most point along the line of the greater curvature (the line of the short gastric vessels) is identified. The apex of the stomach is brought behind the esophagus. Babcock clamps are applied to both sides of the stomach, and the bougie is reintroduced. Using the Babcock clamps, the stomach is "shoeshined" at both ends around the distal esophagus to ensure correct alignment, contour, tension, and placement of the wrap. One should see a straight line between both upper edges of the wrap. The fat pad is removed well away from the greater curvature in the area of the GEJ to prevent vagal injury in a medial-to-lateral direction to enable better adhesion of the stomach to the esophagus. We routinely wrap the stomach around a bougie to ensure that the wrap is not too tight. The length of our fundoplication is 2 to 2.5 cm and typically consists of three or four nonabsorbable Tevdek 2-0 stitches (Fig. 39-9). The first three stitches to close the wrap

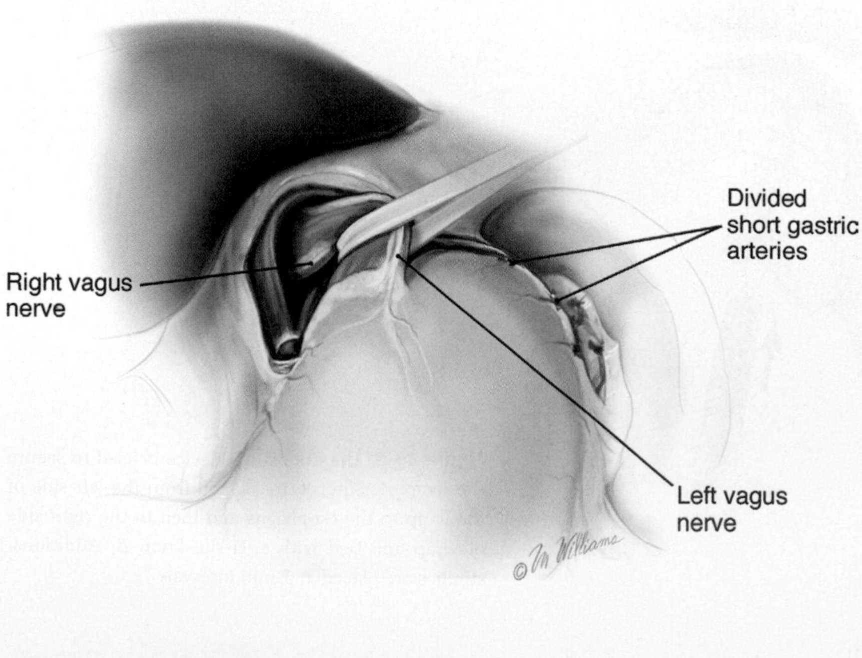

Figure 39-8. The anterior vagus is identified on the left and the posterior vagus is identified on the right side of the esophagus.

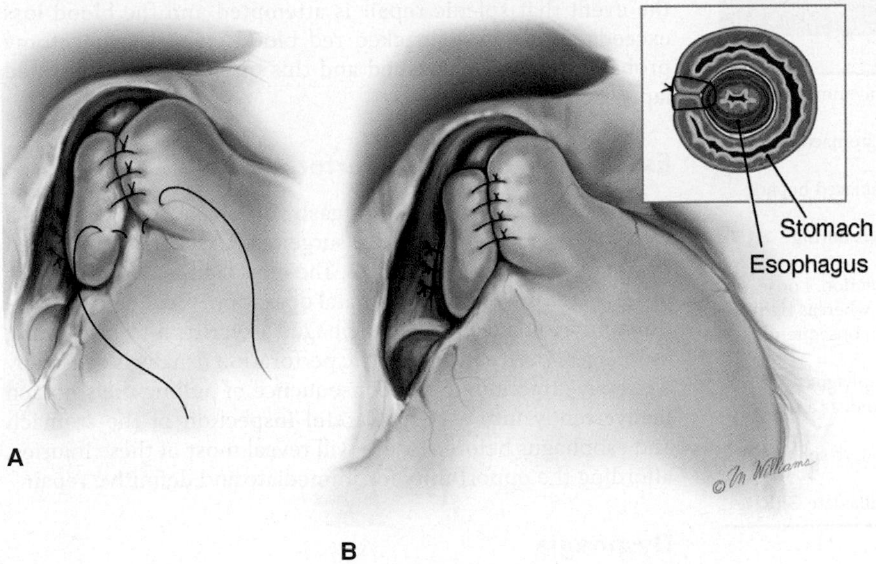

Figure 39-9. A 2- to 2.5-cm fundoplication is created. *A.* The first three stitches close the wrap and traverse all three layers: stomach-esophagus-stomach. *B.* The last stitch is made from stomach to stomach.

traverse all three layers: stomach–esophagus–stomach. Full-thickness bites of esophagus that incorporate the underlying mucosal layer are avoided. Avoiding the mucosal layer when stitching is important because the latter, if tied too tightly, can necrose and leak. The last stitch is made from stomach to stomach. To gauge the tightness of the wrap after the bougie is removed, we place an 18F nasogastric tube through the reinforced esophagus. If the fit is proper, the surgeon should be able to pass the fifth digit under the wrap (Fig. 39-10). Proper esophageal length prevents the wrap from slipping into the chest. Proper patient selection (adequate esophageal length), good technique, and correct placement of stomach and esophageal sutures will prevent the wrap from slipping in the caudal direction. If caudal slippage occurs, the stomach will constrict and assume an "hourglass" appearance, producing a partial obstruction (Fig. 39-11). This can be avoided by adhering to the aforementioned principles.

Abdominal Closure

After assuring hemostasis, the retractors are removed, and pads and instruments are counted. The abdominal fascia is closed with two 1-0 PDS loop sutures, with attention to the corners of the incision and 1 × 1 cm bites of fascia. The subcutaneous layer is not closed. The skin is closed with a stapler or a running 3-0 Vicryl intracuticular stitch. The patient is aroused, extubated, and taken to the postoperative recovery room.

With adequate knowledge of the operative pitfalls, many technical errors can be avoided. These are summarized in Table 39-3.

POSTOPERATIVE MANAGEMENT

The patient is maintained on IV fluids. Pain medication is administered through patient-controlled analgesia and later with an oral analgesic cocktail. The patient is kept NPO with a nasogastric tube in place on the first postoperative day, but the tube is removed the following morning to

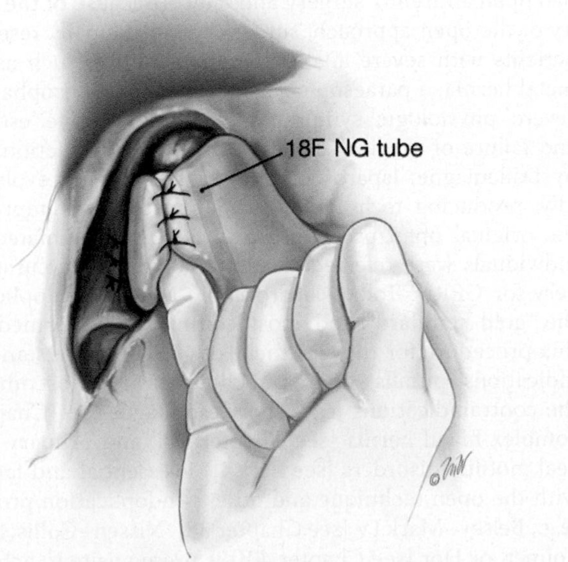

Figure 39-10. A finger is slipped under the wrap to test it.

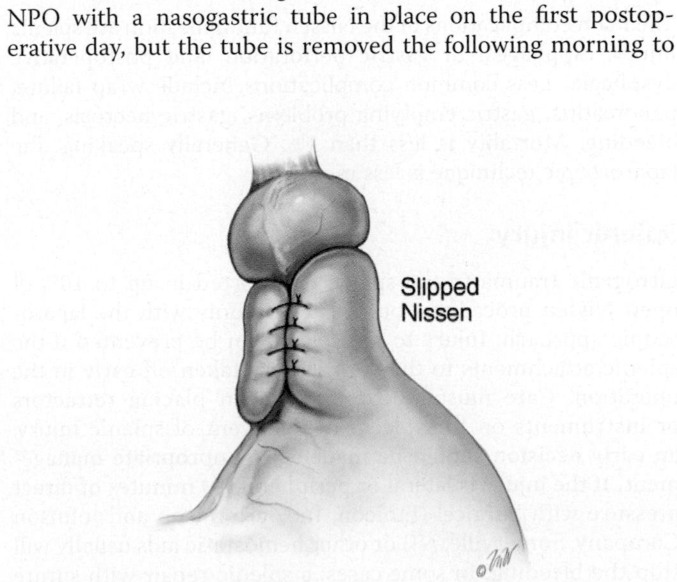

Figure 39-11. Caudal slippage produces an "hourglass" appearance to the stomach and partial obstruction.

Table 39-3

OPERATIVE PITFALLS

Splenic laceration usually involving traction injuries (uncommon with laparoscopic approach).
Injury to the vagus nerve or to vagal branches near the stomach in the gastrohepatic ligament.
Vascular injury to the left gastric artery or injury to a replaced hepatic artery.
Unidentified perforation of the stomach or the esophagus during retraction or dissection.
Improper hiatal closure owing to incomplete hiatal dissection. Loose hiatal closure may lead to postoperative hiatal hernia, whereas tight hiatal closure may lead to esophageal obstruction and consequently achalasia.
Inadequate mobilization of gastric fundus and distal esophagus leading to suboptimal position of the fundoplication and, as a result, inadequate function.
A fundoplication that is too long or too tight will result in dysphagia, gas bloating, and a functional obstruction.
A fundoplication that is too short or too loose will not alleviate GERD.

prevent postoperative emesis because this has been linked to early wrap failure. A swallow study to rule out leak can be ordered in selected patients on postoperative day 1 or 2. We advocate early ambulation and begin the patient on a clear liquid diet the morning after surgery. The patient is discharged on this diet on postoperative day 2 or 3 and seen in follow-up at 2 weeks (when the diet is advanced as tolerated), at 6 weeks, and thereafter as needed while avoiding certain foods, such as bread, leafy vegetables, and carbonated beverages. The patient is encouraged to cut food into small pieces, chew well and slowly, avoid "chugging and gulping," eat multiple small meals; becoming a "grazer" as opposed to eating one to two large meals a day. This behavior modification requires education, patient by-in, and compliance. Recently, a number of groups have reported laparoscopic fundoplication as an outpatient procedure. At this time we caution against this practice.

PROCEDURE-SPECIFIC COMPLICATIONS

The main complications of the Nissen fundoplication are splenic injury, esophageal or gastric perforation, and postoperative dysphagia. Less common complications include wrap failure, pancreatitis, gastric emptying problems, gastric necrosis, and bleeding. Mortality is less than 1%. Generally speaking, the laparoscopic technique is less morbid.

Splenic Injury

Iatrogenic trauma to the spleen is reported in up to 10% of open Nissen procedures but less commonly with the laparoscopic approach. Injury to the spleen can be prevented if the splenic attachments to the stomach are taken off early in the operation. Care must be exercised when placing retractors or instruments on the spleen. In the event of splenic injury, an early decision should be made as to appropriate management. If the injury is lateral or peripheral, 10 minutes of direct pressure with Surgicel (Ethicon, Inc., a Johnson and Johnson Company, Somerville, NJ) or other hemostatic aids usually will stop the bleeding. In some cases, a splenic repair with suture is needed. A splenectomy should be performed if the splenic laceration is extensive or located in the area of the hilum. In the event that splenic repair is attempted and the blood loss exceeds two units of packed red blood cells, a splenectomy probably should be pursued and this often can be performed laparoscopically.

Esophageal or Gastric Perforation

In a retrospective review of gastroesophageal leaks from a series of over 1000 antireflux surgeries, Urschel[13] determined the incidence of leak to be 1.2%. The most significant predisposing risk factor was previous hiatal operation. Careful identification and avoidance of the esophagus are critical to preventing esophageal perforation. Gastric perforation usually is caused by aggressive traction or as a consequence of pulling the stomach inadvertently into a port. Careful inspection of the stomach and esophagus before closure will reveal most of these injuries, affording the opportunity for immediate and definitive repair.

Dysphagia

Early nausea and vomiting have been associated with wrap failure and must be proactively prevented or recognized and treated. Transient mild dysphagia is commonly reported during the first few postoperative weeks. It is usually caused by postoperative edema localized to the area of the wrap. A number of other possible causes have been reported, including tight hiatal closure (avoided by calibration), long fundoplication wrap (avoided by measuring it), slipped wrap (owing to a foreshortened esophagus or trauma), and impaction of food (owing to improper diet). However, if the dysphagia existed preoperatively, the possibility of a misdiagnosed esophageal motility disorder also must be considered.[14–18]

SUMMARY

The number of patients seeking surgical treatment for early-stage GERD has increased dramatically since the popularization of laparoscopy. Before the era of laparoscopic antireflux procedures, despite a 30-year experience and documented 10-year success rate of approximately 90%,[1] only about 13,000 patients had open antireflux surgery annually.[19] Because of the morbidity of the open approach, surgery was principally reserved for patients with severe anatomic comorbidities, such as a large hiatal hernia, a paraesophageal hernia, a short esophagus, and severe physiologic symptoms including erosive esophagitis and failure of medical therapy. After its introduction in 1991 by Dallemagne, laparoscopic antireflux surgery evolved rapidly, producing techniques that simulated and improved on the original open procedures. By 2004, an estimated 70,000 individuals were referred for minimally invasive curative surgery for GERD. Today, laparoscopic Nissen fundoplication is the "gold standard" and most commonly performed antireflux procedure for the treatment of GERD. Understanding the indications, pitfalls, surgical technique, and most important, the contraindications (e.g., short esophagus [see Chapter 42], complex hiatal hernia [see Chapter 46], and primary esophageal motility disorders [see Part 4]) is essential and familiarity with the open technique and other fundoplication procedures (e.g., Belsey–Mark IV [see Chapter 38], Nissen–Collis, and Hill, Toupet, or Dor [see Chapter 40]) is prerequisite to achieving a satisfactory outcome.

CASE HISTORY

A 45-year-old man, in general, having good health presented with a long-standing history of GERD that was treated with PPIs with good symptomatic response but ultimately was limited by poor compliance. He had a previous history of multiple abdominal operations, including appendectomy for perforated appendicitis, negative laparotomy after a motor vehicle accident, and mesh repair for postoperative ventral hernia. Physical examination was remarkable only for multiple laparotomy incisions. He underwent evaluation that included normal findings on EGD (i.e., normal esophageal length, absence of Barrett esophagus, and no evidence of peptic disease or other pathology) and a pH study that documented multiple episodes of acid reflux with a DeMeester score of 120. Manometry showed normal esophageal contractions and motility. An upper gastrointestinal study was normal. The patient was referred for a laparoscopic Nissen fundoplication, which was uneventful. The patient had an uneventful postoperative course and is without recurrence of GERD for 2.5 years. The patient does not take any medication for GERD.

EDITOR'S COMMENT

Careful attention to all the details and precise anatomical delineation during surgery are critical for good outcome. Calibration with a bougie is important and should be balanced, in my opinion, toward looser wraps to avoid debilitating dysphagia. In that scenario, patients who fail repeated dilatation and have an adequate wrap will ultimately improve after conversion to a less than 360-degree wrap.

—Raphael Bueno

References

1. DeMeester TR, Bonavina L, Albertucci M. Nissen fundoplication for gastroesophageal reflux disease: evaluation of primary repair in 100 consecutive patients. *Ann Surg.* 1986;204:9–20.
2. Nissen R. Eine einfache operation zur beeinflussung der reflux oesophagitis. *Schweiz Med Wochenschr.* 1956;86:590–592.
3. Dallemagne B, Weerts JM, Jehaes C, et al. Laparoscopic Nissen fundoplication: preliminary report. *Surg Laparosc Endosc.* 1991;1:138–143.
4. Voitk A, Joffe J, Alvarez C, et al. Factors contributing to laparoscopic failure during the learning curve for laparoscopic Nissen fundoplication in a community hospital. *J Laparoendosc Adv Surg Tech A.* 1999;9:243–248.
5. Endzinas Z, Maleckas A, Mickevicius A, et al. [Follow-up results and learning curve in laparoscopic gastrofundoplications]. *Zentralbl Chir.* 2002;127:939–943.
6. Watson DI, Baigrie RJ, Jamieson GG. A learning curve for laparoscopic fundoplication: definable, avoidable, or a waste of time? *Ann Surg.* 1996;224:198–203.
7. Hwang H, Turner LJ, Blair NP. Examining the learning curve of laparoscopic fundoplications at an urban community hospital. *Am J Surg.* 2005;189:522–526; discussion 526.
8. Engström C, Cai W, Irvine T, et al. Twenty years of experience with laparoscopic antireflux surgery. *Br J Surg.* 2012;99:1415–1421.
9. Prachand VN, Alverdy JC. Gastroesophageal reflux disease and severe obesity: fundoplication or bariatric surgery? *World J Gastroenterol.* 2010;16(30):3757–3761.
10. Yang S. *Esophageal Function Tests.* St Louis, MO: Mosby; 1998:1–8.
11. Kessing BF, Smout AJPM, Bredenoord AJ. Clinical applications of esophageal impedance monitoring and high-resolution manometry. *Curr Gastroenterol Rep.* 2012;14:197–205.
12. DeMeester FK. Preoperative evaluation of gastroesophageal reflux. *Curr Ther Cardiothorac Surg.* 1989;217–220.
13. Urschel JD. Gastroesophageal leaks after antireflux operations. *Ann Thorac Surg.* 1994;57:1229–1232.
14. Bais JE, Wijnhoven BP, Masclee AA, et al. Analysis and surgical treatment of persistent dysphagia after Nissen fundoplication. *Br J Surg.* 2001;88:569–576.
15. Herron DM, Swanstrom LL, Ramzi N, et al. Factors predictive of dysphagia after laparoscopic Nissen fundoplication. *Surg Endosc.* 1999;13:1180–1183.
16. Hunter JG, Swanstrom L, Waring JP. Dysphagia after laparoscopic antireflux surgery: the impact of operative technique. *Ann Surg.* 1996;224:51–57.
17. Patterson EJ, Herron DM, Hansen PD, et al. Effect of an esophageal bougie on the incidence of dysphagia following nissen fundoplication: a prospective, blinded, randomized clinical trial. *Arch Surg.* 2000;135:1055–1061; discussion 1061–1062.
18. Polk HC Jr. Fundoplication for reflux esophagitis: misadventures with the operation of choice. *Ann Surg.* 1976;183:645–652.
19. Centers for Disease Control and Prevention. Detailed diagnoses and procedures. 2005, www/cdc.gov/nchs.

40 Other Reflux Procedures (Toupet, Dor, and Hill)

W. Coosemans, Philippe Nafteux, and Toni Lerut

Keywords: Dor fundoplication, Toupet fundoplication, Hill fundoplication, antireflux surgery, gastroesophageal reflux disease (GERD)

TOUPET FUNDOPLICATION

The ideal therapy for gastroesophageal reflux disease (GERD) is a tailored approach with a short, floppy Nissen total fundoplication. This is the current "gold standard" for patients with GERD and normal esophageal motility. However, total fundoplication may result in unacceptable rates of postoperative dysphagia in the subset of patients with GERD and disorders of esophageal motility, a spectrum of benign disorders associated with delayed esophageal clearance. Most surgeons prefer a Toupet 270-degree partial posterior fundoplication for patients in this group.[1] Some surgeons advocate partial fundoplication for all patients to minimize the undesirable side effects of a 360-degree wrap.[2,3]

Laparoscopic Technique

The operation is performed with the standard laparoscopic equipment using a 5- or 10-mm, 0- or 30-degree laparoscope. With the patient in the lithotomy reverse Trendelenburg position, the surgeon stands between the patient's legs. The two assistants are on the patient's left and right sides. Five trocars for proper port placement are required (Fig. 40-1).

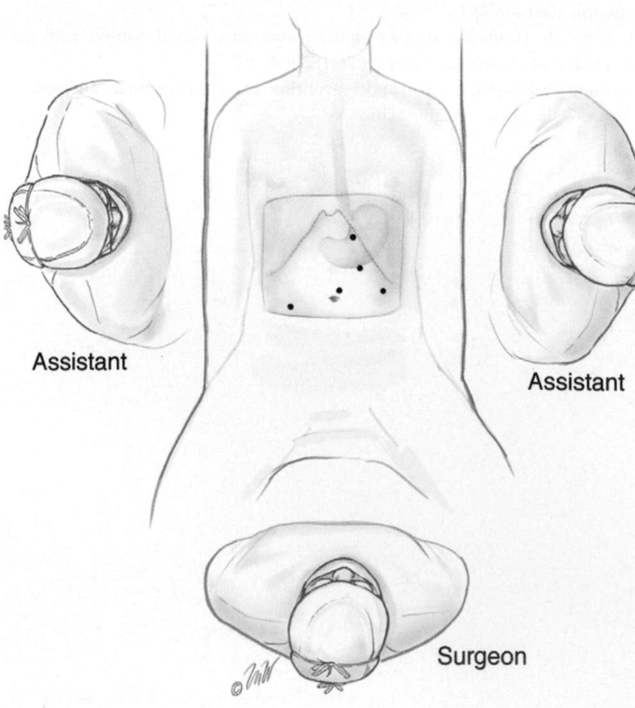

Figure 40-1. Trocar placement.

After the left lobe of the liver has been retracted and the hiatal hernia reduced by pulling at the anterior part of the stomach, the surgeon gains access to the hiatal region and the right crus by opening the lesser omentum. Attention is paid to an accessory left hepatic artery, which is spared if present. The hepatic branches of the anterior vagus are preserved to avoid impaired gallbladder motility and to reduce the risk of wrapping the gastric fundus around the stomach instead of the esophagus (Fig. 40-2).

The phrenoesophageal membrane is detached from both pillars of the right crus circumferentially. Care should be taken to avoid stripping the peritoneal covering of the pillars because this will compromise subsequent suture repair. The gastrophrenic ligament is incised. Working from the right side, a retroesophageal window is created, and the esophagus is encircled with a Penrose drain. The mediastinal esophagus is freed circumferentially for a length of about 10 cm with blunt and sharp dissection to obtain a 3 to 4cm length of tension-free intra-abdominal distal esophagus.

Both the anterior and posterior vagal nerves are identified but not isolated to avoid the risk of delayed gastric emptying with gas bloat syndrome. Although not described in the original Toupet fundoplication, the medial part of the upper short gastric vessels is divided to create a fundoplication without undue circumferential tension around the distal esophagus. Temporarily, a 30-degree scope is used. This maneuver also permits direct access to the retrogastric attachments, which are divided.

Upward traction on the sling provides good access to the V-shaped junction of the pillars (Fig. 40-2). A loose, nonobstructing hiatal closure is performed, leaving a 2-cm retroesophageal space. Unlike the originally described Toupet repair, in which the posterior wrap was sutured to the right and left pillars, the approximation of the pillars is performed with one to three big-bite 0 nonabsorbable sutures tied snugly with an extracorporeal knot. Some surgeons advocate using a 54 to 58F bougie to calibrate the degree of closure. We do not recommend the Maloney bougie in this situation for fear of causing a perforation.

The gastric fundus is passed behind the esophagus. Three to four interrupted 0 nonabsorbable sutures are placed from the esophagus to the left and right anterior edges of the fundus at the 2 o'clock and 10 o'clock positions, respectively to create a posterior wrap over a 3 to 4 cm length. Two or three additional sutures are placed from the right side of the wrap to the corresponding pillar. The final result should be a tension-free 270-degree posterior fundoplication securely fixed to the diaphragm and leaving the anterior part of the esophagus free (Fig. 40-3). The abdomen is deinsufflated and all 10-mm fascial defects are closed.

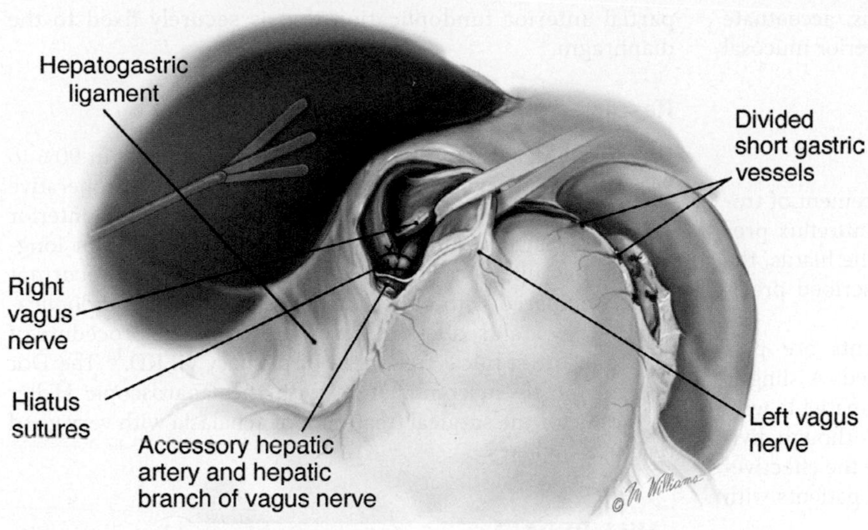

Figure 40-2. Exposure for performing the Toupet fundoplication.

Results

The 270-degree laparoscopic Toupet fundoplication is associated with good early results. In one study it produced a good result in 80% to 90% of patients at 2 years follow-up.[4] Temporary dysphagia, abdominal discomfort, and gas bloat syndrome were infrequent. However, despite achieving adequate fundoplication for most patients, the late results are not as satisfactory, with signs of weakness reported with this repair on follow-up manometry and pH monitoring testing. Particularly for patients with normal esophageal motility, the repair seems to afford a generally less competent antireflux mechanism, with a failure rate of up to 50% on 24-hour pH testing, yet half of such patients remain asymptomatic.[4,5] While these signs of deterioration are concerning, heuristic end points such as symptom resolution, duration of convalescence, satisfaction, well-being, and quality of life bear more weight clinically than outcomes measured with manometry and pH monitoring.[6] Support for this procedure stems from experience in the subset of patients who have delayed esophageal clearance secondary to esophageal motility disorder. Although the results have not been documented independently, many surgeons are of the opinion that the 360-degree total fundoplication creates an unacceptable rate of postoperative dysphagia for this patient group, and they are willing to accept the possibility of a higher rate of postoperative reflux long term.[7,8] This view persists, despite reports that both approaches to fundoplication maintain good reflux control over time and that with time the reported differences in mechanical side effects disappear.[3] Some surgeons prefer this approach for all patients.

DOR FUNDOPLICATION

The Dor fundoplication procedure consists of a 180-degree anterior fundoplication. This type of fundoplication is particularly indicated in patients with severe impairment of esophageal body motility. The principle of this operation is to restore

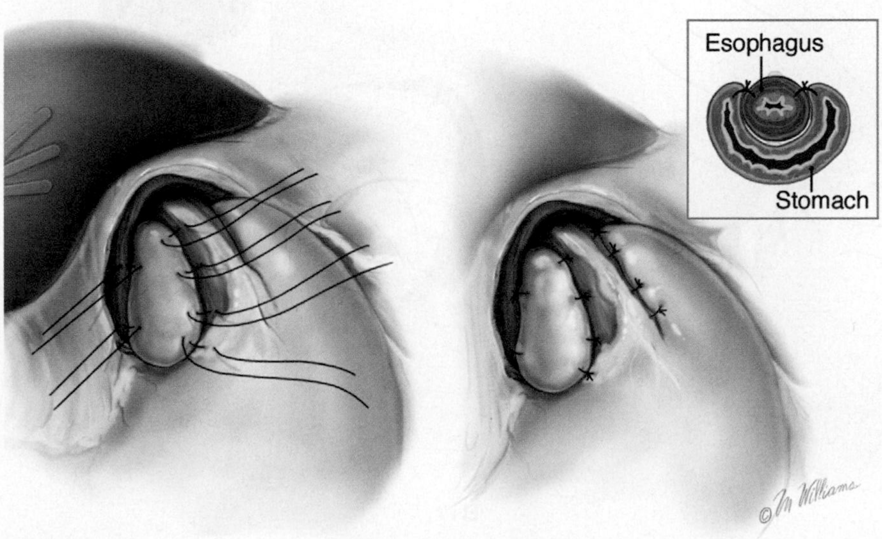

Figure 40-3. Toupet fundoplication. *A.* Right-side wrap fixation. *B.* Left wrap fixation.

an intra-abdominal segment of distal esophagus, accentuate the angle of His, and as a result, create a long anterior mucosal valve at the gastroesophageal junction (GEJ).

Laparoscopic Technique

Surgical equipment, patient positioning, and placement of trocars are the same as for all other laparoscopic antireflux procedures. The anterior and lateral dissections of the hiatus, the crura, and the esophagus are performed as described previously for the Toupet procedure.

The posterior phrenoesophageal attachments are preserved and no retroesophageal window is created. A sling is not used. This operation cannot be performed in patients with foreshortened esophagus or large hiatal hernia. Although division of the upper short gastric vessels may reduce the effectiveness of the fundoplication, it is still preferable in patients with tension expected on the repair.

Fundamental features of this operation are the restoration of at least 5 cm of esophagus in the abdomen and fixation of the gastric fundus (gastropexy) to the diaphragmatic crura. The gastric fundus is sutured to the left margin of the esophagus with four interrupted 0 nonabsorbable sutures extending upward to re-create the angle of His. A most proximal fifth suture fixes the fundus to the left margin of the hiatus (Fig. 40-4A).

The left part of the gastric fundus is folded over the anterior aspect of the esophagus and fixed with one suture to the anterior right side of the esophagus and one suture to the superior margin of the hiatus. The folded fundus is then secured downward with four stitches to the right margin of the esophagus to a point immediately below the esophagogastric junction. These sutures are secured to the right crus (Fig. 40-4B). The upper end of the gastric fundoplication additionally is fixed to the diaphragm, resulting in closure of the anterior part of the hiatus. The final result is a 180-degree partial anterior fundoplication that is securely fixed to the diaphragm.[9]

Results

Early and intermediate-term results are satisfactory in 90% to 94% of patients, with a very low frequency of postoperative dysphagia (0%–2%).[10,11] However, both the Watson anterior 90-degree partial fundoplication and the Dor repair at long-term follow-up appear to have a higher incidence of recurrent reflux compared with either a 270- or 360-degree fundoplication.[12] They are used less frequently today as the procedure of choice in the surgical treatment of primary GERD.[12] The Dor is used mostly in combination with the laparoscopic Heller myotomy for the surgical treatment of achalasia with very good results.[13]

HILL REPAIR

This technique re-creates the angle of His, restores the gastroesophageal valve, and augments the lower esophageal sphincter pressure. Moreover, the GEJ with the restored 180-degree gastroesophageal valve is anchored to the preaortic fascia, which is important for restoring esophageal clearance. Intraoperative manometry to evaluate the antireflux pressure barrier is recommended.[14]

Laparoscopic Technique

Laparoscopic equipment, patient positioning, and the pneumoperitoneum are identical to the previously described Toupet and Dor fundoplications. The left lobe of the liver is retracted cephalad.

With incision of the gastrohepatic ligament, but preservation of the hepatic vagal branches, the right crus is exposed.

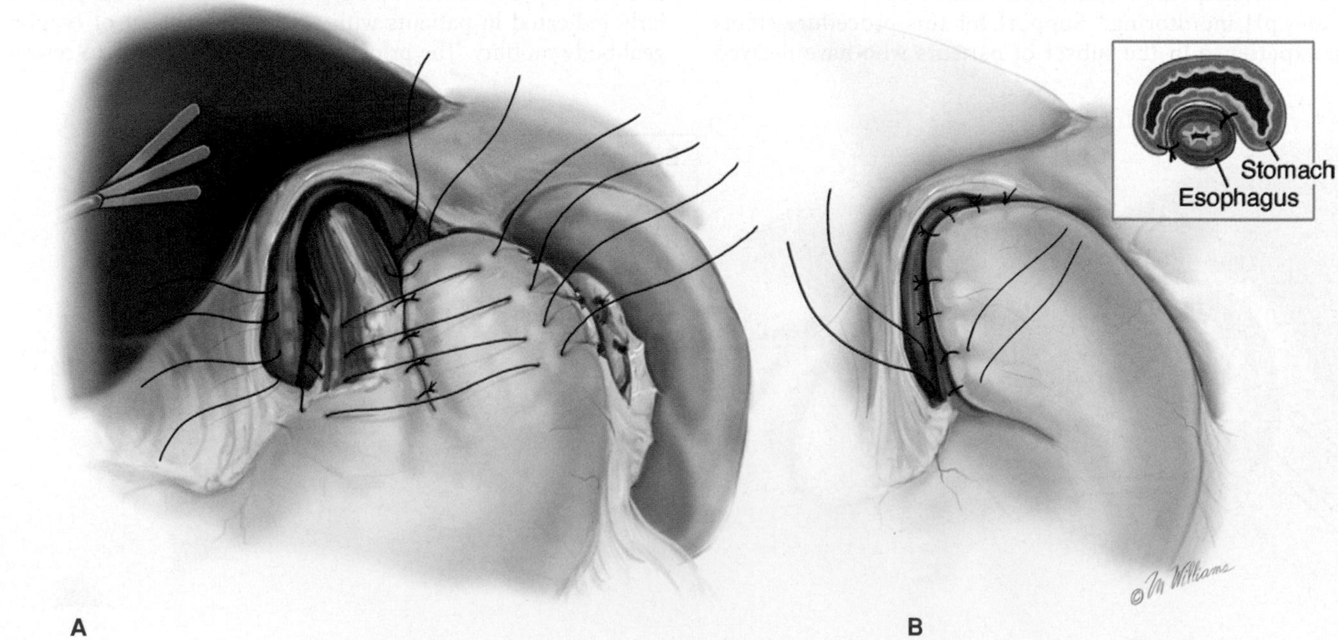

Figure 40-4. Dor fundoplication. *A.* Left wrap fixation. *B.* Completed procedure.

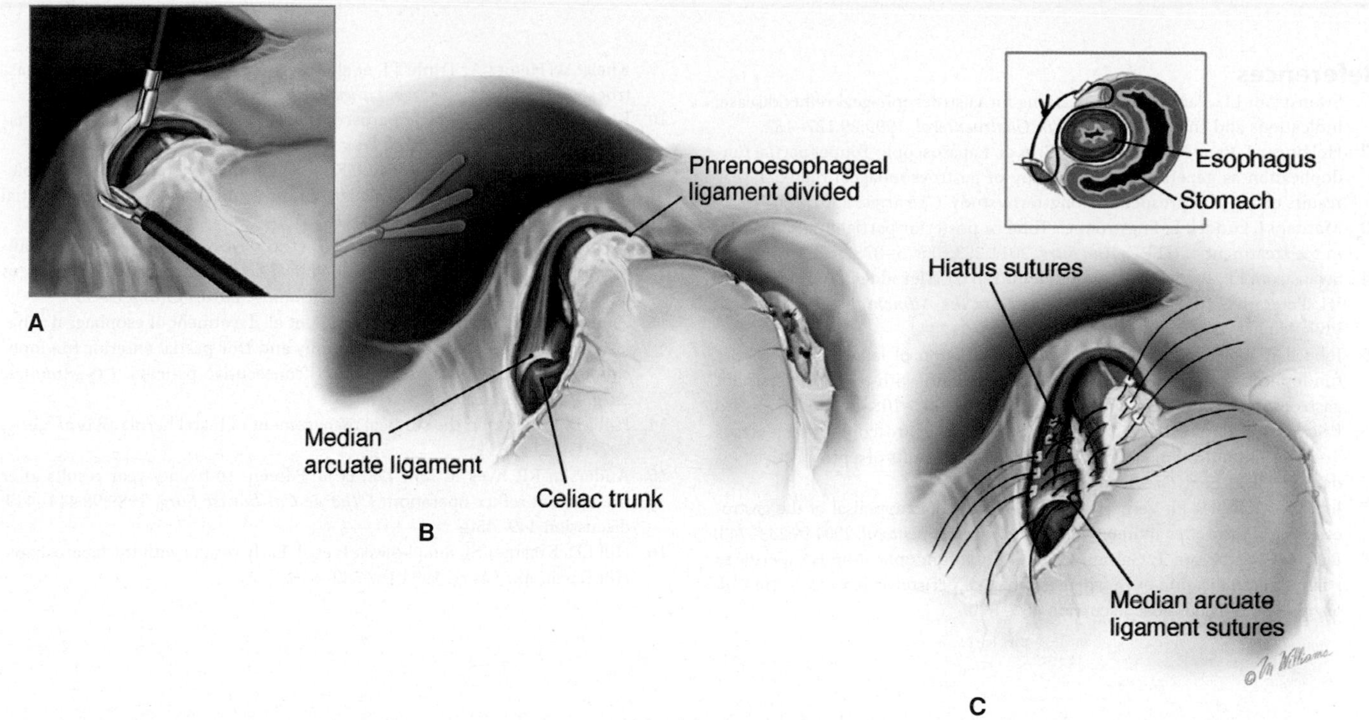

Figure 40-5. Hill repair. *A*. Incision of the phrenoesophageal ligament. *B*. Preaortic fascia and celiac axis. *C*. Sutures in place. The inset shows the posterior phrenoesophageal bundle and right pillar on the left and the anterior phrenoesophageal bundle on the right.

Gentle downward traction on the stomach reduces the hernia when present. Incision of the phrenoesophageal ligament at its diaphragmatic origin exposes the anterior part of the esophagus (Fig. 40-5A). This maneuver preserves the substantial phrenoesophageal bundles, which are of major importance for the subsequent repair. The phrenogastric attachments are divided, and one or two superior short gastric vessels are secured. With blunt dissection of the junction of the pillars of the right crus and the posterior part of the left pillar, a retroesophageal window is created. Any adhesions are divided, giving access to the most caudal portion of the preaortic fascia, the median arcuate ligament and the celiac axis at its aortic origin (Fig. 40-5B).

With circumferential dissection of the esophagus in the posterior mediastinum, a tension-free 3 to 4 cm length of intra-abdominal esophagus is obtained. The vagal nerves are identified but not isolated. The pillars of the hiatus are loosely approximated with at least two size 0 nonabsorbable sutures (with or without Teflon pledgets) including peritoneum, muscle, and fascia.

The previously described anterior and posterior phrenoesophageal bundles are exposed. From the cephalad part of the angle of His, three deep-bite sutures with Teflon pledgets are placed in caudal direction through the anterior bundle, the seromuscular layer of the stomach, the posterior bundle, and the preaortic fascia; two other sutures without pledgets are placed through the median arcuate ligament (Fig. 40-5C). To prevent tears in the aorta, anterior elevation with a grasper separates the fascia, the ligament, and the aorta. To provide a barrier to reflux that is adequate, but not excessive, sutures are tightened gradually until a pressure range of 25 to 35 mm Hg is obtained on intraoperative manometry. Three to five additional sutures from the fundus to the hiatus prevent a recurrent hernia and further augment the valve.

Results

With the use of intraoperative manometry, long term results in open surgery are categorized as good to excellent in 96% of patients over 5 years and 90% of patients followed for an average of 18 years.[15] Comparable early results were achieved with the laparoscopic approach, with 97% good-to-excellent clinical control at 1-year follow-up.[16] The occurrence of dysphagia and gas bloat is uncommon with this 180-degree valve. Major disadvantages are the potential injury of the aorta and celiac trunk, the need for intraoperative manometry, and the steep learning curve.

EDITOR'S COMMENT

This chapter reviews the standard approaches for nonstandard operations for reflux. These should be part of the armamentarium of every esophageal surgeon. Additional modifications may be made for redo surgery or for surgery in conjunction with other procedures. For example, when converting a Nissen fundoplication to a Toupet, the wrap is already attached to the posterior esophageal window. All that needs to be done is to connect the gastric edge to the right crus. In the case of a Dor fundoplication associated with a Heller myotomy, the esophageal muscle should be included in the bites, and fewer stitches may be required.

—Raphael Bueno

References

1. Swanstrom LL. Partial fundoplications for gastroesophageal reflux disease: indications and current status. *J Clin Gastroenterol.* 1999;29:127–132.
2. Holzinger F, Banz M, Tscharner GG, et al. Laparoscopic Toupet partial fundoplication as general surgical therapy of gastroesophageal reflux: 1-year results of a 5-year prospective long-term study. *Chirurgie.* 2001;72:6–13.
3. Mardani J, Lundell L, Engström C. Total or posterior partial fundoplication in the treatment of GERD. *Ann Surg.* 2011;253(5):875–878.
4. Swanstrom LL. Partial fundoplication. In: Yeo CJ, McFadden DW, Pemberton JH, Peters JH, eds. *Shackelford's Surgery of the Alimentary Tract.* 6th ed. Philadelphia, PA: Saunders Elsevier; 2007:276–284.
5. Jobe BA, Wallace J, Hansen PD, et al. Evaluation of laparoscopic Toupet fundoplication as a primary repair for all patients with medically resistant gastroesophageal reflux. *Surg Endosc.* 1997;11:1080–1083.
6. Koch OO, Kaindlstorfer A, Antoniou SA, et al. Laparoscopic Nissen versus Toupet fundoplication: objective and subjective results of a prospective randomized trial. *Surg Endosc.* 2012;26(2):413–422.
7. Jobe BA, Kahrilas PJ, Vernon AH, et al. Endoscopic appraisal of the gastroesophageal valve after antireflux surgery. *Am J Gastroenterol.* 2004;99:233–243.
8. Patti MG, Robinson T, Galvani C, et al. Total fundoplication is superior to partial fundoplication even when esophageal peristalsis is weak. *J Am Coll Surg.* 2004;198:863–869; discussion 869–870.
9. Kneist W, Heintz A, Trinh TT, et al. Anterior partial fundoplication for gastroesophageal reflux disease. *Langenbecks Arch Surg.* 2003;388:174–180.
10. Kleimann E, Halbfass H. Laparoscopic anti-reflux surgery in gastroesophageal reflux. *Langenbecks Arch Surg.* 1998;115:1520–1522.
11. Watson DI, Jamieson GG, Pike GK, et al. Prospective randomized double-blind trial between laparoscopic Nissen fundoplication and anterior partial fundoplication. *Br J Surg.* 1999;86:123–130.
12. Nijjar RS, Watson DI, Jamieson GG, et al. Five-year follow-up of a multicenter, double-blind randomized clinical trial of laparoscopic Nissen vs anterior 90° partial fundoplication. *Arch Surg.* 2010;145(6):552–557.
13. Zaninotto G, Costantini M, Molena D, et al. Treatment of esophageal achalasia with laparoscopic Heller myotomy and Dor partial anterior fundoplication: prospective evaluation of 100 consecutive patients. *J Gastrointest Surg.* 2000;4:282–289.
14. Hill LD. Progress in the surgical management of hiatal hernia. *World J Surg.* 1977;1:425–436.
15. Anderson RP, Ilves R, Low DE, et al. Fifteen- to twenty-year results after the Hill antireflux operation. *J Thorac Cardiovasc Surg.* 1989;98:444–449; discussion 449–450.
16. Hill LD, Kraemer SJ, Snopkowski P, et al. Early results with the laparoscopic Hill repair. *Am J Surg.* 1994;167:542–546.

41 Surgery and Endoscopic Interventions for Barrett Esophagus

Edward D. Auyang and Brant K. Oelschlager

Keywords: Esophageal adenocarcinoma, gastroduodenal reflux, Barrett metaplasia, intestinal metaplasia, antireflux surgery

INTRODUCTION

Barrett esophagus (BE) is a condition in which the stratified squamous epithelium of the esophagus is replaced by intestinal columnar epithelium, a process called intestinal metaplasia (IM). Dr. Norman Barrett, an Australian thoracic surgeon, characterized the findings in an article that he published in 1950.[1] In 1953, the association was made between BE and gastroesophageal reflux disease (GERD) by the English thoracic surgeon Dr. Philip Allison.[2] The etiology of BE is accepted to be due to chronic exposure of the esophageal epithelium to gastroduodenal refluxate. The importance of BE is its potential to progress and develop into adenocarcinoma. The association between BE and esophageal adenocarcinoma was established in a case report in 1975 by Dr. Alan Farnsworth, a cardiac surgeon, in which he identified adenocarcinoma in a segment of BE.[3]

Multiple factors have been identified that lead to an increased risk of developing BE. These include age over 50 years, male gender, white race, elevated body mass index (BMI), intra-abdominal distribution of body fat, hiatal hernia, and chronic GERD.[4] BE is diagnosed by endoscopic biopsy and histologic examination which identifies the IM (Fig. 41-1).

Progression of BE to cancer is recognized as a continuum through dysplasia to cancer. As such, the histologic examination of this disease is often classified into BE without dysplasia, BE with low-grade dysplasia (LGD), and BE with high-grade dysplasia (HGD). Progressive severity of dysplasia leads to a higher risk for the development of esophageal cancer. BE without dysplasia has a 0.5% per year risk of developing into esophageal cancer, whereas BE with LGD has a 1.4% per year risk and BE with HGD has a 6% per year risk.[5] It is this strong association between BE and esophageal adenocarcinoma that has driven the aggressive surveillance and treatment of BE.

SURVEILLANCE

The goal of surveillance is to reduce mortality of a disease by early diagnosis. In the case of BE, the goal of surveillance is to reduce the mortality due to esophageal cancer. The risk of developing esophageal cancer in the general Western population is low; therefore, routine endoscopic screening has not been recommended. For patients who have risk factors for BE as described earlier, there is some data supporting screening endoscopy. Therefore, the American College of Gastroenterology recommends that screening endoscopy in this patient population should be individualized.[6]

For patients already diagnosed with BE, it is a common practice to perform endoscopic surveillance to search for

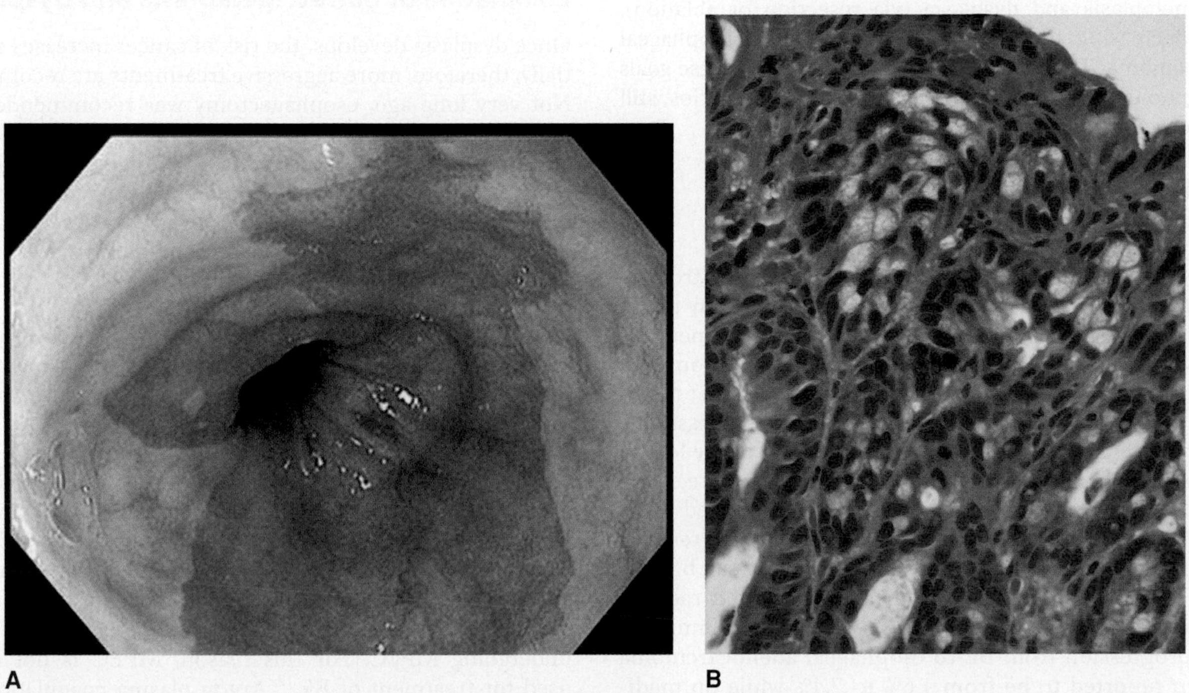

Figure 41-1. Barrett esophagus: EGD and histology.

Table 41-1
RECOMMENDED ENDOSCOPIC SURVEILLANCE SCHEDULE

SEVERITY OF BARRETT ESOPHAGUS (BE)	SURVEILLANCE INTERVAL
BE without dysplasia	Every 3–5 years
BE with low-grade dysplasia	Every 6–12 months
BE with high-grade dysplasia	Every 3 months (Intervention recommended)

signs of progression to cancer. Although this makes intuitive sense, there is a lack of randomized clinical trials to identify the true effectiveness of endoscopic surveillance in patients with BE. There have, however, been population studies that have shown the practice to lead to earlier detection and associated improved survival rates of esophageal adenocarcinoma in patients with BE who had endoscopy prior to diagnosis of cancer.[7] Therefore, the current recommendations by the American Gastroenterological Association (AGA) are as follows: for patients with BE without dysplasia, endoscopic surveillance should be performed every 3 to 5 years. For patients with BE and LGD, endoscopic surveillance is recommended every 6 to 12 months. For patients with BE and HGD who do not undergo intervention, surveillance is recommended every 3 months.[6] It should be noted that in order for endoscopic surveillance to be effective, adequate surveillance involves taking four quadrant biopsies every 1 to 2 cm along the affected length of esophagus in addition to biopsies of any irregular appearing mucosa (Table 41-1).

TREATMENT OF BARRETT ESOPHAGUS

The goals for treatment of BE are (1) to decrease or eliminate gastroduodenal reflux into the esophagus, primarily to improve the associated symptoms of GERD and potentially to limit progression or cause regression of BE and (2) to directly eliminate Barrett metaplasia and dysplasia (via resection or ablation), thereby decreasing the risk for development of esophageal adenocarcinoma. The methods by which to achieve these goals are continuously evolving and in certain clinical scenarios, still remain somewhat controversial.

Control of Reflux

Medical Therapy

There are several ways to reduce and eliminate gastroduodenal reflux. Medical therapy, in the form of proton pump inhibitors, has been shown to be very effective for neutralizing gastric acid and controlling acid reflux symptoms. In addition, there are several studies that have shown that medical therapy can cause modest regression of BE. Regression is often defined in several ways, including decrease in the length of BE, down-grading of Barrett dysplasia, and complete elimination of IM. The regression rates have been reported to be from 19% to 41% depending on the definition of regression. Practitioners should be aware, however, that there can be progression of BE while on medical therapy. Reported rates of progression to dysplasia range from 1.8% up to 31%. Similarly, rates of progression from BE to esophageal adenocarcinoma have been reported to be from 1.6% to 7.4% while on medical therapy. Therefore, acid and symptom control with proton pump inhibitors alone should be used in conjunction with endoscopic surveillance to monitor for regression or progression of disease.

Antireflux Surgery

Antireflux surgery has been offered to patients who have failed medical treatment, usually defined as breakthrough symptoms, or progression or continuation of esophageal damage due to reflux. The technical details of the various types of antireflux operations are discussed in detail in other chapters. Laparoscopic Nissen fundoplication is the most common operation performed, but all operations described for the treatment of GERD may be used in patients with BE.

The use of antireflux surgery to change the natural history of BE is controversial. While there are no randomized controlled trials that show superiority of laparoscopic antireflux surgery over medical therapy for causing regression of BE or preventing the development of esophageal adenocarcinoma, there are some retrospective studies that suggest there may be a benefit of surgery.[8] In a recent review of the literature, we found that on average, 11.1% of patients who underwent medical therapy progressed to dysplasia compared to only 3.4% of patients who had antireflux surgery.[9] Similarly, 4.1% of patients undergoing medical therapy for BE progressed to adenocarcinoma compared to only 0.7% of patients who had antireflux surgery. Although these are selective case studies and few were established to compare medical and surgical therapy, the trends do suggest a possible benefit from antireflux surgery. Despite the improved symptomatic responses to surgery compared to medical therapy and the apparent decreased rates of regression of BE and progression to adenocarcinoma, the regression is still incomplete and progression to adenocarcinoma still occurs.[10] Therefore, surveillance endoscopy should still remain as an important component of treatment for BE after antireflux surgery (Table 41-2).

Elimination of Barrett Metaplasia and Dysplasia

Once dysplasia develops, the risk of cancer increases exponentially, therefore, more aggressive treatments are recommended. Not very long ago, esophagectomy was recommended as the only treatment of choice in patients with BE and HGD and still appears in the Society of Thoracic Surgeons guidelines.[11] In the last decade, however, advanced endoscopic tools have been developed that can provide less invasive ways to adequately treat BE and have made esophagectomy rarely necessary.

Endoscopic Ablation

Endoscopic ablation therapy for BE was first reported in 1992. Laser therapy was studied early on, yet remains largely experimental, given its ineffectiveness in treating large areas of disease, associated perforation rate, and need for multiple treatments to achieve elimination. Multipolar electrocoagulation (MPEC) involves application of a 50-watt probe to an area of metaplasia until a coagulum forms. Studies have shown high success rates for eliminating nondysplastic BE ranging from 89% to 100%, but also have associated high complication rates. Dysphagia occurred in approximately 19% of patients and odynophagia occurred in approximately 16% of patients undergoing MPEC. For this reason, MPEC is not routinely used for treatment of BE.[12] Argon plasma coagulation (APC) is a cauterization tool that uses ionized argon gas to transmit a

Table 41-2

MEDICATION VERSUS LAPAROSCOPIC ANTIREFLUX SURGERY FOR BE

PUBLICATION	NUMBER OF PATIENTS	FOLLOW-UP (YEARS)	ADENOCARCINOMA	DYSPLASIA	REGRESSION
		Medical therapy			
Hillman 2004	279	4.7	7	5	NA
Cooper 2006	188	5.1	3	6	NA
Nguyen 2009	231	7.6	17	53	NA
Heath 2007	82	0.9	6	9	34
Horwhat 2007	67	3.8	2	21	13
Total	847	4.4	35 (4.1%)	94 (11.1%)	47 (31.5%)
		Surgery			
Hofstetter 2001	79	5.0	0	4	16
Bowers 2002	64	4.6	0	1	31
Mabrut 2003	13	3.8	0	0	6
Oelschlager 2003	90	2.6	1	3	30
Desai 2003	50	3.1	0	1	9
O'Riordan 2004	57	3.8	2	2	14
Abbas 2004	33	1.5	1	2	13
Zaninotto 2005	35	2.3	0	0	6
Ozmen 2006	37	1.6	0	1	6
Biertho 2007	70	4.2	0	3	23
Biertho 2009	23	4.5	0	0	14
Total	551	3.4	4 (0.7%)	17 (3.4%)	168 (30.5%)

Adapted from Wassenaar EB, Oelschlager BK. Effect of medical and surgical treatment of Barrett's metaplasia. *World J Gastroenterol.* 2010;16(30):3773–3779.

constant current to a superficial layer of mucosa. Results have shown 89% to 100% elimination of Barrett mucosa, but also a high 3% to 11% recurrence rate after treatment. This is thought to be due to the relatively low depth (2–3 mm) of treatment. Although the penetration depth prevents complications such as perforations from occurring, there have been reports of "buried dysplasia/neoplasia." Given better alternative endoscopic ablation technologies on the market, APC is not frequently performed.[12] Photodynamic therapy (PDT) involves administration of a systemic light-sensitizing agent (porfimer sodium or 5-aminolevulinic acid) followed by endoscopic application of diffusing fiber optics against the target tissue to create necrosis. PDT has been compared with APC in a randomized trial. The result showed only 50% complete eradication of BE compared to 97% for APC.[13] In addition, a higher stricture rate was seen with PDT ranging from 30% overall to 50% after receiving two treatments[12] (Fig. 41-2).

Radiofrequency ablation (RFA) has been shown to be an effective method to destroy dysplastic Barrett's epithelium, and is currently the most common method to do so. A randomized controlled multicenter clinical trial recently showed that ablation can both reduce progression and permanently eliminate Barrett's metaplasia.[14] In this study, there was 90.5% complete eradication of dysplasia in patients with LGD compared to 22.7% of patients who had a sham procedure. For patients with HGD, 81% of patients had complete eradication compared to 19.0% in the sham group. Patients who had RFA also had less disease progression (3.6% vs. 16.3%) and fewer cancers (1.2% vs. 9.3%) compared to sham procedures. It is also a relatively safe procedure with one multicenter prospective study that reported no strictures 2.5 years after having focal ablation.[15] Although there is an apparent high success rate, several limitations exist. Large surface areas of BE and circumferential BE are difficult to treat with RFA compared with focal BE because

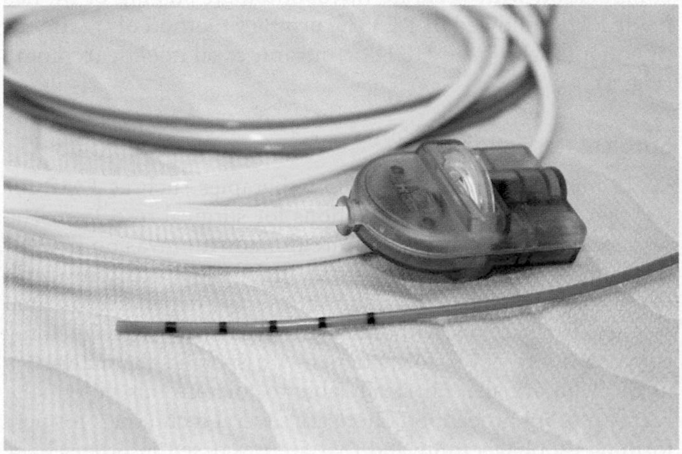

A

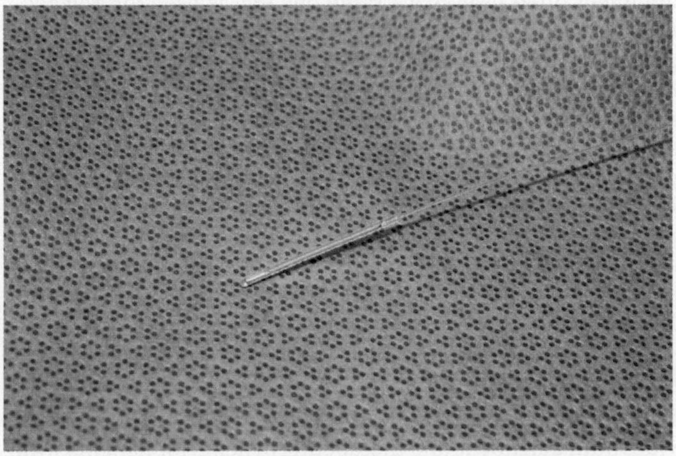

B

Figure 41-2. Multipolar electrocoagulation *(A)* and photodynamic therapy *(B)* devices.

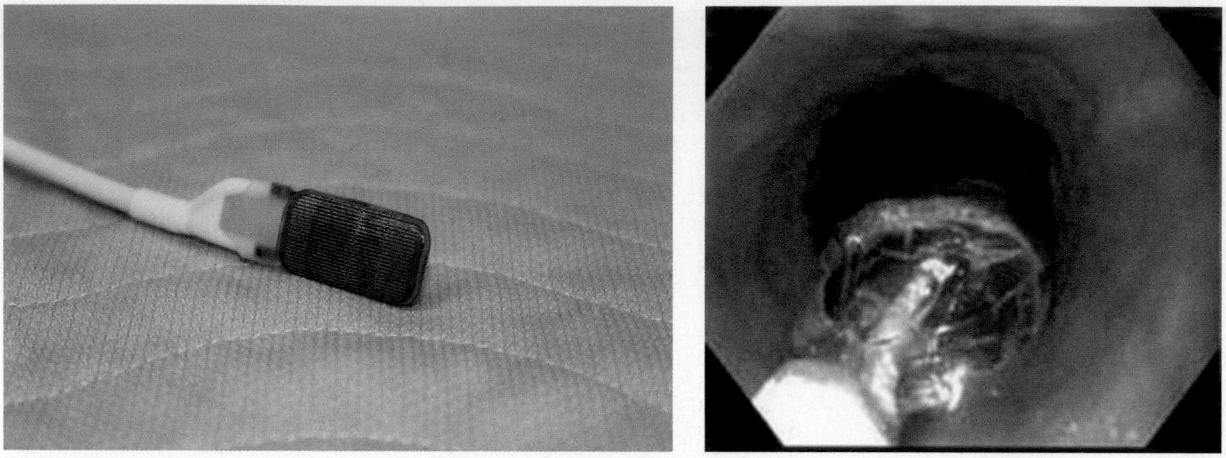

Figure 41-3. Radiofrequency ablation.

of the potential for postablation strictures. In addition, some reports have suggested that Barrett tissue that is deeper than the treatment depth of RFA may become "buried" and overgrown with normal squamous epithelium, thus harboring a deeper focus of dysplastic cells that cannot be accessed with surveillance biopsies. Although this is rare and has not been seen as commonly compared to APC, it is still a concern with this treatment modality (Fig. 41-3).

Cryoablation is a newer technology originally introduced in 1997, which has undergone some recent refinements that holds some promise for ablation of Barrett tissue. This technique involves using liquid nitrogen to freeze the tissue resulting in intracellular destruction while preserving the extracellular matrix, and may allow for deeper, submucosal ablation. A recent study showed 97% complete eradication of HGD, 87% had eradication of all dysplasia, and 57% complete resolution of BE.[16] Randomized clinical trials are currently in progress to evaluate its efficacy compared to other ablative therapies.

Endoscopic Ablation for Nondysplastic BE

Ablation as an alternative for surveillance may be considered for nondysplastic BE. This practice is controversial, but the argument often used is the same one that is used for polypectomy for colonic adenomas—it is a lesion that has some propensity for progressing to cancer; therefore, if the lesion can be safely eradicated, then the risk of cancer can be modified. A multicenter cohort study that followed patients with a diagnosis of nondysplastic BE found that 0.5% per patient-year progressed to esophageal adenocarcinoma.[17] Given the relatively low risk of complications related to RFA and the potential sampling error related to surveillance, ablation may be presented as a reasonable alternative to surveillance.[15] In addition, several studies have reported complete clinical response (no residual IM) with RFA for nondysplastic BE.[18]

Endoscopic Mucosal Resection

Endoscopic mucosal resection (EMR) is a technique that provides both diagnostic and therapeutic benefits for patients with BE. The EMR technique is described in detail in Chapter 173. By taking full mucosal resections of esophageal mucosa, depth and extent of metaplasia and dysplasia can be accurately assessed. This is a clear benefit over ablative therapies in which histopathologic specimens are not obtainable. In patients who undergo EMR for HGD or early cancer, depth of invasion and surgical staging can be performed. In patients who have early-stage esophageal cancer that is confined to the mucosa, EMR has been shown to be an acceptable curative tool, given the low rate of lymph node metastases in these lesions. EMR does bear the risk of causing strictures in up to 50% of patients in addition to causing bleeding or perforation. Therefore, patients with long-segment BE (>3 cm in length) or multifocal BE spanning across a larger distance are typically not amenable to EMR, given the very high likelihood of developing strictures.

EMR in conjunction with RFA has been shown to have excellent results while maintaining a lower complication profile. EMR with RFA was shown to completely eliminate BE with HGD or intramucosal adenocarcinoma in excess of 94% of patients.[12] A recent multicenter trial demonstrated complete eradication of BE in 96% of patients who underwent EMR with RFA, but had only a stricture rate of 14% compared to a stricture rate of 88% for patients who underwent widespread EMR for eradication of BE.[19] This high success rate in combination with accurate histopathologic staging of BE has made EMR followed by RFA the primary method of treatment in patients who have HGD or intramucosal adenocarcinoma (Fig. 41-4).

Surgical Resection

With improvement in endoscopic therapies such as EMR for BE, there became fewer indications for surgical resection. The presence of esophageal adenocarcinoma with invasion beyond the mucosa is currently an indication for esophagectomy, with or without neoadjuvant or adjuvant therapy depending on final staging. For patients without invasive cancer, esophagectomy is becoming reserved for patients with specific characteristics of BE, who are also physically able to tolerate this potentially highly morbid procedure. There are several techniques for performing esophagectomy and that are discussed in other chapters. We will discuss specific scenarios when esophagectomy may be indicated for BE.

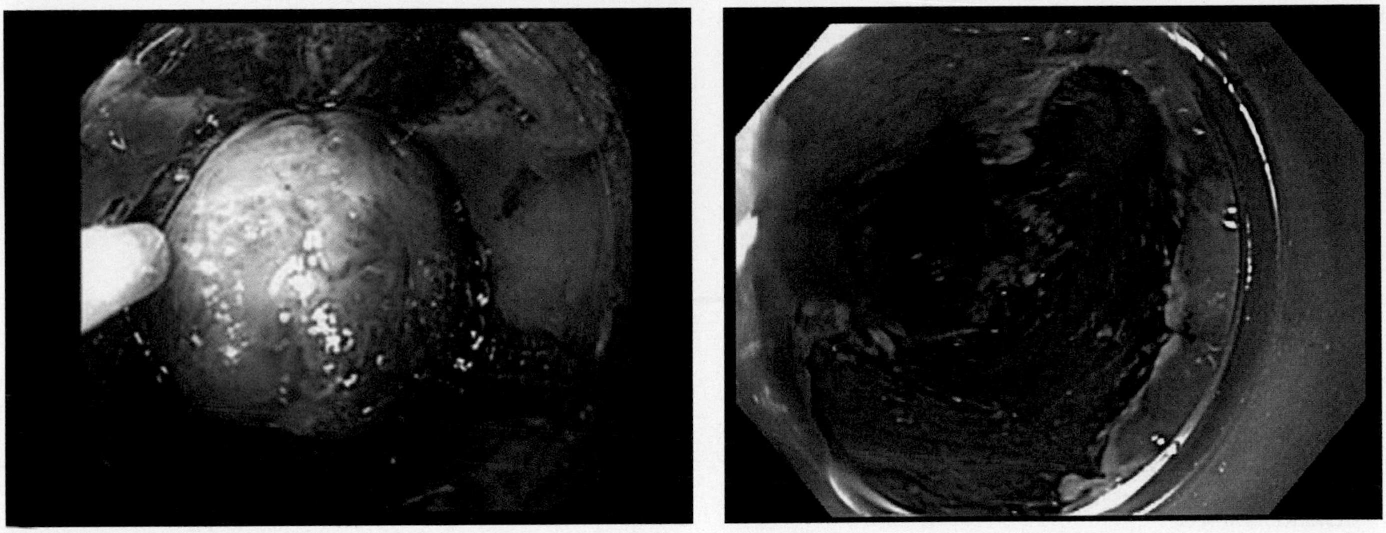

A B

Figure 41-4. Endoscopic mucosal resection.

UNIQUE CLINICAL SCENARIOS WARRANTING ESOPHAGECTOMY

Long-Segment BE with High-Grade Dysplasia

Long-segment BE is defined as involvement of a segment of esophagus that is greater than 3 cm in length. It has been shown that long segment BE has a higher risk for metachronous neoplasms. For this reason, surveillance is difficult for patients with long-segment BE. In addition, the increased segment length is associated with a higher complication rate, thus endoscopic treatment is less ideal. To eliminate a long segment, ablation or EMR must be performed over a long longitudinal distance. Therefore, the stricture rate already associated with endoscopic techniques becomes magnified.[4] For this reason, esophagectomy should be considered for patients with long-segment BE with HGD and who are young or healthy enough to tolerate this operation, especially if the HGD is multifocal.

Multifocal Barrett Esophagus with High-Grade Dysplasia

Multifocal BE, like long-segment BE, has been shown to have a higher risk for metachronous neoplasms. It also presents an endoscopic challenge for all the same reasons. Accurate surveillance is technically challenging because the multifocality of the disease may result in underdiagnosing involved segments of BE. The rate of stricture with endoscopic therapies is mirrored as in long-segment BE; the rates are increased, given the multiple sites need for EMR and ablation. Therefore, esophagectomy should also be considered for patients with multifocal BE with HGD, barring any physical reasons for which the patient would be unable to undergo surgery.

Nodular BE

Nodular has been shown to have a higher incidence of concurrent esophageal cancer. The depth of penetration of nodular Barrett also makes it difficult to adequately treat with EMR, ablation, and even a combination of both. These techniques all have elevated risks as they are applied to deeper and deeper layers of tissue. This does not preclude endoscopic therapy, however. Given the higher cancer rate and difficulty to completely eradicate nodular with endoscopic techniques, esophagectomy should be considered in these patients, especially for recurrent esophageal nodules in areas of resection or ablation.

SUMMARY

Treatment of BE has evolved significantly in the last 15 years. Surveillance for BE is still debated, though it is agreed upon that once Barrett's has been identified, surveillance be continued in a systematic fashion to identify progression to dysplasia and to detect early esophageal adenocarcinoma. The role of antireflux surgery for controlling reflux-associated symptoms, and decreasing disease progression remains widely debated, but should be considered primarily for controlling symptoms.

Barrett metaplasia without dysplasia or neoplasia can be treated with both medical therapy and antireflux surgery. Both methods have shown similar rates of disease regression. There is some evidence to support antireflux surgery to limitation of progression of BE to dysplasia and neoplasia, though there are no definitive randomized clinically conducted trials to support this (nor are there likely to be any).

Endoscopic therapy has become the treatment of choice for with HGD over the last decade. These new endoscopic technologies have entered the field and has replaced esophagectomy as effective and less morbid treatment strategies. The current treatment of choice that has the most data to support its effectiveness is EMR followed by RFA to control all of the abnormal epithelium.

Although becoming increasingly rare, there are still certain unique clinical scenarios in which esophagectomy for BE is indicated. These typically are young patients with multifocal, long-segment BE with HGD, and nodular BE.

EDITOR'S COMMENT

Barrett esophagus or esophagitis is a complication of reflux disease and arguably an indication for both antireflux surgery and life-long surveillance. There is more than one type of BE, each with a different propensity for developing cancer and different long-term sequelae. Treatment therefore must be individualized and longer-term studies are needed to better inform the medical community as to the best treatments. In the meantime, patients with BE need to be educated about the disease, its risks, and the therapeutic options. Esophageal surgeons should be familiar with current therapies for BE so they can provide the best options for their patients.

—Raphael Bueno

References

1. Barrett NR. Chronic peptic ulcer of the oesophagus and 'oesophagitis'. *Br J Surg.* 1950;38(150):175–182.
2. Allison PR, Johnstone AS. The oesophagus lined with gastric mucous membrane. *Thorax.* 1953;8(2):87–101.
3. Farnsworth AE. Adenocarcinoma in a Barrett oesophagus. *Med J Austr.* 1975;1(15):470–472.
4. Spechler SJ, Sharma P, Souza RF, et al. American Gastroenterological Association technical review on the management of Barrett's esophagus. *Gastroenterology.* 2011;140(3):e18–e52.
5. Bhat S, Coleman HG, Yousef F, et al. Risk of malignant progression in Barrett's esophagus patients: results from a large population-based study. *J Natl Cancer Inst.* 2011;103:1049–1057.
6. Wang KK, Sampliner RE, Practice Parameters Committee of the American College of Gastroenterology. Updated guidelines 2008 for the diagnosis, surveillance, and therapy of Barrett's esophagus. *Am J Gastroenterol.* 2008;103:788–797.
7. Cooper GS, Kou TD, Chak A. Receipt of previous diagnoses and endoscopy and outcome from esophageal adenocarcinoma: a population-based study with temporal trends. *Am J Gastroenterol.* 2009;104:1356–1362.
8. Rees JR, Lao-Sirieix P, Wong A, et al. Treatment for Barrett's oesophagus. *Cochrane Database Syst Rev.* 2010;20(1):CD004060.
9. Wassenaar EB, Oelschlager BK. Effect of medical and surgical treatment of Barrett's metaplasia. *World J Gastroenterol.* 2010;16(30):3773–3779.
10. Oelschlager BK, Barreca M, Chang L, et al. Clinical and pathologic response of Barrett's esophagus to laparoscopic antireflux surgery. *Ann Surg.* 2003; 238:458–464; discussion 464–466.
11. Fernando HC, Murthy SC, Hofstetter W, et al. The Society of Thoracic Surgeons practice guideline series: guidelines for the management of Barrett's esophagus with high-grade dysplasia. *Ann Thorac Surg.* 2009;87:1993–2002.
12. Nealis TB, Washington K, Keswani RN. Endoscopic therapy of esophageal premalignancy and early malignancy. *J Natl Compr Canc Netw.* 2011;9(8):890–899.
13. Kelty CJ, Ackroyd R, Brown NJ, et al. Endoscopic ablation of Barrett's oesophagus: a randomized-controlled trial of photodynamic therapy vs. argon plasma coagulation. *Aliment Pharmacol Ther.* 2004;20:1289–1296.
14. Shaheen NJ, Sharma P, Overholt BF, et al. Radiofrequency ablation in Barrett's esophagus with dysplasia. *N Engl J Med.* 2009;360(22):2277–2288.
15. Fleischer DE, Overholt BF, Sharma VK, et al. Endoscopic ablation of Barrett's esophagus: a multicenter study with 2.5-year follow-up. *Gastrointest Endosc.* 2008;68(5):867–876.
16. Shaheen NJ, Greenwald BD, Peery AF, et al. Safety and efficacy of endoscopic spray cryotherapy for Barrett's esophagus with high-grade dysplasia. *Gastrointest Endosc.* 2010;71:680–685.
17. Sharma P, Falk GW, Weston AP, et al. Dysplasia and cancer in a large multicenter cohort of patients with Barrett's esophagus. *Clin Gastroenterol Hepatol.* 2006;4:566–572.
18. Lyday WD, Corbett FS, Kuperman DA, et al. Radiofrequency ablation of Barrett's esophagus: outcomes of 429 patients from a multicenter community practice registry. *Endoscopy.* 2010;42(4):272–278.
19. van Vilsteren FG, Pouw RE, Seewald S, et al. Stepwise radical endoscopic resection versus radiofrequency ablation for Barrett's oesophagus with high-grade dysplasia or early cancer: a multicentre randomised trial. *Gut.* 2011;60:765–773.

42 Management of Shortened Esophagus

Abraham Lebenthal and Raphael Bueno

Keywords: Paraesophageal hernia, gastroesophageal junction, esophageal stricture, esophageal lengthening, extensive mediastinal mobilization of esophagus, Collis gastroplasty, laparoscopic Nissen fundoplication

For many years, there has been a controversy in the surgical literature regarding the existence or relevance of the short esophagus to gastroesophageal reflux disease (GERD) and antireflux surgery.[1–5] A center that performs a high volume of antireflux procedures reported the prevalence to be approximately 14% in patients presenting for surgical treatment of GERD or paraesophageal hernia.[2] The normal esophagus is 39 to 41 cm from the incisors and has an abdominal component of approximately 2 to 3 cm in length. In patients with short esophagus, the abdominal component is less than 2.5 cm. A battery of preoperative tests and intraoperative findings enable the surgeon to recognize the short esophagus.

The etiology of esophageal shortening is multifactorial. Chronic inflammation, which causes scarring and fibrosis, may be the culprit of intrinsic esophageal shortening.[3] Extrinsic short esophagus may be due to proximal displacement of the esophagus secondary to an enlarging hiatal hernia.[5] Surgical esophageal lengthening can be accomplished by extensive mediastinal mobilization with or without a Collis gastroplasty.[6] The goal of Collis surgery is to obtain adequate esophageal length below the hiatus. There is general consensus that an unrecognized short esophagus can cause tension on the surgical wrap, resulting in wrap failure secondary to herniation, slippage, or wrap disruption. Experts differ on the incidence, impact, and correct therapy for short esophagus, and opinions vary widely in the literature. There are those who espouse the liberal use of esophageal lengthening,[1,2] some recommend extensive mediastinal mobilization with selective lengthening,[3] and others "never lengthen" based on the belief that short esophagus is a surgical myth.[4] It is noteworthy that some have changed their views over time.[2,3] Swanstrom et al.,[2] initially estimated that laparoscopic mediastinal mobilization alone was the adequate treatment for only 30% of patients with short esophagus. Recently, however, they have taken the opposite view—that aggressive mediastinal dissection and esophageal mobilization are adequate for most patients and liberal use of Collis gastroplasty is never indicated. Among other benefits, the Collis gastroplasty is known to minimize the incidence of postoperative dysphagia, postoperative acid reflux, and hiatal hernia recurrence.[3] The exact percentage of patients who truly need a Collis gastroplasty is unknown.

In our practice, a significant number of patients referred for failed antireflux procedures are found to have a short esophagus at reoperation. This finding, together with the knowledge that there is little controversy about the need for a tension-free hernia repair, forms the basis of our liberal use of esophageal lengthening procedures when extensive mobilization is not sufficient.

EVALUATION AND DIAGNOSIS OF PATIENTS

At our institution, all patients with GERD symptoms undergo routine endoscopy, upper gastrointestinal study, pH probe analysis (see Chapter 37), and manometry (see Chapters 33 and 37) as part of the preoperative evaluation. Patients with paraesophageal hernia are evaluated according to the severity of their symptoms (Chapter 46). In the emergent setting (e.g., incarceration), manometry and pH probe analysis are not performed. In the elective and semielective settings (e.g., subacute intermittent volvulus), we order manometry without pH probe analysis. Manometry is the essential tool for deciding whether to perform a full or partial wrap because it provides definitive information about the status of the lower esophageal sphincter (LES) and presence of an esophageal motility disorder.[7] During endoscopy, the length of the esophagus should be measured and recorded (distance from the incisors to the Z-line). Endoscopy also provides information about the existence and type of hiatal hernia (see Chapters 37 and 45).

The gastroesophageal junction (GEJ) is a high-pressure zone in the distal esophagus that enables swallowing and prevents reflux. Its proper function is multifactorial, depending on anatomic location as well as physiologic function. It is well established that approximately 2.5 cm of abdominal esophageal length is needed for the GEJ to function properly. Findings on endoscopy of a large hiatal hernia (>5 cm), Barrett esophagus (BE), stricture, or total esophageal length of less than 38 cm should raise suspicion of possible esophageal shortening and the need for Collis gastroplasty.[8–10] The upper gastrointestinal study complements esophagogastroduodenoscopy (EGD) with radiographic images that further our understanding of the patient's anatomy. Ultimately, the decision to lengthen the esophagus can only be made intraoperatively, after full esophageal mediastinal mobilization, abdominal dissection, and fat pad medialization have been performed. Consequently, informed consent to perform an esophageal lengthening procedure should be obtained preoperatively from all patients with possible short esophagus.

ETIOLOGY

Chronic inflammation secondary to the recurrent noxious stimulation of acid reflux and possibly bile can lead to chronic injury, scarring of the distal esophagus, and axial shortening (Fig. 42-1). Short esophagus with GEJ displacement can precipitate the development of a paraesophageal hernia. The severity of reflux or presence of extensive esophageal fibrosis may lead to reversible or irreversible changes in esophageal function.

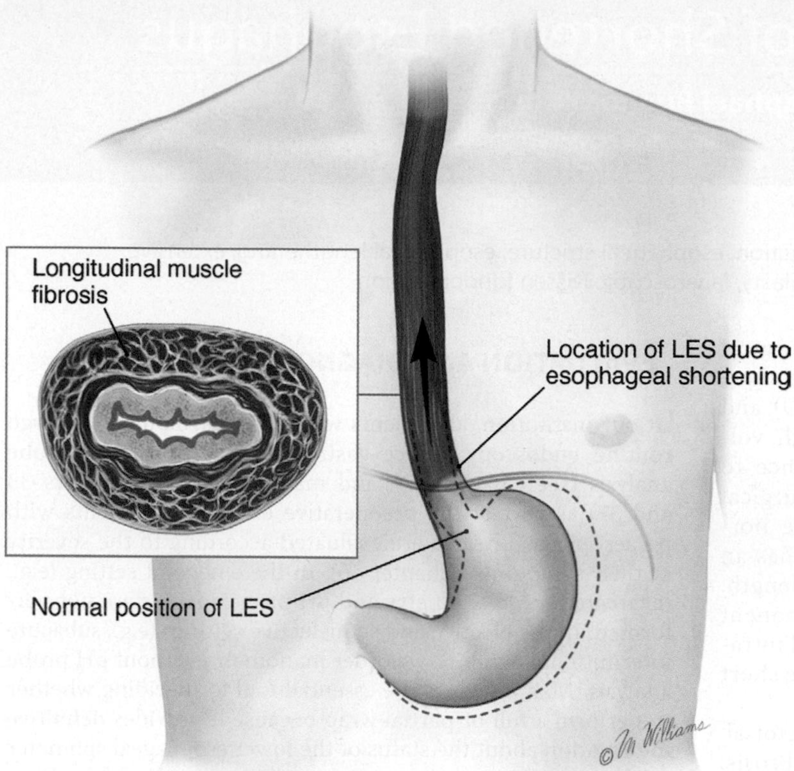

Figure 42-1. Physiologic effect and anatomy of shortened esophagus.

The esophagus will respond to the removal of noxious stimuli in most patients. Rarely is the damage irreversible such that it causes permanent dysmotility necessitating esophagectomy. However, since most patients regain esophageal function after removal of the noxious stimuli, it is our practice always to offer an antireflux procedure at the outset.

Esophageal fibrosis and a lack of elasticity predispose to mechanical wrap failure because increased tension and recoil eventually lead to wrap herniation. Short esophagus has been implicated in the failure of laparoscopic Nissen fundoplication, which should be performed tension-free around the distal intra-abdominal esophagus. If this is not possible, esophageal lengthening maneuvers are indicated. These include mediastinal dissection and laparoscopic Collis gastroplasty. Some argue that high mediastinal esophageal dissection in patients with short esophagus can achieve a tension-free fundoplication with optimal results. Others argue that these circumstances call for a combined approach and advocate a more liberal use of Collis gastroplasty in this subgroup. Unfortunately, there are no prospective, randomized studies that can answer this question definitively.

CHOOSING THE CORRECT OPERATIVE APPROACH

Preoperative evaluation enables operative planning that will alert the surgeon to the possibility of short esophagus and other motility disorders. Our preferred operative approach for treating the short esophagus is laparoscopy. In the rare case of a hostile abdomen, we advocate surgical repair via left thoracotomy. The surgical success depends on tailoring the correct procedure to meet the patient's individual circumstances. Mediastinal esophageal mobilization dissection is classified as type 1, when the circumferential dissection measures less than 5 cm, and type 2, when it is 5 to 10 cm.

There is general consensus about the need to perform type 1 mediastinal mobilization of the short esophagus to obtain maximal esophageal length and perform a tension-free operation. The controversy concerns whether there is an additional need to perform esophageal lengthening or Collis gastroplasty.[3] In 1957, Collis described the procedure known as *open gastroplasty,* the formation of a short neoesophagus by tabularization of the proximal stomach. In addition, he stated that extended transthoracic mediastinal mobilization attained adequate esophageal length in most patients with short esophagus.[6] In 1993, Swanstrom et al.,[2] described the first minimally invasive Collis gastroplasty, which they performed by a combined right thoracoscopy and laparoscopic approach. Johnson et al.,[11] then introduced a laparoscopic Collis procedure in which they used a circular stapler to create a window below the angle of His to facilitate stapling of a gastric wedge. This procedure was associated with ischemia of the gastric apex. Thus, when reticulating staplers were introduced, the laparoscopic procedure was again modified and the standard procedure is currently used.[12] We believe that the controversy about esophageal lengthening is, in part, due to the transient increased morbidity that has been associated with the evolution of this new laparoscopic technique.

Collis gastroplasty combined with Nissen fundoplication is an effective procedure for patients with a short esophagus. Patient satisfaction, postoperative quality of life, and improvement in quality of life in reflux and dyspepsia score after laparoscopic Nissen–Collis fundoplication are comparable to values observed in patients treated with Nissen fundoplication alone.[13] In addition, the Nissen–Collis procedure was shown to be safe with 7-year follow-up in a small subset of patients with short esophagus and complicated severe reflux disease.[14]

Historically, the variability in the use of the Collis gastroplasty to treat giant paraesophageal hernia repair was associated with short-term recurrence rates of 12% to 42%. Laparoscopic Nissen–Collis fundoplication repair of giant or recurrent paraesophageal hernia with mesh reinforcement was shown to minimize short-term recurrence to 4.7%. Most patients reported excellent symptomatic results when evaluated with the GERD Health-Related Quality of Life questionnaire.[15] Recently, Luketich et al., reported that they performed laparoscopic Nissen–Collis fundoplication in 52.5% of patients who underwent reoperation for recurrent GERD. The quality of life and patient satisfaction after Collis gastroplasty with fundoplication were good in 82% of this cohort.[16] Thus, in our large-volume practice, we liberally perform laparoscopic Nissen–Collis fundoplication.

SURGICAL TECHNIQUE

On complete evaluation of the patient, a tailored approach is offered to treat short esophagus. Surgeons who perform redo antireflux procedures should be familiar with the full scope of fundoplication procedures (see Chapters 38–40 and 42), because the patient's unique circumstances will warrant a tailored approach.[17]

We prefer the abdominal approach, when possible. Laparoscopic Nissen fundoplication is the "gold standard" for GERD or paraesophageal hernia. However, up to 14% of patients will require a Collis lengthening procedure, with or without hiatal repair. Rarely, we use other operations, such as Toupet or Dor (see Chapter 40), with a partial wrap for coexisting dysmotility. Regardless of the number of prior surgeries or techniques used (open vs. laparoscopic), we approach all antireflux operations using minimally invasive technique. Rarely, a frozen abdomen is encountered, rendering the abdominal approach technically prohibitive, and we offer a Belsey–Collis procedure instead (see Chapter 38). In our experience, over 95% of these surgeries can be completed minimally invasively without resort to open technique.

The patient is induced using combined anesthesia (i.e., general anesthesia with endotracheal intubation and epidural analgesia). Endoscopy is performed. The patient is placed supine in the lithotomy position. Both arms are tucked in at the sides, and the bed is placed in a shallow anti-Trendelenburg position. A nasogastric tube is inserted for drainage and decompression of the stomach. The stages of the operation are identical to those described in Chapter 39 (Nissen fundoplication). Briefly, these include placement of the camera port using Hassan technique, followed by placement of four additional ports, division of the short gastric vessels with the anterior and posterior gastrosplenic ligaments, opening of the left gastrophrenic ligament with exposure of the left crus, opening of the gastrohepatic ligament, division of the peritoneum over the right crus, and opening of the overlying peritoneum to expose its edge. *We do not attempt to directly identify the esophagus before opening the crura because of the risk of perforation.* The esophagus is revealed by its orientation, longitudinal muscle fibers, and the vagus nerves, which lie medial to the crura. We avoid dividing any structure that could be confused with the vagus nerves until both nerves have been identified. The right crus is dissected from its confluence to the median arcuate ligament, where it joins the left crus. Great care to prevent perforation of the esophagus or stomach should be taken during mobilization of the GEJ. The esophagus is retracted upward, and a window is opened and widened bluntly to reveal the left side of the abdomen. Finally, we open the superior esophagophrenic ligament.

Esophageal Mobilization

The esophagus in our opinion should be mobilized high in the mediastinum to obtain adequate esophageal length. An understanding of thoracic esophageal anatomy is essential when performing mediastinal mobilization (Fig. 42-2). Care should be taken not to injure the left and right vagus nerves (12–3 o'clock and 6–9 o'clock), the aorta and aortic esophageal branches (6 o'clock), the posterior membranous wall or the left mainstem bronchus (deep 2 o'clock), the azygos vein (deep 10 o'clock), the pleura (bilateral), and the pericardium (12–3 o'clock). In general, caution should be taken when performing this dissection because serious injury may result if the surgeon loses anatomic orientation.

Practically speaking, once the esophagus has been dissected free of the crural elements, we grasp the fat pad and pull it caudally to the patient's left. Through another port, we retract the right crus away from the esophagus using a Kittner to allow blunt and sharp dissection of the esophagus high into the mediastinum. The dissection proceeds in a clockwise fashion by appropriate retraction. In this way, the esophagus can be freed at least 5 to 7 cm proximal to the hiatus, which usually provides sufficient length for a "no-tension" wrap. This maneuver requires experience, and care must be taken to avoid injury to the vagii or aorta and to avoid entering the pleurae. On occasion, one should expect the patient to have subcutaneous

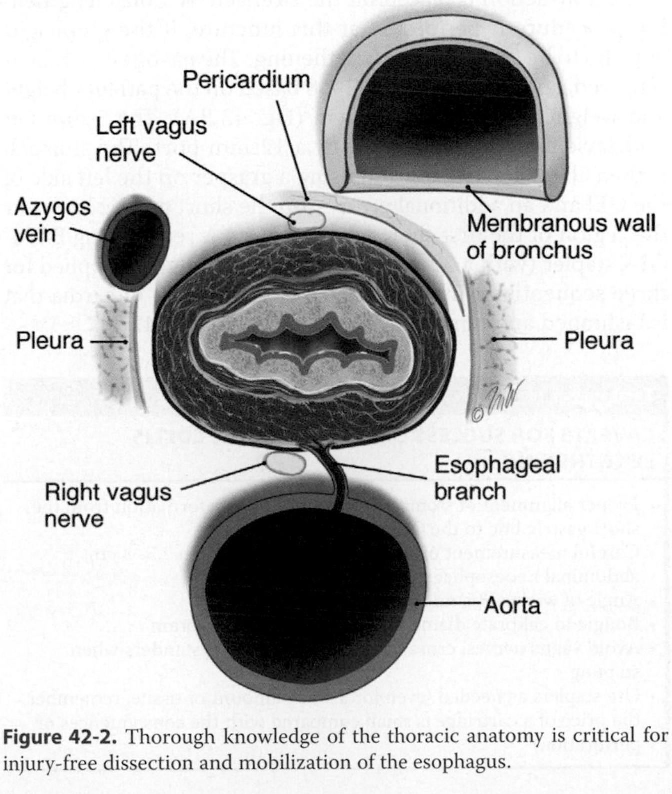

Figure 42-2. Thorough knowledge of the thoracic anatomy is critical for injury-free dissection and mobilization of the esophagus.

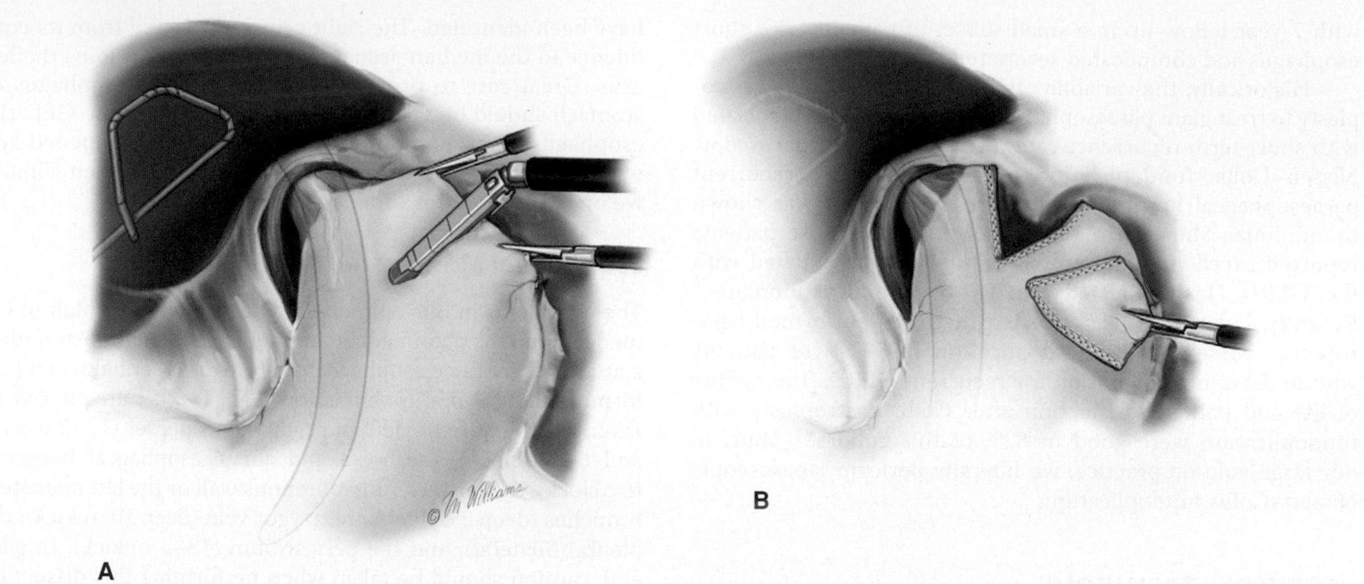

Figure 42-3. *A.* Collis lengthening procedure. Graspers are used to stabilize the stomach. *B.* A reticulating Endo-GIA stapler is used to form a wedge of gastric cardia.

emphysema or neck discomfort postoperatively due to dissection of CO_2 in the mediastinum.

Assessing Esophageal Length

After esophageal mobilization is complete, the fat pad is medialized (taking care not to injure the anterior vagus nerve). This facilitates an accurate tension-free assessment of the level of the GEJ. In making this assessment, one considers the esophageal length measured during intraoperative endoscopy, findings on barium swallow, and the visualized location of the GEJ when no traction is placed on the stomach. A Collis lengthening procedure is performed at this juncture, if the esophagus appears to be short despite lengthening. The nasogastric tube is removed, and a bougie (size 52–58 based on the patient's height and weight) is inserted to 50 cm (Fig. 42-3A). The 5-mm left midclavicular port is replaced by a 12-mm port. The stomach is then aligned and stabilized using a grasper on the left side of the GEJ and an additional grasper on the short gastric line near the region of the first short gastric artery. A reticulating Endo-GIA stapler (with a 30-mm blue staple cartridge) is applied for three sequential firings, forming a gastric wedge of cardia that is fashioned and removed (Fig. 42-3B and Table 42-1).

Table 42-1

CAVEATS FOR SUCCESS OF LAPAROSCOPIC COLLIS LENGTHENING

- Proper alignment of stomach to facilitate wedge formation from the short gastric line to the GEJ
- Careful measurement of the wedge (targeted length 2.5–3 cm; abdominal neoesophagus can use Endo-GIA)
- Angle of wedge (45, not 90 degrees)
- Bougie to calibrate diameter of stomach tubularization
- Avoid vagus nerves, crura, and other innocent bystanders when stapling
- Use staplers as needed (even for a small amount of tissue, remember the price of a cartridge is small compared with the consequences of perforation)

Hiatal Closure and Wrap Formation

After the gastroplasty is complete, the bougie is withdrawn to 25 cm. We routinely close the crura using an Endostitch device (Auto Suture, Norwalk, CT) and a Ti-rite knot (Ti-rite Knot Device, Wilson-Cook Medical, Winston-Salem, NC). With access from the left midclavicular port, the esophagus is elevated, exposing the crura, which are visually assessed for strength. If they appear weak or the patient has a large paraesophageal hernia, we request rehydration of a biodegradable collagen mesh (SurgAssist System, Power Medical Interventions, New Hope, PA) by the scrub nurse on the back table. Typically, at least three stitches are needed for crural closure. The first is placed beyond the crural confluence (V, similar to a vascular anastomosis). Before tying the last stitch, the bougie is reintroduced to 50 cm and the hiatal closure is assessed. Optimally, there should be a few millimeters between the esophagus and the diaphragm. If a mesh reinforcement of the crura is indicated, the mesh is cut to size and sutured anteriorly to itself and to the diaphragm and then posteriorly to itself and the hiatus. Securing the mesh in this manner prevents migration and provides a biologic scaffold, thereby reducing the incidence of recurrence owing to hiatal hernia.

The choice of fundoplication depends on the results of preoperative manometry testing. We perform a laparoscopic Nissen–Collis fundoplication for most patients with short esophagus. This procedure is similar to the laparoscopic Nissen fundoplication described in Chapter 39. The apical point of the staple line is brought under the esophagus and "shoe-shined" with the greater curvature (Fig. 42-4A). This operation is similar to the laparoscopic Nissen fundoplication with one important exception: the target point of the stitch (wrap-"esophagus"-wrap) used to secure the wrap in the Nissen–Collis procedure is the Collis gastroplasty or neoesophagus (Fig. 42-4B). The bougie then is removed. A nasogastric tube is placed, and the ports are closed laparoscopically. After gaining consciousness, the patient is extubated and taken to recovery.

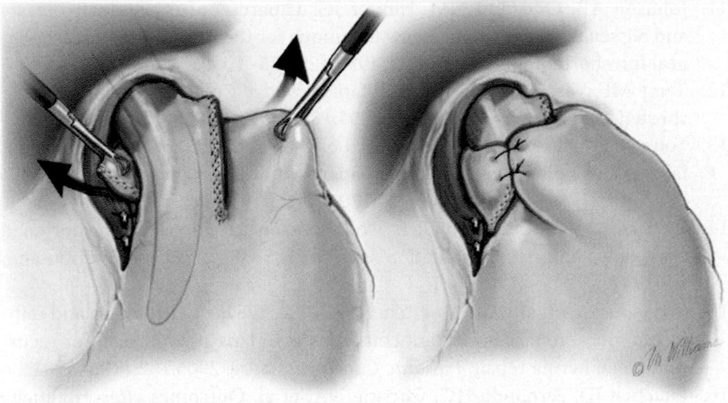

Figure 42-4. *A.* The apical point of the staple line is brought under the esophagus and "shoeshined" with the greater curvature. *B.* The target point of the stitch that secures the fundoplication is the Collis gastroplasty or neoesophagus.

POSTOPERATIVE MANAGEMENT

On postoperative day 1, we routinely obtain a barium swallow to rule out perforation or leak after Collis gastroplasty. If the swallow is normal, we remove the nasogastric tube and slowly advance the diet to clear oral fluids. Early prevention of postoperative nausea and vomiting is important to decrease the rate of wrap failure. In our experience, postoperative nausea and delayed motility are more common in patients with short esophagus. Symptoms usually can be abated by administering Reglan and/or erythromycin. Patients are discharged after they are able to tolerate enough daily liquids to prevent dehydration. Postoperatively, we educate our patients to eat slowly and in small amounts. Patients are sent home on a full liquid diet for 2 weeks. If problems are not encountered, they are advanced to a regular diet devoid of bread and carbonated beverages. Postoperative dysphagia is common and can persist for a variable length of time.

PROCEDURE-SPECIFIC COMPLICATIONS

The major pitfalls of short esophagus include all the pitfalls and dangers described for the laparoscopic Nissen fundoplication (see Chapter 39). In addition, patients undergoing surgery for short esophagus experience poorer overall outcome compared with patients undergoing primary simple antireflux procedures, because they typically suffer from long-standing disease and have more pronounced pathology that may be less reversible in nature. Patient selection is key because at the completion of surgery, the patient's esophagus must reach normal length as the result of mobilization or Collis gastroplasty. Preoperative esophageal motility tests will dictate the preferred wrap (e.g., no history of achalasia, diffuse esophageal spasm, or scleroderma).

Important operative danger points include:

- Unidentified perforation or damage to the hollow viscus, stomach, or esophagus during retraction or dissection and mobilization of the esophagus.
- Improper hiatal closure due to (1) incomplete or loose hiatal closure that may lead to postoperative hiatal hernia or (2) tight hiatal closure that may lead to esophageal obstruction and consequently achalasia.
- Mediastinal esophageal mobilization increases the risk of uncontrolled bleeding in the thorax, pneumothorax, and injury to the vagus nerves.
- Inadequate mobilization of gastric fundus and distal esophagus may lead to suboptimal position of the fundoplication and, as a result, inadequate function.

SUMMARY

The diagnosis and treatment of the short esophagus are controversial. Esophageal shortening is associated with chronic esophageal disease and complicated GERD (e.g., presence of large hiatal hernia, BE, esophageal stricture, or long-standing disease). Preoperative evaluation may suggest the possibility of short esophagus; however, its predictive value for gastroplasty is low. Operative assessment after complete mediastinal esophageal mobilization is used by some to identify short esophagus of a degree that requires the formation of a Collis gastroplasty. The extent of mediastinal esophageal mobilization and the need for Collis gastroplasty are controversial. It is probable that with greater experience and confidence in esophageal mobilization, the requirement for surgical extension decreases. With improvements in laparoscopic skills and equipment over the last 15 years, the laparoscopic Nissen–Collis fundoplication has evolved. Lacking prospective randomized trials, the indication for esophageal lengthening is surgeon-dependent. Most patients undergoing antireflux surgery for GERD or paraesophageal hernias will not require an esophageal lengthening procedure to reduce the GEJ below the esophageal hiatus.

EDITOR'S COMMENT

The incidence of short esophagus is probably related to the degree and duration of reflux or paraesophageal hernia. Collis gastroplasty is particularly useful in patients with BE, long-standing giant paraesophageal hernias, obesity, and those undergoing reoperation for a failed fundoplication. Surgeons who are reluctant to perform a Collis extension should remember that the success of a Nissen–Collis will always be greater than that of a redo Nissen, which is often required when a short esophagus is not sufficiently addressed at the time of initial operation.

—Raphael Bueno

References

1. Luketich JD, Grondin SC, Pearson FG. Minimally invasive approaches to acquired shortening of the esophagus: laparoscopic Collis-Nissen gastroplasty. *Semin Thorac Cardiovasc Surg.* 2000;12:173–178.
2. Swanstrom LL, Marcus DR, Galloway GQ. Laparoscopic Collis gastroplasty is the treatment of choice for the shortened esophagus. *Am J Surg.* 1996;171:477–481.

3. O'Rourke RW, Khajanchee YS, Urbach DR, et al. Extended transmediastinal dissection: an alternative to gastroplasty for short esophagus. *Arch Surg.* 2003;138:735–740.
4. Madan AK, Frantzides CT, Patsavas KL. The myth of the short esophagus. *Surg Endosc.* 2004;18:31–34.
5. Terry M, Smith CD, Branum GD, et al. Outcomes of laparoscopic fundoplication for gastroesophageal reflux disease and paraesophageal hernia. *Surg Endosc.* 2001;15:691–699.
6. Collis J. An operation for hiatus hernia with short oesophagus. *Thorax.* 1957;12:181–188.
7. Livingston CD, Jones HL Jr, Askew RE Jr, et al. Laparoscopic hiatal hernia repair in patients with poor esophageal motility or paraesophageal herniation. *Am Surg.* 2001;67:987–991.
8. Bremner R, Crookes P, Costantini M, et al. The relationship of esophageal length to hiatal hernia in GERD (abstract). *Gastroenterology.* 1992;102:A45.
9. Gastal OL, Hagen JA, Peters JH, et al. Short esophagus: analysis of predictors and clinical implications. *Arch Surg.* 1999;134:633–636; discussion 637–638.
10. Urbach DR, Khajanchee YS, Glasgow RE, et al. Preoperative determinants of an esophageal lengthening procedure in laparoscopic antireflux surgery. *Surg Endosc.* 2001;15:1408–1412.
11. Johnson AB, Oddsdottir M, Hunter JG. Laparoscopic Collis gastroplasty and Nissen fundoplication: a new technique for the management of esophageal foreshortening. *Surg Endosc.* 1998;12:1055–1060.
12. Terry ML, Vernon A, Hunter JG. Stapled-wedge Collis gastroplasty for the shortened esophagus. *Am J Surg.* 2004;188:195–199.
13. Youssef YK, Shekar N, Lutfi R, et al. Long-term evaluation of patient satisfaction and reflux symptoms after laparoscopic fundoplication with Collis gastroplasty. *Surg Endosc.* 2006;20:1702–1705.
14. Richardson JD, Richardson RL. Collis-Nissen gastroplasty for shortened esophagus: long-term evaluation. *Ann Surg.* 1998;227:735–740; discussion 740–742.
15. Whitson BA, Hoang CD, Boettcher AK, et al. Wedge gastroplasty and reinforced crural repair: important components of laparoscopic giant or recurrent hiatal hernia repair. *J Thorac Cardiovasc Surg.* 2006;132:1196–1202.
16. Luketich JD, Fernando HC, Christie NA, et al. Outcomes after minimally invasive reoperation for gastroesophageal reflux disease. *Ann Thorac Surg.* 2002;74:328–331; discussion 331–332.
17. Kauer WK, Peters JH, DeMeester TR, et al. A tailored approach to antireflux surgery. *J Thorac Cardiovasc Surg.* 1995;110:141–146; discussion 146–147.

43 Management of the Failed Reflux Operation

Abraham Lebenthal and Raphael Bueno

Keywords: Slipped wrap, recurrent gastroesophageal reflux disease (GERD), reoperation for reflux, short esophagus, postfundoplication symptoms, delayed gastric emptying, esophageal motility disorder, esophageal lengthening procedure

Management of the failed reflux operation is emerging as an important challenge in modern surgical foregut practice. Over the last decade and a half, the number of patients referred for antireflux surgery has increased eightfold. Approximately 70,000 operations are performed annually in the United States.[1] The increased use of minimally invasive techniques to treat gastroesophageal reflux disease (GERD) has resulted from the lower perceived morbidity associated with laparoscopy in comparison with the open approach.

Most patients who undergo laparoscopic antireflux surgery experience good long-term outcome. Specialty centers report 90% to 95% "sustained benefit" after initial surgery, although not all centers see their own complications.[2,3] The results published by the broader surgical community are less favorable.[3,4] This finding is similar for laparoscopic and open surgery. However, the results are subjective and depend on the definition of failure and the experience of the surgeon.[5–9]

The failure of antireflux surgery may occur early or late. The etiology of the failure is associated with and is sometimes revealed by the timing of symptoms. Early failures can be attributed to poor patient selection and technical error.[9] For example, the misdiagnosis of an unrecognized primary esophageal motility disorder (PEMD) may lead to improper choice of surgical procedure, which dooms the procedure to fail.[10,11] Late failures may be secondary to the progression of underlying disease or attributed to the length of the procedure.[12]

After several decades of experience, multiple reports of transient increases in failed antireflux procedures have ascribed these failures to the initial learning-curve effect,[13–15] modifications of surgical technique during the initial transition to laparoscopic approach,[16] and relaxation of patient selection criteria. With growing experience in the thoracic community, however, these sorts of failures are expected to diminish.

Despite good surgical results after initial operation, some patients present with recurrent symptoms or mechanical failure. Most of these patients can be managed medically with good results. However, 4% to 10% of patients become or remain symptomatic with a poor quality of life and seek additional surgical therapy.[2,10,17–21] Success rates for reoperations range between 50% and 89%.[6] Second and third reoperations traditionally are associated with lower success rates, decreasing as much as 20% with each subsequent operation.[22] The technical difficulty of reoperation has led some surgeons to advocate an open approach.[23] Evidence supporting the safety and efficacy of laparoscopic reoperation, however, is increasing.[1,2,6,24] In our experience, the laparoscopic approach to reoperation is feasible in over 95% of patients regardless of the approach used for the primary or previous surgeries (e.g., open or laparoscopic, thoracic, or abdominal).

REEVALUATION AND DIAGNOSIS

Determining the cause is the difficult aspect of reevaluating patients with recurrent reflux. First, one must establish whether the patient's reflux or procedure-related symptoms are from surgical failure or attributable to some other etiology. In this regard, the diagnosis always should be reexamined to rule out previously undiagnosed or misdiagnosed conditions such as PEMD.

A thorough history is essential to distinguishing the patient's current symptoms from symptoms experienced preoperatively. The relevant symptoms include heartburn, dysphagia (e.g., generalized liquids or solids), postprandial pain, and respiratory symptoms, in particular, recurrent pneumonia and aspiration. If the patient has chest pain, it should be evaluated to discern whether it is secondary to reflux or to some other cause of typical or atypical chest pain (Table 43-1). In our practice, several patients referred for antireflux surgery were found on preoperative workup to have postprandial angina. Another common cause of chest pain is dysphagia that often can be fixed with endoscopic dilatation.

It is essential to understand the mechanics of the patient's previous antireflux procedure by obtaining the operative report and previous diagnostic studies. Understanding the neoanatomy and expected physiologic change is vital to interpreting new diagnostic examinations and procedures. Possible reasons

Table 43-1

DIFFERENT DIAGNOSIS FOR CHEST PAIN

ETIOLOGY	SYMPTOMS
Cardiac	Angina pectoris Myocardial infarction Prinzmetal angina
Pulmonary	Pneumonia Empyema Pleuritic
Musculoskeletal	Myositis Rib fractures Collagen-vascular diseases (e.g., scleroderma)
Peptic disease	Gastric and duodenal ulcer Gastritis and duodenitis
Esophageal disease	Esophagitis PEMDs
Neurologic	Thoracic neuropathies
Vascular	Dissecting thoracic aortic aneurysm

PEMD, primary esophageal motility disorders (e.g., achalasia, nutcracker esophagus, hypertonic, diffuse esophageal spasm [DES]).

for postoperative reflux include failure of surgical technique or incorrect choice of surgical procedure for the patient's initial problem. The failure in surgical technique may take many forms: obstruction (e.g., hiatus, wrap too tight, wrap too long, or wrap poorly placed), herniation (e.g., hiatus not closed adequately or short esophagus), dehiscence (e.g., poor stitch placement, knot tie, and depth), and poor gastric emptying secondary to vagal injury. Consequently, the surgeon performing the evaluation should be familiar not only with the technical details of the patient's original operation but also with all of the procedure-related pitfalls and late complications.

Hinder et al.[5] described four failure patterns after open fundoplication: the slipped or misplaced fundoplication, the disrupted fundoplication, the herniated fundoplication, and the excessively tight or long fundoplication. Two additional failure patterns have emerged in the laparoscopic era: the twisted fundoplication and the two-compartment stomach[9] (Fig. 43-1). The incidence of wrap failure linked to cause is variable. In our opinion, it is usually related to surgical technique and largely preventable. For example, routine hiatal repair at initial operation has been shown to reduce the incidence of recurrent herniation by 80%, and this practice has become standard of care.[2]

The evaluation of patients with recurrent reflux at our institution includes the four standard studies used for GERD: 24-hour esophageal pH probe study, manometry, esophagogastroduodenoscopy (EGD), and esophagram or cine. In addition, for patients with recurrent reflux, we routinely obtain esophageal and gastric emptying studies (i.e., nuclear scintigraphy). If nonacid reflux is suspected, an impedance study is also obtained.

The aim of the evaluation is to differentiate the anatomic versus physiologic cause of the patient's symptoms. Tailoring an effective surgical solution depends on this evaluation. Problems to look for include the presence of a previously undiagnosed PEMD, other esophageal anomaly, postoperative obstruction at the gastroesophageal junction (GEJ), or a primary delayed gastric emptying disorder. A large series of 104 patients demonstrated that a thorough preoperative evaluation can predict the mechanism of postfundoplication failure found at reoperation

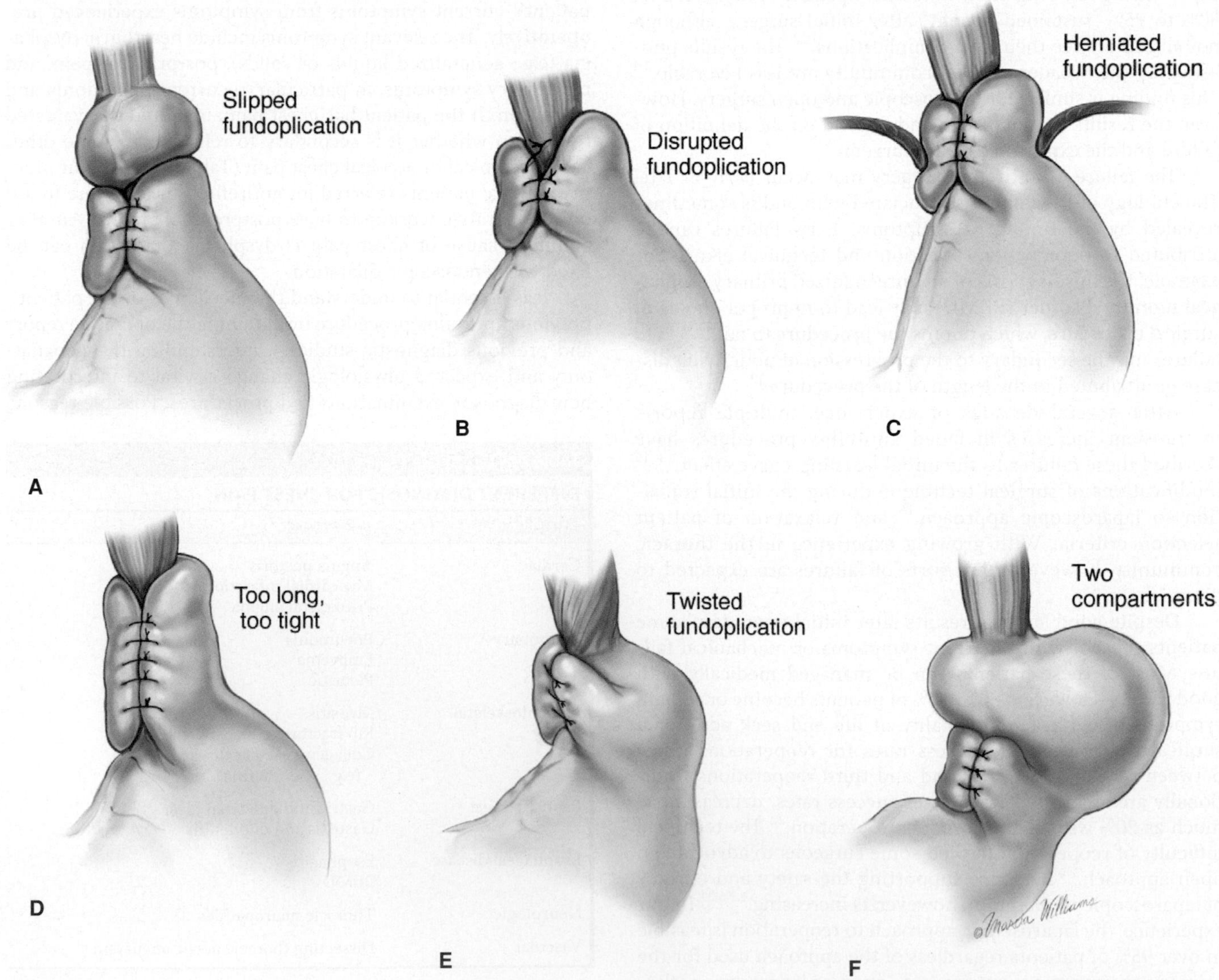

Figure 43-1. Classification of failed fundoplication. *A*. Slipped or misplaced fundoplication. *B*. Disrupted fundoplication. *C*. Herniated fundoplication. *D*. Excessively tight or too long fundoplication. *E*. Twisted fundoplication. *F*. Two stomach compartments.

Table 43-2

MECHANISMS OF POSTFUNDOPLICATION FAILURE

	N (%)
Hiatus closure failure	57 (55)
Crus closure disruption	52 (50)
Stenosis[a]	5 (4.8)
Too tight closure	0
Fundoplication failure	88 (85)
Partial disruption	36 (35)
Complete disruption	7 (6.7)
Hypertensive	24 (23)
Twisted	
Two-compartment stomach	
Relative to esophageal dysmotility	
Fibrosis of fundoplication[b]	
Slipped[c]	18 (17)
Intrathoracic fundoplication	
Paraesophageal component	
Intra-abdominal fundoplication	
Paraesophageal component	
Hourglass[d]	
Gastric body fundoplication	
Too loose	2 (1.9)
Inadequate esophageal length, short[e]	16 (15)
Postoperative gastroparesis	2 (1.9)
Inadvertent vagotomy	
Gas bloat syndrome	
Fistula formation	0
Internal	
External	
Incorrect diagnosis	1 (1)
Achalasia	
Visceral hyperalgesia	
Gastric or esophageal cancer	1 (1)
Gastric hypersecretion	
Gastric outlet obstruction	
Gastroparesis	

Note: The percentages do not add to 100% as many patients had multiple mechanisms of failure.
[a]Dense fibrous scar formation.
[b]Secondary to pledget erosion or suture perforation.
[c]Two centimeters or more gastric mucosa above fundoplication.
[d]Intrathoracic fundus, fundoplication in abdomen.
[e]GEJ less than 3 cm below arch of crus after esophageal mobilization during laparoscopic reoperation.
Source: Reproduced, with permission, from Iqbal A, Awad Z, Simkins J, et al. Repair of 104 failed anti-reflux operations. *Ann Surg.* 2006;244(1):42–51.

in 78% of patients.[1] Mechanisms of postfundoplication failure in this cohort are summarized in Table 43-2.

PREOPERATIVE ASSESSMENT

The preoperative risk-benefit assessment should take into account the patient's underlying health condition, symptoms, quality of life, and disability. The evaluation also must weigh the benefits of a second operation in terms of the surgical risk and higher failure rate. Overall symptom resolution after reoperation is significantly lower (~70%) than after an initial antireflux procedure. This finding may be secondary to the presence of more complex or advanced disease. Reoperation, regardless of the surgeon's experience, is technically more demanding. Adhesions from previous surgery can obscure the anatomy and increase the chance of operative perforation of the esophagus or stomach, pneumothorax, diaphragmatic injury, vagal nerve injury, splenic trauma, and bleeding. Reoperation is associated with an elevated morbidity (15%–40%) and mortality (0%–2%).

TECHNIQUE FOR MINIMALLY INVASIVE LAPAROSCOPIC REPAIR OF FAILED ANTIREFLUX SURGERY

All patients are offered a tailored surgical approach based on the preoperative evaluation. Consequently, surgeons who perform redo antireflux procedures should have experience with the complete range of antireflux operations (see Chapters 38–40). We routinely perform intraoperative EGD before making an incision to confirm the preoperative evaluation and assess esophageal length, structural changes, hiatal hernia, active peptic disease, and other concurrent pathologies that would delay, contraindicate, or alter the planned reoperative approach.

We prefer to use the abdominal approach whenever possible. Laparoscopic Nissen fundoplication remains the "gold standard" for reoperation on recurrent GERD; however, approximately 8% to 20% of patients will require a Collis lengthening procedure, with or without hiatal repair, as described in Chapter 42. Rarely, we use other operations, such as Toupet or Dor, with a partial wrap if the patient has dysmotility (see Chapter 40). Regardless of the number of prior surgeries or the technique used (open versus laparoscopic), we approach all reoperations for failed antireflux surgery using minimally invasive technique. Rarely, a frozen abdomen is encountered, rendering the abdominal approach technically prohibitive, and we offer a Belsey–Collis procedure (see Chapter 38). Since procedure length can vary from 1.5 to 8 hours, cases should be scheduled early in the morning. In our experience, over 95% of these surgeries can be completed minimally invasively without resort to open technique.

Abdominal Approach

The patient is induced using combined anesthesia (i.e., general anesthesia with endotracheal intubation and epidural analgesia). Endoscopy is performed. The patient is placed supine in the lithotomy position. Both arms are tucked in at the sides, and the bed is placed in a shallow anti-Trendelenburg position. A nasogastric tube is inserted for drainage and decompression of the stomach. Our reoperative approach is a synthesis of antireflux procedures mentioned in previous chapters.

Approach Through The Left Chest

A left thoracotomy approach can be used for patients with recurrent failure of fundoplication. The esophagus usually is less adhesed and easier to control and dissect from this approach. As in the abdomen, the surgeon must be able to tolerate some bleeding from the liver during the dissection. The same parameters are addressed as in the abdominal approach. The old wrap is taken down, and the cause of the recurrence is identified and fixed. Collis extension is used liberally. The repair can be performed using the Belsey–Mark IV operation or the Nissen operation.

Practices That Differ From Initial Antireflux Repair

Scope Insertion, Trocar Placement, and Adhesiolysis

We place an 11-mm camera port using a modified Hassan technique to minimize inadvertent injury to the abdominal viscera. Placing a periumbilical trocar in a previously operated patient can be technically challenging. If this is not possible because of adhesions, an alternate initial camera port can be placed. After abdominal insufflation with CO_2 (the insufflation pressure is 15 mm Hg; when needed, a maximal pressure of 20 mm Hg can be used transiently), a 10-mm laparoscope with a deflectable tip capable of 360-degree angulation is inserted.

To minimize cosmetic scarring, we attempt to use original port scars for trocar placement, but alternate sites can be used if the original ports are improperly placed or densely adhesed. If the abdomen has multiple adhesions, we attempt to place one of the four remaining ports in the least adhesed region of the abdomen in its intended location under direct visualization. Careful dissection of adhesions using scissors, ligature, or hook so that all working ports are inserted is paramount. The remaining ports are inserted sequentially. In our experience, the liberal use of an additional 5-mm port placed in an area free of adhesions can save time, aid in the dissection, and may decrease operative morbidity. Rarely, adhesions are so dense that port relocation is not possible, and the abdominal procedure must be terminated. Care should be taken to avoid inadvertent bowel injury. If this occurs, however, the bowel often can be repaired primarily laparoscopically.

Adhesiolysis is a crucial stage in reoperation; safety depends on retraction, visualization, and identification of the avascular planes. Unfortunately, the time required to perform adhesiolysis cannot be assessed preoperatively. In our experience, it can range from a few minutes to several hours. Care should be taken to avoid known pitfalls of antireflux surgery, such as bleeding, perforation, and vagal injury. Thus we perform surgery in a systematic manner (described below) to minimize these pitfalls. If they occur, most can be managed laparoscopically.

Dissection and Wrap Takedown

The conduct and design of the operation are similar to those described in Chapter 39 on laparoscopic Nissen fundoplication. However, greater care must be taken to avoid traction injuries that lead to bleeding or perforation of visceral organs. Especially relevant are the fibrous bands that attach to the spleen and dissection around the wrap and posterior distal esophagus. If the patient had a previous wrap, it typically will be adhesed to the left side of the liver or herniated into the chest. During this phase of the operation, an understanding of why the previous operation failed must be attained. Thus meticulous attention to detail during dissection is essential.

Dissection of the Gastrosplenic Ligament

Typically, dissection is begun by dividing the gastrosplenic ligament. This is carried out sequentially, anteriorly first and then posteriorly, using a 5-mm LigaSure (Valleylab, Boulder, CO) device. The highest two or three short gastric arteries are divided, if not already divided during the initial operation. After reaching the left GEJ, the left gastrophrenic ligament is opened, exposing the left crus. If a hiatal hernia is identified, its contents are reduced into the abdomen, and the peritoneal sac is amputated and removed.

Mobilization of the Distal Esophagus and Proximal Stomach on the Right

Prior fundoplication typically causes dense adhesion between the wrap and the left lobe of the liver. Dissection in this region can be technically challenging. Perforation of the stomach or esophagus and injury to the vagus nerve must be avoided at all costs. The gastrohepatic ligament is opened above the caudate lobe in an avascular region (near the liver), avoiding the left gastric artery, the possibility of a replaced hepatic artery, and vagal branches. The anatomy may be difficult to navigate because of the prior surgery and presence of adhesions. When separating the wrap from the liver, we find it is safer to err on the side of the liver as opposed to causing visceral injury to the stomach. Any bleeding is usually short-lived and easily controlled with retraction. The right crus is identified, and the overlying peritoneum is opened exposing its edge. *We do not attempt to directly identify the esophagus before opening the crura because of the risk of perforation.* In addition, the vagi are always found medial to the crura. The right crus is dissected from its confluence to the median arcuate ligament, where it joins the left crus. Dissection is done meticulously, taking only a thin layer of peritoneum.

The esophagus is revealed by its orientation, longitudinal muscle fibers, and the vagus. We routinely divide the esophagophrenic attachments and peritoneum over the crura in a semicircular fashion down to the median arcuate ligament, taking care to avoid injuring the anterior and posterior branches of the vagus. Finally, the wrap is opened along the plane where it was sewn in the previous operation. This is a difficult step because defining the plane may be technically challenging and remaining within that plane while not causing a perforation may be difficult. Occasionally, the general location of the suture line can be stapled to separate the wrap. Great care to prevent perforation of the esophagus or stomach should be taken during mobilization of the GEJ. The esophagus is retracted upward, and a window is opened and widened bluntly to reveal the left side of the abdomen. We avoid dividing any structure that could be the vagus until the two nerves are identified.

Assessing Esophageal Length

The fat pad is medialized (taking care not to injure the anterior vagus nerve) to accurately assess the level of the GEJ. This determination is made in the context of the esophageal length measurements that were made during intraoperative endoscopy, barium swallow, and the visualized location of the GEJ when no traction is placed on the stomach. If the patient is found to have a short esophagus, the Collis lengthening procedure is performed at this juncture (see Chapter 42).

Integration of Knowledge

A crucial step in the operation is the moment when the operating surgeon integrates all the preoperative and operative findings and determines the cause of the failed antireflux procedure. In this regard, it is important to dissect the old wrap completely because this usually will verify the cause of the failure. An excellent summary of this decision-making process was published by Swanstrom et al.[24] A standard redo wrap then is fashioned, taking into account any lessons learned from the patient's preoperative workup or the intraoperative findings. For example, if the wrap is too loose, a small bougie can be used to calibrate the opening. If there is a short esophagus, a Collis extension is performed. If the wrap was "shoeshined" inadequately at the first operation, an attempt should be made to fashion a more accurate configuration. If the surgeon fails to determine the cause of the previous failure, chances are that the redo procedure also will fail to deliver good long-term palliation.

In addition, when performing a redo procedure, we tend to take a maximal approach when doubt exists. For example, if the esophagus is of equivocal length, we lengthen it. If the crura are of questionable strength, we reinforce them with bioabsorbable mesh, and if gastric emptying is delayed or vagal injury is suspected, we place a percutaneous gastrostomy tube (PEG).

For all redo procedures, we place a Jackson-Pratt no. 10 drain to the left of the wrap because in our experience the postoperative risk of leak is greater with redo surgery.

Closure of Hiatus

The hiatus is often fused and does not need to be closed. When it does require closure, we use the method described in previous chapters for simple closure or crural reinforcement (see Chapters 39 and 42). Choice of fundoplication depends on information gathered during the preoperative evaluation and intraoperative findings. The techniques for the various wraps also have been described in previous chapters.

Some patients who present with reflux after multiple surgeries are found to have a nearly frozen GEJ. In these patients we are often unable to completely dissect off the wrap but instead are able to tighten it anteriorly over a bougie by taking additional stitches to bunch it up. We find that the incidence of gastric leaks in these patients is higher. Rather than risk having to come back emergently, we leave Jackson-Pratt drains around the GEJ and insert a PEG to control the gastric output.

POSTOPERATIVE MANAGEMENT

We routinely obtain a barium swallow to rule out leak after reoperation because of the higher incidence of esophageal perforation. If a Jackson-Pratt drain was placed in the OR, it is removed on the day of discharge, provided that the patient does not have a leak on barium swallow and is able to tolerate clear liquids. The Jackson-Pratt drain is removed on the day of discharge if the patient does not have a leak. In the event of a leak, the drain is left in place for 6 weeks. This enables a controlled fistula to develop, thus alleviating the need for reoperation in the event of a leak.

In all other respects, postoperative management is the same whether the patient is being operated on for the first time or the *n*th time for failed reflux. In our experience, postoperative nausea and delayed motility are more common in patients undergoing reoperation. Symptoms usually can be abated with Reglan or erythromycin or both. Patients are discharged after they are able to tolerate enough daily liquids to prevent dehydration. Postoperatively, we educate patients to eat slowly and small amounts, and patients are sent home on a full liquid diet for 2 weeks. If problems are not encountered, patients are advanced to a regular diet devoid of bread and carbonated beverages. The literature states that postoperative dysphagia is common and can be present for many months, but most patients will prefer some dysphagia to reflux.

PROCEDURE-SPECIFIC COMPLICATIONS

The complications associated with redo laparoscopic Nissen fundoplication for recurrent or persistent reflux are, for the most part, identical to procedural complications for primary Nissen fundoplication (see Chapter 39). Briefly, these include splenic injury, esophageal or gastric perforation, and postoperative dysphagia. Less common complications include wrap failure, pancreatitis, gastric emptying problems, gastric necrosis, and bleeding. Generally speaking, the laparoscopic technique is less morbid, which underscores our preference for the laparoscopic approach even with complex reoperations.

SUMMARY

Exponential growth of laparoscopic Nissen fundoplication over the last decade has caused a dramatic increase in the number of patients presenting with recurrent or persistent reflux symptoms owing to failure of their primary antireflux surgery. The causes of surgical failure are multifactorial. A thorough evaluation and diagnostic workup are necessary to discern the etiology and identify a tailored, effective surgical solution. All patients should be counseled that reoperation carries a greater risk for complications and poorer overall outcome than a primary antireflux procedure. However, approximately 70% of patients report symptom resolution, and overall patient satisfaction is 7 on a scale of 1 to 10. Patient selection is key to successful outcome. All patients must have an esophagus that is of normal length, or steps must be taken to create a normal-length esophagus, and the esophagus must exhibit normal motility (i.e., without evidence of achalasia, DES, or scleroderma). During reoperation, a clear understanding of the mechanics of the failed procedure is paramount, and the importance of fully unwrapping the prior fundoplication cannot be overstated. A tailored approach to this complex reoperation is necessary and should be based on the preoperative evaluation and intraoperative findings. Reoperation can be accomplished safely by means of minimally invasive technique in most patients regardless of the previous mode of surgery and is the preferred approach at our institution.

EDITOR'S COMMENT

The patient must understand that the results of redo surgery may be less than perfect because of the potential for vagal injury or imperfect calibration of the wrap. On occasion, postoperative dysphagia can be managed with repeated endoscopic dilatations.

—Raphael Bueno

References

1. Iqbal A, Awad Z, Simkins J, et al. Repair of 104 failed anti-reflux operations. *Ann Surg.* 2006;244:42–51.
2. Pessaux P, Arnaud JP, Delattre JF, et al. Laparoscopic antireflux surgery: five-year results and beyond in 1340 patients. *Arch Surg.* 2005;140:946–951.
3. Carlson MA, Frantzides CT. Complications and results of primary minimally invasive antireflux procedures: a review of 10,735 reported cases. *J Am Coll Surg.* 2001;193:428–439.
4. Spechler SJ. Medical or invasive therapy for GERD: an acidulous analysis. *Clin Gastroenterol Hepatol.* 2003;1:81–88.

5. Hinder RA, Klingler PJ, Perdikis G, et al. Management of the failed antireflux operation. *Surg Clin North Am.* 1997;77:1083–1098.
6. Hunter JG, Smith CD, Branum GD, et al. Laparoscopic fundoplication failures: patterns of failure and response to fundoplication revision. *Ann Surg.* 1999;230:595–604; discussion 604–606.
7. Hiebert CA, O'Mara CS. The Belsey operation for hiatal hernia: a twenty-year experience. *Am J Surg.* 1979;137:532–535.
8. DePaula AL, Hashiba K, Bafutto M, et al. Laparoscopic reoperations after failed and complicated antireflux operations. *Surg Endosc.* 1995;9:681–686.
9. Cushieri A, Hunger J, Wolfe B, et al. Multicenter prospective evaluation of laparoscopic antireflux surgery. *Surg Endosc.* 1995;7:505–510.
10. Hunter JG, Trus TL, Branum GD, et al. A physiologic approach to laparoscopic fundoplication for gastroesophageal reflux disease. *Ann Surg.* 1996;223:673–685; discussion 685–687.
11. Kauer WK, Peters JH, DeMeester TR, et al. A tailored approach to antireflux surgery. *J Thorac Cardiovasc Surg.* 1995;110:141–146; discussion 146–147.
12. Coelho JC, Goncalves CG, Claus CM, et al. Late laparoscopic reoperation of failed antireflux procedures. *Surg Laparosc Endosc Percutan Tech.* 2004;14:113–117.
13. Voitk A, Joffe J, Alvarez C, et al. Factors contributing to laparoscopic failure during the learning curve for laparoscopic Nissen fundoplication in a community hospital. *J Laparoendosc Adv Surg Tech A.* 1999;9:243–248.
14. Watson DI, Baigrie RJ, Jamieson GG. A learning curve for laparoscopic fundoplication: definable, avoidable, or a waste of time? *Ann Surg.* 1996;224:198–203.
15. Hwang H, Turner LJ, Blair NP. Examining the learning curve of laparoscopic fundoplications at an urban community hospital. *Am J Surg.* 2005;189:522–526; discussion 526.
16. Watson DI, Jamieson GG, Devitt PG, et al. Paraoesophageal hiatus hernia: an important complication of laparoscopic Nissen fundoplication. *Br J Surg.* 1995;82:521–523.
17. Cowgill SM, Gillman R, Kraemer E, et al. Ten-year follow-up after laparoscopic Nissen fundoplication for gastroesophageal reflux disease. *Am Surg.* 2007;73:748–752; discussion 752–753.
18. Lafullarde T, Watson DI, Jamieson GG, et al. Laparoscopic Nissen fundoplication: five-year results and beyond. *Arch Surg.* 2001;136:180–184.
19. Graziano K, Teitelbaum DH, McLean K, et al. Recurrence after laparoscopic and open Nissen fundoplication: a comparison of the mechanisms of failure. *Surg Endosc.* 2003;17:704–707.
20. Heniford BT, Matthews BD, Kercher KW, et al. Surgical experience in fifty-five consecutive reoperative fundoplications. *Am Surg.* 2002;68:949–954; discussion 954.
21. Luketich JD, Fernando HC, Christie NA, et al. Outcomes after minimally invasive reoperation for gastroesophageal reflux disease. *Ann Thorac Surg.* 2002;74:328–331; discussion 331–332.
22. Little AG, Ferguson MK, Skinner DB. Reoperation for failed antireflux operations. *J Thorac Cardiovasc Surg.* 1986;91:511–517.
23. Ohnmacht GA, Deschamps C, Cassivi SD, et al Failed antireflux surgery: results after reoperation. *Ann Thorac Surg.* 2006;81:2050–2053; discussion 2053–2054.
24. Khajanchee YS, O'Rourke R, Cassera MA, et al. Laparoscopic reintervention for failed antireflux surgery: subjective and objective outcomes in 176 consecutive patients. *Arch Surg.* 2007;142:785–791; discussion 791–792.

44 Techniques for Dilation of Benign Esophageal Stricture

Majed A. Al-Mourgi and Raphael Bueno

Keywords: Benign esophageal stricture, benign peptic esophageal stricture, esophageal motility disorders, gastroesophageal reflux disease (GERD)

Benign strictures of the esophagus usually result from scarring and subsequent tissue contraction secondary to esophageal wall injury. This pathology is caused in most cases by long-standing gastroesophageal reflux disease (GERD), often in association with one of the esophageal motility disorders (e.g., achalasia, diffuse esophageal spasm, or aperistalsis).[1,2] Endoscopic dilation of benign esophageal strictures that are refractory to medical management is a less morbid alternative to surgery. Approximately 20% to 30% of cases are unrelated to GERD, and their treatment usually is more challenging. Examples include strictures arising from complications of surgical anastomosis,[3] injuries caused by caustic ingestions, early and late consequences of external-beam radiation, esophageal sclerotherapy, laser or photodynamic therapy, medication- or pill-induced esophagitis that is associated with numerous medications (e.g., alendronate, ferrous sulfate, nonsteroidal anti-inflammatory drugs, phenytoin, potassium chloride, quinidine, tetracycline, and ascorbic acid) but most often aspirin, and rare dermatologic diseases, including epidermolysis bullosa dystrophica, among others.

Benign strictures also may result from external compression of the esophagus caused by mediastinal fibrosis induced by tuberculosis, fungal infection, radiation therapy, or idiopathic fibrosing mediastinitis. These conditions may give rise to long, narrow strictures that are difficult to dilate and in which dilation may be associated with a higher rate of complications.

CLINICAL PRESENTATION

Dysphagia is the most common presenting symptom of benign esophageal stricture. The degree of dysphagia is proportional to the scope (e.g., length) of the stricture and the luminal diameter of the esophagus (<13-mm diameter is associated with dysphagia to solids, >18-mm luminal diameter for normal swallowing). As the stenosis worsens over time, the dysphagia progresses from solid to semisolid to liquid foods. The etiology of the esophageal stricture usually can be identified using radiographic modalities and is confirmed by endoscopic visualization and tissue biopsy. Manometry is the defining diagnostic procedure when esophageal dysmotility is suspected as the primary inciting process. CT scan and endoscopic ultrasound are valuable diagnostic aids that can distinguish benign from malignant strictures. Fortunately, most benign esophageal strictures are amenable to single or combined pharmacologic, endoscopic, or surgical intervention.

MANAGEMENT

The goal of therapy for benign esophageal stricture is twofold: to relieve the patient's dysphagia and to prevent recurrence of the stricture.[4] Conservative and surgical approaches to management are recommended depending on the etiology of the inciting injury. Surgical and medical issues related to esophageal dilation in patients with primary esophageal motility disorders are discussed in Part 4 (see Chapter 33). Medical and surgical issues related to GERD are the topic of this part and are summarized in the Overview (see Chapter 37). This chapter focuses on surgical instrumentation and techniques for the less common or complex benign esophageal stricture.

DIAGNOSIS

Dysphagia is the cardinal symptom of esophageal stricture. In most cases, when a stricture is suspected, the patient is evaluated radiographically with a barium swallow. The goals of this imaging modality are to establish the location, length, and number of strictures; to determine the maximal or minimal luminal diameter in normal and strictured regions; and to identify the presence of associated pathologies, such as esophageal diverticula, including Zenker diverticula, or hiatal hernia. This information is helpful for selecting instrumentation, devising strategies for treatment, estimating the number of sessions that will be required to relieve the patient's symptoms, and counseling patients about the expected risks of dilation. If barium studies raise suspicion for malignancy, a diagnostic endoscopy may be required. Usually, however, endoscopy and dilation are combined in the initial session.

CONTRAINDICATIONS TO DILATION

In addition to specific features of esophageal stricture that contraindicate dilation (e.g., extremely long and tortuous strictures), several comorbidities also can increase the patient's risk. Dilation should not be attempted in the setting of an acute or incompletely healed esophageal perforation. As with any other surgical procedure, the benefits of esophageal dilation should outweigh the risks of the procedure in all patients with bleeding disorders or severe pulmonary or cardiovascular disease. Such patients may not tolerate endoscopy, with or without dilation. Dilation should be performed cautiously in patients with a pharyngeal or cervical deformity, recent surgery, a large thoracic aneurysm, or an impacted food bolus.

INSTRUMENTATION

There are two basic types of dilators, mechanical and balloon, and each may be fitted with a guidewire (Figs. 44-1 and 44-2). Studies comparing mechanical (bougie) and balloon dilation have reported varying results.[5,6] The success of one instrument

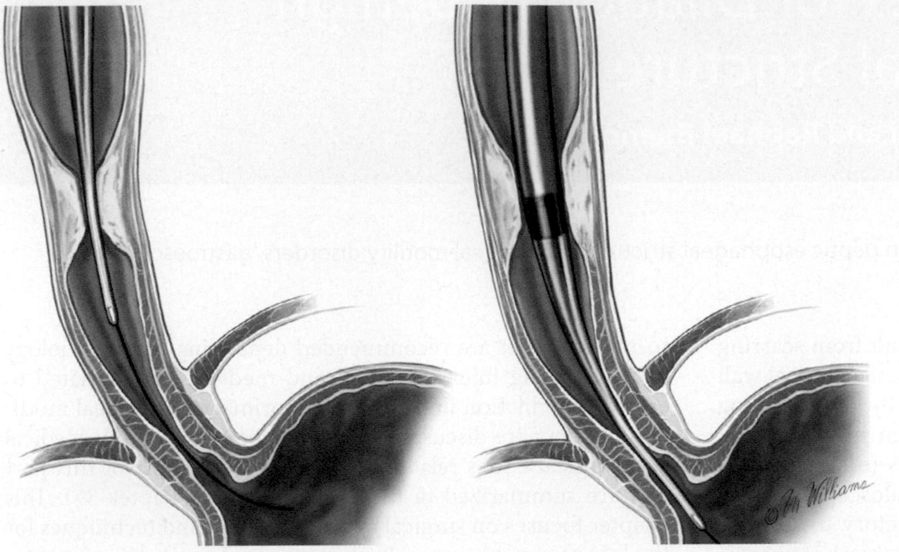

A B

Figure 44-1. Mechanical dilator.

over the other depends largely on the endoscopist's experience and familiarity with a particular product. However, for strictures with complex features, a guidewire-based mechanical or balloon dilating system, such as the Savary esophageal dilator (Wilson-Cook Medical, Inc., Winston-Salem, NC), should be used exclusively. The mechanics of esophageal luminal dilation are not known precisely, but the results probably are affected by circumferential stretching or frank splitting of the stricture. Mechanical and balloon dilators differ in the way they accomplish this goal. Mechanical dilators exert a longitudinal and radial force, dilating progressively from the proximal to the distal extent of the stricture. In contrast, balloon dilators deliver the force radially and uniformly across the entire length of the stricture, which significantly reduces shear stress.

Mechanical Dilators

Mechanical dilators are classified as those that can be passed freely through the stricture and those that are inserted over a guidewire. The Maloney dilator (Medovations, Inc., Germantown, WI) is the most commonly used freehand dilator.[5] Maloney dilators have a tapered heavy tip and come in multiple sizes. Several versions of guidewire-assisted dilators are available, but the Savary-Gilliard device (Wilson-Cook, Inc., Winston-Salem, NC) is probably used most commonly. This dilator is made from plastic, has a tapered tip, and comes in multiple sizes. Bard Interventional Products, Inc. (Tewksbury, MA), has a similar product called the American Dilatation System. An older system, the Eder-Puestow Olive dilators (Eder Instruments Co., Chicago, IL), uses progressively larger elliptical metal dilators that are passed over a guidewire. We prefer the Savary dilators for their flexibility and ease of use in our practice, and these generally have supplanted the metal Olive dilators.

Balloon Dilators

The first variety of balloon devices is the through-the-scope balloon dilator (multiple manufacturers), which is passed directly

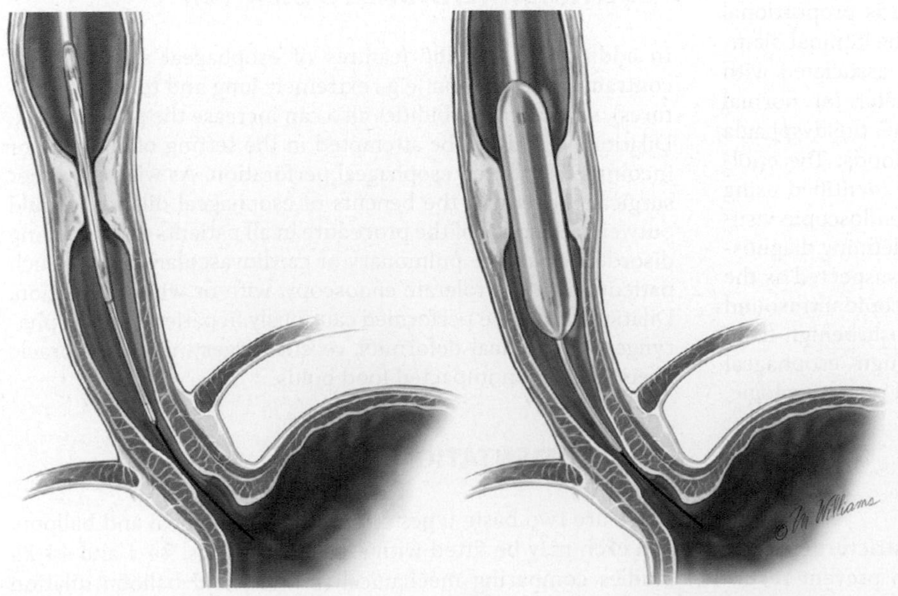

A B

Figure 44-2. Balloon dilator.

through the biopsy channel of the endoscope. The other variety is the over-the-guidewire balloon dilator (Boston Scientific Corp., Natick, MA). Compared with predecessor models, the newer balloons are capable of exerting greater radial forces and more predictably attaining maximum diameter on expansion.

MATCHING INSTRUMENTATION TO LESION CHARACTERISTICS

Simple esophageal strictures typically are related to prolonged reflux esophagitis (i.e., peptic strictures). These strictures have a smooth surface and are short and straight. They are usually located in the distal esophagus and are large enough to be traversed with the endoscope (i.e., stricture diameter is more than 10 mm). In such cases, it is usually unnecessary to resort to a guidewire or balloon system. A freely passed dilator, such as the Maloney dilator, can readily accomplish effective and safe dilation in a simple esophageal stricture.

Strictures that are long, narrow, or tortuous or strictures associated with other pathologies such as a large hiatal hernia, esophageal diverticula, or tracheoesophageal fistula are better managed with a guidewire- or balloon-based system. Attempting to maneuver a freely passed dilator through a tortuous or anomalous esophagus can be problematic because the tip may fail to enter the stomach or may even perforate the esophagus.

SURGICAL TECHNIQUE

Esophageal dilation typically is performed in an outpatient (ambulatory) facility using conscious sedation and topical pharyngeal anesthesia or general anesthesia. Some patients requiring multiple dilations may tolerate the procedure well without sedation. Patients who require frequent dilations even may be given Maloney dilators to take home for self-dilation. Patients are required to fast before dilation to ensure a clear view of the esophageal lumen and prevent aspiration. Patients should be instructed to avoid antiplatelet agents (e.g., aspirin) for 5 to 7 days before the procedure. Antibiotic prophylaxis is given to patients at high risk for bacterial endocarditis. Choice of the initial dilator size is based on the stricture diameter, which can be estimated during radiography or by comparing the stricture to the outer diameter of the endoscope. Dilation usually is performed in the supine position in the sleeping patient or in the decubitus position in the awake patient.

Use of Fluoroscopy

Dilation can be performed without endoscopy, during endoscopy alone, during endoscopy aided by fluoroscopy, or with fluoroscopic guidance alone depending on the clinical circumstances and preference of the endoscopist. As an example, some endoscopists routinely use fluoroscopy when passing a guidewire through a narrow stricture. Others will pass a guidewire through the stricture during endoscopy without fluoroscopy if the patient has undergone prior endoscopy or the passage into the stomach is clear. This would not be recommended when there is a high index of suspicion for unexpected pathology or anatomic variation distal to the view of the endoscope.

Number of Dilators per Session

It is a generally accepted rule that no more than three dilators of progressively increasing diameter should be passed in a single session and that the luminal stenosis should be increased by no more than 2 mm (6F). One or two dilators, at most, are recommended for very tight or very long strictures. These general principles help to reduce the likelihood of adverse sequelae that can arise from overexuberant dilation.

Repeated Sessions

The frequency of repeated dilation sessions depends on the success of initial dilation and the patient's past response to dilation. Patients undergoing esophageal dilation for the first time may require multiple sessions, especially if the stricture has a narrow diameter and exhibits significant resistance during dilation. Such patients may require repeated sessions every 5 to 7 days. After sufficient progress has been achieved, less frequent sessions may be satisfactory. In some patients, however, symptoms tend to recur rapidly after dilation. Such patients require more frequent dilations based on symptoms.

Through-the-Scope Balloon Dilation

Prospective comparisons of through-the-scope balloon dilators with mechanical dilators suggest that they are equally safe for dilating esophageal strictures. In addition, one study suggested that stricture recurrence may be less during the second year after through-the-scope compared with mechanical dilation. Through-the-scope balloon dilators are passed through the channel of the endoscope into the stricture under direct vision or during fluoroscopy. To prevent proximal migration of the balloon during inflation, the endoscope should be positioned just behind the proximal end of the balloon while holding the balloon sheath tightly. The optimal number and duration of inflations have not been established. Most endoscopists perform two dilations of 30 to 60 seconds duration in each session.

ENDPOINT OF DILATION

The size of the lumen after dilation is directly related to the level of symptom relief the patient experiences and the need for recurrent dilation. Although there is no firm or fast rule, in our experience, a luminal diameter of 18 mm (54F) generally is sufficient for normal swallowing and permits intake of a regular diet unless there is a coexisting motility disturbance. Patients with an esophageal lumen of less than 13 mm in diameter (39F) usually will experience dysphagia to solid foods. Some strictures are more difficult to dilate, and such patients may have to accept less than optimal results. Patients dilated to a diameter of 15 mm (45F), for example, are still able to eat a regular, if modified, diet but should be instructed to eat slowly and chew their food well.

COMPLICATIONS

Esophageal perforation is the major and most dreaded complication of esophageal dilation. The incidence of perforation is influenced by the etiology of the stricture and factors related to technique, operator experience, and equipment. Several risk factors for esophageal perforation have been recognized, although the magnitude of risk is uncertain. These factors include malignant stricture, severe esophagitis, prior radiation therapy, history of caustic ingestion, eosinophilic esophagitis, complex (tortuous) or long strictures, presence of esophageal diverticulum, inexperienced operator, large hiatal hernia, use of high inflation pressures with balloon dilation, and a history of previous esophageal perforation or prior esophageal surgery, such as for trauma or a congenital abnormality. (Techniques for the management of esophageal perforation are described in Chapter 48.)

Bacteremia

Esophageal dilation has the highest incidence of bacteremia of all gastrointestinal endoscopic procedures. Nonetheless, complications of bacteremia, such as endocarditis, are rare. Antibiotic prophylaxis is not warranted in most patients undergoing esophageal dilation except for those with a recognized risk for endocarditis.

Chest Pain

Chest pain is sometimes observed after stricture dilation. It is usually mild, self-limited, and requires no specific therapy. Rare patients require a period of a liquid diet and analgesics. However, the development of chest pain (or any signs of clinical deterioration) can signal the development of a perforation. If there is any concern for impending perforation, a water-soluble contrast study should be obtained before discharge. Such patients also may require hospitalization and observation for brief periods, during which the patient should be maintained nothing by mouth.

Hemorrhage

Significant hemorrhage related to esophageal dilation is uncommon except when the patient is anticoagulated. Recent experience suggests that when hemorrhage occurs, it is unrelated to the type of dilator used. Appropriate measures should be taken to prevent bleeding in patients taking medications that affect their coagulation status or platelet function.

Miscellaneous Complications

Other complications of esophageal dilation are related mostly to conscious sedation and endoscopy and include aspiration pneumonia, respiratory failure, and cardiac arrhythmias.

EMERGING TECHNOLOGY

Increasing experience suggests that temporarily placed nonmetal expandable stents can be effective for the management of benign strictures that are refractory to dilation by other current systems. One such silicone-coated stent (Polyflex stent, Rusch International, distributed by Boston Scientific Corporation, Natick, MA) has been approved for use in patients. Clinical experience with this stent in benign strictures has suggested a problem with stent migration.

The general incidence of complications with expandable metal stents is also high, including migration, stent-induced trauma leading to perforation, and tracheoesophageal fistula.[7] Furthermore, approximately 40% of patients have experienced stent-induced stenosis caused by granulation tissue and fibrosis. Consequently, we do not recommend expandable metal stents for benign esophageal strictures in our clinical practice unless they are placed for a limited time only. Other nonmetal stents continue to be developed. A prototype biodegradable esophageal stent made from a coil of poly-L-lactide (Instent, Inc., Eden Praire, MN) has been used in a patient with benign refractory stricture after radiation therapy. This patient experienced short-term relief of dysphagia.

OTHER SURGICAL OPTIONS

Surgical options should be discussed with young patients with peptic strictures who require frequent dilations or who depend on chronic proton pump inhibitor therapy. An antireflux operation is applicable when the stricture cannot be dilated adequately. With significant shortening of the esophagus, a Collis gastroplasty (see Chapter 38) combined with fundoplication is more likely to give a satisfactory result. Resection naturally should be reserved for patients whose strictures cannot be dilated adequately or in whom simpler procedures have failed.[3] The options for restoring continuity of the esophagus after resection include esophagogastrostomy, colon interposition, and jejunal interposition (see Chapter 33).

Patients with proximal strictures related to previous surgery or radiation therapy for head and neck tumors present a special surgical challenge. The proximal nature of these strictures, on occasion, makes them difficult to access via standard endoscopy. We have previously reported a novel approach for dilation of these strictures.[8] The stomach is accessed endoscopically through a gastrostomy site, which is usually present for feeding, and the endoscope is advanced retrogradely into the esophagus under fluoroscopic guidance until the stricture is visualized from below and cannulated with the guidewire. The guidewire is advanced, pulled out from the mouth, and used to advance Savary dilators in the antegrade direction.

SUMMARY

Although dysphagia is the cardinal symptom of esophageal stricture, it should prompt one to look for other causative pathologies, such as GERD, primary esophageal motility disturbances, infection, malignancy, and esophageal webs or rings. Although treatment of some of these conditions may involve esophageal dilation, the techniques differ, requiring accurate diagnosis and appropriate treatment planning before embarking on the procedure.

EDITOR'S COMMENT

The dilatation of a known esophageal carcinoma is more hazardous than that of a benign stricture. A perforation may upstage the patient's cancer and mandate an emergent esophagectomy. Therefore, I prefer to stent patients with obstruction related to carcinoma or provide them with a jejunostomy tube during neoadjuvant therapy.

When sequentially dilating a patient's stricture, I recommend stopping as soon as blood appears on the stent. It is also wise to finish every dilatation procedure by performing a final endoscopy to make sure there is no perforation.

—Raphael Bueno

References

1. Ahtaridis G, Snape WJ Jr, Cohen S. Clinical and manometric findings in benign peptic strictures of the esophagus. *Dig Dis Sci.* 1979;24:858–861.
2. Adler DG, Romero Y. Primary esophageal motility disorders. *Mayo Clin Proc.* 2001;76:195–200.
3. Bender EM, Walbaum PR. Esophagogastrectomy for benign esophageal stricture: fate of the esophagogastric anastomosis. *Ann Surg.* 1987;205:385–388.
4. Said A, Brust DJ, Gaumnitz EA, et al. Predictors of early recurrence of benign esophageal strictures. *Am J Gastroenterol.* 2003;98:1252–1256.
5. Hernandez LV, Jacobson JW, Harris MS. Comparison among the perforation rates of Maloney, balloon, and Savary dilation of esophageal strictures. *Gastrointest Endosc.* 2000;51:460–462.
6. Scolapio JS, Pasha TM, Gostout CJ, et al. A randomized, prospective study comparing rigid to balloon dilators for benign esophageal strictures and rings. *Gastrointest Endosc.* 1999;50:13–17.
7. Song HY, Jung HY, Park SI, et al. Covered retrievable expandable nitinol stents in patients with benign esophageal strictures: initial experience. *Radiology.* 2000;217:551–557.
8. Bueno R, Swanson SJ, Jaklitsch MT, et al. Combined antegrade and retrograde dilation: a new endoscopic technique in the management of complex esophageal obstruction. *Gastrointest Endosc.* 2001;54:368–372.

45 Endoscopic Techniques in Antireflux Surgery

Jon O. Wee

Keywords: Gastroesophageal reflux disease (GERD), transoral incisionless fundoplication, EsophyX

INTRODUCTION

Gastroesophageal reflux disease (GERD) is a clinical condition that can lead to esophagitis, esophageal strictures, aspiration, pneumonia, vocal cord inflammation, pulmonary dysfunction, Barrett esophagus, and esophageal cancer among others. Forty-four percent of the general population has some reflux and up to 10% of the population has daily reflux symptoms.[1,2] Several factors have been known to contribute to GERD including LES function, hiatal hernias, esophageal dysmotility, and gastric delayed emptying. Surgical correction of reflux disease has demonstrated improvement in patient symptoms, correction of some pulmonary dysfunction, and may have a role in reducing the incidence of esophageal cancer.[3] The most common surgical approach today is the laparoscopic Nissen fundoplication (Chapter 39), although other approaches such as the Toupet (Chapter 40) and the transthoracic Belsey (Chapter 38) procedures also have been utilized. Endoscopic treatment for reflux, however, has lagged both in terms of efficacy and durability. We review the attempted endoscopic approaches and the future outlook of endoscopic antireflux surgery.

ENDOSCOPIC THERAPIES

Most endoscopic therapies have focused on trying to increase the resistance at the gastroesophageal (GE) junction.

The Stretta system uses radiofrequency ablation of the GE junction. This method utilizes a flexible catheter with a balloon. Four electrodes are placed into the surrounding tissue at the level of the LES. The probes reach the level of the submucosa and radiofrequency energy is applied, elevating the submucosal temperature to 85°C whereas a cold water infusion in the balloon keeps the mucosal temperature at 50°C. The procedure is repeated. The energy creates thermal lesions in the submucosa which cause scarring and tightening around the LES. In essence, a stricture is created at the LES, increasing resistance at the GE junction. Unfortunately, a randomized sham trial did not demonstrate any difference in any objective measure of reflux in these patients, although some did report a reduction in heartburn symptoms.[4]

Additional studies, to date, all have been characterized by short-term follow-ups of 6 to 12 months, small numbers of patients, and variable improvements in objective symptoms.[5] Aziz et al.[6] in 2010 reported on 30 patients with improvement in health-related quality-of-life (HRQL) scores, LES pressure, and pH scores of those patients off medication, although some patients experienced some delayed gastric emptying. Coron et al.[7] in 2008 demonstrated that 18 of 20 patients were able to stop proton pump inhibitor (PPI) use, although there was no change in esophageal acid exposure.

One prospective nonrandomized comparison of the Stretta system with laparoscopic fundoplication demonstrated a superior outcome with the laparoscopic procedure. Patients in both groups had improvement of their quality of life and symptoms, but only 58% of patients in the Stretta group were able to discontinue medication compared to 97% of patients following the laparoscopic procedure, despite the fact that the Stretta group patients had less severe disease.[8]

Bard Endocinch and the NDO Plication System use sutures placed with a proprietary device to tighten the LES. Although some studies have demonstrated some efficacy, there have been concerns about its durability. Schwartz conducted a double-blind randomized sham-controlled trial with the Endocinch that demonstrated less PPI in the treatment group (65%) compared to the observation group (0%), but there was no difference in esophageal acid exposure in the treatment group versus the sham group.[9] Montgomery et al.,[10] in a randomized placebo controlled trial, likewise determined that there was no difference in esophageal acid exposure at 3 and 12 months.

With regard to the plication system, results have been more promising. A randomized single blind prospective multicenter trial in 2006 did demonstrate greater cessation of PPI treatment in the treatment arm compared to sham (50% vs. 20%, $p = 0.002$) and with greater improvement in esophageal pH compared to sham.[11] von Renteln in 2009 demonstrated 63% of patients had symptomatic improvement.[12] Daily PPI use was eliminated in 69% of patients at 12 months. Khajanchee performed a meta-analysis of 266 patients that demonstrated a decreased in DeMeester score with 32% of patients resulting in a normal range. However, the company lost funding, and the device is no longer available.[13]

Injection of inert products into the LES also has been tried. Plexiglas, Gatekeeper Reflux Repair System, and the Enteryx are some of the products in this category. Plexiglas inserted polymethylmethacrylate (PMMA) into the submucosa of the LES to decrease transient relaxation of the sphincter. Enteryx injected 8% ethylene vinyl alcohol in dimethyl sulfoxide and micronized tantalum powder into the muscular layer of the LES.[14] The compound hardened after injection. This procedure was associated with serious complications including injection into the mediastinum, embolization to the kidney, pericarditis, and aortoesophageal fistula, which resulted in withdrawal from the market. The Gatekeeper used a soft, pliable, biocompatible, hydrophilic prosthesis into the submucosa of the LES. Upon insertion, it absorbs water and expands, creating bulk and decreasing compliance of the LES. A randomized sham-controlled blinded multicenter study demonstrated no improvement in outcomes at 6 months.[15] This, too, was withdrawn from the market.

Endoscopic Partial Fundoplication

The most recent entry into the endoscopic antireflux therapy is the EsophyX device by endogastric solutions. The goal of this device is to produce a 270-degree partial fundoplication. A large tubular device is placed over the endoscope and through the mouth into the esophagus. Once in the stomach, the end of the device is advanced and the tip closed such that it is facing the GE junction. A helical device is anchored to the Z-line. Using this anchor, the GE junction is then pulled into the open device and closed. The gastric fundus is approximated to the distal intra-abdominal lumen by the device. Two stylets are used to deploy two polypropylene H-shaped fasteners that are supposed to traverse from the gastric mucosa to the esophageal mucosa, thereby securing the shape. The device is opened and then rotated, and the sequence repeated until fasteners are placed from the posterior lesser curvature to the anterior lesser curvature and an omega-shaped 270-degree wrap is formed, ideally of 2 cm length. Small hiatal hernias can also reportedly be reduced by using suction traction on the device.

Over 30 peer-reviewed publications have evaluated the EsophyX device. Cadiere et al.[16] were the first to publish their experience in a prospective multicenter trial of 84 patients in 2008. At 12 months, they demonstrated that 73% of patients had greater than or equal to 50% improvement of the GERD-HRQL score, 85% discontinuation of daily PPI use, and 37% normalization of esophageal acid exposure. Resting LES pressure was improved by 53%. There were two esophageal perforations during the insertion of the device and one patient required a four unit blood transfusion from postoperative bleeding. GERD was considered cured in 56% of patients. Pre- and postoperative esophageal pH monitoring demonstrated a significant reduction in DeMeester score from 34 to 28 ($p < 0.001$) at 12-month follow-up. A 2-year feasibility follow-up of 14 patients by the same group in 2009 indicated that the GERD-HRQL score remained favorable and 86% of patients were satisfied with the outcome of the procedure. Ten of fourteen patients remained successfully off of PPI.[17]

Hoppo et al. published a multicenter study involving one American and two Australian institutions in 2010 and 19 patients with GERD. At 10.8 months, 5 of 19 patients had discontinued their PPI and 3 of 19 had reduced their dose. However, 10 of 19 eventually underwent laparoscopic Nissen fundoplication for recurrent reflux symptoms. Three major complications occurred including an esophageal perforation, bleeding requiring transfusions, and one permanent numbness of the tongue.[18]

Demyttenaere et al. reported on 26 patients that demonstrated that only 45% of patients had ≥50% decreased in the GERD-HRQL score and of 45% of patients were satisfied with the procedure while 30% were dissatisfied. Three patients required conversion to a laparoscopic Nissen procedure. Repici in 2010 reported on 20 patients after the transoral incisionless fundoplication (TIF) procedure. Four patients required conversion to a laparoscopic Nissen fundoplication in the first year and only 16.6% of patients demonstrated improved in esophageal acid exposure while in 66.7% it worsened.[19]

Velanovich in 2010 reported on 26 patients. In two patients, the device was not able to be passed. Four patients had a prior Nissen fundoplication and had recurrent symptoms. At 7 weeks follow-up, 19 of 24 patients were satisfied with symptom control and the mediastinal GERD-HRQL scores improved from 25 to 5 ($p = 0.0004$).[20]

Barnes et al. in 2011 reported a US multicenter retrospective evaluation of endoscopic fundoplication in 110 patients at a median follow-up of 7 months. Median GERD-HRQL scores were significantly reduced from 28 to 2 ($p < 0.001$), and median reflux symptom index scores were reduced from 29 to 4 ($p < 0.001$). There were significant benefits for the typical symptoms of heartburn, regurgitation, and dysphagia as well as the atypical symptoms of hoarseness, clearing of the throat, cough, and globus sensation. A total of 102 of 110 patients were able to get off PPI treatment.[21]

Bell and Freeman in 2011 reported their retrospective experience of 37 patients. At 6 months follow-up, 64% of patients with atypical symptoms and 70% of typical patients demonstrated improvement. Five patients required additional intervention including two with redo endoscopic fundoplication and three with a laparoscopic Nissen fundoplication.[22]

A single-center randomized trial comparing the TIF to laparoscopic Nissen fundoplication was published from the Czech republic. The TIF arm had a combined experience of the plicator and the EsophyX. Both arms demonstrated significant improvement in the GERD-HRQL scores although the mean hospital stay was shorter for the endoscopic arm at 2.9 days compared to 6.4 days, $p < 0.0001$.[23]

Muls reported a 3-year follow-up of 66 patients. In all, 61% of patients discontinued daily PPI use. However, only 9 of 23 patients on intention to treat analysis demonstrated a normal pH.[24] Likewise Witteman et al.[25] reported 38 patients at 36 months follow-up and demonstrated that 56% had hiatal hernia reduction and 47% has resolution of esophagitis. However, there was no improvement in esophageal acid exposure. Multiple additional studies have demonstrated improvement in patient symptoms, about 60% to 80% of patients mostly off of PPI medication, and improvement in GERD-HRQL scores. However, the objective esophageal acid exposure data have remained lacking or unchanged. Comparison of pH exposure following EsophyX versus laparoscopic Nissen fundoplication demonstrated only 50% of cases with normalized esophageal acid exposure compared to 100% in the Nissen group.[26]

CONCLUSION

Endoscopic antireflux procedures have evolved over time. Current data suggest that endoscopic fundoplication, with products such as the EsophyX, carries the most promise; however, durability has not yet been demonstrated. The overall results still remain inferior to the laparoscopic approach, but this may change as the technology advances. Currently, a prospective randomized study, the RESPECT trial, comparing the EsophyX to a sham placebo control is under way. Results of this study may help determine its overall efficacy. If durable improvement in symptoms, PPI use, and objective acid exposure can be demonstrated, indications for treatment may favor endoscopic treatment. However, the current literature not only lacks long-term follow-up, but also the cohorts remain small and outcomes variable.

EDITOR'S COMMENT

The proliferation of less invasive methods to treat reflux will continue because the potential market is enormous and surgical repair is not perfect. These approaches will need to be compared to fundoplication both in terms of early and late results. While it is important for esophageal surgeons to participate in the development and implementation of these devices, it is equally important to insist on legitimate data and appropriately inform patients of the experimental nature of such devices.

—Raphael Bueno

References

1. Dent J, El-Serag HB, Wallander MA, et al. Epidemiology of gastro-oesophageal reflux disease: a systematic review. *Gut*. 2005;54(5):710–717.
2. Everhart JE, Ruhl CE. Burden of digestive diseases in the United States part I: overall and upper gastrointestinal diseases. *Gastroenterology*. 2009;136(2):376–386.
3. Chang EY, Morris CD, Seltman AK, et al. The effect of antireflux surgery on esophageal carcinogenesis in patients with Barrett esophagus: a systematic review. *Ann Surg*. 2007;246(1):11–21.
4. Corley DA, Katz P, Wo JM, et al. Improvement of gastroesophageal reflux symptoms after radiofrequency energy: a randomized, sham-controlled trial. *Gastroenterology*. 2003;125(3):668–676.
5. Triadafilopoulos G, DiBaise JK, Nostrant TT, et al. The Stretta procedure for the treatment of GERD: 6 and 12 month follow-up of the U.S. open label trial. *Gastrointest Endosc*. 2002;55(2):149–156.
6. Aziz AM, El-Khayat HR, Sadek A, et al. A prospective randomized trial of sham, single-dose Stretta, and double-dose Stretta for the treatment of gastroesophageal reflux disease. *Surg Endosc*. 2010;24(4):818–825.
7. Coron E, Sebille V, Cadiot G, et al. Clinical trial: radiofrequency energy delivery in proton pump inhibitor-dependent gastro-oesophageal reflux disease patients. *Aliment Pharmacol Ther*. 2008;28(9):1147–1158.
8. Richards WO, Houston HL, Torquati A, et al. Paradigm shift in the management of gastroesophageal reflux disease. *Ann Surg*. 2003;237(5):638–647; discussion 648–649.
9. Schwartz MP, Wellink H, Gooszen HG, et al. Endoscopic gastroplication for the treatment of gastro-oesophageal reflux disease: a randomised, sham-controlled trial. *Gut*. 2007;56(1):20–28.
10. Montgomery M, Håkanson B, Ljungqvist O, et al. Twelve months' follow-up after treatment with the EndoCinch endoscopic technique for gastro-oesophageal reflux disease: a randomized, placebo-controlled study. *Scand J Gastroenterol*. 2006;41(12):1382–1389.
11. Rothstein R, Filipi C, Caca K, et al. Endoscopic full-thickness plication for the treatment of gastroesophageal reflux disease: a randomized, sham-controlled trial. *Gastroenterology*. 2006;131(3):704–712.
12. von Renteln D, Schiefke I, Fuchs KH, et al. Endoscopic full-thickness plication for the treatment of gastroesophageal reflux disease using multiple Plicator implants: 12-month multicenter study results. *Surg Endosc*. 2009;23(8):1866–1875.
13. Khajanchee YS, Ujiki M, Dunst CM, et al. Patient factors predictive of 24-h pH normalization following endoluminal gastroplication for GERD. *Surg Endosc*. 2009;23(11):2525–2530.
14. Deviere J, Costamagna G, Neuhaus H, et al. Nonresorbable copolymer implantation for gastroesophageal reflux disease: a randomized sham-controlled multicenter trial. *Gastroenterology*. 2005;128(3):532–540.
15. Fockens P, Cohen L, Edmundowicz SA, et al. Prospective randomized controlled trial of an injectable esophageal prosthesis versus a sham procedure for endoscopic treatment of gastroesophageal reflux disease. *Surg Endosc*. 2010;24(6):1387–1397.
16. Cadiere GB, Buset M, Muls V, et al. Antireflux transoral incisionless fundoplication using EsophyX: 12-month results of a prospective multicenter study. *World J Surg*. 2008;32(8):1676–1688.
17. Cadiere GB, Van Sante N, Graves JE, et al. Two-year results of a feasibility study on antireflux transoral incisionless fundoplication using EsophyX. *Surg Endosc*. 2009;23(5):957–964.
18. Hoppo T, Immanuel A, Schuchert M, et al. Transoral incisionless fundoplication 2.0 procedure using EsophyX for gastroesophageal reflux disease. *J Gastrointest Surg*. 2010;14(12):1895–1901.
19. Demyttenaere SV, Bergman S, Pham T, et al. Transoral incisionless fundoplication for gastroesophageal reflux disease in an unselected patient population. *Surg Endosc*. 2010;24(4):854–858.
20. Velanovich V. Endoscopic, endoluminal fundoplication for gastroesophageal reflux disease: initial experience and lessons learned. *Surgery*. 2010;148(4):646–651;discussion 651–653.
21. Barnes WE, Hoddinott KM, Mundy S, et al. Transoral incisionless fundoplication offers high patient satisfaction and relief of therapy-resistant typical and atypical symptoms of GERD in community practice. *Surg Innov*. 2011;18(2):119–129.
22. Bell RC, Freeman KD. Clinical and pH-metric outcomes of transoral esophagogastric fundoplication for the treatment of gastroesophageal reflux disease. *Surg Endosc*. 2011;25(6):1975–1984.
23. Svoboda P, Kantorová I, Kozumplík L, et al. Our experience with transoral incisionless plication of gastroesophageal reflux disease: NOTES procedure. *Hepatogastroenterology*. 2011;58(109):1208–1213.
24. Muls V, Eckardt AJ, Marchese M, et al. Three-year results of a multicenter prospective study of transoral incisionless fundoplication. *Surg Innov*. 2013;20(4):321–330.
25. Witteman BP, Strijkers R, de Vries E, et al. Transoral incisionless fundoplication for treatment of gastroesophageal reflux disease in clinical practice. *Surg Endosc*. 2012;26(11):3307–3315.
26. Frazzoni M, Conigliaro R, Manta R, et al. Reflux parameters as modified by EsophyX or laparoscopic fundoplication in refractory GERD. *Aliment Pharmacol Ther*. 2011;34(1):67–75.

46 Techniques for Repair of Paraesophageal Hiatal Hernia

Toni Lerut and Claude Deschamps

Keywords: Giant paraesophageal hernia, parahiatal hernia, intrathoracic stomach, rolling hernia, sliding hiatal hernia

INTRODUCTION

A multiplicity of terms has been used over the years to describe paraesophageal hernia. These reflect the considerable confusion that persists to this day concerning its pathophysiology and treatment. Terms like up-side-down stomach, rolling hernia, intrathoracic stomach, parahiatal, and paraesophageal hernia have all been used to describe this clinical condition. Any herniation of the fundus and/or body of the stomach into the chest anterior or lateral to the esophagus is considered to be a paraesophageal hernia. Once considered an immediate indication for surgical repair, the role of surgery in this operation is changing and patients receive treatment appropriate to their complaints. Persistent symptoms, in particular, those related to the mechanical effects of paraesophageal hernia, eventually will result in an indication for surgery.

PATHOPHYSIOLOGY AND CLASSIFICATION

The common classification for paraesophageal hernia distinguishes four types (Table 46-1). The sliding type hiatal hernia (Type I) is the most common. It occurs when the gastroesophageal junction (GEJ), along with a leading portion of the gastric cardia, slides through the esophageal hiatus into the mediastinum. The sliding hernia may progress to a rolling hernia. As the muscles of the hiatus weaken, the hiatus becomes wider, causing an ever increasing portion of the stomach along with the GEJ to slip through the opening, until the entire greater curvature rolls into the posterior mediastinum (hence the name rolling hernia). A rolling hernia is therefore seen as a progression from a small sliding hernia to complete herniation of the greater curvature of the stomach. It is now generally accepted that most paraesophageal hernias begin as sliding hiatal hernias.

In rare cases, the GEJ may remain in its normal intra-abdominal position. This is called the "true" paraesophageal hernia (Type II). Here a portion of the stomach and sometimes other parts of the abdominal viscera migrate into the mediastinum either through the esophageal hiatus or through an adjacent defect in the diaphragm.

Table 46-1

CLASSIFICATION OF HIATAL HERNIA

I	Sliding hernia
II	True paraesophageal hernia with the GEJ in place intra-abdominally
III	Organoaxial volvulus of the stomach into the mediastinum
IV	Organoaxial volvulus of the stomach with migration of other abdominal viscera into the mediastinum

Occasionally, the stomach may further migrate into the chest causing organoaxial volvulus, in which usually more than half the stomach lies in the mediastinum, a condition known as "giant" paraesophageal hernia (Type III). The lesser curvature remains in the abdomen, fixed by the gastrohepatic omentum and the left gastric vessels, which explains the asymmetric displacement of the stomach generally observed. With organoaxial volvulus, the fundus folds over anteriorly to the esophagus and toward the right side of the mediastinum.

Less frequently, if the defect becomes very large, colon together with omentum, spleen, and eventually small bowel may migrate into the chest, together with the stomach (Type IV).

Types III and IV are most commonly seen in elderly patients. Aging is associated with diminished muscle tone and loss of strength and elasticity of the connective tissues in the phrenoesophageal membrane, which predispose to thinning and widening of the esophageal hiatus. In addition, elderly patients often develop kyphosis. The resultant change in posture may further stretch and weaken the diaphragmatic structures. Finally, obesity can be a predisposing factor because it causes an increase of intra-abdominal pressure on the stomach.

If the herniated stomach becomes trapped between the margin of the esophageal hiatus and the esophagus, this may result in an unreducible incarcerated hernia. This condition may eventually lead to life-threatening complications, such as dilatation of the intrathoracic stomach with partial or complete obstruction, ischemia of a strangulated intrathoracic stomach with subsequent necrosis and perforation, and soiling of the mediastinum or pleural space with gastric contents resulting in infection. Localized pressure ulceration at the margin of the hiatus may result in bleeding (often occult) and anemia.

The anatomical derangements associated with the full spectrum of paraesophageal hernias are summarized in Fig. 46-1.

GENERAL THERAPEUTIC PRINCIPLES

Medical Management

Paraesophageal hernias are usually discovered on diagnostic radiographic images in patients with symptoms of heartburn and chest pain. They also may be discovered incidentally in asymptomatic individuals. After careful questioning to rule out potential life-threatening pathology, treatment appropriate to the patient's symptoms is recommended. Patients without symptoms do not need any treatment. Patients with symptoms of reflux are treated *lege artis.* Moderate dysphagia can be remediated by small meals of semisolid consistency. A prokinetic, for example, metoclopramide, is helpful for treating symptoms of early satiety and fullness. The presence of moderate anemia requires iron replacement. If there is a high index of suspicion for incarceration, the introduction of a nasogastric tube will

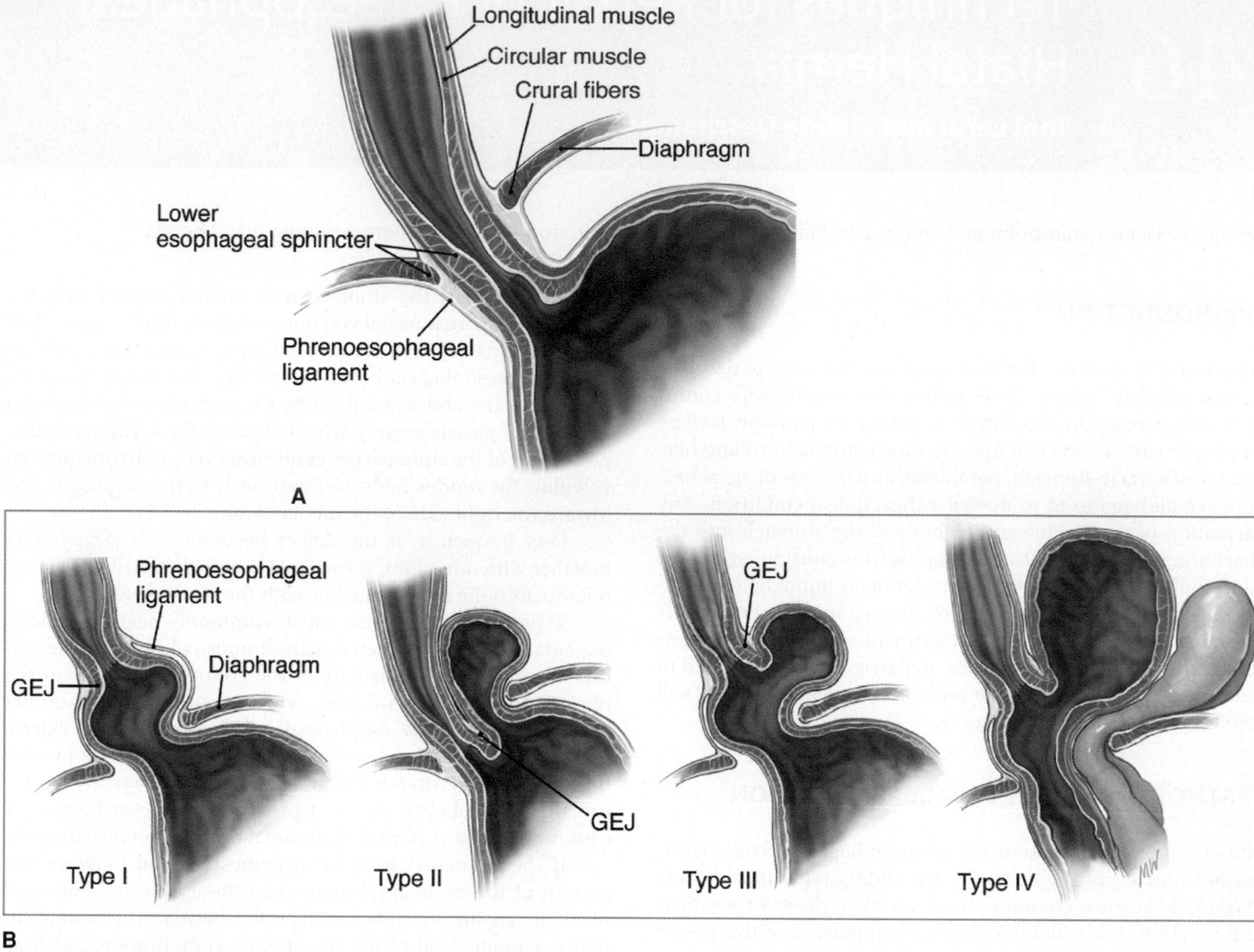

Figure 46-1. *A.* Normal paraesophageal anatomy. *B.* Classification of paraesophageal hernias.

provide relief. However, persistence of symptoms, in particular, those related to the mechanical effects of paraesophageal hernia, eventually will result in an indication for surgery.

Surgical Management

In 1967, Skinner and Belsey published a classic paper[1] that drew attention to the potentially life-threatening complications of symptomatic paraesophageal hernias. In their series, over 25% of patients with a paraesophageal hernia treated with medical therapy died of catastrophic complications, chiefly, aspiration-related pneumonia. This led to the long-standing practice of treating hernias surgically, even those with minimal symptoms. That practice has been challenged over the past several decades with the advent of improved diagnostic procedures, minimally invasive approaches, and long-term outcome data from clinical studies. Even so, giant paraesophageal hernias are more complex than the garden variety sliding hernia, and this influences both surgical approach and outcome. Besides the more complex technical aspects of the surgery, itself, these interventions carry a higher rate of postoperative mortality and morbidity, even in expert hands, causing some surgeons to challenge the necessity of surgical intervention for many large or giant paraesophageal hernias.

A study by Allen et al.[2] from the Mayo Clinic in 1993 reported on 147 patients, 23 of which were not operated but instead followed for a median of 6.5 years. Not a single patient of this series developed life-threatening complications. In four patients, symptoms progressed resulting in elective surgery in two.

In 2002, using a Markov Monte Carlo decision analytic model, Stylopoulos et al.[3] calculated that for the many patients who have only minor symptoms, such as heartburn, bloating, and so on, a policy of watchful waiting entails a lifetime risk of only 1.1% per year for the development of acute symptoms requiring surgery, with mortality related to emergency surgery of only 5.4%.[3] This means that the overall lifetime risk of death is approximately 1% which is less than the reported 30-day mortality in series from high volume centers. Moreover, the older the patient, the higher the postoperative mortality. In the series published by Luketich et al.,[4] the 30-day mortality in patients older than 80 years was 8%.

Given the fact that progression toward life-threatening symptoms/complications is low and occurs mostly in elderly populations, elderly patients with mild symptoms should not undergo surgery. Therefore, for every patient, the advantages of repair should always be carefully weighed against the risks of surgery.

An attempt should always be made to decompress the herniated stomach in patients presenting with symptoms of incarceration. This avoids the necessity of performing an emergency procedure, which is associated with high mortality, and gives adequate time, subsequently, for a thorough preoperative investigation and preparation for elective surgery under optimal conditions, for example, correction of anemia, treatment of aspiration-related pneumonia.

In cases involving clear incarceration that cannot be decompressed, gastric ischemia due to strangulation, massive bleeding, and perforation, emergency surgery is unavoidable. Depending on the experience of the surgeon, an open transthoracic or transabdominal or laparoscopic approach can be used.

The rate for conversion to open surgery, laparotomy, or thoracotomy is up to 15% in laparoscopic cases.[5] Emergency repair in octogenarians is high (up to 16%) in the series reported by Poulose et al.[6]

PREOPERATIVE EVALUATION

Signs and Symptoms

Symptoms that accompany paraesophageal hernias are either related to reflux or to the mechanical aspects of the herniation. It is important to acquire a complete history and physical examination to elicit the typical symptoms of gastroesophageal reflux disease (heartburn and regurgitation) and dysphagia. A detailed discussion of the symptoms related to reflux is provided in Chapter 36.

Many patients with paraesophageal hernias remain asymptomatic for years or have only vague, intermittent symptoms. Although patients may initially deny symptoms, careful questioning can reveal complaints that are related to the esophagus, for example, dysphagia, epigastric or substernal pain, postprandial substernal fullness, nausea, and hiccupping.

Symptoms related to intermittent incarceration are postprandial distress or early satiety and fullness, epigastric pain, intermittent vomiting, or regurgitation. A very large volvulus may cause dyspnea, and on occasion, in this respect, atelectasis may be seen on chest CT.

Anemia and iron deficiency are usually the result of chronic occult bleeding from a pressure ulcer at the margin of the hiatus. In such cases, the patient may present with complaints of exercise-related dyspnea, fatigue, weakness, palpations, and in the case of concomitant coronary disease, angina pectoris. Painful ulceration of the herniated fundus with perforation and massive bleeding may occasionally occur. The perforation may extend into the pleura, mediastinum, or pericardium. When volvulus is present, complete obstruction of food passage may occur.

A posteroanterior and lateral chest x-ray often will show air or an air–fluid level in the mediastinum posterior to the heart indicating the presence of a herniated stomach.

Diagnostic Evaluation

The barium swallow is the gold standard diagnostic study for paraesophageal hernias (Fig. 46-2). It reveals the anatomy and

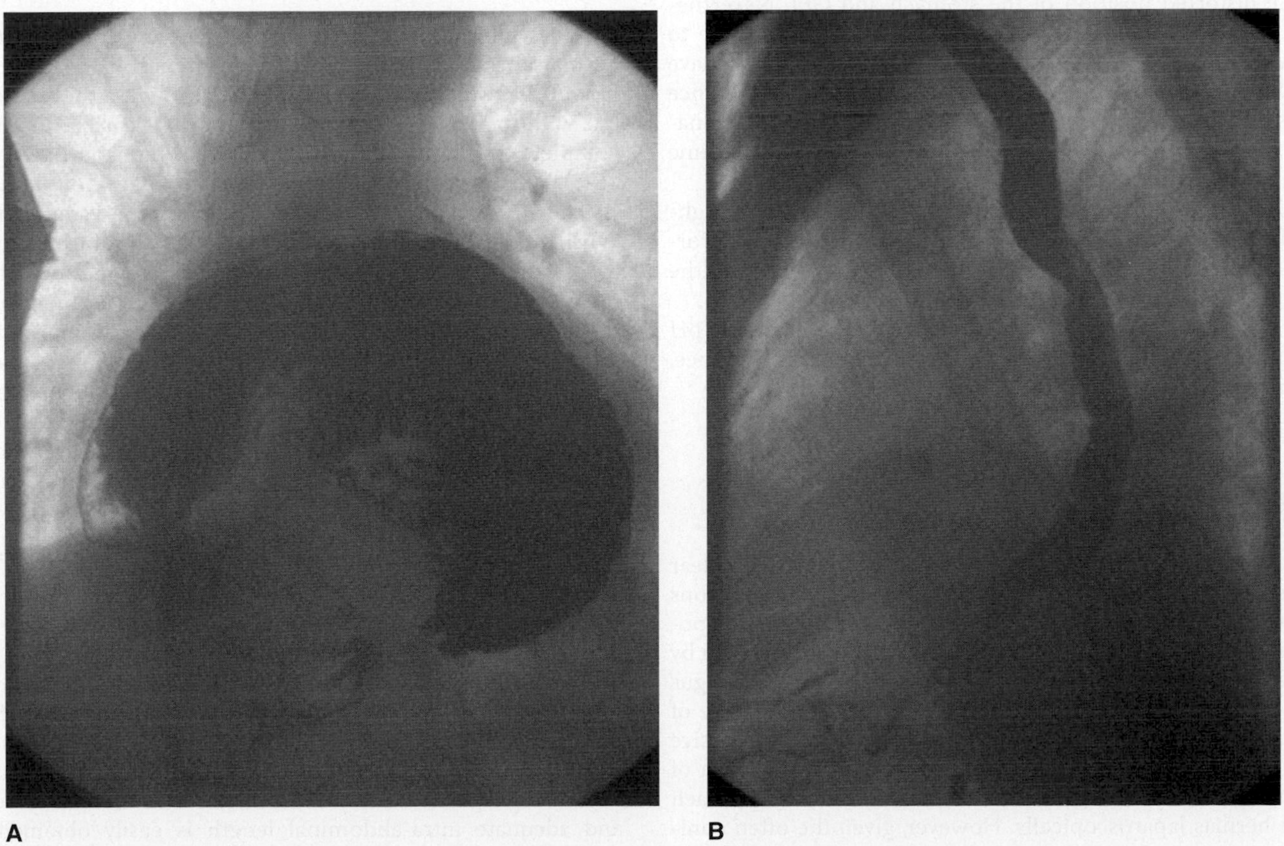

Figure 46-2. Preoperative (*A*) and postoperative (*B*) chest radiographs from a patient with giant paraesophageal hiatal hernia. The anteroposterior chest radiograph (*A*) demonstrates the preoperative intrathoracic stomach with the GEJ in the normal subdiaphragmatic location in a patient with Type II paraesophageal hernia. The lateral chest radiograph (*B*) demonstrates the postoperative appearance after a barium swallow. Note the absence of tension on the distal esophagus, lack of obstruction of esophageal emptying, and fundic wrap below the diaphragm.

relationship of the esophagus and stomach. It also will reveal whether there is free passage of contrast material (this may include a more solid contrast bolus) into the stomach. Less often, it may be helpful in locating the GEJ in relation to the diaphragm. This study reveals the anatomy and relationship of the esophagus and stomach. It also will reveal whether there is free passage of the contrast material (this may include a more solid contrast bolus) into the stomach. Often, it may be helpful in locating the GEJ in relation to the diaphragm. CT scan may be used to assess the extent of volvulus and the size of the hiatus or in identifying other abdominal organs that have migrated into the chest. Contrast studies may also reveal esophageal motility disorders, strictures, endoluminal masses, or diverticula.

Esophagoscopy is critically important; however, in cases involving a large volvulus it might be very difficult if not impossible to pass the endoscope beyond the herniated and distorted gastric pouch, into the antrum, down to the pylorus.

Endoscopy more precisely identifies the location of the GEJ in relation to the hiatus and permits evaluation for the presence and severity of esophagitis, Barrett metaplasia, or cancer to be confirmed or ruled out by biopsy. Equally important, endoscopy makes it possible to measure the distance between the GEJ and the hiatus. If this distance is >5 cm, a strong case can be made for acquired short esophagus, which calls for a different treatment approach. The patient must be awake and breathing during the endoscopy to correctly identify impingement of the hiatus.

Manometry may be useful. However, the study may be difficult to perform in patients with large hiatal hernia because of the distorted position of the stomach and GEJ. Nevertheless, through manometric studies, Maziak et al.[7] were able to show that patients presenting with paraesophageal hernia have a significantly shorter intersphincteric length (i.e., the distance measured on manometry between the upper and lower esophageal sphincter). This has an important consequence at the time of surgical repair.

Manometry and the more recently introduced high-resolution manometry (HRM) will also provide valuable information on the motor function of the esophageal body and the function of the lower esophageal sphincter.

A 24-hour pH study and multichannel impedance pH monitoring, if technically possible, will document the presence, nature, and severity of reflux.[8]

SURGICAL TECHNIQUE

As to the surgical approach and technique, there are no clear guidelines and several controversies persist. Many surgeons prefer laparotomy, whereas others prefer thoracotomy. Proponents of thoracotomy claim that the wide exposure afforded by this approach permits maximal mobilization of the esophagus in the event that a short esophagus is revealed at the time of surgery, or if the patient is found at surgery to have a massive nonreducible Type III or IV hernia. Since the introduction of minimally invasive surgery, the trend has been to approach these hernias laparoscopically. However, given the often complex presentation of these cases, conversion to open surgery may become necessary and the surgeon should be familiar with all surgical approaches before undertaking this repair to tailor the intervention to the patient's individual situation.

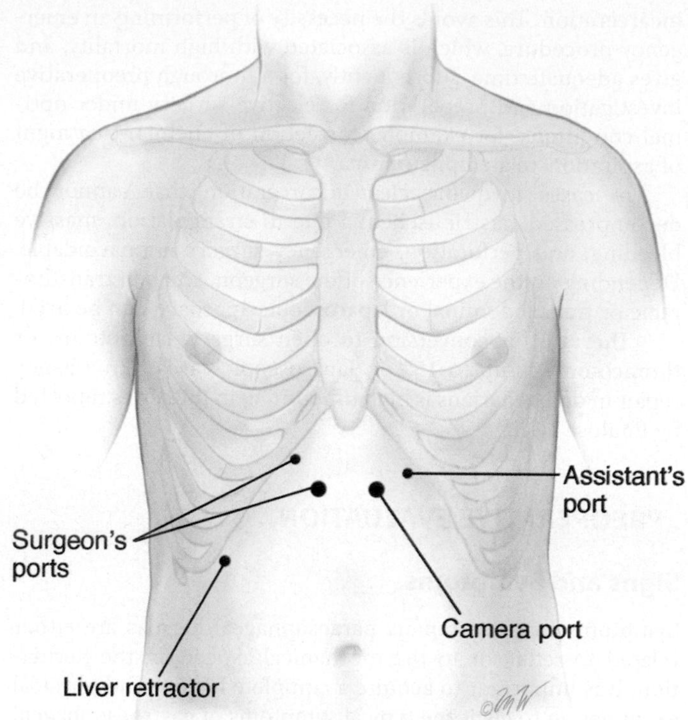

Figure 46-3. Surgeon and port placement.

It is now well accepted that a complete excision of the hernia sac is mandatory to avoid recurrence of the hernia.[9,10] It is probably easier to excise the sac through a thoracotomy, but with increasing experience, it appears feasible to obtain complete excision through a laparoscopic approach (Fig. 46-3). Whatever the route of access, it is of paramount importance to resect the sac without damaging the vagus nerves. With the laparoscopic approach, the sac should be excised before mobilizing the esophagus and by staying away from the esophagus (Fig. 46-4A,B). This can be done by everting the sac at the beginning of the intervention and incising the sac at the border of the hiatus but avoiding damage to the crural muscle. After entering the mediastinum, the sac is further dissected and pulled down allowing both vagi to be identified. It is also important to identify the pleura to avoid inadvertent opening of the pleural sac, which may result in hemodynamic instability due to tension pneumothorax. It is also important to keep the peritoneal covering of the crura intact, or it will be difficult to obtain successful primary closure of the hiatus.

Once the hernia is reduced (Fig. 46-5), the next step is to mobilize the esophagus in the posterior mediastinum. This step is essential to achieving adequate esophageal intra-abdominal length. In particular, full mobilization up to the level of the carina is mandatory in patients who present with a suspicion of short esophagus. In some of these patients, the presumed short esophagus is simply the result of loss of elastic recoil and adequate intra-abdominal length is easily obtained. In patients with a true shortening of the esophagus, adequate length may be difficult to achieve. For these cases, it can be helpful to completely mobilize the fat pad off the stomach and the distal esophagus, again taking great care not to damage the

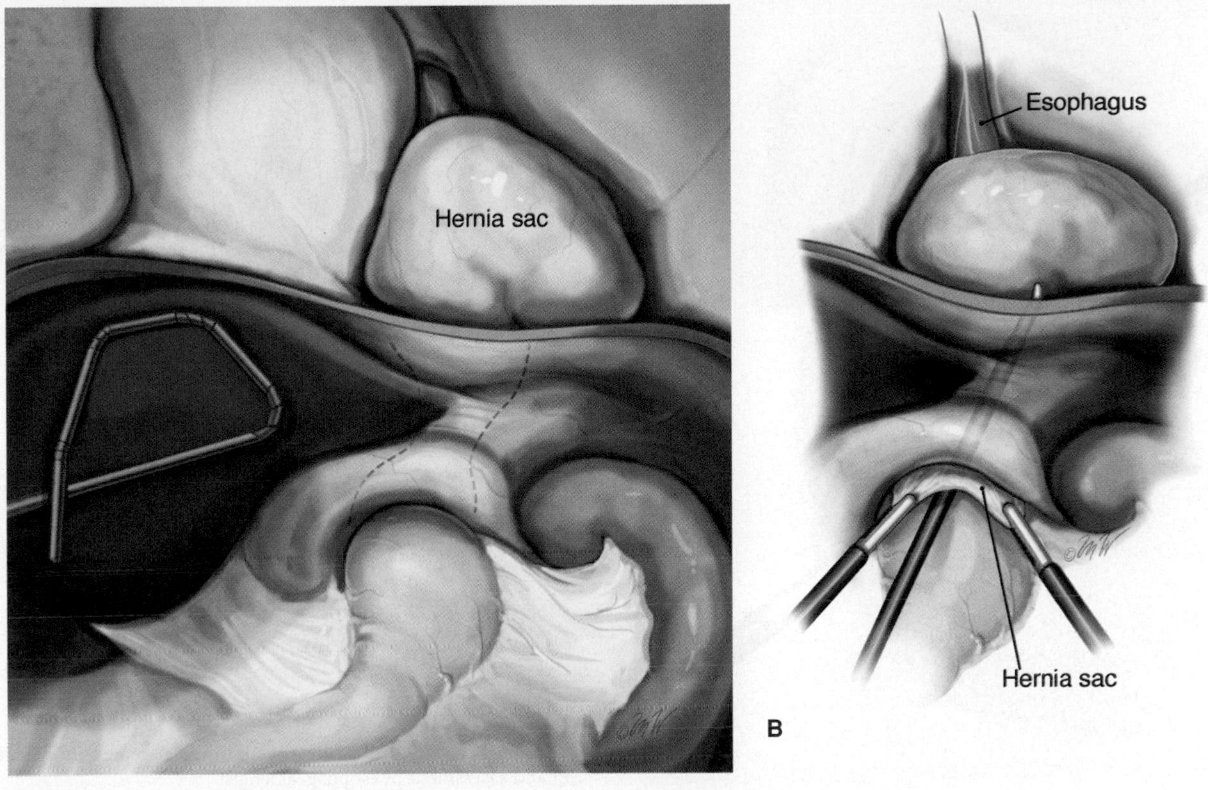

Figure 46-4. Reducing the hernia sac.

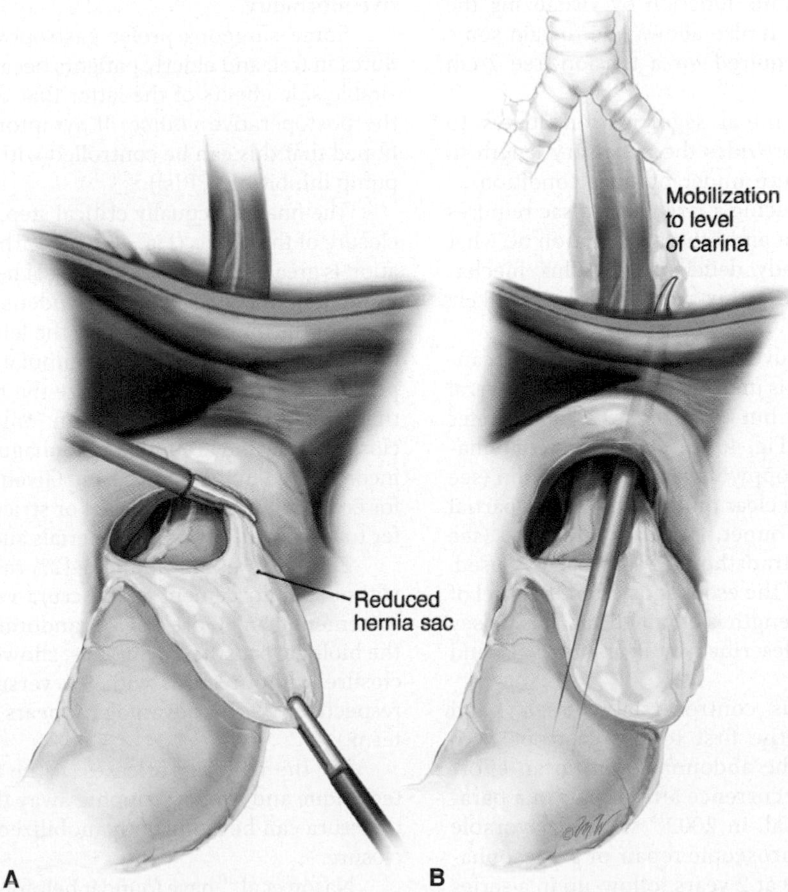

Figure 46-5. An intraperitoneal stomach is established after the hernia sac has been reduced.

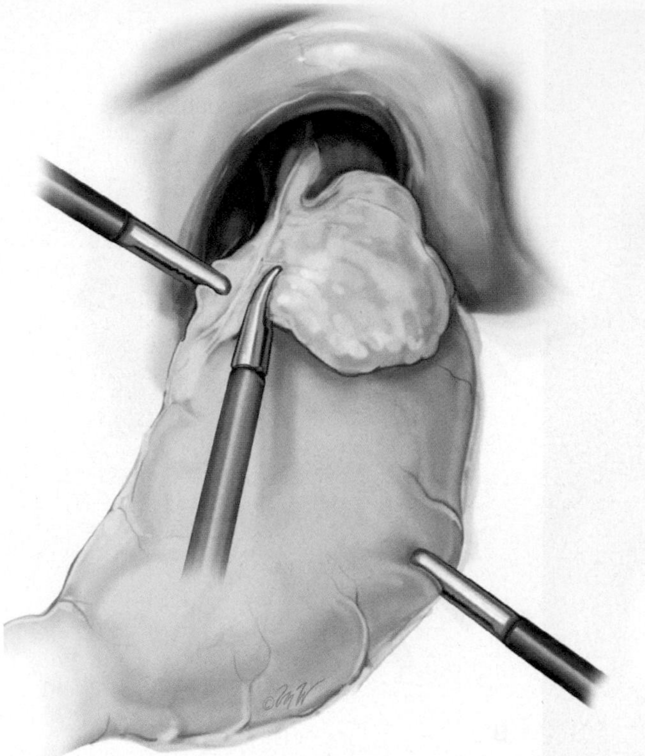

Figure 46-6. The esophageal fat pad is identified and mobilized at the GEJ.

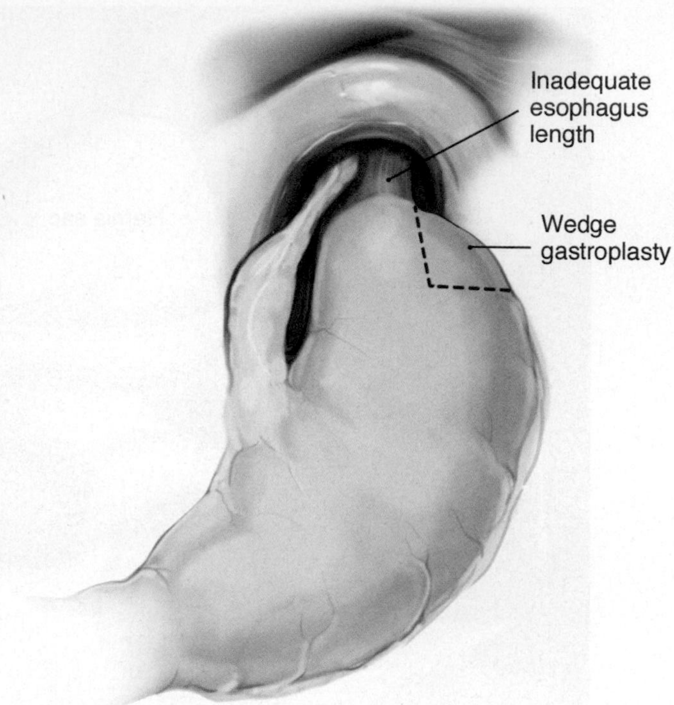

Figure 46-7. Complete mobilization of the fat pad permits visualization of GEJ and assessment of esophageal length.

vagus nerves (Fig. 46-6). This maneuver allows one to identify more precisely the true anatomic junction by visualizing the longitudinal esophageal fibers. It also allows one to gain some additional length, which is required for a tension-free 2-cm intra-abdominal length.

Although this intra-abdominal segment contributes to the antireflux barrier, it also provides the necessary length to perform an antireflux procedure under optimal conditions.[11] Indeed, given the fact that reducing a large hernia sac requires extensive esophageal dissection and causes disruption of, what is for most patients, an already deficient antireflux mechanism, significant postoperative reflux will be the most likely consequence.

If, despite all these maneuvers, the necessary 2 cm cannot be obtained, a gastroplasty is unavoidable. There are several ways to perform a gastroplasty, but today most surgeons prefer the wedge Collis gastroplasty (Fig. 46-7),[12] usually in combination with a 360-degree short floppy Nissen fundoplication (see Chapter 39). If the patient has a clear motility disorder, a partial fundoplication, for example, Toupet, is usually preferred (see Chapter 40). When an open transthoracic approach is used, and if, after full mobilization of the esophagus up to the level of the aortic arch, an insufficient length is obtained, a Collis Belsey gastroplasty is performed as described by Pearson et al.[7] and illustrated in Chapter 38.

The use of gastropexy is controversial. Nissen[13] and Boerema and Germs[14] were the first to use gastropexy to anchor the stomach against the abdominal wall in an effort to decrease the incidence of recurrence after repair of a paraesophageal hernia. Ponsky et al. in 2003[15] showed favorable results of gastropexy after laparoscopic repair of paraesophageal hernia with no recurrence at 2 years follow-up in a series of 28 patients. However, Larusson[16] found gastropexy to be one of the variables associated with an increase in postoperative morbidity.

Some surgeons prefer gastropexy over antireflux procedures in frail and elderly patients because of the potential undesirable side effects of the latter that eventually may jeopardize the postoperative course. If symptomatic reflux occurs, it is hoped that this can be controlled with medical therapy (proton pump inhibitors [PPIs]).

The final but equally critical step of this intervention is the closure of the hiatus (Fig. 46-8A,B). The risk for recurrent herniation is greater with paraesophageal hernia compared with Type I sliding hernia, because of the widening of the hiatus and weakening of the muscles, especially the left crus, caused by the large herniated stomach. This has stimulated some surgeons to use prosthetic materials to minimize the risk of recurrence.[17] Prosthetic material can be used as an "onlay mesh" draped over the closed pillars and around the esophagus or actually as a "curtain" incorporated in the hiatus itself. Given the presumed higher risk for erosion into the esophagus or stricture formation, most prefer to use Gore-Tex or biomaterials such as Surgisis.

Zaninotto et al.[18] found a 42% recurrence rate after repair without reinforcement of the crura versus 9% with mesh reinforcement using Gore-Tex. A randomized controlled trial using the biologic prosthesis, Surgisis, showed initial superiority over closure without mesh with 9% versus 24% recurrence rates, respectively.[19] This advantage appears to diminish over the long term.

For the majority of cases, if the surgeon uses meticulous technique and avoids stripping away the overlying peritoneum, the crura can be sufficiently mobilized to permit a tension-free closure.

Nason et al.[10] have found it helpful to create a pneumothorax on the left side by introducing a pigtail catheter. This results in a

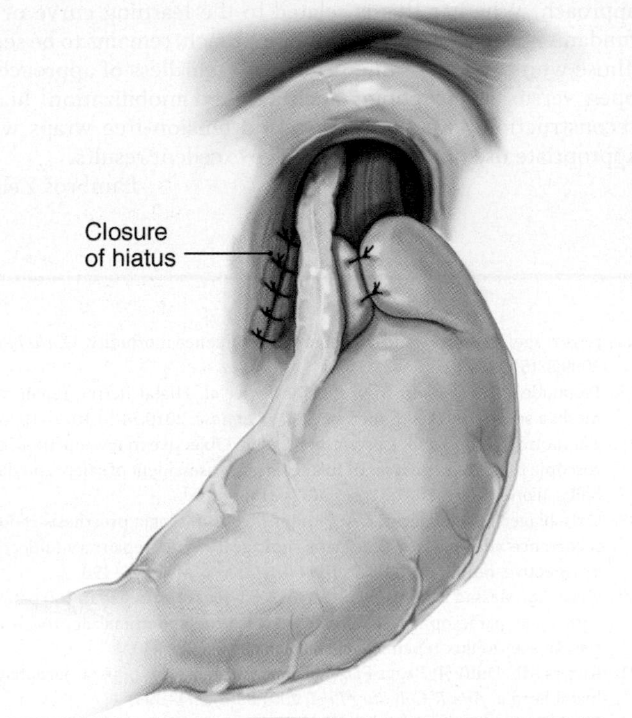

Figure 46-8. Tension-free hiatal closure.

laxity of the left pillar as the diaphragm becomes floppy. Usually three to four stitches will suffice, and to avoid too much anterior displacement, additional sutures in front of the esophagus may be necessary to obtain sufficient narrowing of the hiatus.

POSTOPERATIVE CARE

When the surgery is completed, most patients will be extubated without any difficulty and observed in the recovery room. However, depending on the comorbidities and/or advanced age, some patients may require transfer to the ICU for either a prolonged period of ventilation or further observation. Other aspects that may contribute to a possible admission to the ICU are nonelective technical difficulties at surgery, and/or prolonged duration of the surgery and blood loss.

In the series of 662 laparoscopic repairs published by Luketich et al.,[4] in 29% of the cases, the surgery lasted more than 260 minutes and about one in three patients was admitted to the ICU. These figures again reflect the difficult and complex nature of paraesophageal hernia repair.

If the postoperative course is uneventful, an upper gastrointestinal (GI) contrast study with water-soluble contrast is advised to exclude the possibility of a leak on the esophagus or at the wrap, as well as the possibility of an early intrathoracic recurrence. Small contained leaks can be managed by conservative treatment, that is, NPO and antibiotics for several days until the leak has been resolved on a control contrast study. Larger leaks reflecting a larger tear as well as recurrent herniation in the chest will require reintervention. Other possible reasons for early reintervention include wound infection, paraesophageal hematoma in the residual former hernia cavity, and empyema.

In the absence of leak or herniation on the contrast study, oral alimentation is resumed on postoperative day 1 starting with liquids and soft diet after the nasogastric tube has been removed. For some patients, however, it may take longer for the stomach to regain its peristaltic activity, resulting in prolonged drainage of large amounts of gastric contents via the nasogastric tube. Such patients need to be kept NPO or only sips of water and their nasogastric tube needs to be kept in place for several days until sufficient peristaltic activity has resumed and the gastric drainage level falls below 200 cc. When the postoperative course is uneventful, patients usually can be discharged on day 2 or 3.

PROCEDURE-SPECIFIC COMPLICATIONS

The most commonly encountered complication after hernia repair is dysphagia for solid foods. In most patients, this is a temporary phenomenon related to postoperative edema of the tissues resulting in a too tight wrap, but usually this will subside after 3 to 4 months. In the event of persistent dysphagia, Savary bougie, or eventually pneumatic dilatations, may become necessary to resolve the problem. In a few cases (1%–2%), redo surgery is needed to remediate the problem.[4]

A number of patients will suffer from reflux and in most of them lifelong medical therapy with PPIs will suffice to control the symptoms. In a few patients, redo surgery will be necessary but only after objective documentation of the reflux and its degree of severity.

Further long-term follow-up with quality-of-life questionnaires is advocated by most authors, such as the SF-56 (a commonly used general measure of health-related quality of life) and the Gastrointestinal Quality of Life Index (GIQLI). Over time, a risk of recurrent symptoms as well as recurrent hernia has been documented. Anatomical recurrence has been noted in 10% to 30% according to the literature, but fortunately, most of these are small and asymptomatic.

Other more rare procedure-related complications include gas bloating, postvagotomy diarrhea or dumping, and small bowel herniation in the chest causing obstruction.

OUTCOME

Numerous articles have been published about the surgical repair of paraesophageal hernia.[20–31] The durability of the surgical repair is difficult to assess, as a consequence of inconsistent reporting of follow-up intervals and/or lack of objective data. In most published series, the follow-up interval is rather short. Some papers describe symptom control only, whereas others combine symptomatic outcome with objective assessments such as endoscopy, barium swallow, 24-hour pH monitoring, and manometry. Some studies focus solely on the incidence of anatomic recurrence. In general, open surgery, which is usually performed via transthoracic approach, produces good-to-excellent long-term results in 85% to 99% of patients, with a median follow-up of 2 to 4 years. Laparoscopic repair is associated with a higher rate of anatomic recurrence (15%–40%), but for the most part, these recurrences remain asymptomatic. Patients repaired laparoscopically rarely experience reincarceration, and if the patient does experience gastroesophageal reflux postoperatively, it is generally well managed by PPI therapy. Consequently, the incidence of reoperation with paraesophageal hernia repair is low (3%–4%) even with the laparoscopic approach. Clearly, longer and better follow-up reports are needed to assess the true success rate of surgery for these complex hernias, and definitely these problems should be dealt with by expert surgeons.

EDITOR'S COMMENT

Laparoscopic surgery has revolutionized the field of hiatal hernia management and has increased the volume of cases referred to surgeons. There is still some concern about long-term recurrence, which some series have noted with the laparoscopic approach. Whether this is related to the learning curve or to fundamental shortcomings of this approach, remains to be seen. Those who apply the same principles regardless of approach—open versus laparoscopic—such as good mobilization, hiatal reconstruction with buttressing, and tension-free wraps with appropriate use of gastroplasty, have excellent results.

—Lambros Zellos

References

1. Skinner DB, Belsey RH. Surgical management of esophageal reflux and hiatus hernia. Long-term results with 1,030 patients. *J Thorac Cardiovasc Surg.* 1967;53(1):33–54.
2. Allen MS, Trastek VF, Deschamps C, et al. Intrathoracic stomach. Presentation and results of operation. *J Thorac Cardiovasc Surg.* 1993;105(2):253–258; discussion 8–9.
3. Stylopoulos N, Gazelle GS, Rattner DW. Paraesophageal hernias: operation or observation? *Ann Surg.* 2002;236(4):492–500; discussion 500–501.
4. Luketich JD, Raja S, Fernando HC, et al. Laparoscopic repair of giant paraesophageal hernia: 100 consecutive cases. *Ann Surg.* 2000;232(4):608–618.
5. Bawahab M, Mitchell P, Church N, et al. Management of acute paraesophageal hernia. *Surg Endosc.* 2009;23(2):255–259.
6. Poulose BK, Gosen C, Marks JM, et al. Inpatient mortality analysis of paraesophageal hernia repair in octogenarians. *J Gastrointest Surg.* 2008;12(11):1888–1892.
7. Maziak DE, Todd TR, Pearson FG. Massive hiatus hernia: evaluation and surgical management. *J Thorac Cardiovasc Surg.* 1998;115(1):53–60; discussion 1–2.
8. Walther B, DeMeester TR, Lafontaine E, et al. Effect of paraesophageal hernia on sphincter function and its implication on surgical therapy. *Am J Surg.* 1984;147(1):111–116.
9. Watson DI, Davies N, Devitt PG, et al. Importance of dissection of the hernial sac in laparoscopic surgery for large hiatal hernias. *Arch Surg.* 1999;134(10):1069–1073.
10. Nason KS, Luketich JD, Witteman BP, et al. The laparoscopic approach to paraesophageal hernia repair. *J Gastrointest Surg.* 2012;16(2):417–426.
11. DeMeester TR, Wernly JA, Bryant GH, et al. Clinical and in vitro analysis of determinants of gastroesophageal competence. A study of the principles of antireflux surgery. *Am J Surg.* 1979;137(1):39–46.
12. Collis JL. An operation for hiatus hernia with short esophagus. *J Thorac Surg.* 1957;34(6):768–773; discussion 74–78.
13. Nissen R. Gastropexy as the lone procedure in the surgical repair of hiatus hernia. *Am J Surg.* 1956;92(3):389–392.
14. Boerema I. Hiatus hernia: repair by right-sided, subhepatic, anterior gastropexy. *Surgery.* 1969;65:884–893.
15. Ponsky J, Rosen M, Fanning A, et al. Anterior gastropexy may reduce the recurrence rate after laparoscopic paraesophageal hernia repair. *Surg Endosc.* 2003;17(7):1036–1041.
16. Larusson HJ, Zingg U, Hahnloser D, et al. Predictive factors for morbidity and mortality in patients undergoing laparoscopic paraesophageal hernia repair: age, ASA score and operation type influence morbidity. *World J Surg.* 2009;33(5):980–985.
17. Frantzides CT, Carlson MA, Loizides S, et al. Hiatal hernia repair with mesh: a survey of SAGES members. *Surg Endosc.* 2010;24(5):1017–1024.
18. Zaninotto G, Portale G, Costantini M, et al. Objective follow-up after laparoscopic repair of large type III hiatal hernia. Assessment of safety and durability. *World J Surg.* 2007;31(11):2177–2183.
19. Oelschlager BK, Pellegrini CA, Hunter J, et al. Biologic prosthesis reduces recurrence after laparoscopic paraesophageal hernia repair: a multicenter, prospective, randomized trial. *Ann Surg.* 2006;244(4):481–490.
20. Geha AS, Massad MG, Snow NJ, et al. A 32-year experience in 100 patients with giant paraesophageal hernia: the case for abdominal approach and selective antireflux repair. *Surgery.* 2000;128(4):623–630.
21. Rogers ML, Duffy JP, Beggs FD, et al. Surgical treatment of para-oesophageal hiatal hernia. *Ann R Coll Surg Engl.* 2001;83(6):394–398.
22. Patel HJ, Tan BB, Yee J, et al. A 25-year experience with open primary transthoracic repair of paraesophageal hiatal hernia. *J Thorac Cardiovasc Surg.* 2004;127(3):843–849.
23. Low DE, Unger T. Open repair of paraesophageal hernia: reassessment of subjective and objective outcomes. *Ann Thorac Surg.* 2005;80(1):287–294.
24. McLean TR, Haller CC, Lowry S. The need for flexibility in the operative management of type III paraesophageal hernias. *Am J Surg.* 2006;192(5):e32–e36.
25. Yano F, Stadlhuber RJ, Tsuboi K, et al. Outcomes of surgical treatment of intrathoracic stomach. *Dis Esophagus.* 2009;22(3):284–288.
26. Aly A, Munt J, Jamieson GG, et al. Laparoscopic repair of large hiatal hernias. *Br J Surg.* 2005;92(5):648–653.
27. Gangopadhyay N, Perrone JM, Soper NJ, et al. Outcomes of laparoscopic paraesophageal hernia repair in elderly and high-risk patients. *Surgery.* 2006;140(4):491–498; discussion 498–499.
28. Morino M, Giaccone C, Pellegrino L, et al. Laparoscopic management of giant hiatal hernia: factors influencing long-term outcome. *Surg Endosc.* 2006;20(7):1011–1016.
29. Boushey RP, Moloo H, Burpee S, et al. Laparoscopic repair of paraesophageal hernias: a Canadian experience. *Can J Surg.* 2008;51(5):355–360.
30. Hazebroek EJ, Ganandha S, Koak Y, et al. Laparoscopic paraesophageal hernia repair: quality of life outcomes in the elderly. *Dis Esophagus.* 2008;21(8):737–741.
31. White BC, Jeansonne LO, Morgenthal CB, et al. Do recurrences after paraesophageal hernia repair matter?: ten-year follow-up after laparoscopic repair. *Surg Endosc.* 2008;22(4):1107–1111.

PART 6

ESOPHAGEAL TRAUMA

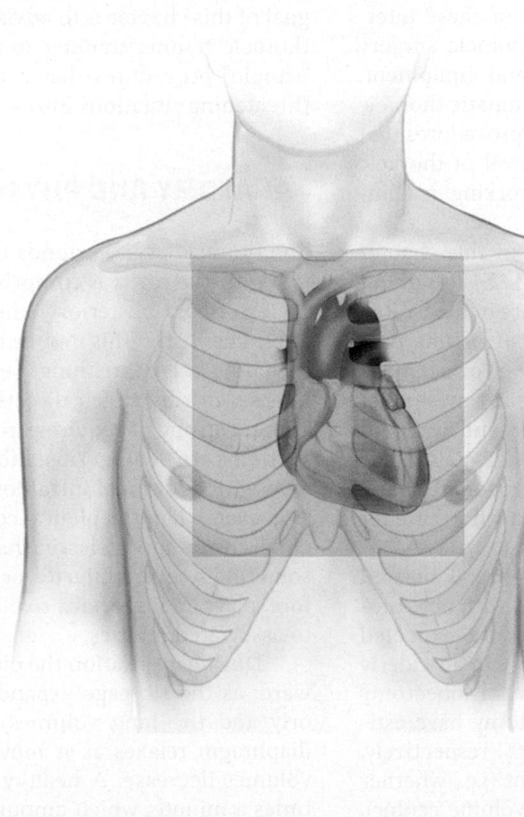

47 Treating Traumatic Chest Injuries in a Limited Resource Setting

Abraham Lebenthal and Urs von Holzen

Keywords: Blunt and penetrating injuries, tension pneumothorax, airway obstruction, pericardial tamponade, chest tube

Trauma is the leading cause of death in individuals between the ages of 1 and 44. In the Western world, motor vehicle accidents account for the majority of these deaths. In a post 9/11 world, it is difficult to argue that practicing thoracic surgeons should not attain a core level of competency in advanced trauma life support techniques. Traumatic injuries are categorized as blunt, penetrating, or caustic. Surgical techniques for blunt and penetrating esophageal trauma are described in Chapters 48 and 49. Corrosive esophageal injury is discussed in Chapter 50. This chapter concerns the management of blunt and penetrating chest injury in an emergent setting, whether in the field, at a disaster relief facility, a community hospital, or other rural setting, where the thoracic surgeon may be called upon to help manage an acute patient with traumatic thoracic injuries.

Morbidity and mortality from thoracic injuries may be categorized as immediate, within minutes to hours, and late. Pattern recognition and aggressive early treatment are crucial to saving lives, and early proactive interventions can significantly improve immediate and late outcomes. Many of these interventions are considered routine in modern thoracic surgery practice, but require a high level of training and equipment. This chapter reviews the pathophysiology of traumatic thoracic injury and presents some urgent and emergent procedures that can be performed by providers with a basic level of thoracic surgery training and associated competencies working in a limited resource setting.

The principles and procedures described in this chapter follow the Advanced Trauma Life Support (ATLS) Program.[1] Over the past decades, the delivery of trauma care in the United States has greatly benefited by the development of this program, as well as by the development of a system for accrediting regional level I trauma centers. A level 1 facility must meet certain objective parameters of service, expertise, and availability of resources. Unfortunately, the majority of hospitals in the United States remain unaccredited for trauma care or are designated at the lowest level (III). Nevertheless, the need to care for trauma victims at less than a level I setting persists.

Most general thoracic surgical procedures are associated with a higher morbidity and mortality compared with non-thoracic surgical procedures. In the United States, the expected mortality from multiple rib fractures is 3% to 5% in an elderly patient, compared with the estimated mortality for lobectomy of 1% to 5%. Pneumonectomy and esophagectomy have estimated mortalities of 4% to 20% and 2% to 20%, respectively, and all of these values are experience-dependent (i.e., whether the treatment is performed at a high- vs. low-volume center). Hence, successful complex general thoracic procedures should be performed by an experienced team, with expertise in perioperative management, in a well-equipped and well-staffed operating facility. These include, but are not limited to, a surgeon with general thoracic experience; an anesthesia team familiar with one-lung ventilation and epidural anesthesia for pain control; blood bank capabilities; chest imaging; continuous pulse oximetry; oxygen supplementation; intensive as well as intermediate care units; dedicated nursing and physical therapy, as well as respiratory therapy.

The fundamentals of attaining good patient outcomes include accuracy of diagnosis, volume restriction before, during, and after the surgical procedure, excellent pain control, and early ambulation. *Volume restriction is critical to preventing right heart failure for which there is no effective treatment.* Pain control in the perioperative period is critical to encouraging cough, which aids clearance of secretions to prevent atelectasis and pneumonia, both major causes of postoperative morbidity and mortality.

Therefore, when working in the field or a community hospital with an inexperienced team, poor support systems, and limited resources, major thoracic procedures should only be performed when no other therapeutic option is available. The goal of this chapter is to advise the surgeon with minimal or no thoracic trauma training to recognize "patterns" and identify "simple" procedures that can be used to convert urgent life-threatening situations into salvageable and stable conditions.

ANATOMY AND PHYSIOLOGY

The thoracic cavity extends from the thoracic inlet to the diaphragm. The cavity is comprised of 12 ribs anchored to the thoracic vertebra posteriorly and the sternum and costochondral angle anteriorly. This mobile bony cage protects vital structures including the heart, lungs, esophagus, and great vessels. The first seven ribs attach directly to the sternum. The first rib is flat and strong: it requires great force to fracture. The 11th and 12th ribs are floating ribs. Rib fractures in adults can be associated with additional intrathoracic injuries such as lung contusion even when the pleural covering is intact. The ribs of small children are more elastic than adults and thus moderate and sometimes severe injuries occur without fracture. Age, therefore, plays an important role in recognizing patterns that point to associated injuries.

During inspiration the diaphragm contracts moving downward; as the rib cage expands, the sternum is pushed anteriorly and the lung volumes increase. During expiration the diaphragm relaxes as it moves up the rib cage and the lung volumes decrease. A healthy adult breathes approximately 12 times a minute, which amounts to about 17,280 breaths a day. The respiratory rate typically increases with injury. Thus, a disturbance of the respiratory mechanics by trauma, iatrogenic injury, or other reason is a major source of thoracic morbidity and mortality. This is fully addressed in the sections on rib fractures and postoperative pain management below.

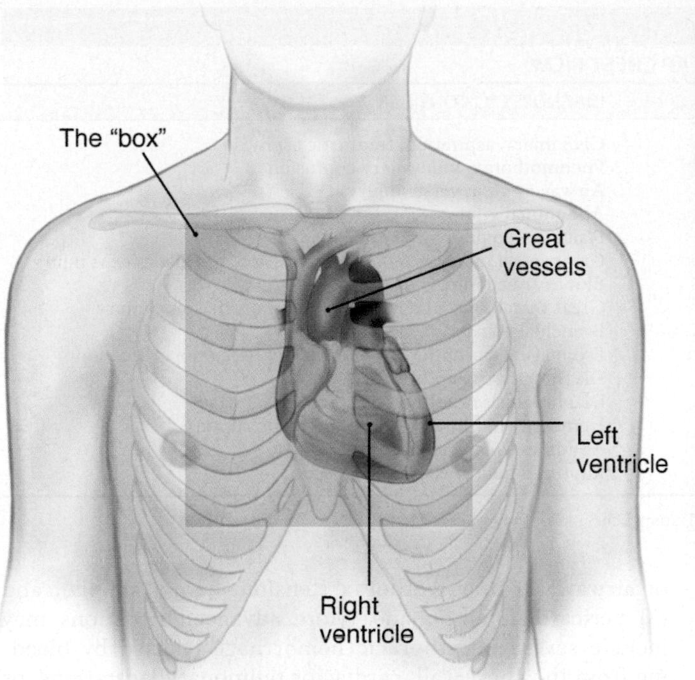

Figure 47-1. The heart surrounded by pericardium and great vessels is found in the middle of the mediastinum. The right ventricle is anterior and thus more susceptible than left ventricle during trauma. The posterior mediastinum contains the esophagus and vertebra. In penetrating trauma, an injury to the central area (between the nipples); referred to as "the box," should trigger a low threshold for surgical exploration.

The trachea enters the thoracic inlet anterior to the esophagus. In a normal adult, it is approximately 12 cm in length. The carina lies directly behind the angle of Louis. The proximal third can be easily accessed from the neck, the distal third is best accessed from the right chest, while the middle third is difficult to reach and is best accessed with sternotomy. The left mainstem bronchus is 4 cm long and has an acute angle from the carina; it lies between the aortic arch and the pulmonary artery.

During surgery, the anesthesiologist prepares the patient for one-lung ventilation with collapse of the operative lung. This is critical to facilitating a workspace during chest surgery. Additionally, while the lung is collapsed, the blood flows preferentially to the opposite lung, thereby increasing the overall oxygenation of blood during surgery. This physiologic shunting is also important for decreasing the blood loss during surgical procedures on the unventilated lung.

Any injury to the central mediastinal area, often referred to as the "box" (Fig. 47-1), should trigger a low threshold for surgical exploration. It is prudent to remember that young healthy adults have great cardiopulmonary reserve. In the setting of serious trauma, the young adult often may appear to be remarkably "stable," their body compensating for the injury, only to suddenly collapse and rapidly die.

DIAGNOSTIC IMAGING

Ultrasound, chest x-ray, fluoroscopy, and chest computed tomography (CT) may be the only imaging modalities available.

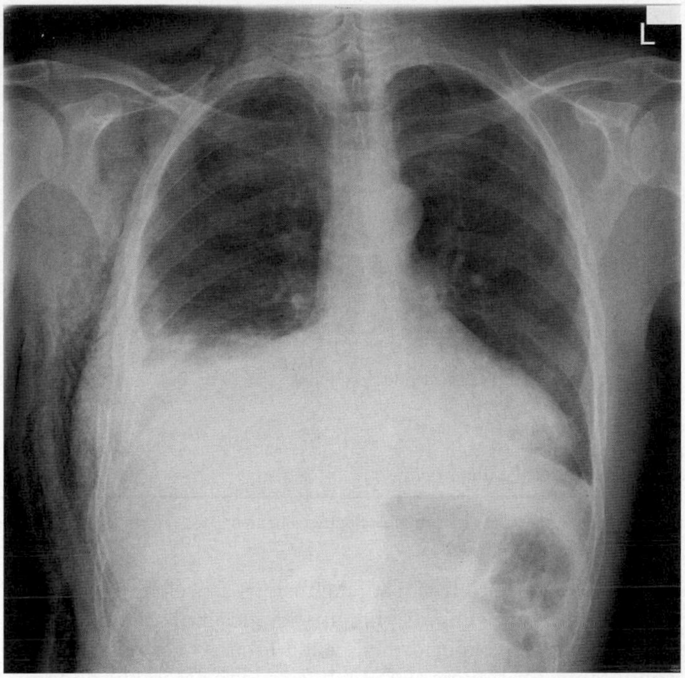

Figure 47-2. Chest x-ray showing partial whiteout of the chest signifying hemothorax in a patient with right-sided trauma. The chest x-ray shows a large right effusion with partial whiteout, subcutaneous emphysema and multiple rib fractures.

Plain Chest Films

The chest x-ray has been used since 1895 to diagnose diseases of the chest (Fig. 47-2). It is useful for assessing the lungs, heart, chest wall, diaphragm, major vessels, and spinal column as well as soft tissue. The lungs can be assessed for nodules or masses, cavitary lesions, and pleural and pericardial effusions. Additionally, it enables assessment of the great vessels, mediastinal structures, and chest wall. Typically, two types of exams exist:

- The *PA and lateral* exam consists of two x-rays; the PA or posteroanterior view, where the patient faces the x-ray film, and the lateral view where the patient is turned sideways. Having two views enables more precise recognition and localization of abnormalities. When only a PA view is available, consideration of anatomic landmarks, such as fissures and selective obscuration of anatomic structures, may be adequate for localizing pathology.
- The pleural cavity is examined for pneumo- or hemothorax, with attention to deepening or blunting of the costophrenic angles. The heart and pericardium are assessed for contour; a large contour may be a sign of hemopericardium. Next, the position of the diaphragm is evaluated and the abdominal cavity is examined for free intraperitoneal air and the aeration of the abdominal contents. The bony structures are examined for fracture. The mediastinum is assessed for size as are the great vessel notches and air (Table 47-1).

Ultrasonography

Ultrasound has limited utility in the chest because ultrasonic waves are interrupted by air in the lung. The amplification of ultrasound passing through fluid, however, can provide

Table 47-1

DIAGNOSTIC CONSIDERATIONS ASSOCIATED WITH FINDINGS ON AP CHEST FILM[a]

FINDINGS	DIAGNOSES TO CONSIDER
Respiratory distress without x-ray findings	CNS injury, aspiration, traumatic asphyxia
Any rib fracture	Pneumothorax, pulmonary contusion
Fracture first 3 ribs or sternoclavicular fracture-dislocation	Airway or great vessel injury
Fracture lower ribs 9–12	Abdominal injury
Two or more rib fractures in 2 or more places	Flail chest, pulmonary contusion
Scapular fracture	Great vessel injury, pulmonary contusion, brachial plexus injury
Sternal fracture	Blunt cardiac injury
Mediastinal widening	Great vessel injury, sternal fracture, thoracic spine injury
Persistent large pneumothorax or air leak after chest tube insertion	Bronchial tear
Mediastinal air	Esophageal disruption, tracheal injury, pneumoperitoneum
GI gas pattern in the chest (loculated air)	Diaphragmatic rupture
NG tube in the chest	Diaphragmatic rupture or ruptured esophagus
Air–fluid level in the chest	Hemopneumothorax or diaphragmatic rupture
Disrupted diaphragm	Abdominal visceral injury
Free air under the diaphragm	Ruptured hollow abdominal viscus

[a]This table summarizes radiographic findings and associated injuries from Advanced Trauma Life Support Program for Doctors.[1]

superior visualization of pleural effusions as well as physiologic information regarding diaphragmatic and cardiac function. In trauma, a study is performed called focused assessment with sonography for trauma (FAST). It is used to assess the abdominal cavity and the pericardium for the presence of blood. The pericardial window is the most sensitive window for blood around the heart. Furthermore, a skilled examiner can also find air or blood in the costophrenic angle as mentioned above.

Fluoroscopy

Fluoroscopy is useful for assessing the esophagus, great vessels, and the diaphragm. Fluoroscopy is a dynamic examination and therefore provides information about the function of the organs examined.

Computed Tomography

CT is the standard examination for chest pathologies today. If available, a chest CT (especially with 3D reconstruction) in a stable patient can accurately diagnose and determine the extent of a traumatic chest injury and is useful for surgical planning.

Management of Thoracic Trauma

When assessing treatment options, triage is critical. The decision to treat or transfer a patient should be based on the provider's level of experience, resources available, and the availability and accessibility to more specialized care. When possible, the immediate emphasis should be on "damage control" as opposed to definitive care. Whenever possible, damage control can and should be expediently performed for life-threatening injuries (e.g., tension pneumothorax) that can be safely and successfully converted to a stable non-life-threatening condition. For other conditions, it may be best to stabilize locally and then transfer the patient to a level I trauma center where he/she can receive a higher level of care.

Thoracic trauma is a significant cause of immediate and delayed patient mortality. There are two major types of thoracic trauma: blunt and penetrating trauma. In contrast to other diseases encountered by a general surgeon, reaction time and pattern recognition are critical for obtaining optimal outcomes.

Basic life-threatening injuries that should be recognized and converted to stable conditions are: (1) loss or obstruction of airway, (2) pneumothorax (tension, hemo, simple), and (3) pericardial tamponade. More advanced situations may include severe intrathoracic hemorrhage (caused by bleeding from the chest wall, cardiac or pulmonary lacerations, or injury to the great vessels). Some injuries like those to the great vessels, especially in the setting of limited resources, might be unsalvageable; whereas a simple laceration of the right ventricle may be easily repaired. Thus, in a minimal resource setting, triage should account for surgical expertise, facilities, equipment, and support needed to salvage the patient. Few patients with thoracic trauma will require a thoracotomy (<10% for blunt injuries, 15%–30% for penetrating injuries). In general, blunt trauma causes more extensive injuries that are harder to repair, while penetrating trauma (especially a stab wound) is easier to repair.

Chest trauma typically leads to lung injury (i.e., contusion, consolidation, and atelectasis) and disruption of chest wall mechanics (i.e., rib fractures, diaphragmatic injuries, muscle contusions, and pain). Over time, this can lead to a vicious cycle of hypoxia, hypercarbia, and acidosis. The majority of patients who suffer from thoracic trauma and reach a medical care facility alive can be managed with small lifesaving interventions. Examples include: (1) surgical airway, (2) tube thoracostomy, and (3) pericardial window. These simple interventions are easy to master and can convert an unstable patient with a life-threatening injury to a stable patient. The late sequelae of chest trauma, particularly rib fracture, lung contusion, and pneumonia, are associated with late preventable deaths in many trauma victims.

The management of thoracic trauma focuses on the principles taught by the ATLS Program for Doctors.[1] The ABC (airway–breathing–circulation) priority is universally important: establishing and maintaining a patent airway, ensuring breathing (i.e., relief of pneumothorax, tension pneumothorax, hemothorax) with external ventilatory support as needed, and aiding circulation (i.e., hemorrhage control, volume resuscitation, relief of tamponade, etc.). Hypoxia is the most serious result of chest injury. It can be due to loss of airway or altered breathing and must be treated immediately. Patients with chest trauma should be examined according to ATLS guidelines:

1. Primary survey
2. Resuscitation and vitals

3. Secondary survey
4. Definitive care

Blunt trauma frequently occurs as a result of motor vehicle accidents and falls. The mechanism of injury and time elapsed will shed light on the severity of the injury as well as the organs likely affected. On examination, the patient's vital signs (pulse, blood pressure, and respiratory rate) and mental status will give an indication of the severity of injury. On physical examination, the trachea should be central in the neck. If the trachea is deviated, pneumothorax should be suspected. The rib cage is examined by pressing along the ribs bilaterally. If a step, instability, or tenderness is found, fractures are suspected. Subcutaneous emphysema, rib fractures, or hemodynamic instability suggest significant injury to the lung (e.g., contusion), possible pneumothorax, and possible significant hemothorax. The lungs as well as heart are auscultated. If the respiratory sounds are distant or nonexistent in one hemithorax or region, a pneumothorax or hemothorax should be suspected. If the patient has distant heart sounds, a narrow pulse pressure, and distended neck veins, a cardiac tamponade should be suspected. It is important to remember that anoxia (and shock) will lead to anxiety, combative behavior, and confusion, which must be managed appropriately by treating the underlying cause and by administering supplemental oxygen, thereby improving oxygenation. Additionally, it is important to remember that patients can exsanguinate into the chest cavity. For all injuries that occur in the field, the question of need for antibiotic coverage should be addressed, as well as tetanus vaccination status and need for vaccination.

URGENT SURGICAL EMERGENCIES AND SOLUTIONS

Airway

A secure airway must be established swiftly to prevent brain damage from hypoxia (Fig. 47-3).

Foreign-Body Removal

Ingestion of a foreign body is a common life-threatening condition. When a foreign body is lodged within the trachea or bronchial tree proximal to the carina, the patient presents with labored breathing associated with dyspnea and/or fixed wheezing (on inspiration and expiration). This most typically is found in the toddler population as a result of foreign-body aspiration. When the occlusion is complete, it can result in rapid demise leading to respiratory arrest. The initial treatment is to dislodge the object by delivering a succession of forceful blows to the back (i.e., palm slaps between the scapulae) or a Heimlich maneuver (i.e., physician stands behind the patient with fist pressed deeply on epigastrium to induce a rapid increase in intrathoracic pressure which causes the foreign body to dislodge so that it can be coughed up by the patient).

Rigid Bronchoscopy

If these maneuvers fail and the provider is experienced in rigid bronchoscopy, an attempt can be made to remove the object bronchoscopically. Position the patient with his/her head at the edge of the bed, and then anesthetize intravenously with an anesthetic agent such as ketamine. Insert the rigid bronchoscope (a straight hollow tube with light source) perpendicular to the mouth and tongue elevating the epiglottis. Then perform a full extension of the head and cannulation of the trachea. Advance the scope gently into the trachea; the foreign body can be removed piecemeal using a grasper or it can be pushed into the scope and then removed with the scope. If neither is possible, and complete obstruction occurs, the foreign body can be pushed distally into a mainstem bronchus to enable ventilation of one lung, thereby stabilizing the patient.

During rigid bronchoscopy, care must be taken not to break any teeth. Adequate relaxation is crucial. This is a technically demanding procedure that should be performed only by those with proper training or when no other solution exists for reestablishing an airway. In the stable patient, soft tissue x-rays of the neck may aid in viewing a foreign body in the airway.

Caution: When a foreign body causes incomplete occlusion of the trachea and cannot be dislodged by simple noninvasive means and the surgeon is inexperienced in rigid bronchoscopy or does not have the necessary instruments or materials, it may be easier and safer to perform tracheostomy and then apply suction to remove the object through the stoma as described below.

Jet Ventilation

If attempts to remove a foreign body or establish a secure airway are unsuccessful, jet ventilation can be used as a temporary

The airway must be reestablished expediently to prevent permanent brain damage.

a) Anatomy: Oropharynx, larynx, and trachea.
b) Presentation: Variable but can include trauma to the above-named anatomical structures, aspiration (foreign body or gastrointestinal contents) or neurologic injury.
c) Signs and symptoms: Stridor, inability to phonate, peripheral, and then central cyanosis, combative behavior, coma, absence of breath sounds, pulmonary followed by cardiac arrest.
d) Remedy: Immediate reestablishment of airway patency.
    a. Clearing (suction or removal) of oral secretions.
    b. Chin lift or jaw thrust maneuver.
    c. Pull out tongue and insert oral airway.
    d. Intubation (oral or nasal) with endotracheal tube.
    e. Surgical airway: Rigid bronchoscopy and removal of foreign body, direct tracheal cannulation (cricothyroidotomy vs. tracheostomy), tracheal laceration, and repair. Injury to oropharynx, larynx, or trachea preventing maintenance of patent airway by less invasive means (a–d covered in detail elsewhere in this text).

Figure 47-3. Airway.

treatment until a secure airway is established. A needle or IV catheter is placed through the cricothyroid membrane and high flow oxygen is administered.

Direct Tracheal Cannulation

Cricothyroidotomy Cricothyroidotomy is performed by opening an urgent surgical airway through the cricothyroid cartilage. This is the quickest, safest, and least technically demanding procedure for relieving a proximal airway obstruction and reestablishing a surgical airway. The cricothyroid cartilage lies anteriorly between the larynx and the first tracheal ring. It is easy to palpate. Pressure in this region causes discomfort. This is the most cranial portion of the trachea. It is also the narrowest portion of the trachea. Cricothyroidotomy should not be performed in children younger than the age of 8 years unless no other option is available, because the first tracheal ring is a complete cartilage ring. Cricothyroidotomy above this level can lead to long-term disability secondary to stricture. Prior to procedure, if possible, the patient should be preoxygenated using a bag mask with jaw maneuver and concentrated oxygen if available.

Equipment needed: #11 blade, endotracheal or tracheotomy tube. Pulse oximetry is suggested. If oximetry is not available, the surgeon must remember that central cyanosis (seen with lip discoloration) correlates with a saturation level <85% in whites but may not be detected until SO_2 drops below 75% in patients with dark skin. Ambo-bag and suction.

Positioning: If the cervical spine has been cleared of injury, a shoulder roll (or 1 L IV fluid bag) is placed horizontally between the scapulae, the patient is positioned supine, and the neck is fully extended. If the cervical spine has not been cleared, the procedure is performed with in-line stabilization.

Procedure: The region of the cricothyroid membrane is avascular. Typically, there is little between the skin and the membrane. A 1 cm vertical midline incision is made in the skin and carried down to the trachea. The cricothyroid membrane is identified and incised horizontally, the stoma is dilated, and the cricothyroidotomy cannula is inserted through the stoma. The cannula is then fixed to the skin using multiple sutures. This procedure has been performed in field situations with improvised means such as using a jack-knife to make the hole and then inserting a car key horizontally and then vertically to stent open the trachea, or using a pen to stab into the cricothyroid ring and then removing the ink carrying cartridge to establish the airway.

Tracheostomy A tracheostomy is a stoma or opening of the trachea that enables direct ventilation, by bypassing the oropharynx, larynx, and proximal trachea. It is the classical approach for acute access to a proximally obstructed airway, or chronic access for long-term ventilatory support, pulmonary toilet, or bypass of a proximal tumor or stricture. A tracheostomy can be performed on individuals of all ages. In the event of prior surgery for a head and neck tumor, where a proximal surgical resection is performed and the proximal trachea is resected, a tracheostoma can be performed in the lower neck or chest. This may require tracheal release maneuvers and is beyond the scope of this chapter. Pitfalls of tracheostomy include loss of airway, injury to posterior membranous wall and or esophagus, tracheo-innominate fistula.

The procedure can be performed at the bedside or in an operating room.

Equipment needed includes: a knife, surgical sutures, needle driver, retractors (two Army–Navy retractors) (Fig. 47-4), a curved snap, a tracheal dilator (or instrument for this purpose), an Ambo-bag, suction, a pulse oximeter (preferred), and tracheostomy cannula. Sterile drapes, antiseptic wash, bovie coagulator, or silver nitrate sticks.

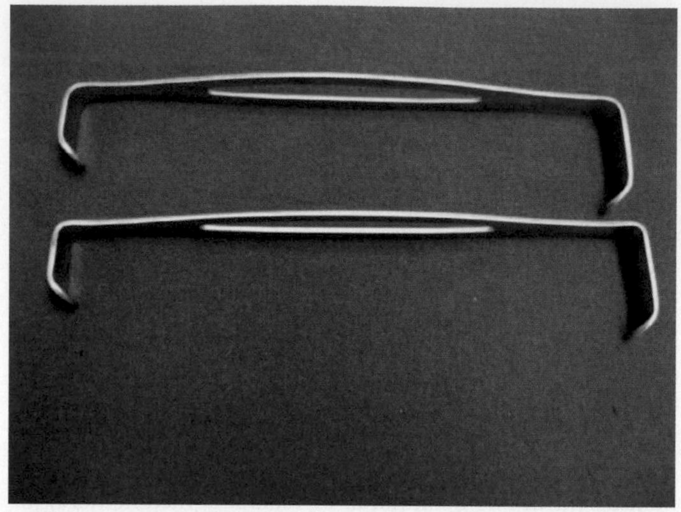

Figure 47-4. Army–Navy retractors.

The tracheostomy cannula will usually be cuffed and have a removable cleanable inner cannula. For the average adult, an internal diameter of 8 is adequate; the normal length would be approximately 8 cm. The inner size of the tube should be similar to that of an endotracheal tube. This can be estimated by comparing it to the diameter of the patient's pinky finger. If a tracheostomy tube is not available, an endotracheal tube can be cut above the balloon insufflation tubing and then used as a cannula. The balloon should be tested by inflation and then pressure to assess proper function prior to starting the procedure.

Positioning: see *Cricothyroidotomy*

Procedure: The neck and upper chest are prepped and draped as is customary. A 1.5-cm incision is made one finger breadth above the sternal notch. This incision can be vertical or horizontal. My preference is horizontal. The skin, the subcutaneous tissue, and the platysma are divided. The long blades of the Army–Navy retractors are now inserted to retract the tissue. The median raphe is divided in the avascular plane. The retractor blades are advanced to retract the strap muscles. The trachea is visualized and elevated by toeing in and pulling up on the retractors. The isthmus of the thyroid is elevated off the trachea to avoid damage to the inferior thyroid vein. Alternatively, the isthmus can be divided, and the vessel ligated. The third tracheal ring is identified. In the event that the patient is being ventilated with a high FiO_2, the FiO_2 is now decreased to less than 40 to prevent airway fire. An anterior portion of the third tracheal ring is resected. Hemostasis is performed using the Bovie or silver nitrate. The tracheostomy is dilated and the tracheostomy tube is inserted. The balloon is inflated, and the patient is ventilated through the newly placed cannula. Meticulous hemostasis is performed; the tube is sutured in place. Ideally, flexible bronchoscopy is performed to confirm correct placement of the cannula (Table 47-2).

Breathing

Breathing must be reestablished expediently to prevent permanent brain damage and respiratory as well as circulatory arrest (Fig. 47-5).

Table 47-2

PITFALLS OF TRACHEOSTOMY

PITFALL	RISK CAN BE REDUCED OR PREVENTED BY
Loss of patent airway	Ensuring good exposure (avoidance of blood vessels, midline dissection, meticulous hemostasis, adherence to anatomical planes of dissection), and proper insertion of cannula to avoid plugging of cannula with secretions
High tracheostomy	Proper placement of tracheostomy avoids risk of tracheal stenosis after decannulation
Metal tracheostomy cannula	A metal cannula creates a risk of posterior membranous wall perforation with erosion into the innominate artery
Incorrect length of tracheostomy cannula	If the tracheal cannula is too long it may cause injury to the carina or slippage into the bronchus resulting in single-lung ventilation If too short it may migrate out of the trachea causing loss of the airway
Incorrect balloon pressure or location	May cause erosion into the innominate artery or necrosis of the serum membranous wall and esophagus resulting in tracheoesophageal fistula

The surgeon must have a high index of suspicion for conditions that prevent breathing in patients with an otherwise patent airway. The most serious of these conditions is tension pneumothorax. When identified, it must be immediately converted from a life-threatening to non-life-threatening condition. Clinical signs of tension pneumothorax include: air hunger, dyspnea, cyanosis, distention of neck veins, tracheal deviation, diminished breath sounds on the side of tracheal deviation, tachycardia or bradycardia, hypotension, severe anxiety, confusion, and combative behavior. Immediate treatment consists of needle decompression.

Once tension pneumothorax is identified, the physician performs a needle decompression. A strong gush of air should immediately exit the chest and the patient should immediately stabilize from a cardiovascular standpoint. If the patient does not completely stabilize, an additional needle can be inserted. If the patient stabilizes, the physician should continue the primary survey according to ATLS protocol, placing a chest tube during the resuscitation phase. Alternatively, if the patient does not stabilize, a chest tube must be immediately placed.

Surgical Therapy for Tension Pneumothorax

Needle Decompression This is the quickest, safest, and least technically demanding procedure for converting a life-threatening tension pneumothorax to a simple pneumothorax. It should be done immediately upon diagnosis.

Equipment needed: A 14- or 16-French IV cannula and an alcohol swab.

Positioning: Supine.

Procedure: The area just under the second rib on the midclavicular line of the affected side is cleaned with an alcohol swab. A 14- or 16-French IV cannula is inserted. An air gush is heard; in the event that the patient does not stabilize, an additional catheter is placed. If this fails to achieve stabilization of the patient, a chest tube is placed.

Caution: Needle decompression of a tension pneumothorax is an emergency measure facilitating temporary stabilization of the patient. This should never be used as the only treatment. Once carried out, a tube thoracostomy set should be opened, prepared, and a chest tube should be placed during the resuscitation phase upon completion of the primary survey.

Tube Thoracostomy The indications and urgency for placing a chest tube must factor into the speed with which the tube is placed (Fig. 47-6). The procedure can be performed anywhere by anyone with proper equipment and training.

A patient suffering from a symptomatic tension pneumothorax which has not been relieved by needle decompression needs an urgent tube placement. The treating doctor must work quickly, focusing only on vital steps (i.e., alcohol swab, incision [larger], relief of tension, placement of tube, and tube anchoring with heavy suture). This is in contrast to a tube placed to drain a chronic effusion or empyema, where proper protocol is followed (see Chapter 9).

Breathing must be reestablished expediently to prevent permanent brain damage and respiratory as well as circulatory arrest.

a) Anatomy: thoracic trauma. Associated with rib fractures, lung injury.
b) Presentation: Variable. Can lead to respiratory arrest.
c) Signs and symptoms: Dyspnea, shortness of breath, air hunger, chest pain, distension of neck veins, tracheal deviation, subcutaneous emphysema, sensitivity over chest wall (with or without instability), unilateral absence of breath sounds, cyanosis, tachycardia then bradycardia, hypotension, anxiety, combative behavior, comatose, pulmonary, and then cardiac arrest.
d) Diagnosis:
Tension pneumothorax, sucking chest wound, flail chest, and massive hemothorax.
e) Treatment: Immediate diagnosis and symptom-reversing therapy.
 a. Percutaneous needle decompression.
 b. Chest tube placement.
 c. Closure of sucking wound (after chest tube placement).
 d. Stabilization of chest- intubation if needed.
 e. Urgent exploration for massive hemothorax.

Figure 47-5. Breathing.

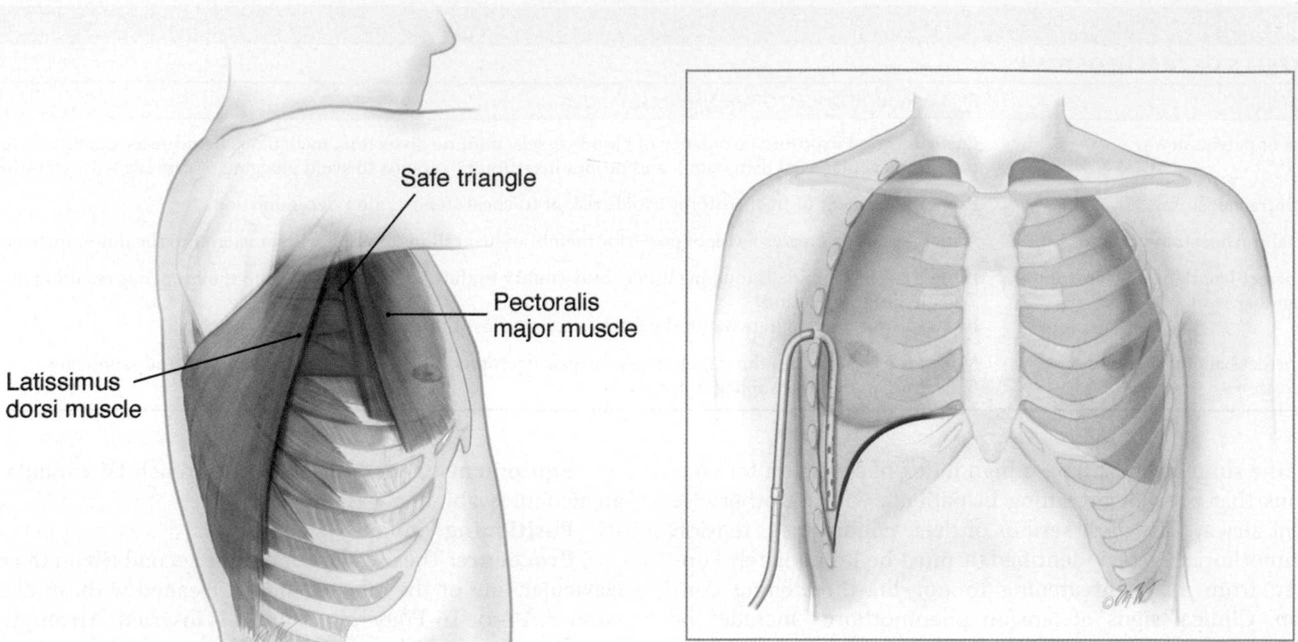

Figure 47-6. Proper placement of chest tube ensures adequate drainage.

A chest tube is a long plastic tube with multiple holes around the circumference of the tip of the tube. Chest tubes come in two shapes: straight or with a right angle. Straight tubes are primarily used to drain air and blood, while right-angle tubes are primarily used to drain pus. Chest tubes are sized according to their diameter, which is recorded in units called French. Straight chest tubes sometimes contain an inner needle or trocar. Typically for adults, a 28-French chest tube will evacuate air, while a 32- to 36-French chest tube would be needed to evacuate blood. Chest tubes are marked with a centimeter scale down the side of the tube. Note: the "zero" does not mark the end of the tube but the last hole. Typically, a straight chest tube should be inserted to the 20 cm mark (from the skin) for an adult female and to the 24 cm for an adult male to assure that it reaches the apex. The tube can always be pulled back, but space contamination can occur if the tube is advanced after initial insertion. The tube is then connected to a drainage system.

After insertion, it is preferable to connect the chest tube to a collecting system on suction. When wall suction is not available alternative suction methods are available (Table 47-3).

Drainage Systems Both open and closed systems may be used for chest tube drainage, but a closed system is preferred because it decreases the likelihood of external infection. With an open system, the chest tube drains openly or into an open bag or canister. Simple systems actively evacuate the effusion by suction, but there is no control over the strength of the suction, and they lack the advantage of water-seal systems. On the other hand, an open system may be the only option available in a minimal resource setting, and it is easy to assemble from reusable glass jars and tubing.

The advantages of more complex closed systems are (1) they separate the patient from the suction by using a water seal (A, B, or C), (2) they have adjustable suction control (B and C), and (3) they have separate drainage and water-seal bottles making it easier to remove the drainage bottle (C) (Fig. 47-7).

Table 47-3

PITFALLS OF CHEST TUBE PLACEMENT

PITFALL	RISK CAN BE REDUCED OR PREVENTED BY
Extrathoracic tube (tube travels outside the chest wall)	Use a larger incision and make sure the patient is receiving adequate analgesia.
Harpooning of spleen or liver	This may occur if the chest tube is placed too low, or if the hemidiaphragm is elevated. If not timely recognized, the chest tube may be forced into a visceral organ causing damage and bleeding. The remedy is proper placement of the chest tube.
Laceration of lung or heart due to presence of multiple adhesions	This can be prevented by placing a finger into the chest and palpating before inserting the chest tube.
Incomplete drainage of infection	The chest tube inserts; however, it does not completely drain the cavity due positioning of the tube and presence of loculations.
Incomplete drainage of air	This may occur if too few chest tubes were placed, or there is inadequate positioning of the tube. Check tube placement and increase the number of chest tubes.

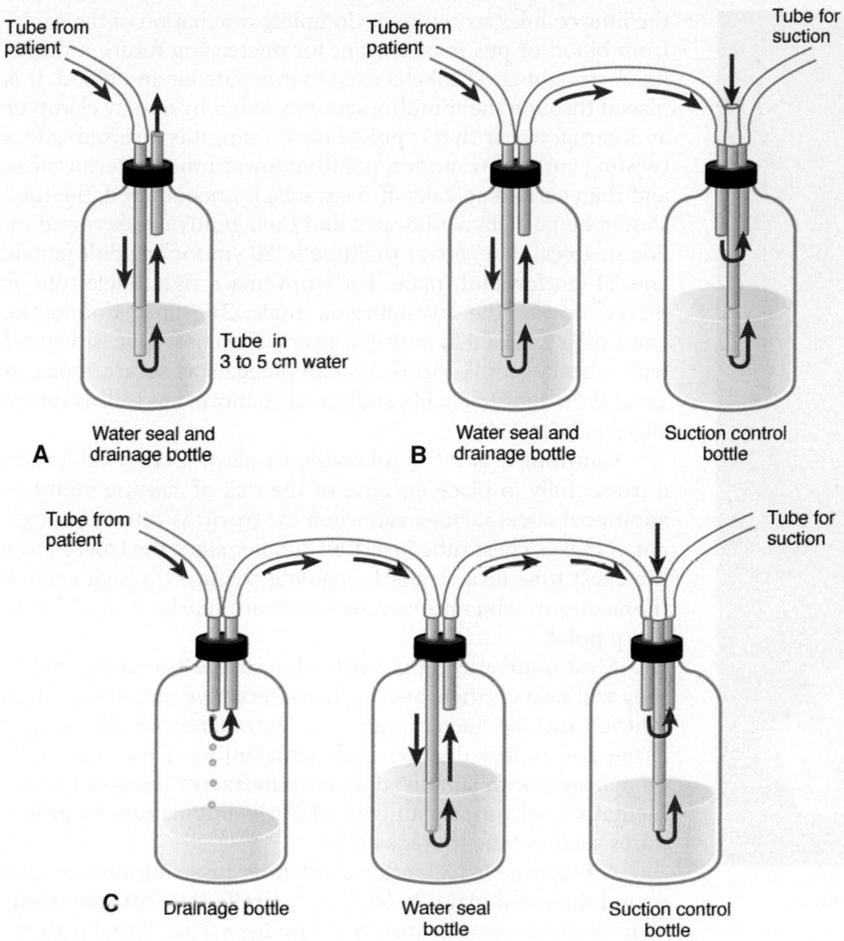

Figure 47-7. Chest tube drainage system using reusable bottles. (**A**), a single bottle is used both for collection of the drainage and water seal without suction. In (**B**), a second bottle has been added for suction. In (**C**) three bottles are used, respectively.

The addition of a water column enables one to calibrate the suction simply by increasing or decreasing the water column.

We prefer commercially available systems such as Atrium (Fig. 47-8). However, when suction and collection system are not available, draining the tube effluent through a Heimlich valve into a bag is the best option (Fig. 47-9). The Heimlich valve is a one-way flutter valve invented by Henry Heimlich in 1963. It enables air and liquids to evacuate the pleural cavity and then collect in a bag preventing suctioning of external contents into the pleural cavity.

If neither a suction device nor Heimlich valve is available, one has to improvise. The middle finger of a surgical glove can be cut off at the base. Using heavy silk, the "finger" is tied to the end of the chest tube and the distal tip of the finger is removed. The chest tube is then inserted into the middle of a drainage bag and the bag is secured to the chest tube, thus achieving an improvised closed one-way system.

Surgical Therapy Chest Tube Placement

Equipment needed: a knife, Metzenbaum scissors, strong surgical sutures (#1 or 2 silk), needle driver, two Kelly clamps, sterile drapes, and antiseptic wash; 10 to 20 cc of 1% lidocaine. A 10-cc syringe and a 21-gauge long needle.

Anesthesia: Local anesthesia is injected subcutaneously by the surgeon and rib blocks are placed. If available, the patient can receive a small amount of IV conscious sedation.

Antibiotics: Two grams Ancef are given for coverage of skin flora. When treating injury in the field with less sanitary conditions, a broader coverage may be needed.

Positioning: The patient is positioned supine and a folded sheet is placed under the affected side to obtain a 20 to 30 degree elevation. The arm on the affected side is either flexed over the head and taped or strapped straight next to the body in a way that will ensure noninterference during the procedure.

Procedure: A fully gowned, gloved, and masked surgeon preps the chest widely with an alcohol-based solution. The chest is then draped in the area of the fifth intercostal space anterior axillary line. The edge of the nipple is left in view. Three towels are placed to form a triangle. The fifth rib is palpated just posterior to the anterior axillary line, lidocaine is injected under the skin in this area, and then into the deep tissue. Lidocaine (2–3 cc) is now injected just inferior to the lower border of the posterior fourth and fifth ribs. Care is taken to avoid injury to the vein–artery–nerve (VAN) complex. A horizontal incision at least 2½ times the diameter of the chest tube is made through the skin. If the patient is unstable, muscular or obese, or if placement is difficult, the skin incision should be widened (a prudent surgeon would make a larger incision from the start for these patients). Metzenbaum scissors are used to spread the subcutaneous tissue vertically to avoid the thoracodorsal and long thoracic vessels. The apical portion of the fifth rib is palpated and the intercostal muscles anchored into this rib are divided using Metzenbaum scissors. The dissection should be bloodless; all sources of bleeding including inadvertent intercostal injury must be controlled.

It is much easier for a novice to place a chest tube at a 90-degree angle with respect to the skin and ribs. Do not attempt to tunnel the tube. A Kelly clamp is used to split the

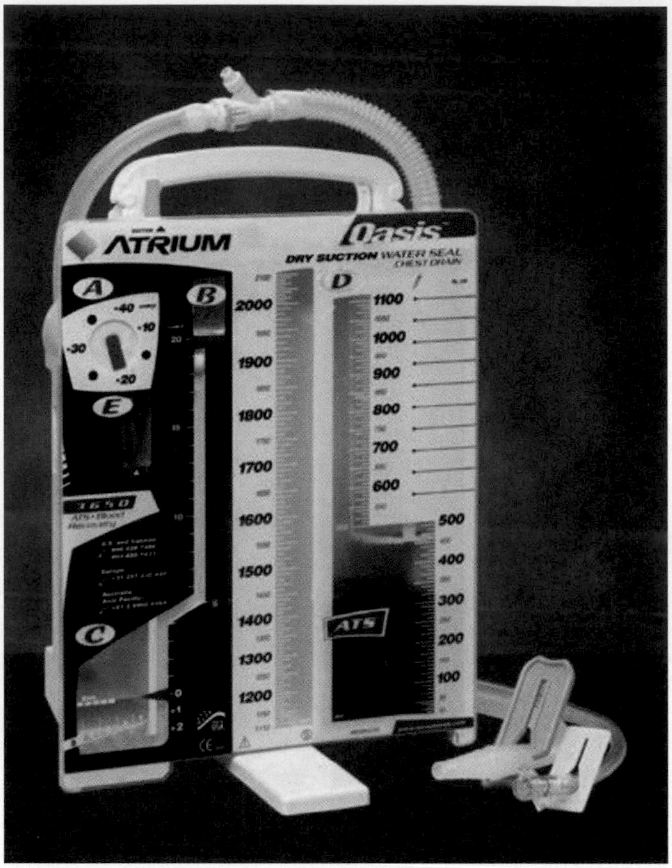

Figure 47-8. Commercially available sucction system.

intercostal muscles along the lower rib. In the event of simple or tension pneumothorax, a rush of air should be heard. In the event of hemothorax, blood and clots will evacuate. In empyema, pus will discharge. If culture or Gram stain is available, the exudate should be removed sterilely in a 10-cc syringe. Empyema as well as effusions can be loculated. Insert a gloved finger into the thoracostomy, feel the lung and chest wall, and rule out significant adhesions. Loculations can be gently broken up using a Yankauer suction. However, care must be taken to avoid causing major bleeding while doing so (by carrying it into the lung or hilar structures). Complete evacuation of the cavity from blood or pus is important for decreasing future morbidity. A straight chest tube is used to evacuate air and blood. It is placed through the minithoracotomy aided by a Kelly clamp or an internal trocar that is pulled back 1 cm. It is inserted with a twisting corkscrew motion pointing toward the posterior chest and then carried apically. If resistance is encountered, the tube should be partially withdrawn and then gently corkscrewed in. For an apical tube, insert the tube to 20 cm for an adult female and 24 cm for adult male. For empyema a right angle tube is placed toward the costophrenic angle. The area around the chest tube is closed in multiple layers. The chest tube is secured with a heavy #2 silk suture, and an omega stay suture is placed around the tube to enable additional anchoring as well as future closure if desired.

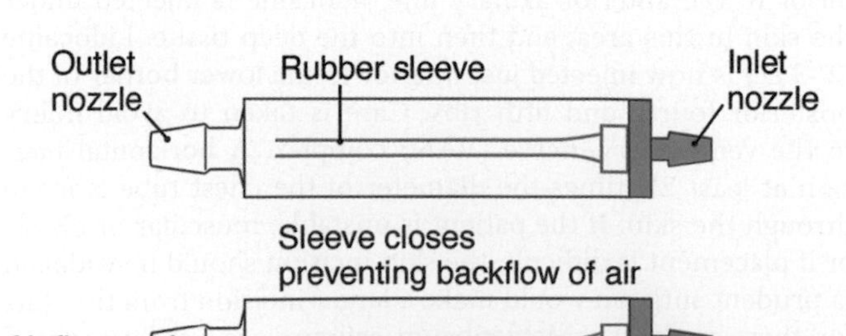

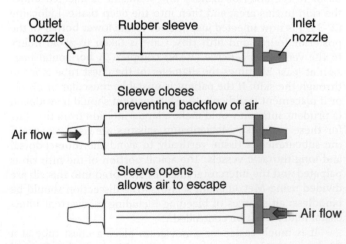

Figure 47-9. One-way flutter valve. The valve has a blue connector toward the patient (blue = sky).

Caution: It is NOT advisable to place a chest tube with a trocar fully in place because of the risk of causing injury to additional viscera. However, when the trocar is withdrawn by 1 cm, it makes chest tube insertion simpler since the trocar gives the chest tube firm strength enabling passage through a small thoracotomy, while preventing insertion injuries caused by its sharp point.

Most traumatic injuries of the lung are self-limiting, that is, they will heal on their own with conservative measures. These injuries include lung contusions, intraparenchymal hemorrhage, and air leak due to parenchymal injury. They can usually be managed with simple supportive measures (oxygen supplementation, adequate pain control, early ambulation) or procedures such as tube thoracostomy.

A massive air leak after chest tube insertion may be due to an injury to a major bronchus, typically the proximal mainstem bronchus near its insertion into the carina. These patients present with massive subcutaneous emphysema and tension pneumothorax. Chest tube insertion demonstrates continuous five-column air leak. On chest x-ray, the lung does not reinflate. Additional chest tubes are placed. If despite placement of these tubes the lung does not reinflate, an airway injury is suspected. This is now confirmed with a chest x-ray demonstrating a *"dropped lung"* despite multiple functioning tubes. The repair is surgical debridement and reimplantation through a posterior lateral approach with interrupted suture.

Rib Fractures Rib fractures may occur in isolation or associated with additional injuries. Multiple rib fractures, even when they represent the sole injury, are associated with an unacceptably high mortality rate of 3% to 5% in elderly patients. This is higher than the expected mortality from an elective lobectomy (range: 1%–5%). Rib fractures are usually accompanied by lung contusion. In addition, they may be associated with hemo-/pneumothorax, parenchymal injury to the liver or spleen, or a major vascular injury. Often rib fractures are diagnosed by a finding of tenderness on physical examination or as a result of findings on chest x-ray. On initial presentation, rib fractures may produce only slight tenderness. Over time (hours to days after injury), however, the broken ribs continue to rub on the exposed periosteum (>17,000 times a day) and the pain cycle gradually increases, leading to decreased lung volumes and splinting of the chest wall. If not treated appropriately, atelectasis can lead to lung consolidation. Ultimately, this may become infected, causing pneumonia.

This cycle should be anticipated and treated prophylactically with an aggressive cocktail of pain medications immediately upon diagnosis. Do not wait for the pain to develop. This cocktail typically includes Tylenol q.6, Motrin q.8, and an opiate for breakthrough pain. If the oral cocktail fails to achieve pain relief, a lidoderm patch can be added and IV non-steroidal anti-inflammatory drugs (NSAIDs) can be given (if kidney function is normal). Alternatively, a thoracic epidural catheter may be placed and epidural patient-controlled anesthesia (EPCA) is initiated or multiple rib blocks are performed. In the setting of multiple rib fractures, an IV PCA drip is suboptimal since it can lead to somnolence and increased respiratory complications. Early ambulation is critical as is the ability to breathe deeply and cough. This will not be possible if the pain is inadequately controlled. These patients should be hospitalized and ambulated aggressively to prevent the known sequelae of multiple rib fractures. This proactive approach has been shown to decrease mortality with multiple fractures.

A subset of patients with rib fractures has instability of the chest. A smaller number experience paradoxical chest wall motion breathing known as "flail chest" (see Chapter 137). This is typically found on physical examination. These patients will need very aggressive pain control to prevent pneumonia. If available, an epidural catheter should be placed and the patient should receive bolus or patient-controlled analgesia for a number of days. Alternatively, multiple rib blocks can be performed, later transitioning to a strong oral cocktail (e.g., Tramadol 75 mg TID, Motrin 600 mg TID, and Tylenol 650 mg QID.). A subset of these patients will require positive pressure ventilation to stabilize the rib cage. Currently, at our medical center, we stabilize the chest wall of patients with flail chest or multiple fractures when the fractures do not involve the most posterior one-third of the rib, since this area is hard to fixate. Typically, this is done through a muscle-preserving posterolateral thoracotomy using metal fixation plates and surgical screws (see Chapter 137). Early results of this technique appear promising in a select subset of patients.

Circulation

Hypovolemic shock is a life-threatening condition in patients with thoracic injuries. To stabilize the patient, one must first identify the mechanism of injury. A number of intrathoracic injuries may lead to hypovolemic shock, including injuries to the great vessels, heart, lungs, and chest wall. Patients with injuries involving the great vessels usually die at the scene. Even in a controlled clinical setting, the repair is complex and beyond the scope of this chapter. A stab wound in "the box" (Fig. 47-1), however, in a hypotensive patient warrants immediate exploration.

The lungs function in a low-pressure system. Therefore, injuries to the lungs generally are more survivable than injuries to the great vessels. Chest wall injuries, including rib fractures, can lead to significant intrathoracic bleeding as well as injury to the lung parenchyma. Undrained blood in the thorax can lead to chronic fibrothorax and may serve as a medium to encourage thoracic space infections. Bleeding within the thoracic space can be caused by rupture of the intercostal vessels, lung laceration, intraparenchymal bleeding, cardiac laceration, and great vessel injury.

Physical examination may show various levels of shock depending on the amount of bleeding the patient has experienced by the time of examination. The patient may be tachycardic or bradycardic, normotensive or hypotensive, or may have cold and clammy extremities and pallor. Anxiety and combative behavior are ominous signs of profound shock. A flail chest, chest wall instability, or tenderness should alert the provider to the presence of possible significant intrathoracic trauma. Decreased and muffled breath sounds may be found with hemothorax. Heart sounds may be distant if the patient has pericardial tamponade secondary to hemopericardium. Volume resuscitation should be limited to the goal of permissive hypotension to optimize the patient's ability to repair his or her injuries.

According to ATLS protocol, two wide-bore IVs are placed peripherally. During the resuscitative phase, a chest x-ray as well as ultrasound is obtained when available. If clinical suspicion exists for hemorrhage into a pleural cavity, with or without imaging, a thoracostomy tube should be expediently placed as previously described. Output on insertion should be recorded as well as hourly output thereafter.

Indications for immediate exploration of the chest include:

- Stable patient with >1500 cc upon initial chest tube insertion or more than one-third the patient's calculated blood volume.
- Persistent blood requirements despite receiving blood products and output greater than 250 cc an hour for a few hours.
- Penetrating trauma to the "box"; medial to the nipple line or scapular tip line.
- Unstable patient with significant hemothorax.

Cardiac Tamponade

Cardiac tamponade is accompanied by Beck's triad, consisting of muffled heart sounds, elevated venous pressure, and decreased arterial pressure. The FAST examination is very sensitive to the detection of pericardial fluid which, in the trauma setting, is assumed to be blood until proved otherwise. In penetrating trauma to the left of the sternum, a left anterior thoracotomy would be the incision of choice. For a right-sided penetrating trauma, a midline sternotomy is recommended.

Cardiac Laceration

Cardiac laceration from anterior penetrating trauma typically involves the right ventricle. It can be approached through an anterolateral thoracotomy or midline sternotomy. The pericardium is opened, and the laceration is repaired with double-armed monofilament pledgeted 2/0 mattress stitches. Care is taken when sewing a beating heart to time the suture with diastole. It is essential to slide the needle smoothly through the tissue to avoid enlarging the hole. If additional stitches are needed, they are placed until complete hemostasis is obtained. Great care must be taken to avoid injury to the coronary vessels.

Emergency Room Thoracotomy: Anterolateral Thoracotomy

Indication: Penetrating trauma, leading to severe shock or witnessed recent loss of signs of life (Fig. 47-10).

Aim: Urgent cross-clamp of aorta, enabling volume resuscitation and rapid control of bleeding source.

Equipment: Alcohol or Betadine, sterile drapes, major thoracotomy tray.

Essential elements include: a large knife, long Metzenbaum scissors, Mayo scissors, DeBakey forceps, mid and long needle drivers, aortic clamps (straight and curved), a large Finochietto retractor, large egg beater retractor. Large laparotomy pads and

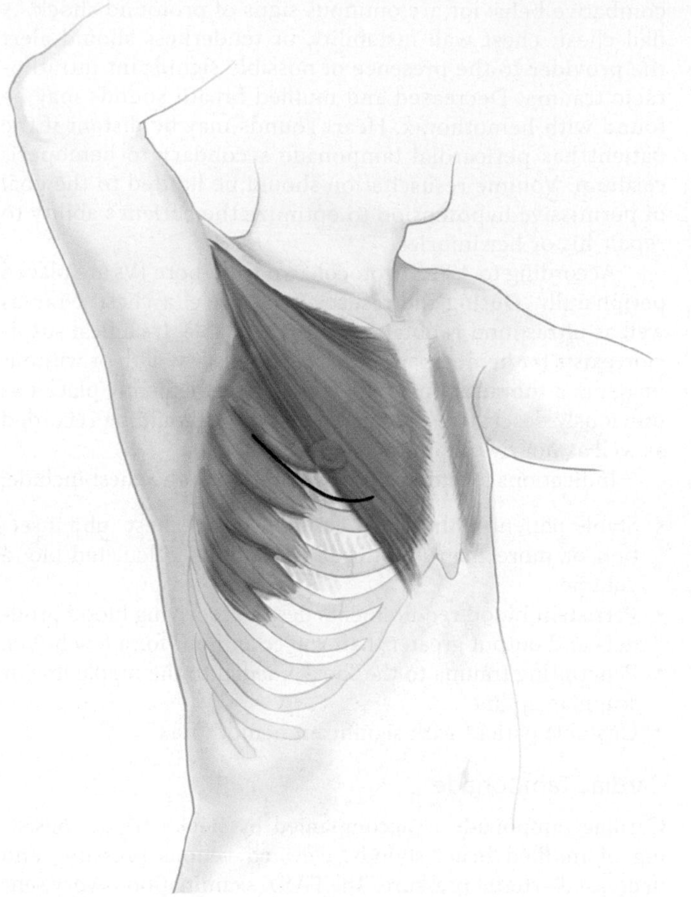

Figure 47-10. Anterolateral thoracotomy. ATLS program (seventh edition) teaches, "Thoracotomy is not indicated unless the surgeon, qualified by training and experience, is present."

strong working suction device, cell recycler if possible. Sutures and ties, Teflon pledgets if available (if not pericardium can be used), large chest tubes, and/or Blake tubes (or soft drainage tubes). Underwater (closed) chest tube collecting system (preferably with suction).

Optional but beneficial: linear staplers with reloads (preferably endoGIA staplers), vascular as well as heavy tissue loads.

Technique: The surgeon stands to the patient's left. Using a large blade (22) the surgeon incises the skin rapidly down to the intercostal muscle. In females, the cut is made along the inferior mammary fold, elevating the breast off the inferior aspect of the pectoralis muscle. Next the intercostal muscle is divided along the apical portion of the sixth rib. The chest is entered and a large Finochietto retractor is placed. Using Yankauer suction, blood is removed from the chest, the chest is packed, the injury is systematically assessed, and appropriate action is taken to repair the injury.

The pericardium is incised with Metzenbaum scissors parallel and above the phrenic nerve, taking into account the beating heart to time the surgical actions appropriately. The volume of the resuscitation can be assessed by observing whether the heart is distended or collapsed. If the patient is in extremis and the descending aorta can be dissected circumferentially, this is done by opening the pleura with Metzenbaum scissors. The surgeon then bluntly dissects around the aorta with the index finger taking care not to inadvertently injure the esophagus or directly avulse the intercostal perforators. A straight aortic clamp is placed temporarily enabling rapid resuscitation and providing a short window of opportunity during which the bleeding that led to hypovolemic shock can be controlled.

Modification for Additional Cardiac Exposure

The incision can be extended medially (horizontally) into or beyond the sternum using heavy curved Mayo scissors (Table 47-4).

Table 47-4

PITFALLS OF ANTEROLATERAL THORACOTOMY

PITFALL	RISK MAY BE REDUCED OR AVOIDED BY
Transection of small arteries leading to unrecognized, delayed bleeding	Meticulous hemostasis to avoid unnecessary bleeding and possible long-term disability caused by injury to internal mammary, thoracodorsal, long thoracic, and intercostal vessels.
Lung injury incurred on entering the chest	These injuries may arise from continued ventilation (patient still on double-lung ventilation), improper placement of a double-lumen tube, lung adhesions to the chest wall, and a lung that is slow to collapse. Anesthesia verifies the proper tube placement after repositioning. One-lung ventilation is instituted from a skin incision. Surgeon carefully enters the intercostal space visualizing and cutting along a protective finger or Yankauer suction. The lung that is not ventilated may need to be suctioned out by anesthesia.
Phrenic nerve injury upon opening the pericardium	Attention to anatomy: The phrenic nerve runs anterolaterally from the thoracic inlet, sloping along the pericardium posterior to the hilar structures.
Cardiac injury incurred by opening the pericardium	Care is taken when sewing a beating heart to time the suture with diastole.
Esophageal injury	Esophageal injury when getting around aorta to clamp.
Traumatic diaphragmatic disruption	More frequent on the left than right, typically associated with an additional injuries. Surgical repair is possible by thoracotomy or laparotomy. The diaphragm is often repaired after reducing herniated contents and then placing multiple interrupted pledgeted mattress stitches (2/0). The phrenic nerve originate in the 3 o'clock position, center of the diaphragm, midaxillary line just lateral to the crura, they then fan out circumferentially peripherally. The vessels originate as direct branches off of the aorta and superior vena cava and follow the nerves. A similar pattern occurs on the right at the 9 o'clock hour in the inferior lateral region of the IVC. The neurovascular bundle must be avoided during the repair to prevent additional injury.

Surgical Technique Thoracic Procedures

Posterolateral Thoracotomy The two major operations in the chest are the anterolateral thoracotomy, described above, and the posterolateral thoracotomy described here.

Posterolateral thoracotomy provides the best exposure to the lungs, as well as hilum, distal trachea, and bronchial tree and is considered the workhorse of thoracic surgery. On the right, it provides good exposure to the esophagus, azygos vein, and distal trachea.

The patient is placed in full lateral decubitus position which takes time to set up. It requires lung isolation (blocker or double-lumen tube), suboptimal in the acute setting.

The skin incision extends from the anterior axillary line beyond the tip of the scapula. Typically, the latissimus muscle is divided and the serratus muscle is spared. The incision into the intercostal space depends on the planned surgery. The third intercostal space is used for injuries near the thoracic inlet, the fourth intercostal space for injuries of the upper lobes, the fifth for injuries of the lower lobes, and sixth for injuries of the lower esophagus.

Staff Requirements Surgeon and assistant, anesthesiologist, two nurses or operating room technicians (one scrubbed and the other circulating).

Equipment Operating room, adjustable lighting, headlight (the most important light source in thoracic surgery). An adjustable operating room table that enables jackknifing (lateral flexing at hips) of the patient. This fully opens the intercostal spaces for optimal exposure. Beanbag or two round pillows for lateral decubitus positioning. Armrests enabling arm of operated side to be placed in "swimmers position" elevating the scapula and exposing the intercostal spaces. Blankets to wrap lower body and proactively prevent hypothermia. Strong working wall suction device.

Alcohol or Betadine, Sterile Drapes A major thoracotomy tray. Essential elements include: a large knife, long Metzenbaum scissors, Mayo scissors, DeBakey forceps, mid and long needle drivers, multiple long straight and curved clamps, lung compression clamp, aortic clamps (straight and curved), a large Finochietto retractor, large egg beater retractor.

Multiple large laparotomy pads. Large chest tubes and/or Blakes (or soft drainage tubes). Underwater chest tube collecting system (preferably with suction).

Optional but beneficial: Electrocautery, linear staplers with reloads (preferably endoGIA), vascular (30 mm) as well as heavy tissue loads (45–60 mm).

Sutures and Ties (Open as Needed) Availability of monofilament 2/0, 3/0, and 4/0 4 vascular ligation or repair; 2/0 and 3/0 chromic or Vicryl for lung parenchymal resection. Long- and medium-sized clips (if available).

For closure: #1 or 2 Vicryl for rib reapproximation, 0 Vicryl for muscle reapproximation, 2/0 Vicryl for deep subcutaneous tissue closure. For skin closure: skin stapler or absorbable 3/0 suture or 3/0 nylon. A heavy silk suture for securing chest tube to the chest wall.

Anesthesia notes: General or combined.

A mechanical ventilator should be available with ability to give oxygen at increased FiO_2.

The anesthetist requires expertise in positioning a double-lumen endotracheal tube (Note: left-sided tubes are easier to position and work well for most patients or a bronchial blocker, when neither is available). A smaller endotracheal tube can be placed directly in the left mainstem bronchus. This can enable right-sided surgery, with one-lung ventilation. However, it does not allow suctioning of the right lung to hasten collapse. One lung intubation on the right (for left-sided surgery) is problematic, since secure tube placement would necessitate blockage of the right upper lobe and thus lead to suboptimal ventilation during surgery. A fibrotic bronchoscope facilitates accurate placement of tube. Tube placement without fiberoptic guidance can be done with clinical examination and reexamination; however, this is suboptimal to using a bronchoscope. The endotracheal tube is placed by anesthesia with patient in supine position and then affixed appropriately. Thereafter, the patient is turned to lateral decubitus position and tube placement must be reconfirmed.

Remember: The left mainstem bronchus is long and sharply angled. The right mainstem bronchus is short and the right upper lobe typically originates 5 to 15 mm from the carina. Identification of the right upper lobe is made by identifying the three segmental bronchi that have the appearance of a "Mercedes Benz" sign. An epidural catheter can improve the ability to give balanced anesthesia and decreases the need in the postoperative setting for opioids, significantly improving pain management. An epidural should be used for all major general thoracic procedures when possible.

Lines and tubes: Two peripheral wide bore IVs, Foley catheter with urinometer, and nasogastric tube. Optional when needed and if available; arterial line and CVP.

Caution: Any case that would require a Swan-Ganz catheter (marginal patient or extensive procedure) should not be done in the setting of limited resources.

Intraoperative continuous monitoring: O_2 saturation with pulse oximeter, blood pressure with noninvasive cuff on nonoperative arm, cardiac rate and rhythm with EKG.

Fluids

Lactated Ringer's solution or Normosol. Blood products should be available including whole blood or packed red cells and fresh frozen plasma (FFP).

Positioning: On the operating table, place a beanbag covered with a sheet in the area of the patient's chest or two Curlex rolls fully opened, folded in half, and then covered by a bed sheet. The patient is initially positioned supine on the table.

After general anesthesia has been induced, and after placement and confirmation of the double-lumen tube as well as lines and continuous monitoring devices, the patient is turned. This requires four people and is coordinated by anesthesia to assure that the endotracheal tube does not migrate out of position. The patient is moved so the downside is in the middle of the long axis of the operative bed and then the patient is rotated 90 degrees. The patient is lifted and an axillary roll (1 L IV bag) is placed just caudal to the axilla. The beanbag is suctioned or soft rolls are placed in the Curlex. The patient is then slightly elevated and the Curlex tied around the rolls. The lower leg is flexed; a pillow is placed between the legs and the upper leg is left straight. Using heavy tape extending from one side of the bed to the other, the iliac crest is taped and stabilized. The arm on the operative side is placed on an arm board and extended in "swimmers position." The lower arm is placed on the extended arm board attached the bed or bent upward in a 90-degree angle. Care should be taken to properly pad all possible pressure points and avoid iatrogenic positioning injuries. The bed is now jackknifed to facilitate maximal opening of the intercostal spaces. A grounding pad is placed on the buttocks or thigh. The lower body is covered with blankets or a bear hugger if available.

Prophylaxis: IV antibiotics are given by anesthesia to cover the skin flora (Ancef 2 g or an equivalent) within an hour prior to skin incision. These are redosed by anesthesia as needed, typically every 4 hours. Five thousand units of subcutaneous heparin is given for DVT prophylaxis for all thoracotomies if available. In addition, when available, sequential venous dilators should be placed on the patient's legs.

Technique: The patient is prepped and draped in standard fashion. Wearing headlamps, the surgeon stands at the patient's back.

An electrocautery unit (if available) and two large Yankauer suctions are prepared and the operating lights are adjusted, while anesthesia institutes single-lung ventilation to cease ventilation of the operative lung. It takes approximately 15 to 20 minutes for the nonventilated lung to fully collapse.

A posterolateral incision is made using a large (22) blade to cut a lazy "S" incision along the sixth interspace from the anterior axillary line to beyond the scapular tip. The incision is started one fingerbreadth beneath the tip of the scapula. The skin and the subcutaneous tissues are divided. When dividing the latissimus muscle, it is important to coagulate or tie any vascular bundles encountered. The serratus anterior is mobilized and retracted to spare the muscle. Next, a scapula retractor is placed under the scapula, and the assistant elevates the scapula while the surgeon counts the ribs. The first rib is a flat rib and must be identified to assure that the count as correct. The interspace for entry into the chest is chosen based on the location of injury. The third intercostal space is best for approaching structures near the thoracic inlet (i.e., SVC, subclavian vessels, proximal thoracic trachea, and esophagus). The fourth intercostal space is best for accessing the upper and middle lobes of the lung. The fifth intercostal space is best for accessing injury near the midesophagus and lower lobe. The sixth intercostal space is best for accessing injuries in the region of the diaphragm.

It is important to remember to cut the intercostal muscle fibers along the lower rib of the interspace and not along the upper rib to avoid injury to the VAN bundle which lies beneath the rib. Care should be taken upon initial entrance into the thoracic cavity to avoid lung injury. For most general thoracic cases, incision is made along the fourth or fifth intercostal space. A Finochietto retractor can be placed to open the chest cavity. It should be opened slowly. If additional exposure is needed, the incision can be opened internally by dividing the intercostal muscle insertion along the lower rib medially as well as in the posterior direction. On posterior extension, care must be taken to elevate the erector spinous ligaments from the intercostal muscle so that these are not divided. The retractor is then opened further. If the exposure is still not adequate, a rib can be "shingled" by removing 1 cm of posterior rib. The rib that is shingled is above or below the incision depending on where one needs to gain maximal additional exposure.

Modifications of Standard Incisions for Additional Exposures

Extending the Incision

Standard incisions can be extended in two ways. The incision can be extended internally by medial as well as posterior division of the intercostal muscle along the rib space or the incision can be extended externally by extending the skin incision medially or posteroapically just lateral to the posterior scapula.

Shingling a Rib

If the exposure is not adequate, a rib can be "shingled" by removing 1 cm of posterior rib. The rib that is shingled can be above or below the incision depending on where one needs to gain maximal additional exposure (Table 47-5).

Table 47-5

PITFALLS ASSOCIATED WITH RIB SHINGLING

PITFALL	RISK MAY BE REDUCED OR AVOIDED BY
Transection of small arteries leading to unrecognized, delayed bleeding	Meticulous hemostasis.
Aggressive opening of rib spreader leading to broken ribs	Opening the rib spreader more slowly, with attention to tension and larger incision or rib shingling as needed.
Injury to intercostal vein–artery–nerve (VAN) bundle while entering the intercostal space, leading to chronic postthoracotomy pain	Attention to surgical technique. The VAN bundle is located underneath each rib. This injury will occur if the incision is made just "below" rather than just "above" the rib.
Cardiac injury when opening the pericardium	Care is taken when sewing a beating heart to time the suture with diastole.
Esophageal injury incurred by maneuvering around the aorta to place a clamp	
Traumatic diaphragmatic disruption	More frequent on the left than right, typically associated with additional injuries. Surgical repair is possible by thoracotomy or laparotomy. The diaphragm is often repaired after reducing the herniated contents and then placing multiple interrupted pledgeted mattress stitches (2/0). The phrenic nerve originates in the 3 o'clock position, center of the diaphragm, midaxillary line just lateral to the crura. The branches of the phrenic nerve fan out circumferentially and peripherally. The vessels originate as direct branches off of the aorta and superior vena cava and follow the nerves. A similar pattern occurs on the right at the 9 o'clock hour in the inferior lateral region of the IVC. The neurovascular bundle must be avoided during the repair to prevent additional injury.
Lung injury incurred on entering the chest	These injuries may arise from continued ventilation (patient still on double-lung ventilation), improper placement of a double-lumen tube, lung adhesions to the chest wall, and a lung that is slow to collapse. Anesthesia verifies the proper tube placement after repositioning. One-lung ventilation is instituted from a skin incision. Surgeon carefully enters the intercostal space visualizing and cutting along a protective finger or Yankauer suction. The lung that is not ventilated may need to be suctioned out by anesthesia.

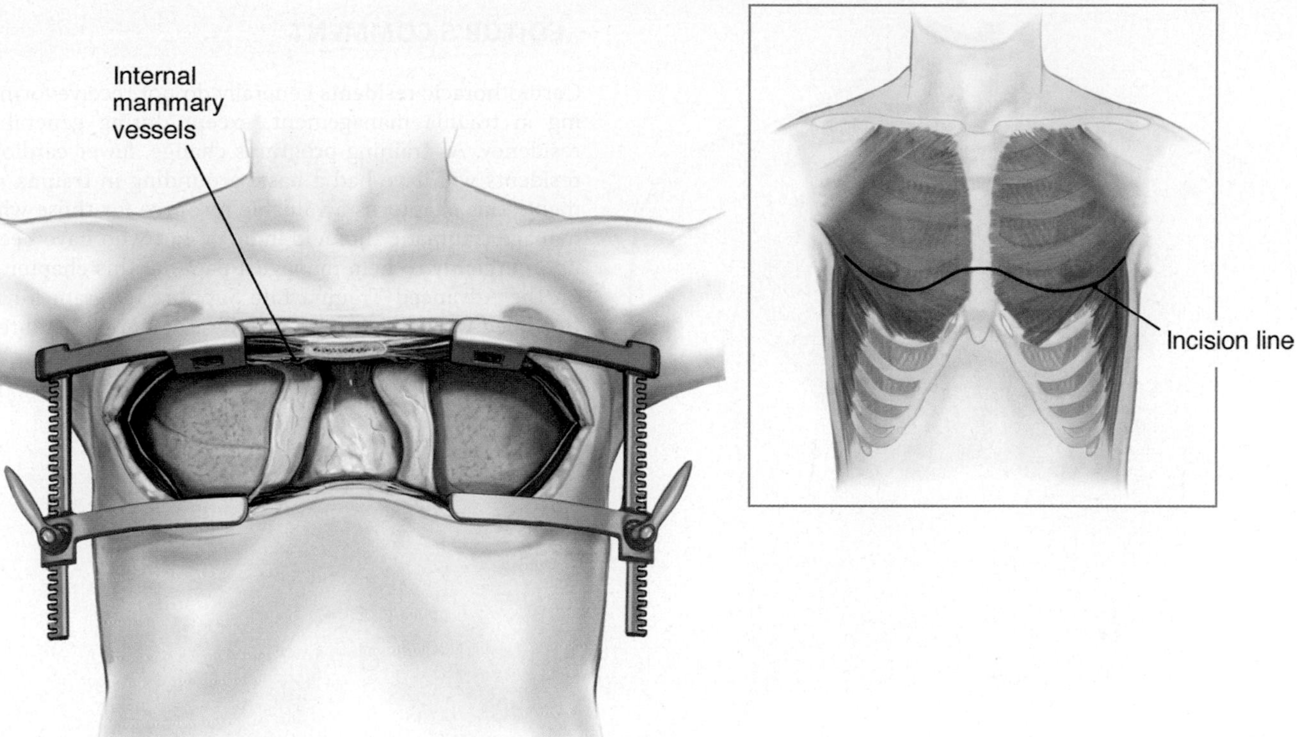

Figure 47-11. Clamshell exposure. A curvilinear incision, along the fourth intercostal space (top of fifth rib), spanning between both anterior axillary lines. The mammary vessels are ligated and two Finochietto retractors are used. Provides rapid and excellent exposure to the lungs, heart, great vessels.

Clam Shell Incision

The clam shell incision (Fig. 47-11) is a curvilinear incision made along the fourth intercostal space (top of fifth rib) and spans between both anterior axillary lines. The mammary vessels are ligated and two Finochietto retractors are used. The incision provides rapid and excellent exposure to the lungs, heart, and great vessels.

Midline Sternotomy

The midline sternotomy (Fig. 47-12) is the workhorse of cardiac surgery. It extends from a point just above the sternal notch down past the xiphoid. This is the classic cardiac surgery incision because it provides excellent exposure to the heart, ascending aorta, aortic arch and its branches, main pulmonary artery trunk, IVC and SVC, innominate artery, and vein. Its only weakness is poor exposure of the left subclavian artery.

Trapdoor Thoracotomy

The so-called trapdoor thoracotomy is a C-shaped incision (Fig. 47-13) that provides optimal exposure to the left subclavian artery. It involves incision along the left clavicle and then curves to the midline along the superior portion of the sternum and then laterally along the fourth rib. A ministernotomy is made from the sternal notch down to the third intercostal space followed by lateral division of the pectoralis and intercostal muscles along the cranial portion of the fourth rib. The incision creates a block consisting of sternum, clavicle, and ribs, which is then retracted laterally, resembling a "trap door."

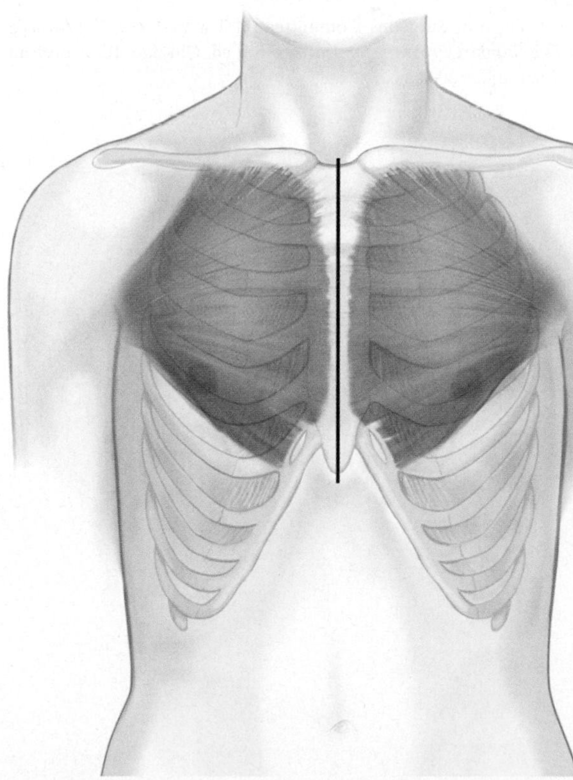

Figure 47-12. Midline sternotomy. Extends from above the sternal notch down past the xiphoid. Classic cardiac surgery incision because it provides excellent exposure to the heart, ascending aorta, aortic arch and its branches, main pulmonary artery trunk, IVC and SVC, innominate artery, and vein. Its only weakness is poor exposure of the left subclavian artery.

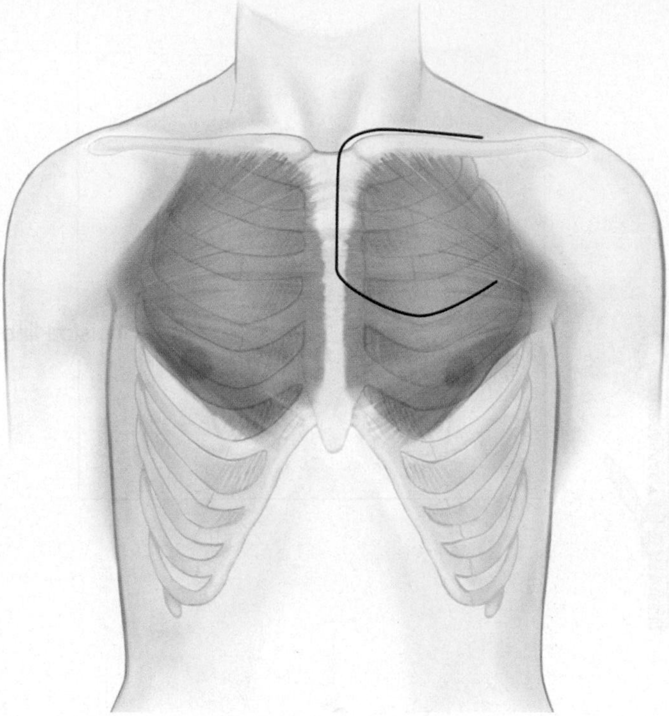

Figure 47-13. Trapdoor incision.

EDITOR'S COMMENT

Cardiothoracic residents generally do not receive formal training in trauma management, except during general surgery residency. As training programs change, fewer cardiothoracic residents will have had a basic grounding in trauma management. This chapter is a valuable resource for those who rarely manage traumatic thoracic injuries, but who have been called upon urgently to help manage a patient. This chapter is based on the Advanced Trauma Life Support Program for doctors. It is filled with simple practical life-saving tips that are quickly located in an emergent situation.

—Michael T. Jaklitsch

Reference

1. American College of Surgeons Committee on Trauma. *ATLS: Advanced Trauma Life Support Program for Doctors*. 8th ed. Chicago, IL: American College of Surgeons; 2008.

48 Management of Esophageal Perforation

Justin D. Blasberg and Cameron D. Wright

Keywords: Thoracic esophageal perforation, cervical esophageal perforation, iatrogenic perforation, blunt and penetrating perforation, barogenic perforation, endoscopic stent

Esophageal perforation is a challenging clinical condition that requires prompt diagnosis and management. Delay in identification and/or treatment results in high rates of morbidity and mortality. There are sharp differences in etiology, presentation, treatment, and outcome of cervical versus thoracic perforation of the esophagus. Most cervical perforations respond well to simple drainage alone. Although the treatment of thoracic esophageal perforations is individualized, most patients are candidates for primary repair regardless of the time to presentation or intervention. Improvements in endoscopic stent technology and increased experience with placement support this modality as a viable treatment option in cases of benign, malignant, and iatrogenic esophageal perforation.

ETIOLOGY

Esophageal perforation usually is the result of iatrogenic injury caused by instrumentation (e.g., esophagoscopy, bougienage, and achalasia dilation)[1–3] (Table 48-1). The most common site for perforation of the normal esophagus is at its most proximal location, immediately above the cricopharyngeus muscle and below the inferior pharyngeal constrictor (Killian's triangle). Injury at this location is most often caused by attempted forceful intubation of the esophagus for endoscopy (rigid or flexible) in a patient who is not sufficiently anesthetized. Other common sites of perforation include those in which the esophagus is normally narrowed (the distal esophagus), pathologically narrowed, or anatomically abnormal. Occasionally, intramural perforation can occur when the mucosa is sheared off the muscularis during endoscopy or bougienage. These conditions are not perforations in the truest sense, but present in a similar fashion and must be differentiated from frank perforation. *Spontaneous* perforation is a misnomer; it is more accurately termed *barogenic perforation* (Boerhaave syndrome). Blunt and penetrating trauma contributes only a small number of perforations.[4] Foreign bodies, infections, and operative injuries are additional, although rare, causes worth noting.[5]

Table 48-1

ETIOLOGY OF ESOPHAGEAL PERFORATION

Iatrogenic	Esophagoscopy, dilation, sclerotherapy, pneumatic dilation, laser therapy, biopsy, stent placement, nasogastric tubes, endotracheal tubes, transesophageal echocardiography (TEE), and esophageal ultrasound
Barogenic	Boerhaave syndrome, childbirth
Trauma	Blunt, penetrating, high-pressure gas (through the oral cavity)
Operative	Cervical spine surgery, pulmonary resection, resection of pleural or mediastinal masses, esophageal surgery, vagotomy, antireflux surgery
Foreign ingestion	Foreign body, caustic ingestion
Tumor	Esophageal cancer, mediastinal invasion of periesophageal tumors or lung cancer
Infection	Necrotizing infections

DIAGNOSIS

Pain is the most common complaint in patients presenting with esophageal perforation. In addition, cervical perforations can present with dysphagia, odynophagia, and dysphonia. Subcutaneous emphysema is often palpable in the neck. Pain from an intrathoracic perforation may be localized initially to the subxiphoid region, and hence may be misinterpreted as a myocardial infarction, aortic dissection, perforated duodenal ulcer, or pancreatitis. The pain also may be substernal, referred to the back, or poorly localized, and is usually severe. Dyspnea and anxiety are common associated findings. Tachycardia is also common, and fever develops early in the clinical course. Shock is rarely seen after cervical perforation because of local containment, whereas with free perforation into the pleural space, as often occurs with Boerhaave syndrome, rapid progression to shock may occur within 24 hours. Perforation by balloon dilation of achalasia similarly may result in a rapid and disastrous course if treatment is delayed. A small instrumental perforation, on the other hand, confined to the wall of the esophagus or situated in the mediastinum, may lead to a much slower development of symptoms. The key feature in the diagnosis of all esophageal perforations is a high index of suspicion. Prompt evaluation of patients with any of these findings or symptoms after endoscopy is most important because early diagnosis improves outcome.

RADIOLOGIC EVALUATION

A lateral plain neck film typically demonstrates air in the prevertebral space even early after cervical perforation (Fig. 48-1). Chest radiographs may show a pleural effusion, subcutaneous emphysema, pneumomediastinum, or pneumothorax. Radiographs soon after the event may be normal, although 75% of patients have abnormal films within 12 hours of presentation. Examination of the esophagus with contrast material is preferably done with water-soluble medium (Figs. 48-2 to 48-5). If the diagnosis is unclear or the definition is inadequate, dilute

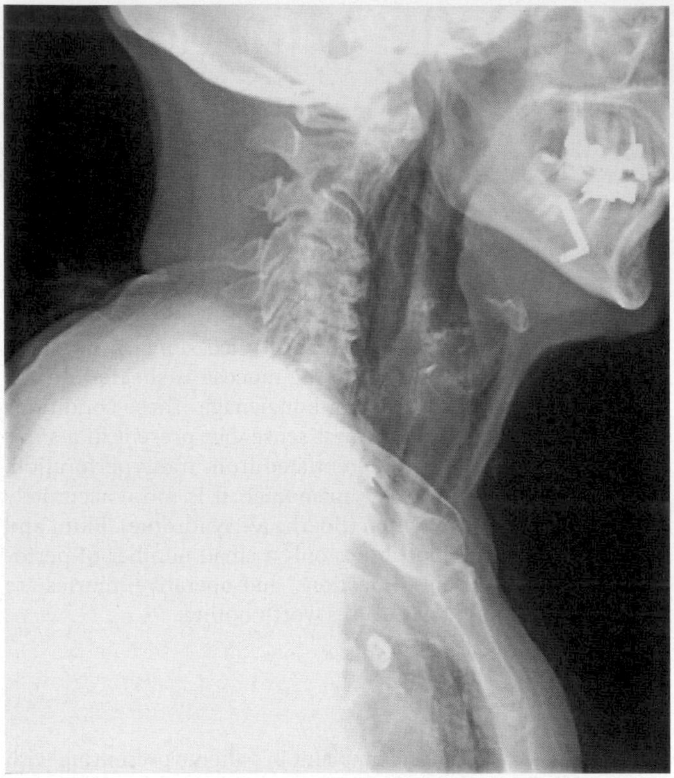

Figure 48-1. Lateral plain film of the neck with soft tissue technique. The patient is a 77-year-old woman who had an attempted esophageal ultrasound, but the probe could not be passed into the esophagus. She complained of neck pain 4 hours after the procedure.

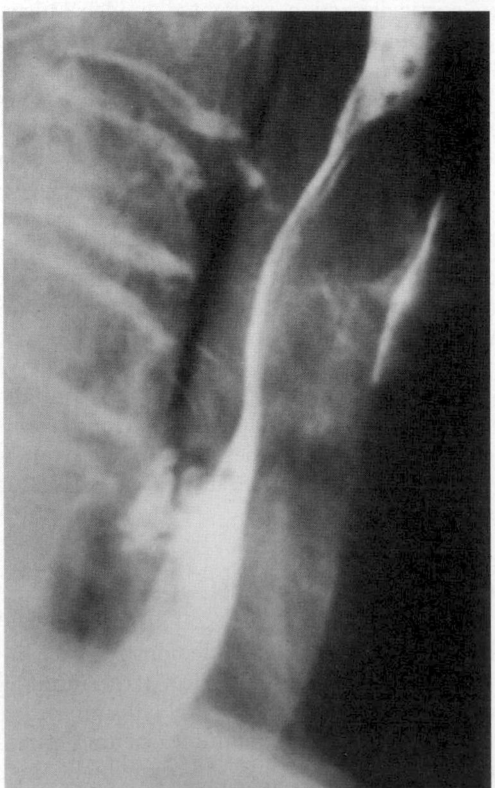

Figure 48-2. Lateral view of a barium swallow of a 66-year-old man who had an upper endoscopy. He complained of pain and trouble swallowing soon after the endoscopy.

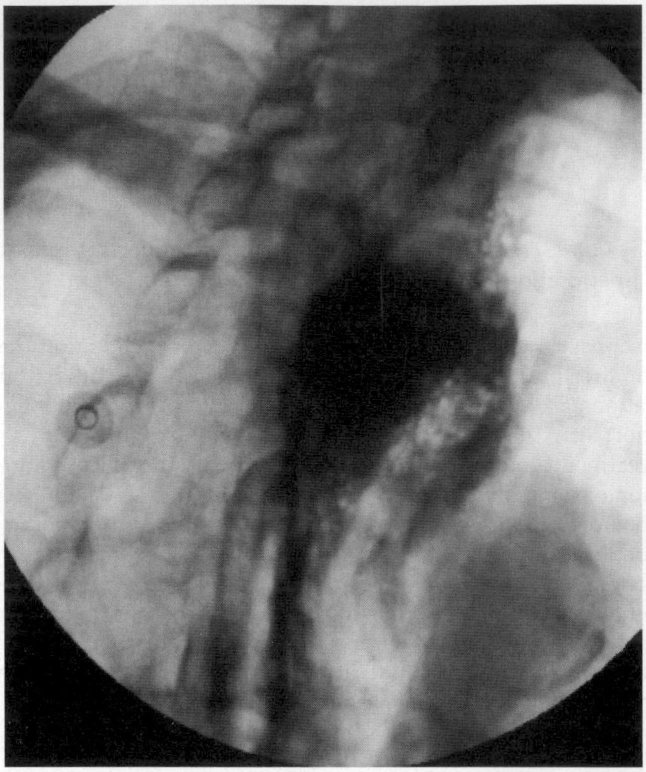

Figure 48-3. Barium swallow of the patient in Figure 48-1 with large, fairly poorly contained perforation at the level of the cricopharyngeus.

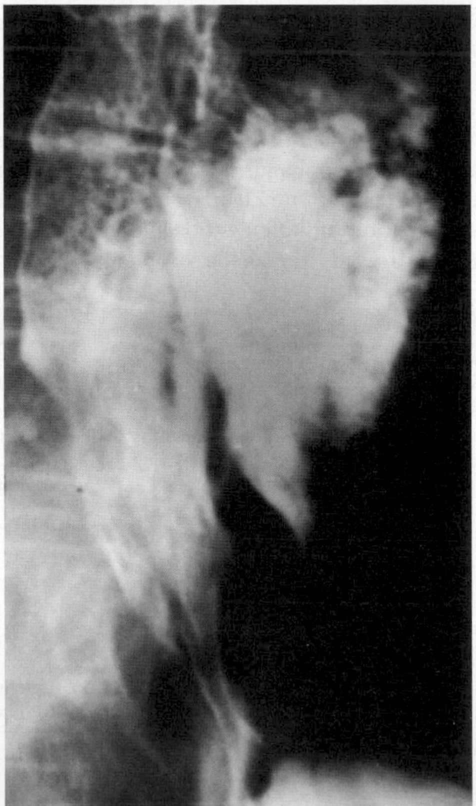

Figure 48-4. Barogenic perforation of the distal esophagus minimally contained by the mediastinal pleura with a large extraluminal contrast cavity. The perforation was closed successfully with primary repair and an intercostal muscle tissue buttress.

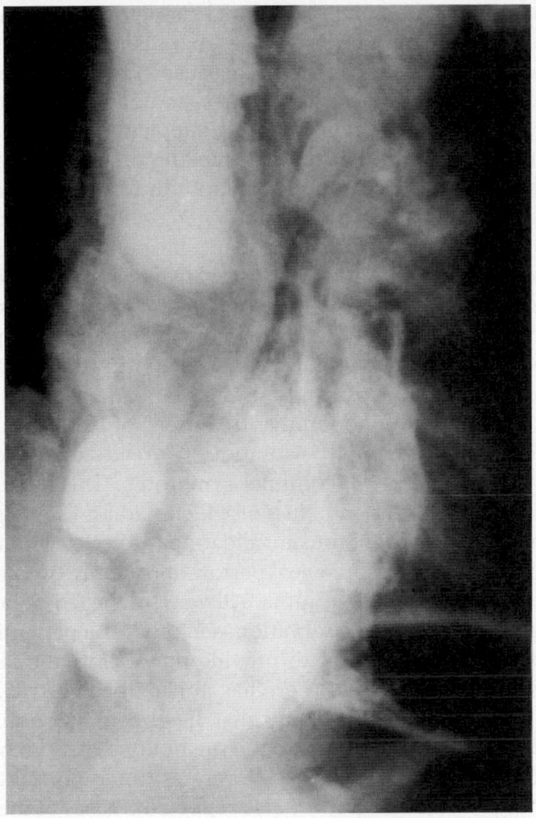

Figure 48-5. Perforation of the distal esophagus in a 77-year-old woman with chronic achalasia after pneumatic dilation. The perforation is poorly contained and into the pleural space. The perforation was closed with primary repair with an intercostal muscle tissue buttress. A myotomy on the opposite side of the esophagus was done to eliminate distal obstruction.

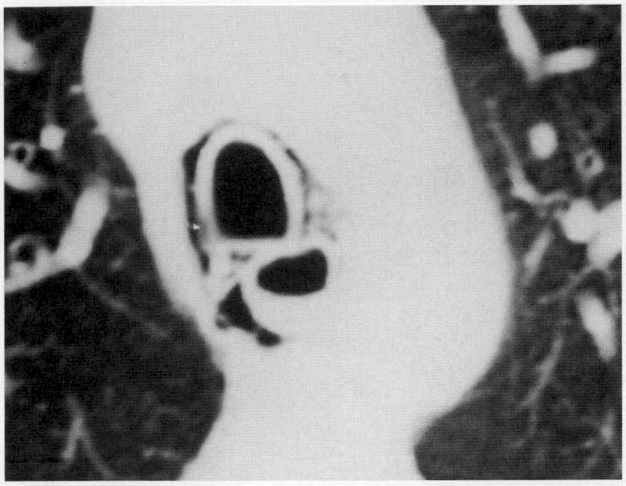

Figure 48-6. CT scan of a patient who had deep posterior chest pain after vomiting. The initial chest radiograph and barium swallow were negative. This CT scan made the diagnosis by demonstrating pneumomediastinum. A repeat contrast examination with barium with the patient almost prone confirmed a small, contained distal perforation.

barium may be used sparingly. The overall false-negative rate in this setting is at least 10%.[3] If perforation is still strongly suspected, a swallow study should be repeated several hours later, or another modality of investigation might prove more helpful. CT scans can aid in the diagnosis of esophageal perforation and identify late sequelae[6]; evidence of perforation may include extraluminal air, extravasation of contrast material, esophageal thickening, and communication of the air-filled esophagus with adjacent structures (Fig. 48-6). Oral or nasogastric tube contrast material can be administered just prior to CT scan, increasing its sensitivity. Planning the diagnostic evaluation with a radiologist is recommended to avoid the administration of contrast material that may delay the use of CT. Endoscopy is occasionally helpful, either to diagnose a perforation (usually in the context of trauma) or to assess the status of the esophagus in planning operative repair. Important information that can be determined by endoscopy includes the exact location of the tear, the presence of a stricture, or the extent of a carcinoma. If carefully performed with a flexible endoscope by an experienced endoscopist/surgeon, there is no additional risk to performing esophagoscopy when potentially important information can be gained.

Intramural perforations can be a source of confusion to the inexperienced radiologist or surgeon. These are usually caused by instrumentation; the mucosa is inadvertently sheared off the muscularis at the cricopharyngeus or a pathologically narrowed area. Intense pain is a common symptom. Barium swallow frequently demonstrates two lumens: the true lumen in which contrast material readily passes downward and a false lumen with contrast pooled in a dependent pouch (Fig. 48-7). CT imaging can help to clarify this diagnosis (Fig. 48-8). Critical to the early detection of esophageal perforation is the physician's awareness of the possibility. Where instrumentation has

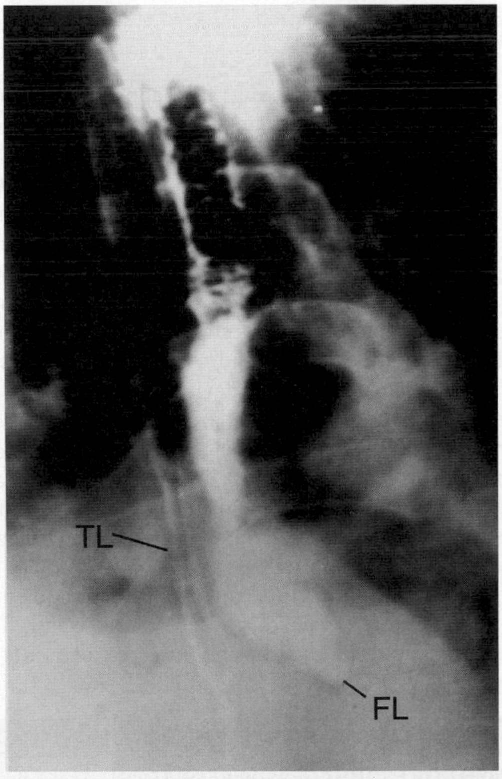

Figure 48-7. Barium swallow of a patient with an intramural perforation originating in the cervical esophagus at a tight congenital stricture. The gastroenterologist noted that it was very difficult to pass the endoscope, lost the mucosal surface, and saw blood and then stopped the endoscopy. The patient complained of severe pain and inability to swallow. The true lumen is denoted by *TL*, and the false lumen containing pooled contrast material ending in a blind pouch is denoted by *FL*.

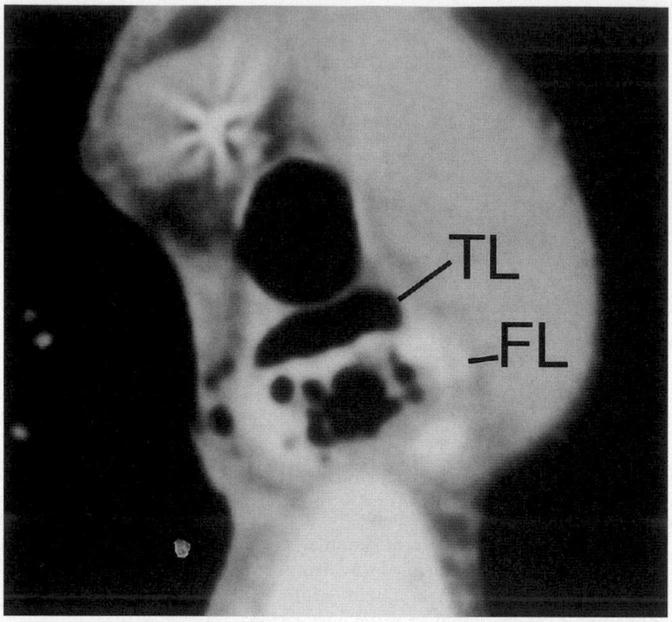

Figure 48-8. CT scan of the patient in Figure 48-7 with an intramural perforation. The true lumen is anterior marked with *TL*, and the false lumen filled with contrast material is marked with *FL*.

preceded the development of any signs or symptoms, perforation must be suspected until proven otherwise.

TREATMENT

Factors important to selecting the appropriate treatment include the location, etiology, and status of the native esophagus. In addition, the severity of contamination, often associated with delay in seeking treatment, can significantly alter the treatment plan (Table 48-2). Management always involves vigorous general support of the patient including resuscitation, broad-spectrum antibiotics, and nutritional optimization. The general principles of treatment are to control or eliminate the esophageal leak, maintain or reestablish gastrointestinal tract continuity, eliminate infection and/or obstruction (if any), and drain or debride collections and devitalized tissue.

Cervical perforations usually are best managed by immediate drainage of the retroesophageal space. This procedure is performed via an oblique neck incision along the anterior border of the sternocleidomastoid muscle. The carotid sheath contents are retracted laterally and the visceral compartment medially. A left-sided approach is preferred to reduce the risk of recurrent nerve injury. Instrumental perforations are typically located directly posterior and are found easily. The cavity of contrast material, saliva, and infected contents should be irrigated and drained. Additional tissue planes should not be opened if they are undisturbed. There is no need to search for the offending mucosal tear because the perforation will heal with proper drainage, antibiotics, and nutritional support. Generally, a Penrose drain is placed, supplemented with active suction if dependent mediastinal tracking of infection is present. The patient is kept nothing by mouth for a period of 5 to 7 days depending on clinical status. Drains may be removed either in the hospital or an outpatient setting.

Table 48-2
TREATMENT OF ESOPHAGEAL PERFORATION
Nonoperative treatment
Primary repair
Resection
Drainage
Exclusion
Stents

In thoracic perforations, conservative management is considered in two situations: (1) a contained perforation, demonstrated by contrast study, which has already undergone a period of observation with no ill effects and (2) an intramural perforation between the mucosa and muscularis. Cameron et al.[7] suggested criteria for nonoperative treatment of esophageal perforation: (1) a contained perforation, (2) ready drainage back into the lumen, and (3) minimal symptoms. This series only reported on eight patients, five of which had an esophagogastric leak after resection, thus invalidating the series with regard to treatment of true esophageal perforations. Only two patients suffered from barogenic trauma. All were managed nonoperatively after a period of observation, such that the patients were self-selected. The decision to provide nonoperative treatment is more compelling when there has already been a trial, so to speak, of supportive care only that has been successful. Far more difficult is the decision to pursue nonoperative treatment immediately after diagnosis. Altorjay et al.[8] reported on 15 transmural perforations (they also reported 6 cases of intramural perforations) treated nonoperatively. In all, 70% were early perforations, and 50% were cervical. Four patients deteriorated and required operation; 2 of 14 patients died (14% mortality). These authors essentially endorsed Cameron's criteria but also added additional recommendations: (1) circumscribed perforation; (2) contrast material flows back into lumen; (3) no cancer, obstruction, or abdominal esophageal leak; and (4) minimal signs and symptoms.

For most perforations of the thoracic esophagus that are diagnosed *early* (<24 hours), there is general agreement that operative repair is best.[9–12] A thoracotomy is performed on the side of the perforation at the expected interspace of the tear. The pleural space is thoroughly cleansed and the lung decorticated. The esophageal laceration is debrided in conservative fashion, the mucosa is meticulously closed with interrupted sutures, and the muscularis is similarly closed as a second layer[12] (Fig. 48-9). An alternative closure technique is to use a linear stapling device to close the mucosal tear[11] (Fig. 48-10). This tear often extends beyond that of the muscularis such that the surgeon must ensure the two ends are well exposed. (This may necessitate extending the muscle tear by incising it to fully expose the underlying mucosal tear.)

Buttressing, even of a fresh perforation, with healthy vascularized tissue of good consistency is advisable. The repair should be checked with instillation of a large volume of methylene blue-tinted saline injected into the esophagus via the nasogastric tube after completion of the suture lines. An optimal buttress is a pedicled intercostal muscle flap, preferably elevated at the time of entry into the chest, such that the vasculature to the muscle is intact. It should be sutured down as if it were being anastomosed to the esophageal wall rather than simply "tacked" over the closure. Other flaps that have been used include the pericardial fat pad, diaphragm, chest wall muscle, omentum, and stomach wall folded over a low perforation. The pleura is *not*

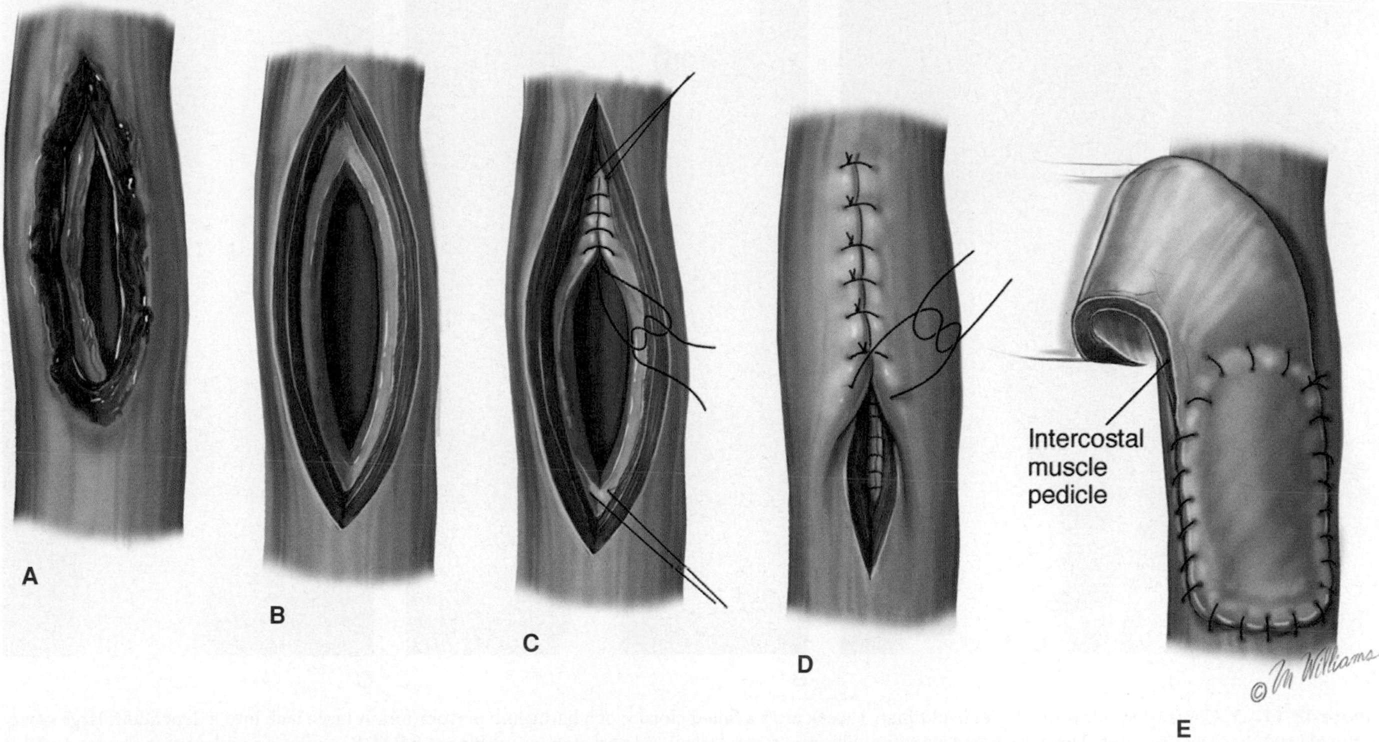

Figure 48-9. Technique of primary repair and intercostal muscle buttress of a typical thoracic esophageal perforation. *A*. The mucosa is often torn further underneath the muscle tear. *B*. The muscle tear is opened further to expose the limits of the mucosal tear, and both are debrided back to healthy tissue. *C*. The mucosa is closed with fine 4-0 absorbable sutures with knots tied on the inside. *D*. The muscle is closed in a second layer. *E*. An intercostal muscle is carefully sutured around the circumference of the repair site to provide a third layer of protection.

thickened sufficiently by inflammation in early perforation to be used effectively as a flap, although this has been mistakenly advised. Intercostal muscle has been used successfully as a primary patch, rather than as a buttress, in patients with rupture after balloon dilation for achalasia, in whom myotomy could not be employed and esophageal closure was impossible. The pleural space is well drained, and large suction tubes placed immediately adjacent to the repair site is recommended.

Drains should be left in place until a postoperative contrast swallow is completed. Gastrostomy and jejunostomy are advisable, the first to keep the stomach empty and prevent reflux into the esophagus, and the latter for long-term feeding. Any

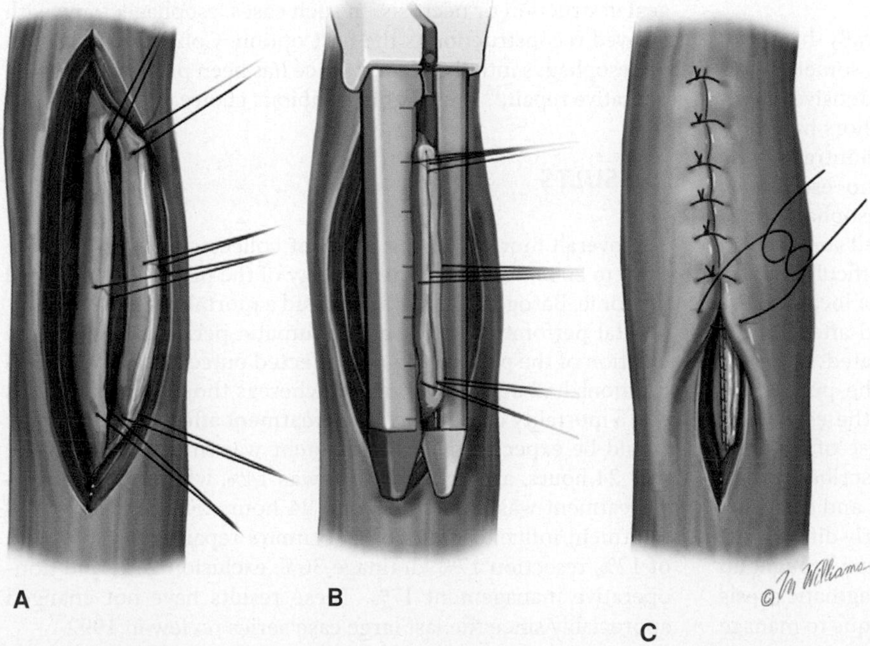

Figure 48-10. Technique of repair of a thoracic esophageal perforation using a GIA stapler. *A*. Stay sutures elevate tissue into the jaws of the GIA stapler. *B*. The muscle is closed as a second layer after the stapler is fired to close the mucosal layer.

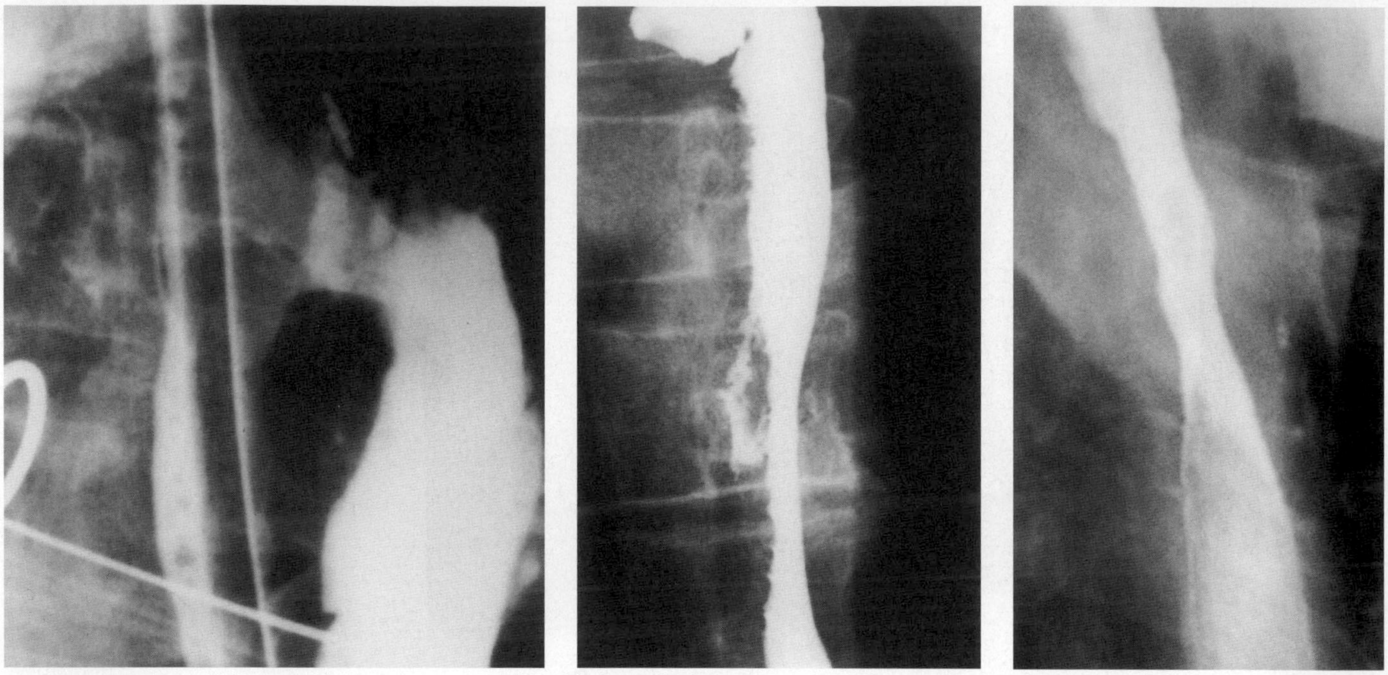

A B C

Figure 48-11. *A*. Contrast swallow of a 56-year-old man 1 week after a failed closure of a barogenic perforation. A large leak into a dependent large cavity in the pleural space was present. The patient had a continued septic state. Attempted percutaneous drainage failed. Reoperation with repeat closure and this time an intercostal muscle buttress was performed. *B*. Contrast swallow 1 week after repeat closure demonstrates a small contained leak at the closure site. Delayed views show that all the contrast material drained into the lumen. *C*. Contrast swallow 1 week later confirms a healed repair.

esophageal or pyloric obstruction *must be* relieved at operation or reperforation is more likely to occur.

In the case of an achalasia patient who is perforated during dilation, the closure should be accomplished in the usual two layers and then a myotomy performed on the opposite side of the esophagus. The standard perforation repair patient is kept nothing by mouth for at least a week, after which a contrast swallow is performed to ascertain whether the repair has been successful. If there is a small, contained leak after repair that is asymptomatic, continued observation and maintenance of the nothing by mouth status is advisable (Fig. 48-11).

Resection for esophageal perforation generally has been restricted to presentation involving a carcinoma, sometimes as a result of biopsy or dilation, or in rare cases of extensive necrosis of the esophagus from infection.[13,14] Some authors have proposed this technique as primary treatment for all intrathoracic perforations. This seems inadvisable because no esophageal substitute ever functions as well as the native esophagus. We believe that *late* perforations also should be treated surgically in almost every case. Surgery may be vastly more difficult because of inflammation, contamination, and induration of localized tissues. However, the mucosa usually can be closed after limited debridement of its edges. Closure of the indurated muscular wall provides, at best, provisional closure for the purpose of accomplishing the surgery. Definitive sealing of the esophagus from the pleural space is accomplished by the use of a sturdy, well-vascularized tissue buttress applied as described previously. Full expansion of the lung by decortication and cleansing of the pleural space is also essential. In a particularly difficult situation, the diaphragm may be opened and omentum brought up as an additional buttress. The risk of transdiaphragmatic sepsis appears to be small in these cases. Another technique to manage late perforation involves insertion of a large T-tube in the esophagus with the sidearm brought out through the chest wall. This is rarely necessary, and results are not predictable. Esophageal diversion is almost never desirable. This allegedly reversible procedure often prevents salvage of a functional native esophagus, which is far superior to any eventual replacement. Diversion was initially a recommended option because of the high incidence of releakage after primary repair, especially in late cases.[15] Use of primary repair with meticulous buttressing obviates the need for diversion, except in a rare case of extensive esophageal destruction or necrosis. In such cases, esophagectomy with delayed reconstruction is the best option. Continued irrigation per esophagus into the pleural space has been proposed to avoid operative repair.[16] This seems a dubious choice.

RESULTS

The overall mortality from a recent collected case series from 1990 to 2003 was 18%.[3] The etiology of the perforation affected outcome. Barogenic perforations had a mortality of 36%, instrumental perforations 19%, and traumatic perforations 7%. The location of the perforation also affected outcome. Cervical perforations had a mortality of 6%, whereas thoracic perforations had a mortality of 27%. Delay in treatment affected outcome, as would be expected. When treatment was initiated within the first 24 hours, average mortality was 14%, whereas it was 27% if treatment was delayed beyond 24 hours. Finally, the type of treatment influenced outcome. Primary repair had a mortality of 12%, resection 17%, drainage 36%, exclusion 24%, and nonoperative management 17%. These results have not changed appreciably since the last large case series review in 1992.[1]

Older series suggested a benefit to using a tissue buttress, with reduced leak rates and mortality after primary repair.[1] More recent series have reported good results without use of a tissue buttress.[11] Our feeling is that adding a tissue buttress may help contain a small postoperative leak and that the morbidity of taking an intercostal muscle for a flap is minimal. Of greater importance is complete exposure of the mucosal tear with meticulous and secure closure of both the mucosa and muscularis. Older series also suggested that primary repair should be undertaken only for early perforations and that exclusion or resection be the mainstay of management for late perforations. Again, recent reports suggest that primary repair is applicable whether performed early or late. As expected, results are better with early repair, although most patients with late repairs also did well.

STENTS

Despite advancements in diagnostic imaging, surgical technique, and postoperative care, open surgical repair for esophageal perforation continues to be associated with significant morbidity and mortality, particularly in cases of delayed presentation (>24 hours). Nonoperative management of esophageal perforation was classically reserved for poor surgical candidates due to associated comorbidities precluding surgical repair, or as palliation for perforations associated with malignant disease. The introduction of expandable bare-metal stents changed the management paradigm in this patient population; protocols of supportive care including nothing per mouth, drainage, broad spectrum antibiotics, and total parenteral nutrition matured to include expeditious stent placement, early resumption of oral intake, and timely hospital discharge. These initial series were difficult to interpret; they included heterogeneous patient populations, a variety of stent types, and varying management protocols, although they uniformly demonstrated good success rates (60%–90%). Increased experience with stents led to expanded use in patients presenting with iatrogenic perforations, particularly after delayed presentation and in those with significant associated mediastinal/pleural contamination. Although their initial use was problematic due to difficulties associated with removal of uncovered metal stents (mucosal ingrowth), several small prospective series demonstrated the utility of stents as a primary treatment option for these patients. This indication has been expanded to included patients following early presentation who traditionally have reasonable outcomes with open surgical repair. The introduction of covered removable self-expanding stent technology, which are easily deployed, restrict mucosal ingrowth, and are adjustable if migration does occur, have led to widespread use by thoracic surgeons for both iatrogenic and benign esophageal perforations.

Although stent deployment for esophageal perforation is a less invasive model, appropriate use mandates equivalent management goals performed during open repair. Namely, rapid closure of the perforation, drainage of associated infection within the pleural space or mediastinum, and enteral access for nutrition during recovery are a necessity. Optimally, stent placement would minimize morbidity and mortality associated with thoracotomy and esophageal repair.

Freeman et al. managed 17 patients following iatrogenic intrathoracic esophageal perforation with silicone stent placement as initial therapy concurrently with mediastinal/pleural drainage by VATS or tube thoracostomy (in cases of delayed presentation or evidence of extraesophageal contamination). Leak occlusion was successful in 94% of patients, and 82% were able to initiate oral intake within 72 hours of stent placement. Only one patient was ineffectively controlled by stent placement and required operative repair. Stent migration required replacement or repositioning in three patients, and all stents were removed within 2 months without stent-related complications. Interestingly, this study included a significant number of sick patients; 65% displayed symptoms of mediastinitis, and 24% of sepsis. Average time from perforation to stent placement was 39 hours. These results are certainly impressive considering the delayed presentation of most patients and evidence of mediastinal contamination. Follow-up endoscopy revealed no evidence of postoperative stricture, likely due to the intrinsic properties of the stent that acts as a rapid manifold for tissue healing.[17]

In a subsequent assessment by Freeman et al. of 19 patients with spontaneous esophageal perforations (Boerhaave syndrome), also managed with silicone stent placement, leak occlusion was successful in 89% of patients, and 79% of patients initiated PO intake within 72 hours of stent placement. Mean time for onset of symptoms to stent placement was 22 hours. This study included patients without significant underlying medical problems but high rates of mediastinitis (68%), sepsis (16%), and obesity; contributing factors that increase risk for open surgical morbidity and mortality. Two patients with leaks at the gastroesophageal (GE) junction failed stent management and required operative repair. Four patients required repositioning or stent replacement due to migration. This migration rate was higher than Freeman's previous study, although not unexpected due to stent placement in proximity to the GE junction. Stent removal was individualized based on cause of perforation, anatomic location, patient's nutritional status, and resolution of any associated infection, and was completed in all patients within 1 month of placement with an overall success rate of 79%. Again, no postoperative strictures were reported. These results were surprisingly good considering the difficulty associated with placing/maintaining stent position in proximity to the GE junction.[18]

In a similar fashion, D'Cunha et al. managed 15 patients with silicone stent placement in lieu of surgical management for esophageal perforation. Almost 60% of patients were stented within 24 hours of diagnosis, and 45% of patients underwent drainage procedures for source control. Overall success was 60% with mean 27 days to resolution. Median time to return of PO intake was 3 days. All stents were removed without complication and no postoperative strictures were noted. Stent migration occurred in 13% of patients. Most notably an 88% success rate was achieved in their final 17 patients as the author's experience matured. In their final nine cases, all patients were successfully managed with stent placement after diagnosis, with resumption of PO intake by postoperative day 1.[19]

Fisher et al. managed 15 patients with spontaneous and iatrogenic esophageal perforations, placing self-expandable metal stents in both groups. Patients were stratified into two groups based on time to intervention: (1) those stented within 45 minutes of perforation (iatrogenic following endoscopic procedures) or (2) patients stented on average 123 hours following injury (Boerhaave's, laparoscopic fundoplication, esophageal diverticulectomy). Patients in the early treatment cohort were managed successfully with stent placement alone and were discharged by hospital day 5. Only one patient required a drainage procedure for fluid accumulation close to the perforation site. In the second group, postoperative management was complicated in some cases by sepsis and multiorgan failure, including one patient death, with an average length of stay of 44 days. Stent extraction was accomplished in 12 patients between 10 days and 8 weeks postoperatively.[20]

In our own institution, we treated a 63-year-old gentleman who underwent endoluminal stent grafting of a thoracic aortic aneurysm, complicated by an aortoesophageal fistula 4 weeks postoperatively. The patient underwent exploration and an isolated perforation in the esophagus was repaired primarily; buttressed with an intercostal muscle flap. In addition, latissimus dorsi was mobilized and ultimately interposed between the aneurysm sac and the esophageal repair. Postoperatively, the patient developed evidence of sepsis, renal failure, and respiratory failure requiring intubation. A gastrografin swallow demonstrated contrast extravasation from the esophagus (Fig. 48-12A). The patient was brought back to the operating room for endoscopic evaluation, stent placement, and mediastinal/pleural drainage (Fig. 48-12B). Postoperatively he responded to antibiotics, resumed oral intake, and ultimately was discharged to a rehabilitation facility. Contrast esophagram at 1 week demonstrated esophageal coverage and resolution of leak (Fig. 48-12C).

These studies demonstrated that esophageal stents are a viable primary treatment option for patients presenting immediately after esophageal perforation. Likewise, prolonged time to presentation following esophageal perforation and the presence of sepsis or shock from associated contamination does not preclude the use of esophageal stents as primary management. Drainage of associated contamination by VATS or percutaneous tube thoracostomy is suggested in these cases. The time point at which percutaneous or operative drainage is necessary has not been well defined. Because this is a vital component of therapy and ultimately impacts outcome, its use should be strongly considered in all patients with any evidence of contamination or for those presenting in a delayed fashion. Stent extraction after healing should always be performed due to complications associated with long-term treatment. This has been facilitated by the ease of removal inherent to covered/silicone stents. The potential for stent migration requires postoperative monitoring with chest x-ray to ensure adequate positioning; covered stents are inherently resistant to mucosal ingrowth and allow for repositioning or replacement without significant difficulty.

Mandatory to the successful management of esophageal perforation with stents is the fundamental premise that the goals achieved during open surgery are accomplished in an equivalent fashion: closure of the esophageal perforation, drainage of contamination, broad spectrum antibiotics, and prompt resumption of enteral nutrition to enhance healing. Stricture rates of 10% to 50% historically are noted following operative esophageal repair, necessitating further endoscopic procedures, dilatations, and risk. This is an obvious advantage of stent therapy. Success ultimately depends on a uniform approach that includes appropriate patient selection, experience with stent placement, and appropriate postoperative care. Endoscopy remains a critical component in the management of esophageal perforation: at presentation, to document leak resolution, and for follow-up evaluation.

EDITOR'S COMMENT

Esophageal perforations are not a single disease, but separate diseases with different symptoms and management dependent upon the mechanism and location of injury. The authors make

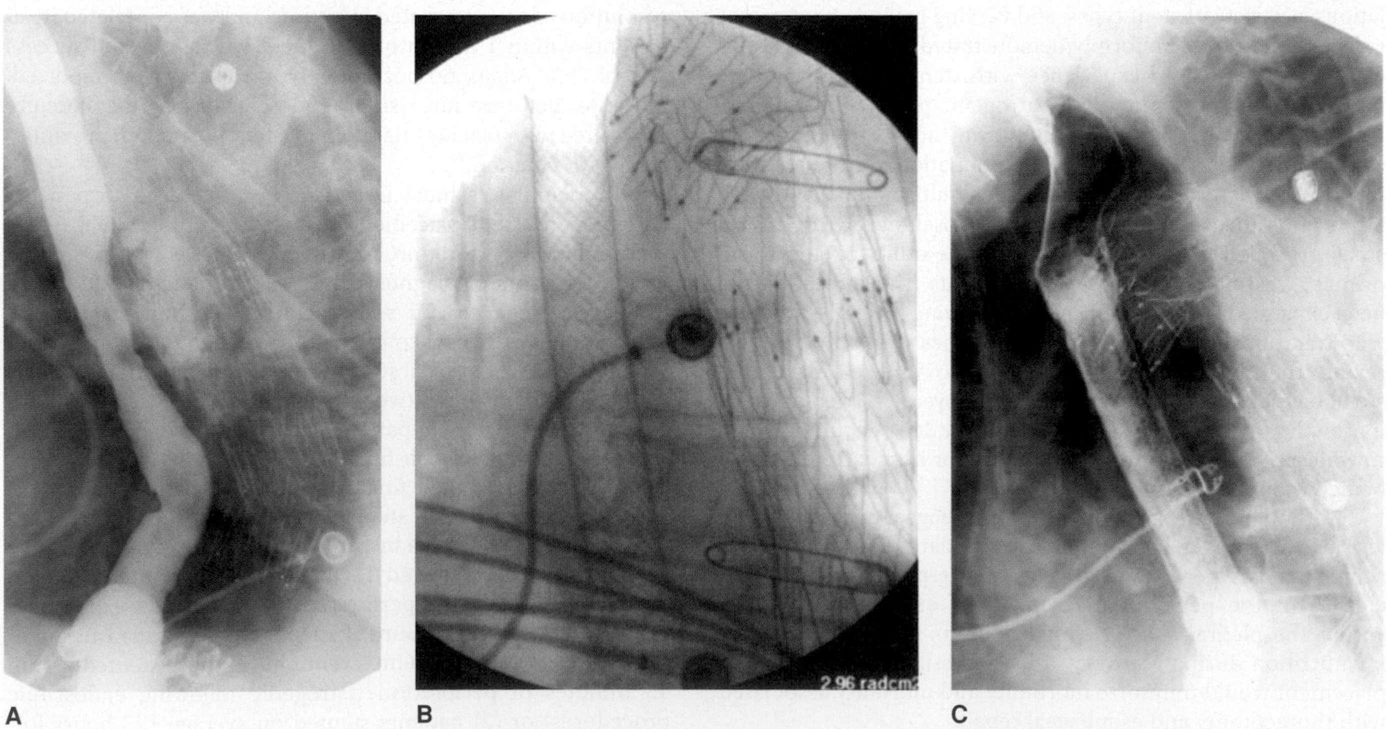

A B C

Figure 48-12. *A.* Contrast swallow of a 63-year-old gentleman 4 weeks after failed closure of an aortoesophageal fistula. *B.* The patient was brought back to the operating room for endoscopic evaluation, stent placement, and mediastinal/pleural drainage. *C.* Contrast swallow 1 week later confirms esophageal coverage and resolution of leak.

this clear. I endorse their observation that the mucosal injury in a cervical esophageal perforation does not have to be specifically closed, but that the perforation needs to be adequately drained. I also appreciate the numerous surgical pearls of wisdom included in the descriptions of the operative repairs. I would point out to the reader that I have personally found either a T-tube repair or esophageal diversion to be helpful for the occasional patient with a late perforation and poor tissue quality. Edematous tissue that cannot adequately hold a stitch can be treated well with either of these two strategies.

This chapter makes a significant contribution in specifically addressing intramural perforations. It also presents a very good discussion of the risks and potential benefits of conservative management for carefully selected patients. It is important to note that esophageal perforation remains a life-threatening disease with double digit 30-day mortality within all subgroups. The discussion of the use of stents is balanced and fair. I agree with the authors that this may dramatically affect the management of perforations in the near future. The observation that stents are less successful with GE junction perforations is an important point, and mimics our experience. We no longer use stents for GE junction perforations but approach them laparoscopically. Also, the need to drain any fluid collection in addition to stent placement cannot be emphasized enough. Finally, the anecdotal report of using a stent to salvage a leak following an open repair suggests one possible strategy for the integration of this new technology to improve the outcome of this highly lethal disease.

—Michael T. Jaklitsch

References

1. Jones WG 2nd, Ginsberg RJ. Esophageal perforation: a continuing challenge. *Ann Thorac Surg.* 1992;53:534–543.
2. Port JL, Kent MS, Korst RJ, et al. Thoracic esophageal perforations: a decade of experience. *Ann Thorac Surg.* 2003;75:1071–1074.
3. Brinster CJ, Singhal S, Lee L, et al. Evolving options in the management of esophageal perforation. *Ann Thorac Surg.* 2004;77:1475–1483.
4. Weiman DS, Walker WA, Brosnan KM, et al. Noniatrogenic esophageal trauma. *Ann Thorac Surg.* 1995;59:845–849.
5. Gaissert HA, Roper CL, Patterson GA, et al. Infectious necrotizing esophagitis: outcome after medical and surgical intervention. *Ann Thorac Surg.* 2003;75:342–347.
6. Fadoo F, Ruiz DE, Dawn SK, et al. Helical CT esophagography for the evaluation of suspected esophageal perforation or rupture. *Am J Roentgenol.* 2004;182:1177–1179.
7. Cameron JL, Kieffer RF, Hendrix TR, et al. Selective nonoperative management of contained intrathoracic esophageal disruptions. *Ann Thorac Surg.* 1979;27:404–408.
8. Altorjay A, Kiss J, Voros A, et al. Nonoperative management of esophageal perforations: is it justified? *Ann Surg.* 1997;225:415–421.
9. Lawrence DR, Ohri SK, Moxon RE, et al. Primary esophageal repair for Boerhaave's syndrome. *Ann Thorac Surg.* 1999;67:818–820.
10. Wang N, Razzouk AJ, Safavi A, et al. Delayed primary repair of intrathoracic esophageal perforation: is it safe? *J Thorac Cardiovasc Surg.* 1996;111: 114–121.
11. Whyte RI, Iannettoni MD, Orringer MB. Intrathoracic esophageal perforation: the merit of primary repair. *J Thorac Cardiovasc Surg.* 1995;109:140–144.
12. Wright CD, Mathisen DJ, Wain JC, et al. Reinforced primary repair of thoracic esophageal perforation. *Ann Thorac Surg.* 1995;60:245–248.
13. Altorjay A, Kiss J, Voros A, et al. The role of esophagectomy in the management of esophageal perforations. *Ann Thorac Surg.* 1998;65:1433–1436.
14. Orringer MB, Stirling MC. Esophagectomy for esophageal disruption. *Ann Thorac Surg.* 1990;49:35–42.
15. Santos GH, Frater RW. Transesophageal irrigation for the treatment of mediastinitis produced by esophageal rupture. *J Thorac Cardiovasc Surg.* 1986;91:57–62.
16. Urschel HC Jr, Razzuk MA, Wood RE, et al. Improved management of esophageal perforation: exclusion and diversion in continuity. *Ann Surg.* 1974;179:587–591.
17. Freeman RK, Van Woerkom JM, Ascioti AJ. Esophageal stent placement for the treatment of iatrogenic intrathoracic esophageal perforation. *Ann Thorac Surg.* 2007;83:2003–2008.
18. Freeman RK, Van Woerkom JM, Vyverberg A, et al. Esophageal stent placement for the treatment of spontaneous esophageal perforations. *Ann Thorac Surg.* 2009;88:194–198.
19. D'Cunha J, Rueth NM, Groth SS, et al. Esophageal stents for anastomotic leaks and perforations. *J Thorac Cardiovasc Surg.* 2011;142(1):39–46.e1.
20. Fischer A, Thomusch O, Benz S, et al. Nonoperative treatment of 15 benign esophageal perforations with self-expandable covered metal stents. *Ann Thorac Surg.* 2006;81:467–472.

49 Blunt and Penetrating Esophageal Trauma

Subroto Paul and Michael Y. Chang

Keywords: Blunt and penetrating esophageal trauma, esophageal rupture (Boerhaave syndrome), iatrogenic injury, esophageal perforation

Esophageal trauma can result from numerous etiologies, including iatrogenic injuries from endoscopic instrumentation or other thoracic surgical procedures, penetrating or blunt trauma, caustic ingestion during suicide attempts, and even spontaneously with forceful vomiting or retching (Boerhaave syndrome).[1–3] These traumatic episodes can lead to esophageal perforation—a medical emergency that requires prompt attention. Any delay in diagnosis or treatment leads to increased patient morbidity and mortality. The signs and symptoms of esophageal trauma are presented in this chapter along with recommendations for management.

CLINICAL CHARACTERISTICS

Esophageal perforation can result from multiple etiologies. Iatrogenic injury is the most common and results as a complication of esophageal instrumentation (50%–70% in modern series).[3] Spontaneous rupture, or Boerhaave syndrome, can also occur, typically after prolonged vomiting or retching. Both blunt and penetrating injuries can lead to esophageal perforation (see Chapter 49). For the normal esophagus, the cervical portion is the most common site of injury during instrumentation.[3–7] Middle and distal esophageal injuries usually result from endoscopic stenting or dilation procedures. Iatrogenic injury sustained during endoscopic procedures such as esophagogastroduodenoscopy and transesophageal echocardiography typically are diagnosed more rapidly because the patient is under direct medical observation at the time of the injury. Although rare, esophageal perforation also can result from nasogastric tube placement, esophageal intubation with an endotracheal tube, and nonesophageal surgical procedures performed in proximity to the esophagus, such as tracheostomy, thyroidectomy, various spinal procedures, and mediastinal lymph node dissection during pulmonary resectional procedures.

Spontaneous esophageal rupture, or Boerhaave syndrome, is caused by prolonged forceful vomiting or from abrupt Valsalva-type maneuvers that abruptly increase intrathoracic pressure.[1,3] The perforation in spontaneous cases occurs in the lower esophagus posteriorly into the left chest.

Penetrating injuries to the neck can also lead to esophageal perforation. Owing to proximity to the carotid artery and trachea, penetrating esophageal injury is rarely isolated. Typically, it is associated with more immediate, life-threatening injuries to these adjacent structures.[6] Blunt neck trauma, which can occur with either powerful direct blows to the neck or more commonly from high-speed motor vehicle accidents, usually causes an intramucosal esophageal hematoma and subsequent dysphagia but rarely perforation. Intramucosal hematomas resolve with expectant management. Full-thickness esophageal injuries can be life threatening and often are missed in this setting, clouded by other more life-threatening injuries with consequent higher morbidity and mortality.[4,6] Full-thickness esophageal injuries are associated with concurrent airway injury. A high index of suspicion is needed when evaluating trauma patients because unrecognized esophageal injury can have disastrous consequences.

Caustic esophageal injury (discussed in detail in Chapter 50) is a form of "chemically" penetrating trauma. It often results from suicide attempts, and the severity of the injury depends on the type, quantity, duration, and for children, taste of the chemical ingested. Alkaline exposure (e.g., lye) is typically more severe than acid (e.g., battery acid or bleach) exposure because alkaline agents cause a liquefactive necrosis, whereas acidic agents lead to a coagulative necrosis.[2,4,8] Treatment of caustic injuries must be expedient to prevent early- and late-term morbidity of this often-fatal injury.

PREOPERATIVE ASSESSMENT

The clinical manifestations of esophageal perforation secondary to blunt or penetrating trauma are nonspecific and depend on the location (i.e., cervical, thoracic, or abdominal esophagus) of injury rather than mechanism. Tachycardia, fever, subcutaneous air, pain, dysphagia, shortness of breath, and listlessness are all nonspecific signs and symptoms of esophageal perforation. Cervical esophageal perforation typically is heralded by neck pain and subcutaneous emphysema involving the neck or upper thorax. Patients with abdominal and thoracic esophageal perforation typically complain of subxiphoid or epigastric pain as well as retrosternal pain occasionally radiating to the back. Tachycardia and dyspnea are uniformly present, leading inevitably to hypotension and shock if the condition is left undiagnosed and untreated.

The need for diagnostic studies depends on the degree of clinical suspicion. In cases of iatrogenic injury, especially those occurring during endoscopy, no further diagnostic studies are needed because the injury is directly visualized. When the presence or nature of esophageal injury is not known, various diagnostic studies can be helpful. In over 90% of patients, chest radiographs will suggest the presence of esophageal injury, with findings of pneumomediastinum, subcutaneous emphysema, and left-sided pleural effusion suggestive of perforation. These findings are nonspecific, however, and an upper gastrointestinal series or chest CT scan with oral contrast material can confirm the diagnosis in over 90% of patients. Water-soluble contrast material is recommended for the upper gastrointestinal series because barium in the mediastinum can cause chemical mediastinitis. Of the two modalities, chest CT scanning is the more sensitive, having been reported to be over 95% sensitive for the diagnosis of esophageal perforation.

Esophagogastroduodenoscopy is used in most cases after the injury has been diagnosed by upper gastrointestinal series or chest CT scan.[3,5] Esophagogastroduodenoscopy alone may miss small injuries and potentially can exacerbate the perforation as well as increase mediastinal contamination with air insufflation. Hence its use is limited to the operating room, where it serves as a diagnostic adjunct to precisely map out the area of injury immediately before definitive surgical repair.

Diagnosis of caustic injury rests on the history because it typically occurs after a suicide attempt or accidental ingestion by an infant. Oropharyngeal pain, emesis, and dysphagia are the predominant signs and symptoms. Diagnosis of perforation is made with an upper gastrointestinal series or chest CT scan. If no perforation is seen on upper gastrointestinal series or chest CT scan, esophagoscopy should be performed 12 to 24 hours after initial presentation to examine the extent of esophageal involvement and depth of injury.

MANAGEMENT AND TECHNIQUE

The management of esophageal perforation depends on multiple factors, but chief among these are the etiology, location, and time from injury to diagnosis. Progressive delay in diagnosis results in a worsened prognosis because of continued contamination, release of inflammatory mediators, and resulting septic physiology. As expected, iatrogenic perforation typically has the best prognosis because diagnosis is immediate, whereas spontaneous and trauma-related perforations carry the worst prognosis because the diagnosis is often missed and treatment delayed.

Management and survival are both influenced by the anatomic location of the perforation. Cervical esophageal perforations are better contained with less spillage and result in a mortality rate of less than 10%, especially when there is no contamination of the mediastinum. Thoracic and abdominal perforations with widespread contamination of the mediastinum, pleura, and peritoneum have a historical mortality rate of over 50% in most series.[1,3,5,7–10] More recent series quote a mortality rate of 20% to 25% resulting from improved surgical critical care and operative technique.[1,3,5,7–9]

Initial management of esophageal perforation involves resuscitation of the patient. The regimen includes administration of intravenous fluids, proton pump inhibitors to reduce gastric acid secretion, broad-spectrum antibiotics to cover oral and gastrointestinal flora (including fungal organisms), and restriction of oral intake. Nasogastric tube placement is avoided initially to prevent worsening the injury, especially if an operative intervention is anticipated. If conservative measures are to be used, a nasogastric tube is carefully placed for gastric decompression.

Surgical treatment for esophageal perforation is the mainstay of therapy; however, nonoperative treatment can be substituted in some situations. Historically, nonoperative management alone with antibiotics and parental hyperalimentation carries a 20% to 40% mortality.[1,3,5,7–13] In selected patients who have well-contained or internally drained perforations and are without septic physiology, nonoperative management may be attempted, especially in those who are poor operative candidates. Many cervical esophageal leaks can be managed this way. However, most thoracic and abdominal leaks require an operative intervention.

Operative intervention consists of four modalities: (1) primary repair, (2) diversion and exclusion, (3) T-tube drainage, (4) esophagectomy with immediate or staged reconstruction, and (5) endoscopic repair with or without associated mediastinal debridement.[3–5,7,12,14–20] The main principles of each of these operative interventions entail controlling the perforation and draining the area of contamination.

Primary repair of esophageal perforation is possible when the tissue quality of the esophagus and surrounding tissues lends itself to repair (see Chapter 48). Hence there is minimal edema and devitalized tissue in the area, permitting proper tissue approximation. Primary repair is pursued in patients with minimal comorbidity who are diagnosed within 24 hours of injury. Usually, cervical esophageal injuries can be repaired primarily because the contamination tends to be minimal, it is contained within the surrounding neck tissues, and the repair can be well drained.[3,6,8,10] Primary repair for thoracic and abdominal perforations is considered in good surgical candidates who have minimal mediastinal and intra-abdominal contamination and devitalized tissue and are stable hemodynamically. Primary repairs should be reinforced with viable tissues such as intercostal or platysmal muscle, pleura, pericardium, or adjacent stomach. When repairing thoracic esophageal injuries, it is prudent to debride and drain the entire mediastinum.

The esophagus is mobilized around the area of perforation. It is important to open the muscle layers over the perforation to identify the full extent of the injury, which can be subtle. A two-layer repair is recommended, with reapproximation of the mucosa with absorbable suture material (such as Vicryl or PDS [polydioxanone] suture; Ethicon, Somerville, NJ) and closure with the muscularis propria using either absorbable or nonabsorbable suture. The repair then is reinforced with intercostal muscle or other viable tissues.[3,8,10,12] (Fig. 49-1). The chest is thoroughly irrigated and extensively drained. In the case of very low intra-abdominal esophageal perforations, a fundoplication or a Thal patch of stomach can be used to buttress the repair as well.[3,5,7–9,12] If presented with extensive contamination and devitalized esophageal tissue, which can accompany late diagnosis or extensive injuries, surgical options include exclusion

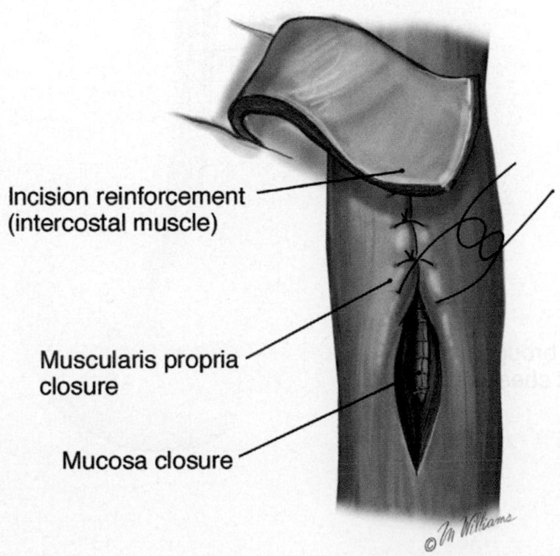

Figure 49-1. The esophageal perforation is repaired and reinforced with intercostal muscle or other viable tissues.

and diversion, T-tube drainage, and esophagectomy.[3,5,7,9,12] Exclusion and diversion techniques involve a cervical esophageal fistula and a gastrostomy, one to divert the oral flow and the other to minimize reflux of gastric contents into the esophagus (see Chapter 31). A jejunostomy is placed for feeding. The mediastinum is also debrided before the repair. The perforation is repaired, and the flow of saliva and bile are diverted to protect the repair. Placement of gastrointestinal conduit is delayed 6 months to 1 year. A modification of this technique involves intrathoracic esophageal repair with drainage, followed by stapling of the esophagus (without division) below the injury and creation of a cervical loop esophagostomy to protect the repair. Esophageal peristalsis permits recanalization of the distal staple line, whereas only the proximal staple line needs to be reversed, which often can be performed under local anesthesia without the need for additional major reconstruction.[3,7,14]

Another technique to contain mediastinal contamination from a perforated esophagus uses a Silastic biliary T-tube positioned inside the perforation and brought out of the chest (Fig. 49-2). This form of drainage creates a controlled esophagocutaneous fistula. This technique is especially useful if the esophageal tissues are too edematous to hold sutures. The T-tube then is withdrawn slowly 6 months to 1 year later after resolution of the sepsis. The patient is reevaluated and the esophagus studied to see if any reconstructive options are needed.

An esophagectomy, with or without immediate reconstruction, should be considered for esophageal perforations in the setting of cancer, severe stricture, or dilated megaesophagus from achalasia. These complex surgeries are presented in Chapters 15–23 and 34. Reconstruction should be delayed if the patient is unstable. However, if the patient is stable and the surrounding tissues are of good viability with minimal edema, reconstructive options include creating a conduit from the stomach or colon. The jejunum is rarely used in this setting. The stomach is preferred but may not be possible if injured, as in cases of caustic ingestion. If reconstruction is to be delayed, a cervical esophageal fistula and gastrostomy and jejunostomy are created as in the diversion with exclusion technique.

Endoscopic repair of esophageal perforations has been reported as well. Repairs include esophageal stenting of small perforations, endoscopic suturing of partial- and full-thickness injuries, and fibrin glue repair.[14–20] Of these techniques, endoscopic stenting with covered stents has been the most widely utilized. Endoscopic stenting of esophageal repair has been combined with mediastinal debridement performed either thoracoscopically or through a thoracotomy in order to avoid diversion and salvage the injured esophagus. Initial reports of esophageal stenting for perforation were in patients deemed high risk for surgery. However, more recent reports have extended treatment to patients deemed to have acceptable operative risk. No large randomized trials have been performed, to date, and most reports are from small single institutional case series. The results of these studies are mixed. Esophageal leakage and contamination of surrounding tissues can be contained with stenting, particularly for small tears which are less than 6 cm. However, in many cases, it does not eliminate the need for debridement of devitalized local tissue and the clearance of a cervical, intrathoracic, or abdominal abscess. As definitive repair is avoided, surveillance with repeated endoscopies or radiographic studies is needed to assess stent migration and closure of the seal. Although esophageal stenting for perforation may be effective in some

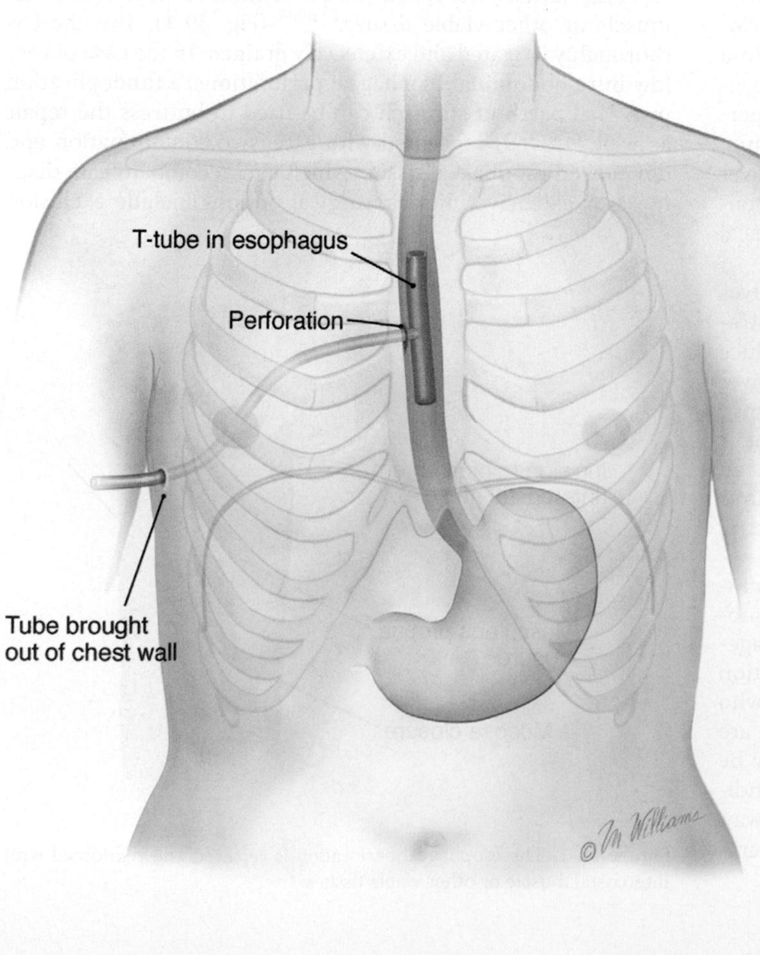

Figure 49-2. A Silastic biliary T-tube is positioned inside the perforation and brought out of the chest to control contamination from a severely perforated esophagus.

cases, in many others it delays definitive treatment.[14–20] As no large studies have been conducted, to date, the efficacy of these approaches remains to be determined before they can be routinely recommended.

POSTOPERATIVE CARE

Postoperative management of patients with esophageal perforations is often precarious because the initial inflammatory insult leads to a septic physiology that is maintained 24 to 48 hours postoperatively; and therefore requires attention to fluid resuscitation and vasopressor requirements. After this phase has passed, nutrition is paramount and is maintained entirely through feeding gastrostomies or jejunostomies or parenteral nutrition if there is an ileus. The primarily repaired or reconstructed neoesophagus is studied with a water-soluble upper gastrointestinal series. The exact timing of this contrast evaluation depends on the patient's clinical course, but typically the evaluation is performed a few days to 1 week after surgery.

Late complications of esophageal injury that result from primary repair and caustic injury include tracheoesophageal fistula and strictures. Esophageal strictures are treated symptomatically with dilation or occasionally stenting, but severe caustic strictures often require esophagectomy and reconstruction. Tracheoesophageal fistula also requires operative intervention, as outlined in Chapter 58.

PROCEDURE-SPECIFIC COMPLICATIONS

The incidence of complications after operative intervention for esophageal perforation depends on the quality of tissues repaired and the overall condition of the patient. If primary repair or T-tube drainage of the esophageal perforation fails and there is widespread contamination with septic physiology, the esophagus must be diverted and excluded, as described earlier.[3–5,7,10,12,14,15] Often there are no physiologic signs of sepsis, but radiologic study (either an esophagram or chest CT scan) reveals a contained esophageal perforation with contrast material exiting and reentering into the esophagus. This scenario typically can be managed conservatively by restricting oral intake and starting IV antibiotics. The contrast study is repeated in 7 days to assess for healing. If there is clinical deterioration, the patient must be explored and the esophagus excluded or diverted and any abscess collection drained.

An intra-abdominal or intrathoracic abscess can be seen with any of the four previously described surgical techniques, causing fever, an elevated white blood cell count, or failure to thrive. Any abscess must be drained, either surgically or with percutaneous CT-guided drainage, when feasible.[3–5,7,10,12,14,15] If repair, T-tube drainage, or exclusion techniques along with drainage fail to contain the perforation and nidus for sepsis, or if the native esophagus is completely necrotic, esophagectomy with delayed reconstruction is the last surgical resort. If a necrotic esophagus is suspected, esophagectomy should not be delayed.

SUMMARY

Esophageal trauma may be caused by blunt or penetrating injury. Most injuries are iatrogenic and occur during endoscopic instrumentation of the esophagus. Untreated, esophageal trauma carries a high morbidity and mortality. Treatment can be conservative in selected patients with high operative risk, but typically a surgical intervention is required. Surgical intervention depends on the location and extent of injury, with options including (1) primary repair, (2) diversion and exclusion, (3) T-tube drainage, (4) esophagectomy, and (5) endoscopic stenting in selected cases.

EDITOR'S COMMENT

There is little time for preparation when it comes to dealing with esophageal perforation or trauma. A thorough knowledge of the fundamental principles and techniques cannot be overemphasized. It is paramount for the surgeon to endoscope the patient just before deciding the course of surgery. Often, the diagnostic imaging is not accurate as to the site of injury or perforation, nor to the state of the esophagus. Careful observation of the patient's injury and consideration of all possible therapeutic options and approaches is recommended before determining the final exposure, sequence, and method of surgical treatment.

It is often the wish of a surgeon to avoid diversion. However, this may lead to multiple attempts at repair, drainage, and stenting followed by recurrent sepsis and long hospitalization. The surgeon must be realistic and use definitive therapy early on whenever appropriate and avoid wishful thinking that less surgery is always better.

—Raphael Bueno

References

1. Vial CM, Whyte RI. Boerhaave's syndrome: diagnosis and treatment. *Surg Clin North Am.* 2005;85:515–524.
2. Zwischenberger JB, Savage C, Bidani A. Surgical aspects of esophageal disease: perforation and caustic injury. *Am J Respir Crit Care Med.* 2002;165: 1037–1040.
3. Brinster CJ, Singhal S, Lee L, et al. Evolving options in the management of esophageal perforation. *Ann Thorac Surg.* 2004;77:1475–1483.
4. Graeber GM, Murray GF. Injuries of the esophagus. *Semin Thorac Cardiovasc Surg.* 1992;4:247–254.
5. Jones WG 2nd, Ginsberg RJ. Esophageal perforation: a continuing challenge. *Ann Thorac Surg.* 1992;53:534–543.
6. Thompson EC, Porter JM, Fernandez LG. Penetrating neck trauma: an overview of management. *J Oral Maxillofac Surg.* 2002;60:918–923.
7. Tomaselli F, Maier A, Pinter H, et al. Management of iatrogenous esophagus perforation. *Thorac Cardiovasc Surg.* 2002;50:168–173.
8. Goudy SL, Miller FB, Bumpous JM. Neck crepitance: evaluation and management of suspected upper aerodigestive tract injury. *Laryngoscope.* 2002;112:791–795.
9. Iannettoni MD, Vlessis AA, Whyte RI, et al. Functional outcome after surgical treatment of esophageal perforation. *Ann Thorac Surg.* 1997;64: 1606–1609; discussion 1609–1610.
10. Kim-Deobald J, Kozarek RA. Esophageal perforation: an 8-year review of a multispecialty clinic's experience. *Am J Gastroenterol.* 1992;87:1112–1119.

11. Crestanello JA, Deschamps C, Cassivi SD, et al. Selective management of intrathoracic anastomotic leak after esophagectomy. *J Thorac Cardiovasc Surg*. 2005;129:254–260.
12. Wright CD, Mathisen DJ, Wain JC, et al. Reinforced primary repair of thoracic esophageal perforation. *Ann Thorac Surg*. 1995;60:245–248; discussion 248–249.
13. Salo JA, Isolauri JO, Heikkila LJ, et al. Management of delayed esophageal perforation with mediastinal sepsis. Esophagectomy or primary repair? *J Thorac Cardiovasc Surg*. 1993;106:1088–1091.
14. Koniaris LG, Spector SA, Staveley-O'Carroll KF. Complete esophageal diversion: a simplified, easily reversible technique. *J Am Coll Surg*. 2004;199:991–993.
15. Sokolov VV, Bagirov MM. Reconstructive surgery for combined tracheoesophageal injuries and their sequelae. *Eur J Cardiothorac Surg*. 2001;20:1025–1029.
16. Koivukangas V, Biancari F, Meriläinen S, et al. Esophageal stenting for spontaneous esophageal perforation. *J Trauma Acute Care Surg*. 2012;73(4):1011–1013.
17. Freeman RK, Ascioti AJ, Giannini T, et al. Analysis of unsuccessful esophageal stent placements for esophageal perforation, fistula, or anastomotic leak. *Ann Thorac Surg*. 2012;94(3):959–964.
18. Dai Y, Chopra SS, Kneif S, et al. Management of esophageal anastomotic leaks, perforations, and fistulae with self-expanding plastic stents. *J Thorac Cardiovasc Surg*. 2011;141(5):1213–1217.
19. David EA, Kim MP, Blackmon SH. Esophageal salvage with removable covered self-expanding metal stents in the setting of intrathoracic esophageal leakage. *Am J Surg*. 2011;202(6):796–801.
20. D'Cunha J. Esophageal stents for leaks and perforations. *Semin Thorac Cardiovasc Surg*. 2011;23(2):163–167.

50 Surgical Management of Corrosive Injury to the Esophagus

Stacey Su and Jeanne M. Lukanich

Keywords: Caustic burn injury, attempted suicide, coagulative necrosis, liquefactive necrosis, surgical treatment, esophageal perforation, esophageal stricture, esophageal bypass

While accidental ingestion of caustic materials is more common in children, intentional ingestion is the leading cause of caustic esophageal injury in adults. The diagnosis should be suspected in all patients brought to the emergency ward for attempted suicide. The injury may be fatal and warrants immediate treatment. Identifying the nature of the ingested substance is paramount to proper management because the severity and nature of the injury are related to the chemical and physical properties of the caustic agent (i.e., acid vs. base, solid vs. liquid, concentration, quantity, and duration of contact with esophageal tissues).[1] These exposures cause injuries ranging in severity from first-, second-, or third-degree burn to full-thickness necrosis and frank perforation, often requiring surgical treatment.

ANATOMY

In chemical burn injuries, the esophageal sites most susceptible are the three areas of normal anatomic narrowing (Fig. 50-1). These are the upper esophagus at the cricopharyngeus, the midesophagus where the aortic arch and left mainstem bronchus cross, and the distal esophagus proximal to the lower esophageal sphincter (LES). Passage of the ingested material is delayed through these regions, increasing the duration of exposure and potential for injury. Reflux-associated LES hypotension causes prolonged exposure of the distal esophagus to the caustic agent. This is exacerbated by pylorospasm, particularly associated with alkali ingestion, which propagates the injury by causing regurgitation of caustic contents back into the esophagus.[2] Although there may be relative tolerance of the esophageal squamous epithelium to ingested acid, pylorospasm may lead to pooling of acid, severe gastritis, and full-thickness necrosis with perforation.

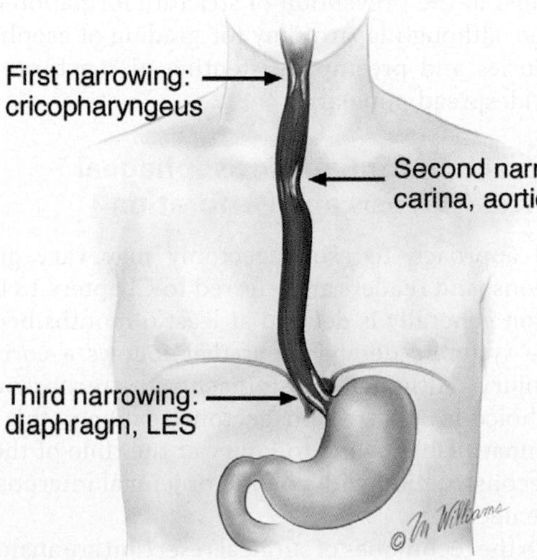

Figure 50-1. Anatomy of the esophagus showing areas of normal anatomic narrowing.

ETIOLOGY

Acids cause coagulation necrosis, which is characterized by the formation of eschar. This deposition of dead black tissue often limits the injury to the superficial esophageal lining. Alkaline exposure causes liquefactive necrosis, which allows the caustic agent to penetrate the esophageal wall more deeply, thereby escalating the severity of the injury.[3] Since the degree of injury is also associated with duration of exposure, it is important to determine whether the ingested material is a solid or a liquid. Solid alkali tends to adhere to the oropharyngeal region, whereas liquid alkali passes more quickly, causing greater esophageal and gastric injury.[4,5] The three phases of chemical injury are (1) inflammation/necrosis, (2) sloughing and ulceration, and (3) fibrosis with stricture formation. Management is guided by early flexible esophagoscopy to grade the degree and location of injury. Chemical burns are graded according to Zargar's 6-point classification of caustic mucosal injury as assessed from endoscopy.[6] First-degree burn (Grade 1) is characterized by hyperemia and edema; second-degree burn (Grade 2A, 2B), by ulceration; and third-degree burn (Grade 3A, 3B), by black or gray discoloration indicative of necrosis.[7] First-degree esophageal burns generally require observation alone because these injuries do not cause perforation or strictures. Second- and third-degree burns of the esophagus require ongoing monitoring for perforation or progression to generalized necrosis. Perforation or near-perforation requires immediate surgical intervention (see Chapter 48), whereas the absence of full-thickness necrosis and perforation necessitates frequent reevaluation and investigation over a prolonged time period.

ACUTE PRESENTATION

The symptoms of caustic ingestion include oral pain, drooling, inability, or refusal to swallow secondary to pain, and hematemesis. Hoarseness, stridor, or dyspnea suggests a laryngeal or supralaryngeal injury. Airway management is of paramount importance because of possible associated burns to the larynx. Intubation guided by fiberoptic or rigid bronchoscopy should be performed. One should be prepared to perform a surgical airway if required. After the airway is addressed, a thorough history and physical examination is completed. History includes verification of the caustic agent and documentation of the time between exposure and treatment. Symptoms of acute perforation include progressive neck, substernal, back, or abdominal pain. Signs of acute perforation are tachycardia, fever, subcutaneous emphysema, pericardial crunch, and chest dullness to percussion. Absence of symptoms does not entirely exclude significant injury, but the number of signs and symptoms present correlates with severity of injury.

Radiologic evaluation may include chest x-ray and CT scans to rule out pneumomediastinum or free intraperitoneal air. Initial CT scans of the neck, chest, and abdomen may be performed without contrast agents, although the administration of water-soluble contrast material improves the predictive value of the scans. Barium esophagram is of limited utility in the initial evaluation as it carries a 30% to 60% false-negative rate.[8]

All caustic ingestion patients are monitored with telemetry and resuscitated with IV fluids. Patients are kept nothing by mouth and given prophylactic IV H_2-blockers or proton pump inhibitors for both symptom relief and to treat reflux.[9] Flexible esophagoscopy is used for evaluation in nearly every patient with esophageal caustic injury. There is controversy regarding the optimal timing for initial endoscopic evaluation.[10] In the past, there was a tendency to wait at least 24 hours of injury, after the patient had been medically stabilized. Most agree that flexible esophagogastroduodenoscopy for complete evaluation should be carried out between 12 and 24 hours after injury (see Chapter 14). Endoscopy past 48 hours is discouraged due to the increased risk of perforation attributable to progressive wall weakening. Esophagogastroduodenoscopy may be impossible to complete depending on the severity of the patient's injury. The flexible scope may be carefully advanced past a site of mild injury but should be stopped at the site of circumferential Grade 2 and 3 injuries. Endoscopy distal to the site of first injury risks iatrogenic perforation.

CONSERVATIVE MANAGEMENT

Patients with first-degree burn are observed for at least 48 hours while their oral diet is advanced cautiously. Patients with second- or third-degree injuries without perforation should be admitted to the ICU and treated with broad-spectrum antibiotics and possibly steroids. While controversial, the administration of antibiotics and steroids may help to lessen gastrointestinal bacterial translocation and to decrease inflammation, respectively.[11–13] This may decrease the frequency and severity of stricture formation, as well as the necessity of multiple subsequent esophageal dilations, although the side effects of steroids with regard to increased susceptibility to infection should be carefully considered. Steroid administration also may relieve airway obstruction owing to mucosal edema and bronchospasm in the acute setting.[7] Reflux secondary to impaired esophageal function at the LES may also increase the potential for stricture formation. Proton pump inhibitors are employed to reduce reflux. Patients are monitored with serial chest x-rays. NPO status is maintained until the patient is able to swallow saliva without pain. A means for either enteral or parenteral nutrition is established. Rigid endoscopy is recommended for the safe placement of nasogastric tube, which serves both to stent the area of injury as well as to provide enteral nutrition. An initial esophagram with water-soluble contrast material is obtained within 48 hours and may be repeated at intervals as clinically indicated. Consideration may be given to various surgical treatments (discussed below) throughout the patient's hospital course.

Intermediate-term follow-up at 3 to 4 weeks, 3 months, and 6 months is necessary to monitor for stricture formation, gastric outlet obstruction, and the development of hourglass esophagus or linitis plastica.[1,10,14] After 6 months, long-term follow-up is required to monitor for the development of esophageal dysmotility or esophageal squamous cell carcinoma.

SURGICAL MANAGEMENT

Surgical management of chemical and burn injuries of the esophagus includes several broad categories of procedures and operations. Initial diagnostic procedures include bronchoscopy and esophagogastroduodenoscopy. Exploratory laparotomy, esophageal stenting, and enteral feeding tube insertion or parenteral feeding access are surgical procedures used often during the initial hospitalization of a chemical burn injury patient. Surgical intervention in the acute setting is rare but may be indicated for a full-thickness injury that results in esophageal perforation or diffuse necrosis evidenced by a systemic inflammatory response. Surgical techniques employed in this setting include esophageal resection and diversion, as is applied in severe cases of necrotizing esophageal perforation (see Chapters 48, 51, and 58).

In the subacute phase, esophageal dilation is often required for the treatment of strictures. Surgical resection with reconstruction may be considered in the chronic phase of injury after a severely strictured esophagus has failed repeated dilations. Esophagectomy ultimately may be required to reduce the risk of late carcinoma, which approaches 40% and manifests after a delay of 20 to 50 years.[15,16]

Exploratory Laparotomy

Exploratory laparotomy has been reported by Estrera and colleagues as an adjunct to esophagoscopic assessment for patients with Grade 2 and 3 injuries seen on esophagoscopy. In this approach, all patients with burns and full-thickness necrosis undergo radical esophagogastrectomy, cervical esophagostomy, and feeding jejunostomy. Patients without full-thickness necrosis undergo intraluminal stent placement for 21 days to prevent obliteration of the esophageal lumen and as a scaffold to promote epithelial ingrowth. Estrera and colleagues have reported excellent results in the prevention of stricture formation using this technique, although laparotomy for grading of esophageal corrosive injuries and preemptive stenting of strictures have not gained widespread popularity.[10]

Surgical Resection for Caustic Esophageal Full-Thickness Necrosis and Perforation

The surgical approach to esophagectomy may vary greatly among surgeons, and readers are referred to Chapters 13 to 27. Reconstruction generally is delayed at least 6 months because of the severe systemic derangement that follows a corrosive esophageal injury.[1] Although the stomach is the reconstructive conduit of choice in most esophagectomy patients, this conduit may be unavailable owing to injury at the time of the initial insult. Reconstruction with colonic or jejunal interposition grafts may be necessary.

Although the techniques of surgical resection are analogous to those used for malignant esophageal disease, the decision to resect for chemical burn-associated esophageal injuries can be more challenging.[17] Full-thickness biopsies of the esophageal wall are not possible, and other data obtained with procedures such as esophagoscopy are incomplete. Changes over time in the endoscopic or radiographic appearance of the esophagus and the patient's clinical status are the most helpful indicators of irreversible necrosis of the esophagus.

The surgical management of caustic esophageal perforation depends on many factors: the size and location of the perforation, the state of neighboring tissues, and the patient's overall clinical status.[18] Extensive full-thickness esophageal and gastric necrosis is treated urgently with total esophagogastrectomy with diverting cervical esophagostomy. In this manner, oropharyngeal secretions are diverted from the site of the perforation.[17] This procedure involves resection (often transhiatal) and diversion; the details of the surgical conduct of this procedure are described in several esophagectomy technique chapters in Part 2 and in Chapter 48 on esophageal perforation. In the setting of extensive esophageal necrosis, diversion without resection is not an option for definitive treatment. The necrotic esophagus in this situation leads to ongoing mediastinal soilage, systemic inflammatory response, and sepsis. It is therefore rarely left in situ once necrosis or perforation has occurred.

The critically ill status of the patient requiring esophageal resection for necrotizing corrosive injury precludes esophageal reconstruction in the acute setting. After the patient has been clinically stabilized, esophageal replacement may be electively planned.

Surgery for Caustic Esophageal Strictures

Esophageal stricture formation is the most frequent sequela of second- or third-degree esophageal burn. Steroids have no proven benefit in the prevention of stricture formation.[9] The time to development of strictures is variable and can occur days to as long as months after the injury. Most commonly, strictures develop between 3 weeks and 3 months after caustic ingestion, with the peak at 2 months.[14,19] Many strictures are mild to moderate in nature and will respond to dilation, often without recurrence. These strictures can be dilated using the standard methods (e.g., Savary, bougienage, or pneumatic) described in detail in Chapter 44.

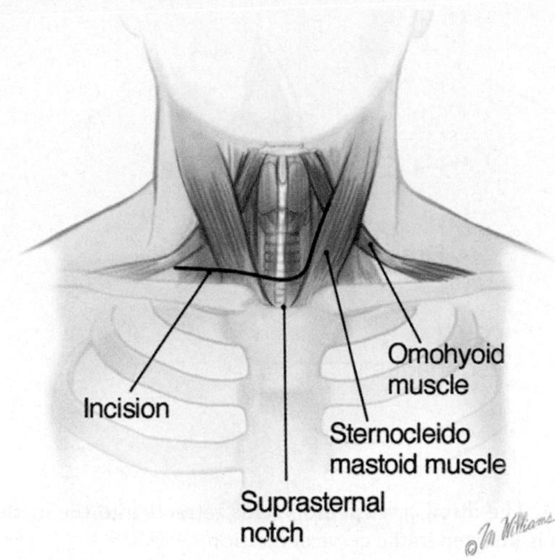

Figure 50-2. Collar incision for esophageal bypass.

Other strictures that occur after caustic esophageal exposure present a greater therapeutic challenge, making it difficult to dilate, and can recur quickly. Since there is no single uniformly effective treatment, many strategies have been suggested and are practiced. One strategy to prevent these strictures involves early bougienage, with treatment performed daily for several weeks before being decreased to every other day for several weeks and then weekly for months. This practice has not been proved to eliminate strictures but may lead to earlier resolution of strictures, although the incidence of perforation and associated morbidity is high. Many surgeons, however, do not perform esophageal dilations until 3 to 6 weeks after injury. Long (>1.5 cm) and eccentric strictures require dilation under fluoroscopic guidance.[7] An in-situ tube (e.g., Dobhoff, nasogastric, or string or bead chain) provides a guide through the esophageal stricture(s) and allows for dilation of tight strictures by preventing complete esophageal luminal obliteration. A nasogastric string or stainless steel bead chain, along with a gastrostomy tube, may facilitate retrograde dilation of strictures and is used commonly in pediatric patients. Local injection of

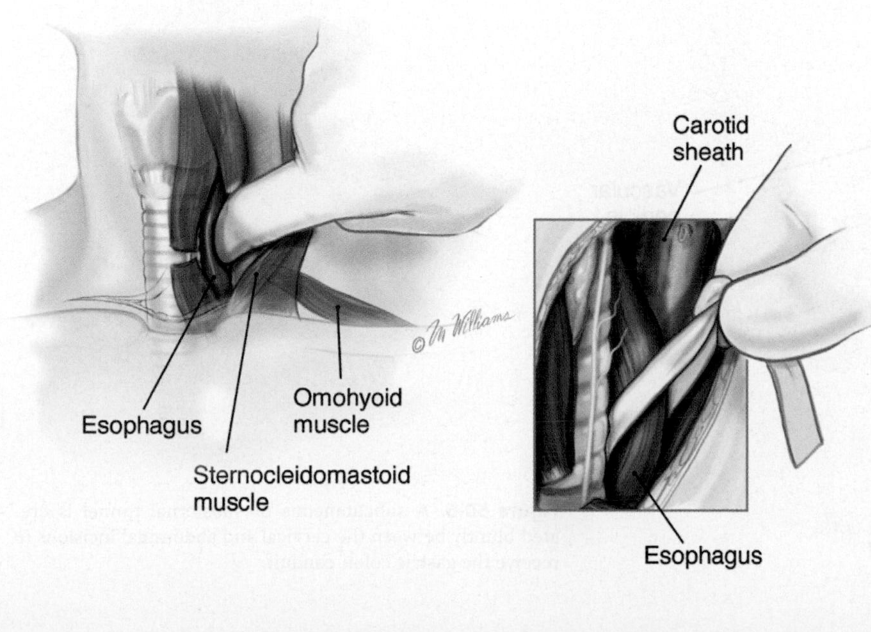

Figure 50-3. Omohyoid and strap muscles are divided as needed. Carotid sheath and jugular vein are retracted laterally.

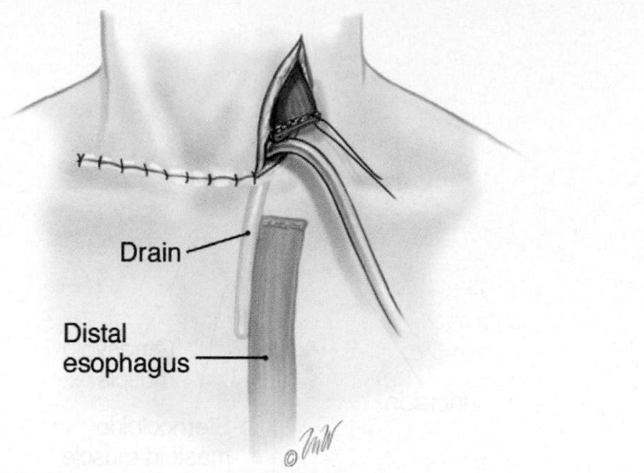

Figure 50-4. The distal cervical esophagus retracts into the mediastinum, and a drain is inserted in the cervical incision.

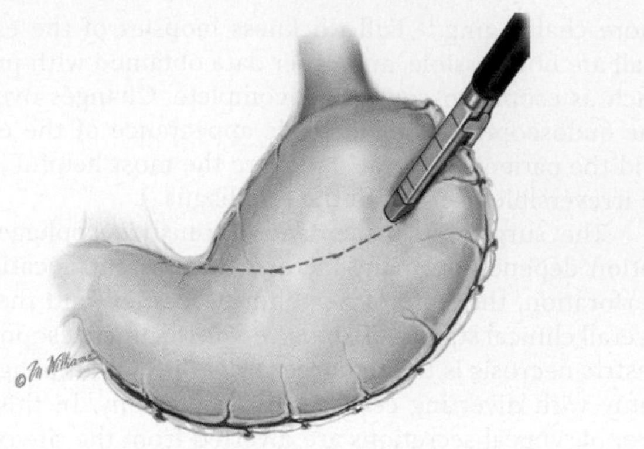

Figure 50-5. The gastric conduit is prepared. The stomach is divided from the top of the fundus to a point between the branches of the right and left gastric vessels.

corticosteroids via gastroscopy and followed by bougienage also can be a useful strategy for managing recalcitrant postcaustic injury esophageal strictures.[1] Another strategy is placement of self-expanding intraluminal stents. Stents have found limited success and may not be applicable for severe strictures, except as a temporizing measure.[20] Some may advocate placement of stents to avoid repeated dilations. Apart from case series, there are no studies to validate schedules for dilation of caustic strictures, or to guide management of caustic strictures with stents.

For the definitive treatment of refractory caustic strictures, elective esophagectomy with reconstruction may be indicated. The use of a gastric tube replacement conduit for severe stricture may be an option in selected patients. Rarely, the severity of initial injury associated with caustic ingestion causes obliteration of the esophagus with mediastinal fibrosis, necessitating passage of the conduit (e.g., colon, stomach) through an alternate route (i.e., subcutaneous, retrosternal, transthoracic). Details regarding these operative techniques can be found in the chapters in Part 2 as well as in Chapter 51.

Esophageal Bypass

Esophageal bypass is performed in patients with benign or malignant strictures of the esophagus, unresectable esophageal

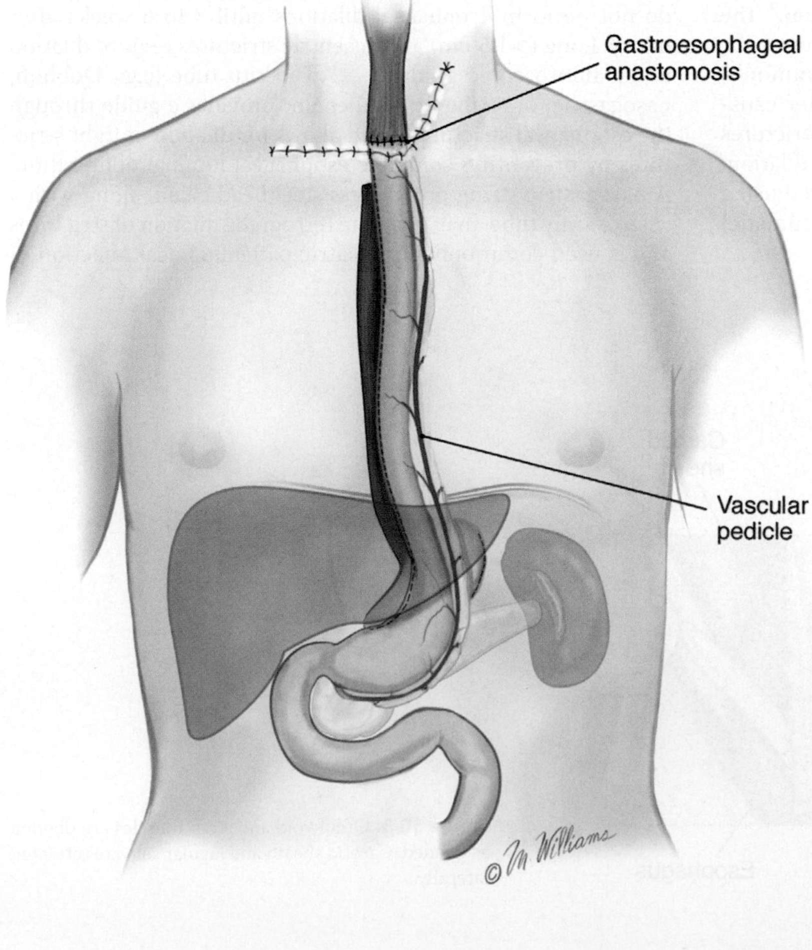

Figure 50-6. A subcutaneous or substernal tunnel is created bluntly between the cervical and abdominal incisions to receive the gastric colon conduit.

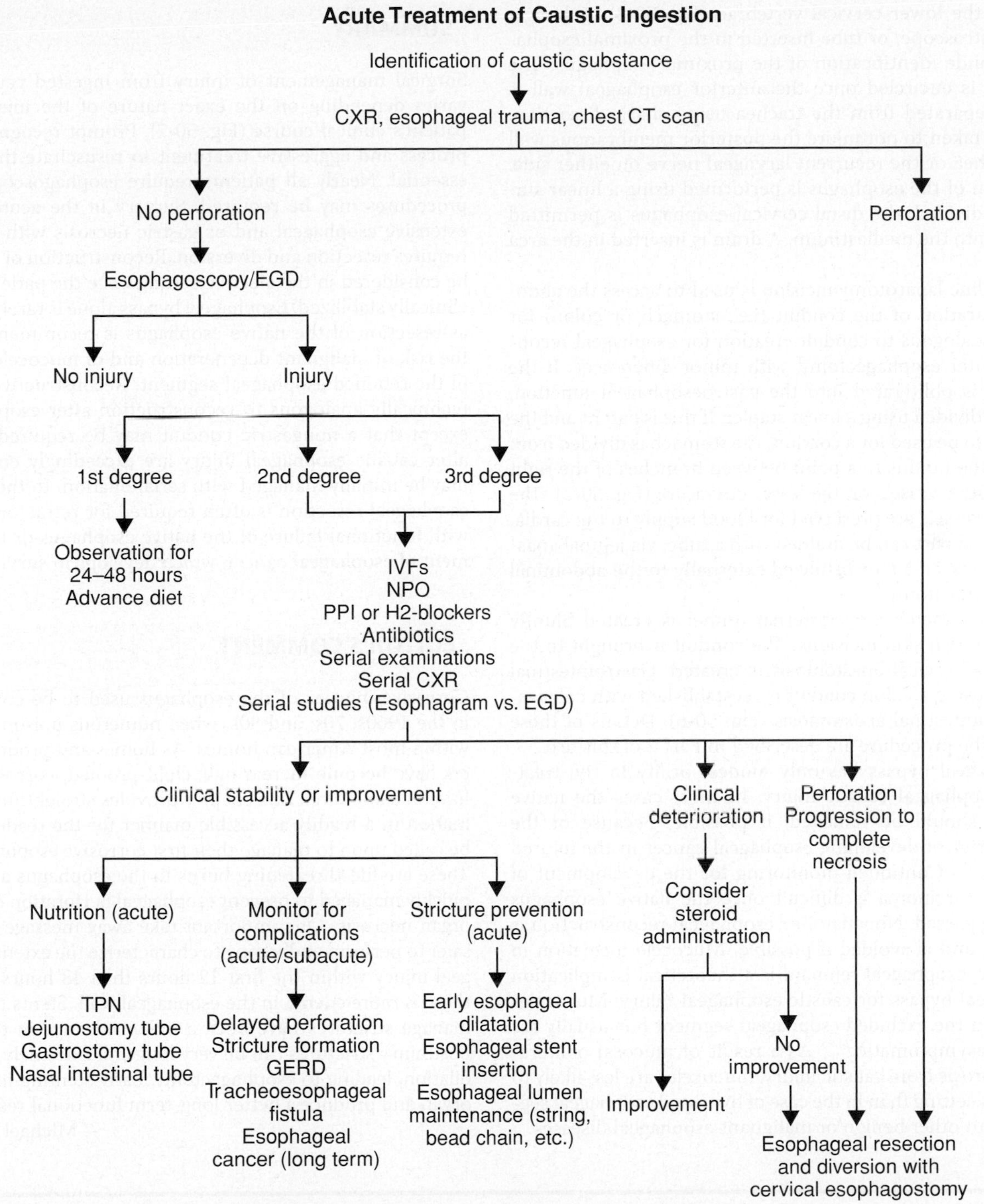

Figure 50-7. Algorithm for acute treatment of caustic ingestion.

cancer, esophageal perforation, and malignant or congenital tracheoesophageal fistula. Variations in surgical technique abound, but the result of surgery is orointestinal continuity and a bypassed esophagus left in situ that is excluded from the gastrointestinal system at both ends. A gastric or colon conduit is used most commonly for the bypassed esophagus.[21,22] In recent years, the use of esophageal bypass particularly in the setting of malignant esophageal disease has been replaced by the widespread use of esophageal stents. However it remains a valuable technique to maintain within one's armamentarium.

Preoperatively, the patient undergoes bowel preparation via an in situ feeding tube, if applicable. Perioperative antibiotics are administered. The patient is placed in the supine position with modest neck extension, and the neck, chest, and abdomen are prepped and draped in the usual sterile fashion. A collar incision 1 cm above the suprasternal notch is extended leftward and parallel to the anterior border of the sternocleidomastoid muscle to access the deep cervical space (Fig. 50-2). The omohyoid and other strap muscles are divided as needed, and the carotid sheath and jugular vein are retracted laterally. Blunt dissection is used to mobilize the posterior esophageal wall from the lower cervical vertebrae (Fig. 50-3). A bougie dilator, gastroscope, or tube inserted in the proximal esophagus may guide identification of the proximal esophagus. The esophagus is encircled once the anterior esophageal wall is carefully separated from the trachea using sharp dissection. Caution is taken to not injure the posterior membranous wall of the trachea or the recurrent laryngeal nerve on either side. Transection of the esophagus is performed using a linear stapler. Now divided, the distal cervical esophagus is permitted to retract into the mediastinum. A drain is inserted in the area (Fig. 50-4).

A midline laparotomy incision is used to access the abdomen. Preparation of the conduit (i.e., stomach or colon) for bypass is analogous to conduit creation for esophageal reconstruction after esophagectomy, with minor differences. If the esophagus is obliterated into the gastroesophageal junction, this can be divided using a linear stapler. If this is patent and the stomach is to be used for a conduit, the stomach is divided from the top of the fundus to a point between branches of the right and left gastric vessels on the lesser curvature (Fig. 50-5). The left gastric vessels are preserved for blood supply to the cardia. This excluded part can be drained with a tube, via jejunal anastomosis (Roux-en-Y), or fistulized externally to the abdominal wall as a cardiostomy.[23]

A subcutaneous or substernal tunnel is created bluntly between the two skin incisions. The conduit is brought to the neck, and a cervical anastomosis is created. Gastrointestinal continuity using a colon conduit is reestablished with cologastric or colointestinal anastomosis (Fig. 50-6). Details of these aspects of the procedure are described in Part 2 of this text.

Esophageal bypass has only modest utility in the treatment of esophageal caustic injury. In most cases the native esophagus should be removed, if possible, because of the long-term risk of developing esophageal cancer in the injured esophagus.[15,16] Continued monitoring for the development of esophageal carcinoma is difficult once the native esophagus has been bypassed. Nonanatomic esophageal reconstruction is suboptimal and is avoided if possible. Mucocele formation in the retained esophageal remnant is a theoretical complication of esophageal bypass for caustic esophageal injury. Mucoceles may form in the excluded esophageal segment but usually are small and asymptomatic.[24,25] As a result of mucosal obliteration and fibrosis from caustic injury, mucoceles are less likely to form in this setting than in the case of bypassed esophageal segments due to other benign or malignant esophageal diseases.

SUMMARY

Surgical management of injury from ingested caustic agents varies depending on the exact nature of the injury and the patient's clinical course (Fig. 50-7). Prompt recognition of the process and aggressive treatment to resuscitate the patient is essential. Nearly all patients require esophagoscopy. Adjunct procedures may be required. Surgery in the acute setting of extensive esophageal and/or gastric necrosis with perforation requires resection and diversion. Reconstruction or bypass may be considered in the elective setting once the patient has been clinically stabilized. Esophageal bypass alone is rarely employed, as resection of the native esophagus is recommended due to the risk of malignant degeneration and of mucocele formation in the retained esophageal segment. Reconstructive surgery is technically analogous to reconstruction after esophagectomy, except that a nongastric conduit may be required. Strictures after caustic esophageal injury are exceedingly common and may be initially managed with serial dilation. In the long term, esophageal resection is often required for refractory strictures with functional failure of the native esophagus or for management of esophageal cancer, which develops in survivors.

EDITOR'S COMMENT

Corrosive injuries of the esophagus used to be commonplace in the 1960s, 70s, and 80s, when numerous poisons were kept within most American homes. As homes and product containers have become increasingly child-proofed, corrosive injuries have become rare. This chapter provides straightforward information in a readily accessible manner for the reader who may be called upon to manage their first corrosive esophageal injury. These are life-threatening burns to the esophagus and must be quickly managed to prevent esophageal perforation or extensive organ necrosis. One important take away message is that it is safer to perform endoscopy to characterize the extent of esophageal injury within the first 12 hours than 48 hours later when there is more edema in the esophageal wall. Stents to open and manage strictures have been a major advance in this disease. Postinjury strictures can be very long and extremely resistant to dilation, leading to esophagectomy. Early stenting may save the organ and produce a better long-term functional result.

—Michael T. Jaklitsch

References

1. Kikendall JW. Caustic ingestion injuries. *Gastroenterol Clin North Am.* 1991;20:847–857.
2. Cattan P, Munoz-Bongrand N, Berney T, et al. Extensive abdominal surgery after caustic ingestion. *Ann Surg.* 2000;231:519–523.
3. DiPalma J. Esophageal disorders. In: Civetta J, Taylor R, Kirby R, eds. *Critical Care.* Philadelphia, PA: Lippincott-Raven; 1997:2071–2077.
4. Kirsh MM, Ritter F. Caustic ingestion and subsequent damage to the oropharyngeal and digestive passages. *Ann Thorac Surg.* 1976;21:74–82.
5. Greenberg R, Bank S, Blumstein M, et al. Common gastrointestinal disorders in the intensive care unit. In: Bone R, ed. *Pulmonary and Critical Care Medicine.* 2nd ed. Chicago, IL: Mosby; 1993:1–27.
6. Zargar SA, Kochhar R, Mehta S, et al. The role of fiberoptic endoscopy in the management of corrosive ingestion and modified endoscopic classification of burns. *Gastrointest Endosc.* 1991;37:165–169.
7. Zwischenberger JB, Savage C, Bidani A. Surgical aspects of esophageal disease: perforation and caustic injury. *Am J Respir Crit Care Med.* 2002;165: 1037–1040.
8. Schaffer SB, Hebert AF. Caustic ingestion. *J La State Med Soc.* 2000;152: 590–596.
9. Fulton JA, Hoffman RS. Steroids in second degree caustic burns of the esophagus: a systematic pooled analysis of fifty years of human data: 1956–2006. *Clin Toxicol (Phila).* 2007;45:402–408.
10. Estrera A, Taylor W, Mills LJ, et al. Corrosive burns of the esophagus and stomach: a recommendation for an aggressive surgical approach. *Ann Thorac Surg.* 1986;41:276–283.
11. Anderson KD, Rouse TM, Randolph JG. A controlled trial of corticosteroids in children with corrosive injury of the esophagus. *N Engl J Med.* 1990;323:637–640.

12. Ramasamy K, Gumaste VV. Corrosive ingestion in adults. *J Clin Gastroenterol.* 2003;37:119–124.
13. Pelclova D, Navratil T. Do corticosteroids prevent oesophageal stricture after corrosive ingestion? *Toxicol Rev.* 2005;24:125–129.
14. Nagi B, Kochhar R, Thapa BR, et al. Radiological spectrum of late sequelae of corrosive injury to upper gastrointestinal tract. A pictorial review. *Acta Radiol.* 2004;45:7–12.
15. Qureshi R, Norton R. Squamous cell carcinoma in esophageal remnant after 24 years: lessons learnt from esophageal bypass surgery. *Dis Esophagus.* 2000;13:245–247.
16. Genc O, Knight RK, Nicholson AG, et al. Adenocarcinoma arising in a retained esophageal remnant. *Ann Thorac Surg.* 2001;72:2117–2119.
17. Kim YT, Sung SW, Kim JH. Is it necessary to resect the diseased esophagus in performing reconstruction for corrosive esophageal stricture? *Eur J Cardiothorac Surg.* 2001;20:1–6.
18. Linden PA, Bueno R, Mentzer SJ, et al. Modified T-tube repair of delayed esophageal perforation results in a low mortality rate similar to that seen with acute perforations. *Ann Thorac Surg.* 2007;83:1129–1133.
19. Han Y, Cheng QS, Li XF, et al. Surgical management of esophageal strictures after caustic burns: a 30 years of experience. *World J Gastroenterol.* 2004;10:2846–2849.
20. de Jong AL, Macdonald R, Ein S, et al. Corrosive esophagitis in children: a 30-year review. *Int J Pediatr Otorhinolaryngol.* 2001;57:203–211.
21. Dosios T, Karavokyros I, Felekouras E, et al. Presternal gastric bypass for late postpneumonectomy esophagopleural fistula. *Dis Esophagus.* 2005;18:202–203.
22. Reed MF, Mathisen DJ. Tracheoesophageal fistula. *Chest Surg Clin N Am.* 2003;13:271–289.
23. Seto Y, Yamada K, Fukuda T, et al. Esophageal bypass using a gastric tube and a cardiostomy for malignant esophagorespiratory fistula. *Am J Surg.* 2007;193:792–793.
24. van Till JW, van Sandick JW, Cardozo ML, et al. Symptomatic mucocele of a surgically excluded esophagus. *Dis Esophagus.* 2002;15:96–98.
25. Frese S, Stein RM, Kuster JR, et al. A large mediastinal tumor with spontaneous regression 30 years after esophageal bypass surgery. *Ann Thorac Surg.* 2002;74:1711–1712.

PART 7

CONGENITAL ESOPHAGEAL SURGERY

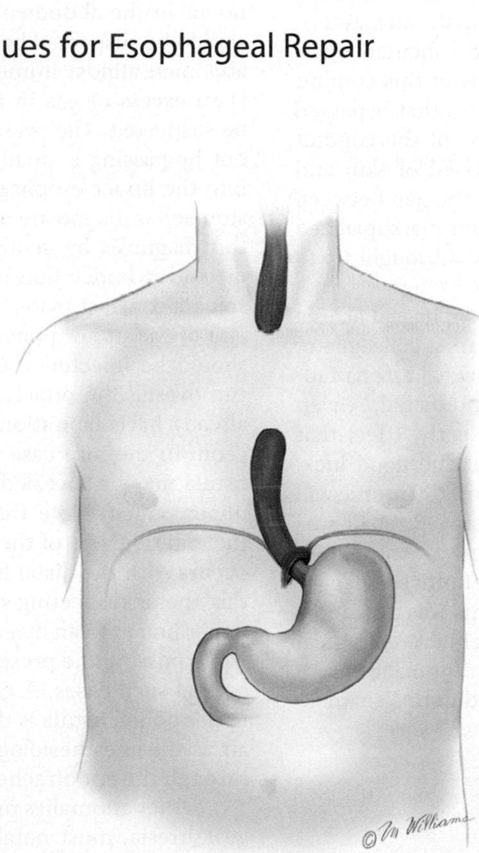

51 Congenital Disorders of the Esophagus in Infants and Children

W. Hardy Hendren III and Christopher B. Weldon

Keywords: Achalasia, congenital esophageal anomalies, esophageal atresia, tracheoesophageal fistula (TEF), clefts, mediastinal cysts, esophageal duplications, vascular rings, hiatal hernia, esophageal stenosis

This chapter presents the most common congenital malformations of the esophagus that require surgical correction in infants and children. Today, most of these entities can be corrected, and a child can lead a normal life after surgery. That was not true until 1939, when Logan Leven of Minneapolis[1] and William E. Ladd of Boston[2] independently saved a newborn with esophageal atresia on the same date! The operation consisted of dividing the tracheoesophageal fistula (TEF), marsupializing the blindly ending upper esophageal pouch, and feeding the baby temporarily through a gastrostomy. Later, a multistaged reconstruction was performed to make an antethoracic esophageal substitute, which was placed subcutaneously anterior to the sternum. The lower two-thirds of this conduit consisted of a Roux-en-Y loop of upper jejunum that bypassed the stomach and duodenum. The upper third of the conduit was a tubularized full-thickness graft comprised of skin and subcutaneous tissue. This was used to bridge the gap between the upper esophageal segment, which had been marsupialized in the neck, and the Roux-en-Y loop, which was brought up to the level of the upper sternum.

An important milestone in surgery for esophageal atresia was an insightful paper by Dr. Thomas Lanman, a colleague of Ladd, in 1940 describing a series of 32 esophageal atresia failures at Children's Hospital Boston.[3] Lanman predicted, "Given a suitable case in which the patient is seen early, I feel that with greater experience, improved technique, and good luck, the successful outcome of a direct anastomosis can and will be reported in the near future." This type of staged repair was abandoned in 1943 when Dr. Cameron Haight[4] of Ann Arbor, Michigan, was first to report the primary definitive repair of esophageal atresia and TEF in the neonate. This was an important step in thoracic surgery for infants and children. Surgical treatments for other congenital esophageal anomalies were developed subsequently and are also described in this chapter.

ESOPHAGEAL ATRESIA AND TRACHEOESOPHAGEAL FISTULA

The spectrum of pathology in infants with esophageal atresia, with or without TEF, is illustrated in Fig. 51-1. These include esophageal atresia with distal TEF, without TEF, with proximal TEF, and with double (proximal and distal) TEF. Isolated TEF without esophageal atresia, so-called H-fistula that usually occurs in the neck rather than midmediastinum, is also encountered. In most infants, esophageal atresia occurs with a single TEF. This form is observed in approximately 85% of affected infants. The upper esophageal pouch ends blindly, and there is a gap between it and the lower esophageal segment. The fistula from the lower esophageal segment usually enters the trachea just above its bifurcation. The blind upper pouch actually may overlap the nearby lower esophageal segment, or the two ends may be separated by a centimeter or more. Esophageal atresia without TEF is the next most common form and is seen in approximately 8% of infants.

Diagnosis

A newborn in respiratory distress should be evaluated immediately for esophageal atresia with or without TEF. If there is no air in the abdomen, isolated "long gap" esophageal atresia should be suspected because a neonate normally has gas in the abdomen almost immediately after birth. Conversely, if there is an excess of gas in the stomach and intestine, TEF should be suspected. The presence of esophageal atresia can be ruled out by passing a small soft plastic catheter through the nose into the upper esophagus. Failure of the tube to pass into the stomach is diagnostic of esophageal atresia. One also can make this diagnosis by gently blowing air into the upper pouch to distend it under fluoroscopy. A *very small amount* of water-soluble contrast material is passed into the tube until the distal end of the upper pouch is visualized. Contrast material never should be injected without fluoroscopic guidance because it can overfill the pouch, causing aspiration. These babies often already have aspiration pneumonia before referral to the surgeon. In the rare case (see Fig. 51-1*C* or *D*), an upper pouch fistula may be revealed when contrast material is put into the upper pouch. Note that the upper pouch fistula arises from the anterior wall of the blind upper esophagus, not its end, as occurs with the distal fistula. The clinical importance of this is that the unsuspecting surgeon in such a case may mobilize the upper pouch to an extent sufficient to perform the anastomosis while missing the presence of the second fistula. We have seen several such cases. A clinical clue to the presence of a second upper pouch fistula is the intermittent filling of the pouch with air as the anesthesiologist applies positive-pressure anesthesia through the endotracheal tube.

Other anomalies may be present in a neonate with esophageal atresia, most notably imperforate anus, which is a broad spectrum of anorectal anomalies and congenital heart disease. Appropriate consultation with a pediatric cardiologist may be indicated, particularly today, when the ideal time to repair many congenital cardiac defects, which are soon fatal, may be in the neonatal period.

Surgical Technique

Esophageal Atresia

The surgical approach to esophageal atresia is made through the right chest in most patients. Rarely, if there is a right descending arch, it may be easier to approach the repair through the left

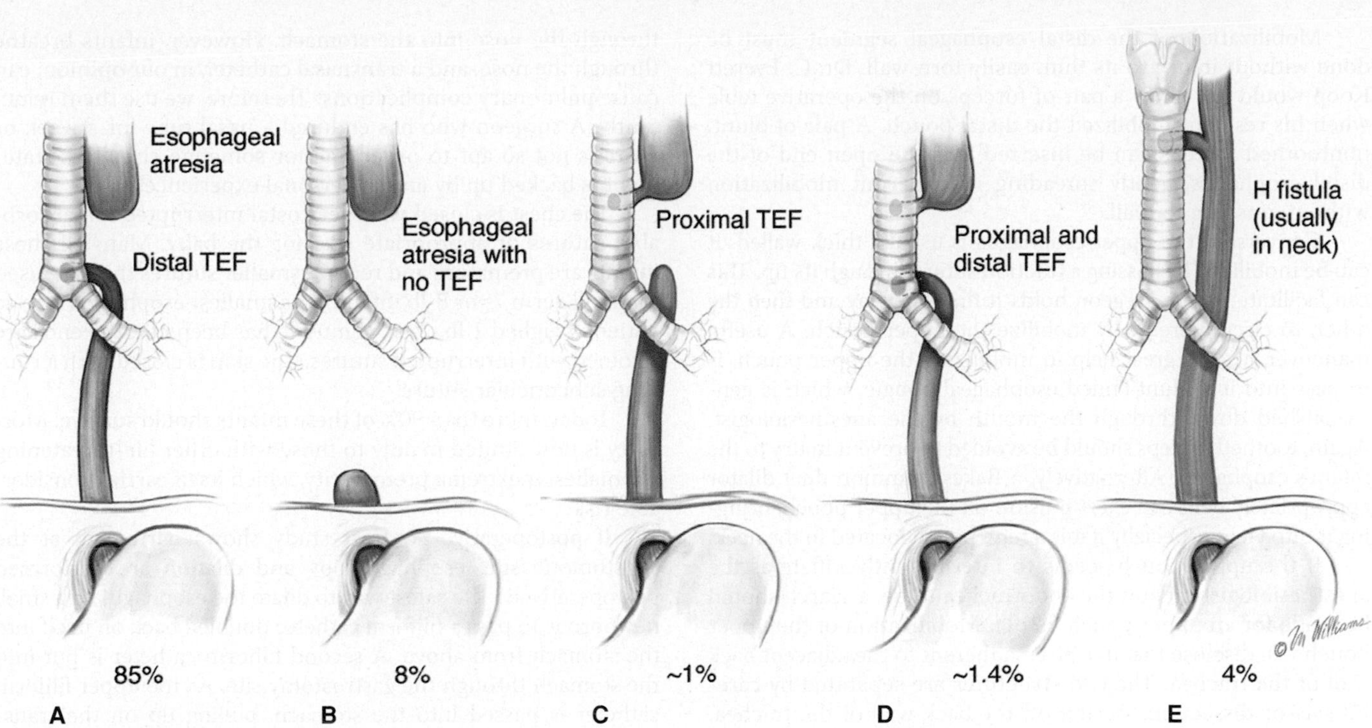

Figure 51-1. Types and frequencies of esophageal atresia with and without TEF.

chest. Neonatal thoracotomy, which transects the chest wall muscles, can result in impaired growth of the thorax on that side as the child matures. An incision that minimizes muscle cutting is that used by the late David Waterston at the Hospital for Sick Children, London, and is our preference. This is a vertical skin incision beginning just below the axilla and moving downward. The chest wall muscles are retracted upward to enter the fourth interspace. Spending a few minutes to bluntly separate the thoracic wall pleura off of the endothorax, keeping it intact, permits a posterolateral extrapleural exposure of the anatomy to be repaired. It is an important safety feature to locate the esophageal anastomosis extrapleurally to avoid widespread mediastinitis if a leak does occur.

There must be constant, close communication between the anesthesiologist and the surgeon because retraction of the mediastinal structures forward may embarrass cardiopulmonary function. Thus the anesthesiologist should warn the surgeon to release the hand-held retractors if there is any sign of cardiac slowing or if blood gas measurements show deteriorating levels. It is best to anticipate the possibility of these events, which proceed much more rapidly in a frail infant than in older patients. Anticipating a possible cardiac arrest in a baby is better than treating the actual event, which is not always salvageable. The surgeon who undertakes major chest surgery in a small baby must be gentle and must work with an experienced pediatric anesthesiologist.

The azygos vein usually is divided to permit the approach to the esophagus, although we have done this surgery by mobilizing the azygos vein and maintaining it intact. If the vein is large and the baby is small, it is advisable to keep the azygos vein intact.

Early in the operation, the lower esophageal pouch should be identified. The vagus nerves will be seen coming from above and running along the sides of the distal pouch. They should be spared. As soon as the entry of the lower pouch into the back wall of the trachea is identified, it should be encircled with a ligature to stop the air blowing down from the trachea into the distal esophagus and from there into the stomach. If the stomach is already greatly overinflated with air from the fistula, we generally decompress it by placing a mushroom catheter into the anterior wall of the stomach through a minilaparotomy using a vertical incision in the midline approximately 2 to 3 cm in length. If a gastrostomy is used to decompress the stomach, we use the Stamm technique with two purse-string sutures of fine nonabsorbable material.

The tube should be brought out through *a separate stab wound* lateral to the laparotomy incision, with the added precaution of suturing the stomach to the abdominal wall. We have seen death occur when the stomach was not sutured and a leakage occurred at the gastrostomy site causing the stomach contents to spill into the upper abdomen. This is entirely preventable by anticipating this possibility. Regarding use of a stab wound, we have seen several infants die because infection occurred in the minilaparotomy incision when a tube traversed the wound. Infection caused a wide fistula between the stomach and the outside world, an entirely preventable event. Some of our teachers brought tubes through the main laparotomy incision. However, the surgeon who has seen that result in a major gastric fistula will prefer use of a stab incision for the tube.

We prefer simple ligation of the distal fistula, flush with the back wall of the trachea, and usually use a single ligature of 3-0 or 4-0 size. If the fistula is not ligated flush with the trachea, it leaves a tracheal diverticulum, which can cause intermittent episodes of pneumonitis. We have reexplored several infants in whom such a pouch had been left, another complication preventable by thinking of its possibility when doing the fistula interruption. An alternative method for closing the defect in the trachea is to close it with a row of fine interrupted sutures. The suture must have a tiny needle; otherwise, this closure can leak, whereas a ligature should not.

Mobilization of the distal esophageal segment must be done without injury to its thin, easily torn wall. Dr. C. Everett Koop would not allow a pair of forceps on the operative table when his resident mobilized the distal pouch. A pair of blunt, nontoothed forceps can be inserted into the open end of the distal esophagus, gently spreading it to permit mobilization without grasping its wall.

Conversely, the upper esophagus is usually thick walled. It can be mobilized by passing a traction suture through its tip. This can facilitate, as the surgeon holds it first one way and then the other, to circumferentially mobilize the upper pouch. A useful maneuver, also of great help in mobilizing the upper pouch, is to pass into it a blunt-ended esophageal bougie, which is gently pushed down through the mouth by the anesthesiologist. Again, toothed forceps should be avoided to prevent injury to the infant's esophagus. Alternatively, a Bakes' common duct dilator appropriately bent can exert pulsion on the upper pouch, bringing it into view, especially if it is a high pouch located in the neck.

If the upper pouch seems to intermittently inflate as the anesthesiologist inflates the endotracheal tube, a search should be made for an upper pouch fistula. Mobilization of the upper pouch will disclose that it is often adherent to the adjacent back wall of the trachea. The two structures are separated by careful scissor dissection, staying off the back wall of the trachea, which is thin and easily entered. The esophagus is a much better developed structure because it has been obstructed in utero and is not easily transgressed. If a traction suture has been used on the end of the upper pouch, that part should be excised when the anastomosis is performed.

Early in the development of surgery for esophageal atresia, a two-layer anastomosis was used by many surgeons. The two-layer anastomosis consisted of a full thickness of the delicate distal esophageal opening to the mucosa of the upper pouch imbricating with a second layer of muscle from the upper pouch to the esophageal wall of the lower pouch. Today we prefer a single-layer anastomosis using the cut end of both upper and lower pouches. The back row of sutures is placed using 5-0 or 6-0 nonabsorbable sutures with the knots tied in the lumen of the two ends of esophagus. In practice, we place all those sutures first and defer tying them until the entire back row is in place. The assistant then grasps with large blunt forceps the two ends of esophagus, holding them gently together while the surgeon ties all the sutures with no tension. Most of the anterior wall sutures are then placed and tied simultaneously, again without tension on the end courtesy of the assistant. The last two or three sutures then are necessarily placed such that the tie will be on the outside. At the completion of the anastomosis, we generally place two or three sutures in the muscular wall of the upper pouch to exert gentle traction downward to avoid tugging on the two ends of the anastomosis.

A small flap of mediastinal tissue can be used to cover the ligated and divided fistula at its tracheal end. A soft plastic catheter is placed in the mediastinal gutter well lateral to the anastomosis. Hence, if leakage occurs, it will track out along the tube. We anchor the tip of that tube in the upper gutter because many years ago we had a tube migrate into the esophageal lumen, which was a disaster.

If the postoperative course is uneventful, we obtain an oral contrast study at 7 to 10 days. If the anastomosis is intact, the chest tube is removed from the gutter, and feedings are begun by mouth. Some surgeons prefer to avoid using a gastrostomy tube and postoperatively leave a transanastomotic plastic tube through the nose into the stomach. However, infants breathe through the nose, and a transnasal catheter, in our opinion, can cause pulmonary complications. Therefore, we use them reluctantly. A surgeon who has endured a nasal tube for a week or more is not so apt to order one for someone else. This statement is backed up by ample personal experience!

The chest is closed with pericostal interrupted nonabsorbable sutures of appropriate size for the baby. Many of these infants are premature and require smaller sutures than are used for a full-term 7- or 8-lb infant. Our smallest esophageal atresia patient weighed 1 lb, 2 oz. If muscle has been cut, the ends are rejoined with interrupted sutures. The skin is closed with a running subcuticular suture.

Today, more than 90% of these infants should survive. Mortality is now limited mainly to those with other life-threatening anomalies or extreme prematurity, which itself carries considerable risk.

If postoperative contrast study shows narrowing at the anastomotic site, esophagoscopy and dilation are performed postoperatively. The safest way to dilate the esophagus in a small newborn is to pass a filiform catheter doubled back on itself into the stomach from above. A second filiform catheter is put into the stomach through the gastrostomy site. As the upper filiform catheter is passed into the stomach, pulling up on the transgastric filiform catheter usually will grab the tip of that passed from above, bringing it out of the gastrostomy site. Followers of increasing size then can be brought down from above through the anastomosis to dilate it. One must be careful not to overdilate the anastomosis, for we have had the unhappy experience of splitting a new anastomosis longitudinally, requiring reoperation.

There is a high (approximately 25%) incidence of gastroesophageal reflux in babies after surgery for esophageal atresia. In part, this may be related to excessive mobilization of the distal esophagus when the gap between the distal and proximal ends is longer than usual. Principally, however, the reflux is related to esophageal dysmotility that is common in these patients. An antireflux operation may be indicated if gastroesophageal reflux persists. One of our patients developed carcinoma of the distal esophagus secondary to reflux at an age of 20 years.[5] She was treated by distal esophagectomy with thoracoabdominal replacement using transverse colon on left colic pedicle (see Fig. 51-2). The patient is now 39 years old and in excellent health and swallowing normally.

Long-gap Esophageal Atresia

Long-gap esophageal atresia (see Fig. 51-1*B*) is a special problem. It is possible to stretch the two ends of the esophagus by various means. The upper pouch can be elongated by passing blunt esophageal bougies from above several times daily. The principal problem with leaving the upper pouch intact, instead of marsupializing it, is the risk of aspiration if it is not suctioned dry many times each day. Stretching the lower end is a more difficult problem. A bougie can be passed through the gastrostomy site, but that is not as satisfactory as dilating the upper pouch. Alternatively, a Bakes' dilator can be used with ultrasound guidance to visualize its passage into the lower pouch. The late Fritz Rehbein[6] of Germany described a method that involved passing sutures through the ends in such a manner as to gradually bring them together. In 1976, we, along with Dr. Richard Hale of the National Magnet Laboratory at Massachusetts Institute of Technology, described an electromagnetic technique to bring the long-gap ends together.[7] We put a metal bullet into each end

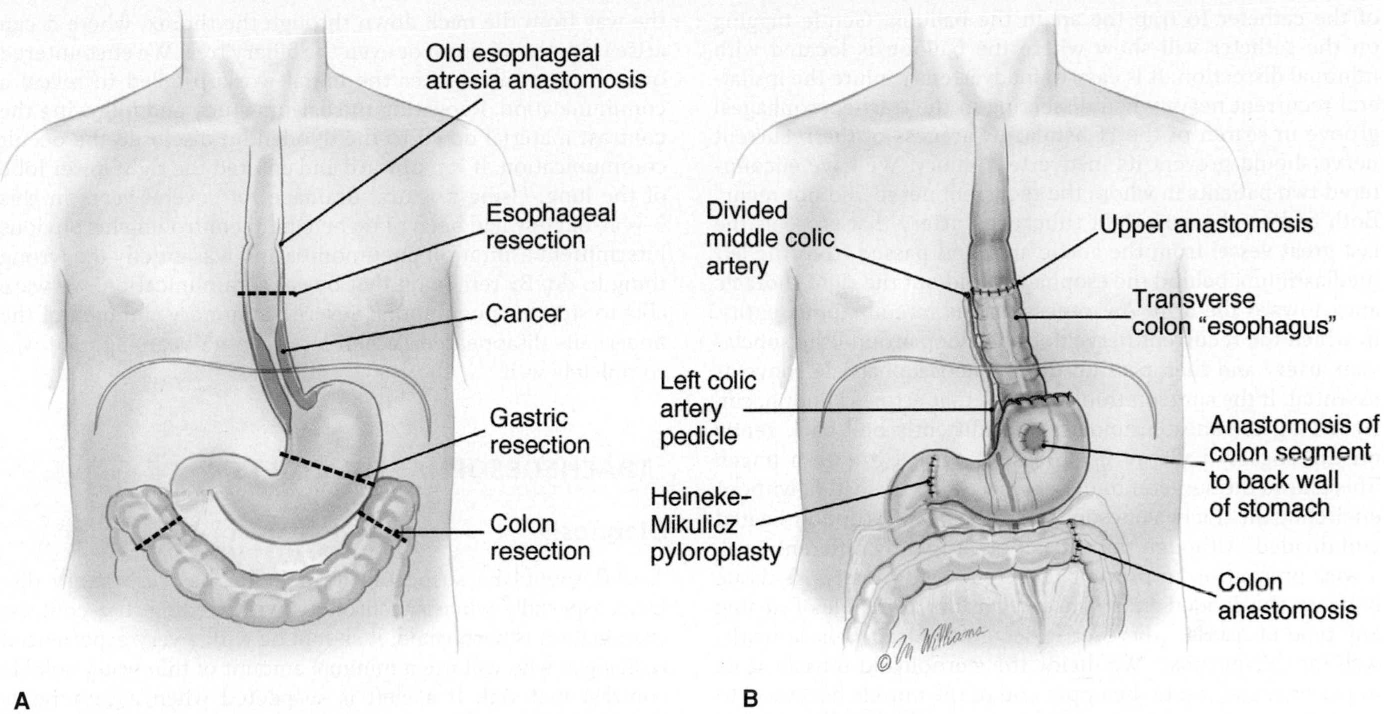

Figure 51-2. *A.* Adenocarcinoma in a 20-year-old patient after original esophageal atresia repair. *B.* Resection and restoration of continuity.

of the esophagus and placed the baby in an electromagnetic field (Fig. 51-3). Intermittently, we turned the magnet on, pulling the bullets together until the blind ends of the esophagus were apposed. Although this was shown to be effective, reluctance of certain members of the nursing service to participate in this activity led us to discontinue this treatment. The objection raised was the need to keep the infant restrained during the treatment, which lasted 4 to 6 weeks. Therefore, for three decades we used colon esophageal interposition by the technique of Mr. David Waterston, with whom we worked in 1962. Prof. Gunther H. Willital of Munster, Germany, has reported an extensive series of patients treated using electromagnetic bougienage.[8]

Tracheoesophageal fistula without Esophageal Atresia (H-fistula)

Isolated TEF (see Fig. 51-1E) often escapes clinical recognition during infancy. The history is usually one of intermittent respiratory infections. A contrast swallow with films in the lateral or oblique view can make the diagnosis. Sometimes the fistula is not seen, however, especially if the radiologist has scant experience looking for fistulas. Endoscopy can be diagnostic. Searching the back wall of the trachea with a 30-degree endoscope (this can be either a bronchoscope or even a cystoscope without water) will reveal the tracheal side of the fistula on the back wall of the trachea. It is usually located in the lower neck, not at the level of the carina, as in the most common type of esophageal atresia with TEF. A small catheter passed through the endoscope and through the fistula will prove its presence. A useful maneuver when the tracheal end of the fistula is not obvious is to place an endotracheal tube to intermittently inflate the trachea with positive pressure while searching the anterior wall of the esophagus for telltale signs of air entering the anterior wall of the esophagus. A drop or two of methylene blue placed into the tracheal lumen can further help to reveal its point of entry in the anterior wall of the esophagus.

The isolated fistula is exposed using a transverse cervical incision just above the clavicle. We pass a Fogarty catheter through the fistula, which runs obliquely from the trachea down to the esophagus. The Fogarty balloon is inflated and maintained in the inflated position by cross-clamping the upper end

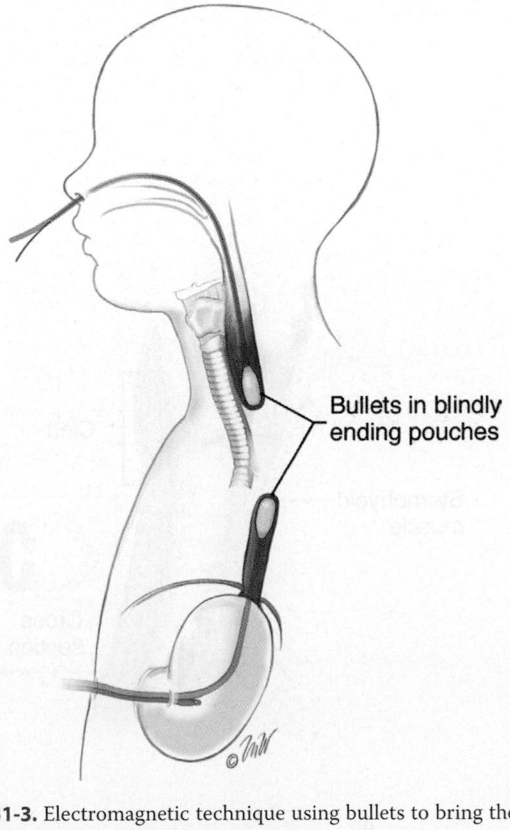

Figure 51-3. Electromagnetic technique using bullets to bring the ends of the esophagus together in long-gap atresia.

of the catheter to trap the air in the balloon. Gentle tugging on the catheter will show where the balloon is located with minimal dissection. It is easy to inadvertently injure the ipsilateral recurrent nerve when dissecting in the tracheoesophageal groove in search of the H-fistula. Awareness of the recurrent nerve should prevent its inadvertent injury. We have encountered two patients in whom the recurrent nerve "did not recur." Both had an aberrant right subclavian artery that arose as the last great vessel from the aortic arch and passed from the left mediastinum, behind the esophagus, and out the right thoracic apex toward the arm. Awareness of this rare anatomic entity, in which the recurrent nerve does not loop around the subclavian artery and then pass up the tracheoesophageal groove, is essential. If the surgeon thinks of this, that error will not occur. By having the anesthesiologist intermittently pull back gently on the Fogarty balloon, it is possible to feel it with a finger. This allows the surgeon to dissect exactly to the fistula without encircling the trachea or esophagus. The fistula is doubly ligated and divided. Although the ends are at a slightly different level, a wise precaution to prevent recurrence is to interpose tissue between the divided ends. This is a cardinal principle of closing any type of fistula, wherever it occurs. A strap muscle works well for this purpose. We divide the sternohyoid muscle at its upper end, and rotate the upper end of the muscle backward to cover the esophageal ligature. This takes only a few minutes and provides great safety against recurrence.[9] The outlook after this surgery should be a normal baby. We have treated one patient who was 10 years old before the diagnosis was made.

There is another rare communication between the gut and the tracheobronchial tree that should be mentioned. The trachea and the primitive gut are adjacent to each other early in development. If there is a persisting communication between the two, as the gut lengthens, that communication can be stretched all the way from the neck down through the thorax, where it can arise from the jejunum or even the biliary tree. We encountered one of these cases, after the initial workup failed to reveal a communication. Repeating the barium study and following the contrast material down to the duodenum disclosed the occult communication. It ran upward and entered the right lower lobe of the lung. Using postural drainage for several years in this 5-year-old boy had been of no benefit in controlling his obvious intermittent aspiration pneumonitis and was exactly the wrong thing to do. By removing that bowel communication, we were able to stop his pneumonia. Severe pulmonary clubbing of the fingernails disappeared. When last seen 45 years ago, he was completely well.[10]

TRACHEOESOPHAGEAL CLEFTS

Diagnosis

A cleft should be suspected if an infant has respiratory distress, especially when synchronous with feeding. If a contrast examination is performed, it should be with a very experienced radiologist who will use a minimal amount of thin water-soluble contrast material. If a cleft is suspected when a catheter is passed, it is probably safer to make a diagnosis endoscopically under anesthesia rather than attempting to show it radiographically. We believe that this is a difficult surgery and that experienced help should be sought for one of these rare lesions. Failure to respect this tenet is likely to be followed by recurrence.

Clefts between the trachea and esophagus are much rarer than simple TEFs. They can assume many anatomic configurations. Two are shown in Figs. 51-4 and 51-5. A small one may be difficult to see both radiographically and endoscopically.

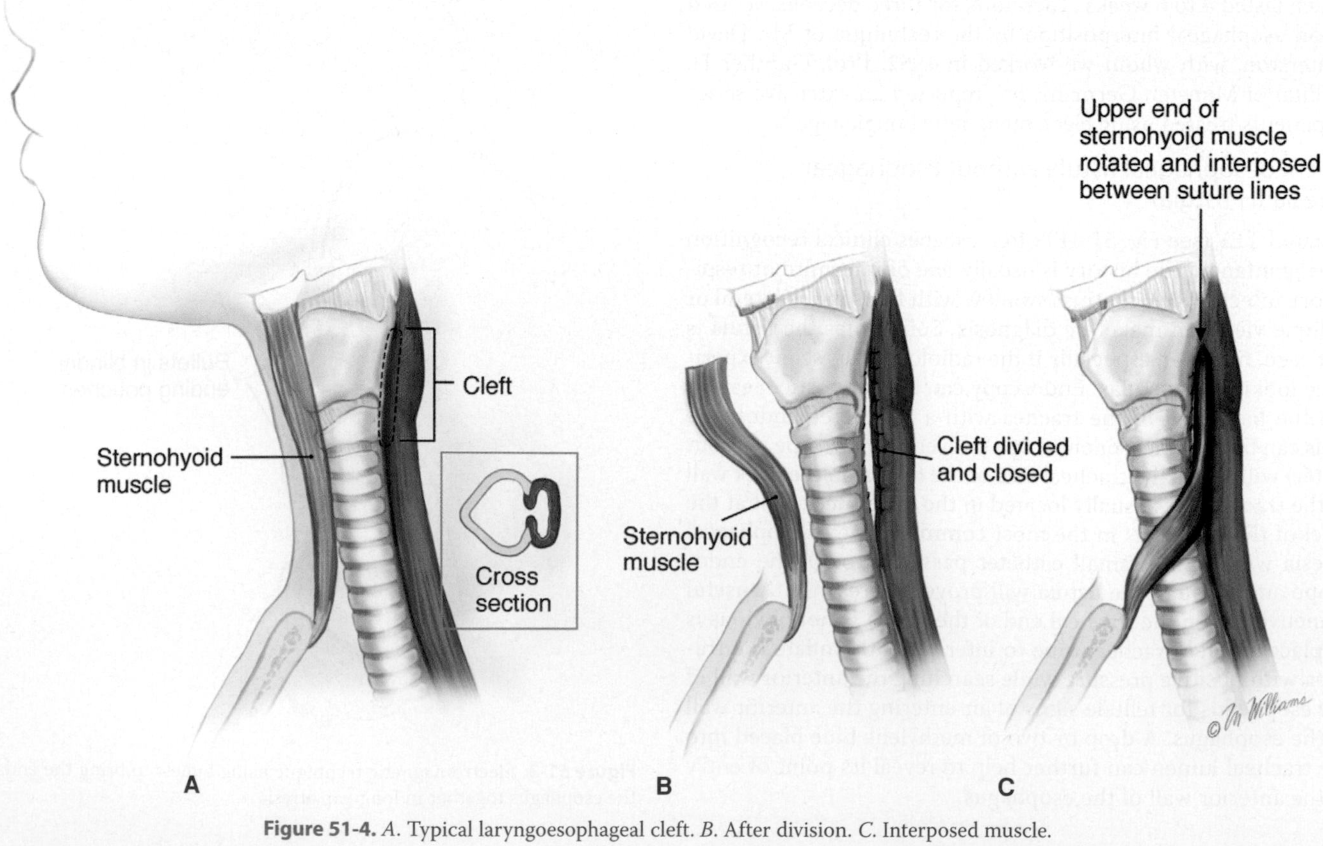

Figure 51-4. *A.* Typical laryngoesophageal cleft. *B.* After division. *C.* Interposed muscle.

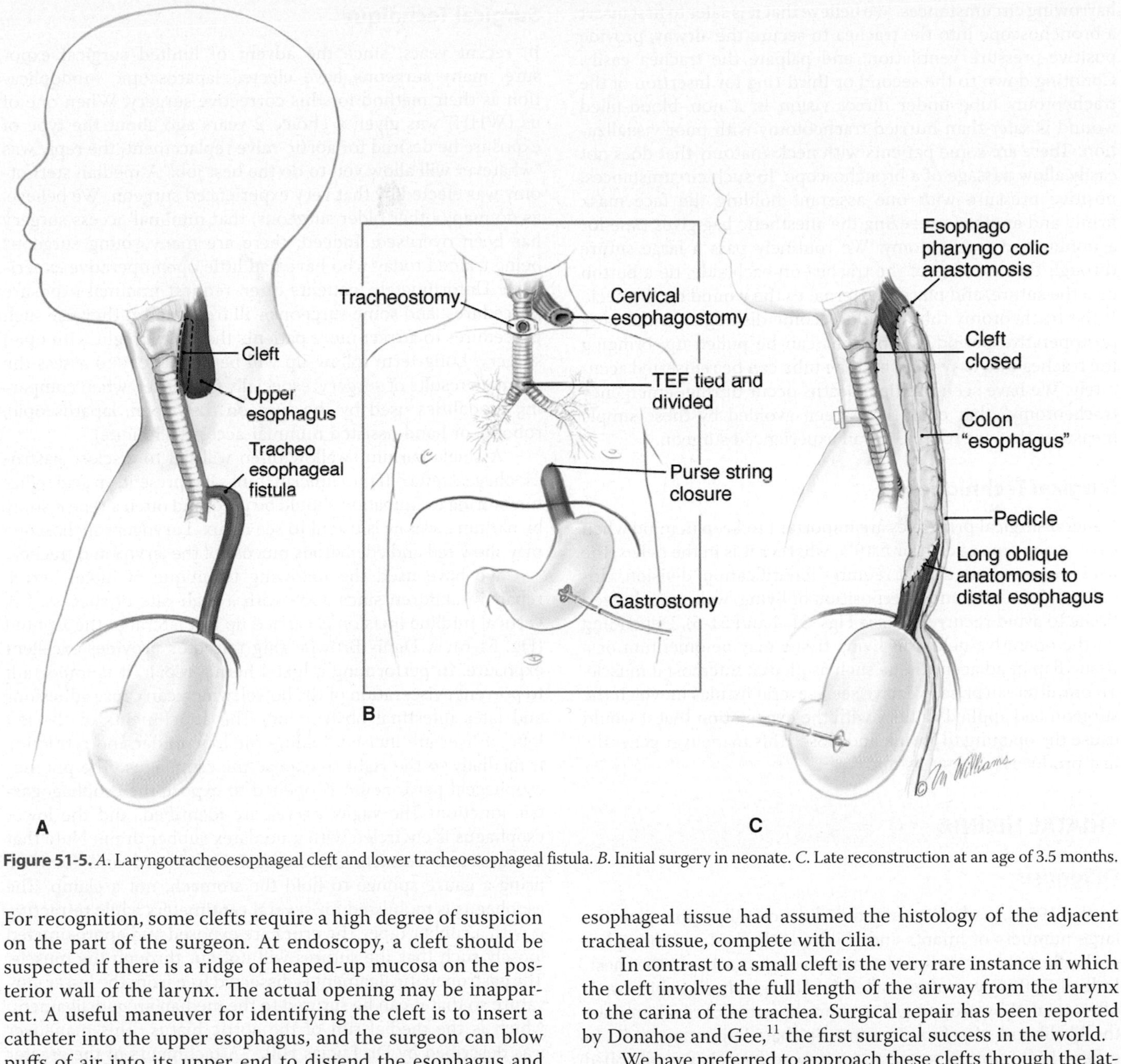

Figure 51-5. *A.* Laryngotracheoesophageal cleft and lower tracheoesophageal fistula. *B.* Initial surgery in neonate. *C.* Late reconstruction at an age of 3.5 months.

For recognition, some clefts require a high degree of suspicion on the part of the surgeon. At endoscopy, a cleft should be suspected if there is a ridge of heaped-up mucosa on the posterior wall of the larynx. The actual opening may be inapparent. A useful maneuver for identifying the cleft is to insert a catheter into the upper esophagus, and the surgeon can blow puffs of air into its upper end to distend the esophagus and open the cleft as air leaks from the esophagus into the trachea. Another useful trick is to insert a Fogarty balloon catheter through the endoscope, probing the possible cleft to demonstrate its presence. If it is a small fistula or an especially small cleft, inflating and gently pulling back on the balloon can reveal its exact location. The Fogarty balloon also facilitates finding its exact location when exploring through the neck with minimal dissection.

When separating and closing a cleft, either congenital or posttraumatic, it is best to leave a margin of esophageal edges on the tracheal tissue. This will prevent the creation of tracheal stenosis by closing the trachea to itself yet will not compromise the esophagus when using a little of its circumference to augment the trachea. In one case (see Fig. 51-5), the child died after discharge. We traveled to that hospital and participated in the postmortem examination that was consistent with aspiration pneumonitis. Of considerable interest was the microscopic cross section of the trachea. It showed that the rim of esophageal tissue had assumed the histology of the adjacent tracheal tissue, complete with cilia.

In contrast to a small cleft is the very rare instance in which the cleft involves the full length of the airway from the larynx to the carina of the trachea. Surgical repair has been reported by Donahoe and Gee,[11] the first surgical success in the world.

We have preferred to approach these clefts through the lateral neck, exercising great caution to avoid injury to the recurrent laryngeal nerve in the tracheoesophageal groove. Some surgeons prefer an anterior approach by splitting the larynx and upper trachea in the midline to approach the pathology from inside the airway. Our preference for a lateral approach is predicated by our preference to insert a strap muscle between the closure suture lines. We have not had a recurrence when that maneuver was used (see Fig. 51-4).

We have seen acquired clefts in several patients after trauma. One was in a youngster with severe head trauma whose airway was intubated with a large endotracheal tube that lay next to a large esophageal tube that had been used for tube feedings. Two large tubes adjacent to each other in an unconscious patient can lead to pressure necrosis of the posterior wall of the trachea and anterior wall of the esophagus. We also have seen an inadvertent opening made in the posterior wall of the trachea and anterior wall of the esophagus by a surgeon attempting to do an emergency tracheotomy under harrowing circumstances. We believe that it is safer to first insert a bronchoscope into the trachea to secure the airway, provide positive-pressure ventilation, and palpate the trachea easily. Counting down to the second or third ring for insertion of the tracheotomy tube under direct vision in a non–blood-filled wound is safer than hurried tracheotomy with poor visualization. There are some patients with neck anatomy that does not easily allow passage of a bronchoscope. In such circumstances, positive pressure with one assistant holding the face mask firmly and another squeezing the anesthetic bag gives time for a nonhurried tracheotomy. We routinely pass a large suture through the cut edge of the trachea on each side, tie a button into the suture, and place it external to the wound on the neck. If the tracheotomy tube should become dislodged in the early postoperative period, the buttons can be pulled up, bringing the trachea into easy view, and the tube can be reinserted accurately. We have seen multiple deaths occur during "emergency tracheotomy" that could have been avoided by these simple measures that are routine for an experienced surgeon.

Surgical Technique

General surgical principles are important to keep in mind when closing any type of cleft or fistula, whether it is in the pelvis, the neck, or anywhere else. It requires identification, division, closure of both ends, and interposition of living, well-vascularized tissue to avoid recurrence (see Figs. 51-4 and 51-5). Depending on the operative field, this living tissue may be omentum or a tissue flap of adjacent tissue such as pleura, intercostal muscle. To our utter surprise, we have seen several fistulas in which the surgeon had applied cautery with the expectation that it would cause the opening to shrink and close. This maneuver generally just produces a bigger fistula!

HIATAL HERNIA

Diagnosis

In the 1950s, pediatric surgeons did not fully appreciate the large numbers of infants and children who had gastroesophageal reflux with or without herniation of stomach into the chest. Indeed, reflux was often called "chalasia." Those babies were often treated by propping them upright in their cribs to reduce the likelihood of reflux. In some, it abated spontaneously. In others, it did not. In recent years, newer drugs have controlled gastroesophageal reflux in many cases and controlled gastric acidity, which, with reflux, can be devastating to the esophagus and lungs. Gastroenterologists and surgeons do not all agree regarding if and when corrective surgery should be used. There are indications, however, that most would agree should prompt surgical correction. Persistent failure to thrive is a strong indication. Another is reflux esophagitis, which can stricture the lower esophagus to a degree that resection and replacement are needed. Recurrent aspiration pneumonitis is another potentially serious complication. We have seen it lead to bronchiectasis. Waiting too long and coping with severe complications is not "conservative therapy" but borders on malpractice. The physician who refers a child for an operation should know what kind of operation the surgeon performs, what the complications are, and what the success rate is. Surgeons select other surgeons for their own family based on these important parameters. Other people's children deserve the same consideration.

Surgical Technique

In recent years, since the advent of limited surgical exposure, many surgeons have elected laparoscopic fundoplication as their method for this corrective surgery. When one of us (WHH) was given a choice 2 years ago about the type of exposure he desired for aortic valve replacement, the reply was "whatever will allow you to do the best job." A median sternotomy was elected by that very experienced surgeon. We believe, as do many other older surgeons, that minimal-access surgery has been overused. Indeed, there are many young surgeons being trained today who have had little open operative experience. Unfortunately, patients often request minimal-exposure procedures, and some surgeons will freely admit they use such procedures to attract more patients than they might with open surgery. Long-term follow-up will be mandatory to assess the ultimate results of surgery, especially for cancer, when comparing modalities used by the surgeon (i.e., open, laparoscopic, robotic, or hand-assisted minimal-access technique).

A single barium swallow often will fail to disclose gastroesophageal reflux. If the clinician thinks it is present, an acid reflux monitoring examination should be used, and often a repeat study by barium swallow is useful to see reflux. Laryngobronchoscopy may show red and edematous mucosa of the larynx and trachea.

We have used the following technique of hiatal hernia repair in children since 1959 with a high rate of success.[12] A vertical midline incision is carried up just lateral to the xiphoid (Fig. 51-6). A Denis Browne ring retractor provides excellent exposure. In performing a hiatal hernia repair, it is important to prevent evisceration of the bowel, which can cause adhesions and later intestinal obstruction. The attachments of the left lobe of liver are incised, folding the lobe under and retracting it medially to the right to expose the esophagus. The phrenoesophageal peritoneum is opened to expose the esophagogastric junction. The vagus nerves are identified, and the lower esophagus is encircled with a nonlatex rubber drain. Note that the assistant retracts the stomach downward and forward, using a gauze sponge to hold the stomach, not a clamp. The esophagus is mobilized for several centimeters while retracting it with a rubber tape. The crura are exposed and approximated loosely such that the sutures will not cut through the muscle. The gastrohepatic ligament is dissected free from the lesser curvature so that it can be sutured to the median arcuate ligament, which is the medial rim of the aortic hiatus. This maneuver was described by Dr. Lucias Hill.[13] Attachments of the greater curvature and short gastric vessels are opened to prepare for fundoplication. The fundus is brought behind the esophagus. It is not a completely circumferential wrap. The esophagogastric junction along the lesser curvature is fastened to the median arcuate ligament using pledgets to help bolster the fixation. Note the use of many fine sutures to tack the esophagus to its hiatus. The anterior aspect of stomach is fixed to the undersurface of the diaphragm. We have not used a complete wrap as described by Dr. Rudolph Nissen.[14]

REPLACEMENT OF THE ESOPHAGUS USING COLON

This is an area in which there are several equally effective approaches. Also, the pathology requiring colon replacement of the esophagus in childhood is variable; some patients are children

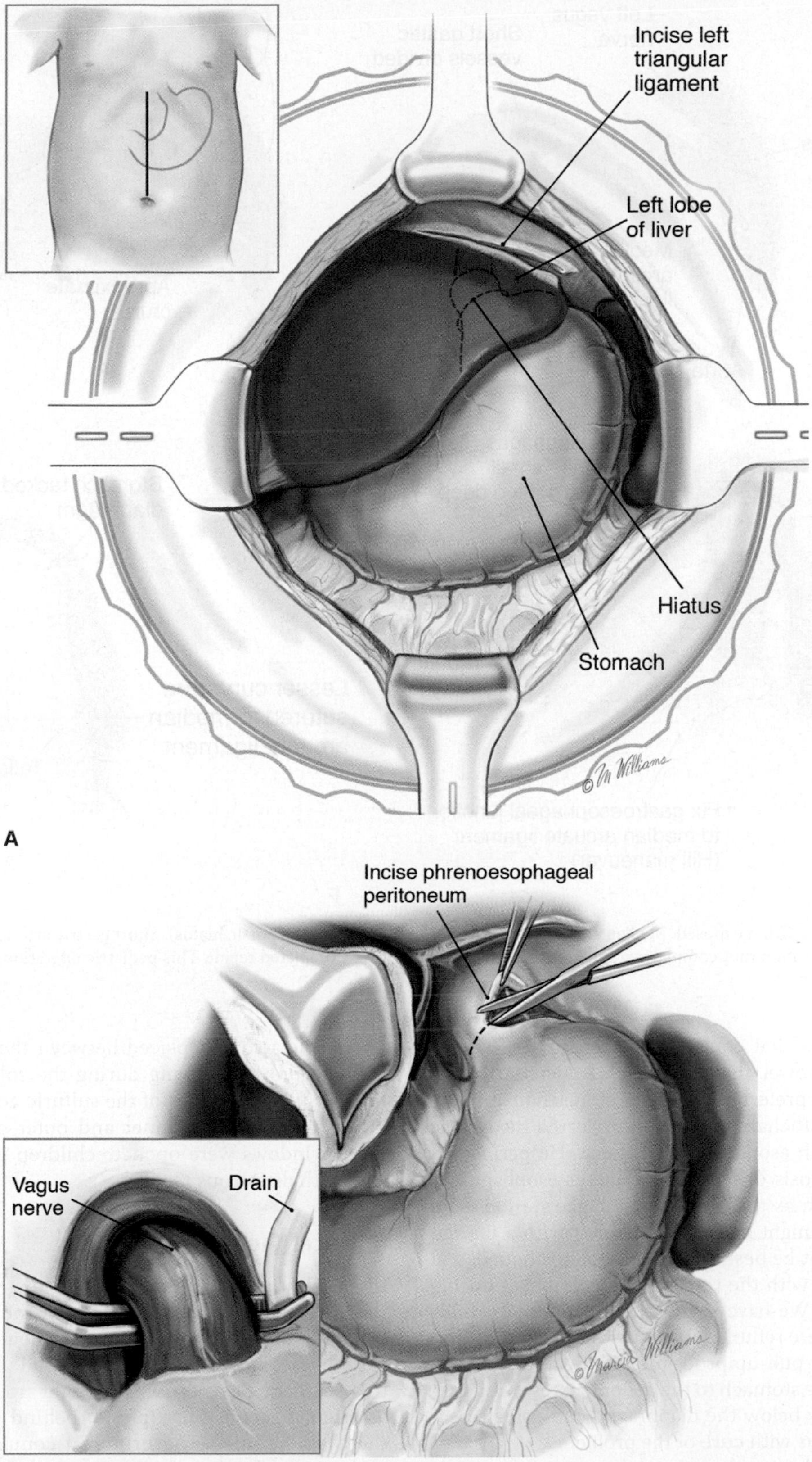

Figure 51-6. Surgery for gastroesophageal reflux. *A*. Exposure of the cardia. Midline incision (inset). *B*. Exposing the gastroesophageal junction and encircling the esophagus. (*continued*)

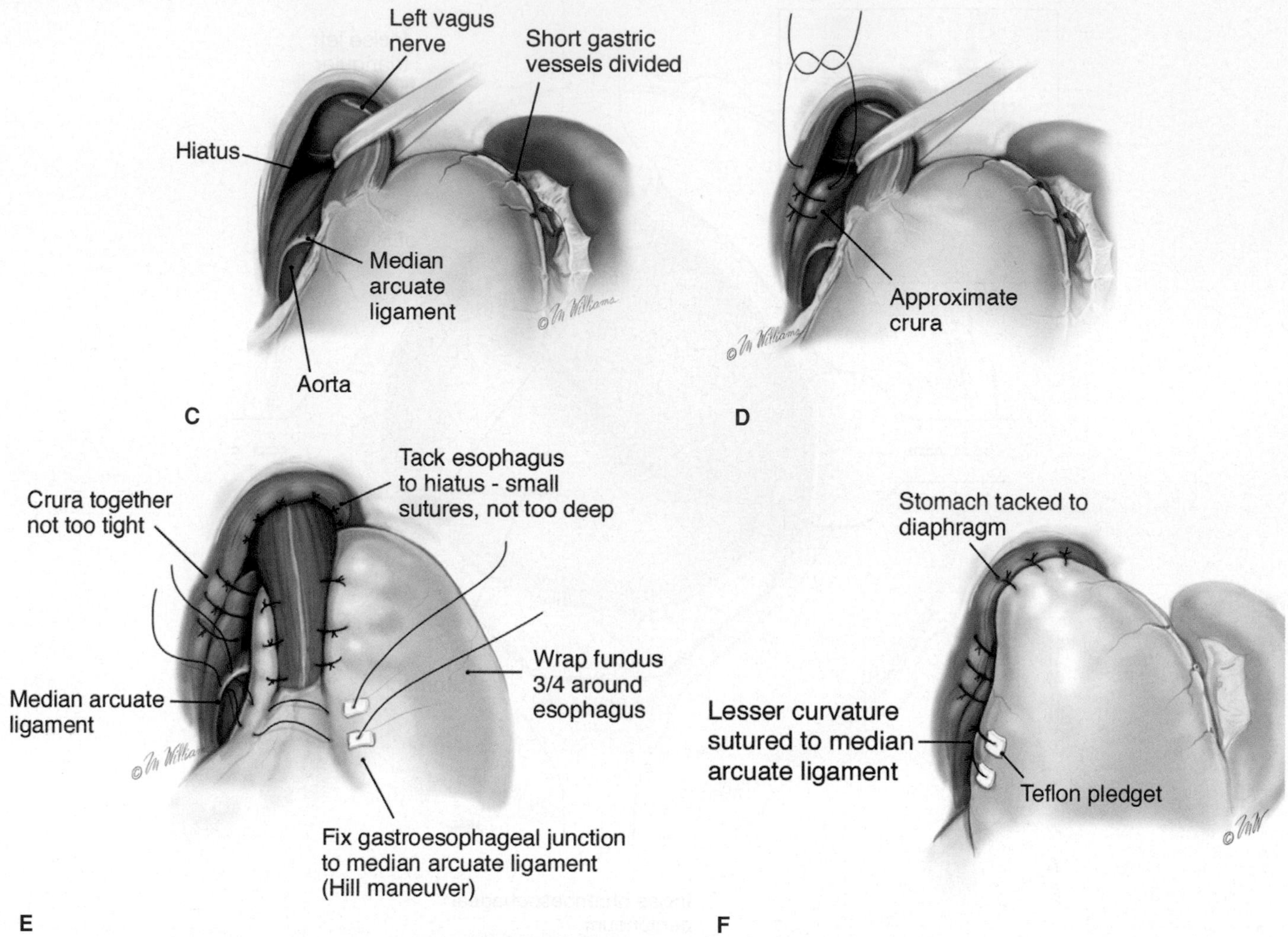

Figure 51-6. (*Continued*) *C.* Crura exposed. Median arcuate ligament exposed (medial rim of aortic hiatus). Short gastric arteries divided. *D.* Crura closed, not too tightly! *E.* Fundoplication (not complete wrap). Prepare for Hill maneuver. *F.* Completed repair. This pediatric operation is similar to the Hill repair described in Part 4, Chapter 33.

with esophageal atresia that could not be repaired except by interposing a tube of bowel. In recent years, Anderson,[15] Spitz et al.,[16] and others have preferred to pull the stomach up into the chest. Indeed, the late Richard H. Sweet[17] preferred the gastric pull-up in patients with esophageal carcinoma. He performed a supraaortic anastomosis of stomach to upper esophagus or an anastomosis as high as the pharynx for higher lesions. On the other hand, what might be best in an adult with a limited life expectancy may not be best in a child who, it is hoped, will live an entire life span with the repair a surgeon makes during infancy or childhood. We have seen several patients in childhood who develop severe reflux esophagitis with ulceration and stricture after a gastric pull-up procedure. Those patients were treated by returning the stomach to the abdomen, restoring gastrointestinal continuity below the diaphragm, and using a secondary colon esophagus with cure of the problem.

Caustic burns of the esophagus are also one of the prime indications for esophageal replacement. Most of these unfortunate children suffer because of adults not keeping caustic solutions out of their reach. Such operations had their advent in America in the mid-1950s. In Europe, especially Russia, this started earlier with the frequent ingestion of sulfuric acid by Russian children at winter's end. In many houses, a container of sulfuric acid was placed between the inner and outer windows to prevent fogging during the cold winter months. The hygroscopic properties of the sulfuric acid prevented moisture buildup between the inner and outer glass panes. In spring, when windows were opened, children got their hands on the acid with disastrous results.

Surgical Technique

In our initial experience with colon replacement, we used the right colon rotated upward on the midcolic pedicle and brought the cecum and terminal ileum to the neck for an easy anastomosis with the cervical esophagus. Generally, this segment of colon was brought up in the anterior mediastinum, beneath the xiphoid, behind the stomach, and out the thoracic inlet. The principal complication seen in these patients was late onset of tortuosity of the retrosternal colon. To straighten the colon in these cases, we used a median sternotomy approach.

In 1962, we adopted the technique described by Mr. David Waterston[18] of the Hospital for Sick Children, London. It is shown in Fig. 51-7.[19] The patient is positioned either with the left side straight up or partially upright. A wide prep and drape

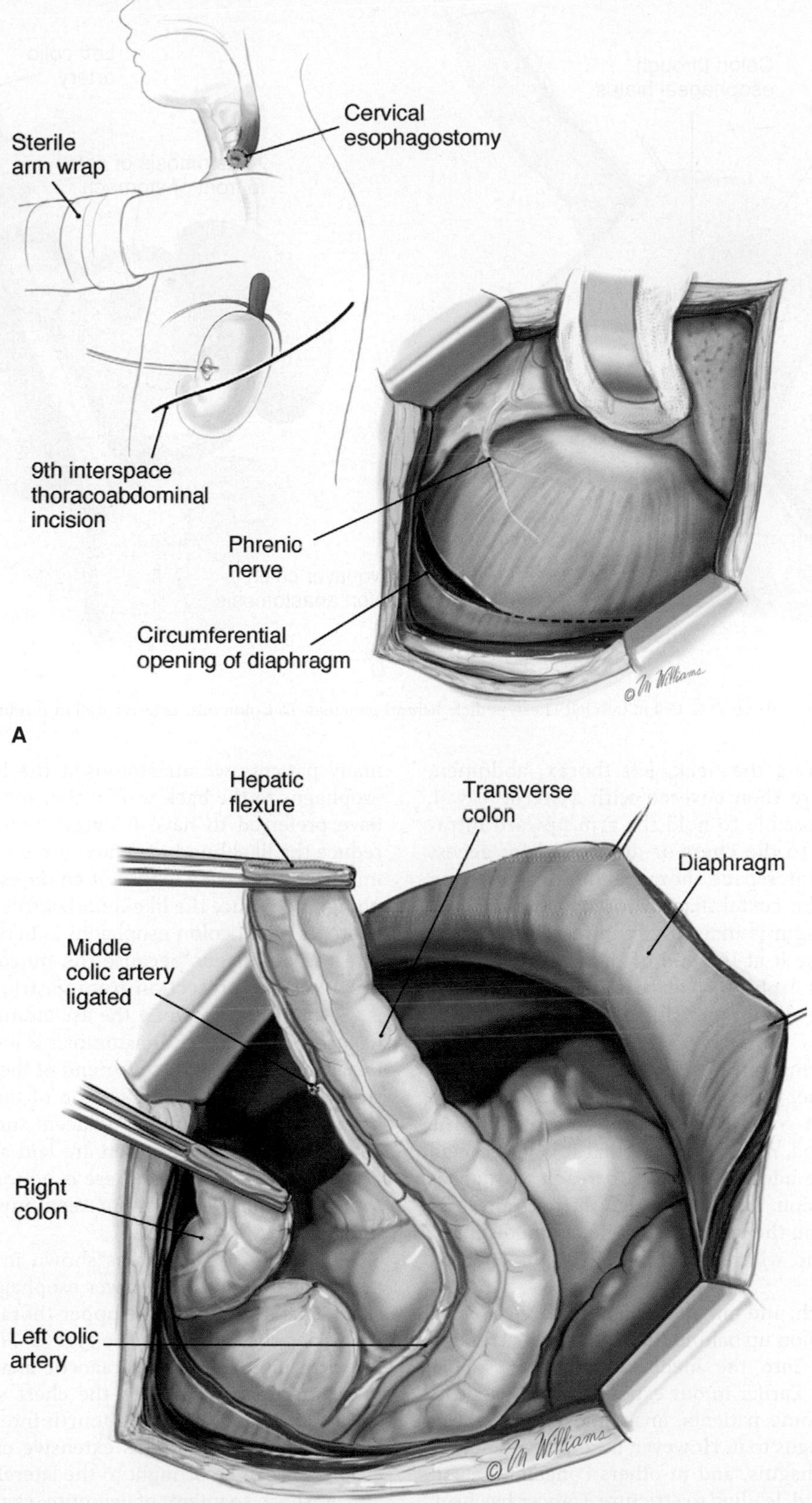

Figure 51-7. *A.* Colon esophagus operation. *B.* Mobilizing transverse colon over left colic artery. (*continued*)

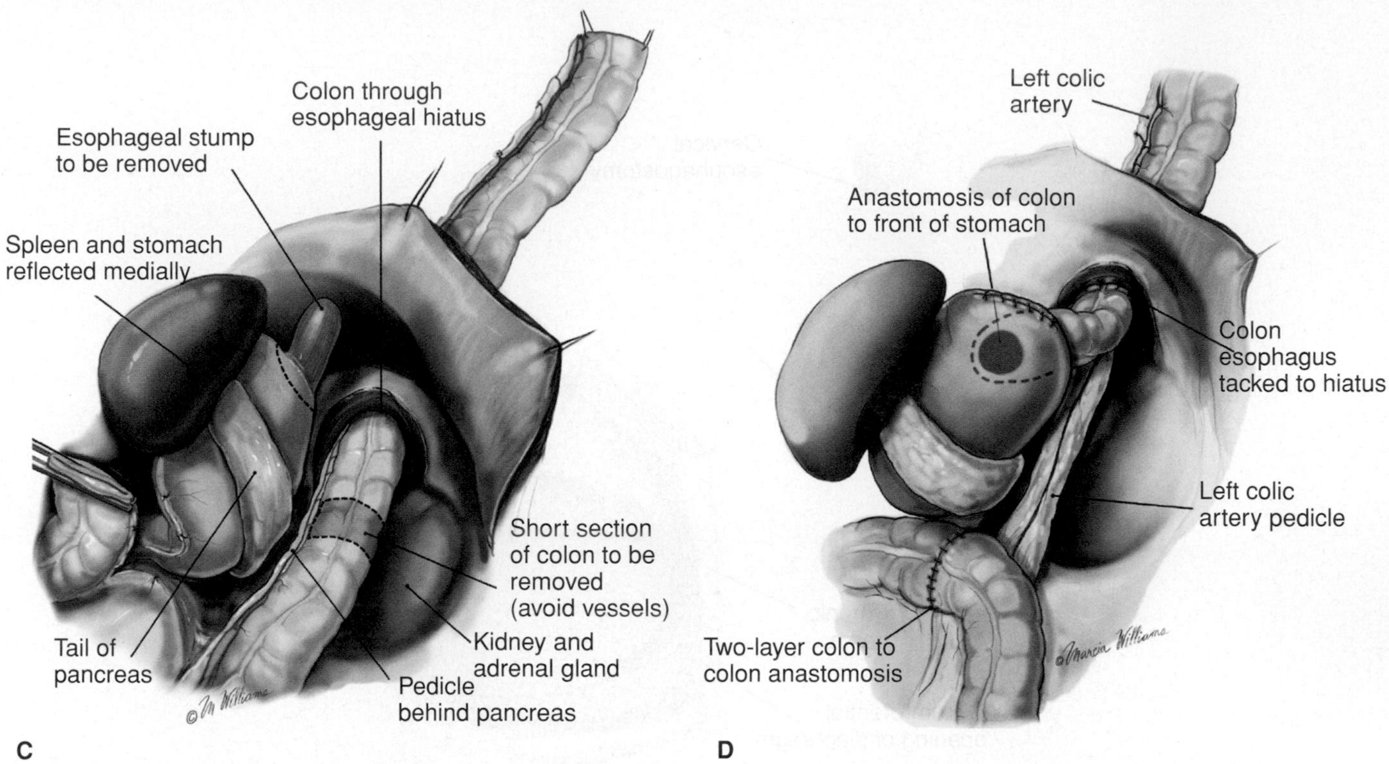

Figure 51-7. (*Continued*) *C*. Colon into left chest, pedicle behind pancreas. *D*. Colon into anterior wall of fundus. (*continued*)

are performed, including the neck, left thorax, abdomen, and left arm, which are then covered with a sterile towel. In this fashion, it is possible to hold the arm upward intraoperatively for access to the chest or downward for access to the neck. A ninth interspace thoracoabdominal incision is made, transecting the costal margin to expose the upper abdomen. The diaphragm is incised circumferentially, leaving a small rim to close it at the end of the operation. This technique preserves the phrenic nerve, which is cut when the surgeon opens the diaphragm through its dome out to the costal margin.

A Denis Browne ring retractor provides excellent exposure, as can several other types of retractors. Reaching across the abdomen, the right colon can be reflected medially. The hepatic flexure is divided, making certain that it is far enough to the right to provide adequate length to reach as high as necessary without tension. In our experience, the transverse colon, rotated upward on the left colic pedicle of blood supply, dividing the middle colic, will reach all the way to the pharynx if necessary.

The spleen, stomach, and tail of the pancreas are reflected medially to bring the colon up behind those structures through the esophageal hiatus into the mediastinum. The esophageal stump is removed. Earlier in our experience, we used the esophageal stump in some patients, anastomosing the lower end of the colon esophagus to it. However, in some patients the stump had reflux esophagitis, and in others congenital cartilaginous rests were found, leading to stricture. Cancer has been reported in a rudimentary stump, probably from severe chronic inflammation.

The straight left colon lies just behind the lung hilum, with left colic vessels tacked to the adjacent mediastinal tissues. In many patients we anastomosed the lower end of the colon esophagus to the back wall of the stomach. More recently, we have preferred to have it enter anteriorly because this may reduce the likelihood of reflux in the recumbent position. It is important to have a length of colon esophagus below the diaphragm to reduce the likelihood of free reflux. Reflux of gastric contents into a colon esophagus is better tolerated than reflux into the esophagus because the mucous glands of the colon provide some protection from gastric acid. Colon continuity is reestablished between the ascending colon and the splenic flexure. Note that the anastomosis is located at a distance from the anastomosis of the lower end of the colon esophagus to the stomach because a short section of the intervening colon has been removed. This avoids adjacent suture lines. Spleen, tail of pancreas, and stomach then are laid anterior to the left colic artery pedicle, on which there is no tension. In this retroperitoneal position we have not seen anything herniate beneath the pedicle.

In some cases, such as shown in Fig. 51-2, the replacement was limited to the lower esophagus. In others, the colon esophagus must reach the upper thorax to be anastomosed in the upper chest or neck (see Fig. 51-7*F*). A maneuver used by Sweet facilitated a high paraaortic anastomosis. This involved tunneling upward beneath the chest wall muscles to make a second thoracotomy in the fourth interspace (see Fig. 51-7*G*). In extreme cases, such as extensive caustic burns, the colon esophagus can be brought to the lateral pharynx.[20]

A short segment of jejunum can be rotated upward to replace the lower esophagus instead of using a segment of colon. It may be less prone to reflux when placed isoperistaltically because of the small bowel's inherent peristaltic waves, which are more effective than those of the colon. Many of our

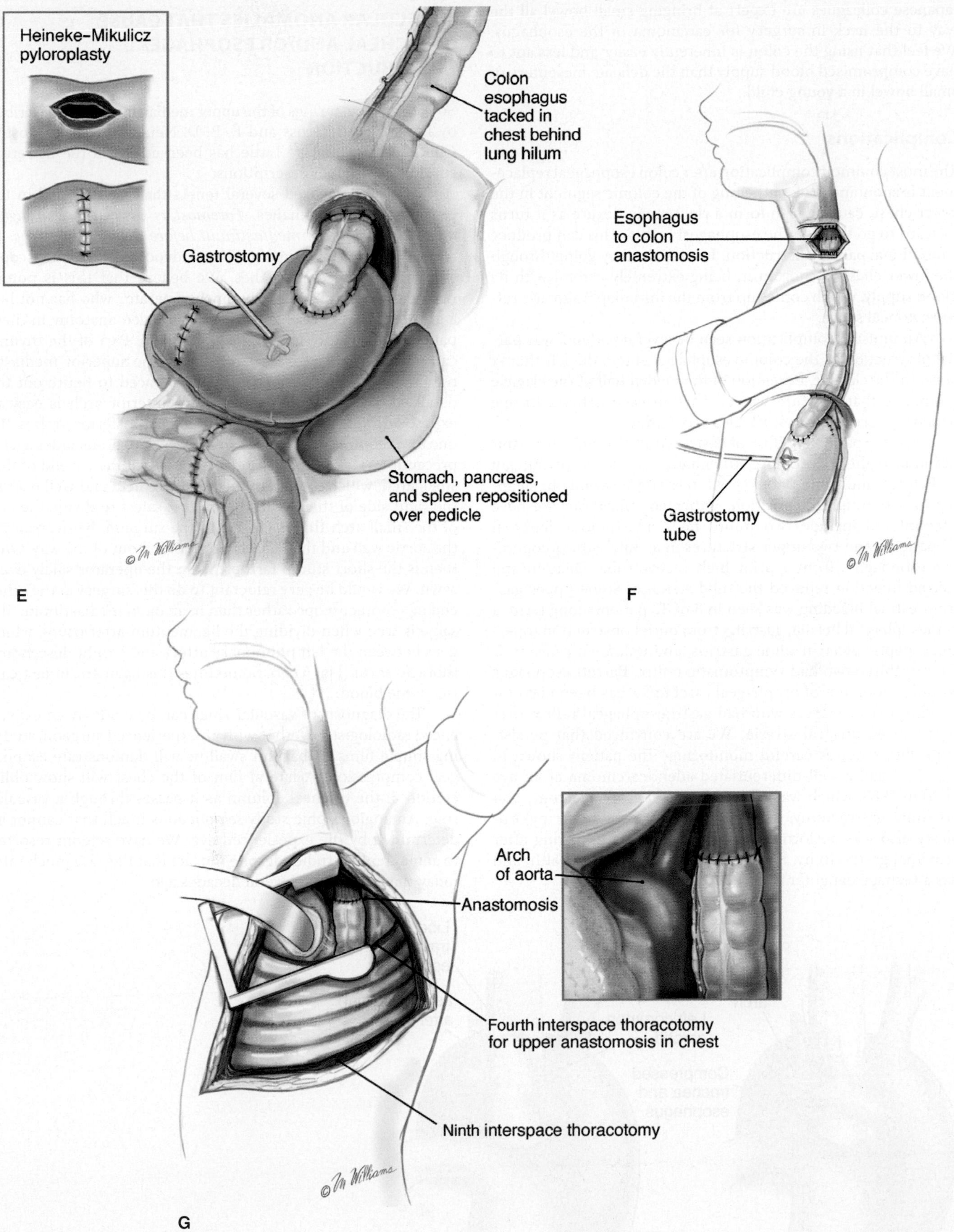

Figure 51-7. (*Continued*) *E.* Completed lower reconstruction. *F.* Typical upper anastomosis in neck. *G.* Paraaortic anastomosis in upper thorax.

Japanese colleagues are expert at bringing small bowel all the way to the neck in surgery for carcinoma of the esophagus. We feel that using the colon is inherently easier and less apt to have compromised blood supply than the delicate mesentery of small bowel in a young child.

Complications

The most common complication after colon esophageal replacement is spontaneous lengthening of the colonic segment in the lower chest, causing it to form a right-angle flexure as it turns forward to go through the esophageal hiatus. This can produce a functional partial obstruction. It is repaired by going through the lower chest to shorten it, being extremely careful with its blood supply, which comes up from the infradiaphragmatic retroperitoneal space.

An unusual complication seen in several patients was partial obstruction as the colonic esophagus enters the left thorax beneath the clavicle. Resection of the medial half of the clavicle to enlarge that aperture was curative in each patient. In one patient, a part of the first rib also was removed.

In some patients, reflux of gastric contents can cause aspiration at night. Pyloroplasty to enhance gastric emptying can be helpful, and some patients will respond favorably to sleeping in a semiupright position. Other complications we have encountered include two minor neck anastomotic leaks in 32 patients and two upper strictures in a child with preoperative esophagitis from a prior high gastric tube. Dilation and steroid injection relieved the mild stenosis. Some upper gastrointestinal bleeding was seen in 8 of 32 patients long term, a paraesophageal hernia, gastritis from outlet obstruction (operated), peptic ulcer, alkaline gastritis, and unknown cause in 2. Four of thirty-two had symptomatic reflux. Barrett esophagus with development of esophageal carcinoma has been encountered in two teenagers who had gastroesophageal reflux after repair of esophageal atresia. We are convinced that persisting reflux requires careful monitoring. The patient shown in Fig. 51-2 had a well-differentiated adenocarcinoma at an age of 20 in 1988, which was treated by distal esophagectomy and proximal gastrectomy, as shown. Heineke–Mikulicz pyloroplasty also was performed to enhance gastric emptying after proximal gastrectomy. She is now age 39, in good health, and has a teenage daughter.

VASCULAR ANOMALIES THAT CAUSE TRACHEAL AND/OR ESOPHAGEAL OBSTRUCTION

So-called vascular rings of the upper mediastinum were described by Dr. Robert E. Gross and E. B. D. Neuhauser at the Boston Children's Hospital.[3,21] Little has been added in the literature since these original descriptions.

Gross emphasized several tenets that are essential in the repair of these anomalies. *Foremost is dissecting thoroughly all the vessels of the mediastinum before dividing anything.* In recent years, some surgeons have advocated a thoracoscopic approach to these anomalies. We believe that this is potentially dangerous, particularly for the operator who has not had a great deal of experience with the deranged anatomy in these patients. A left thoracotomy is performed. Part of the thymus can be removed to give extra room in the superior mediastinum. Each of the vessels then can be traced to figure out the details of the case at hand. A small anterior arch is easy to expose and divide (Fig. 51-8). When the posterior arch is the one that requires division, it can be very dangerous unless great precaution is taken to have secure control of the far end of that small arch, which is deep in the operative field and well over to the right side of the mediastinum. It is safest to divide the end of the small arch that is closest to the surgeon, by oversewing the aortic wall and then gently retracting it out of the way. Only then is the short stump farthest from the operator safely oversewn. We would be very reluctant to do this surgery at the other end of a thoracoscope rather than in an open mediastinum. The same is true when dividing the ligamentum arteriosum, which goes between the left pulmonary artery and a right descending thoracic aorta (Fig. 51-9). Sometimes this ligament in fact carries some blood.

The diagnosis of vascular rings can be made by an experienced radiologist, together with an experienced surgeon, studying simple films. A barium swallow will demonstrate esophageal compression. A lateral film of the chest will show obliteration of the tracheal column as it passes through a vascular ring. An angiographic study *seldom* adds much that cannot be determined by the experienced eye. We have seldom resorted to angiographic studies despite the fact that they are much safer today than they were several decades ago.

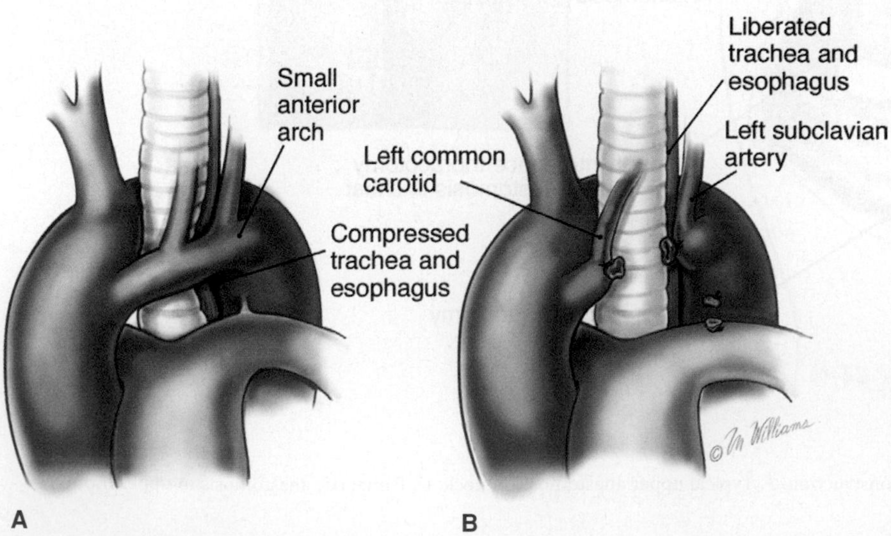

Figure 51-8. Great vessel anomalies. *A*. Typical vascular rings with small arch anteriorly. *B*. Ring divided and ligamentum released.

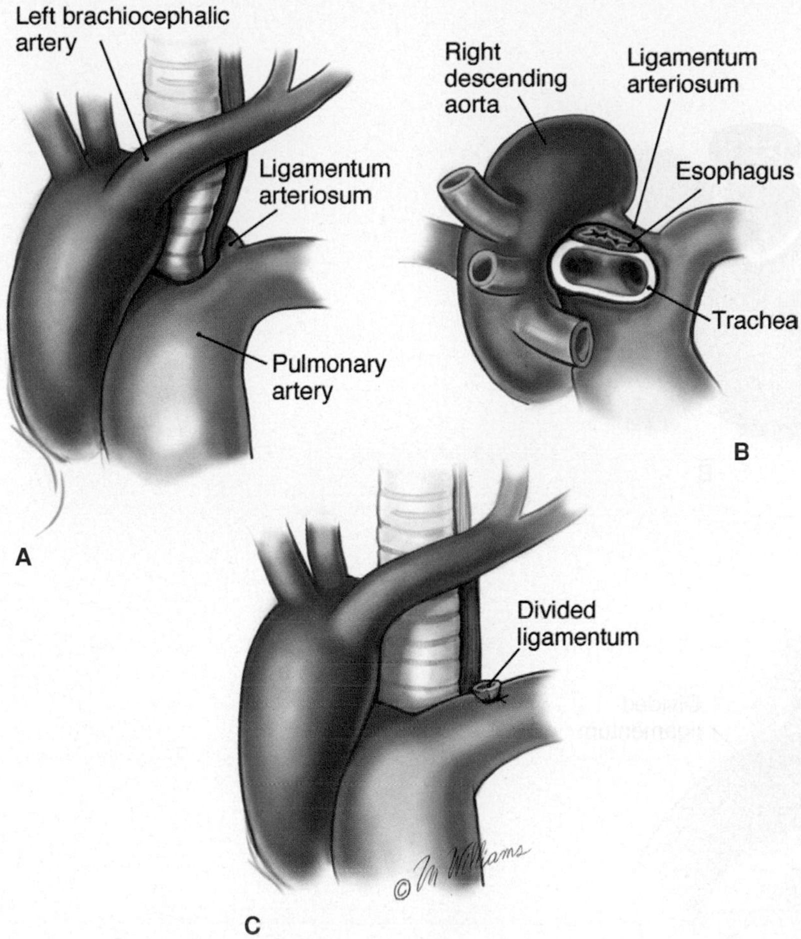

Figure 51-9. *A.* Right descending aorta after left ligamentum arteriosum. *B.* View from above. *C.* After release.

Surgical Technique

Vascular anomalies of the great vessels in the thorax should be meticulously dissected to avoid injury to the esophagus or trachea. Figs. 51-8 to 51-13 illustrate the most common or important types that can cause compression of the trachea and esophagus. A double aortic arch with a small arch in front of the trachea and a larger arch behind the esophagus is illustrated in Fig. 51-8*A.* To relieve this vascular compression, the small arch is divided as shown in Fig. 51-8*B.* Also, the ligamentum arteriosum is divided to allow the left pulmonary artery to move forward and the descending arch to move back.

The anomaly shown in Fig. 51-9 is a descending right aortic arch that is tethered to the left pulmonary artery by the ligamentum arteriosum, which passes behind the esophagus to the left pulmonary artery. It is curative to divide the ligamentum arteriosum that "springs open" the compressive vascular ring. In this and all these types of obstructions, after the causative vessel is divided, the surgeon must visualize the formerly compressed trachea and/or esophagus to make absolutely clear that there is no residual problem. We have done reoperative surgery for several of these children when the first surgeon did not follow these precepts outlined 60 years ago by Gross.

A case involving compression of the trachea by an innominate artery that arises more distal on the aortic arch than usual is presented in Fig. 51-10. Note the vascular "crotch" between the medial wall of the innominate artery and the medial wall of the left common carotid artery. The ligamentum arteriosum is also short and tethers upward to the left pulmonary artery. Fig. 51-10*B* shows this interesting anatomy in cross section. Relief of pressure on the trachea can be affected by thoroughly dissecting the great vessels of the arch and suspending the base of the innominate artery forward to the back wall of the sternum, as shown in Fig. 51-10*C.* This is done by placing Teflon pledgets on the anterior wall of the innominate artery so that fine sutures placed through the *adventitia* will not cut through. The ligamentum is also divided.

A case involving an aberrant right subclavian artery is illustrated in Fig. 51-11. Note that the right subclavian artery arises from the distal arch, passing behind the esophagus and traversing the apex of the right chest to emerge behind the clavicle. This is a common anomaly. It was described in 1794 in London.[22] It is easily diagnosed with a barium swallow that shows the typical indentation of the back wall of the esophagus by the subclavian vessel that traverses upward and to the right, compressing the esophagus. There is a beaklike deformity on the esophagram in which the esophagus drapes over this vessel. It can be dissected free and divided in the thorax on the left side. Alternatively, in several cases we have dissected the vessel in the right lower neck anteriorly, following the vessel proximally into the posterior mediastinum, where it is ligated and divided, letting the ends retract away from the esophagus.

The right recurrent nerve to the larynx does not recur in these cases, where there is no subclavian artery around which it normally passes. Instead, the nerve enters high in the larynx from above. In several instances when operating for an isolated

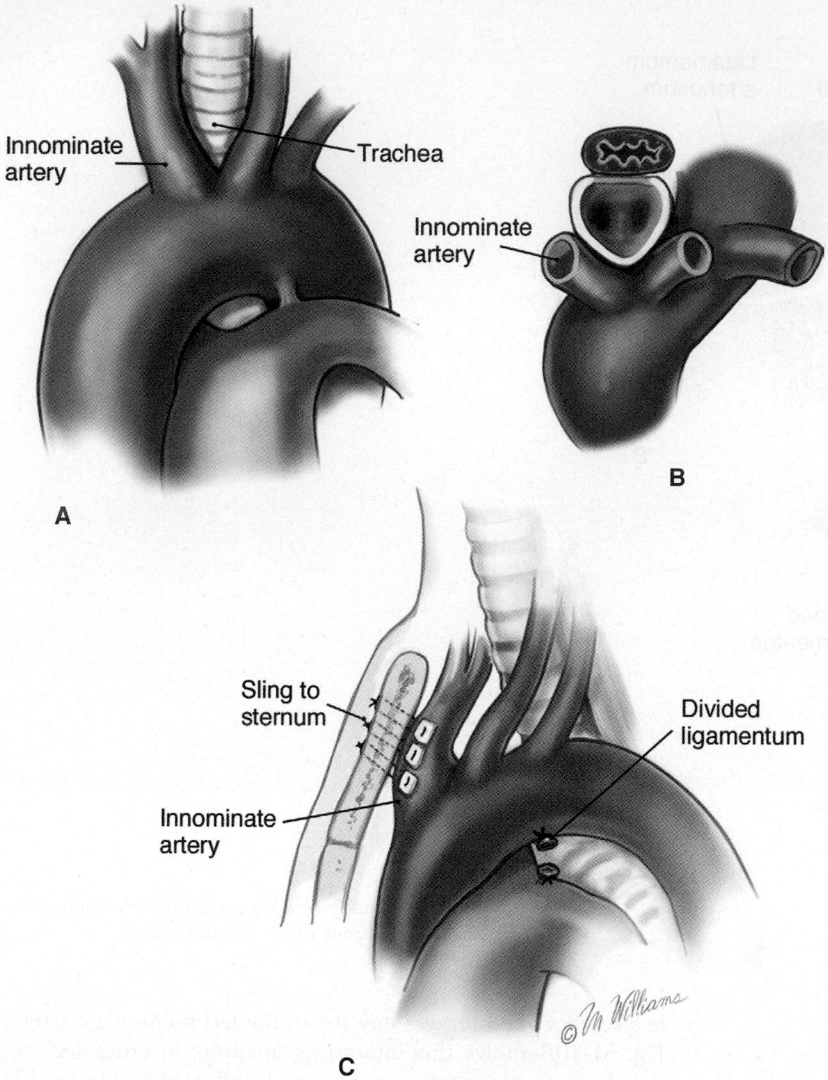

Figure 51-10. *A.* Anomalous innominate. *B.* View from above. *C.* Aorta suspended anteriorly.

cervical TEF, we have seen and divided an anomalous right subclavian artery from the right neck incision. Obviously, the vessel must be secured and suture-ligated proximally before it is divided because retraction into the mediastinum through a short supraclavicular incision would be disastrous.

A double aortic arch with the smaller arch in back and larger one anteriorly is depicted in Fig. 51-12. This is the most dangerous type of arch to divide because the small posterior arch is usually *very short,* making it difficult to simply ligate and divide. We prefer to divide this arch between vascular clamps, leaving only a very short amount of the base nearer to the operator. That side then can be sewn over and over to control it, removing the proximal clamp. That segment of the large arch is retracted forward. If most of the posterior arch is retained on the far side of the mediastinum, as viewed by the surgeon, additional safety is afforded to oversew it deep in the mediastinum. If it should escape the clamp before it is oversewn, it can be very difficult to access the released segment deep in the mediastinum. Precaution is essential in dealing with this special anomaly.

Fig. 51-13 shows an anomalous left pulmonary artery, often termed *pulmonary sling.* Note that the right pulmonary artery is normal, but the left pulmonary artery comes off superiorly, wrapping around the trachea and esophagus to then reach the left lung hilum. We believe that the safest way to approach this is through an upper sternal split, using temporary cardiopulmonary bypass. The anomalous left pulmonary artery is divided and reimplanted on the lateral aspect of the left main pulmonary artery. The trachea itself may be compromised by its severe compression. It may require sleeve resection. Happily, this is a very rare anomaly.

OTHER NONMALIGNANT CONGENITAL ESOPHAGEAL ANOMALIES

Achalasia

Achalasia is a rare esophageal motility disorder (see Chapter 33) that affects 5 in 1 million individuals of all ages. Only 5% of those are children under age 15.[23] The underlying pathology, which consists of nonrelaxation of the lower esophageal sphincter and a markedly distended esophageal body, produces ineffective peristalsis and difficulty in swallowing. The presenting symptoms include weight loss, failure to thrive, superimposed dysphagia, and often regurgitation. On barium

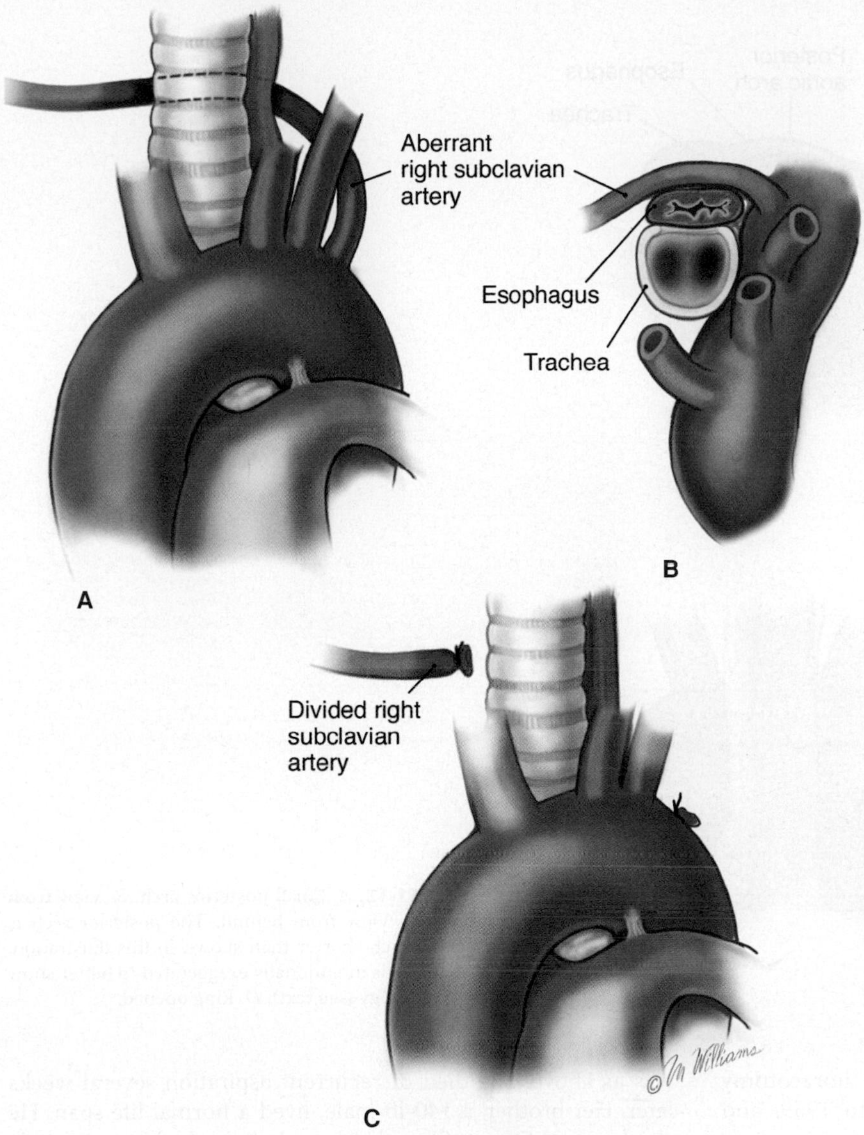

Figure 51-11. *A.* Anomalous right subclavian artery. *B.* View from above. *C.* After release.

swallow, the esophagus has a wide body that tapers in cone-like fashion to a very small distal segment. An air-fluid level is often observed. Esophageal manometry studies reveal ineffective and discoordinated peristaltic waves in the dilated esophagus and high pressure in the lower esophageal sphincter, where pressures exceed 40 mm Hg. As with any hollow viscus, the dilated walls fail to coapt, causing discoordinated peristaltic waves and an inability to propel a food bolus. This phenomenon can be seen in other conditions, such as megaureter and dilated colon in Hirschsprung disease, where the lower colon does not relax. Achalasia is a progressive disorder. Medical therapy has included calcium channel blockers (e.g., nifedipine) and botulinum toxin injected endoscopically into the nonrelaxing lower esophageal sphincter. However, neither of these modalities has had satisfactory long-term results in children.[24,25] Endoscopic balloon dilation was described more than 50 years ago by Gross[26] as being effective in some children. Today, many physicians make several attempts to dilate the lower esophageal sphincter before referring a child for surgery.[27] We believe that most young patients are best treated for this disorder surgically.

Surgical Technique

The technique as performed in adults with achalasia is described in Chapter 34. Although the technique can be performed using open or minimally invasive technique, we prefer the laparotomy approach, as illustrated in Fig. 51-6. The procedure is performed with the tapered end of a Maloney rubber dilator inserted through the esophagus into the stomach. A soft nonlatex rubber drain is placed around the lower esophagus to free the esophagus through its hiatus. The myotomy begins several centimeters above the spastic segment, at or above the level of the inferior pulmonary vein, and is extended at least 1 to 2 cm onto the anterior wall of the stomach (cardia) to prevent postoperative reflux. After the myotomy, it is important to inspect the mucosa for evidence of perforation. This can be done by inflating the esophagus with air or saline through a nasogastric tube. The procedure then is followed as described in Fig. 51-6, including a pyloroplasty to prevent reflux. Some pediatric surgeons have performed this operation thoracoscopically. Experience with this approach is limited, and these children should be followed for postoperative

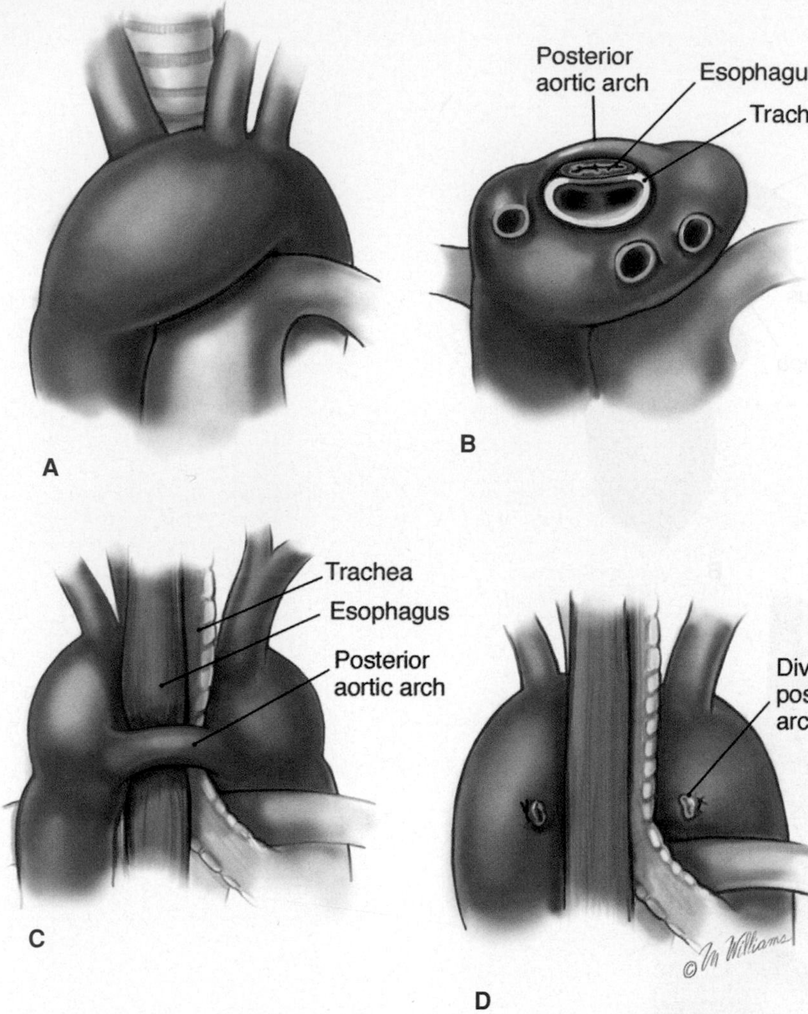

Figure 51-12. *A.* Small posterior arch. *B.* View from above. *C.* View from behind. The posterior arch is always much shorter than shown in this illustration. The image is intentionally exaggerated to better show this pathology (see text). *D.* Ring opened.

gastroesophageal reflux. Our results using the thoracotomy approach have been satisfactory dating back to 1959, and reflux has not been a problem in our practice.

Of incidental interest, one of us has operated on three dogs with achalasia of the esophagus. The first was a female German shepherd puppy belonging to our family. The operation was as above. She died of recurrent aspiration several weeks later. Her brother, a 140-lb male, lived a normal life span. He sired several litters of healthy pups, but one had bowel atresia and one female had achalasia. She was operated on as above and lived a normal life span as a family member. This successful outcome was attributed to long-term loving postoperative care

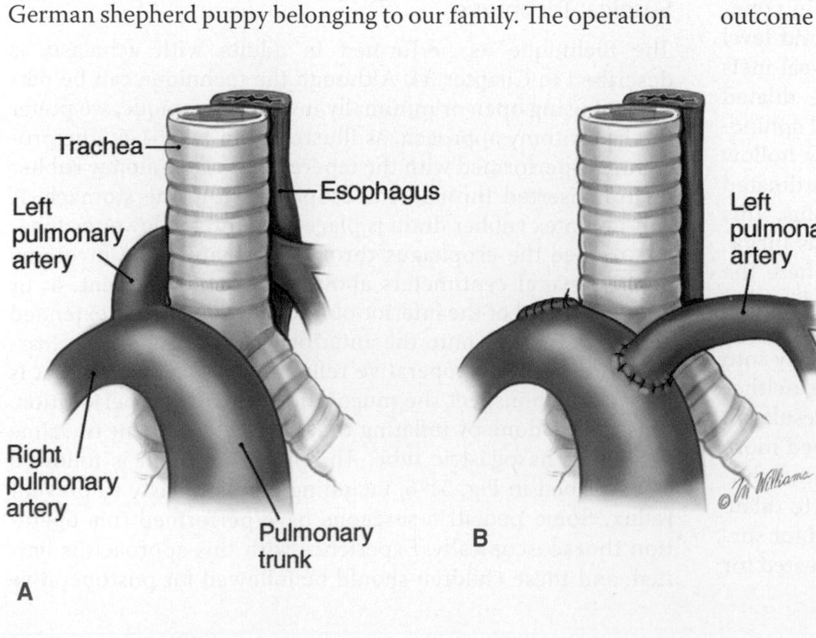

Figure 51-13. *A.* Pulmonary artery "sling." *B.* Pulmonary artery replanted with patient on cardiopulmonary bypass. Bronchial anatomy assessed and sleeve resection performed if needed.

by the surgeon's wife who fed the dog in an upright position for several months and gave supplemental feedings through a gastrostomy tube. The tube was hidden from the puppy, as well as her mother, by a dressing incorporating all the neighbors' discarded pantyhose. The third case was a Schnauzer who succumbed early postoperatively in the animal hospital where the procedure was performed by a pediatric surgical team.

Congenital Esophageal Stenosis

Congenital esophageal stenosis is a rare problem that occurs at a rate of 1 in 25,000 births.[28] Thirty percent of these children have associated anomalies of the gastrointestinal tract, heart, or axial skeleton.[29] The three known variants differ in embryogenesis and location. The first variant consists of a membranous web or diaphragm that typically is found in the middle third of the esophagus. It is thought to be an incomplete form of esophageal atresia and is the rarest type. The second variant is characterized by congenital fibromuscular hyperplasia. It is also found in the middle third of the esophagus and is the most common type, caused by submucosal smooth muscle and fibrous tissue proliferation and hypertrophy. The third form arises from ectopic tracheobronchial remnants, which are usually found in the distal third of the esophagus. This variant is thought to arise from tracheobronchial remnants improperly sequestered in the esophageal wall during the fourth week of gestation as the trachea separates from the esophagus.

Symptoms of congenital esophageal stenosis include both respiratory and gastrointestinal components, with vomiting, dysphagia, and feeding intolerance being most common. Reactive airway disease and recurrent tracheobronchiolitis are also seen often and may cloud the true nature of the problem unless the clinician has a high index of suspicion. Symptoms generally are progressive, and there is often a delay in diagnosis. A barium swallow should show the site of stenosis, but it may not elucidate the precise etiology. Esophagoscopy with endoscopic ultrasound is now used commonly to define the true nature of the problem. For esophageal webs or fibromuscular hyperplasia, endoscopic intervention with catheter-directed balloon-assisted dilation is the first mode of treatment. For many years, bougienage was used for dilation, but pneumatic balloon dilation techniques are now used more often.[30]

Surgical Technique

Patients with tracheobronchial remnants or with fibromuscular hyperplasia and recurrent obstruction after multiple dilations should have segmental esophagectomy and anastomosis unless the segment is too long. Two layers of fine monofilament sutures are used to reconstruct the defect. Midesophageal lesions are best approached through a right thoracotomy, whereas distal lesions are best approached from the left side. If the lesion involves the intraabdominal esophagus, one should consider buttressing the repair with a partial fundoplication to prevent postoperative gastroesophageal reflux. Long-term outcomes have been excellent. Occasionally, a long-segment stenosis will require substitution with colon or small bowel.

Mediastinal Cysts and Esophageal Duplications

Several types of cystic masses occur in the mediastinum of infants and children. Some are neoplastic, and some are congenital.[31] Teratoma, lymphangioma, and thymic cysts are found most commonly in the anterior mediastinum. Bronchogenic cysts are found more commonly in the middle mediastinum. In the posterior mediastinum it is more common to see esophageal duplications. Tumors of neural origin are found in the paravertebral region; sometimes these ganglioneuromas and neuroblastomas can extend into adjacent intervertebral foramina to involve the spinal canal. Some mediastinal masses are symptomatic, depending on their size and location. Others are picked up incidentally on routine chest x-ray.

Esophageal duplications represent 10% to 20% of all gastrointestinal duplications. They are rarely found in the cervical esophagus, yet we have seen upper airway obstruction caused by foregut cysts of the hypopharynx that block the inlet to the larynx.[31] The mucosal lining may be entirely inappropriate for that level of the gastrointestinal tract where the duplication is found. This is an interesting feature common to all gastrointestinal duplications. The gastric mucosa can occur at any level from the neck to the pararectal region. Colonic mucosa similarly has been seen in duplications at any level of the gastrointestinal tract from the pharynx to the rectum.

There are two general types of esophageal duplications: enteric and intramural. Enteric lesions are most commonly tubular structures that result from incomplete separation of the primitive notochord from the endoderm during embryogenesis. If a defect such as a bony cleft is found anywhere in the vertebral column from the neck to the pelvis, one should consider a tubular duplication in the differential diagnosis. We have encountered several of these duplications traversing from the right thorax below the diaphragm up to the cervical region. These require formidable dissection in the neck, chest, and below the diaphragm, where the duplication may connect with the gastrointestinal tract or even the biliary tract. Intramural esophageal duplications are somewhat more straightforward. They are usually contained completely within the walls of the esophagus and probably result from incomplete vacuolization during development of the early esophagus. They seldom connect with the adjacent lumen, although if gastric mucosa is present, they can erode into the adjacent esophagus. Preoperative evaluation of these patients usually includes a barium swallow, which may demonstrate partial obstruction of the adjacent normal esophageal lumen from compression caused by the adjacent duplication. Chest CT scan after intravenous contrast material injection is also obtained routinely. If there is a vertebral defect, MRI also can add useful information.

During the surgical procedure, it is useful to gently pass a soft rubber bougie into the normal esophagus, if it passes easily, and then excise the adjacent duplication. The esophageal wall, which may be stretched over the duplication, is incised vertically, shelling out the duplication and taking care not to injure the underlying normal esophageal mucosa. In adults, it is not uncommon to follow a patient with a small esophageal duplication or an asymptomatic bronchogenic cyst with serial x-rays, although the anomaly can be removed easily thoracoscopically. In children with long life expectancy, however, there are several reasons these cysts should be removed.[32,33] First, they may progressively secrete fluid and enlarge to sufficient size to produce respiratory symptoms. Second, they may become infected. Occasionally, a cyst may undergo malignant degeneration. If the cyst has a gastric lining, it may erode, causing hemorrhage or perforation. In the rare occurrence of a connection between the lumen of an esophageal duplication and the lumen of the adjacent esophagus, that opening should be closed with great care, before closing the esophageal muscular wall overlying the defect.

SUMMARY

Historically, major thoracic surgery in infants and children came to the forefront when Robert Gross became the first to successfully ligate a patent ductus arteriosus in a 7-year-old girl named Lorraine Sweeney. Gross was then the chief resident in surgery at the Boston Children's Hospital. His chief, William E. Ladd, was out of town. Ladd never forgave him for that surgical coup. Gross felt that Ladd would not have approved that risky venture. Today (2008), at age 78 years, Lorraine is alive and well and 70 years postoperative. This case exemplifies the aim of pediatric surgery, which is to make possible an entire life that otherwise might have ended in infancy or childhood.

EDITOR'S COMMENT

Many of the congenital esophageal disorders have been routinely addressed in infancy or childhood with great success. As a consequence, adult patients who had surgery as babies will occasionally present with long-term complications of the original procedure or anatomical challenges resulting from these procedures. For example, I have treated patients who have a substernal colonic conduit that was divided during an emergency CABG as an adult, as well as patients with diverticulitis in their intrathoracic colon esophageal replacement. It is therefore incumbent on all thoracic surgeons to familiarize themselves with the various anatomic repairs of the congenital esophageal disorders. As for the current approaches to esophageal surgery in the pediatric population, these are evolving inexorably to less invasive methods, which require the same expertise and attention to details as the open approaches.

—Raphael Bueno

References

1. Leven N. Congenital atresia of the esophagus with tracheoesophageal fistula: report of fistulous communication and cervical esophagostomy. *J Thorac Surg.* 1941;10:648–657.
2. Ladd W. The surgical treatment of esophageal atresia and tracheoesophageal fistulas. *N Engl J Med.* 1944;230:625.
3. Lanman T. Congenital atresia of the esophagus: a study of thirty-two cases. *Arch Surg.* 1940;41:1060.
4. Haight C, Towsley H. Congenital atresia of the esophagus with tracheoesophageal fistula: extrapleural ligation of fistula and end-to-end anastomosis of esophageal segments. *Surg Gynecol Obstet.* 1943;76:672–688.
5. Adzick NS, Fisher JH, Winter HS, et al. Esophageal adenocarcinoma 20 years after esophageal atresia repair. *J Pediatr Surg.* 1989;24:741–744.
6. Rehbein F, Schweder N. Reconstruction of the esophagus without colon transplantation in cases of atresia. *J Pediatr Surg.* 1971;6:746–752.
7. Hendren WH, Hale JR. Esophageal atresia treated by electromagnetic bougienage and subsequent repair. *J Pediatr Surg.* 1976;11:713–722.
8. Willital G. Long gap esophageal atresia: esophageal reconstruction by double esophageal segmental elongation (magnetically or mechanically) and also anastomosis. In: Willital GH, Kiely E, Gohary AM, et al., eds. *Atlas of Child Surgery.* Berlin: Pabst; 2005:62–66.
9. Hendren WH. Repair of laryngotracheoesophageal cleft using interposition of a strap muscle. *J Pediatr Surg.* 1976;11:425–429.
10. Hendren WH. Case records of the Massachusetts General Hospital. Duodenobronchial fistula, congenital, in a 5-year-old boy. *N Engl J Med.* 1961;264: 936–940.
11. Donahoe PK, Gee PE. Complete laryngotracheoesophageal cleft: management and repair. *J Pediatr Surg.* 1984;19:143–148.
12. Kim SH, Hendren WH, Donahoe PK. Gastroesophageal reflux and hiatus hernia in children: experience with 70 cases. *J Pediatr Surg.* 1980;15:443–451.
13. Hill LD. An effective operation for hiatal hernia: an eight year appraisal. *Ann Surg.* 1967;166:681–692.
14. Nissen R. Reminiscences: reflux esophagitis and hiatal hernia. *Rev Surg.* 1970;27:307–314.
15. Anderson K. Replacement of the esophagus. In: Welch KD, Randolph JG, Ravitch MM, eds. *Pediatric Surgery.* Chicago, IL: Mosby-Year Book; 1986. Chapter 70.
16. Spitz L, Kiely E, Sparnon T. Gastric transposition for esophageal replacement in children. *Ann Surg.* 1987;206:69–73.
17. Sweet RH. The results of radical surgical extirpation in the treatment of carcinoma of the esophagus and cardia with five year survival statistics. *Surg Gynecol Obstet.* 1952;94:46–52.
18. Waterston D. Colonic replacement of esophagus (intrathoracic). *Surg Clin North Am.* 1964;44:1441.
19. Hendren WH, Hendren WG. Colon interposition for esophagus in children. *J Pediatr Surg.* 1985;20:829–839.
20. Choi RS, Lillehei CW, Lund DP, et al. Esophageal replacement in children who have caustic pharyngoesophageal strictures. *J Pediatr Surg.* 1997;32:1083–1087; discussion 1087–1088.
21. Gross R. Surgical relief for tracheal obstruction from a vascular ring. *N Engl J Med.* 1945;233:586–590.
22. Bayford D. An account of a singular case of deglutition. *Mem Med Soc Lond.* 1794;2:275.
23. Karnak I, Senocak ME, Tanyel FC, et al. Achalasia in childhood: surgical treatment and outcome. *Eur J Pediatr Surg.* 2001;11:223–229.
24. Khoshoo V, LaGarde DC, Udall JN, Jr. Intrasphincteric injection of botulinum toxin for treating achalasia in children. *J Pediatr Gastroenterol Nutr.* 1997;24:439–441.
25. Glassman MS, Medow MS, Berezin S, et al. Spectrum of esophageal disorders in children with chest pain. *Dig Dis Sci.* 1992;37:663–666.
26. Gross R. *The Surgery of Infancy and Childhood.* Philadelphia, PA: Saunders; 1953.
27. Emblem R, Stringer MD, Hall CM, et al. Current results of surgery for achalasia of the cardia. *Arch Dis Child.* 1993;68:749–751.
28. Nishina T, Tsuchida Y, Saito S. Congenital esophageal stenosis due to tracheobronchial remnants and its associated anomalies. *J Pediatr Surg.* 1981;16:190–193.
29. Nihoul-Fekete C, Backer A, Lortat-Jacob S. Congenital esophageal stenosis. *Pediatr Surg Int.* 1987;2:86.
30. Takamizawa S, Tsugawa C, Mouri N, et al. Congenital esophageal stenosis: therapeutic strategy based on etiology. *J Pediatr Surg.* 2002;37:197–201.
31. Canty TG, Hendren WH. Upper airway obstruction from foregut cysts of the hypopharynx. *J Pediatr Surg.* 1975;10:807–812.
32. Read CA, Moront M, Carangelo R, et al. Recurrent bronchogenic cyst: an argument for complete surgical excision. *Arch Surg.* 1991;126:1306–1308.
33. Suen HC, Mathisen DJ, Grillo HC, et al. Surgical management and radiological characteristics of bronchogenic cysts. *Ann Thorac Surg.* 1993;55: 476–481.

52 Minimally Invasive Techniques for Esophageal Repair

Biren P. Modi and Christopher B. Weldon

Keyword: Minimally invasive, MIS, VATS, thoracoscopy, esophageal atresia, foregut duplication cysts

INTRODUCTION

While minimally invasive techniques have been used to alleviate esophageal symptoms, such as thoracoscopic release of vascular rings causing esophageal obstruction or laparoscopic fundoplication for gastroesophageal reflux disease (GERD), this chapter focuses on minimally invasive methods for direct surgical repair of congenital esophageal anomalies: esophageal atresia (EA) with or without tracheoesophageal fistula (TEF) and foregut duplication cysts.

As described in the previous chapter, the advent of successful surgical intervention for EA in the 1930s and 1940s was a hallmark event for pediatric surgery, changing a universally fatal anomaly into one that could be surgically repaired with an expectation for long-term success. With the development of minimally invasive techniques and the rapid advance of both supporting technology and surgical skill and experience, thoracoscopic approaches to esophageal repair have been proposed. Since the first report of a primary thoracoscopic repair of congenital EA in 1999 and EA with TEF in 2000, the use of this technique has gained traction and now is being performed at many, if not most, centers with advanced pediatric surgery capabilities.[1]

The novelty of reports describing the thoracoscopic technique for repair of EA/TEF, not to mention that the operation is performed on some of our most fragile patients, is likely responsible for the delay in widespread acceptance of this approach. It ranks among the most technically demanding of pediatric minimally invasive procedures and requires advanced thoracoscopic surgical skill.[1,2] Multiple centers, however, now have reported their experience with this approach to treating EA with or without TEF, and as experience and longer-term outcomes accumulate, its place in the field of pediatric surgery will be determined.

On the other hand, the excision of foregut duplication cysts, specifically esophageal duplication cysts, is particularly suited to minimally invasive techniques, and this procedure now is routinely performed thoracoscopically. In contrast to newborns with EA in all its various forms, patients with foregut duplication cysts generally are older, more healthy, and rarely present with comorbid conditions. The absence of comorbidity perhaps is most responsible for the ready acceptance of the thoracoscopic approach to excising foregut duplication cysts.

ESOPHAGEAL ATRESIA WITH AND WITHOUT TRACHEOESOPHAGEAL FISTULA

EA occurs in 1 in 5000 births. It can develop in many forms, with the most common being the "Type C" atresia, comprised of EA with a distal TEF (see Fig. 52-1). The second most common scenario is EA without TEF, so-called pure EA. Although other forms exist, these two forms are most amenable to the thoracoscopic approach to esophageal repair. Since the first reporting of thoracoscopic repair of pure EA in 1999[3] and EA with distal TEF in 2000,[4] this approach has become increasingly used, and multi-institutional experiences have been reported.[1]

General Principles

As with any intestinal anastomosis, the key surgical principle of the thoracoscopic esophageal repair in EA is to perform the procedure with the same high standards as one would follow when performing open surgery. Paramount in this procedure is healthy tissue, placed together with minimal tension. Some technical principles are detailed below, but are highlighted by the need to handle tissue gently and to incorporate sturdy, full-thickness bites including mucosa into the anastomosis without creating undue tension. As with all minimally invasive techniques, ergonomics and surgeon comfort during the procedure are important to prevent fatigue and allow for fine, delicate movements in the dissection of fragile structures. In addition, although we tend to use intracorporeal knot-tying techniques, extracorporeal techniques using a knot pusher are also well described. Finally, although the surgical techniques may be modified, it is paramount that the surgeon not compromise the quality of the operation to achieve a successful minimally invasive procedure.

The key clinical characteristic that defines thoracoscopic surgery, in antithesis to its open counterpart, is the significantly

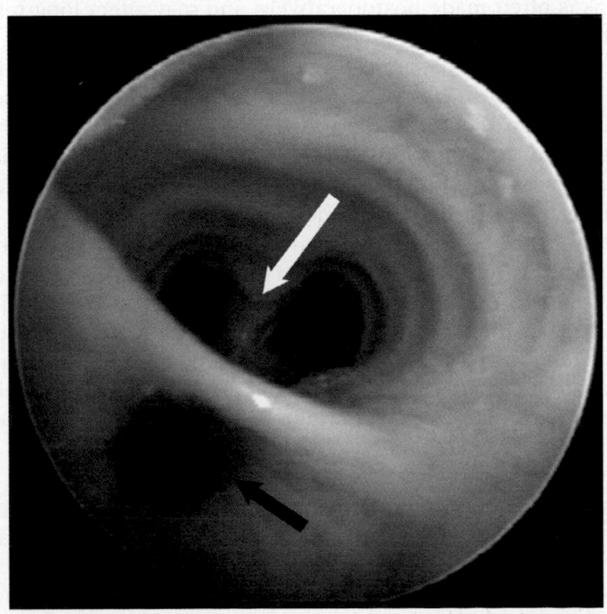

Figure 52-1. Rigid bronchoscopic view of a large tracheoesophageal fistula. Note the tracheal rings anteriorly and the fistula (black arrow), located in the usual position in the posterior membranous portion of the trachea just above the carina (white arrow).

reduced morbidity related to the incision(s). In the immediate postoperative period, the drastically reduced pain associated with thoracoscopic surgery allows for faster recovery and decreased pulmonary complications in children who may already be at risk for other conditions such as congenital cardiac disease (see below). In addition, patients, especially newborns, are at particular risk for sequelae of open thoracotomy, including musculoskeletal deformities such as "winged" scapula, muscular atrophy with resultant asymmetry, and/or scoliosis.[1]

Timing of surgery depends on the patient's underlying diagnosis (pure EA vs. EA/TEF) and their stability. Pure EA patients can undergo thoracoscopic repair in a delayed fashion, after initial tube gastrostomy and a period of growth on enteral nutrition. Patients with EA/TEF are generally repaired within the first 24 hours of life assuming appropriate size, hemodynamic stability, and the absence of more pressing concomitant congenital defects.

Preoperative Assessment and Patient Selection

Since the various forms of EA can all be a component of the VACTERL (**V**ertebral anomalies, **A**norectal anomalies, **C**ardiac defects, **T**racheo-**E**sophageal anomalies, **R**enal anomalies, **L**imb defects) association, appropriate screening tests should be performed on all patients found to have EA. These include echocardiogram, spine ultrasound and plain films, and renal ultrasound. Chief among these, and the only one necessary prior to operative intervention for EA/TEF, is the echocardiogram. This allows for identification of intracardiac defects, such as ventricular septal defects or tetralogy of Fallot, and for identification of a potential right-sided aortic arch. In most cases, the surgical approach for repair of EA/TEF is through the right chest. A right-sided aortic arch, however, will prompt most surgeons to change to the left chest. Another common association involving EA is the cleverly but somewhat incompletely named CHARGE syndrome (**C**oloboma, **H**eart defects, choanal **A**tresia, **R**etardation, **G**enital hypoplasia, **E**ar abnormalities). This diagnosis is often made postoperatively, and may affect long-term outcomes.

While hemodynamically unstable patients and very premature or growth restricted newborns (<1500 g) should likely not undergo thoracoscopic repair of EA/TEF, there are other relative contraindications. These include significant congenital heart disease and smaller infants (less than 2.5 kg). One additional feature which should be assessed is the expectation of relative "gap" between the proximal esophageal pouch and the fistula in TEF or the distal pouch in pure EA. Plain films can help determine the location of the proximal pouch, with its coiled nasogastric tube, and obviously, the presence of a distal fistula based on the presence of bowel gas. Meanwhile, bronchoscopic evaluation can assess the level of the fistula (e.g., location relative to the carina). In cases of pure EA, most patients receive a gastrostomy at birth followed by delayed esophageal repair. In these cases, a preoperative gap assessment can be obtained by placing a radiopaque instrument such as a Bakes dilator via the gastrostomy and transorally, and obtaining fluoroscopic imaging while placing moderate pressure on the dilators. This technique can also be used intraoperatively for easy identification of the esophageal ends.

Each individual patient's qualifications for a thoracoscopic approach must be assessed using a combination of these multiple variables. As surgeons (and anesthesiologists) gain more experience and confidence, these boundaries will continue to be tested.[1,5]

Technique

Evaluation of the Fistula

We prefer to perform rigid bronchoscopy on all children with suspected EA (see Fig. 52-1), to identify and locate the TEF and also to potentially control it with the use of a balloon-tipped catheter which can be lodged within the proximal fistula and allow for the safer administration of positive-pressure ventilation during the initial stages of anesthesia prior to operative control of the fistula. While this is our chosen technique, not all surgeons perform this step.

Rigid bronchoscopy requires cervical extension in the supine position and the gentle use of an appropriately sized rigid ventilating bronchoscope. Important findings to note should include the assessment of vocal cord function for documentation prior to potential surgery on and around the vagus nerves, assessment for location of the distal fistula, a thorough and methodical evaluation of the posterior membranous trachea to rule out the possibility of multiple TEFs, and the assessment of tracheal stability with the presence or absence of significant tracheobronchomalacia. We then place a Fogarty-type balloon catheter transorally and bronchoscopically direct it into the fistula, inflating the balloon just inside the fistula itself. At the conclusion of bronchoscopy, the patient is orotracheally intubated with the goals of maintaining spontaneous ventilation if possible and avoiding intubation of the fistula which could result in disastrous decompensation. All of these steps are similar for both the open and thoracoscopic techniques.

Anesthetic Considerations and Lung Isolation

The anesthetic technique employed and full two-way communication between the anesthesia and surgery teams are essential to the successful completion of a thoracoscopic procedure in a neonate.[1] The team must be efficient to limit anesthetic time, limit time on positive-pressure ventilation prior to fistula control and maximize the amount of work accomplished during (essentially) single-lung ventilation.

Neonates with pure EA or EA/TEF typically undergo inhalational induction followed by bronchoscopy and balloon control of the fistula. Appropriate IV access is then obtained, typically in the form of 2 to 3 peripheral intravenous catheters and an arterial line for both monitoring of blood pressure and access to obtain blood for laboratory measurements. Transfusion intraoperatively is generally not warranted, and most patients are provided with hourly maintenance isotonic solution as well as 20 to 40 mL/kg of intravenous fluid boluses. Patients have safely been maintained on neuromuscular blockade without significant risk of gastric overdistention, even without preoperative balloon control of the fistula.[6] Orotracheal intubation usually suffices, though some practitioners will attempt blind or fiberoptic-guided left mainstem intubation. Adequate lung deflation can be achieved by gentle carbon dioxide (CO_2) insufflation using a low flow (1 L/min) and low pressures (4–5 mm Hg).[5]

One key physiologic point is the expected immediate decompensation upon entry into the chest, when the patient is subjected, essentially, to single-lung ventilation. The anesthesia and surgery teams should expect relative hypoxia and hypercarbia, which are usually transient and recover within minutes as intrinsic physiologic mechanisms compensate for the loss of ventilation in the lung on the operative side and thus recover more normal matching of ventilation and perfusion. The frequent evaluation of blood gas measurements will allow for monitoring of this trend. In addition, should the patient not tolerate CO_2 insufflation or lung retraction, both of these may be reversed instantaneously by the surgeons to allow the anesthesiologist to recruit the lung and improve the patient's status. Ultimately, the free-flowing discussion between the surgeons and anesthesiologists allows for ongoing decision-making regarding proceeding with thoracoscopic repair or converting to an open approach.

Positioning of Patient and Port Placement

Following bronchoscopy and anesthetic preparation, most surgeons prefer a modified prone position (see Fig. 52-2), with the patient's right chest elevated 45 degrees. This positioning allows the lung and anterior mediastinal structures to fall anteriorly with gravity retraction, thus giving the surgeon excellent exposure to the posterior mediastinum, airway, and esophagus.

With this positioning, the surgeon and assistant stand on the anterior side of the patient, while the monitor is placed at eye level on the posterior side of the patient alongside the scrub nurse.

Three access sites are necessary for the procedure. An initial camera port (generally 4 mm) is placed just inferoposterior to the scapula, usually coinciding with the fifth intercostal space. We use a cut-down type approach, making an appropriate skin incision followed by blunt dissection above the rib using a straight Jacobson dissector. Lung ventilation is held when the pleura is encountered and the pleural space is entered bluntly. The chest wall defect is dilated to the appropriate size and the 4-mm trocar inserted. We use metal trocars fitted with a sleeve (a cut portion of an 18Fr red rubber catheter), which is sewn to the skin to prevent trocar migration.

Two additional ports are placed under direct visualization (Fig. 52-2). One is placed 1 to 2 intercostal spaces above the first port, and more in the midaxillary line (this generally falls in the middle of the axilla). If endoclips are to be used to control the TEF, this should be a 5-mm port. The 5-mm port also has the benefit of allowing for direct passage of suture with needles (e.g., 5-0 Vicryl or PDS on a TF needle). Otherwise, if ligature control is to be used, a 3- or 4-mm port may be used and suture passed directly through the chest wall when necessary. The third port, usually 3 mm, is placed 1 to 2 intercostal spaces below the first port, in the posterior to midaxillary line. Ideally, the second and third trocars placed, corresponding to the right and left hand working ports, will allow for the instruments to meet at a right angle at the level of the fistula and anastomosis.[5,7] Should gravity and CO_2 insufflation not provide adequate exposure, additional lung retraction can be achieved by the placement of another trocar or stab incision inferiorly for the use of an instrument by the surgical assistant solely for anterior lung retraction.

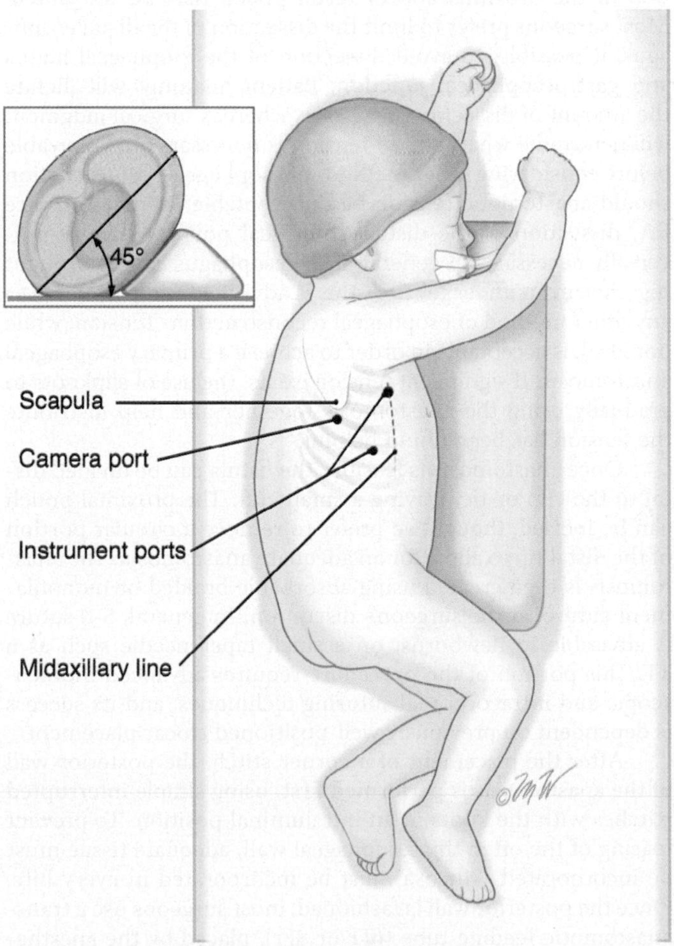

Figure 52-2. Illustration of modified prone positioning in thoracoscopic EA/TEF repair and the usual trocar placement.

Identification and Ligation of the Fistula

Upon port placement, CO_2 insufflation is achieved and the posterior pleural space should be readily visible. The azygos vein is identified, mobilized with blunt dissection and generally sacrificed either with hook cautery or division between ties (Fig. 52-3). Ligation and division of the azygos makes the underlying distal esophagus readily evident (Fig. 52-4). In cases

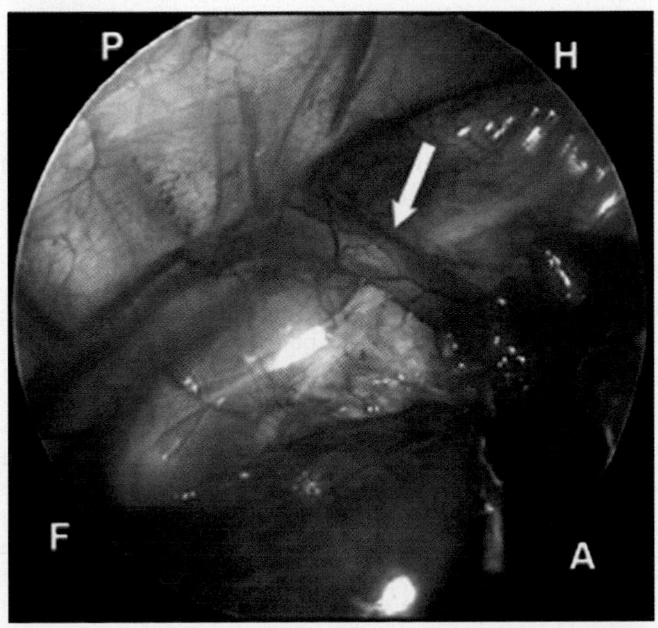

Figure 52-3. Intraoperative image demonstrating the initial view of the posterior pleural space. Note the azygos system and the azygos vein (white arrow) coursing anteromedially. The lung is compressed from CO_2 insufflation with excellent visualization of the posterior mediastinum. Orientation: H, head; F, feet; P, posterior; A, anterior.

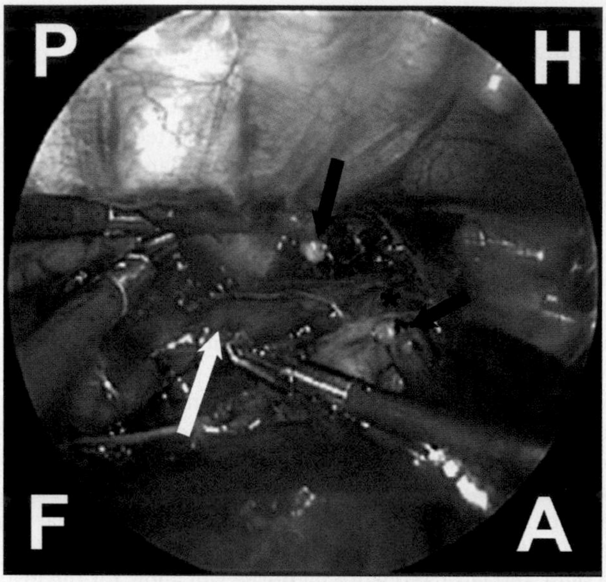

Figure 52-4. Intraoperative image demonstrating the identification and mobilization of the distal esophagus and tracheoesophageal fistula (white arrow) as it enters into the trachea (asterisk). Note the ligated ends of the azygos vein (black arrows) with the fistula directly beneath. Orientation: H, head; F, feet; P, posterior; A, anterior.

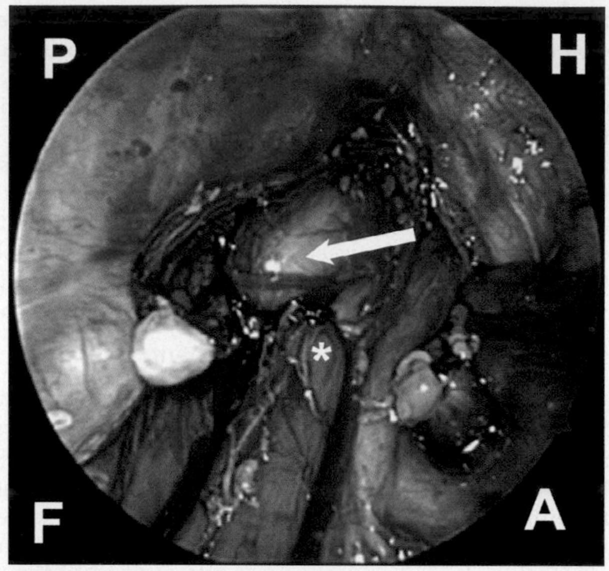

Figure 52-5. Intraoperative image demonstrating the proximal esophageal pouch (white arrow) as it appears in the thoracic inlet when the anesthesiologist places inward pressure on the nasogastric tube. Note in this case the fistula has already been ligated (asterisk), and it is possible to obtain a sense of the feasibility of primary anastomosis between the two ends. Orientation: H, head; F, feet; P, posterior; A, anterior.

of EA/TEF, this usually corresponds to the entry of the fistula into the membranous portion of the trachea just above the carina. The excellent view through a surgical telescope generally makes identification of the distal esophagus easy. For EA/TEF, blunt and sharp dissection with the use of curved dissectors and laparoscopic scissors are used to follow the fistula to its entry into the posterior trachea where the fistula can be ligated using an endoclip or ligature. During this dissection, care is taken to avoid injury to the vagus nerve. Ligation flush with the trachea is important to prevent formation of a tracheal diverticulum which could pool secretions and lead to soiling of the lungs in the future. Once ligation of the fistula is achieved, the "pressure is off" in terms of concern regarding the use of positive-pressure ventilation and the risk of gastric overdistention. Prior to division of the fistula, it is sometimes useful to mobilize the upper esophageal pouch to prevent retraction of the distal esophageal pouch prior to creation of the anastomosis.

Identification and Mobilization of the Proximal Esophageal Pouch

With the anesthesiologist placing pressure on the nasogastric tube, the proximal esophageal pouch is evident (Fig. 52-5). Blunt and sharp dissection with judicious electrocautery can be used to then free the proximal pouch all the way to the thoracic inlet. The surgeon should work on all sides simultaneously, though always saving the dissection of the common wall with the trachea for times when maximal tension is evident due to dissection of the other sides. This common wall is typically dissected sharply with some electrocautery if needed. Some surgeons prefer to place a traction suture through the distal tip of the pouch to provide a sturdy handle for manipulation of the proximal pouch during this dissection.

Anastomosis

At this point, traction on the proximal pouch should be able to demonstrate the ability to achieve an adequate primary anastomosis under minimal tension. If not, additional dissection of the proximal and/or distal pouch may be warranted. Most surgeons prefer to limit the dissection of the distal esophagus, if possible, to avoid dissection of the esophageal hiatus and gastroesophageal junction. Patient anatomy will dictate the amount of dissection necessary, whereas surgical judgment will determine what level of tension is necessary and allowable before considering other methods of esophageal reconstruction should anastomotic tension be unacceptable. In cases of pure EA, dissection of the distal esophageal pouch is nearly universally necessary. In general, if the esophagus can be brought together, even under tension, this is advisable and preferable to any other method of esophageal reconstruction. Tension, while not ideal, is acceptable in order to achieve a primary esophageal anastomosis. If significant tension exists, the use of slipknots to gradually bring the anastomosis together and help distribute the tension has been found helpful.[8,9]

Once anastomosis is feasible, the fistula can be divided distal to the clip or tie, leaving a small cuff. The proximal pouch can be incised, though we prefer to remove a circular portion of the distal tip to allow for an adequate anastomosis. The anastomosis is then created using absorbable braided or monofilament suture, at the surgeon's discretion. In general, 5-0 suture is advisable in newborns, on a small taper needle such as a TF. This portion of the procedure requires advanced thoracoscopic and intracorporeal suturing techniques, and its success is dependent on previously well-positioned trocar placement.

After the placement of a corner stitch, the posterior wall of the anastomosis is performed first, using simple interrupted stitches with the knots in an intraluminal position. To prevent tearing of the often thin esophageal wall, adequate tissue must be incorporated. Mucosa must be incorporated in every bite. Once the posterior wall is fashioned, most surgeons use a trans-anastomotic feeding tube (6Fr or 8Fr), placed by the anesthesiologist transnasally and guided into the distal esophagus and stomach thoracoscopically (Fig. 52-6).

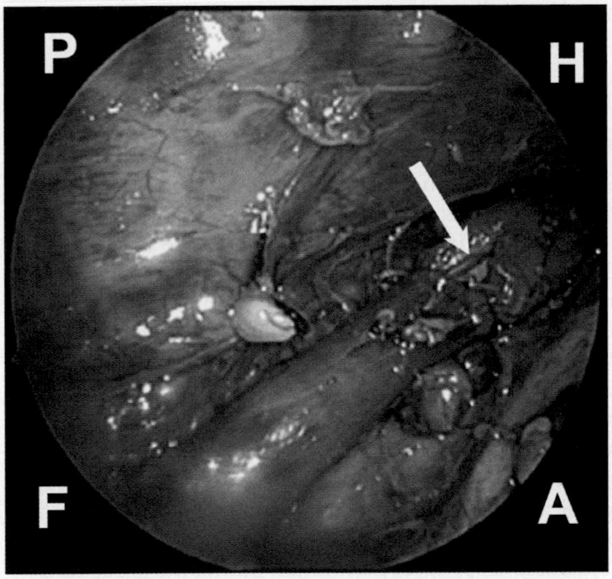

Figure 52-6. Intraoperative image demonstrating completion of the posterior row of sutures and the placement of a transanastomotic feeding tube (orange tube, white arrow). Orientation: H, head; F, feet; P, posterior; A, anterior.

The anterior wall is then fashioned in the same manner, with the transanastomotic feeding tube allowing for large bites without concern for incorporation of the posterior wall of the esophageal lumen. After completion of the anastomosis (Fig. 52-7), hemostasis is verified.

Completion of Procedure

An air leak test can be performed by instilling a small amount of saline, retracting the lung, and asking for a Valsalva maneuver from the anesthesiologist while visualizing the tracheal fistula tie or clip. If desired, some viable tissue (e.g., end of azygos, pleural flap) can be placed between the esophagus and trachea to reinforce the fistula ligation and help prevent recurrence of the TEF. Alternatively, a piece of treated bovine pericardium may be used as a biologic barrier to prevent reformation of the TEF and can be placed between the esophageal suture line and the clip/ligature on the tracheal side of the fistula ligation (Fig. 52-7). A 12Fr chest tube can then be placed through the left hand working port site, positioned lateral to the anastomosis and secured to the skin. The lung is then observed to inflate during normal breathing to verify no injury to the trachea or right mainstem bronchus, and the ports are then removed. Local anesthetic can be administered at the start or finish of the case. The incisions are closed with small absorbable sutures for the muscular fascia, deep dermal and subcuticular layers and sterile dressings are applied. The chest tube is generally placed to low suction (–10 cm H_2O).

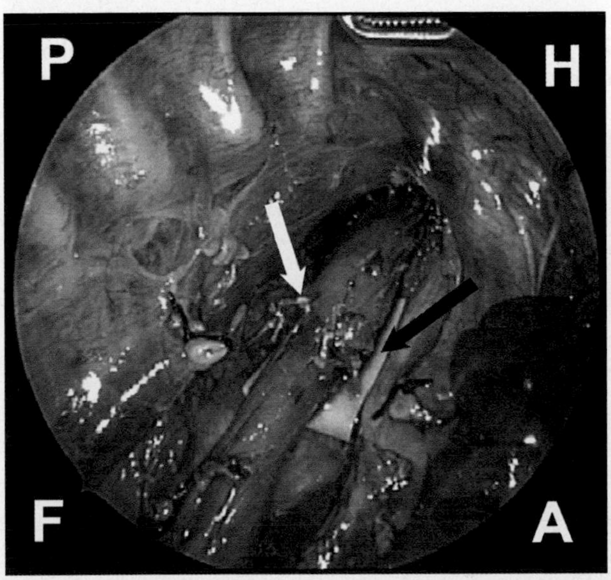

Figure 52-7. Intraoperative image demonstrating the completed anastomosis. Note the use by this surgeon of a pericardial patch only (black arrow) to create a barrier between the anastomotic suture line (white arrow) and the underlying tie on the site of the tracheal fistula. Orientation: H, head; F, feet; P, posterior; A, anterior.

Postoperative Management

The patient is generally left intubated and slowly weaned from the ventilator over the next day or several days. In cases of significant anastomotic tension, additional precautions may be taken, including longer-term sedation and even paralysis to prevent additional tension from being placed on the anastomosis.[9] Care must be taken to avoid aggressive endotracheal suctioning which could injure the recently dissected trachea or dislodge the controlling clip or ligature on the fistula. In addition, should reintubation be required, it should be performed by a practitioner familiar with the anatomy involved and cognizant of the risks of both deep tracheal intubation and accidental esophageal intubation. Many surgeons have horror stories of disrupted tracheal or esophageal suture lines as a result of unfortunate events during emergent reintubation.

Feeding via the nasogastric tube is based on surgeon preference. All patients are placed on aggressive acid-reducing regimens, usually at a maximal dose of proton pump inhibitors. The high incidence of gastroesophageal reflux, coupled with esophageal dysmotility and injury to the anastomosis from refluxed acid, make this an important adjunct therapy.

Chest tube output is monitored for the possibility of lymphatic leak or for evidence of oral secretions which would be concerning for anastomotic leak. An esophagram is obtained, usually around postoperative day 7. If no leakage is demonstrated, oral feedings can be initiated and the chest tube can be removed. Evidence of leak is usually localized or controlled by the chest tube, in which case a repeat contrast study can be obtained after another week to assess for seal of the leak which will occur in most cases.

Outcomes and Complications

Though pediatric surgeons are relatively early in their experience with thoracoscopic repair of EA and TEF, short-term outcomes reported by centers known for excellence in minimally invasive surgery are encouraging. One notable report of 104 patients, involving several centers from multiple countries, outlines a success rate of thoracoscopic repair of nearly 95%. Complications in these patients included leak (8%), stricture (4%), and recurrent fistula (2%). Nearly 32% of patients required at least one esophageal dilation. Three patients died in this series, two from unrelated causes and one from tracheal fistula closure disruption during reintubation.[1] These outcomes are remarkably similar to those obtained in similar series of patients repaired through open thoracotomy. Long-term follow-up of these patients will allow for comparison of musculoskeletal complications which may demonstrate a significant benefit of the minimally invasive technique.

Important in the interpretation of these data, however, is the fact that the minimally invasive series represents the work of surgeons skilled in very high-level minimally invasive surgery. They noted a significant learning curve and the need for surgical expertise in performing this operation thoracoscopically.

Summary

Thoracoscopic repair of EA and TEF is feasible in most patients with standard anatomy, with outcomes similar to open repair when performed by skilled minimally invasive surgeons. As experience with this technique grows, and a new generation of surgeons is trained in advanced minimally invasive techniques, this will likely become a routine procedure in the armamentarium of the pediatric surgeon.

FOREGUT DUPLICATION CYSTS

Foregut duplication cysts occur as a mishap of the normal ventral budding process of the lung primordium off the foregut. Their location as posterior mediastinal cystic structures usually results in symptoms of recurrent respiratory problems such as cough or wheeze (usually in the case of bronchogenic cysts) or partial esophageal obstruction resulting in feeding difficulty or dysphagia (in the case of esophageal duplication cysts). As abnormalities of development, these lesions do not regress, and surgical excision is therefore required to prevent or treat these symptoms. Reports of malignant degeneration lend additional credence to the practice of routine surgical excision.

General Principles

The thoracoscopic excision of foregut duplication cysts has become relatively routine as overall surgical experience and comfort with thoracoscopy in young children continues to grow. In contrast to patients with EA, patients undergoing surgery for foregut duplication cysts are generally larger and older and have less comorbidities. This makes the preoperative comfort level with thoracoscopy that much higher. Nonetheless, thoracoscopic surgery in these cases involves the use of advanced minimally invasive techniques, including suturing in a tight space to repair the esophagus or close a hole in the airway, such that a high level of surgical skill is still warranted before undertaking these procedures.

Preoperative Assessment and Patient Selection

As mentioned, most patients with these lesions are relatively healthy and can tolerate thoracoscopy well. If significant airway obstruction is present resulting in overinflation of one or the other lung, visualization may be impaired and thoracotomy may be required. Likewise, if inflammatory changes from infection of the lesion make resection significantly difficult, conversion to an open procedure may be warranted.

Otherwise, most patients are candidates for thoracoscopic resection. Preoperative imaging with chest computed tomography helps to identify the lesion and plan the procedure. In the case of esophageal duplication cysts, an esophagram may be of use to determine the nature of the lesion's relationship to the esophageal lumen. In most cases, these cysts are located within the muscular wall of the esophagus, sharing a common wall with the esophageal lumen.

Technique

Anesthetic Considerations and Lung Isolation

Almost all cases will be approached through the right chest, though ultimately preoperative imaging may lead the surgeon to choose the left side instead. This is usually in the case of carinal bronchogenic cysts that may be affecting the left mainstem more than the right. Most patients benefit from anesthetic lung isolation. If a double-lumen endotracheal tube is not feasible due to patient size, a bronchial blocker can be used to isolate the right lung. In addition, CO_2 insufflation during the procedure will assist with compression of the lung. Peripheral intravenous access and a monitoring arterial line are used. In addition, an appropriate sized esophageal bougie is used in the case of esophageal duplication cysts to help with dissection of the cyst and its common wall with the esophageal mucosa and with identification of possible esophageal perforation during the procedure.

Positioning of Patient and Port Placement

Similar to the EA repair, the patient is placed in a modified prone position, with the right chest elevated approximately 45 degrees. Again the surgeon and assistant both stand to the anterior side of the patient. An initial, usually 5 mm, port can be placed in the axilla, in the mid- to posterior axillary line, and low-flow, low-pressure CO_2 insufflation instilled. Visualization of the lesion (Fig. 52-8) can then help to best place two additional ports in the mid- to anterior axillary line, with the aim to have the instruments meet at an approximate right angle at the lesion.

Cyst Excision

For esophageal duplication cysts, the esophagus and cyst are mobilized by incising the overlying pleura and using a combination of blunt and sharp dissection with judicious electrocautery. The esophageal muscular wall is split bluntly and the cyst raised out of the muscular wall in a submucosal plane (Fig. 52-9). Performing the entire dissection off the muscular wall before then finally dissecting the common wall with the esophageal mucosa maximizes the visualization during this more risky portion of

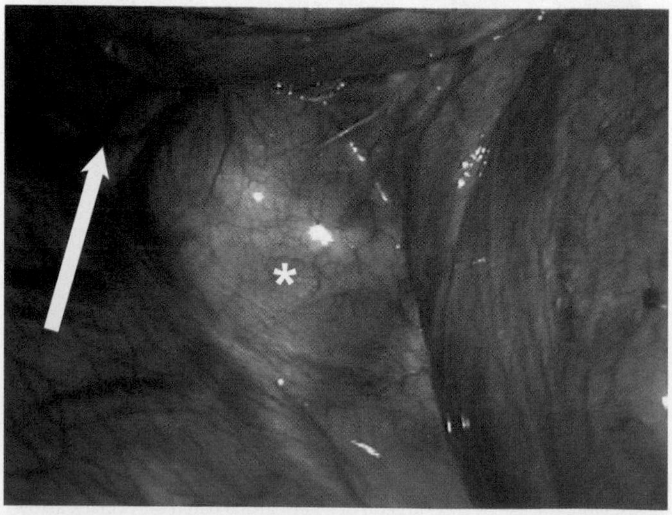

Figure 52-8. Intraoperative image demonstrating appearance of an esophageal duplication cyst (asterisk) upon thoracoscopic entry. Note the azygos venous system and azygos vein (white arrow) similar to the anatomy seen during EA/TEF repair.

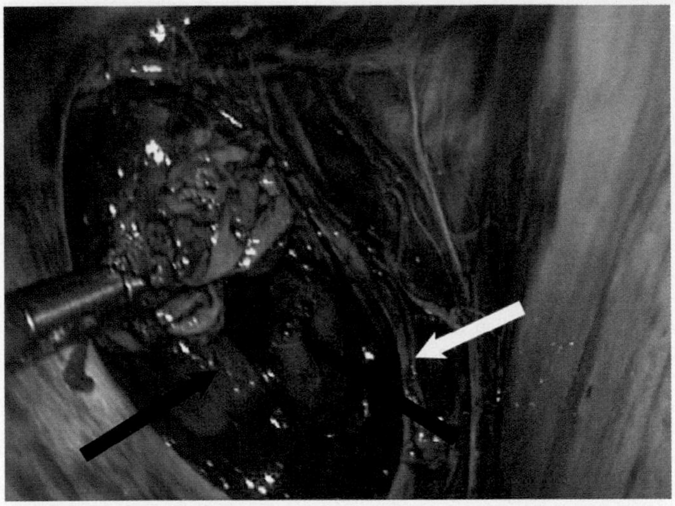

Figure 52-9. Intraoperative image demonstrating excision of the esophageal duplication cyst in a submucosal plane. Note the parietal pleura (white arrow) with the underlying esophagus. The esophageal muscle has been split longitudinally (black arrows), and the cyst is being excised from within the esophageal wall. An oroesophageal bougie (not visible) provides feedback for the location of the underlying mucosa and esophageal lumen.

the procedure. If the lumen is entered, absorbable suture is used to close the defect in an interrupted fashion. After excision of the cyst, we prefer to close the muscular wall, again using interrupted sutures (Fig. 52-10).

Excision of bronchogenic cysts is similar to that of esophageal duplication cysts. These lesions, however, are typically not within the wall of the airway and can be separately dissected free. They are often large and can be needle decompressed to assist with visualization, though leaving the lesion tense can sometimes assist with the dissection by helping to clearly delineate the cyst. These cysts often have a stalk connecting them to the airway, usually at the carina. This stalk should in general be ligated or sutured to assure satisfactory closure of the airway. Postexcision air test under saline can assist with identification of a residual air leak.

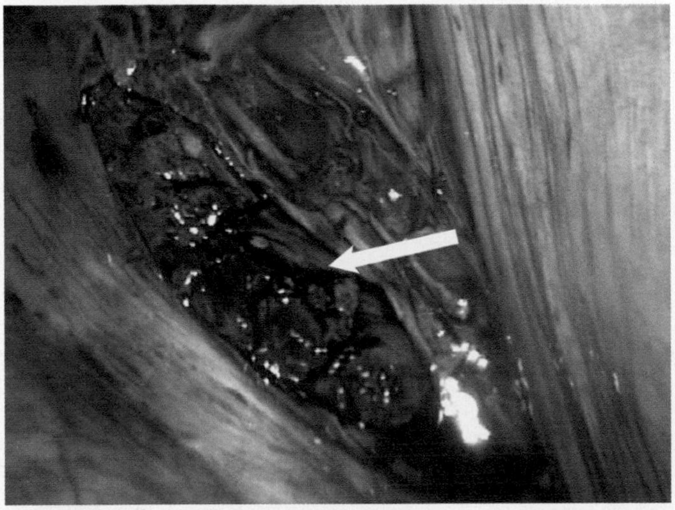

Figure 52-10. Intraoperative image demonstrating the completed repair of the esophageal wall. Note the reapproximation of the previously split edges of the esophageal muscular wall with interrupted sutures. The surgeon in this case has chosen braided nonabsorbable suture, though we typically prefer braided or monofilament absorbable suture.

For any lesion in which a common wall exists, the dissection may be made safer by leaving the wall intact and stripping the cyst mucosa. Small mucosal remnants should be fulgurated. After excision, the cyst can be removed through the thoracoscopic ports, sometimes in pieces.

Completion of Procedure

Given the potential communication with the airway or esophageal lumen, a chest tube is left in place through one of the ports. The lung is observed to verify reinflation. After removal of the ports, the incisions are closed in layers with absorbable sutures, dressings applied, and the chest tube placed to suction drainage.

Postoperative Management

In general, the patients can be extubated in the operating room. Chest tube drainage is short-term, to verify no evidence of air leak or esophageal leak. For esophageal duplication cysts, if the esophagus required closure due to intraoperative perforation, an esophagram is obtained on postoperative day 5 to 7 to verify patency without leak and the chest tube is then removed and oral feeds resumed. Otherwise, the patient can be started on a soft diet on postoperative day 1 and discharged once routine discharge criteria are met. Many surgeons prefer to maintain the patients on a soft diet for several weeks to allow for satisfactory healing of the esophagus.

Complications

The complications associated with surgery on foregut duplication cysts include persistent air leak, or even bronchopleural fistula, and esophageal leak. Multiple single-institution series have reported acceptable rates of these complications for the thoracoscopic approach, in the 5% to 10% range.[10,11] In contrast, however, the length of stay for patients undergoing thoracoscopic surgery is days less than that of patients undergoing open thoracotomy.

Summary

Thoracoscopic resection of foregut duplication cysts has become relatively universal except in rare circumstances. Nonetheless, advanced minimally invasive techniques, skills, and comfort level are required on the part of the surgeon. Outcomes are favorable.

EDITOR'S COMMENT

As expected, minimally invasive surgery continues to permeate the field of pediatric surgery. It is important for the adult surgeon to understand the congenital anatomy and the techniques of pediatric repair as these may impact surgery in unexpected manner. For example, I once operated on a patient with a large hiatal hernia who as a baby underwent a repair of coarctation of the aorta by Dr. Blalock. In the process of the dissection, I discovered that the celiac axis was at the level of the diaphragmatic hiatus as a consequence of the original surgery, thus complicating the repair. Furthermore, congenital defects that were not too symptomatic in childhood may present for therapy in adulthood requiring collaboration with pediatric surgeons for the best repair strategies.

—Raphael Bueno

References

1. Holcomb GW 3rd, Rothenberg SS, Bax KM, et al. Thoracoscopic repair of esophageal atresia and tracheoesophageal fistula a multi-institutional analysis. *Ann Surg.* 2005;242(3):422–428; discussion 428–430.
2. Sinha CK, Paramalingam S, Patel S, et al. Feasibility of complex minimally invasive surgery in neonates. *Pediatr Surg Int.* 2009;25(3):217–221.
3. Lobe TE, Rothenberg SS, Waldschmidt J, et al. Thoracoscopic repair of esophageal atresia in an infant: a surgical first. *Pediatr Endosurg Innov Tech.* 1999;3:141–148.
4. Rothenberg SS. Thoracoscopic repair of a tracheoesophageal fistula in a neonate. *Pediatr Endosurg Innov Tech.* 2000;4:150–156.
5. Rothenberg SS. Thoracoscopic repair of esophageal atresia and tracheo-esophageal fistula in neonates: evolution of a technique. *J Laparoendosc Adv Surg Tech A.* 2012;22(2):195–199.
6. Krosnar S, Baxter A. Thoracoscopic repair of esophageal atresia with tracheoesophageal fistula: anesthetic and intensive care management of a series of eight neonates. *Paediatr Anaesth.* 2005;15(7):541–546.
7. Rothenberg SS. Thoracoscopic repair of esophageal atresia and tracheo-esophageal fistula. *Semin Pediatr Surg.* 2005;14(1):2–7.
8. Martinez-Ferro M. Thoracoscopic repair of esophageal atresia without tracheoesophageal atresia. In: Holcomb GW 3rd, Georgeson KE, Rothenberg SS, eds. *Atlas of Pediatric Laparoscopy and Thoracoscopy*. Philadelphia, PA: Saunders; 2008;291–296.
9. Rothenberg SS. Thoracoscopic repair of esophageal atresia and tracheo-esophageal fistula. In: Holcomb GW 3rd, Georgeson KE, Rothenberg SS, eds. *Atlas of Pediatric Laparoscopy and Thoracoscopy*. Philadelphia, PA: Saunders; 2008, 285–290.
10. Michel JL, Revillon Y, Montupet P, et al. Thoracoscopic treatment of mediastinal cysts in children. *J Pediatr Surg.* 1998;33(12):1745–1748.
11. Partrick DA, Rothenberg SS. Thoracoscopic resection of mediastinal masses in infants and children: an evaluation of technique and results. *J Pediatr Surg.* 2001;36(8):1165–1167.

PART 8

BENIGN UPPER AIRWAYS CONDITIONS

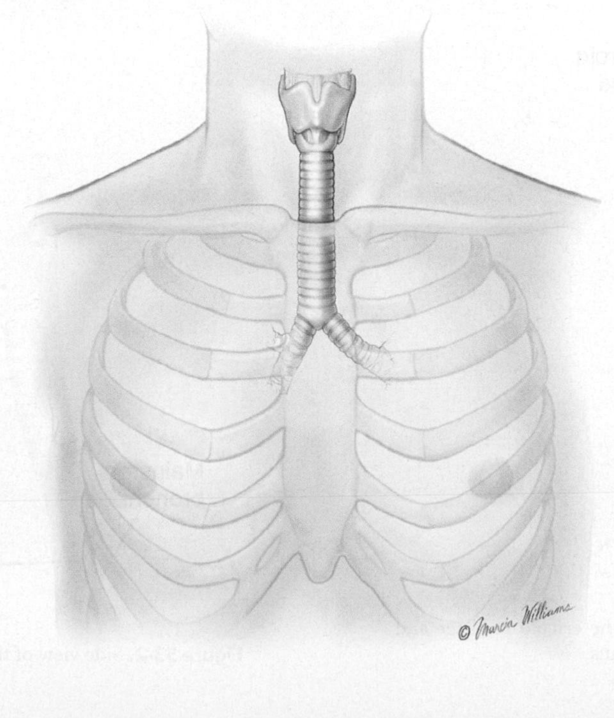

53 Overview of Benign Disorders of the Upper Airways

Zane T. Hammoud and Michael J. Liptay

Keywords: Upper airways, benign tumors, chondroma, granular cell tumor (GST), squamous cell papilloma, glomus tumor, neurofibromas, extrinsic compression, vascular rings, congenital tracheal stenosis, postpneumonectomy syndrome, posttraumatic disorders

The upper airways are defined as the trachea and mainstem bronchi. Functionally, the upper airways serve as conduits for ventilation. Anatomically and physiologically, however, they represent complex structures that are susceptible to a wide variety of processes. Involvement of the trachea, mainstem bronchi, or both in various disease processes, although rare, present challenging problems for both physician and patient.

ANATOMY AND PHYSIOLOGY

The adult human trachea begins at the level of the cricoid cartilage and extends to the bifurcation of the mainstem bronchi (Figs. 53-1 and 53-2). The carinal spur is a useful landmark that denotes the distal extent of the trachea. On average, the adult human trachea measures 11 cm in length, with some variation in proportion to the height of the individual patient. There are approximately two tracheal rings per centimeter of trachea. Thus, on average, the total number of tracheal rings ranges from 18 to 22, with the cricoid forming the only complete tracheal ring. The potential for presentation of the trachea in the neck is a major factor permitting relatively easy surgical access. In a young, nonobese adult, hyperextension of the neck may deliver more than 50% of the trachea into the neck, thereby greatly facilitating any attempt at resection and reconstruction. From a nearly subcutaneous position at the level of the cricoid, the trachea courses posteriorly and caudally at an angle, resting against the esophagus and vertebral column at the level of the carina.

The blood supply of the trachea is vital to successful resection and reconstruction. The upper trachea is principally supplied by branches of the inferior thyroid artery, whereas the lower trachea is supplied by branches of the bronchial artery as well as by branches of the subclavian, supreme intercostals, internal thoracic, and innominate arteries (Fig. 53-3)[1]. These vessels supply the trachea through lateral pedicles of tissue, and the longitudinal anastomoses between the vessels are very thin. Excessive disruption of these lateral vessels by circumferential dissection of the trachea may compromise blood supply and lead to complications, such as stenosis and anastomotic dehiscence. At the level of the second and third tracheal rings, the thyroid isthmus crosses the trachea anteriorly. The recurrent

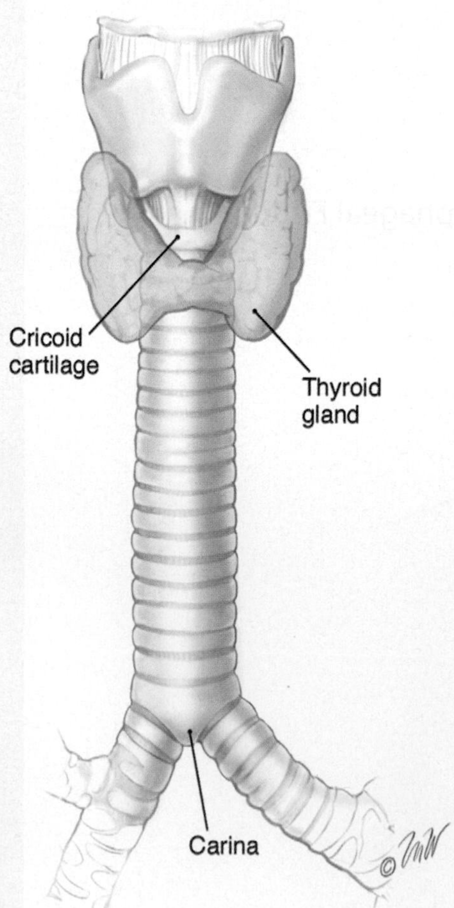

Figure 53-1. The trachea begins at the level of the cricoid cartilage and extends to the bifurcation of the mainstem bronchus.

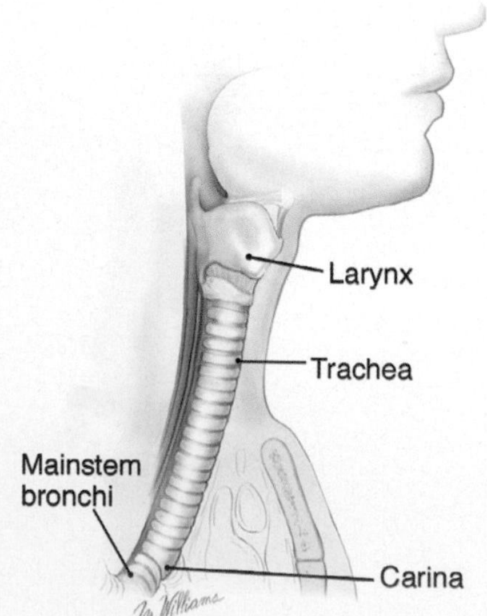

Figure 53-2. Side view of the extent of the trachea.

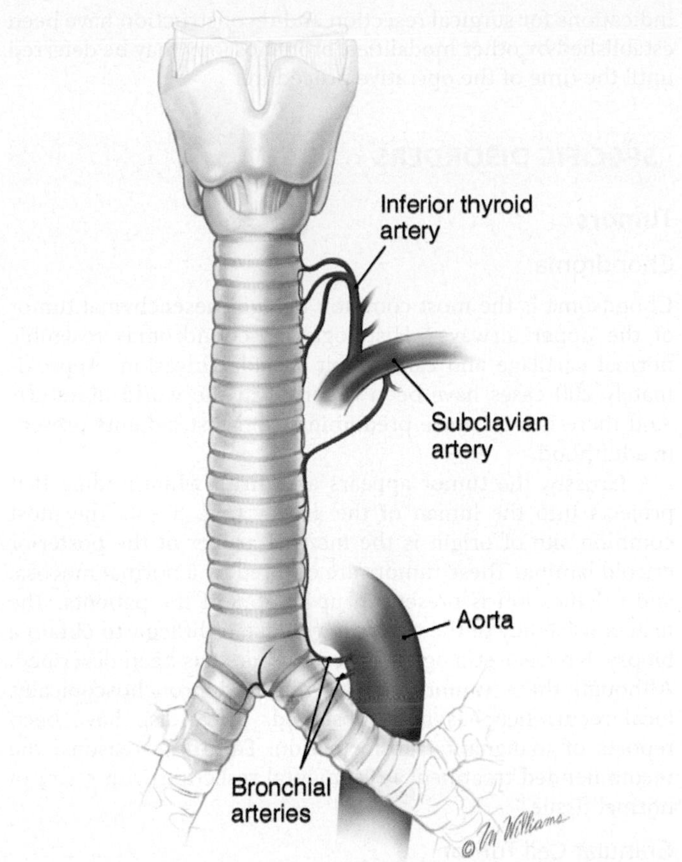

Figure 53-3. The blood supply of the upper trachea is supplied by branches of the inferior thyroid artery, whereas the lower trachea is supplied by branches of the bronchial artery as well as by branches of the subclavian, supreme intercostals, internal thoracic, and innominate arteries.

laryngeal nerves course in a groove between the trachea and the esophagus (Fig. 53-4). The nerves enter the larynx between the cricoid and thyroid cartilages.

The trachea bifurcates into the right and left mainstem bronchi in the region of the fifth through seventh thoracic vertebra. The right mainstem bronchus arises in a direct line with the trachea, whereas the left mainstem bronchus arises at a sharper angle. This anatomy helps to explain the more frequent right-sided location of aspirated material(s).

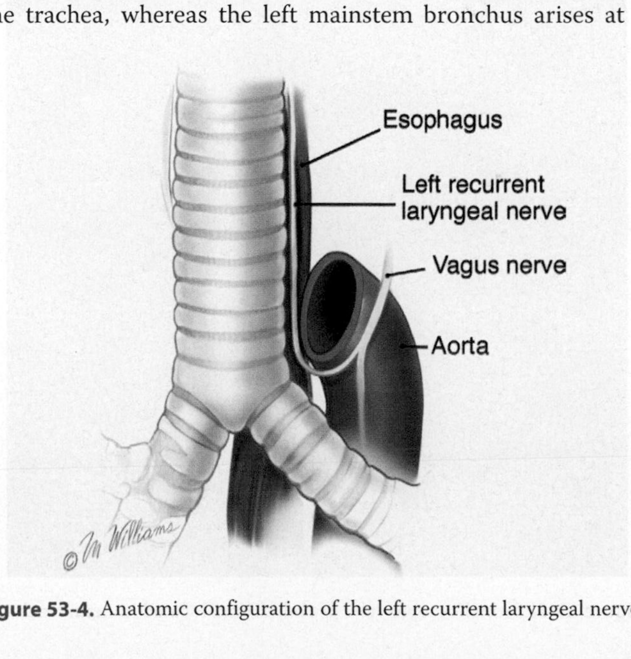

Figure 53-4. Anatomic configuration of the left recurrent laryngeal nerve.

The length of the right mainstem bronchus from the trachea to the point of the takeoff of the right upper lobe bronchus is approximately 1.2 cm. The length of the left mainstem bronchus is approximately 4 to 6 cm from the trachea to the takeoff of the left upper lobe bronchus. Both mainstem bronchi are supplied directly by bronchial arteries.

Most commonly, the trachea is approached through a cervical neck incision. As noted earlier, up to 50% of the entire trachea may be accessed in this manner. The right and left mainstem bronchi are usually approached through a right posterolateral thoracotomy. The carina may be approached through a right posterolateral thoracotomy, a clam shell incision, or a median sternotomy.

ETIOLOGY AND NATURAL HISTORY

Diseases affecting the upper airways are rare. Tumors of the trachea and mainstem bronchi occur most commonly in adults. Most of the primary tumors are malignant, with the majority representing adenoid cystic carcinoma or squamous cell carcinoma. Benign tumors occur most commonly before the seventh decade of life. They tend to occur sporadically and lead to symptoms secondary to progressive airway obstruction. Nonneoplastic diseases, such as infection, are less common than tumors, although the precise incidence is difficult to discern. Left untreated, diseases affecting the upper airways cause significant morbidity and, in some cases, mortality from airway obstruction.

PRESENTING SIGNS AND SYMPTOMS

Symptoms of upper airway pathology are often subtle and insidious in onset. The rarity of upper airway diseases may delay the suspicion of airway pathology as the cause of an individual patient's symptoms. Shortness of breath is the most common symptom experienced by patients who are affected by disease of the upper airways.[2] When a tumor or mass is present, dyspnea occurs after the effective airway lumen has been narrowed by approximately one-third. Even in the face of significant airway narrowing, the patient will have an apparently normal chest x-ray and often is diagnosed as suffering from "asthma." At times, these patients are treated with steroids for prolonged periods of time before a specific diagnosis, such as a tracheal tumor, is established. As the airway narrows further, the classic symptom of wheezing becomes more prominent. The presence of stridor indicates severe compromise of the airway. Failure to improve on steroid therapy often leads to further workup, at which time a specific upper airway diagnosis is established. Cough is another common symptom and may be secondary to irritation or to ineffective clearance of secretions, leading to pneumonia.

DIFFERENTIAL DIAGNOSIS

The symptoms caused by diseases of the upper airways are common to many processes. Other causes of dyspnea must be considered. These include cardiac causes, such as congestive heart failure, as well as pulmonary causes, such as pulmonary embolus. In addition, a myriad of other common processes, such as chronic obstructive pulmonary disease, must be considered. Wheezing is most commonly a sign of primary reactive airways disease, whereas cough may be caused by pneumonia as well as other processes that irritate the airways. It is important to remember, however, that it is the potentially numerous and far more common processes that produce symptoms similar to those of upper airway diseases that often lead to the delay in diagnosis of upper airways disease.

DIAGNOSTIC TECHNIQUES

The overpenetrated posteroanterior chest x-ray is often the most useful means by which to obtain an excellent view of the trachea and mainstem bronchi. The presence of a mass and extent of luminal narrowing may be seen by careful inspection of the tracheal air column. Deviation from midline of the tracheal air column also may be noted on a standard chest film. Furthermore, postobstructive pneumonia may be seen. Although not universally available, tracheal tomograms, as described by Weber and Grillo,[3] provide excellent visualization of the entire upper airways. These are particularly useful in planning for resection and reconstruction. These are no longer necessary in the era of CT scans and three-dimensional (3D) reconstruction.

CT scanning permits cross-sectional visualization of the upper airways. The presence of an intraluminal mass is often clearly identified by CT scan. Furthermore, by knowing the distance between cuts, or utilizing spiral CTs, one often can accurately estimate the size of the mass as well as the length of airway involved. 3D helical CT scanning and reconstructed axial imaging are used to obtain virtual bronchoscopic views of the upper airways, thereby permitting an accurate assessment of airway pathology. The presence of an extrinsic mass that is compressing the airways is also best identified by CT scan. MRI may supply additional information, but it is rarely more helpful than the information obtained by CT scan.

On occasion, especially in cases of extrinsic compression of the airway, a barium esophagram may be useful. Rarely, arteriography may be useful in defining compression of the airway by vascular structures.

Functional studies may provide useful information in the diagnosis of upper airway disease. Pulmonary function studies may point to airway obstruction. A decrease in peak flow rates, as well as a flattening of the expiratory flow-volume loop, may lead to suspicion of an obstructive process if clinical signs have been overlooked. Furthermore, pulmonary function studies may provide information regarding the status of the pulmonary parenchyma. While this may not alter the decision to perform surgery, it may alter the conduct of a given operation, for example, whether or not single-lung ventilation will be tolerated.

Bronchoscopy is mandatory in the evaluation of upper airway disease. If a mass is noted in the airway, bronchoscopy is essential to establishing a histologic diagnosis (i.e., biopsy) and for determining the extent of the mass. If it is necessary to establish an adequate airway by removing a portion of a tumor or to obtain more adequate tissue for diagnosis, then rigid bronchoscopy may be preferable. Bronchoscopy always should be performed by experienced individuals and with appropriate precautions for the possibility of airway compromise. When the indications for surgical resection and reconstruction have been established by other modalities, bronchoscopy may be deferred until the time of the operative procedure.

SPECIFIC DISORDERS

Tumors

Chondroma

Chondroma is the most common benign mesenchymal tumor of the upper airways.[4] Histologically, chondromas resemble normal cartilage and can exhibit vascular invasion. Approximately 200 cases have been reported in the world literature. And there is a 5:1 male predominance. Most patients present in adulthood.

Grossly, the tumor appears as a firm, white nodule that projects into the lumen of the airway (Fig. 53-5). The most common site of origin is the internal aspect of the posterior cricoid lamina. These tumors are covered by a normal mucosa, and calcification is present in up to 75% of the patients. The firm consistency of the tumor may make it difficult to obtain a biopsy. No clear etiology for these tumors has been described. Although these tumors can be removed bronchoscopically, local recurrence has been observed. There also have been reports of malignant transformation. For these reasons, the recommended treatment is segmental resection with a rim of normal tissue.[5]

Granular Cell Tumor

Granular cell tumors (GSTs) can occur in any organ. The most common site of occurrence is the tongue. Burton et al.[6] conducted a 50-year review of the literature and reported only 30 cases of tracheal GST. In a 10-year review of all reported cases in the Netherlands, only four cases of upper airway GSTs were found.[7] These tumors occur predominately in women, with a racial predominance in blacks. In the airway, the majority of

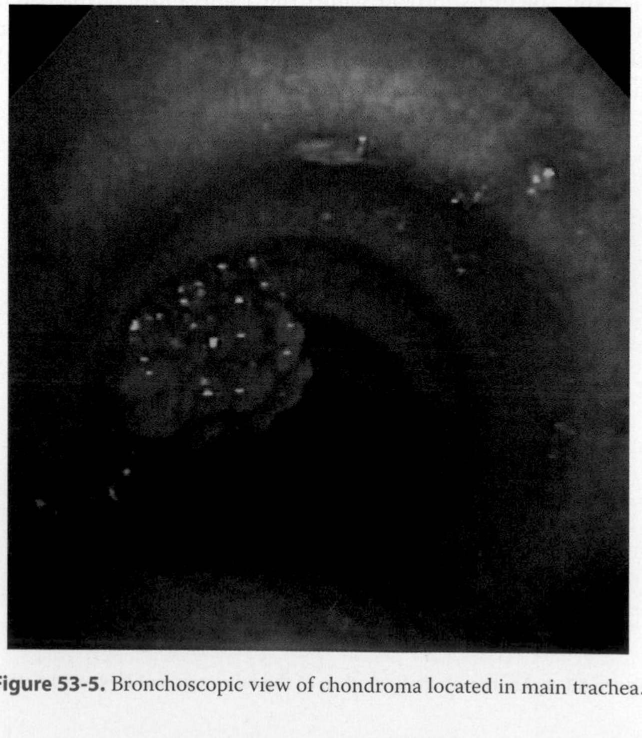

Figure 53-5. Bronchoscopic view of chondroma located in main trachea.

GSTs are located in the cervical trachea. The tumors are solitary in 80% of patients.

Although originally thought to be derived from skeletal muscle, GSTs are now thought to be of neurogenic origin, probably from the Schwann cell. Histologically, these tumors consist of round cells with centrally placed nuclei. Characteristically, these tumors stain positive for the S-100 protein, a protein found in the central nervous system, primarily in neurons. They also have a distinct tendency for local invasion into surrounding tissues, and malignant transformation has been reported in 1% to 2% of GSTs. However, malignant transformation has never been reported in the trachea.

The mainstay of therapy for GSTs of the upper airways is surgical excision. However, there is no clear agreement regarding the extent of excision. Daniel et al.[8] found that tumors larger than 1 cm had an increased risk for full-thickness wall involvement and therefore an increased risk of local recurrence after bronchoscopic excision. Therefore, they recommend segmental airway resection for GSTs larger than 1 cm. Because of the risk of recurrence, all patients with excised GSTs should undergo serial bronchoscopic examination for several years.

Squamous Cell Papilloma

Solitary squamous cell papilloma arising in the upper airways is quite rare. Although it is the most common benign tumor of the larynx, the largest review of the literature reported only 55 cases involving the tracheobronchial tree.[9] These tumors occur predominately in males, and there is a strong association with a history of smoking. Papillomas are easily excised bronchoscopically, and this is the preferred method of excision. Surgical resection is reserved for patients in whom the tumor is wide based, there is suspicion of malignancy, or the tumor is located in an area that makes endoscopic removal difficult.

Glomus Tumor

These tumors most commonly involve the skin of the extremities. When located in the tracheobronchial tree, the trachea is the most frequent site of involvement. The most recent review of the world literature revealed only 16 reported cases of glomus tumor of the trachea.[10] These tumors are composed of smooth muscle cells, which are similar to those of the glomus body. Although there are malignant variants, these tumors are benign in most of the reported cases. There is a male predominance, and the average age at diagnosis is 58 years. The preferred treatment is segmental resection with primary reconstruction.

Neurofibromas

Only 23 cases of tracheobronchial neurofibromas have been reported.[11] These tumors are usually multiple, not encapsulated, occur within the nerve sheath, and contain neuritis. They are frequently associated with von Recklinghausen's neurofibromatosis, and up to 12% may undergo malignant transformation. Small tumors may be excised bronchoscopically, with or without laser ablation of the base of the tumor. However, larger tumors or those that appear to invade or obstruct should be removed by formal surgical resection.

Other Tumors

A number of other rare tumors have been reported in the upper airways. Hemangioma may be found in the trachea. Often, hemangiomas will regress spontaneously and require no treatment. However, small doses of both radiation and steroids have been used to cause regression. Fibrous histiocytoma is a histologically benign tumor that can be locally invasive. The term inflammatory pseudotumor is sometimes used to describe this tumor as a consequence of the associated prominent inflammatory component. Although fibrous histiocytoma tends to have a benign behavior in the upper airways, resection is recommended owing to its local infiltration. Lipoma, hamartoma (Fig. 53-6), and leiomyoma also have been reported in the upper airway. Case reports of tracheal myxoma as well as intratracheal thyroid have been published.

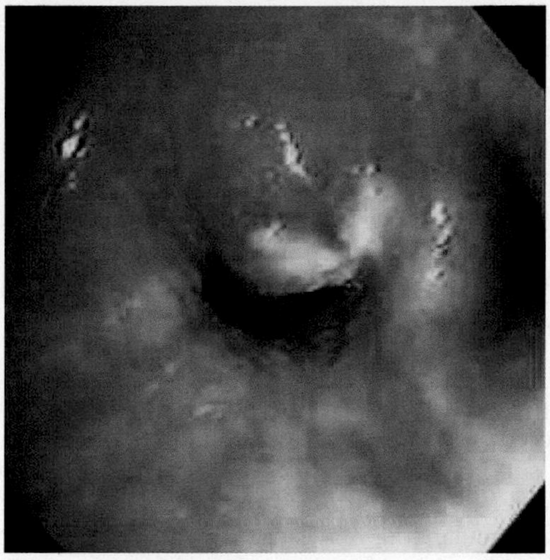

Figure 53-6. Bronchoscopic view of hamartoma in segmental bronchus.

INFECTIOUS/INFLAMMATORY DISEASE

The upper airways may become involved in a variety of disease processes, often secondary to a more systemic illness. Relapsing polychondritis is a disease of unknown origin in which any cartilaginous structure in the body may be affected, most commonly the nose and ears. When the upper airways are involved, patients experience progressive airway obstruction and difficulty in clearing secretions. The disease has a variable course, and therapy is usually limited to palliative stenting.

Wegener's granulomatosis is a systemic inflammatory disease that may involve the upper airways and lead to obstruction. Treatment is focused primarily on the systemic disease. Similarly, amyloidosis at times may affect the upper airways, leading to obstruction. Sarcoidosis may affect the upper airways by causing extrinsic compression from enlarged mediastinal lymph nodes or by causing extensive fibrotic changes within the airway, leading to stenosis and obstruction. Treatment is focused on the underlying condition because the airway process is usually too extensive and diffuse to permit surgical resection. Tracheopathia osteoplastica is a variant condition characterized by the formation of calcified nodules beneath the mucosa adjacent to but not involving the cartilages. It has a variable course and rarely requires surgical treatment.

Tuberculosis may involve the upper airways. Acutely, patients may be affected by tracheitis; as this process heals after medical treatment, a stenosis may develop. On rare occasions, segmental resection may become necessary. However, this should be performed only long after the active process is controlled. Histoplasmosis also may affect the upper airways, principally by causing extrinsic compression. The dense mediastinal fibrosis, as well as the enlarged and hardened mediastinal lymph nodes, may lead to compression of the distal trachea, carina, and mainstem bronchi. In addition, broncholiths may be seen within the airway as a result of erosion of a lymph node. Involvement of the upper airways by cicatricial pemphigoid also has been reported.

Extrinsic Compression

Vascular Rings

A number of congenital vascular anomalies may lead to extrinsic compression of the upper airways. These anomalies typically present in infants or young children and nearly always require surgical correction because of airway obstruction (see Chapter 39). A double aortic arch is the most common complete vascular ring that causes tracheal compression. Anatomically, this anomaly is characterized by an ascending aorta that divides into two arches. The two arches pass around the esophagus and trachea and then rejoin posteriorly to form the descending aorta. Usually, one of the arches is dominant, most commonly the right one. Affected patients typically present in the first year of life with stridor, respiratory distress, and a characteristic seal bark cough. The diagnosis is made by barium esophagram in the appropriate clinical setting. In addition, a CT scan or MRI may be obtained. The treatment is surgical division of the nondominant portion of the double arch at its insertion into the descending aorta, thereby releasing the complete ring. The ligamentum arteriosum, as well as any adhesions around the trachea and esophagus, is also divided. The results of surgery are excellent, with complete resolution of both respiratory and esophageal symptoms.

A right aortic arch with a left ligamentum arteriosum also may form a complete ring and lead to compression of the airway and esophagus. In this anomaly, which may have several variations, the compression is not as severe as with double aortic arch; this may lead to a later onset of symptoms and therefore presentation. The diagnosis is established in a similar manner to double arch. Treatment is also surgical, with division of the ligamentum and release of the ring. Results are excellent, and nearly all patients are relieved of their symptoms one year after treatment.

Rarely, the innominate artery may cause anterior compression of the trachea. This anomaly is seen when the innominate appears to originate from a more posterior location on a normally located aortic arch. The diagnosis is usually suspected on CT scan and can be confirmed by rigid bronchoscopy. Surgical treatment, when indicated, attempts to achieve relief of the anterior compression by suspending the innominate artery to the posterior aspect of the sternum.

A pulmonary artery sling is characterized by a left pulmonary artery that originates from the right pulmonary artery. As the anomalous pulmonary artery courses anteriorly to the esophagus to the hilum of the left lung, a ring is formed that encircles the right mainstem bronchus and distal trachea. In addition to the extrinsic compression, approximately 50% of patients with this anomaly will have complete tracheal rings, leading to severe airway stenosis. Nearly all patients with pulmonary artery sling present in early infancy with respiratory distress, which may be particularly severe if complete tracheal rings are also present. The diagnosis is suspected by the observation of hyperaeration of the right lung on plain chest radiograph as well as with anterior compression of the esophagus on barium esophagram (all other lesions show posterior compression). Both CT scan and MRI may confirm the diagnosis. However, echocardiography is the current modality of choice for making the diagnosis. Echocardiography has been shown to be very accurate and obviates the need for any sedation in an infant whose respiratory status may be tenuous at best. Treatment is always surgical. Although several approaches have been described, surgical correction is usually achieved using cardiopulmonary bypass.[12] The left pulmonary artery is divided and reimplanted into the main pulmonary artery anterior to the trachea. In the presence of complete tracheal rings, a simultaneous tracheoplasty may be performed.

Congenital Tracheal Stenosis

Congenital tracheal stenosis is a rare but life-threatening disorder characterized by congenital absence of the membranous trachea. The trachea is composed of complete cartilaginous O rings, and although the length may vary, this most frequently leads to long-segment tracheal stenosis. The type of stenosis is classified into three categories and may involve the mainstem bronchi as well. In one report, the medical management of this entity resulted in a greater than 40% mortality.[13]

The diagnosis is suspected on clinical grounds. These patients present in the first months of life with severe respiratory distress. The diagnosis is confirmed and the extent of airway involved is assessed by rigid bronchoscopy. Since these patients frequently have other malformations, such as pulmonary artery sling and/or cardiac abnormalities, it is important to perform a thorough diagnostic evaluation before undertaking any surgical repair of the airway.

As alluded to earlier, treatment is surgical correction. For short-segment stenosis, segmental resection and reconstruction are sufficient to achieve long-term patency of the airway. Wright et al.[14] have reported that resection of more than 30% of the pediatric airway results in a substantial failure rate. For long-segment stenosis, a number of surgical options have been devised, including pericardial patch tracheoplasty and slide tracheoplasty. Surgical correction of the stenosis may be made more difficult by the need to correct other anomalies in the same setting (e.g., pulmonary artery sling).

Goiter

Large goiters, particularly those with a significant posterior component, may compress the airway. The goiter may alter the shape of the airway over a prolonged period of time, leading to some compromise in the lumen of the airway. In rare instances, the compression may lead to softening of the tracheal cartilages, resulting in a malacic airway. The diagnosis of compression is made by bronchoscopy. Surgical resection of the compressing goiter results in significant improvement in respiratory symptoms. However, if malacia has occurred, care must be exercised, for removal of the goiter actually may remove an element of support for the airway and therefore lead to airway collapse.

Postpneumonectomy Syndrome

This rare entity occurs most commonly after right pneumonectomy. The mediastinum shifts to the right and may lead to angulation and compression of the remaining airway. Typically, the carina and left mainstem bronchus are compressed by the left pulmonary artery anteriorly and the aorta or vertebral column posteriorly. The syndrome also may occur in a reverse

diameters, length (of both proximal and distal portions of the device), angle, and presence or absence of an inner cannula or fenestrations. The size of the tracheostomy appliance should be large enough to provide adequate bronchoscopic pulmonary toilet if this is a consideration, bearing in mind that larger cannulas lead to higher rates of tracheal stenosis and smaller cannulas are associated with increased airway resistance.[5,6] A 7- or 8-mm diameter (inner circumference) tube typically is used because it is the smallest diameter that will allow for adequate pulmonary toilet. Appliance length usually is fixed but adjustable. Adjustable alternative-length devices are available for patients with anatomic features that do not accommodate standard-length devices. For example, the cannula may be too short, such that it abuts the posterior tracheal membrane, or it may be too long, such that it abuts the carina, leading to partial airway obstruction. The optimal length should place the end of the tracheal cannula 3 to 4 cm above the carina. The high-volume low-pressure cuff is currently preferred because it leads to fewer airway complications while providing substantial airway resistance to airflow around the cuff. When the tracheostomy is still required after the cuff is no longer needed for ventilatory support, the tracheostomy appliance should be replaced with a cuffless or fenestrated variety. If there is sufficient airflow around the deflated cuff, patients with intermittent ventilatory requirements can be fitted with a one-way Passey–Muir valve to permit speech when the patient is not being ventilated. Extreme caution is required, however, because the Passey–Muir valve increases the airway resistance. Failure to deflate the cuff before attaching the one-way valve can result in respiratory failure and death of the patient. Fenestrated appliances decrease airway resistance by permitting airflow through the fenestrations, which, in turn, allows the patient to speak when the tracheostomy is capped and the fenestrations are open. However, a closed inner cannula and inflated balloon must be present to mechanically ventilate these patients, and the fenestrations can make suctioning more difficult and increase granulation tissue in the airway in some instances. Inner cannulas decrease the risk of tracheal occlusion secondary to the accumulation of secretions within the outer cannula. For this reason, inner cannulas are preferred for permanent or long-term tracheostomies. Another option includes placement of a tracheal T-tube through the tracheotomy opening for those who require stenting of upper airway obstruction, either temporary or permanent. Selecting the appropriate appliance requires careful consideration on a case-by-case basis. When patients have recovered sufficiently and no longer need a tracheostomy, the appliance is either removed completely or replaced with a smaller, noncuffed variety for pulmonary toilet. The stoma is covered, and the patient is instructed to hold the stoma closed during coughing. With time, most tracheostomies close spontaneously, although there occasionally can be excessive granulation tissue around the stoma site requiring surgical debridement and closure in the OR.

TECHNIQUES

Surgical Tracheostomy

Surgical tracheostomy usually is performed under general anesthesia in the OR. The key steps are outlined in Table 54-2. The patient is placed in the supine position with the neck extended. Neck extension is facilitated by placing a towel roll under the patient's shoulders. Neck extension facilitates tracheostomy by elevating the trachea out of the thorax into the operative field. Care must be taken to avoid hyperextending the neck. In younger patients, overelevating the trachea creates the possibility of placing the tracheostomy too low in the trachea. Trauma victims and elderly patients are also particularly vulnerable to hyperextension injuries. Neck extension should not be performed in patients with a history of known or suspected cervical spine injury, and it may not be possible in patients with severe kyphosis, arthritis, or spinal fusion. In these patients, tracheal exposure can be aided by using a tracheal hook or by dividing the thyroid isthmus.

Table 54-2

TEN STEPS OF A SURGICAL TRACHEOSTOMY

1. Position the patient supine with neck extended.
2. Make a transverse skin incision 1–2 cm above the suprasternal notch and below the cricoid cartilage.
3. Divide the platysma transversely until the midline strap muscles are reached.
4. Separate the strap muscles in the midline to identify the pretracheal fascia.
5. Divide the thyroid isthmus or reflect it superiorly with retractors to approach the anterior trachea.
6. Count the tracheal rings from the cricoid cartilage, and place stay sutures laterally at the second or third tracheal ring.
7. Minimize FIO_2, incise the ring interspace with a number 15 blade, avoid cautery, and dilate the ring interspace with a tracheal dilator.
8. Place the prelubricated and pretested tracheostomy appliance into the airway and rotate it into position under direct vision.
9. Confirm ventilation with anesthesia by auscultation and by measuring end-tidal PCO_2. Consider bronchoscopic verification at the end of the case.
10. Secure the tracheostomy appliance to the skin with sutures.

After the sterile operative field is prepared with standard surgical techniques, a 2- to 3-cm transverse incision is made 1 to 2 cm above the suprasternal notch (Fig. 54-1). The actual location of the incision may vary depending on anatomic features, such as the location of the cricoid cartilage or a history of prior neck surgery or trauma. After the subcutaneous tissues and the platysma are divided transversely, the anterior superficial cervical fascia is divided longitudinally, which brings the strap muscles into view. The median raphe between the strap muscles (i.e., sternohyoid and sternothyroid) is developed, with hemostasis of the small venous branches by means of cautery. This brings the thyroid gland and pretracheal fascia into view. The pretracheal fascia and tissue below the thyroid isthmus are incised, bringing the anterior surface of the trachea into the operative field. Occasionally, it is necessary to divide the thyroid isthmus, but usually it can be elevated away exposing the superior portion of the trachea with the aid of retractors. When neck extension is not optimal or cannot be performed safely, the isthmus can be divided between clamps and suture-ligated to improve tracheal exposure. The thyroid internal mammary artery, if present and in the operative field, is ligated and divided at this time.

After ensuring complete hemostasis of the operative field, several preparative steps should be taken before performing the tracheostomy: (1) The tracheostomy appliance, which has been selected on the basis of indications for use and size of the trachea, is placed on the field, (2) the tracheostomy cuff is tested under water to confirm that it is intact, (3) the tracheostomy

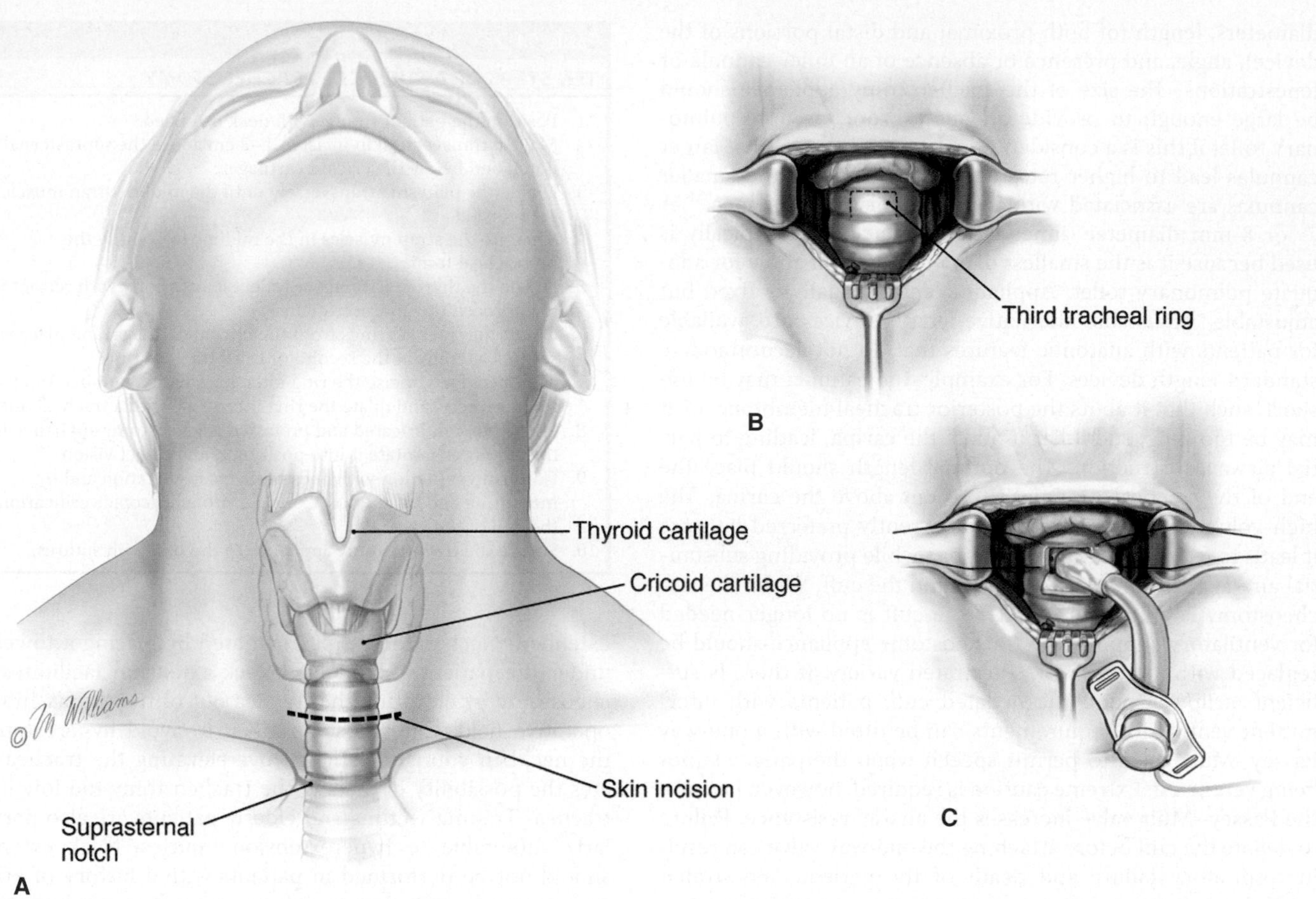

Figure 54-1. Tracheostomy. *A.* Location of incision 1 to 2 cm above the suprasternal notch. *B.* Division of the median raphe between the strap muscles with identification of the thyroid isthmus. *C.* Opening made in the trachea at the third tracheal ring. Under direct visualization, the endotracheal tube is withdrawn to just above the tracheal opening before attempting to insert the tracheostomy appliance.

appliance is well lubricated, and the tracheal obturator is inserted into the appliance, (4) the surgeon confirms that the tracheal rings have been identified and are readily accessible, and (5) before the operation begins, the surgeon also should confer with the anesthesia team to ensure that the airway has been suctioned and is ready for airway exchange.

Tracheal exposure in obese patients or in those with suboptimal neck extension can be optimized further using the tracheal hook to secure the superior trachea near the cricoid cartilage and to elevate the trachea superiorly. Traction sutures also can be placed laterally around the second and third tracheal rings to elevate the trachea superiorly and anteriorly. These sutures also can be used in the immediate postoperative period to facilitate reinsertion of the tracheostomy appliance if it becomes inadvertently dislodged.

After the tracheal rings are counted and proper visualization of the trachea is ensured, a number 15 blade is used to incise the space horizontally between the second and third tracheal rings. Most surgeons subsequently divide the third ring in the midline (cruciate) bilaterally, creating a Bjork flap,[16,17] and excise the flap, making a small hole in the trachea (see Fig. 54-1*C*). Proper positioning of the tracheostomy is critical. The location of the tracheostomy is based on identification of the third tracheal ring. It is impossible to establish a set distance from the suprasternal notch because the trachea is a mobile structure. High placement of the tracheostomy can lead to injury of the cricoid cartilage and subsequent subglottic stenosis. Low placement predisposes to the development of tracheoinnominate fistula, which results when the tracheostomy tube or cuff lies against the innominate artery. Low placement also causes the tracheostomy appliance to abut the carina, which predisposes to granulation tissue formation with subsequent potential for airway obstruction. Ventilation is held, O_2 is minimized, and Bovie cautery is avoided while the trachea is opened because of the risk of causing an airway fire.

When both the anesthesiologist and surgeon are ready to place the tracheostomy, the endotracheal tube is slowly removed by the anesthesia team with direct visualization by the surgeon until the tube is above the tracheostomy. (If a fire occurs, the oxygen must be turned off and the endotracheal tube and tracheostomy removed immediately and taken away from the patient and operative field.) The tracheal opening is enlarged by gentle dilation, and the tracheostomy tube is placed laterally through this opening into the trachea under direct vision and rotated into the correct position with extreme care to avoid a false anterior passage or injury to the membranous portion of the trachea. The cuff is inflated and ventilation resumed at the previous F_{IO_2} requirement. Proper placement of the tracheostomy tube is confirmed by chest expansion, auscultation, ease of ventilation, and confirmation of end tidal of P_{CO_2}. The tracheostomy tube is secured to the skin using nonabsorbable sutures in all four quadrants, in addition to placing a tracheal tie around the neck. Bronchoscopy is performed routinely at the end of the procedure to confirm proper placement of the tracheostomy tube and to clear any secretions or blood that may have accumulated in the airways during the procedure.

Percutaneous Tracheostomy

Percutaneous tracheostomy techniques, which can be performed at the bedside, reportedly saving the cost of OR time, have gained in popularity. Three percutaneous techniques have been described: (1) a translaryngeal technique, (2) a dilation technique using forceps, and (3) a dilation technique using serial dilators in Seldinger fashion. This section describes the third technique only because it is performed most commonly.[7–9,13,18–20] Dilational percutaneous tracheostomy with the aid of serial dilators was described originally in 1969 but modified and popularized by Pasquale Ciaglia in 1985.[21] Relative contraindications for this procedure include an airway emergency, obesity with an inability to palpate landmarks, an enlarged thyroid, and prior tracheostomy or neck surgery. Patients undergoing this procedure are ventilated with 100% oxygen and typically given a nondepolarizing neuromuscular blocker in addition to narcotic analgesics and sedatives. The patient is placed supine with the neck in extension, and the surgical field is prepared. A 1-cm skin incision halfway between the cricoid cartilage and the suprasternal notch is made to permit passage of the dilators, although a traditional tracheostomy incision can be made with dissection of subcutaneous tissues to better define tracheostomy positioning. A bronchoscope is inserted through the endotracheal tube, and the endotracheal tube is withdrawn from the airway and placed above the first tracheal ring. An 18-gauge needle then is inserted into the space between the first and second ring under bronchoscopic guidance. Using Seldinger technique, a J-tube guidewire is placed through the needle into the airway, and the needle is withdrawn. The tract is now dilated with sequential dilators over the guidewire or with a single large curved dilator, as has been advocated by some, with bronchoscopic visualization.[8,18,19] When the tracheal opening has been dilated to an appropriate size, a tracheostomy tube is placed through the opening over the guidewire and subsequently secured once placement is confirmed by the bronchoscope. Multiple variations of this basic technique have been described, some without use of a bronchoscope. We advocate bronchoscopic guidance in our practice, however, because it prevents technical misadventures, such as impalement of the endotracheal tube, puncture of the posterior membranous trachea, or malposition of the tracheostomy.

Numerous studies have compared the relative benefits of percutaneous tracheostomy versus standard surgical techniques. Most of these studies are difficult to interpret because they are nonstandardized and combine various percutaneous techniques. Several recent studies comparing standard surgical techniques with dilational percutaneous tracheostomy suggest lower rates of peristomal bleeding and infection and potential cost benefits with percutaneous technique.[7–9,13,15,18–20,22,23] Other studies have not shown these benefits, and increased complications have been reported often with percutaneous techniques. The likely scenario is that with proper patient selection, surgical expertise, and clinical setting, percutaneous techniques are equivalent to standard surgical techniques in a subset of patients.

The minitracheostomy is an extension of the serial dilation technique and is advocated by some for the management of excessive pulmonary secretions. Originally developed by Matthews and Hopkinson in 1984, it involves the placement of a small 4-mm tracheostomy cannula through the cricothyroid membrane into the trachea.[6,14] The procedure is performed usually in sedated but awake patients using local anesthesia with the placement of a small incision over the cricothyroid membrane and subsequent cannulation of the membrane with an introducer and the small tracheostomy catheter. Minitracheostomies also may be placed at the end of major thoracic procedures in patients in whom secretions are anticipated to be a problem or in critical care patients in whom retained secretions are known to be a problem. A similar procedure is used for placement of subcutaneous original oxygen protocol (SCOOP) catheters, whereby patients with end-stage lung disease can receive higher FIO_2 support via endotracheal delivery than is possible via nasal cannula. However, the SCOOP catheter is usually placed below the cricoid.

Cricothyroidotomy

Cricothyroidotomy typically is performed in emergency situations when translaryngeal intubation has failed or is not possible. Although tracheostomy can be performed in this setting, cricothyroidotomy is preferred because of the simplicity and rapidity with which the technique can be performed compared with tracheostomy. The procedure is performed either through a vertical midline neck incision or through a horizontal incision centered on the palpated cricothyroid membrane once the neck is prepared in a sterile field. A vertical incision is advocated by some to avoid injury to the anterior jugular veins because bleeding may obscure the field and make the procedure more difficult. Others advocate a horizontal incision because it is the most familiar approach for practitioners accustomed to performing standard tracheostomies. Regardless of the incision chosen, exposure is facilitated by placement of a towel roll under the shoulders to extend and hence displace the trachea superiorly and anteriorly. Once the skin incision has been made, blunt dissection is used until the cricothyroid membrane is reached. The membrane then is incised and gently dilated to facilitate the passage of a small endotracheal tube or tracheostomy tube, if available. Placement of a tracheal hook below the thyroid cartilage may provide better exposure of the cricothyroid membrane and allow easier cannulation. Care should be taken to avoid injury, especially fracture of the cricoid ring, because this can require subsequent surgical reconstruction. Once the tube position is confirmed, visually by chest motion and by auscultation and end-tidal PCO_2 return, the tube is secured. Cricothyroidotomy can be performed electively through a horizontal incision as a means of permanent airway access, but this usually is not done because cricothyroidotomy has been associated with a higher rate of subglottic stenosis. Hence, although controversial, an elective cricothyroidotomy usually is converted to a standard tracheostomy in 48 to 72 hours if ventilatory support airway access will be required.

COMPLICATIONS

The various described techniques of tracheostomy are associated with similar complications. Bleeding and infection are the most common problems. Bleeding can occur from multiple sources. Minor bleeding can originate from small vessels of the skin or the tracheal mucosa. Most such bleeding resolves with gentle pressure and time. Occasionally, cautery is required. Bleeding that occurs 2 to 3 weeks after a tracheostomy, especially if arterial in nature, is worrisome for a tracheoinnominate fistula. The incidence of this complication is less than 1%, but it can be lethal if not treated promptly.[4,6,11,22,24] Often, the first indication of a tracheoinnominate fistula is a minor "sentinel" bleed that heralds the subsequent massive hemorrhage that occurs if the fistula is not diagnosed and repaired immediately. Diagnosis of tracheoinnominate fistula is best done by bronchoscopy through the mouth, which often reveals bleeding either from the site where the balloon has eroded into the artery or more often from the lower edge of the stoma where a low tracheal cannula has eroded into the artery. Other diagnostic methods that can be useful are CT scanning of the neck with intravenous contrast material or MRI, although direct examination in the OR is usually the safest and fastest approach if there is sufficient concern

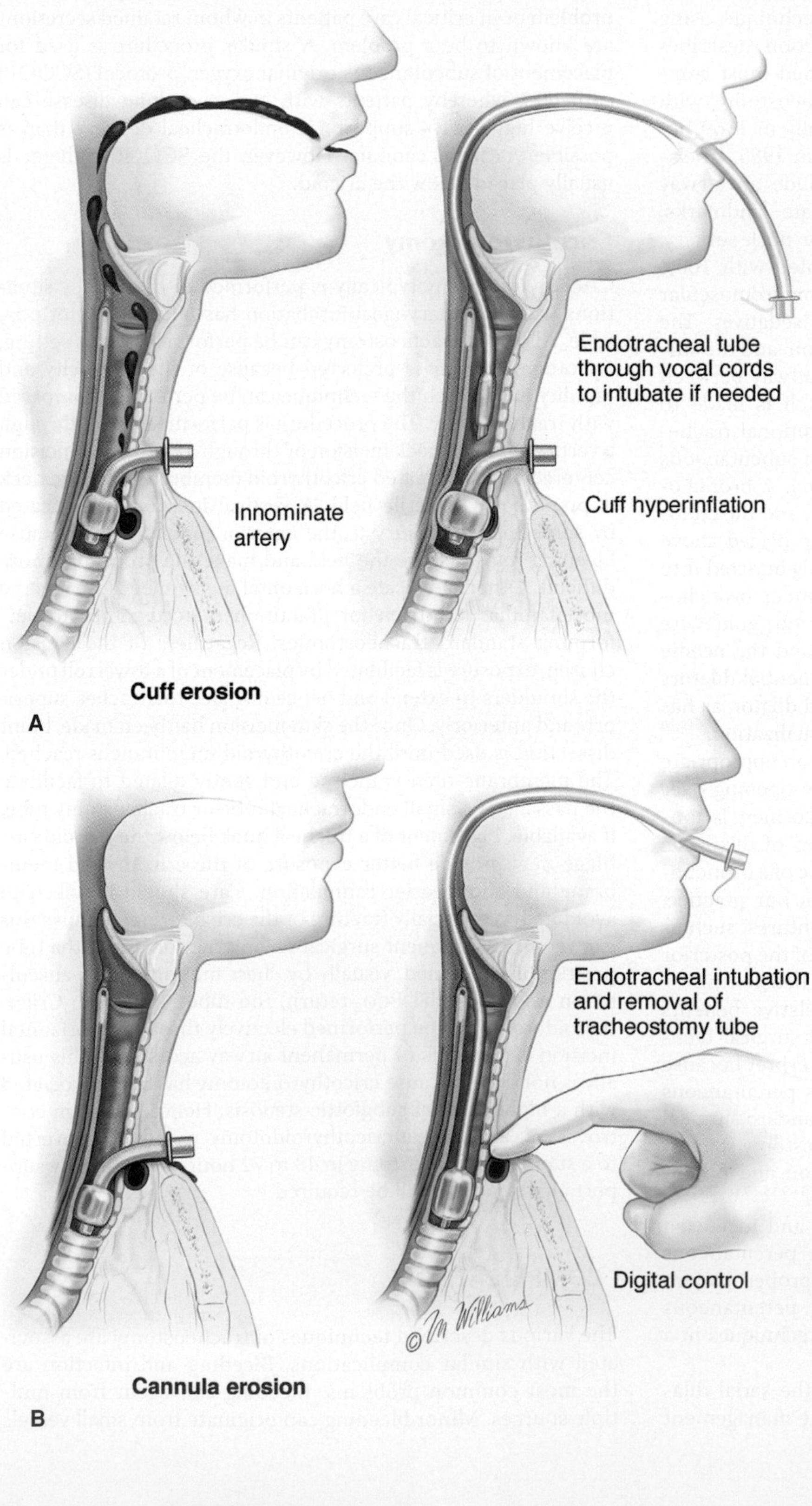

Figure 54-2. Etiology and management of tracheoinnominate fistula. Tracheoinnominate fistula may arise from erosion of the tracheostomy balloon into the innominate artery posteriorly (*A*) or direct erosion of the tracheostomy cannula into the innominate artery (*B*). In both cases, control of the airway with ventilation and protection of the lungs during transport to the OR are the principal goals.

for tracheoinnominate fistula. Immediate temporizing management of an actively bleeding tracheoinnominate fistula requires hyperinflation of the tracheal cuff if the fistula is secondary to cuff erosion (Fig. 54-2). If unsuccessful, or if the fistula is the result of cannula erosion, orotracheal intubation should be performed, followed by removal of the tracheal cannula and insertion of a digit into the stoma to apply manual pressure against the sternum, thereby tamponading the bleeding fistula on the way to the OR. Operative repair of the tracheoinnominate fistula is required immediately, occasionally with the aid of cardiopulmonary bypass. Particularly in cases of infection, repair may be best accomplished by division and ligation of the innominate artery. Endovascular stenting of the innominate artery has also been described to control the fistula by less invasive means. The long-term success of this method is not known but this technique considerably reduces the morbidity of repair in an already medically comprised group of patients.[25,26] Similarly, a tracheoesophageal fistula can develop and typically presents with either gastric dilatation or aspirated tube feeds or food through the tracheostomy. These are best diagnosed by bronchoscopy. If small, these can be temporized by esophageal or airway stenting before definitive surgical repair. Ironically, tracheal stenosis also can result from a tracheostomy, although this is rare and often difficult to distinguish from the injury that occurs secondary to prolonged translaryngeal intubation. Symptomatic tracheal stenosis in patients who have been decannulated often requires tracheal resection if dilation techniques fail to resolve symptoms. Other minor complications include local infection of the tracheostomy stoma site, which usually resolves with proper skin care and antibiotics for cellulitis.

SUMMARY

Tracheostomy is a common surgical procedure that is performed mainly to facilitate the care of chronically ventilated patients. Standard surgical and percutaneous techniques are described to perform a tracheostomy. If performed in appropriate clinical settings by those with adequate experience, both approaches are associated with a low morbidity. Similar complications can occur as a result of tracheostomy and prolonged ventilatory support regardless of the surgical approach, and therefore, all surgeons should be familiar with the diagnosis and the management of these complications.

EDITOR'S COMMENT

The indications for tracheostomy include (1) management of the critically ill patient with respiratory failure to facilitate weaning, (2) bypass of airway obstruction, and (3) airway protection for chronic aspiration to allow for suction. It may also be part of a surgical extirpative procedure such as laryngectomy. I prefer to incise above the third ring transversely, cut the ring anteriorly, grasp with a snap each of the lateral portions of the third ring, elevate them to the skin, dilate the opening, and then advance the tracheostomy under total control. This prevents the most feared complication of tracheostomy—losing the airway. I do not place sutures on the trachea because the message to our residents is that should the tracheostomy tube fall out, the patient should be intubated via the orotracheal route, which is safer and less likely to result in a mediastinal dissection.

—Raphael Bueno

References

1. Pahor AL. Ear, nose and throat in ancient Egypt, part III. *J Laryngol Otol.* 1992;106:863–873.
2. Pahor AL. Ear, nose and throat in ancient Egypt, part II. *J Laryngol Otol.* 1992;106:773–779.
3. Pahor AL. Ear, nose and throat in ancient Egypt, part I. *J Laryngol Otol.* 1992;106:677–687.
4. Heffner JE, Hess D. Tracheostomy management in the chronically ventilated patient. *Clin Chest Med.* 2001;22:55–69.
5. Heffner JE. Tracheotomy application and timing. *Clin Chest Med.* 2003; 24:389–398.
6. Walts PA, Murthy SC, DeCamp MM. Techniques of surgical tracheostomy. *Clin Chest Med.* 2003;24:413–422.
7. Angel LF, Simpson CB. Comparison of surgical and percutaneous dilational tracheostomy. *Clin Chest Med.* 2003;24:423–429.
8. Ernst A, Critchlow J. Percutaneous tracheostomy: special considerations. *Clin Chest Med.* 2003;24:409–412.
9. Bowen TR, Miller F, Mackenzie W. Comparison of oxygen consumption measurements in children with cerebral palsy to children with muscular dystrophy. *J Pediatr Orthop.* 1999;19:133–136.
10. Kane TD, Rodriguez JL, Luchette FA. Early versus late tracheostomy in the trauma patient. *Respir Care Clin N Am.* 1997;3:1–20.
11. Lewis RJ. Tracheostomies: indications, timing, and complications. *Clin Chest Med.* 1992;13:137–149.
12. Marsh HM, Gillespie DJ, Baumgartner AE. Timing of tracheostomy in the critically ill patient. *Chest.* 1989;96:190–193.
13. deBoisblanc BP. Percutaneous dilational tracheostomy techniques. *Clin Chest Med.* 2003;24:399–407.
14. Wright CD. Minitracheostomy. *Clin Chest Med.* 2003;24:431–435.
15. Rumbak MJ, Newton M, Truncale T, et al. A prospective, randomized study comparing early percutaneous dilational tracheotomy to prolonged translaryngeal intubation (delayed tracheotomy) in critically ill medical patients. *Crit Care Med.* 2004;32:1689–1694.
16. McGregor IA, Neill RS. Tracheostomy and the Bjork flap. *Lancet.* 1983;2:1259.
17. Malata CM, Foo IT, Simpson KH, et al. An audit of Bjork flap tracheostomies in head and neck plastic surgery. *Br J Oral Maxillofac Surg.* 1996;34:42–46.
18. Freeman BD, Isabella K, Lin N, et al. A meta-analysis of prospective trials comparing percutaneous and surgical tracheostomy in critically ill patients. *Chest.* 2000;118:1412–1418.
19. Freeman BD, Isabella K, Cobb JP, et al. A prospective, randomized study comparing percutaneous with surgical tracheostomy in critically ill patients. *Crit Care Med.* 2001;29:926–930.
20. Heikkinen M, Aarnio P, Hannukainen J. Percutaneous dilational tracheostomy or conventional surgical tracheostomy? *Crit Care Med.* 2000;28: 1399–1402.
21. Ciaglia P, Firsching R, Syniec C. Elective percutaneous dilatational tracheostomy: a new simple bedside procedure; preliminary report. *Chest.* 1985; 87:715–719.
22. Friedman Y, Fildes J, Mizock B, et al. Comparison of percutaneous and surgical tracheostomies. *Chest.* 1996;110:480–485.
23. Polderman KH, Spijkstra JJ, de Bree R, et al. Percutaneous dilational tracheostomy in the ICU: optimal organization, low complication rates, and description of a new complication. *Chest.* 2003;123:1595–1602.
24. Kremer B, Botos-Kremer AI, Eckel HE, et al. Indications, complications, and surgical techniques for pediatric tracheostomies: an update. *J Pediatr Surg.* 2002;37:1556–1562.
25. Hamaguchi S, Nakajima Y. Two cases of tracheoinnominate artery fistula following tracheostomy treated successfully by endovascular embolization of the innominate artery. *J Vasc Surg.* 2011;55(2):545–547.
26. Shepard PM, Phillips JM, Tefera G, et al. Tracheoinnominate fistula: successful management with endovascular stenting. *Ear Nose Throat J.* 2011; 90(7):310–312.

55 Endoscopic Treatments for Benign Major Upper Airways Disease

Siva Raja and Sudish C. Murthy

Keywords: Upper airways stenosis and malacia, endobronchial surgery, flexible and rigid bronchoscopy, tracheomalacia, benign subglottic or tracheal stenosis

In highly selected patient populations, flexible and rigid endoscopic (endobronchial) management offers effective treatment options for benign major airway disease (e.g., stenosis and malacia). These treatments are associated with less morbidity than traditional surgical interventions. Selection criteria focus primarily on candidacy for more definitive surgical therapy, as patients can be deemed inappropriate candidates for classic resection/reconstruction for a variety of reasons: etiology, extent of disease, failed prior operation, confounding medical comorbidities, and patient preference. Lack of technical expertise at a given institution also may be a factor. Since each institution carries its own bias with respect to these parameters, a patient determined inoperable at one center, in fact, may be considered a reasonable candidate at another.

Clearly, some individuals will benefit greatly from less invasive management of their airway disease. Only rarely is acute life-threatening airway compromise (≥75% luminal compromise) encountered in clinical practice. Moreover, as an alternative to tracheostomy, immediate endoscopic palliation of a high-grade stenosis may be part of a treatment strategy that ultimately incorporates an elective *staged* resection.

Symptomatic subglottic and tracheal stenoses and tracheomalacias are indications for endoscopic therapy in benign upper airways disease. These etiologies are listed in Table 55-1. Whether used as the primary therapy or as an adjunct to definitive surgery, the goal of endobronchial intervention is to restore airway patency and to provide a durable response, while limiting morbidity. Procedures often involve collaboration between surgeons and interventional bronchoscopists. Critical elements of endoscopic treatments are appropriate patient selection, choice of a specific endobronchial intervention based on indication, focused postoperative care (often including steroid therapy and mucolytics), and anticipation of possible repeated interventions.

Table 55-1

ETIOLOGY OF AIRWAY STENOSIS/MALACIA

LOCATION	TYPE	DISEASE
Subglottic	Congenital	Closed first ring Membranous web Cartilage deformity
	Acquired	External trauma Endoluminal trauma Systemic illness
Tracheal	Congenital	Membranous web Vascular anomaly Congenital malacia
	Acquired	External trauma Endoluminal trauma Systemic illness Infection Prior airway intervention

The goal of the endoscopic approach is to preserve the respiratory epithelium, while minimizing radial thermal and mechanical injury to the airway. Many procedures can be performed through an adult flexible bronchoscope (video or fiberoptic), although because of the frequent requirement for rigid bronchoscopy, skill with rigid instrumentation is mandatory and must be actively maintained. General anesthesia is generally indicated, although it is possible to perform limited interventions in a bronchoscopy suite with conscious sedation and topical analgesia. Availability of a suitable procedure room (interventional bronchoscopy suite) or an operative room to perform interventions is essential. The suite should contain several high-resolution monitors, endobronchial ultrasound capability (EBUS), mobile flexible bronchoscopy towers, and fluoroscopic capability.

BENIGN SUBGLOTTIC STENOSIS

The subglottis lies between the vocal cords and the proximal trachea. Congenital subglottic stenosis generally presents early in life and is characterized by an audible biphasic stridor or a persistent or recurrent croup-type cough. Historically, congenital subglottic stenosis required tracheotomy in over 40% of patients as an early palliative maneuver.[1]

Acquired subglottic stenosis is commonly associated with antecedent trauma, either externally (e.g., blunt-force injury to the anterior neck) or, more frequently, internally. There is little doubt that this process represents an important, often delayed, morbidity of laryngotracheal intubation. Internal airway injury can occur as a result of direct mucosal trauma sustained during intubation, endotracheal tube cuff pressure ischemia and mucosal necrosis, constant tube motion and mechanical abrasion, and associated tracheitis.[2] Percutaneous dilatational tracheostomy and laryngotracheal reflux also have been implicated.[3]

Acquired systemic diseases such as amyloidosis, papillomatosis, tuberculosis, and granulomatosis with polyangiitis (GPA), formerly Wegener's granulomatosis, also may include subglottic stenosis as a component of the patient's symptom complex. There is also a rare idiopathic/cryptogenic syndrome, seen almost exclusively in younger women, that manifests as an obstructing subglottic web.[4,5]

BENIGN TRACHEAL STENOSIS

Fortunately, congenital causes of benign tracheal stenosis are quite rare and include extrinsic narrowing or incomplete development secondary to vascular rings or partial vascular

Table 55-2

CLASSIFICATION OF TRACHEAL STENOSIS AFTER TRACHEOTOMY

RELATIONSHIP TO TRACHEOSTOMA	CAUSE
Proximal	High tracheostomy and erosion into the anterior wall
At the stoma	Interaction polyps Granulation tissue
Immediately distal to stoma	Excessive granulation response cuff necrosis
Distal to the endotracheal tube	Excessive motion or pressure of the tracheostomy tube

Adapted from references[1,6,7].

slings. Acquired diseases account for the majority of occurrences. Specifically, intrinsic injuries caused by endotracheal intubation or tracheotomy are the most common and best characterized. Table 55-2 summarizes the four most common locations related to posttracheotomy stenosis.[2,6,7] Healing from direct trauma to the airway can result in a complex, asymmetric scar that can be difficult to palliate. The classic "A-Type" deformity (as opposed to the normal C shape of the trachea) can result from anterior collapse of the proximal trachea at the site of a prior tracheostoma. In addition, some stenoses are accompanied by tracheomalacia, which further complicates their management.

ENDOBRONCHIAL AND ENDOSCOPIC INTERVENTIONS

Numerous techniques can be used to relieve central airway stenosis (Table 55-3). Historically, rigid tracheoplasty (dilatation) was the first option for high-grade proximal airway narrowing. More recently, however, although rigid instrumentation is still a critical element in the management of these conditions, endoscopic treatments have become far more common because of the improved optics of flexible bronchoscopes and the development of a vast array of therapies that can be easily used through them. In addition, since a reduced skill-set is required for flexible approaches, dissemination has occurred quite rapidly. Often procedures become an amalgam of both flexible and rigid techniques as rigid scopes provide ventilatory support and stable airway access, whereas flexible scopes are passed within them and provide improved optics.

Table 55-3

ENDOBRONCHIAL AND ENDOSCOPIC INTERVENTIONS FOR BENIGN AIRWAY STENOSIS

CONDUIT	TYPE	EFFECT
Flexible bronchoscope	Electrocautery	Thermal
	Argon plasma coagulation	Thermal
	Laser (CO_2 or Nd:YAG)	Thermal
	Cryotherapy	Thermal
	Pneumatic tracheoplasty	Mechanical
	Self-expanding metallic stent	Mechanical
Rigid bronchoscope	Rigid tracheoplasty	Mechanical
	Silastic stent	Mechanical
	Microdebrider	Mechanical
Suspension laryngoscope	All[a]	Both

[a]Primarily for subglottic and proximal tracheal therapies.

DILATATION

By far the most common endobronchial intervention, dilatation is seldom performed without another therapy. Depending on the complexity of the stenosis, however, repeated endobronchial dilatations alone may be sufficient to effectively palliate an inoperable airway stenosis. Bougienage (passing a series of graduated bougie tubes through a suspension laryngoscope) is an effective therapy for most simple (web-like) stenoses of the subglottis and proximal trachea. Since the tubes are relatively compliant, this form of rigid tracheoplasty is gentler on the airway than a rigid bronchoscope used to affect the same result. As the complexity of the stenosis increases (i.e., asymmetric, denser scar, component of malacia, and lengthier), rigid tracheoplasty alone becomes far less effective, and its use may lead to significant airway injury. Consequently, prior to any intervention, a thorough assessment of the pathology is mandated.

Unintended disruption of the airway can occur during dilatation because mechanical forces may not be equally distributed during rigid dilatation. If the membranous airway is spared by the pathology, it will be the point of least resistance and may split during the procedure while leaving the stenosis intact. Other weak points in the airway are the membranous–cartilaginous junctions which can dislocate during an undirected rigid dilatation. This potential problem often is overcome by pretreating the stenosis with ablation therapy to create a more controlled dilatation (see below).

With the development of graduated endobronchial balloons, pneumatic tracheoplasty can be performed bronchoscopically. Although this is a seemingly less traumatic approach, endobronchial balloons are inflated well above atmospheric pressure during dilatation, and if used improperly, are no less traumatic than standard rigid dilatation. However, because pneumatic dilatation can be performed more precisely and in a much more gradual fashion, the results are more predictable and often better.

ENDOSCOPIC ABLATION THERAPIES

Thermal energy to disrupt or ablate diseased tissue has been used for over 50 years. Its application within the respiratory system was limited until more recently as technologic advancements have facilitated access. A number of delivery vehicles now are available for airway applications. For benign airway stenoses, there are two main goals of ablative therapies. First, endoscopic resection and vaporization of obstructing granulation tissue or scar can be accomplished. Second, dense focal scars can be incised to create pathways of least resistance so that subsequent rigid or pneumatic dilatations can be more predictably and safely performed.

Several energy sources can create thermal injury and result in tissue ablation. The choice of source depends on the nature of the stenosis, and includes location, cause, thickness, and length of airway involvement. Having the gamut of technologies is essential. The spectrum of ablative interventions, as well as flexible and rigid video bronchoscopes (telescopes) should be available within the designated interventional suite.

Laser

The development of lasers with short wavelengths that can be transmitted through thin quartz filaments has made endoscopic application possible. The carbon dioxide laser operates at a longer wavelength (10.6 μm), which limits its use to superficial structures.[7] The neodymium-doped yttrium aluminum garnet (Nd:YAG) laser, however, operates at wavelengths one-tenth as long, making it the more common source. Fine fiberoptic fibers can be passed through the working channel of a standard flexible bronchoscope and can be manipulated with a high degree of accuracy. Stenoses can be endoscopically resected primarily by vaporization of tissues. Since Nd:YAG laser light is poorly absorbed by both water and hemoglobin; it penetrates more deeply into surrounding tissues than other ablative therapies. Accordingly, the risk of airway perforation and injury to adjacent structures is higher. However, the wider energy dispersion field results in effective coagulation.[8]

A rare but important complication of endoscopic ablative therapies is airway ignition.[8] This is more commonly associated with laser procedures performed through the flexible bronchoscope than through a rigid scope. Reduction of inspired FIO_2 to <40%, avoidance of flammable endotracheal tubes (although there currently is no "laser-safe" endotracheal tube on the market), and use of reinforced endotracheal tubes or LMA are preferred during any thermal procedure. Awareness of this rare complication is critical.

Electrocautery and Argon Plasma Coagulation

Endoscopic electrocautery (diathermy) offers the ability to rapidly snare and remove large granulomas or polyps bypassing the tedious process of vaporization. Alternatively, cautery can be used similarly to the laser. Risk of airway ignition is slightly less with electrocautery because less heat is generated by electrocautery device. The depth of penetration of the thermal injury depends on contact time with tissues and, consequently, is perhaps, slightly better controlled with electrocautery than with other thermal devices.

The flow of electrons through tissues generates heat for coagulation because of the high resistance within the target tissue. Electrocautery probes require direct contact with the target tissue to initiate this effect. Argon plasma coagulation (APC) uses ionized argon gas to conduct electrons into the target, providing a noncontact mode of treatment (lightning effect).[8] Argon gas flows flexibly, and therefore, can travel in a nonlinear fashion to the desired target (i.e., bend around corners). Moreover, as tissues are coagulated, their intrinsic resistance rises, redirecting the argon beam to adjacent, nontreated, lower-resistance tissues.[8] This feature distinguishes APC from the laser. Also, APC can treat more superficial tissues than either laser or diathermy. Argon gas is pressurized and there is some small risk of gas emboli reaching the systemic circulation if the tip of the APC probe is kept too close to an active bleeding source.

Cryotherapy

Cryotherapy has been commonly used in dermatology, otolaryngology, and gastroenterology applications. More recently it was introduced for endobronchial treatment of both malignant and benign lesions. The mechanism of action is cellular necrosis caused by intracellular crystallization from freeze–thaw cycles.[9,10] Initially, there can be some edema following therapy, but subsequent sloughing of treated tissue (with or without balloon dilatation) results in recanalization of the airway lumen. There is very little bleeding encountered at the time of cryoablation, and the resulting microvascular thrombosis permits only minimal delayed bleeding even after tissue is sloughed and regardless of concomitant or subsequent balloon dilatation.[11]

Histological analysis posttreatment has shown sloughing of the epithelium and deeper tissues to include the submucosal glands with preservation of the connective tissue. This appears to reepithelialize the radial margin of the injury.[12] The use of this therapy has been limited by the cryoprobe design, which was somewhat cumbersome. Recent advances have included development of noncontact cryotherapy with liquid nitrogen. This permits more uniform application of the cryogen.[12] Given the advances in this technology, conventional probe-delivered cryotherapy is useful for debulking endoluminal masses (benign and malignant), treating asymmetric scar, and foreign-body (and retained clot) extraction. Importantly, cryotherapy has no potential for airway fire. Spray cryotherapy is currently under active investigation, although its introduction into practice will be complicated by the need for highly pressurized cryogen (liquid nitrogen) which may lead to gas emboli and pneumothorax.

Microdebrider Therapy

Microdebrider therapy is another newer modality useful in the endoscopic management of subglottic and tracheal cicatricial stenosis and malignant or granulation tissue-related airway obstruction. A microdebrider is a rotary cutting tool that attaches to a suction source that simultaneously debrides and evacuates tissue to recanalize the obstructed airway. Recently, this device has become popular for removing obstructing subglottic glands, airway papillomas, tracheal scars, as well as obstructing airway cancers.[13] The suction component of the device continually clears debris and maintains visualization of the lumen. Nevertheless, the limitations of the technology remain accidental injury to normal tissue and bleeding from the raw debrided surface which may ultimately require thermal (or cryo) cauterization.[9] The microdebrider probe must be passed through a rigid scope and visualized with a telescope or flexible video bronchoscope. This current setup does reduce the degrees of freedom of microdebrider movement.

Topical Agents

In addition to the above-described endoscopic modalities, topical agents have been used as an adjunct to dilatational and ablative strategies. Topical endoscopic application of mitomycin C (~0.4 mg/mL) appears to be a safe and moderately efficacious adjuvant therapy, although limited experimental[14] and clinical data[15–17] exist. Mitomycin C can be applied topically to the treated areas, and surprisingly, this does not appear to affect epithelial regrowth; rather, it mainly interferes with refibrosis.[10] Treated areas should be surveyed regularly for squamous metaplasia. Similarly, some data support the use of intralesional steroid therapy to modulate the local inflammatory process, and this may have some benefit in the management of tracheal stenosis.[18] It is common to use mitomycin C and intralesional steroids alternately during chronic endoscopic palliation of a recurrent tracheal stenosis. Although the data is scant on these topical treatments, no appreciable complications have been reported in the literature.

TECHNIQUE

Successful endoscopic management of benign central airway stenosis involves a combination of endobronchial therapies. As discussed previously, dilatation alone generally is insufficient to provide meaningful palliation. After identifying the appropriateness of the candidate for therapy, control of the airway is the initial step. Usually, general anesthesia will be required. Although rare, conscious sedation may be sufficient for some patients. The airway can be controlled by suspension laryngoscope (Fig. 55-1), rigid bronchoscope (Fig. 55-2), endotracheal tube, or laryngeal mask airway (LMA). The choice is predicated on location, etiology, and magnitude of the stenosis. For high-grade stenoses, rigid control of the airway is preferred and can be changed to endotracheal tube or LMA once the airway has been partially recanalized and safely controlled. If a subglottic lesion exists, suspension laryngoscopy provides excellent access. Open tracheostomy supplies should always be close at hand in case a surgical airway is emergently required.

Patients are ventilated with intermittent apnea or jet techniques, and permissive hypercapnea is surprisingly well tolerated by most patients. Ventilating rigid bronchoscopes are useful for this purpose. A thorough assessment of the airway is made, and if more than a simple web-like stenosis exists, an ablative therapy usually will be required. The choice of ablative therapy is often guided by availability at a given institution. Laser, electrocautery, APC, and cryoprobes are designed to fit within the working channel of a standard adult bronchoscope.[19]

Ablative therapies are used for three different purposes. Endoscopic photoresection (i.e., laser and electrocautery) is reserved for dense cicatricial stenoses (Fig. 55-3) or obstructing granulation tissue. The obstruction is vaporized or charred

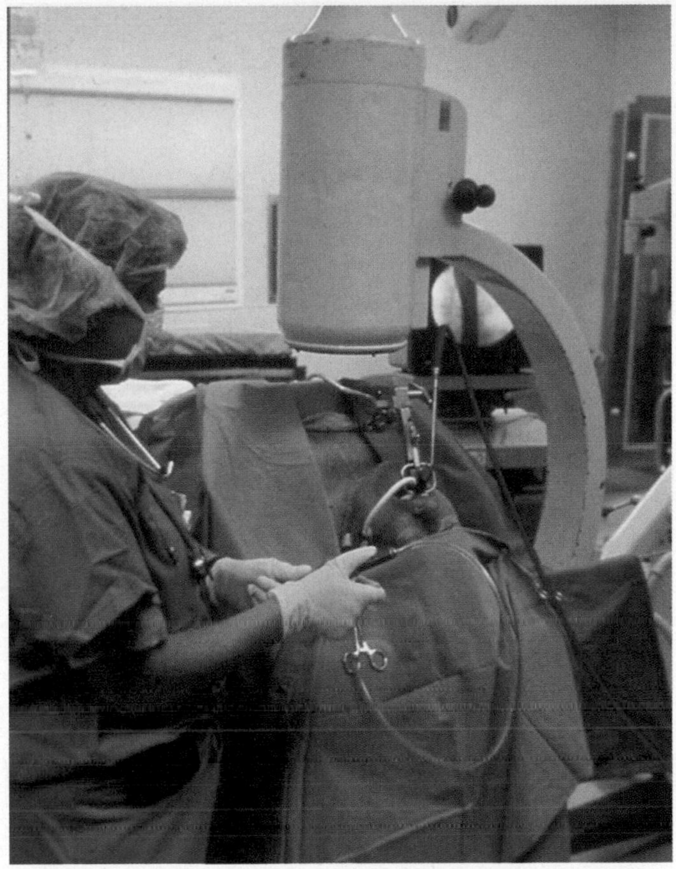

Figure 55-1. The airway can be controlled by suspension laryngoscope, rigid bronchoscope, endotracheal tube, or laryngeal mask airway.

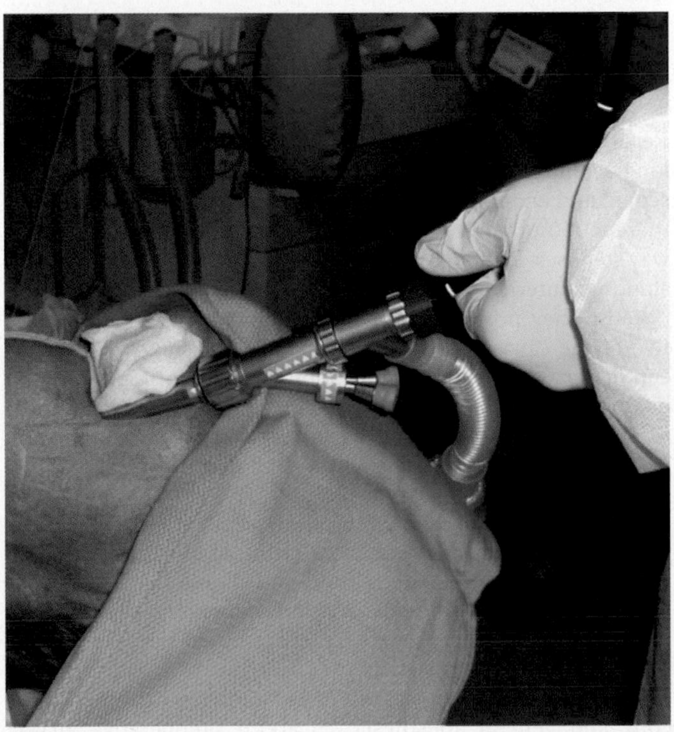

A

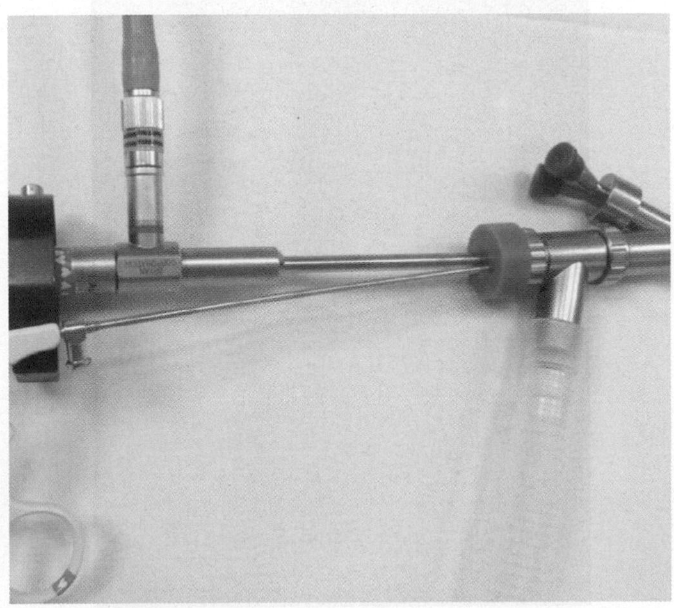

B

Figure 55-2. Rigid bronchoscope.

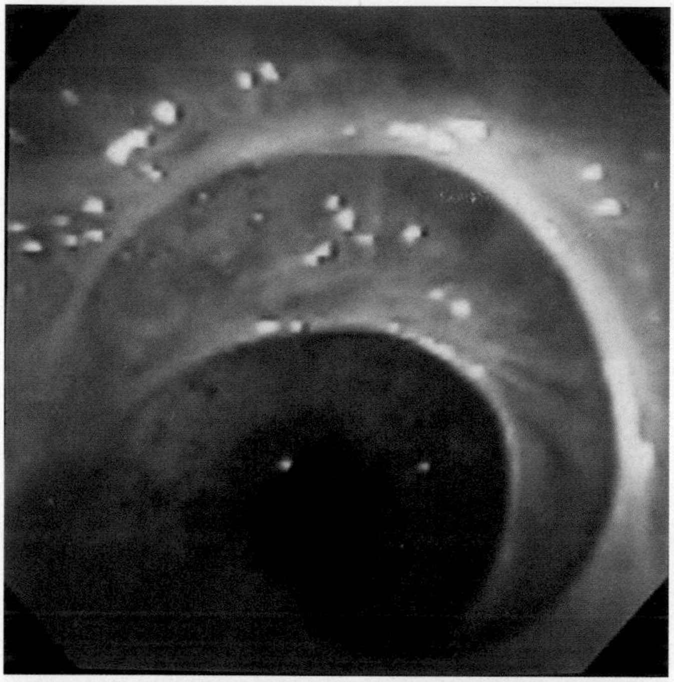

Figure 55-3. Rigid cicatricial stenosis.

then debrided with biopsy forceps. Radial incisions (i.e., laser and electrocautery) (Fig. 55-4) can be made along suspected lines of tension to help guide the direction of fracture of the stenosis during subsequent dilatation (Fig. 55-5). Care should be taken to avoid making these incisions on the membranous trachea. Two or three full-thickness incisions are made after the

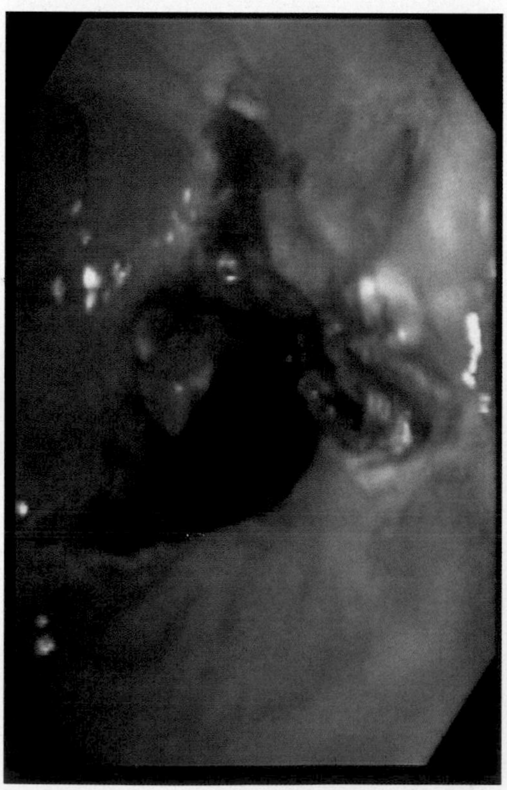

Figure 55-4. Radial incisions with electrocautery. Care must be taken to avoid incisions on the membranous trachea.

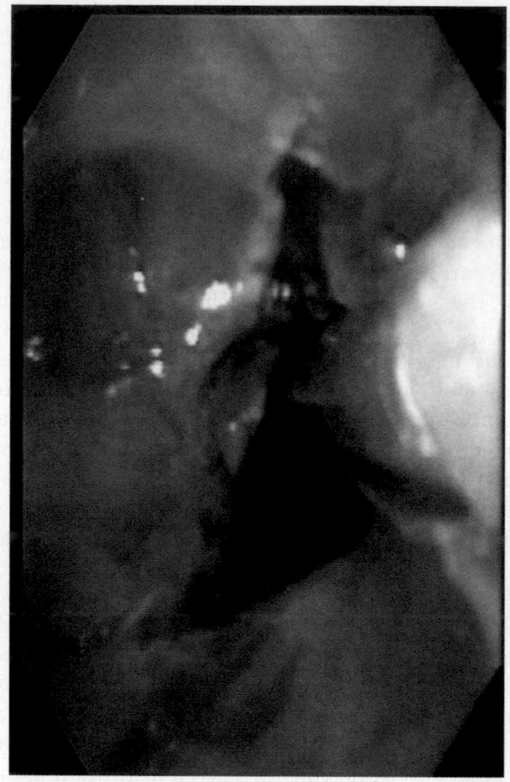

Figure 55-5. Balloon tracheoplasty after radial incisions.

orientation of the airway has been established, and either endoscopic pneumatic dilatation or rigid dilatation follows. Endoscopic coagulation (APC) is used to treat diffuse superficial processes, such as benign polyposis. Regardless of the therapy, airway perforation and ignition are risks.

TRACHEOBRONCHOMALACIA

Regardless of etiology, limited surgical procedures exist for long-segment central airway malacia. Consequently, endoscopic and endobronchial therapies have emerged as the main therapeutic options for these difficult-to-treat functional airway stenoses. Principal among these therapies is endobronchial stenting. Internal airway stents are ideal for airway collapse because they provide support for airway structures irrespective of the cause of malacia. Unfortunately, stents themselves can lead to numerous complications related to migration and host foreign-body reactions. For long-segment and intractable malacia syndromes, T-Tube placement as a destination therapy is reasonable and serves as an important option for these unfortunate patients.

In the context of benign disease, stents can be deployed as primary treatment for malacia or as an adjuvant after benign stenoses have been ablated. There are numerous stents from which to choose, although it is now apparent that silicone stents, as opposed to metallic stents, should be used for the treatment of benign disease.[20]

Placement of most silicone stents requires rigid bronchoscopy and general anesthesia.[21] Careful preoperative airway measurement is required to properly size the stent. To this end, a chest CT scan with three-dimensional reconstruction of the airway is useful. Patients usually are treated with steroids to reduce the chance of bronchospasm during and immediately after the procedure.

It is important to schedule frequent follow-up visits for patients with endobronchial stents. Follow-up visits should include surveillance flexible bronchoscopy. This is necessary because stent-related complications such as migration, mucous impaction, and granulation tissue occur frequently. All patients should be managed with mucolytic therapy (via nebulizer) two or three times daily. Patients also should be instructed that for any decline in respiratory function or development of a new wheeze, medical attention should be sought immediately. Asphyxia can occur with stent migration or occlusion.

SUMMARY

Endoscopic therapies are critical for the comprehensive management of benign airway stenosis and malacia. A multidisciplinary team, including airway surgeon and interventional pulmonologist, is necessary to identify candidates and perform procedures. An institutional commitment to secure appropriate instrumentation and technical support is also required. The threshold for transferring complex patients to more experienced centers should be low.

EDITOR'S COMMENT

Every thoracic surgeon should be familiar with the techniques for endoscopic management of obstructed airways with flexible or rigid bronchoscopes. Each institution should have a minimum supply of flexible and rigid endoscopes available, as well as at least one or two of the other modalities summarized in Table 55-3. The type of modality may vary based on the experience of the hospital and the surgeon, as well as financial considerations. The more options and surgical experience the center has to offer, the better it is for patients. Elective patients should be referred to centers of excellence where sufficient expertise exists.

As rigid bronchoscopy becomes less common, surgeons should practice to maintain their skills. In cases where it is difficult to identify the vocal cords with the rigid scope, consider placing a guidewire or small intubating bougie down the airway via an LMA and use it to guide the rigid scope.

—Raphael Bueno

References

1. Holinger PH, Kutnick SL, Schild JA, et al. Subglottic stenosis in infants and children. *Ann Otol Rhinol Laryngol.* 1976;85(5 Pt 1):591–599.
2. Mehta AC, Harris RJ, De Boer GE. Endoscopic management of benign airway stenosis. *Clin Chest Med.* 1995;16(3):401–413.
3. Lorenz RR. Adult laryngotracheal stenosis: etiology and surgical management. *Curr Opin Otolaryngol Head Neck Surg.* 2003;11(6):467–472.
4. Ashiku SK, Mathisen DJ. Idiopathic laryngotracheal stenosis. *Chest Surg Clin N Am.* 2003;13(2):257–269.
5. Dedo HH, Catten MD. Idiopathic progressive subglottic stenosis: findings and treatment in 52 patients. *Ann Otol Rhinol Laryngol.* 2001;110(4):305–311.
6. Montgomery WW. Current modifications of the salivary bypass tube and tracheal T-tube. *Ann Otol Rhinol Laryngol.* 1986;95(2 Pt 1):121–125.
7. Ossoff RH, Tucker GF, Jr, Duncavage JA, et al. Efficacy of bronchoscopic carbon dioxide laser surgery for benign strictures of the trachea. *Laryngoscope.* 1985;95(10):1220–1223.
8. Mehta AC. *Laser Application in Respiratory Care.* 1st ed. Ontario, Canada: Decker; 1988.
9. Yarmus L, Ernst A, Feller-Kopman D. Emerging technologies for the thorax: indications, management and complications. *Respirology.* 2010;15(2):208–219.
10. Gompelmann D, Eberhardt R, Herth FJ. Advanced malignant lung disease: what the specialist can offer. *Respiration.* 2011;82(2):111–123.
11. Krimsky WS, Rodrigues MP, Malayaman N, et al. Spray cryotherapy for the treatment of glottic and subglottic stenosis. *Laryngoscope.* 2010;120(3): 473–477.
12. Krimsky WS, Broussard JN, Sarkar SA, et al. Bronchoscopic spray cryotherapy: assessment of safety and depth of airway injury. *J Thorac Cardiovasc Surg.* 2010;139(3):781–782.
13. Lunn W, Garland R, Ashiku S, et al. Microdebrider bronchoscopy: a new tool for the interventional bronchoscopist. *Ann Thorac Surg.* 2005;80(4): 1485–1488.
14. Cincik H, Gungor A, Cakmak A, et al. The effects of mitomycin C and 5-fluorouracil/triamcinolone on fibrosis/scar tissue formation secondary to subglottic trauma (experimental study). *Am J Otolaryngol.* 2005;26(1): 45–50.
15. Schweinfurth JM. Endoscopic treatment of severe tracheal stenosis. *Ann Otol Rhinol Laryngol.* 2006;115(1):30–34.
16. Penafiel A, Lee P, Hsu A, et al. Topical mitomycin-C for obstructing endobronchial granuloma. *Ann Thorac Surg.* 2006;82(3):e22–e23.
17. Simpson CB, James JC. The efficacy of mitomycin-C in the treatment of laryngotracheal stenosis. *Laryngoscope.* 2006;116(10):1923–1925.
18. Hirshoren N, Eliashar R. Wound-healing modulation in upper airway stenosis-Myths and facts. *Head Neck.* 2009;31(1):111–126.
19. Bolliger CT, Sutedja TG, Strausz J, et al. Therapeutic bronchoscopy with immediate effect: laser, electrocautery, argon plasma coagulation and stents. *Eur Respir J.* 2006;27(6):1258–1271.
20. Murthy SC, Gildea TR, Mehta AC. Removal of self-expandable metallic stents: is it possible? *Semin Respir Crit Care Med.* 2004;25(4):381–385.
21. Dumon JF. A dedicated tracheobronchial stent. *Chest.* 1990;97(2):328–332.

56 Use of Tracheobronchial Stents

Raphael Bueno

Keywords: Tracheobronchial stents, tracheobronchial stricture, recurrent tumor, tracheobronchial malacia, silicone stents, self-expanding metal stents, bioabsorbable stents

A number of benign and malignant disorders of the upper airways can cause tracheobronchial narrowing, stricture, compression, or collapse (i.e., tracheobronchial malacia), ultimately leading to symptomatic and potentially life-threatening dyspnea. These tracheobronchial compromises can be managed with endobronchial dilation in addition to placement of endotracheal, bronchial, or tracheobronchial stents. Generally, stent placement can be accomplished safely and provides immediate relief of symptoms in the acute setting. Over the long term, stent placement has been shown to improve the patient's quality of life. The use of endobronchial stents has accelerated recently as a result of the proliferation of new biocompatible materials, novel stent designs, and easier techniques for deployment.

Although stents have been described in reports dating back to the 1800s, the concept of using stents to relieve acute tracheobronchial obstruction was not reported until the mid-1950s.[1] Dumon[2] designed a dedicated endoluminal upper airway stent in the late 1990s, and it remains today one of the most commonly used silicone stents. The self-expanding metal stents manufactured from biocompatible metal alloys also were pioneered in the 1990s using technology initially developed for vascular and coronary stents.[3,4] The ideal tracheobronchial stent has yet to be perfected, and there are potentially life-threatening risks associated with all stents currently on the market. Making the correct stent selection therefore is critical for the well-being of the patient.

INDICATIONS FOR ENDOBRONCHIAL STENTS

The indications for deployment of airway stents include (1) extrinsic compression of the central airways with or without intraluminal components owing to malignant or benign disorders; (2) complex, inoperable tracheobronchial strictures; (3) tracheobronchial malacia; (4) palliation for recurrent intraluminal tumor growth; and (5) central airway fistulas (i.e., esophagus, mediastinum, or pleura).

Presenting signs and findings may include dyspnea, cough, hemoptysis, recurrent lung infections, wheezing, and stridor. On occasion, a patient may be referred for evaluation of findings made on a screening CT scan. Since many types of endobronchial therapies are available for patients with airway disorders, it is important to recognize that stenting is just one such modality and the patient may benefit from a combination of treatments.

Desirable Stent Characteristics

The ideal stent should be easy to insert and remove yet resistant to migration. It should be sufficiently strong to support the airway yet flexible enough to withstand (and collapse with) cough without fracturing, narrowing, or moving. The material from which the stent is made should be biologically inert to minimize the formation of granulation tissues. The stent should not change in size when collapsed, or a scar may form at its two ends. The stent should be available in a variety of lengths and sizes, and its walls should be as thin as possible for a maximal intraluminal diameter to prevent retention of secretions. The stent should permit movement of secretions across its surface to prevent inspissation of secretions that could obstruct the stent, yet prevent any accumulation of secretions within it or distal to it. Finally, the stent should perfectly appose the airway wall to cover defects and prevent the ingrowth of tissues that may obstruct its lumen without causing airway ischemia or injury.

CLASSIFICATION OF STENTS

Tracheobronchial stents are classified according to their material composition (i.e., plastic, metal, or mixed) (Table 56-1). Plastic tracheobronchial stents usually are made of silicone, which is inexpensive and inert. They have solid walls, which prevent luminal obstruction secondary to tissue ingrowth, and they are removed easily, although rigid bronchoscopy usually is required for their insertion and removal. As a consequence of their relative mobility, plastic stents have a higher rate of migration (~10%). They are also somewhat thicker than metallic stents, which limits the intraluminal diameter and increases the probability of having retained airway secretions, particularly with smaller caliber stents.

The large number of metallic stents are composed of substances such as stainless steel, alloys that incorporate cobalt and chromium, and Nitinol, a biologically inert titanium and

Table 56-1

CLASSIFICATION OF STENTS

Metallic stents
Balloon-expandable metallic stents
Palmaz stent
Strecker stent
Self-expanding metallic stents
Gianturco-Z stent
Wallstent
Nitinol/InStent/Ultraflex stent
Silicone stents
Dumon stent
Hood stent
Montgomery T-tube
Combination stents
Reynder stent
Dynamic stent
Polyflex
Novastent
AERO® Tracheobronchial stent

nickel alloy. Some of these metals are calibrated to expand maximally at body temperature. The most commonly used are the self-expandable metallic stents (SEMS). These stents are stored in the collapsed state and revert to the fully expanded state on release in the correct airway location. Deployment mechanisms vary among SEMS. The walls of SEMS are thinner than plastic, yielding a larger intraluminal diameter, which permits deployment of smaller stents. The stents are quite strong and are designed to last a lifetime. Because the delivery systems are smaller, they can be inserted with a flexible bronchoscope, sparing the necessity of general anesthesia.

SEMS are available in two forms: covered and uncovered. The benefit of the uncovered variety is that within 3 to 4 months of placement, the stent becomes incorporated in the walls of the trachea or bronchus and lined with a new ciliated epithelial tissue layer, which facilitates the patient's ability to clear secretions. The uncovered metal stent is, for all practical purposes, a permanent prosthesis that permits tissue ingrowth between the metallic components, making it extremely difficult to remove the stent if it fails. For this reason, uncovered SEMS often are not recommended for benign tracheobronchial processes or for patients who are expected to survive for a long time. Covered SEMS were developed specifically to deal with the complication of tumor ingrowth. These are usually coated with Silastic or polyurethane and are essentially identical to the uncovered variety.

Since neither the metallic nor plastic stents have all the desired characteristics of the ideal stent, a number of manufacturers recently have introduced combination stents. These are made partly of metal and partly of silicone or other plastic materials. Nitinol is a component of many of the combination stents. The metal in the stent provides strength and helps reduce migration, while the plastic material provides contiguous coverage and helps maintain its shape.

SPECIFIC FEATURES OF SOME COMMONLY USED STENTS

The two most commonly used balloon-expandable metallic stents are the Palmaz stent and the Strecker stent. The Palmaz stent (Johnson & Johnson, New Brunswick, NJ, and Interventional Systems, Warren, NJ) is reportedly the device used most commonly in children, in part, because of its small size. The stent consists of a 150-μm diameter slotted stainless steel mesh tube. It is available in lengths ranging from 10 to 40 mm. A balloon 6 to 10 mm in diameter fits inside the stent for manual expansion by as much as 6 to 12 mm. An appropriate size for expansion in children is 8 mm for the trachea and 6 mm for the bronchus. After balloon expansion, the stent ceases to exert outward pressure on the airway wall. The stent has been used in primary tracheomalacia or bronchomalacia, external compression of the trachea or bronchi, and collapse of the trachea or bronchi from previous surgery. Occasionally, it needs to be re-expanded, particularly after a violent coughing fit. The Strecker stent is made of a tantalum filament that is fashioned into a cylindrical wire mesh. The stent is flexible, whether compressed or expanded. When expanded, the stent does not change in length. The Strecker stent is 2 to 4 cm long and can be expanded by 8 to 11 mm. This stent has been used successfully in patients with tracheobronchial obstruction.

Specific examples of the SEMS include the Gianturco-Z (William Cook, Bjaeverskov, Denmark), the Wallstent (Boston

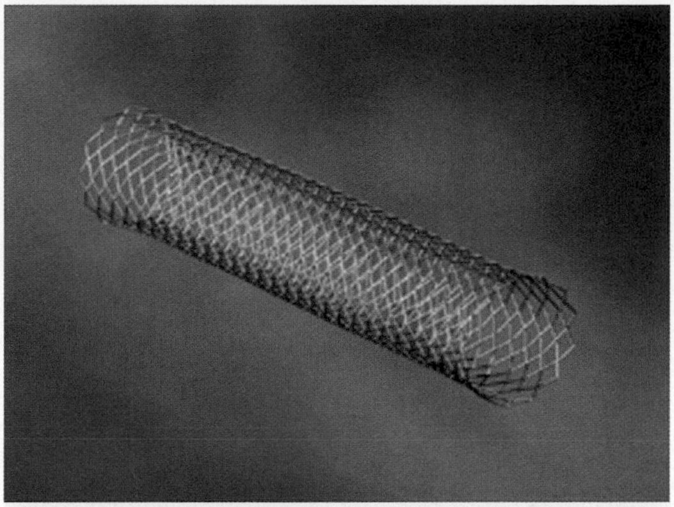

Figure 56-1. Uncovered Wallstent.

Scientific Corporation, Natick, MA), and the Ultraflex stent (Boston Scientific Corporation, Natick, MA). The Gianturco-Z is composed of 460-μm stainless steel filaments that are arranged in a zigzag configuration. The diameter of the stent when expanded is 15 to 40 mm.[5] The stent is available in 2- and 2.5-cm lengths. In its original design, it has metal hooks to prevent migration. The Gianturco-Z stent has been used to expand the tracheobronchial region in benign disease (e.g., posterior anastomotic strictures, tracheal stenosis, and tracheobronchomalacia). The stent exerts adequate radial force and does not shorten when deployed. It does have a tendency to spring forward if released too quickly. Complications are sometimes reported, including breakdown or unraveling of the stent and fatal hemoptysis after erosion into the pulmonary artery.

The Wallstent (originally the Schneider stent) is a stainless steel device composed of approximately 15 to 20 braided (100-μm diameter) filaments (Fig. 56-1). The filaments are arranged in a crisscross fashion to form a cylindrical mesh. Stent diameters range from 6 to 25 mm; lengths range from 2 to 7 cm. The stent exerts adequate radial force and is flexible. However, it can shorten to 20% to 40% of its original size on deployment. An important advantage of using the Wallstent is the ability one has to cut small openings into the mesh when the stent traverses bronchial openings. A disadvantage is that it changes length whenever it is compressed, potentially causing scars and stenosis at its edges.

Stents made of Nitinol (e.g., Nitinol, InStent, and Ultraflex stent) are thermally triggered and change shape in response to temperature changes (Marmen effect).[6] The Nitinol wire is heated, made into a helical shape, and then cooled for deployment. With release into the target site, the high body temperature causes the stent to coil back into its original helical shape. Alternatively, a current of 1.5 to 3 A or 3 to 5 V can be applied to the stent for 1 to 2 seconds until it reaches a temperature of 40°C, causing it to convert to the fully expanded state. Ultraflex stents are configured such that the wire backbone is perpendicular to the airway wall, which prevents substantial shortening or lengthening with changes in airway width and lends considerable stability to the stent (Fig. 56-2).

Silicone Stents

The Dumon stent (Boston Medical Products, Westborough, MA) is a cylindrical silicone stent with external studs that are

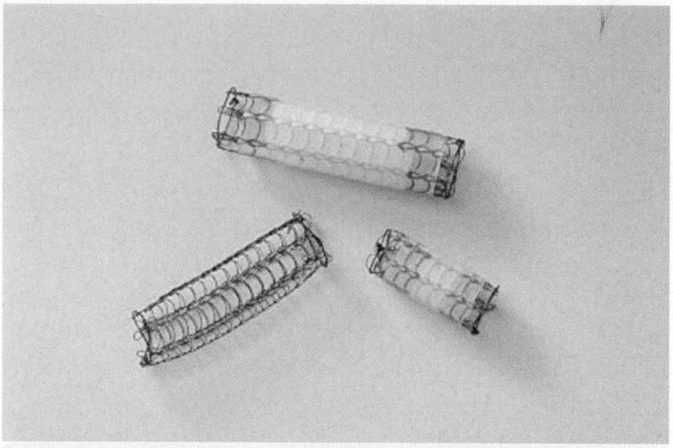

A

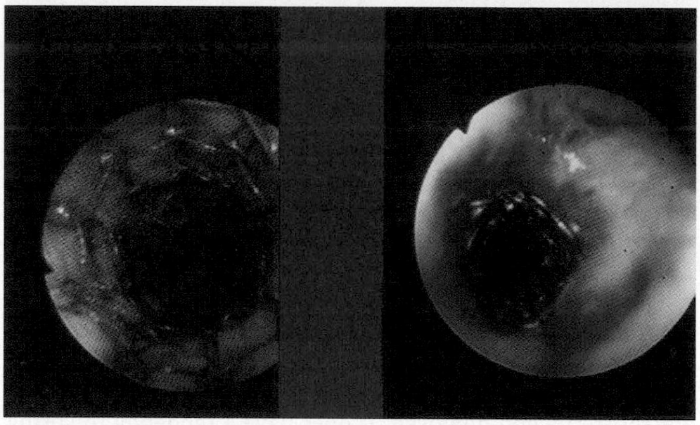

B

Figure 56-2. Ultraflex stents.

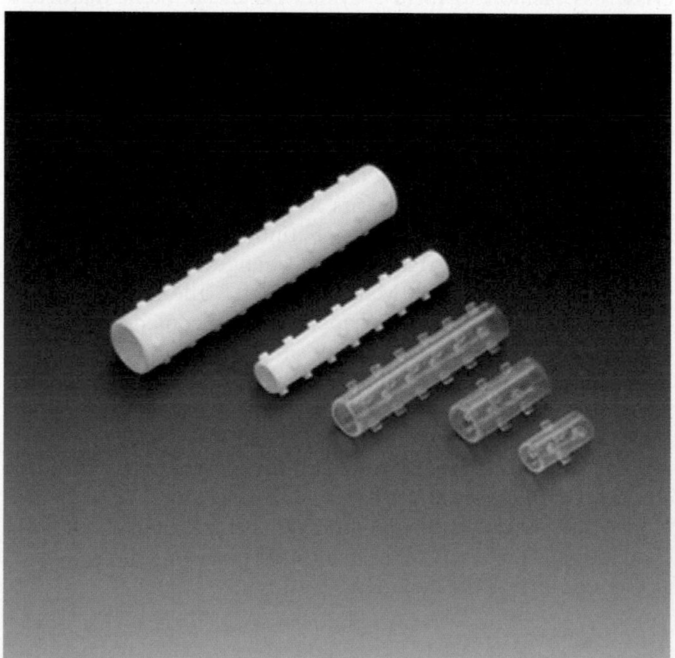

Figure 56-3. Dumon stents.

placed at regular intervals to prevent migration and limit contact with the airway wall, thereby reducing mucosal ischemia (Fig. 56-3). Several other varieties of silicone stents are currently available from Hood (Hood Laboratories, Pembroke, MA) (Figs. 56-4 and 56-5) in the United States and other manufacturers worldwide that have slightly different types of posts or rings to reduce migration. All these silicone stents are less expensive than metallic stents, are available in many sizes, and even can be custom manufactured within a few days. Y stents adjusted to cover the distal trachea and both mainstem bronchi are also available from most of these manufacturers and can be custom made with respect to sizes and angles. Once placed in the airway, the stent can be adjusted with a forceps and bronchoscope.

The Montgomery T-tube, which was introduced in the mid-1960s to support the trachea after laryngotracheoplasty (Fig. 56-6), also can be used for a number of stenting applications. In its original form, the device was an uncuffed silicone

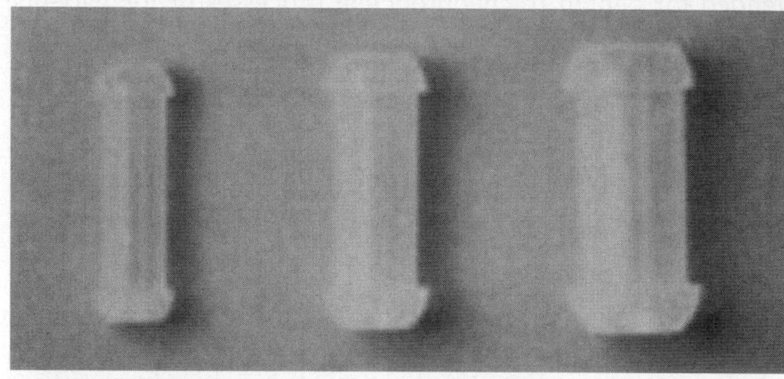

A

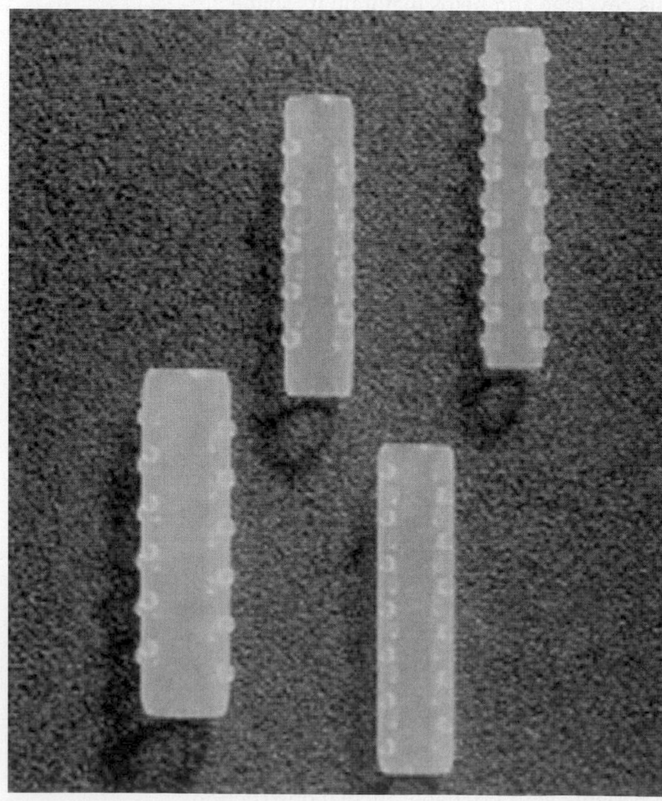

B

Figure 56-4. Hood stents.

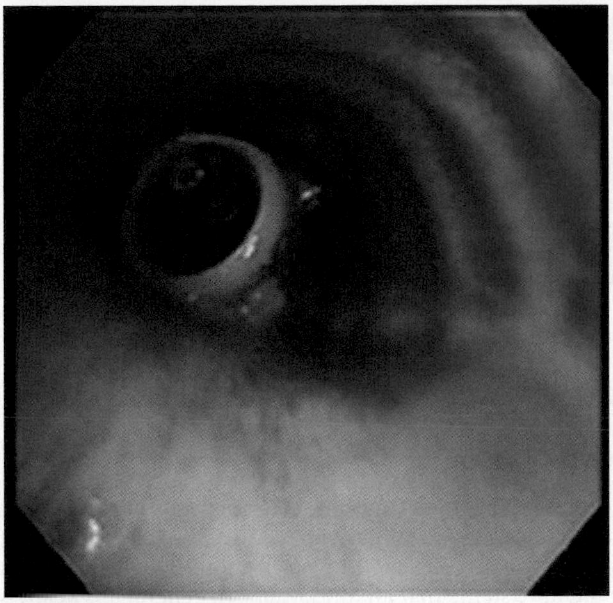

Figure 56-5. Hood stent in bronchus.

T-tube that was inserted with the long limb in the distal trachea, a short limb in the proximal trachea (or in some patients even through the vocal cords), and the T limb projecting through the tracheostomy stoma. Several modifications have been made in the original design to allow for a proximal cuff and other extras, such as a T-Y stent. The T-tube is supplied in sizes ranging from 4.5 to 16 mm (external diameter) and can be custom made as well. Smaller sizes (4.5–8 mm in external diameter) are available for pediatric use.

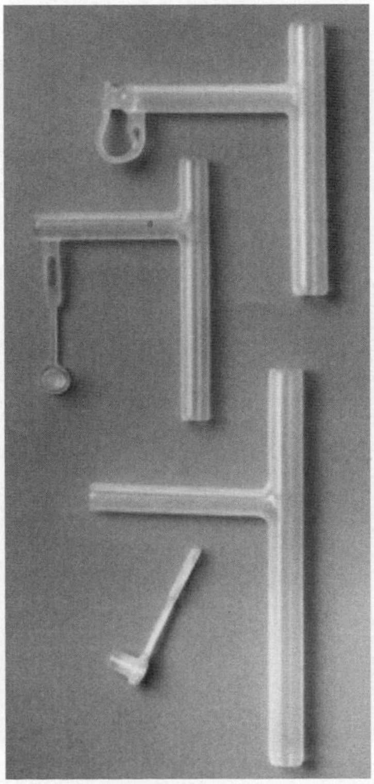

Figure 56-6. Montgomery T-tubes.

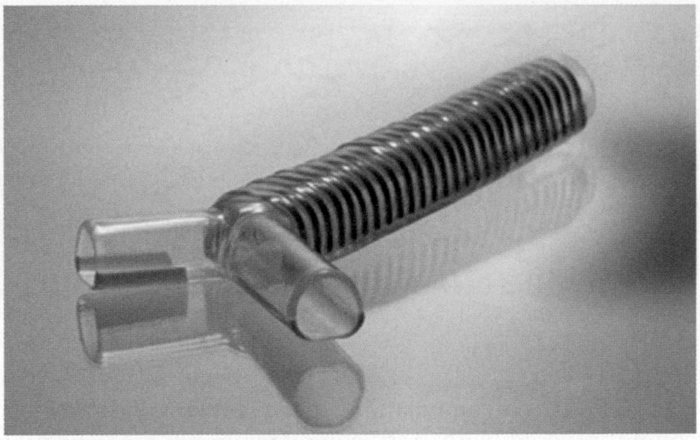

Figure 56-7. Dynamic Y stent.

Other plastic and combination stents include the Reynder stent (Reynder's Medical Supply, Lennik, Belgium), a cylindrical silicone prosthesis that is more rigid than a regular silicone tube but requires a special introducer and a bronchoscope for placement. The Dynamic stent (Rusch AG, Duluth, GA) is a silicone Y stent with anterior and lateral walls that are reinforced with metal to simulate the tracheal wall. Special forceps are available for insertion within the rigid laryngoscope (Fig. 56-7). The Polyflex (Rusch AG, Duluth, GA) is a self-expandable stent made of polyester wire mesh within layers of silicone (Fig. 56-8). Essentially, this is a silicone stent that can be deployed with flexible bronchoscopy, but rigid bronchoscopy is required for removal. Novastent (Novadis, Saint-Victoret, France) is a thin silicone sheet that contains a small metallic hoop of Nitinol alloy. The silicone bands on the ends are designed to prevent migration.

The AERO™ stent (manufactured by MERIT ENDOTEK™, a division of Merit Medical Systems, Inc., South Jordan, Utah) is another recent addition to the family of composite stents

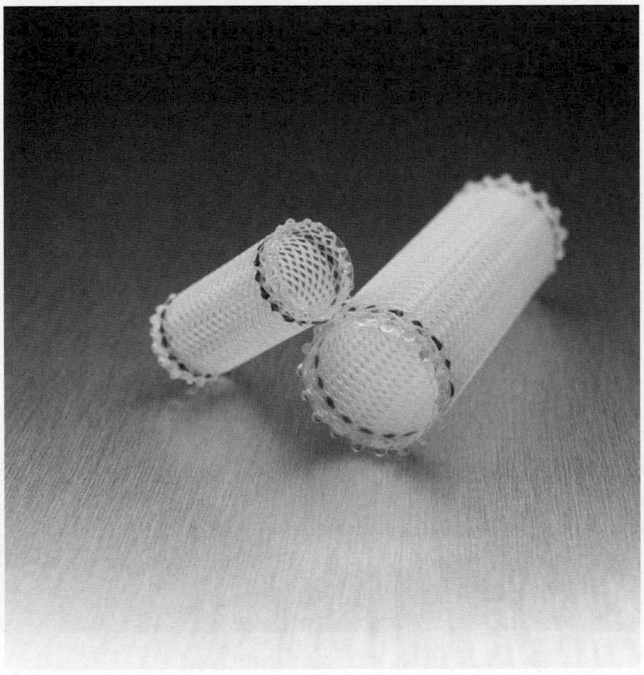

Figure 56-8. Polyflex stents.

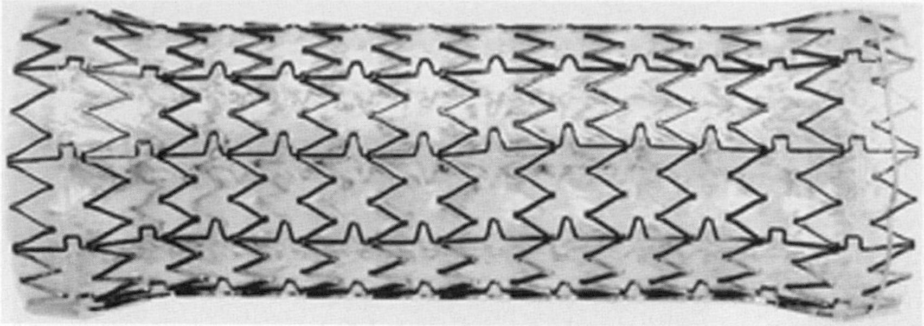

Figure 56-9. AERO™ Tracheobronchial stent system. Manufactured by MERIT ENDOTEK™, a division of Merit Medical Systems, Inc., South Jordan, Utah.

(Fig. 56-9). It is a combination stent made of a Nitinol metal scaffold covered with a silicone-containing biocompatible membrane to minimize the possibility of tissue ingrowth and granuloma formation. The stent does not foreshorten on delivery, and the hydrophilic coating on the inner lumen of the stent minimizes the possibility of mucous adherence and accumulation.

Although we have attempted to review most of the stents that are or have been on the market, one should take account that additional stents are constantly invented and manufactured and the companies making them are bought and sold to larger device companies consistent with the observation that most do not solve all current clinical problems.

PREPROCEDURE ASSESSMENT

Patients should have a chest CT scan for identification of the lesion and measurement of the diameter of the bronchus below and above the area of obstruction, as well as the distance between the desired distal and proximal ends of the stent (Fig. 56-10). The status of the lesion is also assessed via bronchoscopy.

STENT PLACEMENT TECHNIQUE

Stent Selection

The most important factor in selecting an appropriate stent is the indication. Patients with benign disorders and cancer patients who are expected to survive longer than 1 to 2 years should have stents that are removable. In general it is ill advised to place a SEMS for nearly any benign condition. The reasoning is that after a few weeks, SEMS incorporate in the tissues, are quite difficult (although possible) to remove, and may perforate into adjacent structures with time.

Patients who undergo stenting for palliation of advanced cancer are candidates for covered stents only, preferably ones that do not migrate readily. The anatomic position of the lesion sometimes dictates the type of stent to be used. For example, a Y stent or a Dynamic stent is required for lesions affecting the carina (Fig. 56-11). It is currently our practice to place either SEMS or combination stents for all malignant cases. A special example is the malignant inoperable tracheoesophageal fistula. Our preference is to stent the esophagus first with an SEMS or combination stent because this usually solves the problem.

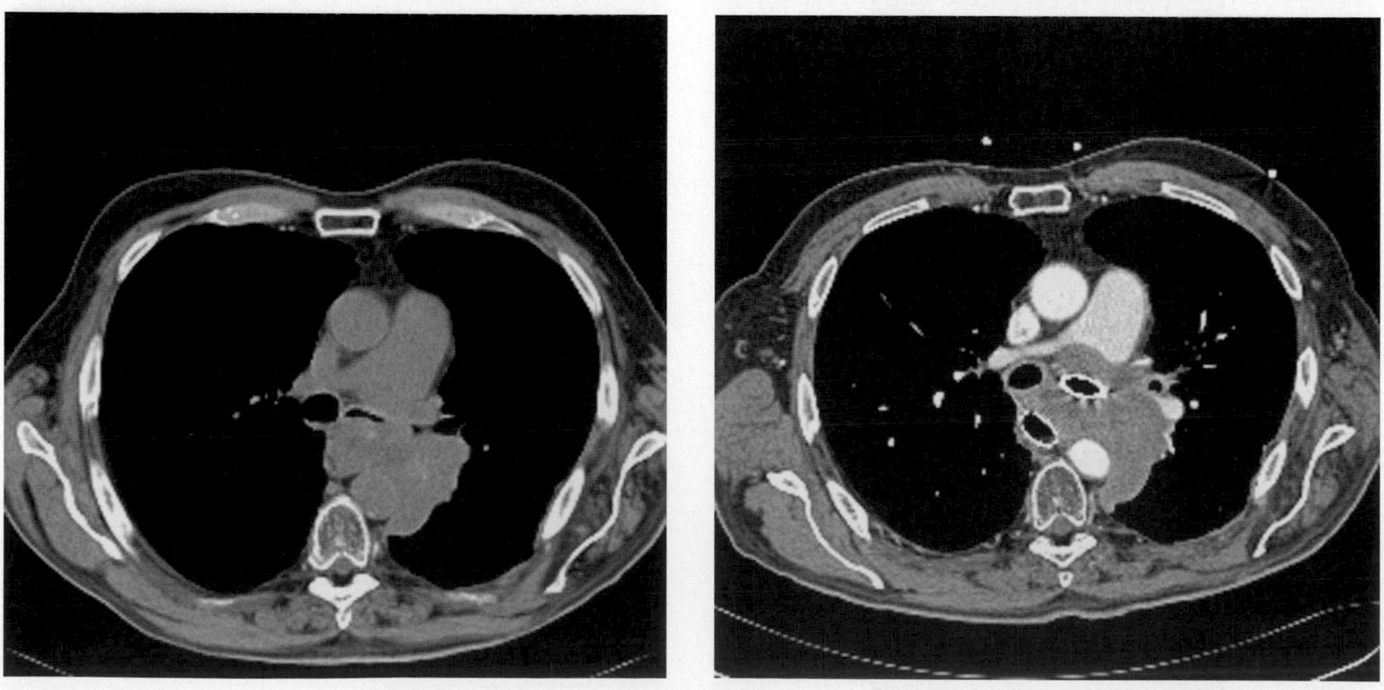

A B

Figure 56-10. CT scanning is used to identify the lesion and size the stent. *A*. Before deployment. *B*. After deployment.

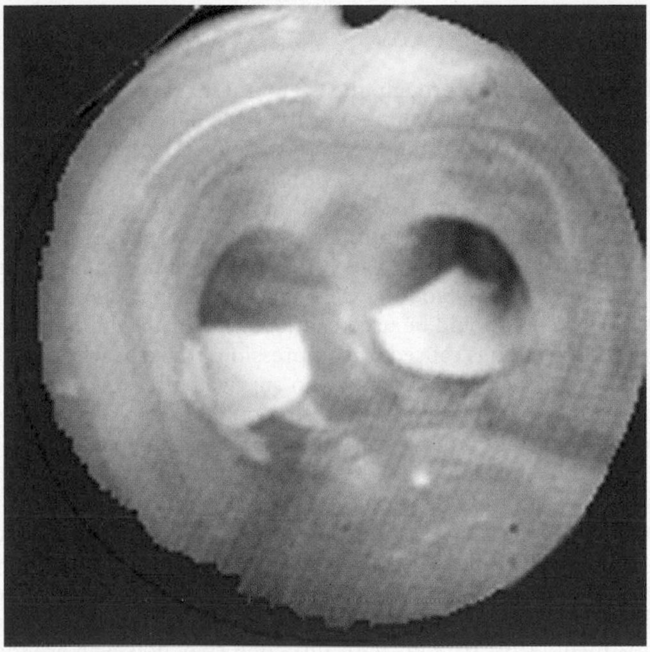

Figure 56-11. Dynamic stent in situ.

If the problem persists, the airway also can be stented with an equivalent stent.

Finally, size matters. Silicone stents generally are thicker than metallic stents and are more likely to get obstructed with secretions in patients who require a smaller sized stent. This problem is encountered more frequently with bronchial applications, such as the difficult situation of stenting a distal short stricture without obstructing other bronchi in locations such as the bronchus intermedius. For some patients, there is no good solution, and surgeons should consider cutting a combination stent to the correct size to customize the stent for the patient. However, this should be considered only by an expert and under patient consent because this approach is not sanctioned by the FDA. The new proliferation of 3D printing may ultimately allow for truly customized stents.

Ideally, the surgeon placing the stent should foresee the potential complications and have available a variety of options for managing immediate complications. Thus, in our opinion, expertise with rigid bronchoscopy is mandatory, and a team experienced in the management of airway disorders is very helpful. Patients who require rigid bronchoscopy for stent placement must have general anesthesia, whereas those undergoing stent placement via flexible bronchoscopy do not always require intubation but do require IV sedation. It is our preferred practice to perform stent placement with the support of an anesthetist to keep all options open.

Fluoroscopy is quite helpful in stent placement but not absolutely mandatory. Most stents are marked with radiopaque markers to show distal, proximal, and midstent locations, which can be identified when stents are placed under fluoroscopic guidance. Guidewires usually can be used to guide most stents into the correct position for deployment by a variety of mechanisms depending on the stent that has been selected. A guidewire with a flexible tip is preferred because it is less likely to perforate the bronchus. It is best, if possible, to deploy the stent such that the middle of the stent is in line with the middle of the shelf of obstruction or narrowing (Fig. 56-12). This reduces

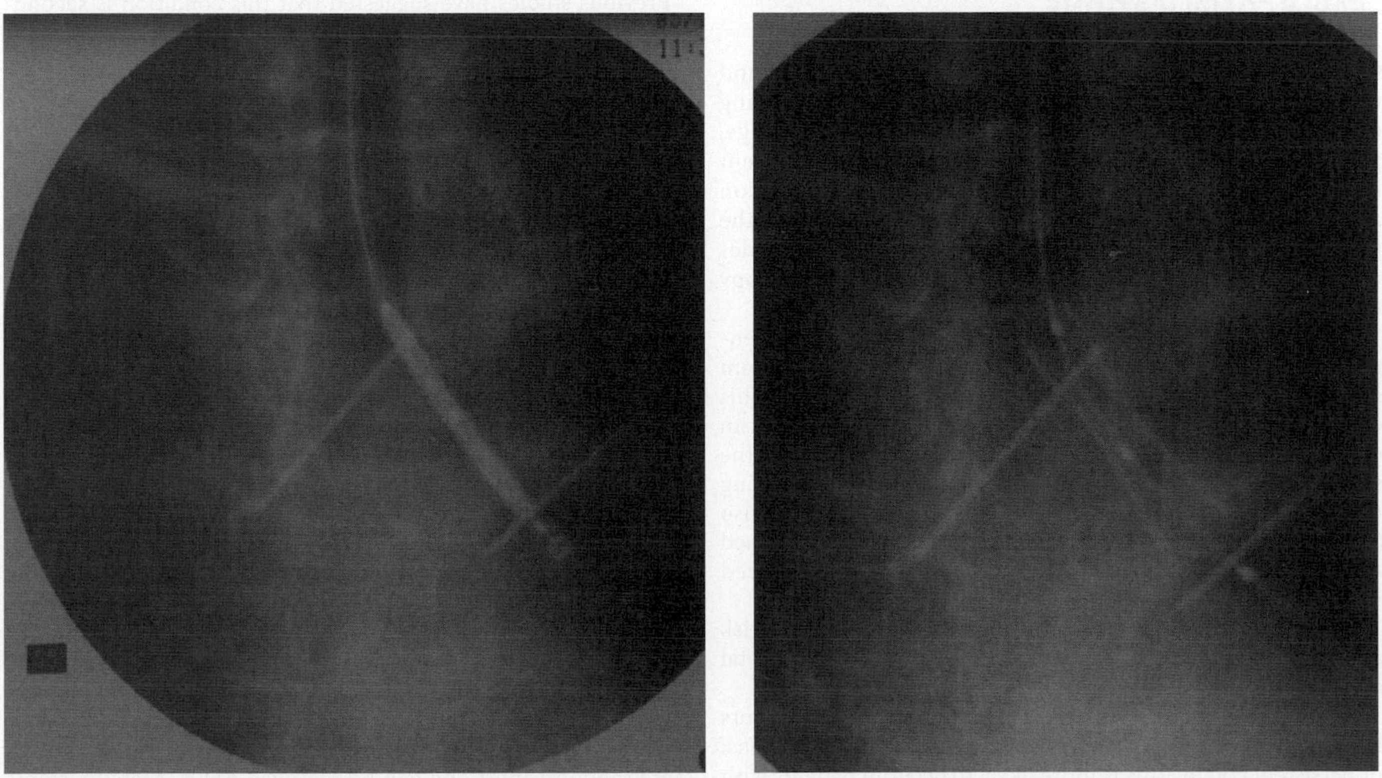

A B

Figure 56-12. Deployment under fluoroscopic guidance.

the risk of migration because the stricture itself will hold the stent in place. Silicone stents usually require specific delivery devices for deployment through the rigid bronchoscope which exist even for large Y stents. These cost approximately $10,000 but are useful to have in expert centers.

Once the stent is positioned in the airway, it can be pulled back using a biopsy forceps. This can be done by either rigid or flexible bronchoscopy (utilizing "Rat Tooth" forceps). It is far easier to place the stent slightly distal to its target location and then pull the stent back into desired position rather than attempt to push the stent into position. It is important to confirm the position of the stent with bronchoscopy, but we do not recommend using an adult bronchoscope for testing any stent with a diameter of less than 12 mm because of the risk of it becoming dislodged.

Once the stent is in position, the patient should get a chest radiograph followed by bronchoscopy within the next 2 to 4 weeks or earlier if the patient has new symptoms. We recommend a perioperative course of antibiotics as well as daily humidification to reduce the accumulation of inspissated, concreted secretions. Mucomyst and DNase may be added as necessary, as well as steroids, when airway trauma is suspected during stent deployment.

T-tube type stents (and these exist as T and T-Y) are usually placed through a tracheostomy. They can and should be custom made for the patient based on CT measurements to maximize the diameter. The distal limb is placed first with a rigid bronchoscope or flexible bronchoscope through an LMA for observation at the cords. Then the proximal limb is placed and straightened. These should be capped and carefully cleaned by removing the stent according to a specific schedule.

EARLY COMPLICATIONS

Cough is a common side effect after stent placement and usually disappears. It responds well to codeine-containing elixirs. Excessive coughing can cause the stent to dislodge, particularly when there is no stricture shelf to hold the stent in place. Although generally not dangerous, stent migration and dislodgment are quite traumatic and terrifying to the patient. Cough also can indicate an obstructed or inadequately placed stent and may require a repeat bronchoscopy for assessment.

Obstruction of the bronchial orifices is another potential complication of stent placement and usually results from incorrect preoperative estimation of length or diameter. This condition is often asymptomatic, although on occasion it can cause localized wheezing as air passes through the mesh of the stent. The stent may become impacted with secretions, giving rise to dyspnea owing to mucous plugging. Patients are also at increased risk of developing pneumonia. The malpositioned stent should be removed and replaced with a correctly sized stent to avoid further complications.

Iatrogenic perforation of the airway wall is always a risk and warrants caution and careful follow-up. It is often a fatal complication.

Stent migration may occur, particularly if undersized stents have been used, and can lead to airway obstruction, infections, or persistent cough. This is more likely to occur in patients with malacia or other nonstricture diseases, where the stent is not held firmly in place.

LATE COMPLICATIONS

Tumor regrowth through the stent mesh causing recurrent obstruction is more common with malignant processes and can be avoided by using a covered stent. Proximal migration of the stent is more common with fixed-diameter stents (e.g., the Palmaz stent) and is observed more often in patients who receive radiation and chemotherapy after stent placement.

Rigid metal stents (e.g., Strecker or Palmaz stents) can erode into nearby blood vessels causing hemoptysis. For this reason, stents should be used cautiously, if at all, when the airway obstruction is caused by compression from a nearby vessel. We have treated two patients who survived after developing a fistula from an airway stent into the pulmonary artery merely by placing a pulmonary artery stent to cover the hole.[7]

Although aneurysmal disease, previous aortic surgery, and neoplasm are the most common causes of aortobronchial fistula, chronic inflammation from an indwelling endobronchial stent, as well as bronchomalacia from recurrent infection, may predispose to the formation of fistulas. Formal graft repair of the aorta with or without pulmonary resection is the classic treatment. Most patients with this condition, however, are too high risk for such an extensive procedure. Although there is risk of infection, endovascular exclusion of the fistula provides a safe and effective alternative for high-risk patients.

Granuloma formation at either end of the stent or growing through the interstices of the stent is the most common complication of expandable metallic stent placement and probably results from an inflammatory response. These granulomata can be ablated using the neodymium:yttrium-aluminum-garnet laser therapy delivered by means of a flexible bronchoscope.

Halitosis is a distressing and difficult complication to resolve. Previous studies have suggested that this condition is secondary to chronic bacterial infection of the stent. Madden et al.[8] found that patients with halitosis usually have covered stents, which may provide a suitable environment for bacterial growth and prevent effective mucociliary clearance.

The cause of chronic chest pain is not fully understood, but it could be attributed to the presence of a foreign body (i.e., the stent) within the airway lumen leading to chronic irritation or polychondritis of the tracheal rings.

SUMMARY

Recent years have seen a proliferation of stents available for airway application. However, no single stent is perfect for all indications. It is therefore important to develop some expertise with various types of stents rather than placing the same brand in every patient notwithstanding the patient's diagnosis. Stent placement can provide immediate relief of symptoms for the acute management of tracheobronchial obstruction irrespective of cause and demonstrates long-term improvement in quality of life. It is one of many endoluminal therapies of the airways, and those interested in placing stents should become educated about alternative therapies as well as potential complications. Of the three major types of stents (i.e., silicone, metal, and combination), silicone stents are the most inert and can be removed easily. Metallic stents are very easy to deploy but can cause long-term irreversible complications. Since the ideal tracheobronchial stent suitable

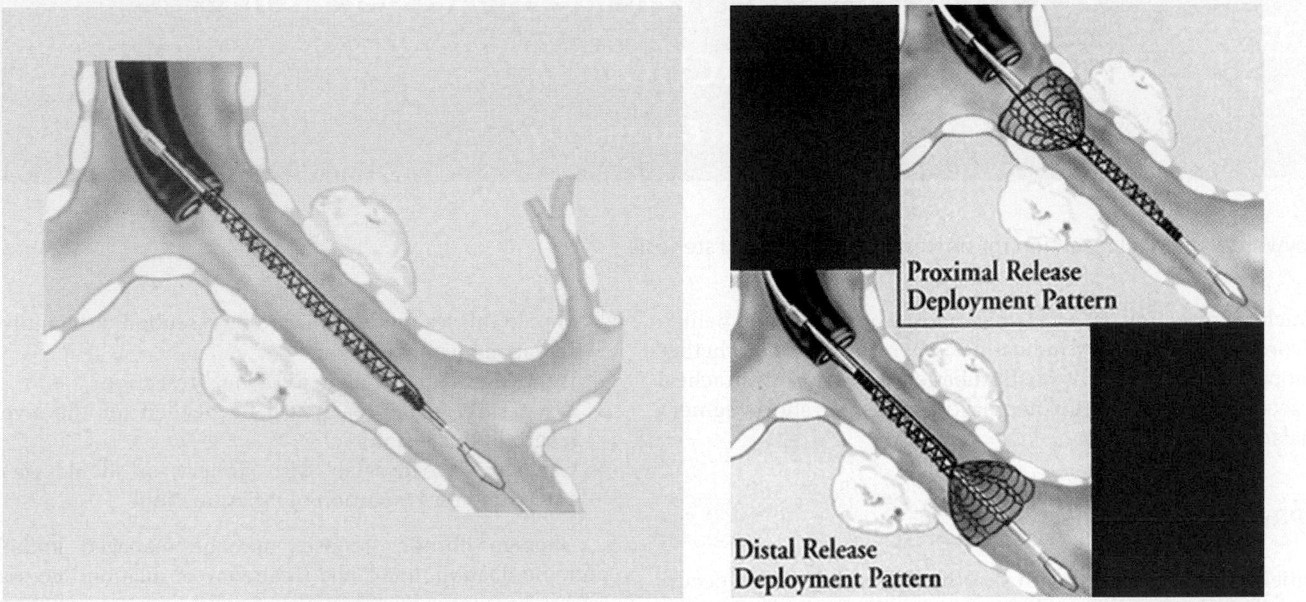

A B

Figure 56-13. Ultraflex stent deployment system.

for all purposes is yet to be developed, selection continues to be based on patient factors, surgeon preference, and characteristics of the underlying pathology.

CASE HISTORY

A 62-year-old man with a history of locally advanced lung cancer (stage IIIB) previously treated with chemotherapy and radiation therapy presented with dysphagia and dyspnea. On examination, he had left-sided wheezing. His chest CT scan demonstrated severe narrowing of the left mainstem bronchus and esophagus. Bronchoscopy confirmed these findings. He underwent placement of an Ultraflex covered endobronchial stent and an Ultraflex esophageal stent with resolution of symptoms, enabling him to tolerate additional chemotherapy (Fig. 56-13).

EDITOR'S COMMENT

Airway stents differ from vascular stents because ironically while the blood can be thinned, secretions cannot be effectively thinned. Therefore, the positioning of stents is limited to the trachea, mainstem bronchi, and perhaps the bronchus intermedius. While it is technically possible to stent individual bronchi, usually the stent gets plugged up, causes too much coughing, or becomes easily dislodged. Patients with malignancy for some reason do much better with stents than patients with benign diseases, underscoring the temporary efficacy of stents. In tracheobronchomalacia, for example, stents can be used to establish the diagnosis and confirm whether or not the patient is a candidate for tracheal surgery, but most will not tolerate these stents for life. Some patients may not be candidates for stents and instead benefit from life-long tracheostomy.

—Raphael Bueno

References

1. Sterioff S. Etymology of the world "stent". *Mayo Clin Proc.* 1997;72:377–379.
2. Dumon JF. A dedicated tracheobronchial stent. *Chest.* 1990;97:328–332.
3. Wright K, Walace S, Charnsangavej C, et al. Percutaneous endovascular stents: an experimental evaluation. *Radiology.* 1985;156:69–72.
4. Stohr S, Bollinger C. Stents in the management of malignant airway obstruction. *Monaldi Arch Chest Dis.* 1999;54:264–268.
5. Duprat G Jr, Wright KC, Charnsangavej C, et al. Self-expanding metallic stents for small vessels: an experimental evaluation. *Radiology.* 1987;162: 469–472.
6. Wayman C, Shimizu K. The shape memory (Marmen) effect in alloys. *Metal Sci J.* 1972;6:175–183.
7. Davison BD, Ring DH, Bueno R, et al. Endovascular stent-graft repair of a pulmonary artery-bronchial fistula. *J Vasc Intervent Radiol.* 2003;14: 929–932.
8. Madden BP, Loke TK, Sheth AC. Do expandable metallic airway stents have a role in the management of patients with benign tracheobronchial disease? *Ann Thorac Surg.* 2006;82:274–278.

57 Techniques of Tracheal Resection and Reconstruction

Thomas K. Waddell and Karl Fabian L. Uy

Keywords: Tracheal resection for benign disease, tracheal stenosis

Tracheal resection is performed most commonly for benign disorders. The primary indication is fibrotic stenosis, whether idiopathic, traumatic, or postintubation. Occasionally, tracheal resection is indicated for neoplastic disease or short-segment malacia.

PRESENTATION

Patients usually present with shortness of breath, which occurs initially only on exertion but in more advanced cases it may even occur at rest. There is often a history of treatment with numerous bronchodilators or steroids for presumed asthma. Occasionally, previous endotracheal intubation or tracheostomy has prompted imaging studies and an earlier referral to a thoracic surgeon. It is important in the history to delve into any previous airway interventions, such as tracheostomy, previous intubations, as well as previously diagnosed malignancies, especially of the head and neck. On examination, patients generally are comfortable at rest but manifest stridor, which usually is inspiratory in nature but occasionally expiratory. Even with severe tracheal stenosis, patients still may have acceptable oxygen saturation. Symptoms usually do not manifest until there is quite a significant degree of stenosis, on the order of a residual 5-mm lumen.

PREOPERATIVE ASSESSMENT

Imaging is a necessary part of the preoperative preparation. Except for patients with acute airway compromise, imaging studies always can be done before the endoscopic assessment or operative intervention. Detailed CT scans of the neck and chest are performed routinely (Fig. 57-1), with three-dimensional reconstruction, if possible (Fig. 57-2). These studies aid in planning for airway management and endoscopic assessment and warn of possible surprises, such as severe distal tracheal or bilateral proximal bronchial stenoses, which may not show on x-rays.

Except for the extremely fragile patient, most will be able to tolerate a tracheal resection if it does not require a thoracotomy. The endoscopic assessment therefore is pursued with a possible resection foremost in mind. This evaluation should be performed independent of surgery because repeat dilations of cicatricial stenoses can delay or obviate the need for surgery altogether.

The bronchoscopy should be conducted in the operating theater, with both flexible and rigid bronchoscopes of varying sizes available, as well as dilators and equipment for tracheostomy or tracheal-tube (T-tube) insertion. The questions to be answered include:

1. Should this lesion be managed by resection or by more conservative means?
2. Is the lesion amenable to a tracheal resection?
3. What surgical approach will be needed for the level and length of this lesion?
4. Can we proceed safely with surgery, or should we allow some time for resolution of inflammation?

Benign fibrotic stenoses may be managed initially by periodic dilation, but if the frequency of dilation necessary to relieve symptoms becomes unacceptable, a resection should be performed. Naturally, for neoplastic disease, resection should be considered as soon as the diagnosis is made. Tracheal resections are always done electively and should be well planned. If the stricture is secondary to intubation or trauma, enough time should be given for the scar to stabilize and assume its final length, a period of 3 to 6 months. If the initial bronchoscopy shows significant inflammation, which is often due to pooling of infected secretions beyond a point of obstruction, the obstruction should be relieved by dilation or bypassed by a tracheostomy or T-tube. In all instances, inflammation should be reduced to the lowest achievable level to avoid anastomotic complications. Oral steroids have been used occasionally to reduce inflammation (but should be reduced in dosage prior to surgery). In the unusual situation where the obstructing neoplasm cannot be bypassed with a tracheostomy, the difficult decision must be made whether to proceed with tracheal resection in the presence of a tracheitis or first core out the tumor. We favor the latter approach rather than risk an anastomotic disruption.

TECHNIQUE

Position

In most situations, the patient is placed supine with the neck hyperextended and a deflatable shoulder bag in place. Arms may be tucked in or abducted. If abducted, 45 degrees is preferable so that the surgeon can stand above or below the arm.

Endoscopy

The surgery always should begin with a full endoscopic assessment, including assessment of vocal cord function and measurement of the length of the lesion. The choice of incision and type of operation depend predominantly on the level and length of the lesion.

Airway Management

Orotracheal intubation is the usual manner of airway control, with dilation as needed to accommodate the usually small

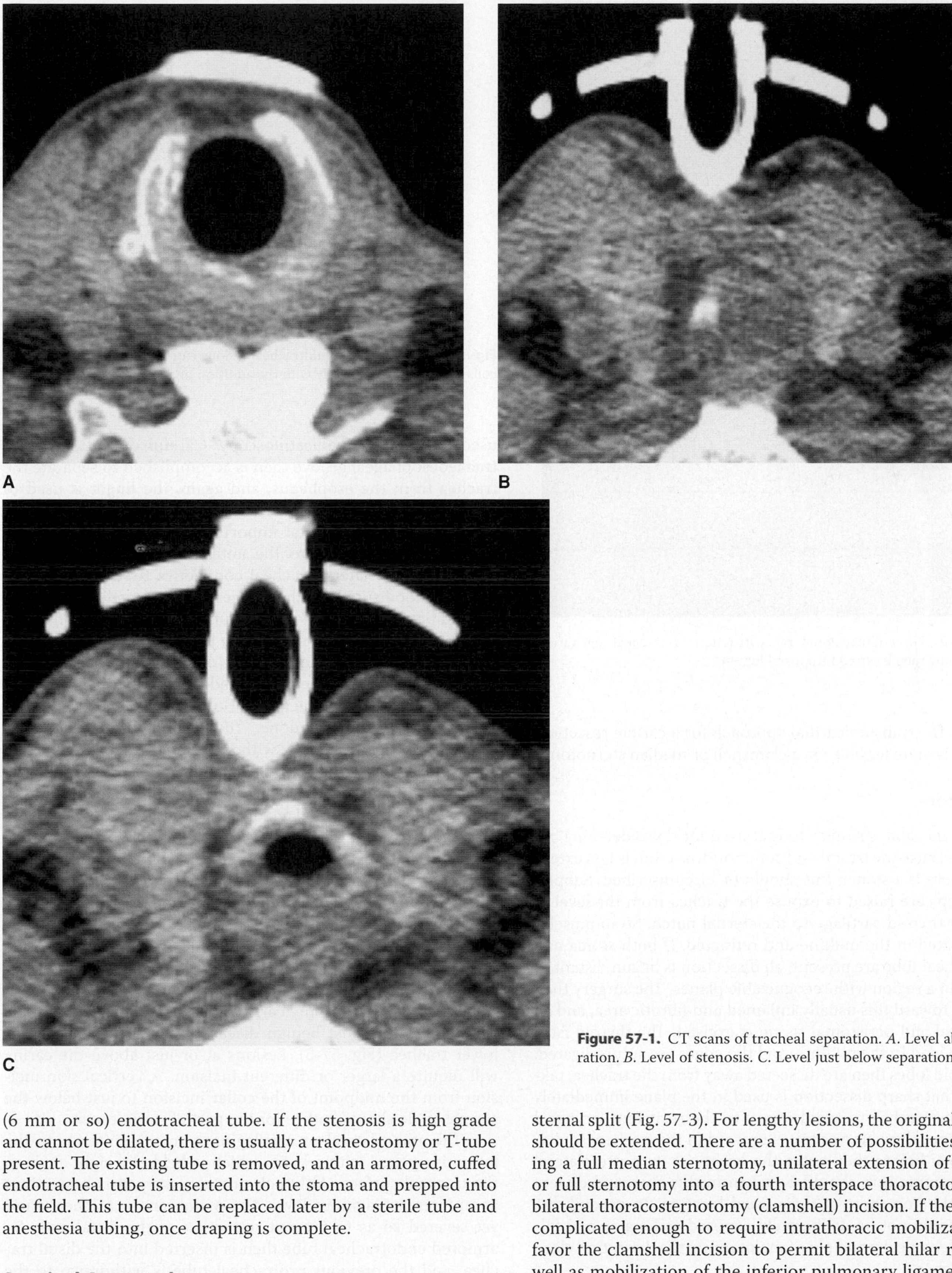

Figure 57-1. CT scans of tracheal separation. *A.* Level above separation. *B.* Level of stenosis. *C.* Level just below separation.

(6 mm or so) endotracheal tube. If the stenosis is high grade and cannot be dilated, there is usually a tracheostomy or T-tube present. The existing tube is removed, and an armored, cuffed endotracheal tube is inserted into the stoma and prepped into the field. This tube can be replaced later by a sterile tube and anesthesia tubing, once draping is complete.

Surgical Approach

Upper and midtracheal lesions can be approached via a low-collar incision, occasionally with the addition of a partial sternal split (Fig. 57-3). For lengthy lesions, the original incision should be extended. There are a number of possibilities, including a full median sternotomy, unilateral extension of a partial or full sternotomy into a fourth interspace thoracotomy, or a bilateral thoracosternotomy (clamshell) incision. If the lesion is complicated enough to require intrathoracic mobilization, we favor the clamshell incision to permit bilateral hilar release as well as mobilization of the inferior pulmonary ligaments. This approach, that is, neck incision plus clamshell, permits management of all except low tracheal and carinal lesions, which are best handled through a right posterolateral thoracotomy from

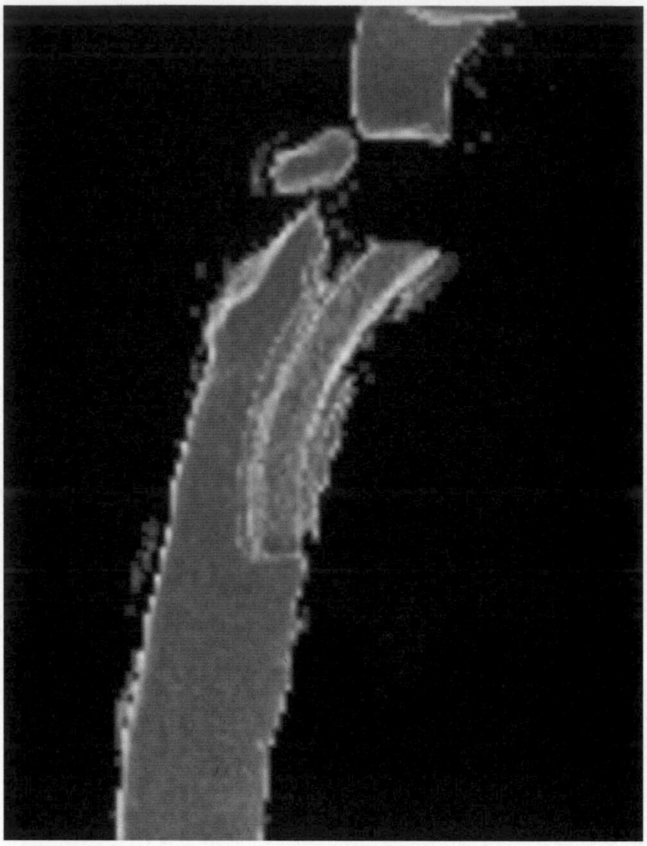

Figure 57-2. Three-dimensional reconstruction of tracheal separation. Tracheostomy tube inserted into distal lumen.

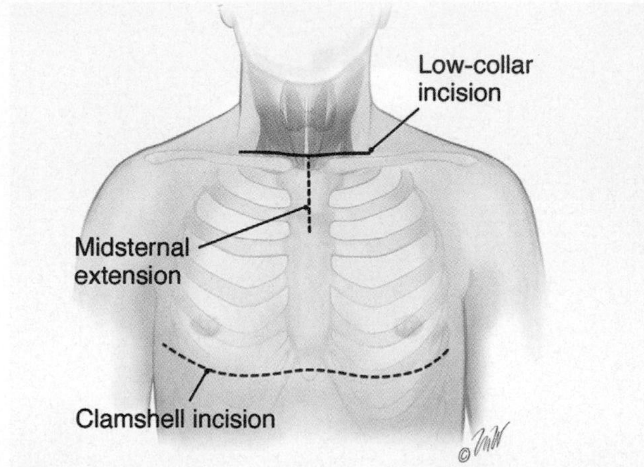

Figure 57-3. Upper and midtracheal lesions can be approached via a low-collar incision, occasionally with the addition of a partial sternal split.

the start. The transpericardial approach for a carinal resection, however, is quite feasible via a clamshell or median sternotomy.

Dissection

The neck incision is similar to that used for thyroidectomy but shorter because the lateral and superior dissection is less extensive. If there is a stoma, this should be circumscribed. Subplatysmal flaps are raised to expose the trachea from the level of the lower thyroid cartilage to the sternal notch. Strap muscles are separated in the midline and retracted. If both stoma and endotracheal tube are present, all dissection is begun distant to this site, in a region with recognizable planes. The surgery then proceeds toward this usually inflamed and fibrotic area, and all pretracheal and peristomal tissue is excised. The thyroid isthmus is divided in the midline, and the edges are suture-ligated. The thyroid lobes then are dissected away from the trachea, taking care that sharp dissection is used in the plane immediately next to the trachea to avoid injury to the recurrent laryngeal nerves. Since these nerves travel upward in the tracheoesophageal groove before they enter the larynx at its posterolateral aspect, extreme care should be taken in this area, and dissection should stop short of their usual location. In general, the nerves should not be deliberately exposed as long as one follows the technical principle of maintaining the dissection close to the trachea.

Once the trachea is exposed, the lesion is evaluated carefully. Mobilization of the anterior trachea is done by blunt finger dissection in the pretracheal space, similar to the technique used for cervical mediastinoscopy. Careful dissection in the tracheoesophageal groove then is accomplished to separate the trachea from the esophagus, and again, the finger is used to bluntly dissect the posterior tracheal plane downward into the mediastinum. It is of vital importance in tracheal surgery to limit these dissections to the anterior and posterior planes to preserve the lateral tracheal connective tissue because the tenuous blood supply to the trachea occurs mostly via laterally located branches (Fig. 57-4).[1] Circumferential dissection of the trachea should be done only at the level of the lesion and 1 to 2 mm beyond the planned margins of resection. These maneuvers should mobilize the trachea adequately so that it can be evaluated for extent of the lesion. Both external and endoscopic assessments should be done. The flexible bronchoscope is inserted through a partially withdrawn endotracheal tube, and using a small needle inserted through the anterior tracheal wall, the proximal and distal extents of the lesion are identified. All gross evidence of external and internal abnormalities should be resected. If a stoma is present, the bronchoscope still should be passed from above through the glottis, and the endotracheal tube in the field should be removed as needed for accurate evaluation. If possible, as it usually is, the stoma is resected along with the lesion.

At this stage of the operation, the surgeon must decide whether to pursue a partial sternal split, a full sternotomy, or a clamshell incision to complete the resection and reconstruction. A partial sternotomy carried just below the sternal angle is sufficient for most benign disease, even for lesions in the lower trachea (Fig. 57-5). Lesions at or just above the carina will require a larger or different incision. A vertical skin incision from the midpoint of the collar incision to just below the sternal angle should suffice for the partial sternotomy.

The anterolateral or cartilaginous trachea inferior to the lesion is opened with a knife, which is held at a right angle to the tracheal surface. Although not necessary, it is best to cut at an intercartilaginous level. The membranous trachea is not yet severed so as to prevent retraction of the distal end. An armored endotracheal tube then is inserted into the distal trachea, and the previous orotracheal tube is withdrawn to the level of the glottis but not removed. It is helpful to place a heavy silk tie through the tip of the endotracheal tube before this is withdrawn to facilitate its removal later in the operation. If a

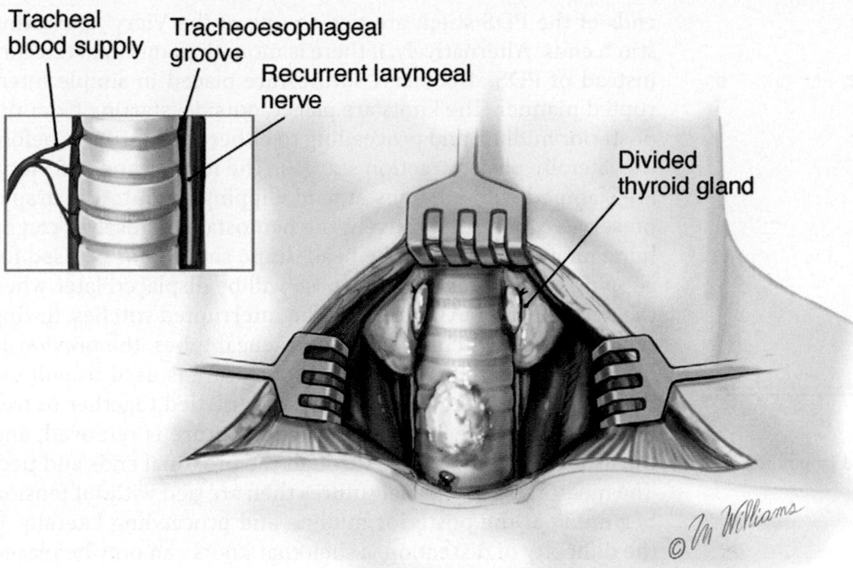

Figure 57-4. Dissection of the trachea should be limited to the anterior and posterior planes to preserve the lateral tracheal connective tissue because the blood supply to the trachea occurs mostly via laterally located branches.

stoma is present, the endotracheal tube is simply transferred to the distal trachea. The interior lumen of the trachea is inspected and confirmed to be grossly free of disease at the cut margin. The proximal margin then is identified in a similar fashion, and the cartilaginous trachea again is opened above this margin. The interior lumen is inspected once more to ensure freedom from gross disease. In this manner, if gross disease is identified at the margin proximally or distally, additional rings can be resected, always from the cartilaginous side only, and sparing the membranous portion to avoid retraction (Fig. 57-6).

Once the final levels are determined, a traction suture is placed at each midlateral position of the distal trachea. We usually use braided polyglactin 910 (Vicryl) 2-0 and apply these sutures around the second cartilage ring away from the cut edge. The needles are left in place. In the case of very proximal lesions, traction sutures may be placed in the midlateral cricoid, but preferably not through and through. The membranous trachea then is sharply transected. The same procedure is followed for the proximal end. Margins may be sent for frozen section as necessary for neoplastic disease.

When the posterior surface of the trachea is difficult to bluntly dissect from the esophagus, the distal end should be completely transected early on and the proximal trachea lifted for better visualization and dissection.

The adequacy of mobilization is assessed by deflating the shoulder bag and asking the anesthetist to flex the neck. Neck flexion is the most important maneuver for release of tension. The traction sutures are used to pull the tracheal edges together and estimate the degree of tension (Fig. 57-7). There is almost

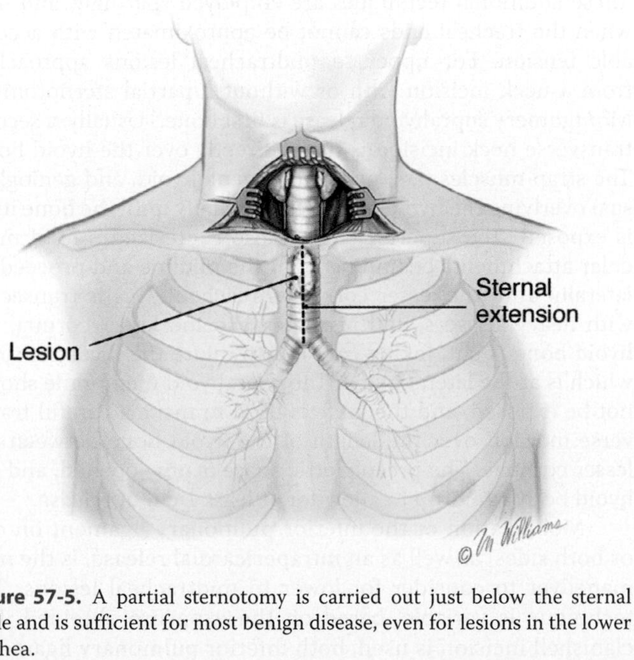

Figure 57-5. A partial sternotomy is carried out just below the sternal angle and is sufficient for most benign disease, even for lesions in the lower trachea.

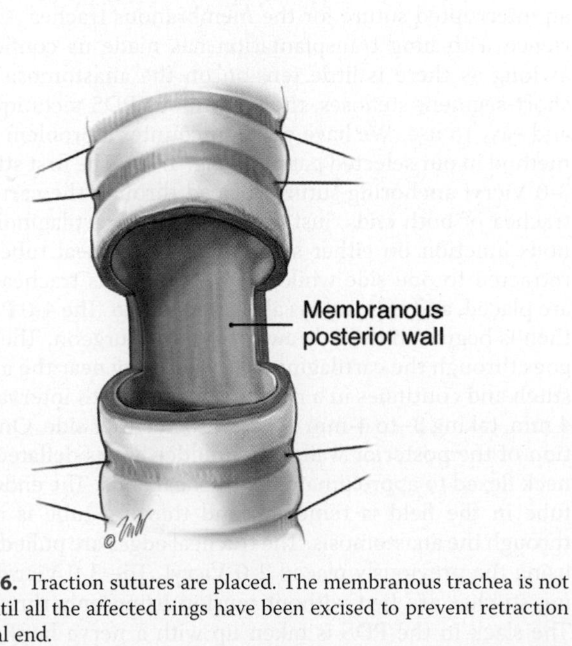

Figure 57-6. Traction sutures are placed. The membranous trachea is not severed until all the affected rings have been excised to prevent retraction of the distal end.

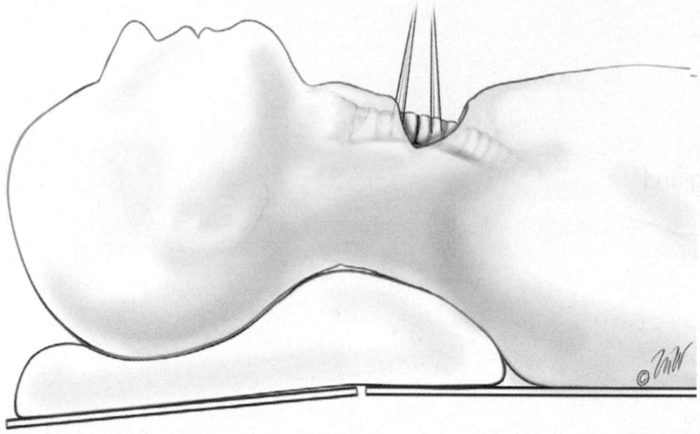

Figure 57-7. After resection, the traction sutures are used to pull the tracheal edges together and estimate the degree of tension.

invariably some tension on the anastomosis, but it should not be excessive. Unfortunately, save for experience and surgical judgment, there is no rule of thumb for determining how much tension is acceptable. If additional mobilization is needed, the shoulder bag is reinflated and additional anterior and posterior dissection is performed. If the level of tension is still unacceptable after maximal dissection, additional release maneuvers can be performed. These are fully described below.

The tracheal anastomosis can be done in a variety of ways, but one unvarying current standard is that the sutures have to be either absorbable sutures of high tensile strength such as Vicryl or polydioxanone (PDS) or nonabsorbable sutures of a nonreactive material such as stainless steel. The knots usually are placed outside the anastomosis, but with stainless steel, these also can be tied inside the lumen without fear of excessive granulation tissue formation. Steel has the advantage of forming a secure knot after only two throws if the knot is square. Hence the size of the intraluminal knot with fine wire is very small.[2]

Our favored technique is as follows: With the neck extended once more, we choose either a running 4-0 PDS or an interrupted suture for the membranous trachea. Our experience with lung transplantation has made us confident that as long as there is little tension on the anastomosis, as with short-segment stenoses, the continuous PDS technique is safe and easy to use. We have yet to encounter a problem with this method in our selected patients (Fig. 57-8). The first stitches are 3-0 Vicryl anchoring sutures placed through the cartilaginous trachea of both ends, just anterior to the cartilaginomembranous junction on either side. The endotracheal tube is easily retracted to one side while the membranous tracheal stitches are placed, and exposure is always adequate. The 4-0 PDS stitch then is begun on the side away from the surgeon. The first bite goes through the cartilaginous trachea very near the anchoring stitch and continues in a running fashion, with intervals of 3 to 4 mm, taking 3- to 4-mm deep bites on either side. On completion of the posterior wall, the shoulder bag is deflated and the neck flexed to approximate the tracheal ends. The endotracheal tube in the field is removed, and the oral tube is advanced through the anastomosis. The tracheal edges are pulled together using the previously placed 2-0 Vicryl. The 3-0 Vicryl anchoring stitches are tied without tension using only three throws. The slack in the PDS is taken up with a nerve hook, and the ends of the PDS stitch are tied to one of the Vicryl anchoring stitch ends. Alternatively, if there is more than minimal tension, instead of PDS, 4-0 Vicryl sutures are placed in simple interrupted manner. The knots are placed outside, starting from the posterior midline and proceeding to either side until just before the laterally placed traction sutures. The long strands of Vicryl are clamped with a hemostat, and clipping them to the drapes preserves order. Alternatively, the hemostats themselves can be hung on a Kelly clamp. The head drape should not be used for clipping the sutures because these will be displaced later when the neck is flexed. After placing the interrupted stitches, flexing the neck, and switching the endotracheal tubes, the previously placed midlateral 2-0 Vicryl traction suture is used to pull the tracheal edges together. They can even be tied together to free up an assistant. The proximal traction suture is removed, and the distal Vicryl is stitched through the proximal ends and tied. The membranous tracheal sutures then are tied without tension beginning at the posterior midline and proceeding laterally. If the difficulty of dissection is such that knots can only be placed inside the lumen, the fine stainless steel wire sutures are easy to place, albeit tying the knots requires some finesse.

Regardless of the technique used for the posterior wall, the anterior sutures of interrupted 4-0 Vicryl now can be placed without difficulty. Occasionally, there is an overlap of the cartilaginous tracheal edges, but this is quite acceptable. The anastomosis then is tested by deflating the endotracheal tube cuff and administering positive pressure. The wound is irrigated, and a small suction drain is left in place at the pretracheal plane (but away from the anastomosis). If a partial sternotomy incision was used, an additional drain is left in the substernal space, and the sternum is approximated with stainless steel wires. The rest of the closure is performed as with any neck surgery.

A stout suture (at least Prolene 2) is placed through the chin at the inferior mandibular angle and then at the anterior chest just above the sternal angle. This is used not to achieve neck flexion but to avoid extension, and is just a reminder stitch.

Release Maneuvers

These additional techniques are employed sparingly, and only when the tracheal ends cannot be approximated with acceptable tension. For upper to midtracheal lesions approached from a neck incision with or without a partial sternotomy, a Montgomery suprahyoid release is first done.[3] Usually, a second transverse neck incision is made directly over the hyoid bone. The strap muscles (i.e., mylohyoid, geniohyoid, and genioglossus) overlying the hyoid are cut horizontally until the bone itself is exposed. The superior edge is also cauterized free of muscular attachments beginning from the midline and proceeding laterally until the lesser cornua is reached. This is transected with heavy scissors, and just lateral to the lesser cornua, the hyoid bone is cut, taking care not to injure the digastric sling, which is at the lateral hyoid. The suprahyoid membrane should not be exposed, and the knife is used to make a careful transverse incision over the length of the hyoid bone between the lesser cornuae. The preepiglottic space is now opened, and the hyoid body can drop to allow for at least 1 cm of release.

Mobilization of the inferior pulmonary ligament on one or both sides, as well as an intrapericardial release, is the next maneuver to consider for lower to midtracheal lesions. The technique is variable, based on the exposure obtained. If a clamshell incision is used, both inferior pulmonary ligaments

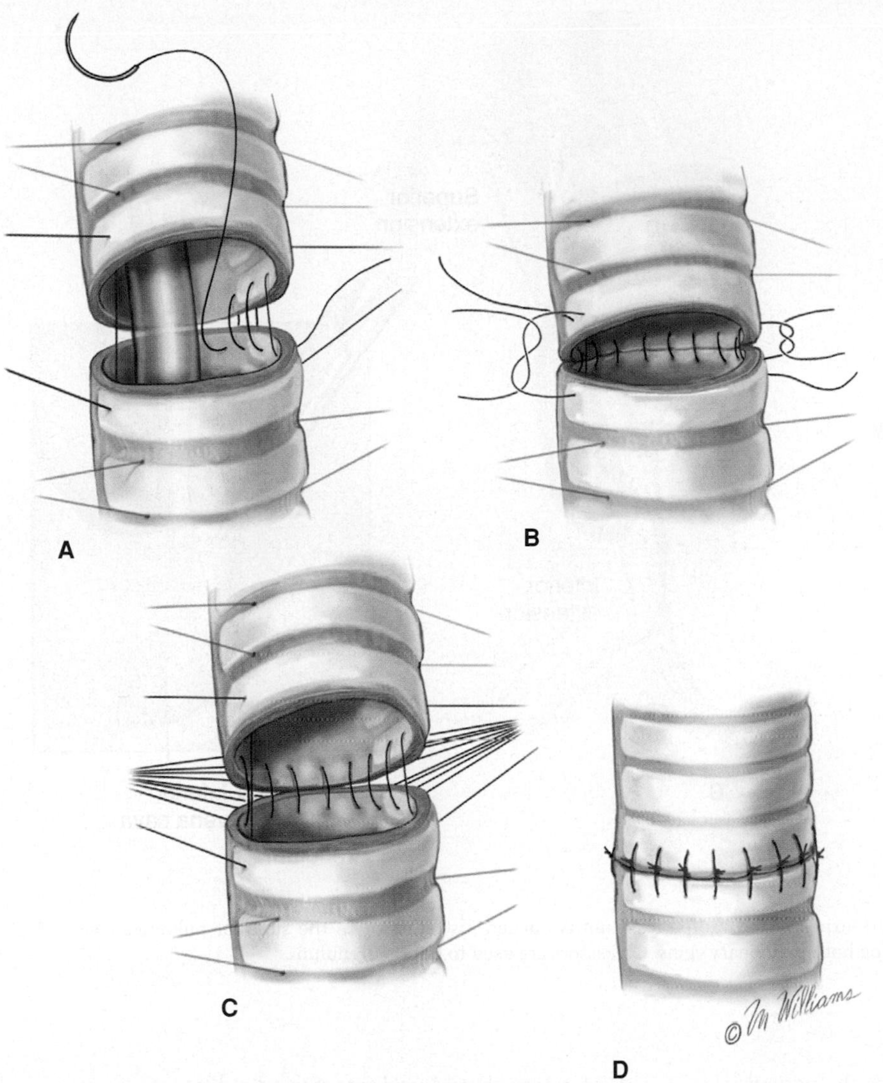

Figure 57-8. *A.* 3-0 Vicryl anchoring sutures are placed through the cartilaginous trachea of both ends. The posterior wall is sutured first. The first bite goes through the cartilaginous trachea and continues in running fashion at intervals of 3 to 4 mm. *B.* On completion of the posterior wall, the tracheal edges are pulled together using the previously placed 2-0 Vicryl, and the 3-0 Vicryl anchoring stitches are tied without tension using only three throws. *C.* The ends of the PDS stitch are tied to one of the Vicryl anchoring stitch ends. Alternatively, if there is more than minimal tension, instead of PDS, 4-0 Vicryl sutures are placed in simple interrupted manner. The knots are placed outside, starting from the posterior midline and proceeding to either side until just before the laterally placed traction sutures. *D.* Regardless of the technique used for the posterior wall, the anterior sutures of interrupted 4-0 Vicryl now can be placed without difficulty.

can be mobilized, and both hila can be subjected to intrapericardial release (Fig. 57-9). On the right side, the pulmonary veins are exposed and the pericardium is opened just anterior to the superior pulmonary vein (Fig. 57-10). Once the pericardium is entered, a circumferential opening is created with scissors, encircling both pulmonary veins, with a release felt on completing the opening. The scissors are used to cut the frenulum, which attaches the inferior vena cava to the pericardium. The superior aspect of the pericardial incision is then carried upward anterior to the pulmonary artery and right mainstem bronchus to expose these structures and isolate them. On the left side, the pulmonary veins cannot be circumscribed, but a pericardial incision is created in a U shape with the two pulmonary veins and the left main pulmonary artery within the U. At least 2 cm of length can be achieved with these maneuvers.

POSTOPERATIVE MANAGEMENT

A bronchoscopy should be done at the end of the procedure for toilet because blood from the field frequently enters the distal airway. Extubation in the OR is almost always possible and is highly desirable. If a complex upper airway resection is performed, or in any patient in whom there is concern about postoperative airway compromise, we favor insertion of a Montgomery T-tube. Apart from its Silastic material, the design of the T-tube renders it far less traumatic to the airway than the tracheostomy tube. Patients should be transported cautiously so as not to disrupt the chin stitch. A recovery room chest x-ray is taken to rule out

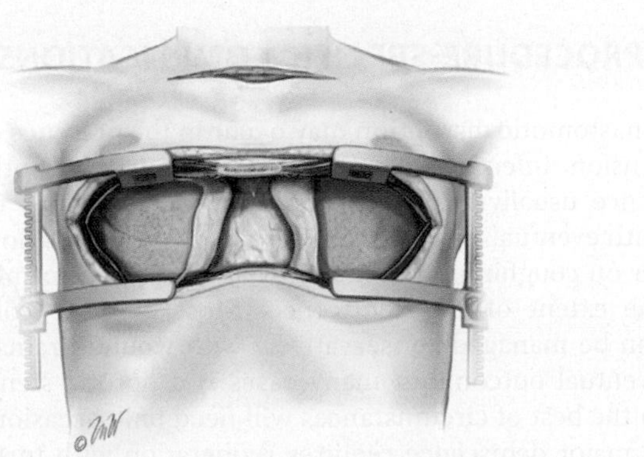

Figure 57-9. With the clamshell incision, both inferior pulmonary ligaments can be mobilized and both hila subjected to intrapericardial release.

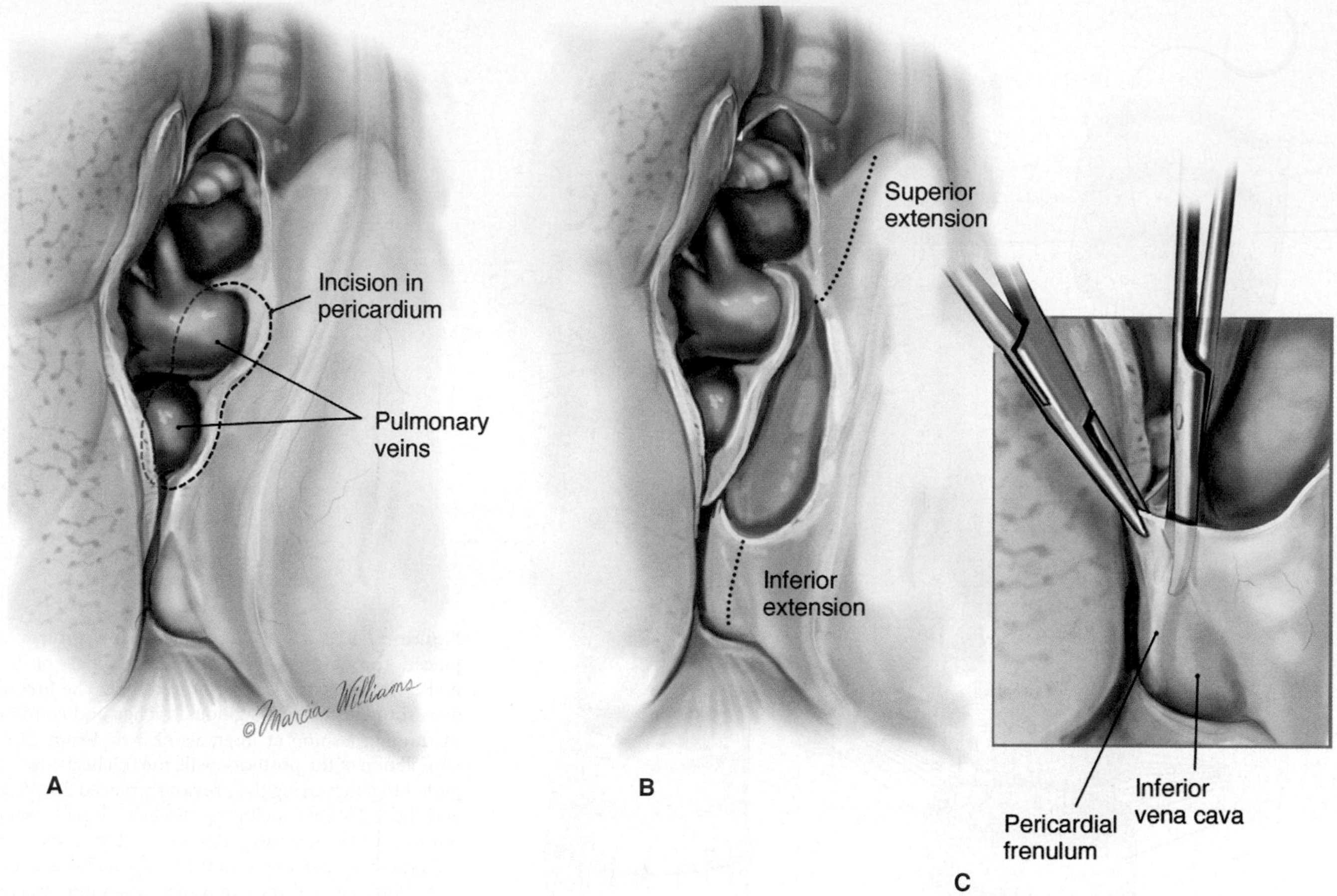

Figure 57-10. *A*. On the right, the pulmonary veins are exposed and the pericardium is opened just anterior to the superior pulmonary vein. *B*. A circumferential opening is created with scissors, encircling both pulmonary veins. C. Scissors are used to cut the frenulum.

pneumothorax. A clear fluid diet starts as soon as the patient is awake and can progress as tolerated. Even with extensive upper airway surgery, it is unusual for persistent aspiration to occur. The suprahyoid release is notorious in this regard, but normal swallowing eventually returns. Drains are removed after 1 to 2 days when output is low, but the chin stitch remains for 7 days. If any chest tubes were inserted, these are removed according to usual criteria. Early mobilization and chest physiotherapy are still important even in the absence of a chest incision to avoid pooling of secretions and a pneumonia or tracheobronchitis.

PROCEDURE-SPECIFIC COMPLICATIONS

Anastomotic disruption may occur in the presence of excessive tension, infection (e.g., tracheobronchitis), or both. A dehiscence usually manifests first as a subcutaneous emphysema with eventual external wound disruption and obvious egress of air on coughing. Bronchoscopy should be performed to assess the extent of the dehiscence. Most of these complications can be managed conservatively with wound drainage, but the eventual outcome in many cases is a fibrotic stenosis, which in the best of circumstances will need only occasional dilation. A major dehiscence requires reoperation with further release maneuvers and reanastomosis if it is technical in etiology. Otherwise, a tracheostomy probably will be required.

Restenoses should undergo periodic dilations, and a reresection is considered only if these are becoming unacceptably frequent. Wound infection usually is minor and responds readily to drainage and antibiotics. Granulation tissue formation usually is observed and can be debrided if overgrowth leads to a significant stenosis, but this is rarely the case.

CASE HISTORY

A 54-year-old man attempted suicide by hanging. He was found and brought to the emergency department in severe stridor, for which he had a lifesaving tracheostomy. Subsequent workup showed that he had a complete tracheal separation. After a year of psychiatric treatment, he was reassessed and found to have a complete tracheal stenosis at the area of separation that was 3 cm long with its proximal end at the subglottis. The tracheostomy was still in situ. Vocal cords were assessed, and the patient was deemed a suitable candidate for a tracheal resection.

He was **anesthetized** with an armored endotracheal tube through the tracheostoma, and a collar incision was made. After meticulous dissection, the trachea was isolated and transected below the lesion and the endotracheal tube transferred. Proximally, a laryngofissure with left posterior arytenoidectomy was performed by our otorhinolaryngology colleagues. The superior extent of the resection included the anterior third of the cricoid. The distal end of the trachea was beveled to fit the proximal end. There was only a moderate amount of tension after mobilization, and the anastomosis was accomplished with a running 4-0 PDS suture at the membranous portion and interrupted 4-0 and 3-0 PDS at the anterior cartilaginous aspect. A size 12 Montgomery T-tube was inserted below the anastomosis, with the upper limb placed through the vocal cords.

The patient's postoperative course was marked by troublesome aspiration, which improved slowly until he was able to tolerate a soft diet on the second week. The T-tube was removed after 2 months.

EDITOR'S COMMENT

I often place a small tracheotomy tube in patients undergoing very proximal tracheolaryngeal resection. These patients are more prone to having difficulty clearing secretions and are more likely to develop significant postoperative swelling at the site of reconstruction. I usually locate the stoma several rings below the anastomotic site and interpose a muscle flap between the stoma and the reconstruction site. A bronchoscopy, awake or through a laryngeal mask airway on or about postoperative day 7, is a reasonable practice to debride any necrotic material that may be sloughing off the anastomosis.

The distal trachea is easily resected and reconstructed via a right posterolateral thoracotomy. Finally, when performing a hilar release maneuver, some authorities suggest that it is better not to make the incision circumferential, but to leave the cephalad portion uncut to avoid disrupting the lymphatic drainage from the lung. Also, the hilar release can be accomplished completely thoracoscopically through two or three incisions on each side. This should be considered as the first step if a complex operation requiring release is planned.

—Raphael Bueno

References

1. Keshavjee S, Pearson F. Tracheal resection. In: Pearson F, Cooper J, Deslauriers J, eds. *Thoracic Surgery*. Philadelphia, PA: Churchill-Livingstone; 2002:409.
2. Salassa JR, Pearson BW, Payne WS. Gross and microscopical blood supply of the trachea. *Ann Thorac Surg*. 1977;24:100–107.
3. Montgomery WW. Suprahyoid release for tracheal anastomosis. *Arch Otolaryngol*. 1974;99:255–260.

58 Surgical Repair of Congenital and Acquired Tracheoesophageal Fistulas

Siva Raja, Albert S. Y. Chang, and David P. Mason

Keywords: Tracheoesophageal fistula (TEF), esophageal atresia, congenital, acquired

The term *tracheoesophageal fistula* (TEF) describes a communication between the gastrointestinal tract and the airway. This defect can present at birth as a congenital anomaly or later in life as an acquired pathology secondary to trauma, malignancy, or inflammation. Management of TEF requires expedient diagnosis with thoughtful planning and implementation of tailored single or multistage therapy. As in all diseases of the esophagus and trachea, patient outcome depends on a clear understanding of the pathophysiology and anatomy of the disease, expert treatment, and sound surgical technique. This chapter focuses on the management of both congenital and acquired TEF.

CONGENITAL

Congenital TEF is most frequently associated with esophageal atresia (EA). Thomas Durston first described EA in 1670. In 1696, Thomas Gibson described TEF with EA. However, it was not until 1939 that Thomas Lanman and Logan Leven reported a successful staged repair. This was soon followed by the first report of a primary repair by Cameron Haight in 1941.[1]

Congenital TEF occurs in about 1 of every 3000 to 4000 live births.[2] The prevalence increases with advancing maternal age and maternal diabetes, and there is a genetic predisposition in children born to affected parents.[3] TEF and EA are believed to develop during the fourth week of gestation after the lung bud has begun to separate from the foregut. This is usually followed by separation of the trachea from the esophagus, which begins at the level of the carina and moves cephalad toward the larynx. It is postulated that abnormal endoderm–mesoderm interactions that occur early in development cause incorrect signaling and inappropriate separation and development of the tracheobronchial tree and esophagus.[4]

Diagnosis and Preoperative Assessment

TEF and EA were first classified by Gross with a lettering system and Ladd with a numbering system. It is now more common to describe them in terms of the anatomic abnormalities of the esophagus and trachea. The most common variant is EA with distal TEF (85%) (Fig. 58-1A), followed by EA alone without TEF (7%) (Fig. 58-1B) and TEF alone without EA (N- or H-type) (4%) (Fig. 58-1C). Other very rare variants include EA with proximal TEF (Fig. 58-1D) and EA with proximal and distal TEF (Fig. 58-1E).[1,2]

With advances in surgical management of TEF and EA, neonates who undergo successful repair can be expected to live near-normal lives. However, both TEF and EA are associated with other congenital abnormalities in 30% to 50% of patients, and these anomalies can have a significant impact on long-term outcomes. Associated defects include cardiac, gastrointestinal, neurologic, skeletal, and genitourinary. The most common cardiac defects are atrial and ventricular septal defects, patent ductus arteriosus, tetralogy of Fallot, and aortic arch abnormalities.[5] The most common gastrointestinal abnormality is imperforate anus, which occurs in 10% of patients.

These patients also may have multiple congenital defects that have been given the acronym *VACTERL* (*V*ertebral, *A*nal, *C*ardiac, *T*racheoesophageal fistula with *E*sophageal atresia, *R*enal, *L*imb). The presence of any three abnormalities determines this designation. The search for additional congenital abnormalities is critical owing to their impact on management strategies and overall survival.[1,2]

Diagnosis

The first sign of possible TEF/EA is typically picked up during prenatal ultrasound with the observation of maternal polyhydramnios and the absence of a fetal stomach bubble. This is especially true with EA alone, in which the fetus is unable to swallow the amniotic fluid as a consequence of the blind proximal esophageal pouch. In patients with TEF alone without EA or the more common EA with distal TEF, polyhydramnios may be absent on account of the distal fistula.[6,7] However, prenatal imaging has only a 44% positive predictive value. Clinical suspicion remains the key to early diagnosis.[8] If not diagnosed prenatally, these patients present soon after birth with excessive drooling and pooling of saliva in the posterior pharynx that is refractory to frequent suctioning. They also have persistent coughing, choking, and cyanosis, especially with the first feeding attempts. In patients with EA with distal TEF, reflux of gastric contents leads to aspiration pneumonitis and respiratory distress with resulting bradycardia, apnea, and sepsis. In patients with TEF without EA, the diagnosis may be delayed. These patients may present later in life as adults, with recurrent coughing and choking while eating and with resulting pneumonia and respiratory infection. Less than 20 adult cases have been reported in the literature.[9]

The simplest means of diagnosis is to insert a firm, radiopaque nasogastric tube (8F in preterm and 10F in term infants). This typically passes no further than 10 to 12 cm in patients with EA, the end of the blind pouch (normal distance to gastric cardia is 17 cm). A chest radiograph and an abdominal radiograph then should be performed to confirm the location of the tube and to estimate the distance of the esophageal gap caused by the atresia. An esophagram can be used cautiously to diagnose TEF without EA, although precautions against aspiration of barium must be taken, with care to suction the airway clear at completion of the procedure. Bronchoscopy and esophagoscopy typically are confirmatory, although the anomaly may be missed at esophagoscopy because of its anterior location and if the fistula is in the proximal third of the esophagus.[9,10]

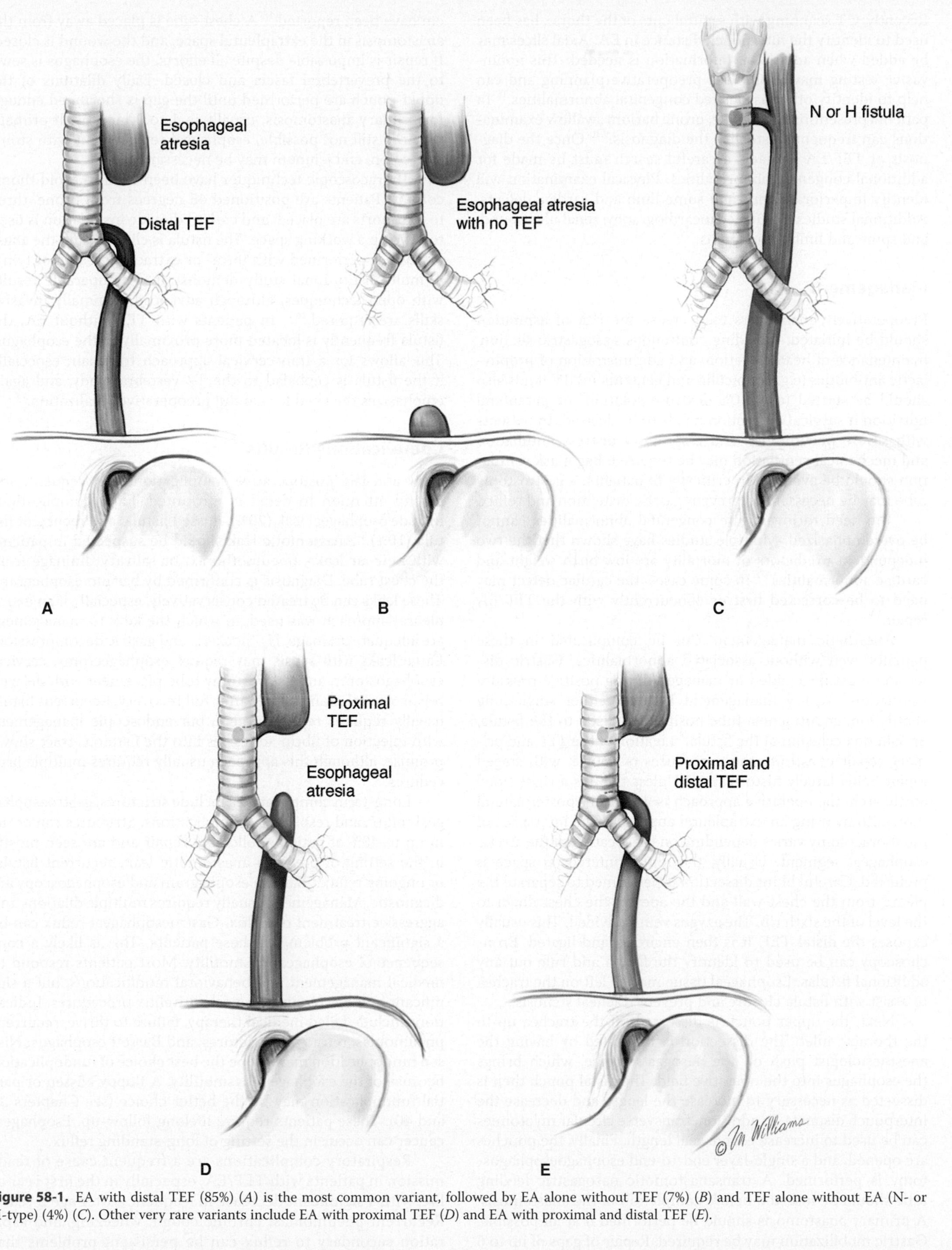

Figure 58-1. EA with distal TEF (85%) (*A*) is the most common variant, followed by EA alone without TEF (7%) (*B*) and TEF alone without EA (N- or H-type) (4%) (*C*). Other very rare variants include EA with proximal TEF (*D*) and EA with proximal and distal TEF (*E*).

Recently, CT scanning with sagittal cuts of the thorax has been used to identify the interpouch distance in EA. Axial slices may be added when additional information is needed. This noninvasive testing may assist with preoperative planning and can help to identify other associated congenital abnormalities.[11] In patients presenting later in life, prone barium swallow examinations can frequently establish the diagnosis.[9,10] Once the diagnosis of TEF/EA is made, a careful search must be made for additional congenital abnormalities. Physical examination will identify imperforate anus and some limb and cardiac defects. Additional studies include echocardiography, renal ultrasound, and spine and limb radiographs.

Management

Preoperatively, maneuvers to decrease the risk of aspiration should be initiated, including continuous nasogastric suction, maintenance of head elevation, and administration of prophylactic antibiotics (e.g., ampicillin and gentamicin). IV fluids also should be started (e.g., 10% dextrose solution) or parenteral nutrition if surgical correction needs to be delayed. In patients with severe pneumonitis and respiratory distress, intubation and mechanical ventilation may be required. Bag mask ventilation should be avoided. In critically ill patients, a gastrostomy tube may be necessary to prevent gastric distention and reflux.

The need to investigate congenital abnormalities cannot be overemphasized. Multiple studies have shown that the two independent predictors of mortality are low birth weight and cardiac abnormalities.[12] In some cases, the cardiac defect may need to be corrected first or concurrently with the TEF/EA repair.[13]

Anesthetic management can be complicated in these patients even without associated abnormalities. Gastric distention must be avoided or managed during positive-pressure ventilation. Airway management includes either single-lung ventilation, endotracheal tube positioning distal to the fistula, or balloon occlusion of the fistula.[8] Ligation of the TEF and primary repair constitute the procedures of choice, with staged repair being largely historical.[12,14] Unless there is a right-sided aortic arch, the operative approach is via a right posterolateral thoracotomy using an extrapleural approach. The interspace of the thoracotomy varies depending on the location of the atretic esophageal segment. Usually, the fourth intercostal space is preferred. Careful blunt dissection is performed to separate the pleura from the chest wall and the apex of the chest down to the level of the sixth rib. The azygos vein is divided. This usually exposes the distal TEF. It is then encircled and ligated. Bronchoscopy can be used to identify the fistula and rule out any additional fistulas. Esophageal tissue may be left on the trachea to assist with fistula closure and prevent tracheal stenosis.

Next, the upper pouch is dissected off the trachea up to the thoracic inlet. The dissection is facilitated by having the anesthesiologist push on the nasogastric tube, which brings the esophagus into the operative field. The distal pouch then is dissected as necessary to increase the length and decrease the interpouch distance. In addition, transverse circular myotomies can be used to increase esophageal length. Finally, the pouches are opened, and a single-layer end-to-end esophagoesophagostomy is performed. A transanastomotic nasogastric feeding tube should be inserted before completion of the anastomosis. A primary anastomosis should be performed if at all possible. Gastric mobilization may be required. Repair of gaps of up to 6 cm have been reported.[15] A chest tube is placed away from the anastomosis in the extrapleural space, and the wound is closed. If repair is impossible despite all efforts, the esophagus is sewn to the prevertebral fascia and closed. Daily dilations of the upper pouch are performed until the gap is shortened enough for primary anastomosis, usually in 1 to 2 months. If primary repair is still not possible, esophageal replacement with stomach, colon, and jejunum may be necessary.

Thoracoscopic techniques have been used to avoid thoracotomy. Patients are positioned 45 degrees from prone, three to four ports are placed, and carbon dioxide insufflation is used to develop a working space. The fistula is clipped, and the anastomosis is performed with intra- or extracorporeal knot tying. A multi-institutional study demonstrated comparable results with open techniques, although advanced minimally invasive skills are required.[16,17] In patients with TEF without EA, the fistula frequently is located more proximally in the esophagus. This allows for a transcervical approach to repair, especially if the fistula is cephalad to the T2 vertebral body, and again emphasizes the need for careful preoperative localization.[18]

Complications/Results

Early and late postoperative complications are frequent, and careful attention to detail is warranted. Early complications include esophageal leak (20%), missed fistula, and recurrent fistula (10%).[2] Anastomotic leak should be suspected in patients with new air leaks, pneumothorax, or salivary drainage from the chest tube. Diagnosis is confirmed by barium esophagram. These leaks can be treated conservatively, especially if an extrapleural approach was used, in which the keys to management are adequate drainage, H_2-blockers, and gastric decompression. Large leaks with sepsis may require esophagectomy, cervical esophagostomy, and gastrostomy tube placement with delayed repair several months later after full recovery. Recurrent fistula usually requires repeat surgery, but endoscopic management with injection of fibrin adhesives into the fistulous tract shows promise, although this approach usually requires multiple procedures.[19]

Long-term complications include strictures, gastroesophageal reflux, and respiratory complications. Strictures can occur in up to 40% of patients following repair and are seen mostly in the setting of previous anastomotic leak, recurrent fistula, or ongoing reflux.[2] Barium esophagram and esophagoscopy are diagnostic. Management usually requires multiple dilations and aggressive treatment of reflux. Gastroesophageal reflux can be a significant problem for these patients. This is likely a consequence of esophageal dysmotility. Most patients respond to medical management and behavioral modifications, but a significant number require surgical antireflux procedures. Indications include failed medical therapy, failure to thrive, recurrent pneumonias, refractory strictures, and Barrett esophagus. Nissen fundoplication may not be the best choice of fundoplication because of the esophageal dysmotility. A floppy Nissen or partial fundoplication may be the better choice (see Chapters 39 and 40). These patients require lifelong follow-up. Esophageal cancer can occur in the setting of long-standing reflux.

Respiratory complications are a frequent cause of readmission in patients with TEF/EA, especially in the first year of life, with a significant decrease in frequency after age 2 years. Recurrent pneumonias, chronic cough, wheezing, and aspiration secondary to reflux can be persistent problems that slowly abate over time. In addition, tracheomalacia is a challenging complication that may develop. Early abnormal tracheal development leads to redundant membranous trachea, predisposing to anteroposterior collapse. Bronchodilators may worsen the condition because of relaxation of the tracheal smooth muscle. While most patients improve with time, a few may require intervention. Aortopexy of the aorta to the posterior aspect of the sternum via a left thoracotomy allows the trachea to be fixed more anteriorly, preventing airway collapse. Tracheal stent placement has been used, but with mixed results. Tracheostomy may be required in refractory cases.[2] Overall, the results have been excellent with primary repair of TEF/EA, with survival approaching 100% in children without associated congenital abnormalities. While the initial care and management in the first two years of life is complicated with frequent emergency room visits, hospital readmissions, multiple surgical procedures, and numerous radiologic imaging studies, most children can look forward to essentially normal lives.[20]

ACQUIRED

Benign

Overview

Historically, the most common cause for benign TEF was endotracheal intubation or tracheostomy tube placement.[21] The advent of high-volume, low-pressure endotracheal cuffs has made tracheal stenosis and TEF far less common albeit the problem has not been eliminated. A recent review from the Mayo Clinic showed that the most common etiologies of TEF in decreasing frequency were esophageal surgery (31%), laryngotracheal trauma (17%), mediastinal granulomatous disease (14%), erosion of indwelling esophageal or tracheal stent (11%), and endotracheal intubation (6%).[22] Symptoms arise secondary to aspiration of oral and gastric contents into the fistulized airway producing sepsis or hemodynamic collapse or from insufflation of air into the esophagus and/or stomach resulting in an inability to ventilate the patient. TEF must be diagnosed quickly and managed aggressively. Management is most challenging in the patient who requires mechanical ventilation.[23]

Diagnosis

The diagnosis of a TEF requires a high index of suspicion on the part of the clinician that must be gleaned from a thorough history. In a nonventilated patient, TEF most commonly presents in the form of recurrent aspiration pneumonias, persistent leukocytosis, or a chronic cough. It is the rare patient who presents with the obvious finding of expectoration of bilious sputum. Since current acquired benign TEFs are most commonly associated with esophageal surgery, this often presents in the perioperative period and less commonly in a delayed fashion up to a decade later. The postoperative patient will likely have an unrecognized injury to the airway or esophagus or an anastomotic leak or conduit tip necrosis. In these cases, as in other etiologies, CT scan can be highly suggestive of TEF as the underlying process. However, bronchoscopy and esophagoscopy are the cornerstones of diagnosis and sometimes management of TEF.

When the TEF is secondary to prolonged endotracheal intubation or tracheostomy, the typical patient suffers from chronic illness, is malnourished, has undergone prolonged ventilation, and has a nasogastric tube in place. TEF develops in the ventilated patient secondary to endotracheal cuff pressure that causes necrosis and erosion of the airway into the esophagus.[24] The nasogastric tube serves as a second foreign body against which the tracheal cuff rides and chafes. Nevertheless, diagnosis of TEF in the ventilated patient should be suspected when the patient's abdomen becomes acutely distended and difficult to ventilate with a significant loss of return of ventilated breaths and accompanying bilious secretions. A presumptive clinical diagnosis of TEF is then made. A plain chest radiograph or CT scan may be performed but its findings are usually nonspecific. Mediastinal air is present occasionally. However, mediastinal inflammation and adhesions usually prevent frank pneumomediastinum and mediastinitis. Endoscopy is usually necessary. Of note, proximal TEF may be missed if the endotracheal tube or tracheostomy appliance is not removed and the proximal membranous trachea is not examined.

The diagnosis of TEF secondary to penetrating injury is usually made early. The location of the injury in the neck or chest usually prompts an aggressive workup including radiologic and endoscopic evaluation. Traumatic TEF also has been documented in the setting of percutaneous dilation tracheostomy where inadvertent injury to the membranous trachea can result in devastating outcome for previously ill patients.[25] As such, percutaneous tracheostomy should always be performed by a skilled practitioner under bronchoscopic guidance. However, diagnosis of TEF after blunt trauma can occur in a delayed fashion. Barium esophagram, CT scanning, and endoscopy are all useful diagnostic tools. TEF should be considered after blunt chest trauma with the appearance of pneumomediastinum or pleural effusion.

Inflammatory processes leading to TEF are often secondary to granulomatous disease. In one small series of TEF, the most frequent etiology was histoplasmosis.[26] The pathology of TEF in this setting provides a technical challenge, particularly when associated with esophageal diverticula. Presentation can be subtle. An esophagram is useful for demonstrating the fistula. Bronchoscopy is critical.

With the advent of tracheal and esophageal stenting for nonmalignant strictures and iatrogenic injuries, TEFs have been seen as a complication of the procedure.[27,28] Possible etiologies include erosion of the stent through the wall, tissue necrosis due to radial force from self-expanding stents and/or avulsion tissue injury from stent changes. TEF in this setting may not be visible until the stent is removed.

Finally, there are several rare causes of benign acquired TEF that include button battery ingestion in children and adults alike and chemical injury after lye ingestion. These etiologies, though rare, can cause significant tissue necrosis resulting in florid sepsis at the time of presentation. In the scenario of button battery ingestion, this is a time dependent factor. Animal studies have shown that in as little as 1 to 4 hours full-thickness esophageal injury can occur.[29,30] In these patients, presumptive diagnosis is made based on history and if unstable, definitive diagnostic tests are deferred in lieu of the need for hemodynamic stabilization.

Management

Initial Management As initial management, the patient must be stabilized and the airway protected from further contamination. In ill patients, this involves orotracheal intubation to prevent further airway contamination. In addition, the stomach must be decompressed. The nasogastric tube must be kept continuously sumping to evacuate air from the stomach. If the patient is ventilator dependent, ventilatory pressures should be reduced to the lowest levels that will support oxygenation and ventilation. This may require pharmacologic sedation and paralysis. The anesthesiologist carefully controls the airway from the head of the bed while the endotracheal tube or tracheostomy appliance is removed over a bronchoscope. The fistula typically is evident a few centimeters distal to the stoma on the membranous wall where the opposing balloon of the tracheostomy was located. The nasogastric tube also is frequently visible through the fistula, making the diagnosis obvious. Alternative modalities for diagnosing TEF are esophagoscopy. However, bronchoscopy is the simplest and fastest way to obtain a diagnosis and also can be used to aid in its treatment.

Once the diagnosis of TEF is made, the next step is to ventilate the patient distal to the fistula. This is simple in principle but frequently difficult in practice. The location of the fistula in the midtrachea leaves little room between the carina and the fistula to place the cuff of the endotracheal tube. A tracheostomy must have a distal arm that is long enough to traverse the fistula but not so long that it produces a mainstem intubation. This is often difficult to find and it may be necessary to use a custom-made or adjustable appliance. Careful bronchoscopic measurements of the distance of the fistula from the carina must be made, as well as measurements of the endotracheal tube and its balloon, to ensure correct placement. The tip of the endotracheal tube should be positioned at the carina or directed just down the left mainstem bronchus, with the Murphy eye of the endotracheal tube directed to the right mainstem bronchus to prevent atelectasis (Fig. 58-2). Confirmatory bronchoscopy must be performed regularly to check position and clear secretions. Sedation or paralysis may be required to prevent the patient from dislodging the endotracheal tube. Once stabilized, the patient should be taken to the OR for placement of a formal drainage gastrostomy tube and/or a feeding jejunostomy tube. The nasogastric tube should then be removed to prevent enlargement of the TEF. However, spontaneous closure of the TEF is unlikely to occur.

After initial stabilization and management, the next more difficult step is definitive management of the fistula. The specific treatment plan is determined by the location of the fistula, length of the fistulous connection, and the quality of the adjacent airway and esophagus. With our ever increasing experience in tracheobronchial and esophageal stenting, it is reasonable to consider this modality as both a bridge to definitive repair and as the definitive therapy. In addition, the clinical condition of the patient should determine if primary repair should be attempted or a staged approach undertaken.

Stenting While the primary objective of closing the fistula frequently can be met, preventing breakdown of the closure is far more difficult to achieve in this debilitated, ventilated group of patients.[31] Attempts at closure while the patient still requires positive-pressure ventilation are almost always doomed to failure, and every attempt should be made to wean the patient from the ventilator first, with a focus on nutrition and the prevention and treatment of airway contamination and nosocomial infection. Airway stenting is our first therapy of choice for all TEFs and that of others.[32] Stenting usually permits coverage of the defect in the membranous airway, and thereby control of airway contamination. In our experience and in other limited published experience, tracheal stents are well suited to cover the defect and prevent contamination of the airway.[33] They are generally well tolerated with few complications. The main morbidity is stent migration, which can be countered with some success by using barbed stents in the distal trachea and percutaneous fixation in the subglottic space.

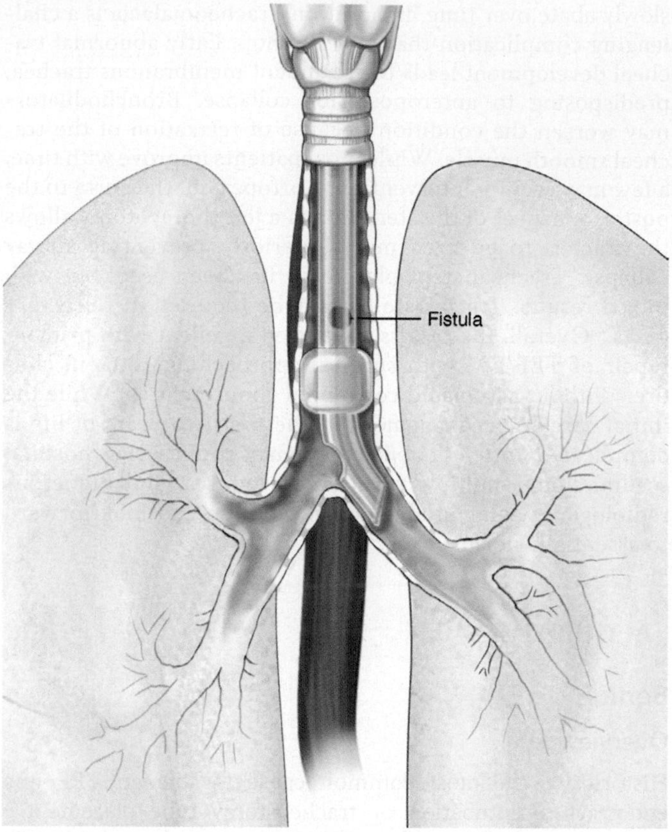

Figure 58-2. A Murphy endotracheal tube is used to ventilate the patient. The tip should be positioned at the carina or directed just down the left mainstem bronchus, with the Murphy eye of the endotracheal tube directed to the right mainstem bronchus to prevent atelectasis.

Similar to airway stenting, TEF also may be treated with esophageal stenting and in rare situations, with dual stenting.[34] Radially expanding esophageal stents can seal the TEF but are more prone to migration in the absence of a mass or a stricture. As such, endoscopists often use endoclips or suture bridles to secure the stent in place. For large fistulas, we advocate double stenting with regular stent exchanges and downsizing (Fig. 58-3). In the Methodist Hospital series, two of four benign TEFs healed with only stenting. Once the spillage of gastric contents into the airway has been controlled and the patient has recovered from the underlying acute event, more definitive repair can be undertaken.

Surgery When conservative measures have been tried and have failed, only then should surgery be considered. The principal surgical objective is closure of the fistula with prevention of breakdown of the airway and esophageal closure. Esophageal diversion should be avoided because of its high morbidity and mortality. However, this may be required if aspiration cannot be controlled. In this setting, the gastroesophageal junction must be divided and an end-cervical esophagostomy performed.

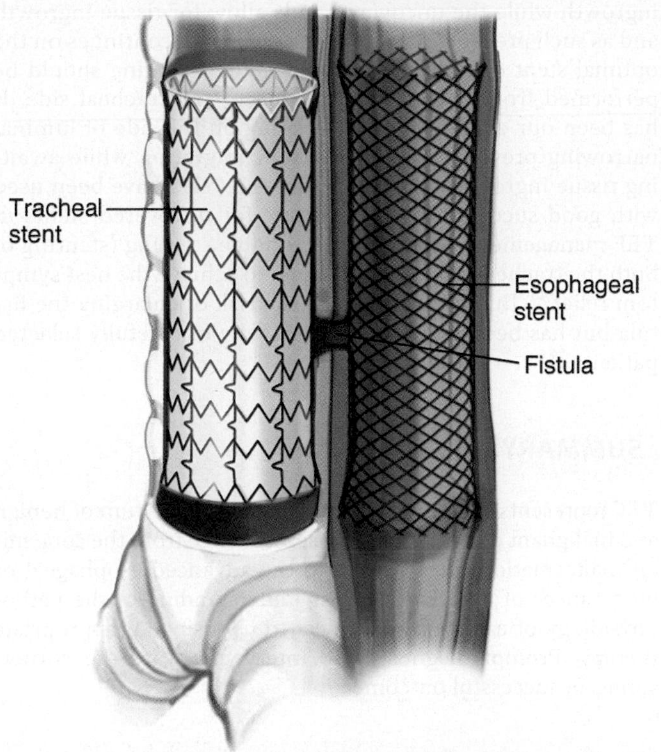

Figure 58-3. Double stenting for large tracheoesophageal fistulas can be an effective approach in selected patients, with opposing stents in the trachea and esophagus.

Upon stabilization, and if the patient can be weaned successfully from the ventilator, definitive surgical repair then can be performed. The surgical approach depends on the location of the fistula. Small fistulas can be addressed through a lateral cervical approach with mobilization of the trachea and direct suture closure of the membranous trachea and esophagus with interposition of a strap muscle (Fig. 58-4). However, most fistulas are large and require tracheal resection with concomitant repair of the esophagus. The most frequently applied approach is an anterior cervical approach with a low-collar incision. An upper sternal split can be performed if more distal exposure to the trachea is necessary. Fistulas close to the carina should be approached through a right posterolateral thoracotomy.

Standard techniques of tracheal resection apply. The trachea is dissected with care circumferentially to preserve the lateral–segmental blood supply and avoid the recurrent laryngeal nerves. Proximal and distal mobilization should be performed only as far as absolutely necessary to bring the trachea together with minimal tension. The airway is transected distally and secured with traction sutures. An armored, flexible endotracheal tube is brought into the field and used to intermittently ventilate the distal trachea. Alternatively, jet ventilation can be used, but this technique is seldom required. With the airway divided, the esophagus is exposed. After carefully defining the mucosal edges, the esophageal defect then can be closed in two layers. Our preference is to use interrupted 4-0 Vicryl sutures for the mucosal layer and silk for the muscular layer. Suture choices vary according to surgeon's preference. A pedicled strap muscle then is mobilized and tacked over the esophageal closure to provide a layer of tissue between the esophageal and tracheal suture lines and prevent breakdown of the repair. The importance of this step cannot be overemphasized. Finally, the trachea is reapproximated using interrupted 4-0 Vicryl suture with removal of the armored tube and careful guidance of the oral–tracheal tube through the anastomosis as the anterior cartilaginous wall is being completed. The neck is flexed to minimize tension on the anastomosis, and a stitch can be brought from the chin to the chest to prevent neck extension in the perioperative period.[24] A nasogastric tube is left in place briefly after the repair and then is removed.

Long TEFs result in large defects, and closure sometimes requires creative solutions. On occasion we have used Allodern® (Life Cell Technologies, Branchburg, NJ) to recreate the membranous trachea when the length of the fistulous opening precludes resection.[35] The material is sewed onto the cartilaginous portion of the airway. It is still important to interpose

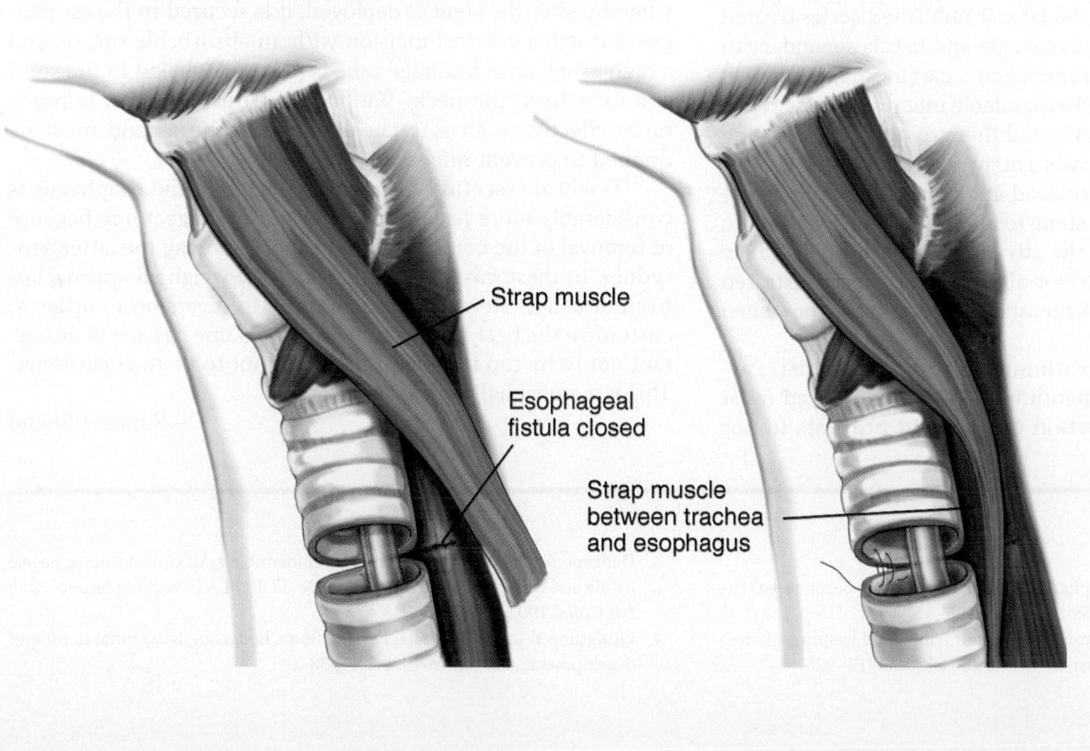

Figure 58-4. Definitive surgical repair of small tracheoesophageal fistula can be addressed through a lateral cervical approach with mobilization of the trachea and direct suture closure of the membranous trachea and esophagus with interposition of a strap muscle.

a muscle flap between the trachea and the esophagus. The tissue ingrowths in this type of acellular matrix decrease the incidence of stenosis. Another solution that has been described in the literature is the use of the in situ esophageal wall as the posterior membranous wall of the trachea. When primary repair of the esophagus is not possible, it can be used to recreate the membranous trachea.[36]

MALIGNANT

Malignant TEF develops in advanced stages of cancer. It is most often due to proximal/midesophageal or bronchogenic carcinoma, although rarely it may be associated with lymphoma. TEF occurs in 10% to 15% of patients with advanced (T4) esophageal cancer and in 1% of patients with bronchogenic carcinoma.[37] The fistula occurs as a result of primary tumor invasion or as an effect of multimodality therapy. Patients undergoing therapies such as esophageal stent placement followed by chemoradiation therapy are at particularly high risk for developing TEF.[38,39]

Patients with malignant TEF have an extremely poor prognosis, with an expected lifespan at diagnosis that is usually measured in weeks. Focus should be on quality of life with symptom control. The primary goals are control of aspiration and establishing or maintaining oral intake. Given the advanced stage of malignancy of patients who present with TEF and the palliative nature of its management, intervention must be carefully individualized. Palliative surgery should remain historic. Some patients may be too ill for any intervention and should be considered for comfort care.

Fortunately, endoscopic management of malignant TEF has improved and shown significant promise. It is minimally invasive and can be tolerated by most patients. Frequently, it can be performed in an outpatient setting. Studies have demonstrated the efficacy of self-expanding metallic stents in palliating TEFs from esophageal or bronchogenic carcinoma.[38,40] Deployment of self-expanding esophageal stents has been shown to prevent aspiration and improve dysphagia in most patients. Complication rates are acceptable, and major complications are unusual. One of the largest published series treated 101 patients with malignant dysphagia and fistula secondary to esophageal malignancy or bronchogenic carcinoma. Success in sealing a fistula using a coated expandable metal stent was 100%. The complication rate was 38%, and the rate of life-threatening complications was 8%. There were no procedure-related deaths. While 99 of 101 patients were dead at a mean follow-up of 201 days, no death was due to a stent-related complication. Rather, this poor survival reflected the advanced stage of malignancy of this patient population.[41] Not all series have demonstrated complete prevention of leakage and reintervention has been needed.[42]

Multiple stent options with multiple materials exist. Partially covered metal self-expanding stents are deployed most commonly. The covered portion of the stent prevents tumor ingrowth while the uncovered ends allow for tissue ingrowth and as such prevents stent migration. Debate continues on the optimal stent choice in terms of whether stenting should be performed from the esophageal side or the tracheal side. It has been our experience that stenting on the side of luminal narrowing prevents immediate stent migration while awaiting tissue ingrowth. Fully covered stents also have been used with good success. There is no role for uncovered stents in TEF management. Some espouse double stenting (stenting of both the trachea and the esophagus) to achieve the best symptom relief.[43] This technique runs the risk of enlarging the fistula but has been employed successfully in carefully selected patients.[44]

SUMMARY

TEF represents the manifestation of a wide spectrum of benign and malignant diseases. These diseases range from the congenital malformation of a neonate to the advanced esophageal or lung cancer of an adult. A clear understanding of the pathophysiology of each TEF is critical to choosing an appropriate therapy. Prompt diagnosis and intervention are the cornerstones of successful outcome.

EDITOR'S COMMENT

Tracheoesophageal fistulas are particularly lethal if left untreated. While it is clear that TEFs of malignant etiology require palliation only, preferably with an esophageal stent, treatment of benign TEFs is more challenging. First one must decide whether the patient is fit (nutritionally and from a pulmonary point of view) to withstand a major surgical repair. Then one must decide whether stenting or surgical repair is the best approach. In our experience, most postoperative TEFs are localized in the esophageal conduit anastomosis and improve with soft covered esophageal stents and drainage. To reduce the rate of stent migration we developed a procedure whereby after the stent is deployed, it is secured to the esophagus through a cervical incision with an absorbable suture, and a high esophageal drainage tube is placed cephalad to the stent and exits from the neck. We find that this approach is much more effective than a tracheal stent but the wound must be drained to prevent infection.

Tracheal resection followed by repair of the esophagus is considerably more hazardous after an esophagectomy because of removal of the combined blood supply during the latter procedure. In these cases one must carefully weigh all approaches from drainage, stent, and reoperation, to diversion in order to customize the best balanced therapy. In some cases it is important not to be too timid and in others not to be too aggressive. This is a truly challenging situation.

—Raphael Bueno

References

1. Myers NA. The history of oesophageal atresia and tracheo-oesophageal fistula–1670–1984. *Prog Pediatr Surg.* 1986;20:106–157.
2. Kovesi T, Rubin S. Long-term complications of congenital esophageal atresia and/or tracheoesophageal fistula. *Chest.* 2004;126(3):915–925.
3. Depaepe A, Dolk H, Lechat MF. The epidemiology of tracheo-oesophageal fistula and oesophageal atresia in Europe. EUROCAT Working Group. *Arch Dis Child.* 1993;68(6):743–748.
4. Litingtung Y, Lei L, Westphal H, et al. Sonic hedgehog is essential to foregut development. *Nat Genet.* 1998;20(1):58–61.

5. Copel JA, Pilu G, Kleinman CS. Congenital heart disease and extracardiac anomalies: associations and indications for fetal echocardiography. *Am J Obstet Gynecol.* 1986;154(5):1121–1132.
6. Kalish RB, Chasen ST, Rosenzweig L, et al. Esophageal atresia and tracheoesophageal fistula: the impact of prenatal suspicion on neonatal outcome in a tertiary care center. *J Perinat Med.* 2003;31(2):111–114.
7. Stringer MD, McKenna KM, Goldstein RB, et al. Prenatal diagnosis of esophageal atresia. *J Pediatr Surg.* 1995;30(9):1258–1263.
8. Broemling N, Campbell F. Anesthetic management of congenital tracheoesophageal fistula. *Paediatr Anaesth.* 2011;21(11):1092–1099.
9. Zacharias J, Genc O, Goldstraw P. Congenital tracheoesophageal fistulas presenting in adults: presentation of two cases and a synopsis of the literature. *J Thorac Cardiovasc Surg.* 2004;128(2):316–318.
10. Hajjar WM, Iftikhar A, Al Nassar SA, et al. Congenital tracheoesophageal fistula: a rare and late presentation in adult patient. *Ann Thorac Med.* 2012;7(1):48–50.
11. Ratan SK, Varshney A, Mullick S, et al. Evaluation of neonates with esophageal atresia using chest CT scan. *Pediatr Surg Int.* 2004;20(10):757–761.
12. Ein SH, Shandling B, Wesson D, et al. Esophageal atresia with distal tracheoesophageal fistula: associated anomalies and prognosis in the 1980s. *J Pediatr Surg.* 1989;24(10):1055–1059.
13. Diaz LK, Akpek EA, Dinavahi R, et al. Tracheoesophageal fistula and associated congenital heart disease: implications for anesthetic management and survival. *Paediatr Anaesth.* 2005;15(10):862–869.
14. Pohlson EC, Schaller RT, Tapper D. Improved survival with primary anastomosis in the low birth weight neonate with esophageal atresia and tracheoesophageal fistula. *J Pediatr Surg.* 1988;23(5):418–421.
15. Allal H, Kalfa N, Lopez M, et al. Benefits of the thoracoscopic approach for short- or long-gap esophageal atresia. *J Laparoendosc Adv Surg Tech A.* 2005;15(6):673–677.
16. Mariano ER, Chu LF, Albanese CT, et al. Successful thoracoscopic repair of esophageal atresia with tracheoesophageal fistula in a newborn with single ventricle physiology. *Anesth Analg.* 2005;101(4):1000–1002, table of contents.
17. Holcomb GW 3rd, Rothenberg SS, Bax KM, et al. Thoracoscopic repair of esophageal atresia and tracheoesophageal fistula: a multi-institutional analysis. *Ann Surg.* 2005;242(3):422–428; discussion 428–430.
18. Killen DA, Greenlee HB. Transcervical repair of H-Type congenital tracheoesophageal fistula: review of the literature. *Ann Surg.* 1965;162:145–150.
19. Meier JD, Sulman CG, Almond PS, et al. Endoscopic management of recurrent congenital tracheoesophageal fistula: a review of techniques and results. *Int J Pediatr Otorhinolaryngol.* 2007;71(5):691–697.
20. Bjornson CL, Mitchell I. Congenital tracheoesophageal fistula and coordination of care: expectations and realities. *Paediatr Child Health.* 2006; 11(7):395–399.
21. Mathisen DJ, Grillo HC, Wain JC, et al. Management of acquired nonmalignant tracheoesophageal fistula. *Ann Thorac Surg.* 1991;52(4):759–765.
22. Shen KR, Allen MS, Cassivi SD, et al. Surgical management of acquired nonmalignant tracheoesophageal and bronchoesophageal fistulae. *Ann Thorac Surg.* 2010;90(3):914–918; discussion 919.
23. Reed MF, Mathisen DJ. Tracheoesophageal fistula. *Chest Surg Clin N Am.* 2003;13(2):271–289.
24. Grillo HC. Surgical treatment of post-intubation lesions of the trachea. *Acta Chir Belg.* 1977;76(3):361–369.
25. Bhatti N, Tatlipinar A, Mirski M, et al. Percutaneous dilation tracheotomy in intensive care unit patients. *Otolaryngol Head Neck Surg.* 2007;136(6):938–941.
26. Mangi AA, Gaissert HA, Wright CD, et al. Benign broncho-esophageal fistula in the adult. *Ann Thorac Surg.* 2002;73(3):911–915.
27. Ladurner R, Schulz C, Jacob P, et al. Surgical management of an esophagotracheal fistula as a severe, late complication of repeated endoscopic stenting treatment. *Endoscopy.* 2007;39 (suppl 1):E341–E342.
28. Han Y, Liu K, Li X, et al. Repair of massive stent-induced tracheoesophageal fistula. *J Thorac Cardiovasc Surg.* 2009;137(4):813–817.
29. Tibballs J, Wall R, Koottayi SV, et al. Tracheo-oesophageal fistula caused by electrolysis of a button battery impacted in the oesophagus. *J Paediatr Child Health.* 2002;38(2):201–203.
30. Slamon NB, Hertzog JH, Penfil SH, et al. An unusual case of button battery-induced traumatic tracheoesophageal fistula. *Pediatr Emerg Care.* 2008;24(5):313–316.
31. Wolf M, Yellin A, Talmi YP, et al. Acquired tracheoesophageal fistula in critically ill patients. *Ann Otol Rhinol Laryngol.* 2000;109(8 Pt 1):731–735.
32. Eleftheriadis E, Kotzampassi K. Temporary stenting of acquired benign tracheoesophageal fistulas in critically ill ventilated patients. *Surg Endosc.* 2005;19(6):811–815.
33. Kim YH, Shin JH, Song HY, et al. Tracheal stricture and fistula: management with a barbed silicone-covered retrievable expandable nitinol stent. *AJR Am J Roentgenol.* 2010;194(2):W232–W237.
34. Blackmon SH, Santora R, Schwarz P, et al. Utility of removable esophageal covered self-expanding metal stents for leak and fistula management. *Ann Thorac Surg.* 2010;89(3):931–936; discussion 936–937.
35. Su JW, Mason DP, Murthy SC, et al. Closure of a large tracheoesophageal fistula using AlloDerm. *J Thorac Cardiovasc Surg.* 2008;135(3):706–707.
36. He J, Chen M, Shao W, et al. Surgical management of huge tracheo-oesophageal fistula with oesophagus segment in situ as replacement of the posterior membranous wall of the trachea. *Eur J Cardiothorac Surg.* 2009; 36(3):600–602.
37. Martini N, Goodner JT, D'Angio GJ, et al. Tracheoesophageal fistula due to cancer. *J Thorac Cardiovasc Surg.* 1970;59(3):319–324.
38. Christie NA, Buenaventura PO, Fernando HC, et al. Results of expandable metal stents for malignant esophageal obstruction in 100 patients: short-term and long-term follow-up. *Ann Thorac Surg.* 2001;71(6):1797–1801; discussion 1801–1792.
39. Spigel DR, Hainsworth JD, Yardley DA, et al. Tracheoesophageal fistula formation in patients with lung cancer treated with chemoradiation and bevacizumab. *J Clin Oncol.* 2010;28(1):43–48.
40. Shin JH, Song HY, Ko GY, et al. Esophagorespiratory fistula: long-term results of palliative treatment with covered expandable metallic stents in 61 patients. *Radiology.* 2004;232(1):252–259.
41. Raijman I, Siddique I, Ajani J, et al. Palliation of malignant dysphagia and fistulae with coated expandable metal stents: experience with 101 patients. *Gastrointest Endosc.* 1998;48(2):172–179.
42. Pennathur A, Chang AC, McGrath KM, et al. Polyflex expandable stents in the treatment of esophageal disease: initial experience. *Ann Thorac Surg.* 2008;85(6):1968–1972; discussion 1973.
43. Herth FJ, Peter S, Baty F, et al. Combined airway and oesophageal stenting in malignant airway-oesophageal fistulas: a prospective study. *Eur Respir J.* 2010;36(6):1370–1374.
44. Freitag L, Tekolf E, Steveling H, et al. Management of malignant esophagotracheal fistulas with airway stenting and double stenting. *Chest.* 1996; 110(5):1155–1160.

59 Tracheobronchial Injuries

Steven J. Mentzer

Keywords: Bronchoscopy, trachea, bronchi, trauma

INTRODUCTION

Tracheobronchial injuries are rare but potentially lethal injuries associated with (1) thoracic trauma, (2) iatrogenic damage, and (3) inhalation injuries.[1] Most traumatic tracheobronchial injuries are associated with a high-energy impact; typically, a motor vehicle accident or fall. These injuries often are associated with significant thoracic compression injuries including fractures to the ribs and clavicle as well as cardiac and pulmonary contusions.

There are several potential traumatic mechanisms for tracheobronchial injury. Based on the types of associated injury, the most likely mechanism is related to shear forces created by rapid deceleration. The highest incidence of airway injury occurs at the sites of mediastinal attachment; that is, within 2.5 cm of the carina. A plausible explanation is that shear develops between restrained and unrestrained airways leading to disruption of the bronchus. Secondary sites of airway injury include the right middle lobe bronchus and the superior segmental bronchi bilaterally. These airways are relatively long and similarly susceptible to differential deceleration forces. Finally, spiral tears of the right mainstem and bronchus intermedius can occur. These injuries are presumably caused by rotational as well as compressive forces.

DIAGNOSIS

The common presenting signs of blunt tracheobronchial injury include dyspnea, subcutaneous emphysema, and hemoptysis. Also, patients with blunt injury commonly present with sternal tenderness or focal rib pain. Patients presenting with these symptoms, in the context of a high-energy impact, should have a chest CT scan and bronchoscopic examination. Stridor is generally restricted to extrathoracic tracheal injuries, subglottic edema, or bilateral vocal cord dysfunction. These patients are typically intubated soon after the development of stridor.

The radiographic findings may include pneumothorax, pneumomediastinum, and fractures of the bony thorax. The chest CT scan in a patient who has survived a high-energy impact may reveal evidence of a pulmonary contusion and mediastinal hematoma, but free rupture of the airway into the pleural space is rare. In most cases, the soft tissues of the mediastinum and hilum contain the rupture. The airway discontinuity is reflected only by a small amount of extraluminal air and edema. These findings are often missed in a patient with multiple associated injuries.

The difficulty of establishing a radiographic diagnosis of tracheobronchial injury mandates bronchoscopy in any patient who has sustained a high-energy impact injury to the thorax and presents with any sign or symptom of intrathoracic injury. The procedure must be performed by an experienced bronchoscopist. The aspiration of blood and mucus in the proximal airways often complicates the initial trauma bronchoscopy; it is common for the airway injury to be missed at the initial bronchoscopy. In addition, airway injuries frequently present as a subtle separation in the airway cartilage that is contained by mediastinal soft tissue. Repeat bronchoscopy is frequently required to unequivocally establish the diagnosis of airway injury.

INDICATIONS FOR SURGERY

The absolute indication for surgery is the free rupture of a proximal bronchus into the pleural space. In most cases, the patient presents with a pneumothorax. The diagnosis of a proximal airway injury is readily established by the large air leak discovered when the tube thoracostomy is placed within the pleural space. In these patients, the airway injury is commonly associated with pulmonary contusion and diminished lung compliance over the ensuing 24 to 72 hours. Prompt repair has the potential advantage of allowing single-lung ventilation during the surgery—an option that may not be tolerated hours later. In addition, the repaired airway will permit greater flexibility in mechanical ventilation strategies as the patient recovers from the acute lung injury.

In general, all contained mainstem bronchial injuries should be repaired as soon as the patient is hemodynamically stabilized and more life-threatening injuries have been excluded. Injuries to the right mainstem bronchus have the potential to rupture into the right pleural space necessitating prolonged or high-pressure mechanical ventilation. In contrast, injuries to the left mainstem bronchus rarely rupture into the pleural space, but are associated with larger gaps in the airway. In both cases, failure to repair the airway can result in functional pneumonectomy secondary to bronchomalacia, stricture, or both. Furthermore, failure to repair the injury promptly can lead to poor airway clearance, chronic infection, and contracted airways, further limiting repair options. Finally, chronic infection can lead to vascular erosion and a fatal bronchovascular fistula.

In patients with severe bilateral pulmonary contusions, hemodynamic and ventilatory instability may preclude any attempt at acute repair of the mainstem bronchus. The only therapeutic option in these patients is to optimize ventilatory support and hope for the opportunity of a late repair.

The indication for repair of a middle lobe or superior segmental airway is less an attempt to salvage distal lung tissue, and more an attempt to prevent secondary complications of stricture and chronic infection. In some patients, the airway separation is minimal and they can be managed without surgery. In other cases, semi-elective repair can be performed when the patient is stabilized and pulmonary compliance has improved. Although mechanical stents have been used successfully in this setting, an ongoing concern is the risk of erosion and bronchovascular fistula.

SURGICAL TECHNIQUE

For patients undergoing surgical repair, anesthetic management must avoid further disruption of the airway caused by endotracheal tube misplacement or high airway ventilatory pressures. In the spontaneously ventilating patient, the transition to positive pressure ventilation may result in sudden rupture and decompression of the airway. Disruption of the airway can lead to massive subcutaneous emphysema, tension pneumothorax, or both. The disrupted bronchial segment must be rapidly and skillfully isolated to maintain adequate lung volumes and gas exchange. In most cases, single-lung ventilation will be required to facilitate repair of the injured airway. Bronchial blockers are typically unhelpful because of the airway injury, and a double-lumen endotracheal tube is used. The skillful fiberoptic placement of a double-lumen endotracheal tube may be required to avoid aggravation of the airway injury.

Surgical repair of the injury requires a posterolateral thoracotomy to gain adequate control of the hilum and proximal airways. Regardless of the level of the injury, we recommend mobilization of an intercostal muscle pedicle to buttress the repair and minimize the risk of a bronchovascular fistula. The intercostal muscle pedicle is best mobilized at the outset of the procedure.

In most cases, the location of the injury is identifiable because of the air dissection and associated soft tissue trauma. Injuries to the right mainstem bronchus typically do not result in displacement of the airway. In contrast, left mainstem bronchial transections can retract several centimeters under the aortic arch—a retraction that can be worsened by rightward displacement of the mediastinum (Fig. 59-1). Despite the problematic appearance of the proximal mainstem bronchus, traction sutures can be used to deliver the bronchus into the field and facilitate the repair. On occasion, injuries of the right mainstem bronchus may extend into the bronchus intermedius reflecting a spiral tear. We have successfully managed these injuries by transecting the mainstem bronchus, separately preparing the proximal and distal airways, and then reconstructing the two repaired airways as a standard end-to-end anastomosis.

The anastomosis of mainstem bronchial injuries is relatively straightforward. The airways do not have the size mismatch problems commonly associated with transplant anastomoses or sleeve reconstructions. Repair of the disrupted airway is typically achieved with a simple end-to-end anastomosis. Whereas absorbable sutures are commonly used, we prefer monofilament sutures in the context of trauma because of the risk of infection, the frequent need for prolonged ventilatory support, and the unpredictable nutritional status of the patient. In addition, we wrap the repair in an intercostal muscle pedicle to minimize pleural contamination and prevent a bronchovascular fistula.

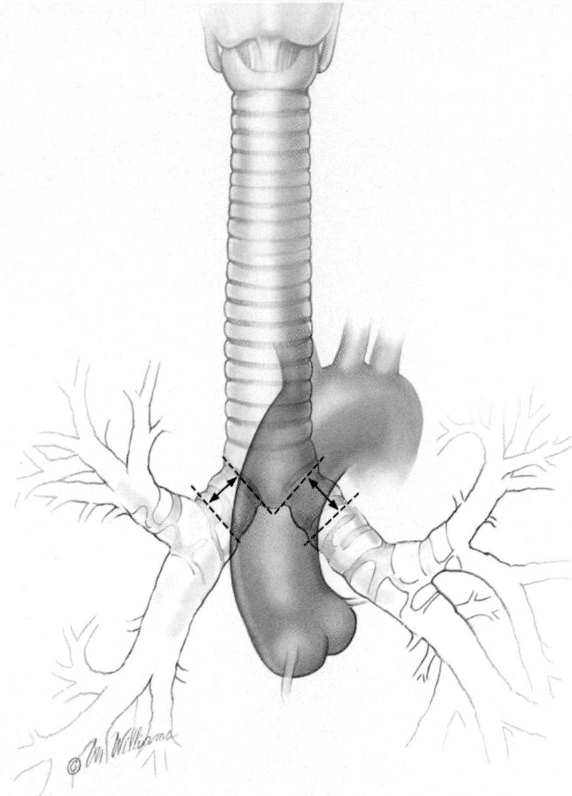

Figure 59-1. Left mainstem bronchial transections can retract several centimeters under the aortic arch, complicating the repair.

EDITOR'S COMMENT

On occasion, the patient undergoing repair of a disrupted airway will desaturate with single-lung ventilation because of fluid resuscitation and lung injuries. I have been able to manage this problem by placing a small catheter through the open side of the double-lumen endotracheal tube and advancing it to the distal lumen of the transected lung, where it is used to deliver oxygen at high flow rates to improve oxygenation.

The intercostal muscle flap should not be used to wrap the repair circumferentially to avoid calcification of the periosteum and late obstruction. I prefer to cover a portion of the repair with the intercostal muscle, and if more is required, to use pericardium or the pericardial fat pad.

Follow-up bronchoscopy is preferred at least a week after the repair to ensure the absence of a stricture or any other complications.

—Raphael Bueno

ACKNOWLEDGMENT

Supported in part by NIH Grant HL47078 and HL75426.

Reference

1. Palade E, Passlick B. [Surgery of traumatic tracheal and tracheobronchial injuries]. *Chirurg.* 2011;82:141–147.

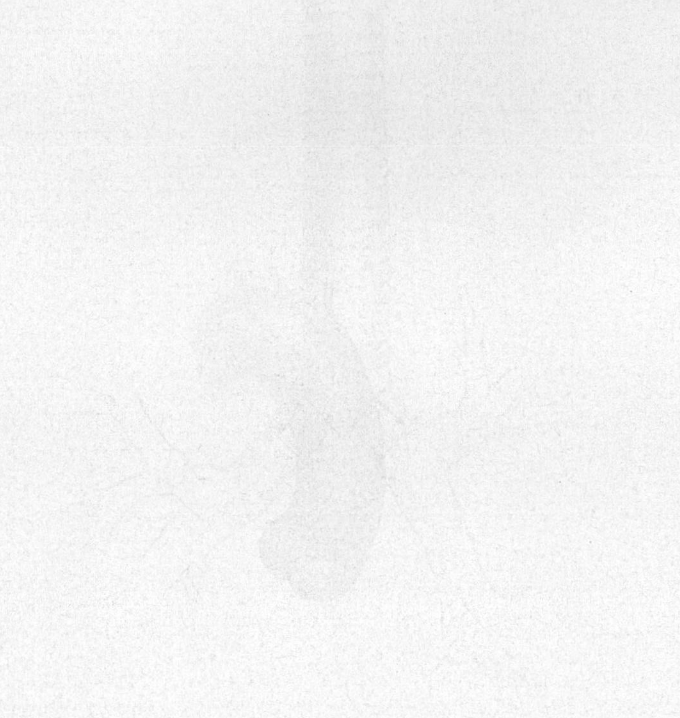

PART 9

CANCER OF THE UPPER AIRWAYS

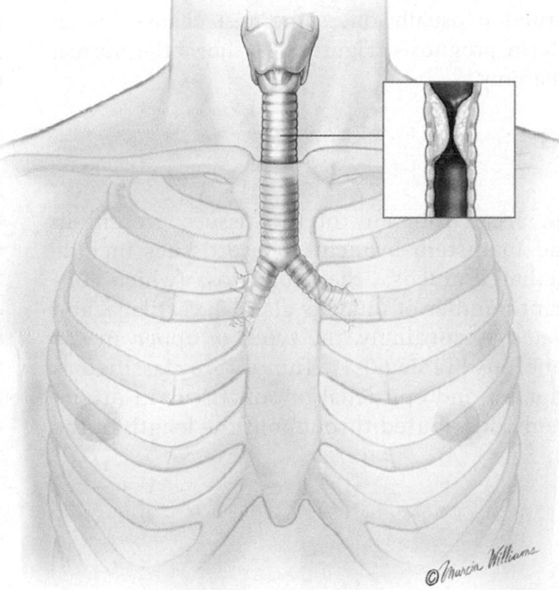

60 Overview

Mark F. Berry and Joseph S. Friedberg

Keywords: Upper airway tumors, neoplasms, trachea, mainstem bronchi, epithelial cell, squamous cell carcinoma (SCC), adenoid cystic carcinoma (ACC), salivary gland, neuroendocrine carcinoid tumors

Upper airway tumors encompass a wide variety of epithelial and soft tissue neoplasms that are relatively rare and usually malignant. Squamous cell and adenoid cystic carcinomas are the most common. Definitive diagnosis is often delayed because the symptoms associated with upper airway tumors are similar to those of more common pulmonary disorders such as chronic obstructive pulmonary disease. Although less invasive palliative treatment modalities are available, surgical resection with airway reconstruction usually offers the best chance for an excellent long-term prognosis. Figure 60-1 shows the normal upper airway anatomy.

ETIOLOGY

Neoplasms can arise from any of the tissues present in the trachea and mainstem bronchi. These tissues include the columnar ciliated mucosa, the submucosa (which contains a significant number of mucous glands), cartilage, and connective tissues. Accordingly, the types of upper airway tumors are numerous (Table 60-1). Tumors are classified as benign or malignant and epithelial or soft tissue in origin. Lesions are evenly distributed throughout the length of the trachea.

In adults, most upper airway tumors are malignant.[1–4] Extremely rare, their incidence is much lower than carcinomas of the larynx and lung. In fact, upper airway tumors account for fewer than 0.2% of all respiratory tract malignancies.[5] The malignant epithelial tumors squamous cell carcinomas (SCCs) and adenoid cystic carcinomas (ACCs) are the most common primary tracheal malignancies, followed by carcinoid and mucoepidermoid carcinomas.[1–4,6–12] Benign tumors represent a wide variety of histologic types. The most common are squamous papilloma, pleomorphic adenoma, and benign cartilaginous tumors.[3]

Squamous Cell Carcinoma

Although SCC usually occurs in lobar and segmental bronchi, it is the most common neoplasm of the trachea and mainstem bronchi.[3,8,13] SCC of the trachea occurs most commonly in males between the ages of 50 and 70 years and is associated with cigarette smoking.[2,3,14] SCC has papillary and basaloid variants and usually appears as a well-localized, exophytic, ulcerated lesion. SCC also can occur as a focally invasive component of a squamous papilloma. The cancer may spread to regional tracheal lymph nodes and directly into mediastinal structures. Approximately one-third of patients have infiltrative

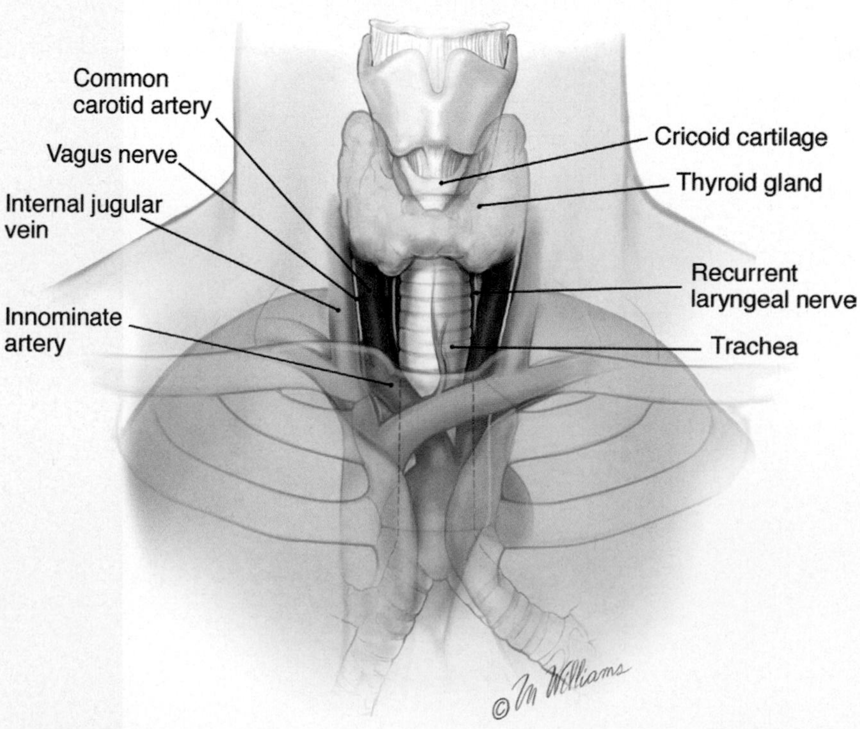

Figure 60-1. Anatomy of the upper airway.

Table 60-1

UPPER AIRWAY TUMORS

	BENIGN	MALIGNANT
Epithelial	Papilloma	Squamous cell carcinoma
	Mucous gland adenoma	Adenoid cystic carcinoma
		Carcinoid tumors
	Pleomorphic adenoma	Mucoepidermoid carcinoma
	Monomorphic adenoma	Adenocarcinoma
	Myoepithelioma	Small cell carcinoma
	Epithelial–myoepithelial tumor	Combined small cell carcinoma
	Oncocytoma	Large cell carcinoma
		Large cell neuroendocrine carcinoma
		Acinic cell carcinoma
		Malignant salivary gland-type mixed tumors
		Pleomorphic carcinoma
		Spindle cell carcinoma
		Giant cell carcinoma
		Carcinosarcoma
		Pulmonary blastoma
		Myoepithelial carcinoma
Soft tissue	Chondroma	Chondrosarcoma
	Glomus tumor	Angiosarcoma
	Hemangioma	Kaposi's sarcoma
	Hemangioendothelioma	Leiomyosarcoma
		Rhabdomyosarcoma
	Granular cell tumor	Liposarcoma
	Hamartoma	Fibrosarcoma
	Leiomyoma	Hemangiopericytoma
	Lipoma	Malignant fibrous histiocytoma
	Neurofibroma	Neurogenic sarcoma
		Osteosarcoma
	Schwannoma	Synovial sarcoma
Miscellaneous	Inflammatory pseudotumor	Malignant lymphoma
	Inflammatory myofibroblastic tumor	Primary pulmonary melanoma
	Castleman disease	Metastases

local extension and mediastinal or pulmonary metastasis at the time of diagnosis.[6]

Adenoid Cystic Carcinoma

ACC, a salivary gland type, is the second most common primary upper airway malignancy.[3,8,13] The mean age for patients with tracheal ACC is 44 years.[15] ACC appears to be unrelated to smoking and is evenly distributed between males and females.[3,7,14] These neoplasms, which can have cribriform, tubular, or solid histologic features, generally have a much slower growth pattern and more insidious onset than SCC. Although histologic pattern is important, prognosis appears to be more a function of disease stage.[16]

ACC growth patterns are either nodular, infiltrative (in which the tumors grow submucosally without producing a distinct mass), or of mixed nodular and infiltrative type.[7,17] Tumors can spread along the airways and involve a long length of trachea by submucosal and perineural spread without involving adjacent mediastinal structures.[15] The microscopic level of invasion often exceeds that which is grossly apparent. Negative resection margins can be difficult to achieve, although long-term disease control has been reported with positive surgical margins.[2,15] Tumors also can spread radially into adjacent parenchyma and lymph nodes. These tumors tend to displace rather than invade mediastinal structures.[17] Approximately 10% of ACC metastasize to regional lymph nodes.[3,12,14] When these tumors metastasize, they locate predominantly in the lung, bone, and liver. Patients can have extended survival despite the presence of pulmonary metastases, which tend to progress very slowly.[1,15]

Carcinoid Tumors

Carcinoid tumors are malignant neuroendocrine tumors that make up to 4% of all primary lung tumors.[18,19] Although most bronchial carcinoid tumors arise in lobar bronchi or the lung periphery, 10% originate in the mainstem bronchi.[20] Carcinoid tumors appear as fleshy, highly vascular masses. Typical carcinoid tumors are low-grade malignancies with no necrosis and fewer than 2 mitoses per 2 mm^2. Typical carcinoids occur equally in men and women, most commonly around age 50, and are not associated with smoking or any other toxic exposure.[7] Hilar and mediastinal lymph node metastases occur in 5% to 10% of patients but are not necessarily associated with poor survival.[21] Atypical carcinoids, which comprise approximately 10% to 20% of all carcinoids, have 2 to 10 mitoses per 2 mm^2 or a foci of coagulative necrosis. The atypical carcinoids are consistently associated with smoking and 30% to 75% incidence of lymph node metastases.[21] Patients with pulmonary carcinoid tumors, typical and atypical combined, usually present with obstructive-type symptoms. Carcinoid syndrome symptoms are uncommon with pulmonary carcinoid tumors.

Salivary Gland-Type Tumors

Salivary gland-type tumors, other than ACC, also can arise from the mixed submucosal seromucinous glands and ducts. These tumors are found in the trachea and mainstem bronchi but occur much more frequently in lobar bronchi.[7] Patients usually present with wheezing or hemoptysis caused by airway tumor growth. Tracheobronchial salivary gland-type tumors are histologically indistinguishable from those arising in the major salivary glands. Benign tumors include mucous gland adenomas, pleomorphic adenomas (also known as benign mixed tumors), oncocytoma, monomorphic adenomas, myoepitheliomas, and epithelial–myoepithelial tumors. Malignant salivary gland-type carcinomas, in addition to ACC described earlier, include low- and high-grade mucoepidermoid carcinomas, acinic cell carcinoma, and salivary gland-type mixed tumors. Other rare salivary gland-type carcinomas that can occur in endobronchial locations are pleomorphic carcinoma, spindle cell carcinoma, giant cell carcinoma, carcinosarcoma, and pulmonary blastoma.

Other Epithelial Neoplasms

Papillomas are benign tracheobronchial epithelial tumors composed of connective tissue with an overlying epithelial surface. Tracheobronchial papillomas generally have an exophytic growth pattern, and their appearance, endoscopically and grossly, resembles a sessile cauliflower-like mass occupying the airway lumen.[22] Papillomas are subclassified as squamous cell, glandular, or mixed depending on the type of epithelial lining contained in the tumor.[7] Squamous cell papillomas, by far the most common type, are associated with human papillomavirus types 6 and 11 and can be either solitary or multiple (squamous papillomatosis).[22,23] The epithelium in these tumors can become dysplastic and progress to carcinoma.

Endobronchial Carcinomas

Although most pulmonary adenocarcinomas are peripheral and involve the larger airways secondarily, endobronchial adenocarcinomas that are histologically distinct from the salivary gland-type tumors do exist.[24] These polypoid lesions have a similar prognosis to the more common peripheral adenocarcinomas.[7] Similarly, one can encounter endobronchial small cell, combined small cell, large cell, and large cell neuroendocrine carcinomas. Combined small cell carcinoma is defined as a small cell carcinoma with an additional component of any nonsmall cell carcinoma histologic type. Large cell carcinoma lacks squamous or glandular differentiation and small cell carcinoma cytologic features; large cell neuroendocrine carcinoma is a variant of large cell carcinoma with neuroendocrine differentiation.

Soft Tissue Neoplasms

The fibroconnective tissues of the trachea and bronchi, which include cartilage, smooth muscle cells, fibroblasts, adipocytes, nerves, lymphatics, and blood vessels, all can give rise to a variety of benign and malignant soft tissue tumors. These tumors are rarer than primary epithelial malignancies of the airway. Hamartoma, the most common benign lung tumor, is a mesenchymal neoplasm that contains adipose tissue, fibrous tissue, and cartilage. These tumors occur mostly in the lung parenchyma, although approximately 10% present in an endobronchial location.[7] Chondromas and chondrosarcomas arise in the cartilaginous rings of the large bronchi or trachea. Glomus tumors are lesions with smooth muscle features that arise from the posterior membranous trachea. Granular cell tumors are polypoid endobronchial lesions that can invade peribronchial structures.

Vascular tumors such as hemangiomas, hemangioendotheliomas, angiosarcomas, and Kaposi's sarcoma occur rarely. Similarly, primary pulmonary leiomyomas, leiomyosarcomas, rhabdomyosarcomas, lipomas, liposarcomas, and osteosarcomas are rare tumors that have been found endobronchially. Other sarcomas, such as fibrosarcoma, hemangiopericytoma, malignant fibrous histiocytoma, and synovial sarcoma, have been reported but occur primarily in the lung periphery.[7] Nerve sheath tumors such as neurofibroma, schwannoma, and neurogenic sarcoma also can occur endotracheally, although these lesions are found far more often in the posterior mediastinum.[7]

Miscellaneous Tumors

Inflammatory pseudotumor and inflammatory myofibroblastic tumors are lesions composed of a spectrum of fibroblastic or myofibroblastic proliferations with a varying infiltrate of inflammatory cells that can occur as endobronchial and endotracheal masses as well as in the lung parenchyma.[7] The airways also can be involved with lymphoma, either from disseminated disease from a nodal lymphoma or from a primary pulmonary lymphoma arising in bronchial-associated lymphoid tissue. Melanoma, whether in the form of metastatic disease or much more uncommonly a primary pulmonary melanoma, can occur in a similar manner. Thyroid and laryngeal carcinomas can involve the upper trachea by direct extension. Tracheal and mainstem bronchi invasion also can result from metastasis from other primary malignancies, including primary pulmonary adenocarcinomas, malignant mesothelioma, and breast, colon, and renal cell adenocarcinomas.

CLINICAL PRESENTATION

Patients with upper airway neoplasms typically present with slowly progressive respiratory symptoms such as dyspnea, cough, hemoptysis, wheezing, stridor, excessive secretions, and recurrent pneumonia (Table 60-2).[7,10,11,14] The rate of progression of symptoms tends to be slower with benign tumors and ACC and more rapid with bronchogenic cancers. Because tracheal neoplasms tend to be slow growing, symptoms owing to upper airway obstruction, irritation, or ulceration can continue for months or even years. Acute life-threatening airway emergencies secondary to near-complete airway occlusion are uncommon but can occur. Symptoms related to involvement of adjacent structures, such as hoarseness and dysphagia, are generally less frequent but also can occur. The peak incidence range of the more common upper airway neoplasms is between the ages of 40 and 60 years. Tumors other than SCC and ACC have a scattered age distribution but tend to occur more commonly in young adults.[5]

The more common pulmonary conditions, including pneumonia, asthma, and chronic obstructive pulmonary disease, are usually suspected on initial presentation. Medical treatments often are attempted for a period of time for presumed parenchymal disease before a tracheal tumor is correctly diagnosed, especially because most patients have a normal initial chest x-ray report. A high index of suspicion therefore is needed to diagnose tracheal neoplasms at an early stage. Any patient with adult-onset asthma, and especially any patient with unilateral wheezing on physical examination, should be suspected immediately of having an upper airway tumor. Diagnoses usually are made more rapidly when patients have hemoptysis, which is most common with SCC, because bronchoscopy generally will be performed even with a normal chest x-ray.[14] Tumors often are locally advanced at the time of diagnosis owing to the slow progression of symptoms. Patients with a short duration of symptoms thus are more likely to be resectable.

Table 60-2

SYMPTOMS OF UPPER AIRWAY NEOPLASMS
Cough
Dyspnea
Recurrent pneumonia
Hemoptysis
Wheezing
Stridor
Excessive secretions
Hoarseness
Dysphagia
Acute respiratory difficulty

DIAGNOSIS AND STAGING

The evaluation of patients with tracheal tumors typically starts with a chest x-ray. Tracheal narrowing, postobstructive atelectasis or pneumonia, or abnormal calcification on chest x-ray can suggest the presence of a tracheal tumor. Fewer than half of tracheal tumors are identified by an initial chest radiograph, which, as mentioned earlier, often leads to a delay in diagnosis. Pulmonary function tests are often used to evaluate the presenting symptoms, and flow-volume loops can indicate upper airway obstruction with plateauing of the inspiratory or expiratory phase in the presence of an upper airway neoplasm. An obstructive pattern with no response to bronchodilators suggests a fixed upper airway obstruction. Pulmonary function tests are also useful for preoperative evaluation and to predict postoperative lung function. Laboratory tests are not helpful in the diagnosis of tracheal tumors.

CT scan of the chest and endoscopic airway evaluation by bronchoscopy should be initiated early in the evaluation of any patient suspected of having an upper airway lesion. Chest CT scanning is capable of demonstrating a tracheal mass, local tumor extent such as mediastinal involvement either by enlarged lymph nodes or by direct tumor extension into adjacent structures, and distant disease spread. Although chest CT scanning historically was thought to identify great vessel invasion, it did not reliably predict tumor length or esophageal invasion. Helical CT scanning is the preferred method for assessing both tumor growth and longitudinal extent along the tracheal or bronchial wall.[17]

Bronchoscopy is essential to confirm the diagnosis and extent of intraluminal involvement. It is used for precise measurement and biopsy to define the margins of the lesion. This information is essential for planning the surgical resection because tumor length is a key component in determining resectability. Endobronchial ultrasound also can be performed during bronchoscopy to further evaluate local tumor extent. Endobronchial ultrasound gives visualization of the airway wall to evaluate for tumor invasion into surrounding structures, as well as peritracheal and peribronchial lymph nodes.[25,26] Flexible bronchoscopy is used primarily to evaluate tracheal tumors and to obtain biopsy. However, flexible bronchoscopy is ineffective for establishing airway control, and rigid bronchoscopy should be used to establish a patent airway in patients with life-threatening conditions such as significant upper airway obstruction or massive hemoptysis. Tracheotomy may complicate any subsequent resection attempt and should be avoided whenever possible for acute airway emergencies. As discussed below, local treatment of tracheal tumors can be performed during both flexible and rigid bronchoscopy as both palliative and curative efforts. Caution is required, however, because bronchoscopic manipulation of airway tumors can lead to complete airway compromise. Biopsy is also contraindicated if the tumor appears to be highly vascular.

Further staging workup should be initiated as needed if a malignant lesion is diagnosed. Laryngoscopy is performed if the tumor involves the subglottic airway or if there is vocal cord dysfunction. Other studies to evaluate regional and distant metastases can include head CT scanning, brain MRI, bone scanning, and positron-emission tomography (PET) scanning. Mediastinoscopy is used to stage bronchogenic carcinoma and also can be useful for direct evaluation of extraluminal spread. As described elsewhere, mediastinoscopy should be done at the time of planned resection to aid in tissue dissection.[9]

SURGICAL TREATMENT OPTIONS

The optimal therapy for upper airway tumors is airway surgical resection and reconstruction. The underlying goal is to preserve as much lung tissue as possible. Excessive longitudinal extent that precludes safe reconstruction, macroscopic mediastinal nodal metastases, and distant metastases are the key elements that make upper airway cancers unresectable. Direct invasion of mediastinal structures, such as the aorta and the esophagus, precludes resection if the involved mediastinal structure cannot be repaired primarily. Unfortunately, early diagnosis is uncommon owing to the lack of early symptoms and because regional spread beyond the trachea often has occurred by the time of detection. The true percentage of unresectable upper airway cancers is unknown. The reported resectability rates vary from 9% to 74%.[2,27,28] Advances in tracheal mobilization likely have increased the number of resectable tumors, and all reasonable surgical candidates should have operative exploration if resectability is in question. Patients expected to require chronic postoperative mechanical ventilation have significant morbidity and mortality and should not undergo attempted resection.[8] A useful guide for resectability is the predicted postoperative forced expiratory volume in 1 second. Although absolute values, such as a minimum value of 800 mL, have been used to determine suitable candidates for surgery in the past, the percent predicted value based in part on patient age, size, and gender is a more clinically useful measurement. A predicted postoperative percent predicted value of forced expiratory volume in 1 second of less than 40% indicates increased perioperative resection risk.[29] The predicted postoperative percent predicted value of the diffusion capacity of the lung to carbon monoxide is another useful parameter to consider when evaluating a patient's suitability for resection, with a value of less than 40% again predicting increased perioperative risk. However, careful surgical judgment that considers objective pulmonary function values but also medical comorbidities and qualitative assessment of functional status is needed to determine whether a patient is an acceptable surgical candidate.

Prognosis generally depends on tumor histology, stage, and overall patient status.[12,30–33] Patients with complete resection of benign or low-grade tracheal tumors are likely to have recurrence-free long-term survival. The overall prognosis for malignant lesions historically is poor, with a median survival of 6 months and a 10% to 20% 2-year survival.[30] Overall survival after tracheal tumor resection is 36% to 79% at 5 years and 27% to 57% at 10 years. Surgical resection is associated with 5-year survival rates of 13% to 50% for SCC and 52% to 80% for ACC.[14,15,30,33,34]

Positive lymph nodes and positive resection margins are much worse prognostic factors for SCC than for ACC.[2,15] Local invasion into the thyroid gland also appears to be a very poor prognostic sign for patients with SCC.[35] After resection, typical carcinoid tumors have 5- and 10-year survival rates of 95% and 90%, respectively, whereas atypical carcinoids have a worse prognosis, with 5- and 10-year survival rates of 61% and 35%, respectively.[7] Median survival rates in patients with unresectable malignant tumors who are treated primarily with radiation ranges from 6 to 31 months, and the 5-year survival rate is 8% to 27%.[28,30–32]

Operative mortality generally depends on both the physiologic impact of the procedure and the length of the airway resection and has improved dramatically over time as surgical judgment and techniques have been refined. Overall operative mortality is 5% to 10% and is expected to be lowest in centers where tracheal surgery is performed commonly.[2,14,15] Operative mortality after tracheal resection has been reported to be as low as 1%, with a 12% to 15% mortality after carinal resection.[2,33] Predominant predictors of operative death after carinal resection include postoperative mechanical ventilation, length of resected airway, and development of anastomotic complications.[9] Anastomotic complications have been observed in 17% of patients undergoing carinal resection and almost always result in death or require surgical reintervention.[9] Early anastomotic complications include necrosis. Late anastomotic complications include stenosis and formation of excessive granulation tissue. Other relatively common complications after resection include atrial arrhythmias and pneumonia.

Illustrated techniques for surgical management of upper airways cancers are presented in Chapters 62 to 66. Endoscopic management is covered in Chapter 67.

NONRESECTIONAL MANAGEMENT

Treatment modalities for patients with unresectable tumors or for those who cannot tolerate or refuse surgery include external-beam radiation therapy and several bronchoscope-based tumor ablation techniques. Chemotherapy generally is not useful for treating upper airway neoplasms, although it is used often in combination with radiation for bronchogenic tumors. Bronchoscopic destructive techniques include mechanical debridement, laser treatment, cryotherapy, brachytherapy, airway stent placement, photodynamic therapy, and argon plasma coagulation. These endoscopic treatments generally are designed to ensure airway patency and are performed either for palliation alone or with curative intent depending on the modality. Tumor resectability ideally should be determined before instituting any of these treatment modalities because they can preclude future safe resection. Preoperative radiation in particular may compromise anastomotic healing and make subsequent resection riskier. These techniques may be used, if necessary, to stabilize a patient's airway. They also permit better preoperative preparation and staging, including local downstaging of tumor, permitting subsequent resection.[27] Nonsurgical and endoscopic treatments for patients with acute airway compromise and patients who are not candidates for surgical resection are broadly categorized as curative or palliative. Modalities used with curative intent include external-beam radiation therapy, brachytherapy, and photodynamic therapy. Bronchoscopic techniques used for palliation include endobronchial debridement or mechanical core out using a rigid bronchoscopy, laser treatment, cryotherapy, argon plasma coagulation, and airway stent placement.

Curative Intent

External-beam radiation may be used postoperatively to prevent local disease recurrence, especially with positive or close margins. Resection combined with postoperative radiation results in the best local tumor control rate.[36] Radiation also has a use for inoperable patients either for palliation or with curative intent. ACC appears to be more radiosensitive than SCC. Higher-dose radiation (>60 Gy) is needed for prolonged local control and long-term survival but is also associated with more complications.[28,30,32] Common acute complications are cough and dysphagia, although tracheal necrosis also has been reported.[28] Late complications include radiation pneumonitis, tracheoesophageal fistula, and esophageal stricture.[30,32,36]

Brachytherapy involves the implantation or temporary placement of radioactive material in the airway to deliver relatively high-dose radiation to the tumor and immediately adjacent tissue with minimal dose to surrounding structures.[37] Brachytherapy may be used as a primary treatment, to improve local control after either resection or external-beam therapy, and for recurrent tumors, especially those already treated with primary radiation therapy.[28,30,31] A catheter is placed using the flexible bronchoscope with fluoroscopic guidance and secured in place. Dummy seeds with radiopaque markers are used to confirm proper catheter position. Radioactive seeds containing a high-dose–rate source, such as a high activity iridium-192 radioisotope, then are implanted into the catheter. Most patients are treated with one to six fractions over several days to weeks on an outpatient basis. Endobronchial brachytherapy is generally well tolerated, although late complications can include radiation bronchitis, stenosis, and massive hemoptysis owing to bronchovascular fistula.

Photodynamic therapy is used with both curative intent and for palliation to destroy airway tumor while maintaining the structural integrity of surrounding tissues.[38] A photosensitizing drug containing hematoporphyrin is administered and accumulates in malignant tissue. The subsequent exposure to activating light from a nonthermal laser generates reactive oxygen species that destroy the tumor by a combination of effects, including direct cell kill, destruction of tumor neovascularization, and the resulting immunologic response.[39,40] Photodynamic therapy generally is administered using flexible bronchoscopy under local anesthesia, with cleanup bronchoscopy a few days later to remove the resulting necrotic tissue.

Palliation

Upper airway obstruction secondary to tumor can be relieved by several other bronchoscopic techniques.[39] Tumors can be debrided mechanically by means of rigid bronchoscopy, although this technique can be limited by bleeding. Laser treatment, cryotherapy, and argon plasma coagulation can be administered using flexible or rigid bronchoscopy to cause tumor ablation by means of necrosis, permitting subsequent safer mechanical debridement. Although these techniques are used mostly for palliative purposes in patients who are not surgical candidates, tumor debulking also may permit future resection or limit the extent of a future parenchymal resection in selected patients.[41–43]

Tracheobronchial stents also can be used to provide effective and durable palliation in patients with large-airway obstructions caused by intraluminal tumors.[44] Stents maintain airway patency before or during surgical or radiation treatment or after other endoscopic treatments.[43] The choice of stent, either nonexpandable silicone or expandable metal, is determined by the anatomy of the lesion and the preference of the placing physician. Silicone stents are inexpensive, can be repositioned and removed easily, initiate little tissue reactivity, and are associated with minimal tumor ingrowth. However, silicone stents require rigid bronchoscopy and general anesthesia for delivery and have the potential for dislodgment, migration, and plugging owing to secretions. Expandable metal stents can be delivered more easily using flexible bronchoscopy with local anesthesia and fluoroscopy. Metal stents exhibit better airway conformation and less potential for migration but are also essentially permanent. Metal stents covered with a layer of silicone or polyethylene should be used when the airway mucosa is not intact to prevent recurrent airway obstruction caused by ingrowth of tumor into the stent.

CURRENT CHALLENGES

Lack of a suitable graft or conduit to reconstruct or replace the native trachea is a problem that has plagued surgeons from the inception of tracheal surgery. It is the only thoracic structure for which a suitable replacement has not been found. Conduits readily used for esophageal surgery such as colon, jejunum, or Dacron graft are too malleable to substitute for the rigid but flexible native organ. Using current methods, only about half the trachea (5 cm) can be resected and still deliver a durable, tension-free anastomosis. Disease that extends to and involves resection of the carina is even more difficult to resect. Since upper airway tumors are rare, slow growing, and initially frequently mistaken for other more common pulmonary disorders, diagnosis is often delayed, and submucosal spread of tumor often exceeds the limits of resectability. Age is another factor that limits accessibility to the lesion. Consequently, meticulous technique (see Chapters 62–66) has evolved to stretch the limits of tracheal resection.

FUTURE DIRECTIONS

A number of studies have been conducted in animal models (e.g., sheep and pig) using vascular grafts toward the goal of finding a suitable substitute for tracheal and carinal reconstructions.[45] In humans, reports describing the use of aortic autograft for long tracheal reconstruction have yielded promising results.[46] Preceding studies in animal models have demonstrated the aortic allograft to have several unique properties that would render it a suitable alternative for long tracheal replacement.[47] It is less immunogenic than other vascular grafts, accounting for the lack of acute or chronic rejection, and it precludes the necessity of long-term immunosuppression, an important factor in survival and quality of life. The graft also appears to be sufficiently rigid to substitute for the native trachea. Most notably, however, it has a demonstrated ability for long-term tracheal regeneration, complete with a stable, viable respiratory endothelial lining. Although it is premature to conclude that aortic allograft will prove to be a suitable reproducible technique for long tracheal reconstruction, the results are promising and bear further scrutiny.[48]

The use of other biomaterials and other tissue engineering techniques to create an airway replacement conduit have also been reported in both preclinical animal studies as well as in patients. These materials include bioartificial nanocomposites seeded with autologous bone-marrow mononuclear cells augmented with bone-marrow stimulating factors, bioabsorbable polymer scaffolds, and autologous cartilage grafts.[49,50] Although the experience is early, the results are encouraging that reliable biomaterials may ultimately be useful in airway reconstruction methods.

EDITOR'S COMMENT

Malignant tumors that involve trachea are often unresectable. This is the case particularly for SCC. Even in cases where the radiographic studies suggest that the tumor can be removed, the patient and the surgeon must be prepared for the possibility that exploration will reveal that the tumor has infiltrated adjacent tissues, including blood vessels, and resection will have to be aborted. Another tumor that commonly involves trachea is thyroid cancer, which invades the trachea by direct extension. If technically possible, this tumor should be excised en bloc with the thyroid, and a tracheal reconstruction should be performed. As to the other endoscopic modalities, these can often be augmented by combinations. For example, photodynamic therapy or laser ablation followed by brachytherapy and/or external-beam radiation may achieve longer durability.

—Raphael Bueno

References

1. Pearson FG, Todd TR, Cooper JD. Experience with primary neoplasms of the trachea and carina. *J Thorac Cardiovasc Surg*. 1984;88:511–518.
2. Grillo HC, Mathisen DJ. Primary tracheal tumors: treatment and results. *Ann Thorac Surg*. 1990;49:69–77.
3. Regnard JF, Fourquier P, Levasseur P. Results and prognostic factors in re-sections of primary tracheal tumors: a multicenter retrospective study. The French Society of Cardiovascular Surgery. *J Thorac Cardiovasc Surg*. 1996;111:808–813.
4. Gaissert HA, Grillo HC, Shadmehr MB, et al. Uncommon primary tracheal tumors. *Ann Thorc Surg*. 2006;82:268–272.
5. Gaissert HA. Primary tracheal tumors. *Chest Surg Clin North Am*. 2003;13:247–256.
6. Allen MS. Malignant tracheal tumors. *Mayo Clin Proc*. 1993;68:680–684.
7. Litzky L. Epithelial and soft tissue tumors of the tracheobronchial tree. *Chest Surg Clin North Am*. 2003;13:1–40.
8. Hazama K, Miyoshi S, Akashi A, et al. Clinicopathological investigation of 20 cases of primary tracheal cancer. *Eur J Cardiothorac Surg*. 2003;23:1–5.
9. Mitchell JD, Mathisen DJ, Wright CD, et al. Clinical experience with carinal resection. *J Thorac Cardiovasc Surg*. 1999;117:39–52.
10. Schneider P, Schirren J, Muley T, et al. Primary tracheal tumors: experience with 14 resected patients. *Eur J Cardiothorac Surg*. 2001;20:12–18.
11. Refaely Y, Weissberg D. Surgical management of tracheal tumors. *Ann Thorac Surg*. 1997;64:1429–1432.
12. Xu LT, Sun ZF, Li ZJ, et al. Clinical and pathologic characteristics in patients with tracheobronchial tumor: report of 50 patients. *Ann Thorac Surg*. 1987;43:276–278.
13. Bhattacharyya N. Contemporary staging and prognosis for primary tracheal malignancies: a population-based analysis. *Otolaryngol Head Neck Surg*. 2004;131:639–642.
14. Gaissert HA, Grillo HC, Shadmehr MB, et al. Long-term survival after resection of primary adenoid cystic and squamous cell carcinoma of the trachea and carina. *Ann Thorac Surg*. 2004;78:1889–1896.
15. Maziak DE, Todd TR, Keshavjee SH, et al. Adenoid cystic carcinoma of the airway: thirty-two-year experience. *J Thorac Cardiovasc Surg*. 1996;112:1522–1531.

16. Moran CA, Suster S, Koss MN. Primary adenoid cystic carcinoma of the lung: a clinicopathologic and immunohistochemical study of 16 cases. *Cancer.* 1994;73:1390–1397.
17. Kwak SH, Lee KS, Chung MJ, et al. Adenoid cystic carcinoma of the airways: helical CT and histopathologic correlation. *AJR.* 2004;183:277–281.
18. Harpole DH Jr, Feldman JM, Buchanan S, et al. Bronchial carcinoid tumors: a retrospective analysis of 126 patients. *Ann Thorac Surg.* 1992;54:50–54.
19. Ribet M, Gosselin B, Gambiez L, et al. Bronchial carcinoids. *Eur J Cardiothorac Surg.* 1993;7:347–350.
20. Davila DG, Dunn WF, Tazelaar HD, et al. Bronchial carcinoid tumors. *Mayo Clin Proc.* 1993;68:795–803.
21. Cardillo G, Sera F, Di Martino M, et al. Bronchial carcinoid tumors: nodal status and long-term survival after resection. *Ann Thorac Surg.* 2004;77:1781–1785.
22. Lam CW, Talbot AR, Yeh KT, et al Human papillomavirus and squamous cell carcinoma in a solitary tracheal papilloma. *Ann Thorac Surg.* 2004;77:2201–2202.
23. Byrne JC, Tsao MS, Fraser RS, et al. Human papillomavirus-11 DNA in a patient with chronic laryngotracheobronchial papillomatosis and metastatic squamous-cell carcinoma of the lung. *N Engl J Med.* 1987;317:873–878.
24. Reed DN Jr, Hassan AA, Wilson RF. Primary mucinous adenocarcinoma of the trachea: the case for complete surgical resection. *J Surg Oncol.* 1985; 28:29–31.
25. Herth F, Becker HD, LoCicero J 3rd, et al. Endobronchial ultrasound in therapeutic bronchoscopy. *Eur Respir J.* 2002;20:118–121.
26. Kurimoto N, Murayama M, Yoshioka S, et al. Assessment of usefulness of endobronchial ultrasonography in determination of depth of tracheobronchial tumor invasion. *Chest.* 1999;115:1500–1506.
27. Daddi G, Puma F, Avenia N, et al. Resection with curative intent after endoscopic treatment of airway obstruction. *Ann Thorac Surg.* 1998;65: 203–207.
28. Mornex F, Coquard R, Danhier S, et al. Role of radiation therapy in the treatment of primary tracheal carcinoma. *Int J Radiat Oncol Biol Phys.* 1998;41:299–305.
29. Ferguson MK. Preoperative assessment of pulmonary risk. *Chest.* 1999;115: 58S–63S.
30. Chao MW, Smith JG, Laidlaw C, et al. Results of treating primary tumors of the trachea with radiotherapy. *Int J Radiat Oncol Biol Phys.* 1998;41:779–785.
31. Schraube P, Latz D, Wannenmacher M. Treatment of primary squamous cell carcinoma of the trachea: the role of radiation therapy. *Radiother Oncol.* 1994;33:254–258.
32. Jeremic B, Shibamoto Y, Acimovic L, et al. Radiotherapy for primary squamous cell carcinoma of the trachea. *Radiother Oncol.* 1996;41:135–138.
33. Mitchell JD, Mathisen DJ, Wright CD, et al. Resection for bronchogenic carcinoma involving the carina: long-term results and effect of nodal status on outcome. *J Thorac Cardiovasc Surg.* 2001;121:465–471.
34. Prommegger R, Salzer G. Long-term results of surgery for adenoid cystic carcinoma of the trachea and bronchi. *Eur J Surg Oncol.* 1998;24:440–444.
35. Honings J, Gaissert HA, Ruangchira-Urai R, et al. Pathologic characteristics of resected squamous cell carcinoma of the trachea: prognostic factors based on an analysis of 59 cases. *Virchows Arch.* 2009;455:423–429.
36. Chow DC, Komaki R, Libshitz HI, et al. Treatment of primary neoplasms of the trachea: The role of radiation therapy. *Cancer.* 1993;71:2946–2952.
37. Yao M, Koh W. Endobronchial brachytherapy. *Chest Surg Clin North Am.* 2001;11:813–827.
38. McCaughan JS Jr, Williams TE. Photodynamic therapy for endobronchial malignant disease: a prospective fourteen-year study. *J Thorac Cardiovasc Surg.* 1997;114:940–946.
39. Mehrishi S, Raoof S, Mehta AC. Therapeutic flexible bronchoscopy. *Chest Surg Clin North Am.* 2001;11:657–690.
40. Metz JM, Friedberg JS. Endobronchial photodynamic therapy for the treatment of lung cancer. *Chest Surg Clin North Am.* 2001;11:829–839.
41. Mulloy MR, Anderson C, Lao O, et al. Sleeve resection of a transcarinal bronchial carcinoid after laser debulking. *Ann Thorac Surg.* 2004;78:1093–1095.
42. Shankar S, George PJ, Hetzel MR, et al. Elective resection of tumours of the trachea and main carina after endoscopic laser therapy. *Thorax.* 1990;45:493–495.
43. Venuta F, Rendina E, De Giacomo T, et al. Nd:YAG laser resection of lung cancer invading the airway as a bridge to surgery and palliative treatment. *Ann Thorac Surg.* 2002;74:995–998.
44. Wood D. Airway stenting. *Chest Surg Clin North Am.* 2003;13:211–229.
45. Seguin A, Martinod E, Kambouchner M, et al. Carinal replacement with an aortic allograft. *Ann Thorac Surg.* 2006;81:1068–1074.
46. Azorin JF, Bertin F, Martinod E, et al. Tracheal replacement with an aortic autograft. *Eur J Cardiothorac Surg.* 2006;29:261–263.
47. Martinod E, Seguin A, Holder-Espinasse M, et al. Tracheal regeneration following tracheal replacement with an allogenic aorta. *Ann Thorac Surg.* 2005;79:942–948.
48. Wurtz A, Porte H, Conti M, et al. Surgical technique and results of tracheal and carinal replacement with aortic allografts for salivary gland-type carcinoma. *J Thorc Cariodvasc Surg.* 2010;140:387–393
49. Jungebluth P, Alici E, Baiquera S, et al. Tracheobronchial transplantation with a stem-cell-seeded bioartificial noncomposite: a proof-of-concept study. *Lancet.* 2011;338:1997–2004.
50. Tsukada H, Gangadharan S, Garland R, et al. Tracheal replacement with a bioabsorbable scaffold in sheep. *Ann Thorac Surg.* 2010;90:1793–1797.

61 Bronchoscopy, Rigid and Flexible

Steven J. Mentzer

Keywords: **Flexible and rigid bronchoscopy, upper airways strictures or masses, acute upper airway obstruction, massive hemoptysis, biopsy, cancer staging**

Visualization of the airways for diagnosis or treatment can involve the use of either flexible or rigid bronchoscopes. Flexible bronchoscopes generally are used for evaluation and biopsy, whereas rigid bronchoscopes are uniquely capable of establishing and maintaining airway control in a life-threatening situation, such as acute upper airway obstruction or massive hemoptysis. Although these procedures often can be used interchangeably, the rigid bronchoscope is uniquely suitable for applications that require precise airway measurement (e.g., tracheal stricture) or a large working port (e.g., endobronchial tumor).

ANATOMY OF THE TRACHEA AND CONTIGUOUS UPPER AIRWAYS

The trachea extends from the cricoid cartilage at the level of C6 to the origin of the left and right mainstem bronchi at the carina (approximately at the level of T6). In normal adults, the trachea is 12 cm long (range: 9–15 cm). The normal trachea is approximately 16 mm in lateral diameter and 14 mm in anteroposterior diameter. The anterior wall of the trachea is composed of cartilaginous horseshoe-shaped rings, and the posterior wall is a continuous membranous wall (Fig. 61-1).

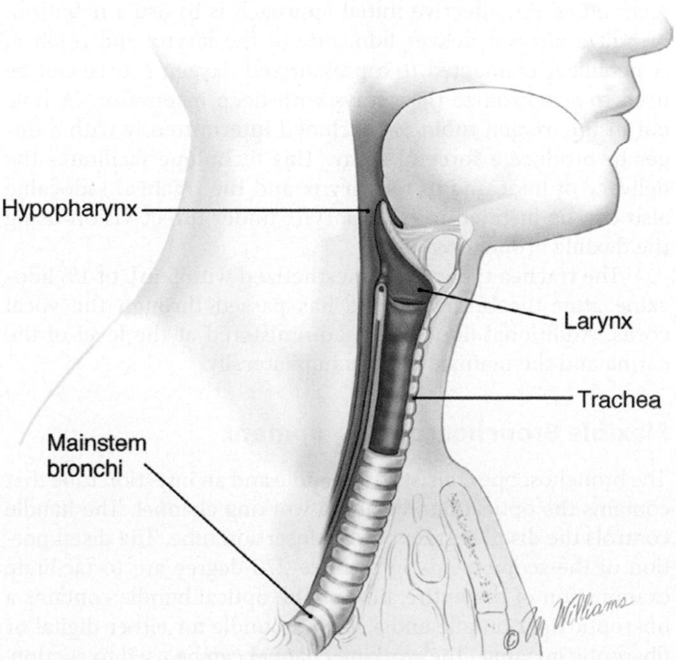

Figure 61-1. Anatomy of the hypopharynx, larynx, and trachea.

The left mainstem bronchus, approximately 4 to 4.5 cm in length, is oriented at 45 degrees to the axis of the trachea. The right mainstem bronchus gives rise to the right upper lobe bronchus near the carina. The right upper lobe has three segments corresponding to the apical (B1), posterior (B2), and anterior (B3) segments. The airway distal to the right upper lobe orifice is the bronchus intermedius. The bronchus intermedius extends 2 cm from the right upper lobe to the middle lobe bronchus. The middle lobe bronchus is 1.2 to 1.5 cm in length and has a diameter of 8 mm. The middle lobe has a medial (B4) and a lateral (B5) segment. The superior segment (B6) of the lower lobe arises at the level of the middle lobe bronchus. The orientation of the basilar segment orifices (B7–10) is variable, and these generally are considered collectively (i.e., composite basilar segmentectomy).

The origin of the left upper lobe bronchus is caudal to that of the right upper lobe bronchus. The left upper lobe orifice branches into upper and lower divisions. The upper division is approximately 1 cm long and gives rise to three segments, two of which are often combined (e.g., B1 + B2 and B3). The lower division is composed of the superior (B4) and inferior (B5) divisions of the lingula. The lower lobe superior segment (B6) has a similar course to the right side. There are only three basilar segments (B8–10; the B7 segment is absent) in the left lower lobe compared with five in the right lower lobe. Similar to the right side, the basilar segments are vertical in orientation and generally considered as a composite structure.

The principal advantages of flexible versus rigid bronchoscopy are detailed in Table 61-1. The diagnostic and therapeutic indications are summarized in Table 61-2.

PREPROCEDURE EVALUATION

Patients undergoing bronchoscopy should have a normal platelet count, prothrombin time, and partial thromboplastin time and no evidence of uremia to minimize the risk of bleeding. Relevant past medical history includes a recent myocardial infarction or documented arrhythmias. Asthma frequently is exacerbated by bronchoscopy and may require pretreatment with bronchodilators.

The label *high-risk bronchoscopy* usually is reserved for patients with a labile PO_2 or evidence of CO_2 retention. Bronchoscopy will decrease arterial PO_2 by 10 to 20 mm Hg under optimal conditions—more if the patient's ventilatory mechanics are impaired.[1,2] It is important to recognize CO_2 retention before the procedure is performed to avoid sedative-related hypercarbic effects. High-risk bronchoscopy should be performed through an endotracheal tube to facilitate positive-pressure ventilation and oxygen delivery if necessary.

Table 61-1

TECHNICAL PRINCIPLES OF BRONCHOSCOPY

	ADVANTAGES	DISADVANTAGES
Flexible	Local anesthesia Good visualization	Small access port Limited suction
Rigid	Large working port Detect tracheal fixation	General anesthesia Limited visualization[a] Requires neck extension

[a]Smaller-diameter rigid scopes not only have smaller distal lumens, but also these scopes bend slightly when examining the left tracheobronchial tree. Visualization can be improved by placing a flexible scope through the rigid scope.

Table 61-2

DIAGNOSTIC AND THERAPEUTIC INDICATIONS FOR BRONCHOSCOPY

INDICATIONS	FLEXIBLE	RIGID
Diagnostic		
Endobronchial symptoms: hemoptysis, chronic cough, atelectasis, obstructive pneumonia, localized wheeze	√	
Tissue diagnosis of lung tumor	√	
Covered brush cultures	√	
Evaluation of burn injury	√	
Placement of endotracheal tube	√	
Precise measurement of tracheal stricture/ tumor		√
Detection of airway fixation		√
Therapeutic		
Intubation	√	
Bronchial toilet (lobar collapse)	√	
Aspiration (diagnosis and treatment)	√	√
Removal of foreign body	±	√
Laser treatment	√	√
Stricture dilatation	√	√
Massive bleeding	±	√

The specific preprocedure evaluation for patients undergoing rigid bronchoscopy includes an examination for concomitant neck injury or cervical disease. In addition, the ventilatory inefficiencies during rigid bronchoscopy make patients with poor lung compliance a particularly high-risk group.

PREMEDICATION

Patients undergoing flexible bronchoscopy benefit from sedation. Although a number of medications have been used, the most common combination used today is an IV narcotic and a benzodiazepine. The most popular benzodiazepine is midazolam (Versed). Midazolam is a short-acting benzodiazepine that decreases anxiety and impairs memory retention. Midazolam is also associated with respiratory depression and hypotension. A typical starting dose is 2 mg IV (1 mg IV in an elderly person).

Fentanyl is the most popular narcotic. A short-acting potent narcotic, fentanyl contributes a sedative effect as well as cough suppression. It is associated with respiratory depression and hypotension as well. A typical starting dose is 50 μg IV (25 μg IV in an elderly person).

MONITORING

All endoscopic procedures carry the risk of cardiac arrhythmia. Although elective outpatient bronchoscopy is rarely associated with arrhythmias, perioperative therapeutic bronchoscopies can be associated with atrial arrhythmias and bradycardias. All patients must have continuous electrocardiographic monitoring for the duration of the procedure. Patients receiving midazolam or fentanyl sedation should have blood pressure monitoring during and after bronchoscopy, and all patients should receive supplemental oxygen and have continuous oxygen saturation monitoring.

FLEXIBLE BRONCHOSCOPY TECHNIQUE

Anesthesia

Flexible bronchoscopy can be performed with topical anesthesia.[3] The medications used are either benzocaine and tetracaine (Cetacaine) or lidocaine (Xylocaine). Cetacaine is a combination of agents that is particularly well suited for bronchoscopy. The rapid onset of Cetacaine is attributable to the action of benzocaine, and its extended duration (typically 30–60 minutes) is owing to the action of butamben and tetracaine. Typically, only four to five sprays are used to avoid inducing methemoglobinemia. Methemoglobinemia occurs when more than 1% of the heme iron is oxidized to the ferric form. The oxidized hemoglobin (i.e., methemoglobin) is incapable of reversibly binding oxygen. Methemoglobinemia is readily treated with an infusion of methylene blue.

To perform a well-tolerated bronchoscopy, three anatomic areas need to be anesthetized: the hypopharynx, larynx, and trachea. The hypopharynx can be anesthetized directly with Cetacaine or lidocaine sprays oriented behind the tongue. Some bronchoscopists prefer to have the patient gargle with lidocaine or swallow Xylocaine jelly.

The larynx can be anesthetized using a combination of techniques. An effective initial approach is to use a nebulizer. Nebulization can deliver lidocaine to the larynx and trachea. A nebulizer connected to a pressurized oxygen source can be used to synchronize the sprays with deep inspiration. A hole cut in the oxygen tubing is occluded intermittently with a finger to produce a forceful spray. This technique facilitates the delivery of lidocaine to the larynx and the trachea. Lidocaine also can be instilled into the larynx under direct vision using the flexible bronchoscope.

The trachea typically is anesthetized with 5 mL of 1% lidocaine after the bronchoscope has passed through the vocal cords. Additional lidocaine is administered at the level of the carina and the mainstem bronchi bilaterally.

Flexible Bronchoscope Equipment

The bronchoscope consists of a handle and an insertion tube that contains the optical bundle and a working channel. The handle controls the distal segment of the insertion tube. The distal portion of the scope bends in a single 270-degree arc to facilitate examination of the entire airway. The optical bundle contains a fiberoptic light bundle and a second bundle for either digital or fiberoptic imaging. The working channel can be used to suction, pass instruments, and lavage the airways.

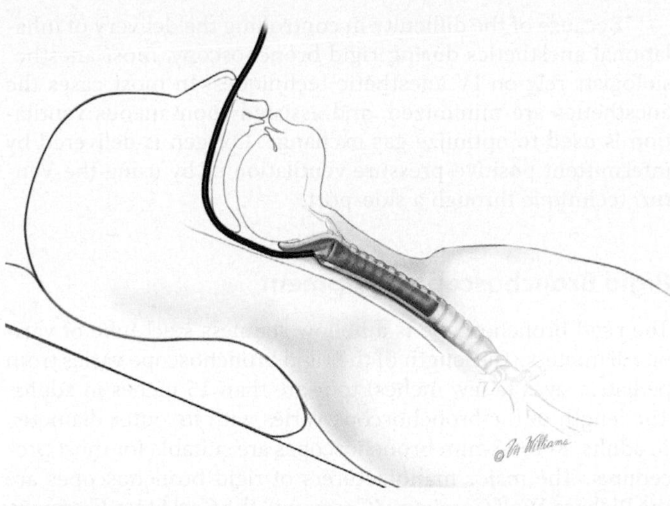

Figure 61-2. Transnasal introduction of the bronchoscope is often used in the outpatient setting because it maintains proper alignment and permits swallowing.

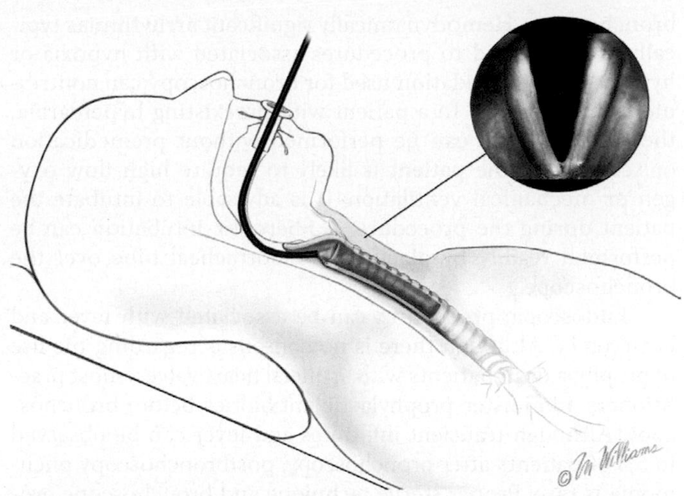

Figure 61-3. Oral introduction, the preferred method for patients with previously traumatized nasal passages or in the presence of a nasogastric tube.

Basic Technique

In the nonintubated patient, the bronchoscope is introduced either through the mouth or through the nose. Transnasal introduction is used commonly as an outpatient procedure (Fig. 61-2). This approach has the advantage of maintaining proper alignment of the bronchoscope as well as permitting the patient to comfortably swallow secretions. After proper application of topical anesthetics, the bronchoscope is gently passed through the nasal passages into the posterior pharynx.

In thoracic surgical patients, previously traumatized nasal passages and the presence of nasogastric tubes make oral introduction the preferred method (Fig. 61-3). The patient is asked to hold a circular bite block in his or her teeth. The bronchoscope is lubricated and the tip curved. Although the operator is looking into the open mouth – not through the bronchoscope – the lighted tip of the bronchoscope is positioned over the glottis. Holding this position in the midline, the operator then looks through the bronchoscope, and the vocal cords are visualized with minimal movements. Then 5 mL of 1% lidocaine is instilled onto the vocal cords. Note the vocal cord mobility with phonation. The bronchoscope is passed through the vocal cords, and another 5 mL of lidocaine is instilled into the trachea. Additional lidocaine may be necessary in the mainstem bronchi.

The trachea should be examined for displacement of the tracheal rings or effacement of the carina. The membranous portion of the trachea should displace anteriorly during expiration and cough. In most cases it is wise to first examine the normal tracheobronchial tree to ensure complete evaluation of the airways. Each segmental orifice must be examined.

Diagnostic procedures can be complicated by bleeding and must be performed in the proper order: washings, brushings, and biopsies. Bronchoalveolar lavage is performed by centering the distal tip of the bronchoscope in a segmental orifice. A volume of normal saline, typically 50 to 150 mL, is instilled into the distal airway while maintaining occlusion of the segmental airway. The patient is asked to take several deep breaths to draw the lavage fluid into the distal airspaces. The lavage fluid then is aspirated into an appropriate container.

Brushings may be directed at either cytologic or bacteriologic diagnoses. Brushings obtained for cytology must be prepared properly to preserve cellular morphology. Similarly, distal airway brushings for bacterial culture also must be performed properly. The so-called covered brush cultures involve a covered sheath with the gelatin plug. The gelatin plug protects the brush from contamination until it is in the distal airway. The plug is expelled, and distal cultures, particularly anaerobic cultures, can be obtained reliably. If the brush is processed properly, quantitative cultures of the distal airway can be obtained.

An important development in bronchoscopy has been the use of complementary imaging techniques; that is, imaging techniques that are implemented simultaneously with the fiberoptic bronchoscopy. There are currently two commonly employed techniques: Endobronchial ultrasound (EBUS) and electromagnetic navigational bronchoscopy (ENB). EBUS is a method for imaging lymph nodes beyond the airway wall—effectively extending the potential for bronchoscopic biopsy to contiguous lymph nodes. EBUS has been associated with low complication rates and false-negative rates between 6% and 9%.[4] A newer imaging modality is ENB. ENB uses spatial correlations between the patient's CT scan and a reference electromagnetic field. Computer correlation between the CT scan and the bronchoscope provides a virtual image of the airway and the surrounding lung. The imaging technology can be used to guide the bronchoscopist and permit a variety of procedures including needle biopsies and placement fiducial markers. Although the accuracy of ENB varies with surgeon experience,[5] continued software improvements are likely to enhance the accuracy of ENB.

Complications

The most predictable complication of bronchoscopy is transient hypoxemia. The PaO_2 routinely drops by 10 to 20 mm Hg during bronchoscopy.[1,2] The relative hypoxemia is worsened by large-volume saline lavage and use of an excessive amount of suction. In most cases the predictable drop in PaO_2 can be prevented with the routine use of supplemental oxygen therapy. Cardiac arrhythmias are unusual during routine bronchoscopy. Hemodynamically significant arrhythmias typically are restricted to procedures associated with hypoxia or hypercarbia. The sedation used for bronchoscopy can contribute to hypercarbia. In a patient with preexisting hypercarbia, the bronchoscopy can be performed without premedication or sedation. If the patient is likely to require high-flow oxygen or mechanical ventilation, it is advisable to intubate the patient during the procedure. A fiberoptic intubation can be performed readily by placing an endotracheal tube over the bronchoscope.

Endoscopic procedures can be associated with fever and bacteremia. Although there is no consensus regarding the use of prophylaxis in patients with artificial heart valves, most practitioners administer prophylactic antibiotics before bronchoscopy. Although transient infiltrates and fever can be observed in 5% of patients after bronchoscopy, postbronchoscopy pneumonia is rare. Proper sterile technique and bronchoscope processing will limit the life-threatening *Pseudomonas* pneumonia associated with a contaminated bronchoscope.

RIGID BRONCHOSCOPY TECHNIQUE

Anesthesia

Patients undergoing rigid bronchoscopy require general anesthesia. Unique to rigid bronchoscopy, the preprocedural examination must include a careful evaluation of the neck. Severe cervical arthritis may prevent neck extension. Patients with micrognathia, protruding teeth, or a small buccal cavity may pose a problem for rigid bronchoscopy. Patients with near-total tracheal obstruction may not tolerate the supine position or sedation. In these patients, awake rigid bronchoscopy can be performed in the sitting position with adequate topical anesthesia.

Because of the difficulty in controlling the delivery of inhalational anesthetics during rigid bronchoscopy, most anesthesiologists rely on IV anesthetic techniques. In most cases the anesthetics are minimized, and assisted spontaneous ventilation is used to optimize gas exchange. Oxygen is delivered by intermittent positive-pressure ventilation or by using the Venturi technique through a side-port.

Rigid Bronchoscope Equipment

The rigid bronchoscope is a hollow stainless steel tube of various diameters. The length of the rigid bronchoscope varies from pediatric sizes (a few inches) to more than 15 inches in adults. The length of the bronchoscope varies with its outer diameter. In adults, 8- to 12-mm bronchoscopes are suitable for most procedures. The major manufacturers of rigid bronchoscopes are the Richard Wolf Company (Germany), the Carl Storz Company (Germany), and the EFER Company (France) (Fig. 61-4).

Most bronchoscopes have a beveled end that facilitates introduction. The Wolf rigid bronchoscopes have an extended flat bevel that facilitates the "coring out" of intraluminal tumor. Most bronchoscopes also have side-ports that permit the introduction of suction catheters or laser fibers. In addition, side-ports can be used to allow ventilation. In some classifications, the presence or absence of a side-port determines whether the bronchoscope is called a ventilating or nonventilating bronchoscope.

Early rigid bronchoscopes used a rigid telescope to facilitate distal viewing. The viewing telescopes were produced at various angles to permit visualization of all the lobar bronchi. The flexible bronchoscope, however, has made the viewing telescope largely obsolete. The flexible bronchoscope can be introduced through the working channel of the rigid bronchoscope to provide not only excellent optical resolution but also a maneuverable end and a working channel.

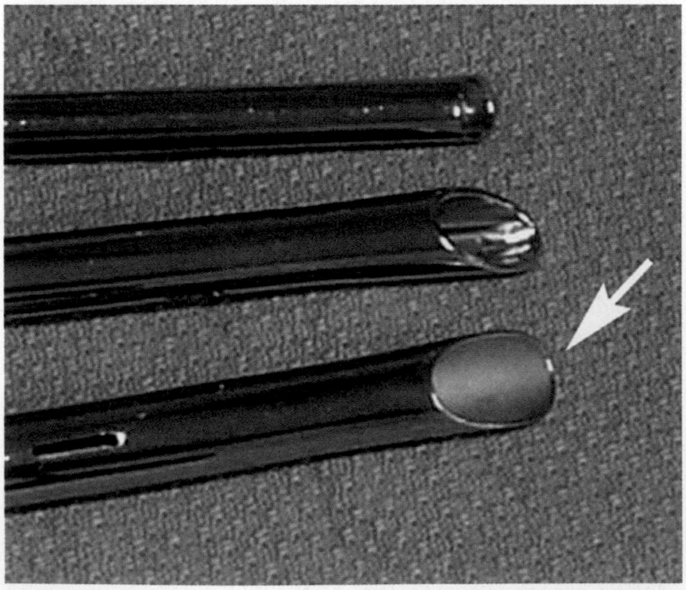

A

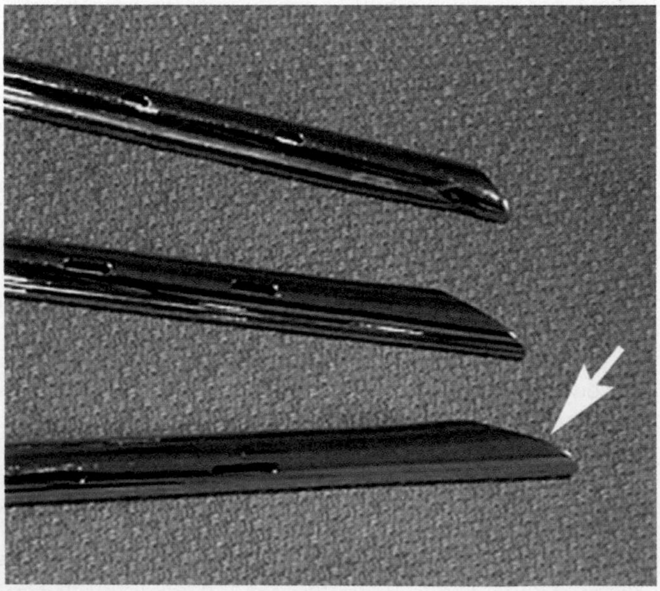

B

Figure 61-4. Rigid bronchoscopes vary in shape and function. *A.* Diagnostic rigid bronchoscopes have a rounded tip that avoids airway injury or mucosal trauma. Therapeutic bronchoscopes are designed for endobronchial strictures and tumors (*arrow*). *B.* Profiles of the different bronchoscopes reflect these functional designs.

Basic Technique

The bronchoscopist stands at the head of the anesthetized patient. The patient is well oxygenated, and pharyngeal secretions are aspirated. The lips, gingiva, and teeth are inspected carefully. Dental structures are protected with the use of rubber guards or folded damp gauze.

Many operators prefer to position the patient in a "sniffing" position for inserting a rigid bronchoscope. The sniffing position displaces the tongue anteriorly. The patient's maxilla is grasped in the left hand, and the thumb is used to protect the incisors and provide a fulcrum for the bronchoscope (Fig. 61-5). The thumb always should be interposed between the bronchoscope and the patient's teeth or gums. The bronchoscope is inserted into the hypopharynx with the distal tip oriented toward the epiglottis. When the epiglottis is visualized, the distal end of the bronchoscope is advanced just beyond the tip of the epiglottis, and the epiglottis/tongue is gently displaced anteriorly. The displacement of the epiglottis/tongue involves gentle rocking of the bronchoscope on the thumb fulcrum. The bronchoscope should not be touching the patient's teeth or gums. This rocking maneuver should bring the vocal cords into view. The rigid bronchoscope is rotated 90 degrees to facilitate passage of the beveled end of the bronchoscope through the vocal cords. Once the bronchoscope is within the lumen of the trachea, it is rotated another 90 degrees so that the distal tip is oriented posteriorly.

Once the bronchoscope has been introduced successfully into the trachea, the sniffing position is converted to cervical hyperextension (Fig. 61-6). To avoid any inadvertent injury to the major airways, the operator should maintain firm control of the patient's head and the bronchoscope with the left hand. The right hand then can be used for biopsy or suctioning.

Complications

The complications of rigid bronchoscopy are related to inadequate preoperative evaluation or poor technique. Cervical injuries or bleeding complications often can be avoided with appropriate preoperative evaluation. Inadequate visualization during insertion can result in trauma to the vocal cords or proximal airway injury. Perforation typically occurs in the posterior wall of the trachea or mainstem bronchi.

A common complication of rigid bronchoscopy is respiratory failure. Assisted ventilation during rigid bronchoscopy does not provide the sustained positive airway pressure that is achieved during endotracheal intubation. Attempts to achieve increased positive airway pressure by packing the mouth or holding the nose and mouth closed generally are ineffective. In the presence of persistent hypoxemia or hypercarbia, it is prudent to remove the rigid bronchoscope and intubate the patient with a standard orotracheal tube. This permits effective

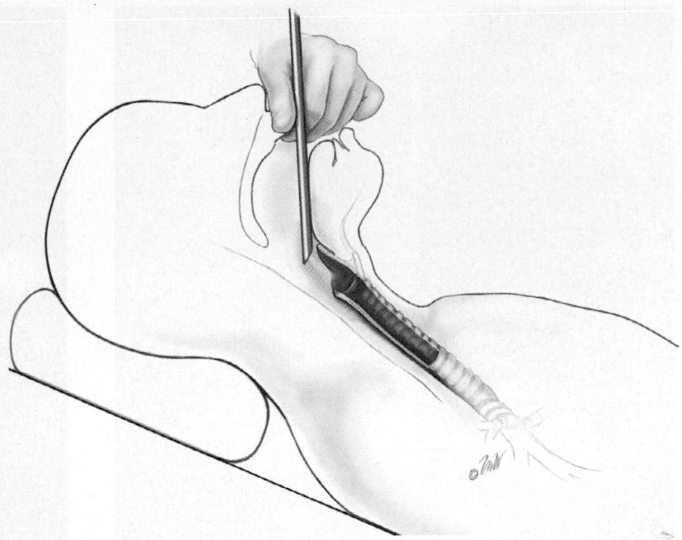

Figure 61-5. The surgeon grasps the patient's maxilla with the left hand whereas the thumb is used to protect the incisors.

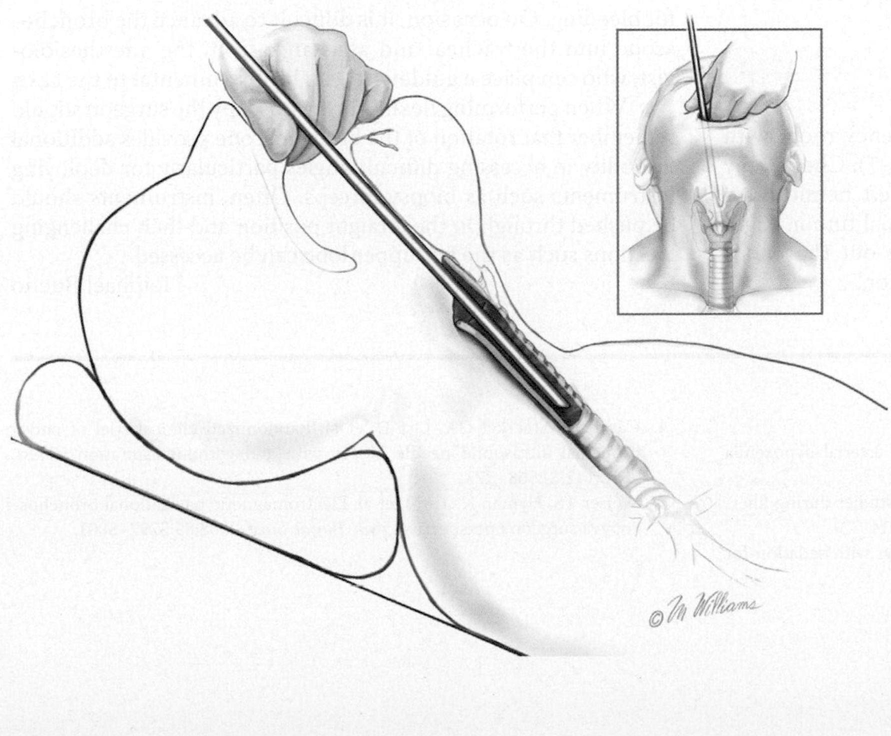

Figure 61-6. Once the bronchoscope has been introduced successfully into the trachea, the "sniffing" position is converted to cervical hyperextension.

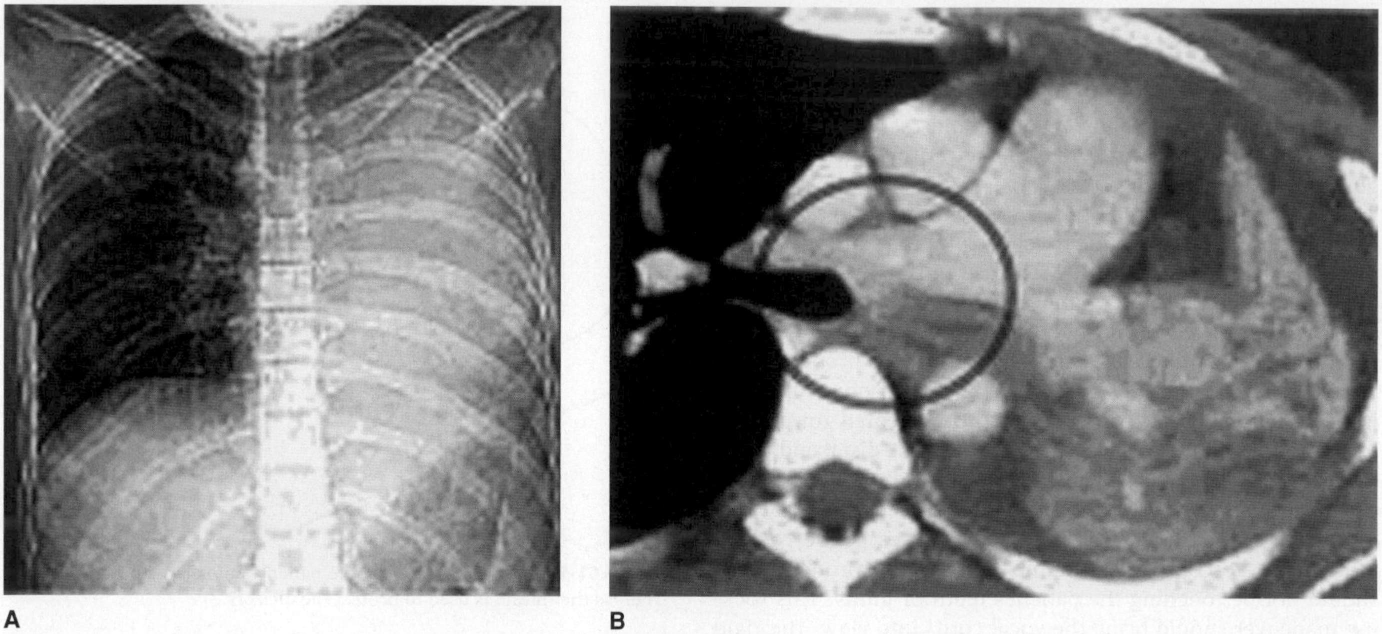

Figure 61-7. *A.* Chest x-ray demonstrating complete opacification of the left hemithorax. *B.* CT scan demonstrating a left mainstem bronchial tumor.

positive-pressure ventilation and the recruitment of adequate lung volumes.

SUMMARY

Rigid and flexible bronchoscopy in the hands of the experienced operator can be an effective and safe diagnostic and therapeutic procedure. Complications are minimized by thorough preoperative assessment. Flexible bronchoscopy has several advantages, including avoidance of general anesthesia. In contrast, the rigid bronchoscopy establishes an adequate airway while providing flexible access to the trachea and mainstem bronchi. The rigid bronchoscope can be combined with flexible bronchoscopy to maximize the advantages of both approaches.

CASE HISTORY

A 54-year-old smoker presented to the emergency room with rapidly progressive shortness of breath (Fig. 61-7). Chest x-ray demonstrated complete opacification of the left hemithorax. CT scan demonstrated a left mainstem bronchial tumor. Rigid bronchoscopy subsequently was used to core out the endobronchial lesion and reestablish left lung inflation.

EDITOR'S COMMENT

These days, rigid bronchoscopy is less often indicated given the ease and availability of flexible bronchoscopy. However, when required, it is critical that all members of the team know their roles. Therefore, frequent in-service training and simulations are important. Rigid bronchoscopy may also be performed through a tracheostomy. On occasion, patients with a small mouth, anterior larynx, or fused neck will require a tracheostomy for access. When trying to access the mainstem airways and beyond, the bronchoscopist on occasion will need to angle the scope outside the patient's body, to the opposite side. Single mainstem bronchial intubation is particularly critical when usual techniques of rigid bronchoscopic tamponade are used for bleeding. On occasion, it is difficult to advance the bronchoscope into the trachea, and assistance from the anesthesiologist, who can place a guidewire, can be instrumental to the case.

When performing flexible bronchoscopy the surgeon should remember that rotation of the bronchoscope provides additional flexibility in accessing difficult angles particularly for deploying instruments such as biopsy forceps. Often, instruments should be pushed through in the straight position and then challenging locations such as the left upper lobe can be accessed.

—Raphael Bueno

References

1. Albertini RE, Harell JH, Moser KM. Management of arterial hypoxemia induced by bronchoscopy. *Chest.* 1975;67:134–135.
2. Kleinholz E, Fussell J, McBrayer R. Arterial blood gas studies during fiberoptic bronchoscopy. *Am Rev Respir Dis.* 1973;108(4):1014.
3. Hirose T, Okuda K, Ishida H, et al. Patient satisfaction with sedation for flexible bronchoscopy. *Respirology.* 2008;13:722–727.
4. Casal RE, Staerkel GA, Ost D, et al. Randomized clinical trial of endobronchial ultrasound needle biopsy with and without aspiration. *Chest.* 2012;142(3):568–573.
5. Weiser TS, Hyman K, Yun J, et al. Electromagnetic navigational bronchoscopy: a surgeon's perspective. *Ann Thorac Surg.* 2008;85:S797–S801.

62 Techniques of Tracheal Resection

Mark F. Berry and Joseph S. Friedberg

Keywords: Trachea, carina, mainstem bronchus, resection and reconstruction

The need for tracheal resection and reconstruction arises with airway obstruction (<5 mm luminal diameter) secondary to postintubation stenosis, primary or secondary benign or malignant tumors, or trauma. Patients who present acutely with symptoms of stridor should be stabilized first by establishing a clear airway. Resection and repair are often delayed to permit adequate time for radiologic and diagnostic studies to aid in surgical planning. Emergency tracheal resection is rarely warranted. Lack of a suitable prosthetic replacement for the trachea limits the amount of this organ that can be resected without placing undue tension on the anastomosis (maximum resection length 5 cm). For this reason, the initial operation must be well planned and executed. Anastomotic dehiscence and other late complications of an unsuccessful first operation are difficult to reverse given the limited material the surgeon has to effect a repair.

GENERAL SURGICAL PRINCIPLES

The surgical approach to an upper airway tumor depends on its location. Proximal tracheal lesions require resection of the trachea and possibly the cricoid cartilage or larynx. Segmental resection of the trachea with direct end-to-end anastomosis is used to remove tracheal main body lesions. Removal of tumors that involve the distal trachea, carina, or mainstem bronchus requires some form of carinal resection, with the extent of airway resection determining the mode of reconstruction. If the disease process involves the lobar orifices, resection can be accomplished by including contiguous resection of the affected lobes.[1,2] Lymph nodes should be resected whenever possible for staging, although extended lymphadenectomy can devascularize remaining airway tissue and should be avoided.

Preoperatively, patients should stop smoking and be weaned from steroids 2 to 4 weeks before resection to avoid deleterious effects on anastomotic healing.[1] Bronchoscopic techniques can be used, if needed, for temporary palliation for patients with severe obstruction while surgery is delayed. The anesthesiologist should place an epidural catheter preoperatively and have experience with complex airway management. Anesthetic management should include inhalation induction and short-acting medications to permit early extubation, which will decrease pressure on the airway anastomosis. For carinal resections, mediastinoscopy should be performed at the time of resection both for staging and to develop the pretracheal plane to improve mobility of the upper airway and lessen the chance of subsequent injury to the left recurrent laryngeal nerve when the distal trachea is dissected free at thoracotomy.[1] Ventilation during airway resection is achieved by distal airway intubation with an armored-type endotracheal tube connected to sterile anesthesia tubing across the surgical field. A sterile camera bag also can be used to house the airway tubing that is passed across the surgical field. The endotracheal tube is pulled back into the proximal airway by the anesthesiologist before airway incision.

After the distal resection margin is incised and the airway is divided circumferentially, the distal airway is intubated by the surgeon while the anesthesia team switches to the sterile circuit. If necessary, both lungs can be ventilated separately for carinal resections.[3] Either a double-lumen endotracheal tube or a long single-lumen tube with selective intubation of the contralateral mainstem bronchus or a bronchial blocker positioned in the ipsilateral bronchus can be employed for mainstem bronchi resections.[4] If necessary, the ipsilateral lung can be ventilated across the operative field if single-lung mobilization is poorly tolerated. The size and inflexibility of double-lumen tubes can present difficulties in procedures that involve carinal resection, and the extra-long single-lumen tube advanced into a mainstem bronchus to provide single-lung ventilation is preferable.[1] The remaining mainstem bronchus is intubated across the operative field as resection proceeds.[1] For carinal resections, the original long endotracheal tube is advanced into the bronchus after the end-to-end tracheobronchial anastomosis is brought together, permitting uninterrupted ventilation during completion of the secondary anastomosis of the remaining bronchus to the trachea.

A great deal of teamwork between the surgeon and the anesthesiologist is required during these cases. Completing tracheal anastomoses will require removing and replacing the endotracheal tube, during which time the anesthesiologist will need to hold ventilation and also be responsible for keeping the surgeon apprised of the patient's status and the estimated timing for reinstituting ventilation. This cycle is repeated until the distal airway is reintubated. In cases where ventilation cannot adequately be performed, such as with near-complete airway obstruction, extracorporeal membrane oxygenation, or cardiopulmonary bypass via peripheral cannulation can be utilized to maintain patient stability during manipulation of the airway.[5,6] Conversely and interestingly, upper airway resection via a cervical approach has been reported in which mechanical ventilation was not utilized at all. Twenty patients have been described as undergoing safe upper airway resection with an average resection length of 4.5 cm while awake and breathing spontaneously with the use of both cervical epidural anesthesia and local anesthesia.[7] However, thus far, this approach has only been reported for the treatment of benign upper airway stenosis and not tracheal tumors or malignancies.

A red rubber catheter can be sutured to the tip of the original endotracheal tube for upper tracheal tumors in cases where withdrawal of the tube proximal to the anastomosis will result in extubation. The profile and hindrance to reconstruction of the red rubber catheter can be further reduced by passing a heavy suture through the tip, which then can be used as a "leader" to guide the tube back through the vocal cords for reintubation of the distal airway from above.

Complete resection at the time of the first operation is the goal to relieve airway obstruction and give the best chance for cure. Since the margins can extend beyond what is grossly visualized and palpable, especially with adenoid cystic carcinoma, intraoperative frozen sections of resection margins are very important. However, upper airway tumor resection involves a compromise between the need to obtain clear margins to prevent postoperative recurrence and preservation of airway length to reduce anastomotic tension and ensure adequate healing. The safe limits of tracheal resection often depend on sound clinical judgment and vary with age, neck mobility, and body weight. Thin patients with long necks generally can tolerate longer lengths of tracheal resection, as can younger patients because of greater tracheal elasticity. Less than complete tumor resection may be acceptable to provide a long period of symptom-free palliation if morbidity risks limit the operative choice, especially for radiosensitive tumors such as adenoid cystic carcinoma.[8–10]

Various techniques have been described for airway anastomosis. Absorbable sutures are used for all airway anastomoses to minimize the potential for granuloma formation. Either silk or Vicryl lateral traction sutures should be placed through the cartilaginous rings on the remaining proximal and distal airway segments as "traction sutures" to take tension off the suture lines when the sutures are tied. Our preferred technique is to use interrupted sutures of 4-0 Vicryl placed in the trachea, with the posterior membranous airway knots placed interiorly (Fig. 62-1A) and the anterior cartilaginous airway knots placed on the outside (Fig. 62-1B).[11] It should be noted that the preferred technique at the Massachusetts General Hospital, where many of the airway surgery procedures were developed, is to use interrupted 4-0 Vicryl sutures, with all knots placed on the outside (Fig. 62-2).[1] Other anastomoses with running sutures or a combination of running and interrupted sutures have been reported. In all likelihood, a successful anastomosis can be constructed if these central tenets are observed: preservation of airway vascular supply, tension-free apposition of the ends (perhaps secondary to the use of proximally and distally placed traction sutures and the appropriate release maneuvers), and accurate tissue approximation with absorbable sutures. Preclinical animal studies have reported that administration of platelet rich plasma and use of hyperbaric oxygen therapy improves anastomotic healing, though benefits of these treatments have not yet been reported in patients.[12,13]

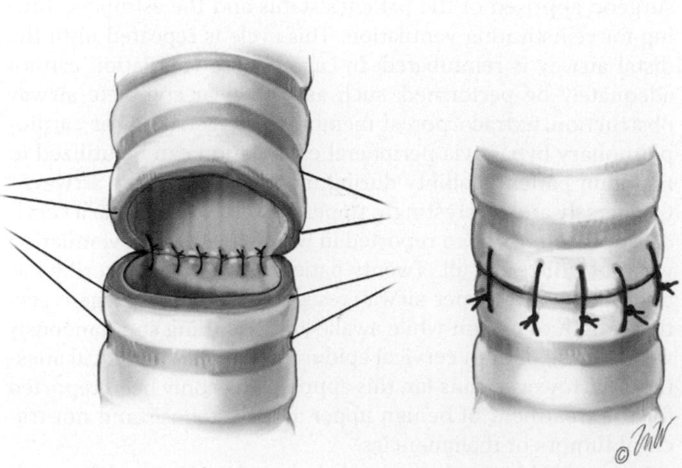

Figure 62-1. Preferred method for anastomotic suture at our institution is to use interrupted sutures of absorbable 4-0 Vicryl (*A*) with the posterior membranous airway knots placed interiorly and (*B*) the anterior cartilaginous airway knots placed exteriorly.

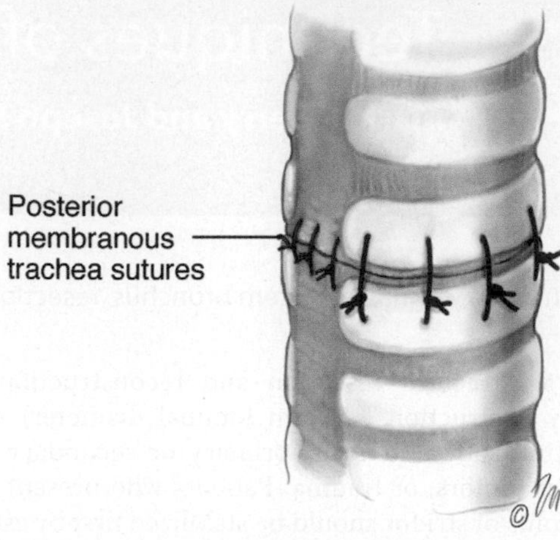

Figure 62-2. Approach used at the Massachusetts General Hospital, with interrupted 4-0 Vicryl sutures, all placed exteriorly.

Almost half the trachea can be removed with a low-tension primary anastomosis when appropriate mobilization techniques are employed. Simple neck flexion may be the most useful single maneuver for reducing anastomotic tension. Dissection of the anterior avascular pretracheal tissue planes while preserving the blood supply in the lateral tissue pedicles, which can be performed via mediastinoscopy, permits some tracheal mobilization, especially distally. Because the tracheal blood supply is segmental, skeletonization of the proximal and distal tracheal ends should be performed for only approximately one tracheal ring, the extent needed to perform the anastomosis. Because extensive lymph node dissection can compromise the trachea and, ultimately, the anastomotic blood supply, it should be avoided. Additional methods can be used if the anastomosis appears to have excessive tension. Suprahyoid laryngeal release by separating the larynx from its thyrohyoid attachments is useful for achieving proximal tracheal mobility for resections that involve the proximal or midtrachea (Fig. 62-3). Postoperative aspiration precautions are needed after laryngeal release because some patients may have initial swallowing difficulties.[8] The distal trachea can be mobilized by inferior pulmonary ligament division and mobilization of the right mainstem bronchus from the pericardium and the right main pulmonary artery and right superior pulmonary vein. The left mainstem bronchus may be divided and reanastomosed end to side with the right mainstem bronchus or bronchus intermedius to provide further mobility. Postoperatively, a heavy suture should be placed loosely from the inferior chin to the anterior chest wall and kept in place for 1 week to prevent inadvertent patient neck extension.[1,11] The use of an orthosis fashioned from a fiberglass splint has also been described to prevent neck extension and alleviate patient discomfort from the tearing sensation that this suture can cause when patients inadvertently try to move their head.[14]

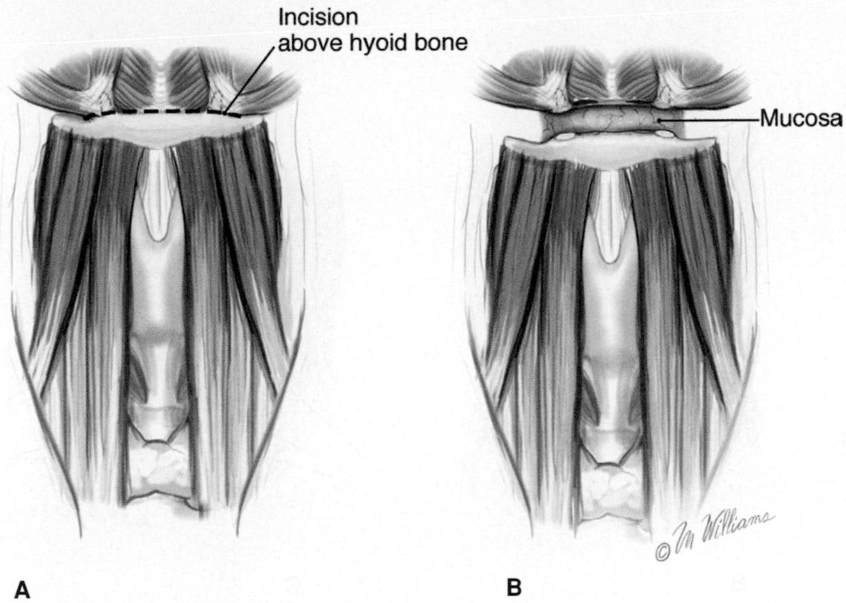

Figure 62-3. *A*. Suprahyoid laryngeal release is performed by separating the larynx from its thyrohyoid attachments to create proximal tracheal mobility for resections of the proximal or midtrachea. *B*. Appearance of trachea after laryngeal release.

SURGICAL TECHNIQUE

Approach to Upper and Middle Tracheal Neoplasms

A cervical approach is used for tumors of the upper third of the trachea.[11,15] The patient's neck and anterior chest are prepared and draped after the patient is placed in the supine position with the neck maximally extended by an inflatable bag behind the shoulders. Neck extension delivers the trachea into the neck. A collar incision is made with platysmal flaps developed to the level of the hyoid bone superiorly and the sternal notch inferiorly. The incision can be extended by making an additional skin incision perpendicular to the collar incision to include a partial or complete median sternotomy if necessary for midtracheal lesions. The strap muscles are separated in the midline, and the dissection is continued to the trachea in the midline. The trachea is mobilized circumferentially at the inferior resection margin, with care taken to avoid injury to the recurrent laryngeal nerves bilaterally and excessive circumferential mobilization that could compromise blood supply to the unresected trachea. The anterior aspect of the trachea is mobilized well into the mediastinum. This is easily accomplished in a virgin mediastinum with digital dissection. The endotracheal tube is pulled back into the proximal trachea by the anesthesiologist. After the distal resection margin is incised and the trachea is divided circumferentially, the sterile armored endotracheal tube is placed into the distal airway. The superior aspect of the divided trachea is grasped with a clamp, and the segment to be resected is mobilized to the level of the proximal resection margin and then removed (Fig. 62-4). A partial laryngeal resection may be required if portions of the cricoid cartilage need to be resected to obtain clear margins, with the trachea tailored to fix the irregular proximal defect.[15] Care should be taken to preserve the recurrent laryngeal nerves, if at all possible. A permanent cervical tracheostomy is performed in patients who require resection of both the trachea and the entire larynx.[8]

The tracheal anastomotic sutures are placed as described earlier. The neck is taken out of extension and flexed with the support of a pillow. The silk stay sutures are pulled toward each other to relieve tension, and the tracheal sutures are tied, starting posteriorly. In addition to the standard anterior tracheal mobilization technique, a suprahyoid release is performed if the suture line appears to be under any tension. The endotracheal tube is advanced and positioned distal to the anastomosis. After closure of the incision, the chin stitch described earlier is placed and kept for 1 week to avoid inadvertent patient neck extension.

Approach to Lower Trachea, Carina, and Mainstem Bronchial Neoplasms

Several approaches can be used for lower airway tumor excision. Tumors of the middle or lower trachea can be removed with either a right posterolateral thoracotomy, entering through the fourth or fifth intercostal space, or a median sternotomy.[8,15] An ipsilateral posterolateral thoracotomy can be used for lesions that involve the mainstem bronchi but not the carina.[4] A bilateral anterior thoracosternotomy (clamshell) incision that gives access to both pleural spaces may be preferable in selected patients, especially those involving a left carinal pneumonectomy.[1] The carina or mainstem bronchus is resected after mobilization of the distal trachea and mainstem bronchi, with ventilation achieved as described earlier.

The mode of subsequent airway reconstruction depends on the relative extent of tracheal and bilateral mainstem bronchi resection.[1] When the lesion is confined solely to a mainstem bronchus, a mainstem bronchial sleeve can be resected with primary anastomosis (Fig. 62-5A). A neocarina can be formed for carinal resections that involve a limited amount of tracheal resection by reapproximation of the right and left mainstem bronchi (Fig. 62-5B). Most of the airway mobilization in this reconstruction comes from the trachea because the aortic arch limits cephalad movement of the newly formed carina, and therefore, this reconstruction is not appropriate when a more extensive amount of trachea is resected. If a moderate amount

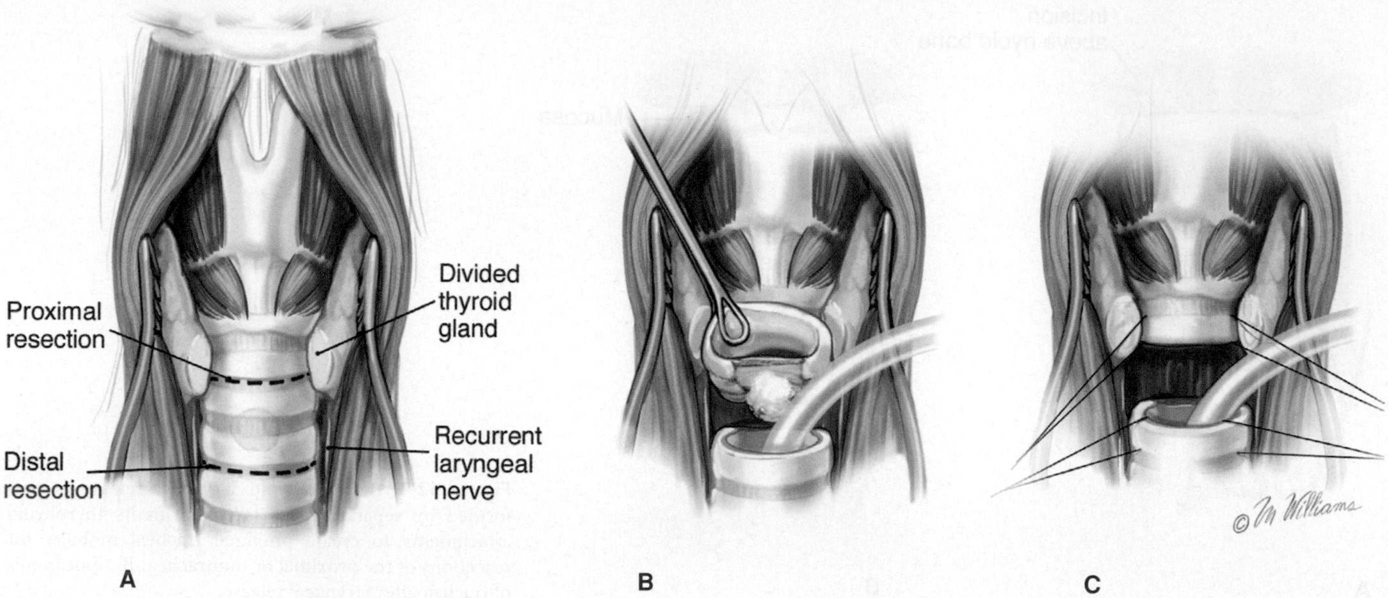

Figure 62-4. *A*. Proximal and distal incision points for the tracheal resection. *B*. Note the sterile armored endotracheal tube, which has been placed into the distal airway after the distal margin has been excised. *C*. The superior aspect of the divided trachea is grasped with a clamp, and the segment to be resected is mobilized to the level of the proximal resection margin and then removed.

of trachea is resected, the trachea is anastomosed end to end with either the right or the left (preferred) mainstem bronchus, with the contralateral bronchus reimplanted into the side of the trachea (Fig. 62-5C). As a general guideline, the extent of airway resection should be limited to less than 4 cm to minimize the risk of anastomotic complication owing to the relative immobility of the left mainstem bronchus when the airway reconstruction involves anastomosis of the left mainstem bronchus to the trachea.[1] If an extensive amount of trachea is resected, the right mainstem bronchus is anastomosed end to end to the trachea, with the left bronchus reimplanted into the bronchus intermedius. The reverse reconstruction (left mainstem end to end to the trachea with the right bronchus reimplanted into the left mainstem bronchus) should be approached with great caution because the immobility of the left mainstem bronchus leads to a significant incidence of anastomotic complications when there is extensive airway resection.

When the lesion involves the orifice of the right upper lobe, a right upper lobe sleeve resection can be performed, with the bronchus intermedius reimplanted to either side of the trachea or the left mainstem bronchus if anastomotic tension is thought to be prohibitive.[1,2] When resection includes both the right upper and middle lobes, the right lower lobe bronchus should be reimplanted into the left mainstem bronchus. If there is either extensive endobronchial involvement, destroyed lung as a result of bronchial obstruction, or involvement of the ipsilateral hilar vessels, a carinal sleeve pneumonectomy with end-to-end anastomosis of the trachea to the remaining mainstem bronchus can be performed.

The end-to-end tracheal–bronchial anastomotic sutures then are placed as described earlier after both margins are examined histologically. The indwelling endotracheal tube is advanced into the bronchus beyond the anastomosis after placement of all sutures. First the traction and then the anastomotic sutures are secured. The anastomosis is tested for air leaks and repaired as needed. The end-to-side anastomosis then is constructed, with the opening created in the side of the trachea or bronchus entirely in the cartilaginous wall to provide rigidity to the anastomosis and at least a centimeter away from the end-to-end anastomosis to avoid devascularization and necrosis of the intervening cartilaginous tissue (Fig. 62-6).[1] All suture lines should be reinforced with circumferential vascularized flaps of pleura, pericardium, omentum, or serratus anterior or intercostal muscle, especially if there is a history of mediastinal irradiation.[16]

POSTOPERATIVE MANAGEMENT

Postoperatively, early ambulation, incentive spirometry, chest physical therapy, and bronchoscopy, as necessary, should be used to help patients clear secretions. Bronchoscopic guidance should be used if reintubation is required in the early postoperative period to avoid lifting the larynx. Postoperative radiation should be used for virtually all malignant lesions, except very superficial tumors.[15] Local control with postoperative radiation is excellent for adenoid cystic carcinoma in particular, making grossly clear but microscopically positive margins acceptable, if necessary. Serial follow-up examinations for benign lesions are recommended, especially when tracheal resection is not performed. Follow-up examination similar to that for lung cancer is appropriate for malignant lesions. Patients who undergo resection of adenoid cystic carcinoma should have extended long-term follow-up, possibly with annual bronchoscopy, because these lesions have been found to recur as long as 17 years after initial resection.[15,17]

POSTOPERATIVE COMPLICATIONS

Operative mortality generally depends on both the physiologic impact of the procedure and the length of the airway resection and has improved dramatically over time as surgical judgment

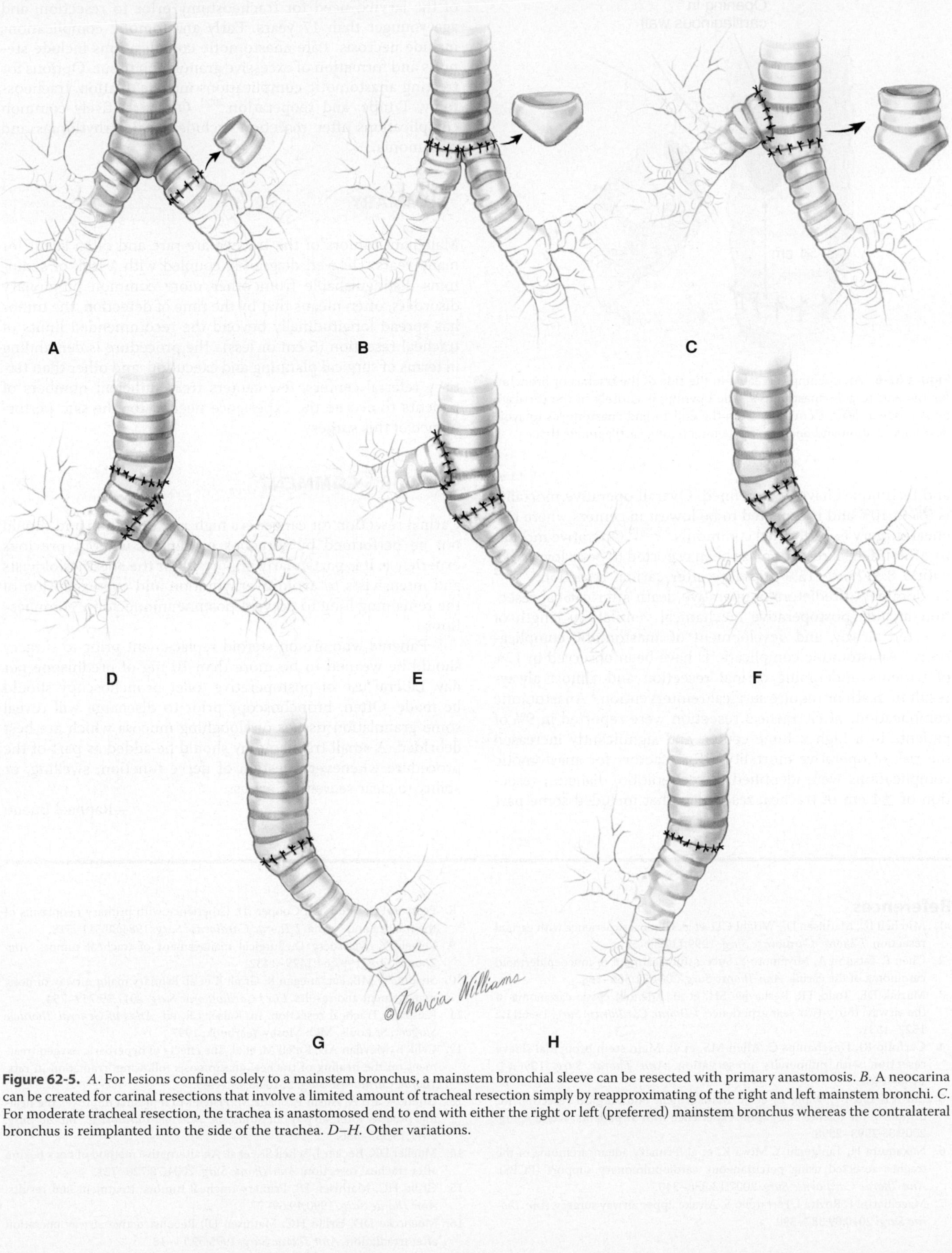

Figure 62-5. *A.* For lesions confined solely to a mainstem bronchus, a mainstem bronchial sleeve can be resected with primary anastomosis. *B.* A neocarina can be created for carinal resections that involve a limited amount of tracheal resection simply by reapproximating of the right and left mainstem bronchi. *C.* For moderate tracheal resection, the trachea is anastomosed end to end with either the right or left (preferred) mainstem bronchus whereas the contralateral bronchus is reimplanted into the side of the trachea. *D–H.* Other variations.

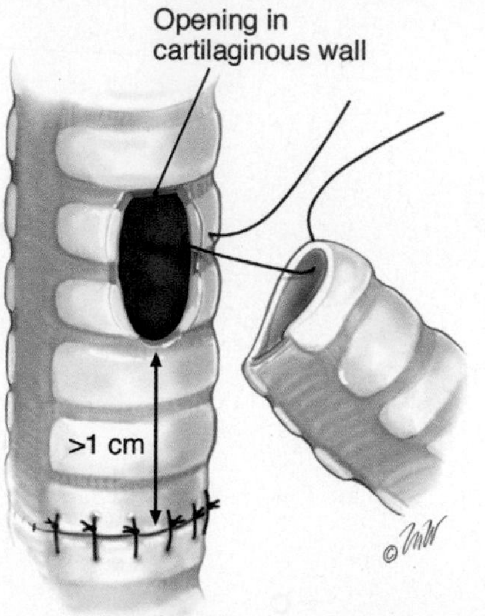

Figure 62-6. An opening is created in the side of the trachea or bronchus for the end-to-side anastomosis. The opening is entirely in the cartilaginous tissue at least 1 cm away from the end-to-end anastomosis to avoid devascularization and necrosis of the intervening cartilaginous tissue.

and techniques have been refined. Overall operative mortality is 5% to 10% and is expected to be lowest in centers where tracheal surgery is performed commonly.[3,5,15,18] Operative mortality after tracheal resection has been reported to be as low as 1%, with a 8.512% to 15% mortality after carinal resection.[15,19–22] Predominant predictors of operative death after carinal resection include postoperative mechanical ventilation, length of resected airway, and development of anastomotic complications.[1] Anastomotic complications have been observed in 17% of patients undergoing carinal resection and almost always result in death or require surgical reintervention.[1] Anastomotic complications after tracheal resection were reported in 9% of patients in a high-volume center, and significantly increased the risk of operative mortality.[20] Risk factors for anastomotic complications were identified as reoperation, diabetes, resection of ≥4 cm of trachea, resections that included some part of the larynx, need for tracheostomy prior to resection, and age younger than 17 years. Early anastomotic complications include necrosis. Late anastomotic complications include stenosis and formation of excessive granulation tissue. Options for treating anastomotic complications include dilation, tracheostomy, T-tube, and reoperation.[20,21] Other relatively common complications after resection include atrial arrhythmias and pneumonia.

SUMMARY

Malignant tumors of the trachea are rare and often silent for many years. Delayed diagnosis, coupled with a lack of symptoms distinguishable from other more common pulmonary disorders, often means that by the time of detection, the tumor has spread longitudinally beyond the recommended limits of tracheal resection (5 cm or less). The procedure is demanding in terms of surgical planning and execution, and other than tertiary referral centers, few centers treat sufficient numbers of patients to accrue the experience needed for the safe performance of this surgery.

EDITOR'S COMMENT

Carinal resection for cancer is a high-risk operation and should not be performed by surgeons or centers without previous experience. It is particularly important for the anesthesiologists and intensivists to avoid overhydration and overexpansion of the remaining lung to prevent postpneumonectomy complications.

Patients who are on steroid replacement prior to surgery should be weaned to no more than 10 mg of prednisone per day. Liberal use of postoperative toilet bronchoscopy should be made. Often, bronchoscopy prior to discharge will reveal some granulation tissues or sloughing mucosa which are best debrided. A small tracheotomy should be added as part of the procedure whenever question of nerve function, swelling, or ability to clear secretions arises.

—Raphael Bueno

References

1. Mitchell JD, Mathisen DJ, Wright CD, et al. Clinical experience with carinal resection. *J Thorac Cardiovasc Surg.* 1999;117:39–52.
2. Chen F, Tatsumi A, Miyamoto Y. Successful treatment of mucoepidermoid carcinoma of the carina. *Ann Thorac Surg.* 2001;71:366–368.
3. Maziak DE, Todd TR, Keshavjee SH, et al. Adenoid cystic carcinoma of the airway: thirty-two-year experience. *J Thorac Cardiovasc Surg.* 1996;112:1522–1531.
4. Cerfolio RJ, Deschamps C, Allen MS, et al. Main stem bronchial sleeve resection with pulmonary preservation. *Ann Thorac Surg.* 1996;61:1458–1462.
5. Liu XY, Liu FY, Wang Z, et al. Management and surgical resection for tumors of the trachea and carina: experience with 32 patients. *World J Surg.* 2009;33:2593–2598.
6. Nakamura H, Taniguchi Y, Miwa K, et al. Primary adenocarcinoma of the trachea resected using percutaneous cardiopulmonary support (PCPS). *Ann Thorac Cardiovasc Surg.* 2007;13:338–340.
7. Macchiarini P, Rovira I, Ferrarello S. Awake upper airway surgery. *Ann Thorac Surg.* 2010;89:387–390.
8. Pearson FG, Todd TR, Cooper JD. Experience with primary neoplasms of the trachea and carina. *J Thorac Cardiovasc Surg.* 1984;88:511–518.
9. Refaely Y, Weissberg D. Surgical management of tracheal tumors. *Ann Thorac Surg.* 1997;64:1429–1432.
10. Shadmehr MB, Farzanegan R, Graili P, et al. Primary major airway tumors; management and results. *Eur J Cardiothorac Surg.* 2011;39:749–754.
11. Kaiser L. Tracheal resection. In: Kaiser LR, ed. *Atlas of General Thoracic Surgery*. St Louis, MO: Mosby Yearbook; 1997.
12. Celik B, Meydan AD, Kefeli M, et al. The effects of hyperbaric oxygen treatment on the healing of tracheal anastomosis following irradiation in rats. *Thorac Cardiovasc Surg.* 2010;58:481–485.
13. Gomez-Caro A, Ausin P, Boada M. Platelet rich plasma improves the healing process after airway anastomosis. *Interact Cardiovasc Thorac Surg.* 2011;13:552–556.
14. Mueller DK, Becker J, Schell SK, et al. An alternative method of neck flexion after tracheal resection. *Ann Thorac Surg.* 2004;78:720–721.
15. Grillo HC, Mathisen DJ. Primary tracheal tumors: treatment and results. *Ann Thorac Surg.* 1990;49:69–77.
16. Muehrcke DD, Grillo HC, Mathisen DJ. Reconstructive airway operation after irradiation. *Ann Thorac Surg.* 1995;59:14–18.

17. Allen MS. Malignant tracheal tumors. *Mayo Clin Proc.* 1993;68:680–684.
18. Gaissert HA, Grillo HC, Shadmehr MB, et al. Long-term survival after resection of primary adenoid cystic and squamous cell carcinoma of the trachea and carina. *Ann Thorac Surg.* 2004;78:1889–1896.
19. Mitchell JD, Mathisen DJ, Wright CD, et al. Resection for bronchogenic carcinoma involving the carina: long-term results and effect of nodal status on outcome. *J Thorac Cardiovasc Surg.* 2001;121:465–471.
20. Wright CD, Grillo HC, Wain JC, et al. Anastomotic complications after tracheal resection: prognostic factors and management. *J Thorac Cardiovasc Surg.* 2004;128:731–739.
21. Mutrie CJ, Eldaif SM, Rutledge CW, et al. Cervical tracheal resection: new lessons learned. *Ann Thorac Surg.* 2011;91:1101–1106.
22. Yamamoto K, Miyamoto Y, Ohsumi A, et al. Results of surgical resection for tracheobronchial cancer involving the tracheal carina. *Gen Thorac Cardiovasc Surg.* 2007;55:231–239.

63 Subglottic Resection of the Airway

Timothy M. Haffey and Robert R. Lorenz

Keywords: Resection and reconstruction of subglottis, cricotracheal resection for subglottic stenosis, squamous cell carcinoma, adenoid cystic carcinoma

INTRODUCTION

The use of cricotracheal resection in the treatment of cancer is rare owing to the rarity of cancers of the subglottis and their lack of confinement to the larynx. Of the three subsites of the larynx, the subglottis is the origin of squamous cell carcinoma (by far the most common cause of laryngeal cancer), in only 1% to 3% of patients.[1] Cricotracheal resection for the treatment of subglottic stenosis is much more common, and the surgical techniques used for treating subglottic stenosis can be applied to surgical resection of the rare neoplasm that remains confined to the subglottis.

The glottis is defined by the American Joint Committee on Cancer as the superior and inferior surfaces of the true vocal cords occupying a horizontal plane 1 cm in thickness extending inferiorly from the lateral margin of the ventricle, including the anterior and posterior commissures. The subglottis is defined as that region which extends from the lower border of the glottis to the lower margin of the cricoid cartilage.[2] On the basis of histologic sectioning of whole larynges, Kirschner[3] was able to demonstrate that the conus elasticus represents the definitive anatomic boundary between the glottis and the subglottis. Tumors above the plane of the conus elasticus tend to behave as glottic tumors and remain within the confines of the larynx, whereas those below the conus spread more easily beyond the borders of the larynx and metastasize more commonly to the prelaryngeal, paratracheal, and mediastinal lymph nodes.[1,4] The epithelial lining also can be used to differentiate the glottis (lined by keratinizing squamous cells) from the subglottis (lined by ciliated respiratory epithelium).

ONCOLOGIC PRINCIPLES

Although squamous cell carcinoma arises in the subglottis in only 1% to 3% of all laryngeal cancers, the subglottis is involved by contiguous spread of tumors of glottic origin in 11% to 33% of patients. These more common tumors are not amenable to cricotracheal resection.[5] Early primary subglottic carcinomas are asymptomatic. Patients generally present with stage T3 or T4 tumors (Table 63-1), and airway obstruction is relatively common. These tumors usually exhibit circumferential growth, early cartilage invasion, and tumor growth beyond the borders of the larynx. Since glottic tumors with subglottic extension are not amenable to cricotracheal resection, and primary tumors of the subglottis of grade T2 or above are not contained within the subglottis, cricotracheal resection for squamous cell carcinoma is only possible for the rare T1 tumor. Otherwise, subglottic squamous cell carcinoma is treated with either radiation therapy or wide-field surgery, such as laryngectomy or laryngopharyngectomy. Tracheal tumors rarely extend superiorly to involve the subglottis. There is also strong evidence that subglottic squamous cell carcinomas should be treated aggressively, as there are poor outcomes published with advanced disease, and there is a propensity for nodal and distant metastasis.[1]

Unlike the glottis, the subglottis contains laryngeal mucous glands and can be the primary site of tumors that arise from these glands. Nonsquamous laryngeal carcinomas make up only 1% to 5% of laryngeal cancers. They consist of adenocarcinoma, adenoid cystic carcinoma, mucoepidermoid carcinoma, neuroendocrine tumors, and cartilaginous tumors. In addition, plasmacytomas, non-Hodgkin lymphoma, and metastatic lesions can arise in the subglottis. Although different tumors require varying margins of resection and may respond to radiation with different efficacies, the selected early nonsquamous cell carcinoma may be resected by cricotracheal resection if the correct conditions exist. Perhaps best suited for cricotracheal resection is the chondroma or chondrosarcoma, the most common laryngeal sarcoma, representing 1% of all laryngeal tumors.[6] Because the low-grade form of chondrosarcoma is easily confused with the benign chondroma, the true incidence is difficult to know. Chondrosarcomas arise from the hyaline cartilages of the larynx, and most commonly arise from the cricoid (70%), especially the posterior lamina, followed by the thyroid cartilage (20%), and the arytenoids (10%).[7] Endoscopically, chondrosarcomas of the posterior cricoid lamina tend to grow into the airway, causing obstruction, and rarely, they extend beyond the confines of the perichondrium. As a consequence of the unresponsiveness of low-grade chondrosarcomas to radiation therapy and their confined growth patterns, cricotracheal resection with voice preservation can be accomplished.[8] This often occurs after multiple endoscopic resections have failed to ameliorate the recurring airway obstruction. Paragangliomas and granular cell tumors of the subglottis are also amenable to cricotracheal resection.

Table 63-1

AJCC STAGING OF SUBGLOTTIC CARCINOMA[2]

T1	Tumor limited to the subglottis
T2	Tumor extends to the vocal cord(s) with normal or impaired mobility
T3	Tumor limited to larynx with vocal cord fixation
T4a	Moderately advanced local disease; tumor invades cricoid or thyroid cartilage and/or invades tissues beyond the larynx (e.g., trachea, soft tissues of neck, including deep extrinsic muscles of the tongue, strap muscles, thyroid, or esophagus)
T4b	Very advanced local disease; tumor invades prevertebral space, encases the carotid artery, or invades mediastinal structures

AJCC, American Joint Committee on Cancer.

Laryngotracheal invasion by thyroid carcinoma has an incidence of 7%.[9] Invasion of the thyroid and cricoid cartilages occurs through direct extension and represents a rare but important cause of death from well-differentiated thyroid carcinoma. Controversy exists over the treatment of locally invasive thyroid carcinoma. "Shaving" the tumor from the larynx and trachea, followed by treatment with ^{131}I, produces good long-term control of the disease, but this technique is only effective if no gross residual tumor is left behind.[10]

PRINCIPLES OF STENOSIS TREATMENT

Subglottic and superior tracheal stenoses remain the most common indications for cricotracheal resection, and the principles of this technique are easily applied to surgical resection of the rare amenable neoplasm. Mechanical ventilation from endotracheal intubation remains the most common etiology of laryngeal stenosis.[11] Mucosal injury by either the tube or the balloon cuff results in either ischemia from pressure or mucosal tears from movement or placement of the tube. These iatrogenic events can lead to mucosal ulceration, perichondritis, chondritis, and finally, cartilage necrosis. The injury can occur at the glottic, subglottic, or tracheal levels and is largely preventable by early tracheotomy and aggressive adjunctive management, such as antibiotics and proton pump inhibitors. Laryngotracheal stenosis can also be caused by autoimmune diseases, infection, scar formation post tracheotomy, and idiopathic causes. Subglottic stenosis can be found in 16% to 20% of patients with Wegner's granulomatosis.[12] In our own practice, having treated more than 80 patients with Wegner's granulomatosis and subglottic stenosis, we find that endoscopic treatment of the stenosis, including direct injection of steroid and balloon dilation has prevented the necessity of tracheotomy or open airway reconstruction in all patients.[13] In previously treated patients, especially in those who have undergone multiple endoscopic laser excisions, we have had to resort to open laryngotracheal reconstruction.

Tracheal and subglottic damage is often due to tracheotomy tube injuries. Inappropriately high tracheotomies, migration of the tube superiorly, and suprastomal granulation tissue are common causes of failure to decannulate patients after tracheotomy.[14] The cause of the superior migration is unknown but may be due to movement from swallowing or external neckties that pull the tube superiorly. These patients often are amenable to cricotracheal resection but are challenged by extensive damage of the trachea and cricoid from chronic infection caused by microbial colonization of the tracheotomy tube, in addition to the concurrent disease that necessitated the tracheotomy in the first place. Contraindications in our own practice for cricotracheal resection for tracheotomy removal include poorly controlled diabetes, systemic steroid therapy, likely need for intubation in the near future, obstructive sleep apnea, and concomitant pulmonary disease. Similarly, poorly controlled diabetes, systemic steroid therapy, and severe pulmonary disease are contraindications to cricotracheal resection for neoplasms of the subglottis, and nonsurgical treatments such as radiation therapy, chemotherapy, and palliative therapy are best suited to patients with significant comorbidities.

PREOPERATIVE ASSESSMENT

Office assessment of the patient includes flexible nasal fiberoptic endoscopy to exclude glottic involvement, vocal fold fixation and posterior commissural interarytenoid stenosis, and impending airway compromise. Fine-cut CT scan determines cartilage invasion and extralaryngeal spread, as well as cervical lymphadenopathy. Three-dimensional reconstruction and "fly through" radiologic endoscopy can further define the pathologic process. It is our practice to use full-body CT/PET to exclude regional and distant disease. Combined endoscopy under general anesthesia including direct laryngoscopy with biopsy, bronchoscopy, and esophagoscopy permit tissue diagnosis, debulking, determination of the inferior extent of the tumor, and exclusion of esophageal spread posteriorly. Patients should be warned that their voice will be hoarse for some period postoperatively and that the quality of their voice may differ permanently with a decrease of fundamental frequency of approximately 10 Hz. This effect can be even more pronounced in women as shown by Smith et al.[15] with a mean decrease in fundamental frequency of 21 Hz in the 14 women they evaluated having undergone cricotracheal resection. The reason for this decrease in fundamental frequency is that the cricothyroid muscle is resected at its attachment to the anterior cricoid ring, resulting in an inability to tense the vocal fold which is the normal physiologic function of the cricothyroid muscle.

TECHNIQUE

Figure 63-1 demonstrates the common technique of cricotracheal resection for circumferential subglottic stenosis. This technique is described not only for use by surgeons wishing to resect stenoses but also for those wishing to excise tumors of the subglottis, as demonstrated in Figure 63-2. In most cases of subglottic tumor resection, the mucosa and submucosa overlying the posterior plate of the cricoid needs to be resected. In some amenable tumors, partial vertical height of the cricoid must be resected to obtain suitable margins, preserving enough posterior cricoid cartilage superiorly and between the arytenoids to preserve arytenoid stability. If the mucosa is resected up to the interarytenoid area, or if a limited margin exists inferior to the true vocal fold, laterally hindering normal vocal fold movement, a laryngofissure is created not only to permit adequate exposure but also to incorporate the use of a stenting T-tube around which healing occurs, preventing postoperative glottic stenosis (Fig. 63-3).

Stenosis Resection

Figure 63-1 demonstrates the common appearance of circumferential subglottic stenosis with involvement of the upper tracheal rings. Not only is the anterior subglottis narrowed, but also the posterior thickening impedes airway patency. Resection of such lesions is begun with induction of anesthesia by transoral intubation with a small-caliber endotracheal tube, often of an extended length to permit later entrance into the trachea without violating the balloon cuff. If the stenosis is of such caliber that dilation must take place before intubation, jet ventilation is used temporarily during the dilation, which is minimal, to avoid causing too much edema. A previously existing tracheotomy tube can be used for induction but is changed

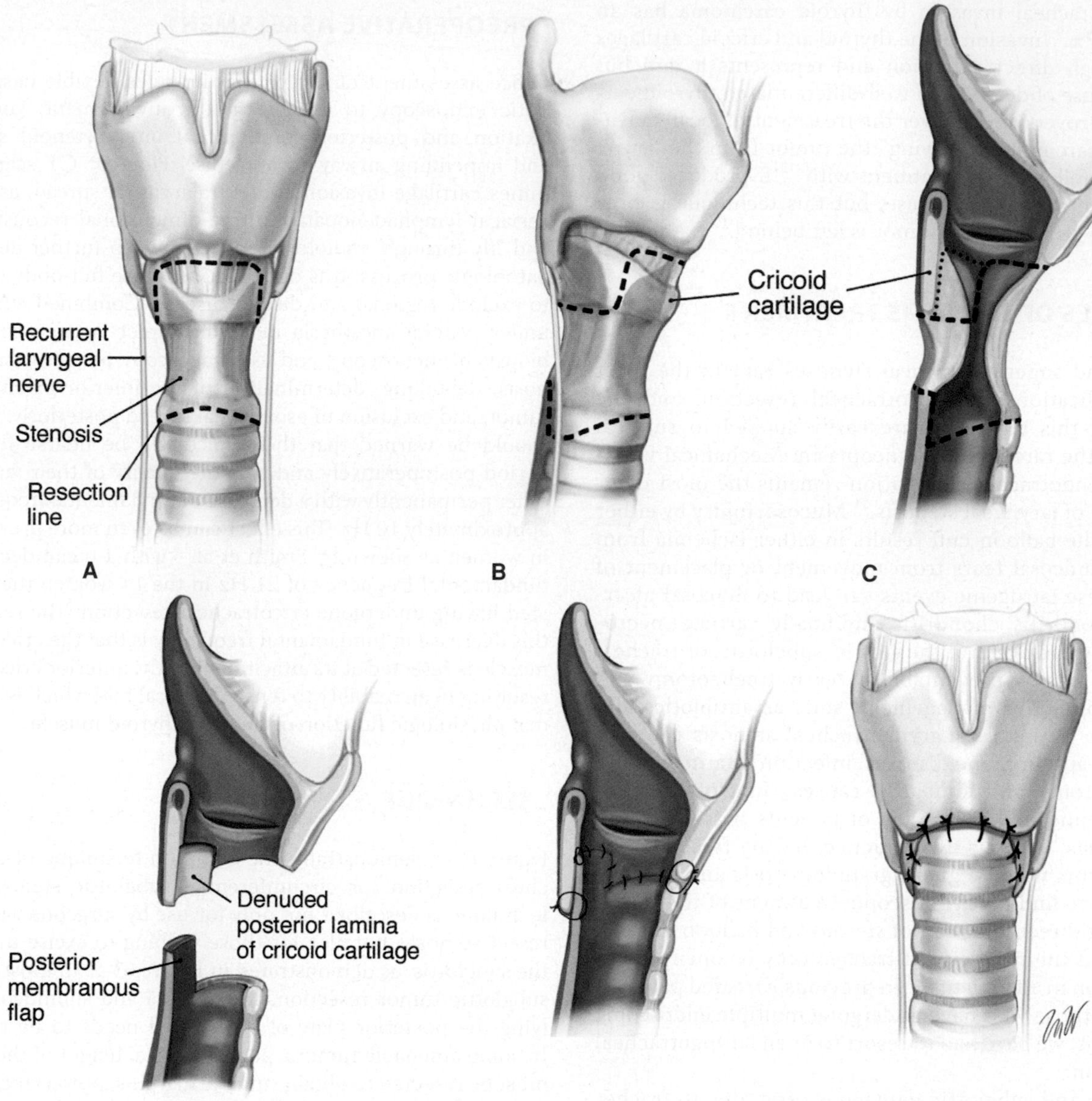

Figure 63-1. *A.* Circumferential stenosis of the subglottis and superior trachea. Dashed lines represent the external extent of resection. A lateral transection through the cricoid lamina allows removal of the anterior cricoid arch while preserving the posterior cricoid lamina, thereby protecting the recurrent laryngeal nerves. A posterior membranous tracheal wall flap is formed distally. *B.* The superior line of resection is through the cricothyroid membrane, curving inferiorly through the lateral cricoid laminae. The first preserved tracheal ring is shaped into an inverted U for anastomosis directly to the thyroid cartilage. If a longer posterior flap is required for reconstruction, the level of tracheal resection may be dropped by an additional ring. *C.* The internal line of resection (dotted line) removes the stenosis involving the posterior cricoid lamina. With neoplasms that involve the cricoid, the posterior lamina may be resected, but the posterior perichondrium and a superior horizontal strut of cartilage should be preserved to maintain arytenoid stability and posterior muscular attachments. *D.* The denuded posterior lamina of the cricoid is covered with the membranous flap from the posterior trachea. The first tracheal ring is shaped to fit the inferior thyroid cartilage resection line. *E.* 4-0 Vicryl is used internally to close the mucosal defect over the posterior cricoid lamina. 3-0 Vicryl suture is used to anastomose the tracheal ring to the thyroid and cricoid cartilages and to anchor the base of the membranous flap to the posterior cricoid cartilage, taking care not to injure the recurrent laryngeal nerves. All knots are tied outside the lumen. *F.* The superior trachea is anastomosed to the thyroid cartilage with 3-0 Vicryl sutures. The most superior tracheal ring has been formed into an inverted U for best fit into the laryngeal defect. Laterally, the cricoid is approximated to the second tracheal ring to minimize the tension on the first preserved tracheal ring.

immediately to translaryngeal intubation such that the tracheostomy tube does not crowd the operative field. After intubation, the head is extended with a shoulder roll, and a transverse incision is made from sternocleidomastoid to sternocleidomastoid superior to the manubrium. The skin flaps are raised subplatysmally superiorly to the hyoid bone and inferiorly to the clavicles. The strap muscles are separated, and the thyroid gland is divided at the isthmus. Neither suprahyoid nor thyrohyoid release maneuvers are routinely used. The trachea is dissected in a pretracheal plane, very close to the cartilaginous rings to avoid damaging the recurrent laryngeal nerves, which we do not identify routinely. The trachea is dissected down to the carina to produce the mobility for future anastomosis, and care is taken to avoid dividing its lateral blood supply.

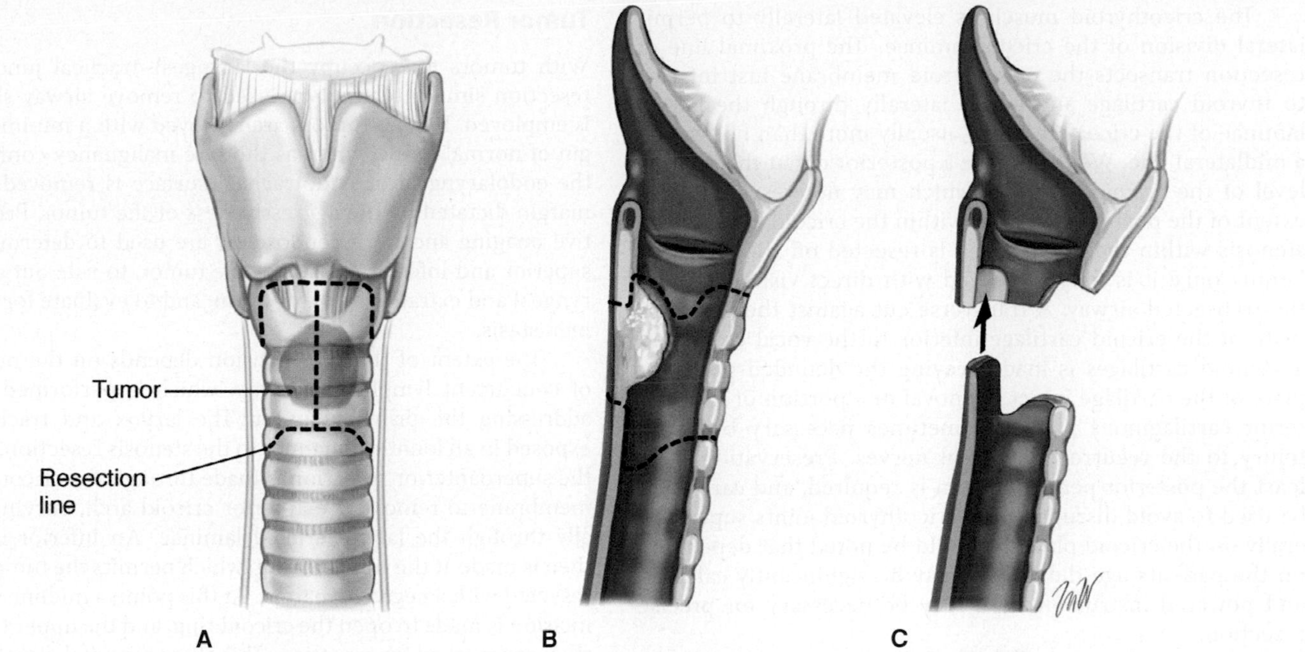

Figure 63-2. *A.* An endolaryngeal tumor occupies the posterior subglottis. The anterior cricoid is separated from the thyroid cartilage in a similar manner as in cricotracheal resection for stenosis. The inferior tracheal resection is performed at a level that obtains a negative margin on the tumor. Lastly, the superior tracheal rings and cricoid arch are divided in the midline for optimal tumor visualization. *B.* Superior and inferior margins are obtained on the tumor. If the posterior cricoid lamina is involved, the cartilage may be resected, but the posterior perichondrium and a strut of cartilage superiorly upon which the arytenoids articulate must be preserved for stability. Additional tracheal rings may be resected to elongate the posterior tracheal flap. *C.* Reconstruction occurs in an identical manner as in stenosis treatment. The denuded posterior cricoid cartilage is covered by the posterior tracheal flap and approximated to the remaining superior mucosa. The first tracheal ring fits like a prow of a ship into the defect of the anterior cricoid arch.

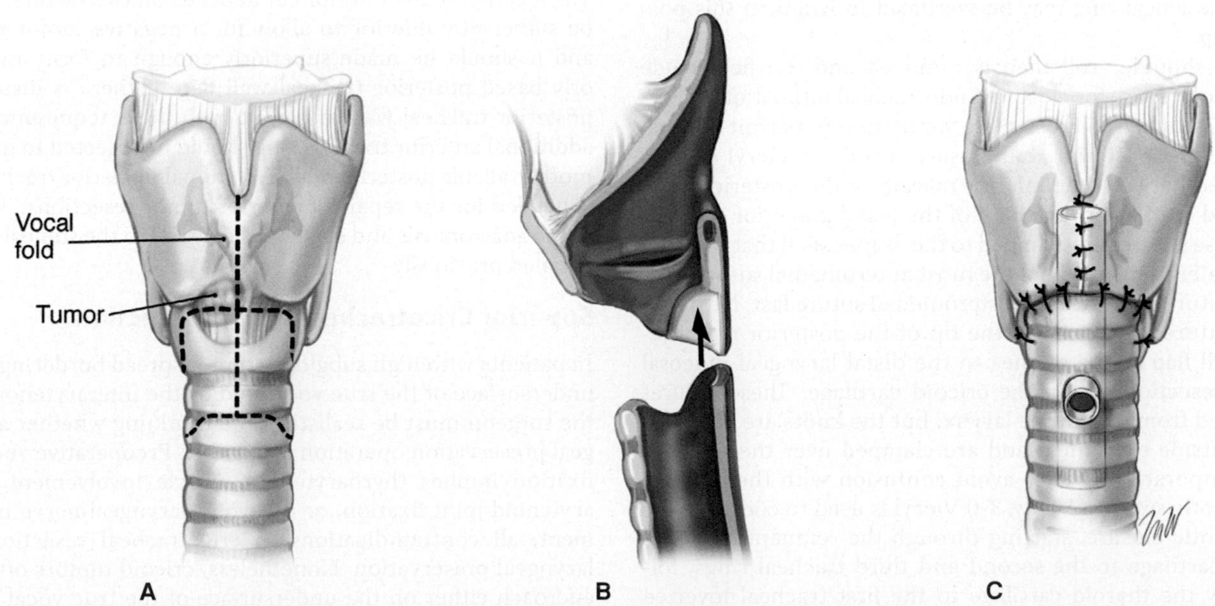

Figure 63-3. *A.* Negative mucosal margins are obtained, with optimal visualization achieved via the laryngofissure. Despite the tumor being superficial, partial thickness of the cricoid cartilage is drilled for an additional deep margin. As much of the interarytenoid mucosa is preserved as possible to maintain arytenoid mobility. *B.* The trachea is advanced into the defect, with the posterior membranous flap approximated directly inferior to the true vocal folds with interrupted 4-0 Vicryl. Less violation of the interarytenoid mucosa is desirable, although postoperative stenting assists in decreasing posterior glottic stenosis. *C.* The temporary T-tube has been placed through a separate tracheotomy two rings inferior to the anastomosis. The superior limb ends superior to the true vocal folds, whereas the inferior limb is short. Other than closure of the laryngofissure, the remainder of the anastomosis is performed in the same manner as in previously described procedures.

The cricothyroid muscle is elevated laterally to permit lateral division of the cricoid laminae. The proximal line of resection transects the cricothyroid membrane just inferior to thyroid cartilage and bevels laterally through the lateral laminae of the cricoid cartilage, usually more than halfway to a midlateral line. We then make a posterior cut at the inferior level of the cricoid cartilage, which may not resect the full extent of the posterior stenosis within the cricoid lamina. The stenosis within the cricoid then is resected off the posterior lamina once it is fully visualized with direct vision through the transected airway. A transverse cut against the posterior plate of the cricoid cartilage inferior to the vocal cords and arytenoid cartilages is made, leaving the denuded posterior plate of the cartilage intact. Removal of a portion of the posterior cartilaginous plate is sometimes necessary but risks injury to the recurrent laryngeal nerves. Preservation of at least the posterior perichondrium is required, and care must be used to avoid disrupting the cricothyroid joints superolaterally on the cricoid plate. It should be noted that depending on the patients age the cricoid may be significantly calcified and powered instrumentation may be necessary for precise resection.

The distal level of resection was determined earlier by endoscopic visualization. If the inferior border of the stenosis or tumor is in question, the initial transection always should be made slightly more superiorly because repeat resection more inferiorly is always possible. The first preserved ring is beveled backward from a high point in the anterior midline to the lower margin of that ring, creating an inverted U, and care is taken not to fracture this ring. At this point, a posterior membranous wall flap is formed to fit over the exposed posterior plate of the cricoid cartilage. The length of flap is determined by the amount of exposed posterior lamina. If needed, an additional anterior tracheal ring may be sacrificed to lengthen this posterior flap.

The shoulder roll then is removed and the field made orderly to prepare for closure. Endotracheal intubation is temporarily switched to cross-table ventilation to permit optimal access to the posterior wall closure. Four 3-0 Vicryl sutures are placed between the inferior margin of the posterior plate of cricoid cartilage to the base of the distal posterior tracheal flap. These sutures are clamped to the drapes such that they can be tied later in the order of the most anteromedial suture first, lateral suture second, and posteromedial suture last. Next, 4-0 Vicryl sutures approximate the tip of the posterior membranous wall flap of the trachea to the distal laryngeal mucosal line of resection within the cricoid cartilage. These sutures are placed from within the larynx, but the knots are arranged to lie outside the lumen and are clamped over the patient's head temporarily so as to avoid confusion with the external anastomotic sutures. Lastly, 3-0 Vicryl is used to complete the anastomotic closure, starting through the remnant of lateral cricoid cartilage to the second and third tracheal rings, followed by the thyroid cartilage to the first tracheal inverted U-ring. Tying of sutures begins after the patient is reintubated transorally and starts with the endolaryngeal 4-0 sutures, continues with the anteromedial sutures, and progresses laterally and posteriorly to the posterior midline. Strap muscles can be approximated over the anastomotic suture line, adding an additional layer of closure. Nonsuction drains are placed, the head is kept in a flexed position, and the patient is extubated immediately.

Tumor Resection

With tumors that occupy the laryngeal–tracheal junction, a resection similar to the type used to remove airway stenoses is employed. Benign tumors are removed with a minimal margin of normal tissue, whereas the rare malignancy confined to the endolaryngeal or endotracheal surface is removed with a margin dictated by the aggressiveness of the tumor. Preoperative imaging and initial endoscopy are used to determine the superior and inferior extents of the tumor, to rule out extralaryngeal and extratracheal extension, and to evaluate for distant metastasis.

The extent of the skin incision depends on the necessity of concurrent lymphadenectomy, which is performed before addressing the primary tumor. The larynx and trachea are exposed in an identical manner to the stenosis resection. Again, the superoanterior resection is made through the cricotracheal membrane to remove the anterior cricoid arch, curving laterally through the lateral cricoid laminae. An inferior incision then is made at the tracheal ring, which permits the tumor to be resected with a negative margin. At this point, a midline vertical incision is made to open the cricoid ring, and the upper tracheal rings are marked for resection. This allows optimal visualization before the posterior cuts are made. Although anterior tumors may be violated by this anterior midline incision, this does not preclude excellent tumor excision, albeit not adhering to the "no touch" tumor technique. In posteriorly placed tumors, the posterosuperior cut is made above the tumor site, with removal of underlying cricoid cartilage if the tumor requires. Again, the most common technique is drilling down the partial thickness of the posterior cricoid plate, although cricoarytenoid stability depends on preservation of the posterior perichondrium and a superior strut of cartilage on which the arytenoid articulates. The location of the inferior cut depends on two factors: it must be sufficiently inferior to allow for a negative tumor margin, and it should be made superiorly enough to form an inferiorly based posterior tracheal wall flap. If there is insufficient posterior tracheal wall to permit both these requirements, an additional anterior tracheal ring should be resected to generate more available posterior wall. A minimal posterior tracheal flap is needed for the repair of anterior tumor resections. The rest of the anastomosis and closure is identical to the stenosis repair detailed previously.

Superior Cricotracheal Tumor Resection

In patients with high subglottic tumor spread bordering on the undersurface of the true vocal fold or the interarytenoid area, the surgeon must be realistic in determining whether a laryngeal preservation operation is possible. Preoperative vocal fold fixation implies thyroarytenoid muscle involvement, cricoarytenoid joint fixation, or recurrent laryngeal nerve involvement, all contraindications to cricotracheal resection with laryngeal preservation. Nonetheless, cricoid tumors often will encroach either on the undersurface of the true vocal fold or the interarytenoid space, and surgical judgment must be used in determining the suitability of candidates for laryngeal preservation surgery. If the tumor is indeed judged to be favorable for resection, three modifications are made to the standard cricotracheal tumor resection technique. The first is a midline laryngofissure. This permits maximal tumor visualization, which is critical in such a location in which adequate margins are needed on the tumor, but postoperative laryngeal function depends on preservation of every millimeter of normal laryngeal structure. The second modification is the formation of a longer distal posterior tracheal wall flap to permit total resurfacing of the denuded posterior cricoid, even between the two arytenoid cartilages if required. This may necessitate resection of additional normal tracheal rings to generate sufficient length to reline the cricoid posterior wall. The last modification is placement of a temporary T-tube through the glottis for the initial 4- to 6-week postoperative period. The tube is placed with the proximal limb lying approximately 0.5 to 1.0 cm superior to the glottic level. The inferior limb can be quite short (2 cm). The horizontal limb is placed through a tracheotomy two rings inferior to the anastomotic line. Strap muscles are approximated to the area around the T-tube during closure to reinforce the airtight seal to prevent postoperative air leaks into the neck.

POSTOPERATIVE CARE

Nonsuction drains and a neck wrap are used to prevent postoperative fluid collections. In cases of cricotracheal resection without T-tube placement, patients are extubated immediately postoperatively. For patients with edema, one to two doses of steroid have been used to decrease swelling without significantly impairing anastomotic healing. Vocal cord function is assessed, and the neck is kept in a flexed position (pillows and strict nursing precautions usually suffice) for 2 weeks postoperatively. Patients are fed via nasogastric tube for 1 to 2 weeks, after which a swallow study is performed before starting an oral diet. Humidified air is used to decrease the risk of mucous plugs forming at the anastomotic suture line. If a laryngofissure and T-tube are used, the T-tube is removed under general anesthesia, during which time the airway is assessed endoscopically for patency and vocal cord motion, and any granulation tissue is removed. Although other authors are more aggressive with oral feeding, we do not start an oral diet until the T-tube has been removed.

PROCEDURE-SPECIFIC COMPLICATIONS

Complications generally involve issues of either stenosis, failure of the anastomosis to heal, or vocal fold dysfunction. When stenosis at the anastomosis occurs, conservative treatment with dilation often can correct the obstruction. Repeat resection and anastomosis may be required if one suspects that a technical error occurred during the initial operation. Posterior glottic stenosis from scarring, from high resection, or from vocal fold immobility is a difficult problem to overcome. Often a laser cordotomy of the less mobile vocal fold will augment the airway sufficiently to permit unlabored breathing, albeit at the cost of good glottic competence, resulting in decreased voice quality. The most emergent and concerning complication is that of a nonhealing anastomosis. Patients with diabetes and those on steroids are the most susceptible to this complication, which, owing to the proximity of the great vessels, can be life threatening. Often the most prudent course of action is to retreat, placing a T-tube and giving antibiotics while the wound progresses, after which the airway is reassessed to determine if a tracheotomy-free airway is possible once the healing process is finished.

FUTURE CONSIDERATIONS

In 1998 Strome et al.[16] led a team in performing the first successful total laryngeal transplantation. This operation was done for complete laryngeal stenosis resulting from trauma and included not only the larynx and pharynx but also the thyroid gland, parathyroid glands, and upper five rings of the trachea. Fourteen years after the transplant, due to a significant decrement in the patient's voice quality, we elected to explant the organ and rehabilitate the voice with a tracheoesophageal puncture.[17] Further laryngeal transplants have been performed since 1998 adding to the body of evidence that this is a viable option for patients unable to undergo organ sparing surgery. Transplantation in the setting of cancer however, remains a barrier as a consequence of malignant potentiation from immunosuppression. Some suggest that the relative risk of developing a cancer while on immunosuppression can be as high as 400 fold that of the general population. The most common malignant lesions seen in transplant recipients are skin cancers, accounting for 37% of posttransplant tumors. The concern of posttransplant malignancy has prompted the development of newer agents with both immunosuppressive efficacy and tumor suppressive properties, such as the rapamycin derivative everolimus (40-O-[2-hydroxyethyl]-rapamycin) (RAD; Novartis Pharma AG, Basel, Switzerland). Everolimus is part of a family of immunosuppressants that targets the mammalian target of rapamycin (mTOR) kinase inhibitors. Its immunosuppressive and antitumor properties have been demonstrated in several animal and human cell lines, including squamous cell carcinoma. The efficacy of everolimus at preventing local and distant spread of cancer has been studied at our own institution, in a murine model, with good results as both a single, or combined agent.[18] Until efforts at biomedical engineering are successful at developing suitable laryngeal replacements for laryngectomees dissatisfied with tracheal puncture, electrolarynges, or esophageal speech, reconstruction with autologous tissue in the setting of malignancy remains the greatest frontier for maximizing function after tumor ablation.

SUMMARY

Cricotracheal resection for the treatment of airway stenosis is a highly effective and successful technique that can be used in the excision of neoplasms. Although squamous cell carcinoma is by far the most common malignancy of the upper aerodigestive tract, it is rarely suitable for resection with the cricotracheal resection method. Squamous cell carcinoma, in particular, should be treated early and aggressively due to a propensity for nodal and distant metastasis, and poorer outcomes with advanced disease. Other malignancies and several benign tumors of the subglottis and upper trachea are especially amenable to cricotracheal resection, and excellent voice, airway, and swallowing results can be achieved. Cricotracheal resection and reconstruction often requires collaboration between otolaryngology and thoracic surgery services, with the main goals being a good oncologic result, while preserving as much normal laryngotracheal anatomy and physiology as possible; including the recurrent laryngeal nerves. Allogenic transplantation is on the horizon of new technologies allowing complete upper aerodigestive tract reconstruction in the face of radical tumor ablation.

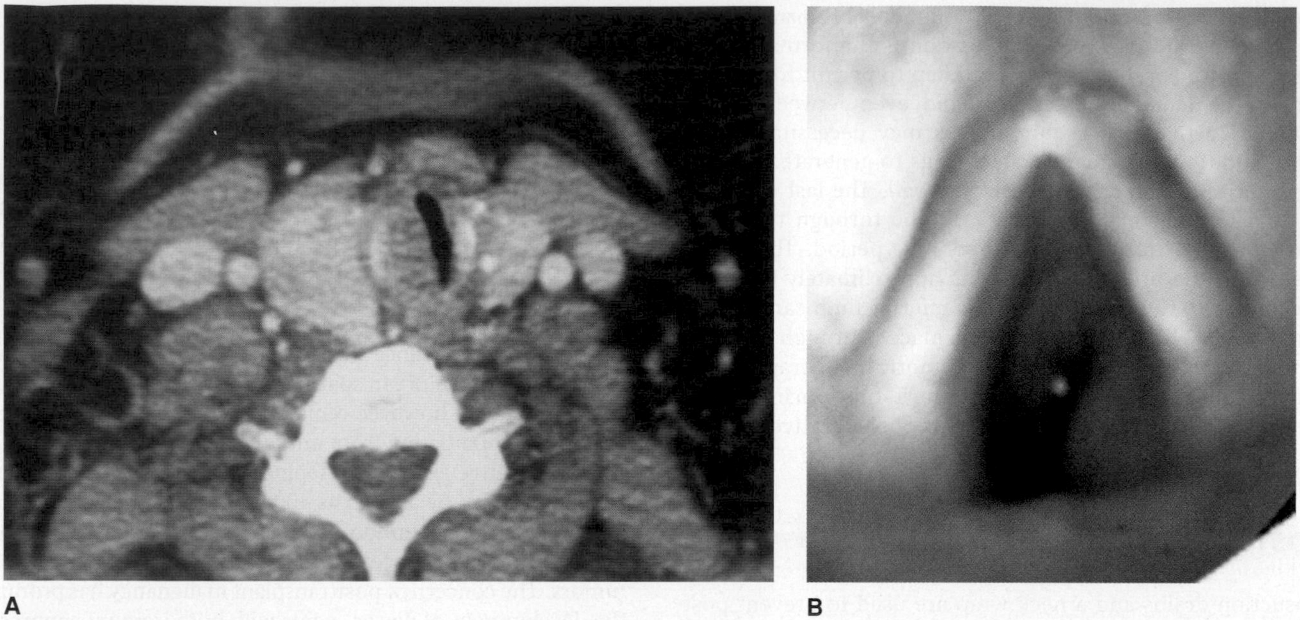

Figure 63-4. *A.* A 62-year-old woman was referred for stridor. Initial presentation suggested a large right-sided substernal goiter with tracheal deviation. Further examination of the CT scan demonstrates a mucosal lesion of the right subglottis. The underlying cricoid cartilage is intact. *B.* Office endoscopy reveals a mucosal fullness to the right posterior cricoid region. Biopsy under general anesthesia demonstrates adenoid cystic carcinoma.

CASE HISTORY

B.J. is a 62-year-old woman who presented with a 1-year history of progressive dyspnea. A CT scan revealed a right-sided thyroid goiter, and she was referred for removal of the mass. On office examination, the patient was not notably hoarse but did demonstrate moderate biphasic stridor. Further review of the CT scan demonstrated a fullness to the right subglottis without destruction of the underlying cricoid cartilage (Fig. 63-4A). Flexible fiberoptic nasal laryngoscopy demonstrated both deviation of the laryngotracheal complex to the left and a narrowed subglottic airway with a lesion on the posterior right subglottis (Fig. 63-4B). Operative management began with direct laryngoscopy and biopsy of the subglottic mass, revealing adenoid cystic carcinoma. A transcervical right thyroid goiter biopsy then was performed, demonstrating a benign thyroid goiter on frozen section.

Since the lesion was present high on the undersurface of the right true vocal fold and posterior cricoid lamina, a cricotracheal resection was accomplished with an accompanying laryngofissure. Partial thickness of the inferior cricoid cartilage was drilled down for an additional deep margin. Division of the thyroid cartilage was performed not only for optimal visualization of the tumor to obtain negative margins but also to allow reconstruction with a posteriorly based tracheal flap and placement of a temporary T-tube (Fig. 63-3). One tracheal ring was resected to obtain total tumor removal and to form a posterior tracheal flap. Level VI (mediastinal) lymph nodes were resected and demonstrated no regional metastases. The patient was allowed to take an oral diet 2 weeks postoperatively without significant dysphagia despite the end of the superior limb of the T-tube lying above the glottic aperture. She received 7200 cGy of radiation to the area starting 4 weeks postoperatively. The T-tube was removed at the end of radiation, and the patient demonstrated a good voice and excellent airway. She was followed postoperatively with routine imaging and fiberoptic examinations to check for local recurrence. Approximately 3 years after surgery she was found to have an asymptomatic lung metastasis on PET scan, and the patient succumbed to her distant disease 7 years after her surgery, with no local recurrence.

EDITOR'S COMMENT

Any resection of the proximal trachea and cricoid likely results in swelling and merits consideration of placing a small uncuffed tracheostomy distal to the anastomosis unless a T-tube is placed. We generally have a thoracic surgeon and otolaryngologist collaborate on these procedures at the Brigham and Women's Hospital to optimize results. A bronchoscopy on postoperative day 7 is useful to clear secretions and evaluate the anastomosis. On occasion we identify early sloughing of mucosa which can be debrided.

The suturing of a posterior mucosal flap on the denuded back wall is challenging technically. The goal is to get the mucosa to attach there, and a few carefully placed sutures suffice.

—Raphael Bueno

References

1. Garas J, McGuirt F. Squamous cell carcinoma of the subglottis. *Am J Otolaryngol.* 2006;27:1–4.
2. Edge S, Byrd D, Compton C. *AJCC Cancer Staging Manual.* 7th ed. New York, NY: Springer-Verlag; 2010.
3. Kirschner J. Growth and spread of laryngeal cancer as related to partial laryngectomy. In: Bryce DP, Albert PW, eds. *Workshops from the Centennial Conference on Laryngeal Cancer.* East Norwalk, CT: Appleton-Century-Crofts; 1976.
4. Smee RI, Williams JR, Bridger GP. The management dilemmas of invasive subglottic carcinoma. *Clin Oncol (R Coll Radiol).* 2008;20:751–756.

5. Stell B, Tobin K. The behavior of cancer affecting the subglottic space. In: Bryce DP, Albert PW, eds. *Workshops from the Centennial Conference on Laryngeal Cancer.* East Norwalk, CT: Appleton-Century-Crofts; 1976.
6. Oestreicher-Kedem Y, Dray TG, Damrose EJ. Endoscopic resection of low grade, subglottic chondrosarcoma. *J Laryngol Otol.* 2009;123:1364–1366.
7. Moisa I, Mahadevia P, Silver C. Unusual tumors of the larynx. In: Silver CE, ed. *Laryngeal Cancer.* New York, NY: Thieme Medical; 1991.
8. Bogdan CJ, Maniglia AJ, Eliachar I, et al. Chondrosarcoma of the larynx: challenges in diagnosis and management. *Head Neck.* 1994;16:127–134.
9. Batsakis JG. Laryngeal involvement by thyroid disease. *Ann Otol Rhinol Laryngol.* 1987;96:718–719.
10. Cody HS 3rd, Shah JP. Locally invasive, well-differentiated thyroid cancer: 22 years' experience at Memorial Sloan-Kettering Cancer Center. *Am J Surg.* 1981;142:480–483.
11. Marques P, Leal L, Spratley J, et al. Tracheal resection with primary anastomosis: 10 years experience. *Am J Otolaryngol.* 2009;30(6):415–418.
12. Langford CA, Sneller MC, Hallahan CW, et al. Clinical features and therapeutic management of subglottic stenosis in patients with Wegener's granulomatosis. *Arthritis Rheum.* 1996;39:1754–1760.
13. Hoffman GS, Thomas-Golbanov CK, Chan J, et al. Treatment of subglottic stenosis, due to Wegener's granulomatosis, with intralesional corticosteroids and dilation. *J Rheumatol.* 2003;30:1017–1021.
14. Lorenz RR. Adult laryngotracheal stenosis: etiology and surgical management. *Curr Opin Otolaryngol Head Neck Surg.* 2003;11:467–472.
15. Smith M, Roy N, Stoddard K, et al. How does cricotracheal resection affect the female voice? *Ann Otol Rhinol Laryngol.* 2008;117(2):85–89.
16. Strome M, Stein J, Esclamado R, et al. Laryngeal transplantation and 40-month follow-up. *N Engl J Med.* 2001;344:1676–1679.
17. Lorenz RR, Strome M. Total laryngeal transplant explanted: 14 years of lessons learned. *Otolaryngol Head Neck Surg.* 2014;150(4):509–511.
18. Shipchandler TZ, Lorenz RR, Lee WT, et al. Laryngeal transplantation in the setting of cancer: a rat model. *Laryngoscope.* 2008;118:2166–2171.

64 Resection of the Carina

Simon K. Ashiku and Malcolm M. DeCamp

Keywords: Carinal tumors, tracheal tumors, carinal pneumonectomy, sleeve pneumonectomy, adenoid cystic carcinoma

Airway neoplasms account for approximately 90% of carinal resections.[1] The incidence of primary tracheal tumors is unclear, but is known to be rare. A recent population-based cancer registry analysis using the SEER database demonstrated an incidence of 2.6 tracheal tumor cases per 1,000,000 people per year.[2] Carinal tumors, as a subcategory of tracheal tumors, are even less common. Most are malignant and can be divided into bronchogenic carcinoma and other airway neoplasms. Bronchogenic carcinomas are by definition malignant; the other airway neoplasms may exhibit a wide range of behavior. As demonstrated in Table 64-1, the most common malignant primary tracheal neoplasms are squamous cell carcinoma (SCC) and adenoid cystic carcinoma (ACC).[3] SCC occurs primarily in smokers in their sixth and seventh decades and may present confined to the trachea or invading into adjacent mediastinal structures. ACC is an exophytic intratracheal lesion, which may involve the tracheal wall to variable extent (Fig. 64-1), and compress mediastinal structures without invading them initially. Lymph node metastases occur, but less commonly than in SCC. A characteristic feature of ACC is its proclivity for extending long distances submucosally and perineurally.

CLINICAL PRESENTATION

Patients commonly present with symptoms and signs of central airway obstruction. They have worsening dyspnea, often progressing to wheezing and/or stridor as the diameter of the airway decreases. Dyspnea on exertion occurs when the airway diameter is less than 8 mm and stridor develops with airways less than 5 mm.[4] Chest radiographs may demonstrate a mass in the tracheobronchial airway column. These findings are often subtle and are usually missed. Consequently, patients are commonly given a diagnosis of adult-onset asthma, and diagnosis is delayed. Patients presenting with either postobstructive pneumonia or a cough with hemoptysis may have their tumors diagnosed more rapidly. Extensive tumors may result in hoarseness, dysphagia or chest discomfort suggesting more diffuse or extensive mediastinal invasion.

DIAGNOSTIC AND STAGING STUDIES

Chest radiographs can appear normal despite significant tracheobronchial obstruction, but careful evaluation often demonstrates the outline of the mass within the airway column. Until recently, carinal tomograms were useful, revealing the location and extent of the lesion, permitting the assessment of the uninvolved proximal and distal airway. Virtually all the essential information was provided in a single view, giving the surgeon an accurate assessment of the lesion's extent. Recently, computerized tomograms have virtually replaced the use of carinal tomograms. The use of high-speed, multidetector helical CT scanners to acquire images combined with the powerful 3D-image reformation software has created impressive two and three dimensional airway reconstructions (Fig. 64-2A,B).

Table 64-1

HISTOLOGIC TYPES OF CARINAL NEOPLASMS FROM A SINGLE INSTITUTION 1962 TO 1996

DIAGNOSIS BY TUMOR TYPE IN PRIMARY CARINAL RESECTION (n = 118)	
Bronchogenic carcinoma (n = 58)	
• Squamous cell carcinoma	42
• Adenocarcinoma	10
• Large cell carcinoma	4
• Small cell carcinoma	1
• Bronchoalveolar carcinoma	1
Other airway neoplasms (n = 60)	
• Adenoid cystic carcinoma	37
• Carcinoid	11
• Mucoepidermoid carcinoma	7
• Malignant fibrosing histiocytoma	2
• Fibrosarcoma	1
• Mixed spindle cell carcinoma	1
• Granular cell tumor	1

From Ashiku SK, Mathisen DJ. Carinal resection. In: Yang ST, Cameron DE, eds. *Current Therapy in Thoracic and Cardiovascular Surgery*. Philadelphia, PA: Mosby; 2004:179.

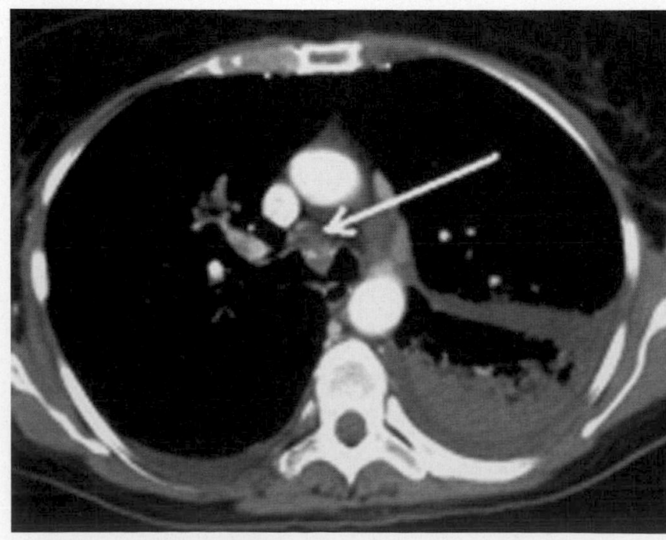

Figure 64-1. Adenoid cystic carcinoma invading through the anterior carinal wall into mediastinal space and abuts the superior vena cava.

In addition, computerized tomograms have proven critical in evaluating extraluminal extension and enlarged regional mediastinal lymph nodes; something conventional tomograms could not provide (Fig. 64-2C).

When a high degree of obstruction exists, the airway can be reopened endoscopically. This palliates acute symptomology and allows a greater degree of preoperative assessment and preparation, as well as the safe delivery of anesthesia. Specifically, patients with postobstructive pneumonia benefit from having the obstruction relieved, the pneumonia treated and the central airways cleared of purulence in advance of definitive resection and reconstruction (Fig. 64-3A–D). This is accomplished using a ventilating rigid bronchoscope under general anesthesia, without respiratory paralysis. Using the tip of the bronchoscope as a coring device, the side with the least obstruction is cleared first. Significant bleeding is rarely a problem, and can be handled with the usual techniques of rigid bronchoscopic tamponade and the judicious use of topical epinephrine solution or iced saline. Unimpeded bronchoscopic examination can then be undertaken.[5]

Metastatic workup is similar to that for lung cancer and should include chest CT, brain MRI, and PET scan to assess extraluminal extension, nodal basins, and distant metastases. Bronchoscopy allows tissue diagnosis and reveals the intraluminal extent of the tumor. Mediastinoscopy is ideally reserved for the day of resection to assess resectability, evaluate regional lymph node status and to begin central airway mobilization. By performing the mediastinoscopy at the time of planned resection, the scarring and decreased mobility associated with a staged approach is avoided. Patients with bronchogenic carcinoma and N2 disease should be considered to have unresectable disease, and surgery should only be performed in a protocol setting. Patients with ACC may benefit from resection despite nodal involvement.[6]

Anesthesia

An experienced anesthesiology team working in close cooperation with the surgical team is essential to achieve successful carinal resection. Placing a patient with a partial airway obstruction under general anesthesia is potentially hazardous. Replacement of spontaneous breathing with positive-pressure ventilation can convert a partially obstructing lesion into a complete obstruction. When maintenance of the airway is a concern, a "breathe down" technique with an inhalation agent is employed and paralytics are given only after the airway is secured. This allows the patient to breath spontaneous during the induction process, maintaining favorable respiratory physiology. Once a stable airway is secured, anesthesia is maintained with total intravenous anesthesia (TIVA) using short-acting agents such as remifentanil and propafenone. This allows immediate extubation at the completion of the procedure and maintains continuous anesthesia during periods when inhalational agents would be interrupted by the apneic intervals necessary to complete the procedure.

The administration of anesthesia through a rigid bronchoscopy during tumor "core-out" can be accomplished with either standard volume ventilation or with "jet" ventilation. Ventilating rigid bronchoscopes do not have balloon cuffs and by necessity have an open top to allow the passage of instruments. With standard volume ventilation there is a substantial air leak around the tip of the bronchoscope and out through the partially open top. Despite the use of a rubber diaphragm

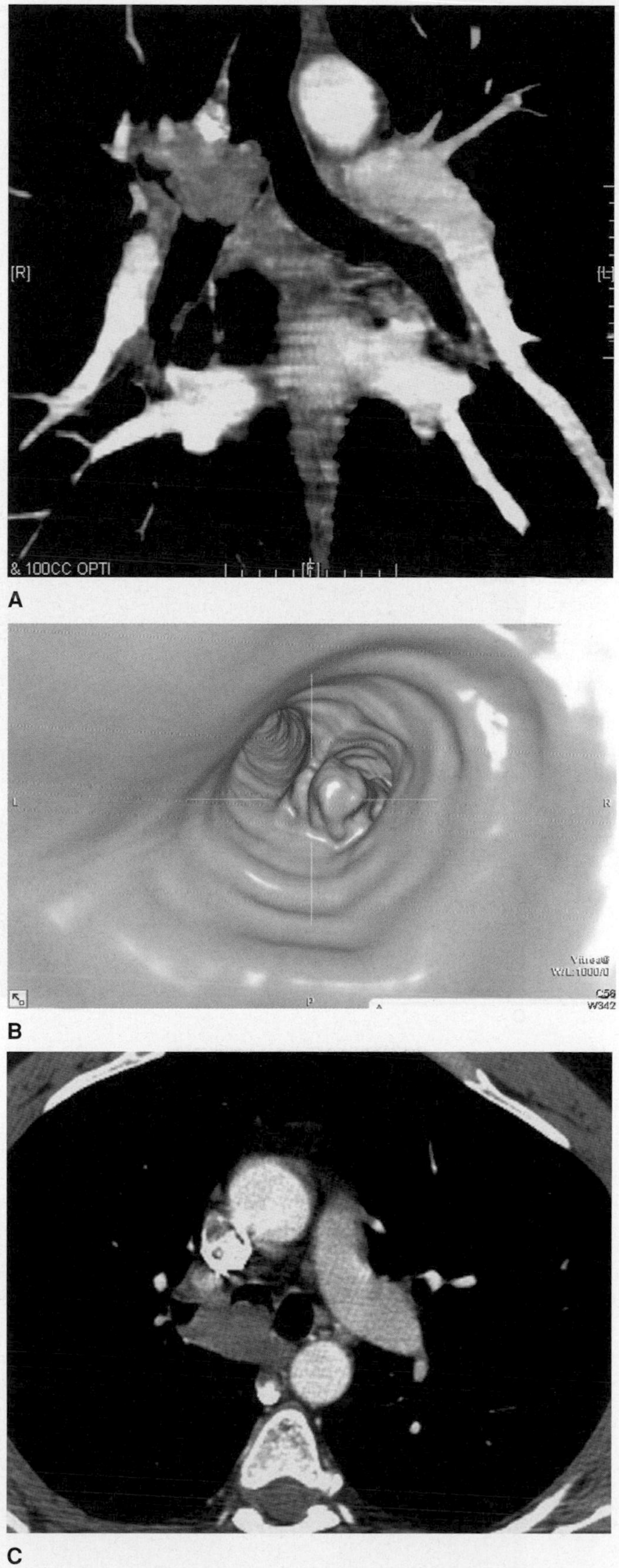

Figure 64-2. *A.* Two-dimensional sagittal airway CT reconstruction showing linear extent of airway extension. *B.* Three-dimensional airway CT reconstruction of same carinal neoplasm as viewed by virtual bronchoscopy. *C.* Computed tomography of carinal neoplasm with involvement of adjacent peribronchial lymph nodes.

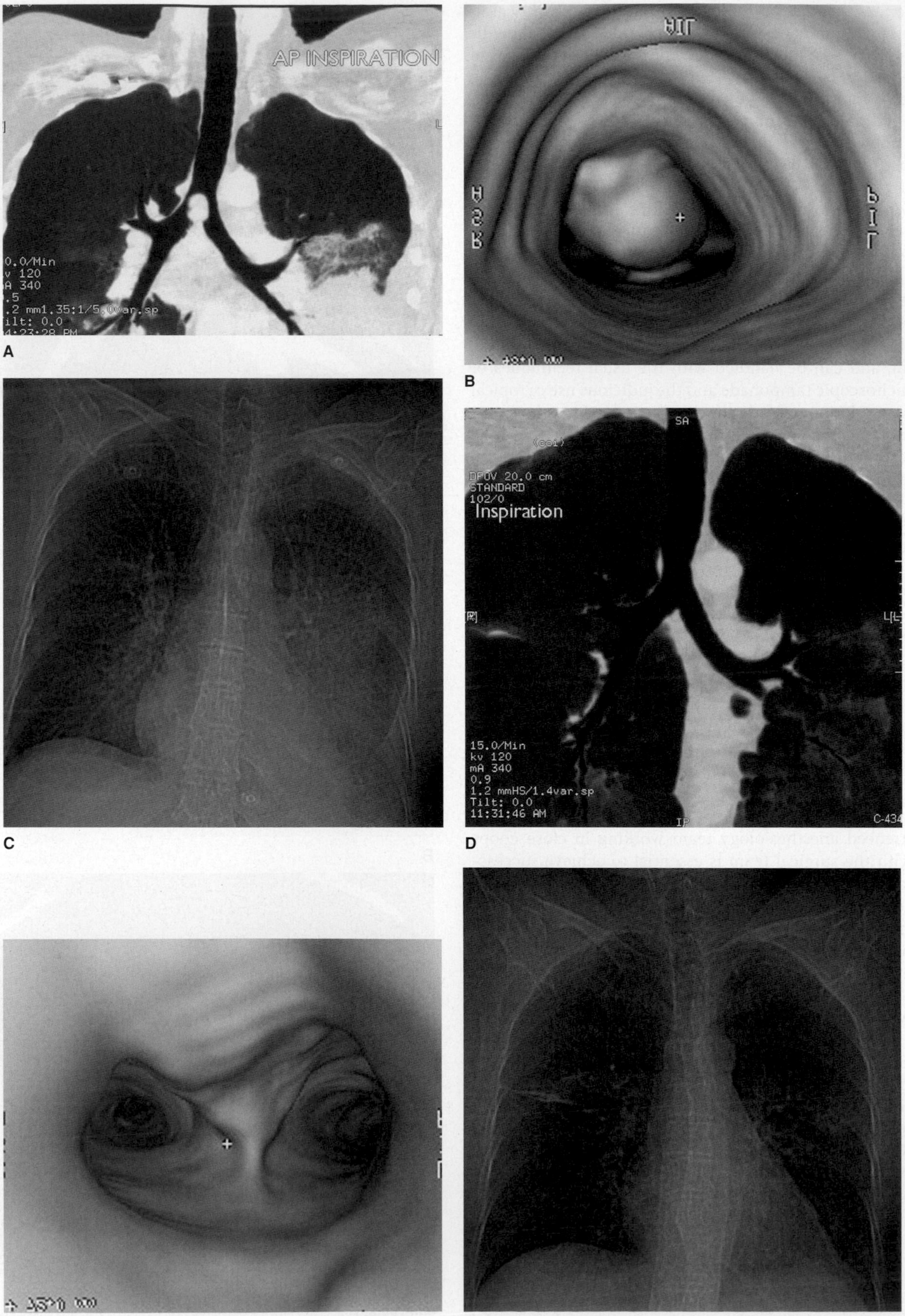

Figure 64-3. *A–C.* Adenoid cystic carcinoma of carina causing a postobstructive pneumonia. *D–F.* Obstruction relieved by bronchoscopic "core-out" of tumor enabling effective treatment of the postobstructive pneumonia.

through which to introduce instruments, the seal is imperfect, and substantial volume is lost. Consequently, higher gas flow is required to compensate for this loss in effective tidal volume. Assessing effectiveness of ventilation is performed by observing adequate chest excursions rather than end-tidal CO_2, since returning gases leak out from the circuit. With "jet" ventilation, gas is delivered at high pressure at the source, resulting in higher flow rates and higher effective tidal volumes. The top of the bronchoscope must be left open to allow venting of excess volume/pressure to reduce the risk of barotrauma. Both methods are safe and effective in experienced hands. When thermoablative devices are employed, special precautions are mandatory to prevent airway fires. Ventilation at low FiO_2 combined with periods of apnea prior to ignition of thermal devices (allows dispersion of oxygen) is employed. Clear communication and precise coordination with the anesthesiologist is essential.

Anesthesia for carinal resection is administered through an extra-long, armored endotracheal tube. Its flexibility allows bronchoscopic placement into one of the mainstem bronchi. After transecting the airway, the orotracheal tube is pulled back into the trachea and intermittent ventilation is performed with sterile cross-field equipment. The orotracheal tube is again advanced once the anastomosis is completed (Fig. 64-4). Occasionally, "jet" ventilation is useful when the left main bronchi is surgically foreshortened and will not accommodate an endotracheal balloon cuff. The small caliber of the tubing and lack of a balloon cuff allow for a less cluttered operative field and improved exposure for suture placement. However, the high-velocity airflow coupled with an open airway allows blood and airway secretions to mix and become sprayed into the lungs and the operative field. This potentially increases the risk of both pleural and pneumonic infections. In addition, the anesthesiology team must be proficient with the techniques of high-frequency "jet" ventilation. Excessive ventilation without time for passive exhalation results in hyperexpansion injury to the lung parenchyma. Inadequate "jet" ventilation results in a slow reduction in FRC as there is no mechanism to provide the PEEP necessary to prevent alveolar collapse. The risk of ARDS is higher when "jet" ventilation is employed.[7]

Cardiopulmonary bypass is generally not helpful, and only introduces unnecessary risks. A rare circumstance may arise where it is required.

Operative Procedure

Mediastinoscopy is performed on the day of proposed surgery not only to assess nodal status and resectability, but to facilitate the resection and reconstruction by mobilizing the pretracheal plane while visualizing the recurrent laryngeal nerve. Scarring of the pretracheal plane from prior mediastinoscopy limits airway mobility, complicates reconstruction, and increases the likelihood of injury to the left recurrent laryngeal nerve. Scar tissue also may be difficult to distinguish from tumor.

Choice of the operative approach is dependent on the type of carinal resection as well as personal preference. Carinal resection alone or carinal resection with right pneumonectomy can be comfortably performed through either a right thoracotomy or median sternotomy. Both approaches have their proponents.[8,9] The bias of the authors is toward the right thoracotomy approach and is discussed below. Carinal resection with left pneumonectomy presents a unique challenge and is discussed later.

A standard right posterolateral thoracotomy in the fourth interspace creates excellent exposure of the carina and allows for most resections through a single incision. When tumor extension down the left main bronchus precludes carinal reconstruction following complete resection, median sternotomy, bilateral thoracotomies, or extended clam-shell incision should be used since they permit sleeve pneumonectomy.

Once the right lung is collapsed and retracted anteriorly, the pleura overlying the carina is incised and the carina exposed. Division of the azygos vein facilitates exposure. The carina should be circumferentially freed by dissecting on the airway and avoiding the left recurrent laryngeal nerve. Dissection should be kept to a minimum and skeletonization of the airway limited to only the diseased segment to be resected (Fig. 64-5). Likewise, a balance must be struck between achieving adequate lymphadenectomy and maintaining tracheobronchial blood supply. Tapes are placed around the trachea and both mainstem bronchi. The inferior pulmonary ligament is released to allow greater mobility of the right lung, and equipment for cross-field

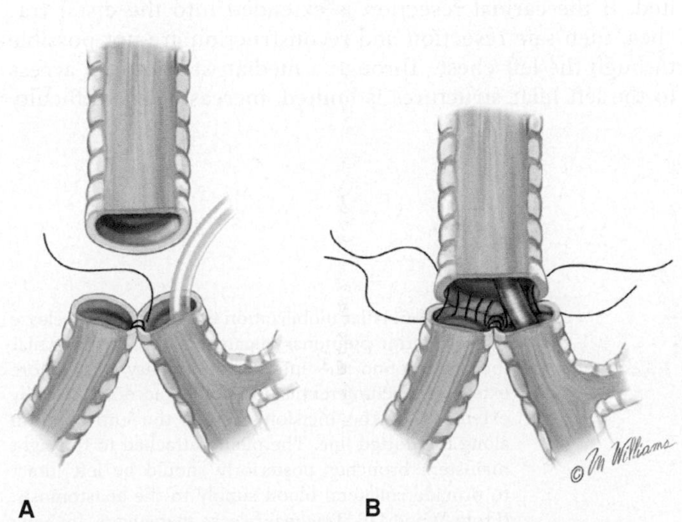

Figure 64-4. *A.* Technique of cross-table ventilation with left main bronchus intubated from the operative field until the anastomosis is nearly complete. *B.* The oral endotracheal tube is advanced by the anesthesiologist.

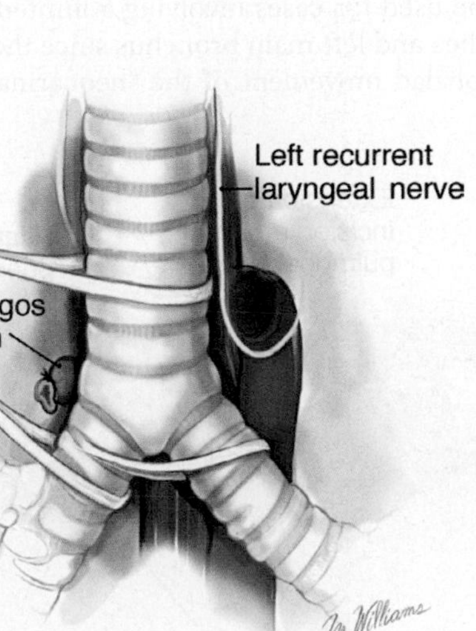

Figure 64-5. Airway dissection is limited to the airway to be resected.

sterile ventilation is prepared. The order of dividing the airway structures varies, but commonly the trachea is divided first. Preoperative bronchoscopic assessment by the surgeon directs the tracheal division to just proximal to the tumor. An adequate margin can then be taken under direct visualization in the form of a complete ring sent separately for intraoperative frozen section. The endotracheal tube is then removed to allow division of both mainstem bronchi under direct endobronchial visualization. Adequate margins are taken of both distal bronchi and sent separately for frozen section. Only the left mainstem bronchus is reintubated, usually across the field, maintaining collapse of the right lung.

If mediastinoscopy was not performed, then airway mobilization should be accomplished in the anterior plane up to the neck proximally and down the left mainstem distally. Additional airway mobility can be obtained by a hilar release. This technique involves making a U-shaped incision in the pericardium below the inferior pulmonary vein (Fig. 64-6). If required, the pericardium can be incised 360 degrees around the hilus for maximal mobility. In this event, the vascular and lymphatic pedicle to the mainstem bronchus is left preserved behind the pericardium. Left-sided hilar release can only be accomplished easily through a median sternotomy by opening the pericardium anteriorly, or bilateral thoracotomies, or an extended clam-shell incision. As with most airway surgery, neck flexion is helpful. Laryngeal release has not been shown to produce meaningful mobility at the level of the carina.[1]

Placement of 2-0 braided absorbable lateral traction sutures in the trachea and both bronchi allows for easy handling of these structures during the reconstruction phase. The optimal mode of carinal reconstruction depends largely on the extent of resection. In the series reported by Mitchell (n = 135), 15 different modes of reconstruction were employed. The three most common methods, arranged in order of frequency, were (1) end-to-end anastomosis of trachea to left mainstem with reimplantation of right into trachea, (2) end-to-end anastomosis of trachea to right mainstem with reimplantation of left into the bronchus intermedius, and (3) anastomosis of trachea to reapproximated left and right mainstem creating a "neocarina" (Fig. 64-7A–C).[10]

The "neocarina" method is the most simple. However, it can only be used for cases involving a limited resection of the distal trachea and left main bronchus since the aortic arch limits the cephalad movement of the "neocarina" (Fig. 64-8A,B). For this reason, end-to-end anastomosis of trachea to the left mainstem with reimplantation of the right into the trachea is more commonly employed (Fig. 64-9A–C). A right hilar release maneuver facilitates this procedure. More extensive resections require end-to-end anastomosis of trachea to the right mainstem with reimplantation of left into the bronchus intermedius. This obviates the need for extensive left mainstem mobility. When there is extensive endobronchial involvement, excessive lung destruction, or invasion of hilar vessels, then carinal (sleeve) pneumonectomy is necessary.

The anastomosis is fashioned with interrupted simple 4-0 polyglycolic acid absorbable sutures placed with knots tied outside the lumen (Fig. 64-10). Once reconstructed, the anastomosis is tested for air tightness to 40 mm Hg. All suture lines are circumferentially wrapped with pedicled flaps of pericardial fat or a broad-based pleural flap. In high-risk patients, especially those who have undergone prior radiotherapy, an intercostal flap stripped of all periosteum or an omentum pedicle is used. These flaps not only buttress the anastomosis, but more importantly, separate them from the hilar vessels, helping to prevent bronchovascular fistulas.

Carinal resection with left pneumonectomy is rarely required and presents a unique and difficult challenge. The long length of the left mainstem allows for most carinal tumors to be resected with sufficient left mainstem remaining for a tension-free anastomosis. However, on rare occasion, a tumor extends distally from the carina to involve a large portion of the left mainstem. In these circumstances, an extended left bronchial airway resection would leave the left lung without sufficient left mainstem to reach around the undersurface of the aortic arch for a tension-free anastomosis. Thus, the left lung cannot be salvaged, and a concomitant left pneumonectomy is required.

There is no single optimal incision to approach a carinal resection with a left pneumonectomy. The carina is best approached via a right thoracotomy or median sternotomy while a left pneumonectomy is best approached via a left thoracotomy. Both single incision approaches, left thoracotomy and median sternotomy, involve compromises in exposure. Through a left thoracotomy, the aortic arch limits access to the carina making resection and reconstruction technically difficult and only possible when the carinal resection is limited. If the carinal resection is extended into the distal trachea, then safe resection and reconstruction are not possible through the left chest. Through a median sternotomy, access to the left hilar structures is limited, increasing the difficulty

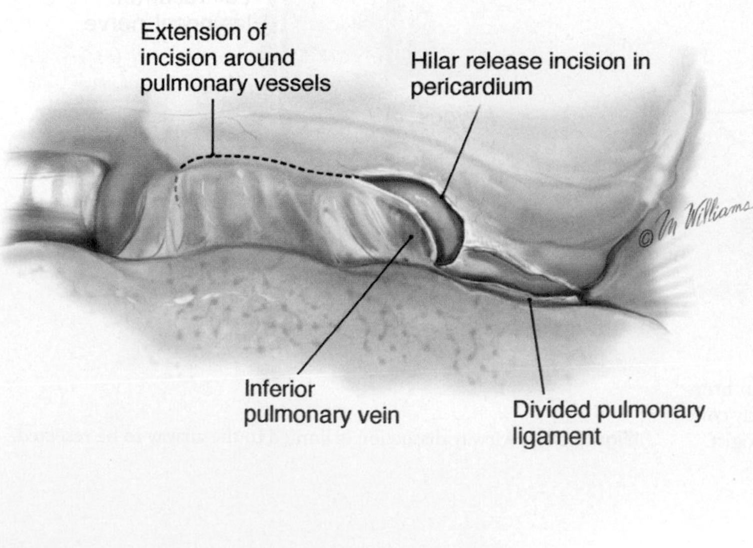

Figure 64-6. Hilar mobilization is performed by release of the inferior pulmonary ligament and a semicircular incision around the inferior pulmonary vein. More extensive circumferential incision is accomplished by extension of the incision around the entire hilum along the dotted line. The pleura attached to the right mainstem bronchus posteriorly should be left intact to provide collateral blood supply to the anastomosis. (From Wood DE. Tracheal release maneuvers. In: Yang ST, Cameron DE, eds. *Current Therapy in Thoracic and Cardiovascular Surgery*. Philadelphia, PA: Mosby; 2004: 129).

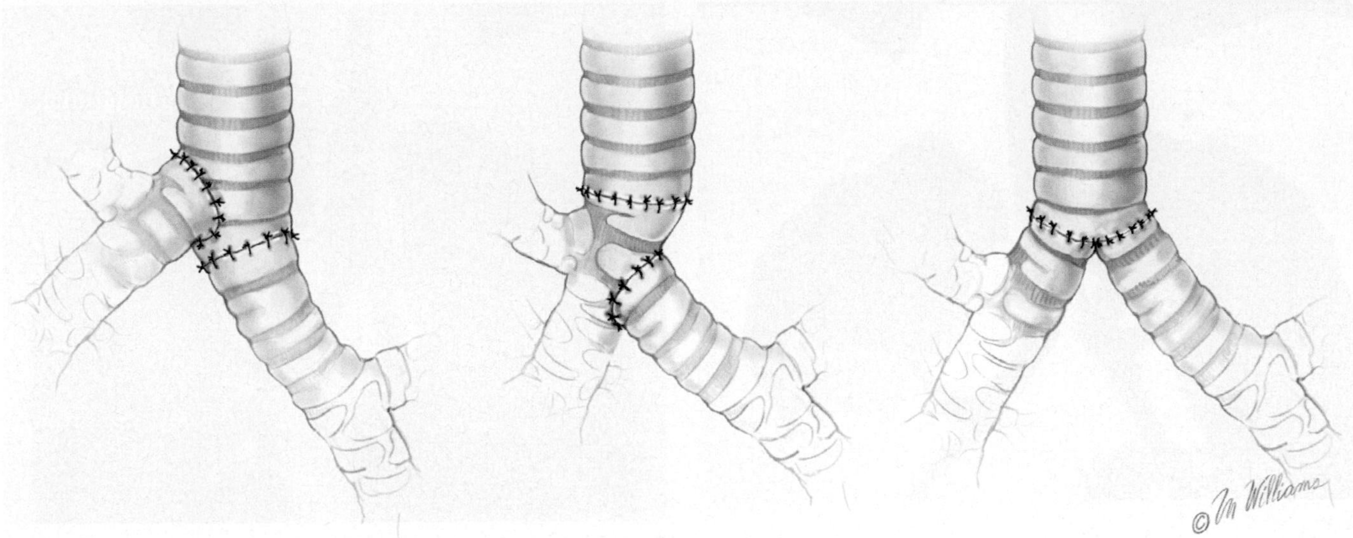

A B C

Figure 64-7. *A.* Most common carinal reconstruction; end-to-end anastomosis of trachea to left mainstem with reimplantation of right into trachea. *B.* Next most common carinal reconstruction; end-to-end anastomosis of trachea to right mainstem with reimplantation of left into the bronchus intermedius. *C.* Anastomosis of trachea to reapproximated left and right mainstem creating a "neocarina" with left main bronchus anastomosed to the trachea, and right main bronchus.

of the pneumonectomy. However, resections extending into the distal trachea are possible. Staged bilateral thoracotomies or bilateral thoracotomies extended across the sternum at the fourth intercostal level (clam shell incision) are less technically demanding for the surgeon, but are more physiologically disruptive to the patient. Recent technical advances may ultimately prove helpful to improve exposure and/or reduce morbidity. Thoracoscopic resection techniques have been employed to limit the morbidity of a stage approach by performing a minimally invasive left pneumonectomy after a right thoracotomy for the carinal resection and airway reconstruction. New suction retractors created for "off pump" coronary artery bypass surgery can be used via a median sternotomy to lift the apex of the beating heart allowing excellent exposure to the left hilar structures, particularly the left inferior pulmonary vein. Regardless of the approach used, carinal resection with left pneumonectomy remains a challenging operation with a high morbidity and mortality.

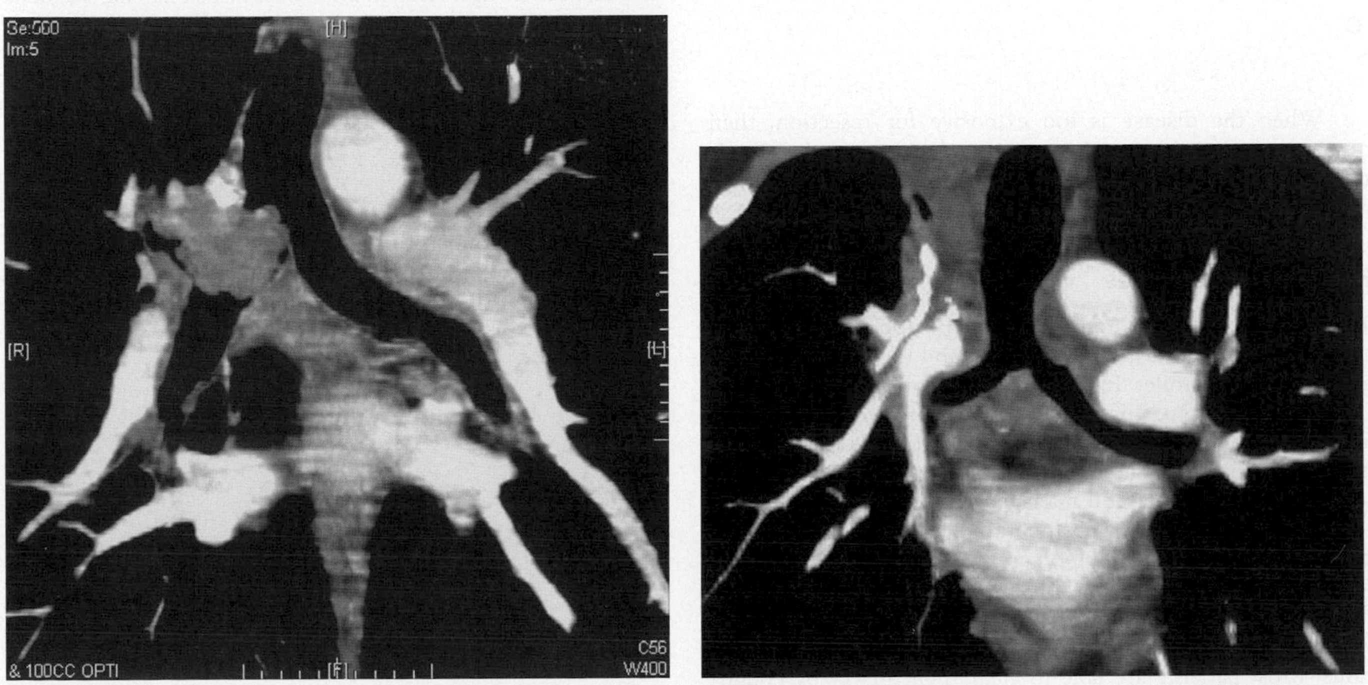

A B

Figure 64-8. *A, B.* Example of tumor requiring minimal resection of left main bronchus allowing for "neocarina"-type reconstruction.

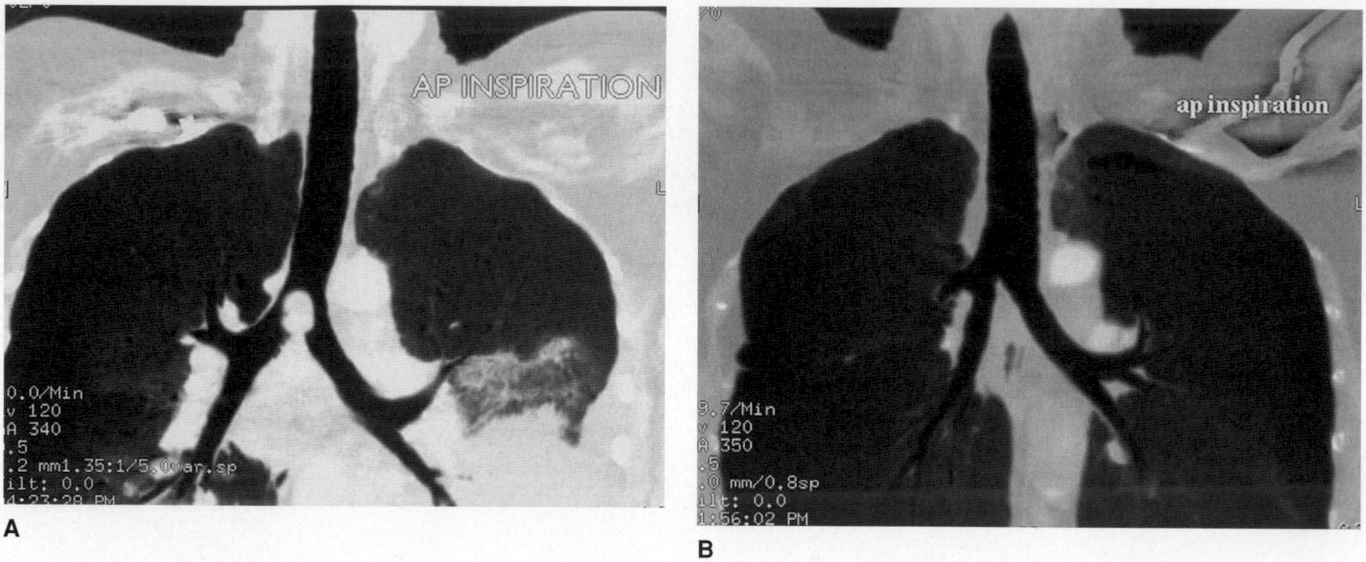

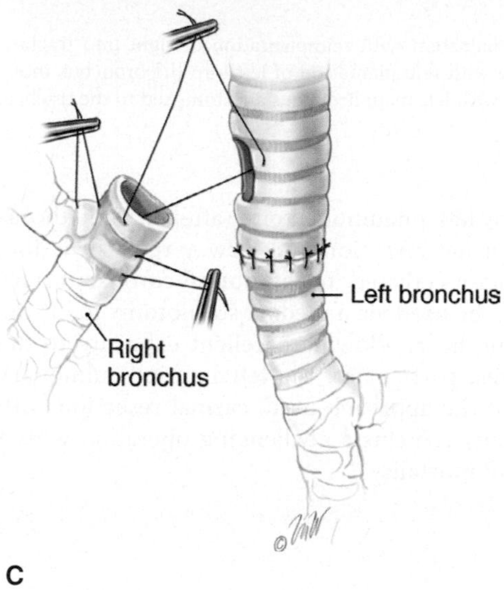

Figure 64-9. *A.* Adenoid cystic carcinoma with submucosal extension beyond carina. *B.* Carinal reconstruction required end-to-end anastomosis of trachea to left mainstem with reimplantation of right into trachea. *C.* Technique for right main bronchus implantation into the side of the trachea.

When the disease is too extensive for resection, then tumor core-out with or without expandable covered stents is often helpful. External beam radiotherapy and brachytherapy remain the standard palliative treatment.

Postoperative Issues

The goals of both intraoperative and postoperative care are the promotion of anastomotic healing and the maintenance of good pulmonary toilet. Ideally, patients should be extubated in the operating room. The need for postoperative ventilation is a relative contraindication to carinal resection as it is a strong predictor of postoperative mortality.[10] Patients with marginal lung function need careful management during the operation to help avoid the need for postoperative ventilation. During the procedure secretions and blood are kept from running distally into the lungs and volume overload is avoided. Postoperatively, fluids are minimized. Postoperatively, patients are supplied with humidity by face mask to facilitate clearance of secretions. Most patients are able to clear their airway by coughing. Frequently, therapeutic flexible bronchoscopy is performed to suction secretions under direct vision. Cervical flexion is

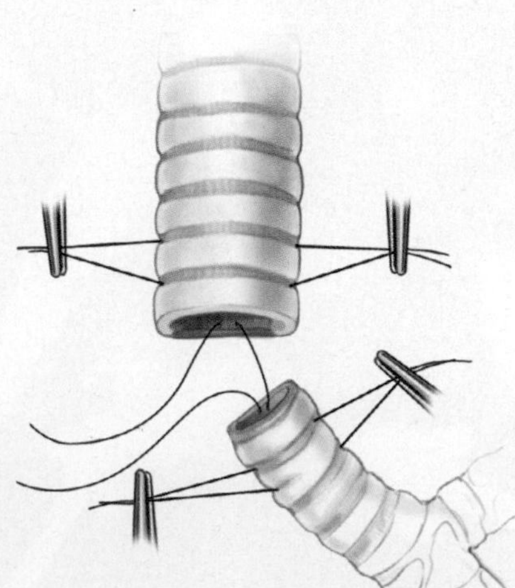

Figure 64-10. Interrupted polyglycolic acid suture placement with knots on the outside of airway.

maintained with the chin-to-chest suture for 5 to 7 days, after which time the patient is advised not to extend the neck for another week. Before removing the chin-to-chest suture, we routinely examine the anastomosis with flexible bronchoscopy to assure normal healing. Oral alimentation is begun cautiously in the first few postoperative days. If there is any concern over a possible injury to the left recurrent laryngeal nerve then a speech and swallowing evaluation, with or without video swallow, is obtained before initiating oral feeding.

Complications

Few centers have reported on a significant experience in carinal resection, and in those who have, the reported experience has been gathered from over several decades. The two largest series were reported by Mitchell (n = 135) and Porhanov (n = 231).[7,10]

In the series reported by Mitchell (1999), the overall mortality for all types of carinal resections over a 32-year period was 12.5%. In the initial 67 patients the mortality was 16.1% and dropped to 9% for the last 67 patients as techniques and perioperative care evolved and outcomes improved. Overall morbidity was 39%. The two major types of complications were anastomosis-related problems and ARDS. Anastomotic complications occurred in 17% of patients. Early complications were necrosis, separation, and mucosal slough. Late complications were stenosis, excessive granulation tissue, and recurrent postobstructive pneumonia. Most of these required intervention. Anastomotic-related complications were associated with a 44% mortality rate. ARDS occurred in 10% of patients, usually following carinal pneumonectomies, and were associated with a 90% mortality rate[10]. The etiology of postpneumonectomy ARDS is unclear, but may result from intraoperative overhydration and lung hyper-inflation. This may induce lung injury and interstitial edema in a lung that already has a disrupted lymphatic drainage system. Major postoperative complications were higher after carinal pneumonectomy than after carinal resection alone, with 30.8% mortality for left carinal pneumonectomy and 15.9% mortality for right carinal pneumonectomies. Complications associated with carinal pneumonectomies accounted for the majority of postoperative deaths.[10]

Similarly, in the series reported by Porhanov (2002), the overall mortality for all types of carinal resections over a 23-year period was 16%. Overall morbidity was 35.6%. Again, the two major types of complications were anastomosis-related problems and ARDS. Anastomotic complications occurred in 25.1% of patients. Dehiscence occurred in 9.1% of patients, all of whom died. Anastomotic-related complications were associated with a 36% mortality rate. ARDS occurred in 4.7% of patients and was associated with an 81% mortality rate. Again, complications associated with carinal pneumonectomies accounted for the majority of postoperative deaths.[7]

ADJUVANT THERAPY

The low incidence of carinal malignancies and their variable histology does not allow for definitive statements about the merits of postoperative radiotherapy and chemotherapy. In the study reported by Regnard, 70/143 patients with SCC, adenocarcinoma, and ACC were treated with radiotherapy postoperatively, whereas 4/143 were treated with combined chemoradiation postoperatively. There was no survival benefit in those with negative operative margins, whereas a significant benefit was found for those with positive surgical margins. No survival benefit was detected for patients with positive lymph nodes treated with postoperative radiotherapy.[11] However, centers with the most experience have recommended the routine use of postoperative radiotherapy in all patients with a resected ACC and bronchogenic carinal neoplasms, regardless of margin or lymph node status.[12,13] The rationale for this approach is based upon the inherently close margins accepted in carinal resections. A compromise is always made between the desire for negative margins with the necessity of a tension-free anastomosis. The role of chemotherapy is even less well understood and no evidence-based consensus can be derived.

PROGNOSIS

Carinal neoplasms are a rare and heterogeneous group, which limits the ability to determine prognostic factors for all histologies. However, limited prognostic data is available for bronchogenic carcinoma as a group and separately for ACC.

The three largest series for which 5-year survival data are available for resected bronchogenic carcinoma of the carina were reported by Dartevelle (1996) (n = 60), Mitchell (2001) (n = 60) and Porhanov (2002) (n = 101). The overall 5-year survival for resected patients was 43%, 42%, and 25%, respectively. The lower overall survival in Porhanov's series partly reflects the inclusion of bronchogenic carcinoma with N2 nodes invasive into the carina, which separately had a 2.6% 5-year survival. In the series reported by Mitchell, 57% presented with N0 disease, 25% had N1 disease, and 18% had N2/N3 disease. Lymph node status strongly influenced survival. The 5-year survival of N0, N1, and N2/N3 patients was 51%, 32%, and 12%, respectively (Fig. 64-3). Microscopically positive margins did not affect survival. Isolated carinal resection resulted in a more favorable prognosis than more extensive resections, with a 5-year survival of 51%.[7,13,14]

SCC make up the majority of bronchogenic carcinomas of the carina. A recent series by Gaissert (2004) carefully evaluated the long-term oncologic outcome of patients with SCC of the trachea and carina. Of 135 patients (90 resected, 45 unresected), 5-year survival was 39.1% in resected and 7.3% in unresected patients. Despite higher mortality in the carinal resection group, overall long-term survival was not significantly different than in the tracheal resection group. Positive nodal disease markedly reduced survival. There were few microscopically positive margins in resected SCC patients, thus, despite an adverse absolute effect on survival, it did not reach statistical significance. Regnard (1996), in a European multicenter retrospective series, reported similar results in 94 patients with resected tracheal and carinal SCC. Survival was 47% at 5 years and 36% at 10 years.[6]

The long-term survival data for resected ACC of the carina has not been as well defined, partly because of its proclivity for late recurrence. The published experience of all tracheal ACC, which includes those involving the carina, suggests a much more favorable prognosis than bronchogenic carcinomas. In the recent series by Gaissert (2004), he reported the long-term outcome of 135 patients with ACC of the trachea and carina as a group. The 5-year survival was 52.4% for the 101 resected patients and 33.3% for the 34 unresected patients.[6]

Positive resection margins adversely affected survival, resulting in a similar 5-year survival as unresected patients. However, there was a survival difference noted at 15 years, with 14.5% alive in the positive resection margins group versus no survivors in unresected patients.

Earlier studies had suggested that nodal status did not adversely affect survival in patient with ACC.[6] However, after longer follow-up of the same ACC patient cohort, nodal status was associated with survival. Median overall survival was 16.8 years in node negative patients and 6.1 years node positive patients. In addition, positive margins again were found to adversely affect survival. Patients with negative margins demonstrated 20.4 years overall median survival, versus 13.3 years for microscopically positive margins, and 6.1 years for grossly positive margins.[15]

Similarly, Regnard (1996) reporting on 65 ACC demonstrated a 5-year survival at 73% and 10-year survival at 57%. Lymph node status was not shown to affect survival. Positive margins did appear to adversely affect survival, but due to low numbers did not reach statistical significance.[11]

CARINAL REPLACEMENT

Over the past century, there have been many efforts directed at replacing the trachea and/or the carina when the disease extent precludes resection and primary reconstruction. Approaches have included the use of foreign materials, autogenous tissue, nonviable tissue, transplantation, and tissue engineering. To date, each approach has been associated with considerable risk for serious complications and death.[16]

In recent years, two methods: nonviable tissue (aortic autograft) and tissue engineering have gone from experimental animal research to human implementation. Martinod et al.[17–19] reported that autologous and allogenic aortic grafts used to replace 5- to 8-cm segments of sheep tracheas and carinas resulted in the regeneration of the airway with new cartilage rings and tracheal epithelium. Jaillard et al.[20] reported on similar results in pigs.

To date, other investigators have not able to reproduce the results of Martinod and Jaillard.[21] Harvested tracheal grafts revealed no evidence of graft incorporation into the surrounding tissue, and there was no histologic evidence of neocartilage within or around the graft. Histologic and radiographic analysis suggested that the grafted aortic grafts underwent necrosis with the integrity of the airway maintained by the intraluminal stent and the paratracheal inflammatory process. The cicatricial scarring resulted in subsequent axial shortening slowly bringing the proximal and distal native tracheas together. It is worth noting that this phenomenon may allow for safe, two-stage end-to-end reconstruction of larger tracheal defects using a first-stage temporary grafting.[22]

In 2006, Martinod et al.[23] reported the first human case of long-segment tracheal replacement with an aortic autograft. The patient died 6 months later from respiratory complications. In 2010, Wurtz et al.[24] reported on six patients who had undergone aortic allografts for extensive airway tumors: three had carinal replacements and three tracheal grafts. All three patients with carinal replacements developed fistulas between the graft and the esophagus, and one died at 26 months as a result. All three patients with trachea-only replacement survived; one had a major complication. One patient died at 45 months of distant recurrence and the remaining four patients were alive and well at the time of reporting with a mean follow-up of 34 months (range: 26–42 months). All required lifelong stenting. Serial bronchoscopies revealed axial shortening of the graft as had been observed in earlier animal data.

The first experimental attempts at creating a tissue engineered trachea were reported by Vacanti et al.[25] in 1994. The technique involves guiding the formation of new tissue by seeding a framework of biodegradable synthetic polymer with cultivated autologous cells. In 2008, Macchiarini et al.[26] reported the first tracheal transplantation with a nonimmunogenic decellularized human donor trachea reseeded with bone-marrow–derived mesenchymal stem cells and respiratory cells. In 2011, he then reported the first human implantation of a fully tissue engineered tracheal and carinal construct.[27] The graft was made of a polymer fabricated into a Y-shaped tube with reinforcing U-shaped rings in matrix. The scaffolding was seeded with autologous bone-marrow mononuclear cells. Six centimeters of distal intrathoracic trachea, the carina, the entire right main bronchus, and the first 2 cm of the left main bronchus were resected and replaced with the engineered graft wrapped with omentum. No stenting was required. At the time of reporting there were no major complications, and the patient was asymptomatic and tumor-free 5 months postoperatively.

Although these techniques hold promise, the gold standard treatment for resectable disease remains surgical resection with primary reconstruction. When presented with unresectable tracheal tumors, palliative therapy with radiation and endoscopic techniques remains the safest approach. However, given the poor 5-year survival of 7.3% for unresectable SCC and 33.3% for unresectable ACC,[6] there remains a need for innovative therapies for tracheal replacement.

SUMMARY

Most carinal resections are performed for either SCC or ACC. Diagnosis and assessment of resectability are accomplished with bronchoscopy and computed tomography reformatted in two and three dimensions. Patients are assessed for metastatic disease with MRI of the brain and total-body PET scans. Mediastinoscopy is employed to assess for regionally advanced disease and for airway mobilization. Regionally advanced disease should be considered unresectable unless performed in a protocol setting. Rigid bronchoscopy and carinal resection create a unique requirement for the delivery of anesthesia requiring an experienced and collaborative team. Most carinal resections can be approached through either a right thoracotomy or a median sternotomy, and should have a low operative mortality. Carinal resection with left pneumonectomy presents a special operative challenge and results in a higher risk of operative mortality. Several methods of airway reconstruction are available and depend upon the extent of airway involvement. In properly selected patients, oncologic outcomes are good, with ACC having a more favorable prognosis then SCC. Postoperative radiotherapy should be considered for all resected patients, regardless of histology or the status of margins. No evidence-based consensus can be derived for the role of chemotherapy.

EDITOR'S COMMENT

Carinal pneumonectomy is a complex and rare procedure that should be performed by experienced surgeons in centers of excellence. Careful preoperative evaluation is required to ascertain the oncologic rationale for this procedure. Attention should be paid to avoid over-hydration or barotraumas from over-lung inflation in the operating room or the rest of the perioperative period. We have found that left VATS mobilization and pericardial release as a first step can help in carinal resection performed from a right thoracotomy approach. As described in the text, it is important to balance the extent of resection versus anastomosis tension and to minimize resection to negative margins. Finally, some patients with squamous cell cancer will have second and third cancers in the lung and head and neck and should be aggressively managed.

—Raphael Bueno

References

1. Grillo HC. Primary tracheal neoplasm. In: Grillo HC, ed. *Surgery of Trachea and Bronchi*. Hamilton, London: BC Decker; 2004:208.
2. Urdaneta AI, Yu JB, Wilson LD. Population based cancer registry analysis of primary tracheal carcinoma. *Am J Clin Oncol.* 2011;34(1):32–37.
3. Ashiku SK, Mathisen DJ. Carinal resection. In: Yang ST, Cameron DE, eds. *Current Therapy in Thoracic and Cardiovascular Surgery*. Philadelphia, PA: Mosby; 2004:179.
4. Hollingsworth HM. Wheezing and stridor. *Clin Chest Med.* 1987;8(2): 231–240.
5. Mathisen DJ, Grillo HC. Endoscopic relief of malignant airway obstruction. *Ann Thorac Surg.* 1989;48:469–473.
6. Gaissert HA, Grillo HC, Shadmehr MB, et al. Long-term survival after resection of primary adenoid cystic and squamous cell carcinoma of the trachea and carina. *Ann Thorac Surg.* 2004;78:1889–1896.
7. Porhanov VA, Poliakov IS, Selvaschuk AP, et al. Indications and results of sleeve carinal resection. *Eur J Cardio-thoracic Surg.* 2002;22:685–694.
8. Pearson FG, Todd TR, Cooper JD. Experience with primary neoplasm of the trachea and carina. *J Thorac Cardiovasc Surg.* 1984;88:511–518.
9. Grillo HC. Carinal reconstruction. *Ann Thorac Surg.* 1982;34:356–373.
10. Mitchell JD, Mathisen DJ, Wright CD, et al. Clinical experience with carinal resection. *J Thorac Cardiovasc Surg.* 1999;117:39–52.
11. Regnard JF, Fourquier P, Levasseur P. Results and prognostic factors in resections of primary tracheal tumors: a multicenter retrospective study. *J Thorac Cardiovasc Surg.* 1996;111:808–813.
12. Grillo HC, Mathisen DJ. Primary tracheal tumors: treatment and results. *Ann Throrac Surg.* 1990;49:69–77.
13. Mitchell JD, Mathisen DJ, Wright CD, et al. Resection of bronchogenic carcinoma involving the carina: long-term results and the effect of nodal status on outcome. *J Thorac Cardiovasc Surg.* 2001;121:465–471.
14. Dartevelle PG. Herbert Sloan lecture. Extended operations for the treatment of lung cancer. *Ann Thorac Surg.* 1997;63:12–19.
15. Honings J, Gaissert HA, Weinberg AC, et al. Prognostic value of pathologic characteristics and resection margins in tracheal adenoid cystic carcinoma. *Eur J Cardiothorac Surg.* 2010;37:1438–1444.
16. Grillo HC. Tracheal replacement: a critical review. *Ann Thorac Surg.* 2002; 73:1995–2004.
17. Martinod E, Seguin A, Pfeuty K, et al. Long-term evaluation of the replacement of the trachea with autologous aortic graft. *Ann Thorac Surg.* 2003;75:1572–1578.
18. Martinod E, Seguin A, Holder-Espinasse M, et al. Tracheal regeneration following tracheal replacement with an allogenic aorta. *Ann Thorac Surg.* 2005;79:942–948.
19. Seguin A, Martinod E, Kambouchner M, et al. Carinal replacement with an aortic allograft. *Ann Thorac Surg.* 2006;81:1068–1074.
20. Jaillard S, Holder-Espinasse M, Hubert T, et al. Tracheal replacement by allogenic aorta in the pig. *Chest.* 2006;130:1397–1404.
21. Tsukada H, Ernst A, Gangadharan S, et al. Tracheal replacement with a silicone-stented, fresh aortic allograft in sheep. *Ann Thorac Surg.* 2010;89(1):253–258.
22. Tsukada H, Majid A, Kent MS, et al. Two-staged end-to-end reconstruction of long segment tracheal defects using a bioabsorbable scaffold grafting technique in a canine model. *Ann Thorac Surg.* 2012;93(4):1088–1092.
23. Azorin JF, Bertin F, Martinod E, et al. Tracheal replacement with an aortic autograft. *Eur J Cardiothorac Surg.* 2006;29(2):261–263.
24. Wurtz A, Porte H, Conti M, et al. Surgical technique and results of tracheal and carinal replacement with aortic allograft for salivary gland-type carcinoma. *J Thorac Cardiovasc Surg.* 2010;140(2):387–393.
25. Vacanti CA, Paige KT, Kim WS, et al. Experimental tracheal replacement using tissue engineered cartilage. *J Pediatr Surg.* 1994;29:201–204.
26. Macchiarini P, Jungebluth P, Go T, et al. Clinical transplantation of a tissue-engineered airway. *Lancet.* 2008;372:2023–2030.
27. Jungebluth P, Alici E, Baiguera S, et al. Tracheobronchial transplantation with a stem-cell-seeded bioartificial nanocomposite: a proof-of-concept study. *Lancet.* 2011;378(9808):1997–2004.

65 Mediastinal Tracheostomy

Daniel G. Nicastri, Jaime Yun, and Scott J. Swanson

Keywords: Aerodigestive tract malignancy, breastplate resection, tracheal division and laryngectomy, transposition of the trachea, tracheocutaneous anastomosis

Despite progress in tracheal surgery over the past 60 years, to date, there is no suitable substitute for the trachea to bridge long gaps after resection. The adult trachea is usually approximately 9 to 13 cm long. Currently, approximately half of the adult trachea can be removed surgically and reanastomosed with various tracheal release and mobilization maneuvers. More extensive tracheal resections are limited by the lack of dependable and predictable replacements. This limitation is quite apparent by the occasional necessity of creating an anterior mediastinal tracheostomy (MT) in palliative, curative, or sometimes emergent or "bail out" procedures.

An anterior MT involves the construction of a tracheostomy stoma on the anterior chest wall using the intrathoracic trachea when there is insufficient length to reanastomose the remaining trachea or to bring the trachea out of the superior mediastinum for a standard suprasternal stoma. The procedure involves laryngectomy (if not done previously) and resection of the upper sternum, the medial third of the clavicles, and the first and usually second ribs. This provides access to the intrathoracic trachea with excellent exposure of the superior mediastinum and brings the chest wall down to the remaining shortened trachea to avoid tension on the stoma. The primary indications for this operation are mostly limited to advanced cervicothoracic neoplasms in the superior mediastinum, although it is done occasionally for benign disease. The indications for this procedure have become less common with the refinement of radiation therapy and tracheal surgery and are confined to very selected clinical scenarios. Tumors in this location that are amenable to resection are quite rare.

Few thoracic surgeons or institutions have any extensive experience with this procedure. MT is a complex procedure that is performed in a difficult, unfamiliar anatomic location and is associated with very high morbidity and mortality. However, as described in multiple series in the literature, curative and palliative resections of advanced or recurrent carcinomas in this region can be accomplished with acceptable outcomes. Often the patient will experience a prolonged recovery with a high risk of associated serious complications. MT requires dedicated postoperative care delivered by experienced medical and nursing teams. With a successful outcome, however, the functional result is the equivalent of laryngectomy.[1] When undertaking this radical procedure, one must show good clinical judgment in patient and case selection. Also, it is imperative to determine whether the procedure is being done for cure or palliation because 1 or 2 cm of length can change the complexion of the procedure.

PATIENT CHARACTERISTICS, INDICATIONS, AND ONCOLOGIC PRINCIPLES

Patient Characteristics

Patients must be selected carefully, and the surgeon's preoperative preparation should be meticulous. The typical patient requiring an anterior MT usually is afflicted with an advanced cervicothoracic malignancy involving either the thyroid, larynx, pharynx, trachea, or esophagus that often invades adjacent structures (Fig. 65-1). It also can be a recurrent tumor at the site where the trachea or larynx was resected previously, such as a recurrence at the site of the tracheal stoma.

An important consideration is whether the patient will need to have restoration of alimentary continuity (Table 65-1) because this adds substantially to the duration, complexity, and stress of the operation. The general condition of the patient should be good enough to tolerate this radical procedure. A thorough history, physical examination, and clinical workup should focus on the following: preoperative nutritional status, weight loss, cardiac and respiratory function, smoking status, and a history of diabetes or steroid dependence. All these conditions should be optimized, and the patient should cease smoking several weeks before surgery. The patient also should undergo preoperative respiratory conditioning, including incentive spirometry and respiratory physical therapy. Other important details include a history of prior abdominal surgery (important to know the esophageal substitution), laryngectomy, tracheal resection, chemotherapy, and radiation therapy. A prior history of radiation therapy will make the neck structures, including the great vessels, more fixed. In addition, tracheal blood supply may be compromised, increasing the risk of ischemic breakdown and delayed healing. Finally, and perhaps most important, it is the surgeon's job to make sure that the patient is psychologically prepared for the morbidity of this procedure (including loss of speech) and a potentially long recovery.

Indications

MT, whether for palliation or for cure, is indicated after tracheal resection, laryngectomy, or laryngopharyngectomy in cases where there is insufficient length of intrathoracic trachea to either reanastomose it superiorly or bring it out suprasternally (Fig. 65-2). This determination depends on various factors, including the patient's anteroposterior diameter (one needs more length in a barrel chest), the effectiveness of tracheal mobilization, and the malleability of the remaining trachea. Some surgeons suggest that the optimal length for MT is

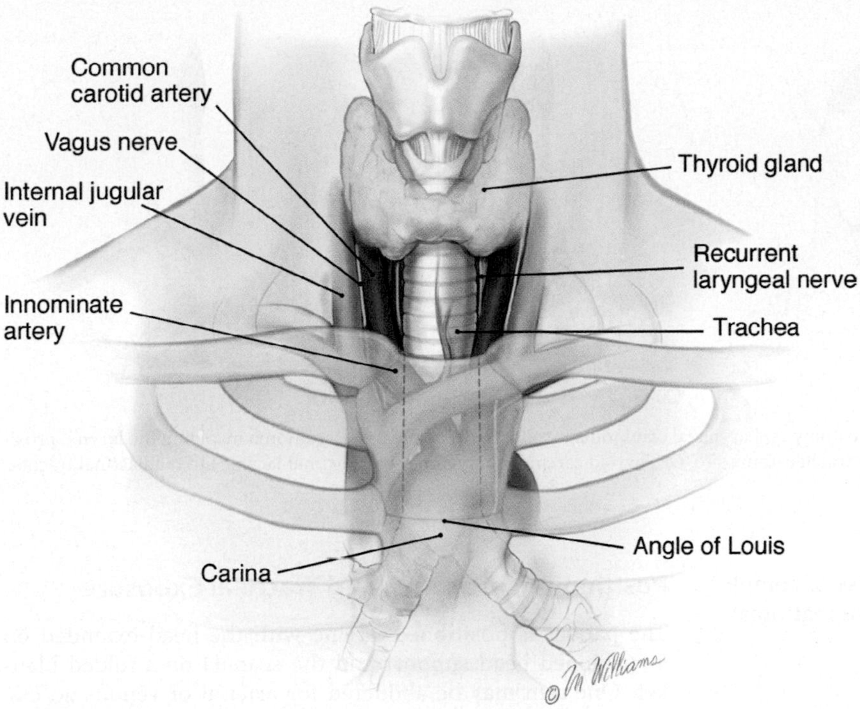

Figure 65-1. Anterior mediastinal anatomy. Note the relationship of the sternal angle of Louis to the carina and inferior trachea.

greater than 5 cm from the carina.[2] The procedure also may be indicated in some patients with a cervicothoracic malignancy and "impending airway obstruction." However, if the disease is unresectable or the patient has significant comorbidities, an airway stent may be more appropriate.

Oncologic Principles

Upper aerodigestive system malignancies severely affect quality of life, and careful consideration must be given not only to cure but also to palliation. The most important oncologic principle is to understand clearly if the goal is cure or palliation. One or two centimeters can change the approach to the procedure. That is, if palliation is the goal, clear margins are not critical, and the additional preserved length may facilitate the procedure. On the other hand, if the procedure is being performed for cure, one must not sacrifice oncologic margin for the sake of tracheal length. Most important, in either case, this procedure must be completed without tension on the anastomosis. Otherwise, neither palliation nor cure may be

Table 65-1

SURGICAL CONSIDERATIONS FOR RESTORATION OF ALIMENTARY CONTINUITY

PROCEDURE	PROCEDURE-SPECIFIC CONSIDERATIONS	COMPLICATIONS
Mediastinal tracheostomy	• Reduce tension intraoperatively with tracheal transposition or innominate artery division	• Innominate artery rupture • Stomal disruption with mediastinitis
	• Avoid circumferential dissection around stoma	• Stomal stenosis (treatment: place sanded end of a Hood silicone salivary tube)[1]
	• Careful dissection around left subclavian vein, and when dividing clavicle, first ribs	• Chyle leak or arm swelling
	• Smoking cessation • Preoperative respiratory exercises	• Poor respiratory dynamics—anterior flail chest or lung herniation[2]
Innominate artery division	• Preoperative arteriogram • Intraoperative electroencephalogram	• Stroke
Thyroidectomy	• Postoperative thyroid function tests • Postoperative cancer monitoring and replacement • Consider partial thyroidectomy • Consider reimplantation of parathyroids	• Hypothyroidism • Hypoparathyroidism
Cervical exenteration with colonic interposition or other esophageal substitute	• Nasogastric tube • Postoperative barium swallow	• Anastomotic leak
	• Preoperative visceral arteriogram • Preoperative colonoscopy, barium enema	• Ischemic colitis • Colon cancer

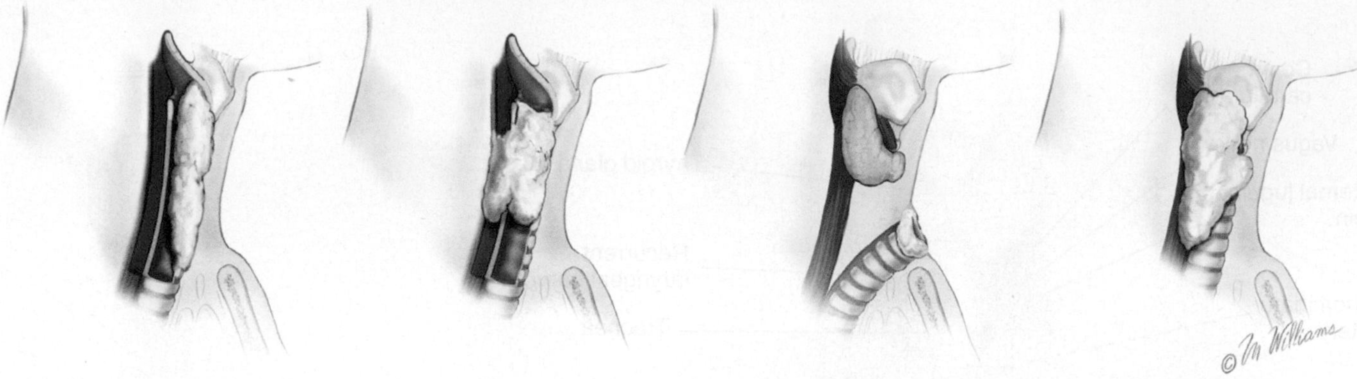

Figure 65-2. Common indications for a mediastinal tracheostomy. *A.* Laryngeal carcinoma involving the trachea. *B.* Carcinoma involving the larynx, proximal trachea, and pharynx. *C.* Recurrence of carcinoma in a tracheostomy site. *D.* Thyroid carcinoma invading the proximal larynx and mediastinal trachea.

achieved. Instead, the patient will be at severe risk of complications such as innominate artery rupture or stomal breakdown with mediastinitis.

PREOPERATIVE ASSESSMENT

Preoperative bronchoscopy, esophagogastroduodenoscopy, computed tomography, and magnetic resonance imaging should be done to assess if the operation is technically possible. The surgeon should assess the length of tumor-free trachea distal to the lesion and the involvement of adjacent vital structures. A metastatic workup is necessary and may include a whole-body positron emission tomography scan, bone scan, and head imaging. MT is not contraindicated in patients with metastatic disease if the goal is palliation. However, with metastatic disease, other therapies, such as airway stents or radiation therapy, may be considered. If there are plans to divide the innominate artery, a preoperative arteriogram assessing the patient's cranial perfusion is important. A visceral arteriogram also may be useful in evaluating the blood supply to the colon as an esophageal substitute. In this case, a barium enema and colonoscopy are recommended to assess the colon as an appropriate conduit. Finally, a bowel preparation should be performed if there is any possibility of esophageal substitution.

TECHNIQUE

The intraoperative preparation depends on the surgeon's technical preferences. For surgeons who consider dividing the innominate artery, arrangements may be made for intraoperative electroencephalography after the artery has been clamped. Arterial line monitoring, nasogastric tube drainage, a Foley catheter, and two large-bore peripheral intravenous lines are ideal. Jugular and subclavian lines may interfere with the operative field. Close coordination between the surgeon and the anesthesiologist is required to safely obtain an airway prior to the surgery. Furthermore, after division of the trachea, it is ideal to have the appropriate tracheostomy available. The tracheostomy used for this procedure has a low-pressure, high-volume balloon with a short distance of tubing distal to that balloon.

Positioning, Incisions, and Tracheal Exposure

The patient is positioned supine with the head extended on a cushioned head support and the scapula on a folded blanket. One arm may be abducted for arterial or venous access. A left-sided radial arterial line is ideal if there is any chance of dividing the innominate artery. Sterile preparation may extend from the chin to the pubis and midaxillary line bilaterally. The abdomen is included if esophageal substitution or omental wrapping of the tracheostomy is planned. The thighs may be prepared as well for a potential split-thickness skin graft or vein graft.

The common incisions used for MT are the extended collar incision and the bipedicled/apron incision (Fig. 65-3).[1,2] When the tracheostomy is being performed for a recurrence in the tracheostomy site, the peristomal skin must be resected and a rotational pectoralis flap is necessary (Fig. 65-3C). The preferred incision is the extended collar incision. However, if there is any hint of tension at the tracheocutaneous anastomosis, we perform a rotational pectoralis flap and prepare the thigh for a split-thickness skin graft for the residual defect.

The surgeon's first goal is to assess the appropriateness of the procedure before proceeding with potentially irrevocable actions such as resecting the breastplate. Occasionally, the surgeon may find either that the tumor is unresectable or that tracheal reanastomosis is possible with adequate mobilization.

Using the extended supraclavicular collar incision (Fig. 65-3A), bilateral subcutaneous platysma flaps are created exposing the strap muscles superiorly. The carotid sheaths, sternum, and hyoid bone are exposed. The sternocleidomastoid muscles and carotid sheaths are displaced laterally. Unilateral vessel involvement by tumor is not a contraindication, because they can be divided and reconstructed. The anterior trachea, posterior trachea, and prevertebral fascia are exposed while preserving the important lateral blood supply of the trachea. For tracheal tumors, the prevertebral space is bluntly dissected, ruling out invasion of the vertebral column and the pharynx superiorly. In general, invasion of the larynx *and* either the esophagus or the trachea *within the thoracic inlet* necessitates an MT to obtain adequate margins for cure.

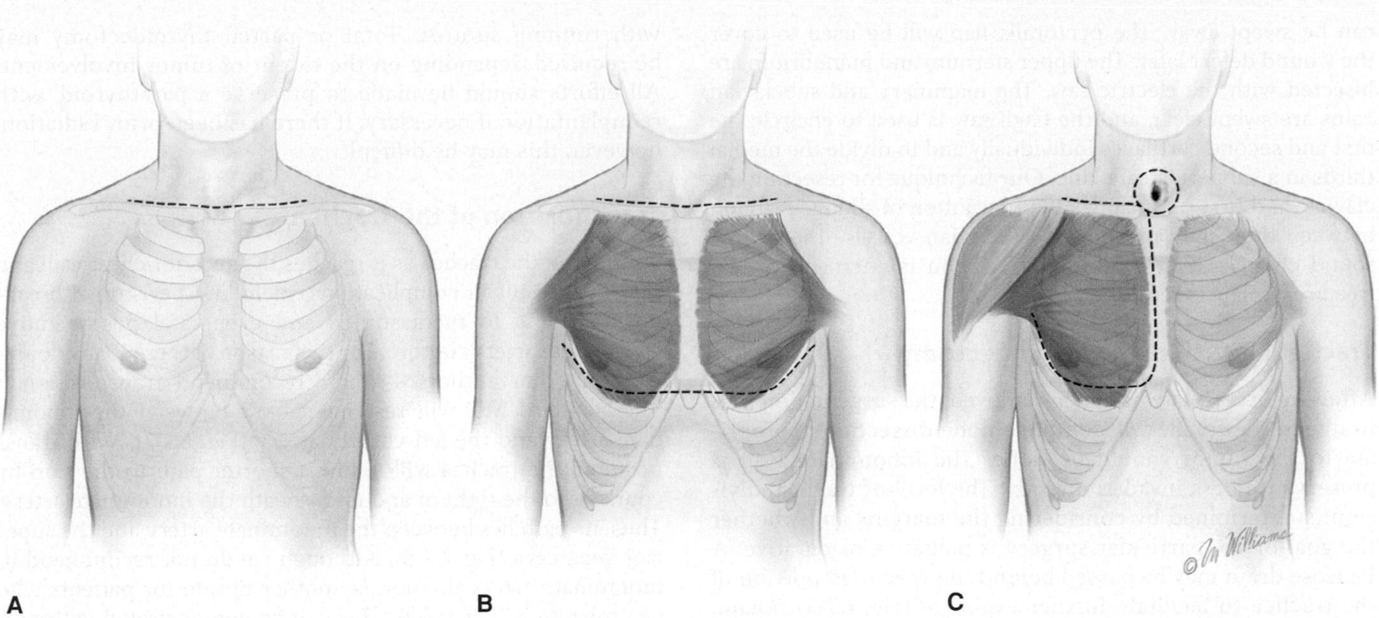

Figure 65-3. Three commonly used incisions. *A.* Collar incision. *B.* Bipedicled (apron) incision. *C.* Pectoralis rotational flap often used for recurrence in a tracheostomy site.

Breastplate Resection

The inferior flap is developed after declaring the need for MT. The goal of this flap is to expose the breastplate, including the upper sternum, clavicle, and the first two ribs (Fig. 65-4). The muscular insertions (i.e., straps and sternocleidomastoid) are divided to expose the sternum, clavicle, and ribs. The decision to extend the resection down to the second rib depends on the level of anticipated tension on the tracheocutaneous anastomosis. If there is any doubt, the upper sternum and second rib should be resected.

First, the mammaries are protected and isolated by locating them at the level of the second rib. Next, the midline pectoralis fascia, from the sternal notch to the angle of Louis, is bisected with electrocautery. The pectoralis muscle then is elevated off the first two medial costochondral joints. The sternum is transected transversely just above the third rib. By elevating the sternum with bone hooks, underlying structures

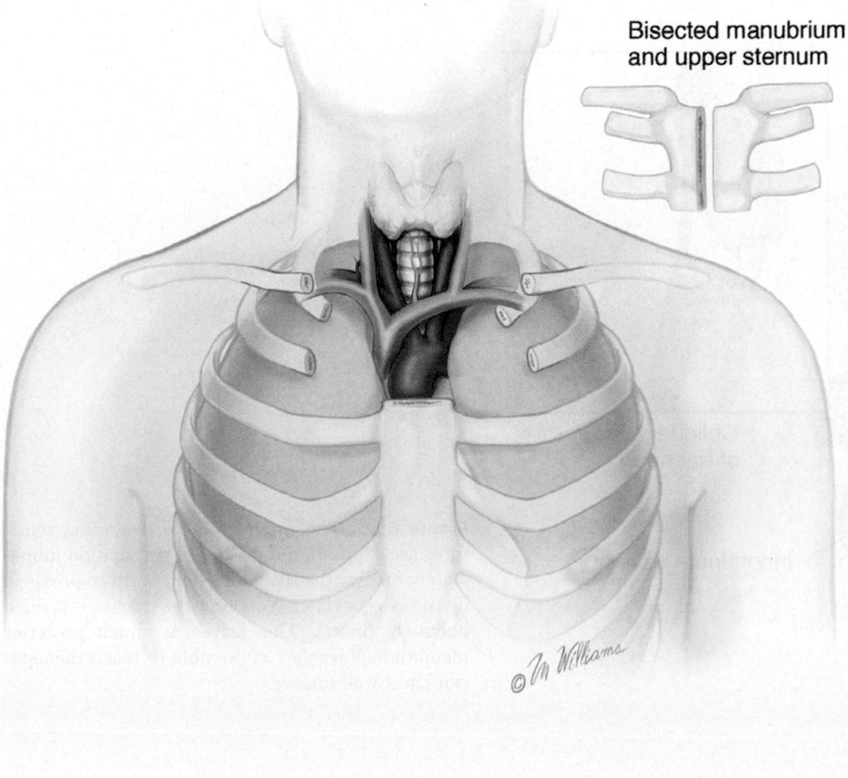

Figure 65-4. The breastplate is resected along with the first one or two ribs. Depending on the final tracheal length, sometimes only the clavicle, manubrium, and first rib are resected. However, it is more usual to include the second rib and the superior portion of the body of the sternum. In the technique shown here, both the manubrium and upper body of the sternum have been resected for better visualization.

can be swept away. The pectoralis flap will be used to cover the wound defect later. The upper sternum and manubrium are bisected with the electric saw. The mammary and subclavian veins are swept clear, and the Gigli saw is used to encircle the first and second cartilages individually and to divide the medial thirds in a subperiosteal plane. Our technique for resecting the clavicle and first rib includes the precaution of sliding a ribbon between the Gigli saw and the subclavian vessels. The sawing sound changes if the "protective" ribbon is encroached. The free breastplate is removed.

Tracheal Division and Laryngectomy

After the breastplate has been removed, the surgeon prepares to divide the trachea. A complete node dissection appropriate to the tumor should be done. The innominate vein is preserved unless invaded directly. The level of tracheal division is determined by considering the margins and whether the goal of the particular surgery is palliative or curative. A Penrose drain may be passed behind the specimen portion of the trachea to facilitate further exposure (Fig. 65-5). Again, attention should be paid to preserving the lateral blood supply of the remaining trachea and stoma (Fig. 65-6, inset). Circumferential devascularization of the trachea (particularly within 1–2 cm of the transected edge) should be avoided to prevent peristomal breakdown and mediastinitis. Prior to division, stay sutures are placed at the inferior tracheal margin. The trachea is divided obliquely at the inferior margin. This facilitates the tracheocutaneous anastomosis such that it may curve anteriorly flush with the skin (Fig. 65-5, inset). After division, it is reintubated (Fig. 65-6) with sterile tubing across the field. The tracheostomy tube is secured with stay sutures to the trachea and to the skin. To preserve the airway, the inferior division is dealt with first. Next, the superior division usually is made at the level of the thyrohyoid membrane, preserving the hyoid bone. The larynx then is oversewn with running sutures. Total or partial thyroidectomy may be required depending on the extent of tumor involvement. All efforts should be made to preserve a parathyroid, with reimplantation if necessary. If there has been prior radiation, however, this may be difficult.

Transposition of the Trachea

Tension on the trachea as it reaches the anterior chest wall and skin may result in complications, including peristomal breakdown leading to mediastinitis and even fatal postoperative innominate artery rupture. For this reason, if there is any doubt, we and other authors strongly recommend transposition.[2,3] The standard MT will rest interposed between the innominate artery and the left carotid artery (Fig. 65-7). With transposition, the trachea will follow a shorter path to the skin by coursing to the right of and underneath the innominate artery. Thus, its path lies between the innominate artery and the superior vena cava (Fig. 65-8). Although we do not recommend it, innominate artery division is another option for patients who can tolerate it (Fig. 65-9). This can be demonstrated with preoperative angiogram or even intraoperative electroencephalogram after clamping for 10 minutes. It may be best suited when the distance from the carina to the end of the remnant trachea is less than 5 cm.[1] After transposition, we recommend wrapping the trachea as it passes underneath the artery with a well-vascularized strap muscle. Other options include omentum or pectoralis muscle. The most important factor, however, is that the trachea is well vascularized and reaches the skin without any tension. Wrapping the trachea will not prevent arterial rupture if there is significant tension.

Tracheocutaneous Anastomosis and Closure

The route of the trachea to the anterior skin must be secured, wrapped, and buttressed by all available tissue. With the

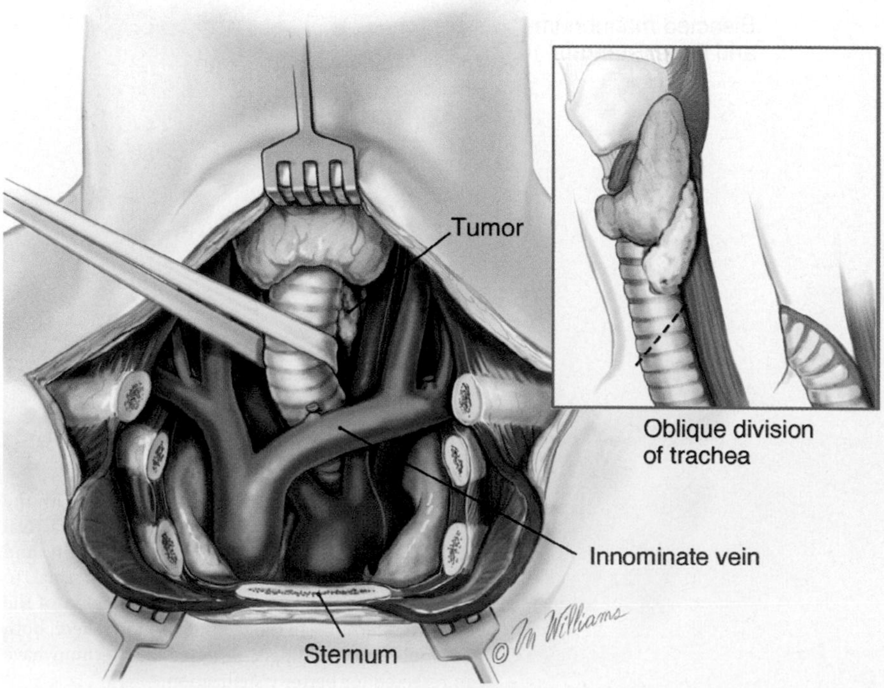

Figure 65-5. The trachea and surrounding structures are exposed and divided. Reintubation immediately follows the distal division, and the proximal division occurs later. Note how the trachea is divided obliquely (inset). This leaves as much posterior membranous trachea as possible to reach the anterior chest wall surface.

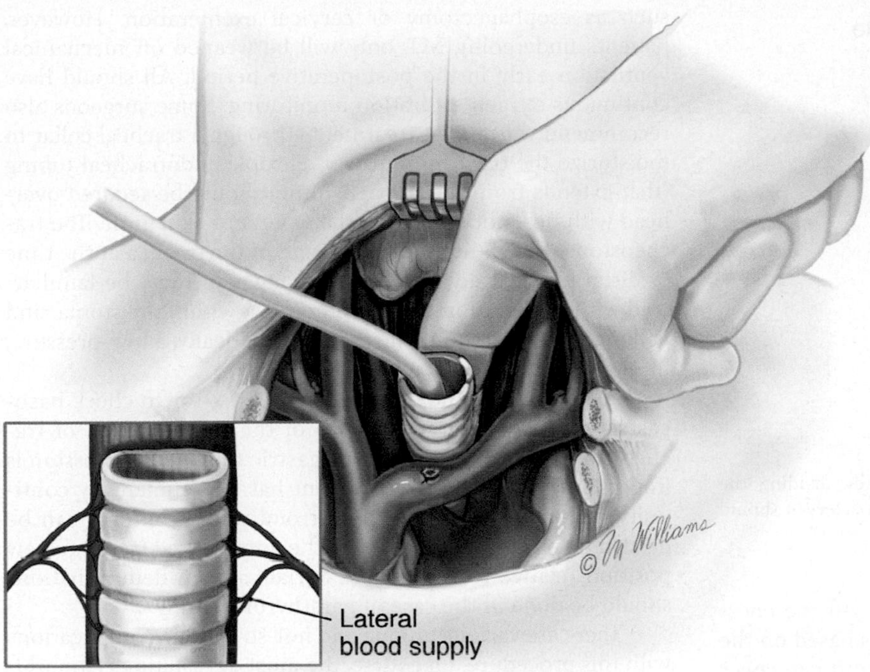

Figure 65-6. After the airway is divided, it is secured with an endotracheal tube. The surgeon bluntly develops the avascular plane posterior to the trachea and anterior to the esophagus. Note how deviation in either direction laterally threatens the blood supply to the mobilized trachea (inset).

exception of the specific strap muscle that protects the innominate artery (in tracheal transposition), all muscles should be reapproximated with interrupted absorbable sutures. As the cervical incision is sutured closed, the tracheocutaneous anastomosis is begun. It must be secured to the skin with full-thickness skin and subcutaneous purchases as well. This is done in an interrupted fashion (Fig. 65-10). A few absorbable sutures may be placed from the subcutaneous tissue to distal trachea to reduce the tension on the tracheocutaneous anastomosis.[1] Drains are placed beneath the inferior and superior flaps and for any alimentary tract anastomoses. If there is a defect in the apron incision, a split-thickness skin graft can be used for coverage (Fig. 65-11).

At this point, if there appears to be any tension, there are several options. A button of skin can be excised below the transverse incision, and the trachea can be brought out through this new defect.[2] In this scenario, we prefer to use the pectoralis rotational flap. Development of the pectoralis flap began when it was lifted off the chest wall before the breastplate resection. This thoracoacromial "nipple" flap (Fig. 65-12) can be done, even in patients without a tracheostomal recurrence.

Rotational Flaps

A thoracoacromial flap is used most often in a patient with laryngeal cancer who suffers recurrence at the stoma site. In these patients, the surrounding skin is resected (Fig. 65-3C). However, it also may be performed after a standard extended collar incision if there is tension at the end of the case. Simply extend the incision inferiorly along the sternum and around the inframammary crease (Fig. 65-3C) to the preferred side. Both

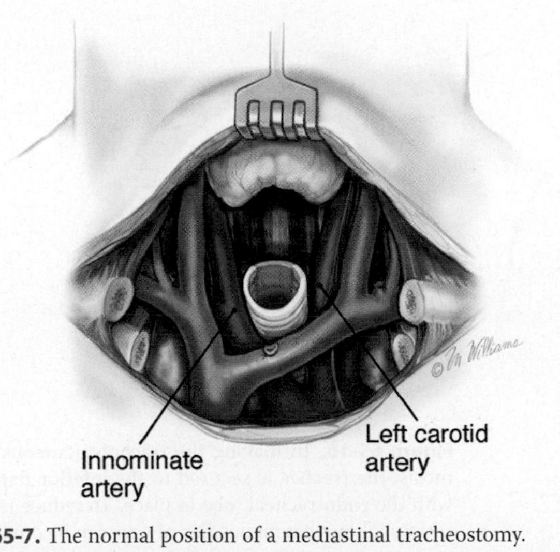

Figure 65-7. The normal position of a mediastinal tracheostomy.

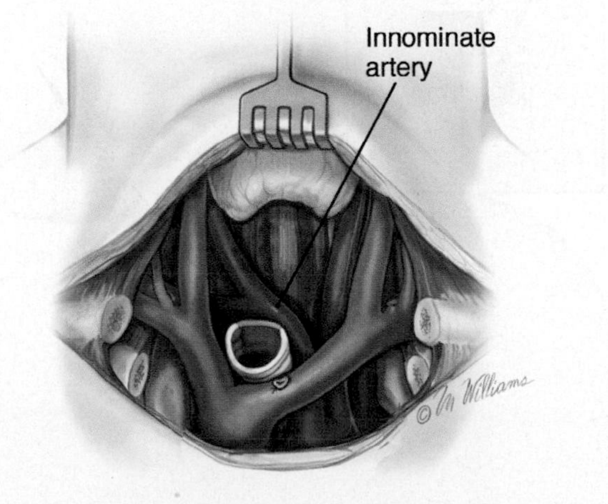

Figure 65-8. If the trachea does not appear to reach the new "depressed" chest wall, then either more sternal body may be resected, or the trachea may be transposed to the right of the innominate artery. The transposed trachea should be wrapped with viable tissue such as a strap muscle to help reduce the likelihood of innominate artery rupture.

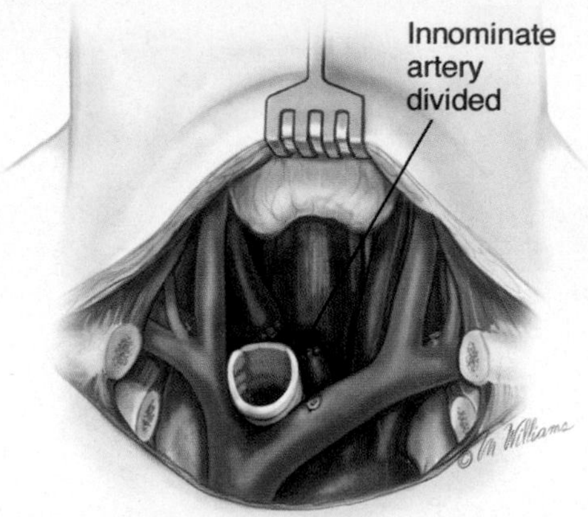

Figure 65-9. Other options to decrease tension include dividing the innominate vein or artery. Before dividing the innominate artery, it should be clamped and tested with electroencephalography.

pectoralis muscles will have already been lifted off the chest wall in the prior dissection. The rotated muscle is based on the thoracoacromial vessels. A split-thickness skin graft can cover the remaining defect (Fig. 65-12).

POSTOPERATIVE CARE, SPECIFIC COMPLICATIONS, AND RESULTS

As with any surgery, postoperative care is very important to a successful outcome. As a unique airway, this surgery requires special attention. ICU care is required for all of these patients at least until postoperative day 1 or 2. Many will be mechanically ventilated if they have undergone a more extensive procedure, such as esophagectomy or cervical exenteration. However, patients undergoing MT only will be weaned off mechanical ventilation early in the postoperative period. All should have continuous oxygen saturation monitoring. Some surgeons also recommend warm mist treatments through a tracheal collar to moisturize the tracheal mucosa.[4] Flexible endotracheal tubing (that extends from the tracheostomy) should be secured overhead with ties, not resting on the wound or skin graft. The tracheostomy tube is sutured to the end of the trachea at the time of distal tracheal division. The nursing staff must be familiarized with the location of the balloon just within the stoma, and balloon pressures should be monitored. Ideally, a low-pressure, high-volume balloon is used.

Postoperative studies include a chest x-ray to check nasogastric tube position and the tip of the short portion of tracheostomy tube. Functional nasogastric tube decompression is imperative, especially if the patient has had alimentary continuity restored. Aspiration of gastrointestinal contents can be devastating and is common with the unprotected trachea's new position relative to the mouth. Serial calcium determinations should be done in the case of parathyroidectomy.

There are various unique and not-so-unique complications with this procedure. Of course, the most devastating is innominate artery rupture. This must be treated with prevention. The importance of creating a tension-free path of the trachea to skin via the innominate artery and aortic arch cannot be overemphasized. Another particular complication is the anterior flail segment (also referred to as lung herniation) from the breastplate resection.[4] For this reason, preoperative respiratory exercises and smoking cessation should be encouraged. Peristomal breakdown also can occur secondary to tension or paroxysmal coughing fits. Depending on adjunct procedures performed, other complications to watch for are hypoparathyroidism, hypothyroidism, perioperative stroke, anastomotic leak, cervical chyle leak, arm swelling (secondary to subclavian vein

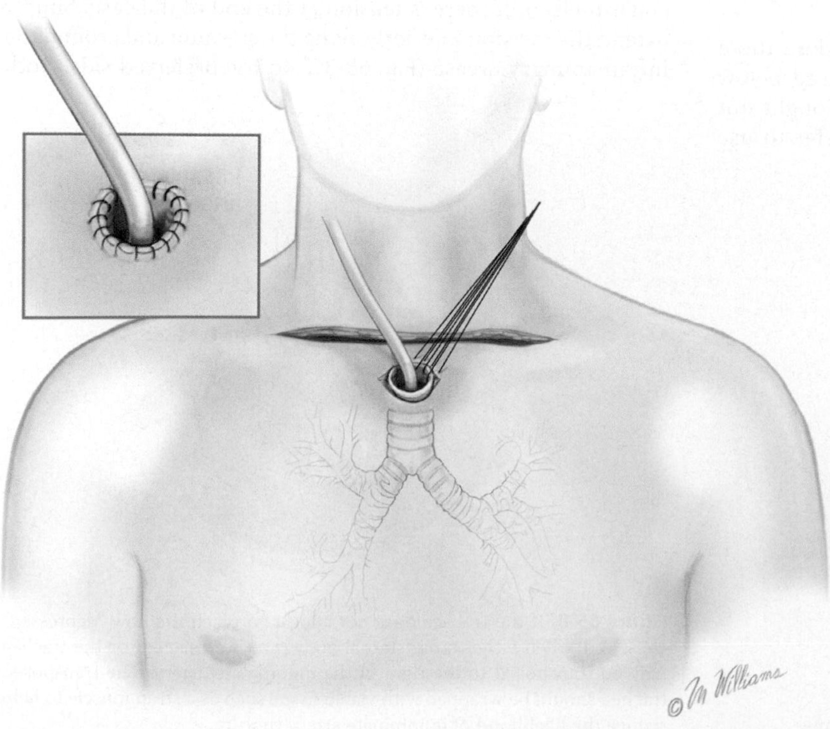

Figure 65-10. In making the tracheocutaneous anastomosis, the trachea is secured to the inferior flap of skin with the endotracheal tube in place. To reduce tension, a rotational myocutaneous flap always can be created.

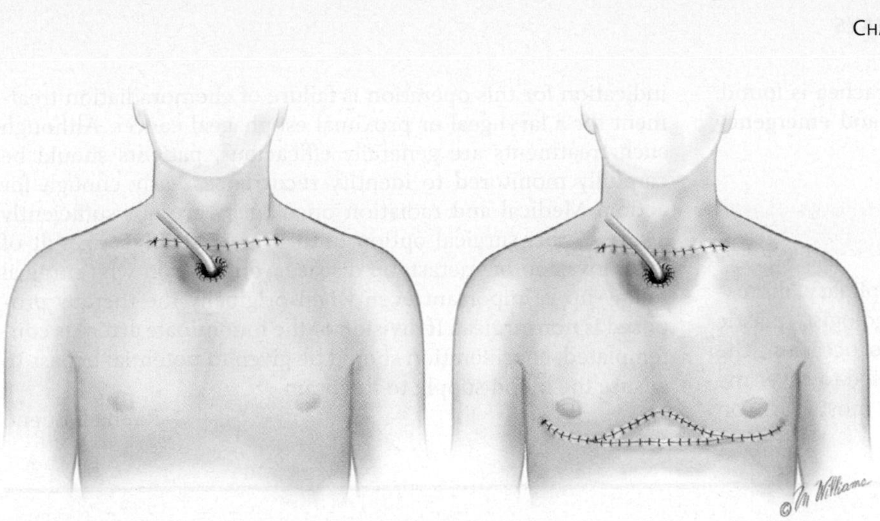

A B

Figure 65-11. Note the depressed chest wall in the closure of the collar incision (*A*) and in the apron incision (*B*). A skin graft can be used to cover the inferior defect in the apron incision.

displacement), and dumping syndrome (secondary to vagus division in esophagectomy).

Perioperative morbidity and mortality are disease- and procedure-specific with regard to MT. In 1996, Orringer reported a 13% mortality in 45 patients. One death was due to innominate artery rupture. He also recorded a secure airway in 100% of patients.[2] Orringer's patient population consisted of 35 patients who underwent MT with concomitant cervical exenteration and esophageal substitution. Grillo and Mathisen reported one perioperative mortality in their series of 18 cervical exenterations with MT. This occurred secondary to ischemic necrosis of the stomach graft used to replace the esophagus.[1]

With regard to loss of speech, some of these patients may learn a form of "esophageal speech" or artificial speech with the latest electrical appliances.

SUMMARY

The MT is a radical procedure that must be performed judiciously. Although, airway security is achieved in almost every case, patients experience a high frequency of complications. Prevention of these complications, in particular, innominate artery rupture, can be achieved through different methods.

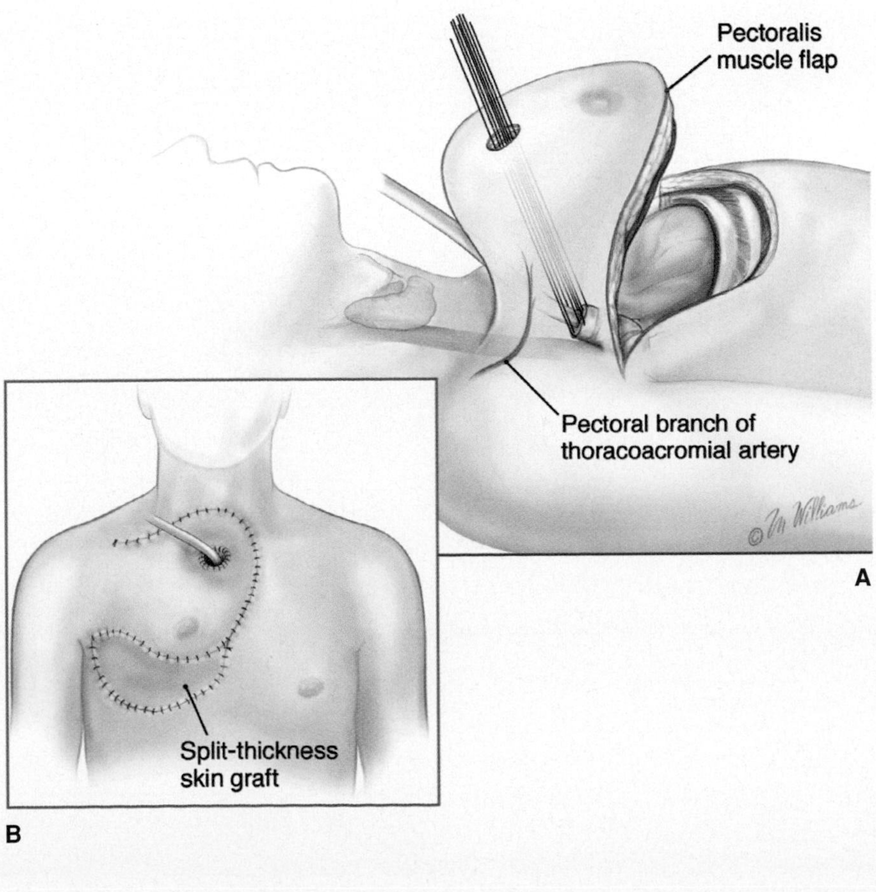

A

B

Figure 65-12. *A*. Rotational myocutaneous flap. This can be used to cover large defects (as in tracheostomal recurrence) or to reduce tension. The blood supply comes from the pectoral branch of the thoracoacromial artery. *B*. A skin graft covers the inferior defect (inset).

Until a safe and reliable replacement for the trachea is found, this will continue to be a palliative, curative, and emergency lifesaving procedure.

EDITOR'S COMMENT

Careful preoperative imaging and multidisciplinary discussions among the thoracic surgeon, otolaryngologist, plastic surgeon, and vascular surgeon are helpful. On occasion, the omentum can be brought up substernally and used to cover the vessels and wrap the tracheostomy. Today, the most common indication for this operation is failure of chemoradiation treatment for a laryngeal or proximal esophageal cancer. Although such treatments are generally efficacious, patients should be carefully monitored to identify recurrences early enough for action. Medical and radiation oncologists are not sufficiently aware of this surgical option until it is too late as a result of local invasion or metastatic disease—one reason why surgical follow-up is important even when originally the therapy proposed is nonsurgical. If division of the innominate artery is contemplated, consideration should be given to potential bypass to ensure the blood supply to the brain.

—Raphael Bueno

References

1. Grillo HC, Mathisen DJ. Cervical exenteration. *Ann Thorac Surg.* 1990;499(3):401–408; discussion 408–409.
2. Orringer MB. Anterior mediastinal tracheostomy. *Chest Surg Clin N Am.* 1996;6(4):701–724.
3. Waddell WR, Cannon B. A technic for subtotal excision of the trachea and establishment of a sternal tracheostomy. *Ann Surg.* 1959;149:1–8.
4. Nesbitt J, Wind G, Orringer M. Thoracic surgical oncology: exposures and techniques. In: Nesbitt JC, Wind GG, eds. *Mediastinal Tracheostomy.* Philadelphia, PA: Lippincott Williams & Wilkins; 2003:237–252.

66 Cancers of the Upper Aerodigestive Tract: Cervical Exenteration

Thomas W. Rice

Keywords: Pharyngo-laryngo-tracheo-esophagectomy

INTRODUCTION

Rarely, locally extensive but nonmetastatic cancers of the upper aerodigestive tract require resection. Cancers of the larynx, cervical trachea, hypopharynx, cervical esophagus, and thyroid can be exenterated with a pharyngo-laryngo-tracheo-esophagectomy as primary therapy, salvage after failed primary therapy, treatment of locally recurrent cancer, treatment of benign complications of successful primary therapy, or long-term palliation. The enormity of these procedures is further overshadowed by the likely possibility of limited survival, the potential for significant complications, and the expected negative impact upon quality of life. However, in curatively resected and properly reconstructed patients, long-lasting effects are little more than that experienced by the laryngectomy patient.

PREOPERATIVE EVALUATION AND PREPARATION

Clinical staging is mandatory to determine the eligibility for exenteration.[1] Distant metastatic cancer (cM1 or ycM1) is excluded by PET/CT and cancer-specific imaging (e.g., thyroid scanning for differentiated thyroid cancers). Regional nodal metastases (cN1 or ycN1) are frequently detected by physical examination and confirmed by cytologic evaluation of fine-needle aspiration (FNA) specimens. However, cervical ultrasonography and FNA may be necessary to better examine and determine regional nodal classification. Local extent of the primary cancer (cT or ycT) is critical in deciding resectability, but is frequently underestimated by preoperative investigations. Regardless, local invasion should be evaluated with particular with respect to particular carotid artery, vertebral body, and mediastinal involvement. This may require multiple imaging modalities (angiography, MRI, fine-cut CT, barium esophagram, bone scan, etc.). The proximal and distal extent of the cancer is assessed by oropharyngoscopy, bronchoscopy, and esophagoscopy (panendoscopy). These endoscopic procedures are accompanied by the appropriate biopsies of the primary cancer and its margins. The skin and subcutaneous tissue overlying and in the vicinity of the primary cancer must be examined to exclude malignant invasion or severe radiation damage if previously administered.

The reconstruction must be planned and prospective organs of replacement/reconstruction evaluated. Vascular insufficiency secondary to smoking accelerated atherosclerosis may necessitate angiographic assessment of these organs and tissues. Gastroscopy and colonoscopy are essential to exclude intrinsic disease if the stomach or colon is being contemplated for replacement. The tissue planned for pedicle or free flaps must be assessed and alternatives considered and evaluated. A mediastinal tracheostomy may be necessary for reconstruction if there is significant length of tracheal involvement. This may require division of the innominate artery to avoid postoperative arterial erosion and ensuing hemorrhagic complications. Therefore, angiographic assessment of cerebral blood supply and patency of the Circle of Willis is compulsory if mediastinal tracheostomy and innominate artery division are planned.

As in all patients undergoing airway and esophageal surgery, cardiopulmonary assessment is essential. Comorbidities must be evaluated and the affected organ systems optimized preoperatively. During this time, the nutritional status and fitness of the patient is maximized.

THE OPERATION

Preparation and Positioning

The patient is positioned supine. Arterial line, oxygen saturation probe, and venous catheter placements are guided by the possibility of division of the innominate artery and sacrifice of the left innominate vein. Similarly EKG pad placement may be affected by resection of the primary cancer or harvesting of reconstructive flaps. EEG leads may be placed for monitoring if there is concern of compromising cerebral perfusion. Techniques and equipment necessary for endotracheal intubation will be determined by the primary cancer and presence of an established tracheostomy. Provisions must be made for cross-table ventilation during surgery.

The operative field is prepared and draped from patient's chin to suprapubic abdomen and bilaterally to midaxillary lines. The thigh and forearm/arm may be included in the field if they will be used for flap harvesting or skin grafting.

Exploration

The operation starts with a collar incision placed above the sternal notch. The incision should be positioned to permit extension laterally, if necessary, over the clavicles and inferior over the manubrium (Fig. 66-1). If a tracheostomy exists, the stoma should be included in the incision. Invaded or radiation-damaged skin is excluded from the flaps, excised, and left attached to the cancer. The superior subcutaneous flap is raised above the hyoid bone, and the inferior flap is lifted to the sternal notch. Cranial, caudal, lateral, and deep invasion are assessed during this mobilization. If uninvolved the strap muscles are then separated in the midline or if invaded they are divided and left attached to the primary cancer. Lateral dissection determines if the carotid sheath is involved by the cancer. The prevertebral space is developed to assure the resection can

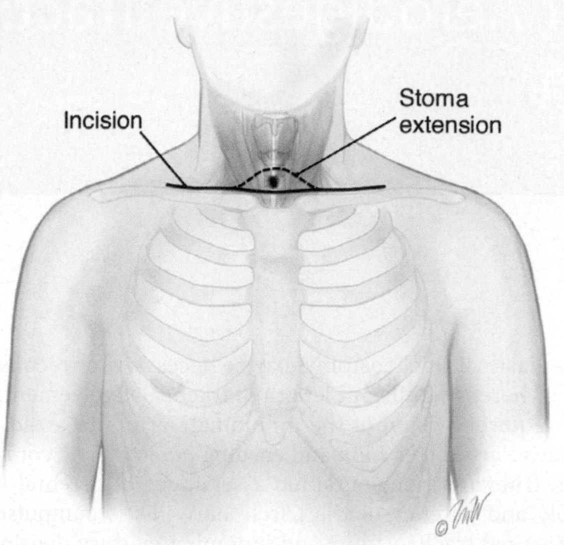

Figure 66-1. A collar incision is made above the sternal notch with inclusion of the tracheostomy stoma if one exists.

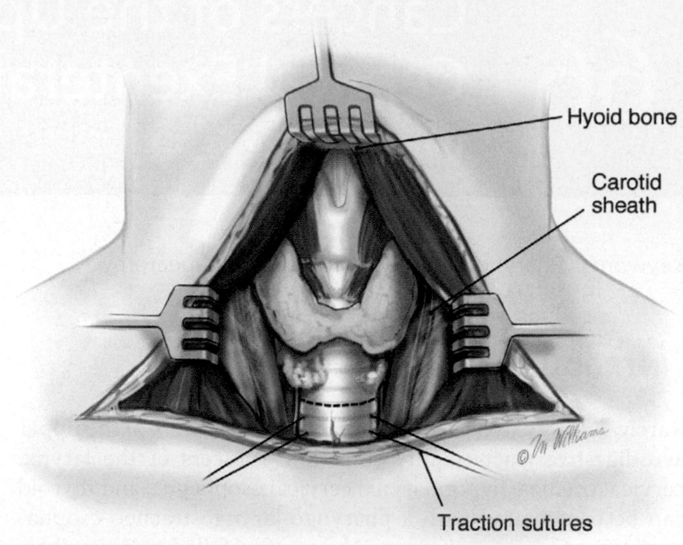

Figure 66-2. The tumor is exposed by raising the superior subcutaneous flap above the hyoid bone and lifting the inferior flap up to the sternal notch. The tumor is inspected for invasion both superiorly and inferiorly. Lateral dissection determines if the carotid sheath is involved by the tumor. The trachea is mobilized circumferentially. Lateral traction sutures are placed in the tracheal wall one cartilage below the anticipated position of tracheal transection.

be completed posteriorly. These steps confirm cancer resectability and to this point no irreversible steps have been taken.

Resection

Typically, the resection begins inferiorly. If a mediastinal tracheostomy is necessary, the incision is extended in the midline inferiorly over the manubrium. The lateral myocutaneous flaps are raised off the bony chest wall, and the manubrium is excised along with the first and second cartilages and the clavicular heads (breast-plate). The level of tracheal division is selected. The trachea is circumferentially mobilized at this site and lateral dissection restricted below this point. Lateral traction sutures are placed in the tracheal wall one cartilage below the anticipated position of tracheal transection (Fig. 66-2). This will stabilize the trachea and facilitate tracheal intubation during cross-field ventilation. Once the trachea has been divided and distal intubation obtained, the tracheal margin is sent for frozen-section analysis. Some thyroid and airway (adenoid cystic carcinoma) cancers may not involve or minimally invade the esophagus, permitting esophageal preservation without compromising the resection. In patients requiring cervical exenteration the point of esophageal transection is determined. The extent of the primary cancer and the method and organ of esophageal reconstruction will dictate this level. If free flap is being used for reconstruction, the esophagus is divided in the low neck and this margin is sent for frozen-section analysis.

The dissection proceeds superiorly. The prevertebral plane, already assessed, is now easily developed. Laterally the dissection is carried along the carotid sheaths. Rarely unilateral sacrifice of the internal jugular vein is required. If unilateral carotid excision is required, arterial reconstruction or bypass will be necessary. If the thyroid is not involved, the isthmus is split and one or both sides are preserved and allowed to remain in the lateral resection margins. If not radiated this practice preserves thyroid and parathyroid function. If possible resected parathyroid tissue that is uninvolved with the primary cancer may be autotransplanted and this position marked with radiopaque clips.

The superior margin of the resection is now defined. The superior border of the hyoid bone is cleared of the attachments of the mylohyoid, geniohyoid, and genioglossus muscles. Lateral muscular attachments of the larynx are divided and the superior laryngeal neurovascular bundle controlled and divided (Fig. 66-3). The pharynx is entered anteriorly and the superior resection proceeds posteriorly. The epiglottis is incorporated in the resection specimen. The superior resection margin is sent for frozen-section analysis.

Reconstruction

The two main methods of pharyngoesophageal reconstruction involve either GI transposition (stomach or colon) or microvascular free flaps (jejunum or myocutaneous). The general approach is to use gastric or colonic transposition for cancers that extend to or below the thoracic inlet and free flaps for the short-length reconstruction required by cancers arising above the thoracic inlet.[2–4] However, in any one institution the experience may be so small that one of these methods may become the reconstruction of choice.

If division of the trachea is well above the sternal notch, a cervical tracheostomy stoma can be constructed. However, if tracheal division is at or below the sternal notch or if the operation is performed for tracheal stomal recurrence, a mediastinal tracheostomy will be necessary.[5,6] The anterior breast-plate is excised. Erosion of the innominate artery, a major complication of mediastinal tracheostomy, can be avoided by separating the tracheal stoma from the innominate artery. If the stoma will be positioned immediately adjacent to the artery, elective division and oversewing of the ends under EEG monitoring has been reported.[7] However, transposing the trachea below and to the right of the innominate artery also has been successfully used to avoid this dreaded complication.[8] Division of the innominate artery must be placed proximal to the carotid-subclavian bifurcation.

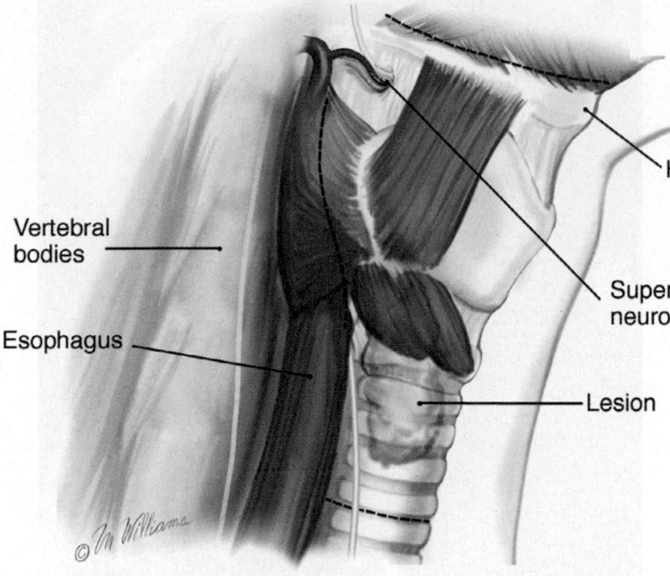

Figure 66-3. The superior margin of the resection is defined, and the superior border of the hyoid bone is cleared of the attachment of the mylohyoid, geniohyoid, and genioglossus muscles. Lateral muscular attachments of the larynx are divided, and the superior laryngeal neurovascular bundle is controlled and divided.

The omentum can be used to cover anastomoses, separate innominate artery stumps from the trachea, and tracheal wrapping below the stoma.[9] If there is significant soft tissue resection and wound closure is problematic a benefit of using myocutaneous free flaps is the ability to reconstruct both GI and soft tissue defects with the flap.[10–12]

POSTOPERATIVE MANAGEMENT

ICU care is mandatory in the initial postoperative management of cervical exenteration patients. Mechanical ventilation is usually required. A customized tracheostomy tube may be necessary for the shortened trachea in patients requiring mediastinal tracheostomy. Trauma to the tracheal stoma should be avoided by careful and secure stabilization of the tracheostomy tube. A low-pressure tracheostomy cuff will protect the edematous and potentially ischemic trachea from necrosis and stricture. Adequate humidification of inspired air/oxygen mixture is important in minimizing pulmonary complications. Vigorous chest physiotherapy and careful pulmonary/tracheostomy care are the major foci of early postoperative care. An NG tube is necessary in patient with gastric reconstruction of the pharyngoesophagus segment, because they are very susceptible to regurgitation. Upright patient positioning is also critical in minimizing aspiration. Nutrition is provided via feeding tubes or parenterally until GI function returns and the pharyngoesophageal replacement has healed. Regardless of parathyroid preservation during resection, careful monitoring of serum calcium and prompt management of postoperative hypocalcemia is required in all patients. The need for long-term thyroid hormone replacement should be assessed.

SPECIFIC COMPLICATIONS AND RESULTS

A common site of complications specific to cervical exenteration is at the GI anastomoses. Varying degrees of anastomotic disruption can occur. This may be as simple as a transient anastomotic leak that can be managed by keeping the patient NPO, providing enteral or parenteral nutrition and locally draining the area. In the extreme there may be graft necrosis necessitating removal of the reconstruction, creating a pharyngostomy, oversewing of the distal GI tract, and constructing a feeding gastrostomy or jejunostomy. Anastomotic strictures are usually managed by repeated dilation. Universally, patients with gastric reconstruction are subject to regurgitation with coughing, reclining, or bending over. This is the result of sacrifice of the upper esophageal sphincter and the high pharyngeal location of the anastomosis. With time and specific maneuvers, such as limiting the size of meals and remaining upright for 2 to 3 hours after eating, this problem can be tolerated. However, this predictable functional disorder has led some to favor the colon over the stomach for GI reconstruction after cervical exenteration.

Tracheocutaneous stomal separation is usually treated conservatively, responding to debridement. Stomal stenosis can be managed with long-term placement of an indwelling tracheostomy tube. Recalcitrant stenosis will require revision of the tracheostomy and possibly conversion of a low cervical tracheostomy to a mediastinal tracheostomy. Vascular complications are common to mediastinal tracheostomy unless the steps mentioned earlier are not taken to separate the stoma from the innominate artery. Cerebrovascular accident not necessarily related to innominate artery division can complicate this extensive resection.

Chylous leakage may complicate extensive dissection about the left subclavian-internal jugular veins. Conservative management using parenteral nutrition and local drainage may not be successful because of the exenteration. Octreotide administration may hasten the resolution of chylous complications. Reexploration with direct ligation of the lymphatic injury or thoracotomy with ligation of the thoracic duct has been used. However, there is increasing experience and use of lymphangiography and x-ray–guided percutaneous embolization of the thoracic duct.

Hepatic failure has complicated the postoperative course of patients with squamous cell carcinoma undergoing cervical exenteration. Alcohol abuse, a factor in development of these cancers, may cause clinically unsuspected cirrhosis that is uncovered in the recovery from this extensive surgery. Pulmonary complications are a common problem in the postoperative course of these patients.

Long-term survival is determined by the underlying cancer.

SUMMARY

Cancers of the upper aerodigestive tract may on rare occasion require resection, typically for salvage following failed primary treatment or long-term palliation. Clinical staging, preoperative evaluation, and operative exploration determine resectability. An en bloc pharyngo-laryngo-tracheo-esophagectomy necessitates (1) reconstruction of the pharynx and esophagus, using gastric or colonic transposition for cancers that extend to or below the thoracic inlet and free flaps for the short-length reconstructions of cancers confined to the neck and (2) a permanent end tracheostomy. Specific complications include (1) varying degrees of GI anastomotic disruption and (2) hemorrhage common to mediastinal tracheostomy unless the steps are not taken to separate the tracheal stoma from the innominate artery. Long-term survival following cervical exenteration is determined by the underlying cancer.

CASE HISTORY

A 65-year-old male, who is a retired army veteran, presented with solid dysphagia and a lump in his left neck. He was found to have a cT4aN1M0 squamous cell carcinoma of the hypopharynx with invasion of the esophagus and a single 2-cm ipsilateral regional nodal metastasis. Prior to therapy, he stopped smoking and reduced his drinking to two glasses of beer a day. He received definitive chemoradiotherapy, three courses of 5-FU (1000 mg/m^2 per day for 4 days) and cisplatin (100 mg/m^2), and concurrent external-beam radiation (60 Gy). His posttreatment course was complicated by dysphagia which responded to two sessions of guided esophageal dilation. He did well for 14 months, but again experienced difficulty swallowing solids and new onset of hoarseness. He was found to have recurrence of squamous cell carcinoma in the anterior wall of the hypopharynx with extension into the cervical esophagus. This was staged as ycT3N0M0.

Clinical examination and imaging suggested this was a local recurrence. He underwent a pharyngo-laryngo-tracheo-esophagectomy (Fig. 66-4). A total esophagectomy was necessary because of involvement of the cervical esophagus and an associated radiation stricture. A pharyngogastric anastomosis was constructed with a single-layer interrupted absorbable suture. The tracheostomy was placed low in his neck just above the sternal notch. An omentum graft was brought substernally to cover the pharyngoesophageal reconstruction and wrap the trachea at the stoma. His postoperative course was complicated by respiratory compromise and a pharyngocutaneous anastomotic fistula. Vigorous chest physiotherapy, frequent suctioning, broad-spectrum antibiotics, meticulous care of his tracheostomy stoma and 3 weeks of mechanical ventilation were necessary for successful treatment of his postoperative pneumonia. Local drainage of the fistula, NG-tube drainage of his stomach, and nutritional support via his j-tube successfully closed the anastomotic fistula in 4 months.

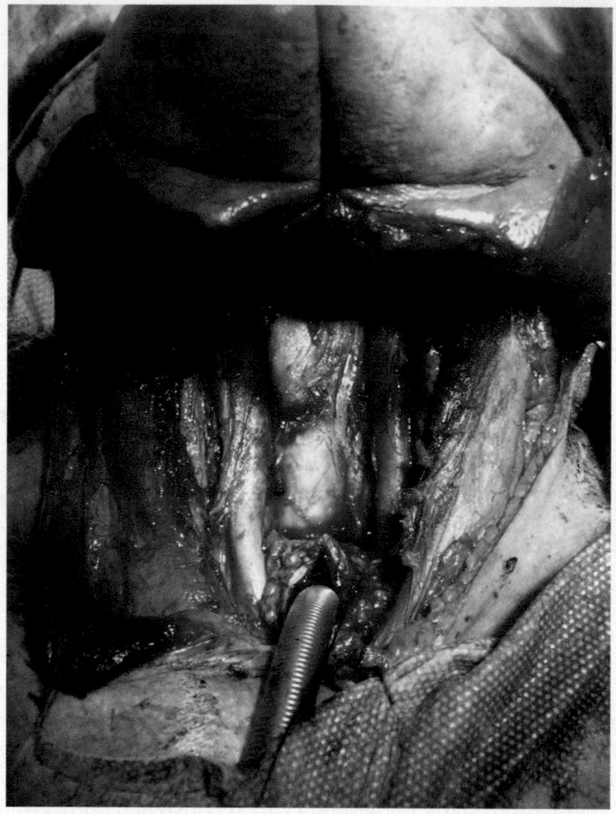

Figure 66-4. An intraoperative photograph after cervical exenteration and before reconstruction. Superiorly, the upper skin flap is retracted toward the patient's chin. Inferiorly, the intubated trachea is seen just above the sternal notch. The intact carotid sheaths border the lateral margins of the resection. The prevertebral fascia can be seen in the deep margin.

Four years after cervical exenteration, he was swallowing well. His tracheostomy stoma was well healed and required only daily tracheostomy care. By physical examination there was no local recurrence of his hypopharyngeal carcinoma. Imaging was proposed at 6-month intervals; however, the scans in the third postoperative year were missed. He was found to have a 2-cm spiculated mass in the upper lobe of his right lung at his fourth year annual CT scan. This was hypermetabolic on FDG-PET examination (SUV 7.3) with no evidence of regional lymph node enlargement or hypermetabolism. FNA proved this to be a squamous cell carcinoma. He received radiosurgery for this presumed cT1aN0M0 metachronous primary squamous cell carcinoma of the lung. After this therapy, 6 years following cervical exenteration, he has remained free of recurrent or metachronous squamous cell cancer.

EDITOR'S COMMENT

Mediastinal exenteration is a formidable operation which is not commonly performed. It is usually performed after failure of chemoradiation making the operation more complex. We often collaborate with an otolaryngologist in this type of procedure to maximize patient benefit. Stomach or colon should usually reach high up, but sometimes, a free flap of jejunum can be used to extend the conduit.

—Raphael Bueno

References

1. American Joint Committee on Cancer. *AJCC Cancer Staging Manual*. 7th ed. New York, NY: Springer; 2010:41–49.
2. de Vries EJ, Stein DW, Johnson JT, et al. Hypopharyngeal reconstruction: a comparison of two alternatives. *Laryngoscope*. 1989;99:614–617.
3. Carlson GW, Schusterman MA, Guillamondegui OM. Total reconstruction of the hypopharynx and cervical esophagus: a 20-year experience. *Ann Plast Surg*. 1992;29:408–412.
4. Pesko P, Sabljak P, Bjelovic M, et al. Surgical treatment and clinical course of patients with hypopharyngeal carcinoma. *Dis Esophagus*. 2006;19:248–253.
5. Gomes MN, Kroll S, Spear SL. Mediastinal tracheostomy. *Ann Thorac Surg*. 1987;43:539–543.
6. Orringer MB. Anterior mediastinal tracheostomy with and without cervical exenteration. *Ann Thorac Surg*. 1992;54:628–637.
7. Grillo HC, Mathisen DJ. Cervical exenteration. *Ann Thorac Surg*. 1990;49:401–409.
8. Orringer MB. As originally published in 1992: Anterior mediastinal tracheostomy with and without cervical exenteration. Updated in 1998. *Ann Thorac Surg*. 1999;67:591.
9. Mathisen DJ, Grillo HC, Vlahakes GJ, et al. The omentum in the management of complicated cardiothoracic problems. *J Thorac Cardiovasc Surg*. 1988;95:677–684.
10. Jinming Z, Xiaoxuan C, Jieren P, et al. The rectus abdominis musculoperitoneal (RAMP) flap for the reconstruction of complicated pharyngoesophageal defects. *Br J Plast Surg*. 2005;58:608–613.
11. Yu P. One-stage reconstruction of complex pharyngoesophageal, tracheal, and anterior neck defects. *Plast Reconstr Surg*. 2005;116:949–956.
12. Vos JD, Burkey BB. Functional outcomes after free flap reconstruction of the upper aerodigestive tract. *Curr Opin Otolaryngol Head Neck Surg*. 2004;12:305–310.

67 Ablative Endoscopic Therapy for Endobronchial Lesions

Armin Ernst

Keywords: Bronchoplasty, electrocautery, argon plasma coagulation, laser therapy, photodynamic therapy, cryotherapy, external beam radiation and brachytherapy, airway stents

Endobronchial lesions are caused by a variety of benign and malignant disease processes. When such lesions obstruct the central airways, trachea, or mainstem bronchi, they quickly turn life threatening. The incidence of central airway obstruction (CAO) has increased largely because of the prevalence of lung cancer. It causes significant morbidity and, without treatment, may lead to suffocation and death. This chapter reviews the gamut of available endobronchial techniques for managing acute CAO, including endobronchial resection with electrocautery, argon plasma coagulation, laser therapy, photodynamic therapy, cryotherapy, external beam radiation and brachytherapy, and airway stents. The most comprehensive use of these techniques should be offered at centers experienced in the management of complex airway disorders with the full array of endoscopic and surgical options at their disposal.

ETIOLOGY/NATURAL HISTORY OF DISEASE

CAO causes significant morbidity and mortality in patients with malignancies that affect the upper airways. Although the precise incidence and prevalence of CAO are unknown, current lung cancer rates suggest that an increasing number of patients experience complications of proximal endobronchial disease.[1] It has been estimated that approximately 20% to 30% of patients with lung cancer develop complications associated with airway obstruction (i.e., atelectasis, pneumonia, or dyspnea)[2] and that up to 40% of lung cancer deaths are caused by locoregional disease.[3] With increased use of temporary artificial airways, such as endotracheal intubation, in a growing elderly population, the incidence of CAO from malignant, nonmalignant, or iatrogenic complications is also predicted to rise.

The most frequent cause of malignant CAO is by direct invasion of an adjacent tumor, chiefly bronchogenic carcinoma, secondarily esophageal and thyroid carcinoma. Primary tumors of the central airway are relatively uncommon. Most primary tracheal tumors are squamous cell carcinoma or adenoid cystic carcinoma. Distal to the carina, the carcinoid tumors account for the majority of primary airway tumors.[4] Distant tumors, such as renal cell, breast, and thyroid, also may metastasize to the airway. Although the epidemiologic data are limited, the most commonly encountered nonmalignant causes of CAO are stenosis from the proliferation of granulation tissue resulting from prior endotracheal or tracheostomy tubes, airway foreign bodies, and tracheo- or bronchomalacia.[5]

PRESENTING SIGNS AND SYMPTOMS

The clinical presentation of patients with CAO secondary to endobronchial lesions depends not only on the underlying disease but also on the location and rate of progression of the airway obstruction, the patient's underlying health status, and other associated symptoms, such as postobstructive sequelae. Mild airway obstructions may have only slight effect on airflow; hence, the patient may be asymptomatic. However, the inflammation associated with even mild respiratory tract infections can cause mucosal swelling and mucous production, which may further occlude the lumen. For this reason, patients sometimes are misdiagnosed with exacerbations of chronic obstructive pulmonary disease or asthma, especially when symptoms such as wheezing and dyspnea improve with therapy aimed at treating the superimposed infection.

Typically, the trachea must be significantly narrowed (<8 mm) before exertional dyspnea is noted. The lumen diameter must be less than 5 mm before symptoms occur at rest.[6] As a consequence of the dramatic loss of lumen diameter necessary for the development of symptoms, there is no forewarning, and up to 54% of patients with tracheal stenosis present in respiratory distress.

DIAGNOSTIC TECHNIQUES

When evaluating patients with suspected CAO, in addition to spirometric tests including forced expiratory volume in 1 second (FEV_1), functional vital capacity (FVC), and FEV_1/FVC ratio, it is crucial to examine the shape of the flow-volume loop. The characteristic blunting of the flow-volume loop that signals the presence of a CAO typically is seen before spirometry yields abnormal results but may not be recognized until the airway is already narrowed to approximately 8 to 10 mm.[7]

Although often obtained as the initial radiologic test, conventional chest radiographs are rarely diagnostic. Recent advances in airway imaging with CT scanning now permit multiplanar and three-dimensional reconstruction with internal (virtual bronchoscopy) and external rendering.[8,9] Excellent image quality can be achieved with low-dose techniques.[10] These new imaging protocols are better able to characterize whether the lesion is intraluminal, extrinsic to the airway, or has features of both. Moreover, with the newer techniques, one can detect whether the airway distal to the obstruction is patent. Measurements of length, diameter, and relationship to other structures such as blood vessels are also more accurate.

PREINTERVENTIONAL ASSESSMENT

Bronchoscopy (either rigid or flexible; see Chapter 54) is a necessary component of the preinterventional workup. Bronchoscopy provides the means for obtaining a tissue diagnosis, and nothing replaces direct visualization to assess the nature and extent of the obstruction. Other information useful for treatment planning, such as the relative amount of intraluminal and extraluminal diseases, is also obtained. Endobronchial ultrasound can be useful for the diagnostic workup of tracheal invasion and can aid in planning therapeutic interventions.[11]

When the obstruction is severe, bronchoscopy may be difficult and potentially dangerous to perform because the instrument further diminishes the diameter of the remaining lumen and does not accommodate ventilatory support. In addition, conscious sedation may depress ventilation and relax the respiratory muscles, causing a relatively stable airway to become unstable. Access to a team skilled in advanced airway management is essential when undertaking flexible bronchoscopy.

THERAPEUTIC TECHNIQUES

Many of the ablative endoscopic techniques presented below are used together clinically. An algorithm is provided for endoscopic management and decision making in CAO (Fig. 67-1).

Bronchoplasty—Dilation of the Airways

In urgent cases, the airways may be dilated using the barrel of the rigid bronchoscope. In more controlled situations, sequential dilation with balloons is preferred. Sequential balloon dilation produces less mucosal trauma and limits the subsequent formation of granulation tissue. The technique has been used successfully for patients with airway stenosis after lung transplantation and surgical resection of the airway, patients with postintubation tracheal stenosis, and patients with malignant airway obstruction. It also has been shown to be safe, effective, and well tolerated in awake patients undergoing flexible bronchoscopy with conscious sedation.

Balloon bronchoplasty is particularly effective in preparing stenotic airways for stent placement, for expanding stents after insertion, and for placement of brachytherapy catheters that otherwise would be impeded by high-grade stenoses. Dilation alone is immediately effective for intrinsic and extrinsic compression, but the results are not sustained. The mucosal trauma itself may lead to granulation and, in fact, accelerate restenosis. For this reason, dilation is commonly followed by laser or stenting procedures.

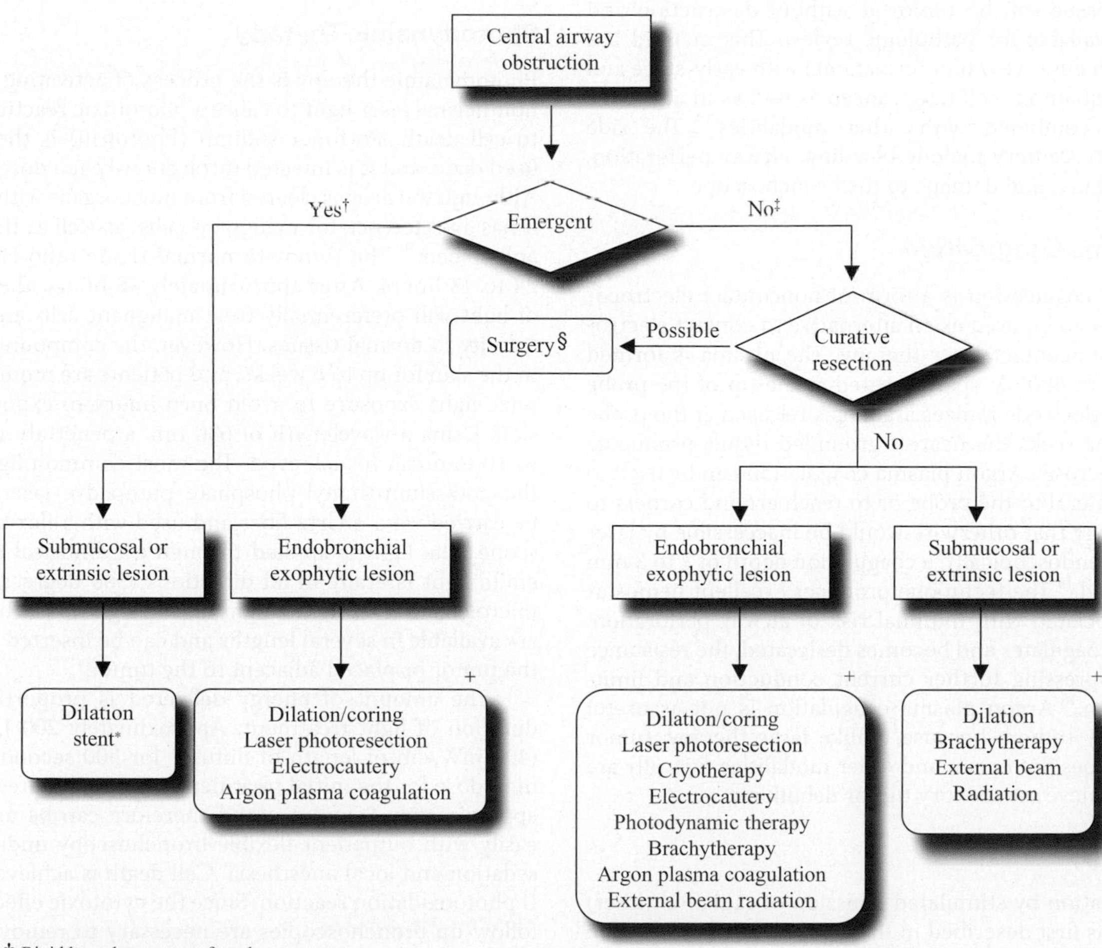

† Rigid bronchoscopy preferred
‡ Careful airway evaluation with airway CT scan, ± flexible bronchoscopy, ± endobronchial ultrasound, ± auto-fluorescence
§ Possibly with pre-surgical endoscopic intervention
+ Can be used singly or in combination, may need stenting
* Silicone / new hybrid stents generally preferred

Figure 67-1. Algorithm for the endoscopic management of central airway obstruction. (Reproduced with permission from Reference 25.)

The microdebrider, a tool borrowed from otorhinolaryngology, can be used to perform mechanical tumor excision in the trachea and mainstem bronchi. The microdebrider has a spinning blade that is contained in a rigid suction catheter and provides the ability to cut with suction to remove blood and tumor or granulation tissue.[12]

Electrocautery

The "active ingredient" of electrocautery is heat, which is generated by passing current from the probe to the tissue. The electric current leaves the body through a grounding plate. The amount and type of current, the characteristics of the tissue, and the contact area between the probe and the tissue all determine the amount of heat generated. The clinical result can vary from simple desiccation to tissue vaporization.

Since most commercially available bronchoscopes are not electrically grounded, the bronchoscopist may "become" the grounding electrode if the unipolar probe tip touches the scope while the current is on.[13] Newer bipolar probes have been developed to eliminate this risk as the current completes the arc through the probe.

Electrocautery with a snare device is well suited for removing pedunculated lesions. By cauterizing the stalk of the lesion, most of the tissue can be removed without destruction and therefore is available for pathologic review. This method has been used with curative intent for patients with early-stage and intraluminal squamous cell lung cancer, as well as in advanced malignancies, combined with other modalities.[14] The side effects of electrocautery include bleeding, airway perforation, endobronchial fire, and damage to the bronchoscope.

Argon Plasma Coagulation

Argon plasma coagulation is a form of noncontact electrocoagulation that can be used as an alternative to contact electrocautery and noncontact laser therapy. The plasma is formed when a 5000- to 6000-V spark created at the tip of the probe by a tungsten electrode ionizes argon gas released at the probe tip. The plasma seeks the nearest grounded tissue, producing coagulative necrosis. Argon plasma coagulation can be used to treat lesions lateral to the probe or to reach around corners to access pathology that otherwise would be inaccessible by laser therapy. Used endoscopically, a coagulation depth of 2 to 3 mm can be achieved.[15] The technique produces excellent hemostasis and is associated with minimal risk of airway perforation. As the tissue coagulates and becomes desiccated, the resistance increases, suppressing further current conduction and limiting penetration.[16] Argon plasma coagulation is not as useful on large, bulky tumors because, unlike laser therapy, tumor vaporization does not occur, and other modalities typically are required to achieve satisfactory tumor debulking.

Laser Therapy

Light amplification by stimulated emission of radiation (laser) technology was first described in the 1960s. With introduction of the neodymium:yttrium-aluminum-garnet (Nd:YAG) laser in 1975, laser tumor debulking became a mainstay of clinical practice. Before that time, CO_2 and argon lasers were the only available options, and for technical reasons, neither could be adapted for use with the bronchoscope. The Nd:YAG laser has a wavelength of 1064 nm and produces an invisible beam that lies in the infrared region and can be used with the flexible bronchoscope.[17] Since there is less absorption by hemoglobin with the Nd:YAG laser, tissue penetration up to 10 mm can be achieved. Less precise than a CO_2 laser, the Nd:YAG laser treats a greater volume of tissue. The laser typically is used at a power of approximately 20 to 40 W. Pulse duration is 0.1 to 1.2 seconds. The laser is always aimed tangentially to the airway. A conservative approach is advised because the depth of penetration is not immediately apparent to the endoscopist, and frequent reanalysis of the lesion and reapplication of the laser are recommended.

The types of lesions most suitable for treatment with laser therapy are central, intrinsic, and short (<4 cm) lesions with a visible distal endobronchial lumen. Lesions that meet these criteria can be obliterated successfully, reestablishing patency of the bronchial lumen in more than 90% of cases.[18]

In experienced hands, the safety record of laser therapy is excellent. Significant complications develop in fewer than 5% of patients. A summary of nearly 7000 laser treatments revealed an overall complication rate of 0.99%.[18] After laser therapy, however, additional treatment with radiation therapy, photodynamic therapy, or stenting is required to prevent local disease recurrence and renewed CAO.

Photodynamic Therapy

Photodynamic therapy is the process of activating a drug with nonthermal laser light to cause a phototoxic reaction that leads to cell death. Porfimer sodium (Photofrin) is the commonly used drug, and it is injected intravenously at a dose of 2 mg/kg. Although the drug is cleared from most organs within 72 hours, it has a preference for malignant cells, as well as the skin, liver, and spleen.[18] The tumor-to-normal-tissue ratio is maximal at 24 to 48 hours. After approximately 48 hours, the application of light will preferentially treat malignant cells and thus limit toxicity to normal tissues. However, the compound is retained in the skin for up to 6 weeks, and patients are required to minimize light exposure to avoid burn injury to exposed areas of skin. Using a wavelength of 630 nm, a penetration depth of 5 to 10 mm can be achieved. The most common light source is the potassium-titanyl-phosphate pump dye laser, which can be carried via a quartz fiber and used with a flexible bronchoscope. The light is applied through a cylindrical diffuser that emits light laterally in all directions (360 degrees) or using a microlens that emits the light in a straight line. The probe tips are available in several lengths and can be inserted directly into the tumor or placed adjacent to the tumor.

The amount of energy delivered is proportional to the duration of light treatment. Approximately 200 J/cm^2 treated (400 mW/cm of length of diffuser for 500 seconds) is a common dose for the initial treatment session. The treatment takes approximately 8 minutes and therefore can be accomplished easily with outpatient flexible bronchoscopy under conscious sedation and local anesthesia. Cell death is achieved via a type II photooxidation reaction. Since the cytotoxic effect is delayed, follow-up bronchoscopies are necessary to remove secretions and cellular debris from the airways.

Photodynamic therapy is an attractive option for treating patients with lung cancer who are unfit for surgery. It can be curative for early-stage lung cancer of the airways, and if used for carcinoma in situ, the complete remission rate may be as high as 83%.[19]

The use of endobronchial ultrasound to help determine the extent of disease before injecting the patient with the photosensitizer also may be beneficial for a more precise delivery of laser light. The major downside to this technique, aside from inducing prolonged photosensitivity in patients with limited life expectancy, is the very high cost of the procedure, the need for multiple endoscopies in a palliative setting, and its ineffectiveness for nonmalignant applications.

Cryotherapy

Cryotherapy or cryosurgery effect tissue or tumor destruction through repeated exposure of the target tissue to freeze-thaw cycles using extremely cold temperature (below −40°C) delivered via nitrous oxide (N_2O) gas. The efficacy of this method depends on the rapidity of the freeze cycle, the lowest temperature attained, the number of freeze-thaw cycles, and the water content of the tissue. Maximal cellular damage is achieved with rapid cooling and slow thawing.

N_2O is stored at room temperature under high pressure. When N_2O is released at the tip of the cryoprobe, the temperature falls to −89°C within several seconds. Although liquid nitrogen also has been used, it peaks early, with maximal negative temperatures reached after 1 to 2 minutes, limiting the cellular injury as compared with N_2O.[20]

Cryotherapy also can be used to remove blood clots and foreign objects with high water content such as grapes. Freezing the object to the probe tip permits the foreign body to be removed along with the cryoprobe and bronchoscope unit from the airways. Cryotherapy is a relatively safe technique. Since freezing and recrystallization depend on cellular water content, and cartilage and fibrous tissue are relatively cryoresistant, the incidence of airway perforation is markedly reduced. Bleeding also tends to be less common because of the hemostatic effects of cryotherapy. In addition, cryotherapy is not associated with the risk of airway fires, electrical accidents, or radiation exposure. The major disadvantage of cryotherapy is that its maximal effects are delayed, and it therefore should not be used to treat patients with acute, severe airway obstruction.

Cryotherapy can be delivered using both the rigid and flexible bronchoscopes. Rigid, semirigid, and flexible probes are available commercially. The size of the probe tip is proportional to the tissue injury. When using the flexible bronchoscope, it is crucial to have the probe protrude several millimeters from the distal tip of the scope so as not to freeze the video chip. Approximately three 60-second freeze-thaw cycles are performed in each area. Generally, however, cryotherapy is considerably less effective than other methods of tissue destruction and therefore is losing importance.

External Beam Radiation and Brachytherapy

External beam radiation to the chest is an established therapy for lung cancer and cancer-related complications. It is minimally effective, however, for cancer-induced airway obstruction. As many as 50% of patients receiving external radiation for local control will develop disease progression within the radiated field.[21] The factor limiting most external beam radiation treatments in the chest is the unwanted exposure of normal tissue (i.e., normal lung parenchyma, heart, spine, and esophagus). Brachytherapy allows radiation to be delivered endobronchially, thus limiting exposure to normal tissues. The term brachytherapy, meaning "short," signifies both the distance of the radiation source from the tissue being treated and the duration of therapy. Brachytherapy typically is performed with the radiation source remaining within the airway. The most commonly used source of radiation is iridium-192 (^{192}Ir), which is delivered via a catheter.

Most endoscopists recommend the afterloading technique. A blind-tipped catheter is placed at the desired position, and thereafter, the radiation source is loaded. A major advantage to this method is the ability to use higher-intensity isotopes without exposing the staff to radiation.

There is no consensus regarding dose rate and cumulative dose in distinguishing low-dose radiation, intermediate-dose radiation, and high-dose radiation brachytherapy. Low-dose radiation therapy has been arbitrarily defined as 75 to 200 cGy/h. The radiation source is placed adjacent to the lesion for 20 to 60 hours. A cumulative dose of 3000 cGy at a radius of 10 mm in the trachea and 5 mm in the bronchi is commonly applied. Low-dose radiation brachytherapy requires hospitalization, and the typical treatment is one session. Intermediate-dose radiation uses fractions of 200 to 1200 cGy/h, with each session lasting 1 to 4 hours and cumulative total doses similar to low-dose radiation. High-dose radiation delivers more than 1000 to 1200 cGy/h.

With brachytherapy, the delivery catheter can be placed in the upper lobe bronchi and segmental bronchi, areas that are typically inaccessible to laser therapy. Endobronchial radiotherapy also has been used successfully in patients with peribronchial disease, and patients often require less retreatment for disease recurrence. Disadvantages to brachytherapy include intolerance of the catheter; excessive radiation-induced bronchitis; cough; fistula formation between the esophagus, pleura, or great vessels; hemorrhage; and infection. The incidence of hemoptysis appears to be associated with the location of the tumor or site of treatment. Treatment of tumors in the right and left upper lobes carries the highest risk for hemoptysis because of the proximity to the great vessels.

Airway Stents

Techniques and products used for tracheobronchial stent placement are presented in Chapter 49. The first dedicated, completely endoluminal airway stent was introduced by Jean-François Dumon in 1990. Since that time, there have been numerous different designs, each of which exhibits various advantages and disadvantages, which were described previously. The importance of airway stents to this discussion is twofold: the necessity of their use after various endoblative therapies to achieve complete tumor debulking, thus limiting local disease recurrence, and the selection of an appropriate stent for benign versus malignant processes.

There are currently two main types of stents: metal and silicone. Although metal stents are placed easily, they can be extremely difficult to extract. Metal stents are available in covered (typically with Silastic or polyurethane) and uncovered varieties. For malignant airway obstruction, the only appropriate metal stents are covered models, which prevent tumor ingrowth. Silicone stents, on the other hand, require rigid bronchoscopy for placement, but they are removed more easily and are significantly less expensive. The rate of stent migration, however, tends to be higher with silicone stents than with metal stents.

The most commonly used metal stents are made from nitinol. Nitinol is a superelastic biomaterial that has the ability to undergo great deformations in size and shape. In addition, nitinol has "shape memory"; that is, at cold temperatures, the stent is easily deformable, and at higher temperatures (i.e., body temperature), it regains its original shape. The risk of airway perforation seems to be lower with nitinol stents because they do not change length once expanded and are flexible enough to change shape with a cough yet have excellent radial strength during constant compression by tumor or stenoses. Nonmetallic stents generally are made from molded silicone and are shaped to prevent migration or contain polyester wire mesh embedded in silicone. Dynamic stents contain metal struts embedded in silicone and are Y-shaped. Silicone stents are commonly placed with the aid of a specially designed stent introducer system in which the stents are preloaded into the introducer and inserted into the stricture with the aid of a stent pusher. The Dumon stent is currently the most widely used stent throughout the world, and some feel that it is the "gold standard" against which future stents will have to be compared.

It is not clear whether stenting may be beneficial for some or all cases of tracheobronchial malacia with symptoms of airway obstruction. The dynamic characteristics of tracheobronchial malacia are quite different from those of static causes of CAO, and therefore, the forces placed on the stents are also different. The shape of the airway in patients with tracheobronchial malacia is different from the normal trachea and also different from the typical cylindrical shape of most stents, thus altering the surface contact dynamics between the stent and airway.

It is crucial that the indications for stent placement are clear, that the appropriate stent is selected, that an endoscopist with significant experience inserts the stent, and that the patient is provided with appropriate education and follow-up. Especially in cases of benign CAO, a metal stent should be placed only when no other therapeutic options, including surgical correction, are available.

PERIOPERATIVE MANAGEMENT

All patients with a history of airway obstruction should carry a card or bracelet identifying them as patients with complicated airways or indwelling airway stents. The presence of a complicated airway, however, does not preclude intubation, if needed. On completion of the procedure used to ablate a malignant obstruction, most patients can be extubated. For patients who experienced respiratory failure for some time prior to the intervention and have limited pulmonary reserve, a brief period of positive-pressure ventilation may be required.

TECHNIQUE

Readers are referred to Chapter 54 for a description of rigid and flexible bronchoscopic techniques. Virtually any technique can be used effectively for endobronchial therapy, provided that the user is experienced.

PROCEDURE-SPECIFIC COMPLICATIONS

Close follow-up of all patients is indicated to identify problems at an early stage. Potential complications include stent migration, airway occlusion by secretions, accumulation of necrotic tissue or granulation tissue, infection, and recurrence of the obstruction caused by progression of the underlying disease. Patients therefore must be educated about symptoms that should prompt further investigation.

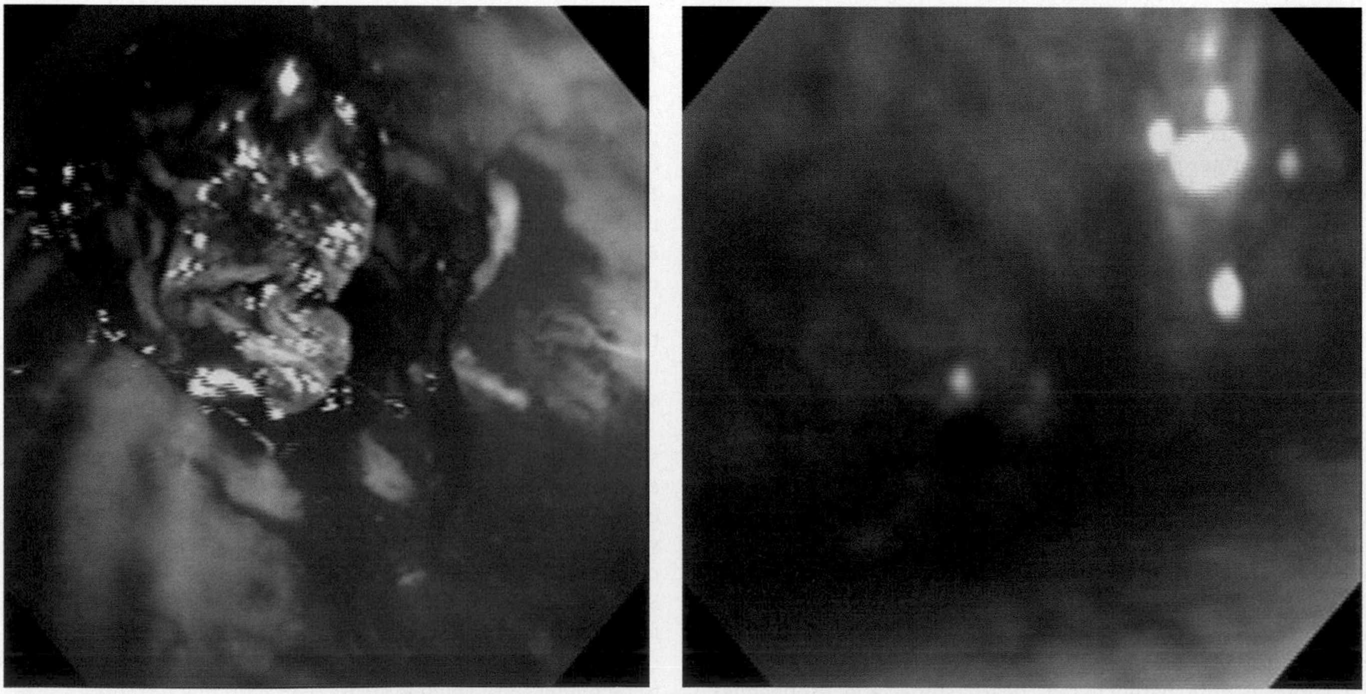

A B

Figure 67-2. *A.* Left mainstem bronchus obstruction due to aspergilloma. *B.* Pinhole opening of a right mainstem bronchus due to sarcoidosis.

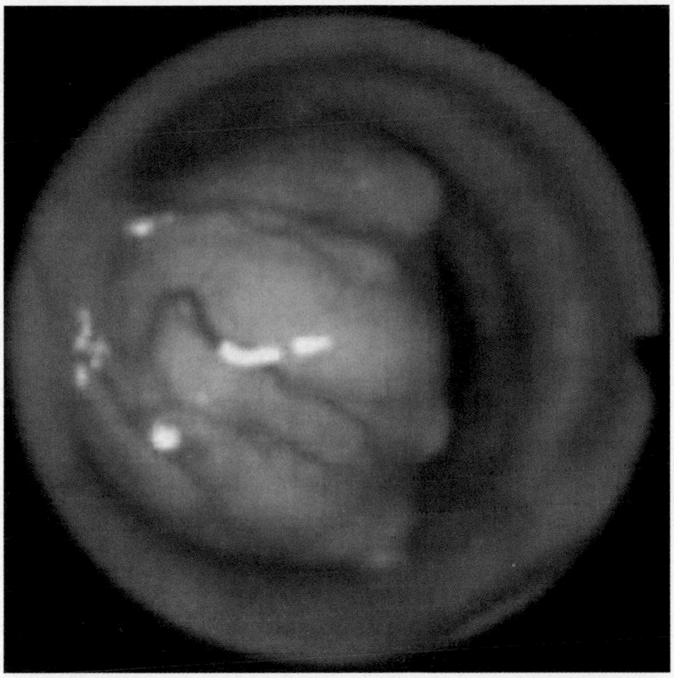

A

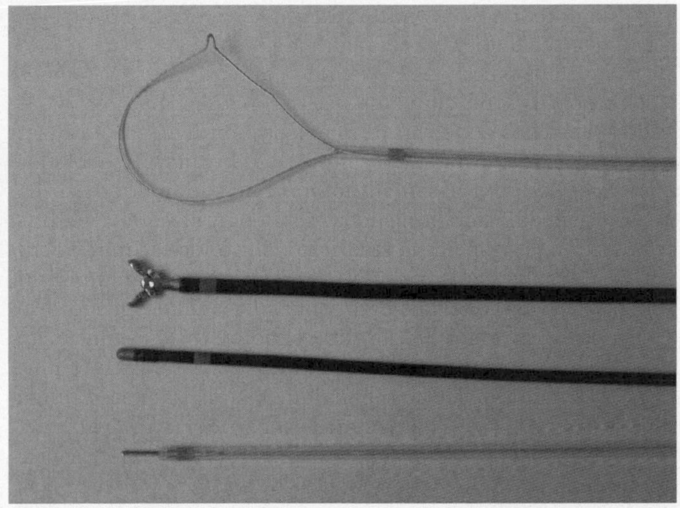

B

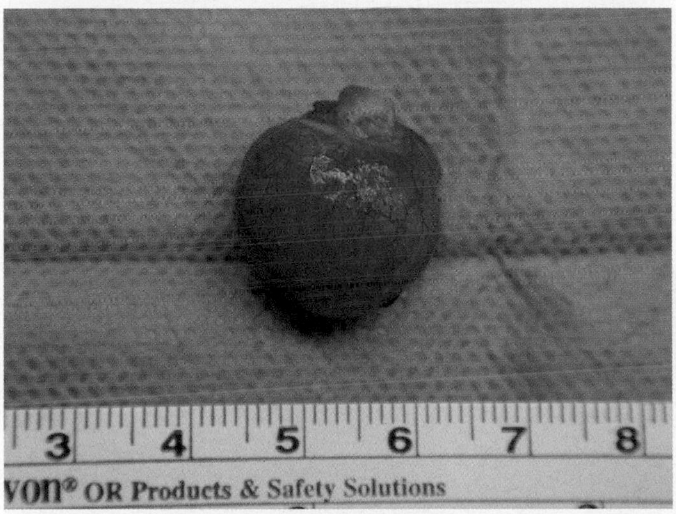

C

Figure 67-3. *A.* High-grade tracheal obstruction due to a pedunculated hamartoma. *B.* Accessories used for endobronchial electrosurgery. *C.* Hamartoma specimen (shown in *A*) removed with the help of an electrosurgery snare.

SUMMARY

CAO caused by endobronchial lesions may be extrinsic, intrinsic, or mixed; fixed or dynamic; and benign or malignant. Patients with CAO present with a number of symptoms ranging from mild shortness of breath to respiratory failure. In the decompensated patient, it is of vital important to restore oxygenation and ventilation immediately. Further interventions are based on the nature of the obstruction, quality-of-life issues, available techniques, and physician expertise. Almost any technique can achieve the desired results if performed by an experienced bronchoscopist.[23] The endoscopic management of CAO can provide successful palliation in over 90% of patients.[24] Often the best therapy includes a combination of several treatment approaches. Interventions should be chosen that leave open other options for further therapy. Although it is essential for all pulmonary and critical care physicians and surgeons to be educated about the diagnosis and initial management of CAO, the most comprehensive assessment and therapy generally are provided by centers with a multidisciplinary airway team that specializes in the management of patients with compromised airways.

CASE HISTORIES

Examples of clinical scenarios necessitating urgent bronchoscopic intervention are presented along with several therapeutic or palliative strategies for managing the underlying disease process. Infectious and neoplastic processes (benign or malignant) causing airway constriction (<5 mm luminal diameter) account for the majority of emergent CAOs (Figs. 67-2 and 67-3).

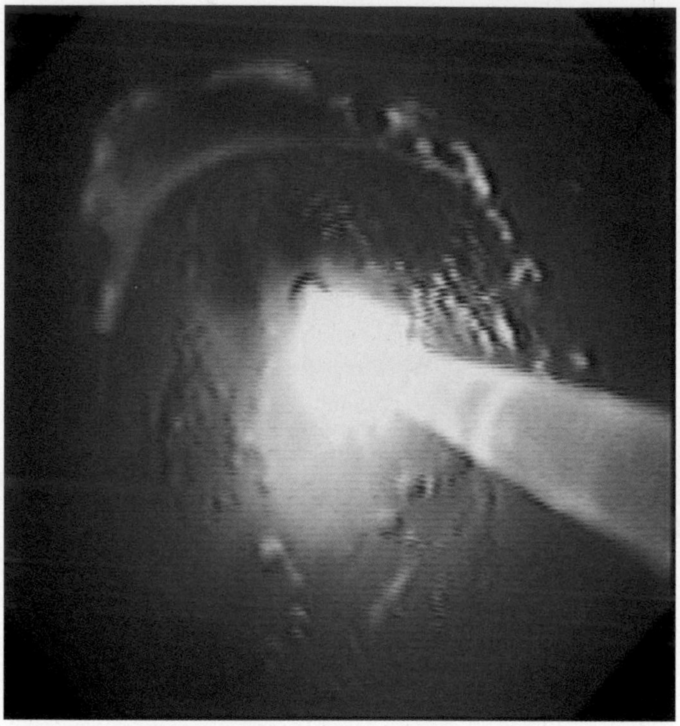

Figure 67-4. Light activation of Photofrin with a KTP laser via a flexible fiber placed in a patient with non–small-cell carcinoma and airway obstruction. The light is reddish in color and cold.

Endobronchial surgery with electrocautery is used for definitive resection of a benign hamartoma (Fig. 67-3B,C). Photodynamic therapy (Fig. 67-4) is delivered to a patient with a CAO secondary to non–small-cell lung cancer.

After relief of the emergent CAO, a patient with a post lung transplant stenosis in the right mainstem, bronchus is implanted with an expanding metal stent (Figs. 67-5 and 67-6).

EDITOR'S COMMENT

Although there are multiple endobronchial techniques for managing tumors that involve the central airways, there are no prospective randomized studies that compare the various treatment strategies. Hence, the specific treatment used for each patient depends on the expertise of the treating physician and available equipment. It is important to consider the simple oncologic principles while treating patients. The first objective is to establish airway patency, the second to establish local control, and the third systemic control. For best long-term results, it is usually necessary to combine multiple modalities.

—Raphael Bueno

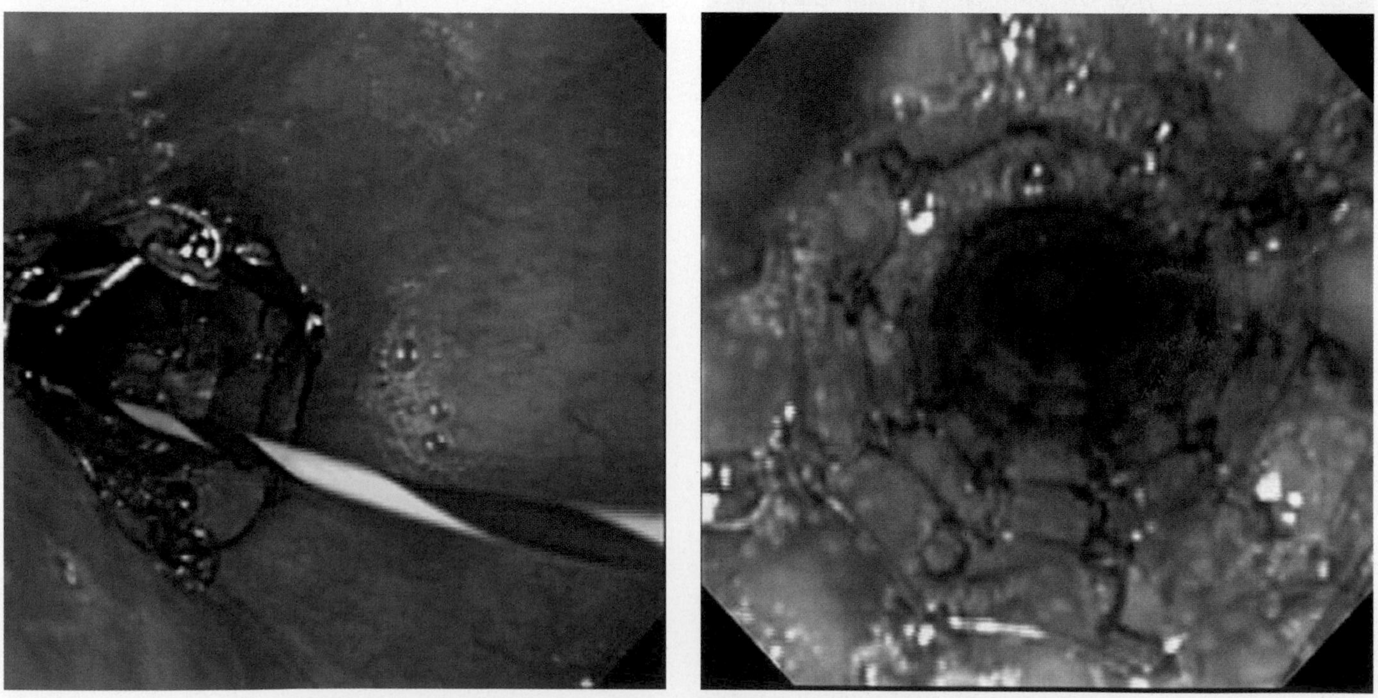

A B

Figure 67-5. Placement of an expandable metal stent. *A*. Shows the guidewire still in place. *B*. Shows a view through the stent.

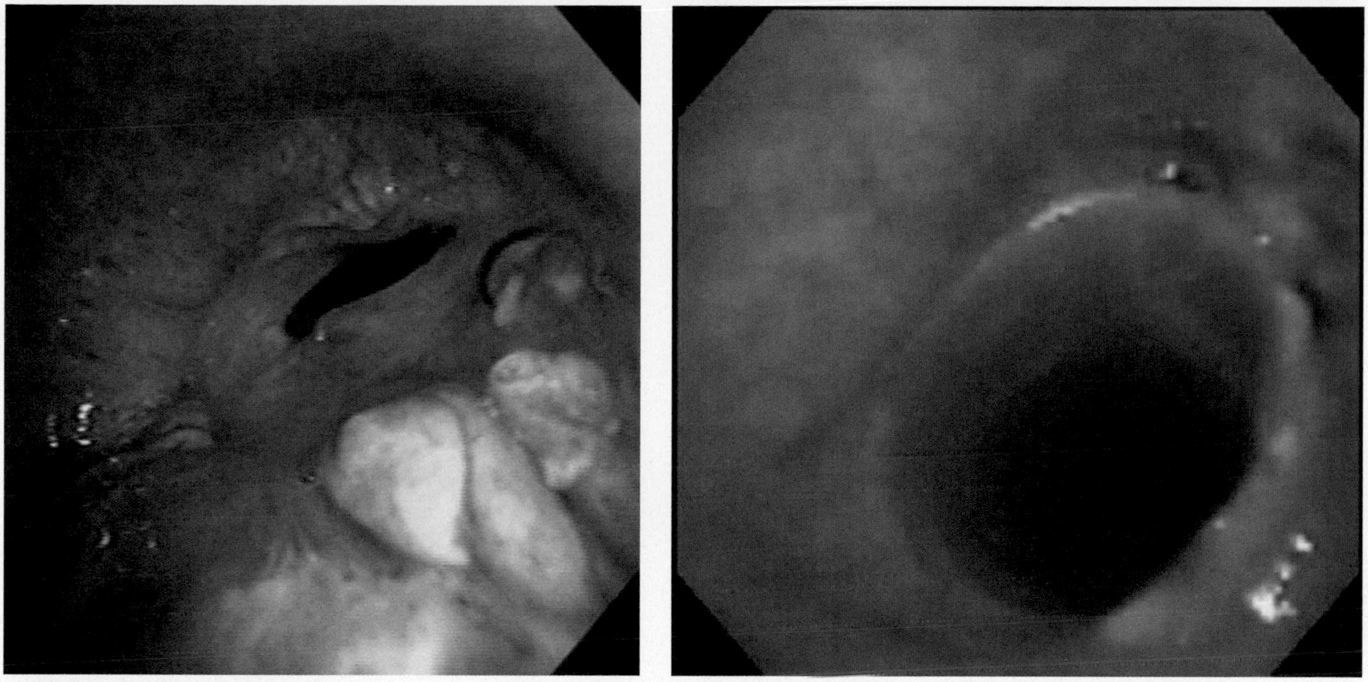

A B

Figure 67-6. *A.* A posttransplant anastomosis of the right mainstem bronchus. *B.* The same patient after dilation and placement of a silicone stent.

References

1. Ayers ML, Beamis JF Jr. Rigid bronchoscopy in the twenty-first century. *Clin Chest Med.* 2001;22:355–364.
2. Ginsberg R, Vokes E, Ruben A. Non-small cell lung cancer. In: DeVita VT, Hellman S, Rosenberg SA, eds. *Cancer: Principles and Practice of Oncology.* Philadelphia, PA: Lippincott-Raven; 1997:858–911.
3. Noppen M, Meysman M, D'Haese J, et al. Interventional bronchoscopy: 5-year experience at the Academic Hospital of Vrije Universiteit Brussel (AZ-VUB). *Acta Clin Belg.* 1997;52:371–380.
4. Wood D. Management of malignant tracheobronchial obstruction. *Surg Clin North Am.* 2002;82:621–642.
5. Geffin B, Grillo HC, Cooper JD, et al. Stenosis following tracheostomy for respiratory care. *JAMA.* 1971;216:1984–1988.
6. Hollingsworth HM. Wheezing and stridor. *Clin Chest Med.* 1987;8:231–240.
7. Stoller JK. Spirometry: a key diagnostic test in pulmonary medicine. *Cleve Clin J Med.* 1992;59:75–78.
8. Boiselle PM, Ernst A. Recent advances in central airway imaging. *Chest.* 2002;121:1651–1660.
9. Boiselle P, Feller-Kopman D, Ashiku S, et al. Tracheobronchomalacia: evolving role of dynamic multislice helical CT. *Radiol Clin North Am.* 2003;41:627–636.
10. Choi YW, McAdams HP, Jeon SC, et al. Low-dose spiral CT: application to surface-rendered three-dimensional imaging of central airways. *J Comput Assist Tomogr.* 2002;26:335–341.
11. Miyazu Y, Miyazawa T, Kurimoto N, et al. Endobronchial ultrasonography in the assessment of centrally located early-stage lung cancer before photodynamic therapy. *Am J Respir Crit Care Med.* 2002;165:832–837.
12. Simoni P, Peters GE, Magnuson JS, et al. Use of the endoscopic microdebrider in the management of airway obstruction from laryngotracheal carcinoma. *Ann Otol Rhinol Laryngol.* 2003;112:11–13.
13. Hooper RG, Jackson FN. Endobronchial electrocautery. *Chest.* 1985;87:712–714.
14. van Boxem T, Westerga J, Venmans B, et al. Tissue effects of bronchoscopic electrocautery: bronchoscopic appearance and histologic changes of bronchial wall after electrocautery. *Chest.* 2000;117:887–891.
15. Reichle G, Freitag L, Kullmann J-J, et al. Argon plasma coagulation in bronchology: a new method—alternative or complementary? *J Bronchol.* 2000;7:109–117.
16. Farin G, Grund KE Technology of argon plasma coagulation with particular regard to endoscopic applications. *Endosc Surg Allied Technol.* 1994;2:71–77.
17. Ramser ER, Beamis JF Jr. Laser bronchoscopy. *Clin Chest Med.* 1995;16:415–426.
18. Cavaliere S, Venuta F, Foccoli P, et al. Endoscopic treatment of malignant airway obstructions in 2008 patients. *Chest.* 1996;110:1536–1542.
19. Kato H, Okunaka T, Shimatani H. Photodynamic therapy for early stage bronchogenic carcinoma. *J Clin Laser Med Surg.* 1996;14:235–238.
20. Maiwand MO, Homasson JP. Cryotherapy for tracheobronchial disorders. *Clin Chest Med.* 1995;16:427–443.
21. Susnerwala SS, Sharma S, Deshpande DD, et al. Endobronchial brachytherapy: a preliminary experience. *J Surg Oncol.* 1992;50:115–117.
22. Villanueva AG, Lo TC, Beamis JF Jr. Endobronchial brachytherapy. *Clin Chest Med.* 1995;16:445–454.
23. Sutedja G, Postmus PE. Bronchoscopic treatment of lung tumors. *Lung Cancer.* 1994;11:1–17.
24. Stephens KE Jr, Wood DE. Bronchoscopic management of central airway obstruction. *J Thorac Cardiovasc Surg.* 2000;119:289–296.
25. Ernst A, Feller-Kopman D, Becker HD, et al. Central airway obstruction. *Am J Respir Crit Care Med.* 2004;169:1278–1297.

PART 10

LUNG CANCER OVERVIEW AND PATHOLOGY

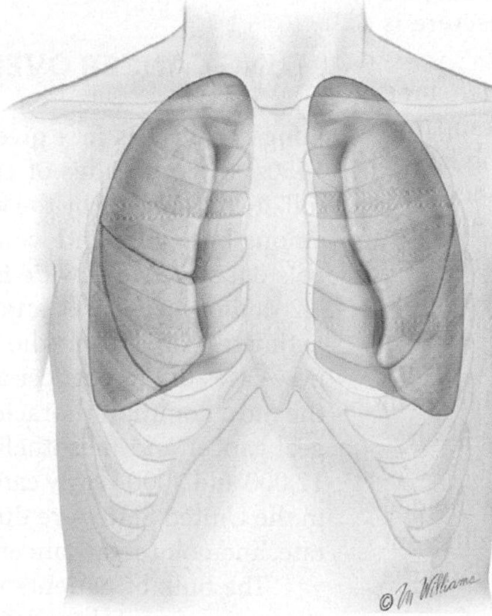

68 Overview of Anatomy and Pathophysiology of Lung Cancer

Ciaran J. McNamee, Ann Adams, and David J. Sugarbaker

Keywords: Small-cell lung cancer (SCLC), non–small-cell lung cancer (NSCLC), adenocarcinoma, carcinoma in situ, large cell carcinoma, squamous cell carcinoma, occult lung cancer, solitary pulmonary nodule, pulmonary resection, TNM staging system for NSCLC, neuroendocrine, mucoepidermoid, survival curves for staging systems, development of surgical techniques

ANATOMY OF THE LUNG AND TRACHEOBRONCHIAL TREE

The chest has two lungs (a right lung and a left lung) (Fig. 68-1). Each lung is divided into independent lobes, with separate segments. Each segment (and therefor each lobe) maintains its own individual vascular and lymphatic network such that removal of a segment or a lobe does not disturb the vascular or lymphatic patterns of neighboring lung segments. Furthermore, tumors that arise in one segment usually follow a separate and individual drainage pattern which allows for the curative removal of subunits of each lung without jeopardizing the viability of the whole lung. Thus knowledge of pulmonary architecture is crucial to the management of lung cancer.

The right lung is marginally larger because the left lung accommodates the heart by having only 8 segments compared with the right lung, which has 10 segments. Each lung has at least one fissure that divides the lung into smaller lobes. The left lung is divided in two by a single horizontal fissure that creates an upper and lower lobe. The right lung has two fissures, one horizontal and one oblique. These fissures delineate three lobes: upper, middle, and lower. A normal anatomic variant includes the presence of an azygos lobe (see Fig. 68-1, inset), which is usually found at the apex of the right lung. This small variant lobe is separated from the upper lobe by a deep fissure-like groove that cradles the azygos vein.

The lobes of the left and right lung, in turn, are divided into segments representing areas of lung served by different bronchioles, as shown in Figure 68-2. This figure also shows the intimate relationship between the lungs and tracheobronchial tree. The trachea lies anterior to the esophagus (not shown). At the bifurcation of the trachea, or carina, the left and right mainstem bronchi branch off, and each branch enters the hilus of its respective lung. These, in turn, divide into progressively smaller airways, called bronchioles that form a root-like network that extends through the sponge-like tissues of the lung. The exterior layer of the bronchi is composed of cartilage with rings of smooth muscle that permit the bronchi to expand and retract on inspiration and expiration. The cartilaginous segments become more irregular at the distal end of this network, and there are none on the bronchioles.

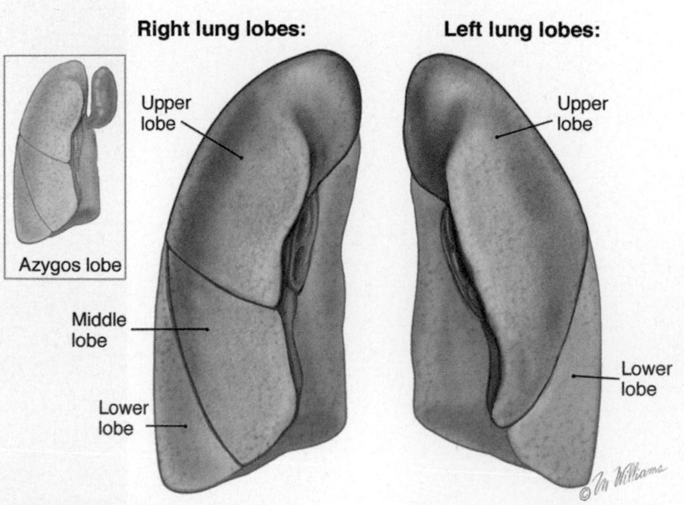

Figure 68-1. Anatomy of the lungs.

LUNG CANCER OVERVIEW

Lung cancer was first given status as a global epidemic in the 1950s, when decades of cigarette smoking began to take their toll. It continues to be the leading cause of cancer-related deaths among both men and women worldwide.[1] Based on best available data, the worldwide incidence of lung cancer accounts for 1.2 million new cases and 1.1 million cancer deaths annually.[2] Estimates for 2012 in the United States alone, project 226,160 new cases of lung cancer and 160,340 lung cancer deaths.[1] It is the most common thoracic malignancy compared with esophageal cancer and mesothelioma that account for approximately 12,000 and 3000 yearly cancer deaths, respectively. More deaths in the United States are due to lung cancer than to breast, prostate, and colorectal cancer combined.[1]

The bulk of patients with lung cancer can be divided into two major groups based on treatment and prognosis: small-cell lung cancer (SCLC) and non–small-cell lung cancer (NSCLC). SCLC is the more aggressive form and usually has spread systemically by the time of diagnosis. Untreated, the mean survival is 2 to 4 months. Median survival with treatment is between 18 and 36 months.

Currently, SCLC accounts for 15% to 20% of new lung cancer cases per year in the United States. The malignancy is characterized by a proliferation of small anaplastic cells. Because of its tendency to early metastasis, the cancer usually is not amenable to surgical resection, and hence, surgery plays only a limited role in its management. It is, however, modestly responsive to systemic treatment with chemotherapy.[3] The combination of etoposide and cisplatin/carboplatin, with radiotherapy as appropriate, remains the standard of care for both limited stage (LS) and extensive stage (ES) disease.[4] Recent innovations, including the addition of thoracic radiation to systemic chemotherapy protocols, increasing the intensity of thoracic radiation, and prophylactic cranial irradiation,[5] have produced some benefits in terms of prolonging disease-free intervals and

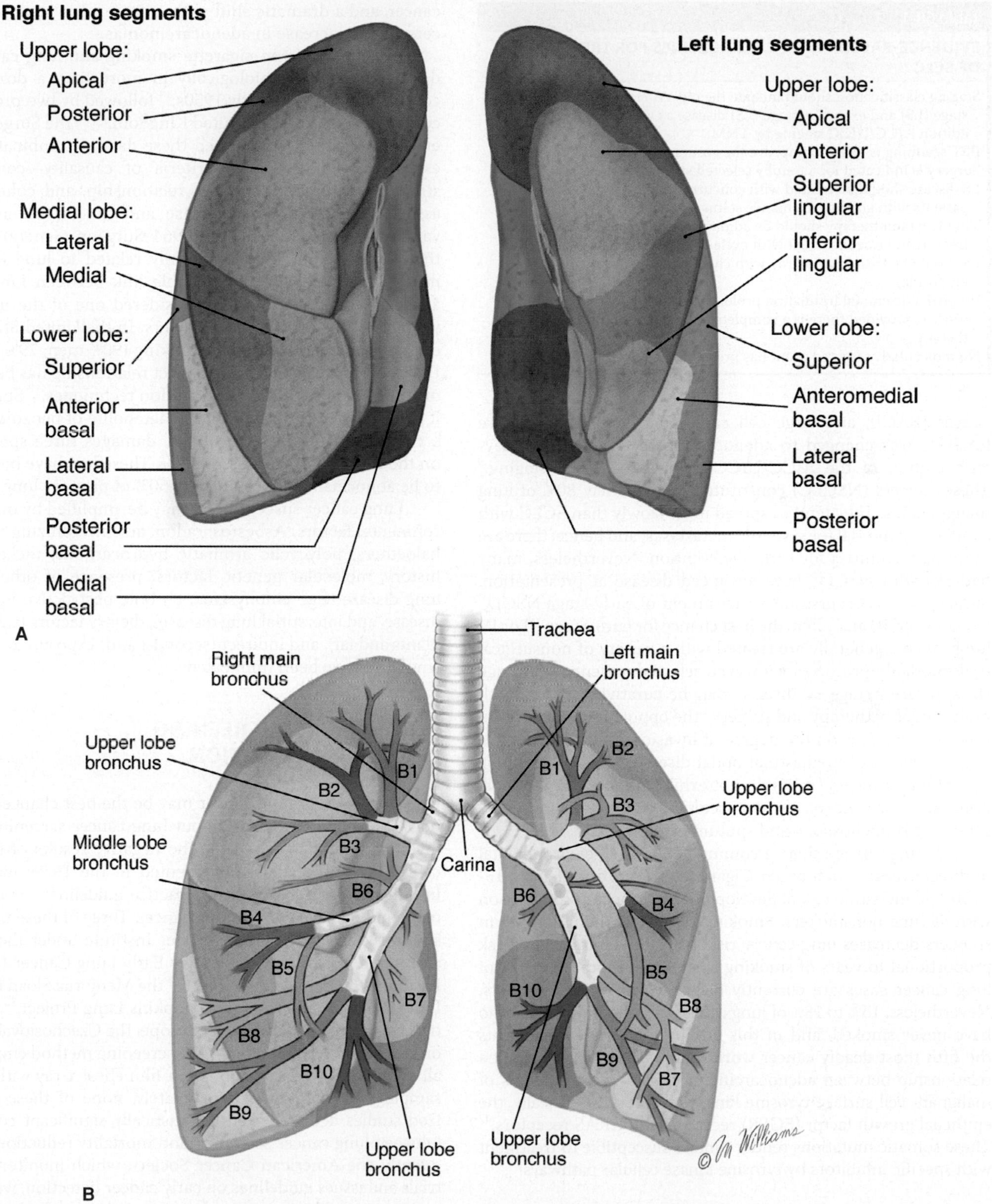

Figure 68-2. *A*. Segments of the left and right lungs. *B*. Tracheobronchial tree.

survival.[6] Current practice guidelines from the American College of Chest Physicians (ACCP) outline the role of each of these modalities (Table 68-1).[7] Surgery may be rarely recommended and may have a survival benefit in carefully selected patients with stage I SCLC, after thorough mediastinal evaluation.[8]

In contrast, the role of surgery in NSCLC is more clearly defined. Surgical treatment of early-stage disease provides the best chance for cure. NSCLC is comprised of three major histopathologic subtypes: squamous cell carcinoma, adenocarcinoma, and adenocarcinoma in situ (formerly bronchioloalveolar

Table 68-1

EVIDENCE-BASED PRACTICE GUIDELINES FOR TREATMENT OF SCLC

Staging classification should include the old VA classification of limited stage (LS) and extensive stage (ES) disease as well as the seventh edition AJCC/UICC staging by TNM
PET scanning is likely to improve the accuracy of staging
Surgery is indicated for carefully selected stage I SCLC patients
LS disease should be treated with concurrent chemoradiotherapy in patients with good performance status
Thoracic radiotherapy should be administered early in the course of treatment, i.e., concurrent with cycle 1 or 2 of chemotherapy
ES should be treated primarily with chemotherapy (cisplatin plus etoposide)
Prophylactic cranial irradiation prolongs survival in both LS and ES disease, provided there is a complete or partial response to initial therapy
No molecularly targeted agent has proved to be effective against SCLC

cancer [BAC]), and large cell carcinoma. The nomenclature for BAC was changed to adenocarcinoma in situ in the seventh edition of the AJCC/UICC manual for TNM staging.[9] These cancers (NSCLC) constitute approximately 80% of lung malignancies. They tend to spread more slowly than SCLC with a reduced potential for systemic metastases, and hence, there are more opportunities for early intervention. Nevertheless, many patients with NSCLC have advanced disease at presentation. Surgery is the cornerstone for treatment of early-stage NSCLC (stages I and II) and offers the best chance for cure. Stage III or IV lung cancers generally are treated with a variety of nonsurgical multimodality protocols. However, selected patients with stage III, and rarely stage IV disease, may be curatively treated with multimodality therapy and surgery. The opportunity for surgical resection depends on the degree of invasion of local structures and the extent of mediastinal nodal disease.[10] A small proportion of lung cancers (<1%) do not exhibit tumors by radiologic criteria. These cancers, termed occult cancers, are diagnosed by screening bronchoscopy and sputum cytology.

All lung cancers share a common etiology in environmental or direct exposure to tobacco. Cigarette smokers experience a 15- to 50-fold increased risk of developing lung cancer in comparison with lifetime nonsmokers. Smoking cessation among long-term smokers decreases lung cancer risk, with the diminution of risk proportional to years of smoking abstinence. More than 50% of lung cancer cases are currently diagnosed in former smokers. Nevertheless, 15% to 18% of lung cancers arise in individuals who have never smoked, and in this group, lung cancer represents the fifth most deadly cancer worldwide.[11] There is a confirmed relationship between adenocarcinoma in situ and mutations of malignant cell surface tyrosine kinase receptors, specifically, the epithelial growth factor (EGFR) receptors and KRAS receptors.[12] These somatic mutations render tumors susceptible to treatment with specific inhibitors by tyrosine kinase cellular pathways.

EPIDEMIOLOGY

Despite an encouraging age-adjusted decline in lung cancer mortality rate in the 1990s, the absolute number of lung cancer deaths in the United States has increased dramatically since the 1950s because of a growing population of increasingly elderly persons (age >70 years).[13] Other characteristics of the lung cancer pool in the United States include a pronounced increase in this cancer in women, now claiming more lives than breast cancer, and a dramatic shift with a decrease in squamous cancers and an increase in adenocarcinomas.

The link between cigarette smoking and lung cancer was demonstrated epidemiologically in more than a dozen case-control studies of the early 1950s,[14] followed by two prospective cohort studies from the United Kingdom.[15,16] The Surgeon General of the United States used these data in combination with established epidemiologic criteria of causality—consistency, strength, specificity, temporal relationship, and coherence of association between the disease and the disease-associated variable—to conclude in the 1964 Surgeon General's Report that "cigarette smoking is causally related to lung cancer in men." Because of the indisputable link between lung cancer and cigarette smoking, it is considered one of the most preventable forms of all human cancers. In the United States, 80% of cases can be attributed to smoking (90% men; 79% women). Direct evidence of this cause–effect relationship has been demonstrated using genetic amplification techniques.[17] Specifically, it has been demonstrated that a metabolite of benzo[α]pyrene, a component of cigarette smoke, damages three specific loci on the p53 tumor suppressor gene. These loci have been found to be abnormal in approximately 60% of primary lung cancers.

Lung cancer susceptibility may be amplified by other environmental factors. Asbestos, radon, arsenic, ionizing radiation, haloethers, polycyclic aromatic hydrocarbons, nickel, family history, molecular genetic factors, presence of other benign lung disease (e.g., emphysema, chronic obstructive pulmonary disease, and interstitial lung disease), dietary factors (e.g., antioxidants and fat), and indirect (second-hand) exposure to cigarette smoke all have been implicated.

LUNG CANCER SCREENING FOR EARLY DETECTION

Early detection of lung cancer may be the best chance for cure, but achieving a consensus about lung cancer screening eluded investigators for many years. The negative results of four lung cancer screening trials implemented in the 1970s had a lasting impact on recommended practice guidelines for the treatment and management of lung cancer. Three of these trials were sponsored by the National Cancer Institute under the aegis of a program called the Cooperative Early Lung Cancer Detection Program: the Mayo Lung Project,[18] the Memorial Sloan Kettering Lung Project,[19] and the Johns Hopkins Lung Project.[20] A fourth trial was conducted in eastern Europe: the Czechoslovakia Study on Lung Cancer Screening.[21] The screening method employed in all these studies consisted of plain-film chest x-ray with sputum sampling for cytology. Unfortunately, none of these randomized studies demonstrated a statistically significant correlation between lung cancer screening and mortality reduction. Consequently, the American Cancer Society, which monitors clinical trials and issues guidelines on early cancer detection, was unable to recommend lung cancer screening as the standard of care.[22]

Disappointing results with chest x-ray and sputum cytology prompted the investigation of low-dose helical computed tomography, which appeared to be more promising as a screening tool than conventional x-ray for the detection of small (<2 cm) pulmonary nodules. The Early Lung Cancer Action Project (ELCAP) was initiated by investigators at Weill Cornell Medical College to evaluate this effort.[23] On the basis of average tumor size in a baseline screening of 1000 high-risk asymptomatic individuals, the ELCAP investigators found that 80% of nodules diagnosed were of clinical stage I. These findings were reported in Lancet in 1999.[23]

In 2002, the National Lung Screening Trial (NLST), a joint effort of the Lung Screening Study (LSS), and the American College of Radiology Imaging Network (ACRIN) began randomly assigning patients to a 3-year course of annual screening with either low-dose CT or chest radiography. Groundbreaking results showing that a 20% mortality reduction could be achieved with low-dose CT were published in the New England Journal of Medicine and in Radiology in 2011.[24,25]

To assess the clinical implications of these findings, the American Association for Thoracic Surgery organized a multispecialty taskforce to create guidelines for the clinical management of patients with high risk of developing lung cancer and for survivors of previous lung cancers.[26,27] The gist of these recommendations is that screening with low-dose CT should be conducted annually in North Americans between 55 and 79 years of age who have a 30 pack-year history of smoking. Long-term cancer survivors should be followed with annual low-dose CT until the age of 79 years. Annual low-dose screening should be offered to individuals starting at age 50 if they have a 20 pack-year history with an additional cumulative risk of 5% or greater over the following 5 years.

Despite the benefits of increased pulmonary nodule detection afforded by low-dose CT, the false-positive rate remains high and better methods of distinguishing benign from malignant nodules are needed to avoid unnecessary surgery and keep the costs of surveillance low. Clinical testing that combines fine-needle aspiration (FNA) biopsy with molecular cytologic testing is one approach currently being investigated to improve the diagnosis of benign versus malignant lesions.[28]

HISTO-CYTO-PATHOLOGIC CLASSIFICATION OF LUNG CANCER

The International Agency for Research on Cancer (IARC) is a specialized branch of the World Health Organization (WHO) that promotes international collaboration in cancer research. Among other works, the IARC publishes the WHO Classification of Tumors, a series of organ and system-specific pathologic tumor classifications that undergo periodic review and update. Relevant to our field, the WHO provides the framework for the pathological classification of lung cancer. Since inception, that framework has relied principally on the pathologic evaluation of routinely stained biopsy specimens and cytologic preparations. In clinical practice, however, pathologists have increasingly relied on additional tests, such as immunohistochemistry, to distinguish cancer subtypes. Classification of lung carcinomas by histopathologic subtype, for example, provides important information about prognosis, improves the stratification of staging with survival, and aids in the selection of optimal treatments. The latest edition, *Pathology and Genetics of Tumours of the Lung, Pleura, Thymus and Heart,* was published in 2004 and incorporates a number of important developments including the recognition of lung carcinoma heterogeneity, the introduction of diagnostic immunohistochemical staining (IHC) techniques for lung cancer subtype determination, and the recognition of newly described entities such as fetal adenocarcinoma, cystic mucinous tumors, and large cell neuroendocrine carcinoma.[29]

In 2011, a multidisciplinary panel of experts from the International Association for the Study of Lung Cancer (IASLC), the American Thoracic Society (ATS), and the European Respiratory Society (ERS) proposed major changes in the way lung adenocarcinoma is diagnosed that alter the pathologic classification of lung cancer in a fundamental way (Table 68-2).[30] For the first time, recommendations were established regarding the classification of resection specimens, biopsies, and cytology specimens, as well as

Table 68-2

PROPOSED NEW HISTOLOGIC CLASSIFICATION OF LUNG CANCER[a]

PREINVASIVE LESIONS
- Squamous dysplasia/carcinoma in situ (CIS)
- Atypical adenomatous hyperplasia (AAH)
- Adenocarcinoma in situ (AIS) (nonmucinous, mucinous, or mixd nonmucinous/mucinous)
- Diffuse idiopathic pulmonary neuroendocrine cell hyperplasia (DIPNECH)

INVASIVE LESIONS
- Squamous cell carcinoma (SCC)
  - Variants
    - Papillary
    - Clear cell
    - Small cell (probably should be discontinued)
    - Basaloid
- Small cell carcinoma
  - Combined small cell carcinoma
- Adenocarcinoma
  - Minimally invasive adenocarcinoma (MIA) (≤ 3 cm lepidic predominant tumor with ≤ 5 mm invasion)
    - nonmucinous, mucinous, mixed mucinous/nonmucinous
  - Invasive adenocarcinoma
    - Lepidic predominant (formerly nonmucinous bronchioloalveolar carcinoma (BAC) pattern, with >5 mm invasion)
    - Acinar predominant
    - Papillary predominant
    - Micropapillary predominant
    - Solid predominant with mucin
  - Variants of invasive adenocarcinoma
    - Invasive mucinous adenocarcinoma (former mucinous BAC)
    - Colloid
    - Fetal (low and high grade)
    - Enteric
- Large cell carcinoma
  - Variants
    - Large cell neuroendocrine carcinoma (LCNEC)
    - Combined LCNEC
    - Basaloid carcinoma
    - Lympho-epithelioma-like carcinoma
    - Clear cell carcinoma
    - Large cell carcinoma with rhabdoid phenotype
  - Adenosquamous carcinoma
  - Sarcomatoid carcinomas
    - Pleomorphic carcinoma
    - Spindle cell carcinoma
    - Giant cell carcinoma
    - Carcinosarcoma
    - Pulmonary blastoma
    - Other
  - Carcinoid tumor
    - Typical carcinoid (TC)
    - Atypical carcinoid (AC)
  - Tumors of the salivary gland type
    - Mucoepidermoid carcinoma
    - Adenoid cystic carcinoma
    - Epimyoepithelial carcinoma

[a]Modified from the 2004 WHO Classification[29] and the 2011 IASLC/ATS/ERS Classification of Lung Adenocarcinoma[30] based on the analysis of Travis, et al.[31] The classification presented in this table primarily addresses the histological classification of resected specimens. Additional classifications have been proposed for small biopsies and cytology specimens and for diagnostic terms and criteria for other major histological subtypes.[31]

Table 68-3

MAJOR DIFFERENCES IN THE HISTOLOGICAL CLASSIFICATION OF LUNG ADENOCARCINOMA BETWEEN WHO CLASSIFICATION OF 2004[1] AND IASLC/ATS/ERS RECOMMENDATIONS OF 2011[2]

CHANGE	REF.
The term 'bronchioloalveolar carcinoma' (BAC) has been replaced by 'carcinoma *in situ*' (CIS).	32
A new category has been created for minimally invasive tumors <5 mm.	32
The term 'lepidic predominant adenocarcinoma' has been adopted to describe mixed tumors with a BAC component.	32
A new limit (<3 cm) has been established for the designation 'noninvasive or minimally invasive' tumor.	32
Any tumor with evidence of lymphatic or pleural invasion or necrosis does not qualify as a 'minimally invasive' tumor.	32
The term "mixed" has been replaced by 'predominant growth pattern.' It is additionally recommended that reporting should include estimates of percentage growth patterns for patients with mixed histology.	32
A new grading system has been proposed.	33
Low grade Non-invasive and minimally invasive tumors	33
Moderate grade Invasive tumors with acinar, papillary, and lepidic growth patterns	33
High grade Tumors with predominant solid, micropapillary, or mucinous growth	33

diagnostic terms and criteria for other major histologic subtypes in addition to adenocarcinoma.[31] These changes respond to the increasing understanding of pathology with respect to the extent of cancer invasion and its impact on personalized medicine, as well as the importance of histologic classification and molecular testing in stratifying patients for specific therapies.[32] A detailed presentation of these changes is beyond the scope of this chapter. Table 68-3 provides a brief summary of the major differences in the classification of lung adenocarcinoma between the WHO classification of 2004 and the recommendations proposed by the IASLC/ATS/ERS.[33,34] Future pathologic systems of lung cancer may incorporate molecular subtyping as a histo-cyto-molecular classification system.

Squamous and SCLCs tend to arise in the central airways, whereas adenocarcinoma and large cell lung cancers tend to locate peripherally. SCLCs arise from neuroendocrine cells that are distributed in small numbers in the normal epithelium. There are four major types of neuroendocrine tumors: small-cell neuroendocrine, large cell neuroendocrine, and typical and atypical carcinoids. Typical carcinoids grow slowly and rarely spread beyond the lungs. Atypical carcinoids, which are rare, exhibit more rapid growth and are more likely to spread to other organs. The location of the carcinoid tumor (i.e., central, peripheral, or endobronchial) dictates the treatment approach; however, prognosis following resection for this tumor depends on an R0 resection (i.e., gross and microscopic complete tumor removal) and regional node dissection.

Squamous cell carcinomas arise from metaplastic squamous cells because squamous cells are absent from the normal epithelium. Adenocarcinomas arise from Clara cells or type 2 pneumocytes, the precursors of bronchioles and alveoli, respectively. Large cell cancers consist of poorly differentiated cells. Mucoepidermoid tumors arise from tracheobronchial mucous glands and have similar cellular features to mucoepidermoid tumors that originate in the salivary glands.

Identifying the specific histologic subtype confirms the diagnosis and can, in addition, provide important information with respect to molecular markers which may impact prognosis and treatment. However the more important distinction for clinical management and treatment outcomes, as mentioned above, is between SCLC and NSCLC. The chapters of Parts 11 and 12 focus on the surgical management of NSCLC.

CLINICAL PRESENTATION NSCLC

Patients are candidates for surgical resection when there is a diagnosis or reasonable probability of NSCLC. Despite the disparate histology, these patients share similar prognosis and are managed with a unique staging system discussed below. Primary NSCLC tumors are often peripheral and grow more slowly than SCLC. Symptomatic manifestations of local disease in NSCLC include cough, hemoptysis, chest pain, dyspnea, wheezing, and pneumonia. Symptoms of locally advanced disease include hoarseness, phrenic nerve paralysis, dysphagia, stridor, superior vena cava syndrome, pleural effusion, pericardial effusion, Pancoast syndrome, evidence of lymphangitic spread, and cancer cachexia. Manifestations of extrathoracic spread include brain metastases, bone metastases, and spread to liver, adrenal glands, and intraabdominal lymph nodes. At clinical presentation, 60% to 75% of patients have cough, weight loss, or dyspnea. Hemoptysis, chest or bone pain, fever, and weakness occur slightly less often.[35] The physical examination foretells advanced disease if, among other signs, there is evidence of lymphadenopathy in the supraclavicular or cervical regions, percussion dullness suggesting a pleural effusion, or neck vein distention from superior vena cava obstruction (Table 68-4).[35]

TNM STAGING SYSTEM FOR LUNG CANCER

All cancers follow a progression from primary tumor to local invasion to systemic metastasis which is achieved through lymphatic, or hematogenous dissemination, or a combination of both. This is particularly relevant to thoracic malignancies because the pulmonary lymphatic system drains in an orderly progression along the bronchi to the hilum and then to the mediastinal nodes. This lends greater accuracy to both staging and prognostic correlation for cancer resections by anatomic lobar dissection with hilar and mediastinal node removal. The confounding difficulty is that skip metastases can occur in up to 25% of patients. The staging system used for NSCLC lung cancers[9] defines the extent of disease based on the size of the tumor (T), the extent of nodal involvement (N) (Fig. 68-3), and the presence of distant metastases (M). The TNM concept was proposed originally by Denoix in the 1940s and later adopted by the American Joint Committee on Cancer and the International Union Against Cancer in 1986. The system has been revised several times in recent years.

The current version (edition 7) was revised by the International Association for the Study of Lung Cancer (IASLC) in

Table 68-4

CLINICAL MANIFESTATIONS OF LUNG CANCER

Symptoms related to primary tumor	
Cough	Central airway cancer causing postobstructive pneumonia or lymph node enlargement
Dyspnea	Early indication of tumor in main airway; may be associated with unilateral wheeze
Hemoptysis	Blood-streaked sputum, rarely severe; usually accompanied by abnormal chest x-ray
Chest pain	Nonspecific, aching pleuritic pain may indicate spread to pleural surface
Symptoms related to intrathoracic spread of primary tumor	
Nerves	Recurrent laryngeal nerve, usually the left side, causes hoarseness with poor expectoration and cough and an increased risk of aspiration
	Phrenic nerve; elevated hemidiaphragm on chest x-ray, breathlessness
	Brachial plexus; Pancoast or superior sulcus tumor; causes pain, muscle wasting, and cutaneous temperature change over the involved nerve root (eighth cervical or first and second thoracic)
	Sympathetic chain and stellate ganglion; Horner syndrome; causes unilateral enophthalmos, ptosis, diminished pupil size, and ipsilateral loss of facial sweating
Chest wall	Dull persistent pain not related to breathing or cough; retrosternal pain indication of massive hilar or mediastinal nodal involvement; severe and localized pain usually indicative of direct invasion of pleural or chest wall by primary or a rib metastasis
Pleura	Pleuritic chest pain, an early sign of malignant pleural effusion; pain disappears after appearance of pleural effusion; identified on physical examination by dullness to percussion and decreased breath sounds; also indicates pleural extension of disease or involvement of mediastinal nodes
SVCO	Superior vena cava obstruction; an indication of a small-cell lung cancer that has invaded the SVC
Heart and pericardium	Usually involves pericardium rather than heart; an indication of metastatic disease by direct lymphatic spread
Esophagus	Enlargement of hilar or mediastinal nodes
Symptoms related to extrathoracic metastatic spread	
Bones	Pain; may occur in any bone but usually involves axial skeleton and proximal long bones
Liver	Weakness and weight loss; rarely produces abnormal liver function tests until there is substantial metastatic involvement
Adrenal	Usually discovered during staging studies or procedures; rarely produces renal insufficiency
Brain and spinal cord	Spinal cord metastases usually also involve brain metastases, which may produce headache, nausea, vomiting, and other neurologic symptoms, including personality change
Lymph nodes and skin	Palpable subcutaneous lymphadenopathy; amenable to fine-needle aspiration

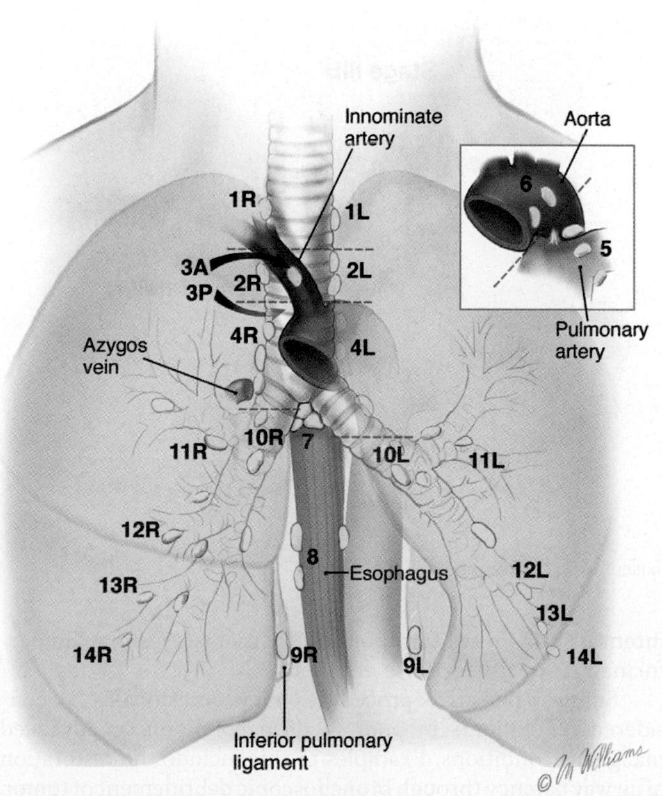

Figure 68-3. Regional lymph node stations.

2010 resulting in several changes in TNM descriptors, which have caused a stage shift for certain patient groups. Caution is warranted when using this system in the clinical setting. There is a common misperception that a change in stage automatically yields a change in disease management. This belief is unfounded as the revised classification system does not provide any direct information about the superiority of one treatment approach over another. It does provide a superior tool for describing tumor characteristics. If properly used, it should aid comparative analysis in clinical research. However, only the results of clinical trials of particular treatments in defined patient populations can remain the basis for selecting optimal treatment approach (Fig. 68-4).

The TNM classification of malignant tumors consists of eight stages from early-stage carcinoma in situ to late-stage disease. These stages are shown in Figure 68-5 and the recommendations for the treatment of lung cancer are based on clinical outcomes which are stage specific. These are reviewed in Chapter 69. Stage I and II: early-stage lung cancer is treated by surgical resection. Patients with stage III tumors (i.e., locally advanced) may be possible surgical candidates on a case-by-case basis. This is primarily determined by the extent of local invasion with respect to T status and node status. Surgery for advanced local invasion with tumor infiltration of mediastinal structures such as the superior vena cava or the carina may be warranted if specific criteria are met. Surgery should be avoided for tumors involving unresectable mediastinal structures such as the great

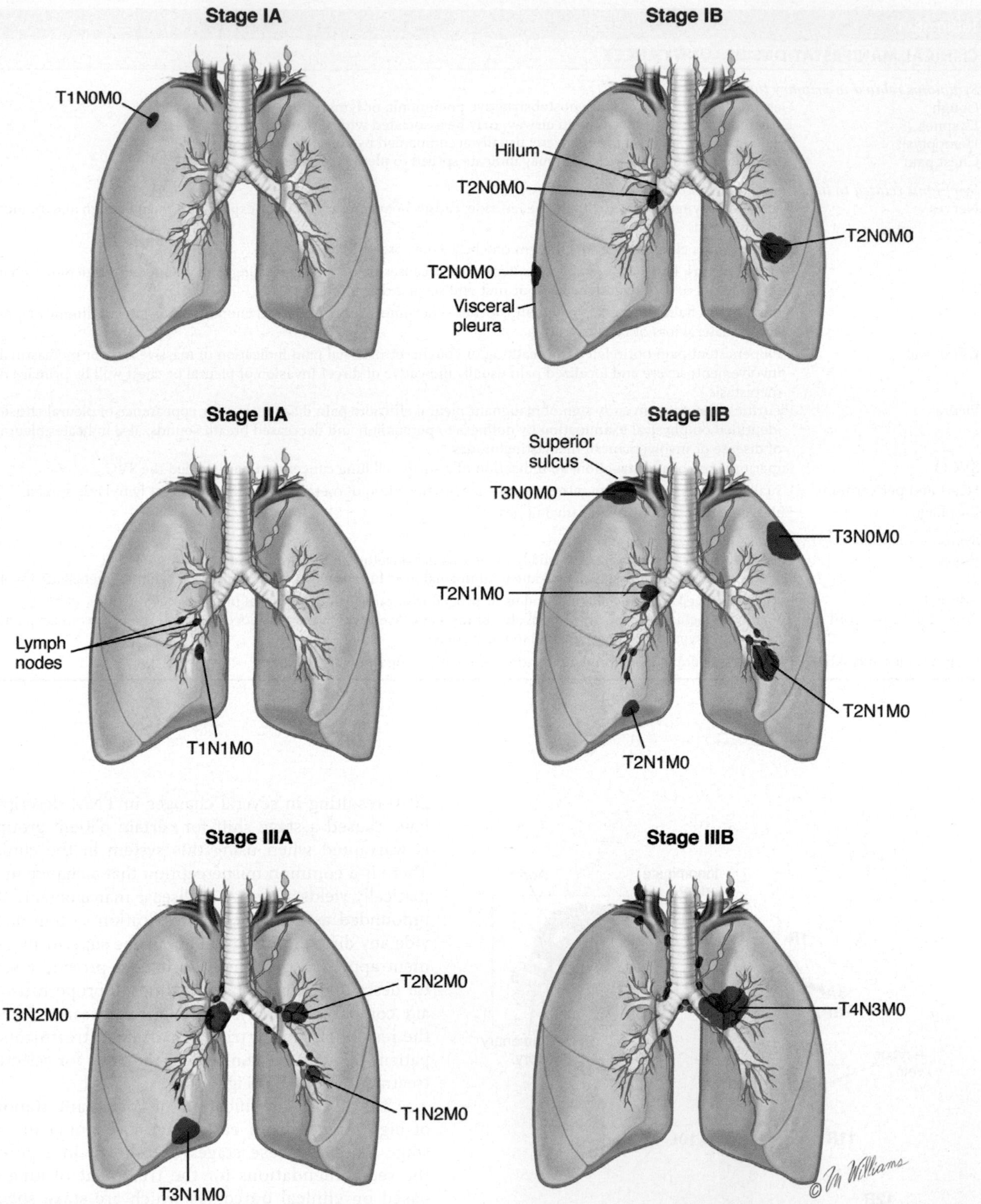

Figure 68-4. Location of tumor based on stage groupings.

vessels, the esophagus, or the heart, or advanced multinodal mediastinal disease. An R0 resection (complete microscopic and macroscopic disease resection) is the goal of all stage I and II resections. Surgical resection for stage IV NSCLC (i.e., extensive metastatic spread) is usually contraindicated except in the uncommon scenario of surgery for oligometastatic disease, whereby resection with curative intent of proven solitary pulmonary metastases may be performed if specific criteria are met.

Surgical palliative procedures may occasionally be considered for patients in poor medical condition or advanced malignant conditions. Examples of this include the restoration of airway patency through bronchoscopic debridement of tumor, photodynamic therapy, airway stenting, or brachytherapy.

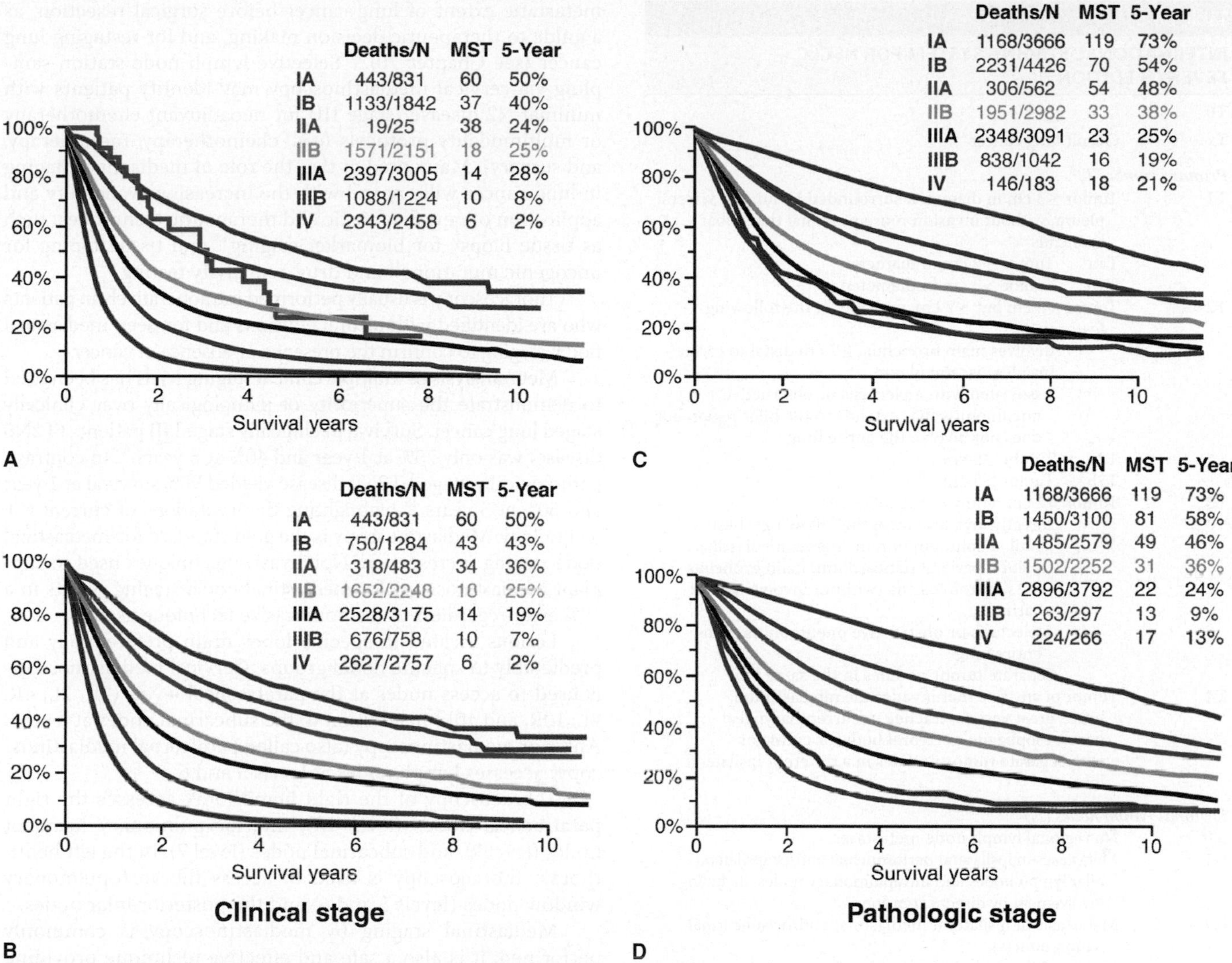

Deaths/N MST 5-Year
IA 443/831 60 50%
IB 1133/1842 37 40%
IIA 19/25 38 24%
IIB 1571/2151 18 25%
IIIA 2397/3005 14 28%
IIIB 1088/1224 10 8%
IV 2343/2458 6 2%
100%
80%
60%
40%
20%
0%
0 2 4 6 8 10
Survival years
A
Deaths/N MST 5-Year
IA 1168/3666 119 73%
IB 2231/4426 70 54%
IIA 306/562 54 48%
IIB 1951/2982 33 38%
IIIA 2348/3091 23 25%
IIIB 838/1042 16 19%
IV 146/183 18 21%
Survival years
C
Deaths/N MST 5-Year
IA 443/831 60 50%
IB 750/1284 43 43%
IIA 318/483 34 36%
IIB 1652/2248 18 25%
IIIA 2528/3175 14 19%
IIIB 676/758 10 7%
IV 2627/2757 6 2%
Survival years
Clinical stage
B
Deaths/N MST 5-Year
IA 1168/3666 119 73%
IB 1450/3100 81 58%
IIA 1485/2579 49 46%
IIB 1502/2252 31 36%
IIIA 2896/3792 22 24%
IIIB 263/297 13 9%
IV 224/266 17 13%
Survival years
Pathologic stage
D

Figure 68-5. Survival curves for clinical and pathologic staging comparing the sixth edition of the TNM Classification of Malignant Tumors with amendments to the seventh edition proposed by the International Association of the Study of Lung Cancer. (Modified with permission from Goldstraw P, Crowley J, Chansky K, et al. The IASLC Lung Cancer Staging Project: proposals for the revision of the TNM stage groupings in the forthcoming (seventh) edition of the TNM classification of malignant tumours. *J Thorac Oncol.* 2007;2:706–714.)

DIAGNOSTIC STUDIES AND STAGING METHODS

Noninvasive radiologic evaluation begins with a chest x-ray and chest CT scan through the adrenal glands to assess and determine the size of the lesion, involvement of surrounding structures, and overall resectability (Table 68-5). The sensitivity of CT scanning for detecting lung cancer is between 50% and 80%. MRI, once thought to hold promise as a diagnostic tool, is usually reserved for advanced anatomic problems when the results of CT scanning are ambiguous and for delineation of CNS metastases.[36] PET scanning has high sensitivity (range: 79%–95%) for detecting lung cancers, particularly distant metastatic disease, but a lower specificity for disease determination. Integrated CT/PET is both sensitive and specific, yielding 98% correct tumor staging compared with final histopathologic staging. These technologies are expanding, but the instruments are expensive and not as widely available as CT.[37] Although CT scanning remains the mainstay of clinical staging, CT scanning alone is inaccurate because it has a limited ability to determine mediastinal nodal involvement, chest wall invasion, mediastinal invasion, and malignancy of pleural effusions.[37,38]

A number of staging and diagnostic procedures have evolved using bronchoscopy. Invasive bronchoscopic procedures include transbronchial needle aspiration, endobronchial ultrasound biopsy (EBUS-FNA), endoesophageal ultrasound fine-needle aspiration (EUS-FNA), and transbronchial and transesophageal needle biopsy. Although radiologic reconstructions of the bronchi and trachea are useful adjuncts to operative planning, bronchoscopy is recommended before every surgical resection as an aid to identifying anatomic abnormalities that might interfere with surgical resection and to confirm the accuracy of noninvasive study by determining the proximal extent of the tumor (i.e., distance from the carina). It is also valuable in identifying occult synchronous disease or anatomic variants of normal.

Invasive preresectional surgical staging, pioneered by the Thoracic Surgical Group of Toronto, is routine practice in many centers.[39,40] Mediastinal staging via mediastinoscopy was conceived originally to spare the morbidity of an exploratory thoracotomy.[39] It is used presently to document the nodal

Table 68-5

INTERNATIONAL STAGING SYSTEM FOR NSCLC, SEVENTH EDITION

T0		
Tx	Occult lung cancer	
Primary tumor (T)		
T1	Tumor ≤3 cm in diameter, surrounded by lung or visceral pleura, without invasion more proximal than lobar bronchus	
	T1a	Tumor ≤2 cm in diameter
	T1b	Tumor >2 cm in diameter
T2	Tumor >3 cm but ≤7 cm, with any of the following features:	
		Involves main bronchus, ≥2 cm distal to carina
		Invades visceral pleura
		Associated with atelectasis or obstructive pneumonitis that extends to the hilar region but does not involve the entire lung
	T2a	Tumor ≤5 cm
	T2b	Tumor >5 cm
T3	Tumor >7 cm or any of the following:	
		Directly invades any of the following: chest wall, diaphragm phrenic nerve, mediastinal pleura, parietal pericardium, main bronchus <2 cm from carina (without involvement of carina)
		Atelectasis or obstructive pneumonitis of the entire lung
		Separate tumor nodules in the same lobe
T4	Tumor of any size that invades the mediastinum, heart, great vessels, trachea, recurrent laryngeal nerve, esophagus, vertebral body, or carina or with separate tumor nodules in a different ipsilateral lobe	
Regional lymph nodes (N)		
N0	No regional lymph node metastases	
N1	Metastases in ipsilateral peribronchial and/or ipsilateral hilar lymph nodes and intrapulmonary nodes, including involvement by direct extension	
N2	Metastasis in ipsilateral mediastinal and/or subcarinal lymph node(s)	
N3	Metastasis in contralateral mediastinal, contralateral hilar, ipsilateral or contralateral scalene, or supraclavicular lymph node(s)	
Distant metastasis (M)		
M0	No distant metastasis	
M1	Distant metastasis	
	M1a	Separate tumor nodule(s) in a contralateral lobe; tumor with pleural nodules or malignant pleural or pericardial effusion
	M1b	Distant metastasis present (includes metastatic tumor nodules in a different lobe from the primary tumor)
Stage groupings of TNM subsets		
Stage IA	T1a–T1bN0M0	
Stage IB	T2aN0M0	
Stage IIA	T1a–T1bN1M0	
	T2bN0M0	
Stage IIB	T2bN1M0	
	T3N0M0	
Stage IIIA	T–T3N2M0	
	T4N0–N1M0	
Stage IIIB	T4N2M0	
	T1a–T4N3M0	
Stage IV	Any T, any N, M1a or M1b	

Source: Adapted from Krivinka R, Kubik A. [Cigarette smoking and the risk of lung cancer]. *Cesk Zdrav.* 1971;19(2):57–61.

metastatic extent of lung cancer before surgical resection, as a guide to therapeutic decision making, and for restaging lung cancer (see Chapter 70).[41] Selective lymph node station sampling via cervical mediastinoscopy may identify patients with minimal N2 disease (stage III) for neoadjuvant chemotherapy or multimodality protocols (e.g., chemotherapy, radiotherapy, and surgery). Many predict that the role of mediastinal staging in lung cancer will expand with the increasing availability and application of new diagnostic and therapeutic techniques, such as tissue biopsy for biomarker staging[42] and tissue typing for oncogenic mutations[43] and drug-sensitivity testing.[44]

Thoracoscopy is usually performed intraoperatively in patients who are identified with pleural effusions and for deep mediastinal nodal staging to confirm the presence or absence of cancer.

Meta-analysis of multiple clinical staging trials has been used to demonstrate the superiority of pathologically over clinically staged lung cancer. Survival in clinically staged IB patients (T2N0 disease) was only 75% at 1 year and 40% at 5 years.[45] In contrast, pathologically staged T2N0 disease yielded 90% survival at 1 year and 60% at 5 years,[45] highlighting the limitations of current CT technology. Mediastinoscopy is the gold standard for mediastinal node staging preresection. Noninvasive techniques used to supplant mediastinoscopy for mediastinal nodal staging results in a 10% error regardless of the noninvasive technique used.

Lesions located in specific lobes drain preferentially and predictably to specific nodal groups. Cervical mediastinoscopy is used to access nodes at the paratracheal levels (2R, 2L, 4R, 4L, 10R, and 10L) in addition to the subcarinal nodes at level 7. Anterior mediastinoscopy (also called parasternal mediastinoscopy) accesses lymph nodes at levels 5 and 6.

Thoracoscopy of the right hemithorax accesses the right paratracheal nodes (level 4R), inferior pulmonary ligament nodes (level 9), and subcarinal nodes (level 7). In the left hemithorax, thoracoscopy is used to access the aortopulmonary window nodes (levels 5 and 6) and the posterior hilar nodes.

Mediastinal staging by mediastinoscopy is commonly performed; it is also a safe and effective technique providing important histologic information with minimal morbidity. It is usually performed on an outpatient basis. It is currently indicated for patients with lung cancer suspected to have spread to the mediastinal nodes to provide accurate histologic lymph node staging and it is used to guide therapy. Patients not suspected of having mediastinal lymph node involvement may be staged with preoperative CT/PET and/or intraoperative thoracoscopic staging if appropriate to confirm the absence of mediastinal malignancy. The drawbacks to preresectional staging with mediastinoscopy are twofold: it requires general anesthesia and delays the surgical resection.

PREOPERATIVE ASSESSMENT

Preoperatively, all patients must undergo pulmonary function testing to assess their overall fitness for surgery and to predict postoperative outcome. These studies include forced vital capacity (FVC), forced expiratory volume in 1 second (FEV_1), and diffusion capacity of carbon monoxide (DLCO). The FEV_1 then is used to calculate the predicted postoperative FEV_1. A $ppoFEV_1$ of 0.8 to 1.0 L or more is desired for lung resection of any kind. This value is the product of FEV_1 and the percent of lung parenchyma that will remain after resection. Residual lung parenchyma can be estimated by the percent of remaining pulmonary lobes (x of 5) or remaining anatomic pulmonary segments (x of 18) or estimated percent of remaining ventilation or perfusion based on the $\dot{V}/\dot{Q}$ scan.

STANDARD PULMONARY RESECTIONS

Depending on the size, location, and extent, the lesion may be resected using an anatomic (e.g., lobectomy, pneumonectomy, bilobectomy, or sleeve lobectomy) or nonanatomic (e.g., segmentectomy, wedge resection, precision cautery, or metastasectomy) resection (Chapters 70–79). These can all be performed by an open technique or with minimal access surgery. Lobectomy is the standard anatomic resection for NSCLC when the lesion occurs within the boundary of an anatomic lobe (see Chapter 71). The most common technique begins with a thoracotomy incision followed by hilar division of the lobar pulmonary arteries, draining pulmonary lobar veins, and associated bronchus. This is followed by meticulous dissection of hilar lymph nodes and lymphatics, which then are removed en bloc with the specimen lobe as a single unit. Alternatively, a sternotomy incision may be used for access to bilateral pleural spaces, mediastinum, and anterior hila in the presence of bilateral pulmonary nodules. This approach and muscle sparing thoracotomies are associated with decreased postoperative pain. They may be used for early-stage I or II NSCLC.

MINIMALLY INVASIVE SURGICAL TECHNIQUES

Less-invasive pulmonary resections using video-assisted thoracic surgery technique, thoracoscopy, and other minimally invasive surgical techniques have improved the morbidity of surgical resection and afford surgery in patients with compromised pulmonary function The benefits of these techniques include shorter postoperative stay, reduced narcotic requirements for postoperative pain management, reduced shoulder dysfunction compared with patients undergoing thoracotomy, and greater patient satisfaction.

LUNG CANCER SURGERY IN THE ELDERLY

More than half of all cancers are diagnosed in patients aged 65 years or older, yet the risk of surgery is greatest in this group. Paradoxically, elderly patients also have a higher rate of early-stage cancer detection compared with younger adults. Lung-sparing resections using minimally invasive techniques, such as limited thoracoscopic wedge resection, are increasingly being offered to elderly patients (age >65 years) who have impaired or diminished respiratory function along with other comorbid conditions that make them unfit for pneumonectomy or lobectomy.[46] Postoperatively, pulmonary complications have been identified as the major cause of morbidity and mortality after surgery in elderly patients. It is reasonable to assume that a reduction in pulmonary complications through the use of less-invasive lung-sparing procedures will lead to a decrease in morbidity and mortality in the elderly age group.

FIVE-YEAR SURVIVAL IN RESECTABLE NSCLC

The importance and value of accurate staging are evident in studies that report cumulative 5-year survival rates for NSCLC. Broadly estimated, average 5-year survival for all stages combined is 16%. This low survival rate has improved only minimally from earlier years despite multiple new modalities of treatment over the last 50 years. For stage I and II disease combined, it is 52%; however, for early-stage disease (stage IA) it may be as high as 80%. Examined individually, these reports demonstrate considerable variability. Reviews published before the 1997 revision of the TNM staging system differ from reports published thereafter, reflecting the expansion of stages I and II (i.e., stage IAB and IIAB) and the reassignment of certain stage III patients to stage IIB based on prognosis. A report published in 1995 estimated that the 5-year cumulative survival rate for patients with stage I (A + B) disease was 64.6%, and for those with stage II disease it was 41.2%.[47] Naruke et al.[48] and Mountain[45] independently evaluated 5-year survival in stage I (A + B) and stage II (A + B) disease using the 1997 revised IASLC. A summary of their findings reveals that the 5-year survival in stage I (A + B) disease combined is between 67% and 75%, whereas the limit of survival in stage IIB disease was no better than 38%. This reduced survival for stage II disease reflects the adverse effect of nodal metastasis, which portends aggressive tumor biology and behavior.

Table 68-6

DIAGNOSTIC PROCEDURES USED FOR LUNG CANCER

Noninvasive	CXR CT PET CT/PET
Minimally invasive	EUS EUS/FNA EBUS EBUS/FNA EUS/FNA + EBUS (replacing mediastinoscopy as "gold standard" at some centers)
Surgical	Mediastinoscopy ("gold standard" for lung cancer staging) Video-assisted thoracic thoracotomy Thoracoscopy

CXR, chest x-ray; CT, computed tomography; PET, positron emission tomography; CT/PET, integrated computed tomography and positron emission tomography; EUS, endoscopic ultrasound; EUS/FNA, endoscopic ultrasound with fine-needle aspiration; EBUS, endobronchial ultrasound; EBUS/FNA, combined endobronchial ultrasound and fine-needle aspiration.

SUMMARY

The importance of having a universally adopted international lung cancer staging system, as we do, is most evident when it comes to estimating survival, which is stage specific. It is also of great value when comparing outcomes of multimodality treatment protocols consisting of combinations of surgery, chemotherapy, radiotherapy, and other innovative treatments. Although surgery alone has been the mainstay of treatment for early-stage NSCLC, there is now compelling evidence from randomized trials that neoadjuvant and adjuvant chemotherapy will improve survival for appropriate stage II and IIIA NSCLC patients. There is as well clear evidence that adjuvant chemotherapy is helpful for stage IB tumors greater than 4 cm in diameter. Meaningful analysis of the numerous multimodality treatment protocols would be impossible without a universal staging system. This reliance is increased with the continuing expansion of new and divergent clinical methods to permit earlier lung cancer detection through screening, when surgery has the greatest chance for cure, or to tailor multimodality treatment protocols capable of preventing recurrence and improving survival.

References

1. Siegel R, Naishadham D, Jemal A. Cancer statistics, 2013. *CA Cancer J Clin.* 2013;63(1):11–30.
2. Ferlay J, Shin HR, Bray F, et al. Estimates of worldwide burden of cancer in 2008: GLOBOCAN 2008. *Int J Cancer.* 2010;127(12):2893–2917.
3. Murray N, Turrisi AT 3rd. A review of first-line treatment for small-cell lung cancer. *J Thorac Oncol.* 2006;1(3):270–278.
4. Okamoto H, Watanabe K, Kunikane H, et al. Randomised phase III trial of carboplatin plus etoposide vs split doses of cisplatin plus etoposide in elderly or poor-risk patients with extensive disease small-cell lung cancer: JCOG 9702. *Br J Cancer.* 2007;97(2):162–169.
5. Aupérin A, Arriagada R, Pignon JP, et al. Prophylactic cranial irradiation for patients with small-cell lung cancer in complete remission. Prophylactic Cranial Irradiation Overview Collaborative Group. *N Engl J Med.* 1999;341(7):476–484.
6. Slotman B, Faivre-Finn C, Kramer G, et al. Prophylactic cranial irradiation in extensive small-cell lung cancer. *N Engl J Med.* 2007;357(7):664–672.
7. Jett JR, Schild SE, Kesler KA, et al. Treatment of small cell lung cancer: diagnosis and management of lung cancer, 3rd ed: American College of Chest Physicians evidence-based clinical practice guidelines. *Chest.* 2013;143(5 suppl):e400S–e419S.
8. Schreiber D, Rineer J, Weedon J, et al. Survival outcomes with the use of surgery in limited-stage small cell lung cancer: should its role be re-evaluated? *Cancer.* 2010;116(5):1350–1357.
9. Detterbeck FC, Boffa DJ, Tanoue LT. The new lung cancer staging system. *Chest.* 2009;136(1):260–271.
10. Jett JR, Schild KE, Keith RL, et al. Treatment of non-small cell lung cancer, stage IIIB: ACCP evidence-based clinical practice guidelines (2nd edition). *Chest.* 2007;132(3 suppl):266S–276S.
11. Alberg AJ, Brock MV, Ford JG, et al. Epidemiology of Lung Cancer: diagnosis and management of lung cancer, 3rd ed: American College of Chest Physicians evidence-based clinical practice guidelines. *Chest.* 2013;143(5 suppl):e1S–e29S.
12. Pao W, Iafrate AJ, Su Z. Genetically informed lung cancer medicine. *J Pathol.* 2011;223(2):230–240.
13. Jemal A, Murray T, Samuels A, et al. Cancer statistics, 2003. *CA Cancer J Clin.* 2003;53(1):5–26.
14. Doll R, Hill AB. Smoking and carcinoma of the lung; preliminary report. *Br Med J.* 1950;2(4682):739–748.
15. Doll R. Bronchial carcinoma: incidence and aetiology. *Med World.* 1954;80(4):370–391.
16. Doll R, Hill AB. Lung cancer and other causes of death in relation to smoking; a second report on the mortality of British doctors. *Br Med J.* 1956;2(5001):1071–1081.
17. Denissenko MF, Pao A, Tang M, et al. Preferential formation of benzo[a] pyrene adducts at lung cancer mutational hotspots in P53. *Science.* 1996;274(5286):430–432.
18. Fontana RS, Sanderson DR, Miller WE, et al. The Mayo Lung Project: preliminary report of "early cancer detection" phase. *Cancer.* 1972;30(5):1373–1382.
19. Martini N. Results of Memorial Sloan-Kettering lung project. *Recent Results Cancer Res.* 1982;82:174–178.
20. Frost JK, Ball WC Jr, Levin ML, et al. Early lung cancer detection: results of the initial (prevalence) radiologic and cytologic screening in the Johns Hopkins study. *Am Rev Respir Dis.* 1984;130(4):549–554.
21. Krivinka R, Kubik A. [Cigarette smoking and the risk of lung cancer]. *Cesk Zdrav.* 1971;19(2):57–61.
22. Smith RA, Metlin CJ, Davis KJ, et al. American Cancer Society guidelines for the early detection of cancer. *CA Cancer J Clin.* 2000;50(1):34–49.
23. Henschke CI, Mccauley DI, Yankelevitz DF, et al. Early Lung Cancer Action Project: overall design and findings from baseline screening. *Lancet.* 1999;354(9173):99–105.
24. National Lung Screening Trial Research Team, Aberle DR, Adams AM, et al. Reduced lung-cancer mortality with low-dose computed tomographic screening. *N Engl J Med.* 2011;365(5):395–409.
25. National Lung Screening Trial Research Team, Aberle DR, Berg CD, et al. The National Lung Screening Trial: overview and study design. *Radiology.* 2011. 258(1):243–253.
26. Jaklitsch MT, Jacobson FL, Austin JH, et al. The American Association for Thoracic Surgery guidelines for lung cancer screening using low-dose computed tomography scans for lung cancer survivors and other high-risk groups. *J Thorac Cardiovasc Surg.* 2012;144(1):33–38.
27. Jacobson FL, Austin JH, Field JK, et al. Development of The American Association for Thoracic Surgery guidelines for low-dose computed tomography scans to screen for lung cancer in North America: recommendations of The American Association for Thoracic Surgery Task Force for Lung Cancer Screening and Surveillance. *J Thorac Cardiovasc Surg.* 2012;144(1):25–32.
28. De Rienzo A, Yeap BY, Cibas ES, et al. Gene expression ratio test distinguishes normal lung from lung tumors in solid tissue and FNA biopsies. *J Mol Diagn.* 2014;16(2):267—272.
29. Travis W, Brambilla E, Müller-Hermelink H, Harris C. (Eds). World Health Organization Classification of Tumours. Pathology and Genetics of Tumors of the Lung, Pleura, Thymus and Heart. Lyon: IARC Press;2004.
30. Travis WD, Brambilla E, Noguchi M, et al. International association for the study of lung cancer/american thoracic society/european respiratory society international multidisciplinary classification of lung adenocarcinoma. *J Thorac Oncol.* 2011;6(2):244–285.
31. Travis WD. Pathology of lung cancer. *Clin Chest Med.* 2011;32(4):669–692.
32. Travis WD, Brambilla E, Riely GJ. New pathologic classification of lung cancer: relevance for clinical practice and clinical trials. *J Clin Oncol.* 2013;31(8):992–1001.
33. Xu L, Tavora F, Burke A. 'Bronchioloalveolar carcinoma': is the term really dead? A critical review of a new classification system for pulmonary adenocarcinomas. *Pathology.* 2012;44(6):497–505.
34. Yoshizawa A, Motoi N, Riely GJ, et al. Impact of proposed IASLC/ATS/ERS classification of lung adenocarcinoma: prognostic subgroups and implications for further revision of staging based on analysis of 514 stage I cases. *Mod Pathol.* 2011;24(5):653–664.
35. Beckles MA, Spiro SG, Colice GL, et al. Initial evaluation of the patient with lung cancer: symptoms, signs, laboratory tests, and paraneoplastic syndromes. *Chest.* 2003;123(1 suppl):97S–104S.
36. Laurent F, Montaudon M, Corneloup O. CT and MRI of lung cancer. *Respiration.* 2006;73(2):133–142.
37. Lardinois D, Weder W, Hany TF, et al. Staging of non-small-cell lung cancer with integrated positron-emission tomography and computed tomography. *N Engl J Med.* 2003;348(25):2500–2507.
38. Antoch G, Stattaus J, Nemat AT, et al. Non-small cell lung cancer: dual-modality PET/CT in preoperative staging. *Radiology.* 2003;229(2):526–533.
39. Pearson FG. Use of mediastinoscopy in selection of patients for lung cancer operations. *Ann Thorac Surg.* 1980;30(3):205–207.
40. Mentzer S. Mediastinal staging prior to surgical resection. *Oper Tech Thorac Cardiovasc Surg.* 2005;6:152–165.
41. Le Chevalier T, Lynch T. Adjuvant treatment of lung cancer: current status and potential applications of new regimens. *Lung Cancer.* 2004;46(suppl 2):S33–S39.
42. Franklin WA, Carbone DP. Molecular staging and pharmacogenomics. Clinical implications: from lab to patients and back. *Lung Cancer.* 2003;41(suppl 1):S147–S154.
43. Oyama T, Osaki T, Baba T, et al. Molecular genetic tumor markers in non-small cell lung cancer. *Anticancer Res.* 2005;25(2B):1193–1196.
44. Perea S, Hidalgo M. Predictors of sensitivity and resistance to epidermal growth factor receptor inhibitors. *Clin Lung Cancer.* 2004;6(suppl 1):S30–S34.
45. Mountain CF. Revisions in the international system for staging lung cancer. *Chest.* 1997;111(6):1710–1717.
46. Jaklitsch MT, Mery CM, Audisio RA. The use of surgery to treat lung cancer in elderly patients. *Lancet Oncol.* 2003;4(8):463–471.
47. Nesbitt JC, Putnam JB Jr, Walsh GL, et al. Survival in early-stage non-small cell lung cancer. *Ann Thorac Surg.* 1995;60(2):466–472.
48. Naruke T, Tsuchiya R, Kondo H, et al. Implications of staging in lung cancer. *Chest.* 1997;112(4 suppl):242S–248S.

69 Role of the Pathologist and Pathology-Specific Treatment of Lung Cancer

Lucian R. Chirieac and Andrea Wolf

Keywords: Immunohistochemistry, epithelial, mesenchymal, adenocarcinoma, squamous cell carcinoma, small-cell lung cancer, non–small-cell lung cancer, neuroendocrine carcinoma, adenocarcinoma in situ, minimally invasive carcinoma, staging, surgery

A pathologist experienced in thoracic oncology is an essential member of the thoracic team. Surgical resection related to lung cancer and other pulmonary pathology accounts for the largest proportion of current thoracic practice. The goals of pathologic analysis of surgical lung specimens are to classify the lung cancer, determine the extent of its invasion (i.e., pleural, lymphovascular, soft tissue, or chest wall), and establish the status of the surgical margins for cancer involvement.[1] Accurate disease identification and staging are of pinnacle importance to the decision-making process and influence the diagnosis (benign or malignant), course of treatment, selection of optimal surgical approach, and pursuit of appropriate adjuvant and neoadjuvant therapies such as chemotherapy, radiation, and other innovative approaches to treatment. Further, determination of the specific molecular abnormalities of the tumor is critical for predicting sensitivity or resistance to a growing number of drugable targets primarily tyrosine kinase inhibitors (TKIs).[2,3] After a malignancy has been identified, the pathologist must determine whether the tumor is primary or metastatic. Most tumors found in the lung represent metastatic foci from distant primaries, such as breast and colon cancer, as opposed to a primary lung malignancy. While the pathologic features of metastatic versus primary adenocarcinoma may be similar, for example, the treatment course is not. Immunohistochemistry (IHC) is required to make the distinction and has proved to be an invaluable diagnostic adjunct. Primary malignant tumors of the lung are most often of epithelial or mesenchymal origin. The epithelial tumors are broadly divided into small-cell lung cancer (SCLC) and non–small-cell lung cancer (NSCLC). NSCLC is further classified as squamous cell carcinoma (SCC), adenocarcinoma, and large-cell carcinoma (LCC).[4] The World Health Organization (WHO) tumor classification system has historically provided the foundation for the classification of lung tumors, including histologic types, clinical features, staging considerations as well as the molecular, genetic, and epidemiologic aspects of lung cancer.[4–6]

The pathologist plays a fundamental role in the preoperative, intraoperative, and postoperative evaluation. The preoperative evaluation includes examination of one of the following specimens: bronchial brushings, bronchial washings, fine-needle aspiration biopsy, core needle biopsy, endobronchial biopsy, and transbronchial biopsy. Because lung tumors demonstrate a great deal of heterogeneity, accurate classification depends on sampling technique: If the pathology sample is limited, sometimes the only categorization that can be made is the distinction between NSCLC and SCLC. The generic term "non–small-cell lung cancer (NSCLC)" should be avoided as a single diagnostic term. In small biopsy samples of poorly differentiated carcinomas where IHC is used, the following terms are acceptable: "NSCLC favor adenocarcinoma" or "NSCLC favor SCC."[6,7] Mutational testing (e.g., epidermal growth factor receptor [EGFR], anaplastic lymphoma kinases [ALKs]) should be performed in this setting. Lymph node status is one of the most important prognostic features in patients with NSCLC.[8,9] Since mediastinoscopy with pathologic examination of lymph nodes remains the "gold standard" for the evaluation of lymph node status in patients with NSCLC, mediastinal lymph nodes are sampled during the preoperative evaluation and provide information important to staging and therapeutic options.[10–13]

The intraoperative evaluation of the surgical pathology specimen is performed by frozen-section examination, which can be analyzed immediately, and findings are communicated to the operating room. Lobectomy or pneumonectomy specimens are routinely evaluated intraoperatively to determine the status of the surgical resection margin, to diagnose incidental nodules discovered at the time of surgery, and to evaluate regional lymph nodes.

The postoperative evaluation reveals pathologic characteristics necessary for classification of tumor type, staging, and prognostic factors. The pathology diagnostic report should include the histologic classification as described by the WHO for carcinomas of the lung with squamous morphology, neuroendocrine differentiation, and other variant carcinomas. The recently published classification of adenocarcinoma should be used for this tumor subtype in resection specimens and small biopsy specimens.[6] Use of bronchioloalveolar carcinoma (BAC) terminology is strongly discouraged. The parameters considered in the surgical pathology report are histologic type, histopathologic grade, visceral pleural invasion (Fig. 69-1), venous/lymphatic vessel invasion (Fig. 69-2), and involvement of mediastinal lymph nodes and TNM stage groupings.[14]

Although the WHO pathologic classification of lung tumors published in 2004 was the basis for categorizing lung tumors,[5] there were a number of pitfalls that made it difficult to utilize the classification system: (1) the term bronchioloalveolar carcinoma (BAC) was used for widely divergent clinical, radiologic, pathologic, and molecular subsets of patients, (2) the "mixed subtype" category accounted for more than 90% of all resected lung adenocarcinomas, despite great heterogeneity in clinical, radiologic, pathologic, and molecular features, and (3) the WHO classification was based primarily on resection specimens, despite the fact that 70% of patients were presenting in advanced stages where the only type of tissue samples were obtained by biopsy or cytology.

The recent tumor classification system issued in 2011,[6] addresses the inadequacies of the 2004 classification and provides the foundation for tumor diagnosis and patient therapy and a critical basis for epidemiologic, molecular, and clinical

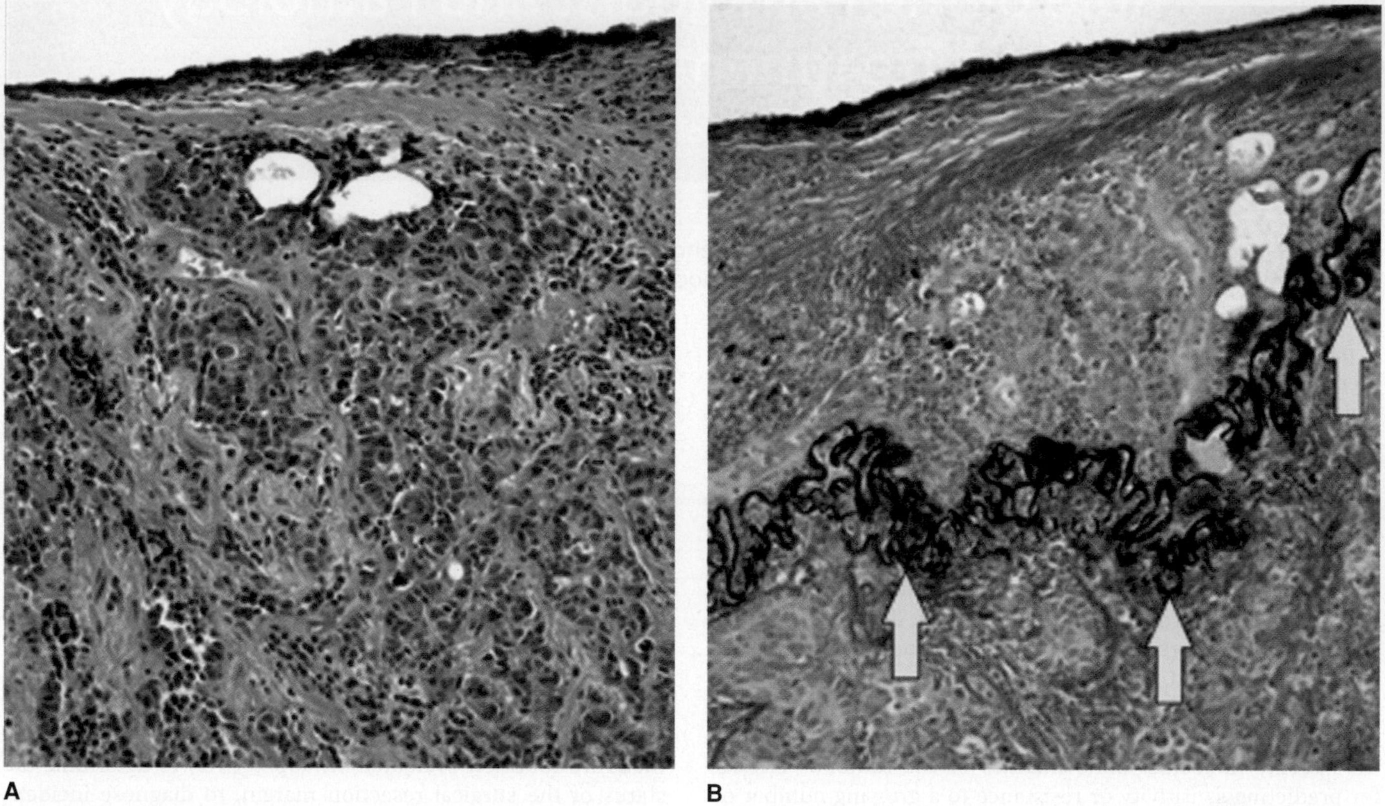

Figure 69-1. Lung adenocarcinoma with invasion of visceral pleura. *A.* Photomicrograph from a lobectomy specimen removed for adenocarcinoma. Tumor cells are invading into the parenchyma and are in the vicinity of the pleura but do not appear to cross over (H&E stain, ×200). *B.* However, an elastic stain highlights the elastic lamina of the visceral pleura (*arrows*) clearly being transected by tumor (elastic Verhoeff stain, ×200).

studies. The most important changes in the 2004 revised classification system were (1) eliminate the term, bronchioloalveolar carcinoma, (2) define the term *adenocarcinoma in situ (AIS)*, (3) define the term *minimally invasive adenocarcinoma (MIA)*, (4) revive the term *lepidic*, (5) promote comprehensive histologic subtyping, (6) emphasize and introduce the term *micropapillary carcinoma*, (7) detach the term mucinous adenocarcinoma, and (8) discourage use of the term NSCLC and subclassify the tumors in as much detail as possible.

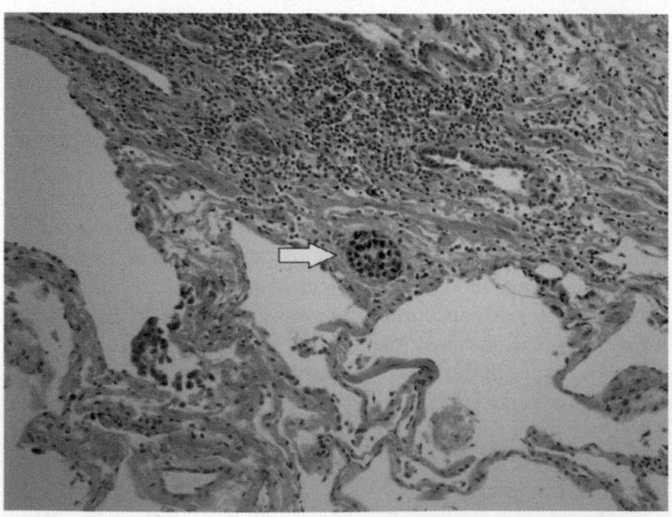

Figure 69-2. Lymphovascular invasion. Photomicrograph from a lobectomy specimen removed for adenocarcinoma illustrating a cluster of tumor cells (*arrow*) present in a vascular space, away from the main tumor mass (H&E stain, ×200).

For the first time in the history of lung cancer evaluation, the classification of lung cancer will be applicable to either (a) resected specimens or (b) small biopsy and cytology specimens. In the revised WHO classification system, (1) lesions attributed to preinvasive lung cancer now include atypical adenomatous hyperplasia (AAH) and AIS (formerly BAC); (2) the term bronchioloalveolar carcinoma (BAC) has been completely eliminated; (3) two new entities, both with favorable prognoses, were added to the category of adenocarcinoma, namely, AIS and MIA; and (4) the formerly known mucinous BAC category was renamed invasive mucinous adenocarcinoma and "shifted" to the category of "Variants of Invasive Adenocarcinoma" (Table 69-1). Since adenocarcinomas are extremely heterogeneous, extensive sampling is necessary to identify each of these histologies in the surgical pathology specimen. The surgical pathology report always should include the histologic classification published by the WHO for carcinomas of the lung (Table 69-2).

In contrast to surgical resections, the biopsy or cytology specimens have a limited amount of tissue and therefore the strategy and prioritization should focus on molecular tests that could identify potentially drugable molecular targets. For tumors that show clear morphologic features of adenocarcinoma or SCC, the standard terms are used. However, if the tumor only shows a carcinoma with no clear squamous or glandular

Table 69-1

ADENOCARCINOMA CLASSIFICATION IN RESECTED SPECIMENS
Preinvasive lesions
Atypical adenomatous hyperplasia
Adenocarcinoma in situ (formerly BAC)
Minimally invasive adenocarcinoma
(≤3 cm lepidic predominant tumor with ≤5 mm invasion)
Nonmucinous, mucinous, mixed mucinous/nonmucinous
Invasive adenocarcinoma
Lepidic predominant (formerly nonmucinous BAC pattern, with >5 mm invasion)
Acinar predominant
Papillary predominant
Micropapillary predominant
Solid predominant
Variants of invasive adenocarcinoma
Invasive mucinous adenocarcinoma (formerly mucinous BAC)
Colloid
Fetal (low and high grade)
Enteric

features (NSCLC-NOS), a minimal immunohistochemical workup is recommended using a single adenocarcinoma marker and squamous marker. At the moment, the best markers for adenocarcinoma and SCC are TTF-1 and p63, respectively.[15] One of the key aspects that potentially impacts radiologists is the need to obtain sufficient tissue not only for diagnosis, but also for molecular studies. This requires a strategic and multidisciplinary approach so the method of biopsy results in either a core biopsy or a cell block from tissue samples obtained for cytology.

LUNG ADENOCARCINOMA

Adenocarcinoma in situ (AIS), formerly BAC, is an important subtype of pulmonary adenocarcinoma. This cancer has received increasing attention in recent years owing to its increasing incidence and rate of sensitivity to epidermal growth factor—TKIs.[16] AIS is a primary lung tumor with a peripheral location, well-differentiated cytology, lepidic growth pattern and a tendency for both aerogenous and lymphatic spread. The key feature is preservation of the underlying architecture of the lung with no invasion.

Minimally invasive adenocarcinoma (MIA) was introduced to define patients with a near 100% 5-year disease-free survival. It is defined as a lepidic predominant tumor measuring 3 cm or less that has an invasive component of 5 mm or less.[17] MIA is characterized by a combination of ground glass opacity (GGO) and a central solid opacity, with the solid component measuring 5 mm or less. Nonmucinous MIA (Fig. 69-3), is more common than mucinous MIA and most often appears as a GGO. Mucinous MIA (Fig. 69-4) appears radiologically as a solid or part-solid nodule.

Invasive adenocarcinoma changes were inserted in the classification of invasive adenocarcinomas. Overtly invasive adenocarcinomas are classified according to the predominant subtype after the use of comprehensive histologic subtyping to estimate the percentages of the various components in a semiquantitative fashion in 5% to 10% increments. The term lepidic predominant adenocarcinoma consists of mixed subtype tumors containing a predominant lepidic growth pattern of type II pneumocytes and/or Clara cells that have an invasive component >5 mm. A micropapillary predominant subtype is added because it has been recognized as a poor prognostic category. Signet ring and clear cell carcinoma subtypes are now recorded as cytologic features whenever present with a comment about the percentage identified.

Table 69-2

WORLD HEALTH ORGANIZATION (WHO) CLASSIFICATION OF LUNG
A. Preinvasive lesions
a. Squamous dysplasia
Carcinoma in situ
b. Atypical adenomatous hyperplasia (AAH)
c. Adenocarcinoma in situ (≤3 cm formerly BAC)
Nonmucinous
Mucinous
Mixed mucinous/nonmucinous
d. Diffuse idiopathic pulmonary neuroendocrine cell hyperplasia
B. Squamous cell carcinoma (SCC)
a. Papillary
b. Clear cell
c. Small cell
d. Basaloid
C. Small-cell lung carcinoma (SCLC)
a. Variant
Combined small-cell carcinoma (small-cell carcinoma and non–small-cell component)
D. Minimally invasive adenocarcinoma (≤3 cm lepidic predominant tumor with ≤5 mm invasion)
a. Nonmucinous
b. Mucinous
c. Mixed mucinous/nonmucinous
E. Adenocarcinoma
a. Lepidic predominant (formerly nonmucinous BAC, with >5 mm invasion)
b. Acinar predominant
c. Papillary predominant
d. Micropapillary predominant
e. Solid predominant with mucin production
F. Variants of invasive adenocarcinoma
a. Invasive mucinous adenocarcinoma (formerly mucinous BAC)
b. Colloid
c. Fetal (low and high grade)
d. Enteric
e. Fetal adenocarcinoma
G. Large-cell carcinoma
Variants
Large-cell neuroendocrine carcinoma
Combined large-cell neuroendocrine carcinoma
Basaloid carcinoma
Lymphoepithelioma-like carcinoma
Clear cell carcinoma
Large-cell carcinoma with rhabdoid phenotype
H. Adenosquamous carcinoma
I. Sarcomatoid carcinoma
Pleomorphic carcinoma
Spindle cell carcinoma
Giant cell carcinoma
Carcinosarcoma
Pulmonary blastoma
J. Carcinoid tumor
Typical carcinoid
Atypical carcinoid
K. Carcinomas of salivary-gland type
Mucoepidermoid carcinoma
Adenoid cystic carcinoma
Others
L. Unclassified carcinoma

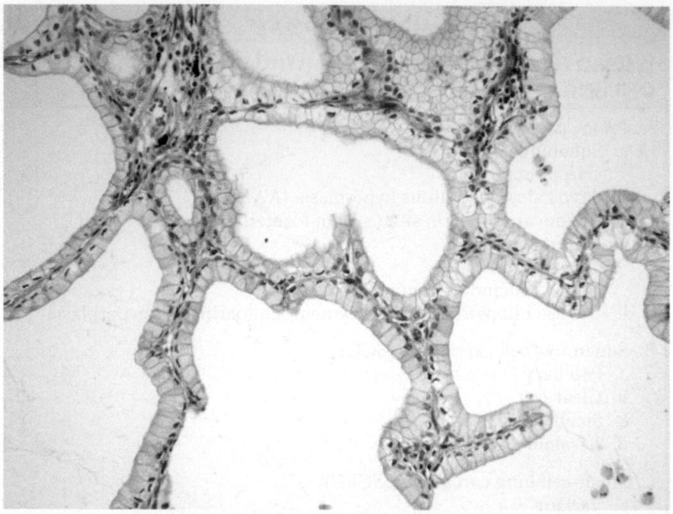

Figure 69-3. Mucinous carcinoma. Respiratory alveoli are lined by malignant mucinous columnar cells arranged in a lepidic growth pattern. The alveolar architecture is preserved (H&E stain, ×200).

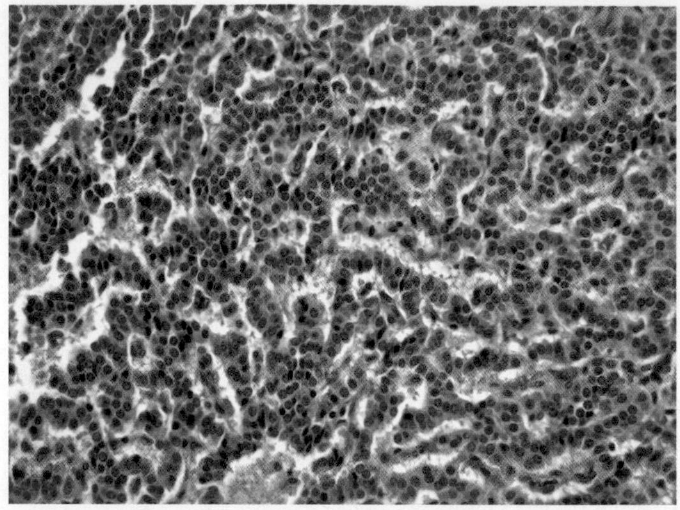

Figure 69-5. Typical carcinoid tumor. This tumor demonstrates cells arranged in cords and tubules with a nesting pattern. The tumor cells have a moderate amount of eosinophilic cytoplasm and nuclei showing finely granular (salt and pepper) chromatin. No necrosis or mitoses are seen (H&E stain, ×400).

Tumors with Neuroendocrine Morphology

Neuroendocrine tumors of the lung are a distinctive subset of lung cancers characterized by varying degrees of neuroendocrine morphologic, immunohistochemical, and ultrastructural features.[18] This category includes a wide spectrum of tumor types: low-grade typical carcinoid (TC) (Fig. 69-5), intermediate-grade atypical carcinoid (AC) (Fig. 69-6), and two high-grade tumors, large-cell neuroendocrine lung carcinoma (LCNEC) (Fig. 69-7) and SCLC (Fig. 69-8).[19] Accurate classification of neuroendocrine tumors has prognostic importance. The grade of malignancy of neuroendocrine tumors progresses in the following order: TC, AC, LCNEC, and SCLC.[19] No prognostic difference was noted between LCNEC and SCLC. The carcinoid nomenclature is preferred by the WHO over terms such as *well-differentiated neuroendocrine carcinoma* because it provides continuity with established terminology familiar to clinicians.[5] In the 2004 WHO classification, TC and AC are categorized together under the heading of *carcinoid tumors;* LCNEC is listed as a subtype of LCC, and SCLC is retained as an independent category. Histologically, the neuroendocrine features consist of an organoid or trabecular growth pattern, peripheral palisading of tumor cells around the periphery of tumor nests, and the formation of rosette structures.

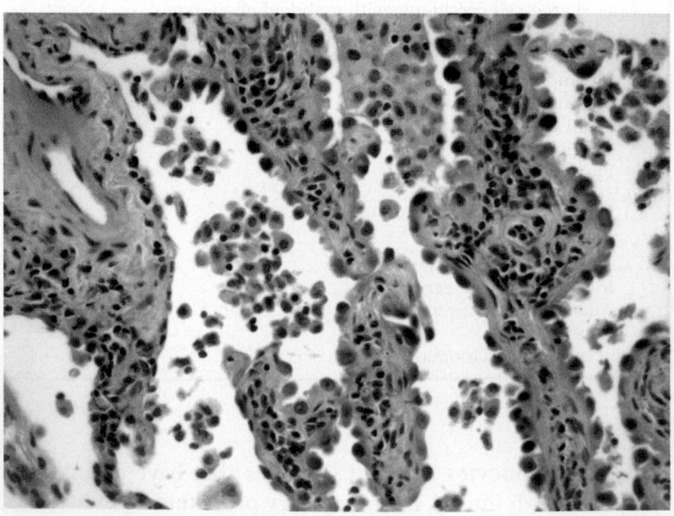

Figure 69-4. Nonmucinous carcinoma. Uniform involvement of the alveolar walls by proliferation of cuboidal cells with severe atypia. The tumor cells have hyperchromatic nuclei with severe atypia protruding into the alveolar spaces in a hobnail growth pattern (H&E stain, ×400).

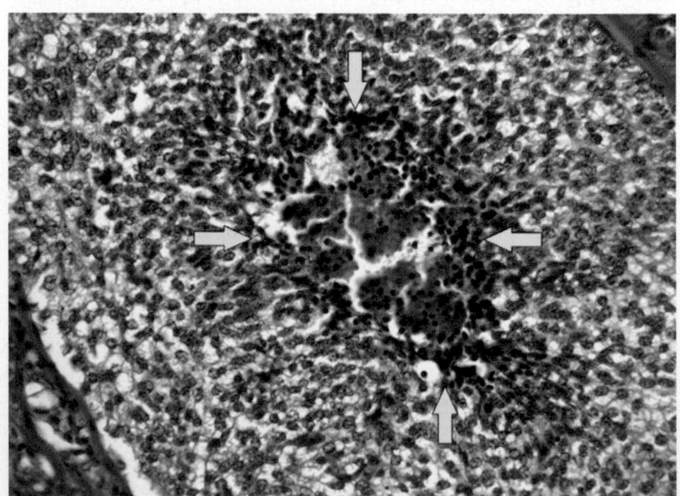

Figure 69-6. Atypical carcinoid tumor. This tumor is defined as a neuroendocrine tumor that meets one of the two criteria: 2 to 10 mitoses per 2 mm^2 or necrosis. Although no mitoses were identified, necrosis was present focally (*arrows*). The tumor cells are atypical, have a moderate amount of eosinophilic cytoplasm, and have nuclei showing finely granular (salt and pepper) chromatin (H&E stain, ×400).

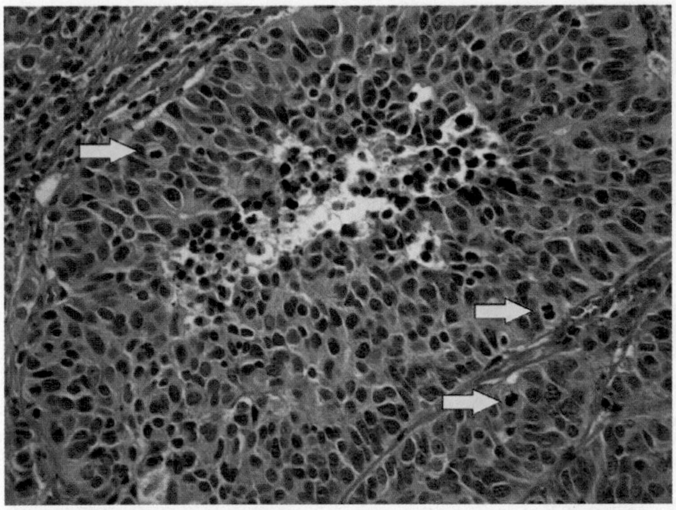

Figure 69-7. LCNEC is defined as a neuroendocrine tumor with greater than 10 mitoses per 2 mm^2 (*arrows*) and cytologic features of large-cell carcinoma. Cells have polygonal shape, abundant cytoplasm, and prominent nucleoli (H&E stain, ×400).

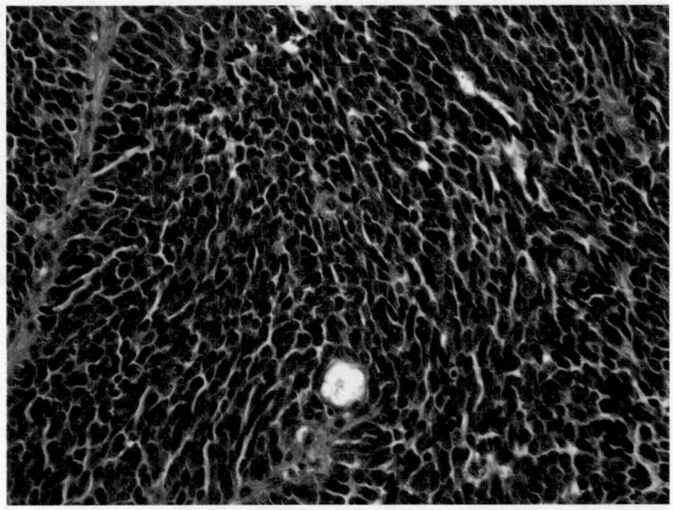

Figure 69-8. Small-cell carcinoma. The tumor consists of sheets of small cells with a brisk mitotic rate, scant cytoplasm, finely granular nuclear chromatin, and inconspicuous or absent nucleoli (H&E stain, ×400).

TC is defined as a neuroendocrine tumor with fewer than 2 mitoses per 2 mm^2 and no necrosis (Fig. 69-5). AC is defined as a neuroendocrine tumor that meets one of the two criteria: 2 to 10 mitoses per 2 mm^2 or necrosis (Fig. 69-6). In contrast to the high-grade neuroendocrine tumors, TC and AC do not occur in combination with other types of carcinoma. The number of mitoses and necrosis may be present only focally within a given tumor. Therefore, accurate classification of carcinoid tumors into TC or AC may not be possible in limited biopsy specimens with scant diagnostic material, and a definite diagnosis may require larger fragments of tumor. In these situations, it is recommended that small biopsies be signed as "carcinoid tumor" and the appropriate classification be performed on thorough examination of the resected specimens.[5,18]

LCNEC is defined as a neuroendocrine tumor with more than 10 mitoses per 2 mm^2 and cytologic features of LCC (Fig. 69-7). These features include cells with polygonal shape, abundant cytoplasm, and prominent nucleoli. Evidence of neuroendocrine differentiation must be demonstrated by performing IHC for the specific neuroendocrine markers chromogranin and synaptophysin.[4] Only tumors that show both neuroendocrine morphology and positive staining should be classified as LCNEC. It is important to note that up to 20% of conventional adenocarcinoma, small-cell carcinoma (SCC), or LCC will stain with neuroendocrine markers. Such tumors have been designated as NSCLC with neuroendocrine differentiation.

SCLC is defined as a neuroendocrine tumor with more than 10 mitoses per 2 mm^2 and small-cell cytologic features (Fig. 69-8). Cells have an oval or vaguely spindled shape and have scant cytoplasm. Nuclei are hyperchromatic and have absent or very small nucleoli (Fig. 69-8). Crush artifact may be prominent on small biopsies, but this is not pathognomonic for the diagnosis of SCC. In larger core biopsies or resected specimens, the cells may appear slightly larger than in a transbronchial biopsy and may have distinct cytoplasm. Numerous prominent nucleoli and large cells should not be seen.

LCNEC and SCLC may occur in combination with other NSCLCs as well as with each other. Such tumors are termed *combined LCNEC*, *combined SCLC*, and *combined SCLC/LCNEC*, respectively.[4,20] While the two high-grade neuroendocrine tumors show numerous similarities, they are retained in separate classifications because LCNEC currently has not been shown to respond to chemotherapy in the same fashion as SCLC. Surgery is the currently preferred treatment for LCNEC, although further studies are ongoing.[21–24]

Immunohistochemical Staining

Although the concordance is generally good between the histologic subtype and the immunophenotype seen in small biopsies compared with surgical resection specimens, caution is advised in attempting to subtype small biopsies with limited material or cases with an ambiguous immunophenotype. IHC should be used to differentiate primary pulmonary adenocarcinoma from SCC or LCC, from metastatic carcinoma, and from malignant mesothelioma; and to determine whether neuroendocrine differentiation is present.[15,25,26] Limited use of IHC studies in small tissue samples is strongly recommended, thereby preserving critical tumor tissue for molecular studies particularly in patients with advanced stage disease. A limited panel of p63 and TTF-1 should suffice for most diagnostic problems.[15]

Differentiation between Primary Pulmonary Adenocarcinoma and Metastatic Adenocarcinoma

The morphologic features of primary adenocarcinoma of the lung may be similar to the features of an adenocarcinoma that is metastatic from a distant primary site. Although the presence of multiple nodules often leads to the presumptive diagnosis of metastases, multifocal adenocarcinoma is not rare and needs to be distinguished from metastases. Furthermore, patients with a solitary pulmonary nodule may have metastatic adenocarcinoma to the lung as the first presentation of disease.

TTF-1 is a homeodomain-containing transcription factor that regulates tissue-specific expression of surfactant apoprotein A, surfactant apoprotein B, surfactant apoprotein C, Clara cell antigen, and T1α. TTF-1 is very important in distinguishing primary from metastatic adenocarcinoma because most of

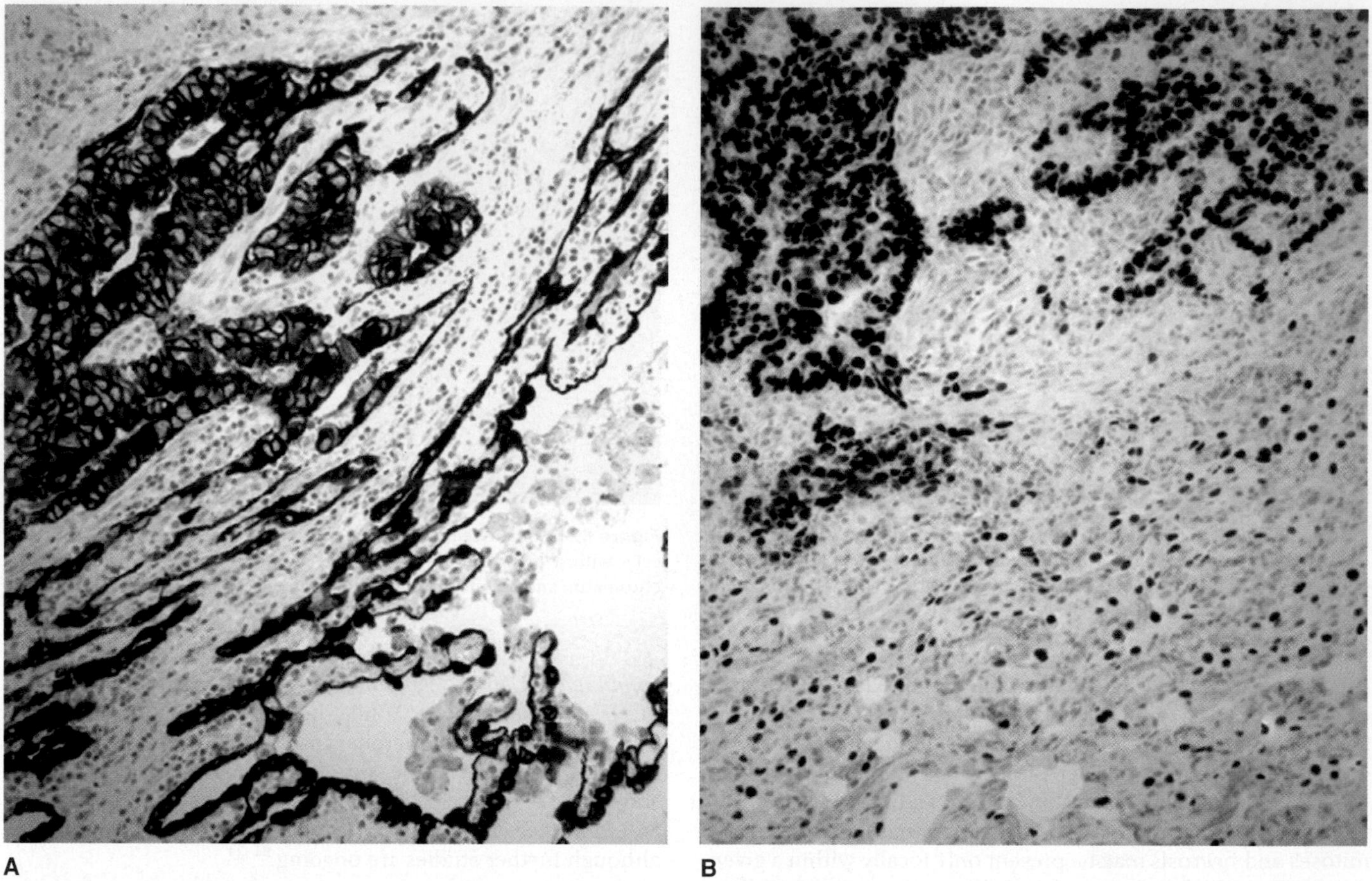

Figure 69-9. Adenocarcinoma from a patient with a solitary lung nodule. The pathologic features of metastatic and primary adenocarcinoma are often indistinguishable. Tumor cells (*upper left corner*) and normal alveolar epithelium (*lower left corner*) are positive for CK7 (*A*) and TTF-1 (*B*).

the cases of primary carcinomas are positive, whereas metastatic adenocarcinoma to lung is virtually always TTF-1 negative (Fig. 69-9A). Lung cancer subtypes have different TTF-1 expression: 75% positive in adenocarcinoma, 85% positive in SCLC, and rarely in the SCC and LCC. Napsin A is an aspartic proteinase expressed in normal type II pneumocytes and in proximal and distal renal tubules and appears to be expressed in >80% of lung adenocarcinomas and may be a useful adjunct to TTF-1.[27] The panel of TTF-1 and p63 (or alternatively p40) may be useful in refining the diagnosis in small biopsy specimens previously classified as NSCLC, not otherwise specified[6] to either adenocarcinoma or SCC.

Although SCC (Fig. 69-10) is usually p63-positive, there is no marker to date that is able to distinguish between primary and metastatic SCC. However, p63 is an important immunostain in cases of poorly differentiated NSCLC, where the distinction between adenocarcinoma and SCC is virtually

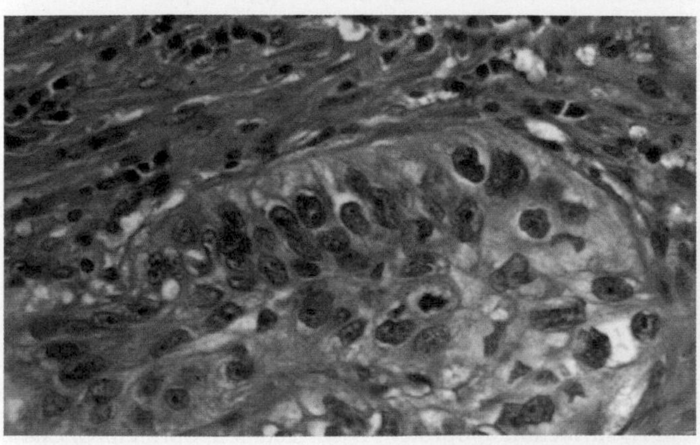

Figure 69-10. Moderately differentiated squamous cell carcinoma (H&E stain, ×200).

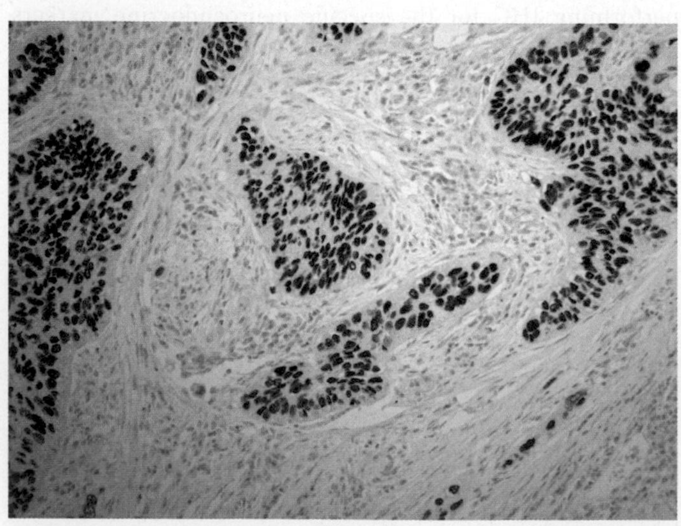

Figure 69-11. In this case of squamous cell carcinoma, the tumor cells are positive for p63 (×200).

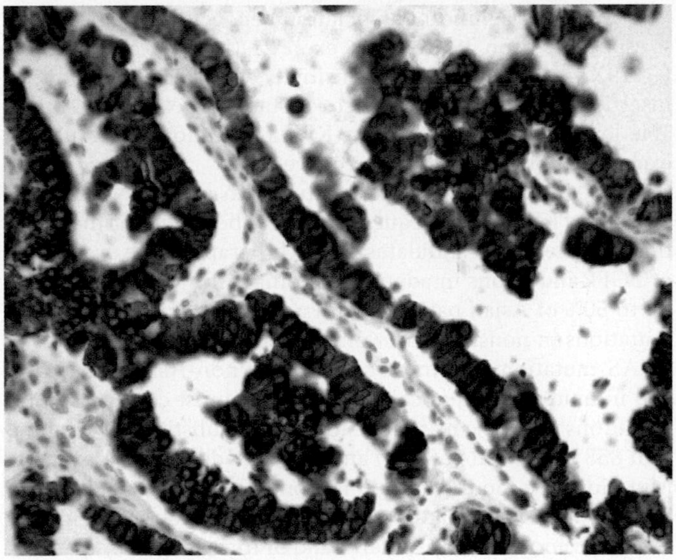

Figure 69-12. Atypical carcinoid tumor positive for synaptophysin (×400).

impossible to make on the basis of H&E-stained slides alone (Fig. 69-11).

CDX-2 is a highly specific and sensitive marker for metastatic gastrointestinal malignancies that could be used to differentiate these gastric entities from primary lung tumors (Fig. 69-9B).

Determining the Neuroendocrine Status of Tumors

CD56, chromogranin (reacts with cytoplasmic neuroendocrine granules), and synaptophysin (reacts with a cell membrane glycoprotein) are used to diagnose the neuroendocrine tumors of the lung. All TC and AC tumors stain with chromogranin and synaptophysin, whereas SCC is negative in 25% of cases (Figs. 69-12 and 69-13). Neuroendocrine markers are valuable in diagnosing *NSCLC with neuroendocrine differentiation,* a specific group of poorly differentiated tumors without a neuroendocrine morphology.

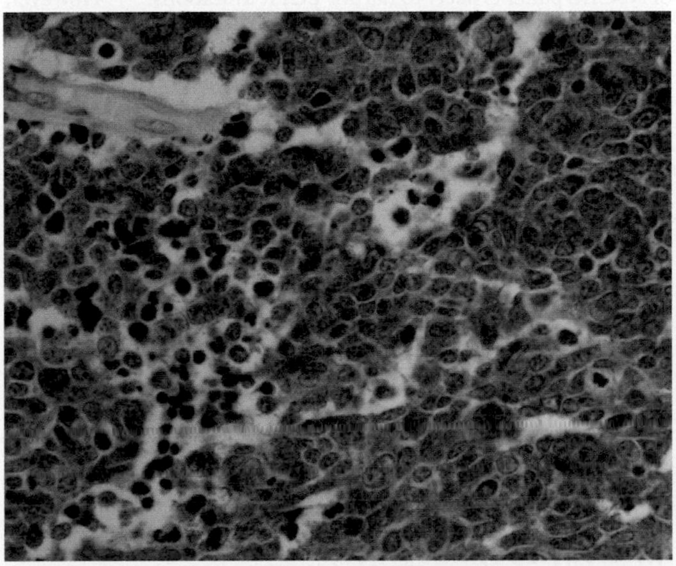

Figure 69-13. Large-cell neuroendocrine carcinoma. Evidence of neuroendocrine differentiation must be demonstrated by performing immunohistochemistry for specific neuroendocrine markers. Tumor cells were positive for synaptophysin (×400).

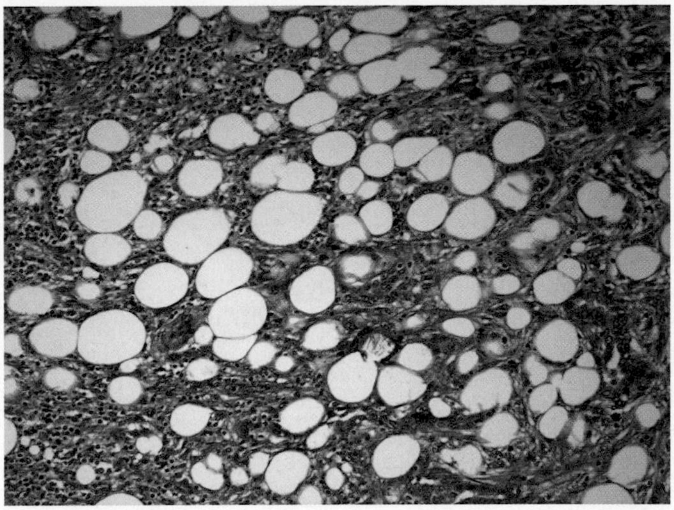

Figure 69-14. Histopathology of diffuse malignant mesothelioma. Malignant tumor cells arranged in tubules and cords invade into the adipose tissue of the chest wall. Invasion into adipose and/or fibrous tissue of the chest wall is an important criterion for the diagnosis of diffuse malignant mesothelioma (H&E stain, ×200).

Distinguishing between Malignant Mesothelioma and Lung Adenocarcinoma

IHC is most valuable in distinguishing between malignant mesothelioma and lung adenocarcinoma. The distinction between pulmonary adenocarcinoma and malignant mesothelioma (epithelioid type) is made by using a panel of markers including two with known immunopositivity in mesothelioma (but negative in adenocarcinoma) and two with known positivity in adenocarcinoma (but negative in mesothelioma).[25] Immunostains relatively sensitive and specific for mesothelioma include WT-1, calretinin, D2–40, HMBE-1, and cytokeratin 5/6 (negative in adenocarcinoma).[28,29] Antibodies immunoreactive in adenocarcinoma include CEA, B72.3, Ber-EP4, MOC-31, CD15, and TTF-1 (negative in mesothelioma). (Figs. 69-14–69-16)[25].

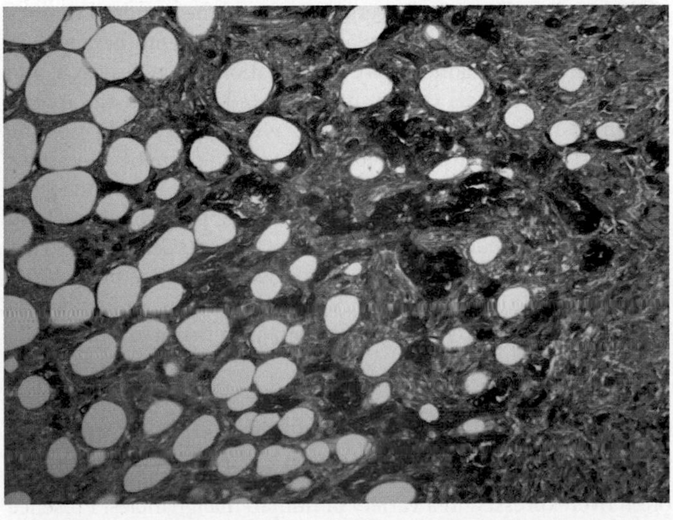

Figure 69-15. In diffuse malignant mesothelioma, the tumor cells are positive for calretinin (×200).

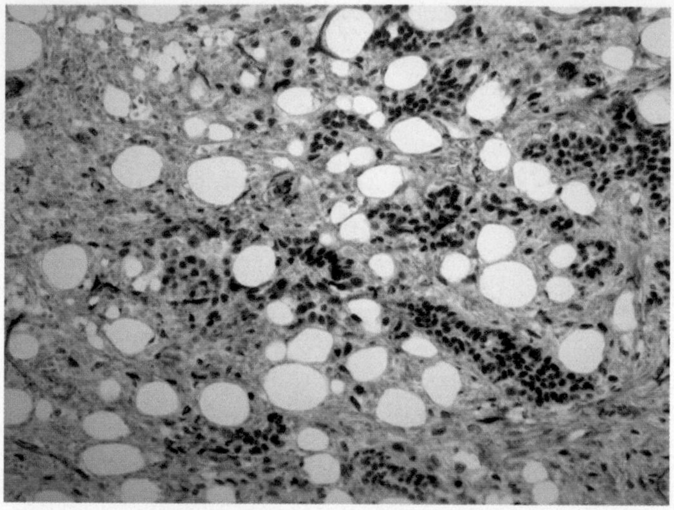

Figure 69-16. Diffuse malignant mesothelioma cells positive for WT-1. Tumor cells have positive nuclear staining (×200).

MOLECULAR DIAGNOSTIC STUDIES IN LUNG CANCER

Discoveries in molecular pathogenetic mechanisms have had a major impact in the field of pulmonary disease, with important implications for the screening, diagnosis, and treatment of lung cancer. Small molecules or chemical compounds modeled on the protein structure of their targets are being actively developed and potentially are powerful therapeutic agents, designed to interfere with critical intracellular signaling pathways.

As a result of all these developments, physicians involved in the care of patients with lung cancer should have an understanding of molecular biology and related techniques to facilitate selection of the most appropriate therapies for their patients, to understand the novel agents and techniques that are under investigation in clinical trials, and to communicate adequately with their increasingly well-informed patients. In addition, it is imperative that institutions and pathology departments bank frozen tissue on a routine basis with patient informed consent because DNA, RNA, and protein extracted from such material is of paramount importance for evaluating genetic information. Lung cancer is one of the most challenging cancers to treat and the standard therapy includes surgical resection, platinum-based chemotherapy, and radiation therapy alone or in combination. New research and ongoing clinical trials involve new targeted therapies and milder treatment regimens that improve survival. Targeted therapeutic agents are based on the concept of discovering genetic alterations and the signaling pathways altered in cancer and have added significantly to our armamentarium to prolong patient survival and minimize drug toxicity. Although improvements seen in the trials are modest, the hope is that an increased number of biomarkers will be available in the near future to help clinicians predict which patients are most likely to benefit from such therapies.

EGFR AND KRAS

EGFR is normally found on the surface of epithelial cells and is often overexpressed in a variety of human malignancies. Presence of EGFR-activating mutations represents a critical biological determinant for proper therapy selection in patients with lung cancer.

There is a significant association between EGFR mutations – especially exon 19 deletion, exon 21 (L858R), and exon 18 (G719X) mutations – and sensitivity to TKIs.[2,30,31] Exon 20 insertion mutation may predict resistance to clinically achievable levels of TKIs. EGFR and KRAS mutations are mutually exclusive in patients with lung cancer.[32]

KRAS mutations are associated with intrinsic TKI resistance, and KRAS gene sequencing could be useful for the selection of patients as candidates for TKI therapy.[33] The prevalence of EGFR mutations in adenocarcinoma is 10% of Western and up to 50% of Asian patients, with a higher frequency of EGFR mutations in nonsmokers, women, and nonmucinous cancers. KRAS mutations are most common in non-Asians, smokers, and in mucinous adenocarcinoma.[34] The most common EGFR mutations result in an arginine for leucine substitution at amino acid 858 in exon 21 (L858R) and in frame deletions at exon 19. Mutations are more common in nonmucinous lung adenocarcinoma with lepidic pattern (formerly BAC pattern) and in lung adenocarcinoma with papillary (and or micropapillary) pattern.

Primary resistance to TKI therapy is associated with KRAS mutation. Acquired resistance is associated with second-site mutations within the EGFR kinase domain, amplification of alternative kinases (such as MET),[35] histologic transformation from NSCLC to SCLC, and epithelial to mesenchymal transition (EMT).

ANAPLASTIC LYMPHOMA KINASE

ALK gene rearrangements[36] represent the fusion between ALK and a variety of partners including echinoderm microtubule-associated protein-like 4 (EML4). ALK fusions have been identified in a subset of patients with NSCLC and represent a unique subset of NSCLC patients for whom ALK inhibitors may be a very effective therapeutic strategy.[37] Crizotinib is an oral ALK inhibitor that was approved by the FDA for patients with locally advanced or metastatic NSCLC who have the ALK gene rearrangement (i.e., ALK positive). ALK NSCLC occurs most commonly in a unique subgroup of NSCLC patients who share many of the clinical features of NSCLC patients likely to harbor EGFR mutations.[38–41] However, for the most part, ALK translocations and EGFR mutations are mutually exclusive.[40] ALK translocations tend to occur in younger patients and in those with more advanced NSCLC while this relationship has not been reported for EGFR mutant NSCLC.[42,43]

The current standard method for detecting ALK NSCLC is fluorescence in situ hybridization (FISH), although other methods are currently being used for rapid screening of lung cancers with ALK rearrangements, including polymerase chain reaction (PCR) and IHC. A big advantage of FISH is that a probe set, developed for the diagnosis of ALK-rearranged anaplastic large-cell leukemia (ALCL), is applicable to the diagnosis of ALK-rearranged lung adenocarcinomas. Recently developed IHC tests are useful for the detection of the majority of ALK-rearranged lung adenocarcinomas.[38,40]

PATHOLOGY-SPECIFIC SURGICAL STRATEGY

Histology-Specific Surgery

Small-cell Lung Cancer

Historically, SCLC has been considered a nonoperative disease. Early randomized studies suggested no benefit to surgery over radiation or chemotherapy only. The Medical Research Council trial published in 1973 evaluated only patients with SCLC involving the bronchus, and complete resection was performed in only 34 of 71 (48%) patients.[44] The Lung Cancer Study Group, Eastern Cooperative Oncology Group (ECOG), and European Organization for Research and Treatment of Cancer published an intergroup trial in 1994, which randomized patients with limited SCLC who had responded to five cycles of chemotherapy (cyclophosphamide, doxorubicin, vincristine), but again these included only patients who had bronchoscopically visible disease. While most of the surgical patients (54 of 70, 77%) underwent complete resection, 35 (50%) surgical patients had cN2 disease, 24 (34%) had pN2 disease, and 12 (17%) were unresectable at the time of surgery.[45] Neither of these studies demonstrating lack of benefit of surgery in "limited" SCLC included patients with early SCLC as defined by modern-day staging techniques, including PET-CT, brain MR, and endobronchial ultrasound (EBUS) or mediastinoscopy for nodal evaluation.

Resection is recommended for early-stage SCLC. Early-stage SCLC comprises a small proportion of an already rare entity. Ten to fifteen percent of lung cancers are SCLC, and only 3% to 7% of these patients present with stage I or II disease, as determined in a SEER database study of all patients diagnosed with lung cancer between 1988 and 2005 and followed for at least 3 months.[46] Resection offers benefit for tumors that prove to be combined or mixed SCLC/NSCLC (10%–30% of SCLC cases). In addition, resection offers the best local control in limited disease. The same SEER database analysis[46] found lobectomy alone (47% 5-year overall survival) to be superior to radiation therapy (17% 5-year overall survival), a finding which was significant on multivariable analysis (HR = 0.56; 95% CI = 0.41–0.76). Other studies have demonstrated similar survival for lobectomy in early-stage SCLC.[47] The National Comprehensive Cancer Network (NCCN) currently recommends lobectomy with mediastinal nodal sampling or dissection for patients with clinical stage I disease to be followed by adjuvant chemotherapy, even if nodes are pathologically negative.[48] Patients treated with complete resection should also undergo prophylactic whole brain irradiation following adjuvant chemotherapy if performance status and neurocognitive function are not impaired, given the high propensity of SCLC to metastasize to the brain.

Carcinoid

Surgical resection is recommended for pulmonary carcinoid, which can be found at all levels from the trachea to the lung periphery.[49] The prognosis for resection of low-grade TC is excellent, with 82% 10-year survival in Wilkins series that spans a 50-year experience[49] as well as in a modern Australian series.[50] Most surgeons advocate a parenchymal-sparing approach, which often mandates sleeve resection (bronchus, carina, or even trachea) to preserve lung for tumors that are frequently central. Peripheral carcinoids can be managed with sublobar resection, including segmentectomy or wedge resection, with good results, as supported by a recent SEER database evaluation of 3270 pulmonary carcinoid patients, in which sublobar resection compared well to lobectomy when assessed for noninferiority in multivariable analysis.[51]

Non–small-cell Lung Cancer

The remaining primary epithelial lung malignancies are NSCLC, including adenocarcinoma, SCC, and others, such as LCC. Treatment for most NSCLCs depends on stage, with surgical resection generally the treatment of choice for early-stage disease. Chapter 71 describes the standard lobectomies for NSCLC isolated to individual lobes. SCCs are frequently central and may necessitate sleeve resection or even pneumonectomy if there is involvement of hilar vessels or bronchi.

In contrast to the other forms of NSCLC, adenocarcinomas are remarkably heterogeneous and recent advancements in molecular genetics, histopathology, and imaging have had significant impact on the treatment of these tumors. Adenocarcinoma represents the most common histology among NSCLC and lung cancer in the United States.[6] Tumors previously identified as BAC, and now defined as AIS or MIA, often demonstrate indolent behavior and favorable long-term survival.[52] Increased understanding of these aspects of tumor biology and the advent of targeted biologic therapy for certain genetic mutations[53] have revolutionized the treatment of patients with AIS, MIA, and adenocarcinoma. These tumors frequently present as nonsolid or subsolid nodules on low-dose chest computed tomography, presenting a conundrum for treating clinicians. Given indolent and multicentric behavior for subsolid nodules, parenchymal-sparing sublobar resection is likely the best surgical approach,[54] but these lesions are frequently not palpable, making wedge resection difficult if possible at all. Anatomic segmentectomy would be preferred, but when a nonsolid adenocarcinoma crosses segmental boundaries, it may necessitate lobectomy, which is suboptimal in the setting of potentially multicentric disease. Whether to follow these preinvasive and early invasive adenocarcinomas with surveillance imaging and when to treat with surgery, radiation, or biologic therapy are areas ripe for further research.[55]

Stage-specific Surgery

Stage I–III NSCLC

Chapter 68 introduced the seventh edition staging system for NSCLC. As discussed above in this chapter, treatment for most early-stage NSCLCs involves surgical resection with lobectomy, segmentectomy, or wedge resection. More advanced stage disease warrants consideration of multimodality therapy, including chemotherapy and external beam radiation.

Adjuvant Chemotherapy Following Surgical Resection

Stage is the major factor influencing whether a patient who undergoes surgical resection for NSCLC should receive adjuvant chemotherapy. Early trials suggested no benefit to adjuvant chemotherapy following resection. The ECOG compared concurrent radiation and cisplatin etoposide with radiation alone following resection of stage II or IIIA NSCLC and found no statistically significant difference in overall survival or recurrence.[56] The Adjuvant Lung Project, Italy randomized 1209 patients who underwent complete resection for stage I, II, or IIIA NSCLC to an adjuvant cisplatin-based regimen (MVP) or observation and likewise found no statistically significant difference in overall or progression-free survival between the two groups[57] following resection for more advanced disease. In the largest randomized-controlled study of adjuvant chemotherapy following surgery, the International Adjuvant Lung Cancer Trial randomized 1867 patients with stage I, II, or III disease to cisplatin-based chemotherapy or observation. Patients receiving adjuvant chemotherapy experienced a significantly higher overall and disease-free survival.[58] Two additional international multicenter randomized studies demonstrated similar benefit for adjuvant cisplatin–vinorelbine doublets: the National Cancer Institute of Canada/National Cancer Institute of the United States Intergroup JBR.10 trial for patients with stage IB or II NSCLC[59] and the Adjuvant Navelbine International Trialist Association (ANITA) Trial for patients with Stage IB, II, or IIIA disease.[60] Of note, the ANITA investigators performed subgroup analyses and survival benefit for adjuvant cisplatin–vinorelbine was only demonstrated with the stage II and IIIA patients (not in stage IA), but the authors felt the numbers were small and the study was not sufficiently powered to evaluate differences for the individual stages.

Therefore, it is generally agreed that for stage II disease (and for those with stage III disease diagnosed upon final pathology following resection), treatment should include anatomic surgical resection followed by adjuvant chemotherapy. Adjuvant chemotherapy is not recommended following resection for stage IA NSCLC. For stage IB disease, the role of adjuvant chemotherapy was evaluated by the Cancer and Leukemia Group B (CALGB) 9633 trial, in which 344 patients with stage IB NSCLC were randomized to receive carboplatin–paclitaxel or observation following lobectomy or pneumonectomy, and no difference in overall survival was found between the groups.[61] On unplanned subgroup analysis, the investigators found a survival benefit of adjuvant chemotherapy for patients with tumors 4 cm or larger, but overall, the study was felt to be underpowered to detect subtle differences in survival given the relatively long survival of these patients compared to those with more advanced disease.

Superior Sulcus (Pancoast) Tumors

Although a few patients with superior sulcus (Pancoast) tumors will have stage II disease (if the lesion is 7 cm or smaller and the hilar and mediastinal nodes are negative), most will have stage IIIA or IIIB disease, depending on the status of the mediastinal nodes. Practice has evolved over time,[62] but superior sulcus tumors are generally treated with induction chemoradiation followed by surgical resection, using the Southwest Oncology Group (SWOG) protocol of cisplatin–etoposide with 45 Gy concurrent radiation followed by en bloc resection of the tumor with lobectomy.[63]

Stage III NSCLC

Stage IIIA NSCLC is a heterogeneous disease that includes four types of pathology: (1) bulky N2 disease; (2) microscopic N2 disease found on preoperative staging; (3) microscopic N2 disease found at the time of or following resection; and (4) T3N1 tumors (hilar nodal disease with tumor involving the chest wall or mainstem bronchus within 2 cm of the carina). Even among individual specialties, such as medical oncology[64] or thoracic surgery,[65] there is little consensus regarding how to treat patients with stage IIIA NSCLC. For patients with bulky N2 disease, this is particularly controversial.

Several randomized trials have been conducted to investigate the best multimodality approach. A recent phase III trial compared radiation to surgery following response to platinum-based induction chemotherapy for patients with histologically proved stage IIIA-N2 NSCLC. Three hundred and thirty-two patients were randomized and results suggested no difference between the two arms, with a median and 5-year overall survival of 16.4 months and 15.7% for resection and 17.5 months and 14% for radiation.[66] The Lung Intergroup Trial 0139 randomized 396 patients with Stage IIIA-N2 NSCLC who underwent two cycles of cisplatin–etoposide with concurrent 45 Gy radiation per the SWOG protocol and deemed fit for surgery to undergo either surgery followed by two more cycles of chemotherapy or additional chemoradiation (for a total of four cycles and 60 Gy). Although progression-free survival was higher for the surgical arm (median 12.8 months vs. 10.5 months, $p = 0.017$), there was no difference in overall survival (23.6 months vs. 22.2 months, for surgery compared to radiation, $p = 0.24$).[67] Nearly all (14 out of 16) of the treatment-related deaths in the surgical arm were following pneumonectomy, prompting a subgroup analysis for patients who underwent lobectomy and not pneumonectomy. In this subgroup, overall survival was higher for patients who underwent lobectomy following induction chemoradiation than for those who underwent definitive chemoradiation. This has led many clinicians to use caution in treating patients with stage IIIA-N2 disease with induction chemoradiation followed by pneumonectomy. The Intergroup 0139 trial also found that a single N2 nodal station (compared to multistation disease) was independently associated with higher survival among surgical patients ($p = 0.009$). This finding suggests that single-station disease behaves differently compared to multistation stage IIIA-N2 disease, supporting the practice of some surgeons to consider primary surgical resection with lymphadenectomy followed by adjuvant chemotherapy or chemoradiation for single-station stage IIIA-N2 disease.

There is even less consensus regarding the treatment of N3 disease, or stage IIIB. A phase II study of a trimodality approach using the SWOG protocol (two cycles of cisplatin–etoposide with concurrent 45 Gy radiotherapy) followed by resection for stable or improved disease was conducted for patients with stage IIIA-N2 and N3 disease.[68] No difference for survival was found for patients with N2 versus N3 disease at diagnosis, with a 3-year survival of 26%, and the strongest predictor of long-term survival was negative nodal status on resection. The SWOG investigators also examined the role of definitive chemoradiation (four cycles of cisplatin–etoposide with concurrent 61 Gy) for patients with stage IIIB NSCLC.[69] The 3-year and 5-year survival percentage for the 50 patients accrued were 17% and 15%, respectively.

A reasonable approach for the four types of N2 disease (Table 69-3) described above is (1) chemoradiation with consideration of surgical resection for bulky N2 disease depending on response to induction therapy; (2) chemotherapy or chemoradiation followed by surgical resection for micrometastatic disease found on preoperative staging; (3) surgical resection followed by chemotherapy or chemoradiation for single-station disease found at the time of surgery (particularly for the left upper lobe and station 4 L) or for multistation disease found

Table 69-3

TREATMENT APPROACH TO NODAL DISEASE IN STAGE IIIA NSCLC

Bulky N2 disease	Chemoradiation with consideration of resection for bulky N2 disease that responds to induction therapy
Microscopic N2 on preoperative staging	Chemotherapy or chemoradiation followed by surgical resection of micrometastatic disease
Microscopic N2 found at time of or following resection	Surgical resection followed by chemotherapy or chemoradiation
T3N1 tumors (hilar nodal disease with tumor involving chest wall or mainstem bronchus within 2 cm of carina)	Chemotherapy or chemoradiation followed by resection if T3N1 disease does not progress on induction therapy

on pathology following resection; and (4) chemotherapy or chemoradiation followed by resection if disease has not progressed for T3N1 disease, with chemoradiation followed by en bloc resection for superior sulcus (Pancoast) tumors.

Stage IV NSCLC

The role of surgery in stage IV disease is traditionally palliative, such as pleurodesis or pleurX catheter placement for NSCLC with malignant pleural effusion. There are particular circumstances, however, in which curative surgery is attempted in the setting of stage IV NSCLC. In a series of 28 patients who underwent extrapleural pneumonectomy (EPP) for pleural dissemination of NSCLC, the median survival for nine patients who had node-negative disease was 52 months (vs. 14 months for those with positive nodes, $p = 0.0003$), suggesting that EPP may prolong survival in NSCLC patients with node-negative malignant pleural effusion (stage IV).[70] Data gathered retrospectively from 14 SWOG trials involving 2531 patients suggest that approximately 7% of patients with metastatic NSCLC present with a solitary metastasis,[71] often called oligometastatic NSCLC. This represents a unique situation in which a multidisciplinary approach of chemotherapy, surgical resection of the lung primary, and treatment of the metastasis with resection, radiotherapy, or both may be used.[72] Generally, this is considered for oligometastases to the brain or the adrenal, but others have reported small series (fewer than 10 patients) of pulmonary resection with metastasectomy for nonbrain, nonadrenal oligometastasis.[73] The data regarding pulmonary resection and oligometastasectomy are retrospective and sparse, with most studies combining metachronous and synchronous presentation of metastases. Whether to perform surgical resection for NSCLC in the setting of oligometastatic disease should be considered on an individual basis in collaboration with other treating physicians and after thorough discussion of treatment options with the patient.

SUMMARY

Surgical excision remains the only therapeutic modality that can cure selected lung cancer patients. The surgical strategy varies depending on histology and stage, in addition to other morphologic and molecular parameters. Pathologists play an important role in the surgical management of patients with lung cancer from preoperative diagnosis and staging, to intraoperative evaluation of the extent of distant disease and margin status, to postoperative assessment of tumor genetic alterations. They offer guidance in selecting appropriate surgical therapies and chemotherapeutic regimens, as well as in identifying morphologic and molecular prognostic markers and predictors of response to therapeutic agents. They are expected to provide accurate diagnosis and classification of the patient's lung cancer. Most important, pathologists are required to provide pathologic staging information in lung resection specimens, surgical resection margin status, and information about lung cancer subtype.

Tumor stage, as determined by current American Joint Committee on Cancer guidelines, is considered to be one of the most important prognostic factors for patients with lung neoplasms. Frozen-section examination of mediastinal lymph nodes obtained by mediastinoscopy is used routinely to determine whether NSCLC patients will undergo tumor excision. Determination of the pT and pN status of the resected surgical pathology specimen determines whether the patient will be treated with postoperative chemotherapy and/or radiation therapy. Furthermore, classification algorithms based on the presence of genetic alterations found in lung cancer can be used to identify drugs or therapeutic agents targeting these alterations.

Investigation and analysis of lung cancer for particular targeted molecular abnormalities expand the expertise of the pulmonary oncologic pathologist, who in addition to conventional pathologic analysis of surgical lung specimens will determine the molecular abnormalities of lung cancer that may be able to predict for sensitivity and resistance to various chemotherapeutic agents and targeted therapies.

EDITOR'S COMMENT

With the new WHO criteria published in 2011, pathologists, pulmonologists, and thoracic surgeons are relearning the nomenclature that defines lung cancer. This is particularly pertinent in the era of molecular targeted therapy, where gene mutations, rather than pathology, better define the treatment to which an individual patient is likely to respond. That said, the differentiation between squamous NSCLC and other nonsquamous pathologies appears to be a crucial first step, as the types of chemotherapy chosen for first-line therapy differ between these entities. Although most surgeons still recommend surgery for all NSCLC patients, there is now an increasing awareness of the potential role of surgery even in some SCLC patients. Likewise, if a patient is found to have NSCLC with neuroendocrine features, some medical oncologists would suggest an SCLC-type regimen in the neoadjuvant or adjuvant setting. An additional area of major change is the reclassification of BAC as AIS, with different degrees of invasion and lepidic spread. This will probably have a huge impact on the management of GGO on radiographic imaging in the future. Finally, use of molecular marker panels are now recommended by NCCN guidelines, at least for patients with metastatic disease, both to determine prognosis and to help choose appropriate chemo/biologic therapy.

—Mark J. Krasna

References

1. Fosella F, Putnam J, Komaki R, eds. *Lung Cancer.* New York, NY: Springer; 2003.
2. Cappuzzo F, Ligorio C, Toschi L, et al. EGFR and HER2 gene copy number and response to first-line chemotherapy in patients with advanced non-small cell lung cancer (NSCLC). *J Thorac Oncol.* 2007;2:423–429.
3. Eberhard DA, Johnson BE, Amler LC, et al. Mutations in the epidermal growth factor receptor and in KRAS are predictive and prognostic indicators in patients with non-small-cell lung cancer treated with chemotherapy alone and in combination with erlotinib. *J Clin Oncol.* 2005;23:5900–5909.
4. Travis WD, Linnoila RI, Tsokos MG, et al. Neuroendocrine tumors of the lung with proposed criteria for large-cell neuroendocrine carcinoma. An ultrastructural, immunohistochemical, and flow cytometric study of 35 cases. *Am J Surg Pathol.* 1991;15:529–553.
5. Travis W, Brambilla E, Muller-Hermelink H, Harris C, eds. Pathology and genetics of tumours of the lung, pleura, thymus and heart. Lyon: International Agency for Research on Cancer (IARC); 2004.
6. Travis WD, Brambilla E, Noguchi M, et al. International association for the study of lung cancer/american thoracic society/european respiratory society international multidisciplinary classification of lung adenocarcinoma. *J Thorac Oncol.* 2011;6:244–285.
7. Travis WD, Brambilla E, Noguchi M, et al. International Association for the Study of Lung Cancer/American Thoracic Society/European Respiratory Society: international multidisciplinary classification of lung adenocarcinoma: executive summary. *Proc Am Thorac Soc.* 2011;8:381–385.
8. Faries MB, Bleicher RJ, Ye X, et al. Lymphatic mapping and sentinel lymphadenectomy for primary and metastatic pulmonary malignant neoplasms. *Arch Surg.* 2004;139:870–876; discussion 6–7.
9. Rea F, Marulli G, Callegaro D, et al. Prognostic significance of main bronchial lymph nodes involvement in non-small cell lung carcinoma: N1 or N2? *Lung Cancer.* 2004;45:215–220.
10. Okubo K, Kato T, Hara A, et al. Imprint cytology for detecting metastasis of lung cancer in mediastinal lymph nodes. *Ann Thorac Surg.* 2004;78:1190–1193.
11. Semik M, Netz B, Schmidt C, Scheld HH. Surgical exploration of the mediastinum: mediastinoscopy and intraoperative staging. *Lung Cancer.* 2004;45 (Suppl 2):S55–S61.
12. Sihoe AD, Yim AP. Lung cancer staging. *J Surg Res.* 2004;117:92–106.
13. Marchevsky AM. Problems in pathologic staging of lung cancer. *Arch Pathol Lab Med.* 2006;130:292–302.
14. Gephardt GN, Baker PB. Lung carcinoma surgical pathology report adequacy: a College of American Pathologists Q-Probes study of over 8300 cases from 464 institutions. *Arch Pathol Lab Med.* 1996;120:922–927.
15. Rekhtman N, Ang DC, Sima CS, et al. Immunohistochemical algorithm for differentiation of lung adenocarcinoma and squamous cell carcinoma based on large series of whole-tissue sections with validation in small specimens. *Mod Pathol.* 2011;24:1348–1359.
16. Jackman DM, Chirieac LR, Janne PA. Bronchioloalveolar carcinoma: a review of the epidemiology, pathology, and treatment. *Semin Respir Crit Care Med.* 2005;26:342–352.
17. Terasaki H, Niki T, Matsuno Y, et al. Lung adenocarcinoma with mixed bronchioloalveolar and invasive components: clinicopathological features, subclassification by extent of invasive foci, and immunohistochemical characterization. *Am J Surg Pathol.* 2003;27:937–951.
18. Beasley MB, Brambilla E, Travis WD. The 2004 World Health Organization classification of lung tumors. *Semin Roentgenol.* 2005;40:90–97.
19. Asamura H, Kameya T, Matsuno Y, et al. Neuroendocrine neoplasms of the lung: a prognostic spectrum. *J Clin Oncol.* 2006;24:70–76.
20. Nicholson SA, Beasley MB, Brambilla E, et al. Small cell lung carcinoma (SCLC): a clinicopathologic study of 100 cases with surgical specimens. *Am J Surg Pathol.* 2002;26:1184–1197.
21. Iyoda A, Hiroshima K, Baba M, et al. Pulmonary large cell carcinomas with neuroendocrine features are high-grade neuroendocrine tumors. *Ann Thorac Surg.* 2002;73:1049–1054.
22. Takei H, Asamura H, Maeshima A, et al. Large cell neuroendocrine carcinoma of the lung: a clinicopathologic study of eighty-seven cases. *J Thorac Cardiovasc Surg.* 2002;124:285–292.
23. Zacharias J, Nicholson AG, Ladas GP, et al. Large cell neuroendocrine carcinoma and large cell carcinomas with neuroendocrine morphology of the lung: prognosis after complete resection and systematic nodal dissection. *Ann Thorac Surg.* 2003;75:348–352.
24. Rossi G, Cavazza A, Marchioni A, et al. Role of chemotherapy and the receptor tyrosine kinases KIT, PDGFRalpha, PDGFRbeta, and Met in large-cell neuroendocrine carcinoma of the lung. *J Clin Oncol.* 2005;23:8774–8785.
25. Husain AN, Colby T, Ordoñez N, et al. Guidelines for pathologic diagnosis of malignant mesothelioma: 2012 update of the consensus statement from the international mesothelioma interest group. *Arch Pathol Lab Med.* 2013.137:647–667.
26. Mukhopadhyay S, Katzenstein AL. Subclassification of non-small cell lung carcinomas lacking morphologic differentiation on biopsy specimens: utility of an immunohistochemical panel containing TTF-1, napsin A, p63, and CK5/6. *Am J Surg Pathol.* 2011;35:15–25.
27. Jagirdar J. Application of immunohistochemistry to the diagnosis of primary and metastatic carcinoma to the lung. *Arch Pathol Lab Med.* 2008;132: 384–396.
28. Chirieac LR, Pinkus GS, Pinkus JL, et al. The immunohistochemical characterization of sarcomatoid malignant mesothelioma of the pleura. *Am J Cancer Res.* 2011;1:14–24.
29. Ordonez NG. D2-40 and podoplanin are highly specific and sensitive immunohistochemical markers of epithelioid malignant mesothelioma. *Hum Pathol.* 2005;36:372–380.
30. Paez JG, Janne PA, Lee JC, et al. EGFR mutations in lung cancer: correlation with clinical response to gefitinib therapy. *Science.* 2004;304:1497–1500.
31. Sequist LV, Joshi VA, Janne PA, et al. Response to treatment and survival of patients with non-small cell lung cancer undergoing somatic EGFR mutation testing. *Oncologist.* 2007;12:90–98.
32. Riely GJ, Politi KA, Miller VA, et al. Update on epidermal growth factor receptor mutations in non-small cell lung cancer. *Clin Cancer Res.* 2006;12:7232–7241.
33. Shigematsu H, Gazdar AF. Somatic mutations of epidermal growth factor receptor signaling pathway in lung cancers. *Int J Cancer.* 2006;118:257–262.
34. Finberg KE, Sequist LV, Joshi VA, et al. Mucinous differentiation correlates with absence of EGFR mutation and presence of KRAS mutation in lung adenocarcinomas with bronchioloalveolar features. *J Mol Diagn.* 2007;9:320–326.
35. Benedettini E, Sholl LM, Peyton M, et al. Met activation in non-small cell lung cancer is associated with de novo resistance to EGFR inhibitors and the development of brain metastasis. *Am J Pathol.* 2010;177:415–423.
36. Cataldo KA, Jalal SM, Law ME, et al. Detection of t(2;5) in anaplastic large cell lymphoma: comparison of immunohistochemical studies, FISH, and RT-PCR in paraffin-embedded tissue. *Am J Surg Pathol.* 1999;23: 1386–1392.
37. Kwak EL, Bang YJ, Camidge DR, et al. Anaplastic lymphoma kinase inhibition in non-small-cell lung cancer. *N Engl J Med.* 2010;363:1693–1703.
38. Mino-Kenudson M, Chirieac LR, Law K, et al. A novel, highly sensitive antibody allows for the routine detection of ALK-rearranged lung adenocarcinomas by standard immunohistochemistry. *Clin Cancer Res.* 2010;16:1561–1571.
39. Sasaki T, Rodig SJ, Chirieac LR, Janne PA. The biology and treatment of EML4-ALK non-small cell lung cancer. *Eur J Cancer.* 2010;46: 1773–1780.
40. Rodig SJ, Mino-Kenudson M, Dacic S, et al. Unique clinicopathologic features characterize ALK-rearranged lung adenocarcinoma in the western population. *Clin Cancer Res.* 2009;15:5216–5223.
41. Shaw AT, Yeap BY, Mino-Kenudson M, et al. Clinical features and outcome of patients with non-small-cell lung cancer who harbor EML4-ALK. *J Clin Oncol.* 2009;27:4247–4253.
42. Inamura K, Takeuchi K, Togashi Y, et al. EML4-ALK lung cancers are characterized by rare other mutations, a TTF-1 cell lineage, an acinar histology, and young onset. *Mod Pathol.* 2009;22:508–515.
43. Wong DW, Leung EL, So KK, et al. The EML4-ALK fusion gene is involved in various histologic types of lung cancers from nonsmokers with wild-type EGFR and KRAS. *Cancer.* 2009;115:1723–1733.
44. Fox W, Scadding JG. Medical Research Council comparative trial of surgery and radiotherapy for primary treatment of small-celled or oat-celled carcinoma of bronchus. *Ten-year follow-up. Lancet.* 1973;2:63–65.
45. Lad T, Piantadosi S, Thomas P, et al. A prospective randomized trial to determine the benefit of surgical resection of residual disease following response of small cell lung cancer to combination chemotherapy. *Chest.* 1994;106:320S–323S.

46. Varlotto JM, Recht A, Flickinger JC, et al. Lobectomy leads to optimal survival in early-stage small cell lung cancer: a retrospective analysis. *J Thorac Cardiovasc Surg*. 2011;142:538–546.
47. Vallieres E, Shepherd FA, Crowley J, et al. The IASLC lung cancer staging project: proposals regarding the relevance of TNM in the pathologic staging of small cell lung cancer in the forthcoming (seventh) edition of the TNM classification for lung cancer. *J Thorac Oncol*. 2009;4:1049–1059.
48. NCCN. Guidelines. In: http://www.nccn.org/professionals/physician_gls/pdf/scic.pdf; 2013.
49. Wilkins EW Jr, Grillo HC, Moncure AC, et al. Changing times in surgical management of bronchopulmonary carcinoid tumor. *Ann Thorac Surg*. 1984;38:339–344.
50. Cao C, Yan TD, Kennedy C, et al. Bronchopulmonary carcinoid tumors: long-term outcomes after resection. *Ann Thorac Surg*. 2011;91:339–343.
51. Fox M, Van Berkel V, Bousamra M 2nd, et al. Surgical management of pulmonary carcinoid tumors: sublobar resection versus lobectomy. *Am J Surg*. 2013;205:200–208.
52. Sakurai H, Maeshima A, Watanabe S, et al. Grade of stromal invasion in small adenocarcinoma of the lung: histopathological minimal invasion and prognosis. *Am J Surg Pathol*. 2004;28:198–206.
53. Lynch TJ, Bell DW, Sordella R, et al. Activating mutations in the epidermal growth factor receptor underlying responsiveness of non-small-cell lung cancer to gefitinib. *N Engl J Med*. 2004;350:2129–2139.
54. Wolf AS, Richards WG, Jaklitsch MT, et al. Lobectomy versus sublobar resection for small (2 cm or less) non-small cell lung cancers. *Ann Thorac Surg*. 2011;92:1819–1823; discussion 24–25.
55. Naidich DP, Bankier AA, MacMahon H, et al. Recommendations for the management of subsolid pulmonary nodules detected at CT: a statement from the Fleischner Society. *Radiology*. 2013;266:304–317.
56. Keller SM, Adak S, Wagner H, et al. A randomized trial of postoperative adjuvant therapy in patients with completely resected stage II or IIIA non-small-cell lung cancer. eastern Cooperative Oncology Group. *N Engl J Med*. 2000;343:1217–1222.
57. Scagliotti GV, Fossati R, Torri V, et al. Randomized study of adjuvant chemotherapy for completely resected stage I, II, or IIIA non-small-cell Lung cancer. *J Natl Cancer Inst*. 2003;95:1453–1461.
58. Arriagada R, Bergman B, Dunant A, et al. Cisplatin-based adjuvant chemotherapy in patients with completely resected non-small-cell lung cancer. *N Engl J Med*. 2004;350:351–360.
59. Winton T, Livingston R, Johnson D, et al. Vinorelbine plus cisplatin vs. observation in resected non-small-cell lung cancer. *N Engl J Med*. 2005; 352:2589–2597.
60. Douillard JY, Rosell R, De Lena M, et al. Adjuvant vinorelbine plus cisplatin versus observation in patients with completely resected stage IB-IIIA non-small-cell lung cancer (Adjuvant Navelbine International Trialist Association [ANITA]): a randomised controlled trial. *Lancet Oncol*. 2006;7: 719–727.
61. Strauss GM, Herndon JE 2nd, Maddaus MA, et al. Adjuvant paclitaxel plus carboplatin compared with observation in stage IB non-small-cell lung cancer: CALGB 9633 with the Cancer and Leukemia Group B, Radiation Therapy Oncology Group, and North Central Cancer Treatment Group Study Groups. *J Clin Oncol*. 2008;26:5043–5051.
62. Attar S, Krasna MJ, Sonett JR, et al. Superior sulcus (Pancoast) tumor: experience with 105 patients. *Ann Thorac Surg*. 1998;66:193–198.
63. Rusch VW, Giroux DJ, Kraut MJ, et al. Induction chemoradiation and surgical resection for superior sulcus non-small-cell lung carcinomas: long-term results of Southwest Oncology Group Trial 9416 (Intergroup Trial 0160). *J Clin Oncol*. 2007;25:313–318.
64. Tanner NT, Gomez M, Rainwater C, et al. Physician preferences for management of patients with stage IIIA NSCLC: impact of bulk of nodal disease on therapy selection. *J Thorac Oncol*. 2012;7:365–369.
65. Veeramachaneni NK, Feins RH, Stephenson BJ, et al. Management of stage IIIA non-small cell lung cancer by thoracic surgeons in North America. *Ann Thorac Surg*. 2012;94:922–926; discussion 6–8.
66. van Meerbeeck JP, Kramer GW, Van Schil PE, et al. Randomized controlled trial of resection versus radiotherapy after induction chemotherapy in stage IIIA-N2 non-small-cell lung cancer. *J Natl Cancer Inst*. 2007;99:442–450.
67. Albain KS, Swann RS, Rusch VW, et al. Radiotherapy plus chemotherapy with or without surgical resection for stage III non-small-cell lung cancer: a phase III randomised controlled trial. *Lancet*. 2009;374:379–386.
68. Albain KS, Rusch VW, Crowley JJ, et al. Concurrent cisplatin/etoposide plus chest radiotherapy followed by surgery for stages IIIA (N2) and IIIB non-small-cell lung cancer: mature results of Southwest Oncology Group phase II study 8805. *J Clin Oncol*. 1995;13:1880–1892.
69. Albain KS, Crowley JJ, Turrisi AT 3rd, et al. Concurrent cisplatin, etoposide, and chest radiotherapy in pathologic stage IIIB non-small-cell lung cancer: a Southwest Oncology Group phase II study, SWOG 9019. *J Clin Oncol*. 2002;20:3454–3460.
70. Sugarbaker D, Tilleman T, Swanson S, et al. The role of extrapleural pneumonectomy in the management of pleural cancers (abstract). *J Clin Oncol*. 2009;27:15 s.
71. Albain KS, Crowley JJ, LeBlanc M, Livingston RB. Survival determinants in extensive-stage non-small-cell lung cancer: the Southwest Oncology Group experience. *J Clin Oncol*. 1991;9:1618–1626.
72. Pfannschmidt J, Dienemann H. Surgical treatment of oligometastatic non-small cell lung cancer. *Lung Cancer*. 2010;69:251–258.
73. Ambrogi V, Tonini G, Mineo TC. Prolonged survival after extracranial metastasectomy from synchronous resectable lung cancer. *Ann Surg Oncol*. 2001;8:663–666.

PART 11

STANDARD PULMONARY RESECTIONS

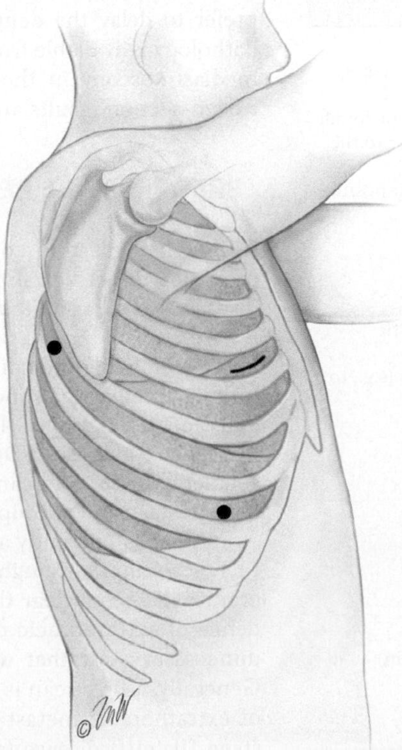

70 Techniques for Staging and Restaging of Lung Cancer

Edward Hong and Michael J. Liptay

Keywords: Mediastinoscopy, endobronchial ultrasound (EBUS), endoscopic esophageal ultrasound (EUS), VATS staging

Lung cancer is the leading cause of cancer death in the United States in both men and women. In 2011, there were an estimated 221,000 new cases of lung cancer and 156,900 estimated deaths owing to the disease.[1] When indicated, surgery is the most effective curative therapy for lung cancer. For patients with limited non–small-cell lung cancer (NSCLC), lung resection remains the therapy of choice, offering the greatest potential for cure and long-term survival. Surgery also may play a limited role in small-cell lung cancer. However, of patients who present initially with lung cancer, 55% have distant metastatic disease, 30% have disease spread to regional lymph nodes, and only 15% have disease confined to the lung.[2] Thus, accurate staging in lung cancer is an essential component of management and prognosis.

After primary tumor diagnosis, in addition to evaluating for distant spread and assessing lung reserve and comorbidities, evaluation of the mediastinum and mediastinal lymph nodes is vital to defining tumor stage and subsequent surgical planning. Despite advances in technology, mediastinoscopy remains an important tool for the thoracic surgeon in the staging of bronchogenic carcinoma, as well as in the diagnosis of disease in the mediastinum, as described in Chapter 156.

Originally described by Carlens in 1959,[3] mediastinoscopy has been the subject of a number of studies. It has been shown to be a safe procedure, with morbidity rates between 0.6% and 3.7% and mortality rates ranging from 0% to 3% in several large series.[4] In comparison with noninvasive diagnostic procedures, such as CT scanning and MRI, studies have shown a sensitivity for cervical mediastinoscopy ranging from 0.44 to 0.92.[5] Specificities and positive predictive values of 1.00 have been described, but this is often secondary to the study design, with reference made to findings during mediastinoscopy, rather than actual disease at various lymph node stations. Although mediastinoscopy is currently the "gold standard" for assessing lymph node status (its negative predictive value is >90%), this chapter also addresses other existing and emerging imaging modalities that can be used to augment staging accuracy. The indications and contraindications to cervical mediastinoscopy are outlined in Table 70-1.

Table 70-1

INDICATIONS AND CONTRAINDICATIONS FOR MEDIASTINOSCOPY

Indications
1. To determine the status of mediastinal lymph nodes in the staging of lung cancer and hence aid in both prognosis and potential treatment. Although some authors advocate mediastinoscopy for all potential surgical cases of lung cancer, others confine its use to the following scenarios:
   a. Biopsy of mediastinal lymph nodes >1 cm on CT scan or positive by PET scan
   b. Central primary tumor
   c. Peripheral tumor with chest wall invasion
   d. Potential need for pneumonectomy
   e. Multiple enlarged N1 lymph nodes
2. To assess tracheal or mediastinal invasion by other neoplastic processes
3. As a diagnostic modality for sampling of mediastinal tissue (e.g., to rule out infectious or other inflammatory disease)

Contraindications
1. Permanent tracheostomies (e.g., after laryngectomy)
2. Relative contraindications:
   a. Aortic arch aneurysm
   b. Innominate artery aneurysm
   c. Previous sternotomy and mediastinitis
   d. Superior vena cava obstruction (SVCO)

Cervical mediastinoscopy complications (~2.5% of cases)[5]
1. Paresis of the left recurrent laryngeal nerve
2. Hemorrhage (most commonly from injury to the azygos vein)
3. Pneumothorax
4. Pneumonia
5. Perforation of the esophagus

PREOPERATIVE ASSESSMENT

Chest x-ray, chest CT scan, pulmonary function tests, and appropriate medical optimization are performed before mediastinoscopy and major lung resection. Although most surgeons prefer to delay the definitive pulmonary resection until final pathology is available from the mediastinoscopy, some perform mediastinoscopy in the setting of definitive resection if the frozen-section results are negative for metastatic tumor.

PREOPERATIVE PET IMAGING

Although mediastinoscopy/otomy has the distinct advantage of providing direct visualization of suspicious mediastinal nodal disease, as well as a tissue diagnosis of such nodes, other studies are available in the preoperative staging repertoire. A noninvasive imaging modality currently in clinical use to evaluate for hilar, mediastinal, and extrathoracic metastases is positron-emission tomography (PET). By using the radioisotope [^{18}F] fluorodeoxyglucose (FDG) to detect metabolically overactive cellular growth, one can more accurately describe a patient's clinical stage and appropriate therapeutic maneuvers.

There is currently no absolute indication for the use of PET scanning, although some guidelines do exist in the literature. It seems clear that for patients who display clear evidence of extrathoracic disease, PET scanning is a costly and unnecessary test that will not change clinical management. Generally, a PET scan is indicated for patients with a question of extrathoracic metastases, those with questionable clinical stage III (cIII) disease (and even cI and cII disease), because surgical management may be altered in at least 8% to 18% of these patients.[6,7]

The data to support these clinical recommendations are substantial. PET scans, when compared with CT scans of the chest, abdomen, and pelvic anatomy, have an increased sensitivity for detecting disease, ranging from 79% to 95% versus 50% to 86% for CT.[8–10] The significance of this is most noticeable in light of evidence that 7.5%, 18%, and 24% of patients with cI, cII, and cIII disease, respectively, will have extrathoracic disease by PET scanning and hence may avoid an unnecessary nontherapeutic resection.[11] The strengths of PET scanning lie in its superior sensitivity and accuracy (>90%).[12] This has led many to provide recommendations about continued operative staging (i.e., mediastinoscopy) depending on PET and CT scanning. Surgical staging may not be necessary in patients with negative CT and PET,[13] negative PET and mediastinal nodes less than 1.5 cm,[14] or if the primary lesion has a PET standardized uptake value (SUV) of less than 2.5 and a negative mediastinum.[15]

Although it has excellent sensitivity, the specificity of PET scanning is unacceptably low. A number of inflammatory and infectious conditions can produce a positive PET scan in the absence of malignancy, thus leading to either unnecessary operative diagnostic procedures or, worse yet, a decision to forego definitive treatment because of a false assumption of metastatic disease (overstaging). This is critical because there are data to suggest that even minimal N2 disease (e.g., ipsilateral mediastinal nodal metastases) can be resected with a primary tumor for a 5-year survival rate of 40% compared with 8% for bulky N2 disease.[11] In addition, since several studies have demonstrated high false-negative and false-positive rates (11%–33% and 15%–52%, respectively, with PET), surgical staging continues to be an important part of the preoperative workup.

Endobronchial Ultrasound and Endoscopic Esophageal Ultrasound in Mediastinal Staging

The introduction of endobronchial ultrasound (EBUS) and endoscopic esophageal ultrasound (EUS) has aided clinicians in determining appropriate candidates for surgical versus nonoperative therapy for lung cancer in a less invasive manner. Endobronchial ultrasound with transbronchial FNA (EBUS-TBNA) can be used to biopsy lymph nodes in stations 1 to 4, 7, and 10 to 12. Accuracy rates of over 90% have been reported by the combined use of EBUS and EUS-FNA biopsy to stage the mediastinum in NSCLC.[16]

To describe the technique of EUS briefly, an endoscope is inserted into the esophagus with sonographic examination of nodal tissue distributed around the esophagus. By passing the endoscope distally, one can assess adrenal lesions and, more frequently, posterior mediastinal lymph nodes, most notably stations 7, 8, and 9. Level 5 nodes in the aortopulmonary window can be accessed, as well as occasionally the levels 2 and 4 paratracheal nodes. In contrast with PET, nodes as small as 3 mm can be visualized, and those 5 mm or larger may be biopsied.[17] The only inaccessible mediastinal nodes are those anterior to the tracheobronchial tree (levels 2, 3, and 4) because air within the proximal airway distorts ultrasound findings.

EUS with FNA has gained considerable acceptance as an adjunct to mediastinoscopy, particularly in evaluating posterior mediastinal nodes at levels 5, 7, 8, and 9. Recent data suggest that EUS with FNA is superior to any other technique in investigating the posterior mediastinum, with sensitivity of 84% to 94%, specificity of 100%, and accuracy of 94% to 98% in determining regional disease.[18–21]

Some have advocated the use of EBUS-TBNA and EUS-FNA as a primary method of staging the mediastinum. This method can be supported by its minimally invasive approach and relatively low risk, coupled with its ability to provide accurate, thorough information about locoregional and distant disease. A randomized controlled multicenter trial assigned 241 patients to either surgical staging alone or combined EBUS-TBNA and EUS-FNA followed by surgical staging if no nodal metastases were found. For patients without evidence of mediastinal metastases following surgical staging in either group, a thoracotomy with complete lymph node dissection was done. This study found that EBUS-TBNA and EUS-FNA improved the detection of nodal metastases and reduced the number of unnecessary thoracotomies by more than half compared with surgical staging alone.[22] In a recent prospective trial, EBUS-TBNA and mediastinoscopy were performed in the same setting in 153 patients, and thoracotomy with pulmonary resection and mediastinal lymphadenectomy were performed on those patients for whom no evidence of N2 or N3 disease was found on EBUS-TBNA or mediastinoscopy.[23] EBUS-TBNA was found to have no statistical difference in sensitivity, negative predictive value, and diagnostic accuracy compared to mediastinoscopy.[24] In fact, such data are so encouraging that some centers have suggested replacing mediastinoscopy with EBUS-TBNA and EUS-FNA as the "gold standard" for staging the mediastinum.

Enthusiasm for EBUS/EUS used either alone or in conjunction with currently accepted surgical staging techniques must be tempered by a number of factors. Much of the current data supporting EBUS/EUS has been compiled at advanced tertiary care centers with significant experience in the technique. The assessment of tissue (mediastinoscopy) versus cytology (EBUS/EUS) also may factor into the accuracy of detecting micrometastases, as well as the ability to provide adequate tissue for tumor marker and mutation analysis.

CERVICAL MEDIASTINOSCOPY TECHNIQUE

Preparation

General anesthesia is induced with a single-lumen endotracheal tube. The patient is positioned supine on the OR table with the occiput of the head at the top of the table. The neck is maximally extended with the aid of an interscapular roll. The back is elevated to 20 to 30 degrees in a reverse Trendelenburg position. The headboard can be lowered to aid in extension, permitting direct access to the suprasternal notch. The endotracheal tube is positioned laterally, away from the operating hand of the surgeon and the mediastinoscope. The table generally is rotated 90 degrees away from the anesthetist. The anterior chest and neck are fully prepped and draped in the event that emergent sternotomy is necessary. Placing a right radial arterial line can be helpful for monitoring, especially dampening of the arterial waveform, which may indicate innominate artery compression.

Technique

A 3-cm incision is made in the midline one fingerbreadth above the sternal notch (Fig. 70-1A). The incision is carried down through the platysma. The midline then is opened vertically between the two layers of strap muscles until the trachea is exposed. Occasionally, the thyroid isthmus needs to be retracted cephalad or even divided to aid in exposure. Rarely, the thyroid artery, internal mammary artery, or branch of the inferior thyroid artery needs to be ligated. The anterior trachea is exposed, and the pretracheal fascia is incised and elevated. A pretracheal tunnel is fashioned with blunt dissection with the index finger (Fig. 70-1B). During the dissection, the dorsal aspect of the finger remains on the trachea, whereas the volar aspect comes in contact with the innominate artery (Fig. 70-1C). A side-to-side sweeping motion is made with the finger to clear the pre- and paratracheal spaces. The mediastinoscope is introduced into the pretracheal tunnel with constant traction anteriorly and a slow rotating motion during the dissection (Fig. 70-2). Care is taken to avoid forcing the scope at any time. Further blunt dissection is performed with a blunt metal suction device.

The mediastinum is inspected by direct vision using the scope. The surgeon proceeds with dissection of the right and left paratracheal regions first, working inferiorly to the tracheobronchial angles and finishing in the subcarinal region. Identification of the azygos vein, tracheal bifurcation, proximal mainstem bronchi, and pulmonary artery aid in anatomic reference. The subcarinal nodes generally are sampled last because bronchial artery and perinodal bleeding can be more difficult to control. The nodes are partially dissected free before biopsy with the aid of blunt dissection using the suction device, thus minimizing bleeding. If there is any doubt that a structure is indeed a lymph node, aspiration with a long needle can be performed. When sufficiently separated, the node is grasped with the aid of a large-cupped laryngeal forceps or similar instrument, and traction is applied under direct vision. If simple pulling and twisting cannot deliver the specimen, further dissection is indicated. Using a suction/cautery device, coagulation of any bronchial or nodal hilar vessels can be accomplished.

Video cervical mediastinoscopy permits precise visualization of small feeding vessels and has improved the safety of teaching the technique to future thoracic surgeons. The video mediastinoscope permits both video screen-aided dissection and dissection by aid of direct visualization down the barrel of the scope.

Nodal Sampling

Determining the ideal number of lymph nodes to biopsy depends on the indication:

1. *Single specimen:* Sarcoidosis, lymphoma, or other mediastinal mass once an adequate sample has been sent or frozen-section confirmation is given.

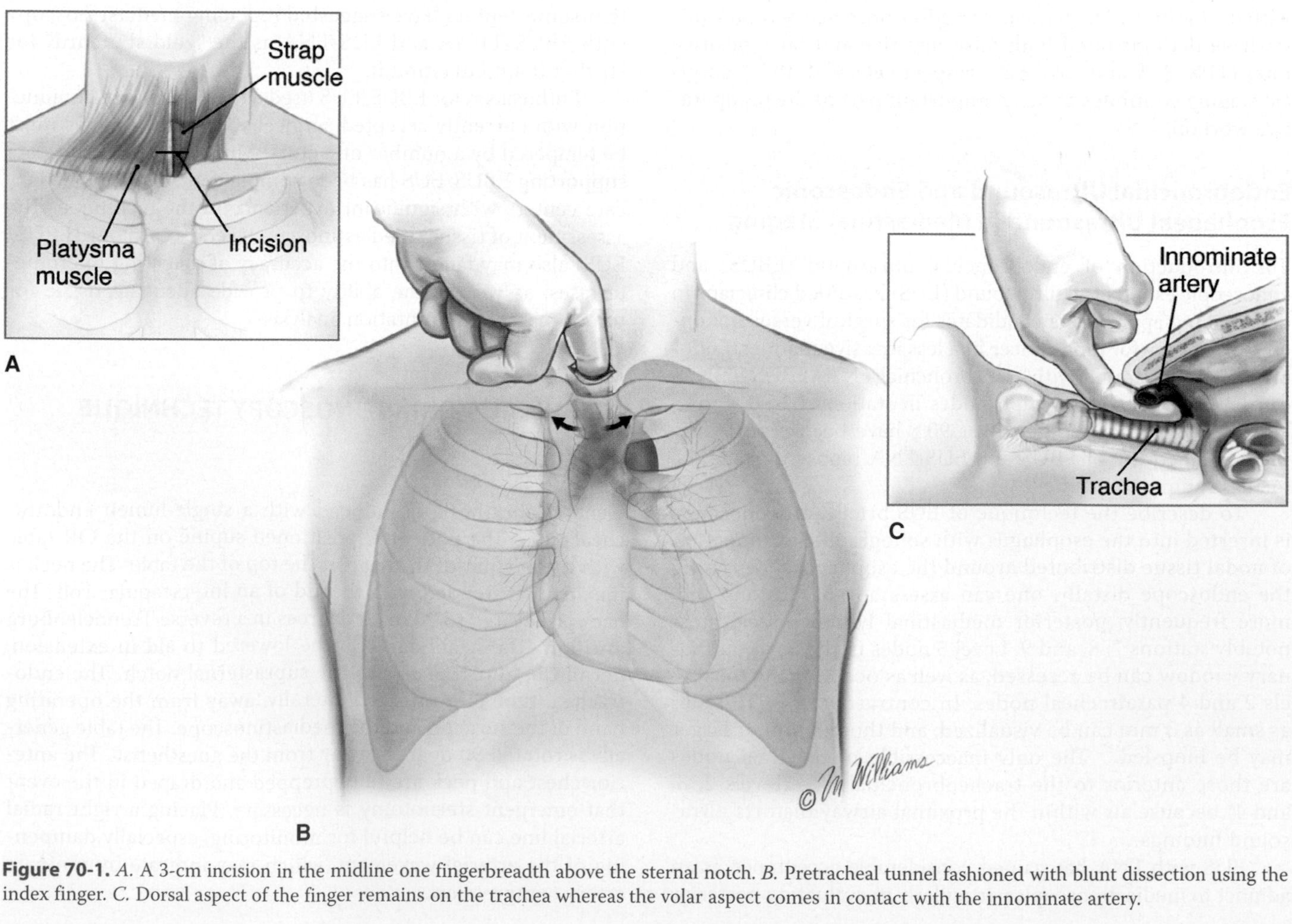

Figure 70-1. *A.* A 3-cm incision in the midline one fingerbreadth above the sternal notch. *B.* Pretracheal tunnel fashioned with blunt dissection using the index finger. *C.* Dorsal aspect of the finger remains on the trachea whereas the volar aspect comes in contact with the innominate artery.

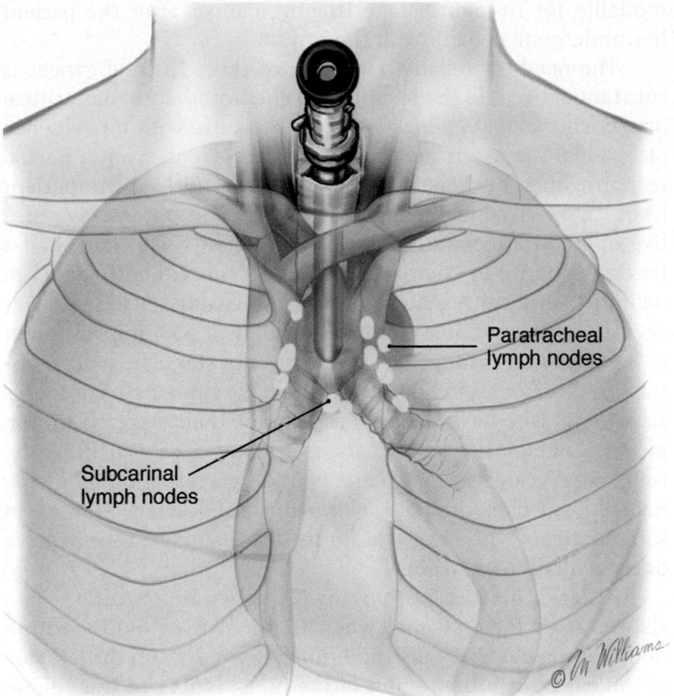

Figure 70-2. The mediastinoscope is introduced into the pretracheal tunnel with constant traction anteriorly and a slow rotating motion during the dissection.

2. *Lung cancer:* High right paratracheal node (2R), low right paratracheal node (4R), tracheobronchial angle (10R, 10L), subcarinal lymph node (7L), and left paratracheal node (4L). Sampling of all accessible lymph node stations is ideal for accurate staging.
3. If pathologically malignant nodal disease is evident on the contralateral side to the primary tumor, other nodes need not be accessed because staging would not be affected. Alternatively, it may be more expedient to sample all the above-mentioned nodes rather than wait for a frozen section if no evidence of gross disease is present.

Aortopulmonary Window/Periaortic Nodal Sampling (Levels 5 and 6)

Left anterior mediastinotomy (Chamberlain procedure) and a VATS approach are both acceptable methods of assessing levels 5 and 6 lymph nodes on the left.

INTRAOPERATIVE COMPLICATIONS

Hemorrhage is by far the most critical potential complication of mediastinoscopy. Once the lymph nodes are sampled, careful attention is turned to hemostasis. A 0.5-in gauze packing strip is used to pack the mediastinum. If copious bleeding is encountered, the first maneuver should be to keep the mediastinoscope engaged in the mediastinum and attempt to pack the wound with the gauze. This almost always temporizes the situation and allows the surgeon to prepare for more extensive surgery and potential increased blood loss. The bleeding is almost always from the bronchial artery, not from the pulmonary artery. Torquing the scope to apply pressure on the actual bleeding site usually will stop the hemorrhage while allowing constant visual inspection. Additional IV access, blood products, and surgical support can be mobilized while the mediastinum is tamponaded with gauze packing with the mediastinoscope in place. Very often, patience and adequate packing can avoid further surgery. Placing epinephrine-soaked gauze in the mediastinum also may stem localized bleeding. On rare occasion, a median sternotomy is required to control the hemorrhage. However, before undertaking a sternotomy to control a pulmonary artery bleeder, consideration may be given to performing an ipsilateral thoracotomy or lobectomy. Rarely, injury to one of the major veins including the innominate and superior vena cava can cause severe bleeding. Likewise, an injury to the azygos vein while performing a biopsy of level 10R LN is possible. When dissection proceeds along the left paratracheal area, care must be taken to avoid left recurrent nerve injury. Hoarseness may occur in 5% to 10% of patients. Avoidance of cautery and traction on the nerve are most important.

POSTOPERATIVE CARE

The strap muscles are closed with simple interrupted or running absorbable suture, whereas the skin is closed with absorbable sutures applied in running subcuticular fashion. Steri-Strips are applied. A chest x-ray is taken by some surgeons after the procedure to rule out pneumothorax or unexpected hemothorax. Assessment for any hoarseness of voice is made. Patients usually are discharged home if only cervical mediastinoscopy was performed. Patients may shower the next day. The most frequent procedure-associated morbidity in our experience has been urinary retention in elderly males likely related to the general anesthetic (10% in men older than 70 years). Generally, anticoagulants and aspirin-containing products are avoided at least 7 days before the procedure and for 72 hours after the procedure.

VATS Staging

Thoracoscopy has become an integral part of thoracic surgery in both diagnostic and therapeutic resections. Most of our planned resections are accomplished with VATS, and a VATS exploration is useful for evaluating the primary tumor and pleura as well as ipsilateral and posterior mediastinal nodes.

VATS staging of the primary tumor and mediastinum has been investigated by a number of groups, with encouraging results reported in the literature. One such study revealed that in 17 patients undergoing VATS staging followed by definitive resection with open lymph node dissection, there was 100% correlation between VATS and open staging.[25] In 52 patients with biopsy-proved NSCLC and mediastinal lymphadenopathy by CT scan, there was a 0% false-negative rate. More important, patients with stage IIIa (44%) or stage IIIb (16%) disease were appropriately identified, thereby obviating the need for initial surgical therapy.[26] These early results would indicate that VATS is a valuable tool in surgical staging, helping to stratify newly diagnosed patients to initial surgical versus medical therapy.

Others have been more precise in applying VATS staging, specifically using a minimally invasive approach to discern stage IIIb disease. Some recent guidelines have suggested that VATS has greater than 90% accuracy in determining such locoregional disease, including diagnosing malignant pleural effusion and contralateral nodal (N3) disease.[27] These recommendations are based on two studies that showed the usefulness of this technique. VATS may upstage initially cytologically negative pleural effusions in 6% to 60% of patients, confirm M1 disease in up to 50%, and downstage disease in up to 30% of patients.[28,29] Most important, 6% to 14% of patients may be downstaged to a "resectable" status, highlighting the value of VATS and the hazard of initial overstaging by imaging studies only.

Despite these encouraging data, however, there remain some limitations to VATS. One study has shown that VATS staging may result in an open operation in up to 22% of patients undergoing the procedure[30] whereas another study has shown that VATS results were unreliable in 38% of patients studied.[31] These data are less impressive than others and may be related to familiarity and skill with VATS. Nonetheless, they make the point that with all new technology and skill sets, education, practice, and a learning curve necessarily accompany any significant movement forward.

Of note, there is additional interest in using thoracoscopic techniques to stage other malignancies in the thorax. Krasna and Jiao, among others, have reported on a VATS and laparoscopic approach to stage esophageal cancer.[32] While this technique is still investigational and not used widely for routine staging of nonpulmonary malignancies, the sophistication of this process may lend itself to more frequent application.

Restaging Stage III Disease

For patients who are diagnosed initially with stage III disease and undergo neoadjuvant chemotherapy with or without radiation therapy to downstage their disease, it may be important to pathologically restage the mediastinum.[33,34] There are at least theoretically increased risks with repeat mediastinoscopy. Safe mediastinoscopy is based on accurate identification of anatomic landmarks and the ability to dissect nodal tissue away from vasculature and vital structures. Obliterated planes and fibrosis from the first procedure and induction therapies can make the second dissection treacherous. Two studies have revealed that a second mediastinoscopy is both safe (no deaths in a series of 279 patients) and effective, with a sensitivity of 87% and an accuracy of 94%.[35,36] These studies aside, the second mediastinoscopy has the potential to be significantly more challenging from a technical standpoint. Concern has been raised that there may be decreased sensitivity with repeat mediastinoscopy, which is a valid issue to address. Patients with persistently positive mediastinal nodes after neoadjuvant therapy may have a significantly worse prognosis than those who respond to chemoradiotherapy, and a false-negative mediastinoscopy would lead to unnecessary surgery.

As an adjunct or alternative to repeat mediastinoscopy, repeat PET scanning is often pursued. The benefits of PET scanning are clear in that using a noninvasive staging technique avoids the necessity of submitting the patient to repeat mediastinoscopy in an environment of adhesions and fibrosis while theoretically providing an equally reliable staging report. Data suggest that repeat PET scanning may accurately down- or upstage disease in up to 37% of patients, ultimately dictating operative versus nonoperative therapy.[37] However, one study has revealed that a repeat PET scan may be far less sensitive than initial staging PET scans.[38] Clearly, more research needs to be done before repeat PET scanning is viewed as a sole modality for restaging stage III lung cancer after the patient has undergone neoadjuvant therapy.[5]

The need for reliable restaging of stage III lung cancer is substantial because the response to chemoradiation has critical prognostic value. While a complete response with no evidence of residual disease is ideal, this is a rare event. Even a partial response may be beneficial, however, permitting the patient to be categorized as having a resectable and potentially curative operation. In numerous studies, patients who have had a partial response to chemoradiation and subsequently undergo definitive surgical resection have demonstrated 5-year survivals in the range of 30% to 50%, as well as a 50% improvement in locoregional control.[39–43] These results stand in sharp contrast to those of nonresponders, who have similar survival rates as patients who have surgery initially for their stage III tumor, in the range of 18% at 3 years and 9% at 5 years. Therefore, we generally suggest that patients undergo restaging following neoadjuvant chemoradiation to avoid unnecessary surgery in some patients who have had no mediastinal clearance or have documented progression.

Anterior mediastinotomy, or Chamberlain procedure, can also be used for restaging when the goal is to biopsy lymph nodes or masses in the aortopulmonary window on the left side of the chest or in the region of the hilus. Nodes in this region filter lymph from the left lung, in particular, the left upper lobe. The technique for anterior mediastinotomy is described in Chapter 156.

SUMMARY

Since the introduction of cervical mediastinoscopy in 1959, many improvements in the diagnosis, staging, and treatment of lung cancer have been introduced. CT/PET scanning has shown promising results that may affect the use of routine mediastinoscopy in all patients with suspected lung cancer. EUS/FNA gives minimally invasive access to areas in the mediastinum inaccessible by mediastinoscopy (e.g., lower subcarinal and inferior mediastinal). That said, the importance of accurate pathologic assessment of lymph nodes remains. Thoracic surgeons need to remain facile in mediastinoscopy to ensure continued accurate pathologic nodal staging for the future.

EDITOR'S COMMENT

Given the importance of pathologic staging, mediastinoscopy and thoracoscopy are crucial tools for lymph node staging. Although PET scanning has revolutionized our ability to predict the nature of pulmonary nodules and identify distant lesions that are suspicious for metastasis, tissue diagnosis is still *mandatory*, since a change in stage will result in a change in treatment. All patients with an identifiable lymph node by CT greater than 5 mm should be offered a noninvasive approach first if this technology and expertise are available. In addition, for those undergoing neoadjuvant treatment for stage III disease, repeat pathologic staging can predict prognosis and help avoid unnecessary resection in high-risk patients who have persistent mediastinal disease. We therefore currently try to obtain a tissue diagnosis by needle biopsy (EUS)/(EBUS) or transbronchial fine needle aspiration (TBNA)/percutaneous needle biopsy (PNB) and reserve mediastinoscopy for restaging.

Alternatively, a repeat mediastinoscopy can be performed with relatively few complications. We do not accept a PET-negative mediastinum as evidence of N0 disease and likewise do not accept a PET-positive mediastinum as evidence of N2 disease. Rather, tissue, by cytology or mediastinoscopy biopsy, is routinely obtained.

The mediastinoscope used should have a rounded tip to avoid injury to vascular structures during insertion. I currently prefer to use the videomediastinoscope as it provides excellent visual acuity (for the surgeon older than 40 years old!) and a great opportunity for teaching this technically demanding procedure to residents and fellows. We routinely have a tray that includes a "box" with five compartments for the upper, lower paratracheal, and subcarinal lymph nodes. In addition, an attempt is made routinely to obtain the right level 10 tracheobronchial lymph node. I personally dissect down to level 7 first without taking any samples to avoid blood draining down and obscuring the view. Alternatively, for patients with a suspicion of lymphoma, for example, we sample "abnormal" lymph nodes as we go and send for frozen sections, stopping once any positive result is obtained.

—Mark J. Krasna

References

1. NCCN. NCCN Practice Guidelines in Oncology, 2014; www.nccn.com/professionals/physician_gls/PDF/nscl.pdf.
2. Edwards BK, Howe HL, Ries LA, et al. Annual report to the nation on the status of cancer, 1973–1999, featuring implications of age and aging on U.S. cancer burden. *Cancer*. 2002;94:2766–2792.
3. Carlens E. Mediastinoscopy: a method for inspection and tissue biopsy in the superior mediastinum. *Dis Chest*. 1959;36:343–352.
4. Park BJ, Flores R, Downey RJ, et al. Management of major hemorrhage during mediastinoscopy. *J Thorac Cardiovasc Surg*. 2003;126:726–731.
5. Kramer H, Groen HJ. Current concepts in the mediastinal lymph node staging of nonsmall cell lung cancer. *Ann Surg*. 2003;238:180–188.
6. Detterbeck FC, Falen S, Rivera MP, et al. Seeking a home for a PET: 2. Defining the appropriate place for positron emission tomography imaging in the staging of patients with suspected lung cancer. *Chest*. 2004;125:2300–2308.
7. MacManus MP, Hicks RJ, Matthews JP, et al. High rate of detection of unsuspected distant metastases by PET in apparent stage III non-small-cell lung cancer: implications for radical radiation therapy. *Int J Radiat Oncol Biol Phys*. 2001;50:287–293.
8. Pozo-Rodriguez F, Martin de Nicolas JL, Sanchez-Nistal MA, et al. Accuracy of helical computed tomography and [18F] fluorodeoxyglucose positron emission tomography for identifying lymph node mediastinal metastases in potentially resectable non-small-cell lung cancer. *J Clin Oncol*. 2005;23:8348–8356.
9. Graeter TP, Hellwig D, Hoffmann K, et al. Mediastinal lymph node staging in suspected lung cancer: comparison of positron emission tomography with F-18-fluorodeoxyglucose and mediastinoscopy. *Ann Thorac Surg*. 2003;75:231–235; discussion 5–6.
10. Luketich JD, Friedman DM, Meltzer CC, et al. The role of positron emission tomography in evaluating mediastinal lymph node metastases in non-small-cell lung cancer. *Clin Lung Cancer*. 2001;2:229–233.
11. Baum RP, Hellwig D, Mezzetti M. Position of nuclear medicine modalities in the diagnostic workup of cancer patients: lung cancer. *Q J Nucl Med Mol Imaging*. 2004;48:119–142.
12. Hellwig D, Ukena D, Paulsen F, et al. [Meta-analysis of the efficacy of positron emission tomography with F-18-fluorodeoxyglucose in lung tumors. Basis for discussion of the German Consensus Conference on PET in Oncology 2000]. *Pneumologie*. 2001;55:367–377.
13. Poncelet A, Lonneux M, Coche E, et al. PET-FDG scan enhances but does not replace pre-operative surgical staging in non-small cell lung carcinoma. *Eur J Cardiothorac Surg*. 2001;20:468–475.
14. De Langen A, Raijmakers P, Riphagen I, et al. The size of mediastinal lymph nodes and its relation with metastatic involvement: a meta-analysis. *Eur J Cardiothorac Surg*. 2006;29:26–29.
15. Kernstine KH, McLaughlin KA, Menda Y, et al. Can FDG-PET reduce the need for mediastinoscopy in potentially resectable nonsmall cell lung cancer? *Ann Thorac Surg*. 2002;73:394–401; discussion 401–402.
16. Eloubeidi MA, Tamhane A, Chen VK, et al. Endoscopic ultrasound-guided fine-needle aspiration in patients with non-small cell lung cancer and prior negative mediastinoscopy. *Ann Thorac Surg*. 2005;80:1231–1239.
17. Fritscher-Ravens A. Endoscopic ultrasound evaluation in the diagnosis and staging of lung cancer. *Lung Cancer*. 2003;41:259–267.
18. Eloubeidi MA, Cerfolio RJ, Chen VK, et al. Endoscopic ultrasound-guided fine needle aspiration of mediastinal lymph node in patients with suspected lung cancer after positron emission tomography and computed tomography scans. *Ann Thorac Surg*. 2005;79:263–268.
19. Annema JT, Versteegh MI, Veselic M, et al. Endoscopic ultrasound-guided fine-needle aspiration in the diagnosis and staging of lung cancer and its impact on surgical staging. *J Clin Oncol*. 2005;23:8357–8361.
20. Caddy G, Conron M, Wright G, et al. The accuracy of EUS-FNA in assessing mediastinal lymphadenopathy and staging patients with NSCLC. *Eur Respir J*. 2005;25:410–415.
21. Annema JT, Versteegh MI, Veselic M, et al. Endoscopic ultrasound added to mediastinoscopy for preoperative staging of patients with lung cancer. *JAMA*. 2005;294:931–936.
22. Annema J, Meerbeeck J, Tournoy K, et al. Mediastinoscopy vs endosonography for mediastinal nodal staging of lung cancer: a randomized trial. *JAMA*. 2010;304:2245–2252.
23. Wallace MB, Ravenel J, Block MI, et al. Endoscopic ultrasound in lung cancer patients with a normal mediastinum on computed tomography. *Ann Thorac Surg*. 2004;77:1763–1768.
24. Yasufuku K, Pierre, A, Keshavjee S, et al. A prospective controlled trial of endobronchial ultrasound-guided transbronchial needle aspiration compared with mediastinoscopy for mediastinal lymph node staging of lung cancer. *J Thorac Cardiovasc Surg*. 2011;142:1393–1400.
25. Champion JK, McKernan JB. Comparison of minimally invasive thoracoscopy versus open thoracotomy for staging lung cancer. *Int Surg*. 1996; 81:235–236.
26. Brega Massone PP, Conti B, Magnani B, et al. Video-assisted thoracoscopic surgery for diagnosis, staging, and management of lung cancer with suspected mediastinal lymphadenopathy. *Surg Laparosc Endosc Percutan Tech*. 2002;12:104–109.
27. Passlick B. Initial surgical staging of lung cancer. *Lung Cancer*. 2003;42: S21–S25.
28. De Giacomo T, Rendina EA, Venuta F, et al. Thoracoscopic staging of IIIB non-small cell lung cancer before neoadjuvant therapy. *Ann Thorac Surg*. 1997;64:1409–1411.
29. Roberts JR, Blum MG, Arildsen R, et al. Prospective comparison of radiologic, thoracoscopic, and pathologic staging in patients with early non-small cell lung cancer. *Ann Thorac Surg*. 1999;68:1154–1158.
30. Rau B, Hunerbein M, Below C, et al. Video-assisted thoracic surgery: staging and management of thoracic tumors. *Surg Endosc*. 1998;12:133–136.
31. Sebastian-Quetglas F, Molins L, Baldo X, et al. Clinical value of video-assisted thoracoscopy for preoperative staging of non-small cell lung cancer: a prospective study of 105 patients. *Lung Cancer*. 2003;42:297–301.
32. Krasna MJ, Jiao X. Thoracoscopic and laparoscopic staging for esophageal cancer. *Semin Thorac Cardiovasc Surg*. 2000;12:186–194.
33. Jaklitsch MT, Gu L, Harpole DH, et al. CALGB thoracic surgeons. Prospective phase II trial of pre-resection thoracoscopic (VATS) restaging following neoadjuvant therapy for IIIA(N2) non-small cell lung cancer (NSCLC): results of CALGB 39803. *J Clin Oncol*, 2005 ASCO Annual Meeting Proceedings. Vol. 23, No. 16 S (June 1 Supplement), 2005: 7065.
34. Jaklitsch MT, Herndon JE 2nd, DeCamp MM Jr., et al. Nodal downstaging predicts survival following induction chemotherapy for stage IIIA (N2) non-small cell lung cancer in CALGB protocol #8935. *J Surg Oncol*. 2006;94:599–606.
35. Stamatis G, Fechner S, Hillejan L, et al. Repeat mediastinoscopy as a restaging procedure. *Pneumologie*. 2005;59:862–866.

36. Pauwels M, Van Schil P, De Backer W, et al. Repeat mediastinoscopy in the staging of lung cancer. *Eur J Cardiothorac Surg.* 1998;14:271–273.
37. Changlai SP, Tsai SC, Chou MC, et al. Whole body 18F-2-deoxyglucose positron emission tomography to restage non-small cell lung cancer. *Oncol Rep.* 2001;8:337–339.
38. Ryu JS, Choi NC, Fischman AJ, et al. FDG-PET in staging and restaging non-small cell lung cancer after neoadjuvant chemoradiotherapy: correlation with histopathology. *Lung Cancer.* 2002;35:179–187.
39. Lorent N, De Leyn P, Lievens Y, et al. Long-term survival of surgically staged IIIA-N2 non-small-cell lung cancer treated with surgical combined modality approach: analysis of a 7-year prospective experience. *Ann Oncol.* 2004;15:1645–1653.
40. DeCamp MM Jr, Ashiku S, Thurer R. The role of surgery in N_2 non-small cell lung cancer. *Clin Cancer Res.* 2005;11:5033s–5037s.
41. Voltolini L, Luzzi L, Ghiribelli C, et al. Results of induction chemotherapy followed by surgical resection in patients with stage IIIA (N_2) non-small cell lung cancer: the importance of the nodal down-staging after chemotherapy. *Eur J Cardiothorac Surg.* 2001;20:1106–1112.
42. Bueno R, Richards WG, Swanson SJ, et al. Nodal stage after induction therapy for stage IIIA lung cancer determines patient survival. *Ann Thorac Surg.* 2000;70:1826–1831.
43. Lewinski T, Zulawski M, Turski C, et al. Small cell lung cancer I-IIIA: cytoreductive chemotherapy followed by resection with continuation of chemotherapy. *Eur J Cardiothorac Surg.* 2001;20:391–398.

71 The Five Lobectomies

John R. Roberts

Keywords: Pulmonary resection, lobectomy, sleeve resection, right upper lobectomy, right middle lobectomy, right lower lobectomy, left upper lobectomy, left lower lobectomy

INTRODUCTION

The ability to select patients appropriately, perform a competent pulmonary lobectomy, and manage patients safely in the postoperative interval epitomizes the skills of a good general thoracic surgeon, more than any other aspect of the job. Lung cancer patients comprise a majority of general thoracic surgical patients, and lobectomy, particularly the extended versions (i.e., sleeve lobectomy and lung and chest wall resection), constitutes most of a general thoracic surgeon's work. In no other endeavor does a thoracic surgeon have more impact on his or her patients.

However, the frequency with which an operation is performed often does not mean that it is well performed. A recent evaluation of the National Cancer Database revealed that many or most lobectomies in the United States were done without checking surgical margins or performing mediastinal lymph node dissections despite extensive evidence that these actions are important for long-term survival after cancer resections.[1]

The reason for this lack of uniformity is not entirely clear but it is probably that many surgeons, both general and cardiac, regard general thoracic surgery as a secondary rather than primary occupation.[2] Whatever the reasons, appropriate performance of this common but potentially dangerous operation is important for our patients.

Lobectomies can be done in many different ways, but the sites of danger usually remain the same. In fact, a surgeon may choose an unusual approach because it lessens the chance of problems for a particular patient compared with the standard approach.

PREOPERATIVE EVALUATION

Staging

Preresection staging should be done for all patients undergoing lung resection. At this time, a complete history and physical examination focusing on involvement of lymph nodes and liver masses, followed by chest CT scan and PET scan, are appropriate. The latter evaluation will rule out distant metastases other than brain metastases. Patients without symptoms of headache are unlikely to have brain metastases, and therefore, head CT scan or MRI is not obligatory.

All patients with lung cancer may have mediastinal metastases. Although PET scans are quite sensitive for identifying mediastinal metastases, they remain less accurate than mediastinoscopy (see Chapter 70). Preoperative mediastinoscopy is indicated for all patients with a PET scan-positive mediastinum and should be considered for certain patients with a PET scan-negative mediastinum (i.e., those with enlarged nodes on CT scan or with hilar lesions). Although the PET scan remains useful for ruling out distant metastases, it should not be the only study performed to evaluate the mediastinum. Many patients have been denied resection because their PET scan was positive in the mediastinum, only to find a more knowledgeable physician who, on mediastinoscopy, diagnosed mediastinal granulomatous disease instead and then successfully resected the patient's stage I cancer (Table 71-1).

Thoracoscopic examination and staging of the pleural space benefit patients undergoing lung resection[3]: Thoracoscopy may identify pleural metastases. Thoracoscopy can be used to determine a suitable incision for resection. Thoracoscopy is not indicated for all patients undergoing routine resection of an apparent stage I cancer but can be used to evaluate small pleural effusions or large cancers believed to be unresectable as a consequence of mediastinal invasion (Table 71-2).

Cardiopulmonary Evaluation (or Minimizing Preoperative Risk)

Immediate perioperative mortality (i.e., death within 2–5 days) is very rare after a lung resection. Most deaths occur within the first week. Postoperative mortality in lung resection patients results mostly from respiratory complications. Predicting perioperative mortality in lung resections relies on identifying those patients who

- might have a perioperative complication and
- might not survive it

Our literature has dealt with this problem primarily by focusing on preoperative lung function or predicted postoperative lung function as a means of identifying patients who would not survive a respiratory complication (Table 71-3).

Table 71-1

CAUSES OF PET POSITIVITY

1. Granulomatous disease
   - Histoplasmosis
   - Tuberculosis
   - Sarcoidosis
   - Other fungal diseases
2. Healing fractures
3. Previous surgical intervention
   - Thoracotomy
   - Talc sclerosis
4. Cancer
5. Other active infections

Table 71-2

PREOPERATIVE OR PRERESECTION STAGING FOR LUNG CANCER PATIENTS

1. Complete history and physical examination
2. Chest CT scan
3. Positron emission tomography
4. Mediastinoscopy
5. Thoracoscopy (for some patients)
6. Brain MRI for those patients with headache or any other neurologic symptoms

SURGICAL TECHNIQUE

Right Upper Lobectomy

Viewed from the patient's side, the anatomy of the right hilum is a triangle with the pulmonary artery (PA) at the apex, the vein anterior, and the bronchus posterior (Fig. 71-1*A*). The azygos vein caps the triangle. It is often adhesed to the bronchus, the artery, or both and can be divided as a first step to gain proximal control of the PA and to perform the paratracheal lymphadenectomy.

Harvesting the mediastinal nodes is an important part of the procedure and can give more proximal exposure to the PA and bronchus, if needed, and is a good first step. The nodes are resected by dividing the azygos vein and harvesting the nodal packet (typically 3 × 1.5 × 1.5 cm) and by, in turn, dividing the mediastinal pleura posterior to the superior vena cava and anterior to the trachea. The nodes extend inferiorly to the PA and superiorly all the way to the subclavian artery at the thoracic inlet (Fig. 71-1*B*). However, overly aggressive manipulation in this area can lead to right true vocal cord paralysis. Consequently, the dissection should stop well inferior of the subclavian artery (Table 71-4).

Although many ascribe importance to the order of division of the hilar structures, there are no studies to confirm either a technologic or an oncologic benefit to a particular sequence. In any case, a small benefit would be superseded by a surgical mishap. Consequently, many do what is most appropriate for the particular patient (usually this means whichever is easiest). My preference is to divide the PA first, then the vein, then the bronchus, and finally the parenchyma, unless the artery is covered by the vein, in which case the vein, then artery, then bronchus are divided in that order. In both cases, the parenchyma is divided last to prevent air leaks.

Table 71-3

PREOPERATIVE CARDIOPULMONARY EVALUATION

1. Complete pulmonary function testing
2. For patients with FEV_1 <1.5 L or 50% of predicted or diffusing capacity (DLCO) below 40%:
   a. Quantitative perfusion scanning, to evaluate lung function on each side
   b. Diffusion capacity evaluation
   c. Oxygen exercise consumption testing
3. Complete history and physical examination—for patients with any history of angina, documented ASCVD, or CHF
   a. Evaluation by cardiologist, with possible stress testing or cardiac echo

ASCVD, atherosclerotic cardiovascular disease; CHF, congestive heart failure.

Table 71-4

POTENTIAL HAZARDS OF RIGHT PARATRACHEAL NODE DISSECTIONS

1. The superior aspect of the right pulmonary artery is present at the inferior aspect of the nodal packet
2. The right recurrent nerve is present at the apex of the nodal packet
3. Small venous branches off the superior vena cava (or the cava itself) can be injured during dissection
4. The pericardium and aorta lie deep to the packet and can be injured in those patients who have received preoperative chemoradiation
5. Any patients with granulomatous disease may have chronic inflammation and calcification which can make nodal dissection even more difficult than those patients who have received chemoradiation

The hilum is first approached by dividing the parietal pleura around the hilum, being careful to avoid the phrenic nerve, which should be swept medially. If the superior vein covers the PA anteriorly, the vein is approached and the middle lobe vein identified and preserved (Fig. 71-2). The vein then may be divided with a stapling device or with ligatures and suture ligatures proximally and distally. Pulmonary vessels should be controlled with two sutures proximally (e.g., either two ties or a tie and suture ligature) or a stapling device (e.g., gray, red, or white). Single ties or suture ligatures are not adequate. Small branches can be doubly clipped (Table 71-5).

After dividing the upper lobe branch of the superior vein and the main upper lobe PA (which may be present as two or three branches), a single small, more inferior branch of the ongoing PA usually ascends superiorly to the upper lobe (Fig. 71-3). This artery must be controlled and divided to complete the upper lobectomy, and often this can be the most challenging part of the procedure. Sometimes the vessel can be identified from the anterior aspect of the dissection, after the main arterial branch to the upper lobe has been divided. Otherwise, it is at risk when the bronchus is dissected and can be identified in the crotch between the takeoff of the right upper lobe bronchus. It should be divided before dissection and division of the bronchus. Small clips are recommended (Table 71-6), but may be avulsed if the parenchyma is subsequently divided with

Table 71-5

POTENTIAL HAZARDS OF RIGHT UPPER LOBECTOMY

1. The pulmonary artery can be injured:
   a. While developing the plane between the right upper lobe bronchus and the pulmonary artery.
   Solution—Open the pericardium and control the right main pulmonary artery during dissection.
   b. Identifying and dividing the recurrent posterior artery.
   Solution—avoid clipping this artery if you plan stapler division of the parenchyma. Instead, tie or use energy for this small vessel.
2. The phrenic nerve can be injured:
   a. While taking down apical adhesions.
   Solution—identify the phrenic nerve in its usual course on the lateral wall of the superior vena cava and track it superiorly.
   b. While dividing the anterior parietal pleura.
   Solution I—the nerve can be encased or trapped in nodes at the takeoff of the phrenic nerve. Carefully mobilize the nerve superior to and inferior to the area of entrapment prior to mobilization away from the base of the superior vein.
   Solution II—leave the nerve in its place, and divide the separate branches of the superior pulmonary vein proximal to the area of entrapment.

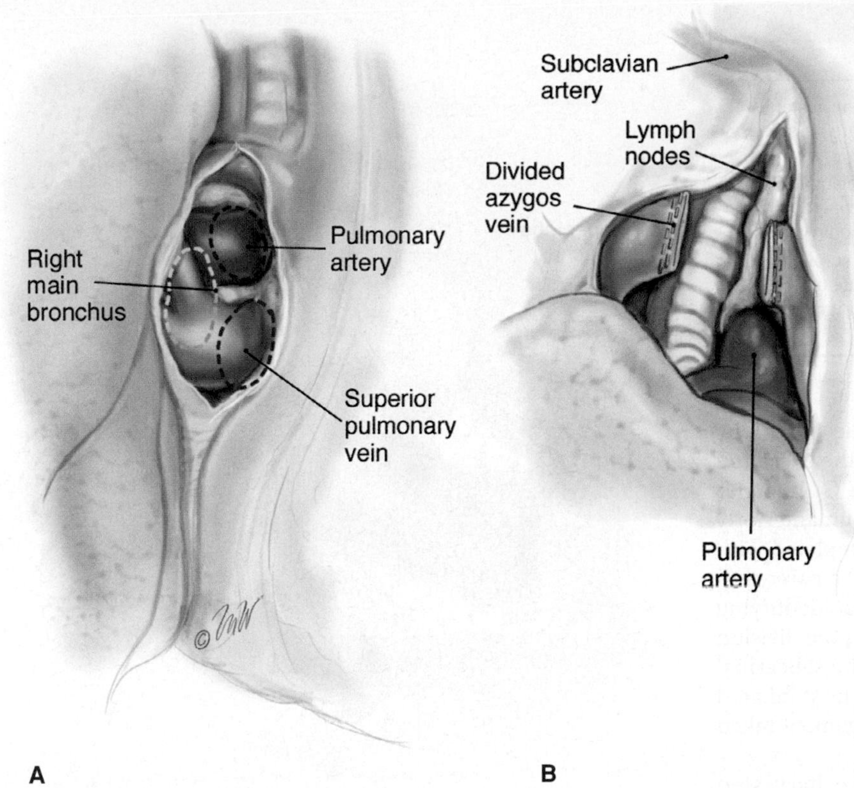

Figure 71-1. Right upper lobectomy: *A.* The anatomy of the hilum viewed from the patient's side forms a triangle. *B.* The azygos vein, which caps the triangle, can be divided to gain proximal control of the pulmonary artery.

stapling devices. More recent experience demonstrates that an energy device (specifically Ligasure) safely divides the small vessel.

Developing the plane between the bronchus and the artery is the most dangerous part of a right upper lobectomy.

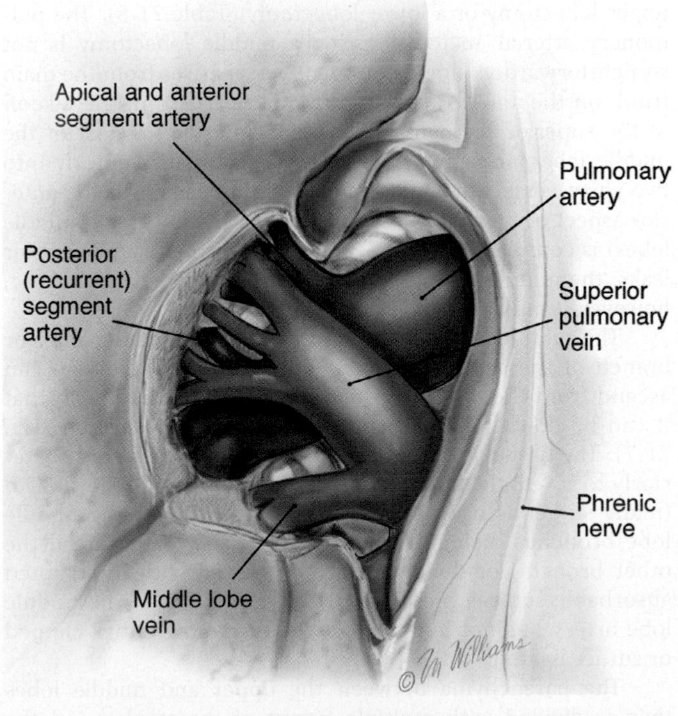

Figure 71-2. Right upper lobectomy: Hilar exposure. If the superior vein lies anterior to the pulmonary artery, the middle lobe vein must be identified and preserved.

Granulomatous disease, preoperative chemoradiation, and even mediastinoscopy may result in adhesions between the posterior wall of the artery and the anterior wall of the bronchus that may lead to injury to the artery. If there is evidence of such adhesions the azygos vein must be divided to obtain proximal control of the PA. The arterial anatomy to the right upper lobe varies significantly, sometimes present as a single large trunk or two or three smaller branches off the main PA (Fig. 71-3). Three single branches to respective segments of the upper lobe is the most unusual presentation, but when present, the branches can be doubly clipped and divided. A large main trunk may either be divided with a stapler or clipped and closed with running Prolene (3-0 or 4-0) or silk (3-0). After the vessels to the right upper lobe segments are identified and divided, a recurrent or posterior ascending branch, usually smaller than the main branches to the upper lobe, can be identified in most patients. Clipping is the best way to control it.

With the vasculature controlled, the bronchus is carefully dissected, first with scissors and then with a finger (Fig. 71-4). Nodes around the bronchus should be harvested both for staging and to permit better closure of the bronchus. The bronchus then can be divided after closure with a stapling device (heavy tissue or green loads should be used), or it can be divided with scissors or blade (being careful to leave enough tissue to close it without tension) and closed with interrupted absorbable sutures (PDS, usually 2-0 or 3-0). If stapled, the stapler's long axis should lie along the axis of the membranous trachea. By doing so, the flexible membranous trachea will seal the cartilaginous trachea.

The parenchyma then is divided and sealed. The anterior (minor) fissure between the upper and lower lobes is sometimes absent or is incomplete. In this case, a stapler can be used to divide the parenchyma between the upper and lower lobes. The middle lobe vein is used as a landmark to identify the

Table 71-6

TYPES OF STAPLERS

1. Vascular staplers, gray, white, or red, usually with a 2.5-mm staple length. They are used to close pulmonary artery or single pulmonary veins.
2. Medium thickness staplers, blue, usually with a 3.5-mm staple length. They are used to divide parenchyma or to control left atrium when tumor approaches close to the origin of the pulmonary vein.
3. Heavy thickness staplers, green, usually with a 4.8-mm staple length, or black with 5-mm staple length designed to close tissue up to 3 mm thick. They are used for thick pulmonary parenchyma or for bronchi.

fissure (Fig. 71-5). After the bronchus is divided, the upper lobe and bronchus should be lifted toward the apex of the chest and the parenchyma divided using multiple fires of a GIA stapler or clamps and then oversewn. The division is begun anteriorly just caudad to the middle lobe vein and then completed with sequential firings of the stapler, first completing the parenchymal division between the upper and middle lobes, identifying and avoiding the artery deep, and then completing the division posteriorly between the upper and lower lobes. The subcarinal and paratracheal nodes should be harvested, the lung inflated to test for air leaks, and the inferior pulmonary ligament taken down.

The paratracheal and subcarinal nodes are harvested and sent to the pathologist. The middle lobe is tacked to the lower lobe with 3-0 Vicryl sutures and the chest policed for bleeding points. Bronchial margins should be checked, at least, before closing the chest to ensure complete resection (Table 71-7).

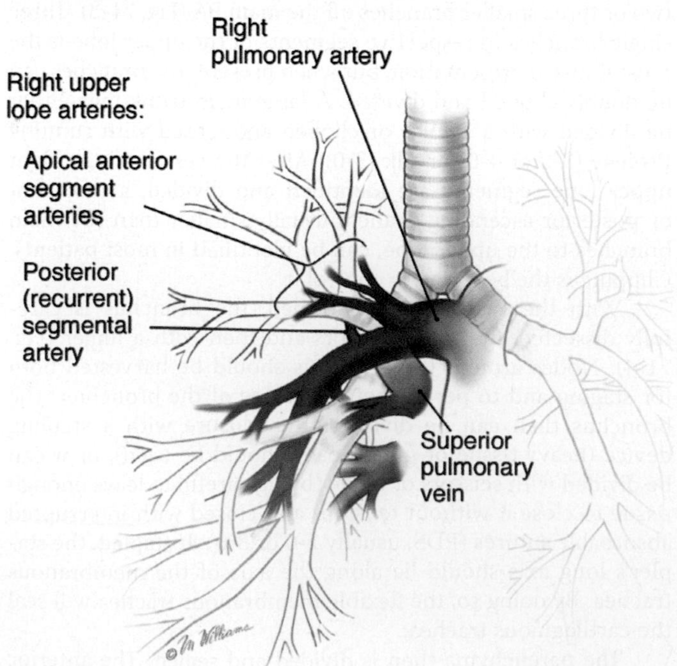

Figure 71-3. Right upper lobectomy: Pulmonary arterial anatomy pertinent to right upper lobectomy. A single more inferior branch of the pulmonary artery usually ascends superiorly to the right upper lobe and must be controlled and divided.

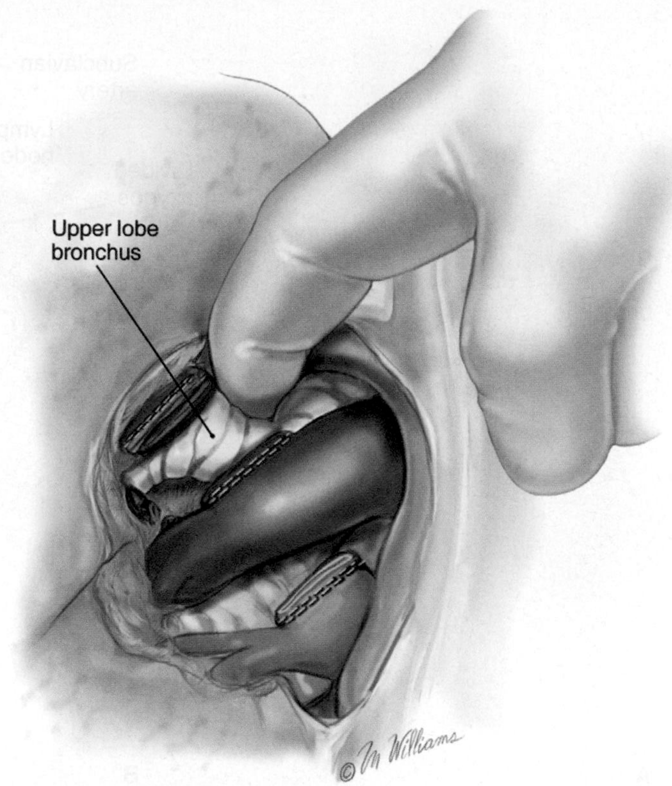

Figure 71-4. Right upper lobectomy: After the vasculature is controlled, the bronchus is dissected.

Right Middle Lobectomy

Right middle lobectomies are rarely done alone and probably are done more commonly as bilobectomies, together with an upper lobectomy or a lower lobectomy (Table 71-8). The pulmonary arterial anatomy during a middle lobectomy is not straightforward. A single dominant vessel arises from the main trunk on the anterior surface directly across from the takeoff of the superior segmental artery and inferior to most of the middle lobe parenchyma (Fig. 71-6). It branches quickly into two short vessels that subsequently branch again. If the anterior aspect of the major fissure (between the lower and middle lobes) is complete or can be completed without significant air leaks, the middle lobe artery often can be divided first. If not, however, it must be divided last.

The middle lobe vein is identified as the smaller inferior branch of the superior vein. Rarely, a middle lobe vein can ascend from the inferior vein. This vein is small enough that it can be doubly clipped and divided or suture ligated (Fig. 71-7). The tissue deep to the vein then should be swept posteriorly to reveal the middle lobe bronchus. It should be stapled (many surgeons use a blue stapler load only for the middle lobe bronchus, using green or thick tissue loads for all the other bronchi) or divided and then closed with interrupted absorbable sutures (2-0 or 3-0 Vicryl or PDS). If the middle lobe artery has not been controlled, it is now either clipped or suture ligated.

The parenchyma between the upper and middle lobes then is divided with multiple firings of the stapler, and the specimen margins are sent to the pathologist. Subcarinal and paratracheal nodes are harvested and the lung inflated to test

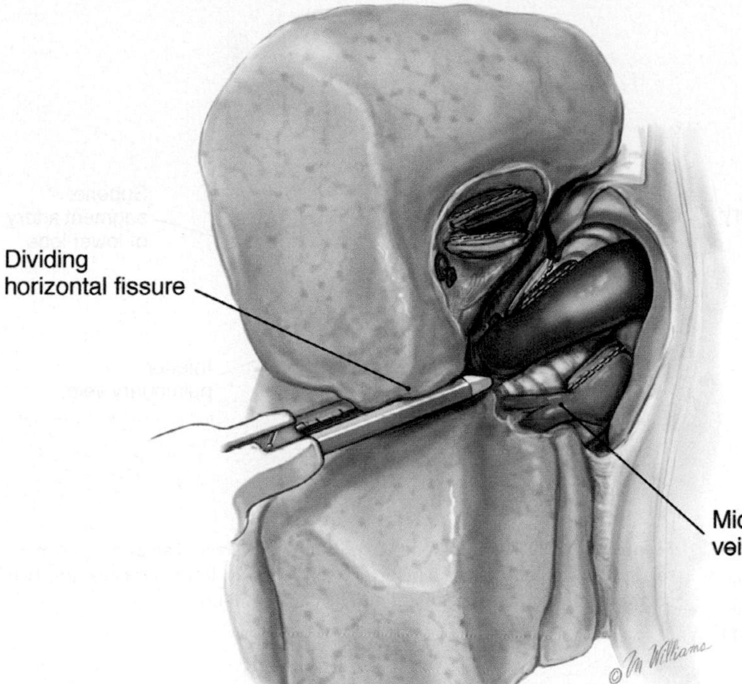

Figure 71-5. Right upper lobectomy: The horizontal fissure is divided using a stapler. Note the middle lobe vein serves as a guide for locating the minor fissure between the upper and lower lobes.

the bronchial and parenchymal closure. The chest should be policed for bleeding points and instrument counts confirmed.

Right Lower Lobectomy

When the major fissure is complete, a right lower lobectomy is the most straightforward of the lobectomies. The artery to the lower lobe, which branches into two trunks – the superior segmental and the basilar segment arteries (Fig. 71-8) – can be identified in the fissure. The takeoff of the middle lobe artery must be identified and preserved, and the lower artery then should be encircled and divided inferior to that takeoff but superior to the superior segmental artery (Fig. 71-9). Alternatively, the basilar segmental artery and superior segmental artery can be divided separately (Table 71-9).

The inferior vein is identified by taking down the inferior pulmonary ligament, harvesting the level 8 and 9 nodes at this time (Fig. 71-10). The phrenic nerve lies close along the anterior aspect of the ligament and must be protected and preserved. The inferior vein then is encircled and either divided with a vascular load stapler or clamped and oversewn with a running Prolene suture.

The parenchyma is divided anteriorly and posteriorly with a stapler (Fig. 71-11). This leaves only the bronchus, which must be divided in such a way as to protect the middle lobe bronchus.

When the fissure is not complete or scarring in the fissure prevents identification of the artery, a lower lobectomy can be done cephalad to caudad. In the right lower lobe, the vein, bronchus, and artery lie almost in a line (from caudad to cephalad) and can be divided in that order. With this approach, the inferior pulmonary ligament is taken down and the vein identified. It is divided and controlled either with a stapler or clamps and sutures, and the lower lobe then is elevated caudad. The pleural reflections anteriorly and posteriorly are divided, and the bronchus now comes into view. In patients with granulomatous

Table 71-7

CHECKING THE MARGINS

1. Check all margins (bronchus, artery, vein, and parenchyma) that appear close
2. Bronchial margins are all that is necessary for most lobectomies
3. Cut your own margins:
   a. To prevent nodal metastases from being read as positive margins
      i. Clean off all nodal tissue from bronchus, artery, or vein
      ii. Wash margin tissue in distilled water to lyse free-floating cells
   b. To ensure that the appropriate tissue is evaluated
4. To prevent "surprise" positive margins, ask your pathologist to "freeze all margins to be subsequently evaluated"
5. Consider additional resection for any positive margin

Table 71-8

POTENTIAL HAZARDS DURING RIGHT MIDDLE LOBECTOMY

1. Injuring the ongoing pulmonary artery:
   a. Manipulating the lung after division of the bronchus and vein.
   b. While dissecting out the middle lobe artery in the main fissure. Solution for both—dissect the main pulmonary artery and obtain control for any unusually difficult dissections. This allows quick control of the artery if there is injury.
2. Compromising the bronchus to the lower lobe while dividing the middle lobe bronchus:
   Solution—clamp the middle lobe bronchus prior to division, and then inflate the lower lobe. If it does not inflate, consider intraoperative bronchoscopy to evaluate the lower lobe bronchus before dividing the bronchus.

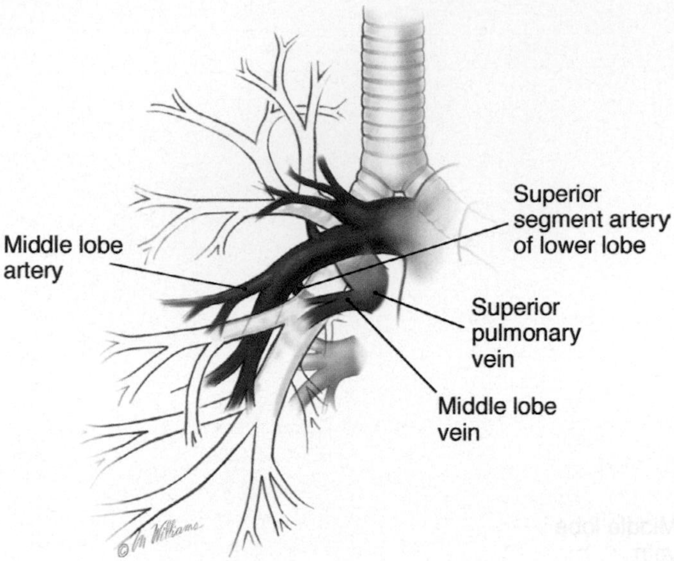

Figure 71-6. Right middle lobectomy: Pulmonary arterial anatomy pertinent to right middle lobectomy. Note the middle lobe artery, a single dominant vessel arising from the main trunk on the anterior surface across from the superior segmental artery.

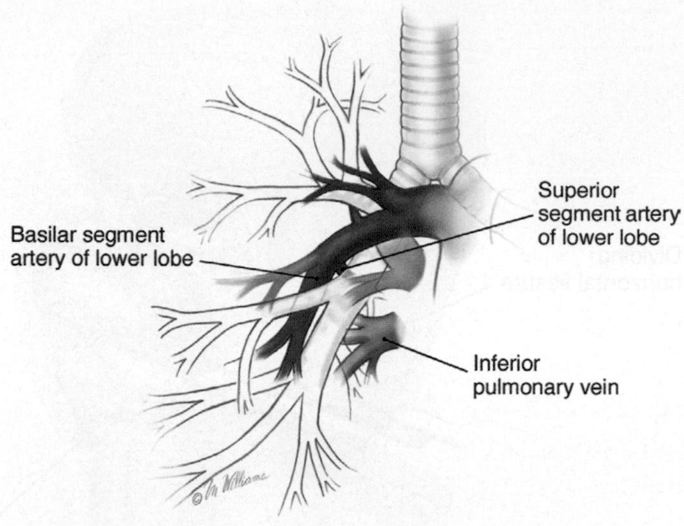

Figure 71-8. Right lower lobectomy: Pulmonary arterial anatomy pertinent to right lower lobectomy. The artery to the lower lobe branches into two segments, the superior segment and basilar segment.

disease or other inflammatory processes, the artery and bronchus will be adhesed. The bronchus must be carefully dissected away from the artery and then divided as described earlier. If the artery can be dissected away from the parenchyma and divided, that is ideal. Alternatively, the vein and bronchus can be retracted inferiorly, and blue (intermediate) stapler loads can be used to divide the parenchyma and artery together. From experience, it is safe to include the artery with parenchyma in an intermediate stapler load, as long as the bronchus has been divided and retracted away.

Pericardiectomy

Rarely, a tumor invading the pericardium around the inferior vein can be resected with an incision in the pericardium

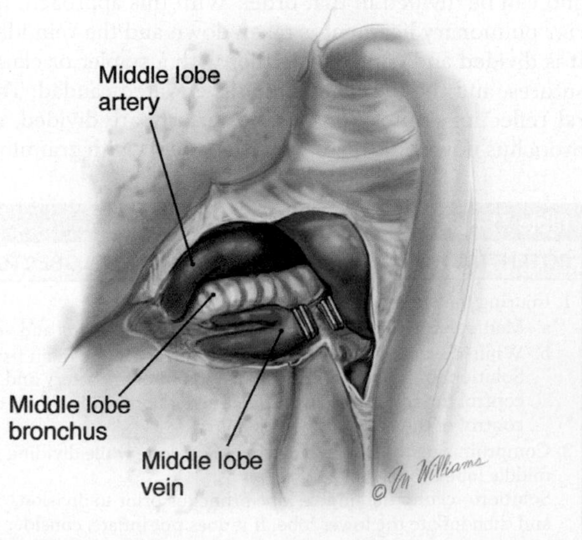

Figure 71-7. Right middle lobectomy: Middle lobe vein is double-clipped and divided, or suture ligated.

that avoids the phrenic nerve. This is usually easy because the phrenic nerve lies farther from the hilum at the level of the inferior vein than at the superior vein. After the pericardium is opened, approximately 1 to 1.5 cm of additional margin on the inferior vein is now available to resect the lower lobe without requiring a pneumonectomy (Fig. 71-12). This intrapericardial approach is more commonly used for pneumonectomy.

Left Upper Lobectomy

A left upper lobectomy truly is done in "tiger country." The main PA appears in the left pleural space from the arch of the aorta. Both are close to the recurrent nerve and to the phrenic nerve (Fig. 71-13 and Table 71-10).

Order of Technique

While the right upper lobe almost always has to be taken from superior to inferior, the left upper lobe can be approached anteriorly, superiorly, posteriorly, or inferiorly. Approached anteriorly, the superior vein is mobilized away from the artery and then divided first. This uncovers the anterior aspect of the PA and allows sequential division of the pulmonary arterial vessels, the anterior and apicoposterior branches of the artery, and the lingular artery (Fig. 71-14). The parenchyma then is divided and finally the bronchus. This approach is best followed when the tumor adheres to the artery and dividing the vein can give better access to the main PA or branches of the PA.

If the mass lies in the lung periphery, a superior approach is usually best for two reasons—the arterial supply can be controlled first, and the fissure can be stapled and sealed easily. For this approach, the pleural reflection is first divided, and then the apicoposterior arterial branch (sometimes both the apicoposterior and anterior branches) is divided after the main PA is encircled with tape to control it (Fig. 71-15). The superior pulmonary vein then is divided. This usually leaves the bronchus and the lingular arteries. Ideally, the arteries and parenchyma should be harvested first and the bronchus last. However, the bronchus can be taken before the arteries if care is taken to avoid avulsing the arteries. As earlier, the bronchi can be closed

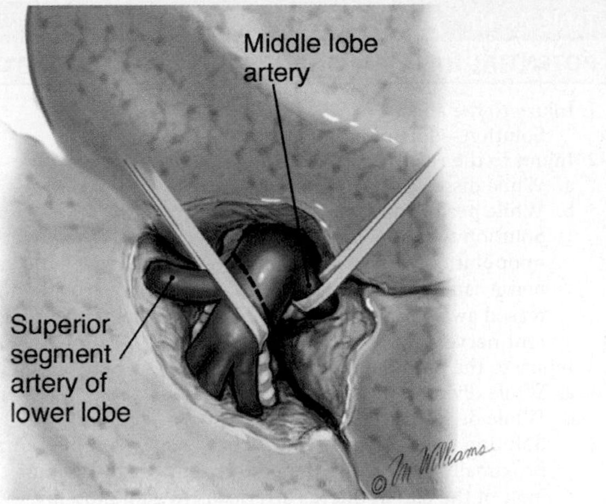

Figure 71-9. Right lower lobectomy: After identifying the middle lobe artery which is preserved, the basilar segmental artery is encircled and then divided.

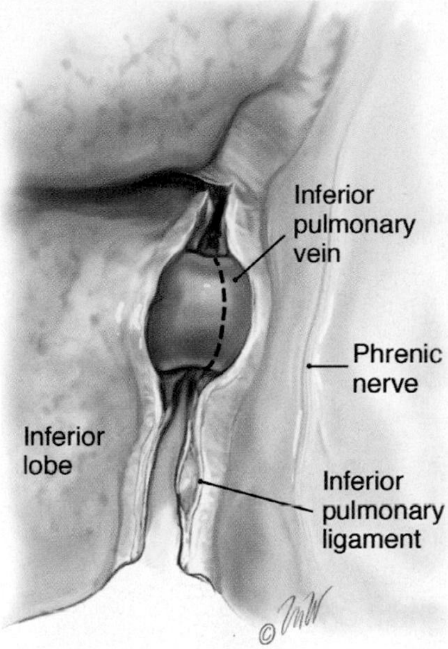

Figure 71-10. Right lower lobectomy: The inferior pulmonary ligament is taken down, with caution to avoid injury to the phrenic nerve, to expose the inferior pulmonary vein. This vein is encircled and divided, or clamped and oversewn.

with a heavy (green load) stapler or can be sewn with interrupted absorbable sutures (Vicryl 3-0 or PDS 3-0). The margins should be checked for evidence of disease, and the aortopulmonary nodes and subcarinal nodes should be harvested.

Problem Areas

Proximity to the aorta: Even tumors arising in the proximal upper lobe approaching the aorta seldom invade the aorta. However, bulk in the window at the origin of the PA can make access to the PA difficult. In this case, the adventitia and pleura that reflect off the aorta toward the PA can be divided and the mass mobilized inferiorly. This allows access to the proximal left PA, which then can be controlled just beyond its takeoff from the main PA. In addition, a large bulky tumor can potentially put torque on the main PA causing an adventitial "crack" which can lead to a full thickness injury and tear. If additional access is needed, two maneuvers can give additional mobility:

- Opening the pericardium
- Dividing the remnant of the patent ductus arteriosus

Either of these maneuvers put the recurrent nerve at risk.

The recurrent nerve: The vagus nerve descends from the neck in the coronal midline and crosses the aorta at the peak of the arch. The recurrent nerve branches off the vagus and curves superiorly toward the neck from the underside of the aorta. It is at risk with any mobilization of the PA and especially with aortopulmonary lymphadenectomy. The nerve should be visualized, and direct resection or injury should be avoided, but one must remember that the nerve is very sensitive to indirect injuries such as distant cautery or even mild traction.

Table 71-9

POTENTIAL HAZARDS DURING RIGHT LOWER LOBECTOMY

1. Injuring the right middle lobe artery during dissection of the lower lobe arteries.
2. Compromising the lumen of the right middle lobe bronchus while dividing the right lower lobe bronchus.
   Solution—clamp the lower lobe bronchus prior to division, and then inflate the right lung to confirm expansion of the middle lobe. If it does not inflate, consider intraoperative bronchoscopy to evaluate the lower lobe bronchus before dividing the bronchus.
3. Injuring the phrenic nerve while dissecting the hilum of the lower lobe.
   Solution—be cognizant that the inferior course of the phrenic nerve may track posteriorly close to the inferior vein.

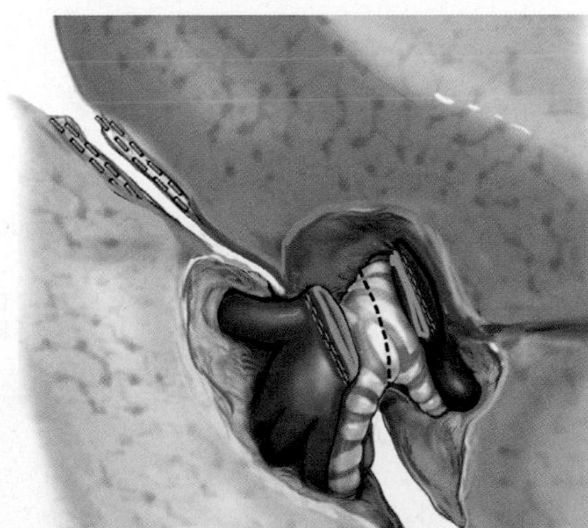

Figure 71-11. Right lower lobectomy: After the vascular has been divided, the parenchyma is divided superior and inferiorly using a stapler, leaving only the bronchus, which is carefully dissected away from the artery, and then divided.

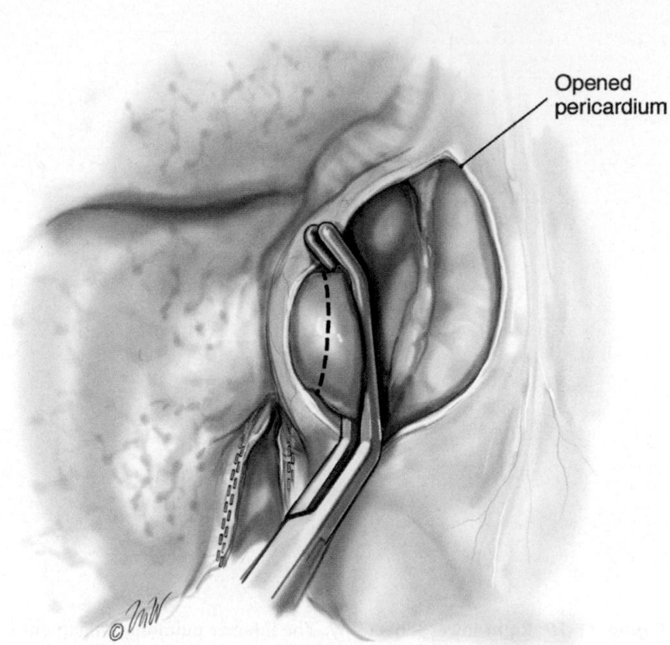

Figure 71-12. Pericardiectomy: A 1- to 1.5-cm margin of inferior pulmonary vein is available for resecting the lower lobe without necessitating pneumonectomy.

Table 71-10
POTENTIAL HAZARDS DURING LEFT UPPER LOBECTOMY
1. Injury to the aorta: Solution—don't do it! 2. Injury to the recurrent nerve: a. While dissecting the pulmonary artery. b. While performing lymphadenectomy. Solution to both—identify the vagus nerve as it courses over the midpoint of the aorta. If suspicious nodes involve the vagus, the nerve can be divided close to the pulmonary artery, and the nodes teased away from the underside of the aorta, preserving the recurrent nerve. 3. Injury to the pulmonary artery: a. While dividing the short arterial vessels. b. While dividing the bronchus. Solution to both—gain control of the left main pulmonary artery proximally by opening the pericardium, or by dividing the remnant of the patent ductus arteriosus to gain mobility.

Postoperative Clinical Note

After left upper lobectomy and nodal dissection, patients should be carefully evaluated for voice strength and potential aspiration within the first 12 hours after surgery. Any suspicious findings (hoarseness or coughing after drinking) should prompt video swallowing evaluation. Those patients with aspiration should not eat or drink until they receive successful swallowing therapy or vocal cord medialization.

Phrenic nerve injury: The phrenic nerve lies just anterior to the hilum and is at risk during dissection or from tumor invasion.

Left Lower Lobectomy: Complete or Nearly Complete Fissure

As with the right lower lobe, the left lower lobe can be approached superiorly if the fissure is complete or nearly so. In this case, the parenchymal division is completed first. The arteries to the superior segment and to the basilar segments in the fissure are divided next. Stapler division with vascular loads or ties with

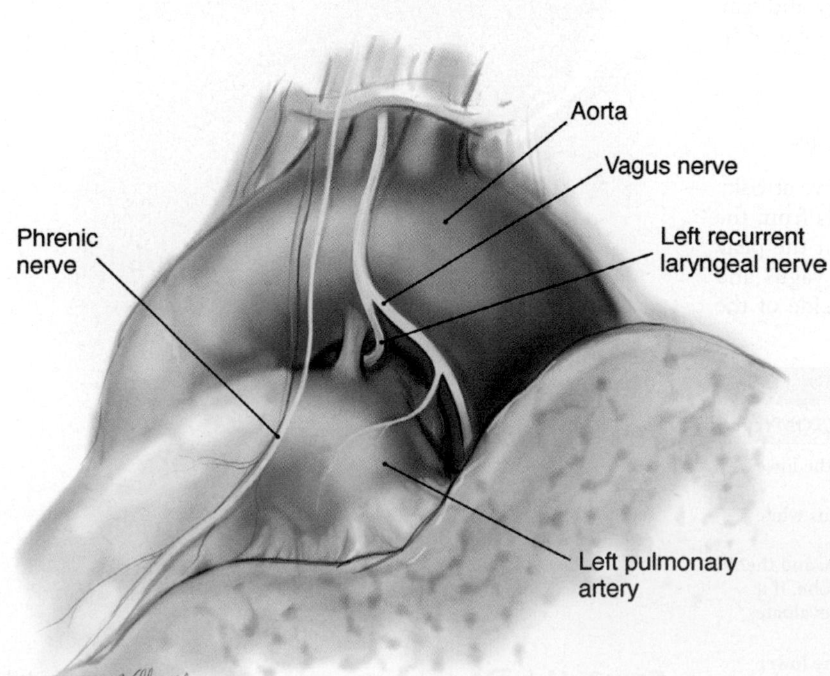

Figure 71-13. Left upper lobectomy: The proximity of the recurrent laryngeal and phrenic nerves and aorta can pose many obstacles to easy left upper lobectomy.

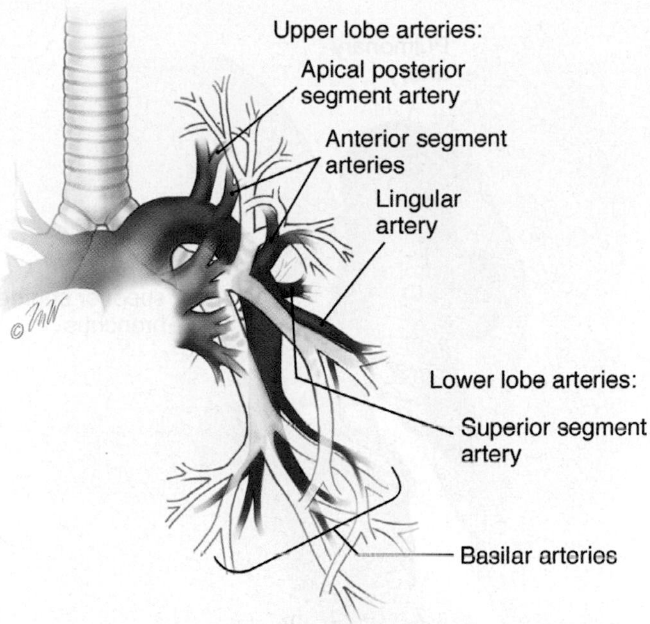

Figure 71-14. Left upper lobectomy: Pulmonary arterial anatomy pertinent to left upper lobectomy, which can be approached anteriorly, superiorly, posteriorly, or inferiorly.

suture transfixation or double ties should be used to control the vessels.

After the arteries are controlled and divided, the vein can be divided in the same fashion as the artery. The vein may be identified posteriorly and dissected away from the bronchus (Fig. 71-16) or identified anteriorly by taking down the inferior ligament and encircling the vein. The vein then is divided in a standard fashion.

The parenchyma between the upper and lower lobes is divided in one of the manners described earlier, and the bronchus is closed either with a stapler or interrupted absorbable sutures (Fig. 71-17).

Left Lower Lobectomy: Absent or Incomplete Fissure

If the fissure is absent or very incomplete, left lower lobectomy can be done from the bottom up—that is, division of vein, bronchus, artery, and parenchyma, in that order. The pulmonary ligament is carefully taken down and the inferior vein is encircled and divided by the preferred method—stapler or suture division. Double ties are seldom used for this vein. The vein is deep to the bronchus which is deep to the artery, which is deep to the parenchyma. The divided vein is retracted inferiorly, and the bronchus, which is adjacent and immediately superior to the vein, is then dissected and divided and then closed either with a stapler or with absorbable sutures. The artery to the lower lobe is divided (being careful to preserve

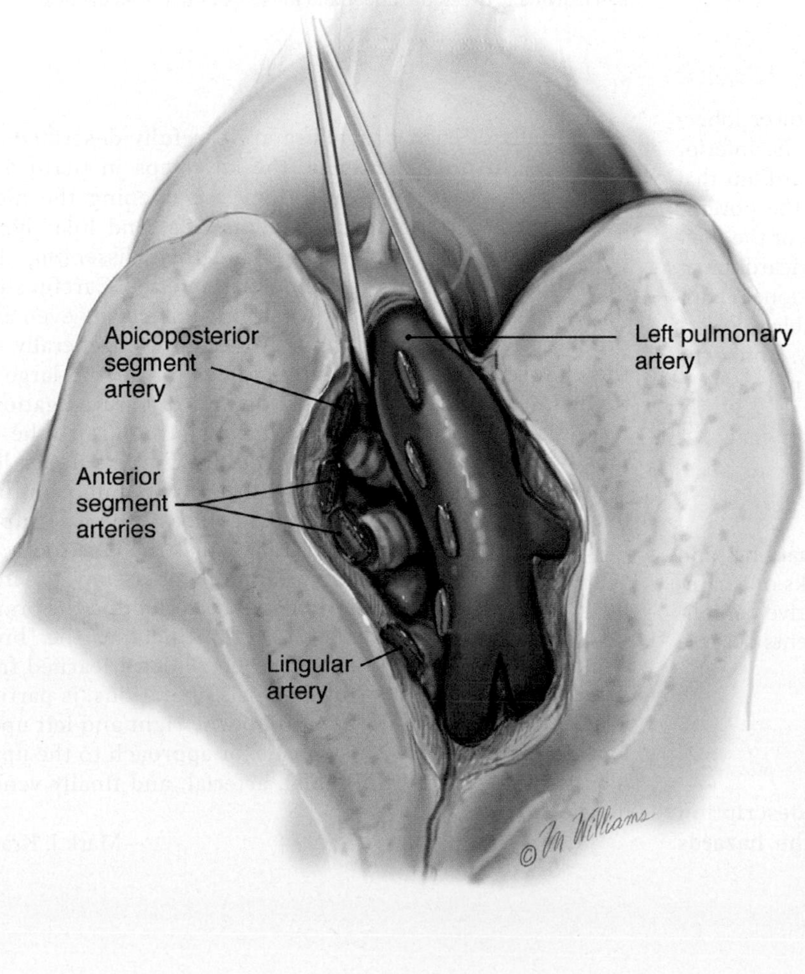

Figure 71-15. Left upper lobectomy: A superior approach to access a peripheral lung mass in the left upper lobe. The main pulmonary artery is encircled with tape to establish control and the apicoposterior and anterior arterial branches are divided.

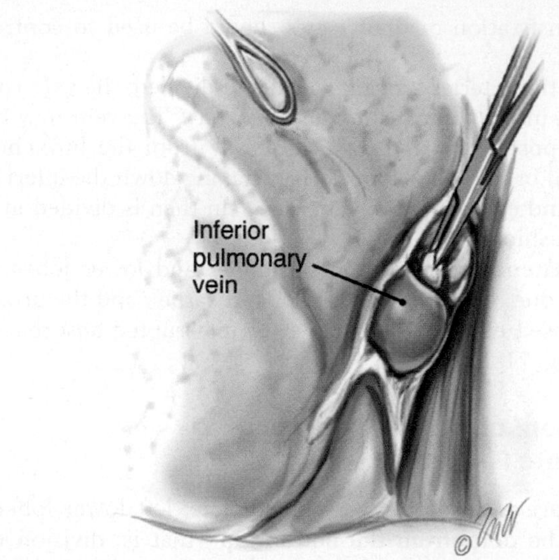

Figure 71-16. Left lower lobectomy: The inferior pulmonary vein is divided in much same fashion as the pulmonary artery. The vein is identified and dissected away from the bronchus.

the lingular artery to the upper lobe), and the parenchyma is divided and sealed with stapler division. Alternatively, the artery and the parenchyma can be mass ligated and divided with staplers (blue loads) without problem. From experience, it is safe to include the artery with parenchyma in an intermediate stapler load, as long as the bronchus has been divided and retracted away.

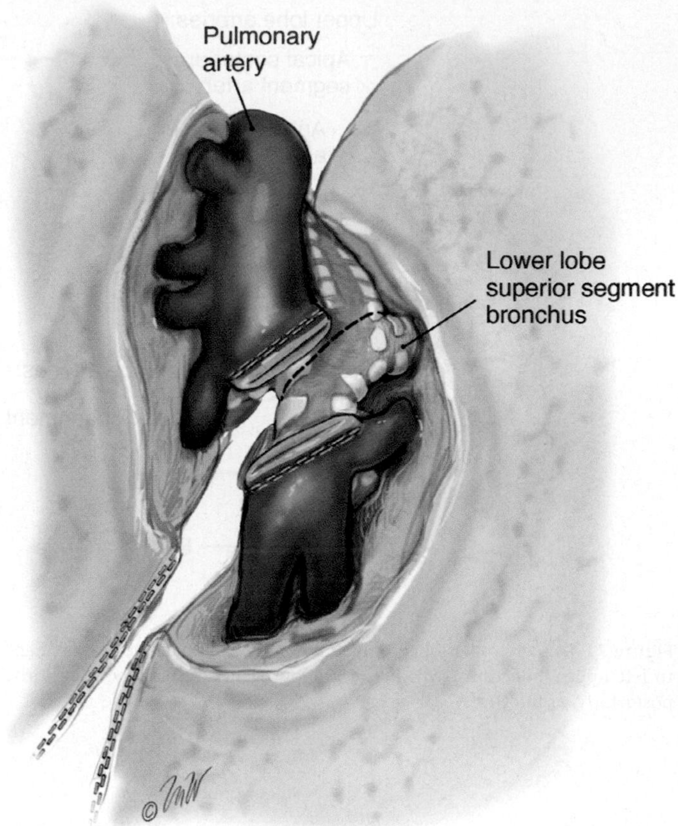

Figure 71-17. Left lower lobectomy: The lower lobe superior segment bronchus is closed with a stapler or interrupted absorbable sutures after the parenchyma between the upper and lower lobes has been divided.

PERICARDIECTOMY

As mentioned above in the description of right lower lobectomy, a tumor invading the pericardium around the inferior vein can be resected with an incision in the pericardium that avoids the phrenic nerve. This is usually easy, as the phrenic nerve lies further away from the hilum at the level of the inferior vein than at the superior vein. After the pericardium is opened, approximately one to one and a half additional centimeters of margin on the inferior vein now are available to resect the lower lobe without requiring a pneumonectomy. Unlike the case with pneumonectomy, the pericardium does not need to be reconstructed when a lobectomy is done.

CONCLUSION

Performing a careful lobectomy, assessing the margins, and completing a thorough lymphadenectomy are marks of a careful thoracic surgeon. Avoiding common postoperative complications are marks of a thorough clinician. Our patients deserve nothing less.

EDITOR'S COMMENT

Dr. Roberts has provided an excellent, detailed description of each of the five lobectomies. Specifically, the hazards and pitfalls of each procedure are carefully described and reviewed. In my experience, the key steps in performing open or thoracoscopic lobectomy are opening the mediastinal pleura, removing the mediastinal and hilar lymph nodes as they are encountered, and then dissecting right onto the adventitia of the pulmonary arteries. Careful sharp dissection can ensure a safe anatomic lobectomy even after preoperative chemoradiation. Although we generally use the endoscopic linear vascular stapler for all the large PA branches, standard double ligation and/or suture ligation is used for smaller vessels to avoid avulsion injury to the PA. Finally, when performing a lobectomy, the left upper lobe PA dissection is the most difficult, in my opinion, as there usually are many short vessels. In contrast, the right upper lobectomy is the most straightforward as the PA usually is a separate trunk. In performing a middle lobectomy, the main pitfall is injury to the underlying main PA behind the branch PA. An option for difficult dissection includes the "bronchus first" approach. This technique, which I learned from surgeons who did many tuberculosis operations, is particularly helpful postchemoradiation in the right and left upper lobe situation. It involves a posterior approach to the upper lobe with sequential bronchial, arterial, and finally venous division.

—Mark J. Krasna

References

1. Goodney PP, Lucas FL, Stukel TA, et al. Surgeon specialty and operative mortality with lung resection. *Ann Surg*. 2005;241(1):179–184.
2. Little AG, Rusch VW, Bonner JA, et al. Patterns of surgical care of lung cancer patients. *Ann Thorac Surg*. 2005;80(6):2051–2056; discussion 2056.
3. Nakamura H, Taniguchi Y, Miwa K, et al. Comparison of the surgical outcomes of thoracoscopic lobectomy, segmentectomy, and wedge resection for clinical stage I non-small cell lung cancer. *Thorac Cardiovasc Surg*. 2011;59(3):137–141.

Selected References

1. Kates M, Swanson S, Wisnivesky JP. Survival following lobectomy and limited resection for the treatment of stage I non-small cell lung cancer <= 1 cm in size: a review of SEER data. *Chest*. 2011;139(3): 491–496.
2. Fan J, Wang L, Jiang GN, et al. Sublobectomy versus lobectomy for stage I non-small-cell lung cancer, a meta-analysis of published studies. *Ann Surg Oncol*. 2012;19(2):661–668.
3. Whitson BA, Groth SS, Andrade RS, et al. Survival after lobectomy versus segmentectomy for stage I non-small cell lung cancer: a population-based analysis. *Ann Thorac Surg*. 2011;92(6):1943–1950.
4. Roberts JR, Blum MG, Arildsen R, et al. Prospective comparison of radiologic, thoracoscopic, and pathologic staging in patients with early non-small cell lung cancer. *Ann Thorac Surg*. 1999;68(4): 1154–1158.

72 Pneumonectomy

John R. Roberts

Keywords: Pulmonary resection, lobectomy, sleeve resection

As long as surgery remains the best curative treatment for lung cancer, patients will continue to require pneumonectomy to treat lung cancer and for other occasional problems.[1] Arguably, no other surgery carries as high a risk for perioperative mortality as pneumonectomy. Operative mortality from pneumonectomy has been reported to be between 5% and 20%.[2–8] In a meta-analysis of 27 studies, 90-day mortality for right pneumonectomy was 20% and left pneumonectomy was 9%, for an overall mortality of 11%.[9] For this reason, appropriate selection, operative technique, and postoperative management of patients who potentially may undergo pneumonectomy is crucial. We say *potentially* because patients scheduled for pneumonectomy ultimately may undergo a sleeve resection or exploration without resection depending on the findings at surgery.

Surprisingly, low preoperative lung function has not been demonstrated consistently to increase the perioperative risk of pneumonectomy, although some authors have found preoperative lung function to be an important factor.[10–12] This finding may result from diligent efforts to identify and eliminate patients with poor pulmonary function from the surgical pool. Some have found poor preoperative lung function to increase the preoperative risk.[13–15] Other factors have included increased age,[7,8,11,14,16,17] right-sided procedures,[8,9,12,14–19] preoperative chemo/radiation,[12,14,20] large intraoperative fluid volumes,[12,20,21] perioperative cardiac dysrhythmias,[16] and immediate preoperative smoking history.[12,22]

This chapter includes discussion of the preoperative evaluation and management of pneumonectomy patients, the decision to perform pneumonectomy rather than sleeve resection, the technical aspects of the operation, and the postoperative management, all with the goal of decreasing perioperative mortality.

PREOPERATIVE EVALUATION AND MANAGEMENT

Staging, Surgical, or PET?

All patients with lung cancer, especially those who may undergo pneumonectomy, should first undergo preoperative staging (Table 72-1). At this time, a complete history and a physical examination that focuses on the identification of lymph nodes and liver masses, followed by a chest CT scan and a PET scan, are appropriate. This evaluation will rule out distant metastases other than brain metastases. Patients without symptoms of headache and with PET-negative mediastinum are unlikely to have brain metastases, so that brain CT scans or MRIs are not obligatory. However, the risk of the procedure supports appropriate evaluation to rule out brain metastases if the surgeon desires.

Table 72-1

PREOPERATIVE AND PRERESECTION STAGING FOR POTENTIAL PNEUMONECTOMY PATIENTS

1. Complete history and physical examination
2. Chest CT scan
3. Positron emission tomography
4. Brain MRI
5. Mediastinoscopy
6. Thoracoscopy

Candidates for pneumonectomy typically have large or hilar masses and thus a high likelihood of mediastinal metastases. Although PET scans are quite sensitive for detecting mediastinal metastases, they remain less accurate than mediastinoscopy[23] (see Chapter 70). For this reason, tissue biopsy (either with endobronchial ultrasound, preoperative mediastinoscopy, or thoracoscopy) is indicated for patients who may undergo pneumonectomy, even if they have a PET-negative mediastinum. PET scans are useful for ruling out distant metastases, but should not be the only study used to evaluate the mediastinum.

Surgical Evaluation

We have discussed the importance of surgical staging of the mediastinum prior to pneumonectomy. Two other surgical evaluations (bronchoscopic and thoracoscopic) should be considered.

Bronchoscopic evaluation of the airway will ensure that a patient with a hilar mass on the right does not also have an endobronchial lesion on the left. The patient could die from the surgery to attempt to cure his right-sided cancer, and even if the surgery is successful, the pneumonectomy would have no impact on the left-sided cancer.

Thoracoscopic examination and staging of the pleural space benefits patients undergoing pneumonectomy in several ways[24]:

1. Thoracoscopy helps to rule out pleural metastases that usually cannot be identified except at exploration.
2. Thoracoscopic nodal sampling or lymphadenectomy can evaluate suspicious nodes in patients who have not had tissue nodal sampling.
3. Thoracoscopy can be used to determine the incision used for resection (see also Chapters 2 and 70).

Cardiopulmonary Evaluation

An extensive but complicated literature describes the various modalities used to evaluate preoperative lung function as a means to predict postoperative complications. A preoperative forced expiratory volume in 1 second (FEV_1) of more than 2 L has been relatively arbitrarily chosen as a threshold for resection without further pulmonary evaluation and has been confirmed by experience.

Table 72-2

PREOPERATIVE CARDIOPULMONARY EVALUATION

1. Complete pulmonary function testing
2. For patients with FEV_1 <2 L or 50% of predicted:
   a. Quantitative perfusion scanning to evaluate lung function on each side
   b. Diffusion capacity evaluation
3. Complete history and physical examination for patients with any history of angina, documented atherosclerotic cardiovascular disease (ASCVD), or congestive heart failure (CHF)
   a. Evaluation by cardiologist, with possible stress testing or echocardiogram

The obstructive nature of cancers that may lead to pneumonectomy assures that many patients will have less than 50% perfusion to the affected lung. Quantitative perfusion scanning has been used successfully for almost 30 years to determine the relative contribution of each lung to the patient's lung function.[6] Patients with a predicted postoperative FEV_1 (better than preoperative FEV_1) of more than 800 mL are considered to have adequate pulmonary reserve to undergo resection. This technique has been found to be accurate in long-term follow-up (up to 5 years),[25] especially with respect to predicting the postoperative FEV_1[26] (Table 72-2). Kim et al.[13] have reported that perfusion less than 35% to the resected lung diminishes the operative risk. These parameters are also currently used in most cooperative group trials including lung resection.

Typical cardiac ischemia evaluations (i.e., stress testing) should be done in all patients with any history of cardiac ischemia (angina, other chest pain, or history of coronary artery bypass) and should be considered in patients with significant peripheral vascular disease.

Left Lung Resection

Left pneumonectomy generally is safer than right pneumonectomy, at least in terms of overall perioperative and postoperative mortality. On the other hand, risks associated with long bronchial stump require careful technical attention to details of resection. However, the procedure may be technically more difficult, especially in patients with large hilar masses.

Left hilar cancers are truly in "tiger country," approaching or involving the aortic arch, recurrent laryngeal nerve, phrenic nerve, pericardium, and the main pulmonary artery before it bifurcates into right and left main pulmonary arteries. (The left main pulmonary artery is very short.) The primary procedures are described separately, since the anatomy and the dissections are different on the left and right sides.

TECHNIQUE

Left Pneumonectomy

The mediastinal pleura is divided circumferentially around the hilum using either scissors or an energy probe, including the inferior pulmonary ligament. Harvesting the lymph nodes in the aortopulmonary window gives better exposure to the proximal pulmonary artery. This must be done carefully to avoid injuring the recurrent laryngeal nerve, which branches off the vagus nerve on the inferior surface of the aortic arch and then dives into the mediastinum immediately inferior and adherent to the arch. Unless it is involved with tumor, the phrenic nerve should also be preserved until a decision is made about sleeve resection. It may abut the anterior aspect of the nodes in the AP window, and so is also at risk.

Harvesting the subcarinal lymph nodes gives better access to the bronchus and allows the surgeon to better palpate the bronchus. Cautery should be used judiciously or not at all in this space, since the blood vessels to the bronchus arise here.

The vagus superior to the aorta or the recurrent nerve can be harvested if either is involved with cancer. However, resection of these nerves will lead to vocal cord paralysis.

Evaluation for Sleeve Resection

The lung is examined carefully to determine whether sleeve resection is possible. Maneuvers that help include:

1. Dividing the pleura circumferentially;
2. Taking down the inferior pulmonary ligament;
3. Complete parenchymal separation of the upper and lower lobes; and
4. Completing the mediastinal lymphadenectomy.

Factors that make sleeve resection difficult include:

1. Tumors that invade the pericardium at either pulmonary vein;
2. Tumors that involve both the main pulmonary artery and the left mainstem bronchus; and
3. Tumors that involve artery or bronchus but extend into the fissure to involve the other lobe. Thus, upper lobe tumors that extend inferiorly to involve the fissure extensively or lower lobe tumors that extend superiorly can be difficult to resect and reconstruct.

The pulmonary artery is dissected away from the vein anteroinferiorly and the bronchus posteriorly (Fig. 72-1). This dissection is made safer by proceeding posteriorly to separate the artery from the bronchus (Fig. 72-2). Quite often this can be done bluntly, either with Kittner dissectors or with an index finger (see Fig. 72-1), and usually can be done before mobilizing or dividing the superior vein. However, in patients with an inferiorly positioned artery or superiorly positioned vein, the vein can be dissected and divided first.

The artery should be occluded with either a vascular clamp, a tourniquet, or a vascular stapler (closed but not fired) for 2 to 3 minutes to ensure that right ventricular failure or pulmonary hypertension will not result after pneumonectomy. After the artery is clamped, systolic blood pressure and oxygenation are assessed, and if stable, indicate that the patient can tolerate pneumonectomy. If hemodynamic instability or hypoxia develops, a pulmonary artery catheter may be inserted to direct pressor treatment, but in most cases, it is necessary to perform a sleeve resection or abandon the procedure altogether. Care should be taken during this maneuver not to "fracture" the PA when temporarily occluding the vessel.

Additional length on the artery (to allow complete resection) can be obtained by two specific maneuvers:

1. Dividing the ligamentum arteriosum (being careful to avoid injury to the recurrent nerve).
2. Opening the pericardium to identify the very short left main pulmonary artery within the pericardium. In this maneuver, it is recommended (obligatory) to test clamp the artery before it is divided because the anatomy may be distorted by the malignancy, which can lead to inadvertent division of the *main* pulmonary artery.

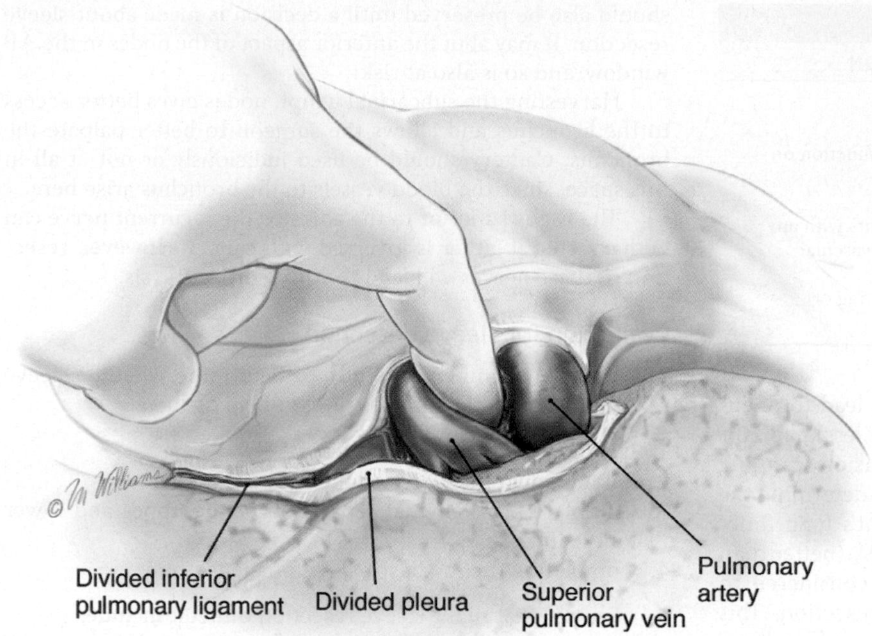

Figure 72-1. Left pneumonectomy. Using a combination of blunt and scissors dissection, the pulmonary artery is dissected away from the pulmonary vein anteroinferiorly.

The artery is divided by one of several techniques: vascular stapler (two fires with division between two stapler lines or with an endostapler that cuts between two stapler lines); vascular clamps proximal and distal, with a double suture line of 5-0 Prolene; or some combination of the above techniques (Fig. 72-3).

The pulmonary veins are now divided. If the tumor invades the pericardium, or if the pericardium has been opened to gain arterial control, the veins can be controlled and divided by extending the pericardial opening inferiorly, just posterior to the phrenic nerve. (The pericardium should be reconstructed if it is opened.) The pulmonary veins form a single branch as they enter the left atrium and can be divided at this level with any of the techniques described for the artery. Blue (3.5 mm) staplers, rather than vascular-load staplers, should be used to control the atrium because vascular loads can fail on this thicker tissue (Fig. 72-4) (Table 72-3).

When dividing the veins outside the pericardium, the superior and inferior veins must be identified separately. The inferior vein begins at the superior edge of the inferior pulmonary

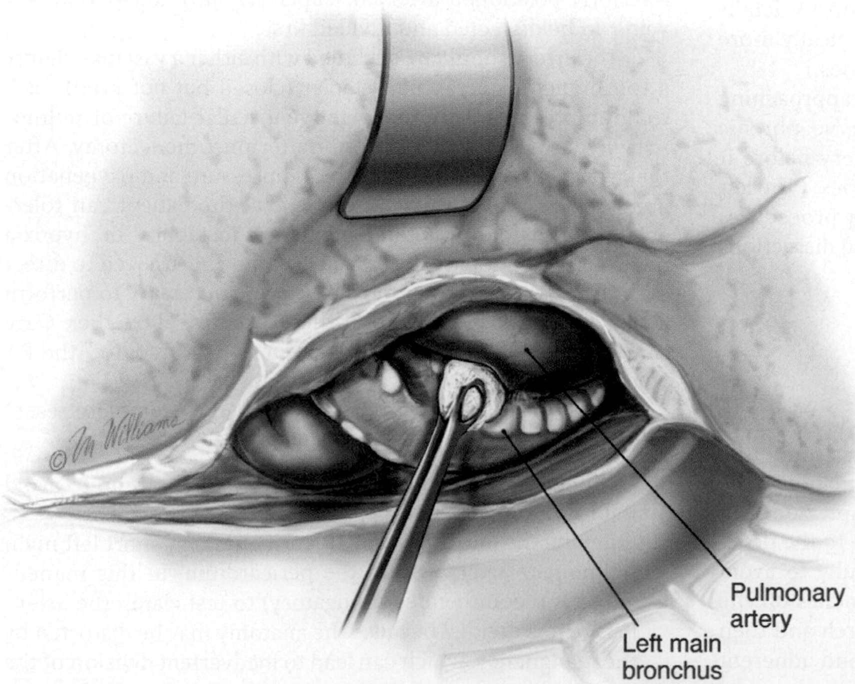

Figure 72-2. The bronchus is dissected away from the pulmonary artery posteriorly.

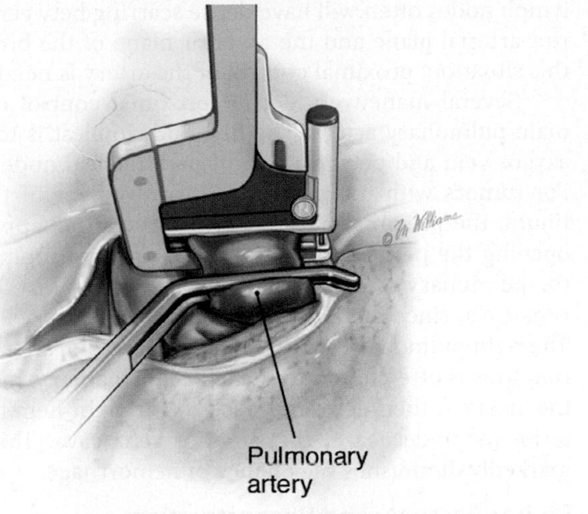

Figure 72-3. A vascular stapler is used to divide the artery. Other techniques may be used, including proximal and distal vascular clamps oversewn with a double suture of 5-0 Prolene.

ligament, and the superior vein is the most anterior structure of the hilum. These veins can be divided with vascular stapler loads or controlled with vascular clamps and oversewn with 4-0 or 5-0 Prolene.

Careful management of the bronchus decreases the chance of bronchial stump leak with its attendant dangers (Table 72-4). The table lists aspects of dissection that can affect the chances of bronchial stump devitalization or devascularization.

The bronchus is usually the last structure divided (Fig. 72-5). The lung is grasped and used to deliver the bronchus inferiorly into the chest, with the goal of dividing the left main bronchus just distal to the carina, while leaving sufficient length to avoid tension on the closure. The anesthesiologist is asked to hold ventilation and to back out the double-lumen tube or blocker used to collapse the left lung. The bronchial clamp or bronchial stapler is positioned across the bronchus to close it in an anterior-to-posterior fashion. If a stapler is used, the heavy load (green) or 4.8-mm stapler is chosen. The bronchus is divided and closed with the stapler or with absorbable suture (typically 2-0 or 3-0 PDS or Vicryl). This can be facilitated by dissection of the subcarinal lymph node packet.

Table 72-3

STAPLER TYPES AND SIZE

1. Vascular staplers, gray, white or red, usually with a 2.5-mm gap. These are used to close pulmonary artery or single pulmonary veins
2. Medium thickness staplers, blue, usually with a 3.5-mm gap. These are used to divide parenchyma or to divide the atrium
3. Heavy thickness staplers, green, usually with a 4.8-mm gap. These are used for thick pulmonary parenchyma or for bronchi

The bronchus must be tested to 30 cm H_2O. If no leak is seen, the bronchus is covered with vascularized tissue. I prefer to use pericardial fat pad or thymus, but vascularized pericardium can be used. Others describe using intercostal muscle. It should be sutured either to the bronchus, itself, or to the tissues around the bronchus.

Right Pneumonectomy

Patients undergoing right pneumonectomy are more likely to die from this procedure than left pneumonectomy patients. Mortality typically is due to the complications of recovering from surgery rather than the surgery itself. Consequently, for right pneumonectomy, postoperative management is crucial.

As on the left side, I perform thoracoscopy to identify any occult pleural metastases. If no metastases are seen, the appropriate incision is selected and the chest opened. The pleura around the hilum is divided and the inferior pulmonary

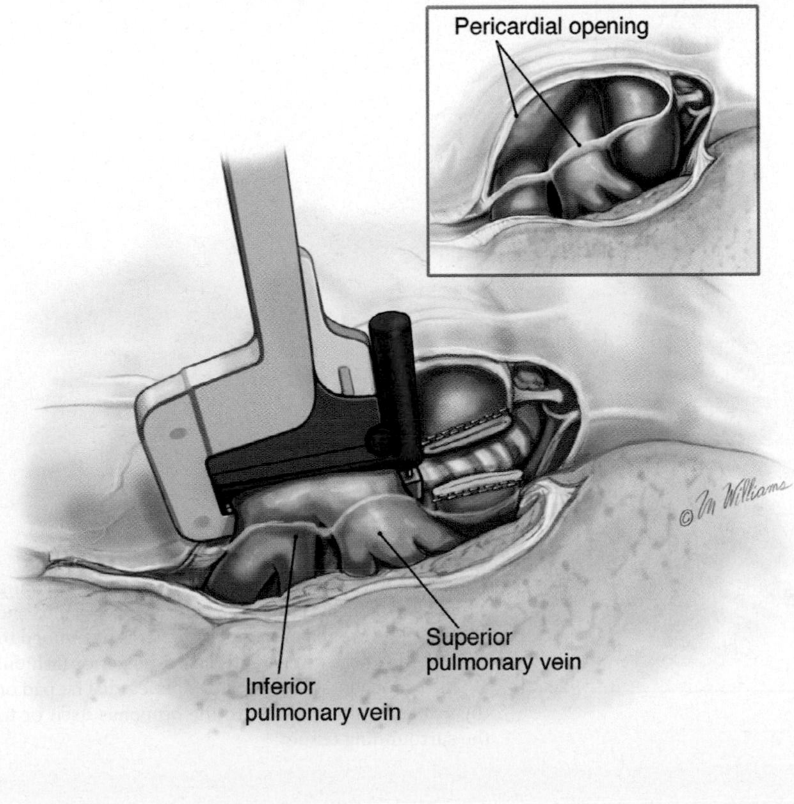

Figure 72-4. The pulmonary veins are divided. If the pericardium has been opened to gain control of the tumor, this incision can be extended to control the pulmonary veins (inset).

Table 72-4

BRONCHIAL STUMP CARE

1. Avoid removal of bronchial adventitia
2. Divide the left bronchus within the aortopulmonary window to yield a short stump
3. Harvesting the subcarinal nodes is important, but use clips or scissors rather than cautery or energy, which increase the chances of devascularization
4. The stump should be closed from an anterior-to-posterior direction, such that the flexible membranous bronchus can move against and seal the more rigid cartilaginous bronchus
5. The bronchus should be covered with vascularized tissue, either pericardium or pericardial fat pad/thymus

ligament is taken down (Fig. 72-6). For lesions in the hilum, dividing the azygos vein and harvesting the right paratracheal nodes first gives better exposure to the proximal pulmonary artery and proximal right mainstem bronchus.

As for left pneumonectomy, the tumor and lung should be evaluated to determine whether sleeve resection, rather than pneumonectomy, can be done. The right upper lobe sleeve is the most straightforward sleeve resection to perform—both the airway and the artery can be sleeved.

Once the decision to proceed to pneumonectomy is made, the artery is dissected away from the bronchus and vein. A patient who has had previous chemoradiation therapy or who has a history of granulomatous disease in the mediastinal lymph nodes often will have dense scarring between the posterior arterial plane and the anterior plane of the bronchus. For this situation, proximal control of the artery is needed.

Several maneuvers permit proximal control of the right main pulmonary artery. The first and simplest is to divide the azygos vein and perform a right paratracheal node dissection. For tumors with more extensive involvement of the mediastinum, the proximal pulmonary artery can be approached by opening the pericardium (Fig. 72-7). If more room is needed, the pulmonary artery can be identified medial to the superior vena cava, since the right main pulmonary artery is very long. The right pulmonary artery can be divided just after its bifurcation (this is often found to the left of the patient's midline), and the artery is then delivered back to the right hemithorax posterior (or underneath) the superior vena cava. This approach markedly diminishes the chance of hemorrhage.

Pericardiectomy and Reconstruction

Some textbooks state that pericardial reconstruction after resection must be done on the right side to prevent cardiac torsion on the axis defined by the superior and inferior vena cavae, but it is not necessary to do so on the left side. I have had patients arrest after left-sided pericardiectomy without reconstruction and believe that the *extent* of resection, rather than the side, is the important factor.

The only goal for reconstruction is to fill the pericardial defect in such a manner as to prevent cardiac herniation. For limited resections (<2 cm in diameter), reconstruction may not

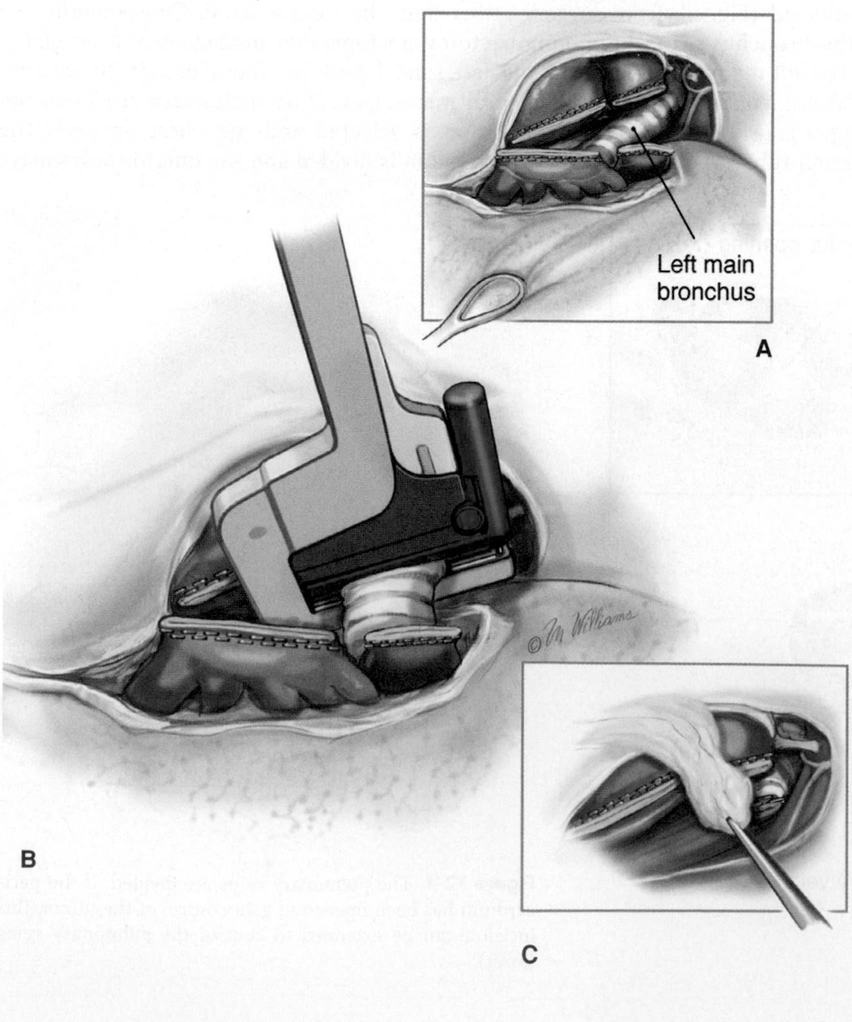

Figure 72-5. *A.* Before dividing the bronchus, the lung is grasped to deliver the bronchus inferiorly into the chest. *B.* The bronchial clamp or stapler is positioned to close the bronchus in an anterior-to-posterior fashion. *C.* The bronchus is covered with a pericardial fat pad or thymus and sutured either to the bronchus itself or to the surrounding tissues.

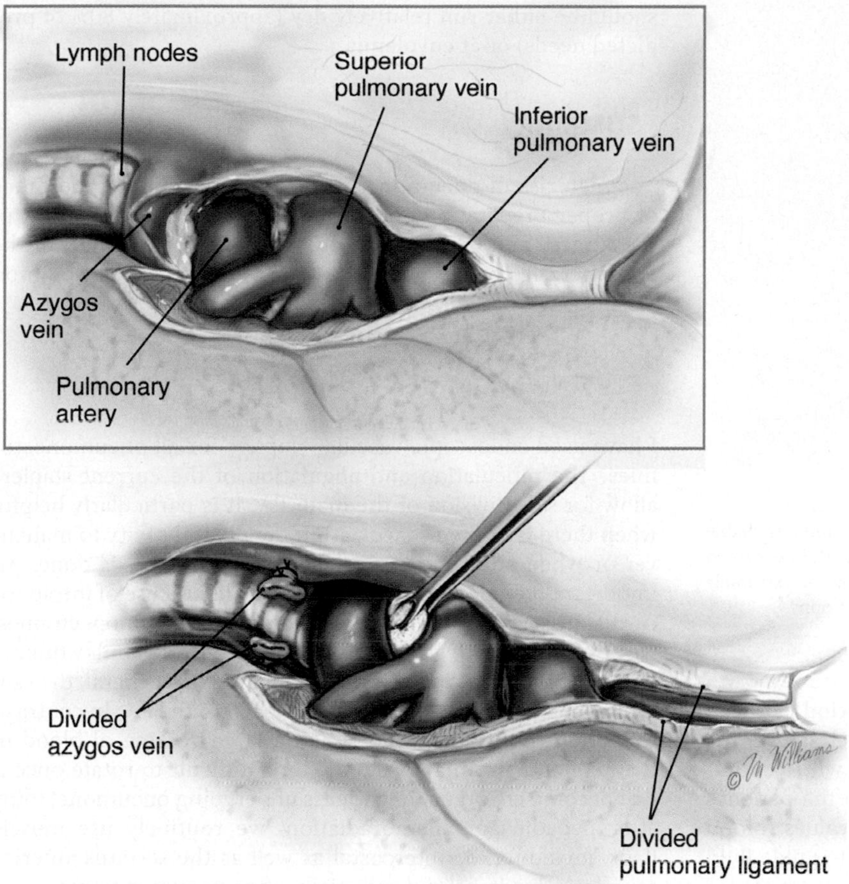

Figure 72-6. Right pneumonectomy. The pleura surrounding the hilum is divided, the inferior pulmonary ligament is taken down, and for tumors in the hilum, the azygos vein is divided, harvesting the right paratracheal nodes first (inset).

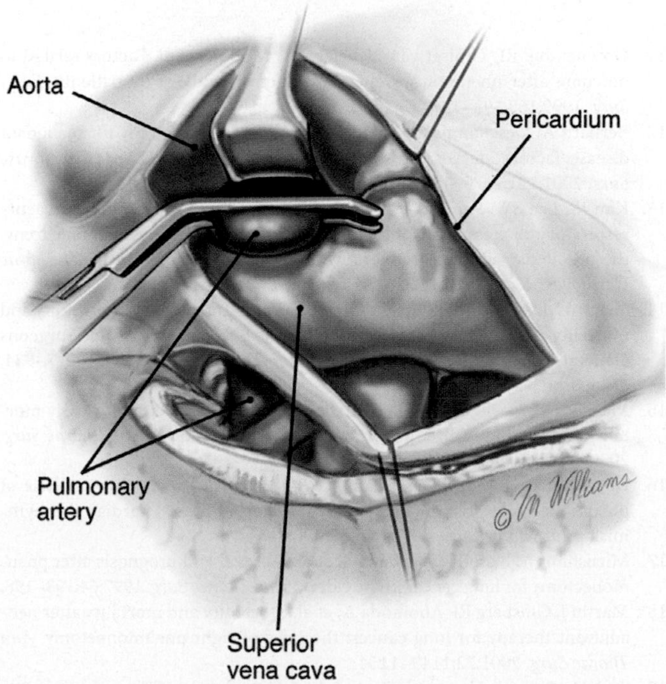

Figure 72-7. When there is extensive mediastinal involvement, the proximal pulmonary artery can be approached medially to the superior vena cava.

be necessary to prevent herniation, but probably is helpful to avoid cardiac irritation and supraventricular tachyarrhythmias. Larger defects sometimes can be filled with the vascularized flap used to buttress the bronchus, especially if a bulky pericardial fat pad is used.

Most surgeons use a nonabsorbable material – PROLENE (Ethicon, Inc., Somerville, NJ) or Gore-Tex® (W.L. Gore and Associates, Flagstaff, AZ) mesh – to reconstruct the pericardium (Fig. 72-8). These patches should be sewn into place using interrupted sutures placed approximately 1 cm or more apart since the goal is to anchor the patch in place but not to make it watertight. The patch should also be loose to avoid constricting the heart, which will assume a different shape and position when the patient is upright. The patch should be loose to the point of being floppy, with special attention to avoid constriction of the superior vena cava. Finally, limited experience indicates that absorbable material, such as Vicryl mesh, can be used to reconstruct pericardial defects.

PERIOPERATIVE MANAGEMENT

There is insufficient space to discuss every aspect of the perioperative management for lung resections. However, fluid management is a key problem that deserves attention and can prevent complications in patients undergoing pneumonectomy. Several studies have been published indicating that

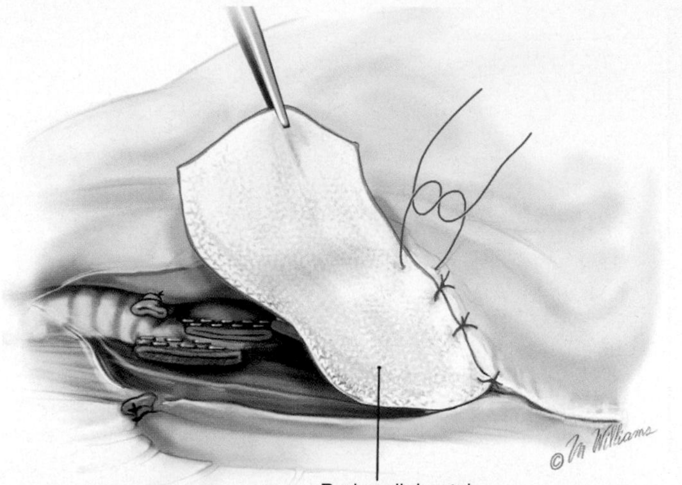

Figure 72-8. The pericardium is reconstructed with nonabsorbable PROLENE or Gore-Tex® mesh. The patch is sewn in place with interrupted sutures approximately 1 cm or more apart. The patch should be extremely loosely fitted to the point that it can be described as being floppy.

excessive fluid given during the perioperative period can lead to increased postoperative mortality. Nevertheless, in the immediate perioperative period, 2 to 5 L of fluid will accumulate in the chest. This amount must be added to the patient's basic needs for fluid. Renal function laboratory values (blood urea nitrogen [BUN] and creatinine) can be used to guide fluid resuscitation, as can urine output. Perhaps the main caveat for these patients is that they do not develop the third-space accumulation that laparotomy or cardiac patients do and therefore should be either run relatively dry (approximately 80% of predicted needs) or at euvolemia.

SUMMARY

The high risk of pneumonectomy underscores the importance of proper preparation and experience in both the conduct of the surgery and the perioperative management. Review of the idiosyncrasies of the pulmonary anatomy and other common pitfalls is warranted.

EDITOR'S COMMENT

I have used endoscopic vascular staplers for all pneumonectomies. The reticulation and angulation of the current staplers allow for safe division of the main PA. It is particularly helpful when there is limited space within the pleural cavity to maneuver or when an intrapericardial pneumonectomy is done. An important technical consideration is the liberal use of intrapericardial dissection, especially with left-sided pneumonectomies; we never hesitate to get better proximal control of bulky tumors both for division of the PA and PV. Likewise, in general, the vein is divided first as it allows a safe approach to the PA. In contrast, this often results in "trapping" of a large volume of blood in the lung and also may make the lung difficult to rotate once it had become engorged. In patients undergoing pneumonectomy after neoadjuvant chemoradiation, we routinely use muscle flaps, including the intercostal as well as the serratus anterior muscles. This is helpful especially after pneumonectomy as it helps fill the space as well as buttressing the bronchial stumps.

—Mark J. Krasna

References

1. Shiraishi Y, Katsuragi N, Nakajima Y, et al. Pneumonectomy for complex aspergilloma: is it still dangerous? *Eur J Cardiothorac Surg.* 2006;29:9–13.
2. Darling GE, Abdurahman A, Yi QL, et al. Risk of a right pneumonectomy: role of bronchopleural fistula. *Ann Thorac Surg.* 2005;79:433–437.
3. Deslauriers J, Gregoire J, Jacques LF, et al. Sleeve lobectomy versus pneumonectomy for lung cancer: a comparative analysis of survival and sites or recurrences. *Ann Thorac Surg.* 2004;77:1152–1156; discussion 1156.
4. Camplese P, Sacco R. Pneumonectomy for lung cancer: technical and general aspects. *Rays.* 2004;29:413–417.
5. Swartz DE, Lachapelle K, Sampalis J, et al. Perioperative mortality after pneumonectomy: analysis of risk factors and review of the literature. *Can J Surg.* 1997;40:437–444.
6. Boysen PG, Block AJ, Olsen GN, et al. Prospective evaluation for pneumonectomy using the 99mtechnetium quantitative perfusion lung scan. *Chest.* 1977;72:422–425.
7. Au J, el-Oakley R, Cameron EW. Pneumonectomy for bronchogenic carcinoma in the elderly. *Eur J Cardiothorac Surg.* 1994;8:247–250.
8. van Meerbeeck JP, Damhuis RA, Vos de Wael ML. High postoperative risk after pneumonectomy in elderly patients with right-sided lung cancer. *Eur Respir J.* 2002;19:141–145.
9. Kim AW, Boffa DJ, Wang Z, et al. An analysis, systematic review, and meta-analysis of the perioperative mortality after neoadjuvant therapy and pneumonectomy for non-small cell lung cancer. *J Thorac Cardiovasc Surg.* 2012;143:55–63.
10. Mitsudomi T, Mizoue T, Yoshimatsu T, et al. Postoperative complications after pneumonectomy for treatment of lung cancer: multivariate analysis. *J Surg Oncol.* 1996;61:218–222.
11. Groenendijk RP, Croiset van Uchelen FA, Mol SJ, et al. Factors related to outcome after pneumonectomy: retrospective study of 62 patients. *Eur J Surg.* 1999;165:193–197.
12. Bernard A, Deschamps C, Allen MS, et al. Pneumonectomy for malignant disease: factors affecting early morbidity and mortality. *J Thorac Cardiovasc Surg.* 2001;121:1076–1082.
13. Kim JB, Lee SW, Park SI, et al. Risk factor analysis for postoperative acute respiratory distress syndrome and early mortality after pneumonectomy: the predictive value of preoperative lung perfusion distribution. *J Thorac Cardiovasc Surg.* 2010;140:26–31.
14. Shapiro M, Swanson SJ, Wright CD, et al. Predictors of major morbidity and mortality after pneumonectomy utilizing the Society for Thoracic Surgeons General Thoracic Surgery Database. *Ann Thorac Surg.* 2010;90:927–934; discussion 34–35.
15. Mansour Z, Kochetkova EA, Santelmo N, et al. Risk factors for early mortality and morbidity after pneumonectomy: a reappraisal. *Ann Thorac Surg.* 2009;88:1737–1743.
16. Harpole DH, Liptay MJ, DeCamp MM, Jr., et al. Prospective analysis of pneumonectomy: risk factors for major morbidity and cardiac dysrhythmias. *Ann Thorac Surg.* 1996;61:977–982.
17. Mizushima Y, Noto H, Sugiyama S, et al. Survival and prognosis after pneumonectomy for lung cancer in the elderly. *Ann Thorac Surg.* 1997;64:193–198.
18. Martin J, Ginsberg RJ, Abolhoda A, et al. Morbidity and mortality after neoadjuvant therapy for lung cancer: the risks of right pneumonectomy. *Ann Thorac Surg.* 2001;72:1149–1154.
19. Stolz A, Pafko P, Harustiak T, et al. Risk factor analysis for early mortality and morbidity following pneumonectomy for non-small cell lung cancer. *Bratisl Lek Listy.* 2011;112:165–169.

20. Parquin F, Marchal M, Mehiri S, et al. Post-pneumonectomy pulmonary edema: analysis and risk factors. *Eur J Cardiothorac Surg.* 1996;10:929–932; discussion 33.
21. Moller AM, Pedersen T, Svendsen PE, et al. Perioperative risk factors in elective pneumonectomy: the impact of excess fluid balance. *Eur J Anaesthesiol.* 2002;19:57–62.
22. Vaporciyan AA, Merriman KW, Ece F, et al. Incidence of major pulmonary morbidity after pneumonectomy: association with timing of smoking cessation. *Ann Thorac Surg.* 2002;73:420–425; discussion 425–426.
23. Konishi J, Yamazaki K, Tsukamoto E, et al. Mediastinal lymph node staging by FDG-PET in patients with non-small cell lung cancer: analysis of false-positive FDG-PET findings. *Respiration.* 2003;70:500–506.
24. Roberts JR, Blum MG, Arildsen R, et al. Prospective comparison of radiologic, thoracoscopic, and pathologic staging in patients with early non-small cell lung cancer. *Ann Thorac Surg.* 1999;68:1154–1158.
25. Boysen PG, Harris JO, Block AJ, Olsen GN. Prospective evaluation for pneumonectomy using perfusion scanning: follow-up beyond one year. *Chest.* 1981;80:163–166.
26. Taube K, Konietzko N. Prediction of postoperative cardiopulmonary function in patients undergoing pneumonectomy. *Thorac Cardiovasc Surg.* 1980;28:348–351.

73 Segmentectomy for Primary Lung Cancer

Dirk Van Raemdonck, Herbert Decaluwé, Paul De Leyn, Shamus R. Carr, and Joseph S. Friedberg

Keywords: pulmonary resection, segmentectomy, lung cancer

INTRODUCTION

Segmentectomy was initially described by Churchill and Belsey[1] in 1939 for the treatment of bronchiectasis. Although the operation is still used to treat suppurative and other nonmalignant processes (e.g., aspergilloma, pulmonary sequestration), other pulmonary infections, pulmonary abscesses, and benign tumors of the lung (hamartomas, papillomas), this chapter concerns its controversial use in early-stage lung cancer.[2] Until 1950, pneumonectomy was the standard of care for lung cancer. However, increasing awareness of the diminution of respiratory function caused by pneumonectomy soon led to interest in lobectomy and other lesser resections for tumors of amenable size and location. In 1973, Jensik et al.[3] reported the first series of segmentectomies for early-stage lung cancer. Since then, limited resection for lung cancer has been a topic of much debate, and the controversy has been plagued by conflicting results between studies comparing segmentectomy and standard lobectomy or pneumonectomy.

GENERAL PRINCIPLES

Segmentectomy is an anatomic sublobar resection that involves the removal of functionally discrete units of the bronchovascular anatomy. The bronchovascular architecture is composed of a series of individual segments. Each segment has a pyramidal structure with its apex at the hilum and its base on the surface of the lung. Individually, the segments are supplied solely, with few collateral connections, by the following structures: (1) a segmental bronchus as a tertiary branch of the bronchial tree; (2) a segmental branch of the pulmonary artery (as well as the bronchial artery); and (3) a segmental (± intersegmental) branch of the pulmonary vein together with lymphatics. Each segment behaves as a discrete anatomical and functional unit that can be removed by segmental resection without affecting the functionality of the remaining lobe or adjoining bronchial segment. In properly selected patients with early-stage non–small-cell lung cancer (NSCLC), segmentectomy can achieve outcomes that are equivalent in overall survival to pneumonectomy and lobectomy.

A thorough knowledge of the human lung anatomy is mandatory for any surgeon undertaking this resection. There are 10 segments in the right lung (3 in upper lobe, 2 in middle lobe, and 5 in lower lobe) and 8 to 10 segments in the left lung (4–5 in upper lobe and 4–5 in lower lobe) (Fig. 73-1).

Several operations fall under the umbrella of sublobar pulmonary resection. These are the wedge, the segmentectomy, and the extended segmentectomy. It is important to note that a *wedge* resection, sometimes called an *atypical* segmentectomy because of its sublobar resection status, is *not* an anatomical resection. Although sometimes preferred because it is less technically demanding than segmentectomy, the wedge resection is associated with numerous pitfalls, including a difficulty in obtaining or identifying a tumor-free resection margin, limited extent of lymph node sampling and excision, high rate of local recurrence, and diminished overall survival. *Segmentectomy,* on the other hand, respects anatomic barriers and is associated with better overall and disease-free survival. *Extended* segmentectomy describes the technique whereby the parenchyma is divided lateral to the intersegmental plane to accommodate a wider resection margin.

PATIENT SELECTION

Two groups of patients with NSCLC may benefit from segmentectomy, those who are able to tolerate lobectomy, but for whom curative resection is likely with a sublobar resection

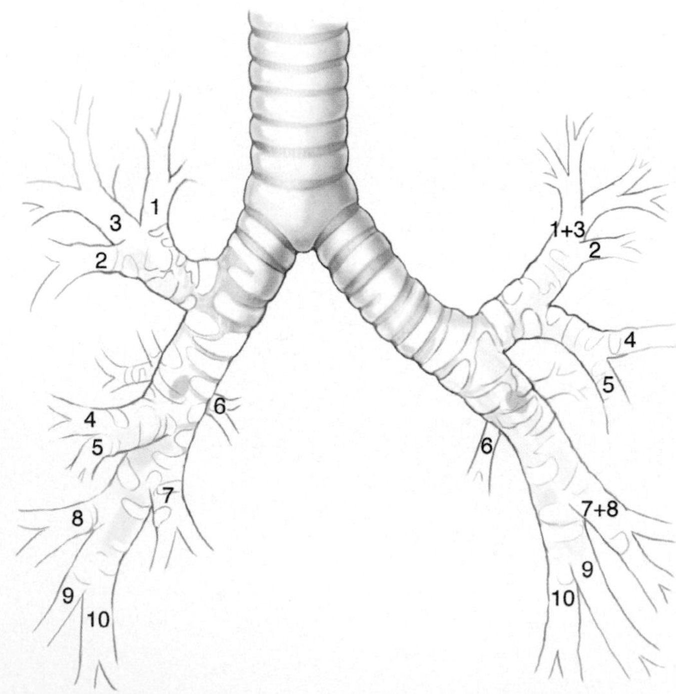

Figure 73-1. A schematic drawing of the different segments of the lungs. Note the right lung has 10 anatomical segments, whereas the left lung has 9 segments only. Anterior view of the distal trachea, carina, right and left bronchial trees. Right upper lobe segments: 1 apical; 2: anterior; 3: posterior. Right middle lobe segments: 4: lateral; 5: medial. Right lower lobe segments: 6: superior; 7: medial basal; 8: anterior basal; 9: lateral basal; 10: posterior basal. Left upper lobe segments: 1 and 3: apical posterior; 2: anterior; 4: superior lingular; 5: inferior lingular. Left lower lobe segments: 6: superior; 7 and 8: anteromedial basal; 9: lateral basal; 10: posterior basal. (Courtesy of Dr. Thomas W. Rice and Joseph A. Pangrace, Cleveland Clinic.)

based on the small size of the tumor and negative nodes. The second group is those who are unable to tolerate lobectomy and for whom a lesser resection constitutes an alternative local cancer treatment. Patients with poor pulmonary reserve (forced expiratory volume in 1 second [FEV_1] less than 50% of predicted) or with multiple resectable lesions may also be considered for a segmental resection if complete resection is likely.

Conventional fractionated radiation therapy has been the alternative local treatment for medically inoperable patients with early-stage NSCLC and is associated with modestly prolonged survival compared to observation. Recently, several nonsurgical treatments have become available, including stereotactic body radiation therapy (SBRT) and percutaneous ablative therapy including radiofrequency, cryotherapy, and microwave (Chapter 85). Although these treatments appear to decrease the risk of respiratory failure, disability, and death, there is currently little evidence of efficacy compared to a parenchymal-sparing surgical resection. In the few trials that are available, all nonoperative modalities have higher recurrence rates over shorter intervals. Currently, two ongoing randomized trials are investigating the value of SBRT versus sublobar resection or lobectomy.

PREOPERATIVE ASSESSMENT

Preoperative workup and evaluation for thoracic surgery is discussed elsewhere in this book in detail (see Chapter 4). The same principles apply for segmentectomy.

The presence of stage I NSCLC should be ensured preoperatively. Combined PET/CT scan is the best radiographic and metabolic test available for ruling out extrathoracic disease, assessing the mediastinal and hilar lymph nodes, and excluding other suspicious nodules in the lung. Endobronchial ultrasound (EBUS) and endoscopic esophageal ultrasound (EUS) are first-line tools for mediastinal staging and should be used followed by videomediastinoscopy to rule out false-negative results when suspicious-looking lymph nodes are detected on radiographic imaging. MRI of the brain with contrast should be considered in all patients with headache or other neurologic symptoms, since a brain metastasis cannot be visualized by PET/CT.

Medical operability should be checked in patients with poor performance status if any surgical procedure is being planned. Algorithms for differentiating risk levels for patients being considered for a lung resection have recently been published.[4] These European guidelines provide cutoff values for subjecting at-risk patients to additional assessment and threshold values to differentiate low-risk from high-risk patients. Cardiology risk stratification and pulmonary function testing including the diffusion capacity of carbon monoxide for the lung (D_{LCO}) are recommended in every patient undergoing pulmonary resection. Further exercise testing with oxygen consumption (VO_2) should be performed in patients with FEV_1 and/or D_{LCO} <80%. Patients with VO_2 max or a predicted postoperative (ppo) value below 10 mL/kg/min or 35% are not candidates for major anatomic resections. In patients with VO_2 max values between 10 and 15 mL/kg/min or between 35% and 75%, ppo FEV_1 and ppo D_{LCO} should be calculated. If both values are >30%, resection can be performed up to the calculated extent. Otherwise, ppoVO_2 max should be calculated.

SURGICAL TECHNIQUE

The patient is placed in lateral decubitus position and intubated under general anesthesia with a double-lumen endotracheal tube. An epidural catheter is placed for pain. The chest is usually entered through the fifth intercostal space or one rib higher if there is a concern for pathology at the lung apex. The operation can be performed using open or video-assisted thoracic surgery (VATS) technique. For the open procedure described later, we routinely perform a muscle-sparing posterolateral thoracotomy with division of the latissimus dorsi and mobilization and retraction of the serratus anterior (see Chapter 2).

After entering the chest, the hemithorax is inspected and lung palpated to rule out evidence of advanced disease that would preclude segmental resection. If there is any uncertainty about the preoperative diagnosis, tissue is obtained for frozen-section analysis before proceeding. Central lesions may be sampled via needle biopsy. Frozen sections then are obtained of N1 and N2. The presence of metastatic disease in any lymph node constitutes an indication to proceed with lobectomy,[5] provided the patient is surgically fit based on the preoperative assessment. Frozen section of the resection margin is also recommended.[6]

Segmentectomy

Although any bronchovascular segment can be removed, certain operations are more commonly performed. These include taking or sparing the superior segment for lower lobe cancers and taking or sparing the lingula for left upper lobe cancers. It is generally easier to remove the superior segment of the lower lobe (S6), the lingular segments (S4 + S5), and the basilar segments of the lower lobe (S7–S10), whereas the individual segments in the upper lobe (S1, S2, S3) and lower lobe (S7, S8, S9, S10) are more challenging. Although the spatial approach and the order of dividing the individual bronchovascular structures may vary depending on the individual segment(s), the overall principles remain the same.

Regardless of which segment is being resected, the fissure is opened first to reveal the pulmonary arterial branch. The appropriate segmental artery(ies) are identified and divided in the usual manner to expose the underlying segmental bronchus. Gentle traction on the segment with an atraumatic clamp may help to expose segmental branches that are hidden deep within the lung parenchyma (Fig. 73-2).

The S4, S5, and S6 segments each have an individual central vein that can be ligated or clipped, whereas the veins in other segments run close to the periphery and cannot be identified until dissection of the intersegmental plane has commenced and drainage into the superior or inferior venous trunks becomes visible. In some cases, early division of the individual central segmental vein can facilitate visualization of the pulmonary artery. However, these veins cannot be identified upon stapling of the parenchyma, so it is important to identify the anatomy of the venous trunks carefully before dividing the segmental vessels to avoid inadvertent ligation of veins draining blood from adjacent segments. This may result in venous thrombosis, lobar infarct, and potentially disastrous complications postoperatively.

Intraoperative bronchoscopy can be very helpful if there is confusion regarding the segmental anatomy or concern about potential compromise of the adjacent segmental bronchial orifice. A pediatric bronchoscope fits easily through the lumen of

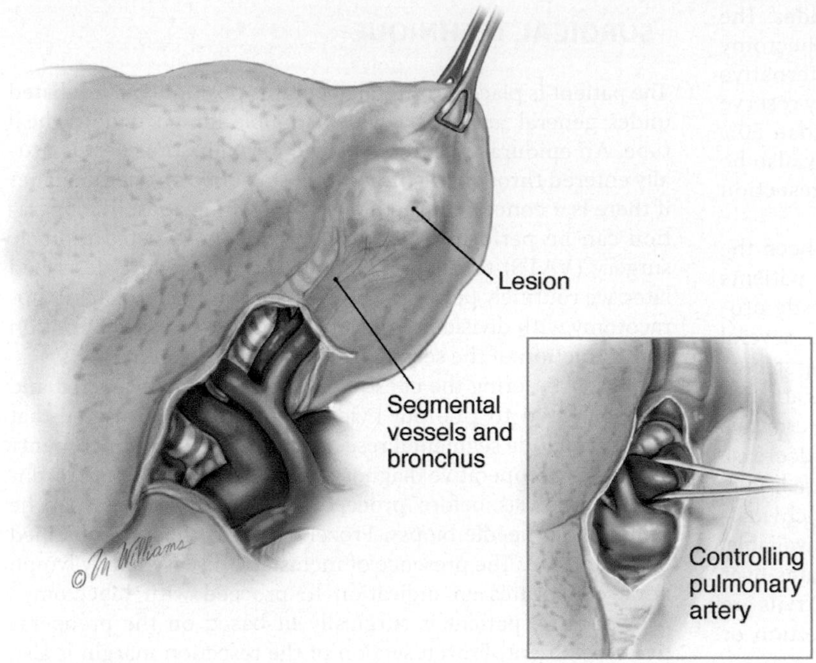

Figure 73-2. Traction on the segment itself can aid in identifying the appropriate arterial branches and segmental bronchus.

a double-lumen endotracheal tube to reveal the endobronchial view. In addition, the light on the scope illuminates the airway which can be visualized from the operative field.

Before dividing the parenchyma, it can be difficult to identify the appropriate plane, especially when VATS techniques are used. Observing the differential ventilation of the individual segments by clamping the segmental bronchus before (or after) full inflation can better delineate the intersegmental plane (Fig. 73-3). The segmental bronchus is then divided with a stapler

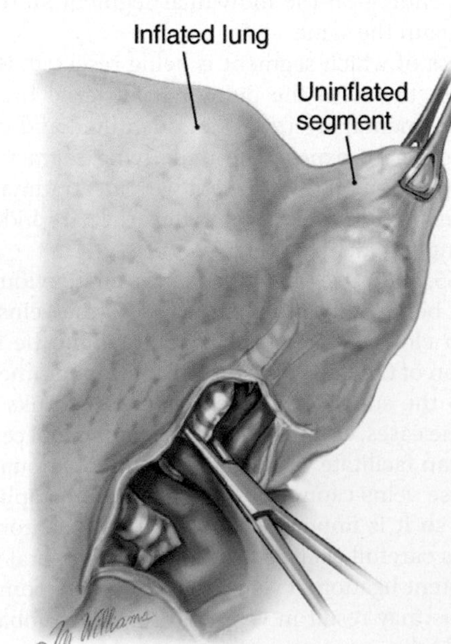

Figure 73-3. A simple technique for determining the appropriate plane for parenchymal division is shown. After the segmental bronchus is clamped, the anesthetist is asked to gently inflate the lung while the surgeon observes the demarcation between the inflated and the deflated segment.

or scalpel and closed in routine fashion. For suturing the bronchial stump, we prefer two over-and-over running 4-0 absorbable monofilament sutures after folding the membranous part inside the lumen of the bronchus and bringing the cartilaginous rings together according to the technique previously described by the Dutch surgeon Klinkenberg. Finally, the parenchyma between the involved and adjacent segments needs to be divided for which two techniques have been described: the open and stapled division.

For the open technique, the intersegmental plane is teased apart by using a clamp to place traction on the stump of the transected segmental bronchus, whereas the rest of the lung is well ventilated. Sharp and blunt finger dissection may also help to open the intersegmental plane (Fig. 73-4). Cautery, harmonic scalpel, or small vascular clips are used to ensure hemostasis. Small air leaks can be oversewn with fine sutures. In addition, the raw surface of the adjacent segment can be covered with pleural or pericardial fat pad. Care has to be taken to avoid compression or kinking of the remaining bronchovascular structures which can result in a nonfunctional lobe thereby eliminating the benefit of segmentectomy versus lobectomy. The advantage of the open technique is that reexpansion of the adjacent parenchyma is maximal, but it carries a higher risk of prolonged air leaks.

For the stapled technique, the virtual fissure is compressed and cut with the aid of a linear stapler. We prefer an endovascular linear cutting stapler. This technique results in better pneumostatic control in the remaining lung but it comes at the expense of volume loss as the visceral pleural layers are drawn together when closing the device. The remaining parenchyma is then somewhat trapped by the individual staplers, which blocks reexpansion of the lobe to its maximum volume (Fig. 73-5). The "extended" segmentectomy is accomplished by deploying the stapler lateral to the intersegmental plane so as to include the adjacent subsegments in the specimen.[7]

VATS segmentectomy is a safe and feasible operation, as confirmed by published reports from several high-volume

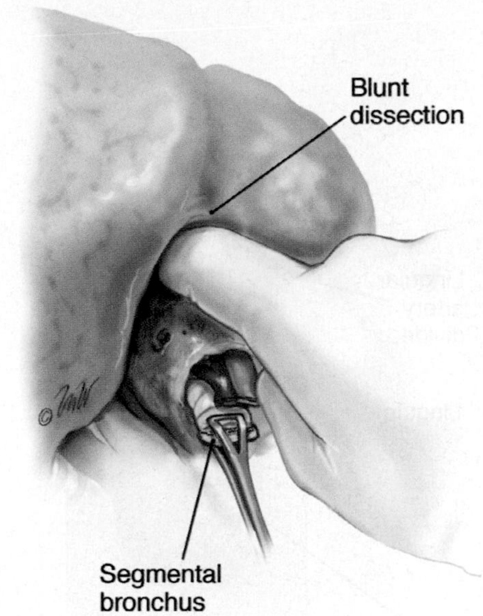

Figure 73-4. For open division of the segmental parenchyma, traction is applied to the distal transected segmental bronchus, and the intersegmental plane is developed sharply or bluntly with finger dissection.

centers. The benefits of using VATS with segmental resection seem to mirror the more robust data available for VATS lobectomy in terms of decreased morbidity, length of stay, postoperative pain, and other metrics. However, caution must be exercised as these resections can be quite challenging and one should always proceed as if performing an open procedure with careful individual dissection and ligation of the bronchial and vascular structures. Port placement can literally make or break VATS segmentectomy. In general, the standard port sites described by McKenna or Flores are the most versatile. McKenna routinely

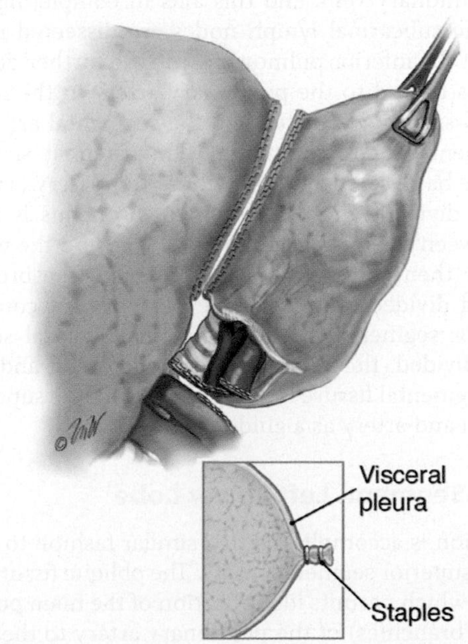

Figure 73-5. The segmental parenchyma is divided using open or staple division. Shown here is the staple technique, which can cause volume loss when the visceral pleural layers are drawn together during the act of stapling.

uses four incisions, whereas Flores[8] describes only three for VATS lobectomies. We have found both to be appropriate for performing segmental resections. There are certainly times when it is quite easy to perform an operation through only three ports, while at other times, the fourth port significantly increases the options and ease of the resection. In general, we start with three and add a fourth port anteriorly, as described by McKenna, or at the scapular tip as needed.

Right Upper Lobe Segments

The *apical segment* dissection begins by incising the mediastinal pleura. The apical branch of the anterior arterial trunk is identified and divided. The apical segmental bronchus is then approached posteriorly and isolated after ligating the bronchial artery branches. For right upper lobe segmentectomy, the vein is usually encompassed in the staple line.

The *anterior segment* is approached from the medial aspect, beginning with incision of the mediastinal pleura. The anterior segmental artery is identified as it branches from the anterior arterial trunk. The anterior segmental vein is likewise identified and ligated, taking care not to compromise other segmental tributaries to the superior pulmonary vein. The horizontal fissure is completed, the anterior segmental bronchus is divided, and the segment is excised.

In performing a *posterior segmentectomy*, the major fissure is opened posteriorly and the pulmonary artery is traced proximally to identify the posterior segmental artery. Once identified, it is ligated. The posterior segmental bronchus is deep and lies slightly medial to the artery. Again, the vein is taken with the intersegmental plane. Alternatively, the artery branch may be ligated after dissection and transection of the segmental bronchus, which can be tracked posteriorly along the right upper lobe bronchus.

Superior Segment, Right Lower Lobe

If the major fissure is well developed, the pulmonary artery can be approached directly in the fissure. If the fissure is incomplete, it must first be developed to expose the artery. The pleura is opened posteriorly at the bifurcation of the right upper lobe bronchus and the bronchus intermedius and continued anteriorly to identify the recurrent artery to the posterior segment of the upper lobe and the superior segmental artery to the lower lobe. With these bifurcations visualized, the posterior portion of the major fissure can be developed. A stapler can be used to divide this parenchyma, taking care to exclude the arteries and bronchi from the jaws of the stapler. Sometimes it is helpful to place a ¼ in Penrose drain through the "window" that has been created and feed the lower jaw of the stapler into the drain. The drain can then be used to guide the stapler through the window without risk of falsely passing the stapler and injuring or dividing a vessel or bronchus. The posterior fissure can be a difficult spot to manipulate the stapler. Passing the stapler through the future chest tube site may afford a more benevolent angle of attack.

Once the posterior portion of the major fissure is opened, the artery can be isolated and divided. This will provide exposure to the bronchus, which runs deep to the artery. The superior segmental vein can usually be identified posteriorly as a separate tributary running into the inferior vein. Again, care must be taken not to compromise the remainder of the vein.

Basal Segment, Right Lower Lobe

This operation begins in the major fissure with dissection of the pulmonary artery to identify the right middle lobe artery, the superior segmental artery, and the basilar segmental artery. Circumferential dissection of the artery allows it to be divided. The basal segmental bronchus lies deep to artery. The inferior pulmonary vein is identified by first taking down the inferior pulmonary ligament. The anterior and posterior hilum is dissected to complete the inferior pulmonary vein isolation. Further dissection into the lung parenchyma permits visualization of the confluence of the segmental pulmonary veins. The bronchus is then dissected and divided. This allows demonstration of the veins deep to the bronchus. The superior segmental vein is identified and the intersegmental plane is completed using this vein as a guide, making sure that it is not compromised.

Left Upper Lobe Upper Division (Lingular Sparing)

Proximal control of the pulmonary artery may facilitate left upper lobe segmentectomy, but it is not mandatory. First, the anterior mediastinal pleura is opened to permit identification of the superior pulmonary vein. The lingular vein is identified and preserved. We begin by dividing the upper division segmental vein. A lymph node is normally encountered at this bifurcation and sent for frozen section. If positive, the segmentectomy should be abandoned in favor of lobectomy. Dividing this vein facilitates identification of the left main pulmonary artery. The dissection is continued distally along the main pulmonary artery to expose the segmental arteries, which are divided. At this point we find it beneficial to complete the oblique fissure. With this accomplished and the arterial branches divided, only the bronchus remains. The upper lobe bronchus can then be dissected up to the bifurcation of the upper division and lingula. This allows the upper division bronchus to be stapled and divided. Placing the stapler along the pulmonary vein from the lingula and heading toward the lingular bronchus, the intrasegmental fissure can be developed and completed.

Lingula

As with most segmental resections, the ease of dissection is a function of the completeness of the fissure. If the fissure is complete, it is quite easy to identify and isolate the artery and all its branches. If the fissure is incomplete, it must first be developed and this is best accomplished by tracing the pulmonary artery into the fissure. Commonly, a plane can be developed between the lobes using sharp dissection or a very low setting on the electrocautery to avoid significant air leaks. If raw parenchyma is encountered as the fissure is developed, we complete the fissure with a stapling device. The lingular arteries may arise separately as a common trunk from the ongoing pulmonary artery. The lingular bronchus will be found under the divided arteries. Care must be taken to avoid compromise of the superior divisional bronchus to the upper lobe when dividing the lingular bronchus. The lung is then retracted posteriorly, and the hilar pleura is incised to expose the superior pulmonary vein. The lingular branch is then identified and divided (Fig. 73-6). Finally, the parenchyma is divided as described for other segments. The other option for this procedure is to begin with identification and division of the lingular vein in the hilum. Attention then

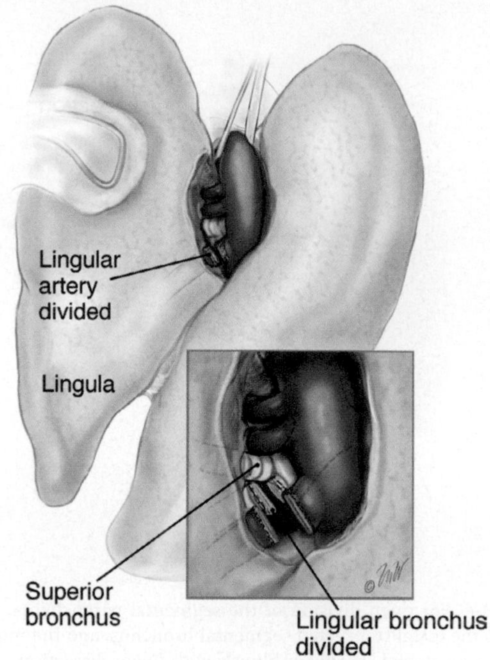

Figure 73-6. The segmental artery to the lingula when arising as common trunk from the pulmonary artery, must be divided first to expose the lingular bronchus.

turns to the fissure for dissection and division of the appropriate branches of the pulmonary artery and bronchus.

Basal Segment, Left Lower Lobe

After releasing the inferior pulmonary ligament, attention is turned to the hilum. The inferior pulmonary vein is identified and circumferentially dissected. There is usually a lymph node that can be dissected from the posterior superior aspect of the inferior pulmonary vein, and this aids in completing the dissection. The subcarinal lymph nodes are dissected next. The branches of the inferior pulmonary vein are further delineated. Attention is turned to the pulmonary artery in the major fissure. The fissure is completed and the segmental artery to the basal segments is circumferentially dissected. It sits directly anterior the basal segmental bronchus. This artery (sometimes arteries) is divided. The basal segment bronchus is then dissected between the inferior pulmonary vein and the bronchus. The stapler then comes from anteriorly and the bronchus is stapled and divided. Care must be made to not compromise the superior segmental bronchus. With the basal segmental bronchus divided, the veins are easily identified and divided. The intersegmental fissure is completed using the superior segmental vein and artery as a guide.

Superior Segment, Left Lower Lobe

This resection is accomplished in a similar fashion to the right lower lobe superior segmentectomy. The oblique fissure is completed first which permits identification of the main pulmonary artery. The branch(es) of the pulmonary artery to the superior segment are then dissected and divided, allowing visualization of the segmental bronchus that lies immediately behind and inferior to the divided pulmonary artery. The segmental bronchus is then dissected out and the N1 lymph nodes are removed. Once this is done, the segmental bronchus is divided. If the segmental vein is identified, it can either be individually ligated or incorporated into the completion of the intersegmental fissure using a staple technique.

POSTOPERATIVE CARE

The postoperative care after segmentectomy is comparable to other patients undergoing pulmonary resection. Upon closure, we usually leave two 28 Fr drains in the chest, the first directed toward the apex and the second above the diaphragm. However, one author (Shamus Carr) only uses a single 24 Fr chest tube directed posteriorly toward the apex with additional holes cut in the tube to aid drainage near the diaphragm. We do not put the drains on suction routinely unless there is an increasing pneumothorax or subcutaneous emphysema due to a large air leak. The focus of postoperative care is directed toward adequate analgesia and pulmonary toilet. A dedicated pain team visits patients daily to monitor the patient-controlled analgesia pumps. Dedicated physiotherapists, early ambulation, regular portable chest x-rays, and a low threshold for bronchoscopy are all helpful to minimizing the risk of pulmonary complications.

SPECIFIC COMPLICATIONS

Morbidity and mortality after segmentectomy are comparable to lobectomy in most reported series. It is unusual to have a residual space problem after segmentectomy compared with lobectomy. However, the postoperative course can be complicated by atelectasis in the remaining segments as a result of sputum impaction, disturbed bronchial anatomy, or by persistent air leaks, especially if stapling devices were not used to divide the intersegmental plane in an attempt to preserve maximum volume of the remaining lung.[2] A hematoma in the adjacent lung parenchyma can sometimes be seen on chest radiographs, but this process usually has begun to resolve prior to discharge and has completely resolved by the first outpatient follow-up visit. Signs of a progressive lobar infiltrate unique to the remaining lobe may be the first sign of lobar infarct. Reexploring the patient may be indicated after appropriate imaging and bronchoscopic workup. Not recognizing this complication may lead to sepsis and increased morbidity and mortality.

RESULTS

The last several decades have seen an increasing number of conflicting reports about the putative benefits of wedge resection versus anatomic lobectomy for the treatment of early-stage NSCLC (Table 73-1), with recent recommendations concerning the benefits of low-dose CT for lung cancer screening, more smaller-sized tumors are being visualized. This has led many surgeons to question the appropriateness of lobectomy for all cases of NSCLC.[7]

A randomized trial of lobectomy versus limited resection by Ginsberg and Rubinstein,[9] on behalf of the Lung Cancer Study Group (LCSG), in patients with a clinical T1N0M0 NSCLC randomized to a lobectomy ($n = 125$) or lesser resection ($n = 122$; wedge resection 67% or segmentectomy 33%) demonstrated a three-fold decrease in locoregional recurrence (6.4% vs. 17.2%) and a reported statistically significant ($p = 0.088$) 5-year survival benefit (65% vs. 44%) in favor of lobectomy, based upon a one-sided p-value. This study published in 1995 established lobectomy with systematic nodal dissection as the "procedure of choice" relative to lesser resections in patients with early-stage NSCLC. Nevertheless, the LCSG study was criticized because wedge resection and segmentectomy were not separated and a high percentage (33%) of patients in the sublobar group underwent wedge resection.

A number of single-institutional retrospective reports, primarily from Japan,[10–12] have demonstrated that segmentectomy might be equivalent to lobectomy in terms of survival for carefully selected patients. Koike et al.[10] compared survival and local recurrences in a retrospective study in patients with tumors smaller than 2 cm. Seventy-four patients underwent limited resection (14 wedge resections, remaining segmentectomies) and 159 patients had lobectomy. There was no difference in local recurrence or survival between these groups. Importantly, postoperative spirometry was significantly better in patients who underwent sublobar resections.

In 2005, Okada et al.[12] reported the results of a large retrospective study in 1272 patients. There was no significant difference in 5-year cancer-specific survival between patients undergoing segmentectomy versus lobectomy for tumors ≤3 cm. However, patients undergoing wedge resection for such tumors had significantly lower survival at 5 years (39.4% vs. 85.7% for lobectomy). On the other hand, for tumors greater

Table 73-1

SELECTED SERIES FROM THE LITERATURE COMPARING OUTCOMES BETWEEN LOBECTOMY AND SUBLOBAR RESECTIONS FOR EARLY-STAGE NSCLC

			LOBECTOMY			SUBLOBAR RESECTION[a]			
AUTHOR (REF)	YEAR	STUDY DESIGN	*N*	REGIONAL RECURRENCE (%)	5-YEAR SURVIVAL (%)	*N*	REGIONAL RECURRENCE (%)	5-YEAR SURVIVAL (%)	*P* VALUE SURVIVAL
LCSG[9]	1995	pro rand	122	6.4	65	125	17	44	0.088
Koike[10]	2003	retro n-rand	159	1.3	90.1	74	2.7	89.1	N.S.
Okada[11]	2006	pro n-rand	305	6.9	89.1	262	4.9	89.6	N.S.
Schuchert[13]	2007	retro n-rand	246	4.9	80	75	7.7	83	N.S.
Wolf[15]	2011	retro n-rand	84	8.0	80	154	16	59	0.003

[a]Including wedge resections and segmentectomy.
NSCLC, non–small-cell lung cancer; pro, prospective; retro, retrospective; (n)-rand, (non)-randomized; N.S., not significant.

than 30 mm in diameter, survivals were 81.3% after lobectomy, 62.9% after segmentectomy, and 0% after wedge resection.

In 2006, Okada et al.[11] reported on a multi-institutional, nonrandomized study over a 9-year period comparing survival and local recurrence for peripheral NSCLC ≤2 cm (90% adenocarcinoma) after sublobar resection in 305 patients (30 wedge resections, remaining segmentectomies) versus 262 patients after lobectomy. Overall 5-year survival, local recurrence, and distant recurrence were 89.6%, 4.9%, and 9.2% in the sublobar group versus 89.1%, 6.9%, and 10.3% in the lobectomy group, respectively.

In a study from the University of Pittsburgh (UPMC) authored by Schuchert et al.,[13] 428 patients underwent resection for Stage IA and IB NSCLC. No significant difference in 5-year survival (80% vs. 83%) or local recurrence (4.9% vs. 7.7%) was found between lobectomy and segmentectomy, respectively. However, when the tumor margin to size ratio was less than 1, the local recurrence rate was higher. When the ratio was greater than 1, the local recurrence rate was 6.2% and not statistically different from lobectomy. However, when the ratio was under 1, the local recurrence rate after segmentectomy was 25%. Although this ratio was easier to achieve with smaller tumors, larger tumors in lower lobe basal segments enjoyed the same benefits.

The same group recently reported[14] similar outcomes in 429 patients with pathologically proven stage 1A tumors only (5-year cancer specific survival 91% vs. 90% for T1a and 78% vs. 82% for T1b and recurrence rates 14.7% vs. 14.0%, respectively). This demonstrated that anatomic segmentectomy achieves equivalent recurrence and survival compared with lobectomy.

Despite favorable results in many studies, a report from Brigham and Women's hospital in Boston[15] of 238 patients who underwent resection for a small (2 cm or less) NSCLC between 2000 and 2005, lobectomy ($n = 84$) was associated with longer overall ($p = 0.0027$) and recurrence-free ($p = 0.0496$) survival, but no statistically significant improvement in rate of local recurrence after sublobar resection (16% vs. 8%, $p = 0.1117$).

From all these nonrandomized studies mentioned earlier, it appears that for tumors less than 2 cm or when a margin to tumor ratio is greater than 1, anatomic segmental resection is justified with excellent results comparable to lobectomy. However, a recent SEER database analysis of 14,473 patients meeting the selection criteria, lobectomy was found to confer a significant survival advantage compared with segmentectomy (excluding wedge resections) for stage I NSCLC.[16] This study has some inherent flaws and caution should be exercised with the interpretation of this study. First, it is a retrospective national database based upon population-based cancer registries where the type of surgery was self-reported. Therefore, it is not clear if all of the segmental resections were actually anatomic or if they represented just very large wedge resections.

Finally, a meta-analysis of published studies with 11,360 patients in total concluded that for stage I patients, sublobar resection causes lower survival than lobectomy, whereas the outcome after segmentectomy is comparable to that after lobectomy for stage IA patients with tumors ≤2 cm.[17]

In an effort to increase the level of evidence to support limited resection for these small (≤2 cm) tumors, two prospective randomized studies are currently ongoing, one in the United States and Canada with an expected enrollment of 1258 patients in 5 years (CALGB-140503) and one in Japan with an accrual of 1100 patients in 3 years (JCOG0802/WJOG4607L). Inclusion criteria in both trials are peripheral small (≤2 cm) NSCLC excluding noninvasive lung cancer on CT (so-called pure ground-glass opacity). In the North American trial, the investigational arm is segmentectomy or wedge resection, whereas in the Japanese trial only segmentectomy is allowed. The results of these trials are hoped to be available within 5 to 10 years from now.

Segmentectomy can also be performed via minimally invasive techniques. Reported series have shown that the outcome after VATS segmentectomy for small lung cancers is quite favorable in terms of perioperative course and intermediate survival.[18–20] VATS segmentectomy was compared to open segmentectomy in two retrospective studies, one from Duke University including 77 patients (48 VATS vs. 29 open)[20] and one from the University of Pittsburgh including 225 patients (104 VATS vs. 121 open).[19] Both series reported a significantly reduced length of stay (4–5 days vs. 7 days), whereas a lower 30-day mortality (0% vs. 6.9%) was observed in the Duke series and a reduced rate of postoperative pulmonary complications (15.4% vs. 29.8%) was found in the Pittsburgh series in favor of the VATS approach. There were no differences in the operative time, estimated blood loss, recurrence, or survival between both groups in the latter series, whereas the survival was significantly ($p = 0.0007$) better in favor of VATS patients in the first series. One study reported by Swanson and colleagues[21] compared segmentectomy ($n = 31$) versus lobectomy ($n = 113$) in patients operated for stage I NSCLC by VATS. Aside from a slightly increased number of patients with prolonged air leaks in the segmentectomy group, no major differences were seen in the length of stay (4 days), local recurrence (3.5%), and 3-year survival (80%). However, VATS segmentectomy can be quite challenging and may not be widely applicable at the current time.

SUMMARY

Segmentectomy has been part of the thoracic surgeon's armamentarium for more than 70 years. In the last four decades, the indication for segmentectomy has shifted from a procedure for infectious etiologies (bronchiectasis, empyema, tuberculosis, and other infectious and nonmalignant lesions) to a surgical option for patients with peripheral stage IA NSCLC with a favorable size (≤2 cm) or with limited cardiopulmonary reserve. The only randomized study published demonstrates lower recurrence rates for lobectomy compared to a sublobar resection. These early published survival results after sublobar resection for lung cancer was tainted by the inclusion of nonanatomic wedge resections. Wedge resection resulted in a higher chance of leaving involved sump nodes behind and exposing the patient to a higher risk of local and regional recurrence. More recent retrospective and single-institutional reports suggest that the outcome in carefully selected patients with small (≤3 cm, and more likely ≤2 cm) peripheral tumors (mainly adenocarcinoma) is excellent after anatomic segmentectomy and comparable to lobectomy. Nevertheless, we must await results from ongoing randomized trials before segmentectomy can be embraced as the standard oncologic procedure for early-stage NSCLC. A VATS approach for sublobar resection has proved feasible, achieving excellent survival results comparable to open segmentectomy, but with shorter hospital stay and lower pulmonary morbidity. Proponents of this approach believe it may well become the future of surgery for lung cancer.[22]

OTHER TECHNIQUES FOR IDENTIFYING THE INTERSEGMENTAL PLANE

A recent article from Japan demonstrated the use of indocyanine green and infrared thoracoscope[23] to identify the intersegmental plane between segments after the segmental pulmonary artery has been ligated. In patients with severe COPD, collateral ventilation between adjacent segments may hinder identification of the intersegmental plane.

ACKNOWLEDGMENT

Dirk Van Raemdonck is a senior clinical investigator supported by the Fund for Research-Flanders (G.3C04.99).

EDITOR'S COMMENT

The first "non lingular" segmentectomy was actually performed by my mentor, Dr. Richard Overholt, at the New England Deaconess hospital in Boston. His "posterior approach," described in 1947 (Overholt RH, Langer L. A new technique for pulmonary resection; its application in the treatment of bronchiectasis. *Surg Gynecol Obstet.* 1947;84:257–268.) used a transcostal approach with dissection in the hilum. This "bronchus" first approach is still useful in patients after prior surgery or pulmonary/pleural infection or inflammation. Once the data from current randomized become available, a rational approach to subcentimeter lesions, found during lung cancer screening can be undertaken. The concept of lung-sparing surgery is paramount to treating patients with a long anticipated survival to minimize pulmonary morbidity. The margin-to-size ratio popularized by the Pittsburgh group promises to be an important determinant of adequacy of resection.

—Mark J. Krasna

References

1. Churchill ED, Belsey R. Segmental pneumonectomy in bronchiectasis: the lingula segment of the left upper lobe. *Ann Surg.* 1939;109(4):481–499.
2. Jones DR, Stiles BM, Denlinger CE, et al. Pulmonary segmentectomy: results and complications. *Ann Thorac Surg.* 2003;76(2):343–348; discussion 348–349.
3. Jensik RJ, Faber LP, Milloy FJ, et al. Segmental resection for lung cancer. A fifteen-year experience. *J Thorac Cardiovasc Surg.* 1973;66(4):563–572.
4. Brunelli A, Charloux A, Bolliger CT, et al. The European Respiratory Society and European Society of Thoracic Surgeons clinical guidelines for evaluating fitness for radical treatment (surgery and chemoradiotherapy) in patients with lung cancer. *Eur J Cardiothorac Surg.* 2009;36(1):181–184.
5. Nomori H, Ohba Y, Shibata H, et al. Required area of lymph node sampling during segmentectomy for clinical stage IA non-small cell lung cancer. *J Thorac Cardiovasc Surg.* 2010;139(1):38–42.
6. Kodama K, Higashiyama M, Takami K, et al. Treatment strategy for patients with small peripheral lung lesion(s): intermediate-term results of prospective study. *Eur J Cardiothorac Surg.* 2008;34(5):1068–1074.
7. Okada M, Yoshikawa K, Hatta T, et al. Is segmentectomy with lymph node assessment an alternative to lobectomy for non-small cell lung cancer of 2 cm or smaller? *Ann Thorac Surg.* 2001;71(3):956–960; discussion 961.
8. Flores RM. Video-assisted thoracic surgery (VATS) lobectomy: focus on technique. *World J Surg.* 2010;34(4):616–620.
9. Ginsberg RJ, Rubinstein LV. Randomized trial of lobectomy versus limited resection for T1 N0 non-small cell lung cancer. Lung Cancer Study Group. *Ann Thorac Surg.* 1995;60(3):615–622; discussion 622–623.
10. Koike T, Yamato Y, Yoshiya K, et al. Intentional limited pulmonary resection for peripheral T1 N0 M0 small-sized lung cancer. *J Thorac Cardiovasc Surg.* 2003;125(4):924–928.
11. Okada M, Koike T, Higashiyama M, et al. Radical sublobar resection for small-sized non–small cell lung cancer: a multicenter study. *J Thorac Cardiovasc Surg.* 2006;132(4):769–775.
12. Okada M, Nishio W, Sakamoto T, et al. Effect of tumor size on prognosis in patients with non-small cell lung cancer: the role of segmentectomy as a type of lesser resection. *J Thorac Cardiovasc Surg.* 2005;129(1):87–93.
13. Schuchert MJ, Pettiford BL, Keeley S, et al. Anatomic segmentectomy in the treatment of stage I non-small cell lung cancer. *Ann Thorac Surg.* 2007;84(3):926–933.
14. Carr SR, Schuchert MJ, Pennathur A, et al. Impact of tumor size on outcomes after anatomic lung resection for stage 1 A non-small cell lung cancer based on the current staging system. *J Thorac Cardiovasc Surg.* 2012;143(2):390–397.
15. Wolf AS, Richards WG, Jaklitsch MT, et al. Lobectomy versus sublobar resection for small (2 cm or less) non-small cell lung cancers. *Ann Thorac Surg.* 2011;92(5):1819–1823; discussion 1824–1825.
16. Whitson BA, Groth SS, Andrade RS, et al. Survival after lobectomy versus segmentectomy for stage I non-small cell lung cancer: a population-based analysis. *Ann Thorac Surg.* 2011;92(6):1943–1950.
17. Fan J, Wang L, Jiang G-N, et al. Sublobectomy versus lobectomy for stage I non-small-cell lung cancer, a meta-analysis of published studies. *Ann Surg Oncol.* 2012;19(2):661–668.
18. Shapiro M, Weiser TS, Wisnivesky JP, et al. Thoracoscopic segmentectomy compares favorably with thoracoscopic lobectomy for patients with small stage I lung cancer. *J Thorac Cardiovasc Surg.* 2009;137(6):1388–1393.
19. Schuchert MJ, Pettiford BL, Pennathur A, et al. Anatomic segmentectomy for stage I non–small-cell lung cancer: comparison of video-assisted thoracic surgery versus open approach. *J Thorac Cardiovasc Surg.* 2009;138(6):1318.e1–1325.e1.
20. Atkins BZ, Harpole DH, Mangum JH, et al. Pulmonary segmentectomy by thoracotomy or thoracoscopy: reduced hospital length of stay with a minimally-invasive approach. *Ann Thorac Surg.* 2007;84(4):1107–1112; discussion 1112–1113.
21. Shapiro M, Swanson SJ, Wright CD, et al. Predictors of major morbidity and mortality after pneumonectomy utilizing the society for thoracic surgeons general thoracic surgery database. *Ann Thorac Surg.* Elsevier Inc; 2010;90(3):927–935.
22. Swanson SJ. Video-assisted thoracic surgery segmentectomy: the future of surgery for lung cancer? *Ann Thorac Surg.* 2010;89(6):S2096–S2097.
23. Misaki N, Chang SS, Igai H, et al. New clinically applicable method for visualizing adjacent lung segments using an infrared thoracoscopy system. *J Thorac Cardiovasc Surg.* 2010;140(4):752–756.

74 VATS Lobectomy

Daniel G. Nicastri and Scott J. Swanson

Keywords: Video-assisted thoracic surgery (VATS), lung cancer, lymph node dissection

Video-assisted thoracic surgery (VATS) lobectomy has been used in the treatment of lung cancer since the early 1990s. While there is evidence that lobectomy is better than wedge resection in most patients, there are no *large* prospective, randomized studies favoring video-assisted lobectomy over conventional lobectomy by thoracotomy.[1] However, there are several series that support the use of VATS lobectomy technique. These include some small ($n \leq 100$) prospective, randomized studies that compare VATS with lobectomy by thoracotomy (Table 74-1). From these data, as well as data from several exclusive VATS series, it is clear that VATS lobectomy is technically feasible and safe and even may provide better quality-of-life outcomes in patients with resectable lung cancer. Despite these efforts, VATS lobectomies represent about 25% to 30% of all lobectomies performed in the United States.[6]

The VATS cancer operation is specifically defined as an anatomic lobectomy (or segmentectomy, when indicated) and consists of individual hilar ligation by means of three or four small incisions and no rib spreading. This anatomic lobectomy should leave the patient with results *identical* to a cancer resection by thoracotomy. That is, the surgeon resects the tumor with negative margins, performing individual vascular and bronchial ligation and division and a complete hilar lymph node dissection. Furthermore, mediastinal lymph node dissection or sampling is performed as appropriate. Certain aspects of the technique, most notably avoidance of rib spreading or the use of a rib retractor, are emphasized, with the goal of improving the patient's postoperative experience. Cosmetic aspects, such as smaller scars (largest incision is usually 5 cm), are also important. One variant, the video-assisted simultaneously stapled lobectomy, does not involve individual hilar ligation. In essence, it is a different operation and is not discussed in this chapter. Nevertheless, some surgeons have achieved excellent results with this technique.[7]

TECHNICAL AND ONCOLOGIC PRINCIPLES

Oncologically, this surgery is equivalent to a lobectomy by thoracotomy. The ultimate measure of success in cancer surgery is long-term survival. Proving that VATS lobectomy is comparable with conventional lobectomy would require a large prospective, randomized multicenter trial. It is unlikely that this will ever occur for lack of sufficient patient accrual. Many

Table 74-1

SELECTED VATS VERSUS THORACOTOMY SERIES

YEAR	AUTHOR	PATIENTS VATS/Thor (n)	COMPLICATIONS	LENGTH OF SURGERY	BLOOD LOSS	LYMPH NODE DISSECTION	PAIN	LENGTH OF STAY
2001	Nomori[31,a]	33/33	NS (no mortality)	NS (VATS > Thor)	NS	NS	Day 0–7: VATS < Thor ($p < 0.05$) and less analgesic requirements ($p < 0.001$) Day 14: NS	NS
1999	Sugiura[5,a]	22/22	NS	NS (VATS > Thor)	VATS < Thor ($p = 0.0089$)	N/A	Day 0–7: Less analgesics and epidural intubation with VATS ($p < 0.05$)	NS
1998	Ohbuchi[3,a]	35/35	N/A	VATS > Thor ($p = 0.04$)	VATS < Thor ($p = 0.03$)	NS	Day 0–7: Less with VATS ($p < 0.0001$)	VATS < Thor ($p < 0.0001$)
1995	Kirby[13,b]	25/30	VATS < Thor ($p < 0.05$)	NS	NS	9.3 (thor) vs. 9.5 (VATS)	NS	NS

Note: These early series suggest that the VATS and thoracotomy approaches have similar safety profiles and efficacy. There may be less pain with the VATS technique in the early postoperative period.

Thor, thoracotomy; NS, not significant; N/A, not applicable.

[a] Case–control study/retrospective.

[b] Randomized, prospective study, but according to authors, rib spreading was used occasionally in removing the specimens.

Table 74-2
SELECTED VATS LOBECTOMY SURVIVAL DATA

YEAR	AUTHOR	NUMBER OF PATIENTS/ POSTOPERATIVE STAGE	OUTCOMES 3-YEAR SURVIVAL	4-YEAR SURVIVAL	5-YEAR SURVIVAL
2004	Roviaro et al.[12]	176/stage I			63%
2004	Ohtsuka et al.[21]	82/stage I	89%		
2003	Walker et al.[15]	117/stage I			78%
2001	Solaini et al.[28]	72/stage I	90%		
2000	Kaseda et al.[14]	50/stage I			97%
1998	McKenna et al.[29]	233/stage I		70%	

Note: These series demonstrate excellent survival outcomes for stage I patients undergoing VATS lobectomy. Five-year survival for stage IA after thoracotomy and lobectomy has been reported to be between 61%[8] and 82%.[14]

patients prefer the minimally invasive technique, and the lack of data of the highest order (i.e., large prospective, randomized series) does not matter to them. Today's patients are well informed, often using resources such as the Internet to choose the optimal technique or surgeon. Several meta-analyses show similar-to-possibly improved survival with VATS lobectomy compared with open lobectomy.[8,9]

SURVIVAL

In lieu of ideal prospective, randomized data, the existing data demonstrate comparable and sometimes better long-term survival rates with VATS lobectomy (Table 74-2). Stage I 5-year VATS survivals can range from 63% to 97%.[12,14,15] Although direct comparison is precluded, indirect comparison of these data with two series of patients undergoing lobectomy by thoracotomy demonstrates a trend for improved survival with VATS lobectomy. Mountain[16] reported 5-year survival in stage IA surgical patients of 61%. Martini et al.[17] reported 5-year survival of 82% in stage IA surgical patients. Some hypothesize that the higher survival range observed with VATS is a result of the decreased presence of inflammatory mediators interleukin 6 and interleukin 8 in VATS patients compared with thoracotomy patients.[18–20] This theoretical decrease in postoperative inflammation may free the immune system to devote more effort to tumor cell surveillance and destruction.

LOCOREGIONAL RECURRENCE

The reported locoregional recurrence rates for VATS lobectomy are comparable with the published standards for lobectomy (Table 74-3). In general, locoregional disease is estimated to recur in 5% to 10% of all patients.[1,17] Port-site and incisional recurrence are extremely rare. Since the use of endoscopic bags for removing tumor became general practice, incisional or port-site recurrence has been reported to be in the low range of 0% to 0.57% of all cases.[6,22]

LYMPH NODE DISSECTION

Lymph node dissection can be accomplished adequately in VATS lobectomy. In fact, several studies have shown that thoracotomy may provide only minimal, if any, advantage in exposing lymph nodes and stations.[23–25] Sagawa et al. reported their experience with standard thoracotomy after VATS lobectomy. This group reported an average increased yield of 1.2 lymph nodes (2%–3%) at follow-up thoracotomy, but without effect as to clinical stage in a single patient. Lymph node sampling was very efficient, with 40 nodes sampled on the right and 37 on the left using the VATS technique alone.[25]

INDICATIONS, PATIENT CHARACTERISTICS, AND PREOPERATIVE ASSESSMENT

The indications for VATS lobectomy are basically the same as those for conventional lobectomy, namely, non–small-cell lung cancer, metastasectomy, and carcinoid tumors. The ideal and typical patient has stage I non–small-cell lung cancer. Absolute contraindications to VATS lobectomy are becoming less frequent and still include the presence of T4 tumors that require a more direct approach to resection such as carinal resection and

Table 74-3
LOCOREGIONAL RECURRENCE

YEAR	AUTHOR	NUMBER OF PATIENTS/ CLINICAL STAGES	LOCOREGIONAL RECURRENCE RATE (%)	FOLLOW-UP
2004	Ohtsuka et al.[21]	106 (stage I)	6	25 mo (median)
2003	Walker et al.[15]	158 (stage I, II)	6	38 mo (mean)
2000	Sugi et al.[34]	48 (stage I)	6	60 mo (median)
1995	Ginsberg and Rubinstein[1]	125 (stage IA)	6.4	54 mo (minimum)

Note: Locoregional occurrence has been reported between 0% and 6% in VATS lobectomy series with various follow-up times. For comparison, Ginsberg and Rubinstein (The Lung Cancer Study Group) reported an incidence of 6.4% for locoregional recurrence in thoracotomy patients.[1]

the presence of N3 disease. Relative contraindications include central hilar tumors, bulky mediastinal or hilar lymphadenopathy and a history of neoadjuvant chemotherapy or radiation. Although these issues can be managed by surgeons experienced in minimally invasive techniques. Incomplete or absent fissures rarely mandate conversion to thoracotomy. Furthermore, segmentectomy can be performed thoracoscopically.[26] Older or more frail patients even may tolerate lobectomy better by VATS than by thoracotomy.[27]

The preoperative studies for VATS lobectomy are those typically performed for a lung cancer workup. These include chest radiograph, CT scan, bronchoscopy, pulmonary function studies, PET scan, and when necessary, other modalities for metastatic workup. In reviewing the CT scan, the surgeon should focus on whether there are any issues, such as bulky lymphadenopathy, that would render the hilar dissection more difficult with VATS.

SURGICAL TECHNIQUE

It is important to perform a safe and effective surgery without compromising any established oncologic principles. Conversion to an open technique should be viewed as a sign of good judgment, not failure. The adequacy of resection should not be jeopardized by the predilection for a VATS approach.

A thoracotomy tray with vascular clamps and chest retractors always should be available in the room. Sponge-stick and dental pledgets also should be ready and available on the field for tamponade of major bleeding sites while a thoracotomy is expeditiously and carefully performed.

Once preoperative evaluation has deemed the patient to be a candidate for VATS lobectomy, the patient is brought to the OR. The patient is anesthetized and intubated. Bronchoscopy is performed to rule out endobronchial lesions that would preclude a VATS approach. Mediastinoscopy is performed when indicated. Lung isolation is obtained with a double-lumen endotracheal tube or bronchial blocker. Good lung isolation is an absolute need throughout the entire case. Once the position of the tube is confirmed, the patient is placed in the lateral decubitus position. The endotracheal tube is reconfirmed via bronchoscopy to ensure that it has not migrated out of position. The ipsilateral lung is immediately collapsed to permit ample time for atelectasis to occur before entering the chest. Suction also may be applied through a suction catheter or bronchoscope to aid in collapse of the isolated lung.

Several different approaches have been described in the literature. Two to four ports which include the incision used to extract the lobe within a bag which is typically about 3 to 5 cm are required to perform a VATS lobectomy. We prefer to use three incisions: an inferior camera port, a posterior working port, and an anterior incision (Fig. 74-1). Avoidance of rib spreading is the key element in VATS lobectomy for preventing postoperative pain and trauma to the intercostal nerve bundles, which are responsible for the postthoracotomy pain syndrome.

By exchanging the camera and instruments and using the angles afforded by the three ports, all visualization and most dissection techniques practiced in open lobectomy procedures can be duplicated. Port placement may vary slightly to account for patient body habitus, location of the tumor, and surgeon preference. However, optimal port placement is important for successful resection. The camera port is created first, and it is usually placed at the seventh or eighth intercostal space. This is the only incision which typically requires a rigid port. Whether to locate it in the anterior, middle, or posterior axillary line depends on multiple factors, including the level of the diaphragm, as determined by review of preoperative chest radiograph, the location of the pathology, and the side of the procedure (left vs. right). Ideally, this port should provide views of the anterior and posterior hilum and should align with the major fissure. We use a 30-degree scope almost exclusively. It provides optimal views not afforded by a 0-degree scope, particularly during the difficult dissection around the superior hilum, and avoids "crowding" of the working instruments. Once the scope is inserted, we inspect the chest cavity and select the ideal position for the remaining two ports. The anterior port should be placed immediately over the hilum because this will be used for vein and artery dissection. Dissection of both the hilum and fissure will be performed through this port. The initial incision is limited to 1 to 2 cm in length. It is not fully extended (i.e., 3–5 cm in length) until the decision is made to proceed with VATS lobectomy. The port is usually created anterior to the latissimus dorsi muscle in the fourth intercostal space for an upper lobectomy and the fifth intercostal space for a lower lobectomy. The third port is usually sited in the fifth intercostal space, either inferior or posterior to the scapular tip. This port usually serves as the lung retraction port. Hemostasis is very important when creating the ports because bleeding from the port sites onto the camera and into the surgical field during the procedure is a nuisance and can prolong the operation significantly.

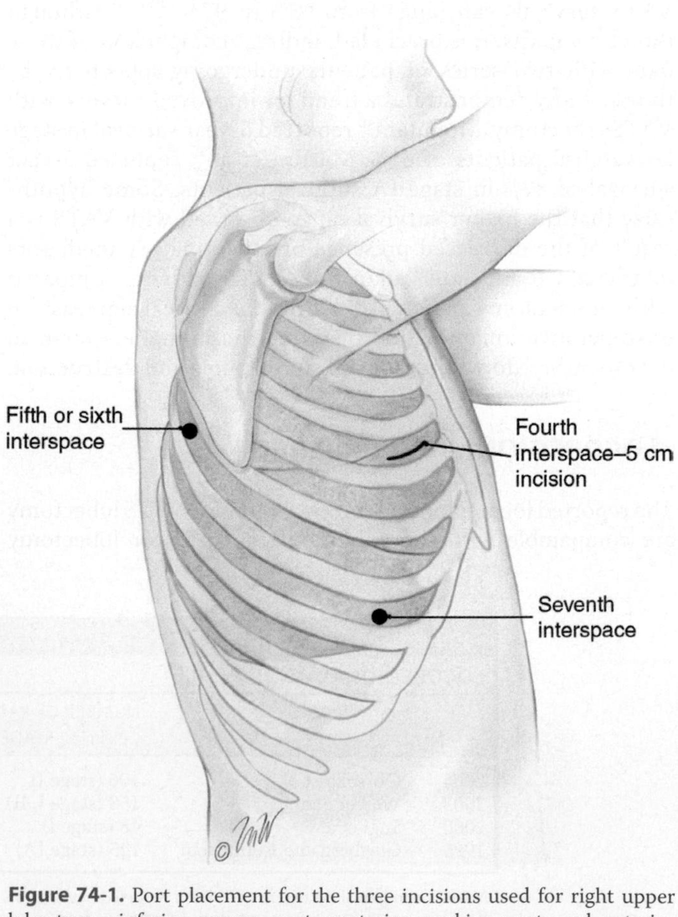

Figure 74-1. Port placement for the three incisions used for right upper lobectomy: inferior camera port, posterior working port, and anterior access/utility incision.

Once all the ports have been created, a more thorough exploration is performed. The pleural surface is inspected for implants. Adhesions may be encountered. These can be lysed and are not a contraindication to proceed with VATS lobectomy. Careful and complete adhesiolysis permits full mobility of the lung. Retraction of the lung is critical to completing the resection. For this reason, the inferior pulmonary ligament is always divided. The discovery of tumor invasion into the chest wall does not preclude a VATS approach. In experienced hands and for relatively limited chest wall involvement, an en bloc chest wall resection can be performed. Digital palpation of the tumor and lung is performed through the anterior access port not only to confirm the location and presence of the tumor but also to rule out additional unsuspected nodules or pathology not identified on preoperative studies. Before resection, the ipsilateral mediastinal lymph nodes are sampled, especially if mediastinoscopy was not performed earlier. If N2 disease is discovered on frozen section, the VATS resection is generally aborted, in keeping with treatment principles for N2 disease and the patient is treated with neoadjuvant therapy. If a preoperative tissue diagnosis has not been determined, a wedge or core biopsy is performed initially, followed by lobectomy if frozen section reveals carcinoma.

A combination of conventional and endoscopic surgical instruments may be used for dissection. We have found the following conventional instruments to be particularly useful in accomplishing VATS lobectomy: ring forceps, right-angle clamps, Harken clamps, Pearson scissors, long Allis clamps, Frazier clamps, biopsy forceps, and a red rubber catheter. Familiarity with the use of these instruments in open techniques translates to facility in their use during the VATS resection.

The order of division of the hilar structures is irrelevant in terms of oncologic outcome. Depending on the lobe, the order of division of the hilar structures differs and is described in detail below. Dissection of the hilar structures is fraught with danger, and one must have a comprehensive understanding of the anatomy and possible variations thereof, especially the pulmonary artery branches. Also, despite improved video technology, one must be aware of the limitations of performing three-dimensional dissections guided by a two-dimensional picture.

Hilar dissection is carried out with instruments placed through the anterior access incision utilizing videoscopic visualization throughout. Using a combination of sharp and blunt dissection, we divide the pleura. The lung is retracted away to aid the dissection. The hilar structures then are divided sequentially with an endovascular stapler. We complete the fissures with serial firings of an endoscopic stapler. The resected specimen then is placed in a heavy laparoscopic extraction sac to prevent tumor seeding of the port and is removed through the anterior access incision without spreading the ribs.

Next, we perform a complete lymph node dissection for accurate staging. This includes levels 2, 4, 7, 8, and 9 on the right and levels 5, 6, 7, 8, and 9 on the left. Finally, we test the stump for pneumostasis under water to a pressure of at least 30 to 35 mm Hg. Hemostasis is checked. Electrocautery of the ports is used sparingly to avoid injury to the neurovascular bundle. A single 24F chest tube is left in the chest for postoperative drainage. We rarely employ an epidural catheter for pain relief but perform a 5-rib block and port-site block using bupivacaine with epinephrine. We also routinely use intravenous anti-inflammatory drugs (ketorolac) for 24 hours. The ports are closed, and the patient is repositioned supine on the OR table. A completion bronchoscopy is performed to check the staple line and for pulmonary toilet before extubating the patient in the OR.

The conduct of the operation for the different lobes is essentially the same and is described below with a few caveats based on experience.

Right Upper Lobectomy

For right upper lobectomies, we usually place the camera port in the seventh intercostal space along the anterior axillary line (Fig. 74-2A). This placement provides good visualization of the anterior and superior hilum, the area of most hazardous dissection. The access port usually is located in the fourth intercostal space anteriorly, just anterior to the anterior border of the latissimus dorsi muscle. The posterior port is placed inferior or posterior to the scapula tip, which usually depends on the morphology of the chest. The orientation of this port should provide a right-angle configuration between instruments in the access and working ports. After initial exploration, the dissection is begun in the anterior hilum. The right upper lobe (and sometimes the middle lobe) is grasped gently with ring forceps and retracted posteriorly. This maneuver creates excellent exposure of the anterior hilum. The superior pulmonary vein is isolated first in the anterior hilum by dividing its pleural covering with a Harmonic scalpel, Pearson scissors, and/or endo-Kittners. The phrenic nerve is carefully dissected away from the hilum to prevent injury. The draining veins of the middle lobe must be identified as well to prevent unintentional division. An oiled 2-0 silk suture then is looped around the superior pulmonary vein (Fig. 74-2B). The vein is divided with an endovascular stapler, usually introduced through the posterior port, which provides the best angle. After division of the superior pulmonary vein, the truncus anterior and its variable number of branches are exposed (Fig. 74-3). They are dissected free individually or as one trunk depending on their configuration and accessibility. They are then *divided* individually or as one trunk using an endovascular stapler. The "endoleader," a rubber catheter, can be used to safely guide the stapler through the tight space around the arterial branches.[25] The arteries are best divided with the endovascular stapler introduced through the camera port, with the camera switched to viewing from the access port (Fig. 74-3, inset). A sponge-stick or dental pledget on a clamp always should be in the scrub technician's hand "at the ready" for tamponade of bleeding from malfunction of the stapler or avulsion of the hilar vessels. This single maneuver bides time for adequate control and conversion to an open thoracotomy, if needed. Once the arterial branches are divided, the next step is to dissect the interlobar main pulmonary artery at the confluence of the fissures. This dissection can be difficult with incomplete fissures. There are several alternatives to address this problem. One maneuver is to partially, but carefully, divide the fissure with a stapler or Harmonic scalpel. This provides better exposure of the interlobar pulmonary artery for dissection. The goal of exposing the interlobar pulmonary artery is to identify the space between the recurrent ascending arterial branch to the posterior segment of the upper lobe and the artery to the superior segment of the lower lobe. This space permits safe division of the recurrent ascending branch and completion of the posterior fissure. The most commonly used option for dealing with the incomplete fissure or for isolating the

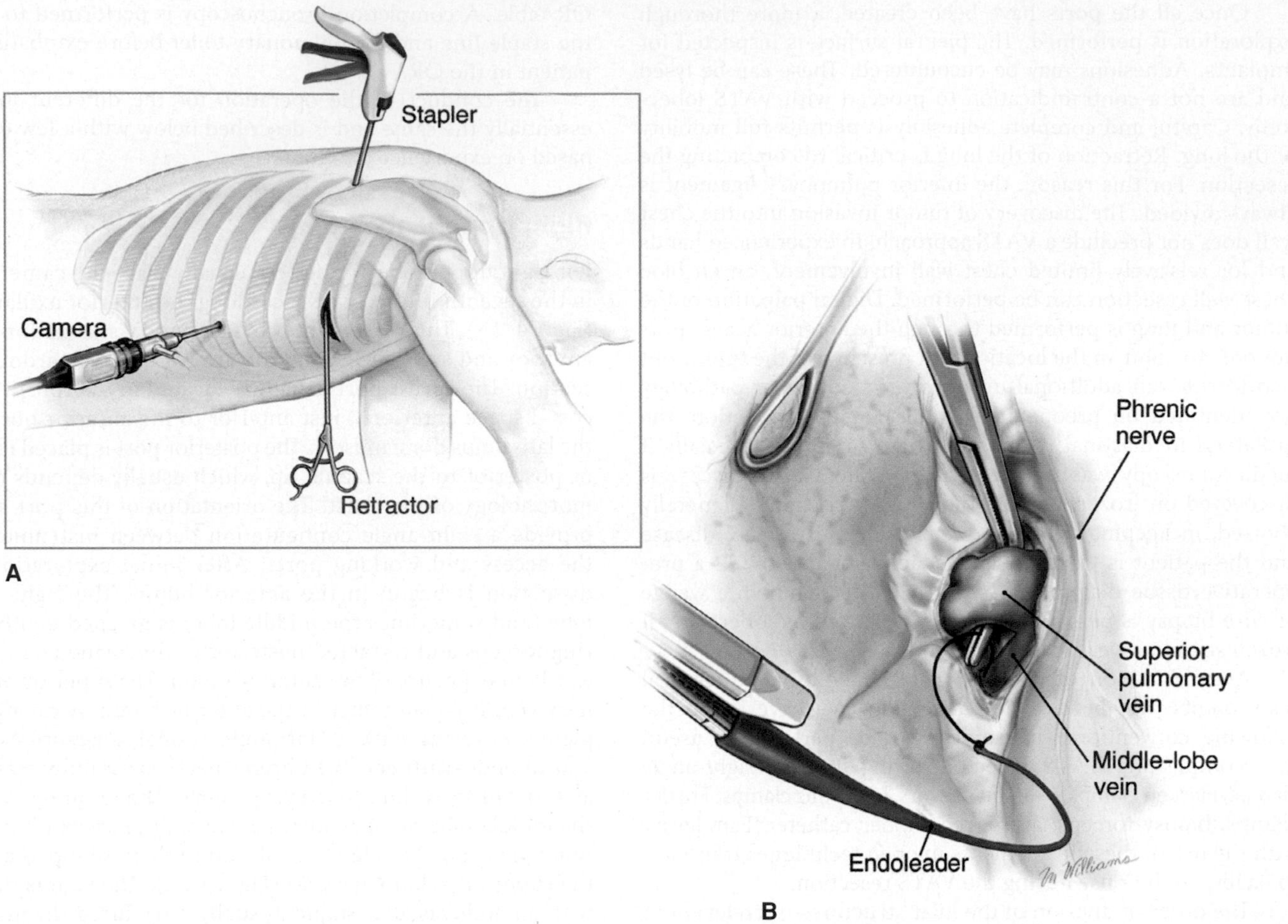

Figure 74-2. An oiled 2-0 silk suture is looped around the superior pulmonary vein, which is divided with an endovascular stapler, usually introduced through the posterior port, which provides the best angle.

recurrent posterior segmental arterial branch is to approach it anteriorly and/or superiorly with the bird's-eye view provided by the 30-degree scope. Once all the arterial branches to the upper lobe are divided, the right upper lobe bronchus is dissected free by sweeping all nodal tissue on the bronchus toward the specimen side (Fig. 74-4). An endoscopic stapler, usually loaded with "thick tissue" staples, then is introduced through the camera port to divide the bronchus, leaving a short, intact stump. The fissure is completed with serial firings of the endoscopic stapler, if not already performed. The specimen lobe then is placed in a heavy laparoscopic extraction sac and is removed through the access incision without rib spreading.

Left Upper Lobectomy

In our opinion, the left upper lobectomy is the most difficult to perform technically because of the variability in the arterial circulation, which can have up to three to eight branches. The order of division of the hilar structures is the same as with the right upper lobe—vein, artery, bronchus. The inferior camera port is placed more posteriorly to avoid obstruction of view by the heart (especially if enlarged) and the pericardial fat pad. In patients with marginal pulmonary function and a small tumor, a lingular-sparing left upper lobectomy, or lingulectomy, as appropriate, should be considered. Anatomically, the lingula can be considered the equivalent of the middle lobe on the left side. The order of hilar structure division is the same as for a right middle lobectomy (see below).

Right Middle Lobectomy

For right middle lobectomy, the camera port usually is placed in the seventh intercostal space along the midaxillary line. This position provides an excellent view of both the anterior hilum and the major fissure. The anterior access port usually is placed in the fourth intercostal space, whereas the working port generally is placed posterior to the scapular tip in the sixth or seventh intercostal space. The right middle lobe is retracted laterally, and the middle lobe veins (usually two branches) are dissected free and divided using the endovascular stapler. The middle lobe bronchus then is exposed. We divide the bronchus first because the bronchus is anterior to the artery. One must be careful not to injure the artery when dissecting around the bronchus. Next, we dissect out the arterial branches to the middle lobe. These are looped and divided with the endovascular stapler. The "endoleader" technique may be helpful in guiding the stapler around these branches.[2] The fissure is completed and the middle lobe is removed in a specimen sac through the access incision.

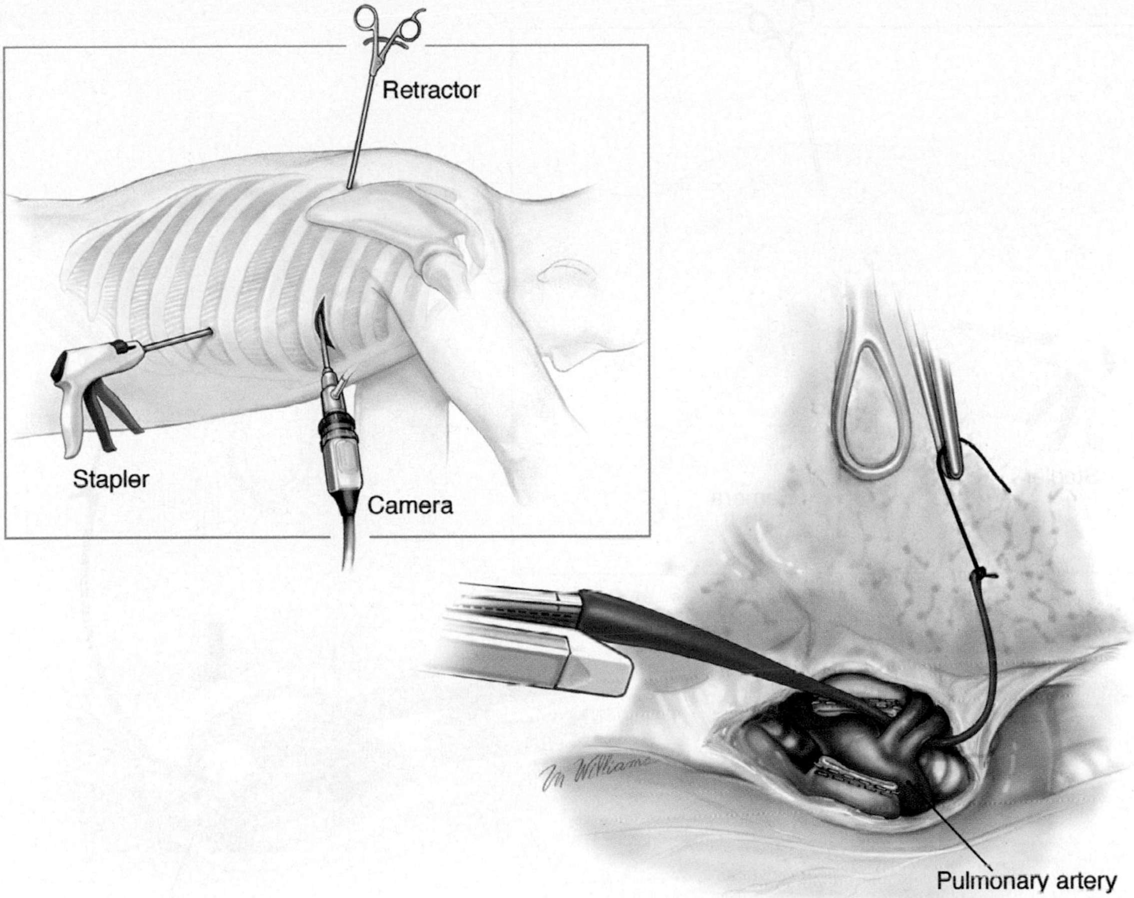

Figure 74-3. The truncus anterior and its variable number of branches are exposed, dissected free, and divided individually or as a trunk depending on configuration and accessibility. Before the arteries are divided, the camera is switched to the anterior access port for better visualization, and the stapler is placed in the inferior port (inset). An endovascular stapler fitted with a rubber "endoleader" for guidance is used to divide the vessels.

Right and Left Lower Lobectomy

The camera ports usually are placed in the eighth interspace to avoid crowding of the instruments. On the right, the camera port generally is positioned in the midaxillary line. On the left, in people with large hearts or "barrel chests," the port is placed more posteriorly to avoid obstruction of the view by the heart. The access port usually is placed anteriorly in the fifth intercostal space. The posterior working port usually is placed posterior to the scapular tip in the sixth or seventh intercostal space. We first divide the inferior pulmonary ligament and sample the level 9 lymph nodes. The lower lobe is retracted superiorly with a ring forceps through the posterior port, putting the ligament under tension. A long-tip electrocautery or ultrasonic scalpel divides the ligament through the access port. The level 9 lymph nodes are removed and sent for frozen section. Next, the interlobar main pulmonary artery is dissected free in the fissure. The basilar trunk and artery to the superior segment are identified, dissected, looped, and divided with the endovascular stapler. Next, the inferior pulmonary vein is dissected free, looped, and then divided with an endovascular stapler. Finally, the bronchus to the lower lobe is dissected and divided with an endoscopic stapler. As in the open technique, care must be observed on the right side to avoid impingement on the middle lobe bronchus. The fissure is completed, and the lobe is removed in a specimen sac through the access incision without any rib spreading.

POSTOPERATIVE ISSUES AND RESULTS

The elements of postoperative care are the same for VATS lobectomy as for conventional lobectomy. Typically, however, the postoperative course can be accelerated with regard to days of chest tube drainage and length of hospital stay (Table 74-4). The same complications occur with VATS lobectomy as with conventional thoracotomy but perhaps with decreased frequency. Morbidity in patients undergoing conventional lobectomy occurs in approximately 28% to 38% based on data reported from several large series.[4,30] Mortality for these same series ranges from 2% to 2.9%. A representative series of VATS lobectomies and segmentectomies has reported major morbidity and mortality rates of 6% to 9% and 0% to 0.9% respectively.[26] The most common postoperative complications are atrial fibrillation and prolonged air leak.

The risk of fatal intraoperative hemorrhage merits special consideration because it may be a barrier to more surgeons using this technique. This risk is clearly related to experience and skill in the videoscopic dissection of the hilum. Regardless, of the perceived difficulty of this dissection, the risk of intraoperative hemorrhage is very low and similar to with open procedures based on reported series. The ability to control bleeding with a sponge-stick or other instrument gives the surgeon ample time to extend the incision and convert to a full thoracotomy.

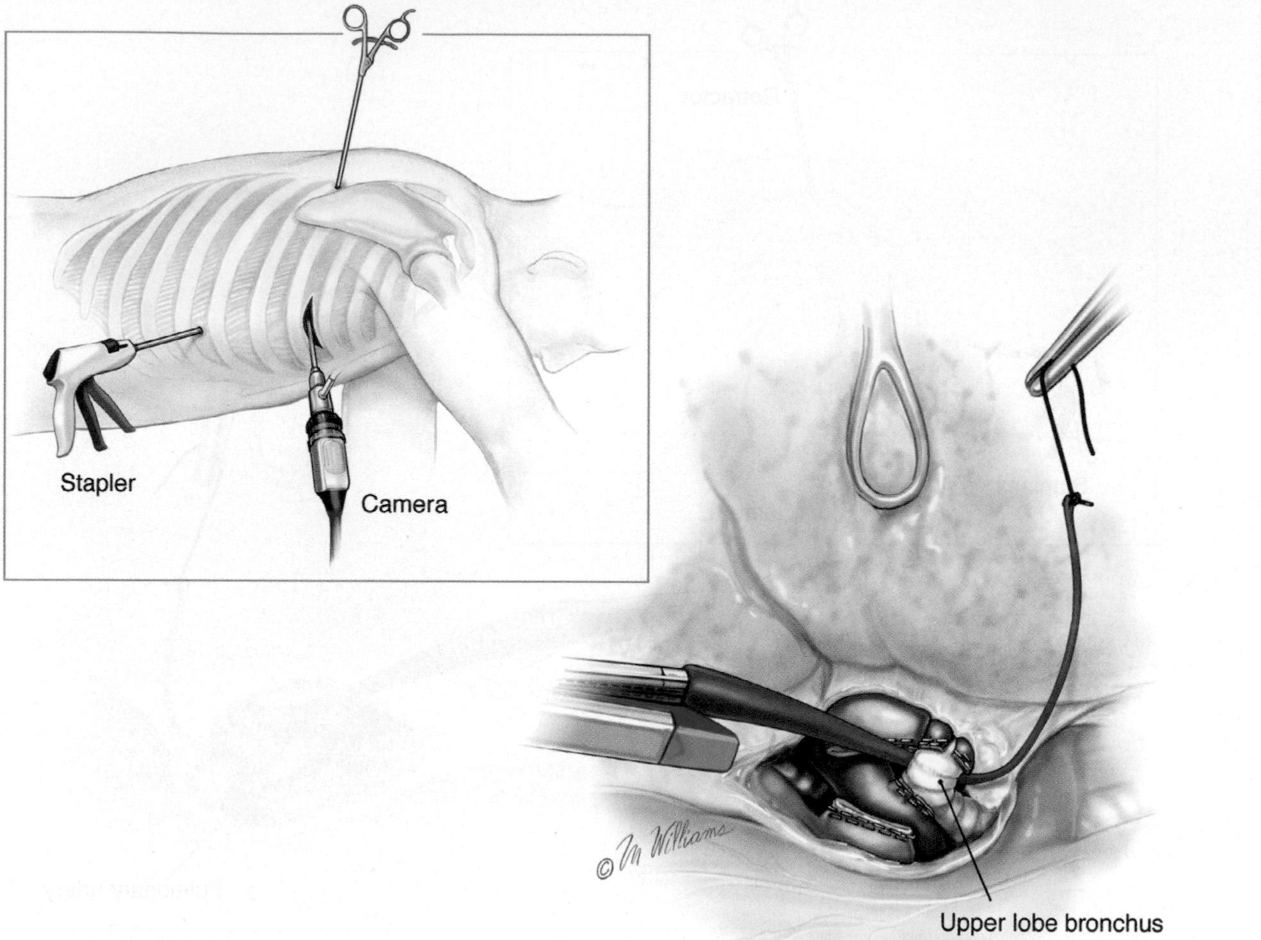

Figure 74-4. The endovascular stapler is switched for an endoscopic stapler. "Thick tissue" staples are used to divide the bronchus, leaving a short, intact stump.

ONCOLOGIC OUTCOMES

Through the many single- and multi-institution series, it has been established that VATS lobectomy can be performed safely. The 3-, 4-, and 5-year survivals for some of the published series in Table 74-2 and the locoregional recurrence data in Table 74-3 demonstrate that this surgery can be performed with good oncologic outcome. The published morbidity and mortality rates are also comparable to or better than those of lobectomy by thoracotomy. Other significant factors, such as those that fall under the expansive category of quality of life, ultimately may validate VATS lobectomy.

Quality of Life

VATS lobectomy may give patients improved quality of life as compared with open lobectomy. Quality of life is measured in terms of psychological and physical effects. Factors that affect patient perception include postoperative morbidity, mortality, pain, independence, and overall oncologic outcome, to name a few.

Table 74-4

SELECTED VATS PERIOPERATIVE DATA

SERIES	SIZE	CONVERSION (%)	COMPLICATIONS	TRANSFUSION	PERIOPERATIVE MORTALITY	LENGTH OF STAY (MEDIAN DAYS)	CHEST TUBE DAYS
McKenna et al.[37]	1100	2.5	15%	4.1%	0.8%	3	N/A
Walker et al.[15]	159	11.2	N/A	N/A	1.8%	6	N/A
Kaseda et al.[24]	128	11.7	N/A	N/A	0.8%	N/A	N/A
Solaini et al.[28]	125	10.4	11.6%	N/A	N/A	N/A	N/A
Nicastri et al.[35]	110	11	24.5%	7.3%	0.9%	4	3
Daniels et al.[36]	110	1.8	19.1%	N/A	3.6%	3	3
Ohtsuka et al.[21]	106	10	9%	N/A	1%	7.6 (mean)	1.1 (mean)

Note: These VATS series demonstrate morbidity and mortality rates with some quality-of-life measures. In the largest series of patients undergoing lobectomy predominantly by thoracotomy, the morbidity ranges from 28% to 38%, and mortality ranges from 2% to 2.9%.[30]

The quality-of-life variable that argues favorably for VATS lobectomy over lobectomy by thoracotomy is the tolerable postoperative course associated with VATS. Avoiding rib spreading theoretically reduces pain. Evidence that VATS causes less pain and is associated with lower analgesia requirements during the early and late postoperative periods has been published (Table 74-1).[3,31–33] This may be related to lack of rib spreading and earlier removal of the chest tube after VATS lobectomy. Patients are often discharged earlier on postoperative days 2 through 4 and may achieve earlier independence. Demmy et al. compared VATS with thoracotomy to determine discharge independence and found that a significantly higher percentage of case-control thoracotomy patients were discharged to nursing facilities, whereas approximately 95% of VATS patients, despite shorter hospital stays, were discharged to home with or without nursing assistance.[26]

Currently, there are several large series that support chemotherapy in early-stage lung cancer patients with stage IB and greater disease.[5,10] However, receiving chemotherapy postoperatively can be fraught with delays and complication. In fact, a recent trial reported that as few as 45% of patients receive full-dose chemotherapy on schedule.[11] The practice of administering chemotherapy in early-stage lung cancer patients has raised a new question—whether minimally invasive (VATS lobectomy) procedures can expedite the chemotherapy course. A quicker recovery from surgery may mean a higher likelihood of completing a full course on schedule. This may translate into improved survival data. The optimal time for chemotherapy is probably in the very early postoperative period, while the tumor burden is lowest, even given the limitations of wound healing.

SUMMARY

Once mastered, VATS lobectomy can be performed safely with excellent perioperative and oncologic results. The frequency with which this operation is performed remains low. The literature continues to show excellent benefit and with time the penetration of this operation is improving

CASE HISTORY

A 66-year-old woman with a significant remote smoking history was found to have a left upper lobe mass on routine preoperative workup for elective orthopedic surgery (Fig. 74-5). A CT/PET scan further delineated the mass with a standardized uptake value of 5.1 (Fig. 74-6). Brain imaging was negative, and pulmonary function tests were excellent. The patient underwent cervical mediastinoscopy, thoracoscopy, and a needle biopsy, which confirmed the diagnosis of non–small-cell lung cancer. The surgeons then proceeded with video-assisted left upper lobectomy and mediastinal lymph node dissection. Her postoperative course was unremarkable, and she was discharged on postoperative day 3. Final pathology results revealed a stage IB lung adenocarcinoma. Postoperative chemotherapy was recommended and begun 3 weeks after surgery. The patient tolerated the full course of chemotherapy on schedule. The patient is now 6 months out of surgery without any evidence of recurrence or change in lifestyle.

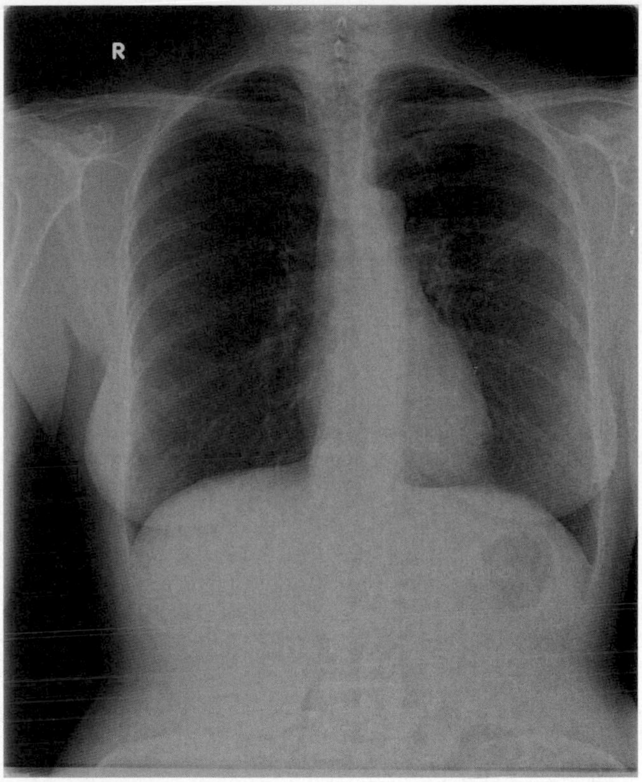

Figure 74-5. A mass is visible overlying the third anterior rib in this chest radiograph.

EDITOR'S COMMENT

Our approach is quite similar to Dr. Swanson's except that we generally perform the VATS lobectomy completely thoracoscopically. That is, we use port access and an operating thoracoscope throughout. This allows a complete lobectomy with truly minimal access incision. The lobe is then placed in a sterile bag and removed through an incision that is just large enough to allow its removal. This has resulted in excellent cosmesis as well as very good functional outcomes. The duration of CT drainage is the sole determinant of discharge.

—Mark J. Krasna

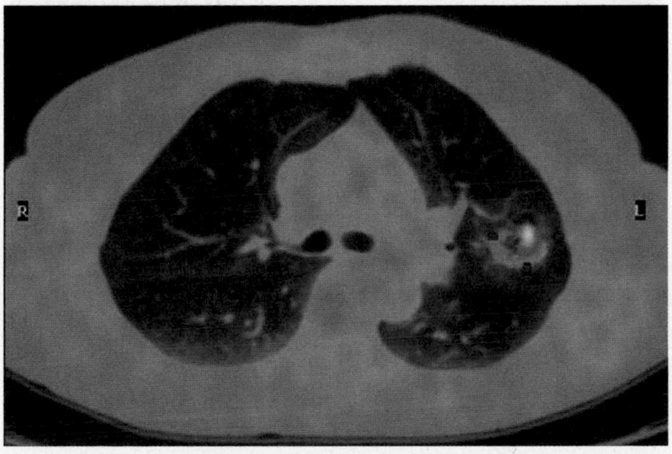

Figure 74-6. This CT/PET scan demonstrates the same left upper lobe lesion with a high standardized uptake value.

References

1. Ginsberg RJ, Rubinstein LV. Randomized trial of lobectomy versus limited resection for T_1N_0 non-small cell lung cancer. Lung Cancer Study Group. *Ann Thorac Surg.* 1995;60:615–622; discussion 622–623.
2. Garcia J, Richards W, Sugarbaker D. Surgical treatment of malignant mesothelioma. In: Kaiser LR, Kron IL, Spray IL, eds. *Mastery of Cardiothoracic Surgery*. Philadelphia, PA: Lippincott-Raven; 1997.
3. Ohbuchi T, Morikawa T, Takeuchi E, et al. Lobectomy: video-assisted thoracic surgery versus posterolateral thoracotomy. *Jpn J Thorac Cardiovasc Surg.* 1998;46:519–522.
4. Deslauriers J, Ginsberg R, Piantadosi S. Prospective assessment of 30-day operative morbidity for surgical resections in lung cancer. *Chest.* 1994;106:329S–330S.
5. Sugiura H, Morikawa T, Kaji M, et al. Long-term benefits for the quality of life after video-assisted thoracoscopic lobectomy in patients with lung cancer. *Surg Laparosc Endosc Percutan Tech.* 1999;9:403–408.
6. Swanson SJ, Meyers BF, Gunnarsson CL, et al. Video-assisted thoracoscopic lobectomy is less costly and morbid than open lobectomy: a retrospective multi-institution database analysis. *Ann Thorac Surg.* 2012;93(4):1027–1032.
7. Lewis RJ, Caccavale RJ, Bocage JP, et al. Video-assisted thoracic surgical non-rib spreading simultaneously stapled lobectomy: a more patient-friendly oncologic resection. *Chest.* 1999;116:1119–1124.
8. Whitson BA, Groth SS, Duval SJ, et al. Surgery for early-stage non-small cell lung cancer: a systematic review of the video-assisted thoracoscopic surgery versus thoracotomy approaches to lobectomy. *Ann Thorac Surg.* 2008;86(6):2008–2016.
9. Yan TD, Black D, Bannon PG, et al. Systematic review and meta-analysis of randomized and nonrandomized trials on safety and efficacy of video-assisted thoracic surgery lobectomy for early-stage non-small cell lung cancer. *J Clin. Oncol.* 2009;27(15):2553–2562.
10. Strauss G, Herndon JE II, Maddaus M. Randomized clinical trial of adjuvant chemotherapy with paclitaxel and carboplatin following resection in stage IV non-small cell lung cancer (NSCLC): report of Cancer and Leukemia Group B (CALGB) Protocol 9633 (abstract 7019). *J Clin Oncol.* 2004;22: 621S.
11. Winton T, Livingston R, Johnson D, et al. Vinorelbine plus cisplatin vs observation in resected non-small-cell lung cancer. *N Engl J Med.* 2005;352:2589–2597.
12. Roviaro G, Varoli F, Vergani C, et al. Long-term survival after videothoracoscopic lobectomy for stage I lung cancer. *Chest.* 2004;126:725–732.
13. Kirby TJ, Mack MJ, Landreneau RJ, et al. Lobectomy: video-assisted thoracic surgery versus muscle-sparing thoracotomy. A randomized trial. *J Thorac Cardiovasc Surg.* 1995;109:997–1001; discussion 1001–1002.
14. Kaseda S, Aoki T, Hangai N, et al. Better pulmonary function and prognosis with video-assisted thoracic surgery than with thoracotomy. *Ann Thorac Surg.* 2000;70:1644–1646.
15. Walker WS, Codispoti M, Soon SY, et al. Long-term outcomes following VATS lobectomy for non-small cell bronchogenic carcinoma. *Eur J Cardiothorac Surg.* 2003;23:397–402.
16. Mountain CF. Revisions in the international system for staging lung cancer. *Chest.* 1997;111:1710–1717.
17. Martini N, Bains MS, Burt ME, et al. Incidence of local recurrence and second primary tumors in resected stage I lung cancer. *J Thorac Cardiovasc Surg.* 1995;109:120–129.
18. Nagahiro I, Andou A, Aoe M, et al. Pulmonary function, postoperative pain, and serum cytokine level after lobectomy: a comparison of VATS and conventional procedure. *Ann Thorac Surg.* 2001;72:362–365.
19. Yim AP, Wan S, Lee TW, et al. VATS lobectomy reduces cytokine responses compared with conventional surgery. *Ann Thorac Surg.* 2000; 70:243–247.
20. Craig SR, Leaver HA, Yap PL, et al. Acute phase responses following minimal access and conventional thoracic surgery. *Eur J Cardiothorac Surg.* 2001; 20:455–463.
21. Ohtsuka T, Nomori H, Horio H, et al. Is major pulmonary resection by video-assisted thoracic surgery an adequate procedure in clinical stage I lung cancer? *Chest.* 2004;125:1742–1746.
22. Swanson S, DeCamp M, Mentzer SJ. Thoracoscopic resection of lung malignancy without port site recurrence: the Brigham and Women's Hospital experience. *Chest.* 1997;112:9S.
23. Kondo T, Sagawa M, Tanita T, et al. Is complete systematic nodal dissection by thoracoscopic surgery possible? A prospective trial of video-assisted lobectomy for cancer of the right lung. *J Thorac Cardiovasc Surg.* 1998;116:651–652.
24. Kaseda S, Hangai N, Yamamoto S, et al. Lobectomy with extended lymph node dissection by video-assisted thoracic surgery for lung cancer. *Surg Endosc.* 1997;11:703–706.
25. Sagawa M, Sato M, Sakurada A, et al. A prospective trial of systematic nodal dissection for lung cancer by video-assisted thoracic surgery: can it be perfect? *Ann Thorac Surg.* 2002;73:900–904.
26. Shapiro M, Weiser TS, Wisnivesky JP, et al. Thoracoscopic segmentectomy compares favorably with thoracoscopic lobectomy for patients with small stage I lung cancer. *J Thorac Cardiovasc Surg.* 2009;137(6):1388–1393.
27. Demmy TL, Curtis JJ. Minimally invasive lobectomy directed toward frail and high-risk patients: a case-control study. *Ann Thorac Surg.* 1999;68:194–200.
28. Solaini L, Prusciano F, Bagioni P, et al. Video-assisted thoracic surgery major pulmonary resections: present experience. *Eur J Cardiothorac Surg.* 2001;20:437–442.
29. McKenna RJ Jr, Wolf RK, Brenner M, et al. Is lobectomy by video-assisted thoracic surgery an adequate cancer operation? *Ann Thorac Surg.* 1998; 66:1903–1908.
30. Allen MS, Darling GE, Pechet TT, et al. Morbidity and mortality of major pulmonary resections in patients with early-stage lung cancer: initial results of the randomized, prospective ACOSOG Z0030 trial. *Ann Thorac Surg.* 2006;81:1013–1019; discussion 1019–1020.
31. Nomori H, Horio H, Naruke T, et al. What is the advantage of a thoracoscopic lobectomy over a limited thoracotomy procedure for lung cancer surgery? *Ann Thorac Surg.* 2001;72:879–884.
32. Stammberger U, Steinacher C, Hillinger S, et al. Early and long-term complaints following video-assisted thoracoscopic surgery: evaluation in 173 patients. *Eur J Cardiothorac Surg.* 2000;18:7–11.
33. Landreneau RJ, Hazelrigg SR, Mack MJ, et al. Postoperative pain-related morbidity: video-assisted thoracic surgery versus thoracotomy. *Ann Thorac Surg.* 1993;56:1285–1289.
34. Sugi K, Kaneda Y, Esato K. Video-assisted thoracoscopic lobectomy achieves a satisfactory long-term prognosis in patients with clinical stage IA lung cancer. *World J Surg.* 2000;24:27–30; discussion 30–1.
35. Nicastri D, Litl V, Yun J. Safety and efficacy of thoracoscopic lobectomy in 110 consecutive patients. Western Thoracic Surgical Association, 2005.
36. Daniels LJ, Balderson SS, Onaitis MW, et al. Thoracoscopic lobectomy: a safe and effective strategy for patients with stage I lung cancer. *Ann Thorac Surg.* 2002;74:860–864.
37. McKenna RJ Jr, Houck W, Fuller CB: Video-assisted thoracic surgery lobectomy: experience with 1100 cases. *Ann Thorac Surg.* 2006;81:421–425.

75 Sleeve Resection/Bronchoplasty for Lung Cancer

Siva Raja, David P. Mason, and Sudish C. Murthy

Keywords: Bronchoplasty, non–small-cell lung cancer (NSCLC), lobectomy, airway reconstruction

The importance of parenchymal preservation during pulmonary surgery was realized over 50 years ago when descriptions of bronchial resection and reconstruction were first published.[1–3] Since then, considerable technical refinement and anatomic insight have expanded indications for lung-sparing operations. Bronchoplastic resections form one category of these procedures with a unique set of indications. These operations are technically more demanding than standard anatomic pulmonary resections, although, the additional time spent performing these procedures is justly rewarded in considerable functional lung preservation.

The terms *bronchoplasty* and *bronchoplastic resection* have been applied to a wide variety of operations of main or lobar bronchi. The operations *usually* involve a concomitant parenchymal resection; resection and reconstruction of the bronchus alone is quite rare. Bronchoplasty refers to resection and reconstruction of a lobar bronchial orifice (e.g., right upper lobe) without removing a segment of main bronchus. This is in contradistinction to a "sleeve" resection in which a circumferential portion (or sleeve) of a central bronchus is included as part of the operation. Because of the gaps that sleeve resections create in the target airways, release maneuvers (to reduce tension on the anastomosis) are usually necessary.

INDICATIONS

The standard indication for bronchoplastic resection is an endobronchial lesion emanating from either the main bronchus itself or a lobar bronchus with main bronchus encroachment. The extent of the diseased area must allow for safe reconstruction when margins are considered. Etiology is often a low-grade neoplasm such as typical carcinoid or mucoepidermoid cancer[4] or, rarely, isolated bronchial stenosis secondary to granulomatous disease, trauma, caustic injury, foreign body, or benign neoplasm.[5,6] Bronchoplastic resections can be applied to more invasive cancers, that is, non–small-cell lung cancer (NSCLC) or metastases, when trying to spare lung parenchyma in a patient with marginal pulmonary function. While lung is preserved, oncologic principles, namely, achieving a complete resection (including a negative margin), must not be compromised.[7] Positive margins are not an acceptable alternative to complete resection.

The issue of N1/N2 lymph node involvement clearly complicates the decision to proceed with a lung-sparing bronchoplastic resection versus pneumonectomy or bilobectomy. To date, there are no data to suggest that larger parenchymal resections provide a higher cure rate for stage II or stage III lung cancer. Therefore, bronchoplasty can be performed for stage II or stage III lung cancer as long as a complete resection can be obtained. In addition, data from several European studies of neoadjuvant chemotherapy and/or radiation therapy suggest that a bronchoplastic resection can be performed without additional morbidity. Of note, radiation therapy completed more than 3 months before the resection considerably increases the technical difficulty and should be considered high risk. Few definitive contraindications exist for bronchoplastic or sleeve resection techniques as long as the patient's performance status allows. One should know in advance whether pneumonectomy is an option in case the sleeve is technically not feasible.

PREPARATION

Bronchoscopy is universally required for operative planning. Flexible video bronchoscopy offers a slightly less morbid alternative for diagnosis and initial palliative therapy than does traditional rigid bronchoscopy, though both are acceptable methods to access and treat the central airways. For patients presenting with obstructing pneumonia, airway patency should be restored using endobronchial techniques (i.e., laser, cautery, pneumatic or rigid dilation); any infection should be effectively drained and treated before proceeding with a planned resection.

Noninvasive imaging includes chest computed tomography scan (CT) and, for NSCLC, a PET scan. To complete the staging process, mediastinoscopy should be performed for all lung cancers before attempting a sleeve. If performed at the same setting as the planned resection, mediastinoscopy can be used to mobilize the mainstem bronchi and trachea and serve as an important release strategy. If N2 lymph node involvement is found (for patients with lung cancer), the patient is usually offered induction therapy before the resection or treated definitively with chemoradiation.

Epidural analgesia is recommended to optimize pain control and pulmonary toilet. Ipsilateral lung isolation usually is obtained with a contralateral double-lumen tube and not a single-lumen tube with bronchial blocker.

TECHNIQUES

All bronchoplastic procedures include reconstruction of the airway. Familiarity with parenchymal and vascular anatomy is essential. No consensus exists regarding the optimal suture type or technique one should use, and personal preference prevails with regard to these details. We favor the use of monofilament material.

Finally, my personal preference is to buttress all bronchoplasty reconstructions. Transposed tissue pedicles include thymic (epicardial) fat pad, pleura, pericardium, and occasionally, muscle flap. The most common muscle pedicle is adjacent intercostal, though some do not recommend wrapping this type of flap circumferentially for anecdotal concern of heterotopic ossification from retained periosteum. Serratus anterior can also be used as a buttress for reconstructions after induction chemoradiation therapy.

Bronchotomy Closure

The most basic bronchoplastic technique is hand-sewn closure of a bronchial stump divided close to its takeoff from the mainstem bronchus. Often, a flap of membranous airway can be turned back over the open stump and sewn in place with interrupted 4-0 monofilament suture (Fig. 75-1). This maneuver is predicated on having enough uninvolved membranous airway. As with all of these procedures, intraoperative frozen section analysis of the margins must be performed. Some short bronchial stumps can be closed by simple anteroposterior reapproximation (Fig. 75-2). The surgeon must assess the quality of the tissue and have a sense of the tension under which the bronchus is reapproximated. Closely spacing the interrupted sutures helps to distribute tension but will not compensate for a marked mismatch. Airway compliance should be assessed carefully before considering a bronchotomy closure. In older patients, calcium within the anterior bronchial rings can make simple closure of a tight bronchial stump more risky, and surprisingly, the more complex sleeve resection is often the safer operation. Conversely, in younger patients, even if a small amount of the mainstem bronchus is plicated during the closure, results are typically excellent. Only rarely should primary closure be attempted after wedge bronchotomy (Fig. 75-3). Although this type of reconstruction can be performed with minimal tension, the resulting kink in the airway can lead to obstruction postoperatively. Intraoperative bronchoscopy is an important tool to assess the geometry of the airway after reconstruction and judge the suitability of the reconstructed anatomy.

Bronchial Sleeve Resection

Most bronchial sleeve resections occur in the context of parenchymal (lobar) resection. Rarely, pathology isolated to the left mainstem bronchus or bronchus intermedius mandates an isolated resection of the airway alone.

Important factors to consider are (1) will the operation result in a *complete resection*, (2) can the repair be constructed *tension-free*, and (3) if not, what are the *fallback options*? To this end, the etiology of the disease becomes important. Specifically, for lung cancer, accurate staging is mandatory. Also, a history of prior chest surgery makes complete mobilization of the lung more difficult, and a previous coronary artery bypass may complicate a hilar release. A mediastinoscopy performed several weeks before will make it difficult to mobilize the carina and distal trachea for right-sided resections. Finally, can the patient tolerate a bilobectomy or pneumonectomy if the planned bronchoplastic resection cannot be completed safely or with an adequate margin?

Any lobar resection can be accompanied by a sleeve of resected bronchus. Left-sided resections are more challenging because the aortic arch and heart tend to limit exposure. Mediastinoscopy is useful not only from a cancer staging standpoint but also in mobilizing the proximal left and right mainstem bronchi and carina. The surgeon must confirm the anatomy of the airway lesion with bronchoscopy.

Right Upper Lobe Sleeve Resection

Right upper lobe sleeve resection is the most common and straightforward sleeve resection. A left-sided double-lumen tube is placed during induction of anesthesia, and the patient is positioned for a lateral thoracotomy. Muscle-sparing techniques can be used to enter the hemithorax at the fourth or fifth interspace. Some trapezius and posterior latissimus musculature may require division if the fourth interspace is entered. An intercostal muscle pedicle can be harvested for later use.

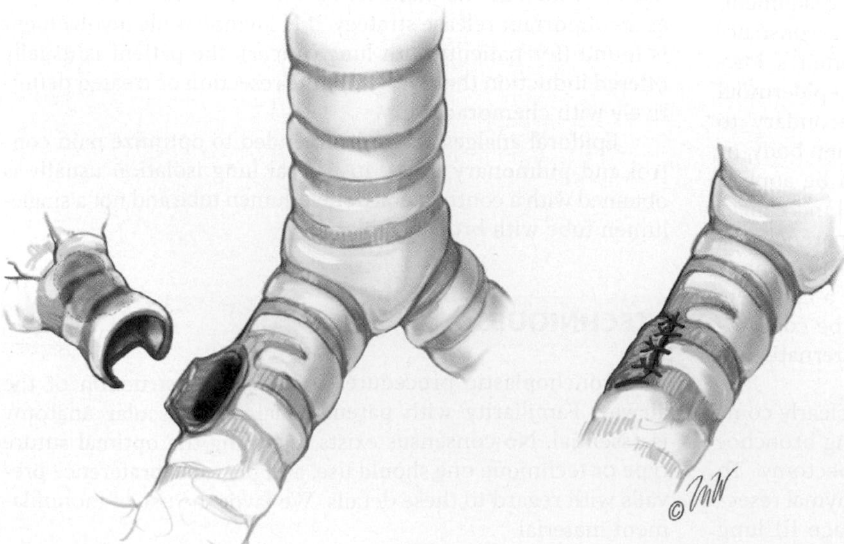

A

B

Figure 75-1. Bronchoplastic removal (*A*) and closure (*B*) of a bronchial stump using a flap of the membranous airway.

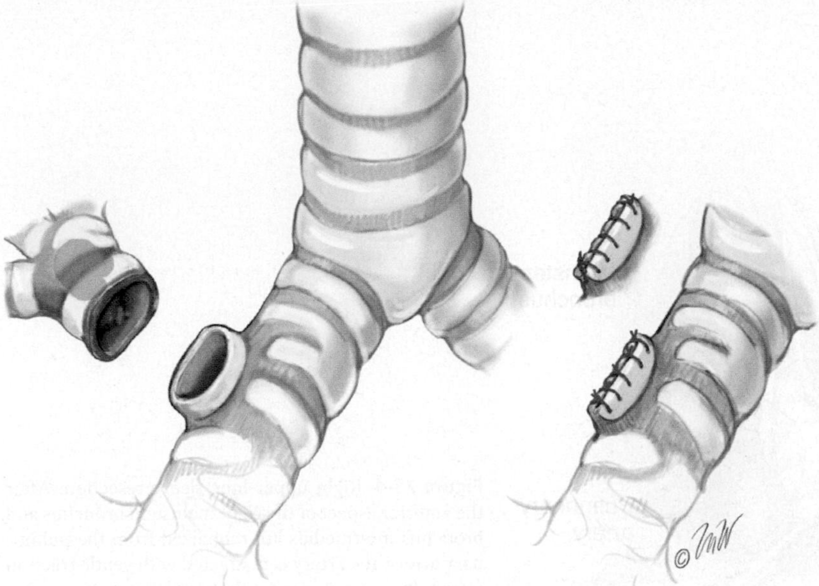

Figure 75-2. Alternative technique for bronchoplastic removal (*A*) and closure (*B*) of a short bronchial stump involving simple suture reapproximation.

The lung must be fully mobilized. The anterior and posterior pleural reflections over the hilum are divided. The inferior pulmonary ligament is divided up to the inferior pulmonary vein. The chest should be surveyed carefully to ensure that no obvious contraindications for the procedure exist (e.g., pleural metastases, interlobar spread). Separation of the pulmonary arterial and venous supplies to the upper lobe and completion of the horizontal fissure and cephalad aspect of the major fissure follow.

Once the lobe is isolated, the subcarinal space is dissected until the pericardium and carina are easily visualized. This entails mobilizing the esophagus from the airway. The subcarinal lymph node packet is removed. The anterior aspect of the right mainstem bronchus and bronchus intermedius are freed from loose fibroareolar attachments of the pulmonary artery. The ongoing pulmonary artery is distracted from the airway with gentle traction inferiorly and anteriorly. Finally, the distal trachea is gently mobilized while preserving the lateral vascular stalks.

Umbilical tapes are passed around the proximal right mainstem bronchus and the bronchus intermedius (Fig. 75-4). Unless disease extends close to the carina, the proximal right mainstem bronchus should not be skeletonized. The azygos vein seldom needs to be divided. The airway is transected in a perpendicular fashion proximally and distally (Fig. 75-4, *inset*). The specimen is sent for margin analysis. Determining the exact location for airway division can be aided by bronchoscopy. To reduce tension on the bronchial anastomosis, proximal and distal release maneuvers are performed. Standard proximal release maneuvers involve dissection of the anterior and, if necessary,

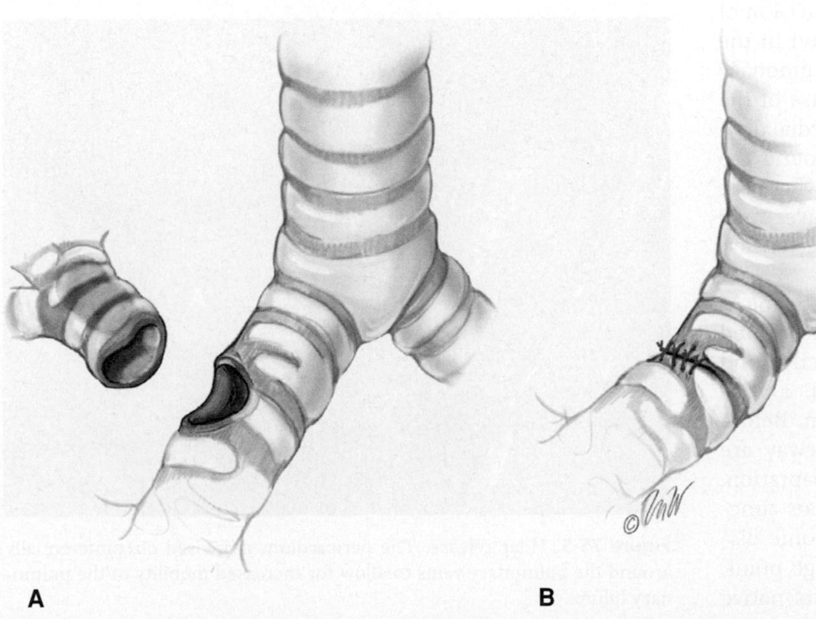

Figure 75-3. Bronchoplastic removal (*A*) and primary closure of a wedge bronchotomy (*B*).

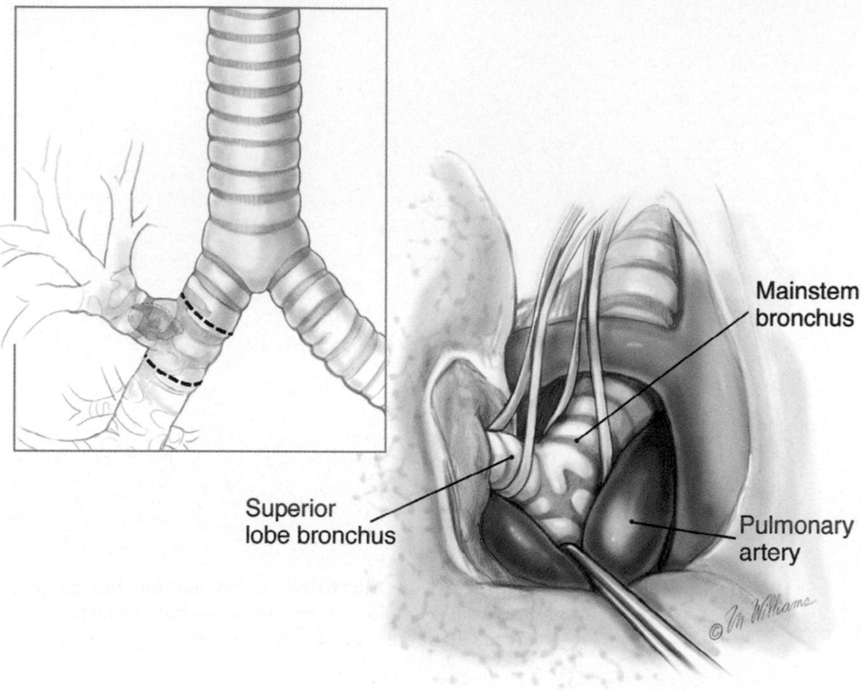

Figure 75-4. Right upper lobe sleeve resection. After the anterior aspect of the right mainstem bronchus and bronchus intermedius are mobilized from the pulmonary artery, the artery is distracted with gentle traction inferiorly and anteriorly. Umbilical tapes are passed around the proximal right mainstem bronchus and the bronchus intermedius *(inset)*. The airway is transected proximally and distally.

posterior mainstem bronchus and trachea from investing fibroalveolar tissues. Since most of the proximal airway vascular supply is segmental and delivered through lateral pedicles, the airway is mobilized circumferentially above and below these lateral attachments without compromising the blood supply. Extensive, *complete* circumferential dissection results in ischemia at the anastomosis. For right-sided bronchoplastic resections, the left mainstem bronchus is easily mobilized by adhering to the same principles. The right mainstem bronchus, however, cannot be easily dissected for left-sided resections. Little is gained by extended (≥5 cm) anterior and posterior mobilization because the proximal airway will remain tethered by its lateral vascular attachments.

For distal release, in addition to completely dividing the inferior pulmonary ligament, a full hilar release may be required (Fig. 75-5). This entails the circumferential division of the pericardium investing the right hilum. An incision in the pericardium is made anteriorly over the superior pulmonary vein and carried out in a caudad fashion until the base of the inferior pulmonary vein has been exposed. The pericardial division is then reflected posteriorly (and superiorly) around the posterior aspect of the left atrium in a C-loop toward where the pulmonary artery exits the pericardium. This maneuver fully mobilizes the hilum and should markedly reduce the tension on the airway anastomosis.

If the resection margins are free of disease, a few choices for reconstructing the airway can be considered. Interrupted suture technique has been demonstrated to be effective and reliable. For anastomoses of well-matched bronchi, a *continuous suture technique* simplifies the reconstruction. Before beginning the anastomosis, the cut ends of the airway are oriented (Fig. 75-6) and tested for a tension-free coaptation. Stay sutures placed at the membranous–cartilaginous junction facilitate coaptation (Fig. 75-7). It is easy to become disoriented because if viewed from posterolateral vantage point, the airway will be rotated almost perpendicular to its native position during the reconstruction. Palpation permits identification of the membranous airway and should be repeated frequently if orientation becomes unclear during the anastomosis. Once proper alignment is established, a running suture (usually 4-0 monofilament) is begun at the *medial* membranous–cartilaginous junction (which will project as the most posterior aspect of the anastomosis from the posterolateral thoracotomy vantage). The anastomosis proceeds in a medial–lateral fashion in both directions. The entire *membranous airway* can be reapproximated with this running suture and tied to a second anchoring suture placed at the lateral cartilaginous–membranous junction. The lateral (corner) stitch then is run medially (to reapproximate the cartilaginous airway) toward the apex

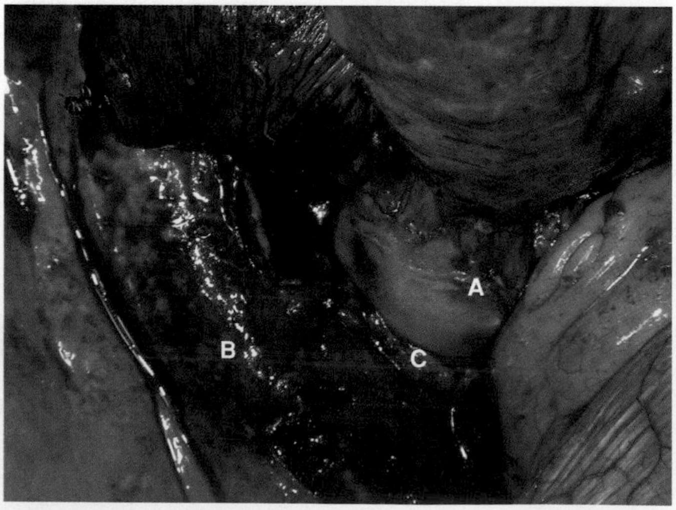

Figure 75-5. Hilar release. The pericardium is incised circumferentially around the pulmonary veins to allow for increased mobility of the pulmonary hilum.

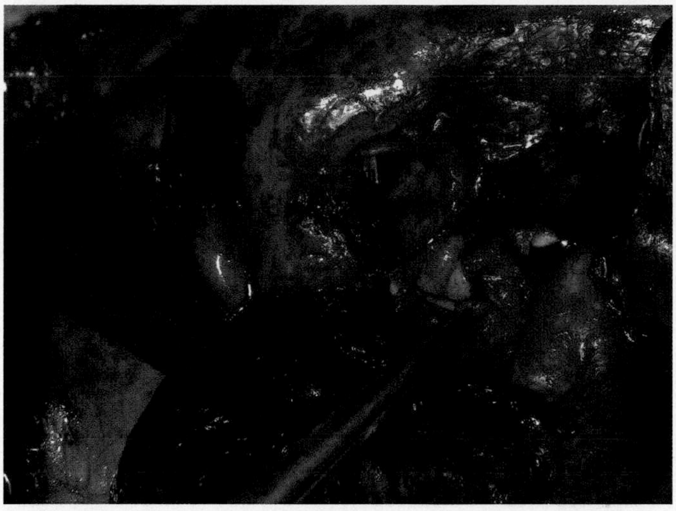

Figure 75-6. Tension-free coaptation of the transected ends of the airway.

of the airway, where it is tied to the running suture sewn in the other direction. Alternatively, the cartilaginous portion is closed with a running suture performed from medial to lateral. The posterior membranous portion can be closed as described above. All knots are kept on the outside of the lumen.

Interrupted suture technique is also an option (particularly for a size mismatch), but the organization of the sutures can become cumbersome and frustrating. When there is a size discrepancy between the right mainstem bronchus and the bronchus intermedius, a telescoping anastomosis can be performed with the membranous portion run and the anterior cartilaginous airway interrupted.

Once the bronchoplasty is completed, the anastomosis is leak tested at 25 to 30 cm H_2O of pressure. No air leak can be tolerated from the reconstructed airway. It is customary to buttress the anastomosis with a pedicled flap of autologous tissue (e.g., thymic fat pad, pleura, or intercostal muscle), although this is of no proven benefit to airway healing. Importantly, buttressing is *not* the solution for lack of pneumostasis of the bronchoplasty and will *not* salvage a poorly constructed anastomosis. Buttressing does, however, separate the anastomosis from the pulmonary artery. This is especially important if bronchial and arterial sleeve resections are performed concomitantly.

Patients should be extubated in the OR. The effectiveness of steroids postoperatively is unproved.[8] Although induction steroids have the theoretical benefit of diminishing edema and maximizing airway patency.

Early postoperative bronchoscopy is rarely required but recommended for unexpected airway leak. Mild pulmonary dysfunction from ipsilateral pulmonary edema is common. Chest tube management is identical to that in nonbronchoplastic resections. We perform bronchoscopy at 6 weeks to assess airway healing. Some surgeons perform bronchoscopies, scheduled at yearly intervals, up to 5 years, for cancer surveillance.

Other Sleeve Resections

Resection of any other lobe can be combined with a bronchoplastic procedure (Fig. 75-8). Although the principles of reconstruction are the same for all, tension-free anastomosis with negative margins, there are slight differences in the anatomic concerns of each.

For tumors of the orifice of the right middle lobe bronchus (usually carcinoid), the position of the involved bronchus and tumor in relation to the superior segmental and composite basilar bronchi becomes important. It can become a very tedious, often treacherous, undertaking to attempt reconstruction if the lower lobe bronchus is cut back to the *orifices* of the segmental bronchi. Scalloping the distal airway in an attempt to save the superior segment complicates and

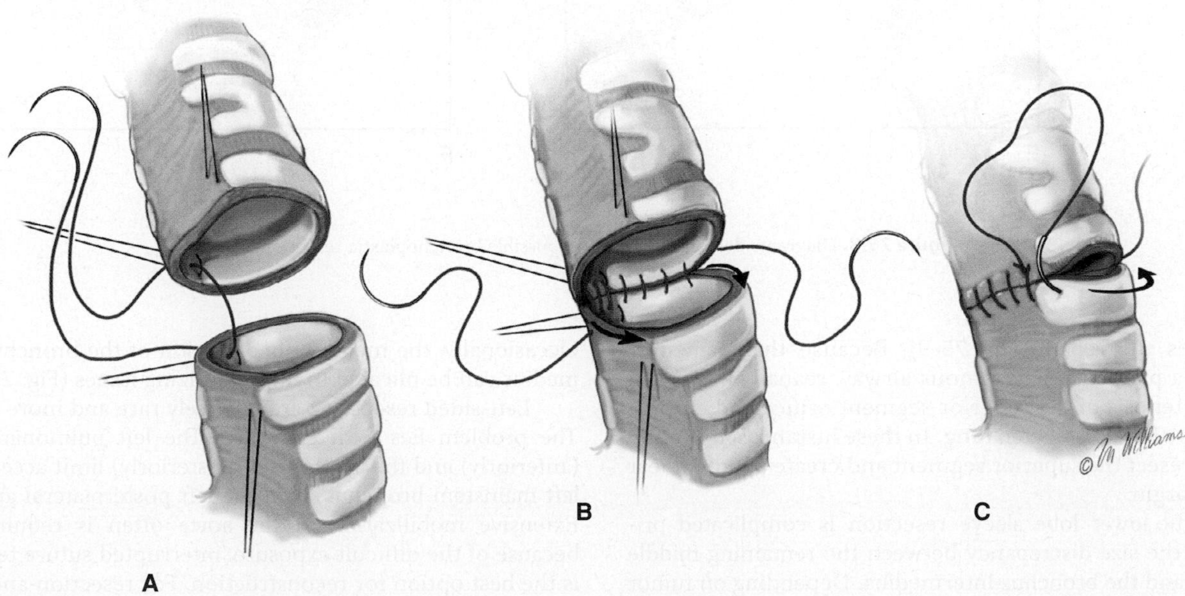

Figure 75-7. Running anastomosis technique. *A.* Stay sutures are placed at the membranous–cartilaginous junction of both proximal and distal airways for orientation purposes. *B.* Running suture technique is begun on the medial aspect of the anastomosis and proceeds laterally (in both directions) to coapt the entire membranous component and the medial half of the cartilaginous airway. *C.* The membranous suture is secured to a lateral anchor stitch, and this second suture is run medially toward the apex of the cartilaginous airway.

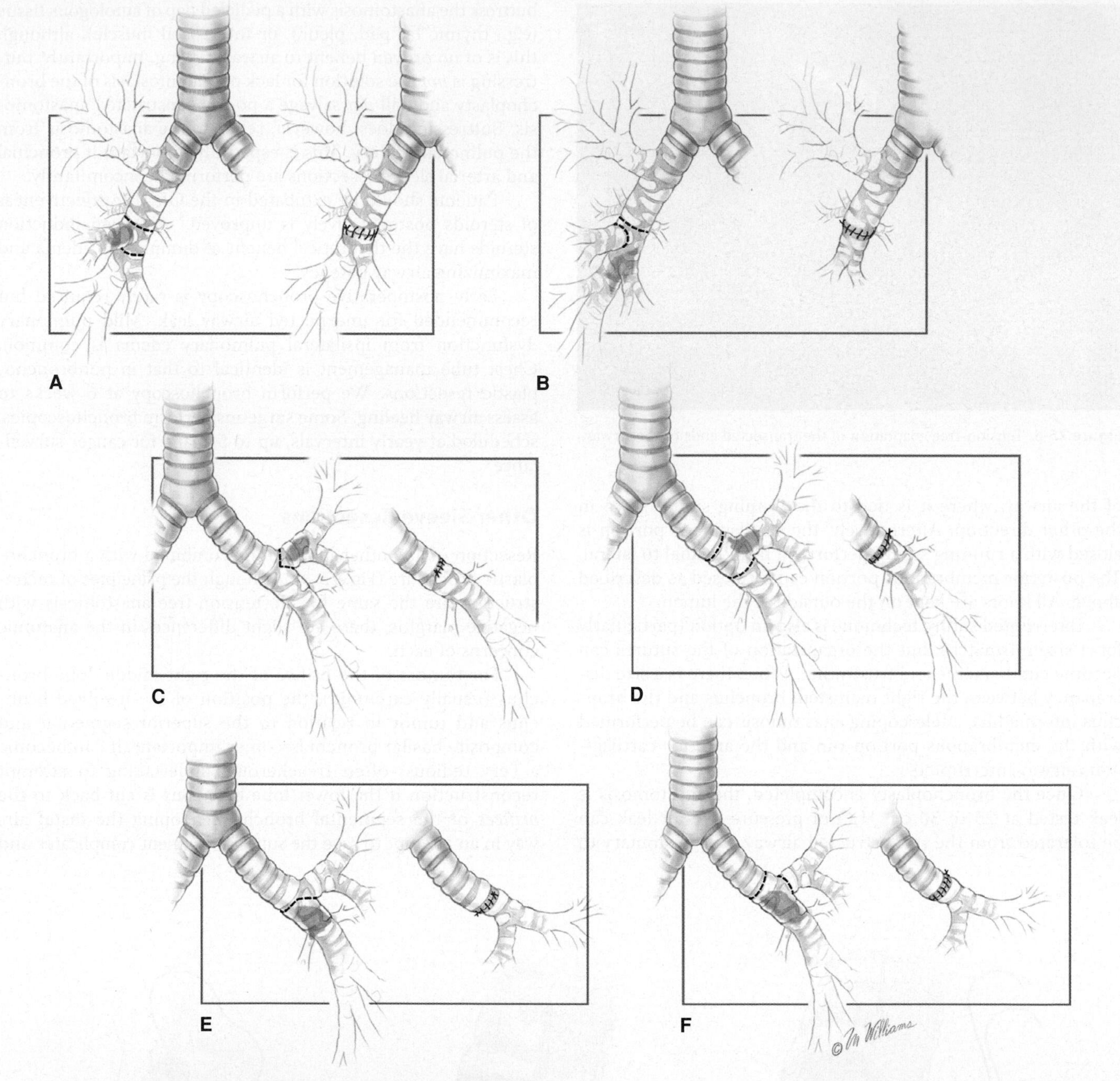

Figure 75-8. Diagrams demonstrating other possible bronchoplastic resections.

jeopardizes the repair (Fig. 75-9). Because this maneuver produces a patulous membranous airway, reanastomosis can result in stenosis of the superior segment orifice and chronic atelectasis of the associated lung. In these instances, it is often better to resect the superior segment and create a more linear sewing margin.

A right lower lobe sleeve resection is complicated primarily by the size discrepancy between the remaining middle bronchus and the bronchus intermedius. Depending on tumor location, a flange of tissue around the middle lobe orifice can be saved and will be a much better size match for reconstruction (Fig. 75-10). When a size mismatch cannot be avoided, a telescoping technique of interrupted sutures can be used. Occasionally, the membranous portion of the bronchus intermedius can be plicated to improve sizing issues (Fig. 75-11).

Left-sided resections are relatively rare and more difficult. The problem lies with exposure. The left pulmonary artery (anteriorly) and the aortic arch (posteriorly) limit access to the left mainstem bronchus from the left posterolateral approach. Extensive mobilization of the aorta often is required, and because of the difficult exposure, interrupted suture technique is the best option for reconstruction. For resection and reconstruction of the left mainstem bronchus, these issues become critical. For an isolated proximal left mainstem tumor, the bronchoplastic procedure can also be performed through a sternotomy, with or without cardiopulmonary bypass. The left

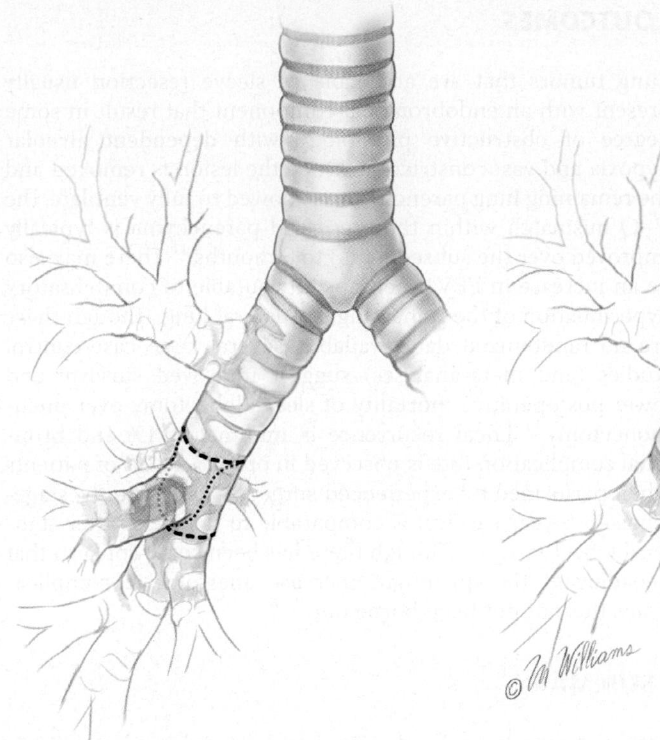

Figure 75-9. *A.* Technical problems can arise when the airway is scalloped to accommodate an inferior takeoff of the right middle lobe during a sleeve resection of the lobe. *B.* Sacrifice of the superior segment may be a better alternative.

mainstem bronchus is located from this exposure through the posterior pericardium just cephalad to the main pulmonary artery and to the left of the ascending aorta. Injury of the left recurrent nerve can complicate *any* left-sided bronchoplastic procedure. Alternatively, a proximal left mainstem bronchial tumor can be approached from a right posterolateral thoracotomy with good exposure to the posterior aspect of the carina and proximal left mainstem. Airway control in this setting can be tedious with the need for cross-table ventilation and a brief ECMO run can facilitate the procedure.

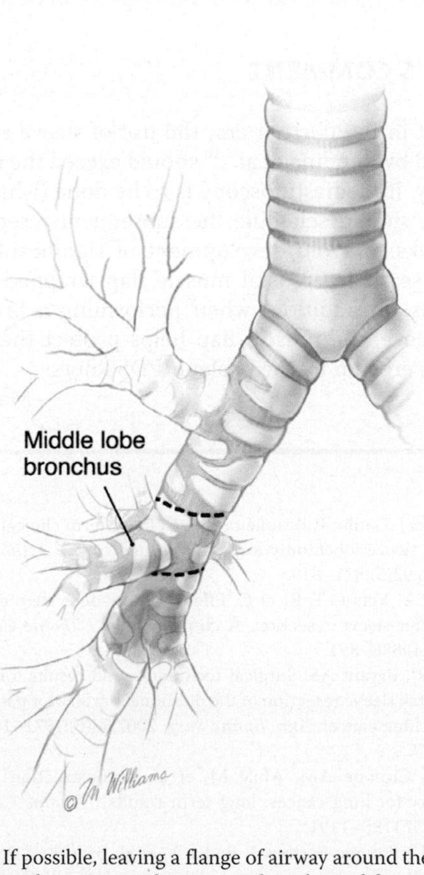

Figure 75-10. If possible, leaving a flange of airway around the middle lobe orifice of intermediate size is a better match and simplifies reconstruction after right lower lobe sleeve resection.

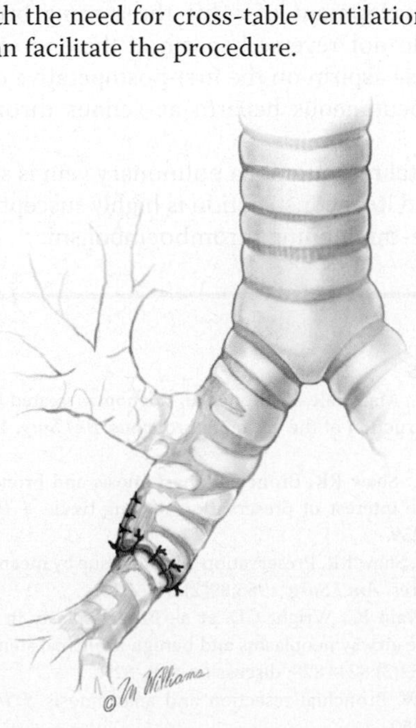

Figure 75-11. Plication of the membranous airway also can reduce a size mismatch.

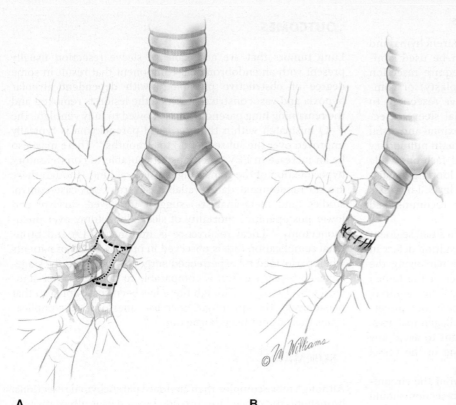

Pulmonary Vascular Sleeve Resections

Sleeve resection of the airway spares lung parenchyma and vascular sleeve of the pulmonary artery can be used similarly when pathology dictates. This might require resection of either a noncircumferential part (arterioplasty) or complete segment of the pulmonary artery (sleeve resection) to be resected. To perform a pulmonary arterial sleeve resection, classic vascular surgical principles of proximal and distal control are required. Proximal control of the main pulmonary artery is best obtained in an intrapericardial fashion, while distal control may be obtained by clamping or looping the distal margin at the appropriate extrapericardial level. Low-dose systemic heparinization before clamping is recommended (2000–3000 units).[9]

A simple arterioplasty might suffice if only a small segment of the pulmonary artery is involved and the resulting defect in the artery can be repaired primarily without narrowing the outflow by greater than 10% to 20%. However, if the lumen compromise is greater, a patch angioplasty will be required. A variety of grafts can be used including native (our preference) or bovine pericardium, decellularized collagen matrices, or autologous vein (e.g., azygos). It is important to avoid any undue laxity in the patch to minimize kinking of the vessel when lung is reexpanded.

When tumors involve a significant portion of the circumference of the pulmonary artery, a segmental resection should be employed. Following resection, a primary anastomosis can be performed with a running 5-0 monofilament nonabsorbable suture. As with any vascular anastomosis, de-airing maneuvers should be performed. Should the resection of a long segment of the artery be necessary, pericardial conduits can be constructed.[10] If a concomitant bronchial sleeve resection is also performed, the arterial anastomosis is usually performed to reperfuse the lung, but care must be taken to avoid traumatizing the newly repaired vessel during the airway reconstruction. Routine use of tissue buttresses is advocated in these cases to minimize development of a life-threatening bronchovascular fistula. We do not reverse heparin at the end of the case and favor low-dose aspirin on the first postoperative day along with standard subcutaneous heparin as venous thromboembolism prophylaxis.

Segmental resection of a pulmonary vein is seldom, if ever, indicated, and its reconstruction is highly susceptible to thrombosis and life-threatening thromboembolism.

OUTCOMES

Lung tumors that are amenable to sleeve resection usually present with an endobronchial component that result in some degree of obstructive physiology with dependent alveolar hypoxia and vasoconstriction. Once the lesion is removed and the remaining lung parenchyma is allowed to fully ventilate, the V–Q mismatch within the preserved parenchyma is typically improved over the subsequent 3 to 8 months.[11] There may also be an increase in FEV1, perhaps attributable to compensatory hyperinflation of the remaining ispsilateral lung. Though there are no randomized data available, several large case-control studies (and meta-analyses) suggest improved survival and lower postoperative mortality of sleeve lobectomy over pneumonectomy.[12] Local recurrence is minimal at 1% and bronchial complication rate is observed in only 1% to 2% of patients when performed by experienced surgeons. Importantly, stage-adjusted 5-year survival is comparable to that seen after standard lobectomy.[13–16] Though there has been some concern that neoadjuvant therapy might increase anastomotic complications, this has not been borne out.[17,18]

SUMMARY

Although more complex than standard parenchymal resections, bronchoplastic procedures provide lung-sparing alternatives to pneumonectomy or bilobectomy without compromised cancer-related outcomes. Patient selection is critical, but in appropriately screened patient populations, and when performed by experienced surgeons, excellent outcomes can be achieved.

EDITOR'S COMMENT

I agree that in the current era, the use of sleeve resections as popularized by Rendina et al.[8,10] should exceed the use of pneumonectomy. If mediastinoscopy is to be done (which I do routinely), one should schedule the subsequent resection in less than 2 weeks to avoid development of significant scarring. I routinely use an intercostal muscle flap wrapped around the anastomosis. In addition, when performing a bronchial and vascular sleeve, the muscle flap helps protect the pulmonary artery from erosion by the prolene/PDS knots.

—Mark J. Krasna

References

1. D'Abreu AL, Mac Hale SJ. Bronchial "adenoma" treated by local resection and reconstruction of the left main bronchus. *Br J Surg*. 1952;39(156):355–357.
2. Paulson DL, Shaw RR. Bronchial anastomosis and bronchoplastic procedures in the interest of preservation of lung tissue. *J Thorac Surg*. 1955; 29(3):238–259.
3. Paulson DL, Shaw RR. Preservation of lung tissue by means of bronchoplastic procedures. *Am J Surg*. 1955;89(2):347–355.
4. Bueno R, Wain JC, Wright CD, et al. Bronchoplasty in the management of low-grade airway neoplasms and benign bronchial stenoses. *Ann Thorac Surg*. 1996;62(3):824–828; discussion 828–829.
5. Gebauer PW. Bronchial resection and anastomosis. *J Thorac Surg*. 1953; 26(3):241–260.
6. Farray D, Mirkovic N, Albain KS. Multimodality therapy for stage III non-small-cell lung cancer. *J Clin Oncol*. 2005;23(14):3257–3269.
7. Deslauriers J, Gaulin P, Beaulieu M, et al. Long-term clinical and functional results of sleeve lobectomy for primary lung cancer. *J Thorac Cardiovasc Surg*. 1986;92(5):871–879.
8. Rendina EA, Venuta F, Ricci C. Effects of low-dose steroids on bronchial healing after sleeve resection. A clinical study. *J Thorac Cardiovasc Surg*. 1992;104(4):888–891.
9. Cerfolio RJ, Bryant AS. Surgical techniques and results for partial or circumferential sleeve resection of the pulmonary artery for patients with non-small cell lung cancer. *Ann Thorac Surg*. 2007;83(6):1971–1976; discussion 1976–1977.
10. Venuta F, Ciccone AM, Anile M, et al. Reconstruction of the pulmonary artery for lung cancer: long-term results. *J Thorac Cardiovasc Surg*. 2009;138(5):1185–1191.
11. Bagan P, Le Pimpec-Barthes F, Badia A, et al. Bronchial sleeve resections: lung function resurrecting procedure. *Eur J Cardiothorac Surg*. 2008; 34(3):484–487.

12. Stallard J, Loberg A, Dunning J, et al. Is a sleeve lobectomy significantly better than a pneumonectomy? *Interact Cardiovasc Thorac Surg.* 2010;11(5):660–666.
13. Lausberg HF, Graeter TP, Tscholl D, et al. Bronchovascular versus bronchial sleeve resection for central lung tumors. *Ann Thorac Surg.* 2005;79(4):1147–1152; discussion 1147–1152.
14. Schirren J, Eberlein M, Fischer A, et al. The role of sleeve resections in advanced nodal disease. *Eur J Cardiothorac Surg.* 2011;40(5):1157–1163.
15. Schirren J, Bölükbas S, Bergmann T, et al. Prospective study on perioperative risks and functional results in bronchial and bronchovascular sleeve resections. *Thorac Cardiovasc Surg.* 2009;57(1):35–41.
16. Bölükbas S, Eberlein MH, Schirren J. Pneumonectomy vs. sleeve resection for non-small cell lung carcinoma in the elderly: analysis of short-term and long-term results. *Thorac Cardiovasc Surg.* 2011;59(3):142–147.
17. Milman S, Kim AW, Warren WH, et al. The incidence of perioperative anastomotic complications after sleeve lobectomy is not increased after neoadjuvant chemoradiotherapy. *Ann Thorac Surg.* 2009;88(3):945–950; discussion 950–941.
18. Bagan P, Berna P, Brian E, et al. Induction chemotherapy before sleeve lobectomy for lung cancer: immediate and long-term results. *Ann Thorac Surg.* 2009;88(6):1732–1735.

76 Radical Lymphadenectomy

Christopher T. Ducko and Michael T. Jaklitsch

Keywords: Staging, non–small-cell lung cancer (NSCLC), lymph node dissection, radical mediastinal lymphadenectomy, N status, survival, prognosis, nseoadjuvant chemotherapy, radiation therapy

When treating patients with non–small-cell lung cancer (NSCLC), it is important to assign an accurate clinical or pathologic stage to the disease at the time of diagnosis. This adds value to the process of selecting the most appropriate therapy for the individual patient, whether it be surgical resection, neoadjuvant chemotherapy or radiotherapy, or definitive chemoradiation. The current cancer staging convention uses the basic descriptors originally proposed by Denoix[1] primary tumor (T), lymph node involvement (N), and tumor metastasis (M). The contemporary classification system was adopted worldwide in 1997 after features of the 1986 combined American Joint Committee on Cancer and the International Union Against Cancer TNM staging system[2] were reconciled with the 1983 American Thoracic Society statement on cancer staging. The organization responsible for updating this system is the International Association for Lung Cancer Staging which revised the staging system in 2009[3] and will do so again in 2016. The value of classifying NSCLC patients according to a uniform staging system that has prognostic implications based on stage grouping is difficult to overstate.

Clinical staging can be determined on the basis of CT scanning, MRI, and CT/PET scanning. Pathologic staging requires biopsy, which can be obtained from cervical or anterior mediastinoscopy, during video-assisted thoracic surgery (VATS) approaches, less commonly by means of open thoracotomy, and more recently by fine-needle aspiration performed during endoscopic or endobronchial ultrasound sampling.[4,5] Lymph node involvement has important implications for surgical treatment strategies for lung cancer.[6–8] Patients without lymph node involvement (N0) or those with limited involvement (N1), which is usually determined at the time of surgery, are candidates for resection based on T and M status. Most patients with contralateral or supraclavicular disease (N3) or T4 involvement are not resectable (stage IIIB). The usual approach in stage IIIA patients with ipsilateral mediastinal nodal involvement (N2) involves either neoadjuvant chemotherapy or chemoradiation, followed by resection if appropriate, when N2 status is determined prior to resection. In some cases, surgically detected N2 disease can be discovered at the time of resection by means of lymph node dissection in conjunction with the pulmonary resection.[9] There is no doubt that sampling of lymph nodes in some fashion is useful for staging and prognostic purposes. However, the extent of lymph node dissection is controversial, and the benefits of systematic sampling versus complete mediastinal lymph node dissection or extended lymph node dissection are still under review.[10–13]

LYMPH NODE MAPPING

To unify the two most widely used systems of lymph node mapping in NSCLC, the American Joint Committee on Cancer and the International Union Against Cancer adopted a standardized method of classifying lymph node stations in 1996. This was outlined in 1997 by Mountain and Dresler based on the work of Naruke and the American Thoracic Society and the North American Lung Cancer Study Group.[14] The most notable difference between these systems was the boundary between peribronchial hilar (N1) and paratracheal mediastinal (N2) lymph nodes comprising stations 4 and 10, respectively. These are now separated by the pleural reflection between the visceral pleura (station 10) and the mediastinal pleura (station 4) (Fig. 76-1). The other definitions remained basically the same. The nodal station descriptions of mediastinal, hilar, and intrapulmonary are designed to be reproducible, and stage groupings are based on studies of prognostic factors, including metastasis.

Regional lymph node stations for lung cancer staging are shown in Figure 76-2. Any double-digit station is classified as N1. Single digit lymph nodes are N2. The anatomic definitions for lymph node mapping are shown in Table 76-1. Involvement

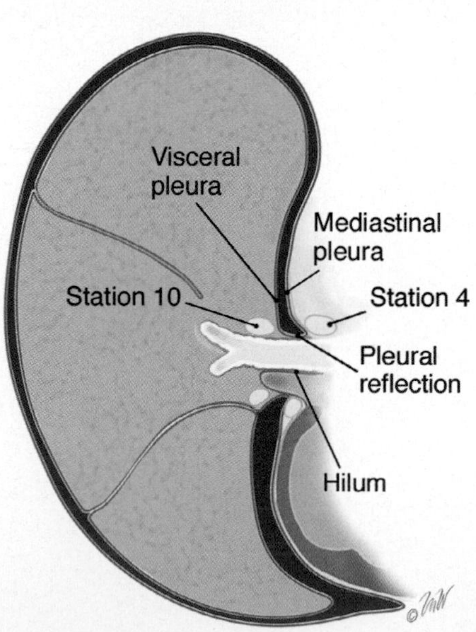

Figure 76-1. In the unified staging system, the peribronchial hilar (N1) and paratracheal mediastinal (N2) lymph nodes are separated by the pleural reflection between the visceral pleura (station 10) and the mediastinal pleura (station 4).

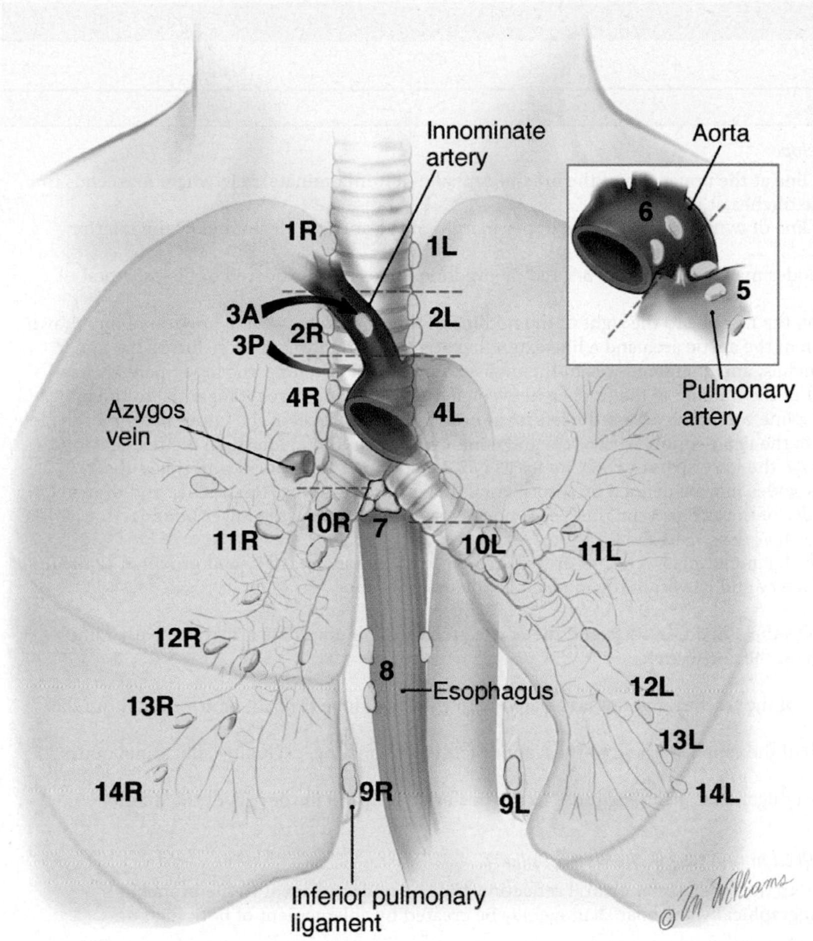

Figure 76-2. Lung cancer lymph node stations map. Note that any double-digit numeral is considered N1 disease. *Inset.* Subaortic (5) and paraaortic (6) lymph nodes. L, left; R, right; A, anterior; P, posterior.

of contralateral mediastinal or hilar stations, as well as ipsilateral supraclavicular or scalene nodes, is considered N3 disease. Survival is inversely proportional to nodal involvement and was validated in a database analysis by Mountain and Dresler.[14]

The distribution and likelihood of lymph node metastasis based on lobar location of the cancer has been described.[15] In Cerfolio and Bryant's study of 954 patients, incidence and location of N2 disease were distributed as shown in Figure 76-3, based on location of the primary lung lesion. This knowledge can help advocates of mediastinal lymph node sampling to target the lymph node stations to be obtained at the time of resection.[16,17] Others perform radical lymphadenectomy routinely with each resection regardless of primary lobar location.[18] This is thought to improve the yield of lymph node sampling, detect noncontiguous lymph node involvement (skip metastases), and improve survival.[11,13,19,20]

SURGICAL TECHNIQUE

The technique of mediastinal lymph node dissection was first described in detail by Cahan et al.[21] in 1951, when simple pneumonectomy was differentiated from radical pneumonectomy, which included hilar and mediastinal lymph nodes in continuity. Prognosis became linked to lymph node involvement, and lymph node mapping for cancer was established. The technique of mediastinal staging preceding surgical resection has been described.[22,23] Mediastinal lymph node dissection at the time of resection will be reviewed herein. While originally performed by means of open thoracotomy, this method of lymph node dissection is now possible by means of VATS technique with a greater technical demand yet comparable results.[24–26] Median sternotomy also can be used for extended lymph node dissections, but is not widely used.[27] A combination of blunt and electrocautery dissection is fairly standard. A fine metal suction tip can sometimes prove invaluable via VATS approaches. Other techniques that make use of the Harmonic Scalpel (Ethicon Endo-Surgery Inc.; Cincinnati, OH) or the LigaSure (Covidien; Boulder, CO) device are safe and effective as well.

In routine practice, it is common to dissect the lymph nodes after pulmonary resection. However, if the decision to proceed with resection would be altered by positive N2 involvement, the lymph node dissection is undertaken first. This is especially true when preoperative imaging studies suggest obvious N2 involvement that was not confirmed with prior staging efforts. Previously, cases that involved "surprise" N2 findings may have warranted chest closure and neoadjuvant treatment before resection or may have limited the extent of intended resection.[28] However, some of this complex decision-making that had been based on mathematical models and inaccurate assumptions has been revisited. It would now appear that patients with unsuspected N2 disease, who have undergone comprehensive preoperative staging, should get resected even if N2 involvement is discovered at the time of surgery.[9] The importance of proper specimen labeling using standard nomenclature cannot be overemphasized. Each lymph node station should be labeled accordingly and submitted separately to avoid confusion among specimens.

Table 76-1

LYMPH NODE MAP DEFINITIONS

NODAL STATION	ANATOMIC LANDMARKS
N2 nodes—all N2 nodes lie within the mediastinal pleural envelope	
1. Highest mediastinal nodes	Nodes lying above a horizontal line at the upper rim of the brachiocephalic (left innominate) vein where it ascends to the left crossing in front of the trachea at its midline
2. Upper paratracheal nodes	Nodes lying above a horizontal line drawn tangential to the upper margin of the aortic arch and below the inferior boundary of No. 1 nodes
3. Prevascular and retrotracheal nodes	Prevascular and retrotracheal nodes may be designated 3A and 3P; midline nodes are considered to be ipsilateral
4. Lower paratracheal nodes	The lower paratracheal nodes on the right lie to the right of the midline of the trachea between a horizontal line drawn tangential to the upper margin of the aortic arch and a line extending across the right main bronchus at the upper margin of the upper lobe bronchus, and contained within the mediastinal pleural envelope; the lower paratracheal nodes on the left lie to the left of the midline of the trachea between a horizontal line drawn tangential to the upper margin of the aortic arch and a line extending across the left main bronchus at the level of the upper margin of the left upper lobe bronchus, medial to the ligamentum arteriosum and contained within the mediastinal pleural envelope Researchers may wish to designate the lower paratracheal nodes as No. 4s (superior) and No. 4i (inferior) subsets for study purposes; the No. 4s nodes may be defined by a horizontal line extending across the trachea and drawn tangential to the cephalic border of the azygos vein; the No. 4i nodes may be defined by the lower boundary of No. 4s and the lower boundary of No. 4, as described above
5. Subaortic (aortopulmonary window)	Subaortic nodes are lateral to the ligamentum arteriosum or the aorta or left pulmonary artery and proximal to the first branch of the left pulmonary artery and lie within the mediastinal pleural envelope
6. Paraaortic nodes (ascending aorta or phrenic)	Nodes lying anterior and lateral to the ascending aorta and the aortic arch or the innominate artery, beneath a line tangential to the upper margin of the aortic arch
7. Subcarinal nodes	Nodes lying caudal to the carina of the trachea, but not associated with the lower lobe bronchi or arteries within the lung
8. Paraesophageal nodes (below carina)	Nodes lying adjacent to the wall of the esophagus and to the right or left of the midline, excluding subcarinal nodes
9. Pulmonary ligament nodes	Nodes lying within the pulmonary ligament, including those in the posterior wall and lower part of the inferior pulmonary vein
N1 nodes—all N1 nodes lie distal to the mediastinal pleural reflection and within the visceral pleura	
10. Hilar nodes	The proximal lobar nodes, distal to the mediastinal pleural reflection and the nodes adjacent to the bronchus intermedius on the right; radiographically, the hilar shadow may be created by enlargement of both hilar and interlobar nodes
11. Interlobar nodes	Nodes lying between the lobar bronchi
12. Lobar nodes	Nodes adjacent to the distal lobar bronchi
13. Segmental nodes	Nodes adjacent to the segmental bronchi
14. Subsegmental nodes	Nodes around the subsegmental bronchi

Source: Reproduced with permission from Mountain CF, Dresler CM. Regional lymph node classification for lung cancer staging. *Chest.* 1997;111:1718–1723.

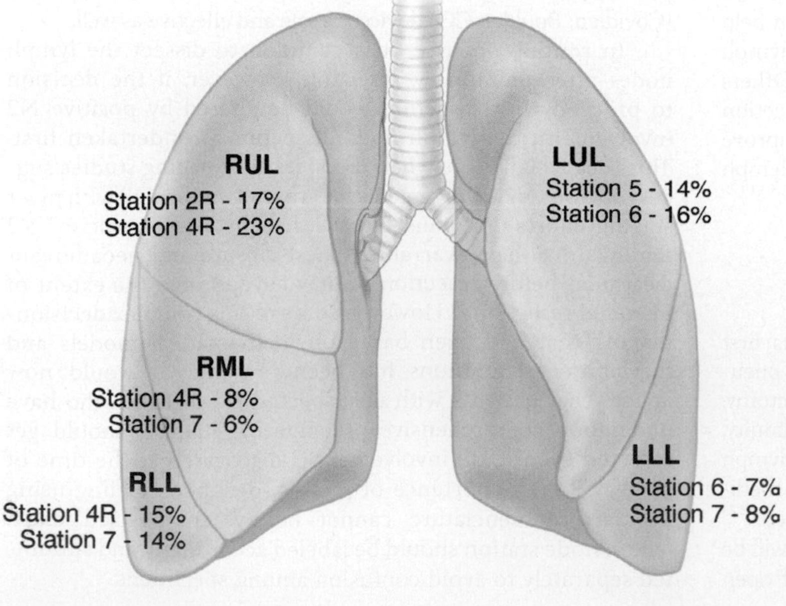

Figure 76-3. Distribution of nodal involvement in patients with N2 disease.

Right-Sided Lymphadenectomy

Nodal stations to be addressed from the right chest include stations 2 and 4, stations 7 to 9, and N1 stations included in the lobar resection, 10 and 11. The boundaries to the paratracheal nodes (stations 2 and 4) include superior vena cava anteriorly, right brachiocephalic vein and subclavian artery superiorly, trachea and right mainstem bronchus medially, azygos vein and pulmonary artery inferiorly, esophagus and vagus nerve posteriorly, and mediastinal pleura laterally.

Resection of this nodal packet begins with exposure via incision in the fourth or fifth intercostal space. The lung is retracted inferiorly, and the pleura overlying the azygos vein is opened sharply using a parallel incision (Fig. 76-4). The azygos vein is mobilized and can be divided or resected for complete exposure. This can be done easily by using a vascular stapling device. The dissection then is performed from caudal to cephalad using an Allis or Babcock clamp to grasp the lymph node packet and sweep it off the medial structures. The inferior paratracheal station 4 nodes are carefully dissected at the tracheobronchial angle just above the pulmonary artery and pericardium. A flap of pleura is reflected further in a cephalad direction over the superior vena cava, avoiding the phrenic nerve anteriorly, and over the trachea posteriorly. The station 4 nodes are dissected en bloc from their paratracheal position behind the superior vena cava, which can be retracted anteriorly with a Cushing vein retractor or dental pledget. Small perforating veins draining anteriorly to the superior vena cava are identified and controlled, usually with clips or careful electrocautery. Care must be taken posteriorly to avoid the esophagus, vagus nerve, and membranous trachea along the posterior aspect of the station 4 nodal packet. The dissection is completed at the apex just above the level of the aortic arch toward the right subclavian artery, where the station 2 nodes are found. The recurrent laryngeal branch of the vagus nerve has its takeoff in this location and should be avoided.

The landmarks associated with the pyramid-shaped subcarinal nodes of station 7 include the tracheal carina superiorly and anteriorly, the esophagus posteriorly, the tracheal bifurcation into the mainstem bronchi laterally, and the pericardium and upper aspect of the inferior pulmonary vein inferiorly. Dissection at this level can be performed from either side, but the left is more challenging owing to the length of the mainstem bronchus and proximity of the aortic arch. The right-sided resection of station 7 subcarinal lymph nodes begins with retraction of the lung anteriorly (Fig. 76-5). The mediastinal pleura is opened posteriorly between the azygos and hilum. The nodal packet is teased out and grasped with a clamp near the lung parenchyma at the bronchus intermedius and superior to the inferior pulmonary vein. The dissection is carried proximally along the mainstem bronchus. Bronchial arterial branches are controlled with clips or careful electrocautery. Proper orientation of the airway must be maintained to avoid inadvertent injury of the left or right mainstem bronchus, and the esophagus is kept retracted posteriorly.

The remainder of the N2 nodes includes stations 8 and 9. These can be approached from either side fairly equally. The paraesophageal nodes (station 8) are inferior to the carina along the esophagus, whereas the station 9 nodes are within the inferior pulmonary ligament (Fig. 76-6). Most lung resections include

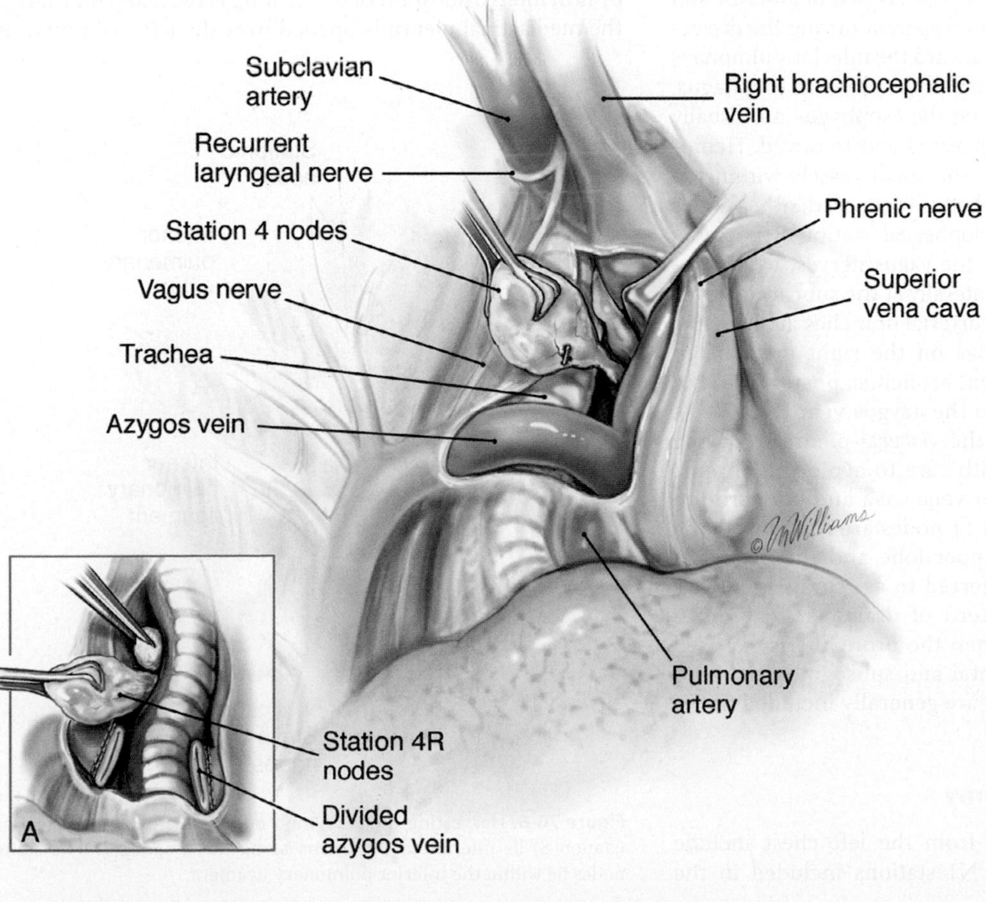

Figure 76-4. Right lymphadenectomy. Harvesting the paratracheal nodes. After the lung is retracted inferiorly and the pleura overlying the azygos vein is opened sharply, the azygos vein is mobilized and can be divided or resected for complete exposure. *A*. An Allis or Babcock clamp is used to grasp the lymph node packet and sweep it off the medial structures.

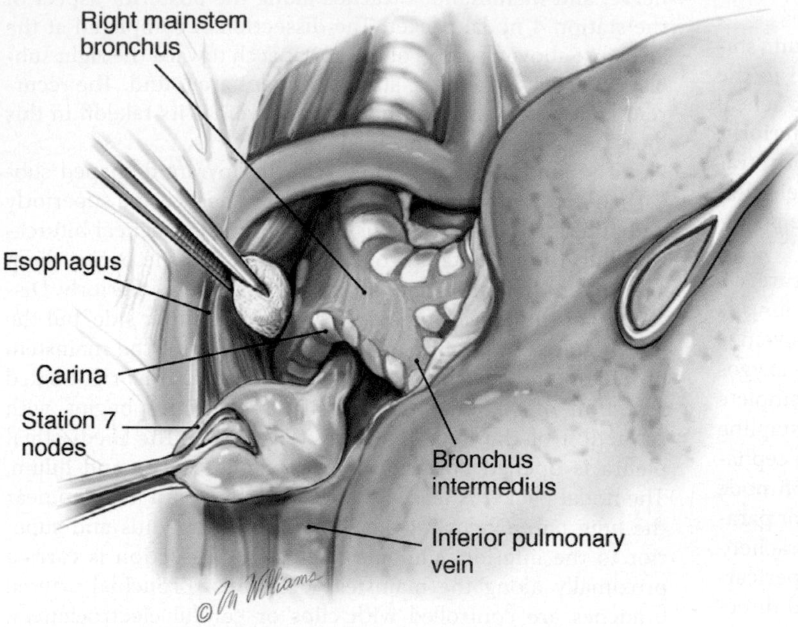

Figure 76-5. Harvesting the station 7 subcarinal lymph nodes. After retracting the lung anteriorly, the mediastinal pleura is opened posteriorly between the azygos and hilum.

mobilization of the inferior ligament either for lower lobe resection or to improve postoperative lung expansion and avoid a residual apical space. Therefore, the approach to dissection of station 9 nodes is straightforward. The lower lobe is oriented such as to put the inferior pulmonary ligament under tension. The ligament then is carefully mobilized in a cephalad direction away from the diaphragm with a combination of blunt and electrocautery dissection. The ligament is composed of anterior and posterior folds, which soon become apparent during the dissection. The mobilization is directed toward the inferior pulmonary vein, with care taken to avoid injury to the adjacent esophagus. Within the areolar tissues overlying the esophagus are usually several station 9 nodes that are elevated and removed. Hemostasis is achieved with control of the small vessels within the ligament inferiorly. Once the esophagus is exposed, other nodes can be sampled from the paraesophageal station 8 position, if present. Care is taken to avoid the vagus nerves, which run along each side of the esophagus laterally at the subcarinal level, as well as bronchial or intercostal arterial branches at all levels.

Station 10 hilar lymph nodes on the right are located overlying the distal right mainstem bronchus, posterior to the pulmonary artery and inferior to the azygos vein (Fig. 76-7). Exposure is gained by opening the visceral pleura overlying the superior hilum anteriorly with care to avoid the phrenic nerve running along the superior vena cava and pericardium anteriorly. The interlobar station 11 nodes are found near the bifurcation between the right upper lobe and the bronchus intermedius. These are often referred to as "sump" nodes as a result of their interlobar pattern of drainage. Station 12 lobar nodes are encountered when the bronchus is exposed and transected, whereas segmental and subsegmental nodes (stations 13 and 14, respectively) are generally included in the lobectomy specimen.

Left-Sided Lymphadenectomy

Nodal stations to be addressed from the left chest include mediastinal stations 4 to 9 and N1 stations included in the lobar resection, 10 to 14. The boundaries for station 5 and 6 nodes include the phrenic nerve anteriorly, the aortic arch and head vessels superiorly, the vagus nerve and descending thoracic aorta posteriorly, the pulmonary artery and pericardium inferiorly, the ascending aorta and trachea medially, and the mediastinal pleura laterally.

Resection of nodes at stations 5 and 6 begins with a fourth or fifth intercostal approach. The lung is retracted inferiorly, and the mediastinal pleura is opened over the left main pulmonary

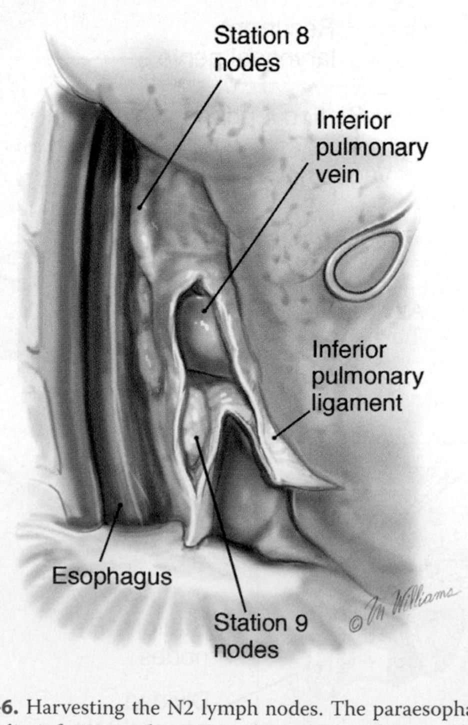

Figure 76-6. Harvesting the N2 lymph nodes. The paraesophageal nodes (station 8) lie inferior to the carina along the esophagus. The station 9 nodes lie within the inferior pulmonary ligament.

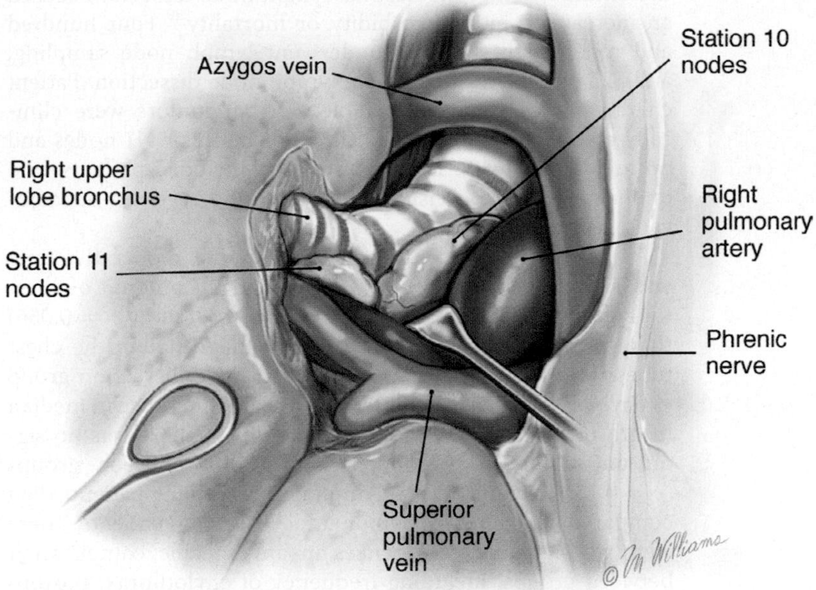

Figure 76-7. The station 10 hilar lymph nodes, which overlie the distal right mainstem bronchus, posterior to the pulmonary artery and inferior to the azygos vein, are exposed by opening the visceral pleura. The interlobar station 11 nodes are located near the bifurcation between the right upper lobe and the bronchus intermedius.

artery between the phrenic and vagus nerves, and a flap is created from the aortopulmonary window in a cephalad direction along the aortic arch (Fig. 76-8). The prevascular station 6 nodes are found in this location. They can be grasped with an Allis or Babcock clamp, with care taken to avoid the surrounding nerves. Bleeding is controlled with clips or ligatures to prevent an injury from electrocautery. The station 5 lymph nodes in the aortopulmonary window are found more posteriorly along the pulmonary artery near the ligamentum arteriosum. This vestige of the ductus arteriosus may be divided for mobilization of the aorta and pulmonary artery, if needed. The left recurrent laryngeal nerve, which branches from the vagus nerve, must be protected along its course under the aortic arch during dissection. Electrocautery must be minimized or avoided outright. When necessary, the left paratracheal nodes are found along the trachea medial to the ligamentum arteriosum (station 4) and further cephalad above the aortic arch between the left brachiocephalic vein and the left subclavian artery (station 2). These stations, along with station 3, alternatively may be approached posterior to the aortic arch and left subclavian artery by opening the pleura posteriorly and retracting the vessels anteriorly. Intercostal arterial branches need to be divided for this exposure. Care must be given to the recurrent laryngeal nerve as it courses cephalad along the trachea near the esophagus. This method is not widely used in North America.

The dissection for station 7 from the left is similar to the approach from the right. The lung is retracted anteriorly, and the posterior mediastinal pleura is opened along the groove anterior to the descending thoracic aorta, which is retracted posteriorly (Fig. 76-9). The left mainstem bronchus is exposed, and the subcarinal nodal packet is grasped with a clamp and removed. Dissection may be done in blunt or sharp fashion,

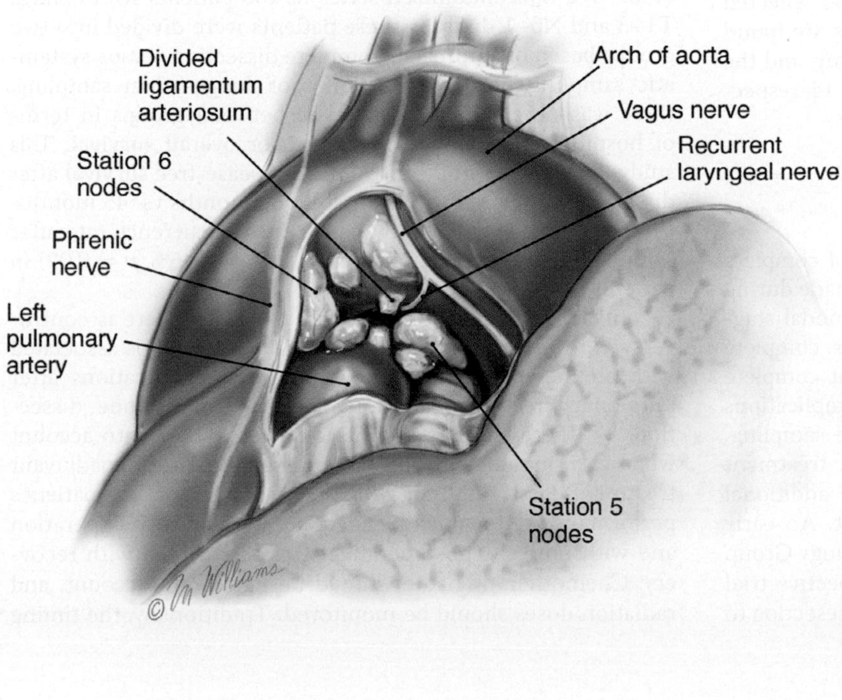

Figure 76-8. Left lymphadenectomy. Station 5 and 6 nodes are accessed through a fourth or fifth intercostal incision. The lung is retracted inferiorly, and the mediastinal pleura is opened over the left main pulmonary artery between the phrenic and vagus nerves.

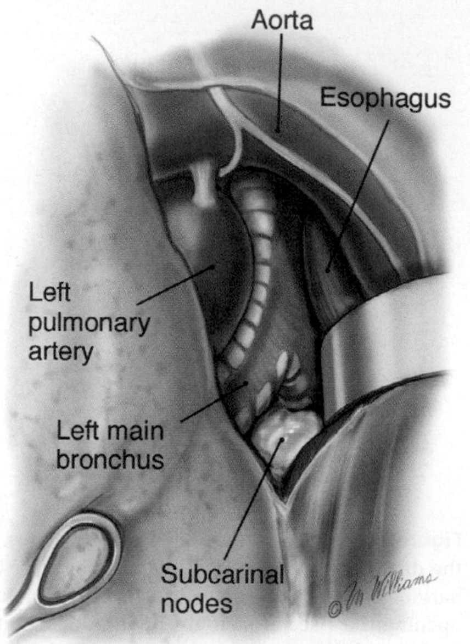

Figure 76-9. Left lymphadenectomy. To access station 7 nodes, the lung is retracted anteriorly and the posterior mediastinal pleura is opened along the groove anterior to the descending thoracic aorta.

during which time attention must be given to hemostasis of the bronchial and intercostal perforating vessels. Care also must be exercised in dissecting the subcarinal nodal packet off the main carina itself and the right mainstem bronchus. The esophagus is deep to the bronchus and is retracted posteriorly with the aorta, whereas the pericardium is found at the anteromedial extent of the dissection and inferiorly at the superior portion of the inferior pulmonary vein.

Samples from the paraesophageal (station 8) and inferior pulmonary ligament (station 9) nodes are obtained in similar fashion as on the right side once the posterior pleura is opened anterior to the descending aorta from the carina to the diaphragm. Station 10 on the left is found inferior to the pulmonary artery and posterior to the superior pulmonary vein at the distal left mainstem bronchus. Interlobar station 11 nodes are approached via the fissure with the left upper lobe reflected anteriorly or superiorly. The station 12 lobar nodes are found during dissection of the bronchus prior to lobectomy, and the segmental and subsegmental nodes (stations 13 and 14, respectively) are usually found within the specimen.

TECHNICAL PITFALLS

While most surgeons understand the importance of complete staging of the mediastinum, including assessment made during lung resection, there is variability in approach to nodal staging at different centers (i.e., lymph node sampling vs. complete dissection). In part, this is due to the concern that complete lymph node dissection may lead to increased complications or mortality compared with selective lymph node sampling. Furthermore, some surgeons hold the belief that treatment outcome or survival may not be altered with the additional knowledge of pathologic lymph node involvement. An early study from the American College of Surgeons Oncology Group Z0030 reported results from a randomized, prospective trial regarding morbidity and mortality after pulmonary resection to determine whether mediastinal lymph node dissection caused an increase in either morbidity or mortality.[29] Four hundred and ninety-eight patients underwent lymph node sampling, and 525 patients had complete lymph node dissection. Patient characteristics were comparable, and all tumors were clinically resectable (T1 or T2) with N0 or nonhilar N1 nodes and no metastases (M0). Exclusion criteria included patients who underwent wedge excision and those who received neoadjuvant treatment.

In the lymph node dissection group, mean operative time was 15 minutes longer ($p < 0.0001$), and the amount of chest tube drainage was greater (1459 mL vs. 1338 mL, $p = 0.056$) than in the lymph node sampling group. Although the chest tubes were left in longer in the lymph node dissection group (5 days vs. 4 days, $p = 0.495$), there was no difference in median length of hospital stay (6 days, $p = 0.404$). There was no significant difference in operative mortality between groups ($p = 0.157$), where 10 (2%) lymph node sampling patients died compared with 4 (0.76%) lymph node dissection patients. There were no significant differences in any specific complication between groups, including frequency of chylothorax, postoperative hemorrhage requiring reoperation, number of patients requiring postoperative transfusion, recurrent nerve injuries, air leaks, or bronchopleural fistulas. While the impact of complete mediastinal node dissection on long-term survival is not known from this study, the added dissection did not create significant additional complications when compared with lymph node sampling in this population.

A recent follow-up to the American College of Surgeons Oncology Group Z0030 Trial has not yet reported any results on survival benefit between lymph node sampling and dissection, but it did prove that lymph node dissection is safe and feasible in any hospital setting.[30] Furthermore, the study provides a benchmark in assessing the adequacy of lymph node harvest and what nodes to routinely collect. Right-sided resections should include nodes from 2R, 4R, 7, 8, 9, and 10R stations, whereas those on the left need to involve 4L, 5, 6, 7, 8, 9, and 10L stations. In this study, a minimum of 6 nodes were resected 99% of the time and there were more than 10 nodes in 90% of patients. Similar findings were reported by Lardinois et al.[13]in a nonrandomized series of 100 patients with clinical T1–3 and N0–1 disease. These patients were divided into two groups based on approach: complete dissection versus systematic sampling. While dissection took longer than sampling, there was no significant difference between groups in terms of hospitalization length, morbidity, or overall survival. This study did show a significantly longer disease-free survival after dissection compared with sampling (60 months vs. 45 months, $p < 0.03$) and a significantly higher local recurrence rate after sampling compared with dissection (13% vs. 45%, $p = 0.02$) in patients with stage I disease.

In patients with more advanced disease, there is controversy as to whether or not neoadjuvant treatment is associated with an increased risk of postoperative complications after pulmonary resection accompanied by lymph node dissection.[31,32] There are certain consequences to take into account when carrying out a lymph node dissection after neoadjuvant treatment. First, the timing of surgery is a factor. The patient's performance status must be adequate to tolerate the operation and withstand the postoperative stress associated with recovery. Chemotherapy nadirs should be taken into account, and radiation doses should be monitored. Traditionally, the timing of resection should be no sooner than 4 to 6 weeks after neoadjuvant treatment to permit the intended response to take effect and avoid acute inflammatory changes and yet not so far removed that postradiation fibrosis changes have begun. The lymph node dissection can be much more tedious after neoadjuvant treatment because, by definition, patients receiving neoadjuvant treatments have bulkier disease to begin with, as well as lymph node sclerosis from the treatment effect. The surgical approach generally is the same as in patients treated primarily, but identifying the proper dissection plane between the nodes and the pulmonary vasculature or airway is often challenging. If the dissection is too technically difficult, the decision to proceed and risk inadvertent injury of surrounding structures should be tampered with realistic considerations of whether or not final lymph node pathology will affect outcome, and if adjuvant treatment will be necessary, offered and/or tolerated.

Additional attention should be paid to the bronchus following neoadjuvant treatment. This is especially true because radiation treatment and nodal dissection can alter bronchial blood supply.[33–35] These associated ischemic changes merit buttressing the bronchial stump to prevent bronchopleural fistula.[36,37] This can be done using any of a number of flaps, including an intercostal muscle pedicle, pericardial or pleural patch, or thymic fat pad.

As with any minimal access surgery, there is a learning curve associated with proficiency in VATS lobectomy. The same holds true for the associated lymph node removal, be it sampling or dissection. However, when the surgeon is versed in open techniques, lymph node dissection by VATS is feasible.[38] Innovations in thoracoscopic equipment and technique have enabled minimally invasive thoracic surgery to advance safely. Using the then recently developed devices such as reticulating endoscissors, miniretractors, endoclips, and Harmonic scalpels, Kaseda et al.[25] performed 36 VATS lobectomies with lymph node dissection. The average number of lymph nodes resected (24, ranging from 10 to 51) was comparable with those from open thoracotomy (22, ranging from 16 to 36). Subsequently, systematic node dissection by VATS was compared with open thoracotomy in 350 patients undergoing pulmonary resection.[26] Although the study was nonrandomized and the cohorts were not entirely matched, there were no significant differences in the number of nodes dissected between the VATS and open thoracotomy groups. Operative mortality and morbidity were comparable.

SUMMARY

Determination of lymph node status is a critical component to the staging and treatment of NSCLC. Whether or not the surgeon performs systematic lymph node sampling or complete lymph node dissection, some level of nodal sampling is important for comprehensive staging. This practice helps to determine prognosis and may affect survival without added surgical morbidity or mortality. A working knowledge of the lymph node anatomy is necessary. Complete subcarinal and inferior pulmonary ligament dissections should be routine. For right-sided lesions, dissection of the paratracheal nodal packet is necessary. On the left side, dissection of the aortopulmonary and paraaortic stations is compulsory. In experienced hands, lymph node dissection can be done using VATS techniques. Despite advances in endoscopic access to lymph nodes for staging, surgeons are encouraged to complement pulmonary resection with lymph node dissection for comprehensive oncologic surgery.

EDITOR'S COMMENT

This chapter updates the important question of the value of lymph node dissection at the time of resection. The technique described herein is safe and reproducible. The importance of lymph node sampling to some degree will become more apparent when the American College of Surgeons Commission on Cancer (ACSCOC) adopts a minimum number of lymph nodes to be resected on all lung cancer surgeries as a prerequisite to qualifying for national standards. These will soon be adopted by the National Quality Forum (NQF). The only other caveat I would make is that in the event that central (levels 2–7) mediastinal lymph nodes are identified unexpectedly at resection, there is some evidence that one should stop and offer neoadjuvant therapy. Then a resection can be undertaken after the completion of therapy if the patient has had a good response. This is my current approach.

—Mark J. Krasna

References

1. Denoix P. Sur l'organisation d'une statisque permanente du cancer. *Bull Inst Natl Hyg (Paris).* 1944;1:67–74.
2. Mountain CF. A new international staging system for lung cancer. *Chest.* 1986;89:225S–233S.
3. Goldstraw P. The 7th Edition of TNM in lung cancer: what now? *J Thorac Oncol.* 2009;4:671–673.
4. Kim E, Bosquee L. The importance of accurate lymph node staging in early and locally advanced non-small cell lung cancer: an update on available techniques. *J Thorac Oncol.* 2007;2:S59–67.
5. Annema JT, van Meerbeeck JP, Rintoul RC, et al. Mediastinoscopy vs endosonography for mediastinal nodal staging of lung cancer: a randomized trial. *JAMA.* 2010;304:2245–2252.
6. Pearson FG. Non-small cell lung cancer: role of surgery for stages I-III. *Chest.* 1999;116:500S–503S.
7. Riquet M, Manac'h D, Le Pimpec-Barthes F, et al. Prognostic significance of surgical-pathologic N1 disease in non-small cell carcinoma of the lung. *Ann Thorac Surg.* 1999;67:1572–1576.
8. Friedel G, Steger V, Kyriss T, et al. Prognosis in N2 NSCLC. *Lung Cancer.* 2004;45(2):S45–S53.
9. Detterbeck F. What to do with "Surprise" N2?: intraoperative management of patients with non-small cell lung cancer. *J Thorac Oncol.* 2008;3:289–302.
10. Izbicki JR, Passlick B, Pantel K, et al. Effectiveness of radical systematic mediastinal lymphadenectomy in patients with resectable non-small cell lung cancer: results of a prospective randomized trial. *Ann Surg.* 1998;227:138–44.
11. Keller SM, Adak S, Wagner H, et al. Mediastinal lymph node dissection improves survival in patients with stages II and IIIa non-small cell lung cancer. Eastern Cooperative Oncology Group. *Ann Thorac Surg.* 2000;70:358–365; discussion 65–66.
12. Doddoli C, Aragon A, Barlesi F, et al. Does the extent of lymph node dissection influence outcome in patients with stage I non-small-cell lung cancer? *Eur J Cardiothorac Surg.* 2005;27:680–685.
13. Lardinois D, Suter H, Hakki H, et al. Morbidity, survival, and site of recurrence after mediastinal lymph-node dissection versus systematic sampling after complete resection for non-small cell lung cancer. *Ann Thorac Surg.* 2005;80:268–274; discussion 74–75.

14. Mountain CF, Dresler CM. Regional lymph node classification for lung cancer staging. *Chest.* 1997;111:1718–1723.
15. Cerfolio RJ, Bryant AS. Distribution and likelihood of lymph node metastasis based on the lobar location of nonsmall-cell lung cancer. *Ann Thorac Surg.* 2006;81:1969–1973; discussion 73.
16. Okada M, Tsubota N, Yoshimura M, et al. Induction therapy for non-small cell lung cancer with involved mediastinal nodes in multiple stations. *Chest.* 2000;118:123–128.
17. Sugi K, Nawata K, Fujita N, et al. Systematic lymph node dissection for clinically diagnosed peripheral non-small-cell lung cancer less than 2 cm in diameter. *World J Surg.* 1998;22:290–294; discussion 4–5.
18. Graham AN, Chan KJ, Pastorino U, et al. Systematic nodal dissection in the intrathoracic staging of patients with non-small cell lung cancer. *J Thorac Cardiovasc Surg.* 1999;117:246–251.
19. Ludwig MS, Goodman M, Miller DL, et al. Postoperative survival and the number of lymph nodes sampled during resection of node-negative non-small cell lung cancer. *Chest.* 2005;128:1545–1550.
20. Bonner JA, Garces YI, Sawyer TE, et al. Frequency of noncontiguous lymph node involvement in patients with resectable nonsmall cell lung carcinoma. *Cancer.* 1999;86:1159–1164.
21. Cahan WG, Watson WL, Pool JL. Radical pneumonectomy. *J Thorac Surg.* 1951;22:449–473.
22. Mentzer S. Mediastinal staging prior to surgical resection. *Oper Tech Thorac Cardiovasc Surg.* 2005;152:152–165.
23. Lerut T, De Leyn P, Coosemans W, et al. Cervical videomediastinoscopy. *Thorac Surg Clin.* 2010;20:195–206.
24. Ramos R, Girard P, Masuet C, et al. Mediastinal lymph node dissection in early-stage non-small cell lung cancer: totally thoracoscopic vs thoracotomy. *Eur J Cardiothorac Surg.* 2012;41:1342–1348; discussion 8.
25. Kaseda S, Hangai N, Yamamoto S, et al. Lobectomy with extended lymph node dissection by video-assisted thoracic surgery for lung cancer. *Surg Endosc.* 1997;11:703–706.
26. Watanabe A, Koyanagi T, Ohsawa H, et al. Systematic node dissection by VATS is not inferior to that through an open thoracotomy: a comparative clinicopathologic retrospective study. *Surgery.* 2005;138:510–517.
27. Watanabe Y, Shimizu J, Oda M, et al. Aggressive surgical intervention in N2 non-small cell cancer of the lung. *Ann Thorac Surg.* 1991;51:253–261.
28. Ferguson MK. Optimal management when unsuspected N2 nodal disease is identified during thoracotomy for lung cancer: cost-effectiveness analysis. *J Thorac Cardiovasc Surg.* 2003;126:1935–1942.
29. Allen MS, Darling GE, Pechet TT, et al. Morbidity and mortality of major pulmonary resections in patients with early-stage lung cancer: initial results of the randomized, prospective ACOSOG Z0030 trial. *Ann Thorac Surg.* 2006;81:1013–1019; discussion 9–20.
30. Darling GE, Allen MS, Decker PA, et al. Randomized trial of mediastinal lymph node sampling versus complete lymphadenectomy during pulmonary resection in the patient with N0 or N1 (less than hilar) non-small cell carcinoma: results of the American College of Surgery Oncology Group Z0030 Trial. *J Thorac Cardiovasc Surg.* 2011;141:662–670.
31. Perrot E, Guibert B, Mulsant P, et al. Preoperative chemotherapy does not increase complications after nonsmall cell lung cancer resection. *Ann Thorac Surg.* 2005;80:423–427.
32. Roberts JR, Eustis C, Devore R, et al. Induction chemotherapy increases perioperative complications in patients undergoing resection for non-small cell lung cancer. *Ann Thorac Surg.* 2001;72:885–888.
33. Yamamoto R, Tada H, Kishi A, et al. Effects of preoperative chemotherapy and radiation therapy on human bronchial blood flow. *J Thorac Cardiovasc Surg.* 2000;119:939–945.
34. Satoh Y, Okumura S, Nakagawa K, et al. Postoperative ischemic change in bronchial stumps after primary lung cancer resection. *Eur J Cardiothorac Surg.* 2006;30:172–176.
35. Levchenko EV, Orlov SV, Lisochkin BG, et al. [Effect of preoperative chemotherapy, mediastinal lymph node dissection and stump cover on bronchial regeneration following experimental pneumonectomy]. *Vopr Onkol.* 2005;51:583–587.
36. Cerfolio RJ, Bryant AS, Yamamuro M. Intercostal muscle flap to buttress the bronchus at risk and the thoracic esophageal-gastric anastomosis. *Ann Thorac Surg.* 2005;80:1017–1020.
37. Taghavi S, Marta GM, Lang G, et al. Bronchial stump coverage with a pedicled pericardial flap: an effective method for prevention of postpneumonectomy bronchopleural fistula. *Ann Thorac Surg.* 2005;79:284–288.
38. McKenna RJ, Jr. Lobectomy by video-assisted thoracic surgery with mediastinal node sampling for lung cancer. *J Thorac Cardiovasc Surg.* 1994;107:879–881; discussion 81–82.

77 Open and VATS Wedge Resection for Lung Cancer

Rodney J. Landreneau and Matthew J. Schuchert

Keywords: Sublobar resection, malignant lung lesion, open thoracotomy, muscle-sparing thoracotomy, anterior minithoracotomy, lobectomy

INTRODUCTION

Nonanatomic, sublobar "wedge" resection of lung cancer is generally considered a "compromise" pulmonary resection for primary treatment of lung cancer directed to the physiologically impaired patient who is at high risk for lobectomy.[1,2] This assessment of the clinical utility of wedge resection is being challenged, particularly for the management of the small peripheral lung cancer where a generous wedge resection can be accomplished with acceptable surgical margins.

The goal of sublobar resection is lung parenchymal preservation, and as with the use of segmental breast-preserving resection of small breast cancers, limitation in the ability to control the tumor locally is appreciated as an important potential drawback. As with breast cancer, surgical margin status is at the heart of the matter of local recurrence. Regional lymph node status and histologic, molecular, and biologic findings suggestive of an aggressive tumor, such as angiolymphatic invasion, visceral pleural invasion, and gene mutational findings appear to be independent predictors of survival from the "resection marginal" status of surgery.

Nevertheless, local recurrence following lung cancer resection is an important problem leading to potential patient morbidities (i.e., bronchial obstruction, chest wall invasion, pleural effusion). Intraoperative measures to avoid local recurrence, such as enhancing surgical margins of resection and the use of intraoperative radiobrachytherapy at the margin of surgical resection, have been explored.[3–5] Postoperative radiotherapy directed to the staple line margins of resection has also been explored in the past.[6]

In this chapter, we review the basic strategies for successful open thoracotomy and VATS wedge resection of peripheral small lung malignancies (i.e., peripheral small primary lung cancer and pulmonary metastasis from remote primary cancers). We also direct attention to the primary uses of wedge resection for the diagnosis of suspicious pulmonary lesions suspected to be malignant (i.e., the indeterminate pulmonary nodule). The outcomes reported in the literature for wedge resection of these pathologic conditions will be reviewed.

PRIMARY PULMONARY LESIONS AMENABLE TO SUBLOBAR (WEDGE) RESECTION

The primary principles for selection of sublobar resection for pulmonary pathologic lesions are noted in Table 77-1. The lesion should be in the outer third of the lung parenchyma and less than 3 cm in diameter, as more deeply seated and larger lesions will require broader resections toward the base of the lobar hilum which may compromise margins of resection or result in loss of the physiologic integrity of the remaining lobe (Fig. 77-1).[7–10] Similarly, if an endobronchial extension of the tumor is identified by bronchoscopic examination, wedge resection with adequate surgical margins is impossible. Upon these basic tenets rest the utility of wedge resection for the management of pulmonary parenchymal lesions, specifically the use of wedge resection for the treatment of lung cancer. Of course, the use of laser or electrocautery precision excision of deeper pulmonary lesions may make possible the resection of small, deeper lesions which are not in close proximity with the segmental bronchial anatomy.[11,12]

Table 77-1

PRIMARY PULMONARY LESIONS AMENABLE TO SUBLOBAR RESECTION
1. Located in outer third of pulmonary parenchyma
2. Small in size (<3 cm diameter)
3. Clear surgical margins accomplished with distance of 1 cm (preferable equivalent to diameter of the pulmonary nodule)
4. No endobronchial involvement by the lesion as noted by bronchoscopic examination

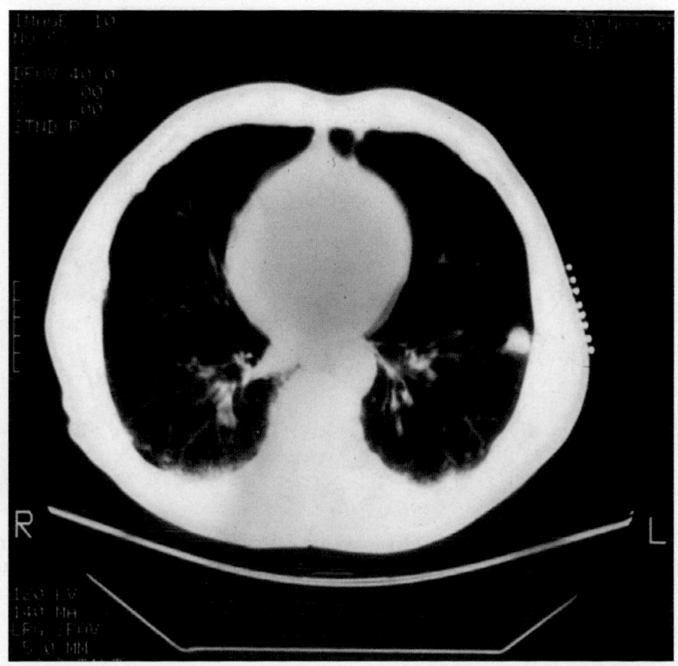

Figure 77-1. Chest CT depicting ideal pulmonary lesion amenable to definitive wedge resection.

TECHNICAL ASPECTS OF OPEN THORACOTOMY APPROACHES TO MALIGNANT LUNG LESIONS

Rather than the "one size fits all" approach to pulmonary resection, common in the day before VATS, open thoracotomy approaches to wedge resection have evolved to minimize the surgical trauma related to the thoracotomy incisional access. Today, open thoracotomy access to accomplish wedge resection should be muscle-sparing, limited in extent, and positioned to provide direct access to the target lesion(s).

A lateral vertical thoracotomy, originally described by Noirclerc, provides excellent exposure for most pulmonary pathology (Fig. 77-2).[13,14] An oblique to vertical incision is used to facilitate entry into the chest at multiple intercostal levels. The fingers of the serratus anterior musculature are separated and the belly elevated to expose the underlying intercostal musculature. Excellent exposure to all lobes of the lung is affected. During the course of resection, it is important to ensure that adequate margins of resection are achieved without "overresecting" the parenchyma which could result in excessive tension along the staple line increasing the risk of staple line dehiscence. After resection, mediastinal and hilar nodal sampling is suggested for more accurate pathologic staging of the malignancy.

Alternatively, a posterior auscultatory triangle, muscle-sparing approach (Fig. 77-3)[15,16] or a lateral thoracotomy approach retracting the serratus musculature anteriorly and the latissimus dorsi posteriorly can provide effective open thoracotomy exposure (Fig. 77-4).[17,18] The anterior thoracotomy approach with the patient in the supine position has been shown to be an effective means of avoiding median sternotomy to achieve bilateral access for pulmonary metastasectomy (Figs. 77-5 and 77-6).[19–23] VATS assistance can be utilized with this approach to visualize and facilitate wedge resection of more posteriorly located lung lesions.

Of course, the use of open thoracotomy is associated with increased perioperative incision-related pain and morbidity compared with the VATS approach to resection.[24–26] However, it does not appear that there is any important difference in chronic postthoracotomy pain between open thoracotomy and VATS approaches to wedge resection.[27]

TECHNICAL ASPECTS OF VATS APPROACHES TO MALIGNANT LUNG LESIONS

During the 1990s, the most effective intercostal access strategies for anatomic lung resection and wedge resection were formalized. It became clear that a mastery of computed tomography (CT) imagery was important to facilitate the accurate localization of the target lesion(s) for resection as bimanual digital palpation of the lung commonly done with open thoracotomy was not possible. Early on, CT-directed needle localization and other localization measures with lipoidal injection into the lung were utilized, however, today, these measures are rarely utilized.[28]

Intercostal access for pulmonary resection is planned with the concept of providing maximal visualization of the intrathoracic anatomy and effective introduction of instrumentation for resection (Fig. 77-7). The concept of triangulation of the target lesion with scope access at a neutral lower intercostal access and anterior and posterior intercostal access for grasping tools and resective devices (staplers, electrocautery units, or laser) is primarily employed. The usual intercostal access for wedge resection is depicted in (Fig. 77-8).[7,10]

The wedge resection is initiated by identifying the location of the pulmonary lesion through visual cues of lesional effacement against the collapsed lung during selective double-lumen tube ventilation and through digital palpation of the

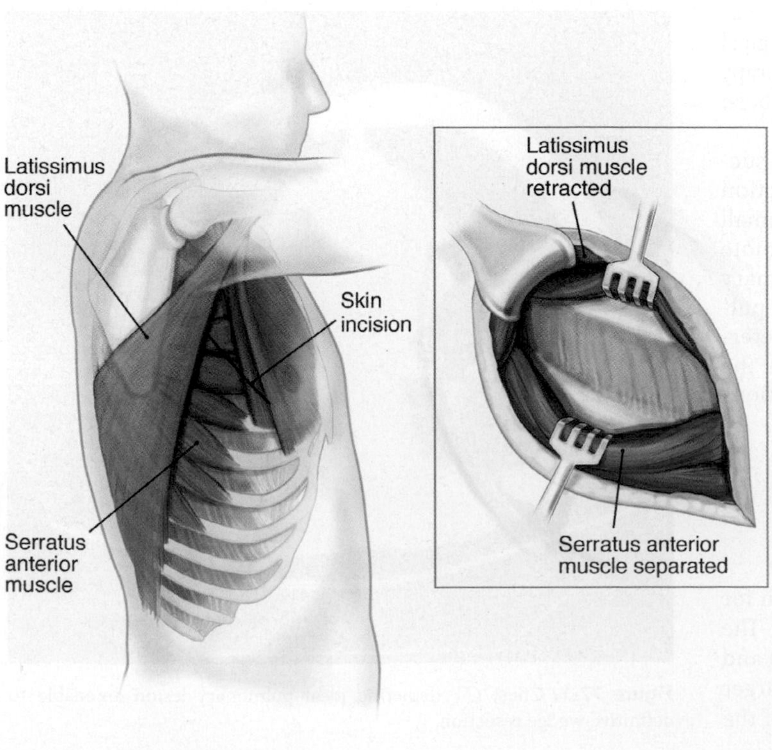

Figure 77-2. Anterior muscle-sparing lateral thoracotomy—French incision.

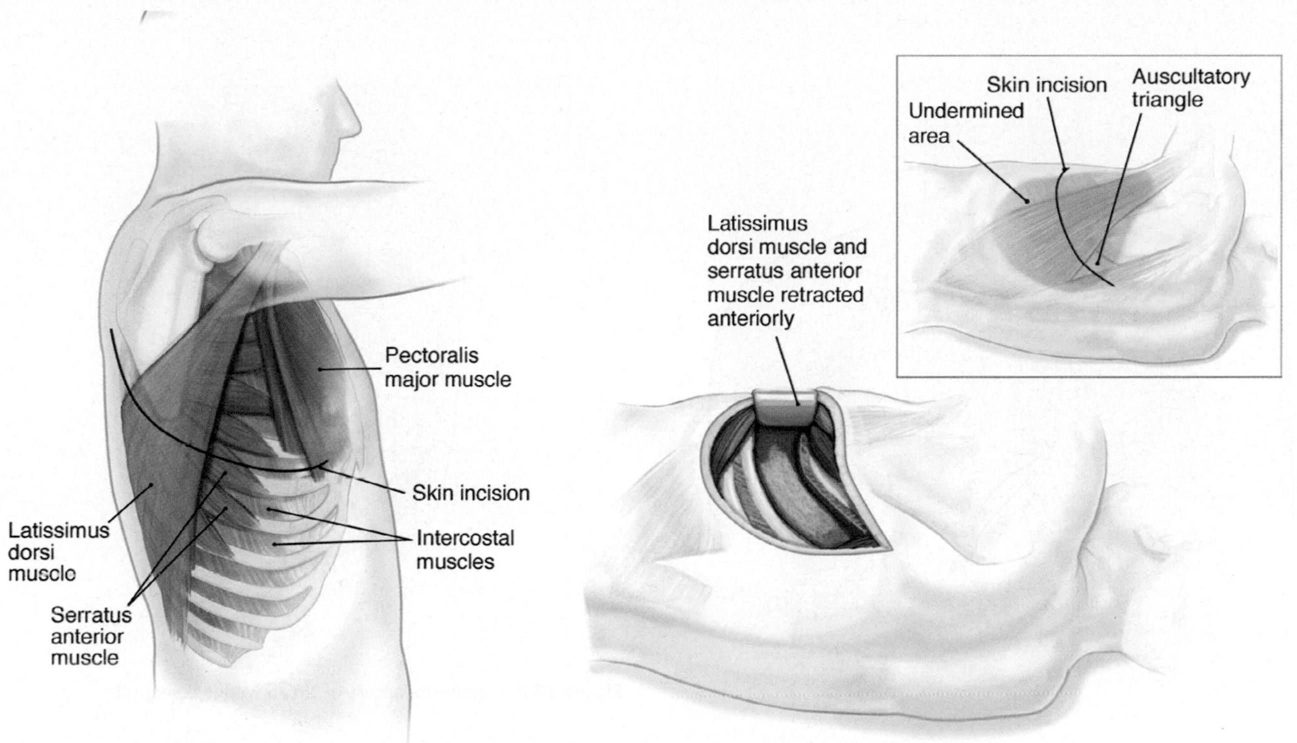

Figure 77-3. Auscultatory posterolateral muscle-sparing thoracotomy.

lung surface through a site of intercostal access in the area of lesion probability based upon CT imaging (Fig. 77-9). The lung is then grasped in the area of the lung lesion and a compressive clamp (Landreneau "Masher"; Starr Medical Inc., NY) is placed beneath the lung lesion along the line of the anticipated stapled surgical margin. If the margin appears acceptable, an endostapler is introduced along this proposed line of dissection and fired.[7,8,10] The integrity of the staple line and the margin are assessed and further application of the stapler beneath the parenchymal line of resection is performed. Alternating the intercostal entry points of the stapler and grasping instrument

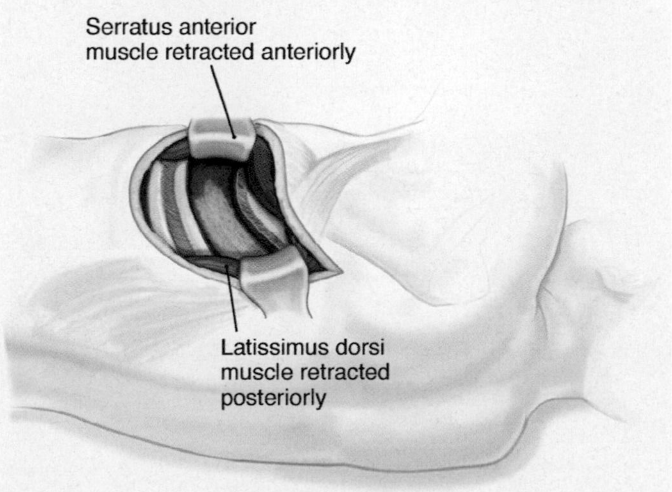

Figure 77-4. Lateral muscle-sparing thoracotomy reflecting serratus anterior and latissimus dorsi muscles.

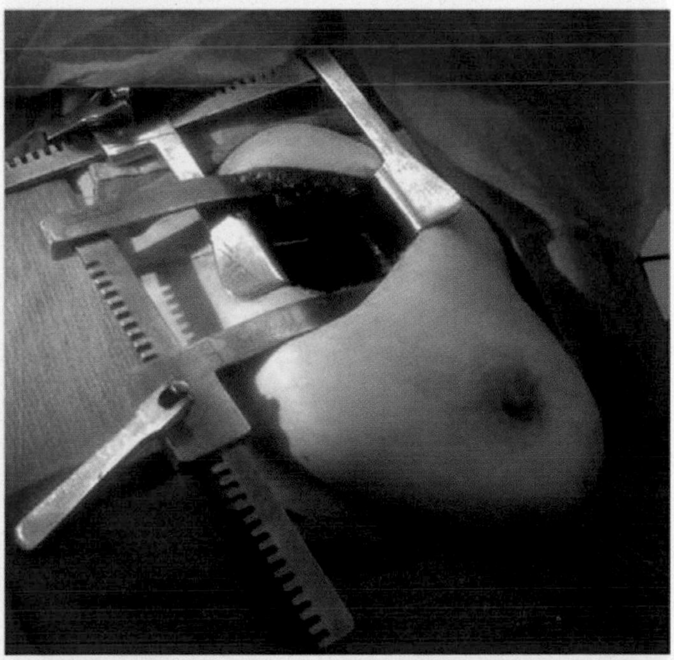

Figure 77-5. Anterior minithoracotomy. Extended Chamberlain Procedure. (Adapted with kind permission from Pettiford BL, Schuchert MJ, Abbas G, et al. Anterior minithoracotomy: a direct approach to the difficult hilum for upper lobectomy, pneumonectomy, and sleeve lobectomy. *Ann Surg Oncol.* 2010;17:123–128, Copyright 2010 Springer Science and Business Media.)

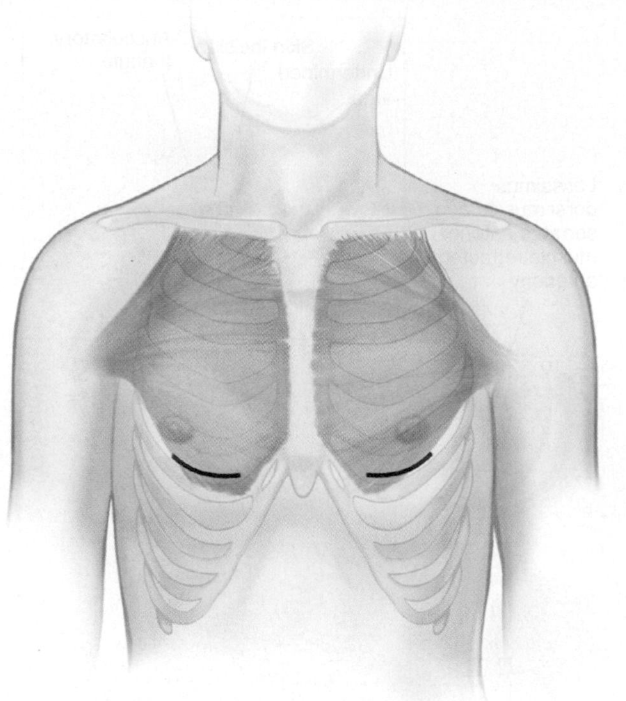

Figure 77-6. Inframammary bilateral mini-thoracotomy.

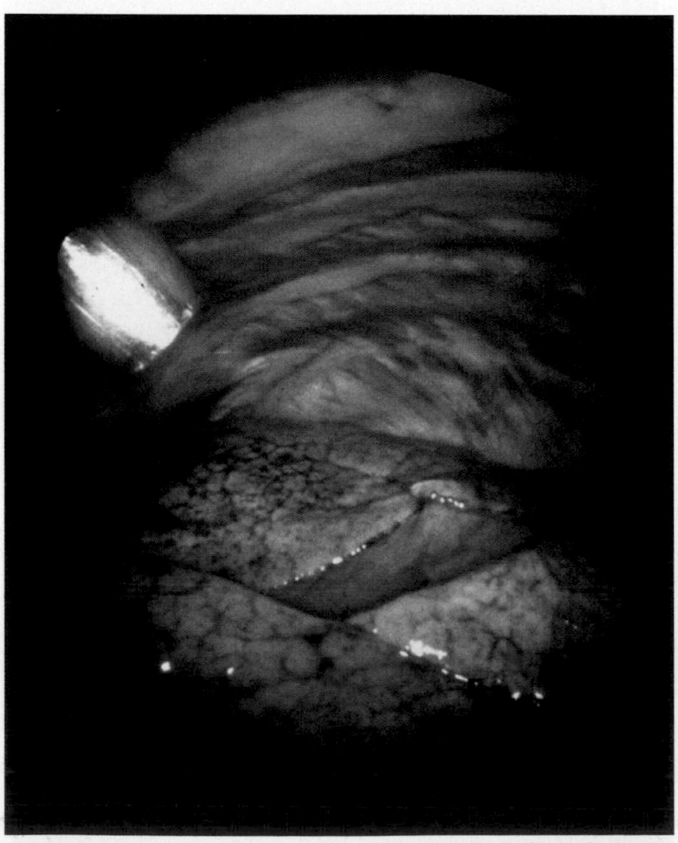

Figure 77-7. Image of pleural access via VATS.

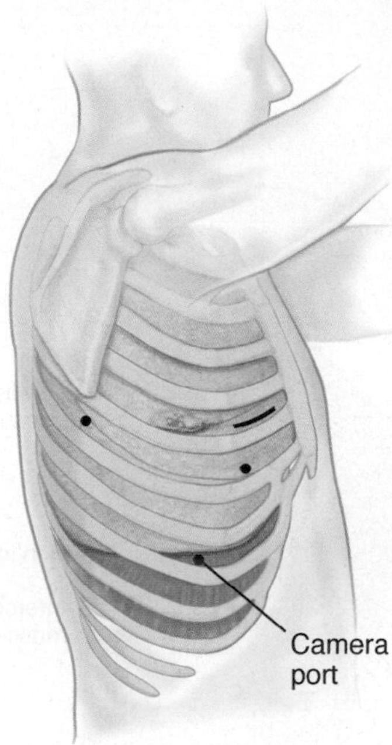

Figure 77-8. Intercostal access of VATS wedge resection.

is also commonly performed to finish the wedge resection and avoid "banana peeling" of the lung along an extended line of stapled resection (Table 77-2 and Figs. 77-10–77-12).[7] As mentioned above, the Nd:YAG laser can be used to accomplish wedge resection of deeper lung lesions where the endostapler is unable to close upon the lung tissue beneath the lesion due to tissue thickness. Figure 77-13 illustrates the technique of combined Nd:YAG laser tissue ablation beneath the target pulmonary lesion with eventual application of the endostapler across the thinner base of lung parenchyma needed to accomplish wedge resection with adequate margins (Fig. 77-13).[29]

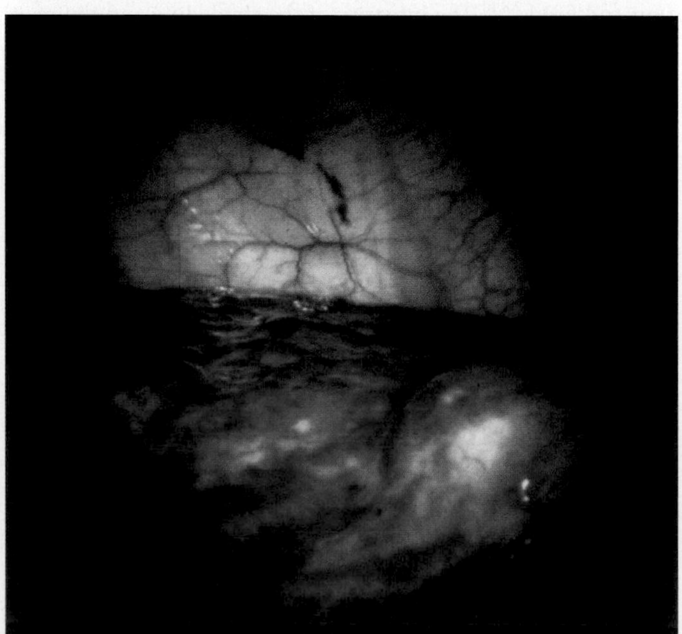

Figure 77-9. Effacement of pulmonary parenchyma against subpleural nodule with lung collapse during selective ventilation.

Table 77-2

PRIMARY POINTS OF CONTROVERSY REGARDING PULMONARY METASTASECTOMY

1. Unilateral versus bilateral thoracic exploration to remove all metastatic disease
2. Open thoracotomy for bimanual palpation of the lung versus VATS approaches directed to disease demonstrable by CT imaging
3. The number of metastatic lesions present that defines the opportunity of a therapeutic resection of disease

USE OF SUBLOBAR RESECTION FOR THE INDETERMINATE PULMONARY NODULE

The risk of cancer in a newly found pulmonary nodule is dependent on a variety of clinical and morphologic circumstances. Recent data resulting from the National Lung Screening Trial (NLST) identified a 20% reduction in lung cancer deaths among those patients who undergo low-dose helical CT surveillance scanning compared with the observation arm of the study undergoing standard chest x-ray alone.[30] Henshke and the I-ELCAP consortium also demonstrated extraordinarily favorable survival (greater than 80% overall and greater than 90% for stage I lung cancers) among patients who underwent surgical resection of lung lesions that were later found to be primary lung cancers.[31]

These compelling data should lead us to recommend early resection of suspicious new lung lesions identified in high-risk patients (i.e., age over 50; impaired pulmonary function; and significant smoking history—greater than 20 pack-years). We should look to remove these lesions with appropriate diagnostic resections, that is, wedge resection or segmentectomy. Schuchert et al.[32] have recently identified the safety and utility of VATS sublobar resection, in this case by anatomic segmentectomy, in the diagnosis of the suspicious indeterminate nodule. Over 85% of indeterminate nodules in this series were found to be malignant in nature. The morbidity and mortality associated with these surgical diagnostic approaches were negligible. In addition, anatomic resection was felt to be definitive therapy among those patients who underwent sublobar resection. Wedge resection with adequate surgical margins should provide similar diagnostic utility as the segmentectomy results reported by Schuchert.

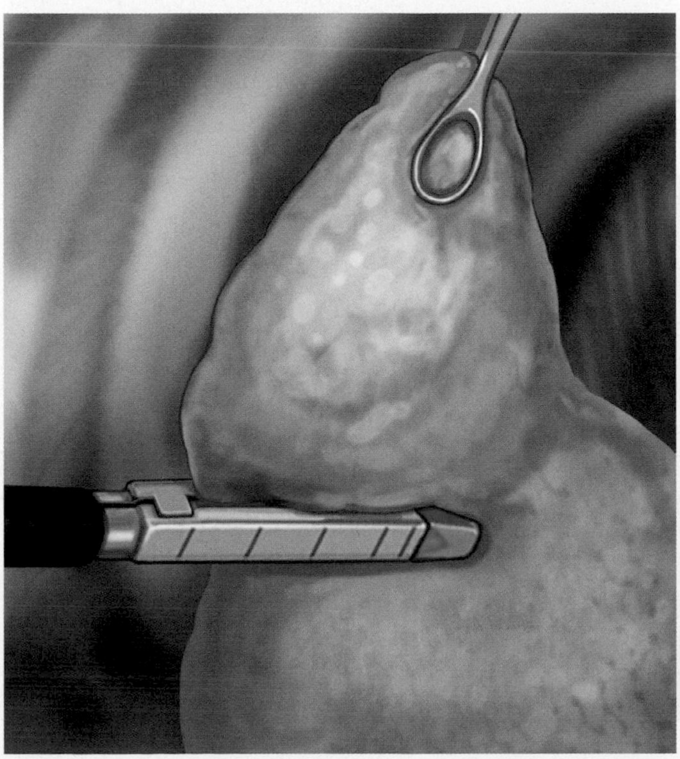

Figure 77-10. Application of stapling device to begin VATS wedge resection.

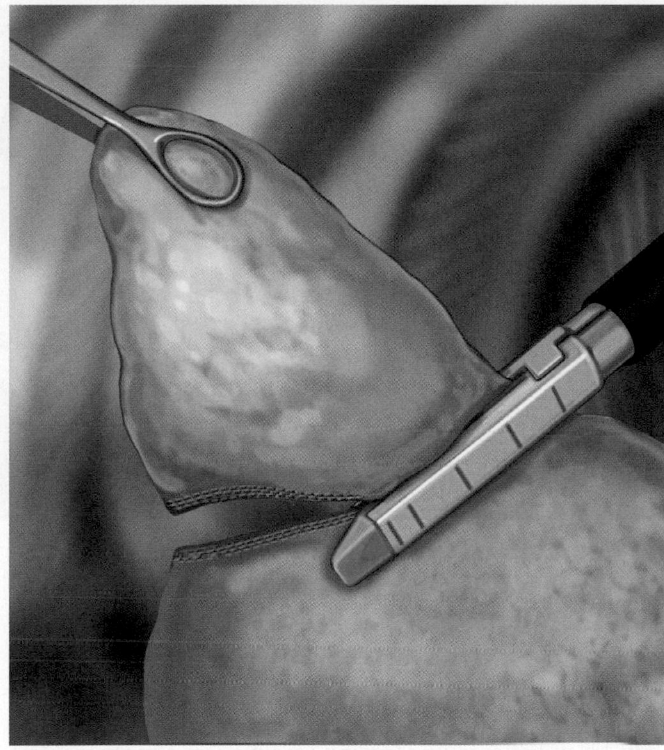

Figure 77-11. Alternate application of endostapler to complete wedge resection.

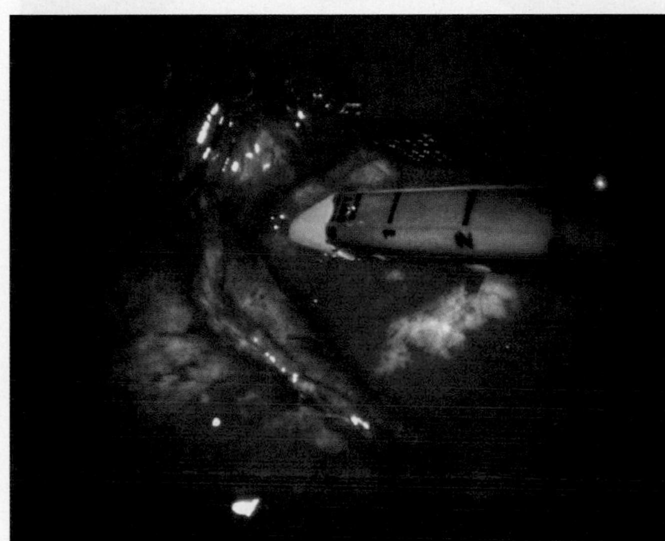

Figure 77-12. VATS wedge resection in progress.

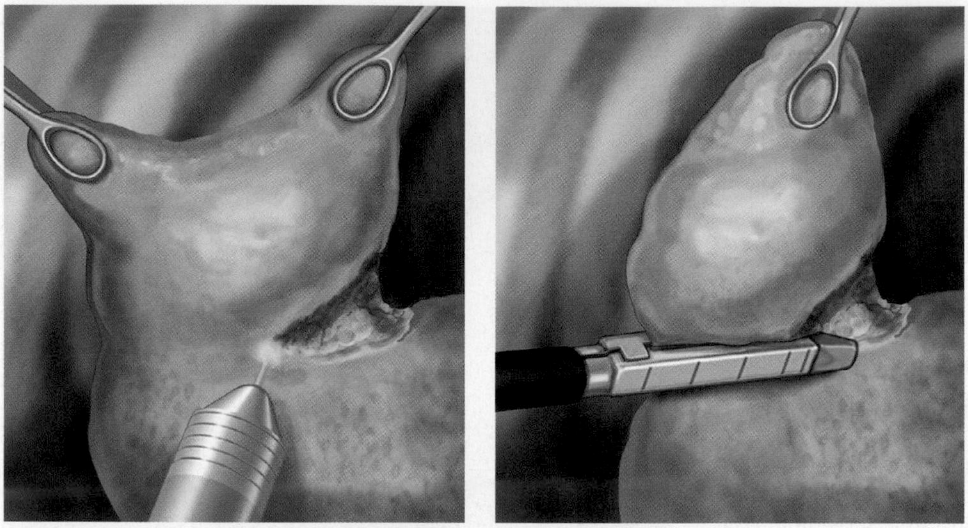

Figure 77-13. Combined Nd:YAG laser and endoscopic stapler wedge resection of lung.

SUBLOBAR RESECTION FOR PULMONARY METASTASES. WHICH IS BETTER—OPEN VERSUS VATS APPROACHES?

Only 1% of patients undergoing resection of remote visceral primary malignancies will be found to have subsequent pulmonary metastases amenable to long-term survival with resection of these pulmonary sites of disease.[33–35] Some would argue that pulmonary metastasectomy and metastasectomy, in general, is merely "chasing the tail" of a systemic disease with a more indolent tumor biology (Fig. 77-14).[36–42] A primary tenet of pulmonary metastasectomy is preservation of lung parenchyma with the use of wedge resection with clear margins for patients who may require re-resection for recurrent disease or subsequent disease progression within the lung impairing lung functional reserve.[22,43–46] Of course, the thoracic surgical dicta related to recommending pulmonary metastasectomy relate to control of the primary remote site of malignancy, oligometastases to the lung, a long interval between primary tumor management and the development of low-volume metastatic burden to the lungs, and no other effective treatment for the pulmonary metastatic lesions other than resection or local ablation.[35,44–46] Indeed, the summary of over 5200 pulmonary metastasectomies within the *International Registry of Lung Metastases* reported by Pastorino et al.[35] estimated that pulmonary metastasectomy may provide benefit in the setting of a single metastasis present, germ cell histology (rarely operated upon today), and a long interval between primary tumor resection and appearance of the pulmonary metastasis. A revealing figure from that analysis summarized the surgical outcomes of patients undergoing metastasectomy with increased risk of metastasectomy failure based upon the

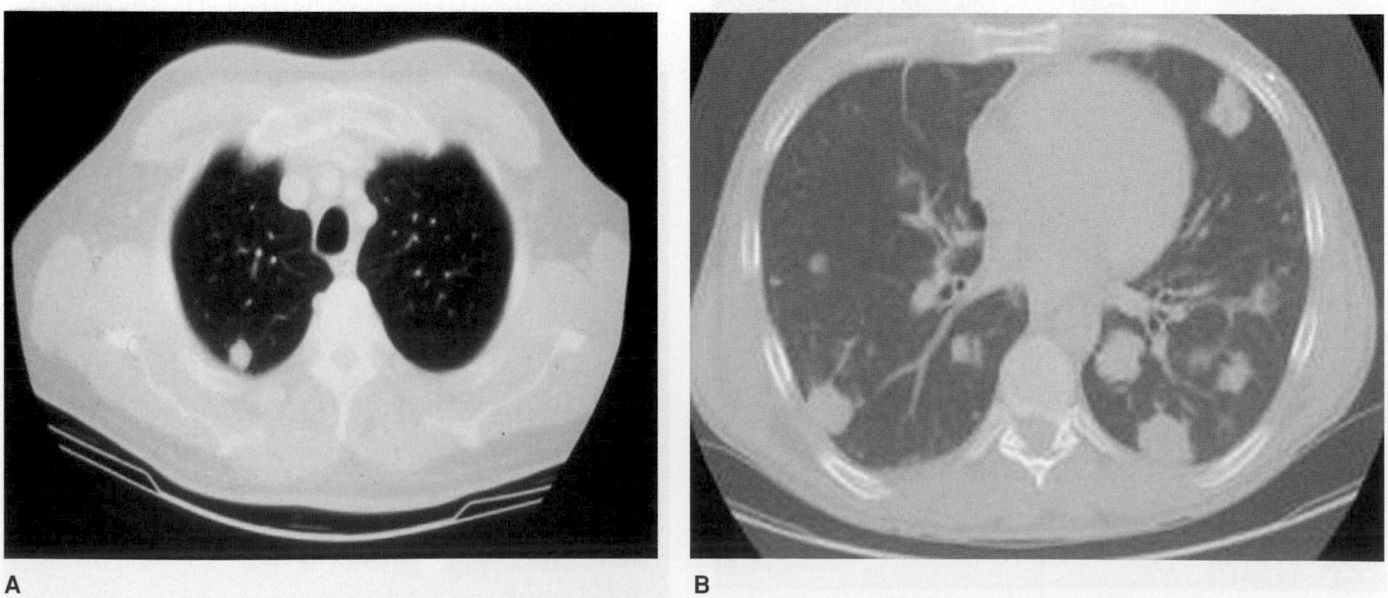

Figure 77-14. *A.* Solitary metastases. (Used with permission from El-Sherif A, Gooding WE, Santos R, et al. Outcomes of sublobar resection versus lobectomy for stage I non-small cell lung cancer: a 13-year analysis. *Ann Thorac Surg.* 2006;82:408–415; discussion 415–406.) *B.* Bilateral metastastic disease.

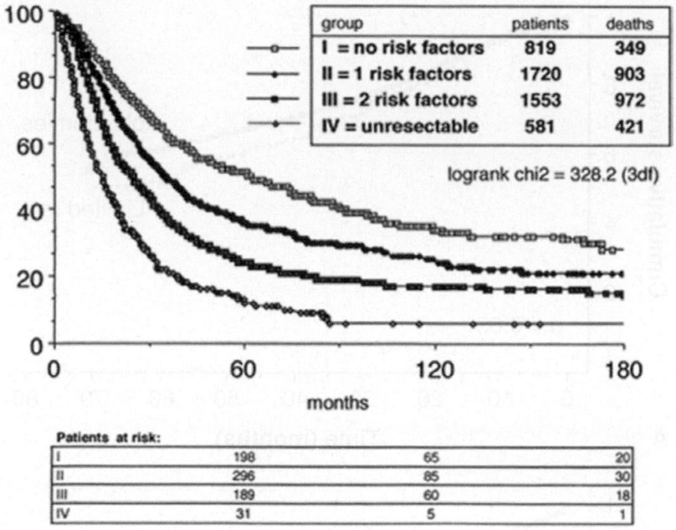

Figure 77-15. Metastasectomy Registry Risk Factor analysis. (Reprinted with permission from Pastorino UBM, Friedel G, Ginsberg RJ, et al. Long-term results of lung metastasectomy: prognostic analyses based on 5206 cases. The International Registry of Lung Metastases. *J Thorac Cardiovasc Surg.* 1997;113:37–49. Copyright 2006 Elsevier.)

variables of number of metastases, completeness of resection, and interval between primary tumor and the appearance of pulmonary metastasis (Fig. 77-15).[35] Four prognostic groups were created among patients in the registry, excluding patients with germ cell tumors from the analysis. Group I included completely resected patients with a disease-free interval (DFI) greater than 36 months and a single metastasis; Group II consisted of patients with one major risk factor—DFI less than 36 months or multiple metastases; Group III were patients with two major risk factors—DFI less than 36 months and multiple metastases resected; and Group IV comprised patients whose tumors were incompletely resected or unresectable.[35] These basic concepts for potential therapeutics still hold today, although many thoracic surgical teams have taken a much more aggressive stance with regard to performance of pulmonary metastasectomy.

The obvious but incalculable influence of metastatic disease biology is at play in the results seen with pulmonary metastasectomy. Radical "metastasectomizers" have argued that accurate evaluation of the lung cannot be accomplished using VATS approaches as limited ability to manually evaluate the entire lung, and remove all suspicious lesions. They exhort that "complete" resection vital to proper metastasectomy principles is potentially violated with the use of VATS.[22,40,41,45] The primary points of controversy are noted in Table 77-3.

Those favoring VATS approaches to metastasectomy rebut these arguments by acknowledging that reliance on CT imaging may not identify all pulmonary lesions palpable, but note that a significant minority of lesions resected based upon manual palpation are found to be benign in nature, and that the finding of multiple lesions, if positive, converts the surgical intervention to one of diagnostic confirmation of poor prognosis only. They also argue that "state of the art" CT imaging does allow accurate assessment of disease burden within the pulmonary parenchyma and also allows for strategic planning for effective VATS resection when a truly oligometastastic process is present.[47,48] Finally, the proponents of the VATS

Table 77-3

UTILITY OF SURGICAL RESECTION IN THE MANAGEMENT OF THE PERIPHERAL, EARLY-STAGE LUNG CANCER

1. Confirmation that treatment is being directed toward truly malignant disease
2. Assurance of complete extirpation of the cancer with acceptable margins of resection
3. Accurate assessment of mediastinal and hilar lymph node involvement which identifies "surprise" node positivity affecting adjuvant therapy decisions
4. Provision of adequate tissue for complete pharmacogenomic evaluation to provide individualized adjuvant therapy for the patient with tumors with aggressive characteristics for recurrence and systemic disease progression

approach to metastasectomy argue that their critics favoring "open thoracotomy" have commonly utilized a unilateral thoracotomy approach to the metastatic process leaving the contralateral lung unexplored, assuming that no disease is present in the contralateral lung.[41,46] Certainly bilateral VATS exploration can be accomplished as an alternative to this unilateral thoracotomy concept with targeted resection based upon CT evidence.[20] Experience with the management of metastatic sarcoma to the lung has identified bilateral metastatic foci in the majority of patients affected by pulmonary spread.[22] These findings of simultaneous or eventual contralateral disease associated with sarcoma metastastic to the lung are also noted over the natural history of most patients with visceral malignancies with lung metastases. The arguments of "unilateral radical metastasectomizers" seem a bit counterintuitive when these issues are examined more closely.

RESULTS OF SUBLOBAR "WEDGE" RESECTION FOR THE SMALL PERIPHERAL PRIMARY LUNG CANCER

Although we prefer anatomic segmentectomy for the management of the peripheral clinical stage I lung cancer, nonanatomic wedge resection with adequate margins of resection and careful hilar and mediastinal nodal staging may have equivalent therapeutic benefit to segmentectomy or lobectomy.[49–51] This brings us to the clinical reasoning behind the use of sublobar resection for the small peripheral lung cancer. The primary motivation for most surgeons considering lesser resections than lobectomy relates to the potential preservation of pulmonary parenchymal reserve with wedge resection or segmentectomy. Many reports of sublobar resection involved its use for patients with impaired lung function with otherwise resectable disease.[2–6,36,52–54] Although the randomized study of sublobar resection compared with lobectomy done by the Lung Cancer Study Group demonstrated an initial postoperative lung functional benefit with sublobar resection compared with lobectomy, these investigators reported similar pulmonary function between sublobar resection and lobectomy a year after surgery.[1] However, the pulmonary functional analysis in this study was flawed in that only 60% of patients in this study actually underwent pulmonary testing. Other surgeons from Asia and North America have demonstrated a sustained preservation in lung function with sublobar resection compared to lobectomy for early-stage lung cancer.[37,38,55]

Another consideration of thoracic surgeons choosing wedge resection instead of pulmonary lobectomy is the relative increase in risk of mortality or major morbidity with lobectomy. Although the modern day mortality associated with lobectomy is small, as noted in the recent report by Allen and the surgeons of ACOSOG,[56] a general consensus is that there is reduced mortality and major morbidity associated with these lesser resections compared with lobectomy.[49,50,55]

So what are the potential disadvantages of wedge resection in the management of the small peripheral lung cancer? Most clinical series of wedge resection for lung cancer reported in the literature have had limited mediastinal and hilar nodal sampling as part of the intraoperative staging evaluation. This is primarily the result of a "peek and shriek" approach to wedge resection being performed in most circumstances, as a "compromise resection" directed toward patients with impaired cardiopulmonary reserve for whom lobectomy was felt to be a prohibitive risk.[2,36,54] By comparison, with anatomic resection systemic mediastinal and hilar node sampling is routinely performed, and not surprisingly, up to 30% of patients may be upstaged at surgical resection from the preoperative clinical stage. This circumstance is true even in this age of advanced diagnostics through PET/CT imaging and endoscopic bronchial ultrasound biopsy (EBUS). In addition, up to 15% of stage I lung cancer patients may be upstaged from a clinically negative mediastinal and hilar lymph node status to a pathologic-positive nodal status.[57–59] This "understaging" of clinically early lung cancer is a serious concern when we consider the new appreciation of the value of adjuvant chemotherapy for resected lung cancer with node positivity.[60–62]

With this background, let us look at the results with wedge resection for small, peripheral lung cancers. Several series have demonstrated equivalent survival with wedge resection or lobectomy for stage I lung cancer,[2,36,54,63] exemplified by the survival curve from Erret et al. (Fig. 77-16).[63] Mery et al. analyzed the survival after sublobar resection compared with lobectomy for stage I and II NSCLC from the national *Surveillance, Epidemiology, and End Results* (SEER) database.[54] Over 14,000 patients' outcomes were reviewed. Mery et al. demonstrated the importance of age with regard to survivorship following resection of early-stage disease. They noted that for patients in their seventh decade of life, sublobar resection conferred equivalent survival to that of lobectomy, however, among younger patients, lobectomy appeared to provide a survival advantage (Fig. 77-17).[36] El-Sherif and associates reviewed a recent 13-year experience with the management of early-stage lung cancer at the University of Pittsburgh. Among patients with stage IA cancers, no difference in survival could be found

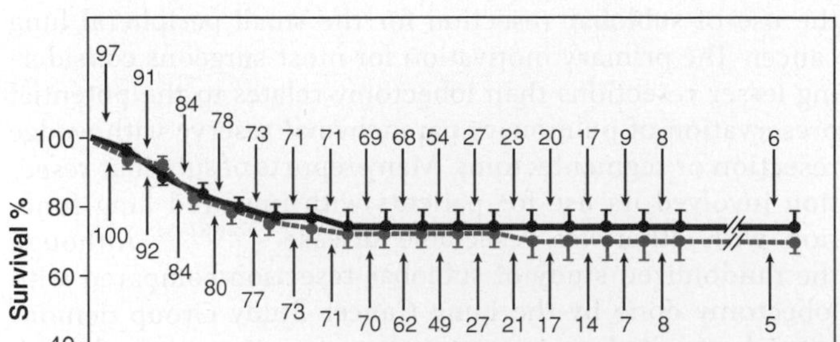

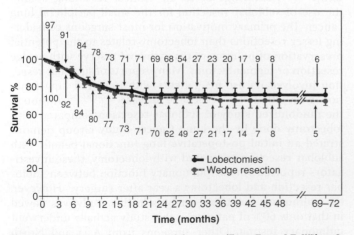

Figure 77-16. Survival wedge versus lobectomy. (From Errett LE, Wilson J, Chiu RC, et al. Wedge resection as an alternative procedure for peripheral bronchogenic carcinoma in poor-risk patients. *J Thorac Cardiovasc Surg.* 1985;90:656–661, Copyright (1985) Elsevier.)

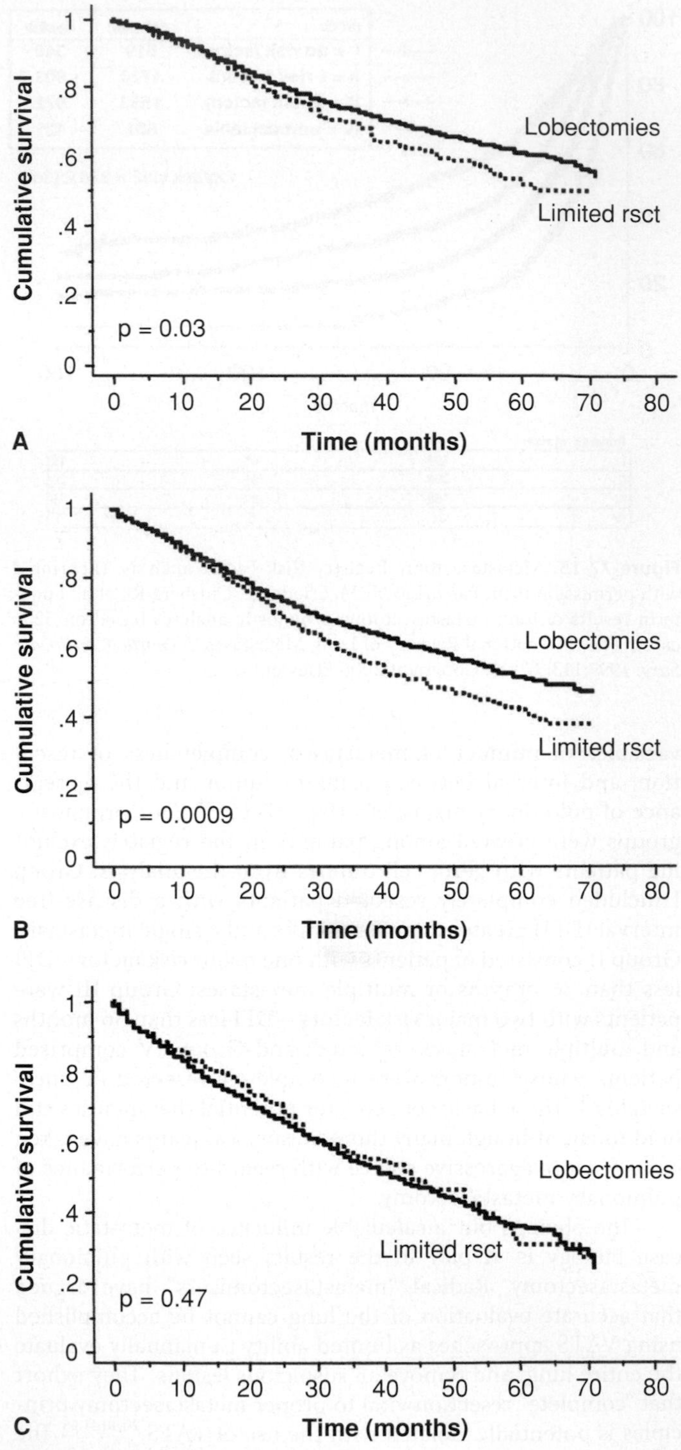

Figure 77-17. *A.* Survival patients less than 65 years—wedge versus lobectomy. *B.* Age 65 to 75 years—wedge versus lobectomy. *C.* Patients greater than 75 years—wedge versus lobectomy. (Reproduced with permission from Mery CM, Pappas AN, Bueno R, et al. Similar long-term survival of elderly patients with non-small cell lung cancer treated with lobectomy or wedge resection within the surveillance, epidemiology, and end results database. *Chest.* 2005;128:237–245. American College of Chest Physicians.)

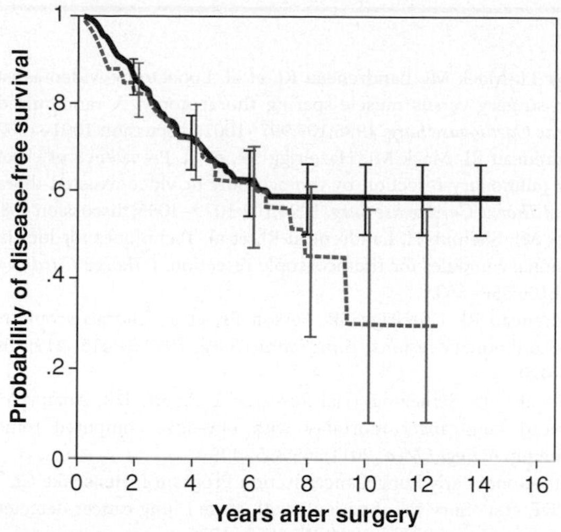

Figure 77-18. Wedge versus lobe survival stage IA NSCLC. (Used with permission from El-Sherif A, Gooding WE, Santos R, et al. Outcomes of sublobar resection versus lobectomy for stage I non-small cell lung cancer: a 13-year analysis. *Ann Thorac Surg.* 2006;82:408–415; discussion 415–406.)

between patients who underwent wedge resection and patients who underwent lobectomy (Fig. 77-18).[36] Landreneau et al. also identified similar survival among stage I NSCLC patients who underwent wedge resection compared with lobectomy when corrected for noncancer-related deaths.[2] Finally, the randomized Lung Cancer Study Group study described earlier could not identify a survival advantage with lobectomy over sublobar resection for patients with stage I lung cancer.[1,64]

The reported results from the studies mentioned emphasize the growing understanding of the importance of comorbid disease, age, and the biology of lung cancer in determining outcome following surgical resection. These factors appear to be more important than extent of parenchymal resection performed for the small peripheral lung cancer.

The importance of tumor biology and the focus upon treating the common occult systemic presence of the cancer was emphasized by breast surgical oncologists in the 1980s.[65] These same thought leaders in breast cancer treatment advocated breast-conserving surgical therapy over more radical extirpation of the "offending organ" popularized by Halsted and his surgical prodigy, which dominated surgical oncologic thought for over seven decades.[66,67] The surgical dogma of radical mastectomy fell to the new concepts of limited, breast-conserving surgery, sentinel axillary node sampling, and frequent use of adjunctive radiotherapy to facilitate local control of the malignant process. Of course, complete removal of the primary cancer and regional involved lymph nodes, a surgical concept respected from the time of John Hunter, continues to be a primary consideration.[68] However, greater focus upon aggressive use of systemic therapy for node-positive breast cancers, maintenance hormonal therapy for hormone receptor-positive tumors, and even prophylactic chemotherapy for high risk, node-negative breast cancers has become the standard of care. Many thoracic surgeons have incorporated the concepts mentioned for the management of breast cancer toward the treatment of the small peripheral lung cancer.[2,52,53,69–78] The biology of these small lung cancers certainly drives survival following resection rather than the extent or radicality of parenchymal resection performed in the local management of the tumor.

As we explore the use of lesser resections for the small peripheral lung cancer, some have begun to ask if alternative ablative approaches, such as focused radiotherapy or thermal ablation of the tumor, may provide equivalent local control to that of surgical resection. They have even questioned the need for excisional biopsy of the small lung lesion clinically suspicious for cancer. Certainly, ablative treatment of benign disease can potentially improve the survival statistics with these approaches.

We argue against such image-guided approaches as primary management of the good-risk patient. Beyond supporting the use of wedge or segmentectomy excision of the lesion to assure that we are dealing with a cancerous lesion, we again, agree with the clinical concepts supporting removal of small primary breast cancers. These advantages of surgical resection are certainly applicable to the management of the early-stage lung cancer. As noted in Table 77-3, these include confirmation of a malignant diagnosis prior to definitive treatment, removal of the entire tumor for improved local control with confirmation of clear surgical margins, accurate assessment of mediastinal and hilar lymph node involvement which identify "surprise" node positivity affecting adjuvant therapy decisions, and provision of adequate tissue for complete pharmacogenomic evaluation to provide individualized adjuvant therapy for patient with tumors with aggressive biologic characteristics for recurrence and systemic disease progression.

CONCLUSIONS

The role of surgery and extent of surgical resection required to affect local control and regional control of the small peripheral lung cancer continues to be evaluated.

Presently, national investigations are underway in North America and Japan randomizing sublobar resection or lobectomy for stage IA (intraoperative pathologic determination of node negativity and lesion size less than 2 cm in diameter) NSCLC will help to answer these surgical approach issues.[79,80]In addition, the completion of trials comparing the results of surgical resection with stereotactic radiotherapy for the peripheral clinical stage I lung cancer is needed to aid the thoracic oncologist in identifying the most effective individualized care of their lung cancer patients.

EDITOR'S COMMENT

This chapter elaborates on the debate regarding standard lobar resection for primary NSCLC and the use of sublobar approaches. In addition, the authors compare the data on open versus VATS resection of pulmonary metastases. Although there is little in the way of randomized data to support one approach over the other, the general approach is to offer lobectomy to patients who can tolerate it as a surgical approach. On the other hand, for patients who are at high risk, in whom a lobar resection may be associated with excessive morbidity or mortality, a sublobar approach or even ablative approach can be considered. This debate has particular applicability now that the data from the NLST are in and lung cancer screening is taking place more frequently. The management of the incidental subcentimeter nodule found on screening CT may prove to be an appropriate area for study in the use of sublobar resection.

—Mark J. Krasna

References

1. Ginsberg RJ, Rubinstein LV. Randomized trial of lobectomy versus limited resection for T1 N0 non-small cell lung cancer. Lung Cancer Study Group. *Ann Thorac Surg.* 1995;60:615–622; discussion 622–623.
2. Landreneau RJ, Sugarbaker DJ, Mack MJ, et al. Wedge resection versus lobectomy for stage I (T1 N0 M0) non-small cell lung cancer. *J Thorac Cardiovasc Surg.* 1997;113:691–698; discussion 698–700.
3. d'Amato TA, Galloway M, Szydlowski G, et al. Intraoperative brachytherapy following thoracoscopic wedge resection of stage I lung cancer. *Chest.* 1998;114:1112–1115.
4. Santos R, Colonias A, Parda D, et al. Comparison between sublobar resection and 125Iodine brachytherapy after sublobar resection in high-risk patients with stage I non-small cell lung cancer. *Surgery.* 2003;134:691–697; discussion 697.
5. Fernando HC, Santos RS, Benfield JR, et al. Lobar and sublobar resection with and without brachytherapy for small stage IA non-small cell lung cancer. *J Thorac Cardiovasc Surg.* 2005;129:261–267.
6. Miller JI, Hatcher CR, Jr. Limited resection of bronchogenic carcinoma in the patient with marked impairment of pulmonary function. *Ann Thorac Surg.* 1987;44:340–343.
7. Dowling RD, Landreneau RJ, Magee MJ, et al. Thoracoscopic wedge resection of the lung. *Surg Rounds.* 1993;16:341–349.
8. Landreneau RJ, Mack MJ, Keenan RJ, et al. Strategic planning for video-assisted thoracic surgery. *Ann Thorac Surg.* 1993;56:615–619.
9. Landreneau RJ, Mack MJ, Hazelrigg SR, et al. Video-assisted thoracic surgery: a minimally invasive approach to thoracic oncology. In: DeVita VT, Hellman S, Rosenberg SA, eds. *Cancer: Principles and Practice of Oncology-Update Series.* 4th ed. Philadelphia, PA: Lippincott; 1994:1–14.
10. Ferson PF, Landreneau RJ, Dowling RD, et al. Comparison of open versus thoracoscopic lung biopsy for diffuse infiltrative pulmonary disease. *J Thorac Cardiovasc Surg.* 1993;106:194–199.
11. Cooper JD, Perelman M, Todd TR, et al. Precision cautery excision of pulmonary lesions. *Ann Thorac Surg.* 1986;41:51–53.
12. Landreneau RJ, Hazelrigg SR, Johnson JA, et al. Neodymium:yttrium-aluminum garnet laser-assisted pulmonary resections. *Ann Thorac Surg.* 1991;51:973–977; discussion 977–978.
13. Noirclerc M, Dor V, Chauvin G, et al. [Extensive lateral thoracotomy without muscle section]. *Ann Chir Thorac Cardiovasc.* 1973;12:181–184.
14. Fry WA. Thoracic incisions. *Chest Surg Clin N Am.* 1995;5:177–188.
15. Horowitz MD, Ancalmo N, Ochsner JL. Thoracotomy through the auscultatory triangle. *Ann Thorac Surg.* 1989;47:782–783.
16. Ashour M. Modified muscle sparing posterolateral thoracotomy. *Thorax.* 1990;45:935–938.
17. Bethencourt DM, Holmes EC. Muscle-sparing posterolateral thoracotomy. *Ann Thorac Surg.* 1988;45:337–339.
18. Hazelrigg SR, Landreneau RJ, Boley TM, et al. The effect of muscle-sparing versus standard posterolateral thoracotomy on pulmonary function, muscle strength, and postoperative pain. *J Thorac Cardiovasc Surg.* 1991;101:394–400; discussion 400–401.
19. Pettiford BL, Schuchert MJ, Abbas G, et al. Anterior minithoracotomy: a direct approach to the difficult hilum for upper lobectomy, pneumonectomy, and sleeve lobectomy. *Ann Surg Oncol.* 2010;17:123–128.
20. d'Amato T, Santucci TS, Macherey RS, et al. Bilateral anterior minithoracotomy with video assistance for lung volume reduction surgery and pulmonary metastasectomy. *Surg Endosc.* 2002;16:364–366.
21. Bains MS, Ginsberg RJ, Jones WG 2nd, et al. The clamshell incision: an improved approach to bilateral pulmonary and mediastinal tumor. *Ann Thorac Surg.* 1994;58:30–32; discussion 33.
22. Roth JA, Pass HI, Wesley MN, et al. Comparison of median sternotomy and thoracotomy for resection of pulmonary metastases in patients with adult soft-tissue sarcomas. *Ann Thorac Surg.* 1986;42:134–138.
23. Meyers BF, Patterson GA. Technical aspects of adult lung transplantation. *Semin Thorac Cardiovasc Surg.* 1998;10:213–220.
24. Landreneau RJ, Hazelrigg SR, Mack MJ, et al. Postoperative pain-related morbidity: video-assisted thoracic surgery versus thoracotomy. *Ann Thorac Surg.* 1993;56:1285–1289.
25. Lemmer JH Jr., Gomez MN, Symreng T, et al. Limited lateral thoracotomy. Improved postoperative pulmonary function. *Arch Surg.* 1990;125:873–877.
26. Kirby TJ, Mack MJ, Landreneau RJ, et al. Lobectomy–video-assisted thoracic surgery versus muscle-sparing thoracotomy. A randomized trial. *J Thorac Cardiovasc Surg.* 1995;109:997–1001; discussion 1001–1002.
27. Landreneau RJ, Mack MJ, Hazelrigg SR, et al. Prevalence of chronic pain after pulmonary resection by thoracotomy or video-assisted thoracic surgery. *J Thorac Cardiovasc Surg.* 1994;107:1079–1085; discussion 1085–1086.
28. Mack MJ, Shennib H, Landreneau RJ, et al. Techniques for localization of pulmonary nodules for thoracoscopic resection. *J Thorac Cardiovasc Surg.* 1993;106:550–553.
29. Landreneau RJ, Hazelrigg SR, Ferson PF, et al. Thoracoscopic resection of 85 pulmonary lesions. *Ann Thorac Surg.* 1992;54:415–419; discussion 419–420.
30. National Lung Screening Trial Research T; Aberle DR, Adams AM, et al. Reduced lung-cancer mortality with low-dose computed tomographic screening. *N Engl J Med.* 2011;365:395–409.
31. International Early Lung Cancer Action Program I; Henschke CI, Yankelevitz DF, et al. Survival of patients with stage I lung cancer detected on CT screening. *N Engl J Med.* 2006;355:1763–1771.
32. Schuchert MJ, Abbas G, Awais O, et al. Anatomic segmentectomy for the solitary pulmonary nodule and early-stage lung cancer. *Ann Thorac Surg.* 2012;93:1780–1785; discussion 1786–1787.
33. Aberg T, Malmberg KA, Nilsson B, et al. The effect of metastasectomy: fact or fiction? *Ann Thorac Surg.* 1980;30:378–384.
34. Aberg T. Selection mechanisms as major determinants of survival after pulmonary metastasectomy. *Ann Thorac Surg.* 1997;63:611–612.
35. Pastorino U BM, Friedel G, Ginsberg RJ, et al. Long-term results of lung metastasectomy: prognostic analyses based on 5206 cases. The International Registry of Lung Metastases. *J Thorac Cardiovasc Surg.* 1997;113:37–49.
36. El-Sherif A, Gooding WE, Santos R, et al. Outcomes of sublobar resection versus lobectomy for stage I non-small cell lung cancer: a 13-year analysis. *Ann Thorac Surg.* 2006;82:408–415; discussion 415–416.
37. Takizawa T, Haga M, Yagi N, et al. Pulmonary function after segmentectomy for small peripheral carcinoma of the lung. *J Thorac Cardiovasc Surg.* 1999;118:536–541.
38. Keenan RJ, Landreneau RJ, Maley RH, Jr., et al. Segmental resection spares pulmonary function in patients with stage I lung cancer. *Ann Thorac Surg.* 2004;78:228–233; discussion 228–233.
39. Treasure T. Pulmonary metastasectomy: a common practice based on weak evidence. *Ann R Coll Surg Engl.* 2007;89:744–748.
40. McCormack PM, Bains MS, Begg CB, et al. Role of video-assisted thoracic surgery in the treatment of pulmonary metastases: results of a prospective trial. *Ann Thorac Surg.* 1996;62:213–216; discussion 216–217.
41. Landreneau RJ. Commentary. *Ann Thorac Surg.* 1996;62:216–217.
42. Horton R. Surgical research or comic opera: questions, but few answers. *Lancet.* 1996;347:984–985.
43. McCormack PM, Burt ME, Bains MS, et al. Lung resection for colorectal metastases. 10-year results. *Arch Surg.* 1992;127:1403–1406.
44. Lin JC, Wiechmann RJ, Szwerc MF, et al. Diagnostic and therapeutic video-assisted thoracic surgery resection of pulmonary metastases. *Surgery.* 1999;126:636–641; discussion 641–642.
45. McCormack PM, Ginsberg KB, Bains MS, et al. Accuracy of lung imaging in metastases with implications for the role of thoracoscopy. *Ann Thorac Surg.* 2001;56:863–865; discussion 865–866.
46. Landreneau RJ. Commentary. *Ann Thorac Surg.* 1993;56:867.
47. Landreneau RJ, De Giacomo T, Mack MJ, et al. Therapeutic video-assisted thoracoscopic surgical resection of colorectal pulmonary metastases. *Eur J Cardiothorac Surg.* 2000;18:671–676; discussion 676–677.
48. Mutsaerts EL, Zoetmulder FA, Meijer S, et al. Outcome of thoracoscopic pulmonary metastasectomy evaluated by confirmatory thoracotomy. *Ann Thorac Surg.* 2001;72:230–233.
49. Schuchert MJ, Pettiford BL, Luketich JD, et al. Parenchymal-sparing resections: why, when, and how. *Thorac Surg Clin.* 2008;18:93–105.
50. Schuchert MJ, Pettiford BL, Keeley S, et al. Anatomic segmentectomy in the treatment of stage I non-small cell lung cancer. *Ann Thorac Surg.* 2007;84:926–932; discussion 932–933.
51. Carr SR, Schuchert MJ, Pennathur A, et al. Impact of tumor size on outcomes after anatomic lung resection for stage 1 A non-small cell lung cancer based on the current staging system. *J Thorac Cardiovasc Surg.* 2012; 143:390–397.

52. Jensik RJ, Faber LP, Milloy FJ, et al. Segmental resection for lung cancer. A fifteen-year experience. *J Thorac Cardiovasc Surg.* 1973;66:563–572.
53. Read RC, Yoder G, Schaeffer RC. Survival after conservative resection for T1 N0 M0 non-small cell lung cancer. *Ann Thorac Surg.* 1990;49:391–398; discussion 399–400.
54. Mery CM, Pappas AN, Bueno R, et al. Similar long-term survival of elderly patients with non-small cell lung cancer treated with lobectomy or wedge resection within the surveillance, epidemiology, and end results database. *Chest.* 2005;128:237–245.
55. Harada H, Okada M, Sakamoto T, et al. Functional advantage after radical segmentectomy versus lobectomy for lung cancer. *Ann Thorac Surg.* 2005;80:2041–2045.
56. Allen MS, Darling GE, Pechet TT, et al. Morbidity and mortality of major pulmonary resections in patients with early-stage lung cancer: initial results of the randomized, prospective ACOSOG Z0030 trial. *Ann Thorac Surg.* 2006;81:1013–1019; discussion 1019–1020.
57. Lopez-Encuentra A, Garcia-Lujan R, Rivas JJ, et al. Comparison between clinical and pathologic staging in 2,994 cases of lung cancer. *Ann Thorac Surg.* 2005;79:974–979; discussion 979.
58. Whitson BA, Groth SS, Maddaus MA. Surgical assessment and intraoperative management of mediastinal lymph nodes in non-small cell lung cancer. *Ann Thorac Surg.* 2007;84:1059–1065.
59. Schuchert MJ, Abbas G, Pennathur A, et al. Anatomic lung resection for clinical stage I non-small cell lung cancer, (NSCLC): equivalent outcomes following anatomic segmentectomy and lobectomy. *Proceedings of the the American College of Chest Physicians.* Vancouver, BC, Canada.
60. Arriagada R, Bergman B, Dunant A, et al. Cisplatin-based adjuvant chemotherapy in patients with completely resected non-small cell lung cancer. *N Engl J Med.* 2004;350:351–360.
61. Winton T, Livingston R, Johnson D, et al. Vinorelbine plus cisplatin vs. observation in resected non-small cell lung cancer. *N Engl J Med.* 2005;352:2589–2597.
62. Douillard JY, Rosell R, De Lena M, et al. Adjuvant vinorelbine plus cisplatin versus observation in patients with completely resected stage IB-IIIA non-small cell lung cancer (Adjuvant Navelbine International Trialist Association [ANITA]): a randomised controlled trial. *Lancet Oncol.* 2006;7:719–727.
63. Errett LE, Wilson J, Chiu RC, et al. Wedge resection as an alternative procedure for peripheral bronchogenic carcinoma in poor-risk patients. *J Thorac Cardiovasc Surg.* 1985;90:656–661.
64. Treasure T. The evidence on which to base practice: different tools for different times. *Eur J Cardiothorac Surg.* 2006;30:819–824.
65. Fisher B, Anderson SJ. The breast cancer alternative hypothesis: is there evidence to justify replacing it? *J Clin Oncol.* 2010;28:366–374.
66. Halsted WS. The results of operations for the cure of cancer of the breast performed at the Johns Hopkins Hospital from June 1889, to January 1894. *Johns Hopkins Med Rep.* 4:297.
67. Imber G. *Genius on the Edge: The Bizarre Double Life of Dr. William Stewart Halsted.* New York, NY: Kaplan Pub.; 2010: x, 389 pp.
68. Moore W. *The Knife Man.* London: Bantam Press; 2005: xiii, 482 pp.
69. Lewis RJ. The role of video-assisted thoracic surgery for carcinoma of the lung: wedge resection to lobectomy by simultaneous individual stapling. *Ann Thorac Surg.* 1993;56:762–768.
70. Ketchedjian A, Daly B, Landreneau R, et al. Sublobar resection for the subcentimeter pulmonary nodule. *Semin Thorac Cardiovasc Surg.* 2005;17: 128–133.
71. Schuchert MJ, Kilic A, Pennathur A, et al. Oncologic outcomes after surgical resection of subcentimeter non-small cell lung cancer. *Ann Thorac Surg.* 2011;91:1681–1687; discussion 1687–1688.
72. Okada M, Koike T, Higashiyama M, et al. Radical sublobar resection for small-sized non-small cell lung cancer: a multicenter study. *J Thorac Cardiovasc Surg.* 2006;132:769–775.
73. Sienel W, Dango S, Kirschbaum A, et al. Sublobar resections in stage IA non-small cell lung cancer: segmentectomies result in significantly better cancer-related survival than wedge resections. *Eur J Cardiothorac Surg.* 2008;33:728–734.
74. Sawabata N, Ohta M, Matsumura A, et al. Optimal distance of malignant negative margin in excision of nonsmall cell lung cancer: a multicenter prospective study. *Ann Thorac Surg.* 2004;77:415–420.
75. El-Sherif A, Fernando HC, Santos R, et al. Margin and local recurrence after sublobar resection of non-small cell lung cancer. *Ann Surg Oncol.* 2007;14:2400–2405.
76. Swanson SJ. Video-assisted thoracic surgery segmentectomy: the future of surgery for lung cancer? *Ann Thorac Surg.* 2010;89:S2096–S2097.
77. Schuchert MJ, Pettiford BL, Pennathur A, et al. Anatomic segmentectomy for stage I non-small-cell lung cancer: comparison of video-assisted thoracic surgery versus open approach. *J Thorac Cardiovasc Surg.* 2009;138:1318–1325. e1311.
78. Kilic A, Schuchert MJ, Pettiford BL, et al. Anatomic segmentectomy for stage I non-small cell lung cancer in the elderly. *Ann Thorac Surg.* 2009;87: 1662–1666; discussion 1667–1668.
79. A phase III randomized trial of lobectomy versus sublobar resection for small (<2 cm) peripheral non-small cell lung cancer. CALGB 140503.Clinical Trials.gov Identifier: NCT00499330.
80. Nakamura K, Saji H, Nakajima R, et al. A phase III randomized trial of lobectomy versus limited resection for small-sized peripheral non-small cell lung cancer (JCOG0802/WJOG4607 L). *Jpn J Clin Oncol.* 2010;40: 271–274.

78 Pulmonary Metastasectomy

Bryan M. Burt, Carlos M. Mery, and Michael T. Jaklitsch

Keywords: Pulmonary metastases, extrathoracic primary tumors, carcinoma, sarcoma, germ cell tumors, melanoma, solitary pulmonary nodule, role of surgical resection

The recognition of pulmonary metastases from an extrathoracic primary tumor is a dramatic and emotional change in the care of the cancer patient. The clinical situation immediately changes from potential cure to the tacit acknowledgment of probable incurability. Goals of therapy change from living without evidence of disease to living, and living well, with systemic disease. We believe that pulmonary metastasectomy in carefully selected patients contributes to quality of life and may give the patient extended periods of time without obvious disease.

Many primary tumors metastasize to specific target organs.[1] In the 1930s, it was noted that patients dying of pulmonary metastases frequently failed to exhibit extrapulmonary disease at autopsy.[2] As a result, several surgeons felt that it would be reasonable to offer surgical resection of these lesions in the hope of prolonging survival. The first reported pulmonary metastasectomy removed a single renal cell metastasis in 1930, and the patient lived for two more decades.[3] Interest in this surgical approach was increased with the development of systemic adjuvant chemotherapy, which appeared to increase survival.

The role of surgical resection of metastatic disease, however, is not universally accepted in the nonsurgical community. No randomized trial has been constructed to establish a survival advantage of pulmonary metastasectomy. In fact, the multitude of variables that would have to be included in the eligibility criteria (e.g., number of metastases, cell type, disease-free interval [DFI], cardiorespiratory reserve) makes it unlikely that a randomized trial of this nature will ever be performed. Without such data, however, some authors remain skeptical that surgical resection adds significant benefit.[4,5] Opponents to this approach point out that larger trials claiming improved survival after metastasectomy have been conducted in heterogeneous populations with tumors of mixed histologic types and mixed doubling times. The patients who benefit the most from surgical resection have a small tumor burden and a long doubling time (DFI), and this group may be able to live a long time with their disease even without surgical resection. The skeptics argue that a hypothetical study population that included slow-growing tumors in 40% of the subjects would produce a 30% 5-year survival after surgery, and that same 30% also would still be alive without an operation.

These arguments highlight the heterogeneity of this patient population and emphasize the need to tailor the surgical approach to each individual patient. Patients with dozens of metastases or rapid recurrence after a previous pulmonary metastasectomy will not gain major benefit from surgery. A very elderly patient with a slow-growing metastasis that would require pneumonectomy for resection might be better treated in other ways. These exceptions still leave many patients with pulmonary metastases that can be removed safely with an anticipated low morbidity and mortality.[6]

A large volume of retrospective data is available to substantiate a significant long-term survival with pulmonary metastasectomy. When these data are compared with those of patients with pulmonary metastases who did not undergo metastasectomy, it is likely that pulmonary metastasectomy affords a distinct survival benefit.[7–13] Furthermore, resection has other advantages. It can prevent further growth and consumption of lung tissue (dyspnea), hemoptysis, and chest wall invasion with subsequent pain.

The International Registry of Lung Metastases was established in 1991 to document long-term results and has accrued data on 5206 cases of pulmonary metastasectomy. The distribution of primary malignancies in this data bank was shown to be 43% carcinoma, 42% sarcoma, 7% germ cell tumors, and 6% melanoma. Actuarial 5- and 10-year survival rates after complete metastasectomy were 36% and 26%, respectively. Determinants of improved survival include complete resection, DFI (time from removal of primary tumor to recognition of pulmonary metastases) of 36 months or greater, and single metastasis. These results provide strong evidence that pulmonary metastasectomy is a safe and potentially curative procedure, because it is highly unlikely that a slow tumor doubling time could produce a 26% 10-year survival rate.[6]

Surgical resection of a single pulmonary metastasis has become a widely accepted treatment modality for properly selected patients. Opinions vary widely, however, regarding the utility of surgical resection in the face of multiple metastases, lung and lymph node metastases, or repeat metastases after a previous pulmonary metastasectomy. Each of these topics is explored in this chapter. We also examine the current indications for pulmonary metastasectomy, outcomes of surgery, prognostic indicators by cell type where data are available, and the approach to treatment of extrathoracic pulmonary metastases.

INDICATIONS

Ehrenhaft et al.[14] published the first "criteria for pulmonary metastasectomy" in 1958. The current indications have remained largely the same but with slight evolution:

1. Control of the primary site
2. No other distant extrapulmonary metastatic disease or, if present, immediate plans to control it with surgery or another treatment modality
3. Pulmonary metastases that are thought to be completely resectable, even if located in both the lungs
4. Adequate cardiopulmonary reserve of the patient
5. A technically feasible operation

Additional criteria for pulmonary metastasectomy have been described and include no other effective treatment except resection, difficulty of differential diagnosis from lung cancer, and symptomatic pulmonary metastases.[15–17] Among patients who do not fulfill the preceding criteria, surgery should proceed only if it will provide ample palliation, such as in situations of bronchial obstruction or distal pulmonary suppuration. The criteria for surgical resection will continue to evolve as we gain a better understanding for cell type-specific tumor biology and as improved systemic treatment becomes available.

Once it is determined that a patient meets the criteria for surgical intervention, the decision to proceed should be made in cooperation with a thoracic surgeon and a medical oncologist. A multidisciplinary approach offers the benefit of coordinating the timing of surgery and systemic treatment both now and in the face of future recurrence.

RADIOLOGIC STAGING

Preoperative staging and operative planning largely depend on cross-sectional imaging. Radiologic staging is inaccurate in a large proportion of patients, however, and underestimates the burden of disease. In many centers, thorough intraoperative staging by open bimanual palpation is performed in every patient to optimize resection of all metastatic deposits, particularly when more than one lesion is identified on preoperative radiographs.[6]

Helical CT scanners are now widely available. They allow thin-section imaging of the chest and detect approximately 20% to 25% more nodules than conventional CT scanning.[18,19] Large retrospective studies comparing high-resolution helical CT scanning with intraoperative detection of lesions by manual palpation have demonstrated sensitivities of 78% to 82% for CT detection. Approximately 22% of patients would have residual malignant deposits detectable by palpation if CT alone was used to guide resection.[20,21] Helical CT scanning may not be sensitive enough to obviate the need for manual lung palpation if the goal is resection of all detectable metastases. The magnitude of survival benefit with removal of deposits so small that they can only be detected by palpation, however, is uncertain. This is an important issue with the availability of minimally invasive thoracoscopic approaches to pulmonary metastasectomy that preclude manual palpation of the lung.

Helical CT scanning is most likely to miss nodules smaller than 6 mm in diameter. Sensitivity of CT scanning decreases in proportion to the size of the metastatic lesion. Sensitivity is 100% for lesions larger than 10 mm but only 66% for lesions between 6 and 10 mm.[21] Manual palpation can detect 2-mm nodules at the surface of the lung and 4-mm nodules in the central part of the lobe. Clearly, a CT scan can preclude surgery if the number of nodules prevents a feasible operation.

There is no pathognomonic radiographic feature that distinguishes metastatic disease from primary lung cancer. That said, metastatic nodules often are observed to be well-circumscribed spherical deposits with smooth margins. They are predominantly subpleural in location or located in the outer third of the lung fields, and when multiple nodules are present, the probability of metastatic disease increases significantly. So-called lollipop nodules, which have the appearance of distinct round nodules at the end of a terminal pulmonary artery branch, also raise suspicion for a metastatic process. Primary bronchogenic lung cancer, conversely, often demonstrates irregular borders and associated linear densities.

The presence of a new radiographic nodule in a patient with prior malignancy represents a cancer in more than two-thirds of cases, probably as a function of nodule size (Table 78-1). For patients with a history of extrathoracic malignancy, the probability of a malignant solitary pulmonary nodule ranges from 67% for subcentimeter nodules to 91% for nodules larger than 3 cm. For all lesions smaller than 3 cm, the chance is essentially equal that the nodule represents a primary lung cancer or extrathoracic metastasis. For nodules larger than 3 cm in size, the probability of a primary lung cancer is greater.[22]

Table 78-1

DIAGNOSIS AS A FUNCTION OF SIZE AMONG PATIENTS WITH A HISTORY OF EXTRATHORACIC MALIGNANCY

TUMOR SIZE (CM)	NO.	BENIGN	LUNG CANCER	METASTASES
<1.0	81	27 (33)	23 (28)	31 (38)
1.0–1.9	103	25 (24)	43 (42)	35 (34)
2.0–2.9	50	4 (8)	23 (46)	23 (46)
≥3.0	54	5 (9)	29 (54)	20 (37)
Total	288	61 (21)	118 (41)	109 (38)

Note: Values as number followed by percent.
Reproduced with permission from reference Monteiro A, Arce N, Bernardo J, et al. Surgical resection of lung metastases from epithelial tumors. *Ann Thorac Surg*. 2004;77:431–437; Extrathoracic Malignancy.

PROGNOSTIC DETERMINANTS

Many patient and tumor factors have been found to predict improved survival after metastasectomy. Most commonly, these include a long DFI after treatment of the primary tumor, a low number of pulmonary metastases, and favorable cell type.[6] The actual determinants may be discordant among different reports, likely owing to variance in definitions, measured endpoints, different grouping of cell types, and perhaps different tumor biology.

One positive predictive element ubiquitous to nearly all reports of pulmonary metastasectomy is the poor consequences of incomplete resection. Complete removal of all metastatic deposits is associated with long-term survival (Fig. 78-1).

DFI is regarded by many authors to be important. However, in a review of 32 retrospective reports of pulmonary metastasectomy, 19 reports determined that DFI was a significant prognostic factor, whereas 13 indicated that it was of no consequence.[23] The heterogeneous and small populations represented in these studies make this point difficult to interpret. The International Registry of Lung Metastases was established in 1991 to answer these types of questions. This registry, reported over 20 years ago, has accumulated its data through voluntary reporting by surgeons throughout the world. DFI is an important prognostic marker in this registry. It is important to note that the DFI is considered in terms of likelihood of achieving long-term disease-free survival but is not an absolute indication or contraindication to surgery.

Studies are evenly divided with respect to whether the number of metastatic lesions affects prognosis after pulmonary metastasectomy. Based on 15 reports in the literature,

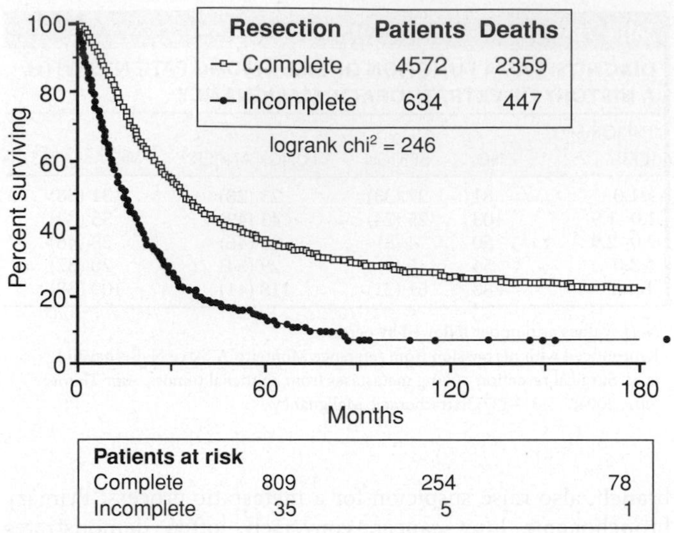

Figure 78-1. Complete resection versus incomplete resection: overall actuarial survival after pulmonary metastasectomy. The number of patients at risk at 5, 10, and 15 years is shown at the bottom of the curve. (Reproduced with permission from Pastorino U, Buyse M, Godehard F, et al. Long-term results of lung metastasectomy: prognostic analyses based on 5206 cases. The International Registry of Lung Metastases. *J Thorac Cardiovasc Surg.* 1997;113:37–49; Fig. 1)

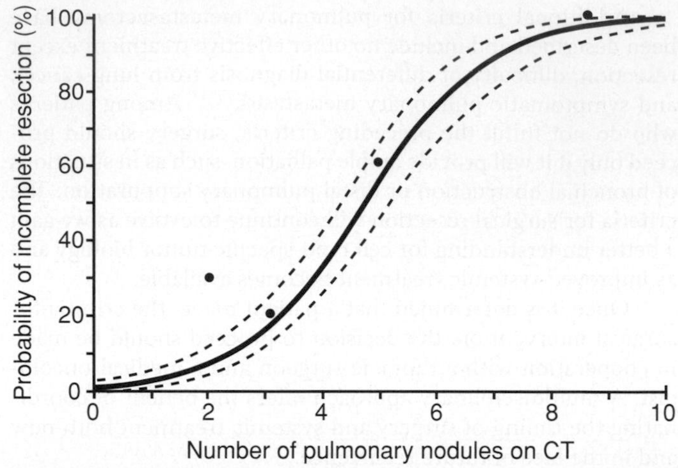

Figure 78-2. Probability of incomplete resection according to the number of pulmonary nodules for metastatic renal cell carcinoma. Filled circles are actuarial probabilities, and the solid line is logistic regression estimate (enclosed within dashed 68% confidence limits). (Reproduced with permission from Murthy SC, Kim K, Rice TW, et al. Can we predict long-term survival after pulmonary metastasectomy for renal cell carcinoma? *Ann Thorac Surg.* 2005;79:996–1003; Fig. 2.)

Todd[23] found that the number of metastatic lesions was a consistent factor for sarcomatous metastases, in which fewer than five lesions was associated with a more favorable outcome.[23] For epithelial tumors, the probability of incomplete resection has been a function of the number of pulmonary nodules (Fig. 78-2)[24] and the presence of more than one lesion may increase the probability of lung metastases to recur.[25] The important issue for the surgeon considering resection of multiple metastases is the feasibility of the operation. If several nodules need to be removed from the same lobe or a central nodule needs to be removed, a lobectomy may be required. As more lung tissue is removed, the perioperative risks increase.

Histology of the tumor itself is remarkable for the extremes of survival benefit. Germ cell tumors are associated with a very good prognosis. The prognosis associated with multiple melanoma metastases, lung primary metastases to the other lung, and pancreatic metastases is so poor that surgery likely will not benefit the patient.[26]

APPROACH TO SURGERY

Two main principles direct the surgical approach for resection of pulmonary metastases: complete resection of malignancy and maximal sparing of normal lung tissue. Complete resection of metastatic disease is not only the goal but also an important predictor of survival in nearly all reported series. All resections are performed conservatively, leaving as much normal parenchyma as possible. For peripheral nodules, this usually means wedge resection. For deeper nodules, segmentectomy may be required. This conservative approach leaves the patient with a greater degree of cardiopulmonary reserve to withstand subsequent treatments, should a recurrence appear, and maintains the patient's quality of life. Mortality rates of pulmonary metastasectomy do not differ from those of resection for lung cancer and range between 0.6% and 2%.[6,27]

Bronchoscopy is indicated in patients with centrally located lesions, in patients with symptoms of airway involvement, and in patients with cell types that are prone to endobronchial involvement, such as breast, colon, and renal cell cancers.[28]

Single-lung anesthesia is used. Complete atelectasis of the lung will ensure adequate palpation of pulmonary parenchyma in open procedures and permits the technique of thoracoscopic exploration and resection.

The choice of incision for unilateral disease is somewhat controversial. Lateral thoracotomy has been the most commonly described approach to pulmonary metastasectomy. This approach offers adequate access to all areas of the hemithorax and permits wedge or anatomic resection under direct vision.

Some authors favor median sternotomy as an approach to unilateral disease. This incision has the advantages of simultaneous examination of both the lungs, identification and treatment of contralateral occult disease, and reduced postoperative discomfort and deficit in pulmonary function. Its disadvantage in pulmonary metastasectomy is difficult exposure of the posterior costovertebral lung fields and the lateral left lower lobe. The bilateral anterior thoracotomy (clamshell incision) provides excellent exposure to the posterior aspect of both lungs, but is complicated by increased postoperative pain.

Inspection of both hemithoraces in treatment of unilateral disease will identify occult tumor deposits in some cases; however, there does not appear to be a survival advantage to this approach compared with lateral thoracotomy.[29] Known bilateral lesions are resected via median sternotomy, the clamshell approach, or two-stage bilateral thoracotomy.

Metastatic lesions involving the diaphragm, chest wall, mediastinum, and pericardium are often resectable. Five-year survival after extended resections including chest wall and diaphragm has been reported to be as high as 25%.[30]

VIDEO-ASSISTED THORACOSCOPIC SURGERY

Video-assisted thoracoscopic surgery (VATS) is a less-invasive alternative to thoracotomy or sternotomy. VATS approaches are applicable for both diagnostic purposes and therapeutic metastasectomy, provided that the lesions are located in the peripheral third of the lung. The advantages of thoracoscopic resection include improved postoperative recovery, shorter hospital stay, and decreased long-term morbidity. Disadvantages include the risk of incomplete resection, which possibly could be alleviated by thoracotomy and direct palpation.

Most pulmonary metastases are located in the peripheral third of the lung and are accessible by a thoracoscopic approach.[31] Generally, the lesion should be small and located in the outer third of the lung, and endobronchial involvement should be absent. Conversion to an open approach is appropriate for lesions located deeper in the lung parenchyma or if all suspicious lesions cannot be identified in a timely manner. To avoid seeding of the intercostal port site, the specimen should be extracted in a sterile specimen bag.

Much of the controversy over the VATS approach to metastasectomy centers on the belief that manual palpation of the deflated lung is essential to identifying all metastatic diseases, a technique precluded by a thoracoscopic approach. Retrospective and prospective studies have concluded that VATS is an inadequate procedure for pulmonary metastasectomy because identification of all metastatic foci is not possible without a complete manual palpation of the entire lung.[32,33] The number of missed lesions on preoperative conventional CT scanning was too high. One prospective trial was closed after 18 metastasectomies begun using a VATS approach and completed with thoracotomy for complete lung palpation, which resulted in 56% failure rate of CT and VATS to detect all lesions. This study has been criticized for the quality and uniformity of CT imaging used, because high-quality CT imaging is vital to success when considering the VATS approach to metastasectomy.

The bigger question concerning manual palpation of the lung and discovery of all occult lesions during the operation is whether this approach has any effect on survival. It is quite possible that the same long-term results can be achieved with repeat metastasectomy by either repeat VATS or thoracotomy, if occult lesions become apparent clinically.

VATS may be a more appropriate operative choice for certain types of tumors, such as colorectal carcinoma, which most often presents with a single metastasis, as confirmed at thoracotomy.[34] It has been shown that the incidence of pulmonary recurrence associated with VATS metastasectomy for colorectal cancer is approximately 20%, which is similar to the findings observed with open approaches.[34]

VATS is an excellent diagnostic approach for differentiating benign lesions, metastases, or a new primary in patients with solitary pulmonary nodules and a history of antecedent cancer. Among patients with no history of cancer, there is a 63% chance that the solitary pulmonary nodule will be malignant. The chance for malignancy is 82% for patients with antecedent lung cancer, with lung cancer being the most common etiology. Patients with a history of extrathoracic malignancy have a 79% probability of malignancy and roughly even odds that the metastasis is from the previous cancer versus a lung cancer.[22] Although CT scan quantification of attenuation, shape, size, and texture characteristics of solitary pulmonary nodules shows promise for accurately differentiating benign from malignant lesions, differentiating metastases from primary lung cancers is not yet possible. In our opinion, resection is the most reliable method for diagnosis and is essential to designing the best therapeutic strategy for maximizing survival. VATS resection is well suited for this objective.

LYMPH NODE INVOLVEMENT

Hilar or mediastinal lymph node involvement sometimes accompanies pulmonary metastases. Determinants of nodal involvement, as well as the prognostic and therapeutic implications, are poorly understood. The frequency with which pulmonary metastases can metastasize to regional lymph nodes is not well characterized and is a subject of debate. In an autopsy series, a 33% incidence of mediastinal lymph node metastases was seen in patients with extrapulmonary carcinoma.[35] Several retrospective reviews have reported the incidence of hilar or mediastinal lymph node metastases to be 5% to 28.6%.[6,36–38] Lymph node metastases are found more commonly with carcinoma than with sarcoma.

Several retrospective reviews have attempted to clarify the importance of systematic regional lymph node dissection during pulmonary metastasectomy.[37,38] Only a few reports have addressed the prognostic value of lymph node metastases in patients undergoing metastasectomy. In some series, it is reported that the only factor affecting survival is the presence of metastatically involved lymph nodes.[37] In a series of nonsarcomatous extrathoracic primary malignancy, lymph node metastases were found in 29% of the 70 patients undergoing complete lymphadenectomy, and tumor recurrence was significantly higher in patients with lymph node metastases. Three-year survival was 38% for those with lymph node metastases versus 69% for those without. The presence of hilar or mediastinal lymph node metastases predicts poor survival in colorectal[39,40] and renal cell metastases.[24] Others have shown a trend rather than a statistically significant difference toward improved survival in patients without involvement of mediastinal lymph nodes when all cell types are studied.[38] Clearly, the relevance of nodal metastases should be explored within each cell type.

Although the standard accepted resection for primary lung cancer is either complete lymphadenectomy or lymph node sampling, this is not true for the treatment of pulmonary metastases. Routine lymph node dissection is not performed uniformly. Some authors recommend consideration of complete mediastinal lymph node dissection at the time of pulmonary metastasectomy to improve staging and guide treatment.[37] We and other authors believe that a pulmonary metastasis will exhibit the same pattern of lymphatic drainage as a primary lung cancer (Fig. 78-3). In other words, pulmonary metastases can metastasize. If a draining node is confirmed to be involved with metastatic disease at the time of surgery, we recommend anatomic resection when possible.[24,39,40] Some authors recommend the same guidelines for assessment as one would use in a patient with a primary lung cancer, including mediastinoscopy and lymph node dissection. We cannot definitively say whether prophylactic regional lymph node dissection at the time of pulmonary metastasectomy contributes to improved survival, although it does allow more accurate oncologic staging and may signal the need for adjuvant therapy.

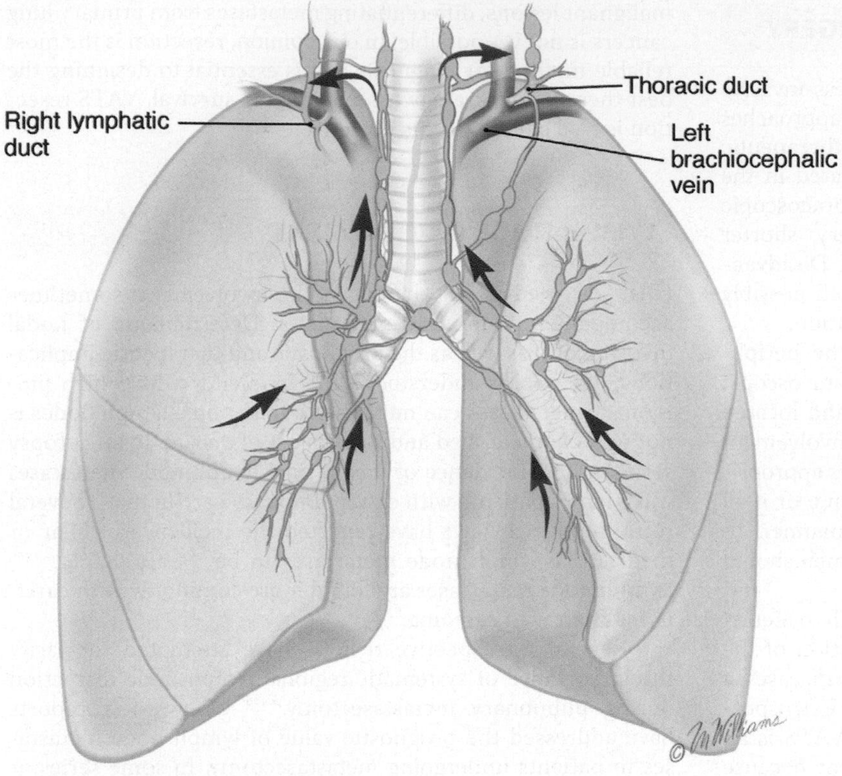

Figure 78-3. Draining lymph nodes that are confirmed to have metastatic involvement by an extrathoracic primary should be resected anatomically, because these foci will exhibit the same pattern of lymphatic drainage as primary lung cancers and also may metastasize.

CELL TYPES AND OUTCOMES

Many retrospective series on pulmonary metastasectomy report overall 5-year survival rates of 30% to 40%.[6,27] Data from the International Registry of Lung Metastases showed that after complete resection, the 5-year survival was 33% for patients with a DFI of 0 to 11 months after control of the primary malignancy and 45% for those with a DFI greater than 36 months. For single lesions, the 5-year survival was 43%, and it was 27% for four or more lesions. Global overall survival was 36% at 5 years, 26% at 10 years, and 22% at 15 years after complete resection. These data represent the gamut of epithelial, sarcoma, melanoma, and germ cell tumors, for which the benefit of resection will depend on specific tumor histology (Fig. 78-4)[6]. The literature on cell type-specific experience with pulmonary metastasectomy is growing.

Colorectal Cancer

Although several new chemotherapeutic agents have shown promising effects on systemic metastases, no standard chemotherapy has been found to improve survival significantly in patients with colorectal metastases to the lung. Encouraging surgical results have led to the acceptance of aggressive surgical management. The overall 5- and 10-year survival rates are approximately 35% to 45% and 20% to 30%, respectively.[41–45] Important prognostic factors include number of pulmonary metastases, carcinoembryonic antigen level, and regional lymph node involvement.[17]

Renal Cell Cancer

Pulmonary resection for renal cell metastases can offer a 20% to 50% 5-year survival.[24,46,47] Larger number and size of nodules, increasing number of lymph node metastases, shorter DFI, and decreased preoperative forced vital capacity are predictive risk factors for death in this population.[24]

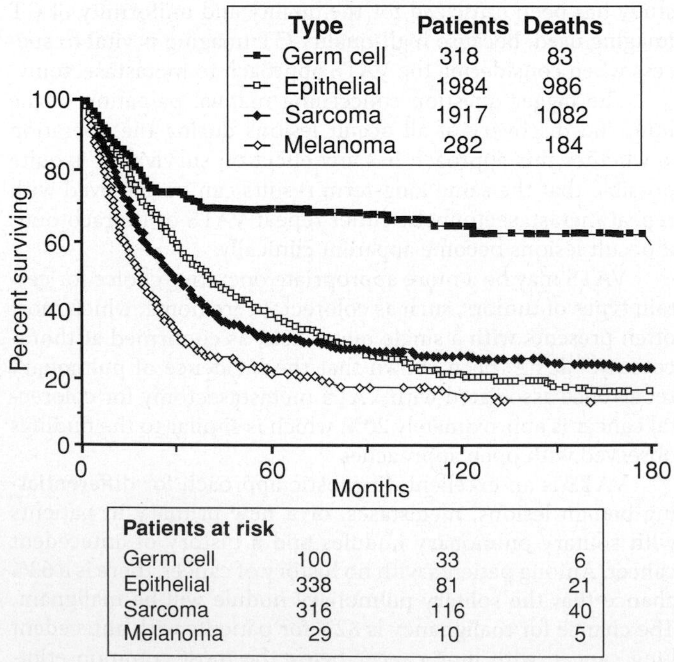

Figure 78-4. Survival of patients following complete resection according to four major tumor types: epithelial, sarcoma, germ cell, and melanoma. (Reproduced with permission from Pastorino U, Buyse M, Godehard F, et al. Long-term results of lung metastasectomy: prognostic analyses based on 5206 cases. The International Registry of Lung Metastases. *J Thorac Cardiovasc Surg.* 1997;113:37–49; Fig. 4.)

Germ Cell Cancers

The advent of effective chemotherapy has changed the management of pulmonary metastases of germ cell tumors dramatically, and chemotherapy is now the first line of treatment. Surgical resection has been relegated to an adjuvant form of therapy and is reserved for patients who have a complete serologic response to chemotherapy with normalization of serum tumor markers and residual primary lesions. Although surgery may benefit patients who have had a decrease in serum markers shy of complete normalization, the patient with continued elevation of markers is likely better served with a change in chemotherapy. For most patients with germ cell cancers, pulmonary resection is no longer used as primary treatment.

Cisplatin-based chemotherapy is essential as initial treatment for nonseminomatous testicular cancer. Pathologic findings of mature teratoma or necrosis in resected pulmonary metastases indicate good prognosis, with only a 5% to 10% relapse rate. Pulmonary resection is used both diagnostically and therapeutically to determine whether active microscopic disease is still present after normalization of tumor markers and to remove residual mature teratoma. The 5-year survival rate for patients who have these tumors is 68% to 82% after pulmonary metastasectomy.[48]

Sarcoma

Sarcoma has a natural tendency to metastasize to the lungs. Isolated pulmonary sarcoma metastases occur in 23% to 54% of patients with sarcoma.[49] Pulmonary metastasectomy is an important method of therapy since most sarcomas are relatively chemoresistent. Several retrospective studies have established 3-year survivals of 20% to 54% for patients with surgical resection of sarcoma lung metastases.[50] Sarcomas are a heterogeneous group with over 50 different histologic subtypes. Among patients with soft-tissue sarcoma that develop pulmonary metastases, the most common histologic findings include malignant fibrous histiocytoma, synovial sarcoma, and leiomyosarcoma.[51]

Osteosarcoma

Operative resection is the only potentially curative treatment for patients with thoracic metastases from osteogenic sarcoma. After the primary tumor has been resected, routine adjuvant chemotherapy can improve the disease-free survival and decrease the burden of metastatic pulmonary disease.[52] The 5-year survival for pulmonary metastases is related to the timing of appearance with respect to the initiation of chemotherapy. Survival when lesions are detected after completion of chemotherapy is significantly better than with the appearance of metastases during chemotherapy.[53] Global 5-year survival rates after pulmonary metastasectomy range from 20% to 50%.[23,28]

Soft-Tissue Sarcoma

Soft-tissue sarcomas are notoriously resistant to chemotherapy and almost always metastasize solely to the lungs. Surgery remains the only potential curative treatment, and the median survival after diagnosis of pulmonary metastases without surgery is 15 months. Reported 5-year survival rates after pulmonary metastasectomy for soft-tissue sarcoma range from 25% to 35%.[54,55] Factors associated with improved survival among different reports include prolonged DFI, low-grade tumor, young age, slow tumor doubling time, low number of nodules, histology of malignant fibrocystic histiocytoma, and unilateral disease.[54,55]

Breast Cancer

Metastatic surgery for breast cancer is highly controversial because of the availability of other effective systemic treatments such as chemotherapy, hormone therapy, and molecular targeting therapy. Dramatic improvements in these treatment options have made pulmonary resection less common. Large retrospective data sets, however, suggest that resection for lung metastases from breast cancer may provide equal or better long-term results than chemotherapy and hormone therapy, with 31% to 50% 5-year survival.[23,56] Postoperative survival is influenced by estrogen receptor status and DFI in some studies.[56,57] We believe that solitary pulmonary nodules in patients with previous breast cancer are best treated with excisional biopsy because differentiation from primary lung cancer is difficult. In general, these patients are worked up in preparation for possible lobectomy, if the tissue diagnosis is consistent with a lung primary. For multiple metastases from breast cancer, medical treatment should be the first-line therapy after establishing a tissue diagnosis.

Gynecologic Cancers

Encouraging results have been reported for pulmonary metastasectomy of uterine cancers. Five-year survival of 47% is reported for squamous cell carcinoma, 33% to 40% for cervical adenocarcinoma, 76% for endometrial adenocarcinoma, and 86% for choriocarcinoma.[58]

Melanoma

Pulmonary metastases from malignant melanoma are associated with poor survival owing to the aggressive behavior of this tumor and its propensity to metastasize systemically to other sites besides the lung. The largest melanoma series, based on 7564 patients, found a 12% incidence of pulmonary metastases in patients with melanoma and an associated 5-year survival rate of 4%. However, of those patients who underwent resection of a solitary pulmonary nodule, 5-year survival was 20%, and patients with two pulmonary nodules undergoing resection fared better than those with three or more nodules. DFI, negative lymph nodes, and treatment with chemotherapy are also associated with a good prognosis.[12]

Head and Neck Cancers

Postoperative survival after resection of pulmonary metastases from head and neck cancer appears to vary by cell type. Five-year survival rates of 34% for squamous cell carcinoma, 64% for glandular tumors, and 84% for adenoid cystic carcinomas are reported.[48]

REPEAT METASTASECTOMY

Multiple pulmonary metastasectomies may be required when there are isolated recurrences in the lung after initial pulmonary metastasectomy, and these can be accomplished in a safe and

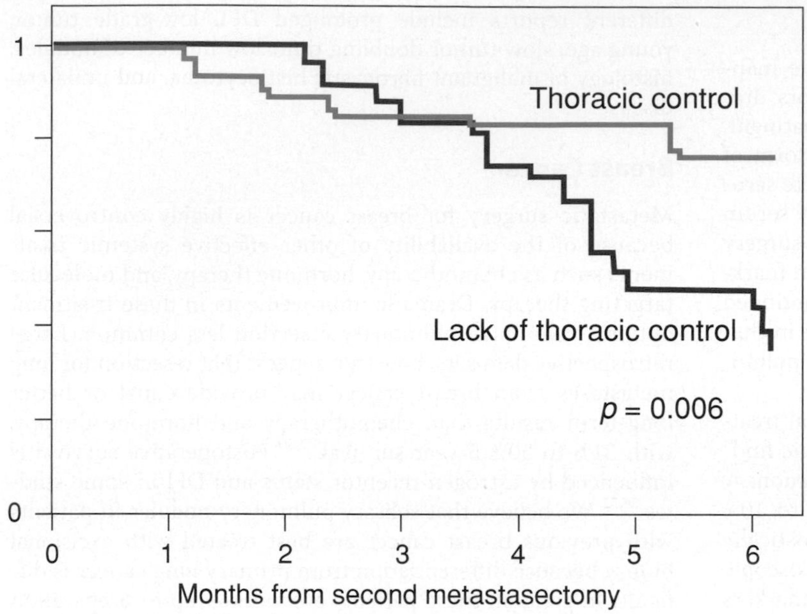

Figure 78-5. Survival benefit in repeat metastasectomy depends on thoracic control of disease with increasing number of metastasectomies.

effective manner.[6,16] After initial pulmonary metastasectomy, a significant number of patients will have recurrence in the lung. In a study of epithelial tumors, after first pulmonary resection, the disease recurred in 68% of patients, with the lung being the first site of recurrence in 38% of patients.[25] After curative resection for metastatic soft-tissue sarcoma, 40% to 80% of patients recurred in the lung. For these patients, there is a clear-cut role for repeat pulmonary metastasectomy.[54]

The role of repeat metastasectomy has been evaluated retrospectively. In the 1997 report from the International Registry of Lung Metastases, 53% of the 5206 patients undergoing pulmonary metastasectomy experienced a recurrence.[6] Five-year survival in these 1042 patients able to undergo a second operation was 44%, and 10-year survival was 29%. Similar 5-year survival rates have been reported by Robert et al.(48%) and Kandioler et al.(50%).[26,59]

In a more recent analysis, 82 patients who underwent surgical resection of pulmonary metastases at the Brigham and Women's Hospital (from 1989 to 2004) were analyzed and 31 (38%) were determined to have leiomyosarcoma. Of these, 15 (48%) had repeated pulmonary metastasectomy. There was no difference in disease-free survival between patients with

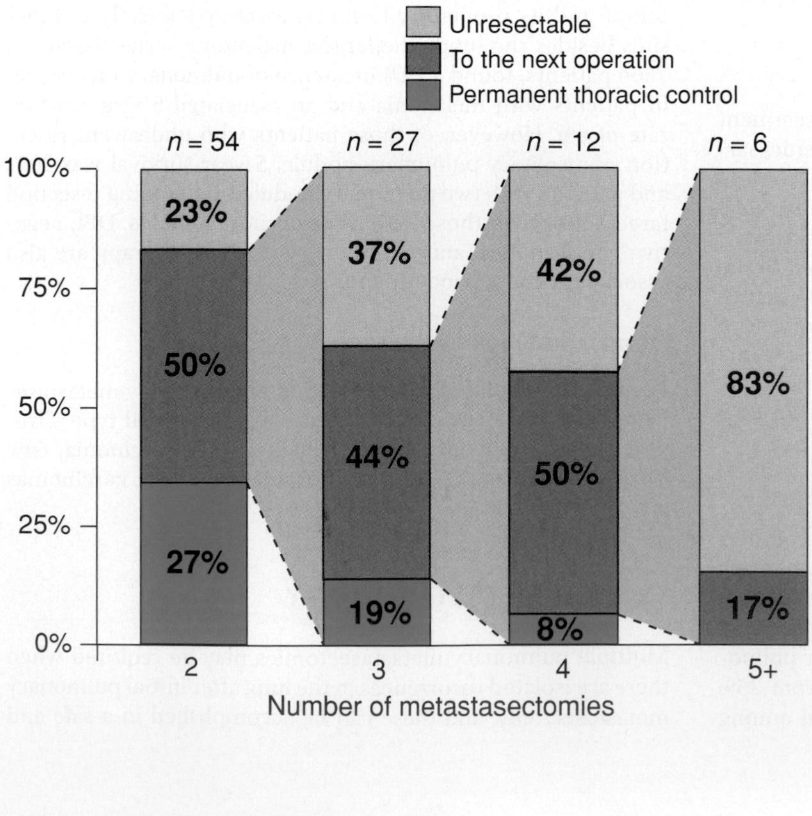

Figure 78-6. Preservation of local control in the chest is associated with a long-term survival after repeat metastasectomy.

leiomyosarcoma and those with other histologic subtypes of sarcoma, but there was a marked improvement in overall survival (70 vs. 24 months; $p = 0.049$). In multivariate analysis, the DFI from primary tumor resection to pulmonary metastases and the DFI from pulmonary metastasectomy to second pulmonary recurrence were identified as independent predictors of survival.[50] The authors concluded that leiomyosarcoma pulmonary metastases behave more indolently than other sarcoma histologic types, and repeat pulmonary resections are warranted.

Survival decreases with the number of repeat resections, and the probability of benefiting from a repeated attempt at thoracic metastasectomy diminishes after each previous operation (Fig. 78-5). For all tissues types, the 5-year survival after the second metastasectomy is 59%; for those undergoing three procedures, it is 38%; and for those undergoing four or more procedures, the survival is 46 months.[16] All deaths are due to recurrent unresectable cancer.

These reports combined suggest that each successful metastasectomy reestablishes the probability for long-term survival by returning the patient to a clinical local control state (Fig. 78-6). Expected survival drops to 8 months, however, after a recurrence can no longer be removed.[16]

We and other authors propose that equal results can be obtained by resecting only radiographically visible lesions without an open search for occult disease by manual palpation, provided that the patient undergoes close imaging follow-up with resection of lesions detected on subsequent scans.[16,50] These patients may achieve equal survival if these metastases can be removed in several minimally invasive operations, provided that the risk of further metastatic spread from the remaining pulmonary focus of cancer is relatively low.

SUMMARY

There is adequate experience in the literature to conclude that resection of pulmonary metastases can be performed with extremely low mortality and minimal morbidity. Resection of pulmonary metastases improves survival in most malignancies if complete resection is performed in the setting of adequate pulmonary reserve. VATS is a useful alternative to thoracotomy for resection of metastases, provided that the patient is followed closely postoperatively. Repeat metastasectomy should be considered in any patient with recurrent metastases who fits the criteria for operation.

EDITOR'S COMMENT

Resection of pulmonary metastasis is generally indicated, provided that the primary tumor is controlled and all resectable disease is removed. Factors such as tumor doubling time and tumor type, among others, have not been shown to affect long-term survival. Recent data support looking for lymph node metastases, especially in colorectal and renal metastases, and if these are found, then pulmonary resection is not performed. Modern day spiral CT scans probably can identify nodules even below 4 mm in size. The need for palpation therefore is questionable and hence VATS resection is feasible. Sequential removal of all lesions identified will probably lead to as good a long-term survival as open palpation and exploration. The tiny lesions that are missed by CT will likely be picked up later on and removed subsequently.

—Mark J. Krasna

References

1. Sugarbaker ED. The organ selectivity of experimentally induced metastases in rats. *Cancer.* 1952;5:606–612.
2. Farrell J. Pulmonary metastasis: a pathological, clinical, roentgenologic study based on 78 cases seen at necropsy. *Radiology.* 1935;24:444–450.
3. Barney J, Churchill EJ. Adenocarcinoma of the kidney with metastases to the lung cured by nephrectomy and lobectomy. *J Urol.* 1939;42:269–276.
4. Aberg T, Malmberg KA, Nilsson B, et al. The effect of metastasectomy: fact or fiction? *Ann Thorac Surg.* 1980;30:378–384.
5. Aberg T. Selection mechanisms as major determinants of survival after pulmonary metastasectomy. *Ann Thorac Surg.* 1997;63:611–612.
6. Pastorino U, Buyse M, Friedel G, et al. Long-term results of lung metastasectomy: prognostic analyses based on 5206 cases. The International Registry of Lung Metastases. *J Thorac Cardiovasc Surg.* 1997;113:37–49.
7. Tafra L, Dale PS, Wanek LA, et al. Resection and adjuvant immunotherapy for melanoma metastatic to the lung and thorax. *J Thorac Cardiovasc Surg.* 1995;110:119–128; discussion 129.
8. Jablons D, Steinberg SM, Roth J, et al. Metastasectomy for soft tissue sarcoma. Further evidence for efficacy and prognostic indicators. *J Thorac Cardiovasc Surg.* 1989;97:695–705.
9. Martini N, Huvos AG, Mike V, et al. Multiple pulmonary resections in the treatment of osteogenic sarcoma. *Ann Thorac Surg.* 1971;12:271–280.
10. Staren ED, Salerno C, Rongione A, et al. Pulmonary resection for metastatic breast cancer. *Arch Surg.* 1992;127:1282–1284.
11. Friedel G, Hurtgen M, Penzenstadler M, et al. Resection of pulmonary metastases from renal cell carcinoma. *Anticancer Res.* 1999;19:1593–1596.
12. Harpole DH Jr, Johnson CM, Wolfe WG, et al. Analysis of 945 cases of pulmonary metastatic melanoma. *J Thorac Cardiovasc Surg.* 1992;103:743–748; discussion 748–750.
13. Marincola FM, Mark JB. Selection factors resulting in improved survival after surgical resection of tumors metastatic to the lungs. *Arch Surg.* 1990;125:1387–1392; discussion 1392–1393.
14. Ehrenhaft JL, Lawrence MS, Sensenig DM. Pulmonary resections for metastatic lesions. *AMA Arch Surg.* 1958;77:606–612.
15. Martini N, McCormack PM. Evolution of the surgical management of pulmonary metastases. *Chest Surg Clin N Am.* 1998;8:13–27.
16. Jaklitsch MT, Mery CM, Lukanich JM, et al. Sequential thoracic metastasectomy prolongs survival by re-establishing local control within the chest. *J Thorac Cardiovasc Surg.* 2001;121:657–667.
17. Kondo H, Okumura T, Ohde Y, et al. Surgical treatment for metastatic malignancies. Pulmonary metastasis: indications and outcomes. *Int J Clin Oncol.* 2005;10:81–85.
18. Collie DA, Wright AR, Williams JR, et al. Comparison of spiral-acquisition computed tomography and conventional computed tomography in the assessment of pulmonary metastatic disease. *Br J Radiol.* 1994;67:436–444.
19. Remy-Jardin M, Remy J, Giraud F, et al. Pulmonary nodules: detection with thick-section spiral CT versus conventional CT. *Radiology.* 1993;187:513–520.
20. Parsons AM, Detterbeck FC, Parker LA. Accuracy of helical CT in the detection of pulmonary metastases: is intraoperative palpation still necessary? *Ann Thorac Surg.* 2004;78:1910–1916; discussion 1916–1918.
21. Margaritora S, Porziella V, D'Andrilli A, et al. Pulmonary metastases: can accurate radiological evaluation avoid thoracotomic approach? *Eur J Cardiothorac Surg.* 2002;21:1111–1114.
22. Mery CM, Pappas AN, Bueno R, et al. Relationship between a history of antecedent cancer and the probability of malignancy for a solitary pulmonary nodule. *Chest.* 2004;125:2175–2181.
23. Todd TR. The surgical treatment of pulmonary metastases. *Chest.* 1997;112:287S–290S.
24. Murthy SC, Kim K, Rice TW, et al. Can we predict long-term survival after pulmonary metastasectomy for renal cell carcinoma? *Ann Thorac Surg.* 2005;79:996–1003.
25. Monteiro A, Arce N, Bernardo J, et al. Surgical resection of lung metastases from epithelial tumors. *Ann Thorac Surg.* 2004;77:431–437.

26. Robert JH, Ambrogi V, Mermillod B, et al. Factors influencing long-term survival after lung metastasectomy. *Ann Thorac Surg.* 1997;63:777–784.
27. Mountain CF, McMurtrey MJ, Hermes KE. Surgery for pulmonary metastasis: a 20-year experience. *Ann Thorac Surg.* 1984;38:323–330.
28. Rusch VW. Pulmonary metastasectomy. Current indications. *Chest.* 1995;107:322S–331S.
29. Roth JA, Pass HI, Wesley MN, et al. Comparison of median sternotomy and thoracotomy for resection of pulmonary metastases in patients with adult soft-tissue sarcomas. *Ann Thorac Surg.* 1986;42:134–138.
30. Putnam JB Jr, Suell DM, Natarajan G, et al. Extended resection of pulmonary metastases: is the risk justified? *Ann Thorac Surg.* 1993;55:1440–1446.
31. Crow J, Slavin G, Kreel L. Pulmonary metastasis: a pathologic and radiologic study. *Cancer.* 1981;47:2595–2602.
32. McCormack PM, Ginsberg KB, Bains MS, et al. Accuracy of lung imaging in metastases with implications for the role of thoracoscopy. *Ann Thorac Surg.* 1993;56:863–865; discussion 865–866.
33. McCormack PM, Bains MS, Begg CB, et al. Role of video-assisted thoracic surgery in the treatment of pulmonary metastases: results of a prospective trial. *Ann Thorac Surg.* 1996;62:213–216; discussion 216–217.
34. De Giacomo T, Rendina EA, Venuta F, et al. Thoracoscopic resection of solitary lung metastases from colorectal cancer is a viable therapeutic option. *Chest.* 1999;115:1441–1443.
35. Abrams HL, Spiro R, Goldstein N. Metastases in carcinoma: analysis of 1000 autopsied cases. *Cancer.* 1950;3:74–85.
36. Thomford NR, Woolner LB, Clagett OT. The surgical treatment of metastatic tumors in the lungs. *J Thorac Cardiovasc Surg.* 1965;49:357–363.
37. Ercan S, Nichols FC 3rd, Trastek VF, et al. Prognostic significance of lymph node metastasis found during pulmonary metastasectomy for extrapulmonary carcinoma. *Ann Thorac Surg.* 2004;77:1786–1791.
38. Loehe F, Kobinger S, Hatz RA, et al. Value of systematic mediastinal lymph node dissection during pulmonary metastasectomy. *Ann Thorac Surg.* 2001;72:225–229.
39. Inoue M, Kotake Y, Nakagawa K, et al. Surgery for pulmonary metastases from colorectal carcinoma. *Ann Thorac Surg.* 2000;70:380–383.
40. Saito Y, Omiya H, Kohno K, et al. Pulmonary metastasectomy for 165 patients with colorectal carcinoma: A prognostic assessment. *J Thorac Cardiovasc Surg.* 2002;124:1007–1013.
41. Okumura S, Kondo H, Tsuboi M, et al. Pulmonary resection for metastatic colorectal cancer: experiences with 159 patients. *J Thorac Cardiovasc Surg.* 1996;112:867–874.
42. Goya T, Miyazawa N, Kondo H, et al. Surgical resection of pulmonary metastases from colorectal cancer: 10-year follow-up. *Cancer.* 1989;64:1418–1421.
43. McCormack PM, Burt ME, Bains MS, et al. Lung resection for colorectal metastases. 10-year results. *Arch Surg.* 1992;127:1403–1406.
44. McAfee MK, Allen MS, Trastek VF, et al. Colorectal lung metastases: results of surgical excision. *Ann Thorac Surg.* 1992;53:780–785; discussion 785–786.
45. Girard P, Ducreux M, Baldeyrou P, et al. Surgery for lung metastases from colorectal cancer: analysis of prognostic factors. *J Clin Oncol.* 1996;14:2047–2053.
46. van der Poel HG, Roukema JA, Horenblas S, et al. Metastasectomy in renal cell carcinoma: a multicenter retrospective analysis. *Eur Urol.* 1999;35:197–203.
47. Cerfolio RJ, Allen MS, Deschamps C, et al. Pulmonary resection of metastatic renal cell carcinoma. *Ann Thorac Surg.* 1994;57:339–344.
48. Liu D, Labow DM, Dang N, et al. Pulmonary metastasectomy for head and neck cancers. *Ann Surg Oncol.* 1999;6:572–578.
49. Blackledge G, Steward WP, Verweij J, et al. Experience with ifosfamide in the EORTC soft tissue and bone sarcoma group. *Semin Oncol.* 1992;19(1 Suppl 1):14–18.
50. Burt BM, Ocejo S, Mery CM, et al. Repeated and aggressive pulmonary resections for leiomyosarcoma metastases extends survival. *Ann Thorac Surg.* 2011;92(4):1202–1207.
51. Blackmon SH, Shah N, Roth JA, et al. Resection of pulmonary and extrapulmonary sarcomatous metastases is associated with long-term survival. *Ann Thorac Surg.* 2009;88(3):877–884; discussion 884–885. doi: 10.1016/j.athoracsur.2009.04.144
52. Goorin AM, Shuster JJ, Baker A, et al. Changing pattern of pulmonary metastases with adjuvant chemotherapy in patients with osteosarcoma: results from the multiinstitutional osteosarcoma study. *J Clin Oncol.* 1991;9:600–605.
53. Tsuchiya H, Kanazawa Y, Abdel-Wanis ME, et al. Effect of timing of pulmonary metastases identification on prognosis of patients with osteosarcoma: the Japanese Musculoskeletal Oncology Group study. *J Clin Oncol.* 2002;20:3470–3477.
54. Temple LK, Brennan MF. The role of pulmonary metastasectomy in soft tissue sarcoma. *Semin Thorac Cardiovasc Surg.* 2002;14:35–44.
55. van Geel AN, Pastorino U, Jauch KW, et al. Surgical treatment of lung metastases: The European Organization for Research and Treatment of Cancer-Soft Tissue and Bone Sarcoma Group study of 255 patients. *Cancer.* 1996;77:675–682.
56. Friedel G, Pastorino U, Ginsberg RJ, et al. Results of lung metastasectomy from breast cancer: prognostic criteria on the basis of 467 cases of the International Registry of Lung Metastases. *Eur J Cardiothorac Surg.* 2002;22:335–344.
57. Ludwig C, Stoelben E, Hasse J. Disease-free survival after resection of lung metastases in patients with breast cancer. *Eur J Surg Oncol.* 2003;29:532–535.
58. Anraku M, Yokoi K, Nakagawa K, et al. Pulmonary metastases from uterine malignancies: results of surgical resection in 133 patients. *J Thorac Cardiovasc Surg.* 2004;127:1107–1112.
59. Kandioler D, Kromer E, Tuchler H, et al. Long-term results after repeated surgical removal of pulmonary metastases. *Ann Thorac Surg.* 1998;65:909–912.

79 Resection of Bronchogenic Carcinoma with Oligometastatic Disease

Mark J. Krasna

Keywords: Non–small-cell lung cancer, craniotomy, stereotactic radiosurgery

The development of brain metastasis in a patient with non–small-cell lung cancer (NSCLC) is an ominous prognostic sign. About 30% of individuals with NSCLC eventually develop brain metastasis.[1] This number increases to about 50% in autopsy series.[2] When the metastases are multiple, palliative treatment in the form of radiation therapy is recommended. Solitary brain metastasis, however, can be approached surgically. The proportion of NSCLC patients that develops brain metastasis amounts to approximately 40,000 patients per year. The magnitude of this problem can be appreciated by comparing this number with the incidence of new primary cancers of the pancreas ($n = 27{,}000$), stomach ($n = 24{,}000$), and esophagus ($n = 13{,}000$). The median survival rate of untreated lung cancer with brain metastasis is approximately 1 month. Steroid therapy increases the median survival by 2 months. Whole-brain radiation increases survival by 3 to 6 months.[3] Recent reports indicate longer survivals when surgical treatment is combined with whole-brain radiation.[4,5] The experience of several large centers that offer a surgical approach to lung cancer with brain metastasis is discussed herein, with an analysis of factors underlying prolonged survival.

In addition, other sites of metastatic disease also commonly present as oligometastases. Patients with lesions to the adrenals, liver, and bone are sometimes amenable to aggressive surgical and multimodality regimens. For the purposes of this chapter, data on brain and adrenal lesions will be presented.

Previous studies have reported 5-year survival rates of 11% to 21% in patients treated with cranial and thoracic resection.[5,6] Despite this, many patients are offered palliative treatment only with chemotherapy or radiotherapy after a brain metastasis has been detected. There is controversy regarding the ideal management of thoracic disease in this patient population, and there are few series that incorporate patients treated with craniotomy or stereotactic radiosurgery (SRS).[7]

THORACIC RESECTION WITH CRANIOTOMY OR STEREOTACTIC RADIOSURGERY—PATIENTS AND METHODS

In our prior series from the University of Maryland, 28 patients with solitary brain metastasis were treated by thoracotomy with resection of lung cancer and craniotomy with excision of brain metastasis or SRS. More recent patients in our series have undergone lung resection and gamma knife stereotactic radiosurgery (GK-SRS). The series consisted of 16 men and 12 women ranging in age from 42 to 70 years, with a mean age of 56.24 years.

The initial presenting symptom was neurologic in 50% of patients. The range of neurologic symptoms included hemiparesis, headaches, monoparesis, ataxia, visual disturbances, seizures, behavioral changes, and mild weakness. In these patients, the onset of the cerebral metastasis was synchronous with the primary in that the pulmonary lesion was identified on the chest x-ray concomitant with the initial presentation of the metastasis. The remainder presented with pulmonary complaints related to their bronchogenic carcinoma, including cough, hoarseness, and chest pain, but later developed symptoms related to both pulmonary and neurologic systems.

Patients with initial neurologic symptoms generally underwent craniotomy or, recently, SRS. After initiating steroid treatment, these patients were referred for initial treatment of their brain lesion. The lung lesion was generally approached later. Patients who were seen primarily for a pulmonary malignancy initially underwent a pulmonary resection. The types of pulmonary resections performed were lobectomy, bilobectomy, pneumonectomy, and wedge resection. A complete dissection of the mediastinal lymph nodes generally was carried out in conjunction with the pulmonary resection. We now use routine bronchoscopy and mediastinoscopy before deciding to proceed with pulmonary resection. Resections generally were considered curative (R0), with no gross tumor left behind. All resection margins were tumor-free microscopically, and the mediastinal nodes were removed.

The tumor cell type was most frequently adenocarcinoma, followed by squamous or adenosquamous, large-cell undifferentiated, or anaplastic carcinoma. In determining the staging of the tumor, only the status of the primary tumor and lymph nodes was considered because of the known presence of a solitary cerebral metastasis. Based on such consideration, in diminishing frequency, tumors were most often stage I, stage II, and stage IIIA.

Radiation therapy after lung resection or adjuvant chemotherapy often was tried. To date, 11 patients are alive and without evidence of recurrent cancer. Seventeen patients have died: 14 died of recurrent cancer, of whom seven died of widespread systemic metastases, four had recurrence in the chest, and three had central nervous system (CNS) metastases. One patient died of multiple-organ failure secondary to sepsis 47 days after lobectomy. One patient died 1 month after a left lower lobectomy of sudden cardiac arrest, and one patient died of respiratory failure complicating severe chronic obstructive pulmonary disease 17 months after craniotomy.

Survival after craniotomy often exceeds 5 years, with a 37% 5-year survival reported in prior studies. The difference in survival between those who received brain irradiation after craniotomy and those who did not was not significant in our series, although this finding has been challenged recently in reports of other similar series. Relief of neurologic symptoms after craniotomy is usually immediate.[7]

In prior series, the following factors were analyzed to determine the effects on survival: age, sex, order of presentation (i.e., cerebral, pulmonary, or synchronous presentation), interval between thoracotomy and craniotomy if the thoracotomy was done first, interval between craniotomy and thoracotomy if the craniotomy was done first, cell type of tumor, type of pulmonary resection (i.e., pneumonectomy, bilobectomy, lobectomy, or wedge resection), curative or palliative resection, T classification of the lung tumor, nodal status (N0, N1 vs. N2) of the lung primary, lung tumor stage, duration of neurologic symptoms prior to craniotomy, location of brain metastasis, brain irradiation after craniotomy versus no irradiation, and use of chemotherapy or radiation therapy for the lung lesion. By univariate analysis, three factors were found to correlate with longer survival: curative pulmonary resection ($p = 0.001$), nodal status ($p = 0.001$), and age less than 55 years ($p = 0.006$). However, when all the factors were analyzed by the Cox multivariate model, only curative resection remained a significant factor for prolonged survival ($p < 0.01$).

ADRENAL METASTASIS

In a series from France, 94 of 4668 patients who underwent lung cancer surgery had oligometastatic disease. Metastasis occurred in brain ($n = 57$), adrenal gland ($n = 12$), bone ($n = 14$), liver ($n = 5$), and skin ($n = 6$). Sixty-nine metastases were resected. The 5-year survival rate was 16% (median, 13 months). Induction therapy, adenocarcinoma, N0 staging, and lobectomy were the criteria of better prognosis, but metastasis resection was not. The authors concluded this pattern may reflect a specific tumor biology in which a solitary metastasis would benefit both from surgical or non-surgical treatment.[8]

Dartevelle's group published a series of 23 patients who underwent complete resection of an isolated adrenal metastasis after surgical treatment of NSCLC. There were 19 men and 4 women, with a mean age of 54 ± 10 years. The diagnosis of adrenal metastasis was synchronous with the diagnosis of NSCLC in 6 patients and metachronous in 17 patients. The median disease-free interval for patients with metachronous metastasis was 12.5 months (range, 4.5–60.1 months). The overall 5-year survival was 23.3%. Univariate and multivariate analysis demonstrated that disease-free interval of greater than 6 months was an independent and significant predictor of increased survival in patients after adrenalectomy. All patients with disease-free interval less than 6 months died within 2 years of the operation. The 5-year survival was 38% after resection of an isolated adrenal metastasis that occurred more than 6 months after lung resection.[8] Although these authors believed that adjuvant therapy and pathologic staging of NSCLC did not affect survival, most physicians would treat with a full chemotherapy regimen to follow.

In a recent meta-analysis consisting of 10 publications that contributed 114 patients, 42% of patients had synchronous metastases and 58% had metachronous metastases. The median DFIs were 0 and 12 months, respectively. Patients in the synchronous group were younger than those in the metachronous group (median age 54 years vs. 68 years). Complications from adrenalectomy were infrequent. Median overall survival was shorter for patients with synchronous metastasis than those with metachronous metastasis (12 months vs. 31 months, generalized Wilcoxon p value < 0.02). However, the 5-year survival estimates were equivalent at 26% and 25%, respectively.[9]

COMMENT

A solitary brain metastasis associated with primary bronchogenic carcinoma can occur without producing any neurologic symptoms. In a recent study, 42 patients with a solitary brain metastasis were treated with GK-SRS from 1993 to 2006. There were 27 men and 15 women, and the median age was 58 years (range, 38–74 years). The median Karnofsky performance status (KPS) was 90 (range, 70–100). Thirty-eight patients (90.5%) presented with symptoms of solitary brain metastasis or were found to have brain metastasis on staging brain MRI within 1 month of histologic diagnosis of their primary NSCLC. The maximum diameter of the single brain metastasis was between 0.5 and 3.5 cm (median, 1.5 cm). Brain lesions were located as follows: parietal lobe (12), frontal lobe (10), temporal lobe (9), occipital lobe (7), cerebellum (3), and thalamus (1). Initial staging to evaluate the extent of thoracic and extracranial disease included CT scans of the chest and abdomen ($n = 42$) and PET scans ($n = 13$).

Surgical staging was performed on 27 of 42 patients using mediastinoscopy, mediastinal dissection, or transbronchial needle aspiration to identify positive hilar and mediastinal lymph nodes. Twenty-two patients (52.4%) had radiographically or pathologically involved hilar (N1) and/or mediastinal (N2/N3) lymphadenopathy; the thoracic disease thus was stage I, stage II, and stage III in 14, 9, and 19 patients, respectively.

The median dose prescribed was 18 Gy to the 50% isodose line (range, 11–25 Gy). Additional whole-brain radiation therapy (WBRT) was delivered to 33 of 42 patients based on physician and/or patient preference. Twenty-one patients had WBRT after GK-SRS and 12 before. WBRT preceded thoracic therapy or chemotherapy in 21 patients, whereas 12 patients received it after thoracic therapy or chemotherapy or at the time of CNS progression.

Patients were considered to have definitive thoracic therapy if they underwent surgical resection or received sequential or concurrent chemotherapy and external beam radiation with definitive intent. Twenty-six patients (62%) completed definitive thoracic therapy: 9 patients had sequential or concurrent chemotherapy and radiation, 12 patients underwent surgical resection with or without preoperative or postoperative therapy, and 5 patients underwent a planned trimodality approach with preoperative chemoradiation followed by surgical resection. The median dose of thoracic radiation delivered to patients treated definitively was 61.2 Gy (range, 45–68.4 Gy). Nondefinitive thoracic therapy ($n = 16$) included chemotherapy alone, palliative radiation therapy at doses greater than 2 Gy per fraction for an abbreviated course, radiation therapy followed by chemotherapy, and no therapy in six, four, three, and three patients, respectively.

The median overall survival for the 42 patients was 18 months (range, 1.5–150 months). The 1-, 2- and 5-year actuarial overall survival rates were 71.3%, 34.1%, and 21%, respectively. Currently, there are 8 patients alive with a median active follow-up of 64.5 months (range, 9–150 months). The cause of death was identified in 20 of 34 patients. Neurologic progression was determined to be the cause of death in 5 of 20 patients (20%). The sites of progression in these five patients were CNS alone (three), CNS and distant (one), and CNS and thoracic (one). Symptomatic radiation necrosis requiring intervention (resection) in the absence of intracranial progression was documented in one patient.

Patients who had definitive thoracic therapy ($n = 26$) versus those who had nondefinitive therapy ($n = 16$) had a median overall survival of 26.4 months (95% confidence interval 16.2–36.6 months) versus 13.1 months (95% confidence interval 4.3–21.8 months) and a 5-year overall survival rate of 34.6% versus 0% ($p < 0.0001$), respectively. There was no statistical difference between patients treated definitively with ($n = 18$) or without ($n = 8$) surgery ($p = 0.369$). Patients with a KPS of 90 or greater had a median overall survival of 27.8 months compared with 13.1 months for those with a KPS of less than 90 ($p < 0.0001$). The prognostic factors significant on multivariate analysis were definitive thoracic therapy (relative risk = 2.97, $p = 0.020$) and KPS (relative risk = 5.85, $p = 0.001$).

Since the brain is affected by metastatic disease in 30% to 50% of patients, routine CT scan or MRI of the brain is recommended by our group in all cases of bronchogenic carcinoma, at least when greater than clinical T1N0. Likewise, many surgeons advocate routine brain CT or MRI for all adenocarcinomas. The diagnosis of brain metastasis in the past was made by nuclear isotope brain scanning or arteriography or both early in the study. CT scanning has been used in all patients since 1976. MRI has been used since 1985. For patients suspected of having cerebral metastases, double-dose delayed CT has proved significantly more sensitive than CT scans obtained immediately after the administration of a lesser dose of iodinated contrast material. Davis et al.[10] reported that MRI with enhancement proved superior to double-dose delayed CT for lesion detection, anatomic localization of lesions, and differentiation of solitary versus multiple lesions.

Brain metastasis has been considered an advanced progression of the disease and has been treated historically with corticosteroids and irradiation. Although corticosteroids produce rapid improvement in the neurologic symptoms, they prolong life for a median of 2 months only. Radiation therapy provides 80% relief of symptoms, but the median survival rate is only 3 to 6 months.[3] Ballantine and Byron[11] in 1948 and Flavell[12] in 1949 were the first to carry out staged surgical excision of a solitary non–small-cell intracranial metastasis with the primary intrathoracic lesion. Magilligan et al.[4] in 1976 introduced the modern approach of combined lung/brain resection with a 5-year survival rate of 21% and a low mortality rate of 3%. Subsequently, large series of patients treated with the combined modality of resection of cerebral metastasis followed by brain radiation were reported. Burt et al.[5] reported 185 consecutive patients undergoing combined therapy. The overall survival rate was 55% at 1 year, 27% at 2 years, 18% at 3 years, and 13% at 5 years, with a median survival of 14 months. Vecht et al.[13] reported 63 patients receiving combined treatment of neurosurgery and WBRT with a median survival rate of 10 months. Lonjon et al.[14] reported 36 patients receiving such treatment with a median survival of 9.6 months.

Our past studies of combined treatment confirm these results. The survival rate of 28 patients undergoing this treatment was 58% at 1 year and 37% at 5 years, with a median survival of 1.60 years. Most of these patients received postoperative WBRT in the range of 3000 to 4500 rads. In 10 patients, a small-field boost of 900 to 2500 rads to the tumor-bearing area was added after completion of the WBRT. Two patients developed radiation fibrosis of the brain, one with incapacitating ataxia and the other with deterioration of memory. The advisability of postoperative WBRT remains unanswered.[6]

Armstrong et al.[15] evaluated 185 patients with NSCLC who underwent resection of brain metastases. Forty-two patients who received preoperative WBRT (23%) were excluded. Sixty-four patients were equally divided into two groups, one ($n = 32$) received no WBRT; the other was prognostically matched to the first group ($n = 32$). A third group consisted of all other WBRT patients ($n = 79$). Most patients received 3000 rads in 10 fractions. Overall brain failures occurred in 38% of the first group, 47% of the second group, and 42% of the third group. The use of WBRT had no apparent impact on survival or on overall brain failure rates. The only impact of WBRT was the reduction of focal failure, defined as failure within the brain adjacent to the site of resected brain metastasis.

However, Vecht et al.[13] compared the effect of neurosurgical excision plus radiotherapy with radiotherapy alone in a prospective, randomized test of 63 patients. WBRT was given in two fractions per day for a total of 4000 rads. The combined treatment compared with radiotherapy alone led to a longer survival. Median survival was 10 months in patients treated with the combined approach and 6 months in patients treated with radiotherapy alone ($p = 0.04$).

The factors contributing to prolonged survival have been addressed by various authors. Magilligan et al.[4] found a wedge resection to be a significant predictor of improved survival; because this type of resection generally is reserved for small peripheral tumors with no hilar or mediastinal adenopathy, it suggests that the size of the primary tumor directly influenced survival. Rossi et al.[16] found that the vigor of the patient, as assessed by Karnofsky and Zubrod scales and absence of nodal disease, influenced survival rate. Burt et al.[5] found no significant difference in age, locoregional stage (TN), or histologic features in patients with synchronous versus metachronous lesions. However, multivariate analysis demonstrated that complete resection of the primary disease significantly prolonged survival. Lonjon et al.[14] found that the postoperative clinical status (Karnofsky score) and the postoperative neurologic grading were significant factors to determine survival. Nakagawa et al.[17] found that the variables significantly associated with a favorable prognosis included surgical excision of the primary lesion, adenocarcinoma as the histologic diagnosis, the use of adjuvant treatment, a preoperative score of over 80% on the Karnofsky scale, and metastasis confined to the brain. Additional but nonsignificant contributors to a good prognosis included younger than 65 or 70 years, early-tumor stage, curative lung cancer surgery, a single metastatic brain tumor, a solid versus cystic tumor, and a supratentorial location of the brain metastasis. Our series agrees with those of Hankins et al.[6] and Burt et al.,[5] namely that the most significant factor in prolonged survival following combined surgery and radiation for solitary brain metastasis was curative excision of the primary lung tumor.

However, despite prolonged survival and improvement in the quality of life after surgery and radiation therapy, recurrence of the brain metastasis contributes to the death of these patients. Patchell et al.[18] reported that the recurrence at the site of the original brain metastasis was 20% in the surgery group and 52% in the radiation group. Nakagawa et al.[17] reported that 19% of patients treated with surgery or radiation died directly because of the brain metastasis, and 3.6% died of treatment-related complications.

Nakagawa et al.[17] recommended that adjuvant treatment generally should follow excision of brain metastasis, considering that metastatic lesions smaller than 1.0 cm, which are not seen on CT scan, can be shown by MRI postoperatively. Radiation-insensitive tumors might disappear on MRI after combined chemotherapy and irradiation owing to enhancement of the radiation effect by chemotherapy. A significantly longer survival was found in patients who received adjuvant treatment than in those who did not. Chemotherapeutic regimens were divided into those involving platinum based nitrosoureas, and other anticancer agents. Patients given platinum had a significantly longer mean survival time (468 days) than patients given other anticancer agents (243 days) ($p < 0.05$). Hypothetically, these patients' tumors have gone through the layers of the brain coverings, and the blood supply as well as the blood-brain barrier have already been compromised. This had led many authors to initiate the use of chemotherapy in addition to localized SBRT or WBRT for treatment of oligometastatic disease. Finally, with the advent of newer agents, especially the tyrosine-kinase inhibitors (TKIs) and other oral agents, delivery of adequate dose of chemosuppressive therapy is possible even to the brain.

Another recent approach to solitary brain metastasis is the use of a gamma knife with precise localization of the tumor by stereotactic method, which is promising, especially in patients who are not good surgical candidates.[19]

Multiple series have demonstrated that thoracic therapy and extent of thoracic disease may have an impact on survival. In a series by Bonnette et al., 99 of 103 patients had surgical resection of their synchronous solitary brain metastasis and primary NSCLC. The median overall survival was 12.4 months, and the 5-year overall survival was 11%.[20] Moreover, Billings et al. reported a median and 5-year overall survival of 24 months and 21.4%, respectively, for 28 patients who underwent surgical resection for their brain and thoracic disease. The superior overall survival in the series of Billings et al. may be attributed to the 15 patients (53.6%) with thoracic stage I disease. Contrary to the series of Bonnette et al., Billings et al. reported a significant improvement in overall survival if there was no pathologic evidence of lymph node metastasis (5-year overall survival 35% vs. 0%, $p = 0.001$).[21] Hu et al. reviewed 84 patients who underwent surgical resection or SRS for their brain metastasis, but only 44 patients received any therapy for their thoracic disease. The median overall survival of 15.5 months was significantly better for those who had thoracic therapy versus 5.9 months for those who did not ($p = 0.046$).[22]

A different approach to minimize brain atrophy and mental deterioration following radiotherapy is the use of intraoperative radiation therapy at the time of surgical intervention. Nakamura et al.[23] reported 1-year survival of 59% in 14 patients undergoing surgery and intraoperative radiation therapy, which is similar to the result obtained in 71 patients receiving surgical excision and whole-brain irradiation. The frequency of remote recurrence after the new therapy was 20% in 1 year, which was almost the same as that of the usual therapy (surgery plus whole-brain irradiation).

The use of hyperthermia plus nitrosoureas has been reported in 17 patients with NSCLC with brain metastasis. Sixteen (94%) responded with clinical improvement, radiologic regression, or disease stabilization. The survival time of the improved patients was 12.7 months.[24]

There is a concern regarding the true cause of the single brain lesion because the majority of patients were diagnosed on MRI without guided biopsy. Patchell et al. found that 11% of patients with abnormal imaging had intracranial disease other than metastasis; however, this study included a heterogeneous collection of malignancies.[18] The frequency of false-positive MRI findings with more modern imaging in patients with NSCLC is probably lower. In addition, KPS, age, extent of thoracic disease, and other patient characteristics may have influenced the decision to offer GK-SRS and/or definitive thoracic therapy in our series.

The results of RTOG 0214 were recently published in *JCO*. Three hundred fifty-six patients were accrued of the targeted 1058. The study was closed early because of slow accrual. There was no significant difference in survival (overall or disease-free) between those receiving prophylactic cranial irradiation (PCI) and those observed (these were the primary endpoints). Interestingly, however, there was a major difference in the incidence of brain metastasis and the number of lesions between the two groups. The 1-year rates of brain metastasis were significantly different, 7.7% versus 18.0% for PCI versus observation ($p < 0.004$). Patients in the observation arm were 2.52 times more likely to develop brain metastasis than those in the PCI arm. Finally, this was achieved with minimal neurologic toxicity.[25]

Another form of SRS recently reported in patients with brain metastases is CyberKnife (CK). In a series from China, clinical symptoms 1 week after CK were evaluated in 40 patients including 26 with lung cancer metastasis. Complete remission (CR), remission, stabilization, and aggravation occurred in 26 of 40 cases, 10 cases, 3 cases, and 1 case, respectively. Three months after CK treatment, CT and MRI showed complete remission, partial remission (PR), no change (NC), and progressive disease (PD) of 32 cases, 21 cases, 11 cases, and 4 cases, respectively, The local control rate was 77.8% (53/68) and the therapeutic effective rate was 94.1 (64/68). All patients were followed for more than 14 months. Four patients died of recurrent brain metastasis and other metastasis, and five patients died of a primary tumor. The 3-month, 6-month, and 1-year survival rates were 97.5% (39/40), 82.5% (33/40), and 67.5% (27/40), respectively. Three months after treatment, 14 patients had neuropathy, a lesion outside the original metastasis, on CT or MRI, a ratio of 35.0% (14/40). Six patients were treated effectively by repeated CK.[26]

The most recent guidelines from the American Society of Therapeutic Radiology and Oncology (ASTRO) 2005 state that based on Level I–III evidence, for selected patients with small (up to 4 cm) brain metastases (up to three in number and four in one randomized trial), the addition of radiosurgery boost to WBRT improves brain control as compared with whole-brain radiotherapy alone. In patients with a single brain metastasis, the radiosurgery boost with whole-brain radiotherapy improves survival. Local and distant brain control is significantly poorer with omission of upfront whole-brain radiotherapy (Level I–III evidence). There was no statistically significant difference in overall toxicity between those treated with radiosurgery alone versus whole-brain radiotherapy and radiosurgery boost based on an interim report from one randomized study.[27]

Despite the potential for long-term survival, many patients are offered only chemotherapy or palliative radiation therapy for their thoracic disease without considering their thoracic stage and performance status. At our center, an aggressive staging and treatment paradigm has been instituted when approaching patients with a synchronous solitary brain metastasis. Patients undergo a brain MRI and CT/PET scan to appropriately determine the extent of intracranial and extracranial disease. Studies have shown that CT scans often underestimate the extent of intracranial disease and that PET scans may identify metastases in approximately 25% of patients thought to have thoracic disease only.[28] Thus, overall survival actually may be improved with PET scanning in all patients.[29] In addition, surgical candidates will undergo surgical mediastinal staging. Patients then are selected for definitive brain and thoracic management based on the extent of intracranial and thoracic disease, presence of involved lymph nodes, and physiologic/performance status. The timing of brain and thoracic therapy also depends on these factors. Patients with a good KPS are often recommended to receive GK-SRS or surgical resection and WBRT. If patients have neurologic symptoms or a large brain metastasis and are not surgical candidates, we recommend GK-SRS and WBRT prior to thoracic therapy or chemotherapy. WBRT may be delivered prior to GK-SRS in order to decrease the volume of the lesion. This may allow a higher GK-SRS dose to be delivered. If the brain lesion is small and asymptomatic, we perform GK-SRS prior to thoracic therapy. If the patients do not progress extracranially, we proceed with WBRT after thoracic therapy or chemotherapy. If patients require further evaluation over a 2- to 3-week period to assess their surgical candidacy and extent of thoracic and extrathoracic disease, we may proceed with WBRT before thoracic therapy for logistical reasons.

SUMMARY

The use of SRS or craniotomy and resection in the treatment paradigm of patients with synchronous solitary brain metastasis from NSCLC is recommended. The median overall survival of 18 months and 5-year overall survival of 21% are similar to surgical series and stage III patients treated with concurrent chemoradiation. Improved KPS at diagnosis and definitive thoracic therapy significantly affected survival. This potential for long-term survival has influenced our treatment approach. Likewise, the management of patients with adrenal metastasis as the only site of disease portends a better survival than other M1b patients.[30] Thus, patients should be considered for definitive thoracic therapy after undergoing SRS or surgical resection of their brain and or adrenal metastasis.

EDITOR'S COMMENT

This is a unique subgroup of lung cancer patients with metastatic disease. Several reports of aggressive treatment of these so-called oligometastatic lesions have shown good local control with reasonable long-term survivals. In the era of SRS for brain lesions, up to three lesions have been treated aggressively, followed by stage-specific local lung cancer treatment. In general, this treatment is offered only to stage I or II patients. On the other hand, stage III patients who recur commonly in the brain after a reasonable time interval also are treated aggressively. The role of prophylactic brain radiation in patients with NSCLC, given the results of the Radiation Therapy Oncology Group (RTOG) protocol 0214, have not changed the standard approach to date, although there were clearly fewer brain metastases in this group.

—Mark J. Krasna

References

1. Deviri E, Schachner A, Halevy A, et al. Carcinoma of lung with a solitary cerebral metastasis. Surgical management and review of the literature. *Cancer.* 1983;52:1507–1509.
2. Galluzzi S, Payne PM. Brain metastases from primary bronchial carcinoma: a statistical study of 741 necropsies. *Br J Cancer.* 1956;10:408–414.
3. Martini N. Rationale for surgical treatment of brain metastasis in non-small cell lung cancer. *Ann Thorac Surg.* 1986;42:357–358.
4. Magilligan DJ Jr, Duvernoy C, Malik G, et al. Surgical approach to lung cancer with solitary cerebral metastasis: twenty-five years' experience. *Ann Thorac Surg.* 1986;42:360–364.
5. Burt M, Wronski M, Arbit E, et al. Resection of brain metastases from non-small-cell lung carcinoma. Results of therapy. Memorial Sloan-Kettering Cancer Center Thoracic Surgical Staff. *J Thorac Cardiovasc Surg.* 1992;103:399–410; discussion 410–411.
6. Hankins JR, Miller JE, Salcman M, et al. Surgical management of lung cancer with solitary cerebral metastasis. *Ann Thorac Surg.* 1988;46:24–28.
7. Flannery TW, Suntharalingam M, Regine WF, et al. Long-term survival in patients with synchronous, solitary brain metastasis from non-small-cell lung cancer treated with radiosurgery. *Int J Radiat Oncol Biol Phys.* 2008;72:19–23.
8. Mercier O, Fadel E, de Perrot M, et al. Surgical treatment of solitary adrenal metastasis from non-small cell lung cancer. *J Thorac Cardiovasc Surg.* 2005;130(1):136–140.
9. Tanvetyanon T, Robinson LA, Schell MJ, et al. Outcomes of adrenalectomy for isolated synchronous versus metachronous adrenal metastases in non-small-cell lung cancer: a systematic review and pooled analysis. *J Clin Oncol.* 2008;26(7):1142–1147.
10. Davis PC, Hudgins PA, Peterman SB, et al. Diagnosis of cerebral metastases: double-dose delayed CT vs contrast-enhanced MR imaging. *AJNR Am J Neuroradiol.* 1991;12:293–300.
11. Ballantine HT Jr, Byron FX. Carcinoma of the lung with intracranial metastasis; successful removal of metastatic and primary lesions. *Arch Surg.* 1948;57:849–854.
12. Flavell G. Solitary cerebral metastases from bronchial carcinomata: their incidence and a case of successful removal. *Br Med J.* 1949;2:736.
13. Vecht CJ, Haaxma-Reiche H, Noordijk EM, et al. Treatment of single brain metastasis: radiotherapy alone or combined with neurosurgery? *Ann Neurol.* 1993;33:583–590.
14. Lonjon M, Paquis P, Michiels JF, et al. [Single cerebral metastasis of bronchopulmonary cancers]. *Rev Neurol (Paris).* 1994;150:216–221.
15. Armstrong JG, Wronski M, Galicich J, et al. Postoperative radiation for lung cancer metastatic to the brain. *J Clin Oncol.* 1994;12:2340–2344.
16. Rossi NP, Zavala DC, VanGilder JC. A combined surgical approach to non-oat-cell pulmonary carcinoma with single cerebral metastasis. *Respiration.* 1987;51:170–178.
17. Nakagawa H, Miyawaki Y, Fujita T, et al. Surgical treatment of brain metastases of lung cancer: retrospective analysis of 89 cases. *J Neurol Neurosurg Psychiatry.* 1994;57:950–956.
18. Patchell RA, Tibbs PA, Walsh JW, et al. A randomized trial of surgery in the treatment of single metastases to the brain. *N Engl J Med.* 1990;322:494–500.
19. Loeffler JS, Shrieve DC, Wen PY, et al. Radiosurgery for intracranial malignancies. *Semin Radiat Oncol.* 1995;5:225–234.
20. Bonnette P, Puyo P, Gabriel C, et al. Surgical management of non-small cell lung cancer with synchronous brain metastases. *Chest.* 2001;119:1469–1475.
21. Billing PS, Miller DL, Allen MS, et al. Surgical treatment of primary lung cancer with synchronous brain metastases. *J Thorac Cardiovasc Surg.* 2001;122:548–553.
22. Hu C, Chang EL, Hassenbusch SJ III, et al. Nonsmall cell lung cancer presenting with synchronous solitary brain metastasis. *Cancer.* 2006;106:1998–2004.
23. Nakamura O, Matsutani M, Shitara N, et al. New treatment protocol by intra-operative radiation therapy for metastatic brain tumours. *Acta Neurochir (Wien).* 1994;131:91–96.
24. Pontiggia P, Duppone Curto F, Rotella G, et al. Hyperthermia in the treatment of brain metastases from lung cancer. Experience on 17 cases. *Anticancer Res.* 1995;15:597–601.

25. Gore EM, Bae K, Wong SJ, et al. Phase III comparison of prophylactic cranial irradiation versus observation in patients with locally advanced non-small-cell lung cancer: primary analysis of radiation therapy oncology group study RTOG 0214. *J Clin Oncol.* 2011;29(3):272–278.
26. Wang Z, Yuan, Z, Zhang W, et al. Brain metastasis treated with Cyberknife. *Chin Med J (Engl).* 2009;122(16):1847–1850.
27. Mehta MP, Tsao MN, Whelan TJ, et al. The American Society for Therapeutic Radiology and Oncology (ASTRO) evidence-based review of the role of radiosurgery for brain metastases. *Int J Radiat Oncol Biol Phys.* 2005;63(1):37–46.
28. Schellinger PD, Meinck HM, Thron A. Diagnostic accuracy of MRI compared to CCT in patients with brain metastases. *J Neurooncol.* 1999; 44:275–281.
29. Schrevens L, Lorent N, Dooms C, et al. The role of PET scan in diagnosis, staging, and management of non-small cell lung cancer. *Oncologist.* 2004;9:633–643.
30. Mordant P, Arame A, De Dominicis F, et al. Which metastasis management allows long-term survival of synchronous solitary M1b non-small cell lung cancer? *Eur J Cardiothorac Surg.* 2012;41(3):617–622.

PART 12

EXTENDED PULMONARY RESECTIONS

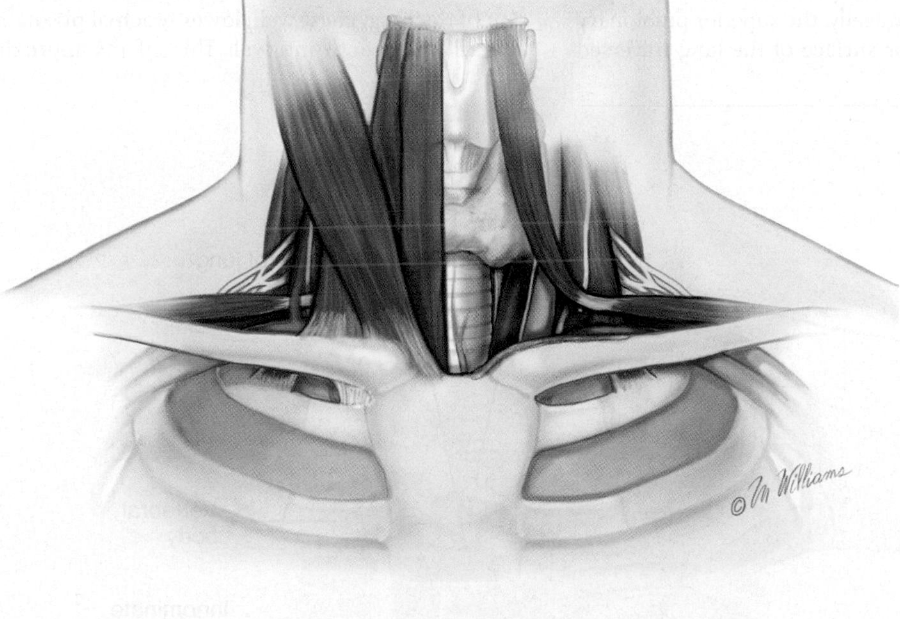

80 Pancoast Syndrome: Extended Resection in Superior Pulmonary Sulcus and Anterior Approach

Harold C. Urschel, Jr.* and Mark J. Krasna

Keywords: Pancoast, superior sulcus tumors, trimodality therapy

INTRODUCTION

Approximately 5% of all non-small cell lung cancers (NSCLC) are located in the extreme apex of the lung, frequently with involvement of some combination of the first and second ribs, brachial plexus, subclavian vessels, and upper thoracic vertebral bodies. This phenomenon is referred to as a superior sulcus carcinoma, indicating tumor location in the uppermost portion of the costovertebral gutter within the chest. Pancoast syndrome refers to superior sulcus tumors along with the triad of (1) shoulder and arm pain, (2) wasting of the hand muscles, and (3) ipsilateral Horner syndrome (i.e., ptosis, miosis, and anhidrosis due invasion of the stellate ganglion). Henry Pancoast was a radiologist who described these findings in 1932 but failed to recognize the pulmonary origin of these tumors. Unaware of Pancoast report, Tobias, an Argentine physician, described similar clinical findings and ascribed them to the presence of peripheral lung tumors. Pancoast–Tobias syndrome is perhaps a more appropriate eponym for this entity. Anatomically, the superior pulmonary sulcus is the area on the superior surface of the lung traversed by the subclavian vessels and encircled by the first rib and spine (Fig. 80-1). It also may be described as the thoracic outlet or thoracic inlet.

For the next 25 years, these tumors were considered unresectable and uniformly fatal. In 1951, during irradiation therapy, a patient of Dr. Robert Shaw developed unbearable pain that precluded continuation of his irradiation therapy. With a threat of suicide, Dr. Shaw performed an en bloc resection of the cancer, with the chest wall, and lower trunk of the brachial plexus. Dr. Shaw did not expect him to live long; however, the patient survived over 40 years (outliving Dr. Shaw).

In 1961, Shaw et al.[1] described successful outcomes in 18 patients undergoing 30 Gy of radiation, followed by resection, and this became the standard of care for the next 20 to 30 years. In over 400 patients with N0 stage I, Urschel found that approximately 35% had a 5-year survival. The treatment of choice since these reports has been preoperative irradiation (3000 rads over 2–3 weeks) followed by surgical en bloc resection of the lung, chest wall, lower brachial plexus, and vertebrae at a 1- to 2-month interval. This effects approximately a 35%

*Deceased

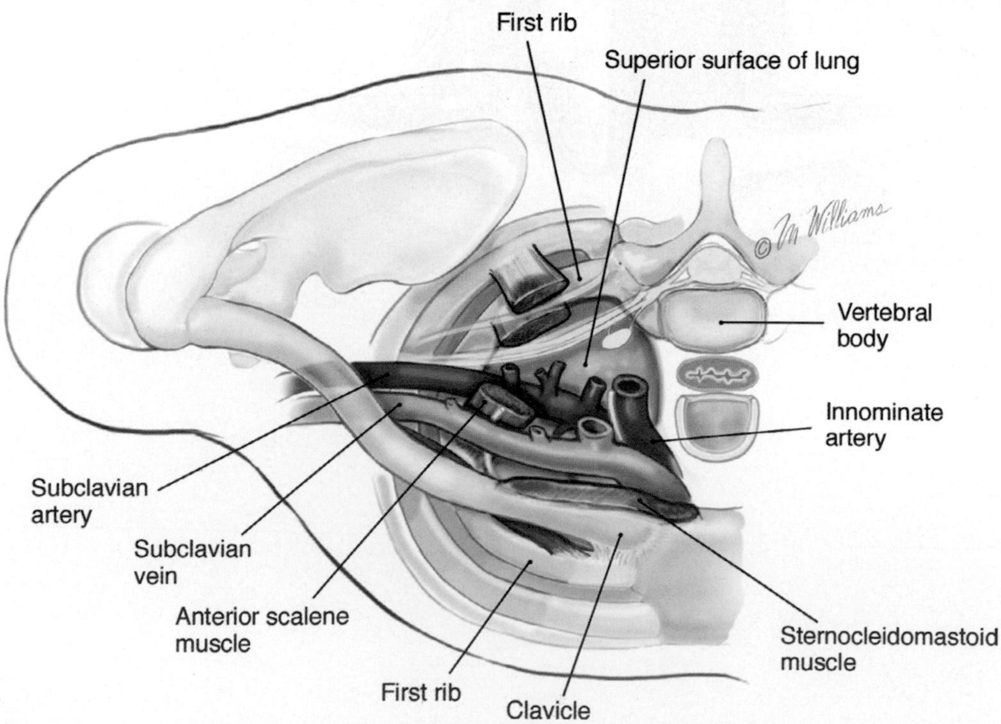

Figure 80-1. Defining anatomy of the superior pulmonary sulcus.

to 50% 5-year survival with N0 stage I patients. Recently, the Intergroup 0160 phase II trial demonstrated superior outcomes by using trimodality therapy for superior sulcus tumors, which now represents the standard of care.[2]

BACKGROUND

Dr. Shaw's initial successful outcome caused our group to treat several other patients in similar fashion with 3000 rads to the tumor and mediastinal lymph nodes over a period of 2 to 3 weeks, followed by a waiting period of 2 to 4 weeks. This delay allows time for the benefits of irradiation, which theoretically include shrinking of the tumor, blocking of the lymphatics, and weakening of the cells that might be left after surgery because the margins are extremely close in such tumor resections. In 1961, 14 patients were reported, with approximately 40% 5-year survival shown.[1] Chardack and MacCallum[3,4] presented a patient in 1953 and 1956 who had been resected and treated successfully with postoperative irradiation therapy. This approach, however, has not been as reproducible in other centers.

GENERAL PRINCIPLES AND PATIENT SELECTION

Factors that predict a favorable outcome after resection of superior sulcus tumors include R0 resection, absence of N2 or N3 metastases,[5] lobectomy rather than limited pulmonary resection,[6] and a complete pathologic response after induction chemoradiotherapy.[7,8] Surprisingly, tumor stage (T3 vs. T4 status) may be less important prognostically in this subset of patients; in the Intergroup 0160 study, this criterion was not a significant determinant of survival. The need for vertebral or subclavian vessel resection should not be considered an absolute contraindication to surgical treatment. Fadel et al.[9] reported 5-year survival rates after resection of 36% in the presence of subclavian artery invasion.

Limited survival benefit occurs with surgical resection alone. Local recurrences are common and extremely debilitating in terms of pain and limb function. Even with induction radiotherapy, complete resection is achieved in only 60% of patients, and overall 5-year survival is no better than 30%. Resectability, local control, and long-term survival have been positively affected by the addition of concurrent chemotherapy, as demonstrated by the long-term results of the phase II multicenter Intergroup 0160 trial.[2] Two cycles of chemotherapy (i.e., cisplatin and etoposide) concurrent with 45 Gy of radiation to the primary tumor, followed by surgical resection 3 to 5 weeks later, with two adjuvant cycles of chemotherapy was well tolerated in 110 patients. This regimen resulted in R0 resection rates of 94% for T3 lesions, 96% for T4 lesions, an overall complete pathologic response rate of 56%, and 5-year survival of 44% (54% for R0 resection). Relapse occurred predominantly in the brain, with local failure in only 10 patients, a significant pattern shift in this disease. Ongoing questions exist about the optimal dose of radiation; our group[8] has used higher radiation doses (median dose 56 Gy) with good tolerance and concomitant increased rates of complete pathologic response. Ideally, higher-dose regimens should be studied in a multicenter study protocol to make sure that these excellent results are generalizable.

Most superior sulcus tumors are approached posteriorly through a posterolateral thoracotomy extending up to the base of the neck, which is appropriate for posteriorly located tumors (Shaw–Paulson posterior approach). Exposure of tumors above the thoracic inlet is suboptimal with a posterior approach, however, and this may explain why there have been incomplete resections in the past. The anterior approach of Dartevelle is preferable for more anteriorly and superiorly located tumors because it provides better access to the subclavian vessels and other cervical structures. Many surgeons favor an anterior exposure when there is a palpable supraclavicular mass, clinical involvement of the C7 or C8 nerve root, Horner syndrome, proven or suspected vascular invasion, or any involvement of the thoracic inlet (or Sibson fascia) and structures superior to it.[10] It is important to be familiar with both the anterior and posterior exposures to permit maximum flexibility while operating.

Given the magnitude of the surgical resections, especially following concurrent chemoradiation, it is important to select patients with satisfactory performance status, as well as adequate cardiac, pulmonary, and renal function (especially for platinum-based regimens). Smoking cessation is also critical. Marginal respiratory status in conjunction with pulmonary and chest wall resection increases perioperative risk. Careful neurologic assessment is critical to determine the extent of brachial plexus involvement. Any neurologic dysfunction higher than the lower trunk of the plexus is likely to lead to significant limb dysfunction after resection; in some rare cases, forequarter amputation may be considered a better palliative option.[11,12] In addition, long-track neurologic symptoms may indicate extensive spinal cord involvement owing to vertebral invasion.

PREOPERATIVE ASSESSMENT

Initial assessment is similar to that for any lung cancer resection. Tissue is almost always obtainable by transthoracic needle aspiration.[13] Of note, tuberculosis and lymphoma have been reported to mimic Pancoast tumors. Tissue diagnosis therefore is critical before commencing multimodality therapy. In addition to chest and upper abdomen CT scanning and CT/PET, it is often helpful to include a neck CT scan to better image the thoracic inlet. To better delineate involvement of the brachial plexus, subclavian vessels, vertebral bodies, or neural foramina, MRI with contrast enhancement is the preferred imaging modality for this region. Involvement of the lower trunks of the brachial plexus may be considered a contraindication to resection because of limb dysfunction; however, resection of the T1 and C8 nerve roots can be easily accomplished. Brain imaging, using CT scanning or MRI, is also recommended as part of a thorough metastatic assessment. Extrathoracic metastases or persistent N2 or N3 disease after induction therapy is considered an absolute oncologic contraindication by most. It is critical to perform a thorough mediastinoscopic evaluation as part of the initial workup[14] or after induction chemoradiation.[8] If persistent postoperative N2 or N3 disease is documented, surgery should be attempted when it is the only satisfactory way to palliate pain because cure cannot be achieved.[15]

Extensive involvement of the subclavian and carotid arteries is not an absolute contraindication to resection (Table 80-1). Doppler ultrasound of the neck vessels and great vessels, including the vertebral artery, is helpful not only for assessment of tumor invasion but also to look for atherosclerotic changes

Table 80-1
CONTRAINDICATIONS TO SURGERY
Inadequate cardiopulmonary reserve
Distant metastases
Persistent N2 or N3 disease after induction therapy
Involvement of trunks of the brachial plexus
Involvement of nerve roots higher than C8

Table 80-2
ADDITIONAL PREOPERATIVE TESTS RECOMMENDED FOR SUPERIOR SULCUS TUMORS
Contrast-enhanced MRI of thoracic inlet/brachial plexus
Doppler ultrasound of neck and great vessels
Electromyography in selected patients

that may affect clamp placement or critical stenosis.[15] Careful neurologic examination and, in some cases, electromyography can help to define brachial plexus involvement, phrenic nerve involvement, and cord involvement. Preoperative neurosurgical consultation is highly recommended if there is any question of brachial plexus involvement or vertebral invasion; a team approach can be very useful intraoperatively (Table 80-2).

DIAGNOSIS

Clinical Presentation

Most patients present with shoulder and elbow pain because of involvement of the lower trunk of the brachial plexus. The discomfort often follows the distribution of the ulnar nerve because of malignant invasion of T1 and C8 nerve roots and extension into the parietal pleura and first rib.[16] Weakness and atrophy of the intrinsic muscles in the hand, along with pain and paresthesias in the medial aspect of the arm and fourth and fifth digits (distribution of the ulnar nerve), sometimes associated with a loss of the triceps reflex, also are caused by C8 and T1 nerve root involvement. Pain may radiate into the neck and head and posteriorly into the scapular area or anteriorly into the chest (Fig. 80-2).

Classically, the patient presents holding the elbow with the opposite arm to support the shoulder and take the pressure off the brachial plexus for symptomatic relief (Fig. 80-3).[16,17] Frequently, the diagnosis is missed because of concentration on cervical osteoarthritis, discs, or other differential diagnoses, often delaying recognition of the true etiology. Horner syndrome classically presents as an ipsilateral ptosis, with narrowing of the palpebral fissure, miosis, and anhidrosis. It is produced by involvement of the sympathetic chain in the area of C7 and C8, the upper two-thirds of the stellate ganglion (Fig. 80-4).[18] Vertebral involvement and spinal cord compression with paralysis (paraplegia) are observed occasionally. Phrenic or recurrent laryngeal nerve invasion is present infrequently, producing diaphragmatic paralysis or hoarseness. Superior vena cava syndrome may result if anterior tumors are present. This syndrome leads to swelling of the face and distention of the neck and upper chest wall veins. Primary pulmonary tumors also may produce the usual symptoms of cough, hemoptysis, dyspnea, wheeze, and weight loss.

Radiographic Findings

Chest roentgenographs (posteroanterior and lateral) are the simplest methods of discerning an apical mass (Fig. 80-5A). Apical lordotic chest views are valuable after the screening procedure. CT scan of the chest provides additional information, particularly about bone invasion (including the first rib) and vertebral involvement (Fig. 80-5B). It also may be used to delineate lung and liver metastases. MRI is particularly helpful in soft tissue areas, such as invasion of the brachial plexus, vascular structures, and chest wall, as well as lymph node metastases in the mediastinum (Fig. 80-5C).[19]

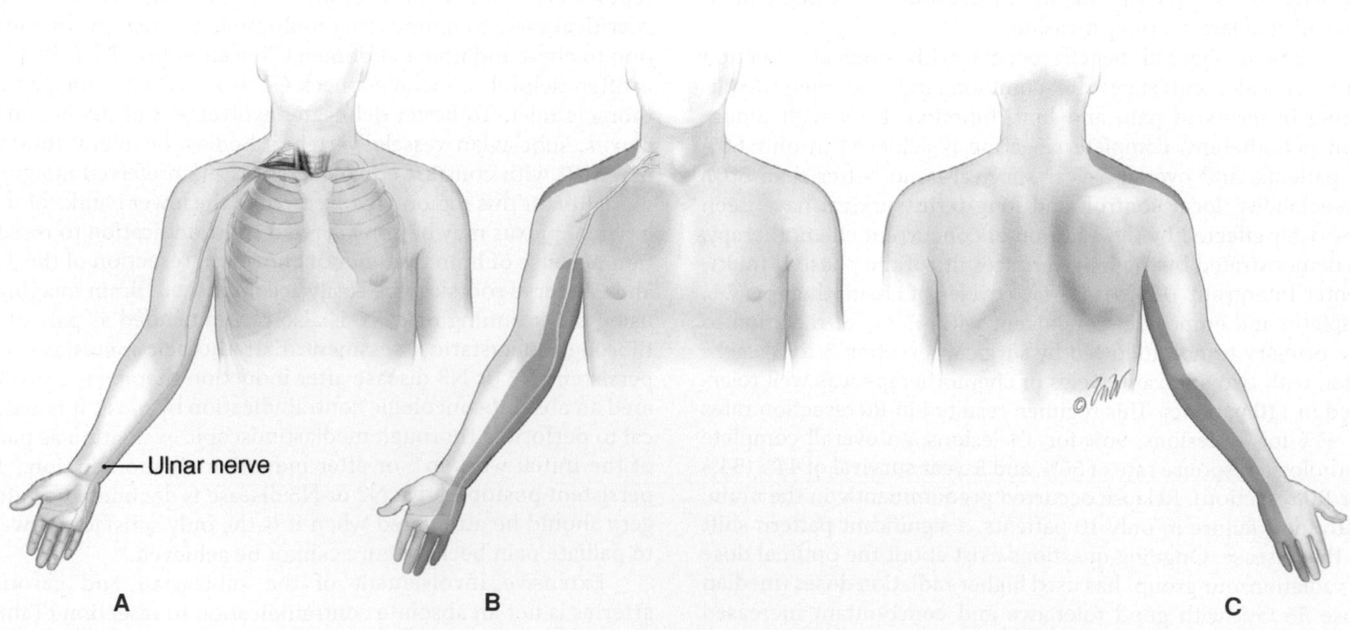

Figure 80-2. Spectrum of presenting symptoms. Patients may experience (*A*) discomfort along the distribution of the ulnar nerve caused by malignant invasion of the T1 and C8 nerve roots, (*B*) weakness and atrophy of the muscles along the ulnar nerve root with pain and paresthesias, and (*C*) pain radiating into the neck, head, posteriorly on the scapula, or anteriorly into the chest.

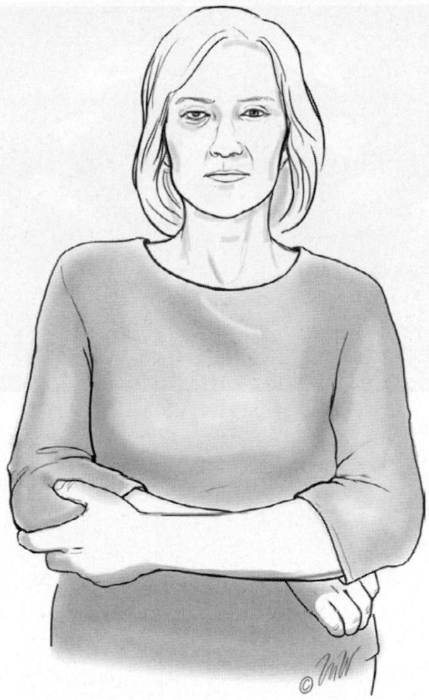

Figure 80-3. Typical clinical presentation includes wasting, pain, paresthesias, and paresis of arm and hand.

Diagnosis Tests

The definitive diagnosis is established by a transthoracic needle biopsy, usually through the supraclavicular space or the posterosuperior chest between the scapula and spine. These small needles are guided by fluoroscopy, ultrasound, or CT in most cases. The first description of transcervical biopsy via the supraclavicular approach was reported by McGoon [20] in 1964. Biopsy may be performed under local or general anesthesia. The diagnostic yield for needle biopsy is greater than 90%. Diagnostic yield from sputum cytology is less than 20%, and for bronchoscopy (fiberoptic or rigid), it is less than 30%.[21] The diagnostic yield of these tests is low because most of these tumors are peripheral.

Staging and Perioperative Assessment

Cervical mediastinal lymph node exploration is necessary before treatment in these patients to establish whether the lymph nodes are positive. The suggestion of enlarged nodes on either the CT scan or MRI may be helpful, but the staging of actual metastases is critical.[22] False positive and false negatives occur frequently and often only supraclavicular lymph nodes are involved. If the mediastinal nodes are positive for a right upper lobe lesion, it is still treated as an operable case because the lymph nodes are assumed to be "regional." Metastasis to the contralateral mediastinal lymph nodes is a poor prognosticator

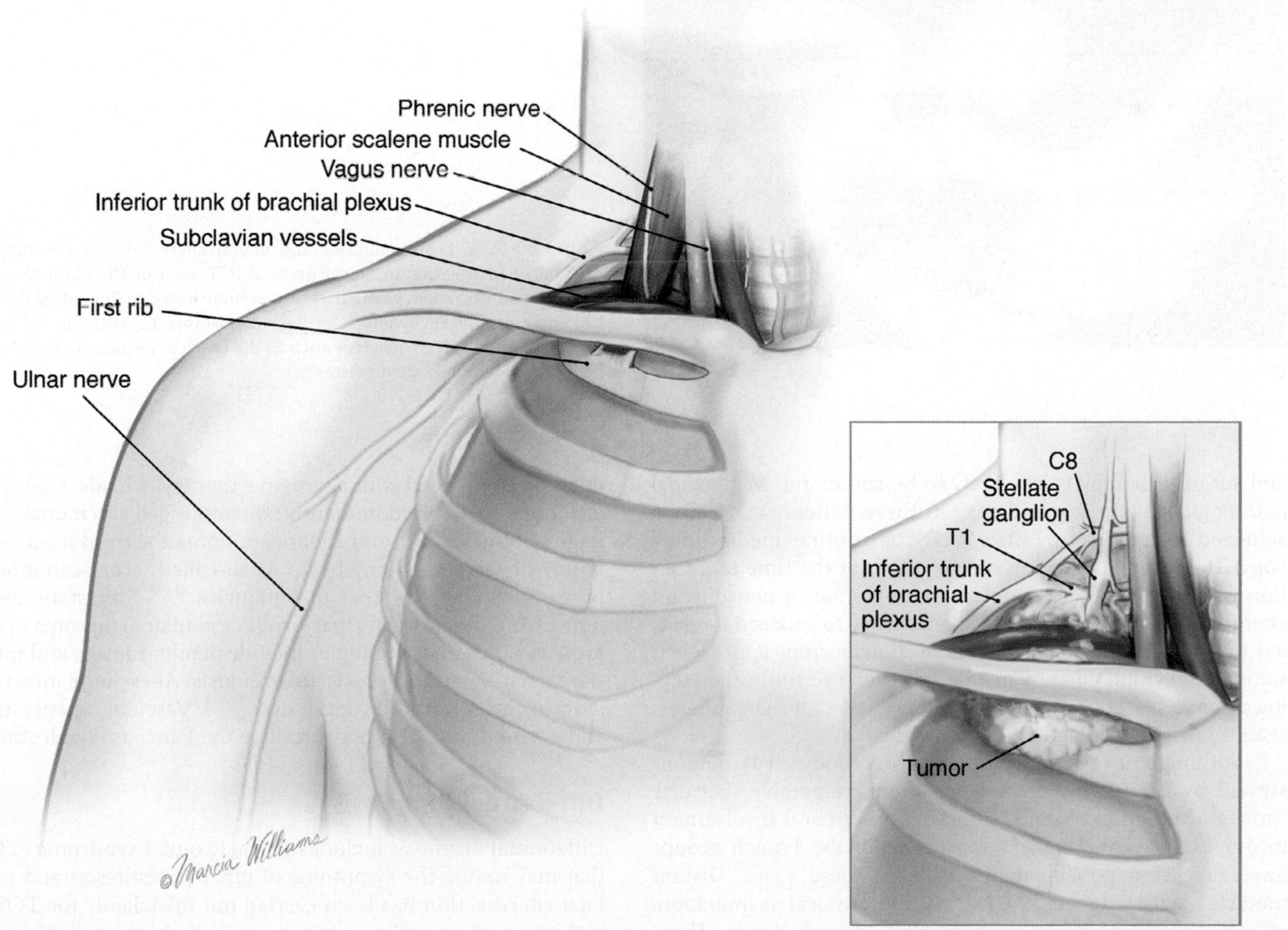

Figure 80-4. Horner syndrome is produced by involvement of the sympathetic chain in the area of C7 and C8 in the upper two-thirds of the stellate ganglion.

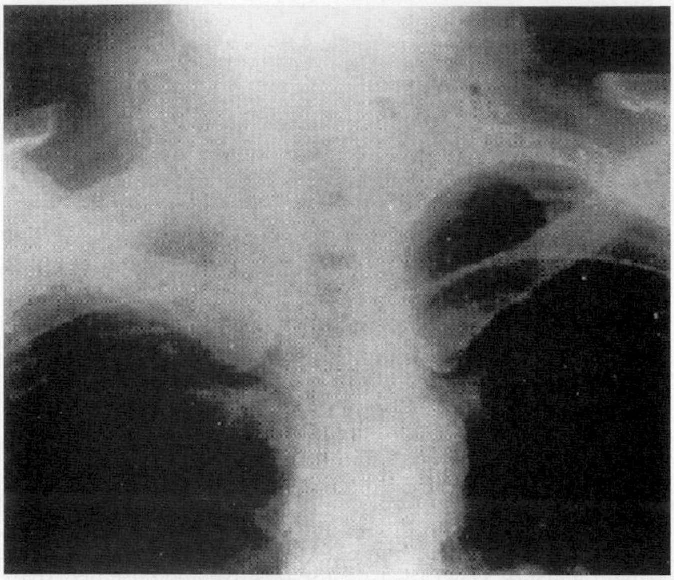

A

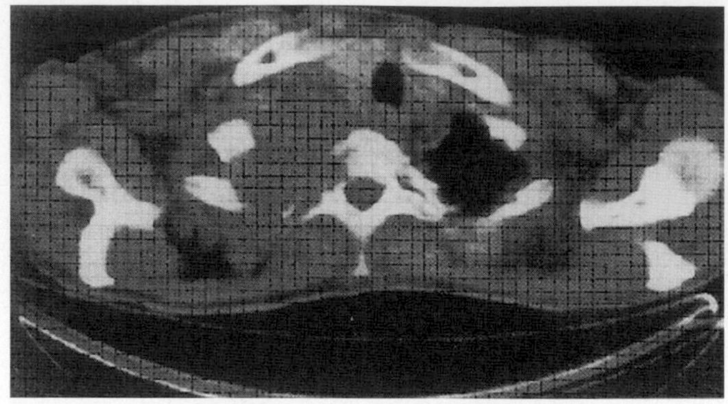

B

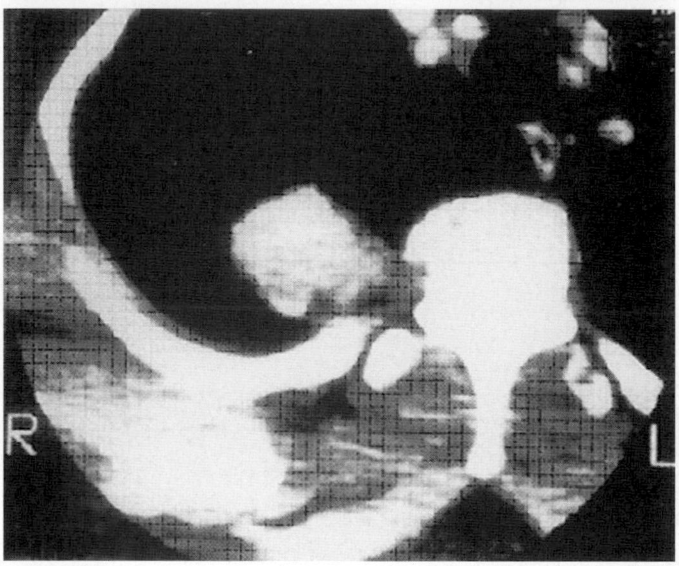

C

Figure 80-5. *A.* Posteroanterior and lateral chest X-ray is the simplest method of identifying an apical mass. *B.* CT scan of the chest provides additional information, particularly about bone invasion (including the first rib) and vertebral involvement or liver metastases. *C.* MRI can aid in the investigation of soft tissue areas such as the brachial plexus, chest wall, and mediastinal lymph node metastases.

and surgical therapy is less likely to be successful. Mediastinal pathologic staging is mandatory in these patients and can be achieved using TBNA/EBUS/VATS or routine mediastinoscopy. The timing of staging can be either at the time of initiation of induction therapy or after completion of neoadjuvant chemoradiation in order to decide whether to proceed if residual positive lymph nodes are found. Our current approach is sample the lymph node by needle and then use surgical restaging prior to resection (where we will not resect if there are persistent positive mediastinal lymph nodes).

Although invasion of the vertebral body (T4) demonstrated by CT usually renders a patient inoperable (because "no reported cures" have resulted with vertebral involvement in our experience[19]); recent reports from the French groups have suggested possible cures even in these cases. Distant metastases are suspected by history and physical examination, as well as retroperitoneum, liver, and adrenal glands. These lesions should be biopsied and metastasis confirmed before a decision to proceed with aggressive therapy is made. Cell types encountered are predominantly squamous cell carcinoma, with large cell the second, and adenocarcinoma the third most commonly observed.[23] Many begin as so-called "scar" carcinomas or are secondary to other malignancies.[24–28] Metastatic carcinoma from other organs may produce similar symptoms in this area. Various other etiologies include benign tumors and infections such as actinomycosis, tuberculosis, Allescheria infection, cryptococcosis, and hydatid cyst.[29–36] Vascular aneurysms[37] and amyloidosis[38] also may produce the Pancoast syndrome.

Differential Diagnosis

Differential diagnosis includes thoracic outlet syndrome (TOS) that may mimic the symptoms of ulnar paresthesias and pain. First rib resection has been carried out mistakenly for TOS in patients with superior sulcus tumor of the lung.[16] Vascular, esophageal, and cardiac disease also can mimic symptoms of superior pulmonary sulcus tumors, and these areas should be ruled out in the differential diagnosis.[16]

Indications for Surgery

If the patient has a tumor in the area of the superior pulmonary sulcus with or without rib involvement and with or without lower brachial plexus involvement, and it is staged as a T3N0 or N1, he or she is operable. N2 disease is operable if it is in the upper lobe and the mediastinal nodes are considered to be ipsilateral metastases. Involvement of the vena cava and subclavian artery or vein is not an absolute contraindication for surgery. These patients should undergo neoadjuvant chemoradiation followed by reassessment of the extent of disease prior to planned resection.

In addition to chest and upper abdomen CT scanning and CT/PET, it is often helpful to include a neck CT scan to better image the thoracic inlet. To better delineate involvement of the brachial plexus, subclavian vessels, vertebral bodies, or neural foramina, MRI with contrast enhancement is the preferred imaging modality for this region. Involvement of the lower trunks of the brachial plexus may be considered a contraindication to resection because of limb dysfunction; however, resection of the T1 and C8 nerve roots can be easily accomplished. Brain imaging, using CT scanning or MRI, is also recommended as part of a thorough metastatic assessment.

Extrathoracic metastases or persistent N2 or N3 disease after induction therapy is considered an absolute oncologic contraindication by most. It is critical to perform a thorough mediastinoscopic evaluation as part of the initial workup[11] or after induction chemoradiation.[5] If persistent postoperative induction N2 or N3 disease is documented, surgery should be attempted when it is the only satisfactory way to palliate pain because cure cannot be achieved.[12]

Although vertebral involvement traditionally has been a contraindication for surgical resection of superior sulcus carcinoma, recent advances in spinal instrumentation have permitted a more complete resection of vertebral body tumor. Gandhi et al. [39] (Garrett Walsh & Associates at MD Anderson) have published good results in 17 patients with vertebral resection of carcinoma extension. Contraindications include extensive involvement of the brachial plexus, mediastinal perinodal involvement, significant invasion of the soft tissues of the neck, and distant metastasis. Palliative resection is performed occasionally for intractable pain.[19] Recent reports by Dartevelle et al.[40,41] and Grunenwald et al.[42] suggest a role for extensive resection with good outcomes in selected patients.

TREATMENT

Preoperative Radiotherapy Followed by Surgery

After preoperative radiotherapy (3000 rads delivered over 2–3 weeks) or chemoradiation followed by a 4-week waiting period, surgical extirpation with an en bloc resection of the pulmonary tumor, chest wall, lower brachial plexus, and vertebrae through the posterior thoracoplasty approach is performed. The en bloc resection of the pulmonary tumor and chest wall is accompanied by resection of the sympathetic chain, the lower trunk of the brachial plexus in most cases (T1 nerve root in most cases; C8 nerve root less frequently), and rarely, the subclavian artery with an interposed graft. A margin of vertebral body is removed with most tumors. A segmentectomy, subsegmental resection, lobectomy, or pneumonectomy is performed to complete the en bloc dissection, although sublobar resections have been reported by some to have a negative impact on local control and long-term survival. Chest wall replacement is required occasionally for anterior tumors but usually not for those lying under the scapula. If six or more ribs are taken, posterior reconstruction with Marlex or other synthetic material is important to keep the scapula from sticking inside the chest.[43]

The anterior cervical approach championed by Dartevelle et al.[41] involves a median sternotomy and cervical resection of the clavicle, as well as en bloc resection of the artery, often the vein, and the tumor.

Chemotherapy and/or Chemoradiation

Induction chemotherapy combined with radiation has markedly improved the treatment of superior sulcus tumors. Wright et al.[44] from Massachusetts General Hospital reported significant improvement in complete resection rate, pathologic response, 2- and 4-year survival, and reduction of local recurrence with CT/radiation induction therapy over induction radiation therapy alone in over 30 patients. Since then, they have treated 15 more patients (total 30), and there have been two distant recurrences. The 5-year survival approaches 50%.

The Southwest Oncology Group reported less good results with combination chemo/radiation induction therapy, but this was a multicenter study in contrast to the preceding study.[45] Recently, Kwong et al.[8] have reported on excellent response rates and long-term survival in a single institution study of neoadjuvant chemoradiation including patients presenting with N2 disease.

TECHNIQUE

Shaw-Posterior Surgical Technique

Routine measures for lung resection should be undertaken, such as use of preoperative antibiotics, deep vein thrombosis prophylaxis, and a double-lumen endotracheal tube. Central venous line placement is prudent for reliable IV access and central venous pressure monitoring and in most patients should be placed on the contralateral side to keep the line out of the surgical field. Radial arterial pressure monitoring is also recommended and also should be placed on the nonoperative side in case subclavian artery manipulation is required. It is also wise to coordinate surgical scheduling with a spine specialist (neurosurgeon of orthopedic) for backup in case of vertebral body or other neurologic involvement.

After induction of general anesthesia, the patient is intubated with a double-lumen endotracheal tube. The patient is placed in the lateral decubitus position with an axillary roll under the "down" side (Fig. 80-6). The incision begins above the angle of the scapula, halfway between it and the spinous processes (i.e., thoracoplasty technique), and extends inferiorly, angling anteriorly around the tip of the scapula. The subcutaneous tissue is divided, followed by trapezius and rhomboid muscles. Although we generally try to spare the posterior superior serratus muscle, occasionally, this too needs to be divided to allow adequate exposure.

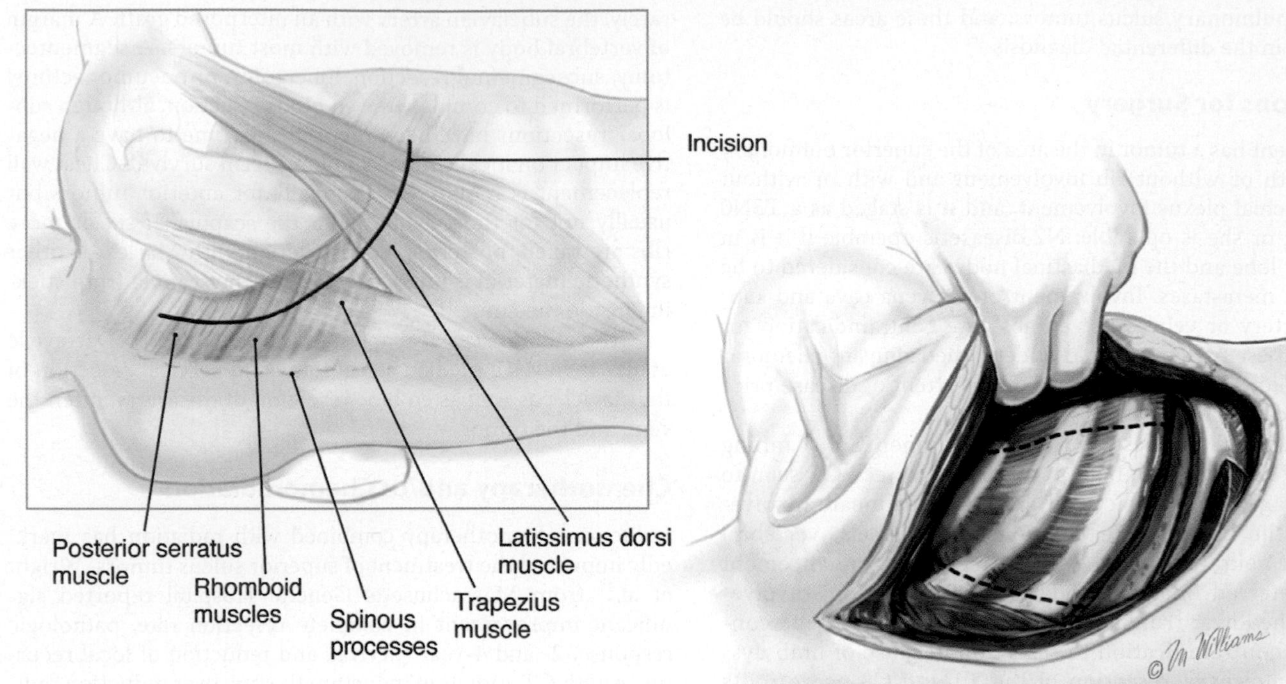

Figure 80-6. (*Inset*) Patient positioning and incision. The subcutaneous tissue and trapezius and rhomboid muscles, followed by the posterior superior serratus, are divided.

The intercostal muscle overlying the fourth rib is incised. A Finochietto retractor is placed between the top of the fourth rib and the scapula superiorly. Since double-lumen intubation is used for the operation, the lung is already collapsed. The fourth interspace is opened. Alternatively, this can be done using the cautery. The surgeon places a hand in the patient's chest to palpate the tumor and determine its extent, the number of ribs involved, and the length of each rib to be resected (Fig. 80-7). If the tumor is large, a lower interspace may be used. If possible we generally try to preserve the intercostal muscle flap thus developed, to use for later reinforcement of the airway stump (especially after induction therapy). Anteriorly, the ribs are divided with the rib shears after ligating, dividing, or clipping the neurovascular bundle under each rib. The dissection is carried up to and through the first rib. Posteriorly, the ribs are sheared off with an osteotome, taking the rib at the level of the transverse processes, disarticulating the ribs or taking a small segment of vertebrae, if necessary. The intercostal bundles may be cauterized or clipped. This is carried through the third, second, and first ribs. Patients with CT evidence of tumor invading the vertebrae are generally considered inoperable. However, if at operation the tumor is found to lie adjacent to the vertebrae, a margin of vertebrae is taken with the osteotome. Preparation by involvement of a neurosurgical or orthopedic team may be prudent in this situation.

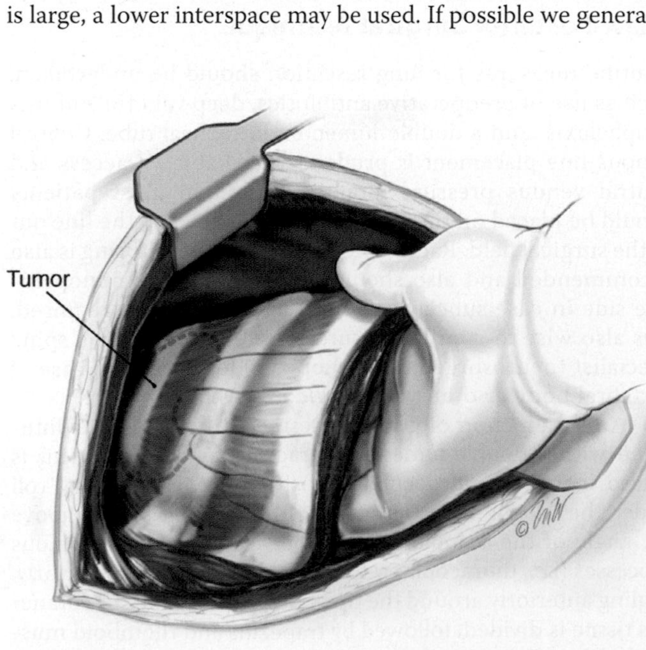

Figure 80-7. The intercostal muscle overlying the fourth rib is incised, the fourth interspace is opened, and the tumor is palpated to determine the extent of resection.

After the first rib is cut anteriorly and posteriorly, the surgeon inserts the index finger from one hand in the front and the index finger from the other hand from the back to palpate the tumor (Fig. 80-8) and identify its relationship to the T1 and C8 nerve roots, the lower trunk of the brachial plexus, and the axillary subclavian artery and vein (Fig. 80-9). The scalenus anticus and medius muscles are divided with the finger holding the en bloc section anteriorly and inferiorly. Caution is taken to avoid injury to the artery or vein. The T1 nerve root is divided posteriorly, and the segment is lifted up with the tumor. The C8 nerve root is visualized and may be divided if necessary. The anterior part of the T1 nerve root is divided. The subclavian artery is dissected from the tumor. If the artery is involved, an interposition graft, such as autogenous saphenous vein, is used. This is usually not the case because the adventitia protects the artery from tumor invasion.

A lobectomy optimally is performed after the en bloc chest wall resection. Segmental resection of the lung can considered

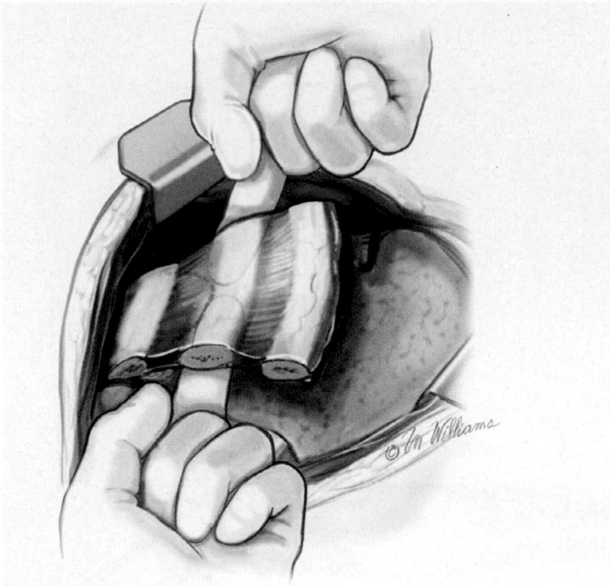

Figure 80-8. After the rib is cut anteriorly, the index fingers are inserted to palpate the tumor.

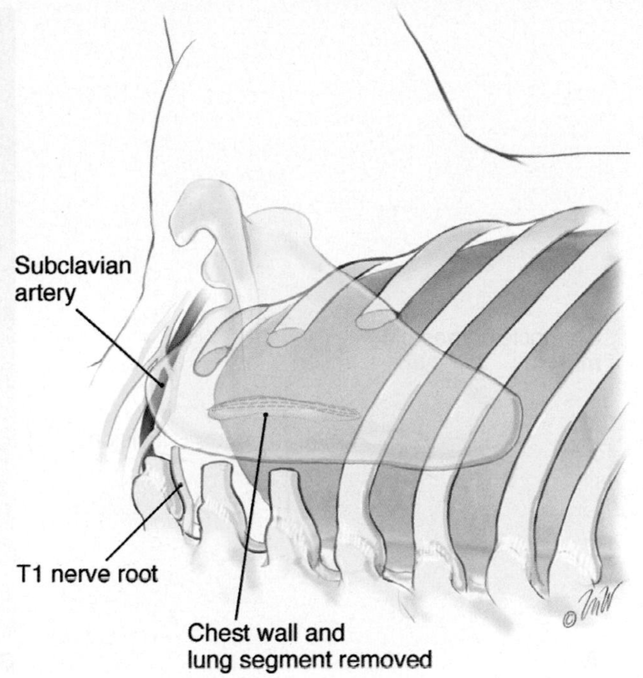

Figure 80-10. After en bloc resection of the chest wall, a lobectomy or segmental resection of the lung is performed. With anterior tumor, the chest wall is reconstructed with Marlex. For posterior tumors, the scapula usually overlies the posterior area of the chest wall and reconstruction with Marlex is not required.

if the patient is very high risk or no residual tumor is found. In general, these patients have had higher incidence of local recurrences. The chest wall is closed with Marlex if anterior in location. For posterior tumors, however, the scapula covers the posterior area, and usually no chest wall reconstruction is necessary (Fig. 80-10). If the fifth rib is removed, the scapula tip may get hooked under the sixth rib. If it appears that this may be a possibility, the tip of the scapula can be excised (Fig. 80-11). The wound is closed in layers with interrupted 0 Nurolon sutures in a figure-of-eight fashion (Tom Jones stitch), running 2-0 Vicryl in the subcutaneous tissues, and skin clips in the skin.

Dartevelle Transclavicular Technique

For the anterior approach as described by Dartevelle et al.,[41] the patient is positioned supine with the neck hyperextended and turned away from the tumor. A rolled towel behind the shoulders helps with exposure of the operative site.[46] The arms can be tucked at the sides, but it may be wise to leave access to the anterolateral chest on the operative side in case an anterolateral thoracotomy is necessary. The patient should be sterilely prepared from the angle of the mandible to below the costal margin and from the midclavicular line of the contralateral chest to the midaxillary line on the side of the tumor and beyond the shoulder superiorly. An L-shaped incision is performed along the anterior border of the sternocleidomastoid

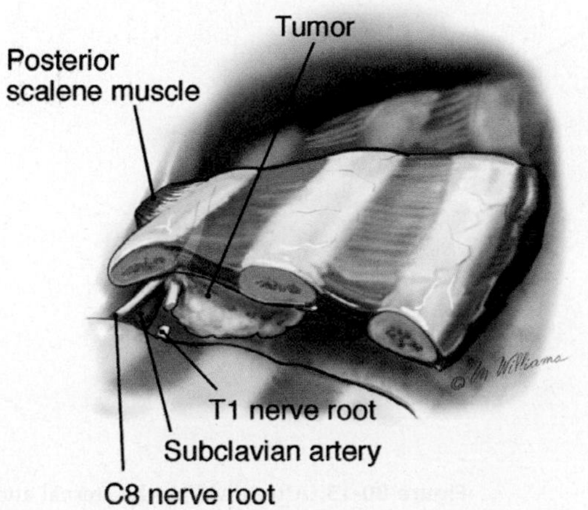

Figure 80-9. Using both index fingers as described, the surgeon determines the relationship of the tumor to the T1 and C8 nerve roots, lower trunk of the brachial plexus, and axillary subclavian artery and veins.

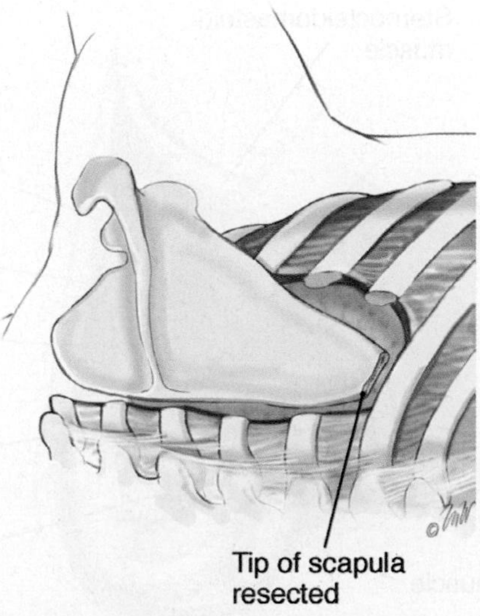

Figure 80-11. If the fifth rib was removed during en bloc chest wall resection and it appears that the tip of the scapula may get hooked under the sixth rib, the tip of the scapula is excised.

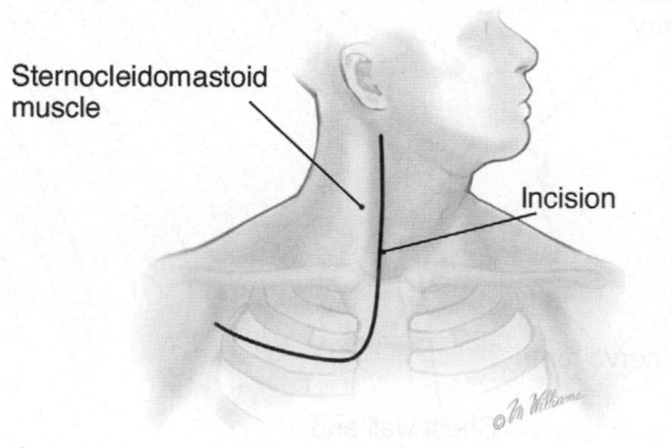

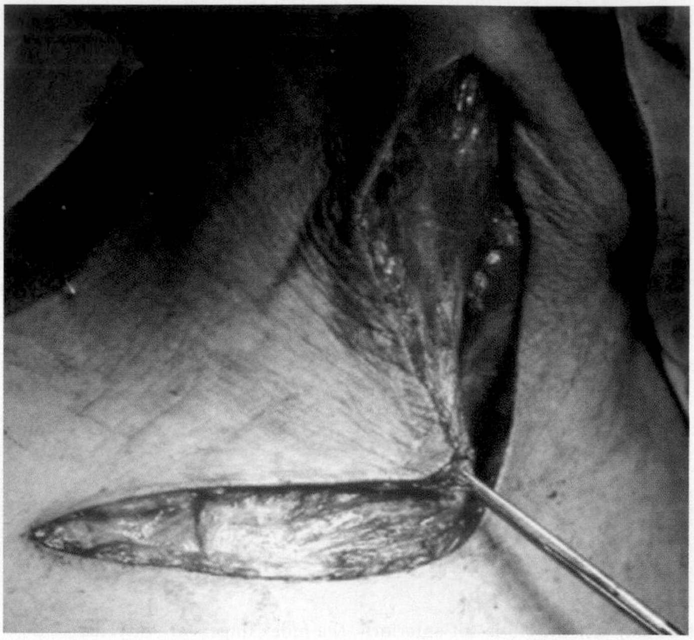

Figure 80-12. *A.* An L-shaped incision is performed along the anterior border of the sternocleidomastoid muscle. Note that the incision is extended horizontally a few centimeters below and parallel to the clavicle into the deltopectoral groove. *B.* Intraoperative photograph.

muscle, extending horizontally a few centimeters below and parallel to the clavicle into the deltopectoral groove (Fig. 80-12). Depending on the planned area of entry into the thoracic cavity, this transverse incision can be placed over the second, third, or fourth intercostal space.

The sternal attachments of the sternocleidomastoid muscles are divided, as are the upper digitations of the pectoral muscle on the clavicle; a myocutaneous flap now can be pulled back to expose the thoracic inlet (Figs. 80-13 and 80-14). The medial half of the clavicle is removed (the sternal or Gigli saw

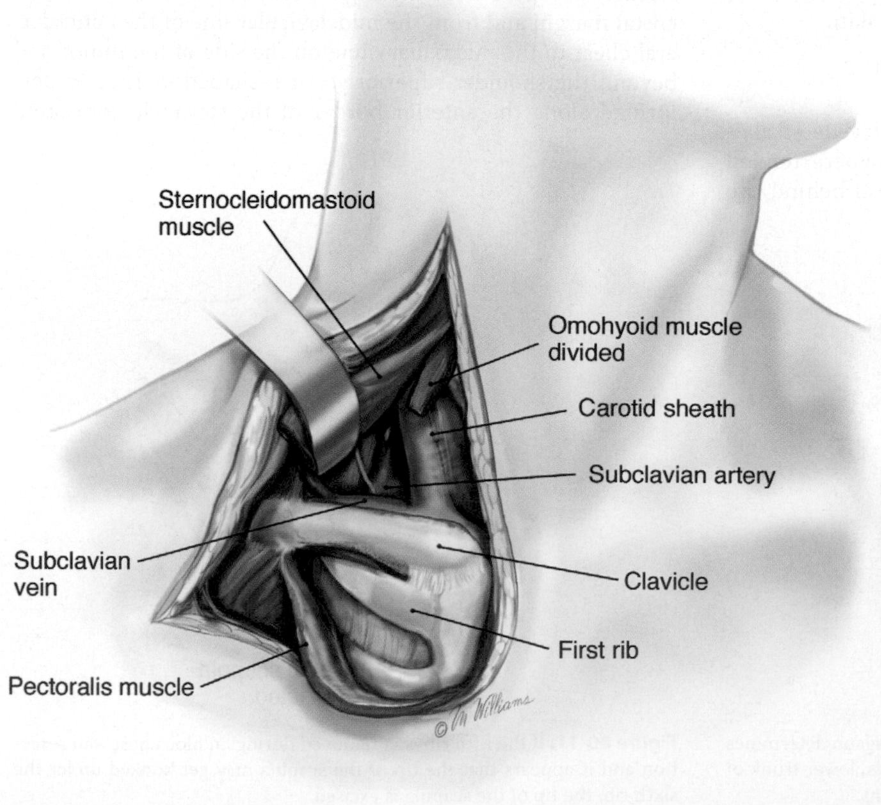

Figure 80-13. After dividing the sternal attachments of the sternocleidomastoid muscles and upper digitations of the pectoral muscle on the clavicle, the myocutaneous flap created by the incision can be pulled back to expose the thoracic inlet.

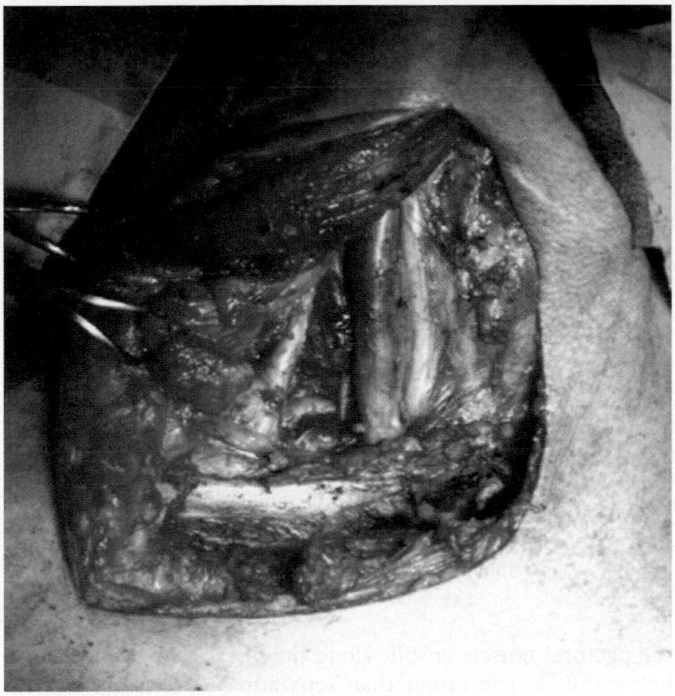

Figure 80-14. Same exposure of the thoracic inlet presented in the intraoperative photograph in Figure 80-12.

works well for this). The omohyoid is divided, if necessary, and the scalene fat pad is removed and checked for metastases. The subclavian vein and its branches, as well as the distal internal jugular vein (depending on the cephalad extent of tumor), are dissected and controlled proximally and distally. On the left it is often necessary to ligate the thoracic duct as it enters the vein. In general, veins should be resected and not reconstructed, realizing that the patient may have edema in that extremity, which can be managed with arm elevation and compression garments. As collaterals develop, the end result is usually not significantly morbid. It can be helpful to divide the anterior, external, and even internal jugular vein to facilitate mobilization and resection of the subclavian vein.

The pleural cavity is entered one interspace below the tumor to assess its intrathoracic extent. Next, the anterior scalene muscle can be divided at the first rib, unless it is grossly invaded, in which case it is better to divide it as proximally as possible, taking care to preserve the phrenic nerve (Fig. 80-15). This is followed by dissection of the subclavian artery and its branches, which all can be divided to facilitate mobilization. The exception is that the vertebral artery should be preserved when possible, but if it is invaded by tumor and there is no significant extracranial carotid vascular disease by preoperative duplex study, it should be taken en bloc with the tumor. If it is not possible to free the tumor from the subclavian artery in a subadventitial plane, then preparations should be made to resect and reconstruct it (see below). Next, the middle scalene muscle is taken as high as necessary to better expose the brachial plexus. It may be helpful to have the neurosurgical team assist with neurolysis of the plexus. Nerve roots can be divided but should not be taken higher than C8 (see Fig. 80-15, *inset*). It is important to ligate the roots to avoid a cerebrospinal fluid leak. If necessary for an R0 resection, the prevertebral muscles along with the paravertebral sympathetic chain and stellate ganglion can be resected safely as well. Many of these patients will have preexisting Horner syndrome, but if not, this possibility should be mentioned when obtaining informed written consent for the operation.

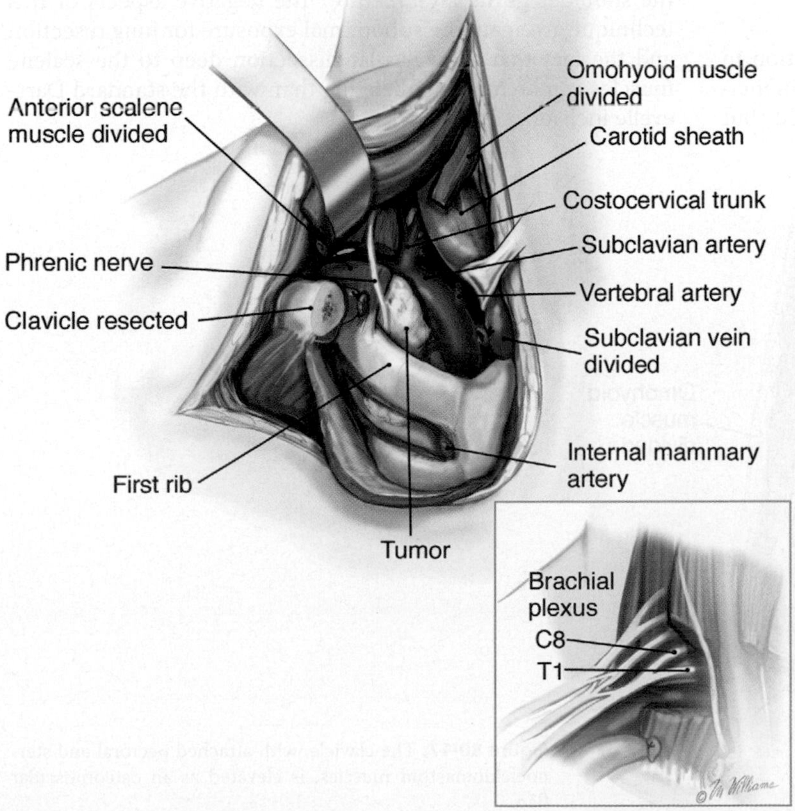

Figure 80-15. The pleural cavity is entered one interspace below the tumor to assess its intrathoracic extent. Assistance from the neurosurgical team is recommended for neurolysis of the plexus. (*Inset*) Nerve roots higher than C8 should not be taken.

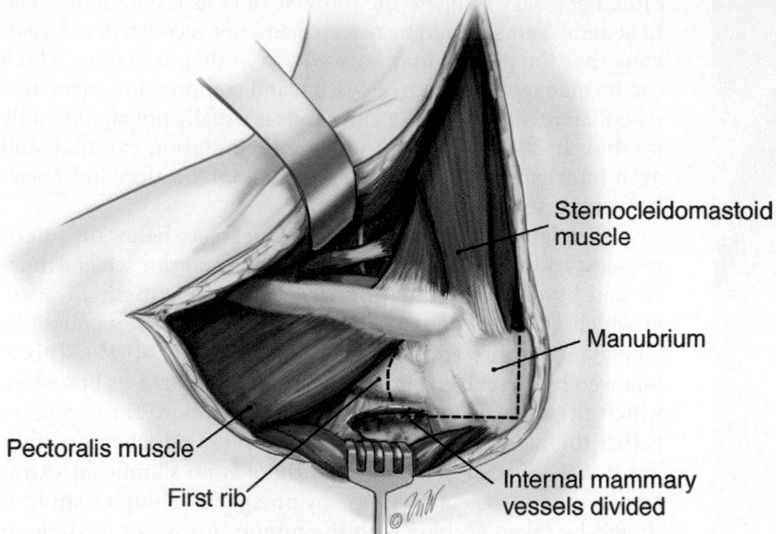

Figure 80-16. Osteomuscular-sparing approach with preservation of the sternoclavicular joint. The pectoral muscle is split along the fibers a few centimeters below the clavicle rather than separating it from the clavicle.

At this point, the first rib can be divided at the transverse process posteriorly and a few centimeters anterior to the tumor or at the costosternal junction. The second and third ribs also can be resected en bloc with the tumor as needed. This provides an entry point into the pleural space through which the upper lobectomy can be performed. In the past, an accessory anterior or in some cases posterolateral thoracotomy (after repositioning and reprepping the patient) has been made, but with videothoracoscopy assistance, and use of long thoracoscopic instruments and staplers, the additional incisions are less often necessary.

Osteomuscular-Sparing Approach

This technique differs from the above-described operation in that the sternoclavicular joint is preserved. The same skin incision is made, and the sternocleidomastoid is mobilized, but the pectoral muscle is split along the fibers a few centimeters below the clavicle rather than separating it from the clavicle (Fig. 80-16). An L-shaped incision is made in the manubrium with the sternal saw to release the upper outer corner adjacent to the sternoclavicular joint. The proximal internal mammary artery is ligated, and the first costal cartilage is resected. Now the clavicle, with attached pectoral and sternocleidomastoid muscles, can be elevated as an "osteomuscular flap" (Fig. 80-17). The remainder of the resection is carried out as described earlier. For closure, the manubrium is reapproximated with two sternal wires. Aesthetic and functional results are reportedly superior to those of claviculectomy owing to preservation of the shoulder girdle architecture. The negative aspects of this technique are again the suboptimal exposure for lung resection and the fact that the vascular dissection deep to the scalene muscles can be more challenging than with the standard Dartevelle incision.[46]

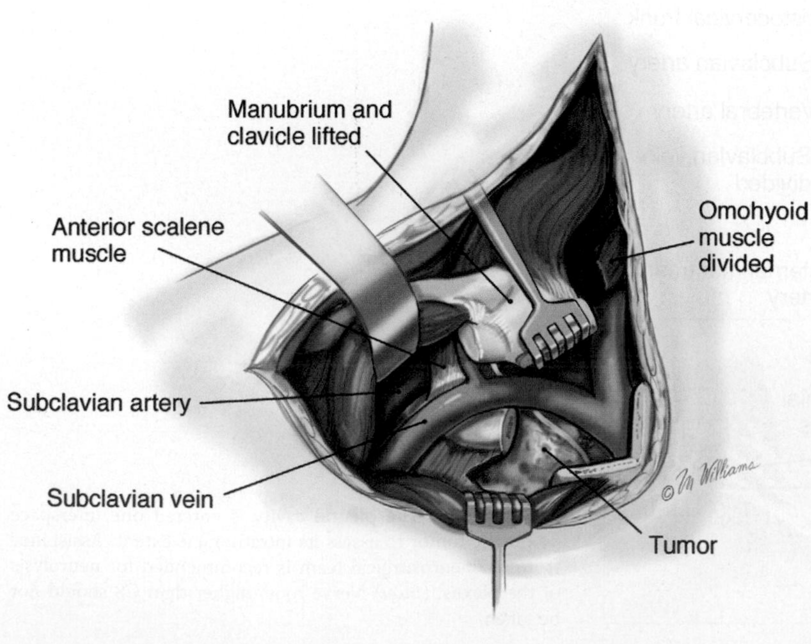

Figure 80-17. The clavicle, with attached pectoral and sternocleidomastoid muscles, is elevated as an osteomuscular flap.

Hemiclamshell or Trapdoor Incision

The hemiclamshell or trapdoor incision (when extended above the clavicle or along the sternocleidomastoid) was proposed originally for trauma to the great vessels or for mediastinal tumors. It provides excellent exposure of the anterior mediastinum and chest apex and has been used with some success for superior sulcus tumors as well. The basic incision consists of a median sternotomy down to the fourth interspace with lateral extension through the intercostals (Fig. 80-18). A standard sternal retractor then may be used to elevate the sternum, or a mammary retractor can be helpful to elevate sternal and intercostal aspects of the incision. Several modifications have been suggested, including extension along the sternocleidomastoid or superior to the clavicle. In this case, the mammary artery should be ligated proximally. Some surgeons recommend resection of the medial clavicle, as in the Dartevelle approach.[46] Another alternative is to resect the first costal cartilage and costoclavicular ligament to preserve the architecture of the shoulder girdle while allowing improved mobility of the anterior chest wall and better exposure and control of the distal subclavian vessels.[47] The incision is closed by wiring the sternum, reapproximating the intercostal space, and then suturing the pectoral muscles if disturbed during the dissection. A major advantage to this incision is better exposure of the pulmonary hilum. However, the posterior aspect of the thoracic inlet is difficult to dissect with this technique; also, the incision maybe excessive for a smaller, anterior, truly apical tumor.

Vascular Resection

Before deciding on the need for vascular resection, the artery should be properly exposed. The vein should be mobilized as described earlier and divided proximal and distal to the tumor if invaded. Next, the artery should be prepared for proximal and distal control by dividing the anterior scalene muscle, preserving the phrenic nerve if not invaded by tumor. The internal mammary artery and ascending cervical artery are divided; the vertebral artery is sacrificed if involved or if the adjacent subclavian artery is involved. In many cases, the tumor can be dissected away from the subclavian artery in the subadventitial plane (Fig. 80-19A). If the media of the artery has been invaded by tumor, steps should be taken for resection (see Fig. 80-19B). Systemic heparinization should be performed, usually with 5000 units of IV heparin. Then the artery can be clamped proximally and distally to permit en bloc resection of the involved portion with the tumor. Reconstruction should be delayed until the rest of the tumor resection is performed. In some cases, it may be helpful to generously wedge the tumor-bearing portion of the upper lobe to be removed with attached ribs and vascular structures so that the vascular reconstruction can be completed immediately, and the heparin then can be reversed. In this way, the completion lobectomy can be performed off heparin. Another option is to give heparin, clamp the artery, complete all the resection en bloc, and then perform the vascular reconstruction, but the vessels will be clamped for a longer period of time.

Reconstruction often can be end-to-end because the distance to traverse is diminished after first rib resection. Otherwise, the material of choice for vascular reconstruction is ringed polytetrafluoroethylene (6 or 8 mm) with end-to-end anastomoses, followed by reversal of heparin with protamine. In the series reported by Fadel et al. [9], the graft length was 1.5 to 4 cm. Shunts were not used. There is no need to place a tissue flap between the vascular graft and the lung. Artery ligation is not an option; if all collaterals are divided during tumor resection and mobilization of the artery, limb ischemia will occur.

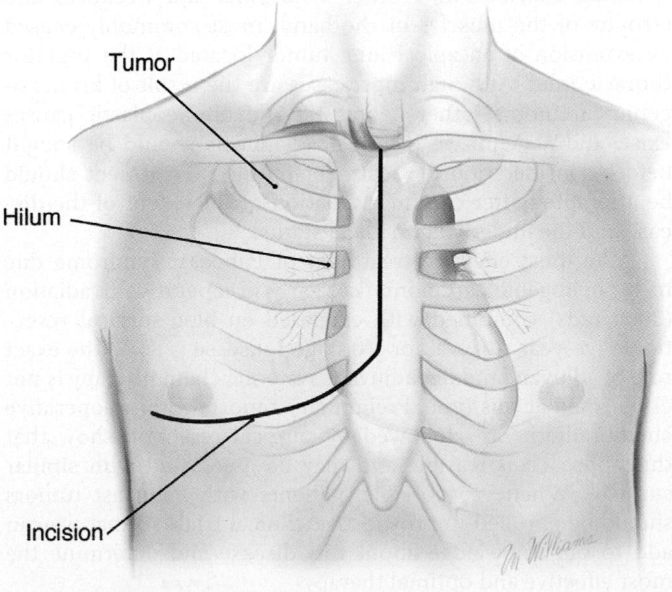

Figure 80-18. Hemiclamshell or trapdoor incision provides excellent exposure of the anterior mediastinum and chest apex. Incision consists of a median sternotomy down to the fourth interspace with lateral extension through the intercostals.

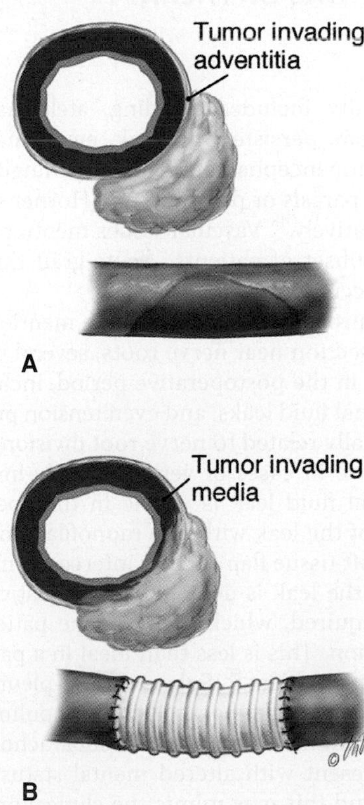

Figure 80-19. *A.* Tumor can be dissected away from the subclavian artery in the subadventitial plane. *B.* If the media of the artery is invaded, the affected portion is reconstructed.

Postoperative Care

Postoperative care is similar to that of any lung resection. With extensive chest wall resection, atelectasis is more common.[45] Good postoperative analgesia, adequate pleural drainage, and aggressive pulmonary toilet cannot be overemphasized. Routine mechanical ventilatory support is not necessary. Special attention must be paid to the involved extremity when vascular resection is required, with hourly vascular checks initially. Some surgeons recommend IV heparinization within 4 to 6 hours postoperatively, and then aspirin, once the patient is ambulatory and continued for 6 months postoperatively.[46] When concomitant venous ligation is necessary, it can be challenging to assess the perfusion of the extremity, and frequent Doppler checks may be reassuring. Arm elevation and lymphatic massage may help to alleviate edema. Wound healing can be more of a problem when extensive collaterals are ligated along the subclavian artery; diligence for this is encouraged, with aggressive debridement if wound necrosis occurs. When the clavicle has been divided and rewired, an arm sling for stabilization for 4 to 6 weeks postoperatively is recommended.

After arterial resection, follow-up duplex studies should be carried out at 3 and 6 months and annually thereafter. In addition, the blood pressure should be measured in both upper extremities at each follow-up visit. If symptoms of arterial insufficiency occur or duplex study suggests significant stenosis (>80%), angiography is recommended.[9] In case of graft occlusion (most often from radiation fibrosis), it may not require intervention in the absence of symptoms. Reported 5-year patency rates are 85%.[7]

COMPLICATIONS OF THERAPY

Surgery

Surgical morbidity includes bleeding, atelectasis, infection, thromboembolism, persistent air leak, empyema, spinal fluid leak with pneumoencephalogram and meningitis, chylothorax, ulnar nerve paresis or paralysis, and Horner syndrome not present preoperatively.[48] Vascular issues mentioned earlier are unique to this subset of patients. Acute graft thrombosis is a possibility but occurs rarely.

Unusual neurologic sequelae deserve mention. Because of resection or dissection near nerve roots, several unusual problems may occur in the postoperative period, including meningitis, cerebrospinal fluid leaks, and even tension pneumocephalus.[49] This is usually related to nerve root division or dissection near the dural sac in cases of vertebral body invasion. Often the cerebrospinal fluid leak is visible in the operating room; careful closure of the leak with fine monofilament suture, buttressed with a soft tissue flap such as intercostal muscle, is usually effective. If the leak is detected postoperatively, a lumbar drain will be required, which confines the patient to bed in the supine position. This is less than ideal in a patient needing vigorous pulmonary toilet.[50] Subarachnoid-pleural fistula has been reported acutely or subacutely when a pulmonary parenchymal air leak communicates with the subarachnoid space.[49,50] Patients may present with altered mental status, seizures, or hyponatremia, and this may mimic the clinical presentation of cerebral metastases. In one patient, reoperation with tissue flap coverage of the leaks was required; in another, expectant management was satisfactory.

Other neurologic sequelae include weakness of intrinsic muscles of the hand after T1 nerve root division, but the hand is usually still functional. When C8 or the lower trunk of the brachial plexus must be divided, permanent paralysis of intrinsic muscles of the hand should be expected.[31] Interestingly enough, taking T1 or even T2 does not seem to produce much of a clinical problem, and even C8 does not give the usual severe problems of ulnar plexus injuries. Possibly this is so because the slow growth of the tumor permits other nerve roots to assume function. Surgical morbidity is 38%, and mortality is between 5% and 10%.[51,52]

Irradiation Therapy

Adverse effects of irradiation therapy include skin fibrosis, fatigue, esophagitis, radiation pneumonitis, pulmonary fibrosis, myelitis, and brachial neuritis, all of which may be extremely devastating to the patient.[53]

Chemotherapy

Complications of chemotherapy include myelosuppression, increased risk of bleeding and infection, peripheral or central neuropathy, renal insufficiency, mucositis, nausea, vomiting, diarrhea, and hypersensitive reaction to secondary malignancies.[54]

Recurrence

There is a significant risk of local or regional recurrence and distant metastases following treatment of superior sulcus tumors, just as there is for any bronchogenic carcinoma. Brain metastasis is one of the most common in younger patients with large cell and adenocarcinoma.[55]

SUMMARY

Pancoast syndrome is a collection of characteristic symptoms and signs that includes shoulder and arm pain in a specific dermatomal distribution, Horner syndrome, and weakness and atrophy of the muscles of the hand, most commonly caused by extension of an apical lung tumor located at the superior thoracic inlet. Although most cases are the result of bronchogenic carcinoma, other neoplastic and nonneoplastic causes exist, and a definitive histologic diagnosis should be sought before consideration of treatment options. Treatment should be attempted after careful evaluation of the extent of the disease and the underlying medical status.

The most effective treatment of Pancoast syndrome due to bronchogenic carcinoma is clearly preoperative irradiation (3000 rads) combined with extended en bloc surgical resection. Five-year survival for N0 stage I disease is 35%. The exact role of adjuvant and neoadjuvant systemic chemotherapy is not established at this time. Preliminary reports with preoperative chemoradiotherapy followed by surgical resection show that this approach is feasible and may be associated with similar survival. Whenever possible, patients with Pancoast tumors should be enrolled in prospective clinical trials so that we can add to our knowledge about this disease and determine the most effective and optimal therapy.

Understanding of the anatomy of the thoracic inlet has led to novel surgical approaches to superior sulcus tumors. Many technical challenges have been overcome, making R0 resection feasible in patients with tumors anterior and superior within the thoracic inlet that previously had been deemed unresectable. Several modifications to Dartevelle technique have either facilitated exposure or improved functional or cosmetic results. The latest data on trimodality therapy in patients with Pancoast–Tobias tumors have further extended the likelihood of prolonged survival. Further refinement of surgical technique, it is hoped, will continue to improve longevity and minimize the morbidity associated with resection.

CASE HISTORY

A 55-year-old white woman with a history of smoking and a cough presented with left-sided shoulder pain. The patient developed numbness, tingling, and discoloration of the left fourth and fifth digits. Chest x-ray was positive for a lesion along the anterior apical superior sulcus with a shadow between the first and second ribs. A CT scan was positive for a tumor that appeared to be invading the first, second, and third ribs, and was questionably involving the subclavian artery and vein and the lower trunk of the brachial plexus. This was followed by MRI, which showed nerve root involvement at T1 with possible involvement of vertebral bodies C6–8. The edge of the subclavian artery was clear, and the edge of the subclavian vein was not.

The patient underwent a percutaneous needle biopsy that was positive for NSCLC. A PET scan was positive for a tumor in the lung and the chest wall with questionable mediastinal lymph nodes. The patient underwent a transbronchial needle aspiration of the paratracheal lymph nodes on the left side, and these were positive for metastatic NSCLC, and the patient was referred for neoadjuvant chemotherapy with carboplatin and taxol with radiation therapy concurrently at 61.2 Gy with a spinal cord dose at 45 Gy. Six weeks after treatment, the patient had repeat CT and PET scans. These both showed shrinkage of the tumor and no uptake in the mediastinum and decreased uptake in the tumor. An MRI of the brain at that time was negative, and the MRI of the chest still showed some questionable involvement of subclavian vessels and the lower trunk of the brachial plexus. The patient underwent a planned bronchoscopy and mediastinoscopy, which was negative for any evidence of persistent mediastinal nodal disease. The patient was explored starting with a left-sided anterior Dartevelle approach. Sparing the clavicle, the T1 nerve root was divided and the first rib was cut anteriorly. The subclavian artery was mobilized successfully without any tumor involvement. However, division of the subclavian vein was necessary. After this was done and full mobilization was achieved, the patient was repositioned in the lateral decubitus position, and the standard posterior Shaw approach was used for resection of the tumor and en bloc chest wall resection of ribs 1, 2, and 3. The chest then was entered from the fourth intercostal space, and a left upper lobectomy with mediastinal lymph dissection was performed. All lymph nodes were negative. The patient had a complete pathologic response on final pathology. An intercostal muscle flap, harvested at the time of posterior chest entry, was placed at the bronchial stump. Postoperatively, the patient developed upper extremity edema, as expected with vein ligation, and this was treated with Jobst stockings and arm elevation.

EDITOR'S COMMENT

This chapter described with my coauthor, Hal Urschel, one of the world's experts in this field who, sadly, passed this year, provides an overview of superior sulcus tumors both from an oncological and technical perspective. Although generally treated with a combination of radiation and surgery, we currently routinely approach these lesions with neoadjuvant chemoradiation followed by surgical resection. After the standard posterior Shaw–Paulson approach is described, the anterior approach is noted. This is especially useful for patients with Pancoast tumors that involve the anterior chest wall and/or the anterior vessels. By using either a classic Dartevelle approach or a modified anterior "hemiclamshell," one can gain excellent access to the upper lobes, sternum, ribs, and vena cava as necessary. We have found that by modifying the location of the incision one can either perform a separate thoracotomy posteriorly or remove the lobe from the same anterior incision.

—Mark J. Krasna

ACKNOWLEDGMENT

Mrs. Rachel Montano is to be highly commended for her dedication and commitment to the completion of this chapter.

References

1. Shaw RR, Paulson DL, Kee JL. Treatment of superior sulcus tumor by irradiation followed by resection. *Ann Surg.* 1961;154:29–40.
2. Rusch VW, Giroux DJ, Kraut MJ, et al. Induction chemoradiation and surgical resection for non-small cell lung carcinomas of the superior sulcus: initial results of Southwest Oncology Group Trial 9416 (Intergroup Trial 0160). *J Thorac Cardiovasc Surg.* 2001;121:472–483.
3. Chardack WM, Maccallum JD. Pancoast tumor; five-year survival without recurrence or metastases following radical resection and postoperative irradiation. *J Thorac Surg.* 1956;31:535–542.
4. Chardack WM, Maccallum JD. Pancoast syndrome due to bronchiogenic carcinoma: successful surgical removal and postoperative irradiation; a case report. *J Thorac Surg.* 1953;25:402–412.
5. Attar S, Krasna MJ, Sonett JR, et al. Superior sulcus (Pancoast) tumor: experience with 105 patients. *Ann Thorac Surg.* 1998;66:193–198.
6. Ginsberg RJ, Rubinstein L. The comparison of limited resection to lobectomy for T1N0 non-small cell lung cancer. LCSG 821. *Chest.* 1994;106:318S–319S.
7. Rusch VW, Giroux DJ, Kraut MJ, et al. Induction chemoradiation and surgical resection for superior sulcus non-small-cell lung carcinomas: long-term results of Southwest Oncology Group Trial 9416 (Intergroup Trial 0160). *J Clin Oncol.* 2007;25:313–318.
8. Kwong KF, Edelman MJ, Suntharalingam M, et al. High-dose radiotherapy in trimodality treatment of Pancoast tumors results in high pathologic complete response rates and excellent long-term survival. *J Thorac Cardiovasc Surg.* 2005;129:1250–1257.
9. Fadel E, Chapelier A, Bacha E, et al. Subclavian artery resection and reconstruction for thoracic inlet cancers. *J Vasc Surg.* 1999;29:581–588.
10. Alifano M, D'Aiuto M, Magdeleinat P, et al. Surgical treatment of superior sulcus tumors: results and prognostic factors. *Chest.* 2003;124:996–1003.
11. Wittig JC, Bickels J, Kollender Y, et al. Palliative forequarter amputation for metastatic carcinoma to the shoulder girdle region: indications, preoperative evaluation, surgical technique, and results. *J Surg Oncol.* 2001;77:105–113; discussion 114.

12. Ferrario T, Palmer P, Karakousis CP. Technique of forequarter (interscapulothoracic) amputation. *Clin Orthop Relat Res.* 2004;423:191–195.
13. Detterbeck FC, DeCamp MM, Jr., American College of Chest Physicians, et al. Lung cancer. Invasive staging: the guidelines. *Chest.* 2003;123:167S–175S.
14. Rusch VW. Management of Pancoast tumours. *Lancet Oncol.* 2006;7:997–1005.
15. Jaklitsch MT, Herndon JE, 2nd, DeCamp MM, Jr., et al. Nodal downstaging predicts survival following induction chemotherapy for stage IIIA (N2) non-small cell lung cancer in CALGB protocol #8935. *J Surg Oncol.* 2006;94:599–606.
16. Urschel HC, Jr. Superior pulmonary sulcus carcinoma. *Surg Clin North Am.* 1988;68:497–509.
17. Grover F, Komaki R. Superior sulcus tumors. In: Roth J, Ruckdeschel J, Weisenburger T, eds. *Thoracic Oncology.* Philadelphia, PA: Saunders; 1995:225–238.
18. Sundaresan N, Hilaris BS, Martini N. The combined neurosurgical-thoracic management of superior sulcus tumors. *J Clin Oncol.* 1987;5:1739–1745.
19. Urschel HC, Jr. New approaches to Pancoast and chest wall tumors. *Chest.* 1993;103:360S–361S.
20. McGoon DC. Transcervical technic for removal of specimen from superior sulcus tumor for pathologic study. *Ann Surg.* 1964;159:407–410.
21. Maxfield RA, Aranda CP. The role of fiberoptic bronchoscopy and transbronchial biopsy in the diagnosis of Pancoast's tumor. *N Y State J Med.* 1987;87:326–329.
22. O'Connell RS, McLoud TC, Wilkins EW. Superior sulcus tumor: radiographic diagnosis and workup. *AJR Am J Roentgenol.* 1983;140:25–30.
23. Fuller DB, Chambers JS. Superior sulcus tumors: combined modality. *Ann Thorac Surg.* 1994;57:1133–1139.
24. Lands RH, Patel N, Maran S, et al. Small cell lung cancer presenting as a Pancoast tumor. *J Tenn Med Assoc.* 1991;84:113–114.
25. Johnson DH, Hainsworth JD, Greco FA. Pancoast's syndrome and small cell lung cancer. *Chest.* 1982;82:602–606.
26. Hatton MQ, Allen MB, Cooke NJ. Pancoast syndrome: an unusual presentation of adenoid cystic carcinoma. *Eur Respir J.* 1993;6:271–272.
27. Chong KM, Hennox SC, Sheppard MN. Primary hemangiopericytoma presenting as a Pancoast tumor. *Ann Thorac Surg.* 1993;55:9.
28. Amin R. Bilateral Pancoast's syndrome in a patient with carcinoma of the cervix. *Gynecol Oncol.* 1986;24:126–128.
29. Gallagher KJ, Jeffrey RR, Kerr KM, et al. Pancoast syndrome: an unusual complication of pulmonary infection by Staphylococcus aureus. *Ann Thorac Surg.* 1992;53:903–904.
30. Vandenplas O, Mercenier C, Trigaux JP, et al. Pancoast's syndrome due to *Pseudomonas aeruginosa* infection of the lung apex. *Thorax.* 1991;46:683–684.
31. Stanley SL, Jr., Lusk RH. Thoracic actinomycosis presenting as a brachial plexus syndrome. *Thorax.* 1985;40:74–75.
32. Collins PW, de Lord C, Newland AC. Pancoast's tumour due to aspergilloma. *Lancet.* 1990;336:1595.
33. Simpson FG, Morgan M, Cooke NJ. Pancoast's syndrome associated with invasive aspergillosis. *Thorax.* 1986;41:156–157.
34. Winston DJ, Jordan MC, Rhodes J. *Allescheria boydii* infections in the immunosuppressed host. *Am J Med.* 1977;63:830–835.
35. Mitchell DH, Sorrell TC. Pancoast's syndrome due to pulmonary infection with *Cryptococcus neoformans* variety gattii. *Clin Infect Dis.* 1992;14:1142–1144.
36. Gotterer N, Lossos I, Breuer R. Pancoast's syndrome caused by primary pulmonary hydatid cyst. *Respir Med.* 1990;84:169–170.
37. Rong SH. Carotid pseudoaneurysm simulating Pancoast tumor. *AJR Am J Roentgenol.* 1984;142:495–496.
38. Gibney RT, Connolly TP. Pulmonary amyloid nodule simulating pancoast tumor. *J Can Assoc Radiol.* 1984;35:90–91.
39. Gandhi S, Walsh GL, Komaki R, et al. A multidisciplinary surgical approach to superior sulcus tumors with vertebral invasion. *Ann Thorac Surg.* 1999;68:1778–1784; discussion 84–85.
40. Dartevelle P, Macchiarini P. Surgical management of superior sulcus tumors. *Oncologist.* 1999;4:398–407.
41. Dartevelle PG, Chapelier AR, Macchiarini P, et al. Anterior transcervical-thoracic approach for radical resection of lung tumors invading the thoracic inlet. *J Thorac Cardiovasc Surg.* 1993;105:1025–1034.
42. Grunenwald D, Spaggiari L, Girard P, et al. Transmanubrial approach to the thoracic inlet. *J Thorac Cardiovasc Surg.* 1997;113:958–959; author reply 60–61.
43. Urschel HC, Jr. Resection of superior sulcus tumor. In: Urschel HC, Jr., Cooper JD, eds. *Atlas of Surgery.* New York, NY: Churchill Livingstone; 1995:190–193.
44. Wright CD, Menard MT, Wain JC, et al. Induction chemoradiation compared with induction radiation for lung cancer involving the superior sulcus. *Ann Thorac Surg.* 2002;73:1541–1544.
45. Narayan S, Thomas CR, Jr. Multimodality therapy for pancoast tumor. *Nat Clin Pract Oncol.* 2006;3:484–491.
46. Macchiarini P. Resection of superior sulcus carcinomas (anterior approach). *Thorac Surg Clin.* 2004;14:229–240.
47. Rusca M, Carbognani P, Bobbio P. The modified "hemi-clamshell" approach for tumors of the cervicothoracic junction. *Ann Thorac Surg.* 2000;69:1961–1963.
48. Ginsberg RJ. Resection of a superior sulcus tumor. *Chest Surg Clin N Am.* 1995;5:315–331.
49. Boyev P, Krasna MJ, White CS, et al. Subarachnoid-pleural fistula after resection of a pancoast tumor with hyponatremia. *Ann Thorac Surg.* 1995;60:683–685.
50. Martin LW, Walsh GL. Vertebral body resection. *Thorac Surg Clin.* 2004;14:241–254.
51. Kanner R, Martini N, Foley K. Incidence of pain and other clinical manifestations of superior pulmonary sulcus (Pancoast) tumors. In: Bonica J, ed. *Advances in Pain Research and Therapy.* New York, NY: Raven Press; 1982:27–39.
52. Martini N. Surgical treatment of non-small cell lung cancer by stage. *Semin Surg Oncol.* 1990;6:248–254.
53. Komaki R, Mountain CF, Holbert JM, et al. Superior sulcus tumors: treatment selection and results for 85 patients without metastasis (Mo) at presentation. *Int J Radiat Oncol Biol Phys.* 1990;19:31–36.
54. Westgate S, Perry M. Toxicity of combined modality therapy. In: Aisner J, ed. *Comprehensive Textbook of Thoracic Oncology.* Baltimore, MD: Williams & Wilkins; 1996:1002–1018.
55. Heelan RT, Demas BE, Caravelli JF, et al. Superior sulcus tumors: CT and MR imaging. *Radiology.* 1989;170:637–641.

81 Cardiopulmonary Bypass for Extended Thoracic Resections

Daniel G. Cuadrado, Marzia Leacche, Eric S. Lambright, and John G. Byrne

Keywords: Cardiopulmonary bypass for thoracic resections, locally advanced lung cancer, resection and reconstruction of the left atrium, thoracic aorta, superior vena cava

INTRODUCTION

Bronchogenic carcinoma remains the most common cause of cancer death in both men and women in the United States. These tumors can exhibit local progression and invasion before metastatic spread has occurred, which does not preclude resection with curative intent. Any contiguous structure within the chest may be involved, with chest wall involvement being the most common. Other potential sites of local invasion include the left atrium, aorta, superior vena cava, vertebral bodies, diaphragm, and esophagus. The increased potential for morbidity and mortality are well documented for these complex extended resections, making appropriate patient selection crucial. Long-term prognosis depends on accurate pretreatment staging to assist in selection of therapy and complete resection. Cardiopulmonary bypass (CPB) may be necessary to allow surgical resection of central, locally advanced malignancies because they involve, or are close to, the heart and/or the great vessels. CPB serves as an alternative to conventional ventilation during extended resections providing oxygenation and hemodynamic support. This chapter will review the role of CPB for the extended resection of lung cancer, as well as the clinical and technical considerations and expected surgical outcomes.

GENERAL PRINCIPLES

For those patients presenting with locally advanced lung cancers, long-term outcome is primarily dependent on the ability to obtain a complete (R0) resection. For non–small-cell lung cancers (NSCLCs) with direct invasion into the mediastinum, Martini et al.[1] found a survival rate of 30% if an R0 resection was obtained in contrast to 14% if the resection was incomplete. Likewise, for tumors invading the heart or the great vessels, 5-year survival rate ranges between 23% and 40% with complete resection versus 0% with incomplete resection.[2,3]

The operative approach is ultimately based on the tumor anatomy, the need for vascular reconstruction, and the urgency with which circulatory support is initiated. To optimize outcomes, one must maintain a flexible strategy with regard to arterial and venous cannulation sites, need for aortic clamping, cardioplegia requirements, and deairing options.

When an injury to a major vascular structure (i.e., pulmonary artery, superior vena cava) occurs during a thoracotomy, CPB support may be required. In the setting of a right thoracotomy approach, cannulation can be achieved via the ascending aorta and the right atrium. In the setting of a left thoracotomy approach, cannulation can be obtained via the descending thoracic aorta and main pulmonary artery.[4]

If the groin is accessible, systemic venous drainage can be achieved by placing a long venous cannula into the right atrium through the femoral vein. In the emergent setting, decompression of the heart with the ability to control blood loss and return shed blood is usually all that is required to enable primary or patch repair of the injury to the central vascular structure.

In the elective setting, standard median sternotomy is the surgical approach used to address lesions involving the central pulmonary arterial system. Standard ascending aorta and right atrial cannulation are used for CPB institution. Reconstruction with pulmonary homograft or autologous pericardium can be readily achieved. In lesions involving the left atrium, median sternotomy is usually satisfactory; however, one must be alert to the issues of deairing and ensure appropriate means of preventing systemic air emboli. Additionally, tumor emboli can occur, and care must be taken to limit tumor manipulation before cardiac decompression and adequate circulation control.[5] If the left thoracotomy is the surgical approach used, it is useful to access the left femoral vein with a small caliber catheter prior to turning the patient to the side.

EFFECT OF CARDIOPULMONARY BYPASS ON CANCER BIOLOGY

Cancer progression is a multistep process including proliferation, migration, vascular invasion, and angiogenesis. The effects of operative stress on cancer cell proliferation have been shown in several in vitro models.[6–8] One such study demonstrated that lung cancer cell proliferation was better in human serum obtained immediately following lung resection when compared with serum drawn preoperatively.[8]

The immunosuppressive effects of extracorporeal circulation have been clearly elucidated. The physiologic stress of CPB has been shown to alter the circulating levels of certain cytokines and growth factors.[9–11] There are also inhibitory effects to both cell-mediated and humoral immunity.[12,13] In a study performed in patients undergoing cardiac surgery with and without CPB, those undergoing CPB had a significantly decreased inhibitory capacity of serum for cancer cell proliferation.[14] Previous series of extended resections have demonstrated an earlier recurrence rate after resection with CPB.[3,15]

Centrally Advanced Tumors

Locally advanced tumors that involve the central pulmonary vasculature or the heart (T4 lesions) are classically considered to be unresectable. Achieving a tumor-free proximal margin or satisfactory proximal vascular control may not be possible with standard (non-CBP) techniques. A small but definable subset of such patients will benefit from surgery if CPB is used to facilitate these complex resections. Accurate preoperative evaluation, including aggressive staging, must be performed to exclude the presence of occult metastatic disease, determine the patient's physiologic fitness, and establish the limits of resection to achieve the optimal long-term survival for each individual patient. Since these tumors are often larger and more centrally located, preoperative imaging should include PET and CT scanning. There should be consideration for magnetic resonance imaging (MRI) of the brain to rule out occult disease. Mediastinoscopy must be performed not only for identifying nodal disease, but also as an assessment of the extent of airway and pulmonary artery involvement.

The role of induction chemotherapy prior to resection of T4 malignancies remains undefined. There are some small series in which preoperative chemotherapy improved resectability.[16–18] In one series, induction chemotherapy prevented 20% of patients from proceeding on to resection due to toxic side effects.[19] Furthermore, there is evidence that induction therapy increases surgical morbidity and mortality.[20–22] In patients undergoing extended surgical resection, induction therapy followed by surgery is associated with an increase in morbidity and mortality when compared to surgery alone.[20] Therefore, decisions for preoperative chemotherapy should be tailored on a case-by-case basis.

Most thoracic surgeons are reluctant to perform pulmonary resections with patients on CPB. Several authors[23–26] have reviewed the results and safety of combined cardiac and pulmonary procedures requiring CPB. Their opinions are varied, and several authors have expressed concerns for the adverse effects of CPB on hemostasis and pulmonary function. Others[4,27,28] with significant institutional experience have written more extensively on the subject, describing the advantages, disadvantages, and parameters for patient selection when CPB is used as an adjunct to conventional thoracic surgical techniques.

Byrne et al.[4] reviewed a decade of experience at Brigham and Women's Hospital and Massachusetts General Hospital in Boston. Between January 1992 and September 2002, CPB was used in 14 patients during planned curative resection of locally advanced thoracic malignancies. In 8 of the 14 patients, CPB use was planned to facilitate resection. In the remaining six patients, CPB was required as an emergent therapy to manage central vascular injury. Indications for planned CPB included tumor involvement of the left atrium, pulmonary artery, and superior vena cava. Complete resection was achieved in 12 patients (86%). There was one operative death from pulmonary embolism. Complications included low cardiac output state (5), stroke (1), pulmonary edema (1), and reoperation for bleeding (3). The overall 1-, 3-, and 5-year survival rates were 57%, 36%, and 21%, respectively. The authors concluded that although CPB is rarely required for thoracic malignancy resection, in appropriate circumstances, it can be used with low morbidity and mortality and may be lifesaving if the surgery is complicated by a central vascular injury. They also concluded that the ability to perform a complete resection influences ultimate survival. In addition, optimal outcome depends on careful patient selection with use of radiographic imaging and thorough intraoperative inspection.

Vaporciyan et al.[28] reported the University of Texas MD Anderson Cancer Center's experience from January 1995 to July 2000 using CPB for resection of metastatic or noncardiac primary malignancies that extended directly into the heart. This series included 19 patients, 11 of whom underwent surgery for curative intent. Complete resection was achieved in 10 of these patients. There were two deaths in the group operated on for palliation. Major complications occurred in the majority of patients (58%) and included acute respiratory distress syndrome, mediastinal hematoma, and pneumonia. The overall 1- and 2-year survival rates were 65% and 45%, respectively. The authors concluded that the use of CPB has a role in selected patients with these central thoracic malignancies if there is confidence that complete resection can be achieved.

VENA CAVA INVOLVEMENT WITH BRONCHOGENIC CARCINOMA

Bronchogenic carcinoma of the right upper lobe can invade the mediastinal pleura and on rare occasions invade the superior vena cava (Fig. 81-1). Involvement of the superior vena cava may also occur as a consequence of metastatic nodal disease, which, when present, is a uniformly poor prognostic indicator. There is an increasing experience in extended resections of pulmonary malignancy with en bloc resection of the superior vena cava. Several authors[2,15,29–31] have suggested a benefit in selected patients, but there is still uncertainty regarding a consistent benefit.

Technical Considerations for Vena Cava Resection and Reconstruction

Optimal exposure to the superior vena cava is achieved through median sternotomy. Bronchogenic tumors are approached through the right chest, which provides excellent visualization of the superior vena cava and the atrium, but limited access to and control of the left brachiocephalic vein. Two techniques can be used for resection and reconstruction of the superior vena cava. If less than a third of the circumference of the vena cava is involved, partial resection with primary or patch closure using autologous pericardium can be performed if there

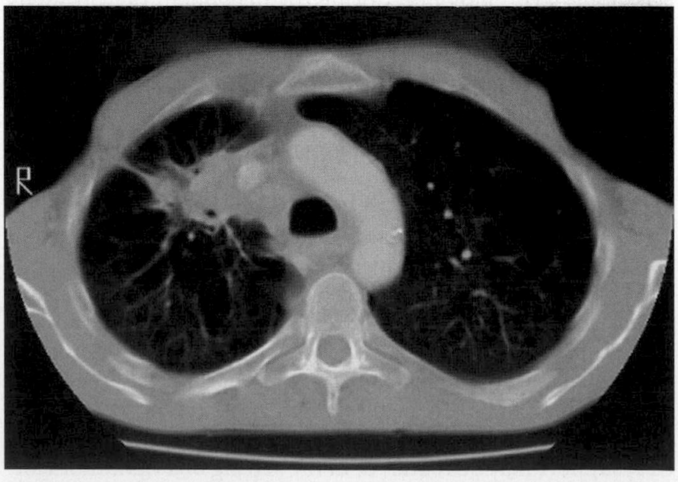

Figure 81-1. Right upper lobe mass abutting superior vena cava. Caval invasion was identified at right thoracotomy. Tangential resection of the superior vena cava with autologous pericardial patch reconstruction was performed.

are concerns regarding stenosis. If there is greater involvement of the superior vena cava, complete resection and reconstruction will be required. Reconstruction can be performed with autogenous venous or prosthetic grafts. Options for autogenous graft replacement include the jugular vein, the superficial femoral vein, or spiral saphenous vein. This option is more limited because the graft diameter must be as great as the brachiocephalic vein for a satisfactory outcome.

Dartevelle[30] has described the use of synthetic polytetrafluoroethylene vascular graft as the material of choice for complete venous replacement. Before the work of Dartevelle, prosthetic graft replacement of the superior vena cava was thought to be a surgical contraindication because of the high rate of thrombosis and infection, as well as the deleterious physiologic effects of clamping the superior vena cava. Specific interventions such as maintaining adequate cerebral perfusion pressure, monitoring cerebral oxygenation, limiting clamp time with efficient reconstruction, paying attention to the prevention of bacterial contamination, using anticoagulation judiciously, and appropriately using shunts or bypass are all required to ensure a satisfactory outcome. Contraindications to superior vena caval resections included complete venous obstruction and involvement by a malignant that is otherwise unresectable.

Results of Combined Pulmonary and Superior Vena Caval Resection

Dartevelle described his experience with combined pulmonary and complete caval resection in 14 patients with NSCLC.[30] These extensive tumors required carinal pneumonectomy in six patients, extended pneumonectomy in seven patients, and one patient received a lobectomy. Six of the 14 patients had ipsilateral mediastinal nodal disease. Major complications were seen in three patients which included bronchopleural fistula in two and extrapericardial cardiac herniation in one. The mortality rate was 7.1%, and 5-year survival rate was 31%. A more recent review of 29 patients undergoing superior vena cava resections over a 25-year period revealed better 5-year survival in patients without carinal involvement (43.2%) and in those with non–squamous-cell carcinoma (51%).[32]

Thomas et al.[29] reviewed their institutional experience in 15 patients, four of whom required complete caval resection. There was one death in the postoperative period and a complication rate of 20%. The authors observed a median survival of 8.5 months with two local recurrences, and the 1-, 2-, and 5-year survival rates were 46.7%, 32%, and 24%, respectively. The authors concluded that extended resection, when feasible, is justified.

Spaggiari et al.[31] reported similar observations in their report on 25 patients in which seven patients had complete resection of the superior vena cava with graft interposition. Ipsilateral mediastinal nodal disease was observed in 56%. Complete resection was achieved in 80% of patients with a perioperative complication rate of 36% and mortality rate of 12%. The observed median survival was 11.5 months, and the 5-year actuarial survival rate was 29% with four long-term survivors. The data were inadequate to differentiate survival according to nodal status, but the authors commented that the survival trends favored node-negative patients. The authors recommended mediastinoscopy in all patients with superior vena caval involvement to exclude N2 patients.

LEFT ATRIAL INVASTION WITH BRONCHOGENIC CARCINOMA

Given the anatomic continuity between the pulmonary hilum and the pulmonary veins, the left atrium is the most common cardiac chamber involved by bronchogenic carcinoma. Left atrial invasion can occur by one of the two mechanisms. The first involves contiguous invasion from the base of the pulmonary vein, whereas the second is via direct invasion by the primary tumor or metastatic lymph node.

The first description of left atrial resection was by Allison in 1946.[33] Initial attempts at this extended resection involved combined pulmonary and left atrial resection with the use of a side-biting vascular clamp.[34] Although the series are small, some of these patients did show long-term benefit. However, with more extensive left atrial involvement and the risk of tumor embolization, this approach may be inappropriate.

Technical Considerations for Left Atrial Resection and Reconstruction

CPB offers the advantage of complete radical resection and reconstruction on an arrested heart. Alternatively, resection and repair can be performed on a beating heart with a clamp applied to a more extensive area of the left atrium. The approach is through a median sternotomy. Standard ascending aortic and bicaval cannulation can be utilized. The left atrium can be opened after aortic cross-clamping and cardioplegic arrest or after the induction of hypothermic ventricular fibrillation in order to avoid air embolism.[35,36]

In cases when a vascular clamp is utilized, there is a risk of massive hemorrhage with clamp dislodgement. One distinct advantage of CPB is that vascular clamp dislodgement and injuries to the left atrial wall during resection and reconstruction can be addressed in a more controlled manner. Reconstruction can typically be performed with autologous or bovine pericardium.

Results of Combined Pulmonary and Left Atrial Resection

In a series of 19 patients undergoing simultaneous pulmonary and left atrial resection, Ratto et al.[37] reported a 5-year survival rate of 14% with a median survival of 25 months. With complete resection, others have found 5-year survivals ranging from 16% to 23%.[34,38] The majority of patients require pneumonectomy along with radical resection to achieve a tumor-free margin. The presence of N2 disease portends a dismal prognosis and should preclude surgical resection.

LUNG TUMORS WITH INFILTRATION OF THE THORACIC AORTA

Left-sided lung cancers may involve the descending thoracic aorta. It is often difficult to determine the presence and extent of aortic invasion on imaging studies (Fig. 81-2). If the fat plane between the aorta and the tumor is absent or there is tumor abutment involving greater than 90 degrees of the aortic circumference, invasion should be suspected. However, ultimate

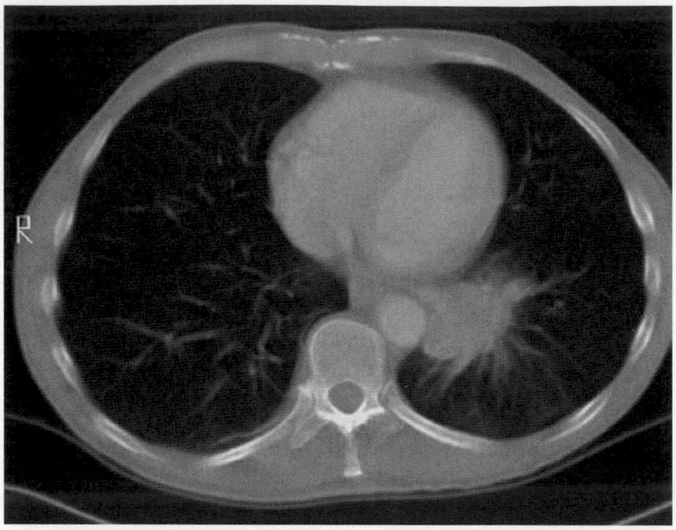

Figure 81-2. Left lower lobe mass abutting the descending thoracic aorta. Aortic adventitial invasion identified at exploration. Tangential resection of the aorta was required.

determination of involvement of the aorta generally is made at the time of exploration. Aortic invasion by bronchogenic carcinoma is usually limited to the adventitia. As with lesions involving the central pulmonary vasculature, these T_4 tumors with full-thickness involvement of the thoracic aorta are classically deemed unresectable. Experience with combined pulmonary and aortic resection is limited and often anecdotal. However, some authors[8–10] have described their experiences with these combined resections. These reviews suggest a favorable impact on survival in highly selected patients; however, the few available reports in the literature make it difficult to draw more generalized conclusions.

Technical Considerations for Aortic Resection and Reconstruction

Different technical methods are needed to manage the aorta that is locally invaded with lung cancer. The options include resection of the tumor in a subadventitial plane, partial resection with patch reconstruction, and complete segmental aortic resection with tube graft reconstruction. The use of a shunt prosthesis has been described between the ascending and descending aorta.[2,15] Venous cannulation can be obtained through the main pulmonary artery or femoral veins with arterial cannulation of the descending aorta. A right radial arterial line should be utilized to gage the adequacy of upper body perfusion. The aorta can then be cross-clamped between the innominate and left common carotid artery.[39] If there is involvement of tumor of the aortic arch proximal to the left common carotid artery, hypothermic circulatory arrest with selective cerebral perfusion may be required.[40,41] Hybrid approaches such as endovascular stent grafting of the thoracic aorta followed by resection of the aortic adventitia and media have been described.[42]

Results of Aortic Resection and Reconstruction

Nakahara et al.[15] reported their results in three patients in whom the aorta was resected at the time of pulmonary resection. One patient was a midterm survivor; however, the other two succumbed to metastatic disease within a year. In 1994, Tsuchiya et al.[2] reported their experience in 28 patients at the National Cancer Hospital in Tokyo. Resection in a subadventitial plane was used in 75% of patients. In those 21 patients, 10 had complete resections, and all patients with incomplete resections did poorly. The authors commented that peeling the adventitia off the aorta is inadequate for lung cancer invading the aorta. Of the seven patients who had a complete aortic resection with tube graft reconstruction, four developed recurrent disease. Only one of the seven patients who were managed with complete aortic resection was a long-term survivor. Klepetko et al.[39] reported similar observations in their experience in seven patients undergoing full-thickness aortic resection with patch or tube graft reconstruction. Perfusion was supported with CPB in six of the operations without apparent untoward events. Long-term survival was achieved in two of the seven patients. Horita et al.[40] reported that only one patient remained alive for more than 5 years following resection of the aortic arch under hypothermic circulatory arrest. These observations regarding pulmonary malignancies with direct aortic invasion support the observation that complete resection and long-term cures are rare, but possible, in appropriately selected patients.

SUMMARY

The management of bronchogenic carcinomas that invade vital structures within the mediastinum and chest requires sound surgical judgment and a pragmatic approach. Many of these lesions are metastatic at the time of presentation, and a thorough evaluation, including surgical staging of the mediastinum, must be performed to ensure that patients who are offered surgery have a realistic expectation of benefit. Since the majority of data regarding these subgroups of patients are case series and anecdotal reports, conclusions are difficult to draw. However, resections and the appropriate use of CPB to provide a margin of safety for these extended operations do offer a potential for curative therapy in an appropriately selected patient. Prognosis for these patients is otherwise dismal.

EDITOR'S COMMENT

This chapter by Byrne et al. is a very important comment on our technical advances in resecting T4 lung cancer. It is clear from the preceding sections that partial or en bloc resections are possible, and may even confer improved survival upon this subgroup of patients. Although all the reported series are small, the literature does support the value of resection. Using an aggressive approach up front offers the patients the best option for cure. One caveat in my own experience is to exclude patients with either N2 or N3 disease as their long-term survival is limited. By performing a mediastinal staging procedure on all these patients, one can determine in whom the risks of these aggressive operations are most worthwhile.

—Mark J. Krasna

References

1. Martini N, Yellin A, Ginsberg RJ, et al. Management of non-small cell lung cancer with direct mediastinal involvement. *Ann Thorac Surg.* 1994;58(5):1447–1451.
2. Tsuchiya R, Asamura H, Kondo H, et al. Extended resection of the left atrium, great vessels, or both for lung cancer. *Ann Thorac Surg.* 1994;57(4):960–965.
3. Fukuse T, Wada H, Hitomi S. Extended operation for non-small cell lung cancer invading great vessels and left atrium. *Eur J Cardiothorac Surg.* 1997;11(4):664–669.
4. Byrne JG, Leacche M, Agnihotri AK, et al. The use of cardiopulmonary bypass during resection of locally advanced thoracic malignancies: a 10-year two-center experience. *Chest.* 2004;125(4):1581–1586.
5. Mansour KA, Malone CE, Craver JM. Left atrial tumor embolization during pulmonary resection: review of literature and report of two cases. *Ann Thorac Surg.* 1988;46(4):455–456.
6. Ikeda M, Furukawa H, Imamura H, et al. Surgery for gastric cancer increases plasma levels of vascular endothelial growth factor and von Willebrand factor. *Gastric Cancer.* 2002;5(3):137–141.
7. Shimizu H, Katano Y, Nagano K, et al. Recurrent hepatocellular carcinoma with rapid growth after cardiac surgery. *Hepatogastroenterology.* 2005;52(66):1863–1866.
8. Yoshimasu T, Oura S, Hirai I, et al. Surgery for lung cancer may affect the metastatic ability of lung cancer cells. *J Jpn Assoc Chest Surg.* 2004;17(7):774–777.
9. Wan S, Marchant A, DeSmet JM, et al. Human cytokine responses to cardiac transplantation and coronary artery bypass grafting. *J Thorac Cardiovasc Surg.* 1996;111(2):469–477.
10. Mayumi H, Zhang Q-W, Nakashima A, et al. Synergistic immunosuppression caused by high-dose methylprednisolone and cardiopulmonary bypass. *Ann Thorac Surg.* 1997;63(1):129–137.
11. Naldini A, Borrelli F, Carraro F, et al. Interleukin 10 production in patients undergoing cardiopulmonary bypass: evidence of inhibition of th-1-type responses. *Cytokine.* 1999;11(1):74–79.
12. Roth JA, Golub SH, Cukingnan RA, et al. Cell-mediated immunity is depressed following cardiopulmonary bypass. *Ann Thorac Surg.* 1981; 31(4):350–356.
13. Grundmann U, Rensing H, Adams H-A, et al. Endotoxin desensitization of human mononuclear cells after cardiopulmonary bypass: role of humoral factors. *Anesthesiology.* 2000;93(2):359–369.
14. Yamamoto S, Yoshimasu T, Nishimura Y, et al. In vitro evaluation of the effect of cardiac surgery on cancer cell proliferation. *Ann Thorac Cardiovasc Surg.* 2011;17(3):260–266.
15. Nakahara K, Ohno K, Mastumura A, et al. Extended operation for lung cancer invading the aortic arch and superior vena cava. *J Thorac Cardiovasc Surg.* 1989;97(3):428–433.
16. Macchiarini P, Chapelier AR, Monnet I, et al. Extended operations after induction therapy for stage IIIb (T4) non-small cell lung cancer. *Ann Thorac Surg.* 1994;57(4):966–973.
17. Rendina EA, Venuta F, De Giacomo T, et al. Induction chemotherapy for T4 centrally located non-small cell lung cancer. *J Thorac Cardiovasc Surg.* 1999;117(2):225–233.
18. Grunenwald DH, Andre F, Le Pechoux C, et al. Benefit of surgery after chemoradiotherapy in stage IIIB (T4 and/or N3) non-small cell lung cancer. *J Thorac Cardiovasc Surg.* 2001;122(4):796–802.
19. Rusch VW, Giroux DJ, Kraut MJ, et al. Induction chemoradiation and surgical resection for non-small cell lung carcinomas of the superior sulcus: initial results of Southwest Oncology Group Trial 9416 (Intergroup Trial 0160). *J Thorac Cardiovasc Surg.* 2001;121(3):472–483.
20. Fowler WC, Langer CJ, Curran WJ Jr, et al. Postoperative complications after combined neoadjuvant treatment of lung cancer. *Ann Thorac Surg.* 1993;55(4):986–989.
21. Roberts JR, Eustis C, Devore R, et al. Induction chemotherapy increases perioperative complications in patients undergoing resection for non-small cell lung cancer. *Ann Thorac Surg.* 2001;72(3):885–888.
22. Matsubara Y, Takeda S-I, Mashimo T. Risk stratification for lung cancer surgery: impact of induction therapy and extended resection. *Chest.* 2005;128(5):3519–3525.
23. Piehler JM, Pairolero PC, Weiland LH, et al. Bronchogenic carcinoma with chest wall invasion: factors affecting survival following en bloc resection. *Ann Thorac Surg.* 1982;34(6):684–691.
24. Ulicny KS Jr, Schmelzer V, Flege JB Jr, et al. Concomitant cardiac and pulmonary operation: the role of cardiopulmonary bypass. *Ann Thorac Surg.* 1992;54(2):289–295.
25. Yokoyama T, Derrick M, Lee A. Cardiac operation with associated pulmonary resection. *J Thorac Cardiovasc Surg.* 1993;105(5):912–916.
26. Miller DL, Orszulak TA, Pairolero PC, et al. Combined operation for lung cancer and cardiac disease. *Ann Thorac Surg.* 1994;58(4):989–994.
27. Gillinov AM, Greene PS, Stuart RS, et al. Cardiopulmonary bypass as an adjunct to pulmonary surgery. *Chest.* 1996;110(2):571–574.
28. Vaporciyan AA, Rice D, Correa AM, et al. Resection of advanced thoracic malignancies requiring cardiopulmonary bypass. *Eur J Cardiothorac Surg.* 2002;22(1):47–52.
29. Thomas P, Magnan PE, Moulin G, et al. Extended operation for lung cancer invading the superior vena cava. *Eur J Cardiothorac Surg.* 1994;8(4):177–182.
30. Dartevelle PG. Extended operations for the treatment of lung cancer. *Ann Thorac Surg.* 1997;63(1):12–19.
31. Spaggiari L, Regnard J-F, Magdeleinat P, et al. Extended resections for bronchogenic carcinoma invading the superior vena cava system. *Ann Thorac Surg.* 2000;69(1):233–236.
32. Yildizeli B, Dartevelle PG, Fadel E, et al. Results of primary surgery with T4 non-small cell lung cancer during a 25-year period in a single center: the benefit is worth the risk. *Ann Thorac Surg.* 2008;86(4):1065–1075.
33. Allison PR. Intrapericardial approach to the lung root in the treatment of bronchial carcinoma by dissection pneumonectomy. *J Thorac Surg.* 1946;15:99–117.
34. Shirakusa T, Kimura M. Partial atrial resection in advanced lung carcinoma with and without cardiopulmonary bypass. *Thorax.* 1991;46(7):484–487.
35. Korst RJ, Rosengart TK. Operative strategies for resection of pulmonary sarcomas extending into the left atrium. *Ann Thorac Surg.* 1999;67(4):1165–1167.
36. Baron O, Jouan J, Sagan C, et al. Resection of bronchopulmonary cancers invading the left atrium – benefit of cardiopulmonary bypass. *Thorac Cardiovasc Surg.* 2003;51(3):159–161.
37. Ratto GB, Costa R, Vassallo G, et al. Twelve-year experience with left atrial resection in the treatment of non-small cell lung cancer. *Ann Thorac Surg.* 2004;78(1):234–237.
38. Kuehnl A, Lindner M, Hornung H-M, et al. Atrial resection for lung cancer: morbidity, mortality, and long-term follow-up. *World J Surg.* 2010; 34(9):2233–2239.
39. Klepetko W, Wisser W, Birsan T, et al. T4 lung tumors with infiltration of the thoracic aorta: is an operation reasonable? *Ann Thorac Surg.* 1999;67(2):340–344.
40. Horita K, Itho T, Ueno T. Radical operation using cardiopulmonary bypass for lung cancer invading the aortic wall. *Thorac Cardiovasc Surg.* 1993;41(2):130–132.
41. Okubo K, Yagi K, Yokomise H, et al. Extensive resection with selective cerebral perfusion for a lung cancer invading the aortic arch. *Eur J Cardiothorac Surg.* 1996;10(5):389–391.
42. Berna P, Bagan P, De Dominicis F, et al. Aortic endostent followed by extended pneumonectomy for T4 lung cancer. *Ann Thorac Surg.* 2011; 91(2):591–593.

PART 13

COMPLICATIONS OF PULMONARY RESECTION

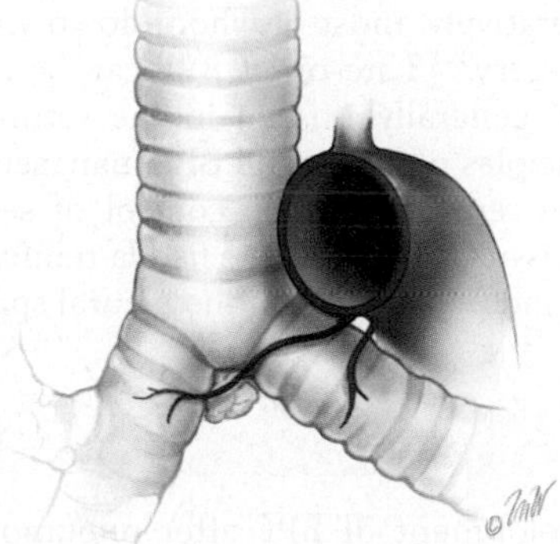

82 Bronchopleural Fistula After Pneumonectomy

Mark F. Berry and David H. Harpole, Jr.

Keywords: Pneumonectomy, morbidity, bronchopleural fistula, empyema

INTRODUCTION

Bronchopleural fistula (BPF) occurs in 1.5% to 7% of patients after pneumonectomy. BPFs can have devastating consequences, with mortality of 25% to 71% and prolonged hospital stays involving multiple procedures for survivors.[1,2] Presentation may be acute or delayed: The majority of patients present within 3 months postoperatively, most of whom do so within the first 12 days after surgery.[2,3] Late-onset BPF can be more difficult to diagnose and generally is seen in the setting of empyema. The basic principles of successful BPF management include protection of the remaining lung, control of sepsis, debridement of necrotic tissue, closure of the fistula reinforced with vascularized tissue, and obliteration of the pleural space.

RISK FACTORS

Risk factors for the development of BPF after pneumonectomy include anatomic, technical, and patient factors (Table 82-1).[4,5] Right pneumonectomy is associated with a fourfold to fivefold higher incidence of BPF than left pneumonectomy, likely related to anatomic differences between the right and left mainstem bronchi.[6] A right pneumonectomy stump has minimal mediastinal coverage of the bronchial stump compared with a left-sided stump, which retracts underneath the aorta into the mediastinum when properly fashioned (Fig. 82-1). The right mainstem bronchus is also oriented much more vertically than the left, which permits secretions to pool in the bronchial stump. Finally, the vascular supply to the left mainstem bronchus is augmented by direct vascular branches as the bronchus passes behind the aorta. The blood supply on the right travels from the trachea via local branches in the subcarinal space, which are often disrupted by dissection and lymph node removal.

Technical factors related to BPF formation include devascularization of the bronchial stump by excessive dissection; a long bronchial stump with increased pooling of secretions and risk of secondary infection that leads to stump breakdown; stump closure with suture instead of staples; and closure under tension, as in the case of a thickened bronchial wall at the point of closure.[4,7] Closure under tension also can be implicated in a predominance of right-sided BPFs because the diameter of the right mainstem bronchus at the point of transection generally is larger than the left. Although excessive bronchial dissection increases the risk of BPF, mediastinal lymphadenectomy has not been shown to increase the risk of BPF.[8]

The primary patient factor associated with BPF is postoperative mechanical ventilation. The overall BPF incidence in a series of 256 patients was 3.1%, which increased to 19.3% in patients requiring postoperative ventilation.[9] Prolonged high airway pressures likely create trauma at the level of the stump that impairs healing. The need for postoperative mechanical ventilation also may explain the association between BPF and severe chronic obstructive pulmonary disease, as well as low forced expiratory volume in 1 second (FEV_1) and the diffusion capacity of the lung to carbon monoxide (D_{LCO}). Other

Table 82-1

RISK FACTORS FOR BRONCHOPLEURAL FISTULA AFTER PNEUMONECTOMY

ANATOMIC
Right pneumonectomy
Completion pneumonectomy after previous ipsilateral lung resection
TECHNICAL
Devascularization of bronchial stump
Long bronchial stump
Tension at stump suture or staple line
Persistent disease at bronchial stump
PATIENT
Surgery for benign disease
Postoperative mechanical ventilation
Poor pulmonary reserve
Low preoperative FEV_1 and D_{LCO}
Diabetes
Malnutrition
Chronic steroid use
Preoperative infectious process or empyema
Preoperative chemotherapy or radiation therapy
Blood transfusion

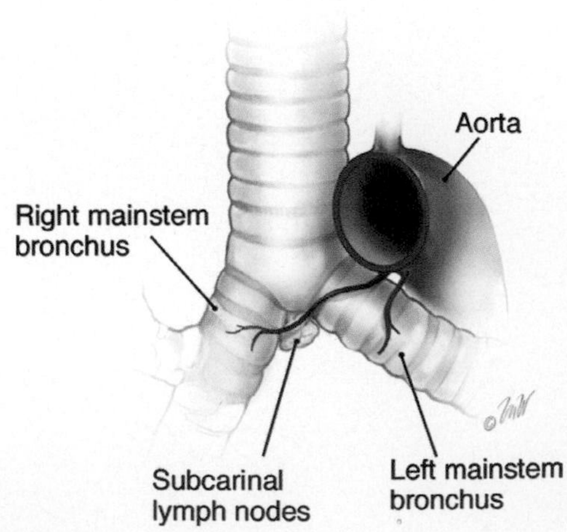

Figure 82-1. Patients with right pneumonectomy are four to five times more likely to develop a BPF owing to the anatomic differences between the right and left mainstem bronchi. The right bronchus has a more vertical orientation, which may permit collection of fluid in the stump and lacks direct vascular branches from the aorta, relying instead on the trachea and local branches in the subcarinal space that are often disrupted during lymph node removal.

patient factors include those that impair wound healing, such as preoperative radiation therapy (>45 Gy), poor nutritional status, and prolonged corticosteroid use. Local infectious processes such as tuberculosis or the presence of empyema also increase the risk of BPF.

Coverage of the bronchial stump may reduce the incidence in patients at an increased risk for developing BPF after pneumonectomy.[4] Bronchial stump coverage with an intercostal muscle flap was associated with a reduction in the incidence of BPF from 8.8% to 0% in a randomized trial involving diabetic patients.[10] Coverage is likely especially important on the right side, where the stump is exposed in the pneumonectomy space. Many groups routinely cover all right-sided stumps, covering left-sided stumps only for patients with increased risk. Coverage can be provided by using a variety of local and distant tissues as vascularized flaps that are tacked over the bronchial stump. Tissues used routinely include pericardial fat pad and intercostal muscle flaps. If these tissues are inadequate, or if the patient is thought to be at extraordinary risk of stump complications, larger muscle or omental flaps are used.

DIAGNOSIS

BPF should be suspected in patients who develop fever, empyema, aspiration pneumonia, an excessively productive cough, or an increasing air leak or amount of pleural air after lung resection. Many patients present early with a fulminant course, including expectoration of large amounts of serous or seropurulent fluid, respiratory distress, and sepsis. Appearance of these symptoms should raise the index of suspicion and be followed by a quick and accurate diagnosis before there is overwhelming aspiration of pleural fluid into the remaining lung. This presentation is most common in large fistulas with abundant drainage of pleural fluid into the tracheobronchial tree. Small fistulas more commonly present with productive cough with serous or purulent sputum, fever, hemoptysis, or subcutaneous emphysema. Findings on chest radiograph suggestive of BPF include progressive subcutaneous or mediastinal emphysema, development of a new air–fluid level in a previously opacified pneumonectomy space, a 2-cm drop in an existing air–fluid level with shift of the mediastinum away from the pneumonectomy space, or new development of multiple air–fluid levels. Late-onset BPF often presents with nonspecific symptoms, including low-grade fever, anorexia, fatigue, and weight loss similar to late postpneumonectomy empyema. Proving the presence of a fistula in these patients can be more problematic because the connection is often small and not identified by bronchoscopy. Nuclear medicine techniques have been used to confirm the presence of radiolabeled inhaled gas in the postpneumonectomy space.

Whether the diagnosis is apparent clinically or radiographically or suggested by advanced testing, all patients should undergo diagnostic bronchoscopy. A large fistula generally can be visualized. Fistulas smaller than 1 to 2 mm may be difficult to identify. Perhaps more important, bronchoscopy provides information about the length of the remaining bronchial stump and the condition of the tissue at the level of the stump that can be helpful in planning definitive repair. In addition, pulmonary toilet can be optimized by aspirating any fluid or secretions in the remaining lung.

SURGICAL TREATMENT

Draining the Pleural Space

Acute management focuses on controlling life-threatening conditions, including postural drainage with the affected lung positioned down in cases of airway flooding, early thorough pleural drainage to prevent sepsis and aspiration pneumonia, and appropriate antibiotic therapy. Adequate nutrition is also paramount to a favorable outcome.

Drainage can be performed at the bedside with a tube thoracostomy under local anesthesia placed to either balanced drainage system or water seal but not suction. Immediate drainage is especially important for patients who present with large fistulas in which a significant volume of pleural contents is draining into the airways, potentially flooding the contralateral lung. Care must be taken to place the tube above the level of the previous thoracotomy incision because the diaphragm will be elevated as part of the normal thoracic remodeling that occurs after pneumonectomy. In addition, the patient should be in the supine position when the thoracostomy tube is placed. Lateral positioning places the remaining lung in a dependent position and encourages further aspiration. Once the tube is in place, further positional maneuvers to prevent aspiration include maintaining the patient in as close to an upright position as possible and rotating the patient such that the pneumonectomy side is down.

Once the urgent situation is controlled and the patient is started on appropriate parenteral antibiotics, the remaining pleural debris and necrotic tissue are removed. Debridement can be accomplished by means of an open thoracic window or thoracotomy. The selection of technique depends on the patient's overall condition. At this stage, debilitated or critically ill patients may tolerate a major thoracic procedure poorly, especially a prolonged procedure involving muscle flaps or other approaches used to definitively address the fistula. These patients often benefit from a period of treatment with a simple open window thoracostomy to permit control of sepsis and nutritional support followed by delayed definitive closure.

Technique for Open Window Thoracostomy

Open window thoracostomy allows open drainage of an infected intrathoracic space by using a U-shaped incision over the most dependent portion of the space (Fig. 82-2). Segments of one or two ribs are removed to limit the tendency of the opening to contract and close. The skin flap then is sutured directly to the parietal pleura with interrupted absorbable sutures to create an epithelialized tract, which both maintains the patency of the window and encourages healing. The window should not be placed too far posteriorly such that it is difficult for the patient to manage. Similar care is taken to avoid placing the window too far inferiorly, where it might interfere with the diaphragm. Other techniques, including placement of large-bore drainage tubes through the window as stents, also will help to maintain patency. Dressing changes with moistened gauze then are performed until the cavity is sterilized. Very small fistulas may close spontaneously once the local sepsis is eradicated. Most, however, require definitive closure. Patients in generally good condition at the time of presentation can proceed directly to simultaneous debridement of the pleural space and definitive closure.

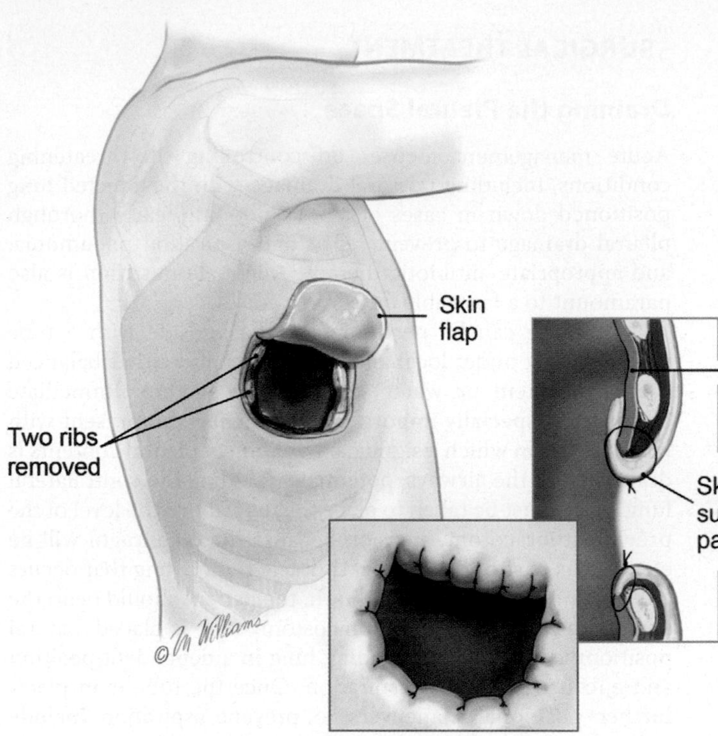

Figure 82-2. Open-window thoracostomy drainage was first proposed by Eloesser. Note the U-shaped incision over the infected space and technique (inset) for securing the skin flap directly to the parietal pleura.

Closing the Bronchopleural Fistula

Most patients can tolerate early exploration and closure of the fistula, and this procedure should be undertaken as soon as the patient is medically stable. Exploration is preferentially performed by means of a posterolateral thoracotomy on the ipsilateral side, with lung isolation via selective intubation of the contralateral mainstem bronchus to prevent further soilage of the remaining lung. If not readily visible, the fistula can be identified with the aid of positive-pressure ventilation while covering the area of the bronchial stump with irrigation. The pleural space is thoroughly irrigated and debrided to remove all necrotic tissue. The bronchial stump is carefully dissected to minimize trauma to its blood supply. All attempts are made to leave a final stump that is less than 1 cm in length measured from the carina (Fig. 82-3). If sufficient length remains on initial exploration, stapling device can be used to reclose the stump. In most cases, there is too much inflammation to permit stapling, however, and the mobilized bronchial stump is reclosed with interrupted monofilament sutures. A balance must be obtained between exposing enough bronchus to avoid tension on the closure and avoiding too much exposure, which could damage the blood supply.

Reinforcing the suture line with vascularized tissue is perhaps the most important aspect of closure. Pedicled flaps of the muscle or omentum are mobilized into the chest and sutured over the bronchial stump.[3,11] Flap choice depends on the quality of the tissue, damage to potential flap muscles from the previous thoracotomy, and the amount of space to be filled. The serratus anterior is used commonly after pneumonectomy. This muscle is often preserved during the initial operation even when an open procedure was done, because of its utility in dealing with potential complications. The flap is based on the vascular pedicle that runs on the lateral undersurface of the scapula. The muscle is mobilized and inserted between the ribs in either the second or third interspace, where it will generally reach the hilum with no tension. If the interspaces are tight and can possibly compromise the vascular supply of the flap, a segment of the third rib can be removed to allow the flap to comfortably enter the pleural space. The flap generally is secured with interrupted absorbable sutures to the peribronchial or mediastinal areolar tissue. This tissue aids in healing and infection control because its blood supply emanates from regions beyond the inflamed field. In cases where the stump is frankly necrotic or densely scarred into the mediastinum, the fistula may not be able to be closed directly. In this event, a muscle or omental flap is sutured to the freshened edges of the open fistula or surrounding mediastinum to occlude the communication and permit healing. An advantage of using a relatively large muscle such as the

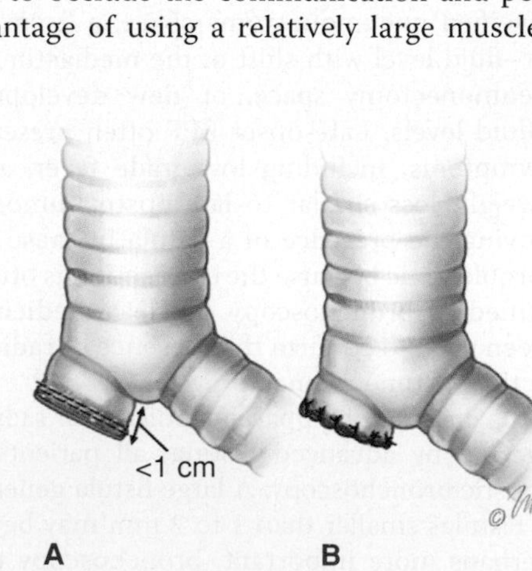

Figure 82-3. Ideally, the length of the bronchial stump should be less than 1 cm. *A.* If there is sufficient length on the stump after initial exploration, a stapling device can be used to reclose the stump. *B.* Often there is too much inflammation to permit stapling, and the mobilized bronchial stump is reclosed with interrupted monofilament sutures.

serratus anterior to close the fistula is that it also contributes bulk to fill some of the dead space in the postpneumonectomy chest.

In severely ill patients with difficult bronchial stumps, simultaneously placing a temporary tracheostomy with a long cuffed tube in the contralateral mainstem bronchus may be useful. The tracheostomy is left in place for several weeks to permit the flap to become fixed over the opening of the fistula without the stress of positive-pressure ventilation, which can slow healing.

Case reports and small case series have also reported successful BPF treatment using endoscopic techniques. The use of bronchoscopic placement of stents, glues, sealants, coils, submucosal tissue expander injection, and devices designed for transcatheter closure of cardiac defects have all been reported to successfully lead to closure of BPFs after pneumonectomy.[3] However, these techniques should likely be considered only when primary repair fails or is not possible because of patient condition. Generally, these only work with smaller BPFs.

Once the fistula is closed, the pleural space must be sterilized. In early-onset BPF, when there has been minimal contamination, thorough operative debridement and irrigation may be sufficient. In more advanced cases with greater contamination, sterilization can be accomplished by creating an open window with dressing changes as described earlier or by closure over irrigation catheters after the fistula has been repaired. Chest tubes or other irrigation catheters can be placed and irrigated either continuously or several times daily with antibiotic solution. When there is no remaining evidence of infection within the space, on the basis of either Gram stain of granulation tissue or culture of irrigation fluid, definitive closure is performed.

More recently, several retrospective studies have reported successful management of empyema cavities using vacuum-assisted closure (VAC) devices, even in the setting of a BPF. Although limited, these studies suggest that VAC, as an adjunct to the standard treatment, can potentially alleviate the morbidity and reduce inpatient length of treatment in patients with empyema after lung resection.[12] Management typically involves filling the intrathoracic cavity with foam to the superficial wound edges. Negative pressure, gradually increased from −25 to −125 mm Hg over time, is applied to clean the wound and support healing. The VAC is generally changed every 2 to 3 days.

Occasionally, it is impossible to access the bronchial stump for effective repair, especially on the left side when the stump is retracted underneath the aorta (Fig. 82-4). In such cases, fistula closure can be approached via median sternotomy.[13] This approach permits exposure of the carina in a previously non-operated field between the superior vena cava and the aorta, and the mainstem bronchus can be redivided and closed in a field free of infection. After median sternotomy, the pericardium is opened, and dissection between the superior vena cava and aorta exposes the carina. If possible, a segment of the mainstem bronchus should be resected to provide a fresh edge for stapling or suture closure and to avoid contamination from the distal bronchial remnant. Another approach to the carina is through the right chest for a left-sided fistula. A right posterolateral thoracotomy is performed in this approach, and the lung is mobilized and retracted anteriorly so the mediastinal pleura can be incised at the level of the subcarinal area. The left bronchial stump can be mobilized, restapled flush with the carina, and covered with a flap of intercostal muscle, pericardial fat, or mediastinal tissue.[14] Central extracorporeal membrane oxygenation (ECMO) can be utilized if necessary if the patient has instability during the attempted repair.

Obliterating the Remaining Pleural Cavity

The final step in the treatment of BPF is obliteration of the remaining pleural space. The patient's overall condition and

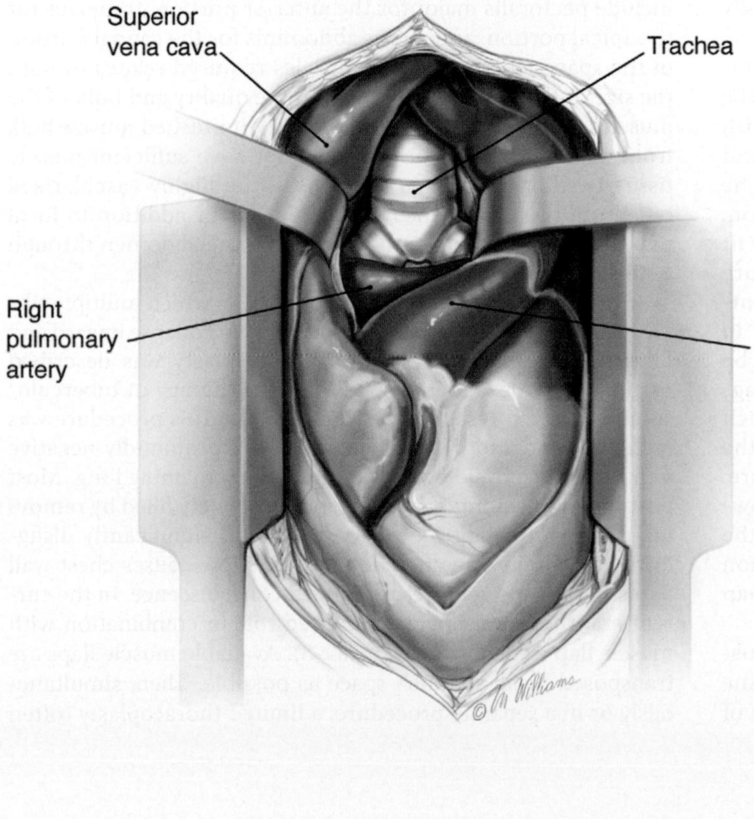

Figure 82-4. A median sternotomy approach can be used when the left mainstem bronchus is retracted underneath the aorta, limiting access to the bronchial stump. This approach exposes the carina between the superior vena cava and the aorta and permits operation in a sterile field.

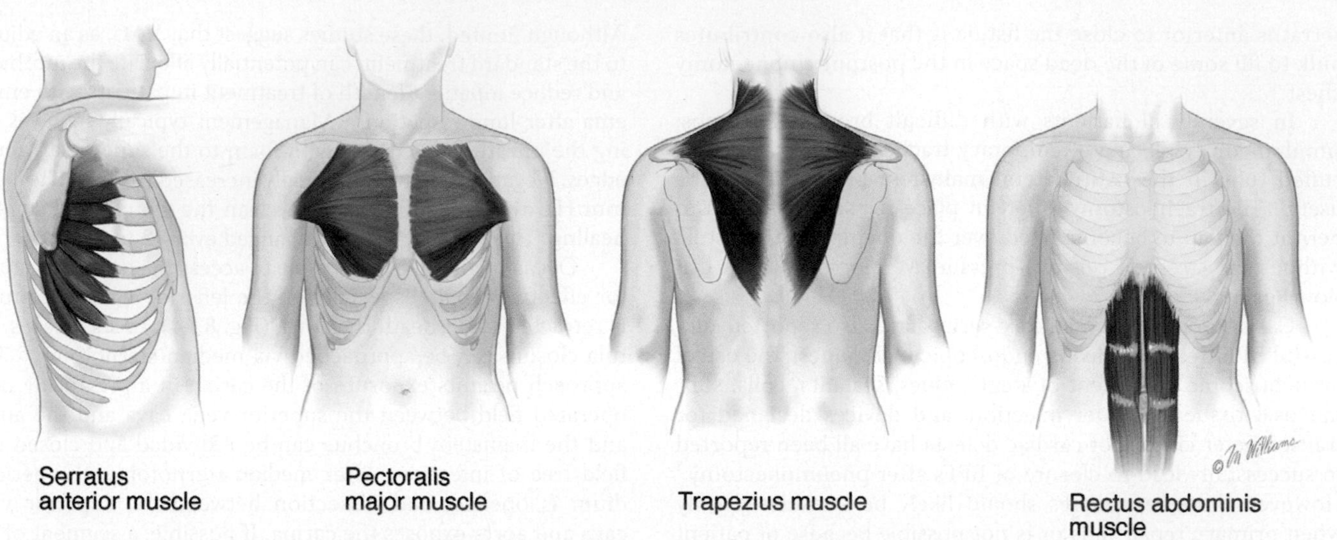

Figure 82-5. Muscle flaps available for transposition into the pleural space. The serratus anterior is ideal for filling small defects, such as BPF. It takes its blood supply from the lateral thoracic artery, and entrance into the chest is made from the primary incision. The pectoralis major receives blood from two sources, the thoracoacromial artery and the internal mammary artery. Entry into the chest is made through a 5-cm rib resection. It is used most commonly for sternal infections and for BPFs that originate from an upper lobe bronchus. The trapezius is used to fill the apical pleural space, and the rectus abdominis provides tissue for the caudal pleural space.

suitability for complete closure must be carefully reevaluated before taking this final step. Most closure failures are related to persistent or recurrent BPF. Patients with a chronic fistula, carcinomatosis within the space, persistent infection within the space, or poor nutritional status should not undergo obliteration maneuvers unless or until these issues have been addressed. A period of treatment with open thoracic window and adequate nutritional support can improve the patient's likelihood of a positive long-term outcome.

Obliteration of the pleural space can be accomplished by one or a combination of three techniques. The first option is to fill the sterilized cavity with antibiotic solution (Clagett maneuver). If the chest was closed initially over irrigation catheters, obliteration is a simple procedure. Antibiotic solution is infused into the cavity until it is completely filled, the irrigation catheters are removed, and the site is suture closed. If the patient was treated initially with an open thoracic window, the skin edges are excised and flaps are mobilized to permit closure without tension. The chest is filled with antibiotic solution in a similar fashion, and the window then is closed in multiple layers to prevent leakage of fluid. Antibiotic selection is tailored to culture and sensitivity tests rather than to a set of standard antibiotics. Excessive doses of intrapleural antibiotics can result in renal failure or other systemic complications and should be avoided. This technique was described originally by Clagett and Geraci[15] in 1963 as a two-stage procedure in which open-window drainage was followed by obliteration of the space with antibiotic fluid without direct fistula closure. The technique is used rarely in its original form today, however, because of recurrences related to persistence of the fistula. The more common approach is the modified version with an intermediate step of fistula closure with muscle flap as described earlier.

The second technique involves transposition of muscle flaps that fill the pleural space with vascularized tissue (Fig. 82-5). Muscle flaps are an excellent choice because of their rich blood supply and ability to extend to almost any region of the pleural space. The choice of flaps depends on the availability and suitability of local muscles. Latissimus dorsi is often the largest muscle available in this location but frequently has been transected at the time of the original thoracotomy. Previously transected latissimus dorsi is unlikely to survive as a transposed flap. Many groups intentionally preserve the serratus anterior at initial operation for later use as a flap (Fig. 82-6). The serratus anterior is mobilized with maintenance of its attachments to the upper scapula and passed into the chest between the ribs or through a window created by resecting a segment of the second or third rib. Other useful local muscles include pectoralis major for the anterior portion, trapezius for the apical portion, and rectus abdominis for the caudal portion of the space. The number of muscles required relates to both the size of the remaining cavity and the quality and bulk of the muscles. Many patients with BPF have diminished muscle bulk from chronic debilitation and may not have sufficient muscle tissue to fill the space. In such cases, the highly vascularized omentum is an excellent replacement for or addition to local muscle flaps and can be mobilized from the abdomen through a substernal tunnel (Fig. 82-7).

The third technique is thoracoplasty, in which multiple ribs are resected to allow chest wall soft tissue to collapse inward and fill the pneumonectomy space. Thoracoplasty was described originally by Alexander[16] in 1937 for the therapy of tuberculosis and involved resection of 10 or 11 ribs. This procedure was highly morbid and disfiguring, and had a profoundly negative impact on the physiologic function of the remaining lung. Most postpneumonectomy spaces can be completely filled by removing ribs two to eight; however, this is still significantly disfiguring, may limit arm and shoulder function, causes chest wall paresthesias, and requires prolonged convalescence. In the current era, thoracoplasty has a limited role in combination with muscle flap transposition (Fig. 82-8). Available muscle flaps are transposed to fill as much space as possible. Then, simultaneously or in a separate procedure, a limited thoracoplasty (often

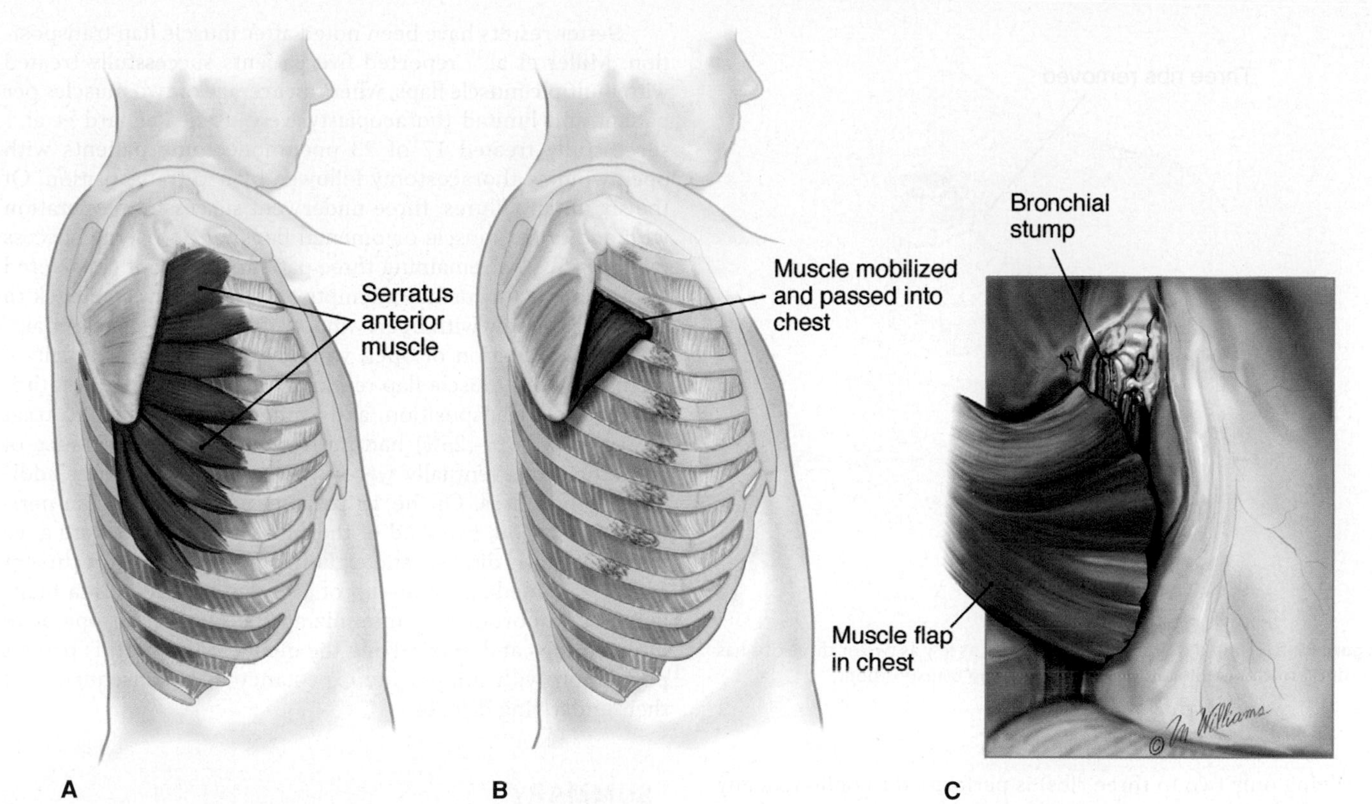

Figure 82-6. The serratus anterior is often preserved at initial operation by maintaining its attachment to the upper scapula and used later as a muscle pedicle. The free end is passed into the chest between the ribs or through a window created by resecting a segment of the rib.

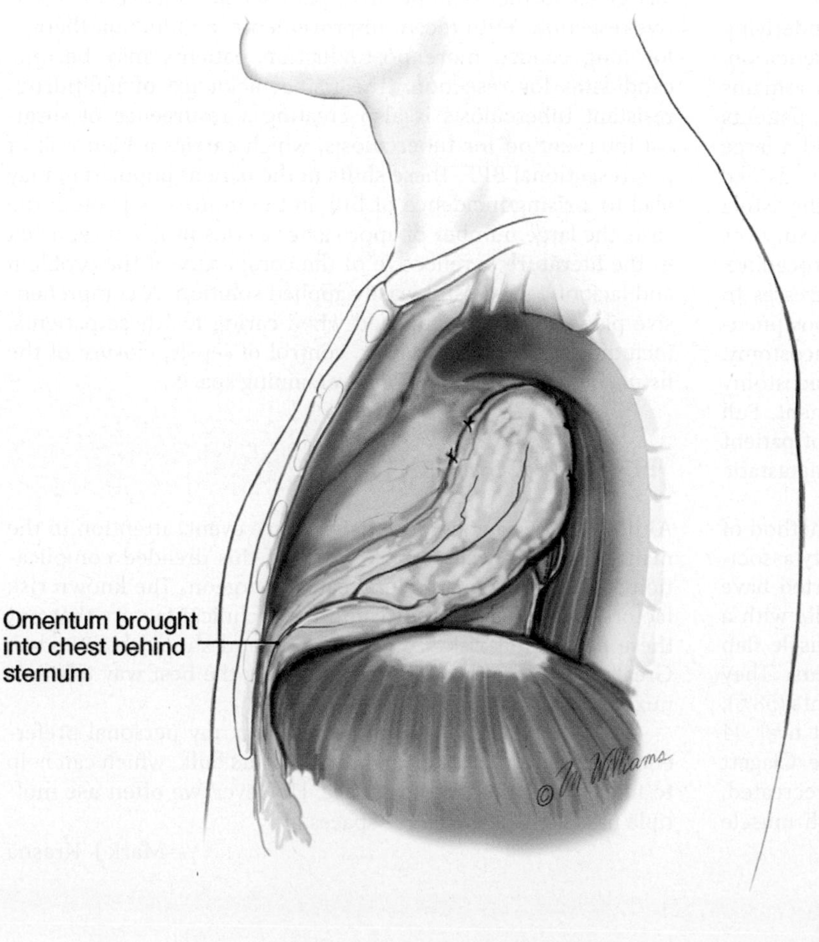

Figure 82-7. Patients with BPF may be severely debilitated from long-term illness that leaves a paucity of muscle bulk. In these patients, the omentum is an excellent substitute for a pedicled muscle flap and has a rich vascular supply. It is mobilized from the abdomen through a substernal tunnel.

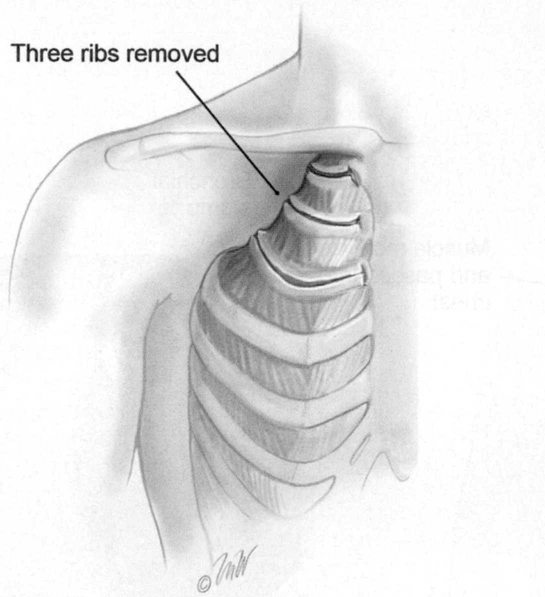

Figure 82-8. Limited thoracoplasty involving as few as two or three ribs has a limited role in combination with muscle flap transposition.

involving only two to three ribs) is performed to obliterate any remaining space.

OUTCOMES

Outcomes after BPF are related most strongly to the underlying disease and condition of the patient at the time of presentation. The reported overall mortality for this complication remains distressingly high. The main cause of death in these patients is aspiration pneumonia of the contralateral side, and a large number never stabilize enough to permit repair of the fistula. Aspiration pneumonia occurs more commonly when the fistula occurs shortly after surgery. A second group of patients survives the initial insult long enough to receive a drainage procedure, such as open window thoracostomy, but never progresses to closure. Regnard et al. described the treatment of 30 postpneumonectomy patients with initial open window thoracostomy. Of those, seven (23%) received open window thoracostomy with dressing changes as their only definitive treatment. Full repair was not accomplished in this group because of patient death, other major illnesses, locally recurrent or metastatic cancer, or patient choice.[17]

The modified Clagett technique is the simplest method of definitive treatment and limits the operative morbidity associated with flap harvest; however, the outcomes reported have been suboptimal. Pairolero et al. reported their results with a three-step modified Clagett procedure including muscle flap reinforcement of the bronchial stump in 45 patients. They reported an ultimately successful outcome in 26 patients (58%), with an average of 5 surgical procedures per patient over 34 hospitalization days and 6 operative deaths.[18] If the Clagett technique fails, the open window thoracostomy is recreated, and a more complex method of closure such as with muscle flap is attempted.

Better results have been noted after muscle flap transposition. Miller et al.[19] reported five patients successfully treated with multiple muscle flaps, where an average of two muscles per patient and limited thoracoplasty were used. Regnard et al.[17] successfully treated 17 of 23 pneumonectomy patients with open window thoracostomy followed by flap transposition. Of the six initial failures, three underwent successful reoperation with additional muscle or omental flaps for an overall success rate of 87%. The remaining three patients were not considered to be suitable for further attempts and were converted back to definitive therapy with open window drainage. Michaels et al.[20] used a combination of open window thoracostomy, repair of the fistula with muscle flap reinforcement, additional intrathoracic muscle transposition, and limited thoracoplasty to treat 16 patients. Four (25%) had initial failure with recurrence of empyema but eventually were treated successfully after additional procedures. Of the 15 patients who survived the perioperative period, five died of their lung cancer, two were alive with metastatic disease, and eight had no evidence of recurrent cancer at a median follow-up of 19 months. These data highlight the importance of minimizing the number of operative interventions and maximizing the quality of life in this patient population with limited life expectancy as a consequence of their underlying disease.

SUMMARY

BPF continues to be a frustrating complication of pneumonectomy that leads to significant morbidity and mortality even in the modern era. Progress in the care of critically ill patients has given formerly inoperative patients the chance for curative resection. With recent improvements in induction therapy for lung cancer, more postinduction patients may become candidates for resection. The rising incidence of multidrug-resistant tuberculosis is also creating a resurgence of surgical intervention for tuberculosis, which carries a high risk of postresectional BPF. These shifts in the patient population may lead to a rising incidence of BPF in the future. As is often the case, the large number of approaches to this problem reported in the literature is reflective of the complexity of the problem and lack of a successful, easily applied solution. A comprehensive plan must be established when caring for these patients, including nutritional support, control of sepsis, closure of the fistula, and obliteration of any remaining space.

EDITOR'S COMMENT

Although BPF in general remains a rare event, attention to the management as well as prevention of this dreaded complication is important for the lung cancer surgeon. The known risk factors for patient disability and the technical factors that put these patients at risk are well known and should be avoided. Great care at the initial surgery remains the best way to minimize the risk of BPF.

Regarding the choice of muscle flap, my personal preference is the serratus anterior, because of its bulk, which can help to fill the pneumonectomy space. However, we often use multiple muscle flaps for larger spaces.

—Mark J. Krasna

References

1. Asamura H, Naruke T, Tsuchiya R, et al. Bronchopleural fistulas associated with lung cancer operations. Univariate and multivariate analysis of risk factors, management, and outcome. *J Thorac Cardiovasc Surg.* 1992;104:1456–1464.
2. Hollaus PH, Lax F, el-Nashef BB, et al. Natural history of bronchopleural fistula after pneumonectomy: a review of 96 cases. *Ann Thorac Surg.* 1997;63:1391–1396.
3. Lois M, Noppen M. Bronchopleural fistulas: an overview of the problem with special focus on endoscopic management. *Chest.* 2005;128:3955–3965.
4. Deschamps C, Bernard A, Nichols FC 3rd, et al. Empyema and bronchopleural fistula after pneumonectomy: factors affecting incidence. *Ann Thorac Surg.* 2001;72:243–247.
5. Alexiou C, Beggs D, Rogers ML, et al. Pneumonectomy for non-small cell lung cancer: predictors of operative mortality and survival. *Eur J Cardiothorac Surg.* 2001;20:476–480.
6. Algar FJ, Alvarez A, Aranda JL, et al. Prediction of early bronchopleural fistula after pneumonectomy: A multivariate analysis. *Ann Thorac Surg.* 2001;72:1662–1667.
7. Panagopoulos ND, Apostolakis E, Koletsis E, et al. Low incidence of bronchopleural fistula after pneumonectomy for lung cancer. *Interact Cardiovasc Thorac Surg.* 2009;9:571–575.
8. Allen MS, Darling GE, Pechet TT, et al. Morbidity and mortality of major pulmonary resections in patients with early-stage lung cancer: initial results of the randomized, prospective ACOSOG Z0030 trial. *Ann Thorac Surg.* 2006;81:1013–1019.
9. Wright CD, Wain JC, Mathisen DJ, Grillo HC. Postpneumonectomy bronchopleural fistula after sutured bronchial closure: incidence, risk factors, and management. *J Thorac Cardiovasc Surg.* 1996;112:1367–1371.
10. Sfyridis PG, Kapetanakis EI, Baltayiannis NE, et al. Bronchial stump buttressing with an intercostal muscle flap in diabetic patients. *Ann Thorac Surg.* 2007;84:967–971.
11. Shrager JB, Wain JC, Wright CD, et al. Omentum is highly effective in the management of complex cardiothoracic surgical problems. *J Thorac Cardiovasc Surg.* 2003;125:526–532.
12. Haghshenasskashani A, Rahnavardi M, Yan TD, et al. Intrathoracic application of a vacuum-assisted device in managing pleural space infection after lung resection: is it an option? *Interact Cardiovasc Thorac Surg.* 2011;13:168–174.
13. Ginsberg RJ, Pearson FG, Cooper JD, et al. Closure of chronic postpneumonectomy bronchopleural fistula using the transsternal transpericardial approach. *Ann Thorac Surg.* 1989;47:231–235.
14. Moreno P, Lang G, Taghavi S, et al. Right-sided approach for management of left-main-bronchial stump problems. *Eur J Cardiothorac Surg.* 2011;40:926–930.
15. Clagett OT, Geraci JE. A procedure for the management of postpneumonectomy empyema. *J Thorac Cardiovasc Surg.* 1963;45:141–145.
16. Alexander J. *The Collapse Therapy of Pulmonary Tuberculosis.* Springfield, MA: Charles C Thomas; 1937.
17. Regnard JF, Alifano M, Puyo P, et al. Open window thoracostomy followed by intrathoracic flap transposition in the treatment of empyema complicating pulmonary resection. *J Thorac Cardiovasc Surg.* 2000;120:270–275.
18. Pairolero PC, Arnold PG, Trastek VF, et al. Postpneumonectomy empyema: the role of intrathoracic muscle transposition. *J Thorac Cardiovasc Surg.* 1990;99:958–966.
19. Miller JI, Mansour KA, Nahai F, et al. Single-stage complete muscle flap closure of the postpneumonectomy empyema space: a new method and possible solution to a disturbing complication. *Ann Thorac Surg.* 1984;38:227–231.
20. Michaels BM, Orgill DP, Decamp MM, et al. Flap closure of postpneumonectomy empyema. *Plast Reconstr Surg.* 1997;99:437–442.

83 Management of Hemoptysis in Lung Cancer

Daniel M. Cohen and Michael T. Jaklitsch

Keywords: Hemoptysis, lung cancer, surgical management, flexible and rigid bronchoscopy, brachytherapy, argon plasma coagulation

Lung cancer is a silent killer. Symptoms are present in only approximately 40% of patients in a population screened for lung cancer who have radiographic changes.[1] Even in those patients with symptoms, these are usually nonspecific, and clues to the existence of an underlying lung cancer may be gleaned only from the patient's history. A history of long-standing cigarette smoking, age greater than 40 years, significant weight loss, and a chronic cough are clinical pointers worth noting.

Although some degree of hemoptysis may be the presenting complaint in 29% of patients with lung cancer, the degree of hemoptysis varies considerably.[2] Most commonly, patients report a discrete episode of blood-streaked sputum at least once before seeing a physician. Often this is attributed to chronic bronchitis, especially in the face of a normal recent chest radiograph. Since a chest computed tomography (CT) scan has been shown to be much more sensitive for detecting underlying pulmonary lesions compared with a plain chest radiograph, a chest CT scan should be obtained in all patients with a history of hemoptysis.[3]

A more severe hemoptysis can be seen with the expectoration of clots after a vigorous coughing episode. It is surprising how many patients will continue to downplay the significance of more severe episodes of hemoptysis or fail to seek urgent medical attention. The expectoration of clots is not considered pathognomonic for lung cancer. Massive hemoptysis (by definition, >200 mL per day), although less common with lung cancer, can occur in up to 20% of patients in whom lung cancer is the cause.[4] Furthermore, it has been reported to be fatal in up to 50% of patients with lung cancer and demands serious and immediate attention in a hospital setting.[5]

The single most common cause of streaky hemoptysis in the United States is acute bronchitis. The most common cause of the expectoration of clot or massive hemoptysis, however, is lung cancer, especially in patients older than 50 years who have a long-standing smoking history. Other causes of hemoptysis, which cannot be ignored, include tuberculosis, chronic bronchitis, bronchiectasis, pneumonia, pulmonary infarction, lung abscess, aspergilloma, arteriovenous malformation of the lung, mitral stenosis, and bronchial adenoma. Lung cancer should be ruled out before considering other causes.

GENERAL PRINCIPLES

Massive hemoptysis must be considered a surgical emergency. The potential for imminent loss of life dictates attention first to preservation of the airway, breathing, and circulation (the ABCs of resuscitation). In the face of massive hemoptysis, the patient should be intubated with a single-lumen endotracheal tube (ET). A plain chest radiograph and urgent flexible bronchoscopy frequently can be used to determine which side of the airway is the source of bleeding. If the ET can be guided selectively into the contralateral airway, it can preserve the life of the patient, even if the ipsilateral airway completely fills with blood and clots. Intravenous (IV) access with two large-bore catheters should be established quickly. A large amount of clot in the proximal airway may necessitate urgent tracheotomy to save the patient from drowning and asphyxiation. This maneuver will facilitate the expeditious removal of large clots and blood from the trachea. Once the ABCs of resuscitation are secured, efforts should be directed toward establishing a diagnosis.

PREOPERATIVE ASSESSMENT

A plain chest radiograph should be obtained in any patient presenting with hemoptysis. The simple fact that disease can be seen within one or the other lung field can provide invaluable information for the ongoing care of the patient. It should be noted, however, that up to 5% of patients with a history of hemoptysis and an underlying cancer may have a normal chest radiograph.[6]

Traditionally, flexible bronchoscopy has been considered as the next diagnostic test to perform in a patient who presents with hemoptysis. The likelihood of localizing a bleeding site is considerably higher if bronchoscopy is undertaken during or within 48 hours of an event.[7] Furthermore, emergency bronchoscopy after intubation can be used to guide the ET into either the left or the right main stem bronchus. In this way, the affected side can be isolated from the healthy lung.[8] Early bronchoscopy does not guarantee that an endobronchial bleeding site will be identified. In one study, no discrete bleeding source was found in approximately half of patients.[8]

A high-resolution chest CT is an important tool for identifying the source of bleeding and possibly may replace bronchoscopy as the first-line procedure.[9] In one study, when the chest radiograph was nonspecific, chest CT was found to be diagnostic in 43% and bronchoscopy in only 14% of patients.[10] In this same study, the site of bleeding was localized by chest CT scan in 52% compared with 23% by bronchoscopy. In reality, bronchoscopy and CT scanning should be viewed as complementary studies when used to identify the source of hemoptysis. While CT scan can visualize parenchymal abnormalities in the periphery of the tracheobronchial tree as well as the presence of extraluminal disease, the bronchoscope is better suited for diagnosing endobronchial tumors and subtle airway abnormalities such as mucosal edema. Some of these bronchoscopic findings may not be obvious on a standard chest CT scan. Thus, CT scanning of the chest and bronchoscopy have greater sensitivity and specificity when used in combination.

TECHNIQUE

The management of hemoptysis depends on the rate of bleeding and the underlying cardiopulmonary status of the patient. In a few cases, bleeding into the airway may be brisk, having the potential to be fatal within minutes. Patients may succumb rapidly, not from exsanguination and shock, but from drowning and asphyxiation. Selecting the appropriate therapeutic maneuvers to institute from the outset requires sound clinical judgment and skill. Practicing the basic maneuvers during training sessions increases the probability of successful management of the airway in the face of massive hemoptysis if the bleeding site is known.

In the face of catastrophic massive hemoptysis, the patient should be positioned with the bleeding lung in a dependent position to protect the normal lung. Once the patient is intubated, the bronchoscope is advanced into the airway in an attempt to keep at least one side of the airway patent and free from occluding clots. In all cases, bronchoscopy is central to the management of these patients. If visualization is completely obscured by blood, the bronchoscope should be passed toward the side opposite from the presumed bleeding. Once passed down to the distal airway, the flexible bronchoscope can serve as a stylet to guide the tip of the ET beyond the carina and to selectively intubate the mainstem bronchus of the nonbleeding lung. The balloon on the ET occludes the unaffected mainstem bronchus, preventing blood from entering the distal airway. In this way, the surgeon establishes control of the patient's airway and breathing. The next step is to support the circulation with IV access and transfused blood as needed.

After the acute situation has been controlled, the patient should be transferred to the OR for additional evaluation and clearance of the airway to the bleeding lung. Once the site of bleeding has been identified, it often can be controlled by suction and clearing of the secretions alone, administration of iced saline lavage through the bronchoscope, or installation of vasoconstrictive agents such as dilute epinephrine. Distal sources of bleeding may require forced installation of saline to dilate the bronchi and permit better visualization or the use of an ultrathin bronchoscope to reach subsegmental bronchi. Bleeding of distal sources also can be controlled by bronchoscopic packing of the distal airway using Surgicel (Ethicon, Inc., a Johnson and Johnson Company, Piscataway, NJ). This is performed by extending the bronchoscopic forceps out of the instrument port and grasping a 2×2 cm^2 of Surgicel before inserting the bronchoscope into the ET. The Surgicel is then guided into the bleeding airway by the biopsy forceps and held in position.[11] Once the bleeding has subsided, obvious abnormalities of the airway can be specifically addressed. Laser coagulation, electrocautery, fibrin glue, or foam tamponade can also be used to achieve emergent hemostasis in the airway.

Once the acute bleeding has been stopped, a rigid bronchoscope is used to clear the airway, provide a conduit for ventilation, and tamponade the source of bleeding. If the bleeding does not stop and the side of origin is known, single-lumen unilateral intubation on the unaffected side alone or in combination with a bronchial blocker to tamponade the bleeding is critical. If the bleeding side cannot be localized because the bleeding is too brisk or visualization is impaired, a double-lumen tube with endobronchial tamponade is a reasonable alternative.

After the patient has been adequately resuscitated, multidetector CT angiography is indicated.[12] This technique provides thin-slice images and multiplanar reconstruction of the vessels and bleeding source. Then, interventional radiologists can perform catheter angiography and selective embolization of a bleeding vessel more expeditiously and accurately. Selective embolization has been applied successfully in 79% to 85% of patients at 1 month; however, the recurrence rate is 20% to 33%.[13,14] External beam radiotherapy or bronchoscopic brachytherapy can be added to reduce the risk of recurrent bleeding once the diagnosis of cancer has been established. The specific technique chosen to control bleeding will depend on the lesion causing the hemoptysis, the availability of the technique, and the expertise of the operating surgeon.

SURGERY

Emergent surgical intervention is recommended when arterial embolization has failed to control the source of hemoptysis. The mortality and morbidity in patients requiring emergent surgery are high. Surgery should be considered only when the source of bleeding is unilateral and has been clearly identified, and then only in patients with adequate pulmonary reserve.[15] Elective surgery may be entertained in patients with hemoptysis after the bleeding has been controlled and when, from an oncologic standpoint, it is appropriate to remove the underlying tumor.

SPECIAL CONSIDERATIONS

Brachytherapy

This is a method of delivering direct radiation within or near the affected tissue. Brachytherapy is useful to palliate malignancies in patients who have already received a maximum dose of external beam radiation. This technique is associated with a reduction of hemoptysis. Some studies, however, have reported an increased late risk of perforation or fatal hemoptysis after high-dose brachytherapy in 10.8% of patients.[16]

Argon Plasma Coagulation

This technique has been found to be effective in treating hemoptysis from primary and metastatic tumors that originate in the tracheobronchial tree.[16] This procedure can be performed in the outpatient setting or at the bedside in an ICU.

SUMMARY

Lung cancer is responsible for 20% of all cases of hemoptysis in the United States. While massive hemoptysis is unusual with lung cancer, the mortality approaches 50%, and it should be considered a medical emergency, demanding immediate attention in a hospital setting. Caregivers should first pay attention to the ABCs of resuscitation and intubate the patient immediately if the airway is compromised. If the plain radiograph fails to demonstrate the site of bleeding, a chest CT scan should be obtained as soon as possible. Urgent flexible bronchoscopy will aid in identifying the side of bleeding and facilitate selective intubation of the unaffected airway to protect the patient from drowning and asphyxia. At this juncture, the patient can either be transferred to the angiography suite for identification of the bleeding source and selective embolization or can go directly to the OR for further evaluation and clearance of clots from the airway. Local maneuvers can be employed through the bronchoscope to stop the bleeding and clear the airway. Emergency open surgery should be considered only if other measures have failed, a unilateral source of bleeding has been identified, and the patient can tolerate resection because of an acceptable pulmonary reserve. Elective surgical resection should be considered only if bleeding has been controlled and it is appropriate to resect the underlying tumor for oncologic reasons.

CASE HISTORY

A 58-year-old woman is presented to the emergency room with a single episode of hemoptysis. She estimated that she had coughed up a half cup of blood in a single cough. She had never had hemoptysis before. Her antecedent history was unremarkable except for smoking one pack of cigarettes a day for the past 40 years and moderate exertional dyspnea over the past 6 months. Physical examination was remarkable for a unilateral wheeze on the right. She had no evidence of blood within the nares, but traces of blood could be seen in the oral cavity. Her vital signs were normal. Portable chest radiograph showed a right hilar mass.

While under evaluation in the emergency ward, the patient again coughed and produced 200 mL of bright red blood. Her heart rate increased to 110 beats per minute, and her systolic blood pressure fell to 90 mm Hg, with a mean arterial pressure of 70 mm Hg. The patient was urgently intubated in a controlled manner, but the ET quickly filled with blood. A flexible bronchoscope was placed down the ET, although nothing but blood could be seen through the scope. The bronchoscope was guided in a blind manner toward the left of the ET and trachea while the patient's head was turned to the right. In this manner, the bronchoscope would have a high probability of advancing into the left main bronchus. The ET was advanced as far as possible over the bronchoscope and selectively intubated the left main bronchus. The balloon was inflated, and additional blood no longer filled the tube. Large-bore IV lines were placed for blood and fluid resuscitation, and an arterial line was placed while the bronchoscope was used to clear the distal left mainstem bronchus. Although a clear narrow passage was created down to the secondary carina between the left upper lobe and the left lower lobe, a large amount of organized clot remained in the airway and could not be removed readily by the flexible bronchoscope.

The patient was taken to the OR. She was still bringing up copious amounts of clot through the ET, and her arterial saturations were in the mid-80% range. A decision was made to perform a tracheotomy to more effectively clear the airway. With the flexible bronchoscope within the lumen of the ET, the balloon was deflated. There was no sign of current bleeding. The ET was withdrawn to the level of the tracheotomy. A Yankauer suction tip and O-ring forceps were passed through the tracheotomy incision into the trachea to remove the organized clot from the airway. A tracheostomy tube was inserted, and the balloon was inflated. Bronchoscopy of the right main airway now was possible, and a soft, friable tumor was seen at the level of the right upper lobe takeoff. A no. 6 Fogarty arterial catheter was passed through the tracheostomy and placed deflated in the right mainstem bronchus. Biopsies and brushings of the tumor were obtained.

EDITOR'S COMMENT

Hemoptysis is a dreaded disorder that is often managed emergently. Maintaining a patent airway, even at the expense of obstructing the diseased airway, is paramount. Although flexible fiberoptic bronchoscopy can be used to guide the ET into the uninvolved bronchus, it may be impossible to do so in the face of true massive hemoptysis. In this situation, rigid bronchoscopy remains a reasonable alternative and is the only way to provide adequate suction to maintain a patent airway. Therapeutic intervention in this setting includes using all available modalities. If a discrete endobronchial lesion is seen, laser or argon plasma coagulation (APC) can be used acutely. Generally, most patients will undergo bronchial artery embolization. This can then be followed by definitive treatment such as resection or external beam radiation.

—Mark J. Krasna

References

1. Fontana RS, Sanderson DR, Taylor WF, et al. Early lung cancer detection: results of the initial (prevalence) radiologic and cytologic screening in the Mayo Clinic Study. *Am Rev Respir Dis.* 1984;130:561–565.
2. Hyde L, Hyde CI. Clinical manifestations of lung cancer. *Chest.* 1974;65:299–306.
3. Sobue T, Moriyama N, Kaneko M, et al. Screening for lung cancer with low-dose helical computed tomography: anti-lung cancer association project. *J Clin Oncol.* 2002;20:911–920.
4. Hirshberg B, Biran I, Glazer M, et al. Hemoptysis: etiology, evaluation, and outcome in a tertiary referral hospital. *Chest.* 1997;112:440–444.
5. Lee TW, Wan S, Choy DK, et al. Management of massive hemoptysis: a single institution experience. *Ann Thorac Cardiovasc Surg.* 2000;6:232–235.
6. Colice GL. Detecting lung cancer as a cause of hemoptysis in patients with a normal chest radiograph: bronchoscopy vs CT. *Chest.* 1997;111:877–884.
7. Ong TH, Eng P. Massive hemoptysis requiring intensive care. *Intensive Care Med.* 2003;29:317–320.
8. McGuinness G, Beacher JR, Harkin TJ, et al. Hemoptysis: prospective high-resolution CT/bronchoscopic correlation. *Chest.* 1994;105:1155–1162.
9. Revel MP, Fournier LS, Hennebicque AS, et al. Can CT replace bronchoscopy in the detection of the site and cause of bleeding in patients with large or massive hemoptysis? *AJR Am J Roentegenol.* 2002;179:1217–1224.
10. Haro M, Jimenez J, Tornero A, et al. [Usefulness of computerized tomography and bronchoscopy in patients with hemoptysis. Analysis of 482 cases.] *Ann Med Interna.*2002;19:59–65.
11. Valipour A, Kreuzer A, Koller H, et al. Bronchoscopy-guided topical hemostatic tamponade therapy for the management of life-threatening hemoptysis. *Chest.* 2005;127:2113–2118.
12. Yildiz AE, Ariyurek OM, Apkinar E, et al. Multidetector CT of bronchial and non-bronchial systemic arteries. *Diagn Interv Radiol.* 2011;17:10–17.
13 Swanson KL, Johnson CM, Prakash UB, et al. Bronchial artery embolization: experience with 54 patients. *Chest.* 2002;121:789–795.
14. Park HS, Kim YI, Kim HY, et al. Bronchial artery and systemic artery embolization in the management of primary lung cancer patients with hemoptysis. *Cardiovasc Intervent Radiol.* 2007;30:638–643.
15. Gollins SW, Ryder WD, Burt PA, et al. Massive haemoptysis death and other morbidity associated with high dose rate intraluminal radiotherapy for carcinoma of the bronchus. *Radiother Oncol.* 1996;39:105–116.
16 Morice RC, Ece T, Ece F, et al. Endobronchial argon plasma coagulation for treatment of hemoptysis and neoplastic airway obstruction. *Chest.* 2001;119:781–787.

PART 14

NONOPERATIVE TREATMENTS FOR LUNG CANCER

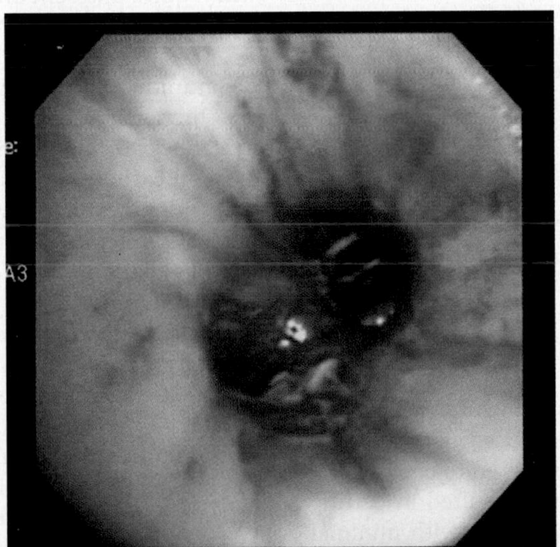

84 Percutaneous Thoracic Tumor Ablation

Jon O. Wee

Keywords: Stage I non–small-cell lung cancer, ablative therapies, radiofrequency ablation

INTRODUCTION

Lung cancer remains the leading cause of cancer death for both men and women.[1] Only one-third of patients diagnosed with lung cancer are stage appropriate for surgical therapy. In addition, the rising population of elders in the United States and other Western countries has caused an increase in the number of patients with comorbidities, making primary surgical and curative therapy more complicated. In fact, a review of the California cancer registry revealed that stage I cancer patients who received no treatment have a median survival of 9 months. Eighty-nine percent of patients who were recommended for treatment but refused died within 5 years, and 78% of these patients died from cancer-specific causes. For T1 lesions, the survival rate for treated cancers was 155 months versus 26 months for untreated cancers.[2] For those patients treated with conventional external radiation alone, 5-year survival is 10% to 30%.[3] Hence, appropriate treatment even for patients with major comorbidities should be available.

Surgical resection remains the gold standard treatment for early-stage lung cancer. In addition, the lung is a frequent site of metastasis in that pulmonary metastases occur in 30% of all malignancies.[1] However, a significant proportion of patients are unable or unwilling to undergo surgery. For these patients, ablative therapy may be an option for localized treatment. The technique of percutaneous tumor ablation has developed through the introduction of multiple modalities including microwave, cryoablation, high-intensity focused ultrasound scan, irreversible electroporation, interstitial laser, and radiofrequency ablation (RFA). The most studied and proven method among these is RFA.

Radiofrequency energy was first used in surgery with the application of cauterization in 1926, introduced by William T. Bovie, after pulsed electrical current was shown to cause coagulation in tissue, while continuous current resulted in cutting of tissue. The technique afforded precision cuts with minimal blood loss. Percutaneous RFA was first reported in 1990 for liver tumor ablation.[4] Since then, the indications have expanded to other organs, such as kidney, bone, and lung. The mechanism of action and outcomes of treatment are reviewed.

MECHANISM OF ACTION

The term, radiofrequency ablation, refers to the therapeutic use of electromagnetic radiation (EMR) for the selective destruction and removal of biologic lesions. Electromagnetic radiation exhibits wave-like behavior corresponding in magnitude to the light spectrum (e.g., microwaves, radio waves, infrared, visible light, ultraviolet, X-rays, gamma rays). RFA uses energy at the frequency and length of radio waves (2–300 Hz).[5] A circuit is created that flows from the tip of the electrode, to a large, diffuse grounding pad placed over the patient's thighs, to an external generator. The small cross-sectional area of the electrode creates a surrounding region of high energy flux. The molecules next to the electrode, usually water, align with the direction of the current. The rapidly alternating current causes the adjacent molecules to vibrate. Molecules farther away from the probe are affected by the other vibrating molecules. The frictional loss of energy between molecules results in a temperature increase.[6] The electrode, itself, is not a source of heat, but creates the electromagnetic field that causes molecular movement, and hence heat generation.

Temperature control is an important issue in RFA. The temperature must be managed to allow energy to be conducted through the tissues. Excessive energy can cause build-up of char around the probe that insulates conduction and limits energy dissipation. With regard to the lung, the parenchyma is thermally insulated by the air-filled alveoli. Tumors within the lung will require different amounts of energy than those attached to the pleura, as the chest wall creates different resistive patterns.[7]

Tissue is sensitive to temperatures above 40°C.[8] Protein denaturation and coagulation occur between 60°C and 100°C. The therapeutic effect of RFA diminishes when temperatures rise above 105°C, at which point the tissue starts to boil, vaporize, and carbonize. Gas formation increases tissue impedance, preventing heat expansion and limiting the ablative area. Carbonization creates insulation around the probe that prevents heat dissipation.

Heat transmission can also be affected by the local anatomy. Approximation to a vessel 3 mm or larger can create enough heat loss from the flow of lower temperature blood to prevent adequate ablation, the so-called "heat sink" effect. This can lead to incomplete or inadequate ablation of tumors in close proximity to vessels. Animal studies of lesions close to the heart and myocardium have demonstrated RFA to be safe with no damage to the myocardium, possibly owing to the loss of heat from the higher blood flows in the heart.[9] Tumors in close proximity to the heart subsequently have higher rates of recurrence with a 69.3% recurrence at 1 mm distance versus 8.6% recurrence at 9 mm.[10]

TECHNIQUE

The typical set-up for an ablation requires a generator, a probe, and a ground. The grounding pad is used to complete the circuit from the patient to the generator. It is often large and applied to both thighs to dissipate the charge without causing local heat effects. The radiofrequency generators are capable of outputting approximately 250 W with high-frequency alternating currents ranging from 460 to 500 kHz.[5] With regard to the electrodes, three commercially available devices are the most

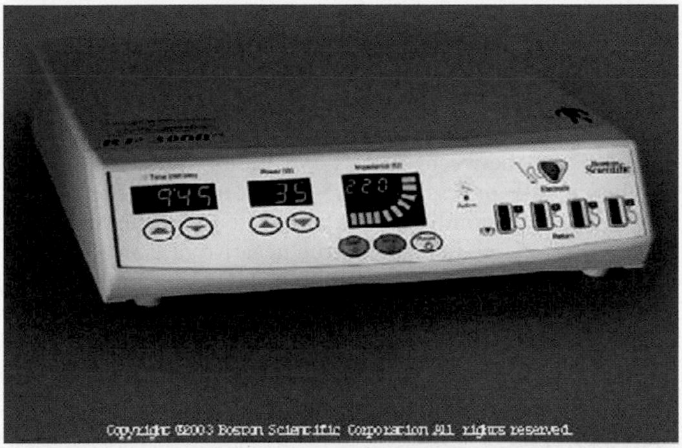

A

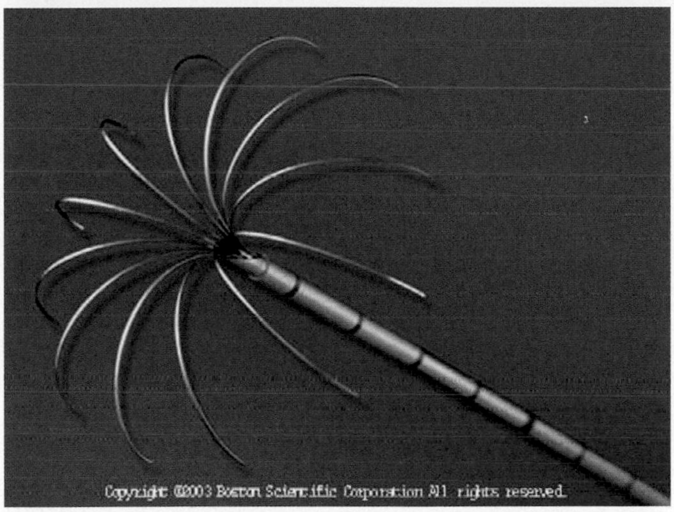

B

Figure 84-1. *A.* Boston Scientific LeVeen ablation system uses an impedance-based feedback system to adjust its energy output. *B.* Distal monopolar electrodes deploy in an umbrella fashion with diameters of 2 to 5 cm. (Reproduced with permission from Boston Scientific, Natick, MA.)

popular. The Boston Scientific LeVeen ablation system uses an impedance-based feedback system to adjust its energy output (Fig. 84-1). The distal monopolar electrodes are deployed in an umbrella fashion with diameters of 2 to 5 cm. Covidien produces the formally Valleylab Cool-tip technology. The catheter is cooled internally with running saline to slow heating of adjacent tissue, thereby reducing tissue resistance. It uses impendence monitoring to adjust its energy output, and multiple electrodes can be clustered to allow for larger ablation zones (Fig. 84-2). Angiodynamics produces the radiofrequency interstitial tissue ablation (RITA) temperature-controlled system. They offer two probes, the StarBurst which has several electrodes that expands like a Christmas tree to a maximum size of 7 cm (Fig. 84-3). Real-time temperature readings at the distal electrodes are utilized to adjust energy output. Their Talon system is similar, but uses saline infusion into the tissue at the electrode tips to reduce charring and to allow for a more uniform distribution of heat.

We prefer the Angiodynamics RITA system with Talon probes. Patients are worked up in the standard fashion including chest CT, PET/CT, and pulmonary function testing (PFT).

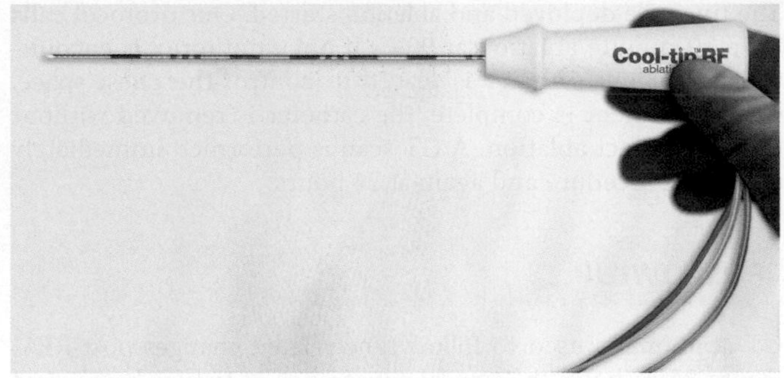

Figure 84-2. Cool-tip RF by Covidien. Covidien currently manufactures the former Valleylab cool-tip technology. (Reproduced with permission from Covidien, Dublin, Ireland.)

Early stage or localized lesions are considered appropriate for treatment. Patients are brought into the CT scanner, placed under conscious sedation with fentanyl and Versed medication, and continuously monitored. A scout scan is performed to identify the lesion. Patients are placed in various positions to allow for the shortest route to the lesion, either supine, lateral decubitus, prone, or some variation thereof. Crossing lung fissures should be avoided to decrease the risk of pneumothorax. Local anesthesia is given on the skin and intercostal space while a straight tract is probed with the needle. Then, using CT fluoroscopic guidance, the electrode is delivered into the tumor.

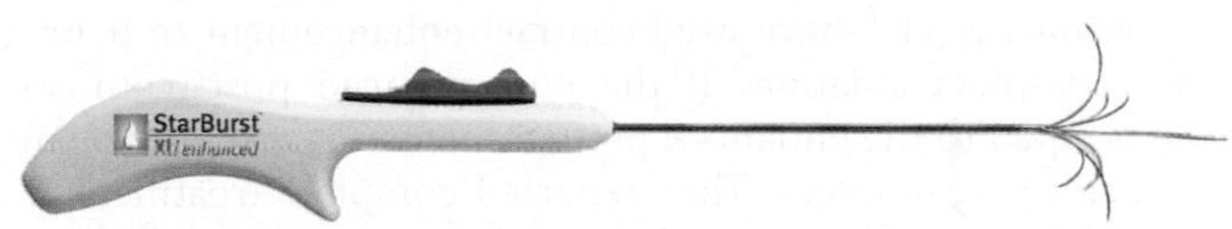

A

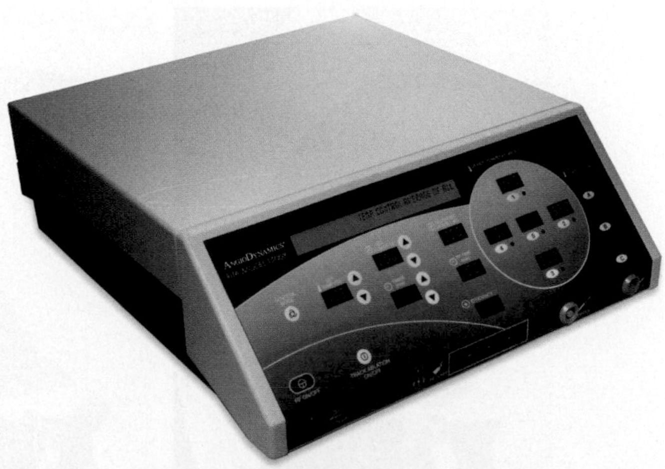

B

Figure 84-3. AngioDynamics' radiofrequency interstitial tissue ablation (RITA) temperature-controlled system offers several probes in the StarBurst family of devices. **A.** The StarBurst family of devices features several electrodes that expand like a Christmas tree with an ablation size ranging from 1 cm to 7 cm depending on the probe selected. **B.** The StarBurst Talon system infuses saline into the tissue at the electrode tips to reduce charring and to allow for a more uniform distribution of heat. (Reproduced with permission from Angiodynamics, Latham, NY.)

The tines are deployed and ablation started. Our protocol calls for a 10-minute ablation at 90°C. If pneumothorax is encountered, a pigtail catheter is placed to control the chest space. Once treatment is complete, the catheter is removed without the use of tract ablation. A CT scan is performed immediately after the procedure and again at 24 hours.

FOLLOW-UP

CT scanning is used to follow time-related changes post-RFA. Figure 84-4 shows the typical appearance of tissues before and after the application of RFA. In a rodent model of normal lung, the appearance of RFA treatment is that of a central density surrounded by a ground-glass opacity. This corresponds to an area of tissue necrosis centrally with a surrounding zone of ongoing necrosis and tissue damage in the ground glass area.[11] In a case report of an ablation followed by resection 3 weeks later, an inner band of thermally coagulated blood, chronic hemostasis, and thrombosis with a focal area of lytic necrosis was seen. Surrounding this was an outer band of hemorrhage associated with lytic necrosis of lung tissue.[12] Initially, the ablation area will increase in size, but then start to condense. A baseline CT scan is advised at 3 months. Following this, the tumor should progressively shrink.[13] Cavitation of the ablated zone can occur in about one-third of all treatments.[14] To detect recurrent or persistent disease, the ablation area must be evaluated for any increase in size. This can lead to some delay. Some have demonstrated that it takes about 7 months to detect an incomplete treatment.[15]

Thanos et al.[16] have used contrast enhancement to determine complete ablation. If the nonenhanced posttreatment scan is equal to the enhanced pretreatment area, the treatment is considered complete. They reported complete treatment in 79% of lesions, with an overall 1-year recurrence rate of 15%.

To mitigate this delay, the feasibility of using PET/CT to detect incomplete ablations has been investigated. PET uses fluorine-18-fluorodeoxyglucose (FDG) uptake to indicate cellular activity. Uptake can increase in the first 3 weeks following ablation as the ablative zone is infiltrated by phagocytes and cellular repair cells.[17] In some studies, FDG uptake was shown to increase for up to 12 months following treatment; hence, differentiation between fibrosis and tumor can be difficult.[18] Residual uptake or less than 60% reduction of uptake relative to baseline at 2 months may be associated with tumor recurrence.[19] Baere et al. reported a true negative rate of 100% with PET/CT in 41 patients followed by PET/CT at 1 month and 3 months. They also noted that in 15% of patients, the central lymph nodes were FDG avid, reportedly related to the inflammatory process.[20]

OUTCOMES

RFA has been used to ablate primary lung tumors as well as a multitude of pulmonary metastases. In fact, most publications reported a mixed bag of pathology. In addition, reported recurrence rates vary in definition. Most surgical publications relating to surgical resection consider regional lymph nodes as a recurrence, whereas, in most radiologic reports, recurrence is only measured at the site of the tumor. Hence, overall recurrence rates must be viewed more closely. A review of 17 publications reported a complete ablation rate of 90% ranging from 38% to 97%.[21] Tumors <2 cm in size had higher rates of complete ablation.[22,23] As tumor sizes increase, rates of tumor ablation tend to decrease. Lee et al.[24] noted ablation rates of 38% in tumors 3 to 5 cm and 8% for those larger than 5 cm. Simon reported a statistically significant difference in tumor progression for tumors <3 cm compared to those >3 cm ($p = 002$).[25] The 1-year progression-free rate was 83% for tumors <3 cm versus 45% for those >3 cm. At 3 years, it was 57% versus 25%. Median time to progression was 12 months for larger tumors versus 45 months. Lee notes that

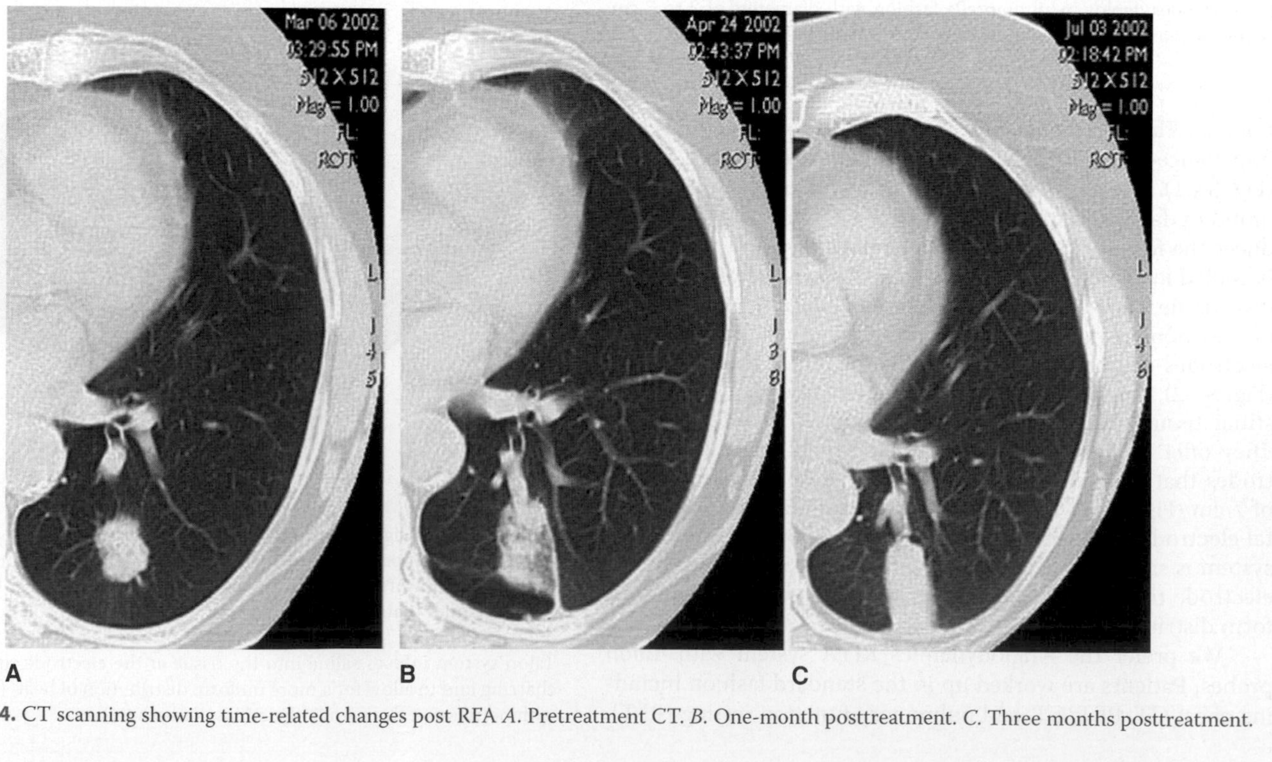

Figure 84-4. CT scanning showing time-related changes post RFA *A*. Pretreatment CT. *B*. One-month posttreatment. *C*. Three months posttreatment.

all tumors <3 cm had a complete response with a survival of 19.7 months in complete responders versus 8.7 months in partial responders.[24] Herrera reported a complete or partial response in 67% of tumors smaller than 5 cm but only 33% control for those >5 cm.[26]

Others have demonstrated that when the ratio of ablation volume to tumor volume was ≥3, the complete ablation rate at 1 year was 83% compared to 61% when the ratio was <3.[22] In fact, a margin of 4.5 mm of ground glass opacity surrounding the tumor zone results in a complete ablation.[27] As most catheters extend to a 5 cm diameter, tumors <3 cm are best treated to provide the 0.5 cm to 1 cm margin of additional tissue ablation. In addition, electrode configuration may have an effect on recurrence with a lower success rate for the straight electrode, such as the LeVeen, compared with the expandable electrode, although this difference may be more related to tumor location than electrode selection.[22]

A prospective multicenter intent to treat study (RAPTURE) was published in 2008.[28] The study included 106 patients with 183 treated tumors. Complete response at 1 year was 88%. Lung cancer patients had 1- and 2-year survivals of 70% and 48%, respectively. Most of these patients were at high risk and died of non–cancer-related diseases. Stage I patients had a 2-year survival of 75% and a cancer-specific survival of 92%.

Simon et al.[25] reported on 75 primary non–small-cell lung cancer (NSCLC) cases, stages IA and IB, treated with RFA. Median survival was 29 months. The 1-, 2-, 3-, 4-, and 5-year survivals were 78%, 57%, 36%, 27%, and 27%, respectively. With smaller tumors <3 cm, the progress-free survival rate was 47% at 5 years. Fernando[29] reported a mean survival of 21 months for NSCLC patients with a median progression-free survival of 18 months. Beland[30] demonstrated a 23-month, disease-free survival. Of the recurrences, 38% were local, 18% intrapulmonary, 18% nodal, and 21% distal. Zemlyak[31] compared RFA to surgical resection for stage I lung cancer. The 3-year survival was 87.1% for surgery and 87.5% for RFA.

Similar survival rates have been reported for metastatic disease, although extrathoracic metastasis is an independent factor in overall survival.[32] Several studies looking at colorectal metastasis reported a 2-year survival rate of 64% to 78%.[15,32] The RAPTURE study reported a 1-year survival of patients with colorectal metastasis of 89% and 2-year survival of 66%.[28] Simon noted a 1-year survival of 87%, and 3- and 5-year survival of 57% for colorectal metastasis.[25] Other studies have demonstrated higher 1-year survival at 95% and 3-year survival at 50%.[33] For sarcoma, renal cell, and head and neck cancers, 5-year survival is in the range of 45% with disease-free survival of 36 months or more.[34]

Overall lung function is preserved. Baere evaluated PFTs at 1 month and showed no difference between pretreatment and posttreatment function.[15] Lencioni also saw no difference in pulmonary function at 12 months.[28] In addition, Lee noted good symptom control in noncurative patients who had hemoptysis (80%), chest pain (36%), and cough (25%).[24]

Lee et al.[35] evaluated the utility of RFA as an adjuvant treatment for lung cancer. Patients with stage III and IV disease were treated with either chemotherapy alone or chemotherapy and RFA. Survival for the chemotherapy alone was 29 months. Those who received both chemotherapy and RFA had a survival of 42 months ($p = 0.03$). Although a small study, there may be some utility in using RFA in the adjuvant setting.

COMPLICATIONS

Pain is the most common postprocedure complaint and is more common in lesions close to the parietal pleura versus those that lie deep in the lung parenchyma. It is generally limited to the periprocedural period. Patients may also experience transient hyperthermia, with temperatures rising to 38°C during the ablation treatment. Pulmonary hemorrhage occurs in approximately 5% of patients, similar to those undergoing core needle biopsy.[36]

Pneumothorax can be seen on CT scan in approximately 50% of treatments.[31,37] However, only 4% to 16% require placement of a chest tube. The rates of delayed and recurrence pneumothorax are reported to be 10.3% and 6.7%, respectively.[38] However, only 4 of 33 patients required intervention with an overall rate of <2%. Fernando reported a 38.9% pneumothorax rate although not all cases required intervention.[29] Risk factors for pneumothorax are age more than 60 years, presence of emphysema, lesions smaller than 1.5 cm, lower lobe lesions, lesions deeper than 2.6 cm, and crossing fissures.[37,39]

Hemoptysis can present in about 15% of patients.[26] Most incidences are minor and self-limited. Severe hemorrhage has been reported with central lesions and tumors in close proximity to major pulmonary vessels.[40] Simon et al.[25] demonstrated a mortality of 2.6% (4 of 153 patients) related to the RFA treatment. Two of the four patients had had prior pneumonectomy.

OTHER TECHNOLOGY

Other thermal techniques include cryotherapy which uses a probe to cause selective freezing. This causes ice crystals to form within the cells, which ruptures the cellular membranes, causing overall cellular damage.[41] The 3-year survival in stage I NSCLC has been reported as 77% with a 37% rate of pneumothorax.[31] Microwave technology has demonstrated a mean diameter of ablation that is 25% larger than single-cooled RFA probes.[42] Combined microwave probes can treat larger volumes. However, studies have not demonstrated the superiority of microwave over RFA. A study of 50 patients noted a 1-year local control rate of 67% with a mean time to recurrence at 16.2 months. The 1-year survival was 65% with a cancer-specific survival of 83%.[43] Certainly, this technology as well as others require further assessment.

CONCLUSION

As patients become older, comorbidity increases and lung function decreases, raising the need for less invasive yet effective therapies for treating pulmonary malignancies. RFA is a cost-effective, minimally invasive option that can be performed on an outpatient basis.[16] Many centers observe patients for 1 or 2 days after the procedure, as is our practice. The indications for RFA include early stage disease, single site recurrence, limited metastases, and palliation for some symptoms. Combination treatment with adjuvant chemotherapy or radiation may improve outcomes and provide further options for patients.

References

1. Smith RA, Glynn TJ. Epidemiology of lung cancer. *Radiol Clin North Am.* 2000;38:453–470.
2. Raz DJ, Zell JA, Ou SH, et al. Natural history of stage I non-small cell lung cancer: implications for early detection. *Chest.* 2007;132:193–199.
3. Casal RF, Tam AL, Eapen GA. Radiofrequency ablation of lung tumors. *Clin Chest Med.* 2010;31:151–163.
4. McGahan JP, Browning PD, Brock JM, et al. Hepatic ablation using radiofrequency electrocautery. *Invest Radiol.* 1990;25:267–270.
5. Hong K, Georgiades C. Radiofrequency ablation: mechanism of action and devices. *J Vasc Interv Radiol.* 2010;21:S179–S186.
6. Organ LW. Electrophysiologic principles of radiofrequency lesion making. *Appl Neurophysiol.* 1976;39:69–76.
7. de Baere T. Lung tumor radiofrequency ablation: where do we stand? *Cardiovasc Intervent Radiol.* 2011;34:241–251.
8. Goldberg SN, Gazelle GS, Mueller PR. Thermal ablation therapy for focal malignancy: a unified approach to underlying principles, techniques, and diagnostic imaging guidance. *AJR Am J Roentgenol.* 2000;174:323–331.
9. Steinke K, Arnold C, Wulf S, et al. Safety of radiofrequency ablation of myocardium and lung adjacent to the heart: an animal study. *J Surg Res.* 2003;114:140–145.
10. Iguchi T, Hiraki T, Gobara H, et al. Percutaneous radiofrequency ablation of lung tumors close to the heart or aorta: evaluation of safety and effectiveness. *J Vasc Interv Radiol.* 2007;18:733–740.
11. Tominaga J, Miyachi H, Takase K, et al. Time-related changes in computed tomographic appearance and pathologic findings after radiofrequency ablation of the rabbit lung: preliminary experimental study. *J Vasc Interv Radiol.* 2005;16:1719–1726.
12. Steinke K, Habicht JM, Thomsen S, et al. CT-guided radiofrequency ablation of a pulmonary metastasis followed by surgical resection. *Cardiovasc Intervent Radiol.* 2002;25:543–546.
13. Steinke K, King J, Glenn D, et al. Radiologic appearance and complications of percutaneous computed tomography-guided radiofrequency-ablated pulmonary metastases from colorectal carcinoma. *J Comput Assist Tomogr.* 2003;27:750–757.
14. Bojarski JD, Dupuy DE, Mayo-Smith WW. CT imaging findings of pulmonary neoplasms after treatment with radiofrequency ablation: results in 32 tumors. *AJR Am J Roentgenol.* 2005;185:466–471.
15. de Baere T, Palussiere J, Auperin A, et al. Midterm local efficacy and survival after radiofrequency ablation of lung tumors with minimum follow-up of 1 year: prospective evaluation. *Radiology.* 2006;240:587–596.
16. Thanos L, Mylona S, Ptohis,N, et al. Percutaneous radiofrequency thermal ablation in the management of lung tumors: presentation of clinical experience on a series of 35 patients. *Diagn Interv Radiol.* 2009;15:290–296.
17. Okuma T, Okamura T, Matsuoka T, et al. Fluorine-18-fluorodeoxyglucose positron emission tomography for assessment of patients with unresectable recurrent or metastatic lung cancers after CT-guided radiofrequency ablation: preliminary results. *Ann Nucl Med.* 2006;20:115–121.
18. Kavanagh BD, McGarry RC, Timmerman RD. Extracranial radiosurgery (stereotactic body radiation therapy) for oligometastases. *Semin Radiat Oncol.* 2006;16:77–84.
19. Higaki F, Okumura Y, Sato S, et al. Preliminary retrospective investigation of FDG-PET/CT timing in follow-up of ablated lung tumor. *Ann Nucl Med.* 2008;22:157–163.
20. Deandreis D, Leboulleux S, Dromain C, et al. Role of FDG PET/CT and chest CT in the follow-up of lung lesions treated with radiofrequency ablation. *Radiology.* 2011;258:270–276.
21. Zhu JC, Yan TD, Morris DL. A systematic review of radiofrequency ablation for lung tumors. *Ann Surg Oncol.* 2008;15:1765–1774.
22. Hiraki T, Sakurai J, Tsuda T, et al. Risk factors for local progression after percutaneous radiofrequency ablation of lung tumors: evaluation based on a preliminary review of 342 tumors. *Cancer.* 2006;107:2873–2880.
23. Nguyen CL, Scott WJ, Young NA, et al. Radiofrequency ablation of primary lung cancer: results from an ablate and resect pilot study. *Chest.* 2005;128:3507–3011.
24. Lee JM, Jin GY, Goldberg SN, et al. Percutaneous radiofrequency ablation for inoperable non-small cell lung cancer and metastases: preliminary report. *Radiology.* 2004;230:125–134.
25. Simon CJ, Dupuy DE, DiPetrillo TA, et al. Pulmonary radiofrequency ablation: long-term safety and efficacy in 153 patients. *Radiology.* 2007;243:268–275.
26. Herrera LJ, Fernando HC, Perry Y, et al. Radiofrequency ablation of pulmonary malignant tumors in nonsurgical candidates. *J Thorac Cardiovasc Surg.* 2003;125:929–937.
27. Anderson EM, Lees WR, Gillams AR. Early indicators of treatment success after percutaneous radiofrequency of pulmonary tumors. *Cardiovasc Intervent Radiol.* 2009;32:478–483.
28. Lencioni R, Crocetti L, Cioni R, et al. Response to radiofrequency ablation of pulmonary tumours: a prospective, intention-to-treat, multicentre clinical trial (the RAPTURE study). *Lancet Oncol.* 2008;9:621–628.
29. Fernando HC, De Hoyos A, Landreneau RJ, et al. Radiofrequency ablation for the treatment of non-small cell lung cancer in marginal surgical candidates. *J Thorac Cardiovasc Surg.* 2005;129:639–644.
30. Beland MD, Wasser EJ, Mayo-Smith WW, et al. Primary non-small cell lung cancer: review of frequency, location, and time of recurrence after radiofrequency ablation. *Radiology.* 2010;254:301–307.
31. Zemlyak A, Moore WH, Bilfinger TV. Comparison of survival after sublobar resections and ablative therapies for stage I non-small cell lung cancer. *J Am Coll Surg.* 2010;211:68–72.
32. Yamakado K, Hase S, Matsuoka T, et al. Radiofrequency ablation for the treatment of unresectable lung metastases in patients with colorectal cancer: a multicenter study in Japan. *J Vasc Interv Radiol.* 2007;18:393–398.
33. Petre EN, Jia X, Thornton RH, et al. Treatment of pulmonary colorectal metastases by radiofrequency ablation. *Clin Colorectal Cancer.* 2013;12:37–44.
34. Friedel G, Pastorino U, Buyse M, et al. [Resection of lung metastases: long-term results and prognostic analysis based on 5206 cases—the International Registry of Lung Metastases]. *Zentralbl Chir.* 1999;124:96–103.
35. Lee H, Jin GY, Han YM, et al. Comparison of survival rate in primary non-small-cell lung cancer among elderly patients treated with radiofrequency ablation, surgery, or chemotherapy. *Cardiovasc Intervent Radiol.* 2012;35:343–350.
36. Steinke K, King J, Glenn D, et al. Pulmonary hemorrhage during percutaneous radiofrequency ablation: a more frequent complication than assumed? *Interact Cardiovasc Thorac Surg.* 2003 2:462–465.
37. Nour-Eldin NE, Naguib NN, Saeed AS, et al. Risk factors involved in the development of pneumothorax during radiofrequency ablation of lung neoplasms. *AJR Am J Roentgenol.* 2009;193:W43–W48.
38. Yoshimatsu R, Yamagami T, Terayama K, et al. Delayed and recurrent pneumothorax after radiofrequency ablation of lung tumors. *Chest.* 2009;135:1002–1009.
39. Hiraki T, Tajiri N, Mimura H, et al. Pneumothorax, pleural effusion, and chest tube placement after radiofrequency ablation of lung tumors: incidence and risk factors. *Radiology.* 2006;241:275–283.
40. Yamakado K, Takaki H, Takao M, et al. Massive hemoptysis from pulmonary artery pseudoaneurysm caused by lung radiofrequency ablation: successful treatment by coil embolization. *Cardiovasc Intervent Radiol.* 2010;33:410–412.
41. Hoffmann NE, Bischof JC. The cryobiology of cryosurgical injury. *Urology.* 2002;60:40–49.
42. Brace CL, Hinshaw JL, Laeseke PF, et al. Pulmonary thermal ablation: comparison of radiofrequency and microwave devices by using gross pathologic and CT findings in a swine model. *Radiology.* 2009;251:705–711.
43. Wolf FJ, Grand DJ, Machan JT, et al. Microwave ablation of lung malignancies: effectiveness, CT findings, and safety in 50 patients. *Radiology.* 2008;247:871–879.

85 Radiotherapy for Inoperable Non–Small Cell Lung Cancer

David J. Sher

Keywords: Radiotherapy, non-small cell lung cancer, inoperable lung cancer, SBRT

INTRODUCTION

The multimodality management of inoperable non–small cell lung cancer (NSCLC) – from early-stage disease to locally advanced presentations – has changed substantially over the past 20 years. With the exception of small, stage I NSCLC, most nonmetastatic patients are treated with both local and systemic therapy, and there is an increasing interest in the integration of all three modalities. Radiation oncology has experienced dramatic technologic innovations over this time, which has allowed for reduced toxicity and consequent improvements in the therapeutic ratio, and in the notable case of stage I NSCLC, significantly higher cure rates.

The purpose of this chapter is to summarize the state of contemporary thoracic radiotherapy as it is used in the management of nonmetastatic, inoperable NSCLC. Inherent to this discussion are the relevant improvements in radiation therapy planning and delivery, which will be outlined in the beginning of this chapter. The remarkably improved efficacy of stereotactic body radiotherapy (SBRT) for stage I NSCLC will then be described, and this discussion will conclude with a focus on locally advanced lung cancer, highlighting three key and controversial issues that are central to the development of a treatment plan: use of chemotherapy, total radiotherapy dose, and the volume of tissue irradiated.

TECHNOLOGIC INNOVATIONS

Brief History of Radiation Therapy

In the early era of radiotherapy, radiation planning was based on external anatomic landmarks and simple measurements of patient thickness.[1] These plans were obviously crude, but the large field size presumably made up for inaccuracies in treatment planning. By the 1960s, fluoroscopic simulators, which emulated treatment machine geometry, were developed commercially, allowing radiation oncologists to design fields based on bony anatomy. Radiation planning was performed in two dimensions following the fluoroscopic simulation, in which plain radiographs were taken in the treatment position. The external contour of the patient was modeled at the isocenter of the field, and relevant internal structures were drawn on the contour by the physician, including the target and critical normal organs. The appropriate location of these structures was determined by their anatomic relationship with bony anatomy. Although the visualization of bony anatomy allowed radiation fields to become more complex, they were still fundamentally limited by an inability to know the three-dimensional (3D) location of the tumor and surrounding normal structures.

The 1970s witnessed the dawn of axial imaging, as computed tomography (CT) and magnetic resonance imaging (MRI) were developed and introduced into medical care.[1] As soon as CT was developed, it became obvious to radiation oncologists and physicists that the technology could revolutionize radiation planning.[2] First, the anatomic detail dramatically improved the physician's knowledge of tumor extent, and theoretically this information would lead to better target coverage. Second, the 3D dataset would allow the radiation planner to create a substantially more sophisticated beam arrangement, using computerized dosimetry and a "beam's eye-view" to optimally cover the tumor and avoid normal structures.[3] Multiple research groups attempted to merge CT technology with radiotherapy planning, and by 1996, several commercial 3D planning systems became available, bringing conformal radiotherapy (CRT) into general practice.[4] Radiotherapy plans created by these systems are termed 3D-conformal radiotherapy (3D-CRT), in contrast to the plans calculated from fluoroscopic simulators, simply termed 2D.[5]

Simulation and Target Delineation

As detailed earlier, the bedrock of modern thoracic radiotherapy is the CT simulation, in which patients are first immobilized and then CT is performed, ideally with intravenous contrast. The immobilization is often performed using a thick plastic bag with beads inside, and a vacuum is created within the bag once the patient is in the appropriate position; the bag is thus held in position once the vacuum is applied. The CT is typically obtained in 2.5- to 3-mm thick slices, though thinner or thicker slices may be used depending on the indication.

Although one of the most obvious benefits of CT simulation is the improvement in target delineation, the information contained in the 3D dataset also has provided tremendous insight into predictors of radiation pneumonitis (RP). Treatment planning software can calculate a *dose–volume histogram (DVH)*, which describes the percent of lung that receives a certain dose, as well as additional statistics such as the mean, maximum, and minimum dose. For example, the percent volume of lung receiving more than 20 Gray (Gy) is called the V20, and similarly the percent volume of lung receiving more than 5 Gy is the V5. Although much work needs to be performed to better predict the risk of this severe complication – particularly in the molecular arena – rough predictors of RP have been devised, such as the V5, V20, and mean lung dose (MLD), and these help guide radiation oncologists as they determine the safety of a given radiotherapy plan.[6,7]

The salient benefit of CT-based planning is the improved delineation of the target. This process has been particularly advanced by the development of four-dimensional CT (4D-CT) simulation, in which the purported fourth "dimension" is time.[8] In brief, during 4D-CT, an external marker is placed on the patient, which is ultimately used to mark the different phases of the respiratory cycle. The scan is performed multiple times at the same couch position, and thus several axial slices are obtained at a given position; these slices are reformatted according to the respiratory cycle at which they are taken, and a "movie" of the tumor during the respiratory cycle is visible. Multiple studies have confirmed that lower lobe primary masses and lymph nodes, particularly in the hilar and subcarinal stations, often move more than 1 cm in the superior to inferior direction.[9,10] Without this patient-specific knowledge, margins around the tumor could be either too small or too large; in comparison, simulation with 4D-CT allows for the optimal margin and improves the therapeutic ratio.

Furthermore, the use of positron emission tomography (PET) and PET-CT has also improved the delineation of primary and lymph node targets. Although a more complete discussion of PET imaging is beyond the scope of this chapter, several studies have shown that PET and/or PET-CT aids the radiation oncologist in distinguishing primary tumor from atelectasis, and malignant from benign adenopathy.[11] For example, DeRuysscher showed that PET-CT radiotherapy planning could increase the total radiation dose by over 20% and keep the toxicity risk the same by virtue of shrinking down the treatment volume based on the metabolic imaging.[12] Similarly, RTOG 0515 prospectively recorded the treatment volumes contoured by the radiation oncologist on CT and PET-CT and found that the gross tumor volumes (GTV) were significantly smaller on PET-CT volumes, and the nodal volumes were changed in 51% of patients.[13] Although not mandatory, the integration of PET-CT information with the CT simulation images has become a standard practice in treatment planning.

Treatment Delivery

Once 3D information became available and treatment planning software developed the computing power and algorithms to calculate dose throughout the treatment volume, beam arrangements became more complex, and physicians were able to maximize dose to the tumor while reducing the dose to the organs-at-risk. Today, the majority of patients are treated with 3D-CRT, although intensity modulated radiation therapy (IMRT) has also been employed in the past several years.

IMRT introduced two new concepts in radiation planning and delivery. The first is termed "inverse planning," in which the physician specifies the dose to tumor volumes and normal structures (e.g., esophagus, spinal cord), and the physicist instructs a computer algorithm to design a plan to meet those constraints. This process is distinctly different than traditional "forward planning," in which the physician first creates the fields and the physicist or dosimetrist then determines the dose distribution. The benefit of the inverse planning algorithm is the ability to carve dose away from multiple normal structures while ensuring a radical dose to the planning target volume (PTV), and it is simply too difficult to accomplish this feat without a sophisticated cost function.

The second main component of IMRT is, as the name implies, intensity modulation. By definition, intensity is the total energy per unit area per unit time.[14] In standard radiotherapy, the intensity across a given beam is basically constant; there is no variation across the field. If a particular beam delivers 100 cGy to a 10×10 cm^2 area at a certain depth, that 100 cm^2 region is essentially all receiving 100 cGy. In contrast, for a given IMRT field, the intensity throughout the field may vary substantially, a dosimetric feat which is typically accomplished through the use of multileaf collimators (MLC), narrow moveable leaves in the head of the linear accelerator.[2] In IMRT, each radiation beam is split into multiple subfields, each with a different arrangement of the MLCs, such that the final delivered dose – the summation of each subfield – is highly variable across its area.

Planning studies have suggested that IMRT can reduce the volume of normal lung receiving radiotherapy, which may lead to a lower risk of pneumonitis and allow for dose-escalation.[15] Moreover, by definition, IMRT is able to push dose away from important normal structures such as the spinal cord, brachial plexus, and esophagus. However, IMRT faces at least three fundamental obstacles for its routine use in thoracic radiotherapy: potential geographic miss due to tumor motion (i.e., "interplay effect"), increased spread of low-dose irradiation to the normal lung, and cost. With respect to the interaction of tumor motion and the treatment beam, consider that the open area of the beam is constantly changing throughout the treatment, and the tumor is constantly moving; thus, if the tumor is moving during respiration to an area where the MLCs are closed, no dose will be delivered for a period of time; that underdosing can build up over the course of treatment, and the tumor may theoretically receive a subtherapeutic dose.[16]

The second concern with IMRT is the increase in low-dose spillage in the lung. Although there are typically four to five beams in a standard 3D-CRT plan, IMRT may utilize seven to nine beams, and consequently there may be a higher V5 (i.e., percent of the lung receiving 5 Gy or more), which could lead to an increased risk of pneumonitis.[17] Although some data refute the hypothesis that IMRT increases the pneumonitis rate and argue that IMRT decreases it, other reports have supported the notion of a higher rate of severe toxicity.[18,19] The final issue with IMRT is cost, as the planning and delivery of the treatment are more complex, time-consuming, and thus expensive. Thus, whether a patient is better served by 3D-CRT of IMRT is patient-specific.

Despite these advances, in some situations, highly mobile tumors require large treatment ports and thus intolerable dose to the normal lung tissue. Although one solution to this dilemma is prescribing a lower dose of radiotherapy, this approach is clearly suboptimal. Thus, additional techniques have been developed to "gate" a mobile tumor; that is, turn on the irradiation only during certain parts of the respiratory cycle (e.g., end inspiration). There are three fundamental approaches to achieve this gating: attach the patient to a respirator-type device and only turn on the beam when a specified volume of air is inhaled (i.e., Active Breathing Control™), use external markers on the patient (or even surface anatomy) that acts as a surrogate for diaphragmatic motion, and only treat when that marker is at a position that represents a given phase of respiration, and insert an internal radio-opaque fiducial into the patient's tumor that is visible on fluoroscopy and use that fiducial as a marker to verify the external marker.[20–22] Whether or not these tools are implemented for a given patient is a function of tumor motion, risk of lung complications, patient tolerance of the gating method, and available technology.

On-Treatment Imaging

A highly precise radiotherapy plan is ultimately useless if the patient is not reproducibly set up each day for the treatment. Patients typically receive permanent small tattoos at simulation, and these tattoos serve as markers for the radiation therapist to place the patient at the isocenter (i.e., the middle of the treatment position) for each treatment. However, skin marks are highly unreliable from a day-to-day standpoint, particularly as patients lose weight during treatment, and thus additional isocenter verification is important, especially as the radiotherapy plan becomes more complex. For many years, the megavoltage beam from the treatment machine itself was used as an imager ("port film"), and radiographs were taken at the isocenter at least one time per week. However, megavoltage radiographs have very poor resolution, and although they are an improvement over simple setup to skin, they still needed improvement.

Over the past 10 years, linear accelerators became equipped with kilovoltage imagers perpendicular to the head of the gantry. This arrangement allowed physicians to obtain diagnostic quality x-rays before each fraction of treatment without adding to the total radiation dose. As a consequence, daily setup was more precise. This concept of using higher-resolution, daily imaging was termed image-guided radiotherapy, or IGRT; in contrast to the acronym IMRT, which defines a very specific type of treatment planning and delivery, IGRT refers to the paradigm of using daily imaging to reduce the treatment margins (and even shrink them over the course of therapy).[23] Image-guided radiotherapy is thus agnostic to the actual radiotherapy delivery technique.

Although daily orthogonal kilovoltage imaging was an improvement over daily megavoltage port films, the real advance in IGRT was the development of cone-beam computed tomography (CBCT), which is a CT scan performed on the linear accelerator, in the treatment position. In comparison to diagnostic CT scans which have multiple rows of detectors, CBCT uses the attached kilovoltage imager (or even the treatment beam as a megavoltage imager) to sweep around the patient, and the data are reformatted at the treatment console into a CT image. Although the quality of the image is far from diagnostic-level, it provides a remarkable improvement over orthogonal imaging, and the key structures (e.g., tumor, spinal cord) are easily visible; the accuracy of patient setup is therefore significantly improved, which allows for the possibility of decreased margins and either a higher total radiation dose or lower lung toxicity.

Stereotactic Body Radiotherapy

The concept of stereotactic radiation treatment was initially devised in the 1960s by neurosurgeon Lars Leksell and physicists Kurt Liden and Borje Larsson, who developed intracranial stereotactic radiosurgery (SRS).[24] Despite minimal to nonexistent axial imaging, SRS was feasible because the highly precise stereotactic frame was screwed into the patient's head, and thus the degree of accuracy of the stereotactic system translated to an equivalent level of accuracy of tumor localization.

However, prior to the very recent development of IGRT, obtaining the same level of setup accuracy in the extracranial body was much more difficult. One of the earliest reports of SBRT to the spine involved surgically fixating the vertebra to the stereotactic coordinate system, but this is not a viable solution for routine practice, and for almost any other body site, a frame cannot be screwed into the body.[25] Thus, as opposed to intracranial SRS, there was no straightforward, highly accurate system of setting the patient up at isocenter. Moreover, the complexities of treatment planning mandated the use of 3D-CRT, as delivering 54 Gy in 3 fractions with SBRT rather than 60 Gy in 30 fractions has a higher risk of significant side effects.

By the 1990s, CT simulation and 3D-CRT became feasible, and extracranial stereotactic frames were designed that allowed for rigid immobilization and stereotactic localization without surgical intervention.[26] Some centers also developed fluoroscopic systems that could image internal fiducial markers in lung tumors to ensure the treatment beam was turned on when the lesion was in the field.[27] These highly precise setup devices finally allowed for high-dose, SBRT, (Fig. 85-1) which is typically delivered using multiple (8–12) noncoplanar beams that converge on the target, leading to a high dose in the tumor margin with sharp falloff dose into the normal lung. Some physicians now promote calling this technique SABR or stereotactic ablative radiotherapy.

Many technological advances have been developed since the original linear accelerators were used to treat thoracic SBRT. For example, treatment planning software has become remarkably more sophisticated, IGRT enables highly accurate setup without requiring an external coordinate system, and other systems such as respiratory gating have been introduced as well. Linear accelerators have been specifically designed for SBRT (e.g., CyberKnife™, Accuray, Sunnydale, CA; Novalis TX™, Varian Medical Systems, Palo Alto, CA), which include unique IGRT systems for improved setup and delivery accuracy.[28] Although there are technical differences between these platforms, such as the typical need for internal gold fiducials for treatment with the CyberKnife, essentially any lesion that can be treated with one system can be treated by another; the key to a successful treatment is physician expertise rather than a particular linear accelerator.[28]

MEDICALLY INOPERABLE STAGE I LUNG CANCER

As detailed in other chapters, the standard-of-care in the management of stage I NSCLC is lobectomy and lymph node dissection. However, given the general medical compromise of this patient population, a nontrivial percentage of individuals are not candidates for this procedure. Although there is controversy surrounding the relative benefits of segmentectomy and wedge resection, until recently there was no viable nonsurgical alternative.

Conventional Results

Indeed, until the mid-2000s, the standard approach for the treatment of medically inoperable stage I NSCLC was conventionally fractionated radiotherapy to 60 to 70 Gy in 30 to 35 fractions. Given the relatively small field, the treatment was tolerable, but it was also associated with unacceptably poor local control. For example, Bradley[29] reported on the outcomes of patients at Washington University in St. Louis with medically inoperable stage I NSCLC treated with RT alone to a median dose of 70 Gy. Although patients with tumors 2 cm or smaller experienced a 2-year local control probability of 83%, the tumors between 2 and 3 cm had a local control probability of only 62%, and that fell to 50% for tumors between 3 and 5 cm. Such poor local control rates are not compatible with long-term survival in this population. Similarly, in the University of Michigan dose-escalation trial of node-negative patients,

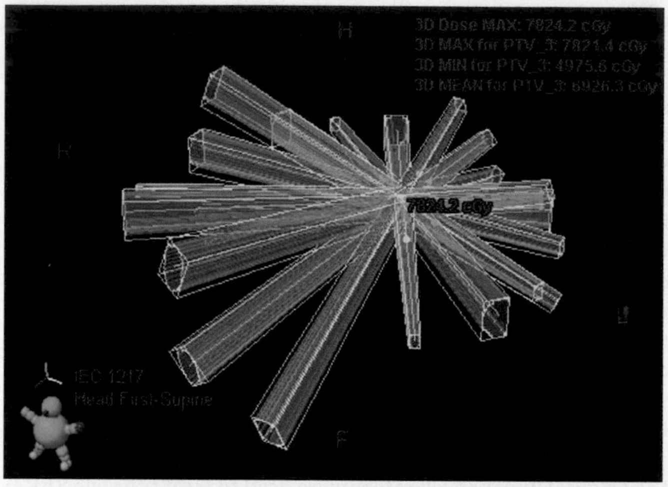

A

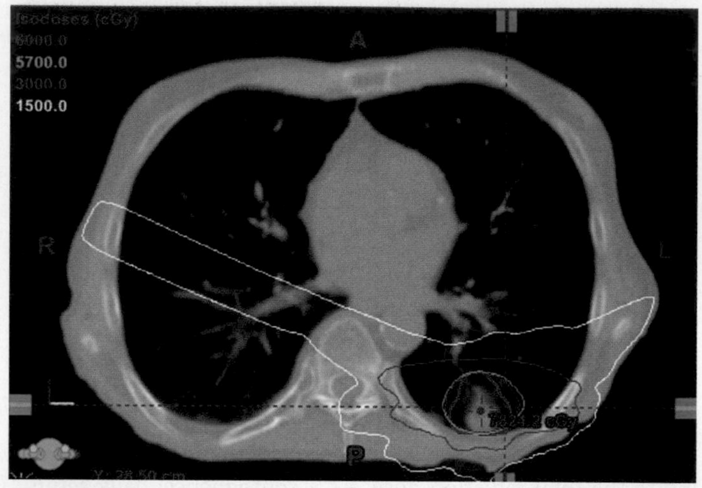

B

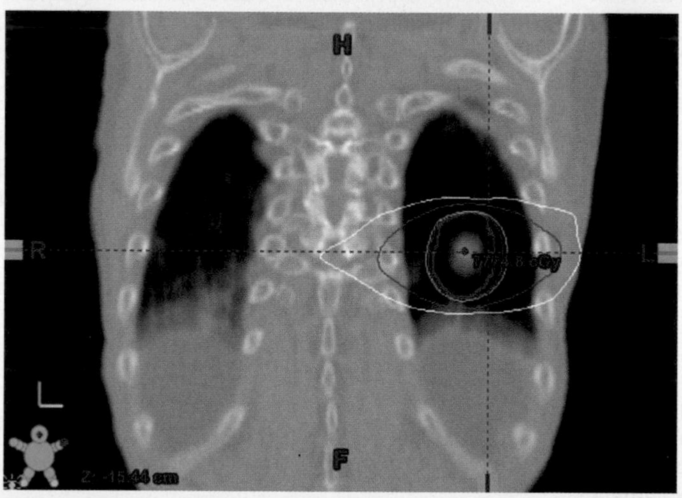

C

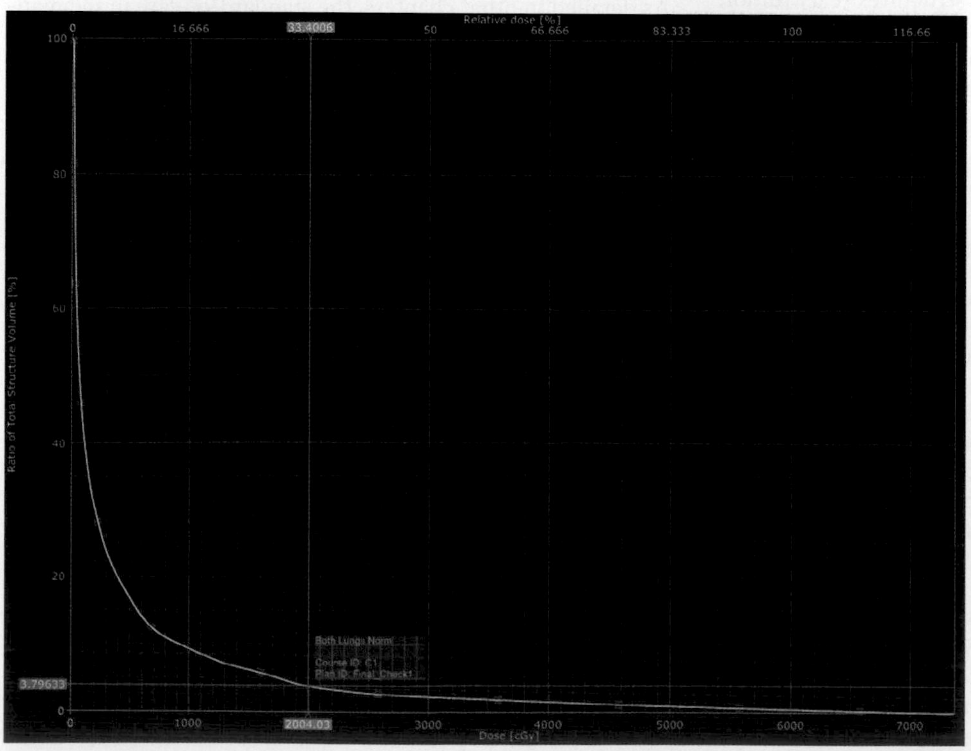

D

Figure 85-1. Stereotactic body radiotherapy (SBRT) plan for a patient with stage I squamous cell carcinoma. This patient has a history of a liver transplant and did not have the performance status to tolerate surgical resection. He was treated with SBRT, to a total dose of 60 Gy in 5 fractions. The 5-fraction treatment was chosen to reduce skin toxicity. *Panel A.* The beam arrangement of 11 beams, including 5 noncoplanar beams, was chosen to reduce dose to the skin and chest wall. *Panel B.* Axial dose distribution. Each line represents tissue receiving a given dose. Notice the dramatic reduction in dose within centimeters of the target (red outline). *Panel C.* Coronal dose distribution. *Panel D.* Dose–volume histogram. Cross-hairs show the "V20," volume of lung receiving 20 Gy or more (in this case, 3.8%).

10 out of 35 patients (29%) developed an in-field recurrence, despite a median total dose of 84 Gy.[30] In a Cochrane review of medically inoperable NSCLC, local recurrence rates ranged from 6% to 70%, with most ranging between 40% and 60%.[31] Nevertheless, it is clear that conventionally radiotherapy is inadequate for treating stage I disease, poor outcomes that are compounded by the inconvenient requirement of 6 to 8 weeks of daily treatment in these regimens.

Stereotactic Body Radiotherapy

The development of SBRT has significantly improved the local control and likely overall survival outcomes in patients with medically inoperable NSCLC, as the very high doses of radiotherapy are thought to overwhelm any underlying radio-resistance of the tumor. Several of the earlier series come from Japan, where patients were initially treated using dosing schemes that were lower than the 54 to 60 Gy in three fractions as is typically done now. The outcomes, such as reported in 2004 by Onishi et al.[32] were promising. In a series that totaled 245 patients, the total local progression probability was only 14.5%. There was a volume–response relationship, though, as the local failure probability for T1 tumors was 9.7% versus 20% for T2 malignancies. Although many other retrospective series showed comparable outcomes, only one phase I dose-escalation trial has been performed.

In this trial, investigators at University of Indiana escalated the total dose from 24 Gy in 3 fractions to 60 Gy in 3 fractions for T1 tumors with any dose-limiting toxicity, and the maximally tolerated dose for T2 tumors was 66 Gy; an unacceptable rate of lung toxicity was seen at 72 Gy.[33] Of note, only 1 local failure was seen in the patients who received over 16 Gy per fraction. The investigators continued to the phase II component of the trial, which found continued excellent local control (95% at 2 years) but a risk of treatment-related mortality in six patients whose lesions were centrally located. Four of these patients died from pneumonia, one from a pericardial effusion, and one from hemoptysis in the context of recurrent tumor. Although the true etiology of these toxicities – that is, unique to SBRT treatment or a stochastic process – are debatable, the Indiana experience has defined the Radiation Therapy Oncology Group (RTOG) eligibility criteria for SBRT, which is at least 2 cm beyond the proximal bronchial tree.

On the heels of this single-institution study, RTOG 0236 was a multi-institutional, phase II study of SBRT for medically inoperable patients with peripheral, stage I NSCLC.[34] The prescription dose was 60 Gy in 3 fractions, comparable to the Indiana experience. This trial showed that SBRT was feasible and highly efficacious in a multi-institutional setting, as the 3-year in-field, in-lobe, and locoregional control probabilities after treatment were 98%, 91%, and 87%, respectively. The 3-year overall survival was an impressive 56%, particularly notable given the underlying severe comorbidities in the cohort. It is important to note that the dose in this trial was 20 Gy × 3, but that this dose was calculated without "heterogeneity corrections," which adjust for the air density of the lungs. As a consequence, the peripheral dose in RTOG 0236 was in effect 54 Gy, and thus 18 Gy × 3 has been essentially adopted as the standard regimen for peripheral lesions.[35] (Table 85-1) displays reported prospective and notable retrospective trials using SBRT. The results have been so promising that a national trial has been activated comparing SBRT

Table 85-1

SUMMARY OF PROSPECTIVE PHASE II CLINICAL STUDIES AND NOTABLE RETROSPECTIVE SERIES STUDYING STEREOTACTIC BODY RADIOTHERAPY (SBRT) FOR STAGE I NON–SMALL CELL LUNG CANCER

INSTITUTION	NUMBER	MEDIAN F/U (months)	DOSE (Gy/# fractions)	LC (Year)	OS (Year)	GRADE 3 TOXICITY (%)	REFERENCES
Prospective							
Indiana	70	50.2	60/3	88.1% (3)	42.7% (3)	16	36
Karolinska	57	35	45/3	92% (3)	60% (3)	30	37
RTOG 0236	59	34.4	60/3	97.6% (3)	55.8% (3)	16.3	34
Kyoto	45	30	48/4	98% (3)	IA: 83% (3) IB: 72	0	38
Retrospective							
VUMC	206	12	60/3, 60/5, 60/8	93% (2)	64% (2)	5	39
Cleveland Clinic Foundation	94	15.3	50/5, 60/3	95% (1.5)	75% (1.5)	0	40
Princess Margaret	108	19.1	50/10, 60/8, 48/4, 54/3, 60/3	89% (4)	30% (4)	6	41

F/U, follow-up; Gy, Gray; LC, local control; OS, overall survival RTOG, Radiation Therapy Oncology Group; VUMC, VU Medical Center, Amsterdam, The Netherlands.

with sublobar resection in medically compromised patients (ACOSOG Z4099 / RTOG 1021).

The most well-known toxicity following SBRT, toxic death after treatment of central lung tumors as seen in the Indiana study, is quite rare, although Song et al.[19] do describe a 33% (3/9 patients) risk of severe bronchial stenosis with subsequent pneumonia and/or death ($n = 1$) and an 88% (8/9 patients) risk of any bronchial stenosis in patients treated with SBRT near the proximal tree. Thus, although it is questionable whether SBRT is associated with lethal side effects in the proximal lesions, at the very least it appears to be more morbid than irradiation of peripherally located lesions. Some single-institutional experiences have successfully treated central lesions with a more gentle fractionation regimen (e.g., 4 to 5 fractions to approximately 50 Gy), without severe lung toxicity.[42,39] RTOG 0819 is currently enrolling patients in a phase I/II dose-escalation trial for patients with centrally based lesions. This study is actively accruing and will define the optimal dose and associated efficacy when using SBRT for central tumors.

Especially, given the fragile population typically treated with SBRT, other lung toxicities such as pneumonitis and pulmonary function test (PFT) decline are generally mild, but they do occur. In busy, experienced radiotherapy clinics, the treatment of peripheral lesions is associated with a risk of grade 2 to 3 pneumonitis between 2% and 11%.[39,–43–45] Indeed, physicians at the Cleveland Clinic Foundation reported no change in the mean PFTs among 92 patients treated with SBRT, although 20% of patients experienced at least a 12.7% decrease of predicted FEV_1, and 20% of patients developed a decline in diffusion capacity of at least 18% of predicted.[43] Interestingly, the risk of these side effects appears to be higher in multi-institutional trials, as the probabilities of grade 2 or 3 to 4 pneumonitis probabilities were 24% and 16%, respectively, in RTOG 0236. This difference may be a function of older planning techniques, as most modern series started treating patients in the mid-2000s.

More recently it has become clear that chest wall toxicity is another potential complication of SBRT, in which patients with peripheral lesions can develop chronic chest wall pain and/or rib fracture. This complication usually occurs between 6 months and 1 year after finishing treatment. It is typically transient, but as shown by Stephans et al.[46] and Dunlap et al.[47], it can occur in 7% to 28% of patients, which can significantly decrease quality-of-life until it resolves. That being said, with careful monitoring of the chest wall dose during planning, the risk of this complication can be significantly decreased, and it is likely that future series which observed this constraint will show a lower risk of chest wall complications.

Locally Advanced Lung Cancer

Locally advanced lung cancer, defined here as stage IIIA or IIIB, comprises over half of the patients who present with nonmetastatic disease, yet further progress in improving overall survival has been relatively stagnant. As described later, the main advance over the past 20 years has been the integration of chemotherapy with radiation treatment, first as induction therapy, and then concurrent treatment, but further investigation into the relative benefit of more intensive radiotherapy has thus far been disappointing.

Integration with Chemotherapy

In the 1980s and early 1990s, locoregional control and overall survival outcomes after radiotherapy alone for locally advanced lung cancer were dismal. Meaningful radiation dose escalation was not feasible due to technical constraints, and with the recognition that lung cancer is typically a systemic disease at presentation, the main strategies to improve survival focused on combination therapy (Table 85-2).

Table 85-2

SUMMARY OF SELECTED PROSPECTIVE CLINICAL STUDIES USING CHEMORADIOTHERAPY FOR STAGE III NON–SMALL CELL LUNG CANCER

TRIAL	NUMBER	CHEMOTHERAPY	RADIATION THERAPY	LC (Year)	OS (Year)	REFERENCES
EORTC—Schaake-Koning	107	Daily cisplatin	55 Gy, split-course	31% (2)	16% (3)	48
Jeremic et al.	65	Daily carboplatin, etoposide	69.6 Gy, BID	42% (4)	23% (4)	49
WJLCG	147	Cisplatin, vindesine, mitomycin	56 Gy	67% (crude)	15.8% (5)	50
GLOT-GFPC	100	Cisplatin, etoposide	66 Gy	69% (crude)	25% (3)	51
CALGB 39801	182	Carboplatin, paclitaxel	66 Gy	64% (crude)	19% (3)	52
RTOG Summary[a]	1,356	Variable	Variable, >60 Gy	48% (5)	15% (5)	53
Auperin meta-analysis	603	Variable	Variable	65% (5)	15.1% (5)	54

LC, local control; OS, overall survival; EORTC, European Organisation for Research and Treatment of Cancer; Gy, Gray; WJLCG, West Japan Lung Cancer Group; GLOT-GFPC, Groupe Lyon-Saint-Etienne d'Oncologie Thoracique-Groupe Français de Pneumo-Cancérologie; CALGB, Cancer and Leukemia Group B; RTOG, Radiation Therapy Oncology Group.
[a]Some patients received induction chemotherapy and radiotherapy alone.

The landmark Dillman[55] trial, published in 1993, compared cisplatin-based induction chemotherapy and radiotherapy with radiotherapy alone, and the results were practice-changing, as the treatment approach was associated with an overall survival benefit of 24% versus 10% at 3 years, and 17% versus 6% at 5 years. This finding was further supported by RTOG 8808/ECOG 4588, which randomized patients between daily RT, BID RT, and cisplatin-based induction chemotherapy followed by daily radiotherapy.[56] Patients in the chemotherapy arm benefitted from significantly superior survival versus the radiotherapy alone arms (median survival 13.8 vs. 12.3 vs. 11.4 months, for the induction, daily RT, and BID RT arms, respectively).

Although induction chemotherapy was associated with a survival benefit, in principle, the use of concurrent chemotherapy may optimize its radiosensitizing properties. Indeed, Schaake-Koning et al.[48] showed that the use of concurrent chemoradiotherapy versus radiotherapy alone was associated with a locoregional control and survival benefit; patients receiving split-course radiotherapy with daily cisplatin experienced superior 2-year locoregional control (31% vs. 19%) and survival (26% vs. 13%) versus radiotherapy alone. Similar results were found by Jeremic et al.[49] using a hyperfractionated radiotherapy regimen, in which patients were randomized to receive 69.6 Gy to radiation alone or radiotherapy with concurrent, daily carboplatin and etoposide, finding a significant 14% absolute difference in overall survival at 4 years in patients who received concurrent treatment.

Given the superiority of induction chemotherapy and radiotherapy over radiotherapy alone, and concurrent chemoradiotherapy over radiotherapy alone, the next logical question is the optimal combination of chemotherapy and radiotherapy: induction, concurrent, or both. RTOG 9410 compared induction chemotherapy and radiotherapy alone with two concurrent radiotherapy arms, one with hyperfractionated radiotherapy (69.6 Gy in 34 1.2 Gy BID fractions) and one with conventional radiotherapy.[57] Although this study has yet to be published, preliminary results have shown a survival benefit with the concurrent chemoradiotherapy arms. Similarly, Furuse et al.[50] randomized 320 patients between induction chemotherapy (cisplatin, vindesine, and mitomycin) followed by daily radiotherapy to 56 Gy, versus the same chemotherapy with concurrent split-course radiation treatment Despite the mandated break during radiotherapy, patients receiving concurrent treatment experienced superior survival (median 16.5 vs. 13.3 months), though curiously there was no demonstrable difference in failure-free recurrence between the two arms. Several other studies have further supported the benefit of concurrent versus induction chemotherapy, and a recent meta-analysis of these studies by Auperin et al. not only showed an absolute benefit of 5.7% with concurrent therapy, but also that the main benefit of concurrent treatment was improved locoregional control (HR 0.77).

Two recent trials attempted to determine the optimal timing of chemotherapy and radiotherapy. Belani et al. performed a phase II randomized trial (Locally Advanced Multimodality Protocol [LAMP]) comparing induction chemotherapy with paclitaxel and carboplatin followed by radiotherapy alone versus induction chemotherapy followed by chemoradiotherapy with weekly paclitaxel and carboplatin versus chemoradiotherapy followed by adjuvant chemotherapy. There were no survival differences between the arms, although the upfront chemoradiotherapy arm appeared to have the highest median survival (16.3 months vs. 13.0 and 12.7 in the induction arms).[58] In CALGB 39801, Vokes et al.[52] compared chemoradiotherapy using 66 Gy with weekly carboplatin and paclitaxel to induction chemotherapy followed by the same chemoradiotherapy. There was no difference in overall survival between the two arms, despite the use of induction chemotherapy; as expected, induction chemotherapy was associated with more grade 4 toxicity. It is notable that 53 patients (15% of entire cohort) never received radiotherapy, which may have influenced the results. Given these two trials, induction chemotherapy prior to chemoradiotherapy is not a common practice unless investigated on clinical trials.

Since chemotherapy clearly extends survival in resected NSCLC and these trials of induction therapy do not, it is possible that the competing risk of locoregional failure after chemoradiotherapy obviates any systemic disease benefit from neoadjuvant or adjuvant chemotherapy, though this question will hopefully be reopened over time as control rates improve with nonoperative therapies.

Radiotherapy Dose

In the radiotherapy community, one of the most controversial issues is the total dose used in the treatment of inoperable NSCLC. Unfortunately, there are few randomized data to address this question. The classic dose-escalation randomized trial, RTOG 7301, randomized patients between 40 Gy delivered as split-course, 40 Gy continuous course, 50 Gy continuous course, and 60 Gy continuous course.[59] No chemotherapy was given, and thus the competing risk of distant recurrence significantly reduces the power to see a survival difference from improved local control. Indeed, although there were no differences in overall survival, there was a significant difference in intrathoracic recurrences with higher-dose radiotherapy: 52% after 40 Gy, 41% after 50 Gy, and 30% after 60 Gy. When the recurrence risks were stratified by tumor size, local relapse rates were higher in the 40 Gy arms in comparison to the higher-dose arms for tumors between 1 and 3 cm, and 4 and 6 cm but not in larger tumors. This trial, published in 1982, essentially established the standard radiotherapy dose for conventionally fractionated radiotherapy that has remained until today.

RTOG 9311 was a more recent dose-escalation study for stage I–III NSCLC, in which the radiation dose was escalated to over 90 Gy using daily fractionation.[60] Despite these high doses, there was no relationship between dose and response, progression-free survival, or overall survival in the 161 patients treated. On the other hand, there was a strong relationship between tumor size and overall survival and progression-free survival on multivariable analysis. RTOG 9311 did not include chemotherapy in the treatment regimen, and thus competing risk of distant metastasis may have eliminated any local control benefit of dose escalation.

Recently, Machtay et al.[53] performed a combined analysis of 7 RTOG chemoradiotherapy trials to analyze whether biologically effective dose (BED), a formula that considers the total dose and dose per fraction, was associated with local control and overall survival. The authors used the patient-specific data on the actual dose received rather than the protocol-specified dose. With a sample size that numbered over 1300 patients, the authors showed that the risk of locoregional failure and overall mortality decreased by 3% and 4%, respectively, for every increase of 1 Gy in the received BED. Although this study is limited by potential confounding between radiation dose and performance status/disease progression (i.e., worse comorbid disease leads to both shortened radiation treatment and life expectancy) the data do suggest that dose is associated with locoregional control and survival.

Several retrospective studies have more recently analyzed the relationship between local control and total radiation dose. For example, Rengan et al.[61] evaluated the Memorial Sloan-Kettering experience with bulky stage III patients and found that compared with patients treated to a lower dose, those irradiated to 64 Gy or higher experienced higher 2-year local control (53% vs. 24%, $p = 0.024$) and a borderline improvement in overall survival (median 20 months vs. 15 months, $p = 0.068$). This group also found a significant relationship between GTV volume and local failure, as doubling the GTV resulted in a 46% increased risk of local failure. Investigators at the Washington University in St. Louis arrived at similar conclusions in analyzing their dataset of 207 patients with inoperable NSCLC; of note, 73% of the population had stage III disease, and almost half of the entire cohort received chemotherapy.[62] Patients who received 70 Gy or more had significantly improved local control and cause-specific survival (absolute benefit of 3 years approximately 20%), but not overall survival. However, GTV volume was much more influential in overall survival and local control, as this variable was significant on multivariable analysis for both outcomes, whereas radiotherapy dose was not.

A more recent randomized controlled trial of 200 patients nominally compared the use of smaller versus larger radiotherapy fields, but in actuality compared 60 to 64 Gy to 68 to 74 Gy, depending on whether a limited or extensive nodal field was delivered.[63] In obvious contrast to RTOG 7301, patients received chemotherapy in both arms, and 3D-CRT was mandated. Local control was significantly greater at 5 years in the high-dose arm (51% vs. 36%). Although there was a visible but nonsignificant trend for improved survival in the high-dose arm ($p = 0.2$), only the survival percentage at 2 years was significantly different (39.4% vs. 25.6%). It is important to note that this study used nonstandard chemotherapy (1 cycle of induction, followed by chemoradiotherapy with 4 to 6 cycles in total) and needs additional follow-up, as the median follow-up at the time of its publication was 27 months. Nevertheless, although this study was not presented as a dose-escalation trial, in fact that is exactly what this paper describes, and for the first time since RTOG 7301, it shows a significant local control benefit to higher dose of radiotherapy in a randomized trial, which may have translated into a survival advantage had the study been appropriately powered.

In summary, it is difficult to abstract any firm conclusions on the relationship between radiotherapy dose and local control and survival. RTOG 7301 was performed in an earlier era using antiquated radiotherapy techniques and staging studies, and patients were treated without chemotherapy. Retrospective studies are limited by selection bias, and although several of the presented analyses suggest a relationship between dose and survival, the fact that GTV volume is consistently related to outcome argues that deliverable dose was more a function of the size of the tumor, and in actuality, any benefit from dose-escalation was a result of confounding; in other words, smaller tumors have a more favorable prognosis, and since the volume is smaller, it is safer to treat them to a higher dose, which is why higher dose appears to confer a more favorable prognosis.

In all likelihood, RTOG 0617 will provide the final word on the optimal radiotherapy dose, as patients are randomized between 60 and 74 Gy of chemoradiotherapy. The study has targeted accrual at 500 (currently standing at 464), which will provide for a power of 80% to see a 7-month median survival improvement with higher-dose radiotherapy. It is arguably the most important trial in locally advanced NSCLC accruing today, with the results expected in several years. Until that is published, doses between 60 and 74 Gy are considered within the standard-of-care, though doses in excess of 70 Gy are best reserved for clinical trials.

Radiotherapy Volume

The vast majority of published clinical trials utilizing thoracic radiotherapy have utilized large treatment fields that treated regional nodal basins that did not contain gross disease; this practice is called "elective nodal irradiation," or ENI, and it is the standard practice in many disease sites in radiation oncology.[64] In principle, lymph nodes with a reasonable chance at harboring occult metastases are treated to a lower but theoretically sterilizing dose (e.g., 50 Gy). In the lung, performing ENI implies irradiating the supraclavicular fossa, bilateral mediastinum and in some situations, bilateral hila. This treatment field significantly increases the dose that the normal lung receives, which can meaningfully increase lung and esophageal toxicity and further, prevent dose-escalation to the primary tumor.

An alternative treatment planning approach is to only treat the known tumor and involved lymph nodes, which is called involved-field radiation therapy (IFRT). Because less normal lung and esophagus are irradiated, the benefits of this strategy include safer dose-escalation to the known gross disease as well as less esophageal toxicity.[65] The obvious risk of this strategy is that occult disease in the lymph nodes is missed in the treatment field, which could lead to regional recurrence, and multiple surgical series have shown the risks of microscopic nodal disease, even in stage I disease, can exceed 35%.[66] Nevertheless, multiple retrospective series and prospective trials, accounting for hundreds if not thousands of patients, have shown that the risk of isolated elective nodal failure – in other words, regional recurrence that could have been prevented with a higher, elective dose to that region – is less than 10%. As detailed earlier, the single randomized trial of ENI versus IFRT, in which dose was escalated in the IFRT arm, favored IFRT in local control, perhaps survival, and toxicity (significantly less pneumonitis, 29% vs. 17%, $p = 0.044$); yet this trial was primarily a question of dose, and whether ENI improves locoregional control when dose is held constant (if technically possible) was not the hypothesis of the trial.[63]

These data showing a low risk of isolated elective nodal failure following radiotherapy conflict with known patterns of microscopic disease in NSCLC. There are several explanations for this finding. It is theoretically possible that the tumors in patients treated with primary RT have a different biology than those patients treated with surgical resection, but this scenario is unlikely.[67] A second possibility is that elective nodes receive a sterilizing dose through incidental radiation to the involved field: "nonelective" elective nodal irradiation. Several investigators have shown that over 50% of nontargeted proximal nodal stations (e.g., subcarina treating a primary tumor and hilum) receive a sterilizing dose of radiotherapy through incidental radiotherapy from IFRT. However, as radiation planning becomes more conformal with IMRT, IGRT, and smaller margins, lower incidental doses are delivered to these elective regions, with the potential for a higher likelihood of elective nodal failure.

The third potential explanation to explain the discrepancy between the likelihood of occult nodal disease and low regional failure rate is the poor locoregional control of known gross disease following with radiotherapy or chemoradiotherapy. There is thus no opportunity to see an elective nodal failure because the patients are first progressing from their gross disease at presentation. In an interesting paper from the University of Pennsylvania, Fernandes et al.[68] showed that while the 2-year probability of isolated elective nodal failure after IFRT was only 4.5%, initially uninvolved nodes still recurred 21% of the time at some point in the treatment course. Such data reinforce the notion that occult nodal disease may actually present clinically if given enough time.

Nevertheless, as of 2011, to my knowledge every cooperative group trial involving NSCLC mandates involved-field radiotherapy and no longer allows ENI, and to the extent that active national studies define the standard-of-care, IFRT would thus be considered the appropriate radiotherapy fields. However, controversy still remains, and every radiation plan must be tailored to the individual patient, based on his own disease characteristics and the predicted likelihood of harboring nodal metastases in any given nodal station. Although the extensive fields that irradiated the thoracic inlet to 5 cm below the carina are no longer delivered, more tailored elective nodal treatment, such as treating an entire ipsilateral level 4 station if an inferior level 4 node is positive on imaging, may be indicated based on the clinical scenario. From a thoracic surgeon's perspective, the concept of involved-field radiotherapy highlights the importance of information obtained from the mediastinoscopy. The additional pathologic information may be very useful for designing the radiotherapy fields in the context of IFRT, even if the overall management paradigm does not change based on the results. Moreover, as systemic and local control improves over time, either with novel chemotherapeutic or radiotherapy advances, the relative benefit of elective nodal irradiation becomes more prominent, and the indications of ENI may need to be addressed again at a later point.

CONCLUSIONS

This chapter has summarized both the technical advances in thoracic radiotherapy as well as treatment innovations in inoperable NSCLC. With respect to early-stage disease, technical improvements in radiation therapy delivery have led to SBRT, which has dramatically improved local control, and presumably survival, in medically inoperable NSCLC.

In locally advanced patients, technical advances have led to better tumor delineation, more accurate patient setup, and more precise and conformal delivery of radiotherapy. These improvements have likely improved the therapeutic ratio, as higher doses of radiotherapy can be delivered with lower toxicity, but the relationship between survival and advanced techniques must still be analyzed. Although survival outcomes have slowly increased over time, this improvement is more a function of chemotherapy delivery rather than improved radiation treatment. Given the combined challenge of eradicating locoregional disease and distant metastases, further research must be performed on optimizing combined modality therapy, with more creative integration of all three core therapies in lung cancer—radiation therapy, chemotherapy, and thoracic surgery.

EDITOR'S COMMENT

This excellent chapter has reviewed the state of the art in radiation therapy for NSCLC. Regarding early-stage disease, the comments concerning the use of SBRT for medically inoperable disease are quite correct. Depending on the results of the current trials for its use in resectable and central disease, one may be able to apply these conclusions to those populations as well. The author gives a very clear review of the status of using radiation therapy for locally advanced inoperable disease, clearly restating the case for concurrent chemoradiation therapy. The current study will finally put to rest questions related to high-dose (60 Gy) versus extra high-dose (70 Gy) radiation therapy. One final point not mentioned here is the role of chemoradiation as neoadjuvant therapy for potentially resectable stage IIIA NSCLC. Although there remains much argument regarding the role of pnuemonectomy in these patients, there is a developing consensus for the role of high-dose chemoradiation followed by surgery when lobectomy is feasible.

—Mark J. Krasna

References

1. Baker GR. Localization: conventional and CT simulation. *Br J Radiol.* 2006;79 Spec No 1:S36–S49.
2. Mah D, Chen CC. Image guidance in radiation oncology treatment planning: the role of imaging technologies on the planning process. *Semin Nucl Med.* 2008;38(2):114–118.
3. Goitein M. Future prospects in planning radiation therapy. *Cancer.* 1985;55(9 suppl):2234–2239.
4. Gunderson LT, Tepper JE, eds. *Clinical Radiation Oncology.* 1st ed. Philadelphia, PA: Churchill Livingstone; 2000.
5. Purdy JA. Current ICRU definitions of volumes: limitations and future directions. *Semin Radiat Oncol.* 2004;14(1):27–40.
6. Graham MV, Purdy JA, Emami B, et al. Clinical dose-volume histogram analysis for pneumonitis after 3D treatment for non-small cell lung cancer (NSCLC). *Int J Radiat Oncol Biol Phys.* 1999;45(2):323–329.
7. Kwa SL, Lebesque JV, Theuws JC, et al. Radiation pneumonitis as a function of mean lung dose: an analysis of pooled data of 540 patients. *Int J Radiat Oncol Biol Phys.* 1998;42(1):1–9.
8. Keall P. 4-dimensional computed tomography imaging and treatment planning. *Semin Radiat Oncol.* 2004;14(1):81–90.
9. Mageras GS, Pevsner A, Yorke ED, et al. Measurement of lung tumor motion using respiration-correlated CT. *Int J Radiat Oncol Biol Phys.* 2004;60(3):933–941.
10. Sher DJ, Wolfgang JA, Niemierko A, et al. Quantification of mediastinal and hilar lymph node movement using four-dimensional computed tomography scan: implications for radiation treatment planning. *Int J Radiat Oncol Biol Phys.* 2007;69(5):1402–1408.
11. De Ruysscher D. PET-CT in radiotherapy for lung cancer. *Methods Mol Biol.* 2011;727:53–58.
12. De Ruysscher D, Wanders S, Minken A, et al. Effects of radiotherapy planning with a dedicated combined PET-CT-simulator of patients with non-small cell lung cancer on dose limiting normal tissues and radiation dose-escalation: a planning study. *Radiother Oncol.* 2005;77(1):5–10.
13. Bradley J, Bae K, Choi N, et al. A phase II comparative study of gross tumor volume definition with or without PET/CT fusion in dosimetric planning for non-small-cell lung cancer (NSCLC): primary analysis of radiation therapy oncology group (RTOG) 0515. *Int J Radiat Oncol Biol Phys.* 2012;82:435–441.
14. Khan F. *The Physics of Radiation Therapy.* Philadelphia, PA: Lippincott Williams and Wilkins; 2003.

15. Yom SS, Liao Z, Liu HH, et al. Initial evaluation of treatment-related pneumonitis in advanced-stage non-small-cell lung cancer patients treated with concurrent chemotherapy and intensity-modulated radiotherapy. *Int J Radiat Oncol Biol Phys*. 2007;68(1):94–102.
16. Court L, Wagar M, Berbeco R, et al. Evaluation of the interplay effect when using RapidArc to treat targets moving in the craniocaudal or right-left direction. *Med Phys*. 2010;37(1):4–11.
17. Mayo CS, Urie MM, Fitzgerald TJ, et al. Hybrid IMRT for treatment of cancers of the lung and esophagus. *Int J Radiat Oncol Biol Phys*. 2008;71(5):1408–1418.
18. Vogelius IS, Westerly DC, Cannon GM, et al. Intensity-modulated radiotherapy might increase pneumonitis risk relative to three-dimensional conformal radiotherapy in patients receiving combined chemotherapy and radiotherapy: a modeling study of dose dumping. *Int J Radiat Oncol Biol Phys*. 2011;80(3):893–899.
19. Song CH, Pyo H, Moon SH, et al. Treatment-related pneumonitis and acute esophagitis in non-small-cell lung cancer patients treated with chemotherapy and helical tomotherapy. *Int J Radiat Oncol Biol Phys*. 2010;78(3):651–658.
20. Korreman SS, Juhler-Nottrup T, Persson GF, et al. The role of image guidance in respiratory gated radiotherapy. *Acta Oncol*. 2008;47(7):1390–1396.
21. Verellen D, Depuydt T, Gevaert T, et al. Gating and tracking, 4D in thoracic tumours. *Cancer Radiother*. 2010;14(6–7):446–454.
22. McNair HA, Brock J, Symonds-Tayler JR, et al. Feasibility of the use of the active breathing co ordinator (ABC) in patients receiving radical radiotherapy for non-small cell lung cancer (NSCLC). *Radiother Oncol*. 2009;93(3):424–429.
23. Chen GT, Sharp GC, Mori S. A review of image-guided radiotherapy. *Radiol Phys Technol*. 2009;2(1):1–12.
24. Lasak JM, Gorecki JP. The history of stereotactic radiosurgery and radiotherapy. *Otolaryngol Clin North Am*. 2009;42(4):593–599.
25. Hamilton AJ, Lulu BA, Fosmire H, et al. LINAC-based spinal stereotactic radiosurgery. *Stereotact Funct Neurosurg*. 1996;66(1–3):1–9.
26. Blomgren H, Lax I, Naslund I, et al. Stereotactic high dose fraction radiation therapy of extracranial tumors using an accelerator. clinical experience of the first thirty-one patients. *Acta Oncol*. 1995;34(6):861–870.
27. Shirato H, Shimizu S, Shimizu T, et al. Real-time tumour-tracking radiotherapy. *Lancet*. 1999;353(9161):1331–1332.
28. Chang BK, Timmerman RD. Stereotactic body radiation therapy: a comprehensive review. *Am J Clin Oncol*. 2007;30(6):637–644.
29. Bradley JD, Wahab S, Lockett MA, et al. Elective nodal failures are uncommon in medically inoperable patients with stage I non-small-cell lung carcinoma treated with limited radiotherapy fields. *Int J Radiat Oncol Biol Phys*. 2003;56(2):342–347.
30. Chen M, Hayman JA, Ten Haken RK, et al. Long-term results of high-dose conformal radiotherapy for patients with medically inoperable T1–3N0 non-small-cell lung cancer: is low incidence of regional failure due to incidental nodal irradiation?. *Int J Radiat Oncol Biol Phys*. 2006;64(1):120–126.
31. Rowell NP, Williams CJ. Radical radiotherapy for stage I/II non-small cell lung cancer in patients not sufficiently fit for or declining surgery (medically inoperable): a systematic review. *Thorax*. 2001;56(8):628–638.
32. Onishi H, Araki T, Shirato H, et al. Stereotactic hypofractionated high-dose irradiation for stage I nonsmall cell lung carcinoma: clinical outcomes in 245 subjects in a japanese multiinstitutional study. *Cancer*. 2004;101(7):1623–1631.
33. McGarry RC, Papiez L, Williams M, et al. Stereotactic body radiation therapy of early-stage non-small-cell lung carcinoma: phase I study. *Int J Radiat Oncol Biol Phys*. 2005;63(4):1010–1015.
34. Timmerman R, Paulus R, Galvin J, et al. Stereotactic body radiation therapy for inoperable early stage lung cancer. *JAMA*. 2010;303(11):1070–1076.
35. Xiao Y, Papiez L, Paulus R, et al. Dosimetric evaluation of heterogeneity corrections for RTOG 0236: Stereotactic body radiotherapy of inoperable stage I-II non-small-cell lung cancer. *Int J Radiat Oncol Biol Phys*. 2009;73(4):1235–1242.
36. Fakiris AJ, McGarry RC, Yiannoutsos CT, et al. Stereotactic body radiation therapy for early-stage non-small-cell lung carcinoma: four-year results of a prospective phase II study. *Int J Radiat Oncol Biol Phys*. 2009;75(3):677–682.
37. Baumann P, Nyman J, Hoyer M, et al. Outcome in a prospective phase II trial of medically inoperable stage I non-small-cell lung cancer patients treated with stereotactic body radiotherapy. *J Clin Oncol*. 2009;27(20):3290–3296.
38. Nagata Y, Takayama K, Matsuo Y, et al. Clinical outcomes of a phase I/II study of 48 Gy of stereotactic body radiotherapy in 4 fractions for primary lung cancer using a stereotactic body frame. *Int J Radiat Oncol Biol Phys*. 2005;63(5):1427–1431.
39. Lagerwaard FJ, Haasbeek CJ, Smit EF, et al. Outcomes of risk-adapted fractionated stereotactic radiotherapy for stage I non-small-cell lung cancer. *Int J Radiat Oncol Biol Phys*. 2008;70(3):685–692.
40. Stephans KL, Djemil T, Reddy CA, et al. A comparison of two stereotactic body radiation fractionation schedules for medically inoperable stage I non-small cell lung cancer: the cleveland clinic experience. *J Thorac Oncol*. 2009;4(8):976–982.
41. Taremi M, Hope A, Dahele M, et al. Stereotactic body radiotherapy for medically inoperable lung cancer: prospective, single-center study of 108 consecutive patients. *Int J Radiat Oncol Biol Phys*. 2012;82:967–973.
42. Chang JY, Balter PA, Dong L, et al. Stereotactic body radiation therapy in centrally and superiorly located stage I or isolated recurrent non-small-cell lung cancer. *Int J Radiat Oncol Biol Phys*. 2008;72(4):967–971.
43. Stephans KL, Djemil T, Reddy CA, et al. Comprehensive analysis of pulmonary function test (PFT) changes after stereotactic body radiotherapy (SBRT) for stage I lung cancer in medically inoperable patients. *J Thorac Oncol*. 2009;4(7):838–844.
44. Grills IS, Mangona VS, Welsh R, et al. Outcomes after stereotactic lung radiotherapy or wedge resection for stage I non-small-cell lung cancer. *J Clin Oncol*. 2010;28(6):928–935.
45. Bradley JD, El Naqa I, Drzymala RE, et al. Stereotactic body radiation therapy for early-stage non-small-cell lung cancer: the pattern of failure is distant. *Int J Radiat Oncol Biol Phys*. 2010;77(4):1146–1150.
46. Stephans KL, Djemil T, Tendulkar RD, et al. Prediction of chest wall toxicity from lung stereotactic body radiotherapy (SBRT). *Int J Radiat Oncol Biol Phys*. 2012;82:974–980.
47. Dunlap NE, Cai J, Biedermann GB, et al. Chest wall volume receiving >30 Gy predicts risk of severe pain and/or rib fracture after lung stereotactic body radiotherapy. *Int J Radiat Oncol Biol Phys*. 2010;76(3):796–801.
48. Schaake-Koning C, van den Bogaert W, Dalesio O, et al. Effects of concomitant cisplatin and radiotherapy on inoperable non-small-cell lung cancer. *N Engl J Med*. 1992;326(8):524–530.
49. Jeremic B, Shibamoto Y, Acimovic L, et al. Hyperfractionated radiation therapy with or without concurrent low-dose daily carboplatin/etoposide for stage III non-small-cell lung cancer: a randomized study. *J Clin Oncol*. 1996;14(4):1065–1070.
50. Furuse K, Fukuoka M, Kawahara M, et al. Phase III study of concurrent versus sequential thoracic radiotherapy in combination with mitomycin, vindesine, and cisplatin in unresectable stage III non-small-cell lung cancer. *J Clin Oncol*. 1999;17(9):2692–2699.
51. Fournel P, Robinet G, Thomas P, et al. Randomized phase III trial of sequential chemoradiotherapy compared with concurrent chemoradiotherapy in locally advanced non-small-cell lung cancer: Groupe lyon-saint-etienne d'oncologie thoracique-groupe francais de pneumo-cancerologie NPC 95–01 study. *J Clin Oncol*. 2005;23(25):5910–5917.
52. Vokes EE, Herndon JE,2 nd, Kelley MJ, et al. Induction chemotherapy followed by chemoradiotherapy compared with chemoradiotherapy alone for regionally advanced unresectable stage III non-small-cell lung cancer: cancer and leukemia group B. *J Clin Oncol*. 2007;25(13):1698–1704.
53. Machtay M, Bae K, Movsas B, et al. Higher biologically effective dose of radiotherapy is associated with improved outcomes for locally advanced non-small cell lung carcinoma treated with chemoradiation: an analysis of the radiation therapy oncology group. *Int J Radiat Oncol Biol Phys*. 2010;82:425–434.
54. Auperin A, Le Pechoux C, Rolland E, et al. Meta-analysis of concomitant versus sequential radiochemotherapy in locally advanced non-small-cell lung cancer. *J Clin Oncol*. 2010;28(13):2181–2190.
55. Dillman RO, Herndon J, Seagren SL, et al. Improved survival in stage III non-small-cell lung cancer: seven-year follow-up of cancer and leukemia group B (CALGB) 8433 trial. *J Natl Cancer Inst*. 1996;88(17):1210–1215.
56. Sause WT, Scott C, Taylor S, et al. Radiation therapy oncology group (RTOG) 88–08 and eastern cooperative oncology group (ECOG) 4588: preliminary results of a phase III trial in regionally advanced, unresectable non-small-cell lung cancer. *J Natl Cancer Inst*. 1995;87(3):198–205.
57. Curran WJ, Scott CB, Langer CJ, et al. Long-term benefit is observed in a phase III comparison of sequential versus concurrent chemo-radiation for patients with unresected stage III NSCLC: RTOG 9410. *Am Soc Clin Oncol*. 2003;22:621.

58. Belani CP, Wang W, Johnson DH, et al. Phase III study of the Eastern Cooperative Oncology Group (ECOG 2597): induction chemotherapy followed by either standard thoracic radiotherapy or hyperfractionated accelerated radiotherapy for patients with unresectable stage IIIA and B non-small-cell lung cancer. *J Clin Oncol.* 2005;23(16):3760–3767.
59. Perez CA, Stanley K, Grundy G, et al. Impact of irradiation technique and tumor extent in tumor control and survival of patients with unresectable non-oat cell carcinoma of the lung: report by the radiation therapy oncology group. *Cancer.* 1982;50(6):1091–1099.
60. Werner-Wasik M, Swann RS, Bradley J, et al. Increasing tumor volume is predictive of poor overall and progression-free survival: secondary analysis of the radiation therapy oncology group 93–11 phase I-II radiation dose-escalation study in patients with inoperable non-small-cell lung cancer. *Int J Radiat Oncol Biol Phys.* 2008;70(2):385–390.
61. Rengan R, Rosenzweig KE, Venkatraman E, et al. Improved local control with higher doses of radiation in large-volume stage III non-small-cell lung cancer. *Int J Radiat Oncol Biol Phys.* 2004;60(3):741–747.
62. Bradley JD, Ieumwananonthachai N, Purdy JA, et al. Gross tumor volume, critical prognostic factor in patients treated with three-dimensional conformal radiation therapy for non-small-cell lung carcinoma. *Int J Radiat Oncol Biol Phys.* 2002;52(1):49–57.
63. Yuan S, Sun X, Li M, et al. A randomized study of involved-field irradiation versus elective nodal irradiation in combination with concurrent chemotherapy for inoperable stage III nonsmall cell lung cancer. *Am J Clin Oncol.* 2007;30(3):239–244.
64. Chang DT, Zlotecki RA, Olivier KR. Re-examining the role of elective nodal irradiation: finding ways to maximize the therapeutic ratio. *Am J Clin Oncol.* 2005;28(6):597–602.
65. Grills IS, Yan D, Martinez AA, et al. Potential for reduced toxicity and dose escalation in the treatment of inoperable non-small-cell lung cancer: a comparison of intensity-modulated radiation therapy (IMRT), 3D conformal radiation, and elective nodal irradiation. *Int J Radiat Oncol Biol Phys.* 2003;57(3):875–890.
66. Jeremic B. Low incidence of isolated nodal failures after involved-field radiation therapy for non small-cell lung cancer: blinded by the light?. *J Clin Oncol.* 2007;25(35):5543–5545.
67. Jeremic B. Incidental irradiation of nodal regions at risk during limited-field radiotherapy (RT) in dose-escalation studies in nonsmall cell lung cancer (NSCLC). enough to convert no-elective into elective nodal irradiation (ENI)?. *Radiother Oncol.* 2004;71(2):123–125.
68. Fernandes AT, Shen J, Finlay J, et al. Elective nodal irradiation (ENI) vs. involved field radiotherapy (IFRT) for locally advanced non-small cell lung cancer (NSCLC): a comparative analysis of toxicities and clinical outcomes. *Radiother Oncol.* 2010;95(2):178–184.

86 Management of Superficial Central Airway Lung Cancers

Todd L. Demmy and Gregory M. Loewen

Keywords: Radiologically occult lung cancer, sputum analysis, photodynamic therapy (PDT), cryotherapy, white-light bronchoscopy (WLB), autofluorescence (AF) bronchoscopy, optical coherence tomography, virtual bronchoscopy, endobronchial ultrasound (EBUS), brachytherapy

INTRODUCTION

Squamous cell lung cancer represents between 25% and 30% of all primary lung malignancy. It is believed that most squamous cell cancers begin in the central airway, and will evolve in a stepwise, predictable way. These cancers are preceded by premalignant lesions that include squamous metaplasia, squamous dysplasia, and carcinoma in situ. Evidence of premalignant change is detected inconsistently in the induced sputum of high-risk individuals. If the carcinogenesis progresses, eventually central airway tumors will shed malignant cells that can be detected in sputum cytology preparations. Early superficial central airway cancers do not shed malignant cells in a reliable way, and the large-scale lung cancer screening trials of the 1970s and 1980s failed to demonstrate a mortality benefit from lung cancer screening with sputum cytology. Nonetheless, a small percentage of patients were identified with positive sputum cytology despite a normal chest x-ray in these trials. Cancers in this category were termed *radiographically occult lung cancers.* Although radiographically occult, many of these cancers were found to be early invasive carcinomas, arising from the segmental bronchi with metastases to adjacent lymph nodes. Diagnoses of these lung cancers were confirmed typically with white-light bronchoscopy (WLB).

The stepwise theory of lung cancer evolution is based in part on sputum obtained from high-risk patients and evidence obtained at autopsy in patients with lung cancer. Recent work suggests that premalignant bronchial epithelial dysplasia may occur frequently adjacent to a primary lung cancer. Further evidences suggest that the presence of dysplastic cells in sputum cytology may even be a marker for peripheral lung cancer.[1] In addition, there appears to be a great deal of biologic variation with some rapid transitions to deep invasion and metastases. The new lung cancer staging system has adopted the designation of "T1 ss" for "superficial-spreading tumor of any size but confined to the wall of the trachea or mainstem bronchus"—in addition to the "Tis" previously designated for carcinoma in situ.[2] Although microinvasion may be present pathologically, these lesions are typically too thin to be detectable with CT or PET scans. The evaluation and treatment of this group of malignancies are the focus of this chapter.

GENERAL PRINCIPLES

Timed observations also support the progression of the disease—from occult sputum-positive malignancy to the radiographically detectable image 2 years later.[3] This still represents a relatively late stage in the process of oncogenesis. For instance, a 3- to 5-mm nodule contains over 500 million cells.[3] It may be possible to detect small nodules like this by studying the epithelium at sites distant from primary tumors. Monoclonal patches (only 200–400 cells) can be detected that have characteristics very similar to the primary tumor.[4] Given the oncogenesis and field cancerization hypotheses, exfoliated tumor cells may survive longer in the sputum because of their resistance to apoptosis once separated from the tissue.[3] Tempering this enthusiasm is the fact that the bronchial mucosa is a dynamic system where premalignant or malignant conditions can either follow an indolent course or resolve spontaneously. For instance, careful step sectioning of lung specimens from heavy smokers (>2 packs per day) revealed three or more cell rows of atypical cells in 76.2% and frank carcinoma in situ in 11.4% of specimens. Such values are higher than the expected lung cancer prevalence rate for this subpopulation.[5] Biopsy of small early lesions failed to yield any tumor on subsequent resection or bronchoscopic evaluation. It is possible that some of these lesions were small enough to be removed by the actual biopsy or, alternatively, were destined to resolve spontaneously.

DIAGNOSTIC METHODS

Although sputum cytology has failed to lower lung cancer mortality in the screening trials of the 1970s, sputum surveillance is used occasionally in high-risk groups, and this typically leads to bronchoscopy for the detection of early superficial airway cancer. Bronchoscopic evaluation subsequent to positive sputum cytology most frequently detects superficial central airway cancer (T1 ss) or carcinoma in situ (Tis). Recovery of malignant cells from the same site on two separate bronchoscopic examinations is considered an adequate indication for surgical resection or an endobronchial intervention.

Sputum cytology can be specific for small cell lung cancer, but is less helpful in distinguishing cell types of non–small-cell lung cancer. In comparative studies, 20% of squamous cell carcinomas determined by resection histology were interpreted as large cell and undifferentiated carcinomas on sputum cytology.[6] Sputum showing small cell carcinoma almost always will have a concordant diagnosis with biopsied tissue. In contrast, a specific diagnosis of adenocarcinoma will be made in only two-thirds of patients with cytologically positive sputum samples.[6]

Various factors influence the incidence of positive sputum. In patients producing sputum, three positive samples will achieve a correct cell type 90% of the time.[6] Tumors (especially squamous cell) that approach T_2 size yield a high sputum sensitivity, and this finding appears to be amplified in patients with severe obstructive disease, as defined by a forced expiratory volume in 1 second (FEV_1) value of less than 50% of vital capacity.[6] Centrally located tumors are more likely to produce positive cytologic diagnoses.

Sputum cytology screening might hold the promise of detecting potentially curable lung cancer with the use of automated analysis or morphometrics. Automated quantitative cytometry has been used prospectively in 561 current or former smokers. Of the total population, 423 patients proved to have sputum atypia, defined as the presence of five or more cells with abnormal DNA content, using automated quantitative cytometry.[1] Such systems have done a good job of identifying clearly positive cases, as well as premalignant changes including squamous metaplasia and squamous dysplasia. Some specimens are still flagged for review because of metaplastic changes and inflammatory-based alterations in the cytology. Occasionally, false-positive sputum cytology can occur as a result of severe acute inflammation or even in cases of pulmonary infarction. Tissue confirmation is necessary, and advanced bronchoscopic techniques (such as autofluorescence [AF]) are now used to identify treatable superficial central airway cancers.

Bronchoscopic Evaluation (White Light and High Magnification)

Advances in endoscopic imaging have changed the management of sputum-positive lung cancers. Before 1970, patients required rigid bronchoscopy that often missed peripheral lesions. When fiberoptic bronchoscopy became available, it localized 66% of sputum-positive lung cancers detected by screening or clinical suspicion at the first examination. Using one to five bronchoscopic evaluations, 93% of cases were detected within 1 year. Accordingly, sedation and local anesthesia became preferred for the first bronchoscopy to determine lesion visibility. Currently, 25% of radiographically occult sputum-positive lung cancers remain undetected by traditional bronchoscopy.

During routine WLB, early bronchoscopic mucosal changes of squamous cell carcinoma include paleness, dullness, roughening, and microgranularity. An example is shown in Figure 86-1. These changes may be subtle or absent. Before AF bronchoscopy, the workup of positive sputum cytology in a patient with normal imaging studies began with WLB under general anesthesia by obtaining cytology brush samples from each normal appearing bronchial segment. Cytotechnologist assistance during sampling ensures accurate labeling and optimal specimen processing. If a brushing from an unremarkable appearing segment demonstrates malignant cells, repeat site sampling 2 weeks later confirms the diagnosis by excluding false-positive results or contamination by cells from another region. This tedious approach generally has been replaced with AF bronchoscopy.

Even if the cancer source is visible by bronchoscopy, some recommend that radiographically occult lung cancer patients undergo routine brushing of all segmental bronchi or enhanced endoscopic imaging techniques (described below). This is because additional primary malignancies have been discovered in 12.6% of lung segments distant from the visible carcinoma.[7] However, this finding was not replicated in recent AF imaging studies.

The cytological quality of cells obtained by multiple-brushing methods is crucial. Single cancer cells or those with degenerated cytoplasm are misleading because they can disperse widely to contaminate remote segments. Instead, medium to large clusters of cancer cells having basophilic cytoplasm without degeneration are diagnostic. Irrigating the bronchoscopic channel before and after each brushing and careful specimen handling limit cross-contamination.

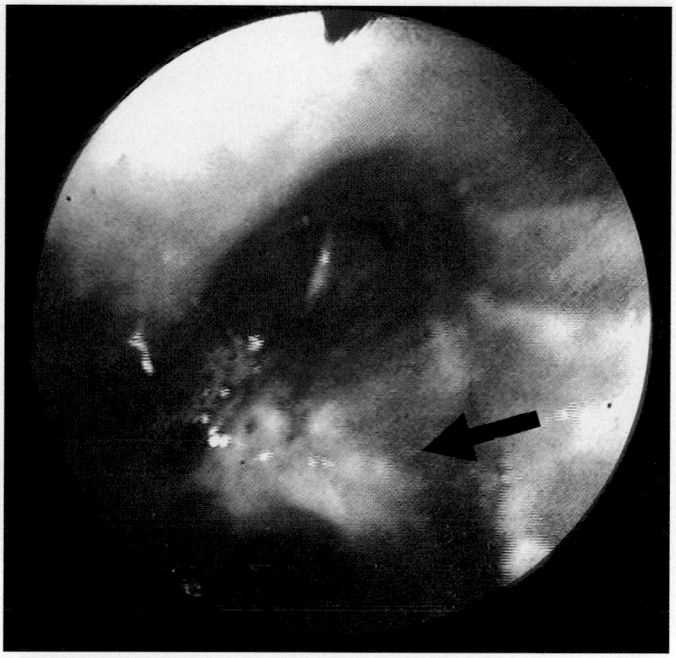

Figure 86-1. Bronchoscopic appearance of early-stage lung cancer. Erythema and nodular necrotic material at the tertiary carina of the left upper lobe (arrow).

Special Staining to Detect Superficial Airway Malignancies

Over the years, various chemicals improved the detection of bronchial mucosal lesions. Examples of these chemicals are: toluidine blue, eosin, berberine sulfate, fluorescein, tetracycline, acridine orange, and hematoporphyrin compounds.

Methylene blue stains malignant bronchial tumors very dark blue, whereas normal mucous membranes remain unchanged. This procedure was termed *chromobronchoscopy*. More recent experiences show that methylene blue can achieve a sensitivity of 86% and a specificity of 89% or better.

The use of hematoporphyrin derivatives to detect early neoplastic lesions in bronchial mucosa preceded its use for therapeutic ablation. Prior to the development of AF bronchoscopy, Lam et al. reported the use of hematoporphyrin derivative at a dose of 0.25 mg/kg, in conjunction with detection of reduced green and red fluorescence from neoplastic tissue in contrast to the robust fluorescence of the normal bronchial epithelium.[8] This differential in tissue fluorescence led to bronchoscopy imaging systems that ultimately did not require administration of a systemic photosensitizer, thus avoiding skin photosensitization.

AF Bronchoscopy and Narrow Band Imaging

Both AF and narrow band imaging (NBI) bronchoscopy are advanced techniques capable to identify Tss as well as premalignant changes in the bronchial mucosa. Both types of systems are available commercially in the United States. NBI bronchoscopy generates mucosal images using two light bandwidths absorbed differentially by superficial capillaries and by blood vessels below the mucosal capillaries. NBI bronchoscopy

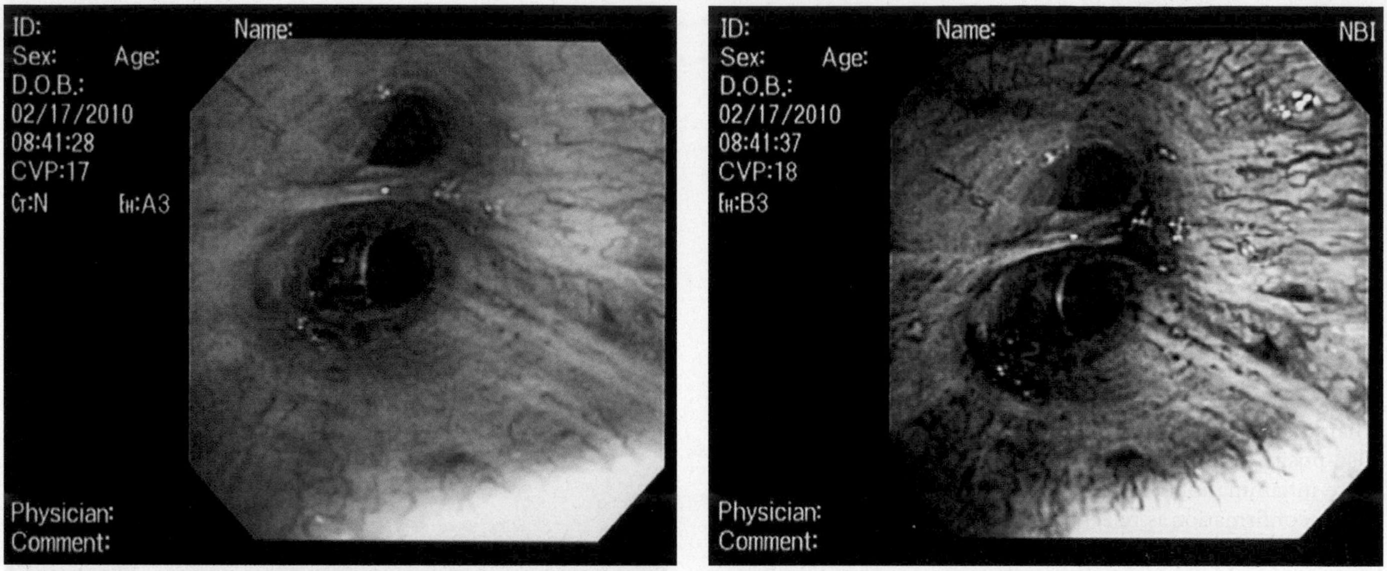

A B

Figure 86-2. NBI image of squamous dysplasia/carcinoma in situ. *A.* WL Bronchoscopy image *B.* NBI bronchoscopy image.

highlights abnormal nests of capillary blood vessels as occurs with angiogenic dysplasia and such resolution increases diagnostic yield NBI imaging also improves the sensitivity of intraepithelial neoplasia detection over WLB alone[9]; however, it does not improve the specificity in a profound way.[10] Figure 86-2 shows an abnormal NBI image of the mucosa in the right middle lobe, which on biopsy revealed squamous dysplasia and carcinoma in situ. NBI has been studied less widely than AF bronchoscopy.

Rather than depending on macroscopic changes in capillary density, AF imaging exploits the native fluorescence of the bronchial epithelium. Figure 86-3 shows the fluorescence spectra of both normal and carcinoma in situ mucosae exposed to a helium–cadmium laser-emitting monochromatic light in the 442-nm range. Figure 86-4 illustrates a superficial central carcinoma detected with AF bronchoscopy. When using the Pinpoint system (Novadaq, Bonita Springs, FL), the lesions appear dark, in contrast to the green appearance of normal mucosa. Other commercially available systems vary slightly in their color scheme but the basic imaging principles are similar

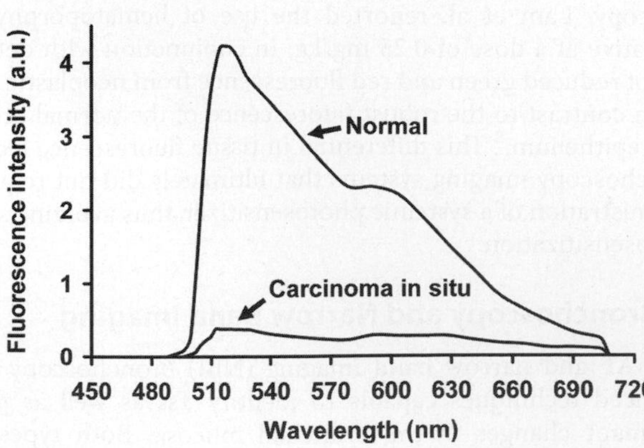

Figure 86-3. Autofluorescence bronchoscopy spectra of both normal and carcinoma in situ mucosa. (Adapted with permission from Hung J, Lam S, LeRiche JC, et al. Autofluorescence of normal and malignant bronchial tissue. *Lasers Surg Med.* 1991;11:99–105.)

(Stortz, Pentax, Wolf). In general, AF bronchoscopy effectively augments WLB in the detection of intraepithelial premalignant lesions. In a meta-analysis of over 1000 cases, AF combined with conventional WLB was 80% sensitive for the detection of preinvasive epithelial neoplasms.[11] In a more recent meta-analysis of over 3000 cases, the sensitivity of AF bronchoscopy plus WLB was double that of WLB alone.[8] The diagnostic sensitivity of AF bronchoscopy or WLB is limited to directly visible lesions in the central airways and does not extend to peripheral lesions that may be identified with CT screening techniques.[12]

AF bronchoscopy also detects hyperplasia and metaplasia (as well as dysplasia and carcinoma in situ) at a 3.75 times higher rate than WLB in an early report by Vermylen et al.[13] Extensive experience with AF bronchoscopy at the British Columbia Cancer Agency Research Centre found that autofluorescence doubled the detection rate of pre invasive lesions from 40% to 80%.[13] In this group of heavy smokers or former smokers with sputum atypia, the carcinoma in situ rate was 1.6%, with moderate-to-severe dysplasia occurring in another 19% of patients. The lesions were relatively small and over half measured less than 1.6 mm in greatest dimension. Investigators found AF bronchoscopy to be superior to standard WLB in Japanese patients with suspicious sputum cytology obtained for symptoms or mass screening. One center compared the accuracy rate of AF bronchoscopy with their formerly employed method of brushing and washing all bronchi and segmental bronchi. Although this was only a historical comparison, a much higher detection rate was seen with AF bronchoscopy.[14]

More convincing evidence was observed in a study of patients with previous lung cancer or abnormal sputum cytology with high-risk factors. In this study, both the bronchoscopist and the order in which the procedures were performed were randomized. AF bronchoscopy detected moderate dysplasia (or more severe lesions) better than WLB (68% versus 22%).[15] Procedure order did not make any difference, and AF bronchoscopy detected angiogenic squamous dysplasia particularly well.

When AF bronchoscopy is combined with low-dose spiral CT (LDSCT) for the early detection of lung cancers, the effect

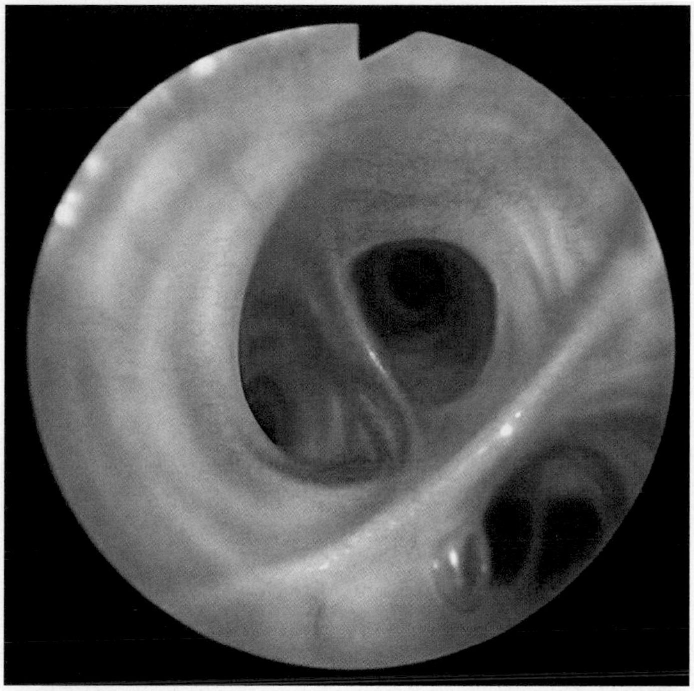

A

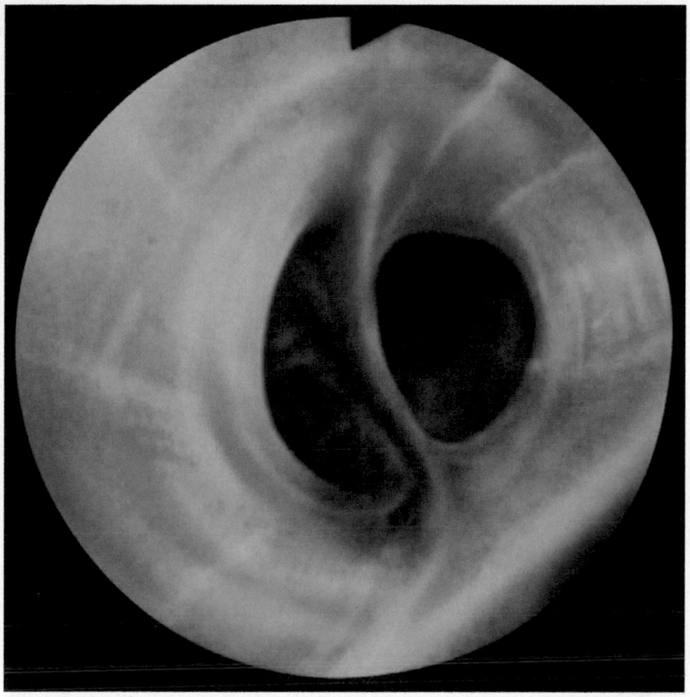

B

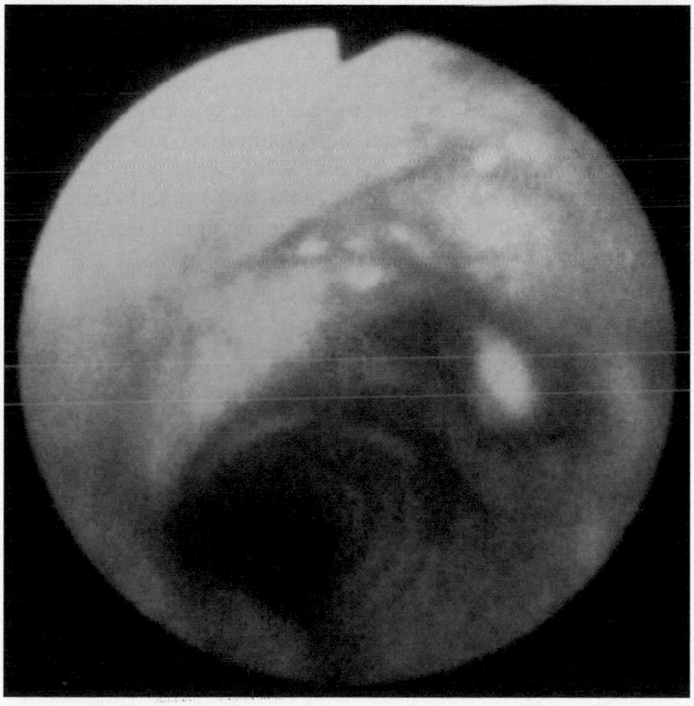

C

Figure 86-4. Autofluorescence bronchoscopy image, normal airways. *A.* White light. *B.* AF bronchoscopy images. *C.* Microinvasive squamous cell carcinoma, proximal trachea.

is additive—malignancies are identified by bronchoscopy that are missed by LDSCT.[16] A strategy incorporating LDSCT with AF bronchoscopy is under investigation in a Pan-Canadian lung cancer screening trial, and this strategy holds promise for detection of Tss in high-risk patients.

AF bronchoscopy has a potential preoperative role in confirmed operable early-stage lung cancer patients. AF bronchoscopy detected additional synchronous preinvasive neoplasms or occult cancers in 23% of such patients and enabled the bronchoscopist to "map" endobronchial lesions before undertaking endobronchial therapies, such as photodynamic therapy (PDT).[17]

Despite no universally accepted guidelines for AF bronchoscopy, it is reasonable to use it for investigating high-grade sputum atypia/malignancy in patients without radiographic abnormalities, or for surveillance of high-risk individuals combined with LDSCT. The role of AF bronchoscopy for surveillance in high-risk scenarios[18,19] is feasible, and further work is needed to see if this strategy will have a salutary effect on lung cancer mortality like LDSCT.

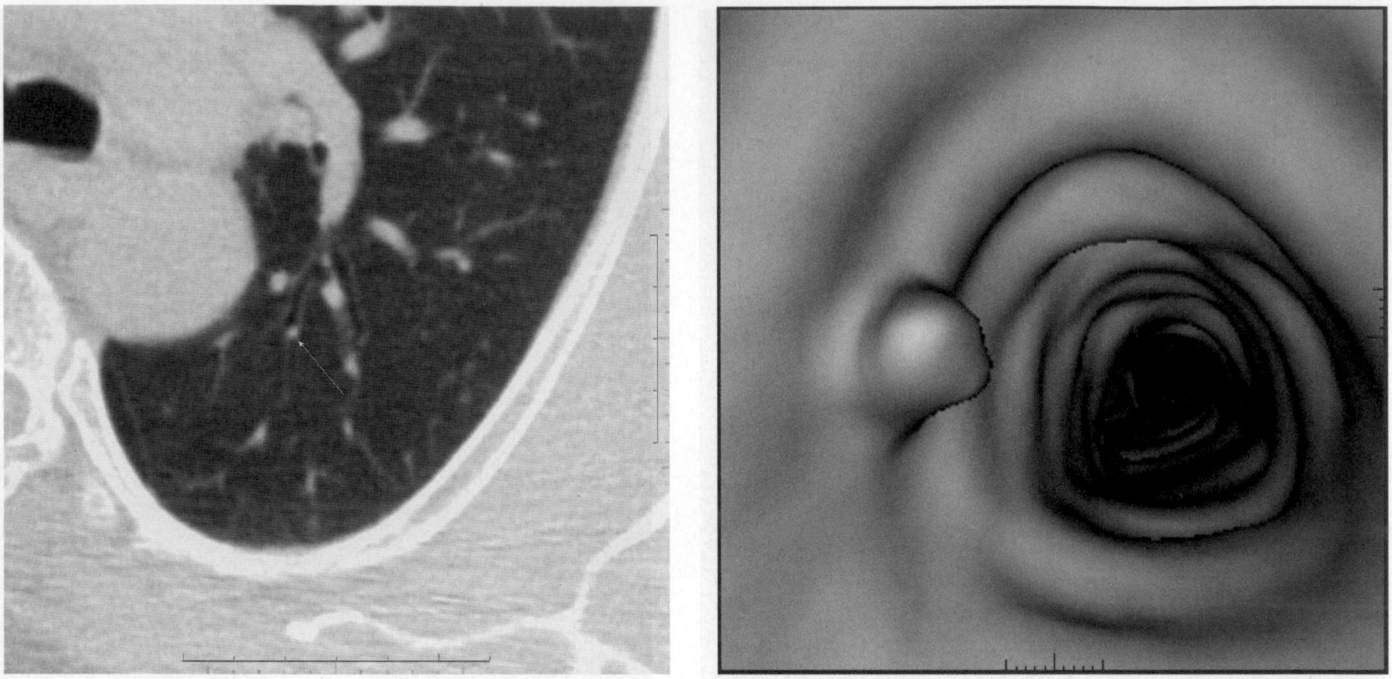

A B

Figure 86-5. Virtual bronchoscopy images. Enhanced thin-slice CT image (*A*) that with similar images is used to create virtual bronchoscopy image showing mucosal irregularity (*B*). (Courtesy of Alan Litwin, M.D., Roswell Park Cancer Institute.)

Optical Coherence Tomography and Confocal Microendoscopy

Although AF bronchoscopy improves sensitivity for the detection of intraepithelial neoplasia, it is far from specific. Many abnormal or suspicious sites seen on AF bronchoscopy turn out to be intraepithelial fibrosis or inflammation. Optical coherence tomography (OCT) is a new technology that permits real-time microscopic imaging. OCT has been used in conjunction with AF bronchoscopy for imaging premalignant lesions and carcinoma in situ.[20] In such systems, a miniaturized confocal microscope is added to a fiberoptic platform like a bronchoscope as an enhanced method to visualize the bronchial epithelium. Optical spectroscopy also attempts to improve the specificity of AF bronchoscopy-detected lesions.

Virtual Bronchoscopy

Advanced modeling of the airway by reconstruction of thin slice CT images has become a popular, noninvasive way to study the proximal tracheobronchial tree (Fig. 86-5). Although promising, it cannot yet detect subtle changes in bronchial mucosa apparent by bronchoscopy. However, improved CT computing resolution fused with imaging that assesses mucosal metabolic activity, like positron emission tomography (PET), will require frequent reassessment of this dynamic technology. In the meantime, thin airway lesions are not detected reliably by virtual bronchoscopy.

PET Scanning

In a study of 22 patients with preinvasive central lung cancer, investigators found that the sensitivity of PET scanning was 73% with a specificity of 85%.[21] These lesions typically represent a smaller size than the accepted threshold for peripheral lung nodules, accounting for the reduced sensitivity. However, meaningful information can be obtained by this imaging if occult advanced disease is present. While we obtain PET scans on patients with positive sputum cytology or superficial central lung cancer routinely, fiberoptic imaging should not be omitted, even if PET scan results are negative.

Endobronchial Ultrasound

Endobronchial ultrasound (EBUS) is a ubiquitous new technology that may make it easier to determine the depth of bronchial wall invasion for superficial central carcinomas. The depth of invasion can predict whether or not endobronchial treatment strategies are feasible. Radial probe EBUS relies on a contact balloon to achieve sonic transmission to demonstrate a five-layered image of the bronchus (Fig. 86-6). There is a 95% EBUS concordance with histologic findings on resected specimens. In the comparison of EBUS with CT findings, there was a diagnostic accuracy of 94% for EBUS compared with only 51% accuracy for chest CT.[22] EBUS has been used prospectively to evaluate the depth of penetration in superficial squamous cell carcinomas considered for PDT. EBUS was used in 18 biopsy-proved superficial squamous cell carcinomas (including three carcinomas in situ), and nine lesions proved to have imaging evidence of intracartilaginous tumor without penetration and were treated successfully by PDT. The remaining nine patients were proved to have extracartilaginous tumors by EBUS imaging and were considered candidates for other therapies, such as surgical resection, chemotherapy, and radiotherapy.[23] Although routine chest CT scanning is not useful for identifying de novo cases of early endobronchial squamous cell carcinoma, investigators have tried to correlate retrospective CT findings with superficial squamous cell carcinoma and also have used thin-slice CT scanning to gauge the depth of penetration with success.

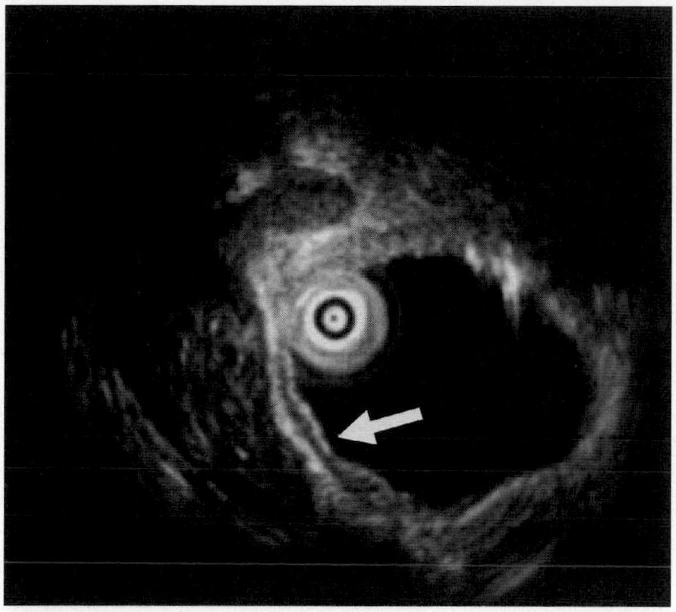

Figure 86-6. Endobronchial ultrasound. Arrow has been added to indicate mucosal layer. (Reproduced with permission from Herth F, Ernst A, Schulz M, et al. Endobronchial ultrasound reliably differentiates between airway infiltration and compression by tumor. *Chest.* 2003;123:458–462.)

Head and Neck Examination

Sputum cytology returns positive in two-thirds of patients with cancer of the larynx or hypopharynx. Accordingly, patients with radiographically occult sputum-positive lung cancer should undergo a head and neck evaluation. Because of the similar risk factors leading to these diseases, the head and neck region may be the actual tumor site, or alternatively, lung cancer may appear years after treatment of a head and neck malignancy.

TREATMENT METHODS FOR SPUTUM-POSITIVE LUNG CANCER

A number of factors complicate the selection of best therapy for a patient with radiographically occult sputum-positive lung cancer. Patients with isolated stage I lung cancer who have good performance status and isolated disease are treated best by surgical resection. To review minimally invasive and traditional methods to control early-stage lung cancer, see Part 8.

However, as the disease becomes more multicentric, or when there is a severe degree of lung impairment such that lung capacity preservation is compelling, other therapies may be safer. Figure 86-7 presents an algorithm for the management of early-stage sputum-positive lung cancer. The sections that follow describe methods that ablate localized lung cancer or premalignant lesions.

Some have argued that squamous cell carcinoma in situ represents a "pseudodisease" associated with overdiagnosis bias. This argument is supported by the indolent tumor biology of some malignancies. It is clear that not all cases of carcinoma in situ progress to invasive squamous cell carcinoma, but many do. Moreover, even preneoplastic lesions (e.g., squamous metaplasia and dysplasia) have been shown to progress when followed by AF bronchoscopy over a period of years, and this issue is currently under investigation in the setting of a national

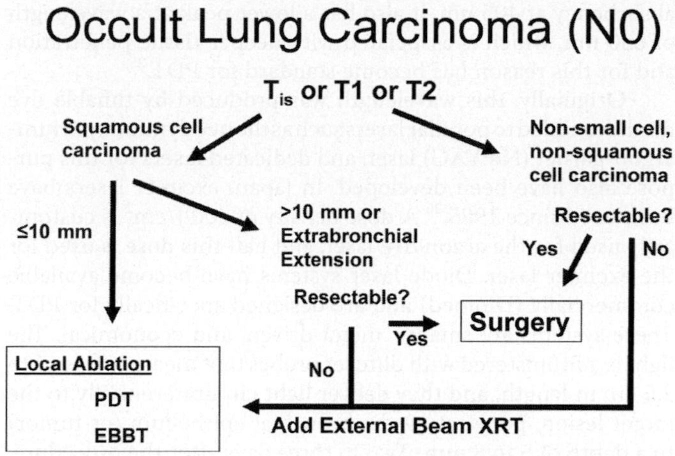

Figure 86-7. Treatment flow diagram for management of superficial central lung cancers. Given institutional experience, other forms of ablative therapy could be used for small mucosal lesions. EBBT, endobronchial brachytherapy; PDT. photodynamic therapy; XRT, radiation therapy.

registry. Carcinoma in situ of the lung has a much higher frequency of stromal invasion than carcinoma in situ of the cervix. When 44 sputum-positive patients from a large-scale screening study who refused intervention were followed prospectively, two-thirds died within 10 years of lung cancer, whereas there was a greater than 90% survival in treated patients. Therefore, sputum-positive patients with normal anticipated longevity should be treated definitively, but the management of frail patients with intermediate-risk lesions is uncertain.

Lesion characteristics aid in selection of the proper approach. A symptomatic lesion warrants treatment to improve quality of life, but over half of patients have no new complaints.[24] Concerns about lymph node metastasis suggest a resectional approach that would permit concomitant nodal resection. Lesions less than 3 mm thick and less than 20 mm in length typically remain node negative.[25] If there is mucosal invasion (approximately 5 mm thickness), there is an 8% incidence of N1 disease, and if the bronchial wall is invaded, the chance is 78%. Another criterion is whether the lesion is visible by WLB. For lesions that are not seen on chest x-ray or bronchoscopy, the risk of nodal metastasis is low. Radiographically occult lesions that are visible by bronchoscopy have a 23% chance of nodal metastasis.

Photodynamic Therapy

PDT is a treatment modality for surface cancers that combines a photosensitizer with a specific light wavelength to achieve a nonthermal photochemical reaction that destroys tumor cells. This technique is facilitated by the relative concentration gradient of the photosensitizer within the tumor compared with normal bronchial epithelium following a systemic bolus. Success of this technology has required parallel advancements in laser technology that allow targeted delivery of specific wavelengths of light and in the refinement of the photosensitizer compounds. Currently, porfimer sodium (Photofrin) is the only photosensitizer approved by the Food and Drug Administration for PDT, and it is designated for use in the palliation of central airway obstruction from endobronchial tumor, as well as for ablation of small endobronchial microinvasive carcinomas with curative intent. Although this compound has peak absorbency at 405 nm, it also has a lower peak at a wavelength of 630 nm, which is associated with deeper tissue penetration and for this reason has become standard for PDT.[25]

Originally, this wavelength was produced by tunable dye modules added to popular lasers such as the neodymium:yttrium-argon-garnet (Nd:YAG) laser, and dedicated lasers for this purpose also have been developed. In Japan, excimer lasers have been used since 1985.[26] A dose density of 200 J/cm^2 is customarily used for the argon dye laser, and half this dose is used for the excimer laser. Diode laser systems have become available commercially (Diomed) and are designed specifically for PDT. These systems are smaller, menu-driven, and economical. The light is administered with diffuser probes that measure from 1 to 2.5 cm in length, and they deliver light circumferentially to the target lesion, penetrating the bronchial epithelium (or tumor) to a depth of 5 to 8 mm. Two to three days after the procedure, a "clean-out" bronchoscopy is necessary to remove necrotic tissue. The debris sometimes can be removed en masse by first loosening it circumferentially with biopsy forceps and then withdrawing the scope while dragging the plug behind. Rigid bronchoscopy permits the use of large forceps, or alternatively, a small cryoprobe can be placed within the debris, activated, and withdrawn with the frozen coagulum attached. At that time, an additional dose of PDT also can be given if there is residual tumor. The primary side effect of porfimer administration is profound skin photosensitivity, which persists for 4 to 6 weeks. Patients can completely avoid the skin rash or sunburn if they observe careful sunlight precautions during this period; however, normal room light exposure hastens the departure of the compound. This side effect may be obviated with new investigational compounds such as 2-(1-hexyloxyethyl)-2-devinyl pyropheophorbide-a (HPPH or Photochlor).[27]

The early reports of the use of PDT for endobronchial therapy were limited by variations in light delivery as well as heterogeneous patient groups. Such an experience cited a complete response rate of only 30%. Selective use on thin neoplasms with visible distal margins by bronchoscopy yielded complete response rates exceeding 90%.[25,26] Table 86-1 shows the relation of tumor size and distal margin to complete response rate. Edell and Cortese reported a group of 13 patients with 14 early-stage lung cancers.[28] These patients received 200 to 400 J/cm^2 of 630-nm irradiation 2 to 4 days following injection of 2.5 mg hematoporphyrin derivative. Eleven tumors showed a complete response after a single treatment and the remaining three after a second treatment; 77% of the tumors showed no recurrence after 7 to 49 months. No substantial complications were observed in these patients. Three patients had a mild sunburn reaction. The authors conclude that PDT may be an alternative to surgery for patients with early squamous cell carcinoma. Kato et al. described a study involving use of Photofrin PDT on 95 lesions in 75 patients with early lung cancer.[26] The complete response rate was related to the tumor size, with a complete response rate of 96.8% for lesions less than 0.5 cm but only 37.5% for those greater than 2 cm. The overall 5-year survival rate for all 75 patients predicted according to Kaplan–Meier analysis was 68.4%.

Table 86-1

PDT SUCCESS AND LESION CHARACTERISTICS

TUMOR CHARACTERISTICS	NUMBER OF LESIONS	CR (RATE)	PR	REC
Size (cm)				
<0.5	31	30 (96.8%)	1	2
0.5–0.9	38	35 (92.1%)	3	3
0.9–1.9	10	8 (80.0%)	2	1
≥2.0	16	6 (37.5%)	10	
Total	95	79 (83.2%)	16	6
Distal margin				
Visible	67	59 (86.8%)	8	5
Invisible	28	20 (71.4%)	8	1
Total	95	79 (83.2%)	16	6

CR, complete response; PR, partial response; REC, recurred.
Source: Aapted with permission from Weigel TL, Martini N. Occult lung cancer treatment. *Chest Surg Clin North Am.* 2000;10:751–762.

If patients are referred for the treatment of radiologically occult lung cancer, then high-resolution CT scanning and AF bronchoscopy should be used before an endobronchial-based therapy such as PDT. AF bronchoscopy permits pretreatment "mapping" of the flat, sometimes poorly visible early endobronchial cancers. At one center, 70% of patients had the endobronchial procedure aborted because of these findings and the treatment switched to resection for cure or palliative intent.[4]

For other patients, however, PDT may be a second-line consideration for cure by avoiding resection or to make a lesser resection surgically feasible.[25] In situations where tumor control is suboptimal, it is generally occult extrabronchial disease and inadequate light delivery that account for the failure.[4] In an updated series from Edell and Cortese, the patients who received PDT had a high complete response rate (93%), and 77% were spared an operation[28]; however, 15% of patients developed recurrence and required surgery. At another center, 44 of 45 patients with a tumor size of less than 1 cm had a complete response. Figure 86-8 illustrates the use of PDT in a patient with superficial central squamous cell carcinoma that was localized to the superficial mucosa of the right upper lobe (RB2).

Skin toxicity from porfimer sodium includes a sunburn-like reaction that may resemble second-degree burns in severe cases. Skin toxicity generally can be eliminated if patients carefully observe sunlight precautions and avoid full-spectrum light. Patients of darker skin, including African Americans, may experience further darkening of the skin with porfimer. Local toxicity from PDT effect is seen in all patients; this includes endobronchial erythema with tenacious mucus formation in the area of treatment. The patient's ability to tolerate this local reaction must be weighed against the severity of the underlying lung disease (e.g., chronic obstructive pulmonary disease) before PDT is considered. Other toxicities of porfimer are uncommon and generally are grade 2 or less and include rises in aspartate aminotransferase/alanine aminotransferase (AST/ALT) levels, pleural effusion, and allergies. Posttreatment chest soreness or mild-to-moderate pain is seen occasionally and resolves quickly with oral analgesics. Most of these studies were dominated by men with squamous cell carcinoma cell types.[26] Bronchial stenosis from PDT is rare and is not a feature of any of the major series that have been reported in lung cancer.

Current research in PDT includes new methods of light delivery and new photosensitizers, as described earlier. For example, investigators are examining the delivery of light more distally throughout the branched airway structures using substances of various refractive indices.[29] In summary, PDT has been used more extensively than any other endobronchial modality for the treatment of microinvasive endobronchial carcinoma and carcinoma in situ and has the advantage of being

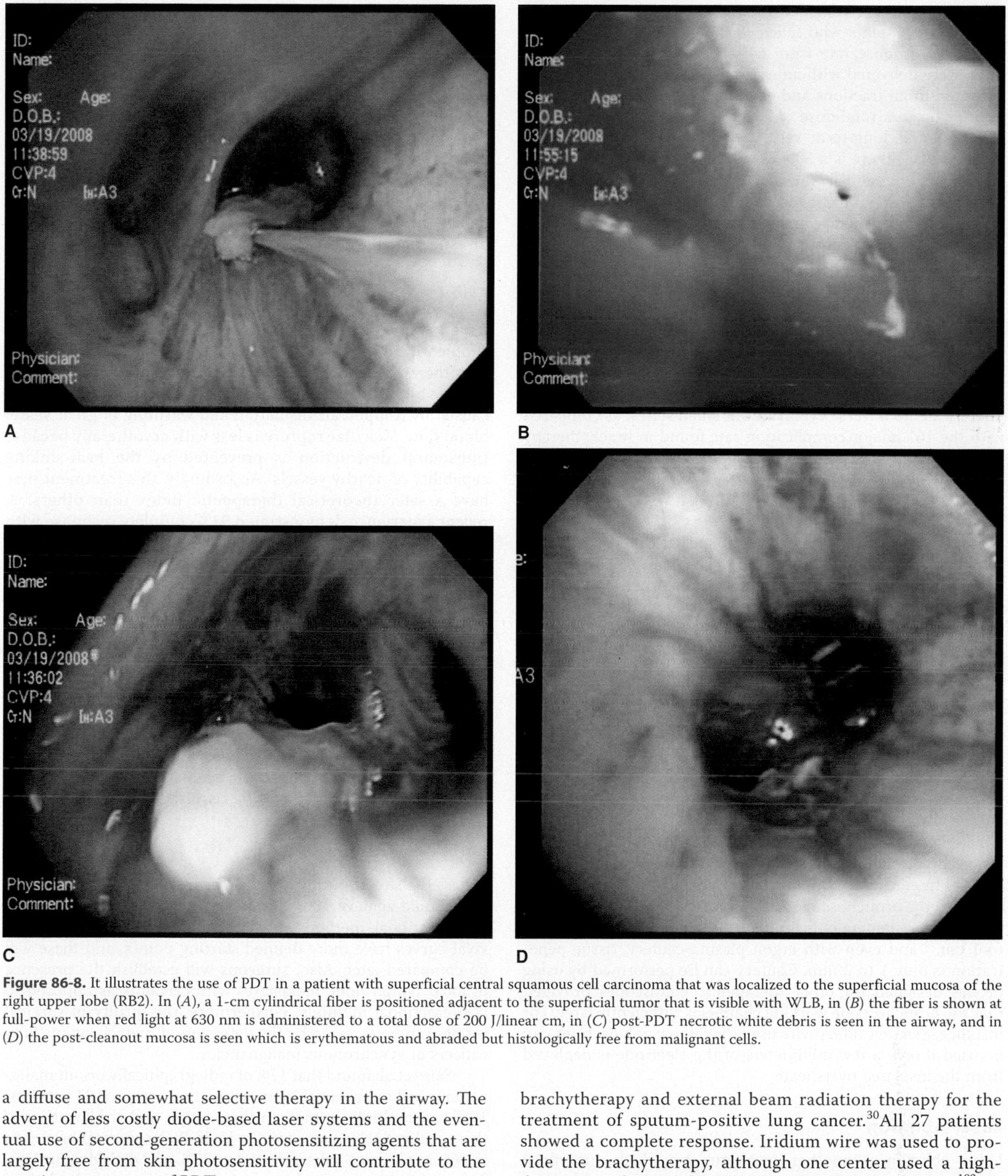

Figure 86-8. It illustrates the use of PDT in a patient with superficial central squamous cell carcinoma that was localized to the superficial mucosa of the right upper lobe (RB2). In (*A*), a 1-cm cylindrical fiber is positioned adjacent to the superficial tumor that is visible with WLB, in (*B*) the fiber is shown at full-power when red light at 630 nm is administered to a total dose of 200 J/linear cm, in (*C*) post-PDT necrotic white debris is seen in the airway, and in (*D*) the post-cleanout mucosa is seen which is erythematous and abraded but histologically free from malignant cells.

a diffuse and somewhat selective therapy in the airway. The advent of less costly diode-based laser systems and the eventual use of second-generation photosensitizing agents that are largely free from skin photosensitivity will contribute to the growing acceptance of PDT.

Brachytherapy

There is less experience with radiation therapy, but early reports using new treatment techniques have been promising. Two centers reported the use of a combination of brachytherapy and external beam radiation therapy for the treatment of sputum-positive lung cancer.[30] All 27 patients showed a complete response. Iridium wire was used to provide the brachytherapy, although one center used a high-dose rate, whereas the other used a low-dose rate (^{192}Ir). Unfortunately, many of these patients sustained a severe bronchial stenosis or other serious complications generally not observed with PDT. Care needs to be taken with brachytherapy for early-stage lung cancer because of the difficulty of positioning a radiation dose wire at the optimal distance from the targeted tissue.

Another center decided to use external beam radiation therapy for patients who failed PDT and raised their overall complete response rate from 64% to 90%. These treatments often were delivered with an external dose of a roughly 40 Gy delivered in 20 fractions and escalating intraluminal therapies of 5 Gy up to a total dose of 25 Gy.[25] Although the complete response and long-term results of brachytherapy approach those of PDT, there is a 50% asymptomatic bronchial stenosis rate and an occasionally unexpected fatal complication such as hemoptysis.[25] PDT has been combined in a sequential manner with high-dose–rate brachytherapy for palliation of bulky tumor central airway obstruction, but this strategy has not been reported for microinvasive disease or carcinoma in situ.

Brachytherapy has allowed treatments to areas invisible to conventional imaging, such as needed by the radiation oncologist for external beam planning. This problem has been addressed by use of endoscopically guided three-dimensional conformal radiation planning where the bronchoscope was used to mark the radiographically occult tumors in four patients.[31] There were no adverse events in this small series, as compared with the 16% major complication rate found in brachytherapy trials probably caused by suboptimal catheter positioning.[32]

Coagulation Techniques

Since PDT historically has required special expertise, expensive light sources, and a systemic dose of an expensive drug to achieve ablation at a localized level, less expensive technology that delivers similar local tissue destruction is appealing. In a pilot investigation, van Boxem et al. studied 13 patients using 30 W of high-frequency electrocautery to cause nonselective tissue destruction. Cautery was applied until all visible tumor showed necrosis. An 80% complete response rate was observed. In the three patients who did not achieve a complete response, PDT was attempted and also failed.[33] Recently, argon plasma coagulation guided by AF bronchoscopy has been used to ablate radiographically occult lung cancer. Since these therapies are less expensive and do not cause photosensitivity, they will be watched with interest as more experience accumulates. Unlike PDT, this method relies on delivering therapy to areas visible by bronchoscopy and is a focal treatment rather than diffuse. In contrast, PDT may affect small tumor patches not visible to the bronchoscope and can treat a much wider disease area. Cautery generally is limited to lesions less than or equal to 1 cm,[25] and even with argon plasma cautery, tissue penetration is only 1 to 2 mm. Cautery can be performed by using probes designed for other therapeutic endoscopes provided that the bronchoscope working channel is sufficiently large. For instance, a snare cautery wire used for colonic polypectomy can be used if only a few millimeters of the electrode is deployed from the insulated oversheath.

Laser Ablation

Laser ablation is another technique by which superficial mucosa is destroyed. Some centers use a laser with rigid bronchoscopy because the larger available forceps expedite debridement. In general, the technique employs an Nd:YAG laser in which the initial beam of radiation (<30 W) is applied to the tumor for coagulation. Then a power setting near 50 W can vaporize residual superficial tumor. For a subset of early neoplasms from a large palliative laser report, a complete response rate was achieved in all 23 patients with no evidence of recurrence.[34] In contrast to other ablative techniques, this type of ablative therapy may be more risky because of a deeper penetration potential of certain laser wavelengths. This is generally not a problem during the ablation of bulky tumors that occlude the airway—a commonly accepted indication for laser bronchoscopy. However, it may be a problem when full-thickness bronchial penetration occurs without the "protection" afforded by tumor encasement. Because of this concern and the other options available, the Nd:YAG laser for superficial malignancy is not recommended and may be best saved for investigational use.

Cryotherapy

Cryotherapy provides another potentially economical and simple way in which to treat radiologically occult lung cancer. Cryotherapy was once used to treat large pulmonary malignancies but was limited by the variations in heat transmission caused by trapped air insulation and warming of great vessel blood flow. Vascular rupture is less with cryotherapy because transmural destruction is prevented by the heat-sinking capability of nearby vessels. Accordingly, this treatment may have a safer theoretical therapeutic index than others. A recent experience demonstrated 91% complete response with no adverse events,[35] but long-term effects, including bronchial stenosis, have not been explored. Cryotherapy usually is performed by flexible bronchoscopy, but it also may be performed by rigid bronchoscopy because it allows introduction of a nitrous oxide cooled cryoprobe. Three cycles of freezing and thawing are performed on each lesion, and each cold application lasts approximately 20 seconds. The tumor surface is treated with a marginal area of 5 mm of normal mucosa around the tumor.[35] If the lesion occurs on a carina, the cryoprobe is applied to each side of the carina and then to the tip itself. About 2 weeks following the initial cryotherapy, an additional bronchoscopic evaluation is necessary, and multiple treatments also may be required.

Lung Resection

Unless the site of occult lung cancer is missed, surgical resection should achieve 100% complete response compared to the nonresectional methods described earlier. Accordingly, survival curves have more defined starting points, and these will be compared later. Also, surgeons will establish the presence of lobar lymph node metastases with certainty as opposed to nonresectional methods. Furthermore, the quality of surgical results can be assessed by the detection of metachronous lung cancers or synchronous malignancies.

Saito et al. found that 17% of radiographically occult malignancies had extrabronchial invasion. In a series of 94 patients, 10% had multiple primary malignancies, and the location of these malignancies was found to be in the segmental bronchus in 36% of patients, subsegmental in 20%, and divisional in 18%. The remainder appeared in more distal sites or tracheal sites. Most of these patients were detected by sputum cytology found in large-scale screening. Of 127 patients in their subsequent report, 97 were either T1N0M0 or earlier stage; only 8 of the entire group had N1 or N2 nodes.[36] The techniques and results of lung resection for various stages of lung cancer are described in Part 8.

Medical Treatment for Sputum-Positive Lung Cancer

For the various chemotherapy options for patients with invasive lung cancer, the reader is referred to Chapter 76. *Secondary chemoprevention* actually refers to the medical treatment of premalignant bronchial epithelial lesions, including metaplasia and dysplasia but not including carcinoma in situ. There have been multiple secondary chemoprevention trials for patients with premalignant lesions (Table 86-2). Lee conducted a secondary chemoprevention trial in 152 smokers with biopsy-confirmed metaplasia or dysplasia of the lung epithelium and found that isotretinoin (13-cRA; 1 mg/kg) did not cause regression of the lesion when compared with placebo.[37] In a more recent study from the same institution, 9-*cis*-retinoic acid was compared with 13-cRA plus α-tocopherol or placebo. This group of 226 former smokers was randomly assigned to treatment groups and re-evaluated in 3 months. Six biopsies from predetermined sites were evaluated. The results showed that while neither treatment affected the histology of the sites, 9-*cis*-retinoic acid did restore the retinoic acid β receptor (RARβ) in a significant number of lesions. Other compounds that have been tried in this effort include fenretinide, etretinate, β-carotene with retinol, anethole dithiolethione, vitamin B_{12}, budesonide, and folic acid. The only trials that have shown a beneficial effect in the histology of the bronchial epithelium were those that used AF bronchoscopy for detection of the endpoint (see Table 86-2). Oral prostacyclin has shown potential benefit in the treatment of endobronchial dysplasia. In a multicenter double-blind, randomized, phase II placebo-controlled trial of 125 patients with dysplasia, oral iloprost improved the dysplasia index in former (but not current) smokers over a 6-month treatment period.[38] Other chemoprevention agents under investigation include targeted agents (e.g., gefitinib and erlotinib), COX-2 inhibitors (e.g., exisulind and celecoxib), and antiproliferative agents (e.g., vitamin D). The success of retinoids in the prevention of head and neck malignancies is proof in principle that such a strategy may be useful in the secondary chemoprevention of lung cancer. Ultimately, if any of these agents proves to be effective for premalignant lesions, it also potentially may find application in the treatment of carcinoma in situ.

Summary of Treatment Options

Surgery is considered the optimal therapy for patients with late- to early-stage sputum-positive lung cancer. However, patients who have sputum-positive lung cancer seem to have notable differences. Generally, survival for these patients is better than that in the stage I lung carcinoma population, with survival rates between 81% and 90%.[36] In one screening population, the overall survival rate was 74% in those resected for cure and 55% when combining those receiving radiation and/or surgical therapy.[46] This is much greater than an overall expected survival of unscreened patients, which is expected to be about 17%.

Because of a selection effect, these patients have 4% per year or higher rates of developing secondary lung carcinomas, many of which are also occult. This is double the rate of a general population. In addition, the survival rate falls from 90% to 59% if the patients have multiple sites of malignancy rather than a solitary site detected by sputum.[36] In one center, the operative mortality was double that of other patients receiving lobectomy, possibly because of the increased incidence of airflow obstruction and other comorbidities associated with higher rates of sputum positivity. We have found that there is a direct relationship between the degree of airway obstruction and the presence of premalignant lesions in the airway.[47]

For the other therapies listed earlier, such as PDT, radiation (with brachytherapy), electrocautery, and cryotherapy, approximately 30% to 35% of patients suffer recurrences 1 to 5 years following the initial therapy.[26,28,48] This, combined with the repetitive application of such therapies, makes it difficult to construct clean survival curves like those after a definitive event such as surgical resection. For patients in whom surgery is not an option because of multicentricity or the need to conserve pulmonary function, PDT is a good option that has the most experience to support it, and because it can be repeated in the event of local recurrence. The other therapies listed earlier are considered alternative options with less supporting evidence. A recent review suggested that Nd:YAG laser therapy has the weakest evidence to support it and carries a relative high risk of perforation.[48]

Table 86-2

SELECTED SECONDARY CHEMOPREVENTION TRIALS IN LUNG CANCER

AUTHOR	ENDPOINT	METHOD	COMPOUND	RESULT	*N*
Lee et al.[37]	Dysplasia/metaplasia index	WLB	Isotretinoin	Neg	152
Kurie et al.[39]	Metaplasia and dysplasia	WLB	4HP retinamide	Neg[a]	139
Lam et al.[40]	Dysplasia grade	AFB	ADT	Pos[b]	112
Kurie et al.[41]	Metaplasia and RARβ expression	WLB	9-*cis*-retinoic acid	Pos[c]	226
Lam et al.[42]	Dysplasia and MI	AFB	Retinol	Neg	81
Kohlhaufl et al.[43]	Metaplasia and dysplasia	AFB	Inhaled retinol	Pos	11
Ayoub et al.[44]	RARβ	WLB	13-*cis*-retinoic acid	Pos[d]	44
Lam et al.[45]	Dysplasia	AFB	Budesonide	Neg	112
Keith et al.[38]	Dysplasia	AFB	Iloprost	Pos	152

AF, autofluorescence; B, bronchoscopy; Pos, positive study; Neg, negative study; RARβ, retinoic acid receptor beta; WL, white light.

[a]Although 4HPR did not reverse bronchial epithelial histology, it did modulate expression of hTERT.

[b]ADT (anethole dithiolethione) did not affect nuclear morphometry index (MI).

[c]Only 6.9% of the subjects had metaplasia at baseline.

[d]Effect on dysplasia and metaplasia not reported.

Source: Adapted from Lee JS, Lippman SM, Benner SE, et al. Randomized placebo-controlled trial of isotretinoin in chemoprevention of bronchial squamous metaplasia. *J Clin Oncol*. 1994;12:937–945.

SURVEILLANCE OPTIONS

Patients who have sputum-positive lung cancer probably have a higher incidence of subsequent lung cancer, many of which are also radiographically occult. Sometimes these early lung cancers can be synchronous (9.3%). Patients who have multiple synchronous cancers may have a worse prognosis, although cure of each cancer can be achieved if definitive treatment is possible. While the risk for new cancers is about 1% to 2% per year in the general population, the rate is higher (perhaps double) for centrally located early-stage cancer. One study found 13% metachronous primaries.[49] Recently published results of the National Lung Screening Trial (NLST) have provided proof-in-principle that early detection of lung cancer is a strategy that can lower mortality.[50] In this pivotal study, 53,454 current or former smokers were randomized to undergo either low-dose CT of the chest or posterior/anterior and lateral chest radiography on a yearly basis for 3 years. Lung cancer screening with CT resulted in a 20% decrease in mortality from lung cancer, compared with the control group. In the extreme high-risk population of patients previously cured of lung cancer, we believe that patients should have annual CT scans to detect new cancers. Since limited data are available to guide decision making for unusual patients treated for sputum-positive cancer, it is reasonable to consider screening or surveillance with AF bronchoscopy, which has better sensitivity than sputum cytology. This is so because subsequent lesions tend to be multicentric and radiologically occult. Alternatively, a more sophisticated surveillance technology such as AF bronchoscopy may be selected if available.

In patients who have had ablative therapy using PDT or other methods, surveillance should be determined by the degree of response to the original lesion, as well as by the presence of other suspicious lesions. Generally, serial follow-up evaluations every 3 to 4 months for 1 to 2 years are needed at a minimum. Occasionally, lesions may appear to be resected and return later as advanced node-positive disease despite this surveillance.

SUMMARY

Superficial spreading lung cancer confined to the wall of the trachea or mainstem bronchus, as well as carcinoma in situ represent an uncommon subset of lung cancer. Figure 86-7 represents a treatment flow diagram for management of superficial central lung cancers. These patients may present with sputum-positive, radiographically occult lung cancer at an early stage with a potentially better prognosis. Accordingly, some of these patients with small lesions can undergo limited ablative therapies to achieve cancer control without sacrificing vital lung capacity. Most of these patients are subsequently at high risk of upper aerodigestive malignancies and require careful long-term surveillance.

CASE HISTORY

A 45-year-old woman with a 60 pack-year smoking history underwent an empirical course of antibiotics for a persistent cough for the presumed diagnosis of bronchitis. She was otherwise healthy and had few complaints except for occasional exercise intolerance. Both her parents had died of lung cancer in their sixth decade. Physical examination was normal except for scattered wheezes and evidence of recent tobacco use. A chest roentgenogram was interpreted as normal, and this was followed by a CT scan that was likewise unremarkable except for two peripheral 3-mm nodules. A 3-day collection of sputum showed suspicious cytology and WLB show scattered areas of mild mucosal changes, some of which showed dysplasia on endobronchial biopsy. The patient was referred for AF bronchoscopy that revealed a 5-mm patch of carcinoma in situ in the right upper lobe orifice with a visible distal margin. No other abnormal areas were diagnosed. After a discussion of relative risks for various procedures, including pulmonary resection, the patient selected PDT. Two days after a systemic administration of porfimer sodium, the patient received 200 J/cm^2 of 630-nm light to this mucosal lesion, and a repeat examination several days later demonstrated inflammation and coagulum over the site of the lesion. In 3 months there was no tumor visible at that site. Four years later, the patient had ceased her smoking habit and had no bronchoscopic abnormalities but developed a peripheral left upper lobe nodule on surveillance CT scan that was active by PET imaging. A video-assisted thoracic surgery (VATS) wedge biopsy confirmed adenocarcinoma, and a minimally invasive lobectomy treated what was determined ultimately to be stage IA disease.

EDITOR'S COMMENT

Sputum-positive but radiographically occult lung cancers are rare. Patients presenting with this scenario require careful evaluation and close follow-up with chest CT and interval bronchoscopies until detection of the tumor and for a lifetime thereafter. It is unclear whether AF bronchoscopy impacts survival in these patients. Nevertheless, it is certainly a diagnostic option. Unlike esophageal cancer and Barrett's esophagitis, high-grade dysplasia and carcinoma in situ in the airways are not always indications for aggressive therapy.

–Mark J. Krasna

References

1. McWilliams A, Mayo J, MacDonald S, et al. Lung cancer screening: a different paradigm. *Am J Respir Crit Care Med.* 2003;168:1167–1173.
2. Detterbeck FC, Boffa DJ, Tanoue LT, et al. Details and difficulties regarding the new lung cancer staging system. *Chest,* 2010;137(5):1172–1180.
3. Tockman MS, Mulshine JL. The early detection of occult lung cancer. *Chest Surg Clin N Am.* 2000;10:737–749.
4. Woolner LB, Fontana RS, Cortese DA, et al. Roentgenographically occult lung cancer: pathologic findings and frequency of multicentricity during a 10-year period. *Mayo Clin Proc.* 1984;59:453–466.
5. Auerbach O, Hammond EC, Garfinkel L. Changes in bronchial epithelium in relation to cigarette smoking, 1955–1960 vs. 1970–1977. *N Engl J Med.* 1979;300:381–385.
6. Johnston WW, Bossen EH. Ten years of respiratory cytopathology at Duke University Medical Center. II. The cytopathologic diagnosis of lung cancer during the years 1970 to 1974, with a comparison between cytopathology and histopathology in the typing of lung cancer. *Acta Cytol.* 1981;25:499–505.
7. Sato M, Saito Y, Nagamoto N, et al. Diagnostic value of differential brushing of all 'branches of the bronchi in patients with sputum positive or suspected positive for lung cancer. *Acta Cytol.* 1993;37:879–883.

8. Lam S, Palcic B, McLean D, et al. Detection of early lung cancer using low dose Photofrin II. *Chest.* 1990;97:333–337.
9. Herth FJ, Eberhardt R, Anantham D, et al. Narrow-band imaging bronchoscopy increases the specificity of bronchoscopic early lung cancer detection. *J Thorac Oncol.* 2009;4(9):1060–1065.
10. Zaric B, Perin B, Becker HD, et al. Combination of narrow band imaging (NBI and autofluorescence imaging (AFI) videobronchoscopy in endoscopic assessment of lunch cancer extension. *Med Oncol.* 2012;29(3):1638–1642 .
11. Lam S, MacAulay C, Leriche JC, et al. Detection and localization of early lung cancer by fluorescence bronchoscopy. *Cancer.* 2000;89:2468–2473.
12. Schreiber G, McCrory D. Performance characteristics of different modalities for diagnosis of suspected lung cancer: summary of published evidence. *Chest.* 2003;123:115S–128S.
13. Vermylen P, Pierard P, Roufosse C, et al. Detection of bronchial preneoplastic lesions and early lung cancer with fluorescence bronchoscopy: a study about its ambulatory feasibility under local anaesthesis. *Lung Cancer.* 1999;25:161–168.
14. Sato M, Sakurada A, Sagawa M, et al. Diagnostic results before and after introduction of autofluorescence bronchoscopy in patients suspected of having lung cancer detected by sputum cytology in lung cancer mass screening. *Lung Cancer.* 2001;32:247–253.
15. Hirsch FR, Prindiville SA, Miller YE, et al. Fluorescence versus white-light bronchoscopy for detection of preneoplastic lesions: a randomized study. *J Natl Cancer Inst.* 2001;93:1385–1391.
16. McWilliams AM, Jaoy JR, Ahn MI, et al. Lung cancer screening using multislice thin-section computed tomography and autofluorescence bronchoscopy. *J Thorac Oncol.* 2006;1(1):61–68.
17. Pierard P, Faber J, Hutsebaut J, et al. Synchronous lesions detected by autofluorescence bronchoscopy in patients with high-grade preinvasive lesions and occult invasive squamous cell carcinoma of the proximal airways. *Lung Cancer.* 2004;46:341–347.
18. Jeremy George P, Banerjee AK, Read CA, et al. Surveillance for the detection of early lung cancer in patients with bronchial dysplasia. *Thorax.* 2007;62(1):43–50.
19. Loewen G, Natarajan N, Tan D, et al. Autofluorescence bronchoscopy for lunch cancer surveillance based on risk assessment. *Thorax.* 62(4):2007;335–340.
20. Thiberville L, Moreno-Swirc LS, Vercauteren T, et al. *In vivo* imaging of the bronchial wall microstructure using fibered confocal fluorescence microscopy. *Am J Respir Crit Care Med.* 2007;175:22–31.
21. Pasic A, Brokx HA, Comans EF, et al. Detection and staging of preinvasive lesions and occult lung cancer in the central airways with 18F-fluorodeoxyglucose positron emission tomography: a pilot study. *Clin Cancer Res.* 2005;11(17):6186–6189.
22. Herth F, Ernst A, Schulz M, et al. Endobronchial ultrasound reliably differentiates between airway infiltration and compression by tumor. *Chest.* 2003;123:458–462.
23. Miyazu Y, Miyazawa T, Kurimoto N, et al. Endobronchial ultrasonography in the assessment of centrally located early-stage lung cancer before photodynamic therapy. *Am J Respir Crit Care Med.* 2002;165:832–837.
24. Breuer RH, Pasic A, Smit EF, et al. The natural course of preneoplastic lesions in bronchial epithelium. *Clin Cancer Res.* 2005;11:537–543.
25. Weigel TL, Martini N. Occult lung cancer treatment. *Chest Surg Clin N Am.* 2000;10:751–762.
26. Kato H, Okunaka T, Shimatani H. Photodynamic therapy for early stage bronchogenic carcinoma. *J Clin Laser Med Surg.* 1996;14:235–238.
27. Loewen GM, Ravi P, Bellnier D, et al. Endobronchial photodynamic therapy for lung cancer. *Lasers Surg Med.* 2006;38:364–370.
28. Edell ES, Cortese DA. Photodynamic therapy in the management of early superficial squamous cell carcinoma as an alternative to surgical resection. *Chest.* 1992;102:1319–1322.
29. Friedberg JS, Skema C, Burdick J, et al. A novel technique for light delivery through branched or bent anatomic structures. *J Thorac Cardiovasc Surg.* 2003;126:1963–1967.
30. Fuwa N, Ito Y, Matsumoto A, et al. The treatment results of 40 patients with localized endobronchial cancer with external beam irradiation and intraluminal irradiation using low dose rate ^{192}Ir thin wires with a new catheter. *Radiother Oncol.* 2000;56:189–195.
31. Tavecchio L, Gramaglia A, Mancini A, et al. Bronchoscopically-guided conformal radiation therapy for radiographically occult lung carcinoma. *Radiother Oncol.* 2001;58:269–271.
32. Perol M, Caliandro R, Pommier P, et al. Curative irradiation of limited endobronchial carcinomas with high-dose rate brachytherapy: results of a pilot study. *Chest.* 1997;111:1417–1423.
33. van Boxem T, Venmans B, Schramel F, et al. Radiographically occult lung cancer treated with fiberoptic bronchoscopic electrocautery: a pilot study of a simple and inexpensive technique. *Eur Respir J.* 1998;11:169–172.
34. Cavaliere S, Venuta F, Foccoli P, et al. Endoscopic treatment of malignant airway obstructions in 2,008 patients. *Chest.* 1996;110:1536–1542.
35. Deygas N, Froudarakis M, Ozenne G, et al. Cryotherapy in early superficial bronchogenic carcinoma. *Chest.* 2001;120:26–31.
36. Saito Y, Sato M, Sagawa M, et al. Multicentricity in resected occult bronchogenic squamous cell carcinoma. *Ann Thorac Surg.* 1994;57:1200–1205.
37. Lee JS, Lippman SM, Benner SE, et al. Randomized placebo-controlled trial of isotretinoin in chemoprevention of bronchial squamous metaplasia. *J Clin Oncol.* 1994;12:937–945.
38. Keith RL, Blatchford PJ, Kittelson J, et al. Oral iloprost improves endobronchial dysplasia in former smokers. *Cancer Prev Res (Phila).* 2011;4(6): 793–802.
39. Kurie JM, Lee JS, Khuri FR, et al. N-(4-hydroxyphenyl)retinamide in the chemoprevention of squamous metaplasia and dysplasia of the bronchial epithelium. *Clin Cancer Res.* 2000;6:2973–2979.
40. Lam S, MacAulay C, LeRiche JC, et al. A randomized phase IIb trial of anethole dithiolethione in smokers with bronchial dysplasia. *J Natl Cancer Inst.* 2002;94:1001–1009.
41. Kurie JM, Lotan R, Lee JJ, et al. Treatment of former smokers with 9-cisretinoic acid reverses loss of retinoic acid receptor-beta expression in the bronchial epithelium: results from a randomized placebo-controlled trial. *J Natl Cancer Inst.* 2003;95:206–214.
42. Lam S, Xu X, Parker-Kelin H, et al. Surrogate end-point biomarker analysis in a retinol chemoprevention trial in current and former smokers with bronchial dysplasia. *Int J Oncol.* 2003;23:1607–1613.
43. Kohlhaufl M, Haussinger K, Stanzel F. Inhalation of aerosolized Vitamin A: reversibility of metaplasia and dysplasia of human respiratory epithelia—a prospective pilot study. *Eur J Med Res.* 2002;7:72–78.
44. Ayoub J, Jean-Francois R, Cormier Y, et al. Placebo-controlled trial of 13-cisretinoic acid activity on retinoic acid receptor-beta expression in a population at high risk: implications for chemoprevention of lung cancer. *J Clin Oncol.* 1999;17:3546–3552.
45. Lam S, LeRiche JC, McWilliams A, et al. A randomized phase IIb trial of pulmicort turbuhaler (budesonide) in people with dysplasia of the bronchial epithelium. *Clin Cancer Res.* 2004;10:6502–6511.
46. Bechtel JJ, Petty TL, Saccomanno G. Five year survival and later outcome of patients with x-ray occult lung cancer detected by sputum cytology. *Lung Cancer.* 2000;30:1–7.
47. Jayaprakash V, Loewen G, Menezes R, et al. "Spirometric Surveillance for Intraepithelial Neoplasia". *American College of Chest Physicians* Annual Meeting, Salt Lake City, Utah, October, 2006.
48. Mathur PN, Edell E, Sutedja T, et al. Treatment of early stage non-small cell lung cancer. *Chest.* 2003;123:176S–180S.
49. Koike T, Terashima M, Takizawa T, et al. Surgical results for centrally-located early stage lung cancer. *Ann Thorac Surg.* 2000;70:1176–1179; discussion 1179–1180.
50. National Screening Research Team; Aberle DR, Adams AM, Berg CD, et al. Reduced lung cancer mortality with low-dose computed tomographic screening. *N Engl J Med.* 2011;365(5):395–409.

PART 15

MULTIMODALITY MANAGEMENT OF NON–SMALL-CELL LUNG CANCER

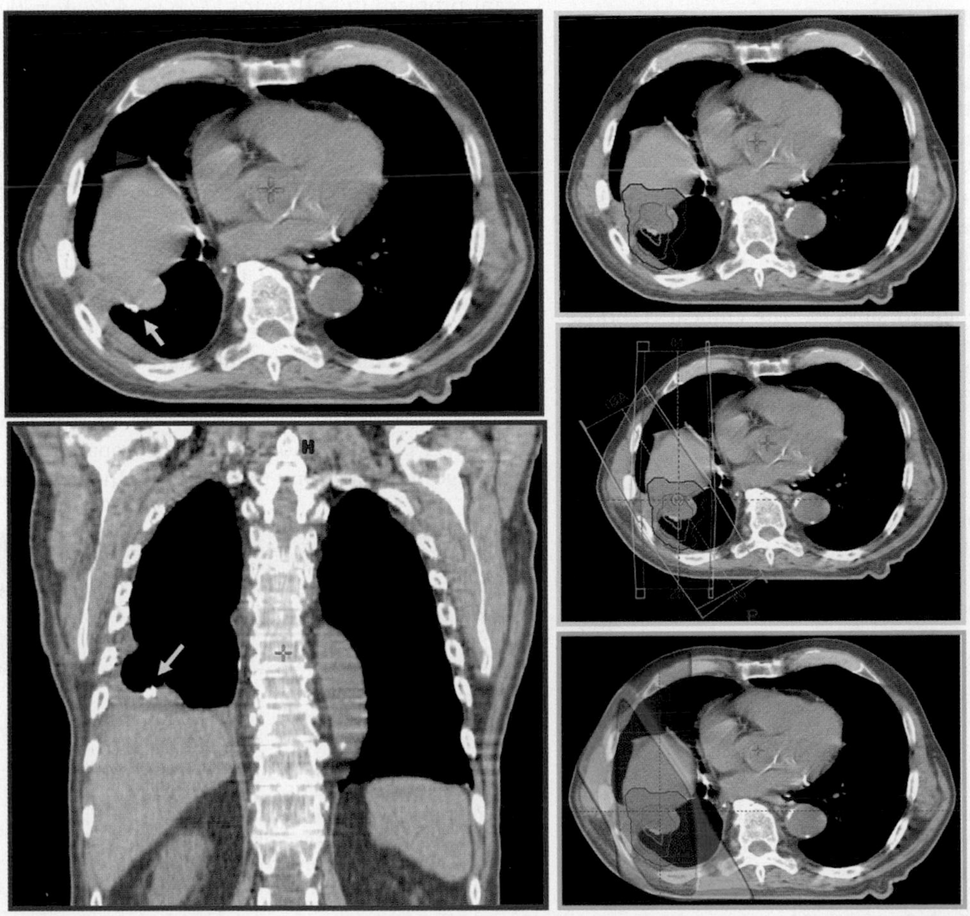

87 Neoadjuvant and Adjuvant Radiation Therapy in Lung Cancer

Raymond H. Mak and Elizabeth H. Baldini

Keywords: Radiation therapy, neoadjuvant, adjuvant, locally advanced NSCLC

INTRODUCTION

Radiation therapy (RT) plays an important role in the management of locally advanced non–small-cell lung cancer (NSCLC). In the neoadjuvant (preoperative) setting, thoracic RT with concurrent chemotherapy (CT) can be an effective means for downstaging mediastinal disease and improving the likelihood of complete resection. In the adjuvant (postoperative) setting, RT may decrease the risk of locoregional recurrence for patients with high-risk disease such as pathologic N2 involvement and/or positive margins. Modern techniques of radiation treatment planning and delivery have improved the safety profile and efficacy of thoracic RT.

NEOADJUVANT RT

Neoadjuvant Concurrent CT and RT

In patients with stage IIIA, locally advanced NSCLC, neoadjuvant RT with concurrent CT (CT/RT) can play an important role in downstaging mediastinal disease and increasing the likelihood of an R0 resection. Neoadjuvant CT/RT has been studied systematically in the past several decades in the cooperative group setting. The Southwestern Oncology Group (SWOG) conducted a phase-II study (SWOG 88-05) of preoperative RT to 45 Gy with two cycles of concurrent "EP50/50" chemotherapy (cisplatin 50 mg/m^2 on days 1, 8, 29, and 36 and etoposide 50 mg/m^2 on days 1–5 and days 29–33) in 126 patients with stage IIIA/B NSCLC with either biopsy-proven positive N2 or N3 nodes, or T4 primary lesions.[1] Patients with a response or stable disease proceeded to surgery. The clinical response rate to neoadjuvant therapy was 59%, and the resectability rate was 85% for patients with stage IIIA and 80% for patients with stage IIIB disease. The pathologic complete response rate was 21%. With a median follow-up of 2.4 years, the 3-year overall survival was 26%. While the locoregional recurrence rate was a promising 11%, the distant recurrence rate was 61%. Of interest, the strongest predictor of survival was clearance of mediastinal nodal (N2) disease by neoadjuvant treatment. The study reported a 3-year overall survival of 44% in patients with complete clearance of nodal disease (ypN0) and 18% in patients without nodal clearance (ypN+). Outcomes were particularly poor in patients with N3 disease by the presence of contralateral lymph nodes with a 3-year overall survival of 0%. However, the 3-year overall survival in patients with N3 disease due to the presence of supraclavicular lymph nodes was 35%. Treatment was relatively well tolerated, but concurrent CT/RT did result in grade 4 toxicity in 13% of patients and grade 5 toxicity in 10% of patients. However, this trial was conducted in an era when RT was delivered using fluoroscopic planning instead of modern computed tomography-based approaches.

Given the promising results of SWOG 88-05, this trimodality approach was compared against concurrent CT/RT alone in the Intergroup 0139 trial. This trial randomized 396 patients with initially unresectable T1-3, pathologic N2 NSCLC to preoperative concurrent CT/RT followed by surgery versus concurrent CT/RT alone.[2] Treatment in the trimodality arm was similar to the SWOG 88-05 regimen and included 45 Gy of preoperative RT with two cycles of concurrent EP50/50 followed by surgery 3 to 5 weeks afterwards, but added two cycles of consolidative CT after surgery. The treatment in the CT/RT alone arm consisted of radiation to 61 Gy with two cycles of concurrent EP50/50 and two cycles of consolidative CT. In the trimodality arm, there was an 18% pathologic complete response rate and clearance of mediastinal nodal disease (ypN0) occurred in 47% of patients. With a median follow-up of 22.5 months, in comparison to concurrent CT/RT alone, trimodality therapy significantly improved local recurrence (10% vs. 22%; $p = 0.002$) and 5-year progression-free survival (22% vs. 11%; $p = 0.017$). Despite the addition of two cycles of consolidative CT, distant metastatic recurrence remained a significant problem in both arms (37% vs. 42%; $p = 0.32$). There was no significant difference in overall survival between trimodality therapy and concurrent CT/RT alone with a 5-year overall survival of 27% versus 20% and median survival of 23.6 months versus 22 months ($p = 0.24$). In an unplanned subset analysis of patients by nodal status after preoperative therapy, patients with ypN0 disease (47% of patients) had a 5-year overall survival of 41% compared to 24% for patients with ypN+ disease (42% of patients). Patients who did not proceed to surgery after neoadjuvant CT/RT had a much worse prognosis with a 5-year overall survival of 8%. The lack of a statistically significant difference in survival between the two arms may have been due to a higher rate of treatment-related mortality in the trimodality arm (7.9% vs. 2.1%). In particular, patients receiving pneumonectomy in the trimodality arm of this study had a 26% (14 of 54 patients) mortality rate compared to 1% for patients undergoing lobectomy (Table 87-1). In an unplanned analysis,

Table 87-1

MORTALITY RATE BY SURGERY TYPE IN THE TRIMODALITY ARM OF THE INTERGROUP 0139 TRIAL

SURGERY TYPE	TOTAL ($n = 202$)	DEATHS *N* (%)
None	38	1 (3)
Exploration only	9	0 (0)
Wedge	3	0 (0)
Lobectomy	98	1 (1)
Any pneumonectomy	54	14 (26)
Right complex pneumonectomy	12	6 (50)
Right simple pneumonectomy	17	5 (29)
Left complex pneumonectomy	19	3 (16)
Left simple pneumonectomy	6	0 (0)

patients undergoing lobectomy had a 5-year overall survival of 36% compared to 18% ($p = 0.002$) in a matched group of patients undergoing concurrent CT/RT alone. In contrast, patients undergoing pneumonectomy did not have a significantly different 5-year overall survival (22% vs. 24%) compared to a matched group of patients undergoing concurrent CT/RT.

The results of the Intergroup 0139 trial suggest that trimodality therapy improves local control and progression-free survival, but does not significantly improve overall survival. However, the high mortality rate for patients who underwent pneumonectomy, particularly complex right pneumonectomy, may have diminished the potential survival benefit due to the addition of surgery. In a hypothesis generating subset analysis, it appeared that patients who were eligible to undergo a lobectomy after neoadjuvant CT/RT may have had the biggest benefit in overall survival from trimodality therapy compared to concurrent CT/RT alone.

Interestingly, since the publication of the results of Intergroup 0139, multiple retrospective series of patients treated with a pneumonectomy as part of trimodality therapy have shown lower mortality rates. For instance, a series of 73 patients from Brigham and Women's Hospital and Dana-Farber Cancer Institute who underwent pneumonectomy (62% left-sided and 38% right-sided) after preoperative RT demonstrated 30- and 100-day mortality rates of 6% and 10%, respectively.[3] The mortality rate was 11% in the 28 patients who underwent complex pneumonectomy versus 9% in the 45 patients who underwent simple pneumonectomy, and 4% in the 45 patients who underwent left pneumonectomy versus 18% in the 28 patients who underwent right pneumonectomy. Other single institutional studies have demonstrated comparable mortality rates of 5% to 15%,[4,5] which are lower than the 26% mortality rate seen in the Intergroup 0139 study. Thus, trimodality therapy that includes pneumonectomy may be feasible with acceptable toxicity rates in centers with a high case volume.

With the development of more modern RT techniques and based on positive experiences reported at the University of Maryland,[6,7] the Radiation Therapy Oncology Group (RTOG) conducted a Phase II, multi-institutional pilot study (RTOG 0229) of dose escalated preoperative RT to 61.2 Gy in 34 fractions with concurrent weekly carboplatin and paclitaxel prior to lobectomy or pneumonectomy in patients with resectable stage III disease.[8] The primary endpoint of the study and the reason for testing a high preoperative RT dose was to increase the mediastinal nodal clearance rate from 47% as observed in the Intergroup 0139 trial to 50%–70%. Given the higher preoperative RT dose compared to Intergroup 0139 (~33% higher), the study mandated placement of a muscle flap on the bronchial stump to buttress the bronchus and minimal intravenous fluid use in the immediate postoperative period (<1500 mL per day for the first 4 days). The study also encouraged diuretic therapy in the postoperative period (furosemide 20 mg twice daily).

The eligibility criteria included stage T1-3, N2-3 (excluding patients with supraclavicular nodes, performance status 0–1, and FEV1 > 2 L or predicted postoperative FEV1 > 0.8 L. The study enrolled 60 patients with 57 patients eligible for analysis. The neoadjuvant treatment was delivered as intended in the majority of patients with 91% receiving neoadjuvant CT and RT as per protocol.

Thirty-seven (65%) of the 56 patients who completed neoadjuvant CT/RT underwent surgery (34 lobectomies, 3 pneumonectomies), iresulting in 74% R0 and 26% R1 resections. An additional six patients had surgical staging of the mediastinal nodes after neoadjuvant therapy, and overall 63% (27/43) achieved complete mediastinal nodal clearance (ypN0). With a median follow-up of 24.4 months, the median OS was 26.6 months with a 2-year OS of 54%. The median PFS was 12.9 months with a 2-year PFS of 33%. In an unplanned subgroup analysis of ypN0 versus ypN+ versus no surgery, the 2-year OS estimates were 75%, 52%, and 23%, respectively ($p < 0.0002$) and the 2-year PFS estimates were 56%, 26%, and 8%, respectively ($p < 0.0001$). The incidence of grade 3 postoperative pulmonary complications was 14% (5/37), and there was one postoperative grade 5 event due to pulmonary edema in a patient who underwent pneumonectomy.

Thus, this RTOG 0229 study demonstrated that pulmonary resection can be safely performed after neoadjuvant CT with full-dose RT in the multi-institutional setting with a higher rate of complete mediastinal nodal clearance compared to historical controls from Intergroup 0139. The study also demonstrated a low incidence of postoperative mortality overall with careful surgical techniques and postoperative care.

Neoadjuvant Concurrent CT and RT versus Neoadjuvant CT with Adjuvant RT

A potential alternative to neoadjuvant concurrent CT/RT is neoadjuvant CT alone followed by resection and postoperative RT as described in Chapter 88. While there are no data from randomized trials directly comparing the two neoadjuvant approaches, a German randomized trial does provide some insights. In this German study, 524 patients with stage IIIA and IIIB NSCLC were treated with three cycles of neoadjuvant CT (cisplatin and etoposide) and then randomized to neoadjuvant concurrent CT/RT followed by surgery or immediate surgery followed by adjuvant RT.[9] In essence, the trial compares different sequencing of the three treatment modalities after initial neoadjuvant CT: either neoadjuvant concurrent CT/RT followed by resection or neoadjuvant CT alone followed by resection and postoperative adjuvant RT. The concurrent neoadjuvant CT/RT consisted of three cycles of carboplatin and vindesine with hyperfractionated, twice daily RT (total dose 45 Gy with 1.5 Gy delivered twice a day followed by a 24 Gy boost if inoperable or R1/R2 resection), which are approaches not commonly used in the United States. Patients in the neoadjuvant CT alone arm received adjuvant RT consisting of 54 Gy in 30 daily fractions after R0 resection or 68.4 Gy in 38 fractions after R1/R2 resection or in inoperable patients. With a median follow-up of 70 months, this study demonstrated no significant difference between the neoadjuvant CT followed by neoadjuvant CT/RT arm versus the neoadjuvant CT alone followed by resection and adjuvant RT arm in 5-year overall survival (18% vs. 21%; $p = 0.97$) or progression-free survival (14% vs. 16%; $p = 0.087$). The therapy in both arms was relatively well tolerated with a low rate of treatment-related deaths (5.8% vs. 6.4%, respectively). For the patients who underwent pneumonectomy (35%), the mortality rate was not significantly different between the neoadjuvant CT followed by CT/RT arm versus the neoadjuvant CT alone followed by resection and adjuvant RT arm (14% vs. 6%); moreover, the mortality rate in both arms was lower than that in the Intergroup 0139 study. Among the patients who underwent resection, neoadjuvant concurrent CT/RT was superior to neoadjuvant CT alone followed by resection and adjuvant RT; complete (R0) resection rates were

75% versus 60% ($p = 0.008$), and mediastinal downstaging rates were 46% versus 29% ($p = 0.02$).

This study demonstrated that the addition of neoadjuvant concurrent CT/RT to initial neoadjuvant CT does not impact survival compared to a strategy of sequencing RT after neoadjuvant CT and surgery, but the concurrent neoadjuvant CT/RT approach does result in increased downstaging of both the primary and mediastinal diseases. In unplanned subset analyses of these patients, there was no increase in overall survival for patients with either mediastinal downstaging or complete resection, but the small numbers of patients in these subgroups likely underpowered this analysis. Furthermore, this study's results must be interpreted with caution since the hyperfractionated RT approach utilized in the neoadjuvant CT/RT arm is not commonly used in the United States, and both arms received three cycles of upfront neoadjuvant CT. Thus, while there is no conclusive evidence regarding the optimal neoadjuvant approach, it does appear that neoadjuvant concurrent CT/RT may have an important role in improving the likelihood of mediastinal nodal clearance and achieving R0 resections, which are both surrogate outcomes that may be associated with improved survival.

Neoadjuvant Concurrent CT and RT for Superior Sulcus Tumors

Neoadjuvant concurrent CT/RT may play a particularly important role in the management of superior sulcus tumors. A multi-institutional phase II trial led by SWOG (Intergroup 0160/SWOG 9416) demonstrated the efficacy of neoadjuvant CT/RT in 95 patients with T3-4, N0-1 NSCLC involving the superior sulcus.[10] The neoadjuvant concurrent CT/RT was identical to the Intergroup 0139 study (45 Gy and concurrent cisplatin and etoposide), but radiation treatment planning was performed using three-dimensional (3D) computed tomography rather than two-dimensional (2D) techniques. Of the 95 patients, 83 (87%) were able to undergo thoracotomy and an impressive 76 (92%) of these patients had a complete resection. Additionally, 63% of the patients undergoing surgery had a pathologic complete response or minimal microscopic residual disease. With a median follow-up of 82 months, the 5-year overall survival was 44% and the 5-year overall survival in patients who underwent a complete resection was 54%. Treatment was well tolerated with treatment-related deaths observed in 2.7% of patients. Regarding patterns of failure, local failure was seen in only 17 (18%) of 95 patients, and distant recurrence occurred in 26 (27%) of 95 patients, with brain metastases the most common site of failure. Overall, this study demonstrated that neoadjuvant concurrent CT/RT for patients with superior sulcus tumors produced excellent resection rates and outcomes with minimal toxicity.

Neoadjuvant Concurrent CT and RT Summary

Prospective trials of neoadjuvant concurrent CT/RT followed by surgery have demonstrated that this approach is well tolerated and results in improved local control and progression-free survival compared to definitive concurrent CT/RT alone. In these studies, clearance of mediastinal nodal disease by neoadjuvant therapy was an important favorable prognostic factor for overall survival. The Intergroup 0139 randomized trial demonstrated a survival benefit for patients who underwent lobectomy after neoadjuvant therapy, but a higher mortality rate was seen for patients who underwent pneumonectomy (particularly right-sided complex pneumonectomy). However, multiple single institution centers have demonstrated lower mortality rates with pneumonectomy after neoadjuvant therapy, suggesting that this approach may be feasible at centers with high surgical volume and experience with the trimodality approach. Additionally, the Phase II RTOG 0229 trial demonstrated that dose escalation of preoperative RT is feasible and well-tolerated using modern RT techniques and careful surgical technique, and results in high likelihood of mediastinal nodal clearance. However, further study is required and high dose preoperative RT approaches should be conducted only at surgical centers with significant experience with this approach. Despite the excellent local control rates seen with trimodality therapy, distant recurrence remains a significant problem, and underscores the need to identify better systemic agents.

Neoadjuvant RT and CT Recommendations

It is our practice at Brigham and Women's Hospital and Dana-Farber Cancer Institute to offer neoadjuvant concurrent CT/RT to patients with stage IIIA NSCLC who are good candidates for surgery. Surgery is also sometimes considered for select patients with stage IIIB disease (such as those who are young, have an excellent performance status, have a low bulk of nodal disease and achieve nodal downstaging following neoadjuvant therapy). Successful delivery of trimodality therapy requires close interdisciplinary communication and coordination of care between the thoracic surgeon, medical oncologist, and radiation oncologist. Typically, we recommend neoadjuvant concurrent CT/RT and the CT options include the SWOG/Intergroup 0139 regimen of cisplatin and etoposide for patients who are in good health or weekly carboplatin and paclitaxel for older patients or those with comorbidities as described in Chapter 88. A few weeks following completion of neoadjuvant therapy, restaging studies such as chest computed tomography or positron emission tomography (PET) are obtained and resection is performed approximately 4 to 6 weeks after completion of RT in eligible candidates. Patients who are deemed to be "marginally resectable" at initial trimodality consultation undergo a carefully timed reevaluation toward the end of neoadjuvant concurrent CT/RT. Specifically, about 1 to 2 weeks before the completion of neoadjuvant therapy, restaging studies are obtained and reviewed by the thoracic surgeon to assess for tumor response and resectability. Patients eligible for resection complete the neoadjuvant treatment course and then proceed to surgery, whereas those judged to be unresectable continue concurrent CT/RT to a higher dose without a treatment break. Consolidation CT after surgery is an option for patients who tolerate trimodality therapy well.

Neoadjuvant RT Techniques

Our RT planning process for neoadjuvant concurrent CT/RT includes four-dimensional (4D) computed tomography imaging that accounts for tumor motion during the respiratory cycle, fusion of PET images for precise tumor and nodal localization, and incorporation of any additional clinical or pathologic information from bronchoscopy and mediastinoscopy. We limit our target volumes to the primary tumor, grossly involved lymph nodes as delineated by PET, chest computed tomography, and/or mediastinoscopy (Fig. 87-1A). We treat these target volumes with a margin to account for microscopic tumor spread and

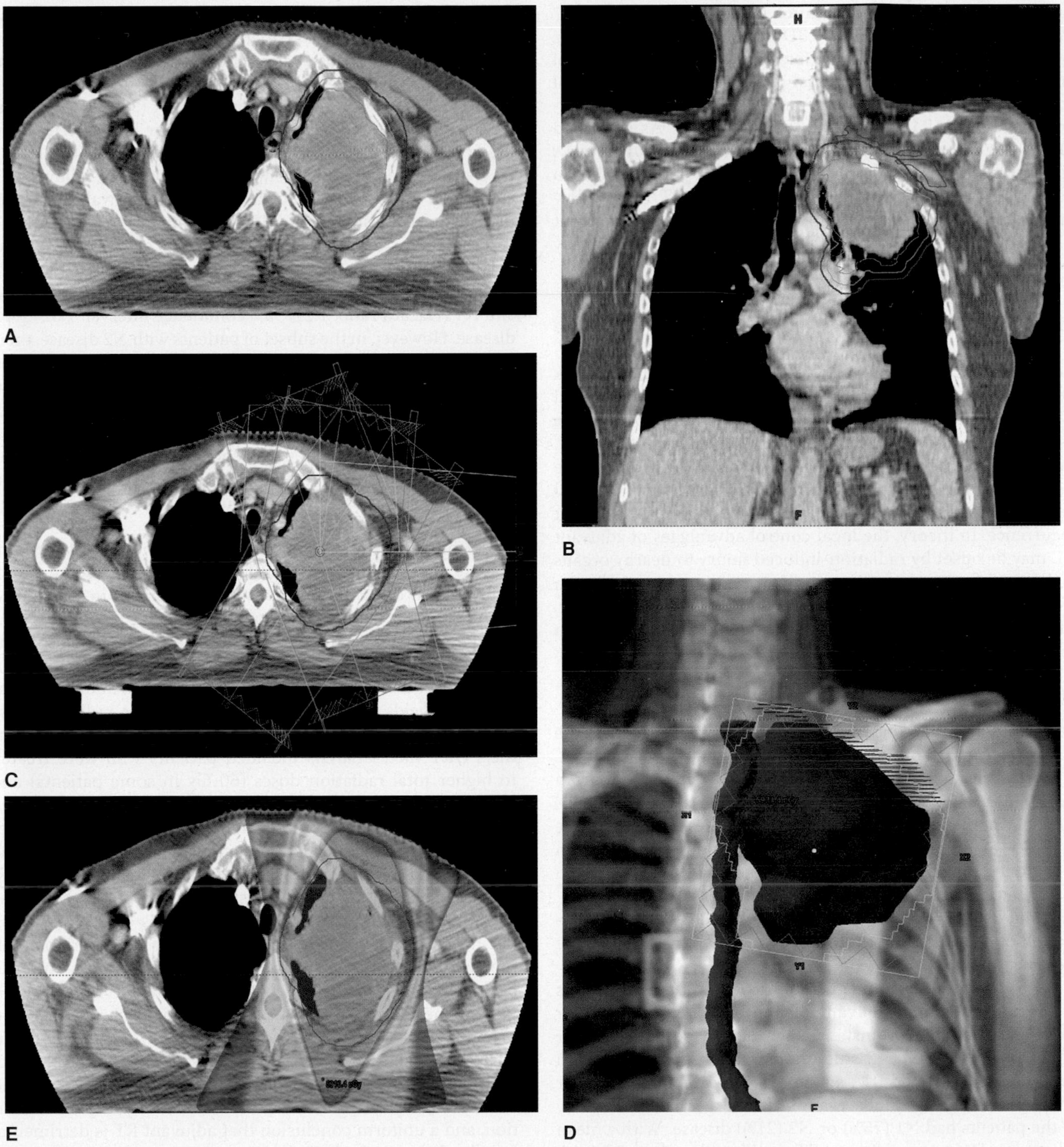

Figure 87-1. Neoadjuvant radiation therapy planning images for a patient with stage IIIA non–small-cell lung cancer including a $9.2 \times 8.4 \times 6.3$ cm left upper lobe apical primary and an AP window lymph node. The patient was treated with neoadjuvant CT and radiation to a dose of 54 Gy. This was followed by left upper lobectomy and mediastinal nodal dissection that showed no evidence of residual disease. (*A*) Axial and (*B*) coronal images from the radiation planning computed tomography scan demonstrating the delineated tumor target volumes including gross tumor volume (*pink*), clinical target volume, a volumetric expansion that includes potential microscopic disease (*green*), final planning target volume, a volumetric expansion that provides a margin for setup uncertainties (*red*), and normal organs at risk including the esophagus (*purple*) and the brachial plexus (*blue*); (*C*) axial image from the planning scan showing the intensity-modulated radiation therapy plan's beam arrangements including three anterior oblique fields and two posterior oblique fields that encompass the tumor planning target volume (*red*); (*D*) "Beam's eye view" of one of the anterior oblique radiation treatment beam projected onto a digitally reconstructed radiograph that demonstrates shaping of the beam around the tumor planning target volume (*red*), and shielding (*yellow lines*) of the normal structures including the esophagus (*purple*) and the brachial plexus (*blue wire*); (*E*) axial image with radiation dose distribution overlaid using a color wash scheme with *red* representing full prescription dose (54 Gy), *green* representing intermediate dose (40 Gy), and *blue* representing the low-dose region (20 Gy). The tumor planning target volume is well covered by the full prescription dose, and there is a steep fall-off of dose medially.

daily treatment setup uncertainties to a dose of 54 Gy in 27 fractions. We typically utilize 3D conformal RT techniques, but in select cases where radiation dose constraints to critical organs such as the lungs, brachial plexus, esophagus, or spinal cord cannot be met, we utilize an intensity-modulated radiation therapy (IMRT) technique (Fig. 87-1C–E). As described earlier, eligible patients then proceed to surgery 4 to 6 weeks after completion of neoadjuvant CT/RT. For patients who do not have a sufficient response to neoadjuvant CT/RT to allow for resection, we typically recommend continuing concurrent CT/RT to a higher, definitive dose (~60–66 Gy) without any treatment break from the first course of therapy.

ADJUVANT RT

Adjuvant RT can play an important role in decreasing the risk of local recurrence after surgical resection of locally advanced NSCLC with high-risk features, but the evidence supporting the use of adjuvant RT in specific subgroups remains controversial. In general, the therapeutic gain for adjuvant RT in reducing the risk of local recurrence is significant, but the overall survival benefit is likely modest due to the competing risks of distant recurrence. In theory, the local control advantages of adjuvant RT may be offset by radiation-induced injury to nearby organs including the lungs and heart. However, modern radiation techniques have increased the safety profile of this treatment, and thus, adjuvant RT is generally considered to be beneficial in select patients with high-risk features.

Historical Outcomes with Adjuvant RT

To understand the controversy surrounding adjuvant RT, the historical context of adjuvant RT studies must be reviewed. Historical series and prospective studies of adjuvant RT from the 1970s to 1990s generally produced poor results with substantial morbidity and high mortality rates. However, the majority of these older studies utilized antiquated radiation techniques including Cobalt machines which produce much higher entrance dose compared with modern linear accelerators and 2D fluoroscopic planning which did not allow visualization of dose distribution to critical normal organs and large treatment portals.

Despite these technological limitations, studies from this era demonstrated that adjuvant RT improved local control after surgical resection. For instance, the landmark Lung Cancer Study Group (LCSG) 773 study randomized 210 patients with pathologic stage II and IIIA squamous-cell carcinoma to either adjuvant RT to 50 Gy or observation after surgery.[11] The majority of the patients had N1 (75%) or N2 (21%) disease. With a mean follow-up of 3.5 years, adjuvant RT significantly reduced the risk of any local recurrence (3% in the adjuvant RT arm vs. 41% in the surgery alone arm) as well as local recurrence as the first site of failure (1% vs. 20%, respectively). However, this improvement in local control did not translate to improved survival with a 5-year overall survival of 38% in both arms. Of note, 75% of the recurrences occurred outside the radiation field, which included the bronchial stump, ipsilateral hilum, and mediastinum.

In contrast to the LCSG 773 study, other prospective randomized trials from this era demonstrated that adjuvant RT improved locoregional control, but was detrimental to survival because of higher rates of radiation-related toxicity such as radiation pneumonitis[12] and a higher risk of intercurrent death[13] in the adjuvant RT arms. Furthermore, a PORT (postoperative RT) meta-analysis of 2128 patients in nine randomized trials of adjuvant RT versus observation demonstrated a similar overall survival detriment.[14] This meta-analysis included patients with stage I (26%), stage II (34%), and stage IIIA (38%) NSCLC who were treated with either cobalt-60-based or linear accelerator-based RT from 1966 to 1995 with a range of doses from 30 to 60 Gy and different target volumes. In all patients, adjuvant RT resulted in a 21% relative decrease in overall survival with 2-year overall survival estimates of 48% for patients treated with RT versus 55% for those treated with surgery alone. This survival detriment was even higher in the subset of patients with pathologic N0 (Hazard ratio: 1.41; 95% confidence interval: 1.09–1.83) and N1 (Hazard ratio: 1.21; 95% confidence interval: 1.02–1.44) disease. However, in the subset of patients with N2 disease, there was no difference in overall survival between the two groups, and there was a potential trend toward improved overall survival favoring adjuvant RT (Hazard ratio: 0.96; 95% confidence interval: 0.79–1.17). Furthermore, adjuvant RT resulted in a lower risk of locoregional recurrence with 276 (29.1%) locoregional failures in the patients who received surgery alone versus 195 (20.7%) locoregional failures in the patients who received adjuvant RT.

While the studies and literature from this era demonstrated a concerning survival detriment related to the use of adjuvant RT, these findings must be interpreted in the context of the radiation delivery technologies available during this time period. For instance, the PORT meta-analysis included patients who were treated with cobalt-60 treatment machines, 2D planning approaches, and large treatment fields including the use of lateral fields that likely resulted in higher radiation dose to the lungs, heart, and other normal tissues. Furthermore, the PORT meta-analysis included patients who were treated to higher total radiation doses (60 Gy in some patients) and with higher dose per fraction (2.5 Gy in some patients) than commonly used today. These outdated techniques and doses likely increased the morbidity of adjuvant RT in this prior era. A recent Surveillance, Epidemiology, and End Results (SEER) study demonstrated an excess risk of death from heart disease in patients treated with adjuvant RT in this era (1983–1988); but this excess risk decreased over a later time period when modern RT techniques including linear accelerators and CT-based planning became widely adopted (1989–1993).[15]

Furthermore, many of the studies in this era included patients with pathologic N0 disease (25% in the PORT meta-analysis), which likely further decreased the ability to detect any potential therapeutic benefit. Thus, the results of trials and the meta-analyses from this era must be interpreted with caution, and a uniform conclusion that adjuvant RT is detrimental for all patients with NSCLC is inappropriate.

Outcomes with Adjuvant RT Using Modern Radiation Treatment Techniques

Mature data from randomized studies of adjuvant RT versus observation utilizing modern radiation treatment techniques including CT-based planning, 3D calculation of radiation dose distributions, and incorporation of respiratory motion are currently not available. However, there are nonrandomized data that suggest the decrement in overall survival observed in older studies may no longer be applicable with modern treatment techniques. For instance, Lally et al.[16] utilized the SEER database to study outcomes after adjuvant RT versus observation from 1988 to 2002, an era where radiation was predominantly delivered with modern techniques. In 7565 patients with stage II and III NSCLC who had undergone lobectomy or pneumonectomy, the study observed that 47% of the patients in this era received adjuvant RT. In this SEER cohort, there was no difference in overall survival for patients who received adjuvant RT versus those who did not, but subset analyses demonstrated improved overall survival in patients with pathologic N2 disease (5-year overall survival 27% vs. 20%; $p = 0.03$). However, adjuvant RT resulted in a significant decrease in overall survival in patients with pathologic N0 (5-year overall survival 31% vs. 41%; $p < 0.001$) and pathologic N1 diseases (5-year overall survival 30% vs. 34%; $p < 0.001$).

Additional data supporting the safety of modern radiation treatment techniques in delivering adjuvant RT and the efficacy of this approach in comparison to observation are limited to two large single-institution experiences. All patients in these two studies were treated with modern treatment planning techniques and linear accelerators using energies of 6 MV or higher. Sawyer et al.[17] described 224 patients with pathologic N2 disease who underwent surgery at the Mayo Clinic and either underwent observation or adjuvant RT with modern techniques to a median dose of 50.4 Gy. The study showed that adjuvant RT resulted in improved 4-year overall survival (43% vs. 22%) and locoregional control (83% vs. 40%) compared to observation alone, with the greatest benefit seen in patients with high-risk features (defined in this study as multiple N2 nodes). Complementing the results of this Mayo series, Machtay et al.[18] demonstrated in a series of 202 patients treated with modern adjuvant RT at the University of Pennsylvania that the risk of death from intercurrent disease for patients receiving less than 54 Gy of adjuvant RT was only 2%, which underscores the improved toxicity profile of modern radiation treatment techniques.

Modern Prospective Studies of Adjuvant RT with or without CT

While adjuvant RT can reduce the risk of locoregional recurrence, particularly in patients with pathologic N2 disease, the overall survival benefits observed in the studies described earlier have been modest. Distant recurrence remains a substantial problem in patients with locally advanced disease, and more recent prospective studies have studied combining adjuvant RT with either sequential or concurrent adjuvant CT in an effort to address the risks of both local and distant diseases.

The Eastern Cooperative Group (ECOG) led a large intergroup, phase III study (Intergroup 0115/ECOG3590) that randomized 488 patients with resected stage II or IIIA NSCLC to adjuvant RT or adjuvant RT with four cycles of concurrent cisplatin (60 mg/m^2) and etoposide (120 mg/m^2) every 28 days.[19] The RT dose was 50.4 Gy in 28 fractions with an additional boost of 10.8 Gy in six fractions for patients with extracapsular nodal extension. In comparison to adjuvant RT alone, the addition of CT to adjuvant RT did not significantly improve overall survival (median survival 39 vs. 38 months), risk of in-field recurrence (12% vs. 13%), or overall recurrences (53% vs. 56%).

Concurrent CT increased the risk of grade 3 to 4 toxicity including esophagitis and leukopenia, but the rate of grade 5 toxicity was low in both groups (1.2% vs. 1.6%). A subsequent unplanned analysis of cause of death in this study by Wakelee et al. demonstrated no difference in the risk of death in patients with intercurrent disease in the adjuvant RT (4-year rate of 12.3%) and the adjuvant RT and CT (4-year rate of 13.7%) groups compared to age- and gender-matched controls (4-year rate 10.1%).[20] The results of this study demonstrate the safety and efficacy of adjuvant RT in a more modern treatment era, but disappointingly showed no improvement in outcomes with the addition of CT.

The Radiation Therapy Oncology Group (RTOG) also studied adjuvant RT with concurrent CT in a phase II study (RTOG 97-05) of 88 patients with stage II and stage IIIA NSCLC.[21] The RT consisted of 50.4 Gy in 28 fractions to the mediastinum and ipsilateral hilum with a boost of 10.8 Gy for extracapsular nodal extension or T3 disease. In contrast to the Intergroup/ECOG study, the CT consisted of four cycles of carboplatin and paclitaxel. With a median follow-up of 56.7 months, the median survival was 56.3 months with a 3-year overall survival of 61%. The study demonstrated a 3-year progression survival of 50% and a local failure rate of 15%. The acute toxicity rates were acceptable with ≥grade 3 esophagitis in 16% of patients, and acute respiratory toxicity in 6%. Late toxicity included a 6% crude incidence of late ≥grade 3 pulmonary toxicity and 5% crude incidence of cardiac toxicity. The authors concluded that the outcomes and toxicity of this phase II study were comparable to the Intergroup/ECOG study, and worthy of further study.

The Role of Modern Adjuvant RT after Adjuvant CT

As described in Chapter 88, recent studies have demonstrated an overall survival benefit of adjuvant CT after surgical resection in patients with stage II and III NSCLC. Despite this improved survival, locoregional recurrence may occur in ~20% to 30% of patients after adjuvant CT.[22] These findings have stimulated renewed interest in exploring the role of adjuvant RT with modern 3D conformal RT techniques in combination with adjuvant CT.

The CALGB attempted to address this question in a Phase III study (CALGB 9734) that randomized patients with completely resected stage IIIA NSCLC who had received four cycles of adjuvant CT to either adjuvant RT or observation.[23] The CT consisted of four cycles of carboplatin and paclitaxel, and the RT involved treating the ipsilateral hilum, mediastinum, and supraclavicular fossae to 50 Gy. Unfortunately, the study was closed early due to slow accrual after enrolling only 44 out of a planned 480 patients. The study showed no significant difference between observation and adjuvant RT in median failure-free survival (16.8 vs. 33.7 months; $p = 0.7$), 1-year overall survival (72% vs. 74%; $p = 0.91$), or rate of any recurrence (67% vs. 47%; $p = 0.32$) including both local and distant recurrences. However, these results are difficult to interpret since the study did not fully accrue and was underpowered.

Additionally, an unplanned secondary analysis of the Adjuvant Navelbine International Trialist Association (ANITA) trial provides further evidence supporting the potential role of adjuvant RT after adjuvant CT in select high-risk patients. The ANITA trial, which is described in further detail in Chapter 88, was a randomized phase III trial of four cycles of adjuvant cisplatin and vinorelbine versus observation in 804 patients with completely resected stage I–IIIA NSCLC.[24] In this study, adjuvant RT to 45 to 60 Gy using 2 Gy per fraction daily with

Table 87-2

SECONDARY ANALYSIS OF CRUDE LOCOREGIONAL RECURRENCE RATES IN THE ANITA TRIAL BY USE OF AJDUVANT RADIATION THERAPY (RT), ADJUVANT CHEMOTHERAPY (CT), AND PATHOLOGIC NODAL STATUS

ANY LOCOREGIONAL RECURRENCE	ALL PATIENTS (n = 840)	PATHOLOGIC N0 (n = 367)	PATHOLOGIC N1 (n = 243)	PATHOLOGIC N2 (n = 224)
No CT/no RT	75 (26.2%)	37 (21.5%)	22 (29.0%)	16 (42.1%)
No CT/+adjuvant RT	29 (20.1%)	1 (6.3%)	13 (22.7%)	15 (22.1%)
+CT/no RT	58 (18.4%)	29 (17.7%)	11 (13.4%)	18 (25.7%)
+CT/+adjuvant RT	16 (18.2%)	3 (20.0%)	5 (20.0%)	7 (14.6%)

a high-energy linear accelerator was recommended, but not mandated for patients with nodal disease. The RT was delivered per local institutional policies using techniques at the discretion of the treating clinician. An unplanned secondary analysis of this study demonstrated that 232 (28% of the study population) patients received adjuvant RT with 13.4%, 36.6%, and 50% of patients with pathologic N0, N1, and N2 disease receiving this treatment, respectively.[19] Of note, more patients randomized to the observation (no adjuvant CT arm) received adjuvant RT (33.3% vs. 21.6%). Adjuvant RT appeared to reduce the crude risk of locoregional recurrence, particularly in patients with N2 disease (Table 87-2). Moreover, when examining the potential interactions between pathologic nodal status and the use of CT, the authors identified potential subgroups that may have a survival benefit from adjuvant RT (Table 87-3). Of note, adjuvant RT improved overall survival in patients with pathologic N2 disease in both the adjuvant CT and no CT arms of the trial. However, in patients with pathologic N1 disease, those who were randomized to the adjuvant CT arm had decreased overall survival with adjuvant RT, while those who were randomized to no CT had improved survival with adjuvant RT. These hypothesis-generating results indicate a potential role for adjuvant RT in patients with high-risk disease (pathologic N2 or pathologic N1 in the absence of adjuvant CT), but the results must be confirmed in a randomized trial.

Summary of Adjuvant RT

In conclusion, modern adjuvant RT appears to be relatively well tolerated compared to treatment techniques utilized in older eras and provides a local control benefit in multiple retrospective series and secondary analyses. Furthermore, a SEER analysis and a secondary analysis of the ANITA study demonstrate a potential survival benefit for adjuvant RT in the subset of patients with pathologic N2 disease. While there is currently no level I evidence supporting the use of adjuvant RT, there is an ongoing multi-institutional European trial (EORTC/IFCT LUNG ART) evaluating the role of adjuvant RT in patients with completely resected N2 disease who have received either neoadjuvant or adjuvant CT.

Adjuvant RT Recommendations

Until the LUNG ART randomized trial has accrued and results have matured, our practice at the Brigham and Women's Hospital and Dana-Farber Cancer Institute is to consider the role of adjuvant RT on a case-by-case basis. Our indications for adjuvant RT include: (1) positive margins; (2) pathologic N2 disease; (3) high-risk pathologic N1 disease with either bulky or numerous nodes involved and/or cases without mediastinal dissection or with limited nodal dissection. Typically, in patients with pathologic N2 disease or high-risk N1 disease, we sequence adjuvant RT after adjuvant CT. In patients with positive margins, we consider adjuvant RT with concurrent CT, and typically adopt the treatment approaches outlined in the ECOG and RTOG trials of adjuvant concurrent CT and RT.

Adjuvant RT Techniques

Our radiation treatment techniques include using 4D CT planning that accounts for respiratory motion and incorporation of data from presurgical PET operative reports, discussion with the thoracic surgeon, and pathology results. We limit our target volumes to the regions at highest risk of recurrence, including the bronchial stump/hilum and high-risk mediastinal nodal stations (Fig. 87-2A, B). We do not treat the primary tumor bed unless there were positive or close margins. Treatment is typically delivered using a 3D conformal RT plan (Fig. 87-2C) that incorporates dose constraints for critical normal tissues, and we commonly utilize a radiation dose of 50.4 to 54.0 Gy using 1.8 to 2.0 Gy per fraction, and with a boost to 10.8 Gy for extracapsular nodal extension or positive margins. We utilize tight constraints on the radiation dose to the remaining lung tissue (with particular attention to the contralateral lung in patients who have undergone a pneumonectomy), heart, and other critical organs (Fig. 87-2D, E). In cases where positive or close margins are a concern, it is

Table 87-3

SECONDARY ANALYSIS OF 5-YEAR OVERALL SURVIVAL IN THE ANITA TRIAL BY USE OF ADJUVANT RADIATION THERAPY (RT), ADJUVANT CHEMOTHERAPY (CT), AND PATHOLOGIC NODAL STATUS

5-YEAR OS	ALL PATIENTS (n = 840) (%)	PATHOLOGIC N0 (n = 367) (%)	PATHOLOGIC N1 (n = 243) (%)	PATHOLOGIC N2 (n = 224) (%)
No CT/no RT	43	62	31	17
No CT/+adjuvant RT	33	44	43	21
+CT/no RT	51	60	56	34
+CT/+adjuvant RT	45	44	40	47

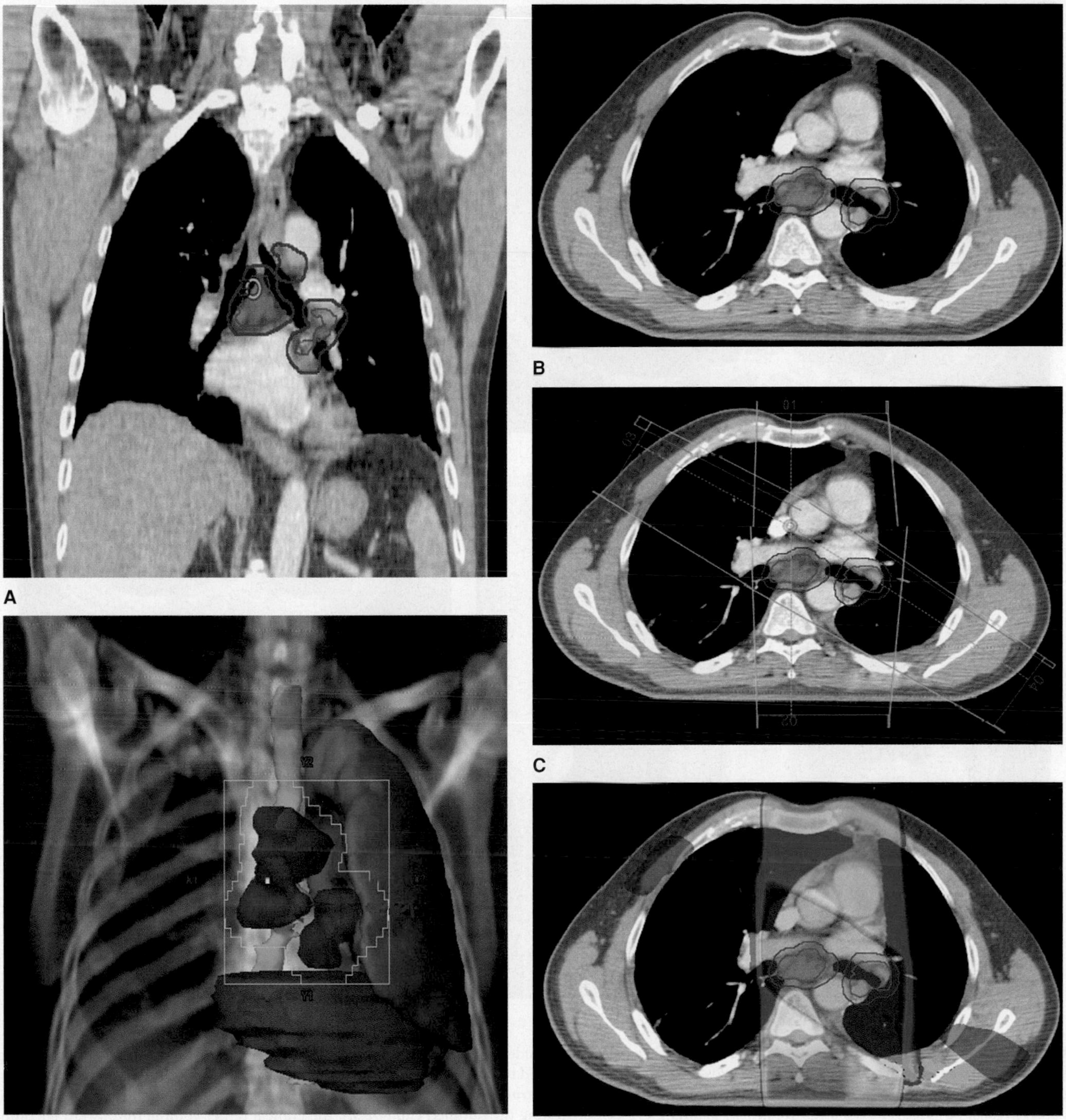

A B C D E

Figure 87-2. Adjuvant radiation therapy for a patient with pT1bN2M0, stage IIIA non–small-cell lung cancer who underwent VATS left lower lobectomy for 2.7 cm primary lung adenocarcinoma with negative margins, but with unexpectedly positive left hilar, subcarinal, and AP window lymph nodes on mediastinal lymph node dissection. (*A*) Coronal and (*B*) axial images from the radiation planning computed tomography scan demonstrating the delineation of the clinical target volume (*pink*) including the involved nodal stations and planning target volume (*red*) that includes a volumetric expansion to account for treatment setup uncertainties; (*C*) radiation beam arrangements including two anterior–posterior and two lateral–oblique fields covering the nodal target volumes; (*D*) "Beam's eye view" of the anterior radiation field projected on a digitally reconstructed radiograph that demonstrates coverage of the nodal planning target volume (*red*) and blocking (*yellow lines*) of normal organs including the lung (*blue*), esophagus (*cyan*), and heart (*brown*); (*E*) radiation dose distribution on an axial image from the planning CT demonstrating full 50.4 Gy dose coverage (*red color wash*) of the nodal planning target volumes, and lower dose levels including 40 Gy (*green*) and 20 Gy (*blue*).

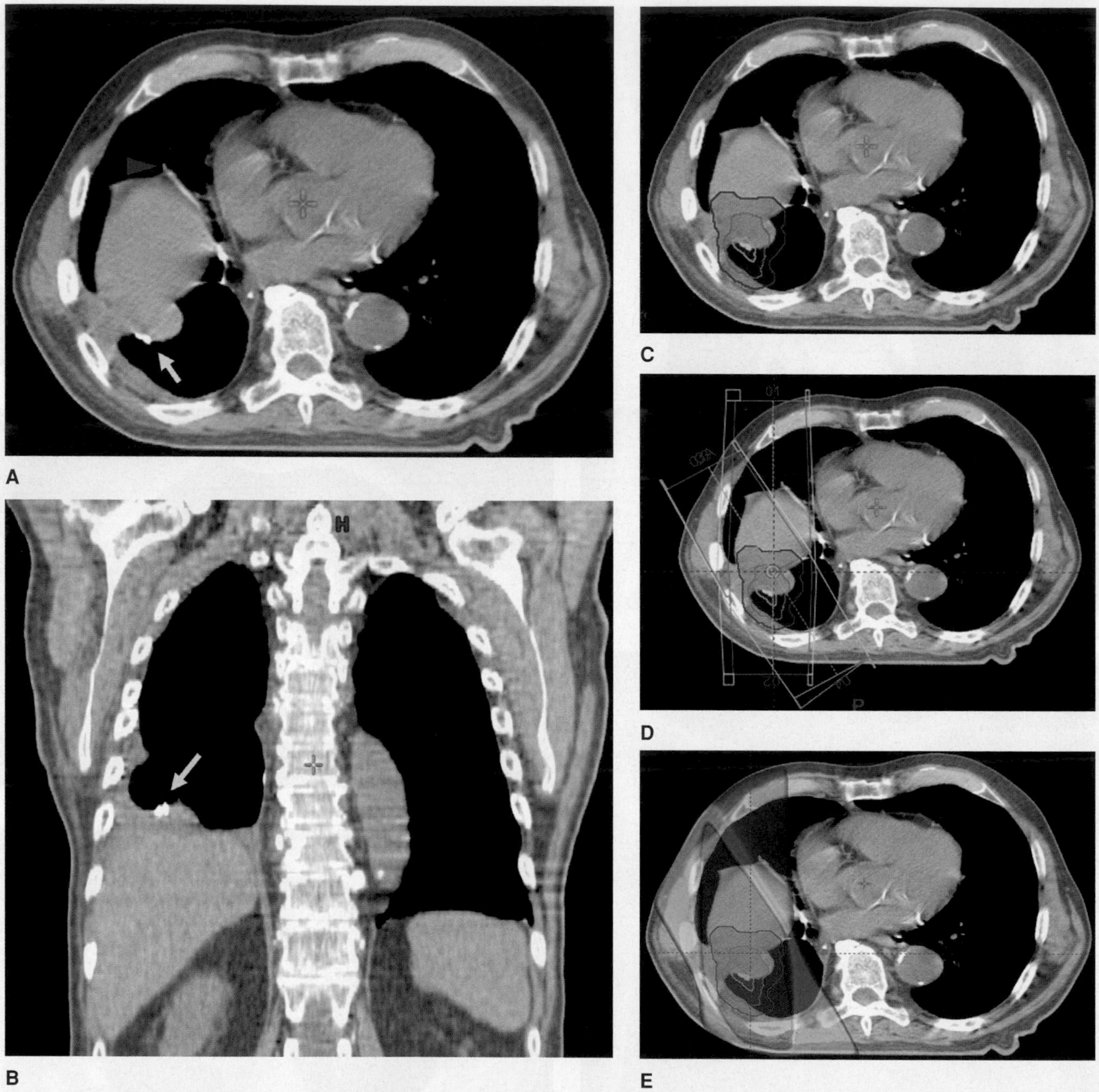

Figure 87-3. Surgical clips aiding adjuvant radiation therapy in a patient who underwent right middle and lower lobectomy with the intraoperative finding of extension of disease to involve the diaphragm. (*A*) Postoperative axial computed tomography images demonstrate surgical clips placed at the site of positive margins on the diaphragm (*blue arrow*), and the lobectomy suture line (*red arrow head*); (*B*) postoperative coronal CT images demonstrating the surgical clip (*blue arrow*); (*C*) adjuvant radiation treatment planning CT demonstrating the outlined clip (*green*), the clinical target volume (*orange*) to encompass the tumor bed, and the planning target volume (*red*) which includes a margin for daily setup variation; (*D*) orientation of adjuvant radiation therapy treatment fields to cover the planning target volume including an anterior–posterior, posterior–anterior, and two oblique fields; (*E*) radiation dose distribution covering the target volumes on axial CT images including full dose (*red* = 60 Gy), intermediate dose (*green* = 40 Gy), and lower dose (*blue* = 20 Gy) regions.

very helpful for RT planning when the thoracic surgeon places surgical clips to delineate the regions at highest risk of recurrence (Fig. 87-3).

SUMMARY

RT using modern techniques can play an important role in both neoadjuvant and adjuvant treatment approaches for patients with locally advanced NSCLC. Neoadjuvant concurrent CT/RT can increase the likelihood of both downstaging mediastinal nodal disease and achieving a complete resection. Adjuvant RT improves local control and may improve survival in select patients with high-risk disease. Overall, with improvements in RT delivery techniques, both neoadjuvant and adjuvant RT are well tolerated and efficacious components of our armamentarium to treat locally advanced NSCLC.

EDITOR'S COMMENT

This chapter provides an excellent review of the role of radiation in the neoadjuvant and adjuvant settings. A previous chapter described the role of definitive chemoradiation for nonresectable locoregional (stage IIIa and IIIb disease). The discussion above points out the value of neoadjuvant therapy to incite a pathologic complete response or at least mediastinal nodal clearance. The recent RTOG 0229 study showed the value of full-dose chemoradiation in the neoadjuvant setting in a phase II study. Like the BWH group, my philosophy is to be selective in choosing patients for resection after neoadjuvant therapy. While I think the decision to proceed with trimodality therapy should be made as a team upfront, the final decision whether or not to offer resection depends on patient physiologic factors, as well as the likelihood of residual lymph node disease. As was described in the past by Bueno et al., I repeat the mediastinal lymph node staging with a mediastinosocopy, remediastinoscopy, or repeat TBNA. If persistent lymph node disease is found (especially if it is on the contralateral side), I generally do not offer resection unless in unique situations.

—Mark J. Krasna

References

1. Albain KS, Rusch VW, Crowley JJ, et al. Concurrent cisplatin/etoposide plus chest radiotherapy followed by surgery for stages IIIA (N2) and IIIB non-small-cell lung cancer: mature results of Southwest Oncology Group phase II study 8805. *J Clin Oncol.* 1995;13(8):1880–1892.
2. Albain KS, Swann RS, Rusch VW, et al. Radiotherapy plus chemotherapy with or without surgical resection for stage III non-small-cell lung cancer: a phase III randomised controlled trial. *Lancet.* 2009;374(9687):379–386.
3. Allen AM, Mentzer SJ, Yeap BY, et al. Pneumonectomy after chemoradiation: the Dana-Farber Cancer Institute/Brigham and Women's Hospital experience. *Cancer.* 2008;112(5):1106–1113.
4. d'Amato TA, Ashrafi AS, Schuchert MJ, et al. Risk of pneumonectomy after induction therapy for locally advanced non-small cell lung cancer. *Ann Thorac Sur.* 2009;88(4):1079–1085.
5. Kim AW, Faber LP, Warren WH, et al. Pneumonectomy after chemoradiation therapy for non-small cell lung cancer: does "side" really matter? *Ann Thorac Sur.* 2009;88(3):937–943.
6. Sonett JR, Krasna MJ, Suntharalingam M, et al. Safe pulmonary resection after chemotherapy and high-dose thoracic radiation. *Ann Thorac Surg.* 1999;68:316–320.
7. Sonett JR, Suntharalingam M, Edelman MJ, et al. Pulmonary resection after curative intent radiotherapy (>59 Gy) and concurrent chemotherapy in non-small-cell lung cancer. *Ann Thorac Surg.* 2004;78:1200–1205.
8. Suntharalingam et al. *Int J Radiat Oncol Biol Phys* 2012;84(2):456-63.
9. Thomas M, Rube C, Hoffknecht P, et al. Effect of preoperative chemoradiation in addition to preoperative chemotherapy: a randomised trial in stage III non-small-cell lung cancer. *Lancet Oncol.* 2008;9(7):636–648.
10. Rusch VW, Giroux DJ, Kraut MJ, et al. Induction chemoradiation and surgical resection for superior sulcus non-small-cell lung carcinomas: long-term results of Southwest Oncology Group Trial 9416 (Intergroup Trial 0160). *J Clin Oncol.* 2007;25(3):313–318.
11. Weisenburger TH. Effects of postoperative mediastinal radiation on completely resected stage II and stage III epidermoid cancer of the lung. LCSG 773. *Chest.* 1994;106(6 Suppl):297S–301S.
12. Van Houtte P, Rocmans P, Smets P, et al. Postoperative radiation therapy in lung cancer: a controlled trial after resection of curative design. *Int J Radiat Oncol Biol Phys.* 1980;6(8):983–986.
13. Dautzenberg B, Arriagada R, Chammard AB, et al. A controlled study of postoperative radiotherapy for patients with completely resected non-small cell lung carcinoma. Groupe d'Etude et de Traitement des Cancers Bronchiques. *Cancer.* 1999;86(2):265–273.
14. PORT Meta-analysis Trialists Group. Postoperative radiotherapy for non-small cell lung cancer. *Cochrane Database Syst Rev.* 2000;(2):CD002142.
15. Lally BE, Detterbeck FC, Geiger AM, et al. The risk of death from heart disease in patients with nonsmall cell lung cancer who receive postoperative radiotherapy: analysis of the Surveillance, Epidemiology, and End Results database. *Cancer.* 2007;110(4):911–917.
16. Lally BE, Zelterman D, Colasanto JM, et al. Postoperative radiotherapy for stage II or III non-small-cell lung cancer using the surveillance, epidemiology, and end results database. *J Clin Oncol.* 2006;24(19):2998–3006.
17. Sawyer TE, Bonner JA, Gould PM, et al. The impact of surgical adjuvant thoracic radiation therapy for patients with nonsmall cell lung carcinoma with ipsilateral mediastinal lymph node involvement. *Cancer.* 1997;80(8):1399–1408.
18. Machtay M, Lee JH, Shrager JB, et al. Risk of death from intercurrent disease is not excessively increased by modern postoperative radiotherapy for high-risk resected non-small-cell lung carcinoma. *J Clin Oncol.* 2001;19(19):3912–3917.
19. Keller SM, Adak S, Wagner H, et al. A randomized trial of postoperative adjuvant therapy in patients with completely resected stage II or IIIA non-small-cell lung cancer. Eastern Cooperative Oncology Group. *N Engl J Med.* 2000;343(17):1217–1222.
20. Wakelee HA, Stephenson P, Keller SM, et al. Post-operative radiotherapy (PORT) or chemoradiotherapy (CPORT) following resection of stages II and IIIA non-small cell lung cancer (NSCLC) does not increase the expected risk of death from intercurrent disease (DID) in Eastern Cooperative Oncology Group (ECOG) trial E3590. *Lung Cancer.* 2005;48(3):389–397.
21. Bradley JD, Paulus R, Graham MV, et al. Phase II trial of postoperative adjuvant paclitaxel/carboplatin and thoracic radiotherapy in resected stage II and IIIA non-small-cell lung cancer: promising long-term results of the Radiation Therapy Oncology Group–RTOG 9705. *J Clin Oncol.* 2005;23(15):3480–3487.
22. Douillard JY, Rosell R, De Lena M, et al. Impact of postoperative radiation therapy on survival in patients with complete resection and stage I, II, or IIIA non-small-cell lung cancer treated with adjuvant chemotherapy: the Adjuvant Navelbine International Trialist Association (ANITA) randomized trial. *Int J Radiat Oncol Biol Phys.* 2008;72(3):695–701.
23. Perry MC, Kohman LJ, Bonner JA, et al. A phase III study of surgical resection and paclitaxel/carboplatin chemotherapy with or without adjuvant radiation therapy for resected stage III non-small-cell lung cancer: cancer and leukemia group B 9734. *Clin Lung Cancer.* 2007;8(4):268–272.
24. Douillard JY, Rosell R, De Lena M, et al. Adjuvant vinorelbine plus cisplatin versus observation in patients with completely resected stage IB-IIIA non-small-cell lung cancer (Adjuvant Navelbine International Trialist Association [ANITA]): a randomised controlled trial. *Lancet Oncol.* 2006;7(9):719–727.

88 Innovative Radiation Techniques: Role of Brachytherapy and Intraoperative Radiotherapy in Treatment of Lung Cancer

Nitika Thawani, Subhakar Mutyala, Itai M. Pashtan, and Phillip M. Devlin

Keywords: Lung cancer, early-stage non–small-cell lung cancer, brachytherapy, intraoperative radiation therapy, endobronchial brachytherapy

Brachytherapy, the use of radioactive isotopes placed directly on the desired target tissues during surgery or placed endoluminally, can be used for treatment of lung cancer. It offers several theoretic advantages when compared with traditional radiotherapy. Direct surgical placement of the radiation source allows for specific targeting and uniform delivery of the radiation minimizing the amount of normal lung in the radiation field. This potentially limits radiation side effects and ensures patient compliance which has been a major disadvantage of external beam radiation therapy.

EARLY STAGE LUNG CANCER

It has been established that lobectomy offers the best chance of cure for early-stage non–small-cell lung cancer. According to the Lung Cancer Study Group, sublobar or wedge resection is not as effective as lobectomy or pneumonectomy because it is associated with a high incidence of local recurrence.[1] However, a large resection requires the patient to have a reasonable residual forced expiratory volume in 1 second (FEV_1) of 0.8 to 1.2 L and a ventilation–perfusion scan corresponding to adequate breathing in other lung segments. Patients who have long histories of smoking commonly fail to have these advantageous characteristics. Techniques that combine sublobar resection with radiotherapy delivered intraoperatively or through the implantation of radioactive ^{125}I seeds at the lung resection margin have shown promising results (see section "planar seed experience"). This procedure has been reported to reduce local disease recurrence and improve palliation of symptoms. Additionally, it provides a treatment option for patients who are not physically capable of undergoing lobectomy or pneumonectomy or who are considered high-risk surgical candidates consequent to other comorbidities.

Varying systems for radiation delivery are presently used in clinical practice. Three techniques have been described for use following sublobar resection all of which are compatible with thoracoscopy.

PLANAR SEED IMPLANT TECHNIQUE

There are several reports of wedge resection procedures for stage I tumors that have been performed in conjunction with planar ^{125}I seed implants. This procedure has been reported to reduce local disease recurrence and improve local control.

After the wedge resection, the surgeon must measure the area at risk for length and width to determine the dimension of the implant. The implant is made of two components. The source material, called the Seed-in-Carrier, available through the Oncura Company (Plymouth Meeting, PA), consists of ^{125}I seeds that are embedded in strands of absorbable Vicryl suture. A second isotope recently became commercially available, using ^{131}Cs, from Isoray Medical (Richland, WA). There are 10 seeds in each strand, and each seed and strand is spaced 1 cm apart center to center. The individual seed measures 0.7 × 4 mm in dimension. The source material is attached to an absorbable mesh material made of either Dacron or Vicryl that is custom trimmed to fit the area at risk. Before trimming, 1 cm is added to the overall dimension to ensure an adequate margin for suturing. Parallel lines spaced 1 cm apart are drawn longitudinally on the mesh patch. The radioactive strands then are stitched to the mesh along these lines. The radioactive strands and suture should be handled with care using forceps only (Fig. 88-1). The source material is anchored on each side of the implant with a small staple, and any excess source material should be cut and disposed of properly in accordance with radiation disposal guidelines (Fig. 88-2). The custom mesh then is placed over the area of interest and sutured into place, using extreme care not to puncture the seeds (Fig. 88-3). Previously the mesh was prepared in the operating room; however, a prefabricated mesh construct is now available, in either ^{125}I or ^{131}Cs, which simplifies this step (Fig. 88-4). After the operation is concluded and the patient is stable (or at some future date), a postoperative CT scan is obtained over the area of interest to verify and document the final dose.

A novel technique of delivering radiation has also been developed at Brown University, where a ^{169}Yb brachytherapy

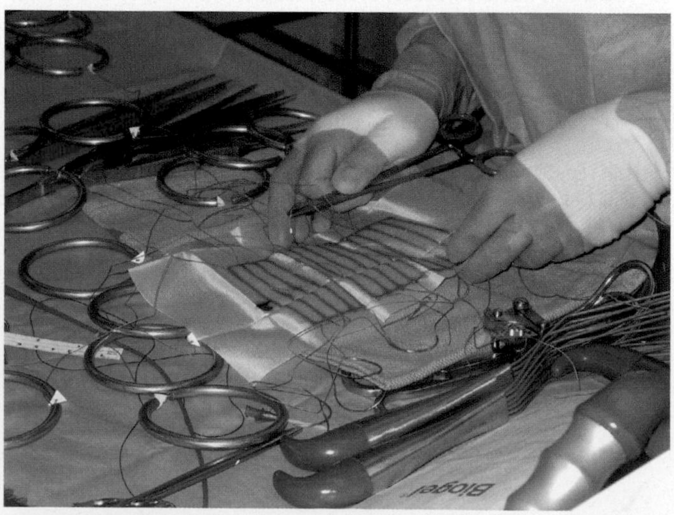

Figure 88-1. The commercial source for the brachytherapy seeds used in our patients is called a Seed-in-Carrier and consists of ^{125}I seeds embedded in strands (10 seeds per strand) of absorbable Vicryl suture. The radioactive strands and suture should be handled with caution using forceps only.

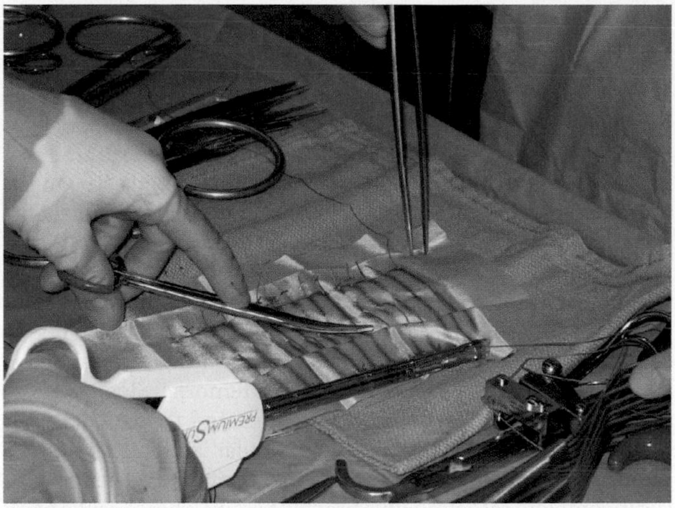

Figure 88-2. Excess source material is cut and disposed off properly in accordance with radiation disposal guidelines.

source delivery system has been developed which can be used in conjunction with commercially available surgical stapling instruments (Fig. 88-5). This includes a radioactive ^{169}Yb seed sealed within titanium tube 0.28 mm in diameter and then capped and resealed by titanium wires laser welded to the tube to serve as legs of a tissue-fastening system. The use of these in patients is subject of future study.[2]

Planar Implant Experience

Santos et al.[3] from Allegheny General Hospital published a large series using this technique. Their retrospective study of 101 patients with sublobar resection and planar seed implants at the suture line was compared with 102 similar patients with sublobar resection alone. Patients were surgically resected using video-assisted thoracic surgery (VATS) technique. The implants were made using Vicryl mesh. A planned dose of 100

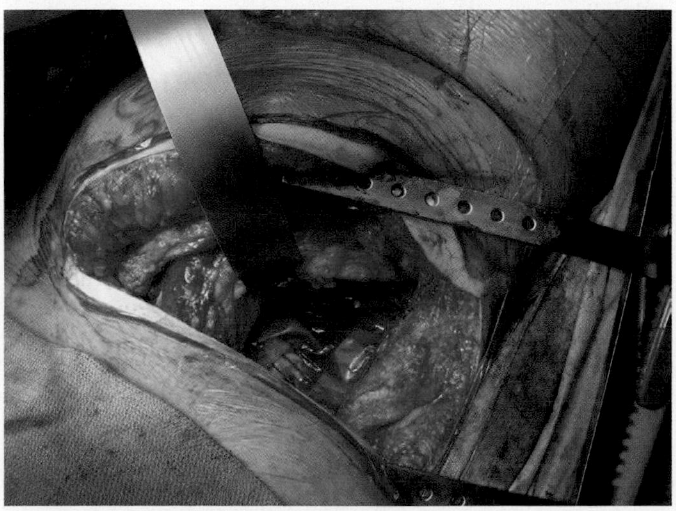

Figure 88-3. The source material is attached to Dacron or Vicryl absorbable mesh and trimmed to the treatment area. One centimeter is added to the overall dimension before trimming to leave an adequate margin for suturing. Intraoperatively, the custom mesh is placed over the treatment area and sutured in place, taking great care to avoid puncturing the radioactive seeds.

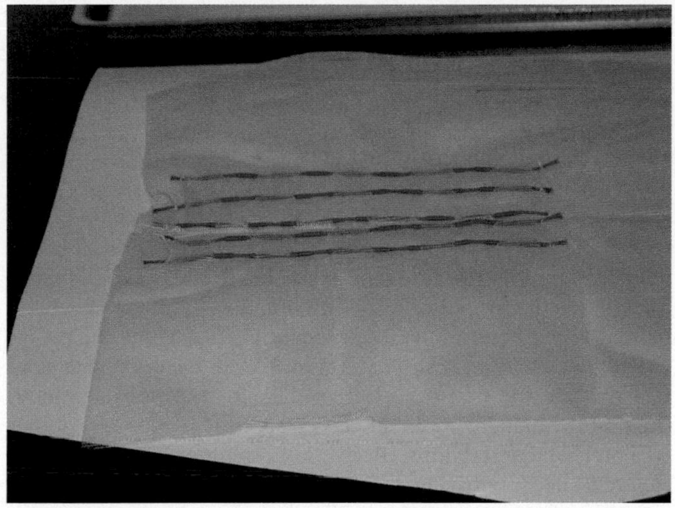

Figure 88-4. The source is preloaded in Vicryl suture and mesh. The implant is sterile and can be immediately implanted. Pictured is ^{131}Cs, but ^{125}I is also available.

to 120 Gy was delivered to a depth of 0.5 cm. The mesh then was sutured to the staple line. The local relapse rate was 2% for seeds (at 18 months) versus 18.6% for sublobar resection alone (at 24 months, $p = 0.0001$). Age and FEV1 were similar in each group, but the group with the implants had more stage IB patients ($n = 23$) than the group undergoing surgery alone ($n = 0$). Overall 4-year survival was 60% for surgery alone and 67% for surgery plus seed implants. The results were not statistically significant.

The New England Medical Hospital and Tufts University published a series of 33 patients who underwent a wedge resection (or segmental resection) with seed implants at the lung margins.[4] The strands of seed in this series were implanted directly on the suture line without mesh. The planned dose was 125 to 140 Gy delivered to a depth of 1 cm. There was recurrence at the suture line in 2 of 33 (6%) patients (median follow-up 51 months), and the 5-year projected survival was 47%. The cancer-specific 5-year survival was 61%.

A multicenter retrospective study[5] compared lobar and sublobar resection in stage I non–small-cell lung carcinoma and examined the use of adjuvant brachytherapy with sublobar

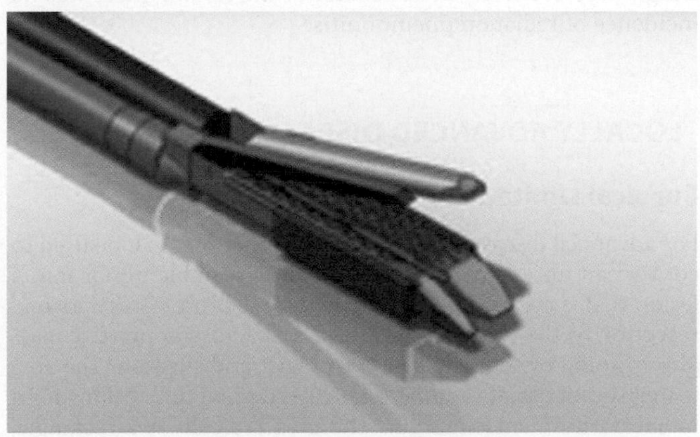

Figure 88-5. Gammaclip is a ^{169}Yb isotope imbedded in a surgical clip. The surgical clip can be used "sidecar" with commercially available staple devices.

resection. A total of 291 patients with T1N0 disease were evaluated, 124 treated with sublobar resection and 167 with lobectomy. Within the sublobar resection cohort, 60 out of 124 were treated with adjuvant Vicryl mesh brachytherapy with a significant decrease in local recurrence rate from 17.2% to 3.3% at a mean follow-up of 34.5 months in the mesh patient group. The American College of Surgeons Oncology Group (ACOSOG) has recently completed a phase III clinical trial ACOSOC Z4032 comparing sublobar resection alone and sublobar resection with adjuvant mesh brachytherapy. The early toxicity results for pulmonary function and dyspnea have been published.[6,7] These show no significant change from baseline on either PFT or dypnea scores. The outcome results of this trial will provide the first prospective data for the use of brachytherapy to augment sublobar resection.

Stereotactic Ablative Body Radiotherapy (SABR) or stereotactic body radiation therapy (SBRT) has also emerged as an option for treatment in medically inoperable patients with early-stage lung cancer. Another prospective ACOSOG study, ACOSOG Z4099/RTOG1021, is specifically for high-risk operable patients and randomly assigns patients to either sublobar resection with mesh implant brachytherapy or SABR.

Volume Tumor Implanting

For patients unable to tolerate surgery, the seeds can be implanted directly in the tumor using a variation of this technique called volume implanting. Although this technique yields an inferior result to surgery, for inoperable patients, this may be an option for increasing the radiation dose. The radioactive seeds, usually ^{125}I, are implanted in the tumor and any other area of gross disease. After the needle is inserted into the tumor, the seeds are deposited individually or in a line. The seeds are placed to cover a volume of disease, in contrast to the planar technique, which targets the resection cavity and margin. Clinicians at the Memorial Sloan Kettering Cancer Center of New York reported 65% locoregional control in their experience with volume implants.[8] Another study from the Norris Cancer Center describes the volume implant technique used in 14 patients.[9] All patients underwent surgical lymph node staging before the procedure. ^{125}I seeds were used to implant the tumor. The local control rate was 71% with a 15-month median follow-up. All the relapses occurred in patients with stage III cancers. A dose of 80 Gy was delivered at the periphery, with a high dose of 200 Gy in the center of the tumor. There was no incidence of radiation pneumonitis.

LOCALLY ADVANCED DISEASE

Surgical Limitations

For advanced disease, brachytherapy sometimes can be used to convert an unresectable or marginally resectable tumor into a lesion that is acceptable for oncologic resection. After maximal resection by the surgeon, the area at risk (close or positive margin) is noted by the radiation oncologist and surgeon. The area is measured, usually adding 0.5 to 1 cm to all dimensions for a radiation dosimetric margin. The area typically is a rectangle, but can be any shape. This area then is treated with brachytherapy. One way to clear this margin is to place a permanent planar implant.

Planar Seed Experience for Locally Advanced Disease

Dana-Farber Cancer Institute published their experience of patients with a total of 48 implants.[10] The implant model we used consisted of ^{125}I seeds in suture that were then sutured to a mesh patch and implanted in high-risk surgical beds. The mean follow-up in our series was 21 months. Local control was maintained in 81%. There were three patients (6%) with grade 3 to 4 toxicity, one with a tracheoesophageal fistula, one with esophageal perforation, and one with persistent pneumothorax. Both patients with esophageal problems had partial-thickness resection of their esophagus with seeds placed on the surgical bed.[11]

A retrospective series from the Memorial Sloan Kettering Cancer Center demonstrated that stage III patients with mediastinal involvement exhibited similar median (16 vs. 17 months) and 5-year survival (15%) for complete resection versus incomplete resection plus brachytherapy. These results were superior to brachytherapy alone without resection and neither resection nor brachytherapy.[12] The Memorial Sloan Kettering Cancer Center reported another series of patients with all lung cancer stages. This series had a 50% increase in median survival (8–12 months) with brachytherapy after incomplete resection compared with no surgery.[13] This was compared with a 17-month median survival for complete resection. New York Hospital looked at this technique in a prospective study.[14] Twelve patients with stage III non–small-cell lung cancer who had gross or microscopically positive margins after resection were implanted using the planar technique. The implants were composed of either ^{125}I or ^{103} Pd embedded in a Gelfoam plaque. The dose prescribed was a 1-cm margin around the area of positive margins. All patients received either preoperative or postoperative external beam radiation at a dose range of 45 to 60 Gy. The results showed 82% local control with addition of brachytherapy for positive margins after surgery. The 2-year overall and cancer-specific survivals were 45% and 56%, respectively. In another series, the Memorial Sloan Kettering Cancer Center also reported 75% locoregional control with partial resection and implant compared with 86% locoregional control with full resection.[15]

Intraoperative Radiation Therapy (IORT) and Afterloading Catheters

Radiation delivered intraoperatively also can be used for treating close and positive resection margins. Two methods can be used: afterloading and IORT. Afterloading is delivered by placing hollow blind-ended plastic catheters along the area at risk, after which the radiation is loaded into the catheters. The catheters are spaced 1 cm apart in parallel lines. The open end of the catheter is directed out of the skin. Care must be taken to prevent kinking or sharp angles, which would prevent loading. The patient is permitted to stabilize for a period and then sent to the radiation department for loading. IORT is delivered more conventionally using a mobile accelerator in a specially equipped operating room (OR).

Afterloading

Afterloading can be delivered by a low-dose-rate (LDR) or high-dose-rate (HDR) method. With the LDR method, radioactive sources on a string are loaded into the catheters, where they remain for several days. During the interval, the patient

Table 88-1

PUBLISHED EXPERIENCE WITH INTRAOPERATIVE RADIATION THERAPY (IORT)

INSTITUTION	NUMBER OF PATIENTS	RADIATION SCHEME	RESULTS
NCI[18]	4	IORT 0, 20, 30, 40 Gy	25% 5-yr OS, toxicity over 25 Gy
Graz University[19]	14	IORT 10–20 Gy + EBRT 46–56 Gy	5-yr OS 15%, recurrence-free 5 yr 53%
Montpellier[20]	17	IORT 10–20 GY + 45 Gy EBRT	Actuarial survival at 11 yrs 18%, median survival 36 mo
Allegheny University[17]	21	IORT 10 Gy + EBRT 45–59.4 Gy (pre or postop)	5-yr actuarial survival 33%
Instituto Madrileno[21] (Madrid, Spain)	18	IORT +EBRT (per or postop)	5-yr actuarial survival 22%, cause-specific 33%

must remain isolated in a radiation-safe room with full radiation precautions. After an appropriate interval, the catheters are removed and radiation precautions are withdrawn. A newer version of this technique, HDR afterloading, uses a remote-control device. Catheters are placed, as with the LDR method. However, the radiation is delivered using a single computer-controlled source that can be placed at various positions and dwell times. This flexibility permits greater dose conformation, termed dose optimization. All treatments are delivered in a shielded room, which reduces incidental dose exposure to the technical staff. Both techniques are considered radiobiologically equivalent. The Memorial Sloan Kettering Cancer Center has used the afterloading technique (LDR) in the mediastinum with good local control and 2-year actuarial survivals of 76% and 51%, respectively, for N2 disease. Another group from Seattle also demonstrated good local control with the addition of brachytherapy.[16]

Intraoperative Radiation Therapy

Specialized equipment is needed for IORT. The radiation can be delivered using a mobile accelerator in a shielded OR or in the radiation department, where the radiation vault is also a functional OR. After surgical resection, the area at risk must be demarcated by the surgeon. The normal tissue can be moved out of the field or shielded with thin strips of lead. The cone from the linear accelerator is inserted into the patient, or applicators for HDR brachytherapy are placed. All personnel must leave the room when the radiation is delivered, which usually takes several minutes.

IORT Experience

Several series have used this technique. The largest series in the literature is from the University Clinic of Navarra, Pamplona, Spain.[17] Calvo and colleagues retrospectively reported findings in 104 patients treated between 1984 and 1993, all of whom had stage IIIA or IIIB cancers. Between 1984 and 1989, 22 patients had surgery and IORT followed by endobronchial brachytherapy (EBRT). Between 1989 and 1993, 82 patients had neoadjuvant chemotherapy. Responders (46 patients) had surgery, IORT, and EBRT; nonresponders had chemoradiation, surgery, with IORT as a final boost. Their technique used a dose of 10 to 15 Gy (18–20 Gy unresectable). The series reported local control rates for patients with microscopic residual disease of 66% (33 of 50) and 35% (15 of 42) for patients with macroscopic residual disease. The best results were observed with Pancoast tumors, which demonstrated a local control rate of 92% (11 of 12) and 100% (5 of 5) for microscopic and macroscopic disease, respectively. The most common toxic event was grade III–IV esophagitis in 25%. Other reported toxicities were symptomatic pneumonitis, transient neuropathy, and lung fibrosis. Other series are listed in Table 88-1.

Complications

Complications from any of these techniques are similar and minimal compared with the surgery itself. Poor wound healing or abscess formation can occur but is very rare. The most concerning toxicity is fistula formation. Care must be used to avoid placing the seeds directly on any injured organ, such as the esophagus or blood vessels.[11] Intact tissue can tolerate very-low-dose-rate (VLDR) radiation well; however, any injury to the organ, whether caused by the tumor or as a consequence of the surgery, can predispose to a fistula. This complication can be avoided when implantation is necessary by adding another layer of luminal protection for the blood vessels of the esophagus using biologic or artificial technique. However, if there has been extensive dissection in the subcarinal space or partial esophageal wall resection, we do not recommend permanent seed implantation because of the predisposition to fistula formation, necessitating further surgery. We have reported two cases of mediastinal carcinoid tumors in patients who had been treated previously with chemoradiation. In both instances, the tumor was adherent to the esophageal muscularis, and an esophageal fistula developed, necessitating additional surgical repair.[22]

Recurrence or Metastasis

Tumor recurrence or metastasis can be treated with brachytherapy. Brachytherapy has the advantage that it can be used for patients and tumors that have already received radiation. Care must be taken in reirradiating the heart, spinal cord, or esophagus; the other organs can tolerate reirradiation with brachytherapy. Depending on the location and surgical resection, any of the previously described techniques can be used, from permanent seeds, to afterloading catheters, to IORT. Sometimes seed implants are preferred because of their slower rate of delivery. The slower the rate, the larger is the dose of reirradiation the patient can tolerate. LDR and VLDR techniques are better tolerated than HDR techniques in certain risky organs.

ENDOBRONCHIAL LESIONS

Endobronchial Primary

Some data exist regarding the use of endobronchial therapy as a boost or alternative to external beam therapy for definitive treatment. Although, theoretically, the addition of endobronchial therapy should escalate the dose, there are no prospective data showing that this therapy prolongs survival or increases local control. One retrospective study shows good control from definitive EBRT.[23] The majority of data of endobronchial radiation shows reduction of symptoms.

Palliation

One of the most common uses of brachytherapy is EBRT for palliation. Patients with lung disease commonly experience obstructive pneumonia, hemoptysis, or both. These symptoms can drastically affect quality of life or even be life threatening. Radiation can be administered for palliation, either with external beam or brachytherapy. Brachytherapy provides a benefit because higher doses can be delivered directly to the tumor, sparing the normal lung. The only disadvantage of brachytherapy is the necessity of putting the patient through another procedure, which some end-stage patients might not be able to tolerate.

Technique

The patient is bronchoscoped under conscious sedation or general anesthesia. After the tumor is visualized, a brachytherapy catheter is threaded through the bronchoscope. The proximal end remains outside the patient, and the distal end lies distal to the tumor. The proximal and distal extents of the tumor in relation to the catheter should be noted for treatment planning, usually under fluoroscopy. The radiation source then is placed in the catheter, usually with an HDR afterloader, but LDR also can be used. The catheter could be used for multiple fractions if it can be secured safely and the patient has been admitted to the hospital. Otherwise, the entire procedure should be repeated for two-to-three fractions for full palliation.

Experience

The M. D. Anderson Cancer Center published[24] its 10-year experience with EBRT for palliation in a series of 175 patients, 160 of whom received previous external beam therapy. The treatment regimen was 15 Gy × 2 at 6 mm from the catheter for a total dose of 30 Gy. The results showed a rate of 66% subjective improvement (34% slight improvement, 32% significant improvement) and 78% objective improvement on repeat bronchoscopy. The complication rate was 11%. The rate of major complications (e.g., massive hemoptysis) was 5%. Table 88-2 summarizes the published series on EBRT.

Complications

The major complications from EBRT, aside from procedural events relating to bronchoscopy, are massive hemoptysis and bronchial necrosis. Whether the etiology of hemoptysis is a consequence of the treatment or the tumor is a controversial issue. However, by fractionating the treatment, toxicity can be avoided. Langendijk et al. showed that treatment doses of 7.5 or 10 Gy yielded 11% mortality from hemoptysis, similar to controls,[29,30] whereas 15 Gy at 1 cm was associated with almost 50% mortality from hemoptysis. Similar results were reported by Muto et al. from Italy. They found that fractionating the dose from 10 Gy × 1, 7 Gy × 2, and 5 Gy × 3 (all prescribed to a depth of 1 cm) yielded a similar response, but there were fewer side effects with the greater number of fractions.[31]

SUMMARY

The goal of these innovative radiation therapies is locoregional control because not all patients are suitable candidates for lobectomy or pneumonectomy, and sublobar resections are associated with an increased rate of local recurrence. Since virtually every study comparing the effectiveness of lobectomy or pneumonectomy versus wedge resection favors the lobectomy, and many patients cannot tolerate a full surgical resection, the combination of limited resection and brachytherapy may have widespread application in future clinical studies.[14] Other circumstances that favor the use of a limited resection with targeted brachytherapy include advanced age, poor pulmonary function, presence of other high-risk comorbidities, unresectable tumor mass, need for palliation, tumor reduction to render a mass oncologically resectable, and so forth.

EDITOR'S COMMENT

Although this technique is well accepted for endobronchial disease in high-risk individuals, it has only occasionally been used as a routine for unresectable tumors or suspicious margins. The recently completed American College of Surgeons' Oncology Study Group (ACOSOG) Z40 study and subsequent other trials, seek to evaluate the role of brachytherapy seeds used after wedge resection in high-risk individuals to improve local control and perhaps disease-free survival. This study will show the safety and efficacy of this technique. Other high-dose techniques, including intraoperative radiation, are also discussed comprehensively.

—Mark J. Krasna

Table 88-2

PUBLISHED EXPERIENCE WITH ENDOBRONCHIAL BRACHYTHERAPY (EBBT)

INSTITUTION	PATIENTS	DOSE	EBRT	RESULTS
M.D. Anderson[24]	175	15 Gy at 6 mm	Yes (160)	66% subjective improvement 78% objective improvement
Hackensack University[25]	117	5 Gy at 1 cm times 3	Yes, 37.5 Gy	72% resolution of symptoms 54% bronchoscopic response
Defense military service, Madrid[26]	81	5 Gy times 4 at 0.5–1 cm	no	85% symptomatic complete response 56% broncoscopic complete response
Ankara University[27]	95	7.5 Gy times 3 or 10 Gy times 2 at 1 cm	Some patients with history of EBRT	All symptoms responded (details not given)
Clinique Sainte Catherine[28]	189	8–10 Gy times 3–4 at 1 cm	Some patients with history of EBRT (69.3%)	Responses: Hemoptysis 74% Dyspnea 54% Cough 54%

References

1. Ginsberg RJ, Rubinstein LV. Randomized trial of lobectomy versus limited resection for T1N0 non-small cell lung cancer. Lung cancer study group. *Ann Thorac Surg*. 1995;60:615–22; discussion 622–623.
2. Leonard KL, Depetrillo TA, Munro JJ, et al. A novel ytterbium-169 brachytherapy source and delivery system for use in conjunction with minimally invasive wedge resection of early-stage lung cancer. *Brachytherapy*. 2011; 10(2):163–169.
3. Santos R, Colonias A, Parda D, et al. Comparison between sublobar resection and iodine-125 brachytherapy after sublobar resection in high-risk patients with stage I non-small-cell lung cancer. *Surgery*. 2003;134:691–697; discussion 697.
4. Lee W, Daly BD, DiPetrillo TA, et al. Limited resection for non-small cell lung cancer: observed local control with implantation of I-125 brachytherapy seeds. *Ann Thorac Surg*. 2003;75:237–242; discussion 242–243.
5. Fernando HC, Santos RS, Benfield JR, et al. Lobar and sublobar resection with and without brachytherapy for small stage IA non-small cell lung cancer. *J Thorac Cardiovasc Surg*. 2005;129(2):261–267.
6. Fernando HC, Landreneau RJ, Mandrekar SJ, et al. The impact of adjuvant brachytherapy with sublobar resection on pulmonary function and dyspnea in high-risk patients with operable disease: preliminary results from the American College of Surgeons Oncology Group Z4032 trial. *J Thorac Cardiovasc Surg*. 2011;142(3):554–562.
7. Fernando HC, Landreneau RJ, Mandrekar SJ, et al. Thirty- and ninety-day outcomes after sublobar resection with and without brachytherapy for non-small cell lung cancer: results from a multicenter phase III study. *J Thorac Cardiovasc Surg*. 2011;142(5):1143–1151.
8. Hilaris BS, Nori D, Beattie EJ Jr, et al. Value of perioperative brachytherapy in the management of non-oat cell carcinoma of the lung. *Int J Radiat Oncol Biol Phys*. 1983;9:1161–1166.
9. Fleischman EH, Kagan AR, Streeter OE, et al. Iodine-125 interstitial brachytherapy in the treatment of carcinoma of the lung. *J Surg Oncol*. 1992;49: 25–28.
10. Mutyala S, Stewart A, Khan AJ, et al. Permanent iodine-125 interstitial planar seed brachytherapy for close or positive margins for thoracic malignancies. *Int J Radiat Oncol Biol Phys*. 2010;76(4):1114–1120.
11. Stewart A, O'Farrell D, Kazakin J. Esophageal fistula formation following partial esophageal wall resection and permanent radioactive seed implantation for mediastinal carcinoid tumors. *Radiother Oncol*. 2004;71: S139–S140.
12. Burt ME, Pomerantz AH, Bains MS, et al. Results of surgical treatment of stage III lung cancer invading the mediastinum. *Surg Clin North Am*. 1987; 67:987–1000.
13. Hilaris BS, Martini N. The current state of intraoperative interstitial brachytherapy in lung cancer. *Int J Radiat Oncol Biol Phys*. 1988;15:1347–1354.
14. Nori D, Pugkhem T. Intraoperative brachytherapy using Gelfoam radioactive plaque implants for resected stage III non-small cell lung cancer with positive margin: a pilot study. *J Surg Oncol*. 1995;60:257–261.
15. Hilaris BS, Martini N. Interstitial brachytherapy in cancer of the lung: a 20-year experience. *Int J Radiat Oncol Biol Phys*. 1979;5:1951–1956.
16. Aye RW, Mate TP, Anderson HN, et al. Extending the limits of lung cancer resection. *Am J Surg*. 1993;165:572–576.
17. Calvo FA, Ortiz de Urbina D, Abuchaibe O, et al. Intraoperative radiotherapy during lung cancer surgery: technical description and early clinical results. *Int J Radiat Oncol Biol Phys*. 1990;19:103–109.
18. Pass HI, Sindelar WF, Kinsella TJ, et al. Delivery of intraoperative radiation therapy after pneumonectomy: experimental observations and early clinical results. *Ann Thorac Surg*. 1987;44:14–20.
19. Juettner FM, Arian-Schad K, Porsch G, et al. Intraoperative radiation therapy combined with external irradiation in nonresectable non-small-cell lung cancer: preliminary report. *Int J Radiat Oncol Biol Phys*. 1990;18:1143–1150.
20. Fisher S, Fallahnejad M, Lisker S. Role of intraoperative radiation therapy (IORT) for stage III non-small cell lung cancer. *Hepatogastroenterology*. 1994;41:15.
21. Aristu J, Rebollo J, Martinez-Monge R, et al. Cisplatin, mitomycin, and vindesine followed by intraoperative and postoperative radiotherapy for stage III non-small cell lung cancer: final results of a phase II study. *Am J Clin Oncol*. 1997;20:276–281.
22. Stewart AJ, O'Farrell DA, Mutyala S, et al. Severe toxicity after permanent radioactive seed implantation for mediastinal carcinoid tumors. *Brachytherapy*. 2007;6:58–61.
23. Aumont-le Guilcher M, Prevost B, Sunyach MP, et al. High dose rate for non-small cell lung carcinoma: a retrospective study of 226 patients. *Int J Radiat Oncol Biol Phys*. 2011;79(4):1112–1116. Epub 2010 May 25.
24. Kelly JF, Delclos ME, Morice RC, et al. High-dose-rate endobronchial brachytherapy effectively palliates symptoms due to airway tumors: the 10-year M. D. Anderson cancer center experience. *Int J Radiat Oncol Biol Phys*. 2000;48:697–702.
25. Gejerman G, Mullokandov EA, Bagiella E, et al. Endobronchial brachytherapy and external-beam radiotherapy in patients with endobronchial obstruction and extrabronchial extension. *Brachytherapy*. 2002;1:204–210.
26. Escobar-Sacristan JA, Granda-Orive JI, Gutierrez Jimenez T, et al. Endo bronchial brachytherapy in the treatment of malignant lung tumours. *Eur Respir J*. 2004;24:348–352.
27. Celebioglu B, Gurkan OU, Erdogan S, et al. High dose rate endobronchial brachytherapy effectively palliates symptoms due to inoperable lung cancer. *Jpn J Clin Oncol*. 2002;32:443–448.
28. Taulelle M, Chauvet B, Vincent P, et al: High dose rate endobronchial brachytherapy: results and complications in 189 patients. *Eur Respir J*. 1998;11: 162–168.
29. Langendijk JA, Tjwa MK, de Jong JM, et al. Massive haemoptysis after radiotherapy in inoperable non-small cell lung carcinoma: is endobronchial brachytherapy really a risk factor? *Radiother Oncol*. 1998;49:175–183.
30. Langendijk H, de Jong J, Tjwa M, et al. External irradiation versus external irradiation plus endobronchial brachytherapy in inoperable non-small cell lung cancer: a prospective randomized study. *Radiother Oncol*. 2001; 58:257–268.
31. Muto P, Ravo V, Panelli G, et al. High-dose rate brachytherapy of bronchial cancer: treatment optimization using three schemes of therapy. *Oncologist*. 2000;5:209–214.

89 Adjuvant and Neoadjuvant Chemotherapy

Stephanie Cardarella and Bruce E. Johnson

Keywords: Adjuvant, neoadjuvant, chemotherapy

The most effective treatment for early-stage (I–IIIA) non-small-cell lung cancer (NSCLC) is surgical resection. Despite optimal surgical techniques employed for the resections, a substantial percentage of patients with stage I–IIIA NSCLC subsequently relapse and die from their lung cancer.[1] Studies that suggested adjuvant chemotherapy could prolong survival for some patients with early-stage lung cancer began to emerge. A number of trials have since documented that the use of chemotherapy in both the preoperative (neoadjuvant) and postoperative (adjuvant) settings can prolong survival. This chapter summarizes the evidence showing the benefit from adjuvant and neoadjuvant therapy for specific subgroups of patients with early-stage NSCLC.

ADJUVANT CHEMOTHERAPY

Randomized trials including 29 to 841 patients with early-stage NSCLC performed over the last 30 years were jointly analyzed in an individual patient data meta-analysis published by the Non-Small Cell Lung Cancer Collaborative Group (NSCLCCG) in 1995.[2] This analysis, involving more than 4300 patients, showed a strong trend toward improved survival of approximately 5% at 5 years for patients with surgically resected early-stage NSCLC treated with adjuvant cisplatin-based chemotherapy compared with those on observation alone (hazard ratio [HR] = 0.87; 95% confidence interval [CI], 0.74 to 1.02; $p = 0.08$). These results prompted a new generation of larger randomized controlled trials to attempt to validate the observations made in the meta-analysis. The patient, treatment, and outcome information from the studies enrolling more than 300 patients and comparing surgery alone to surgery followed by chemotherapy is presented in Table 89-1. This chapter does not address the use of postoperative tegafur and uracil (UFT). Although Japanese trials have demonstrated a survival benefit with adjuvant UFT, there have been no confirmatory trials in Western populations, and this agent is not presently available in the United States so is not included in this chapter.[9]

Adjuvant Therapy Trials Showing a Difference in Survival

All of the six trials were initiated between 1994 and 1996 when the information from the meta-analysis became available. With the exception of the Big Lung Trial (BLT), which had only about 20% power to detect a 5% improvement in survival with adjuvant chemotherapy, five of the six trials had adequate power to detect up to a 13% difference in survival between the surgery alone and the chemotherapy arms. Three of the six trials listed in Table 89-1 reported a statistically significant survival advantage in the patients treated with chemotherapy after their resection. In the initial study referred to as the International Adjuvant Lung Trial (IALT), 1867 patients with stage I–IIIA NSCLC who underwent a complete resection of their tumor were randomly assigned to either observation or cisplatin given for three to four cycles in combination with etoposide, vinblastine, vinorelbine, or vindesine.[4] Investigators from each institution had the option of administering chest radiotherapy after the completion of surgery and/or chemotherapy for patients with node-positive disease according to their institutional policy. Although

Table 89-1

OVERVIEW OF THE ADJUVANT CHEMOTHERAPY TRIALS ENROLLING MORE THAN 300 PATIENTS, PUBLISHED AFTER THE 1995 NON–SMALL-CELL LUNG CANCER META-ANALYSIS

	ALPI[3]	IALT[4]	BLT[5]	JBR.10[6]	CALGB 9633[7]	ANITA[8]
Study dates	1994–1999	1995–2000	1995–2001	1994—2001	1996–2003	1994–2000
No. of patients	1088	1867	381	482	344	840
Stage eligibility	I–IIIA	I–III	I–III	IB–II	IB	IB–IIIA
Chemotherapy regimen	Mitomycin, vindesine and cisplatin	Cisplatin plus a vinca alkaloid or etoposide	Cisplatin-based[a]	Cisplatin and vinorelbine	Carboplatin and paclitaxel	Cisplatin and vinorelbine
No. of cycles planned	3	3 or 4	3	4	4	4
Pneumonectomy, no. (%)	274 (25%)	648 (35%)	NA	114 (24%)	37 (11%)	310 (37%)
Postoperative radiotherapy	Optional	Optional	Optional	None	None	Optional
Median follow-up, years	5.4	4.7	NA	5.1	6.2	6.3
Hazard ratio for death	0.96	0.86	1.02	0.69	0.83	0.8
95% confidence interval	0.81–1.13	0.76–0.98	0.77–1.35	0.52–0.91	0.64–1.08	0.66–0.96
p-value	0.589	<0.03	0.9	0.04	0.125	0.017
Absolute difference in 5-year survival	1%	4.1%	NA	15%	2%	8.6%

[a]One of four regimens—cisplatin/vindesine, mitomycin/ifosfamide/cisplatin, mitomycin/vinblastine/cisplatin, or vinorelbine/cisplatin.
NA, not available.

the study was terminated early because of slow accrual (3300 patients initially planned), there was a significant improvement in survival in favor of the chemotherapy arm (HR = 0.86; 95% CI, 0.76 to 0.98; $p < 0.03$), translating into an absolute gain of 4.1% at 5 years (from 40.4% to 44.5%). An updated report after 7 years of follow-up, however, revealed that the overall survival advantage was no longer significant (HR = 0.91; 95% CI, 0.81 to 1.02; $p = 0.10$).[10] This late loss of survival benefit appeared to be due to an excess of non–cancer-related deaths in the chemotherapy arm and an increased mortality rate from other causes in this smoking population.

The National Cancer Institute of Canada Clinical Trials Group reported another adjuvant chemotherapy trial (JBR.10) showing a difference in patient outcome.[6] In this trial, 482 completely resected stage IB or II NSCLC patients were randomized to postoperative observation or to vinorelbine, 25 mg/m^2 weekly and cisplatin, 50 mg/m^2 on days 1 and 8 of a 4-week cycle for four cycles. No chest radiotherapy was administered. After a median follow-up of 5.1 years, overall survival was significantly prolonged for the patients treated with surgery plus chemotherapy compared with those treated with surgical resection alone (HR for death = 0.69; 95% CI, 0.52 to 0.91; $p = 0.04$). Five-year survival rates were 69% and 54%, respectively. An updated survival analysis of the JBR.10 trial reported a persistent survival advantage for patients treated with adjuvant chemotherapy after more than 9 years of follow-up.[11] Notably, in both these reports, the benefit was restricted to patients with resected stage II disease and was not seen in the subjects with stage IA and IB NSCLC.

The Adjuvant Navelbine International Trialist Association (ANITA) study also examined adjuvant vinorelbine and cisplatin following resection of the participants' lung cancer.[8] Eight hundred forty patients with stage IB–IIIA NSCLC who had undergone a successful surgical resection were randomly assigned to either observation or chemotherapy. Patients on both arms of the study could receive chest radiation therapy at the discretion of the treating physician. Adjuvant treatment with cisplatin and vinorelbine was associated with significantly improved survival (HR = 0.80; 95% CI, 0.66 to 0.96; $p = 0.017$). The survival benefit for patients randomized to receive chemotherapy compared with controls was 8.6% at 5 years and was maintained at 7 years (8.4%). Again, this benefit was observed in patients with stage II and IIIA NSCLC.

Negative Adjuvant Therapy Trials

The benefits of postoperative chemotherapy demonstrated in the three adjuvant therapy trials that showed a survival advantage for the patients treated with chemotherapy after resection were challenged by three other randomized trials completed after the 1995 meta-analysis, which all failed to show a significant survival advantage with adjuvant chemotherapy. The Adjuvant Lung Project Italy (ALPI) studied patients with resected stage I–IIIA NSCLC by randomly allocating them to treatment with mitomycin, vindesine, and cisplatin (MVP) every 3 weeks for three cycles or to observation after complete surgical resection.[3] Postoperative thoracic radiation was allowed at the discretion of each participating site. One thousand eighty-eight patients were analyzed after a median follow-up period of 64.5 months. In the chemotherapy arm, 69% of patients completed the MVP treatment and half of them required dose modifications or omission of part of the planned regimen. There was no difference between the outcome of patients treated with resection plus chemotherapy versus those treated with surgery alone (HR for death = 0.96; 95% CI, 0.81 to 1.13; $p = 0.589$). The use of the chemotherapy regimen of MVP is considered inferior by today's standards, which may have led to the high death rates during the first year after randomization and the poor compliance with chemotherapy, two strong criticisms of the study. Similarly, the BLT, a randomized trial conducted in the United Kingdom, investigated cisplatin-based chemotherapy in patients deemed potentially resectable or who had undergone resection of their lung cancer.[5] The patients could be treated before (3%) or after (97%) surgical resection with cisplatin for three cycles combined with one of four different regimens (mitomycin and ifosfamide, mitomycin and vinblastine, vindesine, or vinorelbine) or observed without a course of chemotherapy. No benefit from adjuvant chemotherapy was seen among 381 patients. However, the trial was underpowered to detect the magnitude of difference in survival observed in the other trials, and a considerable proportion (15%) of patients had microscopically incomplete surgical resection, which was unlike the other trials.

The CALGB 9633 trial was unique in limiting enrollment to patients with resected stage IB NSCLC who were randomized to treatment with paclitaxel and carboplatin every 3 weeks for four cycles or to observation.[7] The study was terminated early when an interim analysis in 2004 suggested a significantly higher survival rate with adjuvant therapy. After additional follow-up and reanalysis of the data in 2006, the survival benefit still favored chemotherapy but was no longer significant in the overall population (HR = 0.83; 90% CI, 0.64 to 1.08; $p = 0.12$), although the reduction in the hazard ratio of death was of a magnitude similar to that seen in the IALT (HR = 0.86) and ANITA (HR = 0.80) trials. With 344 patients, CALGB 9633 may have lacked statistical power to detect small but clinically meaningful improvements in survival in this relatively good risk population. Further, the use of a carboplatin regimen as opposed to a cisplatin backbone may have affected the results, as a recent meta-analysis demonstrated cisplatin-based chemotherapy to be slightly superior to carboplatin regimens in advanced NSCLC.[12] The role of postoperative chemotherapy in surgically resected stage I NSCLC is discussed further later in this section.

META-ANALYSES

A meta-analysis (Lung Adjuvant Cisplatin Evaluation or LACE) combining individual patient data from the five large adjuvant cisplatin-chemotherapy trials reviewed in this section (ALPI, BLT, IALT, ANITA, and JBR.10) has been published.[13] This analysis has provided insights into the subsets of patients likely to benefit from adjuvant chemotherapy following resection of their NSCLC. In this pooled analysis, data were available on 4584 patients from the trials described earlier in this chapter. The pooled analyses confirmed a statistically significant benefit on overall survival for chemotherapy compared with observation (HR = 0.89; 95% CI, 0.82 to 0.96; $p = 0.005$), corresponding to an absolute gain of 5.4% at 5 years. The benefits of chemotherapy were confined to patients with resected stage II or III disease (HR = 0.83; 95% CI, 0.73 to 0.95, and HR = 0.83; 95% CI, 0.72 to 0.94, respectively). There was suggestion of a worse outcome with adjuvant chemotherapy for the

347 patients with stage IA disease (HR = 1.40; 95% CI, 0.95 to 2.06) and 183 patients with an Eastern Cooperative Oncology Group performance status of two. The LACE meta-analysis also found a trend for longer survival for the patients treated with cisplatin plus vinorelbine compared to cisplatin plus one or two other drugs. However, the higher planned doses of cisplatin in the cisplatin- and vinorelbine-treated patients may be responsible for the observations. Finally, an update of the 1995 meta-analysis presented at the 2007 Annual Meeting of the American Society of Clinical Oncology, involving greater than 8000 patients, showed a convincing and consistent benefit with adjuvant chemotherapy for surgically resected NSCLC, with an overall significant benefit of 4% at 5 years (HR = 0.86; 95% CI, 0.81 to 0.93; $p < 0.000001$).[14]

Stage I NSCLC

The data from the adjuvant trials and meta-analyses support the use of chemotherapy for resected stage II and IIIA NSCLC. However, the data for stage I NSCLC are less clear. Few patients with stage IA disease were included in the reviewed studies. The LACE meta-analysis showed that the benefit of adjuvant chemotherapy varied significantly with stage, with a potential detriment for those with stage IA NSCLC, although data were available on fewer than 350 patients. Similarly, evidence is not yet available from the randomized trials or the LACE meta-analysis to routinely recommend adjuvant chemotherapy for resected stage IB disease. Stage IB NSCLC comprises a heterogeneous group of node-negative tumors, encompassing a wide range of tumor sizes (more than 3 cm but 7 cm or less) and considerable variability in prognosis. The CALGB 9633 was composed exclusively of stage IB patients. The study design showed that patients given paclitaxel and carboplatin lived a bit longer but did not reach a significant survival benefit for the overall population because of the modest antitumor activity of the adjuvant carboplatin and paclitaxel and the lack of power due to the small patient numbers. However, in an unplanned subset analysis, the trial reported significant disease-free and overall survival benefits in favor of postoperative chemotherapy in patients with tumors ≥4 cm in diameter (HR for death = 0.69; $p = 0.043$). In a similar exploratory subgroup analysis of the JBR.10 trial, stage IB patients with tumors 4 cm or greater showed a nonsignificant trend toward improved survival rates with adjuvant chemotherapy.[11] However, there are currently no prospectively validated data supporting a survival benefit with adjuvant chemotherapy in stage IB patients with larger tumors. Likewise, the presence of visceral pleural invasion identifies a group of stage IB patients with poorer prognosis. In a large retrospective analysis of 9758 patients who underwent surgical resection of their NSCLC, the Japanese Joint Committee for Cancer Registration demonstrated poorer survival of resected T2 tumors with visceral pleural invasion (5-year overall survival rate, 53.0%) compared with T2 tumors without visceral pleural invasion (61.6%; $p < 0.001$).[15] However, no analyses have yet reported on the impact of adjuvant chemotherapy in node-negative T2 tumors based on visceral pleural involvement.

RECOMMENDATIONS

Three randomized controlled trials of postoperative cisplatin-based chemotherapy (IALT, JBR.10, and ANITA) and two large individual patient data meta-analyses have convincingly demonstrated that cisplatin-doublet adjuvant chemotherapy causes a statistically significant and clinically meaningful survival advantage for patients with adequately resected early-stage NSCLC. The most consistent benefit from adjuvant chemotherapy has been reported in patients with surgically resected stage II and IIIA NSCLC. Based on this evidence, postoperative adjuvant cisplatin-based chemotherapy is now the standard of care for the management of completely resected stage II and IIIA NSCLC.[16] Data are not specifically available from the randomized trials or the LACE meta-analysis to inform the use of adjuvant chemotherapy in patients with separate tumor nodule(s) in the same lobe as the primary tumor, without lymph node involvement. Tumors with same-lobe nodules were reclassified as T3 instead of T4 on the basis of similar survival rates in the 7th edition of the tumor node metastasis (TNM) staging system for lung cancer of the American Joint Committee on Cancer (AJCC).[1] Our de facto practice is to consider these patients with T3 tumors with separate tumor nodule(s) in the same lobe for cisplatin-based adjuvant chemotherapy based on their similar survival to patients with T3 tumors without satellite nodule and data supporting adjuvant systemic therapy for resected stage IIB NSCLC. The benefit of adjuvant chemotherapy in patients with resected stage IB NSCLC is less concrete. There is incomplete data in studies of NSCLC patients with stage IB disease. Given the currently available information, we recommend strongly considering the stage IB patients with larger tumors (>4 cm) for cisplatin-based adjuvant chemotherapy in an individualized manner, after careful discussion of the risks and perceived modest benefits. Adjuvant systemic therapy may also reasonably be considered in patients with resected node-negative T2 tumors with visceral pleural invasion given their poorer prognosis for survival, although data from adjuvant trials are not yet available in this subgroup. Adjuvant chemotherapy is not recommended for patients with resected stage IA NSCLC. These recommendations are summarized in Table 89-2.

Two of the positive adjuvant therapy trials (JBR.10 and ANITA) used cisplatin and vinorelbine as the adjuvant regimen, and the LACE meta-analysis found that the effect of cisplatin plus vinorelbine was marginally better than the effect of other drug combinations. There are no prospective data suggesting a benefit of carboplatin-based adjuvant chemotherapy. Thus, based on the available evidence, the recommended chemotherapy in the adjuvant setting is cisplatin and vinorelbine. It remains to be determined whether a cisplatin doublet combined with more contemporary cytotoxic agents that have been shown to be more active in patients with stage IV NSCLC (gemcitabine, docetaxel, or pemetrexed) can be substituted

Table 89-2

RECOMMENDATIONS FOR ADJUVANT CISPLATIN-BASED CHEMOTHERAPY FOR SURGICALLY RESECTED NON–SMALL-CELL LUNG CANCER

STAGE	RECOMMENDATION
IA	Adjuvant chemotherapy is not recommended
IB	Adjuvant cisplatin-based chemotherapy is not recommended for routine use[a]
II	Adjuvant cisplatin-based chemotherapy is recommended
IIIA	Adjuvant cisplatin-based chemotherapy is recommended

[a]May consider in select stage IB patients with adverse prognostic factors, such as primary tumor ≥4.0 cm, or visceral pleural invasion (see text).

Table 89-3

ONGOING MULTICENTER CLINICAL TRIALS OF ADJUVANT SYSTEMIC THERAPY IN RESECTED EARLY-STAGE NSCLC

STUDY SPONSOR	IDENTIFIER	TRIAL DESIGN	NOTABLE ELIGIBILITY CRITERIA	SITES
ECOG	NCT00324805	Phase III, cisplatin-based adjuvant chemotherapy with or without bevacizumab after surgical resection	Resected stage IB (>4 cm)-IIIA	United States
CALGB	NCT00863512	Phase III, cisplatin-based adjuvant chemotherapy versus observation after surgical resection	Resected stage T1 a-T2bN0, tumor ≥2.0 cm but ≤7.0 cm	United States
GlaxoSmithKline	NCT00480025	Phase III, adjuvant MAGE-A3 ASCI versus observation after surgical resection +/− adjuvant chemotherapy	Resected stage IB-IIIA, tumor expression of MAGE-A3 by IHC	International
Spanish Lung Cancer Group	NCT00478699	Phase III, customized adjuvant chemotherapy based on BRCA1 mRNA levels after surgical resection	Resected stage II-IIIA	Spain
Intergroupe Francophone de Cancerologie Thoracique	NCT00775385	Phase II/III, standard versus customized adjuvant systemic therapy based on ERCC1 levels and EGFR mutations after surgical resection	Resected stage II-IIIA (non-N2), non-squamous	France
Intergroupe Francophone de Cancerologie Thoracique	NCT00775307	Phase II/III, adjuvant pazopanib versus placebo after surgical resection	Resected stage I (≤5 cm)	France
Chinese Lung Cancer Surgical Group	NCT01410214	Phase II, adjuvant erlotinib versus cisplatin/vinorelbine after surgical resection	Resected stage IIIA, EGFR mutation[a]	China
Massachusetts General Hospital	NCT00567359	Phase II, single arm, erlotinib after surgical resection +/− adjuvant chemotherapy	Resected stage I-IIIA lung adenocarcinoma, EGFR mutation[b]	United States
Massachusetts General Hospital	NCT01746251	Phase II, single arm, afatinib after surgical resection	Resected stage I-III NSCLC, EGFR mutation	United States

[a]EGFR activating mutation in exon 19 or 21.
[b]EGFR exon 19 deletion or the point mutation L858R in exon 21.
ECOG, Eastern Cooperative Oncology Group; CALGB, Cancer and Leukemia Group B; ASCI, antigen-specific cancer immunotherapeutic; IHC, immunohistochemistry; EGFR, epidermal growth factor receptor.

for cisplatin and vinorelbine with similar or more favorable results. The prevailing assumption is that the efficacy of modern cisplatin-based combinations in advanced NSCLC will likely translate to similar efficacy in the adjuvant setting. Correspondingly, the ongoing ECOG 1505 trial (NCT00324805) incorporates adjuvant chemotherapy regimens of cisplatin combined with vinorelbine, gemcitabine, docetaxel, or pemetrexed. The use of these four agents in combination with cisplatin reflects the consensus of the experienced investigators putting together the study. Given that it takes 7 to 10 years from the start of the study to get meaningful survival information, one begins to extrapolate information coming from the trials for patients with advanced disease before the information from the randomized adjuvant chemotherapy trials becomes available.

FUTURE DIRECTIONS

Current research efforts aim at identifying subsets of patients who derive the greatest benefit from adjuvant chemotherapy and those who do not benefit from adjuvant therapy by employing pharmacogenomic approaches to help assess potential efficacy and predict toxicity. In addition, there are ongoing efforts to use gene-expression profiling to identify individuals who are potential candidates for adjuvant systemic treatment for resected NSCLC patients. An example of this is expression of ERCC1 determined by mRNA expression or immunohistochemistry. ERCC1 is a key enzyme involved in DNA repair after cisplatin damage. This was specifically examined in the IALT Biology (IALT Bio) study, where adjuvant chemotherapy did not seem to confer a survival advantage in patients whose tumors had high expression of ERCC1.[17] The predictive value of ERCC1 expression on the effect of adjuvant chemotherapy is being prospectively evaluated in the Tailored Post-Surgical Therapy in Early Stage (TASTE) trial, conducted in Europe (NCT00775385; Table 89-3). Moreover, modern adjuvant therapy trials are attempting to integrate novel biological therapeutics, such as bevacizumab, into standard treatment paradigms. The addition of bevacizumab to paclitaxel and carboplatin has been successful in advanced NSCLC, and is now being investigated in the early-stage setting within the context of a large, phase III randomized controlled trial in the United States (NCT00324805; Table 89-3). The optimal adjuvant therapy for patients whose tumors harbor activating mutations of the epidermal growth factor (EGFR) is also being studied. Subjects with resected NSCLC and EGFR mutations are being treated with adjuvant chemotherapy with or without erlotinib (Table 89-3). Whether these approaches will improve upon the current standard of adjuvant cisplatin-based doublet chemotherapy remains to be determined.

NEOADJUVANT CHEMOTHERAPY

The role of chemotherapy prior to surgery has also been explored in patients deemed to have resectable NSCLC. The potential advantages of neoadjuvant chemotherapy over adjuvant administration include a reduction in tumor size thereby facilitating surgical resection, early eradication of micrometastases, in vivo assessment of the chemosensitivity of the cytotoxic regimen, and improved patient tolerability. However, neoadjuvant chemotherapy might delay potentially curative surgery.

In the early 1990s, two small, randomized trials generated marked interest in the role of neoadjuvant chemotherapy. These two trials, each of which involved 60 patients, compared surgery alone with surgery plus cisplatin-based preoperative or perioperative chemotherapy in patients with stage IIIA (T3 and/or N2) NSCLC.[18,19] Early stopping rules were applied in both studies after interim analyses. Both trials found improved

Table 89-4

OVERVIEW OF THE NEOADJUVANT CHEMOTHERAPY TRIALS ENROLLING MORE THAN 300 PATIENTS

	DEPIERRE ET AL.[20]	MRC LU22[21]	S9900[22]
Study dates	1991–1997	1997—2005	1999—2004
No. of patients	355	519	387
Clinical stage eligibility	IB-IIIA	I-III	IB-IIIA
Chemotherapy regimen and cisplatin carboplatin-based[a]	Mitomycin, ifosfamide Cisplatin or Carboplatin and paclitaxel		
No. of cycles planned	2 preoperatively (plus 2 postoperatively if response)	3	3
Radiographic response rate	64%	49%	41%
Postoperative radiotherapy	Yes if pT3, pN2 and/or incomplete resection	Optional	Not reported
Median follow-up, years	6.7	NA	5.3
Hazard ratio for death	0.80	1.02	0.79
95% confidence interval	0.61–1.04	0.80–1.31	0.60–1.06
p-value	0.089	0.86	0.11
Absolute difference in survival	8.6% at 4 years	Minus 1% at 5 years	9% at 5 years

[a]One of six regimens—cisplatin/mitomycin/vinblastine, cisplatin/mitomycin/ifosfamide, cisplatin/vinorelbine, cisplatin/gemcitabine, carboplatin/paclitaxel, or carboplatin/docetaxel.

NA, not available.

survival rates in patients receiving chemotherapy, although criticisms of these studies include their small size and unusually poor survival of the patients in the control arms. Nonetheless, these trials suggested a need for further research to address the role of neoadjuvant chemotherapy in resectable NSCLC.

Since publication of these early small studies demonstrating the feasibility and potential efficacy of neoadjuvant chemotherapy, a number of large randomized controlled trials have been conducted to evaluate the impact of preoperative chemotherapy for early-stage NSCLC. Summaries of the studies enrolling more than 300 patients are presented in Table 89-4. In the French study by Depierre et al., 355 patients with clinical stage IB–IIIA NSCLC were randomly assigned to undergo immediate surgery or to receive two cycles of mitomycin, ifosfamide, and cisplatin before surgical resection.[20] Patients who responded to preoperative chemotherapy received an additional two cycles postoperatively. In both arms, patients with pT3 or pN2 disease and/or those who had incomplete surgical resection received chest radiotherapy ($n = 113$) after either surgery or postoperative chemotherapy. Median (37 vs. 26 months; $p = 0.15$) and 4-year (43.9% vs. 35.3%) survival were prolonged for patients in the chemotherapy arm compared with those in the surgery alone arm, although these differences did not reach statistical significance. There was a nonsignificant excess of postoperative morbidity and mortality in the chemotherapy arm compared with the primary surgical arm (8.9% vs. 5.1%; $p = 0.16$). A subset analysis suggested that the benefit of chemotherapy was restricted to patients with N0/N1 disease.

In the largest trial reported to date, 519 patients (of 600 planned) with potentially resectable NSCLC were randomized to surgery alone or to receive three cycles of platinum-based chemotherapy (one of six regimens: cisplatin/mitomycin/vinblastine, cisplatin/mitomycin/ifosfamide, cisplatin/vinorelbine, cisplatin/gemcitabine, carboplatin/paclitaxel, or carboplatin/docetaxel) followed by surgery.[21] This trial, referred to as MRC LU22, was stopped early after compelling evidence supporting adjuvant chemotherapy emerged, establishing a new standard of care for resectable NSCLC. Most patients in LU22 had clinical stage I disease (61%), with 31% stage II and only 7% of patients with stage III NSCLC. Postoperative complications were similar between the two groups. No overall survival benefit was seen with neoadjuvant chemotherapy (HR = 1.02; 95% CI, 0.80 to 1.31; $p = 0.86$). Similar to the MRC LU22 trial, the North American S9900 trial closed prematurely after accruing 354 of 600 planned patients. This randomized phase III study evaluated the benefit of three cycles of preoperative carboplatin/paclitaxel followed by surgery with surgery alone in patients with clinical stage IB–IIIA NSCLC (excluding N2 disease).[22] After a median follow-up of 64 months, there was a nonsignificant trend in survival benefit in favor of preoperative chemotherapy (HR = 0.79; 95% CI, 0.60 to 1.06; $p = 0.11$), equivalent to an absolute gain of 9% at 5 years (50% vs. 41%). This magnitude of benefit is similar to that seen with adjuvant chemotherapy administered after the surgical resection. No interaction between treatment and stage was found in this study.

Meta-Analyses

The efficacy of neoadjuvant chemotherapy in resectable NSCLC has also been examined in large meta-analyses.[23–25] Two of the three published meta-analyses were based on pooled data from manuscripts and abstracts, a method considered inferior to a meta-analysis of individual patient data.[23,24] The NSCLCCG recently reported a systematic review and meta-analysis combining individual patient data from fifteen randomized controlled trials, involving 2385 patients, that evaluated the addition of preoperative chemotherapy to surgery versus surgery alone.[25] Seven of the fifteen trials used cisplatin-based chemotherapy, four carboplatin-based combinations, and three either cisplatin or carboplatin-based chemotherapy; the remaining trial employed docetaxel alone. Although all trials randomly assigned patients to neoadjuvant chemotherapy followed by surgery versus surgery alone, there was heterogeneity in the treatments given postoperatively, including five trials that used postoperative chemotherapy in the preoperative arm, usually in responders. Most patients had clinical stage IB-IIIA disease (IB, 44%; II, 27%; IIIA, 22%). The meta-analysis found a significant survival benefit to chemotherapy given before surgery over surgery alone, with a HR of 0.87 (95% CI, 0.78 to 0.96; $p = 0.007$), equivalent to an absolute improvement in survival of 5% at 5 years, similar to the magnitude of benefit observed for adjuvant chemotherapy administered after surgical resection. There was no evidence of a difference in the effect on survival by chemotherapy regimen, platinum agent used, or clinical stage.

ADJUVANT VERSUS NEOADJUVANT CHEMOTHERAPY

The adjuvant and neoadjuvant approaches were compared in the Neoadjuvant/Adjuvant Taxol Carboplatin Hope (NATCH) study, the first randomized controlled trial of preoperative versus postoperative chemotherapy in early-stage NSCLC. This three-arm trial, which accrued 624 patients, compared disease-free survival with surgery alone versus three cycles of preoperative or postoperative carboplatin and paclitaxel chemotherapy in resectable clinical stage I (tumor size > 2 cm), II, and T3N1 NSCLC.[26] Ninety percent of the patients in the neoadjuvant arm received their planned chemotherapy versus 66% in the adjuvant chemotherapy arm. Complete resection rates, surgical procedures, and postoperative mortality were similar across the three arms. After a median follow-up of 51 months, no significant differences in 5-year disease-free or overall survival were detected when preoperative or adjuvant chemotherapy was added to surgery. The study has been criticized for lacking statistical power to detect clinically meaningful differences about the outcome of patients treated with chemotherapy before or after surgery with only 200 patients per group. The numbers of patients needed to observe a 5% difference would need to be similar to the 400 to 900 patients on each arm of the IALT and ANITA studies. Further, despite broad stage eligibility, 75% of the patients had clinical stage I disease, a group in whom the benefit of systemic therapy is not firmly established. Finally, a meta-analysis comparing the efficacy of adjuvant versus neoadjuvant chemotherapy for early-stage NSCLC in 32 randomized trials (22 postoperative and 10 preoperative) involving over 10,000 patients has been published.[27] No significant differences in overall and disease-free survival were observed between the two groups.

Thus, the available evidence suggests that the relative effects of neoadjuvant and adjuvant systemic therapy are likely similar, with comparable hazard ratios for death in published meta-analyses: 0.89 for the adjuvant individual patient data (IPD) LACE meta-analysis, 0.86 for the updated adjuvant IPD NSCLCCG meta-analysis, and 0.87 for the IPD NSCLCCG meta-analysis of neoadjuvant chemotherapy. However, a more convincing body of evidence exists overall from large randomized controlled trials and meta-analyses for the efficacy and tolerability of postoperative chemotherapy than for preoperative chemotherapy. Thus, it is generally recommended that surgery, the most important treatment modality for early-stage NSCLC, not be delayed and that systemic treatment, if indicated, be administered postoperatively.

SUMMARY

The treatment of early-stage NSCLC has undergone a paradigm shift over the past 7 to 8 years with the addition of systemic therapy to local therapy. Several large randomized controlled trials and two meta-analyses have demonstrated a survival advantage for patients with stage II and IIIA NSCLC treated with adjuvant chemotherapy compared with those who underwent observation. Adjuvant platinum-based chemotherapy is now considered the standard of care for patients with stage II to IIIA NSCLC and may be considered an option for select stage IB patients with adverse prognostic factors (primary tumor greater than 4 cm, T2 tumor with visceral pleural invasion). The efficacy of preoperative chemotherapy in patients with early-stage NSCLC has also been analyzed in randomized trials and meta-analyses. Although meta-analyses suggest survival benefits comparable to those seen with postoperative chemotherapy, the majority of individual trials have found no statistically significant differences. However, the recruitment of a high percentage of patients with stage I disease, for whom the benefit of systemic therapy is not yet firmly established, variability of the chemotherapy regimens used, and early trial closure might be responsible for the negative results of individual studies. Further, an important limitation of neoadjuvant trials lies in the challenge to properly stage patients prior to surgical resection, especially stage II patients. Thus, based on clinical trials data, stronger evidence exists supporting the use of postoperative chemotherapy in patients with resectable NSCLC. In this era of personalized targeted therapy, research is ongoing to individualize systemic therapy in early-stage NSCLC and to integrate novel biological therapeutics into the treatment paradigm.

EDITOR'S COMMENT

This chapter provides a comprehensive update on the role of adjuvant therapy for NSCLC. Although there are some proponents of neoadjuvant chemotherapy for early stage disease, this treatment is mostly reserved for advanced stage IIA disease followed by surgical resection. There is a general consensus that chemotherapy with or without targeted therapy, for example, tyrosine kinase inhibitors (TKIs), should be used after stage T1-2, N1, and, of course, Tx N2 disease. The role in stage T3 disease is less clear with the group from New England Medical Center advocating use of a neoadjuvant chemotherapy regimen, which I advocate as well. Likewise, the use of neoadjuvant chemotherapy or chemoradiation therapy for stage T3 N1 is gaining popularity. The main area of controversy is whether patients with T2 N0 disease should also get routine chemotherapy after surgery. The preliminary data from the CALGB 9633 would suggest that this is the case, at least for stage T2 >4 cm lesions.

—Mark J. Krasna

References

1. Goldstraw P, Crowley J, Chansky K, et al. The IASLC Lung Cancer Staging Project: proposals for the revision of the TNM stage groupings in the forthcoming (seventh) edition of the TNM Classification of malignant tumours. *J Thorac Oncol*. 2007;2(8):706–714.
2. Chemotherapy in non-small cell lung cancer: a meta-analysis using updated data on individual patients from 52 randomised clinical trials. Non-small Cell Lung Cancer Collaborative Group. *BMJ*. 1995;311(7010):899–909.

3. Scagliotti GV, Fossati R, Torri V, et al. Randomized study of adjuvant chemotherapy for completely resected stage I, II, or IIIA non-small-cell Lung cancer. *J Natl Cancer Inst.* 2003;95(19):1453–1461.
4. Arriagada R, Bergman B, Dunant A, et al. Cisplatin-based adjuvant chemotherapy in patients with completely resected non-small-cell lung cancer. *N Engl J Med.* 2004;350(4):351–360.
5. Waller D, Peake MD, Stephens RJ, et al. Chemotherapy for patients with non-small cell lung cancer: the surgical setting of the Big Lung Trial. *Eur J Cardiothorac Surg.* 2004;26(1):173–182.
6. Winton T, Livingston R, Johnson D, et al. Vinorelbine plus cisplatin vs. observation in resected non-small-cell lung cancer. *N Engl J Med.* 2005; 352(25):2589–2597.
7. Strauss GM, Herndon JE 2nd, Maddaus MA, et al. Adjuvant paclitaxel plus carboplatin compared with observation in stage IB non-small-cell lung cancer: CALGB 9633 with the Cancer and Leukemia Group B, Radiation Therapy Oncology Group, and North Central Cancer Treatment Group Study Groups. *J Clin Oncol.* 2008;26(31):5043–5051.
8. Douillard JY, Rosell R, De Lena M, et al. Adjuvant vinorelbine plus cisplatin versus observation in patients with completely resected stage IB-IIIA non-small-cell lung cancer (Adjuvant Navelbine International Trialist Association [ANITA]): a randomised controlled trial. *Lancet Oncol.* 2006;7(9):719–727.
9. Kato H, Ichinose Y, Ohta M, et al. A randomized trial of adjuvant chemotherapy with uracil-tegafur for adenocarcinoma of the lung. *N Engl J Med.* 2004;350(17):1713–1721.
10. Arriagada R, Dunant A, Pignon JP, et al. Long-term results of the international adjuvant lung cancer trial evaluating adjuvant Cisplatin-based chemotherapy in resected lung cancer. *J Clin Oncol.* 2010;28(1):35–42.
11. Butts CA, Ding K, Seymour L, et al. Randomized phase III trial of vinorelbine plus cisplatin compared with observation in completely resected stage IB and II non-small-cell lung cancer: updated survival analysis of JBR-10. *J Clin Oncol.* 2010;28(1):29–34.
12. Ardizzoni A, Boni L, Tiseo M, et al. Cisplatin- versus carboplatin-based chemotherapy in first-line treatment of advanced non-small-cell lung cancer: an individual patient data meta-analysis. *J Natl Cancer Inst.* 2007;99(11): 847–857.
13. Pignon JP, Tribodet H, Scagliotti GV, et al. Lung adjuvant cisplatin evaluation: a pooled analysis by the LACE Collaborative Group. *J Clin Oncol.* 2008;26(21):3552–3559.
14. Stewart LA, Burdett S, Tierney JF, Pignon J; on behalf of the NSCLC Collaborative Group. Surgery and adjuvant chemotherapy (CT) compared to surgery alone in non-small cell lung cancer (NSCLC): a meta-analysis using individual patient data (IPD) from randomized clinical trials (RCT). *ASCO Meeting Abstracts.* 2007;25(18 Suppl):7552.
15. Yoshida J, Nagai K, Asamura H, et al. Visceral pleura invasion impact on non-small cell lung cancer patient survival: its implications for the forthcoming TNM staging based on a large-scale nation-wide database. *J Thorac Oncol.* 2009;4(8):959–963.
16. Pisters KM, Evans WK, Azzoli CG, et al. Cancer Care Ontario and American Society of Clinical Oncology adjuvant chemotherapy and adjuvant radiation therapy for stages I-IIIA resectable non small-cell lung cancer guideline. *J Clin Oncol.* 2007;25(34):5506–5518.
17. Olaussen KA, Dunant A, Fouret P, et al. DNA repair by ERCC1 in non-small-cell lung cancer and cisplatin-based adjuvant chemotherapy. *N Engl J Med.* 2006;355(10):983–991.
18. Rosell R, Gomez-Codina J, Camps C, et al. A randomized trial comparing preoperative chemotherapy plus surgery with surgery alone in patients with non-small-cell lung cancer. *N Engl J Med.* 1994;330(3):153–158.
19. Roth JA, Fossella F, Komaki R, et al. A randomized trial comparing perioperative chemotherapy and surgery with surgery alone in resectable stage IIIA non-small-cell lung cancer. *J Natl Cancer Inst.* 1994;86(9): 673–680.
20. Depierre A, Milleron B, Moro-Sibilot D, et al. Preoperative chemotherapy followed by surgery compared with primary surgery in resectable stage I (except T1N0), II, and IIIa non-small-cell lung cancer. *J Clin Oncol.* 2002; 20(1):247–253.
21. Gilligan D, Nicolson M, Smith I, et al. Preoperative chemotherapy in patients with resectable non-small cell lung cancer: results of the MRC LU22/NVALT 2/EORTC 08012 multicentre randomised trial and update of systematic review. *Lancet.* 2007;369(9577):1929–1937.
22. Pisters KM, Vallieres E, Crowley JJ, et al. Surgery with or without preoperative paclitaxel and carboplatin in early-stage non-small-cell lung cancer: Southwest Oncology Group Trial S9900, an intergroup, randomized, phase III trial. *J Clin Oncol.* 2010;28(11):1843–1849.
23. Burdett S, Stewart LA, Rydzewska L. A systematic review and meta-analysis of the literature: chemotherapy and surgery versus surgery alone in non-small cell lung cancer. *J Thorac Oncol.* 2006;1(7):611–621.
24. Song WA, Zhou NK, Wang W, et al. Survival benefit of neoadjuvant chemotherapy in non-small cell lung cancer: an updated meta-analysis of 13 randomized control trials. *J Thorac Oncol.* 2010;5(4):510–516.
25. NSCLC Meta-analysis Collaborative Group. Preoperative chemotherapy for non-small cell lung cancer: a systematic review and meta-analysis of individual participant data. *Lancet.* 2014;383(9928):1561–1571.
26. Felip E, Rosell R, Maestre JA, et al. Preoperative chemotherapy plus surgery versus surgery plus adjuvant chemotherapy versus surgery alone in early-stage non-small-cell lung cancer. *J Clin Oncol.* 2010;28(19):3138–3145.
27. Lim E, Harris G, Patel A, et al. Preoperative versus postoperative chemotherapy in patients with resectable non-small cell lung cancer: systematic review and indirect comparison meta-analysis of randomized trials. *J Thorac Oncol.* 2009;4(11):1380–1388.

PART 16

BENIGN LUNG DISEASE

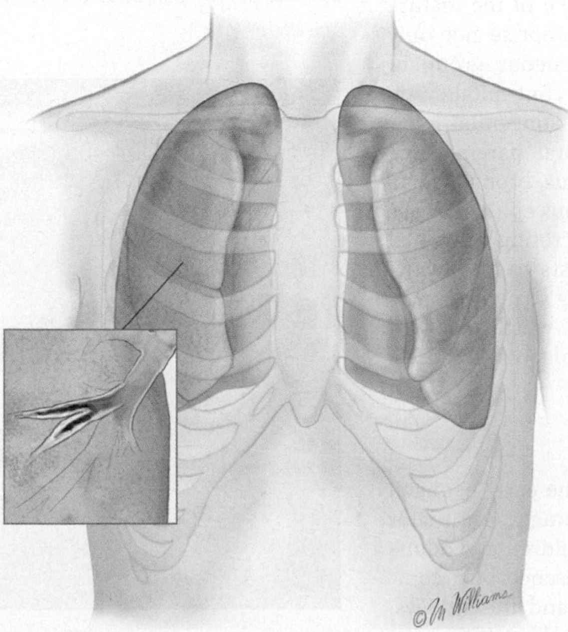

90 Overview of Benign Lung Disease: Anatomy and Pathophysiology

Mirco Santini, Giorgio Cavallesco, and William Grossi

Keywords: Benign, congenital, bronchogenic cyst, pulmonary hamartoma, pulmonary sequestration, bronchiectasis, arteriovenous malformation

Benign tumor, bronchogenic cyst, pulmonary hamartoma, pulmonary sequestration, bronchiectasis, and arteriovenous malformation (AVM) are the principal benign and acquired conditions of the lung encountered in thoracic surgery. This chapter reviews the etiology, clinical presentation, diagnosis, and therapeutic modalities for each of these benign and acquired conditions. Established surgical techniques are described in the ensuing chapters of this section.

BRONCHOGENIC CYSTS

Definition

Bronchogenic cysts are the most common cystic masses in the mediastinum. They are thought to be congenital lesions arising from the primitive foregut. Usually, they are found within the mediastinum or lungs. The mediastinal lesions may be found in close proximity to the carina, mainstem bronchi, trachea, esophagus, or pericardium. Bronchogenic cysts of the skin and subcutaneous tissue also have been reported.

Etiology

The precise embryonic pathway leading to the development of bronchogenic cysts remains unknown. The respiratory tree develops by an outpouching of the primitive foregut during the first 16 weeks of development. Some have theorized that this process fails when a cyst develops in place of the mature structure. These congenital cystic lesions comprise not only the bronchogenic cyst, but also a heterogeneous group of bronchopulmonary malformations, including congenital cystic adenomatoid malformations, sequestrations, congenital lobar emphysema, bronchial atresia, and congenital parenchymal cysts.[1] As with other structures of the bronchus, bronchogenic cysts are lined by ciliated columnar or squamous epithelial cells (respiratory and gastrointestinal). Mucus-secreting bronchial glands found in the epithelium cause the cysts to fill. As the cysts grow, they exert pressure on surrounding structures, particularly the membranous trachea or bronchi, which may lead to severe respiratory obstruction. Cartilage and smooth muscle cells also are found in the cyst wall.

Clinical Features

These cystic malformations may present in the early neonatal period or they may remain entirely asymptomatic until later in life.[1] Symptoms may be evident in both children and adults depending on many factors such as the presence of a communication between the lumen of the cyst and the airways, infection of the fluid within the cyst, and bleeding. If the cyst grows large enough to cause mediastinal shift[1] and obstruction in adjacent structures, the main symptoms will be cough, dyspnea, dysphagia, and chest pain of varying degrees as a result of irritation of the airways and esophagus or inflammation of the mediastinal or parietal pleura. Infectious complications may cause symptoms of fever, elevated leukocyte count, and cough with purulent sputum. Pneumonia localized to the pericystic parenchyma may accompany chronically recurring cysts. Hemoptysis is a sign of an ulcerative process in the cyst wall. Rare complications include cardiac arrhythmias, superior vena cava syndrome, and cancer.

Diagnosis

Plain chest radiographs are diagnostic only when the cavity of the cyst contains an air–fluid level. This finding, especially when the cyst is located in the mediastinum, excludes enterogenous cysts from the differential diagnosis. Plain chest radiography alone can diagnose accurately approximately 80% to 90% of cases and is useful for initial screening.[2]

CT scanning and MRI give greater detail regarding anatomic and topographic localization, especially with respect to surrounding structures. These imaging modalities also provide detail about wall composition and content of the cyst (Fig. 90-1).

Ultrasound is useful when the cyst is close to the chest wall because it may give information about wall thickness and internal content. Transesophageal endoscopic ultrasound is indicated with paraesophageal cysts. Moreover, the widespread use of prenatal ultrasonography and improvements in

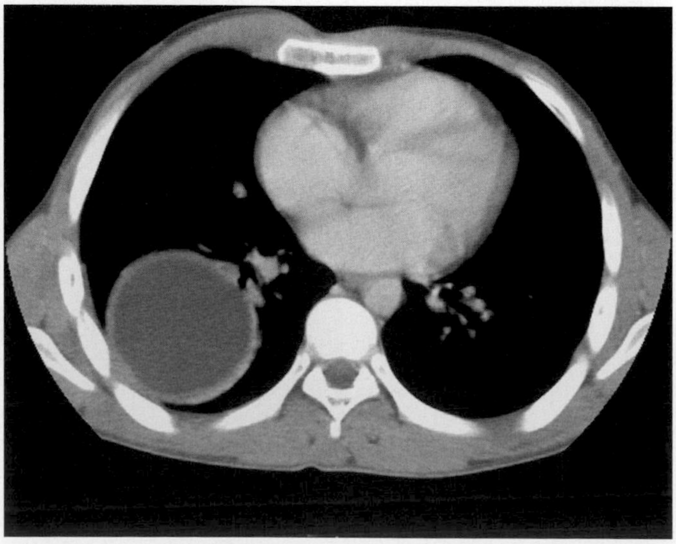

Figure 90-1. CT scan showing a large bronchogenic cyst of the right lower lobe.

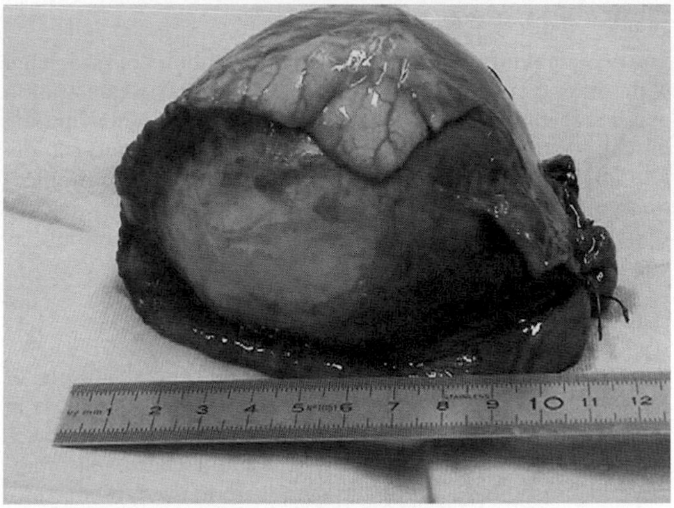

Figure 90-2. Intraoperative specimen: right lower lobe after excision. A large bronchogenic cyst is visible on the pleural surface.

the resolution of echography have progressed to the point that many patients with these lesions are identified *in utero*.[1]

Bronchoscopy performed as part of the diagnostic workup for a bronchogenic cyst usually reveals extrinsic bronchial compression. Occasionally, there is evidence of a fistulous communication between the cyst and the bronchial tree.

Any patient who presents with clinical findings suggestive of bronchogenic cyst will require a plain chest radiograph followed by a CT scan of the chest. However, despite advances in diagnostic imaging, a definite diagnosis of mediastinal bronchogenic cyst is ultimately made based exclusively on the results of a biopsy of the surgically resected tissue specimens.[3]

Therapy

Elective treatment by surgical excision is justified to relieve symptoms in symptomatic patients and to prevent complications in asymptomatic patients. Generally, the excision is technically feasible and easy to perform. However, if there are tight adhesions to the membranous portion of the trachea or mainstem bronchus, or if there is severe inflammation, the excision could be challenging.[4] Video-assisted thoracoscopic surgical (VATS) resection of bronchogenic cysts is now easily performed and can be considered standard therapy for peripheral lesions[3] In cases of intrapericardial bronchogenic cysts, the robotic-assisted approach is particularly suitable. Intrapericardial lesions require meticulous dissection and optimal visualization, both of which are significantly improved with a robotic-assisted approach as compared to a standard video thoracoscopic approach[5] Other techniques, such as aspiration, cyst wall biopsy, and instillation of sclerosant, can be done with mediastinoscopy. Complete resection is preferred over aspiration because removing the entire cyst prevents recurrences and the possibility of malignant degeneration[4] (Fig. 90-2).

PULMONARY HAMARTOMAS

Definition

Pulmonary hamartomas are benign biphasic lesions consisting of epithelial and mesenchymal tissues.

Etiology

Hamartomas arise more often in men than in women. The lesions exhibit extremely slow growth. Although often arising in young adulthood, they usually are not detected until the sixth or seventh decade. Most individuals have a history of smoking.

Clinical Features

Most pulmonary nodules are located peripherally in the lung without preference for a particular lobe. In this location, they are generally asymptomatic. Central endobronchial hamartomas are less common and are associated with signs and symptoms of obstruction that mimic malignant neoplasms or other benign conditions, including pneumonia or atelectasis. The typical hamartoma is less than 2.5 cm in diameter (range 1–8 cm) and contains fat or calcification with fat. Rare giant hamartomas have been reported,[6] and instances of multiple endobronchial hamartomas also have been reported.[7]

Diagnosis

Pulmonary hamartoma may exhibit distinct characteristics on high-resolution CT scanning that can often distinguish it from lung cancer nodules. The endobronchial hamartoma appears as an endobronchial mass with or without signs of obstructive pneumonia or atelectasia. CT scan is of considerable diagnostic aid in cases of endobronchial hamartoma with high fat content. Stey et al. considered highly indicative the presence on CT scan of a mass at high fat density without contrast uptake. At bronchoscopic examination, the endobronchial hamartoma appears as a polypoid or pedunculated neoplasm, well-circumscribed, with a smooth and yellowish surface, without signs of submucosal infiltration. Biopsy is necessary for the differential diagnosis from other benign neoplasms and from carcinoid. Histology would usually detect the coexistence of connective, epithelial, bone, muscle, fat, and cartilage tissues, the latter usually in high prevalence.[8]

Fine-needle aspirates also have been used as a diagnostic tool. The differential diagnosis for peripheral hamartomas includes other benign or malignant lung tumors, secondary metastasis, infectious granulomas, amyloidoma, or Carney's triad (i.e., gastric epithelioid leiomyosarcoma, extra-adrenal paraganglioma, or pulmonary chondroma). The differential diagnosis for endobronchial hamartomas includes bronchogenic carcinoma, papilloma, granular cell tumor, adenoid cystic carcinoma, mucoepidermoid carcinoma, carcinoid tumor, leiomyoma, lipoma, tracheobronchopathia osteochondroplastica, and secondary metastasis.

Therapy

Elective treatment by surgical excision is justified to relieve symptoms in symptomatic patients and to rule out malignancy or prevent complications, if deemed likely, in asymptomatic patients. Peripheral nodules can be removed surgically via thoracotomy or VATS wedge resection. Endobronchial lesions are removed bronchoscopically.[8] Laser treatment through rigid bronchoscopy is considered the gold standard treatment for symptomatic patients with bulky masses on radiological examination. The surgical treatment for endobronchial hamartoma is currently indicated only in cases where the endobronchial lesion cannot be approached through endoscopy, or when lung resection is indicated owing to irreversible parenchymal damage from longstanding airway obstruction.[9] Rarely, hamartomas are observed to undergo malignant transformation, reinforcing the need for surgical resection.

PULMONARY SEQUESTRATIONS

Definition

Pulmonary sequestrations are rare congenital malformations of the lung (see Chapter 93). They consist of masses of nonfunctioning pulmonary tissues that lack normal communication with the bronchial tree.[10] The condition may occur within the lobar lung tissue (intralobar sequestration) or external to the lobe (extralobar sequestrations), but each type has a direct arterial blood supply from the thoracic or abdominal aorta or from one or more of the intercostal branches of the aorta. Extralobar sequestrations are peculiar because they can be surrounded by pleura, similar to an accessory pulmonary lobe; differentiation is based on the lack of normal communications with the bronchial tree. Although there is no single unifying embryonic hypothesis, it is nonetheless thought that these lesions arise as an accessory bud that then migrates with the developing esophagus. Others have suggested an acquired etiology (inflammatory) for pulmonary sequestrations.

Congenital cystic adenomatoid malformations have been observed within extralobar pulmonary sequestrations, suggesting similar etiologic factors. Eighty-five percent of pulmonary sequestrations are localized in the lower lung zones, more often on the left side. Twenty-eight percent of intralobar sequestrations have a homogeneous appearance, 33% are inhomogeneous, and 39% are cystic. Seventy-seven percent of extralobar sequestrations are homogeneous, and 23% are cystic. Extralobar sequestrations sometimes are associated with diaphragmatic hernias (16%), lung hypoplasia (25%), bronchogenic cysts, and cardiovascular malformations.

Pathophysiology

The macroscopic characteristics of intralobar sequestrations do not differ from those of the normal surrounding tissues. Sequestration is suspected when severe adhesions between mediastinal or diaphragmatic structures or parietal pleura and lung are found. Extrapulmonary sequestrations have a more typical pathologic appearance consisting of a pyramidal or ovoid lesion of approximately 0.5 to 15 cm in length surrounded by its own pleura. Cystic lesions secondary to chronic inflammation and fibrosis that replaces normal lung tissue may be observed in the extralobar sequestration.

The inner layer of the cyst consists of respiratory epithelium or, on rare occasion, squamous epithelium with an eosinophilic amorphous fluid-filled center. In extralobar sequestrations, bronchus/alveolar-like structures lined with respiratory epithelium may be observed. Both types have their own systemic arterial supply, but venous flow occurs through the pulmonary veins for the intralobar type and through the systemic veins for the extralobar type. The arteries that supply the sequestrations have a large caliber (up to 0.5 cm in diameter). In 80% of cases, they arise both from the thoracic and abdominal aorta. In this event, the arteries run through the triangular ligament toward the lower lobes. Abnormal origin in a sequestration arising from the coronary artery has been reported.[11]

Clinical Features

The two main forms of pulmonary sequestration are associated with different symptoms. In elderly patients, sequestration may be asymptomatic and observed as an incidental finding on chest radiographs, especially the extralobar sequestration. The intralobar types, because of their bronchial communications, may lead to recurrent pneumonia and respiratory distress symptoms (i.e., dyspnea, cyanosis). Hemoptysis is rare but has been reported as an acute symptom.

Diagnosis

Plain chest radiography is nonspecific in the diagnosis of sequestration. Sometimes it shows the presence of a mass in the lower lobes or, if there is communication with the tracheobronchial tree, a cystic lesion. CT scan of the chest is the standard diagnostic tool, and it can demonstrate the presence of a systemic artery supplying the sequestration. Ultrasonography is noninvasive and safe, making its use ideal in prenatal and postnatal settings.[10] Duplex Doppler ultrasound may be used to demonstrate the abnormal systemic vessel that feeds the sequestration. MRI can be useful in the differential diagnosis (bronchogenic cyst versus bronchiectasis versus solitary lung abscess) and for demonstrating mediastinal structures.

Therapy

Medical therapy is based on anti-inflammatory and antimicrobial drugs. Elective treatment is surgical. Anatomic lobectomy is the treatment for intralobar sequestrations. Posterolateral thoracotomy through the lower intercostal spaces is performed for sequestrations of the lower lobes, although a VATS approach has been reported.[12] Retroperitoneal or abdominal sequestrations may require a laparotomy or a thoracoabdominal approach. Robots have been introduced into surgical procedures in an attempt to facilitate surgical performance. The three-dimensional view with depth perception is a marked improvement over the conventional thoracoscopic camera view. All of this creates images with increased resolution, which when combined with the increased degrees of freedom and enhanced dexterity, could enhance the dissection of anomalous vessels.[13–14]

BRONCHIECTASIS

Definition

Bronchiectasis was first described by Laennec (Paris, France) in the 1800 s as a bronchial dilatation. This definition is still valid, but it must be added that it is always associated with an alteration of the structural layers of the bronchial wall. The surgical management of bronchiectasis is presented in Chapter 94.

Pathophysiology

Various congenital and acquired disease processes can lead to bronchiectasis. During pulmonary infections, obstructive endobronchial processes localized to the peripheral lung may cause bronchial dilatation. Repeated infections damage the epithelial cilia, mucoelastic tissue, and even cartilage. Healing and replacement of these tissues with fibrous tissue results in loss of elasticity with contraction of the peribronchial tissues and traction on the bronchial tree leading to bronchial dilatation.[15] True

Table 90-1

CONGENITAL AND FAMILIAL DISEASES THAT CAUSE BRONCHIECTASIS

ETIOLOGY	SYNDROMES AND DISEASES
Bronchial malformations	Primitive tracheomalacia Williams–Campbell syndrome
Vascular and lymphatic malformations	Sequestration Yellow nails syndrome
Chest malformations	Kyphoscoliosis Phrenic eventration/relaxation
Systemic diseases	Cystic fibrosis α_1-Antitrypsin deficiency
Bronchiectasis in other complex syndromes	Kartagener syndrome (primary ciliary dyskinesia) Mounier-Kuhn syndrome

bronchiectasis is distinct from pseudobronchiectasis (bronchocele). This latter form of bronchial dilatation is reversible and lasts only a few weeks or months after an episode of bronchopneumonia. The epithelial damage is not severe and is without necrosis.

Sometimes bronchiectasis is caused by bronchial obstruction. The obstruction is created by tiny aspirated endoluminal foreign bodies,[16] benign lymphoadenomatoid-bronchial syndromes, or slow-growth tumorlets such as carcinoids.[17]

Bronchial obstruction also can be caused by extrinsic compression from the peribronchial lymph nodes (middle lobe or lingula) in the case of neoplasms or by chronic infections (e.g., histoplasmosis, coccidioidomycosis, aspergillosis, tuberculosis, and AIDS-related infections); see Chapters 102 and 103.[18] Three steps are implicated in the pathophysiology of extrinsic obstruction, namely, secretion retention, chronic infection, and bronchiectasis, as seen before.

Congenital and familial diseases are an uncommon cause of bronchiectasis (Table 90-1). The most important is Kartagener syndrome, or primary ciliary dyskinesia, a rare autosomal recessive disorder involving the combination of situs inversus, bronchiectasis, and sinusitis. A dynein deficiency leads to ciliary dyskinesia. The yellow nail syndrome is a rare clinical entity that combines three main features: yellow discoloration of the nails, chronic lymphedema, and pleural effusion. This syndrome is often complicated by bronchiectasis.[19] The classification of bronchiectasis is morphologic, consisting of three types: (1) cylindrical or tubular, (2) saccular or cystic, and (3) varicose. Cylindrical bronchiectasis has a uniform caliber of dilatation and often is associated with tuberculosis. Saccular bronchiectasis is characterized by an evident dilatation at the distal end, often associated with postinfectious and postobstructive bronchiectasis. Varicose bronchiectasis is a mixed form and presents with alternating areas of saccular and cylindrical dilatation. The subclassification of bronchiectasis is based on blood perfusion. Two types of bronchiectasis are recognized: perfused and nonperfused. Whereas perfused bronchiectasis has intact pulmonary artery flow and cylindrical bronchiectatic changes, the nonperfused type is characterized by a lack of pulmonary artery flow, retrograde filling of the pulmonary artery through the systemic circulation, and cystic bronchiectatic changes.

The location of the bronchiectasis may reveal its pathogenesis. Bronchiectasis related to congenital and familial diseases is always bilateral and involves different segments of the lung. Bronchiectasis related to tuberculosis is located primarily in the upper lobes. Obstructive and inflammatory bronchiectasis is found in the lower lobes. The middle lobe syndrome is a selective localized form of bronchiectasis. The middle lobe bronchus arises with a 30-degree downward open angle from the intermediate bronchus and runs for approximately 2 cm. Lymph node hypertrophy of the angle can easily compress the middle bronchus, leading to atelectasis and bronchiectasis.[20]

Clinical Features

Bronchiectasis may be symptomatic or asymptomatic.[21] Bronchiectasis should be considered in all adults who have persistent productive cough (>90% of patients).

Factors favoring further investigation are any one of the following:

- Young age at presentation
- History of symptoms over many years
- Absence of smoking history
- Daily expectoration of sputum (the volume of sputum produced may vary widely with mean/median daily volumes of 300, 567, and 200 mL)
- Sputum colonization with Pseudomonas aeruginosa
- Nonproductive cough or unexplained hemoptysis. This latter symptom, even if rare, may occur and has been reported as a symptom of the type of bronchiectasis associated with coronary fistula.[22]

Physical examination of the chest may reveal coarse expiratory rhonchi and dullness over localized areas, especially during periods of acute infectious exacerbation.

Diagnosis

Standard chest radiography is often not useful because it shows only nonspecific inflammatory radiographic signs (Fig. 90-3). In the past, the ideal radiographic method was, and in some cases still is, a bronchogram. This procedure provides information about the morphology, localization, and extent of the bronchiectasis (Fig. 90-4). High-resolution, fine-cut CT scan is the procedure of choice for the diagnosis of bronchiectasis.[21]

CT is able to show the extent of the disease bilaterally and gives information about the walls of the bronchioles, including

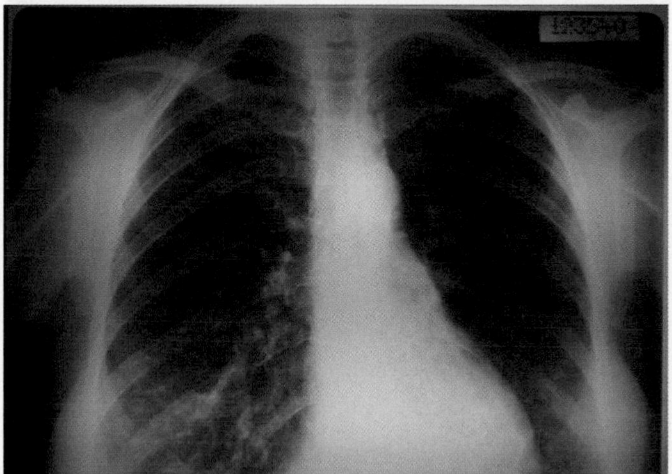

Figure 90-3. Chest radiograph showing bronchiectasis.

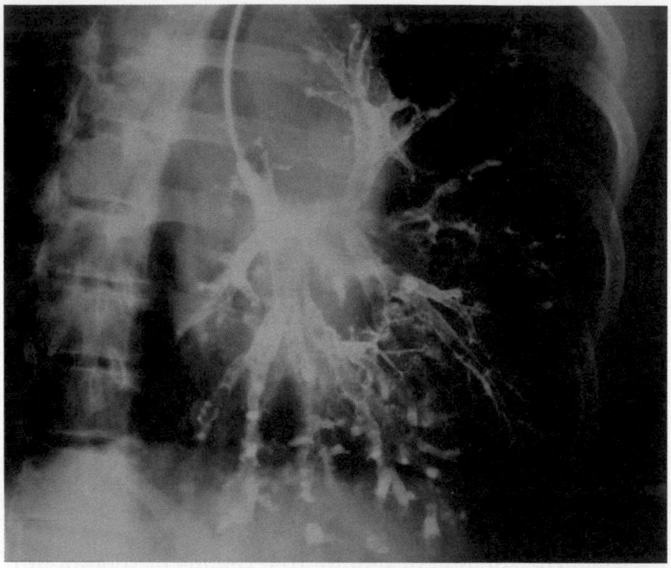

Figure 90-4. Bronchograms of bronchiectasis of the lower lobe.

the presence of peribronchial inflammation and parenchymal disease (Fig. 90-5).

Flexible fiberoptic bronchoscopy is useful for evaluating bronchial neoplasms and endoluminal foreign bodies or obtaining samples for bacterial culture to start specific antibiotic therapy. Bronchoscopy permits biopsy of the respiratory mucosa for the diagnosis of hereditary mucociliary disorders.

Therapy

The treatment aims in adult care are to control symptoms and thus enhance quality of life, reduce exacerbations, and maintain pulmonary function. The evidence is clear that patients with bronchiectasis who have more frequent exacerbations have a worse quality of life.[21]

Medical

Postural drainage is the most effective treatment for mobilizing the thick bronchial secretions but it requires the skills of a trained respiratory physiotherapist. To treat infections, a sputum culture should be performed. Targeted antibiotic therapy is started if an acute infection of the lung is present or for a preoperative workup. Patients with primary or secondary immune deficiency should be under joint care with a clinical immunologist.[21]

The conservative therapeutic approach should be continued for several months. Annual vaccination against influenza and pneumococcus is recommended.

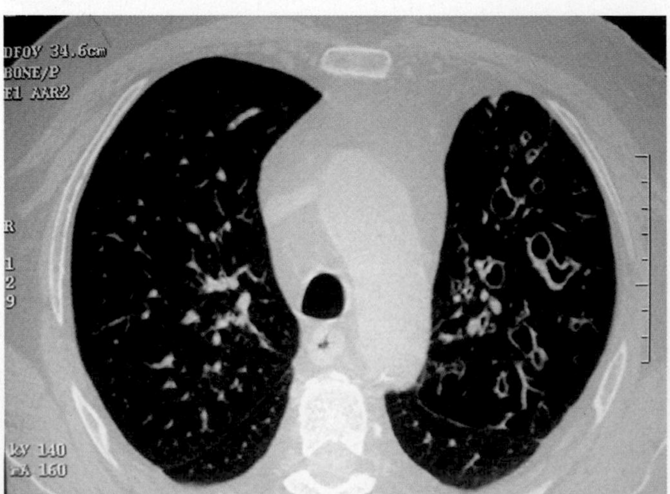

Figure 90-5. High-resolution spiral CT scan of diffuse cylindrical bronchiectasis. (Courtesy of Dr. Nunzio Calia.)

Surgical

Indications for surgery reported in the literature have included failure of medical/conservative therapy, recurrent respiratory infections, persistent sputum production, hemoptysis, chronic cough, and persistent lung abscess.[21,23–26]

Complete excision of the bronchiectatic parenchyma is the goal of surgery. Patients considered candidates for surgical resection must meet the following criteria: (1) localized bronchiectasis that is completely resectable, (2) adequate respiratory reserve, (3) irreversible process versus an early treatable condition, (4) significant symptoms with a continued chronic productive cough, significant hemoptysis, major recurring episodes of pneumonia sufficiently severe to warrant surgery, and (5) failed prolonged attempts at medical therapy.[27]

For massive pulmonary hemorrhage, endobronchial suction with balloon tamponade, embolization of the bleeding vessel (usually a bronchial artery), or emergency resection can be lifesaving. The surgical approach involves anatomic resection of all targeted areas. The anatomic resection depends on the origin of the bronchiectasis. Tuberculous bronchiectasis typically requires resection of the upper lobes, whereas postinfective bronchiectasis usually involves resection of the lower lobes or lingula (Fig. 90-6). Abundant mucopurulent secretions must be treated with particular attention to prevent contamination of the normal airways. Lung transplantation is available for end-stage cardiopulmonary disease in children and adults, although there is a paucity of literature on bronchiectasis specifically. As a general guideline, patients are evaluated for lung transplantation if the FEV_1 is <30% or if there is rapid, progressive respiratory deterioration despite optimal medical management. The following additional factors should lower the threshold for considering referral for transplantation assessment: massive hemoptysis, severe secondary pulmonary hypertension, multiple ICU admissions, or respiratory failure (particularly if requiring noninvasive ventilation). It should be

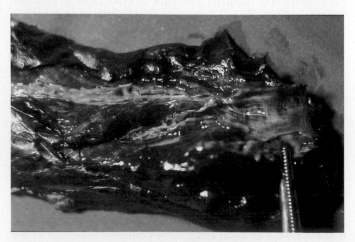

Figure 90-6. Resected lingular lobe with bronchiectasis.

Table 90-2

RESULTS OF SURGICAL RESECTION FOR BRONCHIECTASIS

REFERENCE	PATIENTS	MORTALITY RATE (%)	MORBIDITY RATE (%)
Kutlay et al.[26]	166	1.7	10.5
Agasthian et al.[41]	134	2.2	24.0
Dogan et al.[42]	487	3.5	11.0

noted that antibody deficiency is not an absolute contraindication to transplantation.[21,28–29]

Surgical treatment of bronchiectasis is more effective in patients with localized disease. Excision in such patients is satisfactory with an acceptable rate of morbidity and mortality. Mortality and morbidity rates range from 1.7% to 3.5% in different case series (Table 90-2).

Surgical treatment of bronchiectasis is used widely, but there appear to be no randomized, controlled trials. It is not possible to provide an unbiased estimate of its benefit compared with conservative therapy.[30] Addition of a vascularized muscle flap should be considered to prevent postoperative infection.

PULMONARY ARTERIOVENOUS MALFORMATION

Definition

Pulmonary AVMs are caused by abnormal communications between pulmonary arteries and pulmonary veins and are most commonly congenital in nature (see Chapter 95). Although these lesions are quite uncommon, they are an important part of the differential diagnosis of common pulmonary problems such as hypoxemia and pulmonary nodules. Since their first description at autopsy in 1897, these abnormal communications have been given various names, including pulmonary arteriovenous fistulas, pulmonary arteriovenous aneurysms, hemangiomas of the lung, cavernous angiomas of the lung, pulmonary telangiectasias, and pulmonary AVMs. Abnormal communications among blood vessels of the lung also may be found in a variety of acquired conditions. Right-to-left shunting as a result of communications between pulmonary arteries and pulmonary veins has been reported in many diseases. Communications between bronchial arteries and pulmonary arteries causing left-to-right shunting can develop in chronic inflammatory conditions such as bronchiectasis. Many patients with pulmonary AVMs have hereditary hemorrhagic telangiectasia.

Embryology

By the fourth week of gestation, the respiratory tract can be seen as a groove in the ventral wall of the foregut. The blood vessels of the lung are derived from two sources, namely, the plexiform network of vessels that develops in the pulmonary mesenchyme and the heart. Like bronchi, the vessels may vary in their course based on the eventual development of channels from the preexisting mesenchymal network. During blood vessel development, primitive arteriovenous connections form to initiate the flow of blood. Subsequent vascular remodeling results in normal vessel development. AVMs result from unknown stimuli during the stage of arteriovenous communications in the retiform plexus.

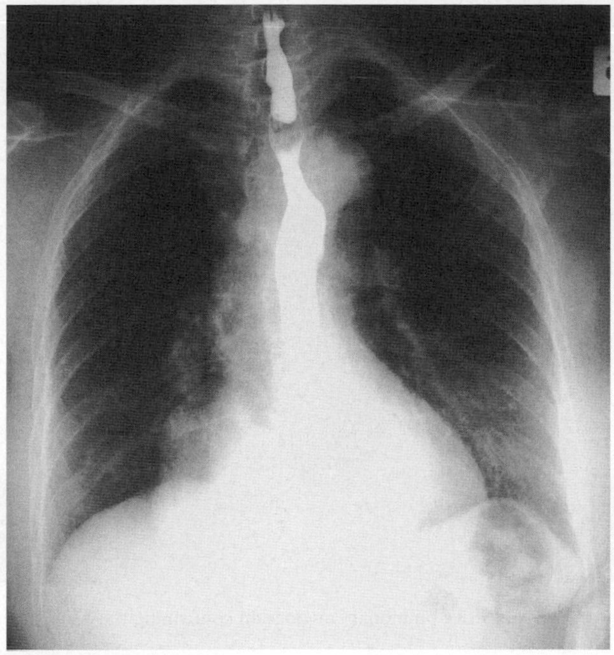

Figure 90-7. Chest radiograph showing a round mediastinal mass of uniform density in the right lower lobe.

Diagnosis and Clinical Features

Clinical symptoms of AVM are based on the grade of the right-to-left shunt. Hemoptysis,[31] dyspnea on exertion, congestive heart failure, or a major neurologic event such as stroke or cerebral abscess may be present.[32] In patients with Rendu–Osler–Weber syndrome, cutaneous and mucosal spider angiomas are present.[33–34]

On physical examination of the thorax, a continuous murmur may be heard over the involved area of the thorax, especially if the AVM is quite large. Standard chest radiographs may reveal a solid round or oval mass of uniform density, frequently lobulated but sharply defined, more commonly located in the lower lobes, and ranging from 1 to 5 cm in diameter. As such, it may be difficult to differentiate from a lung tumor (Fig. 90-7).

CT scan of the chest may provide information about the vascular origin of the mass (Fig. 90-8), but a selective angiogram

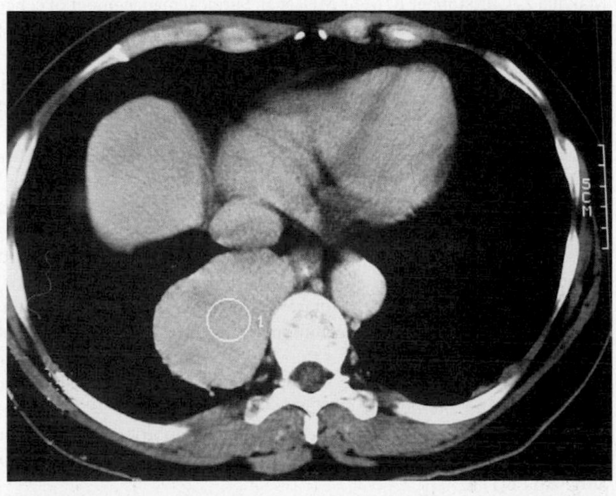

Figure 90-8. CT scan front section confirming the AVM of the right lower branch of the pulmonary artery.

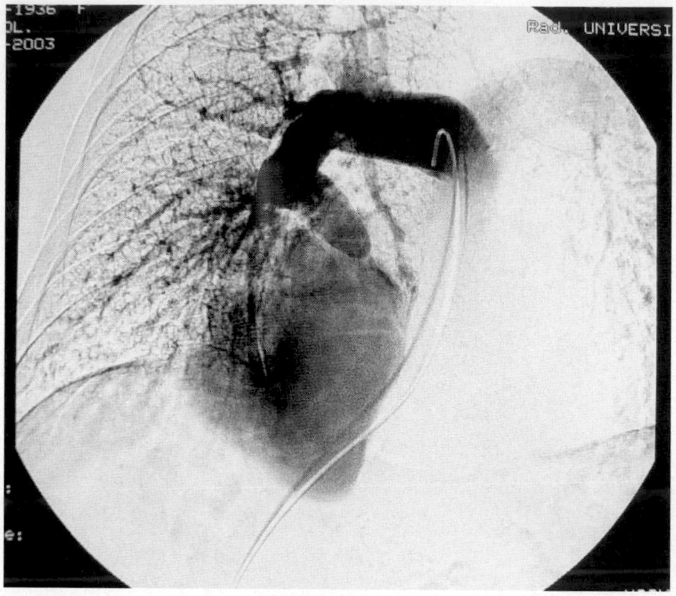

Figure 90-9. Selective pulmonary angiogram confirming the AVM.

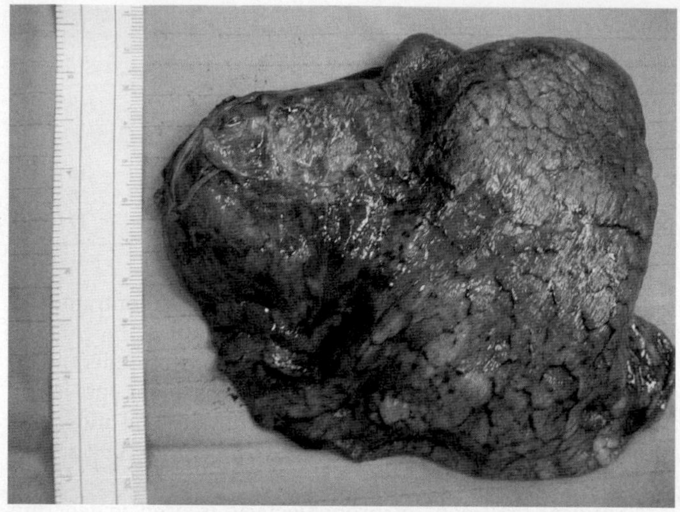

Figure 90-10. Large AVM of the right lower lobe after complete surgical excision.

of the pulmonary artery is essential to localize the AVM, determine its extent, map the AVM for preoperative workup and consideration for therapeutic embolization (Fig. 90-9). Right-to-left shunt entities may be measured by radionuclide perfusion scans of the lung.

Therapy

A small quiescent AVM may be managed conservatively, using the "watch and wait" approach. If the AVM becomes symptomatic, however, the treatment options are embolization or surgery. Localized and large AVMs require a surgical approach. Surgical resection as a mode of treatment for pulmonary AVM carries (at least) the same risks as any other thoracic operation. Surgical resection is not feasible as a primary treatment in patients with masses that are too large and have an overly extensive blood supply. In such cases, preoperative embolization may help to reduce blood flow within the vascular mass and thereby prevent life-threatening intraoperative bleeding. On the downside, lesions that are incompletely excised have a higher risk of recurrence.[35]

Lobectomy (Fig. 90-10) or wedge resection[36] via thoracotomy or VATS is the standard procedure when surgical resection is indicated.[37] Multiple bilateral AVMs may require a bilateral approach and multiple resections.[38] Small or multiple pulmonary AVMs may be treated conservatively with angiographic embolization using different techniques such as balloons, springs, coils, and thrombogenic materials.[39–40]

This section on benign lung diseases concludes with a review of benign and metastatic pediatric pulmonary tumors (Chapter 96).

References

1. Makhija Z, Christopher R, Moir MD, et al. Surgical management of congenital cystic lung malformations in older patients. *Ann Thorac Surg.* 2011;91: 1568–1573.
2. Suen HC, Mathisen DJ, Grillo HC, et al. Surgical management and radiological characteristics of bronchogenic cysts. *Ann Thorac Surg.* 1993;55: 476–481.
3. Takashi M., Mie S., Motohiko F. et al. Thoracoscopic resection of mediastinal bronchogenic cysts in adults. *Asian J Surg.* 2011;34(1):11–14.
4. Granato F, Voltolini L, Ghiribelli C, et al. Surgery for bronchogenic cysts: always easy?. *Asian Cardiovasc Thorac Ann.* 2009;17:467–471.
5. Ross ER Schwartz GS. et al. Robotic-assisted resection of an intrapericardial bronchogenic cyst. *J Robotic Surg.* 2011;5:141–143.
6. Hutter J, Reich-Weinberger S, Hutarew G, et al. Giant pulmonary hamartoma: a rare presentation of a common tumor. *Ann Thorac Surg.* 2006;82: e5–e7.
7. Kang MW, Han JH, Yu JH, et al. Multiple central endobronchial chondroid hamartoma. *Ann Thorac Surg.* 2007;83:691–693.
8. Mondello B, Lentini S, Buda C, et al. Giant endobronchial hamartoma resected by fiberoptic bronchoscopy electrosurgical snaring. *J Cardiothorac Surg.* 2011;6(1):97.
9. Na W, Shinn SH, Paik SS. Dumbbell shaped exophytic and endobronchial lipomatous hamartoma. *Thorac Cardiovasc Surg.* 2009;57(2):122–124.
10. Yong W, Fan L. Pulmonary sequestration: a retrospective analysis of 2625 cases in China. *Eur J Cardiothorac Surg.* 2011;40:e39–e42.
11. Van Langenhove G, Convens C, Seynaeve P, et al. Intralobar pulmonary sequestration supplied by the right coronary artery. *Catheter Cardiovasc Intervent.* 1999;47:218–220.
12. Della Porta M, Galli A, Rebuffat C. Videothoracoscopic approach in the treatment of intralobar pulmonary sequestration: report of a case. *Chir Ital.* 2000;52:299–302.
13. Melfi FMA, Viti. A, Davini F, et al. Robot-assisted resection of pulmonary sequestrations. *Eur J Cardiothorac Surg.* 2011;40:1025–1026.
14. Melfi FM, Mussi A. Robotically assisted lobectomy: learning curve and complications. *Thorac Surg Clin.* 2008;18(3):289–295.
15. King PT. The pathophysiology of bronchiectasis. *Int J Chron Obstruct Pulmon Dis.* 2009;4:411–419.
16. Adegboye VO, Osinowo O, Adebo OA. Bronchiectasis consequent upon prolonged foreign body retention. *Cent Afr J Med.* 2003;49:53–58.
17. Canessa PA, Santini D, Zanelli M, et al. Pulmonary tumourlets and microcarcinoids in bronchiectasis. *Monaldi Arch Chest Dis.* 1997;52:138–139.
18. Allen D, Ng S, Beaton K, et al. Sternal osteomyelitis caused by Aspergillus fumigatus in a patient with previously treated Hodgkin's disease. *J Clin Pathol.* 2002;55:616–618.
19. Rigau NC, Daele JJ. The yellow nail syndrome. *Acta Otorhinolaryngol Belg.* 2003;57:221–224.

20. Akilov K, Ismailov D, Madatov K. Treatment of middle-lobe syndrome. *Khirurgiia (Mosk).* 2003;(5):17–18.
21. Pasteur MC, Bilton D, Hill AT British thoracic society guideline for non-CF bronchiectasis. *Thorax.* 2010;65:1–58.
22. Jim MH, Lee SW, Lam L. Localized bronchiectasis is a definite association of coronarobronchial artery fistula. *J Invas Cardiol.* 2003;15:554–556.
23. Balkanli K, Genc O, Dakak M, et al. Surgical management of bronchiectasis: analysis and short-term results in 238 patients. *Eur J Cardiothorac Surg.* 2003;24:699–702.
24. Mazie`res J, Murris M, Didier A, et al: Limited operation for severe multisegmental bilateral bronchiectasis. *Ann Thorac Surg.* 2003;75:382–387.
25. Prieto D, Bernardo J, Matos MJ, et al. Surgery for bronchiectasis. *Eur J Cardiothorac Surg.* 2001;20:19–23; discussion 23–24.
26. Kutlay H, Cangir AK, Enon S, et al. Surgical treatment in bronchiectasis: analysis of 166 patients. *Eur J Cardiothorac Surg.* 2002;21:634–637.
27. Hodder V, Cameron R, Todd T. *Bacterial Infections.* New York, NY: Churchill-Livingstone; 1995:463.
28. Anon. International guidelines for the selection of lung transplant candidates. The American Society for Transplant Physicians (ASTP)/American Thoracic Society(ATS)/European Respiratory Society(ERS)/International Society for Heart and Lung Transplantation(ISHLT). *Am J Respir Crit Care Med.* 1998;158;335–339.
29. Sweet SC. Pediatric lung transplantation: update 2003. *Pediatr Clin North Am.* 2003;50:1393–1417.
30. Corless J, Warburton C. Surgery vs. non-surgical treatment for bronchiectasis. *Cochrane Database Syst Rev.* 2000;CD002180.
31. Thung KH, Sihoe AD, Wan IY, et al. Hemoptysis from an unusual pulmonary arteriovenous malformation. *Ann Thorac Surg.* 2003;76:1730–1733.
32. Shioya H, Kikuchi K, Suda Y, et al. Recurrent brain abscess associated with congenital pulmonary arteriovenous fistula: a case report. *No Shinkei Geka.* 2004;32:57–63.
33. Marchesani F, Cecarini L, Pela R, et al. Pulmonary arteriovenous fistula in a patient with Rendu-Osler-Weber syndrome. *Respiration.* 1997;64:367–370.
34. Sung-Yuan Hu, Cheng-Han Tsai, Yu-Tse Tsan. Pulmonary arteriovenous malformation in Osler-Weber-Rendu syndrome. *Eur J Cardiothorac Surg.* 2009;36:395.
35. Tennyson C, Routledge T, Chambers A, et al. Arteriovenous malformation in the anterior mediastinum. *Ann Thorac Surg.* 2010;90:9–10.
36. Morikawa T, Kaji M, Ohtake S, et al. Video-assisted anatomic mediobasal segmentectomy of lung. *Surg Endosc.* 2003;17:1678.
37. Storck M, Mickley V, Abendroth D, et al. Pulmonary arteriovenous malformations: aspects of surgical therapy. *Vasa.* 1996;25:54–59.
38. Matsuda S, Hamada M, Sumimoto T, et al. A case of surgical treatment of multiple bilateral pulmonary arteriovenous fistulas in a senile patient. *Nihon Kyobu Shikkan Gakkai Zasshi.* 1990;28:1348–1352.
39. Takahashi K, Fukuoka K, Konishi M, et al. A case of pulmonary arteriovenous malformation treated by transcatheter embolization using coils. *Nihon Kokyuki Gakkai Zasshi.* 2002;40:900–904.
40. Ghani M, Yusuf W, Sdringola S, et al. Percutaneous coil embolization of multiple arteriovenous malformations in left lung causing persistent hypoxia. *Circulation.* 2000;102:E118.
41. Agasthian T, Deschamps C, Trastek VF, et al. Surgical managements of bronchiectasis. *Ann Thorac Surg.* 1996;62:976–978.
42. Dogan R, Alp M, Kaya S

91 Benign Lung Masses

Mark W. Hennon and Chumy E. Nwogu

Keywords: Hamartoma, adenoma, papilloma, solitary pulmonary nodule, video-assisted thoracic surgery (VATS)

Benign lung masses comprise a heterogeneous group of tumors that are defined by their lack of malignant features histologically and their nonaggressive clinical behavior. This is evidenced by the absence of invasion into surrounding tissue planes or metastatic spread to other structures. In a classic study, Martini[1], who investigated the Memorial Sloan Kettering experience, demonstrated that less than 1% of resected lung lesions are benign. More recent reports have shown that despite advances in preoperative imaging and assessment, up to 9% of nodules suspected of being malignant prior to resection are found to be benign.[2] Increasing utilization of CT scanning for lung cancer screening as well as for other cardiopulmonary diagnostic purposes has led to an increase in the number of patients being identified with pulmonary nodules. Given the overall low incidence of these tumors, differentiating a benign from a malignant lung mass can sometimes be difficult. Using a combination of clinical tools including a detailed history and physical examination, laboratory workup, radiographic imaging, and tissue sampling techniques, it is often possible to achieve an accurate assessment of a benign lung mass. It is this evaluation and correct characterization of an indeterminate pulmonary nodule that is invaluable in guiding treatment planning as well as assessing the overall prognosis of the patient.

THE INDETERMINATE SOLITARY PULMONARY NODULE

The solitary pulmonary nodule is a rounded lesion with well-demarcated margins. Its size may vary from a few millimeters to a few centimeters. Two features are particularly helpful in making the distinction between benign and malignant lesions: (1) Nodules with doubling times of less than 10 days or more than 450 days are most likely benign, and (2) calcifications seen on a chest radiograph or CT scan with fine cuts through the tumor that exhibit a central, diffuse, speckled, laminar, or popcorn pattern most likely reflect a benign mass, whereas eccentric calcifications are more characteristic of malignancy. Various diagnostic modalities are available and used to differentiate between benign and malignant lung lesions presenting as a solitary pulmonary nodule.

CT

Often performed early in the evaluation of a pulmonary nodule, the radiographic appearance of a mass on CT can help identify differences between primary lung cancers and benign nodules. Cancers will often have ill-defined tumor margins and spiculation, will involve bronchi or vessels, and will enlarge more rapidly than benign tumors.[3] CT also can be used for guided percutaneous core needle biopsy of accessible pulmonary nodules. In a study of 60 patients with benign pulmonary lesions, percutaneous core needle biopsy was able to provide a definitive diagnosis in 81.7% of cases as opposed to fine-needle aspiration, in which a specific benign diagnosis was made in only 16.7% of cases.[4] Reports also have shown that 1-mm-thick slices on high-resolution CT can be used to differentiate between benign and malignant solitary pulmonary nodules with a sensitivity of 91.4%.[5] Continued improvements in technology with quantitative first pass 320 detector row perfusion CT scanning have led to reports of accuracy and specificity that can rival PET/CT.[6]

MRI

Diffusion-weighted imaging (DWI) MRI is a modality that reflects the diffusion of water protons in tissues, producing different contrasts in different kinds of tissues. Malignant lesions show stronger enhancement and higher maximum signal intensity than benign lesions. Reported sensitivity, specificity, and accuracy have been 88.9%, 61.1%, and 79.6%, respectively.[7] Although not routinely used in the evaluation of the solitary pulmonary nodule, MRI can have application in select instances.

PET/CT

The use of fluorodeoxyglucose PET combined with low-dose CT (PET/CT) scanning has facilitated the determination of malignancy in nodules as small as 6 mm.[6] If the nodule is glucose-avid and has a standardized uptake value of 2.5 or greater, it has a greater than 90% probability of being malignant. PET scanning can distinguish malignant from benign nodules with a sensitivity of 90%.[8] Although sensitivity seems to decrease for nodules smaller than 6 mm in size, and false positives can occur with infectious and inflammatory lesions, PET/CT scanning remains an excellent tool for the diagnosis and staging of patients with thoracic malignancies, and it has been shown to be superior to CT in this respect.[9]

Other Nuclear Medicine Studies

Somatostatin-receptor scintigraphy with the new somatostatin analog technetium-99m depreotide has shown significant promise for discriminating between malignant and benign lung lesions. In a pilot study, 17 of 21 patients with high focal uptake of the marker were found to have a malignancy.[10]

Biomarkers

Many potential markers of malignant behavior have been evaluated by immunohistochemistry in an attempt to better classify neoplastic proliferations, but their clinical utility remains unclear. 15-Lipoxygenase-2, for example, is an arachidonic acid-metabolizing enzyme with expression levels that show an inverse correlation with tumor grade in several subtypes of lung carcinoma. This relationship suggests potential utility in differentiating benign from malignant epithelial lesions.[11] Similar results also were obtained with glutathione-metabolizing enzymes.

Moreover, serum biomarker assays show promise as an adjunct to imaging and other screening studies. In one report, serum immunoassays targeting cytokeratin fragment marker (CYFRA 21-1) and neuron-specific enolase (NSE) exhibited a specificity of 100% in differentiating benign from malignant solitary pulmonary nodules,[12] and the combination of these two tumor markers with carcinoembryonic antigen resulted in greater sensitivity and diagnostic accuracy. Although tumor markers, alone or in combination with the new imaging techniques, brought no additional benefits in terms of sensitivity and accuracy over imaging methods alone, they did exhibit a far superior specificity.[13] Progastrin-releasing peptide is another promising tumor marker for the detection and monitoring of small-cell lung carcinoma, and an enzyme-linked immunoassay for its convenient measurement exists. A recent report evaluating a variety of tumor markers including ProGRP, CEA, SCC, CA 125, CYFRA 21-1, and NSE noted that abnormal tumor marker serum levels (excluding CA 125) were found in less than 5.3% of patients with benign lung nodules.[14]

Serum proteomic screening is another modality currently under investigation. Patient serum samples are examined for circulating protein tumor markers. Tumor protein expression patterns and markers may be detected and analyzed using a variety of techniques, including two-dimensional (2-D) gel electrophoresis, antibody-based microarray, and mass spectrometry.[15] Spectrometry in particular has been used successfully in screen-blinded serum samples to identify lung cancer patients with a sensitivity of 93% and a specificity of 97%.[16]

Proteomic analysis has also shown value in the classification and subclassification of tumors after tissue is obtained. While the current focus is largely on pulmonary malignancy, the ability to classify lesions by their protein expression patterns (e.g., protein types, quantities, and posttranslational modifications) ultimately may aid in identifying benign tumors. The techniques generally are the same as those used in serum screening. Spectrometry is often accomplished by surface-enhanced laser desorption/ionization mass spectrometry or matrix-assisted laser desorption/ionization time-of-flight methods. The difference in these systems is beyond the scope of this chapter, but they have been clearly reviewed in the literature.[17] Matrix-assisted laser desorption/ionization time-of-flight methods permit direct analysis of frozen tissue sections, which are irradiated by laser beams in preselected areas of tumor. The protein signature generated is compared with protein profile databases from known tumors to help classify the unknown lesion.

Detection of malignancy by sputum screening also may be facilitated by molecular markers. The utility of heterogeneous ribonuclear protein B1 expression, for example, has been examined for its value in distinguishing benign from malignant lung masses because it appears to be overexpressed in a variety of lung carcinomas.[18] In addition, transforming growth factor α has been shown to stimulate production of the erbB gene products at a much higher level in tumorigenic as compared with nontumorigenic lung epithelial cells.

Electromagnetic Navigational Bronchoscopy

Evolving technology associated with flexible bronchoscopy has allowed for another option when assessing lung nodules. Electromagnetic navigational bronchoscopy (ENB) with biopsy has enhanced the yield of flexible bronchoscopy, which is often limited by the size and location of the lung nodule of interest. Smaller, more peripheral lung nodules can be successfully targeted for biopsy or placement of fiducial markers using the ENB system. This system consists of computer software that creates a 3-D virtual bronchoscopy reconstruction from CT images, along with the necessary endobronchial guide and electromagnetic location board that emits a low-dose electromagnetic field. In a recent study, the overall diagnostic yield of ENB was 67% in a series of 92 lung lesions from 89 patients. The sensitivity, specificity, positive predictive value, and negative predictive value for benign disease were 91%, 100%, 100%, and 97%, respectively.[19]

Video-Assisted Thoracic Surgery

Definitive diagnosis can be achieved only with excisional biopsy via VATS or thoracotomy. Nodules larger than 10 mm that are suggestive of malignancy or are indeterminate by other means of morphologic analysis have to be defined by surgical excision. Recent advances in minimally invasive surgery instrumentation make the possibility of obtaining a definitive diagnosis with complete resection less daunting for both the patient and the surgeon.

In this chapter, we have tried to approach the multitude of benign lung masses in a systematic way. We have divided lesions into those that occur primarily in an endobronchial location and those that are found mostly in an intraparenchymal position. Hamartomas are examined separately because of their high incidence compared with other benign lung lesions and because they occur both endobronchially and intraparenchymally. In the study of each tumor type, an effort has been made to analyze it on the basis of demographics, clinical presentation, histology, imaging or bronchoscopic appearance, and finally, treatment options. Also, within each major division, we have further categorized the tumors according to the type of cell from which they originated.

HAMARTOMA

The most common benign lesion of the lung is the hamartoma. It accounts for more than 70% of all benign lung tumors.[20] On rare occasion, a pulmonary hamartoma is found with a gastric leiomyosarcoma and a functioning extra-adrenal paraganglioma comprising what is known as Carney's triad. Hamartomas represent abnormal arrangements of mature mesenchymal tissue types normally found in the lung. Most commonly, pulmonary hamartomas include a cartilaginous component, but fibrous elements, adipose tissue, and smooth muscle are also seen (Fig. 91-1).

Radiographically, hamartomas appear as smooth, lobulated, well-circumscribed solitary peripheral lesions most often located in the lower lung fields with diameters ranging from 1 to 3 cm and increasing at a mean rate of 3 to 5 mm per year (Fig. 91-2). Popcorn-like or diffuse calcifications can be seen in 10% to 30% of radiographs of hamartomas. Endobronchial lesions, which occur in 3% to 20% of cases, are seldom detected radiographically, unless there are concomitant lung parenchymal

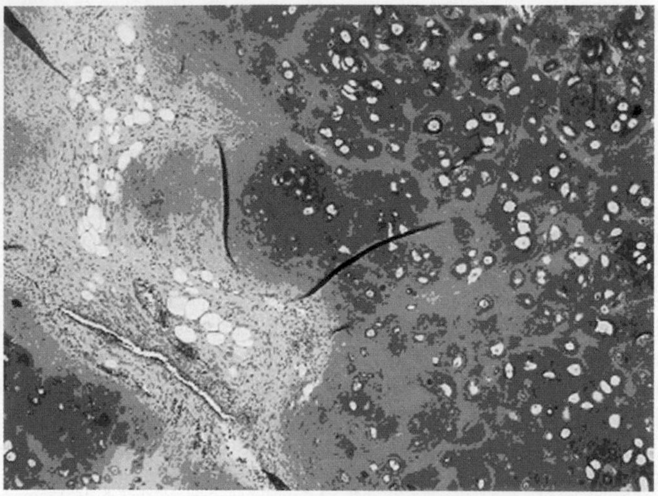

Figure 91-1. Photomicrograph of a hamartoma indicating the presence of cartilage.

changes such as atelectasis, pneumonia, or abscess formation (Fig. 91-3).

On CT scan, calcifications associated with hamartomas are detected only 5% of the time. The presence of fatty tissue in a peripheral solitary lesion identified on CT scan is highly suggestive of hamartoma. However, fatty tissue identification occurs in only 50% of cases. The general appearance of hamartoma on CT scan is consistent with a smoothly marginated mass with mixed fat and soft-tissue attenuation. The treatment of hamartomas is described separately.

BENIGN TUMORS OF THE LUNG WITH A PREDOMINANTLY ENDOBRONCHIAL LOCATION

Tumors of Epithelial Origin

Papilloma

A papilloma most commonly presents as a solitary endobronchial tumor less than 1.5 cm in size in men with an extensive

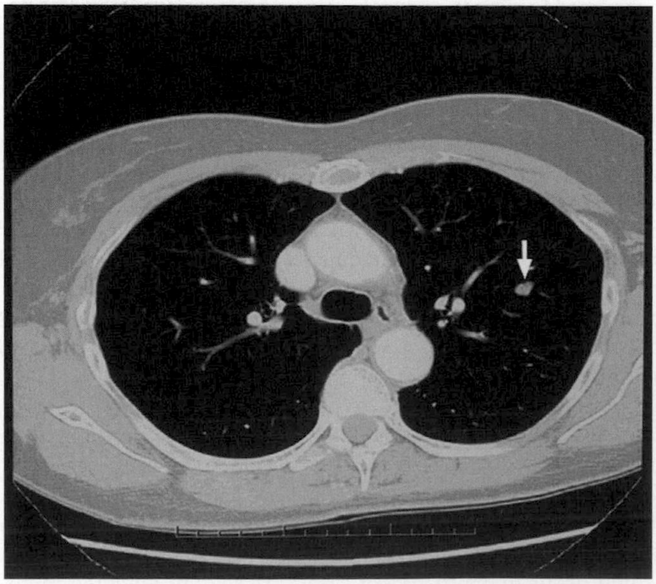

Figure 91-2. A left upper lobe hamartoma.

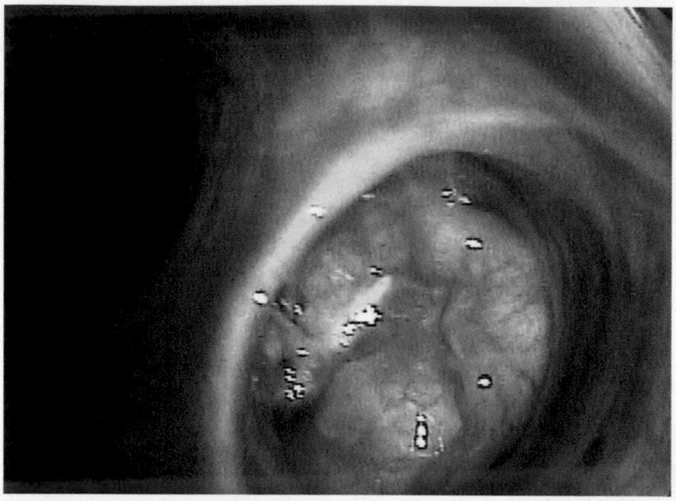

Figure 91-3. Endobronchial hamartoma.

smoking history, usually in the fifth and sixth decades of life. These lesions are usually located endobronchially and produce obstructive symptoms. In children, on the other hand, they are usually seen in association with laryngeal papillomatosis involving the vocal cords or the trachea. They present as multiple squamous papillomas that carry a risk of malignant degeneration and usually require surgical excision. Human papillomavirus serotypes 16 and 18 have been implicated as etiologic factors (Fig. 91-4).[21]

Papillomas can be divided into three histologic categories based on their epithelial surface: squamous, glandular (columnar), and mixed. Most respiratory tract papillomas are of the squamous type. Papillomas associated with human papillomavirus serotypes 16 and 18 tend to show dysplasia and an increased tendency to become malignant. Furthermore, the lesions of viral respiratory tract papillomatosis are more likely to invade local tissues. Glandular papillomas must be distinguished from well-differentiated adenocarcinoma.

Papillomas are diagnosed bronchoscopically from their typical papillary appearance. Treatment is usually laser ablation or endoscopic removal unless malignancy develops, which usually requires bronchotomy and a sleeve resection.

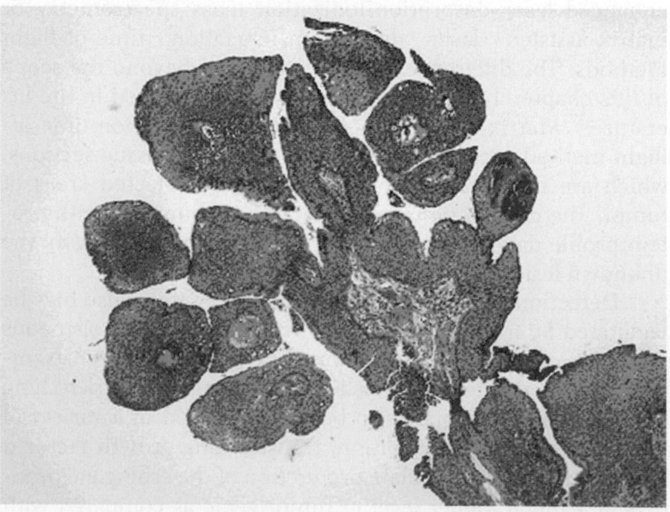

Figure 91-4. Photomicrograph of a right mainstem bronchial papilloma.

Photodynamic therapy also has been used with some success to treat multiple laryngotracheobronchial papillomas. A nonresectional treatment approach mandates regular bronchoscopic follow-up with biopsies.

Mucous Gland Adenoma

This lesion arises primarily from the submucosal mucous glands of a lobar or segmental bronchus of the lower lobes and can be seen in both children and adults. These tumors usually are encapsulated and easily separated from the bronchus. Most patients are symptomatic and present with fever, hemoptysis, chest pain, recurrent pneumonia, or persistent cough. If there is no bronchial obstruction, the patient is asymptomatic.

Cystic change is a critical diagnostic feature of these lesions with cysts containing mucinous or serous contents. Other criteria for diagnosis include an endobronchial location, exophytic growth superficial to the cartilaginous plate, and the presence of at least some normal-appearing bronchial gland mucinous epithelium. Mucoepidermoid carcinoma sometimes can mimic a benign mucous gland adenoma. The immunophenotype varies from tumor to tumor, but epithelial membrane antigen, blood group substances, and keratin are frequently identifiable in the epithelium. Tumors also may express aberrant B blood group antigen (ABO system) in A- or O-type patients.[22]

On chest radiograph, adenomas appear as round, dense, well-demarcated nodules or as postobstructive pneumonitis, atelectasis, or consolidation. In some patients, the chest radiograph appears normal. On CT scan, they appear as round or oval masses that are heterogeneously low in attenuation and can be multicystic. Their size is widely variable, from as small as 2 cm to as large as 6 cm in diameter. Lesions can demonstrate an air-meniscus sign that suggests their expansive and endobronchial nature. Endoscopically, they appear as firm pink nodules with intact overlying epithelium or as lobulated, usually pedunculated endobronchial masses. A gelatinous coating over the surface of the tumor helps to distinguish it bronchoscopically from other lesions. Definitive diagnosis, however, can only be made with pathologic examination of the tissue.

Treatment is usually endoscopic removal with laser, cryotherapy, or curettage. Surgical resection is performed only if bronchoscopic removal is incomplete or if the distal lung parenchyma is destroyed. Wedge resection is commonly performed, but lobectomy may be necessary if there is irreversible damage to the distal lung tissue. Pneumonectomy should be avoided in children because it can interfere with the normal development of the thorax.[23]

Tumors of Mesenchymal Origin

Benign Endobronchial Histiocytoma

Benign endobronchial histiocytoma is a rare endobronchial lesion that occurs most commonly in children or young adults. In many cases, these tumors belong to the broader category of inflammatory pseudotumor and may be composed of varying amounts of storiform fibroblasts, plasma cells, foamy histiocytes, and other inflammatory cells. They have no distinguishing radiographic features, and their exact incidence is unknown as a result of their rarity. They usually present with hemoptysis and can be associated with cavitation. Wide local excision is recommended owing to their low-grade potential for malignant degeneration.[24] Bronchoplastic resection has been used successfully to treat these tumors.

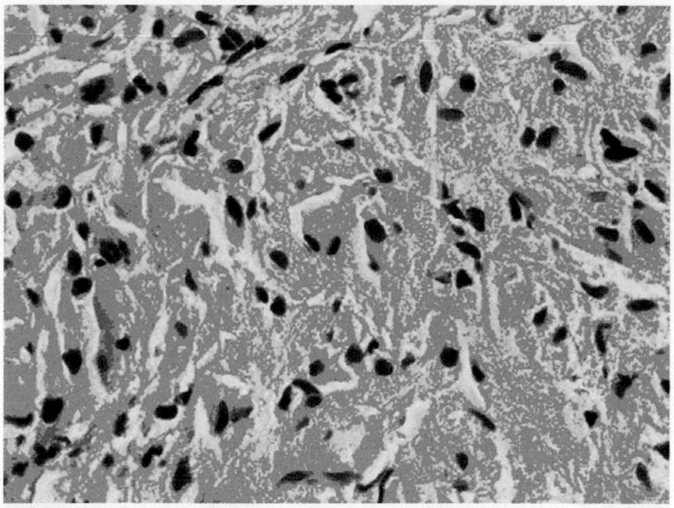

Figure 91-5. Granular cell tumor photomicrograph.

Tumors of Miscellaneous Origin

Granular Cell Tumor

Granular cell tumors are rare benign tumors of the lung (Fig. 91-5). Approximately 75% of these tumors are solitary, 15% are solitary but found in association with multiple skin lesions, and 10% are multiple. In approximately 50% of patients, these tumors are discovered incidentally. In the other half, the tumors usually cause bronchial obstruction that leads to atelectasis, hemoptysis, or pneumonia. Granular cell tumors usually are sessile polyps that grow within the trachea or a central bronchus and are now known to be neural in differentiation. Although they are usually seen as tracheal or bronchial polyps, rare peripheral examples also have been reported. Histologically, the cells are usually polygonal and demonstrate ample eosinophilic cytoplasm with coarse granularity and small, bland nuclei. Ultrastructural and immunohistochemical evidence suggests schwannian differentiation, with positive immunohistochemical staining for neural markers such as S100, CD56, and myelin basic protein.[25] The cytoplasm is filled almost entirely with secondary and tertiary lysosomes, which impart the classic pink cytoplasmic color on hematoxylin and eosin staining and can be identified by electron microscopy.

On chest radiographs or CT scans they appear as coin lesions and may cause lobar infiltrates or lobar atelectasis (Fig. 91-6). They are usually circumscribed but not encapsulated and range in size from 0.3 to 5.0 cm. Treatment is conservative resection. Curative resection of recurrences also has been reported. More recently, laser therapy has been used with success for certain obstructing tumors.

BENIGN LUNG TUMORS WITH PREDOMINANTLY PARENCHYMAL LOCATION

Tumors of Epithelial Origin

Mucinous Cystadenoma

This lesion is usually peripheral in location and appears with approximately equal frequency in both men and women who have a history of heavy smoking. It appears to have a predilection

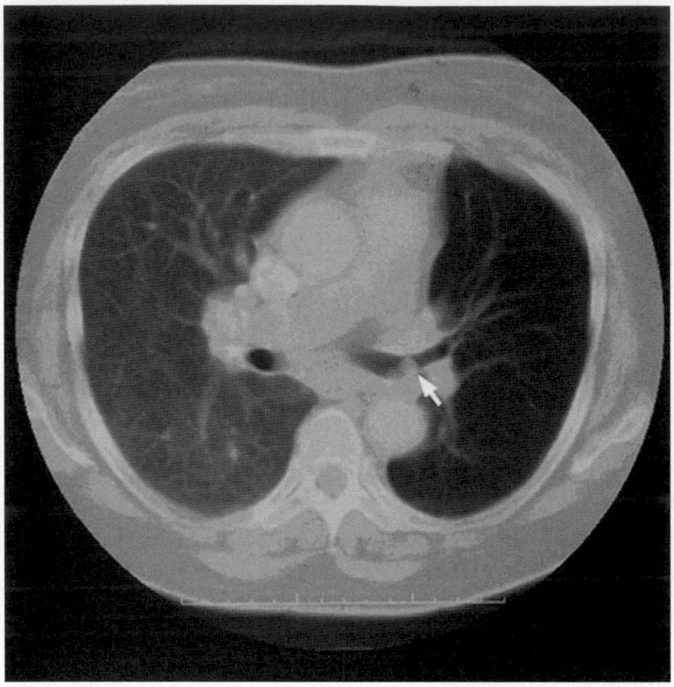

Figure 91-6. CT image of a granular cell tumor.

for the right lung. It occurs in the fifth or sixth decade of life and usually is discovered incidentally on a chest radiograph.

This is a unilocular cystic lesion with a fibrous wall and mucinous contents. The relatively bland, cuboidal-to-columnar mucinous epithelium may be sparse or detached. There is no association of cystadenoma with larger airways, and it lacks the ciliated lining, bronchial glands, and cartilage of a bronchogenic cyst. Immunophenotypic and ultrastructural characteristics are nonspecific and of limited utility in the differential diagnosis. A cytokeratin 7-positive, cytokeratin 20-negative phenotype, however, may help to distinguish it from metastatic disease (Fig. 91-7).

On chest radiograph, cystadenomas are well-demarcated singular cystic masses located mostly in the periphery of the lung parenchyma. On CT scan, they appear as homogeneous masses with a smooth margin (Fig. 91-8).

Treatment is complete surgical excision with excellent prognosis. Since these lesions may harbor areas of cellular

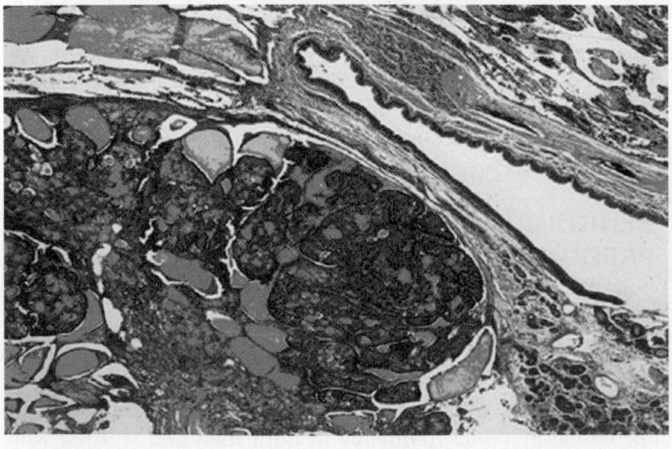

Figure 91-7. Photomicrograph of a mucinous cystadenoma.

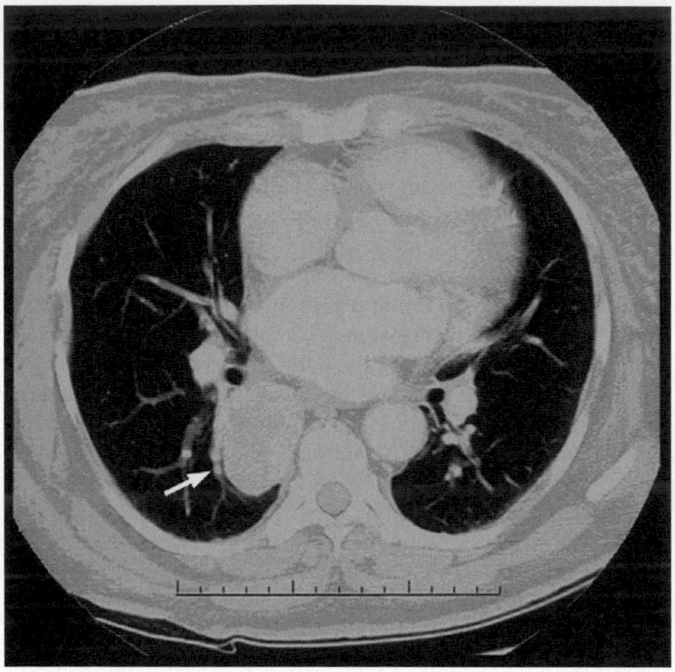

Figure 91-8. CT image of a mucinous cystadenoma.

atypia, in situ malignancy, or invasive adenocarcinoma, complete excision is necessary, and careful postoperative histopathologic examination is imperative.[26]

Alveolar Adenoma

Alveolar adenomas are very rare, and the largest series reported in the literature consists of only a few patients. These tumors are, on average, 2 cm in diameter, well encapsulated, and can be shelled out easily from the surrounding lung parenchyma. They present more commonly in women between the fifth and seventh decades of life. Usually asymptomatic, most are discovered on routine chest radiograph. Patients can present with chronic, insidious cough, usually nonproductive, but shortness of breath or obstructive symptoms are rare.

These benign lesions arise from a joint proliferation of alveolar epithelium and septal mesenchymal cells. Grossly and microscopically, they are well circumscribed and multicystic. The epithelium is predominantly composed of type II pneumocytes. It is still unclear whether the mechanism of origin involves proliferation of a single primitive cell with dual differentiation or independent proliferation of both cell types. Alveolar adenoma must be distinguished clinicopathologically from atypical adenomatous hyperplasia (a preneoplastic lesion also confusingly called bronchioloalveolar adenoma), lymphangioma, and congenital adenomatoid malformation.

Alveolar adenomas usually are identified on routine chest radiographs as solitary nodules located in the midlung fields. The tumor margins are well demarcated, and they are usually noncalcified. On CT scan, they appear as small, homogeneous nodular areas of ground-glass opacity. A cystic component to the tumor sometimes can be seen on CT scan.

Definitive diagnosis by bronchoscopy is difficult because of the peripheral location of most tumors. Because the radiographic presentation of the tumor is nonspecific, definitive diagnosis requires accurate recognition of the characteristic histologic features of the tumor.

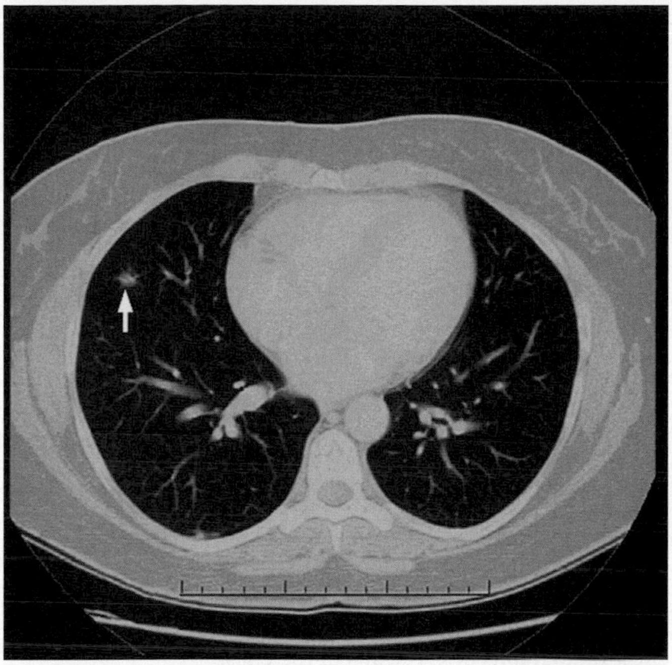

Figure 91-9. CT image of an alveolar adenoma.

Surgical excision via VATS (preferably) or open thoracotomy appears to be curative. Wedge resection is the procedure of choice, but lobectomy also has been reported (Fig. 91-9).

Tumors of Mesenchymal Origin

Leiomyoma

These benign tumors of the lung comprise 2% of all benign lung lesions and are found half the time in an endotracheal or endobronchial location and half the time in a parenchymal location. They are more common in females and in young adults.

Most endobronchial leiomyomas cause hemoptysis, which leads to their discovery. The parenchymal ones are usually discovered incidentally on a chest radiograph. The parenchymal lesions are solitary masses that have variable sizes. As in leiomyomas of other organs, pulmonary tumors show sweeping fascicles of bland spindle cells with moderate eosinophilic cytoplasm and cigar-shaped nuclei. They are typically well circumscribed (Fig. 91-10).

Occasionally, leiomyomas are observed in young women with uterine leiomyomas, but in these cases, they are considered to be evidence of metastatic disease and can even prove fatal. Recent studies have demonstrated the presence of unique periglandular cells in the stroma of these metastasizing leiomyomas. These cells lack the conventional immunohistochemical characteristics of normal lung smooth muscle cells but stain positively for a variety of unique markers such as CD 10, CD 34, alpha smooth muscle actin, estrogen receptor, and progesterone receptor. It has been speculated that interactions of such cells actually may induce glandular metaplasia in the entrapped pulmonary epithelium seen in these tumors.

Treatment of metastasizing pulmonary leiomyomas requires surgical removal, chemotherapy, and hormonal manipulation. Recent approaches to hormonal manipulation with estrogen-receptor modulators and aromatase inhibitors have proved successful and have obviated the need for oophorectomy.

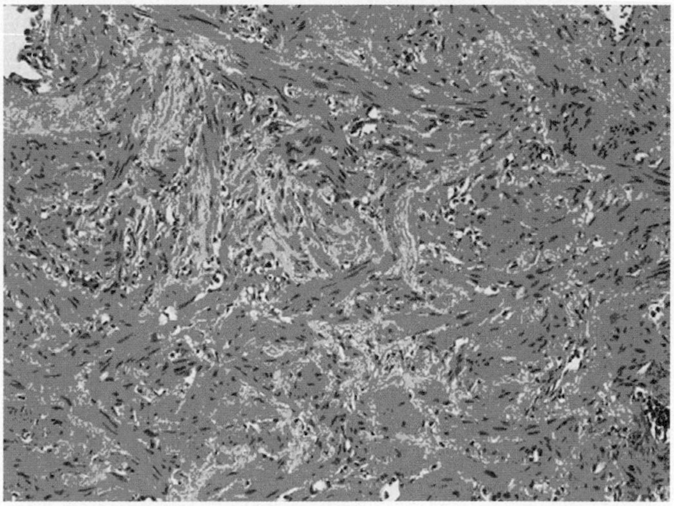

Figure 91-10. Photomicrograph of leiomyoma at 100× magnification. The presence of smooth muscle cells is characteristic.

Nonsurgical treatment is preferred if the nodules are multiple and diffuse.

The more common, nonmetastasizing endobronchial lesions are treated with endoscopic laser ablation, simple endoscopic removal, or sleeve bronchoplasty, provided that the distal lung tissue is not destroyed. Parenchymal leiomyomas are treated with complete surgical resection.

Intrapulmonary Fibrous Tumor

This tumor arises from the mesenchymal layer of the visceral pleura and extends into the lung parenchyma. These tumors, however, are not derived from the mesothelium, are not related to asbestos exposure, and do not show mesothelial differentiation. Nonetheless, when an intrapulmonary fibrous tumor is encountered, mesothelioma is the main differential diagnostic consideration.

These intrapulmonary fibrous lesions tend to be well circumscribed, with firm white cut surfaces. Histologic examination reveals that the tumors are composed of spindle cells with oval nuclei and diffuse fine chromatin, surrounded by dense bundles of collagen in less cellular areas. Variable cellularity and branching or "staghorn" blood vessels are common features helpful in the identification of intrapulmonary fibrous tumor. The cells stain for vimentin and CD 34, the latter of which is particularly helpful in excluding mesothelioma from the differential diagnosis.[27]

The most characteristic radiographic finding of these lesions is the obtuse angle that they make with the chest wall, thus revealing that they arise from the pleura and not the lung. In fact, they have also been reported in the retroperitoneum, mediastinum, and on the parietal surface of the stomach or intestine. They can become quite large, although most are less than 10 cm in diameter.

Treatment is usually surgical resection, which is considered curative. Most commonly, resection is done with VATS because most tumors are pedunculated, and their complete removal is easy. It is important to examine the resected tumor carefully after surgical excision because a malignant variant has been reported.

Hemangiomas

Cavernous Hemangioma

These are rare lung tumors that are thought to form from pulmonary arteriovenous malformations, and their presence raises suspicion of the possibility of hereditary hemorrhagic telangiectasia (Osler–Weber–Rendu syndrome). MRI is the most accurate way to detect and evaluate them. Solitary lesions are surgically excised. If the lesion is endobronchial, a sleeve resection of the involved bronchus is indicated.

Sclerosing Hemangioma

This rare benign lung tumor, most likely of epithelial origin, demonstrates evidence of bronchiolar and alveolar pneumocyte differentiation. The tumor can present between the second and seventh decades of life and has a strong predilection for middle-aged women. It is usually asymptomatic (75% of cases), but symptomatic patients present with chest pain, dyspnea, or hemoptysis. The tumor appears as a solitary nodule on chest radiography and is found most commonly in the lower lobes.

Typically sharply circumscribed, variants of the tumor also may demonstrate multifocality, satellite nodules surrounding a large central lesion, or even nodal metastases. Under the microscope, four basic architectural patterns may be identified: papillary, sclerotic, solid, and hemorrhagic. Round stromal cells and surface lining cells are present, and both may show immunoreactivity to epithelial membrane antigen. Complete surgical resection is curative, and although a minority may metastasize to regional lymph nodes, this does not seem to affect the overall prognosis.

Pulmonary Capillary Hemangiomatosis

This condition represents an aggressive benign tumor of the lung that consists of multiple capillaries proliferating slowly but diffusely in the lung parenchyma, involving the pulmonary vessels and the smaller airways in this proliferation. This results in the development of pulmonary hypertension and eventually in right-sided heart failure. The diagnosis can be made radiographically by observing the typical reticulonodular pattern that characterizes the affected lung. The only treatment available is bilateral lung transplantation because single-lung transplantation has been reported to be inadequate for treating this process.[28]

Tumors of Inflammatory Origin

Inflammatory Pseudotumor (Inflammatory Myofibroblastic Tumor)

Inflammatory myofibroblastic tumor is an uncommon lesion of borderline malignant potential (low-grade malignancy). It is most likely caused by an excessive inflammatory response to tissue injury and it is frequently preceded by an upper respiratory tract infection. In fact, an organizing pneumonia can function as the nidus for formation of the pseudotumor. The lung is the most common site of occurrence, but it may be seen in the small and large bowel mesentery, omentum, mediastinum, retroperitoneum, and other locations.

Inflammatory myofibroblastic tumor usually presents in children and young adults with no sex or racial predilection. In appearance, it is a firm, nonencapsulated, white or yellow mass. Patients can present with cough, dyspnea, chest pain, wheezing, or hemoptysis. Forty percent of cases are asymptomatic and can be detected by finding solitary nodules on routine chest radiographs or CT scans of the chest.

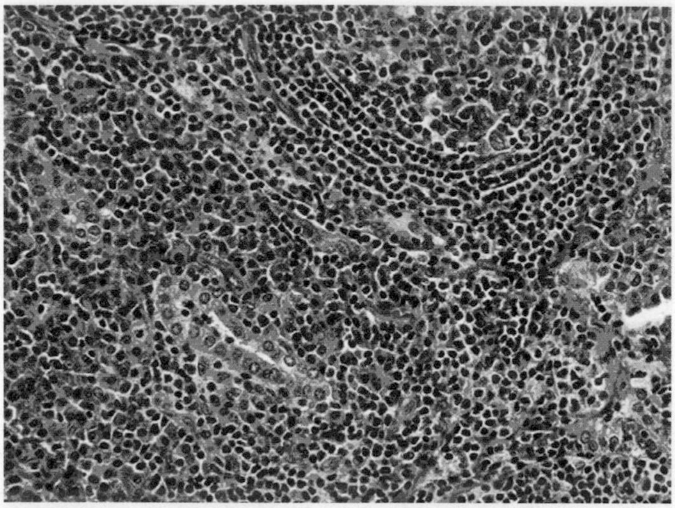

Figure 91-11. Photomicrograph of an inflammatory pseudotumor.

The mass size varies from 1 to 10 cm, and sometimes it is accompanied by hilar or mediastinal lymphadenopathy, pleural effusion, or distal atelectasis resembling bronchogenic carcinoma. Nevertheless, unlike bronchogenic carcinoma, inflammatory pseudotumors tend to be well circumscribed. Definitive diagnosis usually requires surgical biopsy.

Histologically, they are characterized by a mixture of spindle and inflammatory cells, including plasma cells. Immunohistochemically, the spindle cells express smooth muscle actin, vimentin, and sometimes activin-like kinase receptor 1 (ALK1). The inflammatory cells are polyclonal, which is a critical point in separating these tumors from lymphoma or plasmacytoma (Fig. 91-11).

The tumors seem to follow two patterns of biologic behavior. One tumor group is aggressive, attains large sizes, has a higher number of inflammatory cells on histologic examination, and tends to invade adjacent structures such as the pulmonary vessels or the diaphragm. The other, more common, group consists of tumors that tend to remain small, do not invade local tissues, and have a smaller number of inflammatory cells.

Treatment is complete surgical excision. Incomplete removal of the tumor may lead to recurrence. Overall prognosis is excellent. For unresectable or multiple lesions, radiation, chemotherapy, or steroids can be used with variable success. Spontaneous regression is seen occasionally in children.

Hyalinizing Granuloma

Hyalinizing granuloma is a rare benign pulmonary tumor of dense hyalinized connective tissue that develops in response to inflammation. Most patients have a previous history of fungal or mycobacterial infections that could induce tumor formation or a history of some autoimmune disease. The presence of hyalinizing granulomata also can follow systemic diseases such as multiple sclerosis or systemic idiopathic fibrosis. They can occur at any age from young adults to the elderly, and there is no sex predilection.

Patients either can be asymptomatic or present with a combination of cough, chest pain, dyspnea, and occasionally, weight loss. Lesions can be solitary or multiple but are usually

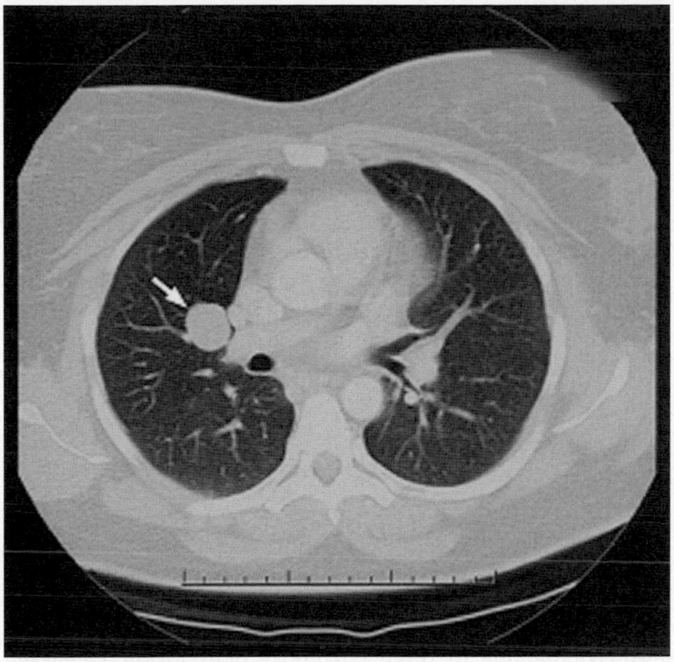

Figure 91-12. CT image of a hyalinizing granuloma.

bilateral. The tumor size is also highly variable from a few millimeters to several centimeters. Treatment is usually surgical excision (Fig. 91-12).

Tumors of Miscellaneous Origin

Nodular Amyloid

Nodular amyloid is part of a spectrum of amyloid lesions associated with the lung that includes a tracheobronchial amyloid type and a diffuse interstitial pulmonary amyloid type. Nodular amyloid is found most commonly in the lower lobes as single or multiple nodules of amyloid surrounded by giant cells and is not associated with systemic amyloidosis. Lesions also can be asymmetric and bilateral. Both sexes are equally affected, and the disease can present at any age, with the sixth and seventh decades of life being most common. The histologic appearance reveals eosinophilic deposits with "apple green" birefringence after staining with Congo Red and examination under polarized light. The nodules may calcify, or metaplastic bone or cartilage formation may occur, and inflammatory cells are often present in the background (Fig. 91-13).

Patients are usually asymptomatic, and the nodules are discovered incidentally on chest radiograph. However, the disease is rarely associated with multiple myeloma, and the presence of nodular amyloid always should raise suspicion and induce appropriate diagnostic workup for multiple myeloma (Fig. 91-14).

The lesion size can range from 0.4 to 15 cm, with an average size of 3 cm. Diagnosis can be established with bronchoscopic lung biopsy, although these patients do have an increased risk of postbiopsy bleeding.[29]

Surgical excision is considered curative. Long-term follow-up is necessary because of the reported association of nodular amyloid with macroglobulinemia and lymphoma. Laser therapy also has been used successfully when patients with tracheobronchial amyloidosis present with obstructive symptoms.

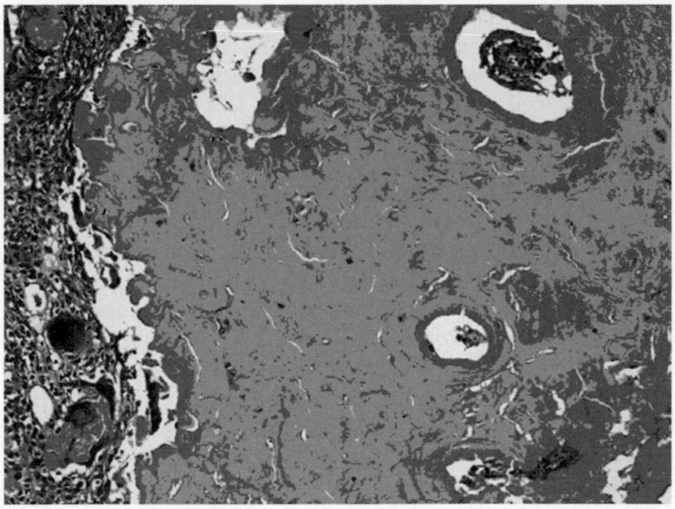

Figure 91-13. Nodular amyloid (H&E stain; 100×). Nodular deposits of amorphous, eosinophilic amyloid material (right) are surrounded by inflammatory cells, including multinucleate giant cells (bottom left).

Primary Pulmonary Thymoma

Primary pulmonary thymoma is a very rare tumor that arises in the lung of a patient with a normal thymus gland. The tumor most likely arises from embryologic descent of thymic tissue to a position more inferior than normal, but on occasion, it may arise from developmentally immature cells. The tumor exhibits a slight female preponderance and tends to occur in older patients with a mean age of 55 years. There is also some association with myasthenia gravis. Primary pulmonary thymomas can present with fever, retrosternal pain, nonproductive cough, malaise, and hemoptysis, but most patients are asymptomatic, and the tumor is often discovered incidentally on routine chest radiograph.

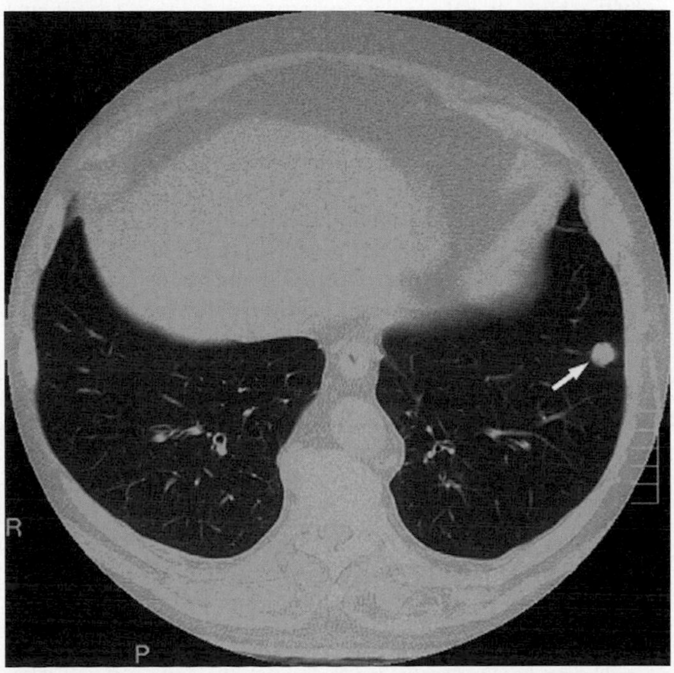

Figure 91-14. CT image of a left lower lobe nodular amyloid lesion.

Intrapulmonary thymoma is identical histologically to a thymoma that arises in the mediastinum. Diagnosis is facilitated by immunohistochemistry, which permits identification of thymic-type T-cell antigens (CD3 and/or CD5) and other markers of immaturity (CD1a, TdT, or CD99). The epithelial component of the thymoma expresses cytokeratin, endomysial antibodies, and sometimes CD5. This epithelial and lymphoid immunophenotype can be critical in distinguishing primary pulmonary thymoma from other tumors in the differential diagnosis, namely, lymphoma or lymphoepithelial-like carcinoma of the lung.

Intrapulmonary thymomas can be located centrally, in a hilar location, or peripherally. The size of the lesion ranges from 1.7 to 12 cm. As in mediastinal thymomas, extension beyond the capsule suggests invasive behavior. Primary pulmonary thymoma has no distinctive radiographic features but appears as a well-circumscribed lesion confined in the lung. They are slow-growing lesions that remain asymptomatic until they cause bronchial obstruction.

Treatment is surgical excision. Prognosis is good in well-circumscribed, encapsulated lesions that are resected completely. The presence of an effusion does not preclude cure unless the pleura is directly involved by the tumor. In the rare case of an extensive, unresectable tumor involving the pleura, radiation therapy can be used with good results.

BENIGN PULMONARY TUMOR WITH MALIGNANT POTENTIAL

Pleomorphic Adenoma (Mixed Tumor) of the Lung

Pulmonary mixed tumors show a predilection for women, can appear at any age between the fifth and eighth decades of life, and usually have a parenchymal location but also can be endobronchial. The most common presenting symptoms include obstructive symptoms such as productive cough and fever. They tend to be slow growing and can reach significant size before they cause symptoms.

Histologically, they contain both stromal and epithelial components and are also found in the salivary glands. Although overexpression of oncogenes and tumor suppressor genes have been reported for the salivary gland variant, there is a relative scarcity of such reports for pulmonary pleomorphic adenomas. A high proliferative index and immunoreactivity to tumor suppressor gene *p16* have been documented in one lung example.[30]

Chest radiography usually reveals a sharply defined density. CT scan or MRI reveals a well-circumscribed, homogeneous lesion ranging from 1.5 to 16 cm in size, usually with no mediastinal or hilar lymphadenopathy. Definitive diagnosis can be established with transbronchial biopsy.

Treatment of choice is complete surgical excision because if nests of tumor are left behind, they tend to recur. Recurrence can be seen as late as 9 years after apparent complete tumor clearance and can present as either a recurrent lung lesion or as distant metastases, usually to the spine, liver, or breast. Implantation of tumor cells during the operation is considered to be one reason for this rare occurrence. Therefore, long-term surveillance is necessary. The treatment of choice for metastases in accessible sites appears to be surgical excision because the metastases are slow growing and may remain solitary for a long time. Radiation therapy can be used for palliation from bone metastases, but the tumor itself shows low susceptibility to radiation.

SUMMARY

Despite their multitude, benign masses of the lung are rare and constitute only 1% of lung lesions resected. They are often clinically silent and are discovered incidentally on a chest radiograph. The most critical issue with a solitary pulmonary nodule is to differentiate it from a possible malignancy. In fact, benign lesions of the lung are often a diagnosis of exclusion during the evaluation of an indeterminate solitary pulmonary nodule. With improved imaging and an assortment of diagnostic techniques, significant progress has been made in our ability to perform this differentiation. Contrast-enhanced and high-resolution CT scanning, dynamic MRI, and PET scanning, along with the discovery of highly specific tumor markers and the recent use of serum proteomics, have allowed us to identify benign masses of the lung with much greater accuracy than ever before. This has led to greater confidence when we decide to observe a patient rather than proceed directly to an excisional biopsy. However, in many cases it is still necessary to perform either diagnostic or therapeutic surgical resection. In these patients, the recent advances in minimally invasive thoracic surgery that diminish morbidity have made this prospect much less daunting for both the surgeon and the patient.

EDITOR'S COMMENT

The authors have provided a thorough review of the etiology, evaluation, and management of the wide variety of benign (and low malignant potential) lung tumors. Although rare, most thoracic surgeons encounter a number of these during their career and thus it is important for one to be familiar with these tumors so as to consider lung-sparing surgical options whenever possible.

—Yolonda L. Colson

References

1. Martini N. Results of Memorial Sloan-Kettering lung project. *Recent Results Cancer Res*. 1982;82:174–178.
2. Smith MA, Battafarano RJ, Meyers BF, et al. Prevalence of benign disease in patients undergoing resection for suspected lung cancer. *Ann Thorac Surg*. 2006;81:1824–1829.
3. Ohtsuka T, Nomori H, Horio H, et al. Radiological examination for peripheral lung cancers and benign nodules less than 10 mm. *Lung Cancer*. 2003; 42:291–296.
4. Greif J, Marmor S, Schwarz Y, et al. Percutaneous core needle biopsy vs fine needle aspiration in diagnosing benign lung lesions. *Acta Cytol*. 1999; 43:756–760.
5. Iwano S, Makino N, Ikeda M, et al. Solitary pulmonary nodules: optimal slice thickness of high-resolution CT in differentiating malignant from benign. *Clin Imaging*. 2004;28:322–328.
6. Ohno Y, Koyama H, Matsumota K et al. Differentiation of malignant and benign pulmonary nodules with quantitative first-pass 320-detector row perfusion CT versus FDG PET/CT. *Radiology*. 2011;258(2):599–609.

7. Satoh S, Kitazume Y, Ohdama S, et al. Can malignant and benign pulmonary nodules be differentiated with diffusion-weighted MRI? *Am J Roentgenol.* 2008;191:464–470.
8. Sarinas PS, Chitkara RK. PET and SPECT in the management of lung cancer. *Curr Opin Pulm Med.* 2002;8:257–264.
9. Bury T, Dowlati A, Paulus P, et al. Evaluation of the solitary pulmonary nodule by positron emission tomography imaging. *Eur Respir J.* 1996;9:410–414.
10. Baath M, Kolbeck KG, Danielsson R. Somatostatin receptor scintigraphy with 99m Tc-depreotide (NeoSpect) in discriminating between malignant and benign lesions in the diagnosis of lung cancer: a pilot study. *Acta Radiol.* 2004;45:833–839.
11. Gonzalez AL, Roberts RL, Massion PP et al. 15-Lipoxygenase-2 expression in benign and neoplastic lung: an immunohistochemical study and correlation with tumor grade and proliferation. *Hum Pathol.* 2004;35:840–849.
12. Seemann MD, Beinert T, Furst H, Fink U. An evaluation of the tumour markers, carcinoembryonic antigen (CEA), cytokeratin marker (CYFRA 21-1) and neuron-specific enolase (NSE) in the differentiation of malignant from benign solitary pulmonary lesions. *Lung Cancer.* 1999;26:149–155.
13. Seemann MD, Seemann O, Dienemann H, et al. Diagnostic value of chest radiography, computed tomography and tumour markers in the differentiation of malignant from benign solitary pulmonary lesions. *Eur J Med Res.* 1999;4:313–327.
14. Molina R, Auge JM, Bosch X et al. Usefulness of serum tumor markers, including progastrin-releasing peptide, in patients with lung cancer: correlation with histology. *Tumour Biol.* 2009;30(3):121–129.
15. Maciel CM, Paschoal ME, Kawamura MT, et al. Serum protein profiling of lung cancer patients. *J Exp Ther Oncol.* 2004;4:327–334.
16. Xiao X, Liu D, Tang Y, et al. Development of proteomic patterns for detecting lung cancer. *Dis Markers.* 2003;19:33–39.
17. Meyerson M, Carbone D. Genomic and proteomic profiling of lung cancers: lung cancer classification in the age of targeted therapy. *J Clin Oncol.* 2005;23:3219–3226.
18. Snead DR, Perunovic B, Cullen N, et al. hnRNP B1 expression in benign and malignant lung disease. *J Pathol.* 2003;200:88–94.
19. Eberhardt R, Anantham D, Herth F, Feller-Kopman D, Ernst A. Electromagnetic navigation diagnostic bronchoscopy in peripheral lung lesions. *Chest.* 2007;131:1800–1805.
20. Arrigoni MG, Woolner LB, Bernatz PE, et al. Benign tumors of the lung: a ten-year surgical experience. *J Thorac Cardiovasc Surg.* 1970;60:589–599.
21. Popper HH, el-Shabrawi Y, Wockel W, et al. Prognostic importance of human papilloma virus typing in squamous cell papilloma of the bronchus: comparison of in situ hybridization and the polymerase chain reaction. *Hum Pathol.* 1994;25:1191–1197.
22. England DM, Hochholzer L. Truly benign "bronchial adenoma": report of 10 cases of mucous gland adenoma with immunohistochemical and ultrastructural findings. *Am J Surg Pathol.* 1995;19:887–899.
23. Lack EE, Harris GB, Eraklis AJ, Vawter GF. Primary bronchial tumors in childhood: a clinicopathologic study of six cases. *Cancer.* 1983;51:492–497.
24. Bueno R, Wain JC, Wright CD, et al. Bronchoplasty in the management of low-grade airway neoplasms and benign bronchial stenoses. *Ann Thorac Surg.* 1996;62:824–828; discussion 828–829.
25. Deavers M, Guinee D, Koss MN, Travis WD. Granular cell tumors of the lung: clinicopathologic study of 20 cases. *Am J Surg Pathol.* 1995;19:627–635.
26. Traub B. Mucinous cystadenoma of the lung. *Arch Pathol Lab Med.* 1991;115:740–741.
27. Chang YL, Lee YC, Wu CT. Thoracic solitary fibrous tumor: clinical and pathological diversity. *Lung Cancer.* 1999;23:53–60.
28. Eltorky MA, Headley AS, Winer-Muram H, et al. Pulmonary capillary hemangiomatosis: a clinicopathologic review. *Ann Thorac Surg.* 1994;57:772–776.
29. Strange C, Heffner JE, Collins BS, et al. Pulmonary hemorrhage and air embolism complicating transbronchial biopsy in pulmonary amyloidosis. *Chest.* 1987;92:367–369.
30. Ang KL, Dhannapuneni VR, Morgan WE, Soomro IN. Primary pulmonary pleomorphic adenoma: an immunohistochemical study and review of the literature. *Arch Pathol Lab Med.* 2003;127:621–622.

92 Bronchoplasty for Benign Lung Lesions

Kazunori Okabe

Keywords: Tracheobronchomalacia, bronchial stenosis after anastomosis, bronchial disruption, benign endobronchial tumor, endobronchial inflammatory polyp, pulmonary tuberculosis, hamartoma

Although bronchoplasty for malignant lung lesions is common, bronchoplasty for benign lung lesions is relatively rare. In most instances, these lesions are published as individual case reports, and various approaches and procedures have been performed. In this chapter, selected case reports of bronchoplasty for benign lung lesions are used to illustrate each disease entity. Specific entities discussed in this chapter include bronchoplasty for tracheobronchomalacia, tuberculous bronchial lesions, endobronchial benign tumors, endobronchial inflammatory polyps, bronchial stenosis after bronchial anastomosis, and bronchial disruption.

TRACHEOBRONCHOMALACIA

Tracheobronchomalacia is characterized by weakness of the tracheobronchial wall and supporting cartilage. Collapsing airways due to tracheobronchomalacia have been stabilized with a variety of external splints; for example, autologous rib or various types of prostheses. A new technique has been reported in which a ringed polytetrafluoroethylene (PTFE) graft splint was placed for a serious case of tracheobronchomalacia.[1] The patient was a 55-year-old man with grade 3 tracheobronchomalacia (Johnson's classification) (Table 92-1).[2] Chest CT scan showed a crescent deformity of the trachea (Fig. 92-1A). Bronchoscopy revealed crescent-type stenosis (Fig. 92-1B). Matsuoka et al.[1] cut the 12-mm diameter ringed PTFE graft to a length of 2.5 cm (Fig. 92-2A). The prosthesis was divided longitudinally and spread. The rings were cut at various points to fit the membranous portion of the trachea and bronchi (Fig. 92-2B), after which the prosthesis was sutured to the cartilage and membranous portion with 4-0 PDS-II sutures (Fig. 92-2C). This process was repeated from the trachea to the bilateral bronchi. The patient's symptoms were markedly improved after surgery. Postoperative chest CT scan showed that the caliber of the trachea was well preserved (Fig. 92-3).

Table 92-1

JOHNSON'S CLASSIFICATION OF TRACHEOMALACIA

DEGREE OF TRACHEAL COLLAPSE	
First degree	Collapse of 1/2 to 3/4 of trachea with coughing
Second degree	Collapse of 3/4 to complete collapse of trachea with coughing
Third degree	Complete collapse of the trachea with coughing
Fourth degree	Complete collapse of trachea with coughing and ectasia at rest

TUBERCULOUS BRONCHIAL LESIONS

Endobronchial tuberculosis is often associated with significant tracheobronchial stenosis. The incidence of strictures in females is remarkably higher than in males.[3,4] The left main bronchus is affected most often.[3,4] If the stricture is an active tuberculous lesion and the patient has symptoms due to the stenosis, antituberculosis medication should be given, and laser ablation, balloon dilation, and/or stenting should be performed.[3–5] Surgical bronchoplasty is indicated for nonactive tuberculous lesions with symptoms and/or repeated infections.[3–5] Case reports of sleeve resection of the left main bronchus, sleeve left upper lobectomy, balloon dilation, and Dumon stent placement have been published.[6–8]

Sleeve Resection of Left Main Bronchus

A 31-year-old woman came to the hospital with left chest pain and dyspnea after medical therapy for pulmonary tuberculosis.[6] Chest x-ray showed atelectasis of the left lower lobe and mediastinal deviation to the left (Fig. 92-4A). Bronchoscopy revealed a cicatricial obstruction of the left main bronchial orifice (Fig. 92-4B). By MRI, it was concluded that the left upper lobe and lower lobe bronchi were patent. Sleeve resection of the left mainstem bronchus was performed from the carina to the left second carina. The anastomosis was done by interrupted 4-0 absorbable suture, and it was reinforced by two mattress stitches of 4-0 nonabsorbable suture. Virtual CT endoscopy showed no anastomotic stenosis 1 year and 9 months after the operation (Fig. 92-5).

Sleeve Left Upper Lobectomy

A 33-year-old man presented with a past medical history of pulmonary tuberculosis.[7] He developed left pneumonia, and chest x-ray showed left atelectasis. Stenosis of the left mainstem bronchus could be seen at bronchoscopy, and balloon dilation was performed twice. However, stenosis and pneumonia recurred frequently. Therefore, he was admitted for surgery. Chest x-ray showed patchy and granular shadows due to the repeated pneumonia (Fig. 92-6). Chest tomogram showed a 15-mm obstruction of the left mainstem bronchus, and the left upper lobe bronchus was not seen. Stenosis of the left mainstem bronchus was clearly observed by three-dimensional CT scan (Fig. 92-7A). Bronchoscopy revealed occlusion of the left mainstem bronchus two rings from the carina (Fig. 92-7B). At thoracotomy, via the fourth intercostal space, the left upper lobe was found to be damaged by tuberculosis. Therefore, a left upper sleeve lobectomy was performed. The total left mainstem bronchus was resected, and the carina and the left lower lobe

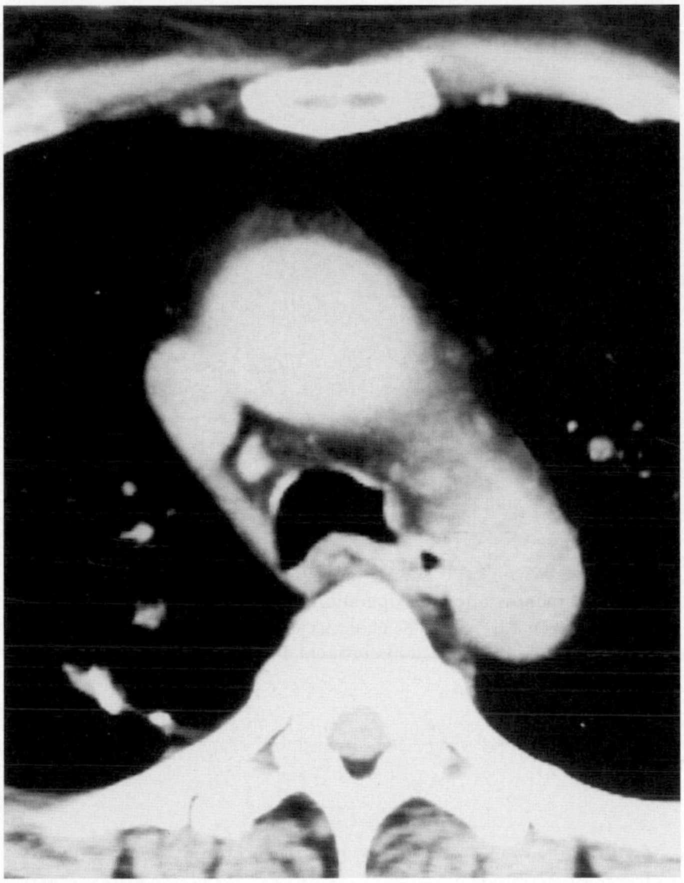

A

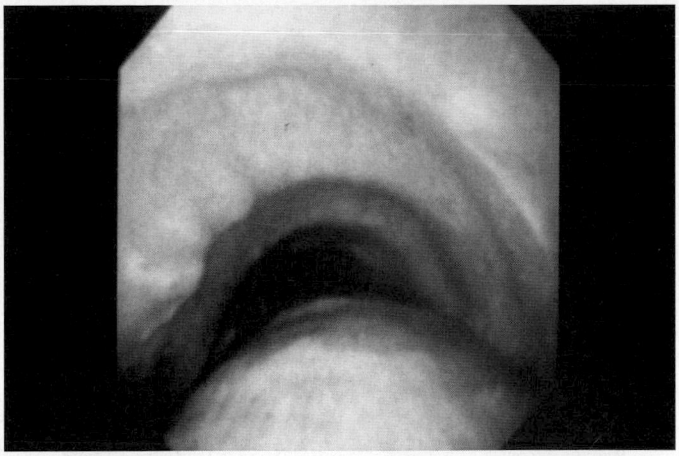

B

Figure 92-1. *A*. Chest CT scan revealed a crescent deformity of the trachea. (Used with permission from Matsuoka H, Nishio W, Sakamoto T, et al. Use of span plasty with ringed PTFE for serious tracheobronchomalacia. *Jpn J Chest Surg.* 2002;16:602.) *B*. Bronchofiberscopic findings revealing a slit-like stenosis of crescent type. (Used with permission from Matsuoka H, Nishio W, Sakamoto T, et al.: Use of span plasty with ringed PTFE for serious tracheobronchomalacia. *Jpn J Chest Surg.* 2002;16:602.).

bronchus were anastomosed with 4-0 PDS interrupted sutures. Postoperative bronchoscopy revealed an excellent anastomosis (Fig. 92-7C).

Balloon Dilation and Dumon Stent

Kobayashi et al.[8] reported that balloon dilation alone for tuberculous bronchial stenosis resulted in dilation failure and recommended implantation of a Dumon stent instead. Figure 92-8A illustrates severe stenosis of the left mainstem bronchus before balloon dilation. Nine months after the seventh balloon dilation, the stenosis still remained (Fig. 92-8B). Figure 92-8C shows the condition of the left mainstem bronchus 6 months after the placement of a 10-mm diameter Dumon stent (Novatech, Grasse, France). Because granulation formation was seen at the distal edge of the stent, it was removed. Nineteen months after stent removal, the granulation disappeared completely (Fig. 92-8D), and the lumen was reestablished without further need for dilations.

ENDOBRONCHIAL BENIGN TUMOR

Benign tumors of the airways are much less common than those with malignant potential. In particular, benign endobronchial tumors are extremely rare. Benign neoplasms

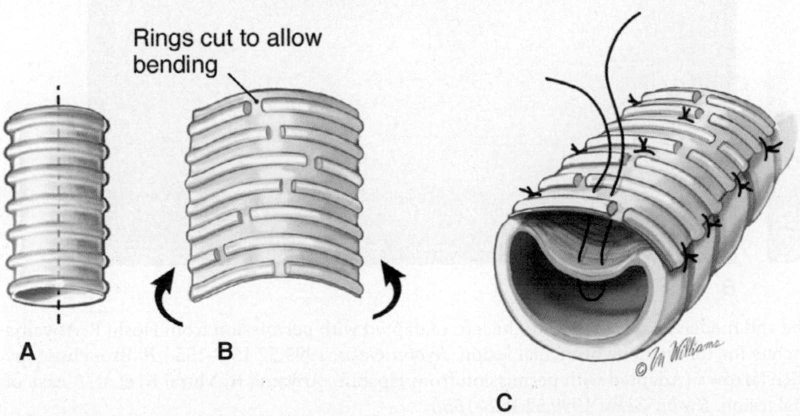

Figure 92-2. *A*. A ringed PTFE with a diameter of 12 mm is cut to a length of 2.5 cm. *B*. After dividing the prosthesis longitudinally, it is spread. The rings are cut in various places to fit the membranous portion of the trachea and bronchi. *C*. The reinforcement is first sutured to the edge of the cartilaginous rings with 4-0 PDS-II. It is then sutured in a similar fashion at the proximal, distal, and central points of the membranous portion.

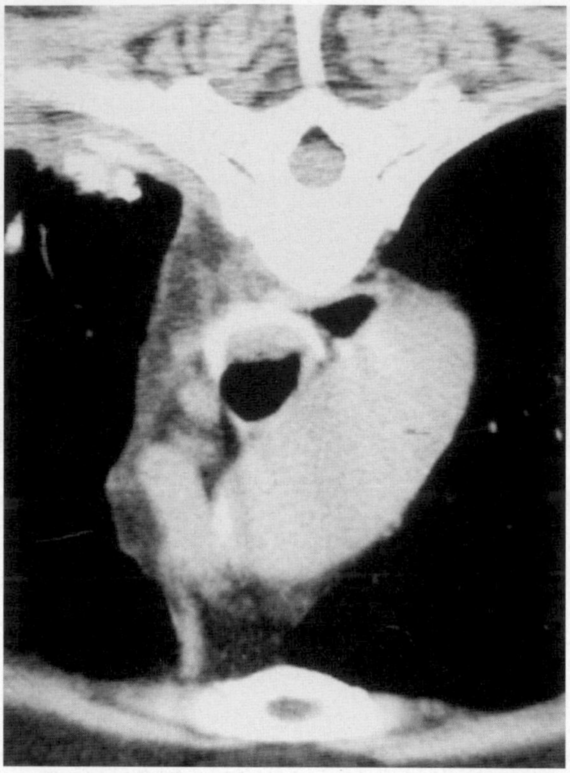

Figure 92-3. Postoperatively, the caliber of the trachea was well preserved. (Used with permission from Matsuoka H, Nishio W, Sakamoto T, et al. Use of span plasty with ringed PTFE for serious tracheobronchomalacia. *Jpn J Chest Surg.* 2002;16:602.)

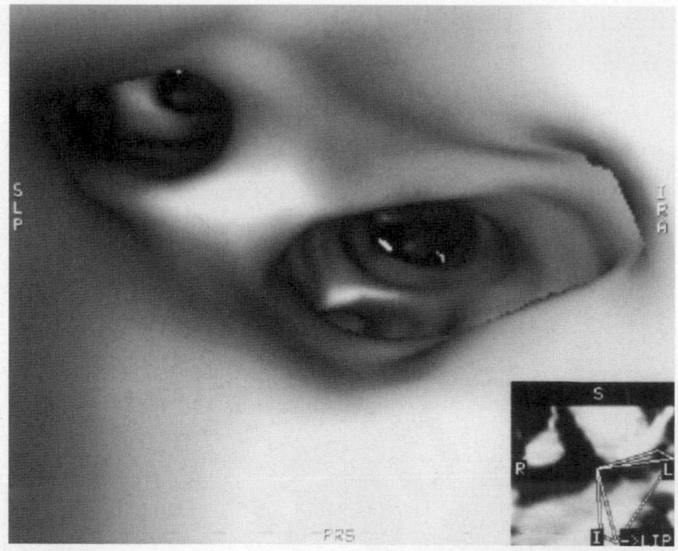

Figure 92-5. Virtual CT endoscopy showed no anastomotic stenosis 1 year and 9 months after the operation. (Adapted with permission from Hoshi E, Aoyama K, Murai K, et al. A case of sleeve resection of the left main bronchus for tuberculous bronchial lesion. *Kyobu Geka.* 1999;52:152–155.)

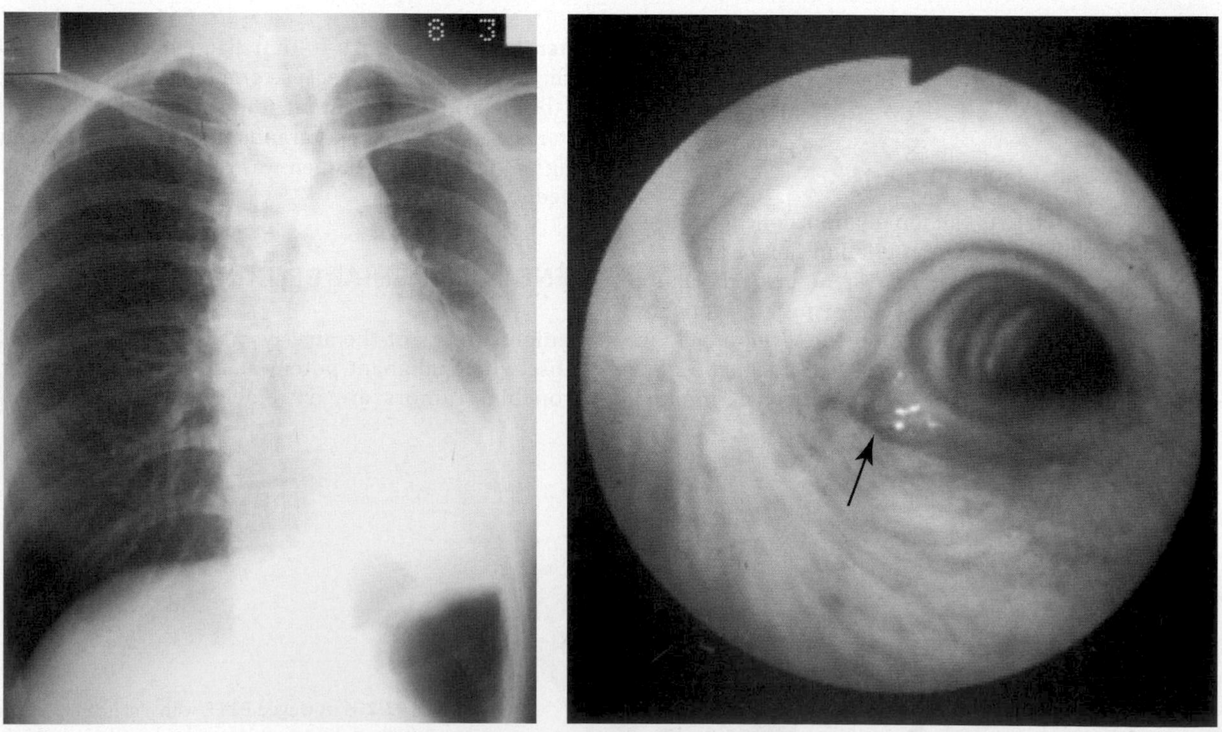

A B

Figure 92-4. *A.* Chest x-ray showed atelectasis of the left lower lobe and mediastinal deviation to the left. (Adapted with permission from Hoshi E, Aoyama K, Murai K, et al. A case of sleeve resection of the left main bronchus for tuberculous bronchial lesion. *Kyobu Geka.* 1999;52:152–155.) *B.* Bronchoscopy revealed cicatricial obstruction of the left mainstem bronchial orifice (arrow). (Adapted with permission from Hoshi E, Aoyama K, Murai K, et al. A case of sleeve resection of the left main bronchus for tuberculous bronchial lesion. *Kyobu Geka.* 1999;52:152–155.)

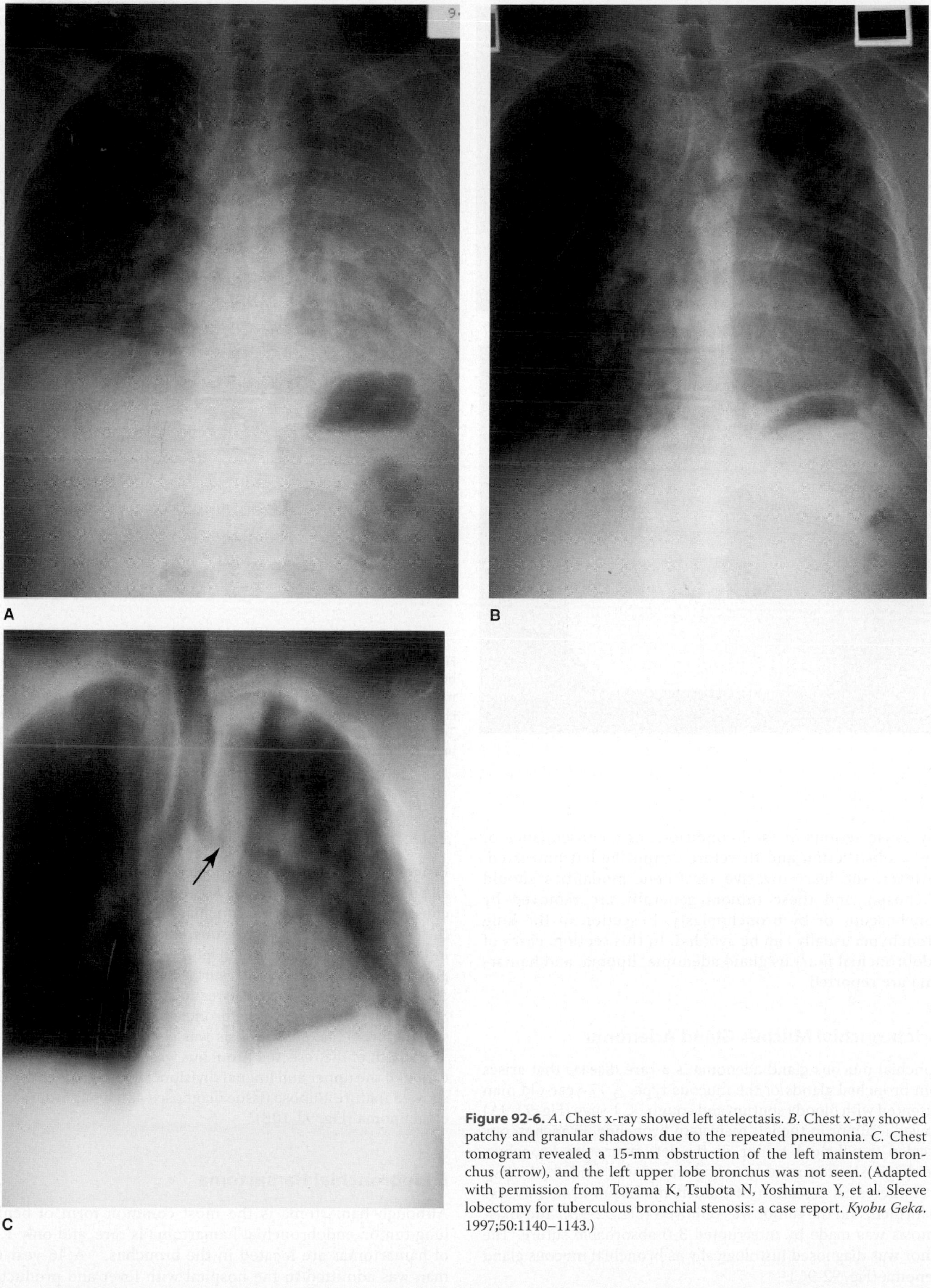

Figure 92-6. *A*. Chest x-ray showed left atelectasis. *B*. Chest x-ray showed patchy and granular shadows due to the repeated pneumonia. *C*. Chest tomogram revealed a 15-mm obstruction of the left mainstem bronchus (arrow), and the left upper lobe bronchus was not seen. (Adapted with permission from Toyama K, Tsubota N, Yoshimura Y, et al. Sleeve lobectomy for tuberculous bronchial stenosis: a case report. *Kyobu Geka*. 1997;50:1140–1143.)

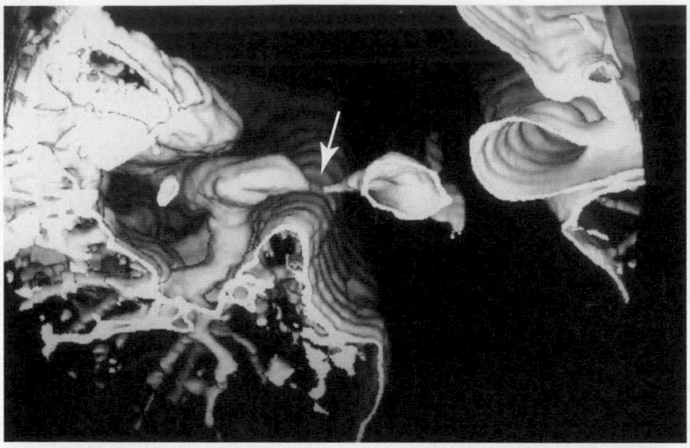

A

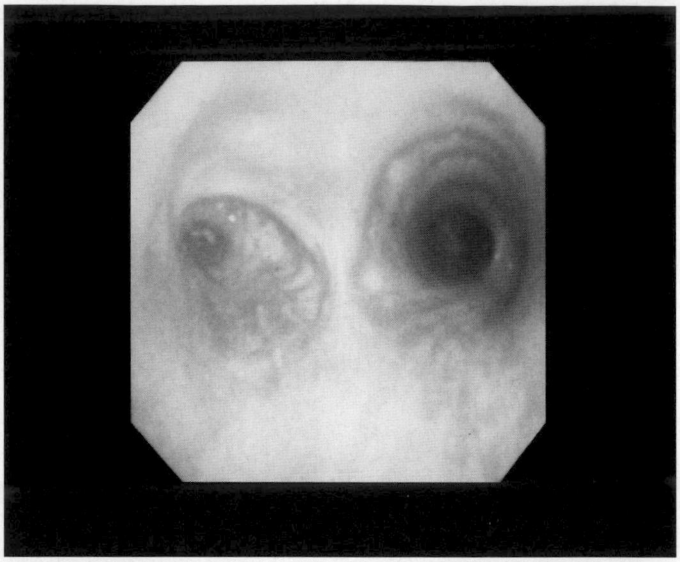

B

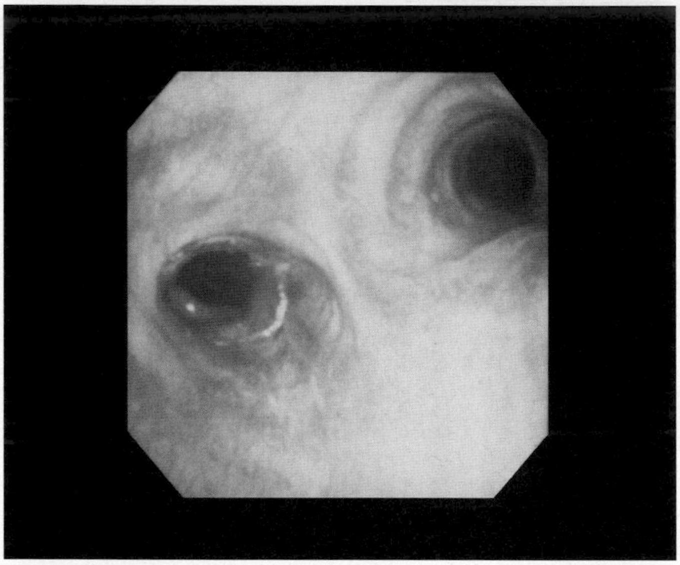

C

Figure 92-7. *A*. Three-dimensional CT scan revealed the left mainstem bronchial stenosis (arrow). *B*. Bronchoscopy revealed occlusion of the left mainstem bronchus two rings from the carina. *C*. Postoperative bronchoscopy revealed excellent anastomosis. (Adapted with permission from Toyama K, Tsubota N, Yoshimura Y, et al. Sleeve lobectomy for tuberculous bronchial stenosis: a case report. *Kyobu Geka*. 1997;50:1140–1143.)

may cause serious or fatal conditions as a consequence of airway obstruction and therefore cannot be left untreated. However, the least invasive treatment modalities should be chosen, and these tumors generally are removed by bronchoscopy or by bronchoplasty. Resection of the lung parenchyma usually can be avoided. In this section, cases of endobronchial mucous gland adenoma, lipoma, and hamartoma are reported.

Endobronchial Mucous Gland Adenoma

Bronchial mucous gland adenoma is a rare disease that arises from bronchial glands of the mucous type. A 77-year-old man presented with bloody sputum and cough.[9] CT scan (Fig. 92-9A) showed a tumor in the left mainstem bronchus. Bronchoscopy revealed a polypoid tumor in the left mainstem bronchus. The diagnosis of mucous gland adenoma was made by biopsy. Circumferential resection of the left mainstem bronchus was performed, and the tumor was removed (Fig. 92-9B). The anastomosis was made by interrupted 3-0 absorbable suture. The tumor was diagnosed histologically as bronchial mucous gland adenoma (Fig. 92-9C).

Endobronchial Lipoma

Bronchial lipoma is rare and makes up approximately 0.1% of all pulmonary tumors.[10] A 72-year-old man was found by bronchoscopy to have an endobronchial lipoma in the bronchus of the lingula accompanied by squamous cell carcinoma (SCC) in the lower lobe bronchus.[11] Figure 92-10A shows a yellowish polypoid tumor with smooth surface at the orifice of the bronchus of the lingula. A left lower lobectomy was done for the SCC. Sleeve resection of the bronchus of the lingula with telescoping bronchial anastomosis was performed for the lipoma. The length of the resected bronchus was 10 mm from the bifurcation of the upper and lingual division. Histologic examination showed mature adipose tissue diagnosed as a benign endobronchial lipoma (Fig. 92-10B).

Endobronchial Hamartoma

Although hamartoma is the most common form of benign lung tumor, endobronchial hamartoma is rare, and only 1.4% of hamartomas are located in the bronchus.[12] A 46-year-old man was admitted to the hospital with fever and productive

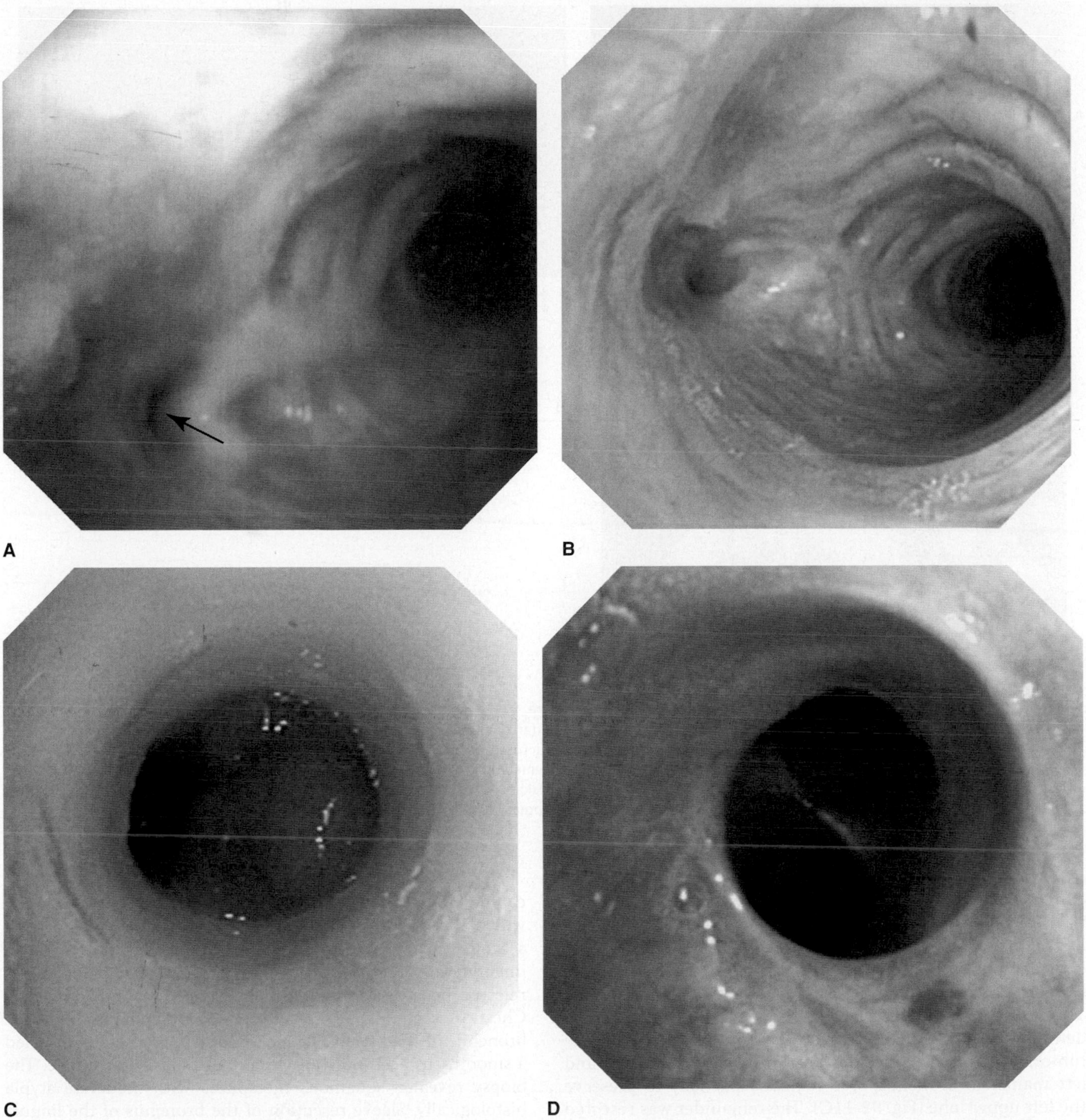

Figure 92-8. *A*. Bronchoscopy showed severe stenosis of the left mainstem bronchus (arrow) before balloon dilation. *B*. The stenosis of the left mainstem bronchus still remained 9 months after the seventh balloon dilation. *C*. Bronchoscopy showed the Dumon stent, which was placed in the left mainstem bronchus 6 months ago. The distal edge of the stent became stenotic owing to granulation tissue. *D*. The granulation tissue regressed 19 months after the stent removal. (Adapted with permission from Kobayashi M, Matsui K, Masuda N, et al. Treatment of tuberculous bronchial stenosis. *JJSRE*. 2001;23:381.)

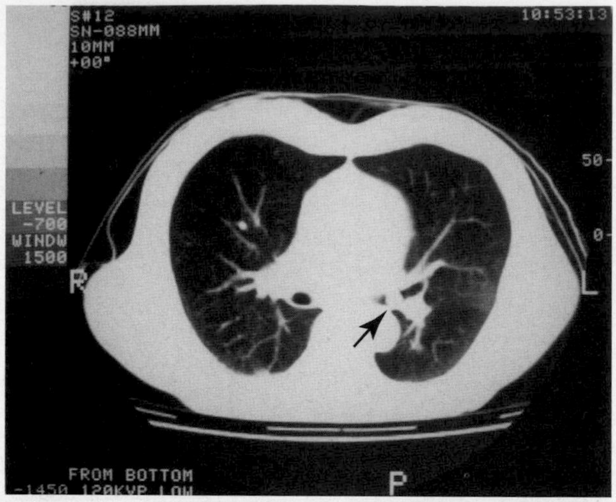

A

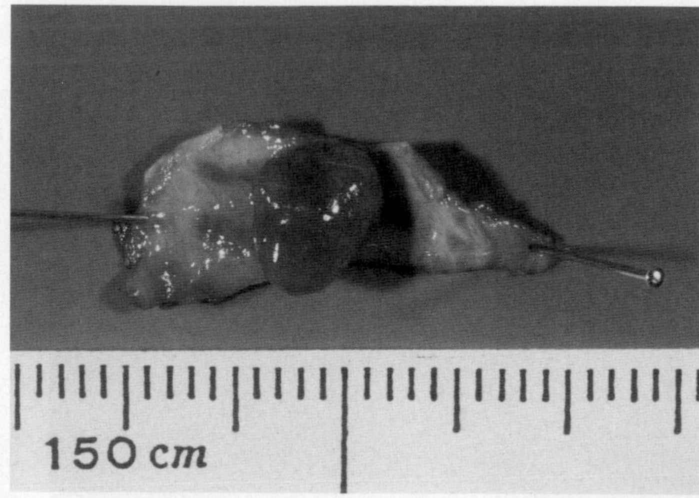

B

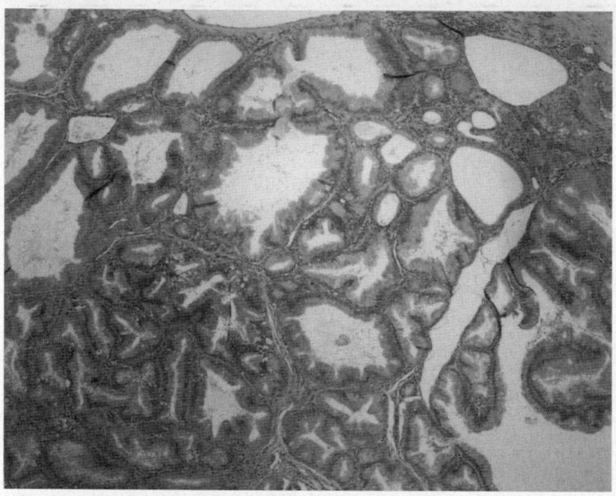

C

Figure 92-9. *A*. CT scan showed the tumor in the left mainstem bronchus (arrow). *B*. Macroscopic findings of the resected bronchus and tumor. *C*. Microscopic findings of the tumor. The tumor is diagnosed histologically as bronchial mucous gland adenoma. (Used with permission from Okabe K, Aoe M, Nakata M, et al: A case of bronchial mucous gland adenoma with cancer in adenoma. *JJSRE*. 1991;13:82.)

cough.[13] Chest x-ray and CT scan (Fig. 92-11A) showed partial atelectasis of the left lung. A 20 × 17 mm mass in the left mainstem bronchus was observed by CT scan. Bronchoscopy demonstrated complete obstruction of the left mainstem bronchus by a hard tumor with a smooth surface (Fig. 92-11B). The tumor was too hard to get a good biopsy specimen for definitive diagnosis. By thoracotomy and bronchotomy, the tumor, which obstructed the left upper lobe bronchus and left mainstem bronchus, was removed partially to preserve the left upper lobe (Fig. 92-11C). The remainder was resected completely by transbronchial electrosurgery snare and neodymium: yttrium-aluminum-garnet (Nd:YAG) laser 2 weeks after the thoracotomy. The tumor was 35 × 15 × 15 mm in diameter and was diagnosed as a hamartoma. No finding of recurrence was seen by bronchoscopy at follow-up 3 years after the resection.

ENDOBRONCHIAL INFLAMMATORY POLYP

Inflammatory bronchial polyp is a rare, benign, and nontumorous lesion similar to inflammatory polyps of the nasal cavities. It is composed of inflammatory granulation tissue. It can be treated bronchoscopically and/or surgically. Resection with a forceps, hot snare, and Nd:YAG laser is available using a bronchoscope. A case of sleeve bronchial resection for an inflammatory polyp is reported here.[14] A 60-year-old man was referred because cancer was suspected by sputum cytology. Chest CT scan (Fig. 92-12A) revealed a polypoid lesion in the bronchus of the lingula. Bronchoscopy (Fig. 92-12B) revealed a smooth-surfaced polypoid lesion at the lingular orifice. The biopsy revealed squamous metaplasia with moderate atypia histologically. Sleeve resection of the bronchus of the lingula was performed, and the lesion was resected (Fig. 92-12C). The superior bronchus and inferior bronchus of the lingular division were anastomosed, respectively, to the upper lobe bronchus by interrupted 5-0 absorbable sutures. The pathologic diagnosis of the resected specimen was inflammatory bronchial polyp (Fig. 92-12D).

BRONCHIAL STENOSIS AFTER BRONCHIAL ANASTOMOSIS

Bronchial stenosis may occur after bronchial wedge resections, sleeve resection, or lung transplantation. Treatments

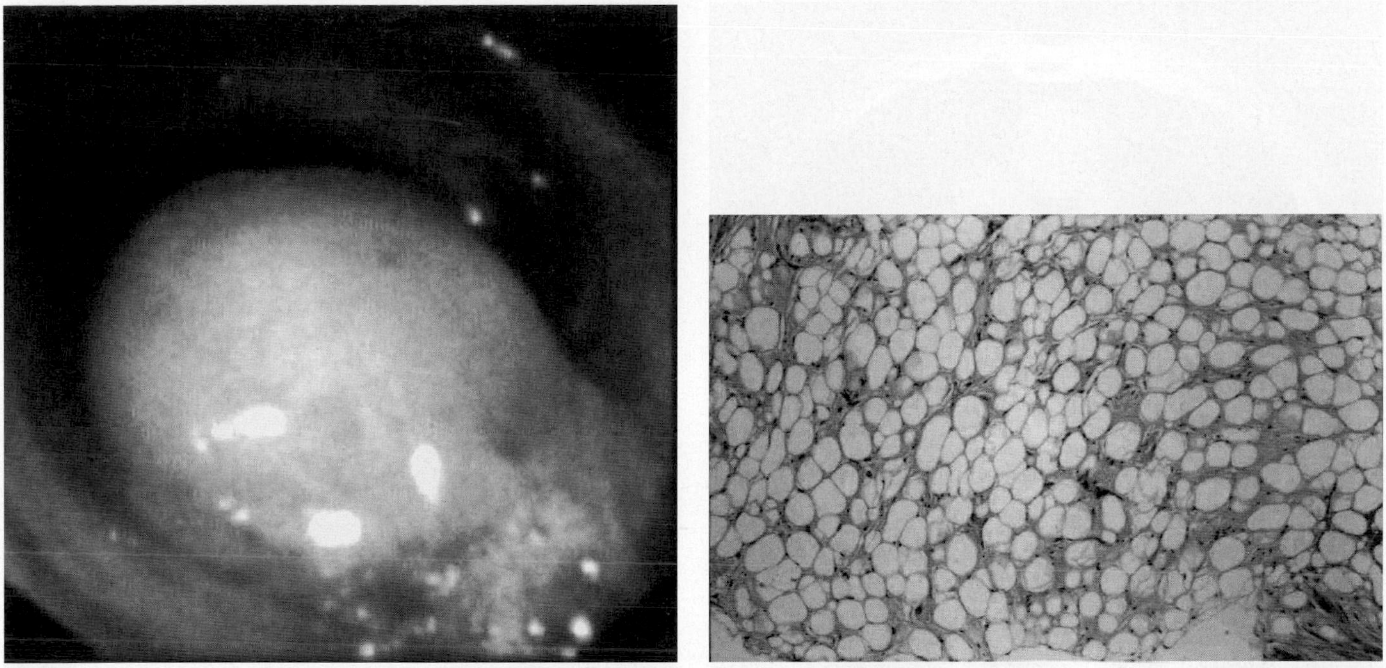

A B

Figure 92-10. *A*. A bronchoscopic examination revealed a yellowish polypoid tumor with a smooth surface at the orifice of the bronchus of the lingula. *B*. Histologic examination showing mature adipose tissue diagnosed as a benign endobronchial lipoma. (Adapted with permission from Kamiyoshihara M, Sakata K, Otani Y, et al. Endobronchial lipoma accompanied with primary lung cancer. *Surg Today*. 2002;32:402–405.)

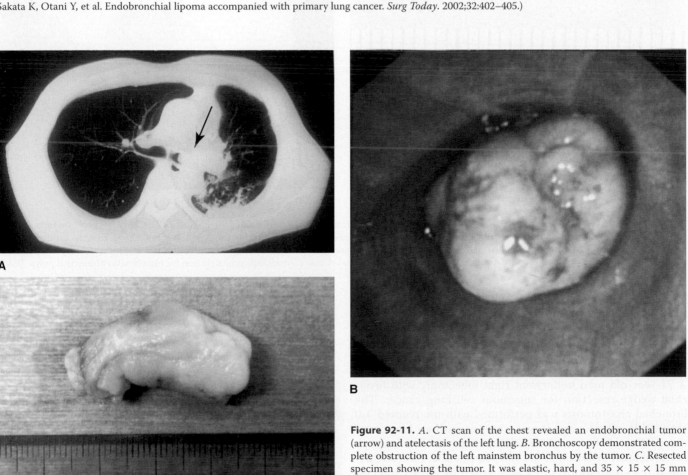

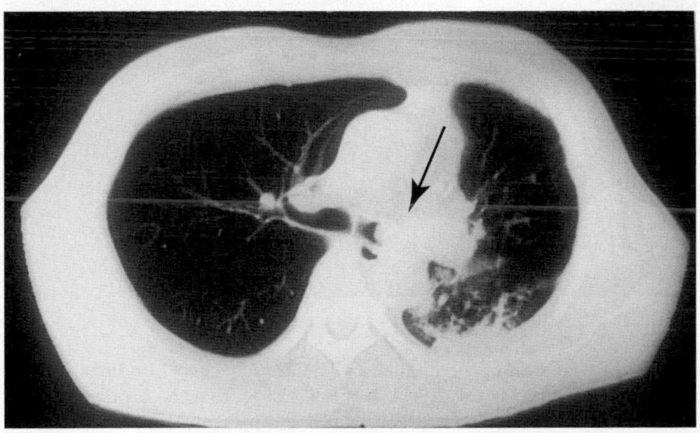

A

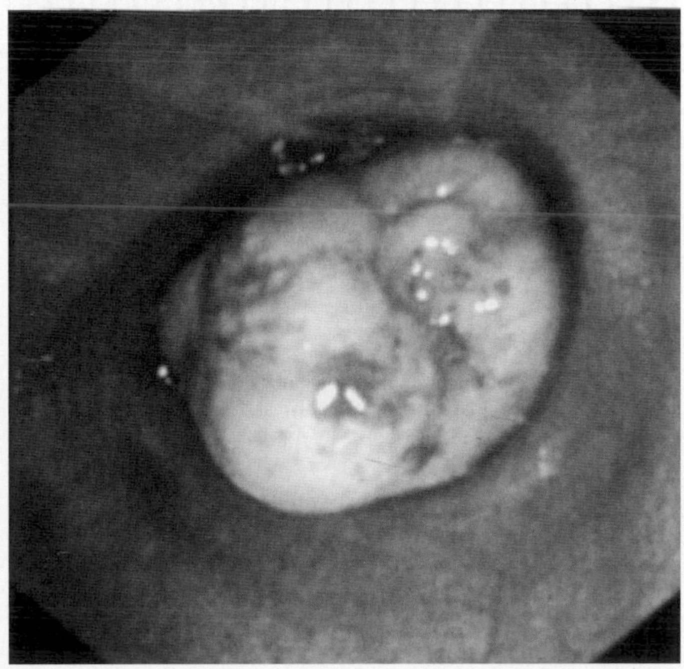

B

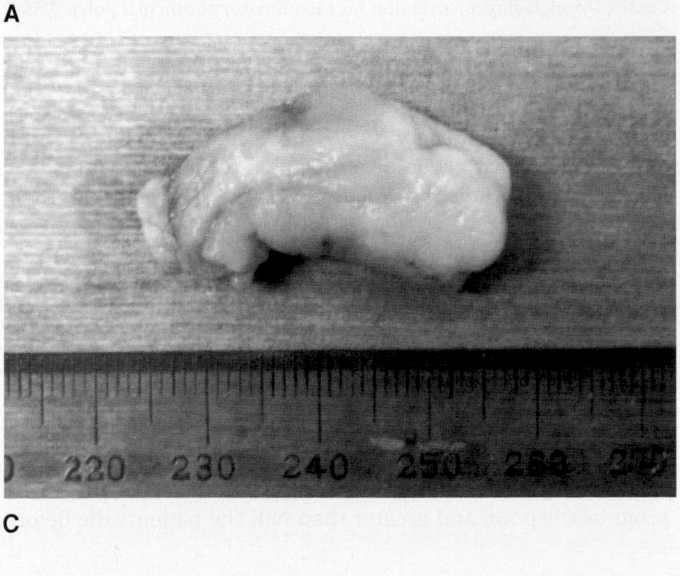

C

Figure 92-11. *A*. CT scan of the chest revealed an endobronchial tumor (arrow) and atelectasis of the left lung. *B*. Bronchoscopy demonstrated complete obstruction of the left mainstem bronchus by the tumor. *C*. Resected specimen showing the tumor. It was elastic, hard, and 35 × 15 × 15 mm in diameter and was diagnosed as hamartoma. (Adapted with permission from Ishibashi H, Akamatsu H, Kikuchi M, et al. Resection of endobronchial hamartoma by bronchoplasty and transbronchial endoscopic surgery. *Ann Thorac Surg*. 2003;75:1300–1302.)

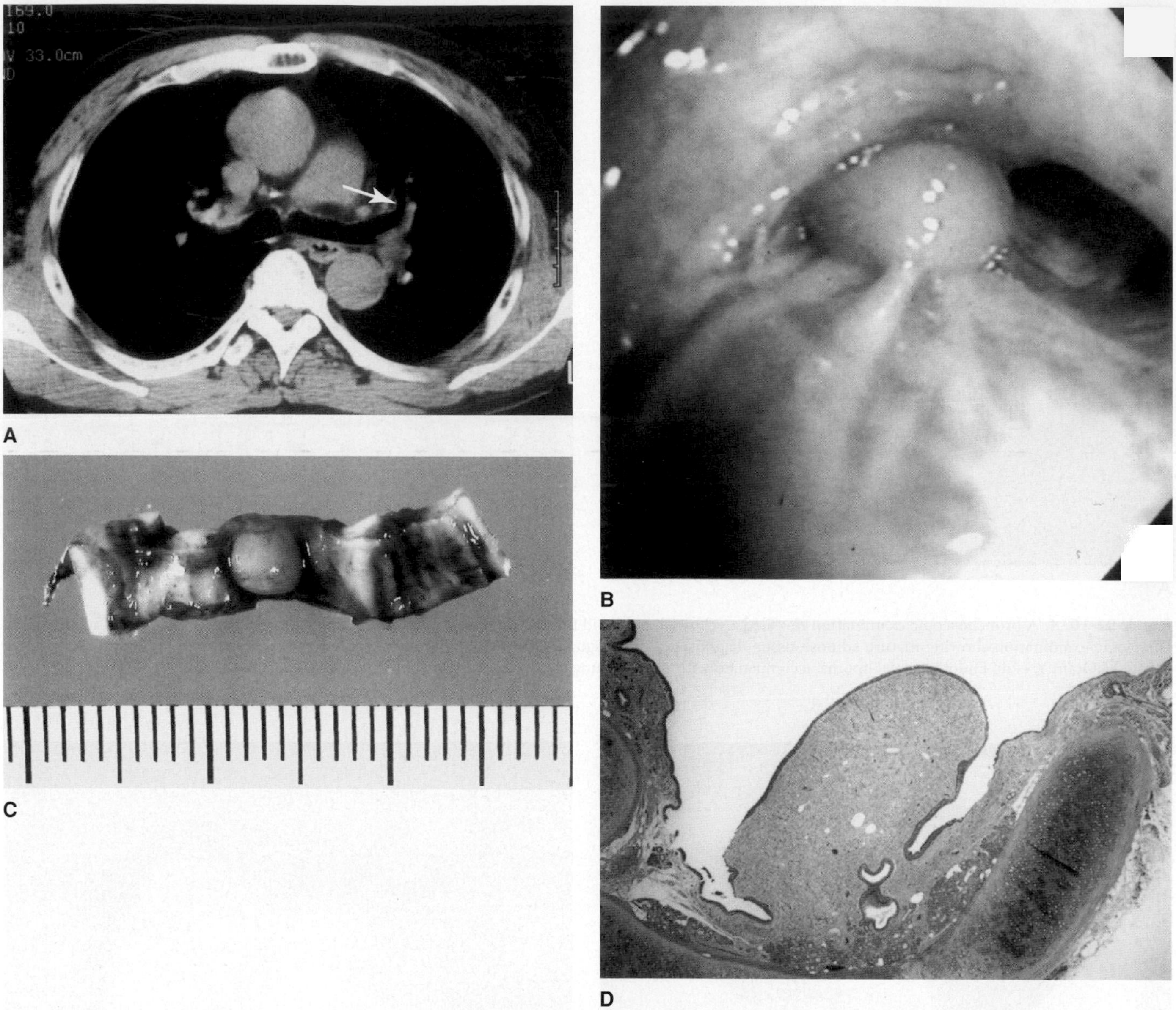

Figure 92-12. *A.* Chest CT scan on admission showed a polypoid shadow (arrow) in the bronchus of the lingula. *B.* The bronchoscopic findings showed a smooth-surfaced polypoid lesion in the bronchus of the lingula. *C.* The resected specimen showing the polypoid mass arising from the bronchus of the lingula. *D.* Microscopic findings of the polyp showing fibrous connective tissue covered by columnar ciliated epithelium and inflammatory infiltration of neutrophils. (Used with permission from Mizobuchi T, Iwai N, Nomoto Y, et al. A case of bronchial reconstruction for inflammatory bronchial polyp. *JJSRE.* 2000;22:505.)

include surgical resection and reanastomosis, debridement by forceps, laser resection, balloon dilation, and stent placement. As an example, a case of debridement by forceps, laser resection, and stent placement for anastomotic stenosis after right upper wedge lobectomy is reported here.[15] A 71-year-old man underwent right lobectomy with bronchial wedge resection for squamous cell lung cancer. The bronchial anastomosis was performed with interrupted 3-0 absorbable sutures, and it was wrapped with an intercostal muscle flap. A few weeks after the surgery, bronchoscopy revealed local infection at the anastomotic site. Necrotic tissue at the anastomotic site was removed by biopsy forceps. Methicillin-resistant *Staphylococcus aureus* was detected in the bronchial lavage fluid, and vancomycin was given. Six months after surgery, bronchoscopy was done because of increased breathing difficulty, and severe anastomotic stricture was found. Figure 92-13A shows the stenosis of 2 mm and inflammatory granulation tissue. Three-dimensional CT scan revealed a serious anastomotic stenosis (Fig. 92-13B). Therefore, Nd:YAG laser resection for the inflammatory granulation was performed, and a self-expanding metallic stent (Ultraflex stent, Boston Scientific, Natick, MA) was placed successfully. Figures 92-13C and D show the placed stent and widely opened anastomosis.

BRONCHIAL DISRUPTION

Bronchial disruption secondary to blunt trauma is unusual. The prognosis is poor, and greater than half the patients die before

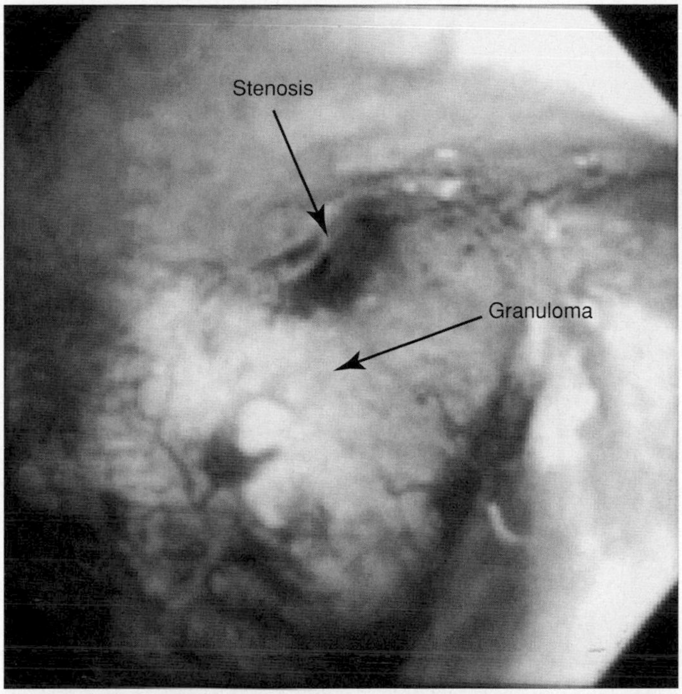

A

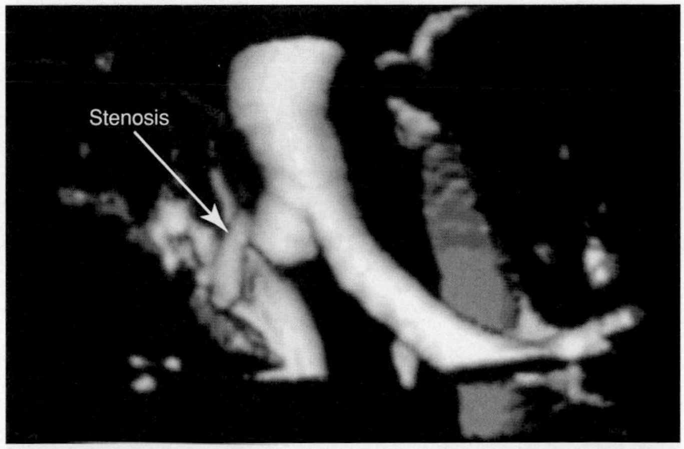

B

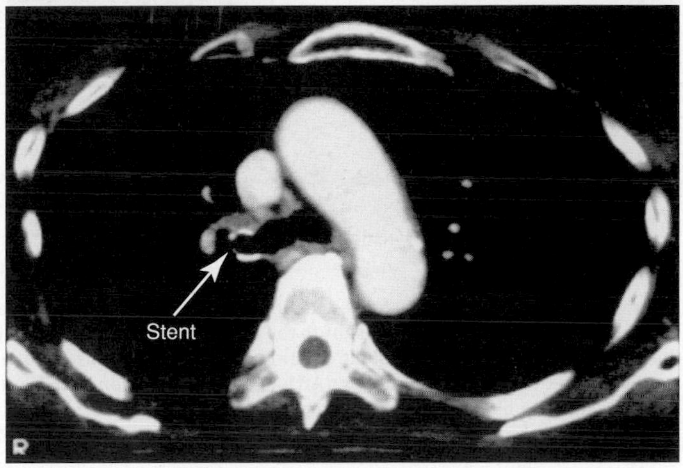

D

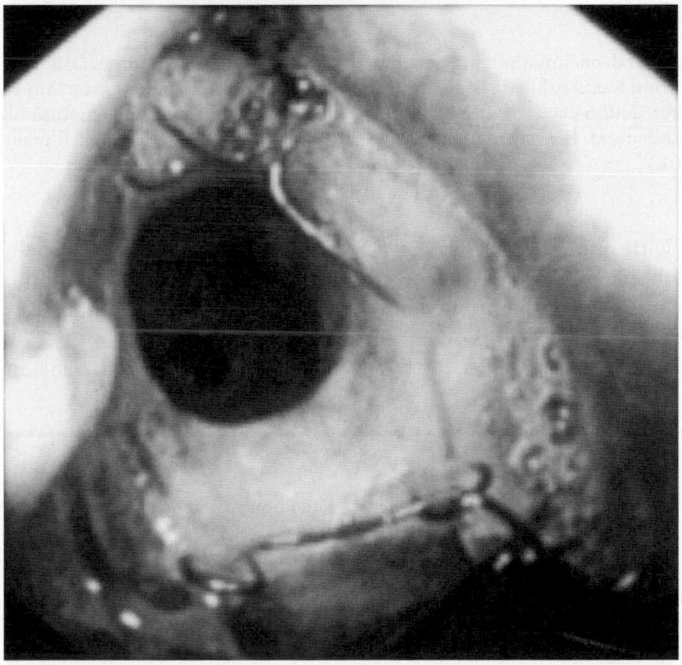

C

Figure 92-13. *A.* Bronchoscopy revealed severe stenosis and inflammatory granuloma at the anastomotic lesion. *B.* Chest three-dimensional CT scan revealed a severe anastomotic stenosis. *C.* Bronchoscopy showed the inserted stent and the improved bronchial mucosa. *D.* CT scan revealed good position and dilation of the inserted stent. (Adapted with permission from Inoue S, Fujino S, Sawai S, et al. Experience with self-expanding metallic stents (SEMS, Ultraflex stent) for postoperative bronchial stenosis. *JJSRE.* 2001;23:454.)

arriving at a hospital.[16] It is important to suspect the condition by clinical and radiographic findings. Early bronchoscopy is strongly recommended to get a definitive diagnosis. More than 80% of tracheobronchial disruptions are within 2.5 cm of the carina.[16] If bronchial disruption is found, immediate surgical repair should be performed. A case of complete transection of the left mainstem bronchus due to blunt chest trauma has been reported.[17] A 62-year-old man was hit by a car and brought to an emergency center. Severe subcutaneous emphysema was present in the neck and chest. Breath sounds were reduced in the left chest. Chest x-ray (Fig. 92-14A) after bilateral chest tube placements showed bilateral pneumothoraces, subcutaneous emphysema, pneumomediastinum, multiple rib fractures, and tracheal shift to the right. Chest CT scan (Fig. 92-14B) revealed bilateral lung contusion in addition to the chest x-ray findings. Because of a massive air leak from the left chest tube, bronchoscopy was done. It demonstrated complete transection of the left mainstem bronchus at two rings from the carina. Emergency thoracotomy was performed, and an end-to-end anastomosis was carried out with interrupted 4-0 absorbable sutures. The anastomosis was wrapped with a fifth intercostal muscle flap.

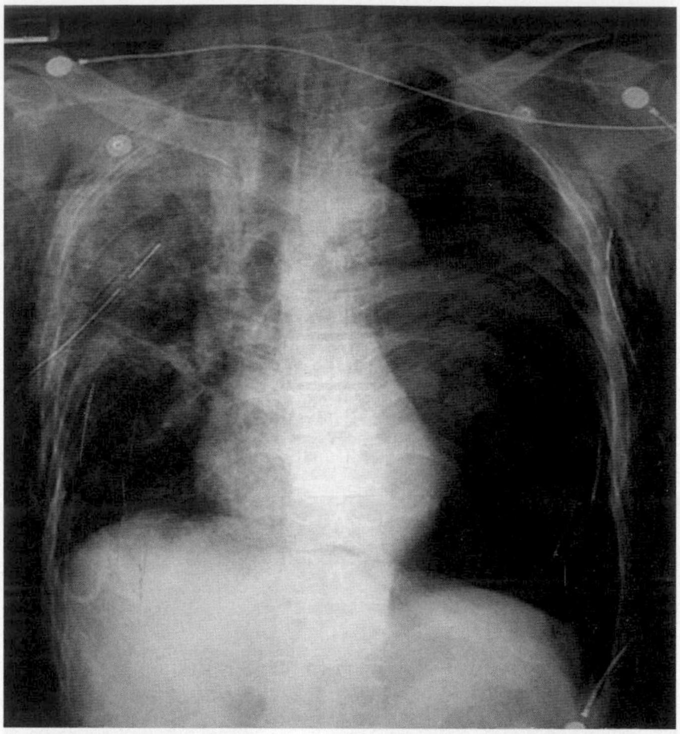

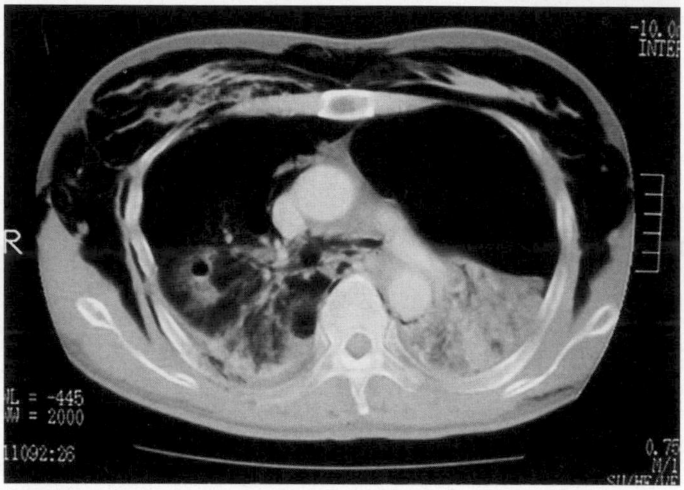

Figure 92-14. *A*. Chest x-ray after bilateral chest tube placements showed bilateral pneumothorax, subcutaneous emphysema, pneumomediastinum, multiple rib fractures, and tracheal shift to the right. (Adapted with permission from Kamiyoshihara M, Ishikawa S, Ihara N, et al. Complete transection of the left main bronchus due to a blunt chest trauma: report of a case. *Kyobu Geka*. 2001;54:603–605.) *B*. Chest CT scan revealed bilateral lung contusions in addition to the chest x-ray findings. (Adapted with permission from Kamiyoshihara M, Ishikawa S, Ihara N, et al: Complete transection of the left main bronchus due to a blunt chest trauma: Report of a case. Kyobu Geka 54:603, 2001.)

EDITOR'S COMMENT

Although bronchoplasty for benign disease is not commonly performed, the importance of maintaining bronchial patency with minimal loss of lung parenchyma is paramount. As such, these cases are particularly challenging and understanding the full range of therapeutic options, as presented in this chapter, is important for all thoracic surgeons.

—Yolonda L. Colson

References

1. Matsuoka H, Nishio W, Sakamoto T, et al. Use of span plasty with ringed PTFE for serious tracheobronchomalacia. *Jpn J Chest Surg*. 2002;16:692.
2. Johnson T, Mikita J, Wilson R, et al. Acquired tracheomalacia. *Radiology*. 1973;109:576–580.
3. Kawamura M, Watanabe M, Kobayashi K. Surgical treatment for tuberculous tracheobronchial stenosis. *Kekkaku*. 1999;74:891–896.
4. Nakajima Y, Shiraishi Y. Surgical treatment and endobronchial stent placement for tuberculous tracheobronchial strictures. *Kekkaku*. 1999;74: 897–905.
5. Yamamoto H, Kanzaki M, Obara T, et al. Treatment for tuberculous bronchial stricture [In Japanese]. *JJSRE*. 2001;23:375.
6. Hoshi E, Aoyama K, Murai K, et al. A case of sleeve resection of the left main bronchus for tuberculous bronchial lesion. *Kyobu Geka*. 1999;52:152–155.
7. Toyama K, Tsubota N, Yoshimura Y, et al. Sleeve lobectomy for tuberculous bronchial stenosis: a case report. *Kyobu Geka*. 1997;50:1140–1143.
8. Kobayashi M, Matsui K, Masuda N, et al. Treatment of tuberculous bronchial stenosis [In Japanese]. *JJSRE*. 2001;23:381.
9. Okabe K, Aoe M, Nakata M, et al. A case of bronchial mucous gland adenoma with cancer in adenoma [In Japanese]. *JJSRE*. 1991;13:82.
10. Schraufnagel D, Morin J, Wang N. Endobronchial lipoma. *Chest*. 1979;75: 97–99.
11. Kamiyoshihara M, Sakata K, Otani Y, et al. Endobronchial lipoma accompanied with primary lung cancer. *Surg Today*. 2002;32:402–405.
12. Gjevre J, Myers J, Prakash U. Pulmonary hamartomas. *Mayo Clin Proc*. 1996; 71:14–20.
13. Ishibashi H, Akamatsu H, Kikuchi M, et al. Resection of endobronchial hamartoma by bronchoplasty and transbronchial endoscopic surgery. *Ann Thorac Surg*. 2003;75:1300–1302.
14. Mizobuchi T, Iwai N, Nomoto Y, et al. A case of bronchial reconstruction for inflammatory bronchial polyp [In Japanese]. *JJSRE*. 2000;22:505.
15. Inoue S, Fujino S, Sawai S, et al. Experience with self-expanding metallic stents (SEMS, Ultraflex Stent) for postoperative bronchial stenosis [In Japanese]. *JJSRE*. 2001;23:454.
16. Mills S, Johnston F, Hudspeth A, et al. Clinical spectrum of blunt tracheobronchial disruption illustrated by seven cases. *J Thorac Cardiovasc Surg*. 1982;84:49–58.
17. Kamiyoshihara M, Ishikawa S, Ihara N, et al. Complete transection of the left main bronchus due to a blunt chest trauma: report of a case. *Kyobu Geka*. 2001;54:603–605.

93 Pulmonary Sequestration

Lambros Zellos

Keywords: Hemoptysis, pulmonary infection, intralobar, extralobar

Pulmonary sequestration is a congenital syndrome characterized by abnormal systemic blood supply to the lung, usually the lower lobe. The anomaly causes a predisposition for pulmonary complications such as infection and hemoptysis. There are two types of sequestrations, intralobar and extralobar. As the name implies, the intralobar sequestration is located within the normal lung (Fig. 93-1), whereas the extralobar sequestration is separate from the normal lung, enclosed in its own pleural envelope (Fig. 93-2). One should be aware of the various other associated anomalies, such as abnormal communication of the bronchial tree, systemic venous drainage, rare communication to the foregut, and diaphragmatic hernia (Table 93-1). In addition, the aberrant systemic vessel can arise from any systemic intrathoracic or upper abdominal vessel, such as the aorta, the subclavian artery, and even the coronary arteries. While they are found most commonly in the lower lobes, left more often than right, sequestrations also can occur in the right or left upper lobe.

CLINICAL PRESENTATION

Extralobar pulmonary sequestrations tend to present at an early age with respiratory distress because they are associated with other congenital anomalies, such as diaphragmatic hernias. They have systemic venous drainage and no bronchial communication. In contrast, intralobar sequestrations are commonly diagnosed in adulthood, present with frequent pulmonary infections or hemoptysis, have pulmonary venous drainage and a normal bronchial communication, and are rarely associated with other anomalies.[1–3] Fever, cough, multiple pulmonary infections, and hemoptysis can occur, although up to 13% can be asymptomatic.[4] The affected lobe tends to develop chronic changes owing to recurrent infections with eventual cystic destruction of the parenchyma. A chest x-ray that reveals consolidation along the medial aspect of the lower lobe should arouse suspicion of a sequestration. A chest computed tomography (CT) scan can confirm the diagnosis of the sequestration, and angiography is not necessary. The treatment of choice for sequestration is

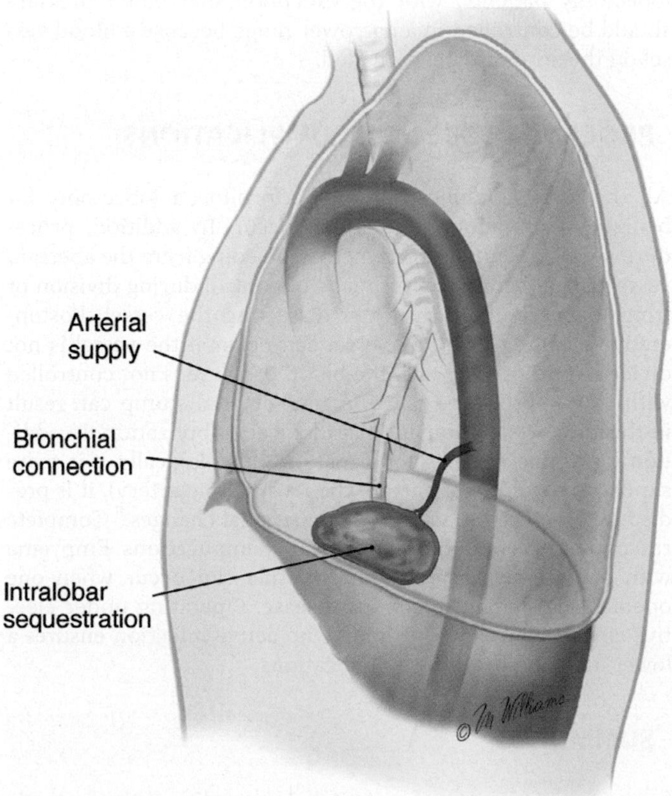

Figure 93-1. Intralobar pulmonary sequestration.

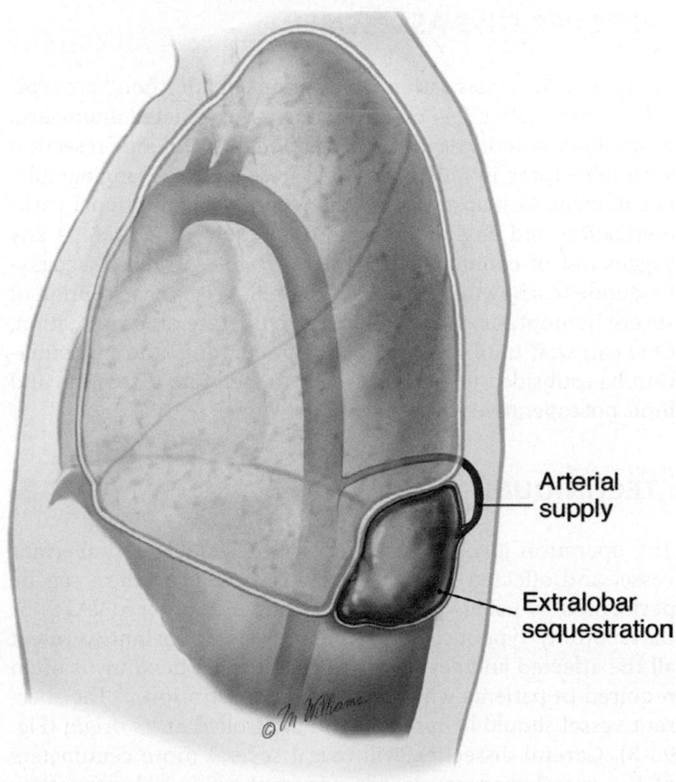

Figure 93-2. Extralobar pulmonary sequestration.

Table 93-1

DISTINGUISHING CHARACTERISTICS OF ELS VERSUS ILS

CHARACTERISTICS	ELS	ILS
Incidence	Rare	Uncommon
Sex predominance	4:1 M:F	1.5:1 M:F
Laterality	Left > right	Left > right
Pleural involvement	Yes	No
Arterial supply	Systemic; rare pulmonary	Systemic
Venous drainage	Systemic	Pulmonary
Communication		
Bronchial	No	Yes
Foregut	No	No
Associated anomalies	>50%	Rare
Diaphragmatic hernia	30%	Isolated
Clinical aspects		
Age at recognition	Neonate	Adolescent, young adult
Symptoms	Respiratory distress	Cough, fever
Radiograph	Triangular mass lesion	Lower lobe abscess
Pathology	Spongy, cystic	Abscess cavity

ELS, extralobar pulmonary sequestration; ILS, intralobar pulmonary sequestration. *Source:* Ferguson TB Jr., Ferguson TB. Congenital lesions of the lung and emphysema. In: Sabiston DC Jr., Spencer FC, eds. *Gibbon's Surgery of the Chest.* 5th ed. Ch. 24. New York, NY: Mosby; 1995:822–884.

resection. There are occasional reports of embolization with coils or Amplatz occlusion devices, but the durability and long-term sequelae of embolization remain unknown.[5,6]

IDEAL PATIENT CHARACTERISTICS AND PREOPERATIVE ASSESSMENT

Patients with sequestration who present in adulthood are typically young with a few comorbidities or associated anomalies. Pulmonary function is more than adequate to tolerate resection with lobectomy in most patients. CT scan or CT angiography is sufficient to map the aberrant vessel, and traditional catheterization and angiography are not required. If there is any suggestion of communication with the foregut, esophagogastroduodenoscopy may be needed as well. With the exception of severe hemoptysis, there is no need to operate on presentation. One can wait until the last bout of pneumonia and inflammation has subsided for several weeks to facilitate dissection and limit postoperative empyema.

TECHNIQUE

The operation involves resection of the sequestered aberrant vessel and affected lung parenchyma. The procedure can be performed by using video-assisted thoracic surgery (VATS) or thoracotomy-type incisions.[1,7,8] Since it is important to resect all the affected and destroyed lung tissue, a lobectomy is often required in patients with intralobar sequestration.[1,3] The aberrant vessel should be resected and controlled at its origin (Fig. 93-3). Careful dissection will reveal several more centimeters of the vessel than are readily apparent on initial inspection. Since the venous return also may be anomalous, attention should be paid during dissection to avoid inadvertent injury

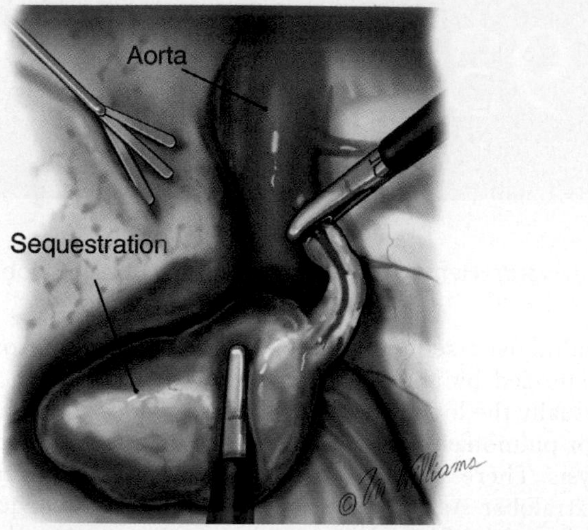

Figure 93-3. The aberrant vessel is dissected, controlled, and divided at its origin.

and uncontrolled bleeding. Communication to the foregut also can exist, and care should be taken to avoid leaving an open viscus unattended. Finally, the destroyed parenchyma has to be resected completely to avoid a nidus of infection and hemoptysis. Flap buttress of the bronchus may be considered to avoid bronchial dehiscence in patients with extensive inflammation.

POSTOPERATIVE CARE

Postoperative care in these patients is similar to that in other lobectomy patients, with the exception that blood pressure should be controlled in a narrower range because a blood vessel off the aorta has been divided.

PROCEDURE-SPECIFIC COMPLICATIONS

All the usual complications of performing a lobectomy for benign inflammatory lesions can occur. In addition, procedure-specific complications include bleeding from the aberrant vessels intraoperatively from lack of control during division or from inadvertent injury when dissecting the vessel. Postoperative bleeding from the vessel can occur if the vessel is not divided appropriately or if the blood pressure is not controlled within an appropriate range. A long arterial stump can result in thrombus formation and paradoxical embolization. In addition, since this vessel is abnormal (i.e., histologically, it is more similar to a pulmonary artery than a systemic artery), it is predisposed to atheromatous and aneurysmal changes.[9] Complete resection is warranted to avoid future complications. Empyema with or without bronchopleural fistula can occur when one operates for benign infectious disease. Operating under elective circumstances when there is no active infection ensures a lower incidence of these complications.

SUMMARY

Sequestration is a rare congenital abnormality of the systemic blood supply to part of the lung. In adults, the condition is heralded by recurrent infections and/or hemoptysis. Treatment

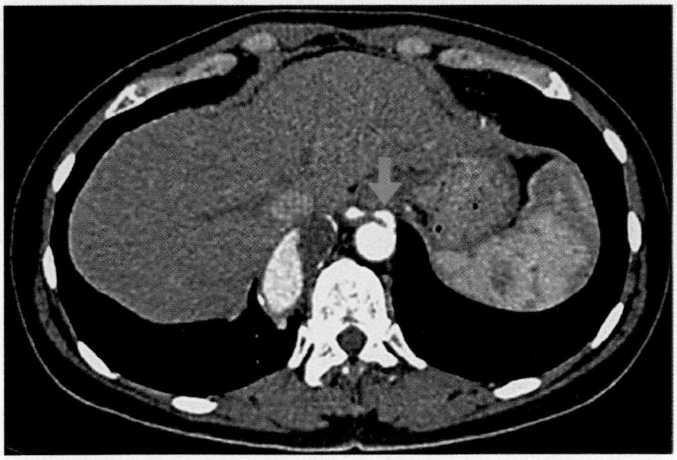

Figure 93-4. CT angiogram shows the origin of the aberrant vessel from the descending thoracic aorta (arrow) as well as the aneurysmal dilation of the aberrant vessel within the sequestration. (Modified image used with permission from Tatli S, Yucel EK, Couper GS, et al. Aneurysm of an aberrant systemic artery to the lung. *AJR Am J Roentgenol.* 2005;184: 1241–1244.)

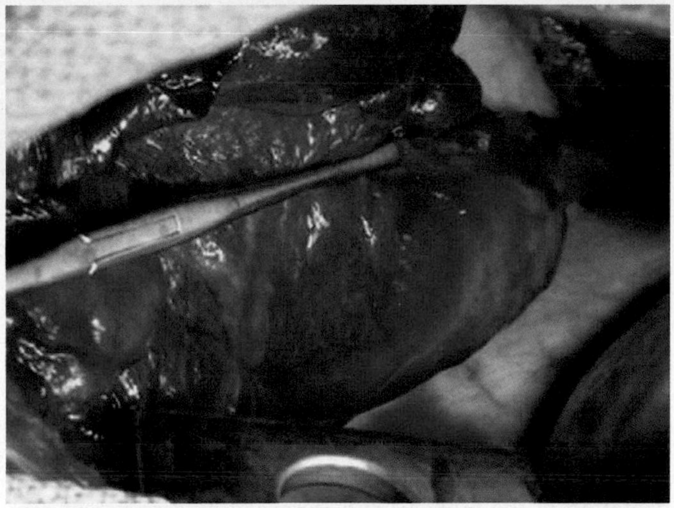

Figure 93-5. Intraoperative picture shows right lower lobe with sequestration and the aberrant artery arising from the aorta in the upper right corner. (Used with permission from Tatli S, Yucel EK, Couper GS, et al. Aneurysm of an aberrant systemic artery to the lung. *AJR Am J Roentgenol.* 2005;184:1241–1244.)

involves resection of the aberrant vessel and affected lung parenchyma, preferably under elective circumstances. Preoperative identification of the aberrant vessel and of any associated abnormalities assists in the planning of the operation and prevention of complications.

CASE HISTORY

A 47-year-old woman underwent a CT scan as workup for back pain and was found to have a sequestration to the right lower lobe. The aberrant vessel originated in the descending thoracic aorta and had become aneurysmal. The patient had a CT angiogram to better define the vessel (Fig. 93-4). At thoracotomy, she was found to have an intralobar sequestration with an aneurysm of the aberrant vessel (Fig. 93-5). A right lower lobectomy was done with division of the aberrant vessel at its origin from the aorta with an endovascular GIA stapler.

EDITOR'S COMMENT

This chapter provides a clear and concise discussion of the differential characteristics, presentation, and management of extralobar and intralobar sequestrations. The critical teaching points highlighted are to identify and control the aberrant systemic arterial blood supply, minimize infection at the time of operation, and if possible, spare lung parenchyma. Successful operation has been reported by both thoracotomy and VATS approaches depending on the degree of inflammation and parenchymal destruction encountered at the time of surgery.

—Yolonda L. Colson

References

1. Louie HW, Martin SM, Mulder DG. Pulmonary sequestration: 17-year experience at UCLA. *Am Surg.* 1993;59:801–805.
2. Bratu I, Flageole H, Chen MF, et al. The multiple facets of pulmonary sequestration. *J Pediatr Surg.* 2001;36:784–790.
3. Van Raemdonck D, De Boeck K, Devlieger H, et al. Pulmonary sequestration: a comparison between pediatric and adult patients. *Eur J Cardiothorac Surg.* 2001;19:388–395.
4. Wei Y, Li F. Pulmonary sequestration: a retrospective analysis of 2625 cases in China. *Eur J Cardiothorac Surg.* 2011;40(1):e39–e42.
5. Lee KH, Sung KB, Yoon HK, et al. Transcatheter arterial embolization of pulmonary sequestration in neonates: long-term follow-up results. *J Vasc Intervent Radiol.* 2003;14:363–367.
6. Marine LM, Valdes FE, Mertens RM, et al. Endovascular treatment of symptomatic pulmonary sequestration. *Ann Vasc Surg.* 2011;25(5):696.e11–e15.
7. Halkic N, Cuenoud P, Corthesy M, et al. Pulmonary sequestration: a review of 26 cases. *Eur J Cardiothorac Surg.* 1998;14:127–133.
8. Nakamura H, Makihara K, Taniguchi Y, et al. Thoracoscopic surgery for intralobar pulmonary sequestration. *Ann Thorac Cardiovasc Surg.* 1999;5: 405–407.
9. Tatli S, Yucel EK, Couper GS, et al. Aneurysm of an aberrant systemic artery to the lung. *AJR Am J Roentgenol.* 2005;184:1241–1244.

94 Surgery for Bronchiectasis

David C. Mauchley and John D. Mitchell

Keywords: Lobectomy, segmentectomy, pulmonary infections, congenital and acquired etiologies, video-assisted thoracic surgery (VATS)

INTRODUCTION

Since the first description by Laennec in 1819, bronchiectasis has continued to be recognized as a considerable cause of respiratory illness worldwide. It is defined by the permanent dilatation of the bronchi[1] and is caused by a recurrent process of transmural infection and inflammation. Patients suffer from chronic cough, excessive sputum production, a progressive decline in respiratory function despite prolonged antibiotic treatment, and occasionally life-threatening hemoptysis once the disease is entrenched. The majority of patients with this ailment can be treated medically, but those who fail or become intolerant of medical therapy are eligible for surgical intervention.

Early attempts at surgical treatment of bronchiectasis were fraught with complications. Postoperative bronchopleural fistula (BPF) and empyema were common, and perioperative mortality rates were high. The introduction of effective antibiotics in the 1950s paired with improvements in surgical technique led to a decline in perioperative morbidity and mortality. Currently, surgical intervention is mainly reserved for patients with focal disease and persistent symptoms despite optimal medical management. The diffuse form of the disease is best treated with bilateral lung transplantation and will not be discussed extensively in this chapter.

GENERAL PRINCIPLES AND PATIENT SELECTION

Bronchiectasis is subdivided into specific types based on the pathologic or radiographic appearance of the airways (Fig. 94-1). Cylindrical or tubular bronchiectasis is defined by dilated, slightly tapered airways and often is seen in patients with tuberculosis infections. Varicose bronchiectasis resembles the chronic venous state of the same name, with areas of dilatation and narrowing. Saccular or cystic bronchiectasis is characterized by progressive dilatation of the airways which end in sac-like cystic structures that resemble a cluster of grapes. This subtype is more common after obstruction or bacterial infection. Regardless of the subtype, thick mucoid secretions often are seen pooled in the dilated airways causing a chronic, transmural inflammatory state involving the wall of the airway. Lung parenchyma distal to the dilated, ectatic airways is often damaged as well, with fibrosis and emphysematous changes present. The accompanying bronchial circulation and lymph nodes may be engorged and hypertrophied. The left lower lobe is most commonly affected (Fig. 94-2), followed by the lingula and right middle lobe (Fig. 94-3). Occasionally, the process may progress to multilobe involvement with cavitation and parenchymal destruction, requiring pneumonectomy (Fig. 94-4).

The etiology of bronchiectasis can be divided into obstructive and nonobstructive types (Table 94-1). Obstruction of the airways due to foreign body inhalation is most common in children and shows a predilection for the right lower lobe and posterior segment of the right upper lobe. Both intrinsic narrowing and extrinsic compression of the airway by tumors can lead to bronchiectasis as well. The right middle lobe bronchus is at particular risk because of its relatively narrow lumen. Recurrent mucous plugging can lead to bronchiectasis and is most commonly associated with allergic bronchopulmonary aspergillosis (ABPA).

Infectious agents, both viral and bacterial, make up the most common etiology for the development of bronchiectasis. Children who suffer from measles, adenovirus, or pertussis are at risk of developing bronchiectasis later in life. Viral infections can lead to bronchiectatic airways both through direct infection and through a reduction in host defenses. Bacterial infections, particularly those involving potentially necrotizing agents such as *Staphylococcus aureus*, *Pseudomonas aeruginosa*, *Streptococcus pneumoniae*, and various anaerobes, remain important causes of bronchiectasis, particularly when there is a delay in treatment or other factors that prevent eradication of the infection.

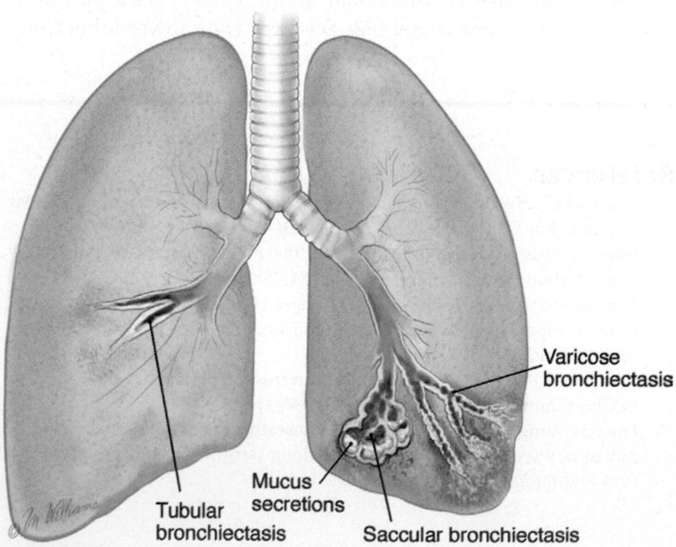

Figure 94-1. The three basic forms of bronchiectasis are depicted. Cylindrical or tubular bronchiectasis gives rise to tapered airways. Varicose bronchiectasis is characterized by areas of dilatation and narrowing. Saccular or cystic bronchiectasis causes progressively dilated airways that end in sac-like cystic structures that resemble clusters of grapes.

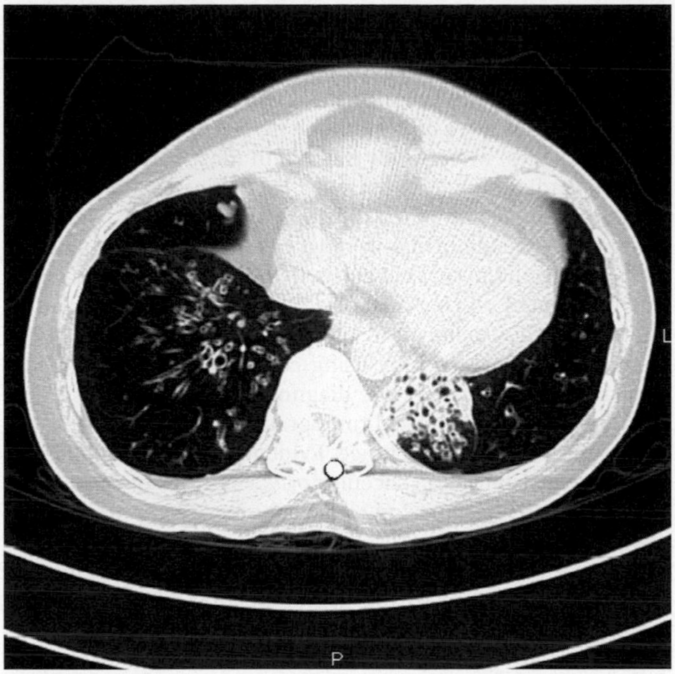

Figure 94-2. CT appearance of severe left lower lobe bronchiectasis, with destruction and contraction of the lobe. The right lower lobe is affected to a lesser degree.

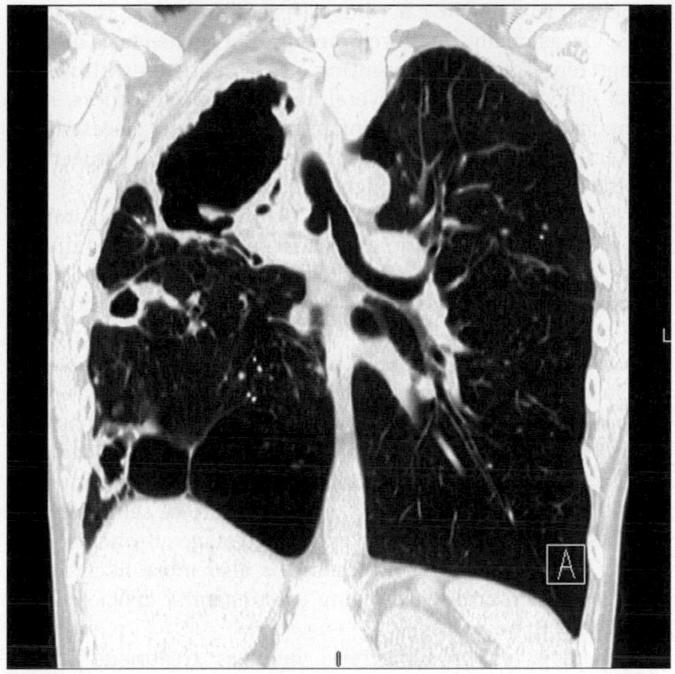

Figure 94-4. CT appearance of a largely destroyed right lung, with bronchiectasis and multilobar cavitation.

Bronchiectasis in patients with ABPA is caused by an immune reaction to the fungal organism, with production of inflammatory mediators and subsequent direct airway invasion by the fungus. Tuberculosis remains an important cause worldwide, but now is less common in North America. Nontuberculous mycobacterial (NTM) infections represent an important cause of bronchiectasis that is currently on the rise in the United States as well as throughout the world. Primary ciliary dyskinesia and various immune deficiencies such as hypogammaglobulinemia are examples of congenital disorders that lead to bronchiectasis through impairment in host defense mechanisms. Cystic fibrosis is an important cause of

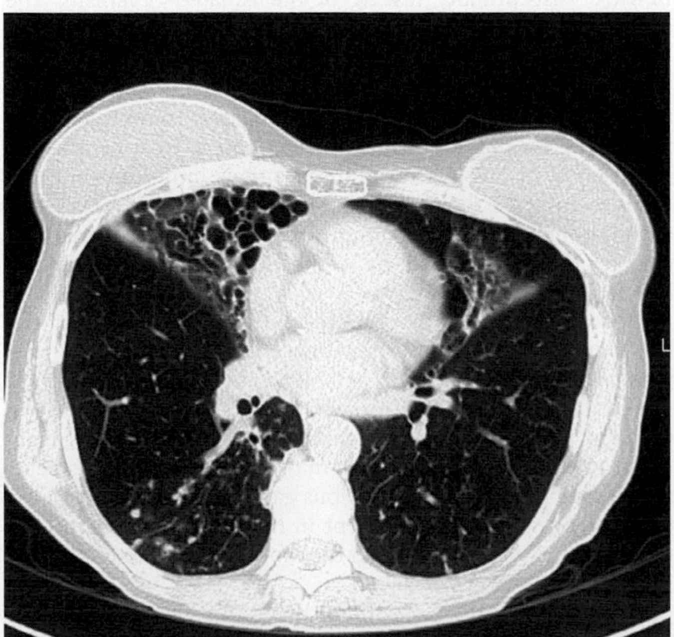

Figure 94-3. CT appearance of right middle lobe and lingular bronchiectasis.

Table 94-1 ETIOLOGY OF BRONCHIECTASIS
Obstructive
Foreign Body Aspiration
Tumors
Carcinoid Tumors
Endobronchial chondromas and lipomas
Extrinsic Compression
Mucous Plugs
ABPA
Nonobstructive
Post-infectious
Viral
Measles
Adenovirus
Pertussis
Bacterial
Staphylococcus aureus
Streptococcus pneumonia
Pseudomonas aeruginosa
Haemophilus influenzae
Nontuberculous mycobacterium
Mucociliary abnormalities
Cystic fibrosis
Primary ciliary dyskinesia
Immunologic abnormalities
Hypogammagloulinemia (IgA and IgG)
Neutrophil function abnormalities
Ataxia telangiectasia
Associated with systemic disease
Rheumatoid arthritis
α_1-antitrypsin deficiency
Inflammatory bowel disease

bronchiectasis, and it can show a predilection for the upper lobes. Occasionally, the development of bronchiectasis in middle age represents the presenting sign in patients with milder forms of cystic fibrosis. Several autoimmune disorders, such as rheumatoid arthritis and inflammatory bowel disease, have been linked to the presence of recurrent pulmonary infections and the development of bronchiectasis.

For the purposes of surgical planning, it is also important to distinguish the etiologies that lead to focal and diffuse forms of bronchiectasis. The focal variety is often associated with an isolated abnormality causing relative or complete bronchial obstruction. An aspirated foreign body, a slowly growing tumor, and broncholith are examples. Rarely, bronchial compression (as seen with middle lobe syndrome) or angulation of the bronchus (after surgical lobectomy) produces obstruction leading to recurrent infection and the development of localized disease. The process of infection, bronchial inflammation and dilatation, and parenchymal scarring tends to be self-renewing once established, leading to further damage. Bronchiectasis arising from post-infectious causes is also more likely to be localized, whereas disease owing to congenital deficiencies is more likely to be diffuse.

Therapy for bronchiectasis involves treatment of the underlying disorder (if possible), suppression of the bacterial load through appropriate use of antibiotics, encouragement of proper pulmonary hygiene (including the routine use of bronchodilators, mucolytic agents, and postural drainage), and surgery in selected patients. The role of surgery is threefold. First, patients with focal areas of disease that cause unremitting symptoms, associated with localized lung parenchymal destruction, are candidates for resection therapy, usually by means of segmentectomy or lobectomy. Second, the rare patient who presents with massive hemoptysis should be considered for surgical therapy even if less invasive temporizing maneuvers such as bronchial artery embolization are successful. Finally, some patients with end-stage bronchiectasis may be candidates for lung transplantation. As with other patients with end-stage suppurative lung disease, sequential double-lung transplantation is indicated to avoid contamination of the new lung grafts.

Several features or characteristics make a patient with focal bronchiectasis an ideal candidate for resectional therapy. First, the disease should be truly localized and amenable to anatomic lung resection. Nonanatomic or wedge resections should be avoided because they leave behind more proximal dilated bronchi with pooled secretions that, over time, serve to further contaminate adjacent lung parenchyma. Second, adequate pulmonary reserve for the planned resection should be present. This is usually not a major issue because the heavily diseased lung segments tend to contribute little to the patient's overall lung function. Finally, it is preferable to minimize the bacterial load present within the bronchi and lung tissue at the time of surgery with appropriate antimicrobial therapy, often initiated months in advance. This is particularly true in the setting of mycobacterial disease to minimize the risk of subsequent complications such as BPF.

PREOPERATIVE ASSESSMENT AND PREPARATION

Patients with bronchiectasis present with recurrent pulmonary infections characterized by dyspnea and an unremitting chronic cough productive of thick, tenacious, purulent sputum. Hemoptysis is common and on rare occasion can be massive when there is erosion into the enlarged bronchial vessels. Occasionally, patients with bronchiectasis will describe a nonproductive cough, indicative of upper lobe involvement. Auscultation reveals crackles, wheezes, or rhonchi in most patients.

The radiographic findings in bronchiectasis are understandably important in establishing the diagnosis. Standard radiographs are abnormal in most cases, demonstrating focal areas of consolidation, atelectasis, evidence of thickened bronchi (best noted as ring shadows when seen on end), and in advanced cases, delineation of the dilated cystic changes in the airway. Bronchography using contrast medium, once the standard for establishing the diagnosis of bronchiectasis, has been replaced by computed tomography (CT) scanning as the diagnostic procedure of choice. Evidence of airway dilatation, changes consistent with saccules or varicosities of the airway, and lack of airway tapering toward the periphery are all consistent with bronchiectasis. Evidence of cavitary disease also may be seen. The severity of bronchial wall thickening on CT scan has been linked to the degree of lung impairment and subsequent functional decline.[2,3] Upper lobe involvement suggests the diagnosis of cystic fibrosis or ABPA. Middle lobe and lingular disease is more typical of nontuberculous (environmental) mycobacterial infection such as Mycobacterial avium complex, and lower lobe predominance suggests bacterial involvement.

As mentioned earlier, initiation of targeted antimicrobial therapy before the planned surgical date is crucial to the success of the procedure. This is particularly true in the setting of mycobacterial disease, such as *Mycobacterium tuberculosis* and the various nontuberculous (previously termed "atypical", "MOTT", or "environmental") mycobacterial species now more common in the United States. For example, patients at our institution with focal bronchiectasis and *Mycobacterium avium* complex infection are typically started on a three- or four-drug regimen for 2 to 3 months before surgery based on in vitro susceptibility testing of the isolated organism. The regimen is continued through the hospital stay and for several months thereafter, often to a total of 24 months.[4] The preoperative antibiotic treatment, of course, will vary considerably depending on the offending organisms; routine bacterial pathogens do not require the preoperative treatment duration typical in mycobacterial disease. It is important in most cases to reimage the patient before surgery because effective antimicrobial therapy may improve areas of parenchymal and cavitary disease, particularly in those with normal (noncystic fibrosis) genotypes.[5]

Most patients with chronic suppurative disease of the lungs are malnourished, often to a considerable degree, as a result of the long-standing catabolic state these patients experience. If malnutrition is present, an aggressive preoperative regimen of nutritional supplementation is advised. In many cases, nutritional augmentation may require use of a nasojejunal feeding tube or a percutaneous gastrostomy. In our experience, preoperative improvement in nutritional status in these debilitated patients may lessen the morbidity of the subsequent procedure.[6]

At our institution, all patients being considered for surgical management of bronchiectasis or other infectious disease are discussed at a weekly multidisciplinary conference. The conference is attended by surgeons, pulmonologists, and infectious disease physicians with specialization in respiratory infectious disease. Similar to a multidisciplinary approach common in thoracic oncology, this helps ensure that patients receive the appropriate antimicrobial therapy and helps delineate the optimal timing of surgical intervention. Allowing time for antibiotic therapy to produce a bacterial nadir at the time of surgery minimizes the risk profile in the perioperative period.

SURGICAL TECHNIQUE

Anesthesia

A standard anesthetic technique typical for thoracic surgical procedures is used. Single-lung ventilation is achieved with placement of a double-lumen tube. A thoracic epidural catheter is employed when an open (thoracotomy) approach is planned. In patients in whom a thoracoscopic lobectomy or segmentectomy is performed, the epidural is usually omitted. An arterial line and urinary catheter are placed. Fluid administration is limited, as with other forms of major lung resection. Extubation at the end of the operation is planned.

Bronchoscopy

Preoperative bronchoscopic examination of the airway is essential. Bronchial obstruction owing to tumor or an aspirated foreign body should be ruled out. If severe inflammation of the airway mucosa is found, it may be best to defer definitive resection until better infection control is obtained. Finally, normal variations in bronchial anatomy make preoperative bronchoscopy by the surgeon advisable, particularly if a segmental resection is planned.

Surgical Approach

Our approach to surgical resection for bronchiectasis has been previously reported.[6–8] Traditionally, anatomic lung resection for bronchiectasis (e.g., segmentectomy, lobectomy, pneumonectomy) has been performed via open thoracotomy. The acceptance of a video-assisted thoracoscopic (VATS) approach has been delayed by the impression that dense pleural adhesions, perihilar lymphadenopathy, and a hypertrophic bronchial circulation would make VATS resection unnecessarily challenging and potentially unsafe. However, in the last decade there have been several reports of successful resection using such an approach. We recommend a standard VATS technique utilizing two 10-mm ports and a 3- to 4-cm utility incision based over a rib space in the anterior axillary line (Fig. 94-5). No rib spreading is used. Typically, the initial two ports are placed—one in the seventh intercostal space, anterior axillary line, and the other just posterior to the scapular tip—and the safety and feasibility of a VATS approach are confirmed. The utility incision then can be made, centered over an interspace (usually fourth or fifth) to allow easy access to the area of dissection. The serratus muscle fibers are separated along the axis of the utility incision. The exact placement of the ports and the utility incision depends in part on the planned resection. Muscle transposition (latissimus dorsi, intercostal) is feasible using a thoracoscopic approach.

For patients in whom extensive extrapleural dissection is needed, an open approach is used. A lateral thoracotomy affords excellent exposure to all planned resections, with the possible exception of completion pneumonectomy, where a posterolateral incision is preferred. If possible, the latissimus dorsi muscle should be spared for possible transposition later, if needed.

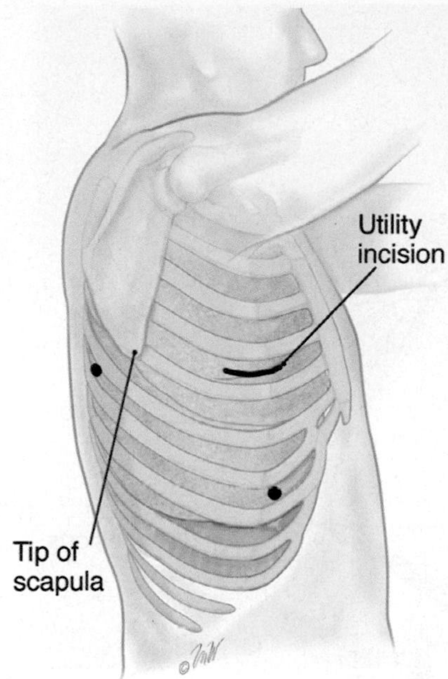

Figure 94-5. Target port placement for a standard VATS approach. Initially, two 10-mm ports are placed, one in the seventh intercostal space along the anterior axillary line and the second posterior to the scapular tip. A 5-cm utility incision is placed over the area of dissection, which is usually at the fourth or fifth interspace.

Extent of Resection

After access is achieved, the anatomic resection is completed in a standard fashion, with individual ligation of the vessels and bronchus to the target lobe or segment. The resection technique is the same whether the approach is VATS or open, although stapling devices are usually mandatory when a VATS approach is used. Situations in which there is concern regarding the bronchial closure, particularly pneumonectomy, may suggest the need for an open approach to facilitate a tailored suture closure of the bronchus and tissue transposition. The diseased segment or lobe often has considerable pleural adhesions that are lysed with cautery, taking care to avoid the usually adjacent phrenic nerve (Fig. 94-6). There is usually considerable bronchial artery hypertrophy and lymphadenopathy surrounding the involved pulmonary hilum, consistent with the chronic infectious state. It is important to achieve complete resection of the diseased bronchi and associated lung tissue, if possible. We prefer in these patients to divide the lung parenchyma (e.g., along the fissures), erring on the side of the uninvolved lobe and thus ensuring complete removal of diseased tissue. In VATS cases, the soft tissues at the utility incision should be retracted and protected from contamination, and the diseased tissue removed with the use of a deployable bag or similar device. As with resections for lung cancer, this latter technique is imperative; certain NTM organisms such as *Mycobacterium abscessus* can cause devastating chest wall infections if a careless method is adopted for removal of the specimen.

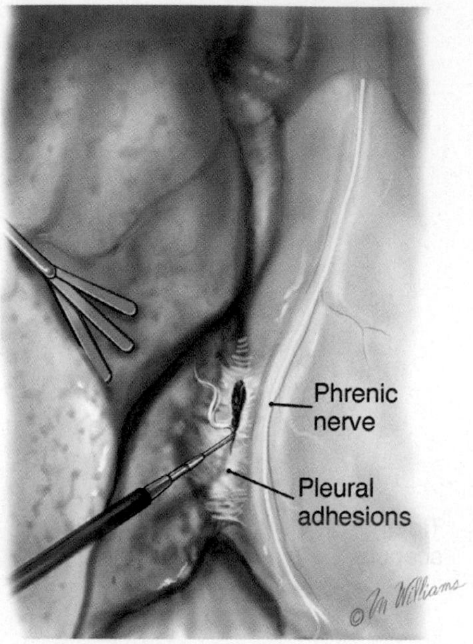

Figure 94-6. Dense pleural adhesions are lysed to facilitate bronchial closure during an open pneumonectomy, with care to avoid the phrenic nerve.

Once the specimen is removed from the field, it is divided on the back table for appropriate cultures to guide subsequent antimicrobial therapy. We typically "double culture" specimens at two different laboratories to minimize sampling or contamination error. The intrathoracic space typically is drained with one or two 28 F thoracostomy tubes.

Use of Tissue Flaps

Tissue transposition is indicated if there is risk of potential breakdown of the bronchial stump or when a significant intrathoracic "space" is present after resection. Postoperative BPFs are more common in the setting of certain poorly controlled infections, such as multidrug-resistant *M. tuberculosis*, or after certain resections, such as right pneumonectomy. We favor use of either a latissimus dorsi or intercostal muscle flap for bronchial stump coverage in routine circumstances and use of omentum after pneumonectomy, particularly after a right-sided resection.[9] Use of the serratus anterior muscle is often problematic because of winged scapula-related problems of wound healing and skin necrosis in these chronically malnourished patients.

Mobilization of the latissimus dorsi muscle is completed at the initiation of the procedure, and the muscle is transposed into the chest through the second or third intercostal space after resection. The omentum is mobilized before thoracotomy via laparoscopy or a limited midline abdominal incision, based on the right gastroepiploic artery and vein, and tacked to the undersurface of the appropriate hemidiaphragm for retrieval later after lung resection.

The presence of a significant intrathoracic "space" appears to be more common after major lung resection for infectious lung disease such as bronchiectasis compared with other indications for surgery. The use of transposed muscle such as latissimus dorsi minimizes the potential complications in this setting, including postresection empyema or prolonged air leak.

POSTOPERATIVE MANAGEMENT

With few exceptions, patient management after lung resection for bronchiectasis is routine. Appropriate antimicrobial coverage is continued in the postoperative period and often for several months afterwards, as described earlier, depending on the isolated organisms. Special emphasis is placed on pulmonary toilet, chest physiotherapy, early postoperative mobilization, and nutritional supplementation. Postoperative bronchoscopy may be needed to aid secretion clearance. Chest tube management is typical of other indications for lung resection. Most patients after VATS resection are ready for discharge by the second or third postoperative day, whereas patients undergoing more extensive resections by means of open thoracotomy may require hospitalization for 5 to 7 days.

COMPLICATIONS

The complications that accompany lung resection for bronchiectasis mirror those that follow similar resections for other indications with a few exceptions. Morbidity following resection ranges from 9% to 20% (Table 94-2). BPF and space problems are more common after resection for bronchiectasis and are discussed in further detail below.

Bronchopleural Fistula

In our practice, development of BPF after segmental or lobar resection is rare. It remains a considerable source of morbidity after pneumonectomy, particularly after right or completion pneumonectomy or in the setting of persistently smear-positive patients with organisms such as multidrug-resistant *M. tuberculosis*. In these patients, prevention is the key: Appropriate antimicrobial coverage before surgery, a tailored hand-sewn bronchial closure, and use of muscle or omental coverage of the bronchial stump may minimize this disastrous complication.

When a BPF occurs, it will present in a manner similar to that seen after lung resection for other indications. Fever, cough productive of serous followed by purulent sputum, contralateral lung infiltrates, and a dropping air–fluid level on chest radiograph are typical findings. Drainage of the infected space is a key initial step to limit damage to the remaining lung. BPFs noted very early after the initial resection may be treated with primary reclosure and rebuttressing of the stump; later BPFs usually require rib resection and creation of an Eloesser flap, followed by BPF closure (usually with omental transposition, if not used previously) and subsequent Clagett procedure, for successful treatment (see Chapter 82).

Space Problems and Empyema

As mentioned previously, space problems are somewhat more common after lung resection for infectious lung disease than after resection for lung carcinoma. This is due to the relative inability of the remaining lung to fully expand to minimize the residual space, perhaps because of chronic granulomatous changes in the other lobes. In most cases, the space is well tolerated and does not cause problems if the residual lung is fully expanded. However, in difficult resections in which significant pleural soilage or parenchymal injury is observed, the space may lead to a prolonged air leak or, worse, an empyema.

Table 94-2
OPEN RESECTION FOR BRONCHIECTASIS

REFERENCE	PROLONGED AIR-LEAK/SPACE ISSUES (%)	ATELECTASIS (%)	EMPYEMA/BPF (%)	BLEEDING (%)	ARRHYTHMIA (%)	OVERALL MORBIDITY (%)	OVERALL MORTALITY (%)
Zhang et al.[10]	2.7	2.0	1.0	1.1	4.0	16.2	1.1
Fujimoto et al.[11]	5.6	6.7	6.7	1.1	0	19.6	0
Prieto et al.[12]	5.9	0	0	3.4	3.4	15	0
Kutlay et al.[13]	1.7	2.3	1.2	1.7	0	10.5	1.7
Balkanli et al.[14]	2.5	2.9	1.7	1.7	0	8.8	0

Again, prevention is the key: significant space problems should be anticipated, with avoidance of complications through careful dissection technique and liberal use of autologous tissue flaps.

RESULTS

Several large series of open resectional therapy for bronchiectasis have been published in the last decade.[10–14] They report encouraging results, with operative mortality rates of 0% to 1.7% and morbidity rates of 9% to 20% (Table 94-2). The most common reported complications include atelectasis requiring therapeutic bronchoscopy, prolonged air leak, cardiac arrhythmias, space problems, empyema, and BPF. Completion pneumonectomy remains a formidable operation for bronchiectasis with reported mortality as high as 23%.[9] Failure of medical therapy (recurrent infections despite repeated courses of antibiotics) is the most commonly reported indication for surgical intervention, with only a small percentage of patients presenting with significant hemoptysis or lung abscess. A minority of patients have bilateral disease. All authors stressed the importance of localized disease, early surgical referral and intervention, and complete resection as the keys to successful surgical therapy.

Multiple studies have demonstrated improved safety and shorter hospital stays with a thoracoscopic (VATS) approach to lobectomy and segmentectomy in oncology patients.[15–19] Three series in the last decade[8,20,21] have specifically analyzed the outcomes of patients who undergo a VATS resection for bronchiectasis. Weber et al.[20] reported a five trocar method of performing thoracoscopic lobectomy in 76 patients with benign lung disease. The majority of these patients either had bronchiectasis or chronic lung infection alone. They reported a mortality rate of 0%, morbidity rate of 18.7%, and conversion to open procedure in 15.3%. Conversion was mainly due to dense pleural adhesive disease or upper lobe-predominant disease. Compared to a cohort of patients who underwent planned open lobectomy during the same time period, those who underwent a VATS resection suffered fewer post-operative complications, had less blood loss, and had a shorter hospital stay. Zhang et al.[21] reported 52 patients who underwent VATS lobectomy using two ports and a utility incision. Their results were similar with no mortality, a morbidity of 15.4%, and a conversion rate of 13.5%. Pain was assessed in these patients with an 11 point scale and was significantly lower than that was accessed in a cohort of patients undergoing open lobectomy in the same timeframe. Finally, we have recently reported the experience in VATS resection for bronchiectasis.[8] It included 212 resections in 171 patients, with a mortality rate of 0%, a complication rate of 9%, a conversion rate of 4.7%, and a mean hospital stay of 3.7 days. The results of the above reports clearly indicate that pulmonary resection for bronchiectasis can feasibly be carried out with a VATS approach with negligible mortality, lower morbidity, shorter hospital stay, and less pain when compared to open thoracotomy.

SUMMARY

Surgical treatment of bronchiectasis is usually successful and can be accomplished with minimal morbidity or mortality. Keys to successful surgical intervention are (1) presence of localized disease, (2) relatively early intervention to minimize development of resistant organisms and involvement of dependent lung segments, (3) successful identification of the predominant organisms involved, with targeted antimicrobial therapy based on in vitro sensitivities initiated prior to surgery and continued postoperatively, (4) assessment of preoperative nutritional status and nutritional supplementation where indicated, (5) complete resection of the involved segments of lung containing bronchiectatic airway, and (6) anticipation of potential complications and alteration of the operative plan to minimize subsequent morbidity.

CASE HISTORY

A 62-year-old woman with a long history of pulmonary infections, bronchiectasis, and mycobacterial superinfection was referred for further evaluation and treatment. Previous sputum cultures had yielded *M. avium* complex. At the time of her initial *M. avium* complex diagnosis, she had been treated with a three-drug regimen (i.e., clarithromycin, ethambutol, and rifampin) for 18 months. At the time of presentation, she complained of chronic fatigue and dyspnea on exertion and a variably productive cough. Born in New York, she resided for the past decade in Florida. She was a nonsmoker, had no pets, and did not have either a hot tub or a pool. Her family history was notable for a sister also with bronchiectasis and *M. avium* complex infection, who died of respiratory complications the year before.

A positive sputum smear was obtained at presentation, and cultures grew *pan sensitive M. avium* complex. Thin-cut CT scan of the chest demonstrated parenchymal destruction and coarse bronchiectasis of the right middle lobe, with minor involvement of the dependent right lower lobe superior segment (Fig. 94-7A to C). Her pulmonary function tests revealed an FEV_1 of 77% and an FVC of 86% of predicted. Although the patient was thin, initial studies did not suggest malnutrition.

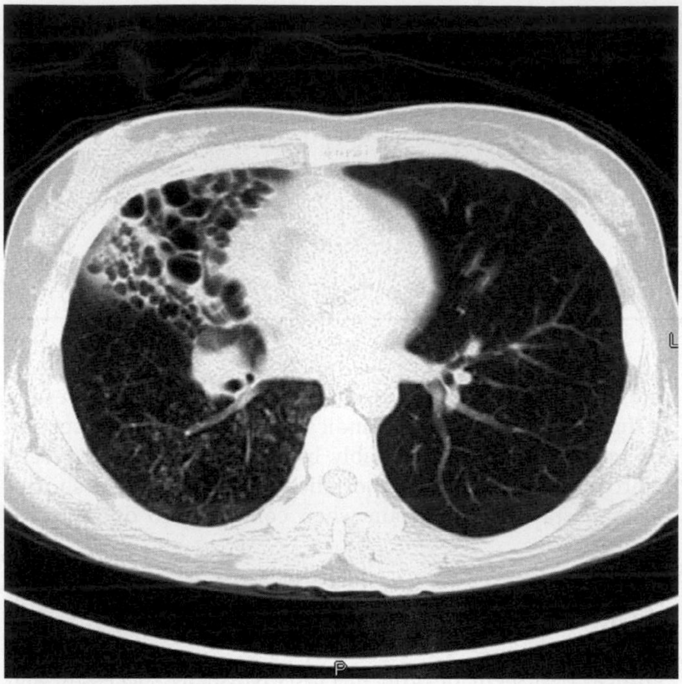

A

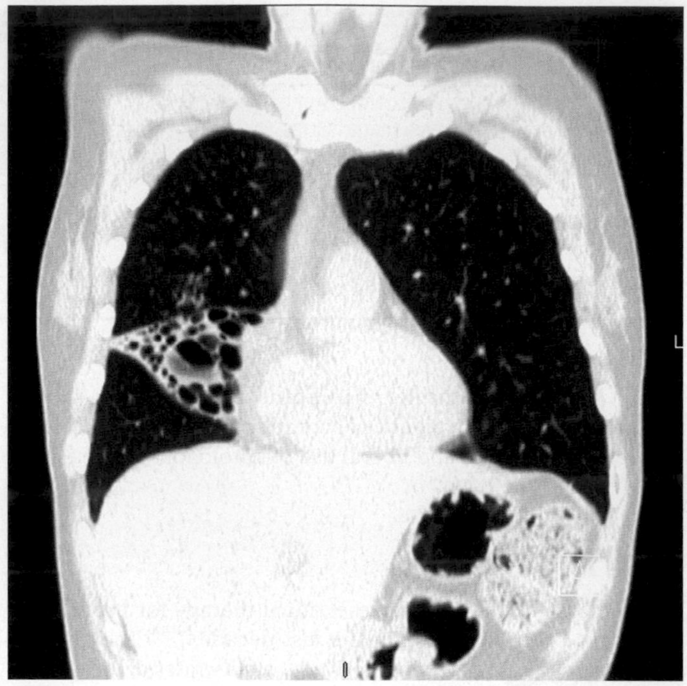

B

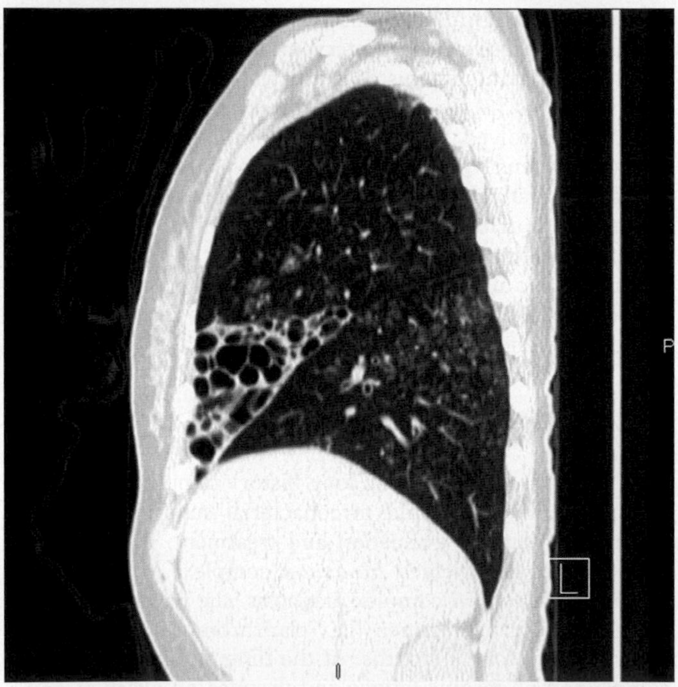

C

Figure 94-7. Axial (*A*), coronal (*B*), and sagittal (*C*) views of a patient with severe right middle lobe bronchiectasis, with minor involvement of the right lower lobe.

The patient was placed on a three-drug outpatient regimen based on in vitro drug sensitivities, in addition to intravenous amikacin 8 weeks before surgery. She underwent an uncomplicated VATS right middle lobectomy, with discharge on the third postoperative day. Her antibiotics were continued through the hospitalization. The surgical specimen demonstrated severe bronchiectasis and chronic granulomatous inflammation consistent with her history of NTM disease. The intravenous antibiotic (amikacin) was stopped following the surgery, and her oral antimicrobial coverage was adjusted based on intraoperative cultures obtained at surgery. Antibiotic coverage was continued for an additional 12 months once she was noted to be sputum culture negative. She remains alive and well and is essentially asymptomatic with respect to her pulmonary disease.

EDITOR'S COMMENT

This is an excellent review on the etiology, management, and indications for surgical intervention in bronchiectasis. The authors have clearly outlined the role of limited anatomic surgical resection in unremitting localized disease or massive hemoptysis and potential double-lung transplantation for end-stage disease. The detailed description of the surgical approach and common pitfalls highlights that this chapter is written by surgeons for surgeons.

—Yolonda L. Colson

References

1. Reid LM. Reduction in bronchial subdivision in bronchiectasis. *Thorax.* 1950;5:233–247.
2. Sheehan RE, Wells AU, Copley SJ, et al. A comparison of serial computed tomography and functional change in bronchiectasis. *Eur Respir J.* 2002; 20:581–587.
3. Ooi GC, Khong PL, Chan-Yeung M, et al. High-resolution CT quantification of bronchiectasis: clinical and functional correlation. *Radiology.* 2002; 225:663–672.
4. Iseman MD. Medical management of pulmonary disease caused by *Mycobacterium avium* complex. *Clin Chest Med.* 2002;23:633–641.
5. Kim JS, Tanaka N, Newell JD, et al. Nontuberculous mycobacterial infection: CT scan findings, genotype, and treatment responsiveness. *Chest.* 2005; 128:3863–3869.
6. Mitchell JD, Bishop A, Cafaro A, et al. Anatomic lung resection for nontuberculous mycobacterial disease. *Ann Thorac Surg.* 2008;85(6):1887–1893.
7. Yu JA, Pomerantz M, Bishop A, et al. Lady Windermere revisited: treatment with thoracoscopic lobectomy/segmentectomy for right middle lobe and lingular bronchiectasis associated with non-tuberculous mycobacterial disease. *Eur J Cardiothorac Surg.* 2011;40(3):671–675.
8. Mitchell JD, Yu JA, Bishop A, et al. Thoracoscopic lobectomy and segmentectomy for infectious lung disease. *Ann Thorac Surg.* 2012;93(4): 1033–1039.
9. Sherwood JT, Mitchell JD, Pomerantz M. Completion pneumonectomy for chronic mycobacterial disease. *J Thorac Cardiovasc Surg.* 2005;129:1258–1265.
10. Zhang P, Jiang G, Ding J, et al. Surgical treatment of bronchiectasis: a retrospective analysis of 790 patients. *Ann Thor Surg.* 2010;90(1):246–250.
11. Fujimoto T, Hillejan L, Stamatis G. Current strategy for surgical management of bronchiectasis. *Ann Thorac Surg.* 2001;72:1711–1715.
12. Prieto D, Bernardo J, Matos MJ, et al. Surgery for bronchiectasis. *Eur J Cardiothorac Surg.* 2001;20:19–23, discussion 23–24.
13. Kutlay H, Cangir AK, Enon S, et al. Surgical treatment in bronchiectasis: analysis of 166 patients. *Eur J Cardiothorac Surg.* 2002;21:634–637.
14. Balkanli K, Genc O, Dakak M, et al. Surgical management of bronchiectasis: analysis and short-term results in 238 patients. *Eur J Cardiothorac Surg.* 2003;24:699–702.
15. Leshnower BG, Miller DL, Fernandez FG, et al. Video-assisted thoracoscopic surgery segmentectomy: a safe and effective procedure. *Ann Thorac Surg.* 2010;89(5):1571–1576.
16. Onaitis M, Petersen R, Balderson S, et al. Thoracoscopic lobectomy is a safe and versatile procedure. Experience with 500 cases. *Ann Surg.* 2006;244: 420–425.
17. Paul S, Altorki NK, Sheng S, et al. Thoracoscopic lobectomy is associated with lower morbidity than open lobectomy: a propensity-matched analysis from the STS database. *J Thorac Cardiovasc Surg.* 2010;139(2): 366–378.
18. Villamizar NR, Darrabie MD, Burfeind WR, et al. Thoracoscopic lobectomy is associated with lower morbidity compared with thoracotomy. *J Thorac Cardiovasc Surg.* 2009;138(2):419–425.
19. Atkins BZ, Harpole DH, Jr, Mangum JH, et al. Pulmonary segmentectomy by thoracotomy or thoracoscopy: reduced hospital length of stay with a minimally-invasive approach. *Ann Thorac Surg.* 2007;84(4):1107–1113.
20. Weber A, Stammberger U, Inci I, et al. Thoracoscopic lobectomy for benign disease–a single centre study on 64 cases. *Eur J Cardiothorac Surg.* 2001; 20(3):443–448.
21. Zhang P, Zhang F, Jiang S, et al. Video-assisted thoracic surgery for bronchiectasis. *Ann Thorac Surg.* 2011;91(1):239–243.

95 Pulmonary Arteriovenous Malformation

Lambros Zellos

Keywords: Congenital and acquired etiologies, hereditary hemorrhagic telangiectasia, Rendu–Osler–Weber syndrome, pulmonary angiography, embolization, thoracotomy, video-assisted thoracic surgery, fistulectomy, segmental resection, lobectomy, pneumonectomy

The term pulmonary arteriovenous malformation (AVM) refers to lesions that have abnormal communications between the pulmonary arteries and pulmonary veins. Numerous other names have been used in the past to describe these lesions, such as pulmonary telangiectasias, aneurysms, fistulas, hemangiomas, and cavernous angiomas. These lesions can be congenital, usually as part of the hereditary hemorrhagic telangiectasia, also known as Rendu–Osler–Weber syndrome, or acquired from bronchiectasis, infections, hepatic cirrhosis, mitral stenosis, malignancies, or trauma. AVMs have been described based on number (single vs. multiple), location (unilateral vs. bilateral; parenchymal vs. pleural), and size or type of drainage (simple vs. complex).[1,2]

CLINICAL PRESENTATION

Clinical suspicion for the presence of pulmonary AVM should arise when there is the presence of nonspiculated pulmonary nodule suggestive of AVM; a family history of hereditary hemorrhagic telangiectasia; sequelae of right-to-left shunting such as hypoxemia, dyspnea, clubbing, cyanosis, and polycythemia; and systemic embolism such as cerebral stroke or cerebral abscess. Epistaxis can be reported in up to 85% of patients with hereditary hemorrhagic telangiectasia.[1] A continuous bruit can be auscultated over the lesion. The triad of cyanosis, clubbing, and polycythemia is seen in 20% of patients. Approximately 90% of AVMs are unilateral, and 50% to 67% of patients have a single AVM.[1,2] Rarely, patients may present with massive hemothorax under tension from acute hemorrhage secondary to rupture of the AVM.

IDEAL PATIENT CHARACTERISTICS AND PREOPERATIVE ASSESSMENT

Workup should include a chest computed tomography (CT) scan, which is the most sensitive test, evaluation of the shunt fraction, and pulmonary angiography to assess the feasibility of embolization. Approximately 25% of AVMs tend to enlarge up to a rate of 2 mm per year, and patients who are not treated have a stroke rate of 13% and a brain abscess rate of 11%. Complications are more common in patients who have AVMs greater than 2 cm or afferent vessels greater than 3 mm.[1,2] At minimum, treatment should be offered to these patients, if not to all patients with angiographically accessible lesions.[1]

Embolization of pulmonary AVMs was first described in 1977.[1,2] Pulmonary angiography is performed, and numerous techniques have been described, including coils, balloons, sclerosing agents, and Amplatzer occluding devices.[3] Multiple AVMs may be embolized at a single session or a few weeks apart. Embolization is feasible in most patients with angiographically accessible lesions, although treating patients with multiple feeding vessels can be challenging. Complications after balloon occlusion include balloon migration with distal embolization, balloon deflation, and pulmonary infarction. Long-term follow-up after embolization procedures is sparse. Recurrence after embolization has been reported.

Surgery is reserved for patients who cannot be embolized or who have failed embolization. Surgical techniques used include thoracotomy and video-assisted thoracic surgery, and the extent of resection can range from fistulectomy and segmental resection to lobectomy and even pneumonectomy.[4] While pneumonectomy has been used in the past, most lesions today can be treated with lung-sparing techniques. Preoperative pulmonary function testing is done as indicated based on the anticipated degree of pulmonary resection.

SURGICAL TECHNIQUE

When anatomic resections such as segmentectomy or lobectomy are deemed necessary to resect the AVM, as can be the case for deep fistulas (Fig. 95-1), they are carried out in the standard

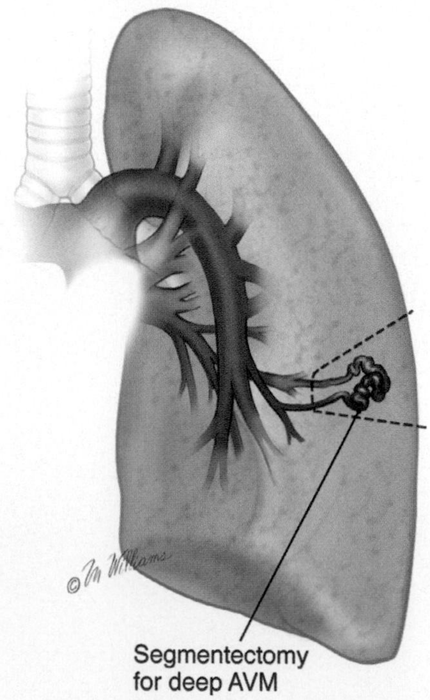

Figure 95-1. When the fistulas are deep, anatomic resection via lobectomy or segmentectomy is required.

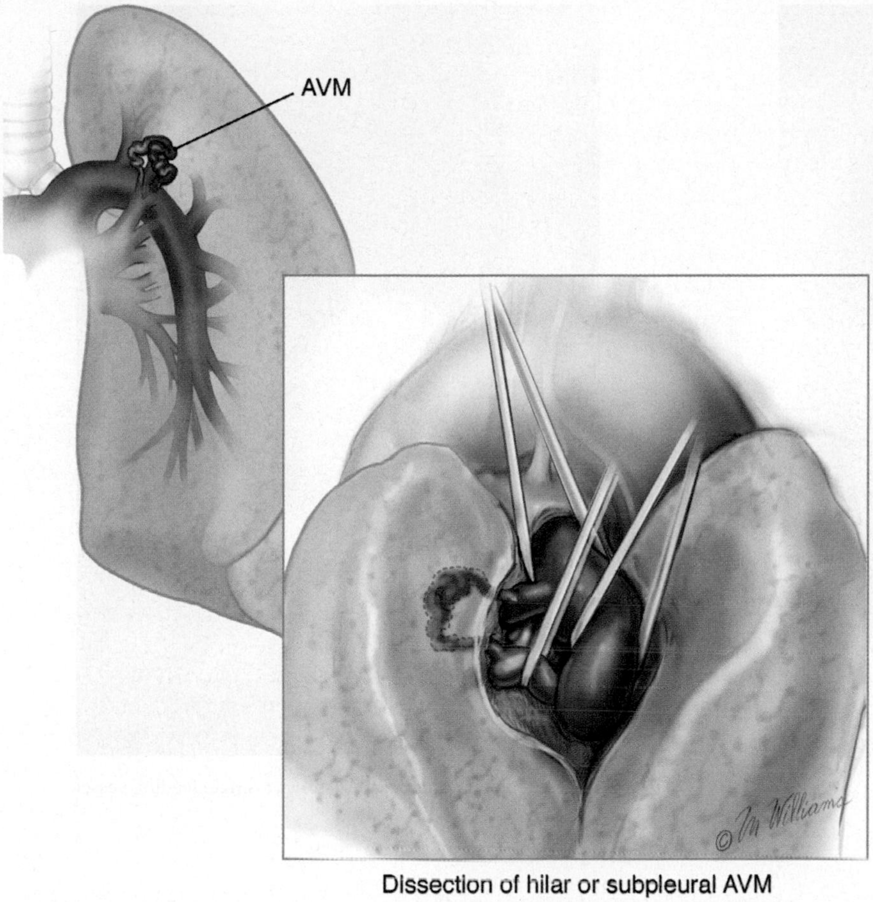

Figure 95-2. Hilar or subpleural AVM requires fistulectomy and careful dissection, ligation, and division of the feeding vessels.

manner. However, when fistulectomy is performed for hilar or subpleural fistulas, then attention must be paid to ensure meticulous dissection, ligation, and division of all feeding vessels and prevention of complications such as thrombosis, air embolism, and bleeding (Fig. 95-2).

A standard thoracotomy is used for exposure. The pulmonary artery and vein proximal and distal to the fistula are dissected and controlled with tourniquets.[4] After systemic heparinization, the tourniquets are cinched. The fistula is then dissected, and all tributaries are identified, ligated, and divided. The main trunk of the fistula can be clipped and divided or resected with the artery, followed by vein repair by means of standard vascular techniques.[5] The pulmonary artery tourniquet and then the pulmonary vein tourniquet are loosened with gentle lung reinflation, as is done with lung transplantation, to flush clot or air before tying the sutures to avoid embolism. If there is concern about proximity of the arterial and venous suture lines, tissue can be positioned between them. However, this is not practical if multiple fistulas are resected. Instead, standard anatomic resection of lung parenchyma, that is, lobectomy or segmentectomy, is carried out either with open technique or thoracoscopically. Arterial blood gas analysis should reveal resolution of the A-a gradient if all fistulas have been resected.

POSTOPERATIVE CARE

The duration of postoperative hospitalization is determined by the size of the incision and the extent of the pulmonary resection. Chest tubes are removed as usual. Routine anticoagulation with systemic heparinization is not advocated. Recurrence after surgical resection is rare.

PROCEDURE-SPECIFIC COMPLICATIONS

Pulmonary or systemic embolism from air or clot and thrombosis at the arterioplasty or venoplasty are the procedure-specific complications. Thrombosis, however, can be insidious and extensive, resulting in pulmonary infarction. Persistent hypoxemia should prompt investigation, especially if all the AVMs were addressed during the surgery. Prevention with systemic heparinization intraoperatively is the best policy. Cerebral embolism is the most serious complication and should be apparent in the immediate postoperative period.

SUMMARY

Pulmonary AVMs remain rare lesions that should be treated to avoid the sequelae of systemic embolization, cerebral abscess, and hypoxemia. Interventional radiology procedures can be used to address most of these lesions, and when surgical intervention is needed, lung-sparing procedures should be used with attention to embolic and thrombotic complications.

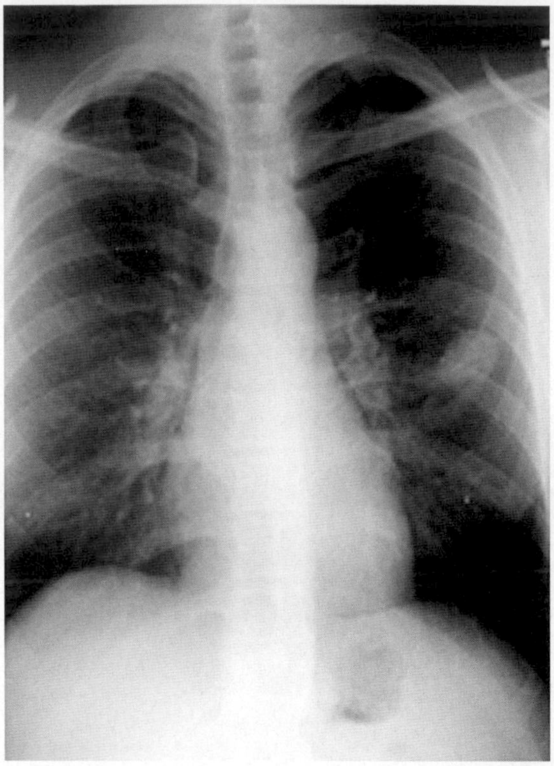

Figure 95-3. Chest x-ray shows a left lower lobe nodule.

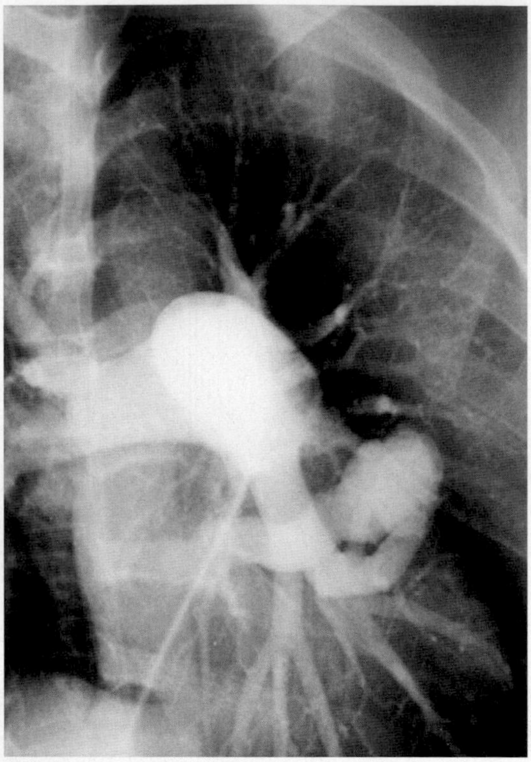

Figure 95-5. Pulmonary angiography shows a single feeding vessel.

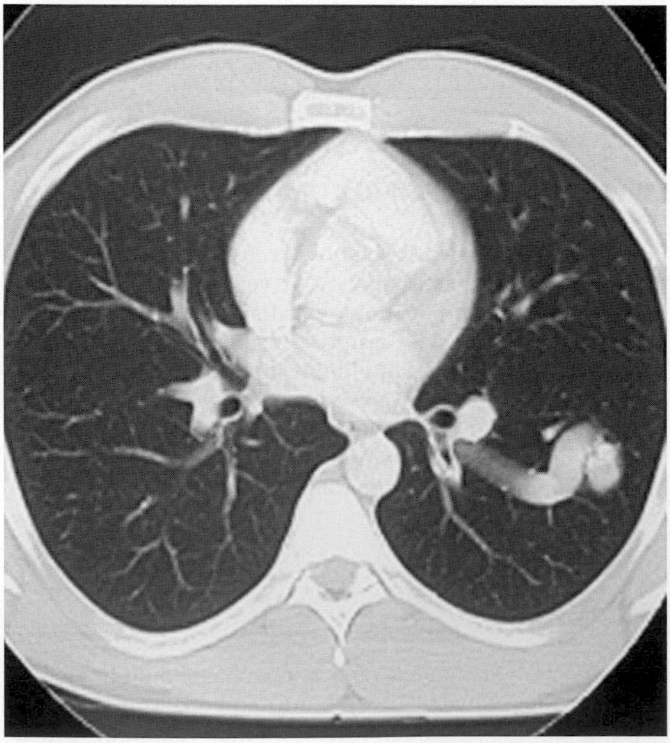

Figure 95-4. Chest CT scan demonstrates a solitary AVM in the left lower lobe.

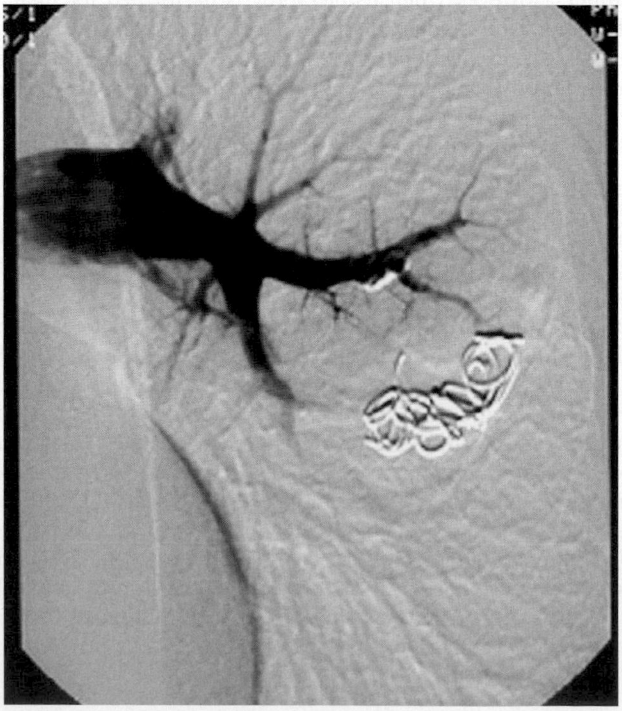

Figure 95-6. The AVM was embolized successfully.

CASE HISTORY

A 31-year-old man presented with hemoptysis, hypoxia, and a nodule on chest x-ray (Fig. 95-3). A chest CT scan was done that revealed a pulmonary AVM (Fig. 95-4). Angiography and embolization were performed without complications (Figs. 95-5 and 95-6).

EDITOR'S COMMENT

Although many AVMs can be successfully treated via embolization, for those lesions that are not angiographically accessible or have failed embolization, understanding the surgical management of these lesions is critically important so as to avoid potentially serious complications such as thrombosis with resultant pulmonary infarct or embolic stroke.

—Yolonda L. Colson

References

1. Gossage JR, Kanj G. Pulmonary arteriovenous malformations: a state of the art review. *Am J Respir Crit Care Med.* 1998;158(2):643–661.
2. Shields TW. Congenital vascular lesions of the lung. In: Shields TW, LoCicero J III, Ponn RB, eds. *General Thoracic Surgery*. 5th ed. Philadelphia, PA: Lippincott Williams & Wilkins; 2000;975–985.
3. Hart JL, Aldin Z, Braude P, et al. Embolization of pulmonary arteriovenous malformations using the Amplatzer vascular plug: successful treatment of 69 consecutive patients. *Eur Radiol.* 2010;20(11):2663—2670. Epub 2010 Jun 24.
4. Puskas JD, Allen MS, Moncure AC, et al. Pulmonary arteriovenous malformations: therapeutic options. *Ann Thorac Surg.* 1993;56(2):253–257; discussion 257–258.
5. Schroder C, Frohlich G, Harms CP, et al. Fistulectomy as an alternative to segmentectomy for pulmonary arteriovenous fistula. *J Thorac Cardiovasc Surg.* 2001;122(2):386–388.

96 Pediatric Primary and Secondary Lung Tumors

Christopher B. Weldon and Robert C. Shamberger

Keywords: Pediatric, lung, tumor, benign, malignant

INTRODUCTION

Pediatric pulmonary tumors are extremely uncommon entities without a unifying presenting symptomatology, clear diagnostic strategy, or definitive therapeutic regimens. Patients may present with all manner of symptoms or complaints, and these concerns are almost always nonspecific. Secondary to their rarity and the heterogeneous nature of the presenting findings, tumors are seldom thought of as the causative factor for a child presenting to a primary care provider with respiratory complaints, especially in light of the prevalence of other, far more common diseases in young patients such as reactive airway disease, upper and lower respiratory infections, or even inhaled/ingested aerodigestive foreign bodies. The published data document that the proportion of benign lesions to metastatic lesions to primary malignancies is on the order of 60:5:1.[1,2] As such, the most critical factor in diagnosing these lesions is a high index of suspicion, especially if symptoms do not abate with the intended treatment strategies directed at the suspected underlying causative agent (i.e., asthma that is refractory to standard therapies or the respiratory infection that fails to resolve in a timely fashion with appropriate antimicrobial drugs). There is often a significant delay then, from the initial presentation to a healthcare provider and definitive histopathologic diagnosis. Staging, treatment strategies, and outcomes will be tumor-specific, but surgery generally plays a critical role if cure is to be achieved in all lesions.

GENERAL CONSIDERATIONS

Presentation/Evaluation

Presenting symptoms in pediatric patients can range from the incidentally found tumor or lesion in the asymptomatic child to the child who presents *in extremis* with severe hemorrhage or cardiorespiratory collapse from parenchymal or mediastinal compression or invasion. The size, location, number, degree of vascularity, specific tracheobronchial anatomic location, associated organ (heart, great vessels) or structure (trachea) involvement (directly or indirectly), and malignant potential all are factors known to influence the precise constellation of presenting symptoms. Patients presenting with benign tumors are most commonly asymptomatic (24%).[3,4] However, when patients with benign tumors do present with symptoms, fever, cough, and pneumonitis have been documented to have the highest reported frequency (~10%) in this cohort. Those pediatric patients who are found to have metastatic lung cancers are also most commonly asymptomatic, as these lesions are generally small, numerous, and peripherally located on staging studies. Seldom does the child with pulmonary metastases present with pulmonary symptoms as the initial physical complaint. Primary malignant tumors in children generally do present with symptoms, however, and two large series found only 6% of children were asymptomatic upon presentation.[3,4] In fact, these reports document that one-third of patients present with a refractory cough, and a not so insignificant number (10%–25% per symptom) also present with evidence of fever, pneumonitis, respiratory distress, or hemoptysis.

As previously stated, however, these symptoms are nonspecific, and definitive diagnosis is almost always delayed. A high index of suspicion with close, diligent follow-up is mandated in all patients who do not respond to appropriate interventions directed at the suspected disease process that could be masking the presence of a mass. An algorithm has been published[5] documenting at least one approach that may be used in the treatment of pediatric patients suspected of harboring a pulmonary tumor (Fig. 96-1). Ideally, the patient is evaluated at presentation and a baseline history and physical examination is conducted with acquisition of chest radiographs (two views) and disease-appropriate laboratory evaluations. A close interval follow-up examination (2–4 weeks) is generally recommended to ensure the symptoms have resolved or responded to treatment. For persistent, recurrent, or ongoing symptoms refractory to treatment interventions, a return visit with further studies, including a chest computed tomogram (CT) should be entertained if there is any question on the interpretation of the data collected during the prior visit. Although the risks of secondary malignancies from radiation exposure in children are not trivial,[6] missing a tumor is of even more concern since extirpation is always a component of cure and if the lesion is discovered when small, parenchymal preservation approaches with negative margins and reduced rates of lymph node metastases would be expected. Although other imaging modalities, including magnetic resonance imaging and positron emission tomography, have been described in pediatric pulmonary tumors, their widespread application and utility remain unproved. An early referral to a pediatric pulmonologist also may be warranted to provide for another opinion on the child with refractory pulmonary symptoms and to investigate the utility of bronchoscopic evaluation. Again, close-interval follow-up is warranted to ensure symptom resolution. If a lesion is found on chest CT or bronchoscopy and is amenable to resection without undue perioperative morbidity or mortality, then resection is warranted after appropriate staging studies are performed. Preoperative pulmonary function testing also may be desired in cases where pneumonectomy and/or combined chest wall resection may be indicated so as to have a baseline to predict postoperative recovery and function. A biopsy procedure (bronchoscopically, image-guided, or surgical) can be entertained and discussed, especially in the case of large, central, or invasive tumors that are not amenable to upfront resection without

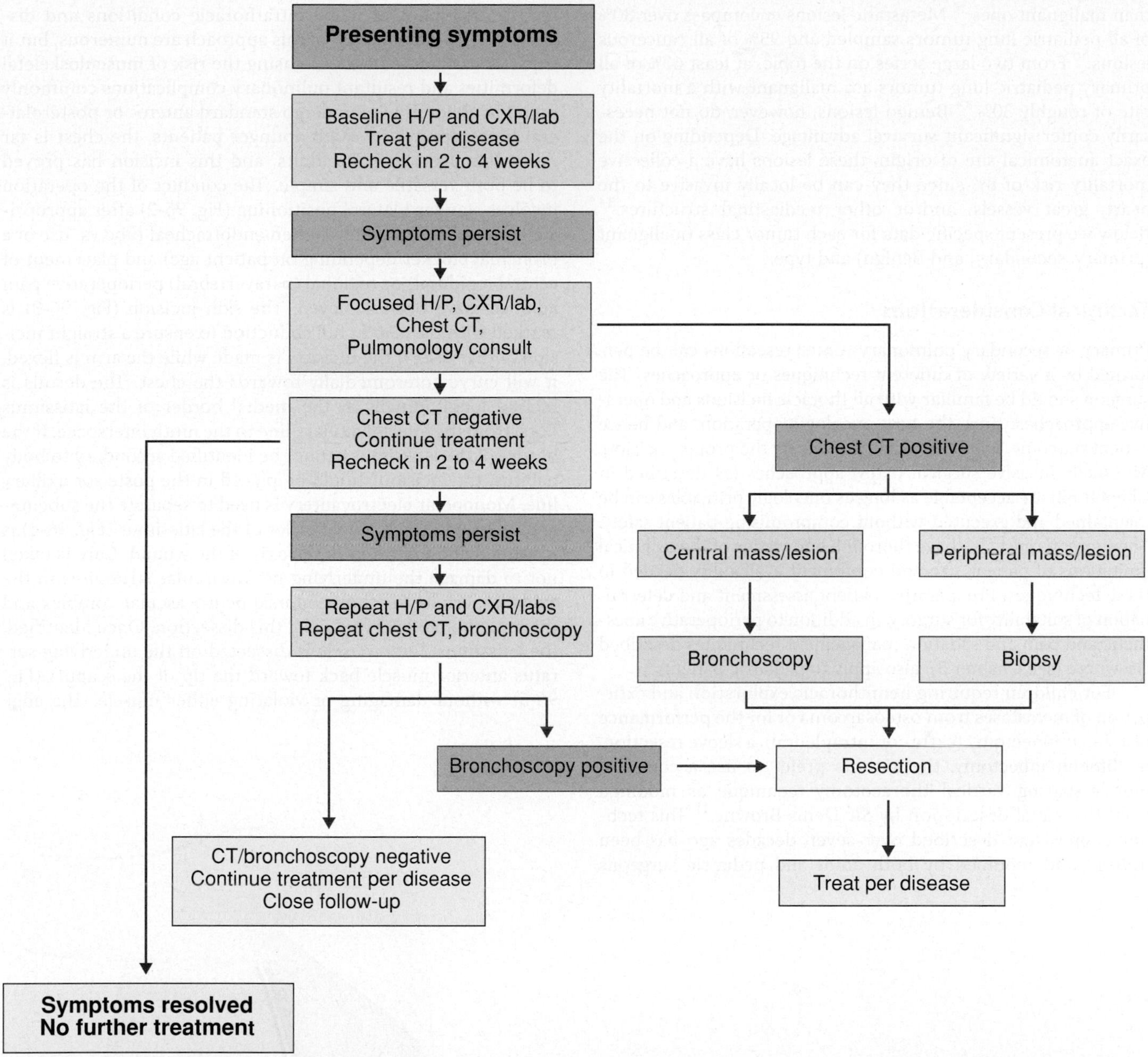

Figure 96-1. This algorithm demonstrates the proposed evaluation of a patient with respiratory symptoms. A baseline work-up should be undertaken as a first step, including a history and physical exam (H/P), chest radiograph (CXR), and laboratory evaluations (LABS). The most likely underlying disease process should be treated with the appropriate medical therapy, and then there should be close follow-up within 2-4 weeks. If symptoms persist, then a repeat work-up should be performed with the addition of a chest computed tomogram (CT) and pulmonology consult. If this work-up, including the chest CT and pulmonology consults are nondiagnostic, then further medical therapy should be administered with close follow-up. If the patient becomes asymptomatic, then no further therapy is warranted. But if the symptoms persists, then a repeat work-up should be ordered, including a bronchoscopy and another chest CT. If this work-up is again negative, then medical management should be continued with close follow-up. If the chest CT and/or bronchoscopy demonstrate a lesion, then the work-up should proceed as if these studies were positive from the first encounter. If the lesion is peripheral on a CT scan and amenable to a biopsy, then this should be considered prior to resection and disease-specific treatment. If the lesion is centrally located, then a bronchoscopy should be performed, prior to resection and further disease-specific treatment.

significant perioperative risk. One must be careful in this setting, however, since soiling the pleural space with tumor may be detrimental in specific subtypes, and there is a significant risk of peribronchoscopic hemorrhage with mortal outcomes in the setting of endobronchial lesions.[7–9] While commonplace in the adult literature, definitive therapeutic bronchoscopically directed strategies are not recommended treatment modalities in children with endobronchial pulmonary tumors because there can be significant technical limitations in small patients and the ability to achieve a wide local resection with negative margins using these techniques is often not possible.

Biology/Epidemiology

Benign and malignant pediatric pulmonary tumors are rare entities overall, but benign lesions are tenfold more common than malignant ones.[10] Metastatic lesions encompass over 80% of all pediatric lung tumors sampled and 95% of all cancerous lesions.[10] From two large series on the topic, at least 60% of all primary pediatric lung tumors are malignant with a mortality rate of roughly 30%.[3,4] Benign lesions, however, do not necessarily confer significant survival advantage. Depending on the exact anatomical site of origin, these lesions have a collective mortality risk of 8% since they can be locally invasive to the heart, great vessels, and/or other mediastinal structures.[3,4] Below we present specific data for each tumor class (malignant [primary, secondary] and benign) and type.

Technical Considerations

Primary or secondary pulmonary tumor resections can be performed by a variety of different techniques or approaches. The surgeon should be familiar with all thoracic incisions and operative approaches, since the best oncologic operation, and hence patient outcome, will be facilitated by using the proper incision. Minimally invasive surgical (MIS) approaches (as described in Chapter 52) are acceptable as long as oncologic principles can be maintained and executed without compromising patient safety. The surgeon must also have thorough knowledge of the technical limitations of patient size and equipment availability needed in these techniques. Preoperative patient assessment and determination of suitability for surgery, in addition to perioperative anesthetic and pain and sedation management techniques described elsewhere (see Chapter 5), also apply to pediatric patients.

For children requiring hemithoracic exploration and extirpation of metastases from osteosarcoma or for the performance of a pneumonectomy (extra- or intrapleural), a sleeve resection, or difficult lobectomy, the authors prefer to use a complete muscle-sparing vertical thoracotomy technique as modified from the initial description by Sir Denis Browne.[11] This technique since first described over seven decades ago has been utilized and modified by both adult and pediatric surgeons for the treatment of many intrathoracic conditions and diseases.[12–16] The advantages of this approach are numerous, but it is particularly noted for decreasing the risk of musculoskeletal deformities and resultant pulmonary complications commonly found in children who undergo standard antero- or posterolateral thoracotomy.[17–20] With younger patients, the chest is far more compliant than in adults, and this incision has proved to be both versatile and simple. The conduct of the operation involves standard lateral positioning (Fig. 96-2) after appropriate lung isolation (double-lumen endotracheal tube vs. use of a bronchial blocker depending on patient age) and placement of central (epidural) or regional (paravertebral) perioperative pain adjuncts have been achieved. The skin incision (Fig. 96-3) is marked with the arm in full abduction to ensure a straight incision. Otherwise, if the incision is made while the arm is flexed, it will curve anteromedially towards the chest. The dermis is incised longitudinally at the medial border of the latissimus dorsi from the inferior axillary line to the ninth interspace. If the border of the latissimus cannot be identified secondary to body habitus, the incision should be placed in the posterior axillary line. Monopolar electrocautery is used to separate the subcutaneous tissues. The medial border of the latissimus (Fig. 96-4) is identified and dissected in the axis of the wound. Care is taken not to damage the underlying neurovascular structures in the axilla, especially the thoracodorsal neurovascular complex and the long thoracic nerve during this dissection. Once identified, the latissimus dorsi muscle is dissected off the underlying serratus anterior muscle back toward the tip of the scapula (Fig. 96-5) without damaging or violating either muscle. The edge

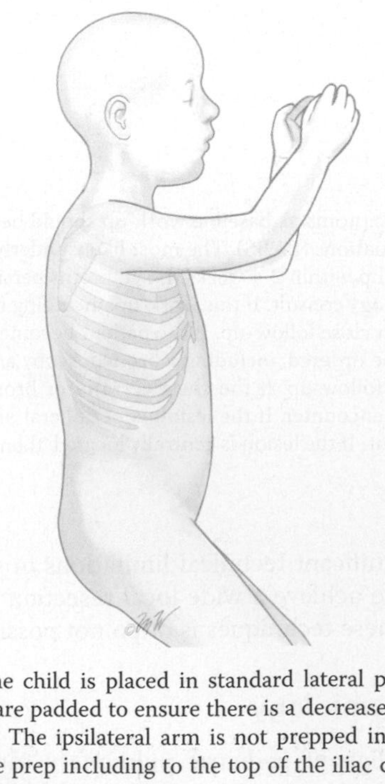

Figure 96-2. The child is placed in standard lateral positioning, and all pressure points are padded to ensure there is a decreased risk of decubitus ulcer formation. The ipsilateral arm is not prepped into the field, but it should be a wide prep including to the top of the iliac crest, and from the spine to the sternum.

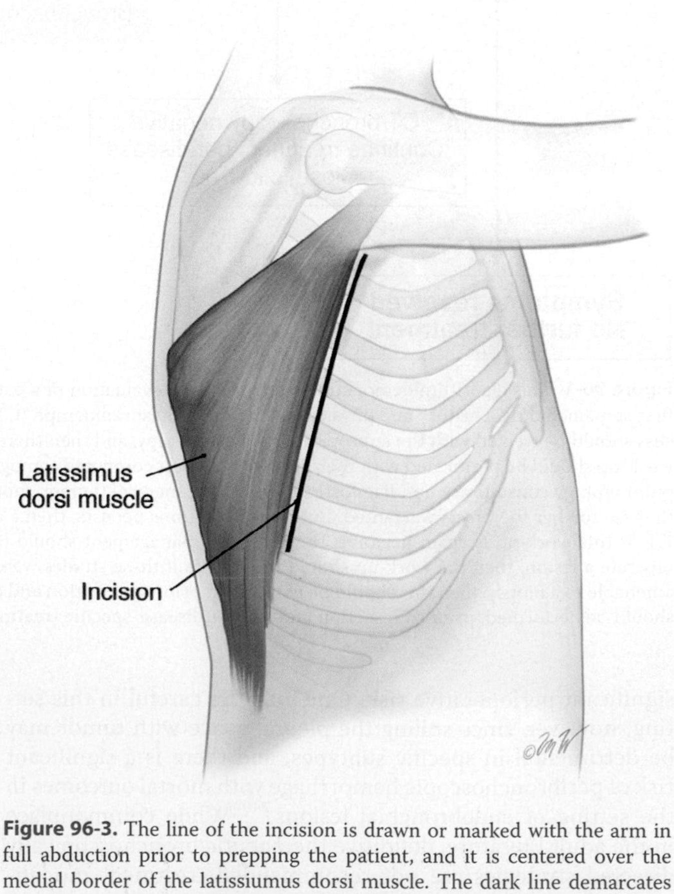

Figure 96-3. The line of the incision is drawn or marked with the arm in full abduction prior to prepping the patient, and it is centered over the medial border of the latissiumus dorsi muscle. The dark line demarcates the skin incision in relation to the border of the latissimus in the figure

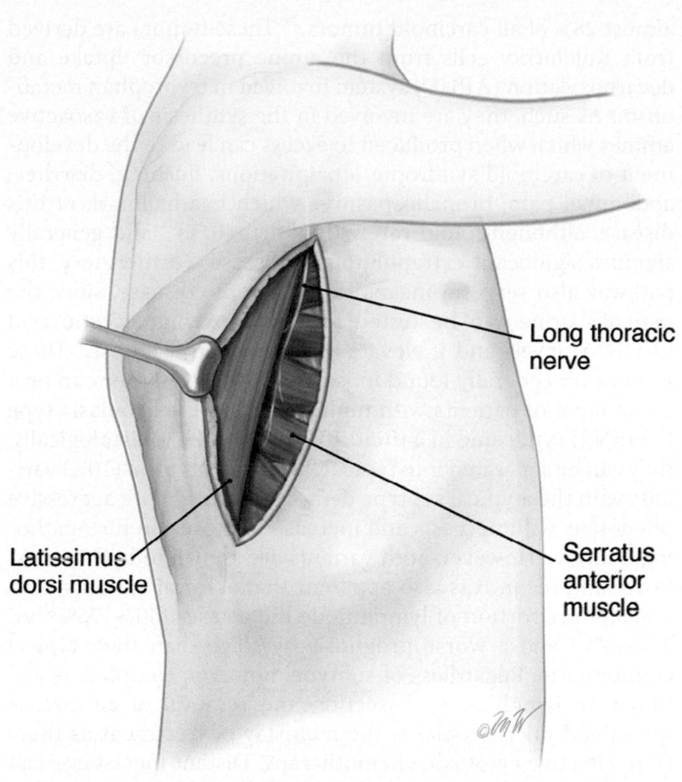

Figure 96-4. Once the skin and subcutaneous tissues are dissected, the medial border of the latissimus is identified, and the fascia is incised and dissected a long the entire length of the medial border of the muscle being careful not to damage the long thoracic or the thoracodorsal nerves.

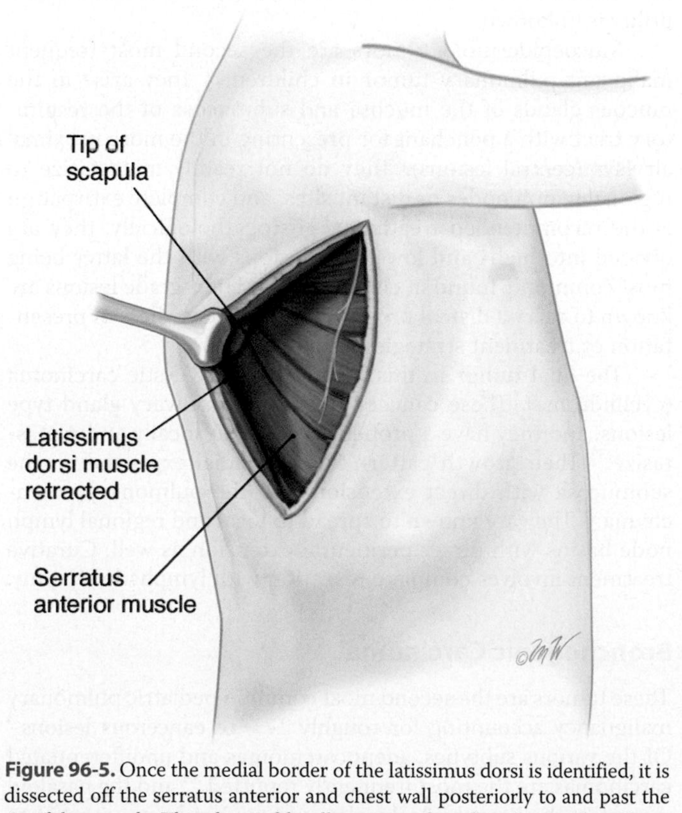

Figure 96-5. Once the medial border of the latissimus dorsi is identified, it is dissected off the serratus anterior and chest wall posteriorly to and past the tip of the scapula. This plane is bloodless except for a few chest wall perforating vessels. Once cleared, the tip of the scapula marks the border of the serratus anterior muscle which can then be used to dissect it off the chest wall.

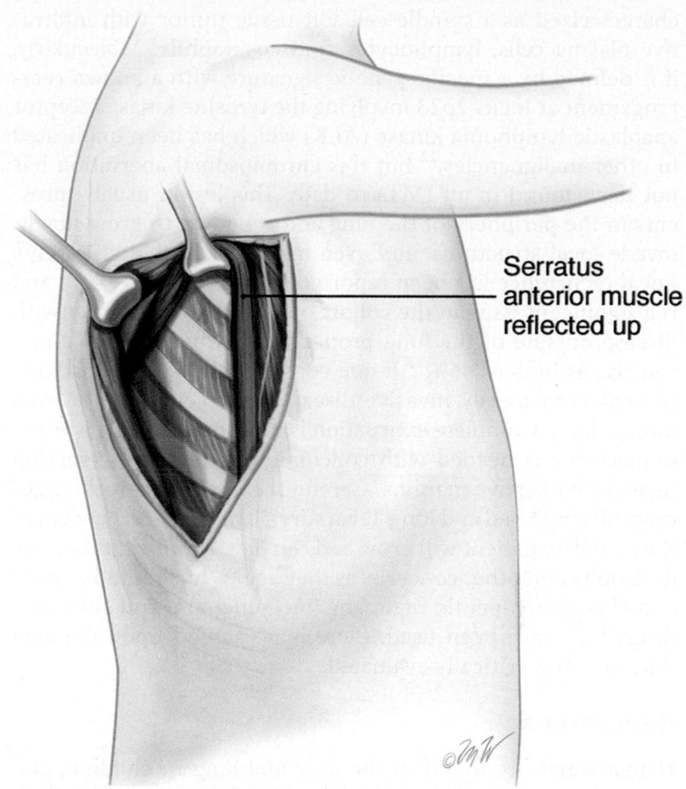

Figure 96-6. This figure demonstrated the chest wall directly under the dissected serratus anterior muscle. Once encountered, blunt dissection defining the rib space necessary for entry into the thorax commences.

of the serratus anterior muscle is then located at its insertion on the tip of the scapula and the fascial plane connecting it to the chest wall is incised sharply (Fig. 96-6). Once this plane is entered, the serratus is dissected off the chest wall medially, rostrally, and caudally until it is completely separated. Caution must be exercised to avoid damage to the muscle or the neurovascular structures in the area, and once free, a blunt dissection can take place to identify the appropriate intercostal space to enter for the proposed operation as is standard for all thoracotomies. Once the chest is entered, the required pulmonary or thoracic operation can be performed as described elsewhere in this text. The wound is closed by reapproximating the intercostal space and all muscle, subcutaneous and dermal layers, with absorbable sutures.

BENIGN TUMORS

Inflammatory Myofibroblastic Tumor

The most common benign pediatric pulmonary tumor is an inflammatory myofibroblastic tumor (IMT). Some caution must be utilized in describing this lesion against the known literature; however, as the terminology describing this tumor has only recently been codified and previous reports over several decades may have misinterpreted or even misrepresented this tumor. Nevertheless, we do know that it was found in over 50% of all benign tumors resected in the two largest series to date,[3,4] and it was recently classified by the World Health Organization (WHO) as an intermediary lesion.[21] Microscopically, it is characterized as a spindle cell soft tissue tumor with infiltrative plasma cells, lymphocytes, and eosinophils. Molecularly, it is defined by a specific genetic signature with a known rearrangement at locus 2p23 involving the tyrosine kinase receptor anaplastic lymphoma kinase (ALK) which has been implicated in other malignancies,[22] but this chromosomal aberration has not been found in all IMTs to date. This lesion usually presents in the periphery of the lung and is known to grow slowly, invade local structures, and even metastasize (though rarely). Local recurrence has been reported to be as high as 14%[23] and is a significant issue in the cohort of patients who present with disease outside of the lung proper where the recurrence rate can rise as high as 46%.[23] If one considers that 27% of patients present with locally invasive disease, this fact becomes even more telling. Complete extirpation is warranted, even if a pneumonectomy is needed with concomitant chest wall resection to achieve negative margins. Careful reconstructive techniques must be employed and long-term surveillance will be needed, as the pediatric patient will grow and can have significant thoracic dystrophy and other concerns as they age. While radiotherapy[24] and chemotherapeutic regimens (including anti-inflammatory drugs)[25–27] have been used, there is no agreed upon regimen that has been critically evaluated.

Hamartoma

Hamartomas are found in the liver and lung in children, and they are the second most common benign pediatric pulmonary tumor. These tumors are formed by normal parenchymal components arranged in a haphazard and disorganized fashion. Both cartilaginous and gland-like clusters of cells are irregularly arranged and grow unchecked without the benefit of capsule or pseudocapsule. Macroscopically, they are found to be well demarcated from the normal, surrounding lung with glandular tissue separated by septae of fibrous tissue. These lesions represent roughly 20% of all benign pediatric pulmonary tumors,[3,4] and in the minority of cases (no more than 25%) they present with the pathognomonic stippled popcorn calcification on chest radiograph.[28] They tend to start in the periphery, but they can grow to become quite large and pose operative challenges during resection with deaths reported at surgery secondary to their size and location.[4] Complete resection is warranted in all cases, and parenchymal preserving approaches should be considered if possible. Finally, this disease may also serve as a harbinger of the presence of Carney triad[29] (gastrointestinal stromal tumor, paraganglioma and/or pheochromocytoma, pulmonary hamartoma) in the afflicted patient. Hence, when found, referral to a geneticist and pediatric oncologist may be warranted to investigate the presence of this disease and treatment of other tumors if discovered.

MALIGNANT TUMORS

Bronchial Adenomas

Bronchial adenomas encompass three distinct tumor types: carcinoid tumors, mucoepidermoid carcinomas, and adenoid cystic carcinomas. Combined, they comprise approximately 40% of malignant pediatric pulmonary lesions[3,4] and are the largest group of cancerous tumors encountered in children.

Carcinoid tumors are the most prevalent cancerous pulmonary tumor in children, and pulmonary tumors account for almost 28% of all carcinoid tumors.[30] These tumors are derived from Kulchitsky cells from the amine precursor uptake and decarboxylation (APUD) system involved in tryptophan metabolism. As such, they are involved in the synthesis of vasoactive amines which when produced to excess can lead to the development of carcinoid syndrome – palpitations, flushing, diarrhea, abdominal pain, bronchospasm – which is a hallmark of this disease, although found rarely (less than 10%)[31] and generally signifies significant extrapulmonary disease. Furthermore, this pathway also serves a means to test for the disease, since the patient's urine can be tested for 5-hydroxyindoleacetic acid (5-HIAA) levels and if elevated, confirm the diagnosis. These tumors are generally found in isolation, although they can be a component of patients with multiple endocrine neoplasia type I (MEN I) syndrome in a minority of cases (4%). Histologically, they can be separated into typical (90%) and atypical (10%) variants with the atypical subtype demonstrating a more aggressive phenotype with necrosis and increased mitoses on histopathologic review. However, both variants are known to both metastasize and recur. It is also apparent that atypical variants have a higher proportion of lymph node metastases (30%–75%[32] vs. 5%–10%[8]) and a worse prognosis by stage than their typical counterparts. Regardless of subtype, however, complete resection with lymph node dissection and removal of all disease (gross and microscopic) is the mainstay of treatment as there is no effective cytotoxic chemotherapy. Distant metastases can be treated with metastasectomy or other local control measures (radiofrequency ablation, chemoembolization) in combination with adjuvant therapies (chemotherapy, radiotherapy, somatostatin analogues) to treat symptoms of excess vasoactive amine production. The widespread use of these techniques in children, however, is not necessarily recommended as their utility is unknown.

Mucoepidermoid tumors are the second most frequent malignant pulmonary tumor in children.[3,4] They arise in the mucous glands of the mucosa and submucosa of the respiratory tract with a penchant for presenting in the more proximal airways (central lesions). They do not readily metastasize to regional lymph nodes or distant sites, and complete extirpation is the recommended treatment. Histopathologically, they are divided into high- and low-grade lesions with the latter being most commonly found in children.[7,33–35] High-grade lesions are known to carry a dismal prognosis almost regardless of presentation or treatment strategies employed.[36]

The final tumor in this class is adenoid cystic carcinoma (cyclindroma). These cancers are deemed salivary gland-type lesions, and they have a propensity to recur locally and metastasize.[32] Their growth pattern is slow, radial expansion in the submucosa with direct extension into the pulmonary parenchyma.[32] They are known to spread to local and regional lymph node basins with direct perineural extension as well. Curative treatment involves complete resection with lymphadenectomy.

Bronchogenic Carcinoma

These tumors are the second most common pediatric pulmonary malignancy accounting for roughly 17% of cancerous lesions.[3] Of the various subtypes, adenocarcinomas and undifferentiated carcinomas are the most frequently reported,[3,4] and the basaloid variant of the bronchioloalveolar subtype has been reported to have a better prognosis.[37] In comparison to adults, these cancers are extremely rare in children with an incidence of 0.16% in the first decade of life, 0.9% in the second decade of life, and only 1.2% under the age of 40 years.[38,39] Treatment mirrors the adult regimens described elsewhere, and outcome data in children demonstrate that these lesions typically present late in the course of their disease and generally have an ominous prognosis.[4] Of note, however, these cancers have been reported to arise from and/or coexist in embryological cystic pediatric lung lesions (bronchogenic cysts, cystic pulmonary adenomatoid malformations [CPAMs]).[40,41] Hence, any child presenting antenatally or postnatally with a cystic lung lesion should be evaluated for complete operative extirpation within the first year of life.

Pleuropulmonary Blastoma

Pleuropulmonary blastoma (PPB) accounts for approximately 16% of childhood pediatric lung cancers and was ultimately histopathologically characterized in 1988.[42] Prior to this report, it was a confusing lesion that was called many different names secondary to the fact that it is composed of mesenchymal elements and embryonic stroma, but lacking a neoplastic epithelial component. It is thought to be derived from somatopleural mesoderm or thoracic splanchnopleura, and the tumors have been subclassified based on the degree of cystic elements present (Type I: all cyst, Type III: no cyst, and Type II: mixed).[43] As with bronchogenic carcinomas, these lesions have been reported to coexist or arise from congenital cystic lung lesions,[44] and one series reported almost one-third of PPBs were found with congenital pulmonary lesions.[45] These lesions are typically quite aggressive and prognosis is poor, regardless of subtype with a 10-year 8% survival rate reported in one large series.[46] Treatment involves complete extirpation of all disease if possible at diagnosis, but if not, neoadjuvant chemoradiation is recommended with surgery thereafter. Unfortunately, there is no agreed upon regimen to treat these tumors, and they tend to be quite large involving the lung, mediastinal structures, and chest wall when diagnosed.

METASTATIC TUMORS

The surgical treatment of pediatric pulmonary metastases is a field whereby sound data are lacking. There exist no large randomized prospective studies documenting its utility in any one disease. Data do exist in regard to specific tumor types, but these studies are usually case series from a single institution with a broad range of patients treated over a long period of time and often with varying regimens. Kayton[47] published the best work to date summarizing the most relevant and applicable data, but this work can only be considered a guide and not an absolute recommendation. Despite this dearth of knowledge, however, there are four principles that must be accounted for prior to undertaking pulmonary metastasectomy in the pediatric patient. First, the pathology of the primary tumor and accurate staging must be established and the data in regard to the timing and utility of pulmonary metastasectomy measured against this knowledge. Some tumors are readily responsive to adjuvant therapies and resection is not warranted except to confirm the presence (or absence) of pulmonary disease so as to guide therapy. Furthermore, the existence of other metastatic sites may temper the need to attempt pulmonary metastasectomy. Therefore, knowledge and confirmation of the primary tumor type and stage is critical to understanding the benefits and limitations of surgical therapies for the pulmonary disease. Second, the primary tumor site should be treated first and adequate disease control – surgical, medical – established prior to entertaining pulmonary metastasectomy as a component of cure. Third, the primary tumor site should have effective adjuvant therapies available so that micrometastatic disease can be treated in and around the timing of the pulmonary metastasectomy. Last, the type of surgery (thoracoscopic vs. thoracotomy), degree of resection (wedges vs. anatomic resection), and approach (sternotomy, uni- vs. bilateral and/or anterior vs. posterior thoracotomy) must also be considered on a case-by-case basis, tempered by the underlying disease and surgeon preference. The goal would be to preserve as much lung function as possible with the least morbidity in the fewest operations. Some tumors (osteosarcoma, adrenocortical carcinoma) mandate very aggressive approaches, while others do not. Ultimately, extensive discussions with the oncology, pulmonary, anesthesia, and critical care teams must commence early in the course of the patient's disease process so all are prepared and ready for any possible clinical course and to ensure the best possible outcome.

Technical Considerations

Pulmonary metastasectomy can be performed safely with minimal morbidity and a mortality rate of less than 1% as documented in the International Registry of Lung Metastases.[48] The type of pulmonary resection can be either anatomic or nonanatomic ("wedge"), but the majority of pulmonary metastasectomies performed in children are "wedge resections" where the lesion is completely excised with a small rim of normal lung parenchyma (<5 mm). Collective studies document the success of this procedure without the need for formal lung resection along anatomic boundaries.[48–53]

The use of MIS approaches for the resection of pulmonary lesions has been described in several studies.[54–59] It has become an established technique, except in the case of osteosarcoma where multidetector CT scanning has been shown to underestimate the number of lesions and formal thoracotomy has been recommended.[60] Therefore, staged or sequential bilateral thoracotomies or bilateral thoracic exploration through a sternotomy are recommended in patients with osteosarcoma, although this approach has not been shown in a prospective study to prolong either event-free survival or overall survival. Ultimately, the decision about the precise approach utilized in the treatment of a child with a pulmonary metastasis will be surgeon dependent.

Adrenocortical Carcinoma

Pulmonary metastases from adrenocortical carcinoma should be resected and every effort should be made to control the disease for both symptom control and for attempted cure. Effective adjuvant therapies are not available as the 5-year event-free survival was only 54% as reported in the International Pediatric Adrenocortical Tumor Registry.[61] While the authors of this work could not postulate on the effectiveness of metastasectomy because of data analysis issues, several series[62–65] have documented the utility of initial and subsequent pulmonary metastasectomy in these patients. Of note, however, these studies dealt primarily with adult patients and the assumption that the biology of these tumors is the same as that in children may not be true.

Differentiated Thyroid Cancer

Pulmonary metastases from differentiated thyroid cancer should be sampled to confirm the underlying nature of the lesion, but they should not be aggressively resected since adjuvant medical therapies exist that are both effective and well tolerated. The largest series exploring this question was reported by Demidchik et al.[66] who reviewed the records of 740 children presenting with differentiated thyroid cancer. Roughly 18% of patients had evidence of pulmonary metastases at presentation and all were treated with radioactive iodine therapy. The 10-year survival rate in this cohort was 98.8% with only five children succumbing to their disease at 115 months from last report. As this is an indolent disease, however, continued diligent follow-up is warranted in these children even into adulthood.

Germ Cell Tumors

Pulmonary metastases from gonadal germ cell tumors (GCTs) should be considered for resection not so much for local disease control and treatment, but for the histopathologic evaluation of residual disease in order to help guide future therapies. Although GCTs are chemoresponsive and have known tumor markers that can be monitored, radiographically identifiable disease at the conclusion of therapy may harbor live, active tumor even in the setting of negative tumor markers in up to 40% of patients.[67–71] The existence of active disease at the conclusion of standard adjuvant treatments would then warrant the initiation of second-line adjuvant therapies to eradicate the disease and give the best chance at cure.

Hepatoblastoma

Pulmonary metastases from hepatoblastoma should be considered for resection at the conclusion of adjuvant therapies if radiographically identifiable lesions persist. The data[72–74] supporting this statement are drawn from the observation of several reports documenting that patients who did not undergo resection of identifiable disease at the conclusion of treatment had worse outcomes than those who did undergo metastasectomy as sustained disease response to chemotherapy alone was no greater than 26%. In fact, in the same cohort of patients reviewed, the majority of long-term survivors had surgery and adjuvant chemotherapy for their disease.

Neuroblastoma

Pulmonary metastases in neuroblastoma are an ominous finding that generally signifies very aggressive disease with near certain lethality in a short time.[75,76] The role of surgery in these cases is simply to confirm that the lesions identified on imaging studies are not due to an infection or some other nononcologic cause that may influence the overall treatment strategy.

Nephroblastoma

Pulmonary metastasectomy in the setting of nephroblastoma should only be performed to confirm that the lesions present on imaging studies are in fact cancers. Several reports[77–79] have documented the effectiveness of adjuvant chemotherapy and locally directed radiotherapy in the treatment of pulmonary metastases in this disease. However, the importance of confirming that metastases truly exist prior to the initiation of adjuvant radiotherapy was recently highlighted by Ehrlich et al.[80] who reported that almost one-third of patients with small (<1 cm) nodules found on CT did not have histopathologic evidence of cancer when biopsied. Hence, the practitioner must be cautious in this setting so as not to overtreat patients.

Osteosarcomas

Pulmonary metastasectomy in the setting of osteosarcoma is a well-established practice that dates back to the first report by Martini et al.[81] over four decades ago. Numerous other reports[82,83] have documented the utility of repeated, open thoracic explorations for the removal of all evidence of disease as this confers a survival advantage. Unfortunately, these metastases are often quite small (<2 mm) and can be significantly underrepresented by conventional radiologic studies,[60] hence the need and importance of direct inspection and palpation of the entire lung to locate and remove all evidence of disease. Parenchymal preserving approaches should be utilized in all cases, as patients may develop repeated metastatic foci that mandate subsequent resections. Finally, these operations should not take place, however, until there is definitive disease control at the primary site and in the absence of other metastatic sites.

References

1. Cohen MC, Kaschula ROC. Primary pulmonary tumors in childhood: a literature review of 31 years; experience and the literature. *Pediatr Pulmonol.* 1992;14:222–232.
2. Crisei KL, Greenberg SB, Wolfson BJ. Cardiopulmonary and thoracic tumors of childhood. *Radiol Clin North Am.* 1997;35:1341–1366.
3. Hancock BJ, DiLorenzo M, Youssef S, et al. Childhood primary pulmonary neoplasms. *J Pediatr Surg.* 1993;28:1133.
4. Hartman GE, Shochat SJ. Primary pulmonary neoplasms of childhood: a review. *Ann Thorac Surg.* 1983;36:108.
5. Weldon CB, Shamberger RC. Pediatric pulmonary tumors: primary and metastatic. *Sem Ped Surg.* 2008;17:17–29.
6. Brenner DJ, Hall EJ. Computed tomography—an increasing source of radiation exposure. *N ENgl J Med.* 2007;357:2277–2284.
7. Hause DW, Harvey JC. Endobronchial carcinoid and mucoepidermoid carcinoma in children. *J Surg Oncol.* 1991;46:270–272.
8. Schreurs AJ, Westerman CJ, Van der Bosch JM. A twenty-five year follow-up of ninety-three resected typical carcinoid tumors of the lung. *J Thorac Cardiovasc Surg.* 1992;104:1470–1475.
9. Wellons HA, Eggleston P, Golden GT. Bronchial adenoma in childhood: two case reports and review of the literature. *Am J Dis Child.* 1976;130:301–304.
10. Welsh JH, Maxson T, Jaksic T. Tracheobronchial mucoepidermoid carcinoma in childhood and adolescence: case report and review of the literature. *Int J Pediatr Otorhinolaryngol.* 1998;45:265–273.
11. Browne DJ. Patent ductus arteriosus. *Proc Roy Soc Med.* 1952;45:719–722.
12. Baeza OR, Forster ED. Vertical axillary thoracotomy: a functional and cosmetically appealing incision. *Ann Thorac Surg.* 1976;22:287–288.
13. Bethancourt DM, Holmes EC. Muscle-sparing posterolateral thoracotomy. *Ann Thorac Surg.* 1988;45:337–339.
14. Mitchell R, Angell W, Wuerflein R, et al. Simplified lateral chest incision for most thoracotomies other than sternotomy. *Ann Thorac Surg.* 1976;22:284–286.
15. Rothenberg SS, Porkorny WJ. Experience with a total muscle sparing approach to thoracotomy in neonates, infants and children. *J Pediat Surg.* 1992;27:1157–1159.
16. Soucy P, Bass J, Mark E. The muscle sparing thoracotomy in infants and children. *J Pediat Surg.* 1991;26:1323–1325.

17. Cherup LL, Siewers RD, Futrell JW. Breast and pectoral muscle maldevelopment after anterolateral and posterolateral thoracotomies in children. *Ann Thorac Surg*. 1986;41:492–497.
18. Durning RP, Scoles PV, Fox OD. Scoliosis after thoracotomy in tracheo-oesophageal fistula patients. *J Bone Joint Surg*. 1980;62:1156–1159.
19. Freeman NV, Walkden J. Previously unreported shoulder deformity following right lateral thoractomy for oesophageal atresia. *J Pediat Surg*. 1969;4:627–636.
20. Jaurequizia E, Vazquez J, Murcia J. Morbid musculoskeletal sequelae of thoracotomy for tracheo-oesophageal atresia. *J Pediat Surg*. 1985;20:511–514.
21. Kemperson RL, Fletcher CD, Evans HL, et al. Tumors of the soft tissues. In: *Armed Forces Institute of Pathology Tumor Series*. 3rd ed. Washington, DC: Armed Forces Institute of Pathology; 2001.
22. Griffin CA, Hawkins AK, Dvorak C, et al. Recurrent involvement of 2p23 in inflammatory myofibroblastic tumors. *Cancer Res*. 1999;59:2776–2780.
23. Janik JS, Janik JP, Lovell MA. Recurrent inflammatory pseudotumors in children. *J Pediatr Surg*. 2003;38:1491–1495.
24. Maier HC, Sommers SC. Recurrent and metastatic pulmonary fibrous histiocytoma/plasma cell granuloma in a child. *Cancer*. 1987;60:1073–1076.
25. Su W, Ko A, O'Connell TX, et al. Treatment of pseudotumors with nonsteroidal anti-inflammatory drugs. *J Pediatr Surg*. 2000;35:1635.
26. Hoer J, Steinau G, Fuzesi L, et al. Inflammatory pseudotumor of the diaphragm. *Pediatr Surg Int*. 1999;15:387–390.
27. Aru GM, Abramowsky CR, Ricketts RR. Inflammatory pseudotumor of the spleen in a young child. *Pediatr Surg Int*. 1997;12:299–301.
28. Eggli KD, Newman B. Nodules, masses and pseudo-masses in the pediatric lung. *Radiol Clin North Am*. 1993;31:651.
29. Carney JA. The triad of gastric epithelioid leiomyosarcoma, functioning extra-adrenal paraganglioma, and pulmonary chondroma. *Cancer*. 1979;43:374–382.
30. Raut CP, Kulke MH, Glickman JN, et al. Carcinoid tumors. *Curr Probl Surg*. 2006;43:383–450.
31. Ganti S, Milton R, Davidson L, et al. Facial flushing due to recurrent bronchial carcinoid. *Ann Thorac Surg*. 2007;83:1196–1197.
32. Litzky L. Epithelial and soft tissue tumors of the tracheobronchial tree. *Chest Surg Clin North Am*. 2003;13:1–40.
33. Al-Qahtani AR, Dilorenzo M, Yazbeck S. Endobronchial tumors in children: institutional experience and literature review. *J Pediatr Surg*. 2003;38:733–736.
34. Curtis JM, Lacey D, Smyth R, et al. Endobronchial tumors in childhood. *Eur J Radiol*. 1998;29:11–20.
35. Tsuchiya H, Nagashima K, Ohashi S, et al. Childhood bronchial mucoepidermoid tumors. *J Pediatr Surg*. 1997;32:106–109.
36. Heitmiller RF, Mathiesen DJ, Ferry JA, et al. Mucoepidermoid lung tumors. *Ann Thorac Surg*. 1989;47:394–399.
37. Ohye RG, Cohen DM, Caldwell S, et al. Pediatric bronchioloalveolar carcinoma: a favorable pediatric malignancy? *J Pediatr Surg*. 1989;33:730–732.
38. Fonenelle LJ. Primary adenocarcinoma of the lung in a child: review of the literature. *Am Surg*. 1976;42:296–299.
39. Jubelirer SJ, Wilson RA. Lung cancer in patients younger than 40 years of age. *Cancer* 1991;67:1436–1438.
40. Granate C, Gambini C, Balducci T, et al. Bronchioalveolar carcinoma arising in a cystic adenomatoid malformation in a child: a case report and review on malignancies originating in congenital adenomatoid malformations. *Pediatr Pulmonol*. 1998:62–66.
41. MacSweeney F, Papagiannopoulos K, Goldstraw P, et al. Assessment of the expanded classification of congenital cystic adenomatoid malformations and their relationship to malignant transformation. *Am J Surg Pathol*. 2003;27:1139.
42. Manivel JC, Priest JR, Watterson J, et al. Pleuropulmonary blastoma. The so-called pulmonary blastoma of childhood. *Cancer*. 1988:1516–1526.
43. Dehner LP, Watterson J, Priest J. Pleuropulmonary blastoma. A unique intrathoracic pulmonary neoplasm of childhood. *Perspect Pediatr Pathologe*. 1995;18:214–216.
44. Weinblatt ME, Siegel SE, Isaacs H. Pulmonary blastoma associated with cystic lung disease. *Cancer*. 1982;49:669.
45. Tagge EP, Mulvihill D, Chandler JC, et al. Childhood pleuropulmonary blastoma: caution against nonoperative management of congenital lung cysts. *J Pediatr Surg*. 1996;31:187.
46. Priest JR, McDermott MB, Bathia S, et al. Pleuropulmonary blastoma. A clinicopathological study of 50 cases. *Cancer*. 1997;80:147–161.
47. Kayton ML. Pulmonary metastasectomy in pediatric patients. *Thorac Surg Clin*. 2006;16:167–183.
48. Pastorino U. History of the surgical management of pulmonary metastases and development of the International Registry. *Semin Thorac Cardiovasc Surg*. 2002;14:18–28.
49. Karnak I, Senocak ME, Kutluk T, et al. Pulmonary metastases in children: an analysis of surgical spectrum. *Eur J Pediatr Surg*. 2002;12:15.
50. Rusch VW. Pulmonary metastasectomy. Current indications. *Chest*. 1995;107:322S–331S.
51. Kilman JW, Kronenberg MW, O'Neill JA Jr., et al. Surgical resection for pulmonary metastases in children. *Arch Surg*. 1969;99:158–165.
52. Baldeyrou P, Lemoine G, Zucker JM, et al. Pulmonary metastases in children: the place of surgery. A study of 134 patients. *J Pediatr Surg*. 1984;19:121–125.
53. Abel RM, Brown J, Moreland B, et al. Pulmonary metastasectomy for pediatric solid tumors. *Pediatr Surg Int*. 2004;20:630–632.
54. Gilbert JC, Powell DM, Hartman GE, et al. Video-assisted thoracic surgery (VATS) for children with pulmonary metastases from osteosarcoma. *Ann Surg Oncol*. 1996;3:539–542.
55. Hardaway BW, Hoffer FA, Rao BN. Needle localization of small pediatric tumors for surgical biopsy. *Pediatr Radiol*. 2000;30:318–322.
56. Waldhausen JH, Shaw DW, Hall DG, et al. Needle localization for thoracoscopic resection of small pulmonary nodules in children. *J Pediatr Surg*. 1997;32:1624–1625.
57. Partrick DA, Bensard DD, Teitelbaum DH, et al. Successful thoracoscopic lung biopsy in children utilizing preoperative CT-guided localization. *J Pediatr Surg*. 2002;37:970–973.
58. Scorpio RJ, Stokes K, Grattan-Smith D, et al. Percutaneous localization of small pulmonary metastases, enabling limited resection. *J Pediatr Surg*. 1994;29:685–687.
59. McConnell PI, Feola GP, Meyers RL. Methylene blue-stained autologous blood for needle localization and thoracoscopic resection of deep pulmonary nodules. *J Pediatr Surg*. 2002;37:1729–1731.
60. Kayton ML, Huvos AG, Casher J, et al. Computed tomographic scan of the chest underestimates the number of metastatic lesions in osteosarcoma. *J Pediatr Surg*. 2006;41:200–206.
61. Michalkiewicz E, Sandrini R, Figueiredo B, et al. Clinical and outcome characteristics of children with adrenocortical tumors: a report from the International Pediatric Adrenocortical Tumor Registry. *J Clin Oncol*. 2004;22:838–845.
62. Appelqvist P, Kostianinen S. Multiple thoracotomy combined with chemotherapy in metastatic adrenal cortical carcinoma: a case report and review of the literature. *J Surg Oncol*. 1983;24:1–4.
63. De Leon DD, Lange BJ, Walterhouse D, et al. Long-term (15 years) outcome in an infant with metastatic adrenocortical carcinoma. *J Clin Endocrinol Metab*. 2002;87:4452–4456.
64. Kwauk S, Burt M. Pulmonary metastases from adrenal cortical carcinoma: results of resection. *J Surg Oncol*. 1993;53:243–246.
65. Schulick RD, Brennan MF. Long-term survival after complete resection and repeat resection in patients with adrenocortical carcinoma. *Ann Surg Oncol*. 1999;6:719–726.
66. Demidchik YE, Demidchik EP, Reiners C, et al. Comprehensive clinical assessment of 740 cases of surgically treated thyroid cancer in children of Belarus. *Ann Surg*. 2006;243:525–532.
67. Cagini L, Nicholson AG, Horwich A, et al. Thoracic metastasectomy for germ cell tumours: long term survival and prognostic factors. *Ann Oncol*. 1998;9:1185–1191.
68. Liu D, Abolhoda A, Burt ME, et al. Pulmonary metastasectomy for testicular germ cell tumors: a 28-year experience. *Ann Thorac Surg*. 1998;66:1709–1714.
69. Horvath LG, McCaughan BC, Stockle M, et al. Resection of residual pulmonary masses after chemotherapy in patients with metastatic non-seminomatous germ cell tumours. *Intern Med J* 2002;32:79–83.
70. Kesler KA, Wilson JL, Cosgrove JA, et al. Surgical salvage therapy for malignant intrathoracic metastases from nonseminomatous germ cell cancer of testicular origin: analysis of a single-institution experience. *J Thorac Cardiovasc Surg*. 2005;130:408–415.
71. Pfannschmidt J, Zabeck H, Muley T, et al. Pulmonary metastasectomy following chemotherapy in patients with testicular tumors: experience in 52 patients. *Thorac Cardiovasc Surg*. 2006;54:484–488.
72. Feusner JH, Krailo MD, Haas JE, et al. Treatment of pulmonary metastases of initial stage I hepatoblastoma in childhood. Report from the Childrens Cancer Group. *Cancer* 1993;71:859–864.
73. Perilongo G, Brown J, Shafford E, et al. Hepatoblastoma presenting with lung metastases: treatment results of the first cooperative, prospective

study of the International Society of Paediatric Oncology on childhood liver tumors. *Cancer.* 2000;89:1845–1853.
74. Schnater J, Aronson D, Plaschkes J et al. Surgical view of the treatment of patients with hepatoblastoma: results from the first prospective trial of the International Society of Pediatric Oncology Liver Tumor Study Group. *Cancer.* 2002;94:1111–1120.
75. DuBois SG, Kalika Y, Lukens JN, et al. Metastatic sites in stage IV and IVS neuroblastoma correlate with age, tumor biology, and survival. *J Pediatr Hematol Oncol.* 1999;21:181–189.
76. Kammen BF, Matthay KK, Pacharn P, et al. Pulmonary metastases at diagnosis of neuroblastoma in pediatric patients: CT findings and prognosis. *AJR Am J Roentgenol.* 2001;176:755–759.
77. Green DM, Breslow N, Ii Y, et al. The role of surgical excision in the management of relapsed Wilms' tumor patients with pulmonary metastases: a report from the National Wilms' Tumor Study. *J Pediatr Surg.* 1991;26:728.
78. Green DM, Beckwith JB, Breslow NE, et al. Treatment of children with stages II to IV anaplastic Wilms' tumor: a report from the National Wilms' Tumor Study Group. *J Clin Oncol.* 1994;12:2126–2131.
79. Green DM, Breslow NE, Beckwith JB, et al. Comparison between single-dose and divided-dose administration of dactinomycin and doxorubicin for patients with Wilms' tumor: a report from the National Wilms' Tumor Study Group. *J Clin Oncol.* 1998;16:237–245.
80. Ehrlich PF, Hamilton TE, Grundy P, et al. The value of surgery in directing therapy for patients with Wilms' tumor with pulmonary disease. A report from the National Wilms' Tumor Study Group (National Wilms' Tumor Study 5). *J Pediatr Surg.* 2006;41:162–167.
81. Martini N, Huvos AG, Mike V, et al. Multiple pulmonary resections in the treatment of osteogenic sarcoma. *Ann Thorac Surg.* 1971;12:271–280.
82. Harting MT, Blakely ML. Management of osteosarcoma pulmonary metastases. *Semin Pediatr Surg.* 2006;15:25–29.
83. Harting MT, Blakely ML, Jaffe N, et al. Long-term survival after aggressive resection of pulmonary metastases among children and adolescents with osteosarcoma. *J Pediatr Surg.* 2006;41:194–199.

PART 17

CHRONIC OBSTRUCTIVE PULMONARY DISEASE

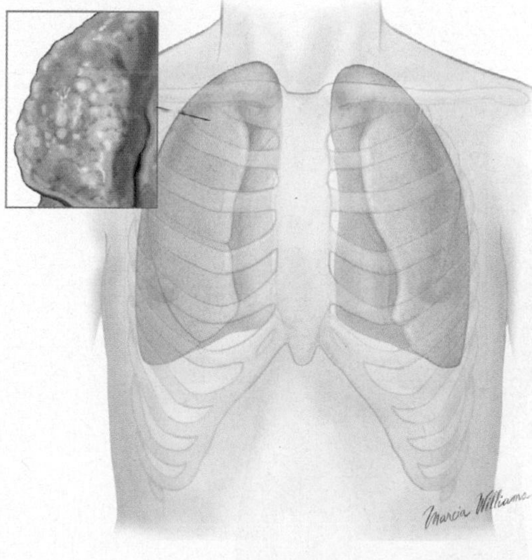

97 Overview of Chronic Obstructive Pulmonary Disease

Michael H. Cho and Christopher H. Fanta

Keywords: Anti-inflammatory therapies in COPD, antibiotics in COPD, asthma, chronic bronchitis, chronic obstructive pulmonary disease (COPD), emphysema, forced expiratory volume in one second (FEV_1), forced vital capacity (FVC), global initiative for chronic obstructive lung disease (GOLD), hypercapnia, long-acting bronchodilators, respiratory bronchiolitis, short-acting bronchodilators, small airways disease, smoking cessation, spirometry

Chronic obstructive pulmonary disease (COPD) is defined by the Global Initiative for Chronic Obstructive Lung Disease (GOLD)[1] as persistent, usually progressive airflow limitation associated with an enhanced inflammatory response, generally in response to noxious stimuli, such as cigarette smoking. COPD is one of the few major diseases with a rising burden; it is now the third leading cause of death in the United States.[2] Worldwide, an increasing prevalence of cigarette smoking, other exposures such as to biomass fuel, a reduction in other causes of early mortality, and an aging population are expected to lead to an increase in the global burden of COPD, and its rise from the fifth to the fourth most common cause of mortality (Fig. 97-1).[3]

COPD is a common comorbid condition in patients presenting for thoracic surgical evaluation, in large part due to shared risk factors of age and cigarette smoking. In addition, increasing evidence suggests that COPD itself may be an independent risk factor for lung cancer[4] and cardiovascular disease.[5,6] COPD is commonly underdiagnosed.[7] The presence of COPD has substantial impact on thoracic surgical outcomes.[8,9]

This chapter reviews some of the diagnostic and management considerations of COPD related to thoracic surgery, specifically:

1. Diagnosis and severity of COPD.
2. Management of stable COPD, with the goal of identifying comorbidities and optimizing pulmonary function prior to surgery.
3. Management of exacerbations.

Assessment of preoperative pulmonary risk is covered in Chapter 4. Surgical management of COPD is discussed in the ensuing Chapters 97 to 100.

DIAGNOSIS AND SEVERITY OF COPD

The diagnosis of COPD should be considered in any patient who has persistent dyspnea, chronic cough or sputum, and/or a history of exposure to risk factors for disease (generally at least 10–20 pack-years of cigarette smoking).[1,10] The GOLD definition of COPD is deliberately simple: airflow obstruction

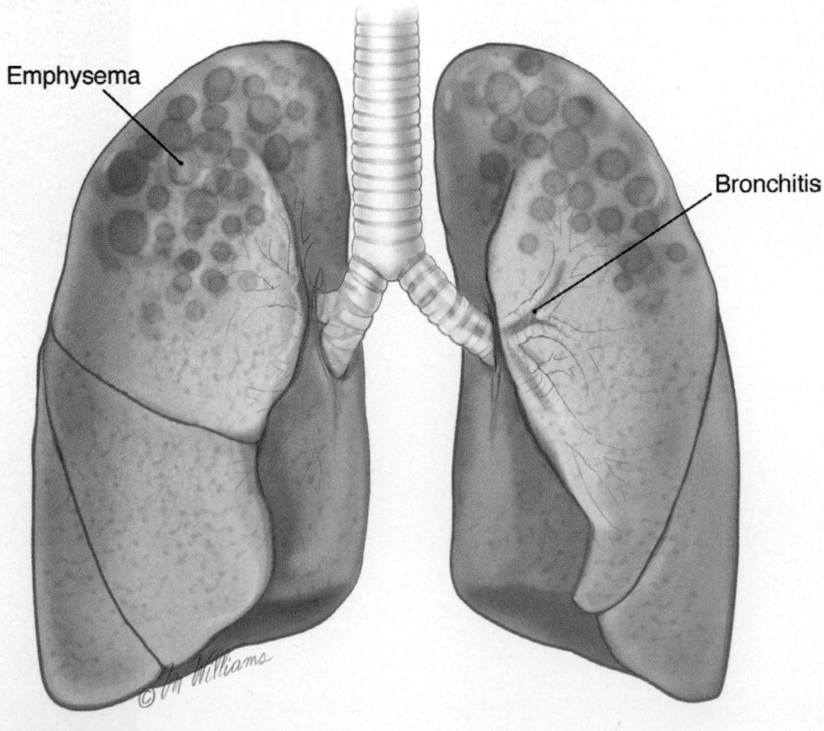

Figure 97-1. Regions of lung affected in chronic bronchitis and emphysema. These conditions are present in the majority of patients with COPD in the United States.

is identified by a reduced forced expiratory volume in 1 second (FEV_1) together with a reduced FEV_1 to forced vital capacity (FEV_1/FVC) ratio <0.7, and thus can be diagnosed in the appropriate setting by spirometry and bronchodilator testing. The use of the fixed ratio of FEV_1/FVC is chosen for simplicity but may lead to underdiagnosis in young patients and more conspicuously, potential overdiagnosis in elderly patients,[11] because of the normal decline in FEV_1/FVC with age, as demonstrated in population-based studies of healthy normal controls. Of interest, older subjects potentially misclassified as having obstruction have been shown to have worse outcomes, suggesting that using a fixed ratio is acceptable.[12,13]

Despite the simplicity of making a diagnosis of COPD based on spirometry and fixed-ratio definition of airflow obstruction, underdiagnosis is common because many patients with COPD are asymptomatic or minimally symptomatic.[7] Conversely, a large fraction of patients who carry a diagnosis of COPD either do not have obstruction on spirometry or have never had spirometry.[14,15] Dyspnea together with a history of cigarette smoking is insufficient to establish a diagnosis of COPD: only a minority of long-term cigarette smokers develops airflow obstruction and COPD. Even in the presence of compatible spirometry, the differential diagnosis of airflow obstruction is broad, and many diseases can masquerade as COPD or be present in addition to COPD (e.g., asthma, congestive heart failure, bronchiectasis, tuberculosis, and bronchiolitis).[1]

COPD is a complex disease that incorporates three other disease states: emphysema, small airways disease (respiratory bronchiolitis), and chronic bronchitis.[16] Airflow obstruction in COPD results from emphysema and small airways disease. Emphysema is defined anatomically as parenchymal destruction due to abnormal and permanent enlargement of the airspaces distal to the terminal bronchioles without obvious fibrosis. Emphysema leads to airflow obstruction through loss of lung elastic recoil and flow limitation, although a substantial portion of subjects with emphysema by CT scan do not have airflow obstruction.[17] Small airways disease is the major cause of airflow limitation in COPD, and detailed studies have demonstrated that narrowing and loss of these small airways precedes emphysematous destruction.[18] Chronic bronchitis, the consequence of mucous gland hyperplasia and hypertrophy in larger, more central airways, is defined by symptoms of chronic cough productive of phlegm for at least 3 months out of the year for at least 2 years.[19] While these symptoms frequently overlap with conditions causing airflow obstruction, a substantial fraction of patients with chronic bronchitis do not have chronic airflow obstruction.[20] Nonetheless, chronic mucous hypersecretion is an independent risk factor for postsurgical respiratory complications, including hypoxemia and pneumonia.[21]

These components of COPD lead to several pathophysiologic consequences. The most typical finding in COPD is chronic airflow obstruction. During exhalation, airflow is determined by the balance of elastic recoil of the lungs and airway resistance, both of which are impaired in COPD. Hyperinflation is a consequence of airflow obstruction and reduced elastic recoil. It serves as a compensatory mechanism to increase lung volumes and expiratory flow rates. However, hyperinflation also leads to a disadvantageous position of the diaphragm and increased work of inspiration, increased sensation of dyspnea, decreased exercise capacity, and impaired cardiac function.[22] Gas exchange abnormalities are largely a consequence of ventilation–perfusion mismatch,[23] although significant hypoxemia at rest may be absent even in patients with severe airflow obstruction and associated dyspnea. In the absence of respiratory depressant medications, hypercapnia develops in a minority of patients and only in the presence of severe airflow obstruction (FEV_1 less than approximately 1.5 L).[24]

The major risk factor for COPD is cigarette smoking, and smoking cessation is the single most effective measure to reduce the risk of further decline in lung function. There is a dose-response curve with smoking, such that each pack-year increases the risk of COPD.[25] Ongoing smoking increases the rate of decline in lung function, and smoking cessation reduces the rate of lung function decline.[26] Exposures to noxious particles other than cigarette smoke, either through occupation[27] or in the home,[28] are also potential contributors to COPD. A substantial contribution of genetic factors has been identified in family based studies, although most of these factors have yet to be determined.[29] An exception is the small and under-recognized fraction of patients with COPD who have a specific genetic predisposition—alpha-1 antitrypsin deficiency. These patients are important to identify as they may benefit from genetic counseling and weekly infusions of purified alpha-1 antitrypsin protein (augmentation therapy).[30] Other risk factors include asthma and developmental or early lung disease. Asthma and COPD generally have different underlying causes of inflammation. However, long-standing asthma frequently leads to irreversible airflow obstruction[31] and these two diseases can have substantial overlap, particularly in the setting of cigarette exposure. Airways hyperresponsiveness – bronchoconstriction in response to external triggers – in patients without a clinical diagnosis of asthma is also a risk factor for chronic airflow obstruction.[32] Factors related to lung growth and development – and subsequent reduced maximally attained lung function – are also likely important. In epidemiologic studies, birth weight is associated with FEV_1.[33] More specifically, in prematurely born infants, bronchopulmonary dysplasia is associated with risk for emphysema and airways obstruction,[34] although the characteristics of bronchopulmonary dysplasia are changing.[35]

The severity of COPD is most commonly characterized according to GOLD grade (formerly stage), which utilizes the degree of airflow obstruction based on postbronchodilator spirometry (Table 97-1). FEV_1 is a simple metric that has been associated with symptoms of dyspnea, other measures of disease severity (such as degree of emphysema[36] and exacerbations,[37]) and importantly, overall survival.[38,39] However, other metrics such as the BODE index,[40] which combines body mass index (BMI), airflow obstruction (FEV_1), dyspnea (Medical Research Council Dyspnea Score), and exercise capacity (6-minute walk), have been demonstrated to provide better prediction of mortality than FEV_1 alone. Recent GOLD guidelines suggest a combined COPD assessment, based on GOLD spirometric classification and Modified British Medical Research Council dyspnea score or COPD Assessment Test (www.catestonline.org).[1,41] Biochemical markers are being sought that can further characterize COPD phenotypes and improve predictive models of COPD mortality.[42]

COPD is a highly morbid disease, with predictably greater mortality at higher stages of airflow obstruction (Table 97-2). The decline in lung function in COPD is also generally progressive, with a mean decline of FEV_1 of approximately 30 to 40 mL per year,[43,44] but highly variable. A large-scale, 3-year, multi-center observational study of COPD, called "Evaluation of COPD Longitudinally to Identify Predictive Surrogate Endpoints" (ECLIPSE), found that approximately one-third of subjects had a decline of FEV_1 of <20 mL per year, while

Table 97-1

COMBINED COPD ASSESSMENT IN GOLD

GOLD GRADE			EXACERBATION HISTORY
1	A	B	0
2			1
3	C	D	≥2
4			≥2
Symptoms →	mMRC 0–1 CAT < 10	mMRC ≥ 2 CAT ≥ 10	

one-third of subjects had a decline of >40 mL per year. Rate of decline was inversely proportional to initial FEV_1. Risk factors for accelerated decline were current smoking, emphysema, and bronchodilator reversibility[44]; the former two of these risk factors have been identified in multiple other studies.[26,45]

COPD has been increasingly recognized as a systemic disease with multiple comorbidities. While the majority of these likely arise due to shared risk factors (e.g., age and cigarette smoking), there is increasing evidence that COPD itself may be an independent risk factor for the development of these comorbid conditions, through either shared inflammatory mechanisms[4] or altered physiology.[47] Cardiovascular disease frequently coexists with COPD and is an important cause of mortality,[48] yet some evidence suggests that coronary artery disease[49] and heart failure[50] are underdiagnosed. Pulmonary hypertension is common, particularly in more severe COPD. A selected group of patients have pulmonary artery pressures disproportionate to the degree of airflow obstruction,[51] and it is possible that some of these patients may be candidates for pulmonary vasodilator therapy in a very limited number of settings.[52] Reduced BMI and osteoporosis are associated with COPD and in particular with the degree of emphysema.[53] Anxiety and depression are common in COPD and associated with a worse prognosis.[54,55] Other common comorbidities are anemia and diabetes.[56] In an analysis of the cause-specific mortality among patients with COPD followed in a 3-year clinical trial, 27% died of cardiovascular diseases and 21% died of cancer.[48]

In summary, COPD is deliberately simple to diagnose, yet represents a complex syndrome, with varying contributions from different risk factors, pathophysiologic manifestations, and comorbidities. Testing to consider in the diagnosis and evaluation of the COPD patient is listed in Table 97-3.

MANAGEMENT OF STABLE COPD

Smoking Cessation

In patients who continue to smoke, smoking cessation is the intervention with the greatest capacity to affect outcome in COPD. Smoking cessation is associated with reduced rate of lung function decline in COPD[26] and is one of the few modalities that affects mortality from COPD.[59] Smoking is an important risk factor for postoperative complications in thoracic surgery.[60] In a series of randomized trials in a variety of surgical disciplines, smoking cessation decreased the overall rate of complications by 41%, including pulmonary and wound healing complications,[61,62] with longer periods of cessation resulting in an increase in effect. Nevertheless, success is challenging; nicotine addiction is a chronic disease, and relapse is common. Long-term quit rates are often less than 25%.[63,64]

Aids to facilitate a patient's smoking cessation efforts generally consist of two components: (1) counseling and (2) pharmacotherapy. Even brief periods of counseling can increase quit rates, and there is a dose–response relationship with repeated counseling.[65,66] A five-step intervention program (the 5 A's: Ask about smoking; Advise smokers to quit; Assess willingness to attempt to quit; Assist with treatment and referrals; Arrange follow-up) can form a useful framework for intervention, and three types of counseling – practical, and social support both as a part of treatment and outside of treatment – can be effective.[67] Successful programs provide information about the health effects of smoking, the medical basis of nicotine addiction, and guidance for recognizing and addressing the risk factors for relapse.[68]

Nicotine replacement products (gum, inhaler, spray, patch, or lozenge) form the basis for most pharmacotherapy, and they successfully increase abstinence rates. Patients should be educated about the proper use of the product. The patch is the easiest and most widely used form of replacement: patients smoking more than half a pack of cigarettes per day should use the 21-mg dose and taper over 6 to 8 weeks. Patients opting for the gum should be instructed to chew the gum intermittently, as continuous chewing results in enhanced absorption and subsequent nausea. Bupropion, a mildly stimulating medication thought to act through noradrenergic and dopaminergic release, can approximately double the rate of smoking cessation compared with placebo.[69] Bupropion can reduce the seizure threshold and therefore is contraindicated in persons with a history of seizures. Varenicline is a centrally acting partial nicotine receptor agonist that has also been demonstrated to be effective versus placebo (approximately 2.3-fold increase in relative risk of quitting) and more effective than bupropion (relative risk approximately 1.52).[70] Concerns have been raised about a possible association between neuropsychiatric side effects – and in particular, suicidal and self-injurious behavior – for both bupropion and varenicline. Patients should be monitored closely for adverse effects, and the drug should be discontinued with evidence of unusual behavior or mood symptoms. Varenicline has also been associated with a possible increase in cardiovascular events.[71,72] Although this effect appears to be small

Table 97-2

GOLD CLASSIFICATION OF SEVERITY OF AIRFLOW LIMITATION[1]

GRADE	DESCRIPTION	FEV_1% PREDICTED	EXACERBATIONS PER YEAR[37,43,46]	3-YEAR MORTALITY[43,46]
1	Mild	≥80%	?	?
2	Moderate	≥50%–<80%	0.7–0.9	11%
3	Severe	≥30%–<50%	1.1–1.3	15%
4	Very severe	<30%	1.2–2.0	24%

Postbronchodilator FEV_1, in the setting of FEV_1/FVC <0.7.

Table 97-3

ADDITIONAL STUDIES IN COPD

TEST	RATIONALE
Chest x-ray	Exclude other diagnoses, assess for concomitant comorbidities (e.g., kyphoscoliosis, congestive heart failure)[57]
Chest CT	As above; assess for degree and distribution of emphysema, airway disease.
Lung volumes, Diffusion capacity (DLCO)	Characterize severity of COPD; assess presence of concomitant pulmonary disease (e.g., restriction/pulmonary hypertension) especially if discordant with spirometry.
Pulse oximetry, Arterial blood gas	Assessment for hypoxemia and need for supplemental oxygen. Assess for degree of hypercapnia (particularly if SpO_2 <92%).[1]
Alpha-1 antitrypsin protein level	Consider for all patients[58] but particularly in the setting of younger age, lower lobe emphysema, family history.
Exercise testing, Composite scores (e.g., BODE)[40]	May be useful for preoperative risk stratification, prognosis.
EKG, Cardiac stress test, Echocardiogram	Assess for cardiac comorbidities including coronary artery disease, cardiomyopathy, pulmonary hypertension, particularly in the setting of other findings (e.g., dyspnea, reduced DLCO, hypoxemia disproportionate to degree of airflow obstruction).

and likely outweighed by the long-term benefits of smoking cessation, these data may be important to consider when choosing smoking cessation modalities. Electronic cigarette-shaped devices ("e-cigarettes") provide a vapor for inhalation and allow smokers to mimic the behavior of smoking tobacco. However, the complete biochemical contents of the inhaled vapor from e-cigarettes are uncertain and unregulated, and the long-term safety of these devices has not been proved.[73]

Bronchodilators

Bronchodilators are the current mainstay of management for COPD. These medications can improve lung emptying, reduce dynamic hyperinflation, and improve exercise performance. Importantly, bronchodilator responsiveness in COPD is not predicted by a single spirometric measurement. In one study, using American Thoracic Society (ATS) criteria for defining bronchodilator responsiveness, over 50% of patients changed status (bronchodilator responsive vs. nonresponsive) between visits.[74] Furthermore, the extent of improvement in symptoms and functional capacity is not predicted from bronchodilator testing or changes in FEV_1.[1,75] Inhaled bronchodilators are generally preferred, although proper technique is critical for effectiveness. There are two major classes of bronchodilators, $beta_2$-agonist and anticholinergic, both of which are available in both short- and long-acting formulations (Table 97-4). Combination of different pharmacologic classes (e.g., $beta_2$-agonist and anticholinergic) may be more effective and decrease side effects compared with monotherapy.[76]

Short-acting bronchodilators (e.g., $beta_2$-agonists such as albuterol or anticholinergics such as ipratropium) can be useful for acute relief of symptoms or rescue therapy, with some data suggesting a greater effectiveness for anticholinergics.[77] However, long-acting bronchodilators are more effective at improving FEV_1, dyspnea, quality of life, and exacerbation rate and should generally be used for all but the most minimally impaired patients (e.g., FEV_1 >80%). These medications are also more convenient, as they are available in both twice-daily (beta-agonists salmeterol, formoterol) and once-daily (beta-agonists indacaterol and vilanterol, anticholinergics tiotropium and umeclidinium) dosing. Large, randomized controlled trials have demonstrated effectiveness of both long-acting $beta_2$-agonists and long-acting anticholinergics.[43,78] Adverse effects

Table 97-4

INHALED BRONCHODILATORS AVAILABLE FOR TREATMENT OF COPD

DURATION OF ACTION	CATEGORY	GENERIC NAME	BRAND NAMES	FORMULATIONS
Short duration of action (4–6 h)	$Beta_2$-agonist	Albuterol	ProAir, Proventil, Ventolin	Metered-dose inhaler; liquid for nebulization
		Levalbuterol	Xopenex	Metered-dose inhaler; liquid for nebulization
		Pirbuterol	Maxair	Metered-dose inhaler
	Anticholinergic	Ipratropium	Atrovent	Metered-dose inhaler, liquid for nebulization
	Combination $beta_2$-agonist and anticholinergic	Albuterol and ipratropium	Combivent, Duoneb	Metered-dose inhaler, liquid for nebulization
Long duration of action (12–24 h)	$Beta_2$-agonist	Salmeterol	Serevent	Multi-dose dry-powder inhaler
		Formoterol	Foradil, Perforomist	Single-dose dry-powder inhaler; liquid for nebulization
		Arformoterol	Brovana	Liquid for nebulization
		Indacaterol	Arcapta	Single-dose dry-powder inhaler
	Anticholinergic	Tiotropium	Spiriva	Single-dose dry-powder inhaler
	$Beta_2$-agonist combined with an inhaled corticosteroid	Salmeterol and fluticasone	Advair	Metered-dose inhaler and multi-dose dry-powder inhaler
		Formoterol and budesonide	Symbicort	Metered-dose inhaler
		Formoterol and mometasone	Dulera	Metered-dose inhaler
	Ultra-long-acting $beta_2$-agonist combined with an inhaled corticosteroid	Vilanterol and fluticasone furoate	Breo	Multi-dose dry-powder inhaler
	$Beta_2$-agonist combined with anticholinergic	Vilanterol and umeclidinium	Anoro	Multi-dose dry-powder inhaler

of these medications are generally minimal. In patients with asthma, use of long-acting betaagonists (LABAs) alone (without an inhaled corticosteroid) has been associated with worse outcomes compared to placebo. However, similar concerns do not apply to COPD.[79] Tachycardia and cardiac rhythm disturbances can occur with both categories of bronchodilator medications, although relief of obstruction and dyspnea generally outweighs the negative effects.[77,80] Initial concern for possible adverse cardiovascular effects of tiotropium was not substantiated in a large, randomized, controlled clinical trial.[43,81] No clear data favor the choice of one long-acting bronchodilator over another.[1,10] In one study, tiotropium was superior to the LABA, salmeterol, in reducing exacerbations, although the difference was small,[82] and tiotropium has the advantage of once-daily dosing. Indacaterol, a newer once-daily LABA, appears at least as effective as tiotropium in effecting sustained bronchodilation.[83,84]

Theophylline is an oral methylxanthine with nonspecific phosphodiesterase and adenosine receptor antagonist activity. It produces a modest bronchodilator effect compared with placebo and in combination with inhaled bronchodilators.[85,86] Theophylline also has potential nonbronchodilator effects that may improve symptoms in COPD.[87] The use of theophylline has generally been limited, due to a low therapeutic index and risk of interactions with other medications through the cytochrome P450 system; toxicity can include nausea, vomiting, tremor, arrhythmia, and seizures. Thus, use of theophylline is generally relegated to a select group of patients who may be refractory to other therapies.

Anti-inflammatory Medication

In contrast to the success of inhaled and oral corticosteroids in controlling asthma, the response in COPD is substantially less dramatic. Nevertheless, in patients with moderately severe disease (FEV_1 <60% predicted),[78] inhaled corticosteroids can improve lung function, improve quality of life, and reduce the frequency of exacerbations. An effect on rate of decline in lung function is unclear with some studies finding a modest benefit, and others showing no difference.[78,88] Although generally well tolerated, adverse effects can include oral candidiasis, hoarseness, easy bruising, and a small but significantly increased risk of pneumonia.[89] While significant, this latter risk may be outweighed by the reduction in exacerbations.[90] Use of oral steroids for stable COPD is generally not recommended, given the substantial side effects from long-term use and lack of convincing evidence of benefit.[91] In addition, no data support the value of the response to a short course of oral corticosteroids in predicting the subsequent response to inhaled steroids.

Inhaled corticosteroids are generally not used as monotherapy in COPD; inhaled long-acting bronchodilators have greater benefits and fewer adverse effects. However, in selected patients (see below) combination therapy involving inhaled corticosteroids and LABAs appears to be effective in further improving lung function, health status, and exacerbations versus either medication alone.[78,92] One study involving more than 6000 subjects with moderate-to-severe COPD found a trend toward reduction in all-cause mortality after 3 years of combination high-dose inhaled steroids and long-acting beta agonists (LABAs) compared with placebo.[78] The specific combination of inhaled corticosteroids and long-acting anticholinergic bronchodilator (without a LABA) has not been studied. However, limited evidence suggests that therapy with all three medication classes – inhaled corticosteroid, LABA, and long-acting anticholinergic – may further improve lung function and quality of life,[93–95] though further data are needed.[96]

Roflumilast is an oral, once-daily, phosphodiesterase-4 inhibitor, a new class of medication designed to reduce inflammation by inhibiting the breakdown of intracellular cAMP. In two randomized controlled trials of patients with chronic bronchitis, severe COPD, a history of exacerbations, and receiving inhaled bronchodilators, roflumilast reduced moderate and severe exacerbations by approximately 17%,[97] and modestly but significantly improved FEV_1. Side effects include nausea, reduced appetite, and abdominal pain; caution is advised in depressed and underweight patients, and weight monitoring during treatment is recommended. Roflumilast should not be given with theophylline.

Other Therapies

Vaccinations should be considered for all COPD patients. Influenza vaccination reduces serious illness and death and should be given annually to all patients. In a small, randomized, controlled trial in patients with COPD, vaccination was associated with a relative reduction in influenza of 0.24[98]; and another study demonstrated that influenza vaccination did not provoke COPD exacerbations.[99] Pneumococcal vaccine is recommended for all patients older than 65 years, and in younger patients with severe disease or other comorbid conditions.[1]

The role of long-term antibiotics for stable COPD is not clear. Several recent studies have demonstrated a benefit of antibiotics in reducing exacerbations, particularly of macrolides, which may also have beneficial nonantibacterial effects.[100,101] However, the outcomes of this treatment for longer than 1 year are unknown, and benefits need to be weighed against the risks of medication side effects (such as hearing loss) and increasing bacterial resistance. Chronic antibiotics are not currently recommended by GOLD.[1] The mucolytics, carbocysteine and n-acetylcysteine, also have antioxidant properties. Limited evidence suggests that some patients, particularly those not on inhaled corticosteroids, may benefit from their use.[102–104]

Pulmonary rehabilitation has been shown to have substantial benefits in COPD.[105] A course of at least 6 weeks of rehabilitation – with longer periods generally conferring greater benefit – can lead to improvements in exercise capacity and quality of life and a reduction in hospitalizations.[106] Some observational studies appear to show an effect on mortality, although this effect has not been consistently demonstrated.[107,108] For patients unable to participate in structured programs, encouragement of general physical activity is recommended, though it has not been specifically studied. The benefits of pulmonary rehabilitation appear to decrease over time, though maintenance programs, including self-monitoring, can improve retention.[109,110]

Comprehensive outpatient pulmonary rehabilitation programs include: (1) exercise training, (2) disease education, and (3) discussion of nutrition. Lower extremity training is the cornerstone of pulmonary rehabilitation and has been the most well-studied form of exercise in COPD; upper extremity training[111] may be of limited additional benefit. Education is believed to improve compliance, disease understanding, and recognition of symptoms. Attention to nutrition is important in severe COPD, where approximately 20% to 30%[112] of patients have a reduction in BMI and fat-free mass index. A reduced BMI is an independent risk factor for mortality.[113]

Supplemental oxygen is one of the few treatments that has an effect on survival in COPD. In two randomized controlled trials, continuous oxygen (15 hours or more each day) in patients with chronic hypoxemia reduced 5-year mortality by approximately half.[114,115] Based on these and subsequent studies, oxygen is recommended for patients with a resting PaO_2 ≤55 or SpO_2 ≤88% (confirmed twice over a 3-week period) or PaO_2 55 to 60 with secondary evidence of chronic hypoxemia (pulmonary hypertension, polycythemia, or cor pulmonale).

A subset of patients without chronic hypoxemia at rest have oxygen desaturation during exercise, sleep, or air travel. Supplemental oxygen can improve breathlessness in subjects with COPD,[116,117] and may be prescribed for PaO_2 <55 or SaO_2 <88% during exercise. Coexisting sleep apnea is common in COPD, and the presence of this or other sleep-related breathing disorders should be assessed. Even in the absence of these disorders, nocturnal hypoxemia is not uncommon. Oxygen prescribed in this setting may improve sleep[118] and reduce pulmonary arterial pressures[119] and may be prescribed for hypoxemia, or a fall in PaO_2 > 10 mm Hg or a fall in SaO_2 >5% with signs and symptoms of hypoxemia (impaired cognitive process, restlessness, or insomnia). Nevertheless, in contrast to continuous oxygen administration for chronic hypoxemia at rest, neither of these indications has been demonstrated to improve survival, and the long-term benefits, if any, are unclear.[120,121] Most current guidelines recommend supplemental oxygen for air travel in those patients who would be expected to become significantly hypoxemic (PaO_2 <50 mm Hg) at an altitude of approximately 7000 feet, the typical cabin pressure in a commercial airplane when at its cruising altitude. Hypoxemic challenge tests can be used to identify these patients,[122] though some experts have also advocated for the use of prediction equations.[121]

Surgical treatments for COPD include bullectomy, lung volume reduction surgery (LVRS), and lung transplantation. These therapies are discussed further in Chapters 98, 99, and 108 to 112. Novel, bronchoscopic approaches to lung volume reduction are also being developed, including placement of endobronchial one-way valves, instillation of biologic tissue sealants[123] and insertion of preformed wire coils.[124] These are discussed in Chapter 100.

General and Subgroup-Specific Guidelines

Management of COPD includes recommendations for all patients and those specific to certain subgroups. All patients with COPD should have potential exposures identified and reduced. For the majority of patients, this exposure is smoking, and smoking cessation counseling and potentially pharmacotherapy should be offered. For others, it may include occupational or other environmental exposures. Influenza and pneumococcal vaccination should be administered as described earlier. Physical activity should be encouraged, and nutritional counseling offered when appropriate. Patients with hypoxemia should be offered supplemental oxygen, provided it can be administered safely (active cigarette smoking being a relative contraindication). Patients with alpha-1 antitrypsin deficiency should be considered for replacement therapy.

Use of specific bronchodilator and anti-inflammatory therapies are based on disease severity. The recently updated GOLD guidelines[1] are based on a combination of lung function and symptoms (Table 97-5). For minimally affected patients in Group A, a short-acting bronchodilator is sufficient in most cases. This choice can be either a short-acting beta-agonist (e.g., albuterol) or short-acting anticholinergic (e.g., ipratropium). Alternatively, a combination of the two short-acting medications, or a LABA or anticholinergic can be given. For Group B and above, short-acting bronchodilators (generally beta-agonist, unless the patient is not on a long-acting anticholinergic) can be added for immediate relief of symptoms, and pulmonary rehabilitation is recommended. Long-acting bronchodilators either single (first line) or in combination (second line) are recommended for Group B. An inhaled corticosteroid combined with a LABA, or a long-acting anticholinergic is recommended for Groups C and D. An alternative for Group C is a combination of any two of these agents. An alternative for Group D is any combination of two or three of these agents. Phosphodiesterase inhibitors are an alternative particularly in Group D but also in Group C in patients with chronic bronchitis and frequent exacerbations.

Table 97-5

GUIDELINES FOR THE MANAGEMENT OF COPD

THERAPY	GOLD[1]	ACP/ACCP/ATS/ERS[10]
Short-acting bronchodilators	Group A	FEV_1 60%–80% FEV_1 <60%
Long-acting bronchodilators	Group B, C, D	FEV_1 <60% with symptoms
Long-acting bronchodilator combination	Group B (Alternative) Group C, D	FEV_1 <60% with symptoms
Long-acting beta-agonist + inhaled corticosteroid	Group C, D	FEV_1 <60% with symptoms
Pulmonary rehabilitation	Group B, C, D	FEV_1 <50% FEV_1 >50% with symptoms

The older ACP/ACCP/ATS/ERS guidelines[10] differ slightly, and do not use the updated GOLD groups. Patients with very mild obstruction (FEV_1 ≥80% predicted) generally have minimal symptoms attributable to airflow obstruction. Most studies of COPD treatment have not included patients with this mild degree of severity, and instead have generally focused on Stage 2 and above. Thus, these guidelines do not find evidence to support treatment of this group, or for asymptomatic patients with up to moderate airflow obstruction. Weak evidence suggests that inhaled bronchodilators may be used for patients with an FEV_1 60% to 80% predicted. Conversely, strong evidence supports long-acting bronchodilators in patients with an FEV_1 <60% predicted. Combination therapy can be added for symptomatic patients with an FEV_1 <60% predicted. Pulmonary rehabilitation should be prescribed for symptomatic or exercise-limited patients with an FEV_1 <50% predicted, and may also be appropriate for symptomatic patients with less severe airflow obstruction.

Stable COPD in the Perioperative Setting

Postoperative patients frequently are unable to perform proper technique for use of a metered-dose or dry-powder inhaler. In these cases, repeated administration of nebulized short-acting bronchodilators can be used to replace the patient's preoperative medications. While data suggest that patients receiving inhaled corticosteroids, particularly in high doses, may have relative adrenal axis impairment,[125] there are no data that support the routine use of "stress-dose" steroids for this population in the perioperative setting.

COPD EXACERBATIONS

A COPD exacerbation is a worsening of respiratory symptoms beyond the patient's normal day-to-day variability that leads to a change in medication. Exacerbations accelerate the decline of lung function and are associated with significant morbidity and mortality. Most COPD patients with at least moderate disease will suffer exacerbations, with above 2 per year considered frequent. The diagnosis of an exacerbation is essentially one of exclusion, as the differential diagnosis of increased dyspnea in COPD is broad, and many conditions (e.g., congestive heart failure, pulmonary embolism)[126] have the potential to mimic or aggravate underlying COPD.[127] The most common etiology of exacerbations appears to be respiratory tract infections, either viral or bacterial.

The initial evaluation and location for treatment for a COPD exacerbation should be based on the medical history and clinical signs of severity. Mild exacerbations can be treated as an outpatient, while severe exacerbations may require hospitalization or even ICU admission. Potentially useful tests to evaluate the etiology and severity of the exacerbation include pulse oximetry, chest radiograph, chest CT or CT angiogram, arterial blood gas, electrocardiogram, and complete blood count. Indications for hospitalization can include marked increase in symptoms, severe underlying COPD (e.g., GOLD Grade 3 or 4) or other comorbidities (e.g., cardiovascular disease), onset of new symptoms, and failure of outpatient treatment. Persistent severe dyspnea or gas exchange abnormalities, hemodynamic instability, or altered mental status necessitate ICU admission.

Management of a COPD exacerbation includes three classes of medications – bronchodilators, corticosteroids, and antibiotics – as well as consideration of ventilatory support. For acute exacerbations requiring emergency room visitation or hospitalization, frequent short-acting anticholinergic and beta-agonist bronchodilators are generally used in combination. No clinical studies have evaluated the role of long-acting bronchodilators in this setting. Bronchodilators delivered by nebulization may be more effective than by metered-dose inhaler, since patients are often too dyspneic to use inhalers correctly.

Systemic corticosteroids shorten recovery time and reduce the duration of hospitalization; in a double-blind, placebo-controlled trial, corticosteroids reduced the absolute rate of treatment failure (defined as death, need for intubation, readmission, or intensification of drug therapy) by approximately 10%.[128] This trial demonstrated no additional benefit to a prolonged course of systemic steroids (8 weeks vs. 2 weeks). Strong evidence to support specific steroid dosing is lacking.[129,130] Observational studies suggest that oral therapy in non-critically ill patients is generally preferred,[131] though intravenous steroids may be needed in patients unable to tolerate oral medication or those who are critically ill.[132] A dose of 30 to 40 mg of prednisone or the equivalent for 10 to 14 days is recommended by GOLD, although a recent clinical trial found that a 5-day course of oral corticosteroids may be sufficient.[1]

While bacterial infections appear to be responsible for a large fraction of exacerbations, the benefit of antibiotic use has been only demonstrated in patients who have an increase in either sputum purulence or volume, or require mechanical ventilation.[133–135] Sputum cultures should not be performed routinely, given the likelihood of failure to identify a specific pathogen and the delay in return of results. An exception can be made for patients at higher risk for resistant organisms and/or *Pseudomonas*, such as those with more severe disease or recently hospitalized. The specific choice of antibiotic should be guided by local and patient resistance patterns for likely bacterial pathogens (e.g., *Haemophilus influenzae, Moraxella catarrhalis*, and *Streptococcus pneumoniae* in most patients; pseudomonas in patients with more severe COPD).[127]

Many patients will require supplemental oxygen. Excess administration of oxygen should be avoided as it may precipitate hypercapnia through multiple mechanisms, including increasing perfusion to low V/Q units, the Haldane effect, and decreased respiratory drive.[136,137] A target SpO_2 of 90% to 95% is preferable in the chronically hypercapnic patient rather than providing higher inspired oxygen concentrations to achieve SpO_2 values >95%.

Ventilatory support is an important component in the management of moderate to severe exacerbations. Particularly in more severe exacerbations, arterial blood gas determination should generally be performed, because unlike pulse oximetry it provides an assessment of the severity of hypercapnia and acidosis. Noninvasive ventilation can reduce intubation rates and mortality,[138] and should be considered in patients with severe dyspnea or respiratory acidosis who are not in immediate need of intubation and are candidates for noninvasive ventilation after a careful review of contraindications. A recent meta-analysis of 14 studies, including over 700 patients, found that noninvasive ventilation in hypercapnia ($PaCO_2$ >45 mm Hg) reduced the need for intubation and mortality each by approximately half.[139] This benefit may be present only in those with more severe disease (pH <7.30 or hospital mortality >10%).[140] For intubated COPD patients, mechanical ventilation parameters to consider include maximizing exhalation time and attention to auto-PEEP and cycling-off criteria. Noninvasive ventilation can again be considered to facilitate successful extubation. Further discussion of mechanical ventilation is provided in Chapter 7.

Most patients will begin to recover from an exacerbation within several days, with a median time to recovery to baseline function in one study of 10 to 14 days.[141] Hospitalized patients who are clinically stable for 24 hours, able to return to their baseline long-acting medication with need for short-acting agents less than every 4 hours and lack of nocturnal awakening due to dyspnea can be considered for discharge, with follow-up assessment in 4 to 6 weeks.[1] Patients scheduled for surgery can be reevaluated at this time, though the duration of recovery varies, with a small set of patients never recovering to their baseline.[142]

SUMMARY

COPD is characterized by persistent and usually progressive airflow limitation. While simple to diagnose, misdiagnosis is common. There is substantial heterogeneity in disease both pathophysiologically (with varying components of emphysema, small airways disease, and chronic bronchitis) and in course and outcome (such as degree of lung function impairment, dyspnea, comorbidities, and rates of exacerbations and lung function decline). GOLD-based airflow obstruction grades and groups based on symptoms and exacerbations can be useful in determining severity of disease and appropriate treatment.

Management of stable COPD in the outpatient setting is primarily based on relieving symptoms, improving quality of life, and reducing exacerbations. Only two medically based interventions – smoking cessation and oxygen therapy for subjects who have resting hypoxemia – have been demonstrated to alter the course of disease and improve mortality. Standard medical therapy, usually consisting of inhaled bronchodilators and potentially inhaled steroids, has not been convincingly shown to alter the rate of lung function decline, although one study found a trend toward reduced all-cause mortality.[78] Long-acting bronchodilators should generally be prescribed for at least moderately severe disease. Combination therapy with a second long-acting bronchodilator and/or inhaled corticosteroid should be considered in subjects with more severe symptoms. Pulmonary rehabilitation is an important therapeutic consideration for most symptomatic patients.

COPD exacerbations are defined by an acute worsening of respiratory symptoms that leads to a change in medication, and are a major contributor to morbidity, hospitalizations, and mortality in COPD. The most common trigger for a COPD exacerbation is infection, but many causes of dyspnea can mimic or worsen COPD. Intensified bronchodilator treatment and systemic corticosteroids are the mainstay of therapy. Patients with increased sputum purulence and/or volume or suffering severe exacerbations requiring ventilatory support should receive antibiotics. Noninvasive ventilation in selected patients with hypercapnia has been associated with reduced mortality in exacerbations.

EDITOR'S COMMENT

Clinically relevant disease classifications should ideally provide both an explanation of the mechanism of disease as well as a prediction of the clinical course and response to therapy. An important result of the experience with LVRS is that the best predictor of a good response to LVRS – namely, apical predominant emphysema – is not incorporated into most current classification schemes. This observation suggests we need to fundamentally reevaluate our assumptions about the development and treatment of emphysema.

—Steven J. Mentzer

References

1. Vestob J, Hurd SS, Agustí AG, et al. Global strategy for the diagnosis, management, and prevention of chronic obstructive pulmonary disease: GOLD executive summary. *Am J Respir Crit Care Med.* 2013;187(4):347–65. doi: 10.1164/rccm.201204-0596PP.
2. Miniño AM, Xu J, Kochanek KD. *National Vital Statistics Reports: Deaths: Preliminary Data for 2008.* Hyattsville, MD: National Center for Health Statistics; 2010.
3. Mathers CD, Loncar D. Projections of global mortality and burden of disease from 2002 to 2030. *PLoS Med.* 2006;3:e442.
4. Houghton AM, Mouded M, Shapiro SD. Common origins of lung cancer and COPD. *Nat Med.* 2008;14:1023–1024.
5. Sin DD, Wu L, Man SF. The relationship between reduced lung function and cardiovascular mortality: a population-based study and a systematic review of the literature. *Chest.* 2005;127:1952–1959.
6. Finkelstein J, Cha E, Scharf SM. Chronic obstructive pulmonary disease as an independent risk factor for cardiovascular morbidity. *Int J Chron Obstruct Pulmon Dis.* 2009;4:337–349.
7. Soriano JB, Rigo F, Guerrero D, et al. High prevalence of undiagnosed airflow limitation in patients with cardiovascular disease. *Chest.* 2010;137:333–340.
8. Sekine Y, Yamada Y, Chiyo M, et al. Association of chronic obstructive pulmonary disease and tumor recurrence in patients with stage IA lung cancer after complete resection. *Ann Thorac Surg.* 2007;84:946–950.
9. Turner MC, Chen Y, Krewski D, et al. Chronic obstructive pulmonary disease is associated with lung cancer mortality in a prospective study of never smokers. *Am J Respir Crit Care Med.* 2007;176:285–290.
10. Qaseem A, Snow V, Shekelle P, et al. Diagnosis and management of stable chronic obstructive pulmonary disease: a clinical practice guideline from the American College of Physicians. *Ann Intern Med.* 2007;147:633–638.
11. Roberts SD, Farber MO, Knox KS, et al. FEV1/FVC ratio of 70% misclassifies patients with obstruction at the extremes of age. *Chest.* 2006;130:200–206.
12. Mannino DM, Sonia Buist A, Vollmer WM. Chronic obstructive pulmonary disease in the older adult: what defines abnormal lung function? *Thorax.* 2007;62:237–241.
13. Mannino DM, Diaz-Guzman E. Interpreting lung function data using 80% predicted and fixed thresholds identifies patients at increased risk of mortality. *Chest.* 2011;141:73–80.
14. Cooke CE, Sidel M, Belletti DA, et al. Review: clinical inertia in the management of chronic obstructive pulmonary disease. *COPD.* 2012;9:73–80.
15. Walters JA, Walters EH, Nelson M, et al. Factors associated with misdiagnosis of COPD in primary care. *Prim Care Respir J.* 2011;20:396–402.
16. Rennard SI. COPD: overview of definitions, epidemiology, and factors influencing its development. *Chest.* 1998;113:235S-241S.
17. Wilson DO, Weissfeld JL, Balkan A, et al. Association of radiographic emphysema and airflow obstruction with lung cancer. *Am J Respir Crit Care Med.* 2008;178:738–744.
18. McDonough JE, Yuan R, Suzuki M, et al. Small-airway obstruction and emphysema in chronic obstructive pulmonary disease. *N Engl J Med.* 2011;365:1567–1575.
19. Definition and classification of chronic bronchitis for clinical and epidemiological purposes. A report to the Medical Research Council by their Committee on the Aetiology of Chronic Bronchitis. *Lancet.* 1965;1:775–779.
20. de Oca MM, Halbert RJ, Lopez MV, et al. Chronic bronchitis phenotype in subjects with and without COPD: the PLATINO study. *Eur Respir J.* 2012;40:28–36.
21. Barisione G, Rovida S, Gazzaniga GM, et al. Upper abdominal surgery: does a lung function test exist to predict early severe postoperative respiratory complications? *Eur Respir J.* 1997;10:1301–1308.
22. O'Donnell DE. Hyperinflation, dyspnea, and exercise intolerance in chronic obstructive pulmonary disease. *Proc Am Thorac Soc.* 2006;3:180–184.
23. Wagner PD, Dantzker DR, Dueck R, et al. Ventilation-perfusion inequality in chronic obstructive pulmonary disease. *J Clin Invest.* 1977;59:203–216.
24. Lane DJ, Howell JB, Giblin B. Relation between airways obstruction and CO_2 tension in chronic obstructive airways disease. *Br Med J.* 1968;3:707–709.
25. Burrows B, Knudson RJ, Cline MG, et al. Quantitative relationships between cigarette smoking and ventilatory function. *Am Rev Respir Dis.* 1977;115:195–205.
26. Anthonisen NR, Connett JE, Kiley JP, et al. Effects of smoking intervention and the use of an inhaled anticholinergic bronchodilator on the rate of decline of FEV1. The Lung Health Study. *JAMA.* 1994;272:1497–1505.
27. Balmes J, Becklake M, Blanc P, et al. American Thoracic Society Statement: occupational contribution to the burden of airway disease. *Am J Respir Crit Care Med.* 2003;167:787–797.
28. Torres-Duque C, Maldonado D, Perez-Padilla R, et al. Biomass fuels and respiratory diseases: a review of the evidence. *Proc Am Thorac Soc.* 2008;5:577–590.
29. Cho MH, Castaldi PJ, Wan ES, et al. A genome-wide association study of COPD identifies a susceptibility locus on chromosome 19q13. *Hum Mol Genet.* 2011;21:947–957.
30. Silverman EK, Sandhaus RA. Clinical practice. Alpha1-antitrypsin deficiency. *N Engl J Med.* 2009;360:2749–2757.
31. Vonk JM, Jongepier H, Panhuysen CI, et al. Risk factors associated with the presence of irreversible airflow limitation and reduced transfer coefficient in patients with asthma after 26 years of follow up. *Thorax.* 2003;58:322–327.

32. O'Connor GT, Sparrow D, Weiss ST. A prospective longitudinal study of methacholine airway responsiveness as a predictor of pulmonary-function decline: the Normative Aging Study. *Am J Respir Crit Care Med.* 1995;152:87–92.
33. Lawlor DA, Ebrahim S, Davey Smith G. Association of birth weight with adult lung function: findings from the British Women's Heart and Health Study and a meta-analysis. *Thorax.* 2005;60:851–858.
34. Northway WH, Jr., Moss RB, Carlisle KB, et al. Late pulmonary sequelae of bronchopulmonary dysplasia. *N Engl J Med.* 1990;323:1793–1799.
35. Baraldi E, Filippone M. Chronic lung disease after premature birth. *N Engl J Med.* 2007;357:1946–1955.
36. Washko GR, Criner GJ, Mohsenifar Z, et al. Computed tomographic-based quantification of emphysema and correlation to pulmonary function and mechanics. *COPD.* 2008;5:177–186.
37. Hurst JR, Vestbo J, Anzueto A, et al. Susceptibility to exacerbation in chronic obstructive pulmonary disease. *N Engl J Med.* 2010;363:1128–1138.
38. Celli B, Decramer M, Kesten S, et al. Mortality in the 4-year trial of tiotropium (UPLIFT) in patients with chronic obstructive pulmonary disease. *Am J Respir Crit Care Med.* 2009;180:948–955.
39. Traver GA, Cline MG, Burrows B. Predictors of mortality in chronic obstructive pulmonary disease. A 15-year follow-up study. *Am Rev Respir Dis.* 1979;119:895–902.
40. Celli BR, Cote CG, Marin JM, et al. The body-mass index, airflow obstruction, dyspnea, and exercise capacity index in chronic obstructive pulmonary disease. *N Engl J Med.* 2004;350:1005–1012.
41. Jones PW, Harding G, Berry P, et al. Development and first validation of the COPD Assessment Test. *Eur Respir J.* 2009;34:648–654.
42. Celli BR, Locantore N, Yates J, et al. Inflammatory biomarkers improve clinical prediction of mortality in chronic obstructive pulmonary disease. *Am J Respir Crit Care Med.* 2012;185:1065–1072.
43. Tashkin DP, Celli B, Senn S, et al. A 4-year trial of tiotropium in chronic obstructive pulmonary disease. *N Engl J Med.* 2008;359:1543–1554.
44. Vestbo J, Edwards LD, Scanlon PD, et al. Changes in forced expiratory volume in 1 second over time in COPD. *N Engl J Med.* 2011;365:1184–1192.
45. Nishimura M, Makita H, Nagai K, et al. Annual change in pulmonary function and clinical phenotype in chronic obstructive pulmonary disease. *Am J Respir Crit Care Med.* 2012;185:44–52.
46. Calverley P, Pauwels R, Vestbo J, et al. Combined salmeterol and fluticasone in the treatment of chronic obstructive pulmonary disease: a randomised controlled trial. *Lancet.* 2003;361:449–456.
47. Barr RG, Bluemke DA, Ahmed FS, et al. Percent emphysema, airflow obstruction, and impaired left ventricular filling. *N Engl J Med.* 2010;362:217–227.
48. McGarvey LP, John M, Anderson JA, et al. Ascertainment of cause-specific mortality in COPD: operations of the TORCH Clinical Endpoint Committee. *Thorax.* 2007;62:411–415.
49. Brekke PH, Omland T, Smith P, et al. Underdiagnosis of myocardial infarction in COPD - Cardiac Infarction Injury Score (CIIS) in patients hospitalised for COPD exacerbation. *Respir Med.* 2008;102:1243–1247.
50. Rutten FH, Cramer MJ, Grobbee DE, et al. Unrecognized heart failure in elderly patients with stable chronic obstructive pulmonary disease. *Eur Heart J.* 2005;26:1887–1894.
51. Thabut G, Dauriat G, Stern JB, et al. Pulmonary hemodynamics in advanced COPD candidates for lung volume reduction surgery or lung transplantation. *Chest.* 2005;127:1531–1536.
52. Blanco I, Gimeno E, Munoz PA, et al. Hemodynamic and gas exchange effects of sildenafil in patients with chronic obstructive pulmonary disease and pulmonary hypertension. *Am J Respir Crit Care Med.* 2009;181:270–278.
53. Bon J, Fuhrman CR, Weissfeld JL, et al. Radiographic emphysema predicts low bone mineral density in a tobacco-exposed cohort. *Am J Respir Crit Care Med.* 2010;183:885–890.
54. Hanania NA, Mullerova H, Locantore NW, et al. Determinants of depression in the ECLIPSE chronic obstructive pulmonary disease cohort. *Am J Respir Crit Care Med.* 2010;183:604–611.
55. Ng TP, Niti M, Fones C, et al. Co-morbid association of depression and COPD: a population-based study. *Respir Med.* 2009;103:895–901.
56. Barnes PJ, Celli BR. Systemic manifestations and comorbidities of COPD. *Eur Respir J.* 2009;33:1165–1185.
57. Macchia A, Rodriguez Moncalvo JJ, Kleinert M, et al. Unrecognised ventricular dysfunction in COPD. *Eur Respir J.* 2012;39:51–58.
58. American Thoracic Society/European Respiratory Society statement: standards for the diagnosis and management of individuals with alpha-1 antitrypsin deficiency. *Am J Respir Crit Care Med.* 2003;168:818–900.
59. Anthonisen NR, Skeans MA, Wise RA, et al. The effects of a smoking cessation intervention on 14.5-year mortality: a randomized clinical trial. *Ann Intern Med.* 2005;142:233–239.
60. Birim O, Zuydendorp HM, Maat AP, et al. Lung resection for non-small-cell lung cancer in patients older than 70: mortality, morbidity, and late survival compared with the general population. *Ann Thorac Surg.* 2003;76:1796–1801.
61. Mills E, Eyawo O, Lockhart I, et al. Smoking cessation reduces postoperative complications: a systematic review and meta-analysis. *Am J Med.* 2011;124:144–154.e8.
62. Silverstein P. Smoking and wound healing. *Am J Med.* 1992;93:22S–24S.
63. Gonzales D, Rennard SI, Nides M, et al. Varenicline, an alpha4beta2 nicotinic acetylcholine receptor partial agonist, vs sustained-release bupropion and placebo for smoking cessation: a randomized controlled trial. *JAMA.* 2006;296:47–55.
64. Jorenby DE, Hays JT, Rigotti NA, et al. Efficacy of varenicline, an alpha4beta2 nicotinic acetylcholine receptor partial agonist, vs placebo or sustained-release bupropion for smoking cessation: a randomized controlled trial. *JAMA.* 2006;296:56–63.
65. Wilson DH, Wakefield MA, Steven ID, et al. "Sick of Smoking": evaluation of a targeted minimal smoking cessation intervention in general practice. *Med J Aust.* 1990;152:518–521.
66. Kottke TE, Battista RN, DeFriese GH, et al. Attributes of successful smoking cessation interventions in medical practice. A meta-analysis of 39 controlled trials. *JAMA.* 1988;259:2883–2889.
67. A clinical practice guideline for treating tobacco use and dependence: A US Public Health Service report. The Tobacco Use and Dependence Clinical Practice Guideline Panel, Staff, and Consortium Representatives. *JAMA.* 2000;283:3244–3254.
68. Stead LF, Bergson G, Lancaster T. Physician advice for smoking cessation. *Cochrane Database Syst Rev.* 2008;CD000165.
69. Jorenby DE, Leischow SJ, Nides MA, et al. A controlled trial of sustained-release bupropion, a nicotine patch, or both for smoking cessation. *N Engl J Med.* 1999;340:685–691.
70. Cahill K, Stead LF, Lancaster T. Nicotine receptor partial agonists for smoking cessation. *Cochrane Database Syst Rev.* 2011;CD006103.
71. Rigotti NA, Pipe AL, Benowitz NL, et al. Efficacy and safety of varenicline for smoking cessation in patients with cardiovascular disease: a randomized trial. *Circulation.* 2010;121:221–229.
72. Singh S, Loke YK, Spangler JG, et al. Risk of serious adverse cardiovascular events associated with varenicline: a systematic review and meta-analysis. *CMAJ.* 2011;183:1359–1366.
73. Cobb NK, Abrams DB. E-cigarette or drug-delivery device? Regulating novel nicotine products. *N Engl J Med.* 2011;365:193–195.
74. Calverley PM, Burge PS, Spencer S, et al. Bronchodilator reversibility testing in chronic obstructive pulmonary disease. *Thorax.* 2003;58:659–664.
75. Tashkin D, Kesten S. Long-term treatment benefits with tiotropium in COPD patients with and without short-term bronchodilator responses. *Chest.* 2003;123:1441–1449.
76. In chronic obstructive pulmonary disease, a combination of ipratropium and albuterol is more effective than either agent alone. An 85-day multicenter trial. COMBIVENT Inhalation Aerosol Study Group. *Chest.* 1994;105:1411–1419.
77. Braun SR, Levy SF. Comparison of ipratropium bromide and albuterol in chronic obstructive pulmonary disease: a three-center study. *Am J Med.* 1991;91:28S–32S.
78. Calverley PM, Anderson JA, Celli B, et al. Salmeterol and fluticasone propionate and survival in chronic obstructive pulmonary disease. *N Engl J Med.* 2007;356:775–789.
79. Rodrigo GJ, Nannini LJ, Rodriguez-Roisin R. Safety of long-acting beta-agonists in stable COPD: a systematic review. *Chest.* 2008;133:1079–1087.
80. Khorfan FM, Smith P, Watt S, et al. Effects of nebulized bronchodilator therapy on heart rate and arrhythmias in critically ill adult patients. *Chest.* 2011;140:1466–1472.
81. Michele TM, Pinheiro S, Iyasu S. The safety of tiotropium–the FDA's conclusions. *N Engl J Med.* 2010;363:1097–1099.
82. Vogelmeier C, Hederer B, Glaab T, et al. Tiotropium versus salmeterol for the prevention of exacerbations of COPD. *N Engl J Med.* 2011;364:1093–1103.
83. Donohue JF, Fogarty C, Lotvall J, et al. Once-daily bronchodilators for chronic obstructive pulmonary disease: indacaterol versus tiotropium. *Am J Respir Crit Care Med.* 2010;182:155–162.

84. Buhl R, Dunn LJ, Disdier C, et al. Blinded 12-week comparison of once-daily indacaterol and tiotropium in COPD. *Eur Respir J*. 2011;38:797–803.
85. Zhou Y, Wang X, Zeng X, et al. Positive benefits of theophylline in a randomized, double-blind, parallel-group, placebo-controlled study of low-dose, slow-release theophylline in the treatment of COPD for 1 year. *Respirology*. 2006;11:603–610.
86. ZuWallack RL, Mahler DA, Reilly D, et al. Salmeterol plus theophylline combination therapy in the treatment of COPD. *Chest*. 2001;119:1661–1670.
87. Murciano D, Auclair MH, Pariente R, et al. A randomized, controlled trial of theophylline in patients with severe chronic obstructive pulmonary disease. *N Engl J Med*. 1989;320:1521–1525.
88. Highland KB, Strange C, Heffner JE. Long-term effects of inhaled corticosteroids on FEV1 in patients with chronic obstructive pulmonary disease. A meta-analysis. *Ann Intern Med*. 2003;138:969–973.
89. Crim C, Calverley PM, Anderson JA, et al. Pneumonia risk in COPD patients receiving inhaled corticosteroids alone or in combination: TORCH study results. *Eur Respir J*. 2009;34:641–647.
90. Calverley PM, Stockley RA, Seemungal TA, et al. Reported pneumonia in patients with COPD: findings from the INSPIRE study. *Chest*. 2010;139: 505–512.
91. Rice KL, Rubins JB, Lebahn F, et al. Withdrawal of chronic systemic corticosteroids in patients with COPD: a randomized trial. *Am J Respir Crit Care Med*. 2000;162:174–178.
92. Nannini LJ, Cates CJ, Lasserson TJ, et al. Combined corticosteroid and long-acting beta-agonist in one inhaler versus long-acting beta-agonists for chronic obstructive pulmonary disease. *Cochrane Database Syst Rev*. 2007:CD006829.
93. Aaron SD, Vandemheen KL, Fergusson D, et al. Tiotropium in combination with placebo, salmeterol, or fluticasone-salmeterol for treatment of chronic obstructive pulmonary disease: a randomized trial. *Ann Intern Med*. 2007;146:545–555.
94. Welte T, Miravitlles M, Hernandez P, et al. Efficacy and tolerability of budesonide/formoterol added to tiotropium in patients with chronic obstructive pulmonary disease. *Am J Respir Crit Care Med*. 2009;180:741–750.
95. Short PM, Williamson PA, Elder DH, et al. The impact of tiotropium on mortality and exacerbations when added to inhaled corticosteroids and long-acting beta-agonist therapy in COPD. *Chest*. 2011;141:81–86.
96. Karner C, Cates CJ. The effect of adding inhaled corticosteroids to tiotropium and long-acting beta(2)-agonists for chronic obstructive pulmonary disease. *Cochrane Database Syst Rev*. 2011;9:CD009039.
97. Calverley PM, Rabe KF, Goehring UM, et al. Roflumilast in symptomatic chronic obstructive pulmonary disease: two randomised clinical trials. *Lancet*. 2009;374:685–694.
98. Wongsurakiat P, Maranetra KN, Wasi C, et al. Acute respiratory illness in patients with COPD and the effectiveness of influenza vaccination: a randomized controlled study. *Chest*. 2004;125:2011–2020.
99. Tata LJ, West J, Harrison T, et al. Does influenza vaccination increase consultations, corticosteroid prescriptions, or exacerbations in subjects with asthma or chronic obstructive pulmonary disease? *Thorax*. 2003;58: 835–839.
100. Seemungal TA, Wilkinson TM, Hurst JR, et al. Long-term erythromycin therapy is associated with decreased chronic obstructive pulmonary disease exacerbations. *Am J Respir Crit Care Med*. 2008;178:1139–1147.
101. Albert RK, Connett J, Bailey WC, et al. Azithromycin for prevention of exacerbations of COPD. *N Engl J Med*. 2011;365:689–698.
102. Decramer M, Rutten-van Molken M, Dekhuijzen PN, et al. Effects of N-acetylcysteine on outcomes in chronic obstructive pulmonary disease (Bronchitis Randomized on NAC Cost-Utility Study, BRONCUS): a randomised placebo-controlled trial. *Lancet*. 2005;365:1552–1560.
103. Zheng JP, Kang J, Huang SG, et al. Effect of carbocisteine on acute exacerbation of chronic obstructive pulmonary disease (PEACE Study): a randomised placebo-controlled study. *Lancet*. 2008;371:2013–2018.
104. Poole P, Black PN, Cates CJ. Mucolytic agents for chronic bronchitis or chronic obstructive pulmonary disease. *Cochrane Database Syst Rev*. 2010: CD001287.
105. Lacasse Y, Martin S, Lasserson TJ, et al. Meta-analysis of respiratory rehabilitation in chronic obstructive pulmonary disease. A Cochrane systematic review. *Eura Medicophys*. 2007;43:475–485.
106. Nici L, Donner C, Wouters E, et al. American Thoracic Society/European Respiratory Society statement on pulmonary rehabilitation. *Am J Respir Crit Care Med*. 2006;173:1390–1413.
107. Puhan MA, Scharplatz M, Troosters T, et al. Respiratory rehabilitation after acute exacerbation of COPD may reduce risk for readmission and mortality – a systematic review. *Respir Res*. 2005;6:54.
108. Ries AL, Make BJ, Lee SM, et al. The effects of pulmonary rehabilitation in the national emphysema treatment trial. *Chest*. 2005;128:3799–3809.
109. Weiner P, Magadle R, Beckerman M, et al. Maintenance of inspiratory muscle training in COPD patients: one year follow-up. *Eur Respir J*. 2004;23: 61–65.
110. Ringbaek T, Brondum E, Martinez G, et al. Rehabilitation in COPD: the long-term effect of a supervised 7-week program succeeded by a self-monitored walking program. *Chron Respir Dis*. 2008;5:75–80.
111. Janaudis-Ferreira T, Hill K, Goldstein RS, et al. Resistance arm training in patients with COPD: a randomized controlled trial. *Chest*. 2010;139: 151–158.
112. Cano NJ, Roth H, Court-Ortune I, et al. Nutritional depletion in patients on long-term oxygen therapy and/or home mechanical ventilation. *Eur Respir J*. 2002;20:30–37.
113. Schols AM, Slangen J, Volovics L, et al. Weight loss is a reversible factor in the prognosis of chronic obstructive pulmonary disease. *Am J Respir Crit Care Med*. 1998;157:1791–1797.
114. Continuous or nocturnal oxygen therapy in hypoxemic chronic obstructive lung disease: a clinical trial. Nocturnal Oxygen Therapy Trial Group. *Ann Intern Med*. 1980;93:391–398.
115. Long term domiciliary oxygen therapy in chronic hypoxic cor pulmonale complicating chronic bronchitis and emphysema. Report of the Medical Research Council Working Party. *Lancet*. 1981;1:681–686.
116. Emtner M, Porszasz J, Burns M, et al. Benefits of supplemental oxygen in exercise training in nonhypoxemic chronic obstructive pulmonary disease patients. *Am J Respir Crit Care Med*. 2003;168:1034–1042.
117. Dean NC, Brown JK, Himelman RB, et al. Oxygen may improve dyspnea and endurance in patients with chronic obstructive pulmonary disease and only mild hypoxemia. *Am Rev Respir Dis*. 1992;146:941–945.
118. Calverley PM, Brezinova V, Douglas NJ, . The effect of oxygenation on sleep quality in chronic bronchitis and emphysema. *Am Rev Respir Dis*. 1982;126:206–210.
119. Fletcher EC, Luckett RA, Goodnight-White S, et al. A double-blind trial of nocturnal supplemental oxygen for sleep desaturation in patients with chronic obstructive pulmonary disease and a daytime PaO2 above 60 mm Hg. *Am Rev Respir Dis*. 1992;145:1070–1076.
120. Nonoyama ML, Brooks D, Guyatt GH, et al. Effect of oxygen on health quality of life in patients with chronic obstructive pulmonary disease with transient exertional hypoxemia. *Am J Respir Crit Care Med*. 2007;176: 343–349.
121. Kim V, Benditt JO, Wise RA, et al. Oxygen therapy in chronic obstructive pulmonary disease. *Proc Am Thorac Soc*. 2008;5:513–518.
122. Shrikrishna D, Coker RK. Managing passengers with stable respiratory disease planning air travel: British Thoracic Society recommendations. *Thorax*. 2011;66:831–833.
123. Ingenito EP, Wood DE, Utz JP. Bronchoscopic lung volume reduction in severe emphysema. *Proc Am Thorac Soc*. 2008;5:454–460.
124. Slebos DJ, Klooster K, Ernst A, et al. Bronchoscopic lung volume reduction coil treatment of patients with severe heterogeneous emphysema. *Chest*. 2011;142(3):574-582.
125. Masoli M, Weatherall M, Holt S, et al. Inhaled fluticasone propionate and adrenal effects in adult asthma: systematic review and meta-analysis. *Eur Respir J*. 2006;28:960–967.
126. Rizkallah J, Man SF, Sin DD. Prevalence of pulmonary embolism in acute exacerbations of COPD: a systematic review and metaanalysis. *Chest*. 2009;135:786–793.
127. Wedzicha JA, Seemungal TA. COPD exacerbations: defining their cause and prevention. *Lancet*. 2007;370:786–796.
128. Niewoehner DE, Erbland ML, Deupree RH, et al. Effect of systemic glucocorticoids on exacerbations of chronic obstructive pulmonary disease. Department of Veterans Affairs Cooperative Study Group. *N Engl J Med*. 1999;340:1941–1947.
129. Walters JA, Gibson PG, Wood-Baker R, et al. Systemic corticosteroids for acute exacerbations of chronic obstructive pulmonary disease. *Cochrane Database Syst Rev*. 2009;CD001288.
130. Walters JA, Wang W, Morley C, et al. Different durations of corticosteroid therapy for exacerbations of chronic obstructive pulmonary disease. *Cochrane Database Syst Rev*. 2011;CD006897.

131. Lindenauer PK, Pekow PS, Lahti MC, et al. Association of corticosteroid dose and route of administration with risk of treatment failure in acute exacerbation of chronic obstructive pulmonary disease. *JAMA*. 2010;303:2359–2367.
132. Alia I, de la Cal MA, Esteban A, et al. Efficacy of corticosteroid therapy in patients with an acute exacerbation of chronic obstructive pulmonary disease receiving ventilatory support. *Arch Intern Med*. 2011;171:1939–1946.
133. Ram FS, Rodriguez-Roisin R, Granados-Navarrete A, et al. Antibiotics for exacerbations of chronic obstructive pulmonary disease. *Cochrane Database Syst Rev*. 2006:CD004403.
134. Quon BS, Gan WQ, Sin DD. Contemporary management of acute exacerbations of COPD: a systematic review and metaanalysis. *Chest*. 2008;133:756–766.
135. Nouira S, Marghli S, Belghith M, et al. Once daily oral ofloxacin in chronic obstructive pulmonary disease exacerbation requiring mechanical ventilation: a randomised placebo-controlled trial. *Lancet*. 2001;358:2020–2025.
136. Aubier M, Murciano D, Milic-Emili J, et al. Effects of the administration of O_2 on ventilation and blood gases in patients with chronic obstructive pulmonary disease during acute respiratory failure. *Am Rev Respir Dis*. 1980;122:747–754.
137. Malhotra A, Schwartz DR, Ayas N, et al. Treatment of oxygen-induced hypercapnia. *Lancet*. 2001;357:884–885.
138. Brochard L, Mancebo J, Wysocki M, et al. Noninvasive ventilation for acute exacerbations of chronic obstructive pulmonary disease. *N Engl J Med*. 1995;333:817–822.
139. Ram FS, Picot J, Lightowler J, et al. Non-invasive positive pressure ventilation for treatment of respiratory failure due to exacerbations of chronic obstructive pulmonary disease. *Cochrane Database Syst Rev*. 2004;CD004104.
140. Keenan SP, Sinuff T, Cook DJ, et al. Which patients with acute exacerbation of chronic obstructive pulmonary disease benefit from noninvasive positive-pressure ventilation? A systematic review of the literature. *Ann Intern Med*. 2003;138:861–870.
141. Aaron SD, Donaldson GC, Whitmore GA, et al. Time course and pattern of COPD exacerbation onset. *Thorax*. 2012;67:238–243.
142. Seemungal TA, Donaldson GC, Bhowmik A, et al. Time course and recovery of exacerbations in patients with chronic obstructive pulmonary disease. *Am J Respir Crit Care Med*. 2000;161:1608–1613.

98 Resection of Blebs, Bullae, and Giant Bullae

Joshua R. Sonett

Keywords: Blebs, giant bullae, bullous disease, emphysema, spontaneous pneumothorax, bullectomy

The pulmonary bleb is a small subpleural collection of air located within the layers of the visceral pleura. Such lesions usually present symptomatically, heralded by a spontaneous pneumothorax. Blebs represent the coalescence of air from small ruptures of terminal alveoli that have dissected through the interstitium to form a small subpleural collection. Lesions that result in spontaneous pneumothorax are located predominantly in the apex of the upper lobe or the apex of the superior segment. Multiple blebs are often identified. Most patients with blebs are without significant underlying lung disease. Pathologically, bleb formation occurs secondary to mechanical stress from increased intrathoracic pressure in the lung tissue that is predisposed to deformation by congenital weakness of the connective tissue. The bleb often forms at the lung apex, where there is increased mechanical stress.[1] Surgical therapy thus is oriented to the apex of the lung.

The bulla is a larger (>1 cm) airspace collection that forms within the parenchyma. The bulla has a fibrous wall and remnants of lung parenchyma, as evidenced by septations and fragments of the alveolar septa. A significant bulla usually presents with symptoms of dyspnea; however, patients also may have pneumothorax, infection, or carcinoma. The practical classification of bullous disease separates patients into two primary groups: those with normal underlying lung and a predominant single bulla versus those with diffuse underlying emphysema and very often multiple bullae. A large single bulla that encompasses more than 30% of the hemithorax is defined as a giant bulla.

The physiology of bulla growth is associated with a parenchymal weakness in the lung that fills preferentially with air. Secondarily, the force of elastic recoil in adjacent lung produces retraction of the surrounding lung and further enlargement of the bulla.[2] Thus, the adjacent nonbullous lung tissue becomes atelectatic and nonfunctional. *Identification and restoration of this potentially normal underlying lung are keys to patient selection and surgical therapy.*

GENERAL PRINCIPLES AND PATIENT SELECTION

Virtually, all operative interventions for blebs, bullae, and giant bullae should now be performed using minimally invasive thoracoscopic techniques.

Operative procedures for bleb resection are primarily indicated secondary to the pneumothorax. Thus, the operative principle involves identification of the pulmonary bleb, stapled resection, and a procedure to increase pleural symphysis. Initial treatment of patients with spontaneous pneumothorax should be nonoperative therapy, with chest tube placement. Smaller percutaneous tubes are now available that may function as well as larger tubes and are less painful for the patient. Swift resolution of the pneumothorax and air leak should follow, permitting rapid removal of the tube. Failure of the pneumothorax or air leak to resolve in 4 to 7 days warrants consideration of operative intervention. Pneumothorax recurs at a rate of 20% to 30% with nonoperative therapy, with the greatest incidence in the first 2 years.[3] Patients who present with recurrent pneumothorax should have surgical intervention because the recurrence rate after failure of initial conservative therapy approaches 50%. Occasionally, patients with high-risk occupations, such as pilots and scuba divers, may be considered for surgical resection at initial presentation. This author does not believe any evidence exits to support operative intervention at the initial presentation until the patient has failed conservative therapy. In addition, there is no evidence to support pre-emptive thoracoscopy on the contralateral side that has been unaffected by pneumothorax.

While patients with bulla (single or multiple) may present with pneumothorax or dyspnea, patients with giant bulla are more likely to present with dyspnea alone. Surgical resection with therapy for pleural symphysis should be offered to patients who present with pneumothorax and a previously identified bulla. Patients presenting with dyspnea, however, require careful and deliberate preoperative evaluation to quantify the risks and potential benefits of resection. Determining the extent and viability of compromised nonbullous lung tissue is essential to this evaluation because the primary goal of resection is to return gas exchange to more normal values, improve mechanical pulmonary function, and preserve normal lung parenchyma.

Bullous lesions can be easily approached with thoracoscopy. Studies of bleb resection and pleural abrasion have documented similar results for thoracoscopy and thoracotomy, and the feasibility of giant bulla resection with thoracoscopy is well documented.[4–6] In addition to reducing pain in the postoperative interval and permitting a more rapid recovery, thoracoscopy may enhance operative examination of the lung and diaphragm. Essential elements of the horoscopic approach include the use of buttressed stapling lines in patients with bullous disease or giant bulla, port placement that avoids injury to the intercostal nerve bundles, and removal of lung tissue from the chest in a protected specimen bag to avoid seeding of potentially occult carcinoma.

PREOPERATIVE ASSESSMENT

Preoperative assessment of patients presenting with bleb disease and spontaneous pneumothorax may be limited. Presently, however, given the low-dose nature of CT scans, all patients presenting with spontaneous pneumothorax should have CT assessment. In younger patients without risk factors, such as smoking, CT is used to rule out congenital lesions and/or high-risk bilateral blebs or bullae. In older patients or those with a significant smoking history, CT scan of the chest should be performed to rule out possible occult carcinoma or bulla. Patients with any evidence of interstitial lung disease or an inflammatory process also should undergo CT scan evaluation and preoperative assessment to discern any possible predisposing medical conditions, such as lymphangiomyotosis (LAM), sarcoid, and other connective tissue disorders. Patients who are immunocompromised (e.g., by immunosuppression or HIV infection) or who have a high suspicion of Pneumocystis pneumonia or other infectious disease should be investigated and treated before operative intervention.

Female patients with recurrent pneumothorax should be evaluated in regard to the timing of their menstrual cycle to assess the possibility of catamenial pneumothorax. If the patient has had recurrent pneumothoraces or pain associated in a regular manner with their menses, then endometriosis and/or systemic hormonal effects may be an important causative agent in the pneumothorax. This is critically important to determine preoperatively, as the treatments, both medical and surgical, are substantially changed if catamenial pneumothorax is suspected. In patients with catamenial pneumothorax, operative intervention is directed at the diaphragm to rule out fenestration defects.

For surgery to be successful in patients with giant bullae, the atelectatic lung must be able to expand and regain function after resection of the bulla or bullous disease. Thus, patients who have a single giant bulla with relatively normal although atelectatic residual lung are ideal candidates for bullectomy. Unfortunately, most patients with bullous disease also have varying degrees of underlying emphysema and compromised lung parenchyma. Radiographic and physiologic testing is used to quantify the extent and viability of the nonbullous compromised lung tissue to define suitable candidates for bullectomy.[7] A CT angiogram may facilitate the identification of lung parenchyma and vasculature that is viable but compressed. Quantitative ventilation/perfusion determination should be used to help quantify hypoperfusion to the target areas of bullectomy and flow to the relatively compressed viable lung tissue. Patients with no evidence of viable lung tissue, the so-called vanishing lung, are not candidates for bullectomy. Patients who experience hypercarbia and hypoxia with exercise have been shown in general to have less benefit.[8] However, definitive results are best predicted by anatomy, and ideal anatomy may trump even very low forced expiratory volume in 1 second (FEV_1) (e.g., <20%). Diffusing capacity of the lung for carbon monoxide (D_{LCO}) is a predictable reflection of the viability of nonbullous lung tissue, and patients with preserved D_{LCO} tend to have better results.[9] Finally, complete cardiopulmonary exercise testing and distance walked in 6 minutes may help to quantitate the preoperative reserve of the patient and further assess the risk of the procedure. Patients undergoing elective surgery should undergo pulmonary rehabilitation and should not be active smokers.

TECHNIQUES

Anesthesia

All patients require double-lumen endotracheal intubation for single-lung ventilation. Patients with bullous disease who have underlying emphysema should have an epidural catheter placed preoperatively; ideally, the catheter should be used during the procedure. Patients with emphysema also should undergo bronchoscopy before the endotracheal tube is placed to clear the airway of significant secretions before the procedure. Great care should be taken by the anesthesiologist to avoid high peak airway pressures and barotrauma. This may require permissive hypercapnia as well as tolerance of hypoxemia. It is critical and should be the expectation of the operative team that patients will be extubated in the OR, thus avoiding continued positive-pressure ventilation that exacerbates pulmonary air leak.

Surgical Management

Thoracoscopy is ideally suited for the resection of blebs, bullae, and giant bullous disease. All patients should be in the lateral decubitus position and optimally flexed at the hip to maximize rib separation. The superior arm should be supported above the plane of the shoulder to permit access to the chest anterior to the scapula with access to the axillary fold. In general, ports should be placed as far anteriorly as possible to take advantage of the wider intercostal interspaces on the anterior chest wall, thus decreasing torsion injury to the intercostal nerves. I almost never place port access posterior to the scapula. Before the ports are placed, Marcaine and epinephrine should be used for intercostal nerve block to limit the nuisance of blood dripping from the port sites and to enhance pain control. A general depiction of port placement is given below; however, after initial camera port placement, definitive placement of the manipulating port and stapling ports should be directed by the thoracoscopic exploration. This can be done by placing a needle into the chest at the proposed port access sites. An additional caveat: Lung tissue that is not intended for resection should never be grasped during the conduct of the operation because of the risk of inadvertent air leaks caused by manual manipulation.

SURGICAL TECHNIQUES FOR SPONTANEOUS PNEUMOTHORAX

Bleb Resection

Figure 98-1 illustrates possible port placement for patients presenting with spontaneous pneumothorax. Note that the "operative triangle" is placed in the anterior axillary region; the largest stapling port is placed in the anterior position. Exploration is begun with a 5-mm, 30-degree scope. The posterior axillary port may either be a 5-mm port or an incision to place a curved sponge stick. This access port is used to manipulate the lung for exploration. Examination of the entire lung parenchyma is undertaken with explicit attention to the apical segment of the upper lobe and the superior segment of the lower lobe. Identified blebs are stapled using a 35-mm device with 3.5-mm "blue" stapler loads and with resection of minimal lung tissue.

In a multi-institutional study reported by Naunheim et al.,[10] blebs were identified in more than one lobe in 10% of the patients, and in 9% of patients, no bleb could be identified. When no discrete bleb is identified, great care should be taken to look for areas of scarring or visceral pleural changes on the lung that could represent changes from a decompressed bleb. Even if no abnormalities are found, apical stapling of the upper lobe still should be performed. It is important to resect as little normal lung as possible, especially taking note that in young patients the elastic recoil of the lung is so effective that seemingly small resections can result

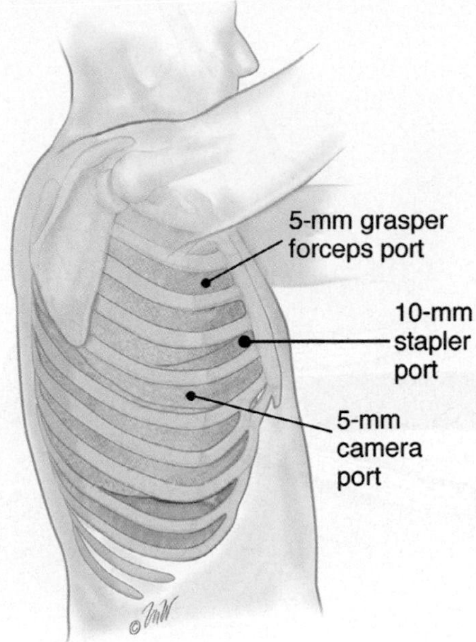

Figure 98-1. Port placement for spontaneous pneumothorax. The operative triangle is located in the anterior axillary region, with largest stapling port in the anterior position.

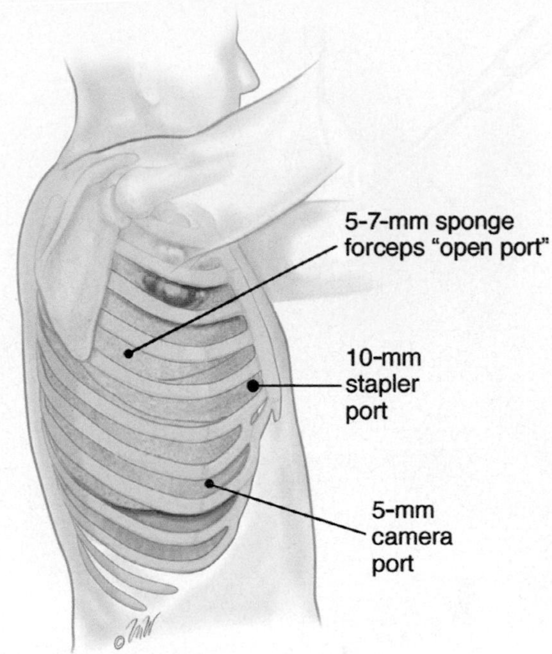

Figure 98-2. Port placement for giant bullous disease. The operative triangle is shifted caudad but still maintains an anterior orientation.

in a significant loss of lung volume. Specimens are removed from the chest either in a protected bag or within the confines of the largest port. Pleural abrasion then should be performed; my present preference is to perform an apical pleurectomy, and this can easily be performed thoracoscopically.

Mechanical abrasion with the aid of a folded Bovie scratch pad or endoscopic peanut can complete the procedure for the lower lateral chest cavity. Talc insufflation should be avoided because the long-term effects are not well defined, and the severe granulomatous reaction may impede future possible thoracic interventions. A single no. 24 chest tube is placed into the most inferior (5-mm) port; thoracoscopic visualization of the tube placement is always performed. To minimize barotrauma to the dependent lung, the contralateral "down" lung is clamped during reexpansion of the operative lung. Active expansion of the lung during ventilation is observed. The chest tube is placed on suction and kept on suction during postoperative day 1 to help promote pleural symphysis. The tube may be removed and the patient discharged on postoperative day 2, provided there are no persistent air leaks.

Resection of Bullous and Giant Bullous Disease

After initial placement of the double-lumen tube, single-lung ventilation should commence as soon as possible to avoid further hyperinflation of the bullous disease on the operative side and to facilitate decompression of the bulla. Figure 98-2 illustrates operative port placement for giant bullous disease (Fig. 98-3). Note that the "operative triangle" is shifted more caudad but still maintains an anterior orientation. If the bullous lesion is based in an inferior portion of the chest, the triangle may be shifted even lower. Again, a 5-mm, 30-degree scope is placed to explore the chest initially. Relatively normal or spared lung should become atelectatic at a faster rate than lung tissue with bullous disease, exaggerating the demarcation between the most diseased and the relatively normal lung parenchyma. The operative course is enhanced by early decompression of the giant bulla or bullous area using a long Bovie-tip electrocautery (Fig. 98-4). The now deflated bulla is grasped at its apex, and the demarcation between bullous and nonbullous disease is delineated with either a sponge stick or thoracoscopic Landreneau masher (Pilling

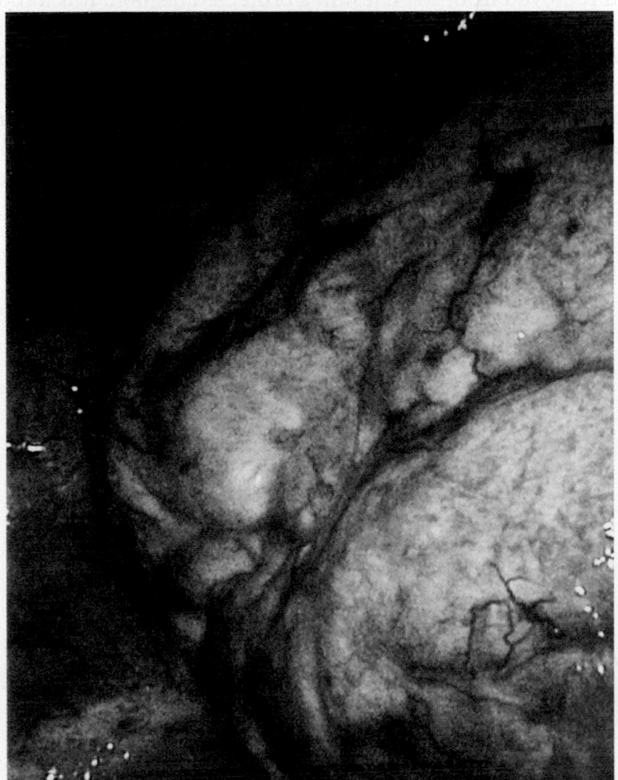

Figure 98-3. Intraoperative photograph of giant bulla.

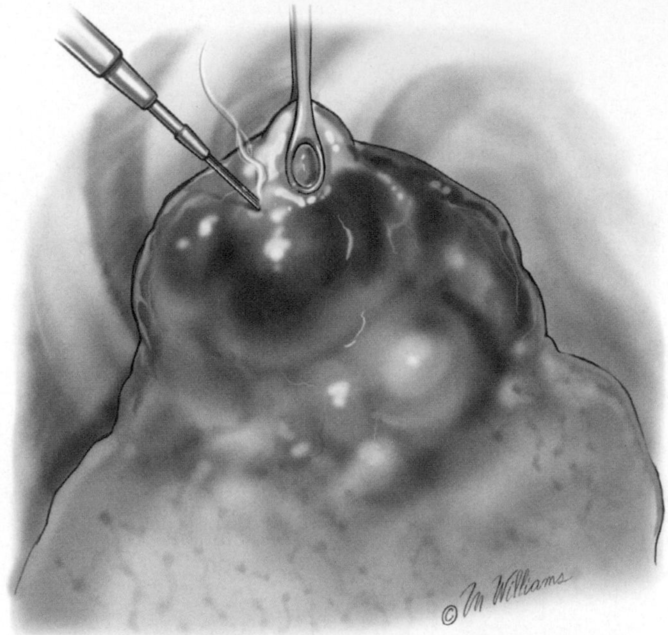

Figure 98-4. The giant bulla or bullous area is decompressed using a long Bovie-tip electrocautery.

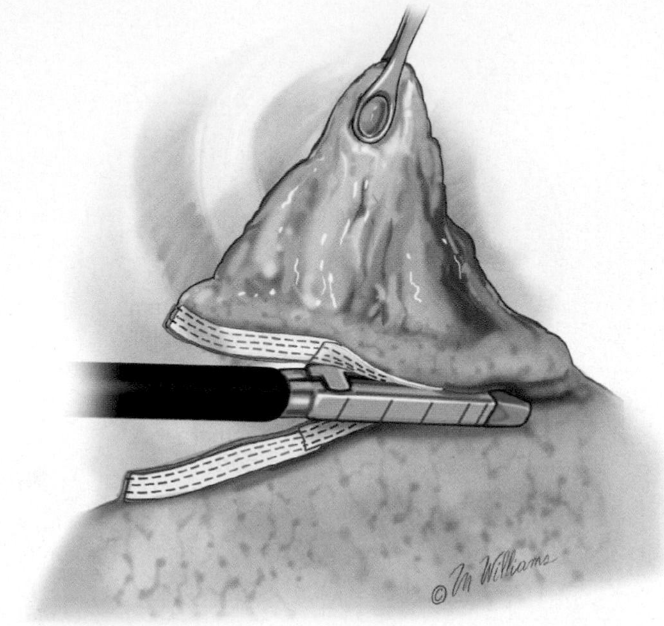

Figure 98-6. The base of the bulla then is plicated using a 45-mm long linear stapler with buttressed support.

Surgical, Teleflex, Inc., Research Triangle Park, NC) (Fig. 98-5). The base of the bulla then is plicated using a 45-mm long linear stapler with buttressed support (Fig. 98-6).

Great care is taken to plicate the bulla completely to avoid any residuum while retaining as much normal tissue as possible. The resected bulla then is placed in an endoscopic bag and removed from the chest in a protected fashion. It is important to remove the tissue in this manner to avoid seeding the chest or chest wall in the case of occult carcinoma or infection. Pleural management with apical pleurectomy and inferior abrasion then should be performed. In patients with limited lung reexpansion, consideration may be given to the development of an apical pleural tent. One 24 chest tube is left in place;

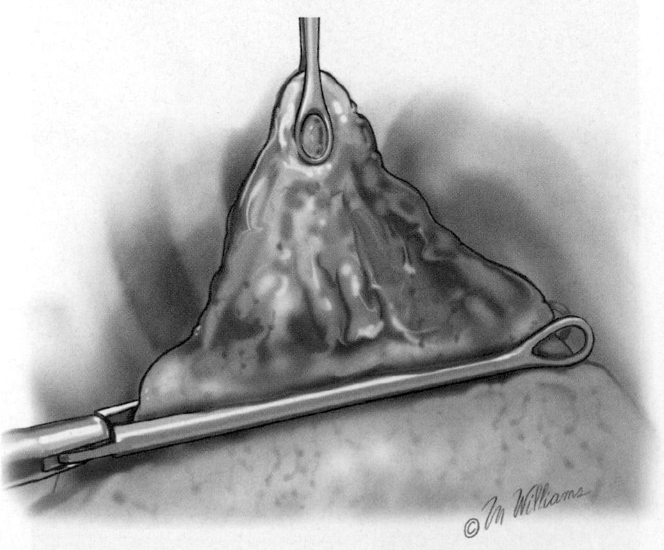

Figure 98-5. After deflating the bulla, it is grasped at its apex. The line between bullous and nonbullous disease is delineated with the aid of a sponge stick or Landreneau masher (latter shown in figure).

preferentially, this should be placed on water seal. Bullae present in the mid to lower lung field (Fig. 98-7) can appear to be intraparenchymal. However, the resection principle is similar to the giant bullae in the apex (Fig. 98-8).

Catamenial Pneumothorax

It is important to note that the surgical approach to recurrent pneumothorax due to catamenial pneumothorax is significantly different from a standard bleb resection. Treating these

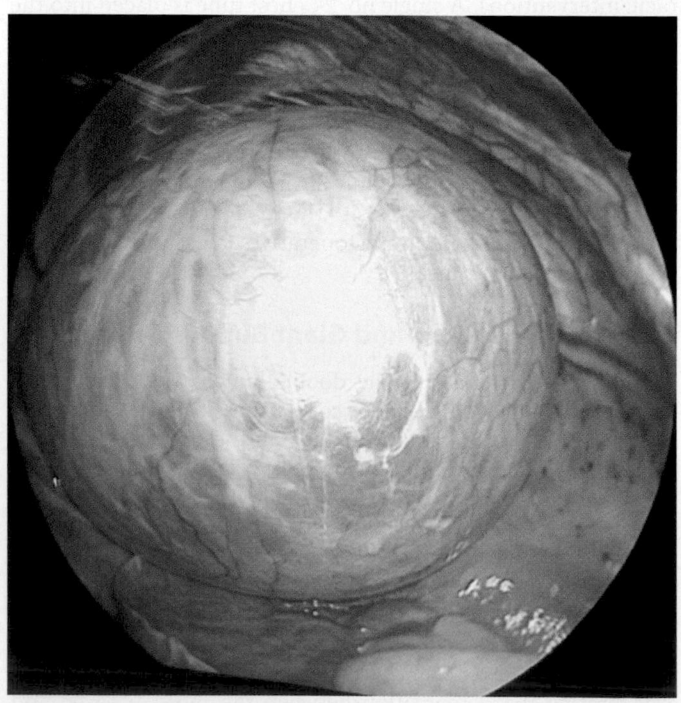

Figure 98-7. Photograph of bulla.

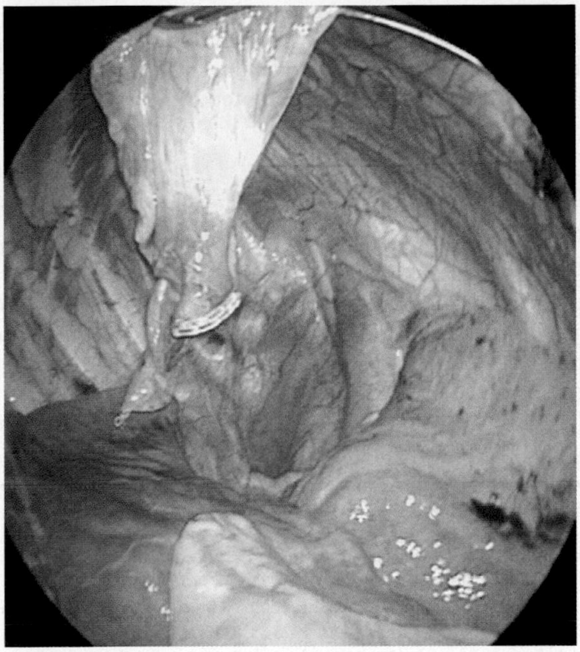

Figure 98-8. Photograph of bulla postresection.

patients in the traditional manner will predictably fail. Initial consideration in these patients is ovulation suppression with hormonal therapy, such as birth control pills. I routinely refer these patients to a GYN specialist in this regard. This may be an appealing approach to patients nearing menopause. In regard to surgical therapy, although a thorough exploration of blebs and/or endometrial lung implants is performed, the primary pathology tends to be diaphragmatic fenestrations. These should be approached thoracoscopically with primary repair of any fenestrations, and then placement of biologic patch on the diaphragmatic surface. The initial ports are placed low on the chest cavity to enable better access to the diaphragm.

POSTOPERATIVE MANAGEMENT

Postoperative management is straightforward for primary bleb resection for pneumothorax. In these patients, the chest tube is left on suction during postoperative day 1 to promote pleural symphysis. The tube may be removed on postoperative day 2 if no leak is apparent, and the patient can be discharged to home. The patient is instructed to limit activities that significantly increase intrathoracic pressure for 4 weeks.

The postoperative care of patients with bullous or giant bullous disease may be more challenging depending on the extent of the underlying emphysema. The operative and anesthetic plan should provide for extubation in the OR. Postoperative hypercarbia should be tolerated unless it is accompanied by systemic acidosis. Oxygen supplementation should be used only as needed to keep saturations above 90%. Excellent pain control, preferably with an epidural, is essential to avoid splinting, atelectasis, and retained secretions. Intravenous nonsteroidal anti-inflammatory medication may enhance pain control significantly. The patient should be mobilized out of bed as early as possible starting on the day of surgery, and physical therapy should begin on postoperative day 1. *The chest tubes are preferentially placed on water seal as long as there is pleural apposition on chest x-ray.* For patients with extensive air leaks, early placement of the chest tube to Heimlich valve may facilitate resolution of the leak. Patients with persistent leak with Heimlich valve in place may be discharged to home and assessed on a weekly basis.

COMPLICATIONS

Prolonged air leak is the primary morbidity of patients undergoing significant bullectomy and occurs in 30% to 50% of patients. Intraoperative techniques, including the use of buttressed sutures and strict adherence to a no-touch technique with respect to all lung tissue that is not intended for resection, may help to decrease the severity and duration of air leaks. Early placement to water seal and Heimlich valve will facilitate earlier resolution of air leaks. Frequently, significant air leaks are accompanied by subcutaneous emphysema. Subcutaneous emphysema is a benign process predominantly, but it can be palliated by placing the chest tubes to suction. In severe cases, subcutaneous emphysema also may be palliated by venting/incising the skin and decompressing the patient. With time, air leaks virtually always resolve, and one should be able to avoid reoperation.

Respiratory failure may occur postoperatively and primarily reflects high-risk patients with lower FEV_1 and/or low D_{LCO} values. Patients with a bronchial component to their symptoms may require frequent postoperative bronchoscopy and may have a higher incidence of respiratory complications. Pneumonia is often encountered during an extended hospital course and should be treated aggressively. Other common complications include atrial fibrillation and bowel complications. Gastrointestinal complications may include Ogilvie type colonic distention, ischemic colitis, and Clostridium difficile colitis. Aggressive early intervention and attention to these issues may reduce potential morbidity and mortality significantly. Adequate pain control is an essential component of the patient's postoperative pulmonary function and airway clearance. Even with thoracoscopy, a well-functioning epidural is essential.

Uncommon complications may include bleeding, reexpansion pulmonary edema,[11] and even chronic pain. These complications may be avoided with careful surgical technique and gentle reexpansion of the lung. Most chronic pain can be avoided by placing the ports in anterior portions of the chest to take advantage of wider interspaces and by placing torque on the intercostal vessels and nerves.

RESULTS

The results of treatment of spontaneous pneumothorax are well documented. Present-day techniques with video-assisted thoracic surgery (VATS) should be considered the standard of care. Naunhiem et al.[10] have reported their early results using VATS. Of 113 patients, there were no deaths, no episodes of postoperative bleeding, and the incidence of recurrent pneumothorax was only 4.1%. The only predictor for recurrence was failure to identify and ablate a bleb at operation, resulting in a 23% recurrence rate versus 1.8% when the bleb was identified properly and ablated. A larger and more recent publication by Liu et al.[12] reported 757 patients treated using VATS for spontaneous pneumothorax. In 49 patients of this series, no blebs or bullae were identified. A recurrence rate of 2.1% was reported for the entire cohort. Increased recurrence was documented in patients with no blebs identified at initial operation and, to a lesser extent, for patients with multiple blebs.

The group at Barnes-Jewish Hospital in St. Louis, Missouri, has reported outcomes after resection of giant emphysematous bulla.[13] Forty-three patients with giant emphysematous bullae were reported, with a mean patient follow-up of 4.5 years. Reflecting the severity of the underlying lung disease in these patients, 79% had nonfatal complications, consisting predominantly of air leak. One patient died (4.3%). Physiologic results included an increase in FEV_1 from 32% at baseline to 55% at 1 year and 49% at 3 years. D_{LCO} and distance walked in 6 minutes increased significantly at 6 months and 3 years. Continuous use of oxygen decreased from 42% at baseline to 7% at 6 months and 21% at 3 years. Dyspnea score also was reported, with 86% reporting relief of dyspnea at 1 year and 81% at 3 years. Similar increases in pulmonary function values using minimally invasive techniques have been documented by Divisi et al.[4]

EDITOR'S COMMENT

The local anatomic changes can be very similar in both normal and emphysematous patients. In addition to reducing the risk of pneumothorax, resecting bullous disease removes nonfunctioning lung tissue and allows the expansion of more functional regions of the lung. This principle can be similarly applied to lung volume reduction surgery.

—Steven J. Mentzer

References

1. Ohata M, Suzuki H. Pathogenesis of spontaneous pneumothorax. With special reference to the ultrastructure of emphysematous bullae. *Chest.* 1980;77:771–776.
2. Morgan MD, Edwards CW, Morris J, et al. Origin and behaviour of emphysematous bullae. *Thorax.* 1989;44:533–538.
3. Clagett OT. The management of spontaneous pneumothorax. *J Thorac Cardiovasc Surg.* 1968;55:761–762.
4. Divisi D, Battaglia C, Di Francescantonio W, et al. Giant bullous emphysema resection by VATS. analysis of laser and stapler techniques. *Eur J Cardiothorac Surg.* 2002;22:990–994.
5. Ishida T, Kohdono S, Fukuyama Y, et al. Video-assisted thoracoscopic surgery of bullous and bleb disorders of the lung using endoscopic stapling device. *Surg Laparosc Endosc.* 1995;5:349–353.
6. Greenberg JA, Singhal S, Kaiser LR. Giant bullous lung disease: evaluation, selection, techniques, and outcomes. *Chest Surg Clin N Am.* 2003;13:631–649.
7. Mehran RJ, Deslauriers J. Indications for surgery and patient work-up for bullectomy. *Chest Surg Clin N Am.* 1995;5:717–734.
8. Hugh-Jones P, Whimster W. The etiology and management of disabling emphysema. *Am Rev Respir Dis.* 1978;117:343–378.
9. Nakahara K, Nakaoka K, Ohno K, et al. Functional indications for bullectomy of giant bulla. *Ann Thorac Surg.* 1983;35:480–487.
10. Naunheim KS, Mack MJ, Hazelrigg SR, et al. Safety and efficacy of video-assisted thoracic surgical techniques for the treatment of spontaneous pneumothorax. *J Thorac Cardiovasc Surg.* 1995;109:1198–203; discussion 1203–1204.
11. McCoskey EH, McKinney LM, Byrd RP Jr, et al. Re-expansion pulmonary edema following puncture of a giant bulla. *J Am Osteopath Assoc.* 2000; 100:788–791.
12. Liu HP, Yim AP, Izzat MB, et al. Thoracoscopic surgery for spontaneous pneumothorax. *World J Surg.* 1999;23:1133–1136.
13. Schipper PH, Meyers BF, Battafarano RJ, et al. Outcomes after resection of giant emphysematous bullae. *Ann Thorac Surg.* 2004;78:976–982; discussion 982.

99 Lung Volume Reduction Surgery

Victor van Berkel and Bryan F. Meyers

Keywords: Emphysema, lung volume reduction surgery (LVRS), median sternotomy

Lung volume reduction surgery (LVRS) is one of the most interesting and controversial areas in thoracic surgery. The purpose of the operation is to palliate dyspnea and improve functional status and quality of life for highly selected patients with emphysema. Chronic obstructive pulmonary disease (COPD) affects approximately 16 million Americans and is the fourth leading cause of death in the United States.[1] Worldwide there are estimated to be a billion smokers and, thanks to a global increase in the number of smokers each year, COPD is projected to be the third leading cause of death by the year 2020.[2] When pulmonary function tests demonstrate a forced expiratory volume in one second (FEV_1) of less than 30% of predicted values, a patient's 3-year mortality risk has been estimated at 40% to 50%. While medical therapy remains the mainstay of treatment for these patients,[3] no medical therapy is able to improve pulmonary function or reverse the progressive nature of the disease. Three situations have emerged in which surgery is useful to palliate emphysema: lung transplantation, bullectomy, and LVRS. This chapter addresses the LVRS strategy.

The goal of LVRS is to palliate some of the distressing symptoms and limitations imposed by end-stage emphysema. Past controversy around this operation has focused on the procedure, interpretation of the results of trials and case series, issues about how new surgical procedures should be introduced and scientifically evaluated, and questions about how they should be funded by health care providers. Ideal candidates for LVRS have marked hyperinflation and significant regions of severe destruction with other distinct areas of more well-preserved lung parenchyma. The areas to be removed, frequently referred to as "target areas," are usually, but not always, located in the upper lobes and have little pulmonary perfusion when studied with contrast CT or nuclear medicine perfusion scans. Surgical excision of these areas improves respiratory mechanics and function of the remaining lung. Clinically, the anticipated benefits are a reduction in dyspnea and improved exercise tolerance. A subset of highly selected patients may experience a survival benefit as well.[4]

PATHOPHYSIOLOGY OF EMPHYSEMA

Emphysema is characterized by abnormal permanent enlargement of air spaces distal to the terminal bronchiole accompanied by destruction of the airspace walls in the absence of obvious fibrosis.[5] The destruction of pulmonary parenchyma causes a decreased mass of functioning lung tissue and also decreases the amount of gas exchange that can take place. As the lung tissue is destroyed, the lung loses elastic recoil and expands in volume. This leads to the typical hyperexpanded chest seen in emphysema patients with common findings including flattened diaphragms, widened intercostal spaces, and horizontal ribs. The increased distensibility of emphysematous lung results in a lung that is easily inflated but tends to remain pathologically inflated throughout the breathing cycle. An important consequence of this defect is that portions of severely emphysematous lung act as nonfunctional, volume-occupying areas. These anatomic changes result in the loss of mechanical advantages exploited in normal breathing and thus lead to an increased work of breathing and dyspnea.[6] When the destruction and expansion occur in a nonuniform manner, the most affected lung tissue can expand disproportionally to compress and crowd the relatively spared lung tissue and thus impair ventilation of the functioning lung. Finally, there is obstruction in the small airways, likely caused by a combination of reversible bronchospasm and irreversible loss of elastic recoil by adjacent lung parenchyma. The suitability of a given patient for surgical treatment of emphysema depends in part on the relative contributions of lung destruction, lung compression, and small airways obstruction to the overall physiologic impairment of that patient. Sputum production, and the impact of excessive sputum on lung health and quality of life, would also play a role in predicting outcomes of LVRS.

RATIONALE FOR LUNG VOLUME REDUCTION SURGERY

The removal of severely diseased, poorly ventilated, and expanded lung tissue may decrease hyperinflation and improve the mechanical function of the diaphragm and thoracic cage. If the most severely diseased lung can be identified and resected, hyperinflation is reduced and overall breathing function will improve by restoring elastic recoil of the remaining lung. This will result in increased expiratory flow rates and allow the more normal lung to function without compression. LVRS may improve alveolar gas exchange and improve ventilation/perfusion mismatch. The end result is a marked improvement in respiratory mechanics and a decreased work of breathing, both of which help patients to function more normally and avoid the sensation of dyspnea. It is interesting to note that the true etiology or etiologies for dyspnea remain poorly understood. Although dyspnea is associated with severe airflow limitation, it is also linked to hyperinflation, respiratory muscle dysfunction, increases in respiratory drive, and abnormalities in alveolar gas exchange. Unfortunately, the correlation between the symptom of breathlessness and routinely measured physiologic parameters of pulmonary function are imprecise.[7]

HISTORY OF SURGERY FOR EMPHYSEMA

The debilitating symptoms of pulmonary emphysema have attracted the interest of surgeons throughout the 20th century. Many creative but ineffective operations have been devised to treat the dyspnea caused by this disease. Costochondrectomy, phrenic crush, pneumoperitoneum, pleural abrasion, lung denervation, and thoracoplasty all have been offered up as surgical treatments for the hyperexpanded and poorly perfused emphysematous lung.[8] As Laforet[9] explained: "The alleged benefits of these maneuvers were frequently lost on patients whose worsening dyspnea left them with little energy to debate with their surgeons."

LVRS was proposed by Brantigan[10] in conjunction with lung denervation. Among 33 patients having the operation, there were 6 operative deaths (18% mortality) and no objective data to support the claim that survivors were subjectively better. LVRS was thus discarded after this initial experience showed the operation to be too risky with uncertain benefit. Over the following four decades, different groups attempted variations on Brantigan procedure with limited success. Observations about the physiologic behavior of emphysema patients during and after lung transplantation led to the reconsideration of volume reduction by Cooper.[11] Similar to Brantigan procedure, Cooper removed approximately 30% of the patient's lung volume by performing peripheral resection of the most emphysematous portions. However, the new approach used linear cutting/stapling devices and was performed as a bilateral procedure via median sternotomy. The procedure was designed to reduce dyspnea, increase exercise tolerance and performance in activities of daily living, and to improve quality of life.

Following this sentinel report by Cooper et al., LVRS enjoyed widespread application within the United States. A critical analysis of Medicare patients undergoing the procedure, however, revealed an unacceptably high mortality associated with the procedure, 23% at 12 months.[12] This led to cessation of Medicare funding for the operation and a decrease in enthusiasm for the procedure. As a way to rigorously evaluate the benefit of the operation, the National Institutes of Health sponsored a large, multicenter trial that began enrolling patients in 1999.[13] The trial, called the National Emphysema Treatment Trial (NETT), was a prospective randomized study of 1218 patients and it has provided strong evidence for the efficacy, safety, and durability of LVRS.[4,14] The outcomes from the NETT analysis, in conjunction with data from earlier trials, help provide the criteria for defining which patients will benefit from LVRS.

PATIENT SELECTION

History and Physical Examination

The evaluation of candidates for LVRS should be aimed at identifying patients with a physiologic profile that is most likely to respond to LVRS (Table 99-1). This includes patients with severe hyperinflation and reduced elastic recoil but less-pronounced airway disease, relatively well-preserved gas exchange, and no major comorbidities that carry an unacceptable perioperative risk.[15] Because LVRS is a palliative procedure, the first evaluation step is to assess symptoms and the degree of quality of life impairment attributable to emphysema. The medical history needs to be thorough and include questions on daily activities and limitations caused by symptoms. The Medical Research Council (MRC) dyspnea score allows standardized grading of symptoms. Patients considered for LVRS typically have severe, incapacitating emphysema. They must have stopped smoking for at least 6 months and have received optimal medical management for their COPD, which includes pulmonary rehabilitation and nutritional support if necessary. Patients must be highly motivated to undergo surgical treatment and be willing to accept the risk associated with LVRS. The evaluation needs to differentiate COPD with predominant airways disease (chronic bronchitis and bronchiectasis) from COPD with predominant features of emphysema. Because the mean age of candidates is in the mid-60s, medical comorbidities are common and cardiovascular disease, cerebrovascular disease, obesity, and cachexia deserve particular attention. Patients with cardiovascular disease may be difficult to evaluate by elicited symptoms or signs as their emphysema limits their ability to induce anginal symptoms. It is important to note that exercise testing is often not useful because of the patient's inability to exercise to heart rate limits. Echocardiography may be limited by chest hyperinflation resulting in poor visualization of the heart. The use of dipyridamole or adenosine during cardiac testing is limited due to concern for inducing bronchoconstriction. Ultimately, because of the barriers to noninvasive evaluation, many candidates for LVRS undergo cardiac catheterization to obtain a definitive answer regarding their cardiovascular risk.

Pulmonary Function

The cornerstone of pulmonary function testing is spirometry. It is used to quantify the degree of airflow obstruction as well as its reversibility with bronchodilator drugs. Airflow obstruction is the most significant abnormality with emphysema and it can be estimated accurately by forced expiratory maneuvers. Lung volumes are measured by plethysmography rather than by dilution techniques because the latter measurements tend to underestimate the degree of trapped gas and residual volume. Additional parameters of pulmonary function that are assessed include resting and formal exercise arterial blood gas analysis.

Table 99-1

PATIENT PROFILE ELIGIBLE FOR LVRS

CRITERIA	METHOD
Disabling COPD	History, QOL survey, MRC dyspnea index, intensive pulmonary rehabilitation
Severe airflow obstruction	PFTs with FEV_1 and lung volumes
Emphysema	CT scan
Hyperinflation	Chest radiograph, plethysmography
Surgically accessible "target areas"	CT scan, V/Q scan
Prediction of adequate remaining lung tissue after LVRS	Resting PaO_2, supplemental oxygen with exercise D_{LCO}
Preserved respiratory muscle function	Normal or minimally elevated $PaCO_2$

COPD, chronic obstructive pulmonary disease; QOL, quality of life; MRC, maximal respiratory capacity; PFT, pulmonary function tests; FEV_1, forced expiratory volume in 1 second; V/Q scan, ventilation–perfusion scan; D_{LCO}, carbon monoxide diffusing capacity.

These are indicative of the patient's pulmonary reserve and reflect their potential for recovery after surgery. In addition, diffusing capacity, as measured by D_{LCO} values, estimates the severity of damage to the pulmonary capillary bed.

Exercise Capacity

The distance walked in 6 minutes is frequently used to assess exercise capacity. This test evaluates cardiopulmonary function and documents the amount of supplemental oxygen necessary to maintain oxygen saturation above 90%. It is also a useful parameter for the objective documentation of functional improvement following LVRS. Other approaches, including that used by the NETT, have used formal cardiopulmonary testing which results in a maximal exercise capacity expressed in Watts to provide an objective measure of functional capacity.

Radiologic Evaluation

The purpose of imaging in patient selection is to identify findings favorable for LVRS. The presence of hyperinflation, the severity of emphysema, and the distribution of emphysema are the main features to assess. These features are important based on the rationale for LVRS as well as to understand the relationship of preoperative radiographic findings with postoperative outcomes.[16]

The presence of hyperinflation is accurately assessed from inspiratory posteroanterior and lateral chest radiographs (Fig. 99-1A,B). Paired inspiratory and expiratory views show the maximum achievable diaphragm excursion and subjectively estimate the potential for improvement in diaphragm function if the lung volume is reduced by LVRS. The main indicators of hyperinflation are a low, flat diaphragm, increased AP diameter, and increased width of the intercostal spaces. Hyperinflated upper lobes may expand anterior to the upper mediastinum and increase the retrosternal space. Hyperinflation does not occur until emphysema is moderately severe and is a relatively specific sign for emphysema. Although hyperinflation should be present in a patient being considered for LVRS, there is no convincing evidence that the degree of hyperinflation predicts the surgical outcome.

The severity and distribution of emphysema on imaging studies correlates with clinical outcome after surgery. The best outcomes, as demonstrated by improvements in FEV_1 and exercise capacity, tend to occur in patients with more severe, heterogeneous disease that predominates in the upper lobes.[17,18] The most severe extreme of heterogeneous target areas is a giant bulla, but the term LVRS refers to lesser degrees of focal destruction in which some lung tissue is present that needs to be excised. The standard chest computed tomography (CT) examination is the most accurate means of evaluating the severity and distribution of emphysema (Fig. 99-2A,B). Unfortunately, there is considerable variation in the interpretation of CT scans in these patients, since the entire lung is affected to some degree by emphysema, and it may be difficult to assess the heterogeneity of the disease. Studies have demonstrated considerable interobserver variability in interpretation of the

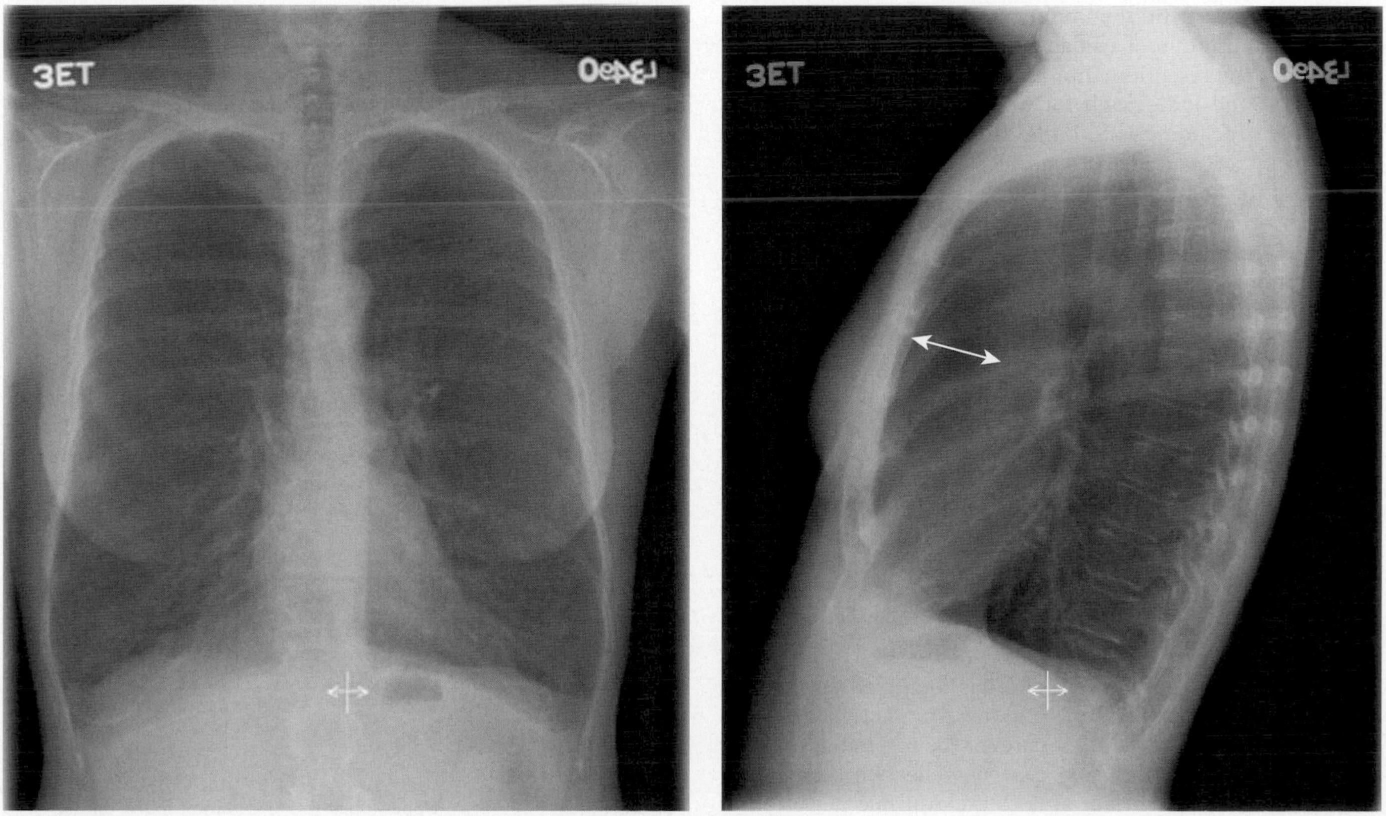

A B

Figure 99-1. Hyperinflation in emphysema These preoperative posteroanterior (*A*) and lateral (*B*) inspiratory radiographs reveal severe hyperinflation. In (*A*), the dome of the diaphragm is flattened and the costal diaphragmatic insertions are visible. In (*B*), the diaphragm appears flat and the upper lobes have expanded anterior to the mediastinum, widening the retrosternal space.

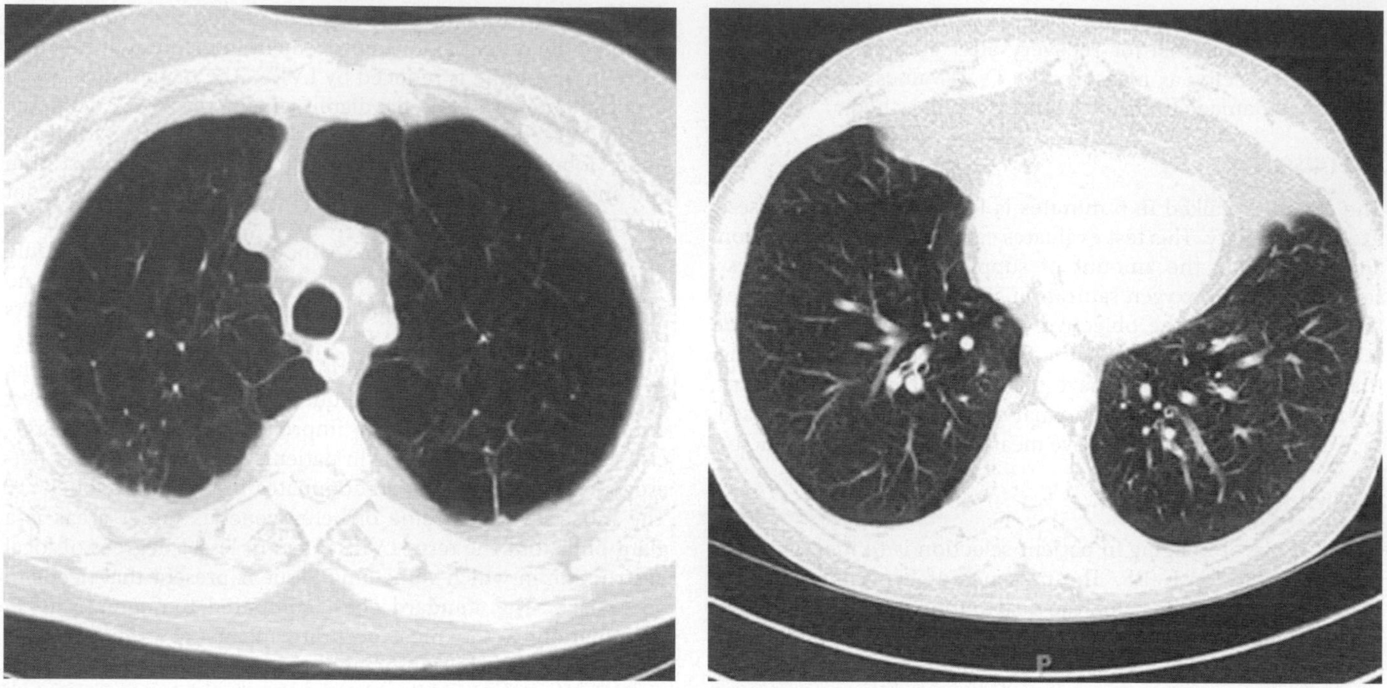

A B

Figure 99-2. Computed tomography cuts taken from a patient selected for LVRS surgery. The apex in (*A*) shows severe emphysematous destruction while the base of the lung in (*B*) shows relative preservation of the lung parenchyma and pulmonary vascular structures.

distribution of emphysema on CT scan.[19] Despite this, the CT scan remains the central component of preoperative imaging. It is the most useful tool available for identification of potential target areas for resection, and also serves as a more rigorous screen than the radiograph for other underlying pathologies that would preclude LVRS. Lung cancer has been discovered in 2% to 8% of candidates for LVRS and some patients are candidates for combined cancer resection and volume reduction.[20,21] Pleural thickening and calcification raise concern for adhesions. In addition, bronchiectasis, inflammatory disease or asymptomatic infiltrates, and pulmonary hypertension may also be identified or suggested by CT and require additional investigation.

Nuclear medicine ventilation-perfusion lung scans depicting regional blood flow patterns provide a valuable roadmap for surgery. Although the absolute severity of emphysema is not accurately assessed, the presence of diffuse or upper or lower lobe predominant disease can be identified. Importantly, a right- or left-sided predominance of lung function may direct surgery toward a unilateral approach if corroborated by CT.

PREDICTORS OF OUTCOMES

Review of surgical results of LVRS has identified risk factors for surgical mortality (Table 99-2). These predictors appear to reflect the function of different parts of the respiratory system. A markedly reduced diffusing capacity reflects a poor distribution of ventilation surface area to the available perfusion of the lung. The greater degrees of severity of disease are usually associated with a significant supplemental oxygen requirement and may indicate that the lung is too impaired to support the patient postoperatively. An elevated $PaCO_2$ indicates excessive work of breathing and chronic muscle fatigue and is a significant risk factor for complications after general anesthesia for any reason. It is not clear why upper lobe predominance has a better outcome than lower lobe resection. This is independent of the etiology for emphysema (smoking vs. $alpha_1$ – antitrypsin deficiency) and may be explained by the fact that the lower lobes comprise a larger volume of lung parenchyma compared to the upper lobes. Other markers of increased risk or poorer outcome include male gender, increasing age, and markedly reduced lung function with FEV_1 less than 20% of predicted values.

SURGICAL TECHNIQUE

Historically, LVRS was accomplished via a median sternotomy. This is an approach that provides excellent exposure and a minimum of incisional morbidity. However, as comfort with thoracoscopic approaches to disease has increased, the majority of these procedures are now done via a VATS approach. We describe here

Table 99-2

PREDICTORS OF OUTCOME FOLLOWING LVRS

PARAMETER	FAVORABLE RESULT	POORER RESULT
Age (years)	<70	>70
FEV_1 (% predicted)	>20	<15
$PaCO_2$	<45	>60
PaO_2	>50	<40
Target area	Upper lobes	Lower lobes, diffuse
Ideal body weight	70–120%	<60%, >130%
(% predicted)	>20	<15

FEV_1, forced expiratory volume in 1 second; $PaCO_2$, partial pressure of carbon dioxide in arterial blood; PaO_2, partial pressure of oxygen in arterial blood.

a technique for performing a bilateral VATS in the supine patient, using buttressed staple lines. It is worth noting, however, that fairly uniform results have been obtained using a wide array of surgical strategies, including bilateral and unilateral approaches, open and thoracoscopic operations, and buttressed or unbuttressed staplers.

Many patients with severe emphysema have a significant element of chronic bronchitis with increased sputum production. Following induction of anesthesia, a single lumen tube is placed and flexible bronchoscopy is carried out to suction secretions and obtain a specimen for culture and for rapid gram stain to guide perioperative antibiotics. If thick, tenacious secretions are encountered, a minitracheostomy may be inserted at the end of the operative procedure to facilitate postoperative pulmonary toilet. Following bronchoscopy, the single lumen endotracheal tube is replaced with a left-sided double lumen tube.

The patient is positioned on the table with a padded roll beneath the shoulders, hips, and along the spine. The arms are then suspended, padded carefully above the patient's head, and affixed to a support bar. This position provides sufficient access to allow placement of three thoracoscopic ports; a camera port in the midaxillary line at the ninth interspace, an assistant port in the posterior axillary line at the eighth interspace, and a working port just medial to the anterior axillary line in the fifth interspace (Fig. 99-3).

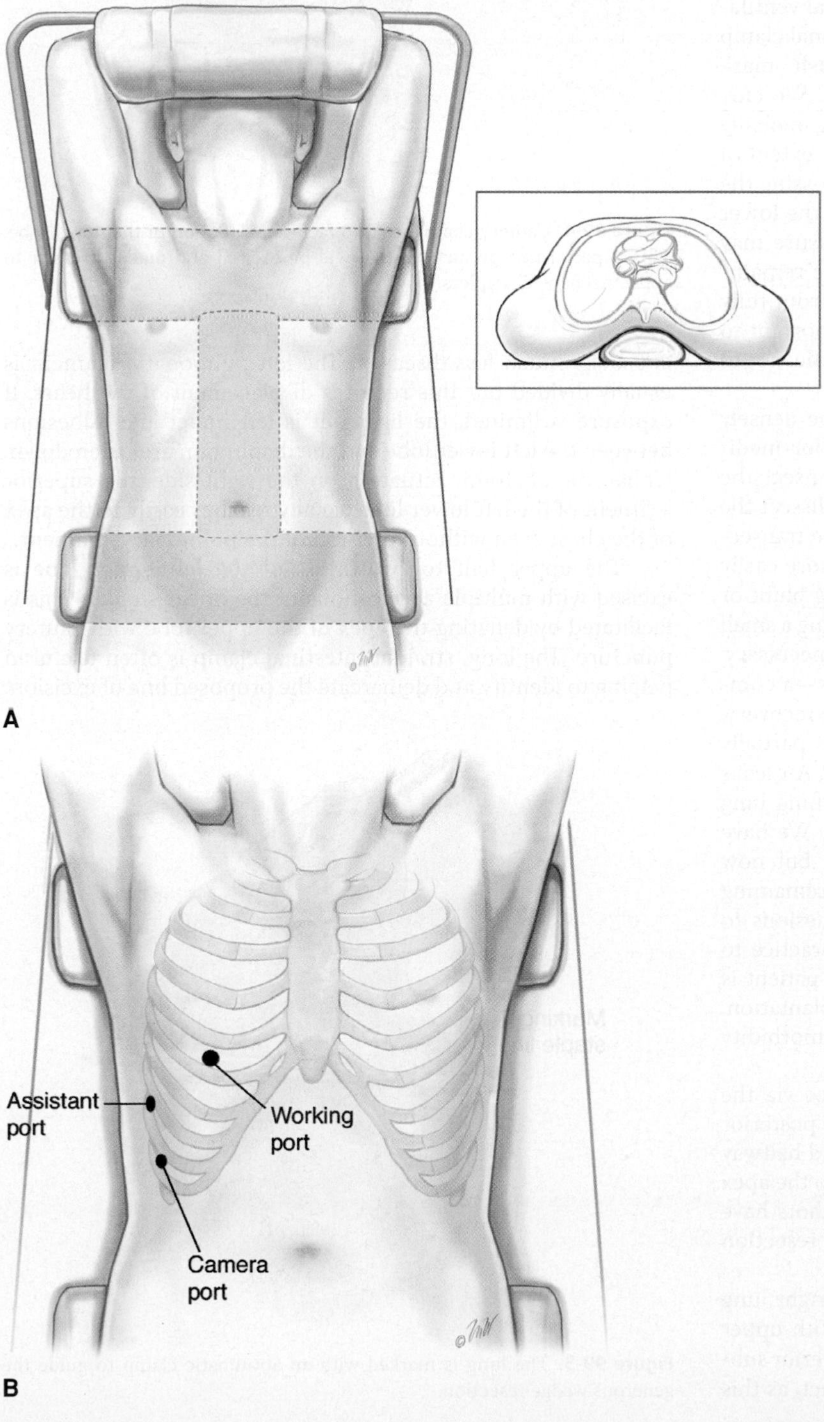

Figure 99-3. *A.* Patient positioning for bilateral VATS LVRS. With the arms protected above the patient's head, and rolls placed beneath the patient's shoulders, hips, and spine, access to both pleural spaces can be accomplished without repositioning. *B.* Three thoracoscopic ports are placed; a camera port in the midaxillary line at the ninth interspace, an assistant port in the posterior axillary line at the eighth interspace, and a working port just medial to the anterior axillary line in the fifth interspace.

Most candidates for LVRS have upper lobe predominant disease. Several minutes after ventilation is suspended to the right lung, the right middle and lower lobes are usually well deflated and become progressively atelectatic. The pulmonary ligament is divided and adhesions are taken down under direct vision. Dense adhesions are not common but may be encountered if there have been prior episodes of pneumonia. We, very rarely, might use an extrapleural dissection adjacent to adhesions to avoid injuring the fragile lung parenchyma.

For upper lobe disease, 70% to 80% of the right upper lobe is excised with multiple applications of a linear stapler buttressed with strips of bovine pericardium. It is often easier to apply the stapler to the deflated lung and this can rapidly be accomplished by using the cautery to fenestrate the apex of the right upper lobe (Fig. 99-4). The marked collateral ventilation leads to prompt collapse. A long, straight intestinal clamp can be applied to the lung to create a linear "crush" mark before application of the linear stapler (Fig. 99-5). We currently staple straight across the upper lobe beginning medially above the hilum and ending up just above the upper extent of the oblique fissure. Care should be taken to avoid crossing the fissure as this may damage the superior segment of the lower lobe (Fig. 99-6). In addition, stapling across the fissure may tether the superior segment of the lower lobe to the remaining upper lobe and prevent the superior segment from fully expanding and filling the apex of the chest. It is important to remember that the goal is to adequately reduce volume, not to remove all of the diseased lung.

Occasionally, the apex of the upper lobe will be densely adherent to the apex of the chest and to the superior mediastinum. In such cases, it may be easier to first transect the upper lobe as described above before attempting to dissect the apical and mediastinal adhesions (Fig. 99-7). Once the transection has been accomplished, the specimen can be more easily detached from the chest wall and mediastinum using blunt or sharp dissection, cautery, or even a linear stapler leaving a small remnant of the lung attached to the mediastinum if necessary. It is imperative to avoid injury to the phrenic nerves—a complication that will severely compromise postoperative recovery.

Following the upper lobe resection, the chest is partially filled with warm saline and the lung is gently inflated. Air leaks at this time are unusual but the reexpanded, remaining lung often does not completely fill the apex of the chest. We have explored the use of a pleural tent in this situation but now reserve it for rare instances, in particular when the remaining lung remains tethered in the chest by virtue of adhesions to the chest wall or diaphragm. It has not been our practice to perform mechanical or talc pleurodesis, even if the patient is not a potential candidate for subsequent lung transplantation. The efficacy of pleurodesis is questionable and the morbidity can be burdensome.

Two chest tubes are placed in the pleural space via the anterior and middle axillary port sites (Fig. 99-8). The posterior tube is brought across the dome of the diaphragm and halfway up the posterior chest. The anterior tube is brought to the apex of the chest near the mediastinum. Recently, the authors have been using a single chest tube after a straightforward resection with no intraoperative air leaks identified.

Ventilation is shifted from the left lung to the right lung and similar port sites are placed on the left side. With upper lobe predominant disease, the goal is to excise the superior subdivision of the left upper lobe leaving the lingula intact, as this is usually much less diseased. The left pulmonary ligament is usually divided but this requires displacement of the heart. If exposure is limited, the ligament is left intact and adhesions between the left lower lobe and the diaphragm are taken down. Unlike the anatomic situation on the right side, the superior segment of the left lower lobe usually reaches easily to the apex of the chest even without division of the pulmonary ligament.

The upper half to two-thirds of the left upper lobe is excised with multiple applications of the linear stapler. This is facilitated by deflating the apex of the upper lobe with cautery puncture. The long, straight intestinal clamp is often useful in helping to identify and demarcate the proposed line of excision.

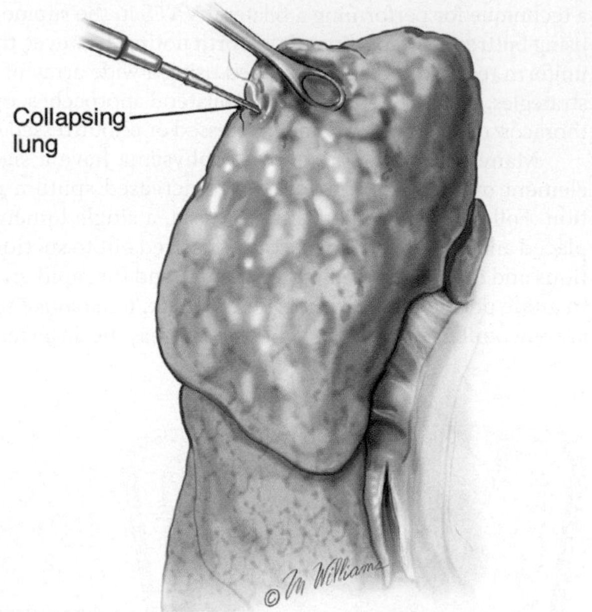

Figure 99-4. Cautery can be used to facilitate deflation of the upper lobe. This is performed on an area that will be excised and makes it easier to apply mechanical staplers.

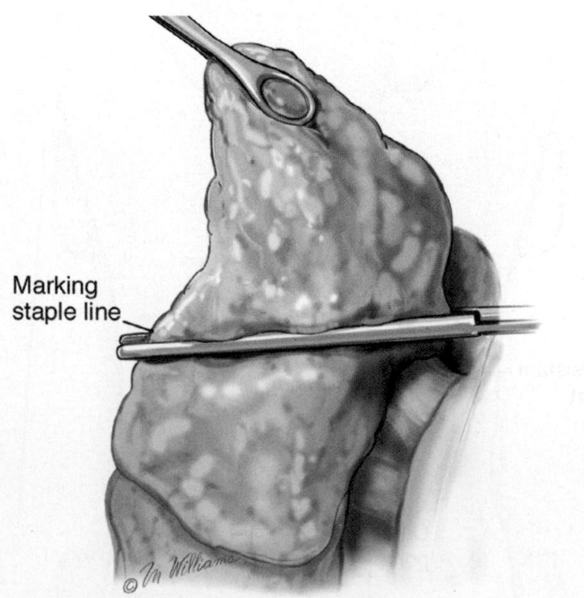

Figure 99-5. The lung is marked with an atraumatic clamp to guide the generous wedge resection.

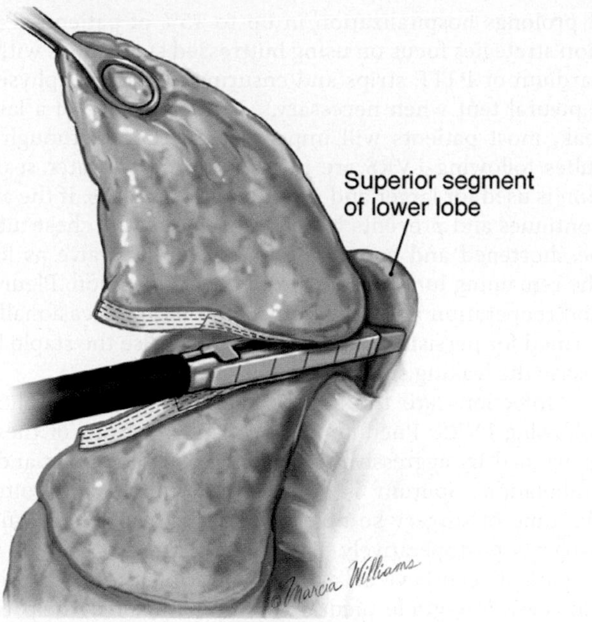

Figure 99-6. The wedge is performed with a buttressed stapler with all due care to avoid injury of the superior segment of the lower lobe.

The line of excision is nearly parallel to the oblique fissure separating the upper and lower lobes. Similar to the right side, care is taken to avoid stapling across the fissure into the superior segment of the left upper lobe (Fig. 99-9).

Following left upper lobe excision, the lung is reinflated and inspected for air leaks. Two chest tubes are placed in a similar manner to the right-sided tubes. Virtually all patients are extubated in the operating room. If excessive secretions are present following the procedure or during the initial bronchoscopy, a 4-mm diameter minitracheostomy is inserted at the time of extubation to facilitate aggressive pulmonary toilet.

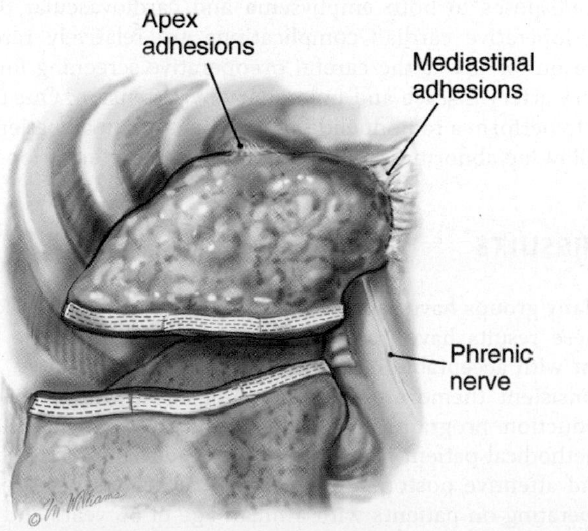

Figure 99-7. It is sometimes easier to perform the wedge resection before separating the pleural adhesions. If there are dense mediastinal adhesions, the phrenic nerve must be identified and protected. A paralyzed diaphragm is catastrophic in these patients. If the adhesions are so dense that the phrenic nerve is not well identified, it is better to leave a little lung parenchyma attached to the mediastinal pleura.

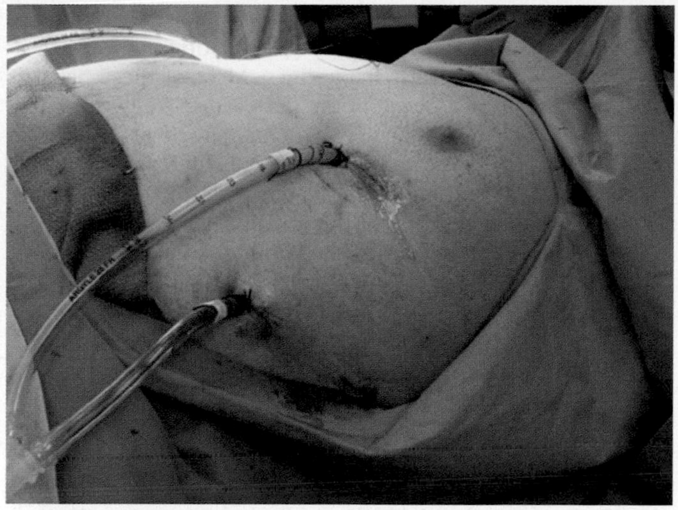

Figure 99-8. Chest tube position at the completion of the procedure.

ANESTHESIA CONCERNS

Pain control is essential to ensure adequate postoperative respiratory function. An epidural catheter is placed and it is imperative to confirm that a bilateral block has been established before beginning the procedure. Although this is not absolutely necessary, we use fluoroscopy to allow placement of the catheter at the tip of T4. During induction, hypotension can result from air trapping as well as pneumothorax. Air trapping leading to "pulmonary tamponade" is treated by removing the patient from the ventilator and allowing them to exhale to the atmosphere. Bronchodilators and prolonged exhalation times are also helpful but it is often necessary to remove the patient from the ventilator during exhalation.

During the procedure, our anesthesiologists avoid narcotics and limit the use of benzodiazepines to limit long-term

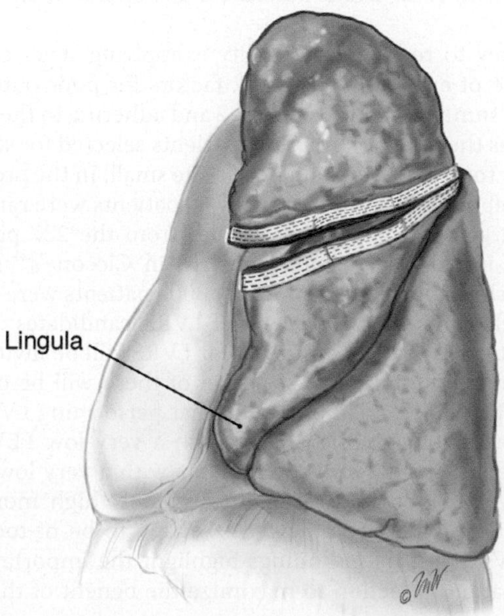

Figure 99-9. A generous left upper lobe wedge is shown. Most of the lingula is left in place.

respiratory depression. The inspiratory pressures are limited to 15 to 20 cm of water during one lung ventilation to avoid excessive pressure on the fresh staple lines. Most of these patients have an element of CO_2 retention and permissive hypercapnia is tolerated. During emergence, patients may be drowsy and it is not unusual to have the initial $PaCO_2$ as high as 90 mm Hg. This is transient and will come down as the patient receives nebulizers and chest physical therapy in the recovery room. It is important not to overreact and intubate, thus risking barotrauma, air leaks, and an unnecessary period of mechanical ventilation.

PERIOPERATIVE MANAGEMENT

Contrary to the management of most patients following pulmonary resection, the chest tubes following LVRS are immediately placed to water seal without the application of suction. The loss of elastic recoil, the obstructive physiology of the remaining lung, and the fragile nature of the tissue makes the lungs more susceptible to hyperinflation caused by chest tube suction. The keys to postoperative management are adequate pain relief, aggressive chest physiotherapy, early ambulation, and management of secretions. Inhaled bronchodilators and systemic steroids during the perioperative period can be very beneficial in reducing airway reactivity.

COMPLICATIONS

The value of LVRS as a palliative procedure is clearly dependent on the surgeon's ability to minimize the frequency and severity of postoperative complications.[22] The true mortality is difficult to assess due to bias in publishing case series with favorable results. Furthermore, individual case series often have an unintentional positive bias as patients that experience good outcomes are more likely to return for follow-up. Despite these caveats, it is noted that most of the published reports on the outcomes of LVRS describe a perioperative mortality under 8%.

The key to reducing morbidity is applying strict criteria at the time of evaluation. The risk factors for poor outcomes have been summarized in Table 99-2 and adhering to these criteria makes the selection fraction (patients selected for surgery divided by total patients evaluated) quite small. In the prospective trial reported by Pompeo,[23] only 60 patients were randomized to surgery or medical treatment, from the 237 patients that were initially evaluated. Similarly, in Ciccone's[24] report out of Washington University, nearly 3000 patients were evaluated to select the first 250 bilateral LVRS candidates. Fewer than one-third of patients referred for LVRS will be invited for onsite evaluation and only a fraction of these will be offered surgery. The NETT[25] demonstrated that performing LVRS on two high-risk subgroups: patients with a very low FEV_1 and homogeneous emphysema and patients with a very low FEV_1 and a low D_{LCO} resulted in an unacceptably high mortality. These patients have been viewed by many to be of too high risk for LVRS and these findings highlight the importance of prudent patient selection to maximize the benefit of this palliative procedure.

The most common complication following LVRS is a parenchyma air leak. Most patients have an initial air leak and it prolongs hospitalization in up to 15% of patients. Prevention strategies focus on using buttressed staple lines with pericardium or PTFE strips and ensuring pleural symphysis with a pleural tent when necessary.[26] In the absence of a large air leak, most patients will improve with time. Although chest tubes following LVRS are initially placed to water seal, suction is used for larger and symptomatic air leaks. If the air leak continues and prevents hospital discharge, the chest tube can be shortened and connected to a Heimlich valve as long as the remaining lung remains expanded off suction. Pleurodesis and reoperation are rarely indicated but are occasionally performed for persistent large air leaks to revise the staple line or excise the leaking site.

Infections are the second major class of complications following LVRS. Pneumonia is the most serious of these and is avoided by aggressive management of secretions and early ambulation. Sputum is routinely submitted for culture at the time of surgery so objective data is available if infiltrates progress postoperatively. Empyema is rare but may be severe as patients can have an air leak and a pleural space problem. However, low-grade pleural contamination may help to promote pleural fusion.

Respiratory decompensation and mucus plugging are a major problem following LVRS. Prevention measures focus on early ambulation and good respiratory therapy. High-risk patients with thick copious sputum are carefully scrutinized during their evaluation. If history and preoperative bronchoscopy are concerning in this regard, a minitracheostomy is placed following extubation in the operating room. If preoperative bronchoscopy reveals heavy, purulent sputum then the procedure should be canceled with a plan to reschedule after a course of antibiotics and reassessment.

Gastrointestinal complications are notable in patients following LVRS.[27] The link between emphysema and gastrointestinal complications is uncertain but many reports have noted a higher rate of intestinal ischemia, perforation, and ileus. We favor early colonoscopy to treat pseudo-obstruction and rule out mucosal ischemia. Despite the fact that cigarette smoking predisposes to both emphysema and cardiovascular disease, perioperative cardiac complications are relatively rare. The reason for this is the careful preoperative screening for coronary artery disease and pulmonary hypertension. Our routine is to perform a radionuclide ventriculogram on all patients and follow-up abnormal results with cardiac catheterization.

RESULTS

Many groups have reported preliminary results for LVRS, and these results have consistently shown benefit to the recipient with acceptable mortality and varying morbidity.[28–33] The consistent theme among reports of successful lung volume reduction programs has been meticulous patient selection, methodical patient preparation with reduction of risk factors, and attentive postoperative care. Most groups have reported operating on patients with a mean age of 65 years and a preoperative FEV_1 of 600 to 800 mL. The typical postoperative length of stay is 8 to 14 days with almost half the patients being detained due to persistent air leaks. Mortality ranges from 0% to 7% for the initial hospitalization. The expected benefits of the operation vary according to whether a unilateral or bilateral approach has been utilized, but gains of 20% to 35% in the FEV_1

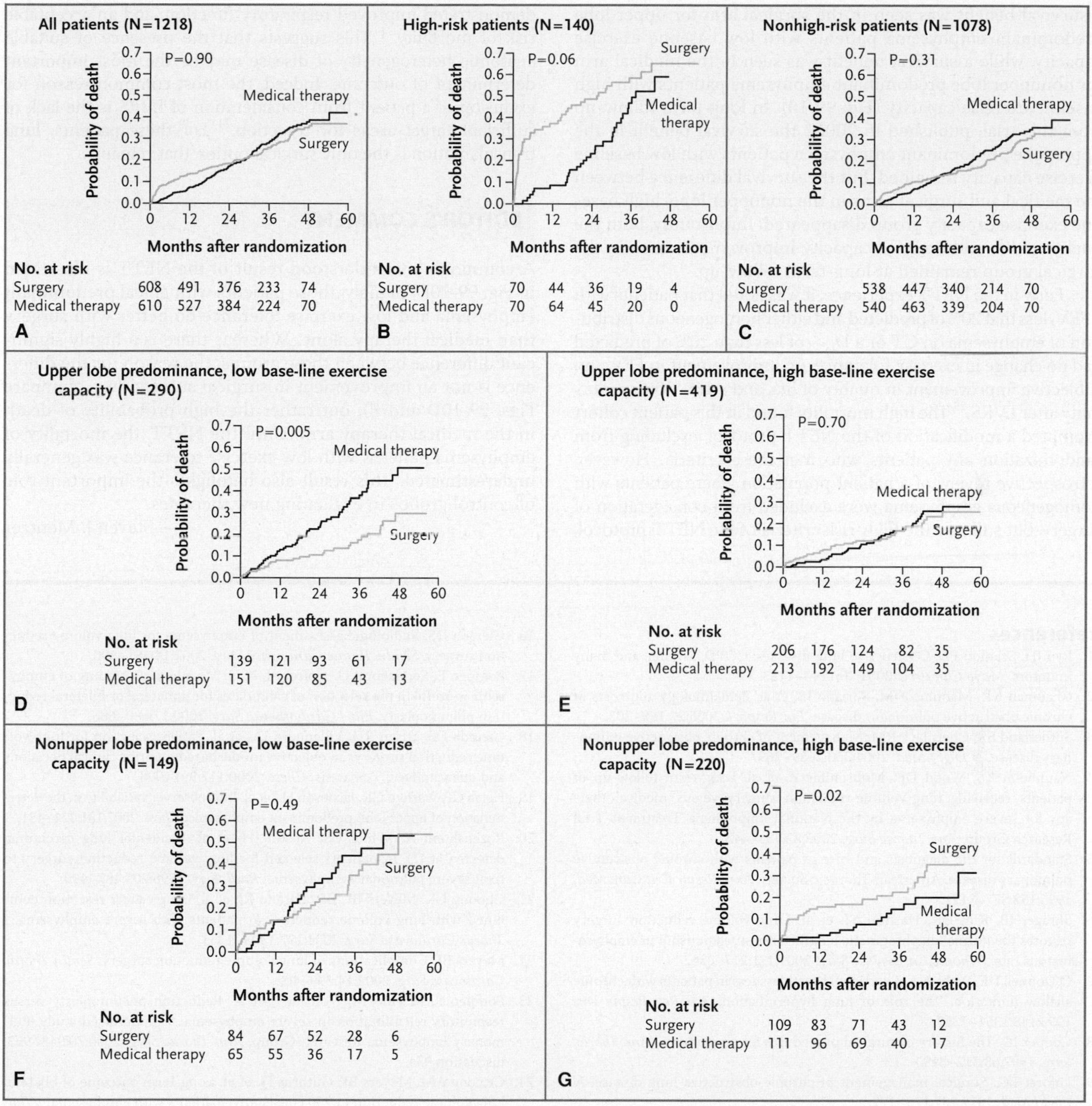

Figure 99-10. Results from the NETT trial (With permission from Fishman A, Martinez F, Naunheim K, et al. A randomized trial comparing lung-volume-reduction surgery with medical therapy for severe emphysema. *N Engl J Med.* 2003;348:2059–2073.).

have been reported for unilateral operations and gains of 40% to 80% are seen with bilateral operations. Most authors also report substantial gains in exercise tolerance, freedom from oxygen use, freedom from steroid use, and subjective quality of life.

As an example of the results reported from an individual institution, Ciccone[24] reported long-term results in 250 bilateral LVRS recipients. After a median follow-up of 4.4 years, the 5-year survival was estimated to be 68%. Eighteen of the 250 patients in that report proceeded to lung transplantation after a median interval of 4.3 years. Five years after surgery, the mean FEV_1 was 7% higher than that prior to surgery and half of the individual patients continued to demonstrate improvement over their preoperative FEV_1 values.

In 2003, the NETT reported the main results of a 5-year effort. This trial included 1218 patients randomized between LVRS and medical therapy between January 1998 and July 2002.[4] In the entire cohort of patients, there was no difference in overall mortality between the surgical group and the medical therapy group. The surgical group did show significant improvement in exercise capacity, 6-minute walk distance, FEV_1, and quality of life measures. In subgroup analysis, a survival benefit was seen in the surgical arm for upper lobe predominant emphysema patients with low baseline exercise capacity, while a survival benefit was seen in the medical arm for nonupper lobe predominant emphysema patients with high baseline exercise capacity (Fig. 99-10). In long-term follow-up from this trial, published in 2006,[4] the survival benefit in the upper lobe predominant emphysema patients with low baseline exercise capacity remained, but the survival difference between the medical and surgical arms in the nonupper lobe, high baseline exercise capacity group disappeared. Importantly, both the quality of life and exercise capacity improvements seen in the surgical group remained at long-term follow-up.

Early in the NETT experience, it was noted that patients with a FEV_1 less that 20% of predicted and either homogeneous distribution of emphysema on CT or a D_{LCO} of less than 20% of predicted had no change in exercise tolerance, no improvement in FEV_1, no subjective improvement in quality of life, and a 16% 30-day mortality after LVRS.[25] The high mortality found in this patient cohort prompted a modification of the NETT protocol, excluding from randomization any patients who met these criteria. However, retrospective review of a patient population where patients with homogeneous emphysema were excluded from consideration of surgery, but still met the high-risk criteria of the NETT protocol, demonstrated improved respiratory function, and an acceptable risk of mortality.[34] This suggests that the presence of suitable anatomic heterogeneity of disease may be the most important determinant of outcome. Indeed, the most common reason for exclusion of a patient from consideration of LVRS is the lack of sufficient target areas for resection.[24] For these patients, lung transplantation is the only surgical option that remains.

EDITOR'S COMMENT

A commonly misunderstood result of the NETT is illustrated in Fig. 99-10D; namely, those patients with apical predominant emphysema and low exercise tolerance do better with surgery than medical therapy alone. Whereas there is a highly significant difference between these groups, the reason for the difference is not an improvement in surgical survival (e.g., compare Figs. 99-10D and E), but rather the high probability of death in the medical therapy arm. Until the NETT, the mortality of emphysema patients with low exercise tolerance was generally underestimated. This result also highlights the important role of control groups in evaluating new therapies.

—Steven J. Mentzer

References

1. Ryu JH, Scanlon PD. Obstructive lung diseases: COPD, asthma, and many imitators. *Mayo Clin Proc.* 2001;76:1144–1153.
2. Chapman KR, Mannino DM, Soriano JB, et al. Epidemiology and costs of chronic obstructive pulmonary disease. *Eur Respir J.* 2006;27:188–207.
3. Sutherland ER, Cherniack RM. Management of chronic obstructive pulmonary disease. *N Engl J Med.* 2004;350:2689–2697.
4. Naunheim KS, Wood DE, Mohsenifar Z, et al. Long-term follow-up of patients receiving lung-volume-reduction surgery versus medical therapy for severe emphysema by the National Emphysema Treatment Trial Research Group. *Ann Thorac Surg.* 2006;82:431–443.
5. Standards for the diagnosis and care of patients with chronic obstructive pulmonary disease. American Thoracic Society. *Am J Respir Crit Care Med.* 1995;152:S77–S121.
6. Shrager JB, Kim DK, Hashmi YJ, et al. Lung volume reduction surgery restores the normal diaphragmatic length-tension relationship in emphysematous rats. *J Thorac Cardiovasc Surg.* 2001;121:217–224.
7. O'Donnell DE, Webb KA. Exertional breathlessness in patients with chronic airflow limitation. The role of lung hyperinflation. *Am Rev Respir Dis.* 1993;148:1351–1357.
8. Cooper JD. The history of surgical procedures for emphysema. *Ann Thorac Surg.* 1997;63:312–319.
9. Laforet EG. Surgical management of chronic obstructive lung disease. *N Engl J Med.* 1972;287:175–177.
10. Brantigan OC, Mueller E, Kress MB. A surgical approach to pulmonary emphysema. *Am Rev Respir Dis.* 1959;80:194–206.
11. Cooper JD, Trulock EP, Triantafillou AN, et al. Bilateral pneumectomy (volume reduction) for chronic obstructive pulmonary disease. *J Thorac Cardiovasc Surg.* 1995;109:106–116; discussion 116–119.
12. Administration HCF. *Report to Congress: Lung Volume Reduction Surgery and Medicare coverage policy-implications of recently published evidence.* Washington DC: CA Services DoHaH; 1998.
13. Rationale and design of the National Emphysema Treatment Trial (NETT): a prospective randomized trial of lung volume reduction surgery. *J Thorac Cardiovasc Surg.* 1999;118:518–528.
14. Fishman A, Martinez F, Naunheim K, et al. A randomized trial comparing lung-volume-reduction surgery with medical therapy for severe emphysema. *N Engl J Med.* 2003;348:2059–2073.
15. Bloch KE, Russi EW, Weder W. Patient selection for lung volume reduction surgery: is outcome predictable? *Semin Thorac Cardiovasc Surg.* 2002;14:371–380.
16. Gierada DS. Radiologic assessment of emphysema for lung volume reduction surgery. *Semin Thorac Cardiovasc Surg.* 2002;14:381–390.
17. Pompeo E, Sergiacomi G, Nofroni I, et al. Morphologic grading of emphysema is useful in the selection of candidates for unilateral or bilateral reduction pneumoplasty. *Eur J Cardiothorac Surg.* 2000;17:680–686.
18. Gierada DS, Yusen RD, Villanueva IA, et al. Patient selection for lung volume reduction surgery: an objective model based on prior clinical decisions and quantitative CT analysis. *Chest.* 2000;117:991–998.
19. Hersh CP, Washko GR, Jacobson FL, et al. Interobserver variability in the determination of upper lobe-predominant emphysema. *Chest.* 2007;131:424–431.
20. Rozenshtein A, White CS, Austin JH, et al. Incidental lung carcinoma detected at CT in patients selected for lung volume reduction surgery to treat severe pulmonary emphysema. *Radiology.* 1998;207:487–490.
21. Choong CK, Meyers BF, Battafarano RJ, et al. Lung cancer resection combined with lung volume reduction in patients with severe emphysema. *J Thorac Cardiovasc Surg.* 2004;127:1323–1331.
22. Meyers BF. Complications of lung volume reduction surgery. *Semin Thorac Cardiovasc Surg.* 2002;14:399–402.
23. Pompeo E, Marino M, Nofroni I, et al. Reduction pneumoplasty versus respiratory rehabilitation in severe emphysema: a randomized study. Pulmonary Emphysema Research Group. *Ann Thorac Surg.* 2000;70:948–953; discussion 954.
24. Ciccone AM, Meyers BF, Guthrie TJ, et al. Long-term outcome of bilateral lung volume reduction in 250 consecutive patients with emphysema. *J Thorac Cardiovasc Surg.* 2003;125:513–525.
25. National Emphysema Treatment Trial Research Group. Patients at high risk of death after lung-volume-reduction surgery. *N Engl J Med.* 2001;345:1075–1083.
26. Brunelli A, Al Refai M, Muti M, et al. Pleural tent after upper lobectomy: a prospective randomized study. *Ann Thorac Surg.* 2000;69:1722–1724.
27. Cetindag IB, Boley TM, Magee MJ, et al. Postoperative gastrointestinal complications after lung volume reduction operations. *Ann Thorac Surg.* 1999;68:1029–1033.
28. Argenziano M, Moazami N, Thomashow B, et al. Extended indications for lung volume reduction surgery in advanced emphysema. *Ann Thorac Surg.* 1996;62:1588–1597.
29. Bissinger R, Zollinger A, Hauser M, et al. Bilateral volume reduction surgery for diffuse pulmonary emphysema by video-assisted thoracoscopy. *J Thorac Cardiovasc Surg.* 1996;112:875–882.
30. Cooper JD, Patterson GA, Sundaresan RS, et al. Results of 150 consecutive bilateral lung volume reduction procedures in patients with severe emphysema. *J Thorac Cardiovasc Surg.* 1996;112:1319–1329; discussion 1329–1330.

31. Gaissert HA, Trulock EP, Cooper JD, et al. Comparison of early functional results after volume reduction or lung transplantation for chronic obstructive pulmonary disease. *J Thorac Cardiovasc Surg*. 1996;111:296–306; discussion 307.
32. McKenna RJ Jr., Brenner M, Fischel RJ, et al. Should lung volume reduction for emphysema be unilateral or bilateral? *J Thorac Cardiovasc Surg*. 1996;112:1331–1338; discussion 1338–1339.
33. Naunheim KS, Keller CA, Krucylak PE, et al. Unilateral video-assisted thoracic surgical lung reduction. *Annals of Thoracic Surgery*. 1996;61: 1092–1098.
34. Wefel JS, Lenzi R, Theriault RL, et al. The cognitive sequelae of standard-dose adjuvant chemotherapy in women with breast carcinoma: results of a prospective, randomized, longitudinal trial. *Cancer*. 2004;100: 2292–2299.

100 Minimally Invasive Methods of Managing Giant Bullae: Monaldi Procedure

Hasan F. Batirel and Lambros Zellos

Keywords: Giant bullae, minimally invasive bullectomy

Giant bullae are space-occupying lesions that cause compression of the surrounding lung parenchyma with impairment of lung function. The bullae arise from emphysematous projections of destroyed lung tissue. Hence they differ from blebs, which are localized collections of air between visceral pleural layers without underlying parenchymal disease.[1] Giant bullae can be classified as three basic morphologic types: Type I bullae have a narrow neck and are superficial, type II are superficial as well but have a broad neck, and type III are both broad and deep.[2] Giant bullae usually require surgical resection. A wide range of procedures from open excision to plication, drainage, video-assisted bullectomy, and lung resection can be applied.[3] Developments in anesthesia and surgery have enabled surgeons to operate on patients with very limited pulmonary function; however, there is a subgroup of patients who carry a significant risk of prolonged air leak and respiratory complications following resection of giant bullae. In this group of patients a minimally invasive method, known as the Monaldi procedure, can be performed. The Monaldi procedure, named after the surgeon who first applied this technique, was used in the mid and late 20th century for drainage of apically located tuberculous cavities, lung abscesses, and subsequently of giant bullae.[4]

CLINICAL PRESENTATION

Most patients who undergo this procedure are heavy smokers of middle to advanced age with a prolonged history of medical treatment. The most common symptoms are dyspnea and chest pain. Giant bullae occupy a significant portion of the intrathoracic space, causing significant compression of adjacent healthy lung tissue. As a result, the physiologic dead space increases and the presence of these bullae aggravate the patient's symptoms of dyspnea in generalized emphysema.

Secondary pneumothorax and hemoptysis can be the initial presenting complications. If the bulla becomes infected, fever, cough, and increased sputum production may accompany the clinical picture. Preliminary evaluation usually begins with a plain chest radiograph. Giant bullae usually have a concave contour at the base, which can be used to differentiate a bulla from pneumothorax (Fig. 100-1). If the bulla is infected, an air–fluid level is seen. The chest x-ray also may demonstrate a generalized heterogeneous emphysema, areas of scarring secondary to previous infections, and interstitial fibrosis (Fig. 100-2). Standard chest computed tomography (CT) is the best study for delineating the extent of the bulla and the degree of compression of surrounding lung tissue.

Patient Selection and Preoperative Assessment

The indication for treatment is defined as the presence of symptoms in a space-occupying bulla that is compressing the surrounding lung parenchyma. Ideally, the bulla should occupy greater than one-third of the hemithorax to be suitable for resection. CT

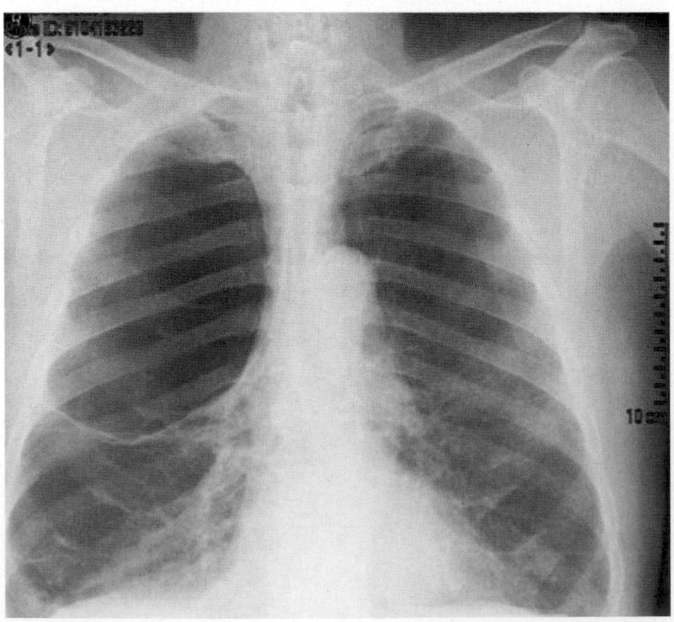

Figure 100-1. A giant bulla in the right upper zone of the chest. This bulla originated from the middle lobe and extended to the pulmonary hilum. It was treated with middle lobectomy.

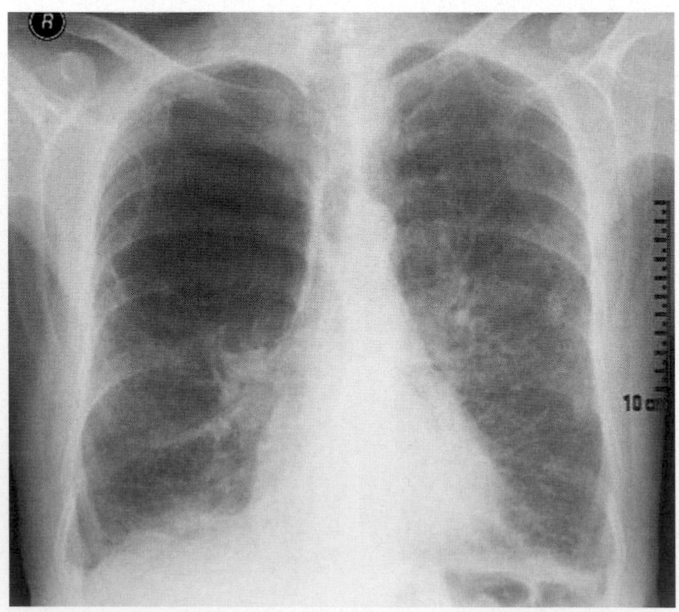

Figure 100-2. A patient with a giant right upper lobe bulla, generalized emphysema, and interstitial fibrosis of the lung. His pulmonary function was severely limited with an FEV_1 of 0.90 L (29%) and FVC of 1.84 L (48%). This patient is an ideal candidate for the Mondaldi procedure.

scan is the preferred imaging modality for preoperative planning. In addition to visualizing the full extent of the bulla, it can demonstrate pleural and parenchymal scarring, interstitial fibrosis, and the general condition of the remaining lung tissue. Ventilation perfusion scintigraphy also may be helpful.

Pulmonary function testing is conducted to determine the extent of the patient's obstructive pathology. Those with markedly decreased forced vital capacity (FVC), forced expiratory volume in 1 second (FEV_1), or diminished diffusion capacity of the lung for carbon monoxide (DL_{CO}) with evidence of hypoxemia and hypercarbia are at increased risk for perioperative complications, and may fail to improve or even worsen with resection. The ideal candidate for surgery is a patient with a peripheral bulla, FEV_1 greater than 500 mL, and carbon dioxide tension less than 6.5 kPa who would not tolerate prolonged anesthesia and major open surgery.

Similar to the Monaldi procedure, percutaneous or endoscopic drainage of infected lung bullae also has been performed successfully in very sick patients resulting in spontaneous resolution of bullae.[5,6] Individuals with better pulmonary reserve have several options available, and bullectomy by means of video-assisted thoracic surgery (VATS) may be the most appropriate procedure for these patients.

The Monaldi procedure has several advantages. First, no lung tissue is removed. This is especially important in patients with limited lung function. Second, suturing and stapling, which commonly results in prolonged air leak and healing problems in emphysematous lung tissue, is avoided. Third, the procedure can be performed through a limited incision with brief anesthesia which is certainly advantageous in patients with poor lung function.[7]

MONALDI TECHNIQUE AND PITFALLS

The Brompton group provides the best description of this technique.[7,8] Initially, they described a two-stage procedure.[9] During the first phase, an extrapleural iodine pack is inserted to induce pleural adhesions. Three weeks later, the bulla is drained. Later, they switched to a single-stage procedure, in which a sclerosing agent is instilled into the bulla and pleural cavity. If pleural sclerosis ensues, the procedure can be performed under local anesthesia. Otherwise the operation is performed in the OR with general anesthesia.

The incisions are planned based on the preoperative chest CT scan (Fig. 100-3). The incision is placed at the point where the bulla lies closest to the chest wall (Fig. 100-4), provided the angle of attack is not awkward for the surgeon, such as over the scapula or so far posteriorly that it would interfere with chest tube placement. The incision should be positioned at the base of the bulla. The patient is positioned to optimize access to the planned incision. A small incision is made at the predetermined site. The underlying rib is resected. The visceral pleura is entered, and purse-string sutures are placed on the visceral pleura (Fig. 100-5). Any septations present inside the bulla are divided under direct vision or with the assistance of a camera to ensure free drainage of the entire bulla.[6] Two drains are used in this procedure: A 32 F Foley catheter is placed inside the bullous cavity, and a chest tube is placed in the pleural space

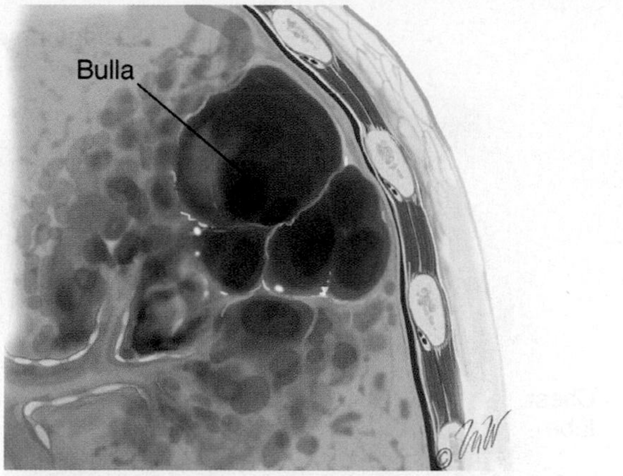

Figure 100-4. Whenever possible, the incision is placed at the site where the bulla comes closest to the chest wall.

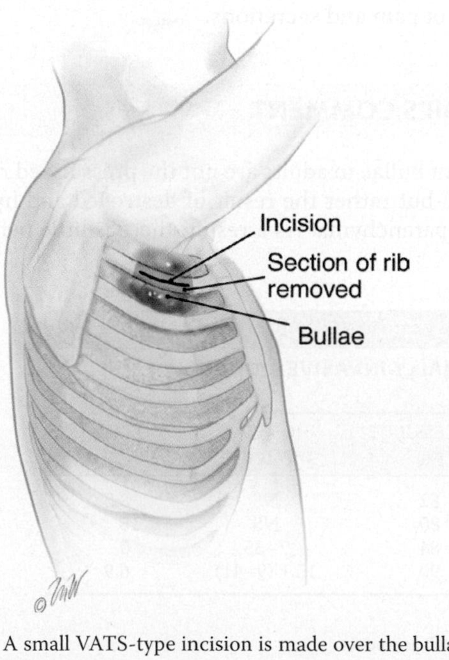

Figure 100-3. A small VATS-type incision is made over the bulla.

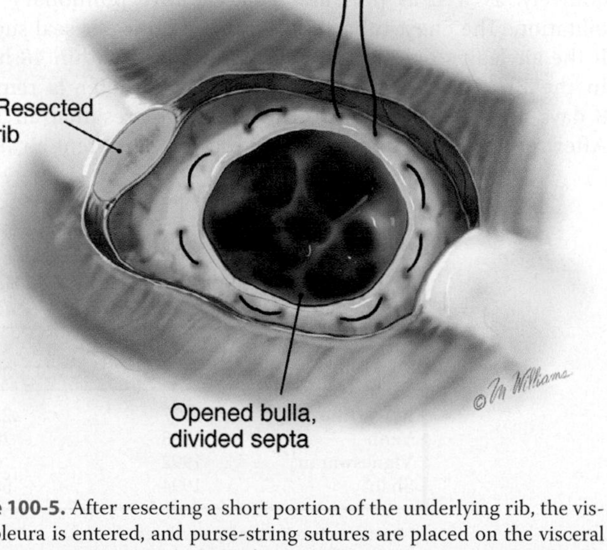

Figure 100-5. After resecting a short portion of the underlying rib, the visceral pleura is entered, and purse-string sutures are placed on the visceral pleura. Septations within the bulla are divided to ensure complete drainage.

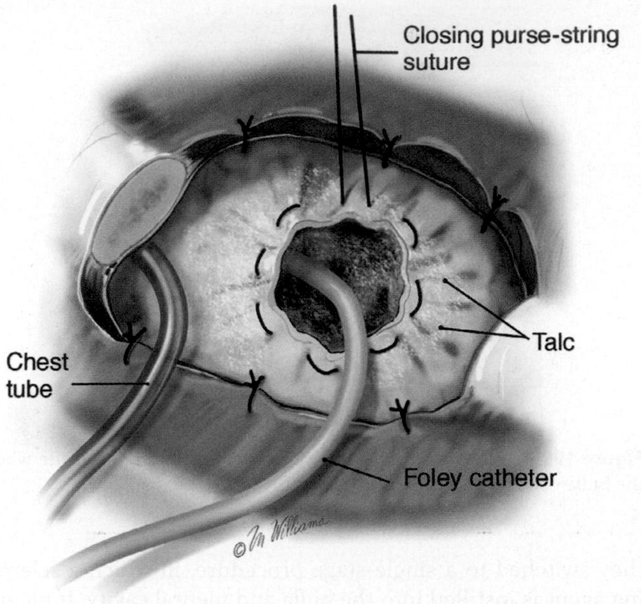

Figure 100-6. A Foley catheter is placed inside the bullous cavity, and a chest tube is placed in the pleural space for drainage. After the bulla is completely drained, the bullous cavity and intrapleural space are insufflated with talc, and the purse-string suture in the visceral pleura is closed over the resected bulla.

(Fig. 100-6). Talc is insufflated into both the bullous cavity and intrapleural space to enhance pleural apposition and symphysis. Following inflation of the balloon with 30 to 40 mL of air, slight traction on the intrapulmonary drain causes the bulla to lie adjacent to the chest wall. The chest tube is placed on suction and the Foley catheter is placed on water seal. The incisions are closed in a standard manner.

POSTOPERATIVE CARE

The postoperative care should adhere to the same principles that apply to any patient with poor pulmonary function. All patients should undergo a smoking cessation program preoperatively, as well as pre- and postoperative pulmonary rehabilitation. The chest tube should remain on water seal suction. If the air leak stops, the catheter is removed within 48 hours. In the Brompton experience, the Foley catheter is removed 8 days after the procedure, irrespective of residual air leak.[7] After removing the chest drain, if there is persistent air leak, a bronchocutaneous fistula will develop. However, the fistula usually closes in 24 to 48 hours. Bronchodilators, chest physiotherapy, early ambulation, and pain control are crucial.

FUNCTIONAL RESULTS AND COMPLICATIONS

The results of the Monaldi procedure in different series are shown in Table 100-1. The success rate is above 80% in all series and improvement in FEV_1 is 22% accompanied by a 26% reduction in residual volume in a single series.[7]

Pneumonias, prolonged air leaks, and frequent need for toilet bronchoscopy are the typical complications in this group of patients. A rare case of cerebral air embolism originating from air in the pulmonary venous system also has been reported following continuous drainage of an infected lung bulla.[10] Recurrence of bullae at the same location or in other areas of the lung was observed in 20% of patients.[7] The Brompton experience, which is the largest single-institution series in the modern era, reports a mortality rate of 6.9% in 58 patients.[8] Mortality is usually due to bronchopneumonia and respiratory failure.

SUMMARY

The Monaldi procedure is an additional option for managing patients with giant bullae. Although VATS excision has become the standard approach in most clinical situations, the Monaldi procedure has several distinct advantages, namely, no lung tissue is removed and no sutures or staplers are applied to the severely emphysematous lung tissue. Hence, it may be an option for patients who have end-stage lung disease, bullous compressive pathology, or bullae that extend to the hilum which are technically difficult or impossible to resect using VATS technique. For patients who can tolerate this procedure, the perioperative management is similar to that for any other end-stage lung disease patient who undergoes a thoracic procedure, with particular attention to early ambulation and management of pain and secretions.

EDITOR'S COMMENT

Most giant bullae in adults are not the pressurized result of "gas trapping," but rather the result of destroyed and hypercompliant lung parenchyma. As a result, there is little benefit to tube

Table 100-1

THE OUTCOME OF SURGICAL SERIES THAT USED THE MINIMALLY INVASIVE MONALDI PROCEDURE IN THE TREATMENT OF GIANT BULLAE

AUTHORS	YEAR	NUMBER OF PATIENTS	SUCCESS RATE (%)	HOSPITAL STAY (DAYS)	MORTALITY (%)
Macarthur[9]	1977	23[a]	82	NS	8.7
Venn[7]	1988	20	80	NS	15
Vigneswaran[11]	1992	6[b]	84	7–35	0
Shah[8]	1994	58	90	15.1 (9–41)	6.9

[a]4 patients had bilateral procedures.
[b]Overall 22 patients were treated for bullous lung disease and only 6 had Monaldi procedure.

drainage unless the bulla is infected. Nonetheless, the Monaldi procedure illustrates a technique that can be applied to other thoracic surgical problems; namely, the creation of a functional pleurocutaneous fistula. As suggested by the Monaldi procedure, symphysis of the surrounding pleura is the important step that permits the management of air leaks with a soft catheter or even without a tube.

—Steven J. Mentzer

References

1. Zellos L. Giant bullectomy. In: L'enfant C, ed. *Lung Biology in Health and Disease*. New York, NY: Marcel Dekkar, 2003:301–308.
2. Deslauriers J. History of surgery for emphysema. *Semin Thorac Cardiovasc Surg*. 1996;8:43–51.
3. Greenberg JA, Singhal S, Kaiser LR. Giant bullous lung disease: evaluation, selection, techniques, and outcomes. *Chest Surg Clin N Am*. 2003;13(4):631–649.
4. Monaldi V. Endocavitary aspiration in the treatment of lung abscess. *Dis Chest*. 1956;29(2):193–201.
5. Chandra D, Rose SR, Carter RB, et al. Fluid-containing emphysematous bullae: a spectrum of illness. *Eur Respir J*. 2008;32(2):303–306.
6. Takanami I. Endoscopic drainage of an infected giant bulla. *Interact Cardiovasc Thorac Surg*. 2006;5(6):794–795.
7. Venn GE, Williams PR, Goldstraw P. Intracavitary drainage for bullous, emphysematous lung disease: experience with the Brompton technique. *Thorax*. 1988;43:998–1002.
8. Shah SS, Goldstraw P. Surgical treatment of bullous emphysema: experience with the Brompton technique. *Ann Thorac Surg*. 1994;58:1452–1456.
9. Macarthur AM, Fountain SW. Intracavitary suction and drainage in the treatment of emphysematous bullae. *Thorax*. 1977;32:668–672.
10. Takizawa S, Tokuoka K, Ohnuki Y, et al. Chronological changes in cerebral air embolism that occurred during continuous drainage of infected lung bullae. *Cerebrovasc Dis*. 2000;10(5):409–412.
11. Vigneswaran WT, Townsend ER, Fountain SW. Surgery for bullous disease of the lung. *Eur J Cardiothorac Surg*. 1992;6(8):427–430.

101 Endoscopic Approaches for Treatment of Emphysema

Carolyn E. Come and George R. Washko

Keywords: Chronic obstructive pulmonary disease (COPD), emphysema, bronchoscopy, lung volume reduction

Treatment of patients with chronic obstructive pulmonary disease (COPD) traditionally has been the task of the internal medicine physician. Global Initiative for Chronic Obstructive Lung Disease recommendations for treatment of COPD include the use of bronchodilators, anti-inflammatory agents, oxygen therapy, aids to assist with smoking cessation, and pulmonary rehabilitation.[1] While pharmacotherapy improves lung function, symptoms, quality of life, and exacerbation rates in COPD, no medical therapies have been shown to improve emphysema, where the primary abnormality is destruction of alveoli with loss of elastic recoil, and subsequent lung hyperinflation. The National Emphysema Treatment Trial (NETT), a large multicenter randomized clinical trial to evaluate the effectiveness of lung volume reduction surgery (LVRS) for the treatment of emphysema, suggested that surgical lung volume reduction, which directly addresses the problem of lung hyperinflation through resection of the most damaged tissue, should be considered for selected patients with emphysema. The findings of this trial, while applicable to a defined subset of COPD patients with advanced upper lobe predominant (ULP) emphysema and reduced exercise capacity, clearly indicate that LVRS can affect lung physiology, symptoms, and even mortality for this disease.[2]

LVRS alters respiratory physiology in several ways—accordingly, posttreatment improvement is multifactorial.[3–10] As originally proposed by Brantigan and Mueller in the 1950s[11] and convincingly demonstrated by Fessler and Permutt,[4] LVRS partially normalizes the mechanical relationship between the hyperinflated emphysematous lung and the surrounding chest wall by increasing the vital capacity and isovolume transpulmonary recoil pressures. Moreover, by reducing the overall size of the hyperinflated lung, LVRS produces space within the less compliant chest cavity for the remaining lung to expand and function.

While this "resizing" process appears to be the primary mechanism responsible for improvements after lung reduction, other factors play a role. Increased recoil pressures cause an increase in airway conductance in a subset of patients, presumably by raising airway isovolume transmural pressures and increasing airway dimensions.[12,13] The reduction in lung size after LVRS normalizes diaphragmatic and chest wall dimensions and improves ventilatory capacity by shortening the operating length over which the respiratory muscles contract.[8–10] In a smaller number of patients, temporary improvements in oxygenation have been observed as a result of local changes in lung impedance that act to normalize ventilation/perfusion matching. LVRS also may improve dynamic lung mechanics by eliminating lung zones with the longest expiratory time constants, not only reducing the tendency for gas trapping and dynamic hyperinflation during exercise but also increasing the inspiratory capacity.[14] Emerging evidence further indicates that the benefits of LVRS go beyond primary respiratory effects; LVRS may in fact improve the compromised cardiac function that is a common comorbidity in this population.[15–17]

Although LVRS provides a treatment option for many patients with advanced emphysema, it is a major procedure performed in a sick population and is associated with substantial morbidity and mortality. Procedural (90-day) mortality was 5.5% in NETT. In that trial, serious complications were observed in 59% of patients (i.e., respiratory failure, prolonged air leak, pneumonia, and cardiac morbidity).[18] Furthermore, when expressed in terms of quality-adjusted life-years, LVRS is more expensive than other currently accepted surgical interventions that improve quality of life for individuals with end-stage disease, such as coronary artery bypass grafting, cardiac transplantation, and lung transplantation.[19] Due to the risks and costs associated with LVRS, fewer than 200 procedures are estimated to be performed annually in the United States,[20] and as a result, a great deal of effort has been spent to devise safer, less invasive, and less costly alternatives. Several different approaches have been and are being tested in clinical trials in the United States and elsewhere. Initial results suggest that the physiologic basis for symptomatic improvement after "nonsurgical lung volume reduction" may not be the same for each of these new methods and may, in fact, be distinct from the effect of LVRS itself. In this chapter, we summarize the technology, methodology, published experiences, and limitations of each approach (Table 101-1).

NONSURGICAL METHODS FOR LUNG VOLUME REDUCTION

The work of Fessler and colleagues[4] and Ingenito and colleagues[6] has shown that lung volume reduction therapy improves respiratory function in emphysema primarily by reducing the size of the hyperinflated lung within the rigid chest cavity. Thus, any process that eliminates areas of hyperinflated lung could potentially achieve the same effect as surgical resection. A variety of nonsurgical techniques have been developed in an attempt to accomplish this including primarily, one-way valves, endobronchial coils, tissue sealants, thermal airway ablation, and airway bypass.

One-way Valve Devices

Lung volume reduction, in principle, could be accomplished by placing a device in a proximal airway, thereby impeding distal gas flow. Theoretically, gas "trapped" beyond the obstructing device would eventually be absorbed and the lung would collapse. Endobronchial plugs and blockers were the original method developed to promote resorption atelectasis.[21,22] However, the high rate of postobstructive pneumonia, pneumothoraces, and

Table 101-1

BRONCHOSCOPIC LUNG VOLUME REDUCTION THERAPIES

TECHNOLOGY	PRODUCT NAME	TARGET PATIENTS	DATA
One-way valve	Zephyr® endobronchial valve (Pulmonx, formerly Emphasys Medical)	Heterogeneous emphysema with low collateral ventilation	Multicenter registry:[26] 98 patients; variable treatment strategies At 3 mos, there were statistically significant improvements in RV, FEV_1, FVC, and 6MWD, but only 6MWD met MCID Most common complications: pneumothoraces, COPD exacerbations, and pneumonia in untreated lobes VENT (pivotal):[27] 220 randomized to unilateral EBV therapy, 101 to medical care At 6 mos, EBV treated patients had modest improvements in FEV_1, 6MWD, and SGRQ that failed to meet MCID Severe COPD exacerbations and hemoptysis significantly more frequent in treated patients. Pneumothorax and pneumonia (including postobstructive) also more common in treated patients.
	Spiration® IBV valve (Olympus Corp., formerly Spiration, Inc.)	Heterogeneous (studies only in ULP) emphysema with low collateral ventilation	3 prospective case series:[31,33,34] 30, 57, and 91 patients; bilateral IBV therapy >50% of patients had clinically significant improvements in SGRQ out to 12 mos but no significant change in pulmonary function or exercise capacity Shift in lobar volume from treated to untreated lobes Pneumothorax was the most common adverse event Pivotal (results only available abstract form):[36–38] 142 randomized to IBV therapy, 135 to sham bronchoscopy At 6 mos, 32% of IBV-treated patients had SGRQ MCID and 19% had a CT lobe volume response (decreased volume of upper lobes and ≥10% increase in nonupper lobes); no difference in lung function or exercise capacity between the groups Significantly more SAEs in treatment vs. control group, in particular pneumothoraces and episodes of respiratory failure
Coil	RePneu® lung volume reduction coil (PneumRx, Inc.)	Heterogeneous or homogeneous emphysema	Pilot:[42] 16 patients with heterogeneous emphysema; 4 treated unilaterally, 12 bilaterally At 6 mos, statistically significant improvements in SGRQ (79% with MCID), FEV_1 (64% with MCID), FVC, RV, and 6MWD (86% with MCID) Most common AEs within 30 d of treatment: COPD exacerbation, mild hemoptysis RESET (small RCT)[45]: ULP, LLP, or homogeneous emphysema; 23 randomized to LVRC treatment (21 treated bilaterally), 24 to medical care At 3 mos, improvement in SGRQ significantly greater in treatment group with 65% achieving MCID. Improvements in FEV_1, RV, and 6MWD (74% with MCID) also significantly greater in treatment group At 30 d, more SAEs in treatment group (COPD exacerbations, pneumothoraces, lower respiratory tract infections); no difference between groups after 30 d Pivotal trial (RENEW) ongoing: 315 patients to be randomized to bilateral LVRC treatment or optimal medical therapy Primary endpoint: mean absolute change in 6MWD at 12 mos Treated patients will be followed for 5 yrs.
Tissue sealant	AeriSeal® emhysematous lung sealant system(Aeris Therapeutics, Inc.)	Heterogeneous ULP or homogeneous with decreased upper lobe perfusion	Pilot:[53] 10 patients with ULP emphysema, 10 with homogeneous disease and decreased upper lobe perfusion; treated bilaterally At 3 mos, statistically significant decrease in upper lobe lung volume, as well as statistically significant improvements in FEV_1 (clinically significant), FVC, RV, MRCD (clinically significant), and SGRQ (clinically significant) that persisted to 1 yr Improvements were greatest in patients with ULP emphysema Self-limited post treatment inflammatory response was the most common adverse event Pivotal trial (ASPIRE) ongoing: 300 patients with ULP emphysema will be randomized to bilateral AeriSeal® treatment vs. medical therapy Primary endpoint: mean change from baseline to 12 mos in postbronchodilator FEV_1 Treated patients to be followed for 5 yrs
Bronchoscopic thermal vapor ablation	InterVapor™ System (Uptake Medical Corp.)	Heterogeneous ULP emphysema	Pilot:[54, 55] 44 patients; treated unilaterally At 6 mos, significant volume loss in treated lobe, as well as significant increases in FEV_1 (55% achieved MCID), SGRQ (73% achieved MCID), RV, 6MWD, and mMRC (63% achieved MCID) At 12 mos follow-up, changes in lobar volumes were similar but improvements in physiologic and clinical measures were smaller in magnitude (46% met FEV_1 MCID, 68% exceeded SGRQ MCID) 11 SAEs in first 30 d, 29 over 6 mos including 1 death; most SAEs were respiratory-related (COPD exacerbation, infection)

(continued)

Table 101-1 (*Continued*)

BRONCHOSCOPIC LUNG VOLUME REDUCTION THERAPIES			
TECHNOLOGY	PRODUCT NAME	TARGET PATIENTS	DATA
Airway bypass	Exhale® drug-eluting stents (Broncus Technologies, Inc.)	Homogeneous emphysema	Pilot:[58] 35 patients; treated bilaterally At 1 mo, there were statistically significant improvements in RV, TLC, FVC, FEV_1, mMRC, 6MWD, and SGRQ. But, at 6 mos, only statistically significant improvements in RV and mMRC (not clinically significant) Three intraoperative SAEs including one death due to major bleeding into the airway. Postoperatively, COPD exacerbations and infection were common EASE (pivotal):[59] 208 patients randomized to airway bypass, 107 to sham bronchoscopy Early improvements in treatment group short-lived; no difference between arms in coprimary efficacy endpoint (FVC increase ≥12% and decrease in mMRC score by ≥1 point) at 6 mos Stent expectoration and passage occlusion Higher rate of SAEs in treatment group in first 7 d

AE, adverse event; COPD, chronic obstructive pulmonary disease; CT, computed tomography; EBV, endobronchial valve; FEV_1, forced expiratory volume in 1 second; FVC, forced vital capacity; IBV, intrabronchial valve; LLP, lower lobe predominant; LVRC, lung volume reduction coil; MCID, minimal clinically important difference; mMRC, modified Medical Research Council dyspnea score; MRCD, Medical Research Council dyspnea score; RCT, randomized controlled trial; RV, residual volume; SAE, serious adverse event; SGRQ, St. George's Respiratory Questionnaire; TLC, total lung capacity; ULP, upper lobe predominant; 6MWD, 6-minute walk distance.

device migration led to their abandonment. One-way valves are an evolution of this concept. They are deployed in the proximal airway through a flexible bronchoscope. Once positioned, these devices are designed to block air from entering the target area during inhalation, while allowing gas to escape during exhalation, leading to volume reduction by promoting progressive deflation and atelectasis in distal emphysematous lung. These valves also allow drainage of mucus, reducing the potential for postobstructive pneumonia.

Two one-way valve systems have been developed, both intended primarily for treatment of heterogeneous ULP emphysema: the endobronchial valve (EBV) and the intrabronchial valve (IBV). The EBV, manufactured by Pulmonx (formerly Emphasys Medical), is designed with a nitinol skeleton and a silicone body with a "duckbill" valve on the proximal end. Originally deployed over a guide wire, the most recent version – the Zephyr® EBV (Fig. 101-1) – is deployed through the working channel of a bronchoscope under direct vision. The deployment catheter also functions as a sizing mechanism so that the valve which best fits the bronchus can be chosen. Several studies,[23–26] including a randomized controlled trial,[27] have investigated the use of these valves in patients with severe heterogeneous emphysema.

In a retrospective analysis from a prospective multicenter registry, Wan et al.[26] reported the experience of the first 98 patients treated with EBVs (Emphasys EBV). In the registry, four valves were delivered on average per patient using several different treatment strategies—unilateral (predominant approach) versus bilateral, lobar versus nonlobar exclusion, upper lobe (most common) versus lower lobe. There were modest but statistically significant improvements in residual volume (RV: −350 ± 970 mL, −4.9 ± 17.4%, $p = 0.025$), forced expiratory volume in 1 second (FEV_1: +60 ± 210 mL, 10.7 ± 26.2%, $p = 0.007$), forced vital capacity (FVC: +120 ± 470 mL, 9.0 ± 23.9%, $p = 0.024$), and 6-minute walk distance (6MWD: +36.9 ± 90 m, $p < 0.001$) at 90-day follow-up. Patients with lobar exclusion and unilateral treatment had the greatest benefit. Eight patients (8.2%; one death) had serious complications, the majority of which were pneumothoraces thought secondary to lung volume changes rather than iatrogenic injury. Thirty patients had other complications including COPD exacerbations and pneumonia in nontreated lobes. Importantly, postobstructive pneumonia was not seen as with the earlier generation endobronchial plug devices.

The Endobronchial Valve for Emphysema Palliation Trial (VENT)[27] was a multicenter, prospective, randomized controlled trial designed to evaluate the safety and efficacy of unilateral EBV therapy with the newer Zephyr® valves (deployed through an internal bronchoscope channel rather than over guidewire). Three hundred and twenty-one patients were randomized to EBV therapy ($n = 220$) or optimal medical care (control, $n = 101$). Patients in the EBV group underwent unilateral and unilobar treatment with the aim of completely isolating the target—most diseased lobe (upper in 76.6% of patients). Again, four valves, on average, were placed per patient. At 6 months, there was a 34.5 mL increase (95% CI 10.8 to 58.3) in FEV_1 in the EBV group compared with a 25.4 mL decrease (95% CI −48.3 to −2.6) in the control group ($p = 0.002$ for between-group difference). The 6MWD increased by 9.3 m (95% CI −0.5 to 19.1) in the EBV group and decreased by 10.7 m (95% CI −29.6 to 8.1) in the control group ($p = 0.02$ for between-group difference). Functional outcomes were not as good as those in the multicenter registry. There were also modest (not clinically significant) improvements in disease-specific quality of life (measured by the St. George's Respiratory Questionnaire, SGRQ) and dyspnea (measured by the Modified Medical Research Council scale, mMRC). Further analysis revealed greatest benefit in patients with computed tomographic (CT) complete fissures (i.e., absent interlobar collaterals), complete lobar isolation, and greater emphysema heterogeneity and paralleled findings in the European VENT cohort.[28] At 6 months, there was a trend toward more major complications in the EBV versus control group (6.1% vs. 1.2%, respectively, $p = 0.08$), though this was less apparent between 6 and 12 months (4.7% vs. 4.6%). The most common adverse events (AEs) in the EBV group included postobstructive pneumonia, hemoptysis, and pneumothorax. Severe COPD exacerbations were significantly more common in the EBV group than the control group during the first 90 days, but there was no difference in severe exacerbations after 90 days. At 6 months, 67/194 (34.5%) patients with CT imaging were found to have evidence of valve malposition.

A smaller, longitudinal, single-center study[29] of 40 patients with a median follow-up of 32 months (up to 5 years) suggested a lasting benefit of EBV treatment. While 40% of patients died

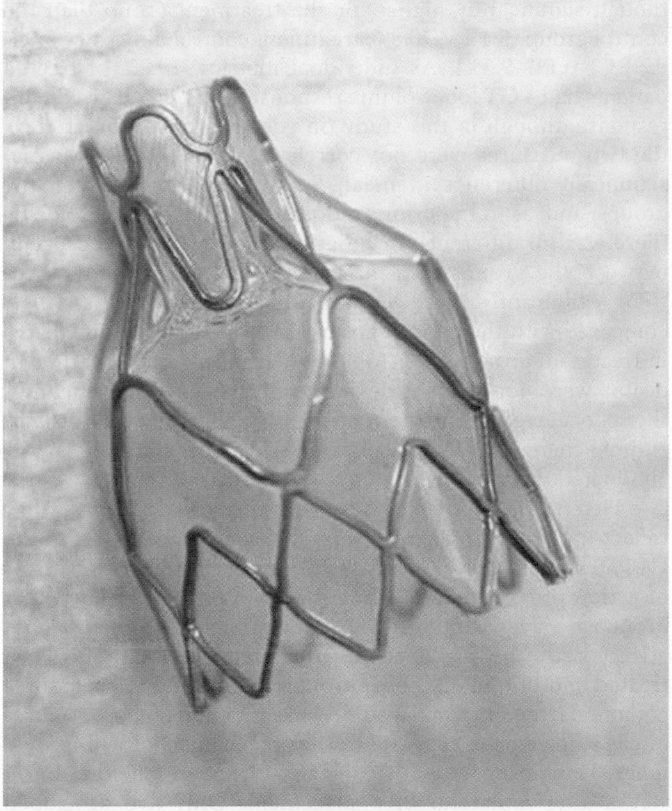

A

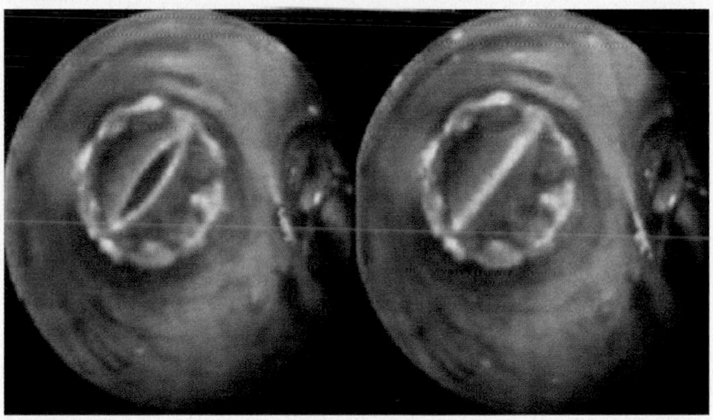

B

Figure 101-1. *A.* Zephyr® Endobronchial Valve. *B.* Implanted Zephyr® Endobronchial Valve end view showing the valve venting during exhalation (left) and sealing during inhalation (right). Reproduced from *BMC Pulmonary Medicine.* 2007;7:10.

during the follow-up, no deaths were procedure-related and this proportion can be contrasted with a projected mortality rate in excess of 40% at 5 years in patients with similar COPD severity.[30] There were statistically and clinically significant improvements in FEV_1, 6MWD, and dyspnea score that persisted out to 5 years.

The second type of one-way valve – Spiration IBV® Valve (Olympus Corp., formerly Spiration, Inc.; Fig. 101-2) – has an umbrella design in which an elastomeric covering is stretched over a nitinol wire frame that anchors the device in place. Air (and mucus) can escape from the lung around the edges of the flexible covering as the umbrella-shaped frame partially collapses, but is prevented from flowing in the forward direction.

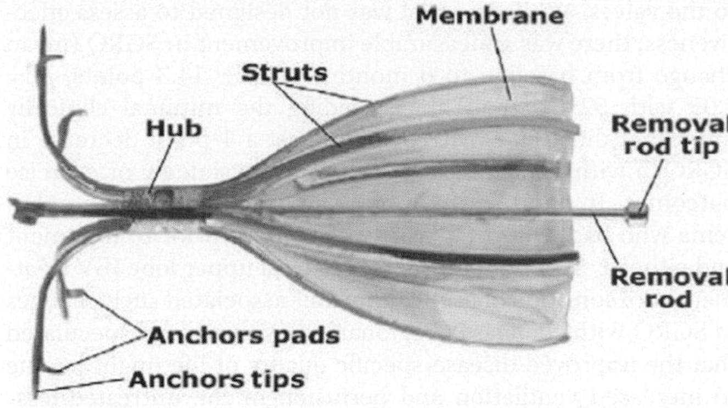

A

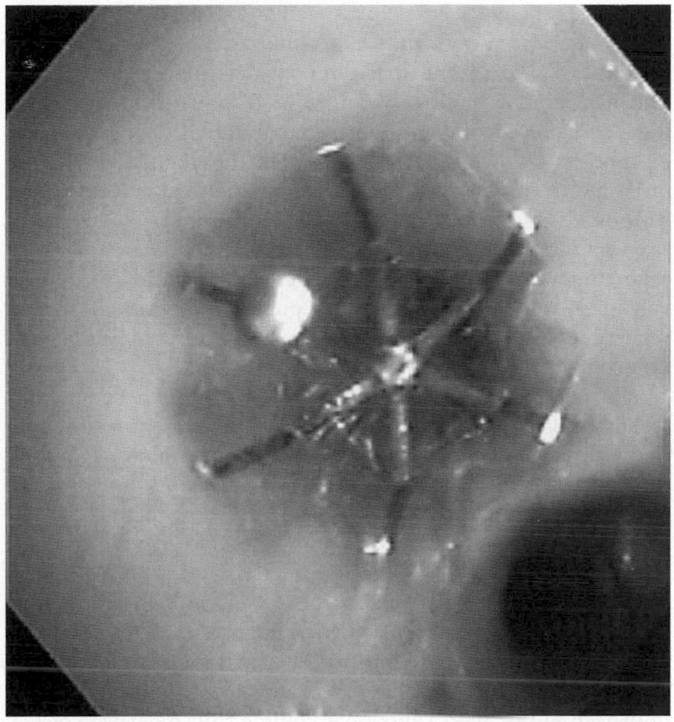

B

Figure 101-2. *A.* Spiration IBV® Valve. *B.* Intrabronchial valve seated in an airway. Reproduced from *J Thorac Cardiovasc Surg.* 2007;133:65–73.e2.

As with the EBV, the IBV can be deployed through the working channel of a flexible bronchoscope under direct visualization and is designed for placement in segmental or subsegmental bronchi. A calibrated balloon is used to determine the valve with the best fit for the target airway.

A number of studies have shown the ability of IBVs to improve perceived quality of life though associated improvements in anatomic lung inflation patterns are variably affected and physiological measures remain unchanged. Moreover, it remains unclear as to the percentage of patients who actually receive benefit or the persistence of treatment. In an initial safety evaluation, Wood et al.[31] reported the results of a multicenter, prospective, open-enrollment cohort study of 30 patients with severe to very severe airflow obstruction, hyperinflation, and ULP emphysema who underwent bilateral upper lobe treatment with IBVs. A mean of 6.5 valves were placed per patient. The procedure was well tolerated with few reported in-hospital or 30-day AEs and no late complications attributed to the valves. While the trial was not designed to assess effectiveness, there was a measurable improvement in SGRQ (mean change from baseline to 6 months: −6.8 ± 14.3 points, p = 0.05 with 52% of patients exceeding the minimal clinically important difference [MCID] of at least a 4-point decrease in SGRQ[32]) with no significant change in physiologic or exercise outcomes. In another study of 57 subjects with ULP emphysema who had paired CT assessments both prior to treatment and either 1, 3, or 6 months after bilateral upper lobe IBV treatment, Coxson and colleagues[33] further associated such changes in SGRQ with changes in regional lung volume and speculated that the improved disease-specific quality of life might be due to increased ventilation and perfusion of the untreated/less-diseased nonupper lobes.

A larger, multicenter, prospective, open-enrollment case series[34] of 91 patients with ULP emphysema who underwent bilateral IBV treatment (mean of 6.7 valves placed per patient) also had similar findings with >50% of patients demonstrating a clinically significant improvement in SGRQ at 1, 3, 6, and 12 months following device placement (no change in FEV_1 or 6MWD). In this larger study, seven patients had device-related serious adverse events (SAEs) in the first 3 months. Pneumothorax was the most common complication particularly when all segments within a lobe were occluded and 16 patients required valve removal (44 valves total; for pneumonia, bronchospasm, recurrent COPD exacerbations, or pneumothorax). There were no occurrences of valve migration or erosion.

In two subsequent multicenter, sham bronchoscopy-controlled trials of IBV treatment (first 73 patients, reported; [35] second 277 patients, completed) SGRQ again improved, though there were fewer responders. In the first study, 73 patients with ULP emphysema were randomized to IBV placement (n = 37) versus sham bronchoscopy (n = 36). To avoid complete occlusion of the upper lobes, lobar atelectasis, and potential pneumothorax, one segment (or subsegment) of the right upper lobe and the lingula were left untreated. A mean number of 7.3 valves were placed per patient in the treatment group. At 3 months, there were 8 (24%) responders (composite endpoint: ≥4-point improvement in SGRQ and lobar volume shift measured by CT with a decrease in upper lobe volume and a volume increase of ≥7.5% in nontreated lobes) in the treatment group versus none in the sham group (p = 0.002). In the treatment group, upper lobe volume decreased by 7.3 ± 9.0% and lower lobe volume increased by 6.7 ± 14.5%; these volume shifts persisted at 6 months. At 3 months, both groups had statistically significant mean improvements in SGRQ compared to baseline (treatment: −4.3 ± 16.2 points, control: −3.6 ± 10.7 points; there was no difference between groups, p = 0.8), though mean change in SGRQ only exceed the MCID in the treatment group. At 6 months, treated patients had further improvement in SGRQ (mean change from baseline: −10.9 ± 18.2 points). There were no significant improvements in pulmonary function tests, dyspnea, or exercise capacity. There were also no differences in procedural AEs or hospital length of stay between groups, indicating that as a whole, IBV treatment appeared safe, though effective in only a subset of patients.

In the second larger study (IBV treatment, n = 142 vs. sham bronchoscopy, n = 135; reported as abstracts[36–38]), the responder rate was again low overall (responder defined as having both an improvement in SGRQ of ≥4 points and regional lung volume changes on CT [decreased volume of the upper lobes and ≥10% increase in nonupper lobes] at 6 months) though significantly higher for the treatment group than the control group (5.1% vs. 0.8%; treatment control difference 5.0%, 95% CI 0.1%–9.5%). As individual metrics, 19.2% of treated patients had a CT lobe volume response and 32.2% had a SGRQ response, though in this study (in contrast to Coxson et al.[33]), the two measures were not correlated. Further, there was no significant difference in mean SGRQ response between the groups, and, as in the prior randomized controlled trial (RCT), there was no difference in lung function or exercise capacity between the groups at 6 months. In this larger study, there were significantly more SAEs in the treatment group (27%) compared with the control group (13%) including more deaths in treatment group (six vs. one, borderline significant), though deaths were not thought device-related. Also, while pneumothorax occurred in three out of the first 37 patients, early algorithmic changes to leave an untreated right upper lobe airway eliminated this AE.

Heterogeneity in trial results and patient response may reflect underlying and unaccounted for heterogeneities in the COPD population as well as the multifactorial mechanisms of action of treatments. While it was initially postulated that bronchial valves would lead to improvement by causing lobar atelectasis,[23] the presence of collateral ventilation between treated and untreated lobes through incomplete lobar fissures confounds regional collapse and treatment response. Subsequent studies have suggested other mechanisms for improvement. Hopkinson et al.[39] evaluated 19 patients before and 4 weeks after unilateral EBV placement. Only five developed visible atelectasis on CT, four of whom had improvements in exercise capacity. However, one-third of patients with no atelectasis on CT also had improved exercise capacity which was attributed to reduced dynamic hyperinflation (end-expiratory lung volume at isotime was reduced in patients with and without atelectasis). Collateral resistance is likely important in this phenomenon[40]—in patients with relatively low resistance collateral channels, the region distal to a valve may still hyperinflate under certain conditions such as exercise; as resistance increases, this dynamic hyperinflation of distal lung tissue decreases as ventilation is directed toward more normal lung units; with even higher collateral resistance, atelectasis occurs and lung mechanics improve through the same mechanisms as LVRS. Another potential mechanism for improvement after valve placement is interlobar ventilatory shifts and improved ventilation perfusion matching as proposed by Coxson et al.[33]

The limited improvements observed in patients with significant collateral ventilation (CV) have led to the development of new techniques for determining the amount of CV in a given segment or subsegment such as the Chartis® Pulmonary Assessment System (Pulmonx). This specialized catheter with a balloon at the distal tip is inserted via the working channel of a bronchoscope. Once inflated, the balloon blocks the airway permitting air to only flow out from the target compartment through the catheter's central lumen allowing airway flow and pressure to be measured. As a result, airway resistance and compartmental CV can be calculated. In an observational study,[41] 80 patients were evaluated for CV with this system prior to unilateral placement of Zephyr® EBVs (either upper or lower lobe). Fifty-one subjects had no evidence of CV. Of those without CV, 71% had a significant improvement in target lobe volume reduction (TLVR, the primary outcome measure) at 30 days as compared to only 17% of those with CV. Moreover, of TLVR responders without CV, 39% had a low degree of heterogeneity between target and nontarget lobes. Clinical responses were better in those without than with CV and were even better in those without CV who achieved TLVR. While an observational study, these findings suggest absence of CV may be more important in predicting response to valve-based therapies than emphysema heterogeneity, at the same time expanding and refining the population who may benefit from such therapies. Additional prospective studies evaluating the effects of Zephyr® EBVs in patients evaluated pretreatment with the Chartis® system are ongoing.

Coils

Lung volume reduction coils (LVRC) are thought to work by (1) compressing diseased tissue, allowing expansion of better-functioning areas of lung; (2) retensioning adjacent lung tissue so that the lung contracts more efficiently during breathing; and (3) tethering open small airways to prevent air trapping. The RePneu® LVRC (Fig. 101-3), manufactured by PneumRx, Inc., is made from nitinol. It is delivered bronchoscopically into subsegmental airways and regains its predetermined shape upon deployment. For placement, a guidewire is advanced into the airway under fluoroscopic guidance and a catheter is passed over the wire and aligned with its distal tip. The airway length is measured with radiopaque markers to choose the appropriate coil size. The guidewire is then removed and a straightened coil is pushed through the catheter into position. Finally, the catheter is removed and the coil regains its original shape (coiling up the surrounding airway and tensioning the adjacent parenchyma).

In a pilot study, Slebos and colleagues[42] evaluated the safety and effectiveness of LVRCs in 16 patients with heterogeneous emphysema. Four patients were treated unilaterally in a single procedure and 12 patients were treated bilaterally in two sequential procedures (28 total procedures performed). A median of 10 coils were placed per lung. AEs possibly related to the device or the procedure within 30 days of treatment included pneumothorax (1), pneumonia (2), COPD exacerbation (6), chest pain (4), and mild (<5 mL) self-limited hemoptysis (21). Between 30 days and 6 months, the main AEs were pneumonia (3) and COPD exacerbations (14). There were no life-threatening events. At 6 months, there were significant improvements in SGRQ, the primary efficacy endpoint (−14.9 ± 12.1 points, $p < 0.001$; 79% of patients exceeded the MCID), FEV_1 (+14.9 ± 17.0%, $p = 0.004$; 64% exceeded the MCID[43]), FVC (+13.4 ± 12.9%, $p = 0.002$), RV (−11.4 ± 9.0%, $p < 0.001$), and 6MWD (+84.4 ± 73.4 m, $p < 0.001$; 86% exceeded the MCID[44]). Outcomes were better in patients who received bilateral treatment.

In a small prospective randomized control trial (RESET)[45] at three centers in the United Kingdom, 47 patients with severe emphysema (ULP, lower lobe predominant [LLP], or homogeneous emphysema) were randomized to LVRC treatment (n = 23) or optimal medical care (control, n = 24). The majority of treated patients underwent treatment of the contralateral lung at 1 month (n = 21). Coils were placed in segmental airways of the most affected lobe or lobes (on average, 18.5 coils per bilaterally treated patient). Improvement in SGRQ was significantly greater in the treated group (−8.11 points [95% CI −13.83 to −2.39] vs. 0.25 [95% CI −5.58 to 6.07] in the control group; p = 0.04 for between-group difference) with 65% of treated patients having an MCID versus only 22% of control patients ($p = 0.01$). At 90 days, mean improvements in FEV_1 and RV were significantly greater in the treated group (14.2 vs. 3.6%, $p = 0.03$; and −0.51 L vs. −0.20 L, $p = 0.03$; respectively). 6MWD increased by an average of 51.2 m in the treated group but decreased by 12.4 m in the control group ($p < 0.001$ for between-group difference) with 74% of treated patients exceeding the MCID. In the first 30 days, there were more SAEs in the treatment group (two COPD exacerbations, two pneumothoraces, and two lower respiratory tract infections) than the control group (one COPD exacerbation). There was no between-group difference in SAEs from 30 to 90 days, and there were no deaths in either group.

While awaiting more definitive trials, the LVRC system has already demonstrated a number of attractive features, despite its need for fluoroscopy. Firstly, LVRC is unaffected

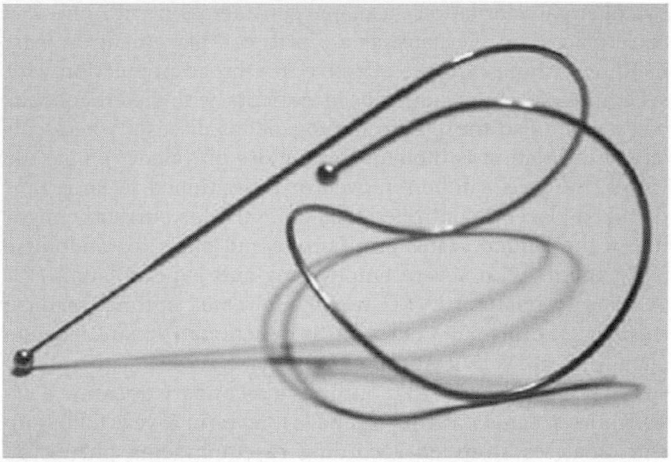

A

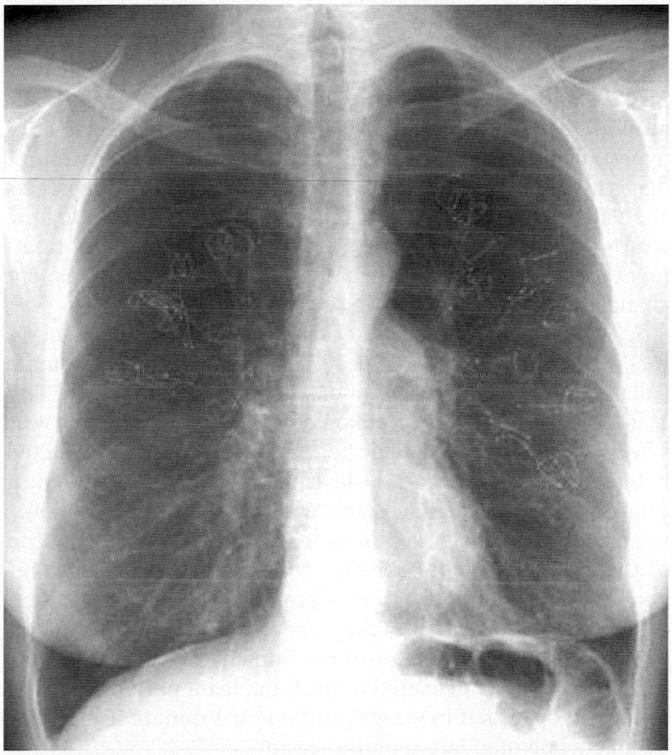

B

Figure 101-3. *A.* RePneu® Lung Volume Reduction Coil. *B.* Posterior–anterior chest radiograph demonstrating coils positioned bilaterally in upper lobe segments. Reproduced from *Chest.* 2012;142:574–582.

by collateral ventilation—a major consideration with one-way valve placement. Perhaps, as a result, coil placement (at least in RESET) appears to be effective in a broad population with severe emphysema, not only in patients with heterogeneous disease but also those with homogeneous disease (where collateral ventilation is thought to be more prevalent[46]). Like the valves, the coils can be removed or repositioned. A large randomized placebo-controlled trial (RENEW) is currently ongoing in the United States and Europe and plans to randomize 315 patients with severe emphysema and hyperinflation (RV ≥225%) to bilateral LVRC treatment versus optimal medical therapy. The primary outcome is functional (mean absolute change in 6MWD from baseline to 12 months) with subjective SGRQ changes at 12 months as a secondary outcome. Furthermore, treated patients will have long term 5-year follow-up with analyses stratified according to emphysema phenotype (heterogeneous or homogeneous).

Tissue Sealant

Like the one-way valves, tissue sealants are designed to directly reduce lung volume by collapsing and sealing damaged areas of hyperinflated lung. The site and mechanism of action are fundamentally different from the valves, however. This system acts at an alveolar rather than an airway level, thus overcoming the issue of collateral ventilation. Unlike valves and coils, this treatment is not reversible—it is intended to produce a permanent change in tissue configuration similar to LVRS.

The initial tissue sealant, developed by Aeris Therapeutics, Inc., used a series of biologically active reagents to promote collapse and scar formation in damaged regions of lung. Phase 1 and 2 trials[47–49] showed biologic lung volume reduction was safe and provided physiologic benefits in appropriately selected patients. Subsequently, Aeris developed the AeriSeal® System, a synthetic polymer foam sealant, which is delivered as follows: the treatment catheter is positioned 2 to 4 cm beyond the end of the bronchoscope under direct visualization; sealant components (5 mL) and air (15 mL) are mixed to generate 20 mL of liquid foam, which is rapidly injected through the catheter while maintaining wedge position; immediately post injection, the 30 mL of air is delivered to push the foam peripherally; the bronchoscope is left in wedge position for 1 minute to allow for complete polymerization of the sealant.

Three open-label, single-arm multicenter trials of the AeriSeal® System have been conducted in Europe and Israel. In the first,[50] 25 patients with heterogeneous ULP emphysema underwent unilateral unilobar treatment (upper lobe or superior segment lower lobe) of up to 6 subsegments over one to two treatment sessions. There were no serious procedural complications. Three patients had spillage of the material into central airways, but it was easily suctioned out. All patients experienced an inflammatory flu-like reaction beginning 8 to 24 hours following treatment that was generally mild and responsive to supportive care; this reaction was more significant in patients treated at four sites versus two to three sites in a single session. Short-term side effects were also more frequent among patients who received treatment at adjacent subsegments. There were eight treatment-related severe COPD exacerbations. Late treatment-related complications (>90 days post treatment) were not seen. There was no evidence of treatment-related mediastinal or pleural pathology. At 3 months, mean change in the ratio of residual volume to total lung capacity (RV/TLC, the primary endpoint) was $-3.4 \pm 9.2\%$, $p = 0.09$ ($-4.7 \pm 9.5\%$, $p = 0.04$ at 6 months) and the percentage of patients with clinically meaningful improvements in FEV_1, FVC, Medical Research Council Dyspnea score (MRCD)[51], 6MWD, and SGRQ was 41%, 41%, 33%, 38%, and 50%, respectively. Similar results were seen at 6 months.

The second study[52] included 56 patients with ULP ($n = 19$), LLP ($n = 7$), or homogeneous emphysema ($n = 30$). To reduce posttreatment acute inflammation, patients received steroids and antibiotics periprocedure. In addition, AeriSeal® System therapy was limited to nonadjacent subsegments. Patients received an initial treatment at two subsegments in one lobe and were eligible for repeat treatment after 12 weeks at 2 or 3 additional subsegments in the contralateral lung (39/56 subjects underwent a second treatment session). The modified protocol reduced acute and subacute side effects substantially (posttreatment inflammation decreased >60% and incidence of all-cause severe COPD exacerbations in the first 90 days decreased from 44% to 9%). Patients with a diffusing capacity for carbon monoxide (DLCO) between 20% and 60% predicted who were treated in the upper lobes (either ULP or homogeneous with reduced perfusion to the upper lobes) had significantly improved lung function, gas trapping, and respiratory-related quality of life at 3 months. For unclear reasons, patients treated in the lower lobes did not improve.

Based on these results, a third prospective study[53] was performed, incorporating both modified protocol and patient selection criteria based on the earlier findings. Twenty patients with a baseline DLCO between 20% and 60% predicted and ULP ($n = 10$) or homogeneous disease with decreased upper lobe perfusion ($n = 10$) received bilateral upper lobe treatment (two nonadjacent subsegments/upper lobe) with the AeriSeal® System. At 3 months, there was a significant reduction in upper lobe lung volume on CT (-895 ± 484 mL, $p < 0.001$ = primary endpoint) that was durable out to 1 year. Treatment was also associated with significant improvements in FEV_1 (265 ± 248 mL, $28.9 \pm 30.6\%$, $p = 0.003$), FVC (251 ± 405 mL, $11.8 \pm 19.4\%$, $p = 0.033$), RV (-639 ± 894 mL, $-10.9 \pm 18.2\%$, $p = 0.036$), dyspnea [ΔMRCD -1 (-1 to 1), $p = 0.011$], and SGRQ (-9.1 ± 12.9 points, $p = 0.016$) at 3 months that also persisted to 1 year. TLVR as well as clinical improvements were greater in patients with heterogeneous ULP disease (Fig. 101-4). There was one serious procedural complication and seven all-cause significant respiratory AEs over 17 patient-years of follow-up.

ASPIRE, a multicenter randomized controlled trial of AeriSeal® System treatment plus optimal medical therapy compared to optimal medical therapy alone in patients with advanced ULP heterogeneous emphysema, is currently underway in the US, Europe, and Israel. Approximately 300 patients will be randomized 3:2 to treatment versus medical therapy. The primary endpoint is the mean change from baseline in postbronchodilator FEV_1 at 12 months; other objective as well as subjective secondary measures include change in CT upper lobe volume and 6MWD as well as the proportion of patients achieving a MCID in SGRQ and MRCD. Long-term follow-up will continue through 5 years in treated patients.

Bronchial Thermal Vapor Ablation

Like a tissue sealant, bronchial thermal vapor ablation (BTVA) causes lung volume reduction by producing irreversible fibrosis

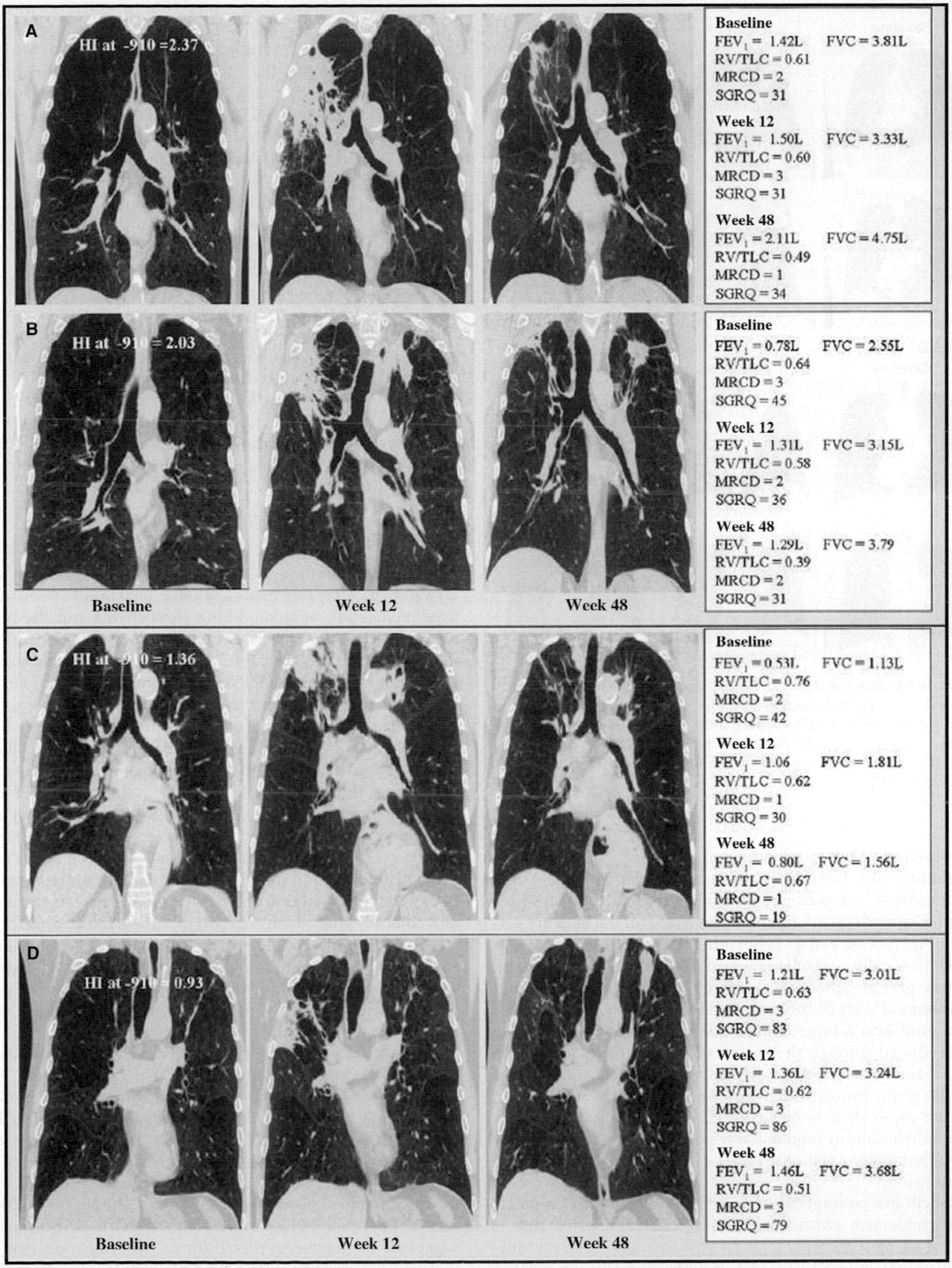

Figure 101-4. Coronal chest CT images pre and post AeriSeal® System treatment with corresponding physiologic and functional data at baseline, 12, and 48 weeks (four patients). Baseline heterogeneity was measured with the heterogeneity index (HI = [% voxels in right upper lobe + left upper lobe < −910 Hounsfield units]/[% voxels in right lower lobe + left lower lobe < −910 Hounsfield units]), where higher values indicate increased heterogeneity and upper lobe predominant emphysema. *A*. Patient A, HI 2.37. *B*. Patient B, HI 2.03. *C*. Patient C, HI 1.36. *D*. Patient D, HI 0.93. FEV_1, forced expiratory volume in one second; FVC, forced vital capacity; RV, residual volume, TLC, total lung capacity; MRCD, Medical Research Council dyspnea score; SGRQ, St. George Respiratory Questionnaire. Reproduced with permission from *Chest*. 2012; 142:1111–1117.

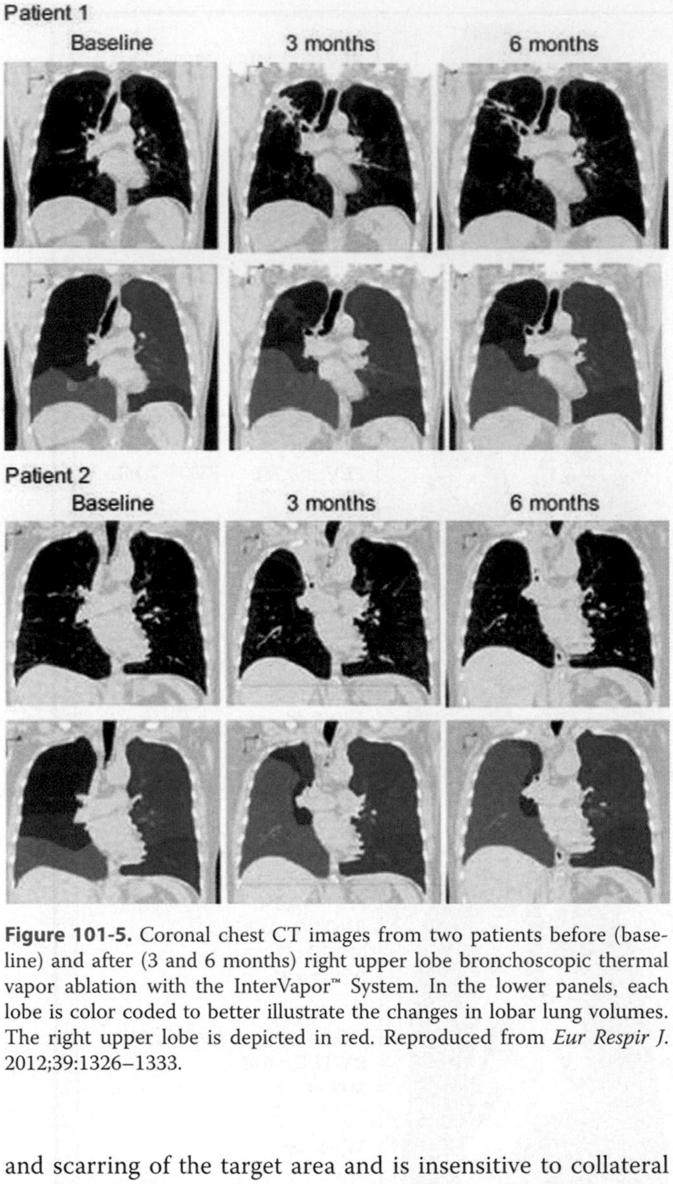

Figure 101-5. Coronal chest CT images from two patients before (baseline) and after (3 and 6 months) right upper lobe bronchoscopic thermal vapor ablation with the InterVapor™ System. In the lower panels, each lobe is color coded to better illustrate the changes in lobar lung volumes. The right upper lobe is depicted in red. Reproduced from *Eur Respir J.* 2012;39:1326–1333.

and scarring of the target area and is insensitive to collateral ventilation. The InterVapor® System (Uptake Medical Corp) includes three components: an application that provides preferred treatment locations and times based on the patient's CT, a vapor generator, and a vapor catheter. The vapor generator is an electronically controlled pressure vessel that generates and delivers precise amounts of energy (heated vapor) through the vapor catheter (flexible shaft with occlusion balloon at the distal end) into a targeted lung segment. The vapor catheter is introduced through the bronchoscope to the airway of the lung segment selected for treatment. An occlusion balloon is inflated (to protect other airways from the heated vapor), and the vapor dose is delivered. The heated vapor induces a thermal reaction in targeted areas of lung leading to a localized inflammatory response followed by fibrosis of airways and parenchyma.

Snell and colleagues[54] reported the results of two open-label, single-arm efficacy and safety clinical studies with a total of 44 patients with ULP emphysema who received unilateral upper lobe BTVA. At 6 months, the average volume loss in the treated lobe (measured by CT) was 715.5 ± 99.4 mL ($p < 0.001$), a 48% reduction in lobar volume (Fig. 101-5). The mean increase in FEV_1 at 6 months (coprimary efficacy endpoint) was 140.8 ± 26.3 mL, 17% ($p < 0.001$) with 55% of patients achieving the MCID. SGRQ (coprimary efficacy endpoint) improved by 14 ± 2.4 points ($p < 0.001$) with 73% of patients exceeding the MCID. There were also significant improvements in RV (−406 ± 112.9 mL, $p < 0.001$), 6MWD (46.5 ± 10.6 m, $p < 0.001$), and mMRC dyspnea score (−0.9 ± 0.17 points, $p < 0.001$ with 63% of patients exceeding the MCID[51]). There were no AEs during the procedure. In the first 30 days, there were 11 SAEs, and 29 over 6 months including one death. The majority of SAEs at both time points were respiratory-related. A posttreatment inflammatory reaction (elevated inflammatory markers ± symptoms) peaked within 2 to 4 weeks and resolved within 8 to 12 weeks.

Herth and colleagues[55] followed the above cohort out to 12 months. Changes from baseline in treated upper lobe and ipsilateral lower lobe volumes were similar; however, improvements in physiologic and clinical measures were smaller in magnitude than those seen at 6 months (ΔFEV_1 86.2 ± 173.8 mL (10%), $p < 0.05$, 46% achieved a MCID compared with baseline; ΔSGRQ −11 ± 14 units, $p = 0.05$, 68% met MCID from baseline). Responses were greater in patients with higher versus lower heterogeneity indices. Incidence of SAEs diminished over time with only 10 between 6 and 12 months.

Airway Bypass

Instead of attempting to collapse damaged regions of lung, airway bypass creates extra-anatomic passages between damaged, collaterally ventilated lung parenchyma and the central airways. This approach is designed to bypass small, collapsible, high-resistance airways in damaged emphysematous lung by creating low-impedance pathways into the central airways, resulting in more effective emptying and improved respiratory mechanics. While this procedure should theoretically be useful in heterogeneous or homogeneous emphysema with collateral ventilation, trials have focused on homogeneous disease where collateral ventilation is prevalent. The procedure is performed by passing a flexible bronchoscope into an area of known emphysema and using a Doppler probe to identify an area free of blood vessels. Next the bronchial wall is pierced with a transbronchial needle and dilating balloon. Finally, a stent is placed to expand and maintain the new passage between the airway and adjacent lung tissue (Fig. 101-6). The Exhale® drug-eluting stent (Broncus Technologies, Inc.) is composed of stainless steel and silicone and contains paclitaxel, which is intended to inhibit fibrotic responses and improve long-term passage patency (in previous animal studies, non-drug-eluting stents became occluded within 1 week of placement).[56,57]

In a multicenter pilot study,[58] 35 patients received bilateral upper lobe airway bypass with the Exhale® Emphysema Treatment System. Ninety-four percent of patients had homogeneous emphysema. A median of eight stents were placed per patient. At 1-month follow-up, there were statistically significant improvements in RV, TLC, FVC, FEV_1, mMRC, 6MWD, and SGRQ. But, at 6 months, only improvements in RV and mMRC remained significant (−400 mL [−6.6%], $p = 0.04$ and −0.5 points, $p = 0.025$, respectively). A retrospective analysis suggested the degree of pretreatment hyperinflation may predict which patients achieve the best results, as patients with an RV/TLC ratio above the median of 0.67 had greater benefit (though results still only significant for RV (−870 mL [−14.1%], $p = 0.022$) and mMRC [−0.5 points, $p = 0.035$] at 6 months).

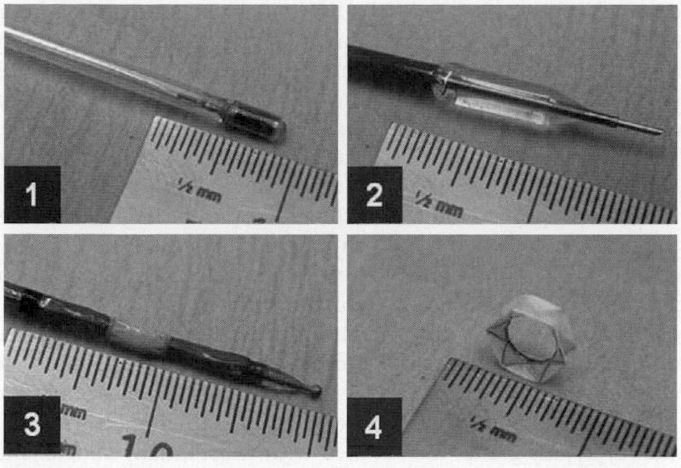

A

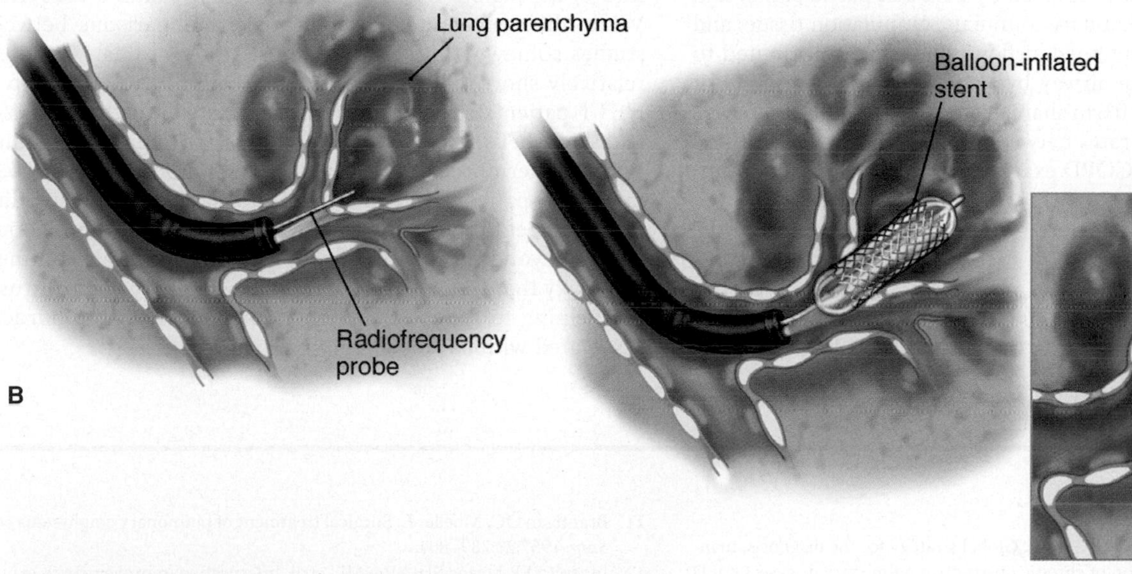

B

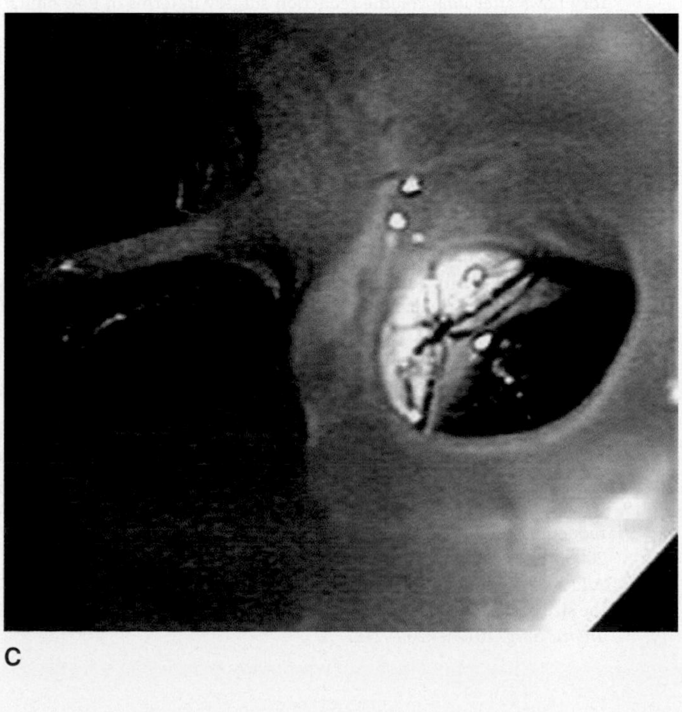

C

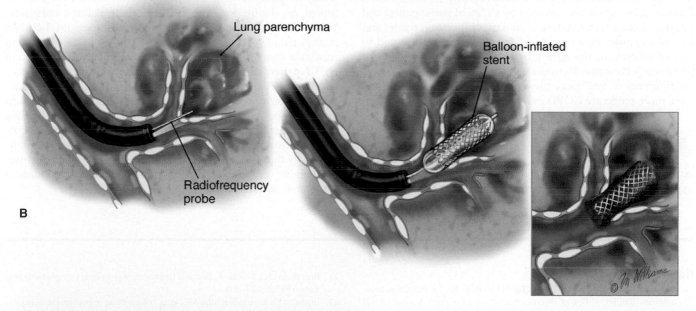

Figure 101-6. *A.* Devices used for airway bypass: (1) Exhale® Doppler Probe, (2) Exhale® Transbronchial Balloon Dilation Needle, (3) Exhale® Drug-Eluting Stent mounted on delivery catheter, (4) Exhale® Drug-Eluting Stent deployed. *B.* Cartoon of a technique for insertion of bronchopulmonary stents: flexible bronchoscope is inserted to the level of the segmental bronchus, a blood vessel-free location is identified with a Doppler probe (step not shown), bronchial wall is fenestrated with the transbronchial needle and dilating balloon (or radiofrequency probe), paclitaxel-eluting stent is placed to expand and maintain the new passage between the airway and adjacent lung tissue. *C.* Implanted stent at follow-up bronchoscopic examination. Parts *A* and *C* reproduced with permission from *J Thorac Cardiovasc Surg.* 2007;134:974–981.

For less hyperinflated patients, no outcome measures were significant at 6 months. In a subset of patients, bronchoscopic exam at 6 months revealed 18/26 (69%) of the stents were patent. There were three intraoperative SAEs including one death due to major bleeding into the airway and two episodes of pneumomediastinum/subcutaneous emphysema. Postoperatively, 22 patients experienced SAEs, most commonly COPD exacerbations and infection. Despite antibiotic prophylaxis, five patients had respiratory infections in the first week.

Exhale® airway stents for emphysema (EASE)[59] was a multicenter, double-blind, randomized controlled trial in which 315 patients with severe hyperinflation (RV/TLC ≥0.65) and homogeneous emphysema were randomized to airway bypass (208) or sham bronchoscopy (107). Patients were followed for 12 months. A mean of 4.7 stents were placed per patient. While there were early improvements in the airway bypass group, the benefits declined by 1 month. At 6 months, there was no difference between arms in the coprimary efficacy endpoint (FVC increase ≥12% and decrease in mMRC score by ≥1 point). Stent expectoration (clinically reported by 11.5% of participants) and passage occlusion (secondary to mucus, granulation tissue, and lack of adequate, maintained airflow) may have contributed to lack of efficacy. In the airway bypass group, the 7-day rate of SAEs was 3.4% versus 0% in sham group. At 6 months, there was no difference in SAE rates between the groups; however, there were more moderate COPD exacerbations in the bypass group.

SUMMARY

Lung volume reduction surgery removes emphysematous, hyperinflated lung tissue, thereby improving the mechanical relationship between the lung and the surrounding chest wall and allowing the remaining more normal lung to expand and function better. Beyond smoking cessation and oxygen therapy, LVRS is the only treatment that definitively prolongs survival in patients with emphysema. However, given the substantial morbidity and mortality associated with major thoracic surgery in an already sick population, less invasive bronchoscopic strategies capable of achieving similar benefits have been sought. Although none of these technologies (one-way valves, coils, tissue sealant, bronchial thermal vapor ablation, and airway bypass procedures) are FDA-approved to date, all are approved for clinical use outside the United States. Despite diverse mechanisms of action, all procedures can be performed via flexible bronchoscopy (typically under moderate sedation rather than general anesthesia) and are associated with substantially shorter inpatient stays than LVRS and lower procedural mortality. In addition, nontraditional LVRS candidates (i.e., those with nonULP or homogeneous emphysema) or patients with significant comorbidities may, in the future, be eligible for bronchoscopic lung volume reduction. While differences in endpoints make comparisons between studies somewhat difficult and most studies to date have had relatively short follow-up compared with 5-year follow-up of NETT patients,[60] evidence to date suggests differential efficacy and safety between types of bronchoscopic lung volume reduction. Furthermore, it is clear that certain modalities work best in certain patients and improved mechanistic understanding and therapeutic targeting may well be a way to improve outcomes beyond device modifications alone. As trials continue, it is likely that some of these methods will prove clinically useful, helping to reduce the tremendous suffering and burdens associated with advanced emphysema.

References

1. Vestbo J, Hurd SS, Agusti AG, et al. Global strategy for the diagnosis, management, and prevention of chronic obstructive pulmonary disease: GOLD executive summary. *Am J Respir Crit Care Med.* 2013;187:347–365.
2. Fishman A, Martinez F, Naunheim K, et al. A randomized trial comparing lung-volume-reduction surgery with medical therapy for severe emphysema. *N Engl J Med.* 2003;348:2059–2073.
3. Gelb AF, Zamel N, McKenna RJ, Jr, et al. Mechanism of short-term improvement in lung function after emphysema resection. *Am J Respir Crit Care Med.* 1996;154:945–951.
4. Fessler HE, Permutt S. Lung volume reduction surgery and airflow limitation. *Am J Respir Crit Care Med.* 1998;157:715–722.
5. Fessler HE, Scharf SM, Permutt S. Improvement in spirometry following lung volume reduction surgery: application of a physiologic model. *Am J Respir Crit Care Med.* 2002;165:34–40.
6. Ingenito EP, Loring SH, Moy ML, et al. Physiological characterization of variability in response to lung volume reduction surgery. *J Appl Physiol.* 2003;94:20–30.
7. Celli BR, Montes de Oca M, Mendez R, et al. Lung reduction surgery in severe COPD decreases central drive and ventilatory response to CO2. *Chest.* 1997;112:902–906.
8. Bloch KE, Li Y, Zhang J, et al. Effect of surgical lung volume reduction on breathing patterns in severe pulmonary emphysema. *Am J Respir Crit Care Med.* 1997;156:553–560.
9. Lando Y, Boiselle PM, Shade D, et al. Effect of lung volume reduction surgery on diaphragm length in severe chronic obstructive pulmonary disease. *Am J Respir Crit Care Med.* 1999;159:796–805.
10. Gorman RB, McKenzie DK, Butler JE, et al. Diaphragm length and neural drive after lung volume reduction surgery. *Am J Respir Crit Care Med.* 2005;172:1259–1266.
11. Brantigan OC, Mueller E. Surgical treatment of pulmonary emphysema. *Am Surg.* 1957;23:789–804.
12. Ingenito EP, Loring SH, Moy ML, et al. Interpreting improvement in expiratory flows after lung volume reduction surgery in terms of flow limitation theory. *Am J Respir Crit Care Med.* 2001;163:1074–1080.
13. Sciurba FC, Rogers RM, Keenan RJ, et al. Improvement in pulmonary function and elastic recoil after lung-reduction surgery for diffuse emphysema. *N Engl J Med.* 1996;334:1095–1099.
14. Martinez FJ, de Oca MM, Whyte RI, et al. Lung-volume reduction improves dyspnea, dynamic hyperinflation, and respiratory muscle function. *Am J Respir Crit Care Med.* 1997;155:1984–1990.
15. Jorgensen K, Houltz E, Westfelt U, et al. Effects of lung volume reduction surgery on left ventricular diastolic filling and dimensions in patients with severe emphysema. *Chest.* 2003;124:1863–1870.
16. Come CE, Divo MJ, San Jose Estepar R, et al. Lung deflation and oxygen pulse in COPD: results from the NETT randomized trial. *Respir Med.* 2012;106:109–119.
17. Mineo TC, Pompeo E, Rogliani P, et al. Effect of lung volume reduction surgery for severe emphysema on right ventricular function. *Am J Respir Crit Care Med.* 2002;165:489–494.
18. Naunheim KS, Wood DE, Krasna MJ, et al. Predictors of operative mortality and cardiopulmonary morbidity in the National Emphysema Treatment Trial. *J Thorac Cardiovasc Surg.* 2006;131:43–53.
19. Ramsey SD, Berry K, Etzioni R, et al. Cost effectiveness of lung-volume-reduction surgery for patients with severe emphysema. *N Engl J Med.* 2003;348:2092–2102.
20. Akuthota P, Litmanovich D, Zutler M, et al. An evidence-based estimate on the size of the potential patient pool for lung volume reduction surgery. *Ann Thorac Surg.* 2012;94:205–211.

21. Watanabe S, Shimokawa S, Yotsumoto G, et al. The use of a Dumon stent for the treatment of a bronchopleural fistula. *Ann Thorac Surg.* 2001;72:276–278.
22. Sabanathan S, Richardson J, Pieri-Davies S. Bronchoscopic lung volume reduction. *J Cardiovasc Surg (Torino).* 2003;44:101–108.
23. Toma TP, Hopkinson NS, Hillier J, et al. Bronchoscopic volume reduction with valve implants in patients with severe emphysema. *Lancet.* 2003;361:931–933.
24. Snell GI, Holsworth L, Borrill ZL, et al. The potential for bronchoscopic lung volume reduction using bronchial prostheses: a pilot study. *Chest.* 2003;124:1073–1080.
25. Venuta F, de Giacomo T, Rendina EA, et al. Bronchoscopic lung-volume reduction with one-way valves in patients with heterogenous emphysema. *Ann Thorac Surg.* 2005;79:411–416; discussion 6–7.
26. Wan IY, Toma TP, Geddes DM, et al. Bronchoscopic lung volume reduction for end-stage emphysema: report on the first 98 patients. *Chest.* 2006;129:518–526.
27. Sciurba FC, Ernst A, Herth FJ, et al. A randomized study of endobronchial valves for advanced emphysema. *N Engl J Med.* 2010;363:1233–1244.
28. Herth FJ, Noppen M, Valipour A, et al. Efficacy predictors of lung volume reduction with Zephyr valves in a European cohort. *Eur Respir J.* 2012;39:1334–1342.
29. Venuta F, Anile M, Diso D, et al. Long-term follow-up after bronchoscopic lung volume reduction in patients with emphysema. *Eur Respir J.* 2012;39:1084–1089.
30. Celli BR, Cote CG, Marin JM, et al. The body-mass index, airflow obstruction, dyspnea, and exercise capacity index in chronic obstructive pulmonary disease. *N Engl J Med.* 2004;350:1005–1012.
31. Wood DE, McKenna RJ Jr, Yusen RD, et al. A multicenter trial of an intrabronchial valve for treatment of severe emphysema. *J Thorac Cardiovasc Surg.* 2007;133:65–73.
32. Jones PW. Interpreting thresholds for a clinically significant change in health status in asthma and COPD. *Eur Respir J.* 2002;19:398–404.
33. Coxson HO, Nasute Fauerbach PV, Storness-Bliss C, et al. Computed tomography assessment of lung volume changes after bronchial valve treatment. *Eur Respir J.* 2008;32:1443–1450.
34. Sterman DH, Mehta AC, Wood DE, et al. A multicenter pilot study of a bronchial valve for the treatment of severe emphysema. *Respiration.* 2010;79:222–233.
35. Ninane V, Geltner C, Bezzi M, et al. Multicentre European study for the treatment of advanced emphysema with bronchial valves. *Eur Respir J.* 2012;39:1319–1325.
36. Wood DE, Nader D, Elstad MR, et al. Bronchial valve treatment of emphysema: results and conclusions from a double-blind randomized trial. *Am J Respir Crit Care Med.* 2012;185:A5348.
37. Coxson HO, Springmeyer SC, Nader D, et al. Bronchial valve treatment of emphysema: lung volume reduction in a double-blind randomized trial. *Am J Respir Crit Care Med.* 2012;185:A2903.
38. Elstad MR, Mehta AC, Nader D, et al. Bronchial valve treatment of emphysema: procedure and device safety results from a double-blind randomized trial. *Am J Respir Crit Care Med.* 2012;185:A1112.
39. Hopkinson NS, Toma TP, Hansell DM, et al. Effect of bronchoscopic lung volume reduction on dynamic hyperinflation and exercise in emphysema. *Am J Respir Crit Care Med.* 2005;171:453–460.
40. Fessler HE. Collateral ventilation, the bane of bronchoscopic volume reduction. *Am J Respir Crit Care Med.* 2005;171:423–424.
41. Herth FJ, Eberhardt R, Gompelmann D, et al. Radiological and clinical outcomes of using Chartis to plan endobronchial valve treatment. *Eur Respir J.* 2013;41:302–308.
42. Slebos DJ, Klooster K, Ernst A, et al. Bronchoscopic lung volume reduction coil treatment of patients with severe heterogeneous emphysema. *Chest.* 2012;142:574–582.
43. Donohue JF. Minimal clinically important differences in COPD lung function. *COPD.* 2005;2:111–124.
44. Puhan MA, Chandra D, Mosenifar Z, et al. The minimal important difference of exercise tests in severe COPD. *Eur Respir J.* 2011;37:784–790.
45. Shah PL, Zoumot Z, Singh S, et al. Endobronchial coils for the treatment of severe emphysema with hyperinflation (RESET): a randomized controlled trial. *Lancet Respir Med.* 2013;1:233–240.
46. Higuchi T, Reed A, Oto T, et al. Relation of interlobar collaterals to radiological heterogeneity in severe emphysema. *Thorax.* 2006;61:409–413.
47. Reilly J, Washko G, Pinto-Plata V, et al. Biological lung volume reduction: a new bronchoscopic therapy for advanced emphysema. *Chest.* 2007;131:1108–1113.
48. Criner GJ, Pinto-Plata V, Strange C, et al. Biologic lung volume reduction in advanced upper lobe emphysema: phase 2 results. *Am J Respir Crit Care Med.* 2009;179:791–798.
49. Refaely Y, Dransfield M, Kramer MR, et al. Biologic lung volume reduction therapy for advanced homogeneous emphysema. *Eur Respir J.* 2010;36:20–27.
50. Herth FJ, Gompelmann D, Stanzel F, et al. Treatment of advanced emphysema with emphysematous lung sealant (AeriSeal(R)). *Respiration.* 2011;82:36–45.
51. Gross NJ. Chronic obstructive pulmonary disease outcome measurements: what's important? What's useful? *Proc Am Thorac Soc.* 2005;2:267–271; discussion 90–91.
52. Herth FJ, Eberhardt R, Ingenito EP, et al. Assessment of a novel lung sealant for performing endoscopic volume reduction therapy in patients with advanced emphysema. *Expert Rev Med Devices.* 2011;8:307–312.
53. Kramer MR, Refaely Y, Maimon N, et al. Bilateral endoscopic sealant lung volume reduction therapy for advanced emphysema. *Chest.* 2012;142:1111–1117.
54. Snell G, Herth FJ, Hopkins P, et al. Bronchoscopic thermal vapour ablation therapy in the management of heterogeneous emphysema. *Eur Respir J.* 2012;39:1326–1333.
55. Herth FJ, Ernst A, Baker KM, et al. Characterization of outcomes 1 year after endoscopic thermal vapor ablation for patients with heterogeneous emphysema. *Int J Chron Obstruct Pulmon Dis.* 2012;7:397–405.
56. Choong CK, Phan L, Massetti P, et al. Prolongation of patency of airway bypass stents with use of drug-eluting stents. *J Thorac Cardiovasc Surg.* 2006;131:60–64.
57. Choong CK, Haddad FJ, Gee EY, et al. Feasibility and safety of airway bypass stent placement and influence of topical mitomycin C on stent patency. *J Thorac Cardiovasc Surg.* 2005;129:632–638.
58. Cardoso PF, Snell GI, Hopkins P, et al. Clinical application of airway bypass with paclitaxel-eluting stents: early results. *J Thorac Cardiovasc Surg.* 2007;134:974–981.
59. Shah PL, Slebos DJ, Cardoso PF, et al. Bronchoscopic lung-volume reduction with Exhale airway stents for emphysema (EASE trial): randomised, sham-controlled, multicentre trial. *Lancet.* 2011;378:997–1005.
60. Naunheim KS, Wood DE, Mohsenifar Z, et al. Long-term follow-up of patients receiving lung-volume-reduction surgery versus medical therapy for severe emphysema by the National Emphysema Treatment Trial Research Group. *Ann Thorac Surg.* 2006;82:431–443.

PART 18

LUNG INFECTION

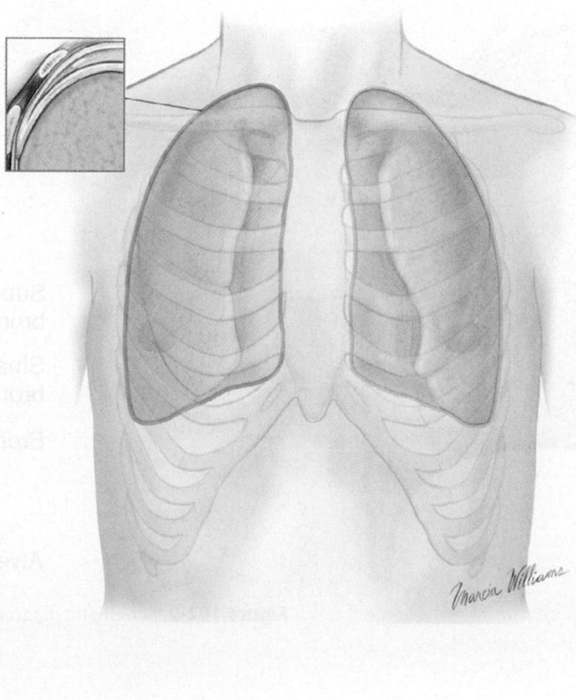

102 Lung Infections and Interstitial Lung Disease: Overview and General Approach

Nicolas C. Issa and Lindsey R. Baden

Keywords: Infection, host defense mechanisms, cystic fibrosis, neutropenia, hematologic malignancies, hematopoietic stem cell transplantation, lung transplantation, lung abscess

ANATOMY AND PATHOPHYSIOLOGY OF NORMAL HOST DEFENSE MECHANISMS

The respiratory tract (Fig. 102-1) is in constant contact with the environment and exposed to direct inoculation by infectious and noninfectious agents. To defend itself against these agents, the respiratory tract is equipped with several types of defense mechanisms including both mechanical and immune-mediated mechanisms. Large size airborne particles (>5 microns) are filtered by the nose and are trapped by the nasal cilia. Intermediate size (1–5 microns) particles are deposited in the trachea and bronchi, and small size particles (0.01–1 microns) and infectious agents often are deposited in the bronchioles and the alveolar space (Fig. 102-2).

The respiratory tract from the trachea to the bronchioles is lined with ciliary cells and goblet cells that secrete a thin layer of mucus. The rhythmic beat of the cilia move the mucus-trapped material upward, which is then cleared externally by the cough mechanism or swallowed interiorly and eliminated by the gastrointestinal tract. This mechanism is called the mucociliary escalator (Fig. 102-3) and is a very important defense mechanism that plays a major role in clearing infectious and noninfectious particles from the respiratory tract.

The alveolar macrophages are another important line of defense. Macrophages clear bacteria and nonliving particles that reach the alveolar space through phagocytosis and digestion by cellular lysosomes. Opsonization, which involves coating of the invading agents by antibodies secreted by lymphocytes present in the mucosa, can further enhance phagocytosis. The alveolar macrophages also secret cytokines upon interaction with foreign particles that help recruit and activate neutrophils, lymphocytes, and other inflammatory cells to clear the foreign material.

The lungs and pleura are also richly supplied by an extensive lymphatic drainage system that helps transport phagocytosed particles and infectious agents out of the lungs to the

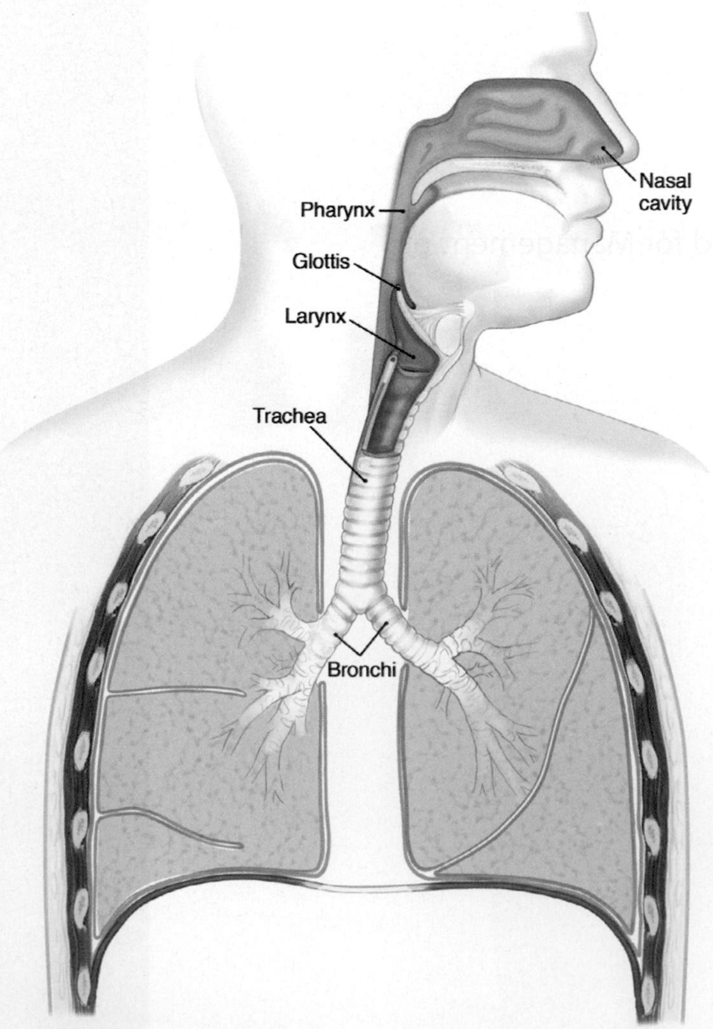

Figure 102-1. Anatomy of the respiratory tract.

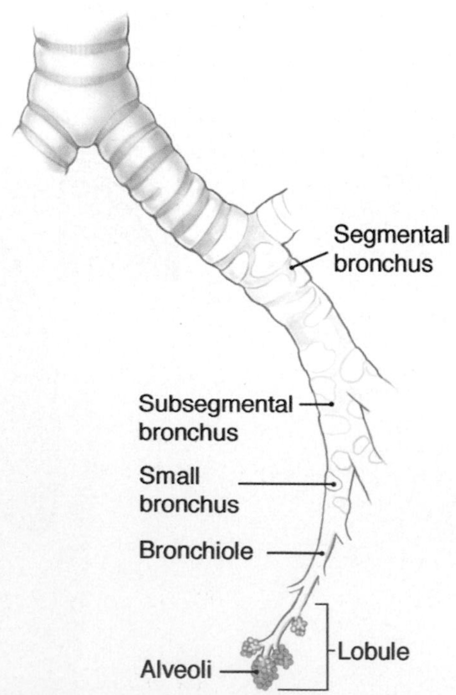

Figure 102-2. Schematic diagram of the airway.

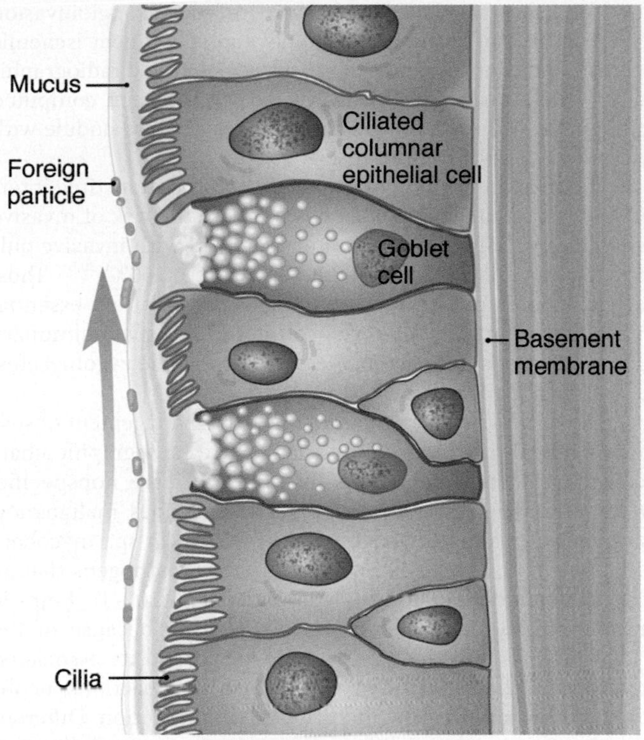

Figure 102-3. Mucociliary escalator.

regional lymph nodes where certain infectious agents (mycobacteria, fungi) can remain in a latent phase potentially for prolonged periods of time.

The interaction between host and pathogen factors determines if an infection is established or cleared. Certain host factors or conditions like altered mental status and alcoholism, for example, may predispose to the development of aspiration pneumonia as a result of the absence of protective gag reflexes. Other factors like endotracheal intubation or chest tube placement may predispose to ventilator-associated pneumonia and surgical wound infection, respectively, by bypassing normal host defenses. Infection could also be initiated when pathogen virulence factors overwhelm the host defense mechanisms.

In this chapter, we discuss lung infections associated with impaired host defense mechanisms and the important role of the thoracic surgeon in the approach to and management of these infections either through procurement of tissue specimens that help establish histopathological and/or microbiological diagnosis or through curative surgical resection of the infected tissue.

INFECTIONS ASSOCIATED WITH IMPAIRED HOST DEFENSE MECHANISMS

Infections Associated with Mucociliary Clearance Dysfunction

The importance of the mucociliary clearance as a key host defense mechanism is highlighted in patients with primary ciliary dyskinesia where failure of the mucociliary escalator function (see Fig. 102-3) leads to chronic suppurative lung disease.[1] Inhibition of the mucociliary clearance mechanism plays a significant role in allowing certain pathogens to establish persistent and recurrent infections in patients with cystic fibrosis (CF), bronchiectasis, and chronic obstructive pulmonary disease (COPD). The course of the disease in these patients is often marked by frequent and recurrent exacerbations due to the intense inflammatory response associated with the infectious process that results in parenchymal destruction and ultimately respiratory failure.

Cystic Fibrosis

CF is an autosomal recessive multisystem disease that was first described as a clinical syndrome in 1938.[2] Inadequate hydration of luminal secretions due to abnormal ion transport leads to accumulation of viscous mucus which compromises the mucociliary clearance mechanism.[3–5] At the base of this defect is a mutation in the cystic fibrosis transmembrane conductance regulator (CFTR) gene.[3–5] The concentrated mucus present in CF airways favors bacterial colonization and persistence. There is also intense neutrophilic inflammation in the airways of CF patients associated with the presence of bacterial pathogens.[6–8] Initial colonization of the airways of CF patients occurs early and is followed by persistent infection. *Pseudomonas aeruginosa* and *Staphylococcus aureus* are common bacterial pathogens that cause colonization and infection in CF patients.[9–12] Biofilm production by these pathogens makes eradication difficult.[13–15] Other important pathogens include *Burkholderia cepacia* complex,[16,17] *Stenotrophomonas maltophilia*,[18] respiratory viral infections, and nontuberculous mycobacteria.[19,20] Various species of fungi also may cause infection and allergy in the airways. Frequent exacerbations in CF patients due to recurrent infections are associated with intense inflammation which results in airway wall damage and lung parenchymal destruction, ultimately leading to respiratory failure.[10,21] Aggressive treatment of pulmonary bacterial infections is an important and effective intervention in the treatment of CF patients. Antimicrobial resistance is common and varies between institutions. Antimicrobial treatment of CF exacerbations could be challenging because of drug resistance and should be guided by antimicrobial susceptibility data.

Thoracic surgeons often are involved in the care of CF patients when respiratory function deteriorates significantly and lung transplantation is considered (see Chapter 108 for an overview of lung transplantation). Eligibility for lung transplantation usually is reviewed by a multidisciplinary team prior to transplantation to optimize perioperative management and help improve transplantation outcome. Perioperative antimicrobials that target known pathogens isolated from the most recent respiratory cultures, guided by antimicrobial sensitivities, often are used to help prevent seeding of the pleural space upon explantation of the native lungs. Such treatment also helps to prevent infection of the anastomotic site, as well as surgical site infection and postoperative infectious complications. The choice of perioperative antimicrobials should be guided preferably by an infectious disease or pulmonary specialist experienced in the treatment of CF. Certain organisms pose increased risk in the lung transplant setting such as *Burkholderia cenocepacia*, thus requiring special consideration when transplantation is being considered in patients colonized pre-transplantation.[22,23]

Infections Associated with Innate and Adaptive Immune System Dysfunction

The human immune system is a complex array of innate and adaptive processes geared toward defending the body against pathogens. The immune system has layered defense mechanisms against infections. Physical barriers (skin, mucosal surfaces) constitute the first line of defense against potential pathogens. The *innate immune system* is the second defense mechanism and provides an immediate but nonspecific immune response through several mechanisms including inflammation, complement system activation, macrophages, dendritic cells, neutrophils, and natural killer cell activation. On the other hand, the *adaptive immune system* is a highly sophisticated defense mechanism that has evolved over millions of years and involves an antigen-specific immune response capable of recognizing "non-self" antigens. It also has the ability to generate memory cells that permit a quick and tailored response to pathogens previously encountered. Both the innate and the adaptive immune systems are interconnected. The innate immune system plays an important role in the activation of the adaptive immune system.

Immunodeficiency could result from either a genetic abnormality (e.g., severe combined immunodeficiency) or could be acquired. The most common causes of acquired immunodeficiency syndromes are due to human immunodeficiency virus (HIV) infection or are secondary to immunosuppressive agents (chemotherapy, biological agents, monoclonal antibodies such as against T and B cells) administered after organ transplantation or for the treatment of chronic inflammatory disease or malignancy.

The resulting net state of immunosuppression can predispose the host to certain types of lung infections depending on the affected component of the immune system. Neutropenia, for example, will predispose the host to infections due to bacterial (*S. aureus, P. aeruginosa*) and fungal pathogens (*Aspergillus*, Zygomycetes, *Candida*), whereas T cell immunodeficiency (HIV, steroids, alemtuzumab, thymoglobulins) predisposes the host predominantly to viral infections (cytomegalovirus [CMV], Epstein–Barr virus [EBV], herpes simplex virus, varicella zoster virus) and fungal infections (*Pneumocystis jirovecii* pneumonia [PCP], *Aspergillus*, Zygomycetes, *Candida*). B cell immunodeficiency (rituximab, hypogammaglobulinemia) predisposes the host to infection by such pathogens as bacterial encapsulated organisms and some viral infections (such as hepatitis B). The use of tumor necrosis factor (TNF) inhibitors (etanercept, infliximab, adalimumab) is particularly associated with mycobacterial (including TB) and fungal infections.[24]

Infections Associated with Chemotherapy-induced Neutropenia in Patients with Solid Tumors and Hematologic Malignancies

Patients with chemotherapy-induced neutropenia are at increased risk for a range of lung infections including bacterial, viral, and fungal infections. Up to 60% of patients with neutropenia develop pulmonary infiltrate at some point during the course of their disease and often with severe consequences.[25,26] Bacterial infections are the most common and are due mainly to gram-negative organisms (*P. aeruginosa, Escherichia coli*, and other gram-negative rods), *S. aureus*, and other bacterial pathogens.[27] Community respiratory viruses also are common and include respiratory syncytial virus (RSV), influenza viruses, parainfluenza viruses, picornaviruses, and adenoviruses.[28] Invasive pulmonary aspergillosis is an important fungal infection in neutropenic patients. Inhaled *Aspergillus* conidia are usually phagocytosed by lung macrophages, and the hyphal growth required for tissue invasion is prevented by neutrophils. In neutropenic patients, however, failure to control hyphal growth leads to angioinvasion with occlusion of tissue blood supply and subsequent ischemic necrosis of the lung parenchyma. This is manifested radiographically by the classic signs of invasive aspergillosis on computed tomography (CT) scan of the chest, that is, a dense nodule with a halo sign or cavitary lesions (Fig. 102-4).

The total duration of neutropenia and the short time interval between neutropenic episodes increase the risk of invasive aspergillosis.[29] The mortality rate associated with invasive pulmonary aspergillosis is high (in the range of 60%).[30,31] Thus, early diagnosis and prompt antifungal treatment are essential in reducing mortality. Other encountered invasive pulmonary fungal infections in neutropenic patients include zygomycetes, fusarium, dematiaceous mold, and other fungi.

The role of the thoracic surgeon in the management of suspected fungal infection is important since radiographic characteristics of the lung lesions in most cases are nonspecific. Differential diagnosis of a lung nodule includes malignancy, various bacterial pathogens including *Nocardia* sp., mycobacterial infection, as well as a variety of fungal pathogens that all may exhibit nodular and/or halo signs (Fig. 102-4). Empiric antimicrobial treatment often is not feasible because of the wide range of pathogens possibly involved and its associated adverse side effects including hypersensitivity reactions, nephrotoxicity, hepatotoxicity, and drug–drug interaction. Different fungal pathogens have different antifungal susceptibility patterns. Obtaining tissue for definitive diagnosis is consequently of utmost importance. This can be done through different approaches including fine-needle aspiration, biopsy, or wedge resection via video-assisted thoracoscopic surgery (VATS). In some instances, resection of the pulmonary lesion when feasible allows for both diagnostic and therapeutic purposes and may significantly reduce the duration of antimicrobial therapy and its associated toxicity. Early surgical intervention also could be life saving, since fungal infections are often angioinvasive and depending on location and proximity to great vessels could erode through vessel walls and cause hemoptysis or exsanguination.

Infections in Hematopoietic Stem Cell Transplant Recipients

Hematopoietic stem cell transplant (HSCT) recipients are at increased risk for severe infectious complications as a result of a combination of factors including underlying disease, the type of conditioning regimen (myeloablative versus nonmyeloablative), the type of HSCT (autologous transplantation versus allogeneic transplantation), and its associated risk of graft versus host disease (GVHD), and its treatment. The timing of infection post-HSCT and the type of pathogens involved vary depending on the type of HSCT and the way it was performed.

In autologous stem cell transplantation, the patient's own stem cells are collected prior to transplantation and cryopreserved to permit intense chemotherapy targeting the underlying disease and then reinfused after conditioning—as stem cell rescue. The time to engraftment (blood counts recovery) in autologous HSCT is relatively short and thus the risk of infection is less compared to allogeneic HSCT.

In allogeneic HSCT, stem cells are collected from family members, volunteers, or from banked cord blood cells. HLA matching is required to decrease the risk of GVHD. To decrease the risk of infectious complications after HSCT, prophylactic or

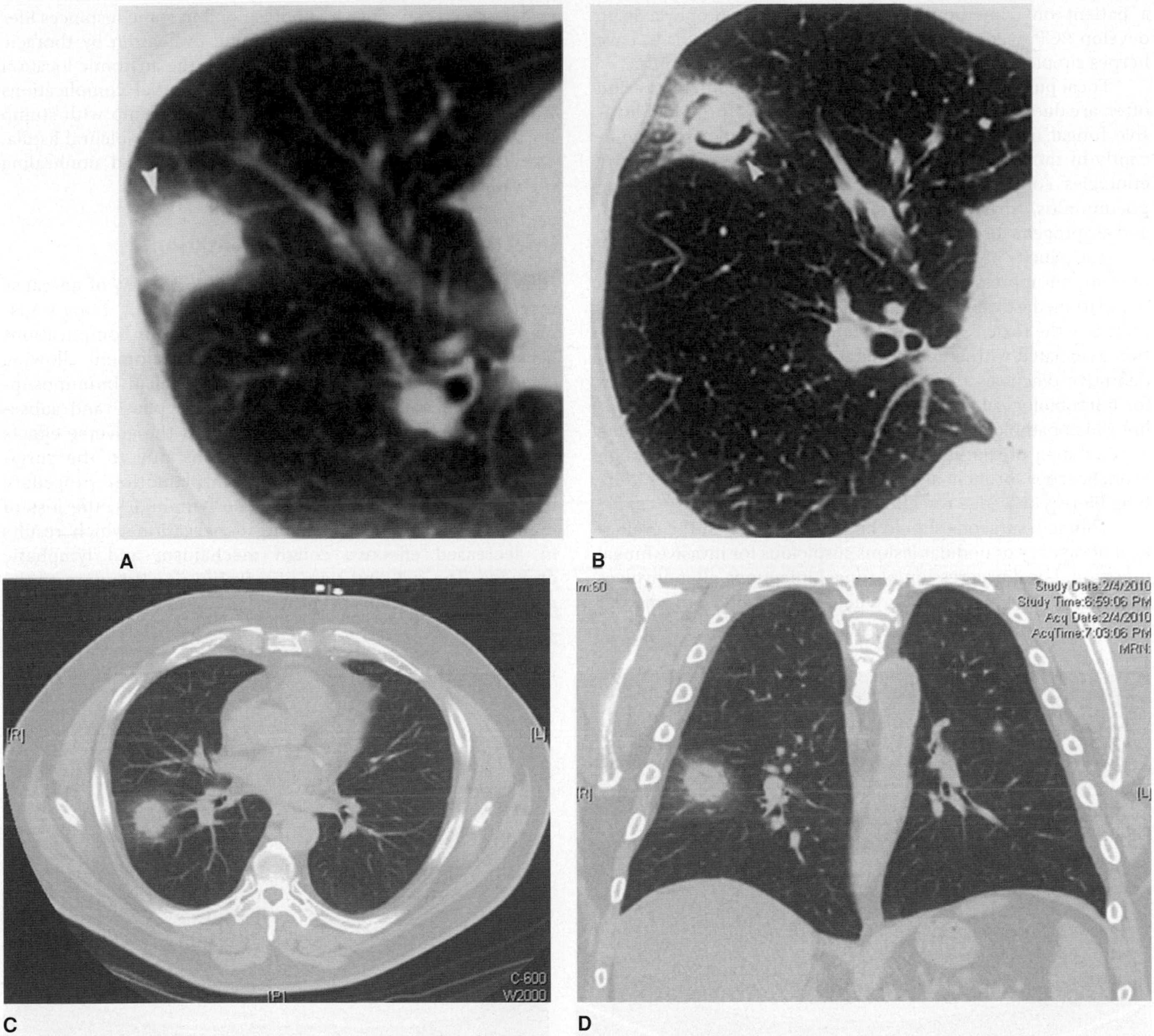

Figure 102-4. *A.* Halo and *(B)* crescent signs typically seen in invasive pulmonary aspergillosis. *C, D.* Halo sign seen with bacterial infection.

pre-emptive antimicrobials using antibacterials, antivirals, and sometimes antifungal agents are often used but the type and duration of prophylactic strategies vary between procedures and institutions based upon patient risk profile for infection.

GVHD occurs when the donor cells (graft) recognize the recipient (host) as "non-self" and attempt to reject it. The treatment of acute GVHD requires the use of intense immunosuppression including high-dose steroids, monoclonal antibodies, or TNF-receptor blockers, all of which increase significantly the risk of opportunistic infections. To decrease the risk of GVHD after allogeneic HSCT, prophylaxis using immunosuppressive regimens targeting T cell activation is often employed.

Pneumonic syndromes are common after HSCT and could be due to either an infectious or noninfectious etiology depending on the timing of onset of signs and symptoms and the nature and duration of antimicrobial prophylaxis.[32] Imaging of the chest using high-resolution CT scan is a very sensitive method to detect and characterize pulmonary infiltrates.[33,34] When evaluating HSCT recipients with lung infiltrates or a focal lung lesion, it is important to note the type of HSCT, the timing of onset of the lung infiltrates or lesion, its radiologic appearance (diffuse, focal, nodular), the current immunosuppressive regimen, whether GVHD is present or absent, and the prophylactic regimen that the patient is taking.

In early postengraftment period, diffuse bilateral pulmonary infiltrates (pneumonitis) could equally be due to infectious or noninfectious etiologies. Infectious etiologies include respiratory viruses (respiratory syncytial virus, influenza viruses, parainfluenza viruses, picornaviruses and adenoviruses),[28,35–38] legionella, CMV, or PCP. Knowledge of the type of prophylactic antimicrobial regimen that the patient is taking helps narrow the differential diagnosis. For example, it is unlikely for a patient on trimethoprim-sulfamethoxazole prophylaxis to develop PCP or for a patient on acyclovir prophylaxis to have herpes simplex virus or varicella zoster virus pneumonitis.

Focal pulmonary infiltrates in the postengraftment period often are due to bacterial or fungal infections. The risk of invasive fungal infections, mainly aspergillosis, increases significantly in the presence of GVHD.[39,40] However, noninfectious etiologies could also be a possibility. Idiopathic interstitial pneumonitis, alveolar hemorrhage, bronchiolitis obliterans, and cryptogenic organizing pneumonia are often encountered.

The paucity of symptoms often encountered in the context of immunosuppression, the broad differential diagnosis in this population, the likelihood of noninfectious etiologies of the lung infiltrate, the toxicity, and the potential for drug–drug interaction associated with empiric therapy, often mandate early and definitive diagnosis through procurement of clinical samples for microbiological diagnosis and preferably tissue samples for both histopathological and microbiological diagnosis from the affected area of the lungs. Samples can be obtained through bronchoscopy, bronchoalveolar lavage, fine-needle aspiration, lung biopsy, or wedge resection via VATS.

Thoracic surgeons should be involved early in the evaluation of cavitary or nodular lesions suspicious for invasive fungal infection. Local progression of fungal infections often involves angioinvasive features and a predilection to erode into adjacent vessels which can cause hemoptysis and in some instances life-threatening massive bleeding. Careful evaluation by thoracic surgeons should take into consideration the anatomic location and resectability of the lung lesion. Potential complications from surgery include inability to close the stump with stump breakdown and the risk of developing a bronchopleural fistula, bleeding due to thrombocytopenia, and wound nonhealing (neutropenia) (Fig. 102-5).

Infections after Lung Transplantation

Infectious complications account for up to 20% of all-cause mortality at 5 years after lung transplantation.[41] Lung transplant recipients are at high risk for infectious complications because of constant exposure to the environment allowing direct pathogen inoculation, the high level of immunosuppression especially during the induction phase and subsequently with treatment of rejection, and the adverse effects on the local host defense mechanisms due to the surgical procedure itself. The lung transplantation procedure is associated with disruption of the lymphatics, the loss of mucociliary clearance, and lung denervation which results in decreased effective cough mechanism and lymphatic drainage. The risk and type of infection is a function of the nature and duration of prophylactic regimens employed,

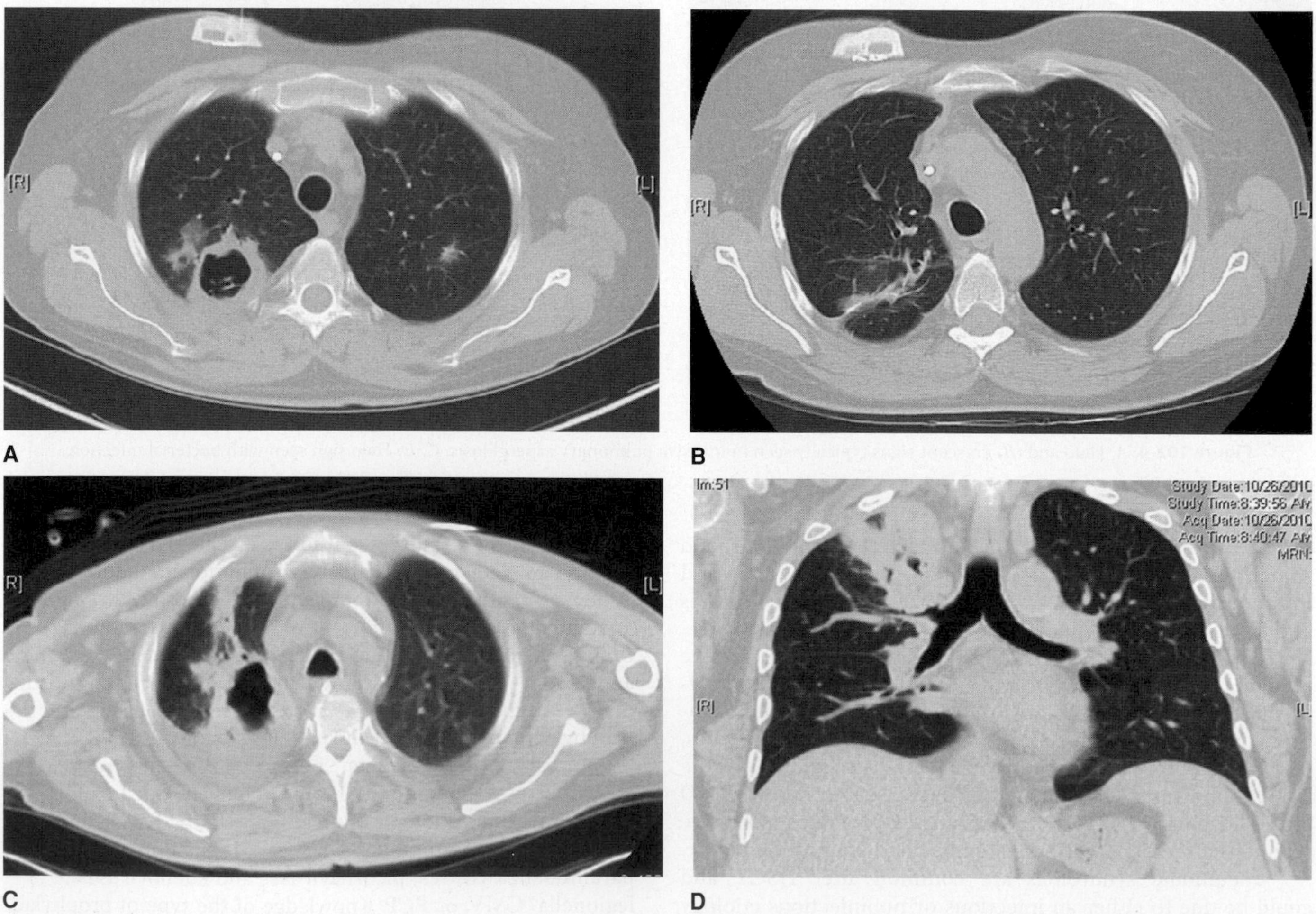

Figure 102-5. *A, B.* Invasive fungal infection due to *Aspergillus* sp. before and after surgical resection. *C, D.* Nonresectable invasive fungal infection due to *Rhizopus* sp. Note proximity to trachea and great vessels.

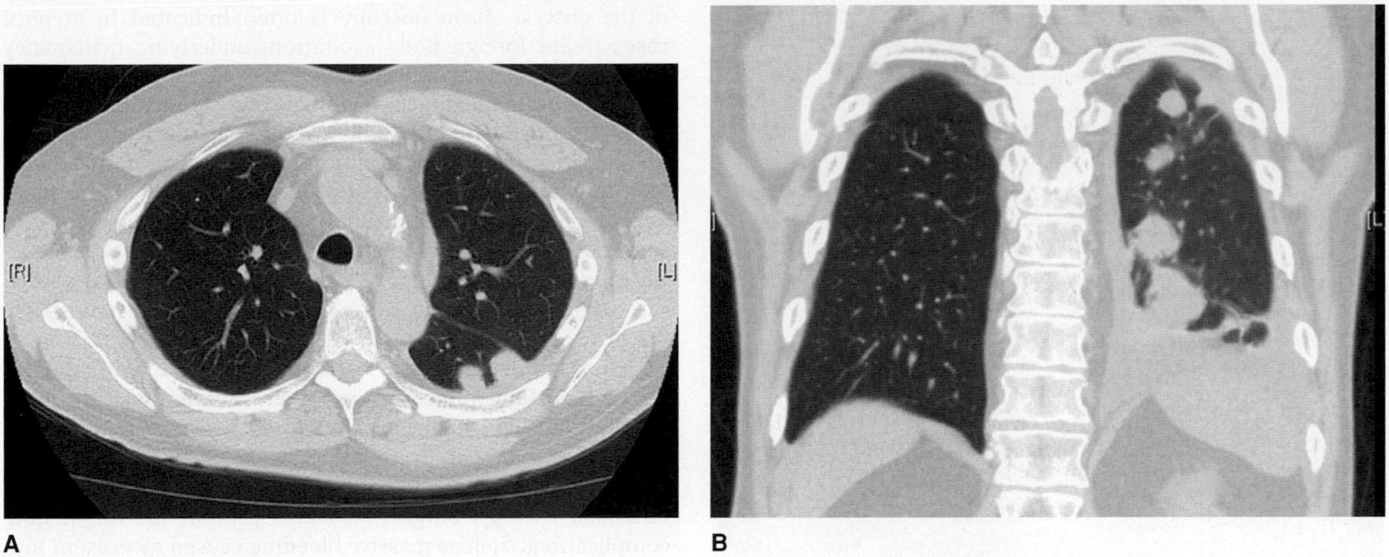

Figure 102-6. Post-transplant lymphoproliferative disease (PTLD) in a lung transplant recipient.

the degree of immunosuppression (presence or absence of rejection), and the timing after transplantation. The most commonly encountered pathogens are *P. aeruginosa*, CMV, community-acquired respiratory viruses, and *Aspergillus* sp.[42] Colonization preceding transplantation, especially in CF and bronchiectasis patients, may play a major role in subsequent infections. Prophylactic regimens targeting known colonizing organisms administered peri-transplantation help decrease the rate of infections after transplantation.

During the early post-transplant period (<1 month after surgery), the most commonly encountered infections include donor and/or recipient-derived infections and nosocomial infections associated with hospitalization and surgery. Most of these infections are caused by bacterial pathogens, but *Candida* infection is also common in the absence of prophylaxis. The period between 1 and 6 months after transplantation is marked by the development of opportunistic infections, mainly CMV, PCP (in the absence of prophylaxis), *Aspergillus* pneumonia, as well as post-transplant lymphoproliferative disease (PTLD) induced by EBV.

Bacterial, viral, fungal, and mycobacterial infections all occur at an increased frequency after lung transplantation.[42] Pleural effusions diagnosed within 3 months of transplantation could represent infection and warrant further investigation particularly if the patient has systemic signs of infection.[43] This often requires intervention by the thoracic surgeon to drain the empyema with placement of chest tubes, pleurodesis, and decortication.

Infectious complications after lung transplantation are important to manage adequately since they may be associated with the development of bronchiolitis obliterans and contribute to allograft loss of function.[44,45]

Diagnostic evaluation of lung infection after lung transplantation includes early and aggressive evaluation. Bronchoscopy (with bronchoalveolar lavage) and transbronchial biopsy are warranted to establish a definitive microbiological and histopathologic diagnosis and to rule out rejection and malignancy (PTLD). Often the management differs significantly depending on the underlying etiology. An opportunistic infection (CMV pneumonia, fungal infection) or PTLD diagnosis, for example, requires decreasing immunosuppression, whereas rejection requires increasing immunosuppression. PTLD is often difficult to differentiate radiographically from an infectious process (bacterial, fungal infections) and a diagnostic procedure is often required (Fig. 102-6). Whenever significant rejection treatment is initiated, antimicrobial prophylaxis against CMV and PCP should be restarted.

Management of Lung Abscess

Lung abscess results from necrosis of the lung parenchyma caused by microbial infection. In most cases, the lung abscess is due to aspiration of oral flora into the lungs as a result of altered mental status, alcoholism, or dysphagia. In the case of multiple lung abscesses, septic emboli are usually suspected. Septic emboli could be due to *S. aureus* bacteremia secondary to tricuspid valve endocarditis or indwelling vascular catheter, or in the case of Lemierre's syndrome could arise from suppurative thrombophlebitis of the internal jugular vein due to an infection by *Fusobacterium necrophorum*.

Lung abscesses may be caused by polymicrobial infection predominantly involving oral anaerobes (*Peptostreptococcus, Prevotella, Bacteroides, Fusobacterium*) or microaerophilic streptococci (*Streptococcus milleri*).[46,47] Lung abscess could be also due to monomicrobial infection. The most common bacteria include *S. aureus, Klebsiella pneumoniae, Streptococcus pyogenes, Haemophilus influenzae* type B, *Legionella, Nocardia, and Actinomyces*.[48–50] In the immunocompromised host, infections due to *P. aeruginosa, Enterobacteriaceae, Nocardia, Aspergillus* are more common. Most patients with lung abscess present with indolent symptoms that evolve over weeks or months. Fever, night sweats, weight loss, and putrid sputum are the most common symptoms. The radiographic features of lung abscess include a cavity with air fluid level (Fig. 102-7).

The treatment of lung abscess in most cases is medical and involves prolonged administration of antimicrobials targeting anaerobes for several months and until radiologic resolution

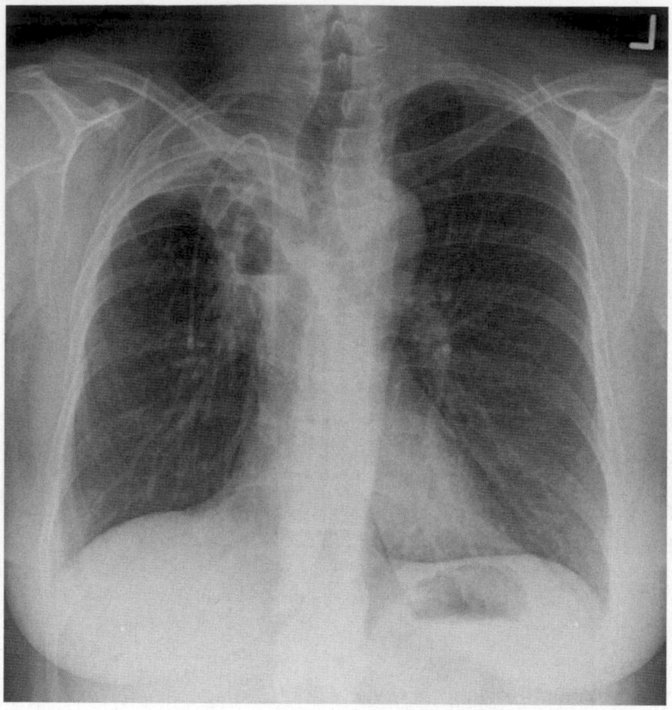

Figure 102-7. Lung abscess with air fluid level in a patient with lung cancer after radiation therapy.

of the abscess. Bronchoscopy is often indicated in atypical cases where foreign body aspiration, underlying malignancy or mycobacterial infection is suspected. Bronchoscopy is also useful in obtaining clinical specimens for culture and allow for biopsy for histopathologic diagnosis in cases where malignancy is suspected. Surgical intervention is rarely required in patients with uncomplicated lung abscess. Indications for surgery include failure to respond to medical treatment, bleeding and suspected malignancy. In patients considered to be poor surgical candidates, placement of percutaneous drain with special care to prevent contamination of pleural space or endoscopic drainage could be attempted.[51,52]

Thoracic surgeons play a pivotal role in the optimal management of lung infections. Surgical interventions are often required to help establish early and definitive diagnosis especially in immunocompromised patients. Surgical procedures are often curative and allow for reduced use of prolonged antimicrobial therapy. Surgery can also prevent life-threatening complications such as massive bleeding caused by erosion into major blood vessels by uncontrolled invasive fungal infections. When evaluating lung infections, a good understanding by the thoracic surgeon of the underlying medical conditions, the host–pathogen interaction, and the complex variables often at play are essential to the decision-making process and to assessing the risks associated with surgical intervention in a particular patient population.

References

1. Regnis JA, Zeman KL, Noone PG, et al. Prolonged airway retention of insoluble particles in cystic fibrosis versus primary ciliary dyskinesia. *Exp Lung Res*. 2000;26(3):149–162.
2. Andersen D. Cystic fibrosis of the pancreas and its relation to celiac disease: a clinical and pathologic study. *Am J Dis Child*. 1938;56:344–399.
3. Rommens JM, Iannuzzi MC, Kerem B, et al. Identification of the cystic fibrosis gene: chromosome walking and jumping. *Science*. 1989;245(4922):1059–1065.
4. Kerem B, Rommens JM, Buchanan JA, et al. Identification of the cystic fibrosis gene: genetic analysis. *Science*. 1989;245(4922):1073–1080.
5. Riordan JR, Rommens JM, Kerem B, et al. Identification of the cystic fibrosis gene: cloning and characterization of complementary DNA. *Science*. 1989;245(4922):1066–1073.
6. Davis PB. Cystic fibrosis since 1938. *Am J Respir Crit Care Med*. 2006;173(5):475–482.
7. Chmiel JF, Davis PB. State of the art: why do the lungs of patients with cystic fibrosis become infected and why can't they clear the infection? *Respir Res*. 2003;4:8.
8. Muhlebach MS, Stewart PW, Leigh MW, et al. Quantitation of inflammatory responses to bacteria in young cystic fibrosis and control patients. *Am J Respir Crit Care Med*. 1999;160(1):186–191.
9. Burns JL, Emerson J, Stapp JR, et al. Microbiology of sputum from patients at cystic fibrosis centers in the United States. *Clin Infect Dis*. 1998;27(1):158–163.
10. Armstrong DS, Grimwood K, Carlin JB, et al. Lower airway inflammation in infants and young children with cystic fibrosis. *Am J Respir Crit Care Med*. 1997;156(4 Pt 1):1197–1204.
11. Gibson RL, Burns JL, Ramsey BW. Pathophysiology and management of pulmonary infections in cystic fibrosis. *Am J Respir Crit Care Med*. 2003;168(8):918–951.
12. Cramton SE, Ulrich M, Gotz F, et al. Anaerobic conditions induce expression of polysaccharide intercellular adhesin in *Staphylococcus aureus* and *Staphylococcus epidermidis*. *Infect Immun*. 2001;69(6):4079–4085.
13. Costerton JW, Stewart PS, Greenberg EP. Bacterial biofilms: a common cause of persistent infections. *Science*. 1999;284(5418):1318–1322.
14. Lyczak JB, Cannon CL, Pier GB. Lung infections associated with cystic fibrosis. *Clin Microbiol Rev*. 2002;15(2):194–222.
15. Murray TS, Egan M, Kazmierczak BI. *Pseudomonas aeruginosa* chronic colonization in cystic fibrosis patients. *Curr Opin Pediatr*. 2007;19(1):83–88.
16. Mahenthiralingam E, Baldwin A, Vandamme P. *Burkholderia cepacia* complex infection in patients with cystic fibrosis. *J Med Microbiol*. 2002;51(7):533–538.
17. Mahenthiralingam E, Vandamme P. Taxonomy and pathogenesis of the *Burkholderia cepacia* complex. *Chron Respir Dis*. 2005;2(4):209–217.
18. Demko CA, Stern RC, Doershuk CF. *Stenotrophomonas maltophilia* in cystic fibrosis: incidence and prevalence. *Pediatr Pulmonol*. 1998;25(5):304–308.
19. Olivier KN, Weber DJ, Lee JH, et al. Nontuberculous mycobacteria. II: nested-cohort study of impact on cystic fibrosis lung disease. *Am J Respir Crit Care Med*. 2003;167(6):835–840.
20. Olivier KN, Weber DJ, Wallace RJ Jr, et al. Nontuberculous mycobacteria. I: multicenter prevalence study in cystic fibrosis. *Am J Respir Crit Care Med*. 2003;167(6):828–834.
21. Balough K, McCubbin M, Weinberger M, et al. The relationship between infection and inflammation in the early stages of lung disease from cystic fibrosis. *Pediatr Pulmonol*. 1995;20(2):63–70.
22. De Soyza A, Archer L, McDowell A, et al. Lung transplantation for cystic fibrosis; the effect of *B. cepacia* genomovars on post transplant outcomes. *J Heart Lung Transplant*. 2001;20(2):158.
23. De Soyza A, McDowell A, Archer L, Dark JH, Elborn SJ, Mahenthiralingam E, et al. *Burkholderia cepacia* complex genomovars and pulmonary transplantation outcomes in patients with cystic fibrosis. *Lancet*. 2001;358(9295):1780–1781.
24. Koo S, Marty FM, Baden LR. Infectious complications associated with immunomodulating biologic agents. *Infect Dis Clin North Am*. 2010;24(2):285–306.
25. Maschmeyer G, Link H, Hiddemann W,et al. Pulmonary infiltrations in febrile patients with neutropenia. Risk factors and outcome under empirical antimicrobial therapy in a randomized multicenter study. *Cancer*. 1994;73(9):2296–2304.

26. Nováková IR, Donnelly JP, De Pauw B. Potential sites of infection that develop in febrile neutropenic patients. *Leuk Lymphoma*. 1993;10(6):461–467.
27. Jain P, Sandur S, Meli Y, et al. Role of flexible bronchoscopy in immunocompromised patients with lung infiltrates. *Chest*. 2004;125(2):712–722.
28. Whimbey E, Englund JA, Couch RB. Community respiratory virus infections in immunocompromised patients with cancer. *Am J Med*. 1997;102(3A):10–18; discussion 25–26.
29. Muhlemann K, Wenger C, Zenhausern R, et al. Risk factors for invasive aspergillosis in neutropenic patients with hematologic malignancies. *Leukemia*. 2005;19(4):545–550.
30. Nivoix Y, Velten M, Letscher-Bru V, et al. Factors associated with overall and attributable mortality in invasive aspergillosis. *Clin Infect Dis*. 2008;47(9):1176–1184.
31. Caballero E, Drobnic ME, Perez MT, et al. Anti-*Pseudomonas aeruginosa* antibody detection in patients with bronchiectasis without cystic fibrosis. *Thorax*. 2001;56(9):669–674.
32. Gosselin MV, Adams RH. Pulmonary complications in bone marrow transplantation. *J Thorac Imaging*. 2002;17(2):132–144.
33. Conces DJ Jr. Noninfectious lung disease in immunocompromised patients. *J Thorac Imaging*. 1999;14(1):9–24.
34. Heussel CP, Kauczor HU, Heussel G, et al. Early detection of pneumonia in febrile neutropenic patients: use of thin-section CT. *AJR Am J Roentgenol*. 1997;169(5):1347–1353.
35. Ljungman P. Respiratory virus infections in bone marrow transplant recipients: the European perspective. *Am J Med*. 1997;102(3A):44–47.
36. Lewis VA, Champlin R, Englund J, et al. Respiratory disease due to parainfluenza virus in adult bone marrow transplant recipients. *Clin Infect Dis*. 1996;23(5):1033–1037.
37. Englund JA, Piedra PA, Jewell A, et al. Rapid diagnosis of respiratory syncytial virus infections in immunocompromised adults. *J Clin Microbiol*. 1996;34(7):1649–1653.
38. Ljungman P. Respiratory virus infections in stem cell transplant patients: the European experience. *Biol Blood Marrow Transplant*. 2001; (7 Suppl): 5S–7S.
39. De La Rosa GR, Champlin RE, Kontoyiannis DP. Risk factors for the development of invasive fungal infections in allogeneic blood and marrow transplant recipients. *Transpl Infect Dis*. 2002;4(1):3–9.
40. Fukuda T, Boeckh M, Carter RA, et al. Risks and outcomes of invasive fungal infections in recipients of allogeneic hematopoietic stem cell transplants after nonmyeloablative conditioning. *Blood*. 2003;102(3):827–833.
41. Aurora P, Edwards LB, Christie J, et al. Registry of the International Society for Heart and Lung Transplantation: eleventh official pediatric lung and heart/lung transplantation report—2008. *J Heart Lung Transplant*. 2008;27(9):978–983.
42. Remund KF, Best M, Egan JJ. Infections relevant to lung transplantation. *Proc Am Thorac Soc*. 2009;6(1):94–100.
43. Wahidi MM, Willner DA, Snyder LD, et al. Diagnosis and outcome of early pleural space infection following lung transplantation. *Chest*. 2009;135(2):484–491.
44. Husain S, Singh N. Bronchiolitis obliterans and lung transplantation: evidence for an infectious etiology. *Semin Respir Infect*. 2002;17(4): 310–314.
45. Weigt SS, Elashoff RM, Huang C, et al. Aspergillus colonization of the lung allograft is a risk factor for bronchiolitis obliterans syndrome. *Am J Transplant*. 2009;9(8):1903–1911.
46. Bartlett JG. Anaerobic bacterial infections of the lung. *Chest*. 1987;91(6):901–909.
47. Bartlett JG. The role of anaerobic bacteria in lung abscess. *Clin Infect Dis*. 2005;40(7):923–925.
48. Francis JS, Doherty MC, Lopatin U, et al. Severe community-onset pneumonia in healthy adults caused by methicillin-resistant *Staphylococcus aureus* carrying the Panton-Valentine leukocidin genes. *Clin Infect Dis*. 2005;40(1):100–107.
49. Gillet Y, Issartel B, Vanhems P, et al. Association between *Staphylococcus aureus* strains carrying gene for Panton-Valentine leukocidin and highly lethal necrotising pneumonia in young immunocompetent patients. *Lancet*. 2002;359(9308):753–759.
50. Wang JL, Chen KY, Fang CT, . Changing bacteriology of adult community-acquired lung abscess in Taiwan: *Klebsiella pneumoniae* versus anaerobes. *Clin Infect Dis*. 2005;40(7):915–922.
51. Weissberg D. Percutaneous drainage of lung abscess. *J Thorac Cardiovasc Surg*. 1984;87(2):308–312.
52. Herth F, Ernst A, Becker HD. Endoscopic drainage of lung abscesses: technique and outcome. *Chest*. 2005;127(4):1378–1381.

103 Surgical Treatment of Thoracic Fungal Infections

Ann Adams, Ritu R. Gill, and Ciaran J. McNamee

Keywords: Pulmonary fungal infections, aspergillosis, blastomycosis, *Cryptococcus gattii*, Candida, coccidioidomycosis, histoplasmosis, paracoccidioidomycosis, sporotrichosis (*Sporothrix schenckii*), penicilliosis

Thoracic fungal infections have a complex and variable presentation, ranging from benign self-limited processes, which spontaneously resolve, to severe life-threatening infections associated with disabling morbidity and high mortality. Persistent fungal infections in normal individuals may either resolve without producing symptoms, or worsen leading to severe complications of hemoptysis, mediastinal fibrosis, empyema, and meningitis. Immune-compromised hosts demonstrate greater susceptibility to fungi than normal individuals and have more severe outcomes including vascular invasion, septicemia with fungal dissemination, organ infarction, and death. Adding to this complexity, the epidemiology of fungal disease is constantly changing as species emerge or relocate or increase in virulence. Early intervention can improve survival and in some cases obviate the necessity of surgery. It is critical therefore to recognize the clinical manifestations of thoracic fungal infection early in its clinical course. Fortunately, recent advances in knowledge concerning fungal biology including the functional genome, the structure of the cell wall and membrane, and the use of molecular and epidemiologic techniques have led to rapid identification of pathogens and the institution of effective, less toxic antifungal agents.[1]

INFECTION, TRANSMISSION, EXPOSURE

Fungi that are implicated in pulmonary pathology consist primarily of dimorphic organisms. They begin as airborne spores and later convert to yeast forms after entering the pulmonary system. The lung is a common portal of entry and represents the primary portal and site of infection in both immune-competent and immune-suppressed individuals. Opportunistic hospital-acquired infections generally arise in ICU patients with indwelling vascular or catheter instrumentation or following solid organ or hematopoietic stem cell transplantation.[2] Occasionally, infection may occur by nonpulmonary portals such as cutaneous inoculation, for example, sporotrichosis. Human-to-human transmission is extremely rare and primarily occurs in the organ transplant population.

Opportunistic fungal organisms may also persist in a chronic latent state, allowing possible future activation and infection if there is compromise of the immune system. As humans are often colonized with fungal organisms, the distinction between colonization and infection may be diagnostically challenging, and outcomes from fungal infection may vary depending on the degree and extent of fungal invasion based on a balance of factors between the host and organism.

The presence of endemic fungal infection in at-risk individuals may initially be suspected by a history of travel to niche areas of fungal prevalence (Fig. 103-1).[3] However, with current global travel opportunities, latent fungal reactivation can occur following distant past travel which may require extensive individual interrogation as to possible fungal exposure from prevalent areas. It is also important to remain vigilant as fungal infections can resemble or coexist with malignant disease.

EPIDEMIOLOGY

The epidemiology of thoracic fungal infections is constantly changing. The pace of this change has accelerated in recent decades, and four factors have been identified to account for this rapid change: an increasingly mobile world population, the aging population in Western countries, climatic environmental changes, and increased immune suppression for organ transplantation. The recognition and treatment of fungal infection is also dependent on microbiologic reclassification patterns. Actinomycosis and nocardia, for example, are no longer classified as fungal infections, since the source of infection recently has been identified as bacterial.[4] Emerging and opportunistic infections undergo epidemiologic changes associated with climactic changes which alter current endemic fungal niches allowing for the emergence of new pathogens. In addition, alterations in immune pharmacologic management with new biologic immunosuppressant agents (e.g., TNF-alpha inhibitors), potent transplant rejection drugs, or chronic steroid use for chronic pulmonary conditions influence host predisposition for fungal infections.[4]

Thoracic fungal infections are categorized by host factors (immune competence and host defenses) or by invading organisms which are based on geography and virulence factors. Host defense categories include the following subpopulations: immune-competent or immune-deficient individuals with or without defective pulmonary defenses. Fungal invasion factors involve endemic versus opportunistic fungal organisms. Opportunistic fungi serve as common pathogens primarily for immune-suppressed individuals who also remain susceptible to endemic fungi. These individuals are additionally at risk of infection by saprophytic fungi (i.e., fungi that grow on dead organic matter) and emerging (mostly opportunistic) fungi.

DIAGNOSIS

Individuals presenting with clinical disease due to fungal infection are categorized by their immune status: immune-competent versus immune-suppressed. The latter group is comprised of transplant recipients, patients receiving biologic immunosuppressive agents, and patients with malignant and/or hematologic conditions or acute debilitating injuries which suppress the individual's immune state. Most fungal infections that afflict immune-suppressed hospitalized patients occur in the ICU setting or in the immediate

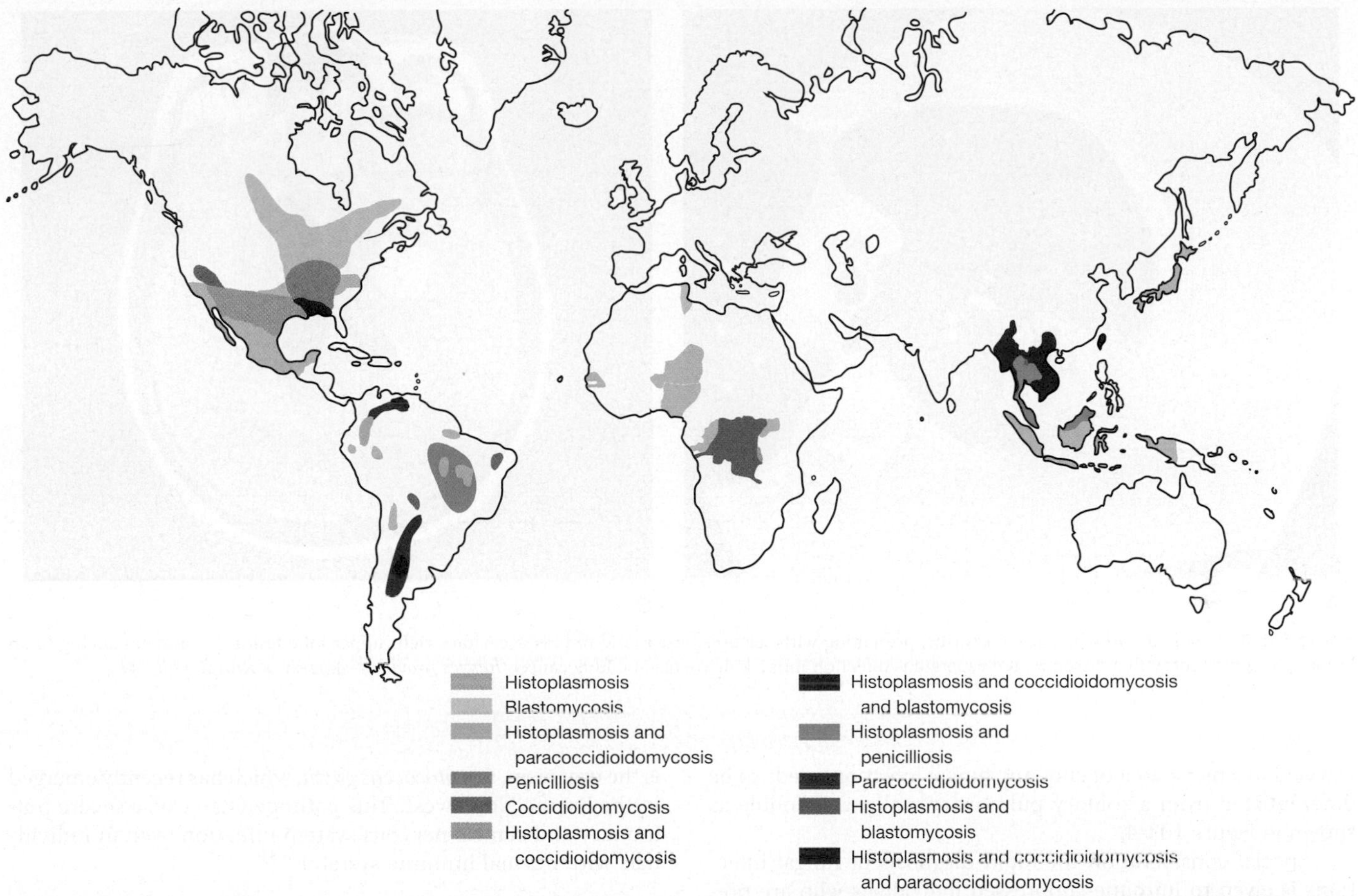

Figure 103-1. Endemic niche areas for fungal prevalence. (Adapted with permission from: Hsu LY, Ng ES, Koh LP. Common and emerging fungal pulmonary infections. *Infect Dis Clin North Am*. 2010;24(3):557–577.)

post-transplant recipient. Therefore, early determination of the patient's immune status will help to establish the individual's exposure risk for well-defined geographically prevalent areas of fungal infection (see Fig. 103-1).[3]

Radiography has an important role in diagnosing fungal disease since the radiographic abnormalities observed with fungal infection overlap with the radiographic signs of thoracic malignancy. For example, both entities may exhibit signs of patchy parenchymal infiltrates, pulmonary nodules, consolidation, cavitation, and pleural effusion. In addition, patients with endemic fungal disease may have unilateral or bilateral mediastinal adenopathy. The presence of a halo or a reversed halo sign on a lung CT, often seen in thoracic malignancy, is also a common sign of mucormycosis and may suggest fungal parenchymal disease (Fig. 103-2). Chest CT along with a heightened index of clinical suspicion has a prominent role in the diagnosis and separation of fungal infections. Marom and Kontoyiannis[5] demonstrated a survival advantage when early CT was performed in immune-compromised patients with neutropenic fever.

A fungal infection may also be multicentric, having the appearance of a metastatic process. For example, a case of disseminated aspergillosis, shown in Figure 103-3, was initially mistaken for a metastatic cancer. An incidental pulmonary nodule arising in a patient who resides in or has recently

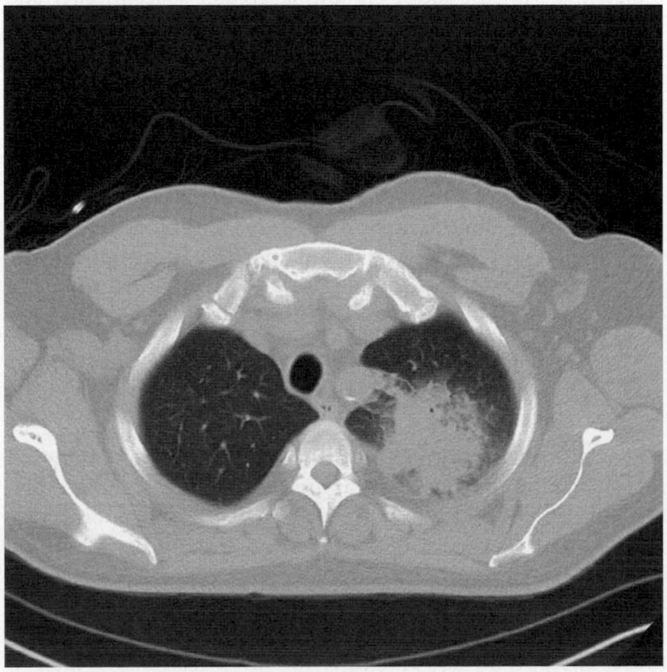

Figure 103-2. Bilateral lung nodules with halo sign (i.e., presence of ground glass opacity on chest CT surrounding a pulmonary nodule or mass representing hemorrhage). *Image provided courtesy of Rachna Madan, MD.*

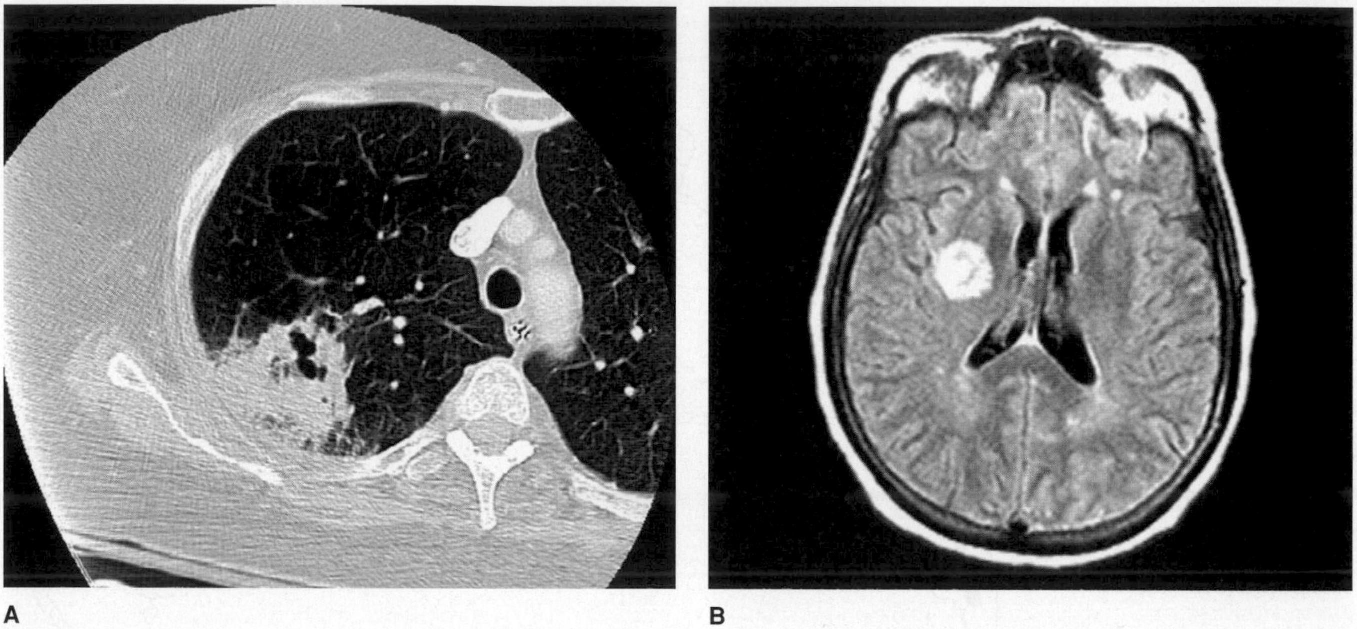

Figure 103-3. A patient with rhematoid arthritis, presenting with seizures, was found to have a cavitary right upper lobe lesion (*A*) and enhancing brain lesions (*B*) consistent with a disseminated aspergillus infection mimicking metastatic lung cancer. *Images provided courtesy of Ritu R. Gill, MD.*

traveled to a niche area of endemic fungal infection needs to be differentiated from a solitary pulmonary malignant nodule as shown in Figure 103-4.

Special consideration for rapid diagnosis of fungal infections is given to immune-suppressed individuals who are predisposed to opportunistic infection. Moreover, there are clear differences in disease severity and survival between groups of transplant recipients, for example, solid organ transplant recipients (SOT) versus hematologic stem cell transplant (HSCT) recipients, with the latter exhibiting greater susceptibility and mortality to fungal infections.[6] Subgroup differences also may be found within these subpopulations.

ROLE OF SURGERY

Although surgical therapy for fungal lung disease is uncommon, given the development of effective antimicrobial agents, the thoracic surgeon may be called upon to perform diagnostic lung biopsies, and occasionally for the primary treatment of complications of fungal infections (see Table 103-1).[7]

ENDEMIC FUNGAL INFECTIONS

The endemic fungal infections that affect immune-competent individuals in areas of geographic fungal prevalence are histoplasmosis, coccidioidomycosis (Fig. 103-4), blastomycosis (Fig. 103-5), paracoccidioidomycosis (previously identified as South American blastomycosis), and penicilliosis. Sporotrichosis is found chiefly in tropical and subtropical areas. Immune-suppressed individuals in endemic areas may be more susceptible to endemic fungal infections, which if acquired are more virulent with higher mortality in this at-risk population. Immune-competent individuals generally experience subclinical disease and often are able to deal with these organisms independent of antifungal therapy. One exception is the organism, *Cryptococcus gattii*, which has recently emerged in the Pacific Northwest. This pathogen can cause severe pulmonary and central nervous system infection even in individuals with normal immune systems.[3,8,9]

Histoplasmosis

The most common endemic fungal infection worldwide, histoplasmosis, may be caused by one of the two organisms: *Histoplasma capsulatum* or *Histoplasma duboisii*. The *H. capsulatum* variety has a worldwide distribution. In the United States it is found primarily in the Ohio and Mississippi Valley regions. The *H. duboisii* variety coexists with *H. capsulatum* in central and Western sub-Sahara and has a special tropism for cutaneous and skeletal structure but lacks the ability for thoracic diseases associated with *H. capsulatum*. Histoplasmosis is primarily a soil dweller and arises from bird and bat droppings. Inhalation of the microconidia from this fungus is a classic model for endemic fungal dissemination and infection within the pulmonary system. The clinical presentation and disease severity following fungal inoculum exposure is entirely dependent on the balance between the number of inhaled organisms and the immune status of the individual.

Inhalation of spores of this fungus into the lower respiratory tract leads to phagocytosis by alveolar macrophages with internal macrophage conversion of the organism to yeast forms and subsequent spread throughout the reticuloendothelial system. Dendritic airway cells limit disease progression by both ingesting and killing yeast organisms and then presenting histoplasma antigens to stimulate naïve T lymphocytes which activate macrophages to destroy intracellular yeast infections. This orchestrated response occurs 2 to 3 weeks following histoplasma inoculation, and in the majority of patients will limit the disease process. Less than 1% of immune-competent patients may develop the following complications: Pericarditis, granulomatous mediastinitis, histoplasmoma, broncholithiasis, and mediastinal fibrosis. Chronic cavitary disease may occur in

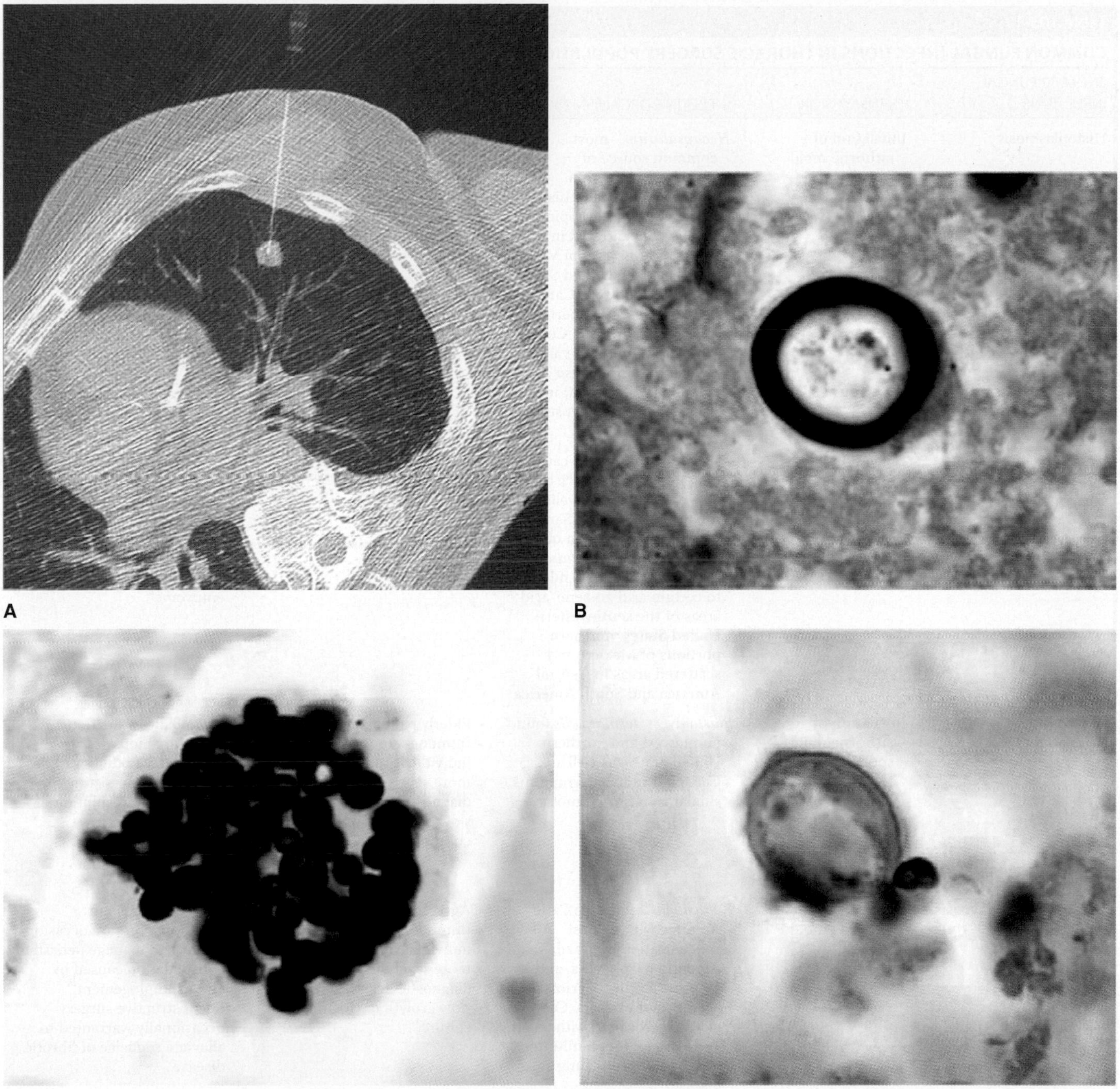

Figure 103-4. An incidental left upper lobe pulmonary nodule in a liver transplant patient was biopsied and determined to be coccidioidomycosis. (*A*) CT appearance of pulmonary nodule. Pathology (*B, C, D*). *Images provided courtesy of Ritu R. Gill, MD.*

older patients with COPD. This condition is both progressive and life threatening without treatment.[3]

Immune-suppressed individuals who are exposed to histoplasmosis generally present with acute, severe pneumonia which manifests with the radiographic appearance of diffuse pulmonary infiltrates and hilar lymphadenopathy. If the immune response is inadequate to deal with the organisms, further progressive dissemination may lead to organ failure and death.

Diagnostic tests for histoplasmosis include culture testing (may be too slow for fungus recovery), antibody assays in immune-competent individuals, and urine antigen testing. Treatment includes antifungal therapy for both acute and progressive disease states (i.e., acute pulmonary histoplasmosis, chronic cavitary pulmonary histoplasmosis, progressive disseminated histoplasmosis, and mediastinal lymphadenitis). Routine antifungal therapy in the absence of steroid therapy is not recommended for delayed complications, such as pulmonary nodules, mediastinal granuloma, mediastinal fibrosis, broncholithiasis, and inflammatory syndromes (i.e., pericarditis, arthritis, and erythema nodosum). Surgery is rarely required other than for differentiation of malignancy from histoplasmoma and to deal with complications from broncholithiasis or cavitary disease.[3,10] Mediastinal disease with recurrent pericardial effusions or vascular fibrosis rarely requires surgical treatment.[7]

Table 103-1

COMMON FUNGAL INFECTIONS IN THORACIC SURGERY POPULATIONS

ENDEMIC FUNGAL INFECTIONS	TRANSMISSION	INFECTING ORGANISM NICHE	AT-RISK POPULATIONS	ROLE OF SURGICAL TREATMENT
Histoplasmosis	Inhalation of airborne mold spores	*H. capsulatum*—most common source of respiratory infection. Inhabits soil contaminated by bird and bat droppings. Highly concentrated in the Ohio and Mississippi Valley regions of the United States and also in Eastern Canada, Mexico, Central America, and South America. Coexists with the *H. duboisii* variety (which does not cause pulmonary infection) in Central and Western sub-Saharan regions	• Patients with preexisting COPD • Immune-deficient hosts, e.g., patients infected with AIDS • Elderly patients	• Diagnostic procedure to differentiate malignancy from histoplasmoma • Pulmonary resection of infected cavitary lesions with or without antifungal therapy[a] • Surgical removal of broncholiths by open resection, minimally invasive VATS, or bronchoplastic procedures[b]
Coccidioidomycosis	Inhalation of airborne mold spores	*Coccidioides immitis*—causes lung infection in more than 60% of cases. Soil dwelling fungus native to the San Joaquin Valley region of California. The *Coccidioides posadasii* variant is endemic to certain arid-to-semi-arid areas of the southwestern United States, northern portions of Mexico, and scattered areas in Central America and South America	• Immune-deficient hosts • Elderly patients	• Diagnostic evaluation of pulmonary nodules, symptomatic nonresponsive cavitary disease, and complications of infection, including effusion, pneumothorax, and empyema[b]
Blastomycosis	Inhalation of airborne mold spores	*Blastomyces dermatitidis* found in midwest and northern United States, as well as Canada. Produces symptoms similar to Histoplasmosis	• Elderly patients • Immune-suppressed individuals may experience more severe disease due to diagnostic delays caused by slow growth of organism in culture	• Diagnostic evaluation including biopsy of pulmonary nodules or hilar adenopathy persisting for months after resolution of infection • Surgical treatment of empyema following infection[b]
Paracoccidioidomycosis	Inhalation of airborne mold spores	*P. brasiliensis* found in Latin America with highest concentration in Brazil, Argentina, Colombia, and Venezuela. Infects primarily agricultural workers. Chronic disease associated with fever and bilateral lung infiltrates leading to fibrotic lung disease.	• Agricultural workers • Immune-suppressed individuals may experience more severe disease due to diagnostic delays caused by slow growth or organism in culture.	• Surgery to rule out carcinoma on rare occasions. • Surgery to manage persistent consolidation caused by airway impingement[b] • Reconstructive surgery occasionally warranted to alleviate sequelae of fibrotic disease
Penicillosis	Inhalation of airborne mold spores	*Penicillium marneffei* found primarily in tropical Asia	• Immune-deficient hosts with HIV and low CD4 counts more commonly affected than other immune-suppressed individuals	
Spirotrochosis	Cutaneous contact with organism	*Sporothrix schenckii* is found in tropical and temperate zones worldwide, but unlike other endemic mycoses, the infection occurs by a cutaneous route through contact with the organism in the soil and in moss	• Patients with preexisting COPD • Immune-deficient hosts with HIV and low CD4 counts more commonly affected than other immune-suppressed individuals • Culture results return rapidly; serology is helpful for diagnosis	• Diagnostic evaluation • Surgical resection may be required to treat fibrotic lung disease in compromised COPD patients • Resection may be required to correct air space problems[b]

Table 103-1 (*Continued*)

COMMON FUNGAL INFECTIONS IN THORACIC SURGERY POPULATIONS

RARE AND EMERGING FUNGAL INFECTIONS[c]	TRANSMISSION	INFECTING ORGANISM NICHE	AT-RISK POPULATIONS	ROLE OF SURGICAL TREATMENT
Zygomycosis[b]	Inhalation of airborne mold spores	Zygomycetes (i.e., *Rhizopus,* mucormycosis, Cunninghamella and others) are molds found in decaying vegetation and soil worldwide	• Diabetes, hematologic malignancy with transplantation, solid organ transplantation, treatment of iron overload states, AIDS, and immune-compromised patients using voraconazole or posaconazole, a new class of drugs with broad antifungal activity	• Angioinvasive fungi cause rapid necrosis leading to extensive destruction and death • Treatment requires urgent pulmonary resection with removal of all devitalized tissue, up to and including pneumonectomy[b]
Hyalohyphomycosis	Inhalation of airborne mold spores	Hyalohyphomycoses (i.e., Fusarium, Scedosporium) are dematiaceous (black) molds responsible for an increase of pneumonia in transplant recipients and in patients with hematologic malignancies. Caused by inhalation of mold spores. Appearance is similar to Aspergillus on histologic examination. Differentiation relies on culture speciation. Have unique ability to sporulate in vivo leading to vascular invasion with yeast dissemination	• Immune-suppressed transplant recipients and patients with hematologic malignancies • Scedosporium is second most common mold to colonize airways of cystic fibrosis patients	• Dematiaceous molds produce abscesses and infected cavities difficult to eradicate with antimicrobials alone • Surgical excision for localized disease may be indicated given poor response of organism to antifungal therapy
Phaeohyphomycosis	Inhalation of airborne spores or inoculation of black molds	Phaeohyphomycosis (i.e., Curvularia, Bipolaris, Exophiala, and Alternaria) is caused by inhalation or inoculation of species of black molds leading to allergic bronchopulmonary disease (ABPD) associated with eosinophil elevations	• Non-allergic pulmonary disease occurs in immunocompromised individuals and represents tissue invasion of this fungus which is a common airway colonizer • Invasive phaeohyphomycosis may manifest as pneumonias or parenchymal or endobronchial nodules	May cause severe, life-threatening infections in immune-deficient, as well as immune-competent hosts
Trichosporon		Trichosporon and adiaspiromycosis caused by *Emmonsia crescens* cause significant fulminant, often fatal disease		
OPPORTUNISTIC FUNGAL INFECTIONS	**TRANSMISSION**	**INFECTING ORGANISM**	**AT-RISK POPULATIONS**	**ROLE OF SURGICAL TREATMENT**
Candidiasis	Endogenous exposure	Most common infecting organism in ICU. Majority of infections arise in patients with vascular access devices *Candida nonalbicans* associated with higher mortality and rising more rapidly than *Candida albicans*	• Transplant recipients. Most common infection of SOT • (SOT and HSOT) • Cancer patients (hematologic malignancies and chemotherapy induced immune-suppression) • Long-term immunosuppression with steroids, Sirolimus, lympholytic treatment; or Infliximab • Patients with other debilitating disease (Lupus, Crohn's)	• Rarely required for *Candida albicans* • Recent cases of candida empyema have been reported, some fatal[b]
Aspergillosis	Ubiquitous molds found in organic matter. Endogenous exposure is primary mode of severe life-threatening illness	The majority of illness is caused by *Aspergillus fumigatus* and *Aspergillus niger* and, less frequently, *Aspergillus flavus* and *Aspergillus clavatus.* The aspergillosis species causes 4 main syndromes: • aspergilloma	• Patients with chronic neutropenia • Nonneutropenic patients who are immune deficient secondary to steroid use • Solid organ transplant recipients with chronic pulmonary damage	• Surgical resection may be considered in patients with CNPA that is refractory to prolonged antifungal therapy

(*continued*)

Table 103-1 (*Continued*)

COMMON FUNGAL INFECTIONS IN THORACIC SURGERY POPULATIONS

OPPORTUNISTIC FUNGAL INFECTIONS	TRANSMISSION	INFECTING ORGANISM	AT-RISK POPULATIONS	ROLE OF SURGICAL TREATMENT
		• allergic bronchopulmonary aspergillosis (ABPA) • localized chronic necrotizing Aspergillus pneumonia (chronic necrotizing pulmonary aspergillosis [CNPA]), • invasive aspergillosis (IPA)	• Invasive aspergillosis is the most common organism in HSOT recipients. • Cystic fibrosis • Organisms proliferate in a preexisting cavity in an immune-competent host • Organisms invade the vasculature in immune-deficient host	• Patients with aspergilloma may have massive hemoptysis for which surgical resection may be considered • Immune-suppressed patients with IPA at risk of pulmonary artery invasion
Emerging fungal infections (see above)				
Cryptococcus	Although widely disseminated in nature, endogenous exposure is primary mode of severe life-threatening infection	Infection with *Cryptococcus neoformans* may lead to neurologic sequelae	HIV Transplant recipients	• *Cryptococcus* infection may cause pleural effusion • Thoracoscopic management has been reported for a case of fibrinopurulent cryptococcal empyema
Pneumocystis jirovecii [d](previously *Pneumocystis carinii*)	Airborn innoculation	*Pneumocystosis jirovecii*	HIV Immunosuppressed individuals	Diagnosis of organism

[a]Sutaria MK, Polk JW, Reddy P, et al. Surgical aspects of pulmonary histoplasmosis. A series of 110 cases. *Thorax*. 1970;25(1):31–40.
[b]LoCicero J, 3rd, Shaw JP, Lazzaro RS. Surgery for other pulmonary fungal infections, Actinomyces, and Nocardia. *Thorac Surg Clin*. 2012;22(3):363–374.
[c]Rare and emerging fungal infection tends to require more surgical involvement compared with common fungal infections because of the limited availability of effective antimicrobial therapies.
[d] D'Avignon LC, Schofield CM, Hospenthal DR. Pneumocystis pneumonia. *Semin Respir Crit Care Med* 2008;29:132–140.

Coccidioidomycosis

The coccidioidomycosis (see Fig. 103-4) organism occupies a geographic area within the southwest of the United States and Northwestern Mexico. Sixty percent of infected patients are asymptomatic with subclinical disease that is detectable only by a cellular reaction to coccidioidal antigen.[11] The remaining 40% of patients primarily demonstrate three varieties of pulmonary clinical syndromes (described below) other than the disseminated form of the disease which is more likely to occur in immune-compromised individuals, Filipinos, and African Americans.[3,12]

The pulmonary disease states due to this organism consist of two syndromes. The first is acute pulmonary coccidioidomycosis with lung infiltrates or consolidation, hilar adenopathy, and possibly pleural effusion. The extent of disease from coccidioidomycosis, much like histoplasmosis, is dependent upon the balance between the numbers of invading organisms and the immune status of the individual. The second is the chronic form of pulmonary coccidioidomycosis, which affects less than 5% of patients. These patients may experience pulmonary nodules or cavities or a chronic progressive pneumonia which may be associated with either diabetes mellitus or preexisting pulmonary fibrosis. This entity, like the above clinical states, may resemble tuberculosis both radiographically and clinically.

Diagnostic tests for coccidioidomycosis include culture testing, antibody serology testing for immune-competent individuals, and antigen testing. Treatment for chronic fibrocavitary medically refractory disease or pleural space infection may include surgical resection which may also be performed for the diagnosis of nodular disease.[7] Prophylaxis for immune-suppressed individuals is controversial, but transplant candidates and recipients visiting or living in endemic areas may benefit from targeted prophylactic therapy.[3,12]

Blastomycosis

Similar to coccidioidomycosis, blastomycosis (see Fig. 103-5) is clinically silent in greater than 50% of individuals. Symptomatic patients often present late after exposure (30–45 days).[13] Acute pulmonary involvement in immune-competent individuals resembles bacterial pneumonia with lobar consolidation. The disease is often identified in the chronic phase with lung

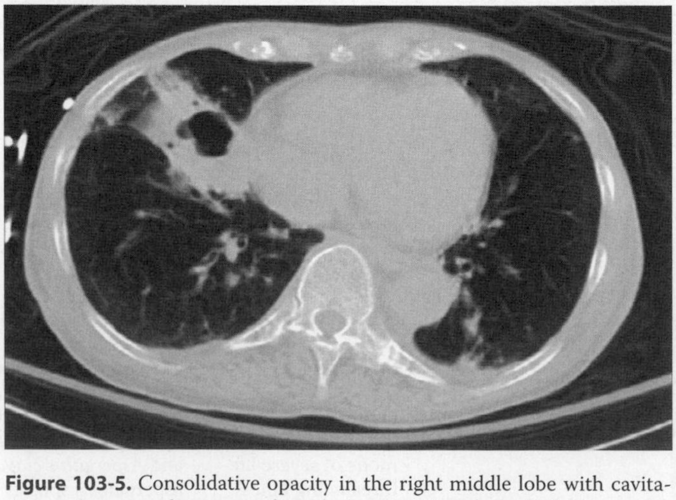

Figure 103-5. Consolidative opacity in the right middle lobe with cavitation and surrounding parenchymal changes. Transbronchial biopsy was consistent with blastomycosis. *Images provided courtesy of Ritu R. Gill, MD.*

masses, cavities, or infiltrates which may be accompanied by cutaneous and subcutaneous lesions.[3,13] Immune-suppressed individuals, who may acquire this infection either from new acquisition or reactivation, suffer disease consequences with greater severity and higher mortality.[3,13]

Culture results may be delayed for 4 to 6 weeks following testing which may complicate treatment in severe disease states that require immediate treatment.[3,13] Treatment guidelines for all individuals recommend antifungal therapy to prevent extrapulmonary dissemination.[14] Surgical involvement is for nodular disease identification or pleural space infections.[7]

Paracoccidioidomycosis

This organism has a Latin American geographic distribution, although Brazil is primarily affected, and the organism *Paracoccidioides brasiliensis* includes at least three species distinguished by nationally based infection which occurs primarily in agricultural workers. Chronic disease leads to systemic symptoms of a febrile illness with bilateral infiltrates leading to fibrotic lung disease.[3] As with blastomycoses, positive culture returns may be delayed and the diagnosis may depend on serologic tests. Immune-suppressed individuals may experience more severe forms of the disease and have increased risk because of diagnostic delays due to slow culture growth of this organism. Surgical therapy is rare other than differentiation from malignancy and for reconstructive therapy for chronic disease.[7]

Penicilliosis

Penicillium marneffei is an emerging opportunistic endemic mycosis located primarily in tropical Asia. Immune-competent individuals may suffer subclinical infection. HIV patients with low CD4 counts are more commonly affected in comparison with other immune-suppressed individuals. Chronic disease manifests with diffuse pulmonary infiltrates and generalized lymphadenopathy and cutaneous lesions. Without treatment it is progressive and fatal.[3]

Sporotrichosis

Infection with *Sporothrix schenckii* occurs in tropical and temperate zones worldwide, but unlike the other endemic mycoses, the infection occurs by a cutaneous route through contact with the organism in the soil and in moss. Exposure by this route leads to cutaneous or lymphatic disease with later progression to the lungs and systemic dissemination. Significant spore aeration can result in disseminated pulmonary disease leading to cavitary fibrotic lung disease or hilar or mediastinal adenopathy for which surgery may be required.[7] Culture results for Sporotrichosis are returned reasonably rapidly and serology testing is helpful for diagnosis.[15]

EMERGING FUNGAL INFECTIONS

There are three main groups of important molds in this category: Zygomycosis, Hyaline septated molds, and dematiaceous molds.

Zygomycosis

This term zygomycosis (used interchangeably with mucormycosis) (Fig. 103-6) includes saprophytic molds that occur in a worldwide distribution in decaying plants and animals.

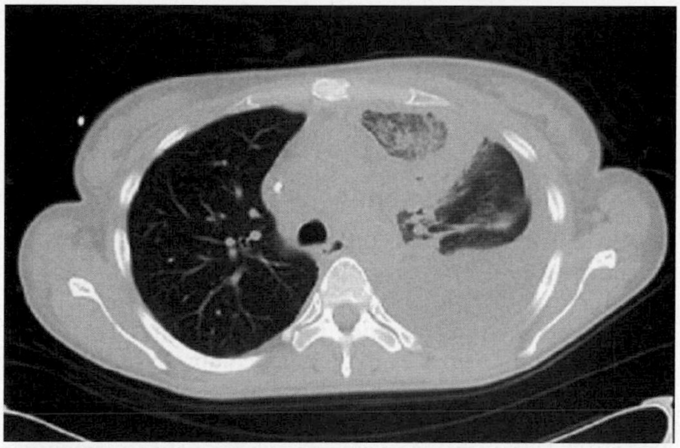

Figure 103-6. Consolidative opacity in the left upper lobe with central ground glass opacity and peripheral solid component representing the "reverse halo sign" seen in zygomycosis (aka mucormycosis). *Images provided courtesy of Ritu R. Gill, MD.*

Mucorales infection occurs by spore inhalation and the disease is progressive in individuals with diabetes, hematologic malignancy with transplantation, solid organ transplantation, treatment of iron overload states, AIDS, and immune-compromised patients using voraconazole or posaconazole, a new class of drugs with broad antifungal activity.[1]

The most common species associated with angio-invasion are organisms of the rhizopus species which infect the sinuses, brain, lung, GI tract, and kidneys. This is a lethal infection that may lead to massive and fatal hemoptysis from pulmonary vessel invasion.[16] Surgical treatment for this highly aggressive organism may include extensive debridement and resection of involved tissues.[7]

Hyalohyphomycosis

The most common form of disease from molds in this group include Fusariosis and Scedosporium infections which are responsible for an increased pneumonia presence in transplant recipients and patients with hematologic malignancies.[1]

Fusariosis organisms resemble aspergillus on histologic examination; differentiation depends on culture speciation. These organisms are unique in their ability to sporulate in vivo leading to vascular invasion with yeast dissemination.[3,17,18] Transplant recipients manifest differences in disease response and outcome between SOT and HSCT recipients. These differences are likely causally associated with neutropenia in HSCT recipients who experience disseminated infections (commonly with pulmonary involvement) as compared to localized disease in SOT recipients. Immune reconstitution is important for treatment, since prolonged neutropenia with infection has a high mortality.[3,17]

Scedoporium is the second most common mold after aspergillus to colonize the airway of cystic fibrosis patients, and like Fusariosis, has the ability to undergo adventitious sporulation. Moreover, the disease severity is worse for HSCT recipients as compared to SOT recipients. Surgical excision for localized disease may be a component of therapy given the poor response of this organism to antifungal therapy.[3,17]

Phaeohyphomycosis

This disease is caused by inhalation or inoculation of species of black molds leading to allergic bronchopulmonary disease

(ABPD) associated with eosinophil elevations. Nonallergic pulmonary disease occurs in immune-compromised individuals and represents tissue invasion of this fungus which is a common airway colonizer. Invasive phaeohyphomycosis may manifest as pneumonias or parenchymal or endobronchial nodules.

Opportunistic Fungal Infections

Opportunistic fungal infections are caused by the following organisms: *Candida*, *Aspergillus*, emerging fungal organisms (noted above), *Cryptococcus*, and *Pneumocystis jirovecii* (previously *Pneumocystis carinii*). Infections from these fungal organisms occur primarily in immune-compromised individuals and fall into several easily recognizable groups (infections are worsened by the presence of diabetes in all groups) (see Table 103-1): transplant recipients, cancer patients, immune-suppressed populations, and patients with other debilitating disease, including Lupus and Crohn disease.

Differences occur between the above groups and are accentuated in the transplant recipients as noted in a recent report using data from the Transplant Associated Infections Surveillance Program (TRANSNET)[19]: Invasive aspergillosis has replaced Candida as the most common invasive fungal infection in the HSCT population. There is a low 1-year survival for invasive fungal infections in HSCT recipients (6% for Fusarium infections, 25% for invasive aspergillus, 28% for zygomycosis, and 34% for invasive candidiasis). Invasive fungal infections in HSCT recipients increase as the donor match differs from the recipient (increasing infection rates for autologous and allogenic [matched, unrelated, mismatched]). Candida is still the most common infection of SOT recipients except for lung transplant recipients where Aspergillus infections predominate.[18]

Candida

This organism is the most common opportunistic fungal infection in ICU patients and SOT recipients (excluding lung transplants due to tracheobronchial or anastomotic Aspergillus infections).[2,18,20] Other patient groups that may be affected by this organism are patients with solid tumors and hematologic malignancies at risk for neutrophil defects as opposed to T-cell deficiencies. As compared to the other fungal infections noted above, infections from this organism typically arise from endogenous sources, and the majority of infections occur in the presence of vascular access devices (Fig. 103-7). Candida nonalbicans infections as compared with Candida albicans are rising rapidly in frequency and carry a higher mortality.[2,18,20] Pulmonary consolidation may be difficult to diagnose as candida pneumonia owing to candida colonization of the airway. Furthermore this organism may predispose to pulmonary bacterial infections.[20] Surgery is rarely required for this organism other than to deal with pleural or pericardial space infections.

Aspergillus

Aspergillus is ubiquitous in nature and is the most common opportunistic mold to cause pulmonary infection. Host factors allowing aspergillus hyphae invasion include prior structural lung disease or defects in immune resistance. However, severe infection most often arises in immune-deficient patient populations comprising two groups: Patients with chronic neutropenia and nonneutropenic patients secondary to steroids or SOT recipients with chronic pulmonary damage.

Patients with normal immune systems are at risk for any of the following Aspergillus infections as shown in Figure 103-8. Aspergillus colonization is common in all patients (50% of cystic fibrosis patients are colonized with aspergillus); the presence of this organism may lead to recurrent episodes of hemoptysis.

Immune-suppressed patients differ with respect to this organism related to the individual suppression type. In SOT, specifically lung transplant patients, aspergillus colonization rarely leads to invasion, whereas in HSCT recipients or patients with hematologic malignancies it has a high predictive value for invasion.[18] With respect to lung transplantation, the following clinical Aspergillus infections can occur: Standard colonization, pseudomembranous necrotizing tracheobronchilitis, invasive aspergillosis, and ABPA.

Bronchial mucosa disruptions occurring in lung transplant patients and aspergillus colonization has made aspergillus the most common fungal infection in lung transplant recipients in comparison with other SOT recipients, suggesting the use of routine antifungal therapy until bronchial remodeling is complete (Fig. 103-9).[18,21] Aspergillus anastomotic infections carry significant mortality as does invasive aspergillosis as seen in Table 103-2.

Surgical therapy for Aspergillus infections is indicated for immune-competent symptomatic medically refractory patients with adequate pulmonary reserve; lung resection is required for parenchymal disease and possibly thoracoplasty for pleural disease. Immune-suppressed patients have a high mortality (30%–80%) from invasive pulmonary aspergillosis owing to massive hemoptysis. Lobectomy is indicated in these high risk individuals with radiographic suggestions of pulmonary artery involvement.[22]

Cryptococcus Neoformans

This organism (Fig. 103-10) is ubiquitous in the environment and infection may lead to neurologic infection and involvement with pathologic processes. Inhalation of spores from this organism with subsequent macrophage internalization may lead to yeast germination inside host macrophages. These infected macrophages may then disseminate yeast infections according to a Trojan horse model of infection of distant organs.[23] The groups at risk with this organism are HIV individuals and transplant recipients.[9]

Pneumocystis Jirovecii

This organism previously named *P. carinii* is thought to be transmitted via an airborne route leading to either colonization or clearance depending on the status of host T lymphocytes. Certain at-risk groups suffer higher colonization rates by this organism: HIV infected patients, COPD patients, diabetes, myeloma, chronic lymphocytic leukemia (CLL), and sarcoidosis. With the introduction of highly active antiretroviral therapy (HAART) medications and Pneumocystis pneumonia (PCP) prophylaxis, patients without HIV now constitute the majority of current PCP infections. This patient population includes immune-deficient states, malignancies (hematologic and solid organ), and transplant recipients.

The disease presentation includes symptoms of pneumonia and respiratory distress without physical signs of pneumonia. The organism is not easily cultured and diagnosis relies on microscopic visualization in pulmonary secretions. Mortality is still high for all infected groups revealing the value of prevention.

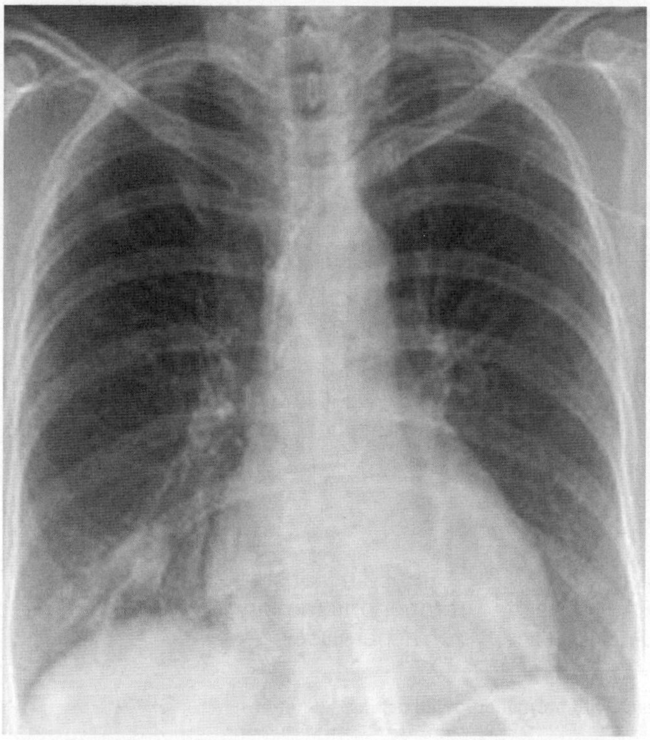

A

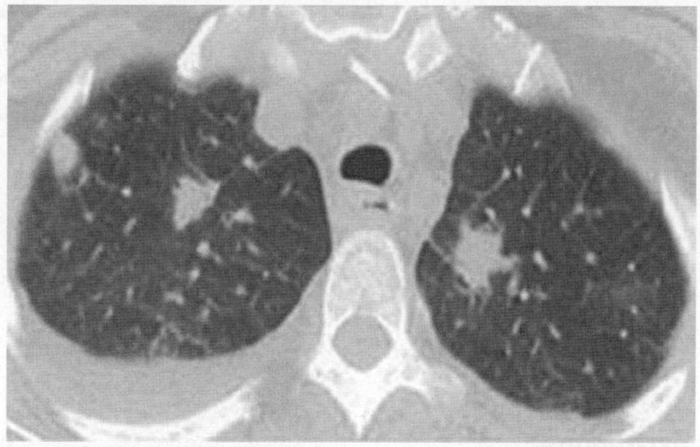

B

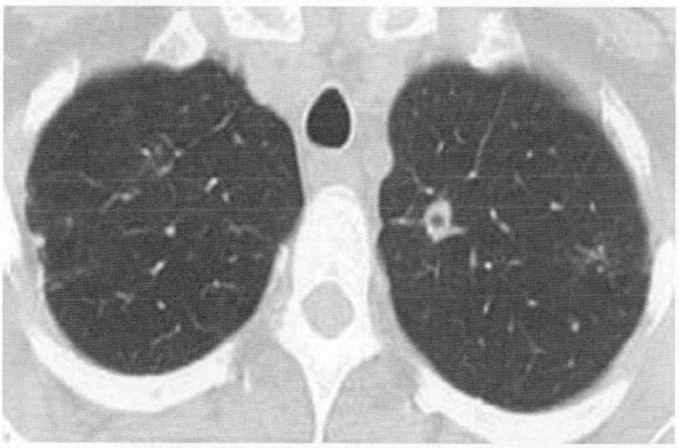

C

Figure 103-7. (*A*) CT scan images (*B, C*) show multiple nodules in an egocentric distribution with and without cavitation secondary to hematogenous dissemination of Candida from a central line. *Images provided courtesy of Ritu R. Gill, MD.*

Table 103-2

EPIDEMIOLOGIC CHARACTERISTICS OF INVASIVE ASPERGILLOSIS (IA) IN SOLID ORGAN TRANSPLANT RECIPIENTS[a]

TYPE OF TRANSPLANT	MEAN INCIDENCE (% AND INTERVAL)	MEAN TIME TO ONSET (IN DAYS AND INTERVAL)	% DISSEMINATED ASPERGILLOSIS	MORTALITY (%)
Liver	2 (1–8)	17 (6–1.107)	50–60	87
Lung	6 (3–14)	120 (4–1.410)	15–20	68
Heart	5.2 (1–15)	45 (12–365)	20–35	78
Kidney	0.7 (0–4)	82 (20–801)	9–36	77
Pancreas	1.1–2.9	NA	NA	100
Small bowel	2.2 (0–10)	289 (10–956)	66	66
Allogenic stem cell	10 (5–26)	78 (46–120)	27–30	78–92
Autologous stem cell	4.8 (2–6)	20 (7–456)	10–20	78–92
Nonmyeloablative stem cell	11 (8–23)	107 (4–282)	34	63–67

[a]Adapted from Singh N, Patterson DL. Aspergillus infections in transplant recipients. *Medicine (Baltimore).* 1999;78:123–128.; Gangneux JP, Camus C, Philippe B. Epidemiologie et facteurs de risque de l'aspergillose invasive du suget non neutropenique (full text in English on www.em-consulte.com/revue/rmr). *Rev Mal Respir.* 2008;25:139–153. doi: RMR-02-2008-25-2-01761-8425-101019-200802945 [Table 1].

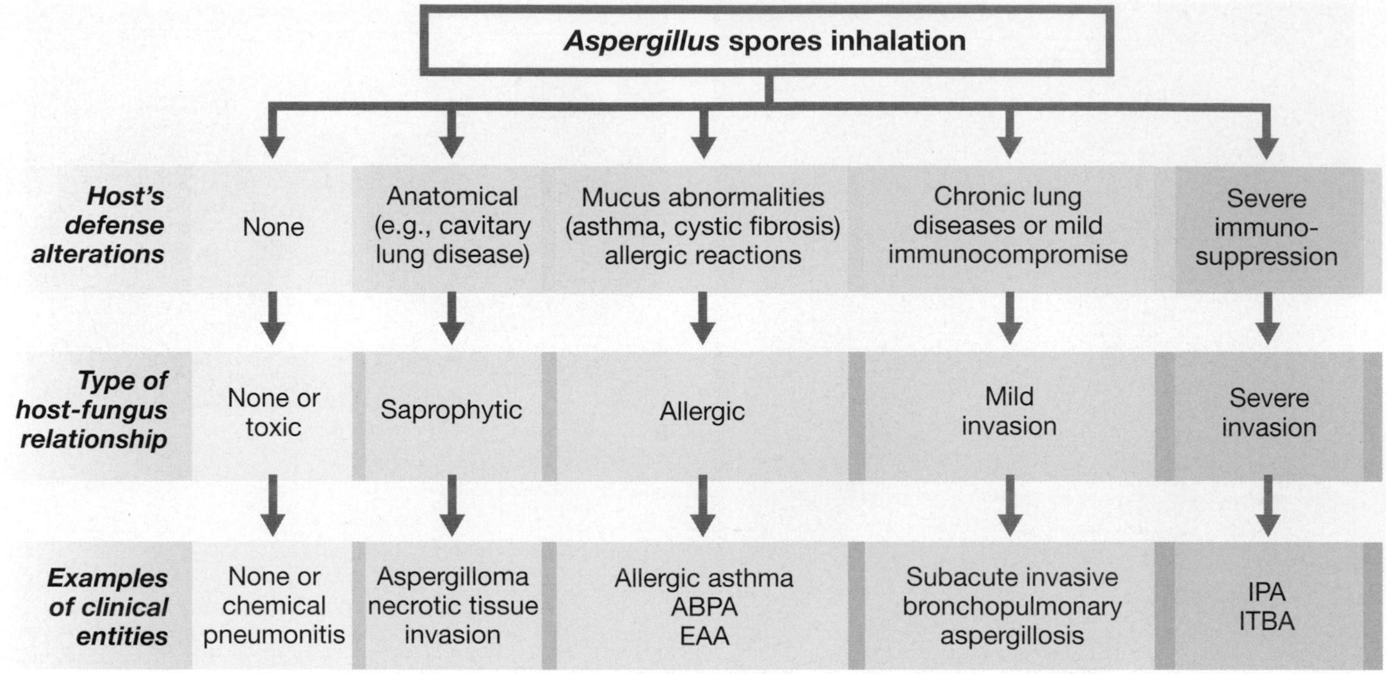

Figure 103-8. Aspergillus infections found in patients with normal or varied defense alterations.

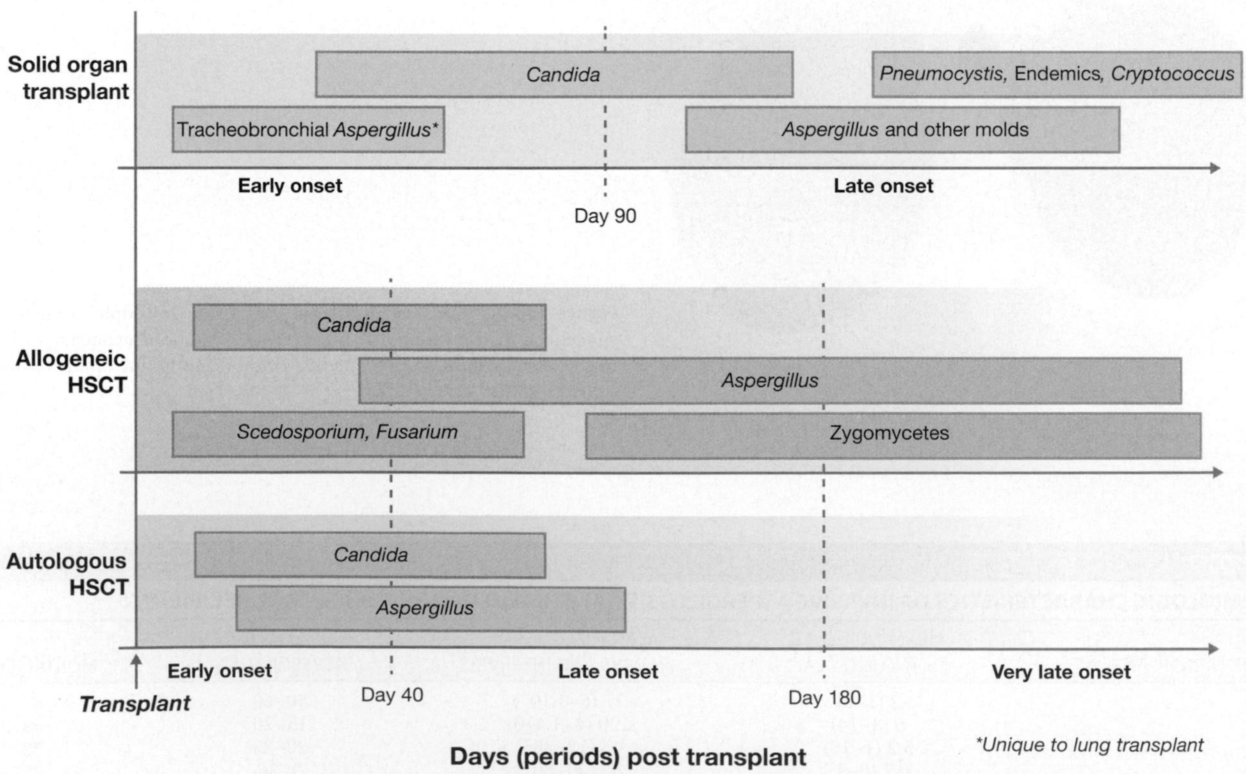

Figure 103-9. Timing of fungal infection in transplant recipients.

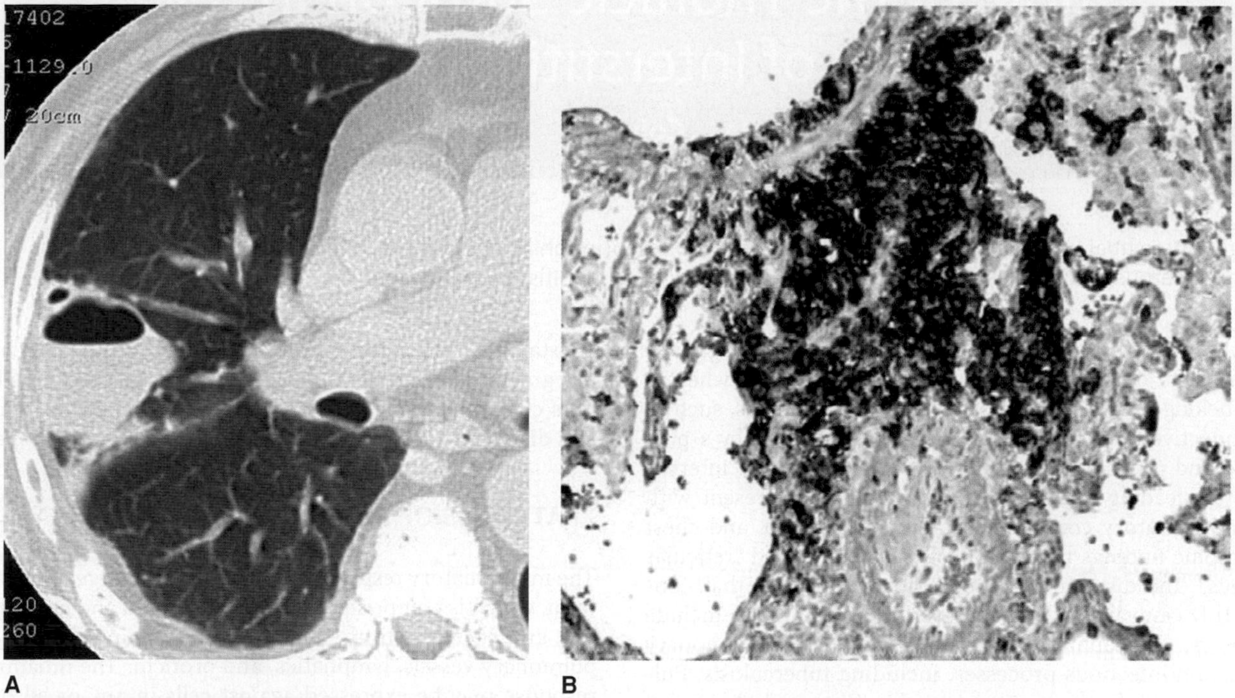

Figure 103-10. Axial CT scan image (*A*) and pathology image (*B*) consistent with *Cryptococcus neoformans* infection in the right middle lobe. *Images provided courtesy of Ritu R. Gill, MD.*

EDITOR'S COMMENT

Thoracic fungal infections are an important clinical consideration, not because the diseases are common, but because they are commonly confused with thoracic malignancy. As more effective antifungal therapies are developed, it will be increasingly important to recognize the clinical and radiologic features of thoracic fungal infections to avoid unnecessary surgical intervention.

—Steven J. Mentzer

References

1. Smith JA, Kauffman CA. Pulmonary fungal infections. *Respirology*. 2012;17(6):913–926.
2. Morace G, Borghi E. Fungal infections in ICU patients: epidemiology and the role of diagnostics. *Minerva Anestesiol*. 2010;76(11):950–956.
3. Hsu LY, Ng ES, Koh LP. Common and emerging fungal pulmonary infections. *Infect Dis Clin North Am*. 2010;24(3):557–577.
4. Sullivan DC, Chapman SW. Bacteria that masquerade as fungi: actinomycosis/nocardia. *Proc Am Thorac Soc*. 2010;7(3):216–221.
5. Marom EM, Kontoyiannis DP. Imaging studies for diagnosing invasive fungal pneumonia in immunocompromised patients. *Curr Opin Infect Dis*. 2011;24(4):309–314.
6. Baddley Y, Andres DR, Mark Ka, et al. Factors associated with mortality in transplant patients with invasive aspergillosis. *Clin Infect Dis*. 2010;50:1559–1567.
7. LoCicero J, 3rd, Shaw JP, Lazzaro RS. Surgery for other pulmonary fungal infections, Actinomyces, and Nocardia. *Thorac Surg Clin*. 2012;22(3):363–374.
8. Byrnes EJ, 3rd, Bartlett KH, Perfect JR, et al. *Cryptococcus gattii*: an emerging fungal pathogen infecting humans and animals. *Microbes Infect*. 2011;13(11):895–907.
9. Li SS, Mody CH. *Cryptococcus*. *Proc Am Thorac Soc*. 2010;7(3):186–196.
10. Knox KS, Hage CA. Histoplasmosis. *Proc Am Thorac Soc*. 2010;7(3):169–172.
11. Ampel NM. New perspectives on coccidioidomycosis. *Proc Am Thorac Soc*. 2010;7(3):181–185.
12. Vikram HR, Dosanjh A, Blair JE. Coccidioidomycosis and lung transplantation. *Transplantation*. 2011;92(7):717–721.
13. Smith JA, Kauffman CA. Blastomycosis. *Proc Am Thorac Soc*. 2010;7(3):173–180.
14. Chapman SW, Dismukes WE, Proia LA, et al. Clinical practice guidelines for the management of blastomycosis: 2008 update by the Infectious Diseases Society of America. *Clin Infect Dis*. 2008;46(12):1801–1812.
15. Ramos-e-Silva M, Vasconcelos C, Carneiro S, et al. Sporotrichosis. *Clin Dermatol*. 2007;25(2):181–187.
16. Gupta KL, Khullar DK, Behera D, et al. Pulmonary mucormycosis presenting as fatal massive haemoptysis in a renal transplant recipient. *Nephrol Dial Transplant*. 1998;13(12):3258–3260.
17. Nishi SP, Valentine VG, Duncan S. Emerging bacterial, fungal, and viral respiratory infections in transplantation. *Infect Dis Clin North Am*. 2010;24(3):541–555.
18. Person AK, Kontoyiannis DP, Alexander BD. Fungal infections in transplant and oncology patients. *Infect Dis Clin North Am*. 2010;24(2):439–459.
19. Lockhart SR, Wagner D, Iqbal N, et al. Comparison of in vitro susceptibility characteristics of *Candida* species from cases of invasive candidiasis in solid organ and stem cell transplant recipients: Transplant-Associated Infections Surveillance Network (TRANSNET), 2001 to 2006. *J Clin Microbiol*. 2011;49(7):2404–2410.
20. Evans SE. Coping with *Candida* infections. *Proc Am Thorac Soc*. 2010;7(3):197–203.
21. Gangneux JP, Camus C, Philippe B. Epidemiology of invasive aspergillosis and risk factors in non neutropaenic patients. *Rev Mal Respir*. 2010;27(8):e34–e46.
22. Pages PB, Abou Hanna H, Caillot D, et al. [Place of surgery in pulmonary aspergillosis and other pulmonary mycotic infections]. *Rev Pneumol Clin*. 2012;68(2):67–76.
23. Botts MR, Hull CM. Dueling in the lung: how *Cryptococcus* spores race the host for survival. *Curr Opin Microbiol*. 2010;13(4):437–442.

104 Role of the Thoracic Surgeon in the Diagnosis of Interstitial Lung Disease

Subroto Paul and Yolonda L. Colson

Keywords: Interstitial lung disease, granulomatosis, sarcoidosis, eosinophilic pneumonia, idiopathic pulmonary fibrosis, granulomatous vasculitides, tuberculosis, hypersensitivity pneumonitis, idiopathic interstitial pneumonia

Interstitial lung disease (ILD) represents over 200 diagnostic entities. Some are distinct clinicopathologic disorders, whereas others belong to a broader class of clinical syndromes, such as the connective tissue diseases. ILD is characterized by a progressive and diffuse inflammation of the pulmonary interstitium often leading to fibrosis. Patients typically present with chronic respiratory complaints, including dyspnea, and chest radiographic findings that demonstrate pronounced "reticular markings." The distinct clinicopathologic disorders that constitute ILD can vary widely in presentation. Examples include sarcoidosis, eosinophilic pneumonias, idiopathic pulmonary fibrosis, and infectious processes, including tuberculosis. Pulmonary fungal infections are reviewed in Chapter 102.

The primary goal of the thoracic surgeon in the evaluation of patients with symptoms and radiologic findings consistent with ILD is to facilitate an expedient diagnosis. The least invasive diagnostic modalities include bronchoscopy, bronchoalveolar lavage, and chest CT scanning. However, lung biopsy by transbronchial, open, or video-assisted thoracic surgery (VATS) techniques remains the most definitive and expeditious means of establishing the diagnosis. Development of VATS techniques has greatly reduced the morbidity associated with lung biopsy. This chapter provides an overview of the spectrum of disease and diagnostic approach to ILD from the surgical perspective.

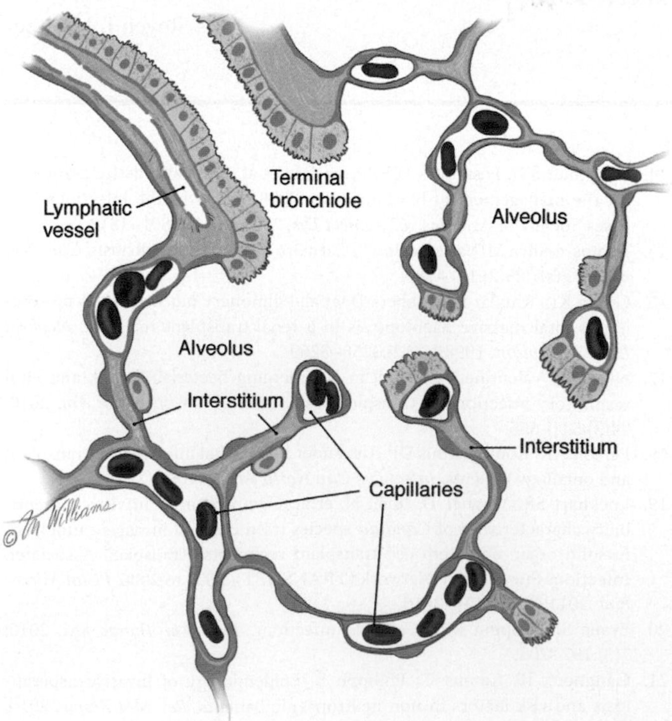

Figure 104-1. Morphologically, the lung parenchyma has two general components: airspace and interstitium. The airspace is comprised of the respiratory bronchioles, alveolar ducts, and alveoli. The interstitium consists of the fibrous septa, alveolar walls, and connective tissues that surround the vascular and bronchial lumina.

PATTERNS OF INTERSTITIAL LUNG DISEASE

The inflammatory response observed in ILD targets the interstitium, which is comprised of the fibrous septa and alveolar walls that give structure to the lungs. Within the interstitium lie the pulmonary vessels, lymphatics, and bronchi. The inflammatory response may be expressed against cells in any or all of these structures (Fig. 104-1). Often it is focused on one component of the interstitium, permitting a loose categorization of two patterns of injury: granulomatous and alveolitic (Table 104-1).[1,2]

Granulomatous Pattern

The pattern of disease injury denoted as granulomatous is initiated by a cell-mediated immune response to a foreign or self-protein, that is antigen, which may or may not be known. The response is initiated by a release of inflammatory cytokines. Activated immune cells, typically macrophages, encircle and engulf the protein that the immune system has failed to recognize in an antigen-specific fashion. The antigen is sequestered and granulomata are formed. This inflammatory process, once activated, can spread to the alveoli, which renders the pattern of injury difficult to discern in end-stage disease. The granulomatous mechanism is expressed in several pulmonary diseases, which are described briefly below.

Infection

Mycobacterium tuberculosis infection is the most common cause of granulomatous lung disease worldwide.[3,4] *Aspergillus*

Table 104-1

CATEGORIZATION OF INTERSTITIAL LUNG DISEASE INTO GRANULOMATOUS AND ALVEOLITIC SUBTYPES

Granulomatous
Infections—tuberculosis, helminths, aspergillosis
Sarcoidosis
Granulomatous vasculitides—Wegener granulomatosis and Churg–Strauss syndrome
Hypersensitivity pneumonitis
Foreign body/Inorganic dust
Eosinophilic pneumonias
Histiocytosis X
Alveolitic
Goodpasture syndrome
Drug-induced injury
Idiopathic interstitial pneumonias

and certain helminths also can lead to pulmonary granulomatous disease (see Chapter 102).[1,2] Diagnosis relies on history, a positive purified protein derivative test, and sputum culture.

Sarcoidosis

Sarcoidosis is a chronic systemic disorder characterized by the presence of granulomata in certain affected organs. The disorder remains poorly understood and the responsible antigen has not yet been identified. Patients with sarcoidosis may have variable and fluctuating symptoms. Classically, patients present with fever, myalgias, chills, fatigue, and weight loss. Angiotensin-converting enzyme levels are often elevated. Diagnosis is often suspected radiographically by the appearance of bilateral hilar and mediastinal lymph node enlargement on plain chest films, sometimes accompanied by a reticulonodular pulmonary pattern. Most patients diagnosed by chest radiography alone are asymptomatic. In patients with mediastinal lymphadenopathy, tissue diagnosis can be made via cervical mediastinoscopy. The rare patient with only interstitial lung pathology, or in patients with progressive lung lesions despite treatment, VATS lung biopsy may be helpful to establish the diagnosis and rule out other etiologies.

Granulomatous Vasculitides

In Wegener granulomatosis and Churg–Strauss syndrome – two representative granulomatous vasculitides – the granulomata form around the pulmonary vessels. Wegener granulomatosis is characterized by the presence of necrotizing granulomata within the pulmonary parenchyma, which often become cavitary and can be confused radiographically with squamous cell lung cancer or other infectious etiologies (Fig. 104-2). The renal vasculature also may be involved, and 90% of patients have antibodies to antineutrophil cytoplasmic antibodies against the PR3 serine proteinase (c-ANCA).[3,5–10] Churg–Strauss syndrome is a rare systemic disorder characterized by eosinophilia and eosinophilic granulomata of the pulmonary vasculature. Diagnosis of both these diseases rests on clinical suspicion, along with the laboratory studies and pathologic findings on lung biopsy or other sites of disease involvement.

Hypersensitivity Pneumonitis

Hypersensitivity pneumonitis is caused by repeated inhalation of dust-containing organic antigens, which leads to diffuse inflammation of the lung parenchyma and airways in previously sensitized patients.[11–13] The most common types of hypersensitivity pneumonitis are Farmer's lung due to chronic exposure to moldy hay, straw, or grain, or Bird fancier's lung due to exposure to avian proteins in feathers and droppings. Although many other antigens have also been implicated, with diseases named after various interesting occupations (e.g., *bagassosis* derived from *bagasse,* or sugarcane dust, *cheese washer's lung* from handling cheese mold, *compost lung*), hypersensitivity pneumonitis has also been described following exposure to fungi or bacteria in humidifiers, heaters, or air conditioning units. Diagnosis lies in careful history taking, especially when a known occupational exposure is suspected. Early parenchymal changes are characterized by neutrophil and macrophage infiltration of the distal bronchioles and alveoli. Progression to granuloma formation and interstitial fibrosis occurs with continued exposure to the antigen. Diagnosis is suspected by exposure history, but tissue biopsy may be required if disease progresses despite contact avoidance.

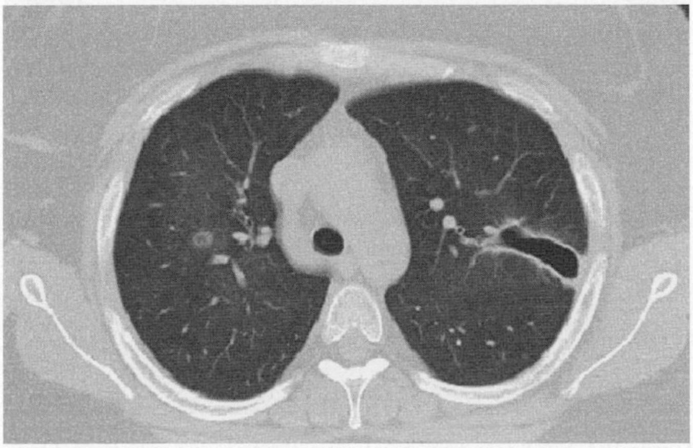

Figure 104-2. CT scan representative of radiographic findings seen in Wegener granulomatosis. Note the large cavitary lesion in the left lung.

Foreign Body/Inorganic Dust

Exposure to small foreign particulate matter or dust, whether organic or inorganic, can lead to a spectrum of pulmonary disease processes such as those associated with chronic exposure to metal dusts (e.g., beryllium, aluminum, and zirconium) or small organic particles leading to hypersensitivity pneumonitis. A common example is silicosis caused by inhalation of crystalline silica dust by miners or sandblasters, or even desert sand, as in Desert lung or Desert storm pneumonitis described in personnel serving in the Gulf War.[14,15] Although now relatively rare in the United States after the introduction of respirator masks and other occupational safety measures, silicosis is still considered to be the most common occupational lung disease worldwide.[16] It is characterized by nodular lesions predominantly in the upper lobes. Patients may be asymptomatic to the initial exposure but later develop symptoms secondary to occult lung injury. Again, diagnosis is based on exposure history but may require tissue to make a definitive diagnosis or for worker's compensation claims.

Eosinophilic Pneumonias

Eosinophilic pneumonia is a pulmonary process characterized by the accumulation of eosinophils within the parenchymal tissues. Eosinophilic pneumonias can be caused by helminth infections, such as *Strongyloides stercoralis* and *Ancylostoma duodenale,* and drug allergies.[8,17] More often than not, the etiology is unknown. Idiopathic eosinophilic pneumonias have three forms: simple, acute, and chronic. Simple eosinophilic pneumonias are rare, characterized pathologically by an interstitial edema that is abundant with eosinophils and typically resolves spontaneously, particularly with smoking cessation. Patients with acute eosinophilic pneumonia present in severe respiratory distress. Their prognosis is poor. The chronic form is more indolent and often found in patients with a history of asthma. Chronic eosinophilic pneumonia is similar in both histology and, in most cases, radiographic appearance to the simple and acute forms. Diagnosis of all these syndromes requires the demonstration of peripheral blood eosinophilia and often a tissue biopsy.[17,18] The disease clears rapidly with steroid treatment, although there is a higher rate of relapse with the acute form.[8,14]

Histiocytosis X

Histiocytosis X is a rare disorder characterized by the peribronchial accumulation of specialized antigen-presenting cells known as *Langerhans cells*. Long-standing disease, also known as *eosinophilic granulomatosis*, can lead to interstitial fibrosis and also may present with skeletal involvement. Tissue biopsy is often required for diagnosis.[19] Spontaneous remission can occur, particularly with smoking cessation, although treatment with steroids may be required.

Alveolitic Pattern

The alveolitic categorization of ILD applies when the injury is directed primarily toward the alveolar wall, resulting in airspace disease. Cellular and humoral components of the immune system may both be involved. Alveolitic mechanisms have been implicated in a variety of pulmonary diseases, summarized below (see Table 104-2).[1,2]

Goodpasture Syndrome

Goodpasture syndrome is a systemic disease process characterized by pulmonary hemorrhage and glomerulonephritis in the setting of anti-glomerular basement membrane antibodies. It is a rare disorder diagnosed predominantly in young males and is linked to the presence of the HLA-DRw2 allele, but it can present in later years with equal sex distribution and a lower incidence of lung hemorrhage. The disease is caused by antibodies directed against a collagen protein found in the alveolar and glomerular membrane, resulting in an antibody-mediated injury.[20–22] Patients present with both hemoptysis and hematuria. Diagnosis is based on clinical symptomatology and usually renal biopsy.[21,22]

Table 104-2

TEN STEPS TO VIDEO-ASSISTED THORACOSCOPIC SURGERY (VATS) LUNG BIOPSY

1. Single-lung ventilation with either placement of double-lumen endotracheal tube or placement of a bronchial blocker together with a single-lumen endotracheal tube (see Fig. 104-5). Bronchoscopic confirmation of correct placement and auscultatory confirmation of lung isolation of the operative side is recommended.
2. Use the chest CT findings to plan the placement of the patient in the full lateral decubitus position with slight flexion of the operating table to widen the lung interspaces.
3. Placement of three 10-mm ports with the idea of triangulating the region of lung targeted for biopsy within the three ports. The camera port should be at the apex of the triangle (see Fig. 104-6).
4. One centimeter skin incisions should be placed in the rib interspaces with Bovie dissection through the soft tissue and intercostal muscles until the endothoracic fascia over the rib is reached. The endothoracic fascia should be divided carefully over the rib to avoid injury to the lung as the thorax is entered.
5. A 10-mm thoracoscopic port then is placed into the chest through this incision.
6. A 10-mm 30-degree camera is inserted through the port into the thoracic cavity, and the thorax is inspected.
7. The other two 10-mm ports then are placed in a similar fashion with direct visualization of entry into the thoracic cavity.
8. With the aid of atraumatic grasping instruments (e.g., O-ring forceps), the lung parenchyma is grasped, inspected, and palpated until the parenchymal lesion(s) of interest is identified (see Fig. 104-7).
9. Endoscopic staplers are used to resect the identified lesion. The lesion then is removed from the thorax within a specimen bag (see Fig. 104-8).
10. After ensuring that hemostasis has been achieved, the ports are removed from the thorax. The thoracoscopic ports then are closed with 2-0 absorbable suture for the soft tissue and 3-0 absorbable suture for the skin.

Drug-induced Injury

Drug-induced lung injury often results in an alveolitic pattern of injury, whether the mechanism of injury is due to a direct cytotoxic, immune-mediated injury, or the dysregulation of cytokine regulated inflammatory cascades. Numerous drugs have been implicated in this disease process, including bleomycin, nitrofurantoin, and amiodarone.[20,23] Drug induced ILD has also been reported with erlotinib and other tyrosine kinase inhibitors used in the treatment of nonsmall cell lung cancer.[24,25] The diagnosis rests on clinical suspicion and correlation with prior drug exposure. Lung biopsy may or may not be helpful as fibrosis becomes apparent in late-stage disease.

Idiopathic Interstitial Pneumonias

Idiopathic interstitial pneumonias encompass a range of pulmonary disorders characterized by infiltration of the pulmonary interstitium with immune cells, leading to alveolitic changes. Continued inflammation eventually results in end-stage pulmonary fibrosis (Fig. 104-3). The multiple terms used in association with this disease reflect the diagnostic confusion that surrounds it, including *Hamman–Rich disease, idiopathic pulmonary fibrosis, usual interstitial pneumonitis,* and *diffuse pulmonary alveolar fibrosis.* Several subclassification schemes have been proposed, which many argue are superfluous because this disorder can be viewed as a continuum. The most common subclassification, proposed by Averill Liebow, divides idiopathic interstitial pneumonias into six categories: (1) usual interstitial pneumonia/idiopathic pulmonary fibrosis, (2) desquamative interstitial pneumonia, (3) nonspecific interstitial pneumonia, (4) acute interstitial pneumonitis, (5) respiratory bronchiolitis-associated ILD, and (6) cryptogenic organizing pneumonia. Patients with this continuum of disorders present with progressive dyspnea in the setting of reticular opacities on plain chest films. Diagnosis of the idiopathic interstitial pneumonia rests on the exclusion of other known disorders and histologic analysis of sufficient lung tissue, making

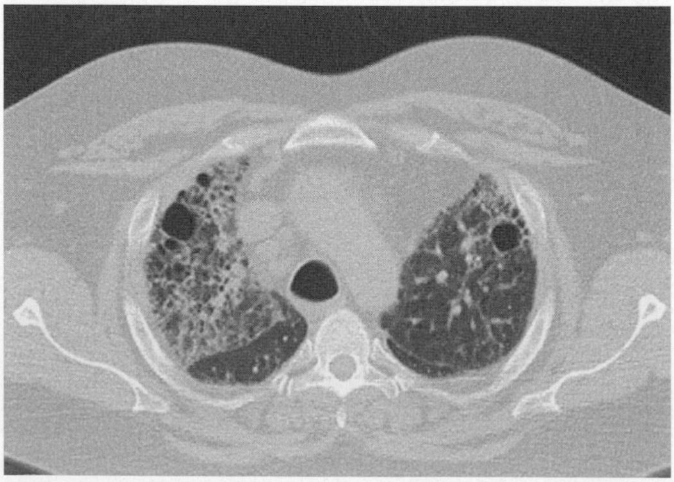

Figure 104-3. CT scan from a patient with idiopathic pulmonary fibrosis. Note the significant fibrotic changes and characteristic honeycomb pattern.

open or VATS lung biopsy usually the preferred approach to tissue diagnosis.[22,26–30] Often, a clear-cut distinction cannot be made between the various subclasses, even with adequate lung tissue. Lymphocytic interstitial pneumonia is often misidentified as belonging to this category because chest radiographs of patients with lymphocytic interstitial pneumonia often show an "interstitial" pattern of disease. However, lymphocytic interstitial pneumonia is a lymphoproliferative disorder with no alveolar injury, and a lung biopsy may be required to exclude this disorder in some patients.[31,32] Patients with progressive disease refractory to immunosuppressive therapy can be treated only by lung transplantation.

CLINICAL PRESENTATION

Patients with ILD typically present with progressive dyspnea, a persistent nonproductive cough, fatigue, and weight loss. Wheezing, hemoptysis, and pleuritic chest pain are rare symptoms in early ILD. Hemoptysis typically is associated with diffuse alveolar hemorrhage syndromes and the granulomatous vasculitides, but not with other forms of ILD. These symptoms occur in the setting of radiographic evidence of interstitial opacities. Although symptoms are typically chronic, an acute presentation is possible, with the allergic responses seen with hypersensitivity pneumonitis, eosinophilic pneumonia, or drug-induced alveolitis.

PATIENT EVALUATION

A thorough history and physical examination are of paramount importance for patients with suspected ILD (Fig. 104-4). The diagnosis is often suggested by a history of environmental/occupational exposures or connective tissue disease. Laboratory studies are used to identify antibodies that might suggest a specific connective tissue disease or the presence of elevated angiotensin-converting enzyme in sarcoidosis.[33] Pulmonary function tests are used to assess the extent of pulmonary dysfunction. ILD is characterized by a restrictive pulmonary physiology with a reduced total lung capacity, functional residual capacity, and residual volume. The diffusing capacity of the lung for carbon monoxide (DLCO) is also impaired. Forced vital capacity and expiratory volume also may be decreased secondary to a low total lung capacity. Chest x-ray and chest CT scan may be helpful in separating "interstitial" from consolidative patterns of disease and in identifying lymphangitic spread of malignancy when additional mass(es) is present.[34] However, chest radiographic findings are nonspecific and are not helpful in discerning the various forms of ILD. Bronchoalveolar lavage can be a useful diagnostic aid for some diseases, including eosinophilic pneumonias and histiocytosis X (Langerhans cells), where a predominant cell type is found in the lavage fluid. However, most patients require lung biopsy to make a definitive diagnosis.[18,29,35]

Lung biopsy can be performed by open, VATS, or transbronchial technique. Transbronchial biopsy typically is attempted first to rule out an infectious etiology or confirm an obvious clinical diagnosis (e.g., Goodpasture syndrome or sarcoidosis), but provides inadequate tissue for diagnosing idiopathic interstitial pneumonia. If the diagnosis remains unclear or if the clinical course or radiographic evidence dictate more aggressive management, surgical biopsy is warranted and is the most effective means of establishing the diagnosis and prognosis. In general biopsy should be obtained from two distinct disease sites, preferably from two different lobes with a margin of normal tissue for comparison to assure adequate sampling of areas of active disease and not just end-stage fibrosis. Some investigators report that lingual or middle lobe biopsy may overrepresent fibrosis and vasculopathy. Others disagree, reporting that lingual or right middle lobe biopsy is equivalent to biopsy of other pulmonary segments, provided that the area selected for biopsy is representative of the disease process present elsewhere in the lung.[36–42] Generally speaking, areas of localized fibrosis or scarring should be avoided and more representative areas selected for biopsy. If an adequate biopsy is performed early in the disease course, before the onset of end-stage fibrosis, the diagnostic accuracy approaches 90%.[43] Other than ruling out infectious etiologies, biopsies of late stage disease or areas of dense fibrosis are much less helpful.

VATS biopsy has proved in most series to be as accurate in establishing a diagnosis as is open-lung biopsy performed through a minithoracotomy.[44,45] VATS lung biopsy typically is done with the patient in the full lateral decubitus position, with single-lung ventilation accomplished through either a double-lumen endotracheal tube or, if not available, insertion of a bronchial blocker through a traditional endotracheal tube (Fig. 104-5). Ports are

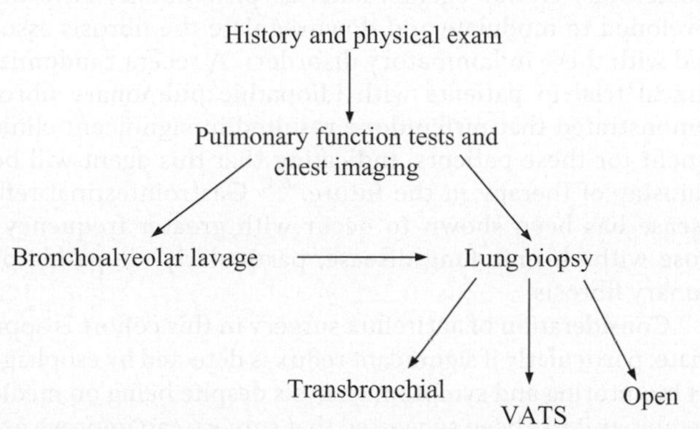

Figure 104-4. Treatment algorithm for interstitial lung disease.

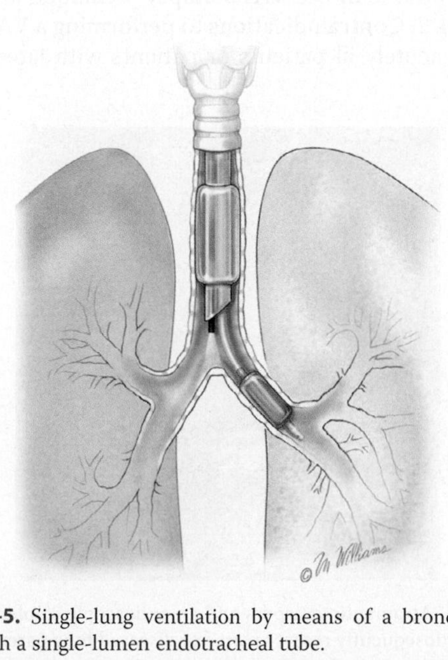

Figure 104-5. Single-lung ventilation by means of a bronchial blocker together with a single-lumen endotracheal tube.

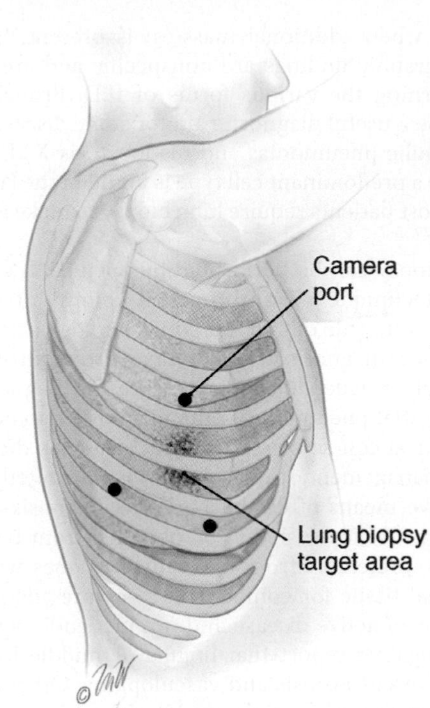

Figure 104-6. Triangulated port placement for VATS lung biopsy of underlying area of involved lung.

placed with the goal of triangulating the area of interest in the lung (Fig. 104-6). Atraumatic graspers are used to localize the representative lesion, and a representative sample of disease lung tissue is resected using endoscopic staplers (Fig. 104-7). It is preferable to divide the lung where the tissue is less involved and compliant, while still including representative active disease in the specimen, in order to avoid subsequent air leaks from the lung parenchyma as positive pressure ventilation and the frequent use of steroids for these conditions can make management of this complication difficult. The lesion then is removed from the thorax within a specimen bag (Fig. 104-8).

After biopsy, hemostasis is achieved and the incisions closed. An outline of the VATS biopsy technique is presented in Table 104-2. Contraindications to performing a VATS biopsy include (1) acutely ill patients or patients with late-stage ILD

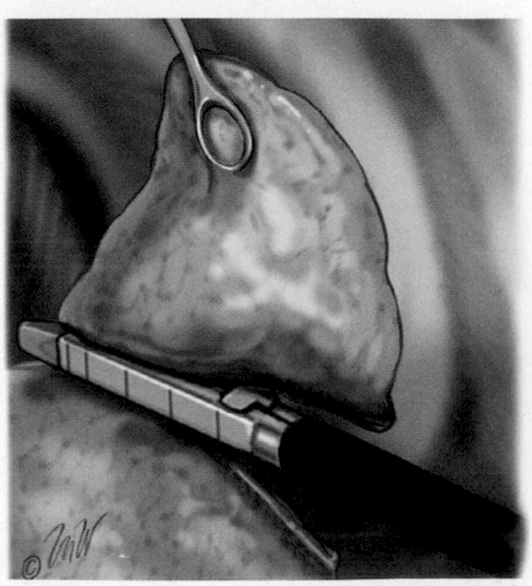

Figure 104-7. Atraumatic graspers and an endoscopic stapler are used to localize and subsequently resect an area of diseased lung parenchyma.

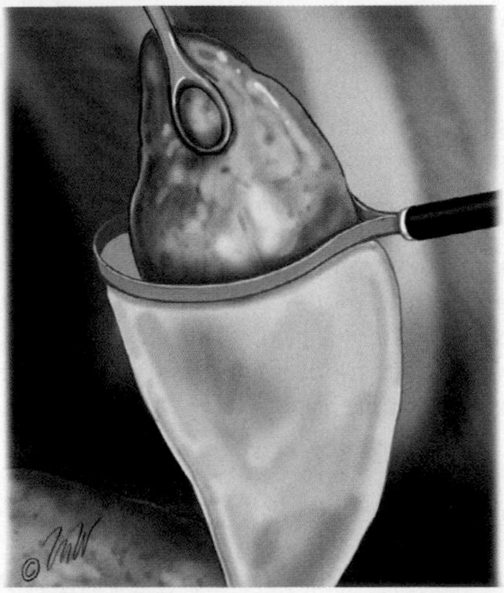

Figure 104-8. The lesion is placed in a specimen bag and removed from the operative field.

with severe fibrosis (for whom definitive diagnosis on biopsy is low), who often have decreased pulmonary compliance and decreased DLCO, precluding general anesthesia even with two-lung ventilation and (2) patients with advanced-stage disease who may not be able to tolerate single-lung ventilation or a full lateral decubitus position. For these later patients, an expedient open-lung biopsy through a minithoracotomy is the best option. As a general principle, lung biopsy is ideally performed during the early stages of ILD because diffuse fibrosis makes both diagnosis and ventilation much more difficult and may even preclude single-lung ventilation and VATS biopsy. The ideal candidate for VATS is an ILD patient who is symptomatic but ambulatory with preserved lung function.

TREATMENT

Treatment options are varied and dependent upon the medical condition of the patient and specific diagnoses suggested clinically and/or included and excluded on histologic analysis. Environmental and drug exposures potentially responsible for the underlying disease are investigated and avoided. Appropriate antimicrobials are started for infectious diseases or superimposed pulmonary infections. However, the mainstay of treatment is directed at suppressing the inflammatory response with immunomodulatory medications, such as corticosteroids. Newer agents, such as pirfenidone, have been developed to modulate and downregulate the fibrosis associated with these inflammatory disorders. A recent randomized clinical trial in patients with idiopathic pulmonary fibrosis demonstrated that pirfenidone resulted in significant clinical benefit for these patients, indicating that this agent will be a mainstay of therapy in the future.[46,47] Gastrointestinal reflux disease has been shown to occur with greater frequency in those with chronic lung disease, particularly idiopathic pulmonary fibrosis.

Consideration of antireflux surgery in this cohort is appropriate, particularly if significant reflux is detected by esophageal pH monitoring and symptom analysis despite being on medical therapy, as it has been suggested that surgery can improve exercise capacity, decrease oxygen requirements and potentially delay disease progression.[48–50] For other appropriate patients with end-stage disease, lung transplantation remains a viable option as described in Chapter 106.

SUMMARY

The thoracic surgeon plays a vital role in the treatment of patients with ILD by safely obtaining the necessary lung tissue to establish a definitive diagnosis, if possible. Although ILD, as a group of over 200 disease entities, is a relatively rare disorder, the symptoms can significantly limit a patient's quality of life, employment options, and future plans, thus warranting a swift and expeditious diagnosis. The number of possible diagnostic entities calls for a thorough understanding of the etiology of ILD and a careful clinical and laboratory evaluation. Although other diagnostic modalities are available, including chest x-ray, CT scan, and bronchoalveolar lavage, lung biopsy preferably done via a VATS approach delivers the most definitive answer in the shortest period of time.

EDITOR'S COMMENT

The group of ILD involves over 200 disease entities that present with overlapping symptomatic and radiographic presentations. Tissue biopsies not only provide positive diagnostic information about the specific disease process, but also negative information that excludes many alternative diagnoses. Even when the histologic findings preclude easy classification, the exclusion of infectious or malignant processes can make a significant clinical contribution and is an underappreciated contribution of surgical biopsies.

—Steven J. Mentzer

References

1. Warren J, Ward P. Immunoglobulin- and complement-mediated immune injury. In: Crystal R, West J, Barnes P, eds. *The Lung: Scientific Foundations.* Philadelphia, PA: Lippincott-Raven; 1977:2411–2419.
2. Paul S, Colson Y. Interstitial lung disease. In: Selke F, Swanson S, Del Nido P, eds. *The Lung: Scientific Foundations.* Philadelphia, PA: Saunders; 2004:151–165.
3. Adams DO. The granulomatous inflammatory response. A review. *Am J Pathol.* 1976;84:164–192.
4. Chan ED, Iseman MD. Current medical treatment for tuberculosis. *Br Med J.* 2002;325:1282–1286.
5. Aberle DR, Gamsu G, Lynch D. Thoracic manifestations of Wegener granulomatosis: diagnosis and course. *Radiology* 1990;174:703–709.
6. Falk RJ, Jennette JC. ANCA small-vessel vasculitis. *J Am Soc Nephrol.* 1997;8:314–322.
7. Faul JL, Kuschner WG. Wegener's granulomatosis and the Churg-Strauss syndrome. *Clin Rev Allergy Immunol.* 2001;21:17–26.
8. Fraser R, Colman N, Muller N, et al. *Goodpasture's Syndrome and Idiopathic Pulmonary Hemorrhage.* Philadelphia, PA: Lippincott-Raven; 1997:1757–1769.
9. Jennette JC, Falk RJ. Small-vessel vasculitis. *N Engl J Med.* 1997;337: 1512–1523.
10. Leavitt RY, Fauci AS. Wegener's granulomatosis. *Curr Opin Rheumatol.* 1991;3:8–14.
11. Bourke S, Dalphin J, Boyd G. Hypersensitivity pneumonitis: current concepts. *Eur Respir J Suppl.* 2001;32:81S–92S.
12. Glazer CS, Rose CS, Lynch DA. Clinical and radiologic manifestations of hypersensitivity pneumonitis. *J Thorac Imaging.* 2002;17:261–272.
13. Moran JV, Greenberger PA, Patterson R. Long-term evaluation of hypersensitivity pneumonitis: a case study follow-up and literature review. *Allergy Asthma Proc.* 2002;23:265–270.
14. Nouh MS. Is the desert lung syndrome (nonoccupational dust pneumoconiosis) a variant of pulmonary alveolar microlithiasis? Report of 4 cases with review of the literature. *Respiration.* 1989;55(2):122–126.
15. Korényi-Both AL, Korényi-Both AL, Molnár AC, et al. Al Eskan disease: Desert Storm pneumonitis. *Mil Med.* 1992;157(9):452–462.
16. Steenland K, Goldsmith DF. Silica exposure and autoimmune diseases. *Am J Ind Med.* 1995;28(5):603–608.
17. Pope-Harman AL, Davis WB, Allen ED, et al. Acute eosinophilic pneumonia: a summary of 15 cases and review of the literature. *Medicine.* 1996;75:334–342.
18. Costabel U, Guzman J. Bronchoalveolar lavage in interstitial lung disease. *Curr Opin Pulm Med.* 2001;7:255–261.
19. Vassallo R, Ryu JH, Schroeder DR, et al. Clinical outcomes of pulmonary Langerhans' cell histiocytosis in adults. *N Engl J Med.* 2002;346:484–490.
20. Ball JA, Young KR Jr. Pulmonary manifestations of Goodpasture's syndrome: antiglomerular basement membrane disease and related disorders. *Clin Chest Med.* 1998;19:777–791.
21. Bolton WK. Goodpasture's syndrome. *Kidney Int.* 1996;50:1753–1766.
22. Fraser R, Colman N. Goodpasture's syndrome and idiopathic pulmonary hemorrhage. In: Fraser RS, Pare RD, eds. *Fraser and Pare's Diagnoses of Diseases of the Chest.* Philadelphia, PA: Saunders; 1999:1757–1769.
23. Martin W. Injury from drugs. In: Crystal R, West J, Barnes P, eds. *The Lung: Scientific Foundations.* Philadelphia, PA: Lippincott-Raven; 1997:2465–2473.
24. ter Heine R, van den Bosch RT, Schaefer-Prokop CM, et al. Fatal interstitial lung disease associated with high erlotinib and metabolite levels. A case report and a review of the literature. *Lung Cancer.* 2012;75(3):391–397.
25. Min JH, Lee HY, Lim H, et al. Drug-induced interstitial lung disease in tyrosine kinase inhibitor therapy for non-small cell lung cancer: a review on current insight. *Cancer Chemother Pharmacol.* 2011;68(5):1099–1109.
26. Fleming MV, Travis WD. Interstitial lung disease. *Pathology (Phila).* 1996; 4:1–21.
27. Hunninghake GW, Zimmerman MB, Schwartz DA, et al. Utility of a lung biopsy for the diagnosis of idiopathic pulmonary fibrosis. *Am J Respir Crit Care Med.* 2001;164:193–196.
28. Katzenstein AL, Myers JL. Idiopathic pulmonary fibrosis: to biopsy or not to biopsy. *Am J Respir Crit Care Med.* 2001;164:185–186.
29. Miller JD, Urschel JD, Cox G, et al. A randomized, controlled trial comparing thoracoscopy and limited thoracotomy for lung biopsy in interstitial lung disease. *Ann Thorac Surg.* 2000;70:1647–1650.
30. Ravini M, Ferraro G, Barbieri B, et al. Changing strategies of lung biopsies in diffuse lung diseases: the impact of video-assisted thoracoscopy. *Eur Respir J.* 1998;11:99–103.
31. Bitterman PB, Rennard SI, Keogh BA, et al. Familial idiopathic pulmonary fibrosis: evidence of lung inflammation in unaffected family members. *N Engl J Med.* 1986;314:1343–1347.
32. Koss MN, Hochholzer L, Langloss JM, et al. Lymphoid interstitial pneumonia: clinicopathological and immunopathological findings in 18 cases. *Pathology.* 1987;19:178–185.
33. Nanki N, Fujita J, Yamaji Y, et al. Nonspecific interstitial pneumonia/fibrosis completely recovered by adding cyclophosphamide to corticosteroids. *Intern Med.* 2002;41:867–870.
34. Dick JA, Morgan WK, Muir DF, et al. The significance of irregular opacities on the chest roentgenogram. *Chest.* 1992;102:251–260.
35. Baughman RP, Drent M. Role of bronchoalveolar lavage in interstitial lung disease. *Clin Chest Med.* 2001;22:331–341.
36. Ayed AK. Video-assisted thoracoscopic lung biopsy in the diagnosis of diffuse interstitial lung disease: a prospective study. *J Cardiovasc Surg (Torino).* 2003;44:115–118.
37. Gaensler EA, Carrington CB. Open biopsy for chronic diffuse infiltrative lung disease: clinical, roentgenographic, and physiological correlations in 502 patients. *Ann Thorac Surg.* 1980;30:411–426.
38. Qureshi RA, Ahmed TA, Grayson AD, et al. Does lung biopsy help patients with interstitial lung disease? *Eur J Cardiothorac Surg.* 2002;21:621–626; discussion 626.

39. Newman SL, Michel RP, Wang NS. Lingular lung biopsy: is it representative? *Am Rev Respir Dis.* 1985;132:1084–1086.
40. Miller RR, Nelems B, Muller NL, et al. Lingular and right middle lobe biopsy in the assessment of diffuse lung disease. *Ann Thorac Surg.* 1987;44:269–273.
41. Wetstein L. Sensitivity and specificity of lingular segmental biopsies of the lung. *Chest.* 1986;90:383–386.
42. Blewett CJ, Bennett WF, Miller JD, et al. Open lung biopsy as an outpatient procedure. *Ann Thorac Surg.* 2001;71:1113–1115.
43. Green FH. Overview of pulmonary fibrosis. *Chest.* 2002;122:334S–339S.
44. Rena O, Casadio C, Leo F, et al. Videothoracoscopic lung biopsy in the diagnosis of interstitial lung disease. *Eur J Cardiothorac Surg.* 1999;16:624–627.
45. Kadokura M, Colby TV, Myers JL, et al. Pathologic comparison of video-assisted thoracic surgical lung biopsy with traditional open lung biopsy. *J Thorac Cardiovasc Surg.* 1995;109:494–498.
46. Noble PW, Albera C, Bradford WZ, et al. Pirfenidone in patients with idiopathic pulmonary fibrosis (CAPACITY): two randomized trials. *Lancet.* 2011;377(9779):1760–1769.
47. Bouros D. Pirfenidone for idiopathic pulmonary fibrosis. *Lancet.* 2011; 377(9779):1727–1729.
48. Pashinsky YY, Jaffin BW, Litle VR. Gastroesophageal reflux disease and idiopathic pulmonary fibrosis. *Mt Sinai J Med.* 2009;76(1):24–29.
49. Fahim A, Crooks M, Hart SP. Gastroesophageal reflux and idiopathic pulmonary fibrosis: a review. *Pulm Med.* 2011;2011:634613.
50. Linden PA, Gilbert RJ, Yeap BY, et al. Laparoscopic fundoplication in patients with end-stage lung disease awaiting transplantation. *J Thorac Cardiovasc Surg.* 2006;131(2):438–446.

105 Adjuvant Surgery for Tuberculosis

Daniel M. Cohen and Ciaran J. McNamee

Keywords: Pulmonary tuberculous diseases, hemoptysis, endobronchial tuberculosis, cavernoma, multidrug-resistant tubercle bacilli

INTRODUCTION

Pulmonary tuberculous diseases are contagious infections caused by bacterial organisms or bacilli of the Mycobacterium family (Mycobacteriaceae). The most common species is tuberculosis but other types produce similar pathologic changes. The disease is spread by the aerolization of respiratory secretions, and infection occurs by inhalation of the tubercle bacilli (TB). Not everyone infected with TB will become sick immediately. Most patients are asymptomatic because of the host's immune-cell-mediated defense mechanisms, which entrap and wall off the bacilli, thereby containing the infection. The isolated bacilli may form granulomas which may lie dormant for years. Others will experience a short illness associated with malaise, low-grade fever, cough, and weight loss. If the body's immunity becomes compromised, a full-blown infection may ensue. Most frequently, these patients will develop extensive pulmonary infiltrates with a febrile illness and dyspnea associated with the concomitant pneumonia. If the walled-off granulomas break down, cavities form and accumulate secretions causing a productive cough. Infection of the pleural lining (pleurisy) may result in chest wall pain or pleural effusions with shortness of breath. Spontaneous pneumothorax may occur as a consequence of excessive coughing and will present with acute dyspnea. Long-standing infections may result in parenchymal destruction, bronchiectasis with erosion into adjacent pulmonary arteries (Rasmussen's aneurysm)[1], and massive hemoptysis.[2] These large cavities may lead to secondary fungal infection with *Aspergillus* (see Chapter 102). In some patients, extensive lung destruction can produce chronic lung collapse and contraction.

INCIDENCE

The World Health Organization estimates that one-third of the world's population is currently infected with TB bacillus and 5% to 10% of those infected become infectious or sick at some stage during their lifetime. Individuals with HIV/AIDS are most at risk for developing the full-blown infection. The largest number of new cases of TB in 2010 occurred in southeast Asia (35%); however, the incidence of new cases in sub-Saharan Africa is nearly twice that of southeast Asia with 350 cases per 100,000 people. In 2009, over 1.7 million individuals died from TB. Although the incidence of TB appears to be stable or falling, adjusted for population growth, the number of new cases is rising annually (Table 105-1).[3]

MEDICAL TREATMENT

The US Food and Drug Administration currently approves 10 drugs for the treatment of TB. Of these, the core first-line treatment for active TB includes isoniazid, rifampin, ethambutol, and pyrazinamide. Regimens have an initial treatment phase of 2 months, followed by a continuation phase of 4 to 7 months. Treatment completion is determined by the number of doses ingested over a given period of time. Modifications to this basic regimen are made under special circumstances including HIV infection, drug resistance, pregnancy, and in pediatric patients.[4]

SURGICAL TREATMENT

The surgical treatment of TB is reserved mainly for treating the complications of the disease arising from previous surgical

Table 105-1

ESTIMATED TB INCIDENCE, PREVALENCE, AND MORTALITY, 2009

	INCIDENCE[a]			PREVALENCE[b]		MORTALITY (EXCLUDING HIV)	
WHO REGION	NO. IN THOUSANDS	% OF GLOBAL TOTAL	RATE PER 100,000 POP[c]	NO. IN THOUSANDS	RATE PER 100,000 POP[c]	NO. IN THOUSANDS	RATE PER 100,000 POP[c]
Africa	2800	30	340	3900	450	430	50
The Americas	270	2.9	29	350	37	20	2.1
Eastern Mediterranean	660	7.1	110	1000	180	99	18
Europe	420	4.5	47	560	63	62	7
Southeast Asia	3300	35	180	4900	280	480	27
Western Pacific	1900	21	110	2900	160	240	13
Global total	9400	100	140	14,000	164	1300	19

[a]Incidence is the number of new cases arising during a defined period.

[b]Prevalence is the number of cases (new and previously occurring) that exists at a given point in time.

[c]Pop indicates population.

treatment or progression of the underlying disease and secondary complications of chronic infection. Occasionally, the diagnosis of TB is an incidental pathologic finding after resection of a pulmonary nodule or mediastinal lymphadenopathy. The surgical treatment of chronic constrictive pericarditis or pleural effusions with or without lung entrapment also may reveal unexpected TB. Strains of multidrug-resistant (MDR) TB have been documented with resistance to all first-line drugs and multiple second-line drugs for which adjuvant surgery may be considered.[5] The remainder of this chapter focuses on surgical treatment specific to the complications of previous operations or secondary complications of chronic infection that necessitate surgical intervention.

Thoracoplasty

Toward the end of the nineteenth century, it was thought that healing of tuberculous cavities would be facilitated by collapse of the lung and thoracoplasty. It was hoped that this operation would promote scar retraction of the tuberculous cavities and subsequent healing. Schede thoracoplasty was widely practiced up to the late 1930s. The thoracoplasty operation is covered in Chapter 106.

The operation, as originally described, became obsolete with the advent of pulmonary resections and drug therapy in the 1940s. In this operation, the infection is controlled by tube thoracostomy drainage or a Clagett window as an initial procedure. Subsequently, the residual space is obliterated by filling the cavity with antibiotics and closing the window or leaving the patient with a permanent window.

In recent years, closure of a residual space or bronchopleural fistula, if present, is accomplished by the interposition of various types of muscle flaps or an omentoplasty.[6] Still, there are some surgeons who continue to perform a limited thoracoplasty with intrathoracic muscle transposition.[7,8] Other investigators have performed a cavernostomy combined with a muscle flap transposition as a single-stage procedure.[9] The overall success rate for the control of infection and obliteration of space issues is about 75% for TB.[10]

Plombage Therapy and its Late Complications

In 1926, Tuffier described a procedure called apicolysis whereby a space was created using an extrapleural or extrafascial dissection and the space was filled with the patient's own fatty tissue. This operation formed the basis of extrapleural plombage collapse therapy, whereby the space was filled with heated paraffin or Lucite balls. Plombage therapy fell out of favor because of long-term complications. These have included infections, migration of these balls with erosion through the chest wall possibly into adjacent lung parenchyma, vascular structures or organs like the esophagus, and compression of the brachial plexus. Plombage therapy has been completely abandoned as a treatment of residual pleural spaces and removal of the foreign material is recommended whenever such patients are identified, as long as the operative risk is acceptable.[11,12] Subsequently, the space is handled by transposition of muscle flaps with or without a limited thoracoplasty.

Lung Destruction, Extensive Bronchiectasis, Residual Disease

Unilateral partial or complete lung destruction is a well-recognized complication of chronic tuberculous lung infection. It is rarely seen in the developed world today but may still be encountered in patients from less developed countries. Usually, it is a consequence of failure of diagnosis, poor compliance, or inadequate medical therapy for primary tuberculosis. It is characterized by extensive scarring with fibrosis and contraction of the underlying lung. The underlying parenchyma is destroyed with multiple cavitations and extensive bronchiectasis. These patients present with general debilitation, productive cough, shortness of breath, and may have massive hemoptysis. The left side is more frequently involved.

Lobectomy or pneumonectomy should be considered when the underlying lung is destroyed, but these are high-risk operations and patients need to be started on adequate antituberculous therapy prior to undertaking surgical resection. Adequate preoperative preparation including nutritional support also must be provided. Careful intraoperative planning and technical expertise is essential. These patients are at high risk for developing a bronchopleural fistula, and satisfactory coverage of the bronchial stump with a muscle flap is imperative. A space issue following resection may necessitate the use of rotational muscle flaps with or without a limited thoracoplasty. Occasionally, the obliteration of the pleural space with extensive scarring and contraction will render an anatomic lobectomy or intrapleural pneumonectomy technically very challenging and high risk. In such circumstances, an extrapleural pneumonectomy should be considered.[13]

A retrospective review of 172 cases of destroyed lung was analyzed by Bai et al.[14] The ages ranged from 7 to 72 years with a median of 38.4 years. The male-to-female ratio was roughly equal. Forty-nine patients had sputum positive for *Mycobacterium tuberculosis* preoperatively yielding a positive TB rate of 28.5%. Of the group, 116 cases had destroyed left and 56 had destroyed right lungs. In all, 110 patients underwent a complete pneumonectomy, 37 an extrapleural pneumonectomy, and 11 lobectomy. Eleven patients developed bronchopleural fistulae and four had subsequent thoracoplasties because of persistent infection or empyema. The overall perioperative mortality rate was 2.9% with an 18.6% complication rate. The sputum negative conversion rate was 87.8% and clinical cure 91.9%.[14]

Drug-Resistant and Other Forms of TB

Although chemotherapy is considered the first-line treatment for pulmonary TB, surgery should be entertained for MDR disease as demonstrated in the Case Report. Usually, these patients have persistent positive sputum with extensive parenchymal disease in the face of appropriate drug therapy over a 3-month period.[15] Operations have included segmentectomy, lobectomy, and pneumonectomy. The complications have included bronchopleural fistulae, especially with right pneumonectomy, and postoperative empyema.[16] Adjuvant therapy is continued for 18 to 24 months after surgery and the mortality has ranged from 0% to 4.3% with a cure rate of 94% to 100%.[17,18] Nontuberculous pulmonary mycobacterial disease, especially *Mycobacterium avium* complex, is encountered more frequently. The introduction of macrolide-containing regimens has improved the outcomes but resistance remains a problem and pulmonary resection during the early stage of the disease should be considered for those patients who are good surgical candidates.[19]

Pleural Disease

Pleural effusions secondary to TB may be seen in young adults with an immunocompromised condition like HIV/AIDS and is associated with 5% of *M. tuberculosis* infections. The diagnosis of TB depends on the demonstration of acid-fast bacilli (AFB) in the sputum, pleural fluid, or pleural biopsy specimens; biochemistry of the fluid (pH <7.2, adenosine deaminase); and PCR testing.[20] For a simple unilocular effusion, tube thoracostomy and antituberculous chemotherapy is all that is necessary. Patients with complex parapneumonic effusions may benefit from the addition of intrapleural fibrinolytics and possibly surgical intervention.[21] True tuberculous empyema is a more chronic condition and is suspected on CT scan findings of a thick, calcified pleural rind associated with loculated pleural fluid positive for acid-fast bacilli. Surgical intervention with decortication to reexpand the entrapped lung and drainage followed by antituberculous chemotherapy is warranted. These operations may be very difficult to perform and often are complicated by bronchopleural fistulae or chronic drainage.[22] The role of steroids for pleural tuberculosis remains controversial.[23]

Hemoptysis

Hemoptysis secondary to pulmonary tuberculosis can be catastrophic and is a common cause of morbidity and occasional mortality. Most often, bleeding occurs because of the bronchial collaterals that feed the infected cavities. Sometimes, pulmonary vessels may become incorporated into the walls of these cavities leading to small dilations (Rasmussen's aneurysms), which may erode. Rarely, bleeding occurs secondary to necrosis of small pulmonary veins or ulcerations of the bronchial mucosa. The management of hemoptysis secondary to tuberculosis does not differ from that described in Chapter 82, *Hemoptysis and Lung Cancer.* Bleeding may be classified as mild (<200 mL/day), moderate (200–400 mL/day), or severe (>600 mL/day). In a study of 59 patients with tuberculosis-related hemoptysis, thoracotomy was performed urgently in 21 with massive bleeding, within 2 days in 22 of 24 with moderate bleeding, and within 4 days in 14 with mild bleeding. Cavitary lesions were demonstrated in all patients with massive bleeding, 22 with moderate bleeding, and 3 with mild persistent bleeding. Four patients had a pneumonectomy, 39 a lobectomy, and 16 a segmentectomy or wedge resection. The overall mortality was 6.8% Three patients developed empyema or bronchopleural fistulae.[24] Others have recommended early surgical resection of persistent tuberculous cavities to avoid life-threatening hemoptysis.[25]

Cavernoma

The presence of cavities in the setting of tuberculosis is thought to be a post primary phenomenon secondary to endobronchial obstruction. It is a rare occurrence today but was often seen in the era prior to the introduction of antibiotics. Cavities begin as an exudative process as a result of obstructive pneumonia and caseating necrosis. Tissue breakdown leads to the formation of cavities.[26] These cavities may be seen in patients who are immunocompromised or who have concomitant tumor. The walls of the cavities are made up of scar in which Rasmussen's aneurysms may form.[1] These cavities may be a site for reactivation and are associated with bleeding or aspergilloma formation. Therefore, surgical intervention is recommended. The operation will depend on the degree of debilitation and may involve resection or cavernostomy with intrathoracic muscle flap transfer. Rarely, a thoracoplasty is used to treat these patients. These operations are high risk and may be associated with cavity reformation, bronchopleural fistulae, and bleeding. The success or failure of the operation is associated with the cavity size, number of bronchopleural fistulae, and drug resistance.[9]

Lung Cancer

Increased risk of developing a lung cancer in a patient with primary tuberculosis has long been suspected. In a population-based cohort study, the incidence of lung cancer was significantly higher in pulmonary tuberculosis patients compared with controls (269 of 100,000 person-years vs. 153 of 100,000 person-years).[27] Another study has demonstrated an 11-fold increase in lung cancer in patients with tuberculosis.[28] More recently, an association has been shown between tumor epidermal growth factor receptor (EGFR) mutation and pulmonary TB in patients with adenocarcinoma of the lungs.[29] Tuberculosis may result in scar formation, and the development of carcinomas is well known. Also, the development of lung cancer in this setting may result from debilitation and the overall immunocompromised state of the patient. Recently, vigilance in patients with a history of tuberculosis has been recommended.

Endobronchial Tuberculosis and Bronchial Obstruction

Endobronchial tuberculosis is defined as an infection of the tracheobronchial tree. It is seen in 10% to 40% of patients with active tuberculosis.[30] It is associated with cough, sputum production, wheezing, dyspnea, and hemoptysis. It may be difficult to diagnose because it is not obvious on chest x-ray. Bronchoscopic sampling is the key to diagnosis. Early treatment of this condition is nonsurgical and involves the eradication of the tubercle bacillus with antibiotics.[31] If this condition goes unrecognized, it can lead to bronchial stenosis which, in the early phase, can be treated with steroids, but further delay results in scarring. How this is managed depends on the extent of the resultant deformity and may involve an endobronchial intervention such as stenting, laser therapy, or surgical intervention with bronchoplastic procedures.[32]

Tracheoesophageal or Bronchioesophageal Fistula

Rarely, tuberculosis can cause erosion of an infected mediastinal lymph node, the airway, or esophagus. Usually these complications can be managed with endobronchial interventions, such as stenting, and antituberculous drugs. More complex lesions may require surgical intervention, which would include closure of the esophageal defect, resection of the involved airway, and tissue interposition.[33]

CASE REPORT

A case of transcontinental spread of MDR *Mycobacterium bovis* in Canada was successfully treated with a combined medical–surgical approach.[5]

A 49-year-old white female from Alberta, Canada traveled to Spain in the spring of 1996 to care for a terminally ill relative with acquired immunodeficiency syndrome (AIDS) complicated by TB. Her visit lasted about 5 weeks, whereupon she returned to Canada. About a year and a half later, in November of 1997, she developed a cough for which she sought medical treatment. The physical exam revealed a healthy-appearing woman with

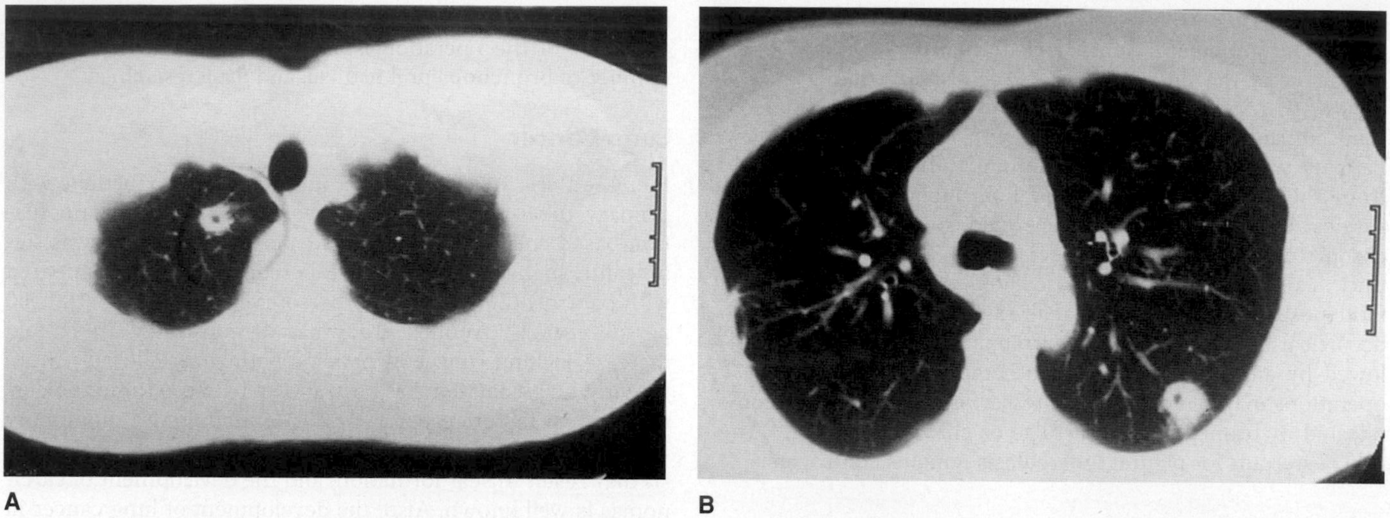

Figure 105-1. This CT scan demonstrates two large nodules, each with a central cavitation (*A*) one in the apical segment of the right upper lobe and (*B*) one in the superior segment of the left lower lobe. Reproduced with permission from Long R, Nobert E, Chomyc S, et al. Transcontinental spread of multidrug-resistant Mycobacterium bovis. *Am J Respir Crit Care Med.* 1999;159:2014–2017.

no predisposing factors for TB, other than the immunocompromising condition of noninsulin-dependent diabetes. HIV serology was negative and CD4 lymphocyte count was normal (1.0×10^9/L). The history was negative for travel other than the previously described visit to Spain. A plain chest x-ray revealed a number of well-defined nodules bilaterally, primarily in the upper lung zones. Chest CT confirmed the presence of at least seven widely distributed nodular lesions, two of which had small central areas of cavitation (Figs. 105-1A,B and 105-2). Nonetheless, direct microscopy of sputum was negative for acid-fast bacilli (AFB). PPD, which had been performed 3 months before and 3 months after travel, and again on presentation in November, was negative. Thoracoscopic biopsy of the right-sided lesions demonstrated caseating granulomas on histopathology. Subsequent tissue and sputum cultures were positive for *M. tuberculosis* on DNA probe (Gen-Probe Accuprobe).

The patient was placed in respiratory isolation and started on standard antituberculous drug therapy consisting of isoniazid 300 mg, rifampin 600 mg, pyrazinamide 1500 mg, and ethambutol 1200 mg together with vitamin B6, 25 mg once daily. Subsequent microbiological study revealed the organism to be *M. bovis.* Drug susceptibility testing indicated resistance to all first-line drugs (*M. bovis* is characteristically resistant to pyrazinamide). Of the 26 available second-line drugs, the isolate was resistant to all except cycloserine and clofazimine.

The patient spent 5 months in respiratory isolation (November 1997–April 1998) where multiple sputa ($n = 12$) were culture-positive for the same isolate. However, all remained negative for AFB on direct microscopy. Repeat CT scan in January revealed two persistent cavitations with localized disease, perhaps accounting for the AFB negativity, that had clearly progressed, albeit slowly, over the past 3 months. Standard therapy was discontinued in February after the second-line susceptibility testing became available, and the patient was started on a new regimen consisting of cycloserine 500 mg twice daily, clofazimine 300 mg once daily, and trimethoprim-sulfamethoxazole, two single strength tablets twice daily.

Given the strength of the patient's resistance to first-line chemotherapy, the relatively weak second-line regimen, and the urgent need to prevent spread of this organism in the community, bilateral wedge resection for organism eradication was planned in two staged procedures, while drug therapy was continued. The surgery was performed under (level 4 biosafety precautions) to prevent nosocomial spread of infection. In mid-March 1998 and mid-April 1998, the left and right thoracotomies were performed, respectively, and all visible disease was resected. Prior to thoracotomy, bronchoscopy was performed to remove secretions. AFB were present on smear and *M. bovis* was cultured from the right apical and left superior segmental lesions, as well as from the right lower lobe lesion. The strain was eventually found to be identical to the strain isolated from the patient's relative in Spain and identical to the *M. bovis* strain documented in multiple HIV-seropositive patients in Spain (Fig. 105-2).

After a 4-month hospitalization, the patient was discharged in May 1998 under direct observation therapy. All sputa collected after the second thoracotomy remained negative for AFB on smear and culture and no new lesions were demonstrable on CT follow-up 1 year later.

None of the patient's 80 known contacts in Canada developed or tested positive for TB at 1 year follow-up. Although sputum-smear-negative cases of pulmonary TB are not likely to infect others, the identification of this MDR strain of *M. bovis* was unprecedented in Canada, and presumably the

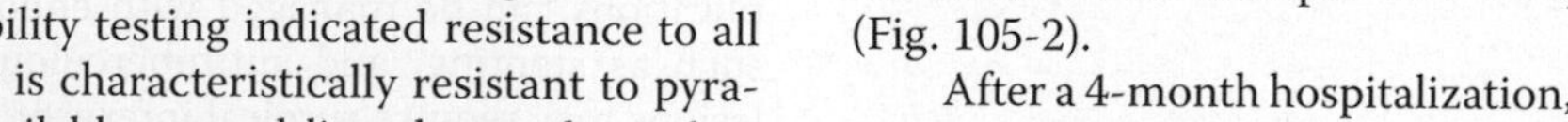

Figure 105-2. Spoligotype of the multidrug-resistant strain *M. bovis* isolated from this patient (*A*) juxtaposed to the outbreak strain isolated from several patients, including the patient's relative in Spain (*B*). Reproduced with permission from Long R, Nobert E, Chomyc S, et al. Transcontinental spread of multidrug-resistant Mycobacterium bovis. *Am J Respir Crit Care Med.* 1999;159:2014–2017.

United States, prompting a conservative approach *with* surgical intervention. In the modern era, pulmonary infections with bacterial organisms or bacilli of the Mycobacterium family are usually amenable to medical treatment with first-line antimycobacterial drugs. The most common species is tuberculosis but other strains produce similar pathologic changes. In strains that involve multiple drug resistance to first and/or second-line agents, surgery is a recognized treatment option, after 3 months of antituberculous drugs.

CONCLUSION

A third of the world's population is currently infected with TB. Individuals with a normal immune system can generally ward off infection by segregating the bacilli, which then lie dormant for the patient's lifetime. Of the approximately 10% to 15% that develop full-blown infection, patients with HIV/AIDS or other conditions that compromise the immune system are most susceptible. Although chemotherapy remains the first-line of therapy, surgery has a role in treating the complications of disease such as those caused by previous surgery (e.g., bronchopleural fistulae), disease progression (e.g., bronchial obstruction), or the secondary complications of a chronic infection (e.g., empyema). Operations may range from simple tube thoracostomy to segmentectomy, lobectomy, or pneumonectomy. Surgeons must be vigilant for exposure to bacilli of the Mycobacterium family during any surgical procedure. For example, TB may be an incidental finding on pathology after resection of a pulmonary nodule or mediastinal lymphadenopathy. TB also may be encountered when treating patients for pleural effusions. Given the urgency of preventing the spread of this infectious disease to the community, adjuvant surgery has an occasional role in patients with MDR TB, after first- and second-line antituberculous therapies have failed.

EDITOR'S COMMENT

Surgical therapy for tuberculosis infections of the lung is primarily for complications of the disease such as hemoptysis, bronchopleural fistula, chronic infections due to resistant organisms or failure of antibiotic therapy to control the disease.

—Editor's Name

References

1. van den Heuvel MM, van Rensburg JJ. Images in clinical medicine. Rasmussen's aneurysm. *N Engl J Med.* 2006;355:e17.
2. Shih SY, Tsai IC, Chang YT, et al. Fatal haemoptysis caused by a ruptured Rasmussen's aneurysm. *Thorax.* 2011;66:553–554.
3. WHO. http://www.who.int/mediacentre/factsheets/fs104/en/
4. CDC. http://wwwcdcgov/tb/?404;http://wwwcdcgov:80/tb/topic/treatment/defauthtm 2013.
5. Long R, Nobert E, Chomyc S, et al. Transcontinental spread of multidrug-resistant *Mycobacterium bovis. Am J Respir Crit Care Med.* 1999;159: 2014–2017.
6. Kitano M. Omentoplasty in thoracic surgery. *Gen Thorac Cardiovasc Surg.* 2008;56:483–489.
7. Botianu PV, Botianu AM, Bacarea V, et al. Thoracodorsal versus reversed mobilisation of the latissimus dorsi muscle for intrathoracic transposition. *Eur J Cardiothorac Surg.* 2010;38:461–465.
8. Krassas A, Grima R, Bagan P, et al. Current indications and results for thoracoplasty and intrathoracic muscle transposition. *Eur J Cardiothorac Surg.* 2010;37:1215–1220.
9. Tseng YL, Wu MH, Lin MY, et al. Intrathoracic muscle flap transposition in the treatment of fibrocavernous tuberculosis. *Eur J Cardiothorac Surg.* 2000;18:666–670.
10. Barker WL. Thoracoplasty. *Chest Surg Clin N Am.* 1994;4:593–615.
11. Massard G, Thomas P, Barsotti P, et al. Long-term complications of extraperiosteal plombage. *Ann Thorac Surg.* 1997;64:220–224; discussion 224–225.
12. Horowitz MD, Otero M, Thurer RJ, et al. Late complications of plombage. *Ann Thorac Surg.* 1992;53:803–806.
13. Brown J, Pomerantz M. Extrapleural pneumonectomy for tuberculosis. *Chest Surg Clin N Am.* 1995;5:289–296.
14. Bai L, Hong Z, Gong C, et al. Surgical treatment efficacy in 172 cases of tuberculosis-destroyed lungs. *Eur J Cardiothorac Surg.* 2012;41:335–340.
15. Pomerantz M, Madsen L, Goble M, et al. Surgical management of resistant mycobacterial tuberculosis and other mycobacterial pulmonary infections. *Ann Thorac Surg.* 1991;52:1108–1111; discussion 1112.
16. Shiraishi Y, Fukushima K, Komatsu H, et al. Early pulmonary resection for localized *Mycobacterium avium* complex disease. *Ann Thorac Surg.* 1998;66:183–186.
17. Mohsen T, Zeid AA, Haj-Yahia S. Lobectomy or pneumonectomy for multidrug-resistant pulmonary tuberculosis can be performed with acceptable morbidity and mortality: a seven-year review of a single institution's experience. *J Thorac Cardiovasc Surg.* 2007;134:194–198.
18. Shiraishi Y. [Surgical treatment of *Mycobacterium avium* complex lung disease]. *Nihon Rinsho.* 2011;69:1458–1461.
19. Shiraishi Y, Nakajima Y, Katsuragi N, et al. Resectional surgery combined with chemotherapy remains the treatment of choice for multidrug-resistant tuberculosis. *J Thorac Cardiovasc Surg.* 2004;128:523 528.
20. Gopi A, Madhavan SM, Sharma SK, et al. Diagnosis and treatment of tuberculous pleural effusion in 2006. *Chest.* 2007;131:880–889.
21. Chapman SJ, Davies RJ. The management of pleural space infections. *Respirology.* 2004;9:4–11.
22. Sahn SA, Iseman MD. Tuberculous empyema. *Semin Respir Infect.* 1999; 14:82–87.
23. Chakrabarti B, Davies PD. Pleural tuberculosis. *Monaldi Arch Chest Dis.* 2006;65:26–33.
24. Erdogan A, Yegin A, Gurses G, et al. Surgical management of tuberculosis-related hemoptysis. *Ann Thorac Surg.* 2005;79:299–302.
25. Brik A, Salem AM, Shoukry A, et al. Surgery for hemoptysis in various pulmonary tuberculous lesions: a prospective study. *Interact Cardiovasc Thorac Surg.* 2011;13:276–279.
26. Hunter RL. On the pathogenesis of post primary tuberculosis: the role of bronchial obstruction in the pathogenesis of cavities. *Tuberculosis (Edinb).* 2011;91(suppl 1):S6–S10.
27. Wu CY, Hu HY, Pu CY, et al. Pulmonary tuberculosis increases the risk of lung cancer: a population-based cohort study. *Cancer.* 2011;117:618–624.
28. Yu YH, Liao CC, Hsu WH, et al. Increased lung cancer risk among patients with pulmonary tuberculosis: a population cohort study. *J Thorac Oncol.* 2011;6:32–37.
29. Luo YH, Wu CH, Wu WS, et al. Association between tumor epidermal growth factor receptor mutation and pulmonary tuberculosis in patients with adenocarcinoma of the lungs. *J Thorac Oncol.* 2012;7:299–305.
30. Kashyap S, Mohapatra PR, Saini V. Endobronchial tuberculosis. *Indian J Chest Dis Allied Sci.* 2003;45:247–256.
31. Um SW, Yoon YS, Lee SM, et al. Predictors of persistent airway stenosis in patients with endobronchial tuberculosis. *Int J Tuberc Lung Dis.* 2008;12:57–62.
32. Rikimaru T. Endobronchial tuberculosis. *Expert Rev Anti Infect Ther.* 2004; 2:245–251.
33. Shen KR, Allen MS, Cassivi SD, et al. Surgical management of acquired nonmalignant tracheoesophageal and bronchoesophageal fistulae. *Ann Thorac Surg.* 2010;90:914–918; discussion 919.

106 Thoracoplasty for Tuberculosis

William A. Cook

Keywords: Empyema, pulmonary cavitary disease, bronchopleural fistula, fungal infection, multiple antituberculous drug resistance, HIV

The specialty of thoracic surgery was born in the convergence of two worldwide plagues. These were tuberculosis, as old as humankind, and avian influenza, which struck a war-wearied world in the winter of 1917 and killed more people than the bubonic plagues of the Middle Ages. Today, with tuberculosis becoming resistant to antituberculous drugs, avian flu beginning to appear around the world, and the world weakened again by war and the new pestilence of AIDS, it seems entirely possible that thoracoplasty may become the once and future operation.

First coming to prominence in Europe in the late nineteenth century for the treatment of chronic infections in the chest with complicating space problems and bronchopleural fistulas, thoracoplasty began to receive greater attention in the United States at the time of the 1917 to 1918 influenza epidemic. The most lethal complication was empyema thoracis. The mortality in some of the 29 army camps surveyed was as high as 70%.[1] A pneumonia commission and subsequently an empyema commission were appointed to study the problem in the clinic and the laboratory. In the amazing period of 1 year, through the efforts of these two commissions, mortality was reduced to an average of 4.3%.[2] As reported by Graham in his insightful book, *Empyema Thoracis,* two early examples of productive research delineated the adverse effects of open pneumothorax on ventilation and the differing pathology between complicating infection with *Streptococcus hemolyticus* or Pneumococcus,[3] the former being much more common. Associated with this pleural disease were a large number of patients with complicating space problems and bronchopleural fistula.

At about the same time, the other impetus for thoracoplasty was developing in the treatment of tuberculous residua when it was recognized that healing could be accelerated by collapse of residual cavities. Many techniques were employed for this, including pneumothorax, pneumoperitoneum, and even the very first videothoracoscopy, which was used to release apical adhesions.[4] Not infrequently, these patients developed infected spaces requiring thoracoplastic procedures, and it was a short step from thoracoplasty for complicating spaces to thoracoplasty as the primary procedure. Enthusiasm for this procedure as an alternative to prolonged, sometimes lifelong commitment to a sanitorium can be imagined from a story told to me by a Greek colleague whose mother had an eleventh rib thoracoplasty performed in three stages by Professor Sauerbruck before World War II using local anesthesia!

The most enthusiastic American proponent of thoracoplasty was John Alexander[5] of the University of Michigan, who applied and evaluated the procedure in a large group of patients. A contemporary tale from this period was shared with me by one of his residents, who, along with this fellow trainee, noted that, paradoxically, the application of thoracoplasty to nontuberculous pulmonary cavities was associated with an increased mortality, a concept he only reluctantly accepted.

Thoracoplasty can be considered in four broad categories:

1. Thoracoplasty with a closed pleural space.
2. Thoracoplasty with open pleural drainage.
3. Thoracoplasty with transposition of a muscle flap into the space either to fill the space or to close a bronchopleural fistula or both.
4. Thoracoplasty done as a preliminary to avoid postresectional space problems.

Contemplation of thoracoplasty in the modern age implies a failure of medical therapy. An open negative cavity or resistant organism with unilateral or bilateral cavitary disease, bilateral disease so extensive that resection is not feasible, and tailoring thoracoplasty to avoid space problems after resection are the probable indications. In these patients, all the precautions observed in the great age of thoracoplasty still apply. First, timing and judgment are more important than the surgery, and thorough understanding of the natural history and pathophysiology of tuberculosis is required for this judgment.[6] This begins with the therapeutic value of rest, fresh air, a high-calorie diet, and patience. Time is on the side of the physician. Between 6 and 12 weeks of preoperative antituberculous medical therapy is favored.

As with any thoracic procedures, the patient should be evaluated for cardiac and pulmonary functions and, if marginal, further assessed with differential $\dot{V}/\dot{Q}$ studies or a $\dot{V}o_{2,max}$ study to see if the intended procedure can be tolerated. Many of these patients will have had bilateral pulmonary disease and, in some cases, prior surgery. An important part of the preoperative care is the bacteriologic analysis and treatment. Many patients are now manifesting resistance to multiple antituberculous drugs, and close collaboration with infectious disease colleagues is mandatory. Another problem here is infection with atypical tuberculosis, especially in patients with HIV infection or otherwise compromised immunity. The presence of cavitary disease in the lung, even if acid-fast bacilli-negative, leads to frequent invasion of the cavity by fungal organisms, the most frequent being *Aspergillus fumigatus.* These organisms or tuberculosis itself can lead to development of mycotic aneurysms in the cavity wall. The rupture of such aneurysms can create one of the true catastrophes in thoracic surgery with massive pulmonary hemorrhage. This possibility alone is reason for an aggressive approach to pulmonary cavitary disease. Finally, in this spectrum are bacterial mixed infections that may have led to bronchopleural fistula or empyema as the presenting problem. Again, the emergence of drug resistance is an ongoing problem. All these areas of consideration are made infinitely more difficult in the presence of infection and HIV infection.

Tuberculosis is best considered as a systemic disease, but when it presents in the lung, it begins as an exudative pneumonia favoring upper and posterior portions. It either goes on to resolution or to destruction of lung tissue with formation of scar or loss of vascular supply with resulting caseating necrosis. It is these foci that persist or excavate and may require surgical attention. Since the inception of antibiotic therapy, there has been a greater tendency to reepithelialization of the bronchocavitary junction with less air trapping. The cavity wall, surrounding parenchymal reaction, and pleural reaction are all less. This pleural reaction is very important because it is usually very vascular, and the adhesions formed are part of the body's attempt to prevent bronchopleural fistula.[7] For this reason, mobilization should be done in the extraperiosteal plane unless resection is contemplated both to avoid bronchopleural fistula and because the systemic vessels are difficult to control and can cause massive operative blood loss. Another suggestion that pertains to adhesions is that although during the period of pneumothorax therapy it was always felt necessary to release apical adhesions when thoracoplasty was anticipated, it is best to preserve them. Dividing them lets the lung fall lower in the chest, thereby requiring resection of more ribs to obtain complete collapse.[5] Before surgery, it is best to decide how many ribs will need resection and what the often compromised patient can tolerate. It may be necessary to stage the resections to reduce morbidity.

TECHNIQUE

Thoracoplasty with Closed Pleural Space

The patient is best positioned in a lateral position, leaning slightly forward. There was some enthusiasm for operation in the prone position previously. Work that my team did on our service at the Albert Einstein College of Medicine in New York City demonstrated that this position, even in healthy volunteers, leads to an average reduction of cardiac output and blood pressure of approximately 25%, and we abandoned it. Use of a double-lumen endotracheal tube will lessen the secretions reaching the dependent lung. However, if the patient is being operated on for pulmonary hemorrhage, I prefer a large-diameter single-lumen tube, which allows for better removal of blood clots. In either case, it is highly advisable to do a bronchoscopic lavage at the end of surgery.

The incision should extend from the spine of the scapula down around its tip and anterior to the anterior axillary line (Fig. 106-1). After division of the trapezius, rhomboids, latissimus dorsi, and serratus anterior muscles, the scapula is elevated. This can be facilitated by placing one blade of a rib retractor on the point of the scapula and one on the chest wall and opening it to its greatest extent. This gives very good exposure of the upper ribs and frees the assistant for more productive activity.

Once the rib cage is exposed, it is necessary to divide the attachments of the serratus posterior, posterior and middle scalenus, serratus anterior, and pectoralis minor muscles to those ribs to be resected (Fig. 106-2). This is required for good collapse to occur. The periosteum is incised on the external surface of the ribs and stripped from them. This must be carried posteriorly to the costovertebral joint for total removal. Division of the costotransverse ligament facilitates this and removal of the transverse process, which is equally important if a posterior gutter is not to be left with incomplete collapse of the lung (Fig. 106-3).

At this point, a decision must be made about the ribs themselves. They may be resected, which often leads to late orthopedic and cosmetic changes.[8] They may be left in place,

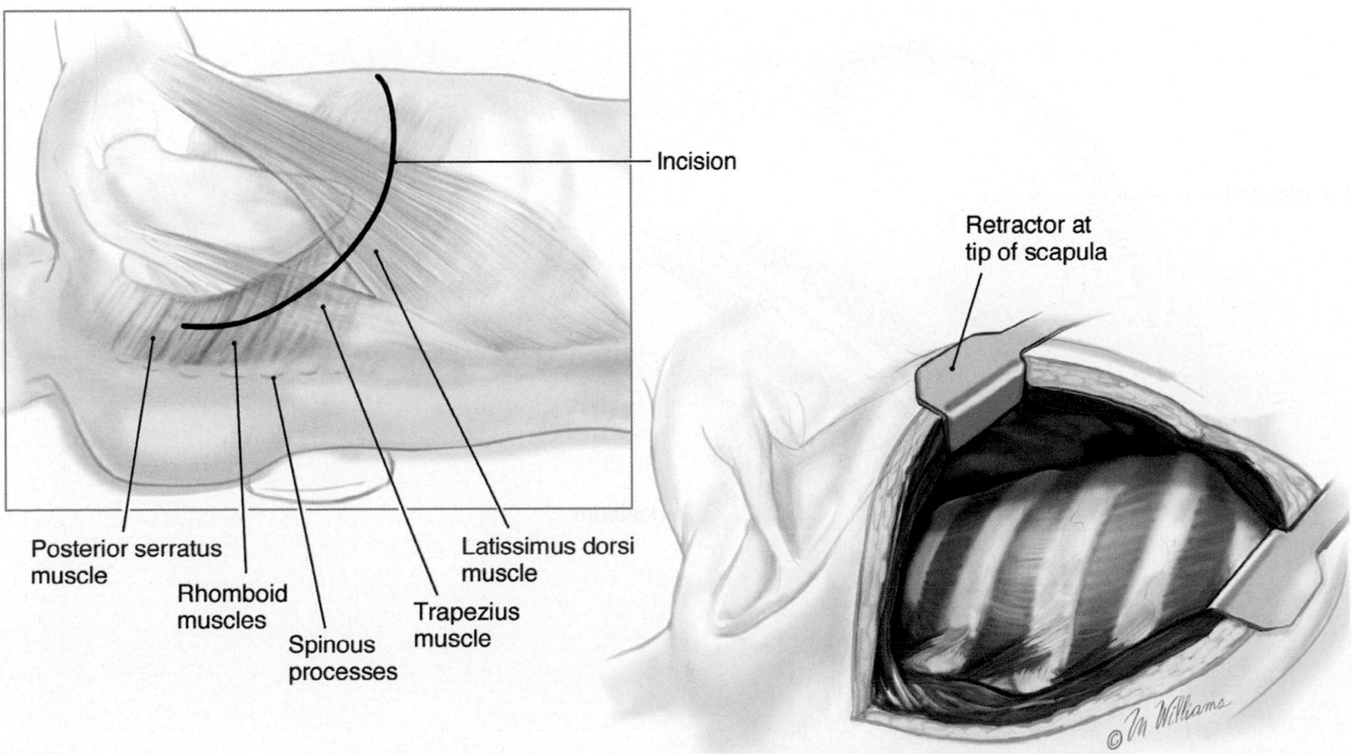

Figure 106-1. *A.* The incision for thoracoplasty should be carried high up posteriorly to access the posterior elements of the upper ribs. *B.* Placing one blade of a rib retractor on the rib cage below and the scapula above permits a stable and wide retraction of the shoulder girdle.

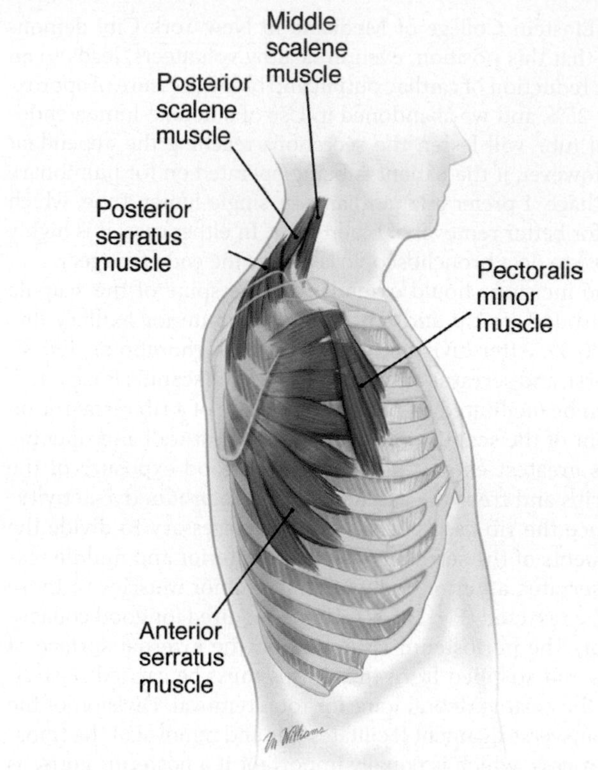

Figure 106-2. Depending on the area of rib cage to be collapsed, it is necessary to divide the muscles inserting on the ribs to be removed.

or they can be rotated 180 degrees and fixed at the ends to act as a plombe. The insertion of various materials between the ribs and the collapsed chest wall to act as a plombe was the cause of many complications and has been abandoned. Once the collapse is complete, the wound is closed in anatomic layers. Sometimes with a six-rib thoracoplasty, the tip of the scapula impinges on the top of the seventh rib, forming a painful bursa. This led some surgeons to do a hemiscapulectomy. This is ill-advised because it leads to rotation of the scapula with added deformity of the shoulder and usually does not solve the problem. It is better to resect a portion of the underlying seventh rib (Fig. 106-4).

Thoracoplasty with Open Pleural Space

In cases where there has been pleural space infection with tuberculosis or mixed infection, there may have been a need for prior drainage. Pure tuberculous infection at times can be treated with aspiration and antituberculous drugs if caught early but has the potential for formation of a pleural peel within 3 to 4 weeks. In the past month, I had such a patient with no parenchymal changes. Early decortication and antituberculous drugs have given a surprisingly good result for him. Although I can find no reference for it, I remember when in the 1960s there was some enthusiasm for steroids in cases of tuberculous pleural and especially pericardial effusions coupled with aspiration and drug therapy.

When conservative measures have failed and early decortication is contraindicated by marginal cardiopulmonary reserve, open drainage is required. This can be accomplished with a small thoracotomy, removal of proteinaceous debris, and insertion of a large-bore mushroom catheter. For more definitive drainage, an Eloesser flap can be created.[9] Using a U-shaped skin incision with the base uppermost and the tip of the flap over the lowest portion of the cavity, portions of the underlying ribs are excised, and the skin flap is turned in and sutured to the upper end of the pleural opening (Fig. 106-5). Total unroofing of the cavity as proposed by Schede[10] has been abandoned. In

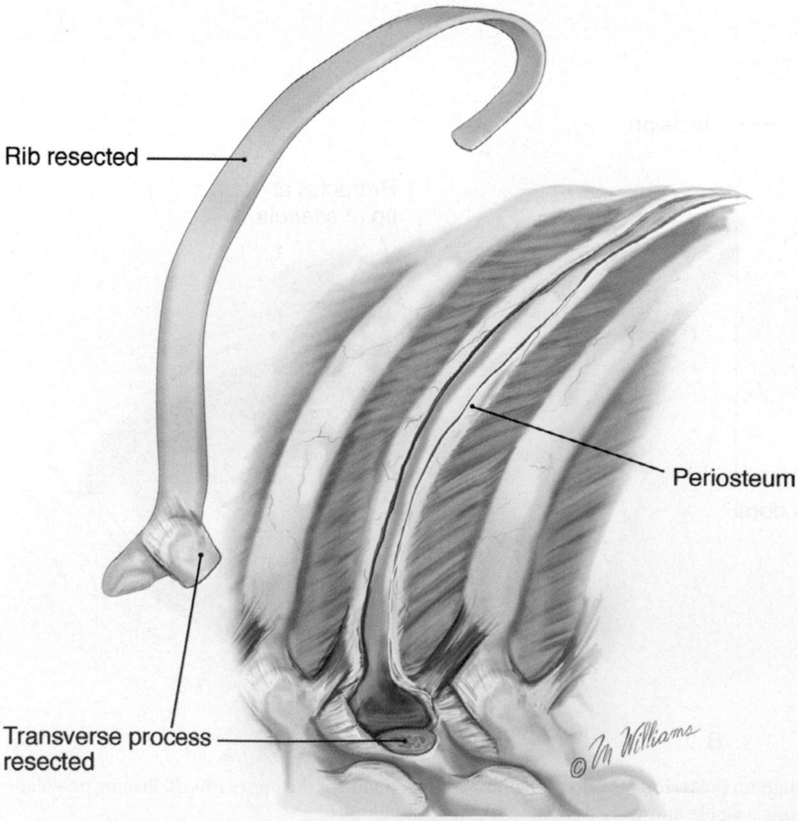

Figure 106-3. It is important to remove all the ribs and the attached transverse processes if the posterior gutter is to be obliterated.

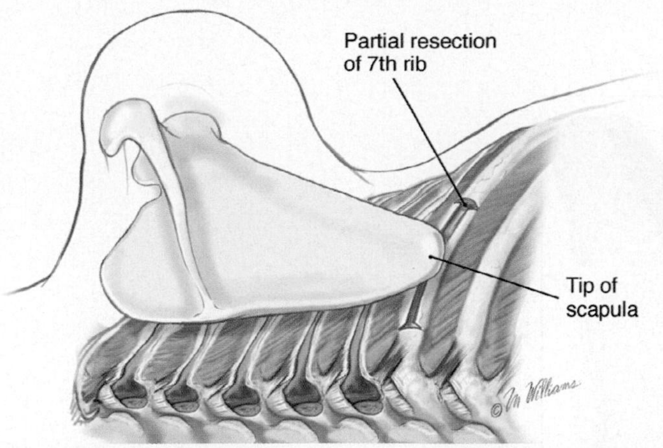

Figure 106-4. Impingement of the scapula tip on the seventh rib can cause a painful bursa to develop. It is better to remove a portion of the rib than to remove a portion of the scapula.

these patients, closure of the space occurs by secondary intention from the periphery of the cavity. This process can be accelerated by a localized extraperiosteal thoracoplasty.

Thoracoplasty with Muscle Flap

The most challenging and debilitating disease occurs when either a primary or postresection space is caused by bronchopleural fistula. It should be noted that postresectional fistulas are encountered most commonly in patients operated on for tuberculous complications before adequate medical treatment has been achieved, such as for active pulmonary hemorrhage. In some of these patients, a combination of drainage, thoracoplasty, and antituberculous drugs will achieve a closure of the fistula. If this does not occur, it will be most helpful to bring in a vascularized muscle flap to apply to the bronchus or the fistula or to completely fill the cavity[11,12] (Fig. 106-6). It can be pointed out here that the vascularized chest wall of a thoracoplasty was the first such myoplasty. Here again, patience is a winning virtue because time must be allowed for maximum medical benefit. Muscle flaps should not be brought into areas of active tuberculous infection. The muscles available are the pectoralis major, serratus anterior, latissimus dorsi, rectus abdominis, and intercostals and should be based on an intact blood supply. These can be introduced directly into a drainage already established or through a small thoracotomy placed to achieve the most direct path through the chest wall to the fistula. They should be sutured around the parenchymal defect or leaking bronchus. Here again, the obliteration of space is a good basic principle and can be achieved by an appropriate thoracoplasty or by filling the space with muscle or both.

Tailoring a Thoracoplasty

In some patients who are candidates for resection of tuberculous residua, the adhesions and scar present in and around the lung that will remain are such that a postoperative space problem is predictable. In this case, a preliminary or synchronous thoracoplasty can be performed as described previously to tailor the thoracic space so that the lung will fill it. Temporal separation of the two procedures has the advantage of less impact on the patient. It also allows for evaluation of the result achieved so that, if needed, an additional rib or two can be conveniently resected at the time of pulmonary resection.

While this discussion has been limited to consideration of thoracoplasty in tuberculosis, it must be noted that the same forces that are leading to an upsurge in typical and atypical tuberculosis are also favoring development of various fungal diseases. The problem of residual space in the thorax is most often associated with aspergillosis, but especially in immune-compromised patients, often fungal disease may invade. In these patients, antifungal medical therapy is not always successful, and surgical intervention is required. All the considerations of maximal medical benefit, careful preoperative assessment,

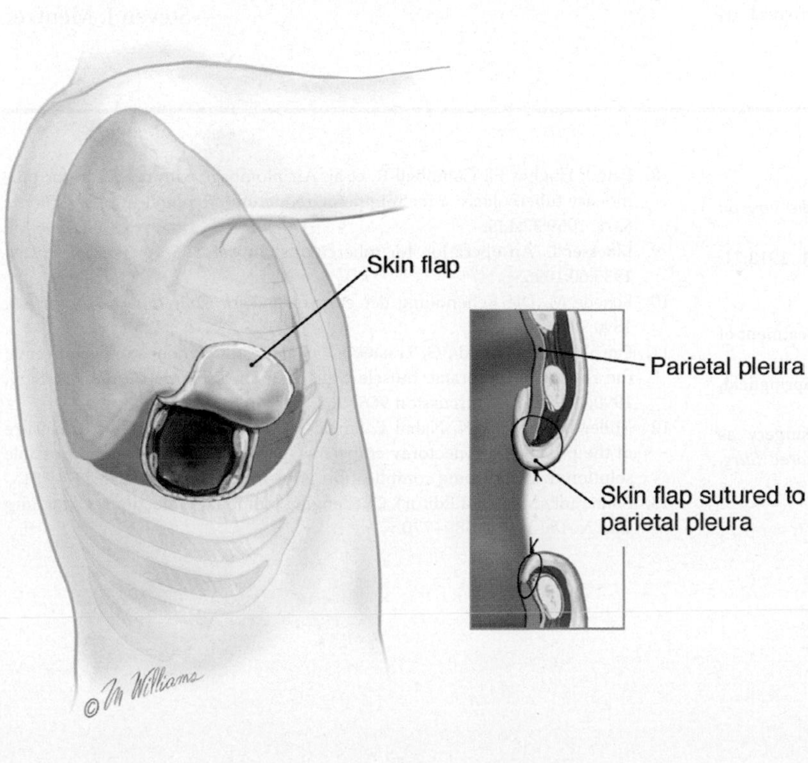

Figure 106-5. For prolonged drainage of a pleural cavity, an Eloesser flap can be fashioned by creating a downward-facing flap, resecting the underlying ribs, and sewing the flap to the parietal pleura.

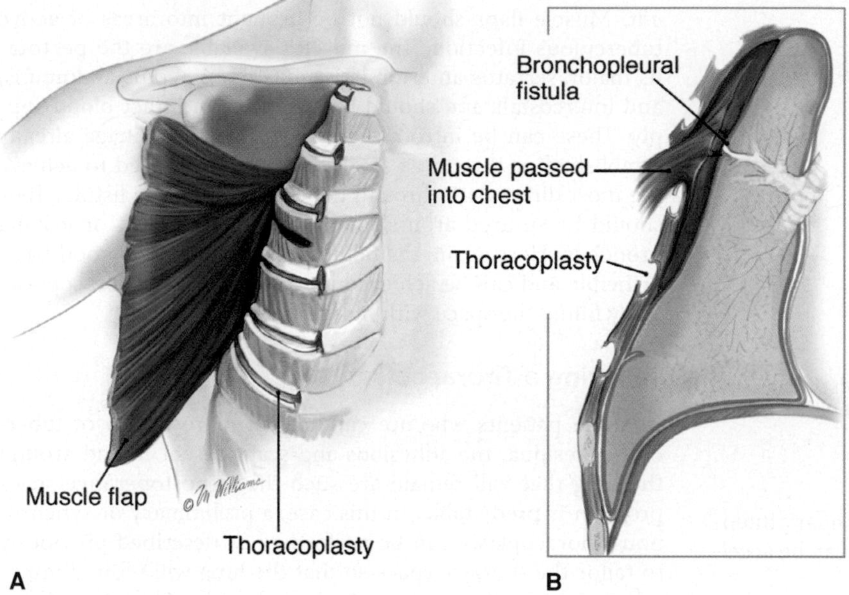

Figure 106-6. Muscles released from the chest wall that is undergoing thoracoplasty (*A*) can be kept well vascularized and brought into the thorax to (*B*) obliterate space or close a bronchopleural fistula.

and strong nutritional support obtain. This topic is too broad for discussion here.[13]

Although the present need for thoracoplasty is infrequent, it seems that all thoracic surgeons should be familiar with its uses, variations, and timing as we move into a period of increasing drug-resistant tuberculosis and a parallel increase in opportunistic infections.

EDITOR'S COMMENT

One use of thoracoplasty in the early- and mid-twentieth century reflected (1) the misguided impression that removal of ribs would prevent overdistention of the remaining lung after pneumonectomy, and (2) an aggressive surgical approach for limiting residual "space" in the chest and minimizing infections. Other surgical options for minimizing the residual thoracic space include complete mobilization of the lung to facilitate expansion into the space, an extrapleural "tent" to eliminate apical space, and maneuvers to facilitate cephalad mobilization of the diaphragm to minimize basilar space (phrenic nerve injection and pneumoperitoneum). In practice, thoracoplasty has been largely replaced by the use of extrathoracic tissue – primarily muscles or omentum – to eliminate intrathoracic space.

—Steven J. Mentzer

References

1. Review of war surgery and medicine. *Reports from the Office of the Surgeon General of the United States.* 1918;1:14–23.
2. Army ECoUS: cases of empyema at Camp Lee Virginia. *JAMA.* 1918;71: 366–443.
3. Graham E. *Empyema Thoracis.* St Louis, MO: Mosby;1925.
4. Jacobaeus H. The cauterizations of adhesions in pneumothorax treatment of tuberculosis. *Acta Tuberc Scand.* 1925;1:62.
5. Alexander J. *The Collapse Therapy of Pulmonary Tuberculosis.* Springfield, IL: Charles C Thomas;1937.
6. Woodruff W, Merkel C, Wright G. Decisions in thoracic surgery as influenced by the knowledge of pulmonary physiology. *J Thorac Surg.* 1953;26:156–183.
7. Woodruff W. Tuberculous empyema. *J Thorac Surg.* 1937;7:420.
8. Pate J, Hughes FJ, Campbell R, et al. Air plombage with resection for pulmonary tuberculosis: a technique for reduction of complications. *J Thorac Surg.* 1959;37:435.
9. Eloesser L. An operation for tuberculous empyema. *Surg Gynecol Obstet.* 1935;60:1096.
10. Schede M. Die Behendlung der empyema. *Verh Cong Innere Med Wiesb.* 1890;9:41.
11. Pairolero PC, Arnold PG, Trastek VF, et al. Postpneumonectomy empyema: the role of intrathoracic muscle transposition. *J Thorac Cardiovasc Surg.* 1990;99:958–966; discussion 966–968.
12. Miller J, Mansour K, Nahai F. Single-stage complete muscle flap closure of the post-pneumonectomy empyema space: a new method and possible solution to a disturbing complication. *Ann Thorac Surg.* 1984;38:227–231.
13. Pomerantz M (Guest Editor). Challenging pulmonary infections. *Chest Surg Clin N Am.* 1993;3:589–770.

107 Surgical Approaches for Chronic Empyema and for Management of Chronic Bronchopleural Fistula

Brian L. Pettiford, James D. Luketich, and Rodney J. Landreneau

Keywords: Bacterial pneumonia, tuberculosis, complications of pneumonectomy, complications of lobectomy, extension of intra-abdominal process, trauma, parapneumonic effusion, thoracentesis, decortication, modified Clagett window, video-assisted thoracic surgery (VATS)

Empyema and bronchopleural fistula (BPF) are two distinct yet intimately related entities. They may occur together or independently, and they share similar etiologies. The management of each process has proved, over several centuries, to be a daunting task that requires sound clinical judgment and a resilient patient.

Hippocrates provided the first clinical description of empyema approximately 2400 years ago. In 229 BC he described the clinical presentation and physical examination findings in patients with empyema. Hippocrates is also credited with the first drainage procedure for empyema. This entailed partial rib resection, drainage, and daily packing.[1] Despite Hippocrates' detailing of the clinical presentation, natural history, and treatment of empyema, it was not until the nineteenth century that significant work on the subject was presented.

In 1843, Trosseau advanced thoracentesis for the treatment of empyema. French surgeon Sedillot described thoracotomy and empyema drainage. More extensive procedures, including thoracoplasty and decortication, were introduced by Estlander (1879) and Fowler (1893), respectively.[2] At the start of the twentieth century, most treatment strategies for acute empyema involved early rib resection and open drainage. Mortality rates with this approach averaged 30%. Graham and Bell, of the United States Army Empyema Commission, made a major advance in the treatment of early empyema. They recommended closed-tube drainage to manage early empyema. This strategy decreased the mortality rate from 30% to 4.3%.[3]

In 1935, Eloesser[4] described an open thoracotomy technique that would permit skin and soft tissue to behave as a valve to allow lung expansion. In 1963, Clagett and Geraci[5] introduced open window drainage for 6 to 8 weeks, followed by empyema cavity obliteration with antibiotic solution and window closure. The Clagett window remains useful in the treatment of chronic empyema. Muscle flap closure of BPF and the postresectional space has become increasingly popular.[6,7] Video-assisted thoracoscopy and fibrinolytic therapy also have roles in the management of empyema.[8,9]

EMPYEMA

Empyema is defined as a purulent pleural collection (Fig. 107-1). Causes include bacterial pneumonia, tuberculosis, postresectional, posttraumatic, and intra-abdominal processes. Approximately 50% of empyemas are caused by bacterial infection. Postresectional causes account for 25%, and an additional 8% to 11% are caused by extension of an intra-abdominal process.[10]

Clinical Presentation

The presenting signs and symptoms of empyema are nonspecific. The most common symptoms are shortness of breath and fever. Patients also may complain of cough and chest pain. Sputum production may or may not be present. These symptoms are also present in patients with pneumonia. Empyema should be considered when a patient manifests these symptoms after a prolonged respiratory illness or a lung resection. Laboratory analysis is also relatively nonspecific and usually includes leukocytosis. C-reactive protein levels that exceed 100 mg/L may be useful as a diagnostic indicator of postpneumonectomy empyema, as described by Icard and colleagues.[11] Physical examination findings may be underwhelming, although in empyema necessitatis an undrained empyema may track through the soft tissues, causing cellulitis in the overlying skin.

Radiographic Evaluation

The radiographic workup of postpneumonic empyema should begin with a posteroanterior and lateral chest x-ray (Fig. 107-2). Hsu and colleagues[12] showed that an empyema appears as a wide air–fluid level on posteroanterior view and has a narrow anteroposterior width on lateral projection. Bilateral decubitus films may provide information regarding a freely flowing or loculated empyema. Radiographs also may differentiate among empyema, BPF, and lung abscess. In BPF, the air–fluid level is most commonly located in the posterior costophrenic sulcus.[13] There is little difference in air–fluid level size between posteroanterior and lateral projections in the case of lung abscess. Schachter and colleagues[14] presented the following qualities

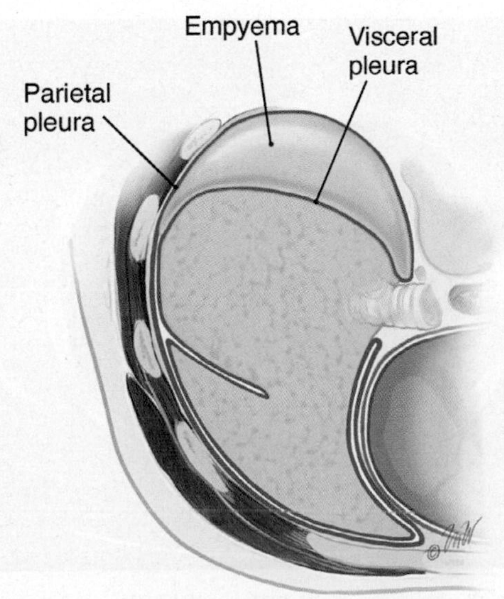

Figure 107-1. Empyema is a purulent pleural collection.

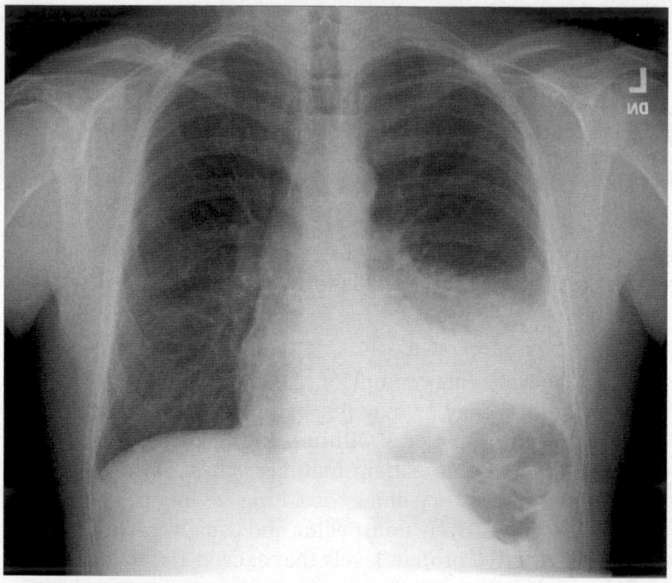

Figure 107-2. This chest film shows a parapneumonic effusion in a patient with left lower lobe pneumonia. The patient ultimately required a left VATS procedure, drainage, and partial decortication.

that distinguish empyema from lung abscess on plain film: (1) The air–fluid level extends to the chest wall; (2) its border tapers near the mediastinum or chest wall; and (3) the air–fluid level crosses the fissure.

Ultrasound also may be used to evaluate empyemic spaces. Major advantages include portability and identification of loculations or pleural fibrosis. This modality also may differentiate transudates from exudates.[15,16] Ultrasound also may guide catheter-based drainage of effusions, although a major limitation is the operator-dependent nature of this modality.

Chest CT scan is the mainstay in the diagnosis and management of empyema and BPF. CT characteristics specific to empyema include a thin, uniform, smooth wall along the exterior surfaces, in contrast with the irregular walls seen in lung abscesses (Fig. 107-3). The "split pleura" sign, which distinguishes the separated visceral and parietal pleural surfaces, can

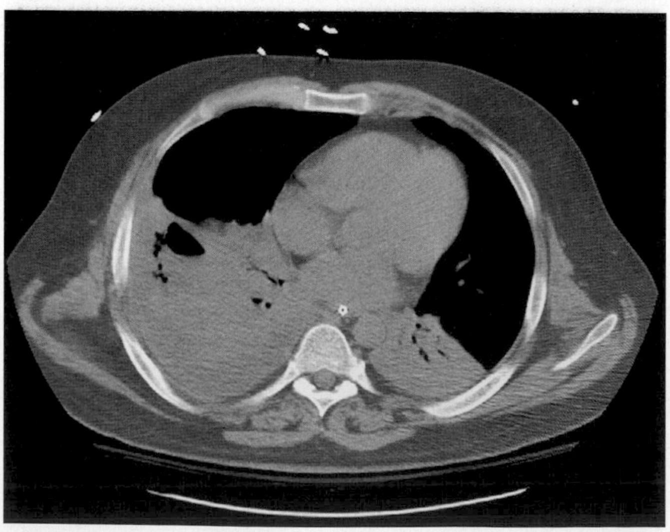

Figure 107-3. Shown here is a right lower lobe abscess in an alcoholic patient with aspiration pneumonia.

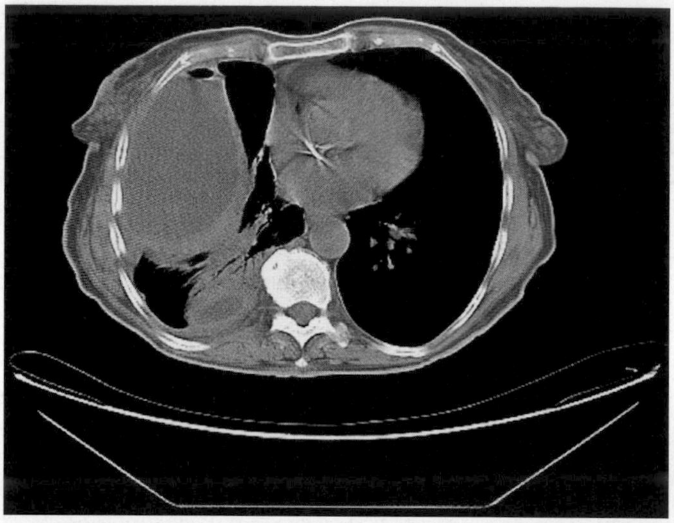

Figure 107-4. Recurrent right empyema in this patient ultimately required right thoracotomy and decortication.

be seen in nearly 70% of empyemas (Fig. 107-4).[17] The presence of empyema fluid separates the two hypervascular surfaces, which are readily identified on contrast-enhanced scans. One major pitfall is the difficulty of differentiating atelectasis or effusion from the diaphragm. Intra-abdominal ascites and subdiaphragmatic abscess also may make proper diagnosis of empyema challenging.

MRI may be applied to the diagnosis of parapneumonic effusions and empyema. The multiplanar imagery provides details specific to the location and relationship of the empyema to pleural structures. In addition, the pleural surfaces can be visualized adequately to identify a split-pleura sign. Even so, given the availability and current use of CT, as well as the cost of MRI, widespread use of MRI is limited as applied to empyema diagnosis.

Parapneumonic Effusions

As mentioned earlier, parapneumonic effusions account for the majority of empyemas. The approach should include plain films. Antibiotic therapy is the treatment of choice if the fluid thickness on decubitus studies is less than 1 cm.[18] Diagnostic and therapeutic thoracentesis is indicated for larger collections and those that persist or enlarge despite medical therapy.

Natural History

The evolution from parapneumonic effusion to empyema involves three stages. Stage 1, the exudative stage, is characterized by freely flowing fluid. At this point, the pleural surfaces are inflamed and quite permeable. This stage corresponds to the uncomplicated parapneumonic effusion described by Light and colleagues.[18] Stage 2, the fibrinopurulent stage, is characterized by bacterial infection and fibrin deposition. The fluid color may progress from clear yellow to purulent. Biochemical fluid analysis can guide management of these fluid collections. A pleural fluid pH of less than 7.00, pleural fluid glucose concentration less than 40 mg/dL, or a positive culture suggests a complicated parapneumonic effusion, and tube thoracostomy is indicated. Frank pus is an indication for tube thoracostomy. The organized phase, stage 3, occurs approximately 1 week after the initial infection. Fibroblastic ingrowth and collagen

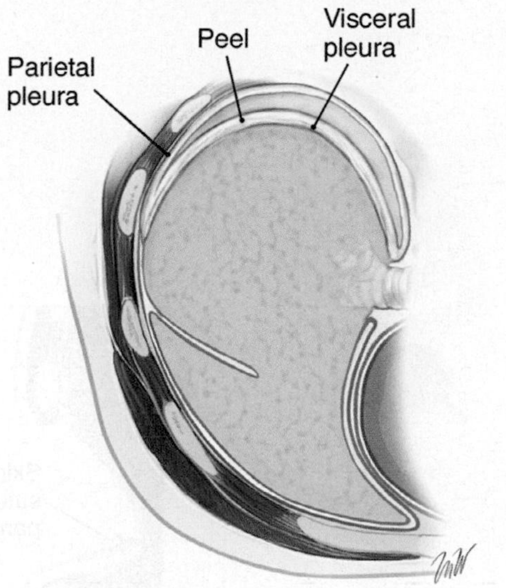

Figure 107-5. In stage 3 empyema, there is fibroblastic ingrowth and collagen deposition that may develop into a thickened membrane, or "peel."

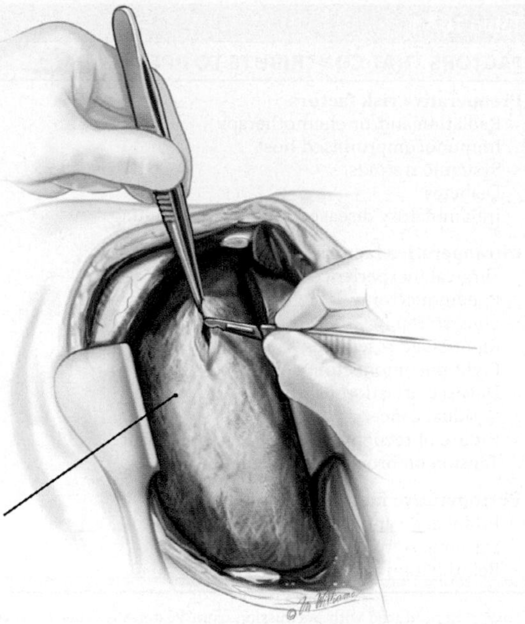

Figure 107-6. Decortication is performed to release the trapped lung. The peel is incised with a no. 15 scalpel blade and then grasped and meticulously excised.

deposition occur. Progression of this phase over a period of 3 to 4 weeks may result in a thickened membrane, or "peel," that results in trapped lung and potentially restricts pulmonary function (Fig. 107-5).

After chest tube placement and drainage, the patient should undergo surveillance chest x-ray and chest CT scan to assess (1) completeness of drainage and (2) lung expansion. If multiple loculations are present on the chest CT scan, intrapleural fibrinolytics or thoracoscopy should be performed. Daily intrapleural streptokinase 250,000 units/100 mL of saline may be administered via the chest tube, followed by chest tube clamping for 4 hours. This therapy can be discontinued when the volume of drainage is low or after lung re-expansion has been demonstrated.[9] Fibrinolytic therapy is most applicable to the fibrinopurulent phase of parapneumonic effusions. Despite the reported success of fibrinolytic therapy, we favor video-assisted thoracic surgery (VATS) over lytic therapy. Thoracoscopy permits adhesiolysis and chest tube positioning under direct vision. In addition, the coagulum may be thoroughly removed, and if necessary, a limited decortication can be performed. The overall condition of the lung also may be assessed and the need for thoracotomy and complete decortication determined.[8] During the fibrinopurulent stage of empyema, VATS offers decreased hospital stay, reduced cost, and improved cosmesis in comparison with thoracotomy.[19]

In the organized phase, a thick fibrous "peel" overlies the visceral pleura. Patients may have a restrictive pattern on pulmonary function testing. Findings suggestive of this phase include the persistence of an empyema cavity after 7 to 10 days of chest tube drainage, failure of full lung expansion on radiographs, and a thick "peel" on chest CT scan or at thoracoscopy.

Preoperative Assessment

In cases of empyema complicated by trapped lung, thoracotomy and decortication are indicated. Preoperative workup should include a chest CT scan and pulmonary function testing. Ventilation/perfusion lung scanning may be useful in selected patients when poor ipsilateral lung function may indicate the need for pneumonectomy.[20] Contraindications to this procedure include a debilitated, moribund patient, adequate drainage and expansion by lesser procedures, severe cardiopulmonary disease, and little or no perfusion to the affected lung.

Surgical Technique

The technique of decortication requires general anesthesia, usually through a double-lumen endobronchial tube. Packed red blood cells should be available perioperatively. The patient is placed in a full lateral decubitus position, and a serratus-sparing posterolateral or vertical axillary thoracotomy incision is made. The pleural cavity is entered through the fifth or sixth interspace after removing a portion of the overlying rib. The peel is incised initially with a no. 15 scalpel blade (Fig. 107-6). The peel is grasped, and a meticulous excision is performed using a combination of blunt and sharp separation of the peel and underlying visceral pleura. Some degree of ventilation to the affected lung will assist with identifying the proper dissection plane. The presence of air leaks indicates an incorrect dissection level. As the fibrinous covering is removed, the underlying lung will readily expand when ventilated. The dissection should be thorough and extend into the fissure and diaphragmatic lung surfaces. This extremely tedious procedure requires patience on the part of the surgeon and anesthesiologist.

Postresection Empyema

Postresectional empyema may occur after pneumonectomy and lesser resections, including wedge biopsy, segmentectomy, and lobectomy. The risk of occurrence is low at 0.01% for wedge resections and up to 2% for lobectomies.[21] Postpneumonectomy empyema is more common, with an incidence of 5% after standard pneumonectomy.[22] The mortality rate is as high as 50%.[23] Empyema from lesser resections usually occurs secondary to persistent parenchymal leak, with a resulting residual space that becomes secondarily infected. Chest tube drainage and directed antibiotic therapy usually are effective management. More extensive procedures, including VATS with

Table 107-1

FACTORS THAT CONTRIBUTE TO PPE

Preoperative risk factors
Radiation and/or chemotherapy
Immunocompromised host
Systemic steroids
Diabetes
Inflammatory diseased lung/destroyed lung
Intraoperative factors
Surgical inexperience
Pneumonectomy
Long stump
Right-sided resections
Right pneumonectomy
Devascularization of stump
Residual cancer at stump
Failure of recognition of BPF before closure
Tension on bronchial closure
Postoperative factors
Prolonged ventilation
Systemic steroids
Reintubation

Source: Reproduced with permission from Vester SR, Faber LP, Kittle CF et al. Bronchopleural fistula after stapled closure of bronchus. *Ann Thorac Surg.* 1991;52:1253–1257; discussion 1257–1258.

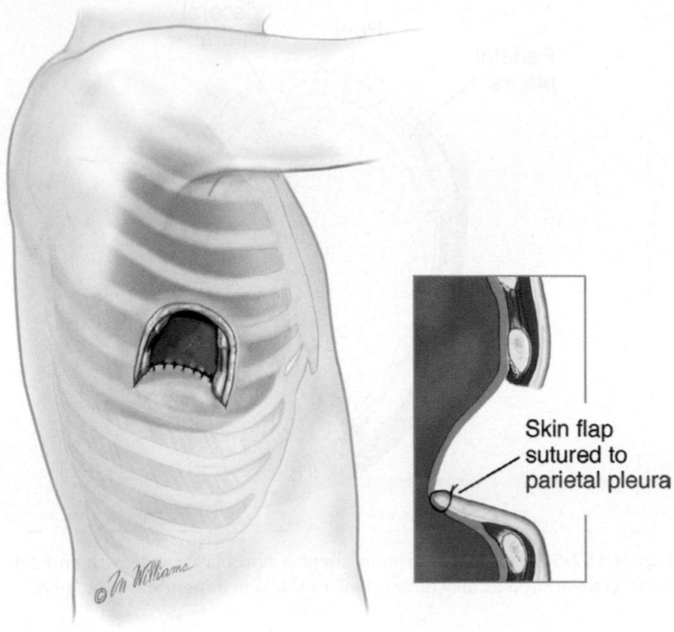

Figure 107-7. Technique for performing a modified Eloesser flap.

drainage, modified Eloesser drainage, and myoplasty, may be needed in refractory cases. Airspace location may determine the muscle type used during myoplasty. Apical airspaces may be obliterated using the pectoralis major, serratus anterior, or latissimus dorsi muscle. The serratus and latissimus also may be used for posterior spaces. The omentum may be mobilized and passed along the anterior diaphragm for inferior spaces.[21]

Postpneumonectomy Empyema

Risk Factors/Presentation/Workup

Postpneumonectomy empyema (PPE) represents a serious complication that may occur early or late after pneumonectomy. PPE is accompanied by BPF in up to 80% of cases. Several risk factors that cause BPF may ultimately lead to PPE, as shown in Table 107-1. Preventive measures should include aggressive preoperative treatment of pleural sepsis with antibiotics and optimization of nutritional status. Perioperative measures include careful dissection around the bronchial stump with preservation of bronchial blood supply, appropriate stump length, minimization of intraoperative spillage, and liberal use of autologous flaps for stump coverage. Right pneumonectomy is associated with a higher rate of stump dehiscence, empyema, and BPF. This is likely because the stump is exposed to the pleural space on the right. The left bronchial stump usually retracts medially and subaortically, providing some degree of protection.

PPE may be insidious in onset. Symptoms of fatigue, cough, weight loss, and pain may be present. Radiographs may be helpful in cases of PPE with concomitant BPF. A decrease in the air–fluid level on plain film in a patient with the preceding complaints and risk factors should prompt further investigation.

Chest CT scan provides information on the volume and homogeneity of the pleural fluid, the position of the ipsilateral diaphragm, and the status of the remaining lung. In cases of PPE with BPF, CT scan may even provide the location of the opening.

Management

Initial management of PPE without BPF is the same as for other types of empyema—tube thoracostomy drainage. Flexible bronchoscopy should be performed to assess bronchial stump integrity. Mediastinal shift and volume loss may alter the dimensions of the pneumonectomy space significantly. Chest CT scan therefore is recommended before tube thoracostomy. Insertion is safest along the fourth interspace in the anterior axillary line.[24] The chest tube should be placed to water seal. If the mediastinum is stable but drainage is inadequate, a modified Eloesser flap can be created, as described by Thourani and colleagues[25] (Fig. 107-7). Between 3 months (for benign disease) and 12 months (for malignant disease), a single-stage complete muscle flap closure may be performed as described by Miller and colleagues.[26] Extrathoracic muscle flaps can be used to close the pleural space. Flaps used in order of decreasing frequency include latissimus dorsi, serratus anterior, pectoralis major, pectoralis minor, and rectus abdominis. Figure 107-8 shows each of these structures with respective blood supplies. The omentum also may be used to obliterate the postpneumonectomy space and may be more useful for bronchial stump coverage in postpneumonectomy BPF.

Nonresectional Postoperative Empyema

Nonresectional postoperative empyema may occur after esophageal surgery with intraoperative spillage or postoperative esophageal leak. Empyema also can complicate intra-abdominal surgery or infection. This may occur after gastric perforation, splenectomy, or pancreatic infection/resection. The management principles are the same as for postresectional empyema.

Tuberculous Empyema

The worldwide prevalence of tuberculosis caused by bacterial infection with *Mycobacterium tuberculosis* deserves mention

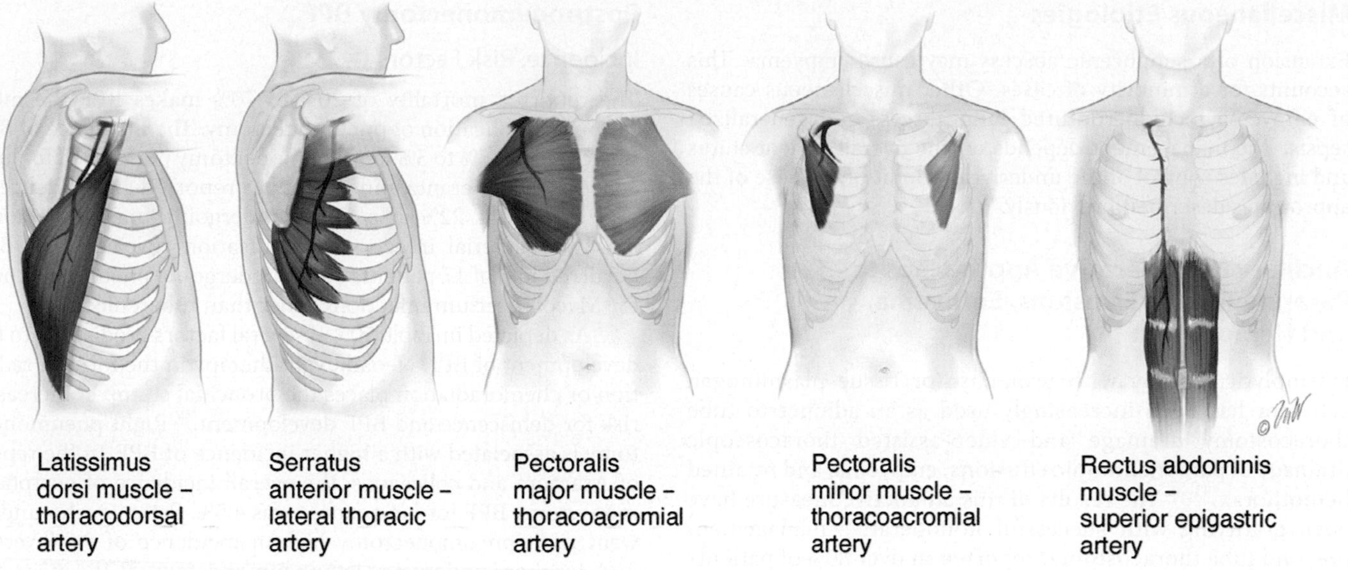

Figure 107-8. Extrathoracic muscle flaps and their respective blood supplies.

because it relates to empyema and BPF. Tuberculosis causes nearly 3 million annual deaths in adults worldwide.[27] In the United States, factors such as HIV infection, IV drug abuse, and immigration patterns led to a 9.4% increase in reported tuberculosis cases in 1990.[28,29] The use of collapse therapy, including intrapleural pneumothorax, plombage, and thoracoplasty, was largely supplanted by antituberculous chemotherapy. The development of multidrug-resistant tuberculosis and its complications has led to a small but renewed role for surgery in the treatment of this disease.

Surgery in Tuberculous Empyema

The preoperative approach should include arterial blood gas determination, pulmonary function testing, and quantitative ventilation/perfusion scans. The latter is particularly helpful in determining the need for lobectomy versus pneumonectomy in the case of destroyed lung. Antituberculous chemotherapy should be administered preoperatively in an effort to produce a negative pleural or sputum culture.[30,31] Tube thoracostomy may be used to successfully drain small BPFs during this time. Empyema may be drained using a window thoracostomy or Clagett procedure. After several months, a thoracomyoplasty may be performed in patients treated initially by open-window thoracostomy.[32] Muscle flap stump closure should be used in all patients undergoing lobectomy with a positive sputum culture, those with anticipated space problems, and all patients undergoing pneumonectomy.[30] The latissimus dorsi muscle is favored and used most commonly for this purpose.

Traumatic Hemothorax

Empyema may complicate traumatic hemothorax associated with blunt or penetrating trauma. Hemothorax also may complicate cardiac surgery, especially if one or both pleural spaces were opened at operation. Although a sterile hemothorax usually is reabsorbed after 1 month, secondary infection poses a significant problem. The initial diagnostic approach should include chest x-ray. Chest CT scan may provide useful information about the amount of hemothorax and the condition of the underlying lung.

Surgical Management

Thoracentesis should be performed if there is a free-flowing hemothorax. In chronic cases, the hemothorax is clotted, and thoracentesis is of no value. It may provide some information about the presence of infection but will result in inadequate drainage. Tube thoracostomy also may prove insufficient for evacuating a clotted hemothorax. We recommend the early resort to VATS for the treatment of hemothorax. Early thoracoscopic management can be used to adequately evacuate large, infected hemothoraces and obviates the need for thoracotomy and decortication.[8] An algorithm for management of empyema and hemothorax is provided in Fig. 107-9.

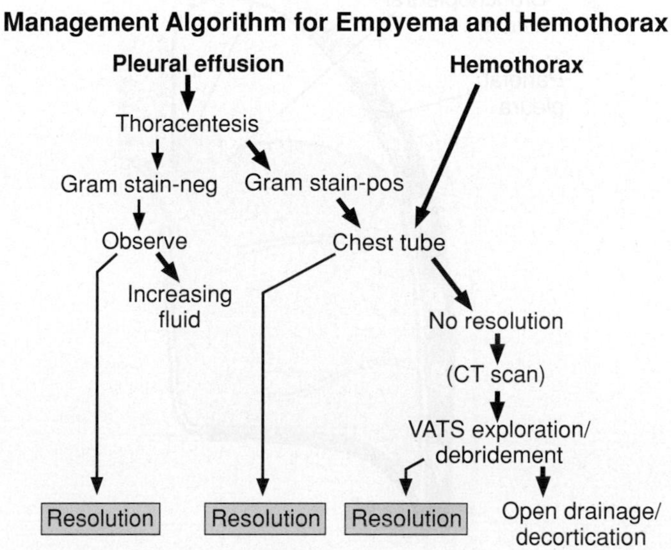

Figure 107-9. Management algorithm for empyema and hemothorax. Reproduced with permission from Landreneau RJ, Keenan RJ, Hazelrigg SR, et al. Thoracoscopy for empyema and hemothorax. *Chest.* 1996;109:18–24.

Miscellaneous Etiologies

Extension of a subphrenic abscess may cause empyema. This accounts for a minority of cases. Other miscellaneous causes of empyema include ruptured lung abscess and generalized sepsis. The management depends on the overall patient status and includes control of the underlying condition and use of the approaches described previously.

Ancillary Nonoperative Approaches to Parapneumonic Effusions, Empyema, and Hemothorax

Fibrinolytic therapy with urokinase or tissue plasminogen activator has been increasingly used as an adjunct to tube thoracostomy drainage and video-assisted thoracoscopic drainage of parapneumonic effusions, empyema, and retained hemothorax.[33–35] The results of this adjunctive measure have been gratifying with successful nonoperative management (beyond tube thoracostomy) reported in over 80% of patients treated. Currently, the use of these fibrinolytic agents appears to have increasing utility in the management of these pleural problems.

BRONCHOPLEURAL FISTULA

Definition/Incidence/Risk Factors

BPF is a communication between the airway and pleural space (Fig. 107-10). The fistula may originate as proximally as the mainstem bronchus or as distally as a segmental bronchus. The incidence of BPF varies based on etiology. Postresectional BPF may occur after lesser resections, such as lobectomy or segmentectomy. The incidence of BPF after lobectomy ranges between 0.5% and 1.2%, and the incidence is 0.3% after segmentectomy.[36,37]

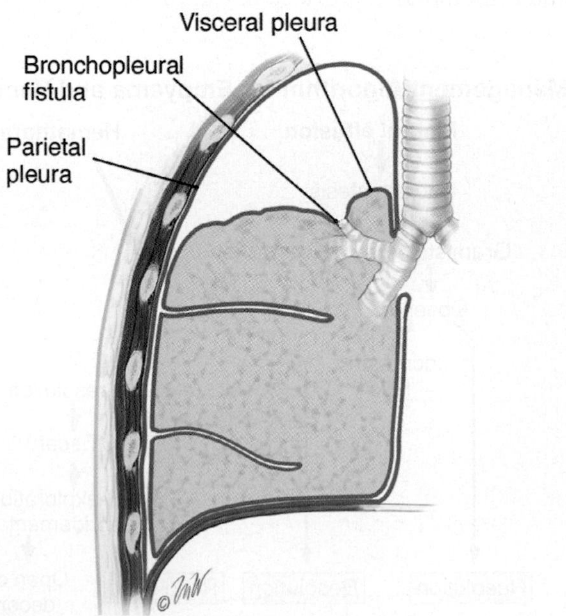

Figure 107-10. A BPF is an anomalous communication between the airway and the pleural space. The communication may be as proximal as the mainstem bronchus or as distal as a segmental bronchus.

Postpneumonectomy BPF

Incidence, Risk Factors

The reported mortality of 20% to 70% makes BPF the most serious complication of pneumonectomy. The incidence of BPF ranges from 1.3% to 5% for pneumonectomy performed for lung cancer.[36,38] Pomerantz and colleagues reported an incidence of BPF as high as 22% in patients undergoing pneumonectomy for mycobacterial infection. Stratification revealed that BPF occurred in 8 of 17 patients (47%) undergoing pneumonectomy for Mycobacterium infections other than tuberculosis.[30]

As depicted in Table 107-1, several factors predispose to the development of BPF. Neoadjuvant therapy in the form of radiation or chemoradiation places the bronchial stump at increased risk for dehiscence and BPF development.[39] Right pneumonectomy is associated with a higher incidence of BPF. In the report of Asamura and colleagues, the overall incidence of postpneumonectomy BPF for lung cancer was 4.5%. Patients who underwent right pneumonectomy had an incidence of 8.6% versus 2.3% for those undergoing left pneumonectomy.[36] The increased risk of BPF after right pneumonectomy has been well explained. Cadaver studies have shown that the right mainstem bronchus usually has one bronchial artery, whereas there are two on the left. The right bronchial stump therefore is at increased risk of ischemia. The left mainstem bronchus retracts below the aortic arch and is buttressed, whereas the right mainstem stump has no coverage and remains exposed in the pleural space. Although pneumonectomy for mycobacterial infections is performed more commonly on the left lung, right pneumonectomy, when performed, is associated with a higher rate of BPF. In a 1991 study of patients undergoing surgery for mycobacterial infection, Pomerantz and colleagues[30] reported that seven of nine patients suffering BPF had undergone right pneumonectomy.

Other factors that predispose to BPF include a long bronchial stump, concomitant infection at the time of pneumonectomy, and prolonged mechanical ventilation. The presence of a long bronchial stump permits pooling of secretions in the stump, which can lead to stump breakdown secondary to chronic inflammation or infection (Fig. 107-11).[40]

Clinical Presentation, Evaluation

The presentation of BPF spans a broad spectrum from vague complaints of fatigue to the massive expectoration of serous pleural fluid with aspiration into the remaining lung. Patients may complain of weakness, loss of appetite, and weight loss.

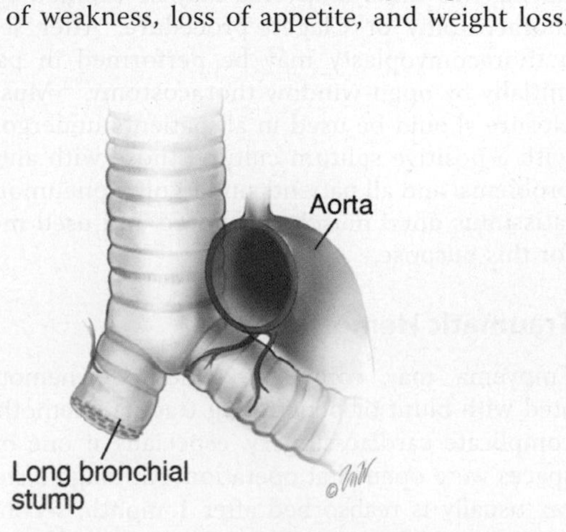

Figure 107-11. Technical factors such as a long bronchial stump after pneumonectomy predispose to the development of BPF.

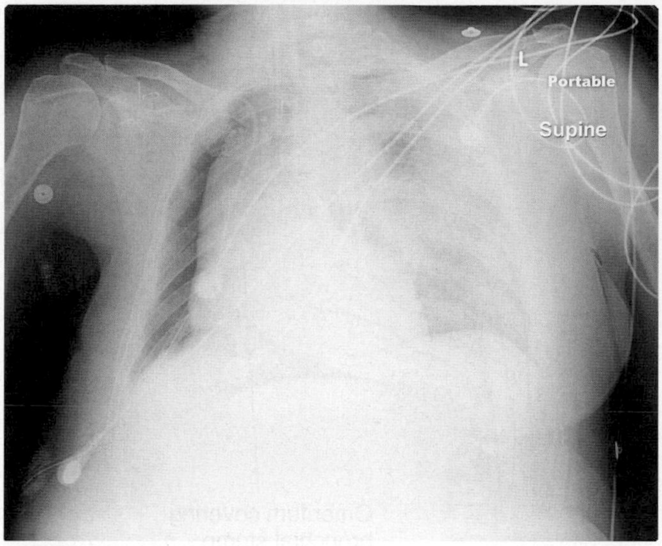

Figure 107-12. Chest x-ray in a patient who developed acute bronchorrhea after right pneumonectomy. Note the absence of fluid in the right pleural space and the mediastinal shift. The left mainstem bronchus has been selectively intubated.

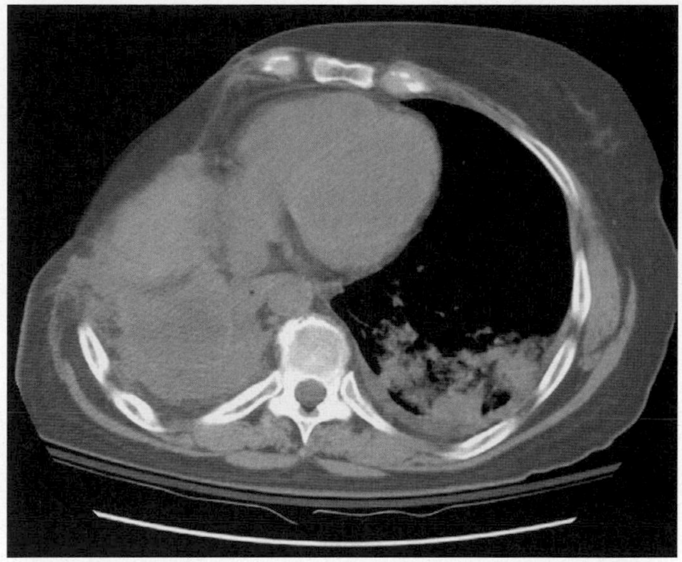

Figure 107-13. Chest CT scan demonstrating muscle flap obliteration of the right pleural space during treatment for postpneumonectomy BPF.

They also may develop a fever and leukocytosis. These symptoms are indistinguishable from those observed in patients with empyema.

A decrease in the air–fluid level or development of a new airspace on chest x-ray may indicate the presence of a BPF (Fig. 107-12). CT scanning may have a role if empyema is suspected and can even identify the fistula is some cases.

Initial Management

If BPF is suspected, flexible bronchoscopy should be performed. The bronchial stump should be inspected closely for erythema, mucosal irregularities, granulation tissue, or the presence of a frank opening. The contralateral airway also should be evaluated, and any secretions should be evacuated and cultured. If the patient manifests a large BPF with massive expectoration of serosanguineous fluid, the pneumonectomy side should be placed dependently, thereby protecting the remaining lung. Concomitantly, the airway should be secured, depending on the degree of respiratory distress. The bronchus to the intact lung should be intubated directly with a single-lumen endotracheal tube. The bronchial portion of a double-lumen tube also can be inserted into the intact bronchus and the cuff inflated for protection. Emergency tube thoracostomy on the pneumonectomy side is performed. If the occurrence is within days of pneumonectomy and there is some question about stability of the mediastinum, the tube is placed to water seal. If several days or weeks have elapsed, special care is taken to place the tube anterior and near the fourth or fifth interspace. This takes into account the mediastinal shift and volume changes within the pleural cavity.

Treatment options for BPF are dictated by the following: (1) time of development in relation to pneumonectomy; (2) side of the BPF; (3) presence of empyema; (4) overall status of the patient; and (5) whether the event is initial or represents a failed attempt at fistula closure.

Surgical Therapy

Recommended management of early postpneumonectomy BPF begins with tube thoracostomy and drainage. This should be followed by thoracotomy, debridement, and identification of the bronchial stump. Saline solution is poured into the pleural space. The pleural cavity then is ventilated under positive pressure. Air bubbles should guide the surgeon to the fistula. The stump should be debrided to viable tissue and a hand-sewn closure performed. Chest tubes then should be placed in superior and dependent positions. Continuous irrigation with antibiotic solution is administered until cultures from the space are sterile.

An alternative approach to chronic BPF and empyema is a two-stage method introduced by Deschamps and colleagues.[41] The first stage involves open pleural drainage and debridement through the prior thoracotomy incision. The fistula is identified and closed at this time. Extrathoracic muscle then is transposed into the pleural cavity to provide stump coverage. If the serratus anterior muscle was spared during the initial thoracotomy, it may be used. The cephalic portion of the previously transacted latissimus dorsi muscle also may be used for coverage (Fig. 107-13). The pectoralis major, rectus abdominis, or omentum also may be used. The wound is then packed, and dressing changes are recommended every 48 hours over a 4- to 6-day period. The second stage may be performed when healthy granulation tissue is present. The cavity is filled with Dab's solution: 0.5 g neomycin, 0.1 g polymyxin B sulfate, and 80 mg gentamicin in 1 L of saline. A watertight wound closure is performed in multiple layers.

Early reoperation and bronchial stump closure are recommended when BPF occurs within 7 days of the initial operation.[21] Wright and colleagues[42] even propose reoperation, stump closure, and coverage in patients who develop BPF fistula within 1 month of pneumonectomy.

Refractory Postpneumonectomy BPF

A less commonly employed but effective means of controlling refractory BPF is a transsternal, transpericardial approach. Originally described in 1960 by Padhi and Lynn[43], this approach provides adequate access to the carina and mainstem bronchi. Ginsberg and Saborio described this technique when a BPF had failed closure attempts via thoracotomy. They advocated its use in patients in whom redo thoracotomy is contraindicated and when carinal resection is necessary at the time of stump closure.[44]

Postlobectomy BPF

As mentioned earlier, the incidence of BPF after lobectomy is less than 1%. The same factors that lead to postpneumonectomy BPF can complicate lobectomy. Patient presentation is the same, ranging from vague complaints of fatigue, chest pain, and fever to an airspace and empyema. Plain film and chest CT scan should be used to characterize the pleural cavity. If an air–fluid space is identified, drainage should be established using tube thoracostomy. If fluid is present, it should be cultured and a biochemical profile sent. Broad-spectrum antibiotics should be given. A flexible bronchoscopy is recommended to assess the integrity of the lobar stump and identify a BPF.

The effectiveness of therapy can be judged by assessing the patient's overall condition, including temperature, white blood cell count, and subjective complaints. Serial chest x-rays and chest CT scans should be performed to determine the adequacy of drainage. If there is no improvement or an increase in the airspace or fluid level, then drainage is inadequate. CT-guided or operative drainage should be performed. After complete drainage of the residual space and documented infection control, steps must be taken to close the fistula. Although BPFs following lesser resections can close spontaneously after treatment with drainage and antibiotics, a plan should be in order for stump closure and space obliteration. Cooper and Miller[21] described the utility of using specific muscle flaps for this purpose. Table 107-2 lists the various flaps that can be used for stump coverage after lobectomy. The pectoralis, latissimus dorsi, or serratus anterior muscle can be used after upper lobectomy. The latissimus, serratus, and omentum may be used to obliterate spaces after lower lobectomy.[21]

Management goals for postlobectomy BPF mirror those for postpneumonectomy BPF: (1) early drainage and antibiotics; (2) stump coverage with extrathoracic muscle, omentum, or other well-vascularized autologous tissue (Fig. 107-14); and (3) obliteration of any residual space with extrathoracic muscle flaps or omentum.

Table 107-2

MUSCLE FLAPS AND BPF

Upper thoracic
Pectoralis major
Latissimus dorsi
Intercostal
Midthoracic
Latissimus dorsi
Serratus anterior
Intercostal
Lower thoracic
Latissimus dorsi
Serratus anterior
Rectus abdominis
Omentum

Source: Reproduced with permission from Cooper WA, Miller JI Jr. Management of bronchopleural fistula after lobectomy. *Semin Thorac Cardiovasc Surg.* 2001;13:8–12.

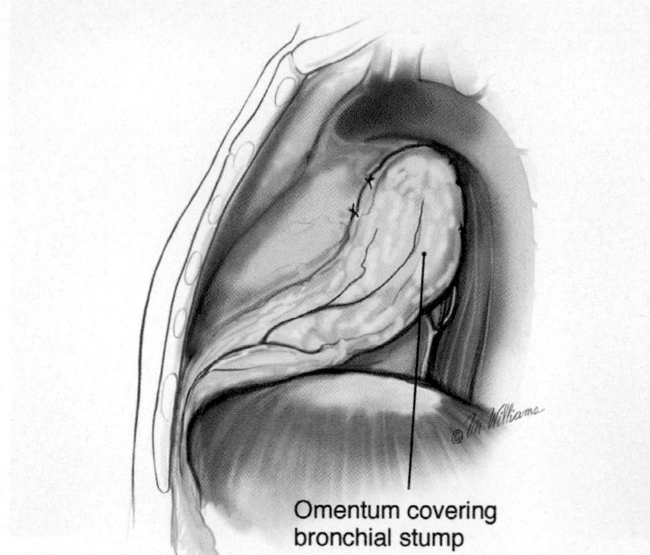

Figure 107-14. Omentum used for autologous tissue coverage in the management of BPF.

Alternative Therapies

Small BPFs may close spontaneously. Persistent BPFs may pose a significant problem in patients who have undergone multiple thoracotomies or median sternotomy. Alternative approaches to control BPFs in this setting have been described. Lin and Ianettoni[45] reported the use of bovine albumin-glutaraldehyde tissue adhesive (Bioglue, Cryolife, Kennesaw, GA) in two patients with refractory BPFs. Hollaus and colleagues retrospectively analyzed bronchoscopic closure of BPFs in 45 patients. They found that small fistulas (<3 mm) are treated effectively by bronchoscopic fibrin glue application. Fistulas that exceed 8 mm are not amenable to this approach.[46]

The experience with covered endobronchial stents for the management of benign and malignant airway stenoses has led some investigators to utilize this approach to right mainstem bronchial stump dehiscence following pneumonectomy.[47,48] In addition, the success noted with removable endobronchial valves for "endoscopic lung volume reduction" for pulmonary emphysema has led to the use of these devices for the management of BPF. Endobronchial valve deployment has been reported with successful control of postresectional bronchial stump dehiscence and peripheral parenchymal BPF.[34,35,49]

SUMMARY

BPF fistula is a dreaded complication of pneumonectomy because of the associated high mortality. The most efficient means of managing this life-threatening complication is prevention. Risk factors should be identified and considered during surgical planning. Flap coverage should be uniformly applied after right pneumonectomy. The use of muscle, pleural, or pericardial flap coverage also should be considered in patients with multiple risk factors.

The strategy for BPF management is greatly influenced by fistula size, time of development relative to the initial resection, availability of tissue for flap coverage, the presence of concomitant empyema, and overall patient condition. Regardless of the approach, certain principles should be adhered to during BPF management: (1) prompt antibiotic therapy; (2) early drainage; (3) infection control if empyema is present; (4) identification and closure of the BPF; (5) stump coverage after closure; and (6) obliteration of any residual space. Empyema and BPF are formidable entities that complicate thoracic surgery. Accurate diagnosis and organized treatment plans can manage these two processes successfully.

EDITOR'S COMMENT

The management of intrathoracic "space" problems has been discussed and debated since the 1920s. Partly because of the rigid thorax, resectional surgery often leaves a portion of the chest unoccupied by normal organs. The result may be impaired ventilatory mechanics, a prolonged air leak, or an empyema. Surgical techniques that limit the residual space are important to minimize, if not prevent, these potentially life-threatening complications.

—Steven J. Mentzer

References

1. Adams F. *The Genuine Works of Hippocrates*. Baltimore, MD: Williams & Wilkins; 1939.
2. Somers J, Faber L. Historical developments in the management of empyema. *Chest Surg Clin N Am*. 1996;6:403–418.
3. Graham E, Bell R. Open pneumothorax: its relation to the treatment of acute empyema. *Am J Med Sci*. 1918;156:839.
4. Eloesser L. An operation for tuberculous empyema. *Surg Gynecol Obstet*. 1935;60:1096.
5. Clagett OT, Geraci JE. A procedure for the management of postpneumonectomy empyema. *J Thorac Cardiovasc Surg*. 1963;45:141–145.
6. Anderson TM, Miller JI Jr. Use of pleura, azygos vein, pericardium, and muscle flaps in tracheobronchial surgery. *Ann Thorac Surg*. 1995;60:729–733.
7. Pairolero PC, Arnold PG, Piehler JM. Intrathoracic transposition of extrathoracic skeletal muscle. *J Thorac Cardiovasc Surg*. 1983;86:809–817.
8. Landreneau RJ, Keenan RJ, Hazelrigg SR, et al. Thoracoscopy for empyema and hemothorax. *Chest*. 1996;109:18–24.
9. Davies RJ, Traill ZC, Gleeson FV. Randomised, controlled trial of intrapleural streptokinase in community acquired pleural infection. *Thorax*. 1997;52:416–421.
10. Ali I, Unruh H. Management of empyema thoracis. *Ann Thorac Surg*. 1990;50:355–359.
11. Icard P, Fleury JP, Regnard JF, et al. Utility of C-reactive protein measurements for empyema diagnosis after pneumonectomy. *Ann Thorac Surg*. 1994;57:933–936.
12. Hsu JT, Bennett GM, Wolff E. Radiologic assessment of bronchopleural fistula with empyema. *Radiology*. 1972;103:41–45.
13. Friedman PJ, Hellekant CA. Radiologic recognition of bronchopleural fistula. *Radiology*. 1977;124:289–295.
14. Schachter EN, Kreisman H, Putman C. Diagnostic problems in suppurative lung disease. *Arch Intern Med*. 1976;136:167–171.
15. Yang PC, Luh KT, Chang DB, et al. Value of sonography in determining the nature of pleural effusion: analysis of 320 cases. *Am J Roentgenol*. 1992;159:29–33.
16. Wiederman H, Rice T. Lung abscess and empyema. *Semin Thorac Cardiovasc Surg*. 1988;96:436.
17. Stark DD, Federle MP, Goodman PC, et al. Differentiating lung abscess and empyema: radiography and computed tomography. *Am J Roentgenol*. 1983;141:163–167.
18. Light R, Girard WM, Jenkinson S. Parapneumonic effusions. *Am J Med*. 1980;69:507–512.
19. Angelillo Mackinlay TA, Lyons GA, Chimondeguy DJ, et al. VATS debridement versus thoracotomy in the treatment of loculated postpneumonia empyema. *Ann Thorac Surg*. 1996;61:1626–1630.
20. Thurer RJ. Decortication in thoracic empyema: indications and surgical technique. *Chest Surg Clin N Am*. 1996;6:461–490.
21. Cooper WA, Miller JI Jr. Management of bronchopleural fistula after lobectomy. *Semin Thorac Cardiovasc Surg*. 2001;13:8–12.
22. al-Kattan K, Goldstraw P. Completion pneumonectomy: indications and outcome. *J Thorac Cardiovasc Surg*. 1995;110:1125–1129.
23. Patel RL, Townsend ER, Fountain SW. Elective pneumonectomy: factors associated with morbidity and operative mortality. *Ann Thorac Surg*. 1992;54:84–88.
24. Wain JC. Management of late postpneumonectomy empyema and bronchopleural fistula. *Chest Surg Clin N Am*. 1996;6:529–541.
25. Thourani VH, Lancaster RT, Mansour KA, et al. Twenty-six years of experience with the modified Eloesser flap. *Ann Thorac Surg*. 2003;76:401–405; discussion 405–406.
26. Miller JI, Mansour KA, Nahai F, et al. Single-stage complete muscle flap closure of the postpneumonectomy empyema space: a new method and possible solution to a disturbing complication. *Ann Thorac Surg*. 1984;38:227–231.
27. World Health Organization. *Global Tuberculosis Control*. Geneva: WHO; 2001.
28. Centers for Disease Control and Prevention. Tuberculosis morbidity—United States, 1992. *Morb Mortal Wkly Rep*. 1993;42:696–697, 703–704.
29. Centers for Disease Control and Prevention. Tuberculosis morbidity in the United States: final data, 1990. *Morb Mortal Wkly Rep CDC Surveill Summ*. 1990;40:23–27.
30. Pomerantz M, Madsen L, Goble M, et al. Surgical management of resistant mycobacterial tuberculosis and other mycobacterial pulmonary infections. *Ann Thorac Surg*. 1991;52:1108–1111; discussion 1112.
31. Treasure RL, Seaworth BJ. Current role of surgery in *Mycobacterium tuberculosis*. *Ann Thorac Surg*. 1995;59:1405–1407; discussion 1408–1409.
32. Garcia-Yuste M, Ramos G, Duque JL, et al. Open-window thoracostomy and thoracomyoplasty to manage chronic pleural empyema. *Ann Thorac Surg*. 1998;65:818–822.
33. Levinson GM, Pennington DW. Intrapleural fibrinolytics combined with image-guided chest tube drainage for pleural infection. *Mayo Clin Proc*. 2007;82:407–413.
34. Ben-Or S, Feins RH, Veeramachaneni NK, et al. Effectiveness and risks associated with intrapleural alteplase by means of tube thoracostomy. *Ann Thorac Surg*. 2011;91:860–863.
35. Thommi G, Shehan JC, Robison KL, et al. A double blind randomized cross over trial comparing rate of decortication and efficacy of intrapleural instillation of alteplase vs placebo in patients with empyemas and complicated parapneumonic effusions. *Respir Med*. 2012;106:716–723.
36. Asamura H, Naruke T, Tsuchiya R, et al. Bronchopleural fistulas associated with lung cancer operations: univariate and multivariate analysis of risk factors, management, and outcome. *J Thorac Cardiovasc Surg*. 1992;104:1456–1464.
37. Vester SR, Faber LP, Kittle CF, et al. Bronchopleural fistula after stapled closure of bronchus. *Ann Thorac Surg*. 1991;52:1253–1257; discussion 1257–1258.
38. al-Kattan K, Cattelani L, Goldstraw P. Bronchopleural fistula after pneumonectomy for lung cancer. *Eur J Cardiothorac Surg*. 1995;9:479–482.
39. Bonomi P, Faber L, Warren W, et al. Postoperative bronchopulmonary complications in stage III lung cancer patients treated with preoperative paclitazel-containing chemotherapy and concurrent radiation. *Semin Oncol*. 1997;24:S12-123–S12-129.
40. Cerfolio R. The incidence, etiology, and prevention of postresectional bronchopleural fistula. *Semin Thorac Cardiovasc Surg*. 2001;13:3–7.
41. Deschamps C, Allen M, Miller D, et al. Management of postpneumonectomy empyema and bronchopleural fistula. *Semin Thorac Cardiovasc Surg*. 2001;13:13–19.
42. Wright CD, Wain JC, Mathisen DJ, et al. Postpneumonectomy bronchopleural fistula after sutured bronchial closure: incidence, risk factors, and management. *J Thorac Cardiovasc Surg*. 1996;112:1367–1371.

43. Padhi R, Lynn R. The management of bronchopleural fistulas. *J Thorac Cardiovasc Surg.* 1960;39:385–393.
44. Ginsberg R, Saborio D. Management of the recalcitrant postpneumonectomy bronchopleural fistula: the transsternal transpericardial approach. *Semin Thorac Cardiovasc Surg.* 2001;13:20–26.
45. Lin J, Iannettoni MD. Closure of bronchopleural fistulas using albumin-glutaraldehyde tissue adhesive. *Ann Thorac Surg.* 2004;77:326–328.
46. Hollaus PH, Lax F, Janakiev D, et al. Endoscopic treatment of postoperative bronchopleural fistula: experience with 45 cases. *Ann Thorac Surg.* 1998;66:923–927.
47. Han X, Wu G, Li Y, et al. A novel approach: treatment of bronchial stump fistula with a plugged, bullet-shaped, angled stent. *Ann Thorac Surg.* 2006;81:1867–1871.
48. Dutau H, Breen DP, Gomez C, et al. The integrated place of tracheobronchial stents in the multidisciplinary management of large post-pneumonectomy fistulas: our experience using a novel customised conical self-expandable metallic stent. *Eur J Cardiothorac Surg.* 2011;39:185–189.
49. Thommi G, Nair CK, Aronow WS, et al. Efficacy and safety of intrapleural instillation of alteplase in the management of complicated pleural effusion or empyema. *Am J Ther.* 2007;14:341–345.

PART 19

LUNG TRANSPLANTATION

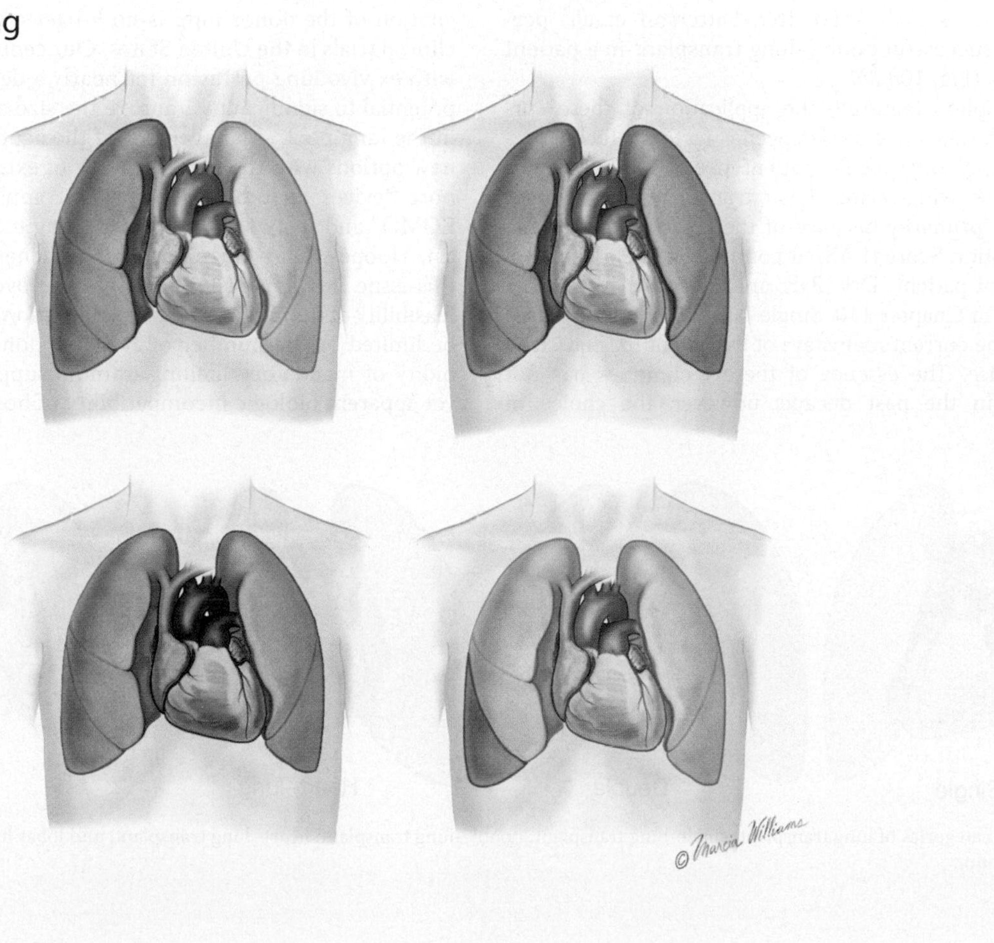

108 Overview of Lung Transplantation with Anatomy and Pathophysiology

Phillip C. Camp, Jr. and Steven J. Mentzer

Keywords: Single-lung transplant, double-lung transplant, heart–lung transplant, end-stage pulmonary disease, idiopathic pulmonary fibrosis, emphysema, chronic obstructive pulmonary disease (COPD), bronchiectasis, α_1-antitrypsin deficiency, bronchiolitis obliterans, primary pulmonary hypertension, cytomegalovirus (CMV), cadaver donor organ, living-related donor organ, artificial lung and mechanical support, living lobar transplant

While there are numerous challenges that face the recipient and practitioner, the field of lung transplantation continues to improve and expand with technical, immunological, and donor-related advancements. The utility of thoracic organ transplantation for end-stage lung disease was not meaningfully realized until the development of cyclosporine in the 1980s. In the preceding decades (1963–1983), fewer than 50 lung transplants were performed worldwide, and no recipient survived for more than 10 months. Early lung transplants failed for four principal reasons: nonfunction of the primary graft, dehiscence of the bronchial anastomosis, acute lung rejection, and pneumonia. Developments in surgical technique, perioperative care, and immunosuppressive drugs culminated in the first successful long-term lung transplant, performed in 1983 in a patient with idiopathic pulmonary fibrosis.[1] The technical highlights of this operation included the concept of using an omental wrap around the bronchial anastomosis to restore bronchial artery circulation and prevent dehiscence, careful patient selection, and effective long-term immunosuppression with cyclosporine. Shortly thereafter, Patterson et al.[2] performed the first successful double-lung transplant in a patient with emphysema (Fig. 108-1).

As the discipline matured, the application of these surgeries changed based on disease-specific factors. Techniques were derived based on specific patient needs as the science progressed. While living-related lobar transplant is no longer in high demand, primarily because of the creation of the current Lung Allocation Score (LAS), it continues to be a vital tool for the occasional patient. Drs. Barr and Starnes have further defined this role in Chapter 110. Single- and double-lung transplantations are the current mainstays of treatment for end-stage pulmonary disease. The essence of these techniques has not changed much in the past decade; however, the choice of operation, sidedness, and advancements are discussed in detail by Drs. Bharat and Patterson in Chapter 109. Combined heart–bilateral lung transplantation for multiple-organ failure in patients with primary pulmonary disease was once a more common surgery until it was observed that transplanting lungs earlier rather than later in these patients could prevent cardiac failure.

The advent of better therapies for pulmonary hypertension, closer monitoring of right heart function, and a better understanding of secondary pulmonary hypertension have had a significant impact on the need for combined heart–lung transplant. Heart–bilateral lung transplantation is now reserved for patients with other coexisting primary pulmonary and cardiac diseases, primarily of a congenital nature. The number of heart–lung transplantation procedures has declined over the years; however, new indications continue to arise for selected patients.

Some of the most exciting areas of advancement are in the mechanical means of supporting both the recipient and the donor lung, as well as a heightened awareness of the immunology of the lung transplant patient. Ex vivo evaluation and resuscitation of the donor lung is no longer a dream and is in full clinical trials in the United States. Our center has been working with ex vivo lung perfusion for nearly a decade, which has the potential to significantly improve the size of acceptable donors in the lung pool.[3] Management of the acutely ill candidate has new options with the expanded use of extracorporeal life support devices including the practical application of "walking ECMO" and the work on artificial lung technology. Drs. Martin, Hoopes, Diaz-Guzman, and Zwischenberger help define this issue in Chapter 113. Despite the overall and improving feasibility of thoracic organ transplantation, its use continues to be limited by the number of available donor organs, the morbidity of mandatory lifelong immunosuppression, and the as yet apparent biologic incompatibility of host and allograft.

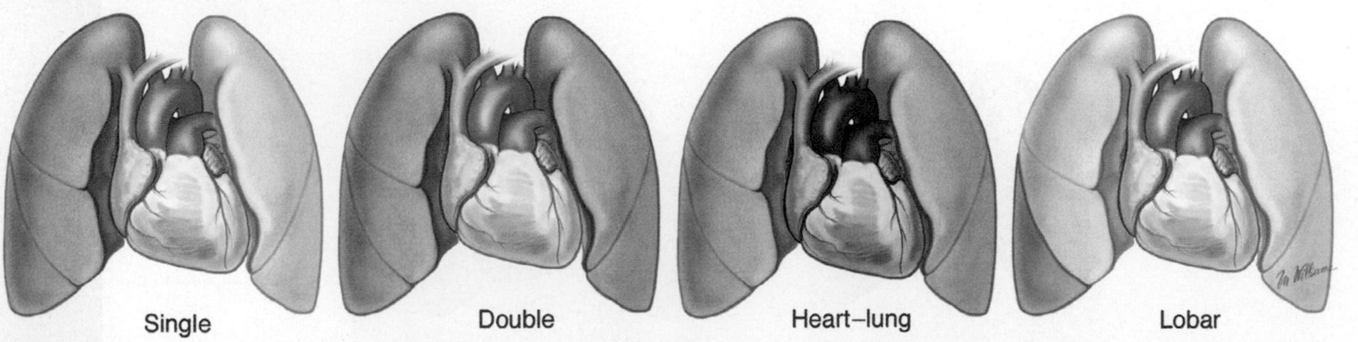

Figure 108-1. Four categories of lung transplant: single-lung transplant, double-lung transplant, heart–lung transplant, and lobar lung transplant including the living-related donor.

ANATOMY AND PHYSIOLOGY

Lung transplantation entails the replacement of a native diseased lung with a cadaver lung (see Chapter 109) or lobar transplant from a living-related donor(s) (see Chapter 110). All adult lung transplants are orthotopic procedures. For most septic diseases and certain pulmonary hypertensive disorders, the extent of disease mandates a bilateral lung transplant. In 2004, 1188 lung transplants were performed in the United States. With improved techniques and improved donor management that number had increased to 1830 for the year ending 2011. While the number of double-lung transplants was virtually equal to single-lung transplants in 2000, it has continued to increase annually and now is double the rate of single-lung transplant.[4,5] Single- and bilateral lung transplants now account for 29.9% (548) and 70.1% (1282) of the total number of transplants, respectively. During this same interval, heart–bilateral lung transplants numbers dropped from 31 to 17 with a peak of 41 in 2010.[4,5]

Lung transplantation surgery involves three major anastomoses: (1) bronchial, (2) pulmonary artery, and (3) atrial. The bronchial anastomosis is associated with the highest complication rate (3%–6%)[6] compared with atrial and arterial anastomoses (<1%). Complications of bronchial anastomosis include dehiscence and stricture. If there is breakdown of the anastomosis, it usually occurs within several weeks of transplantation. Airway obstruction secondary to stricture or malacia manifests within several months. A common area for additional stricture is the postanastomotic donor bronchus. The tissue here is relatively ischemic and remains so for several weeks. Short donor bronchi and overlapping donor/recipient bronchi are techniques used to lessen this area of ischemic injury.

It is interesting to note that certain pulmonary structures (e.g., bronchial and lymphatic vessels) are not routinely reanastomosed after implantation. The bronchial circulation has marked interconnections with the pulmonary arterial circulation.[7] These interconnections result in modest retrograde perfusion of most of the major portions of the airway, with the exception of a "watershed" region in the mid-mainstem bronchus (proximal donor). Attempts to reanastomose the bronchial circulation are technically feasible but have not demonstrated a significant clinical benefit if the watershed region in the mid-mainstem bronchus is excised.[8] No significant difference has been demonstrated in airway healing with intact versus divided bronchial circulation. Similarly, there is no significant difference in the frequency of chronic rejection (bronchiolitis obliterans).

Division of the pulmonary lymphatics does have significance for early posttransplant management. In the normal lung, Starling forces cause 2% of the pulmonary blood flow to be filtered in excess of reabsorption. This excess fluid volume typically is drained by the pulmonary lymphatic system. After lung transplantation, this excess fluid can lead to progressive pulmonary edema, which degrades graft function and must be managed properly. The initial stages of submucosal lymphatic regeneration are not detected until approximately 3 weeks after transplantation.

PRINCIPLES OF TRANSPLANTATION

Immunosuppression

The lung is a mediator of many immunologic processes, serving as an interface between the exogenous and endogenous environments. Consequently, lung transplant patients have required higher levels of immunosuppression than recipients of kidney, heart, or liver. The immunosuppression strategy can be conceptualized as two overlapping phases: (1) induction and (2) maintenance. While there are some variations in the medications used at different lung transplant programs, the approach to immunosuppression is fairly similar. The general concepts are discussed here but are better defined in Chapter 111 by Drs. Goldberg and Camp.

The goal of induction therapy in lung transplantation is to deplete or inactivate the host T cells. The original goal of early aggressive immunosuppression was simply to induce a state of immunologic unresponsiveness or tolerance. In most cases, polyclonal antibodies (e.g., antilymphocyte globulin and antithymocyte globulin) or monoclonal antibodies (e.g., anti-CD3, OKT3, and anti-interleukin 2 receptor) were used to inactivate (or bind) T-lymphocyte antigens. The ability of induction agents to achieve immunologic unresponsiveness, however, proved to be very disappointing. Nonetheless, there remains a practical use for induction therapy in lung transplantation. Because the lungs are relatively edematous after transplantation, aggressive diuresis is commonly used in the postoperative lung transplant recipient to maintain effective gas exchange. In this setting, induction therapy permits potentially nephrotoxic maintenance therapies, such as cyclosporine or tacrolimus, to be minimized during the first postoperative week. Further, during this time following ischemic insult to the donor lungs, the ability of the immune system to multiply the inflammatory result is blunted.

The general approach to maintenance immunosuppression is based on a multiagent regimen composed of calcineurin inhibitors (e.g., cyclosporin A or tacrolimus), cell cycle inhibitors (e.g., azathioprine or mycophenolate), and steroids (Table 108-1). The regimen generally is started at a relatively high dose and tapered over the first 3 months after transplantation. The rate at which the dose of maintenance therapy is tapered depends on the presence and severity of acute rejection episodes experienced by the patient.

Table 108-1

IMMUNOSUPPRESSIVE AGENTS

- Cyclosporin A (CSA) and its intracellular receptor form a complex that binds and inhibits calcineurin. Calcineurin is a component of the lymphocyte signal transduction pathway that regulates interleukin 2 expression. The starting dose is 8 mg/kg/day in two divided doses.
- Tacrolimus (FK-506) is a macrolide compound with a mechanism of action similar to CSA. FK-506 is given intravenously with dosing adjusted to blood levels. Toxicity includes reversible renal dysfunction, hypertension, and neurotoxicity.
- Azathioprine is a purine analog that is converted to several active metabolites, including 6-mercaptopurine. These metabolites inhibit lymphocyte proliferation. Azathioprine is started at a dose of 2 to 2.5 mg/kg/day, and the dose is adjusted to maintain a total white blood cell count of 4000 cells/mm^3.
- Mycophenolate mofetil (MMF) blocks de novo purine synthesis. MMF selectively inhibits lymphocyte proliferation because lymphocytes, in contrast to other cells that use salvage pathways, use only the de novo pathway in purine biosynthesis. MMF is usually given at 1 g PO bid, and the dose is titrated to a white blood cell count greater than 4000 cells/mm^3.
- Corticosteroids have a variety of immunosuppressive effects that are not well understood. Methylprednisolone, prednisolone, and prednisone are all used for transplant immunosuppression.

Table 108-2

REVISED WORKING FORMULATION FOR HISTOPATHOLOGIC CLASSIFICATION AND GRADING OF PULMONARY ALLOGRAFT REJECTION

A:	Acute rejection Grade 0—none Grade 1—minimal Grade 2—mild Grade 3—moderate Grade 4—severe
B:	Airway inflammation Grade 0—none Grade 1R—low grade Grade 2R—high grade Grade X—ungradeable
C:	Chronic airway rejection—obliterative bronchiolitis 0—absent 1—present
D:	Chronic vascular rejection—accelerated graft vascular sclerosis

Note: "R" denotes revised grade to avoid confusion with 1996 scheme.
From Pettersson G, Norgaard MA, Arendrup H, et al. Direct bronchial artery revascularization and en bloc double lung transplantation: Surgical techniques and early outcome. *J Heart Lung Transplant.* 1997;16:320–333.

Acute rejection generally is treated with high-dose steroids. A typical episode of acute rejection is treated with 1 g/day of IV steroids (Solu-Medrol) × 3 doses, followed by a modest taper of oral prednisone to baseline levels.

Acute Rejection

The immune-mediated destruction of the transplanted lung occurs both acutely and chronically. Acute rejection in the lung is often characterized by hypoxemia, fever, and radiographic infiltrates. The presentation of acute rejection can be virtually indistinguishable from acute infection. In contrast, chronic rejection is associated with a slow and progressive decline in pulmonary function.

Acute rejection is an inflammatory reaction initially confined to the perivascular zones. Untreated, the acute rejection will progress to involve not only blood vessels but also airways and interstitium. This pathophysiologic process is reflected in the generally accepted classification of lung allograft rejection (Table 108-2).[9]

Because the signs and symptoms of acute rejection are nonspecific, the diagnosis is often triggered by clinical suspicion and requires histologic confirmation. Many transplant teams use surveillance bronchoscopy, bronchoalveolar lavage, and transbronchial biopsy to evaluate the lung parenchyma and environment. In addition to signs of acute rejection, the lung tissue is evaluated for other sources of inflammation. For example, cytologic inclusion bodies suggest a viral infection, polymorphonuclear leukocytes indicate a possible bacterial infection, and necrosis or hyphae are suggestive of fungal infection.

What has become clear in the past 5 to 10 years is the fact that acute rejection is a much more complex and diverse set of immunologic processes that are both cellular and noncellular mediated and are poorly understood. The recognition of subtle states of rejection has become a very hotly debated topic and which therapeutic modalities, and when, are not yet clearly understood. This topic is of keen interest as there are strong associations between the number and severity of acute rejection episodes, and the development of bronchiolitis obliterans syndrome (BOS) (see below), the common pathologic endpoint of chronic rejection. Early use of newer therapies beyond pulsed doses of maintenance medications

Table 108-3

BOS CLASSIFICATION SYSTEM: 2002

BOS 0	FEV_1 >90% of baseline and $FEF_{25\%-75\%}$ >75% of baseline
BOS 0p	FEV_1 81%–90% of baseline and/or $FEF_{25\%-75\%}$ ≤75% of baseline
BOS 1	FEV_1 66%–80% of baseline
BOS 2	FEV_1 51%–65% of baseline
BOS 3	FEV_1 ≤50% of baseline

Adapted from Estenne M, Maurer JR, Boehler A, et al. Bronchiolitis obliterans syndrome 2001: An update of the diagnostic criteria. *J Heart Lung Transplant.* 2002;21:297–310.

are more commonly used including targeted immunolytic therapies (Antithymocyte, anti-IL2 receptor, anti-CD3), and extracorporeal photopheresis (ECP) to name a few.

Chronic Rejection

Ongoing immune destruction of the lung leads to scarring of the terminal airways, a process known as *bronchiolitis obliterans.* This end-stage process is characterized by the presence of intraluminal polypoid plugs of granulation tissue in the terminal and respiratory bronchioles that cause partial or total obliteration of the lumen of the airway. BOS is the irreversible and final common pathway of a number of lung diseases.

Chronic airway inflammation may be owing to a combination of effects. In some cases, the acute rejection is superimposed on an underlying bronchiolitis obliterans. The ongoing destruction of the airways promotes frequent colonization by bacteria and fungi, and thus a component of inflammatory response actually may reflect infection.

Confirmation of BOS by histologic examination of a transbronchial biopsy is relatively insensitive (60%). However, the histologic severity of bronchiolitis obliterans correlates strongly with airflow obstruction measured by spirometry. Hence the classification system for BOS is based on spirometry (Table 108-3).[10] Patients with bronchiolitis obliterans have a characteristic "scooped" expiratory flow histogram with a marked absolute reduction in forced expiratory volume in 1 second (FEV_1) (Fig. 108-2). Chest radiographs may show hyperinflation secondary to chronic small airway obstruction (Fig. 108-3), and CT scan can show signs of delay in airspace emptying.

Approximately one-third of patients develop histologic evidence of bronchiolitis obliterans within 12 months of lung

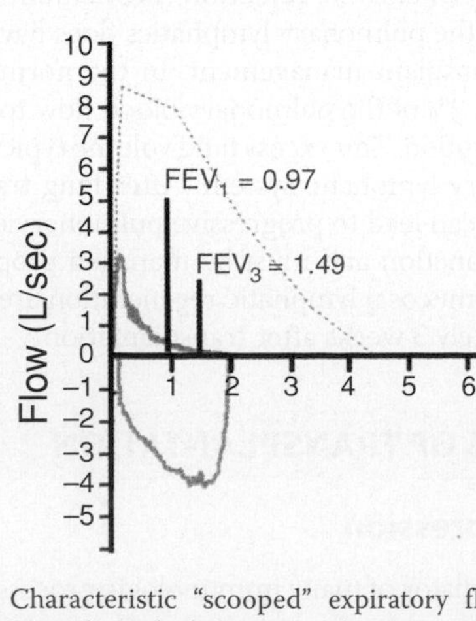

Figure 108-2. Characteristic "scooped" expiratory flow histogram of patients with BOS, with marked absolute reduction in FEV_1.

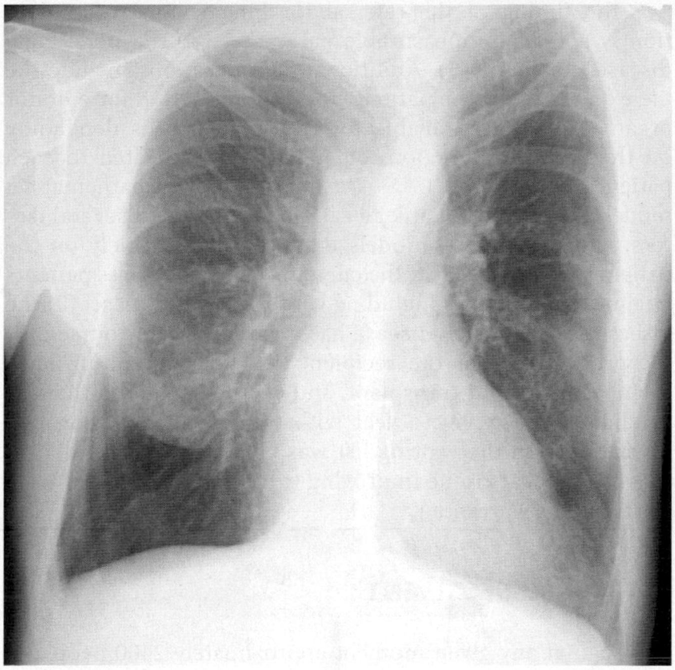

Figure 108-3. Chest radiograph demonstrating hyperinflation secondary to chronic small airway obstruction.

transplant. Although the coincidence of bronchiolitis and chronic infection complicates the analysis, approximately two-thirds of patients ultimately experience a progressive and unrelenting loss of pulmonary function owing to chronic rejection. Multiple therapies are used to arrest or slow this process with varied success. Bronchiolitis obliterans remains the primary obstacle to widespread long-term graft function and survival.

INDICATIONS AND RESULTS

The transplant experience varies depending on approach (single vs. double, heart vs. bilateral lung, cadaver vs. living donor), makeup of the regional transplant recipient/donor pool, and preference and expertise of a particular transplant team. Excellent results can be achieved with differing surgical philosophies, and it can be informative to compare the experience of divergent centers.

The indications for lung transplantation include pulmonary diseases that affect the host lung but will not recur in the transplanted lung. Worldwide, nearly 85% of current candidates for lung transplant have emphysema-related diseases, cystic fibrosis, idiopathic pulmonary fibrosis, or pulmonary hypertension (Fig. 108-4).

The contraindications to lung transplantation include coexisting uncorrectable cardiac disease or other significant extrapulmonary organ dysfunction. Other absolute contraindications for lung transplantation include an active malignancy, HIV infection, hepatitis B antigen positivity, and hepatitis C with histologic evidence of active disease. Patients with active substance abuse, including current smokers, are also contraindicated for lung transplantation.

Relative contraindications to lung transplantation include poor nutritional status (body mass index <17.0 or >35.0), symptomatic osteoporosis, continuous high-dose prednisone, and colonization with panresistant bacteria, fungus, or atypical mycobacteria. Other relative contraindications include the requirement for invasive ventilation as well as psychosocial problems likely to increase postoperative mortality.[11]

Surgical contraindications include the relative concerns related to hemorrhage on cardiopulmonary bypass (CPB) and healing of the airway anastomosis. Patients requiring CPB who have obliterative pleural disease, mediastinal fibrosis, or calcific atria face a markedly elevated risk of perioperative hemorrhage. Patients with a history of mediastinal irradiation may have an increased risk of postoperative airway dehiscence. Right ventricular dysfunction is a relative contraindication to lung transplantation. Pasque and colleagues have shown, however, that some patients with early right-sided heart failure experience improved right ventricular function after transplant.[12] The aforementioned factors are applicable to all transplants, whether the donor organ is from a cadaver or from a living-related donor. Indications unique to the living-related donor are discussed in Chapter 110.

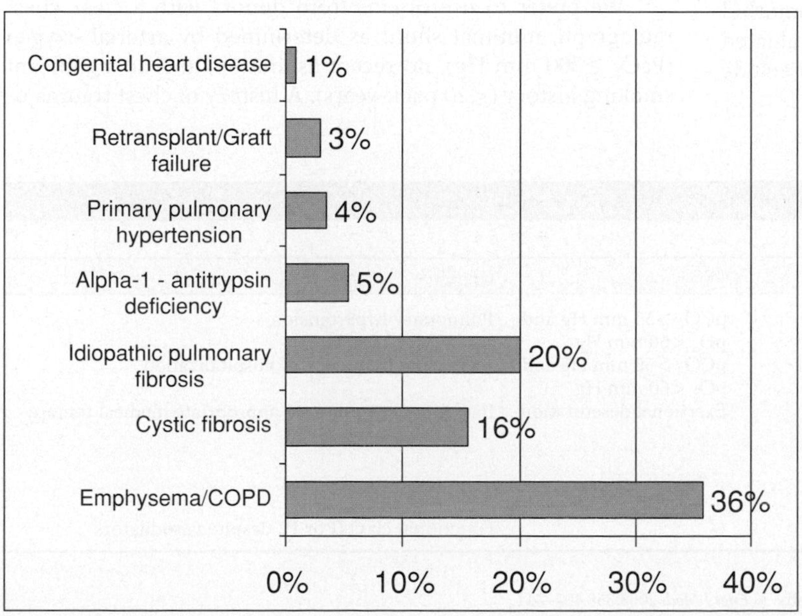

Figure 108-4. Pulmonary diseases treated with either single- or double-lung transplantation worldwide. *(UNOS/ISHLT data as of September 24, 2004.)*

Table 108-4

RECIPIENT SURVIVAL AFTER LUNG TRANSPLANTATION

DISEASE	RECIPIENT SURVIVAL 1 YEAR (%)	3 YEARS (%)
Primary pulmonary hypertension	74.2	59.9
Cystic fibrosis	82.0	64.7
Idiopathic pulmonary fibrosis	71.2	55.9
α_1-Antitrypsin deficiency	73.5	60.3
Emphysema/COPD	83.7	65.2

Note: Survival rates for transplants performed between April 1, 1999 and March 31, 2003 in North America. Based on UNOS/ISHLT data as of September 24, 2004.

In the past 15 years, the 1-year lung transplant survival rate has increased from approximately 70% to 85% as a result of improvements in donor management, airway anastomotic technique, and perioperative recipient management (Table 108-4).[4,5] In contrast, mortality rates after 1 year have remained largely unchanged. These results suggest that the major challenge in lung transplantation is the issue of biologic incompatibility between the donor and recipient and the persistent effect of inflammation in its many forms.

In the first year after lung transplantation, infections are the leading cause of death. Recipients are at high risk for bacterial, fungal, viral, and protozoan infections. Acute infection is rarely seen after the first year. The cause of death after the first year is frequently coexisting chronic rejection (i.e., BOS), infection, and other comorbid diseases.

The functional consequences of lung transplantation vary with the underlying recipient disease and disability. Roughly 80% of patients, however, are able to resume an active lifestyle, including returning to work, and 90% report improved quality of life.

PREPROCEDURE ASSESSMENT

Most patients referred for lung transplantation are younger than 55 to 60 years of age. While age, per se, is not a prognostic factor, it is associated with a rising incidence of comorbid disease. As age advances, recipients are meticulously evaluated to rule out conditions that in and of themselves may preclude transplantation.

The timing of the referral for lung transplant evaluation is guided by measurable parameters of the underlying disease (Table 108-5). Additional considerations include the life expectancy of the patient. The waiting period for a donor organ to become available for transplant varies depending on the geographic region, but it is directly related to each patient's LAS.[4,5] The LAS is a fairly complex mathematical model that is used to rank all candidates based on several factors. Unlike previous models that were based solely on the patient's time on the list, the current model compares patients by numerous factors, including (1) severity of disease, (2) the disease process (each disease has a variable time course), (3) the probability that the recipient will not survive an additional year without transplant, and (4) the likelihood that the candidate will survive a year with transplant. The mortality for patients on the waiting list was once approximately 15%. The LAS appears to be improving this process, but long-term evaluation is warranted.

DONOR ASSESSMENT

Although at any given moment approximately 2400 people in this country are actively waiting for a suitable donor organ, only 7% to 22% of multiorgan donors are suitable for lung donation.[13] In many instances, the donor has been compromised by chest trauma, aspiration pneumonia, ventilator-associated pneumonia, or their own native lung disease. There is hope that ex vivo lung perfusion techniques will be able to help evaluate or resuscitate many currently unusable lungs to improve this very low conversion rate.

Potential recipients for a donor lung are identified initially by ABO blood group compatibility. The size of the donor lungs is estimated using standard reference values derived from age, gender, race, and height.[14] Potential recipient–donor matches should be within 15% to 20% of estimated lung volumes. Donor lungs that are larger, particularly in the setting of double-lung transplantation, may result in cardiac compression with chest closure. Small lungs can function in a larger recipient. Size mismatch is avoided because it disproportionately disadvantages smaller recipients.

We prefer to use organs from donors with a clear chest radiograph, minimal shunt as determined by arterial oxygen (PaO_2 ≥300 mm Hg), no recent aspiration, and no significant smoking history (<20 pack-years). A history of chest trauma or

Table 108-5

GUIDELINES FOR LUNG TRANSPLANT REFERRAL

DISEASE	PULMONARY FUNCTION	ABGS	OTHER
Emphysema	FEV_1 <25% predicted	pCO_2 >55 mm Hg and pO_2 <60 mm Hg	Pulmonary hypertension
Cystic fibrosis	FEV_1 <30% predicted	pCO_2 >55 mm Hg and pO_2 <60 mm Hg	Increasing frequency of hospitalization
IPF	FVC <60% predicted DLCO <60% predicted 10% or greater decrement in FVC or DLCO during 6 months of follow-up	Exertional desaturation	Inadequate response to appropriate medical therapy
Pulmonary hypertension	—	—	Functional class II or IV despite vasodilators

ABG, arterial blood gas; IPF, idiopathic pulmonary fibrosis.
From Starzl T. Immunosuppressive therapy and tolerance of organ allografts. *N Engl J Med.* 2008;358:407–411.

purulent sputum suggests the utility of bronchoscopy to evaluate the airways for blood or evidence of established infection. However, there is a growing movement nationally to extend the criteria for donor acceptability in part because of the dramatic shortage of usable donor lungs. This is a point of considerable academic debate, and the definition of *suitable* will be in flux for some time to come.

It is important to obtain microbiologic cultures of the donor airway to focus the early antibiotic therapy. Prolonged antibiotic use in the setting of aggressive immunosuppression can give rise to opportunistic infections in the early postoperative course.

Donor viral serology is also important for perioperative management. Most transplant programs exclude donors with positive hepatitis C serology because of the risk of hepatitis transmission. In contrast, many donors are CMV positive. CMV causes a complex bidirectional interaction between the donor lung and the recipient. CMV has been associated with acute viral pneumonitis as well as both acute and chronic rejection.[15] When both the donor and recipient are CMV negative, survival is better than any other serologic combination.[4,5] Finally, Epstein–Barr virus (EBV) serology is relevant to later recipient management. EBV-positive donor lungs in an EBV-negative recipient confer a greater risk for posttransplant lymphoproliferative disorders (PTLDs). Each center has a preferred approach to donor assessment. Special considerations apply to the living-related donor and/or heart–bilateral lung cadaver, and these are reviewed in Chapters 109 and 110.

TECHNIQUE

At Brigham and Women's Hospital, we use a standard posterolateral thoracotomy incision placed in the fifth intercostal space for single-lung transplantation. Double or bilateral sequential lung transplants can be performed through a median sternotomy; however, we typically use a transverse thoracotomy. Double-lung transplants generally require CPB to ensure adequate exposure to the left hilum. Techniques for exposure (e.g., bilateral, anterolateral, and clamshell) and preoperative preparation are described in Chapters 109 and 110.

The most important technical aspect of the bronchial anastomosis is the resection of the ischemic portion of the mainstem bronchus. The recipient bronchus is divided at the level of the mediastinal pleura, and the donor bronchus is transected no more than two cartilaginous rings proximal to the lobar carina. If the ischemic mainstem bronchus is resected, the anastomosis should heal properly, regardless of whether a telescoping or end-to-end suture technique is used.

We use a running monofilament suture along the membranous airway to create the bronchial anastomosis. The membranous bronchus is well perfused and is rarely a site of dehiscence or stricture unless there is undue tension of the membranous portion. The tissue is quite thin, and overt tension or poor tissue overlap may place this area at increased risk. In contrast, the medial cartilaginous–membranous junction is the region of airway located farthest from the retrograde pulmonary blood flow and the most likely site of anastomotic separation. Consequently, in this region we use an invaginating or evaginating monofilament mattress suture. Traditionally, the donor bronchus is invaginated into the recipient bronchus. We have recently begun to place the smaller bronchus into the larger bronchus based on best size matching. The technique allows for the least amount of airway narrowing and in the setting of recipient within donor excludes the most ischemic airway outside the well-perfused recipient stump. Our suture technique facilitates (1) a telescoping anastomosis, (2) accommodation of size mismatch, and (3) tight apposition at the area of greatest risk. The anastomosis at the cartilaginous rings generally heals well. We use interrupted absorbable sutures or a continuation of the running monofilament mattress suture.

The completed anastomosis should be airtight. Most patients will require mechanical ventilation for hours to days postoperatively. In addition to complicating the ventilatory management, an anastomotic air leak will contribute to the risk of pleural space infection.

Because of the potential for anastomotic dehiscence, periairway abscess, and the risk of bronchovascular fistula, we recommend interposing donor pericardium, intercostal muscle pedicle, or other vascularized tissue between the pulmonary artery and the bronchial anastomosis. Typically, adequate donor pericardium can be mobilized so that not only are the structures separated, but the bronchial stump also can be wrapped circumferentially.

Mucociliary clearance is impaired in lung transplant patients. Turbulent airflow at the anastomotic transition and mucociliary impairment are among the many potential explanations. To minimize the contribution of suture material to impaired clearance, we ensure that no knots are placed on the intraluminal side of the anastomosis.

The pulmonary artery anastomosis generally is performed using running monofilament suture (e.g., 5-0). The technical issue is to avoid "purse stringing" of the anastomosis. This is typically associated with a large size mismatch, as seen in patients with pulmonary hypertension. Rarely, if the lung donor artery is left too long, it will lead to kinking of the intrapleural portion of the artery. Careful attention to this detail is critical.

The venous anastomosis is constructed last and is more prone to technical complications than the pulmonary artery anastomosis. A short donor atrial cuff and a large size mismatch can lead to torsion-related obstruction of the segmental pulmonary veins. When the atrial anastomosis is even slightly rotated relative to venous inflow, it can lead to increased resistance at the orifice of the pulmonary veins. Even a gradient difficult to quantify by transesophageal echocardiogram can lead to pulmonary edema. Since many patients develop pulmonary edema independent of the atrial anastomotic technique, the surgeon must be confident of the atrial anastomosis before leaving the OR.

As a rule, pulmonary edema that develops in the OR is related to a technical complication. Pulmonary edema that develops 4 hours after the operation generally is attributable to an implantation response. Two aspects of our program to lower the incidence of this lung reperfusion injury are initiation of induction therapy prior to beginning the implantation and controlled perfusion of the first lung during a double-lung transplant, which may help lessen the tissue injury during and following the technical aspects of the implant. Alternative techniques for exposure, bronchial anastomosis, atrial anastomosis, and pulmonary anastomosis are discussed in Chapters 109 and 110.

PERIOPERATIVE MANAGEMENT

The incidence of early graft failure has declined steadily since the first successful long-term lung transplant in 1983.[16] Although many factors likely contribute to this trend, an important element is management of the donor lung. Prior to procurement, the lungs are treated with a pulse of system steroids and 500 μg of prostaglandin just preceding the flush with the chosen perfusate. Donor lungs are routinely anterograde and retrograde flushed in situ to eliminate neutrophils (a source of oxygen-free radicals and inflammatory mediators) and debris, including subclinical pulmonary emboli, fat emboli, and poorly flushed blood. The lungs are inflated with 100% oxygen and stored at 4°C to minimize ischemic injury. Ischemic time has been linked directly to outcome. Hence highly coordinated communication with all surgical teams and transporting agencies minimizes ischemic time and lowers the risk for ischemia–reperfusion injury.

Another trend is the increasing use of CPB during double-lung transplantation. The use of CPB serves three major purposes. It may minimize reperfusion pulmonary edema, which occurs commonly in the first implanted lung during a sequential transplant. Although the etiology is unclear, progressive pulmonary edema occurs in approximately 20% of patients after lung transplantation. This is commonly referred to as the *implantation response,* and patients generally are responsive to diuretics, with the condition resolving within the first 48 to 72 hours.[17] The implantation response can be life-threatening when the pulmonary edema and associated hypoxic vasoconstriction lead to right ventricular dysfunction. Once right-sided heart failure occurs, treatment is limited to extracorporeal membrane oxygenation. The secondary advantage of CPB is time. Patients undergoing lung transplant are often fairly unstable and tolerate manipulation poorly. Initiation of CPB permits maintenance of stable oxygenation and perfusion while allowing for efficient surgical implantation. Third, the maintenance of stable perfusion pressure and metabolite delivery helps to ensure that secondary organ function is preserved, which may improve the stability of the posttransplant course.

Posttransplant pulmonary edema can progress rapidly over the first 4 hours. At Brigham and Women's Hospital, to minimize transplant pulmonary edema, we use aggressive diuretic therapy in the first several hours in the setting of increased filling pressures, poor oxygenation, or evidence of early pulmonary dysfunction, such as ischemia–reperfusion injury. The severity of the implantation response is assessed empirically.

Although nitric oxide (NO) has been used widely in most adult patients, the results have been somewhat disappointing if not inconsistent. The initial use of prophylactic NO to lower the incidence of ischemia–reperfusion injury has not demonstrated a predictable result and often delays the time to initial extubation. However, the postoperative pulmonary hypertension and hypoxemia, when observed in lung transplant recipients, can be ameliorated with NO-mediated treatments, and this should be considered in that clinical setting. The current cost of inhaled NO is very substantial so the use of inhaled prostaglandins has been successfully introduced with a lower cost for the same effect.

Mechanical ventilation is minimized to improve airway clearance and reduce the risk of ventilator-associated pneumonia. Mechanical ventilation is a particular challenge in patients undergoing single-lung transplantation for emphysema. The hypercompliant native lung and the relatively noncompliant transplanted lung yield two distinct mechanical compartments. In this setting, mechanical ventilation may result in hyperinflation of the native lung with suboptimal distending pressures of the transplanted lung. While using a double-lumen tube with two different ventilation pressures is appealing conceptually, it is difficult in practice. The differential mechanical ventilation is hard to synchronize, the double-lumen endotracheal tube position is difficult to maintain, and bronchoscopic airway access is limited to a pediatric bronchoscope. As a result, a more reliable strategy is to optimize the function of the transplanted lung and discontinue mechanical ventilation as soon as possible.

COMPLICATIONS

The long-term surgical complications of lung transplantation that arise more than 6 weeks after surgery are bronchial stricture and malacia. In both cases, these complications are rare if airway length is minimized. A lung donor bronchus is associated with cartilage that is frequently necrotic and colonized with *Aspergillus*. Although anatomic dehiscence may not occur, the healing of this cartilage may be associated with excessive granulation tissue and stricture. Alternatively, the cartilage may lose its structural integrity, and the bronchial malacia may result in poor airway clearance. The clinical course associated with both stricture and malacia is characterized by recurrent infections resulting in bacterial pneumonias that are progressively resistant to antibiotics. Airway strictures can be treated with dilation, laser ablation, or mechanical stents. These measures have variable impact on airway clearance.

Similarly, chronic rejection is frequently associated with chronic infection. The late stages of bronchiolitis obliterans are commonly associated with bronchiectasis, a productive cough, and airway colonization with *Pseudomonas* spp.

Chronic renal insufficiency is a late complication of prolonged calcineurin inhibitor therapy. Both CSA and FK-506 are associated with a progressive decline in glomerular filtration rates.[18]

Chronic immunosuppression is associated with PTLD. Most commonly associated with EBV infection, PTLD can be either polyclonal or monoclonal. Polyclonal PTLD is a relatively benign B-cell proliferative disorder that responds to a reduction in immunosuppression. In contrast, monoclonal proliferative disorders are cytologically indistinguishable from immunoblastic lymphoma. These monoclonal immunoblastic lymphomas rarely respond to even the most aggressive cytotoxic chemotherapy. A thorough review of systemic complications of lung transplantation is provided in Chapter 112.

CURRENT TRENDS

Recent clinical outcome studies of sufficient statistical power have been published to aid the physician–surgeon transplant specialist to manage the supply and demand of a finite number of donor organs. These studies enhance our ability to predict clinical outcome, refine characteristics for patient selection, manage complications, and maximize organ allocation.

While there is general consensus that lung transplantation conveys a survival benefit and improved quality of life for patients with end-stage pulmonary disease,[19] whether this benefit is equal for all diagnostic groups or independent of type of procedure (single-lung transplant vs. double-lung transplant vs. heart–lung transplant) is still being investigated. Over the past 5 years, there has been a significant change in patterns, with double-lung transplantation becoming the most common transplant. Preliminary data seem to support a survival advantage for many patients less than 55 years of age for several disease processes. Mason et al. evaluated outcomes for patients with a higher-risk diagnosis of pulmonary fibrosis. While they noted that survival after lung transplantation for idiopathic pulmonary fibrosis (IPF) is worse than after other indications for transplantation, survival may be improved by double-lung transplant.[20] Chang et al. have been more liberal and found that despite longer median allograft ischemic times, as well as greater patient acuity, as determined by listing diagnosis, overall early and midterm patient survival has remained higher than nationally reported figures. Bilateral lung transplantation in eligible patients is the procedure of choice.[21]

One area of change has been the extended age criteria not only for donors but also for recipients. Traditionally, lung transplant was limited to those younger than 60 years of age, with double-lung transplant being restricted to those younger than 55 years of age. The United Network for Organ Sharing (UNOS) registry currently lists candidates as old as 75 years of age actively awaiting transplant. Not only are age limits being extended but also the role of single- versus double-lung transplant is being evaluated. Nwakanma et al. have examined this issue in the United States. They reviewed UNOS data from 1998 to 2004 and noted that 1656 lung transplant recipients were 60 years of age or older (mean 62.7 ± 2.4 years, median 62 years). Of these, 28% had bilateral and 78% had single-lung transplantation. Survival was not statistically different between the two groups. In the multivariate analysis, bilateral versus single-lung transplantation was not a predictor of mortality. IPF and a *donor* tobacco history of more than 20 pack-years were significantly associated with mortality.[22] There is a very interesting if not problematic trend in lung transplantation based on the current version of the LAS. The modeling currently has significantly increased the percent of older (>65) patients and those with the complex family of interstitial fibrotic lung diseases that are undergoing lung transplantation in the United States. While the rate of patient deaths on the waiting list has improved, there appears to be a suggestion that early postoperative survival may be adversely impacted. We await the final analysis.

The goal of keeping patients alive after referral to the transplant waiting list has generated a series of studies designed explicitly to determine disease-specific survival in the context of organ allocation. One of the pivotal changes in lung transplantation organ allocation in the past several years has been the creation and adoption of the LAS for the ranking of listed lung transplant candidates. Previous methods were based on time on list and did not address the nature of specific disease processes, or the acuity of individual patients. In May 2005, the LAS was implemented to improve the mortality rate for individuals on the waiting list for transplantation, as well as to define a potential best use for this rare resource. A number of key variables have been identified (Table 108-6) as predictive of outcome and are being used to calculate a score that, in essence, does four things: It identifies (1) the specific disease process, each of which has different patterns and clinical risks, (2) the severity of the specific patient's clinical condition, (3) the likelihood of mortality within 1 year based on the individual's current status and medical conditions, and (4) the likelihood of 1-year posttransplant survival given those same factors.

Table 108-6

COMPONENTS OF THE LUNG ALLOCATION SCORE

Age
Body mass index (BMI)
Diagnosis
Pulmonary artery pressure (PAP)
Pulmonary capillary wedge pressure (PCWP)
New York Heart Association (NYHA) functional status
6-Minute walk (6 MW)
Forced vital capacity (FVC)
Supplemental oxygen
Ventilator use
Creatinine
Alveolar-capillary conductance (D_M)
Partial pressure of carbon dioxide (pCO_2)

Use of the LAS has been instrumental in lowering the mortality rate on the waiting list but as noted above has been associated with a higher acuity at the time of transplant. While there was a hope of lower early mortality following transplant, the midterm analysis appears to find some concerns although has not been fully completed. McCue et al.[23] did a small review and found a small but significant 1-year survival advantage among post-LAS implementation patients; however, this was largely due to decreased early mortality in comparison with the control cohort.

Acute and chronic allograft rejection (i.e., bronchiolitis obliterans) remains the major rate-limiting factor for long-term survival after lung transplantation. In a systematic review of published studies from 1990 to 2002, Sharples and colleagues compared the reported risk factors for bronchiolitis obliterans from all transplant centers reporting more than 25 patients. Their work supported the view that bronchiolitis obliterans is an alloimmunologic injury characterized by serial acute rejection episodes that are in some manner mediated by other inflammatory processes (e.g., viral infection or ischemic injury). Burton et al.[24] have demonstrated that the development and progression of chronic allograft rejection after lung transplantation (BOS grades 2 and 3) are associated with a threefold increase in the risk of death at each stage irrespective of whether BOS developed early or late. In general, there are many studies aimed at defining the root causes of BOS, with a common theme being processes related to inflammation. These include pseudomonas infections,[25] use of induction protocols,[26] incidence and severity of viral infections following transplant,[27] the presence of specific inflammatory cell types within the transplant graft,[28] and the presence of gastroesophageal reflux.[29] The association between gastroesophageal reflux and end-stage lung disease is established in patients with IPF. It is reasonable to infer that gastroesophageal reflux disease would have a negative impact on the recipient's posttransplant health and hasten the development of bronchiolitis obliterans.[30] In a retrospective analysis of patients treated at Brigham and Women's Hospital, Linden et al.[31] examined the benefit of performing laparoscopic Nissen fundoplication in patients waiting for lung transplantation. This retrospective analysis revealed 19 of 149 active waiting list recipients with a history of active severe reflux disease who underwent laparoscopic Nissen fundoplication between 2001 and 2005. The technique was shown to be safe and to stabilize oxygen requirements in this subgroup of patients with IPF ($n = 14$). Control patients with IPF who did not undergo the procedure ($n = 31$) had a statistically significant deterioration in oxygen requirements. BOS continues to be the Achilles heel of long-term survival.

In recent years, the indications for recipients have broadened, placing more pressure on the already limited pool of donor organs. As a means of counteracting this shortage, the feasibility of using marginal donor organs has been investigated. In this regard, the Toronto Lung Transplant Group conducted a retrospective review of all their transplant recipients between 1997 and 2000 to compare clinical outcome in standard donors and standard recipients versus marginal donors and extended recipients. Donors were defined as *extended* if they met one or more of the following criteria: age more than 55 years, smoking history longer than 20 pack-years, presence of infiltrate on chest plain film radiograph, PaO_2 of less than 300 mm Hg, and purulent secretion on bronchoscopy. Through the efforts of early studies such as this, it was recognized that suitable donor organs that could impart significant survival benefit likely existed outside the fairly rigid guidelines that directed organ donation. It also has been noted that many donors do not achieve suitable donor status for lung transplantation (17% nationally for all donors) because aggressive early management is not implemented routinely. The notion of reducing waiting list mortality by performing intervening procedures to improve recipient health and chances for long-term graft survival is being actively pursued. Angel and colleagues have shown that a simple algorithm-based protocol was associated with a significant increase in the number of lung donors and transplant procedures without compromising pulmonary function, length of stay, or survival of the recipients.[32] At the national level, the Breakthrough Collaborative for Organ Donation, run by the HRSA, has been championing these and other efforts to improve the pool of suitable donors and improve outcomes in lung transplantation by the use of best practices.

Limited availability of donor organs, as well as morbidity secondary to lifelong immunosuppression and chronic graft rejection, has prompted serious investigation of ways to optimize and extend graft allocation and survival. Literature review and outcomes analysis, as described earlier, provide insight into the purpose and utility of lung transplantation.

FUTURE CHALLENGES

Clinicians and scientists continue to explore the possibility of xenotransplantation, which would provide an unlimited supply of thoracic organs that could be supplied, essentially, on demand.[33] The main barrier to xenotransplantation is immunologic. None of the four distinct immunologic reactions, that is, hyperacute rejection, acute vascular rejection, acute cellular rejection, and chronic rejection, has been conquered in the laboratory. Nonhuman primates (e.g., baboon) and mammals (e.g., pig) present the most promising models; however, societal factors and risk of transferred viral infection preclude the use of organs from nonhuman primates. The pig appears to be the more suitable and acceptable option. Consequently, current guidelines published by the ISHLT focus on the pig model and detail the specific immunologic barriers to overcome. Other options are being explored to extend the role and effectiveness of lung transplantation. Additional novel models of immune suppression are being trialed with early success. The concept often raised by several researchers, including pioneers such as Dr. Thomas Starzl, is the possible development of immune tolerance. Clearly, there are patients who develop tolerance of their grafts and go on to need little or no chronic immune suppression. The process of how to induce such a symbiotic state is the subject of entire books but does raise the exciting idea that chronic immune suppression and the long list of complications associated with it could be eliminated.[34,35]

SUMMARY

Lung transplantation is a lifesaving treatment but is complicated and does not yet impart the same durable outcomes offered by other solid-organ transplants. There have been substantial improvements in the past decade in patient management and understanding of immunology that are making strides towards improved patient outcomes. It serves a clear role in patients with severe, medically maximized lung disease and offers a markedly improved quality of life. Limiting factors for this treatment modality include a limited resource pool and multiple complications that markedly affect the broad and prolonged application of this intervention. Current work is improving the effectiveness of this therapy dramatically, and advanced technique and growing experience allow broader availability to the population as a whole.

EDITOR'S COMMENT

Since the first successful single-lung transplant on November 7, 1983, there has been significant progress in the technical aspects of lung transplantation. Early deaths from acute graft failure and anastomotic dehiscence are now rare complications in the postoperative period. The major barrier to lung transplantation is no longer technical, but rather biologic. The fundamental nature of this barrier is illustrated by the remarkably similar survival curves reported by different transplant groups around the world. The next major advance in lung transplantation will need to address this biologic barrier with the development of new targeted, and possibly lung-specific, immunoregulation.

—Steven J. Mentzer

References

1. Toronto Lung Transplant Group. Unilateral lung transplantation for pulmonary fibrosis. *N Engl J Med.* 1986;314:1140–1145.
2. Patterson GA, Cooper JD, Dark JH, et al. Experimental and clinical double lung transplantation. *J Thorac Cardiovasc Surg.* 1988;95:70–74.
3. Cypel M, Yeung JC, Keshavjee S. Novel approaches to expanding the lung donor pool: Donation after cardiac death and ex vivo conditioning. *Clin Chest Med.* 2011;32:199–211.
4. International Society for Heart and Lung Transplantation. 2013; www.ishlt.org. Accessed January, 2013.
5. UNOS. 2011 Annual Report. http://optn.transplant.hrsa.gov/data/annualReport.asp. Accessed January, 2013.
6. Trulock EP, Christie JD, Edwards LB, et al. Registry of the International Society for Heart and Lung Transplantation: Twenty-fourth official adult lung and heart-lung transplant report-2007. *J Heart Lung Transplant.* 2007;26(8):782–795.

7. Schroder C, Scholl F, Daon E, et al. A modified bronchial anastomosis technique for lung transplantation. *Ann Thorac Surg*. 2003;75:1697–1704.
8. Schraufnagel DE. Microvascular casting of the lung: Bronchial versus pulmonary artery filling. *Scanning Microsc*. 1989;3:575–578.
9. Pettersson G, Norgaard MA, Arendrup H, et al. Direct bronchial artery revascularization and en bloc double lung transplantation: Surgical techniques and early outcome. *J Heart Lung Transplant*. 1997;16: 320–333.
10. Stewart S, Fishbein MC, Snell GI, et al. Revision of the 1996 working formulation for the standardization of nomenclature in the diagnosis of lung rejection. *J Heart Lung Transplant*. 2007;26:1229–1242.
11. Estenne M, Maurer JR, Boehler A, et al. Bronchiolitis obliterans syndrome 2001: An update of the diagnostic criteria. *J Heart Lung Transplant*. 2002;21:297–310.
12. Pasque MK, Trulock EP, Cooper JD, et al. Single lung transplantation for pulmonary hypertension: Single institution experience in 34 patients. *Circulation*. 1995;92:2252–2258.
13. Weill D. Donor criteria in lung transplantation: An issue revisited. *Chest*. 2002;121:2029–2031.
14. Hankinson JL, Odencrantz JR, Fedan KB. Spirometric reference values from a sample of the general US population. *Am J Respir Crit Care Med*. 1999;159:179–187.
15. Westall GP, Michaelides A, Williams TJ, et al. Bronchiolitis obliterans syndrome and early human cytomegalovirus DNAaemia dynamics after lung transplantation. *Transplantation*. 2003;75:2064–2068.
16. Group TTLC. Unilateral lung transplantation for pulmonary fibrosis. Toronto Lung Transplant Group. *N Engl J Med*.1986;314:1140–1145
17. Herman SJ, Rappaport DC, Weisbrod GL, et al. Single-lung transplantation: Imaging features. *Radiology*. 1989;170:89–93.
18. Gill JS, Tonelli M, Mix CH, et al. The effect of maintenance immunosuppression medication on the change in kidney allograft function. *Kidney Int*. 2004;65:692–699.
19. Van Trigt P, Davis RD, Shaeffer GS, et al. Survival benefits of heart and lung transplantation. *Ann Surg*. 1996;223:576–584.
20. Mason D, Brizzio M, Alster J, et al. Lung transplantation for idiopatic pulmonary fibrosis. *Ann Thorac Surg*. 2007;84:1121–1128.
21. Chang A, Chan K, Lonigro R, et al. Surgical patient outcomes after the increased use of bilateral lung transplantation. *J Thorac Cardiovasc Surg*. 2007;133:532–540.
22. Nwakanma L, Simpkins C, Williams J, et al. Impact of bilateral versus single lung transplantation on survival in recipients 60 years of age and older: Analysis of United Network for Organ Sharing database. *J Thorac Cardiovasc Surg*. 2007;133:541–547.
23. McCue J, Mooney J, Quail J, et al. Ninety-day mortality and major complications are not affected by use of lung allocation score. *J Heart Lung Transplant*. 2008;27:192–196.
24. Burton C, Carlsen J, Mortensen J, et al. Long-term survival after lung transplantation depends on development and severity of bronchiolitis obliterans syndrome. *J Heart Lung Transplant*. 2007;26:681–686.
25. Botha P, Archer L, Anderson R, et al. *Pseudomonas aeruginosa* colonization of the allograft after lung transplantation and the risk of bronchiolitis obliterans syndrome. *Transplantation*. 2008;85:771–774.
26. Ailawadi G, Smith P, Oka T, et al. Effects of induction immunosuppression regimen on acute rejection, bronchiolitis obliterans, and survival after lung transplantation. *J Thorac Cardiovasc Surg*. 2008;135:594–602.
27. Chmiel C, Speich R, Hofer M, et al. Ganciclovir/valganciclovir prophylaxis decreases cytomegalovirus-related events and bronchiolitis obliterans syndrome after lung transplantation. *Clin Infect Dis*. 2008;46:831–839.
28. Fildes J, Tunstall K, Walker A, et al. Natural killer cells in peripheral blood and lung tissue are associated with chronic rejection after lung transplantation. *J Heart Lung Transplant*. 2008;27:203–207.
29. Blondeau K, Mertens V, Vanaudenaerde B, et al. Gastro-oesophageal reflux and gastric aspiration in lung transplant patient with or without chronic rejection. *Eur Respir J*. 2008;31:707–713.
30. Hadjiliadis D, Duane Davis R, Steele MP, et al. Gastroesophageal reflux disease in lung transplant recipients. *Clin Transplant*. 2003;17:363–368.
31. Linden PA, Gilbert RJ, Yeap BY, et al. Laparoscopic fundoplication in patients with end stage lung disease awaiting transplantation. *J Thorac Cardiovasc Surg*. 2006;131:438–446.
32. Angel L, Levine DJ, Restrepo MI, Johnson S, Sako E, Carpenter A, Calhoon J, Cornell JE, Adams SG, Chisholm GB, et al. Impact of lung transplantation donor-management protocol on lung donation and recipient outcomes. *AmJ Respir Crit Care Med*. 2006;174:710–716.
33. Cooper DK, Keogh AM, Brink J, et al. Report of the Xenotransplantation Advisory Committee of the International Society for Heart and Lung Transplantation: The present status of xenotransplantation and its potential role in the treatment of end-stage cardiac and pulmonary diseases. *J Heart Lung Transplant*. 2000;19:1125–1165.
34. Starzl T. Acquired immunologic tolerance: With particular reference to transplantation. *Immunol Res*. 2007;38:6–41.
35. Starzl T. Immunosuppressive therapy and tolerance of organ allografts. *N Engl J Med*. 2008;358:407–411.

109 Lung Transplantation Technique

Ankit Bharat and G. Alexander Patterson

Keywords: Single-lung transplant, double-lung transplant, heart–lung transplant, immunosuppression, end-stage pulmonary disease

INTRODUCTION

Since its inception in 1963, over 32,000 lung transplants have been performed globally. For several decades, chronic obstructive pulmonary disease (COPD) was the most common indication for lung transplantation. However, in the United States, the donor lung allocation system has changed the scenario and idiopathic pulmonary fibrosis (IPF) is emerging as a more common indication. IPF accounts for about 25% of lung transplant at our center and 33% nationally.[1] Cystic fibrosis (CF) is the third most common indication.

To be eligible for bilateral lung transplantation, potential transplant recipients should be without significant comorbid disease. Patients with emphysema generally are older than other patient groups (e.g., CF) and thus perhaps are more at risk for cardiovascular or cerebrovascular events. In contrast, CF patients often have occult renal insufficiency secondary to years of antibiotic therapy, particularly with aminoglycosides. Unique infectious concerns are also seen in the CF population because these patients frequently are infected with one or more strains of *Pseudomonas aeruginosa* and often are colonized with mycobacterial or fungal pathogens. Furthermore, CF patients often have a degree of liver disease, pancreatic insufficiency, or both owing to the multiorgan system effects of the CF genetic defect. Patients with primary pulmonary hypertension (PPH) commonly have residual right-sided heart dysfunction immediately after transplantation and need greater attention to cardiac hemodynamics, often requiring an increase of right-sided filling pressures for hemodynamic stability. Finally, the widespread use of IV prostacyclin (Flolan) has permitted many patients with PPH to delay transplantation. Thus, by the time these patients present for transplant, the degree of right-sided heart failure is often quite severe.

CHOICE OF TRANSPLANT

The decision to perform a single-, double-, or heart–lung transplant depends on numerous factors, including recipient characteristics (e.g., disease, age, and comorbidities), institutional bias, organ availability, and the urgency of the transplant. Single-lung transplantation is a good option for patients with IPF.[2] Selected patients with emphysema, specifically those of shorter stature and older age, also can expect good results with single-lung transplantation. Unilateral transplantation is also acceptable for patients with PPH.[3] However, because these cases are challenging and management can be difficult during the first few postoperative days,[4] some programs prefer the double-lung or even combined heart–lung transplantation for patients with PPH. Double-lung transplant is mandatory for patients with CF and bronchiectasis because in both cases the septic native lungs must be excised. When the native disease is accompanied by a pre-existing mycetoma[5] or other chronic fungal or mycobacterial infection, double-lung transplantation is also a better option because it minimizes the post-transplant risk of recurrent infection. The heart–lung transplant is reserved for the rare patient with combined end-stage cardiac and pulmonary disease. Most patients requiring heart–lung transplant have Eisenmenger syndrome with PPH and significant left ventricular dysfunction, perhaps owing to an uncorrected congenital defect. The annual rate of heart–lung transplantation has declined significantly not only because single- or double-lung transplant alone is appropriate in the majority of patients but also because no clear survival advantage has been demonstrated in this patient group.[6] The different types of lung transplantation that are performed currently are shown in Figure 109-1.

We prefer the double-lung transplant at our institution irrespective of disease category. Double-lung transplantation has been documented to produce a superior result in patients with obstructive lung disease,[7] and we find that survival is superior and that early postoperative management is far less complicated with the bilateral approach.

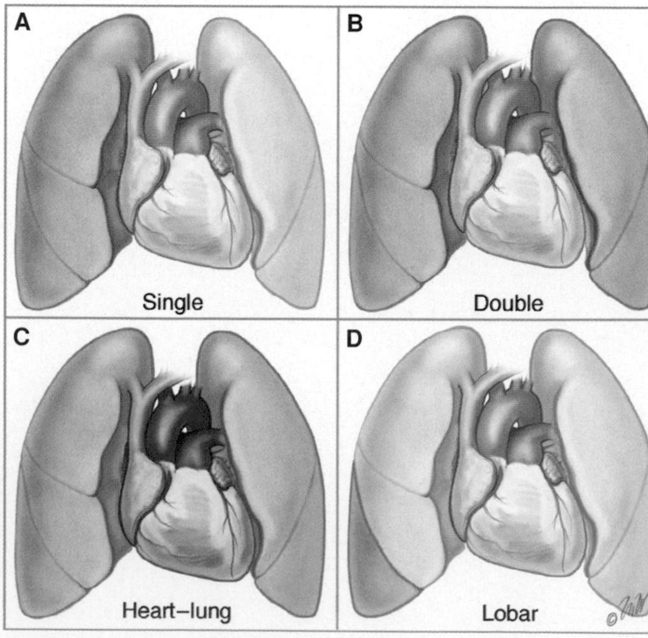

Figure 109-1. Types of lung transplantation performed. *A*. single lung, *B*. double lung, *C*. heart–lung, *D*. lobar.

PROCUREMENT

Donor Lung Procurement

If the initial evaluation (i.e., donor history, chest radiograph, bronchoscopy) reveals no contraindications, we proceed with donor lung procurement. Our technique has been described previously.[8,9] A T-shaped incision centered on the sternal angle is performed over the sternum. After median sternotomy and opening of the pleural spaces, the pericardium is opened, and stay sutures are placed, permitting exposure of the great vessels. The superior vena cava (SVC) is encircled caudal to the azygos vein with silk ties. Alternatively, if heart is also being procured, the azygos vein can be carefully ligated. Usually it is not necessary to encircle the inferior vena cava. The periadventitial tissue overlying the right pulmonary artery (PA) is dissected. The plane between the artery and the SVC is dissected. In similar fashion, the right PA is separated from the posterior aspect of the ascending aorta.

The aorta-pulmonary artery window is dissected in preparation for the aortic cross-clamp. The SVC and aorta are gently retracted laterally, and the posterior pericardium is incised above the right PA, permitting access to the trachea. The plane of the trachea is developed manually and two-thirds of the trachea dissected. We do not encircle the trachea completely at this point to avoid bleeding and inadvertent injury to membranous trachea. Instead of amputating the left atrial appendage, we routinely vent the left heart through the interatrial groove, especially when both heart and lungs are being harvested. This avoids the need of suturing the left atrial appendage after cardiac implantation. In order to do this, the interatrial groove is dissected. After the thoracic dissection is complete, the donor is heparinized with 30,000 units of heparin. The ascending aorta is cannulated with a routine cardioplegia cannula for cardiac preservation. At the bifurcation of the main PA, a Sarns (Ann Arbor, MI) 6.5-mm curved metal cannula is placed and secured with a purse-string suture. If the cannula is placed close to the PA bifurcation, as is in case of heart procurement, the tip of the cannula should face the pulmonic valve to prevent preferential perfusion of any one main PA (Fig. 109-2). After the cannulas have been placed, a bolus dose of prostaglandin E_1 (500 μg) is given directly into the PA using a 16-gauge needle.

Immediately after the prostaglandin E_1 infusion, the SVC is ligated, the interatrial groove is incised and the inferior vena cava is divided, permitting the right and left side of the heart to decompress. The aorta is cross-clamped, and cardioplegia is initiated. The pulmonary flush consisting of several liters (50–75 mL/kg) of cold (4°C) Perfadex® is initiated. The chest cavity is cooled with ice-slush normal saline. Gentle ventilation is continued throughout to prevent hyperinflation or atelectasis and to enhance distribution of the flush solution.

After the cardioplegia and antegrade pulmonary flushes are completed, the cannulas are removed. The heart then is extracted. The inferior vena cava is freed posteriorly and dissected up to the level of the right atrium. Division of the left atrium proceeds from the venting incision in the interatrial groove with the cooperation of the heart and lung teams. The orifices of the superior and inferior pulmonary veins are visualized to leave adequate cuff for lung implantation. The surgeon on the left side of the table can visualize the right vein orifices best and should divide the left atrial cuff over the right pulmonary veins. An appropriate residual atrial cuff should have a rim of left atrial muscle around each of the pulmonary vein orifices. An adequate cuff can be ensured if the interatrial groove is developed on the right (Fig. 109-3). The SVC is transected between ties, followed by both division of the aorta proximal to the cross-clamp and the PA at its bifurcation. The heart then is passed off the field. The appearance of the surgical anatomy after passing off the heart is shown in Figure 109-4.

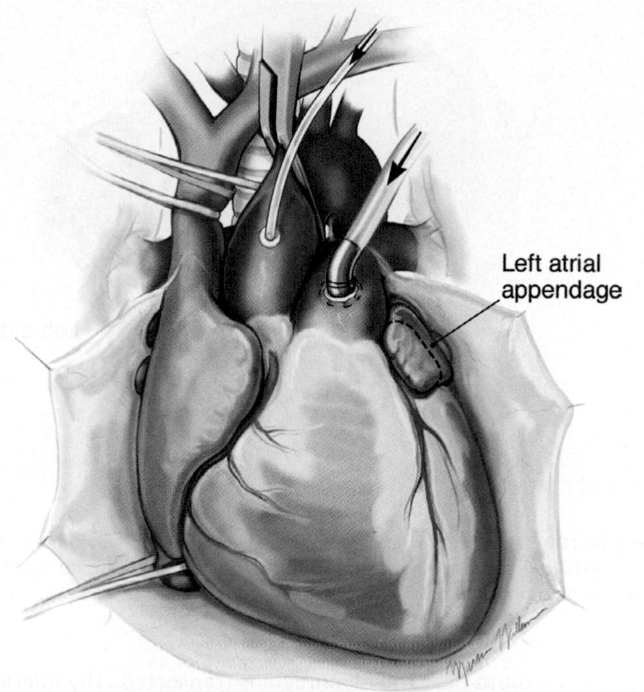

Figure 109-2. Donor heart prepared for explant. Note that the cross-clamp has been placed on the aorta. Venting of the left heart can either be done through left atrial appendage or by incising the interatrial groove (preferred method). A plane of atria is developed if the latter method is used.

After extracting the heart, we use a Foley catheter to deliver a retrograde flush via the pulmonary vein orifices (approximately 250 mL of cold Perfadex® in each orifice). During retrograde flushing, residual blood and small clots are often flushed out of the opened PA bifurcation. Alternatively, this retrograde flush can be done on the back table before departing from the donor site. We incorporated this retrograde flushing procedure into our donor procurements after experimental[10] and clinical research[11] found it to be superior to the antegrade flush, with less pulmonary edema, lower airway resistance, and better oxygenation during the first several hours after transplantation.

We then proceed with en bloc removal of the contents of the thoracic cavity. Removal of the lungs by this technique prevents injury to the membranous trachea, pulmonary arteries, and pulmonary veins. The tracheal dissection is completed at least two to three rings above the carina. The endotracheal tube is opened to atmosphere, and the lungs are permitted to deflate to approximate end-tidal volume while the endotracheal tube is backed into the proximal trachea. The trachea is sealed with a linear stapler and divided at least two rings above the carina (Fig. 109-4). Immediately posteriorly, the esophagus is encircled, stapled, and divided using a linear stapler. While retracting both lungs, heavy scissors are used to divide all the mediastinal tissue down to the spine. Staying directly on the spine, the posterior mediastinal tissue is divided. At this point,

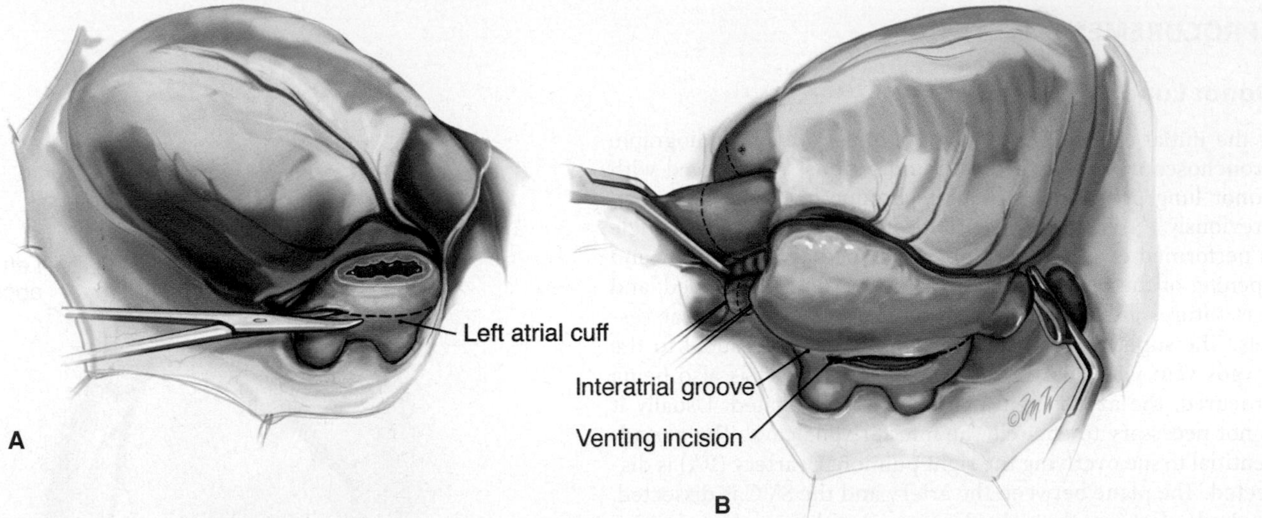

Figure 109-3. The donor heart is explanted along with a sufficient cuff of the left atrium. We prefer to start the incision of the left atrium through the interatrial groove on the right side so that the pulmonary veins are visualized. The incision is continued circumferentially to the left side carefully avoiding the left pulmonary veins on the lung side and the circumflex artery on the heart side.

the pericardium near the diaphragm is transected. The inferior pulmonary ligaments are sharply divided. The lower esophagus is encircled and divided with the linear stapler. Posterior mediastinal tissue is sharply divided to connect with the superior aspect of the dissection. The lungs then are removed en bloc along with the thoracic esophagus and aorta.

If the lungs are returning to the same institution, they are tripled-bagged together with cold preservation solution and transported on ice. Alternatively, if the lungs are to be used at

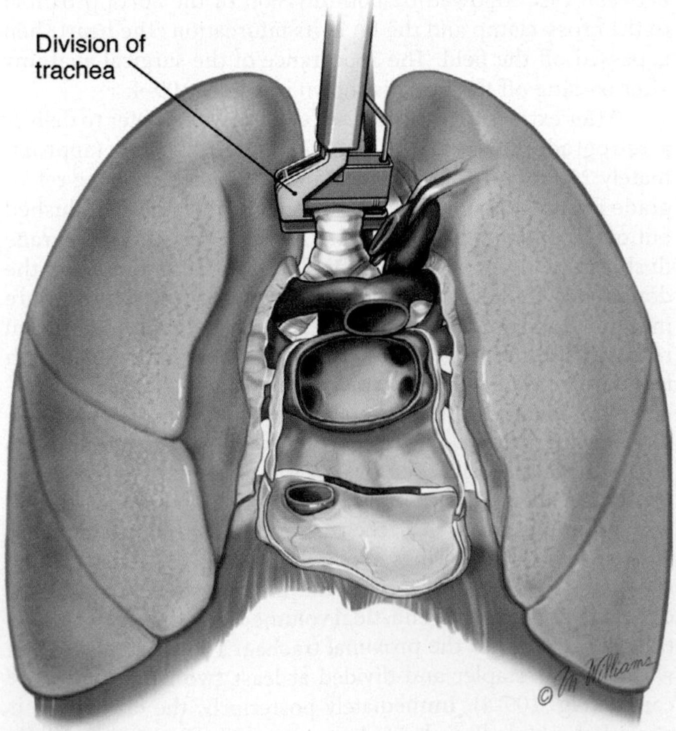

Figure 109-4. Appearance of chest cavity after the donor heart has been removed but before the double-lung bloc has been resected. Esophagectomy has been performed (not shown), and the trachea is being divided.

separate institutions, they are divided on the back table. While the lung bloc is kept in an ice-slush bath, the donor esophagus and aorta are removed, and the pericardium is excised. The lungs are separated by dividing the posterior pericardium, the left atrium between the pulmonary veins, the main PA at the bifurcation, and the left bronchus above the takeoff of the upper lobe bronchus. The left bronchus is divided between staples to maintain the inflation of each lung.

Donor Heart–lung Procurement

The donor harvest procedure for a heart–lung bloc is similar to the separate harvests for heart and lungs, with the exception that the heart and lungs are removed en bloc. After the pulmonary flush and cardioplegia are completed, the SVC is transected between ties, followed by division of the aorta proximal to the cross-clamp. The trachea is completely encircled, doubly stapled, and transected, again permitting the lungs to deflate to approximate end-tidal volume. En bloc removal of the contents of the thoracic cavity proceeds as in the lung procurement technique.

EX VIVO LUNG PERFUSION

It is estimated that only about 15% to 20% of all multiorgan donors are used for clinical lung transplantation.[12] Most lung offers are considered unsuitable due to marginal donor lung function. Injuries from multiple sources such as brain death, ventilator-associated barotrauma, sepsis, and pulmonary edema lead to deterioration of donor lung function. However, such injuries might be reversible and if given time to recover, a proportion of these lungs will ultimately turn out to be acceptable for clinical transplantation. Ex vivo lung perfusion (EVLP) is a novel strategy of differentiating between suitable and suboptimal lung grafts in this donor population with marginal lung function.

There are various protocols being developed for clinical EVLP. Here we discuss briefly the one published recently by the

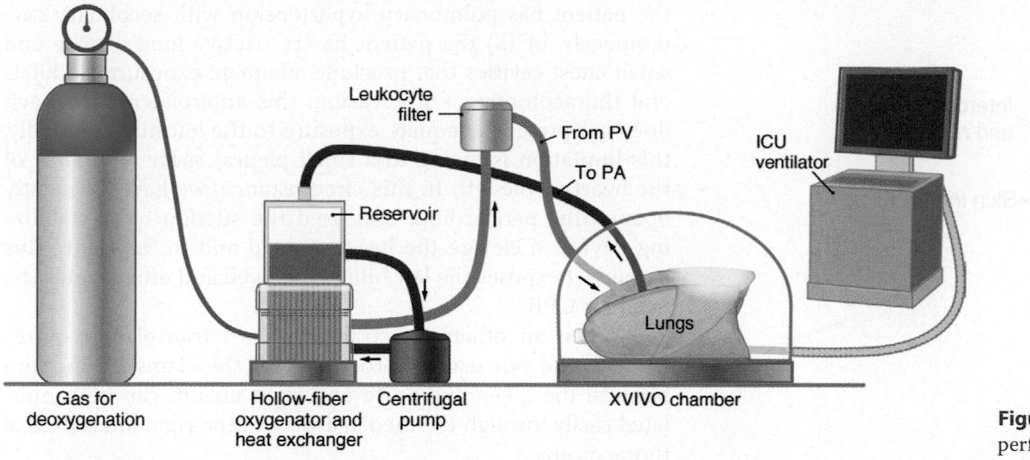

Figure 109-5. Technique of ex vivo lung perfusion (EVLP).

Toronto Lung Transplant Group.[13] The donor lungs are harvested in standard fashion and undergo a period of hypothermic preservation. Subsequently, they are brought to the center for EVLP where they are removed from the hypothermic preservative. The lungs are transferred to the perfusion chamber and the left atrium and PA on the donor lungs cannulated. The lungs are perfused with special acellular perfusate. Retrograde flow is initially performed to de-air the lungs through the PA cannula. The PA cannula is then connected to the circuit and antegrade flow is started with the perfusate at room temperature. As the lungs get warmed to about 32 degrees, ventilation is started and the perfusate flow rate gradually increased. The target maximum maintenance perfusate rate is about 40% of the estimated cardiac output. The flow of gas used to deoxygenate and provide carbon dioxide to the inflow perfusate via a gas exchange membrane is started at 1 L/min. A protective mode of mechanical ventilation is applied using a tidal volume of 7 mL/kg of ideal donor body weight, positive end-expiratory pressure (PEEP) of 5 cm H_2O, and an inspired oxygen fraction (Fio_2) of 21% (Fig. 109-5). The lungs are recruited with a peak airway pressure of 20 cm H_2O every hour.

EVLP is done for 4 hours. Following completion, the lungs are cooled down in the circuit to 10°C over 10 minutes. Subsequently, perfusion and ventilation are stopped and the trachea is clamped to maintain the lungs in an inflated state. The lungs are then preserved at 4°C in Perfadex® until transplantation.

PREPARATION OF THE RECIPIENT

Before anesthesia is induced, most of our patients have epidural catheters placed. If cardiopulmonary bypass (CPB) is planned, we do not place an epidural because of the requirement for heparinization during CPB. Double-lumen endotracheal intubation is routine. When the indication for transplantation is septic lung disease (e.g., CF or bronchiectasis), the patients are intubated initially with a large single-lumen endotracheal tube to permit vigorous suctioning of purulent secretions through an adult fiberoptic bronchoscope. This step maximizes the effective ventilation during independent lung ventilation and decreases the likelihood that CPB will be required.

Routine monitoring devices include a Swan–Ganz catheter, radial and femoral arterial lines, Foley catheter, and a transesophageal echocardiography probe. For bilateral sequential lung transplants, the patient is positioned supine with all extremities padded and arms tucked in at the sides. A pillow is placed behind the knees to prevent hyperextension and peroneal nerve palsy, which can result from prolonged hyperextension of the knees. A heating blanket is placed up to the mid-abdomen. If a posterolateral thoracotomy is used for a single lung transplant recipient, the patient is positioned in the appropriate lateral decubitus position.

CPB is used routinely for children, for lobar transplants, for patients in whom a double-lumen tube cannot be placed (small adults), whenever intracardiac procedures are indicated, and for most patients with pulmonary hypertension. For most of our patients, however, we do not use CPB (but we prepare to do so should it be emergently required). We also do not routinely use the cell saver because the majority of our transplants are performed with less than 500 mL of blood loss.

BILATERAL SEQUENTIAL LUNG TRANSPLANTS

Incisions

Bilateral Anterolateral Thoracotomy

Our standard exposure is the bilateral anterolateral thoracotomy, which prevents the complication of sternal healing associated with the clamshell incision.[14] The skin incision is performed along the inframammary crease at the level of the fourth intercostal space. The skin over the sternum is not divided. The breast tissue and the lower edge of the pectoral muscle are elevated off the chest wall. The chest cavity is entered by dividing the intercostal muscle directly overlying the fifth rib. The internal mammary arteries are identified, isolated, ligated, and divided bilaterally. Alternatively, the internal mammary arteries can be preserved if a 1-cm segment of costal cartilage of the fourth rib is resected at the sternal border, permitting upward mobility of the fourth rib when retracted. More mobility is obtained by dividing the intercostal muscle from within the pleural space to the paraspinal muscles. The serratus anterior muscle and the long thoracic nerve are not divided; rather, they are pulled away from the chest wall to permit access to the posterolateral intercostal space. Optimal exposure then is obtained by appropriate placement of chest

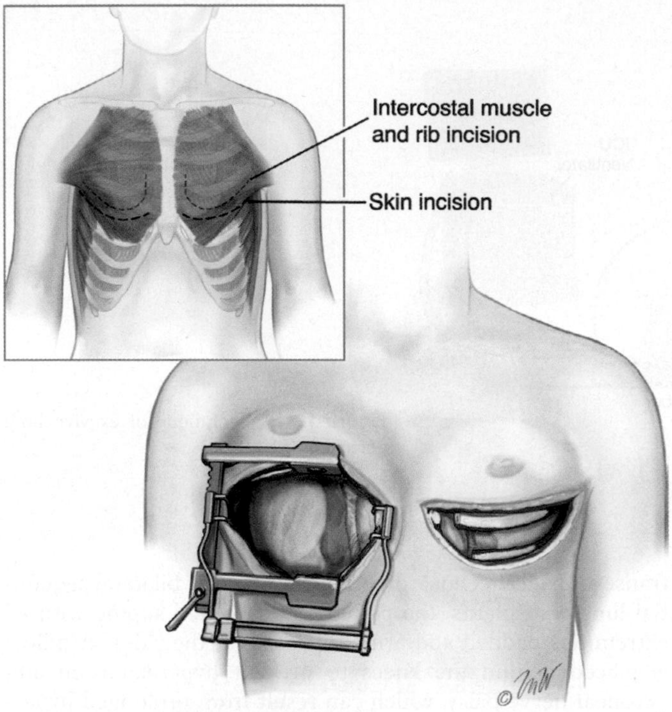

Figure 109-6. Exposure obtained from bilateral anterolateral thoracotomies (sternum sparing).

retractors at 90-degree angles from one another (Fig. 109-6). The table is tilted right or left as necessary to maximize exposure during hilar dissection, lung removal, and implantation.

Transsternal Bilateral Thoracotomy (Thoracosternotomy) Incision

This incision provides excellent exposure to the hilar structures as well as the mediastinum and both pleural spaces (Fig. 109-7). Bilateral retractors are used to elevate the chest wall upward. We resort to the full clamshell incision under the following circumstances: (1) a concomitant heart operation is planned, (2) the patient has pulmonary hypertension with secondary cardiomegaly, or (3) the patient has restrictive lung disease and small chest cavities that preclude adequate exposure via bilateral thoracotomies. On occasion, this anterolateral approach does not provide adequate exposure to the left hilum. Usually, this limitation is owing to a small pleural space with shift of the heart to the left. In this circumstance, we have frequently opened the pericardium and used the suction heart-stabilizing device to elevate the heart upward and to the right. This maneuver exposes the left hilum very well and often avoids the need for CPB.

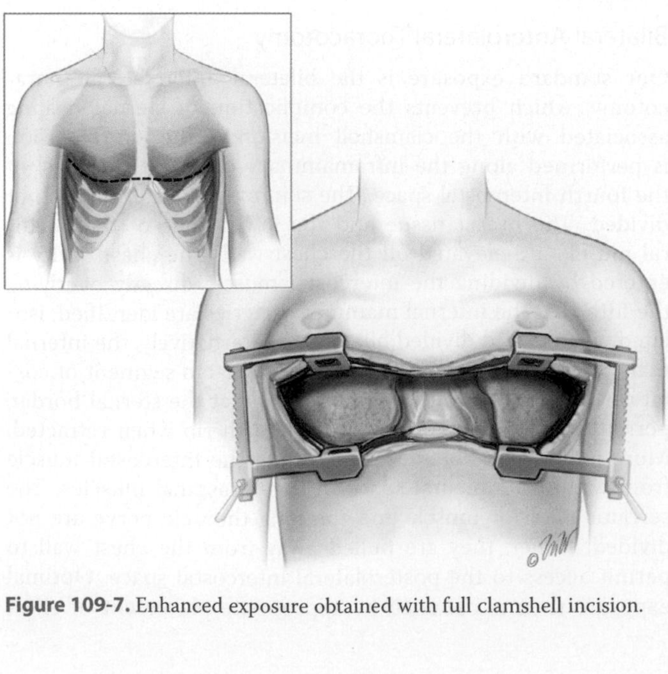

Figure 109-7. Enhanced exposure obtained with full clamshell incision.

When an otherwise straightforward transplant requires CPB, we do not usually proceed with the clamshell incision because the ascending aorta and right atrium can be cannulated easily through the medial aspect of the right anterolateral thoracotomy.

If a transverse sternotomy has been performed, our preference is to reapproximate the sternum with two figure-of-eight no. 7 sternal wires. Other techniques to reapproximate the sternum have been developed.[15]

Posterolateral Thoracotomy and Anterolateral Thoracotomy

Patients with restrictive lung diseases and small chest cavities and patients with secondary pulmonary hypertension and cardiomegaly may present with their heart filling much of the left anterior hemithorax, making access to the left hilum via the anterior approach quite difficult. In these circumstances, CPB can be avoided by performing the left lung transplant first through a left posterolateral thoracotomy. The patient then is turned supine, and the right lung transplant is performed via a right anterolateral approach.

BACK TABLE PREPARATION OF LUNGS

The lungs are removed from the bags and placed on ice and covered with icy laps. First, the tracheal staple line is excised and lungs opened to air. The aorta and esophagus are removed posteriorly. The PA orifice is then examined to the first branch of right and left main PA visualized. The PA is divided by staying right on the raphe at the bifurcation. The atrial cuff is then inspected and divided equally so there is ample sewing ring on both sides. The tissue between the divided PA and atrial cuff is divided to expose the left main bronchus. The left main bronchus is divided distal to the tracheal carina and the lung separated, covered in ice, and labeled. The final preparation of the PA, atrial cuff, and bronchus is done on the operative field in order to make precise assessment of the required length of each structure. Usually, the bronchi are divided such that no more than one ring remains before the secondary carina. A longer donor bronchus predisposes to anastomotic ischemia and stricture.[16] Care is taken to minimize dissection of the donor bronchus to preserve collateral flow through the peribronchial nodal tissue. The PA is also divided fairly close to the first branch as a long and redundant donor PA predisposes to kinking. The PA and left atrial cuffs are freed from any pericardial attachments because these may cause kinking after the anastomosis is completed. The right and left PAs are cleaned back to their first branches and inspected for any injuries or embolic material.

RECIPIENT PNEUMONECTOMY

To reduce the likelihood of requiring CPB, the least functional lung, as determined by preoperative quantitative ventilation/perfusion imaging, is resected and replaced first. An attempt is made to detach all pleural adhesions and fully mobilize the hila of both lungs before the first lung is explanted. Great care is taken to avoid injuring the phrenic nerve as it passes just anterior to the hilum and the vagus nerve that lies posterior to the hilum. This preliminary dissection shortens the time that the first implanted lung is exposed to the entire cardiac output and thus lessens the likelihood of reperfusion edema in that lung. In this respect, both donor lungs should be prepared for implantation before removing the recipient's lungs, if possible.

The pulmonary arteries and pulmonary veins are dissected beyond their primary bifurcations to preserve the length of the main trunks. The pulmonary veins are divided between ties or staple lines at second branch points saving maximal length for the future recipient atrial cuff. The right PA is usually transected between firings of a vascular stapling device 1 cm beyond the ligated first branch to the right upper lobe. Before PA stapling and division, it is important to be sure the PA catheter is not too far peripheral and at risk of division. The left PA is transected between staple lines beyond the second branch to the left upper lobe. The bronchus is transected between cartilaginous rings well into the mediastinum at a site suitable for anastomosis. The posterior bundle of lymphatics and bronchial arteries is exposed and divided with electrocautery or ligated and divided.

The lung is removed from the chest, and the operative field is prepared for implantation of the graft. The PA stump is grasped with atraumatic Duval triangular clamp and mobilized centrally. After sufficient mobilization both anteriorly and posteriorly, the Duval clamp is placed on anterior traction by wrapping a heavy silk tie around it and snapping to the drapes toward the head. The pulmonary vein stumps then are grasped with smaller Duval clamps and retracted laterally to permit circumferential opening of the pericardium. With the pericardium freed, the vein stumps then are retracted and temporarily fixed anteriorly, providing an excellent view of the bronchus. The left-sided, double-lumen endobronchial tube may impair the ability to trim the left bronchus to an appropriately short length, in which case the tube should be backed out a few millimeters. Meticulous hemostasis in the posterior mediastinum is achieved at this point with the knowledge that reaching this portion of the operative field after implantation of the graft lung will be extremely difficult. Finally, a small suction catheter is placed down the appropriate limb of the endotracheal tube to assist in keeping the airway clear by aspiration of blood and iced saline during implantation.

IMPLANTATION

The donor lung is placed within the recipient's chest cavity covered by a cold lap pad. If space permits, a layer of slush is placed in the empty chest cavity first. We find it simplest to perform the anastomoses from posterior to anterior in the following sequence: bronchus, artery, and atrium. A silk traction suture is placed at the midpoint of the anterior bronchus of the recipient and is used to retract the bronchus out of the mediastinum to help with visibility during the anastomosis. Two corner

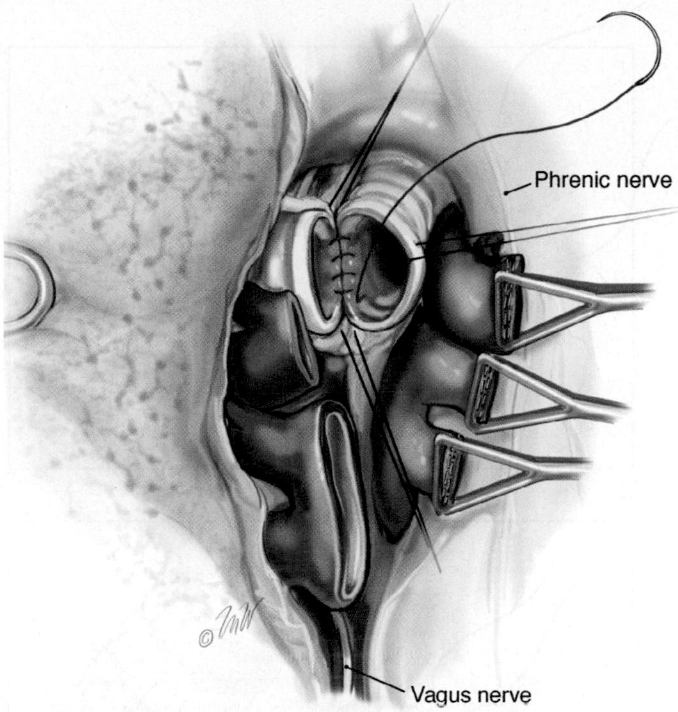

Figure 109-8. A running continuous suture is used for the posterior membranous wall of the bronchial anastomosis.

stitches are placed at the cartilagino-membranous junction of the donor and recipient airway using double armed 4-0 PDS suture and tied down. From one end, the membranous part of the bronchial anastomosis is performed in a running fashion sewing the donor airway to recipient (Fig. 109-8). When the opposite end is reached, the stitch is brought outside either the donor or recipient airway and tied down to the other previously placed corner stitch. From that point, one end of the suture material is used to sew the cartilaginous portion of the bronchi in a running fashion, again, sewing donor to the recipient. Halfway through the cartilaginous anastomosis, the previously placed traction silk stitch in the anterior wall is removed. The other stitch is brought toward the middle from the opposite end and both are tied down to complete the cartilaginous anastomosis. Alternatively, the front cartilaginous wall can be anastomosed in an interrupted fashion using 4-0 PDS or 3-0 Vicryl suture (Fig. 109-9). The bronchial anastomosis is completed by sewing the peribronchial tissue anteriorly over the cartilaginous portion of the airway. If the bronchi are of small caliber, or if there is a size mismatch, which is seen most commonly on the left side, we opt for reapproximating the anterior wall with simple interrupted 3-0 Vicryl sutures to prevent stricturing of the airway. We have stopped reapproximating the posterior peribronchial tissue and we feel that the main purpose of peribronchial tissue is to separate the bronchial and vascular anastomosis and both the PA and vein anastomoses lie anterior to the bronchial anastomosis. Hence, closing the peribronchial tissue anteriorly suffices.

Next, the PAs of the donor and recipient are aligned in proper orientation. The recipient's PA then is clamped centrally with a small Satinsky clamp, with care taken to avoid including the Swan–Ganz catheter in the jaws of the clamp. The vascular staple line is resected at a location that matches

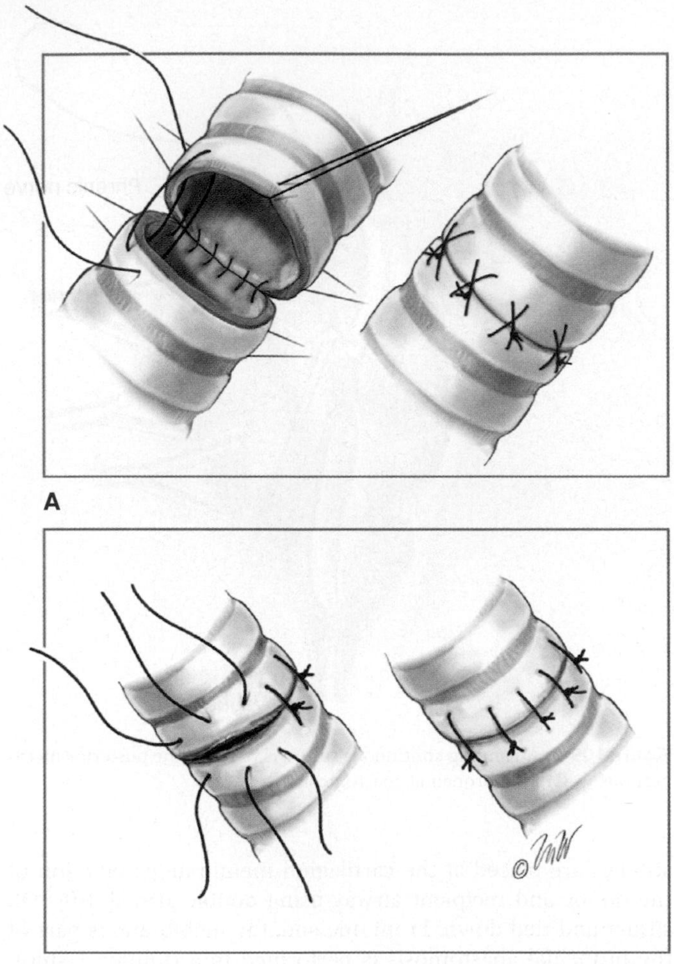

Figure 109-9. *A.* Interrupted figure-of-eight 4-0 PDS suture is used for the anterior wall bronchial anastomosis. *B.* If the bronchus is small, however, we use interrupted 3-0 Vicryl suture for the anterior wall.

the size of the donor and recipient arteries. Both donor and recipient PAs are trimmed to prevent excessive length and possible kinking postoperatively. An end-to-end arterial anastomosis is performed with a running continuous 5-0 polypropylene suture (Fig. 109-10). This anastomosis must be made with precise, small suture bites to avoid anastomotic stenosis.

Both vein stumps then are retracted laterally, and a Satinsky clamp is placed centrally on the recipient's left atrium. Once the clamp is placed, an umbilical tape is used to tie the clamp in closed position to minimize the likelihood of dislodgement during subsequent lateral retraction of the clamp. The vein stumps then are amputated, and the bridge of atrium between vein stumps is divided to create the atrial cuff (Fig. 109-11). Gentle lateral traction on the Satinsky clamp can bring this anastomosis to a more accessible location. Alternatively, a retraction suture placed in the pericardium 2 to 3 cm above the inferior pulmonary vein, with care taken to avoid injury to the phrenic nerve, can be used to partially suspend the heart, providing better exposure to the left atrial anastomosis. The anastomosis is performed with continuous 4-0 polypropylene suture. Sutures are placed using a mattress technique, which achieves good intima-to-intima apposition and excludes all atrial muscle. This limits the thrombogenicity of this suture

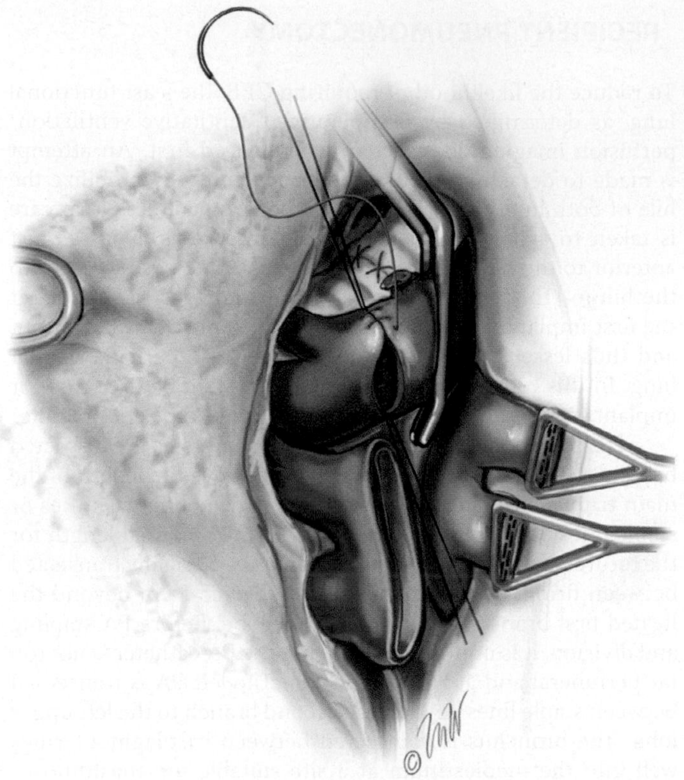

Figure 109-10. A running continuous suture is used for the PA anastomosis.

line. The suture line is left open on its anterior aspect. The lung is partially inflated, and the PA clamp is loosened momentarily. The lung is flushed with the atrial clamp still in place so as to flush out residual pulmonary perfusate solution. The left atrial clamp then is opened momentarily to completely de-air the atrium. The atrial suture line is secured, and the clamps are removed completely. All suture lines, as well as the cut edges

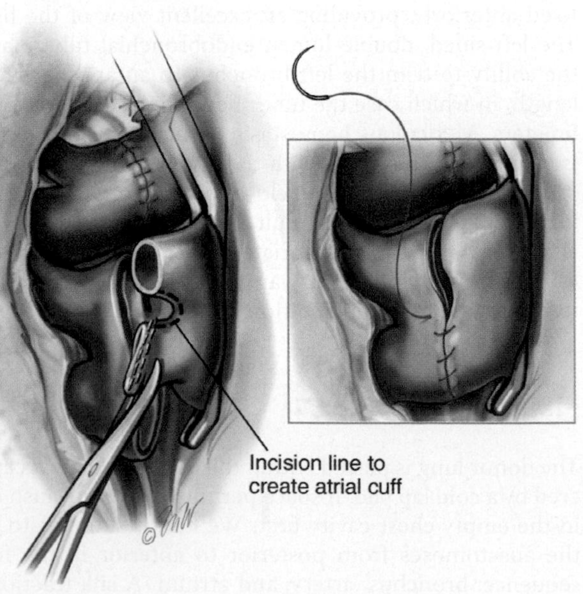

Figure 109-11. The pulmonary vein stumps are individually amputated, and the bridge of tissue in between is divided to permit preservation of cuff length.

of pericardium, then are checked for hemostasis as ventilation and perfusion are restored.

The contralateral transplant is conducted in the same fashion. Traditionally, we have drained the pleural space with two large-caliber chest tubes, one angled and one straight. More recently, if hemostasis during the procedure is excellent, we use two no. 24 Blake drains (Ethicon, Somerville, NJ) in each pleural space, one placed apically and one placed along the diaphragm. The ribs are reapproximated with interrupted figure-of-eight monofilament nonabsorbable suture. The pectoralis muscle and fascia are reapproximated with standard suture material, as is the subcutaneous layer. If a major submammary dissection has been necessary, we drain the submammary space. Staples or a running subcuticular suture is used for the skin, and then sterile dry dressings are applied. Before leaving the OR, bronchoscopy is performed to inspect the bronchial anastomosis and clear away any secretions. The patient is taken while still intubated to the thoracic ICU for postoperative monitoring.

SINGLE-LUNG TRANSPLANTATION

Choice of Side

The choice of side of transplant is based on several factors. Usually, the side with the poorest function determined by preoperative ventilation/perfusion scanning is transplanted. If need for CPB is anticipated, the right side is preferred because cannulation of the ascending aorta and right atrial appendage can be performed easily through the anterior aspect of the thoracotomy. Cannulation of the descending aorta and main PA can be accomplished through the left chest but is somewhat more tedious. We avoid groin cannulation whenever possible. For patients with Eisenmenger syndrome, we prefer the right side to facilitate closure of the coexisting atrial or ventricular septal defects. A patent ductus arteriosus can be repaired in association with a transplant on either side.

Exposure

The standard incision is a generous posterolateral thoracotomy through the fifth interspace. Some groups have recommended the anterior axillary muscle-sparing thoracotomy for emphysema patients.[17] Alternatively, an anterolateral fourth interspace thoracotomy provides excellent exposure, particularly on the right side. This is especially useful if a need for CPB is anticipated.

Pneumonectomy and Implantation

The techniques of pneumonectomy and implantation are identical to those just described for double-lung transplantation.

Use of Cardiopulmonary Bypass in Lung Transplantation

When CPB is planned we prefer to do the majority of the dissection before administration of heparin and cannulation. A two-stage venous cannula is placed in the atrium, and an aortic perfusion cannula is placed in the ascending aorta. We also place a PA vent. After cannulation, the bypass pump is instituted at full flow, and both lungs are excised. After the first lung is implanted, the left atrium is de-aired and the left atrial clamp removed. The PA clamp is left in place. If the left atrial clamp is also left in place, there is often not enough atrium available for clamp placement on the opposite side. The lung is packed in iced saline and slush while the second lung is implanted.

Postoperative Care After Lung Transplantation

Immediately after the surgery, patients are transported intubated to the ICU for constant monitoring. Once stabilized, a standard ventilator pressure-support weaning protocol is initiated. We favor pressure-control ventilation to limit peak airway pressures and prevent barotrauma to the bronchial anastomosis. Plateau pressures should be limited to no more than 35 mm Hg. Fifty percent of lung transplant recipients at our institution are weaned from mechanical ventilation and extubated within 24 hours of transplantation. Patients typically leave the OR on high FiO_2. However, if the initial postoperative arterial blood gas demonstrates a PaO_2 of more than 70 mm Hg and/or saturations greater than 90%, then the FiO_2 is weaned, and repeat measurements of arterial oxygenation are made after each change to minimize the risk of oxygen toxicity. In most patients without significant reperfusion edema, the FiO_2 can be weaned successfully to 40% or less within the first 24 hours of transplantation. Postoperatively, a quantitative lung perfusion scan can be performed to assess patency of vascular anastomosis and graft flow. If a lobar or greater perfusion defect is appreciated, the cause should be further interrogated by angiography or operative exploration.

In single-lung transplant patients with COPD, zero or minimal PEEP is used, along with an adequate expiratory phase of ventilation, to prevent air trapping in the native lung. An expiratory hold maneuver may be useful to detect air trapping in these patients. Careful fluid management is necessary to avoid substantial transplant lung edema, and usually negative fluid balance is attempted within the first 48 hours. Adequate urine output is carefully maintained with combinations of blood, colloid, and diuretics. Recent evidence suggests that lung injury caused by transplantation significantly reduces the ability of the lungs to clear edema fluid.[18] Although often employed in renal doses to facilitate diuresis, the role of low-dose dopamine at 2 to 3 μg/kg/min remains controversial. Overly aggressive diuresis can result in renal insufficiency, which may be exacerbated by high postoperative calcineurin inhibitor levels. Therefore, careful monitoring of immunosuppressive medication levels and renal function is essential in the immediate postoperative period.

Before extubation, patients undergo bronchoscopy to ensure adequate clearance of secretions and viability of the donor bronchi. After extubation, the apical chest tubes are removed in the absence of an air leak, commonly within 48 hours postoperatively. Because of the frequent occurrence and recurrence of pleural effusions postoperatively, especially in bilateral lung transplant recipients, the basal chest tubes remain for several days and usually are removed on postoperative days 5 to 7 (chest tube drainage <150 mL/24 hours).

Vigorous chest physiotherapy, postural drainage, inhaled bronchodilators, and frequent clearance of pulmonary secretions is required in the postoperative care of these patients. Early and constant involvement of the physical therapy team ensures that transplant recipients are out of bed to chair, ambulatory with assistance, and using the treadmill or exercise bikes as soon as possible, even if they remain intubated. In patients with early allograft dysfunction requiring prolonged intubation, early tracheostomy permits easier mobility and better patient comfort, oral hygiene, and clearance of pulmonary secretions.

Adequate pain control is a necessity to prevent atelectasis owing to poor chest movement and inadequate coughing effort secondary to post-thoracotomy incisional pain. An epidural catheter provides an excellent means of achieving pain control with minimal systemic effects. In one study after lung transplantation, use of an epidural catheter was associated with faster extubation and decreased ICU days compared with IV morphine.[19] Patients often require at least some oral narcotics in the first few weeks after transplantation for pain management. Use of oral narcotics or acetaminophen is preferred to nonsteroidal anti-inflammatory drugs that can exacerbate renal insufficiency in these patients already on cyclosporine or other potentially nephrotoxic drugs. Procedure-specific and postoperative complications are reviewed in a different chapter.

HEART–LUNG TRANSPLANTATION

Preparation of Recipient

The recipient undergoes general anesthesia and double-lumen tube is preferred in order to have the option of single-lung ventilation. Routine monitoring devices are the same as those detailed for lung transplantation.

Technique

The type of incision performed is based on surgeon preference with either a median sternotomy or an antero-transsternal (clamshell) thoracotomy, each of which provides excellent exposure. For CPB, arterial cannula is placed in ascending aorta and bicaval cannulation is used for venous drainage. Both pleural spaces are opened, and adhesions are divided. After full bypass, the recipient is cooled to between 28 and 32°C, and mechanical ventilation ceased to permit better exposure. The pericardium around the level of the hilum is excised, and the PA and veins mobilized in the intrapericardial space. The right atrium is excised adjacent to the atrioventricular groove anteriorly, and the excision is extended circumferentially along the atrial septum. The aorta is divided above the aortic valve and retracted superiorly. The remaining PAs, left atrium, and ventricular structures are dissected free from the surrounding mediastinal tissue, and the patient's heart is removed (Fig. 109-12).

The bronchi on each side are mobilized, stapled proximally, and divided. The bronchi are divided beyond the staple line, and both lungs are removed separately. It is important to identify and preserve both phrenic nerves (Fig. 109-13).

The bronchial stumps and tracheal carina are mobilized, and the recipient trachea is divided immediately above the carina (Fig. 109-14). Care must be taken to ensure that bronchial vessels in the subcarinal space are controlled and that hemostasis is ensured before the graft is placed and anastomoses are completed. Exposure to the posterior mediastinum to establish hemostasis after heart–lung implantation is difficult and hazardous. Before the graft is placed, the pericardial openings are extended inferiorly and superiorly to create bilateral openings through which each donor lung can be introduced into its respective pleural space.

The donor heart–lung bloc is brought into the operative field, and each lung is passed through the opening in the pericardium into the pleural cavities posterior to the phrenic nerve–pericardial pedicles. Lick et al.[20] have reported a modified technique in which the lungs are placed anterior to the

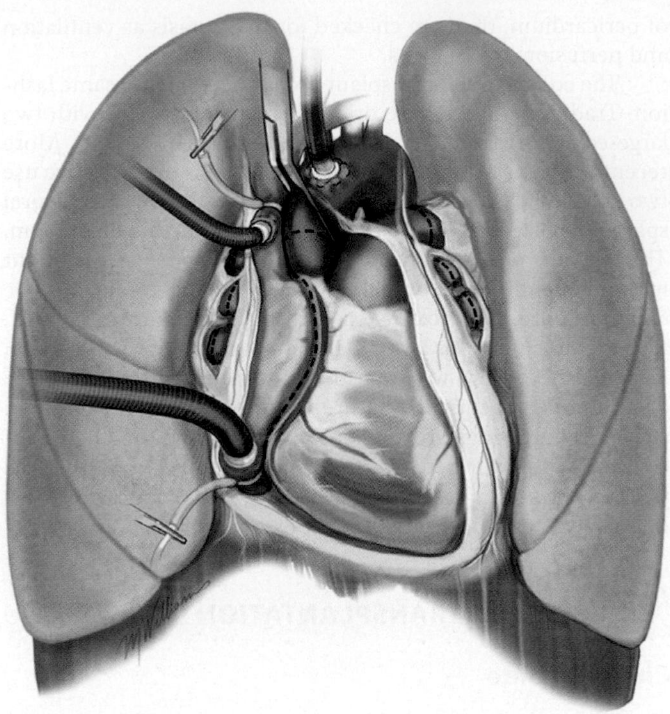

Figure 109-12. Recipient operation for heart–lung transplantation showing removal of the anterior pericardium and dissection of the ascending aorta and both venae cavae. The phrenic nerves are separated on pedicles, providing a space for insertion of the lung grafts. The cannulas for CPB are shown, as are the lines for removal of heart and lungs.

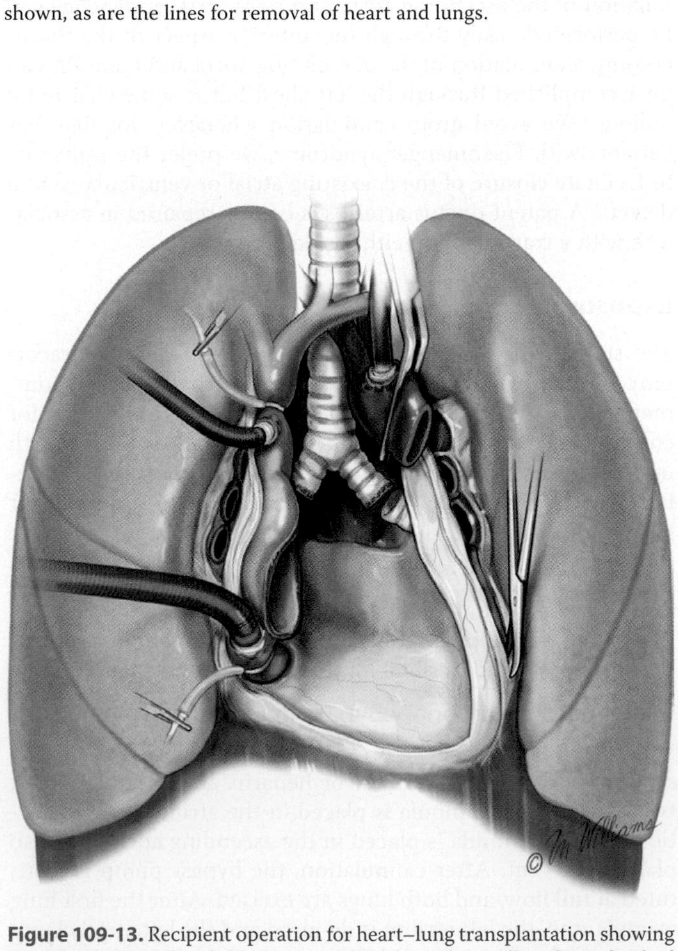

Figure 109-13. Recipient operation for heart–lung transplantation showing the heart removed and the division of the bronchi to allow for individual lung removal.

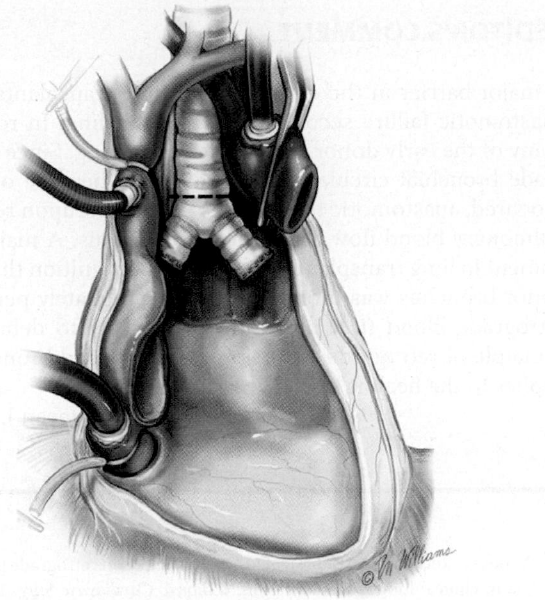

Figure 109-14. After the heart and lungs are removed from the chest, the trachea is divided immediately above the carina to prepare for the tracheal anastomosis.

phrenic nerves into each hemithorax. Placing the hila in front of the phrenic nerves minimizes dissection around and traction on the phrenic nerves and additionally permits the heart–lung bloc to be rotated anteriorly and medially to inspect for hemostasis in the posterior mediastinum after implantation.[20]

The tracheal anastomosis is performed first. We use a running 4-0 monofilament absorbable suture (Fig. 109-15). After

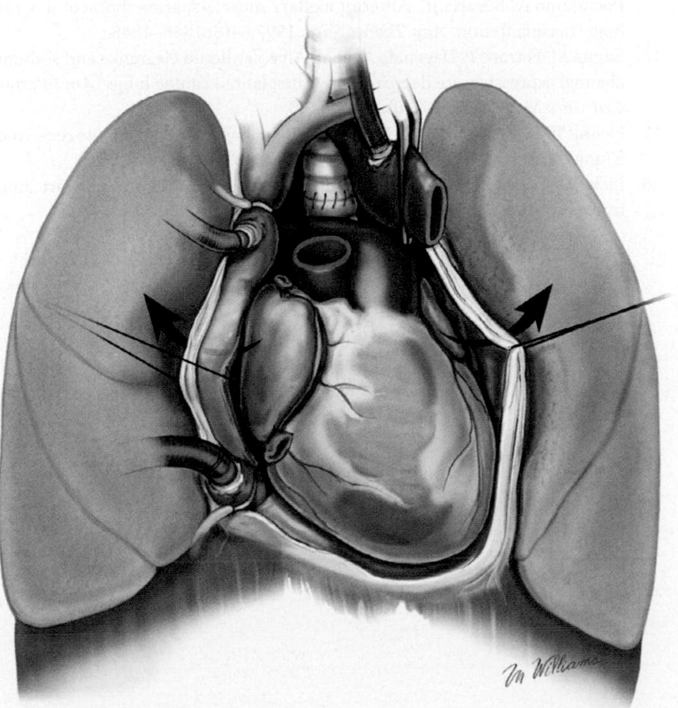

Figure 109-15. The heart–lung graft is brought into the field, and the right lung is passed underneath the right phrenic nerve pedicle. The same is done with the left lung. The tracheal anastomosis is performed first using a continuous 4-0 polypropylene suture.

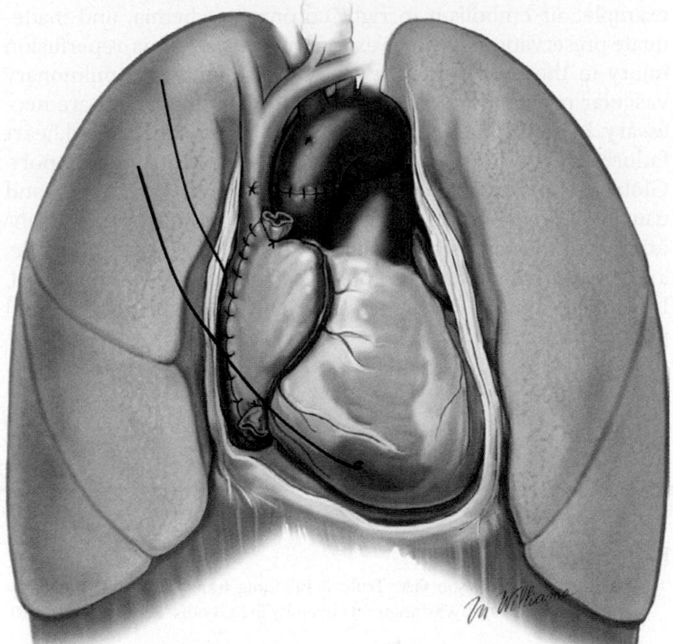

Figure 109-16. Completion of the heart–lung implantation showing the right atrial cuff anastomotic technique (alternatively, bicaval anastomoses can be performed) and the completed aortic anastomosis. The cannulas are removed, and temporary pacing wires are placed.

the tracheal anastomosis, the right atrial anastomosis is performed either by the bicaval technique or by the right cuff technique described by Shumway and Lower.

The aortic anastomosis is performed last while the patient is being rewarmed. Attention to de-airing the heart and aorta is imperative. Transesophageal echocardiography is extremely useful for assessing residual air and for assessing cardiac function. After achieving stable hemodynamics and gas exchange, the patient is weaned from CPB, and the cannulas are removed. Temporary pacing wires are placed on the donor right atrium and ventricle (Fig. 109-16). Appropriate chest tubes are placed in both pleura and mediastinum and the chest closed.

Postoperative Care

While much of the postoperative care for heart–lung graft recipients is similar to that detailed earlier for lung transplant recipients, there are some important points to keep in mind. Between 10% and 20% of heart–lung recipients experience a short period (usually less than 1 week) of transient sinus node dysfunction that perioperatively often presents as sinus bradycardia. Recipients routinely have atrial and ventricular pacing wires placed at the time of the operation, and maintenance of a paced heart rate between 90 and 110 beats/min may be necessary for adequate cardiac output, given the dependency of the denervated heart on rate. Alternatively, isoproterenol (0.005–0.01 μg/kg/min) may be used for the first few days postoperatively to maintain heart rate. Persistence of sinus node dysfunction, although rare, may require a permanent pacemaker. Other dysrhythmias are seen commonly as well and need to be treated appropriately.

Right-sided heart dysfunction can occur in the immediate postoperative period and has several potential causes, for example, air embolism in right coronary, ischemia, and inadequate preservation. It can be exacerbated by ischemia-reperfusion injury in the transplanted lungs with the increased pulmonary vascular resistance. Early identification and treatment are necessary. In addition to pulmonary vasodilators, right-sided heart failure usually is treated successfully with inotropic support. Global depressed myocardial performance also can occur and usually is treated successfully with inotropic support. Contributing causes such as hypovolemia, sepsis, cardiac tamponade, and bradycardia should be considered and treated when found. Inotropic support is weaned gradually over the first several postoperative days.

EDITOR'S COMMENT

A major barrier in the early years of lung transplantation was anastomotic failure secondary to poor healing. In retrospect, many of the early donor airways were too long. Since the antegrade bronchial circulation was divided when the organ was procured, anastomotic healing was dependent upon retrograde pulmonary blood flow to the donor bronchus. A major development in lung transplantation was the recognition that a short donor bronchus was more likely to be adequately perfused by retrograde blood flow and much less likely to dehisce. This principle of retrograde perfusion of the divided bronchus also applies to the healing of sleeve reconstructions.

—Steven J. Mentzer

References

1. Hachem RR, Patterson GA, Trulock EP. Lung transplantation at Barnes-Jewish Hospital and Washington University in St. Louis. *Clin Transpl.* 2010; 227–234.
2. Battafarano RJ, Anderson RC, Meyers BF, et al. Perioperative complications after living donor lobectomy. *J Thorac Cardiovasc Surg.* 2000;120(5):909–915.
3. Pasque MK, Trulock EP, Cooper JD, et al. Single lung transplantation for pulmonary hypertension. Single institution experience in 34 patients. *Circulation.* 1995;92(8):2252–2258.
4. Davis RD Jr., Trulock EP, Manley J, et al. Differences in early results after single-lung transplantation. Washington University Lung Transplant Group. *Ann Thorac Surg.* 1994;58(5):1327–1334; discussion 1334–1335.
5. Hadjiliadis D, Sporn TA, Perfect JR, et al. Outcome of lung transplantation in patients with mycetomas. *Chest.* 2002;121(1):128–134.
6. Trulock EP, Edwards LB, Taylor DO, et al. The Registry of the International Society for Heart and Lung Transplantation: twenty-first official adult lung and heart-lung transplant report–2004. *J Heart Lung Transplant.* 2004; 23(7):804–815.
7. Cassivi SD, Meyers BF, Battafarano RJ, et al. Thirteen-year experience in lung transplantation for emphysema. *Ann Thorac Surg.* 2002;74(5): 1663–1669; discussion 1669–1670.
8. Sundaresan S, Trachiotis GD, Aoe M, et al. Donor lung procurement: assessment and operative technique. *Ann Thorac Surg.* 1993;56(6):1409–1413.
9. Pasque MK. Standardizing thoracic organ procurement for transplantation. *J Thorac Cardiovasc Surg.* 2010;139(1):13–17.
10. Chen CZ, Gallagher RC, Ardery P, et al. Retrograde versus antegrade flush in canine left lung preservation for six hours. *J Heart Lung Transplant.* 1996;15(4):395–403.
11. Venuta F, Rendina EA, Bufi M, et al. Preimplantation retrograde pneumoplegia in clinical lung transplantation. *J Thorac Cardiovasc Surg.* 1999;118(1): 107–114.
12. Pomfret EA, Sung RS, Allan J, et al. Solving the organ shortage crisis: the 7th annual American Society of Transplant Surgeons' State-of-the-Art Winter Symposium. *Am J Transplant.* 2008;8(4):745–752.
13. Cypel M, Yeung JC, Liu M, et al. Normothermic ex vivo lung perfusion in clinical lung transplantation. *N Engl J Med.* 2011;364(15):1431–1440.
14. Meyers BF, Sundaresan RS, Guthrie T, et al. Bilateral sequential lung transplantation without sternal division eliminates posttransplantation sternal complications. *J Thorac Cardiovasc Surg.* 1999;117(2):358–364.
15. Brown RP, Esmore DS, Lawson C. Improved sternal fixation in the transsternal bilateral thoracotomy incision. *J Thorac Cardiovasc Surg.* 1996;112(1): 137–141.
16. van Berkel V, Guthrie TJ, Puri V, et al. Impact of anastomotic techniques on airway complications after lung transplant. *Ann Thorac Surg.* 2011;92(1): 316–320; discussion 320–321.
17. Pochettino A, Bavaria JE. Anterior axillary muscle-sparing thoracotomy for lung transplantation. *Ann Thorac Surg.* 1997;64(6):1846–1848.
18. Sugita M, Ferraro P, Dagenais A, et al. Alveolar liquid clearance and sodium channel expression are decreased in transplanted canine lungs. *Am J Respir Crit Care Med.* 2003;167(10):1440–1450.
19. Heerdt PM, Triantafillou A. Perioperative management of patients receiving a lung transplant. *Anesthesiology.* 1991;75(5):922–923.
20. Lick SD, Copeland JG, Rosado LJ, et al. Simplified technique of heart-lung transplantation. *Ann Thorac Surg.* 1995;59(6):1592–1593.

110 Living Lobar Lung Transplantation

Mark L. Barr and Vaughn A. Starnes

Keywords: Living-related donor, living lobar lung transplant, lobectomy, pneumonectomy

Living lobar lung transplantation was developed as an alternative to deceased donor lung transplantation because of the shortage of acceptable donor organs.[1,2] In living lobar lung transplantation, two healthy donors are selected—one to undergo removal of the right lower lobe and the other to undergo removal of the left lower lobe. These lobes then are implanted in the recipient in place of whole right and left lungs. This technique has proved to be beneficial to a group of patients who otherwise would have succumbed to disease while awaiting lungs from a conventional deceased donor.[3]

GENERAL PRINCIPLES AND PATIENT SELECTION

Living lobar lung transplant candidates should meet the standard criteria for deceased donor lung transplantation and be listed on the Organ Procurement and Transplantation Network lung transplantation waiting list.[4] The expectation for potential recipients should be that they will either die before a deceased donor lung becomes available or become too ill to undergo any sort of organ transplant procedure. In the United States, cystic fibrosis has been the most common indication for living lobar lung transplantation. Other indications have included primary pulmonary arterial hypertension (PAH), pulmonary fibrosis, bronchopulmonary dysplasia, and obliterative bronchiolitis.[2] In Japan, which is the country where the second highest numbers of these cases have been performed and where cystic fibrosis is very rare, the most frequent indications have been PAH, obliterative bronchiolitis (including a subset of patients with prior hematopoietic stem cell transplantation), and interstitial pneumonia.[5]

The goals of donor selection are to identify donors with excellent health, adequate pulmonary reserve for lobar donation, an emotional attachment to the recipient, and a willingness to accept the risks of donation without coercion. Our criteria for donation also include age between 18 and 55 years, no history of thoracic procedures on the side to be donated, and excellent general health. Donors taller than the recipient are favored over donors of the same or lesser height because they have the potential to provide larger lobes. Initially, only the mother and father of the recipient were considered as donors; however, lobes from siblings, extended family members, and unrelated individuals who can demonstrate an emotional attachment to the recipient are also presently considered. A psychosocial interview is conducted. Potential donors are interviewed both separately and with the potential recipient's family to ascertain interpersonal dynamics. Elements of the interview include the motivation to donate, pain tolerance, feelings regarding donation should the recipient expire, and the ability of the potential donor to be separated from family and career obligations. Since an element of coercion always can exist between a potential donor and the recipient and/or the recipient's family, any potential donor who discloses that he or she feels any pressure to donate after careful consultation and explanation of the procedure is denied for unspecified reasons, thus preventing untoward feelings between the family, recipient, and potential donor.

After the psychosocial evaluation, suitable potential donors undergo blood typing for compatibility as well as chest radiography and spirometry to assess lung size and function. This preliminary screening reduces costs because it allows for the evaluation of only a limited number of potential donors. A more thorough medical workup, including routine transplant serologies (i.e., HIV, VDRL, cytomegalovirus, Epstein–Barr virus, and hepatitis), electrocardiogram, echocardiogram, quantitative ventilation/perfusion scanning, and high-resolution chest CT scanning, is conducted after the preliminary screening is completed and found to be acceptable.

After identification of two suitable donors, one is chosen to undergo right lower lobectomy and the other, left lower lobectomy. The right lower lobe is usually selected from the larger donor, whereas the donor with the more complete fissure on the left is chosen to donate that side if the donors are of the same height. Occasionally, an acceptable donor will have a history of prior thoracic procedures, trauma, or infection. In this case, the contralateral side is chosen for donation. Computerized tomography chest scanning and spirometry can be used to estimate the subsequent resulting lung volume in the recipient. Size matching has also been performed utilizing three-dimensional CT volumetric reconstruction imaging.[5] Regardless of whether functional or anatomical methods (or both) are used to determine the appropriate size match between the donor and the recipient, the goal is to avoid the extremes of transplanting an insufficient amount of lung tissue due to undersized lobes versus implanting oversized grafts, the latter of which is a greater risk when the recipient is a child. While human leukocyte antigen (HLA) matching is not required for donor selection, a prospective crossmatch to rule out the presence of anti-HLA antibodies is performed.

OPERATIVE TECHNIQUE

The performance of living lobar lung transplantation involves three simultaneous operations: two donor lobectomies, the recipient bilateral pneumonectomy, and lobar implantation. The operative goals of living-donor lung transplantation are to avoid morbidity to the healthy volunteer lobe donor while providing adequate tissue margins for implantation in the recipient.[6] The lobar vascular and bronchial anatomy of the right and left lower lobes are the most suitable for lobar transplantation.

The Donor Lobectomy

The donors are placed in separate ORs, and epidural catheters are inserted for postoperative pain control. After induction of anesthesia, fiberoptic bronchoscopy is performed to exclude mucosal abnormalities or alterations in bronchial anatomy. The single-lumen endotracheal tube is replaced with a double-lumen tube, and the patient is positioned in the appropriate lateral decubitus position. Prostaglandin E_1 is administered intravenously to dilate the pulmonary bed, and the dosage is adjusted to maintain a systolic blood pressure of 90 to 100 mm Hg. There are important differences in performing a lobectomy for lobar transplantation in comparison with that for cancer or infection. The lobe must be removed with an adequate cuff of bronchus and pulmonary artery and vein to permit successful implantation into the recipient while allowing closure of these structures without compromise in the donor.

Donor Right Lower Lobectomy

The donor lung is deflated, and the chest is entered through a standard posterolateral thoracotomy through the fourth or fifth interspace. The lung is carefully inspected to exclude unsuspected pathology. Excellent exposure is mandatory, allowing dissection of hilar structures without excessive manipulation of the graft. The inferior pulmonary ligament is taken down, and the pleura is opened around the hilum. Dissection in the fissure characterizes anatomic variants and identifies the pulmonary arteries to the right lower and right middle lobes. The relationship between the superior segmental artery to the right lower lobe and middle lobe artery should be visualized (Fig. 110-1). Commonly, the middle lobe has two arteries, with the smaller artery having a more distal origin than the superior segmental artery to the lower lobe. In this case, the smaller artery may be ligated and divided. Ideally, there will be sufficient distance between the takeoff of the middle lobe artery and the superior segmental artery of the right lower lobe to permit placement of a vascular clamp distal to the middle lobe artery, thus enabling a sufficient vascular cuff for the pulmonary arterial anastomosis at implantation.

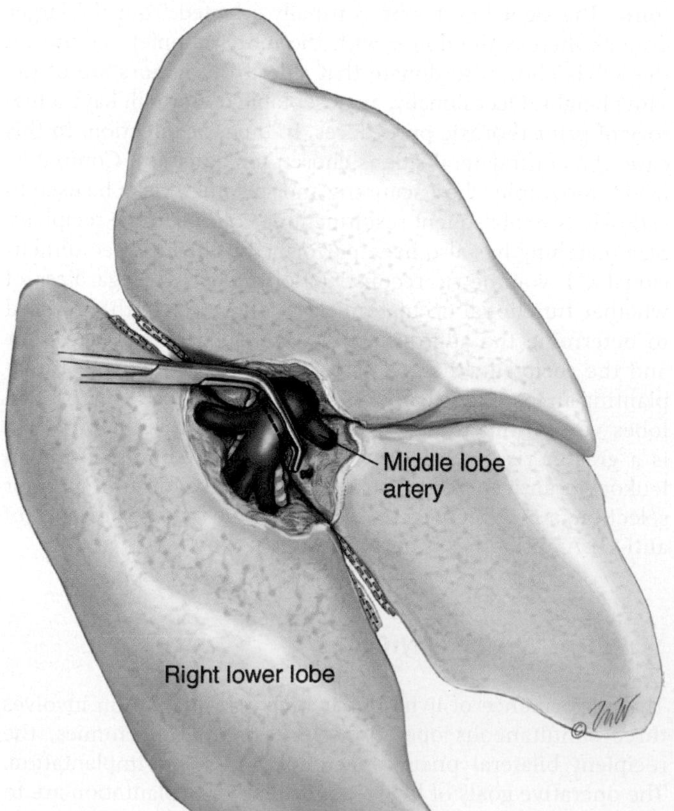

Figure 110-1. Dissection and division of the pulmonary artery for donor right lower lobectomy.

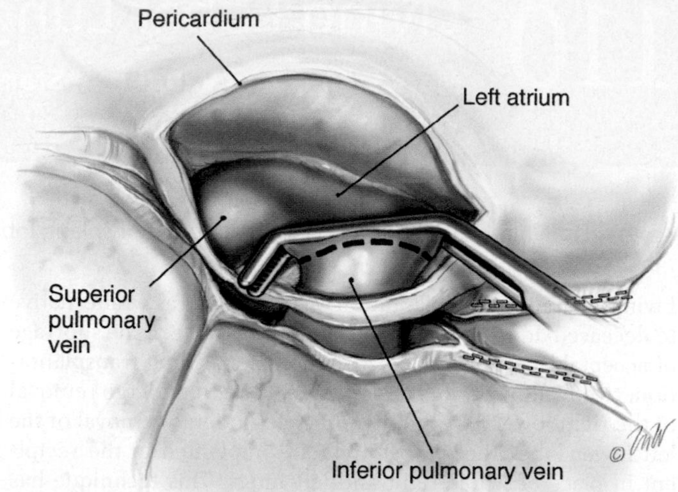

Figure 110-2. Dissection of the right inferior pulmonary vein, permitting placement of a vascular clamp on the intrapericardial left atrium.

After confirming that the inferior pulmonary vein does not receive venous drainage from the right middle lobe, the pericardium surrounding the inferior pulmonary vein is incised. This dissection allows a vascular clamp to be placed on the left atrium and the inferior pulmonary vein to be cut with an adequate cuff on the donor lobe (Fig. 110-2). When the vascular dissections are complete, the fissures are stapled using a 75-mm nonvascular stapler or a 45-mm GIA thoracoscopic stapler. Between 5000 and 10,000 units of heparin and 500-mg methylprednisolone are administered intravenously, and the lung is reinflated and ventilated for 5 to 10 minutes to permit the drugs to circulate through the lung. The lung then is deflated. To avoid vascular congestion of the pulmonary allograft, a vascular clamp is placed first on the pulmonary artery and subsequently on the left atrial side of the inferior pulmonary vein, optimizing the length of the venous cuff for pulmonary venous anastomosis. The pulmonary artery is transected at a point that will leave an adequate vascular cuff for the anastomosis while leaving sufficient length to permit repair without compromising the remaining pulmonary arterial branches. The inferior pulmonary vein is transected with a small cuff of left atrium. The bronchus to the right lower lobe now should be exposed. Minimizing dissection around the bronchus preserves blood supply to both the donor lobe and the remaining lung. The right middle lobe bronchus is identified, and the bronchus to the lower lobe is transected tangentially. The incision begins in the bronchus intermedius above the bronchus to the superior segment of the right lower lobe and moves obliquely to a point just below the takeoff of the right middle lobe bronchus (Fig. 110-3).

Division of the pulmonary vessels and bronchus should be performed expeditiously to limit the warm ischemia time of the

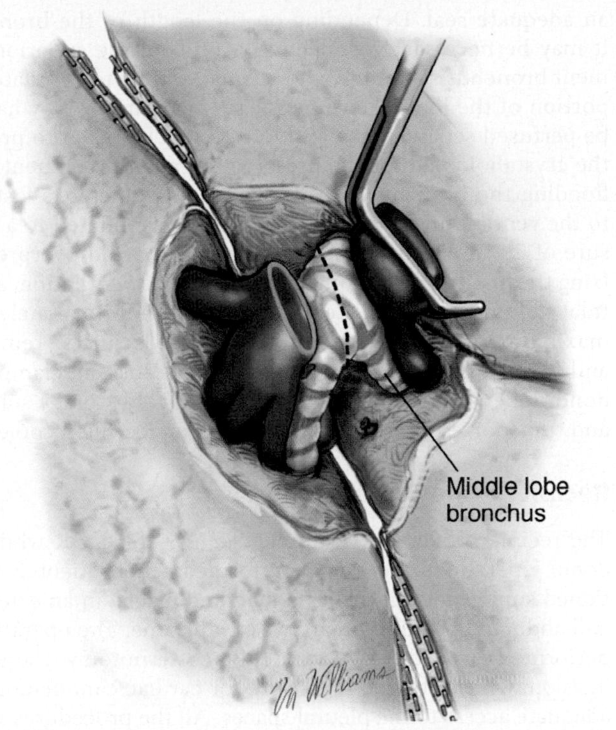

Figure 110-3. Dissection and division of the bronchus to the right lower lobe.

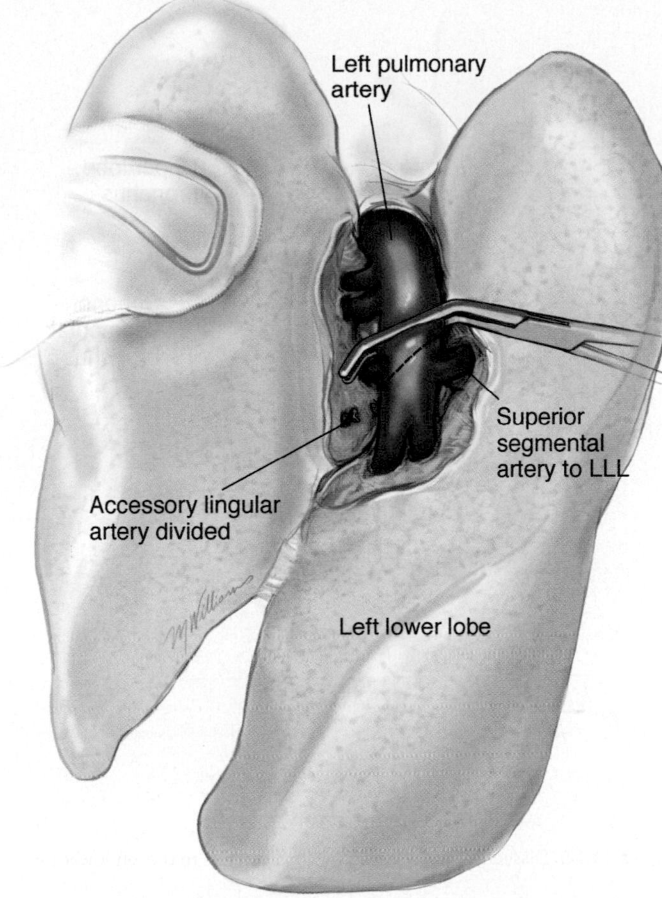

Figure 110-4. Dissection and division of the pulmonary artery for donor left lower lobectomy.

allograft. When separated, the donor lobe is wrapped in a cold, moist sponge and taken to a separate, sterile table for preservation. The donor pulmonary artery is repaired in two layers with a running polypropylene suture, and the pulmonary vein/left atrium is closed in a similar fashion. The bronchus is closed with interrupted polypropylene, being careful to avoid narrowing of the bronchus intermedius or infolding of the middle lobe carina. Resecting a small wedge of cartilage at the orifice of the middle lobe may facilitate closure. The bronchial suture line is covered with a pleural flap to separate the arterial and bronchial suture lines. Two chest tubes are placed in the pleural space, and the chest is closed in the standard fashion.

Donor Left Lower Lobectomy

The chest is opened using a standard posterolateral thoracotomy through the fourth or fifth interspace. The lung is examined in a similar fashion to that described for the right side. The inferior pulmonary ligament is taken down, and the pleura is opened around the hilum. Dissection in the fissure defines the vascular anatomy. The relationship between the superior segmental artery to the lower lobe and the anteriorly positioned lingular artery is evaluated (Fig. 110-4). The lingular artery may be ligated and divided if it is of small size and its origin is too far distal to the artery to the superior segment of the lower lobe. If the significance of this artery is uncertain, the anesthesiologist can inflate and deflate the lung while this artery is occluded. Dissection of the pulmonary artery to the lower lobe should enable placement of a vascular clamp proximal to the artery supplying the superior segment of the lower lobe. The pericardium around the inferior pulmonary vein is opened circumferentially, and the fissures are completed with a nonvascular stapler.

When the dissection is complete, the lung is reinflated and ventilated for 5 to 10 minutes as described for the right side. Heparin and methylprednisolone are administered. The lung is subsequently deflated, and the pulmonary artery and vein are clamped and transected in the sequence described for the right lung. The exposed bronchus is followed upward until the lingular bronchus is identified. Care must be taken to avoid skeletonizing the bronchus because this may compromise healing in the recipient. The tangential transection begins at the base of the upper lobe bronchus and ends superiorly to the bronchus to the superior segment of the left lower lobe (Fig. 110-5). The donor lobe then is taken to a separate table for preservation and storage. The pulmonary vessels and bronchus are repaired in a manner similar to that described earlier.

Allograft Preservation

Preparation of the donor lobe begins at the start of the donor operation with a continuous prostaglandin infusion and meticulous attention to operative technique during the lobectomy. In contrast to standard deceased donor lung explantation, preservation of the lobe in a live donor does not permit in situ flushing and cooling of the graft with cold preservation solutions. Therefore, after the donor lobe is removed, it is taken to a separate, sterile table for cold preservation. The allograft is immersed in cold crystalloid solution. The pulmonary artery and vein are cannulated in an alternating fashion and flushed with 1 to 2 L of cold Perfadex (low potassium, dextran, and glucose) solution until the pulmonary venous and arterial effluents are clear and the parenchyma is blanched white. During

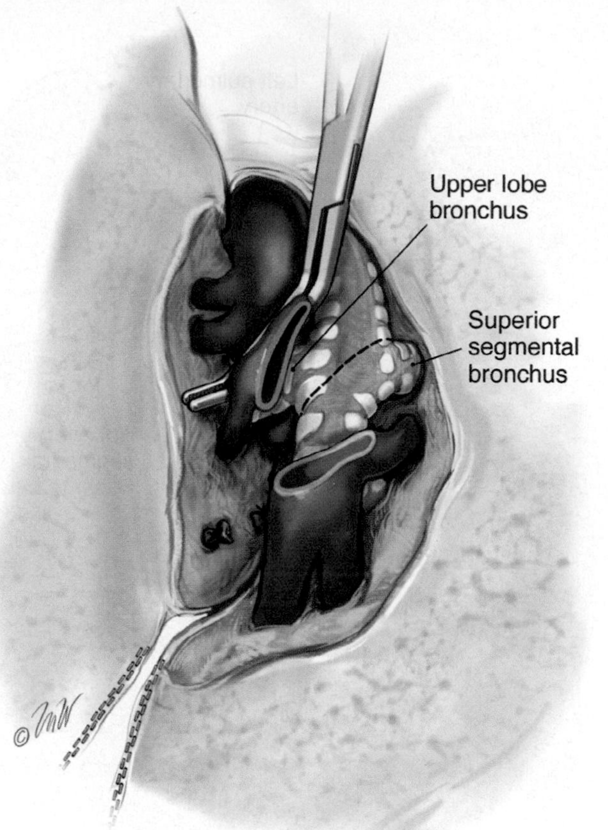

Figure 110-5. Dissection and division of the bronchus to the left lower lobe.

perfusion, the lobe is gently ventilated with room air. A ventilation bag with different size endotracheal tubes should be available. Using an appropriately sized endotracheal tube permits an adequate seal to be formed while ventilating the bronchus and prevents potential damage to the bronchus caused by crushing or squeezing the bronchus in an effort to obtain an adequate seal. Depending on the length of the bronchus, it may be necessary to selectively intubate the superior segment bronchus separately with a smaller tube to ventilate that portion of the lobe. The superior segment artery may have to be perfused separately as well. Care must be taken to prevent the crystalloid bath or the preservation solution effluent from flooding the bronchus. In addition, a manometer is fastened to the ventilation apparatus, and the lobe is inflated to a pressure of 20 to 25 mm Hg, being careful to avoid overpressurizing the lung. After adequate perfusion and ventilation, a final tidal volume is administered to achieve approximately 75% maximum inflation, the endotracheal tube is quickly removed, and the bronchus is occluded with a noncrushing clamp. The donor lobe is placed in a sterile bag with cold storage solution and transported to the recipient OR in an ice-filled cooler.

Recipient Pneumonectomy

The recipient operation commences in a third OR while the donor operations are being performed. The patient is positioned supine and the arms padded and placed in an extended and abducted position on an overhead frame. The operation is performed through a transverse thoracosternotomy (clamshell) incision, which provides exposure for cardiac cannulation and adequate access to the pleural spaces. All the procedures at our center have been preferentially performed while on cardiopulmonary bypass, often because of the recipient's critical condition, as well as to minimize the risk of pulmonary edema while exposing one lobe to the entire cardiac output while the other lobe is implanted. Use of cardiopulmonary bypass prevents spillage of purulent secretions from the second native lung and allows simultaneous reperfusion of both lobes in a controlled fashion. Hilar dissection and lysis of adhesions are completed before heparinization and cardiopulmonary bypass. The pleural cavity of patients with cystic fibrosis is irrigated thoroughly with antibacterial and antifungal solutions. Dissection of the pulmonary artery and veins is performed as distally as possible to optimize cuff length for the anastomoses (Fig. 110-6). When

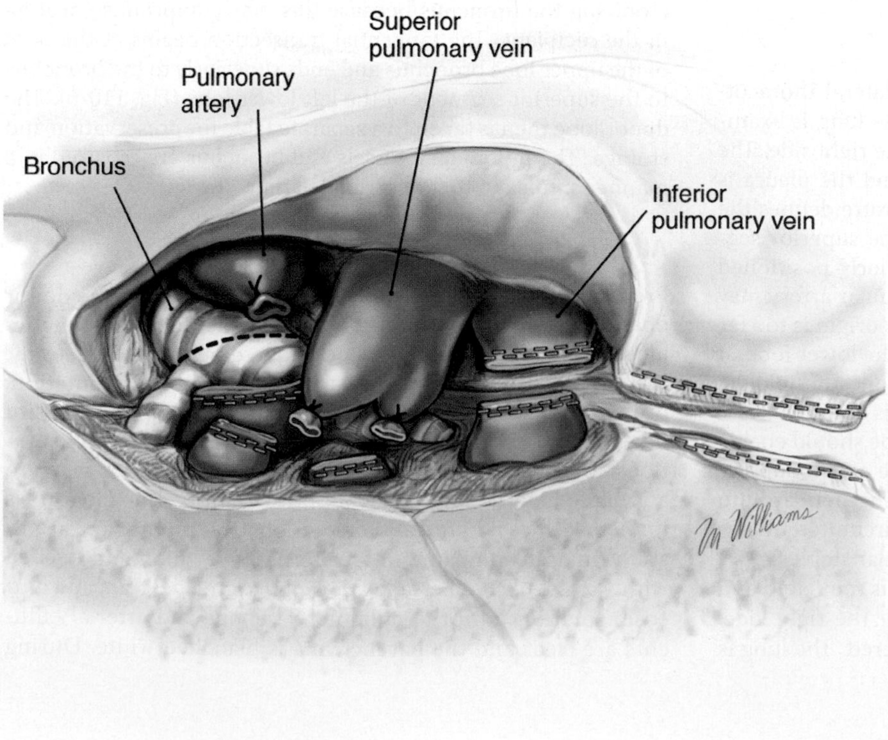

Figure 110-6. Recipient right pneumonectomy.

the dissection is complete, cardiopulmonary bypass is initiated and the pulmonary vasculature is divided. The pulmonary veins are divided between stapling devices while the pulmonary artery is doubly ligated and divided. The bronchus is divided with a stapling device at the level of the takeoff of the upper lobe bronchus. After the onset of bypass, the anesthesiologist suctions the lungs and removes the endotracheal tube.

Allograft Implantation

The first allograft is placed on a cooling jacket within the pleural space, and the exposed lung is wrapped in iced, saline-soaked sponges. The bronchial anastomosis is performed with running 4-0 polypropylene suture. Care is taken to limit the amount of peribronchial dissection. The bronchial anastomosis places the donor lobar vein in close approximation to the superior pulmonary vein of the recipient, and the venous anastomosis is performed in a running fashion with 5-0 polypropylene suture. The short length of the donor vein makes anastomosis directly to the left atrium difficult and underscores the importance of leaving an adequate length of recipient pulmonary vein during pneumonectomy. The pulmonary artery anastomosis is performed end to end with 5-0 polypropylene suture (Fig. 110-7). A similar procedure is performed for the second allograft.

After completing the bilateral implantations, the arterial vascular clamp is slowly removed. The preservation perfusate is permitted to egress from the venous anastomosis before tying the venous sutures, and ventilation is begun gently. Continuous nitric oxide starting at 20 ppm and intermittent aerosolized bronchodilator therapy are both administered via the anesthesia circuit. Blood volume is returned gradually, allowing increased cardiac ejection and pulmonary blood flow to occur with subsequent weaning from cardiopulmonary bypass. At completion of implantation, transesophageal echocardiography to evaluate for patency of the one pulmonary vein on each side draining into the left atrium and bronchoscopy to assess the bronchial anastomoses and for pulmonary toileting are performed. Four chest tubes then are placed, the clamshell incision is closed, and the patient is transported directly to the ICU.

POSTOPERATIVE MANAGEMENT

Donor Management

The donors are transported to the recovery room with epidural catheters in place after the lobectomy. Chest tubes are required until all evidence of air leak has ceased, chest tube output is acceptable, and the remaining lung tissue fills the hemithorax with no significant pneumothorax. Donors receive low-dose enoxaparin and sequential compression devices postoperatively to prevent thromboembolic complications. Oral analgesics are administered on removal of the chest tubes and are continued for a short time at home. Standard postthoracotomy management includes incentive spirometry and physical therapy exercises.

Recipient Management

While immunosuppression, antibiotic therapy and prophylaxis, and long-term management of the lobar recipient are very similar to those for standard deceased-donor lung transplantation, the perioperative management is different given the physiology of lobar transplantation.

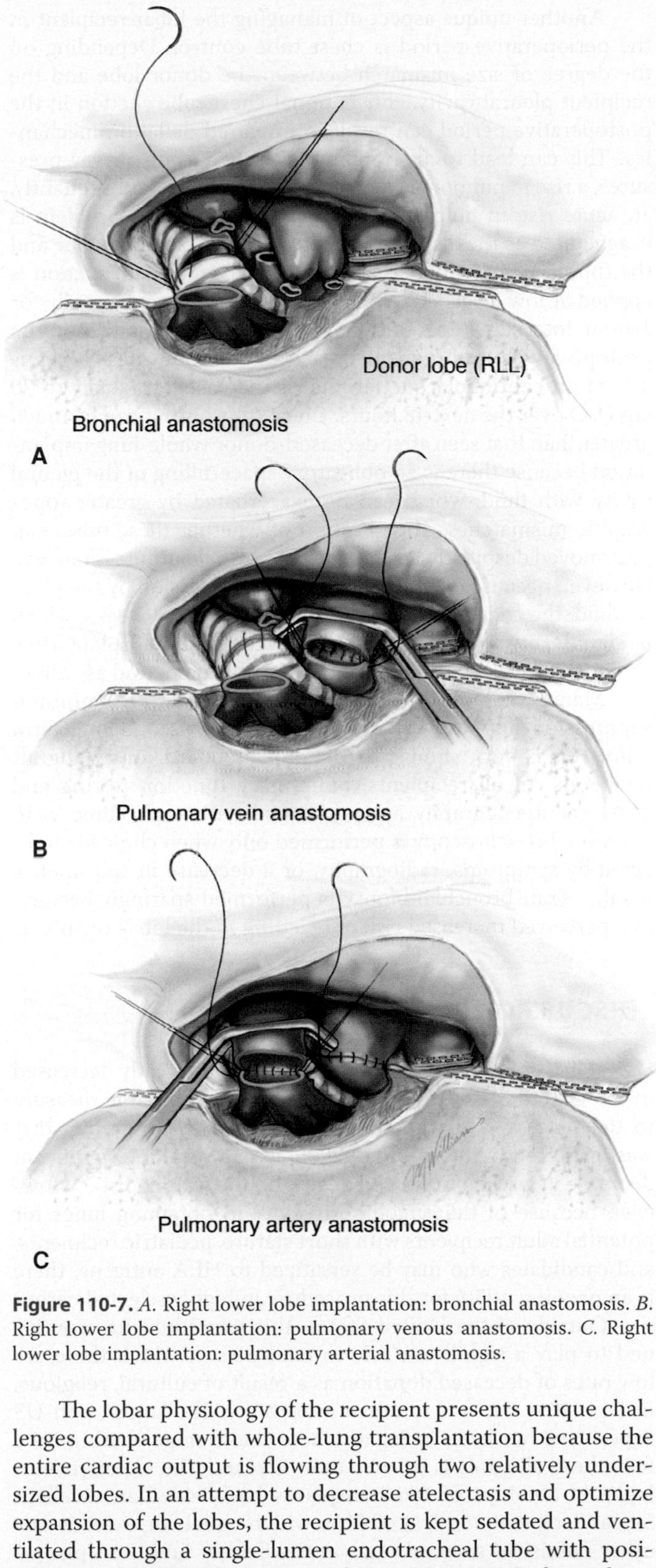

Figure 110-7. *A.* Right lower lobe implantation: bronchial anastomosis. *B.* Right lower lobe implantation: pulmonary venous anastomosis. *C.* Right lower lobe implantation: pulmonary arterial anastomosis.

The lobar physiology of the recipient presents unique challenges compared with whole-lung transplantation because the entire cardiac output is flowing through two relatively undersized lobes. In an attempt to decrease atelectasis and optimize expansion of the lobes, the recipient is kept sedated and ventilated through a single-lumen endotracheal tube with positive end-expiratory pressures of 5 to 10 cm H_2O for at least 48 hours. In addition, efforts are undertaken to decrease pulmonary artery pressures and minimize the risk of reperfusion injury and pulmonary edema. This is accomplished by maintaining the recipient in a relatively hypovolemic state, the use of nitroglycerin infusion, and the use of aerosolized nitric oxide for the first 48 to 72 hours.

Another unique aspect of managing the lobar recipient in the perioperative period is chest tube control. Depending on the degree of size mismatch between the donor lobe and the recipient pleural cavity, conventional chest tube suction in the postoperative period can result in impaired deflation mechanics. This can lead to air trapping with increasing airway pressures, a rise in pulmonary vascular resistance, and subsequently, an acute rise in pulmonary arterial pressure. This problem is exaggerated as the discrepancy between the size of the lobe and the thoracic cavity increases. To avoid this problem, suction is applied at low levels (10 cm H_2O) to each tube sequentially for 1-hour intervals in a rotational fashion for the first 24 hours postoperatively. Subsequently, each of the four chest tubes is placed on continuous suction that is increased gradually to 20 cm H_2O over the next 48 hours. Chest tube output can be much greater than that seen after deceased-donor whole-lung implantation because there is an obligatory space-filling of the pleural cavity with fluid, which can be exacerbated by greater topographic mismatches. The question of whether these tubes can be removed despite these higher than normal outputs is unclear. However, because of concerns of lobe compression by the pleural fluid, the chest tubes are left in place for 2 to 3 weeks, which is significantly longer than for conventional transplantation. Residual air leaks typically resolve in this time period as well.

Management of the lobar recipient in regard to immunosuppression, antibiotic therapy and prophylaxis, and long-term follow-up is very similar to that for standard lung allograft recipients. In all recipients, pulmonary function testing and chest roentgenography are performed with each clinic visit; however, bronchoscopy is performed only when clinically indicated by symptoms, radiography, or a decrease in spirometric results. Transbronchial biopsy is performed sparingly because of a perceived increased risk of bleeding in the lobar recipient.

DISCUSSION

Use of live donors in lung transplantation has greatly decreased in the United States in the past 7 years owing in large measure to the success of the lung allocation score (LAS) system that was instituted in the spring of 2005, with a resulting significant decrease in waiting times and deaths on the waiting list.[7,8] However, because of the ongoing difficulty in obtaining lungs for potential adult recipients with short stature, pediatric recipients, and candidates who may be sensitized to HLA antigens, there is an ongoing utility for this procedure in highly selected cases.

Outside of the United States, this procedure has continued to play a significant role in countries in which there are low rates of deceased donation as a result of cultural, religious, or legislative barriers to organ availability. The largest non-US experience has been in Japan where the average waiting time for a lung allograft is greater than 2 years. The experience in Japan in a cohort of 100 transplants has yielded an excellent 5-year recipient survival of 81%, which equals or exceeds any other published survival rates in the field of lung transplantation, regardless of the donor source.[9]

An additional factor that has contributed to the reduction in the total number of these cases has been concerns regarding both the short-term risks of the surgery on the donor, and the unknown and unstudied long-term outcomes for these living donors. As far as what is known regarding short-term outcomes, the Lung Working Group of the Vancouver Forum compiled and published a retrospective review of 550 live lung donors, which constituted 98% of the global experience as of 2005.[10] The mean age was 38 ± 10 years (range 18–60 years). Sixty percent of the live lung donors were male, 76% were related to the recipient, and 24% were unrelated. Of the related donors, 40% were parents, 29% siblings, 15% uncle/aunt, 9% cousins, 5% son/daughter, and 1% nephew/niece. Of the live donors who were unrelated to the recipients 74% were friends, 20% spouses, and 6% strangers.

In that study, there was no reported perioperative mortality of a lung donor. There were life-threatening complications in three cases (0.5%) including one intraoperative ventricular fibrillation arrest and two having a postoperative pulmonary artery thrombosis. The mean length of the initial hospitalization following the lung lobectomy was 8.5 days (range 3–36). Approximately 4% experienced an intraoperative complication that included ventricular fibrillation arrest (1), the necessity of a right middle lobe sacrifice (7; 1.3%), the necessity of a right middle lobe reimplantation (6; 1.1%), the necessity of a non-autologous packed red blood cell transfusion (5; 0.9%), and a permanent phrenic nerve injury (1). Approximately 5% experienced complications requiring surgical or bronchoscopic intervention. These complications included bleeding, bronchopleural fistula, pleural effusion, empyema, bronchial stricture, pericarditis requiring pericardiectomy, arrhythmias requiring ablation, and chylothorax. There were 14 (2.6%) live lung donors that were readmitted to the hospital because of either a pneumothorax, an arrhythmia, empyema, pericarditis, dyspnea, pleural effusion, bronchial stricture, bronchopleural fistula, pneumonia, hemoptysis, or dehydration. The long-term (defined as greater than 1 year) donor complaints, which were not qualified or quantitated in that study, included chronic incisional pain, dyspnea, pericarditis, and non-productive cough.

In response to the lack of high quality, long-term follow-up information, the National Institute of Allergy and Infectious Diseases (NIAID) is funding an ongoing study of the majority of those individuals who were living lung donors in the United States from 1993 to 2006. The lung portion of the RELIVE consortium is currently characterizing short- and long-term morbidities rates, long-term lung function, and psychosocial outcomes in these patients with study results anticipated in the next year.[11]

The future results of such ongoing studies as well as prior outcomes for the recipients as reported by our group and from Japan are important if this type of procedure is to be considered as an option at more pulmonary transplant centers in view of the institutional, regional, and intra- and international differences in the philosophical, legal, and ethical acceptance of the use of live organ donors for transplantation.[12,13]

EDITOR'S COMMENT

A disappointing finding in lobar transplantation has been the absence of convincing compensatory growth in the transplanted lung. Although the adult lobe expands its volume in a recipient patient, it has been difficult to demonstrate an adaptive increase in lung function. Adaptive regeneration of the lung is an area of active biological research that has many potential disease applications; none of these applications is more important than lobar lung transplantation.

—Steven J. Mentzer

References

1. Starnes VA, Barr ML, Cohen RG. Lobar transplantation. Indications, technique, and outcome. *J Thorac Cardiovasc Surg*. 1994;108:403–410.
2. Starnes VA, Bowdish ME, Woo MS, et al. A decade of living lobar lung transplantation: recipient outcomes. *J Thorac Cardiovasc Surg*. 2004;127:114–122.
3. Bowdish ME, Barr ML, Schenkel FA, et al. A decade of living lobar lung transplantation: perioperative complications after 253 donor lobectomies. *Am J Transplant*. 2004;4:1283–1288.
4. Orens JB, Estenne M, Arcasoy S, et al. International guidelines for the selection of lung transplant candidates: 2006 update—a consensus report from the Pulmonary Scientific Council of the International Society for Heart and Lung Transplantation. *J Heart Lung Transplant*. 2006;25:745–755.
5. Date H. Update on living-donor lobar lung transplantation. *Curr Opin Organ Transplant*. 2011;16:453–457.
6. Bowdish ME, Barr ML, Starnes VA. Living lobar transplantation. *Chest Surg Clin N Am*. 2003;13:505–524.
7. Egan TM, Murray S, Bustami RT, et al. Development of the new lung allocation system in the United States. *Am J Transplant*. 2006;6:1212–1227.
8. http://www.srtr.org/annual_reports/2010/1203_lu.pdf.
9. Egawa H, Tanabe K, Fukushima N, et al. Current status of organ transplantation in Japan. *Am J Transplant*. 2012;12:523–530.
10. Barr ML, Belghiti J, Villamil FG, et al. A report of the Vancouver Forum on the care of the live organ donor: lung, liver, pancreas, and intestine data and medical guidelines. *Transplantation*. 2006;27:1373–1385.
11. Project leader: Barr, Mark L. Project number: 5UO1AI069545-05. http://projectreporter.nih.gov/project_info_description.cfm?aid=7899950&icde=11981871&ddparam=&ddvalue=&ddsub=&cr=1&csb=default&cs=ASC.
12. Barr ML, Schenkel FA, Bowdish ME, et al. Living donor lung transplantation: current status and future directions. *Transplant Proc*. 2005;37:3983–3986.
13. Wells WJ, Barr ML. The ethics of living donor lung transplantation. *Thorac Surg Clin*. 2005;15:519–525.

111 Medical Management of Lung Transplant Patients

Hilary J. Goldberg and Phillip C. Camp

Keywords: End-stage pulmonary disease, lung transplant, medical complications, acute rejection, chronic rejection, infection, immunosuppression, gastroesophageal reflux disease

In addition to representing a significant surgical challenge, successful medical management of the lung transplant patient is a very complex issue. The protocol for medical management has evolved over time. The focus of care in this patient population is fourfold: immunosuppression, graft rejection, complications arising from infection, and other medical complications.

IMMUNOSUPPRESSION

To attenuate graft injury owing to immunologic rejection, all lung transplant patients require lifelong systemic immunosuppression. The morbidity associated with mandatory immunosuppression is a key to the complexity of medical care for this patient group.

Induction Therapy

The risk of acute rejection is 40% to 50% in the first posttransplant year, and 50% of patients will have developed chronic rejection by the fifth posttransplant year.[1] To ameliorate this risk, clinicians have adopted an early and aggressive postoperative immunosuppression strategy using prophylactic T-cell depletion, commonly referred to as induction therapy. Approximately 50% of lung transplant programs utilize some form of induction therapy.[1] In addition to mitigating the incidence of acute rejection, induction therapy also has the advantage of delaying the use of the traditional immunosuppressants (i.e., calcineurin inhibitors) in the immediate postoperative period when the nephrotoxicity induced by these medications is potentially more harmful to the patient.

The standard choices for induction include rabbit and equine polyclonal antithymocyte globulins (thymoglobulin and ATGAM, respectively), murine monoclonal anti-CD3 antibody (OKT3), and interluekin-2 (IL-2) receptor antagonists. Antithymocyte globulin and OKT3 act on the entire T-cell population. IL-2 receptor antibodies (e.g., basiliximab) target the IL-2 receptor alpha chain, which is found selectively on activated T cells. Both antithymocyte globulin and OKT3 work by depleting the number of circulating lymphocytes, resulting in a predictable lymphopenia. Both antibodies are also associated with thrombocytopenia and flu-like illness with fever and chills. A more dramatic release of cytokines (i.e., tumor necrosis factor, IL-2, and γ-interferon) with subsequent cardiovascular collapse has been described with the use of OKT3. All of the induction agents increase the risk of infection. In one study comparing the three main agents, there was no difference in episodes of acute rejection, episodes of bronchiolitis obliterans syndrome (BOS), or survival at 2 years, although there was a statistically significant risk of increased infection with OKT3.[2]

Maintenance Therapy

Long-term immunosuppression is a core component of medical care. Most lung transplant patients are maintained on a three-medication regimen consisting of an oral corticosteroid, a calcineurin inhibitor (i.e., cyclosporine or tacrolimus), and a purine synthesis inhibitor (i.e., azathioprine or mycophenolate mofetil [MMF]).

Most clinicians initiate corticosteroids in the early postoperative period. Intravenous (IV) dosing of moderate-to-high levels of drug is administered during the first week, and patients are thereafter transitioned to oral glucocorticoids, traditionally prednisone. Although lung transplant patients are maintained on glucocorticoids for the long term, attempts are made to minimize the dose to reduce the risk of infection, osteoporosis, glucose intolerance, and mood effects. In our practice, we reduce the corticosteroid dose to 0.5 mg/kg daily on the fifth postoperative day and to 0.3 mg/kg by 3 months posttransplant. Patients are typically maintained on 5 mg prednisone daily.

Calcineurin inhibitors include cyclosporine and tacrolimus. Cyclosporine, a fungal peptide, acts by binding to cytoplasmic proteins and by inhibiting calcineurin. This inhibition causes decreased transcription of many cytokines (IL-2, IL-3, IL-4, IL-5, γ-interferon, and tumor necrosis factor) and decreased activation of T cells. Cyclosporine has a narrow therapeutic window and is highly nephrotoxic. For this reason, close monitoring of cyclosporine blood levels is essential. The published data suggest that the optimal time for this measurement is 2 hours after a dose, although trough levels obtained immediately prior to the dose are more commonly used in clinical practice. The preferential use of tacrolimus over cyclosporine has increased, given recent evidence that tacrolimus is associated with fewer acute episodes of rejection.[3] An additional retrospective study of 29 patients revealed a survival benefit in patients treated with MMF and tacrolimus over those treated with cyclosporine and azathioprine.[4] Tacrolimus appears to have similar nephrotoxicity to cyclosporine but an increased risk of associated glucose intolerance. Both tacrolimus and cyclosporine are metabolized by the cytochrome P450 system. Caution should be used in administering these drugs in combination with other agents affected by this system, particularly azoles and macrolides, which are the commonly used lung transplant recipients.

The third agent, most patients receive is a purine synthesis inhibitor, specifically azathioprine or MMF. These agents decrease B- and T-cell proliferation and result in decreased circulating lymphocytes. The most common toxicities of these agents are bone marrow suppression, gastrointestinal upset, and liver toxicity. Small studies in lung transplantation suggest that MMF may be associated with lower rates of acute rejection than azathioprine.[5–7]

GRAFT REJECTION

Acute Rejection

Despite systemic immunosuppression, acute rejection is common, with studies demonstrating up to 50% of lung transplant recipients having biopsy-proved rejection within the first year.[1] Hypoxemia, fever, infiltrates, lymphocytic pleural effusions, and/or worsening lung function can be seen with acute rejection; however, it also can be clinically silent. Because of an association between episodes of acute rejection and later BOS, many clinicians believe that it is important to diagnose and treat acute rejection in a timely fashion.

In most clinical settings, transbronchial biopsy is the best procedure for establishing the histologic diagnosis. An analysis of 1235 lung biopsies revealed an excellent diagnostic yield when 10 to 12 biopsies were taken either as part of a routine surveillance protocol or in response to clinical changes of concern for acute rejection.[8] Currently, the International Society for Heart and Lung Transplantation has standardized the histologic grading of acute and chronic rejection based on the intensity and distribution of perivascular mononuclear cell infiltrates and bronchiolar and bronchial inflammation.[9] Many institutions, including our own, perform regular surveillance bronchoscopy to evaluate for clinically silent rejection.

Transbronchial biopsies are invasive and do carry a small risk of serious bleeding or infection. Consequently, there have been continued efforts to develop a noninvasive method to diagnose acute rejection. Although many programs use forced expiratory volume in 1 second (FEV_1) values, these are neither sensitive nor specific enough to reliably diagnose acute rejection. A 10% decrease in FEV_1 yields a sensitivity of approximately 50% and a specificity of approximately 70%, with slight variations observed based on the underlying lung disease.[10] Novel techniques including exhaled nitric oxide and serum hepatocyte growth factor have been studied but have not been established as effective clinical tools.

Acute rejection generally is treated with a pulse dose of parenteral corticosteroids, followed by tapering oral corticosteroids over several weeks. Our practice is to administer methylprednisolone (1000 mg) daily for 3 days, followed by tapering oral prednisone over 2 weeks.

Antibody-mediated rejection (AMR) is a newly emerging complication of solid organ transplantation and its relevance and approach to management continue to be elucidated.[11,12] No formal diagnostic criteria have been formulated in lung transplantation, and the approach to this entity is generally extrapolated from kidney transplant literature. The finding of circulating donor-specific antibody in the setting of deteriorating organ function should lead to the suspicion of AMR. Classic pathologic findings include parenchymal vasculitis. The significance of C4 d staining in lung specimens remains controversial. Plasmapheresis and IVIG treatment, along with rituximab therapy, can be considered in the management of AMR.

Chronic Rejection

Chronic allograft rejection manifests pathologically as bronchiolitis obliterans. It occurs in up to 50% of transplant recipients who survive at least 5 years.[1] Patients usually present with progressive dyspnea and obstruction on spirometry without evidence of an alternative diagnosis. Transbronchial biopsy, if performed, can show vascular changes of accelerated atherosclerosis and airway changes indicative of bronchiolitis obliterans. However, in contrast to acute rejection, biopsy is often unrevealing despite a clinical scenario consistent with chronic rejection. Therefore, in 2002, the International Society for Heart and Lung Transplantation updated already established diagnostic and grading guidelines based on changes in FEV_1 in order to establish the diagnosis of BOS in the absence of pathology.[13] For this reason, surveillance spirometry, both in clinic and at home, is an important component of the long-term management of these patients. AMR may also contribute to the development of chronic allograft dysfunction, though the diagnostic and therapeutic approach to this entity remains to be elucidated.

The treatment of BOS is challenging because few of the pathologic features of the syndrome are reversible. The mainstays of therapy traditionally have included changing immunosuppressants within a class, adding a new medication, or initiating novel therapies such as photopheresis.[14,15] A single-center study suggests beneficial effects of alemtuzumab in the treatment of recurrent acute rejection and BOS in antithymocyte globulin refractory patients.[16] Recently, promising data have been published that demonstrate lung function improvements in patients with established BOS after treatment with azithromycin (250 mg three times a week).[17,18] Finally, the importance of occult gastroesophageal reflux disease (GERD) in the propagation of BOS and the beneficial effects of surgical treatment of this problem have been elucidated recently.[19] Our current clinical approach to BOS incorporates both the use of azithromycin and preoperative assessment for the presence of reflux. ECP or alemtuzumab is considered in select patients.

MEDICAL COMPLICATIONS AFTER TRANSPLANT

In addition to graft rejection, transplant recipients are predisposed to other infectious and noninfectious complications that affect all of the major organ systems. These are summarized in Table 111-1 and detailed later.

Infectious Complications

The mandatory use of high-level immunosuppression and constant exposure of the allograft to the environment predisposes lung transplant recipients to increased risk of infection.

Bacterial

The most common site of bacterial infection is pulmonary, and commonly implicated organisms include *Staphylococcus aureus* and *Pseudomonas*.[20] A decrease in early pneumonia has been demonstrated with prophylactic use of antibiotics in the immediate postoperative period, particularly in patients with cystic fibrosis. The upper airways and sinuses can serve as reservoirs for pulmonary infection with colonizing organisms after transplant. We recommend Pneumococcal vaccination for all transplant recipients. Antibiotics should be directed at the organisms that were identified in the recipient's previous cultures or in cultures of the donor's lungs. Empirical coverage should be broad, and tapered rapidly on the basis of available microbiological data. If a patient develops a new infiltrate, early bronchoscopy with bronchoalveolar lavage for Gram stain

Table 111-1

MEDICAL COMPLICATIONS OF LUNG TRANSPLANT AND POTENTIAL THERAPIES

ORGAN SYSTEM	COMPLICATION	THERAPY
Renal	Renal insufficiency secondary to calcineurin inhibitors	Close monitoring of renal function Close monitoring of calcineurin levels Control of hypertension Minimize exposure to nephrotoxins Early evaluation for hemodialysis
Neurologic	Headache Tremor Peripheral neuropathy Posterior leukoencephalopathy Mood changes	Close monitoring of calcineurin levels Monitor for symptoms Consider changing calcineurin inhibitor
Endocrine	Diabetes mellitus Osteoporosis Hyperlipidemia	Steroid-sparing regimens Calcium, vitamin D, and bisphosphonates HMG-CoA reductase inhibitors and others
Hematologic	Leukopenia Thrombocytopenia Anemia	Close monitoring of counts and adjustment of purine synthesis inhibitors Iron supplementation
Oncologic	Posttransplant Lymphoproliferative disorder (PTLD)	Decrease immunosuppression Rituximab Chemotherapy and radiation
Gastrointestinal	Gastroesophageal reflux disease (GERD) Distal intestinal obstruction syndrome	Fundoplication (pre or posttransplant) Aggressive bowel regimen Minimize narcotics

and culture should be performed for a specific diagnosis. Some advocate for the addition of transbronchial biopsy or protected brush specimens to increase the diagnostic yield,[21] but we have rarely found this to be necessary.

In addition to pneumonia, bloodstream infections are common, occurring in up to 25% of patients.[22] The most common bacterial pathogens are *S. aureus* and *Pseudomonas*. *Candida* spp. are the most common fungal organism identified. Lung transplant patients with indwelling central venous catheters are at greatest risk for these infections.

Although still uncommon, nontuberculous mycobacterial (NTM) infections occur more frequently in lung transplant recipients than in the general population.[23,24] In our program's experience, such organisms were isolated from 53 of 237 patients (22.4%) after lung transplantation, but the organisms were pathogenic in only six cases (unpublished data). Rapidly growing NTM were most likely to cause true infection.

Viral

The most frequently encountered viral infection in the transplant population is cytomegalovirus (CMV). The following table outlines the level of risk for the development of CMV infection depending upon the presence of CMV IgG in donor (D) and recipient (R) serum at the time of transplant:

D+/R−: High risk.
D+/R+: Intermediate.
D−/R+: Intermediate.
D−/R−: Low.

In our practice, we administer prophylactic therapy with valganciclovir for 6 to 12 months in intermediate and high-risk lung transplant recipients. Low-risk recipients receive valacyclovir for 6 to 12 months.

CMV active disease can present as either pneumonitis or systemic infection. Patients with CMV pneumonitis present with malaise, dyspnea, cough, and fever. The diagnosis is made when CMV is isolated from bronchoalveolar lavage or biopsy specimens, as well as by classic histopathologic changes demonstrating viral inclusion bodies. A positive CMV viral load in the blood provides supportive evidence of true infection. Additional studies suggest that new, more rapid, and less invasive techniques such as bronchoalveolar lavage viral load may add to the diagnostic yield.[25] Monitoring for systemic infection is achieved by serial studies of CMV antigenemia (as reflected by CMV antigen detected in peripheral leukocytes) or CMV viremia (demonstrated by CMV growth in shell vial culture). The development of antigenemia de novo or a marked increase in titers is consistent with systemic disease.[26] Other end-organ manifestations of CMV disease include retinitis, nephritis, hepatitis, enteritis, and neurologic disease. CMV disease also may be a risk factor for subsequent development of BOS.

The lung transplant patient is predisposed to other viral infections, including herpes simplex virus and Epstein-Barr virus, as well as respiratory viruses such as adenovirus, respiratory syncytial virus, and influenza.[27] We recommend annual influenza vaccine for all of our lung transplantation patients. Infection with Epstein-Barr virus is notable because it is thought to be a risk factor for later development of posttransplant lymphoproliferative disorder (PTLD).[28]

Fungal

Aspergillus and *Candida* are the most common fungal pathogens in the transplant population.[29] Colonization with *Candida* spp. is common, and most patients who are colonized do not develop infection. However, for those who do develop disease, there is significant morbidity and mortality.[30] *Candida* presents most commonly as a bloodstream infection, at the anastomotic site, or as a mediastinitis.[31] These infections can be treated with fluconazole or alternative azole therapy depending upon the candidal species and severity of disease.

Many patients are also colonized with *Aspergillus*; however, this colonization may pose an increased risk of invasive disease.[32] Retrospective studies have demonstrated a decreased incidence of *Aspergillus* infection in patients treated with prophylactic nebulized amphotericin B or itraconazole.[33] All transplant recipients at our institution are placed on inhaled amphotericin postoperatively and remain on treatment for the duration of the initial inpatient stay. Topical prophylaxis may be extended if cultures reveal evidence of fungal colonization. In addition, all bilateral lung transplant recipients are started on micafungin at the time of transplant. IV antifungal therapy is either discontinued if intraoperative and posttransplant cultures are negative or is tailored to the fungal organism that is grown.

Aspergillus infection can take many forms, including disseminated and invasive disease, infection at the anastomotic site, aspergilloma, allergic bronchopulmonary aspergillosis, and semi-invasive tracheobronchitis. Invasive *Aspergillus* infection occurs mainly within the first year; however, up to 15% of cases can occur later in a patient's course, in contrast to other solid-organ transplant populations.[33] Surveillance bronchoscopy is used routinely to assess for infection, particularly at the anastomotic site. Aspergillus infections are treated with topical amphotericin B, voriconazole, or micafungin depending on the severity of disease and the site of infection.

Finally, all patients should receive prophylactic antibiotic treatment for *Pneumocystis jirovecii* particularly in the first year after transplantation. Our practice is to use single-strength trimethoprim-sulfamethoxazole daily or double-strength trimethoprim-sulfamethoxazole three times a week indefinitely. However, some feel that prophylaxis is needed only in the first year or when immunosuppression regimens are increased. For those with allergies to sulfa medications, alternatives include atovaquone, inhaled pentamidine, and dapsone.

Renal Complications

Renal dysfunction is common in lung transplant recipients, with recent data demonstrating a cumulative incidence of chronic renal insufficiency of 24.4% at 1 year, 34.7% at 5 years, and 41.5% at 10 years.[1] Some of these patients eventually require hemodialysis and on rare occasions undergo kidney transplantation for end-stage kidney disease. This high rate of renal dysfunction is largely a manifestation of calcineurin inhibitor toxicity. Calcineurin inhibitors are known to cause acute toxicity and more chronic changes in renal function. The acute toxicity is thought to be due to dysregulation of vascular tone mediators (i.e., endothelin, angiotensin II, and nitric oxide), which results in decreased renal blood flow and impaired glomerular filtration rate.[34] Acute calcineurin toxicity is dose-related and usually is reversible with a decrease in dose or discontinuation of the medication.

In contrast to the acute form, the chronic form of calcineurin toxicity is progressive and often results in end-stage renal disease. In addition to vascular changes, the chronic form is also associated with tubulointerstitial fibrosis and glomerulosclerosis. The chronic toxicity is not thought to be dose-dependent, but there is some evidence, derived from kidney and heart transplant populations, that switching the calcineurin inhibitor leads to some improvement of disease.[35] Both cyclosporine and tacrolimus have been associated with rare presentations of hemolytic-uremic syndrome. In the cases reported, the medication was discontinued and the patient underwent therapy for hemolytic-uremic syndrome. Once clinically stable, the patients were either rechallenged with the initial medication or given an alternative calcineurin inhibitor without return of symptoms of hemolytic-uremic syndrome.

Additional factors promoting renal dysfunction include hypertension, which is common in the posttransplant population. This may be exacerbated by medications, specifically glucocorticoids and calcineurin inhibitors. Furthermore, many of the lung transplant recipients have had exposure to aminoglycosides in both the pretransplant and posttransplant time periods, and most patients will receive ganciclovir or valganciclovir at some point in their treatment course. Both of these agents can be nephrotoxic and, over time, may contribute to the slow decline in glomerular filtration rate which is common in this patient population.

Neurologic Complications

Many of the neurologic complications observed after transplantation are secondary to medications. For example, it is estimated that 10% to 28% of patients who receive cyclosporine experience neurologic changes, and similar events have been described with tacrolimus.[36] Most patients present with mild complaints, such as headache, tremor, or peripheral neuropathy. However, more severe presentations, such as posterior leukoencephalopathy, also have been reported.[37] In these patients, temporary cessation of the specific calcineurin inhibitor or substitution of an alternative agent (e.g., cyclosporine vs. tacrolimus) may be helpful.

Patients who receive glucocorticoids are at risk for neuropsychiatric complications.[38] Patients can present with agitation, mania, or frank psychosis. Symptoms can recur with repeated high doses of steroids.[39] Therapy usually begins with decreasing the dosage, and if symptoms are sufficiently severe, treatment is pursued with lithium, valproic acid, neuroleptics, or other atypical antipsychotics.

Although no literature exists on the neurologic implications of cardiopulmonary bypass in the lung transplant population, there is ample evidence of cognitive impairment when cardiopulmonary bypass is used for patients undergoing cardiac surgery.[40] Many of the transplants in our institution are performed without cardiopulmonary bypass with a resulting decreased risk of neurocognitive effects.

Endocrine and Metabolic Complications

Glucocorticoids, as part of the immunosuppressive regimen, have multiple adverse metabolic effects, including glucose intolerance and diabetes mellitus. These effects are of particular concern in patients with cystic fibrosis, who may already have impaired pancreatic islet cell function. The use of calcineurin inhibitors has been corticosteroid-sparing with subsequent improved glucose control. It is interesting to note that tacrolimus is associated with an increased incidence of new-onset diabetes mellitus based on a meta-analysis of several studies.[41] Glucocorticoids also predispose transplant patients to osteoporosis and decreased bone mineral density. The prevalence of osteoporosis after lung transplantation is as high as 57% to 73%, with a fracture incidence of 18% to 37%.[42] Many patients will have decreased bone mineral density before transplant as a consequence of a smoking history, chronic decreased mobility, and steroid use. Cystic fibrosis patients have further risk factors, including decreased absorption of vitamin D and calcium. In a study of 100 lung transplant patients, the cumulative steroid dose appeared to be the strongest posttransplant determinant of osteoporosis and fracture.[43]

Despite treatment with calcium, vitamin D, and bisphosphonates, many patients continue to have bone loss and are at risk for fracture.[44] In a study of 30 patients, despite aggressive medical management, 37% of patients in their first year posttransplant sustained an atraumatic fracture. Risk factors included female gender, pretransplant corticosteroid use, and low bone mineral density.[45] Our practice is to obtain a bone density study as part of the preoperative evaluation and to administer long-term supplemental vitamin D, calcium, and bisphosphonate.

Although not studied specifically in lung transplant patients, both calcineurin inhibitors and glucocorticoids can contribute to hyperlipidemia. A case-control study recently demonstrated markedly improved survival (91% vs. 54%) in lung transplant patients treated with a HMG-CoA reductase inhibitor for hyperlipidemia compared with patients without hyperlipidemia.[46] This appears to be a potential additional benefit with respect to the development of BOS, separate from its lipid-lowering effects.

Hematologic and Oncologic Complications

One of the most common hematologic complications is mild-to-moderate bone marrow suppression caused by medications. Often this sequela presents as a leukopenia, but thrombocytopenia and anemia are not uncommon. The agents most often associated with this phenomenon include the purine synthesis inhibitors (i.e., azathioprine and MMF), ganciclovir, and trimethoprim-sulfamethoxazole. A slightly increased rate of leukopenia with MMF compared with azathioprine has been reported, but both agents warrant monitoring of white blood cell counts.[47] Our standard of care is to withdraw purine synthesis inhibitors, when the total white blood cell count falls below 2000 or the absolute neutrophil count falls below 1000. Treatment with granulocyte colony-stimulating factor is also considered. During the early posttransplant course, leukopenia and thrombocytopenia are caused most commonly by one of the induction agents (i.e., OKT3, ATGAM, or antithymocyte globulin).

The most concerning hematologic/oncologic complication after transplantation is PTLD. This disorder describes a wide spectrum of B-cell dyscrasias ranging from benign hyperplasia to malignant non-Hodgkin's lymphoma. Most frequently, Epstein-Barr virus infection stimulates a proliferation of B cells that is unregulated in the setting of systemic immunosuppression. The incidence of PTLD in the lung transplant population is reported to be between 1.8% and 7.9%.[48] The presentation of the disease is protean and includes lung nodules and masses, liver lesions, small bowel wall thickening, and lymphadenopathy.[48] Because of the limited understanding of PTLD, therapies for this disorder are still in early stages. Treatment options include decreasing the immunosuppressive regimen and administration of rituximab (anti-CD20 antibody).[49] Refractory PTLD may require treatment with chemotherapy. Death from PTLD is relatively rare in lung transplant recipients (0.1% to 4.8%).[1]

Gastrointestinal Complications

Lung transplant patients are at risk for several gastrointestinal issues related to medications, including peptic ulcer disease, gastritis, perforated bowel, and abdominal infections. Three particular issues deserve special attention.

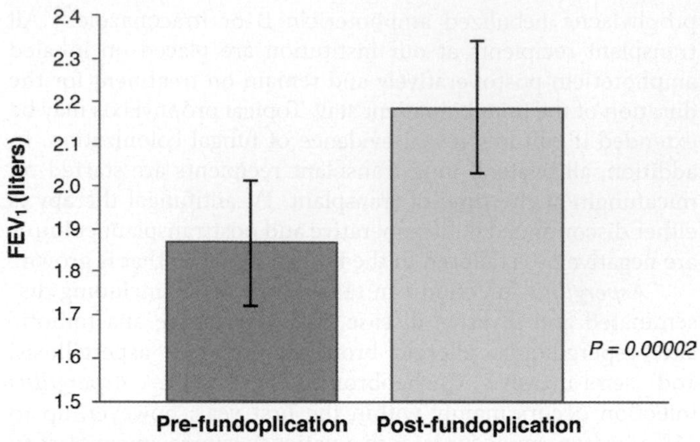

Figure 111-1. Average FEV_1 values before and after fundoplication therapy in patients with GERD.

The first is posttransplant GERD. As discussed earlier, there is emerging evidence of a connection between GERD and BOS. Recent evidence suggests an association between non-acid reflux and the development of BOS.[50] Additionally, improved lung function was noted after these patients were treated surgically with a fundoplication.[19] Because of these findings, it is our practice to screen all patients for GERD preoperatively and to treat affected patients with pretransplantation laparoscopic fundoplication with encouraging results (Fig. 111-1).

The second area of interest is postoperative gastrointestinal disease in the patient with cystic fibrosis. These patients often have preexisting pancreatic insufficiency that may complicate medication absorption postoperatively. Additionally, there is an increased risk of distal intestinal obstruction syndrome, with one report showing an incidence as high as 20%.[51] This is noteworthy because aggressive bowel regimens may prevent distal intestinal obstruction syndrome and eliminate the need for surgical treatment.

Colon and rectal complications are not frequently observed in lung transplant recipients in general.[52] These complications can include abdominal perforation related to diverticulitis, as well as spontaneous perforation. Symptoms can be mild and atypical. Intra-abdominal complications should be suspected in the setting of unexplained abdominal pain, fever, or leukocytosis.

ACKNOWLEDGMENT

The authors acknowledge Dr. Patricia A. Kritek and Dr. Aaron Deykin, who contributed to this chapter in the first edition.

EDITOR'S COMMENT

The lung, like the skin and the gut, is a portal of entry for potential pathogens. Not surprisingly, these organs have been resistant to successful transplantation. As a consequence of their aggressive immunosuppression, medical management of lung transplant recipients requires attention to common transplant-related infections as well as uncommon pulmonary infectious diseases.

—Steven J. Mentzer

References

1. Christie JD, Edwards LB, Kucheryavaya AY, et al. The Registry of the International Society for heart and lung transplantation: twenty-eighth adult Lung and heart-lung transplant report–2011. *J Heart Lung Transplant.* 2011; 30(10):1104–1122.
2. Brock MV, Borja MC, Ferber L, et al. Induction therapy in lung transplantation: a prospective, controlled clinical trial comparing OKT3, anti-thymocyte globulin, and daclizumab. *J Heart Lung Transplant.* 2001;20(12):1282–1290.
3. Fan Y, Xiao YB, Weng YG. Tacrolimus versus cyclosporine for adult lung transplant recipients: a meta-analysis. *Transplant Proc.* 2009;41(5):1821–1824.
4. Izbicki G, Shitrit D, Aravot D, et al. Improved survival after lung transplantation in patients treated with tacrolimus/mycophenolate mofetil as compared with cyclosporine/azathioprine. *Transplantat Proc.* 2002;34(8):3258–3259.
5. O'Hair DP, Cantu E, McGregor C, et al. Preliminary experience with mycophenolate mofetil used after lung transplantation. *J Heart Lung Transplant.* 1998;17(9):864–868.
6. Ross DJ, Waters PF, Levine M, et al. Mycophenolate mofetil versus azathioprine immunosuppressive regimens after lung transplantation: preliminary experience. *J Heart Lung Transplant.* 1998;17(8):768–774.
7. Zuckermann A, Klepetko W, Birsan T, et al. Comparison between mycophenolate mofetil- and azathioprine-based immunosuppressions in clinical lung transplantation. *J Heart Lung Transplant.* 1999;18(5):432–440.
8. Hopkins PM, Aboyoun CL, Chhajed PN, et al. Prospective analysis of 1,235 transbronchial lung biopsies in lung transplant recipients. *J Heart Lung Transplant.* 2002;21(10):1062–1067.
9. Stewart S, Fishbein MC, Snell GI, et al. Revision of the 1996 working formulation for the standardization of nomenclature in the diagnosis of lung rejection. *J Heart Lung Transplant.* 2007;26(12):1229–1242.
10. Becker FS, Martinez FJ, Brunsting LA, et al. Limitations of spirometry in detecting rejection after single-lung transplantation. *Am J Respir Crit Care Med.* 1994;150(1):159–166.
11. Glanville AR. Antibody-mediated rejection in lung transplantation: myth or reality? *J Heart Lung Transplant.* 2010;29(4):395 400.
12. Martinu T, Chen DF, Palmer SM. Acute rejection and humoral sensitization in lung transplant recipients. *Proc Am Thorac Soc.* 2009;6(1):54–65.
13. Estenne M, Maurer JR, Boehler A, et al. Bronchiolitis obliterans syndrome 2001: an update of the diagnostic criteria. *J Heart Lung Transplant.* 2002;21(3):297–310.
14. Lamioni A, Parisi F, Isacchi G, et al. The immunological effects of extracorporeal photopheresis unraveled: induction of tolerogenic dendritic cells in vitro and regulatory T cells in vivo. *Transplantation.* 2005;79(7):846–850.
15. Benden C, Speich R, Hofbauer GF, et al. Extracorporeal photopheresis after lung transplantation: a 10-year single-center experience. *Transplantation.* 2008;86(11):1625–1627.
16. Reams BD, Musselwhite LW, Zaas DW, et al. Alemtuzumab in the treatment of refractory acute rejection and bronchiolitis obliterans syndrome after human lung transplantation. *Am J Transplant.* 2007;7(12):2802–2808.
17. Gerhardt SG, McDyer JF, Girgis RE, et al. Maintenance azithromycin therapy for bronchiolitis obliterans syndrome: results of a pilot study. *Am J Respir Crit Care Med.* 2003;168(1):121–125.
18. Gottlieb J, Szangolies J, Koehnlein T, et al. Long-term azithromycin for bronchiolitis obliterans syndrome after lung transplantation. *Transplantation.* 2008;85(1):36–41.
19. Davis RD Jr, Lau CL, Eubanks S, et al. Improved lung allograft function after fundoplication in patients with gastroesophageal reflux disease undergoing lung transplantation. *J Thorac Cardiovasc Surg.* 2003;125(3):533–542.
20. Campos S, Caramori M, Teixeira R, et al. Bacterial and fungal pneumonias after lung transplantation. *Transplant Proc.* 2008;40(3):822–824.
21. Chan CC, Abi-Saleh WJ, Arroliga AC, et al. Diagnostic yield and therapeutic impact of flexible bronchoscopy in lung transplant recipients. *J Heart Lung Transplant.* 1996;15(2):196–205.
22. Palmer SM, Alexander BD, Sanders LL, et al. Significance of blood stream infection after lung transplantation: analysis in 176 consecutive patients. *Transplantation.* 2000;69(11):2360–2366.
23. Winthrop KL, McNelley E, Kendall B, et al. Pulmonary nontuberculous mycobacterial disease prevalence and clinical features: an emerging public health disease. *Am J Respir Crit Care Med.* 2010;182(7):977–982.
24. Marras TK, Chedore P, Ying AM, et al. Isolation prevalence of pulmonary nontuberculous mycobacteria in Ontario, 1997 2003. *Thorax.* 2007;62(8):661–666.
25. Chemaly RF, Yen-Lieberman B, Castilla EA, et al. Correlation between viral loads of cytomegalovirus in blood and bronchoalveolar lavage specimens from lung transplant recipients determined by histology and immunohistochemistry. *J Clin Microbiol.* 2004;42(5):2168–2172.
26. van der Bij W, Speich R. Management of cytomegalovirus infection and disease after solid-organ transplantation. *Clin Infect Dis.* 2001;33(Suppl 1):S32–S37.
27. Holt ND, Gould FK, Taylor CE, et al. Incidence and significance of noncytomegalovirus viral respiratory infection after adult lung transplantation. *J Heart Lung Transplant.* 1997;16(4):416–419.
28. Aris RM, Maia DM, Neuringer IP, et al. Post-transplantation lymphoproliferative disorder in the Epstein-Barr virus-naive lung transplant recipient. *Am J Respir Crit Care Med.* 1996;154(6 Pt 1):1712–1717.
29. Chan KM, Allen SA. Infectious pulmonary complications in lung transplant recipients. *Semin Respir Infect.* 2002;17(4):291–302.
30. Trulock EP. Lung transplantation. *Am J Respir Crit Care Med.* 1997;155(3): 789–818.
31. Speich R, van der Bij W. Epidemiology and management of infections after lung transplantation. *Clin Infect Dis.* 2001;33(Suppl 1):S58–S65.
32. Cahill BC, Hibbs JR, Savik K, et al. Aspergillus airway colonization and invasive disease after lung transplantation. *Chest.* 1997;112(5):1160–1164.
33. Minari A, Husni R, Avery RK, et al. The incidence of invasive aspergillosis among solid organ transplant recipients and implications for prophylaxis in lung transplants. *Transpl Infect Dis.* 2002;4(4):195–200.
34. Fellstrom B. Cyclosporine nephrotoxicity. *Transplant Proc.* 2004;36(Suppl 2): 220S–223S.
35. Israni A, Brozena S, Pankewycz O, et al. Conversion to tacrolimus for the treatment of cyclosporine-associated nephrotoxicity in heart transplant recipients. *Am J Kidney Dis.* 2002;39(3):E16.
36. Bechstein WO. Neurotoxicity of calcineurin inhibitors: impact and clinical management. *Transpl Int.* 2000;13(5):313–326.
37. Ahn KJ, You WJ, Jeong SL, et al. Atypical manifestations of reversible posterior leukoencephalopathy syndrome: findings on diffusion imaging and ADC mapping. *Neuroradiology.* 2004;46(12):978–983.
38. Fardet L, Petersen I, Nazareth I. Suicidal behavior and severe neuropsychiatric disorders following glucocorticoid therapy in primary care. *Am J Psychiatry.* 2012;169(5):491–497.
39. Wada K, Yamada N, Suzuki H, et al. Recurrent cases of corticosteroid-induced mood disorder: clinical characteristics and treatment. *J Clin Psychiatry.* 2000;61(4):261–267.
40. Vingerhoets G, Van Nooten G, Vermassen F, et al. Short-term and long-term neuropsychological consequences of cardiac surgery with extracorporeal circulation. *Eur J Cardiothorac Surg.* 1997;11(3):424–431.
41. Heisel O, Heisel R, Balshaw R, et al. New onset diabetes mellitus in patients receiving calcineurin inhibitors: a systematic review and meta-analysis. *Am J Transplant.* 2004;4(4):583–595.
42. Cohen A, Sambrook P, Shane E. Management of bone loss after organ transplantation. *J Bone Miner Res.* 2004;19(12):1919–1932.
43. Aris RM, Neuringer IP, Weiner MA, et al. Severe osteoporosis before and after lung transplantation. *Chest.* 1996;109(5):1176–1183.
44. Shane E, Addesso V, Namerow PB, et al. Alendronate versus calcitriol for the prevention of bone loss after cardiac transplantation. *N Engl J Med.* 2004;350(8):767–776.
45. Shane E, Papadopoulos A, Staron RB, et al. Bone loss and fracture after lung transplantation. *Transplantation.* 1999;68(2):220–227.
46. Johnson BA, Iacono AT, Zeevi A, et al. Statin use is associated with improved function and survival of lung allografts. *Am J Respir Crit Care Med.* 2003; 167(9):1271–1278.
47. Wang K, Zhang H, Li Y, et al. Safety of mycophenolate mofetil versus azathioprine in renal transplantation: a systematic review. *Transplant Proc.* 2004; 36(7):2068–2070.
48. Reams BD, McAdams HP, Howell DN, et al. Posttransplant lymphoproliferative disorder: incidence, presentation, and response to treatment in lung transplant recipients. *Chest.* 2003;124(4):1242–1249.
49. Blaes AH, Peterson BA, Bartlett N, et al. Rituximab therapy is effective for posttransplant lymphoproliferative disorders after solid organ transplantation: results of a phase II trial. *Cancer.* 2005;104(8):1661–1667.
50. King BJ, Iyer H, Leidi AA, et al. Gastroesophageal reflux in bronchiolitis obliterans syndrome: a new perspective. *J Heart Lung Transplant.* 2009;28(9):870–875.
51. Gilljam M, Chaparro C, Tullis E, et al. GI complications after lung transplantation in patients with cystic fibrosis. *Chest.* 2003;123(1):37–41.
52. Goldberg HJ, Hertz MI, Ricciardi R, et al. Colon and rectal complications after heart and lung transplantation. *J Am Coll Surg.* 2006;202(1):55–61.

112 Management of Surgical Complications of Lung Transplantation

Jane Yanagawa and Bryan F. Meyers

Keywords: Donor procurement complications, recipient explant complications, posttransplant surgical complications

INTRODUCTION

Recipients of lung transplantation are surviving longer. As a consequence, complications secondary to the procedure (surgical) or resulting from mandatory lifelong immunosuppression (medical) are becoming increasingly evident. These events can lead to significant morbidity and potential mortality if not managed appropriately and in a timely fashion. This chapter focuses on the common surgical complications of lung transplantation.

TECHNICAL COMPLICATIONS

Transplant operations of all types require at minimum two separate surgical procedures: retrieval of the organ from the donor and implantation of the organ into the recipient. Thus technical complications can occur during any phase of either operation. Pitfalls of donor procurement include inadequate harvest of the atrial cuff or iatrogenic injury to the pulmonary artery, pulmonary veins, bronchus, and lung parenchyma. Complications secondary to lung implantation include phrenic nerve injury, hemorrhage, and pulmonary hypertension/hypoxemia.

COMPLICATIONS RELATED TO SUBOPTIMAL DONOR PROCUREMENT

Atrial Cuff and Pulmonary Vein Orifices

Donor procurement is always performed on an emergent basis. Consequently, despite the best efforts of both the heart and lung procurement teams to equitably divide the left atrial cuff and preserve the pulmonary vein orifices, the donor lungs occasionally arrive at the recipient OR in less than optimal condition, with either insufficient left atrial cuff or lacerated pulmonary vein orifices (in particular, the right inferior pulmonary vein). These injuries usually occur as a result of poor visibility or undue haste during division of the left atrial cuff. Laceration of the pulmonary vein orifice is repaired simply by dividing the pericardium overlying the vein and exposing the vessel to the point where it disappears into the lung parenchyma. Small branches of the vein also may require repair if the vein orifice was entered during procurement. These branches should be identified and oversewn to prevent troublesome bleeding after reperfusion.

Casula et al.[1] have described a useful technique for augmenting the pulmonary veins with donor pericardium when the left atrial cuff is found to be inadequate. This method can be used to create a cuff even when the superior and inferior pulmonary veins are completely separated. A running 5-0 polypropylene suture is placed around each vein orifice to tack the intima to the pericardium, thereby creating a "neoatrial cuff." Scissors are used to trim the newly created pericardial cuff and separate it from the other hilar structures. This pericardial cuff substitutes for donor atrium in the atrial anastomosis. Alternatively, donor superior vena cava or redundant donor pulmonary artery can be used for the reconstruction if there is inadequate pericardial tissue.

Pulmonary Artery Injury

The bifurcation of the pulmonary artery always should be taken with the lung graft at the time of procurement. Even when a heart transplant is planned from the same donor, dividing the pulmonary artery at the distal extent of the main trunk proximal to the bifurcation leaves a sufficient and safe length of artery for the heart transplant. Common sites of pulmonary artery injury during donor procurement include the right pulmonary artery as it travels behind the aorta or posterior to the superior vena cava. Because the right pulmonary artery is substantially longer than the left, when injury to this vessel occurs behind the aorta, it rarely requires repair, and the artery simply can be trimmed distal to the laceration. However, when the first branch of the right pulmonary artery is lacerated deep to the superior vena cava, it must be repaired. Usually, the laceration can be repaired with suture, but when reconstruction of the truncus anterior is required, a patch or complete reimplantation may be needed to prevent loss of diameter in the repaired vessel. This sort of repair can be performed with a segment of donor vena cava, azygos vein, or redundant donor pulmonary artery.

Bronchial and Parenchymal Injuries

Traumatic injury to the lung parenchyma or main bronchi during procurement is rarely significant. The worst result is a prolonged air leak after implantation, which eventually resolves. Special care should be taken when the implantation is performed with cardiopulmonary bypass because even small parenchymal injuries may lead to endobronchial bleeding under circumstances of profound anticoagulation for bypass.

On the other hand, atraumatic injury to the lung parenchyma in the form of inadequate cooling and preservation can have grave consequences. For example, technical problems may occur in the delivery of the flush solution used to cool and preserve the lungs during extracorporeal ischemia. Inadequate flushing of the lungs during procurement can lead to profound ischemia–reperfusion injury and poor initial graft function after implantation. We experienced an extreme example of ischemia–reperfusion injury in a bilateral lung transplant performed in a patient with cystic fibrosis. On a routine postoperative ventilation/perfusion scan, no flow was observed perfusing the left lung (Fig. 112-1). A pulmonary arteriogram demonstrated a patent anastomosis without evidence of technical flaws

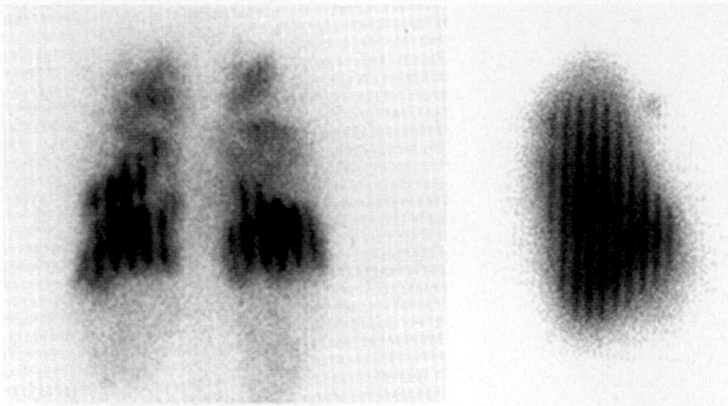

Figure 112-1. Postoperative perfusion scan (*right*) of patient with cystic fibrosis who received a bilateral lung transplant showing absence of perfusion to newly implanted left lung (preoperative perfusion scan on the left showing flow to both lungs for comparison).

to account for the absent blood flow (Fig. 112-2). Reexploration revealed an edematous ischemic lung with severe reperfusion injury that necessitated removal of the graft. Analysis of this case revealed that the flush of preservative solution had been preferentially and exclusively directed down the right pulmonary artery, thus exposing the left lung to a no-reflow phenomenon as a consequence of severe ischemic injury. Our procurement protocol has been developed to minimize this occurrence. When the pulmonary artery cannula used to administer the lung preservation solution is inserted in proximity to the pulmonary artery bifurcation (as required when the heart is also suitable for procurement) and also directed towards the bifurcation, the tip may inadvertently slip into either the left or right pulmonary artery resulting in asymmetric perfusion. We have found that inserting the pulmonary artery cannula near the bifurcation with the tip directed towards the heart provides an adequate and uniform distribution to the bilateral lungs and avoids differential flow. In addition, we look for equal "blanching" of both lungs during the administration of the preservation solution. Finally, after cardiac excision, the remaining perfusion solution is infused into each individual pulmonary vein orifice as a retrograde flush.[2]

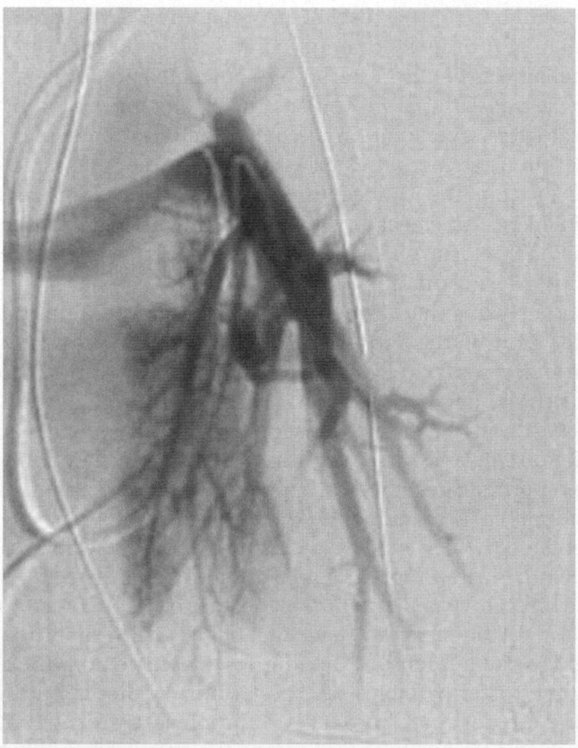

Figure 112-2. Pulmonary artery angiogram performed after postoperative perfusion scan showed no perfusion to newly implanted left lung. A patent left-sided anastomosis is seen without evidence of technical flaws to account for the absent blood flow in the lung. It was concluded in this case that the no-reflow phenomenon secondary to severe ischemic injury was the likely cause for lack of blood flow to the left graft.

COMPLICATIONS RELATED TO RECIPIENT EXPLANT

Phrenic Nerve Injuries

Dense adhesions present at the time of explantation can increase the risk of bleeding as well as the risk of injury to the phrenic and left recurrent nerves. These adhesions are most common in patients with septic lung diseases (e.g., cystic fibrosis and bronchiectasis) and patients who have had previous thoracic surgery. While once rare, it is increasingly common to consider reoperative lung transplantation and the adhesions can be formidable. Particularly dense adhesions have been seen in emphysema patients who have undergone previous lung-volume–reduction surgery. In a multicenter experience of 35 lung transplant patients who had previously undergone lung-volume–reduction surgery, phrenic nerve injury was recorded in two patients (5.7%).[3] We have noted that the phrenic nerve often adheres to the lung-volume–reduction surgery staple line, making dissection of the phrenic nerve both tedious and dangerous. To avoid injury to the phrenic nerve in these patients, we leave the staple line, along with a small amount of residual lung tissue, attached to the phrenic nerve and use a lung stapler to divide the densely attached tissue. Electrocautery to take down mediastinal adhesions should be avoided because it greatly increases the risk of phrenic nerve injury.

If one of the phrenic nerves is injured, little can be done to remedy the situation acutely. The consequences are not as dire with a bilateral transplant, which mitigates the impact of unilateral phrenic injury. The redundant lung ensures an overall acceptable outcome, and consequently, this complication is often underreported. When the phrenic nerve is injured during a unilateral transplant, the benefit of the transplant is greatly diminished. It has been exceedingly rare in our experience or in the reported literature for a patient to require diaphragmatic plication after lung transplantation.

Hemorrhage

Hemorrhage was once a common complication after lung transplantation. Indeed, in the early experience of some programs undertaking heart–lung and en bloc double-lung transplants, approximately 25% of patients required reoperation for postoperative bleeding. However, improved technique and perioperative care have reduced the incidence of life-threatening hemorrhage. While the use of strategic incisions (posterolateral thoracotomy for single-lung transplantation and the clamshell and sternal-sparing clamshell incisions for bilateral lung replacement) has improved surgical exposure and contributed to the prevention of hemorrhage, the availability of a variety of hemostatic agents has played an important role in the control of hemorrhage.[4,5] The use of aprotinin has largely been abandoned due to concerns about toxicity. In contrast, the role of factor concentrates – such as recombinant Factor VII and activated prothrombin complex concentrates – is not as clear. Although small case studies suggest that the use of recombinant Factor VII in lung transplantation is associated with reduced blood loss and decreased need for blood transfusions without the development of thromboembolic complications, further studies are needed to establish the safety and efficacy of such products.[6] At our institution, we consider using factor concentrates when the following occur: (1) bleeding exceeds 500 to 1000 mL/h, (2) hemorrhage is diffuse and cannot be surgically addressed, and (3) bleeding is refractory to pharmacologic agents (DDAVP, aminocaproic acid) and aggressive transfusion of hemostatic components (platelets, fresh frozen plasma, cryoprecipitate).[7]

Pulmonary Hypertension and Hypoxemia

Persistent pulmonary hypertension and unexplained hypoxemia after lung implantation can occur as a result of stenosis at the pulmonary artery anastomosis. A nuclear perfusion scan that demonstrates less than anticipated flow to a single-lung graft or unequal distribution of flow in a bilateral lung recipient can suggest this problem. Occasionally, transesophageal echocardiography can visualize a stenotic vascular anastomosis. Contrast angiography should be performed in any patient for whom there is such a concern. At the time of angiography, the pressure gradient across the pulmonary artery anastomosis should be determined. A gradient of 15 to 20 mm Hg is commonly encountered, especially in single-lung recipients, in whom most of the cardiac output may be directed to the transplanted lung, or in bilateral recipients, who have a high cardiac output. The need for anastomotic revision is dictated by the clinical situation, but this intervention is quite uncommon. Treatment options include observation, reoperation, or angioplasty with or without stent placement if surgical revision is considered too high a risk.[8] Dramatic reduction in flow should not be accepted because the donor bronchus is totally dependent on pulmonary arterial collateral flow.

Compromised flow across the atrial anastomosis also can occur as a result of unsatisfactory anastomotic technique. Impaired venous outflow results in elevated venous pressure and ipsilateral pulmonary edema. Pulmonary artery pressures remain unexpectedly high in this situation, and flow through the graft is less than expected. Transesophageal echocardiography is often used to assess patency and flow through the atrial anastomoses. Contrast studies may be helpful in demonstrating a reduced level of flow through the anastomoses. Open exploration occasionally is necessary to confirm the diagnosis and conduct appropriate repair.

POSTOPERATIVE COMPLICATIONS

Sternal Complications

The bilateral transsternal thoracotomy provides excellent exposure to the hila and pleural spaces, but problems have been reported with poor sternal healing. Brown and colleagues[9] report an institutional prevalence of 36% for sternal disruption

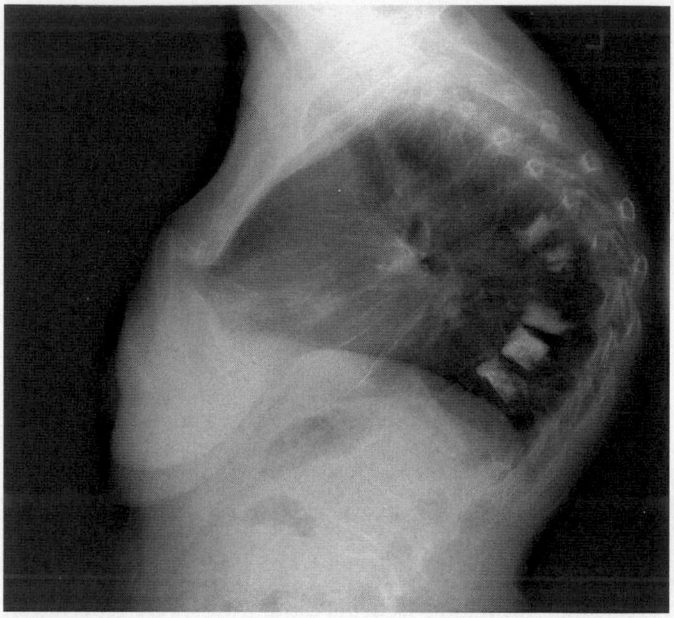

Figure 112-3. Chest radiograph showing a significant angular deformity of the sternum after lung transplantation. This patient also has marked kyphosis and osteopenia (with prior vertebroplasty) and multiple compression fractures.

in transverse bilateral thoracosternotomy for lung transplantation, and they cited disruption rates of 20% to 60% at centers worldwide. Lung transplant recipients are particularly prone to poor sternal healing (Fig. 112-3) owing to their debilitated state and the routine use of postoperative corticosteroids.4 Sternal override is a common complication that results from a tendency of the distal sternum to angulate and displace anteriorly, a translational movement that is not prevented by the sternal wires. The addition of coaxial stabilization, either with long, thin Kirschner wires or with short, stout Steinmann pins placed within the cancellous bone of the sternum, reduces the incidence of sternal override and translational movement at the bony closure. However, these wires have a tendency to migrate, causing other problems (Fig. 112-4). We have removed numerous wires that have migrated from the sternum to various locations in the body. Such retrievals require interventions of various complexity, ranging from the administration of local anesthetic to liberate a wire that has eroded through the anterior chest wall to a laparoscopic procedure under general anesthesia to remove a Kirschner wire from the pouch of Douglas. Case reports suggest that the use of longitudinal titanium plates for sternal fixation may provide improved results for high risk patients or those requiring reclosure after sternal dehiscence. The Synthes Titanium Sternal Fixation System (Synthes, Westchester, PA) involves titanium plates that can be molded to the contour of the sternum, and includes a drill/titanium screw gauging system to ensure that the screws pierce both the anterior and posterior tables of the sternum, without protruding beyond the posterior border.[9] As a prophylactic maneuver, the procedure does add time and cost to the operation, and further studies are needed to define which patients would benefit from such precautions.[10,11]

Deep sternal wound infection is an additional serious complication of transverse sternotomy. We have encountered this problem in several patients, and it has required operative

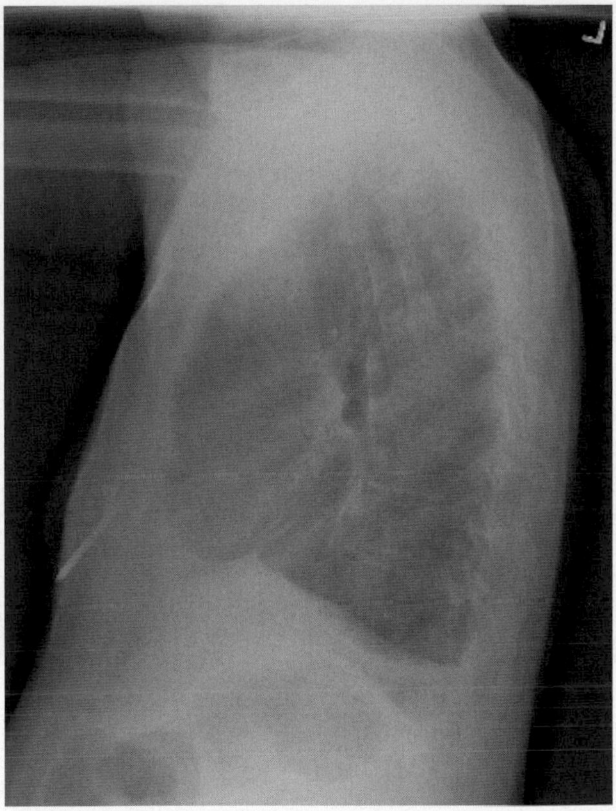

Figure 112-4. Chest radiograph of a lung transplant recipient who had required a clamshell incision for adequate exposure. He presented several months later with a Steinmann pin eroding through his sternum and projecting anteriorly toward his skin. The area was prepped, and the Steinmann pin was simply removed with a small cutdown incision.

and bedside wound debridement with additional antibiotics and a prolonged hospital stay. The estimated prevalence for all sternal closure complications in our historical control group is 34%. With this in mind, we routinely avoid sternal division and have found that adequate exposure in many circumstances can be provided by bilateral anterior thoracotomies alone. Additionally, in rare selected patients, we also advocate modified approaches such as a combined left posterolateral and right anterior thoracotomy to optimize the left hilar exposure without the need for sternal division or separate positioning, preparation, or draping. We have found that the use of a cardiac positioning device designed for off-pump cardiac stabilization (apical suction cup) can be useful to expose the left hilum and avoid sternal division and cardiopulmonary bypass.

Primary Graft Dysfunction

Primary graft dysfunction is one of the most important complications of lung transplantation and represents a common cause of early mortality and prolonged ICU stay. The frequency of primary graft dysfunction at our institution is 23%.[12] The impact of primary graft dysfunction is enormous. Patients experiencing initial graft dysfunction at our institution had a mortality of 28.8% compared with 4.2% in patients without the condition.

Primary graft dysfunction is commonly referred to as ischemia–reperfusion injury. A number of factors such as poor preservation techniques, prolonged ischemic time, and unsuspected donor lung pathology such as contusion, pulmonary thromboembolism, or aspiration all play a role in the development of primary graft dysfunction. Additionally, we have reported a statistically significant difference in the distribution of primary graft dysfunction according to underlying diagnosis leading to transplantation. There appears to be more primary graft dysfunction in patients transplanted for pulmonary hypertension and less in patients transplanted for emphysema. Hyperacute rejection is exceedingly rare, but it must be a consideration in cases of early severe lung dysfunction. Ischemia–reperfusion injury is characterized by noncardiogenic pulmonary edema and progressive lung injury over the first few hours after implantation (Fig. 112-5). Pathologically severe ischemia–reperfusion injury has the appearance of diffuse alveolar damage. Regardless of cause, it is important to establish a diagnosis of early graft dysfunction and to rule out other treatable conditions. We perform open lung biopsy at the time of implantation if graft dysfunction is immediately apparent in the OR. Serologic evaluation for antihuman leukocyte antigen antibodies also may reveal evidence of hyperacute rejection in some patients.

Efforts to prevent primary graft dysfunction have included paying close attention to the inflation and ventilation of the donor lungs as well as the optimization of preservation methods.[13] Considering that lung hyperinflation can produce a striking model of postreperfusion pulmonary edema, we are particularly careful to avoid lung hyperinflation during harvest and storage of the donor lungs.

Extensive research has been devoted to refining the preservation solution to maximally reduce cellular injury during ischemic time. It is clear from experimental[14,15] and clinical work[16] that the low potassium dextran solution provides superior protection compared with the high potassium solution used previously. In addition, experimental work suggests that adding nitroprusside (a potent nitric oxide donor) to the flush solution at the time of harvest provides a preservation advantage.[17]

Other strategies to reduce primary graft dysfunction include controlled reperfusion, a concept that was used originally to reduce cardiac dysfunction after reperfusion of acutely ischemic myocardium at the time of coronary artery revascularization. The clinical use of controlled reperfusion, where recipient blood depleted of leukocytes is administered into the pulmonary arteries of the newly transplanted lungs for the initial reperfusion phase,[18,19] has shown promise as a preventive strategy for ischemia–reperfusion injury.

Ex vivo lung perfusion (EVLP), where harvested lungs are perfused and ventilated ex vivo at body temperature to allow for an evaluation of physiologic integrity, is another novel strategy under intense study. This technique aims to increase lung utilization and improve outcomes by providing time under physiologically protective conditions to adequately assess and optimize suboptimal organs. A prospective clinical trial compared outcomes after high-risk donor lungs ($N = 23$) were subjected to 4 hours of EVLP, after which $N = 20$ were deemed acceptable for transplantation. They found no difference in the incidence of primary graft dysfunction in the high-risk organs that went on to implantation when compared to the control group ($N = 116$) of conventionally selected donor lungs. No conclusion regarding the relationship between EVLP and primary graft dysfunction can be made based on this small and nonrandomized study, but further studies are warranted.[20]

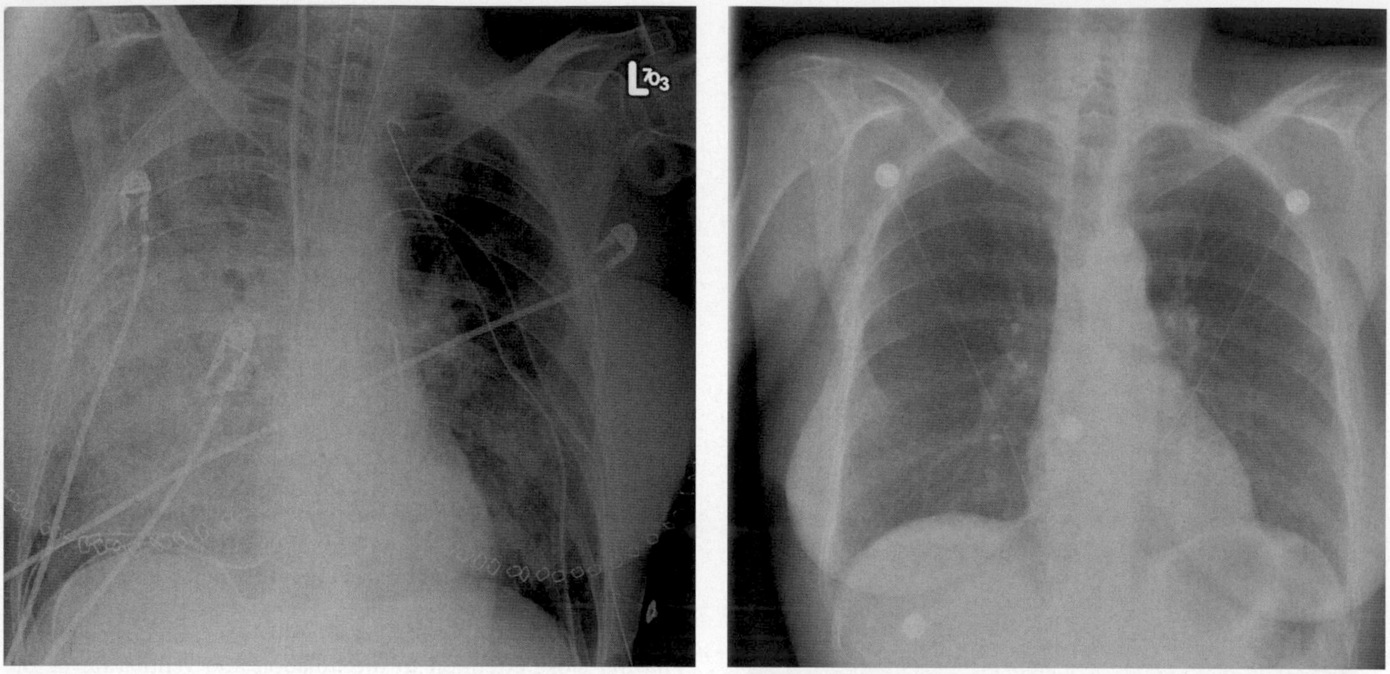

Figure 112-5. *A.* Chest radiograph showing severe right-sided ischemia–reperfusion injury following bilateral lung transplantation. Right lung was implanted first. *B.* Chest radiograph of same patient after resolution of ischemia–reperfusion injury.

In cases of established ischemia–reperfusion injury, treatment is supportive. Management strategies are similar to those utilized for ARDS, and include diuresis and balancing the appropriate ventilatory support without ventilator-induced injury. In most cases, the reperfusion injury peaks and begins to resolve over 24 to 48 hours. We have shown previously that inhaled nitric oxide is beneficial in severe reperfusion injury because it decreases pulmonary artery pressure and improves the PaO_2/FiO_2 ratio.[21] More recently, inhaled prostacyclin has been investigated and shows promise as an economic alternative to nitric oxide.[22,23]

While standard intensive ventilatory and pharmacologic interventions generally suffice, severe graft dysfunction or coexisting cardiac failure may require extracorporeal membrane oxygenation (ECMO) support. We reported the selective use of ECMO after lung transplantation[24] and found satisfactory results when lung failure occurs immediately after transplantation (<24 hours). More recently, Bermudez et al. described the University of Pittsburgh experience with ECMO (7.6% of 763 lung transplantation patients) where support was initiated between 0 and 7 days after transplant. Thirty day survival was 56%. Long-term survival rates in the ECMO patients was significantly worse at 1 year and 5 years than the overall survival rates for the entire cohort (40% and 25% as compared to 82% and 54%, respectively).[25]

An alternative approach to severe, reversible allograft dysfunction has been reported by Eriksson and Steen,[26] who have used core cooling successfully to reduce oxygen requirements and avoid ECMO, giving a chance for the lung to heal. As a last resort, acute retransplantation may be lifesaving. In our series, we have performed a small number of retransplants emergently for primary graft failure (Fig. 112-6).[7] The indications for such expensive and dramatic therapy include the presence of unrelenting lung dysfunction, respiratory failure, and the absence of systemic complications (renal failure, infection) which would greatly diminish the chance of success.

Airway Complications

Airway complications formerly were a major cause of morbidity and mortality after pulmonary transplantation. In the current era of transplantation, airway complications remain a source of morbidity but do not appear to be associated with poorer survival.[7] Using standard methods of implantation, the donor bronchus is rendered ischemic, without reconstitution of its systemic bronchial artery circulation. The donor bronchus relies on collateral pulmonary artery blood flow during the first few days after transplantation. It has been demonstrated that pulmonary collateral flow contributes substantially to bronchial viability at the level of the distal bronchus and lobar origin. A shortened donor bronchial length reduces the length of donor bronchus dependent on collateral flow. Work from our group has shown that a determined effort to shorten the donor bronchus prior to implantation is associated with a decreased rate of anastomotic complications.[27] Superior preservation, improved sepsis prophylaxis, and better immunosuppression have reduced the incidence of airway complication. Across the authors' entire series, the rate of airway anastomotic complications of all degrees of severity is 9.3%.[12]

Airway anastomotic complications include bronchial stenosis, dehiscence, excessive granulation tissue formation, tracheobronchial malacia, fistulas, and infections. Bronchial stenosis represents the most commonly reported problem. Airway complications can be identified in a number of ways. Routine postoperative bronchoscopic surveillance generally provides early evidence of an anastomotic complication. On occasion, CT scan, performed for some other indication, demonstrates an

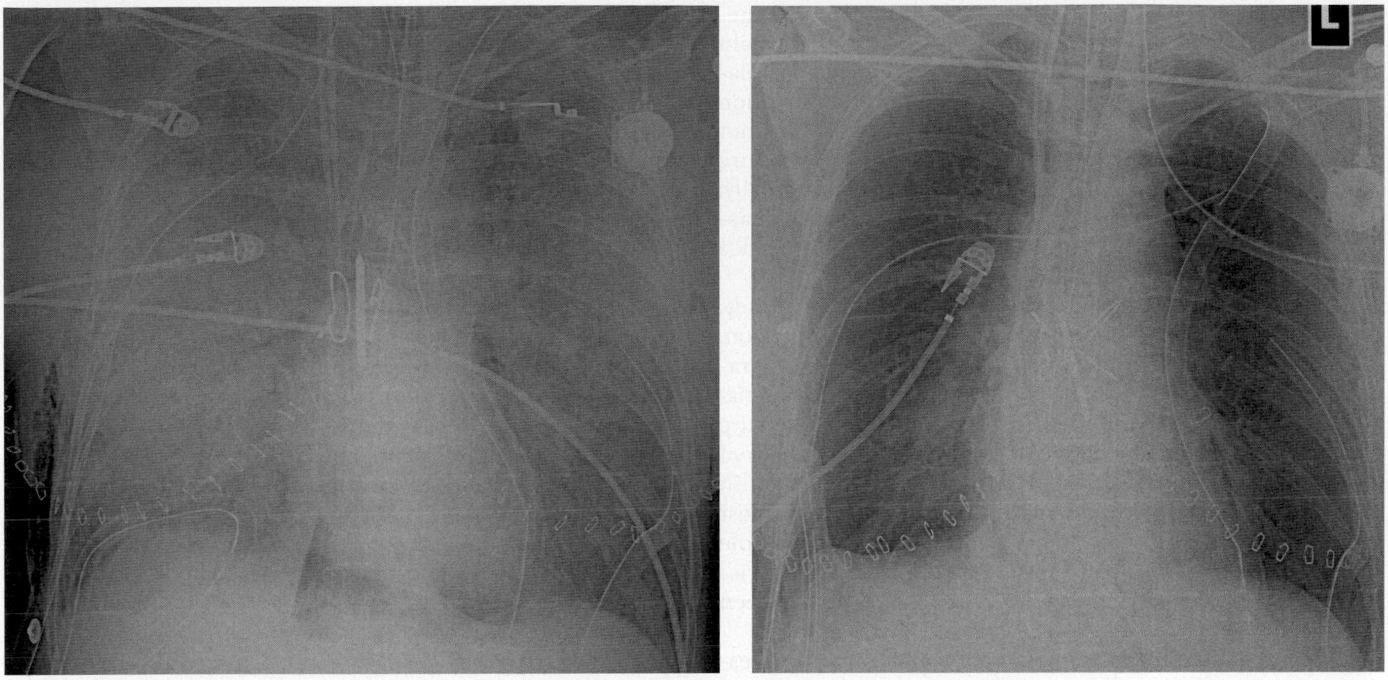

A B

Figure 112-6. *A.* Lung transplant recipient with primary graft failure. *B.* The patient underwent successful emergent retransplantation.

unexpected airway stenosis or dehiscence. In fact, we learned that CT scanning is a useful diagnostic tool for evaluating documented or suspected donor airway complications (Fig. 112-7). Late airway stenoses generally manifest with symptoms of dyspnea, wheeze, or decreased forced expiratory volume in 1 second (FEV_1). Bronchoscopic assessment confirms the diagnosis (Fig. 112-8).

ANASTOMOTIC STENOSIS

Therapeutic options for chronic airway stenosis include observation, balloon bronchoplasty, cryotherapy, electrocautery, laser, brachytherapy, bougie dilation, and stent placement. The nature of the stricture as well as the characteristics of the intervention must be carefully considered when devising a management plan. For example, a right main bronchial anastomotic stricture generally is managed easily by repeated dilation and ultimate placement of an endobronchial stent. There is usually sufficient length to place a right main bronchial orifice stent without impinging on the right upper lobe

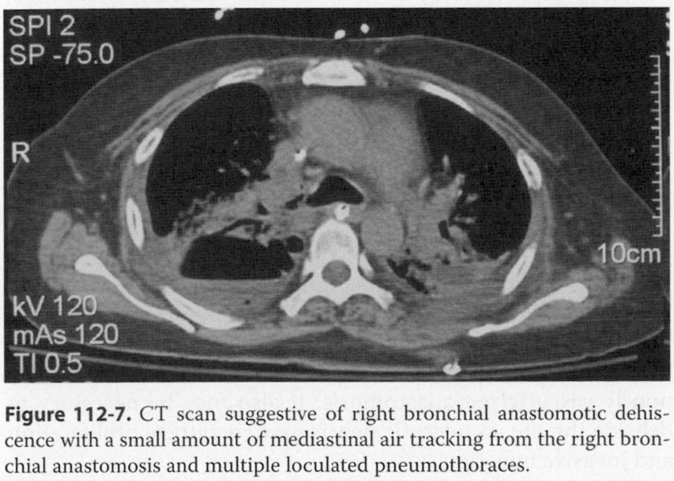

Figure 112-7. CT scan suggestive of right bronchial anastomotic dehiscence with a small amount of mediastinal air tracking from the right bronchial anastomosis and multiple loculated pneumothoraces.

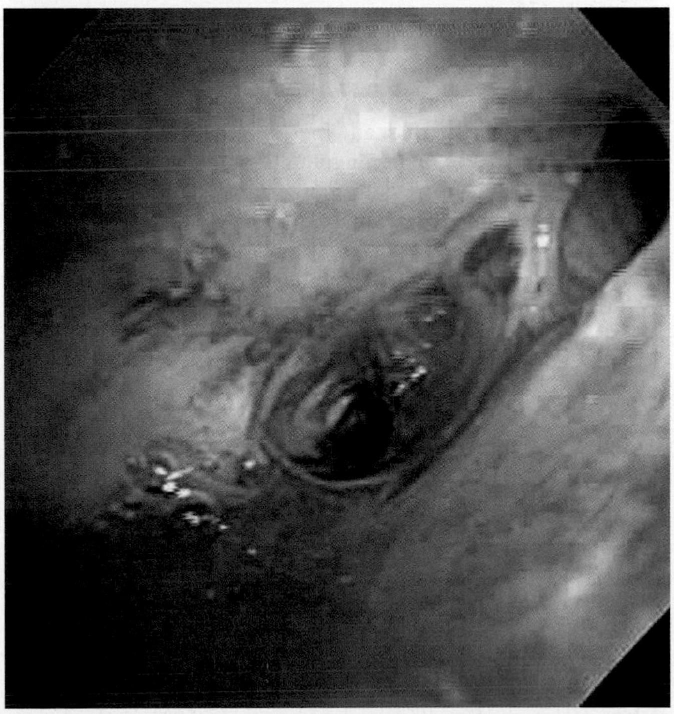

Figure 112-8. Bronchus intermedius stricture occurring after bilateral lung transplantation. On bronchoscopy, the right upper lobe has a widely patent orifice, but the bronchus intermedius appears stenotic. Despite repeated attempts to dilate the stricture, the bronchus intermedius orifice eventually was completely fibrosed.

bronchus. On the left side, however, strictures can be somewhat more difficult to manage. Dilating the distal left main bronchus is technically more difficult because of the angulation of the left bronchus. In addition, the lobar bifurcation immediately distal to the usual site of anastomosis does not provide a suitable length of bronchus distal to the stricture for placement of large-caliber dilating bronchoscopes. Finally, Silastic stents placed across a distal left main bronchial anastomotic stricture may occlude the upper or lower lobe orifice as the stent bridges the stricture.

Dilation is usually the first intervention for mild stenoses. Despite the high (>50%) incidence of complications (infection, granulation tissue overgrowth, mucous plugging, stent migration), stenting is frequently performed as well. Silastic stents are tolerated exceptionally well. However, patients may require daily inhalation of N-acetylcysteine to maintain the patency of the stent. DeHoyos et al.[28] reported dramatic improvement in pulmonary function with the Silastic stent. Fortunately, most stents are required only temporarily. After several months, the stent may be removed, and most stented anastomotic strictures maintain satisfactory patency after the stent has been removed.

Self-expanding metal stents have benefited from impressive technological improvement in recent years. These stents are available in a wide variety of lengths and diameters and are exceptionally easy to insert. Notably, they can be inserted via flexible bronchoscopy, a critical advantage in patients who are intubated. In rare situations, when the airways distal to anastomotic stricture are too small to accept a Silastic stent or when a Silastic stent will obstruct one bronchus while stenting another, the use of a self-expanding metal stent may suit the purpose perfectly. The only caveat is that granulation tissue will rapidly overgrow an uncovered metal mesh stent, sometimes making it impossible to remove.

The most recent addition to this armamentarium is the self-expanding silicone stent without interstices to inhibit the growth of granulation tissue. This stent (Polyflex, Boston Scientific; Boston, MA) theoretically incorporates the advantages of the silicone and self-expanding metallic stents in a single device (Fig. 112-9). Long-term data concerning stability and function of these stents are lacking. However, a small retrospective review of Polyflex stents used for benign airway conditions ($N = 16$, including four airway stenoses after lung transplantation) reported a 75% complication rate, mainly involving stent migration and mucous plugging.[29]

Anastomotic Necrosis and Dehiscence

On bronchoscopy, a normal bronchial anastomotic suture line demonstrates a narrow rim of epithelial slough that ultimately heals. On occasion, one can observe patchy areas of superficial necrosis of donor bronchial epithelium. These areas are generally of no concern and will heal eventually without causing problems. Minor degrees of bronchial dehiscence also have little long-term consequence. Membranous wall defects generally heal without any airway compromise, whereas cartilaginous defects usually result in some degree of late stricture. Significant dehiscence (>50% of the bronchial circumference) may result in compromise of the airway. This problem should be managed expectantly by mechanical debridement of the area to maintain satisfactory airway patency. A stent can be placed only if the distal main airway remains intact. Occasionally, a significant dehiscence results in direct communication with the pleural space, resulting in pneumothorax and a significant air leak following chest tube insertion. If the lung remains completely expanded and the pleural space is evacuated, the leak will seal ultimately, and the airway may heal without significant stenosis. Similarly, a dehiscence may communicate directly with the mediastinum, resulting in significant mediastinal emphysema. If the lung remains completely expanded and the pleural space is filled, adequate drainage of the mediastinum can be achieved by placing a drain in close proximity to the anastomotic line by way of mediastinoscopy. This step also will result in satisfactory healing of the anastomosis, often without stricture. Open surgical repair for reanastomosis, flap bronchoplasty, or retransplantation is reserved for severe cases, as reoperation is associated with poor outcomes.

A high incidence of postoperative airway dehiscence has been reported with the early use of sirolimus (Rapamune, Rapamycin, Wyeth Laboratories, Philadelphia, PA, and Certican, RAD, Everolimus, Rapamycin derivative, Novartis, East Hanover, NJ) in lung transplant recipients.[30] In a series of 15 patients treated in the early postoperative period with sirolimus, four experienced anastomotic dehiscences, and three of these four patients died. The use of sirolimus in the early post-transplant period should be discouraged.

Anastomotic Infections

Because of the requisite immunosuppression and inherent ischemia occurring at the bronchial anastomosis after lung transplantation, anastomotic infections are common and involve opportunistic pathogens. As a result, fungal infections may develop at this site, and Aspergillus and Candida have been identified as potential pathogens that can cause life-threatening bronchial anastomotic infection.[31] Nunley et al.[32] identified 15 (24.6%) saprophytic fungal infections involving bronchial anastomoses in 61 recipients. Most of these infections were due to the *Aspergillus* spp. Stenotic airway complications were seen more frequently in recipients with anastomotic fungal infections (46.7%) compared with those without (8.7%). Specific complications from fungal infections that arose at the bronchial anastomosis included bronchial stenosis, bronchomalacia, and fatal hemorrhage. A number of interventions, including bronchial stenting, balloon dilation, electrocauterization, laser debridement, and radiation brachytherapy, have been used to treat these complications. Additionally, in the series by Nunley and colleagues, three fatalities were associated (4.9%) with saprophytic bronchial anastomotic infections.

Antifungal prophylaxis, bronchoscopic surveillance, and the initiation of early empiric therapy when infection is suspected are all common approaches to reduce the incidence as well as associated morbidity and mortality of fungal infections. If bronchoscopic inspection reveals extensive anastomotic pseudomembranes, a biopsy of the site should be performed to rule out an invasive fungal infection. Success has been reported with a combination of systemic and inhaled antifungal agents. The addition of the inhaled antifungal therapy seems to be justified because aerosolization permits direct drug delivery to the poorly vascularized anastomosis. It also may be necessary to debride the site, as necrotic debris may encourage proliferation and invasive infection.[33,34]

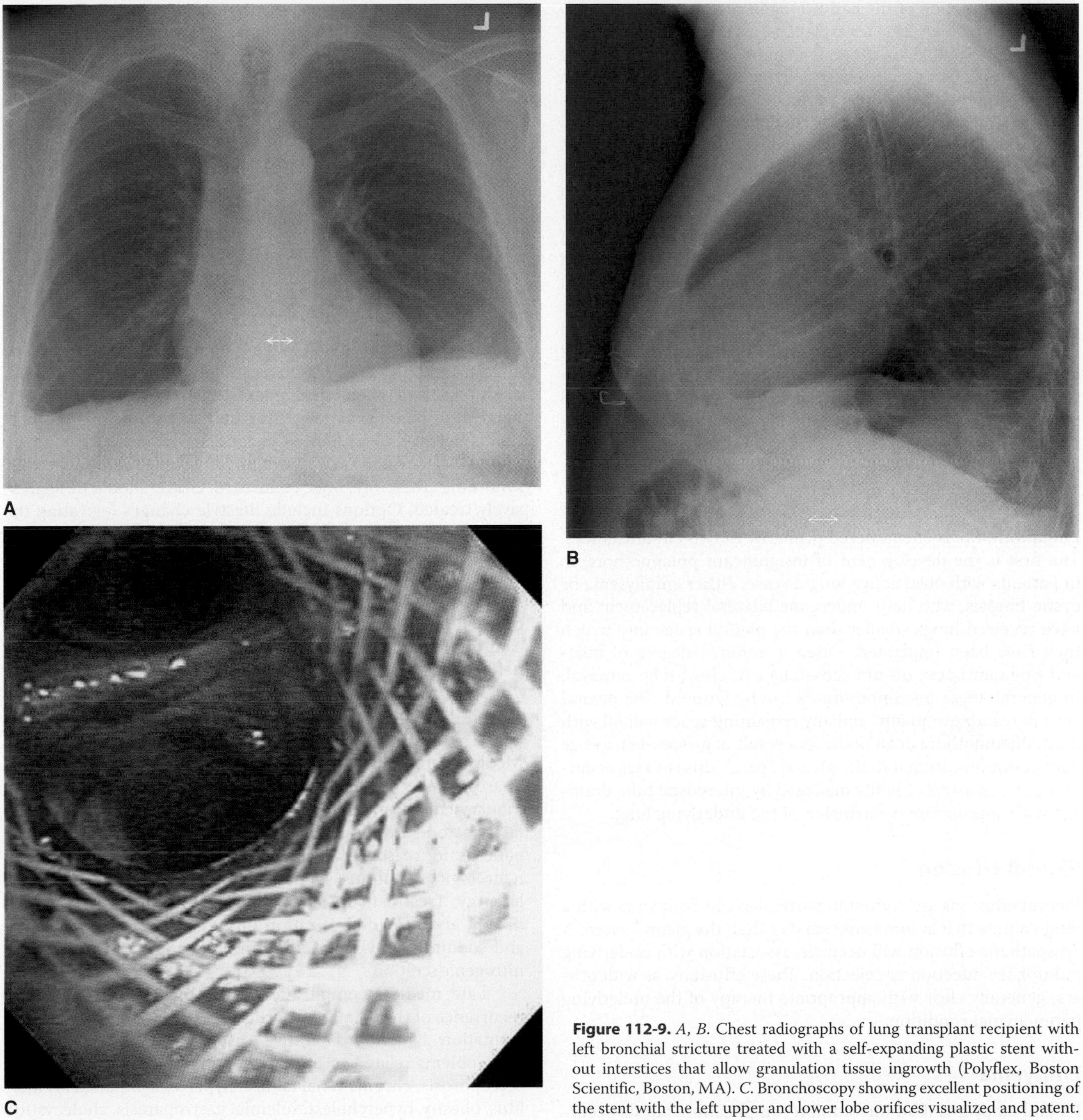

Figure 112-9. *A, B.* Chest radiographs of lung transplant recipient with left bronchial stricture treated with a self-expanding plastic stent without interstices that allow granulation tissue ingrowth (Polyflex, Boston Scientific, Boston, MA). *C.* Bronchoscopy showing excellent positioning of the stent with the left upper and lower lobe orifices visualized and patent.

PLEURAL SPACE COMPLICATIONS

Hyperinflation

Hyperinflation can occur in transplanted lungs as well as the native lung in patients with COPD who undergo single lung transplant. In the context of transplanted lungs, hyperinflation is a particular problem when size mismatch leads to the implantation of undersized lungs. When this occurs, the airway pressure may increase when suction is applied to the chest tubes.[35] The negative pleural pressure presumably inhibits elastic recoil of the lung, leading to detrimental hyperinflation. With hyperinflation, the alveoli do not decompress completely when the patient exhales, resulting in an increase in functional residual capacity. As more mechanical breaths are delivered, a stacking of the breaths occurs, and the lungs function on a flatter portion of the volume–pressure curve. In extreme cases, the residual functional capacity leads to detrimental alveolar hyperexpansion and hemodynamic instability. Awareness of the potential for acute hyperinflation should invoke preventive measures such as avoiding chest tube suction or water seal while the patient is on positive-pressure ventilation.

Hyperinflation of the native lung in recipients with COPD who undergo single lung transplant raises the concern of mediastinal shift leading to allograft compression. This can occur either acutely or as a chronic problem. Strategies to deal with acute native lung hyperinflation include early extubation, ventilation strategies that permit prolonged expiration, and, in dire cases, independent lung ventilation with a double-lumen endotracheal tube. Chronic native lung hyperinflation presents as slowly declining lung function and dyspnea associated with radiographic evidence of mediastinal shift and allograft compression. Reece et al. performed a retrospective review of 206 single-lung transplants performed for COPD, and found that 5% ($N = 10$) had clinically significant hyperinflation and underwent lung-volume–reduction surgery of the native lung. Although those who did well postoperatively enjoyed improved FEV_1 and 6-minute walk values, 20% ($N = 2$) of patients died during their hospitalization.[36] Given the risks associated with surgical intervention, it is critical to rule out other potential diagnoses when patients present with symptoms and imaging findings that suggest graft compression from hyperinflation.

Pneumothorax

Pneumothorax is encountered primarily in two circumstances. The first is the development of insignificant pneumothoraces in patients with obstructive lung disease, either emphysema or cystic fibrosis, who have undergone bilateral replacement and have received lungs smaller than the pleural space into which they have been implanted. Often a minimal degree of bilateral pneumothorax occurs subsequent to chest tube removal. In general, these pneumothoraces can be ignored. The pleural air will resorb eventually, and any remaining space will fill with fluid. Pneumothorax can occur as a result of airway dehiscence with communication into the pleural space. This is a rare occurrence and is usually readily managed by intercostal tube drainage with appropriate reexpansion of the underlying lung.

Pleural Effusion

Pleural effusions are common, particularly in recipients with a lung volume that is somewhat smaller than the pleural space. A sympathetic effusion will occur in association with underlying pulmonary infection or rejection. These effusions, as with others, generally clear with appropriate therapy of the underlying parenchymal condition.

Empyema

Pleural empyema is an uncommon complication, but its occurrence is associated with significant mortality. Spontaneous empyema is rare. It is more common for an empyema to develop after prolonged air leak owing to an open lung biopsy that has been performed on a patient receiving high-dose corticosteroids. Persistent air leak and failure to achieve reexpansion of the lung and subsequent pleurodesis give rise to a chronic pleural space that will become infected eventually. Nunley et al.[37] performed a retrospective review of 392 transplant recipients and found empyema documented in 14 patients (3.6%). In this series, empyemas tended to occur early in the posttransplant period. Four patients with empyema (28.6%) died secondary to infectious complications. No single predominant organism was isolated from the empyemic fluid, which had gram-positive, gram-negative, and saprophytic organisms. There was no relationship between the development of an empyema and the type of transplant performed or whether the transplant was done for a septic or nonseptic lung diagnosis.

We have treated a number of patients who developed empyemas with open drainage or rib resection by creating a Clagett window or Eloesser flap. Of note, an empyema rarely occurs as a result of bronchial dehiscence in communication with the pleural space.

OTHER COMPLICATIONS

Gastroesophageal Reflux

Although prevalent in end-stage lung patients, the occurrence of gastroesophageal reflux increases after lung transplantation, likely related to medication-induced gastroparesis and/or vagal nerve injury during surgery. The resulting chronic microaspiration is believed to lead to airway inflammation and the development of chronic lung rejection or bronchiolitis obliterans syndrome. Therefore, once confirmed, GERD should be aggressively treated. Options include lifestyle changes (elevating the head of the bed and avoiding late night meals), medications (proton-pump inhibitors and prokinetic drugs), and antireflux surgery. Nissen fundoplication has been used successfully to treat lung transplant patients with documented gastroesophageal reflux. This surgical procedure is associated with significant improvements in lung function, particularly if performed before the late stages of the bronchiolitis obliterans syndrome.[38]

Medical Complications

Medical complications that present in the early postoperative phase include acute rejection, atrial dysrhythmias, and pulmonary embolism. Hyperammonemia is a rare and frequently fatal postoperative complication that occurs in lung transplant patients, for reasons that are still unclear. Patients present with neurologic symptoms such as encephalopathy, seizures, and lethargy. Treatment includes hemodialysis, bowel decontamination, and the administration of arginine, sodium benzoate, and sodium phenylacetate to stimulate alternate pathways of nitrogen excretion.[39]

Late medical complications are numerous, and include recurrence of the primary disorder, malignancy, and posttransplantation lymphoproliferative disorders. Long-term medical problems related to immunosuppressive regimens include osteoporosis, chronic renal failure, hypertension, diabetes mellitus, obesity, hypercholesterolemia, gastroparesis, cholecystitis and anemia.

SUMMARY

Complications occur commonly in lung transplant recipients because of their general debilitation and the requirement for lifelong immunosuppression. Prevention and early recognition of these complications are important to control morbidity and mortality in this high-risk population. Focusing on complications can benefit the safe conduct of the initial surgery, as well as identify additional areas that warrant high priority for future investigation.

EDITOR'S COMMENT

In the acute phase after lung transplantation, pulmonary dysfunction can be associated with an interesting mix of potential technical and biologic causes. Pulmonary edema apparent within the first hour generally reflects technical issues (e.g., venous narrowing or atrial torsion) or hyperperfusion of the first lung during sequential single-lung transplants. In contrast, the ischemia–reperfusion response is generally delayed and occurs approximately 4 hours after transplantation. In the absence of a serologic mismatch, immune-mediated pulmonary edema rarely occurs within the first several days of transplantation.

—Steven J. Mentzer

References

1. Casula RP, Stoica SC, Wallwork J, et al. Pulmonary vein augmentation for single lung transplantation. *Ann Thorac Surg.* 2001;71:1373–1374.
2. Pasque MK. Standardizing thoracic organ procurement for transplantation. *J Thorac Cardiovasc Surg.* 2010;139:13–17.
3. Lau C, Guthrie T, Chaparro C, et al. Lung transplantation in recipients with previous lung volume reduction surgery. *J Heart Lung Transplant.* 2003;22:S183.
4. Meyers BF, Patterson GA. Technical aspects of adult lung transplantation. *Semin Thorac Cardiovasc Surg.* 1998;10:213–220.
5. Pasque MK, Cooper JD, Kaiser LR, et al. Improved technique for bilateral lung transplantation: rationale and initial clinical experience. *Ann Thorac Surg.* 1990;49:785–791.
6. Bhaskar B, Zeigenfuss M, Choudhary J, et al. Use of recombinant activated Factor VII for refractory after lung transplant bleeding as an effective strategy to restrict blood transfusion and associated complications. *Transfusion.* 2013;53:798–804.
7. Bui JD, Despotis GD, Trulock EP, et al. Fatal thrombosis after administration of activated prothrombin complex concentrates in a patient supported by extracorporeal membrane oxygenation who had received activated recombinant factor VII. *J Thorac Cardiovasc Surg.* 2002;124:852–854.
8. Shoji T, Hanaoka N, Wada H, et al. Balloon angioplasty for pulmonary artery stenosis after lung transplantation. *Eur J Cardiothorac Surg.* 2008;34:693–694.
9. Brown RP, Esmore DS, Lawson C. Improved sternal fixation in the transsternal bilateral thoracotomy incision. *J Thorac Cardiovasc Surg.* 1996;112:137–141.
10. Gandy KL, Mouston MJ. Sternal plating to prevent malunion of transverse sternotomy in lung transplantation. *Ann Thorac Surg.* 2008;86:1384–1385.
11. Motomura T, Bruckner B, La Francesca S, et al. Experience of sterna secondary closure by means of a titanium fixation system after transverse thoracosternotomy. *Artif Organs.* 2011;35:E168–E173.
12. Meyers BF, de la Morena M, Sweet SC, et al. Primary graft dysfunction and other selected complications of lung transplantation: a single-center experience of 983 patients. *J Thorac Cardiovasc Surg.* 2005;129:1421–1429.
13. Matsuzaki Y, Waddell TK, Puskas JD, et al. Amelioration of post-ischemic lung reperfusion injury by prostaglandin E_1. *Am Rev Respir Dis.* 1993;148:882–889.
14. Keshavjee SH, Yamazaki F, Cardoso PF, et al. A method for safe twelve-hour pulmonary preservation. *J Thorac Cardiovasc Surg.* 1989;98:529–534.
15. Maccherini M, Keshavjee SH, Slutsky AS, et al. The effect of low-potassium-dextran versus Euro-Collins solution for preservation of isolated type II pneumocytes. *Transplantation.* 1991;52:621–626.
16. Fischer S, Matte-Martyn A, De Perrot M, et al. Low-potassium dextran preservation solution improves lung function after human lung transplantation. *J Thorac Cardiovasc Surg.* 2001;121:594–596.
17. Yamashita M, Schmid RA, Ando K, et al. Nitroprusside ameliorates lung allograft reperfusion injury. *Ann Thorac Surg.* 1996;62:791–796.
18. Lick SD, Brown PS Jr, Kurusz M, et al. Technique of controlled reperfusion of the transplanted lung in humans. *Ann Thorac Surg.* 2000;69:910–912.
19. Schnickel GT, Ross DJ, Beygui R, et al. Modified reperfusion in clinical lung transplantation: the results of 100 consecutive cases. *J Thorac Cardiovasc Surg.* 2006;13:218–223.
20. Cypel M, Yeung JC, Liu M, et al. Normothermic ex vivo lung perfusion in clinical lung transplantation. *N Engl J Med.* 2011;364:1431–1440.
21. Date H, Triantafillou AN, Trulock EP, et al. Inhaled nitric oxide reduces human lung allograft dysfunction. *J Thorac Cardiovasc Surg.* 1996;111:913–919.
22. Fiser SM, Cope JT, Kron IL, et al. Aerosolized prostacyclin (epoprostenol) as an alternative to inhaled nitric oxide for patients with reperfusion injury after lung transplantation. *J Thorac Cardiovasc Surg.* 2001;121:981–982.
23. Khan TA, Schnickel G, Ross D, et al. A prospective, randomized, crossover pilot study of inhaled nitric oxide versus inhaled prostacyclin in heart transplant and lung transplant recipients. *J Thorac Cardiovasc Surg.* 2009;138:1417–1424.
24. Meyers BF, Sundt TM 3rd, Henry S, et al. Selective use of extracorporeal membrane oxygenation is warranted after lung transplantation. *J Thorac Cardiovasc Surg.* 2000;120:20–26.
25. Bermudez CA, Adusumilli PS, McCurry KR, et al. Extracorporeal membrance oxygenation for primary graft dysfunction after lung transplantation: long-term survival. *Ann Thorac Surg.* 2009;87:854–860.
26. Eriksson LT, Steen S. Induced hypothermia in critical respiratory failure after lung transplantation. *Ann Thorac Surg.* 1998;65:827–829.
27. Van Berkel V, Guthrie TJ, Puri VP, et al. Impact of anastomotic techniques on airway complications after lung transplant. *Ann Thorac Surg.* 2011;92:316–320.
28. de Hoyos AL, Patterson GA, Maurer JR, et al. Pulmonary transplantation: early and late results. The Toronto Lung Transplant Group. *J Thorac Cardiovasc Surg.* 1992;103:295–306.
29. Gildea TR, Murthy SC, Sahoo D, et al. Performance of a self-expanding silicone stent in palliation of benign airway conditions. *Chest.* 2006;130:1419–1423.
30. King-Biggs MB, Dunitz JM, Park SJ, et al. Airway anastomotic dehiscence associated with use of sirolimus immediately after lung transplantation. *Transplantation.* 2003;75:1437–1443.
31. Kramer MR, Denning DW, Marshall SE, et al. Ulcerative tracheobronchitis after lung transplantation: a new form of invasive aspergillosis. *Am Rev Respir Dis.* 1991;144:552–556.
32. Nunley DR, Gal AA, Vega JD, et al. Saprophytic fungal infections and complications involving the bronchial anastomosis following human lung transplantation. *Chest.* 2002;122:1185–1191.
33. Palmer SM, Perfect JR, Howell DN, et al. Candidal anastomotic infection in lung transplant recipients: successful treatment with a combination of systemic and inhaled antifungal agents. *J Heart Lung Transplant.* 1998;17:1029–1033.
34. Hadjiliadis D, Howell DN, Davis RD, et al. Anastomotic infections in lung transplant recipients. *Ann Transplant.* 2000;5:13–19.
35. Kozower BD, Meyers BF, Ciccone AM, et al. Potential for detrimental hyperinflation after lung transplantation with application of negative pleural pressure to undersized lung grafts. *J Thorac Cardiovasc Surg.* 2003;125:430–432.
36. Reece TB, Mitchell JD, Zamora MR, et al. Native lung volume reduction surgery relieves functional graft compression after single-lung transplantation for chronic obstructive pulmonary disease. *J Thorac Cardiovasc Surg.* 2008;135:931–937.
37. Nunley DR, Grgurich WF, Keenan RJ, et al. Empyema complicating successful lung transplantation. *Chest.* 1999;115:1312–1315.
38. Cantu E, Appel JZ, Hartwig MG, et al. Early fundoplication prevents chronic allograft dysfunction in patients with gastroesophageal reflux disease. *Ann Thorac Surg.* 2004;78:1142–1151.
39. Berry GT, Bridges ND, Nathanson KL, et al. Successful use of alternate waste nitrogen agents and hemodialysis in a patient with hyperammonemic coma after heart-lung transplantation. *Arch Neurol.* 1999;56:481–484.

113 Artificial Lung

Jeremiah T. Martin, Charles W. Hoopes, Enrique Diaz-Guzman, and Joseph B. Zwischenberger

Keywords: Extracorporeal membrane oxygenation (ECMO), end-stage lung disease, respiratory failure, interventional lung assist

INTRODUCTION

Extracorporeal membrane oxygenation (ECMO) has continued to evolve since the pioneers of cardiac surgery, Gibbon and Lillehei, developed cardiopulmonary bypass in the 1950s. The term ECMO applies to the use of an extracorporeal circuit, consisting of tubing, oxygenator and blood pump, in the setting of cardiopulmonary failure. The original ECMO was veno-arterial (VA) as popularized by Bartlett in the early 1980s. Over the last three decades ECMO has evolved into several forms including VA, veno-venous (VV), arterio-venous (AV), right atrium to aorta (RA–Ao), and pulmonary artery to left atrium (PA–LA). ECMO in some form may be indicated for acute cardiac failure, respiratory failure, or a mixed presentation; the specific application of the therapy will depend on the presentation of the patient. Likewise, several programs have developed ambulatory capability of most forms of ECMO to aid recovery or suitability for transplant. Ambulatory ECMO is often referred to as the "artificial lung."

GENERAL PRINCIPLES

Historically, ECMO in the adult was considered "salvage" therapy for patients "dying" from severe respiratory failure despite maximal medical therapy. Some of the oft-quoted trials in the 1980s compared ECMO with conventional medical therapy and failed to show survival advantage. However, there have been significant advances in ECMO, and evidence now favors earlier utilization of the technology to minimize end-organ damage that might occur during prolonged maximal ventilatory and medical support. This is particularly apparent in the case of respiratory failure associated with H1N1 influenza. Survival is approximately 72% for patients placed on ECMO within 6 days of intubation compared with only 30% for patients on ECMO 7 or more days after intubation.[1]

PATIENT SELECTION

ECMO is indicated for the short-to-medium-term management of respiratory failure, cardiac failure, or both. Specifically, patients are evaluated when the native disease process is thought to have an estimated mortality of 50% or greater, is reversible, and/or requires a bridge to transplant. The Extracorporeal Life Support Organization (ELSO) publishes guidelines which cover application of ECMO in the adult. In the case of acute respiratory distress syndrome (ARDS), this would include a PaO_2/FiO_2 ratio of less than 100 despite optimization of ventilator settings.

Special scenarios include H1N1 infection, where early deployment of ECMO is associated with better outcomes, and delay may adversely affect the risk/benefit ratio. In addition, use of ECMO as a bridge-to-transplant for lung recipients should be considered when maximal medical therapy is insufficient. Many programs utilize ambulatory ECMO to improve the respiratory status and conditioning prior to transplant.

ECMO as a bridge to lung transplantation has significantly increased during the last 10 years. A recent analysis of the UNOS database showed that the use of ECMO at the time of lung transplantation has grown 150% in the last 24 months compared to all previous decades (1970–2010). This increase in utilization is reflected in the growing success reported with the use of different ECMO modalities in patients awaiting lung transplantation. We recently submitted our experience with the use of ambulatory ECMO as a bridge to lung transplantation, reporting the use of ECMO in 31 patients with end-stage lung disease. In our series, all of the patients were awake and the vast majority followed an "algorithm-directed" ECMO management program that involved the use of physical therapy and ambulation in preparation for lung transplant. In our series, the 30-day, 1-year, 3-year and 5-year survival was 97%, 92%, 83%, and 66%, respectively.[2] A summary of a modern series of patients bridged to lung transplant while on ECMO is presented in Table 113-1.

PREOPERATIVE ASSESSMENT

ECMO use is now being considered in awake, nonintubated patients to improve oxygenation, to facilitate ambulation, and to improve physical conditioning prior to transplant.

Indications for ECMO

1. Patients with irreversible end-stage lung disease presenting with clinical deterioration (refractory hypoxia or hypercapnia) or lack of response despite the use of invasive or noninvasive mechanical ventilation.
2. Patients with severe pulmonary hypertension refractory to pulmonary vasodilators and/or hemodynamic deterioration caused by right ventricular failure.
3. Patients with severe exercise-induced pulmonary hypertension associated with advanced lung disease, presenting with clinical deterioration and progressive physical decline, and unable to maintain ambulation and good functional status.

Contraindications to the Use of ECMO

1. Active bloodstream infection
2. Acute renal failure not responsive to medical therapy (need for dialysis)

Table 113-1

SUMMARY OF RECENT REPORTS OF THE USE OF ECMO AS BRIDGE TO LUNG TRANSPLANT (SERIES WITH MORE THAN 10 PATIENTS)

REFERENCE	YR	NUMBER OF PATIENTS	DURATION OF ECLS[a] (RANGE)	MODE OF ECLS	% SUCCESSFUL BRIDGE	ONE YR SURVIVAL
Fischer[14]	2006	12	15 ± 8 (4–32)[b]	A-V pumpless	83	80
Cypel[15]	2010	10	5 (1–25)	VA (3), VV (1), AV pumpless (4), PA–LA (4)	100	70
Ricci[16]	2010	12	7.5 (4–48)	AV pumpless	25	NA
Hammainen[17]	2010	16	16.8 ± 19.2[b] (1–59)	VV (7) VA (6)	81	92
Bermudez[9]	2011 (1991–2010)	17	3.2 (1–49)	VV (8) VA (9)	NA	74
Fuenher[18]	2012	26	9 (1–45)	VV(14) VA(12)	77	80 (6 mos)
Lang[11]	2012	34	4.5 (1–63)	VV(18) VA(14) A-V pumpless (1) Combination (4)	76	60
Hoopes[12]	2012	31	11 (2–53)	VV (DLC) (9) VV (Hybrid) (4) VA (9) PA–LA (2) RA–Ao (3) Combination (4)	NA	92

[a]Median duration of ECLS in days.
[b]Mean duration of ECLS in days.

3. Hereditary or acquired coagulation disorders (i.e., blood dyscrasia, heparin-induced thrombocytopenia)
4. Evidence of end-organ failure other than the lung
5. Underlying irreversible neurological or neuromuscular disease

Several studies have shown that the use of mechanical ventilation in patients with idiopathic pulmonary fibrosis is not effective and is associated with high mortality rates. Delaying initiation of ECMO in an attempt to maximize alternative medical treatments may result in worsening physical condition, secondary organ dysfunction, and jeopardize their candidacy for possible lung transplantation.

Areas of Controversy

Advanced age (>65 years) is considered by some a relative contraindication for lung transplantation. Nevertheless, several reports have demonstrated good outcomes in patients >65 years of age. A recent report of the use of ambulatory VV ECMO in patients with cystic fibrosis and hypercapneic respiratory failure suggests that patients with severe bronchiectasis or cystic fibrosis can be successfully bridged to lung transplantation without an increased risk for infectious complications.

TECHNIQUE

There are four categories for ECMO cannulation in the adult:

1. VV ECMO is indicated for management of isolated respiratory failure. The success of this strategy relies on the patient's own hemodynamics and only assists with gas exchange. Blood is withdrawn from the right atrium/inferior vena cava (IVC) via a long peripheral cannula inserted via a central vein. Oxygenated blood is returned via a superior vena cava (SVC) cannula into the right atrium with flow directed at the tricuspid valve. The oxygenated blood is then pumped out the pulmonary artery, through the dysfunctional lungs, and then returned to the left heart where it is pumped to the systemic circulation. The Avalon Elite™ dual lumen cannula (DLC) (Maquet Cardiovascular, San Jose, CA), designed by Wang and Zwischenberger, is a significant advance in the arena of VV ECMO.[3] Single percutaneous access of the right internal jugular vein yields several advantages: single-site cannulation, reduced risk for complications associated with femoral or central cannulation, and the ability to allow ambulation by avoiding the use of the femoral site. Placement of the Avalon cannula may be performed bedside in the intensive care unit (ICU); however, it requires either fluoroscopic or echocardiographic guidance for optimal placement of the return and infusion ports.[4]
2. VA ECMO is indicated in the setting of acute cardiogenic shock or in the setting of a primary respiratory process complicated by diminished cardiac function. Cannulation is performed with venous drainage from the right femoral vein through a long cannula placed such that optimal drainage from the right atrium is achieved. Oxygenated blood is returned via femoral arterial cannula. Cannulas may be placed percutaneously in the ICU or a direct cut-down for access to the femoral vasculature. Blood via the axillary artery by direct anastomosis of a conduit facilitates ambulation. This strategy may be an important consideration in the conversion of ambulatory VV ECMO to VA ECMO as this configuration continues to allow ambulation.[5]

3. AV ECMO/AVCO_2 removal. AV ECMO utilizes the patient's native hemodynamics to drive flow through a low resistance gas exchange device, the goal being CO_2 removal. This configuration is most suited to those patients awaiting lung transplantation whose primary issue is severe CO_2 retention. Sometimes described as pumpless extracorporeal lung assist (pECLA), flow through the circuit is usually 15% to 20% of cardiac output, which limits its use for oxygenation. Central cannulation has also been described.[6,7]
4. Central cannulation refers to placement of ECMO cannulas via thoracotomy or sternotomy. This most commonly refers to placement of ECMO for failure to wean from cardiopulmonary bypass. The disadvantage is the need for full operating room support; however, the full array of ECMO options are available via the great vessels, and complications of peripheral cannulation are avoided.

Significant advances in commercially available oxygenator membranes have resulted in improved durability, including patients bridged to lung transplantation. Currently, most ECMO systems have replaced polypropylene with polymethylpentene (PMP) fibers. PMP membrane oxygenators are smaller, provide efficient gas exchange without plasma leak, and are associated with faster priming (saving blood and valuable time and making CO_2 flushing unnecessary). In addition, the PMP oxygenators are associated with less circuit resistance, are less prone to malfunctioning due to blood trauma or blood clots, and can be functional for several weeks to months. Modern ECMO components, including PMP oxygenators, can be heparin coated, reducing excessive use of heparin, minimizing risk of over-anticoagulation, and reducing the use of blood products. Heparin-coated tubing is also associated with a reduction in the rates of leukocytes, platelets, and complement activation. New centrifugal pumps have been created offering a nonocclusive, demand-regulated pump flow that eliminates the risk of raceway tubing wear and circuit rupture, facilitating patient mobilization and ambulation.

Interventional Lung Assist (Novalung)

The interventional lung assist (iLA), or Novalung, consists of a low resistance PMP membrane designed to allow gas exchange by simple diffusion. The iLA has been successfully used to bridge patients to lung transplantation using a "pumpless" AV mode (pECLA), in which the device is attached to the systemic circulation via femoral artery, although central cannulation has also been reported in patients bridged to lung transplantation (PA–LA or PA–PV). The device is effective for CO_2 removal but is less effective for O_2 augmentation as it only receives approximately 15% to 20% of the cardiac output for extracorporeal gas exchange. Novalung has been compared to other CO_2 removal devices in patients awaiting lung transplantation and all provided similar CO_2 clearance.

Dual Lumen Cannula (Avalon Elite)

A new type of DLC (Fig. 113-1), the Avalon Elite, is placed percutaneously through the internal jugular vein; the drainage lumen is open to both the SVC and IVC, while the infusion lumen is open to the right atrium. The blood from systemic circulation flows through the SVC and IVC into the drainage

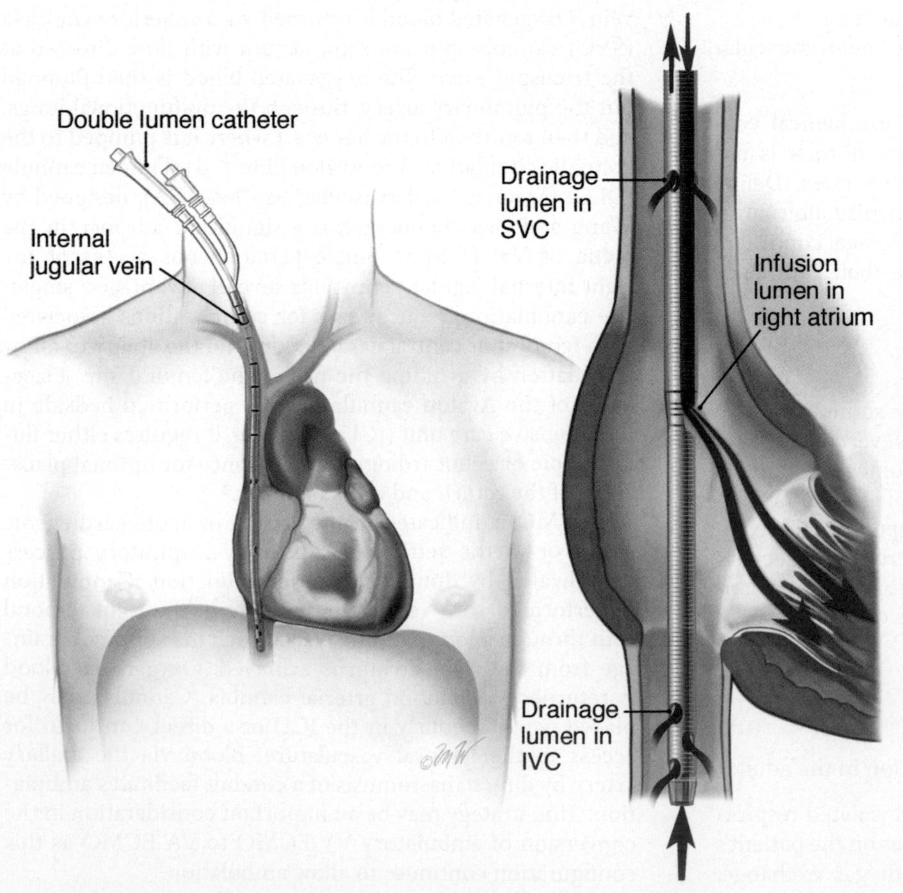

Figure 113-1. Avalon Elite™ double lumen catheter and catheter placement.

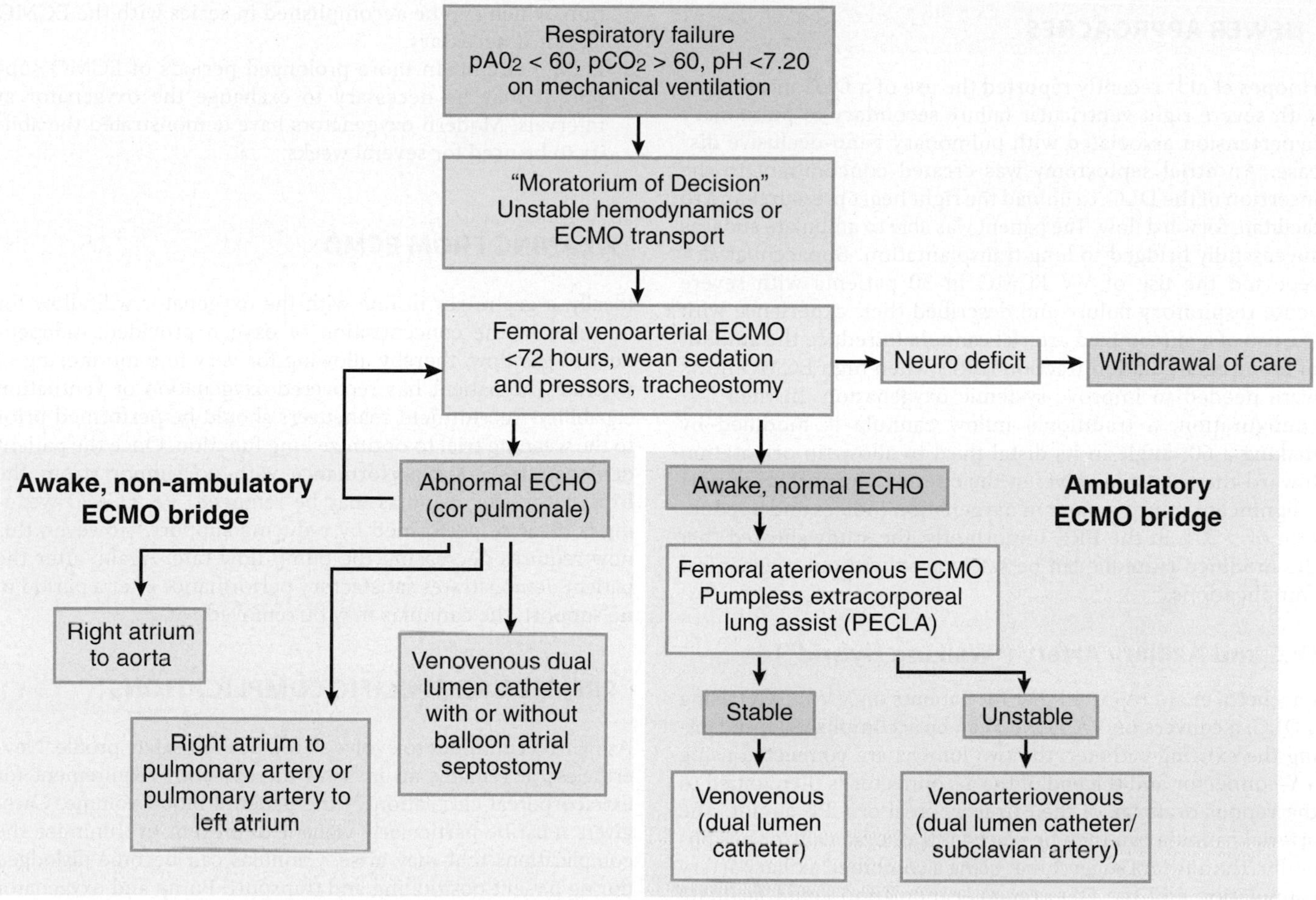

Figure 113-2. Preferred approach for patients bridged to lung transplantation using ECMO.

lumen to the artificial lung device. The blood is oxygenated and returned via the infusion lumen into the right atrium. Compared to traditional ECMO approaches, this device offers important advantages in patients awaiting lung transplantation: it requires single-site cannulation, reduces the risk for complications associated with femoral or central cannulation, and facilitates ambulation by avoiding the use of the femoral site. The DLC has a unique design with improved flexibility (reducing kinking problems associated with rigid cannulas). The infusion lumen of the cannula is an ultra-thin membrane that collapses during insertion to allow space for an atraumatic introducer that facilitates placement. The Avalon DLC has shown recirculation fractions of 2% when fluoroscopy or transthoracic echocardiography guidance is used.

The DLC has been used to facilitate ambulation during ECMO in awake and nonintubated patients. Garcia et al.[8] first reported the use of ambulatory VV ECMO using a DLC in a patient with COPD with refractory hypercapnia. The patient was able to exercise using a treadmill and a stationary bike while on ECMO and was successfully bridged to lung transplantation approximately 19 days later. Subsequent to this report, many other centers have reported similar results and have confirmed the feasibility and safety of the DLC as a bridge to lung transplantation. For VV ECMO, a single-site approach using a DLC was preferred in patients with hypercapnia and preserved oxygenation, whereas a two-site approach was chosen for patients with severe hypoxemia. Bermudez et al.[9] presented their single-center experience with 17 patients that were bridged to lung transplantation. The 30-day, 1-year, and 3-year survival rates were not different when compared to nonsupported patients, and the survival was not affected by ECMO type at 2 years. Hayes et al.[10] reported the use of a DLC to facilitate ambulation and transplant in four patients with cystic fibrosis and hypercapneic respiratory failure. More recently, Lang et al.[11] reported their experience with ECMO as a bridge to lung transplantation in 34 patients, and reported the use of a DLC in two patients.

The cannulation strategy is frequently chosen based on: ability to facilitate ambulation (DLC via internal jugular vein is the preferred route, although central VA ECMO and iLA [PA–LA] can also allow ambulation); hemodynamic instability; and presence of severe pulmonary hypertension and/or right heart failure (central or femoral cannulation for VA ECMO is preferred). Cannulation approaches performed for bridging patients to lung transplantation include femoral vein to internal jugular vein (traditional VV), femoral vein to femoral artery (traditional VA), RA–Ao (central VA), PA–LA, and right internal jugular with DLC (ambulatory VV).

Fig. 113-2 shows our preferred cannulation strategy for ambulatory ECMO as a bridge to lung transplantation.

NEWER APPROACHES

Hoopes et al.[12] recently reported the use of a DLC in a patient with severe right ventricular failure secondary to pulmonary hypertension associated with pulmonary veno-occlusive disease. An atrial septostomy was created concomitant to the insertion of the DLC, to unload the right heart pressures and to facilitate forward flow. The patient was able to ambulate and was successfully bridged to lung transplantation. Bonacchi et al.[13] reported the use of VV ECMO in 30 patients with severe acute respiratory failure and described their experience with the use of a customized arterial cannula to reduce the amount of blood recirculation fraction (BRF) when high ECMO flows were needed to improve systemic oxygenation. In their "χ" configuration, a traditional inflow cannula is modified by making a 60° angle in its distal third to allow tip orientation toward the tricuspid valve. In their series, the authors report a significant improvement in oxygenation indices and a reduction of >20% in the BRF. Importantly, the study showed that the modified cannula can be safely used without mechanical complications.

DLC and Axillary Artery ("Walking Hybrid")

Bacchetta et al.[5] reported that for patients on VV ECMO using a DLC, a conversion VA ECMO can be accomplished by adapting the existing catheter: the two lumens are connected using a Y-connector and the end of the Y-connector is then joined to the venous drainage of the extracorporeal or CPB circuit. The arterial cannula can then be placed intrathoracically or peripherally. The authors suggest that using a combined axillary artery cannulation and the DLC venous cannulation could facilitate ambulation while awaiting lung transplantation.

POSTPROCEDURE CARE/MANAGEMENT OF THE PATIENT ON ECMO

Once ECMO has been established, attention must be directed toward optimizing recovery, minimizing complications, and minimizing end-organ damage.

1. Ventilator: Minimal settings should be employed to minimize barotrauma. FiO_2 should be reduced to 30% or less if possible and $P_{plateau}$ should be maintained below 25.
2. Anticoagulation: Modern ECMO circuits feature heparin-bonded tubing, which will help minimize thrombotic complications; however, the oxygenator requires some level of anticoagulation to be maintained. An activated clotting time (ACT) level of 1.5 times normal should be maintained. Direct monitoring of heparin and other coagulation factors may also be employed.
3. Blood Transfusion: Oxygen carrying capacity must be optimized to make best use of the ECMO circuit, particularly in the VV setting.
4. Hemodynamics: Normal hemodynamics are critical to the performance of VV ECMO. It may be necessary to utilize pressors and occasionally may be necessary to convert to VA ECMO. In the setting of VA ECMO, native cardiac function must be monitored with regular echocardiography to avoid complications. Fluid overload should be aggressively managed with either diuresis or ultrafiltration, which can be accomplished in series with the ECMO circuit if necessary.
5. ECMO circuit: In more prolonged periods of ECMO support it may be necessary to exchange the oxygenator at intervals. Modern oxygenators have demonstrated the ability to be used for several weeks.

WEANING FROM ECMO

Ideally, a gas mixer in line with the oxygenator will allow for decrease in the concentration of oxygen provided, independent of gas flow, thereby allowing for very fine monitoring of whether the patient has recovered oxygenation or ventilation capability. Recruitment maneuvers should be performed prior to the weaning trial to optimize lung function. Once the patient demonstrates good performance with no support from the oxygenator, the cannulas may be removed. VA ECMO weaning is likewise performed by reducing support. However, this now requires decreasing the pump flow rate. Again, after the patient demonstrates satisfactory performance after a period of no support, the cannulas may be removed.

PROCEDURE-SPECIFIC COMPLICATIONS

As ECMO continues to evolve so too does its safety profile. Nevertheless, it remains an invasive therapy with requirement for extracorporeal circulation of the patient's blood volume. Caregivers must be particularly vigilant to prevent or minimize the complications that may arise. Cannulas can become dislodged during patient positioning and transport. Pump and oxygenator may fail, and backups should be readily available. In the case of the commonly used centrifugal pump, a battery backup and hand-crank system should be available at the bedside at all times.

Meticulous hemostasis is a first step to avoid bleeding. ACT may be allowed to run closer to normal for a period to assist with hemostasis. The use of factor transfusion has been described in refractory cases; however, it carries the risk of circuit thrombosis. Cerebral/coronary ischemia is particular to VA ECMO and is most likely to manifest in patients with femoral-only cannulation. Arterial blood is returned from the circuit via the femoral artery and flows retrograde up the descending aorta. In the case of increased native cardiac output, which may occur due to insufficient unloading due to low flow or cannula position, deoxygenated blood may be ejected from the heart to counter the retrograde flow of oxygenated blood from the circuit. If the native ejection is such that the "meeting point" of these two competing blood streams is distal to the left carotid artery, cerebral ischemia will ensue despite excellent distal organ perfusion. It should also be apparent that coronary ischemia is a particular concern. To monitor for this requires right upper extremity pulse oximetry at a minimum, and arterial blood gases should be checked, preferably from the right upper extremity, in addition to echocardiographic monitoring of cardiac function. In some cases it may be necessary to resort to central or peripheral right axillary cannulation.

The recent success of ECMO is a consequence of both significant advances in technology of the components of the circuit as well as available changes in ECMO configuration that allows the use of ECMO in awake and ambulatory patients.

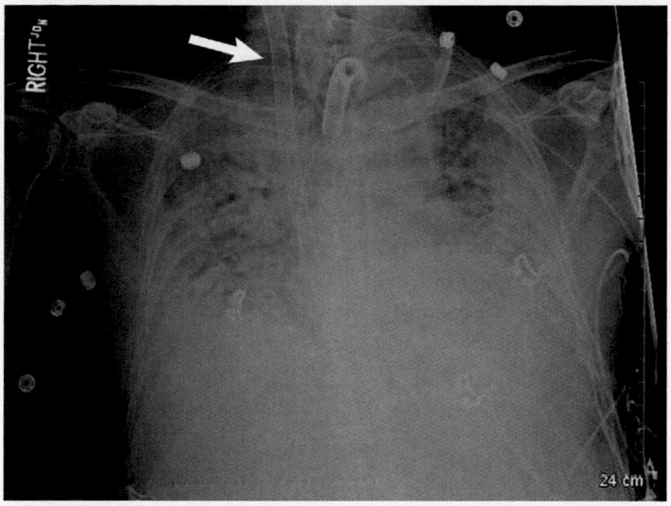

Figure 113-3. Chest radiograph illustrating bilateral diffuse bilateral infiltrates consistent with ARDS and right internal jugular Avalon cannula in place (*arrow*).

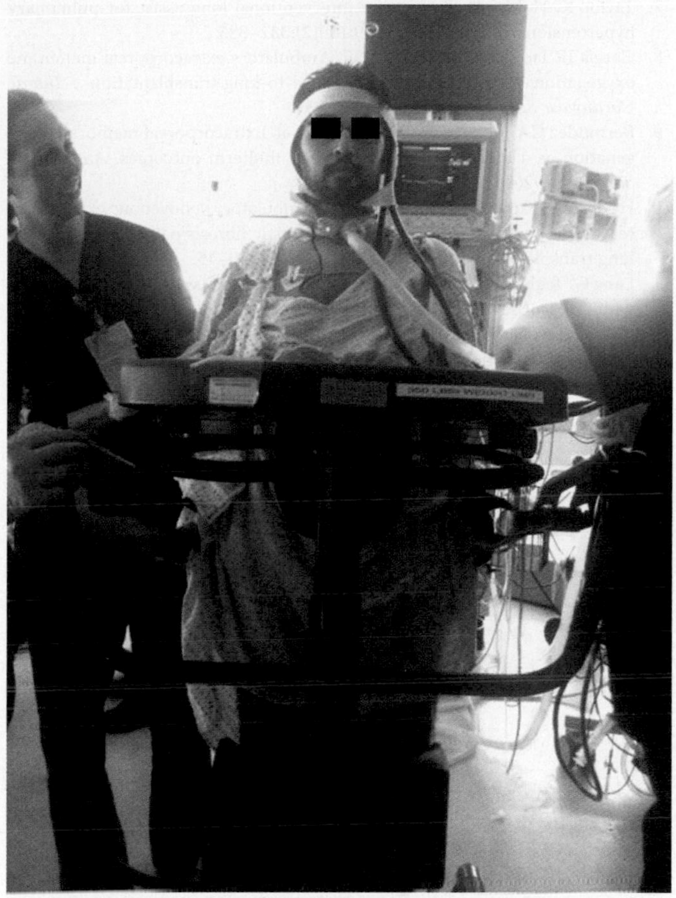

Figure 113-4. Patient performing physical therapy while on VV ECMO.

The objectives are to improve the preoperative condition of the patient by enhancing physical strength, cardiovascular fitness, and reducing the risk for posttransplant complications.

ILLUSTRATED CASE REPORT

A 27-year-old Caucasian male with no significant past medical history was admitted to the ICU after an episode of nonresolving pneumonia complicated by the development of ARDS (Fig. 113-3). The patient deteriorated requiring use of mechanical ventilation. The patient's high airway pressures and decreased lung compliance were treated with continuous sedation and neuromuscular blocking agents. After the patient failed to respond to conventional medical therapy and protective lung ventilation (including use of newer modes of mechanical ventilation such as airway pressure release ventilation [APRV]), he was referred to our institution for consideration of lung transplantation approximately 3 weeks later. As a result of severe deconditioning and profound neuromuscular weakness, the patient was not considered an appropriate candidate for lung transplantation. His poor lung compliance and high oxygen requirements precluded the possibility of achieving ambulation and physical reconditioning. Therefore, ambulatory ECMO as a bridge to lung transplantation was initiated. A 31 French Avalon cannula was inserted in the right internal jugular vein under fluoroscopy and echocardiography guidance (as previously described in the literature).[4] The patient was started on VV ECMO and was weaned from mechanical ventilation within 24 hours. All sedative medications were discontinued and the patient started a program of physical rehabilitation including daily ambulation while on ECMO with a goal of a walk distance of >400 feet (Fig. 113-4). The patient remained on VV ECMO for approximately 49 days and was successfully bridged to a bilateral lung transplant. The patient was discharged home within 2 weeks of transplant with good physical performance and without the use of supplemental oxygen. This case illustrates the value of ECMO for patients with severe end-stage lung failure who are unable to recover from catastrophic lung injury and who are unable to bridge to lung transplantation with the use of conventional mechanical ventilation.

References

1. Extracorporeal Life Support Organization (ELSO). Patient specific supplements to the general guidelines for ECMO centers. April 2009. http://www.elso.med.umich.edu/Guidelines.html. Accessed July 15, 2012.
2. Hoopes C, Diaz-Guzman E, Kukreja J. Ambulatory ECMO as a bridge to lung transplantation. 38th Annual Meeting, Western Thoracic Surgical Association. Maui, Hawaii, 2012.
3. Wang D, Zhou X, Liu X, et al. Wang-Zwische double lumen cannula-toward a percutaneous and ambulatory paracorporeal artificial lung. *ASAIO J.* 2008;54(6):606–611.
4. Javidfar J, Wang D, Zwischenberger JB, et al. Insertion of bicaval dual lumen extracorporeal membrane oxygenation catheter with image guidance. *ASAIO J.* 2011;57(4):203–205.
5. Bacchetta M, Javidfar J, Sonett J, et al. Ease of conversion from venovenous extracorporeal membrane oxygenation to cardiopulmonary bypass and venoarterial extracorporeal membrane oxygenation with a bicaval dual lumen catheter. *ASAIO J.* 2011;57(4):283–285.
6. Pedersen TH, Videm V, Svennevig JL, et al. Extracorporeal membrane oxygenation using a centrifugal pump and a servo regulator to prevent negative inlet pressure. *Ann Thorac Surg.* 1997;63(5):1333–1339.

7. Taylor K, Holtby H. Emergency interventional lung assist for pulmonary hypertension. *Anesth Analg*. 2009;109(2):382–385.
8. Garcia JP, Iacono A, Kon ZN, et al. Ambulatory extracorporeal membrane oxygenation: a new approach for bridge-to-lung transplantation. *J Thorac Cardiovasc Surg*. 2010;139(6):e137–e139.
9. Bermudez CA, Rocha RV, Zaldonis D, et al. Extracorporeal membrane oxygenation as a bridge to lung transplant: midterm outcomes. *Ann Thorac Surg*. 2011;92(4):1226–1231.
10. Hayes D Jr, Kukreja J, Tobias JD, et al. Ambulatory venovenous extracorporeal respiratory support as a bridge for cystic fibrosis patients to emergent lung transplantation. *J Cyst Fibros*. 2012;11(1):40–45.
11. Lang G, Taghavi S, Aigner C, et al. Primary lung transplantation after bridge with extracorporeal membrane oxygenation: a plea for a shift in our paradigms for indications. *Transplantation*. 2012;93(7):729–736.
12. Hoopes CW, Gurley JC, Zwischenberger JB, et al. Mechanical support for pulmonary veno-occlusive disease: combined atrial septostomy and venovenous extracorporeal membrane oxygenation. *Sem Thorac Cardiovas Surg*. 2012;4(3):232–234.
13. Bonacchi M, Harmelin G, Peris A, et al. A novel strategy to improve systemic oxygenation in venovenous extracorporeal membrane oxygenation: the "χ-configuration." *J Thorac Cardiovasc Surg*. 2011;142(5):1197–1204.
14. Fischer S, Simon AR, Welte T, et al. Bridge to lung transplantation with the novel pumpless interventional lung assist device NovaLung. *J Thorac Cardiovasc Surg*. 2006;131(3):719–723.
15. Cypel M, Fischer S, Reynolds S, et al. Safety and efficacy of the Novalung Interventional Lung Assist (iLA) Device as a bridge to lung transplantation. *J Heart Lung Transplant*. 2010;29(Suppl 2):S21.
16. Ricci D, Boffini M, Del Sorbo L, et al. The use of CO_2 removal devices in patients awaiting lung transplantation: an initial experience. *Transplant Proc*. 2010;42(4):1255–1258.
17. Hammainen P, Schersten H, Lemstrom K, et al. Usefulness of extracorporeal membrane oxygenation as a bridge to lung transplantation: a descriptive study. *J Heart Lung Transplant*. 2011;30(1):103–107.
18. Fuehner T, Kuehn C, Hadem J, et al. Extracorporeal membrane oxygenation in awake patients as bridge to lung transplantation. *Am J Respir Crit Care Med*. 2012;185(7):763–768.

PART 20

PLEURAL MALIGNANCY

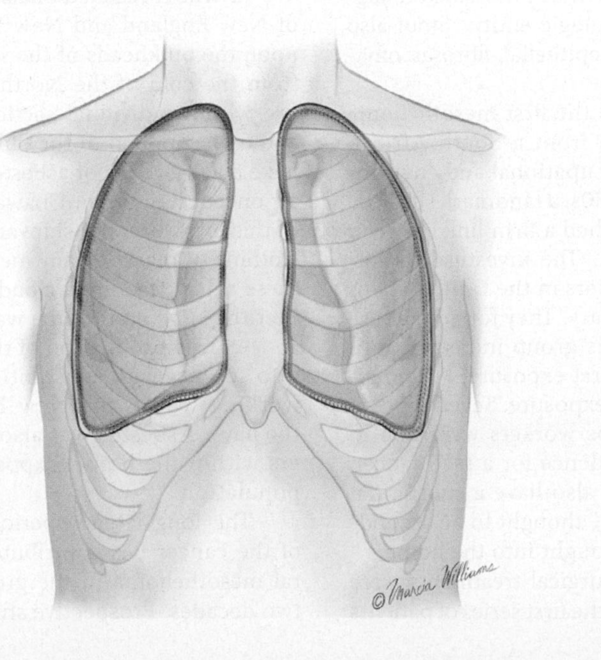

114 Overview and Historical Context of Malignant Pleural Diseases

Michael T. Jaklitsch

INTRODUCTION

Most malignant diseases of the pleura present with a unilateral pleural effusion or thickening. Malignant diseases include the very common secondary malignancy metastatic to the pleura, the less common lung cancer patient with pleural carcinomatosis, and the uncommon patient with primary malignant pleural mesothelioma (MPM). The low morbidity and accuracy of diagnostic thoracoscopy and pleural biopsy have dramatically increased our understanding and treatment of these diseases. This section of chapters provides important details and management of this group of primary malignant and secondary malignant diseases of the pleura.

Ironically, much of our insight has been gained by trying to understand the least common yet deadliest of this group of diseases: pleural mesothelioma. The current incidence of pleural mesothelioma within the United States is 2000 to 3000 cases per year as compared with esophageal and lung cancer, which are at least four and 50 times more common, respectively.[1] Few physicians will treat more than a handful of cases of MPM over the course of their professional careers. Even fewer academic centers in North America and Europe have been able to acquire a collective experience large enough to develop new treatment protocols for this devastating disease. The Brigham and Women's Hospital (BWH) and Dana-Farber Cancer Institute (DFCI) in Boston, Massachusetts, have gained a large experience treating MPM over the last 25 years.

The recognition of mesothelioma as a cancer and the development of treatment options are recent developments in the context of medical history. In 1950, Stout described malignant mesothelioma as a separate pathologic entity.[2] Stout also described the three histologic subsets: epithelial, fibrosarcomatous, and mixed.

In 1960, Wagner et al.[3] published the first mesothelioma case series, reporting on 33 patients from a South African asbestos mining town with known occupational and environmental crocidolite exposure. In the 1970s, a landmark study by Selikoff[4] was published which established a firm link between asbestos exposure and mesothelioma. The investigators followed 17,800 asbestos insulation workers in the United States and Canada for a period of up to 50 years. They found that the incidence of mesothelioma within this group increased rapidly starting 20 to 25 years after the first exposure. Peak incidence occurred at 40 to 45 years after exposure. Seven percent of all deaths in this group of asbestos workers were due to mesothelioma, a shockingly high incidence for a rare cancer. Family members of asbestos workers also have a substantial increased risk, termed "bystander risk," thought to be secondary to exposure to hair and clothes brought into the home.[5]

Early efforts at surgical and nonsurgical treatments were disappointing. Worn[6] published one of the first series of patients undergoing extrapleural pneumonectomy (EPP) in 1974 reporting a 5-year survival rate of 10% and a median survival of 19 months. Butchart et al.[7] published their initial experience with EPP for maximal surgical debulking of pleural mesothelioma in 1976. EPP had previously been used for tuberculous empyema, but was an operative technique that had always been associated with a high perioperative mortality. In Butchart's series, EPP for MPM had a perioperative mortality rate of 31%, a 5-year survival of 3.5%, and a median survival of 10 months. EPP is a technically demanding operation, and details of the operative technique are included in Chapters 120 and 122.

Initial studies investigating adjuvant chemotherapy and radiation therapy repeatedly showed little to no activity against the disease. Median survival of patients enrolled in therapeutic trials varied from 3 to 17 months with the majority falling in the 6 to 10 month range.[8,9]

FREQUENCY OF DISEASE IN NEW ENGLAND

New England has had a rich maritime military history. In August 1776, patriot soldiers from Marblehead and Salem, Massachusetts, rowed George Washington's army to safety across Long Island Sound after the defeat on Brooklyn Heights. Three of the first six frigates built for the fledgling United States Navy were built in New England or New York. The large whaling and cod fishing fleets from New Bedford, Nantucket, and Gloucester were the major oil producers for over 200 years.

The pace of production of United States naval ships during World War II reached one ship per week in the large shipyards of New England and New York. Asbestos slurry was sprayed upon the bulkheads of the ships to insulate the compartments from the cold of the North Sea, as well as insulation against fire within individual sections of the ship. Although quickly and easily applied to the bulkheads, this asbestos slurry would flake and particles of asbestos dust would be suspended in the air once it had dried. Unaware of the long-term complications of this exposure, the shipyard workers did not wear protective clothing or masks. Many mesothelioma patients who served on these ships describe a cloud of white dust below decks whenever the large guns of the warship were fired.

A large proportion of the New England population came into contact with substantial quantities of asbestos by either working within the New England shipyards, or serving in the navy. Asbestos was also commonly used to insulate heaters within the home, exposing an even larger New England population.

The long latency period from exposure to development of the cancer has contributed to the high frequency of pleural mesothelioma in the greater Boston area during the past two decades. Prospective studies following people with known asbestos exposure have demonstrated a rapid rise in the incidence of malignant mesothelioma beginning at 20 years post exposure and a peak incidence of approximately 0.6% per year 40 to 45 years after exposure.

Asbestos continued to be used in manufacturing for many years. In the United States, it wasn't until 1986 that the Toxic Substance Control Act addressed the health risks of asbestos giving the EPA broad authority to regulate the manufacture, use, distribution in commerce, and disposal of the carcinogenic substance.

When one considers the timing of these federal regulations, the latency of the disease, the geographical distribution of asbestos exposure, and the history of asbestos use, it is no coincidence that the BWH has become an epicenter of treatment for MPM.

THE 1980s: DIAGNOSIS AND RECOGNITION OF THE DISEASE

The Sydney Farber Cancer Institute was founded in 1949, and originally served only childhood cancers. In 1969, it expanded its mission to treat adult malignancies, and received federal designation as a regional Comprehensive Cancer Center in 1973. It was renamed the Dana-Farber Cancer Institute in 1983. Located in Boston, Massachusetts, across the street from both the Peter Bent Brigham Hospital (which became the Brigham and Women's Hospital in 1980), and the Harvard Medical School, it soon became a major referral center for both aggressive and unusual malignancies within the New England area. Mesothelioma was among these cancers.

In March of 1980, Antman, et al.[10] published in the *American Journal of Medicine* the experience with the first 40 patients treated at the Sydney Farber Cancer Institute with malignant mesothelioma. These patients had been treated between 1965 and 1978. Thirty-four of the patients had the pleural form of the disease while six patients had peritoneal mesothelioma. Sixty-three percent of these patients reported either an asbestos exposure or were employed in New England shipyards, generally during World War II. In this series, adriamycin-containing chemotherapy regimens induced a partial remission in 40% of the previously untreated patients. Yet, despite these remissions, the majority of patients (78%) ultimately died of local disease. Subtotal resection in this series, and others,[11] resulted in prolonged survival. Specifically, the 10 patients in Antman's review who underwent subtotal resections had a median survival of 15 months, compared to 8.5 months for the 20 patients who underwent only diagnostic operations and other treatments. Further analysis revealed that the median survival was a mere 4.2 months for patients who were diagnosed with limited disease but chose only supportive care. The authors advocated a multimodality approach incorporating maximal surgical resection with adjuvant chemotherapy and radiation therapy.

In 1984 Karen Antman organized a prospective multimodality protocol for MPM at the DFCI. This ambitious protocol started with an EPP, as had been previously described by both Worn and Butchart. Chemotherapy consisted of cyclophosphamide at a dose of 600 mg/m^2, combined with adriamycin 60 mg/m^2, to a cumulative dose of 450 mg/m^2. After 1985, patients also received cisplatinum at 75 mg/m^2 (CAP chemotherapy). Radiation directed at previous sites of bulky disease was given to a dose of 5500 rads after the chemotherapy.

The accurate pathologic diagnosis of malignant mesothelioma versus a primary adenocarcinoma of the lung or a secondary malignancy metastatic to the pleura has been a barrier to treatment development. Stimulated by the need to distinguish between these histologically similar tumors, the Pathology Department at BWH drew on the large source of explanted tumors at our institution to develop a panel of immunohistochemical tests. This work is nicely summarized by two pioneers in this area in Chapter 115: Pathology of Mesothelioma.

THE EARLY 1990s: DEVELOPMENT OF MULTIDISCIPLINARY EXPERTISE

The Division of Thoracic Surgery at the BWH was established in 1988. This separate academic division was to be dedicated to the care of patients with noncardiac thoracic diseases. The work of this surgical division began with Dr. David Sugarbaker's return to Boston from his Toronto General thoracic surgical training. The subsequent congregation of surgeons within a single institution sped the process of technical and clinical modifications, which reduced the expected operative mortality in a short period of time. An early forthright discussion of the operative technique, as well as some of the technical difficulties with the operation, appeared in the 1992 publication by Sugarbaker et al.[12]

The promising results of the BWH program reflected not only the refinement of surgical skill and improvement in perioperative care, but also identification of prognostic variables with a consequent improvement in patient selection.

In 1993, Sugarbaker et al.[13] updated their experience after 52 patients had been treated with EPP in a trimodality setting. This analysis demonstrated significantly longer survival in patients with epithelial histology and node negative disease.

Based on these findings, a Brigham pathologic staging system was proposed.

The original Brigham staging system had four stages. Stage I was comprised of tumors confined within the pleural envelope and without lymph node involvement. Stage II, which would be modified in a few years, also consisted of tumors within the pleural envelope, but with either intraparenchymal (N1) or mediastinal (N2) lymph nodes involved with tumor.[14] Stage III disease was made up of locally aggressive and unresectable tumors beyond the pleural envelope that had invaded into the mediastinum or chest wall, or through the diaphragm, or involved contralateral (N3) nodes. Stage IV disease was defined by distant metastases. This system has recently been replaced with a more predictive staging system that incorporates clinical as well as pathologic parameters, as explained by Dr. William Richards in Chapter 116, The Staging of Malignant Pleural Mesothelioma.

LATE 1990s: DEVELOPMENT OF INTRAOPERATIVE BICAVITARY HEATED CHEMOTHERAPY

Despite these advances in surgical technique and refinement in prognostication and patient selection, the unfortunate fact remained that nearly all patients eventually died of their disease within 10 years of the operation. Recurrences appeared to result by direct extension from the ipsilateral hemithorax. Therefore, in the second half of the 1990s, the BWH group embarked on a new approach to multimodality therapy.

The major treatment plan of the previous 10 years had started with EPP because mesothelioma was predominantly a locoregional disease, and much of the early morbidity was from local spread. Since most patients died as a result of the primary cancer invading the diaphragm, chest wall, and mediastinal organs, initial surgical debulking was chosen prior to the initiation of chemotherapy in order to reverse the aggressive natural progression of this disease.

In 1997, Baldini et al.[15] published a detailed retrospective review of 49 patients who underwent EPP and some combination of adjuvant chemotherapy and/or radiotherapy with a focus on defining patterns of failure. In this series, overall median survival was 22 months and 3-year survival, 34%. Resection margins were microscopically positive in 61% of patients and lymph nodes positive in 29%. Of the 54% of patients with recurrences, 67% percent had the first recurrence within the ipsilateral hemithorax, and 50% had recurrence at some time within the abdomen.

The potential role of intracavitary chemotherapy as a method of improving local regional control had been studied previously in a variety of abdominal malignancies. The local application of chemotherapy allows high cytotoxic levels to reach residual tumor cells by diffusion without the side effects of high dose systemic chemotherapy. Intracavitary chemotherapy with or without hyperthermia had been favorably reported in the literature.

Alberts et al.[16] published a prospective randomized trial in The New England Journal of Medicine in 1996. Intraperitoneal cisplatin was compared to intravenous cisplatin in patients with stage III ovarian cancer following cytoreductive surgery. Among the 654 randomized patients, the estimated median survival was significantly longer in the group receiving intraperitoneal cisplatin (49 months) than in the group receiving intravenous cisplatin (41 months).

The decision to design a phase I dose escalation trial of heated intraoperative cisplatin at the time of EPP had been supported by the BWH, the DFCI, and the leadership of all professional groups who would be involved in patient care. The obstacles to be overcome were formidable. Protocols to maximize both patient and staff safety were designed by a multidisciplinary "heated chemotherapy team" which met once a week to develop guidelines for this novel therapy. Ideas were actively sought from surgeons, anesthesiologists, pharmacists, nurses, scrub technicians, medical oncologists, and respiratory therapists to design the method of drug delivery and disposal in the operating room.

Radical pleurectomy is an attractive alternative for patients who are unsuitable for EPP. This includes patients with a decline in their functional status and elderly patients. A radical pleurectomy leaves the lung, but can remove the central portion of the diaphragm and the ipsilateral pericardium. The technique is well described by Dr. Flores in Chapter 121.

Innovative treatments also include the use of photodynamic therapy as an adjuvant treatment following EPP. Dr. Joseph Friedberg has developed this technique and provides details in Chapter 124.

The development of new chemotherapeutic agents (Chapter 117) with better response rates suggests the potential role of using these agents in a neoadjuvant manner for advanced stage disease. Dr. Walter Weder has been an articulate spokesman of this technique and provides his data in Chapter 125.

The low morbidity associated with thoracoscopic evaluation of the diseased pleural space has opened a new treatment paradigm for malignant effusions, irrespective of cause. A thoracoscope allows the breakdown of loculations and complete drainage of the effusion for palliation of symptoms, provides sufficient histologic material for a definitive diagnosis, and allows therapeutic intervention for long-lasting palliation of symptoms. This aspect of malignant pleural disease is described well in Chapters 119 and 120.

SUMMARY

Malignant pleural disease is a common entity. Initial diagnosis is suspected with unilateral effusion or pleural thickening. Early thoracoscopy provides not only palliation of symptoms, but also allows accurate pathologic diagnosis and assists in staging. No matter the cause of the malignant effusion, several treatment options are currently available, and more are being developed by innovative research. Much remains to be done.

References

1. Connelly RR, Spirtas R, Myers MH, et al. Demographic patterns for mesothelioma in the United States. *J Natl Cancer Inst.* 1987;78:1053–1060.
2. Stout AP. Solitary fibrous mesothelioma of the peritoneum. *Cancer.* 1950;3(5):820–825.
3. Wagner JC, Sleggs CA, Marchand P. Diffuse pleural mesothelioma and asbestos exposure in the North Western Cape Province. *Br J Ind Med.* 1960;17:260–271.
4. Selikoff IJ. Air pollution and asbestos carcinogenesis: investigation of possible synergism. *IARC Sci Publ.* 1977;(16):247–253.
5. Antman KH. Current concepts: malignant mesothelioma. *N Engl J Med.* 1980;303:200–202.
6. Worn H. [Chances and results of surgery of malignant mesothelioma of the pleura (author's transl)]. *Thoraxchir Vask Chir.* 1974;22:391–393.
7. Butchart EG, Ashcroft T, Barnsley WC, et al. Pleuropneumonectomy in the management of diffuse malignant mesothelioma of the pleura. Experience with 29 patients. *Thorax.* 1976;31(1):15–24.
8. Bass P. Chemotherapy for malignant mesothelioma: from doxorubicin to vinorelbine. *Semin Oncol.* 2002;29:62–69.
9. Weissmann LB, Antman KH. Incidence, presentation and promising new treatments for malignant mesothelioma. *Oncology (Huntington).* 1989;3:67–72.
10. Antman KH, Blum RH, Greenberger JS, et al. Multimodality therapy for malignant mesothelioma based on a study of natural history. *Am J Med.* 1980;68:356–362.
11. Legha SS, Muggia FM. Therapeutic approaches in malignant mesothelioma. *Cancer Treat Rev.* 1977;4:13–23.
12. Sugarbaker DJ, Mentzer SJ, Strauss G. Extrapleural pneumonectomy in the treatment of malignant pleural mesothelioma. *Ann Thorac Surg.* 1992; 54:941–946.
13. Sugarbaker DJ, Mentzer SJ, DeCamp M, et al. Extrapleural pneumonectomy in the setting of a multimodality approach to malignant mesothelioma. *Chest.* 1993;103:377S–381S.
14. Sugarbaker DJ, Strauss GM, Lynch TJ, et al. Node status has prognostic significance in the multimodality therapy of diffuse, malignant mesothelioma. *J Clin Oncol.* 1993;11:1172–1178.
15. Baldini EH, Recht A, Strauss GM, et al. Patterns of failure after trimodality therapy for malignant pleural mesothelioma. *Ann Thorac Surg.* 1997;63:334–338.
16. Alberts DS, Liu PY, Hannigan EV, et al. Intraperitoneal cisplatin plus intravenous cyclophosphamide for stage III ovarian cancer. *N Engl J Med.* 1996;335:1950–1955.

115 Pathology of Pleural Malignant Mesothelioma

John J. Godleski and Joseph M. Corson

Keywords: diffuse malignant pleural mesothelioma; cytology; fluorescence in situ hybridization (FISH); immunohistochemistry; epithelial, sarcomatoid, and biphasic histologic cell types; fine needle biopsy; VATS biopsy; frozen section examination (FSE); mediastinoscopy; lymph node biopsy

Malignant mesothelioma (MM) is an uncommon disease with approximately 3000 new cases diagnosed each year in the United States. Most occur in the pleura. However, each year about 300 new cases occur in the peritoneum and many fewer in the pericardium and paratesticular serous membranes. Although most persons with pleural malignant mesothelioma (PMM) are middle-aged males (median 62 years), the disease also occurs in lesser numbers of women and over a wide age range. The presentation is usually with dyspnea secondary to a pleural effusion and/or chest wall pain. Most give a history of occupational exposure to asbestos 20 to 40 years or more earlier. Pathologic diagnosis guides treatment and is generally based on a pleural biopsy obtained by VATS. Prognosis is poor in most cases with few surviving 2 years following diagnosis. However, some recent reports indicate palliation with therapy and present studies aim at cure. This article will focus on the critical role pathology plays[1] as it interfaces with surgery, radiology, and oncology in the management of PMM. We will consider surgical pathology procedures and tissue collection, classification, differential diagnosis, prognostic factors, grading, and causation and pathogenesis of PMM.

SURGICAL PATHOLOGY PROCEDURES AND TISSUE COLLECTION

Important elements in the pathologic diagnosis of PMM are the clinical history, especially the presenting symptom, any history of past or present tumor and relevant radiologic features, especially those seen in the chest x-ray, CT, and/or PET scan. Diffuse nodular pleural thickening or a pleural-based mass are characteristic of PMM. However, in some cases, tumor nodularity is lacking and the pleura is thickened by diffusely fibrotic tumor.

Cytologic examination with cell block examination of pleural fluid is usually one of the first steps after radiologic examination in the workup of patients suspected of PMM. Cytologic examination may establish a diagnosis of adenocarcinoma. In other cases atypical, or even frankly malignant mesothelial cells, may be present. Fluorescence in situ hybridization (FISH) and immunohistochemical studies of pleural fluid specimens may help to establish a malignant diagnosis in some cases. However, tissue invasion, required for the pathologic diagnosis of PMM, is not feasible in pleural fluid specimens. Pathologic diagnosis may be based on a fine needle aspirate or core biopsy, but usually requires examination of a VATS biopsy, or rarely, an open biopsy.

Frozen Section Examination

PMM usually begins in the parietal pleura, rather than in the visceral pleura. This is supported by several observations including those in a thoracoscopic and pathologic prospective study of biopsies of 188 early cases of PMM, which revealed that patients whose tumor was confined to the parietal pleura survived significantly longer (median survival time 32.7 months) than those with involvement of both parietal and visceral pleura (median survival time 7 months). No instances of tumors involving only visceral pleura were encountered.[2] Tumor first appears on gross examination as tiny, 1 to 2 mm gray–white nodules studding the surface of the parietal pleura (Fig. 115-1). Thereafter, tumor nodules enlarge, tumor spreads to the visceral pleura, and visceral and parietal pleural thickening and fusion ensue.[3] Most pleural biopsies are of the parietal pleura. Distinguishing invasive PMM from other lesions on gross examination may be difficult.[4–6] Invasive PMM is characterized by firm, nodular or plaque-like, gray–white thickening of the pleura (Fig. 115-2). In contrast, hyaline pleural plaque, usually identifiable first on radiologic examination, is densely collagenous, hard and white,

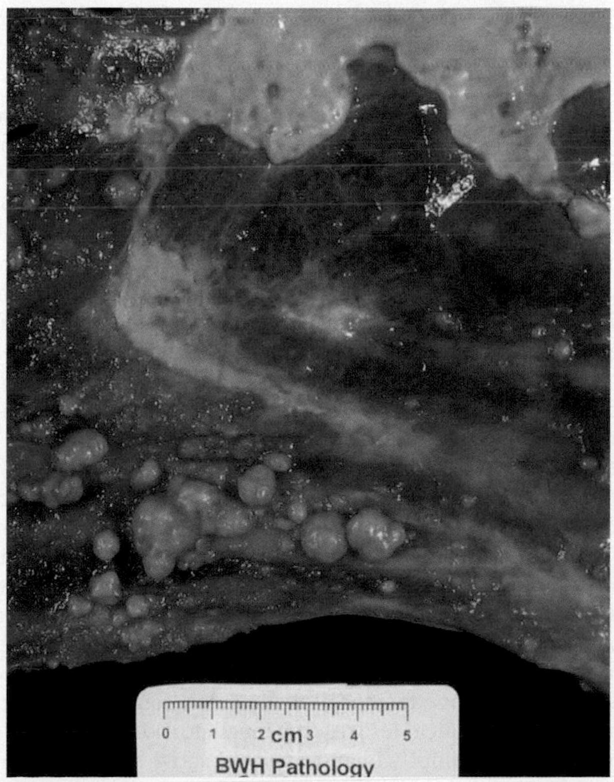

Figure 115-1. Parietal pleura from a pleurectomy specimen with diffuse nodular epithelial type mesothelioma and pleural plaque. The pleural plaque in the top portion of the photo is densely collagenous, hard, and white. In this early lesion, tumor nodules of various sizes are present throughout the pleural surface ranging in size from 1 to 10 mm.

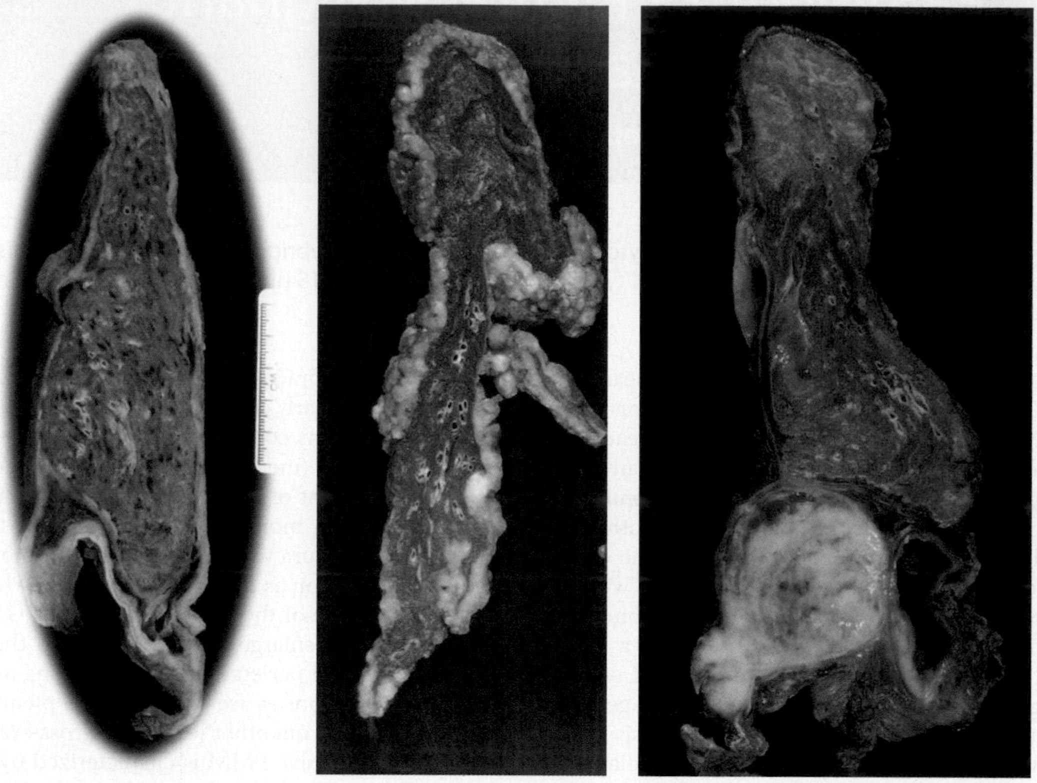

Figure 115-2. *A*. Coronal section of lung and diaphragm. Diffuse PMM tumor thickens and fuses the parietal and visceral pleura along the right lateral surface of the lung. Inferiorly, a hemorrhagic effusion separates minimally thickened visceral pleura from diaphragmatic parietal pleura with diffuse tumor. *B*. Coronal section of lung with diffusely nodular PMM. Parietal and visceral pleural layers are completely fused. *C*. Coronal section of localized PMM. Tumor forms a large supra-diaphragmatic and costophrenic sulcus mass, but the remaining pleura was uninvolved by tumor.

often has a shelf-like border, and may be focally calcified (see Fig. 115-1). Chronic fibrosing pleuritis also thickens the pleura, is firm and gray–white, and often diffuse. It may be difficult to distinguish from the sarcomatoid type of PMM (SPMM), both grossly and microscopically; such cases often require extensive sampling to separate from PMM. Metastatic adenocarcinoma occurs more often in the pleura than PMM and is not distinguishable on radiologic or gross examination. Pleural biopsies are submitted for intraoperative FSE in cases of suspected PMM to establish the presence of tumor in the biopsy. The biopsy should confirm that the tissue taken is adequate for subsequent permanent section examination and diagnosis. Distinction of PMM from metastatic adenocarcinoma is not possible by FSE. PMM is often heterogeneous on histopathologic examination and small biopsies may not be representative.[1] Generous pleural biopsies should be taken, both for diagnosis and for accurate histopathologic typing. The latter provides valuable prognostic information that is utilized in planning therapy. Larger tissue biopsies also may provide nonfrozen tumor for permanent section examination, thus avoiding frozen artifact in the tumor cells that may impede morphologic interpretation and alter immunohistochemical test results. Small portions of tumour in biopsies, fixed promptly in appropriate fixative in the FS room, are recommended to facilitate optimal electron microscopic (EM) examination. EM examination may help to establish a diagnosis, especially in controversial cases. Wedge biopsies to include visceral pleura and biopsies or excisions of lung, chest wall, mediastinal nodules, or other masses suspicious for PMM are occasionally submitted for FSE. They are examined and processed as noted above for pleural biopsies.

Debulking procedures performed to remove grossly visible PMM include Pleurectomy (PP), Parietal Pleurectomy and Decortication (PPD), Extended PPD with resection of diaphragm and/or pericardium, Chest Wall Resection with resection of rib(s), and Extrapleural Pneumonectomy (EPP). In EPP, resection includes parietal and visceral pleura, an entire lung, a portion of pericardium and the ipsilateral hemidiaphragm (Fig. 115-3).

FSE may be utilized to examine margins, and tumor tissue is often taken for special studies, including snap freezing for organ bank preservation. However, the specimens, including pleural, diaphragmatic, and pericardial margins, are usually examined by the pathologist after lung perfusion, fixation, dissection, and extensive tissue sampling, and are performed in the surgical pathology area.[1,6] Digestion studies for quantifying asbestos bodies of fibers in the lung or other tissues may be performed on paraffin tissue blocks. However, it is recommended that formalin-fixed, wet lung tissue (5–10 g) be taken from the periphery of upper and lower lobes and stored as a ready tissue source for quantitative asbestos body/fiber analysis.

Mediastinoscopy with lymph node biopsy, usually performed after a PMM positive pleural biopsy is diagnosed, is a staging procedure; positivity is an adverse prognostic event. Most nodes are not submitted for frozen section examination (FSE); they are best processed for permanent section pathologic examination. However, nodes suspected of infectious

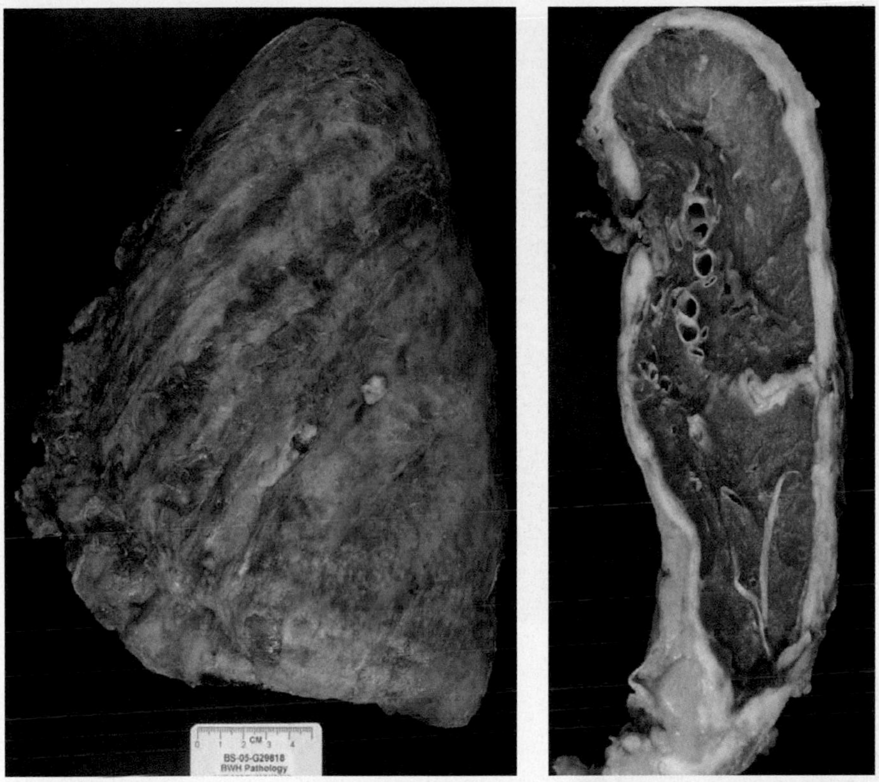

A B

Figure 115-3. *A*. External surface of chest wall parietal pleura of an extrapleural pneumonectomy resection for diffuse PMM. The Pleural is opacified from apex to base by coalescent tumor nodules and pleural plaques. *B*. Coronal section, same specimen as (A), reveals diffusely thickened, faintly nodular, fused parietal and visceral PMM with extension into the major fissure. Lung invasion is not grossly apparent.

disease, or portions thereof, are submitted for culture as well as for permanent section pathologic examination.

CLASSIFICATION OF PLEURAL MALIGNANT MESOTHELIOMA

Pleural mesothelioma is generally considered to be both malignant and diffuse. However, a localized form of PMM (LPMM) that is also malignant has been described and is considered here. It is important to recognize because it has a likelihood of better survival than the diffuse form. Furthermore, a rare form of mesothelioma, previously thought to be restricted to the peritoneum, has been described in the pleura as well differentiated papillary mesothelioma, a solitary or multifocal tumor which has a benign or indolent course. Thus it deserves distinction from the much more common diffuse PMM.

Histopathologic Types

The most widely utilized classification of PMM is a histopathologic classification based on microscopic examination of formalin-fixed, hematoxylin and eosin (H&E) stained tissue sections. The three types of diffuse PMM, recently categorized as subtypes,[4] are epithelial (or epithelioid), sarcomatoid (or sarcomatous), and mixed (or biphasic) (Table 115-1). Histologic features of these subtypes are illustrated in Figure 115-4. The most common type of PMM is epithelial (55% in a large series) with lesser numbers of the mixed type (24%) and of the sarcomatoid type (22%).[4] A desmoplastic malignant mesothelioma is a MM with extensive dense stromal fibrosis (Fig. 115-4D). Usually, but not always, it is of the sarcomatoid type.[1,3–5,7] It is usually classified as a form of sarcomatoid MM, and has a very poor prognosis.

Histopathologic classification by type of PMM is relied on to predict survival, and aid in choosing the course of treatment. Those with epithelial type PMM (EPMM) have the best survival, and those with SPMM, the worst. Mixed forms (MPMM) have a survival intermediate between the other two types. Those with SPMM also are unlikely to exhibit positive cytology on examination of pleural fluid and less likely to respond to multimodality therapy than the other types.

EPMM Variants

EPMM's exhibit numerous histopathologic patterns and most are polymorphous, exhibiting several patterns. These patterns, which have been described as subtypes, variants, categories, and morphologic forms, will be referred to herein as variants. The variants are based on architectural features, for example, tubular, papillary, or solid; or cytologic features, for example, small cell, signet cell,

Table 115-1

HISTOPATHOLOGIC TYPES OF PMM
Epithelial (Epithelioid)
Sarcomatoid (Sarcomatous)
Mixed (Biphasic)
Other Pleural Mesotheliomas (See Text)
Desmoplastic
Localized
Well Differentiated Papillary Mesothelioma

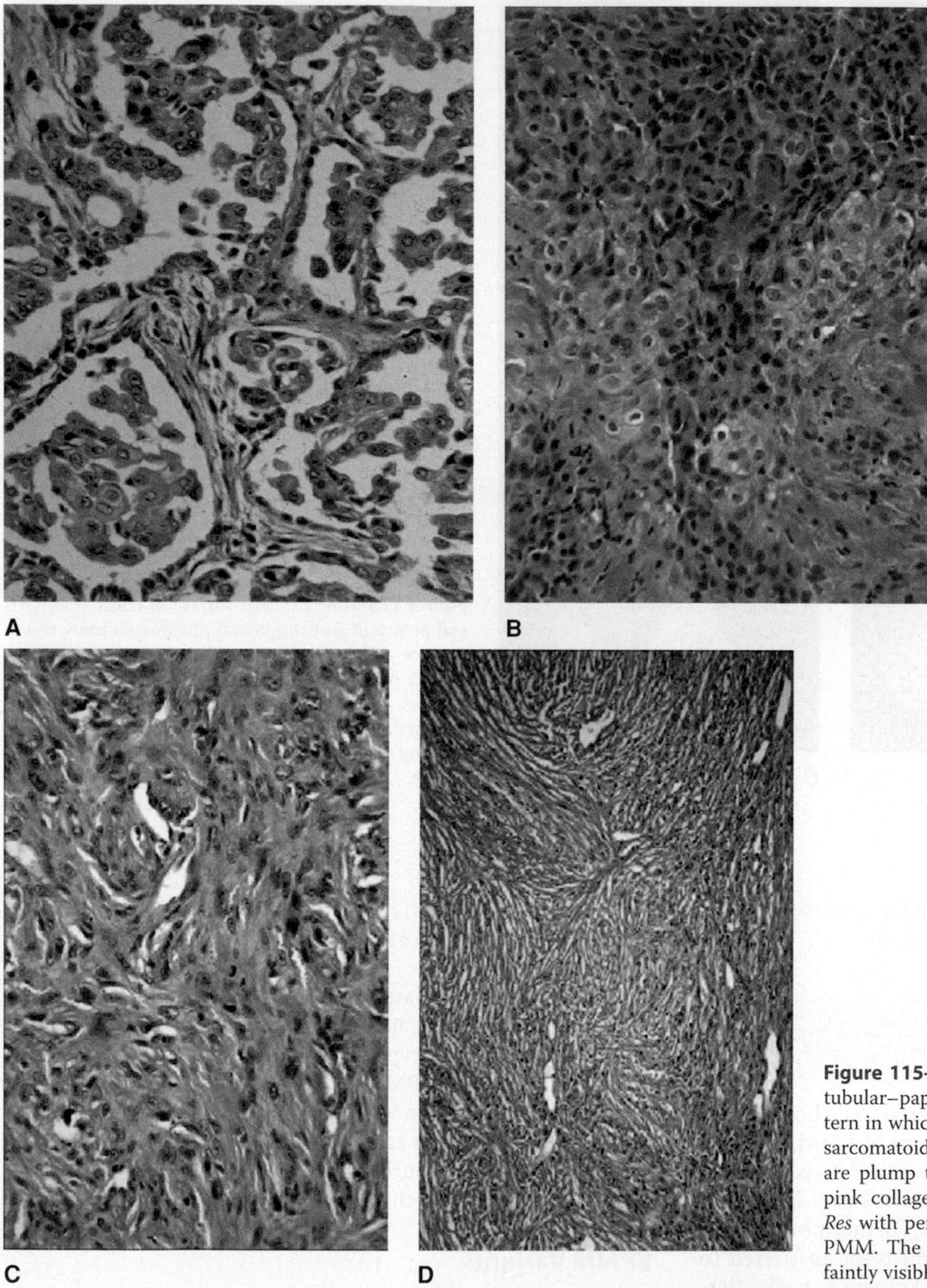

Figure 115-4. *A*. Epithelial (epitheloid) type of PMM with tubular–papillary pattern. *B*. Epithelial type PMM, solid pattern in which tumor forms sheets of uniform cells. *C*. PMM sarcomatoid (sarcomatous) type. The dark tumor cell nuclei are plump to spindled and are haphazardly oriented in a pink collagenous stroma. (Reproduced from *Am J Cancer Res* with permission). *D*. Desmoplastic sarcomatoid type of PMM. The dark nuclei of the sarcomatoid tumor cells are faintly visible in the densely collagenous fibrous stroma.

or deciduoid cell; or stromal, for example, desmoplastic or myxoid. The variants aid in establishing the histopathologic diagnosis. However, they seldom contribute useful prognostic information and hence, are not included in the pathologic diagnosis. More than 20 variants of the epithelial type have been identified.[4,5] The most common variants of the epithelial type variants are tubulopapillary, solid, and microcystic (adenomatoid). An uncommon high grade (undifferentiated) pleomorphic variant of EPMM has been described. It is comprised of clusters and sheets of large, pleomorphic, round cells with hyperchromatic nuclei, frequent mitoses, and necrosis. It resembles a large cell or undifferentiated carcinoma, but may be distinguished by its immunohistochemical reactivity or sometimes by its EM features. Variants of the mixed and sarcomatoid types are far fewer that those of the epithelial type. A few variants have been reported recently to have prognostic value. The myxoid variant was reported to have a prolonged survival (mst. 30 months)[8] and the high grade pleomorphic variant of the epithelial type was reported to have a significantly worse survival than other variants of this histopathologic type.[9] In this large study, 232 cases of EPMM were classified as one of five subtypes. In multivariant analysis, the 34 classified as pleomorphic had an overall worse prognosis (8.1 months survival, $p < 0.001$), compared with the other four subtypes with survivals of 15.8 to 24.9 months; subtype also was an independent predictor of poor survival. Pleomorphic EPMM had a near identical survival curve to the MPMM and no significant difference in overall survival with SPMM, leading the authors to suggest their reclassification to mixed or sarcomatoid type.

It is important to recognize that survival of PMM also varies with pathologic stage. A reliable pathologic staging system is an essential requirement for accurately predicting survival of those with one or more of the many histopathologic variants of PMM.

Localized PMM

LPMM is a rare entity in which the tumor is confined to a solitary pleural mass, of average size about 6 cm (see Fig. 115-2C). The histopathologic, immunohistologic, and EM features are those of PMM; thus, the tumor cannot be distinguished from PMM solely by pathologic examination of a pleural biopsy, but requires careful consideration of radiologic and surgical findings. All three histopathologic types of PMM may occur in LPMM, however, unlike PMM, there is no difference in survival among the three groups. LPMM may recur and metastasize, but diffuse pleural spread does not occur. Importantly, it has a better prognosis than PMM; the largest series reports that 10 of 21 patients with follow-up data were alive and without evidence of recurrence, 18 months to 11 years after diagnosis.[10] However, before concluding that a mass is LPMM, the evidence supporting the localized nature of the PMM should be scrutinized carefully.

Well Differentiated Papillary Mesothelioma (WDPM)

This uncommon papillary epithelioid tumor, which usually occurs in the peritoneum of middle aged women, may occasionally arise in the pleura in a solitary or multiple form.[4,5] Solitary tumors incidental to thoracoscopy or thoracotomy that lack clinical symptoms and effusion attributable to the tumor, and meet certain other criteria are considered benign. The additional criteria are that they are comprised of papillary or club-shaped processes with fibrovascular cores that are covered by a single layer of bland cuboidal mesothelial cells and invasion is not present.[5] Multiple pleural papillary tumors with characteristic histopathologic features of WDPM, pleural effusion or thickening, and minimal or superficial invasion usually pursue a more indolent course than PMM. Rare cases of PMM may contain WDPM-like foci. In such cases, survival of the PMM may be modified, depending on the proportion of the WDPM-like foci in the invasive PMM.

Sarcomatoid PMM (SPMM)

H&E stained sections of this type of PMM reveal spindle cells in a fibrous stroma, separable from the spindled normal pleural stromal cells by the atypical nuclear features and hypercellularity of the tumor cells.[3–5,11] One common pattern in many SPMMs is of small spindled tumor cells with densely hyperchromatic nuclei that vary in size and shape and are arranged in sheets, or form short fascicles. In another common pattern of SPMM, the spindled tumor cells are large and plump with vesicular nuclei, resembling so-called malignant fibrous histiocytoma (undifferentiated spindle cell sarcoma) (Fig. 115-4C). In both variants, interlacing or storiform architectural patterns and necrosis often are present.

Desmoplastic PMM,[3–5] usually occurs as a variant of sarcomatoid mesothelioma and has a poor prognosis. By definition, it contains densely collagenous, hypocellular fibrous tissue with bland nuclei involving 50% or greater of the tumor area. It may be extremely difficult to recognize on FSE due to lack of malignant features such as hyperchromatism, pleomorphism, and hypercellularity in the tissue sampled (Fig. 115-4D). Thus, multiple biopsy samples and pathologic examination of abundant tissue may be required to establish the diagnosis. The presence of a storiform or "patternless" fibrous pattern, and other features, including frankly sarcomatoid areas, or demonstrable invasion of chest wall tissue, for example, invasion of extrapleural adipose or skeletal muscle, serve to distinguish it from its mimic, chronic fibrosing pleuritis (organizing pleurisy, fibrous pleurisy).[4]

Several other variants have been described that are important to recognize; some cases have been diagnosed initially as lymphoma. These include Lymphohistiocytoid PMM, a rare variant constituting less than 1% of MM's, with morphologic features suggesting a lymphoma.[4,5] The prognosis was reported initially to be similar to that of SPMM. However, a recent study of 22 cases reported a prognosis similar to that of EPMM.[12]

Transitional PMM is a rare variant with morphologic features of both EPMM and SPMM[4,5] and a prognosis, based on limited studies, similar to SPMM.[4] Another variant contains heterologous elements, notably osteosarcomatous, chondrosarcomatous, and/or rhabdomyoblastic elements. This variant has clinical, histopathologic, and immunohistochemical features of PMM, but in addition, one or more heterologous elements. In a series of 27 cases, 16 were of sarcomatoid type, 12 were mixed type, and only 1 was EPMM.[13]

The MPMM is comprised of both EPMM and SPMM. The WHO classification of MM defines mixed types as those in which each component represents at least 10% of the tumour.[7] Other experienced pathologists include as mixed types those in which the putative minor component is clearly definable, regardless of its proportion of the tumor in the specimen. The proportion of the epithelial and sarcomatoid element in the PMM appears to be predictive of survival, with the predominantly epithelial type having the better prognosis. Biopsy specimens often do not accurately reflect the proportion of the types of PMM present in the tumor, owing to the polymorphous nature of PMM and the unequal representation of the epithelial and sarcomatoid types in various areas of the tissue. The most accurate predictions of survival come from analysis of larger specimens, such as those from extrapulmonary pneumonectomy, pleurectomy, and chest wall resection.

PLEURAL MALIGNANT MESOTHELIOMA: DIFFERENTIAL DIAGNOSIS (DD)

The distinction of PMM from other tumors is based on evaluation of the clinical, radiologic, and pathologic features. Presenting symptom, history of past or present tumor of other sites, radiologic findings, especially of chest CT and PET scan, and findings at surgery may aid in the distinction. Also, adequacy of the pleural biopsy (see Surgical Pathology Procedures and Tissue Collection) may abet pathologic diagnosis and tumor classification. Morphologic classification based on histopathologic examination and immunohistochemical staining play key roles in the distinction (Fig. 115-5). Furthermore, the results of histochemical stains and/or EM examination also are critical in some cases. Recently, FISH and/or molecular genetics have assumed increasing roles in establishing the pathologic

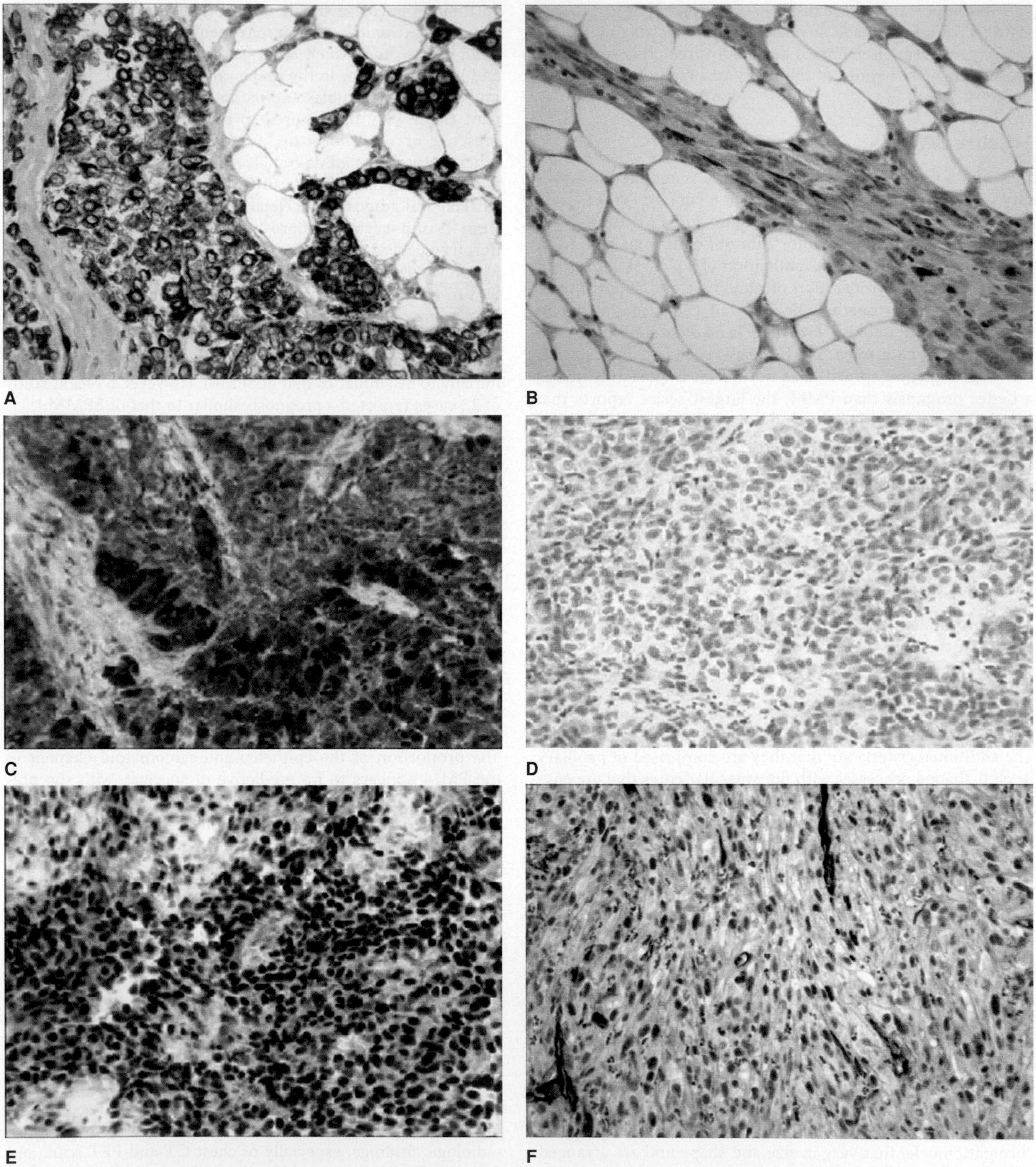

Figure 115-5. Immunohistochemical staining (immunoperoxidase) of PMM. *A*. AE1/AE3 keratin positive tumor cells in cords and nests with strong cytoplasmic staining in an epithelioid tumor. Note the perinuclear accentuation of the staining. Cells of diffuse PMM infiltrate extrapleural adipose tissue. Photo courtesy of Dr. Lucian Chirieac. *B*. Extrapleural adipose tissue is infiltrated by AE1/AE3 keratin positive sarcomatoid PMM. The keratin positivity of the bland appearing spindle cells invading fat offers strong support for the diagnosis of sarcomatoid PMM. Photo courtesy of Dr. Lucian Chirieac. *C*. Calretinin staining of nuclei and cytoplasm is characteristic of an epithelial type PMM. *D*. CEA fails to stain PMM. This solid epithelial type PMM is highly cellular. CEA staining is found in most cases of adenocarcinoma, and thus is an important differentiating negative stain for PMM. *E*. WT-1 strongly stains the nuclei of epithelioid PMM tumor cells. *F*. WT-1 staining of a sarcomatoid PMM supports the diagnosis. Many of the tumor cell nuclei are stained. In addition, cytoplasmic staining of endothelial cells (linear vascular cords) is present and provides a positive internal control. Weak staining of some mesothelioma stromal cells is also apparent. Photo courtesy of Dr. Lucian Chirieac.

Table 115-2
DIFFERENTIAL DIAGNOSIS: EPITHELIAL PMM (EPMM)
Atypical mesothelial proliferation
Adenomatoid tumour
Carcinomas
Desmoplastic small round cell tumor
Epithelioid hemangioendothelioma
Lymphoma
Malignant melanoma
Thymic tumors

diagnosis, for example, FISH when the DD is atypical mesothelial hyperplasia; FISH and molecular genetics when the DD is synovial sarcoma.

The separation of PMM from other tumors of the pleura is closely linked to the histopathologic type of the PMM. The DD of EPMM, which is tabulated in Table 115-2, includes atypical mesothelial hyperplasia and many tumors of primary and metastatic origin. Some of the carcinomas and sarcomas, as well as the rare thymic tumors, may be either primary or secondary. The most common distinctions to be made with diffuse PMM of epithelial type are with atypical mesothelial proliferation and with metastatic adenocarcinoma. Others may be problematic, in part, due to their rare occurrence.

Atypical Mesothelial Proliferation

Proliferations of the squamoid (flat) or cuboidal mesothelial cells that line the pleura have been classified as reactive mesothelial hyperplasia, atypical mesothelial hyperplasia, atypical mesothelial proliferation, and MM in situ.[4,5] This morphologic assessment is based on proliferation of cells with atypical cytologic features, including nuclear hyperchromasia and irregularity of surface cells, and surface mesothelial cell stratification and/or papillary formation. It is important to note that the sequence from hyperplasia to carcinoma that obtains in organs, such as colon and cervix, has not been established for mesothelial cells. Hence, a diagnosis in surface proliferations of MM in situ is reserved for cases in which there is clear evidence of established malignancy, that is, microscopic evidence of bulk tumor on the pleural surface or definite invasion of underlying tissue. Hence, the diagnosis of mesothelioma in situ is considered appropriate only when accompanied by invasive MM.[4,5,14] The distinction between AMP and EPMM may be very difficult on occasion. Pathology consultation, rebiopsy and/or careful follow-up afford several alternatives to the overdiagnosis of EPMM. Recent evaluations of FISH testing performed on paraffin embedded cell blocks or tissue for the presence of homozygous p16 deletions in PMM suggest that such testing may help to distinguish between diffuse PMM and AMP (see section on Cytogenetics and Molecular Genetics, below).

Metastatic Adenocarcinoma

Most of the problems in separating EPMM from its mimics occur in distinguishing it from adenocarcinomas metastatic to the pleura, a much more common occurrence than primary EPMM.[3–5] The most common primary sites of the metastatic carcinomas are lung, breast, ovary, prostate, colon, stomach, kidney, and thyroid gland. Pathologic distinction of PMM from its mimics is based upon clinical information and both conventional H&E and special pathologic tests. For example, the history of the organ site of a known carcinoma may help in selecting the best panel of antibodies for immunohistochemical testing. Histochemical tests for mucins, including mucicarmine, D-PAS, and hyaluronidase alcian blue, utilized for many years, have been replaced largely by immunohistochemical tests of greater sensitivity and specificity. EM examination is not widely used now, but may be invaluable in some cases, especially if tissue has been appropriately fixed at the time of biopsy.

Immunohistochemical tests, performed on paraffin embedded tissue sections, are widely employed for the distinction of adenocarcinoma from EPMM, which has a different immunohistochemical phenotype. However, no single antibody possesses adequate sensitivity and specificity to consistently distinguish PMM and adenocarcinoma. Therefore, panels consisting of a number of antibodies are employed. A panel consisting of two positive and two negative markers for mesothelioma is recommended. Additional antibodies are employed when results are inconclusive. Variation of sensitivity and specificity vary with the laboratory, requiring performance validation of the antibodies employed by each laboratory. Our antibody panel for the distinction of EPMM and adenocarcinoma consists of five antibodies. AE1/AE3 keratin antibody is positive in essentially all EPMM cases (Fig. 115-5A), thereby excluding from the differential diagnosis essentially all metastatic melanomas and lymphomas, excepting ALK positive, large B cell lymphoma. Most adenocarcinomas are also positive. However, the perinuclear-predominant pattern of cytoplasmic staining of mesotheliomas in most cases helps to distinguish them from adenocarcinomas, which typically have a membrane predominant pattern. The two mesothelial positive markers in our panel are calretinin (Fig. 115-5C) and Wilms Tumor Protein-1 (WT-1) (Fig. 115-5E and F). Calretinin is positive in more that 90% of EPMM, and is negative, or only weakly positive in most adenocarcinomas. WT-1 is also present in more than 90% of EPMM's in a nuclear staining pattern, but is also positive in many ovarian serous carcinomas, including those metastatic to the pleura. However, the addition to the panel of PAX 8, positive in most serous adenocarcinomas of the ovary, but negative in PMM, helps in the DD cases of possible metastatic adenocarcinoma in women. Other antibodies employed as positive mesothelioma markers that have been employed include keratin 5/6, thrombomodulin, mesothelin, and D2-40. The two negative markers in our panel are CEA (Fig. 115-5D) and TTF1. CEA is positive in about 75% of metastatic adenocarcinomas, but is negative in adenocarcinomas of the kidney, prostate, and many carcinomas of the thyroid and ovary. In contrast, positive polyclonal CEA staining in mesotheliomas in our laboratory is negative in almost all EPMM. TTF1 is positive in about 70% to 75% of adenocarcinomas of the lung, but is negative in PMM in our laboratory. Negative markers for mesothelioma that have been employed include CD15, BG-8, B72.3, Ber-Ep4, TTF-1, and MOC-31.

Epithelioid hemangioendothelioma (EHE) is a low to medium grade malignant vascular tumor that may occur as a primary or metastatic tumor in the pleura, or as an extension of a lung primary. It may be indistinguishable from EPMM on radiologic examination and on gross and H&E microscopic examination. Histopathologic clues to its possible presence are weak or moderate keratin immunoreactivity and calretinin negativity. It is positive for one or more vascular markers: CD31, CD34, Fli-1, or Factor VIII.

Metastatic renal cell carcinoma (RCC) may be difficult to distinguish from PMM. A recent review concludes that it is important to include at least CD10, RCC marker, PAX2, and PAX8, as positive markers for RCC, in the diagnostic panel.[15]

EM examination of EPMM[3–5] may be helpful in cases with discordant immunohistochemical features, unusual subtypes or poor differentiation. The detection of numerous long, thin, curved microvilli which project from the surface of the cell or into an intracellular lumen, distinguish EPMM from adenocarcinoma. However, the characteristic microscopic villi usually are absent in poorly differentiated EPMM and in SPMM.

In summary, immunohistochemical tests have greatly improved the diagnostic accuracy in PMM. However, consideration of clinical, radiologic and operative features still is important. EM and/or histochemistry may be of help in some cases; some pathologists still rely routinely and heavily on EM. Additional biopsy leads to a definitive diagnosis in some controversial cases.

Differential Diagnosis of SPMM

Included in the differential diagnosis of the sarcomatoid type are benign and malignant tumors and primary and metastatic tumors (Table 115-3).[3–5,11]

Calcific fibrous tumor is a benign tumor that usually occurs in soft tissues, but a few occurring in the visceral pleura and mediastinum have been reported. They may be solitary or multiple, forming a mass up to 12 cm. Dystrophic or psammomatous calcifications, which may be visible on CT scan, are scattered in a collagenous fibrous stroma that is lightly infiltrated by small lymphocytes. Stromal cells are negative for AE/AE3 keratins and CD34, helping to distinguish this tumor from PMM and solitary fibrous tumor (SFT).

Synovial sarcoma may occur in the pleura a primary tumor, as well as metastatic tumor or by extension from a lung primary.[4,5,7] The monophasic spindle cell type of synovial sarcoma, which is in the differential diagnosis of SPMM is usually present as a solitary mass, but diffuse involvement also occurs. On microscopic examination, the cells are usually small, spindled, closely packed, and arranged in interweaving fascicles, a so-called stream of fish pattern, rarely seen in SPMM. AE1/AE3 keratin, usually weak and focal, is present in about two thirds of cases, and it is less extensive than that seen in most cases of sarcomatoid mesothelioma. Cytogenetics in about 90% of cases reveals an X;18 (p11;q11) translocation, considered specific for this tumor. Molecular genetics, using reverse transcriptase polymerase chain reaction (RT-PCR) reveals a SYT-SS1 or SYT-SS2 fusion.

SFT occurs as a benign, occasionally malignant tumor, of the thorax that is thought to derive from submesothelial mesenchyme and is not of mesothelial origin.[4,5,7,11] The usual age range at presentation is the fourth to sixth decade. Most SFT's are discovered as an incidental finding at chest x-ray or CT scan. Rarely, the presenting manifestation is hypoglycemia, secondary to production by the tumor of insulin-like growth factor. Most SFT's are round and smooth-surfaced, with a pushing border and are solitary. They may form a large mass, up to 30 cm or larger. About 80% arise from the visceral pleura, to which they are attached by a peduncle, but others may involve the mediastinum or other intrathoracic sites, including the lung parenchyma. Histopathologic appearance is of bland, slender spindle cells, often in a dense, rope-like collagenous stroma and with branching, staghorn vascular channels. The characteristic immunohistochemical profile is keratin negativity and CD34 positivity. Rarely, malignant SFT's are identifiable by frankly malignant behavior and sarcomatous histopathologic features; however, the prognosis of others with worrisome clinical behavior or pathologic features can be problematic.[4,5]

Table 115-3

DIFFERENTIAL DIAGNOSIS: SARCOMATOID PMM

Calcifying fibrous tumor
Desmoid
Metastatic malignant melanoma
Sarcomas
Angiosarcoma, Synovial sarcoma, other sarcomas
Sarcomatoid carcinoma
Pulmonary, Renal cell, other
Solitary fibrous tumor

ASBESTOS AND PMM

The association of PMM with asbestos exposure is based on landmark epidemiologic studies as well as numerous confirmatory studies including those that quantify asbestos fibers in the lung and tumor (Reviewed in 5,[16]). There is no known threshold limit for asbestos exposure below which there is no risk of PMM.[17] Asbestos fibers induce PMM in animals in chronic inhalation exposure studies, and by direct intrapleural or intraperitoneal injection.[18] Other associations, such as SV-40, have been implicated in the causation of mesothelioma, but these suggest possible cocarcinogenic roles.[19] Asbestos exists as two types of fibers, straight (amphiboles) and curved (serpentine). Amphiboles include the following common fiber types: actinolite, amosite, anthophyllite, crocidolite, and tremolite. Chrysotile is the common serpentine fiber; it usually has a tubular structure, and may be soluble in acids. All fiber types are heat and fire resistant and have insulating properties. All forms of asbestos are fibrous silicates, that is, silicon dioxide with various substituted elements. Available evidence suggests that all asbestos fiber types have carcinogenic potential.[5,16]

Asbestos bodies (asbestos fibers coated with iron and protein) may be observed either in routine histologic sections of lung tissue in heavily exposed individuals or in lung digestion preparations as illustrated in Figure 115-6 A. Asbestos bodies and uncoated fibers may be detected using scanning EM on sections cut from paraffin-embedded tissue or with digested thoracic tissues using transmission or scanning EM. Energy dispersive x-ray analysis may be used with either type of EM as a means to determine the chemical composition and therefore type of fiber identified (Fig. 115-6B). The tissue quantification of asbestos is a critical link in establishing asbestos exposure as etiologically important in specific cases of PMM, and has been correlated to histological type of mesothelioma, survival with mesothelioma, and degree of epigenetic change in cell cycle related genes.[20–23]

Since asbestos has been banned in many countries and its use has declined in most western countries, a decrease in the number of new cases of PMM has been predicted.[24] However, worldwide consumption of asbestos remains surprisingly high in some countries, exceeding consumption levels in the United States of the 1950s through the 1970s. China, Russia, Kazakhstan, India, and Thailand are the current leading consumers

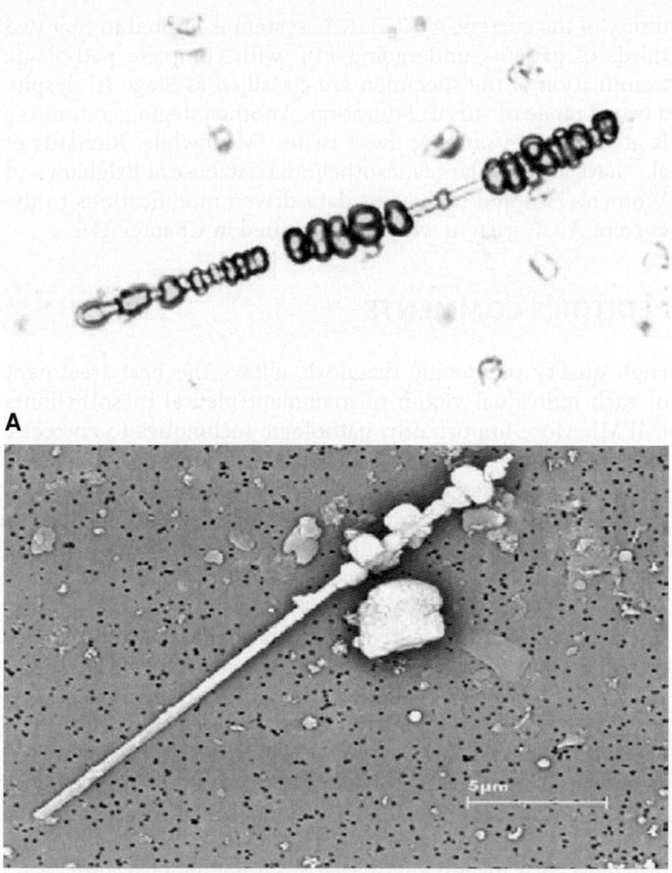

Figure 115-6. *A.* Light microscopic photo of an asbestos body from lung tissue extracted by hypochlorite digestion and mounted on a gridded filter for counting. Note the clear central fiber core and yellow–brown beaded coat rich in iron. The fiber plus the coating define an asbestos body. *B.* Scanning electron microscopy photo of an asbestos body with a fiber that has a small amount of beaded iron and protein in the top portion of the fiber, and the remainder is uncoated. Energy dispersive x-ray analysis capability of the electron microscope can be used to quantify the mineral content of the fiber; this is an amosite fiber based on mineralogical analysis.

of asbestos,[25] and there is little control as to whether asbestos may be included in any products sold in the West by manufacturers in these countries. At the same time, concerns are being expressed that new man-made fiber-like materials, such as multiwalled carbon nanotubules, may have properties that have response similarities to asbestos.[26] Other etiologic factors include irradiation[27] and genetic predisposition.[28,29]

Pathogenetic mechanisms by which asbestos exposure leads to PMM include: (1) asbestos fibers generate free radicals from their surfaces as well as through interactions with cells; (2) asbestos fibers cause a chronic inflammatory reaction leading to prolonged release of reactive oxygen species (ROS), reactive nitrogen species (RNS), cytokines, and growth factors; (3) asbestos fibers damage DNA and interfere physically with mitosis; (4) asbestos fibers and ROS stimulate proliferation of target cells through cell signaling pathways; (5) asbestos fibers and ROS induce apoptosis in cultured mesothelial cells, but PMM cells are highly resistant to apoptosis, thus providing a mechanism for continued growth of malignantly transformed cells; and (6) epigenetic silencing of tumor suppressor genes provides another mechanism that is consistent with the long latency and time course of this malignancy. A detailed recent review of all of these mechanisms has recently been published.[5]

Table 115-4

CYTOGENETICS AND MOLECULAR GENETICS OF MESOTHELIOMA[a]

Karyotype changes:
No specific chromosomal anomaly
Frequently observed changes:
Chromosome Loss at 1p21–22 (85%), 3p21 (65%), 4q33–34, 4q25–26, 4p15.1–15.3, 6q, 6q15–21, 9p21–22, 22q12 (possible tumor suppressor loci)
Chromosome Losses Occurring in Combination: 1p, 3p, 6q, 9p and 22q
Monosomy Chromosomes 4 and 22
Polysomy Chromosomes 5, 7 and 20
Fluorescence In Situ Hybridization
Extra Copies of 1, 3, 6, 7, 11 and 15
Loss of 1p21–22
Loss of Heterozygosity (LOH) at 1p22
Comparative Genomic Hybridization
Losses Detected
9p21 (34%, 22q (32%), 4q31–32 (29%), 4p21–13 (25%), 14q12–24 (23%), 1p21 (21%), 13q12–14 (19%), 3p21 (16%), 6q22 (16%), 10p13-pter (16%), 17;12-pter (16%), 8p21-pter, 15q11.1–21.1, 3p21
Gains Detected
8q22–23 (18%), 1q23/1q32 (16%), 7p14–15 (14%), 15q22–25 (14%) 3p12–13, 7q, 5

[a]Modified from Hicks (2006).

CYTOGENETICS AND MOLECULAR GENETICS

Cytogenetics and molecular genetics have contributed to our capabilities in PMM diagnosis as well as aided in the understanding of the pathogenesis of this malignancy. PMM has been shown to have detectable chromosomal aberrations, and karyotypic analyses can be used for the distinction between reactive mesothelial cells and PMM. However, there is no consistent specific abnormality found in all cases. PMM's have clonal cytogenetic aberrations indicative of malignancy, of which the more common aberrations include deletions of 1p, 3p, 6q, 9p, and 22q, and trisomy 7, 15, and 16. Table 115-4 lists the cytogenetic abnormalities that have been observed.[30] These deletions can be detected by FISH, and they are not observed in benign effusions (Fig. 115-7).[31] Thus, FISH can be a particularly useful adjunct to cytologic assessment of pleural effusions in the consideration of malignant versus benign effusions. FISH can be performed on fixed, interphase cells using probes to the cytogenetic aberrations.

GRADING/STAGING OF PMM

There is no accepted grading system within types of PMM. Although there are differences in prognosis among different types of PMM as noted above, grading systems for within epithelioid or sarcomatoid tumors are an area of active investigation as research groups have more case material with clinical follow-up from which to try to establish differences among features. Ideally, a grading system for each histologic type is needed; the system should be based upon cases treated with the same therapeutic regimen; and the same pathologic staging system should be used for all comparisons. However, at this time staging system of PMM are also problematic. Staging of PMM is reviewed in detail in Chapter 116. Available staging systems

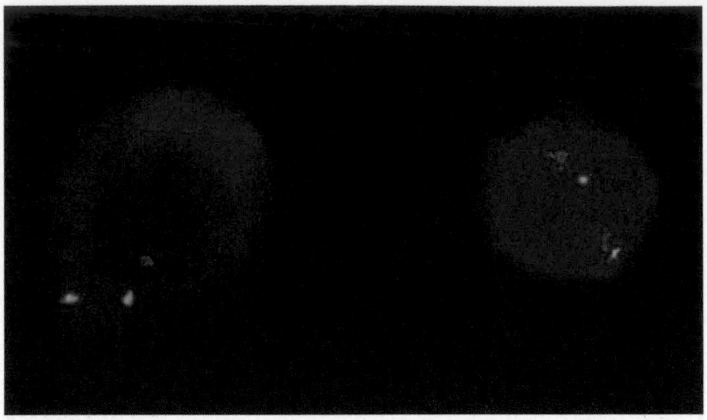

Figure 115-7. Fluorescence in situ hybridization shows a normal cell on the right and a mesothelioma cell on the left. The preparation has been incubated with probes for the centromeric region (green) and the p21 deletion region (red) of chromosome 9. Both cells show two centromeric regions, but the mesothelioma cell has 9p21 deletion. This deletion was seen in 35% of the examined cells. (Photo courtesy of Dr. Edmund Cibas; reproduced from *Cancer Cytopathol* with permission).

include the first clinical system proposed by Butchart et al. in 1976,[32] a modification of that system proposed by investigators at Brigham and Women's Hospital,[33] a tumor-node-metastasis (TNM) based system developed as the International Mesothelioma Interest Group staging system,[34] adopted by the American Joint Commission on Cancer (AJCC) in the 6th edition of its Cancer Staging Manual[35] and by the International Union against Cancer (UICC)[36] which established pathologic staging of PMM in a TNM framework. However, the prognostic utility of the current AJCC/UICC system is limited in that two thirds of patients undergoing EPP with complete pathologic examination of the specimen are classified as Stage III despite a broad range of survival duration. Another staging committee is at work re-evaluating these issues. Meanwhile, Richards et al.[37] have used the large mesothelioma database at Brigham and Women's Hospital to suggest data-driven modifications to the current AJCC system which is described in Chapter 116.

EDITOR'S COMMENTS

High quality pathologic diagnosis allows the best treatment of each individual victim of malignant pleural mesothelioma (MPM). More importantly, pathologic techniques to correctly identify and stage MPM allowed the rapid evolution of disease treatment witnessed over the past 30 years. Being able to distinguish homogeneous groups of patients with the same stage of mesothelioma rapidly expanded the knowledge of a rare disease with only 3000 cases per year diagnosed in the United States. By contrast, there are over 200,000 cases of lung cancer identified in this country yearly. This concise chapter emphasizes the role of the surgeon in providing adequate high quality tissue specimens for H&E stains, FISH, immunohistochemistry, and EM. It describes the methods of differentiating MPM from other differential diagnoses, including chronic fibrosing pleuritis, atypical mesothelial proliferation, primary adenocarcinoma of the lung, metastatic adenocarcinoma, renal carcinoma, and epithelioid hemangioendothelioma. Furthermore, the authors provide a clear discussion of rare mesothelioma variants.

—Michael T. Jaklitsch

References

1. Chirieac LR, Corson JM. Pathologic evaluation of malignant pleural mesothelioma. *Semin Thorac Cardiovasc Surg.* 2009;21:121–124.
2. Boutin C, Rey F, Gouvernet J, et al. Thoracoscopy in pleural malignant mesothelioma: a prospective study of 188 consecutive patients'. Part 2: prognosis and Staging. *Cancer.* 1993;72(2):394–404.
3. Corson JM. Pathology of mesothelioma. *Thorac Surg Clin.* 2004;14:447–460.
4. Churg AC, Cagle PT, Roggli VL. *AFIP Atlas of Tumor Pathology.* Washington, DC: American Registry of Pathology in Collaboration with the Armed Forces Institute of Pathology; 2006.
5. Hammar SP, Henderson DW, Klebe G, et al. Volume II. Neoplastic lung disease: neoplasms of the pleura. In: Tomashefski JF Jr., Cagle PT, Farver CF, et al., eds. *Dail and Hammar's Pulmonary Pathology.* 3rd ed. New York, NY: Springer Science and Business Media, LLC; 2008:558–734.
6. Lester SL. *Manual of Surgical Pathology.* 3rd ed. Philadelphia, PA: Elsevier Saunders; 2010.
7. Churg A, Roggli V, Cagle Ph T, et al. Mesothelioma. In: Travis WD, Brambilla E, Muller-Hermelink HK, et al., eds. *Pathology and Genetics of Tumours of the Lung, Pleura, Thymus and Heart.* Lyon, France: IARE Press; 2004:128–135.
8. Shia J, Qin J, Erlandson RA, et al. Malignant mesothelioma with a pronounced myxoid stroma: a clinical and pathological evaluation of 19 cases. *Virchows Arch.* 2005;447;828–834.
9. Kadota K, Suzuki K, Sima C, et al. Pleomorphic epithelioid diffuse malignant pleural mesothelioma. A clinico pathological review and conceptual proposal to reclassify as biphasic or sarcomatoid mesothelioma. *J Thorac Oncol.* 2011;6(5):896–904.
10. Allen TC, Cagle PT, Churg AM, et al. Localized malignant mesothelioma. *Am J Surg Pathol.* 2005;29(7):866–873.
11. Travis WD. Sarcomatoid neoplasms of the lung and pleura. *Arch Pathol Lab Med.* 2010;134:1645–1658.
12. Gallateau-Salle F, Attanoos R, Gibbs AR, et al. Lymphohistiocytoid variant of malignant mesothelioma of the pleura: a series of 22 cases. *Am J Surg Pathol.* 2007;31:711–716.
13. Cagle PT, Churg A. Differential diagnosis of benign and malignant mesothelial proliferations on pleural biopsies. *Arch Pathol Lab Med.* 2005;129:1421–1427.
14. Klebe S, Mahar A, Henderson DW, et al. Malignant mesothelioma with heterologous elements: clinicopathological correlation and literature review. *Mod Pathol.* 2008;21:1084–1094.
15. Truong LD, Shen SS. Immunohistochemical diagnosis of renal neoplasms. *Arch Pathol Lab Med.* 2011;135(1):92–109.
16. Godleski JJ. Role of asbestos in the etiology of malignant pleural mesothelioma. *Thorac Surg Clin.* 2004;14:479–487
17. Hillerdal G. Mesothelioma: cases associated with non-occupational and low dose exposures. *Occup Environ Med.* 1999;56:505–513.
18. Kane AB. Mechanisms of mineral fibre carcinogenesis. In: Boffetta P, Saracci R, Wilbourn JD, eds. *Mechanisms of Fibre Carcinogenesis.* Lyon: International Agency for Research on Cancer; 1996;11–35, IARC Scientific Publication No. 140.
19. Powers A, Carbone M. The role of environmental carcinogens, viruses and genetic predisposition in the pathogenesis of mesothelioma. *Cancer Biol Ther.* 2002;1:348–353.
20. Klebe S, Brownlee NA, Mahar A, et al. Sarcomatoid mesothelioma: a clinical-pathologic correlation of 326 cases. *Mod Pathol.* 2010;23:470–479.
21. Christensen BC, Godleski JJ, Roelofs CR, et al. Asbestos burden predicts survival in pleural mesothelioma. *Environ Health Perspect.* 2008;116:723–726.
22. Christensen BC, Godleski JJ, Marsit CJ, et al. Asbestos exposure predicts cell cycle control gene promoter methylation in pleural mesothelioma. *Carcinogenesis.* 2008;29:1555–1559.
23. Christensen BC, Houseman EA, Godleski JJ, et al. Epigenetic profiles distinguish pleural mesothelioma from normal pleura and predict lung asbestos burden and clinical outcome. *Cancer Res.* 2009;69(1):227–234.

24. Price B, Ware A. Time trend of mesothelioma incidence in the United States and projection of future cases: an update based on SEER data for 1973 through 2005. *Crit Rev Toxicol.* 2009;39:576–588.
25. Virta RL. Worldwide asbestos supply and consumption trends from 1900 through 2003: U.S. Geological Survey Circular 1298. 2006;80. http://pubs.usgs.gov/circ/2006/1298/c1298.pdf
26. Donaldson K, Murphy FA, Puffin R, et al. Asbestos, carbon nanotubes and the pleural mesothelium: a review of the hypothesis regarding the role of long fibre retention in the parietal pleura, inflammation and mesothelioma. *Part Fibre Toxicol.* 2010;7:5–22.
27. Teta MJ, Lau E, Sceurman BK, et al. Therapeutic radiation for lymphoma. *Cancer.* 2007;109:1432–1438.
28. Hirvonen A, Saarikoski ST, Linnainmaa K, et al. Glutathione S-transferase and N-acetyltransferase genotypes and asbestos-associated pulmonary disorders. *J Natl Cancer Inst.* 1996;88:1853–1856.
29. Roushdy-Hammady I, Siegel J, Emri S, et al. Genetic susceptibility factor and malignant mesothelioma in the Cappadocian region of Turkey. *Lancet.* 2001;357:444–445.
30. Hicks J. Biologic, cytogenetic, and molecular factors in mesothelial proliferations. *Ultrastruct Pathol.* 2006;30:19–30.
31. Factor RE, Dal Cin P, Fletcher JA, et al. Cytogenetics and fluorescence in situ hybridization as adjuncts to cytology in the diagnosis of malignant mesothelioma. *Cancer Cytopathol.* 2009;117:247–253.
32. Butchart EG, Ashcroft T, Barnsley WC, et al. Pleuropneumonectomy in the management of diffuse malignant mesothelioma of the pleura. Experience with 29 patients. *Thorax.* 1976;31:15–24.
33. Sugarbaker DJ, Flores RM, Jaklitsch MT, et al. Resection margins, extrapleural nodal status, and cell type determine postoperative long-term survival in trimodality therapy of malignant pleural mesothelioma: results in 183 patients. *J Thorac Cardiovasc Surg.* 1999;117(1):54–63; discussion 63–55.
34. Rusch VW. A proposed new international TNM staging system for malignant pleural mesothelioma. From the International Mesothelioma Interest Group. *Chest.* 1995;108(4):1132–1138.
35. Greene FL, Page DL, Fleming ID, et al., eds. *AJCC Cancer Staging Manual.* 6th ed. New York: Springer; 2002.
36. UICC International Union Against Cancer: *TNM Classification of Malignant Disease.* 6th ed. New York: Wiley-Liss; 2002.
37. Richards WG, Godleski JJ, Yeap BY, et al. Proposed adjustments to pathologic staging of epithelial malignant pleural mesothelioma based on analysis of 354 cases. *Cancer.* 2010;116:1510–1517.

116 Mesothelioma Staging

William G. Richards

Keywords: Staging, TNM staging system, prognostic models, mesothelioma, lymph node metastasis

CANCER STAGING

Cancer staging systems are intended to assist clinicians to categorize patients diagnosed with a particular malignancy in terms of their life expectancy and potential response to specific therapeutic strategies. Generally speaking, patients categorized as early stage have anatomically localized malignancy associated with a longer life expectancy and better response particularly to local therapies directed at the primary tumor mass. Late stage patients are presumed to have metastatic disease indirectly disseminated to distant anatomical sites associated with shorter life expectancy and requiring systemic therapeutic approaches. A staging system is a set of criteria that defines such categories for a specific malignancy. Stage categories are defined in anatomical terms: How large is the tumor and what anatomical structures have become involved with (i.e., contain invasive proliferations of) tumor cells?

Tumor stage may be used as an eligibility or stratification factor for clinical trials, as a component of algorithms for determining prognosis, and in predicting the efficacy of particular therapeutic strategies for individual patients. Thus, stage serves as an important element of risk–benefit discussions between cancer patients and clinicians. In the context of an aggressive and rapidly fatal malignancy such as malignant pleural mesothelioma (MPM), these issues are critical to clinical, patient, and caregiver decision-making in relation to balancing expected quantity and quality of life. The practical value of any staging system is measured by its ability to separate patients into categories associated with differing expectations in terms of symptom relief, side effects, freedom from disease progression, and/or survival duration in relation to available treatment strategies.

Staging categorizes the physical extent of tumor growth relative to a patient's normal anatomy. Categorical labels typically ranging from stage I to stage IV reflect the progressive nature of the underlying biologic process. Corresponding qualitative descriptions of "local" (stage I), "regional" (stages II–III), and "distant" (stage IV) disease refer, respectively, to a tumor that remains confined to the tissue or organ within which it initially arose, one that extends beyond the initiating tissue or organ either by direct growth to immediately surrounding tissues or by microscopic dissemination via lymphatic vessels to draining lymph nodes, and one that is disseminated via the systemic circulation to establish metastases in remote anatomic locations. For some systems, stage categories are defined directly by lists of criteria. However, the recognition that direct extension of the primary mass and metastasis via lymphatic and systemic routes represent separate and mutually independent classification parameters that may be combined to optimally define stage led to the development and preferential use of the more nuanced tumor-node-metastasis (TNM) classification systems.

Definitive determination of stage requires microscopic evaluation of representative tissue samples from the defining anatomic structures. Accurate staging is therefore only possible when all primary tumors have been surgically resected with an adequate margin, relevant regional lymph nodes and any suspected metastases have been biopsied, and the specimens have been subjected to complete gross and microscopic pathologic examination. The resulting classification is referred to as pathologic stage. Prior to treatment, or when surgical resection is not undertaken, tumor stage may be estimated based on physical examination and noninvasive imaging (clinical stage), alone or in combination with endoscopic or surgical biopsy or exploration with tissue sampling (surgical stage).

STAGING OF MALIGNANT PLEURAL MESOTHELIOMA

It has been challenging to establish a practical staging system for MPM owing to the rarity of the tumor, its anatomical complexity, its histologic heterogeneity (epithelioid, sarcomatoid, biphasic), and the limited availability of effective therapy. All of the staging systems that have been proposed are derived from and primarily applicable to the subset of patients undergoing surgery. However, for the minority of patients with MPM who undergo resection of their tumors, definitive staging based on pathologic assessment of resected MPM specimens is at best modestly correlated with patient outcome. Close apposition of multiple vital structures to pleural surfaces does not permit wide surgical margins to be taken around resected tumor, and this leads to probable underestimation of involvement of adjacent structures in determining pathologic stage. Furthermore, there is poor correspondence between preoperative clinical stage and final pathologic stage. In part, this results from the unique morphology and growth pattern of the primary tumor that render radiographic assessment challenging. The accuracy of clinical staging for the majority of MPM patients who are not treated surgically cannot be directly evaluated, but is likely to be similarly low unless there is unambiguous evidence of metastatic disease.

Staging, therefore, has not been as useful for MPM as it has been for some other malignancies to determine prognosis or inform treatment decisions, particularly whether or not surgical resection should be contemplated. For example, consider non–small-cell lung cancer (NSCLC), for which surgical resection is the standard of care primary therapy for clinical stages I to II, which can be determined with high accuracy by a combination of imaging and mediastinoscopy. A malignant lung tumor typically grows as an expanding, roughly spherical mass that is usually surrounded by lung parenchyma. Its diameter is easily measured radiographically, is predictive of recurrence and prognosis, and thus is a direct determinant of T classification. Lymphatic metastasis occurs in a progressive and predictable pattern based on the location of the primary lesion. By contrast, MPM typically spreads in a nodular pattern over the pleural surfaces. It often encases the ipsilateral lung and may expand to considerable bulk while remaining encapsulated within the pleural envelope, and thus be classified by definition as early disease. On the other hand, the tumor may transgress the pleural boundary in one or more areas to variably involve lung parenchyma, chest wall, pericardium, diaphragm, and/or mediastinal structures, affecting stage classification in ways that are not readily appreciated radiographically. Regional lymph node involvement with tumor is also not accurately assessed using current imaging modalities because nodal size does not correlate well with the presence of metastasis, and because some relevant nodes, particularly hilar and internal thoracic stations, are located in areas that are commonly involved with or immediately adjacent to primary tumor.[1,2]

The establishment of a standard and accurate staging system also has been hampered by the relative rarity and overall poor prognosis of MPM. Only a fraction of patients undergo surgical resection. Consequently, relatively few cases have been available to establish and pathologically validate classification criteria. Surgical series large enough to inform staging have generally been retrospective cohorts from single institutions. Differing degrees of resection, failing to distinguish histologic subtypes, variable application of nonsurgical therapies, and treatment-related morbidity and mortality – each of which may influence outcome independent of stage – have hampered attempts to elucidate more subtle influences of staging criteria on patient prognosis. These factors have led to the proposal over the past several decades of a number of independent staging systems that differ in the significance attributed to specific classification criteria (for review, see Ref. 3).

The earliest MPM staging system proposed by Butchart et al.[4] and later modifications proposed by Mattson[5] and Sugarbaker et al.[6,7] define each stage directly based on specified anatomic criteria and their association with outcome in series of surgically treated patients. TNM staging systems for solid tumors consider tumor size and/or patterns of local invasion (T classification), involvement of regional lymph nodes (N classification), and remote or systemic disease (M classification) in determining stage. Early TNM classification criteria for MPM were proposed by Chahinian.[8] The Cancer Staging Manuals, periodically co-published by the International Union Against Cancer (UICC)[9] and The American Joint Committee on Cancer (AJCC),[10] first included TNM criteria for MPM in their 4th editions. Modified TNM classification (Table 116-1) and stage grouping (Table 116-2) criteria proposed by the International Mesothelioma Interest Group (IMIG)[11] were adopted by the AJCC and UICC and have since remained unchanged through the current (7th) edition.

Table 116-1

NEW INTERNATIONAL STAGING SYSTEM FOR DIFFUSE MALIGNANT PLEURAL MESOTHELIOMA

STAGE	DEFINITION
T1	T1a Tumor limited to the ipsilateral parietal pleura, including mediastinal and diaphragmatic pleura No involvement of the visceral pleura T1b Tumor involving the ipsilateral parietal pleura, including mediastinal and diaphragmatic pleura Scattered foci of tumor also involving the visceral pleura
T2	Tumor involving each of the ipsilateral pleural surfaces (parietal, mediastinal, diaphragmatic, and visceral) with at least one of the following features: • involvement of diaphragmatic muscle • confluent visceral pleural tumor (including the fissures) or extension of tumor from visceral pleura into the underlying pulmonary parenchyma
T3	Describes locally advanced but potentially resectable tumor Tumor involving all of the ipsilateral pleural surfaces (parietal, mediastinal, diaphragmatic, and visceral) with at least one of the following features: • involvement of the endothoracic fascia • extension into the mediastinal fat • solitary, completely resectable focus of tumor extending into the soft tissues of the chest wall • nontransmural involvement of the pericardium
T4	Describes locally advanced technically unresectable tumor Tumor involving all of the ipsilateral pleural surfaces (parietal, mediastinal, diaphragmatic, and visceral) with at least one of the following features: • diffuse extension or multifocal masses of tumor in the chest wall, with or without associated rib destruction • direct transdiaphragmatic extension of tumor to the peritoneum • direct extension of tumor to the contralateral pleura • direct extension of tumor to one or more mediastinal organs • direct extension of tumor into the spine • tumor extending through to the internal surface of the pericardium with or without a pericardial effusion; or tumor involving the myocardium
N—Lymph nodes	
NX	Regional lymph nodes cannot be assessed
NO	No regional lymph node metastases
Nl	Metastases in the ipsilateral bronchopulmonary or hilar lymph nodes
N2	Metastases in the subcarinal or the ipsilateral mediastinal lymph nodes, including the ipsilateral internal mammary nodes
N3	Metastases in the contralateral mediastinal, contralateral internal mammary, ipsilateral, or contralateral supraclavicular lymph nodes
M—Metastases	
MX	Presence of distant metastases cannot be assessed
MO	No distant metastasis
Ml	Distant metastasis present

Source: Reproduced with permission from Rusch VW. A proposed new international TNM staging system for malignant pleural mesothelioma. From the International Mesothelioma Interest Group. *Chest.* 1995;108:1122–1128.

Size Criteria

T classification of malignancies that typically progress as enlarging, approximately spherical masses (e.g., non–small-cell lung carcinoma) is based primarily on tumor size, with upstaging when invasion of specific structures is present. By contrast, tumor size is not easily established for MPM, either clinically or pathologically, owing to the tumor's irregular and highly variable morphology. The difficulty inherent in documenting the size of individual MPM tumors is reflected in the requirement for MPM-specific modification of RECIST criteria for longitudinal assessment of response to therapy.[12] Tumor size is therefore not currently considered when establishing MPM stage. Staging of some other malignancies, particularly those that

Table 116-2

IMIG STAGE GROUPINGS ADOPTED BY UICC/AJCC/IASLC

Stage I	
Ia	T1aN0M0
Ib	T1bN0M0
Stage II	T2N0M0
Stage III	Any T3M0
	Any N1M0
	Any N2M0
Stage IV	Any T4
	Any N3
	Any MN1

Source: Reproduced with permission from Rusch VW. A proposed new international TNM staging system for malignant pleural mesothelioma. From the International Mesothelioma Interest Group. *Chest.* 1995;108:1122–1128.

arise within luminal mucosa (e.g., esophageal, gastric, colorectal carcinoma) or epithelium-lined hollow organs (e.g., bladder cancer) and therefore tend to have irregular rather than spherical morphology, similarly does not include tumor size criteria. For many such tumors, direct invasion into adjacent regular, concentric layers of muscle and vasculature provides a reliable basis for pathologic and endoscopic T classification.

Patterns of Local Invasion

No simple solution exists for MPM, where it is also challenging to accurately determine the degree and pattern of tumor extension into adjacent structures. The pleurae are bordered by the chest wall, diaphragm, pericardium, mediastinal organs, and lung. Commonly, the tumor circumferentially fills the chest cavity creating the potential for concurrent invasion into multiple structures.

According to AJCC/UICC staging criteria, T1 MPM tumors are confined within the ipsilateral pleural surfaces. Boutin et al.[13] described early MPM as arising on the parietal pleura, with subsequent progression to the visceral pleura accompanied by a worsening of prognosis among Buchart stage I patients undergoing thoracoscopy. This observation was the basis for T1 subclassification in the IMIG TNM system. Some authors have questioned whether this distinction is clinically meaningful, because so few T1a tumors are diagnosed.[14,15] Tumors extending into interlobar fissures or involving lung parenchyma or diaphragm muscle are classified T2. Extension of tumor to involve endothoracic fascia or mediastinal adipose tissue, into but not through the pericardium, or chest wall soft tissue at a single focus, constitute T3. Further direct extension of tumor to involve chest wall soft tissue diffusely or at more than one focus, brachial plexus, bone (rib or spine), mediastinal organs, contralateral pleura, or through diaphragm or pericardium, is classified T4.

Even under the best of circumstances, accurate pathologic determination of MPM stage is challenging. The structures that surround the pleura cannot be resected to unambiguously evaluate all margins. Nevertheless, with extensive and systematic sampling, extrapleural pneumonectomy (EPP) specimens may be rigorously staged.[16] This process commonly requires microscopic examination of 20 to 30 sections per specimen. For patients undergoing less complete operative procedures, complete pathologic staging may not be possible as a result of the inability to microscopically evaluate retained tissues.

Lymph Node Metastasis

Regional lymph node staging of MPM uses the same classification system as employed for staging lung cancer.[17] Ipsilateral hilar and intraparenchymal lymph nodes are classified N1. Subcarinal and ipsilateral mediastinal or internal mammary nodes are classified N2. Contralateral mediastinal or internal mammary, or any scalene or supraclavicular nodes, are classified N3.

Lymph node metastasis has long been recognized as an indicator of poor prognosis in MPM.[6] Studies of patients treated with EPP who had complete pathologic analysis have found the presence of N2 metastasis to be among[7] (or the only[18]) significant prognostic factors identified in multivariate analysis. The relationship of N1 and N2 lymph node involvement to prognosis and stage, however, is more complex for MPM than for NSCLC. In the case of lung cancer, these designations are indicative of an orderly peripheral-to-central pulmonary lymphatic drainage pattern that usually results in a predictable metastatic progression through intraparenchymal, hilar, and ultimately, mediastinal nodal stations. By contrast, direct lymphatic drainage from the diaphragmatic pleura to the mediastinal nodal chain[19] allows MPM to metastasize directly to N2 lymph nodes without first affecting N1 stations. Studies consistently report that approximately 40% of patients with N2 metastases do not demonstrate concurrent N1 disease.[18,20,21] Metastasis to only N1 lymph nodes may alternatively arise by direct pleural spread to the hilum or secondary to tumor invasion of lymphatics within lung parenchyma, thence following the pattern characteristic of lung cancer.[22]

Distant Metastasis

MPM has historically been characterized as having a primarily local growth pattern, with only rare distant metastasis.[23] Other studies have suggested that distant disease may be more common than generally appreciated,[24] particularly in the context of surgical removal of the primary, although not all studies of surgical patients have concurred.[25] The distinction between direct and hematogenous metastasis is sometimes problematic because MPM has a tendency to grow through anatomical barriers such as the diaphragm by direct extension to involve "distant" organs such as the liver. Although there is definitive evidence of metastasis to CNS, bone, kidney, adrenal glands, lung, and pleura,[26] the frequency and impact on the natural history is less clear.

Validation and Performance

Staging systems must be periodically reevaluated as therapeutic strategies evolve and new standards of care are established. Such validation involves assessing the ability of staging criteria to stratify outcome in cohorts of patients receiving similar therapy. During more than a decade since publication of the IMIG[11] and revised BWH[7] criteria, multiple therapeutic innovations have been developed and investigated. These range from intravenous chemotherapeutic regimens to intraoperative adjuncts such as hyperthermic intracavitary chemotherapy (HIOC) and photodynamic therapy (PDT) to adjuvant high-dose hemithoracic and intensity-modulated radiation therapy (IMRT). Each staging system has been used in published reports of series of patients treated on- and off-protocol using these strategies. None of the studies has provided validation of either system in terms of stage by stage stratification of outcome. For patients treated without surgery, a much needed standard of care chemotherapy regimen, *combination cisplatin-pemetrexed,* was established with the publication of a landmark multi-institutional phase III trial.[27] Although the stage distribution of patients on trial was reported in a table to demonstrate balance between arms, tumor stage was not among eligibility criteria and patient survival per stage was not reported. A European trial of similar design using another chemically related compound, raltitrexed, which also supported the platinum-antifolate strategy, noted that UICC stage was only barely significant ($p = 0.0466$) in a multivariate prognostic model.[28] Thus the two largest and most influential multi-institutional phase III trials in the MPM treatment literature neither include stage among eligibility criteria nor validate the prognostic utility of current clinical staging.

Richards et al.[15] reported poor stage distribution and survival stratification by pathologic stage among 354 patients with epithelial MPM using either TNM or Brigham criteria. Most patients were classified to stage III by both systems. TNM criteria identified fewer early stage cases, as observed in other studies.[20] The TNM system does consistently identify a significant proportion of patients with stage IV disease with poor prognosis, arguing that current T4 classification criteria are appropriate.

Efforts to Improve Malignant Pleural Mesothelioma Staging

The International Association for the Study of Lung Cancer (IASLC) is conducting a prospective international cohort study of mesothelioma staging to inform potential future adjustment of TNM classification criteria. This effort builds on the IASLC staging committee's data-driven restructuring of NSCLC TNM staging, which was adopted in the AJCC and UICC 7th edition staging manuals. The MPM project was undertaken in two phases, initially focusing on pooling retrospective databases already in existence, while initiating prospective data collection. Initial analysis of the retrospective database that comprised institutional series of surgically managed patients has been published.[29]

The IASLC study confirmed in a large international dataset observations that had been made based on single-institution reports[15,30]: (1) patients with MPM treated with surgery-based therapy experience a broad range of survival from a few months to more than 10 years; (2) the prognostic value of staging depends on the therapy being applied (in this case the extent of macroscopic surgical resection); (3) pathologic TNM stage based on current criteria does not stratify patient survival in a clinically useful way; (4) clinical TNM stage is poorly predictive of pathologic stage; and (5) survival following surgery-based multimodality therapy is more profoundly influenced by tumor histology than by stage.

It is widely recognized that the prognosis of patients with epithelial MPM is more favorable than that of patients with biphasic or sarcomatoid histology tumors. The effect of histology on patient survival is one of considerable magnitude and represents the dominant (and often only) prognostic factor in most published multivariate analyses. Thus in mixed histology cohorts it is difficult to determine the relative influence of factors that are more subtly related to prognosis. The need to stratify by cell type when assessing a survival endpoint in MPM has been recognized,[1,15] but is rarely addressed in practice. Cohort sizes of most MPM studies are small, requiring that all patients be analyzed together to maximize statistical power. This fact, combined with a justifiable desire for parsimony, has resulted in the development of one-size-fits-all staging systems for MPM.

Nevertheless, the divergent clinical and biologic behavior of epithelial and nonepithelial tumors and the low prognostic accuracy of MPM staging require that the possibility of separate or annotated staging strategies be considered. At least, stratification by histology will be required as data analyses intended to inform revisions to staging are undertaken. To the degree that the prognostic models for epithelial and nonepithelial tumors converge, a single staging system should be preferred. However, initial studies have already identified staging parameters that demonstrate histology-dependent relationships to prognosis.

Richards et al.[15] reported on the prognostic significance of individual staging criteria in a large retrospective cohort of patients with surgically treated epithelial MPM. The analysis led to data-driven recommendations for modifying T and N classification for specific features, as well as stage grouping criteria, to optimize prognostication by stage for surgically treated epithelial MPM. Specifically, it was proposed that, relative to current AJCC/UICC classification criteria, tumor involvement of lung parenchyma, diaphragm, and mediastinal fat be upstaged to account for their association with increased hazard for death. It was further proposed that involvement of endothoracic fascia, chest wall at a solitary focus, and pericardium be downstaged, based on their lack of association with outcome Table 116-3).

Subclassification of N2 nodal stations was also recommended, based on differential prognosis associated with involvement at specific N2 stations. For epithelial subtype, Richards et al. observed better prognosis if metastasis is limited to inferior mediastinal lymph nodes, designated N2a, compared to lymph nodes at superior levels, N2b (Table 116-4). This distinction provided for nuanced stage grouping of epithelial MPM (Table 116-5; Fig. 116-1). However, nodal metastasis is less prevalent and has diminished prognostic impact in nonepithelial

Table 116-3

T CLASSIFICATION CRITERIA WITH PROPOSED MODIFICATIONS

T1	Tumor involves any of the ipsilateral pleural surfaces with negative resection margins (>1 mm)
T2	Tumor present within 1 mm of any resection margin, involving endothoracic fascia or chest wall soft tissue (localized), penetrating into but not through pericardium, or involving intralobar fissures
T3	Invasion of chest wall muscle, invasion into but not through diaphragm, invasion of lung parenchyma, or involvement of the apical, anterior, or medial pleural or any diaphragmatic resection margin
T4	Diffuse chest wall invasion, seeding of tumor in a prior chest tube site, transdiaphragmatic invasion, involvement at the bronchial resection margin, invasion of mediastinal organs or adipose tissue, direct extension to contralateral pleura, rib involvement, invasion of spine, extension through pericardium, malignant pleural effusion, invasion of myocardium or brachial plexus

Source: Reproduced with permission from Richards WG, Godleski JJ, Yeap BY, et al. Proposed adjustments to pathologic staging of epithelial malignant pleural mesothelioma based on analysis of 354 cases. *Cancer.* 2010;116:1510–1517.

Table 116-4

PROPOSED ADJUSTMENTS TO N CLASSIFICATION FOR TUMOR INVOLVEMENT AT IPSILATERAL LYMPH NODE LEVELS

LYMPH NODE LEVEL	CURRENT CLASSIFICATION	PROPOSED CLASSIFICATION
Level 2–4	N2	N2b
Level 5–9 + internal mammary lymph nodes	N2	N2a
Level 10–14	N1	N1

Source: Modified with permission from Richards WG, Godleski JJ, Yeap BY, et al. Proposed adjustments to pathologic staging of epithelial malignant pleural mesothelioma based on analysis of 354 cases. *Cancer*. 2010;116:1510–1517.

Table 116-5

PROPOSED TNM STAGE GROUPING

STAGE	TUMOR	NODE	METASTASIS
I	T1-2	N0	M0
	T1	N1-2a	M0
II	T1	N2b	M0
	T2	N1	M0
	T3	N0-1	M0
III	T2-3	N2a	M0
	T4	N0-1	M0
IV	T2-3	N2b	M0
	T4	N2	M0
	T1-4	N3	M0
	T1-4	N0-3	M1

Source: Reproduced with permission from Richards WG, Godleski JJ, Yeap BY, et al. Proposed adjustments to pathologic staging of epithelial malignant pleural mesothelioma based on analysis of 354 cases. *Cancer*. 2010;116:1510–1517.

disease, being essentially absent among sarcomatoid cases. A similar analysis of TNM staging criteria in a cohort of patients with biphasic disease revealed that N2 subclassification is less meaningful given that superior N2 involvement is rare, and that the stage grouping model was found to be more strongly driven by T than N classification.[31] These observations indicate that consideration of tumor histology will be required to improve staging accuracy in future revisions.

If histology-specific staging were to be implemented, a significant logistical challenge may be presented by the low accuracy of current diagnostic procedures to establish the histologic subtype. Open pleural biopsy is the diagnostic procedure of choice for patients under consideration for surgical therapy.[32] It is associated with 93% to 97% sensitivity for the detection of epithelial MPM, but only 31%[33] to 56%[32] specificity. Since only 26% to 56% of cases with nonepithelial histology are recognized at biopsy, the remaining cases are at risk of being misclassified. Cases of nonepithelial MPM are most commonly biphasic, comprising areas of epithelioid and sarcomatoid histology and characterized by regional heterogeneity. Obtaining a larger number of biopsies from regionally distributed areas of involved pleura during these procedures may therefore help to improve diagnostic accuracy. Novel radiographic technologies, such as diffusion magnetic resonance imaging (MRI), hold promise in predicting the presence of biphasic histology,[34] while also providing guidance for the best areas to biopsy in cases of suspected sarcomatoid differentiation.

Another way that staging system performance might be improved is by establishing a more nuanced classification of lymph node metastasis. Current TNM criteria do not distinguish between N1 and N2, which are both grouped in stage III. Several larger studies have demonstrated worse prognosis for N2 than N1, and have recommended changing this aspect of the staging system.[15,21] Various authors have further suggested that staging could be improved by considering the number of positive nodes[20] or the number of involved nodal stations,[21] or by subclassifying specific stations within N2.[15]

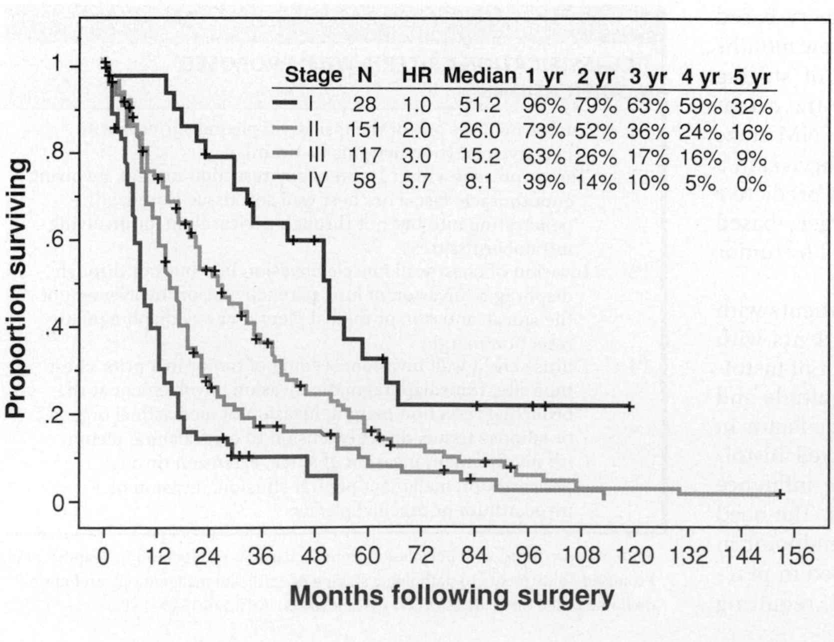

Figure 116-1. Survival by the American Joint Commission on Cancer/International Union Against Cancer staging system. (Reproduced with permission from Richards WG, Godleski JJ, Yeap BY, et al. Proposed adjustments to pathologic staging of epithelial malignant pleural mesothelioma based on analysis of 354 cases. *Cancer*. 2010;116: 1510–1517.)

CLINICAL STAGING

Virtually, all MPM staging systems are based on specific pathologic classification criteria derived from analysis of surgically treated patients. Because most patients diagnosed with MPM will not undergo resection, their stage must be estimated by noninvasive means collectively termed clinical staging. Even those patients who are thought to be potential candidates for surgery-based multimodality treatments are initially staged clinically to determine resectability and predict prognosis. The most common modalities used for clinical staging of MPM are chest computed tomography (CT), MRI, and fluorodeoxyglucose positron emission tomography (FDG-PET). Rarely, when the tumor appears to directly involve the esophagus or celiac axis lymph nodes, endoscopic ultrasound may be useful.[35]

Unfortunately, clinical staging of MPM using current methods does not accurately predict either pathologic stage or prognosis. Pathologic classification is based on microscopic assessment of tumor invasion on a cellular scale that is well below the spatial resolution of current radiographic techniques. Correspondingly, most pathologic classifiers are detected radiologically with low sensitivity. Nakas et al.[36] examined 164 cases of resected MPM with complete IMIG staging data and compared clinical staging by CT with or without MRI to pathologic staging. Clinical staging was found to understage 45% and overstage 11% of patients, leaving only 46% accurately staged. Clinical staging of lymph nodes is particularly inaccurate. Radiographic lymphadenopathy is not correlated with pathologic tumor involvement.[2,37]

Pathologic stage, when available, is itself of dubious prognostic value to individual patients. Thus, apart from cases of either minimal or overtly metastatic disease at presentation, clinical MPM stage has not proved useful for determining prognosis, treatment strategy, or protocol eligibility.

Computed Tomography

Despite its limitations, CT plays a crucial role in determining the extent of disease in patients diagnosed with MPM who are being evaluated for potential surgery. Among imaging modalities used to determine resectability of MPM, CT is the most common first-line choice based on its widespread availability and relative low cost.[38] Overt CT evidence of contralateral or distant metastasis, or of direct tumor extension into the abdomen or diffuse involvement of chest wall, directly contraindicates resection.

However, CT is insensitive for detection of more nuanced anatomical features critical to MPM staging. Focal tumor invasion of chest wall, pericardium, diaphragm, mediastinum, or intralobar fissures is infrequently visualized using CT.[39–41] Studies that have compared CT staging to other radiographic modalities such as MRI and PET have not generally identified sufficient improvement in staging accuracy to justify their incremental cost, except in cases when pivotal findings are equivocal on CT.[42] Recently published guidelines for clinical workup of MPM patients continue to recommend only CT beyond history, physical, and chest x-ray.[43]

Magnetic Resonance Imaging

MRI offers several advantages for imaging asbestos-related pleural disease, MPM in particular. In comparison to CT, high-resolution MRI can provide superior interobserver agreement for detection of pleural thickening, extrapleural fat, pleural effusion, and pleural plaques (although CT is superior for detecting calcification within plaques).[44] In the context of staging MPM, MRI has also been reported to be superior to CT for detecting tumor involvement of bone, interlobar fissures, diaphragm (particularly penetration through to peritoneum)[45], diaphragm muscle, and endothoracic fascia.[42] In general, however, the accuracy of clinical staging using CT and MRI is low, particularly for diagnosing lymph node metastases.[46] Nevertheless, these modalities are usually sufficient to detect advanced disease or potential early disease, and thus are sufficient to rule subsets of patients in or out of consideration for surgical treatment.

Positron Emission Tomography

PET holds promise to improve the accuracy of distinguishing tumor from adjacent normal structures based on a higher level of metabolic activity in tumor tissue. Indeed, early reports noted 94% accuracy for detecting MPM compared to 82% for CT,[47] although small lesions may be PET false-negative. Particularly relevant to patients being considered for surgical therapy, PET has been consistently found to identify extrathoracic metastases that were not recognized using other imaging modalities.[47–49] Consistent with increased PET sensitivity for metastasis, later stage disease (metastatic lesions, extrathoracic spread of tumor) is associated with increased metabolic activity relative to the primary lesion.[50] In this regard, PET may be particularly sensitive for restaging and monitoring for recurrence.

Despite these advantages, PET does not substantially improve the resolution of individual components of T classification, on account of its low anatomical resolution. The advent of integrated PET-CT has improved anatomic interpretation of PET findings, particularly for recognizing advanced stage,[51] but has not impacted the ability to accurately determine the patterns of invasion and breach of specific tissue planes by tumor that are critical to clinical staging. Early studies based on small patient cohorts suggested that PET may be useful to detect mediastinal lymph node metastasis.[49,52] Larger series, however, revealed that the sensitivity of PET for detecting nodal involvement is very low. Sorensen reported that PET-CT had 50% sensitivity and 75% specificity for detecting mediastinal nodal disease (67% accuracy, 17% overstaged, 17% understaged).[53] PET sensitivity for identifying chest wall or mediastinal T4 disease is likewise low (19%), and the maximal standard uptake value (SUV_{max}) is not indicative of T classification. Interestingly, SUV_{max} of the primary was found to correlate with a high likelihood of nodal metastasis,[48] but SUV_{max} and TNM stage were independently prognostic in a multivariate model.[54]

Positive PET findings must be interpreted with caution in patients who have undergone talc pleurodesis as areas of chronic granulomatous talc reaction are commonly PET avid.[55–57] The confounding effect of talc is sufficiently robust that a correction factor for prior talc pleurodesis was required in a prognostic nomogram that incorporates total glycolytic volume as measured by PET imaging.[58]

SURGICAL STAGING

Surgical staging involves obtaining tissue biopsies to assist in determining stage. These methods are more invasive, and most commonly undertaken when primary surgical resection is being considered and would be precluded by a positive biopsy. For example, mediastinoscopy is a common component of surgical staging because mediastinal lymph node involvement is usually taken as an indication for primary systemic therapy. Likewise, areas where there is suspicion of extrathoracic metastasis based on clinical staging may be biopsied via needle aspiration or video-assisted surgery. Current guidelines continue to recommend such procedures,[43] despite mixed reports concerning their accuracy.

Although cervical mediastinoscopy is thought to be more accurate than CT for determining mediastinal lymph node involvement,[37] it provides limited or no access to many mediastinal nodal stations. As a result, reports of the accuracy of the procedure have varied. Rice reported the sensitivity of cervical mediastinoscopy for mediastinal lymph node disease to be as low as 36%.[59] Correspondingly, studies in which mediastinoscopy is routinely performed to stage patients but not used to exclude them from surgery, have not found that the mediastinoscopy result is related to patient outcome.[18] Many authors continue to recommend routine mediastinoscopy despite low negative predictive value[2,20] particularly for patients with epithelial histology tumors based on the poor prognosis of patients who have superior N2-3 nodal metastasis.[15]

Several authors have advocated comprehensive minimally invasive surgical assessment for preoperative identification of advanced disease. Alvarez et al.[60] used contralateral thoracoscopy, laparoscopy, and mediastinoscopy and found disease outside the ipsilateral hemithorax that was not recognized by CT, MRI, and PET in 20% of a cohort of patients. Several authors advocate very aggressive surgical staging using combinations of esophageal ultrasound (EUS) and endobronchial ultrasound (EBUS) to sample stations 8, 9, and 10,[21,61,62] mediastinoscopy or transcervical extended mediastinal lymphadenectomy, and laparoscopy with abdominal lavage.[59,62] Among 18 patients with clinical stage I or II disease by CT, Zielinski et al.[62] found that 8 had involved mediastinal nodes, 8 had abdominal dissemination, and one had chest-wall invasion. Although cytology based on transdermal or endoscopic fine-needle aspiration may be nondiagnostic owing to loss of cellular architecture, molecular tests are being developed to supplement the analysis of aspirated specimens.[63]

PROGNOSTIC MODELS

The inadequacy of staging systems for determining the prognosis of individual patients with MPM has led to the development of a number of prognostic models, based on discerning the prognostic significance of clinical and pathologic factors in cohorts of patients. The European Organization for Research and Treatment of Cancer (EORTC) and the Cancer and Leukemia Group B (CALGB) each identified factors that were prognostic in pooled cohorts of patients treated on prospective chemotherapy treatment trials conducted by the respective groups.[64–66] Common factors identified in models as indicative of poor prognosis include poor performance status, nonepithelial histology, and advanced stage (stage IV). Among these, tumor histology is the only factor that is relevant to patients being considered for surgical resection, for which poor performance status and evidence of advanced disease are standard exclusion criteria.

In addition to histology, a number of demographic, historical, and clinical factors have been reported to have prognostic relevance to surgical MPM patients. These include age and gender,[67,68] CT-derived tumor volume,[30,69] preoperative anemia,[30] and tumor metabolic activity.[70,71] An early report by Benard and colleagues attempted to correlate PET SUV with survival in MPM based on a cut-off at the median value of 4. In this small series of 17 patients, the analysis was confounded in that high SUV patients also had predominantly biphasic and sarcomatoid histology tumors, suggesting that nonepithelial MPM may have higher metabolic activity.[70] However, Flores et al.[48,54] subsequently reported that SUV was not statistically related to histologic subtype, and that the two factors were independently prognostic.

The strong prognostic influence and the strikingly divergent clinical behavior of different tumor histologies have led some authors to stratify patient cohorts by histologic subtype when evaluating other potential prognostic factors. Nowak et al.[58] developed a prognostic nomogram combining weight loss and glycolytic volume (PET SUV integrated with tumor volume, with correction for prior pleurodesis) to predict outcome of patients with nonsarcomatous tumors. PET SUV alone did not significantly stratify survival in their cohort of patients primarily treated with chemotherapy, suggesting that tumor volume provides much of the prognostic information to the model. Gill et al.[30] found that among patients with epithelial tumors undergoing surgical resection, CT-derived tumor volume and preoperative anemia were independently prognostic. An algorithm based on these factors dramatically stratifies the overall survival of patients who have epithelial histology on pleural biopsy and subsequently undergo surgical resection, providing the basis for robust preoperative risk assessment independent of stage.[72] This risk assessment algorithm has been used to identify a homogeneous cohort of patients to assess the effects of specific treatment on survival, a utility which for most cancers is provided by stage.[73]

The success of prognostic models incorporating tumor volume suggests that incorporating this parameter into future staging system versions may provide a practical size criterion to augment T classification and improve staging accuracy. At the time that the prognostic value of tumor volume was originally described by Pass et al.,[69] the methodology for measuring volume using CT scans required specialized equipment and was too time-consuming to be clinically practical. Currently, the availability of FDA-approved commercial software allows volumetric measurements to be integrated with standard radiology workflow. The feasibility of doing so as a standard component of staging is currently being tested in a multi-institutional protocol organized by the IASLC MPM staging panel.

CONCLUSIONS

Apart from identifying overt extrathoracic metastasis, current clinical staging of MPM lacks accuracy in predicting the outcome of patients with MPM under consideration for primary surgical resection and multimodality management. PET-CT demonstrates incremental accuracy advantages over CT alone, but availability and cost considerations may limit its utility in specifying general standards for staging.

Additional surgical staging may be considered where there is suspicion of clinically occult metastatic disease, such as transdiaphragmatic extension or extrapleural lymph node involvement, although the value of routine mediastinoscopy remains controversial. Histologic subtype, tumor volume, preoperative anemia, and other stage-independent prognostic indicators may assist in discriminating risk among patients with apparently unilateral nonmetastatic disease who are otherwise fit for surgical resection.

EDITOR'S COMMENT

Cancer staging systems offer several interrelated benefits: understanding of the disease, guiding therapy, assessing the effectiveness of therapy, researching new treatments, and providing prognosis. Staging systems are traditionally based on the biologic progression of the tumor. One effective staging system is the T (tumor descriptor), N (nodal descriptor), and M (metastatic descriptor) system. In the case of mesothelioma, T is equivalent to local invasion, N correlates with mediastinal nodes, and M describes involvement of additional body cavities. The TNM staging system, however, has not been uniformly successful in guiding therapy and predicting prognosis of mesothelioma. Dr. Richards' work has broken away from the traditional TNM staging system to look at other clinical parameters that are statistically strongly linked with outcomes in this cancer. He describes these as prognostic models. A staging system based on prognostic models has the potential to better characterize homogeneous groups of the disease.

—Michael T. Jaklitsch

References

1. Patz EF Jr, Rusch VW, Heelan R. The proposed new international TNM staging system for malignant pleural mesothelioma: application to imaging. *AJR Am J Roentgenol.* 1996;166:323–327.
2. Pilling JE, Stewart DJ, Martin-Ucar AE, et al. The case for routine cervical mediastinoscopy prior to radical surgery for malignant pleural mesothelioma. *Eur J Cardiothorac Surg.* 2004;25:497–501.
3. Richards WG. Recent advances in mesothelioma staging. *Semin Thorac Cardiovasc Surg.* 2009;21:105–110.
4. Butchart EG, Ashcroft T, Barnsley WC, et al. Pleuropneumonectomy in the management of diffuse malignant mesothelioma of the pleura. Experience with 29 patients. *Thorax.* 1976;31:15–24.
5. Mattson K. Natural history and clinical stage of malignant mesothelioma. *Eur J Respir Dis.* 1982;63:87.
6. Sugarbaker DJ, Strauss GM, Lynch TJ, et al. Node status has prognostic significance in the multimodality therapy of diffuse, malignant mesothelioma. *J Clin Oncol.* 1993;11:1172–1178.
7. Sugarbaker DJ, Flores RM, Jaklitsch MT, et al. Resection margins, extrapleural nodal status, and cell type determine postoperative long-term survival in trimodality therapy of malignant pleural mesothelioma: results in 183 patients. *J Thorac Cardiovasc Surg.* 1999;117:54–63; discussion 63–65.
8. Chahinian AP. Therapeutic modalities in malignant pleural mesothelioma. In: Chretien J, Hirsch A, eds. *Diseases of the Pleura.* New York, NY: Masson; 1983:224–236.
9. International Union Against Cancer (UICC). In: Speissel B, Beahrs OH, Hermanek P, et al., eds. *TNM Atlas.* 3rd ed. Berlin: Springer; 1992.
10. Beahrs OH, Hensen DE, Hutter RVP, et al., eds. *AJCC Manual for Staging of Cancer.* 4th ed. Philadelphia, PA: J.B. Lippincott; 1992.
11. Rusch VW. A proposed new international TNM staging system for malignant pleural mesothelioma. From the International Mesothelioma Interest Group. *Chest.* 1995;108:1122–1128.
12. Byrne MJ, Nowak AK. Modified RECIST criteria for assessment of response in malignant pleural mesothelioma. *Ann Oncol.* 2004;15:257–260.
13. Boutin C, Rey F, Gouvernet J, et al. Thoracoscopy in pleural malignant mesothelioma: a prospective study of 188 consecutive patients. Part 2: Prognosis and staging. *Cancer.* 1993;72:394–404.
14. Hiroshima K, Yusa T, Kameya T, et al. Malignant pleural mesothelioma: clinicopathology of 16 extrapleural pneumonectomy patients with special reference to early stage features. *Pathol Int.* 2009;59:537–545.
15. Richards WG, Godleski JJ, Yeap BY, et al. Proposed adjustments to pathologic staging of epithelial malignant pleural mesothelioma based on analysis of 354 cases. *Cancer.* 2010;116:1510–1517.
16. Lester SL. *Manual of Surgical Pathology.* Boston, MA: Elsevier Churchill Livingstone; 2005.
17. Mountain CF, Dresler CM. Regional lymph node classification for lung cancer staging. *Chest.* 1997;111:1718–1723.
18. de Perrot M, Uy K, Anraku M, et al. Impact of lymph node metastasis on outcome after extrapleural pneumonectomy for malignant pleural mesothelioma. *J Thorac Cardiovasc Surg.* 2007;133:111–116.
19. Okiemy G, Foucault C, Avisse C, et al. Lymphatic drainage of the diaphragmatic pleura to the peritracheobronchial lymph nodes. *Surg Radiol Anat.* 2003;25:32–35.
20. Edwards JG, Stewart DJ, Martin-Ucar A, et al. The pattern of lymph node involvement influences outcome after extrapleural pneumonectomy for malignant mesothelioma. *J Thorac Cardiovasc Surg.* 2006;131:981–987.
21. Flores RM, Routledge T, Seshan VE, et al. The impact of lymph node station on survival in 348 patients with surgically resected malignant pleural mesothelioma: implications for revision of the American Joint Committee on Cancer staging system. *J Thorac Cardiovasc Surg.* 2008;136:605–610.
22. Abdel Rahman AR, Gaafar RM, Baki HA, et al. Prevalence and pattern of lymph node metastasis in malignant pleural mesothelioma. *Ann Thorac Surg.* 2008;86:391–395.
23. Nauta RJ, Osteen RT, Antman KH, et al. Clinical staging and the tendency of malignant pleural mesotheliomas to remain localized. *Ann Thorac Surg.* 1982;34:66–70.
24. Rusch VW, Piantadosi S, Holmes EC. The role of extrapleural pneumonectomy in malignant pleural mesothelioma. A Lung Cancer Study Group trial. *J Thorac Cardiovasc Surg.* 1991;102:1–9.
25. Baldini EH, Recht A, Strauss GM, et al. Patterns of failure after trimodality therapy for malignant pleural mesothelioma. *Ann Thorac Surg.* 1997;63:334–338.
26. Finn RS, Brims FJ, Gandhi A, et al. Post mortem findings of malignant pleural mesothelioma: a two-centre study of 318 patients. *Chest.* 2012;142:1267–1273.
27. Vogelzang NJ, Rusthoven JJ, Symanowski J, et al. Phase III study of pemetrexed in combination with cisplatin versus cisplatin alone in patients with malignant pleural mesothelioma. *J Clin Oncol.* 2003;21:2636–2644.
28. van Meerbeeck JP, Gaafar R, Manegold C, et al. Randomized phase III study of cisplatin with or without raltitrexed in patients with malignant pleural mesothelioma: an intergroup study of the European Organisation for Research and Treatment of Cancer Lung Cancer Group and the National Cancer Institute of Canada. *J Clin Oncol.* 2005;23:6881–6889.
29. Rusch VW, Giroux D, Kennedy C, et al. Initial analysis of the international association for the study of lung cancer mesothelioma database. *J Thorac Oncol.* 2012;7:1631–1639.
30. Gill RR, Richards WG, Yeap BY, et al. Epithelial malignant pleural mesothelioma after extrapleural pneumonectomy: stratification of survival with CT-derived tumor volume. *AJR Am J Roentgenol.* 2012;198:359–363.
31. Richards WG. Applicability of proposed TNM modifications to biphasic mesothelioma. In: 10th International Conference of the International Mesothelioma Interest Group. Kyoto, Japan; 2010.
32. Bueno R, Reblando J, Glickman J, et al. Pleural biopsy: a reliable method for determining the diagnosis but not subtype in mesothelioma. *Ann Thorac Surg.* 2004;78:1774–1776.
33. Kao SC, Yan TD, Lee K, et al. Accuracy of diagnostic biopsy for the histological subtype of malignant pleural mesothelioma. *J Thorac Oncol.* 2011;6:602–605.
34. Gill RR, Umeoka S, Mamata H, et al. Diffusion-weighted MRI of malignant pleural mesothelioma: preliminary assessment of apparent diffusion coefficient in histologic subtypes. *AJR Am J Roentgenol.* 2010;195:W125–W130.

35. Carden CP, Myerson JS, Popat S, et al. Good vibrations and the power of positron thinking: positron emission tomography and endoscopic ultrasound in staging of mesothelioma-two case reports. *J Thorac Oncol.* 2008;3:539–541.
36. Nakas A, Black E, Entwisle J, et al.. Surgical assessment of malignant pleural mesothelioma: have we reached a critical stage? *Eur J Cardiothorac Surg.* 2010;37:1457–1463.
37. Schouwink JH, Kool LS, Rutgers EJ, et al. The value of chest computer tomography and cervical mediastinoscopy in the preoperative assessment of patients with malignant pleural mesothelioma. *Ann Thorac Surg.* 2003;75:1715–1718; discussion 1718–1719.
38. Patz EF Jr, Shaffer K, Piwnica-Worms DR, et al. Malignant pleural mesothelioma: value of CT and MR imaging in predicting resectability. *AJR Am J Roentgenol.* 1992;159:961–966.
39. Rusch VW, Godwin JD, Shuman WP. The role of computed tomography scanning in the initial assessment and the follow-up of malignant pleural mesothelioma. *J Thorac Cardiovasc Surg.* 1988;96:171–177.
40. Ng CS, Munden RF, Libshitz HI. Malignant pleural mesothelioma: the spectrum of manifestations on CT in 70 cases. *Clin Radiol.* 1999;54:415–421.
41. Metintas M, Ucgun I, Elbek O, et al. Computed tomography features in malignant pleural mesothelioma and other commonly seen pleural diseases. *Eur J Radiol.* 2002;41:1–9.
42. Heelan RT, Rusch VW, Begg CB, et al. Staging of malignant pleural mesothelioma: comparison of CT and MR imaging. *AJR Am J Roentgenol.* 1999;172:1039–1047.
43. Stahel RA, Weder W, Lievens Y, et al. Malignant pleural mesothelioma: ESMO Clinical Practice Guidelines for diagnosis, treatment and follow-up. *Ann Oncol.* 2010;21(Suppl 5):v126–v128.
44. Weber MA, Bock M, Plathow C, et al. Asbestos-related pleural disease: value of dedicated magnetic resonance imaging techniques. *Invest Radiol.* 2004;39:554–564.
45. Knuuttila A, Halme M, Kivisaari L, et al. The clinical importance of magnetic resonance imaging versus computed tomography in malignant pleural mesothelioma. *Lung Cancer.* 1998;22:215–225.
46. Heelan R. Staging and response to therapy of malignant pleural mesothelioma. *Lung Cancer.* 2004;45 (Suppl 1):S59–S61.
47. Gerbaudo VH, Sugarbaker DJ, Britz-Cunningham S, et al. Assessment of malignant pleural mesothelioma with (18)F-FDG dual-head gamma-camera coincidence imaging: comparison with histopathology. *J Nucl Med.* 2002; 43:1144–1149.
48. Flores RM, Akhurst T, Gonen M, et al. Positron emission tomography defines metastatic disease but not locoregional disease in patients with malignant pleural mesothelioma. *J Thorac Cardiovasc Surg.* 2003;126:11–16.
49. Schneider DB, Clary-Macy C, Challa S, et al. Positron emission tomography with f18-fluorodeoxyglucose in the staging and preoperative evaluation of malignant pleural mesothelioma. *J Thorac Cardiovasc Surg.* 2000;120:128–133.
50. Gerbaudo VH, Britz-Cunningham S, Sugarbaker DJ, et al. Metabolic significance of the pattern, intensity and kinetics of 18 F-FDG uptake in malignant pleural mesothelioma. *Thorax.* 2003;58:1077–1082.
51. Erasmus JJ, Truong MT, Smythe WR, et al. Integrated computed tomography-positron emission tomography in patients with potentially resectable malignant pleural mesothelioma: staging implications. *J Thorac Cardiovasc Surg.* 2005;129:1364–1370.
52. Benard F, Sterman D, Smith RJ, et al. Metabolic imaging of malignant pleural mesothelioma with fluorodeoxyglucose positron emission tomography. *Chest.* 1998;114:713–722.
53. Sorensen JB, Ravn J, Loft A, et al. Preoperative staging of mesothelioma by 18 F-fluoro-2-deoxy-D-glucose positron emission tomography/computed tomography fused imaging and mediastinoscopy compared to pathological findings after extrapleural pneumonectomy. *Eur J Cardiothorac Surg.* 2008;34:1090–1096.
54. Flores RM, Akhurst T, Gonen M, et al. Positron emission tomography predicts survival in malignant pleural mesothelioma. *J Thorac Cardiovasc Surg.* 2006;132:763–768.
55. Kwek BH, Aquino SL, Fischman AJ. Fluorodeoxyglucose positron emission tomography and CT after talc pleurodesis. *Chest.* 2004;125:2356–2360.
56. Ahmadzadehfar H, Palmedo H, Strunk H, et al. False positive 18 F-FDG-PET/CT in a patient after talc pleurodesis. *Lung Cancer.* 2007;58:418–421.
57. Nguyen NC, Tran I, Hueser CN, et al. F-18 FDG PET/CT characterization of talc pleurodesis-induced pleural changes over time: a retrospective study. *Clin Nucl Med.* 2009;34:886–890.
58. Nowak AK, Francis RJ, Phillips MJ, et al. A novel prognostic model for malignant mesothelioma incorporating quantitative FDG-PET imaging with clinical parameters. *Clin Cancer Res.* 2010;16:2409–2417.
59. Rice DC, Erasmus JJ, Stevens CW, et al. Extended surgical staging for potentially resectable malignant pleural mesothelioma. *Ann Thorac Surg.* 2005;80:1988–1992; discussion 1992–1993.
60. Alvarez JM, Hasani A, Segal A, et al. Bilateral thoracoscopy, mediastinoscopy and laparoscopy, in addition to CT, MRI and PET imaging, are essential to correctly stage and treat patients with mesothelioma prior to trimodality therapy. *ANZ J Surg.* 2009;79:734–738.
61. Rice DC, Steliga MA, Stewart J, et al. Endoscopic ultrasound-guided fine needle aspiration for staging of malignant pleural mesothelioma. *Ann Thorac Surg.* 2009;88:862–868; discussion 868–869.
62. Zielinski M, Hauer J, Hauer L, et al. Staging algorithm for diffuse malignant pleural mesothelioma. *Interact Cardiovasc Thorac Surg.* 2010;10:185–189.
63. Bueno R. Making the case for molecular staging of malignant pleural mesothelioma. *Semin Thorac Cardiovasc Surg.* 2009;21:188–193.
64. Curran D, Sahmoud T, Therasse P, et al. Prognostic factors in patients with pleural mesothelioma: the European Organization for Research and Treatment of Cancer experience. *J Clin Oncol.* 1998;16:145–152.
65. Herndon JE, Green MR, Chahinian AP, et al. Factors predictive of survival among 337 patients with mesothelioma treated between 1984 and 1994 by the Cancer and Leukemia Group B. *Chest.* 1998;113:723–731.
66. Francart J, Vaes E, Henrard S, et al. A prognostic index for progression-free survival in malignant mesothelioma with application to the design of phase II trials: a combined analysis of 10 EORTC trials. *Eur J Cancer.* 2009;45:2304–2311.
67. Sugarbaker DJ, Wolf AS, Chirieac LR, et al. Clinical and pathological features of three-year survivors of malignant pleural mesothelioma following extrapleural pneumonectomy. *Eur J Cardiothorac Surg.* 2011;40:298–303.
68. Wolf AS, Richards WG, Tilleman TR, et al. Characteristics of malignant pleural mesothelioma in women. *Ann Thorac Surg.* 2010;90:949–956; discussion 956.
69. Pass HI, Temeck BK, Kranda K, et al. Preoperative tumor volume is associated with outcome in malignant pleural mesothelioma. *J Thorac Cardiovasc Surg.* 1998;115:310–317; discussion 317–318.
70. Benard F, Sterman D, Smith RJ, et al. Prognostic value of FDG PET imaging in malignant pleural mesothelioma. *J Nucl Med.* 1999;40:1241–1245.
71. Gerbaudo VH, Mamede M, Trotman-Dickenson B, et al. FDG PET/CT patterns of treatment failure of malignant pleural mesothelioma: relationship to histologic type, treatment algorithm, and survival. *Eur J Nucl Med Mol Imaging.* 2011;38:810–821.
72. Gill RR, Yeap BY, Matsuoka S, et al. Stage-independent pre-operative prognostic grouping of surgically-treated patients with epithelial malignant pleural mesothelioma. In: 14th World Conference on Lung Cancer. Amsterdam: Journal of Thoracic Oncology; 2011:S486–S487.
73. Sugarbaker DJ, Gill RR, Yeap BY, et al. Hyperthermic intraoperative pleural cisplatin chemotherapy extends interval to recurrence and survival among low-risk patients with malignant pleural mesothelioma undergoing surgical macroscopic complete resection. *J Thorac Cardiovasc Surg.* 2013;145:955–963.

117 Systemic Chemotherapy for Mesothelioma

David M. Jackman* and Leigh-Anne Cioffredi

Keywords: First line chemotherapy for malignant mesothelioma, second line chemotherapy options for malignant mesothelioma, chemotherapy as part of the multimodality paradigm for potentially resectable malignant mesothelioma, investigational therapies

INTRODUCTION

Mesothelioma is a rare malignancy arising from the mesothelial surfaces of the pleura, peritoneum, pericardium, or tunica vaginalis. There are roughly 2000 to 3000 new cases of mesothelioma annually in the United States.[1] Although the incidence of this disease peaked in the United States about a decade ago, its incidence in many other parts of the world continues to rise, particularly in regions without sufficient asbestos regulation.[2]

Even with aggressive multimodality therapy for seemingly localized disease, disease recurrence or progression occurs in the vast majority of cases. Effective systemic treatment options for mesothelioma are sorely needed. To date, there is only one agent—pemetrexed—that has received specific approval from the U.S. Food and Drug Administration (FDA) for the treatment of mesothelioma. The development of effective systemic therapies for patients with mesothelioma has faced several significant challenges.

The relatively low incidence of this cancer makes accrual to clinical trials—particularly large, randomized trials—challenging. In addition, the relative rarity of this cancer can dampen enthusiasm and limit funding from pharmaceutical companies and funding agencies. As a result, much of the clinical data in this disease consists of smaller, single-arm, investigator-initiated studies. Furthermore, comparisons of outcomes between these smaller studies are complicated by significant variability in staging systems among the trials, as well as by differences in the histologic composition of each trial, which consists of varying percentages of the three main histologic types of mesothelioma: epithelioid, sarcomatoid, and biphasic disease. Epithelioid histology consistently has been associated with a better prognosis. Therefore, differences in the histologic composition of each trial can confound useful comparisons between studies.

Another obstacle to determining treatment efficacy in mesothelioma is the assessment of tumor response: the applicability of standard Response Evaluation Criteria in Solid Tumors (RECIST) has been limited in mesothelioma, particularly with respect to serial assessments of the pleural rind. To address this problem, RECIST have been modified specifically for the assessment of mesothelioma (Table 117-1).[3]

Faced with these challenges and dissuaded by low response rates in early clinical trials of cytotoxic chemotherapy in mesothelioma, drug development in this disease had slowed. More recently, though, the clinical success of agents like pemetrexed and the preclinical activity of novel targeted agents have helped to spur a number of promising clinical trials and have offered a renewed sense of hope for patients suffering from this disease.

*Disclosure: Dr. Jackman is a consultant for Genentech and Foundation Medicine, Inc.

FIRST-LINE CHEMOTHERAPY IN UNRESECTABLE DISEASE

For patients with unresectable mesothelioma, combination with cisplatin plus pemetrexed is the standard first-line therapy and remains the only FDA-labeled treatment option in this disease. Though both cisplatin and antifolate agents were long known to have activity in this disease, the efficacy of this combination in mesothelioma was not demonstrated until 2003.

Cisplatin, an alkylating agent first described in 1845,[4] is an integral component of combination chemotherapy regimens in many cancer types. A meta-analysis of clinical trials reported between 1965 and 2001 highlights the activity of cisplatin in mesothelioma.[5] When used as a single agent, though, activity is modest. Experiences in other cancers had shown that cisplatin is best used in combination with other agents.

Antifolates were also long known to have some efficacy against mesothelioma. This class of agents was among the

Table 117-1

MODIFIED RESPONSE CRITERIA IN SOLID TUMORS (RECIST) FOR ASSESSMENT OF RESPONSE IN MALIGNANT PLEURAL MESOTHELIOMA[3]

Baseline Assessment

- Tumor thickness is measured perpendicular to the chest wall or mediastinum in two positions at three separate levels on transverse cuts of a computed tomography (CT) scan. Transverse cuts at least 1 cm apart and related to anatomical landmarks are used. The sum of these six measurements defines a pleural unidimensional measure.
- In addition, if there is traditionally, bidimensionally measurable disease, such as a lung nodule, the longest diameter of the lesion is measured.
- The total tumor measurement is established as the sum of the pleural unidimensional measure plus the longest diameters of traditionally measurable lesions.

Reassessment

- Pleural thickness is measured at the same position at the same level as on the baseline scans. A pleural unidimenisonal measurement is obtained as previously.
- As before, the total tumor measurement (sum of pleural unidimensional measurement plus the longest diameters of the traditionally measurable lesions) is obtained.

Criteria for Radiographic Response

- Complete response (CR): disappearance of all target lesions with no evidence of tumor elsewhere Partial response (PR): at least a 30% reduction in total tumor measurement. A confirmed response requires repeat observation on two separate occasions at least 4 weeks apart.
- Progressive disease (PD): increase of at least 20% in the total tumor measurement over the nadir measurement, or the appearance of one or more new lesions.
- Stable disease (SD): disease that does not fulfill criteria for either response or progression.

first chemotherapy agents to show activity in mesothelioma. Administration of high-dose methotrexate (3 g/m^2 every 10–21 days) with leucovorin rescue was associated with response in 22 of 60 patients evaluable for response (37%), with a median survival of 11 months.

The development of the multitargeted antifolate pemetrexed in the late 1990s and early 2000s would ultimately establish a new standard for systemic therapy in mesothelioma. This agent inhibits several key enzymes in purine and pyrimidine synthesis: thymidylate synthase, dihydrofolate reductase, and glycinamide ribonucleotide formyltransferase. In a large phase III trial, patients with previously untreated mesothelioma were randomized to receive cisplatin plus pemetrexed or cisplatin alone.[6] The addition of pemetrexed was associated with improvements in response (41.3% vs. 16.7%, $p < 0.0001$), median time to progression (TTP) (5.7 vs. 3.9 months, $p = 0.001$), and median overall survival (OS) (12.1 vs. 9.3 months, $p = 0.02$). The combination of cisplatin plus pemetrexed was generally well tolerated. Although there were three patient deaths in the combination therapy arm that were considered to be treatment-related, all occurred in patients who had not received supplementation with folic acid and vitamin B_{12}. There were no deaths in the vitamin-supplemented group. The most common grade 3 or 4 toxicities in the fully supplemented group included neutropenia (23.2%), nausea (11.9%), vomiting (10.7%), and fatigue (10.1%).

From these results, the combination of cisplatin plus pemetrexed has become the standard first-line therapy in mesothelioma. The agents are delivered intravenously once every 21 days: cisplatin 75 mg/m^2 and pemetrexed 500 mg/m^2. Patients should receive supplementation with vitamin B_{12} (1000 mcg intramuscularly starting 1 week before cycle 1 and then given every 9 weeks thereafter) and folic acid (400 mcg by mouth daily). In addition, patients also typically receive dexamethasone premedication (4 mg PO BID on the day before, day of, and day after chemotherapy) in order to prevent pemetrexed-associated rash. They also receive aggressive antiemetic therapy in light of the emetogenic potential of cisplatin. Restaging scans are recommended after every two to three cycles of treatment to monitor for progression. In the Vogelzang study, patients who tolerated therapy well and who achieved ongoing response or stable disease were continued on treatment. The median number of cycles of combination therapy received in that study was six (range 1–12), with only 7% of fully supplemented patients continuing on eight or more cycles of combination therapy.[6] In practice, the optimum length of therapy has not been established, though extrapolation from other tumor types such as non–small-cell lung cancer has led many investigators to stop combination treatment after four to six cycles.

For those patients whose age, overall condition, and/or medical comorbidities preclude the use of combination therapy with cisplatin plus pemetrexed, treatment with pemetrexed plus carboplatin or with pemetrexed monotherapy could be considered. Although there has been no trial that directly compares pemetrexed-based combinations with cisplatin versus carboplatin, useful data are available from phase II trials as well as from the International Extended Access Program. In a phase II trial of carboplatin plus pemetrexed, 19 out of 102 patients achieved a response (18.6%, 95% CI 11.6%–27.5%), with 48 patients (47%) achieving stable disease.[7] Median TTP was 6.5 months and median OS was 12.7 months, both comparable to the results seen with cisplatin plus pemetrexed in the Vogelzang study. In the Expanded Access Program, patients received carboplatin plus pemetrexed had a response rate of 21.7%, TTP of 6.9 months, and a 1-year survival of 64%.[8]

For those patients for whom combination chemotherapy with a platinum-based agent is deemed intolerable, pemetrexed monotherapy can be considered. A phase II study of pemetrexed monotherapy as well as data from the pemetrexed Expanded Access Program have provided insights into the activity of single-agent activity in mesothelioma. As a single agent, pemetrexed achieves response rates of about 10% to 12%, with median survivals of 10.7 to 14.1 months.[9,10]

SYSTEMIC CHEMOTHERAPY OPTIONS BEYOND FIRST-LINE

Pemetrexed Maintenance or Reinitiation

Just as the optimal duration of first-line therapy is not well established, the role of pemetrexed maintenance therapy is also an area of ongoing investigation. A small phase II study followed 27 patients with nonprogressing disease after six cycles of first-line therapy with a pemetrexed-containing combination. In this study, 13 patients received pemetrexed maintenance versus 14 who did not. Both TTP (8.5 vs. 3.4 months) and OS (17.9 vs. 6.0 months) favored those patients receiving pemetrexed maintenance. Furthermore, treatment was generally well tolerated, with fatigue (15%) as the only non-hematological grade 3 toxicity encountered. A randomized study of the role of maintenance therapy is currently ongoing.

For patients who had received a first-line regimen that did not contain pemetrexed, consideration should be given to pemetrexed as a second-line agent at the time of progression.[11,12] For patients whose disease recurs well after completing first-line therapy with a pemetrexed-containing combination and who had never progressed while on that therapy, physicians can consider reinitiating pemetrexed-based therapy. Though there is no specific trial exploring this indication, it is not unreasonable to return to pemetrexed, given the proven activity of the agent, the existing data for its use in the maintenance setting (see previous), and the general paucity of other commercially available systemic options in mesothelioma.

Other Cytotoxic Chemotherapeutics with Activity in Mesothelioma

Although there are no agents besides pemetrexed that have been specifically FDA-approved for the treatment of mesothelioma, there are existing, commercially available therapies with known activity in this tumor type. The two most commonly considered agents in patients who have progressed on pemetrexed-based therapy are vinorelbine and gemcitabine.

Vinorelbine

Vinorelbine, a semisynthetic vinca alkaloid, also has demonstrated activity against mesothelioma, alone or in combination. In a randomized trial, vinorelbine monotherapy had a response rate of 16% and demonstrated a trend toward improved median OS (9.5 months) compared with active symptom control alone (7.6 months) in previously untreated mesothelioma patients (HR 0.80, 95% CI 0.63%–1.02%; $p = 0.08$).[13] Had the trial not suffered from poor accrual, it might have ultimately attained sufficient power to show a statistically significant benefit for vinorelbine over active symptom control alone. Other phase II trials of vinorelbine monotherapy in mesothelioma have shown similar response rates (16%–24%) and median OSs (9.6–10.6months).[14,15]

Gemcitabine

Gemcitabine, an IV pyrimidine analog, has activity in mesothelioma, both as a single agent and as a part of combination therapy. An early trial of gemcitabine monotherapy reported a 31% response rate, with an additional 40% of patients experiencing significant symptomatic improvement in their disease; however, these results must be viewed with caution owing to the small trial size ($n = 23$) and a high percentage of patients with early-stage disease and epithelial histology.[16] Indeed, two other trials of gemcitabine monotherapy in mesothelioma delivered more sobering results: a multicenter Cancer and Leukemia Group B (CALGB) trial ($n = 17$) had no clinical responses and a median survival of only 4.7 months,[17] whereas a European trial ($n = 27$) showed a response rate of 7% and a median survival of 8 months.[18]

The sentiment for gemcitabine as an agent with clear activity in mesothelioma is perhaps better supported by outcomes exploring its use in combination with platinum. Response rates across six clinical trials that used combination therapy with gemcitabine plus cisplatin have varied from 12% to 48%, with median times to progression that have ranged from about 6 to 8 months.[19–24] In fact, a retrospective review of cases within British Columbia found no difference in median survival between patients treated with cisplatin plus pemetrexed and those treated with cisplatin plus gemcitabine.[25]

Anthracyclines

Along with methotrexate, doxorubicin was among the earliest agents to demonstrate activity in mesothelioma. Clinical trials of single-agent treatment with doxorubicin or epirubicin have demonstrated response rates ranging from 0% to 15%.[26–28] Although anthracycline-based combination regimens also have shown reasonable activity in this disease, cardiotoxicity concerns and the development of other less toxic agents (e.g., pemetrexed) have blunted enthusiasm for further investigation of the anthracyclines in mesothelioma.

CHEMOTHERAPY AS PART OF A MULTIMODALITY APPROACH TO POTENTIALLY RESECTABLE MESOTHELIOMA

Investigators across disciplines continue to explore the role of multimodality approaches in patients with potentially resectable mesothelioma. However, the specific target population, the exact nature and order of the interventions, and the extent of benefit of these aggressive approaches remain undefined. To this point, the only specific intervention that has ever been shown to prolong survival in mesothelioma in a randomized trial is chemotherapy with pemetrexed and cisplatin for patients with unresectable disease. This should not dampen our enthusiasm for exploring newer and better ways of treating localized disease in mesothelioma. Rather, it should challenge us to devise and conduct focused clinical trials to refine our interventions and define our target populations more closely.

Chemotherapy is the only modality ever shown to prolong survival in any randomized trial in mesothelioma. As a consequence, it is considered an important part of multimodality approaches. Based on the experiences in unresectable disease, pemetrexed plus cisplatin is the most common regimen used for localized therapy. Although there are no clinical trials to address whether this is best given before or after surgery, many prospective clinical trials that incorporate chemotherapy have used it neoadjuvantly. In non–small-cell lung cancer, patients were more likely to complete chemotherapy and chemotherapy was more easily tolerated when given neoadjuvantly rather than postoperatively.[29] When one considers the relatively greater potential morbidity of extrapleural pneumonectomy (EPP) for mesothelioma, concerns about tolerability become even more important.

In addition, analysis from a prospective multicenter phase II trial of multimodality therapy suggests that initial response to neoadjuvant chemotherapy may be the most important predictor of survival in patients undergoing trimodality therapy. Seventy-seven patients with T1-3 N0-2 mesothelioma were prospectively enrolled in a trial of four planned cycles of cisplatin plus pemetrexed.[30] Patients with nonprogressing disease then underwent EPP, followed by hemithoracic radiation. Eighty-three percent of patients completed all four cycles of chemotherapy, with an overall response rate of 32.5% (95% CI, 22.2–44.1). Fifty-seven patients proceeded to the operating room, with 54 patients undergoing EPP. Forty-four patients received hemithoracic postoperative radiation, with 40 completing the full planned course. In the context of this planned aggressive approach, median survival in the overall study population was only 16.8 months (95% CI, 13.6 – 23.2 months; censorship, 33.8%). However, it appeared that there was clearly a subset of patients who were more likely to benefit: the 2-year survival on the trial was 37%, and 20% of patients were estimated to live at least 3 years. Univariate analysis of multiple patient and disease factors showed that the only factor associated with prolonged survival was radiologic response to initial chemotherapy. In patients who achieved a complete or partial response to chemotherapy, the median survival was 26 months, whereas those patients who had only stable disease or progressive disease on chemotherapy had a median survival of 13.9 months ($p = 0.05$). Furthermore, patients who were able to complete all three modalities ($n = 40$) had a median survival of 29.1 months and a 2-year survival rate of 61.2%.

With this in mind, if (1) neoadjuvant chemotherapy might be more tolerable than adjuvant treatment and might, therefore, increase the chance of completing all three modalities, and (2) upfront chemotherapy has a potentially prognostic value in determining who might best benefit from aggressive trimodality therapy, it is reasonable to consider chemotherapy upfront for patients with potentially resectable mesothelioma who are being considered for multimodality treatment.

INVESTIGATIONAL THERAPIES

Angiogenesis Inhibition

The potential role of antiangiogenic agents in mesothelioma has provoked significant interest. Preclinical work has detected vascular endothelial growth factor (VEGF) and its receptors VEGFR1 and VEGFR2 in a majority of mesothelioma tumor specimens.[31–33] Moreover, VEGF has been found to stimulate the proliferation of mesothelioma cells *in vitro*, and this growth can be inhibited by the use of purified rabbit polyclonal antibodies targeting VEGF.[33]

Bevacizumab, a humanized monoclonal antibody directed against VEGF, has been shown to increase survival when used in combination therapy in patients with metastatic colon cancer[34] and non–small-cell lung cancer,[35] and it has been shown to prolong TTP in patients with metastatic breast cancer.[36] To study its use in mesothelioma, a phase II trial randomized previously untreated patients to receive cisplatin plus gemcitabine, with or without bevacizumab.[22] The addition of bevacizumab did not result in significant improvements in either response (25% vs. 22%), median progression free survival (PFS) (6.9 vs. 6.0 months), or median OS (15.6 vs. 14.7 months) compared with chemotherapy alone. Subset analysis did show a correlation between higher baseline plasma VEGF levels and shorter PFS and OS, suggesting a basis for further inquiry of bevacizumab in a more selected population.

Cediranib, an oral small molecule inhibitor of VEGF, has also been studied in mesothelioma. In a phase II trial of cediranib in 47 evaluable patients with mesothelioma that had progressed after first-line chemotherapy, four patients had partial responses and 16 patients had stable disease, (disease control rate 42%), with median PFS of 2.6 months and median OS of 9.5 months. [37] A phase I/II trial of cediranib in combination with cisplatin plus pemetrexed as first-line systemic therapy in patients with mesothelioma is currently underway (NCT01064648).

Multitargeted small molecule tyrosine kinase inhibitors (TKIs) with anti-VEGF activity also have been investigated in mesothelioma. Vatalanib, an oral anilinophthalazine that targets VEGFR1 and 2, c-KIT, platelet-derived growth factor receptor (PDGFR), and c-Fms, has been studied in a small phase II trial in previously untreated patients with mesothelioma ($n = 47$).[38] Although there were five objective responses (RR 11%) and median PFS was 4.1 months, the 3-month PFS (55%) did not meet a prespecified primary endpoint of 75%.

Sorafenib, an oral inhibitor of VEGFR2 and 3, ref, PDGFR, and c-KIT, has been studied in a phase II trial for both chemotherapy-naive and previously treated patients with mesothelioma.[39] Although the response rate in this trial was only 4%, the 3-month PFS was 78% and median PFS was 3.7 months, with a median OS of 10.7 months.

In a phase II trial of sunitinib, patients who had progressed after 1 prior therapy received second-line treatment with this oral inhibitor of VEGFR1–3, PDGFR, and c-Kit.[40] Among 22 assessable patients, there were three responses (RR 15%), with a median TTP of 3.5 months and a median OS of 5.9 months. In the face of limited activity for these agents, there are no current plans to develop these agents further in mesothelioma.

Histone Deacetylase Inhibition

Histones serve as a protein spool around which DNA is wound; the wrapping and unwrapping of DNA about these central histones are regulated by histone acetyltransferases and histone deacetylases (HDACs). Inhibitors of HDAC can alter access of transcription factors to DNA, thereby causing increased expression of some genes but repression of others.[41–43] In a phase I trial of vorinostat, an oral HDAC inhibitor, there were 13 patients with mesothelioma. Of these, two patients had objective response to vorinostat monotherapy (RR 15%), and six patients remained on therapy for more than 4 months.[44] From signals of activity for this agent in mesothelioma, an international phase III trial is underway in which patients who have progressed after prior pemetrexed-containing therapy are randomized to receive vorinostat or placebo (NCT00128102).

Anti-Mesothelin Antibodies

Mesothelin is a glycosyl-phosphatidyl inositol-linked (GPI-anchor) cytoplasmic membrane glycoprotein thought to be involved in cell adhesion and is tightly associated with a range of cancers, including mesothelioma.[45] Three anti-mesothelin agents are in clinical development: Morab-009 is a monoclonal anti-mesothelin antibody,[46] SS1P is an anti-mesothelin antibody with a conjugated toxin (*Pseudomonas* exotoxin A),[47] whereas CRS-207 is a mesothelin vaccine derived from attenuated *Listeria monocytogenes* and intended to elicit an antibody response against surface mesothelin.[48] By targeting surface mesothelin, investigators hope to block cell adhesion as well as elicit an antibody-dependent cytotoxicity response against mesothelin-positive tumor cells.[46,49] Separate phase II trials of MORAb-009 (NCT00738582) and SS1P (NCT01445392) in combination with cisplatin plus pemetrexed have completed accrual, but no results have yet been released. A phase I trial of CRS-207 monotherapy has completed accrual, though it appears that its sponsor will be focusing its development in pancreatic cancer at this time.

Other Targets of Interest

In addition to the work mentioned previously, there are ongoing efforts in mesothelioma exploring the efficacy of mammalian target of rapamycin (mTOR) inhibition (NCT00770120), G2 checkpoint abrogation (NCT00700336), human tumor necrosis factor-α (hTNF-α) (NCT01098266), and vaccines targeting the Wilms tumor suppressor gene (WT1) (NCT01265433). Although it is too early to determine the role that these agents will have in the standard treatment of patients with mesothelioma, it is encouraging to see the investment in clinical drug development and infrastructure in this disease.

CONCLUSIONS

Although current systemic treatment options for mesothelioma are limited, many novel agents are being investigated. At this time, first-line therapy with cisplatin plus pemetrexed remains the standard of care. In addition, both gemcitabine and vinorelbine have demonstrated activity in this disease, alone or in combination with cisplatin, and their use is worthy of consideration in patients with mesothelioma who have progressed after pemetrexed-based therapy. Newer agents aimed at the inhibition of targets such as VEGF or HDAC are undergoing further investigation. Despite the modest early clinical results, the use of clinical or biological markers to select a more appropriate treatment group may ultimately result in better outcomes in such refined populations. Additional clinical trials of these and other agents are needed to provide more and better treatment options for patients with mesothelioma, and a greater commitment is required to identify and enroll patients with this disease into appropriate clinical trials.

EDITOR'S COMMENT

The study of mesothelioma in specialized medical centers in the 1980s initiated the search for effective chemotherapy for this diffuse disease of the pleura. The search for a systemic drug has been hampered by the infrequency of the disease (only 3000 cases per year in the United States) and by the inability to accrue homogeneous groups in timely fashion to prospective trials (i.e., groups with mixed histologies or mixed stages). Finally, the variability of staging systems also has hampered the collection of large groups for data analysis. The take-home message of this chapter regarding chemotherapy and mesothelioma is disappointingly simple: few chemotherapeutic agents are effective at this time. Only one drug, the antifolate, pemetrexed, has received FDA approval for malignant mesothelioma. First-line therapy is cis-platinum plus pemetrexed. Although other investigational drugs have been disappointing, to date, many novel agents are being investigated. Historically, chemotherapy was anticipated to have the best probability of success for malignant mesothelioma. The diffuse nature of the disease was thought to preclude surgical therapy. Today, the diffuse nature of the disease requires combinations of multiple modalities of treatment.

—Michael T. Jaklitsch

References

1. Price B, Ware A. Mesothelioma trends in the United States: an update based on Surveillance, Epidemiology, and End Results Program data for 1973 through 2003. *Am J Epidemiol.* 2004;159:107–112.
2. Peto J, Decarli A, La Vecchia C, et al. The European mesothelioma epidemic. *Br J Cancer.* 1999;79:666–672.
3. Byrne MJ, Nowak AK. Modified RECIST criteria for assessment of response in malignant pleural mesothelioma. *Ann Oncol.* 2004;15:257–260.
4. Peyrone M. Ueber die Einwirkung des Ammoniaks auf Platinchlorur. *Ann Chemie Pharm.* 1844;51:1–29.
5. Berghmans T, Paesmans M, Lalami Y, et al. Activity of chemotherapy and immunotherapy on malignant mesothelioma: a systematic review of the literature with meta-analysis. *Lung Cancer.* 2002;38:111–121.
6. Vogelzang NJ, Rusthoven JJ, Symanowski J, et al. Phase III study of pemetrexed in combination with cisplatin versus cisplatin alone in patients with malignant pleural mesothelioma. *J Clin Oncol.* 2003;21:2636–2644.
7. Ceresoli GL, Zucali PA, Favaretto AG, et al. Phase II study of pemetrexed plus carboplatin in malignant pleural mesothelioma. *J Clin Oncol.* 2006;24:1443–1448.
8. Santoro A, O'Brien ME, Stahel RA, et al. Pemetrexed plus cisplatin or pemetrexed plus carboplatin for chemonaive patients with malignant pleural mesothelioma: results of the International Expanded Access Program. *J Thorac Oncol.* 2008;3:756–763.
9. Scagliotti GV, Shin DM, Kindler HL, et al. Phase II study of pemetrexed with and without folic acid and vitamin B12 as front-line therapy in malignant pleural mesothelioma. *J Clin Oncol.* 2003;21:1556–1561.
10. Taylor P, Castagneto B, Dark G, et al. Single-agent pemetrexed for chemonaive and pretreated patients with malignant pleural mesothelioma: results of an International Expanded Access Program. *J Thorac Oncol.* 2008;3:764–771.
11. Janne PA, Wozniak AJ, Belani CP, et al. Pemetrexed alone or in combination with cisplatin in previously treated malignant pleural mesothelioma: outcomes from a phase IIIB expanded access program. *J Thorac Oncol.* 2006;1:506–512.
12. Jassem J, Ramlau R, Santoro A, et al. Phase III trial of pemetrexed plus best supportive care compared with best supportive care in previously treated patients with advanced malignant pleural mesothelioma. *J Clin Oncol.* 2008;26:1698–1704.
13. Muers MF, Stephens RJ, Fisher P, et al. Active symptom control with or without chemotherapy in the treatment of patients with malignant pleural mesothelioma (MS01): a multicentre randomised trial. *Lancet.* 2008;371:1685–1694.
14. Stebbing J, Powles T, McPherson K, et al. The efficacy and safety of weekly vinorelbine in relapsed malignant pleural mesothelioma. *Lung Cancer.* 2009;63:94–97.
15. Steele JP, Shamash J, Evans MT, et al. Phase II study of vinorelbine in patients with malignant pleural mesothelioma. *J Clin Oncol.* 2000;18:3912–3917.
16. Bischoff HG, Manegold C, Knopp M, et al. Gemcitabine (Gemzar) may reduce tumor load and tumor associated symptoms in malignant pleural mesothelioma. *Proc Am Soc Clin Oncol.* 1998;17: abstract 1784.
17. Kindler HL, Millard F, Herndon JE, 2nd, et al. Gemcitabine for malignant mesothelioma: A phase II trial by the Cancer and Leukemia Group B. *Lung Cancer.* 2001;31:311–317.
18. van Meerbeeck JP, Baas P, Debruyne C, et al. A Phase II study of gemcitabine in patients with malignant pleural mesothelioma. European Organization for Research and Treatment of Cancer Lung Cancer Cooperative Group. *Cancer.* 1999;85:2577–2582.
19. Byrne MJ, Davidson JA, Musk AW, et al. Cisplatin and gemcitabine treatment for malignant mesothelioma: a phase II study. *J Clin Oncol.* 1999;17:25–30.
20. Castagneto B, Zai S, Dongiovanni D, et al. Cisplatin and gemcitabine in malignant pleural mesothelioma: a phase II study. *Am J Clin Oncol.* 2005;28:223–226.
21. Kalmadi SR, Rankin C, Kraut MJ, et al. Gemcitabine and cisplatin in unresectable malignant mesothelioma of the pleura: a phase II study of the Southwest Oncology Group (SWOG 9810). *Lung Cancer.* 2008;60:259–263.
22. Karrison T, Kindler HL, Gandara DR, et al. Final analysis of a multi-center, double-blinded, placebo-controlled, randomized phase II trial of gemcitabine/cisplatin (GC) plus bevacizumab (B) or placebo (P) in patients (pts) with malignant mesothelioma (MM). *J Clin Oncol.* 2007;25:391s. In: ASCO; 2007.
23. Nowak AK, Byrne MJ, Williamson R, et al. A multicentre phase II study of cisplatin and gemcitabine for malignant mesothelioma. *Br J Cancer.* 2002;87:491–496.
24. van Haarst JM, Baas P, Manegold C, et al. Multicentre phase II study of gemcitabine and cisplatin in malignant pleural mesothelioma. *Br J Cancer.* 2002;86:342–345.
25. Lee CW, Murray N, Anderson H, et al. Outcomes with first-line platinum based combination chemotherapy for malignant pleural mesothelioma: a review of practice in British Columbia. *Lung Cancer.* 2009;64:308–313.
26. Magri MD, Veronesi A, Foladore S, et al. Epirubicin in the treatment of malignant mesothelioma: a phase II cooperative study. The North-Eastern Italian Oncology Group (GOCCNE)–Mesothelioma Committee. *Tumori.* 1991;77:49–51.
27. Mattson K, Giaccone G, Kirkpatrick A, et al. Epirubicin in malignant mesothelioma: a phase II study of the European Organization for Research and Treatment of Cancer Lung Cancer Cooperative Group. *J Clin Oncol.* 1992;10:824–828.
28. Sorensen PG, Bach F, Bork E, et al. Randomized trial of doxorubicin versus cyclophosphamide in diffuse malignant pleural mesothelioma. *Cancer Treat Rep.* 1985;69:1431–1432.
29. Felip E, Rosell R, Maestre JA, et al. Preoperative chemotherapy plus surgery versus surgery plus adjuvant chemotherapy versus surgery alone in early-stage non-small-cell lung cancer. *J Clin Oncol.* 2010;28:3138–3145.
30. Krug LM, Pass HI, Rusch VW, et al. Multicenter phase II trial of neoadjuvant pemetrexed plus cisplatin followed by extrapleural pneumonectomy and radiation for malignant pleural mesothelioma. *J Clin Oncol.* 2009;27:3007–3013.
31. Konig J, Tolnay E, Wiethege T, et al. Co-expression of vascular endothelial growth factor and its receptor flt-1 in malignant pleural mesothelioma. *Respiration.* 2000;67:36–40.
32. Konig JE, Tolnay E, Wiethege T, et al. Expression of vascular endothelial growth factor in diffuse malignant pleural mesothelioma. *Virchows Arch.* 1999;435:8–12.
33. Strizzi L, Catalano A, Vianale G, et al. Vascular endothelial growth factor is an autocrine growth factor in human malignant mesothelioma. *J Pathol.* 2001;193:468–475.

34. Hurwitz H, Fehrenbacher L, Novotny W, et al. Bevacizumab plus irinotecan, fluorouracil, and leucovorin for metastatic colorectal cancer. *N Engl J Med.* 2004;350:2335–2342.
35. Sandler A, Gray R, Perry MC, et al. Paclitaxel-carboplatin alone or with bevacizumab for non-small-cell lung cancer. *N Engl J Med.* 2006;355:2542–2550.
36. Miller K, Wang M, Gralow J, et al. Paclitaxel plus bevacizumab versus paclitaxel alone for metastatic breast cancer. *N Engl J Med.* 2007;357:2666–2676.
37. Garland LL, Chansky K, Wozniak AJ, et al. Phase II study of cediranib in patients with malignant pleural mesothelioma: SWOG S0509. *J Thorac Oncol.* 2011;6:1938–1945.
38. Jahan TM, Gu L, Wang X, et al. Vatalanib (V) for patients with previously untreated advanced malignant mesothelioma (MM): a phase II study by the Cancer and Leukemia Group B (CALGB 30107). In: ASCO; 2006.
39. Dubey S, Janne PA, Krug L, et al. A phase II study of sorafenib in malignant mesothelioma: results of Cancer and Leukemia Group B 30307. *J Thorac Oncol.* 2010;5(10):1655–1661.
40. Nowak AK, Millward MJ, Francis R, et al. Phase II study of sunitinib as second-line therapy in malignant pleural mesothelioma (MPM). In: ASCO; 2008.
41. Coffey DC, Kutko MC, Glick RD, et al. Histone deacetylase inhibitors and retinoic acids inhibit growth of human neuroblastoma in vitro. *Med Pediatr Oncol.* 2000;35:577–581.
42. Marks PA, Richon VM, Rifkind RA. Histone deacetylase inhibitors: inducers of differentiation or apoptosis of transformed cells. *J Natl Cancer Inst.* 2000;92:1210–1216.
43. Richon VM, Sandhoff TW, Rifkind RA, et al. Histone deacetylase inhibitor selectively induces p21WAF1 expression and gene-associated histone acetylation. *Proc Natl Acad Sci U S A.* 2000;97:10014–10019.
44. Krug LM, Curley T, Schwartz L, et al. Potential role of histone deacetylase inhibitors in mesothelioma: clinical experience with suberoylanilide hydroxamic acid. *Clin Lung Cancer.* 2006;7:257–261.
45. Chang K, Pastan I. Molecular cloning of mesothelin, a differentiation antigen present on mesothelium, mesotheliomas, and ovarian cancers. *Proc Natl Acad Sci U S A.* 1996;93:136–140.
46. Hassan R, Ebel W, Routhier EL, et al. Preclinical evaluation of MORAb-009, a chimeric antibody targeting tumor-associated mesothelin. *Cancer Immun.* 2007;7:20.
47. Li Q, Verschraegen CF, Mendoza J, et al. Cytotoxic activity of the recombinant anti-mesothelin immunotoxin, SS1(dsFv)PE38, towards tumor cell lines established from ascites of patients with peritoneal mesotheliomas. *Anticancer Res.* 2004;24:1327–1335.
48. Hassan R, Ho M. Mesothelin targeted cancer immunotherapy. *Eur J Cancer.* 2008;44:46–53.
49. Thomas AM, Santarsiero LM, Lutz ER, et al. Mesothelin-specific CD8(+) T cell responses provide evidence of in vivo cross-priming by antigen-presenting cells in vaccinated pancreatic cancer patients. *J Exp Med.* 2004;200:297–306.

118 Radiation Therapy for Mesothelioma

Elizabeth H. Baldini

Keywords: Mesothelioma, radiation therapy, intensity modulated radiation therapy (IMRT), electron-photon technique (EPT)

RADIATION THERAPY FOR MALIGNANT PLEURAL MESOTHELIOMA

Treatment of malignant pleural mesothelioma with radiation therapy (RT) is extremely challenging. The target volume for treatment is very large, involving almost the entire hemithorax, and within and adjacent to this treatment volume, there are many normal structures with low tolerances to radiation. Consequently, it is very difficult to create treatment plans that deliver satisfactorily high doses to the complex target volume yet minimal doses to the adjacent radiosensitive normal organs. This chapter will review the history, current approaches, and future ideas for the treatment of pleural mesothelioma with radiotherapy in definitive, adjuvant, and palliative settings.

Definitive Radiation Therapy Alone for Mesothelioma

For the treatment of unresected gross disease, the target volume for RT includes the entire visceral and parietal pleura of one lung. These structures form a circumferential envelope around the lung, extend along fissures between lobes of the lung, and are attached to ipsilateral, pericardial, and diaphragmatic surfaces. A tumoricidal dose of RT for gross disease is >60 Gy, but the normal tissue tolerance of the adjacent organs is much lower. Whole organ tolerances for these structures are as follows: lung, 18 to 20 Gy; heart, 40 Gy; liver, 30 Gy; stomach, 50 Gy; kidney, 18 to 20 Gy; spinal cord, 45 to 50 Gy; and brachial plexus, 50 Gy.[1]

Few reported series address the definitive treatment of unresected pleural mesothelioma, and none show promising results. In 1988, Alberts et al.[2] reported outcome for 262 patients treated with various combinations of RT, pleurectomy, and chemotherapy. RT was delivered to the entire hemithorax with doses of 45 to 80 Gy. All treatment groups had similar outcomes, with a median survival time of 9.6 months; the stepwise addition of treatment modalities was not associated with improved survival. No toxicity data were described. The authors concluded that new agents and approaches were warranted.

In 1990, Ball and Cruickshank[3] reported on a series of 35 patients treated with RT at the Peter MacCallum Institute, 12 of whom received "radical RT." Treatment comprised 40 Gy to the entire hemithorax using AP–PA fields, after which the spinal cord was blocked and the treatment continued to a total dose of 50 Gy. An anterior cardiac block was used for left-sided tumors to limit heart dose to 40 Gy; no shielding was used for lung, liver, or kidney. There were two treatment-related fatalities (17%) due to radiation hepatitis and radiation myelopathy, respectively. Median survival time was 9 months. The authors concluded that there is no role for radical RT given the unacceptable toxicity and lack of demonstrated efficacy.

A third report by Maasilta[4] in 1991, included 34 patients with unresected mesothelioma who were treated to the entire hemithorax with three different high-dose regimens. The spinal cord was shielded after 40 Gy, the liver was partially shielded after 30 Gy, and there was no shielding of the intact lung. The three dose regimens were: 55 Gy in 2.2-Gy fractions (split course) to the hemithorax followed by a boost to gross disease to 70 Gy; 70 Gy to the hemithorax in 1.25-Gy twice-daily fractions (split course); and 35 Gy in 1.25-Gy twice-daily fractions to the hemithorax, with a boost to gross disease using 4-Gy fractions to a total dose of 71 Gy. Radiographic and clinical lung injuries were progressive in all groups and scored as severe by 6 months, very severe by 9 months and compatible with total loss of ipsilateral lung function by 12 months. No local control data were reported.

An interesting recent study from Heidelberg describes experience with "palliative RT" using the modern technique of *intensity modulated radiation therapy* (IMRT).[5] IMRT refers to an advanced RT delivery technique which can achieve more conformal dose distributions around complex target volumes. IMRT divides the RT treatment fields into multiple subfields of varying dose intensities. By using many treatment angles and modulating the beam intensity across apertures, it is possible to partially shield parts of the target volume near a critical structure (and decrease the dose to the normal structure). The end result is a fairly homogeneous dose distribution to the target and shaping of the high-dose lines around and away from surrounding critical structures. The Heidelberg group treated 11 patients with IMRT to target volumes including all gross tumor to doses of 40 to 50 Gy. All patients in that report had recurrent disease at the time of RT, after prior surgery and/or chemotherapy, so the patient group is not directly comparable to those in the above accounts. Median survival following RT was 5 months. Given the small patient number and poor outcome, it is not possible to assess the efficacy or toxicity of this approach. Currently, data are lacking to support RT alone as definitive treatment for mesothelioma and this is not a recommended approach.

Adjuvant Radiation Therapy for Mesothelioma

Adjuvant Radiation Therapy Following Pleurectomy

The delivery of curative adjuvant RT after pleurectomy poses many of the same problems as stated earlier for definitive treatment without resection—namely, it is very difficult to deliver a tumoricidal dose of RT to the complex target of the pleural envelope and fissures given the proximity of many radiosensitive normal structures, including the intact lung.

Several reports of RT after pleurectomy have shown only fair results. The group at Memorial Sloan–Kettering Cancer Center (MSKCC) pioneered a technique using a combination of photons and electrons to treat the hemithorax after pleurectomy.[6,7] The technique consists of treating anterior and posterior photon fields to cover the entire hemithorax and using blocks to protect lung, heart, liver, and stomach. The blocked areas are treated with superficial electrons matched to the photon fields and prescribed to a depth that covers the underlying pleura. Total dose is 42.5 to 45 Gy. This technique is very appealing in theory but, in reality, the cumulative dose distribution is not homogeneous; the result is that some portions of the target volume receive more and some less than the prescription dose, due to imperfect matching of photon and electron fields and other technical factors. Clinical results of patients treated in this fashion initially appeared promising, but an update of 123 patients showed a median survival time of only 13.5 months and 28% had grade 3 to 4 toxicity.[6,8] The authors concluded that this technique of adjuvant RT following pleurectomy is not effective.

Three other studies included subsets of patients treated with pleurectomy and adjuvant radiation. However, the informative value of these studies is limited as treatment and outcome details with respect to RT are not well described.[9–11] Investigators from the University of California at San Francisco reported results for 24 patients treated with pleurectomy followed by a combination of intraoperative electron therapy (median, 15 Gy) and postoperative photon therapy delivered with either a 3-dimensional (3D) conformal approach or IMRT (median, 41.4 Gy).[12] The intraoperative electrons were used to treat the major fissure, pericardium and diaphragm with the goal of improving target coverage and sparing underlying lung. Treatment-related toxicity was considered acceptable and included transient pneumonitis for four patients (17%), pericarditis for one (4%), and esophageal stricture requiring dilatation for one (4%). Median survival time was 18 months.

The use of IMRT in the post pleurectomy setting is potentially appealing. In 2002, Tobler et al.[13] reported on a proposed rotational IMRT technique in which each of multiple beams treats a strip of pleural lining. The resulting dosimetry from this idealized technique showed homogeneous coverage of the circumferential pleural surface. This IMRT approach was considered to be superior to the matched electron–photon technique (EPT) reported by Kutcher et al.,[7] showing both more uniform dose distribution and better sparing of underlying lung. However, this technique does not address treatment of the pleural reflections along the fissures. Rosenzweig et al. at MSKCC have treated 36 patients with IMRT to a median dose of 46.8 Gy, 20 of whom had undergone prior pleurectomy. Results are still preliminary, but acute toxicity has been acceptable.[14] In sum, adjuvant RT following pleurectomy or decortication is associated with moderate toxicity and unclear efficacy. It is not standardly recommended but is worthy of further study.

Adjuvant Radiation Therapy following Extrapleural Pneumonectomy (EPP)

Similar to the above scenarios, the role for adjuvant RT following extrapleural pneumonectomy (EPP) has not been clearly proven. However, there is suggestive evidence in the literature that RT may improve local control in this setting. Local recurrence (LR) rates following EPP alone are as high as 50%, whereas several reports of EPP and postoperative RT have demonstrated LR rates ranging from 16% to 40%.[15–25] Furthermore, Baldini et al.[16] reported a trend for decreased LR among patients who underwent EPP and received adjuvant RT compared to those who did not (9% vs. 27%, respectively). De Perrot et al.[26] also demonstrated that among patients treated with induction chemotherapy and EPP, the use of postoperative RT was associated with lower LR rates. In that study, among patients with N2 disease, LR occurred in 1/11 patients (9%) who received RT compared to 5/9 (56%) who did not; this finding was statistically significant on multivariate analysis. Lastly, in a homogeneous cohort of 88 patients with epithelial mesothelioma who underwent EPP ± chemotherapy at Brigham and Women's Hospital (BWH), the use of postoperative RT was a statistically significant favorable prognostic factor on multivariate analysis (W. G. Richards, personal communication). It is important to note that none of the above reports were randomized comparisons and, as such, all are subject to potential bias. Nonetheless, the data is suggestive of a potential benefit due to adjuvant RT.

In the post EPP setting the absence of the ipsilateral lung simplifies the radiation treatment planning compared to the post pleurectomy/decortication setting, in which the intact lung is in place. Despite this advantage, the design and implementation of RT to the large complex target volume of the hemithorax remains very challenging. Critical remaining normal structures within and adjacent to the target volume include heart, liver, stomach, kidneys, spinal cord, and contralateral lung. Three types of RT techniques following EPP have been implemented with varying success (see Table 118-1). These approaches include a moderate-dose photon technique (MDRT), a high-dose matched EPT, and a high-dose IMRT technique.

The MDRT technique was used at BWH and Dana–Farber Cancer Institute (BWH/DFCI) from 1987 to 2003 and consisted of anterior and posterior photon fields. The large hemithorax field received 30 Gy in 1.5-Gy fractions, the mediastinum received 40 Gy, and any areas of focally positive margins and/or positive nodes were boosted to a dose of 54 Gy using various beam angles.[16] No blocks were placed over the heart, liver, stomach, or kidney. The moderate dose of 30 Gy was chosen because it is within tolerance of all of the relevant normal structures except the ipsilateral kidney, which was acknowledged to be sacrificed. Adequate contralateral kidney function was always documented prior to treatment. Baldini et al. examined the pattern of failure after the combination of EPP; adjuvant cyclophosphamide, doxorubicin, and cisplatin; and MDRT to the hemithorax for patients treated from 1987 to 1993. Treatment-related toxicity was acceptable, and the most common site of failure was the ipsilateral hemithorax, with a LR rate of 35%.[16] Between 1993 and 2003, patients at BWH/DFCI were treated with the MDRT technique with the addition of concurrent chemotherapy (cisplatin, carboplatin/paclitaxel, or paclitaxel). However, local control remained a significant problem, with 12/24 locoregional recurrences reported—seven in the treatment field and five inferior to the field edge (marginal misses).[27] At BWH/DFCI, this MDRT technique has been abandoned for higher-dose techniques which will be described below.

Investigators at MSKCC pioneered a matched EPT to a total dose of 54 Gy.[33] This technique was fully described by Yajnik et al.[33] and involves anterior and posterior photon fields to the entire hemithorax and mediastinum to a dose of 39.6 Gy, after which the spinal cord (and thus, the mediastinum) is blocked and the dose is continued to 54 Gy. Blocks are placed over the abdomen to shield the liver and kidney for right-sided cases and to shield the stomach, kidney, and heart for left-sided cases. These blocked areas are then treated with superficial electron irradiation to cover the area at risk while minimizing

Table 118-1

POST EPP RT TECHNIQUES AND OUTCOMES

AUTHOR, INSTITUTION	*n*	CHEMOTHERAPY (ADJUVANT UNLESS OTHERWISE SPECIFIED)	RT TECHNIQUE, DOSE	LR, %	FATAL PULMONARY TOXICITY POST-MULTIMODALITY THERAPY, %[a]
Baldini et al.[16] BWH/DFCI	46	Cyclophosphamide, doxorubicin, cisplatin	MDRT 30 Gy (± boost to 54 Gy)	35	2
Allen et al.[27] BWH/DFCI	24	Concurrent cisplatin, carboplatin/paclitaxel or paclitaxel	MDRT 30 Gy (± boost to 54 Gy)	50	0
Gupta et al.[25] MSKCC	86	None	EPT 54 Gy	41	ND
Allen et al.[27] BWH/DFCI	15	Cisplatin/gemcitabine or cisplatin/pemetrexed	EPT 54 Gy	27	7
Rea et al.[28] Padua	21	Induction carboplatin/ gemcitabine	EPT 45 Gy (± boost to 55–59 Gy)	35	ND
Rice et al.[24,29] MDACC	63	None	IMRT 50 Gy (± 10 Gy boost)	13	10
Miles et al.[30] Duke	13	Cisplatin/pemetrexed	IMRT 45 Gy	46	8
Allen et al.[31] BWH/DFCI	13	Cisplatin/pemetrexed; intrapleural cisplatin	IMRT 54 Gy	ND	46
Buduhan et al.[21] Swedish Cancer Institute	14	Mostly cisplatin-based induction	IMRT 50.4 Gy	14	ND
van Sandick et al.[32] Netherlands Cancer Institute	15	None	IMRT 54 Gy	33	ND

EPP, extra-pleural pneumonectomy; BWH/DFCI, Brigham and Women's Hospital/Dana–Farber Cancer Institute; MSKCC, Memorial Sloan–Kettering Cancer Institute; MDACC, MD Anderson Cancer Center; RT, radiation therapy; LR, local recurrence; MDRT, moderate dose RT; EPT, matched electron/photon technique; IMRT, intensity modulated radiation therapy; ND, not described.

[a]Some studies described fatal "pneumonias" following completion of all treatment. It is not clear whether these were treatment-related, but they may have been. Furthermore, several studies did not list all causes of death not attributed to mesothelioma; thus fatal pulmonary toxicities may have been inadvertently underappreciated and/or not reported.

the dose to the underlying normal structures. The advantage of this approach is that it delivers an appropriately high dose of RT; the disadvantage is that there are areas at risk that may not be fully covered by the prescription dose. The inferior medial pleura, mediastinum, retrocrural lymph nodes, and portions of the diaphragmatic sulcus are all potentially underdosed. Also, the regions of the match lines between the photon and electron fields contain heterogeneities, with cumulative doses both higher and lower than the prescribed 54 Gy.

Clinical results for EPT are well documented and shown in Table 118-1. The most recent update from MSKCC reported a 41% local and nodal failure rate among 86 patients treated with EPP followed by 45 to 54 Gy.[25] Interestingly, the authors noted that 10 of 15 patients who had a recurrence in local and/or nodal sites and did not have distant failures, recurred in regions of dose inhomogeneity related to the matching of the photons and electrons. Allen et al.[27] reported similar findings for 15 patients treated with this EPT technique at BWH/DFCI; the LR rate was 27% and the treatment was tolerable. Researchers from Padua, Italy, reported a 35% LR rate for 21 patients treated with carboplatin/gemcitabine, EPP and adjuvant RT using EPT.[28] They stated that the RT was well tolerated. The MSKCC matched EPT is a clear improvement over the lower-dose MDRT technique and treatment-related toxicity is acceptable. However, further improvements in dosimetry and local control are still needed.

The third tested RT approach after EPP is IMRT (IMRT is described above in the section Definitive Radiation Therapy Alone for Mesothelioma). This approach for the treatment of mesothelioma after EPP was pioneered by researchers at MD Anderson Cancer Center (MDACC). The radiation oncologists and thoracic surgeons worked together to carefully delineate appropriate target volumes, which included all preoperative pleural surfaces, the ipsilateral mediastinal lymph nodes, the retrocrural space, and the deep margin of the thoracotomy incision.[34,35] Treatment dose was 50 Gy with a potential boost to 60 Gy for areas of positive or close surgical margins. This technique achieved very good dosimetric coverage of the target volumes. Preliminary results for seven patients treated with IMRT showed no LR, but two patients (29%) died of pulmonary complications. In retrospect, it is possible that these were treatment-related deaths.[34,35] An update of 63 patients treated with IMRT after EPP at MDACC showed excellent local control, with a 13% LR rate and acceptable acute toxicity, including nausea for 87%

of patients, weight loss for 86%, mild and transient dyspnea for 24%, and one death due to a bronchopleural fistula and acute respiratory distress syndrome (ARDS).[29] Investigators at Duke reported results for EPP followed by IMRT in 13 patients treated to a median dose of 45 Gy (range, 40–55 Gy).[30] The LR rate was 46% which is higher than seen at MDACC. Twenty three percent of patients developed grade 2 or greater pulmonary toxicity during or within 30 days of IMRT, and one patient (8%) experienced fatal pulmonary toxicity. The authors concluded that 45 Gy IMRT gives reasonable local control, but that treatment-related pulmonary toxicity is a concern, and it is important to exercise caution in the treatment of these patients. Buduhan et al.[21] described a 14% LR rate for 14 patients treated with trimodality therapy including IMRT. In that study, there were no fatal pulmonary toxicities following IMRT. van Sandick et al.[32] detected a 33% LR rate among 15 patients treated with EPP and adjuvant IMRT to a dose of 54 Gy; similarly, no fatal post RT pulmonary toxicities were described.

The EPT and IMRT techniques are both reasonable approaches and it is worthwhile to compare them. It is unclear which is better. Krayenbuehl et al.[36] and Hill-Kayser et al.[37] each performed treatment-planning studies comparing the EPT with the IMRT technique. In both studies, target coverage was *acceptable* for both techniques. Krayenbuehl reported improved target coverage with IMRT whereas Hill-Kayser reported similar coverage for IMRT and EPT. However, both studies showed that the doses to the organs at risk (OAR), especially the contralateral lung, were higher with IMRT compared to EPT. One of the main drawbacks of IMRT is that in order to achieve more conformal dose distributions, it delivers larger volumes of low doses to normal structures. For some tumor sites this is not clinically significant, but for mesothelioma, the increased low dose delivered to the contralateral lung is potentially injurious. Allen et al.[31] at BWH/DFCI treated 13 patients with IMRT after EPP and encountered an unexpected high rate of fatal pneumonitis (46%). Standard dose constraints for the contralateral lung were used: the volume of lung that received 20 Gy (V20) was <20% and the mean lung dose (MLD) was <15 Gy. Detailed analysis revealed that the patients who developed pneumonitis had V20, MLD and V5 (volume of lung that receives 5 Gy) values that were higher than those of the patients who did not develop pneumonitis. The authors concluded that the causes of death were probably multifactorial, but the large volume of contralateral lung that received a very low dose (5 Gy) was likely a significant factor. Treatment plans for the 13 patients were then redone with a restricted field technique and stricter lung constraints (MLD <9.5 Gy and V5 <55%).[38] In all cases, the target volume coverage remained excellent and the new lung constraints were met in all instances except one in which the patient had a V5 of 57.5%. The unexpected BWH/DFCI experience prompted MDACC investigators to re-examine the pulmonary toxicity among their cohort of 63 patients treated with IMRT after EPP; they found a 9.5% incidence of pulmonary-related death (PRD).[24] Univariate analysis showed median V20, V5, and MLD metrics of 9.8%, 92.5%, and 10.2 Gy, respectively, for patients with PRD compared to 3.6%, 70%, and 7.6 Gy for patients without PRD. On multivariate analysis, only V20 was predictive for PRD. The authors concluded that lung metrics should be kept as low as possible; their current goals are MLD <8.5 Gy and V20 <7%.

There have been four prospective trimodality trials using neoadjuvant chemotherapy followed by EPP and adjuvant RT.[18–20,39] The trial conducted by Weder et al. employed RT limited to areas clipped at surgery; the LR rate was not described. The other three trials allowed EPT, IMRT, and 3D conformal RT not otherwise described. Overall LR rates were presented but they were not described according to specific RT technique.

Some as yet untested novel techniques may be applicable to treatment of mesothelioma after EPP. *Helical tomotherapy* is a method of IMRT in which radiation is delivered as a fan beam using a rotating gantry. The patient is moved through the bore of the gantry as it is continuously rotated to deliver a helical dose application. Sterzing et al.[40] conducted a planning study which compared 54 Gy IMRT and helical tomotherapy plans for 10 patients with mesothelioma who had undergone EPP. Both plans produced excellent dose distributions and sparing of OAR. However, the helical tomotherapy plans achieved better target coverage and homogeneity as well as better sparing of the contralateral lung, with MLD <5 Gy compared to 6 Gy for the IMRT plans. Another novel technique employs IMRT and electrons. In a planning study, the group at MSKCC compared IMRT to plans using electrons combined with IMRT for six patients after EPP.[41] Both sets of plans showed excellent target coverage and appropriate sparing of OAR; however, the IMRT plus electron plans demonstrated further dose reductions to liver, kidneys, and heart. Finally, other authors have postulated potential roles for protons, hyperthermia, or boron neutron capture therapy for the treatment of mesothelioma.[42–44]

In sum, the data suggest that adjuvant RT following EPP may be associated with improved local control compared to surgery alone. Both the EPT and IMRT techniques achieve adequate target coverage. Dosimetry and local control rates may be better for IMRT. However, the risk of severe pulmonary toxicity may potentially also be higher with IMRT. On balance, both approaches are acceptable. If IMRT is considered, it should only be employed at experienced centers or on protocol and with strict attention to minimizing contralateral lung doses.

Adjuvant RT to Incision and Drain Sites to Prevent Tumor Seeding

Postoperative RT to surgical incisions and other instrumentation sites is the one area pertaining to RT for malignant pleural mesothelioma in which randomized trials have been performed. Results for the three trials are shown in Table 118-2. The first trial was conducted by Boutin et al.[45] and comprised 40 patients who were randomized to receive or not receive RT

Table 118-2

RANDOMIZED TRIALS OF RT TREATMENT OF SURGICAL INSTRUMENTATION SITES

AUTHOR INSTITUTION	*n*	RT TECHNIQUE AND DOSE	LOCAL RECURRENCE
Boutin et al.[45] Marseille	40	Electrons 21 Gy in 3 fractions	RT 0% No RT 40% $P < 0.001$
Bydder et al.[46] Australia	58	Electrons 10 Gy in 1 fraction	RT 7% No RT 10% $P =$ NS
O'Rourke et al.[47] United Kingdom	61	Electrons or Photons 21 Gy in 3 fractions	RT 23% No RT 10% $P =$ NS

RT, radiation therapy; NS, not statistically significant.

to all scar sites of invasive diagnostic procedures. RT consisted of 21 Gy of electrons given in three fractions with the use of 1 cm of bolus. There were no LRs among patients who received RT compared to 8/20 LRs (40%) among those who did not ($P < 0.001$). The second study, which was reported by Bydder et al.,[46] randomized patients to receive or not receive a single fraction of 10 Gy to procedure sites. No bolus was used. There was no statistically significant difference in the LR rate between treatment arms, and the authors concluded that a single 10 Gy treatment with 9 Mev electrons was ineffective. The third trial was performed in the UK and the RT technique and dose (21 Gy in three fractions) was similar to that used by Boutin et al.[47] That study showed no difference in LR rates between arms and concluded that prophylactic RT to procedure sites does not reduce the incidence of tumor seeding. In sum, given that the data from these randomized trials are conflicting, there is no clear role for prophylactic RT to procedure sites, and such treatment is not standard of care.

Palliative Radiation Therapy for Mesothelioma

As is the case for other malignancies, RT has a role in the palliative treatment of mesothelioma. Provided that the area to be treated is relatively limited (i.e., not the entire hemithorax), RT can ameliorate symptoms such as pain, dyspnea, esophageal symptoms, and superior vena cava syndrome. Several reports have demonstrated symptom relief on the order of 50% to 70%, and there appears to be a dose–response effect. Gordon et al.[48] showed that doses >40 Gy provided pain relief for two thirds of patients in his series. Similarly, Davis et al.[49] documented pain relief for 60% of patients who were treated with regimens of 20 Gy in four fractions or 30 Gy in 10 fractions. de Graaf-Strukowska et al.[50] showed pain relief for 50% of patients treated with 36 Gy in 4-Gy fractions compared to 39% of those treated with fraction sizes smaller than 4 Gy. Lastly, Ball and Cruickshank[3] reported that 70% of patients achieved symptomatic relief following palliative RT. Conventional radiation can also be used for palliation of distant sites such as bone and brain metastases.

SUMMARY

In summary, the role of RT in the curative treatment of malignant pleural mesothelioma remains undefined. There are no data to support treatment of unresected mesothelioma with definitive RT as a single modality. Early reports showed RT was associated with unacceptable toxicity and this approach is not recommended. Adjuvant RT after pleurectomy is also challenging and, similarly, no clear efficacy has been demonstrated. Approaches such as IMRT to the circumferential pleural envelope are intriguing, but long-term data for efficacy and toxicity are lacking. The best setting in which to deliver RT is after EPP, but the large and irregular target volume and multiple, adjacent, sensitive, normal structures render this complex. Treatment with 30 to 40 Gy of MDRT is no longer appropriate, given the greater efficacy of the MSKCC EPT with a dose of 54 Gy. This latter technique achieves adequate but not ideal coverage of the target volume to the prescription dose. Local control rates appear to be better than those seen with the MDRT technique and the toxicity is acceptable. The best dosimetry is achieved using IMRT. However, the pulmonary toxicity profile can be severe, and the relevant predictive factors for complications are not fully understood. For these reasons, physicians should exercise caution, and IMRT after EPP is probably best offered only by experienced teams or on protocol until further data have been gathered. New techniques such as helical tomotherapy and/or IMRT with the addition of electrons may also have a role in treatment in the future. Finally, RT also has a role for palliation of symptoms provided that the disease is confined to a tolerable radiation field.

EDITOR'S COMMENT

Although RT as a single modality treatment does not extend life expectancy in mesothelioma patients, adjuvant radiation as part of a trimodality approach (surgery, radiation, and chemotherapy) does improve life expectancy and quality of life. Delivering radiation to a field that includes an entire hemithorax with adequate dosing in the recesses is very challenging. Even more challenging is the delivery of radiation along tangential lines following pleurectomy when the remaining expanded lung can develop pneumonitis. Indeed it is the patterns of failure within these recesses that led to the development of intraoperative heated chemotherapy protocols noted in Chapter 123. In this chapter, Dr. Baldini provides insight on the application of the newest radiation technologies to mesothelioma, including IMRT, electron beam therapy, and matched EPT.

—Michael T. Jaklitsch

References

1. Emami B, Lyman J, Brown A, et al. Tolerance of normal tissue to therapeutic irradiation. *Int J Radiat Oncol Biol Phys.* 1991;21(1):109–122.
2. Alberts AS, Falkson G, Goedhals L, et al. Malignant pleural mesothelioma: a disease unaffected by current therapeutic maneuvers. *J Clin Oncol.* 1988;6(3):527–535.
3. Ball DL, Cruickshank DG. The treatment of malignant mesothelioma of the pleura: review of a 5-year experience, with special reference to radiotherapy. *Am J Clin Oncol.* 1990;13(1):4–9.
4. Maasilta P. Deterioration in lung function following hemithorax irradiation for pleural mesothelioma. *Int J Radiat Oncol Biol Phys.* 1991;20(3):433–438.
5. Munter MW, Thieke C, Nikoghosyan A, et al. Inverse planned stereotactic intensity modulated radiotherapy (IMRT) in the palliative treatment of malignant mesothelioma of the pleura: the Heidelberg experience. *Lung Cancer.* 2005;49(Suppl 1):S83–S86.
6. Hilaris BS, Nori D, Kwong E, et al. Pleurectomy and intraoperative brachytherapy and postoperative radiation in the treatment of malignant pleural mesothelioma. *Int J Radiat Oncol Biol Phys.* 1984;10(3):325–331.
7. Kutcher GJ, Kestler C, Greenblatt D, et al. Technique for external beam treatment for mesothelioma. *Int J Radiat Oncol Biol Phys.* 1987;13(11):1747–1752.
8. Gupta V, Mychalczak B, Krug L, et al. Hemithoracic radiation therapy after pleurectomy/decortication for malignant pleural mesothelioma. *Int J Radiat Oncol Biol Phys.* 2005;63(4):1045–1052.
9. Achatzy R, Beba W, Ritschler R, et al. The diagnosis, therapy and prognosis of diffuse malignant mesothelioma. *Eur J Cardiothorac Surg.* 1989;3(5):445–447; discussion 48.
10. Soysal O, Karaoglanoglu N, Demiracan S, et al. Pleurectomy/decortication for palliation in malignant pleural mesothelioma: results of surgery. *Eur J Cardiothorac Surg.* 1997;11(2):210–213.

11. Maggi G, Casadio C, Cianci R, et al. Trimodality management of malignant pleural mesothelioma. *Eur J Cardiothorac Surg.* 2001;19(3):346–350.
12. Lee TT, Everett DL, Shu HK, et al. Radical pleurectomy/decortication and intraoperative radiotherapy followed by conformal radiation with or without chemotherapy for malignant pleural mesothelioma. *J Thorac Cardiovasc Surg.* 2002;124(6):1183–1189.
13. Tobler M, Watson G, Leavitt DD. Intensity-modulated photon arc therapy for treatment of pleural mesothelioma. *Med Dosim.* 2002;27(4):255–259.
14. Rosenzweig KE, Zauderer MG, Laser B, et al. Pleural intensity-modulated radiotherapy for malignant pleural mesothelioma. *Int J Radiat Oncol Biol Phys.* 2012;83(4):1278–1283.
15. Janne PA, Baldini EH. Patterns of failure following surgical resection for malignant pleural mesothelioma. *Thorac Surg Clin.* 2004;14(4):567–573.
16. Baldini EH, Recht A, Strauss GM, et al. Patterns of failure after trimodality therapy for malignant pleural mesothelioma. *Ann Thorac Surg.* 1997;63(2):334–338.
17. Rusch VW, Rosenzweig K, Venkatraman E, et al. A phase II trial of surgical resection and adjuvant high-dose hemithoracic radiation for malignant pleural mesothelioma. *J Thorac Cardiovasc Surg.* 2001;122(4):788–795.
18. Krug LM, Pass HI, Rusch VW, et al. Multicenter phase II trial of neoadjuvant pemetrexed plus cisplatin followed by extrapleural pneumonectomy and radiation for malignant pleural mesothelioma. *J Clin Oncol.* 2009;27(18):3007–3013.
19. de Perrot M, Feld R, Cho BC, et al. Trimodality therapy with induction chemotherapy followed by extrapleural pneumonectomy and adjuvant high-dose hemithoracic radiation for malignant pleural mesothelioma. *J Clin Oncol.* 2009;27(9):1413–1418.
20. Van Schil PE, Baas P, Gaafar R, et al. Trimodality therapy for malignant pleural mesothelioma: results from an EORTC phase II multicentre trial. *Eur Respir J.* 2010;36(6):1362–1369.
21. Buduhan G, Menon S, Aye R, et al. Trimodality therapy for malignant pleural mesothelioma. *Ann Thorac Surg.* 2009;88(3):870–875; discussion 76.
22. Okubo K, Sonobe M, Fujinaga T, et al. Survival and relapse pattern after trimodality therapy for malignant pleural mesothelioma. *Gen Thorac Cardiovasc Surg.* 2009;57(11):585–590.
23. Pagan V, Ceron L, Paccagnella A, et al. 5-year prospective results of trimodality treatment for malignant pleural mesothelioma. *J Cardiovasc Surg (Torino).* 2006;47(5):595–601.
24. Rice DC, Smythe WR, Liao Z, et al. Dose-dependent pulmonary toxicity after postoperative intensity-modulated radiotherapy for malignant pleural mesothelioma. *Int J Radiat Oncol Biol Phys.* 2007;69(2):350–357.
25. Gupta V, Krug LM, Laser B, et al. Patterns of local and nodal failure in malignant pleural mesothelioma after extrapleural pneumonectomy and photon-electron radiotherapy. *J Thorac Oncol.* 2009;4(6):746–750.
26. de Perrot M, Uy K, Anraku M, et al. Impact of lymph node metastasis on outcome after extrapleural pneumonectomy for malignant pleural mesothelioma. *J Thorac Cardiovasc Surg.* 2007;133(1):111–116.
27. Allen AM, Den R, Wong JS, et al. Influence of radiotherapy technique and dose on patterns of failure for mesothelioma patients after extrapleural pneumonectomy. *Int J Radiat Oncol Biol Phys.* 2007;68(5):1366–1374.
28. Rea F, Marulli G, Bortolotti L, et al. Induction chemotherapy, extrapleural pneumonectomy (EPP) and adjuvant hemi-thoracic radiation in malignant pleural mesothelioma (MPM): feasibility and results. *Lung Cancer.* 2007;57(1):89–95.
29. Rice DC, Stevens CW, Correa AM, et al. Outcomes after extrapleural pneumonectomy and intensity-modulated radiation therapy for malignant pleural mesothelioma. *Ann Thorac Surg.* 2007;84(5):1685–1692; discussion 92–93.
30. Miles EF, Larrier NA, Kelsey CR, et al. Intensity-modulated radiotherapy for resected mesothelioma: the Duke experience. *Int J Radiat Oncol Biol Phys.* 2008;71(4):1143–1150.
31. Allen AM, Czerminska M, Janne PA, et al. Fatal pneumonitis associated with intensity-modulated radiation therapy for mesothelioma. *Int J Radiat Oncol Biol Phys.* 2006;65(3):640–645.
32. van Sandick JW, Kappers I, Baas P, et al. Surgical treatment in the management of malignant pleural mesothelioma: a single institution's experience. *Ann Surg Oncol.* 2008;15(6):1757–1764.
33. Yajnik S, Rosenzweig KE, Mychalczak B, et al. Hemithoracic radiation after extrapleural pneumonectomy for malignant pleural mesothelioma. *Int J Radiat Oncol Biol Phys.* 2003;56(5):1319–1326.
34. Ahamad A, Stevens CW, Smythe WR, et al. Intensity-modulated radiation therapy: a novel approach to the management of malignant pleural mesothelioma. *Int J Radiat Oncol Biol Phys.* 2003;55(3):768–775.
35. Forster KM, Smythe WR, Starkschall G, et al. Intensity-modulated radiotherapy following extrapleural pneumonectomy for the treatment of malignant mesothelioma: clinical implementation. *Int J Radiat Oncol Biol Phys.* 2003;55(3):606–616.
36. Krayenbuehl J, Oertel S, Davis JB, et al. Combined photon and electron three-dimensional conformal versus intensity-modulated radiotherapy with integrated boost for adjuvant treatment of malignant pleural mesothelioma after pleuropneumonectomy. *Int J Radiat Oncol Biol Phys.* 2007;69(5):1593–1599.
37. Hill-Kayser CE, Avery S, Mesina CF, et al. Hemithoracic radiotherapy after extrapleural pneumonectomy for malignant pleural mesothelioma: a dosimetric comparison of two well-described techniques. *J Thorac Oncol.* 2009;4(11):1431–1437.
38. Allen AM, Schofield D, Hacker F, et al. Restricted field IMRT dramatically enhances IMRT planning for mesothelioma. *Int J Radiat Oncol Biol Phys.* 2007;69(5):1587–1592.
39. Weder W, Stahel RA, Bernhard J, et al. Multicenter trial of neo-adjuvant chemotherapy followed by extrapleural pneumonectomy in malignant pleural mesothelioma. *Ann Oncol.* 2007;18(7):1196–1202.
40. Sterzing F, Sroka-Perez G, Schubert K, et al. Evaluating target coverage and normal tissue sparing in the adjuvant radiotherapy of malignant pleural mesothelioma: helical tomotherapy compared with step-and-shoot IMRT. *Radiother Oncol.* 2008;86(2):251–257.
41. Chan MF, Chui CS, Song Y, et al. A novel radiation therapy technique for malignant pleural mesothelioma combining electrons with intensity-modulated photons. *Radiother Oncol.* 2006;79(2):218–223.
42. Bjelkengren G, Glimelius B. The potential of proton beam radiation therapy in lung cancer (including mesothelioma). *Acta Oncol.* 2005;44(8):881–883.
43. Xia H, Karasawa K, Hanyu N, et al. Hyperthermia combined with intra-thoracic chemotherapy and radiotherapy for malignant pleural mesothelioma. *Int J Hyperthermia.* 2006;22(7):613–621.
44. Suzuki M, Endo K, Satoh H, et al. A novel concept of treatment of diffuse or multiple pleural tumors by boron neutron capture therapy (BNCT). *Radiother Oncol.* 2008;88(2):192–195.
45. Boutin C, Rey F, Viallat JR. Prevention of malignant seeding after invasive diagnostic procedures in patients with pleural mesothelioma. A randomized trial of local radiotherapy. *Chest.* 1995;108(3):754–758.
46. Bydder S, Phillips M, Joseph DJ, et al. A randomised trial of single-dose radiotherapy to prevent procedure tract metastasis by malignant mesothelioma. *Br J Cancer.* 2004;91(1):9–10.
47. O'Rourke N, Garcia JC, Paul J, et al. A randomised controlled trial of intervention site radiotherapy in malignant pleural mesothelioma. *Radiother Oncol.* 2007;84(1):18–22.
48. Gordon W Jr., Antman KH, Greenberger JS, et al. Radiation therapy in the management of patients with mesothelioma. *Int J Radiat Oncol Biol Phys.* 1982;8(1):19–25.
49. Davis SR, Tan L, Ball DL. Radiotherapy in the treatment of malignant mesothelioma of the pleura, with special reference to its use in palliation. *Australas Radiol.* 1994;38(3):212–214.
50. de Graaf-Strukowska L, van der Zee J, van Putten W, et al. Factors influencing the outcome of radiotherapy in malignant mesothelioma of the pleura-a single-institution experience with 189 patients. *Int J Radiat Oncol Biol Phys.* 1999;43(3):511–516.

119 Nonoperative Treatment of Malignant Pleural Effusions

Subroto Paul and Lambros Zellos

Keywords: Thoracentesis, systemic chemotherapy, mechanical pleurodesis, indwelling catheter placement, chest tube placement

Malignant pleural effusions (MPEs) cause considerable morbidity for patients afflicted with cancer. Metastatic breast, lung, and ovarian cancers account for the majority of cases. An estimated 150,000 new patients are diagnosed annually with dyspnea secondary to MPE.[1,2] Initial malignant diagnosis can be established in 50% to 60% of patients by means of a therapeutic thoracentesis.[1,2] However, the malignant effusions often recur, and patients require long-term palliation. The ideal therapy permits expedient, low-cost management of the pleural effusion with minimal morbidity because many of these patients have terminal disease. Operative management includes drainage through the use of video-assisted thoracic surgery (VATS) techniques combined with sclerosis, as well as operative placement of indwelling drainage catheters.[2–4] The operative techniques are described in Chapter 120. Nonoperative management of MPEs, the focus of this chapter, includes systemic chemotherapy and several methods of mechanical drainage, which may be combined with pleural sclerosing agents.

PATHOPHYSIOLOGY

Lung cancer is the leading cause of MPE and accounts for as many as 40% of cases, followed by metastatic breast (25%), ovarian (5%), and gastric cancers (5%). Another 10% of patients have lymphoma-induced effusions, leaving 10% without identifiable primary malignancy.[2,5] Metastatic pleural spread is a complex mechanism that requires a series of mutational events leading to the sequential expression and coordination of numerous growth factors and cell surface adhesion molecules.[6]

Pleural seeding either by direct tumor extension or by hematogenous or lymphangitic spread initiates a series of pathophysiologic events that cause the development of effusions. These mechanisms include (1) the production of angiogenic growth factors that cause increased vascular permeability, including vascular endothelial growth factor, among others, (2) lymphatic obstruction, which perturbs the normal absorption cycle of 2 to 3 L of pleural fluid daily, (3) direct production of fluid by the tumor, which often occurs with ovarian malignancies, and rarely, (4) tumor invasion and blockage of venous structures, which results in venous hypertension and the ensuing alternating Starling's forces that culminate in the effusion.[2]

All or some of these mechanisms contribute to the effusion, which first causes fatigue and lack of interest in activities followed by dyspnea, the principal and most disturbing symptom. The dyspnea tends to be progressive, if untreated, and eventually leads to symptoms at rest, underscoring the need for palliative treatment. The severity or degree of symptoms is related to the underlying cardiopulmonary function, the size of the effusion, or the rate of accumulation. Large effusions compress the lung and alter chest wall compliance, which together cause shortness of breath not only by altering the breathing mechanics, that is, decreasing the forced expiratory volume in 1 second (FEV_1) and tidal volume, but also by stimulating neurologic reflexes that lead to a subjective and uncomfortable sense of shortness of breath.[2]

The development of MPE portends a dismal prognosis because it is a sign of advanced disease. After diagnosis, patients with MPE experience a median survival of only 4 to 6 months. Only 10% to 15% of patients survive beyond a year. Patients with lung and gastrointestinal malignancies have a worse survival rate than those who have breast or hematologic malignancies.[2]

THERAPEUTIC OPTIONS

The treatment of MPE remains an important and at times difficult therapeutic challenge. The primary goal of therapy is to treat patients palliatively by relieving their dyspnea. Careful consideration of multiple factors should determine the optimal therapy. These include performance status, extent of disease, patient comfort and desires, and anatomic factors such as the degree of lung entrapment.

Systemic Therapy

Chemotherapy and Radiation Therapy

Small pleural effusions usually can be treated by malignancy-specific chemotherapy and localized radiation therapy to the primary lung lesion when the effusion is negative for malignancy, especially for those with small-cell lung and breast carcinomas.[2] However, neither of these treatments is effective for moderate to large effusions, and treatment should proceed to local therapies based on symptomatic management. For a detailed discussion of chemotherapy and radiation therapy for lung cancer, see Chapters 88 and 90.

Local Therapy

Thoracentesis

All patients with pleural effusions should undergo therapeutic thoracentesis, if not for the initial diagnosis, then to determine the contribution of the effusion to the patient's dyspneic symptoms. Radiologic assessment with chest x-ray or chest CT scan after thoracentesis can be helpful in determining the extent of the disease and the degree of lung entrapment. If symptoms improve after therapeutic thoracentesis, one is afforded additional time to contemplate a more permanent solution. Failure of symptom improvement should lead to a prompt search for alternative etiologies, such as pulmonary embolus, lymphangitic carcinomatosis, or trapped lung.[2,7]

Thoracentesis is performed by catheter-directed aspiration of the pleural space. Large effusions usually do not need image

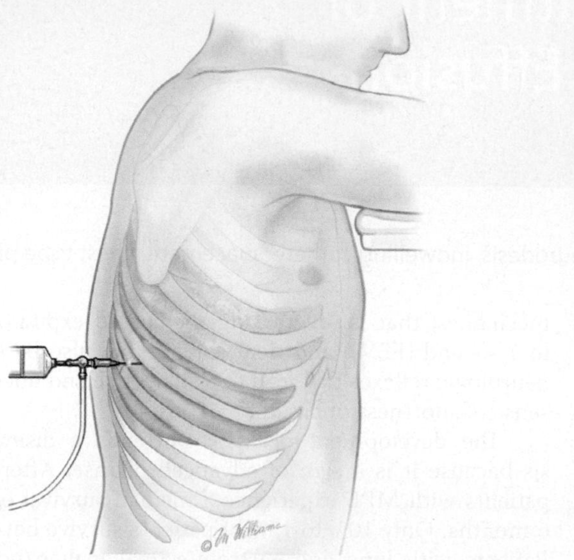

Figure 119-1. The thoracentesis catheter is placed using a catheter-over-needle system. The catheter is placed through the skin, over a rib (to avoid the intercostal neurovascular bundle), and into the chest.

Table 119-1

TREATMENT ALGORITHM FOR PLEURAL EFFUSION

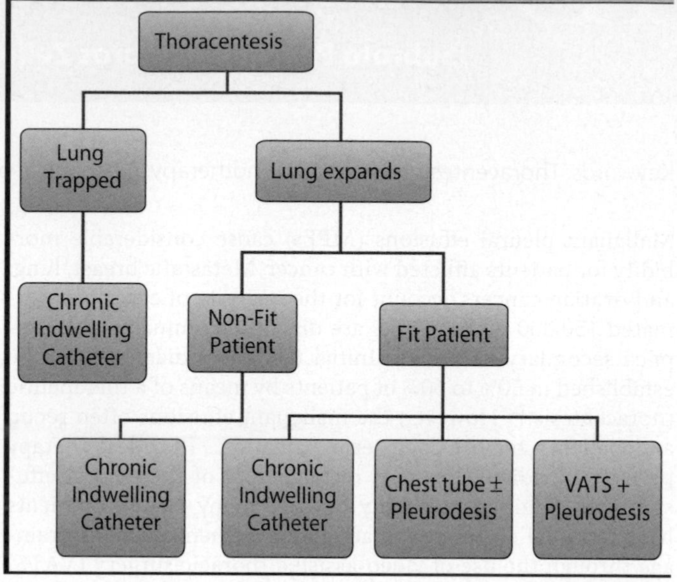

guidance. However, ultrasound-guided catheter aspiration is useful for small to moderate pleural effusions to prevent complications such as pneumothorax or hemothorax, as well as to optimize fluid removal. Several commercial kits are available. The procedure entails the use of a commercial catheter-over-needle system. The catheter is placed through the skin, over a rib (to avoid the intercostal neurovascular bundle), and into the chest (Fig. 119-1). Placement is confirmed by fluid aspiration. Fluid is aspirated manually with a syringe or drawn into a vacuum suction container. Local anesthesia of the chest wall and parietal pleura usually is adequate for pain control in the awake patient.

Complications of these procedures include, as mentioned, pneumothorax from lung puncture or hemothorax from either intercostal vessel injury or injury to other intrathoracic vascular structures, liver, or splenic puncture, which is notably rare. Other complications include reexpansion pulmonary edema, which can occur after large-volume thoracentesis. The exact volume of pleural fluid one can withdraw without developing this condition is unknown, but 2 L is typically the limit for patients with trapped lung or a fixed mediastinum, in whom the pleural pressure increases more dramatically with suction.[2,7] The precise mechanism is unknown, and supportive measures with supplemental oxygen and occasionally diuretics usually will suffice. At times, especially in the elderly or medically compromised patient, the pulmonary edema is so severe that intubation and ventilatory management are required for several days.[8]

Patients with recurrent effusions after thoracentesis can be managed in several ways. Repeat thoracentesis is an option for patients with extremely poor life expectancy (<1 to 2 months) who are either unwilling to undergo further intervention or for whom the anticipated need for fluid removal does not exceed two or three additional treatments. For patients whose symptoms improve with initial thoracentesis, the treatment decision turns on whether the lung expanded after thoracentesis or remained trapped. If the lung expanded fully, the patient may undergo pleurodesis with a chemical sclerosant such as talc, doxycycline, or bleomycin, among many other agents.[2] This option is valid for patients who are medically fit enough to tolerate the inflammatory response that ensues after pleural installation, especially with talc. Talc pleurodesis has been associated with acute respiratory distress syndrome and death and hence must be used with extreme caution in the elderly or medically compromised patient with poor cardiac and pulmonary function.[2] Patients with trapped lung resulting from a long-standing or fibropurulent effusion with fibrin peel formation on the lung surface are not candidates for pleurodesis. Pleural apposition is not possible in this setting, and therefore, the pleural space cannot be obliterated with sclerosing agents. These patients should be managed with a long-term indwelling pleural catheter and possibly decortication if the malignancy is of sufficiently low grade and expected survival sufficiently long to warrant this approach. The treatment algorithm in Table 119-1 was created with the foregoing principles in mind.

For patients with lung reexpansion after thoracentesis, viable options include (1) operative intervention with VATS drainage of the effusion followed by pleurodesis, typically with talc, (2) chest tube placement followed by pleurodesis, and (3) indwelling pleural catheter placement followed by pleurodesis. If the patient has poor pulmonary function and is medically compromised, placement of an indwelling catheter may be the only option.

Chest tube Placement

One of the most basic procedures in thoracic surgery is the placement of a chest tube. Chest tube insertion is an art unto itself. The basic steps for chest tube insertion are summarized in Table 119-2. Briefly, the ideal placement for chest tube insertion varies (especially if there has been previous chest surgery), but for most patients, the anterior or midaxillary line in the fifth or sixth interspace is appropriate. This corresponds to the nipple line in males and just under the breast in females (Fig. 119-2). The precise location is determined by marking the scapular tip, costal margin, and anterior iliac spine. Using these discrete points as a guide, the incision is marked with a felt tip pen and

Table 119-2

CHEST TUBE INSERTION

1. Confirm the side of effusion (right vs. left) clinically and radiologically. Obtain necessary material (i.e., chest tube, chest tube suction unit [e.g., Pleur-evac], chest tube tray, including scalpel blade and handle, Kelly clamps, etc.).
2. Review the chest x-ray or chest CT scan to determine ideal placement of the tube.
3. Position the patient. For most chest tube insertions, the patient should be placed in the lateral decubitus position with the arms secured.
4. The ideal placement for chest tube insertion in most patients is the anterior or midaxillary line in the fifth or sixth interspace, which corresponds to the nipple line in males and just under the breast in females (see Fig. 119-2).
5. Mark the scapular tip, costal margin, and anterior iliac spine with a felt tip pen. Mark the incision to be made (at least 3–4 cm) (see Fig. 119-3).
6. Give appropriate analgesia with IV conscious sedation, if needed, and generous local anesthesia with 1% lidocaine not only in the skin but also into the subcutaneous tissue and tissues just above the pleura.
7. Make the skin incision with a knife, and dissect bluntly or with a knife to a level above the rib.
8. Enter the pleura above the rib by using a blunt Kelly clamp with careful control of its tip. Feel the chest to ensure absence of adhesions.
9. Place a chest tube (28 F right-angle chest tube to base for fluid), and guide to the appropriate position.
10. Secure the chest tube and obtain a chest x-ray.

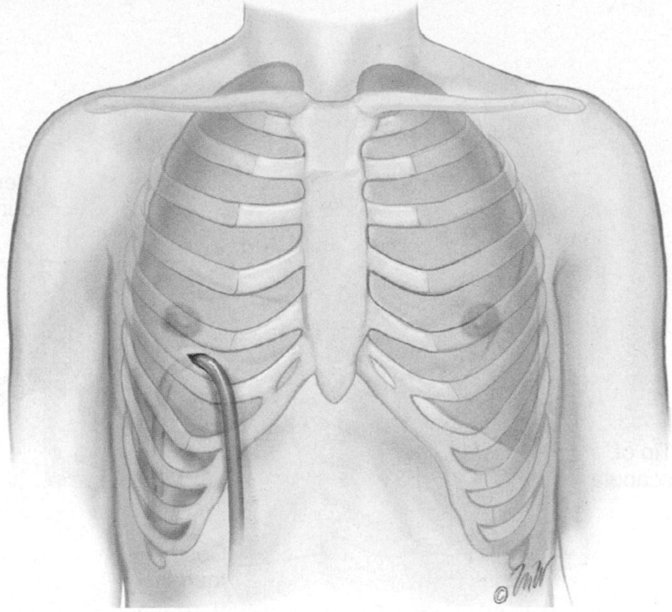

Figure 119-2. The usual position for chest tube placement is below the nipple line in males and below the breast in females.

should be at least 3 to 4 cm in length (Fig. 119-3). The chest tube is inserted over the rib to avoid injury to the neurovascular bundle (*inset*). The tube is left in place for several days until the drainage subsides to 200 mL per day or less. The success rate of chest tube drainage alone is lower compared with chest tube and chemical pleurodesis combined and varies from 10% to 60% depending on the series examined.[2,7] Therefore, if chest tube drainage is performed, pleurodesis is recommended once the lung has fully expanded because efficacy rates of 80% to 90% can be achieved.[2]

Pigtail Catheter Insertion

The technique for catheter-directed drainage is similar to thoracentesis (Fig. 119-4). An 8 to 10 F pigtail catheter is placed and left in the pleural space. The catheter is placed using a Seldinger catheter-over-wire technique after fluid has been aspirated with a needle and syringe. The catheter is placed to suction drainage until the pleural space has been evacuated.[2,4] Drainage with a pigtail catheter has many advantages over chest tube placement, including ease of placement (because it requires only a stab incision), improved patient comfort owing to its small size, and portability, which permits easy home or hospice care. The risks of placement are similar to those of thoracentesis, with pneumothorax with bleeding being the foremost complication. Pneumothorax in this scenario can be treated by suction evacuation of the space after placement. The major disadvantage in this approach is that catheters often become clogged with fibrin debris and hence prevent complete evacuation of the pleural fluid. In patients with full lung reexpansion, pleurodesis can be achieved by instillation of chemical sclerosants through the catheter. Recent studies have demonstrated the utility of this technique, with efficacy rates similar to those of chest tube drainage and chemical pleurodesis but lower associated cost because it can be performed in an ambulatory setting.

Chronic Indwelling Catheter Systems

Chronic indwelling pleural catheters such as the PleurX system (15.5 F) (PleurX Pleural Catheter and drainage systems, Denver Biomedical, Inc., Golden, CO) also have been used to treat chronic pleural effusions. Indwelling catheter placement is similar to pigtail catheter placement and is achieved by means of Seldinger technique,[1,9] although an open technique similar to chest tube placement works as well (Fig. 119-5). The catheter is placed under local anesthesia. These systems, much like pigtail catheters, can be placed in an ambulatory setting. The chief benefits are patient comfort and ease of placement. Because of their large size, indwelling catheters rarely occlude. They are manufactured with a cuff at the skin exit site, which permits tissue incorporation and serves as a barrier to infection. The risks of indwelling catheter placement are similar to those noted for chest tube and pigtail catheter placement. The risk of infection increases with long-term use.[1,9] These catheters have been demonstrated to be safe and effective in relieving symptoms and may be more cost-effective than chest tube pleurodesis. Like chest tubes and pigtail catheters, they can be used to instill sclerosants for pleurodesis.[1,2,9] Current practice recommends placement in patients with trapped lungs or in individuals who otherwise would not tolerate pleurodesis.

Pleurodesis

Chemical pleurodesis serves as an adjunct to mechanical pleural drainage. It should be performed in patients with malignant effusions who have a high likelihood of recurrent effusion after drainage. Pleurodesis is indicated for patients who experience full lung reexpansion after mechanical treatment, which makes pleural apposition possible. Various sclerosing agents are capable of inciting the inflammatory response needed to cause fusion of the visceral and parietal pleurae, thereby obliterating the pleural space and preventing fluid accumulation.

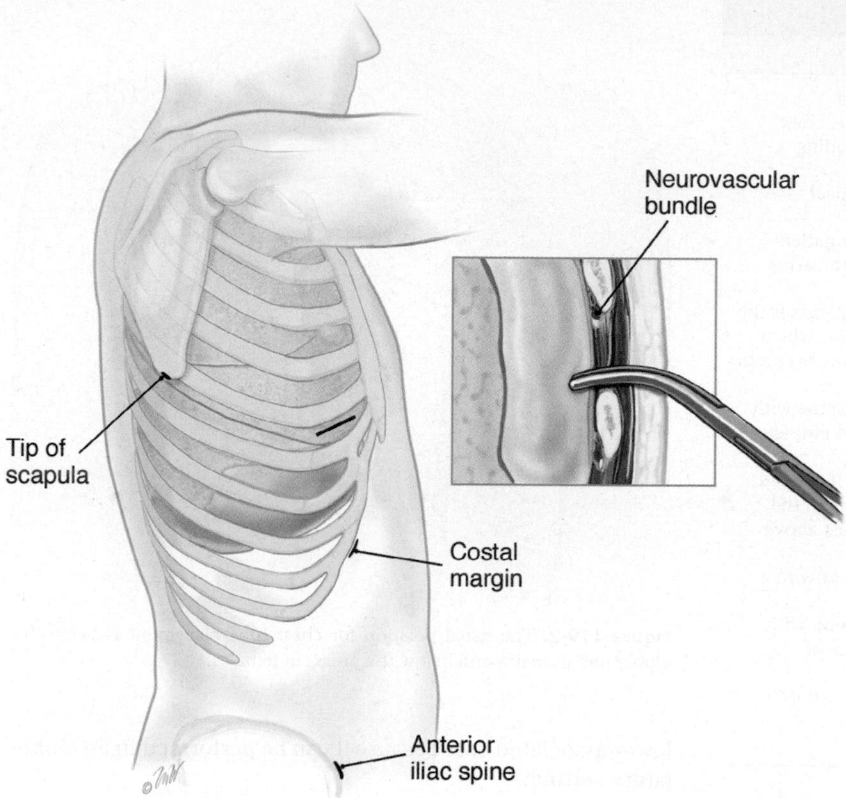

Figure 119-3. Determining the incision site for chest tube insertion.

Several agents have been used, including talc; antibiotics such as doxycycline and tetracycline; chemotherapy agents such as bleomycin and mitomycin C, and even autologous blood or bacteria such as *Corynebacterium parvum*, although the latter is no longer available.[2] Success rates vary for each, but talc is generally regarded as the best agent, with success rates (defined as reaccumulation of pleural fluid within 90 days) of 80% to 95% in most series. As mentioned previously, talc pleurodesis is not without risk because it can cause acute respiratory distress syndrome and death in patients with medical or pulmonary impairment and thus should be used with extreme caution in this group. Our recommendation is to follow the general policy of limiting talc instillation to 2 g for pleurodesis in medically compromised patients and to never exceed 4 g of talc in any patient, irrespective of medical fitness.[2] Pleurodesis is contraindicated in pneumonectomy patients who have developed a pleural effusion on the lung side since the resultant inflammatory response can be lethal. PleurX catheter placement without pleurodesis is the treatment of choice in these patients.

Pleurodesis is performed by instilling the sclerosing agent through the pleural drain (i.e., chest tube, pigtail catheter, or indwelling catheter) using a local anesthetic (e.g., lidocaine or benzocaine) because the ensuing inflammatory response is quite painful. Attention should be paid to the dose of local anesthetic instilled since rapid systemic absorption with complications such as arrhythmias or seizures can occur. Instillation times, varying from

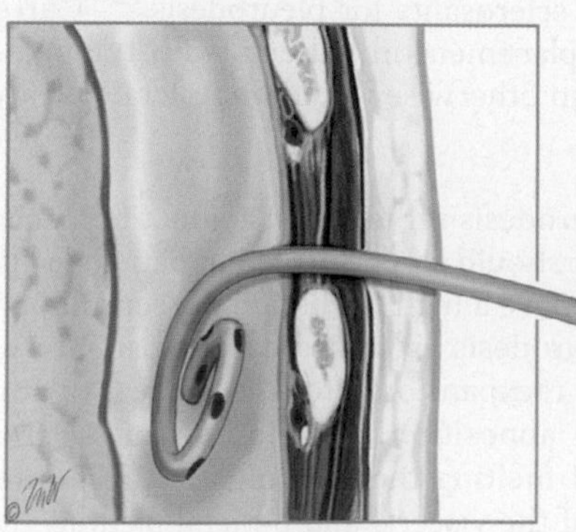

Figure 119-4. Pigtail catheter placement.

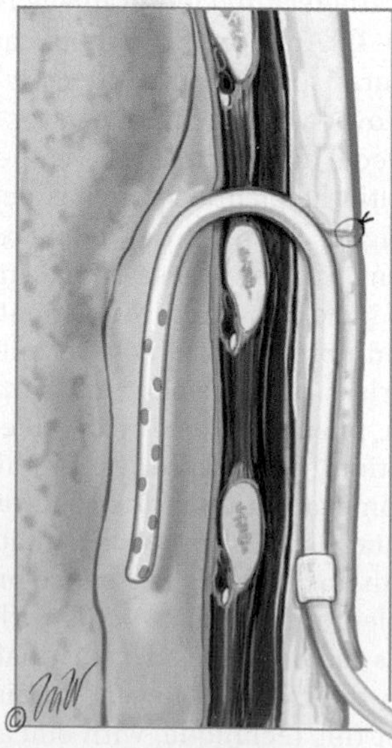

Figure 119-5. PleurX pleural catheter system.

as few as 30 minutes to as many as 4 hours, have been reported with little improvement in efficacy after 1 to 2 hours. Our policy is to administer the sclerosing agent for 1 hour while the patient moves through various positions to ensure even distribution of the slurry. However, these maneuvers are more for comfort than for necessity because spontaneous respiration should disperse the sclerosant evenly. Fever and pain are common and treated accordingly. Pronounced inflammatory reactions are rare and should be monitored during talc instillation, as discussed earlier. For this reason, we avoid performing bilateral pleurodeses in the same setting, preferring to schedule the patient for a second procedure at a later time. After instillation, the pleural drains are placed to suction for 48 to 72 hours. The pleural drain should be removed when pleural drainage is between 200 and 300 mL per day.

FUTURE THERAPIES

Future therapies for recurrent pleural effusion are aimed at treating the mechanisms that underlie malignant effusion formation. Specifically, numerous trials are attempting to determine the efficacy of antiangiogenic therapy. Current phase I and phase II trials are also examining the efficacy of antivascular endothelial growth factor therapy.[6] Efficacy will be determined after adequate trials, but assuredly these therapies will come at an economic price.

SUMMARY

The overriding goal of managing patients with MPE is to treat the dyspnea. In this regard, it is important to select the most cost-effective, low-morbidity regimen available in line with the patient's clinical circumstances. For patients undergoing nonoperative therapies, drainage followed by pleurodesis is the preferred therapy when the lung reexpands after pleural drainage and if the patient is healthy enough to tolerate the inflammatory consequences of pleurodesis. The method used (i.e., chest tube, pigtail catheter, or VATS) is highly dependent on surgeon and institutional preference. For patients unable to tolerate pleurodesis or with persistent lung entrapment after pleural drainage, a chronic indwelling catheter system (e.g., PleurX) may be the best option. The treatment scheme must take into account not only patient comfort but also patient preference in this group of often terminally ill patients.

CASE HISTORY

A 76-year-old woman with stage IV non–small-cell lung cancer was referred by her oncologist for surgical evaluation and treatment of dyspnea. The patient had undergone four cycles of cisplatin-based chemotherapy but continued to have a left pleural effusion, which had increased in size over the last 2 months. She presented with a progressive dyspnea that had worsened significantly over the past 2 weeks. She brought a chest film with her to the appointment (Fig. 119-6) showing clear evidence of a left pleural effusion.

The immediate options included VATS pleurodesis, radiation therapy, ambulatory PleurX catheter placement, and thoracentesis. A decision was made to proceed with thoracentesis both to evaluate the extent to which the effusion contributed to the patient's symptoms and to determine the degree of lung expansion after the effusion had been evacuated. Two liters of fluid was evacuated from the left chest after thoracentesis, and the patient's symptoms improved substantially. On follow-up chest x-ray, there was a large basilar space, indicating incomplete lung reexpansion. The options were placement of a chronic indwelling catheter, intrapleural administration of mitomycin, VATS decortication with talc pleurodesis, or chest tube placement with talc pleurodesis. However, since the left lung did not fully expand in this terminal patient, a chronic indwelling catheter (e.g., PleurX) was recommended.

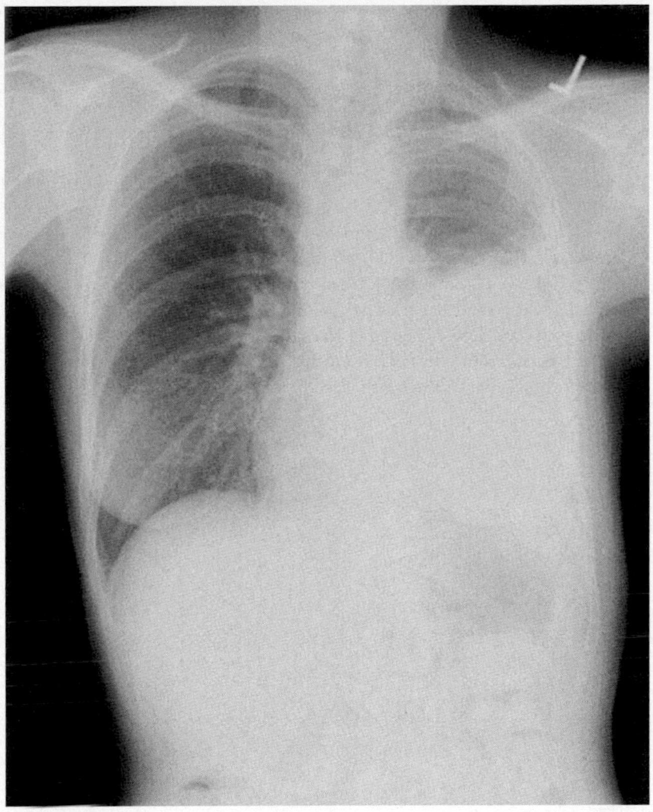

Figure 119-6. Chest x-ray showing evidence of left pleural effusion in a patient with stage IV non–small-cell lung cancer who presented for treatment of dyspnea.

EDITOR'S COMMENT

This is a practical management guide for the low-cost expedient methods of handling symptomatic MPEs. It is important for everyone to remember that the goal of therapy is relief of dyspnea, *not* to produce a perfect x-ray or drain every drop of a loculated effusion. It is beyond the ability of these methods to make the x-ray normal. Yet, they are excellent for palliating dyspnea and hypoxia at rest. Important components of therapy include chemotherapy, diuresis, and heme oxygen therapy. I currently use talc pleurodesis to treat a malignant pleural effusion without lung entrapment in a patient with preserved functional status. Trapped lung patients are better served with pleural catheters and may expand some lung volume over weeks to months. Although catheters can be placed under local anesthesia with sedation, thoracoscopy with single lung ventilation is advisable for sorting out trapped versus untrapped lungs.

—Michael T. Jaklitsch

References

1. Putnam JB Jr, Walsh GL, Swisher SG, et al. Outpatient management of malignant pleural effusion by a chronic indwelling pleural catheter. *Ann Thorac Surg*. 2000;69:369–375.
2. Putnam JB Jr. Malignant pleural effusions. *Surg Clin North Am*. 2002; 82:867–883.
3. Pollak JS. Malignant pleural effusions: treatment with tunneled long-term drainage catheters. *Curr Opin Pulm Med*. 2002;8:302–307.
4. Hingorani AD, Bloomberg TJ. Ultrasound-guided pigtail catheter drainage of malignant pericardial effusions. *Clin Radiol*. 1995;50:15–19.
5. Rodriguez-Panadero F, Borderas Naranjo F, Lopez Mejias J. Pleural metastatic tumours and effusions: frequency and pathogenic mechanisms in a postmortem series. *Eur Respir J*. 1989;2:366–369.
6. Grove CS, Lee YC. Vascular endothelial growth factor: the key mediator in pleural effusion formation. *Curr Opin Pulm Med*. 2002;8:294–301.
7. Tan C, Sedrakyan A, Browne J, et al. The evidence on the effectiveness of management for malignant pleural effusion: a systematic review. *Eur J Cardiothorac Surg*. 2006;29:829–838.
8. Massad I, Halawa SA, Badran I, et al. Negative pressure pulmonary edema: five case reports. *Middle East J Anesthesiol*. 2006;18:977–984.
9. Putnam JB Jr, Light RW, Rodriguez RM, et al. A randomized comparison of indwelling pleural catheter and doxycycline pleurodesis in the management of malignant pleural effusions. *Cancer*. 1999;86:1992–1999.

120 Thoracoscopy with Intrapleural Sclerosis for Malignant Pleural Effusion

Costas S. Bizekis, Michael D. Zervos, and Harvey I. Pass

Keywords: Talc pleurodesis, indwelling pleural catheter, pleuroperitoneal shunt, PleurX catheter

INTRODUCTION

Malignant pleural effusion is a common clinical problem in neoplastic diseases. Approximately half of all patients with metastatic cancer develop a malignant pleural effusion as a consequence of their disease.[1] Although there have been no epidemiologic studies, the annual incidence of malignant pleural effusion in the United States is estimated to be more than 200,000 cases.[2] The main problem that patients who develop such effusions experience is a reduction in the quality of life owing to symptoms such as dyspnea, chest pain (primarily related to involvement of the parietal pleura and chest wall), and cough.[2]

Treatment options for malignant pleural effusions are determined by the symptoms and performance status of the patient, the primary tumor and its response to systemic therapy, lung reexpansion after pleural fluid evacuation, and expected survival. The therapeutic goal of palliative treatment is permanent resolution of the pleural effusion. For patients who are symptomatic from pleural effusions, dramatic improvement or complete resolution of symptoms with remaining or limited recurrence of the effusion can be called a partial success. It must always be remembered that controlling a malignant pleural effusion is a local phenomenon that has no effect on the underlying systemic disease.

A number of different techniques have been used over the past 20 years to treat malignant pleural effusion.[3] The most common method is pleurodesis (i.e., obliteration of the pleural space), effected by instilling a chemical sclerosant in the pleural space after the effusion has been drained completely, either during thoracoscopy (under sedation or general anesthesia) or at bedside thoracostomy.[1,4] There is no single unified approach to thoracoscopy. It can be performed by using flexible or rigid thoracoscopes, with or without video assistance, under local, regional, or general anesthesia, and with or without selective one-lung ventilation.[5] It provides access to the entire pleural cavity, permits biopsy under direct visualization, and by means of a video-assisted procedure, enables optimal preparation of the pleural surface and homogeneous distribution of the sclerosing agent under visual guidance, thereby maximizing the chances for complete pleurodesis.[6,7]

PREOPERATIVE ASSESSMENT

Malignancy must always be in the differential diagnosis of an undiagnosed unilateral or bilateral pleural effusion, and a thoracentesis must be performed. Complete drainage of the effusion is important for evaluating the underlying lung. If the lung remains collapsed after drainage, it usually indicates trapped lung syndrome. Options in cases involving trapped lung are tailored to the individual patient and include either implantation of a chronic indwelling pleural catheter,[8,9] internal drainage from the pleura to peritoneum using a Denver pleuroperitoneal shunt,[10] or pleurectomy (which is performed rarely for effusion control).

It is important to perform bronchoscopy when endobronchial lesions are suspected with accompanying symptoms of hemoptysis and atelectasis, or for large effusions without contralateral mediastinal shift. Moreover, is it important to exclude endobronchial obstruction before attempting a pleurodesis if the entire lung remains collapsed after therapeutic thoracentesis.[11]

To determine the optimal management approach, the patient must be thoroughly examined and evaluated. Because of the limited survival of patients with malignant pleural effusions,[4,8] the selected treatment should have low procedure-related mortality and morbidity.

IDEAL PATIENT CHARACTERISTICS

The ideal patient for sclerotherapy has been recently diagnosed with a malignant pleural effusion and still has a free-flowing effusion without loculations. Failure of sclerotherapy is related to the inability of the lung to reexpand and completely fill the pleural space, and nonexpansion is usually observed with chronic effusions that have been either neglected or drained on multiple occasions. Thickening of the visceral pleura, leading to loss of volume and trapping of the lung, will prevent successful obliteration of the pleural cavity. A large volume pleural tumor is also associated with increased failure of the technique.[4]

TECHNICAL PRINCIPLES

Video-Assisted Thoracoscopic Surgery

For video-assisted thoracoscopic surgery (VATS) procedures, general anesthesia with selective one-lung ventilation via a double-lumen endotracheal tube is commonly preferred.[5,12] However, in some patients with poor cardiac output and increased risk for general anesthesia, conscious sedation consisting of local or locoregional anesthetics and administration of systemic analgesic and sedative medications can be used.[13]

After placing the patient in the lateral decubitus position and instituting selective one-lung ventilation under general anesthesia, the table should be flexed to 30 degrees to widen the intercostal spaces on the operative side. The skin is prepared and draped as for a standard posterolateral thoracotomy. In adult patients, 5- or 10-mm thoracoscopes are often used; however, a smaller 2-mm mini thoracoscope can be used for diagnostic procedures. For general exploration, the first (camera) port is often made in the midaxillary line in the seventh intercostal space. The first port site tunnel is always created bluntly, with

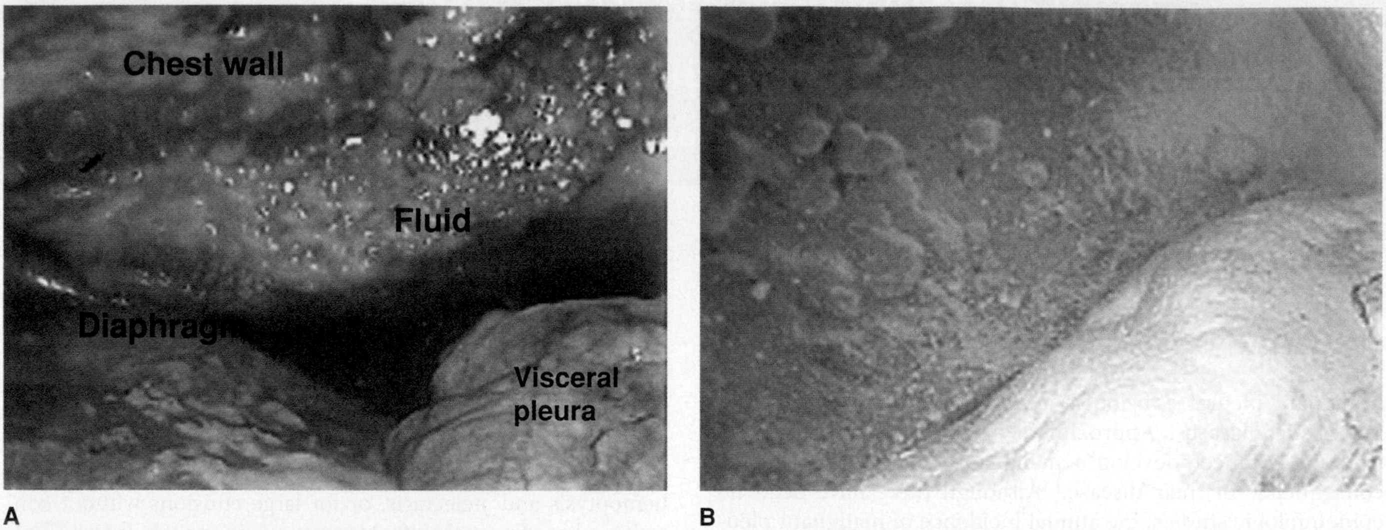

Figure 120-1. *A.* Talc pleurodesis patient with pleural carcinomatosis and malignant pleural effusion prior to aerosolization of talc. *B.* View after talc placement, with all surfaces evenly coated with a thin layer of the powder.

digital exploration performed to detect and release adhesions around the port site before the camera is inserted. Additional trocars are inserted under video guidance. After the pleural fluid has been drained, the pleural cavity is inspected, and directed biopsy specimens are taken. In the presence of adhesions or trapped lung syndrome, adhesiolysis or limited decortication can be done to achieve complete lung reexpansion.

After the lung has been observed to expand and fill the hemithorax, chemical pleurodesis is performed by instilling a chemical irritant such as talc, doxycycline, silver nitrate, or iodopovidone into the pleural space to promote adhesion of the parietal and visceral pleurae.[3] Five grams of sterile purified talc powder (most commonly used) is insufflated through a talc atomizer under video-thoracoscopic vision to ensure that talc covers the entire visceral pleura (Fig. 120-1). At the end of the procedure, usually one or two 28 F chest tubes are inserted. This practice is recommended to maintain complete expansion of the lung after the thoracoscope is withdrawn. Of note, if the pH values decrease below 7.3, the success of thoracoscopic pleurodesis decreases.[14] Also, if the patient undergoing pleurodesis is receiving corticosteroid therapy, the medication should be stopped or the dose, if possible, should be reduced because it may reduce the efficacy of pleurodesis.[11]

POSTOPERATIVE MANAGEMENT

Suction is maintained on the chest tubes for a period of 24 to 48 hours. The drains are removed after radiologic evidence of lung expansion has been obtained and the fluid drainage level diminishes to less than 100 mL per day.[5,12,15,16] For postoperative pain management, nonsteroidal anti-inflammatory drugs can be used,[17] or an epidural catheter can be placed at the time of the operation.

Assessment of Results

Thoracoscopy is a safe and well-tolerated procedure with a low perioperative mortality rate (0.5%).[4] The success rate for VATS pleurodesis (30-day freedom from radiographic evidence of malignant pleural effusion and equal to or greater than 90% expansion of the lung at the time of the procedure) is greater than 90%.[4,15,17] In a large randomized study by Dresler et al.[18] of talc poudrage ($n = 251$) versus talc slurry ($n = 250$), between 68% and 73% of the patients were able to have complete expansion of their lungs at the time of the procedure. Although there were no differences in recurrence among all the patients in the study, there was a slight improvement in the thoracoscopic success of talc poudrage (67%) compared with talc slurry (56%) with respect to complete lung reexpansion ($p = 0.045$). Respiratory complications (atelectasis, pneumonia, or respiratory failure) of thoracoscopic pleurodesis were observed more commonly in patients undergoing thoracoscopic pleurodesis as opposed to talc slurry (14% vs. 6%, respectively, $p = 0.007$), and were the most frequent causes of treatment-related deaths (2% to 3%). Dyspnea and pain are the most common complications of the procedure. Others include postoperative fever, persistent air leak, bleeding, subcutaneous emphysema, reexpansion pulmonary edema, deep vein thrombosis, and port-site recurrence of malignancy. The latter is seen in some mesothelioma patients, and controversy remains as to whether these recurrences can be prevented by postoperative local radiotherapy.[4] In general, it is thought that thoracoscopic pleurodesis has the advantage of assessing lung expansion at the time of the operation and is associated with better results in breast and lung cancer effusions, however, bedside talc slurry injection is a simpler and less invasive technique.

Indwelling Pleural Catheter

The PleurX Catheter System (CareFusion Corp., San Diego, CA) is a soft Silastic chronic indwelling catheter. It is a 66-cm-long, 15.5 F flexible silicone rubber catheter with fenestrations along the distal 24 cm. A valve at the proximal end prevents inadvertent leakage of pleural fluid or entry of air. A polyester cuff is situated approximately 14 cm from the proximal end and lies within a subcutaneous tract to decrease bacterial dislocation and to anchor the catheter in position. Insertion of the PleurX catheter can be accomplished in the outpatient setting under local anesthesia. With careful monitoring, it is possible

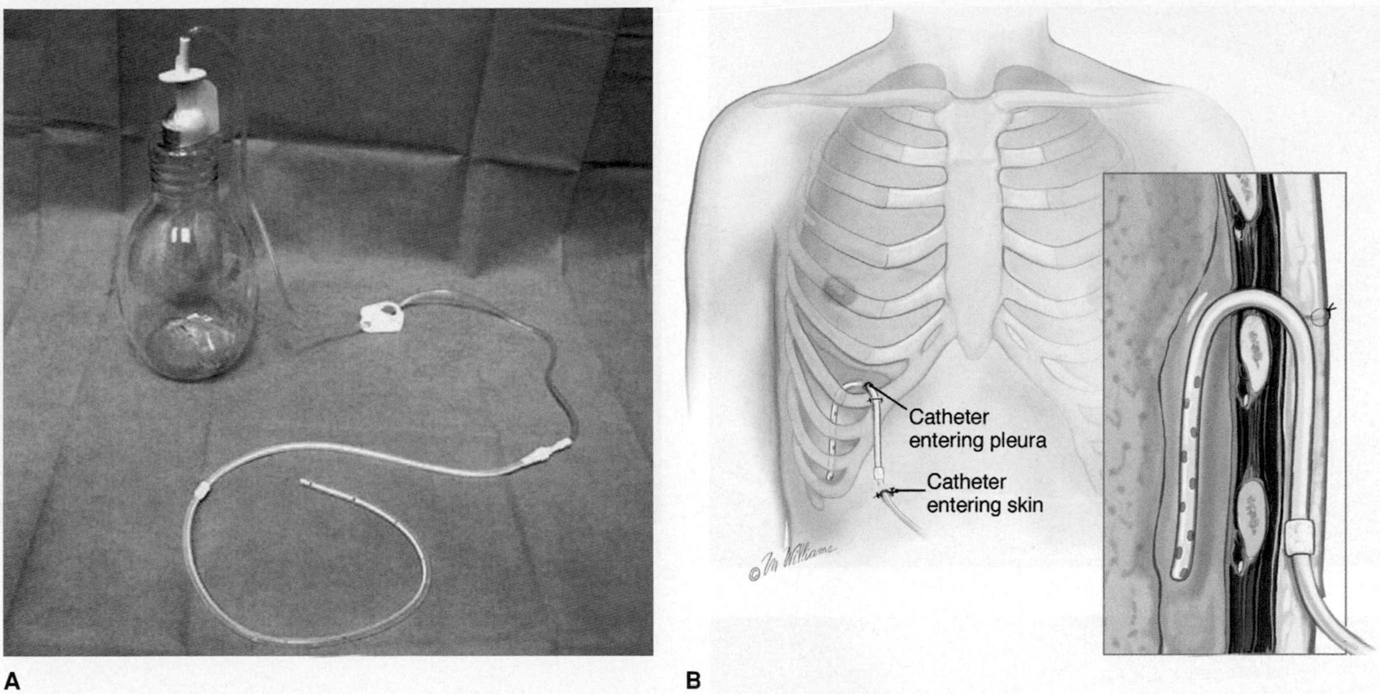

Figure 120-2. *A.* PleurX Catheter System, a vacuum device and setup for home management of recurrent pleural effusions. *B.* Positioning and placement of PleurX catheter for pleural effusions.

to accomplish complete drainage of the effusion at the time of placement. The patient or caregiver then drains the pleural fluid periodically by connecting the tubing to a disposable vacuum container to provide relief of dyspnea and potentially achieve spontaneous pleurodesis (Fig. 120-2A).

After localization of the pleural fluid by needle and administering a local anesthetic, the catheter is inserted using a modified Seldinger technique as follows. A flexible wire is passed through the needle into the thorax, and a 1.5-cm horizontal incision is made at this site (Fig. 120-2B). A counter-horizontal incision is made approximately 5 cm inferiorly and medially to the wire, and a subcutaneous tunnel is created for the pleural catheter. The catheter is drawn through the tunnel, and the Teflon cuff is placed within the tunnel, 1 cm away from the skin edge. A peel-away sheath over a removable stylet (dilator) is inserted over the wire and placed into the thorax. The stylet is withdrawn, and the catheter is threaded through the sheath into the thorax. The peel-away sheath is then withdrawn leaving the catheter in situ. The two skin incisions are closed with interrupted nonabsorbable sutures, and the catheter is secured to the skin. After insertion, 1000 to 1500 mL pleural fluid should be drained. A chest x-ray is obtained to confirm the position of the catheter and to rule out a pneumothorax, after which the patient is sent home.

Detailed written and oral instructions for home catheter care and drainage should be provided to patients and their caregivers. Complications of indwelling pleural catheter placement include local cellulitis, catheter obstruction, and pleural infection. Tumor seeding can be seen in some patients.

At home, patients should drain no more than 1000 to 1500 mL at a time to prevent reexpansion pulmonary edema. Drainage should be performed at a frequency that will prevent or relieve their dyspnea. If over time the output diminishes to less than 50 mL per day for three consecutive days, the catheter can be removed. If the catheter does not drain but the patient is still dyspneic, chest x-ray or CT scan should be performed to rule out a nondraining effusion. By using this method, spontaneous pleurodesis can be achieved in 46% to 70% of patients.[3,8,19,20]

The clinical course in a patient with mesothelioma receiving palliative care for a malignant pleural effusion is depicted in Figure 120-3.

Pleuroperitoneal Shunt

Pleuroperitoneal shunt (Denver Biomedical, Inc., Golden, CO) insertion can provide effective and safe palliation for malignant pleural effusion when associated with the trapped lung syndrome. Since the development and manufacture of the PleurX catheter, use of this shunt has decreased dramatically. This procedure can be done under local or general anesthesia with either VATS or open thoracotomy depending on if there have been multiple previous interventions in the pleura, which may cause pleural adhesions. After the fluid has been drained and the entire pleura thoroughly examined, the degree of lung expansion is assessed. If it is not adequate to fill the entire hemithorax, pleuroperitoneal shunt can be an option for palliation.

A 3-cm transverse incision is made in the ipsilateral rectus sheath to expose the peritoneal cavity. The pleuroperitoneal shunt is tunneled under the skin from the chest to the abdomen, with the pumping chamber lodged in a subcutaneous pocket overlying the costal margin. The pleural and peritoneal limbs are then introduced into the respective cavities under direct vision. Normal saline can be introduced into the pleural space to prime the pump and check shunt function. The site of the pump can be marked on the skin to facilitate pumping by the nurse or the patient.[10] Palliative efficacy should be monitored by chest x-ray films.

Common complications of pleuroperitoneal shunting are shunt occlusion and wound infection. Other complications are

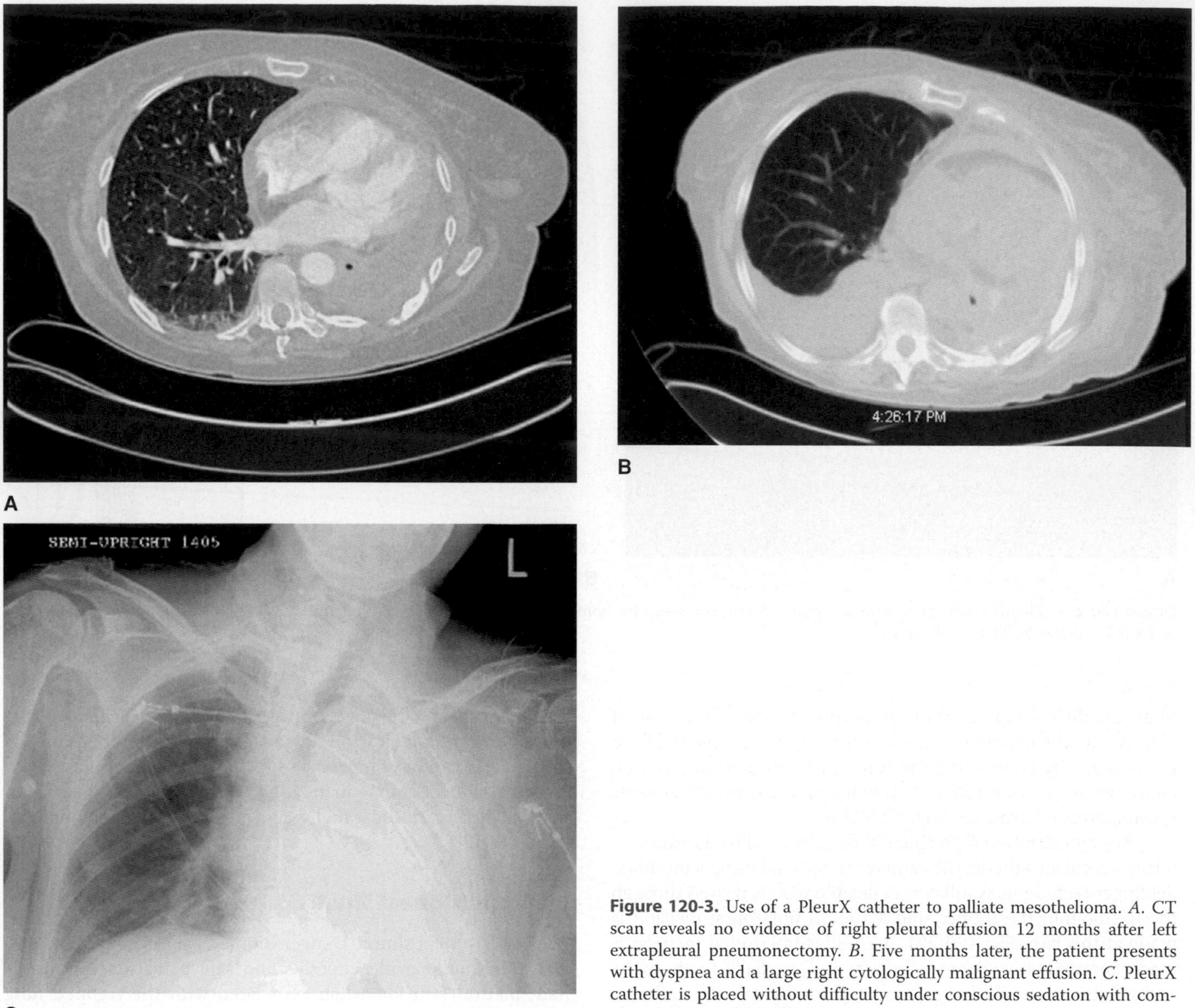

Figure 120-3. Use of a PleurX catheter to palliate mesothelioma. *A.* CT scan reveals no evidence of right pleural effusion 12 months after left extrapleural pneumonectomy. *B.* Five months later, the patient presents with dyspnea and a large right cytologically malignant effusion. *C.* PleurX catheter is placed without difficulty under conscious sedation with complete drainage of the effusion.

owing to surgical technique and anesthesia. Tumor implantation into the peritoneal cavity is rare but can occur.[10,20,21]

SUMMARY

Available data suggest that thoracoscopic pleurodesis with talc may be the optimal technique for pleurodesis in patients with malignant pleural effusion.[1,4,18] The optimal treatment option depends on the patient's situation and whether the patient is fit enough to undergo sedation or general anesthesia. The success rate of thoracoscopic pleurodesis in patients with malignant pleural effusion can be as high as 90%; however, success rates vary with the type of primary malignancy and patient factors such as concomitant steroid use or decreased pleural fluid pH. If pleurodesis fails, indwelling pleural catheters or pleuroperitoneal shunts can provide symptomatic relief.

EDITOR'S COMMENT

Malignant pleural effusions are a common problem. Long-term indwelling pleural catheters have become the most common treatment of malignant pleural effusions. Thoracoscopy with intrapleural sclerosis, however, continues to play a strong role as a consequence of the benefits of the procedure. One advantage of a pleural catheter is that it can be placed at the bedside with local anesthesia and obviates the need for general anesthesia in the frail patient. If the patient is not frail, I believe thoracoscopy should be offered. My standard procedure under general anesthesia is flexible bronchoscopy, exploratory thoracoscopy, drainage of effusion, removal of loculations, pleural biopsy under direct vision, testing of the ability of the underlying lung to expand and fill the chest, placement of the sclerosis agent or pleural catheter (if lung is entrapped), and intercostal nerve block. Although pleural drainage catheters have become popular for a quick and easy way to control the effusion and slowly expand an entrapped lung, there remain several advantages to the thoracoscopy. Thoracoscopy can be combined with single lung anesthesia or a single-lumen endotracheal tube with low tidal volumes or short periods of apnea with lung collapse if a large unilateral effusion allows clear visualization. Thoracoscopy allows for breakdown of loculations, complete drainage of the effusion, and uniform distribution of the sclerosant. If I find an entrapped lung, I leave a pleural catheter. If no entrapment, I add a sclerosant. Although the efficiency of pleural catheters and thoracoscopy are similar, patient satisfaction is higher with the thoracoscopic approach.

—Michael T. Jaklitsch

References

1. Shaw P, Agarwal R. Pleurodesis for malignant pleural effusions. *Cochrane Database Syst Rev.* 2004(1):CD002916.
2. Light RW. Pleural effusions. *Med Clin North Am.* 2011;95(6):1055–1070.
3. Rodriguez-Panadero F, Romero-Romero B. Management of malignant pleural effusions. *Curr Opin Pulm Med.* 2011;17(4):269–273.
4. Antunes G, Neville E, Duffy J, et al. BTS guidelines for the management of malignant pleural effusions. *Thorax.* 2003;58(Suppl 2):ii29–38.
5. Yim AP, Chung SS, Lee TW, et al. Thoracoscopic management of malignant pleural effusions. *Chest.* 1996;109(5):1234–1238.
6. Harris RJ, Kavuru MS, Mehta AC, et al. The impact of thoracoscopy on the management of pleural disease. *Chest.* 1995;107(3):845–852.
7. Schulze M, Boehle AS, Kurdow R, et al. Effective treatment of malignant pleural effusion by minimal invasive thoracic surgery: thoracoscopic talc pleurodesis and pleuroperitoneal shunts in 101 patients. *Ann Thorac Surg.* 2001;71(6):1809–1812.
8. Putnam JB Jr. Malignant pleural effusions. *Surg Clin North Am.* 2002;82(4):867–883.
9. Ohm C, Park D, Vogen M, et al. Use of an indwelling pleural catheter compared with thorascopic talc pleurodesis in the management of malignant pleural effusions. *Am Surg.* 2003;69(3):198–202.
10. Genc O, Petrou M, Ladas G, et al. The long-term morbidity of pleuroperitoneal shunts in the management of recurrent malignant effusions. *Eur J Cardiothorac Surg.* 2000;18(2):143–146.
11. Antony VB, Loddenkemper R, Astoul P, et al. Management of malignant pleural effusions. *Eur Respir J.* 2001;18(2):402–419.
12. Brega-Massone PP, Conti B, Magnani B, et al. Minimally invasive thoracic surgery for diagnostic assessment and palliative treatment in recurrent neoplastic pleural effusion. *Thorac Cardiovasc Surg.* 2004;52(4):191–195.
13. Gravino E, Griffo S, Gentile M, et al. Comparison of two protocols of conscious analgosedation in video-assisted talc pleurodesis. *Minerva Anestesiol.* 2005;71(4):157–165.
14. Crnjac A, Sok M, Kamenik M. Impact of pleural effusion pH on the efficacy of thoracoscopic mechanical pleurodesis in patients with breast carcinoma. *Eur J Cardiothorac Surg.* 2004;26(2):432–436.
15. Cardillo G, Facciolo F, Carbone L, et al. Long-term follow-up of video-assisted talc pleurodesis in malignant recurrent pleural effusions. *Eur J Cardiothorac Surg.* 2002;21(2):302–305.
16. Brega-Massone PP, Lequaglie C, Magnani B, et al. Chemical pleurodesis to improve patients' quality of life in the management of malignant pleural effusions: the 15 year experience of the National Cancer Institute of Milan. *Surg Laparosc Endosc Percutan Tech.* 2004;14(2):73–79.
17. de Campos JR, Vargas FS, de Campos Werebe E, et al. Thoracoscopy talc poudrage : a 15-year experience. *Chest.* 2001;119(3):801–806.
18. Dresler CM, Olak J, Herndon JE, et al. Phase III intergroup study of talc poudrage vs talc slurry sclerosis for malignant pleural effusion. *Chest.* 2005;127(3):909–915.
19. Pollak JS. Malignant pleural effusions: treatment with tunneled long-term drainage catheters. *Curr Opin Pulm Med.* 2002;8(4):302–307.
20. Musani AI, Haas AR, Seijo L, et al. Outpatient management of malignant pleural effusions with small-bore, tunneled pleural catheters. *Respiration.* 2004;71(6):559–566.
21. Ernst A, Hersh CP, Herth F, et al. A novel instrument for the evaluation of the pleural space: an experience in 34 patients. *Chest.* 2002; 122(5):1530–1534.

121 Pleurectomy and Decortication for Malignant Pleural Diseases

Naveed Zeb Alam and Raja M. Flores

Keywords: Malignant pleural mesothelioma, malignant solitary fibrous tumors of the pleura, thymoma, secondary malignancies

Malignant disease of the pleura encompasses a wide scope of clinical presentations ranging from asymptomatic simple pleural effusions to complex tumor masses involving multiple intrathoracic organs. The treatment options are similarly diverse. This chapter focuses on the indications, techniques, and results of pleurectomy and decortication (P/D) in the management of malignant pleural disease.

CLASSIFICATION

Pleural malignancies can be classified as primary, arising from the pleura, or secondary, that is, metastatic. Primary pleural malignancies include malignant pleural mesothelioma (MPM) and malignant localized fibrous tumors of the pleura. Metastatic pleural disease is a common clinical problem. Although lung and breast cancers are the most common primary tumors, virtually any cancer can metastasize to the pleura.

MALIGNANT PLEURAL MESOTHELIOMA

Although primary pleural tumors have been reported since the eighteenth century, the epidemiology of mesothelioma first came to light in 1960 with the report by Wagner et al.[1] of 33 asbestos mine workers from South Africa who developed mesothelioma. Pleural mesothelioma previously was classified as benign or malignant. However, recognition that "benign" or "localized" mesothelioma has a biology that is distinct from MPM led to a change in nomenclature. These benign tumors are now termed *solitary fibrous tumors of the pleura.*

MPM is a rare tumor. Although the geographic distribution of the disease is diverse, taken as a whole, the United States has an incidence just under 1 per 100,000 persons.[2] The incidence has been rising since the 1970s. The male-to-female ratio is 5:1, which is likely reflective of occupational exposure to asbestos.

The clinical presentation of MPM is usually insidious. The most common presenting symptoms are dyspnea and chest pain.

Staging in MPM, as is the case in other aspects of the disease, lacks consensus. Various staging systems exist. The classic system described by Butchart et al. in 1976 is relatively simple and descriptive.[3] The Brigham staging system is based on resectability by extrapleural pneumonectomy (EPP) and may not be of value in patients undergoing P/D.[4] The tumor, node, metastasis (TNM) staging system proposed by the International Mesothelioma Interest Group (IMIG) is the accepted American Joint Commission on Cancer staging system.[5]

Indications for Surgery

In the days before effective systemic therapy, MPM was thought to be uniformly fatal. Surgery was reserved for diagnosis and palliation. In the first reports of "curative" surgery, Butchart et al.[3] performed EPP with a surgical mortality rate of 30%. In the nearly 30 years since the initial report, advances in patient selection, as well as intra- and postoperative management, have decreased the mortality of the operation substantially, as reported by centers with high volumes of mesothelioma surgery. Sugarbaker et al.[6] reported their mortality rate from 183 consecutive EPPs performed at the Brigham and Women's Hospital as 3.8%. At Memorial Sloan-Kettering, Flores reported a 5.2% mortality for EPP.[7] The staggeringly high mortality rate seen in early attempts at EPP led to a movement away from this operation and toward P/D as a method of debulking tumor. The mortality of P/D is reported to be 1.8%,[8] and the lack of evidence demonstrating superiority of EPP over P/D is thought to be a consequence of the upfront mortality increase with the more extensive operation.

There are those who still believe that surgical intervention for purposes other than palliation in mesothelioma is not indicated. Although it is true that there are no randomized controlled trials comparing surgical treatment with supportive care (or other treatments) in these patients, the reality is that these trials likely will never be performed. For those who treat this disease and have a less nihilistic outlook, surgery forms a key component of the treatment algorithm.

Nomenclature

There has been a move in the international mesothelioma community to standardize the terminology associated with the disparate operations performed by various surgeons under the umbrella heading of P/D. This should enable improved analysis of results across various centers and enable more coordinated research efforts, as to date, the majority of reports and studies are single center in origin. Recommendations published jointly by the International Association for the Study of Lung Cancer (IASLC) and the IMIG following a survey suggested that the term P/D be used to denote attempted complete removal of macroscopic tumor from the visceral and parietal pleura and the term extended P/D be used if the diaphragm and pericardium are removed as well.[9]

Indications for P/D

Indications for P/D can be regarded as patient-related or tumor-related. Perhaps the least controversial statement one can make about P/D is that it can be offered to patients who do not have the cardiopulmonary reserve to tolerate pneumonectomy. For patients who can tolerate pneumonectomy, the choice of operation becomes less clear. Some centers perform P/D for patients with early-stage disease, that is, confined to the parietal pleural "capsule" (Butchart I, IMIG T1a or T1b), with the rationale that if no lung parenchyma is involved, the inherent morbidity and mortality risk of adding a pneumonectomy is not warranted. Others disagree, based on the rationale that the absence of lung parenchyma facilitates the administration of postoperative adjuvant radiotherapy.

If one accepts that MPM is a disease where true R0 resections are a theoretical achievement, then the goal of surgery is to remove all gross tumors and serve as a springboard for adjuvant therapy. The choice of operation then is made based on the extent of resection required and the extent of resection the patient can tolerate. Some clinicians believe that with newer methods of radiation administration and ongoing attempts at other local and systemic therapies, the argument that residual lung parenchyma hinders appropriate adjuvant therapy may be less of a factor than it once was.[10]

We reported a retrospective study of 663 patients (385 had EPP and 278 had P/D) which demonstrated a hazard ratio of 1.4 for EPP when controlling for stage, histology, gender, and multimodality therapy. Clearly the study is subject to selection bias, but this reinforces our view that P/D may be the optimal procedure if adequate debulking can be performed by leaving the lung parenchyma in place.[11]

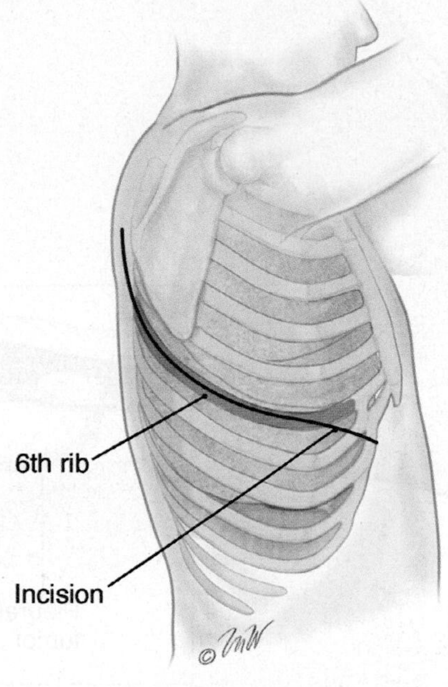

Figure 121-1. S-shaped posterolateral thoracotomy incision extending to the costal margin provides excellent exposure.

Preoperative Evaluation

All patients undergoing consideration for P/D need thorough imaging and cardiopulmonary evaluation. At a minimum, pulmonary function testing should be performed. Quantitative ventilation/perfusion scans may also be indicated if associated lung resections are anticipated or to evaluate the possibility of EPP. Computed tomography (CT) scanning of the thorax and upper abdomen is required, and magnetic resonance imaging (MRI) may be superior in assessing discrete focuses of chest wall invasion or diaphragmatic muscle involvement.[12] However, rarely does MRI change surgical management. Fluorodeoxyglucose positron emission tomography (PET) scanning in MPM can be used to provide stage and prognostic information. In addition to helping to determine the extent of tumor, PET scanning can be used to detect N3 or M_1 disease in 10% of patients.[13,14] The standardized uptake value also can be used to predict the presence of N2 lymphatic spread.[14] High standardized uptake value also has been shown to correlate with poor survival in MPM.[15]

Another controversial question in the preoperative evaluation of patients is the role of mediastinoscopy in MPM. It is useful in determining the N stage of most patients and is more accurate than CT scanning.[16] However, up to 25% of patients have lymph node involvement confined to areas of the hemithorax inaccessible by mediastinoscopy, such as the peridiaphragmatic and internal mammary regions.[7] Furthermore, although N2 disease does negatively impact survival, some feel that it should not be used as the sole reason to deny surgery.

Technique

After the induction of general anesthesia, a double-lumen endotracheal tube should be inserted to facilitate the operation. An arterial line and central venous pressure monitoring are important because blood loss is often significant (approximately 1–2 L). The patient is placed in the lateral decubitus position, and a long S-shaped posterolateral thoracotomy incision extending downward to the costal margin is made (Fig. 121-1). The sixth rib is resected, and the dissection is begun in the plane between the endothoracic fascia and the parietal pleura (Fig. 121-2). The pleural tumor is bluntly dissected away from the chest wall. The plane is then developed in a cephalad direction toward the apex from the posterolateral direction. Care in identifying the subclavian vessels is prudent because a traction injury to these structures is difficult to repair (Fig. 121-3). As each area of dissection is completed, packs are placed to aid in hemostasis because a fair amount of blood loss will result from the blunt dissection. The dissection then is continued inferior and posterior to the incision. After a sufficient area of chest wall has been mobilized, a chest retractor may be inserted.

The pleura now can be mobilized from the mediastinum. Once the upper portion of the lung is completely mobilized from the chest wall, the superior and posterior hilar structures are well exposed. On the left side, the esophagus and aorta must be identified and the dissection around them should be undertaken with care. On the right side, the superior vena cava must be dissected away from the specimen gently. The dissection then continues to the posterior aspect of the pericardium. A plane between the mediastinal pleura and the pericardium is sometimes present. If it is not, the pericardium needs to be *resected en bloc* at a later stage of the operation with subsequent reconstruction. The dissection then is carried toward the posterior diaphragmatic sulcus. If superficial involvement of the diaphragm is found, a partial-thickness resection can be performed. The plane between the tumor and the uninvolved diaphragm can be entered, and the dissection is initiated at the posterior costophrenic angle and carried anteriorly. This is facilitated by strong retraction on the pleura away from the diaphragm. In many patients, deeper involvement of the diaphragm mandates a full-thickness resection of a portion of the muscle. The deep border of the diaphragm then must be dissected from the peritoneum. Care should be taken to avoid entering the abdomen because tumor seeding into the peritoneal cavity is a concern. This is often unavoidable, especially around the central tendon, and any

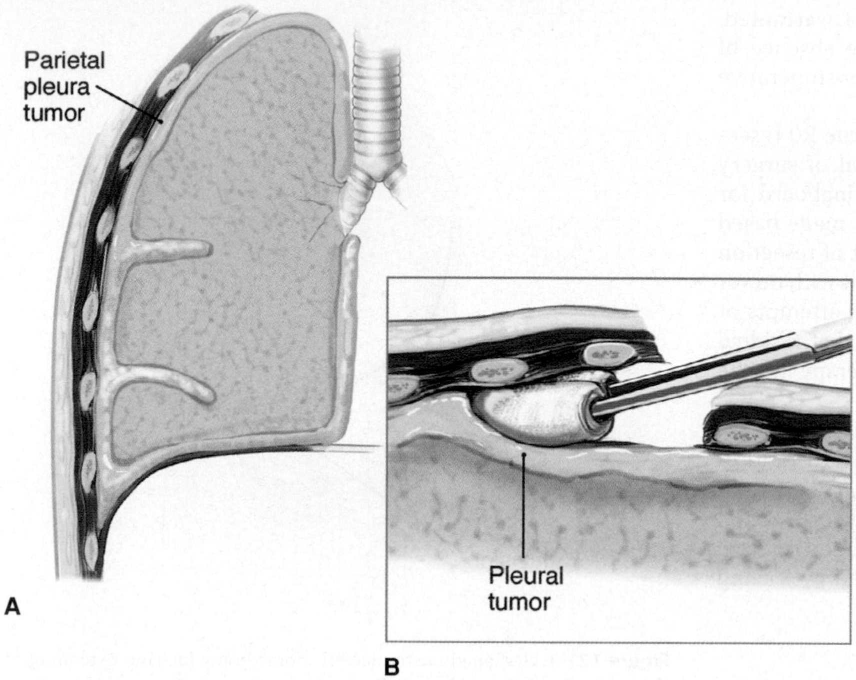

Figure 121-2. **A.** Sagittal section of right lung and pleura. **B.** Pleurectomy is begun between the endothoracic fascia and the parietal pleura using blunt dissection. The plane is developed cephalad.

defect in the peritoneum should be closed immediately. The specimen then is mobilized en bloc back toward the pericardium medially. If resection of the pericardium is required, it is delayed until the tumor is mobilized as much as possible owing to the accompanying arrhythmias from manipulation. The pericardium is opened gradually, and traction sutures are placed on the nonspecimen edge to maintain the position of the heart and to prevent retraction of the pericardium into the opposite hemithorax (Fig. 121-4).

Once the dissection is completed to the hilar structures, the parietal pleura is opened, and the pleural envelope is entered and decortication of the visceral pleura is performed. This is, in some respects, the most technically demanding and tedious component of the operation. Decortication must be performed with care into the fissures because they are often substantially involved with disease (Fig. 121-5). During the decortication, deflation of the lung will minimize blood loss, and inflation will allow better visualization of the plane between the tumor and the visceral pleura or lung parenchyma. Communication with the anesthesiologist about the amount of blood loss is important because most patients require intraoperative transfusion.

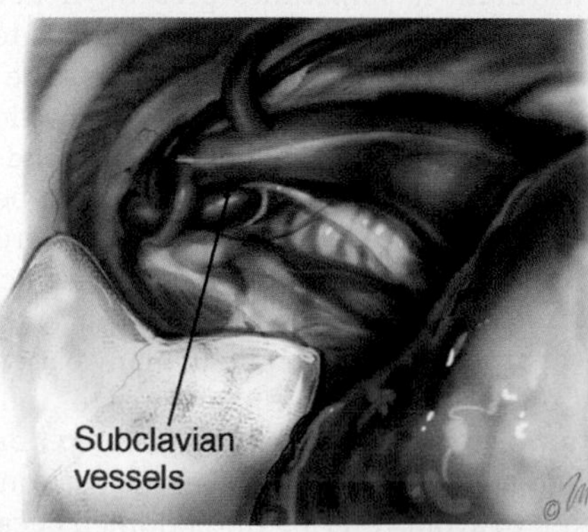

Figure 121-3. Care must be taken in dissecting around the subclavian vessels in the lung apex.

Lymph node dissection should be carried out, and specimens should be labeled and sent separately to the pathologist. The subcarinal lymph nodes should be resected as well as the paratracheal lymph nodes on the right and the aortopulmonary lymph nodes on the left.

Once the gross tumor is removed and the specimen is delivered, reconstruction of the pericardium and diaphragm, if required, is performed. If the diaphragm is largely intact, it can be closed primarily by plication to prevent upward movement and subsequent compression atelectasis of the lower lobe. On the right side, reconstruction of the diaphragm is performed with a double layer of Dexon (United States Surgical, Syneture Division, Norwalk, CT) mesh because the liver prevents herniation of intra-abdominal contents. On the left, 2-mm-thickness Gore-Tex (W.L. Gore and Associates, Flagstaff, AZ) is used because thicker, nonabsorbable material is required to prevent herniation. The prosthesis is secured laterally by placing sutures around the ribs. Posteriorly, it is sutured to the crus or tacked to the prevertebral fascia. The medial aspect is sewn to the remaining edge of the diaphragm at its confluence with the pericardium. The diaphragmatic prosthesis should be made absolutely taut to prevent upward motion of the abdominal contents and subsequent atelectasis of the lower lobe. If the pericardium was resected, it is reconstructed with a single layer of Dexon mesh.

Attention is now turned to obtaining hemostasis. An argon beam electrocoagulator may be used to help control diffuse bleeding from the chest wall. Three chest tubes are placed anteriorly and posteriorly into the apex, and a right-angle tube is placed along the diaphragm. This should permit control of the substantial air leaks that are anticipated and should permit full expansion of the lung. The air leaks tend to resolve after 72 hours if the lung is fully expanded.

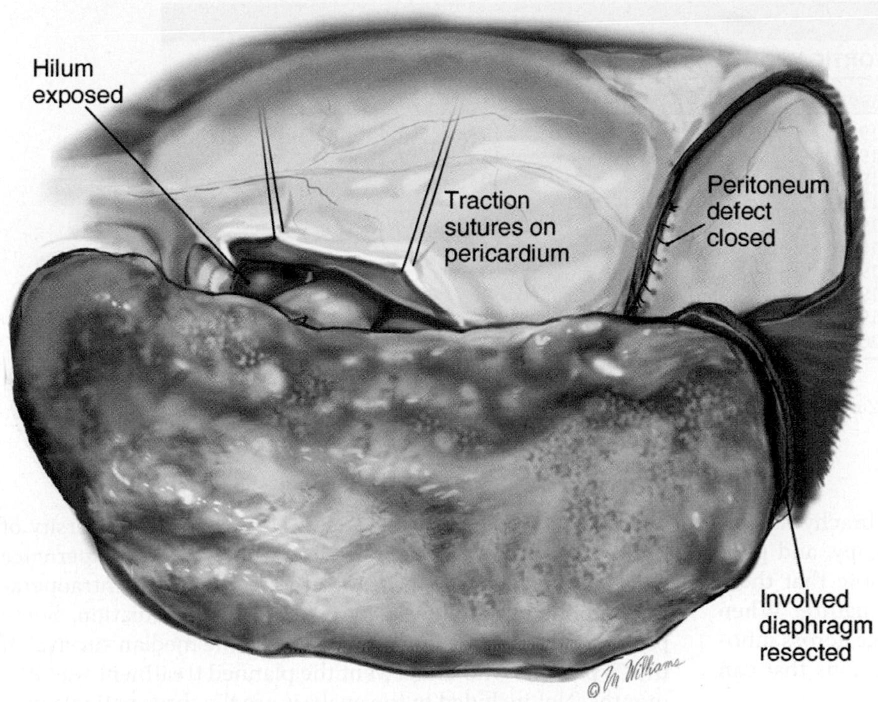

Figure 121-4. The parietal pleura has been stripped from the chest wall, and the lung is ready for decortication. Note the exposed hilar structures, traction sutures on the pericardium, closed peritoneal defect, and resection of involved diaphragm.

Pitfalls

During the dissection, certain areas of particular concern warrant special mention. The subclavian vessels can be injured by traction during the blunt dissection of the apex. On the right, care needs to be taken while dissecting the mediastinal pleura from the superior vena cava. On the left, the plane between the tumor and the adventitia of the aorta, the origins of the intercostal vessels, and the esophagus all should be identified. If the diaphragm is largely left intact and reconstruction is not undertaken, plication is often helpful to prevent elevation and paradoxical motion of the diaphragm and atelectasis of the lower lobe.

Although prior talc pleurodesis is not an absolute contraindication to the operation, it does increase the likelihood of substantial blood loss and air leak.

Insuring adequate lung expansion at the end of the operation is critical. As there will be numerous breaches of lung parenchyma, a substantial degree of postoperative air leak is expected. Failure to re-expand the lung will then result in a fixed space defect in the setting of prolonged air leak—a recipe for substantial postoperative problems including empyema.

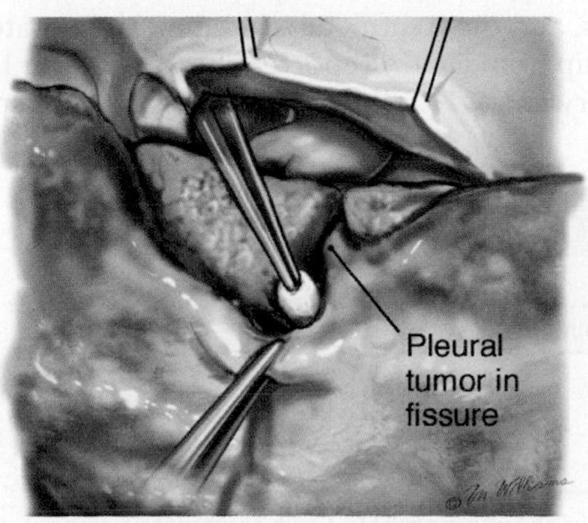

Figure 121-5. Decortication must be performed meticulously in the fissures to remove all gross diseases.

Postoperative Care

As there is usually a substantial degree of air leak in the immediate postoperative period, drains are placed on suction, if tolerated, overnight. As long as there is good lung expansion, the air leak settles down in the first few postoperative days and suction can usually be removed on postoperative day one.

Postoperative complications are similar to most thoracic procedures. Atrial fibrillation rates as high as 17% have been reported.[17] Prolonged air leak due to the inadequate lung expansion and subsequent empyema is particularly difficult to manage especially if a prosthesis is in situ (diaphragmatic or pericardial repair) and would mandate reoperation.

Results

P/D is generally well tolerated, with a mortality rate limited to approximately 1% to 2% when performed at high-volume centers. The most common complication is prolonged air leak, which occurs in 10% of patients. Hemorrhage, pneumonia, and empyema are less common complications.[18] The results of studies examining P/D alone are summarized in Table 121-1. Median survivals range from 9 to 20 months in the literature.

The technical challenge of separating tumor and visceral pleura from the lung parenchyma may result in suboptimal cytoreduction. This is reflected in the observation that the most common site of recurrence is the ipsilateral hemithorax.[29]

Combined-Modality Therapy

Since the results of surgery alone are poor, most recent studies have combined P/D with some form or combination of adjuvant

Table 121-1

STUDIES OF PLEURECTOMY DECORTICATION ALONE

SOURCE	YEAR	PATIENTS (N)	MEDIAN SURVIVAL (MOS)	MORTALITY (%)
Chahinian et al.[19]	1982	30	13	0
Brenner et al.[20]	1982	69	15	N/A
Law et al.[21]	1984	28	20	11
Chailleux et al.[22]	1988	29	14	N/A
Ruffie et al.[23]	1989	63	10	0
Brancatisano et al.[24]	1991	45	16	2
Rusch et al.[25]	1991	26	10	N/A
Allen et al.[26]	1994	56	9	5
Soysal et al.[27]	1997	100	17	1
Ceresoli et al.[28]	2001	38	13	N/A

N/A = not available.
Source: Adapted from Van Ruth S, Baas P, Zoetmulder FA. Surgical treatment of malignant pleural mesothelioma: a review. *Chest.* 2003;123:551–561.

therapy. These have included external radiation, brachytherapy, systemic chemotherapy, intrapleural chemotherapy, and photodynamic therapy (PDT). It is important to note that these studies are almost uniformly observational in nature. When comparisons are performed, they are by and large across inhomogeneous groups, thereby limiting the conclusions that can be drawn about efficacy.

P/D with Radiation

Studies that have used various forms of radiation therapy are summarized in Table 121-2. The earliest experience with combined therapy for MPM was reported by McCormack et al.[8] at the Memorial Sloan-Kettering Cancer Center. The combination of P/D with external radiation and systemic chemotherapy in 18 patients with epithelial mesothelioma produced a median survival of 16 months. In the subsequent 33 patients, brachytherapy was added, and the median survival was 21 months.

In another study at the Memorial Sloan-Kettering Cancer Center, brachytherapy was used in patients who had gross residual disease after P/D, followed by postoperative external beam radiation therapy (median dose of 4200 cGy). Local failure or disease progression occurred in 63% of patients, and median survival was 13 months.[33,34] Alberts et al. evaluated 262 patients with MPM, 26 of whom had P/D followed by radiation and chemotherapy.[30] The median survival for the whole group was 9.6 months and for the subset undergoing surgery survival was 10.9 months, which was not a statistically significant difference.

A Finnish study consisting of 100 patients evaluated five different adjuvant radiation schedules and chemotherapy regimens following pleurectomy.[31] The median survival was 8 months, and the 2-year survival was 20%. The authors found no difference among the groups.

In a more recent study, Lee et al.[32] from the University of California (UCLA), San Francisco reported their experience with 32 patients who had undergone P/D with intraoperative radiotherapy followed by external beam radiation. Some patients received chemotherapy as well. The median survival of the 26 patients who underwent the planned treatment was 18.1 months. Not included in the analysis are the three patients who had unresectable disease, one with recurrent disease and two who had early postoperative deaths.

In patients deemed unfit for EPP who undergo P/D at the Memorial Sloan-Kettering Cancer Center, our current practice is to give adjuvant external beam radiation therapy.[35]

P/D with Intrapleural and/or Systemic Chemotherapy

Studies that have been conducted using intrapleural or systemic chemotherapy are summarized in Table 121-3. Rusch et al.[36] from the Memorial Sloan-Kettering Cancer Center evaluated P/D followed by intrapleural cisplatin and mitomycin followed by systemic cisplatin and mitomycin given 3 to 5 weeks postoperatively. Twenty-eight patients underwent P/D and received intrapleural chemotherapy. There was one postoperative death, and two patients developed grade 4 nephrotoxicity. The median survival was 18 months, and significant morbidity was present in 53% of patients. Local failure was high, with 16 local relapses in 27 patients. The authors were concerned about the potential for serious toxicity.

Rice et al.[37] studied 19 stage I MPM patients who had EPP ($n = 10$) or P/D ($n = 9$) followed by intrapleural administration of cisplatin and mitomycin. The median survival was 13 months, and the treatment related mortality rate was 5%.

A group from UCLA reported their results on 15 patients who underwent P/D followed by intrapleural cisplatin and

Table 121-2

STUDIES OF PLEURECTOMY WITH RADIATION THERAPY

SOURCE	THERAPY	YEAR	PATIENTS (N)	MEDIAN SURVIVAL (MOS)	MORTALITY (%)
McCormack et al.[8]	S, R, C	1982	18	16	2
Alberts et al.[30]	S, R, B	1988	26	11	N/A
Mattson et al.[31]	S, R, C	1992	100	8	N/A
Lee et al.[32]	S, R, ± C	2002	26	18	

S = surgery; R = external radiation; B = brachytherapy; C = systemic chemotherapy; N/A = not available; ± with or without .
Source: Adapted from Van Ruth S, Baas P, Zoetmulder FA. Surgical treatment of malignant pleural mesothelioma: a review. *Chest.* 2003;123:551–561.

Table 121-3

STUDIES OF PLEURECTOMY WITH CHEMOTHERAPY

SOURCE	THERAPY	YEAR	PATIENTS (N)	MEDIAN SURVIVAL (MOS)	MORTALITY (%)
Rusch et al.[36]	S, I, C	1994	28	18	4
Rice et al.[37]	S, I, C	1994	9	13	5
Lee et al.[32]	S, I	1995	15	12	0
Colleoni et al.[38]	S, I, C	1996	20	12	0
Hasturk et al.[39]	S, C	1996	20	12	N/A
Ceresoli et al.[28]	S, C	2001	16	14	N/A
Sugarbaker et al.[43]	S, I	2003	44	9	11

S = surgery; C = systemic chemotherapy; I = intrapleural chemotherapy; N/A = not available.
Source: Adapted from Van Ruth S, Baas P, Zoetmulder FA. Surgical treatment of malignant pleural mesothelioma: a review. *Chest.* 2003;123:551–561.

cytarabine.[32] The median survival was 11.5 months with no treatment-related mortality. A similar study was reported by an Italian group that added systemic chemotherapy to the same regimen of P/D and intrapleural chemotherapy.[38] The 20 patients in this study also had an 11.5-month median survival.

A group from Turkey reported on 20 patients who had P/D followed by systemic chemotherapy consisting of cisplatin, mitomycin, and α-interferon immunotherapy.[39] The median survival was 12 months, and the regimen was well tolerated.

In a more recent study, Ceresoli et at.[28] from Italy retrospectively reviewed their experience with MPM and noted that the 16 patients who had P/D followed by chemotherapy did better than patients who received P/D or chemotherapy alone. The median survivals were 14 months in the combined treatment group, 12 months in the surgery alone group, and 8 months in the chemotherapy alone group. In univariate analysis, this treatment modality had independent prognostic value.

The search for effective therapies to achieve local control in MPM has sparked interest in a number of areas. Hyperthermia has been investigated in combination with surgery. Carry et al.[40] reported the results in three patients with MPM who were given hyperthermic intrapleural mitomycin at 42.6°C for 60 minutes following P/D. The technique was deemed safe.

In a study of similar design, Ratto et al.[41] gave hyperthermic cisplatin (41.5°C) for 60 minutes following P/D (three patients) or EPP (four patients). Patients also received 55 Gy to chest wall incisions. There was no death or toxicity, and the treatment was well tolerated. An interesting finding was that systemic cisplatin levels were significantly higher in the group that had P/D, indicating that the remaining lung plays an important role in the absorption of intrapleural cisplatin.

A group from the Netherlands studied the use of intrapleural hyperthermic (40°C–41°C) cisplatin and doxorubicin after P/D.[42] There was considerable toxicity, with morbidity reported in 47% of patients. The 11 patients had a median survival of 8 months. This group used the same protocol for advanced thymoma patients.

In a dose-escalation study, Sugarbaker et al.[43] performed P/D on 44 patients followed by intraperitoneal and ipsilateral hemithoracic lavage with cisplatin at 42°C. They reported a postoperative mortality rate of 11% and median survival of 9 months.

P/D and Photodynamic Therapy

Studies of PDT, a new modality used to enhance local control, are shown in Table 121-4. A photosensitizer is administered systemically, and then target areas are illuminated with laser to affect cell kill. Moskal et al.[44] from Roswell Park reported their series of 40 patients who had been treated with EPP ($n = 7$), P/D ($n = 28$), or P/D with lobectomy ($n = 5$) followed by PDT.[45] The mortality rate was 6.5%, with two of the deaths in the EPP group. Serious complications arose in 48.3% of patients. The median survival was 15 months.

Pass et al.[46] at the National Institutes of Health performed a randomized study of surgical resection, postoperative cisplatin, interferon, and tamoxifen with or without PDT. Twenty-five patients received PDT (11 P/D and 14 EPP), and 23 patients did not (12 P/D and 11 EPP). The groups were similar, and no survival difference was noted. Median survivals in the PDT group and non-PDT group were 14.4 and 14.1 months, respectively. The conclusion was that there was no value of first-generation PDT when added to multimodality therapy. Further studies with newer photosensitizers and increasing light doses are ongoing.

Table 121-4

STUDIES OF PLEURECTOMY WITH PHOTODYNAMIC THERAPY

SOURCE	THERAPY	YEAR	PATIENTS (N)	MEDIAN SURVIVAL (MOS)	MORTALITY (%)
Pass et al.[46]	S, P, C, I	1997	25	14	4
Moskal et al.[44]	S, P	1998	40	15	7

S = surgery; C = systemic chemotherapy; I = intrapleural chemotherapy; P = photodynamic therapy.
Source: Adapted from Van Ruth S, Baas P, Zoetmulder FA. Surgical treatment of malignant pleural mesothelioma: a review. *Chest.* 2003;123:551–561.

SECONDARY PLEURAL MALIGNANCIES

Almost any cancer can metastasize to the pleural space. The most frequent manifestation of this phenomenon is a pleural effusion. This by and large is an end-stage process, and the goals for these patients are palliative. As such, less invasive measures than P/D can and should be used (see Chapters 119 and 120). Certain cancers can present with localized pleural masses. The most common is lung cancer, locally advanced by definition and not amenable to surgical resection by P/D. Occasionally, recurrences of lung cancers present as isolated pleural masses. There is no evidence to suggest that P/D in these instances offers much in the way of palliation or cure.

A noteworthy exception to the general rule of secondary pleural malignancies is thymoma. Thymomas with drop metastases in the pleura (Masoaka stage IVa) have been treated by some with complete excision of the primary tumor and P/D for the pleural involvement. In highly selected patients, we have performed EPP followed by high-dose hemithoracic irradiation at our center. The rationale for this treatment strategy is that it is generally accepted that the best chance for cure in thymoma is complete resection. Combined-modality approaches are used most often.

Refaely et al.[47] from Israel performed resection followed by hyperthermic perfusion with cisplatin. They evaluated 15 patients with stage IVa thymoma: Five patients had resections with accompanying pleurectomies, one patient had EPP, and nine patients had resections without pleurectomy. They had no mortality and felt that the treatment was safe. Eight of the 15 patients were alive at 60 months.

The greatest difficulty in assessing the literature in this area is related to the extent of pleurectomy performed. Despite descriptions of complete resections for thymomas involving pleura, this may mean local excisions of the pleural disease rather than true P/D. The group from the Netherlands that did use true P/D followed by hyperthermic cisplatin and doxorubicin for mesothelioma also used the same protocol for three patients with stage IVa thymoma.[42] In their short follow-up, all three patients were disease-free at 18 months.

P/D for secondary malignancies is an option in thymoma with pleural metastases, but only as a component of a multimodality management strategy. For other metastatic pleural disease, it has little role.

SUMMARY

The role of surgery in the management of MPM remains controversial. The range of goals of surgery includes diagnosis, palliation of symptoms, debulking of tumor, removal of all gross diseases, and possibly cures. The major approaches in the armamentarium of the mesothelioma surgeon are, in order of increasing complexity, thoracoscopy for biopsy and pleurodesis, partial pleurectomy, radical P/D, and EPP. With no set standards of care or overwhelming evidence to guide the thoracic surgeon, a fair amount of clinical judgment and a frank discussion of goals with the patient and other members of the health care team are required to formulate a comprehensive treatment plan. It is clear that a multimodality approach is required.

In secondary or metastatic pleural disease, the role of surgery is confined largely to diagnosis. A possible exception to this rule is in thymoma, where P/D has been performed in some patients with stage IVa disease with encouraging results.

EDITOR'S COMMENT

Pleurectomy involves the physical removal of the visceral, mediastinal, and parietal pleura while the underlying lung is preserved. Generally, the technique does not remove as much tumor as an EPP, particularly in patients with tumor located deep in the lung fissures or along the attachment of the pleura to the central tendon of the diaphragm and/or the pericardium. Nevertheless, a macroscopic complete resection still can be achieved in some patients using this approach. Since the first edition was published, new terminology has been introduced by an international committee to reflect the various practices of individual surgeons and to improve documentation for better comparative analysis of outcomes. The term P/D has been approved to denote attempted complete removal of macroscopic tumor from the visceral and parietal pleura. The term "extended P/D" should be used if the diaphragm and pericardium are removed as well.[9]

The authors provide several ideas that should be favorably considered by surgeons treating MPM. There is a large difference in the operative mortality between EPP and P/D for mesothelioma, especially in centers without a large operative experience. Furthermore, the quality of life of the mesothelioma patient is improved if the ipsilateral lung has been saved. Pleurectomy, on the other hand, cannot provide the same amount of debulking of the tumor as an EPP. Improved adjuvant therapy at the time of surgery may bring the long-term survival rate of pleurectomy in line with the larger operation of EPP. The authors provide excellent technical details for the operation. Additional details are provided in Chapter 124. I agree with the authors that pleurectomy in secondary malignancies of the pleura has little role except in the treatment of malignant thymoma metastatic to the pleural space.

—Michael T. Jaklitsch

References

1. Wagner JC, Sleggs CA, Marchand P. Diffuse pleural mesothelioma and asbestos exposure in the North Western Cape Province. *Br J Ind Med.* 1960;17:260–271.
2. Verschraegen C. Mesothelioma: incidence and survival rates in the United States. *Proc Am Soc Clin Oncol.* 2003;22:869; abstract 3495.
3. Butchart EG, Ashcroft T, Barnsley WC, et al. Pleuropneumonectomy in the management of diffuse malignant mesothelioma of the pleura. Experience with 29 patients. *Thorax.* 1976;31:15–24.
4. Sugarbaker DJ, Norberto JJ, Swanson SJ. Surgical staging and work-up of patients with diffuse malignant pleural mesothelioma. *Semin Thorac Cardiovasc Surg.* 1997;9:356–360.
5. Rusch VW. A proposed new international TNM staging system for malignant pleural mesothelioma. From the International Mesothelioma Interest Group. *Chest.* 1995;108:1122–1128.
6. Sugarbaker DJ, Flores RM, Jaklitsch MT, et al. Resection margins, extrapleural nodal status, and cell type determine postoperative long-term survival in trimodality therapy of malignant pleural mesothelioma:

results in 183 patients. *J Thorac Cardiovasc Surg.* 1999;117:54–63; discussion 65.
7. Rusch VW, Venkatraman ES. Important prognostic factors in patients with malignant pleural mesothelioma, managed surgically. *Ann Thorac Surg.* 1999;68:1799–1804.
8. McCormack PM, Nagasaki F, Hilaris BS, et al. Surgical treatment of pleural mesothelioma. *J Thorac Cardiovasc Surg.* 1982;84:834–842.
9. Rice D, Rusch V, Pass H, et al. Recommendations for uniform definitions of surgical techniques for malignant pleural mesothelioma: a consensus report of the international association for the study of lung cancer international staging committee and the international mesothelioma interest group. *J Thorac Oncol.* 2011;6(8):1304–1312.
10. Feigen M, Lee ST, Lawford, C, et al. Establishing locoregional control of malignant pleural mesothelioma using high-dose radiotherapy and (18) F-FDG PET/CT scan correlation. *J Med Imaging Radiat Oncol.* 2011;55(3):320–332.
11. Flores RM, Pass HI, Seshan VE, et al. Extrapleural pneumonectomy versus pleurectomy/decortications in the surgical management of malignant pleural mesothelioma: results in 663 patients. *J Thorac Cardiovasc Surg.* 2008;135(3):620–626.
12. Heelan RT, Rusch VW, Begg CB, et al. Staging of malignant pleural mesothelioma: comparison of CT and MR imaging. *AJR Am J Roentgenol.* 1999;172:1039–1047.
13. Benard F, Sterman D, Smith RJ, et al. Metabolic imaging of malignant pleural mesothelioma with fluorodeoxyglucose positron emission tomography. *Chest.* 1998;114:713–722.
14. Flores RM, Akhurst T, Gonen M, et al. Positron emission tomography defines metastatic disease but not locoregional disease in patients with malignant pleural mesothelioma. *J Thorac Cardiovasc Surg.* 2003;126:11–16.
15. Flores R, Akhurst T, Gonen M. FDG-PET predicts survival in patients with malignant pleural mesothelioma. *Proc Am Soc Clin Oncol.* 2003;22:620; abstract 2493.
16. Schouwink JH, Kool LS, Rutgers EJ, et al. The value of chest computer tomography and cervical mediastinoscopy in the preoperative assessment of patients with malignant pleural mesothelioma. *Ann Thorac Surg.* 2003;75:1715–1718; discussion 1718–1719.
17. Neragi-Miandoab S, Weiner S, Sugarbaker DJ. Incidence of atrial fibrillation after extrapleural pneumonectomy vs. pleurectomy in patients with malignant pleural mesothelioma. *Interact Cardiovasc Thorac Surg.* 2008;7(6):1039–1042.
18. Pass HI, Pogrebniak HW. Malignant pleural mesothelioma. *Curr Probl Surg.* 1993;30:921–1012.
19. Chahinian AP, Pajak TF, Holland JF, et al. Diffuse malignant mesothelioma. Prospective evaluation of 69 patients. *Ann Intern Med.* 1982;96:746–755.
20. Brenner J, Sordillo PP, Magill GB, et al. Malignant mesothelioma of the pleura: review of 123 patients. *Cancer.* 1982;49:2431–2435.
21. Law M, Gregor A, Hodson M. Malignant mesothelioma of the pleura: a study of 52 treated and 64 untreated patients. *Thorax.* 1984;39:255–259.
22. Chailleux E, Dabouis G, Pioche D, et al. Prognostic factors in diffuse malignant pleural mesothelioma. A study of 167 patients. *Chest.* 1988;93:159–162.
23. Ruffie P, Feld R, Minkin S, et al. Diffuse malignant mesothelioma of the pleura in Ontario and Quebec: a retrospective study of 332 patients. *J Clin Oncol.* 1989;7:1157–1168.
24. Brancatisano RP, Joseph MG, McCaughan BC. Pleurectomy for mesothelioma. *Med J Aust.* 1991;154:455–457, 460.
25. Rusch VW, Piantadosi S, Holmes EC. The role of extrapleural pneumonectomy in malignant pleural mesothelioma. A Lung Cancer Study Group trial. *J Thorac Cardiovasc Surg.* 1991;102:1–9.
26. Allen KB, Faber LP, Warren WH. Malignant pleural mesothelioma. Extrapleural pneumonectomy and pleurectomy. *Chest Surg Clin N Am.* 1994;4:113–126.
27. Soysal O, Karaoglanoglu N, Demiracan S, et al. Pleurectomy/decortication for palliation in malignant pleural mesothelioma: results of surgery. *Eur J Cardiothorac Surg.* 1997;11:210–213.
28. Ceresoli GL, Locati LD, Ferreri AJ, et al. Therapeutic outcome according to histologic subtype in 121 patients with malignant pleural mesothelioma. *Lung Cancer.* 2001;34:279–287.
29. Rusch VW. Pleurectomy/decortication in the setting of multimodality treatment for diffuse malignant pleural mesothelioma. *Semin Thorac Cardiovasc Surg.* 1997;9:367–372.
30. Alberts AS, Falkson G, Goedhals L, et al. Malignant pleural mesothelioma: a disease unaffected by current therapeutic maneuvers. *J Clin Oncol.* 1988;6:527–535.
31. Mattson K, Holsti LR, Tammilehto L, et al. Multimodality treatment programs for malignant pleural mesothelioma using high-dose hemithorax irradiation. *Int J Radiat Oncol Biol Phys.* 1992;24:643–650.
32. Lee JD, Perez S, Wang HJ, et al. Intrapleural chemotherapy for patients with incompletely resected malignant mesothelioma: the UCLA experience. *J Surg Oncol.* 1995;60:262–267.
33. Mychalczak B, Nori D, Armstrong J. Results of treatment of malignant pleural mesothelioma with surgery, brachytherapy, and external beam irradiation. *Endocurie Hypertherm Oncol.* 1989;5:245.
34. Hilaris BS, Nori D, Kwong E, et al. Pleurectomy and intraoperative brachytherapy and postoperative radiation in the treatment of malignant pleural mesothelioma. *Int J Radiat Oncol Biol Phys.* 1984;10:325–331.
35. Rosenzweig K, Gupta V, Flores R, et al. Hemithoracic radiation therapy and brachytherapy after pleurectomy/decortication for malignant pleural mesothelioma: Results from a 30-year experience. *Am Soc Clin Oncol.* 2005;23:665S–665S; abstract 7180.
36. Rusch V, Saltz L, Venkatraman E, et al. A phase II trial of pleurectomy/decortication followed by intrapleural and systemic chemotherapy for malignant pleural mesothelioma. *J Clin Oncol.* 1994;12:1156–1163.
37. Rice TW, Adelstein DJ, Kirby TJ, et al. Aggressive multimodality therapy for malignant pleural mesothelioma. *Ann Thorac Surg.* 1994;58:24–29.
38. Colleoni M, Sartori F, Calabro F, et al. Surgery followed by intracavitary plus systemic chemotherapy in malignant pleural mesothelioma. *Tumori.* 1996;82:53–56.
39. Hasturk S, Tastepe I, Unlu M, et al. Combined chemotherapy in pleurectomized malignant pleural mesothelioma patients. *J Chemother.* 1996;8:159–164.
40. Carry PY, Brachet A, Gilly FN, et al. A new device for the treatment of pleural malignancies: intrapleural chemohyperthermia preliminary report. *Oncology.* 1993;50:348–352.
41. Ratto GB, Civalleri D, Esposito M, et al. Pleural space perfusion with cisplatin in the multimodality treatment of malignant mesothelioma: a feasibility and pharmacokinetic study. *J Thorac Cardiovasc Surg.* 1999; 117:759–765.
42. de Bree E, van Ruth S, Baas P, et al. Cytoreductive surgery and intraoperative hyperthermic intrathoracic chemotherapy in patients with malignant pleural mesothelioma or pleural metastases of thymoma. *Chest.* 2002;121:480–487.
43. Sugarbaker D, Richards W, Zellos L. Feasibility of pleurectomy and intraoperative bicavitary hyperthermic cisplatin lavage for mesothelioma: a phase I-II study . *Proc Am Soc Clin Oncol.* 2003;22:620; abstract 620.
44. Moskal TL, Dougherty TJ, Urschel JD, et al. Operation and photodynamic therapy for pleural mesothelioma: 6-year follow-up. *Ann Thorac Surg.* 1998;66:1128–1133.
45. Takita H, Mang TS, Loewen GM, et al. Operation and intracavitary photodynamic therapy for malignant pleural mesothelioma: a phase II study. *Ann Thorac Surg.* 1994;58:995–998.
46. Pass HI, Temeck BK, Kranda K, et al. Phase III randomized trial of surgery with or without intraoperative photodynamic therapy and postoperative immunochemotherapy for malignant pleural mesothelioma. *Ann Surg Oncol.* 1997;4:628–633.
47. Refaely Y, Simansky DA, Paley M, et al. Resection and perfusion thermochemotherapy: a new approach for the treatment of thymic malignancies with pleural spread. *Ann Thorac Surg.* 2001;72:366–370.

122 Extrapleural Pneumonectomy for Pleural Malignancies

Jay M. Lee and David J. Sugarbaker

Keywords: Extrapleural pneumonectomy, mesothelioma, pleural malignancy, postoperative complications, revised Brigham staging system, Kaplan–Meier survival curves

Diffuse malignant pleural mesothelioma is a rare aggressive cancer associated with asbestos exposure. Approximately 2000 to 3000 cases occur annually. The natural history is defined by a median survival of 4 to 12 months with no treatment. Difficulties in diagnosis, staging, and treatment have made mesothelioma a challenging entity for most clinicians.

In the 1940s, Sarot[1] first described the technique of extrapleural pneumonectomy (EPP) for tuberculous empyema. In the 1980s, the operation was applied to diffuse malignant pleural mesothelioma and later to other malignancies, including locally advanced lung cancer and thymoma. In 1976, Butchart and associates reported a prohibitive operative mortality of 31%, but other series have reported a mortality range of 6% to 13%.[2] In the 1990s, significant improvements in mortality rates were achieved. In 1999, our institution reported the lowest published operative mortality of 3.8%.[3] A retrospective study of our results from the Brigham and Women's Hospital/Dana Farber Cancer Institute was reported, representing the largest single-institution review of 328 patients with mesothelioma who underwent EPP between 1980 and 2000. With further experience, our operative mortality declined to 3.4%.[4]

PATIENT SELECTION AND PREOPERATIVE ASSESSMENT

The significant improvement in perioperative mortality has been attributed to continuous refinements in technique and aggressive prevention and treatment of complications.[2,4] However, defined criteria for patient selection and comprehensive preoperative assessment also have contributed to the improvement in surgical results.

To be considered a candidate for EPP, a patient must meet several preoperative criteria (Table 122-1). The patient must have a Karnofsky performance status of greater than 70, normal liver and renal function tests, a room air arterial P_{CO_2} of less than 45 mm Hg, and a room air arterial P_{O_2} of greater than 65 mm Hg. While there is no strict age limit, we are hesitant to perform EPP in patients older than 70 years of age. A pulmonary function test that reveals a forced expiratory volume in 1 second (FEV_1) greater than 2 L is considered adequate for pneumonectomy. Quantitative ventilation/perfusion scan is indicated if the FEV_1 is less than 2 L. The combination of ventilation/perfusion scan and preoperative FEV_1 is used to predict postoperative lung function. Patients with a predicted postoperative FEV_1 of greater than 0.8 are acceptable candidates for EPP. Patients with a predicted postoperative FEV_1 of less than 0.8 L are considered for pleurectomy and decortication (see Chapter 121).

Echocardiography provides valuable information, including assessment of ventricular function, chamber size, wall motion abnormalities, valvular disease, and pulmonary artery pressure. Echocardiographic evidence of pulmonary hypertension warrants a right heart catheterization for direct pulmonary artery pressure measurement. The presence of pulmonary hypertension is a contraindication to pneumonectomy. For patients considered to be inoperable on the basis of pulmonary hypertension, temporary balloon occlusion of the ipsilateral main pulmonary artery can be performed during catheterization to simulate pneumonectomy physiology. During balloon occlusion, the patient is monitored for hemodynamic instability.

Preoperative chest MRI and CT scanning are used routinely to determine the extent of disease and to rule out transdiaphragmatic abdominal extension, contralateral hemithorax involvement, and mediastinal invasion. The presence of locally advanced or distant disease to these areas precludes resection. Chest MRI has been shown to be a valuable complement to chest CT scanning in making this determination.[5] However, chest MRI and CT scan can be unreliable in assessing chest wall invasion. As a result, exploration is performed in patients with questionable radiographic evidence of chest wall invasion and no radiographic evidence of distant disease. Extrathoracic chest wall invasion discovered at exploration is a contraindication to resection. Obvious radiologic demonstration of invasion into the chest wall or palpable tumor by examination is considered unresectable, and the patient is not offered exploration.

Chest MRI and CT scan can be misleading in assessing transdiaphragmatic peritoneal invasion because of the difficulty in distinguishing local tumor compression on the diaphragm

Table 122-1

PATIENT SELECTION CRITERIA

Karnofsky performance score	>70
Renal function	Creatinine < 2
Liver function	AST < 80 IU/L, total bilirubin < 1.9 mg/dL, PT < 15 s
Pulmonary function	Postoperative FEV_1 > 0.8 L as per PFTs and quantitative ventilation/perfusion scans
Cardiac function	Grossly normal cardiac function as per ECG and echocardiography (ejection fraction preferably >45%)
Extent of disease	Limited to ipsilateral hemithorax with no transdiaphragmatic, transpericardial, or extensive chest wall involvement

AST = aspartate aminotransferase; PT = prothrombin time, seconds; FEV_1 = forced expiratory volume in 1 s; PFTs = pulmonary function tests; ECG = electrocardiography; EF = ejection fraction.

Adapted with permission from Sugarbaker DJ, Jaklitsch MT, Bueno R, et al. Prevention, early detection, and management of complications after 328 consecutive extrapleural pneumonectomies. *J Thorac Cardiovasc Surg.* 2004;128: 138–146.

versus true transdiaphragmatic invasion. Radiologic evidence of transdiaphragmatic extension, intra-abdominal tumor, or ascites is an indication for diagnostic laparoscopy or exploratory laparotomy to evaluate the peritoneal cavity.

Histologic diagnosis of mesothelioma by pleural biopsy is required before proceeding with resection. Although cytologic diagnosis is possible, the differentiation of mesothelioma from adenocarcinoma or sarcoma can be difficult. Surgical biopsy is considered the gold standard method for definitive diagnosis. Thoracoscopic pleural biopsy is generally performed via a single port along the incision line of the intended future thoracotomy. Radiologic suggestion of contralateral thoracic disease requires tissue confirmation by pleural or lung biopsy from the contralateral chest. Staging cervical mediastinoscopy is performed. If there is metastatic disease to the mediastinal lymph nodes, the patient should undergo induction chemotherapy followed by re-evaluation for surgical resection with restaging radiographic studies for an extent of disease work-up. In the absence of mediastinal involvement, the patient would proceed directly to surgical resection.

TECHNIQUE OF RIGHT EXTRAPLEURAL PNEUMONECTOMY

Anesthesia

A thoracic epidural catheter is placed preoperatively for intraoperative management and postoperative analgesia. Standard monitoring with telemetry, continuous pulse oximetry, central venous access, and urinary Foley catheterization are routinely used. After anesthetic induction, a left-sided double-lumen endotracheal tube is placed for single-lung ventilation, and the patient is positioned in the left lateral decubitus position for an extended right posterolateral thoracotomy. A nasogastric tube is placed, which facilitates identification of the esophagus during extrapleural dissection. It is left in place postoperatively to decompress the stomach and to prevent aspiration.

Surgical Management

EPP is performed in the following order: (1) incision and exposure of the parietal pleura; (2) extrapleural dissection to separate the tumor from the chest wall; (3) en bloc resection of the lung, pleura, pericardium, and diaphragm with division of the hilar structures; (4) radical lymph node dissection; and (5) reconstruction of the diaphragm and pericardium.[2,6,7]

When there is preoperative radiologic evidence suggesting intra-abdominal disease, a limited subcostal incision is made along the line of the thoracotomy incision before proceeding with definitive resection. The diaphragm and peritoneal cavity are inspected for transdiaphragmatic involvement. Laparoscopic evaluation may be used as an alternative approach to an open subcostal incision. If there is evidence of intra-abdominal disease, histologic diagnosis is confirmed by biopsy, and the resection is aborted.

In the absence of intra-abdominal spread, an extended right posterolateral thoracotomy is performed (Fig. 122-1). The incision is started midway between the posterior scapular tip and the spine (*inset*) and extended along the sixth rib to the costochondral junction.[6] The latissimus dorsi and serratus anterior muscles are both divided. The sixth rib is resected.

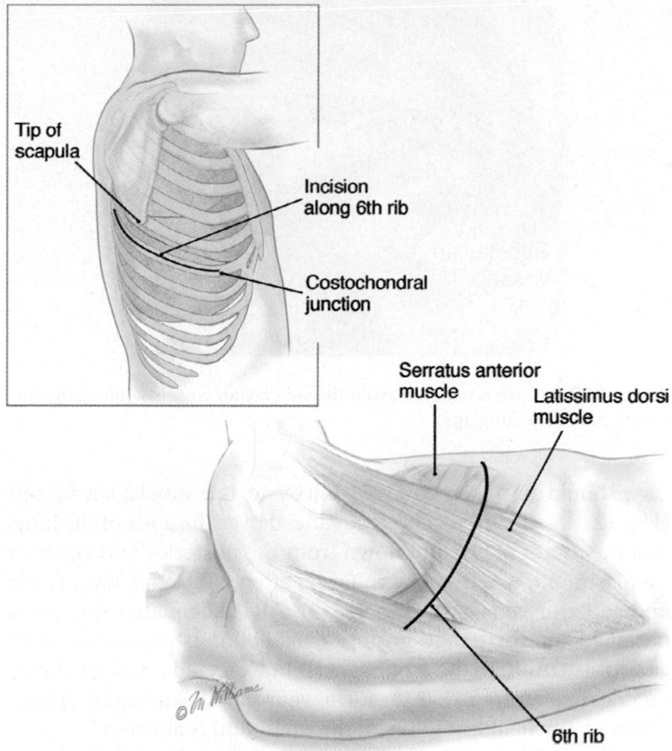

Figure 122-1. Incision and exposure for a right posterolateral thoracotomy.

The posterior periosteum in the bed of the sixth rib is incised, exposing the extrapleural plane.

Extrapleural dissection is performed with the use of blunt and sharp dissections initially in the anterolateral aspect followed by dissection to the apex. Anteriorly, the internal mammary vessels should be identified to prevent avulsion. If extensive chest wall invasion is discovered obliterating the extrapleural plane, surgical resection is precluded. In the absence of chest wall invasion, the extrapleural plane is extended, and previously dissected areas are packed with surgical pads for hemostasis. Along the thoracotomy, two chest retractors are positioned anteriorly and posteriorly to optimize exposure (Fig. 122-2). At the apex,

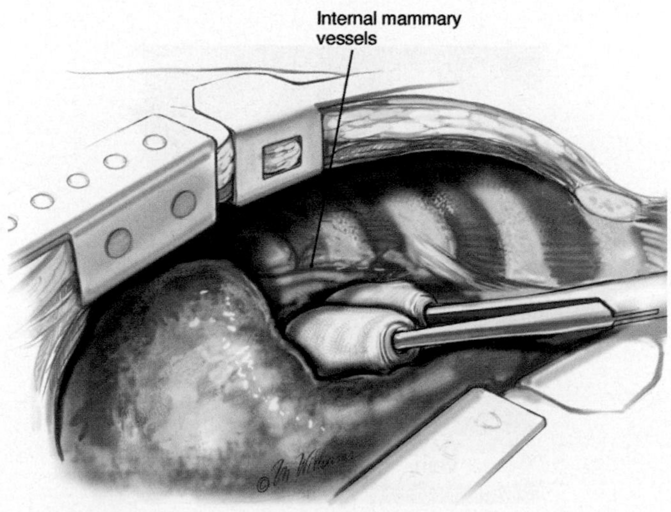

Figure 122-2. Two chest retractors are placed, one anterior and one posterior, to increase the exposure.

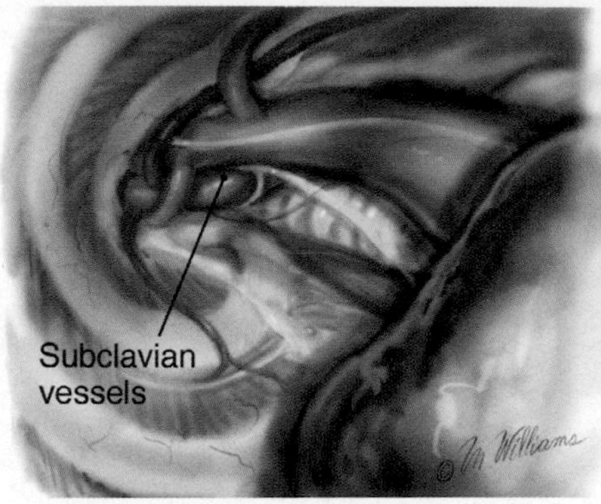

Figure 122-3. Care is taken to avoid the subclavian vessels while dissecting the pleura at the lung apex.

care should be taken to avoid injury to the subclavian vessels (Fig. 122-3). The dissection is advanced over the apex of the lung, and the tumor is brought down from the posterior and superior mediastinum, where care should be attended to the azygos vein and superior vena cava (Fig. 122-4). After adequate exposure is obtained anterolaterally, posterior dissection is performed, with careful attention to the esophagus. If unexpected invasion of vital mediastinal structures (e.g., aorta, vena cava, esophagus, epicardium, or trachea) is identified, the operation is aborted.

The extrapleural dissection is continued until the right upper lobe and right mainstem bronchus are exposed. Resectability is assessed by direct palpation posteriorly for aortic and esophageal invasion. The esophagus is dissected away from the tumor, facilitated by palpation of the nasogastric tube to avoid injury (Fig. 122-5). The pericardium is opened anteriorly, and the pericardial space is palpated to assess for myocardial invasion (Fig. 122-6). In the absence of mediastinal extension, diaphragmatic resection is initiated.

The diaphragm is incised first at its lateral margin, followed by a circumferential resection anteriorly and posteriorly (Fig. 122-7). The diaphragmatic muscle attachments to the chest wall are cauterized or bluntly avulsed (Fig. 122-8). The peritoneum is bluntly dissected off the diaphragm (Fig. 122-9). Dissection is performed at the inferior vena cava and esophageal hiatus with caution (Fig. 122-10). The pericardial incision is extended.

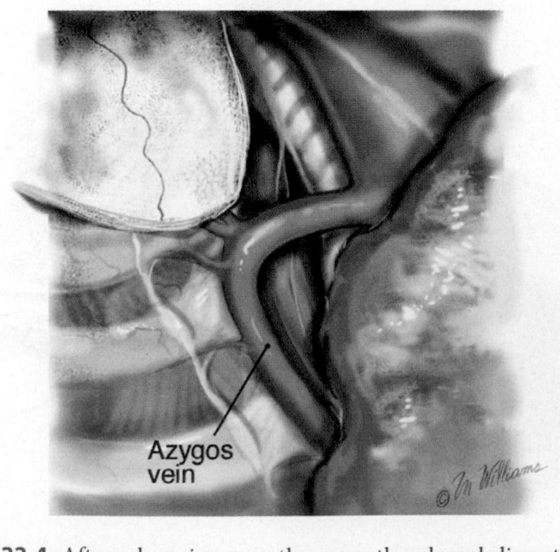

Figure 122-4. After advancing over the apex, the pleural dissection proceeds inferiorly, with attention to the azygos vein and superior vena cava.

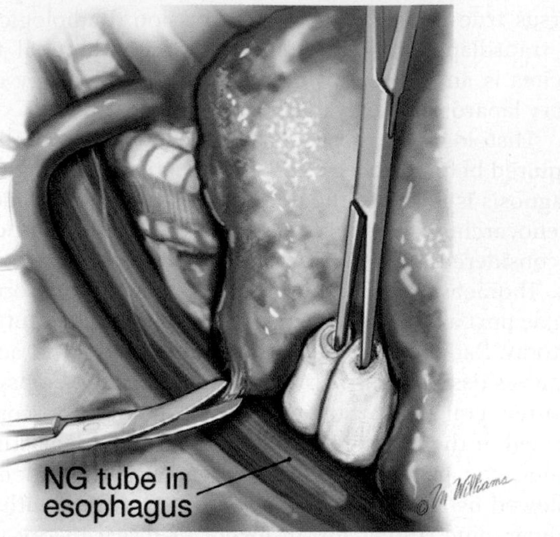

Figure 122-5. A nasogastric tube in the esophagus aids in palpating the esophagus while dissecting the pleura from the esophagus.

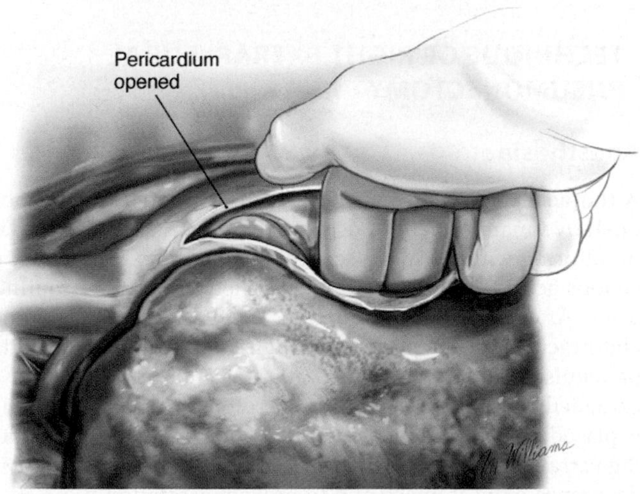

Figure 122-6. The pericardium is opened anteriorly, and the pericardial space is palpated to assess for myocardial invasion.

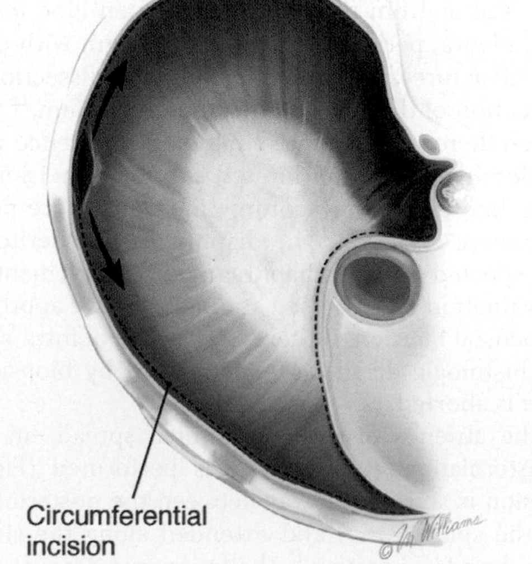

Figure 122-7. The diaphragm is incised circumferentially.

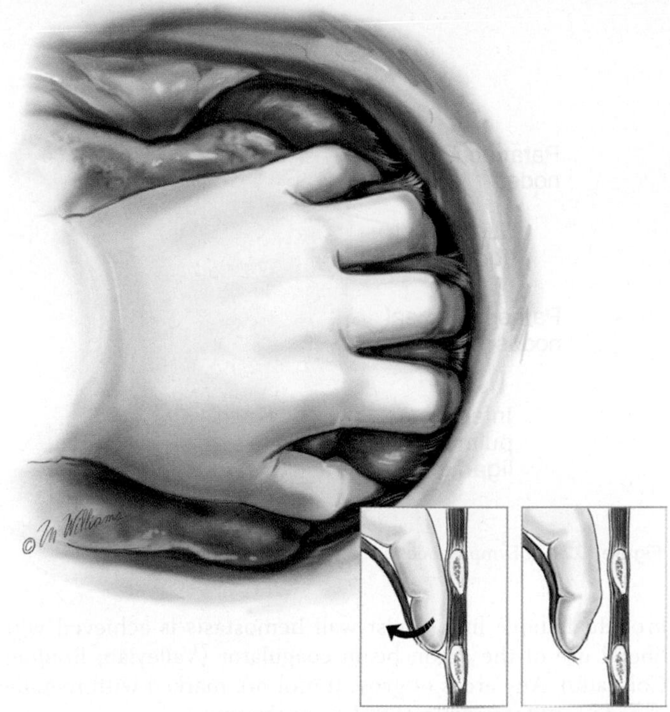

Figure 122-8. The diaphragm is separated bluntly or by avulsion from the chest wall muscular attachments.

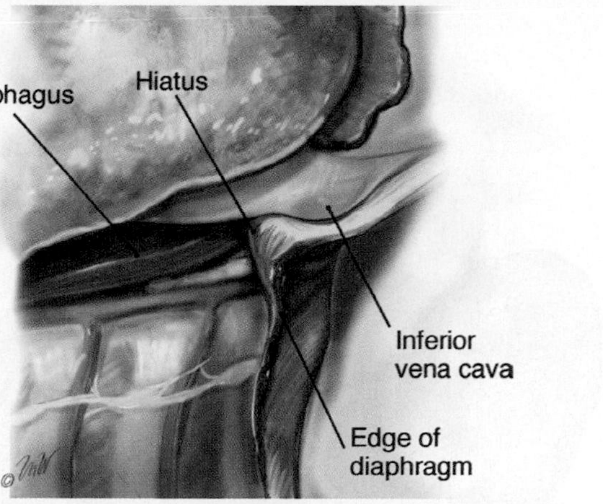

Figure 122-10. Dissection around the esophageal hiatus and inferior vena cava.

The junction of the pericardium and diaphragm and the medial aspect of the diaphragm are divided. With release of the diaphragmatic attachments medially and posteriorly, the esophagus is dissected away from the specimen.

The anterior pericardial incision is extended to the level of the hilum. The main right pulmonary artery is dissected intrapericardially (Fig. 122-11). A soft-flanged catheter (endoleader) is passed around the pulmonary artery to guide the safe passage of the endovascular stapler (United States Surgical, Norwalk, CT), which facilitates division of the pulmonary artery (Fig. 122-12). The superior and inferior pulmonary veins are divided intrapericardially in the same fashion. After division of

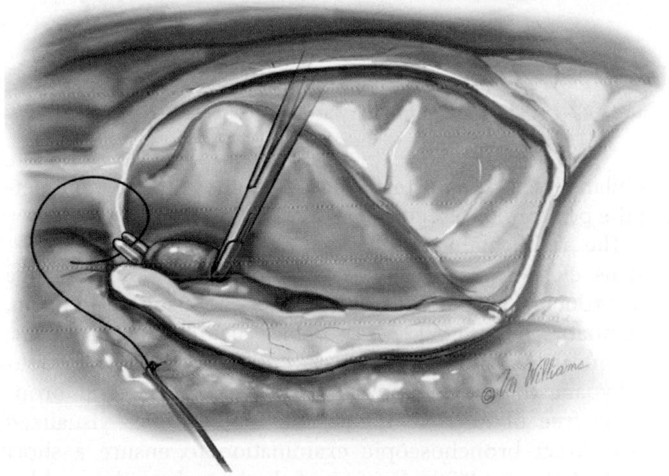

Figure 122-11. The posterior pericardium and medial aspect of the diaphragm are divided.

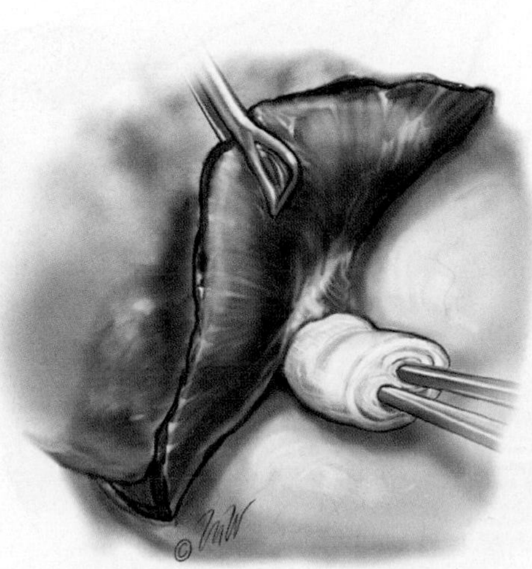

Figure 122-9. The diaphragm is dissected bluntly from the underlying peritoneum.

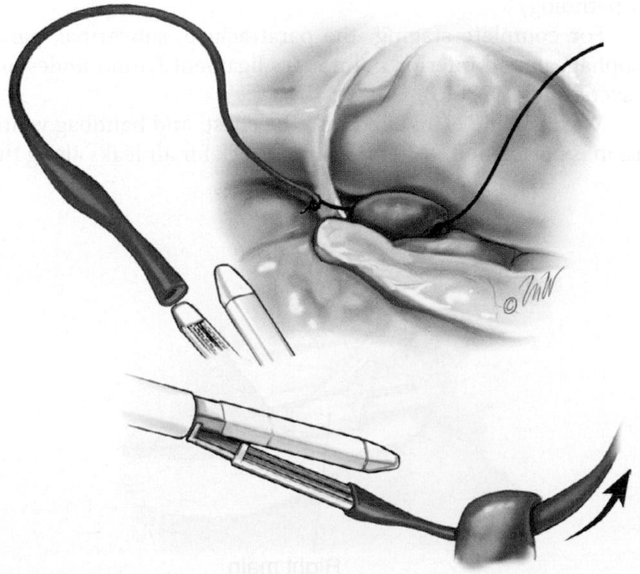

Figure 122-12. An endoleader is passed around the pulmonary artery to guide the safe passage of the endovascular stapler, and the right pulmonary artery is divided.

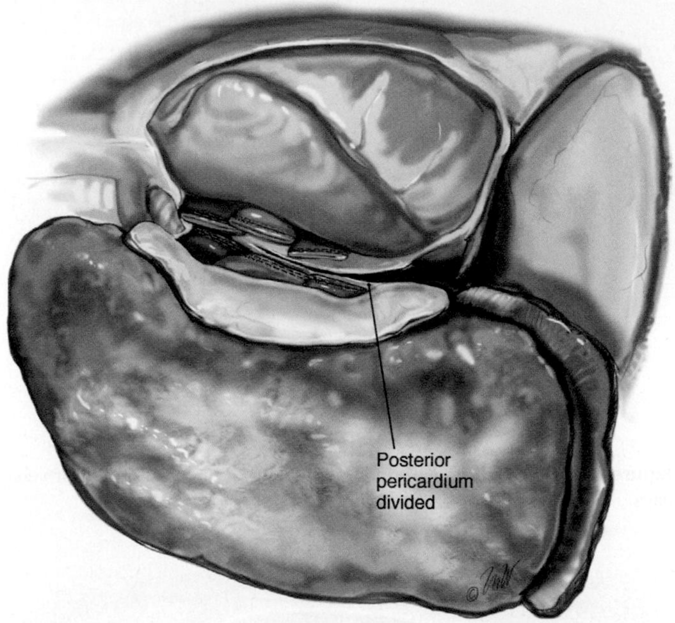

Figure 122-13. The right pulmonary artery is dissected.

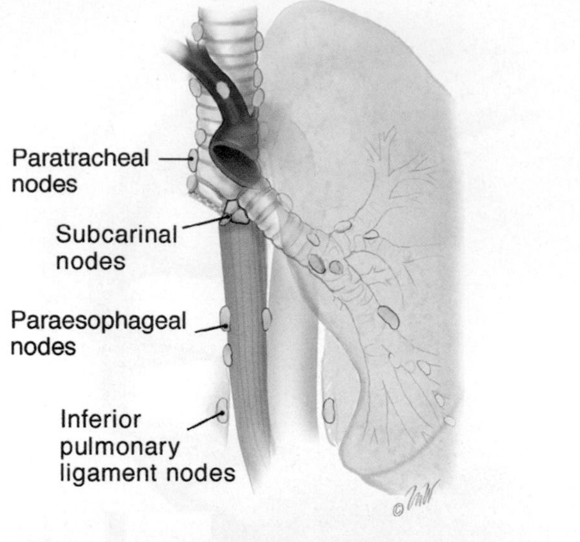

Figure 122-15. Lymph nodes are dissected for clinical staging.

the hilar vessels, the posterior pericardium is incised, completing the pericardial resection (Fig. 122-13).

The right mainstem bronchus is dissected and encircled as close to the carina as possible with a heavy-gauge wire bronchial stapler (TA-30, Ethicon, Johnson & Johnson, Cincinnati, OH) (Fig. 122-14). Before dividing the bronchus, the contralateral lung is handbag ventilated (Valsalva maneuver by anesthesia) to confirm that the contralateral bronchus is free of encroachment, and the stump is visualized under direct bronchoscopic examination to ensure a short bronchial stump. With division of the bronchus, the en bloc resection (i.e., lung, pleura, pericardium, and diaphragm) is complete, and the specimen is removed from the thorax. A frozen-section analysis of the bronchial margin is performed by pathology.

For complete staging, the paratracheal, subcarinal, paraesophageal, and inferior pulmonary ligament lymph nodes are resected (Fig. 122-15).

Warm saline is instilled into the chest, and handbag ventilation is performed to 30 mm Hg to check for air leaks along the bronchial staple line. Chest wall hemostasis is achieved with liberal use of the argon beam coagulator (Valleylab, Boulder, Colorado). Any areas of gross tumor are marked with metallic clips to facilitate adjuvant radiation therapy.

The greater omentum is mobilized off the transverse colon, and the vascular supply is contoured from a pedicle off the gastroepiploic arteries along the greater curvature of the stomach (Fig. 122-16). The omental flap is used later to buttress the bronchial stump.

The diaphragmatic and pericardial defects are reconstructed with Gore-Tex (W.L. Gore and Associates, Flagstaff, Arizona) patches. The diaphragm is reconstructed using two

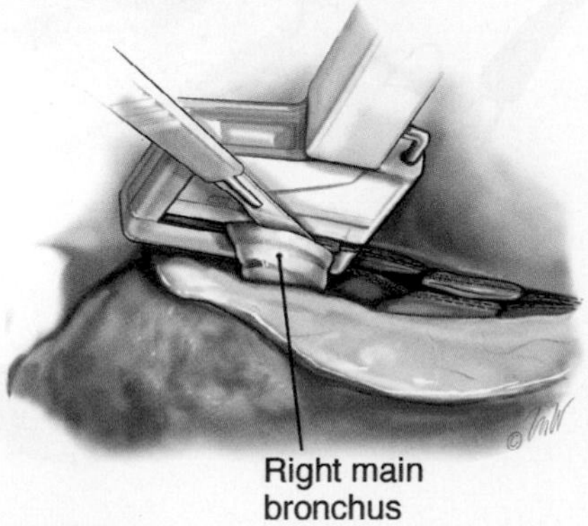

Figure 122-14. The right mainstem bronchus is encircled as close to the carina as possible before division with a heavy-gauge wire bronchial stapler.

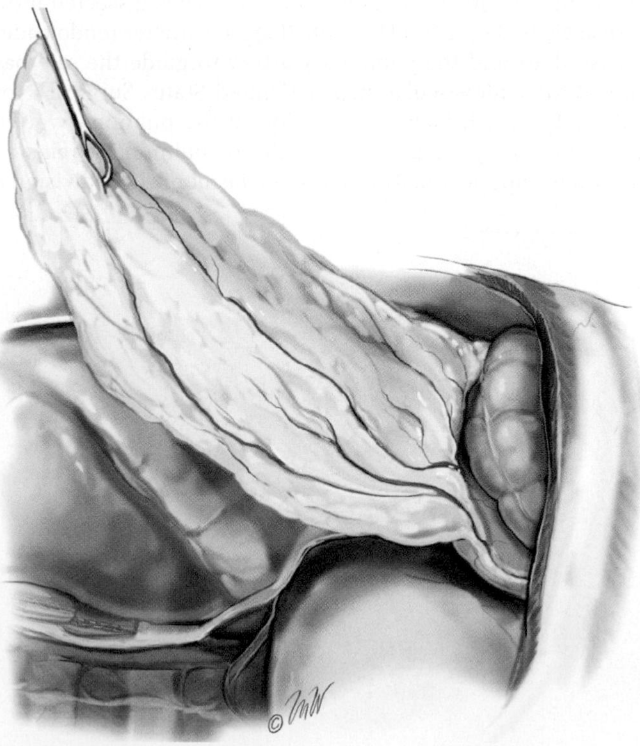

Figure 122-16. The omental flap is harvested for later use as a bronchial buttress.

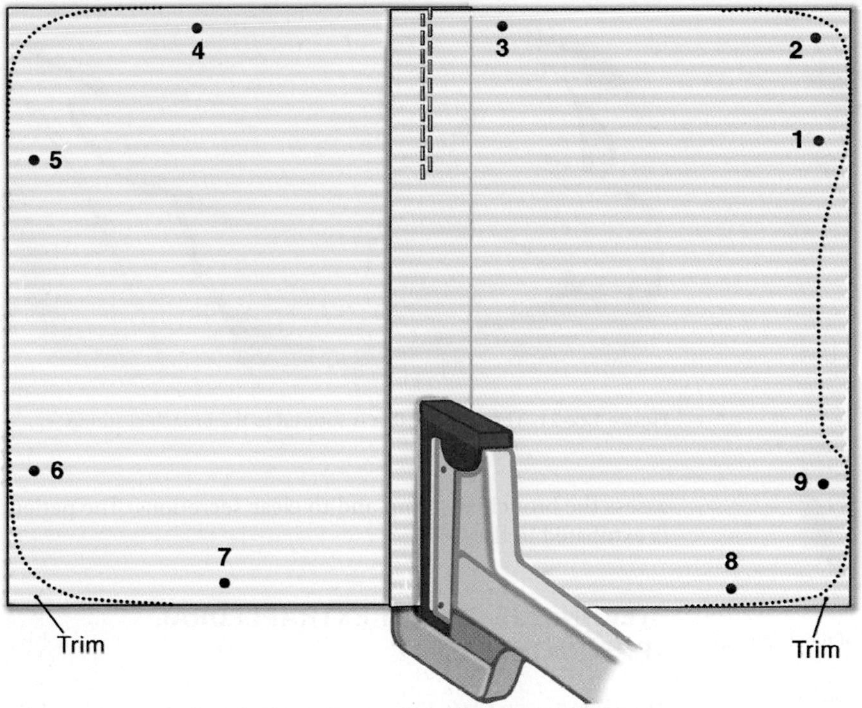

Figure 122-17. The diaphragmatic patch is constructed from two pieces of 2-mm-thick Gore-Tex dual mesh.

pieces (20 cm × 30 cm) of 2-mm-thick Gore-Tex dual patch stapled together in a side-by-side fashion with slight overlap at the center (Fig. 122-17). The patch is contoured to the hemithorax. This creates a loose, floppy patch at the center with less tension along the suture line. This dynamic patch is less likely to be complicated by patch dehiscence from the chest wall and abdominal content herniation into the pneumonectomy cavity. The diaphragmatic patch is sutured anteriorly, laterally, and posteriorly to the chest wall with nine Gore-Tex sutures placed through the patch and intercostal space. Each suture is passed through a 14-mm polypropylene button. The sutures are tied down on the button, buttressing the patch to the chest wall (Fig. 122-18). Before completing the diaphragm reconstruction medially, a small opening is created on the medial mid-portion of the diaphragmatic patch to permit transposition of the omental flap into the pneumonectomy space (Fig. 122-19). The patch is sewn medially to the pericardial edge and diaphragmatic crus. This step in prosthetic reconstruction of the pericardium and diaphragm is critical to prevent intra-abdominal viscus organ herniation into the chest.

The pericardium is reconstructed to prevent cardiac herniation into an empty right hemithorax, a potentially fatal complication. A 15 cm × 20 cm, 0.1-mm-thick, Gore-Tex pericardial patch is fenestrated to prevent development of a pericardial effusion and cardiac tamponade, and sewn to the pericardial edge with interrupted Gore-Tex sutures placed posteriorly first, followed by anterior placement (Fig. 122-20A). Both patches are sutured to the cut edge of the pericardium and to each other medially (Fig. 122-20B). Tension on the pericardial patch should be avoided to prevent dehiscence along the suture line and restriction on the contracting heart.

After the pericardial and diaphragmatic reconstruction is completed, the omental flap is sutured to the bronchial stump to provide coverage and separation from the pulmonary artery staple line (Fig. 122-21). Alternatively, an intercostal muscle or pericardial fat pad may be used. However, we have found that the omentum provides a more reliable vascularized buttress to the bronchial stump.

The thoracotomy is closed in standard fashion. A 12 F red rubber catheter is placed into the pneumonectomy space and

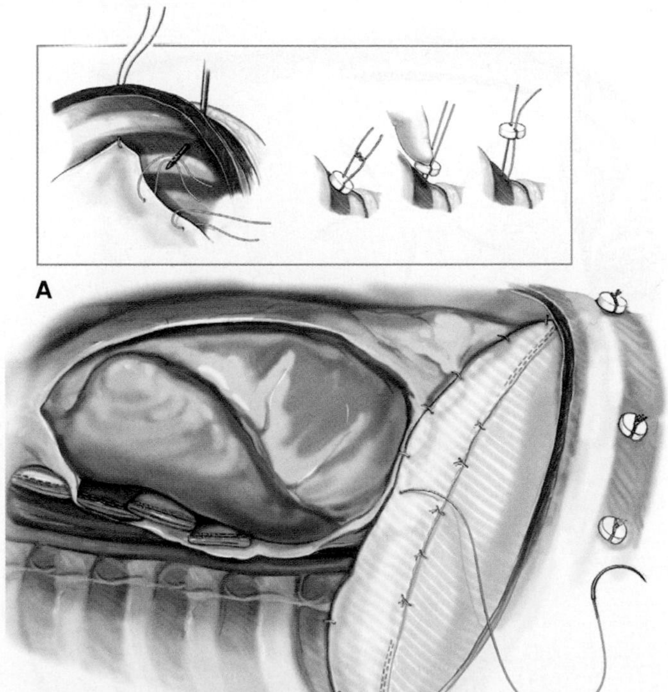

Figure 122-18. Polypropylene buttons (14 mm) (*A*) are used to buttress the (*B*) suture that secures the patch to the chest wall.

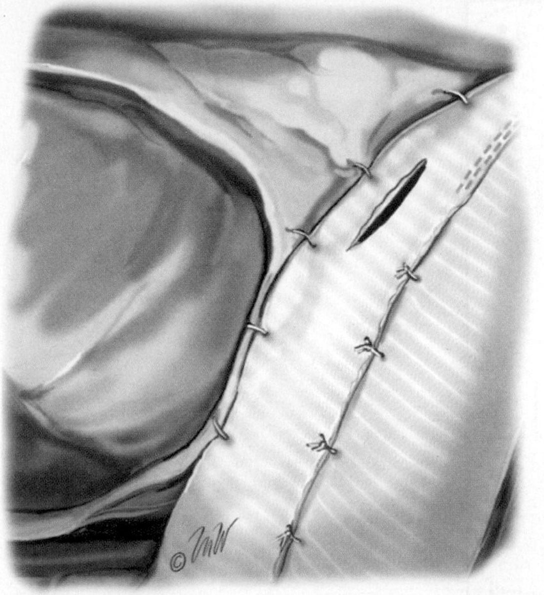

Figure 122-19. A small opening is made in the midportion of the diaphragmatic patch for the omental flap.

brought out on the medial aspect of the incision. The chest wall is closed in multiple layers. The red rubber catheter is connected to a three-way stopcock, and 1000 mL of air in men, or 750 mL in women, is removed, positioning the mediastinum to the midline. After the chest is closed, the patient is placed in the supine position, and flexible bronchoscopy is performed to

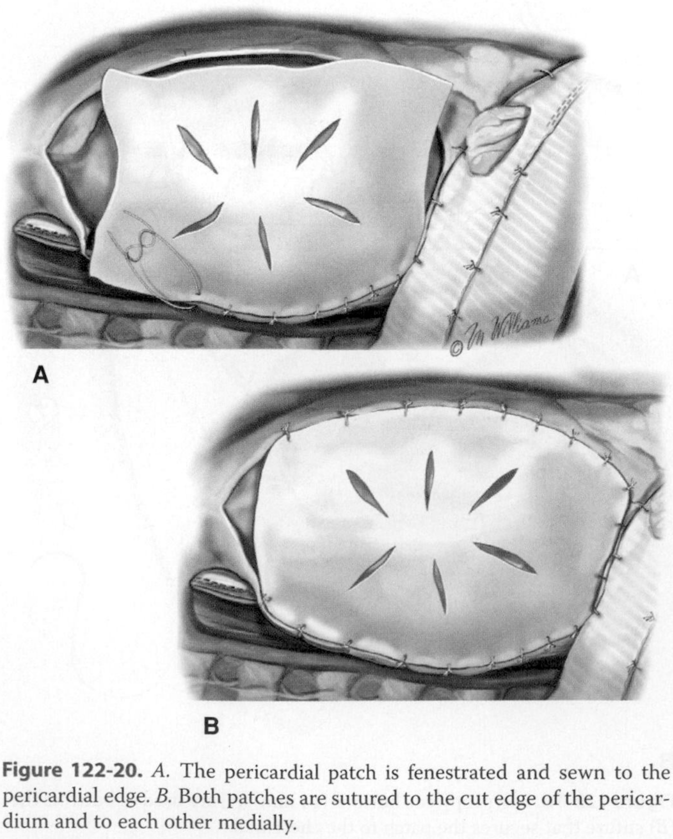

Figure 122-20. *A.* The pericardial patch is fenestrated and sewn to the pericardial edge. *B.* Both patches are sutured to the cut edge of the pericardium and to each other medially.

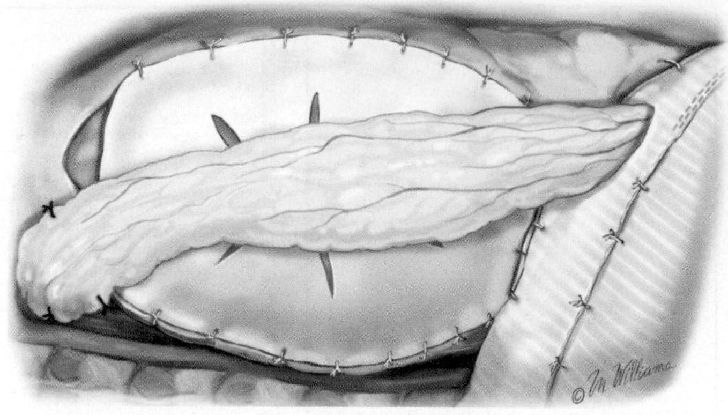

Figure 122-21. The omental flap is sutured to the bronchial stump.

assess the bronchial stump and to clear secretions. The patient is extubated in the OR.

TECHNIQUE OF LEFT EXTRAPLEURAL PNEUMONECTOMY

The technique of left EPP is similar to the technique used for the right side with some key variations.[2,6,7] Important differences in the approach to anesthesia include placement of a right-sided double-lumen endotracheal tube or left-sided endobronchial blocker.

During the posterior extrapleural dissection, it is critical to enter the preaortic plane to prevent inadvertent injury of the intercostal arterial branches. Also, caution should be exercised around the thoracic duct and recurrent laryngeal nerve during dissection in the area of the aortopulmonary window and the subclavian vessel takeoff from the aortic arch (Fig. 122-22). During the diaphragmatic resection, it is imperative to leave

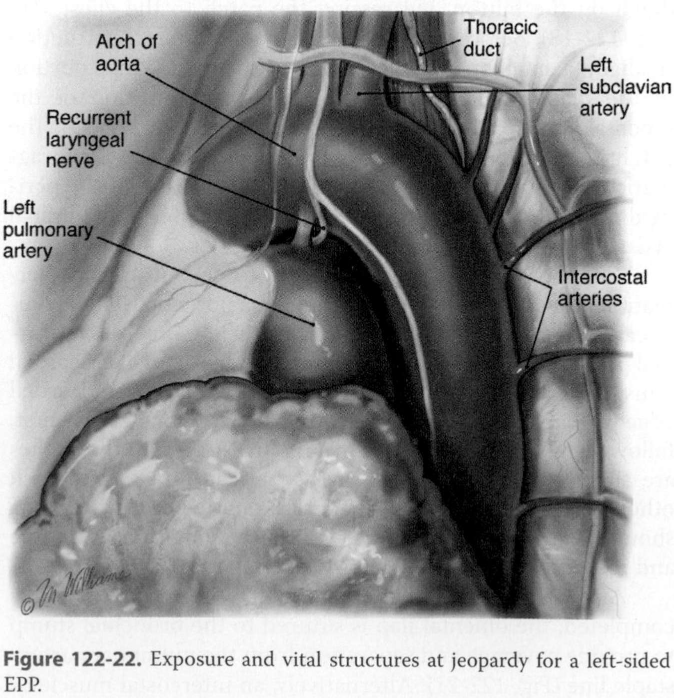

Figure 122-22. Exposure and vital structures at jeopardy for a left-sided EPP.

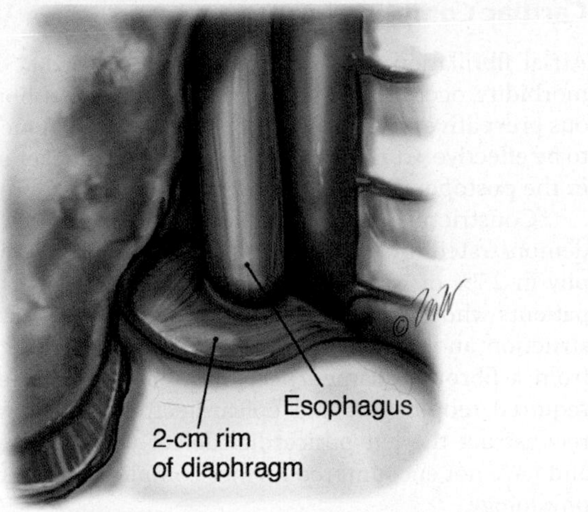

Figure 122-23. Leave 2 cm of diaphragm around the esophagus.

a 2-cm rim of diaphragmatic crus near the gastroesophageal junction (Fig. 122-23). Placement of sutures to this rim of crus to the prosthetic patch during diaphragmatic reconstruction prevents gastric herniation into the pneumonectomy space. Since the left main pulmonary artery is relatively shorter than the right pulmonary artery, it is divided extrapericardially (Fig. 122-24). The left mainstem bronchus should be dissected deep to the aortic arch and as close to the carina as possible. This ensures a short bronchial stump after division. After mediastinal lymph node dissection, the aortopulmonary nodes are removed as well. Although cardiac herniation associated with the pericardial defect is generally not an issue on the left side, we routinely reconstruct the pericardial defect after left EPP to prevent constrictive epicarditis. By using the red rubber catheter, less air is removed from the left pneumonectomy space (750 mL in men and 500 mL in women).

Postoperative Management

As soon as the patient is admitted to the ICU, a standard portable chest radiograph is obtained to confirm placement of the

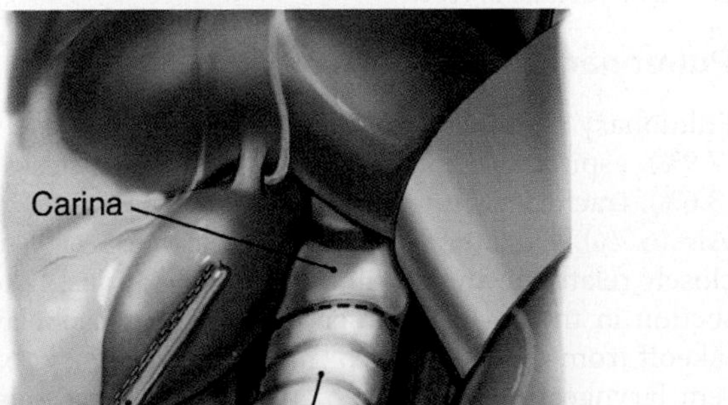

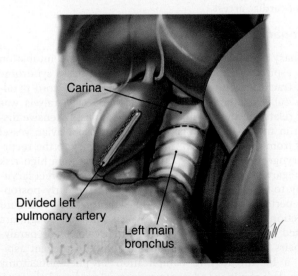

Figure 122-24. The left pulmonary artery is divided extrapericardially because it is shorter in comparison with the right pulmonary artery.

central line, identify appropriate location of the nasogastric and chest tubes, and assess for midline mediastinal position. If a red rubber catheter was placed at surgery, the pressure measurement aids in the postoperative management and is monitored with aspiration of the pleural space, if necessary, to maintain a pleural pressure of less than 10 cm H_2O. This information should always be correlated with the clinical picture. We recommend aspirating no more than 200 to 300 mL per treatment to avoid pulmonary edema or complications of acute respiratory distress syndrome and postpneumonectomy syndrome. Also, additional air may be introduced or removed if the mediastinum is deviated from the midline. Patients are initially managed in the ICU for 2 to 3 days and then transferred to the thoracic intermediate care unit. Patients who have undergone intraoperative, intracavitary heated chemotherapy (see Chapter 123) receive liberal amounts of IV fluids for the initial 24 hours to facilitate renal protection by means of hydration and to prevent hypotension. Otherwise, in patients who have not undergone intraoperative intracavitary heated chemotherapy, fluid is restricted to 1 L per day for 3 to 5 days. Volume requirements are met with colloids and blood transfusions, preferably. The hematocrit is maintained above 30.

Prevention of pulmonary complications, namely, pulmonary embolus and aspiration, is the focus of postoperative management. A thoracic epidural is used routinely for postoperative analgesia for several days until the patient is transitioned to oral pain medications. Chest physiotherapy is encouraged daily. Deep vein thrombosis prophylaxis is achieved with subcutaneous heparin (5000 units) three times per day and pneumatic compression boots. Routine lower extremity noninvasive ultrasound is obtained every 7 days to assess for deep vein thrombosis. Patients remain at bed rest for 48 hours until midline mediastinal stability is achieved. After 48 hours, patients ambulate several times a day. Desaturations are treated aggressively with diuresis and chest physiotherapy. Bedside bronchoscopy under conscious sedation is performed with a low threshold. If pulmonary embolus is suspected, a high-resolution chest CT scan is obtained liberally.

Daily chest radiographs are obtained to assess mediastinal position and surveillance for infiltrates in the remaining lung. Any suggestion of pneumonia clinically or radiologically is treated aggressively with intravenous antibiotics, chest physiotherapy, and bronchoscopy, if indicated.

Nasogastric tubes are used to decompress the stomach and to prevent aspiration. These are removed on postoperative day 2. Oral intake is advanced slowly on resumption of bowel function. The red rubber catheter or chest tube, if placed, is removed on postoperative day 3.

The inability to generate a strong cough or new onset of hoarseness of voice suggests possible vocal cord paresis or paralysis from recurrent laryngeal nerve injury. These clinical signs may not be immediately apparent postoperatively owing to the initial vocal cord swelling associated with prolonged intubation from a long operation and hypervolemia from intraoperative resuscitation. Prompt evaluation with direct laryngoscopy is indicated because these patients are not able to protect their airways and hence are at significant risk of aspiration, nor are they able to appose the vocal cords to generate a cough required to clear endobronchial secretions. If there is vocal cord paresis or paralysis, early vocal cord medialization is indicated.

Table 122-2

POST-EPP MORBIDITIES ($n = 328$)

Age	Median, 58 yrs; range, 28–77 yrs
Length of stay	Median, 10 ds; range, 4–101 ds
Complications[a]	
Minor and major morbidity rate	60.4% (198 of 328)
Atrial fibrillation	44.2% (145 of 328)
Myocardial infarction	1.5% (5 of 328)
Constrictive physiology	2.7% (9 of 328)
Reoperation for constrictive physiology	2.4% (8 of 328)
Tamponade	3.6% (12 of 328)
Cardiac arrest	3% (10 of 338)
Prolonged intubation	7.9% (26 of 328)
Aspiration	2.7% (9 of 328)
Acute respiratory distress syndrome	3.6% (12 of 328)
Tracheostomy	1.8% (6 of 328)
Vocal cord paralysis	6.7% (22 of 328)
Renal failure	2.7% (9 of 328)
Deep vein thrombosis	6.4% (21 of 328)
Pulmonary embolus	1.5% (5 of 328)
Cerebrovascular accident (33 ds postoperative)	0.3% (1 of 328)
Empyema	2.4% (8 of 328)
Bronchopleural fistula	0.6% (2 of 328)
Technical complications (e.g., patch failure or bleeding)	6.1% (20 of 328)
Ischemic colitis, grade II	0.3% (1 of 328)
Ileus	0.9% (3 of 328)
Colectomy for *Clostridium difficile*	0.3% (1 of 328)

[a]Percentage of patients (n/total).

Adapted with permission from Sugarbaker DJ, Jaklitsch MT, Bueno R, et al. Prevention, early detection, and management of complications after 328 consecutive extrapleural pneumonectomies. *J Thorac Cardiovasc Surg.* 2004;128:138–146.

COMPLICATIONS

EPP is a technically challenging operation associated with high morbidity but acceptable mortality. Our results from the Brigham and Women's Hospital/Dana Farber Cancer Institute were reported in a paper describing 328 patients with mesothelioma who underwent EPP.[4] The overall minor and major morbidity rate after EPP was 60.4% (198 of 328 patients) (Table 122-2). Perioperative mortality can be minimized by early detection and aggressive treatment of these complications. This approach has lowered our mortality rate to 3.4% (11 of 328 patients), and the causes of death are listed in Table 122-3.

Table 122-3

CAUSES OF DEATH

CAUSE	NO. OF PATIENTS ($n = 20/496$)
Pulmonary embolus	6
Acute respiratory distress syndrome	4
Myocardial infarction	3
Unknown	3
Cardiac herniation	1
Renal failure	1
Cardiac arrhythmia	1
Heparin-induced thrombocytopenia	1

Adapted with permission from Sugarbaker DJ, Jaklitsch MT, Bueno R, et al. Prevention, early detection, and management of complications after 328 consecutive extrapleural pneumonectomies. *J Thorac Cardiovasc Surg.* 2004;128:138–146.

Cardiac Complications

Atrial fibrillation was the most common cardiac and overall morbidity, occurring in 44.2% of our patients. Although numerous preventive strategies have been attempted, none has proved to be effective. Currently, we are using beta blocker medications in the postoperative period for atrial fibrillation prophylaxis.

Constrictive cardiac physiology owing to epicarditis was demonstrated by cardiac catheterization or echocardiography in 2.7% of patients. Byrne and colleagues reported seven patients who underwent a left EPP with no pericardial reconstruction and later developed constrictive cardiac physiology from a fibrous inflamed peel over the heart.[8] These patients required reoperation and epicardiectomy. We now routinely reconstruct the left pericardial defect with a Gore-Tex patch and have not encountered further complications of constrictive physiology.

Cardiac tamponade was seen in 3.6% of patients. This can occur as a result of retained pericardial effusion from an inadequately fenestrated patch, impaired ventricular filling during diastole from a tight pericardial patch, or impingement of the inferior vena cava from a tight right-sided diaphragmatic patch. An important clue to cardiac tamponade physiology is seen in the OR when the patient becomes hypotensive with elevated central venous pressure on turning from the lateral decubitus to the supine position. The treatment is reoperation and loosening of the pericardial or diaphragmatic patch reconstruction.

Although myocardial infarction was seen only in 1.5% of patients, pericarditis, as demonstrated by ST-segment elevation and elevated cardiac enzymes, was common. Normalization of the electrocardiogram and cardiac markers occurred within 48 hours.

Cardiac arrest was seen in 3% of patients. This occurrence within the immediate 10-day postoperative period requires emergent reopening of the thoracotomy incision, open cardiac massage, and removal of the pericardial patch. Standard chest compression is ineffective in the EPP patient because the mediastinum is dynamic and shifts to the empty pneumonectomy space. After resuscitation, reoperation in the OR is indicated for pulsed irrigation of the opened chest and correction of the cause of cardiac arrest.

Pulmonary Complications

Pulmonary complications included prolonged intubation (7.9%), aspiration (2.7%), acute respiratory distress syndrome (3.6%), tracheostomy placement (1.8%), and vocal cord paralysis (6.7%). Unilateral vocal cord weakness or paralysis was closely related to the pulmonary complications. Extensive dissection in the aortopulmonary window and subclavian vessel takeoff from the aortic arch may result in injury to the recurrent laryngeal nerve. These patients with surgery in high-risk areas, regardless of symptoms, are evaluated with direct laryngoscopy to assess vocal cord movement in the early postoperative period. Patients with obvious symptoms of vocal cord dysfunction, such as hoarseness of voice and poor cough, are evaluated as well. Unilateral vocal cord weakness or paralysis impairs airway protection and the ability to prevent aspiration, a life-threatening complication in pneumonectomy patients. As a result, we advocate early vocal cord medialization with Gelfoam injection to reduce the incidence of aspiration pneumonia.[9] After medialization, swallowing evaluation by speech pathology is required before resumption of oral intake.

Postoperative diuresis is important to prevent pulmonary edema. Chest physiotherapy is used aggressively with frequent ambulation. The bronchoscope is used liberally to clear secretions and during episodes of desaturation.

Excessive mediastinal shift toward the contralateral hemithorax and away from the pneumonectomy side can result in poor lung expansion and atelectasis with resulting respiratory compromise. A red rubber catheter or chest tube is left in place until the third postoperative day and is used to remove fluid from the pneumonectomy space to facilitate midline mediastinal positioning. Excessive bleeding or chylothorax may account for rapid fluid accumulation into the EPP cavity. Chylothorax occurs rarely and can be treated with percutaneous embolization or open ligation of the thoracic duct (see Chapters 131 and 133).

Renal, Hematologic, and Infectious Complications

Renal failure occurred in 2.7% of patients and, in general, was associated with acute respiratory distress syndrome, multiorgan-system failure, and death. Deep vein thrombosis was diagnosed in 6.4% and pulmonary embolus in 1.5% of patients. Pulmonary embolus is a life-threatening complication in pneumonectomy patients. As a result, noninvasive ultrasound of both lower extremities is obtained routinely every 7 days in the postoperative period. Furthermore, a high-resolution pulmonary embolus protocol CT scan is performed with a low threshold in patients with clinical evidence suggestive of a possible pulmonary embolus.

Empyema was seen in 2.4% of post-EPP patients, a catastrophic complication in the presence of prosthetic patches. Clinical evidence of infection is often absent, and the cultures are frequently negative, particularly for anaerobic infections. Our preventive strategy includes intraoperative pulsed irrigation of the pneumonectomy space with 9 L of lavage and a postoperative IV antibiotic regimen for 5 days with cefazolin (Ancef; Smith Kline Beecham, Philadelphia, Pennsylvania), levofloxacin (Levaquin; Ortho-McNeil, Raritan, New Jersey), and metronidazole (Flagyl; Searle, Skokie, Illinois) (Fig. 122-25).[4]

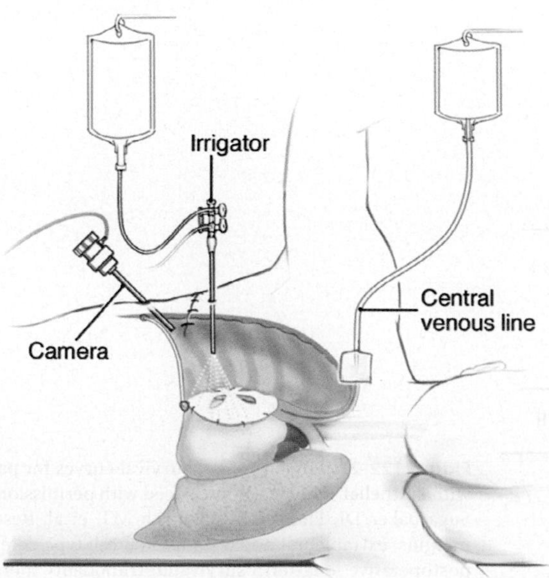

Figure 122-25. Thoracoscopic drainage for early treatment of empyema.

Management of empyema depends on the timing of presentation relative to resection. In patients with empyema in the absence of a bronchopleural fistula during the first postoperative month, we have performed thoracoscopic closed chest treatment with debridement, pulsed irrigation, and removal of patches with success. Postoperative irrigation of the pneumonectomy space is carried out for 5 days. If the severity of the infection is deemed inappropriate for thoracoscopic management or in the presence of a bronchopleural fistula, an Eloesser flap is performed, with the Gore-Tex patches left in place. Staged removal of the patches may prevent mediastinal shift into the pneumonectomy cavity. After 2 to 3 weeks of dressing changes and adequate time for the mediastinum to scar into place, the patches are removed. Patients who present with empyema months to years after resection are managed traditionally with an Eloesser flap and open patch removal at the same time.

Bronchopleural fistula has occurred in 0.6% of patients. The presence of a bronchopleural fistula requires Eloesser flap drainage of the pneumonectomy cavity and patch removal.

RESULTS

The success of EPP in the treatment of mesothelioma has been attributed to defined criteria for patient selection, continuous refinements in technique, and a disciplined approach to the perioperative care with early diagnosis and aggressive treatment of complications. This is exemplified by the reduction in postoperative mortality and improvement in survival.

Our report, from the Brigham and Women's Hospital, of 183 patients who underwent EPP followed by adjuvant chemotherapy and radiation for mesothelioma revealed an overall median survival of 19 months, with 2- and 5-year survivals of 38% and 15%, respectively (Fig. 122-26).[4] The revised Brigham and Women's Hospital staging system for malignant pleural mesothelioma was applied to this cohort of patients (Table 122-4). The staging system had prognostic significance

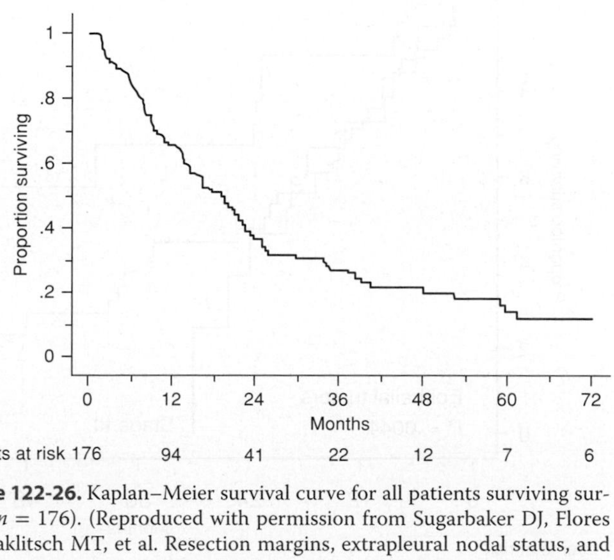

Figure 122-26. Kaplan–Meier survival curve for all patients surviving surgery ($n = 176$). (Reproduced with permission from Sugarbaker DJ, Flores RM, Jaklitsch MT, et al. Resection margins, extrapleural nodal status, and cell type determine postoperative long-term survival in trimodality therapy of malignant pleural mesothelioma: results in 183 patients. *J Thorac Cardiovasc Surg.* 1999;117:54–63.)

Table 122-4

THE REVISED BRIGHAM STAGING SYSTEM FOR MALIGNANT PLEURAL MESOTHELIOMA

STAGE	DEFINITION
I	Disease confined to within the capsule of the parietal pleura; ipsilateral pleura, lung, pericardium, diaphragm, or chest wall disease limited to previous biopsy sites
II	All of stage I with positive intrathoracic (N1 or N2) lymph nodes
III	Local extension of disease into chest wall or mediastinum; heart, or through the diaphragm and peritoneum; with or without extrathoracic or contralateral (N1) lymph node involvement
IV	Distant metastatic disease

Adapted with permission from Sugarbaker DJ, Flores RM, Jaklitsch MT, et al. Resection margins, extrapleural nodal status, and cell type determine postoperative long-term survival in trimodality therapy of malignant pleural mesothelioma: results in 183 patients. *J Thorac Cardiovasc Surg.* 1999;117:54–63; discussion 63–65.

because it significantly stratified long-term survival. Patients with stage I ($n = 66$), II ($n = 41$), and III ($n = 69$) diseases had median survival intervals of 25, 20, and 16 months, respectively.[4] A subset of 31 patients with epithelial cell type, negative resection margins, and negative extrapleural nodal status had a median survival of 51 months, with 2- and 5-year survivals of 68% and 46%, respectively (Fig. 122-27).[4]

SUMMARY

In the last 20 years, the EPP technique has been modified with the incorporation of novel surgical techniques that have led to improved survival, reduced operative time, and a steady reduction in postoperative mortality. The described technique is the culmination of more than 25 years' experience with malignant pleural mesothelioma at the Brigham and Women's Hospital/Dana Farber Cancer Institute.

The successful refinement of the operation, as demonstrated by the current low mortality rate, has allowed application of the procedure to treat other malignancies, such as locally advanced lung cancer, thymic malignancies, and sarcoma. The basic stages of this operation are (1) incision and exposure of the parietal pleura, (2) extrapleural dissection to separate the tumor from the chest wall, (3) en bloc resection of the lung, pleura, pericardium, and diaphragm with division of the hilar structures, (4) radical lymph node dissection, and (5) reconstruction of the diaphragm and pericardium.[2,6,7] This is a complex and challenging operation, as exemplified by an overall morbidity of 60.4%.[4] This operation should be performed only by an experienced surgical team at a high-volume, experienced medical center.[10] The associated complications require a unique management approach with early detection and aggressive treatment in order to achieve a mortality rate of 3.4%.[4]

CLINICAL SCENARIO

A 58-year-old former shipyard worker presented with a several-month history of progressive shortness of breath, nonproductive cough, and 10-lb weight loss. His past medical history was unremarkable except for previous asbestos exposure. The physical examination was remarkable for right-sided decreased breath sounds, dullness to percussion, decreased tactile fremitus, and egophony. A chest x-ray revealed a moderate-sized right pleural effusion, pleural thickening, shrinkage of the ipsilateral hemithorax, and shift of the mediastinum to the right chest. A chest CT scan was obtained that confirmed the chest x-ray findings and also demonstrated diffuse pleural thickening encasing the right lung with questionable chest wall invasion along the sixth and seventh ribs laterally. Chest MRI showed no diaphragmatic or mediastinal invasion.

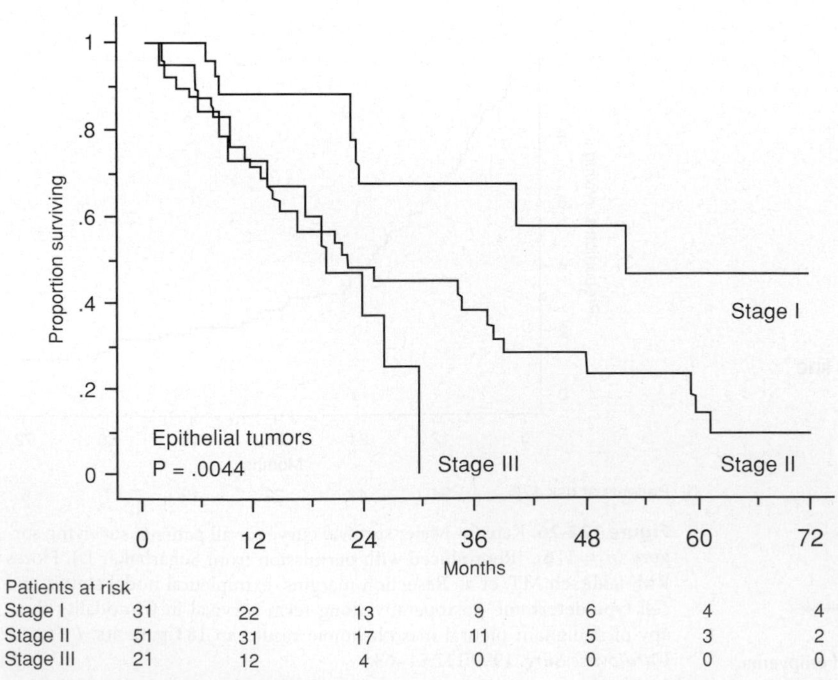

Figure 122-27. Kaplan–Meier survival curves for patients with epithelial subtype. (Reproduced with permission from Sugarbaker DJ, Flores RM, Jaklitsch MT, et al. Resection margins, extrapleural nodal status, and cell type determine postoperative long-term survival in trimodality therapy of malignant pleural mesothelioma: results in 183 patients. *J Thorac Cardiovasc Surg.* 1999;117:54–63.)

Right thoracoscopic drainage of the pleural effusion and pleural biopsy were performed, which revealed no malignant cells on cytology and epithelial mesothelioma on histologic examination. Cervical mediastinoscopy with mediastinal lymph node biopsy demonstrated no evidence of metastatic spread.

Standard laboratory tests, including liver function tests, creatinine, and arterial blood gases, were normal. Pulmonary function testing revealed an FEV_1 of 1.8 L. Ventilation/perfusion scan was performed, which showed lung perfusion to the right lung at 10% and to the left lung at 90%. The predicted postoperative FEV_1 was calculated to be 1.6 L. Echocardiogram demonstrated no evidence of pulmonary hypertension (20 mm Hg plus right atrial pressure) and normal ejection fraction (60%), valvular function, and wall motion.

In the absence of locally advanced or distant disease with a confirmed histologic diagnosis of mesothelioma, an extended right thoracotomy was performed. There was no intraoperative evidence of chest wall invasion because the extrapleural plane was dissected readily. As a result, we proceeded to perform a complete EPP, as described earlier. At the end of the operation, 1000 mL of air was removed via the red rubber catheter. Bronchoscopy revealed a short bronchial stump and retained secretions, which were suctioned. The patient was extubated in the OR and transferred to the ICU. Postoperative chest x-ray revealed that the mediastinum was shifted to the left hemithorax. An additional 400 mL of air was removed via the red rubber catheter, and repeat chest x-ray revealed the mediastinum in the midline position.

On postoperative day 1, the patient was noted to have a hoarse voice. An urgent otolaryngology consult was obtained, and direct laryngoscopy was performed at the bedside, which revealed a paralyzed right vocal cord. The patient was restricted from oral intake and underwent vocal cord medialization with Gelfoam injection the next day. There was significant improvement in his voice thereafter. The nasogastric tube was removed on postoperative day 2, and speech pathology evaluation revealed normal swallowing. The patient was started on an oral diet. Fluid intake was restricted to 1 L per day, and gentle diuresis was initiated.

On postoperative day 3, the red rubber catheter was removed after confirming on a routine daily chest x-ray that the mediastinum was midline in location. The patient was transferred to the stepdown thoracic intensive care unit. Aggressive chest physiotherapy was performed frequently, and the patient ambulated four times a day. On postoperative day 7, the patient underwent routine noninvasive ultrasound of the lower extremities, which revealed no evidence of deep vein thrombosis. On postoperative day 10, the patient was discharged to home with continued improvement. At 7 days from discharge, he was seen in clinic and was noted to be doing well. The final pathology report revealed epithelial mesothelioma in the EPP specimen, and extrapleural lymph nodes revealed no evidence of malignancy. He successfully underwent adjuvant chemotherapy and radiation.

EDITOR'S COMMENT

This chapter includes many technical details for the technique of extrapleural pneumonectomy as developed at the Brigham and Women's Hospital in Boston over the past 30 years. Although there are other published accounts of the technique, details have been constantly added. This description is the most up to date. I would guide less experienced readers to pay particular attention to the selection criteria of patients, the role of contralateral thoracoscopy or laparoscopy to rule out T4 disease, and the use of the omental flap to cover the bronchus. There is an inverse relationship between morbidity and mortality, with the recognition of common morbidities (60%) leading to low mortality (3.4%). The operative mortality of 31% experienced by Butchart and Associates should serve as a warning to new programs with less experience in the operative technique and postoperative management. Both this chapter and Chapter 123 offer important technical details of the operation. There is a difference in fluid management of these patients depending on whether or not intraoperative chemotherapy was used (increase in fluids) or not (restriction of fluids).

—Michael T. Jaklitsch

References

1. Sarot I. Extrapleural pneumonectomy and pleurectomy in pulmonary tuberculosis. *Thorax.* 1949;4:173–223.
2. Chang MY, Sugarbaker DJ. Extrapleural pneumonectomy for diffuse malignant pleural mesothelioma: techniques and complications. *Thorac Surg Clin.* 2004;14:523–530.
3. Sugarbaker DJ, Flores RM, Jaklitsch MT, et al. Resection margins, extrapleural nodal status, and cell type determine postoperative long-term survival in trimodality therapy of malignant pleural mesothelioma: results in 183 patients. *J Thorac Cardiovasc Surg.* 1999;117:54–63; discussion 63–65.
4. Sugarbaker DJ, Jaklitsch MT, Bueno R, et al. Prevention, early detection, and management of complications after 328 consecutive extrapleural pneumonectomies. *J Thorac Cardiovasc Surg.* 2004;128:138–146.
5. Patz EF Jr, Shaffer K, Piwnica-Worms DR, et al. Malignant pleural mesothelioma: value of CT and MR imaging in predicting resectability. *AJR Am J Roentgenol.* 1992;159:961–966.
6. Garcia J, Richards W, Sugarbaker D. *Surgical Treatment of Malignant Mesothelioma.* Philadelphia, PA: Lippincott-Raven; 1998.
7. Argote-Greene L, Chang M, Sugarbaker D. Extrapleural pneumonectomy for malignant pleural mesothelioma. In *Multimedia Manual of Cardiothoracic Surgery (MMCTS).* June 28, 2005. doi:10.1510/mmcts.2004.000133. http://mmcts.ctsnetjournals.org/cgi/content/full/2005/0628/mmcts.2004.000133
8. Byrne JG, Karavas AN, Colson YL, et al. Cardiac decortication (epicardiectomy) for occult constrictive cardiac physiology after left extrapleural pneumonectomy. *Chest.* 2002;122:2256–2259.
9. Bhattacharyya N, Batirel H, Swanson SJ. Improved outcomes with early vocal fold medialization for vocal fold paralysis after thoracic surgery. *Auris Nasus Larynx.* 2003;30:71–75.
10. Bueno R. Multimodality treatments in the management of malignant pleural mesothelioma: an update. *Hematol Oncol Clin North Am.* 2005;19(6):1089–1097.

123 Intracavitary Hyperthermic Chemotherapy for Malignant Mesothelioma

Marcelo C. DaSilva, Paul Sugarbaker, and David J. Sugarbaker

Keywords: Hyperthermic intraoperative chemotherapy lavage (HIOC), thermo-ablation technique, nephrotoxicity, amifostine, sodium thiosulfate, macroscopic complete resection

The rising incidence of malignant mesothelioma worldwide has intensified the search for treatment strategies to extend disease-free survival.[1] To date, the best survival has been observed in patients undergoing multimodality therapy with surgery, either extrapleural pneumonectomy (EPP) or pleurectomy/decortication (P/D), plus chemotherapy and/or radiation therapy.[2–7] Seminal work at the Washington Cancer Center and Brigham and Women's Hospital led to the development of innovative surgical techniques to accomplish macroscopic complete resection, along with intracavitary lavage with hyperthermic platinum-based chemotherapy for local control. The rationale for hyperthermic intraoperative thoracoabdominal chemotherapy has been previously described, with particular emphasis on malignant peritoneal mesothelioma.[8] This chapter describes the thoracic delivery of heated intraoperative chemotherapy for patients with malignant pleural mesothelioma (MPM), along with special advice on perioperative pitfalls and complications.

GENERAL PRINCIPLES

Intracavitary administration of heated chemotherapy (at 42°C) increases the intracellular uptake of drugs, thus minimizing the systemic side effects and maximizing the therapeutic effect. To accomplish maximal delivery of drug at the time of surgery, the chemotherapy lavage is performed after complete macroscopic resection, irrespective of whether the surgeon is operating in the chest or in the abdomen. Factors that may limit the depth of penetration include temperature, residual tumor, fibrinous exudate, excessive bleeding, clotting, and the intracavitary volume of perfusate.

Platinum-based chemotherapy has been used safely in many thoracic and abdominal protocols.[9] The drug binds covalently to various macromolecules, including DNA, the apparent target.[10] The effects of cisplatin on mesothelioma have been studied in the past, and it can be combined with cytoprotective agents or other drugs to minimize toxicity.[11,12] The concentration of the drug with regional administration is up to 50-fold higher than with IV administration. [13] Ratto et al.[14] showed that levels of cisplatin given into the pleura are higher with hyperthermic perfusion than with normothermic perfusion. Heat increases cell permeability, alters cellular metabolism, and improves membrane transport of drugs. This has been demonstrated in animal and human studies.[15,16] A synergistic effect of hyperthermia and cisplatin has been demonstrated.[17,18] Intracavitary cisplatin and its benefits in thoracic malignancies have been studied in the past for both EPP and P/D.[14,19]

Sodium thiosulfate and amifostine provide renal protection during heated chemotherapy. Sodium thiosulfate is a neutralizing agent that has the ability to protect stem cells and reduce the nephrotoxicity of cisplatin. It is thought to bind covalently to cisplatin, forming an inactive complex.[13] The administration of thiosulfate intravenously concurrently with intracavitary platinum-based agents protects against nephrotoxicity.[13,20,21] We favor colloids over crystalloids for volume replacement in the intraoperative and early postoperative period to avoid the development of postpneumonectomy pulmonary edema and renal failure.

PATIENT SELECTION

A careful preoperative assessment of the patient's pulmonary reserve and cardiac function is mandatory. Patient-related factors associated with increased operative risk for pulmonary complications include preexisting pulmonary disease, cardiovascular disease, pulmonary hypertension, dyspnea upon exertion, heavy smoking history, respiratory infection, cough (particularly productive cough), advanced age (>70 years), malnutrition, general debilitation, obesity, and prolonged surgery. Therefore, cessation of smoking 2 weeks (and preferably 6 weeks) before resection is advised. Risk assessment is a complex process for determining the patient's resectability and operability. *Resectability* in patients with malignant pleural mesothelioma refers to the amount of lung tissue (e.g., pneumonectomy) and tumor that can be completely removed without the risk of developing postoperative respiratory insufficiency. It depends directly on the volume of the remaining lung tissue (i.e., pulmonary reserve). *Operability* is the patient's ability to survive the proposed procedure, whether EPP or P/D, and this depends primarily on the patient's comorbid conditions.

PREOPERATIVE ASSESSMENT

While no single test can effectively predict intraoperative and postoperative morbidity and mortality from pulmonary complications, candidates for EPP should have ppoFEV_1 >1000 mL, systolic pulmonary artery pressure <35 mm Hg plus right atrial pressure of approximately 10 mm Hg, and diffusion capacity of the lung for carbon oxide (D_{LCO}) >40. Candidates for P/D should have minimal disease and sufficient cardiopulmonary reserve to withstand the procedure. Both groups of patients must have a glomerular filtration rate (GFR) >60 mL/min/1.73 m^2 (normal range 90–120 mL/min/1.73 m^2) in order to receive the hyperthermic intraoperative chemotherapy lavage (HIOC).

Pulmonary function testing is performed, including a quantitative ventilation/perfusion scan and pulmonary stress test (6-minute walk test). Chest CT scan with intravenous contrast and chest MRI are performed preoperatively to exclude unresectable or metastatic disease. A PET scan can be helpful in demonstrating extrathoracic sites. An echocardiogram is recommended with estimation of the pulmonary systolic pressure to exclude pulmonary hypertension. Surgery is contraindicated in patients who have had a myocardial infarction (MI) within the previous 3 months. Patients with a remote history of MI should undergo a myocardial perfusion study with sestamibi, and cardiac clearance should be obtained. We routinely perform preoperative lower extremity noninvasive Doppler studies to exclude deep vein thrombosis (DVT) and perioperative pulmonary embolism. For patients diagnosed with DVT, an inferior vena cava filter is placed prior to the surgery. Patients receiving heated chemotherapy are admitted the night before surgery and undergo DVT prophylaxis, bowel prep, and overnight intravenous hydration to prevent cisplatin nephrotoxicity.

Pulmonary function testing comprises four elements of the preoperative evaluation: (1) pulmonary spirometry, (2) quantitative ventilation/perfusion (V/Q) scan, (3) pulmonary hemodynamic response testing, (4) exercise testing.

Pulmonary spirometry is affected by height, age, weight, sex, race, and thoracic deformities, as well as arterial oxygenation and diffusion capacity. It is important to remember that although pulmonary spirometry and arterial oxygenation help to predict mortality, they are not good predictors of postoperative complications. D_{LCO} is a more sensitive predictor of postoperative complications. The diffusing capacity is a measure of the conductance of the CO molecule from the alveolar gas to Hb in the pulmonary capillary blood. The transfer of the CO molecule is limited by both perfusion and diffusion. CO (and oxygen) must pass through the alveolar epithelium, tissue interstitium, capillary endothelium, blood plasma, and red cell membrane and cytoplasm before attaching to the Hb molecule. D_{LCO} is directly proportional to VA (alveolar ventilation) in a single breath. Therefore, factors that affect D_{LCO} are low hemoglobin level, low lung volume, previous lung resection, thoracic cage abnormalities (e.g., kyphoscoliosis), as well as patients with chronic obstructive pulmonary disease (COPD), emphysema, chronic pulmonary hypertension, and interstitial lung disease. D_{LCO} may also be reduced temporarily in patients with pneumonia, interstitial infiltrative disorders, and alveolar proteinosis (Table 123-1). The importance of obtaining an inspiratory vital capacity (IVC) greater than 90% of the best measured VC from the day of the test cannot be overemphasized. The inability to achieve an IVC of greater than or equal to 90% of the largest VC measured that day must be noted. Patients with low D_{LCO} should not be considered candidates for extrapleural pneumonectomy. Thus, decreased D_{LCO} is an important and independent predictor of postoperative complications, even in patients without COPD.

Quantitative ventilation/perfusion (V/Q) scan is useful for predicting postoperative lung function. A calculated postoperative FEV_1 (ppo FEV_1%) of <40% is associated with a 50% mortality rate. The absolute minimum ppoFEV_1 in patients undergoing pneumonectomy is 1000 mL.[21]

Pulmonary hemodynamic response testing includes the measurement of pulmonary artery pressure and pulmonary vascular resistance. Pulmonary artery hypertension (PAH) carries a high mortality rate, and therefore it is important to determine its potential reversible causes (Table 123-2). Pulmonary artery pressure can be estimated by a transthoracic or transesophageal echocardiogram, but right heart catheterization may be indicated if the echocardiogram does not produce an accurate measurement. Normal pulmonary artery blood pressure is 20/10 mm Hg (mean 15) at rest at sea level. Pulmonary arterial systolic pressure rises gradually with age, and each 10-mm Hg increase is associated with a 2.7-fold greater risk for mortality.

Table 123-1

PHYSIOLOGICAL AND PATHOLOGICAL CHANGES THAT AFFECT THE CARBON MONOXIDE DIFFUSING CAPACITY OF THE LUNG (D_{LCO})

Extrapulmonary reduction in lung inflation (reduced VA) producing changes in DM or θVc that reduce D_{LCO}
Reduced effort or respiratory muscle weakness
Thoracic deformity preventing full inflation
Diseases that reduce θVc and thus reduce D_{LCO}
Anemia
Pulmonary emboli
Other conditions that reduce θVc and thus reduce D_{LCO}
Hb binding changes (e.g., HbCO, increased FiO_2)
Valsalva maneuver (increased intrathoracic pressure)
Diseases that reduce (in varying degrees) DM and θVc and thus reduce D_{LCO}
Lung resection (however, compensatory recruitment of θ Vc also exists)
Emphysema
Interstitial lung disease (e.g., IPF, sarcoidosis)
Pulmonary edema
Pulmonary vasculitis
Pulmonary hypertension
Diseases that increase θVc and thus increase D_{LCO}
Polycythemia
Left-to-right shunt
Pulmonary hemorrhage (not strictly an increase in θ*Vc*, but effectively an increase in lung Hb)
Asthma
Other conditions that increase θVc and thus increase D_{LCO}
Hb binding changes (e.g., reduced FiO_2)
Muller maneuver (decreased intrathoracic pressure as in asthma, resistance breathing)
Exercise (in addition, a possible DM component)
Supine position (in addition, possibly a slight increase in DM)
Obesity (in addition, a possible DM component)

VA = alveolar volume; DM = membrane conductivity; θ = carbon monoxide (CO)–hemoglobin (Hb) chemical reaction rate; *Vc* = volume of pulmonary capillary blood; FiO_2 = inspired fraction of oxygen; IPF = idiopathic pulmonary fibrosis; Hb = hemoglobin.

Adapted from MacIntyre N, Miller M, Crapo R, et al. Series ATS/ERS Task Force: standardization of lung function testing. *Eur Respir J*. 2005;26:720–735.

Systolic pulmonary artery pressure >35 mm Hg is associated with a 10-fold decrease in survival rate, and pulmonary vascular resistance >190 dyne is associated with a 90% mortality rate.

Maximum exercise testing produces information about the amount of arterial desaturation that occurs during exercise. Patients with maximum oxygen consumption (VO_2 max) <15 mL/kg/min are considered high risk, whereas those with a VO_2 max of 16 to 20 mL/kg/min could probably undergo surgery.

Nevertheless, regular evaluation of patients with pulmonary artery hypertension should focus on variables with established prognostic importance as outlined above. Treatment decisions should be based on parameters that reflect the individual's symptoms and exercise capacity that are relevant in terms of predicting outcome. Not all parameters obtained repeatedly in PAH patients are equally well suited to assessing disease severity and, therefore, are poor predictors. For example, the magnitude of the pulmonary artery pressure (PAP) correlates poorly with symptoms and outcome as it is determined not only by the degree of pulmonary vascular resistance (PVR) increase but also by the performance of right ventricular function (RV). Thus, the PAP alone should not be used for therapeutic decision-making.

Table 123-2

CLINICAL CLASSIFICATION OF PULMONARY HYPERTENSION

GROUP 1
Pulmonary arterial hypertension (PAH)
Idiopathic PAH
Heritable
BMPR2
ALK1, endoglin (with or without hereditary hemorrhagic telangiectasia)
Unknown
Drug and toxin induced
Associated with
Connective tissue disorders
HIV infection
Portal hypertension
Congenital heart disease
Schistosomiasis
Chronic hemolytic anemia
Persistent pulmonary hypertension of the newborn
Pulmonary veno-occlusive disease with left to right shunts and/or pulmonary capillary hemangiomatosis

GROUP 2
Pulmonary arterial hypertension owing to left heart disease
Systolic dysfunction
Diastolic dysfunction
Valvular disease

GROUP 3
Pulmonary arterial hypertension owing to lung disease and/or hypoxemia
COPD
Interstitial lung disease
Other pulmonary diseases with mixed restrictive and obstructive pattern
Sleep-disordered breathing
Alveolar hypoventilation disorders
Chronic exposure to high altitude
Developmental abnormalities

GROUP 4
Chronic thromboembolic pulmonary hypertension

GROUP 5
Pulmonary hypertension with unclear multifactorial mechanisms
Hematologic disorders: myeloproliferative disorders, splenectomy
Systemic disorders: sarcoidosis, pulmonary Langerhans cell histiocytosis: lymphangioleiomyomatosis, neurofibromatosis, vasculitis
Metabolic disorders: glycogen storage disease, Gaucher's disease, thyroid disorders
Others: tumoral obstruction, fibrosing mediastinitis, chronic renal failure on dialysis

Adapted from Goldman L, Schafer AI, eds. *Goldman's Cecil Medicine.* 24th ed. Philadelphia, PA: Elsevier Saunders; 2011.

Table 123-3 lists several parameters of known prognostic importance that are widely used as follow-up tools.

Along with the preoperative testing, radiologic and surgical staging is carried out to determine if the patient is a suitable candidate for surgery (stage I and II), induction chemotherapy (low disease burden but positive mediastinal nodes) followed by surgery, or chemotherapy alone (stages III and IV). Table 123-4 shows an algorithm for the various treatment options for biopsy proven MPM.

HYPERTHERMIC THORACOABDOMINAL CHEMOTHERAPY IN A PATIENT WITH MALIGNANT PLEURAL MESOTHELIOMA

Safety courses are required for all staff participating in a heated chemotherapy procedure. A special method has been designed for drug delivery and disposal in the OR, as outlined below.

The initial preparation and positioning of the patient have been described in the surgical technique chapters on P/D (Chapter 121) and EPP (Chapter 122). After surgical resection is completed, our current protocol requires administration of amifostine at a dose of 910 mg/m^2 for renal protection 30 to 45 minutes prior to the initiation of the lavage. After completing the lavage, the anesthesia team administers an intravenous bolus of sodium thiosulfate (4 g/m^2), followed by a 6-hour infusion of 12 g/m^2 sodium thiosulfate. This protects against intravascular volume depletion and helps to maintain a urine output of 100 mL/h during the lavage and afterwards.

Removing the diaphragm during surgical resection allows entry in the abdominal cavity. Once the tumor and specimen have been removed along with the lymph nodes, the chest is washed with 3 L of normal saline solution and 1 L of sterile water. Next, the chest is packed with Mikulicz's pads and the argon beam cautery is used for hemostasis of both the chest wall and lung surface (the latter for cases involving P/D). Once hemostasis is adequate, the chest is then irrigated with 3 L of warm normal saline solution to remove fibrin and debris before HIOC is initiated.

Special attention should be drawn to areas once laden with dense tumor, such as the costophrenic sulcus or areas that may have been contaminated during the procedure, such as the subscapular region, skin, and soft tissues bordering the incision.

Hemostasis is again ensured before setting up the chemotherapy delivery apparatus (Fig. 123-1). The thoracotomy

Table 123-3

PARAMETERS WITH ESTABLISHED IMPORTANCE FOR ASSESSING DISEASE SEVERITY, STABILITY, AND PROGNOSIS OF PAH.

DETERMINANTS OF PROGNOSIS	WORSE PROGNOSIS	BETTER PROGNOSIS
Clinical evidence of RV failure	Yes	No
Rate of progression of symptoms	Rapid	Slow
Syncope	Yes	No
WHO-FC	IV	I, II
2MWT	Shorter <300 m	Longer >500 m
Cardio-pulmonary exercise testing	O_2 consumption >12 mL/min/kg	O_2 consumption >15 mL/min/kg
BNP/NT-pro-BNP plasma level	Very elevated and rising	Normal or near normal
Echocardiography findings	Pericardial effusion TAPSE <1.5 cm[a]	No pericardial effusion TAPSE >2.0 cm[a]
Hemodynamics	RAP > 15 mm Hg or CI < 2.0 L/min/m^2	RAP < 8 mm Hg and CI > 2.5 L/min/m^2

Abbreviations: 2MWT is two-minute walk test; BNP is B-type natriuretic peptide (BNP) and NT-pro-BNP is N-terminal-pro-BNP; RAP is mean right atrial pressure; RV is right ventricular; WHO-FC is World Health Organization functional class.
[a]The tricuspid annular plane systolic excursion (TAPSE) has been reported to be of prognostic value.

Table 123-4

WORKUP ALGORITHM FOR BIOPSY-PROVEN MPM

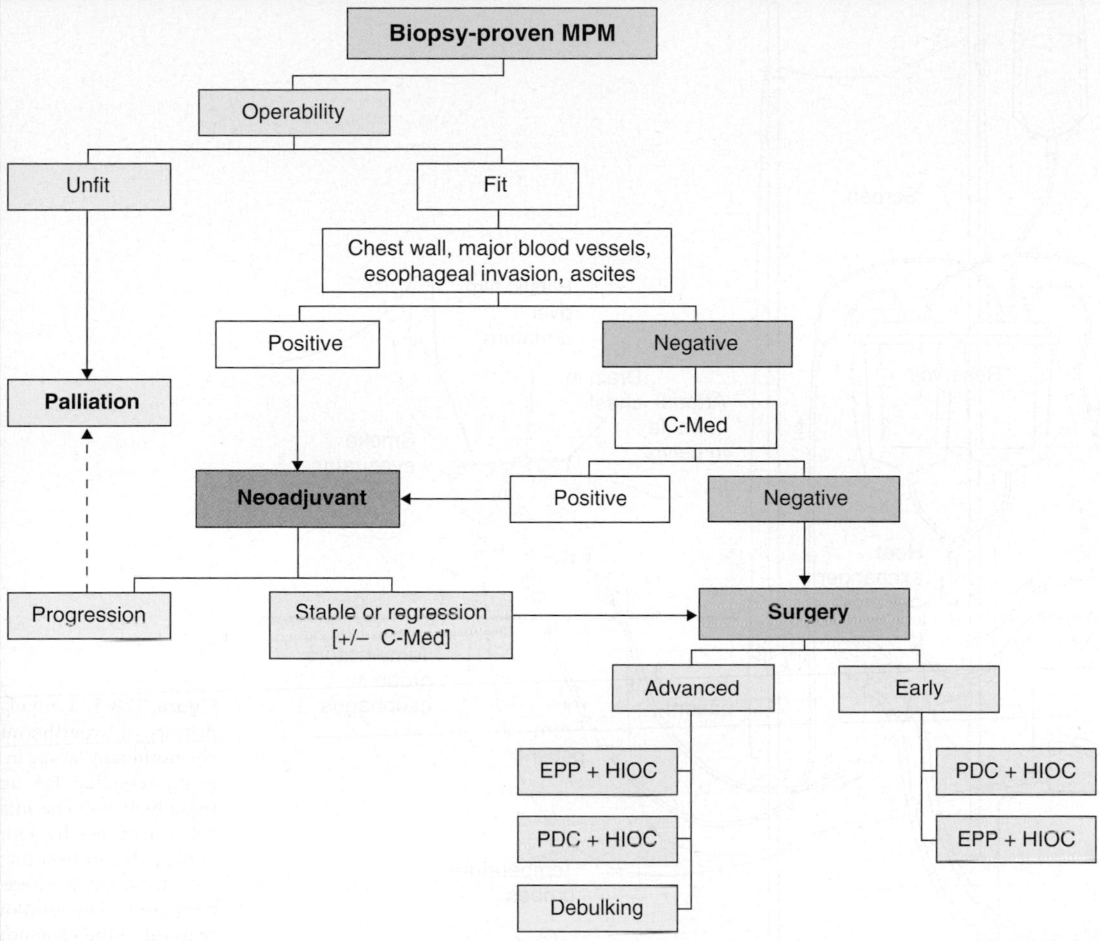

incision is approximated at both ends by using a no. 2 nylon running locking suture, leaving a small aperture in the center of the wound (Fig. 123-2). This permits access for the surgeon to place a double-gloved hand into the thorax and evenly distribute the perfusate. The Omni retractor (Omni-Tract, Minneapolis, MN) is secured to the surgeon's side of the table. Interrupted no. 2 nylon sutures then are placed at selected points along the wound aperture, and the edges of the wound are lifted onto the Omni wishbone arms so as to create a funnel that prevents spillover of the intracavitary chemotherapy.

Two cannulae are placed—the inflow cannula (straight) and the outflow cannula (L-shaped). For right-sided resections, the surgeon places the straight-inflow cannula in the pelvis by holding it in his left hand and pushing it through the wide open thoracoabdominal cavity. For left-sided resections, the surgeon holds the cannula in the right hand and pushes it above the stomach into the pelvis. Special attention is taken not to injure the capsule of the spleen during this maneuver. The L-shaped outflow cannula is placed at the apex of the pleural space to collect the perfusate and return it to the pump. Both drains are then connected to the perfusion pump. Adhesive tapes are used to cover the entire field creating a well. This prevents the lavage fluid from escaping the operative field. A slit is made in the plastic shield, which permits the surgeon to monitor the perfusate level (Fig. 123-3). Once HIOC is initiated, the inflow and outflow perfusate temperatures are monitored constantly and maintained at 42°C. The entire field should be submerged in the solution. The edges of the wound not bathed by the perfusate should be constantly irrigated by the surgeon with a properly labeled bulb syringe that is discarded at the end of the lavage. Constant communication between the surgeon and the perfusionist ensures that the level of the lavage fluid in the chest cavity is appropriate. A smoke evacuator is used to pull air from beneath the plastic cover and pass it through an activated charcoal filter to prevent any possible contamination of air in the OR by chemotherapy aerosols.

After 1 hour of thoracoabdominal lavage, the patient is placed in steep Trendelenburg position, and the perfusate is drained out of the field back into the perfusion circuit. The volume of perfusate returned to the circuit is scrutinized, and different maneuvers are performed to maximize the return of perfusate. These include displacing the omentum or gently sweeping any perfusate retained in the pelvis or in between bowel loops into the field. Leaving behind a significant amount of perfusate will increase the systemic absorption of cisplatin and toxicity and cause prolonged postoperative ileus. At this point, an omental fat pad is fashioned with endovascular staples. It is of paramount importance that the pad reaches the bronchial stump without tension. In the absence of an

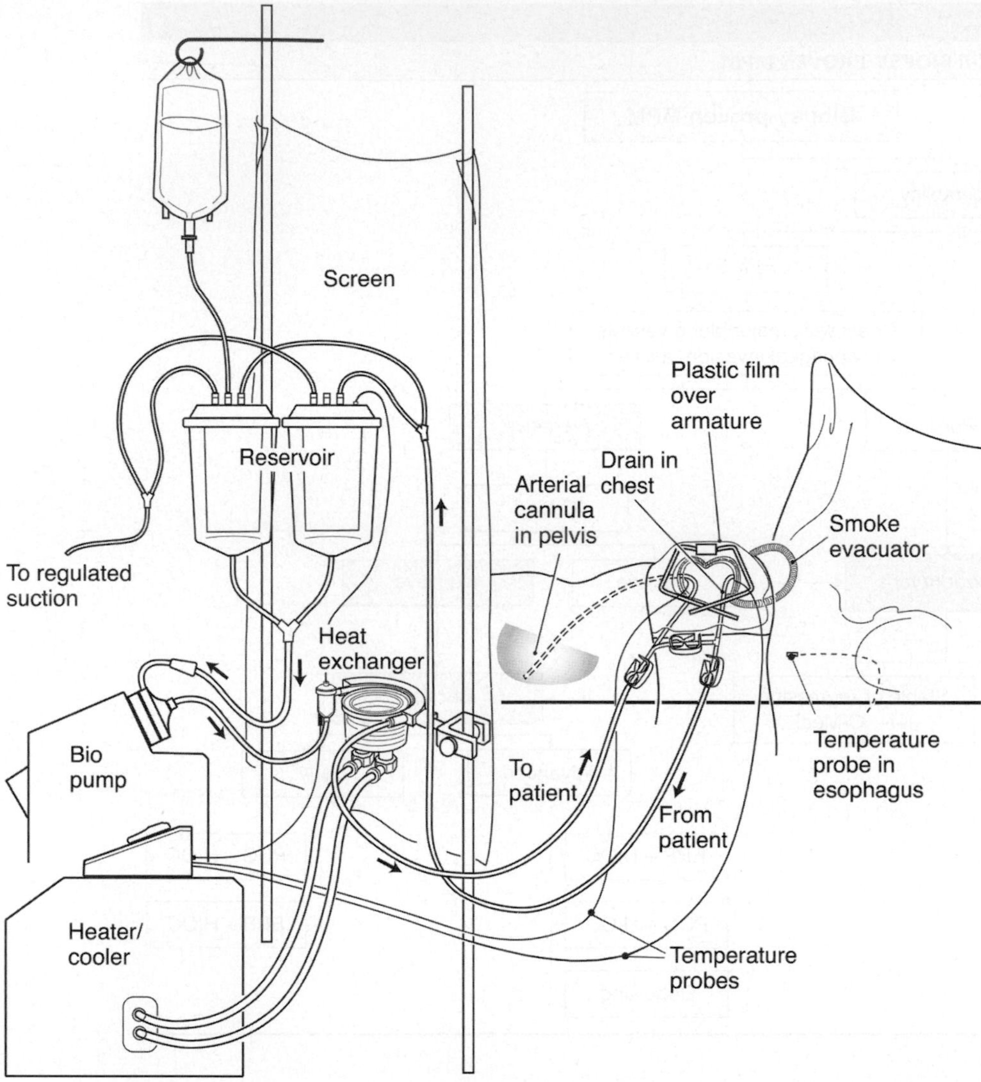

Figure 123-1. Cannula placement for delivery of hyperthermic intraoperative chemotherapy lavage in a patient undergoing resection for malignant pleural mesothelioma. The intake cannula (for delivery of the chemotherapy) is placed in the pelvis or over the diaphragm posteriorly in cases where the diaphragm is spared. The outflow cannula (for removal of the chemotherapy) is placed in the apex of the chest and the patient is placed in slight Trendelenburg position.

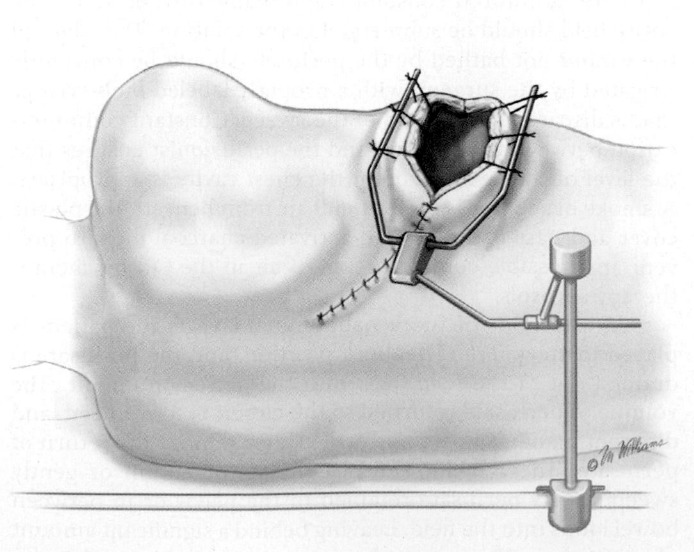

Figure 123-2. The wound is closed with no. 2 running locking nylon sutures from both ends. A thoracic well is created by lifting the edges of the wound over the wishbone arms of the Omni retractor for administration of the lavage.

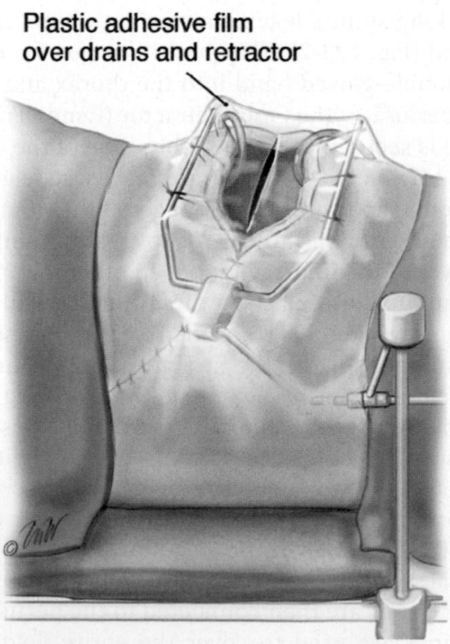

Figure 123-3. The edges of the wound, drains, and retractor are covered with a clear sheet of plastic adhesive.

adequate omental fat pad, one could use pericardial remnant or parathymic fat to buttress the bronchial stump. The chest cavity is once again irrigated with normal saline solution, hemostasis is completed, and the chest is packed with five or six Mikulicz pads.

Next, the diaphragm and pericardium are reconstructed with Gore-Tex patches (W.L. Gore and Associates, Flagstaff, AZ) (Fig. 123-4). For the diaphragm, we routinely use two 2-mm thick patches stapled together. Pericardial reconstruction is carried out with a 0.1-mm fenestrated pericardial patch. An omental flap is constructed most easily by stapling endo-GIA vascular loads (2.9 mm) across parts of the omentum while the abdomen is fully exposed (after the lavage but before the diaphragm patch is undertaken).

Before the incision is closed, a final check for hemostasis is performed. We often use an aerosol 9F fibrin sealant across the thoracic cavity (Evicel, Ethicon, Inc., Somerville, NJ) to assist with firm hemostasis. A 12F Rob-Nel (Dover, Rob-Nel, Kendall, Inc., Mansfield, MA) catheter is left in the thoracic cavity to permit access to the space postoperatively. Once the wound is completely closed, air is withdrawn through the Rob-Nel catheter for medialization of the mediastinum. Current guidelines call for the withdrawal of 750 mL from the right thoracic space in a female and 1000 mL in a male, and 500 mL from the left thoracic space in a female and 750 mL in a male. The preceding serves as a guideline only, however, because the evacuation of air should be aborted early if any suggestion of hemodynamic instability develops as a consequence of excessively negative intrathoracic pressure. Beyond the immediate evacuation of fluid in the OR, the Rob-Nel catheter is used in the ensuing day(s) to withdraw postoperative fluid and correct for mediastinal shift, as well as to reduce intrathoracic pressures. The trend of intrathoracic pressures is monitored, and any sudden rise in pressure should be managed by urgent withdrawal of intrathoracic fluid to avoid potential compression on the mediastinum and vena cava.[23]

Once the patient is turned supine and the double-lumen endotracheal tube is exchanged for a single-lumen tube, bronchoscopy is repeated at the end of the procedure to visualize the bronchial stump and to clear secretions from the remaining dependent lung.

HYPERTHERMIC THORACOABDOMINAL CHEMOTHERAPY FOR INTRA-ABDOMINAL MALIGNANCY

Malignant mesothelioma may affect any of the serous membranes that line the major body cavities (i.e., pleura, peritoneum,

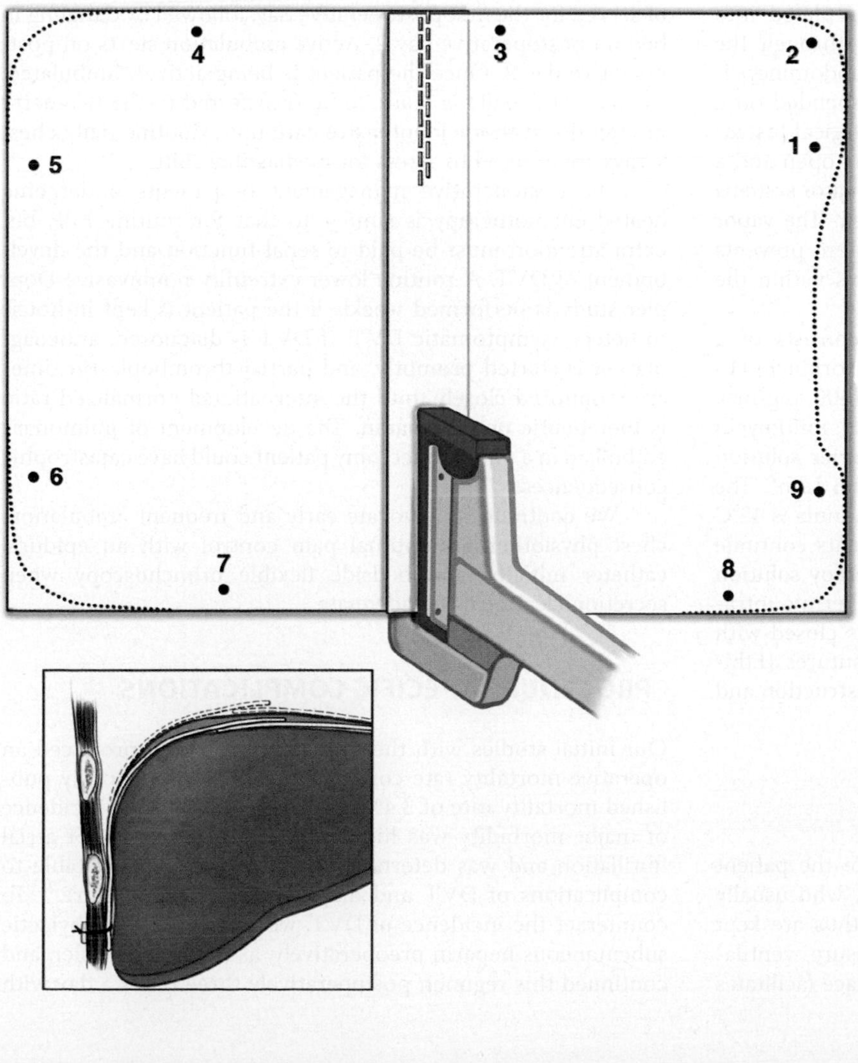

Figure 123-4. Reconstruction of the diaphragm with 2 GORE® DUALMESH® PLUS patches, joined in the middle by two staple lines using a Reloadable Linear Stapler with two staggered rows of titanium staples (60 mm staple line length). The patch is then sewn to the chest wall with 9 ETHIBOND EXCEL™ Polyester Suture 1.

pericardium, tunica vaginalis of the testes). The technique of hyperthermic chemotherapy lavage has been used with good success in patients with malignant peritoneal mesothelioma.[24] Likewise, a pleural mesothelioma may spread to the abdomen or a peritoneal mesothelioma may spread to the chest. When malignant mesothelioma transgresses the diaphragmatic barrier, irrespective of the original site of the cancer, it is important to extend the chemotherapeutic lavage to both body cavities. Thus, intracavitary chemotherapy administration may be part of an abdominal, thoracic, or thoracoabdominal procedure to prevent or to treat pleural or peritoneal metastases from an intra-abdominal malignancy or malignant pleural mesothelioma.

To perform a thoracoabdominal procedure in a patient with malignant peritoneal mesothelioma, as with the thoracic resection described above, after removing all macroscopic disease (cytoreductive surgery) from the peritoneal surface of the abdominal cavity, the diaphragm is carefully inspected. Any small transection of the diaphragm into the pleural space is enlarged to permit free flow of chemotherapy from abdomen to pelvis. Most often in patients with this cancer, there is full thickness invasion of the tendinous midportion of the hemidiaphragm, and it is this portion of the hemidiaphragm that requires resection.

An inflow catheter and four outflow drains are positioned within the abdominopelvic space. A right angle inflow cannula is positioned within the thoracic cavity and connected along with the intra-abdominal drains to the outflow catheter. The hyperthermic chemotherapy solution is circulated into the abdominopelvic space and into the thorax through the open hemidiaphragm. The reservoir within the abdominopelvic space is created by skin traction sutures suspended on a Thompson self-retaining retractor (Thompson Surgical Instruments, Traverse City, MI). The abdomen remains open and a vapor barrier is established using four smoke evacuator systems positioned at the four quadrants of the abdomen. The vapor barrier established by the smoke evacuation system prevents any potential danger from chemotherapy aerosols within the operating room environment.

The intracavitary chemotherapy regimen consists of a combination of mitomycin C (15 mg/m^2) and doxorubicin (15 mg/m^2) combined with systemic fluorouracil (400 mg/m^2). For patients with peritoneal mesothelioma, the mitomycin C is replaced by cisplatin at 50 mg/m^2. The carrier solution is 1.5% dextrose peritoneal dialysis solution at 1.5 L/m^2. The temperature within the abdomen at the inflow cannula is 42°C and at the outflow cannula is 41°C. The treatments continue for 60 minutes. After 60 minutes, the chemotherapy solution is removed. Following completion of the hyperthermic intraoperative chemotherapy lavage, the diaphragm is closed with a series of interrupted and running #1 Vicryl sutures (Ethicon, Cleveland, OH), after which intestinal reconstruction and abdominal closure are performed.

POSTOPERATIVE CARE

The immediate postoperative goal is to extubate the patient in the OR, except for patients undergoing P/D, who usually require some positive-pressure ventilation and thus are kept intubated overnight. Minimizing positive-pressure ventilation and leaving adequate chest tube drains in place facilitates apposition of the lung to chest wall, in turn, reducing the amount of bleeding from raw surfaces of the lung.

The protocol for postoperative management of EPP plus heated chemotherapy patients is similar to the protocol for EPP without heated chemotherapy, with the exception of a few important differences. Heated chemotherapy patients must be well hydrated. For the first 12 hours, the patient receives 100 mL/h of 1 L of sterile water with three ampules of sodium bicarbonate added. For the next 12 hours, the hydration fluid is changed to 100 mL/h of normal saline (D_5/NS). Thereafter, the IV rate and type are tailored to the patient's electrolytes, urine output, and ability to tolerate oral intake.

With heated chemotherapy patients, the nasogastric tube is kept in place until bowel sounds return. The patient's ability to swallow is assessed at bedside before oral intake is instituted. To reduce the risk of aspiration, indirect laryngoscopy and vocal cord visualization occasionally are indicated if there is a suspicion of palsy or paresis. A speech and swallow evaluation is indicated if the patient has a hoarse voice or when aspiration is suspected at bedside swallow evaluation.

The trend of using Rob-Nel catheter pressure measurement aids in postoperative management, with aspiration of the pleural space, if necessary. The need for aspiration should be correlated with the clinical picture. We recommend aspirating no more than 200 to 300 mL at a time to avoid pulmonary edema or complications of acute respiratory distress syndrome. The catheter is usually removed in 2 to 3 days depending on the frequency and necessity of aspiration. Strict bed rest is observed for the first postoperative day, followed by dangling in bed on postoperative day 2. Active ambulation starts on postoperative day 3. Once the patient is being actively ambulated, the patient usually is ready to be transferred to the telemetry or step-down thoracic intensive care unit. Routine daily chest x-rays are ordered to assess for mediastinal shift.

The postoperative management of patients undergoing heated chemotherapy is similar to that for routine EPP, but extra attention must be paid to renal function and the development of DVT. A routine lower extremity noninvasive Doppler study is performed weekly if the patient is kept in-house to detect asymptomatic DVT. If DVT is diagnosed, anticoagulation is started promptly, and partial thromboplastin times are monitored closely until the international normalized ratio is therapeutic on Coumadin. The development of pulmonary embolism in a pneumonectomy patient could have catastrophic consequences.

We continue to advocate early and frequent ambulation, chest physiotherapy, optimal pain control with an epidural catheter initially, and bedside flexible bronchoscopy when secretion clearance is inadequate.

PROCEDURE-SPECIFIC COMPLICATIONS

Our initial studies with the hyperthermic lavage produced an operative mortality rate comparable with our previously published mortality rate of 3.4% for EPP alone.[2,25,26] The incidence of major morbidity was higher in all categories except atrial fibrillation and was determined to be directly attributable to complications of DVT and diaphragmatic patch failure.[27] To counteract the incidence of DVT, we introduced prophylactic subcutaneous heparin preoperatively, as described earlier, and continued this regimen postoperatively three times a day with routine weekly Doppler study.[25] Heated chemotherapy patients are also kept well hydrated commencing immediately after the chemotherapeutic lavage.

Diaphragmatic patch failure can result in herniation of abdominal contents into the thorax. The higher incidence of patch failure may be attributed to violation of the peritoneal cavity (necessary to permit abdominal lavage) and swelling of the abdominal viscera after exposure to hyperthermic chemotherapeutic lavage. Increased cephalad pressure on the patch results in dehiscence. To correct this problem, we doubled the size of the Gore-Tex patch by stapling two patches together, as described in Chapter 122, Figure 122-4. This creates a dynamic patch that permits sufficient upward movement to accommodate for swelling of the abdominal viscera and reduces tension on the sutures to prevent them from pulling away from the chest wall. By using this approach, the diaphragmatic patch failure rate was subsequently reduced from 12% to 3.4%.[25]

For the remainder of the complications, including atrial fibrillation, constrictive pericarditis, cardiac tamponade, cardiac arrest, myocardial infarction, acute respiratory distress syndrome, tracheostomy, pulmonary embolism, vocal cord paralysis, aspiration, and empyema, the difference was not statistically significant between the two groups.

In our phase I–II study, patients who underwent P/D plus hyperthermic chemotherapy lavage had a higher mortality and renal toxicity rate but comparable or better rates for other complications. An apparent dose-related survival benefit was identified and has recently been confirmed in a paper on low-risk patients.[28]

SUMMARY

Hyperthermic thoracoabdominal chemotherapy can be administered safely and effectively in concert with cytoreductive surgery for malignant pleural or peritoneal mesothelioma. In patients with malignant pleural mesothelioma, the treatment can be performed regardless of whether the patient has undergone EPP or P/D. The aim of this treatment is to decrease or delay the rate of recurrence and potentially improve long-term survival in patients with malignant pleural mesothelioma.

References

1. Stayner L, Welch LS, Lemen R. The worldwide pandemic of asbestos-related diseases. *Annu Rev Public Health.* 2013;34:205–216.
2. Sugarbaker DJ, Flores RM, Jaklitsch MT, et al. Resection margins, extrapleural nodal status, and cell type determine postoperative long-term survival in trimodality therapy of malignant pleural mesothelioma: results in 183 patients. *J Thorac Cardiovasc Surg.* 1999;117:54–63; discussion 63–65.
3. Lee YC, Light RW, Musk AW. Management of malignant pleural mesothelioma: a critical review. *Curr Opin Pulm Med.* 2000;6:267–274.
4. Rusch VW, Giroux D, Kennedy C, et al. Initial analysis of the international association for the study of lung cancer mesothelioma database. *J Thorac Oncol.* 2012;7:1631–1639.
5. de Perrot M, Feld R, Cho BC, et al. Trimodality therapy with induction chemotherapy followed by extrapleural pneumonectomy and adjuvant high-dose hemithoracic radiation for malignant pleural mesothelioma. *J Clin Oncol.* 2009;27:1413–1418.
6. Weder W, Opitz I, Stahel R. Multimodality strategies in malignant pleural mesothelioma. *Semin Thorac Cardiovasc Surg.* 2009;21:172–176.
7. Rusch V, Baldini EH, Bueno R, et al. The role of surgical cytoreduction in the treatment of malignant pleural mesothelioma: meeting summary of the International Mesothelioma Interest Group Congress, September 11–14, 2012, Boston, Mass. *J Thorac Cardiovasc Surg.* 2013;145:909–910.
8. Sugarbaker PH, Chang D, Stuart OA. Hyperthermic intraoperative thoracoabdominal chemotherapy. *Gastroenterol Res Pract.* 2012;623–417.
9. Berghmans T, Paesmans M, Lalami Y, et al. Activity of chemotherapy and immunotherapy on malignant mesothelioma: a systematic review of the literature with meta-analysis. *Lung Cancer.* 2002;38:111–121.
10. Pinto AL, Lippard SJ. Binding of the antitumor drug cis-diamminedichloroplatinum(II) (cisplatin) to DNA. *Biochim Biophys Acta.* 1985;780:167–180.
11. Sugarbaker D. Multimodality therapy of malignant mesothelioma. In: Roth J, Ruckdeschel J, Weisenburger T, eds. *Thoracic Oncology*. Philadelphia, PA: Saunders; 1995:538–555.
12. Sugarbaker DJ, Mentzer SJ, DeCamp M, et al. Extrapleural pneumonectomy in the setting of a multimodality approach to malignant mesothelioma. *Chest.* 1993;103:377S–381S.
13. Howell SB, Pfeifle CE, Wung WE, et al. Intraperitoneal cis-diamminedichloroplatinum with systemic thiosulfate protection. *Cancer Res.* 1983;43:1426–1431.
14. Ratto GB, Civalleri D, Esposito M, et al. Pleural space perfusion with cisplatin in the multimodality treatment of malignant mesothelioma: a feasibility and pharmacokinetic study. *J Thorac Cardiovasc Surg.* 1999;117:759–765.
15. Ausmus PL, Wilke AV, Frazier DL. Effects of hyperthermia on blood flow and cis-diamminedichloroplatinum(II) pharmacokinetics in murine mammary adenocarcinomas. *Cancer Res.* 1992;52:4965–4968.
16. Stehlin JS, Giovanella BC, de Ipolyi PD, et al. Results of hyperthermic perfusion for melanoma of the extremities. *Surg Gynecol Obstet.* 1975;140:339–348.
17. Giovanella BC, Stehlin JS, Yim SO. Correlation of the thermosensitivity of cells to their malignant potential. *Ann N Y Acad Sci.* 1980;335:206–214.
18. Azzarelli A. Intra-arterial infusion and perfusion chemotherapy for soft tissue sarcomas of the extremities. *Cancer Treat Res.* 1986;29:103–129.
19. Lee JD, Perez S, Wang HJ, et al. Intrapleural chemotherapy for patients with incompletely resected malignant mesothelioma: the UCLA experience. *J Surg Oncol.* 1995;60:262–267.
20. Markman M, Howell SB, Green MR. Combination intracavitary chemotherapy for malignant pleural disease. *Cancer Drug Deliv.* 1984;1:333–336.
21. Howell SB, Pfeifle CL, Wung WE, et al. Intraperitoneal cisplatin with systemic thiosulfate protection. *Ann Intern Med.* 1982;97:845–851.
22. Kearney DJ, Lee TH, Reilly JJ, et al. Assessment of operative risk in patients undergoing lung resection. Importance of predicted pulmonary function. *Chest.* 1994;105:753–759.
23. Wolf AS, Jacobson FL, Tilleman TR, et al. Managing the pneumonectomy space after extrapleural pneumonectomy: postoperative intrathoracic pressure monitoring. *Eur J Cardiothorac Surg.* 2010;37:770–775.
24. Sugarbaker PH, Chang D, Stuart OA. Hyperthermic intraoperative thoracoabdominal chemotherapy. *Gastroenterol Res Pract.* 2012;2012:623417.
25. Sugarbaker DJ, Jaklitsch MT, Bueno R, et al. Prevention, early detection, and management of complications after 328 consecutive extrapleural pneumonectomies. *J Thorac Cardiovasc Surg.* 2004;128:138–146.
26. Chang M, Sugarbaker D. Innovative therapies: intraoperative intracavitary chemotherapy. *Thorac Surg Clin.* 2004;14:549–556.
27. Alberts DS, Liu PY, Hannigan EV, et al. Intraperitoneal cisplatin plus intravenous cyclophosphamide versus intravenous cisplatin plus intravenous cyclophosphamide for stage III ovarian cancer. *N Engl J Med.* 1996;335:1950–1955.
28. Sugarbaker DJ, Gill RR, Yeap BY, et al. Hyperthermic intraoperative pleural cisplatin chemotherapy extends interval to recurrence and survival among low-risk patients with malignant pleural mesothelioma undergoing surgical macroscopic complete resection. *J Thorac Cardiovasc Surg.* 2013;145:955–963.

124 Photodynamic Therapy in the Management of Pleural Tumors

Joseph S. Friedberg and Shamus R. Carr

Keywords: Mesothelioma, photodynamic therapy, pleural tumors

PLEURAL TUMORS OVERVIEW

Cancer of the pleura is a virulent and lethal malignancy. Primary tumors of the pleura are rare, whereas metastatic tumors, often in the form of malignant pleural effusions, are quite common. Primary tumors of the pleura, malignant pleural mesothelioma being the most common, are typically associated with a life expectancy of less than a year. Metastatic cancers to the pleura, including non–small-cell lung cancer (NSCLC), represent stage IV disease and usually coincide with the most adverse prognosis for the primary cancer that has spread to the pleura.

The most common form of treatment for pleural cancers is systemic therapy and/or palliative care, since the majority of pleural cancers represent metastatic disease. Surgery is not typically considered an effective treatment because of the essentially impossible task of achieving a true negative margin for these cancers that coat every surface of the chest cavity. In an investigational capacity, however, surgery has become the cornerstone of highly aggressive multimodal treatment plans in selected patients, and the most widespread application in malignant pleural mesothelioma.

With the expectation that microscopic disease will remain after even the most aggressive surgical resections, one approach has been to combine an intraoperative adjuvant therapy with systemic therapy and, sometimes, adjuvant external beam radiation. The intraoperative adjuvant therapies include the following: chemotherapy, with or without hyperthermia, heated povidone iodine, radioisotopic radiation, intraoperative photon radiation, and photodynamic therapy (PDT).[1] This chapter focuses on the combination of surgery and PDT and the application of this technique in malignant pleural mesothelioma.

PDT OVERVIEW

PDT is a technique for killing tumors which uses a photosensitizer that is activated by visible light. It has been observed that photosensitizers are preferentially taken up by, or retained in, tumor cells.[2,3] Once inside the cells, the photosensitizer is activated by a laser light with a wavelength specific to the sensitizer's absorption spectrum. Activation of the photosensitizer in the presence of oxygen results in the production of excited species of oxygen capable of inducing cell death. Cell death occurs by apoptosis or from direct destruction of certain cellular elements.[4,5] In addition, PDT may result in neovascular damage that may compromise the tumor's blood supply.[6] Finally, when PDT is used to treat cancer, it appears to enhance the host's immune response to the tumor.[7,8]

In addition to the presence of oxygen, the items needed to perform pleural PDT include the photosensitizer, a light source, and a dosimetry system. PDT is a dose-dependent treatment. That is, without light activation there is no effect on cells that contain the photosensitizer. The overall effect of PDT increases with the amount of activating light delivered. Although photosensitizers may demonstrate some selectivity for neoplastic cells, they also partition into normal tissues and will cause some degree of damage to those tissues when exposed to light. This is critical, especially for pleural PDT, as injury to any structure in the chest can occur absent meticulous attention to light dosimetry.

Photosensitizers

The majority of experience with pleural PDT has been with two photosensitizers, Photofrin and Foscan. Photofrin (dihematoporphyrin derivate) was the first commercially available photosensitizer and has its major excitation wavelengths in the UV region (200–450 nm), the green region (510 nm), and a small absorption peak in the red (630 nm) region of the light spectrum. Meta-tetrahydroxyphenylchloride (Foscan®) is the second drug that has been used for treating mesothelioma.[2] It has major absorption peaks in the UV (200–450 nm) green regions (520 nm), with the highest peak in the red region at 652 nm. Although the shorter wavelengths have higher energy, red light is used for greater tissue penetration, which can be up to several centimeters depending on the absorption and scattering characteristics of the tissue.

Both of these photosensitizers are administered intravenously, preoperatively. As stated previously, photosensitizers may demonstrate some element of selectivity, but will ultimately sensitize all tissues, including the skin. As a result, cutaneous photosensitivity is the primary toxicity associated with administering a photosensitizer.[9,10]

Laser Equipment

To treat large surface areas with PDT, high-power light sources are required. In general, it is necessary to use a laser to supply light at the appropriate wavelength and intensity. Tunable dye lasers, pumped by a larger green light laser with fixed wavelength, are commonly used to produce red light in the 7 W range. These lasers have the advantage of possessing dye modules that can be interchanged to permit production of a broad spectrum of wavelengths. The disadvantage is that they are relatively large and require high-power supplies and water-cooling systems. Recently developed diode lasers are more portable and have power outputs up to 6 W (in the red light waveband). They do not require the use of high-power supplies or water-cooling systems, but have the disadvantage of being fixed at a single wavelength.

Dosimetry

Although photosensitizers may preferentially migrate to tumor tissues, it should be assumed that all tissues are photosensitive. As a result, any structure that is illuminated can be injured. It is crucial, therefore, not to overdose normal tissues with light. Some investigators rely upon "calculated" light doses.[11,12] On the basis of experiments which demonstrate that the measured and calculated light doses may vary widely owing to the unpredictable reflection and refraction patterns of light in vivo,[13] we believe that light dosing should not be empiric and one should rely on measured dosimetry. Consequently, light sensors are placed at strategic positions within the hemithorax and fed into a real-time dosimetry system that has a separate channel for each sensor. During PDT, the light source is moved around the chest cavity until each sensor has measured the desired dose of light.

Currently two types of sensors are used: flat and isotropic. The flat sensors[14] underestimate the light dose delivered to the tissue surfaces in comparison with isotropic detectors.[15] If the type of sensor or photosensitizer is changed, measurements must be made to determine the conversion factor between the sensors or safety studies to determine the safe maximal tolerated dose.[16]

Some investigators fill the hemithorax with diffuse intralipid solution to help scatter light as the light source is moved around the chest cavity.[14,17] This is our preferred method for light delivery regardless of the debulking technique. It assures that there is no shielding of tissue by pooled blood and also permits direct manipulation of the costophrenic recesses, the most difficult areas in which to achieve good light delivery. Others have focused on integral illumination by using a bulb fiber and no light-diffusing medium.[13] This technique is only applicable after a pneumonectomy. In the latter technique, a transparent sterile bag is placed in the chest cavity following pneumonectomy and filled with warm saline to facilitate flattening and expansion of the chest cavity structures. After partial closure of the surgical wound, a single spherical bulb fiber is placed in the center of the bag to allow integral illumination of the entire cavity and enhance the reflection of light. This technique is not compatible with a lung-sparing procedure and may not be applicable if it does not appear that the bag will expand all crevices in the hemithorax. We abandoned this technique when we found that blood was pooling under the bag and preventing light from reaching those areas.

SURGICAL APPROACH

Overview

The concept behind the combination of surgery and PDT for pleural malignancies is that surgery is used to achieve a macroscopic complete resection and PDT is performed after the resection as an intraoperative adjuvant therapy in an effort to treat the residual microscopic disease.[18–21] The two options for achieving a macroscopic complete resection include extrapleural pneumonectomy (Chapter 122) and radical pleurectomy (Chapter 121).

Extrapleural pneumonectomy is defined as the en bloc removal of the lung, parietal pleura, diaphragm, and pericardium. Typically, both the diaphragm and pericardium are reconstructed with prosthetic patches. This operation has the advantage of being standardized with respect to both name and technique. It is almost certainly the technique that results in the least amount of residual microscopic disease, that is, the most complete and reproducible macroscopic complete resection. Finally, without the lung in the chest, radiation can be used as an adjuvant therapy to treat the entire hemithorax.

Radical pleurectomy is a more nebulous operation which, even in the best of hands, almost certainly leaves behind more microscopic disease than an extrapleural pneumonectomy. There is essentially no standardization of this operation and, in fact, the procedure appears in the literature under a multitude of names including pleurectomy, decortication, pleurectomy-decortication, radical pleurectomy-decortication, radical pleurectomy and extended pleurectomy. The intent of the operation also varies, from a palliative debulking of some gross disease to a macroscopic complete resection. This tremendous variability in every aspect of the procedure, including nomenclature, makes it difficult to compare published case series. Finally, the timing of the decision to perform the operation is also variable, ranging from an intraoperative decision based upon intraoperative findings to a preoperative plan. In the former situation, either the bulk of the cancer or the degree of involvement of the cancer with the pulmonary fissures is often cited as the deciding factor as in whether or not the lung can be saved.

For the purposes of the ensuing discussion, radical pleurectomy is the term that we use to describe a lung-sparing operation aimed at achieving a macroscopic complete resection. The goal of each procedure is to save the lung and, if possible, the phrenic nerve and as much of the pericardium and/or diaphragmatic musculature as possible, while still achieving a macroscopic complete resection. Depending upon the degree of invasion, it usually is not necessary to reconstruct the diaphragm. We have found this to be true for the pericardium as well, since the presence of the lung is sufficient to prevent cardiac herniation/torsion. In our hands, radical pleurectomy is a procedure that is planned preoperatively, not an intraoperative decision based upon involvement of the pulmonary fissures, tumor bulk, or other factors.

Thus, with respect to the two types of surgery for malignant pleural mesothelioma, the advantages of extrapleural pneumonectomy include relative standardization and hence comparability of results, the best macroscopic complete resection, the ability to treat with adjuvant radiation and, in our hands, a more expeditious operation than radical pleurectomy. The disadvantages are the consequences of pneumonectomy and, potentially, the need for prosthetic reconstructions. The principal advantage of radical pleurectomy is preservation of the lung and, potentially, the decreased need for prosthetic reconstruction. Preserving the lung not only translates into the potential benefits of preserving quality of life and offering a surgery-based approach to patients who might not be candidates for pneumonectomy, but it may also allow the patient to undergo more aggressive treatment options for their inevitable tumor recurrence. The disadvantages of radical pleurectomy include the presence of more residual microscopic disease, lack of standardization and, in our hands, a longer operation with a more complex postoperative management than with extrapleural pneumonectomy. The ideal surgical approach remains an area of controversy. It may well be that no one approach is correct for every patient. The optimal operative strategy may well be related to the individual patient, characteristics of their particular tumor, and the selection of adjuvant therapies that are going to be used in combination with surgery.

We have performed both extrapleural pneumonectomies and radical pleurectomies for mesothelioma in combination with intraoperative PDT. In a pilot study that compared the outcomes of these two surgical approaches, we found that the

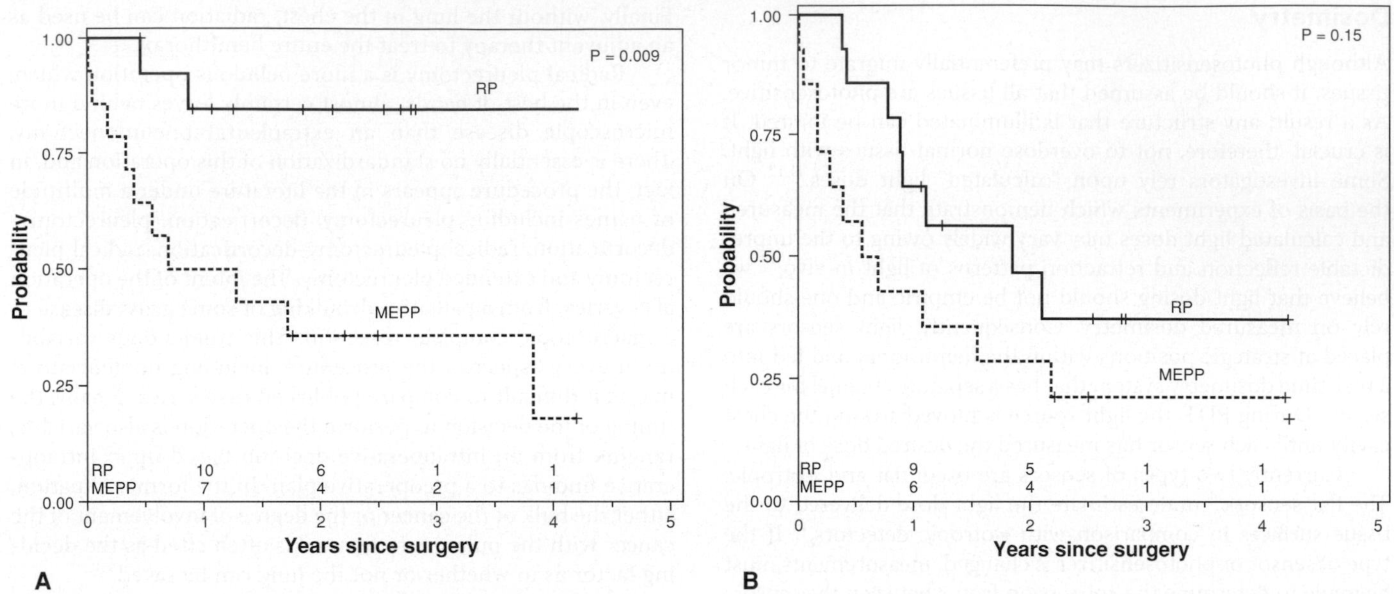

Figure 124-1. *A.* Overall survival for 28 patients (14 in each arm) undergoing intraoperative PDT and either radical pleurectomy (RP) or modified extrapleural pneumonectomy (MEPP). *B.* Disease-free survival for 28 patients (14 in each arm) undergoing intraoperative PDT and RP or MEPP. (Reprinted with permission from Friedberg JS, Mick R, Culligan M, et al. Photodynamic therapy (PDT) and the evolution of a lung sparing surgical treatment for mesothelioma. *Ann Thorac Surg*, 2011; 91(6): 1738–1745.)

patients who underwent radical pleurectomy had longer overall survival compared with patients who underwent pneumonectomy (Fig. 124-1A), despite essentially no difference in disease-free survival (Fig. 124-1B). The term "MEPP" was used in the study cited in Figure 124-1 as the operation involving pneumonectomy preserved the diaphragm, pericardium, and phrenic nerve. The currently accepted definition of extrapleural pneumonectomy is en-bloc resection of the parietal and visceral pleura with the ipsilateral lung, pericardium, and diaphragm. In cases where the pericardium and/or diaphragm are not involved by tumor, these structures may be left intact.[22]

On the basis of this pilot study, we switched exclusively to radical pleurectomy as our surgical approach to malignant pleural mesothelioma. We still, however, will perform an extrapleural pneumonectomy in combination with PDT for NSCLC with pleural dissemination (stage IVa). Although the era of targeted therapies has provided more treatments for patients with this disease, this approach has shown promise as an aggressive option for patients with this cancer.[23] In either case, whether the lung is taken or spared, the light precautions taken during surgery and the performance of PDT are identical.

Patient selection for these procedures takes place in the forum of a multidisciplinary tumor board-type conference with disease limited to one hemithorax as the principal oncologic criteria for consideration as a surgical candidate. Eligible and interested patients undergo an extensive radiographic staging workup and ultimately undergo an invasive staging procedure including bronchoscopy and laparoscopy to rule out radiographically occult metastases. While the presence of ipsilateral mediastinal lymph node metastases (N2 disease) is not currently viewed as an exclusion criterion for radical pleurectomy for mesothelioma, as it is for extrapleural pneumonectomy, this does correlate with a decrease in overall survival and we have started to routinely include endobronchial ultrasound-guided biopsy (EBUS) staging as part of our preoperative evaluation. Contralateral thoracoscopy, to rule out contralateral pleural disease, and mediastinoscopy or EBUS, to rule out N3 disease, are used on a case-by-case basis as dictated by the imaging studies and clinical suspicion. From a safety perspective, the selection criteria are the same as would be used for any major thoracic operation, such as a formal decortication or pneumonectomy, with an added emphasis on nutritional parameters. The PDT superimposes a significant metabolic demand, and malnutrition serves as an exclusion criteria. As part of the informed consent disclosures, it is made clear to all patients that the procedure is investigational and, in addition to the risks of the surgery, there are the superimposed risks of PDT; primarily, cutaneous photosensitivity and a higher incidence of postoperative atrial fibrillation, deep venous thromboses (but not pulmonary embolism), and persistent air leaks in radical pleurectomy patients.

Photosensitizer and Light Precautions

Before surgery, the patient receives the photosensitizer as an outpatient. The patient becomes immediately light sensitive. Therefore, patients should be instructed to bring sunglasses and wear appropriate clothing to cover or shade all exposed skin. With adequate patient education, we have not experienced any problems with sunburning before or after surgery. Once the patient arrives for surgery, hospital light precautions are initiated. This includes no exposure to sunlight through windows or intense overhead lights (fluorescent lights are fine) and probe rotation or spot-checking pulse oximetry. In the operating room the overhead lights and surgical headlights are passed through yellow filters. Yellow represents the portion of the visible light spectrum where the photosensitizers absorb less light, but these are not turned on until the incision is shielded with towels and all skin is protected from these intense light sources (see Fig. 124-2).

Technique of Radical Pleurectomy

General Approach and Strategy

Over the years we have tried multiple techniques in an attempt to develop a standardized approach to radical pleurectomy.

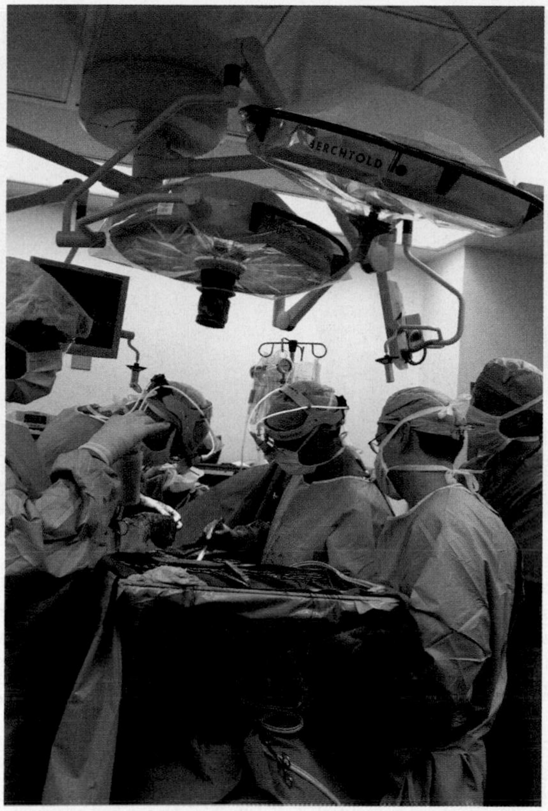

Figure 124-2. The operative field during the pleurectomy. Note the yellow filters on the overhead lights and surgical headlights. Other ongoing light precautions include towels which are sewn to the edges of the incision to prevent direct light exposure to the skin, and continuous rotation of the pulse oximeter to a different finger every 15 minutes.

What follows is a description of our current iteration of this procedure. The general strategy that has resulted in the most reproducible results is to mobilize the entire cancer from the hemithorax, such that it is tethered solely to the lung, and then resect the entire visceral pleura, en bloc with the mobilized cancer. With the proviso that every one of these cancers is different and the surgeon must remain flexible in the approach, the typical order of dissection is bony hemithorax, posterior mediastinum, superior mediastinum, anterior mediastinum, diaphragm, and lung.

Preparation and Incision

Light precautions, as stated above, are taken from the time the patient receives the photosensitizer. Patients undergoing radical pleurectomy will need a central line with one port reserved for total parenteral nutrition, epidural catheter, ipsilateral radial and femoral arterial lines and a nasoenteric tube, peripheral venous access, and a Foley catheter. Once it is confirmed by bronchoscopy that the nasoenteric tube is not in the lungs, it is our routine to give 60 mL of heavy cream spiked with an amp of methylene blue to aid the detection of injury to the thoracic duct during the course of the surgery. The patient is then placed in the lateral decubitus position and a thoracotomy incision is created under operating room fluorescent lights only. The latissimus is divided, but we are usually able to preserve and retract the serratus muscle. Once the chest wall layer is approached, the towels can be sewn to the muscle fascia to shade the skin, and the overhead and surgical headlights can be activated. If there is a rib interspace, the extrapleural plane is approached through the sixth interspace. If the interspace is contracted to the point of rib overlap, or the patient has had previous surgery through the sixth interspace to preclude entry, the seventh rib is removed and the extrapleural plane is approached through the bed of the resected seventh rib.

Chest Wall/Posterior-Superior Mediastinal Mobilization

The initial portion of the operation is the same whether the surgeon is planning to perform a radical pleurectomy or extrapleural pneumonectomy. The first step of the mobilization is to free the cancer from the bony hemithorax, followed by the posterior and superior mediastinum. The plane is identified and entered adjacent to the incision. It is developed bluntly, as much as possible. Blunt finger dissection, working a broad front, causes cleavage in the correct plane. Sharp dissection is more likely to leave behind gross tumor. The argon beam coagulator or Aquamantys® is good for cauterizing the chest wall, from which capillary oozing can lead to significant blood loss. Dissecting the chest wall is the safest portion of the operation and provides a good opportunity for the surgeon to get a sense of how the tumor is interacting with the tissues (Fig. 124-3A,B).

As the dissection is carried to the posterior reflection onto the posterior mediastinum, the surgeon can follow the intercostal veins from the azygos or hemiazygos veins as they traverse the mediastinum to safely transition from the chest wall to the posterior mediastinum. On the right side, the surgeon must take care not to get behind the esophagus; on the left it is the aorta that must be left in place as the pleura is separated from its medial surface. The presence of the nasoenteric tube can aid in identifying the esophagus by palpation, sometimes earlier in the setting of bulky tumors than can be accomplished by vision. In the superior mediastinum, the surgeon must be mindful of the subclavian artery on the left and the vena cava on the right. A 30-degree video thoracoscope for supplemental vision during the dissection is often helpful to assure the correct plane is identified and maintained, especially in the apex of the chest as the thoracic inlet and most superior mediastinal structures are dissected. On the right side, the azygocaval junction is typically approached both superiorly and posteriorly, having followed the azygos vein from behind and the cava from above. A venous injury can occur in this area if the wrong plane is entered.

Anterior Mediastinum

The anterior mediastinum is approached by sweeping off all pericardial fat in an anteroposterior direction, starting in the pericardiosternal recess. The surgeon must take care not to breach the anterior pleural reflection and enter the opposite hemithorax. This portion of the operation is highly variable. Occasionally, nearly the entire pericardium is covered with pericardial fat and removing this fat leaves the pericardium with a macroscopic complete resection. More commonly, the pericardial fat dissection gets the surgeon out of the anterior recess, but most of the pericardium is found to be directly involved with the cancer. Rarely, the tumor will separate, leaving normal appearing pericardium. If that is not the case, an attempt can be made to separate the layers of the pericardium, leaving the serous pericardium intact and resecting the fibrous pericardium en bloc with the cancer and mediastinal pleura. While technically challenging, it is often possible. If the pericardium remains intact, it should be fenestrated after the PDT to avoid postoperative tamponade. If the pericardium is too extensively involved to achieve a macroscopic complete resection, the surgeon has two options: a small area can be resected and the surgeon may

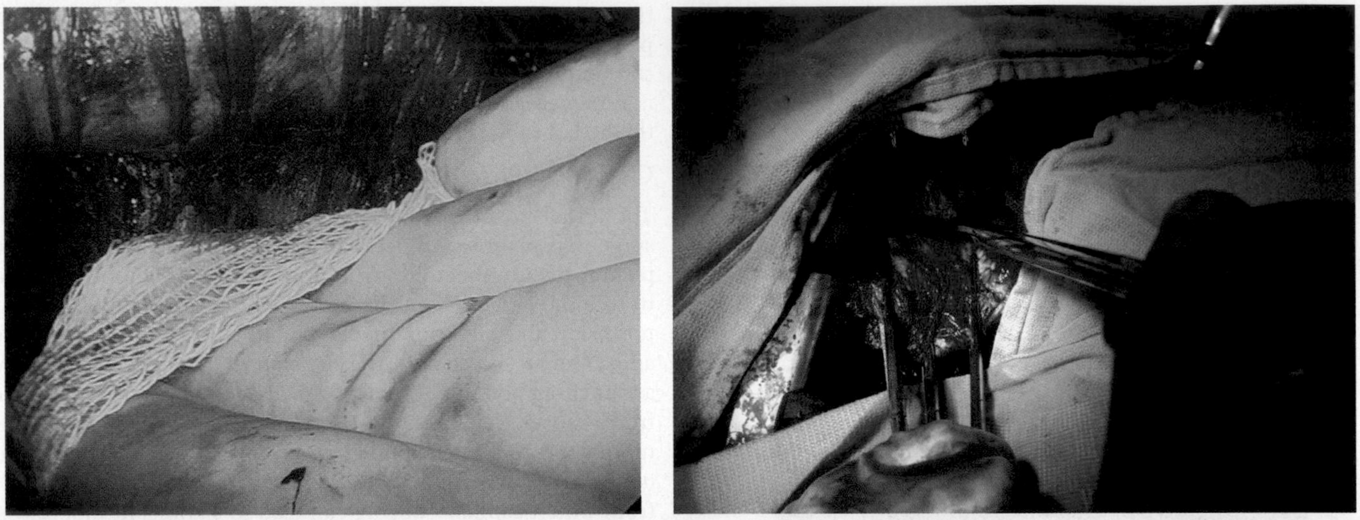

A B

Figure 124-3. *A.* Blunt dissection is performed, sweeping the diaphragm musculature off the tumor, which can be seen at the top portion of the field with residual muscle fibers attached. *B.* Sharp dissection is used to dissect the split thickness of the musculature when blunt dissection does not work. Note the clamps grasping the cast of the sulcus, described by the tumor, as the scissors are allowed to "find the soft plane" which is then sharply incised, harvesting invaded muscle with the tumor and leaving the remaining muscle on the peritoneum. (Reprinted with permission from Friedberg JS. The state of the art in the technical performance of lung-sparing operations for malignant pleural mesothelioma. *Semin Thorac Surg,* 2013; 25:125–143. Figures 2 and 3.)

wish to sew in a prosthetic pericardial patch if there is a concern about potential cardiac herniation, or, for an extensive area, the entire pericardium can be resected. As the lung is being left in place, the pericardium does not have to be reconstructed unless the surgeon is concerned that the patient will be at risk for cardiac torsion or herniation or if it is their preference. Regardless of approach, the goal remains to achieve a macroscopic complete resection. In either case, if there is an area of full thickness involvement of the pericardium that will require resection, that area is left on the pericardium until after the PDT is administered to avoid directly illuminating the heart. After concluding the PDT, the pericardium can be removed with the same options depending on the amount resected as discussed previously. If the surgeon wishes to place a patch, this is done in the same fashion, as with a formal extrapleural pneumonectomy, and it should be pie-crusted or fenestrated to avoid tamponade.

As the dissection is extended posteriorly, ultimately culminating at the anterior hilum of the lung, the phrenic nerve can be identified at the level of the superior mediastinal dissection and skeletonized as it traverses the anterior mediastinum. Whether or not preserving the nerve and the diaphragm without a pleura helps with respiratory function postoperatively is a current area of investigation. It is intuitively attractive and remains our current approach to preserve the phrenic nerve, which is usually possible, even when encased in bulk tumor (Fig. 124-4).

Diaphragm

The diaphragm dissection is started in the costophrenic recess, attempting to bluntly separate the pleura from the underlying bare musculature. Occasionally, rarely, the pleura will separate from the underlying bare musculature. Often, however, this requires sharp dissection and is best accomplished with broad-tipped scissors, allowing the scissors to "find" the plane between the hard cancer and the soft underlying normal tissue (see Fig. 124-3B).

Limited areas of full thickness invasion are resected, leaving only peritoneum, and the diaphragm can be reconstructed primarily with heavy absorbable sutures. Sometimes, especially if the inseparable tumor is a central island and there is sufficient laxity in the remaining debrided diaphragm, the area can be tented away from the abdomen and undercut with a thick tissue

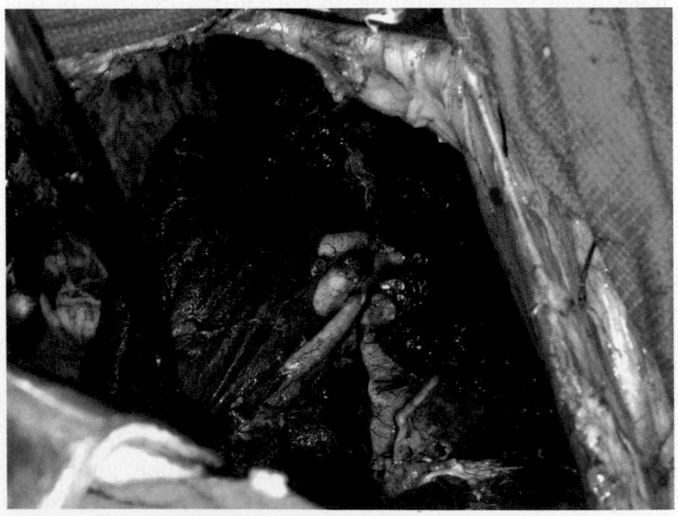

Figure 124-4. Appearance of the right chest after radical pleurectomy. The denuded lung parenchyma is visible with the skeletonized pulmonary artery, with an overlying anthracotic lymph node occupying the central portion of the image. In the lower right corner can be seen residual diaphragm musculature joining with the pericardium, on which can be seen some residual yellow pericardial fat overlying the insertion of the phrenic nerve into the diaphragm. The phrenic nerve then traverses the remaining visible portion of the pericardium. (Reprinted with permission from Friedberg JS. The state of the art in the technical performance of lung-sparing operations for malignant pleural mesothelioma. *Semin Thorac Surg,* 2013; 25:125–143. Figure 10D.)

stapler. Care must be taken to assure that no viscera are caught in the stapler. This is readily done by palpation. The staple line is then oversewn with heavy absorbable sutures as the diaphragmatic muscle, comprising the staple line, can tear and result in a hernia. If too much diaphragm is involved, it must be resected, as with an extrapleural pneumonectomy, and reconstructed with a 2-mm Gore-Tex (W.L. Gore Associates, Inc., Flagstaff, Arizona) patch.

Lung

At this point, in the dissection, the entire tumor is tethered solely to the lung. The anesthesiologist is asked to connect the operative lung to an alternate oxygen supply with an in-line stack of PEEP valves that will allow it to be held under positive pressure ranging from 10 to 30 cm water. The tumor is sharply incised, extending through the visceral pleura (Fig. 124-5A). The plane between the undersurface of the visceral pleura and bare lung parenchyma is developed. Initially, this is best accomplished with a forceps and fine scissors, until at least several millimeters beyond the incision has been liberated. At this point the edge can be better grasped and the bare lung parenchyma can be very gently retracted. The denuded lung is best retracted with a finger and coarse mesh gauze. A well-intentioned assistant can easily plunge a suction catheter into the parenchyma with only minimal pressure and thus should be cautioned, as the lung is devoid of pleura and is astoundingly delicate without the visceral pleura. If this occurs, it will result in air leaks that do not seal very readily. Over the years, the instrument that has proved best suited for further developing the plane is a broad Cobb dissector. Initially, there is often a torrential air leak when the visceral pleura is removed from the parenchyma but, literally, within minutes the leaks nearly abate if the plane has been maintained at the interface of the visceral pleura and parenchyma. In the setting of nodular, rather than planar, cancer the operator simply follows the contour of the tumor as it extends into the lung parenchyma. Often these divots will overlie areas of compressed parenchyma that re-expand when the cancer is separated. Sometimes a cancer will be encountered where

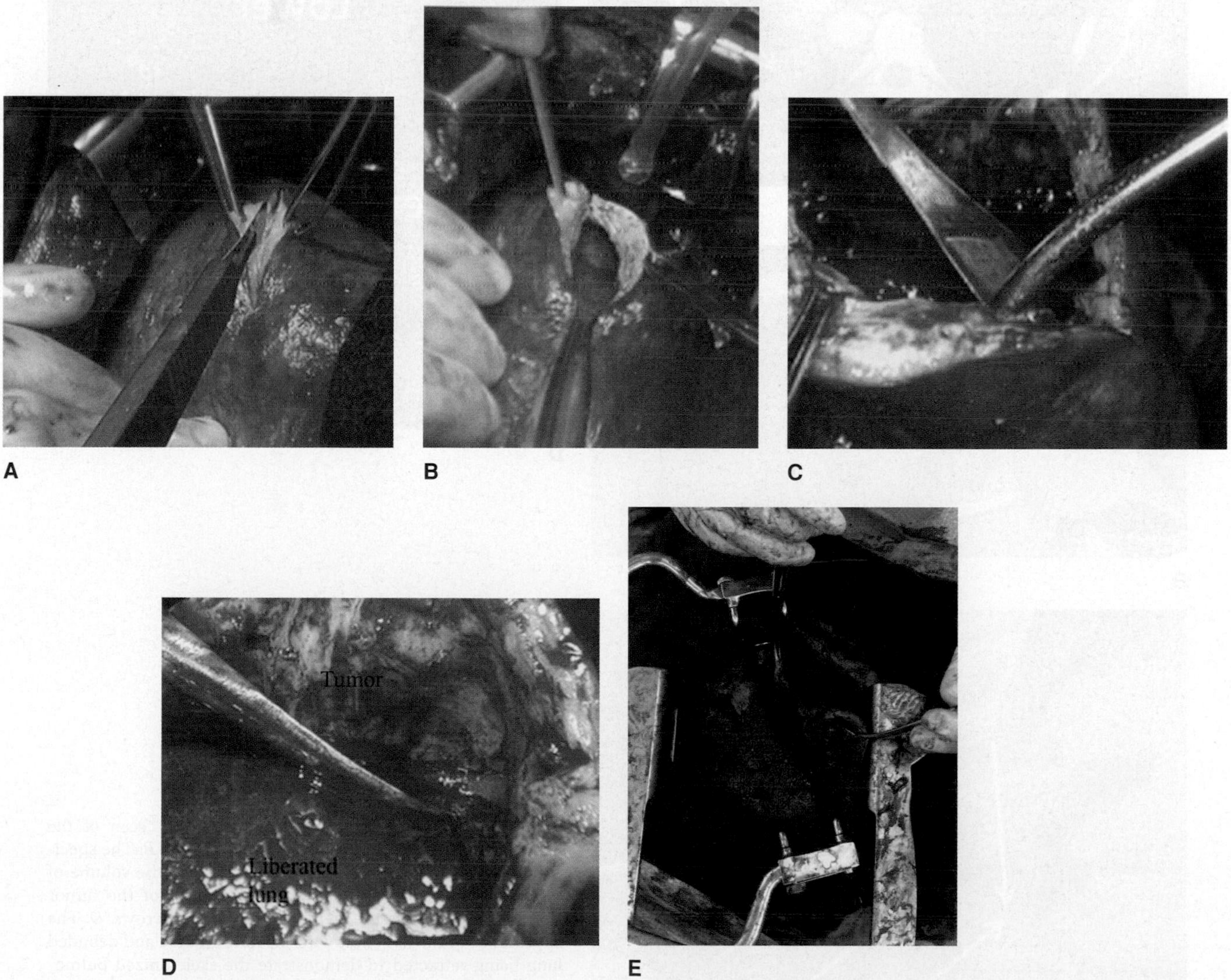

Figure 124-5. Shown here is the technique for separating the cancer from the lung. *A.* The cancer is incised. *B.* The plan is initiated with a Cobb dissector. *C.* The tumor edges are grasped and the plane is extended. *D.* Further separation of the raw parenchyma from the overlying, en bloc, cancer and visceral pleura. *E.* The tumor has been mobilized from either side and is now tethered to the pulmonary artery, from which it is sharply dissected free.

portions, or even the entire lung, will not yield the subpleural plane. In these cases, the electrocautery can be used to open the plane that is visibly evident, but does not yield to cold steel dissection. There are rare cases, often in the setting of mixed histology, when a significant portion of the dissection must be performed with cautery.

A critical element in the lung dissection, and what is often considered a contraindication to lung-sparing surgery, is the requirement to remove tumor from the fissures. This is safely accomplished by saving this part of the lung dissection for last. The cancer is tracked down into the fissure and followed from both sides. Surprisingly, the planes within the fissures are often better preserved and more readily separated than on the other surfaces of the lung. An even level along both sides is maintained as the base of the fissure is approached. At this point the lung is deflated and the surgeon will be able to palpate the deepest portion of the fissure, where the cancer has formed a cast. In any patient with complete fissures, this will typically terminate on the surface of the ongoing pulmonary artery. Under direct vision, the veil-like investing tissue over the artery is sharply divided, thereby releasing the cancer from the fissure. This will often result in skeletonization of the pulmonary artery within the fissure (Fig. 124-6).

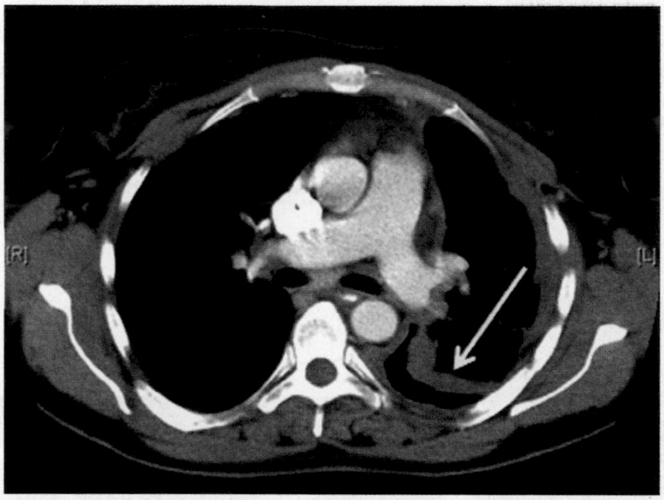

A

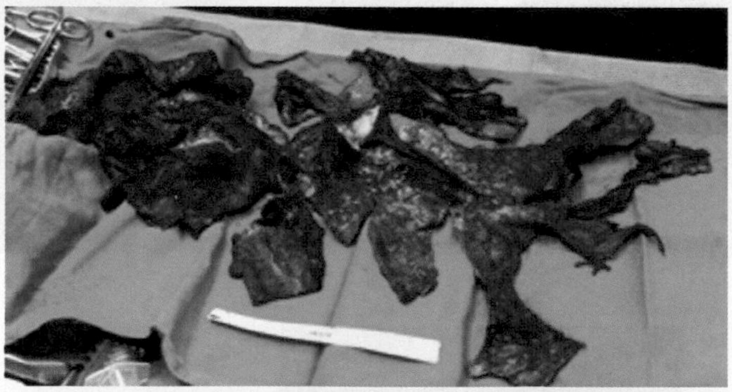

B

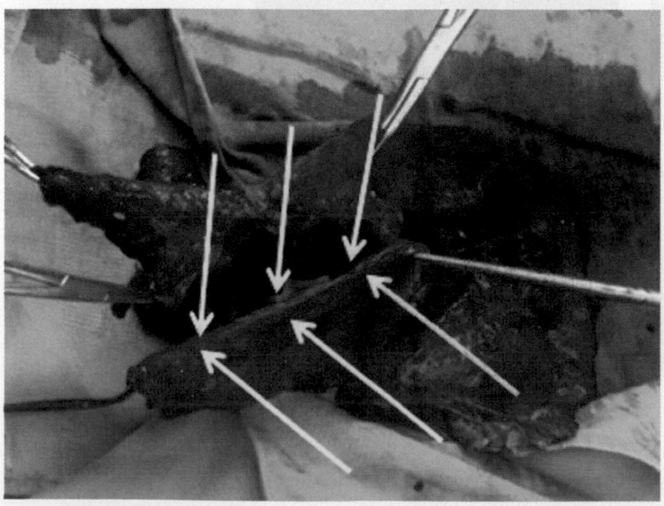

C

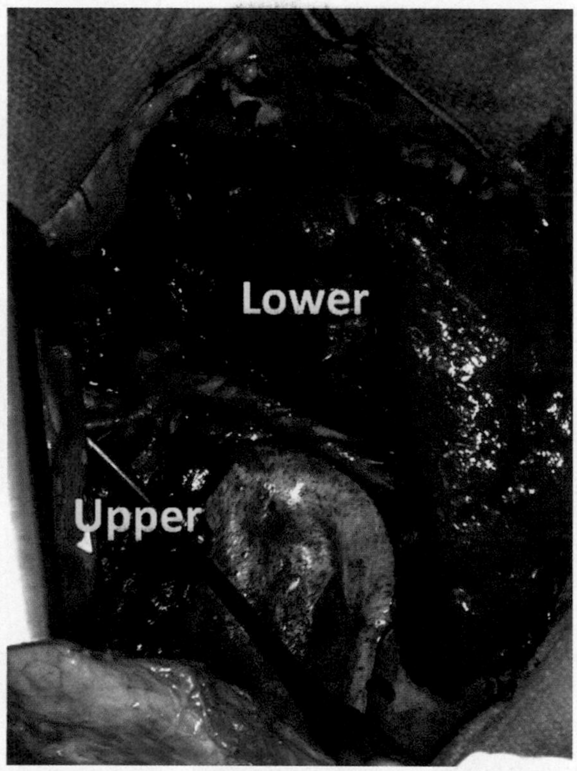

D

Figure 124-6. Left radical pleurectomy. *A.* CT scan of the patient, *arrow* demonstrates tumor in the fissure. *B.* The specimen. The ruler in the foreground is 15 cm and the volume of the tumor exceeded one liter. *C.* The portion of the tumor which invaded the fissure, demonstrated by the arrows. *D.* The appearance of the left chest with the now inflated and denuded lung being retracted to demonstrate the skeletonized pulmonary artery with the pericardium visible in the background. (Reprinted with permission from Friedberg JS. The state of the art in the technical performance of lung-sparing operations for malignant pleural mesothelioma. *Semin Thorac Surg*, 2013; 25:125-143. Figure 11.)

Once the tumor is released in the fissure, the similar investing band of extrapleural tissue can be identified and divided around the hilum, thereby dividing the remaining attachments of the cancer to the patient. In cases where the cancer is pliable, a single large specimen may result. Sometimes, however, the cancer may be so firm that in order to have enough room to work and still preserve the lung, the cancer is better removed piecemeal.

Once the specimen is removed, the chest cavity should be inspected to assure that a macroscopic complete resection has been achieved. Again, video thoracoscope is very useful to help inspect all surfaces and also provides magnification.

Lymphadenectomy

A thoracic lymphadenectomy is then performed dissecting all standard "numbered" nodal stations as well as any phrenic and/or internal mammary nodes. In addition, the author (JF) has been harvesting the posterior intercostal lymph nodes. The significance of these lymph nodes is not established and is an area of active investigation. For the purpose of our publications and analyses, given that these lymph nodes are not described in any current staging schema, we have considered them N1 lymph nodes as we have had multiple instances where these were the only positive lymph nodes. We do, however, have preliminary data suggesting these posterior intercostal nodes may correlate inversely with survival and therefore encourage others to collect these nodes such that their significance can be established. To access them, use electrocautery to incise the posterior interspaces at the level of the rib heads. Often the nodes can be bluntly delivered with a fingertip, like ejecting a pea from a pod, but sometimes it is necessary to reach into the interspace with a Singley forceps. Care must be taken during this maneuver to avoid avulsing the intercostal vessels with which they are associated.

With the lymphadenectomy completed, a final check is done to confirm hemostasis. At this point, preparations are made to start PDT.

Intraoperative PDT

PDT is a dose-dependent treatment. Without any light, the photosensitizer has no effect. With too much light, injury can occur. The key is to precisely measure the amount of light being delivered. By doing this, we are able to routinely deliver intraoperative hemithorax PDT without any direct PDT injuries. There are multiple complications related to the PDT effect, primarily from cytokine release, but we do not experience "burn" injuries that were encountered in the early experience of PDT or are still occasionally witnessed with Phase I dose escalation studies with new photosensitizers. Because the photosensitizer will absorb photons that are directly incident, refracted or reflected, in a complex and moving geographic space like the chest cavity it is impossible to estimate or calculate the light dosage based on time, distance, and power output of the laser. It is by necessity that the amount of delivered light is measured in real time. This is accomplished with light detectors and a dosimetry system.

The first step is to sew in the light detectors. These are isotropic detectors comprised of a small titanium sphere attached to a thin glass fiber (Fig. 124-7A). These detectors are fed into a length of saline-filled sterile intravenous tubing, which is then folded over on the tip and tied with a silk suture. This provides a ready loop for sewing the tubing into the chest cavity (Fig. 124-7B). Typically seven detectors are placed at strategic locations within the hemithorax: anterior and posterior diaphragmatic sulci, apex, anterior and posterior chest wall, pericardium, and posterior mediastinum. These detectors are brought out from the chest cavity (Fig. 124-7C) and connected to the dosimetry system (Fig. 124-7D). This system is composed of the processing box which collects the data and subsequently feeds that information into a laptop computer where the screen gives a real-time read out of both the current fluence rate being seen by each detector and the total cumulative dose measured at each detector (Fig. 124-7E).

Light delivery is accomplished by using an optical fiber, with the tip terminating in a modified endotracheal tube. The tube and the balloon are filled with dilute (10%) intralipid. This accomplishes several objectives. First, it allows the fragile fiber to be easily maneuvered about the chest cavity. Second, it protects the tissues from the actual fiber tip, which is very hot even though it is just visible light that is being delivered. Third, the balloon, in which the tip is centered, helps disperse the light 360 degrees. Once the light detectors are in place and have been tested, PDT can commence. The procedure is quite simple.

Light of the appropriate visible wavelength (porfimer sodium, for instance, absorbs red light at 630 nm) is shined into the chest cavity. Dilute (0.1%) warm intralipid is poured into the chest cavity. This also accomplishes several objectives. First, the fat globules in the intralipid act to reflect the light, which helps to deliver it into all recesses. Second, the intralipid prevents any pooling of blood, which would absorb the light and hence shield the underlying tissue. Third, the intralipid floats the collapsed lung, making it easier to move the tip of the light detector around all surfaces, especially into the fissures of the lung and the hilar regions. The intralipid is constantly turned over during the light delivery, as it becomes blood tinged. Blood absorbs the light and decreases the efficiency of the light delivery. The light is then simply moved around the chest cavity until each of the detectors has recorded the desired dose of light (Fig. 124-7E). A pitfall is not attempting to get all the detectors to register similar dosimetry values at all times. The amount of time required for light delivery depends on the photosensitizer, but is typically an hour or less for an average-sized patient (Fig. 124-8).

Once the PDT is completed, gowns, gloves, and the shielding towels are replaced using a "clean-contaminated" type strategy. Used instruments are not replaced, but are soaked or wiped down with sterile water during the PDT. If a macroscopic complete resection was achieved prior to the PDT, then closure can commence. If a portion of full thickness tumor was left on the diaphragm or pericardium, to avoid directly illuminating the heart or abdominal viscera, it is resected at this point. If the defect in the diaphragm is sufficiently large, a patch can be placed. Most often, however, there is enough laxity in the diaphragm to permit primary closure. If the pericardium was completely debrided, without disruption, it is fenestrated to avoid potential tamponade. If any part of the pericardium requires resection, the tenets and options discussed earlier are followed. Finally, if no chyle leak was detected during the course of the operation, as indicated by the administered cream/methylene blue, then no action need be taken with the thoracic duct. If on the right side the surgeon is concerned about duct disruption, despite the lack of chyle in the field, then the duct can be presumptively ligated at its emergence through the aortic hiatus.

Straight chest tubes are placed anteriorly and posteriorly to the apex. Additional holes should be cut to access air and

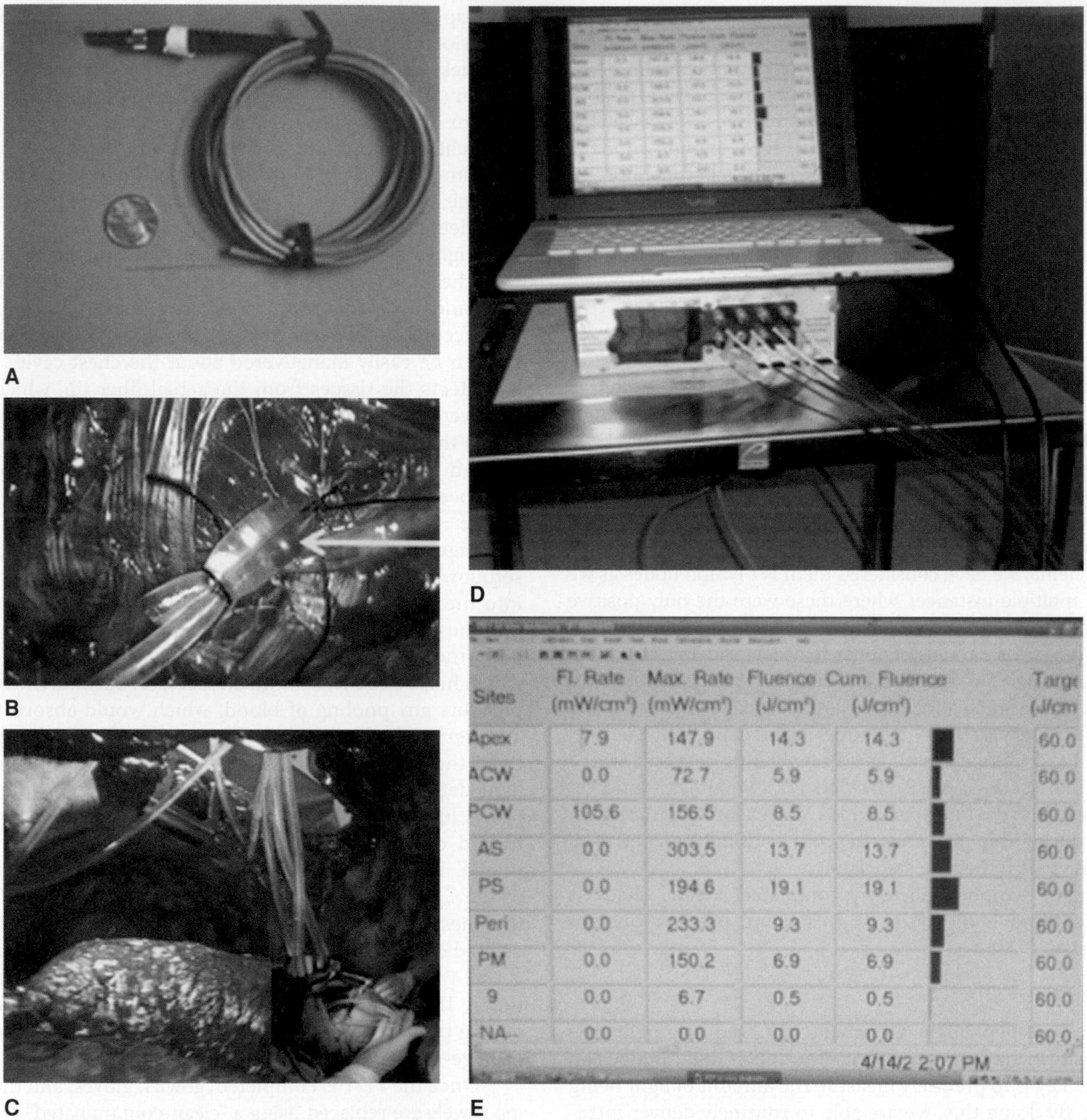

Figure 124-7. *A.* This panel shows the light fiber within its protective sheath. The actual fiber approaches the penny, for size reference. *B.* This panel shows the fiber within the sterile intravenous tubing, sewn to the chest wall. The arrow indicates the light collecting titanium oxide sphere at the tip of the fiber. *C.* This panel shows the light detectors emerging from the chest as viewed from inside. The inset shows the fibers emerging from outside. *D.* This panel shows the fibers connected to the processing box, upon which sits the laptop. *E.* This panel shows a close-up of the laptop screen during PDT, showing both fluence rate and total dose of light.

fluid throughout the entire intrathoracic traverse of the tubes. A rongeur is helpful for making extra holes in the chest tubes, taking care not to cut more than a quarter the diameter of the tube to avoid kinking, and making sure the most proximal hole is cut through the radiopaque marker to assure all holes are intrathoracic. A right angle tube or flexible fluted tube is also placed along the diaphragm, terminating in the posterior costophrenic recess.

Depending upon standard criteria, as well as the surgeon's sense of the need for positive pressure to maintain full lung expansion, the patient can either be extubated or remain on pressure mode ventilation at the end of the operation. There are usually a lot of bloody secretions at the conclusion of these procedures, so the patient should undergo a complete toilet bronchoscopy at the conclusion of the operation and, again prior to extubation if the patient remains intubated. If the patient is extubated, suction should be placed at −20 cm on each chest tube, and even increased if the lung is not fully inflated on the postoperative chest x-ray. There is a premium on achieving full lung expansion and the higher suction to achieve full lung expansion can, counterintuitively, help the air leaks seal more quickly. If the patient is left intubated, usually −10 cm of suction is adequate and can be increased when the patient is extubated. Because of the air leaks, volume calculations on the ventilator are unreliable and the ventilator needs to be adjusted empirically, based upon blood gasses. Typically, patients are hypocarbic, likely

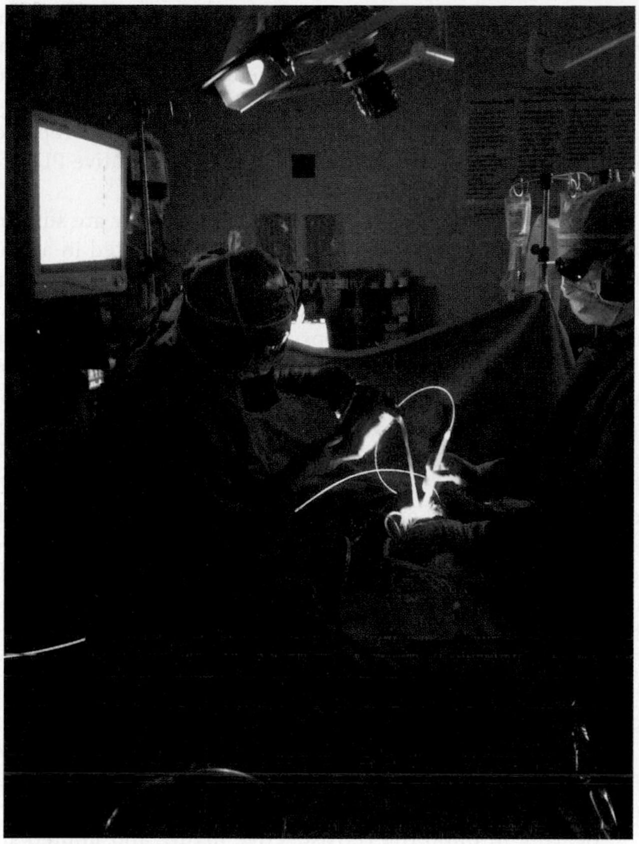

Figure 124-8. Photodynamic therapy being performed. The operator, on the right, is performing the photodynamic therapy by moving the light source, a modified endotracheal tube, around the chest cavity. The assistant, on the left, is pouring in dilute intralipid to serve as a light-dispersing medium.

because of the air leaks. Having all three chest tubes connected to separate collection devices will allow the surgeon to assess leaks and drainage in a more useful manner. If the tubes are still leaking after 2 days, the suction can be decreased as long as the lung remains fully inflated on chest radiograph. Once on water seal, the leaks tend to stop quickly. Tubes are then removed per routine criteria. Despite the enormity of the initial leaks, persistent air leaks occur less than 10% of the time, and we have sent patients home with Heimlich valves, but have never had to reoperate to address a persistent leak.

Attention to nutrition and pulmonary toilet are the critical issues postoperatively. Because most patients will have a compromised diaphragm, even the most motivated patients may have trouble clearing secretions and may require one or several awake bronchoscopies.

Light precautions, depending upon the photosensitizer, must be continued. Perhaps the single most critical postoperative PDT-related consideration is that extreme caution must be taken surrounding the esophagus. PDT causes the esophagus to become very fragile, but it can recover fully and without incident if there is no manipulation. Early in our experience, we had two esophageal perforations that resulted in mortalities. The first was simply from the replacement of a nasogastric tube. The second was from an upper endoscopy performed for upper GI bleeding. Consequently, for the first 6 weeks we are extremely cautious and try to avoid any esophageal manipulation, even replacing a nasogastric tube. With this policy, we have had no additional esophageal complications. Additional postoperative considerations surrounding the addition of PDT to this already sizable operation are primarily related to the inflammatory response and additional metabolic demand. Hence, even patients with normal preoperative albumen will typically drop to half normal levels making the attention to nutrition, starting with immediate postoperative total parenteral nutrition, critical. There is also a large fluid requirement over the first several days and chest tube outputs can be expected to be very high. Our routine is to ideally use colloid for these several days. Patients will also develop some degree of capillary leak syndrome and may become edematous. Concurrent with this fluid shift is a typical pattern of the operative lung being initially clear and subsequently "whiting out" over the first two to three days. This can occasionally involve the contralateral lung. Once the fluid demand begins to abate, diuresis is started.

CLINICAL STUDIES

We have used intraoperative PDT for numerous pleural cancers, both primary and metastatic. Anecdotally, we have seen some excellent results for metastatic breast and ovarian cancer, good results for thymic cancers, and generally poor results for primary or metastatic sarcomas. Our best quantified experience has been with NSCLC with pleural dissemination and mesothelioma.

NSCLC with pleural dissemination, stage IV (M1a), is a difficult clinical problem. We conducted a Phase II trial, when this disease was considered stage IIIB (AJCC 6th ed.). At that time there were no targeted chemotherapeutic agents and the median survival for this form of NSCLC was 6 to 9 months. According to our protocol, patients were treated with preoperative chemotherapy to "best effect" and then restaged. The oncologic eligibility criterion was disease confined to one hemithorax. N3 disease was an exclusionary, but N2 was not. In fact, 90% of the patients in the study had N2 disease. The operation the patients underwent was the appropriate anatomic resection for their primary lesion, which ranged from segmentectomy to pneumonectomy, and a parietal pleurectomy to achieve a macroscopic complete resection. Each patient then underwent PDT as described above with 2 mg/kg porfimer sodium administered 24 hours preoperatively to a measured dose of 30 J/cm^2 (using flat photodiodes which we subsequently correlated sided by side with the current isotropic detectors, which measured almost exactly double the amount of light, 60 J/cm^2). Of the 22 patients enrolled, a macroscopic complete resection and PDT was accomplished in 17, 3 underwent incomplete resection and PDT, and 2 were unresectable. Local control at 6 months, the study objective was 73.3% in the 15 assessable patients. Median overall survival on an intention to treat analysis was 21.7 months. These survivals were calculated from the time of photosensitizer administration, that is, the day before surgery. The results were not calculated from the time of diagnosis or first treatment with chemotherapy (Table 124-1 and Fig. 124-9).[23]

Overall, the results of this study were considered encouraging. Shortly after publication of this article ensued the era of targeted therapies. These therapies have demonstrated significant improvements in survival over previous treatment and hence, referral of patients abated. Subsequently, we have

Table 124-1

THE PATIENT CHARACTERISTICS AND TREATMENTS THEY UNDERWENT FOR NSCLC WITH PLEURAL DISSEMINATION AS PART OF A PHASE II STUDY COMBINING SURGERY AND INTRAOPERATIVE PHOTODYNAMIC THERAPY

PATIENT CHARACTERISTICS ($n = 22$)		
CHARACTERISTIC	NUMBER OF PATIENTS	%
Sex		
Male	9	41
Female	13	59
ECOG status		
0	1	4
1	21	96
Cell type		
Adenocarcinoma	20	92
NSCLC, not specified	1	4
NSCLC, neuroendocrine	1	4
Clinical stage		
T4N0	7	32
T4N1	1	4
T4N2	13	59
Recurrent disease	1	4
Pathologic stage		
T4N0	2	9
T4N2	18	82
No resection	2	9
Minimal pleural disease	1	4
Surgical procedures		
Lobectomy	1	4
Lobectomy or segmentectomy	1	4
Segmentectomy	1	4
Bilobectomy	2	9
Extrapleural pneumonectomy	12	55
Wedge resection	2	9
Pleurectomy alone	1	4
Unresectable	2	9
Preoperative therapy		
Chemotherapy	19	85
Chemoradiotherapy	1	4
None	2	9
Postoperative radiation		
Mediastinal radiation	8	37
Chemoradiation	5	23
Age, years		
Mean	54	
SD	11	
Range	35–72	

NSCLC, non–small cell lung cancer; SD, standard deviation; ECOG, Eastern Cooperative Oncology Group.

Source: Reprinted with permission from Friedberg JS, Mick R, Stevenson JP, et al. Phase II trial of pleural photodynamic therapy and surgery for patients with non-small-cell lung cancer with pleural spread. *J Clin Oncol*, 22(11):2192–2201.

started to see patients who initially had excellent and durable responses to targeted therapies but have recurred or progressed. We have now operated on several of these patients and, anecdotally, are seeing benefit. Obviously, employing surgery for NSCLC remains investigational and should only be considered for highly selected patients under the auspices of a multidisciplinary tumor board in an Institutional Review Board approved protocol.

Malignant pleural mesothelioma remains the disease with which we have the greatest experience. We published a pilot study[22] comparing the results of patients who underwent intraoperative PDT and either extrapleural pneumonectomy or radical pleurectomy. In our hands the radical pleurectomy patients had a significantly longer overall survival, despite little difference in disease-free survival. For that reason we switched exclusively to lung-sparing surgery. Subsequently, we reported our results for lung-sparing surgery and intraoperative PDT for 38 patients with malignant pleural mesothelioma.[24]

The demographics and outcomes of this study are summarized in Table 124-2. A radical pleurectomy resulted in a macroscopic complete resection in 37 of the 38 patients. The one patient in whom a macroscopic complete resection could not be obtained, preoperative biopsy indicated epithelial subtype and a final pathology revealed a large desmoplastic component. Approximately, 20% of the patients had nonepithelial subtypes and 97% had stage III or IV cancer. There was a single postoperative mortality, a stroke. At a median follow-up of 34.4 months, the median survival was 31.7 months for all 38 patients, 41.2 months for the 31/38 epithelial patients, and 6.8 months for the nonepithelial patients. The median overall and progression-free survival for the 20/31 epithelial patients with N2 disease was 31.7 months and 15.1 months, respectively. The median survival for the epithelial patients with N1 or N0 disease was 57.1 months. The median progression-free survival was 9.6 months for all patients, 15.1 months for the epithelial patients, and 4.8 months for the nonepithelial patients. These results are illustrated in Fig. 124-10A–D. All of these survival statistics were calculated from the time of surgery, not the time of diagnosis or time of first treatment.

Bearing in mind the retrospective nature and limited size of this study, these results are very encouraging. Perhaps the most interesting observation was that the disease-free survival was not particularly long but the overall survival, especially for the epithelial subtype patients, was unusually long. This is notable within the context that 97% of these patients had stage III or IV disease and survival calculations were made from the time of surgery, not diagnosis or first treatment, which would have added months to their survival if that were the chosen beginning point. The reason for prolonged survival after recurrence is under investigation. One hypothesis is simply that having two lungs left the patients with more reserve to tolerate adjuvant treatments after recurrence. This is likely a contributing factor, though the survival results in this study were beyond other reported radical pleurectomy series. Given that fact, it suggests that the PDT may have played a role, as that is the distinguishing feature of this radical pleurectomy series. It is known that PDT can induce a tumor-specific immune reaction. Understanding that microscopic disease is left behind after any pleural surgery, and almost certainly more so with radical pleurectomy than extrapleural pneumonectomy, the possibility exists that the residual PDT-treated cells could induce an autologous tumor vaccine effect. This hypothesis is the focus of intense laboratory and clinical investigation at this time.

CONCLUSION

PDT is a unique and interesting cancer treatment. While it acts by a number of mechanisms (direct cell kill, selective destruction of neovasculature, nonspecific and specific immune effects), it can still be combined with essentially any other combination of cancer therapies. Herein, we have detailed the application of

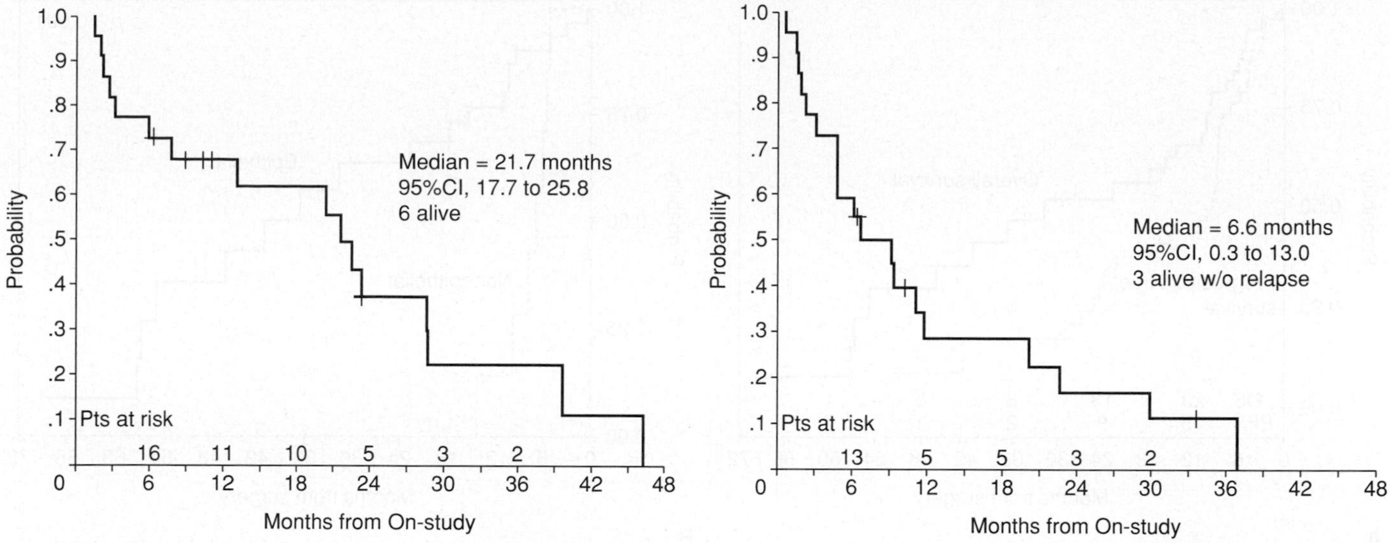

Figure 124-9. Overall (*A*) and progression-free (*B*) survival for all patients ($n = 22$) with NSCLC with pleural dissemination enrolled in a Phase II study combining surgery and intraoperative photodynamic therapy. (Reprinted with permission from Friedberg JS, Mick R, Stevenson JP, et al. Phase II trial of pleural photodynamic therapy and surgery for patients with non-small-cell lung cancer with pleural spread. *J Clin Oncol*, 22(11):2192–2201.)

Table 124-2

DEMOGRAPHICS AND RESULTS SUMMARY FOR 38 PATIENTS WITH MALIGNANT PLEURAL MESOTHELIOMA UNDERGOING RADICAL PLEURECTOMY AND INTRAOPERATIVE PHOTODYNAMIC THERAPY

PATIENT DEMOGRAPHICS AND SURVIVAL OUTCOMES							
		SURVIVAL			PROGRESSION-FREE SURVIVAL		
VARIABLE	*n*	2-YEAR RATE ± SE (%)	MEDIAN (MONTHS)	LOG RANK *P*-VALUE	2-YEAR RATE ± SE (%)	MEDIAN (MONTHS)	LOG-RANK *P*-VALUE
All patients	38	52% ± 9	31.7	...	31 ± 8	9.6	...
Sex							
Male	28	41% ± 10	17.8	0.07	18 ± 8	8.8	0.02
Female	10	79% ± 13	54.7		53 ± 18	28.4	
Age (year)							
>65	18	53% +13	54.7	0.99	27 ± 12	9.0	0 31
±65	20	54% ± 11	31.7		34 ± 11	10.3	
Cell type							
Epithelial	31	64% ± 9%	41.2	<0.001	38 ± 9	15.1	<0.001
Nonepithelial	7	0%	6.8		0%	4.8	
N stage							
N0	9	67% ± 16	57.1	0.10	56 ± 17	26.9	0.21
N+ (4 N1; 24 N2)	28	49% ± 10	22.7		24 ± 9	9.6	
Unknown	1						
AJCC stage							
1	1						
3	28	50% +10	22.7	0.83	30 ± 9	9.2	0.95
4	9	52% ± 18	36.6	3 vs. 4	26 ± 16	10.3	3 vs. 4
Chemotherapy							
None	3	67% ± 27	42.5	...[a]	67 ± 27	Undefined	...[a]
Preoperative	4	0%	2.5		0	5.0	
Postoperative	25	33% ± 10%	9.6		58 ± 10	31.7	
Preoperative and postoperative	6	17% ± 15	10.3		44 ± 22	22.7	
N2 disease only							
Cell type							
Epithelial	20	55 ± 12	31.7	0.001	27 ± 11	15.1	<0.001
Nonepithelial	4	0	6.8		0	4.7	

AJCC, American Joint Committee on Cancer.

[a]No comparison, patients were not randomized to treatment.

Source: Reprinted with permission from Friedberg JS, Culligan M, Mick R, et al. Radical pleurectomy and intraoperative photodynamic therapy for malignant pleural mesothelioma. *Ann Thorac Surg*, 93(5):1658–1667.

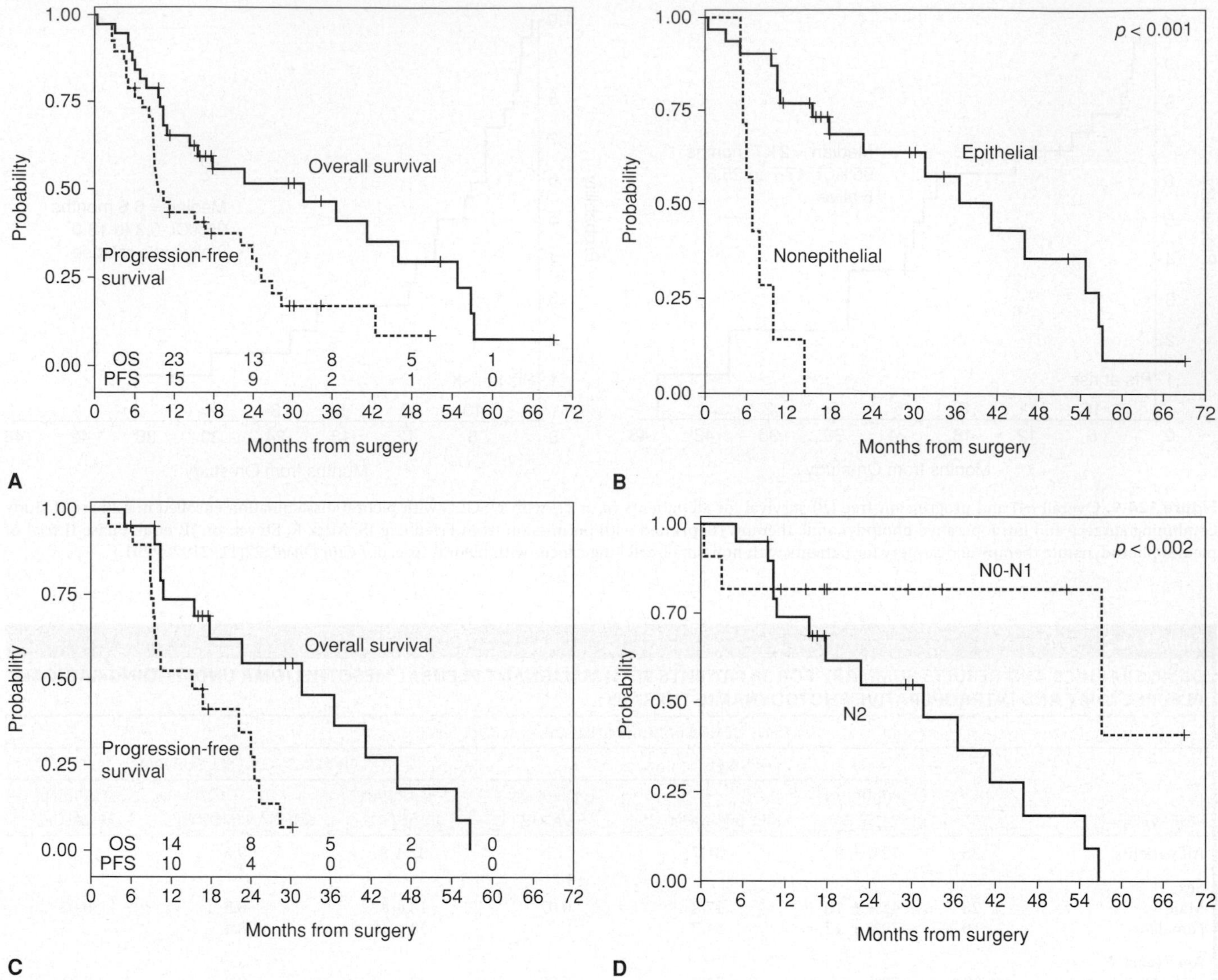

Figure 124-10. *A.* Overall and progression-free survival for 38 patients with malignant pleural mesothelioma undergoing radical pleurectomy and intraoperative photodynamic therapy. *B.* Overall survival for 38 patients with malignant pleural mesothelioma undergoing radical pleurectomy and intraoperative photodynamic therapy, as a function of cellular subtype. *C.* Overall and progression-free survival for 20 patients with malignant pleural mesothelioma undergoing radical pleurectomy and intraoperative photodynamic therapy, who had epithelial subtype and positive N2 disease. *D.* Overall survival for 31 patients with epithelial malignant pleural mesothelioma undergoing radical pleurectomy and intraoperative photodynamic therapy as broken down by the presence or absence of N2 disease. (Reprinted with permission from Friedberg JS, Culligan M, Mick R, et al. Radical pleurectomy and intraoperative photodynamic therapy for malignant pleural mesothelioma. *Ann Thorac Surg,* 93(5):1658–1667.)

combining PDT with surgery for the treatment of pleural cancers. With proper dosimetry, PDT can be performed safely and in a straightforward and easy manner. The fact that PDT effect penetrates several millimeters below the surface is a feature of the treatment that emboldened our group to become increasingly aggressive with saving the lung, to the point where radical pleurectomy is currently our exclusive surgical approach for malignant pleural mesothelioma. With other cancers involving the pleura, such as NSCLC with pleural dissemination, we have shown that PDT can be safely combined with lung resection as well, ranging from segmentectomy to pneumonectomy. The results of using PDT for pleural cancers, especially mesothelioma, are encouraging. The possibility that a PDT-induced tumor-specific immune effect is contributing to the results we have observed is the focus of ongoing investigations and raises the tantalizing prospect of combining immunotherapies with the current approach to amplify this effect.

EDITOR'S COMMENT

Surgical debulking of malignant mesothelioma can be accomplished with extrapleural pneumonectomy or radical pleurectomy. The frequent local recurrence within the same hemithorax, however, suggests that microscopic disease remains after these surgical procedures. Furthermore, the pattern of local recurrence preceding systemic recurrence suggests that any adjuvant therapy that kills the remaining microscopic cells is potentially curative. PDT is an innovative way to destroy cells several centimeters beyond the extrapleural plane of dissection. The authors clearly describe the details of this technique including many of the unforeseen pitfalls for the novice. They have worked out the details of light dosimetry and uniform light delivery. An open hemithorax after pleural resection lends itself particularly well to this technique. I share the authors hope that effective adjuvant therapy would preclude the need to remove the lung and diaphragm, thus providing a better quality of life and potential cure.

—Michael T. Jaklitsch

References

1. Sugarbaker D. Multimodality management of malignant pleural mesothelioma: introduction. *Semin Thorac Cardiovasc Surg.* 2009;21(2):95–96.
2. Friedberg JS, Mick R, Stevenson J, et al. A phase I study of foscan-mediated photodynamic therapy and surgery in patients with mesothelioma. *Ann Thorac Surg.* 2003;75:952–959.
3. Berenbaum MC, Akande SL, Bonnett R, et al. Mesotetra(hydroxyphenyl) porphyrins, a new class of potent tumour photosensitizer with favourable selectivity. *Br J Cancer.* 1986;54:717–725.
4. Young SW, Woodburn KW, Wright M, et al. Lutetium texaphyrin (PCI-0123): a near-infrared, water-soluble photosensitizer. *Photochem Photobiol.* 1996;63:892–897.
5. Godar DE. Light and death: photons and apoptosis. *J Investig Dermatol Symp Proc.* 1999;4(1):17–23.
6. Oleinick NL, Evans HH. The photobiology of photodynamic therapy: cellular targets and mechanisms. *Radiat Res.* 1998;150:146S–156S.
7. Fingar VH. Vascular effects of photodynamic therapy. *J Clin Laser Med Surg.* 1996;14:323–328.
8. Korbelik M. Induction of tumor immunity by photodynamic therapy. *J Clin Laser Med Surg.* 1996;14:329–334.
9. Gollnick SO, Vaughan L, Henderson BW. Generation of effective antitumor vaccines using photodynamic therapy. *Cancer Res.* 2002;62(6):1604–1608.
10. Pass HI, Delaney T, Tochner Z, et al. Intrapleural photodynamic therapy: results of a phase I trial. *Ann Surg Oncol.* 1994;1:28–37.
11. Takita H, Mang TS, Loewen GM, et al. Operation and intracavitary photodynamic therapy for malignant mesothelioma: a phase II study. *Ann Thorac Surg.* 1994;58:995–998.
12. Pinnacle Biologics, Inc. Prescribing information. 2011. Available at http://www.photofrin.com/wp-content/uploads/2013/02/prescribing-info.pdf. Accessed August 1, 2013.
13. Biolitec Pharma Ltd. Summary of products characteristics. 2005. Available at: http://www.biolitecpharma.com/public/smpc.asp?s=foscan. Accessed August 1, 2013.
14. Moskal TL, Dougherty TJ, Urschel JD, et al. Operation and photodynamic therapy for pleural mesothelioma: 6-year follow-up. *Ann Thorac Surg.* 1998;66:1128–1133.
15. Murrer H, Mariginissen HP, Star WM. Ex vivo light dosimetry and Monte Carlo simulations for endobronchial photodynamic therapy. *Phys Med Biol.* 1995;40(11):1807–1817.
16. Friedberg JS, Mick R, Stevenson JP, et al. Phase II trial of pleural photodynamic therapy and surgery for patients with non-small-cell lung cancer with pleural spread. *J Clin Oncol.* 2004;22:2192–2201.
17. Vulcan TG, Zhu TC, Rodriguez CE, et al. Comparison between isotropic and nonisotropic dosimetry systems during intraperitoneal photodynamic therapy. *Lasers Surg Med.* 2000;26:292–301.
18. Schouwink H, Rutgers ET, van der Sijp J, et al. Intraoperative photodynamic therapy after pleuropneumonectomy in patients with malignant pleural mesothelioma: dose finding and toxicity results. *Chest.* 2001;120:1167–1174.
19. Baas P, Murrer L, Zoetmulder FA, et al. Photodynamic therapy as adjuvant in surgically treated pleural malignancies. *Br J Cancer.* 1997;76:819–826.
20. Pass HI, Temecj BK, Kranda K, et al. Phase III randomized trial of surgery with or without intraoperative photodynamic therapy, and postoperative immunochemotherapy for malignant pleural mesothelioma. *Ann Surg Oncol.* 1997;4:628–633.
21. Ris HB, Altermatt HJ, Inderbitzi R, et al. Photodynamic therapy with chlorins for diffuse malignant mesothelioma: initial clinical results. *Br J Cancer.* 1991;64:1116–1120.
22. Ris HB, Altermatt HJ, Nachbur B, et al. Intraoperative photodynamic therapy with mTHPC for chest malignancies. *Lasers Surg Med.* 1996;18:39–45.
23. Friedberg JS, Mick R, Culligan M, et al. Photodynamic therapy (PDT) and the evolution of a lung sparing surgical treatment for mesothelioma. *Ann Thorac Surg.* 2011;91(6):1738–1745.
24. Friedberg JS, Culligan M, Mick R, et al. Radical pleurectomy and intraoperative photodynamic therapy for malignant pleural mesothelioma. *Ann Thorac Surg.* 2012;93:1658–1667.

125 Induction Chemotherapy Followed by Surgery for Malignant Pleural Mesothelioma

Walter Weder and Isabelle Opitz

Keywords: Neoadjuvant chemotherapy, induction chemotherapy, multimodality management

Malignant pleural mesothelioma (MPM) is a rare cancer commonly associated with asbestos exposure.[1] Recently, it was determined that germline mutations in BRCA1-associated protein-1 (BAP1) may predispose to mesothelioma development in nonasbestos-exposed patients.[2] Although basic biologic knowledge about MPM has increased during the past decade, and many new potentially active agents have reached various stages of development, the number of novel treatments that have been approved for MPM patients is limited.

The increasing experience of phase II trials assessing the efficacy of surgery-based multimodal treatment of MPM has reached the point where consistent overall survival data ranging between a median survival of 14 and 25.5 months is demonstrated for extrapleural pneumonectomy (EPP).[3] To date, combined multimodality treatment is the most commonly used treatment for MPM in many centers. One particular approach involves sequencing the surgery to follow induction chemotherapy—a concept that has been adapted from stage III NSCLC with the idea of downstaging the tumor or eradicating the outer tumor layer for better resectability.[4] Further justification for sequencing chemotherapy before surgery is the expectation that the chemotherapy regimen will be better tolerated prior to surgery, and the full required dose will be applied.

GENERAL PRINCIPLES (TECHNICAL, CLINICAL, ONCOLOGIC) THAT SUPPORT THIS APPROACH (EASE AND EFFICIENCY OF CARE)

Recent reviews[5,6] confirm that combined treatment with the antifolate, pemetrexed, and cisplatin achieve best overall survival and quality of life for patients. Therefore, cisplatin plus an antifolate is currently the most frequently used regimen for first line chemotherapy in a neo- or adjuvant setting. The use of induction chemotherapy is supported not only in a response rate of 30% to 40%, but also in convincing resectability rates (up to 74%) for EPP after induction chemotherapy reported in prospective trials.[4,7] Unfortunately, clinical assessment of the chemotherapy treatment response is difficult, and the only available tool for measuring this response is the modified RECIST criteria[8] which are lacking in reliable reproducibility.[9] Therefore, although the exact value of induction chemotherapy may be difficult to assess, the reported outcome after induction chemotherapy followed by EPP described in the following paragraph (MST ranging from 14 to 25.5 months) supports this approach and is definitely not inferior to other multimodal concepts, such as adjuvant chemotherapy after surgery (MST ranging from 13 to 24 months.[3] The fact that MPM does not respond very well to chemotherapy in comparison with other malignancies has been confirmed in all neoadjuvant treatment studies. Nevertheless, there are reports of chemotherapy-induced complete pathological responses in the literature.[10] However, in our experience of 128 EPP after neoadjuvant chemotherapy with cisplatin/gemcitabine or cisplatin/pemetrexed, we have observed only one complete response to date. The strongest argument for induction versus adjuvant chemotherapy is that chemotherapy is often difficult to administer in the postsurgery period after EPP or P/D, and the necessity of dose reduction is not unusual. Not surprisingly, the physical ability to tolerate chemotherapy as well as compliance and motivation of the patient is much better before major surgery.

Regarding the surgical technique for MPM resection, for the time being, there remains no evidence-based answer as to which procedure – P/D or EPP – is the more appropriate technique for achieving long-term survivors. Most studies have studied one or the other technique, and when studied together, P/D was chosen for earlier stages and EPP for more advanced stages, a decision which is often made only in the operating theatre as a consequence of unreliable clinical staging. A large retrospective multicenter study of 663 patients combining the experience of three large centers in the United States, analyzed the outcome after EPP or P/D in MPM patients treated between 1990 and 2006.[11] The authors concluded that the study emphasized the similarities in outcome after EPP or P/D for MPM in a multicenter setting, and they were unable to recommend one surgical approach over the other. In general, patients selected for EPP had locally more advanced disease and P/D was applied in earlier stages. The local recurrence rate was higher for P/D.

The one situation where P/D is clearly advised is for patients with compromised cardiac or pulmonary function, or with certain comorbidities, who are unable to tolerate EPP without excessive risk. If all gross tumor cannot be removed macroscopically especially in stage IV patients, a parenchyma-sparing procedure in the sense of debulking P/D might be recommended.[12] Besides these quite unambiguous situations, the decision to perform P/D or EPP in stage I, II, and III should be individually tailored by combining patients' performance status, personal wish, and the resectability of the tumor load. Furthermore, adjuvant radiotherapy cannot be applied safely after P/D, because radiation of the intact lungs, results most likely in high rates of pneumonitis, even if modern techniques are applied.

EPP has been a matter of recent controversy despite an increasing amount of phase II studies reporting favorable results (Table 125-1). Recently, the MARS trial[13] concluded prematurely that "EPP within trimodal therapy offers no benefit and possibly harms patients" although the trial included 16 patients in the EPP arm only. The study was not designed to answer the question of benefit or not of EPP but rather of the feasibility of such a trial. A definitive answer to this question would need an accrual of 670 patients to identify a survival benefit.[14] Also their criticism of too high morbidity and mortality rate is not supported by recently reported trials for trimodality therapy including EPP

Table 125-1

INDUCTION CHEMOTHERAPY FOLLOWED BY EXTRAPLEURAL PNEUMONECTOMY

	NO OF PAT.	CTX	EPP	MORB.	MORT.	OAS	PFS
Nakas et al.[15]	165	$n = 25$ (NR)	98	68%[a]	7%[a]	14.7[a]	10.7[a]
Treasure et al.[13]	50	$n = 20$: cis + gem $n = 16$: cis + pem $n = 11$: cis + mitomycin + vinblastine $n = 3$: cis + vinorelbine	16	11 (69%)	3 (19%)	14.4	7.6
Van Schil et al.[16]	59	$n = 56$: cis + pem $n = 3$: carbo + pem	42	38 (82.6%)	90 d: 3 (6.5%)	ITT: 18.4 (15.6–32.9) EPP: 21.5 (17.6–NR)	ITT: 13.9 (10.9–17.2)
Buduhan et al.[17]	55	$n = 24$: cis/carbo + pem $n = 23$: cis + methotrexate + vinblastine $n = 5$: cis + gem $n = 3$: other	46	Major: 17 (37%) Minor: 54%	In-hospital: 2 (4.3%)	EPP: 24 (7.2–30.9)	IMRT: 12 EBRT: 7
Krug et al.[18]	77	$n = 77$: cis + pem	54	Atrial fibrillation (10.5%) Pain (7.0%) Dyspnea (5.3%) Anemia (5.5%) Sepsis (3.5%)	2 (3.7%)	ITT: 16.8 (13.6–23.2) EPP: 21.9 (16.8–29.1) EPP + RT: 29.1	ITT: 10.1 (8.6–15.0)
De Perrot et al.[19]	60	$n = 26$: cis + vinorelbine $n = 24$: cis + pem $n = 6$ cis + raltitrexed $n = 4$: cis + gem	45	Major: 15	3 (6.7%)	ITT: 14 EPP: 59	N2: 12 N1: 44 N0: not reached
Rice[20]	100	$n = 5$: systemic agents $n = 1$: intrapleural cis	100	73%	8%	10.2, 14.2	8
Aigner[21]	49	$n = 3$: cis + pem $n = 6$: cis + gem $n = 1$: gem + carboplatin $n = 2$: cis + adriamycin $n = 1$: doxorubicin	49	24 (49%)	5 (10%)	376 d	NR
Schipper[22]	285	$n = 29$ (NR)	73	Major: 50.7% Minor: 34.2%	8.2%	16	NR
Rea et al.[23]	21	$n = 21$: carbo + gem	17	Major: 5 (23.8%) Minor: 6 (28.6%)	No	ITT: 25.5 EPP: 27.5	EPP: 16.3
Weder et al.[24]	61	$n = 58$: cis + gem	45	Major: 16 (35%)	In-hospital: 1 (2.2%)	ITT: 19.8 (14.6–24.5) EPP: 23 (16.6–32.9)	EPP:13.5 (10.2–18.8)
Flores et al.[25]	21	$n = 19$: cis +/ gem	8	Grade 3: 2	No	ITT: 19 EPP: 33.5 No resection: 9.7	NR
Opitz et al.[26]	63	$n = 47$: cis + gem $n = 16$: cis + pem	63	39 (62%)	3.2%	NR	NR
Stewart et al.[27]	74	$n = 15$: cis-based doublet CTX $n = 9$: gemcitabine $n = 5$: pemetrexed $n = 1$: vinorelbine	74	47 (63%)[a]	5 (6.75%)[a]	NR	NR
Weder et al.[28]	19	$n = 18$: cis + gem	16	Major: 6	90 d: 1	ITT: 23	EPP:16.5 (9–29)

[a] Values based on all patients undergoing EPP (regardless of neoadjuvant chemotherapy).

(Table 125-1) showing that mortality can be reduced to 0% to 5% in experienced centers, while taking into account all studies published between 1985 and 2010 it is reduced to 0 to a maximum of 11.8%.[3] Morbidity stays high (22%–82%) but seems to be manageable in terms of improvement in the quality of life for all parameters at 3 months postoperatively.[3]

PATIENT SELECTION

Patients with histologically proved mesothelioma and resectable tumor load who would tolerate the different treatment modalities including surgery are considered for a multimodal approach. The patient selection should be discussed by a multidisciplinary panel, including a medical oncologist and a radio-oncologist in addition to the thoracic surgeon, pathologist, and pulmonologist. The clinical staging and functional assessment is mandatory as a basis for this discussion (see Preprocedure Assessment). In many centers, patients only with the epithelial type of MPM and without N2 lymph node metastases are considered as candidates. However, we propose that N2 nodes in MPM are "local" nodes and therefore should not be an exclusion factor. Furthermore, all types of histologies, as long as they are considered to be resectable tumors, should be included within clinical trials. The final analysis of this extended selection concept is pending.

Regarding prognostic factors with impact on patients' outcome regardless of the treatment, there are no clear recommendations about clinical parameters, although the sarcomatoid histotype is an exclusion criteria in most clinical trials[29] since it is associated with poor prognosis. Data about the role of mediastinal lymph node involvement are conflicting and may be clarified as a result of the new IASLC/IMIG staging project (see below).[7,19]

For the time being no validated predictive markers exist for the assessment of mesothelioma chemotherapy response, although low thymidylate synthase protein levels were predictive for improved survival in a retrospective analysis of patients who received pemetrexed,[30] and NF2 which has been recently used for targeted mTOR therapy selection in preclinical studies,[31] is currently being evaluated in an ongoing clinical trial evaluating everolimus.

PREPROCEDURE ASSESSMENT

For the diagnosis of MPM, the recommendation of the Guidelines of the European Respiratory Society (ERS) and the European Society of Thoracic Surgeons (ESTS)[29] strongly recommend a thoracoscopic pleural biopsy for obtaining multiple, deep tissue biopsies. Cytological assessment of pleural effusion may not be sensitive and specific enough for relevant decision making. Regarding the histological and immunohistochemical evaluation, we refer the reader to Chapter 115. Once the diagnosis is confirmed, several staging investigations and functional assessments are necessary. For clinical staging and assessment of chemotherapy response, several modalities are available including computed tomography (CT), magnetic resonance imaging (MRI), positron emission tomography (PET), and PET/CT.

CT scan is the primary imaging modality. For further treatment and operation planning, the clinical T-stage assessment is mandatory, but unfortunately, chest CT tends to underestimate the extent of MPM. MRI adds some more information about chest wall and diaphragmatic involvement because of its excellent resolution and may increase the precision of CT staging. However, it is not systematically applied because relevant data on its advantages are missing. FDG-PET-CT has not been proved to be more precise in terms of defining the T stage, but it can detect occult distant metastases and permits one to assess tumor metabolism by measuring FDG activity. The latter may also help to interpret tumor response. To complete the staging investigations, a video mediastinoscopy for limited mediastinal lymph node staging should be considered whenever possible. It is important to note, however, that exact staging as for example of the mammarian lymph node – a lymph node station often involved in the mesothelioma-specific tumor spread – is not assessed. According to institutional practice, laparoscopy and contralateral VATS may be performed if clinically indicated.[29]

Response assessment in malignant mesothelioma remains difficult because of the rind-like growth pattern of MPM. Modified RECIST is the standard currently,[8] but was criticized for a high interobserver variability.[32] More sophisticated methods, such as computerized analysis of CT scans to measure tumor volume[33] or PET-CT based algorithms, such as assessment of total glycolytic volume or total lesion glycolysis or decrease in SUV max, have also shown prognostic value and are under evaluation.[34]

Functional assessment includes spirometry for the measurement of FEV1 and diffusion lung perfusion scan can help to select the patients for EPP or P/D.[29] It has been demonstrated that lung function and exercise capacity are not compromised after induction chemotherapy with carbo- or cisplatin and pemetrexed,[35] but we strongly recommend reassessment of the patient's functional capacity, especially the diffusion capacity of the lung, after induction chemotherapy. Cardiac function should be evaluated by ECG and echocardiography (EF>45%, exclusion of pulmonary hypertension). Beside these quantitative assessments, clinical judgment plays a fundamental role and can be underlined quantitatively with ECOG PS and laboratory analyses. With regard to the side effects experienced with platinum-based chemotherapy, appropriate bone marrow function (CBC) and renal function (blood chemistry) should be considered. If reduced hearing capacity, especially in the high frequency range, is mentioned in the medical history, audiometry should be conducted before chemotherapy.

TECHNIQUE

Induction Chemotherapy

Folic acid and vitamin B12 supplementation play an important role in reducing the hematological toxicity of pemetrexed. To reduce platinum-associated side effects, patients should be appropriately hydrated and an antiemesis protocol should be followed. As an alternative to pemetrexed, gemcitabine can be given with good tumoricidal activity. We observed in our patient cohort of 186 patients intended to be treated with induction chemotherapy and EPP, significantly more hematological side effects after cisplatin/gemcitabine chemotherapy (nonrandomized; $n = 63$) in comparison with cisplatin/pemetrexed ($n = 122$) (one patient other) (unpublished data) (Fisher's exact test $p < 0.001$).

Surgery

We consider 4 to 6 weeks after the last cycle of chemotherapy to be a safe time window between induction chemotherapy and radical surgery, either EPP or P/D. Whereas the surgical technique of EPP has been well standardized with *en bloc* resection of the parietal and visceral pleura with the ipsilateral lung, pericardium, and diaphragm,[36] the technique of P/D is not standardized in all centers as demonstrated during the ongoing staging project of the International Mesothelioma Interest Group (IMIG) and the International Association for the Study of Lung Cancer (IASLC).[37] Whereas some surgeons define P/D as macroscopic tumor removal with pleurectomy of the parietal pleura and decortication of the visceral pleura, others include resection of partial pericardium and diaphragm involved by the tumor. The working group now recommends the name extended

PD (EPD) for the latter operation. We refer the reader to Chapters 121 and 122 for a detailed description of both techniques and also to the literature which includes dedicated descriptions including excellent graphic material[36,38]; and therefore we will discuss only some aspects to prevent complications with special relation to induction chemotherapy.

One particular complication is a potentially higher risk for infection, especially after EPP: a postpneumonectomy empyema with or without bronchopleural fistula. Although several groups could not prove a relation between induction chemotherapy and increased morbidity[39,40] in general, the number of empyemas reported initially by our group was high (16%).[26] It seems that this was an unlucky series since the incidence decreased remarkably in the last 5 years despite no specific measures being done.

In addition to irrigating the chest cavity with betadine solution (diluted 1:10 in NaCl 0.9%) at the end of the resection for both its anti-infectious property as well as cytotoxic effect, and standardized IV antibiotics with amoxicillin 2.2 g IV for 5 days after the operation. We do not apply routine bronchial stump coverage for several reasons: a pericardial fat flap is not available in most of the cases because of the radical resection. The tissue available for an intercostal muscle flap is often poor in a retracted hemithorax typical for the nature of mesothelioma disease, as is also the vascularization of such a flap at the end of the operation. To insert an extrathoracic muscle flap into the chest to protect the bronchial stump prophylactically to avoid an insufficiency seems not appropriate to us.

Careful hemostasis is certainly of paramount importance not only to prevent bleeding complications necessitating redo operations but especially to avoid a persistent hemothorax which may harbor an increased risk of later superinfection. For all of these purposes we pack the dissected part of chest during the dissection with betadine-soaked towels which also may reduce blood loss. Repeated meticulous coagulation with the argon beamer to the whole dissection plane of the chest wall is done during the procedure.

Another preventative measure regarding potential respiratory complications should be considered in pleurectomy/decortication: preservation of the phrenic nerve during dissection is important especially for those patients with compromised lung function. Complete tumor resection is a paradigm for every other tumor resection but can become particularly difficult in the context of mesothelioma surgery as the tumor bulk often constricts the phrenic nerve. This operative step has also other consequences since a total resection of the diaphragm should then rather be avoided for maintenance of breathing capacity—certainly only if maximal cytoreduction can be guaranteed.

From the anesthesiological point of care it is important to apply the FiO_2 below 50% if possible to reduce potential oxygen toxicity for prevention of ARDS after platinum-based chemotherapy, which has been reported for induction treatment of lung cancer[41] and is possibly caused by an injury of the alveolar–capillary membrane.[42]

POSTPROCEDURE CARE

Patients are extubated in the OR at the end of the procedure and will be monitored in an intermediate care station until the next morning. Early extubation is not only important to decrease the risk of ventilator-associated pneumonias but also to decrease the extent of air leaks in patients who underwent P/D. Under spontaneous respiration these leaks usually disappear within 48 to 72 hours. Early mobilization of the patient should be done.

Chest drain is maintained after EPP for 24 to 48 hours not only for bleeding monitoring but also for balancing the position of the mediastinum not to compromise the contralateral lung because of mediastinal shift. The relevance of careful fluid administration, early mobilization, and physiotherapy is well described, all of them being important issues for the prevention of respiratory complications.

Thromboembolic complications, such as pulmonary embolism are relevant in most of the series (1.5%–3%)[26,36,43] and life-threatening especially in the setting of EPP. Besides the awareness and sensitive clinical attitude to any oxygen desaturations with a low threshold for CT scan with PE protocol, we recommend oral anticoagulation for a period of 3 months after surgery.

MANAGEMENT OF PROCEDURE-SPECIFIC COMPLICATIONS

Postpneumonectomy empyema rates have been reported between 4% and 16%.[26,43] For the management of empyema variable methods are proposed from drainage of the chest cavity, thoracoscopic procedures including debridement and irrigation, to Clagett window including removal of the prosthetic material used for reconstruction. We introduced a closed chest procedure for empyema management[44] with repeated (two to three times) radical debridement and packing of the chest cavity with povidone-iodine-soaked towels every 48 hours until definitive closure of the chest after filling the cavity with antibiotic solution. If empyema is associated with bronchopleural fistula, management of the fistula is important but should be delayed in this context until major infection in the cavity is controlled. As further resection of the bronchial stump is usually not possible and direct suture of the bronchus difficult, we cover the fistula with vital tissue using a "parachute technique" with latissimus dorsi muscle flap or omentoplasty. With this technique a complete resolution of this complication can be achieved in almost 100% of the cases avoiding open chest procedures which can be harmful for the patient and quality of life.

SUMMARY

MPM remains a clinical challenge and its incidence will continue to increase worldwide. Several aspects of mesothelioma treatment are discussed controversially, in particular, regarding the extent and best type of surgery, radiotherapy, and the role of neoadjuvant or adjuvant treatment. However, the best survival data is reported from groups using multimodality treatment including radical surgery for patients qualifying from the tumor stage and functional reserve. Induction chemotherapy followed by maximal cytoreductive surgery (EPP or P/D) has the advantage of increasing the resectability rate, to induce even sometimes complete pathological responses and to be administered before surgery and therefore to be performed with a high compliance of the patients. Several aspects have to be considered during surgery but morbidity and mortality have not increased in experienced centers since the introduction of induction chemotherapy.

References

1. Park EK, Takahashi K, Hoshuyama T, et al. Global magnitude of reported and unreported mesothelioma. *Environ Health Perspect.* 2011;119(4):514–518.
2. Testa JR, Cheung M, Pei J, et al. Germline BAP1 mutations predispose to malignant mesothelioma. *Nat Genet.* 2011;43(10):1022–1025.
3. Cao CQ, Yan TD, Bannon PG, et al. A systematic review of extrapleural pneumonectomy for malignant pleural mesothelioma. *J Thorac Oncol.* 2010;5(10):1692–1703.
4. Weder W, Stahel R, Bernhard J, et al. Multicenter trial of neo-adjuvant chemotherapy followed by extrapleural pneumonectomy in malignant pleural mesothelioma. *Ann Oncol.* 2007;18(7):1196–1202.
5. Campbell NP, Kindler HL. Update on malignant pleural mesothelioma. *Semin Respir Crit Care Med.* 2011;32(1):102–110.
6. Hollevoet K, Nackaerts K, Thimpont J, et al. Diagnostic performance of soluble mesothelin and megakaryocyte potentiating factor in mesothelioma. *Am J Respir Crit Care Med.* 2010;181(6):620–625.
7. Gupta V, Krug LM, Laser B, et al. Patterns of local and nodal failure in malignant pleural mesothelioma after extrapleural pneumonectomy and photon-electron radiotherapy. *J Thorac Oncol.* 2009;4(6):746–750.
8. Byrne MJ, Nowak AK. Modified RECIST criteria for assessment of response in malignant pleural mesothelioma. *Ann Oncol.* 2004;15(2):257–260.
9. Oxnard GR, Armato SG 3rd, Kindler HL. Modeling of mesothelioma growth demonstrates weaknesses of current response criteria. *Lung Cancer.* 2006;52(2):141–148.
10. Bech C, Sorensen JB. Chemotherapy induced pathologic complete response in malignant pleural mesothelioma: a review and case report. *J Thorac Oncol.* 2010;5(5):735–740.
11. Flores RM, Pass HI, Seshan VE, et al. Extrapleural pneumonectomy versus pleurectomy/decortication in the surgical management of malignant pleural mesothelioma: results in 663 patients. *J Thorac Cardiovasc Surg.* 2008;135(3):620–626.
12. Flores RM. Surgical options in malignant pleural mesothelioma: extrapleural pneumonectomy or pleurectomy/decortication. *Semin Thorac Cardiovasc Surg.* 2009;21(2):149–153.
13. Treasure T, Lang-Lazdunski L, Waller D, et al. Extra-pleural pneumonectomy versus no extra-pleural pneumonectomy for patients with malignant pleural mesothelioma: clinical outcomes of the Mesothelioma and Radical Surgery (MARS) randomised feasibility study. *The Lancet Oncology.* 2011;12(8):763–772.
14. Weder W, Stahel RA, Baas P, et al. The MARS feasibility trial: conclusions not supported by data. *Lancet Oncol.* 2011;12(12):1093–1094.
15. Nakas A, von Meyenfeldt E, Lau K, et al. Long-term survival after lung-sparing total pleurectomy for locally advanced (International Mesothelioma Interest Group Stage T3-T4) non-sarcomatoid malignant pleural mesothelioma. *Eur J Cardiothorac Surg.* 2011;41(5):1031–1036.
16. Van Schil PE, Baas P, Gaafar R, et al. Trimodality therapy for malignant pleural mesothelioma: results from an EORTC phase II multicentre trial. *Eur Respir J.* 2010;36(6):1362–1369.
17. Buduhan G, Menon S, Aye R, et al. Trimodality therapy for malignant pleural mesothelioma. *Ann Thorac Surg.* 2009;88(3):870–875.
18. Krug LM, Pass HI, Rusch VW, et al. Multicenter phase II trial of neoadjuvant pemetrexed plus cisplatin followed by extrapleural pneumonectomy and radiation for malignant pleural mesothelioma. *J Clin Oncol.* 2009;27(18):3007–3013.
19. de Perrot M, Feld R, Cho BC, et al. Trimodality therapy with induction chemotherapy followed by extrapleural pneumonectomy and adjuvant high-dose hemithoracic radiation for malignant pleural mesothelioma. *J Clin Oncol.* 2009;27(9):1413–1418.
20. Rice DC, Stevens CW, Correa AM, et al. Outcomes after extrapleural pneumonectomy and intensity-modulated radiation therapy for malignant pleural mesothelioma. *Ann Thorac Surg.* 2007;84(5):1685–1692.
21. Aigner C, Hoda MA, Lang G, et al. Outcome after extrapleural pneumonectomy for malignant pleural mesothelioma. *Eur J Cardiothorac Surg.* 2008;34(1):204–207.
22. Schipper PH, Nichols FC, Thomse KM, et al. Malignant pleural mesothelioma: surgical management in 285 patients. *Ann Thorac Surg.* 2008;85(1):257–264.
23. Rea F, Marulli G, Bortolotti L, et al. Induction chemotherapy, extrapleural pneumonectomy (EPP) and adjuvant hemi-thoracic radiation in malignant pleural mesothelioma (MPM): feasibility and results. *Lung Cancer.* 2007;57(1):89–95.
24. Weder W, Stahel RA, Bernhard J, et al. Multicenter trial of neo-adjuvant chemotherapy followed by extrapleural pneumonectomy in malignant pleural mesothelioma. *Ann Oncol.* 2007;18(7):1196–1202.
25. Flores RM, Krug LM, Rosenzweig KE, et al. Induction chemotherapy, extrapleural pneumonectomy, and postoperative high-dose radiotherapy for locally advanced malignant pleural mesothelioma: a phase II trial. *J Thorac Oncol.* 2006;1(4):289–295.
26. Opitz I, Kestenholz P, Lardinois D, et al. Incidence and management of complications after neoadjuvant chemotherapy followed by extrapleural pneumonectomy for malignant pleural mesothelioma. *Eur J Cardiothorac Surg.* 2006;29(4):579–584.
27. Stewart DJ, Martin-Ucar AE, Edwards JG, et al. Extra-pleural pneumonectomy for malignant pleural mesothelioma: the risks of induction chemotherapy, right-sided procedures and prolonged operations. *Eur J Cardiothorac Surg.* 2005;27(3):373–378.
28. Weder W, Kestenholz P, Taverna C, et al. Neoadjuvant chemotherapy followed by extrapleural pneumonectomy in malignant pleural mesothelioma. *J Clin Oncol.* 2004;22(17):3451–3457.
29. Scherpereel A, Astoul P, Baas P, et al. Guidelines of the European Respiratory Society and the European Society of Thoracic Surgeons for the management of malignant pleural mesothelioma. *Eur Respir J.* 2010;35(3):479–495.
30. Righi L, Papotti MG, Ceppi P, et al. Thymidylate synthase but not excision repair cross-complementation group 1 tumor expression predicts outcome in patients with malignant pleural mesothelioma treated with pemetrexed-based chemotherapy. *J Clin Oncol.* 2010;28(9):1534–1539.
31. Lopez-Lago MA, Okada T, Murillo MM, et al. Loss of the tumor suppressor gene NF2, encoding merlin, constitutively activates integrin-dependent mTORC1 signaling. *Mol Cell Biol.* 2009;29(15):4235–4249.
32. Armato SG 3rd, Ogarek JL, Starkey A, et al. Variability in mesothelioma tumor response classification. *AJR Am J Roentgenol.* 2006;186(4): 1000–1006.
33. Frauenfelder T, Tutic M, Weder W, et al. Volumetry: an alternative to assess therapy response for malignant pleural mesothelioma? *Eur Respir J.* 2011;38(1):162–168.
34. Ceresoli GL, Chiti A, Zucali PA, et al. Early response evaluation in malignant pleural mesothelioma by positron emission tomography with [18 F] fluorodeoxyglucose. *J Clin Oncol.* 2006;24(28):4587–4593.
35. Marulli G, Rea F, Nicotra S, et al. Effect of induction chemotherapy on lung function and exercise capacity in patients affected by malignant pleural mesothelioma. *Eur J Cardiothorac Surg.* 2010;37(6):1464–1469.
36. Sugarbaker DJ, Jaklitsch MT, Bueno R, et al. Prevention, early detection, and management of complications after 328 consecutive extrapleural pneumonectomies. *Jpn J Thorac Cardiovasc Surg.* 2004;128(1):138–146.
37. Rice D, Rusch V, Pass H, et al. Recommendations for uniform definitions of surgical techniques for malignant pleural mesothelioma: a consensus report of the international association for the study of lung cancer international staging committee and the international mesothelioma interest group. *J Thorac Oncol.* 2011;6(8):1304–1312.
38. Argote-Greene LM, Chang MY, Sugarbaker DJ. Extrapleural pneumonectomy for malignant pleural mesothelioma. *Multimed Man Cardiothorac Surg.* 2005;2005(628):doi: 10.1510/mmcts.2004.000133.
39. Mansour Z, Kochetkova EA, Ducrocq X, et al. Induction chemotherapy does not increase the operative risk of pneumonectomy! *Eur J Cardiothorac Surg.* 2007;31(2):181–185.
40. Stolz AJ, Schutzner J, Harustiak T, et al. [Impact of neoadjuvant chemotherapy on postoperative complications following pneumonectomy]. *Rozhl Chir.* 2009;88(5):225–228.
41. Muraoka M, Oka T, Akamine S, et al. Postoperative complications of pulmonary resection after platinum-based induction chemotherapy for primary lung cancer. *Surg Today.* 2003;33(1):1–6.
42. Leo F, Solli P, Spaggiari L, et al. Respiratory function changes after chemotherapy: an additional risk for postoperative respiratory complications? *Ann Thorac Surg.* 2004;77(1):260–265.
43. de Perrot M, McRae K, Anraku M, et al. Risk factors for major complications after extrapleural pneumonectomy for malignant pleural mesothelioma. *Ann Thorac Surg.* 2008;85(4):1206–1210.
44. Schneiter D, Cassina P, Korom S, et al. Accelerated treatment for early and late postpneumonectomy empyema. *Ann Thorac Surg.* 2001;72(5): 1668–1672.

PART 21

BENIGN PLEURAL CONDITIONS

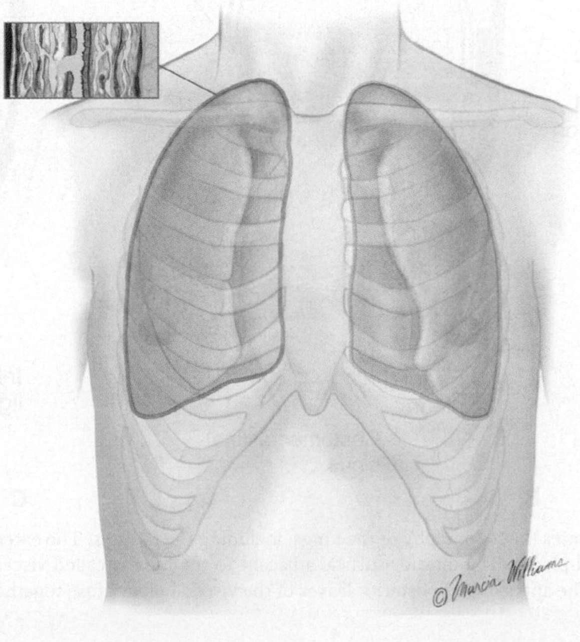

126 Overview of Benign Pleural Conditions: Anatomy and Physiology of Pleura

Sidhu P. Gangadharan

Keywords: Bronchopleural fistula, chylothorax, empyema, exudate, nonmalignant pleural effusion, parietal pleural, pneumomediastinum, pneumothorax, transudate, visceral pleura

The pleural space represents one of the body's potential spaces and can be affected pathologically by liquid, gas, or solid components, all of which can alter respiratory function. These processes may result from benign or malignant conditions, including infectious, inflammatory, or traumatic benign etiologies, as well as primary and secondary malignancies. This chapter provides a brief overview of the clinical presentation, diagnosis, etiology, and treatment of pleural conditions.

ANATOMY AND PHYSIOLOGY

The pleural space lies within the layer of pleura that covers the lung and the pleural layer that lines the chest wall, diaphragm, and mediastinum. The pleural layers are composed of a monolayer of mesothelial cells supported by a thin membrane of collagen and elastin connective tissue.[1] The pleural surfaces are categorized as the visceral and parietal pleurae. The interior surface, termed the visceral pleura, covers the lung. The exterior surface, denoted by the parietal pleura, lines the chest wall, mediastinum, and diaphragm (Fig. 126-1). An analogous representation of this configuration can be created by invaginating an inflated balloon with one's fist (Fig. 126-2). The portion of the balloon that covers the hand is analogous to the visceral pleural surface, and the exterior surface of the balloon represents the parietal pleural surface. The transition from visceral to parietal pleura occurs at the hilum of the lung. Inferior to the hilum, the anterior and posterior leaves of the visceral pleura fuse together at the inferior pulmonary ligament and anchor the medial aspect of the lower lobe to the mediastinum. The sulci, or sinuses, of the pleural space are defined by various structures: the upward bowing of the diaphragm into the hemithorax, the costophrenic sinus, the costomediastinal sinuses anteriorly and posteriorly, and the mediastinophrenic sinus medially. As the diaphragm descends with inspiration, these sinuses are occupied with inflated lung.

The pleural space develops between the fourth and seventh weeks of gestation. The lateral plate of the embryologic mesoderm differentiates into the splanchnopleure, which give rise to the parietal pleura and the somatopleure, which become the visceral pleura. At the end of the seventh week of gestation, the diaphragm has separated the pleural and pericardial compartments from the peritoneal compartment, and over the next month of embryologic development, the pleural space

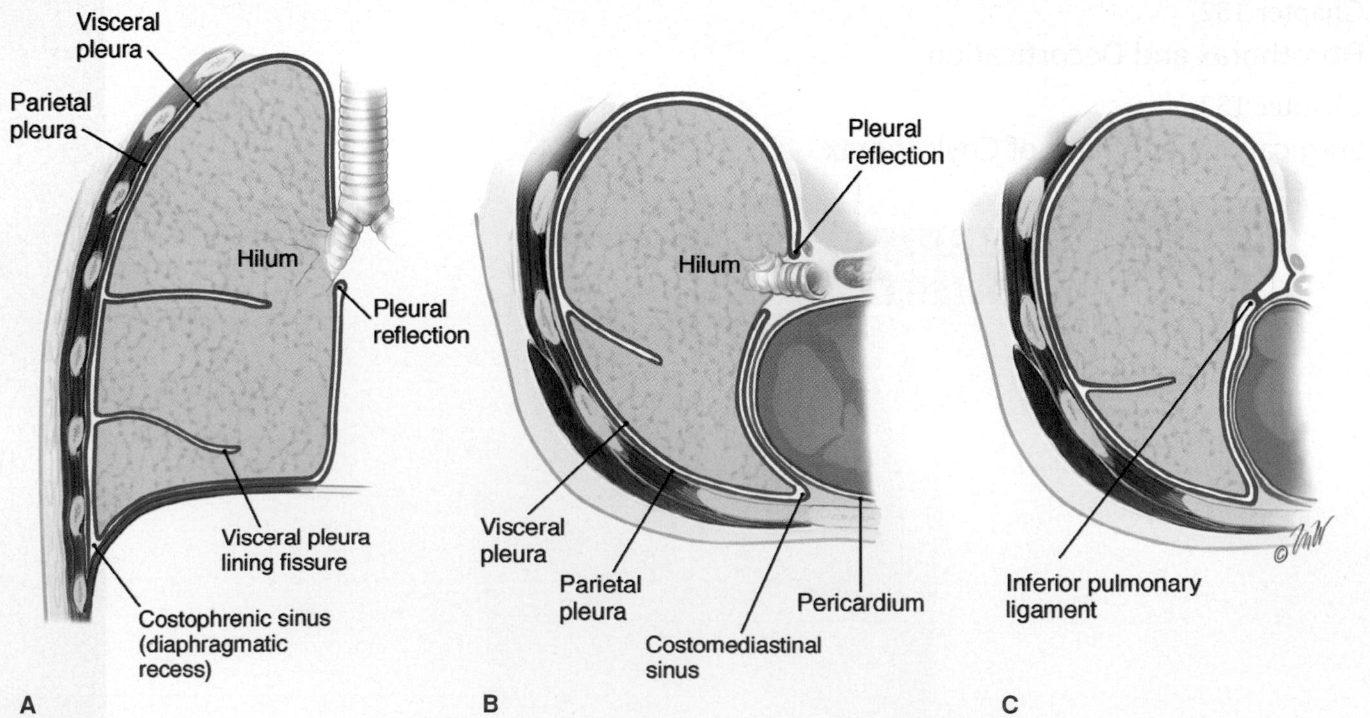

Figure 126-1. *A.* The double-layered pleural sac mimics the topography of the lungs, including the fissures. The exterior surface exposed to the chest wall, diaphragm, and mediastinum is termed the parietal pleura. The interior surface adjacent to the lung is called visceral pleura. *B.* The transition between parietal and visceral pleura occurs at the hilum. *C.* The anterior and posterior leaves of the visceral pleura fuse together at the inferior pulmonary ligament.

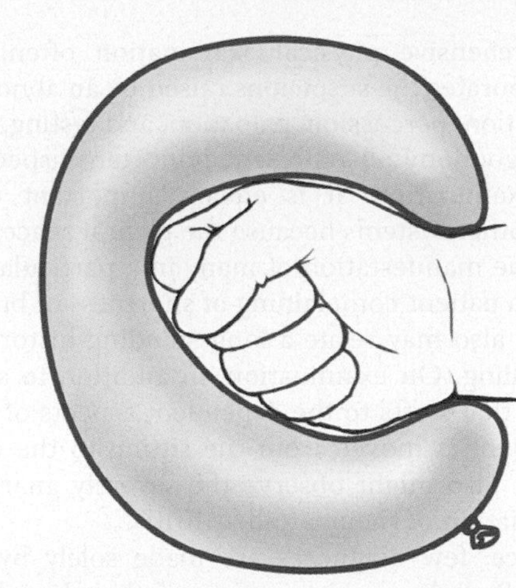

Figure 126-2. There are two pleural sacs, one covering each lobe of the lung. The anatomy of this double-layered structure can be best appreciated by imagining one's fist invaginating a balloon. The hilum is at the wrist.

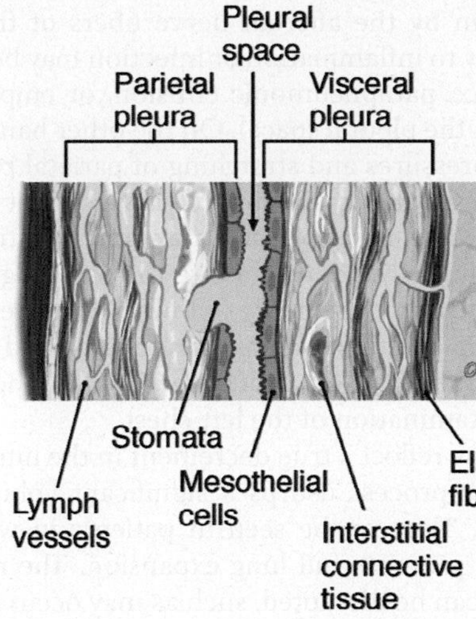

Figure 126-4. A cross-section of the pleural space reveals important features of lymphatic drainage. Note the 1- to 6-μm stomata in the parietal pleura, which facilitate drainage into the submesothelial lymphatic lacunae.

expands cranially and caudally to surround the developing pericardial sac.

As a potential space, the pleural space is capable of transferring the mechanical forces of the expanding hemithorax to the lung, permitting unimpeded inflation. Coupling of chest wall and diaphragmatic forces to the lung across the pleural space is facilitated by the presence of about 1 mL of pleural fluid. Composed primarily of protein, with a smattering of cells (e.g., mesothelial cells, monocytes, and lymphocytes), this physiologic pleural fluid may also facilitate smooth sliding of visceral and parietal pleural surfaces against one another as the lung volume changes.[2–5] Pressure within the pleural space ranges from −2 to −40 cm H_2O as the lung expands from its functional residual capacity to maximum inspiration.[2]

The blood supply of the pleura is divided between the systemic and pulmonary circulations. The parietal pleura is supplied largely by the intercostal arteries, whereas the visceral pleura is supplied by both bronchial and pulmonary arteries (Fig. 126-3).[2,3,6] Similarly, the parietal pleural is innervated by the intercostal nerves.

The lymphatic flux through the pleural space occurs through lymphatic channels within the visceral and parietal pleurae, as well as through the thoracic duct, which conveys the chyle generated by the intestinal lymphatics through the thoracic cavity to drain into the junction of the left jugular and left subclavian veins. The thoracic duct exhibits some variability in its course through the thorax, existing as duplicate ducts or foregoing the usual route between the aorta and azygos vein in the lower right hemithorax before it crosses to the left at the T4 level (see Chapter 133). The lymphatic capillaries of the pleura are found within the submesothelial connective tissue. The parietal pleura also has 1- to 6-μm stomata that facilitate drainage into the submesothelial lymphatic lacunae and from there through intercostal, mammary, and mediastinal lymphatics into the thoracic duct (Fig. 126-4).[7,8]

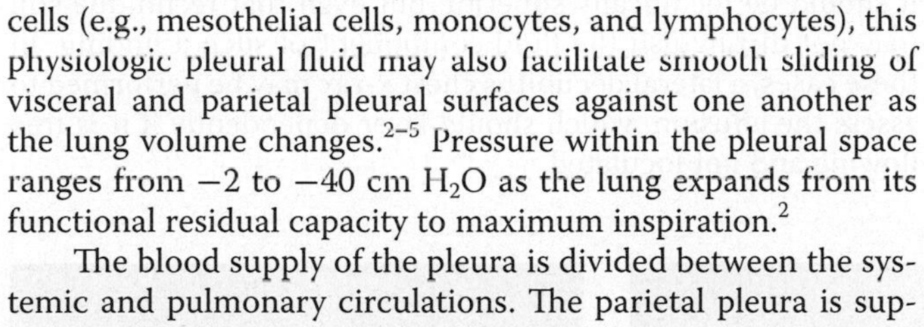

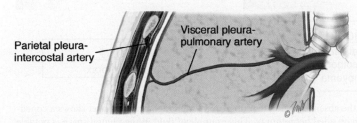

Figure 126-3. The pleura receives its blood supply from two sources. The parietal pleura is sustained by the intercostal arteries, whereas the visceral pleura is sustained by both bronchial and pulmonary arteries.

DIFFERENTIAL DIAGNOSIS

Pleural space diseases can be grouped into abnormalities of liquid, solid, and gas, although there may be some overlap between physical states. Consideration of extrathoracic disease also must be given, since the upper intra-abdominal contents may be located above the level of the costal margin, while still below the dome of the diaphragm, especially after full exhalation. Subphrenic infections, gallbladder inflammation, and splenic rupture all can lead to pain in the lower chest on inspiration. Occasionally, infradiaphragmatic pathology can lead to a pleural process. There have been case reports of gallstones migrating into the pleural space.[9] With the so-called hepatic hydrothorax, a transudate accumulates in the pleural space of cirrhotic patients as ascitic fluid fluxes across the diaphragm, possibly through blebs or fenestrations.[10] Other examples include recurrent pancreatitis that may fistulize to the pleural space.[11]

DIAGNOSTIC WORKUP

The workup of a pleural abnormality begins with a complete history and physical examination. A thorough review of systems should be taken including specific queries about local symptoms such as pain, dyspnea, or cough, as well as more systemic findings such as fevers, weight loss, or neurologic symptoms.

A complaint of chest pain should be explored further—is the pain pleuritic? Was there antecedent trauma? Does the pain radiate to the top of the shoulder or scapula or back? The sensation of pain by the afferent nerve fibers of the parietal pleura secondary to inflammation or infection may be observed with hemothorax, parapneumonic effusion, or empyema (i.e., purulent fluid in the pleural space). On the other hand, changes in intrapleural pressures and stretching of parietal pleural surfaces on the chest wall or diaphragm may account for sensations of discomfort in cases of pneumothorax. The time course of the pain also might yield insight into the pathologic process. For example, a history of retching followed by acute epigastric or substernal pain and then progression to left-sided chest pain would suggest an esophageal rupture with initial mediastinitis followed by contamination of the left chest.

Dyspnea may reflect a true decrement in the lung function if the pathologic process usurps a significant volume within the hemithorax. This can be seen in patients in whom fluid or solid volume prevents full lung expansion. The respiratory mechanics also can be disrupted, such as may occur in cases of pneumothorax, where there is an uncoupling of the mechanical forces of the chest wall and diaphragm from the lung, with a resulting diminution of lung volume caused by the lung's intrinsic elastic recoil. However, dyspnea also may result without a significant loss of lung function. The sensation of incomplete chest expansion that accompanies some pleural processes may lead to dyspnea in the absence of hypoxia or hypoventilation.

A history of cough should be elicited to determine the characteristics of the sputum produced: color, odor, viscosity, amount, and frequency. A period of coughing that is productive of purulent sputum, in conjunction with a fever and chest pain, followed later by a persistent dry cough, may be an indication that a chronic empyema cavity has formed (see Chapter 107). A history of hemoptysis, weight loss, and heavy tobacco use in a patient with a pleural effusion would be suspicious for a malignant effusion or pleural malignancy.

A comprehensive physical examination often, but not always, corroborates the suspicions raised by an abnormal history. Auscultation, percussion, palpation, and testing for tactile fremitus or egophony all represent important aspects of the respiratory examination. It is equally important to detect pathology in other systems because the pleural space may represent only one manifestation of many in a particular disease. For example, a patient complaining of shortness of breath with stair climbing also may relate a long-standing history of joint pain and swelling. On examination, in addition to a dullness to percussion that shifts to the dependent aspects of the chest when the patient is moved from the sitting to the decubitus positions, one also might observe the severely gnarled joints and ulnar deviation of rheumatoid arthritis.

In practice, few diagnoses are made solely by physical examination. Radiologic examination of the pleural space is accomplished with plain chest radiographs, ultrasound, CT scan, and MRI. Plain films are usually the initial investigation of benign conditions from any of the three categories described earlier (Fig. 126-5). The scant volume of pleural fluid present in the healthy state is not visible on chest x-ray, but a pleural effusion of 50 mL should be detectable on a lateral chest film, evidenced as blunting of the posterior costophrenic sinus. A 200-mL effusion is evidenced by blunting of the lateral sulcus.[12] On anteroposterior (portable) films, often the meniscus of the pleural effusion is indistinct, and atelectatic or consolidated lung may contribute to the basilar opacification. An upright posteroanterior and lateral film is preferable because it should be technically superior, but even that technique still may not distinguish the fluid component of such a finding. In these cases, a lateral decubitus chest x-ray may be performed to assess the effusion, which should layer dependently if it is free flowing and not loculated.

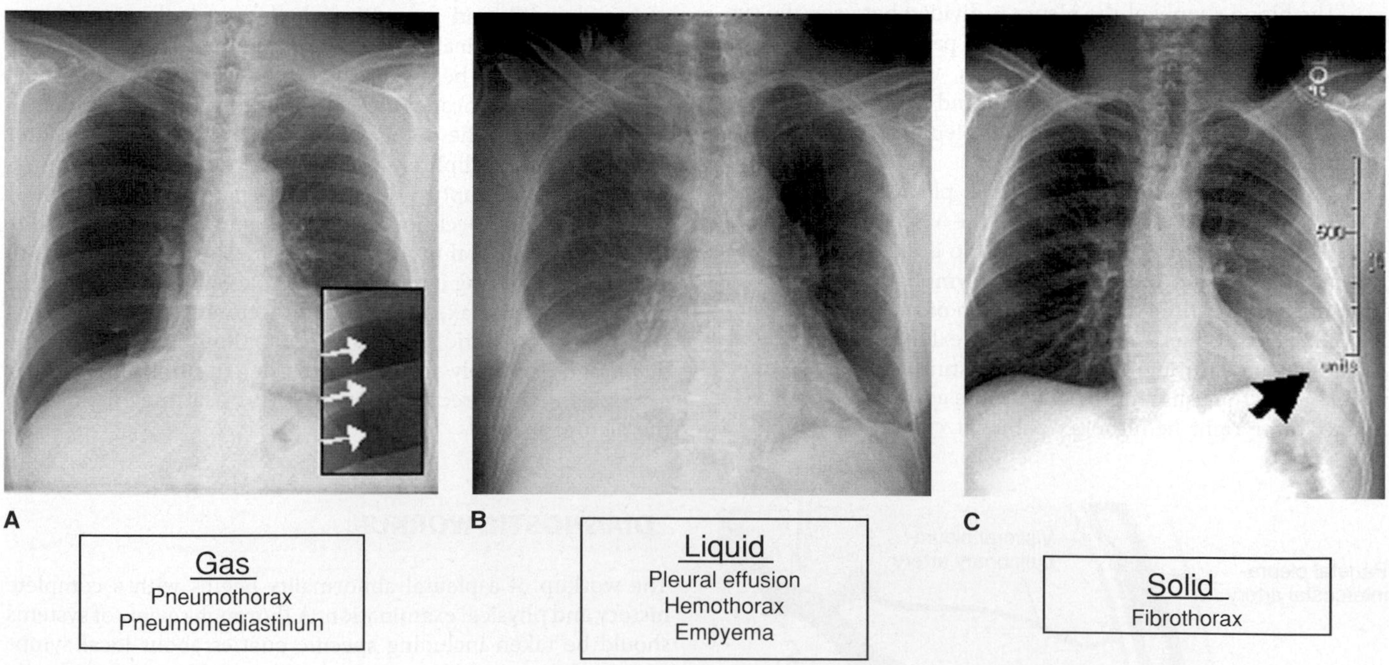

Figure 126-5. *A.* Spontaneous pneumothorax in the right pleural space. Note the absence of lung markings in the right hemithorax. Inset shows a coned-down view of the pleural edge of the collapsed right lung (white arrows). *B.* Right-sided hemothorax. This example of fluid in the pleural space is notable for a meniscus at the costophrenic sulcus. *C.* Fibrothorax. The arrow points to an area of opacification that represents the thickest portion of the chronic empyema cavity. At operation, the full extent of the fibrothorax ranged from the upper third of the hemithorax to the hemidiaphragm, as suggested by the more bland opacity seen on this plain film.

A plain upright chest x-ray is also the mainstay of radiologic evaluation of pneumothorax. Small amounts of air in the pleural space may be detected by observing the visceral pleural line (Fig. 126-5, inset) or noting the absence of lung markings. In an otherwise normal pleural space, the first location of detectable pneumothorax is usually the apex. Thus, in most instances, an upright plain film is the appropriate study to order, although there is experimental evidence from cadaver studies that a lateral decubitus film may be even more sensitive.[13,14] The progressive collapse of the lung with increasing pneumothorax will continue to shorten the radial distances between the visceral pleural surfaces of the pulmonary lobes and the hilum. In a supine patient, the distribution of air within the pleural space is altered, and the pneumothorax may be noted as the "deep sulcus sign," where the lateral sulcus is sharper and more lucent on the affected side or as lucency over the right or left upper quadrants.[15,16]

Chest CT scanning increases the sensitivity of detection of solid, liquid, and gas within the pleural space. Fluid collections can be further characterized by measuring Hounsfield units to distinguish between simple effusions and hemothorax or evolving empyemas.[17] CT scanning is also more sensitive for the detection of pneumothoraces.[18,19] It is worth stating that tension pneumothorax is not a diagnosis that should be made with CT or chest x-ray, but rather clinical assessment. Distinguishing between exudative and transudative pleural effusions is not reliably accomplished with CT scanning alone.[20] In terms of surgical planning, a chest CT scan can be extremely useful in planning video-assisted thoracic surgery (VATS) port sites or even thoracotomy to avoid lung adhesions and obtain optimal access to the intrapleural pathology.

MRI of the chest may be useful in the workup of malignant disease because it demonstrates tumor invasiveness and thus resectability. It has a sensitivity of up to 100% and a specificity of up to 93% in the detection of malignant disease during a workup of pleural masses.[21] Its role in the workup of benign disease is less clear. Although it is not accurate in distinguishing between exudate and transudate, MRI can detect hemothorax reasonably well.[22] In practice, however, it is unlikely to be a necessary adjunct to clinical evaluation.

Ultrasound is less sensitive than CT scanning for the detection of pleural fluid and pneumothorax,[18,19,23] although it may have increased specificity for distinguishing pleural thickening from pleural fluid.[24] Ultrasound is also a portable tool, which has implications in the rapid assessment of critically ill patients in the trauma or intensive care settings. Compared with plain radiography, ultrasound is more sensitive for detecting and quantifying pleural fluid.[25,26] For reasons of safety and efficacy, it is now recommended that procedures for evaluation of pleural effusion (e.g., thoracentesis) be performed with ultrasound guidance.[27]

Thoracentesis represents the first invasive modality in the workup of a pleural effusion. It bears mentioning that thoracentesis typically is not necessary in patients with bilateral pleural effusions and clinical scenarios that point to transudative causes.[28] In one analysis it was found that the clinical judgment of the physician was correct in predicting a transudative effusion in 16 of 16 cases and in 15 of 17 exudative effusions.[29]

The British Thoracic Society guidelines for workup of a unilateral pleural effusion are depicted in Figure 126-6. The first goal of pleural fluid analysis is to distinguish between exudative effusions (e.g., cloudy serum signifying disease of the pleura itself) and transudative effusions (e.g., clear serum but abnormally high concentration). The different diagnoses associated with each type of effusion are listed in Table 126-1. As recommended, the fluid is then sent in three separate tubes for pleural chemistries (e.g., lactate dehydrogenase [LDH], pH, and protein), microbiologic analysis (e.g., aerobic and anaerobic culture, Gram stain, fungal culture, and AFB stain and culture), as well as cytology. Light's criteria are used to determine whether the fluid is transudative or exudative (pleural:serum LDH >0.6, pleural:serum protein >0.5, or pleural LDH >two-thirds of upper normal serum value).[29,30] Whereas other assays have been described to distinguish exudates from transudates, Light's criteria have been validated and in clinical practice remain a mainstay of the workup.[31] It is important to remember that the data may not return as classic profiles of malignant or benign disease. Certain data will "trump" others. For example, the finding of malignant cells on cytology yields a definitive diagnosis of malignant pleural effusion regardless of the protein and LDH levels. Similarly, the finding of pleural food particles suggests viscus (esophageal) perforation, independent of other findings. Other specific analyses can be run on the fluid, depending on the clinical situation. For example, the presence of milky fluid, suggestive of chylous effusion, would prompt the addition of a triglyceride level to the fluid analysis. Amylase levels of the pleural fluid specimen may be determined in suspected cases of pancreatic disease, keeping in mind that malignancy, esophageal rupture, tuberculosis, abdominal trauma, uremia, and radiation pleuritis also have been found to be associated with increased levels of amylase.[32]

In cases of exudative effusion, when the diagnosis is still suspect, a pleural biopsy is warranted.[33] The preferred route at our institution is by means of VATS. This is done under general anesthesia, with single-lung ventilation on the nonaffected side. The exploration and biopsy usually can be accomplished through a single 12-mm port. It is important to bear in mind that the pleural tissue obtained should be sent for both pathologic and microbiologic analyses.

Table 126-1

ETIOLOGIES OF PLEURAL EFFUSION

FREQUENCY	TRANSUDATE	EXUDATE
Very common	Left ventricular failure Cirrhosis Hypoalbuminemia	Malignancy Parapneumonic effusions Empyema
Less common	Hypothyroidism Nephrotic syndrome Mitral stenosis Pulmonary embolism	Lung infarction Rheumatoid arthritis Autoimmune disorders Pancreatitis Benign asbestos effusion Postmyocardial infarction syndrome
Rare	Constrictive pericarditis Urinothorax Superior vena cava syndrome Ovarian hyperstimulation Meigs' syndrome	Yellow nail syndrome Medications Fungal infections

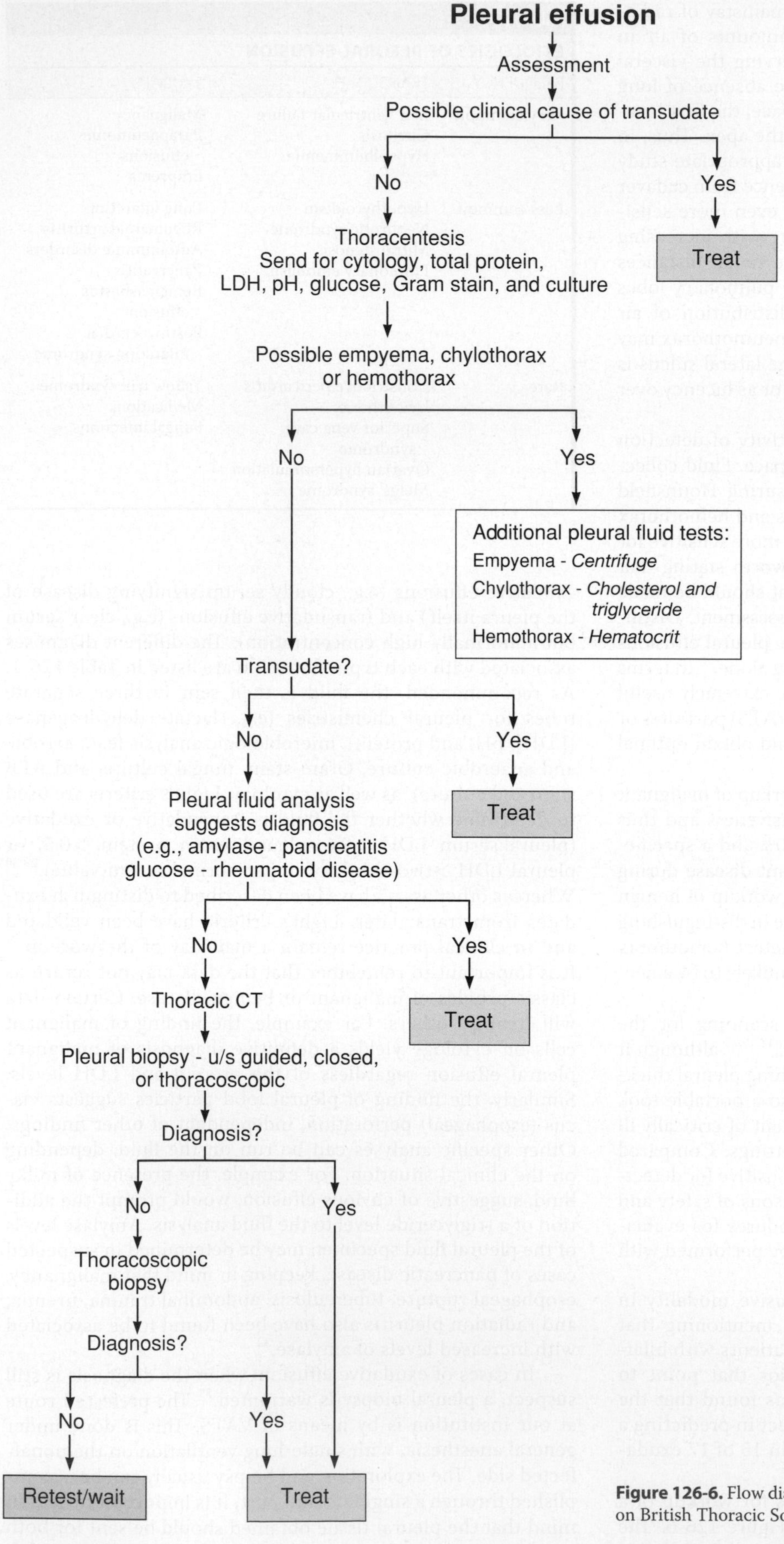

Figure 126-6. Flow diagram for workup of unilateral pleural effusion based on British Thoracic Society guidelines.

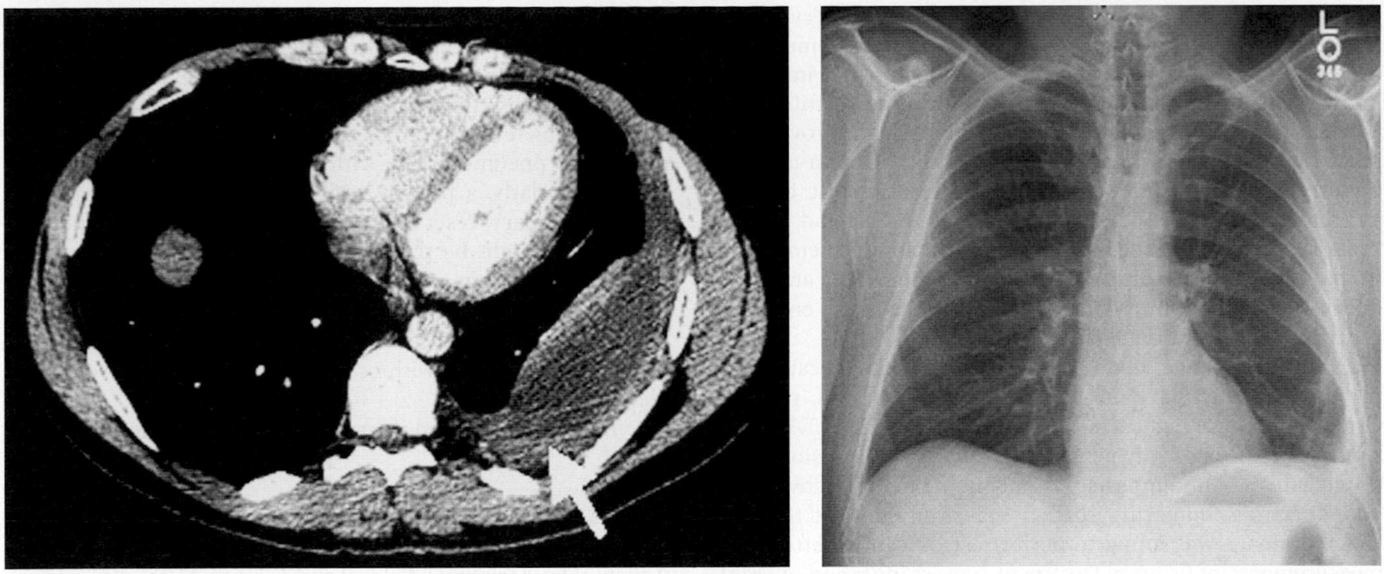

A B

Figure 126-7. Fibrothorax. *A*. CT scan demonstrating the chronic empyema cavity with a hypodense center (fluid) and a thick rind peripherally (white arrow). *B*. Postoperative chest film showing full expansion of the left lung (compare with Fig. 126-5C).

SPECIFIC DIAGNOSES

Empyema

Empyema is defined as a collection of pus in the pleural space. In cases associated with pneumonia, there is a continuum from simple parapneumonic effusion to complex parapneumonic effusion to empyema. Parapneumonic effusion is defined as any effusion found in association with pneumonia.[34] The stages of evolution of these effusions have been described: exudative, fibrinopurulent, and organizing.[35] A simple parapneumonic effusion may resolve with proper antibiotic therapy of the underlying pneumonia. It is worth noting, however, that antibiotic penetration into empyemas is variable and less likely to sterilize anything more advanced than the earliest stages of a developing empyema.[36]

A complex parapneumonic effusion is one that demonstrates a pH greater than 7.20, LDH greater than three times the normal serum LDH value, glucose less than 60 mg/dL, and positive bacterial cultures. These should be drained, but since loculations form inevitably, it is increasingly more difficult to achieve complete drainage with a tube alone. Progression to the thick, fibrous "rind" of the third stage necessitates a decortication procedure to free the lung of the rind and allow full reexpansion (Fig. 126-7). An algorithm to assess and treat patients with pneumonia who are discovered to have a pleural effusion is depicted in Figure 126-8. Thoracentesis should be performed, and pleural chemistries, microbiology, and a postthoracentesis plain radiograph should be assessed to determine whether the effusion demonstrates poor prognostic factors. There exists debate regarding the use of fibrinolytic therapy to optimize drainage of infected pleural fluid. The largest prospective trial (MIST1) was reported in 2005 and randomized 430 patients to receive placebo or intrapleural streptokinase in conjunction with chest tube drainage of infected pleural fluid.[37] There did not appear to be an advantage over placebo in terms of need for surgery, mortality, or length of stay. The MIST2 trial utilized alteplase (a direct plasminogen activator) instead of streptokinase (indirect) but again did not show an improvement

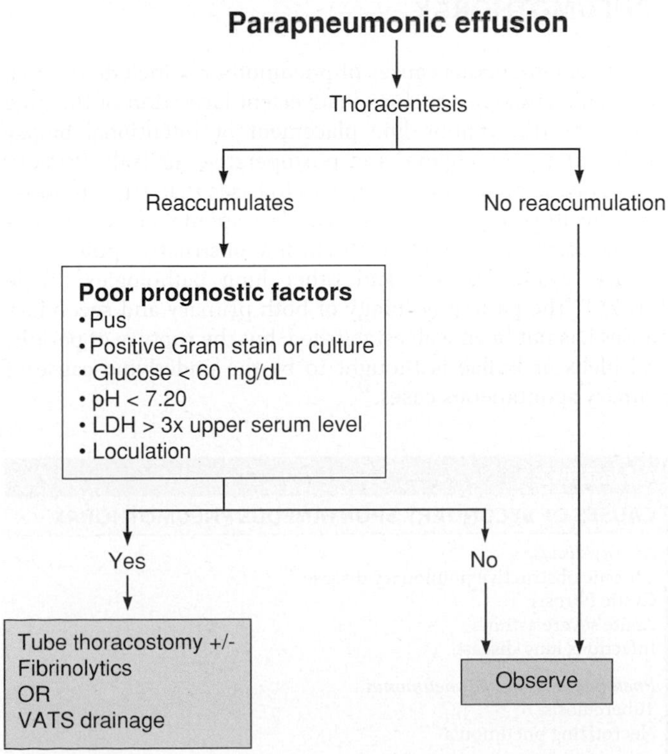

Figure 126-8. Algorithm for workup and treatment of parapneumonic effusion. (Reproduced with permission from Maskell NA, Butland RJ. BTS guidelines for the investigation of a unilateral pleural effusion in adults. *Thorax*. 2003;58:8S–17S.)

over placebo with regard to the rate of surgical intervention, duration of hospitalization, radiographic improvement, or mortality.[38] The MIST2 trial, however, did show an improvement when the enzyme DNase was used in conjunction with alteplase in outcome measures of radiographic improvement, need for surgery, and length of stay. A recent meta-analysis of seven randomized controlled trials on fibrinolytic therapy concluded that despite the recent negative MIST1 and MIST2 trials, there was a benefit of fibrinolytic therapy for empyema when looking at the composite endpoint of mortality and freedom from surgical intervention, as well as the single endpoint of surgical intervention alone.[39]

Our preference is to perform VATS decortication in patients found to have poor prognostic factors (pus, positive Gram stain/culture, glucose <60 mg/dL, pH < 7.20, LDH >3× serum, loculation) with persistent or recurrent effusion after thoracentesis. Although there is only a single prospective, randomized trial comparing surgery versus fibrinolytic therapy, VATS drainage was found to perform significantly better with measurements of primary treatment success, duration of chest tube drainage, and hospital stay.[40]

The medical management of empyema and other nonmalignant pleural effusions is reviewed in Chapter 127.

Other routes of infection of the pleural space exist, including traumatic, direct extension of infectious processes in the abdomen or neck, and iatrogenic (i.e., surgical or interventional). For additional detail about the surgical management of empyema, see Chapter 107. Aggressive drainage remains the key to treatment for most of these conditions.

PNEUMOTHORAX

The nonspontaneous causes of pneumothorax include trauma, iatrogenic etiologies such as inadvertent laceration of the lung during central venous line placement or intentional biopsy of the lung parenchyma, and postoperative air leak. Primary spontaneous pneumothorax refers to cases that arise in previously healthy lungs, whereas secondary spontaneous pneumothorax occurs in patients with chronic obstructive pulmonary disease, cystic fibrosis, and other lung pathologies (Table 126-2).[41] The pathophysiology of both primary and secondary causes has not been well established, but the rupture of peripheral blebs or bullae is thought to be the underlying cause of primary spontaneous cases.[42]

Table 126-2

CAUSES OF SECONDARY SPONTANEOUS PNEUMOTHORAX

Airway disease
Chronic obstructive pulmonary disease
Cystic fibrosis
Acute severe asthma
Infectious lung disease
Pneumocystis carinii pneumonia
Tuberculosis
Necrotizing pneumonia
Interstitial lung disease
Sarcoidosis
Idiopathic pulmonary fibrosis
Connective-tissue disease
Lung cancer

Once identified, pneumothorax must be treated with consideration of the patient's underlying condition. An intubated patient who is subject to positive-pressure ventilation will require closed drainage of the pleural space to prevent an unpredictable evolution of a small pneumothorax into a large or tension pneumothorax with respiratory or hemodynamic effects. Similarly, a patient with underlying lung disease and poor pulmonary reserve may tolerate less well a pneumothorax that might be treated conservatively with observation in a healthy patient with normal lungs. Treatment strategies include observation, aspiration, chest tube drainage, chemical pleurodesis, and surgical resection of the underlying pathology (i.e., blebectomy) with or without mechanical or chemical pleurodesis.[43]

These are discussed in greater detail in Chapter 128.

CHYLOTHORAX

A pleural fluid triglyceride level greater than 110 mg/dL is diagnostic of chylothorax. The fluid is also rich in lymphocytes, as detected on cell counting. It is suggested by the presence of a milky fluid which does not layer on centrifugation, as might be expected with turbid exudative fluid from an empyema.[33] This visual confirmation can be enhanced by feeding the patient a fat-rich meal before the investigation. Once the chylous effusion is in a collecting system, such as that into which a chest tube drains, there is an immiscible quality to it that allows identification of the milky effluent even after the meal has been digested and the lymphatic fluid begins again to run clear. The etiology of chylothorax includes traumatic/iatrogenic sequelae and medical conditions such as lymphoma, chylous ascites, and lymphatic abnormalities.[44]

Conservative management includes closed drainage of the pleural space with a chest tube, strict nonenteral nutrition or medium-chain triglyceride feedings, careful observation of nutrition status, and surveillance for infections. Unfortunately, conservative management may fail in up to 48% of patients.[45] Somatostatin and etilefrine have been used as medical adjuncts to conservative management with some success.[46–48] Percutaneous embolization of the thoracic duct also has been used.[49,50] However, the mainstay of treatment involves VATS ligation of the duct. This technique is discussed in Chapter 133.

SUMMARY

The spectrum of pleural disease is extensive and must be approached with a careful diagnostic algorithm depending on the clinical situation and the type of abnormality encountered—solid, liquid, or gas.

EDITOR'S COMMENT

The pleural space has shaped our surgical approaches to diseases of the chest; a fact that is painfully apparent when the space is obliterated by disease or prior surgery. The function of the pleural space is an intriguing topic for speculation, but a reasonable hypothesis is that this space contributes to the mechanical coupling of respiratory muscle function with alveolar gas exchange.

—Steven J. Mentzer

References

1. Oldmixon EH, Hoppin FG, Jr. Comparison of amounts of collagen and elastin in pleura and parenchyma of dog lung. *J Appl Physiol Respir Environ Exerc Physiol.* 1984;56(5):1383–1388.
2. Agostoni E. Mechanics of the pleural space. *Physiol Rev*. 1972;52(1):57–128.
3. Lai-Fook SJ. Pleural mechanics and fluid exchange. *Physiol Rev*. 2004;84(2):385–410.
4. Light RW, Erozan YS, Ball WC, Jr. Cells in pleural fluid. Their value in differential diagnosis. *Arch Intern Med*. 1973;132(6):854–860.
5. Laurent TC, Fraser JR. Hyaluronan. *Faseb J*. 1992;6(7):2397–2404.
6. Deffebach ME, Charan NB, Lakshminarayan S, et al. The bronchial circulation. Small, but a vital attribute of the lung. *Am Rev Respir Dis*. 1987;135(2):463–481.
7. Wang NS. The preformed stomas connecting the pleural cavity and the lymphatics in the parietal pleura. *Am Rev Respir Dis*. 1975;111(1):12–20.
8. Zocchi L. Physiology and pathophysiology of pleural fluid turnover. *Eur Respir J*. 2002;20(6):1545–1558.
9. Oestmann JW, Bridenbaugh S, Eggeling I. Gallstone migration into the pleural space. *Am J Gastroenterol*. 2000;95(3):836–837.
10. Huang PM, Chang YL, Yang CY, et al. The morphology of diaphragmatic defects in hepatic hydrothorax: thoracoscopic finding. *J Thorac Cardiovasc Surg*. 2005;130(1):141–145.
11. Uchiyama T, Suzuki T, Adachi A, et al. Pancreatic pleural effusion: case report and review of 113 cases in Japan. *Am J Gastroenterol*. 1992;87(3):387–391.
12. Blackmore CC, Black WC, Dallas RV, et al. Pleural fluid volume estimation: a chest radiograph prediction rule. *Acad Radiol*. 1996;3(2):103–109.
13. Beres RA, Goodman LR. Pneumothorax: detection with upright versus decubitus radiography. *Radiology*. 1993;186(1):19–22.
14. Carr JJ, Reed JC, Choplin RH, et al. Plain and computed radiography for detecting experimentally induced pneumothorax in cadavers: implications for detection in patients. *Radiology*. 1992;183(1):193–199.
15. Gordon R. The deep sulcus sign. *Radiology*. 1980;136(1):25–27.
16. Tocino IM, Miller MH, Fairfax WR. Distribution of pneumothorax in the supine and semirecumbent critically ill adult. *AJR Am J Roentgenol*. 1985;144(5):901–905.
17. Kim EA, Lee KS, Shim YM, et al. Radiographic and CT findings in complications following pulmonary resection. *Radiographics*. 2002;22(1):67–86.
18. Rowan KR, Kirkpatrick AW, Liu D, et al. Traumatic pneumothorax detection with thoracic US: correlation with chest radiography and CT–initial experience. *Radiology*. 2002;225(1):210–214.
19. Wall SD, Federle MP, Jeffrey RB, et al. CT diagnosis of unsuspected pneumothorax after blunt abdominal trauma. *AJR Am J Roentgenol*. 1983;141(5):919–921.
20. Nandalur KR, Hardie AH, Bollampally SR, et al. Accuracy of computed tomography attenuation values in the characterization of pleural fluid: an ROC study. *Acad Radiol*. 2005;12(8):987–991.
21. Hierholzer J, Luo L, Bittner RC, et al. MRI and CT in the differential diagnosis of pleural disease. *Chest*. 2000;118(3):604–609.
22. Tscholakoff D, Sechtem U, de Geer G, et al. Evaluation of pleural and pericardial effusions by magnetic resonance imaging. *Eur J Radiol*. 1987;7(3):169–174.
23. Yu CJ, Yang PC, Wu HD, et al. Ultrasound study in unilateral hemithorax opacification. Image comparison with computed tomography. *Am Rev Respir Dis*. 1993;147(2):430–434.
24. Feller-Kopman D. Ultrasound-guided thoracentesis. *Chest*. 2006;129(6):1709–1714.
25. Eibenberger KL, Dock WI, Ammann ME, et al. Quantification of pleural effusions: sonography versus radiography. *Radiology*. 1994;191(3):681–684.
26. Gryminski J, Krakowka P, Lypacewicz G. The diagnosis of pleural effusion by ultrasonic and radiologic techniques. *Chest*. 1976;70(1):33–37.
27. Havelock T, Teoh R, Laws D, et al. Pleural procedures and thoracic ultrasound: British Thoracic Society Pleural Disease Guideline 2010. *Thorax*. 2010;65(Suppl 2):ii61–ii76.
28. Hooper C, Lee YC, Maskell N, et al. Investigation of a unilateral pleural effusion in adults: British Thoracic Society Pleural Disease Guideline 2010. *Thorax*. 2010;65(Suppl 2):ii4–ii17.
29. Scheurich JW, Keuer SP, Graham DY. Pleural effusion: comparison of clinical judgment and Light's criteria in determining the cause. *South Med J*. 1989;82(12):1487–1491.
30. Light RW, Macgregor MI, Luchsinger PC, et al. Pleural effusions: the diagnostic separation of transudates and exudates. *Ann Intern Med*. 1972;77(4):507–513.
31. Heffner JE, Brown LK, Barbieri CA. Diagnostic value of tests that discriminate between exudative and transudative pleural effusions. Primary Study Investigators. *Chest*. 1997;111(4):970–980.
32. Villena V, Perez V, Pozo F, et al. Amylase levels in pleural effusions: a consecutive unselected series of 841 patients. *Chest*. 2002;121(2):470–474.
33. Maskell NA, Butland RJ. BTS guidelines for the investigation of a unilateral pleural effusion in adults. *Thorax*. 2003;58(Suppl 2):ii8–17.
34. Light RW. Parapneumonic effusions and empyema. *Proc Am Thorac Soc*. 2006;3(1):75–80.
35. Andrews NC, Parker EF, Shaw RR, et al. Management of nontuberculous empyema. *Am Rev Respir Dis*. 1962;85:935–936.
36. Teixeira LR, Sasse SA, Villarino MA, et al. Antibiotic levels in empyemic pleural fluid. *Chest*. 2000;117(6):1734–1739.
37. Maskell NA, Davies CW, Nunn AJ, et al. U.K. Controlled trial of intrapleural streptokinase for pleural infection. *N Engl J Med*. 2005;352(9):865–874.
38. Rahman NM, Maskell NA, West A, et al. Intrapleural use of tissue plasminogen activator and DNase in pleural infection. *N Engl J Med*. 2011;365(6):518–526.
39. Janda S, Swiston J. Intrapleural fibrinolytic therapy for treatment of adult parapneumonic effusions and empyemas: a systematic review and meta-analysis. *Chest*. 2012;142(2):401–411.
40. Wait MA, Sharma S, Hohn J, et al. A randomized trial of empyema therapy. *Chest*. 1997;111(6):1548–1551.
41. Tschopp JM, Rami-Porta R, Noppen M, et al. Management of spontaneous pneumothorax: state of the art. *Eur Respir J*. 2006;28(3):637–650.
42. Ayed AK, Chandrasekaran C, Sukumar M. Video-assisted thoracoscopic surgery for primary spontaneous pneumothorax: clinicopathological correlation. *Eur J Cardiothorac Surg*. 2006;29(2):221–225.
43. MacDuff A, Arnold A, Harvey J, et alManagement of spontaneous pneumothorax: British Thoracic Society Pleural Disease Guideline 2010. *Thorax*. 2010;65(Suppl 2):ii18–ii31.
44. Doerr CH, Allen MS, Nichols FC, 3rd, et al. Etiology of chylothorax in 203 patients. *Mayo Clin Proc*. 2005;80(7):867–870.
45. Lapp GC, Brown DH, Gullane PJ, et al. Thoracoscopic management of chylous fistulae. *Am J Otolaryngol*. 1998;19(4):257–262.
46. Cannizzaro V, Frey B, Bernet-Buettiker V. The role of somatostatin in the treatment of persistent chylothorax in children. *Eur J Cardio-thorac Surg*. 2006;30(1):49–53.
47. Rosti L, De Battisti F, Butera G, et al. Octreotide in the management of postoperative chylothorax. *Pediatr Cardiol*. 2005;26(4):440–443.
48. Guillem P, Billeret V, Houcke ML, et al. Successful management of post-esophagectomy chylothorax/chyloperitoneum by etilefrine. *Dis Esophagus*. 1999;12(2):155–156.
49. Cope C. Management of chylothorax via percutaneous embolization. *Curr Opin Pulm Med*. 2004;10(4):311–314.
50. Nadolski GJ, Itkin M. Thoracic duct embolization for nontraumatic chylous effusion: experience in 34 patients. *Chest*. 2013;143(1):158–163.

127 Medical Management of Nonmalignant Pleural Effusions

Rabih Bechara and Armin Ernst

Keywords: Transudate, exudate, hydrothorax, hemothorax, chylothorax, empyema

Pleural effusions can occur as the consequence of a localized disease (exudative), or they can be a manifestation of systemic disease (transudative). They are fairly common, and chest physicians are often asked to diagnose and manage them. This chapter reviews the criteria for exudative and transudative pleural effusions, as well as the diagnostic techniques and medical management of several types of nonmalignant pleural effusions, including parapneumonic, connective tissue disease-related effusions, hepatic hydrothorax, and chylothorax. Therapeutic methods, including ultrasound-guided thoracentesis and the indications for chest tube drainage and pleuroscopy are discussed, as well as the use of thrombolytic therapy.

ETIOLOGY

Four types of fluid can occupy the pleural space: serous fluid (hydrothorax), blood (hemothorax), lipid (chylothorax), and pus (empyema). Once the presence of a pleural effusion is established, it is important to determine whether it is a transudate or an exudate. A transudative pleural effusion indicates the presence of a systemic process, implicating organ systems other than the lung. This transudative pleural effusion is caused by medical conditions that lead to volume overload, such as renal failure, heart failure, and hypoalbuminemia (Table 127-1). In contrast, exudative pleural effusions indicate a local pleural process and necessitate a different treatment approach (Table 127-2). In 1972, Light defined the classic criteria for distinguishing between exudative and transudative pleural effusions.[1] To qualify as an exudate, the pleural effusion must meet one of the following criteria: pleural fluid lactate dehydrogenase (LDH) greater than 200 IU/L, ratio of pleural fluid LDH to serum LDH greater then 0.6, or a ratio of pleural fluid protein to serum protein greater than 0.5 (Table 127-3). These criteria have a high sensitivity and low specificity.

Table 127-1

TRANSUDATIVE PLEURAL EFFUSIONS
Congestive heart failure
albuminemia
Cirrhosis
Urinothorax
Superior vena cava obstruction
Atelectasis
Trapped lung
Peritoneal dialysis
Nephrotic syndrome
Malignancy
Pneumonia

DIAGNOSTIC APPROACHES TO PLEURAL EFFUSIONS

Chest Radiography

The chest radiograph is usually the first diagnostic tool used for assessing a pleural effusion. An effusion that causes blunting of the costophrenic angle in the posteroanterior view usually has a fluid volume of approximately 300 mL. In many cases, decubitus films are also obtained to assess whether the effusion is free flowing or is loculated. It is equally important to look for signs of mediastinal shift. An effusion usually shifts the mediastinum to the contralateral side. When the mediastinum is shifted to the ipsilateral side, other causes are implicated, including atelectasis of the underlying lung secondary to an endobronchial lesion, fixation of the mediastinum by fibrosis, or encasement of the lung by a peel.[2]

Other Imaging Modalities

CT scanning further enhances the abnormalities imaged by chest radiography. Most important, CT scanning differentiates between pulmonary parenchymal and pleural abnormalities. The importance and role of MRI in evaluating pleural effusions are yet to be elucidated.

Ultrasound

Ultrasound has a variety of therapeutic and diagnostic uses, including the ability to image the pleural space at the bedside. It is helpful for determining the presence, size, extent, and location of the pleural effusion. It also can suggest the presence of a complicated and loculated effusion. In complicated effusions, thin echogenic bands appear in the fluid. Ultrasound also can reveal pleural-based masses, which suggest a malignant cause. Therapeutically, ultrasound is used to direct pleural fluid aspiration under visual guidance. Ultrasound guidance decreases the incidence of pneumothorax in nonventilated and ventilated patients.

Thoracentesis

Diagnostic pleural aspiration is essential to the workup. Pleural effusions in patients with congestive heart failure are not usually aspirated; however, the presence of fever or an elevated white blood cell count justifies pleural fluid sampling by means of thoracentesis. The appearance of the thoracentesis sample suggests the etiology of the effusion. The sample is often bloody in patients with trauma, cancer, pulmonary embolism, or tuberculosis. It is milky white in patients with chylothorax and empyema. A yellow-green color suggests rheumatoid pleurisy, and food particles in the pleural fluid suggest esophageal

Table 127-2

EXUDATIVE PLEURAL EFFUSIONS

INFECTIOUS	INFLAMMATORY	LYMPHATIC ABNORMALITIES
Pneumonia (bacterial and mycobacterial)	Pancreatitis	Yellow nail syndrome
Subphrenic abscesses	Radiation Hemothorax Acute respiratory distress syndrome	Lymphangioleiomyomatosis Malignant obstruction
Malignancy (primary lung or metastatic)	Immunologic disorders Lupus pleuritis Rheumatoid pleuritis Wegener granulomatosis Sarcoidosis	Increased negative intrapleural pressure Trapped lung Atelectasis

rupture. Once obtained, the pleural fluid is sent for Gram stain and culture. In addition, cell count with differential, amylase, glucose, protein, LDH, pH, and albumin determinations should to be obtained. Despite all these tests, cultures of infected pleural fluid are still negative in 40% of cases. The presence of pus, organisms, or both on pleural fluid Gram stain indicates empyema and requires drainage of the pleural space. Pleural fluid pH less than 7.2 in the setting of infection also suggests a complicated effusion that should be drained.[3] Reduced glucose (<35 mg/dL) and elevated LDH (>1000 IU/L) levels similarly support the diagnosis of a complicated effusion.

Before being considered for an elective thoracentesis, the patient must have an international normalization ratio of less than or equal to 1.5 and a platelet count of greater than or equal to 50,000 per microliter. The volume of fluid that can be aspirated safely at thoracentesis is still unknown. It is important to monitor pleural pressures as the fluid is being withdrawn and to stop drainage when the pleural pressure reaches −25 cm H_2O or if the patient complains of chest pain and discomfort because both are signs of lung entrapment. Whenever a thoracentesis is performed, however, it is important to withdraw as much fluid volume as is safely possible to avoid the necessity of a repeat procedure.

Relative contraindications to thoracentesis include a bleeding diathesis, anticoagulation, and a small pleural effusion that is difficult to tap. The most significant complication associated with the procedure is pneumothorax. Chest pain is common, occurring in up to 30% of patients, and may be a sign of an intrathoracic "vacuum" resulting from lung entrapment. Cough owing to lung expansion, hypoxemia owing to an increase in the ventilation/perfusion mismatch, vasovagal reactions, bleeding secondary to intercostal artery laceration, infection, and reexpansion pulmonary edema all have been reported as side effects and complications. A chest radiograph is not necessarily needed after a thoracentesis unless the patient is symptomatic but is essential if documentation of lung expansion is required.

Table 127-3

LIGHT CRITERIA FOR EXUDATIVE PLEURAL EFFUSIONS

Fluid/serum protein >0.5
Fluid/serum LDH >0.6
Fluid LDH >two-thirds upper limit of normal

MANAGEMENT OF SPECIFIC DISORDERS

Parapneumonic Effusions and Empyema

Definition/Natural History

Pneumonia accounts for up to 60% of pleural effusions. Most of these effusions are sterile, clear exudates that generally resolve with antibiotic treatment and rarely require tube drainage. Some (5%), however, are complicated with loculations and fibrin deposits. The fluid may be infected, as suggested by a low glucose, an elevated LDH, and a low pH. This stage of pneumonia is not thought to resolve with antibiotics alone and predisposes the patient to complications such as continued pleural sepsis and empyema.

Empyema progresses through three stages: exudative, fibrinopurulent, and organizing. In the exudative stage, the pleural fluid is nonviscous and freely flowing, with minimally inflamed pleural membranes, and the patient is likely to respond to antibiotics. The early fibrinopurulent stage is characterized by increasing viscosity of the fluid, thickening of the pleural membranes, and formations of intrapleural loculations. Patients may respond to antibiotic therapy alone but often require emptying of the pleural space. In the organized stage, more aggressive intervention is indicated, and on many occasions, the patient will require management for the pleural peel that has formed.

All patients with pleural infections should be treated with antibiotics. Depending on the clinical picture, anaerobic coverage is also included. Published guidelines are followed if the culture comes back negative.[4] In designing a specific treatment plan, it is important to recognize that antibiotics penetrate the pleural space to varying degrees. As a rule, aminoglycosides usually are avoided because of their poor pleural space penetration and weak action in an acidic environment.

Drainage Methods

In 2000, a consensus statement was published by the American College of Chest Physicians.[5] The statement proposed the following recommendations for drainage in the management of parapneumonic effusions:

1. Patients with category 1 and 2 effusions are at low risk for poor outcome and do not require drainage.
2. Drainage is recommended for the management of patients with category 3 and 4 parapneumonic effusions because of the increased risk for mortality and need for a second intervention.

3. Therapeutic thoracentesis or tube thoracostomy alone is insufficient for the management of patients with category 3 and 4 parapneumonic effusions.
4. Fibrinolysis and video-assisted thoracic surgery are acceptable approaches for these patients based on mortality and need for a second intervention.

Recurrent Nonmalignant Pleural Effusions

Data that would guide the use of pleurodesis in nonmalignant pleural effusions are scarce. There are no controlled trials comparing various agents and methods of pleurodesis in nonmalignant effusions. In two cohorts,[6,7] the authors studied the outcome of talc poudrage in patients with nonmalignant pleural effusions. Their success rate was 97% during a follow-up period of 1 to 84 months. Side effects included prolonged drainage (50%), reexpansion pulmonary edema (2%), and empyema (2%). Acute respiratory distress syndrome did not develop in any patient. From these limited data, it would appear that the success of pleurodesis in the management of nonmalignant pleural effusions is higher than one would expect. We do not recommend pleurodesis as a first-line treatment, but only after treatment of the causative disease has been fully maximized, if the patient is still experiencing symptoms attributable to the pleural effusion.

Immunologic and Connective Tissue Disorders

The effectiveness of steroid therapy in treating a variety of immunologic and connective tissue disease entities is well established. However, the data used to define the role of steroids in the management of connective tissue disease-related pleural effusions are limited to case reports and small series.

Rheumatoid Pleurisy

Pleural involvement in patients with rheumatoid arthritis is clinically evident in up to 5% of patients. These effusions are characterized by low glucose levels that develop within 5 years of articular manifestations. Once steroid treatment is instituted, the pleural effusion usually resolves within 3 to 4 months. Treatment can be systemic or intrapleural, and the response to therapy is independent of the articular inflammation. Half of these patients, unfortunately, will have a protracted course.

Lupus Pleuritis

Among the connective tissue disorders, systemic lupus erythematosis is the most common cause of pleuritis. Pleuritis in systemic lupus erythematosis presents more often in women than in men, with pleural effusions occurring in up to 30% of patients. The pleural symptoms may antedate other disease manifestations and can be bilateral, unilateral, or alternate from one side to the other. A 60- to 80-mg dose of prednisone daily produces positive results in patients with lupus-related pleural effusions.

Sarcoidosis

Pleural effusion is a rare complication of sarcoidosis. The natural history of sarcoidosis-related pleural effusions is variable; some resolve spontaneously, whereas others resolve with treatment within the same time frame. The approach to a sarcoidosis-related pleural effusion is individualized, and treatment is reserved for symptomatic patients. The dose of prednisone used is variable, ranging between 20 and 40 mg/day with a taper over 3 to 4 weeks.

Postcardiac Injury Syndrome

Postcardiac injury syndrome is an immunologic entity associated with a wide array of manifestations, including pericarditis, fever, leukocytosis, elevated sedimentation rate, pulmonary infiltrates, and pleural effusion. The syndrome can occur days, weeks, and even months after myocardial infarction, cardiac surgery, pacemaker placement, and angioplasty. It is seen more commonly after cardiac surgery, occurring in up to 30% of patients.[8] The effusion is usually treated with antiinflammatory medication and exhibits a variable time course for adequate response. Nonresponders require steroids tapered over 3 to 4 weeks.

Hepatic Hydrothorax

Hepatic hydrothorax is the term for a pleural effusion arising in a patient with cirrhosis. It is usually the result of fluid transfer from the abdomen to the pleural space via defects in the diaphragm. Most often it is right-sided, and ascitic fluid can be absent in many patients. The first-line treatment is the administration of diuretics and sodium restriction. This treatment is given to counteract ascites caused by sodium retention in the kidney. An inappropriate increase in the dose of diuretics can precipitate hepatic encephalopathy in some of these patients, a severe and life-threatening complication. Common diuretics used include spironolactone and furosemide. If these treatment regimens fail, patients may benefit from a transjugular intrahepatic portosystemic shunt procedure. Thoracentesis is reserved for symptomatic patients and patients with fever, to rule out a spontaneous bacterial empyema. Tube thoracostomy with talc pleurodesis attempts have largely been unsuccessful. This therapy can result in prolonged chest tube drainage, excessive protein loss, renal failure, infection, and severe leak at the chest tube site. Treatment failures using this approach are probably secondary to the rapid formation of fluid in the pleural space, which prevents the formation of adhesions between the visceral and parietal pleura. Pleurodesis generally is not recommended for the medical management of hepatic hydrothorax. We have used indwelling drainage catheters in patients with needs for multiple thoracenteses with an overall good success rate. Patients with hepatic hydrothorax nonresponsive to diuretic treatment constitute a difficult population, and the treatment approach must be individualized.

Hemothorax

A hemothorax is defined as bleeding in the pleural space sufficient to raise the pleural space hematocrit to 50%. Independent of cause, large-tube drainage is the primary therapy because large volumes of blood in the pleural space rapidly form intrapleural loculations and increase the risk for empyema and fibrothorax. In some patients with retained intrapleural blood, fibrinolytic agents are instilled with good results.[9] If performed early in the course of the injury, before pleural adhesions form, thoracoscopy can play an important role in the management of patients who sustain traumatic hemothorax complicated by major intrathoracic vessel injury and air leaks.

Chylothorax

Chylothorax, defined as the appearance of lymph and emulsified fat in the pleural effusion, is a rare cause of pleural effusion and is mostly owing to malignancy, thoracic surgical procedures, and chest trauma. A number of cases are associated with diseases such as lymphangioleiomyomatosis and lymphangiectasis. After the underlying cause is determined, specific treatment may be effective for managing the resulting chylothorax. The cornerstone of treatment involves nutritional intervention to prevent protein, vitamin, and lymphocyte loss. Success with a medium-chain triglyceride diet has been variable. Conservative management in a symptomatic patient involves drainage of the chylous effusion by thoracentesis or chest tube placement. Somatostatin has been used successfully in a few cases of chylous effusions refractory to chest tube drainage. Pleurodesis can be successful in the management of chylothoraces, especially if the rate of chyle flow is not high. In refractory cases, embolization and surgical interventions such as ligation, pleuroperitoneal shunting, and fibrin glue application are used.

FUTURE DIRECTIONS IN MEDICAL MANAGEMENT: VASCULAR ENDOTHELIAL GROWTH FACTOR

Knowledge concerning vascular endothelial growth factor (VEGF) and its role in pleural effusions is accumulating rapidly. Evidence gleaned in vitro and in vivo supports the role of VEGF as a potent mediator in pleural fluid accumulation. VEGF is present in large quantities in human pleural effusions[10,11] and consistently higher in exudative than in transudative effusions. VEGF receptors are expressed in pleural tissues in both normal and diseased states.[12] In animal studies,[13] pulmonary edema is induced successfully in mice by delivering VEGF DNA to the respiratory epithelium using an adenovirus vector. In parallel, these effects are abolished by pretreatment with an adenovirus vector expressing the truncated soluble form of the Flt-1 VEGF receptor. Current clinical trials using VEGF tyrosine kinase inhibitor are being conducted to evaluate its ability to prevent pleural effusion and ascites formation. Although all the in vivo studies evaluating the role of VEGF in effusion inhibition are currently being performed on patients with malignant disease, some in vitro evidence suggests that anti-VEGF antibodies decrease *Staphylococcus aureus*-induced mesothelial permeability. These findings are likely to be relevant to the future medical management of pleural effusions.

EDITOR'S COMMENT

For the thoracic surgeon, a patient with bilateral pleural effusions has a medical problem – such as cardiac, renal, or hepatic dysfunction – until proved otherwise. Occasionally, patients with mediastinal lymphatic obstruction or pericardial restriction will develop bilateral pleural effusions and will benefit from an invasive procedure; but these unusual cases require careful assessment of heart, kidney, and liver function prior to any surgical intervention.

—Steven J. Mentzer

References

1. Heffner JE. Evaluating diagnostic tests in the pleural space: differentiating transudates from exudates as a model. *Clin Chest Med.* 1998;19:277–293.
2. Sahn SA. State of the art: the pleura. *Am Rev Respir Dis.* 1988;138:184–234.
3. Heffner JE, Brown LK, Barbieri C, et al. Pleural fluid chemical analysis in parapneumonic effusions: a meta-analysis. *Am J Respir Crit Care Med.* 1995;151:1700–1708.
4. Niederman MS, Mandell LA, Anzueto A, et al. Guidelines for the management of adults with community-acquired pneumonia: diagnosis, assessment of severity, antimicrobial therapy, and prevention. *Am J Respir Crit Care Med.* 2001;163:1730–1754.
5. Colice GL, Curtis A, Deslauriers J, et al. Medical and surgical treatment of parapneumonic effusions: an evidence-based guideline. *Chest.* 2000;118:1158–1171.
6. Vargas FS, Milanez JR, Filomeno LT, et al. Intrapleural talc for the prevention of recurrence in benign or undiagnosed pleural effusions. *Chest.* 1994;106:1771–1775.
7. de Campos JR, Vargas FS, de Campos Werebe E, et al. Thoracoscopy talc poudrage: a 15-year experience. *Chest.* 2001;119:801–806.
8. Soloff LA, Zatuchni J, Janton OH, et al. Reactivation of rheumatic fever following mitral commissurotomy. *Circulation.* 1953;8:481–497.
9. Aye RW, Froese DP, Hill LD. Use of purified streptokinase in empyema and hemothorax. *Am J Surg.* 1991;161:560–562.
10. Mohammed KA, Nasreen N, Hardwick J, et al. Bacterial induction of pleural mesothelial monolayer barrier dysfunction. *Am J Physiol Lung Cell Mol Physiol.* 2001;281:L119–L125.
11. Cheng D, Rodriguez RM, Perkett EA, et al. Vascular endothelial growth factor in pleural fluid. *Chest.* 1999;116:760–765.
12. Thickett DR, Armstrong L, Millar AB. Vascular endothelial growth factor (VEGF) in inflammatory and malignant pleural effusions. *Thorax.* 1999;54:707–710.
13. Kaner RJ, Ladetto JV, Singh R, et al. Lung overexpression of the vascular endothelial growth factor gene induces pulmonary edema. *Am J Respir Cell Mol Biol.* 2000;22:657–664.

128 Pneumothorax and Pneumomediastinum

Ayesha S. Bryant and Robert James Cerfolio

Keywords: Alveolar-pleural fistula, air leak, intrapleural pressure, transpulmonary pressure, iatrogenic or traumatic injury

Pneumothorax is defined as air in the pleural space and is commonly seen after thoracic surgery. *Pneumomediastinum* is defined as air in the mediastinum and is quite rare. Despite their differences, the principles used to treat these two conditions are similar. Successful management requires a thorough understanding of the thoracic anatomy and pathophysiologic mechanisms that cause these conditions. Pneumothorax may signal a life-threatening condition, and pneumomediastinum may be a sign of an innocuous problem that requires no treatment. This chapter provides an overview of the incidence, causes, pathophysiology, symptoms, radiologic signs, diagnostic evaluation, and most importantly, the techniques for treatment of both pneumothorax and pneumomediastinum.

PNEUMOTHORAX

Pneumothorax is a collection of air or gas in the pleural space. It is classified into three subtypes: spontaneous, traumatic, and iatrogenic pneumothorax (Table 128-1). A spontaneous pneumothorax is a collection of air or gas in the chest that causes the lung to collapse. It can be further classified as primary (i.e., collapse of lung for no apparent reason) or secondary (i.e., collapse of the lung secondary to underlying pulmonary pathology), as detailed in Table 128-2. The incidence of all types of pneumothoraces is greater in men than in women. For primary pneumothorax, the incidence is 7.4 per 100,000 per year in men and 1.2 per 100,000 in women. Similarly, the incidence of secondary pneumothorax is 6.3 per 100,000 population per year in men and 2.0 per 100,000 in women. More specifically, the incidence is greatest in tall, thin young males.[1,2]

A tension pneumothorax occurs as a result of a pulmonary parenchymal or bronchial injury that acts as a one-way valve, permitting air to enter the pleural space but not escape. This causes a decrease in venous return and leads to hemodynamic compromise owing to low preload. Iatrogenic pneumothorax occurs as a consequence of inadvertent puncture of the lung during an invasive procedure.

Table 128-1

TYPES OF PNEUMOTHORACES

Spontaneous pneumothorax
Primary-no clinical lung disease
Secondary-complication of lung disease
Traumatic pneumothorax
Penetrating trauma
Blunt trauma
Iatrogenic
Transthoracic needle aspiration or biopsy
Subclavian or jugular vein catheter placement
Thoracentesis

From References 3 and 4.

PATHOPHYSIOLOGY

The lung has an inherent tendency to collapse and the chest wall to expand. Hence the pressure in the pleural space is always negative in relation to atmospheric pressure. The alveolar pressure rises and falls on inspiration and expiration but is always greater than the intrapleural pressure (Fig. 128-1A). Since air flows from an area of higher pressure to an area of lower pressure, when a fistula or air leak or other anomalous communication develops between an alveolus and the pleural space, the air flows down the pressure gradient until an equilibrium is reached or the communication is sealed (see Fig. 128-1*B*). This condition is known as a *pneumothorax*. As the lung becomes smaller, the pneumothorax increases in size. The transpulmonary pressure, also known as *elastic recoil of the lung*, is the difference between alveolar pressure and pleural pressure (Palv–Ppl). When this value equals zero, the lung collapses. The primary physiologic consequence of this process is a decrease in the vital capacity of the lung, a decrease in the partial pressure of oxygen, and if the pressure becomes great enough, compression of the superior vena cava and tension pneumothorax. Young and healthy patients can tolerate these changes fairly well, with minimal changes in vital signs and symptoms, but individuals with underlying lung disease may develop respiratory or hemodynamic distress.

Tension pneumothorax has a far more dangerous outcome. As pressure within the intrapleural space increases, the mediastinum impinges on and compresses the heart and contralateral

Table 128-2

CAUSES OF SECONDARY SPONTANEOUS PNEUMOTHORAX

Disease of airway
Chronic obstructive pulmonary disease
Cystic fibrosis
Acute asthma
Parenchymal lung infection
Pneumocystis jirovecii Pneumonia[a]
Necrotizing infection
Malignancy
Lung cancer
Sarcoma
Metastases
Interstitial lung diseases
Sarcoid
Connective tissue disease
Tuberous sclerosis
Idiopathic interstitial lung disease
Other
Thoracic endometriosis
Lymphangioleiomyomatosis

[a]Previously termed *Pneumocystis carinii.*

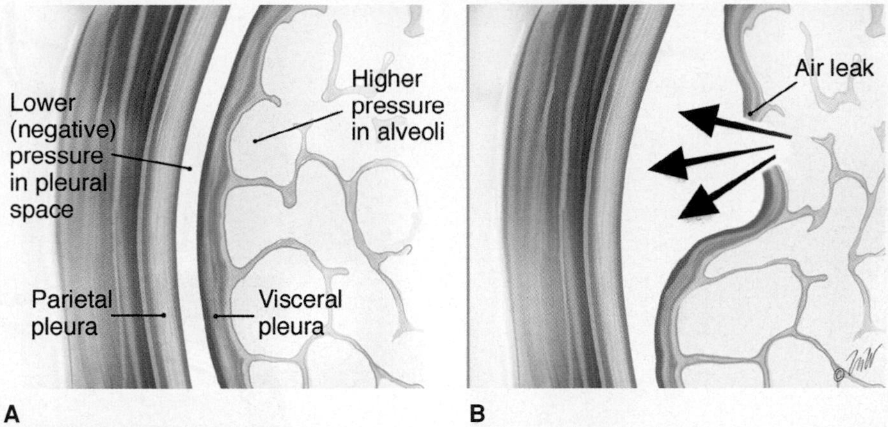

Figure 128-1. *A*. Pressure in the intrapleural space is always negative (just below atmospheric pressure) and always lower than in the alveoli of the lung. *B*. Since air flows from regions of high to low pressure, when there is an anomalous communication between the alveolar tissues and the pleura, air flows down the pressure gradient and collects in the pleural space.

lung, thus decreasing the venous return (Fig. 128-2). Hypoxia results as the collapsed lung on the affected side and the compressed lung on the contralateral side compromise effective gas exchange. The hypoxia and decreased venous return caused by compression of the relatively thin walls of the superior vena cava and atria impair cardiac function. The decrease in cardiac output results in hypotension and may lead to hemodynamic collapse and death, if untreated.

CAUSES

A spontaneous primary pneumothorax is commonly caused by rupture of subpleural apical emphysematous blebs, which are more prevalent in tall, thin males. Different mechanisms have been proposed; however, most concur that this process may occur because alveoli are subjected to a greater mean distending pressure over time, leading to subpleural bleb formation. Since pleural pressure is more negative at the apex of the lung than elsewhere, blebs located at the apex are more likely to rupture and cause pneumothorax.

Another risk factor for pneumothorax is smoking. Smoking increases the risk of spontaneous pneumothorax by 20-fold in men and by nearly 10-fold in women, as compared with similar risks in nonsmokers.[5]

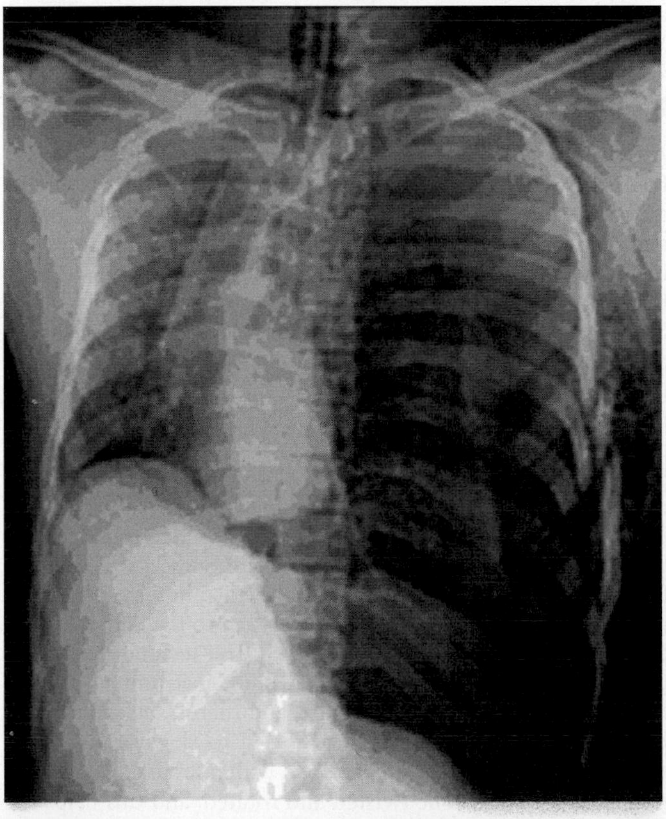

Figure 128-2. Chest x-ray of tension pneumothorax.

MANAGEMENT

The goal of treatment of pneumothorax is to remove air from the pleural space and prevent recurrence. Management depends on the symptoms and the radiologic size of the pneumothorax. Small, asymptomatic pneumothoraces may be followed with chest radiographs alone (Fig. 128-3). For larger pneumothoraces with more severe clinical symptoms and/or iatrogenic etiology, a chest tube should be inserted to protect the pleural space. If the cause is spontaneous, careful follow-up can be chosen.

SURGICAL TECHNIQUE

We prefer surgical intervention when there is persistent air leak (>3 days), large air leak (>expiratory 4[6]), failure of lung reexpansion, and in cases of recurrent spontaneous pneumothorax.[7] Other indications for surgery include a space problem with air leak or occupations that predispose to pneumothorax, such as a pilot or scuba diver. Once the decision to proceed with surgery has been made, several different approaches can be taken, either by open, or by video-assisted thoracoscopic surgery (VATS) or robotic techniques. The latter is preferred by most surgeons because it affords the use of minimally invasive techniques, which can be particularly important when operating on patients with benign disease.[8] However, newer techniques for thoracotomy have made this approach less painful with reduced morbidity. For example, open procedures can be performed using posterolateral muscle-sparing, rib-sparing,

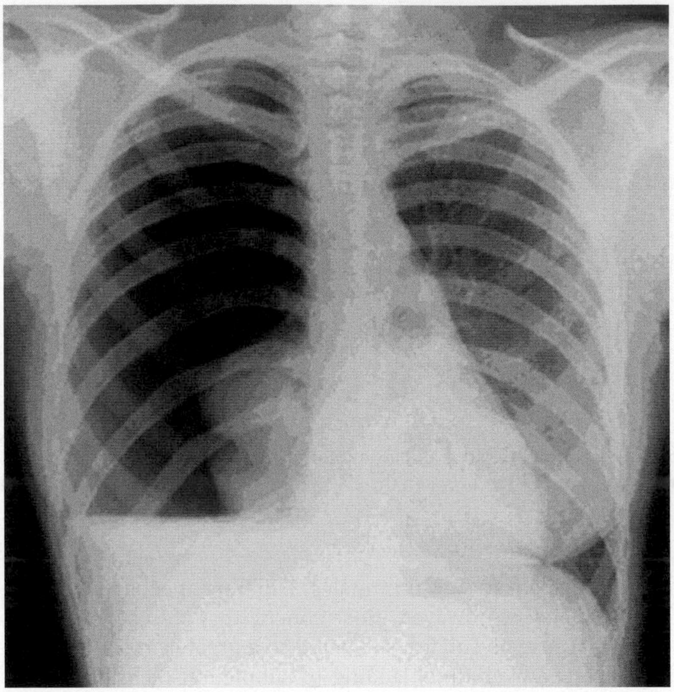

Figure 128-3. Chest x-ray of spontaneous pneumothorax.

and nerve-sparing approaches.[9,10] In addition, because this pathology requires access mainly to the upper hemithorax, axillary thoracotomy is also an option. Since VATS is by far the most common operation used for these patients, we will review the operative steps.

Minimally Invasive Techniques: Video-Assisted Thoracoscopy and Robotic Surgery

The goal of any operation in a patient with a recurrent pneumothorax is to prevent the patient from developing another symptomatic pneumothorax. Thus the conduct of the operation depends on the cause of the pneumothorax. If the patient has one large bleb, it should be resected and the staple line is buttressed with material and a sealant is also applied. Although one may not be able to prevent other parts of the lung from rupturing, the main goal is to prevent significant collapse and thus eliminate the risk of tension pneumothorax as well as shortness of breath. However, even when these goals are met, some patients still will have the sensation of an acute onset of chest pain postoperatively, and this probably signifies a small perforation in the lung. If the pleurodesis is successful, the lung will stay inflated, and the chest roentgenogram should be normal. To achieve these goals, some form of pleurodesis is usually needed. In this regard, we prefer to combine chemical with mechanical pleurodesis. In patients who have had more than one spontaneous pneumothorax every intraoperative technique should be applied to prevent further ones. This includes trying to identify the source of the air leak and removing or stapling it closed, maximizing this staple line from leaking by using buttressing material and a sealant and promoting apposition by performing a parietal pleurectomy and adding chemical pleurodesis in selected patients.

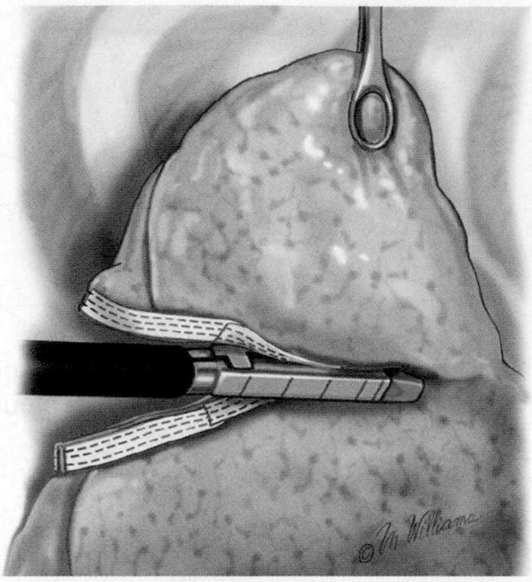

Figure 128-4. A portion of the upper lobe is resected using an endoscopic stapler buttressed with pericardial strips, which help to create adhesions.

Preoperative Care

Patients should have a chest CT scan and pulmonary function testing performed before surgery. A CT scan is ordered to assess the number and severity of blebs, if any, and to ensure there are no indeterminate pulmonary nodules. In older patients with emphysema and hypercapnia, surgery would be ill-advised if numerous large blebs are found on CT scan. These patients should be managed with a chest tube and bedside sclerotherapy. This chapter, however, focuses on the more common phenomenon of a young patient with recurrent pneumothorax. We prefer to use an epidural, even when performing a VATS procedure because the need for pleurectomy as well as mechanical and chemical pleurodesis causes it to be more painful than a VATS wedge resection.

Intraoperative Care

After the induction of general anesthesia, bronchoscopy is performed. A double-lumen endotracheal tube is placed as well as appropriate lines. The patient is positioned with operative side up, and all indwelling chest tubes are removed. Three standard VATS incisions are made. These incisions should be placed in a triangle to permit complete inspection and access to all areas of the chest. The apical segment of the upper lobe and the superior segment of the lower lobe are examined carefully. Even if a bleb cannot be located, we prefer to excise a wedge of the upper lobe and a small part of the lower lobe by using an endoscopic stapler that is buttressed with pericardial strips (Bovine Pericardial Strips, Synovis Surgical Innovations, St. Paul, MN) (Fig. 128-4). The recurrence rate after VATS by means of endoscopic stapler is less than 5%.[9] These strips help to create adhesions. A complete pleurectomy from the mammary artery to the vertebral bodies is performed. It extends from the top of the chest to the diaphragm. The pleura is scraped by attaching a Bovie scratch pad to the end of a long, curved VATS ringed forceps (Fig. 128-5). This technique creates a pleural edge that can be grasped. A blunt instrument, such as a Kittner dissector, a finger to start, and then a sucker (Ethicon Endo-Surgery, Cincinnati, OH) are used to slowly remove the entire pleura. If the pleura is grasped with a long, curved VATS ringed forceps, it can be twisted and rotated, and this helps the operator to perform a complete pleurectomy quickly, usually

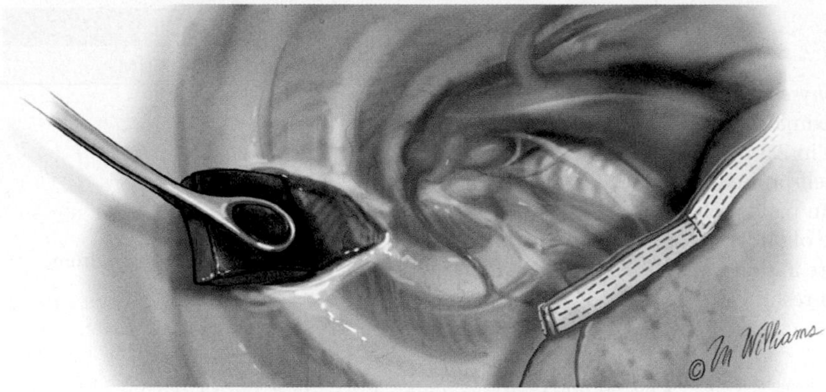

Figure 128-5. A Bovie scratch pad is used to create a pleural edge.

in 15 to 25 minutes (Fig. 128-6). After the pleurectomy is completed, we prefer to add a chemical pleurodesis as well. We do not use talc in these young patients because of some of its potential side effects. The intrapleural injection of talc has resulted in acute respiratory distress syndrome in some patients treated for malignant pleural effusion. In addition, extensive pleural thickening with calcifications can develop many years after intrapleural talc,[11] causing restriction of pulmonary function. Instead we use 500-mg doxycycline in 250-mL normal saline. The intrapleural injection of a tetracycline derivative decreases the recurrence rate for pneumothorax. In a prospective, randomized study of 229 patients with spontaneous pneumothorax, for example, the recurrence rate was 25% in the group treated with intrapleural tetracycline compared with 41% in the control group.[12] Thus we add this to our intraoperative technique. This fluid is instilled in the chest for 10 minutes and then evacuated. Two chest tubes are placed through two more anterior incisions (the most inferior port used for the camera and the most anterior port). We prefer to place two soft 24 F drains. One tube is placed anteroapically, and the other is placed posteroapically.

Postoperative Care

The chest tubes are placed on suction for a few days unless there is an air leak. Although we have written extensively about the benefits of the setting chest tubes to water seal, this applies to patients with an air leak. In patients, often with large and expansive chests, the lungs have difficulty filling this space, and thus we prefer suction. The epidural is removed on postoperative day 2 (or 3), and the patient can be discharged home on day 3 or 4. We usually send the patient home for a week or two with the anterior apical tube in place on a Heimlich valve or, more recently, connected to an Atrium Express (Atrium Medical Corporation, Hudson, NH) device. The patient returns to the outpatient clinic 1 to 2 weeks later. If the device shows no air leak and the radiograph shows no or only a minor pneumothorax, the chest tube is removed. If there is a large pneumothorax that is new, we prefer suction for another few days to help promote visceral–pleural to parietal–pleural apposition. Even if an air leak is present, the tubes can be removed safely if there is no new pneumothorax or subcutaneous emphysema.[13]

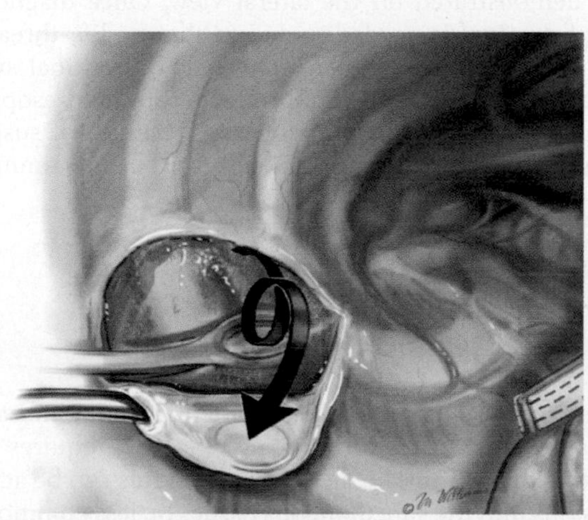

Figure 128-6. The pleural edge is grasped with a long, curved VATS ringed forceps, which is rotated and twisted as shown to facilitate the pleurectomy.

Complications

Chest tube insertion may result in empyema (1%–3%), lung parenchyma perforation (0.2%–0.6%), diaphragmatic perforation (0.4%), and subcutaneous placement (0.6%). In an analysis of 126 chest tube placements by pulmonologists at a teaching hospital, the complication rate was 11%; however, 10 of the 14 reported complications were related to clotting, kinking, or dislodgment of the chest tube.[14]

The most common short-term complication of VATS for a recurrent pneumothorax is an air leak. As described earlier, the initial treatment should be water seal, and if it persists, then outpatient management with an Atrium device is preferred. Persistent air leak commonly occurs in patients with secondary pneumothoraces. Pain is another common complaint after VATS, despite the fact that the ribs are not spread. The pain is usually secondary to impingement of the intercostal nerve. The best management is prevention. We do not use a trocar for the camera or for any of the ports. The trocar can be slipped over the camera once it is introduced into the chest. Pain can lead to inadequate ventilation of the lungs, thus promoting the incidence of atelectasis and pneumonia. Most patients have minimal postoperative discomfort; however, analgesics may be required to achieve adequate control of pain once the epidural is removed.

Recurrence of the pneumothorax is the most frequent and frustrating complication of primary spontaneous pneumothoraces; it occurs in up to 25% to 54% of untreated patients, and most recurrences occur within the first year of the first pneumothorax.[15,16] After VATS, however, the incidence is much less. After a second pneumothorax, the risk of having a third increases by more than 50%.[17] Hemorrhage related to VATS is uncommon. Arrhythmia, which is common after many thoracic procedures, should be managed as described in Chapter 8.

PNEUMOMEDIASTINUM

Pneumomediastinum (also known as *mediastinal emphysema*) is defined as air in the mediastinum. It occurs in approximately 1 per 10,000 hospital admissions per year in adults and in 2.5 per 1000 live births per year.[18] It is generally a benign, self-limited condition. Very few, if any, reports of fatal outcomes in patients with spontaneous pneumomediastinum in the absence of underlying disease exist in the recent literature. These data are in sharp contrast to tension pneumomediastinum, which often results in fatality unless there is immediate surgical intervention.

PATHOPHYSIOLOGY

Pneumomediastinum can be caused by air that originates in the pharynx, the tracheobronchial tree, or the esophagus. Excessive intraalveolar pressure, from a Valsalva type maneuver for example, can lead to rupture of perivascular alveoli (Fig. 128-7). Air escapes into the perivascular connective tissue and subsequently dissects into the mediastinum. From there, the air may dissect superiorly into the visceral, retropharyngeal, and subcutaneous spaces of the neck. From the neck, the subcutaneous compartment is continuous throughout the body; thus air can diffuse widely. Mediastinal air also can pass inferiorly into the retroperitoneum and other extraperitoneal compartments. It even can enter the pericardium and cause pneumopericardium. A study by Clements et al.[19] showed that 85% of patients developed pneumomediastinum after esophageal procedures. When it dissects throughout the body, it usually stops at the level of the inguinal ligament. If the mediastinal pressure rises abruptly, or if decompression is not sufficient, the mediastinal parietal pleura also may rupture, causing pneumothorax (in 10%–18% of patients). Table 128-3 lists the common causes of pneumomediastinum. Mihos et al.[20] have described sports that commonly lead to pneumomediastinum include scuba diving, basketball, and soccer.

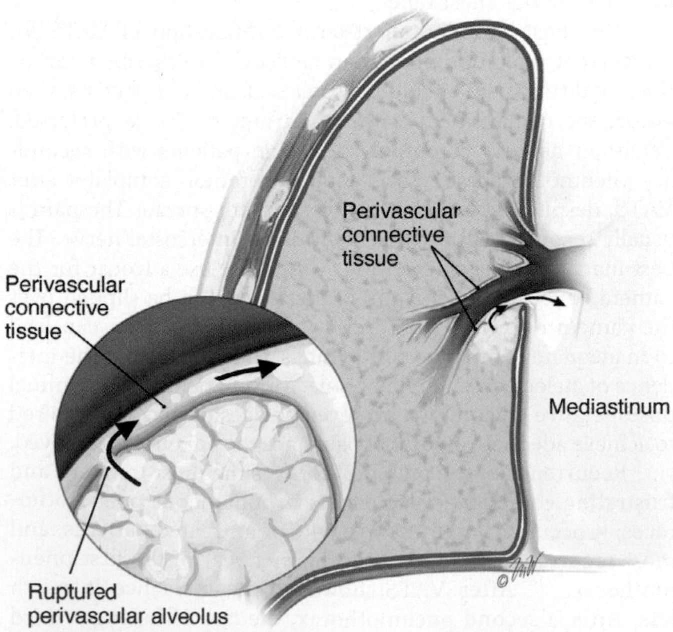

Figure 128-7. In pneumomediastinum, excessive intraalveolar pressure can lead to rupture and escape of air into perivascular connective tissues and eventually mediastinum.

Table 128-3

CAUSES OF SPONTANEOUS PNEUMOMEDIASTINUM
Increased intrathoracic pressure[21,22]
Excessive or forceful coughing
Sneezing
Vomiting
Valsalva maneuvers (childbirth, defecation)
Neonate
Gas trapping associated with neonatal respiratory distress syndrome
Use of mechanical ventilation
Aspiration of meconium or blood
Birth-related trauma
Sports or occupational hazard
Rapid altitude changes (scuba diving, skydiving, pilot)
Basketball
Soccer
Iatrogenic
Laparoscopic surgery (usually esophageal)

A more serious variant of pneumomediastinum, termed *tension pneumomediastinum* (or *malignant* by some), often mimics cardiac tamponade and should be treated immediately with cervical mediastinoscopy.[23] It arises from interference of air in the lung and mediastinum, causing compression of pulmonary and mediastinal vessels and interference with respiration by the splinting action of air in the interstitial tissue of the lung. If unrelieved, it may progress to pulmonary edema and circulatory failure.

SIGNS, SYMPTOMS, AND DIAGNOSIS

The signs and symptoms of pneumomediastinum vary from asymptomatic to severe chest pain below the sternum that may radiate to the neck and arms. Common presentation includes chest pain, subcutaneous emphysema, cough, and neck swelling.[24] The pain may be exacerbated by breathing or swallowing. On examination, subcutaneous air is present in approximately 50% of cases. Hamman sign (i.e., precordial crunching noise synchronous with heartbeat and often accentuated during expiration)[25] is also commonly present. Tension pneumomediastinum is characterized by dyspnea, cyanosis, engorged neck veins, and hypotension.

The diagnosis of pneumomediastinum can be confirmed with a chest x-ray that reveals streaky gas densities along the fascial planes of the mediastinum (Fig. 128-8). This is most clearly demonstrated on the lateral view. Once diagnosed, a thorough workup is needed to ensure that no life-threatening causes have been missed. An upper gastrointestinal swallow and a contrast chest CT scan, bronchoscopy, and esophagoscopy can be performed depending on the index of suspicion. These are all usually normal. VATS also has been recommended but, in our opinion, is rarely necessary.[26]

MANAGEMENT AND SURGICAL TECHNIQUES AND APPROACHES FOR PNEUMOMEDIASTINUM

The treatment of tension pneumomediastinum, most commonly seen in neonates on ventilators,[27] often requires urgent evacuation of air from the mediastinum.[26] This can be achieved by incisions into the subcutaneous tissues or, less commonly, by a cervical mediastinoscopy.[23] Moore et al. used a tube to drain subcutaneous air through a subxiphoid incision in neonates.

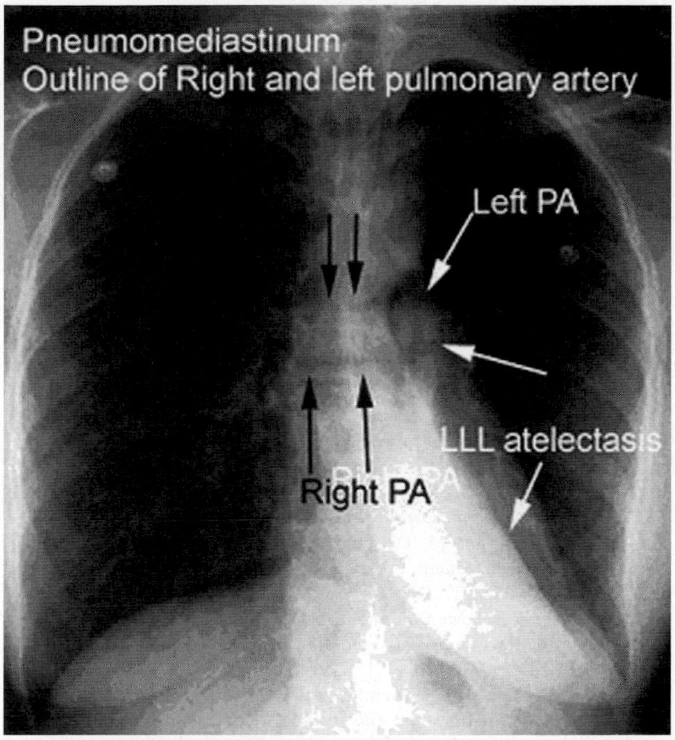

Figure 128-8. X ray of patient with pneumomediastinum showing air around the right and left pulmonary arteries.

The dissection is carried out bluntly along the entire length of the sternum, exposing the anterior mediastinum and the pericardium.[26] Other incisions also have been used for this purpose, such as the transverse suprasternal with or without full sternotomy, infraclavicular,[28] and tracheostomy.[29]

The aim of management of pneumomediastinum is to ensure that a serious underlying cause is not missed. Common causes of pneumomediastinum include asthma exacerbation, emesis, and idiopathic.[24] Most patients with a pneumomediastinum do not require surgical intervention, and in most cases, the condition resolves without intervention.[30,31] A study by Mihos et al. evaluated the treatment course of 25 cases of pneumomediastinum resulting from sports accidents. All patients were treated by observation alone. Complete resorption of the pneumomediastinum occurred in 3 to 8 days in all patients, and hospital stay ranged from 2 to 6 days (mean 3.8 days).[20,24] This experience has led some to avoid the expensive battery of usually normal diagnostic tests. Perhaps in the hemodynamically stable patient observation alone is safe as well as cost-effective.

However, once the need for surgery has been decided, the underlying cause of the pneumomediastinum dictates the surgical approach. If the cause is a ruptured bleb, the previously described approach for pneumothorax should be followed as indicated. If the cause is a perforated esophagus, the location of the tear can be revealed on upper gastrointestinal barium swallow. A posterolateral thoracotomy is performed ipsilateral to the infected effusion. Thus the empyema can be treated and the esophagus repaired. If the tear is limited to the mediastinum and does not drain into a pleural space, surgical intervention may not be needed because the tear is contained. However, if surgery is chosen, the side opposite the aortic arch (usually the right) offers better exposure and greater access to the entire length of the intrathoracic esophagus.

The goal of the operation is to drain the empyema, decorticate the lung to control the pleural space, and if possible, identify and repair the esophageal tear. Importantly, the latter is the least important goal because if there is no distal obstruction, no cancer, and no foreign body, the tear will heal on its own if there is adequate drainage of the infected surrounding space. Patients who have esophageal perforation due to instrumentation or a penetrating injury have a better prognosis than those with spontaneous perforation largely because of earlier diagnosis in the former group.[32] We prefer to identify the tear and close it primarily if the chest is entered within 48 to 72 hours of the injury, depending on the quality of the tissue. Primary repair alone is never enough. The suture line must be reinforced to reduce the risk of esophageal leaks, mediastinitis, and sepsis by buttressing with a pedicled flap.[33] We prefer an intercostal flap that should be harvested before chest retraction.[9] Other options include a diaphragmatic patch, although this has the potential to introduce infection in the subphrenic space. A pericardial fat pad is another option, but its blood supply is not reliable. A pleural flap also can be used, but it is often too thin. The postoperative care depends on the underlying cause and the treatment strategy chosen.

Recurrence of spontaneous untreated pneumomediastinum is rare, although it has been reported in a few smaller series. Abolnik et al.[34] reported a recurrence incidence of 2 in 25 patients over a 2-year period. While the physiologic mechanism of recurrence has not yet been elucidated, some attribute recurrence from a pulmonary cause to a congenital weakness of the alveolar wall.[35]

EDITOR'S COMMENT

To prevent recurrent pneumothorax, surgery must remove the source of the leak; typically a few blebs at the apex of the lung or a rare secondary site (e.g., apical portion of the superior segment). If the site of the pneumothorax is identified and removed, mechanical or chemical pleurodesis is unnecessary. Alternatively, if pleurodesis is performed without removing the source of the pneumothorax, subsequent pneumothoraces may present as basilar air collections (because effective basilar pleurodesis is unlikely with a functioning diaphragm), and these can be difficult to manage with tube thoracostomy or even thoracoscopy.

—Steven J. Mentzer

References

1. Primrose WR. Spontaneous pneumothorax: a retrospective review of aetiology, pathogenesis and management. *Scott Med J.* 1984;29:15–20.
2. Sousa C, Neves J, Sa N, et al. Spontaneous pneumothorax: a 5-year experience. *J Clin Med Res.* 2011;3:111–117.
3. Sahn SA, Heffner JE. Spontaneous pneumothorax. *N Engl J Med.* 2000;342:868–874.
4. Sharma A, Jindal P. Principles of diagnosis and management of traumatic pneumothorax. *J Emerg Trauma Shock.* 2008;1(1):34–41.
5. Bense L, Eklund G, Wiman LG. Smoking and the increased risk of contracting spontaneous pneumothorax. *Chest.* 1987;92:1009–1012.

6. Cerfolio RJ, Bass C, Katholi CR. Prospective randomized trial compares suction versus water seal for air leaks. *Ann Thorac Surg.* 2001;71:1613–1617.
7. Baumann MH, Strange C. Treatment of spontaneous pneumothorax: a more aggressive approach? *Chest.* 1997;112:789–804.
8. Ayed AK, Al-Din HJ. The results of thoracoscopic surgery for primary spontaneous pneumothorax. *Chest.* 2000;118:235–238.
9. Cerfolio RJ, Bryant AS, Patel B, et al. Intercostal muscle flap reduces the pain of thoracotomy: a prospective randomized trial. *J Thorac Cardiovasc Surg.* 2005;130:987–993.
10. Cerfolio RJ, Price TN, Bryant AS, et al. Intracostal sutures decrease the pain of thoracotomy. *Ann Thorac Surg.* 2003;76:407–411; discussion 411–412.
11. Lange P, Mortensen J, Groth S. Lung function 22–35 years after treatment of idiopathic spontaneous pneumothorax with talc poudrage or simple drainage. *Thorax.* 1988;43:559–561.
12. Light RW, O'Hara VS, Moritz TE, et al. Intrapleural tetracycline for the prevention of recurrent spontaneous pneumothorax. Results of a Department of Veterans Affairs cooperative study. *JAMA.* 1990;264:2224–2230.
13. Cerfolio RJ, Bass CS, Pask AH, et al. Predictors and treatment of persistent air leaks. *Ann Thorac Surg.* 2002;73:1727–1730; discussion 1730–1731.
14. Collop NA, Kim S, Sahn SA. Analysis of tube thoracostomy performed by pulmonologists at a teaching hospital. *Chest.* 1997;112:709–713.
15. Light R. *Pleural Diseases.* Philadelphia, PA: Williams & Wilkins; 2001.
16. Sadikot RT, Greene T, Meadows K, et al. Recurrence of primary spontaneous pneumothorax. *Thorax.* 1997;52:805–809.
17. Cran IR, Rumball CA. Survey of spontaneous pneumothoraces in the Royal Air Force. *Thorax.* 1967;22:462–465.
18. Hacking D, Stewart M. Images in clinical medicine. Neonatal pneumomediastinum. *N Engl J Med.* 2001;344:1839.
19. Clements RH, Reddy S, Holzman MD, et al. Incidence and significance of pneumomediastinum after laparoscopic esophageal surgery. *Surg Endosc.* 2000;14:553–555.
20. Mihos P, Potaris K, Gakidis I, et al. Sports-related spontaneous pneumomediastinum. *Ann Thorac Surg.* 2004;78:983–986.
21. Miguil M, Chekairi A. Pneumomediastinum and pneumothorax associated with labour. *Int J Obstet Anesth.* 2004;13:117–119.
22. Ba-Ssalamah A, Schima W, Umek W, et al. Spontaneous pneumomediastinum. *Eur Radiol.* 1999;9:724–727.
23. Beg MH, Reyazuddin, Ansari MM. Traumatic tension pneumomediastinum mimicking cardiac tamponade. *Thorax.* 1988;43:576–577.
24. Caceres M, Ali SZ, Braud R, et al. Spontaneous pneumomediastinum: a comparative study and review of the literature. *Ann Thorac Surg.* 2008;86:962–966.
25. Hamman L. Spontaneous mediastinal emphysema. *Bull Johns Hopkins Hosp.* 1939;64:1–21.
26. Moore JT, Wayne ER, Hanson J. Malignant pneumomediastinum: successful tube mediastinostomy in the neonate. *Am J Surg.* 1987;154:688–691.
27. Rosenfeld DL, Cordell CE, Jadeja N. Retrocardiac pneumomediastinum: radiographic finding and clinical implications. *Pediatrics.* 1990;85:92–97.
28. Shennib HF, Barkun AN, Matouk E, et al. Surgical decompression of a tension pneumomediastinum. A ventilatory complication of status asthmaticus. *Chest.* 1988;93:1301–1302.
29. Kirchner JA. Cervical mediastinal emphysema. *Arch Otolaryngol.* 1980;106:368–375.
30. Miura H, Taira O, Hiraguri S, et al. Clinical features of medical pneumomediastinum. *Ann Thorac Cardiovasc Surg.* 2003;9:188–191.
31. Jougon JB, Ballester M, Delcambre F, et al. Assessment of spontaneous pneumomediastinum: experience with 12 patients. *Ann Thorac Surg.* 2003;75:1711–1714.
32. Bladergroen MR, Lowe JE, Postlethwait RW. Diagnosis and recommended management of esophageal perforation and rupture. *Ann Thorac Surg.* 1986;42:235–239.
33. Wright CD, Mathisen DJ, Wain JC, et al. Reinforced primary repair of thoracic esophageal perforation. *Ann Thorac Surg.* 1995;60:245–248; discussion 248–249.
34. Abolnik I, Lossos IS, Breuer R. Spontaneous pneumomediastinum. A report of 25 cases. *Chest.* 1991;100:93–95.
35. Hamman L. Mediastinal emphysema. *JAMA.* 1945;128:1–6.

129 Benign Tumors of the Pleura

Daniel S. Oh and Ciaran McNamee

Keywords: Solitary fibrous tumors, lipomas, lipoblastomas, adenomatoid tumors, calcifying fibrous tumors

Tumors of the pleura are uncommon, and when they arise, are almost always malignant. Malignant mesothelioma and malignant pleural metastases are far more common than benign pleural tumors. Primary benign tumors of the pleura represent only 5% of all pleural tumors and include solitary fibrous tumors, lipomas and lipoblastomas, adenomatoid tumors, and calcifying fibrous tumors. Of these, solitary fibrous tumors are the most common, and will be the primary focus of this chapter. There have been fewer than a thousand cases of solitary fibrous tumor reported in the published literature since the entity was first described by Klemperer and Rabin in 1931.[1]

GENERAL PRINCIPLES

Solitary fibrous tumor has been known for many decades, but its nomenclature has evolved. In the original description in 1931, Klemperer and Rabin classified mesothelioma as either "localized" or "diffuse."[1] Since that time, solitary fibrous tumor has been previously described as "localized mesothelioma," "benign mesothelioma," "solitary fibrous mesothelioma," or "pleural fibroma." These terms reflected the incorrect assumption that they were related to malignant mesothelioma of the pleura. More recent research has shown that solitary fibrous tumors originate from mesenchymal cells in the subserosal or submesothelial layer of the pleura, not in the mesothelial layer, which is distinct from mesothelioma (Fig. 129-1).[2] Moreover, solitary fibrous tumors are not associated with asbestos exposure, further indicating a unique pathophysiologic process in the origin of these tumors.

Solitary fibrous tumors are rare. A contemporary estimate of an age-adjusted incidence indicates a rate of 0.14 per 100,000[3] in comparison to mesothelioma, which has an incidence of approximately 2 per 100,000.[4] Solitary fibrous tumors occur equally in men and women, and its incidence is highest during the fourth to seventh decades of life. It is asymptomatic in approximately half of the cases. In the other half of patients, solitary fibrous tumors can be associated with either intrathoracic or extrathoracic manifestations. Intrathoracic symptoms are related to the mass effect of the tumor itself on the lungs or chest wall, which can result in dyspnea, chest pain, or a chronic cough. Extrathoracic manifestations are paraneoplastic, and manifest as hypertrophic pulmonary osteoarthropathy or clubbing of the digits in 20% (Pierre–Marie–Bamberg syndrome), hypoglycemia in 5% (Doege–Potter syndrome), gynecomastia, or galactorrhea. Constitutional symptoms may also be present, such as fever, fatigue, and weight loss.

Solitary fibrous tumors most commonly arise on the visceral side of the pleura and are usually ovoid in shape (Figs. 129-2 and 129-3). As the name suggests, these tumors are usually isolated. The tumors usually grow in a pedunculated manner, and the pedicle can be highly vascularized. In addition, large aberrant vessels feeding into the tumor have been described. Due to the pedunculated feature, movement of the mass on x-ray with changing of the patient's position is possible.[5] Invasion of the lung is uncommon, and such tumors are described as an "inverted" solitary fibrous tumor since the bulk of the tumor is intraparenchymal in the lung.

The differential diagnosis of solitary fibrous tumor includes mesothelioma, sarcomas (synovial sarcoma, fibrosarcoma, nerve sheath sarcoma, malignant fibrous histiocytoma), and hemangiopericytoma. The histology of solitary fibrous tumors reveals their mesenchymal origin, and typically consists of a classic "patternless pattern" of whorled, dense fibrous tissue.[6] There are spindle cells mixed with collagen and elastin bundles. Cystic structures can be found within the tumor, as can calcification. Immunohistochemistry can be useful to distinguish them from mesothelioma, as routine histology may not give a definitive diagnosis. Staining characteristics of solitary fibrous tumor include positive staining for vimentin, CD34, and bcl-2, while being negative for keratin.[7]

There is a subset of solitary fibrous tumors that are malignant, but it is difficult to determine this preoperatively. Preoperative needle biopsy usually is not helpful in most cases due to the heterogeneous cellularity of the tumor. Approximately 12% of solitary fibrous tumors are malignant.[2] Furthermore, some tumors contain a mixture of benign and malignant components, indicating that malignant degeneration is possible in

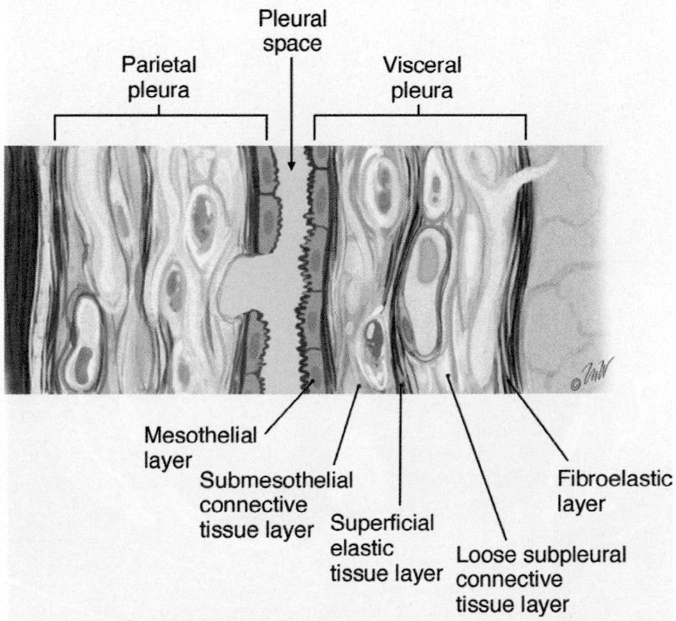

Figure 129-1. Five layers of the pleural membrane: mesothelial layer, submesothelial connective tissue layer, superficial elastic tissue layer, loose subpleural connective tissue layer, and fibroelastic layer.

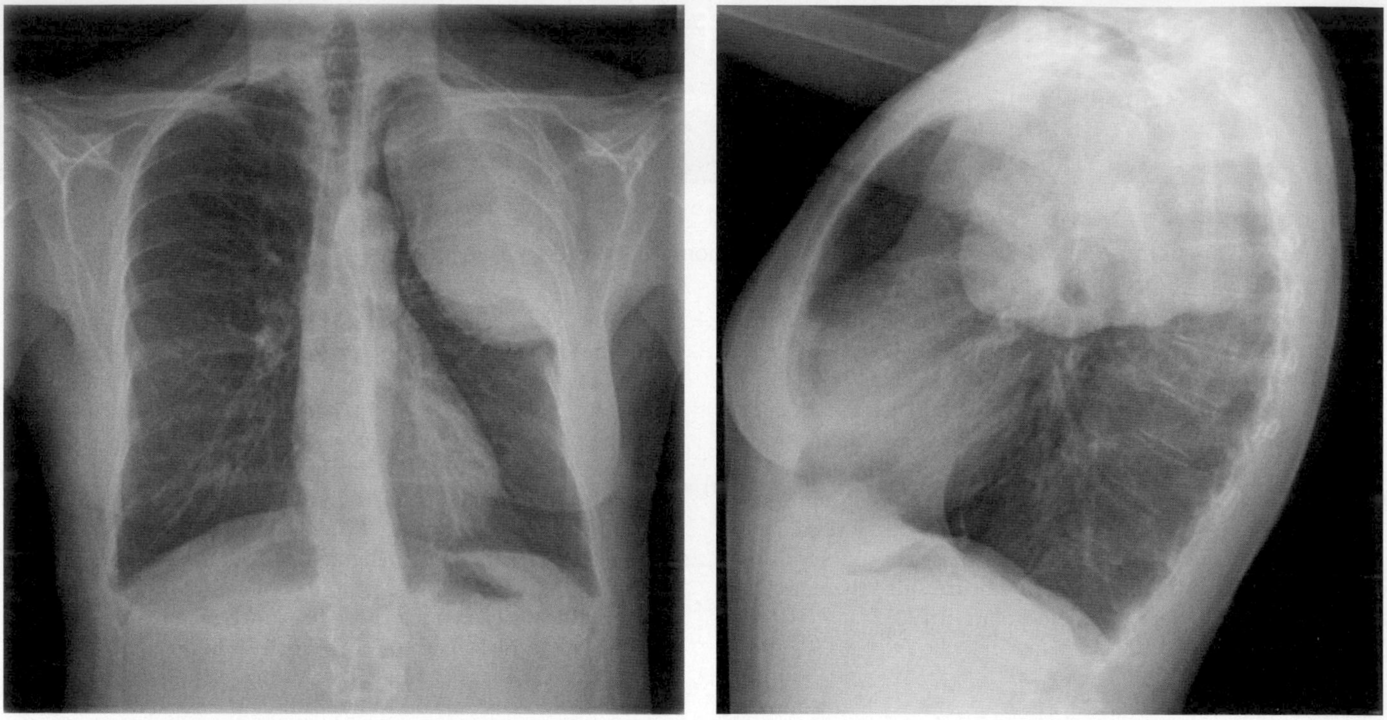

A B

Figure 129-2. Chest x-ray of patient with solitary fibrous tumor of the pleura. Posteroanterior (*A*) and lateral (*B*) chest x-rays. (Courtesy of Dr. Daniel Cohen.)

the natural history of the disease.[7] There are some radiographic criteria that can help distinguish benign and malignant cases of solitary fibrous tumors. Malignant tumors are typically >10 cm, have heterogeneous low attenuation regions of necrosis, hemorrhage, cysts, or myxoid degeneration, and are associated with pleural or pulmonary metastases.[8] Due to their larger size, malignant tumors are more likely to present with symptoms than benign tumors.[6] PET/CT has not generally been found to be helpful for identifying malignant tumors. In one series the positive predictive value was 50% and the negative predictive value was 87.5%.[9]

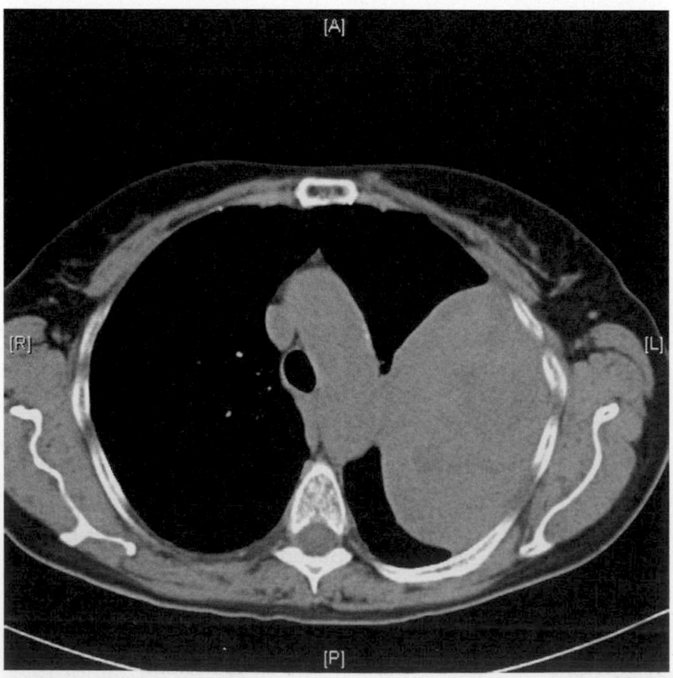

Figure 129-3. CT scan of solitary fibrous tumor of the pleura. Same patient as shown in Figure 129-2. (Courtesy of Dr. Daniel Cohen.)

England et al.[6] provided a histological means of distinguishing benign from malignant solitary fibrous tumors in their landmark 1981 publication, and these criteria continue to be used today. Criteria for malignancy include (1) high mitotic rate >4 mitoses per 10 HPF; (2) high cellularity with crowding and overlapping nuclei; (3) presence of necrosis; and (4) pleomorphism. If any of these four characteristics are present in the tumor, it is classified as malignant. Immunohistochemistry has been attempted to help clarify benign from malignant cases of solitary fibrous tumor, but at this time there is no reliable marker for this purpose. Some malignant tumors lose CD34 staining but always retain bcl-2 positive staining. Ki-67 or proliferating cell nuclear antigen (PCNA) have been examined for distinguishing malignant from benign tumors, but no distinct threshold has been determined.[7] The limitations of this method have been the relative subjectivity of interpreting immunohistochemistry slides and the heterogeneous nature of the tumors, with unequal distribution of cellularity.

De Perrot et al.[7] have further classified solitary fibrous tumors with respect to their malignant potential by categorizing them into four distinct clinical stages (Table 129-1). This system was developed to stratify the risk of recurrence for prognosis based on 185 cases published in the literature. Tumors are classified as either benign or malignant, and either sessile or pedunculated. For benign solitary fibrous tumors,

Table 129-1

DE PERROT CLASSIFICATION OF SOLITARY FIBROUS TUMORS OF THE PLEURA[7]

Stage 0	Benign pedunculated tumor
Stage I	Benign sessile or "inverted" tumor
Stage II	Malignant pedunculated tumor
Stage III	Malignant sessile or "inverted" tumor
Stage IV	Multiple synchronous malignant tumors

there is little prognostic difference in whether the tumor is pedunculated or sessile, with long term survival being 98% versus 92%, respectively. However, for malignant tumors, a pedunculated growth pattern was associated with much better prognosis, with long-term survival being 86% as compared to 37% for sessile tumors. Recurrence occurred in 2% of benign pedunculated tumors, 8% of benign sessile tumors, 14% of malignant pedunculated tumors, and 63% of malignant sessile tumors. Most recurrences occur in the first 24 months following resection. Size has not been shown to be an independent predictor of recurrence.

PREOPERATIVE ASSESSMENT

The preoperative assessment of patients with such tumors is similar to many other thoracic patients. Assessment of pulmonary function should be considered when lung resection is contemplated for tumors arising from the visceral pleura, and is mandatory if an inverted tumor necessitates a formal lobectomy for complete resection. Imaging studies typically consist of a CT scan with intravenous contrast. MRI is often useful in distinguishing soft tissue planes for involvement of the lung and assessing involvement of the chest wall or diaphragm. Preoperative biopsies are helpful when present but not required, as it is common to obtain a paucicellular specimen that is not fully informative. Very large tumors have been found to have significant vascular collaterals, and some have advocated preoperative embolization in these instances to minimize intraoperative blood loss since visualization is often poor during resection.[10–12]

TREATMENT

Complete surgical resection is the mainstay of therapy for solitary fibrous tumor of the pleura. A margin of 1 to 2 cm is recommended with en bloc resection of any involved structures. Pedunculated tumors arising from the lung may include a wedge resection of the lung, but sessile or "inverted" tumors may require lobectomy. Extrapleural dissection may be necessary to resect tumors adherent to the parietal pleura, and chest wall resection is warranted if invasion is encountered. A mediastinal lymph node dissection should be done if the tumor is determined to be malignant, as nodal metastases have been reported.[6] While a minimally invasive approach using video-assisted thoracoscopic surgery (VATS) is possible, often the tumors are too large to remove in this manner and a thoracotomy is required. Resolution of paraneoplastic hypoglycemia (Doege–Potter syndrome) and hypertrophic osteoarthropathy (Pierre–Marie–Bamberg syndrome) can be expected with complete resection.[13]

There is no standardized systemic therapy for the treatment of solitary fibrous tumor. A recent report identified the potential use of imatinib, and PDGFR pathway inhibitor, on tumors that overexpress PDGFR.[14] However, at this time there is no widely accepted or conventional adjuvant therapy for the management of this tumor. Adjuvant chemotherapy and/or radiation can be considered on an individual basis. Following resection, surveillance radiographs are recommended for both benign and malignant solitary fibrous tumors, particularly in the first 24 to 36 months.

EDITOR'S COMMENT

Benign pleural tumors are the exception, along with some breast and uterine tumors, to the general notion that large tumors are malignant. Large smooth-walled tumors in the pleura may only require complete excision to prevent recurrence. Pleural tumors also challenge the notion of what constitutes a "benign" tumor. Although the genetic signature of pleural tumors is likely to provide more detailed insight into potential biologic behavior, our current level of understanding is limited to counting mitoses to estimate the likelihood of local or distant recurrence.

—Steven J. Mentzer

References

1. Klemperer P, Rabin CB. Primary neoplasms of the pleura. *Arch Pathol.* 1931;11:385–412.
2. Briselli M, Mark EJ, Dickersin GR. Solitary fibrous tumors of the pleura: eight new cases and review of 360 cases in the literature. *Cancer.* 1981;47:2678–2689.
3. Thorgeirsson T, Isaksson HJ, Hardardottir H, et al. Solitary fibrous tumors of the pleura: an estimation of population incidence. *Chest.* 2010;137:1005–1006.
4. Weill H, Hughes JM, Churg AM. Changing trends in US mesothelioma incidence. *Occup Environ Med.* 2004;61:438–441.
5. Karabulut N, Goodman LR. Pedunculated solitary fibrous tumor of the interlobar fissure: a wandering chest mass. *Am J Roentgenol.* 1999;173:476–477.
6. England DM, Hochholzer L, McCarthy MJ. Localized benign and malignant fibrous tumors of the pleura: a clinicopathologic review of 223 cases. *Am J Surg Pathol.* 1989;13:640–658.
7. de Perrot M, Fischer S, Brundler M-A, et al. Solitary fibrous tumors of the pleura. *Ann Thorac Surg.* 2002;74:285–293.
8. Song SW, Jung JI, Lee KY, et al. Malignant soiltary fibrous tumor of the pleura: computed tomography-pathological correlation and comparison with computed tomography of benign solitary fibrous tumor of the pleura. *Jpn J Radiol.* 2010;28:602–608.
9. Cardillo G, Carbone L, Carleo F, et al. Solitary fibrous tumors of the pleura: an analysis of 110 patients treated in a single institution. *Ann Thorac Surg.* 2009;88:1632–1637.
10. Palleschi A, Cioffi U, De Simone M, et al. Preoperative embolization for giant thoracic masses. *Interact Cardiovasc Thorac Surg.* 2011;12: 1063–1065.
11. Guo J, Chu Z, Sun Y, et al. Giant solitary fibrous tumor of the pleura: an analysis of five patients. *World J Surg.* 2010;34:2553–2557.
12. Trivino A, Cozar F, Congregardo M, et al. Giant solitary fibrous tumor of the pleura. *Interact Cardiovasc Thorac Surg.* 2011;12:1063–1065.
13. Kalebi AY, Hale MJ, Wong ML, et al. Surgically cured hypoglycemia secondary to pleural solitary fibrous tumor: case report and update review on the Doege-Potter syndrome. *J Cardiothorac Surg.* 2009;4:45–53.
14. Prunotto M, Bosco M, Daniele L, et al. Imatinib inhibits in vitro proliferation of cells derived from a pleural solitary fibrous tumor expressing platelet-derived growth factor receptor-beta. *Lung Cancer.* 2009;64:244–246.

130 Management of Acute Bronchopleural Fistula

Phillip C. Camp Jr. and Steven J. Mentzer

Keywords: Postpneumonectomy empyema, tumor necrosis, lung abscess, necrotizing pneumonia, bacterial, mycobacterial, or fungal infection

There are two types of communications that can develop between the lung parenchyma and the pleural space. Communications that develop in the peripheral lung, typically beyond the cartilaginous airways, are commonly referred to as peripheral air leaks. Peripheral communications generally demonstrate respiratory (phasic) variation in the magnitude of the air leak and will heal with time. In contrast, a communication with the cartilaginous airways is referred to as a bronchopleural fistula (BPF). BPFs are associated with a relatively larger communication. Negative-pressure external drainage usually demonstrates a continuous (nonphasic) air leak. Acute BPF, or communications with proximal airways, frequently require therapeutic intervention.

The etiology of acute BPF may be classified as infectious, malignant, traumatic, iatrogenic, and idiopathic (Table 130-1). The most common types of BPFs are associated with the complications of pulmonary resections. The surgical techniques for managing these problems are described in Chapter 82. The medical management of nonmalignant BPF is discussed in Chapter 127. This chapter summarizes the acute management options for benign BPF.

ACUTE MANAGEMENT

The acute surgical management of BPF depends not only on the etiology but also on the clinical presentation. In general, the main tenets of therapy are (1) the treatment of any systemic infection, (2) drainage of any infected fluid, (3) reexpansion of the lung to eliminate residual pleural space, and (4) treatment of the underlying cause. Specific management is discussed according to etiology.

Nonresectional Benign BPF

The most common nonsurgical etiology for BPF is infection. BPF may be a complicating factor in necrotizing pneumonia or a lung abscess. A variety of bacterial, mycobacterial, and fungal infections have been implicated in benign BPF. Clues to the development of a lung abscess with proximal airway communication include an intractable cough, fever, weight loss, and failure to thrive.[1] Clinical presentation may range from a productive cough to frank sepsis. A pneumothorax may be present as well; however, the presence of intrapleural air does not distinguish between a proximal and peripheral communication. Regardless of the site of communication, the initial management involves the drainage of the pleural space with a chest tube, broad-spectrum antibiotics to treat the underlying infection, and chest physiotherapy to aid drainage. Culture of the drainage fluid permits targeted antibiotic therapy. Surgical intervention is rarely indicated.

Table 130-1

ETIOLOGIES OF ACUTE BPF

Postresectional
Pneumonectomy
Lobectomy
Infectious
Malignant
Traumatic
Other
Bullous disease
Radiation
Acute respiratory distress syndrome
Idiopathic

Malignant BPF is generally the result of the necrosis associated with large tumors in the chest. These may be primary lung carcinomas or metastatic cancers such as sarcomas. Patients may experience shortness of breath as a result of a pneumothorax. Management includes insertion of a chest tube to treat the pneumothorax and bronchoscopy to evaluate the proximal airways. Depending on the stage and location of the tumor, resection may be an option, but usually malignant BPF is associated with advanced disease.

Both penetrating and blunt chest trauma may result in a BPF. Laceration of the peripheral pulmonary parenchyma can be frequently managed by chest tube drainage alone. Failure to reexpand the lung after insertion of chest tubes, particularly in the presence of a continuous (nonphasic) air leak, is an indication for bronchoscopy and possible surgery. Injury to the proximal airway may necessitate thoracotomy with primary repair.

An air leak may be associated with radiation therapy, rupture of bullae, or positive-pressure ventilation. The accumulation of intrapleural air is an indication for insertion of a chest tube. A small leak that rapidly resolves does not require further intervention. A large or continuous air leak may require bronchoscopy to evaluate the proximal airways. In patients on mechanical ventilation for acute respiratory distress syndrome, a number of treatment options have been suggested, including jet ventilation and conventional ventilatory settings.[2]

Postresectional Benign BPF

Incidence

With improved surgical technique and understanding of bronchial healing, the incidence of BPF after pulmonary resection has decreased dramatically over the past several decades.[3] The incidence of BPF ranges from 1.5% to 11.1% after pneumonectomy and 1.5% to 2% after lobectomy. Mortality from BPF has been reported to range from 25% to 71% in the literature.

Risk Factors

Based on univariate and multivariate analyses, several variables have been associated with an increased risk of developing BPF. These factors include advanced age, previous chemotherapy and radiation, postoperative mechanical ventilation, pneumonectomy, and right-sided procedures. Algar et al.[4] studied 242 patients who underwent pneumonectomy for lung cancer. The incidence of BPF was 5.4%. Univariate analysis identified chronic obstructive pulmonary disease, hyperglycemia, hypoalbuminemia, previous steroid use, poor predicted postoperative forced expiratory volume in 1 second (ppo FEV_1), long bronchial stumps, and mechanical ventilation as risk factors. Multiple logistic regression modeling identified bronchial stump coverage, bronchus length, the side of the procedure, ppo FEV_1, chronic obstructive pulmonary disease, and mechanical ventilation as variables influencing the development of BPF.

In a study of 767 patients undergoing lobectomy, 12 (1.6%) developed BPF. Five of twelve (41.7%) died as a result of the BPF. Multivariate analysis identified squamous cell carcinoma, preoperative chemotherapy, lower lobectomy, and middle/lower lobectomy as risk factors for BPF.[5]

Clinical Presentation

The clinical presentation of a patient with a postresectional BPF may range from subtle symptoms of dry cough to fulminant sepsis. BPFs occur most commonly 8 to 12 days postoperatively,[6] although they can be apparent by the first or second postoperative day to several years later.[7]

After pneumonectomy, the pleural space will fill with fluid. A decrease in the fluid level in the postoperative period should raise suspicion for a BPF. Some patients will complain of a dry, nonproductive, persistent cough. Other patients will produce rust-colored sputum reflecting old blood from the postpneumonectomy space. The development of pulmonary consolidation and infiltrate on the contralateral side is also consistent with aspiration of pleural fluid into the remaining lung and should raise the suspicion of a BPF. Symptoms of failure to thrive (e.g., malaise, weight loss, and decreased energy) may be the only complaints of a patient with a BPF. Finally, signs and symptoms of sepsis due to empyema also may be present.

Diagnosis

In a patient with suspected BPF after pneumonectomy, the first step is to rule out empyema by thoracentesis under sterile conditions. Patient positioning is crucial to avoid contamination of the "good" lung. If a stat Gram stain on the pleural fluid is positive or the fluid is grossly suspicious for infection, a chest tube should be inserted immediately to drain the postpneumonectomy space and prevent contamination of the contralateral lung. Broad-spectrum antibiotics should be started until culture and sensitivity results are available.

The patient then should be taken to the OR, where a bronchoscopy should be performed. The bronchial stump should be examined for good apposition of the cartilaginous and membranous walls. A defect may or may not be visible. The length of the bronchial stump also should be noted. If a defect is not identified, there are several maneuvers that can help to identify a fistula. First, saline can be inserted, submerging the staple or suture line. Then air can be inserted via the chest tube in the pleural space and the staple or suture line observed for air bubbling. Others have described instillation of tracer dyes, such as methylene blue, through the bronchoscopy and detection in the chest tube, indicating a BPF.

CT scanning may have a role in the diagnosis and certainly in the evaluation of a peripheral BPF.[8] A ventilation/perfusion scan also may be a helpful noninvasive test, especially in a patient with subacute presentation of failure to thrive.

Treatment

The choice of management depends on the timing and presentation. A BPF diagnosed within the first 48 hours following lobectomy or pneumonectomy is caused by a technical error. The bronchial stump generally should be revised unless very small and amenable to endoscopic treatment. Endoscopic treatment with the use of fibrin glue, cyanoacrylate glue, cellulose, Gelfoam, silver nitrate, and coils has been reported with varying degrees of success. Stents also have been used with some success. For BPF diagnosed beyond 48 hours, traditional teaching has advocated drainage alone. Once the pleural space infection has resolved, the bronchial stump should heal. Wright et al.[3] have suggested that all BPFs occurring within 1 month with minimal pleural contamination should be revised. Most would recommend buttress of the stump with pericardium, thymic fat pad, omentum, or muscle flap. The use of omentum is thought to enhance vascularity and provide fibroblasts to aid in healing. Other options include thoracoplasty and Clagett window. These procedures are discussed in Chapter 82. The application of vacuum-assisted closure (VAC) as an alternative to open window sterilization has recently been reported and was noted to reduce both hospital stay and costs in a patient with acute postpneumonectomy empyema complicated by BPF.[9]

SUMMARY

Acute BPF remains a difficult problem to manage. Optimal therapy depends on specific cause and clinical presentation. Early detection and diagnosis are crucial for successful treatment and satisfactory outcome.

ACKNOWLEDGMENT

The authors wish to acknowledge Aneil A. Mujoomdar who contributed to this chapter in the first edition.

EDITOR'S COMMENT

Postpneumonectomy BPFs are notably life-threatening in two settings: (1) prior to diagnosis and (2) during positive-pressure ventilation. The unrecognized fistula may only produce brown-colored sputum prior to sudden and life-threatening contamination of the contralateral lung. The potential for contralateral pneumonia is the reason that the cavity must be drained urgently. Also, a large proximal fistula will decompress the airways and preclude effective positive-pressure ventilation. General anesthesia can be used, but with either spontaneous ventilation or an occlusive packing (e.g., mineral oil-soaked gauze) in the pneumonectomy space.

—Steven J. Mentzer

References

1. Frytak S, Lee RE, Pairolero PC, et al. Necrotic lung and bronchopleural fistula as complications of therapy in lung cancer. *Cancer Invest.* 1988;6:139–143.
2. Baumann MH, Sahn SA. Medical management and therapy of bronchopleural fistulas in the mechanically ventilated patient. *Chest.* 1990;97:721–728.
3. Wright CD, Wain JC, Mathisen DJ, et al. Postpneumonectomy bronchopleural fistula after sutured bronchial closure: incidence, risk factors, and management. *J Thorac Cardiovasc Surg.* 1996;112:1367–1371.
4. Algar FJ, Alvarez A, Aranda JL, et al. Prediction of early bronchopleural fistula after pneumonectomy: a multivariate analysis. *Ann Thorac Surg.* 2001;72:1662–1667.
5. Nagahiro I, Aoe M, Sano Y, et al. Bronchopleural fistula after lobectomy for lung cancer. *Asian Cardiovasc Thorac Ann.* 2007;15:45–48.
6. Lois M, Noppen M. Bronchopleural fistulas: an overview of the problem with special focus on endoscopic management. *Chest.* 2005;128:3955–3965.
7. Hollaus PH, Lax F, el-Nashef BB, et al. Natural history of bronchopleural fistula after pneumonectomy: a review of 96 cases. *Ann Thorac Surg.* 1997;63:1391–1396.
8. Stern EJ, Sun H, Haramati LB. Peripheral bronchopleural fistulas: CT imaging features. *AJR Am J Roentgenol.* 1996;167:117–120.
9. Han WS, Kim K. Acute postpneumonectomy empyema with bronchopleural fistula treated with vacuum-assisted closure device. *Korean J Thorac Cardiovasc Surg.* 2012;45:260–262.

131 Percutaneous Therapy for Traumatic Chylothorax

Matthew P. Schenker and Richard A. Baum

Keywords: Thoracic duct, cisterna chyli, lymphangiogram, lymphatic puncture, percutaneous embolization

Iatrogenic disruption of the thoracic duct is an uncommon but potentially serious complication of thoracic surgery, particularly esophagectomy.[1] The thoracic duct conveys chyle and lymph from the liver, intestines, abdominal wall, and lower extremities into the systemic venous circulation, and depending on diet and activity, the flow of chyle through the thoracic duct can reach several liters per day.[2] Among other components, this fluid contains essential proteins, lipids, and lymphocytes. The clinical sequelae of unremitting chylous effusions can be severe and life-threatening, including immunosuppression, respiratory compromise, dehydration, cachexia, and death.

Conservative management of chylous pleural effusions includes chest tube drainage, cessation of oral intake, and institution of total parenteral nutrition to decrease the physiologic production of chyle. If lymph production can be minimized, low-output leaks of less than 500 mL per day can sometimes heal spontaneously, although this process may take several weeks, during which time the patient may become nutritionally and immunologically depleted. As a result, some have called for earlier diagnosis and intervention to avoid metabolic compromise.[3,4] Repeat thoracotomy and direct thoracic duct ligation typically are performed early to stop high-output leaks; however, the morbidity and mortality of reoperation in this patient population is a serious consideration, with complication rates approaching 40%.[5]

Recently, percutaneous thoracic duct embolization (TDE) has been introduced as a minimally invasive technique for controlling high-output chylothorax (Fig. 131-1).[6] In this chapter, we review the indications, preprocedural assessment, and techniques of percutaneous TDE.

GENERAL PRINCIPLES

The method of TDE for the control of chylothorax requires a comprehensive understanding of the anatomy of the lymphatic system, especially of the thoracic duct and cisterna chyli and their many anatomical variations. TDE is a two-stage procedure, beginning with pedal lymphangiography which is used to visualize the cisterna chyli or dominant upper lumbar lymphatics for possible cannulation. Alternatively, pelvic intranodal lymphangiography can be employed. Once a suitable retroperitoneal target has been identified, the thoracic duct is accessed percutaneously and embolized, typically from a right anterior oblique transabdominal approach to avoid the aorta, or a right posterior oblique transhepatic approach. If the thoracic duct cannot be cannulated, maceration of the cisterna chyli and upper lumbar lymphatics is undertaken to divert the flow of chyle into the retroperitoneum. One variation of TDE entails retrograde cannulation of the thoracic duct via its ostium near the left angulus venosus, using a coaxial catheter system delivered from a left brachial or basilic vein approach. The retrograde transvenous approach is less reliable, however, owing to the difficulties encountered in locating and seating a catheter in the ostium of the thoracic duct under fluoroscopy and the complexity of passing a wire and microcatheter through its competent terminal valves.

PATIENT SELECTION

The primary indication for TDE is an incessant chylous pleural effusion arising in the setting of suspected traumatic thoracic duct disruption. TDE is generally ineffective for managing nontraumatic chylothorax secondary to infiltrative, obstructive, or malignant disease. True chylous effusions must also be distinguished from pseudochylous effusions, which can result from tuberculosis or rheumatoid disease. A true chylous effusion will contain chylomicrons and exhibit triglyceride levels greater than 110 mg/dL, whereas a pseudochylous effusion will have cholesterol as the dominant lipid component (greater than 200 mg/dL) and chylomicrons will be absent.[7,8]

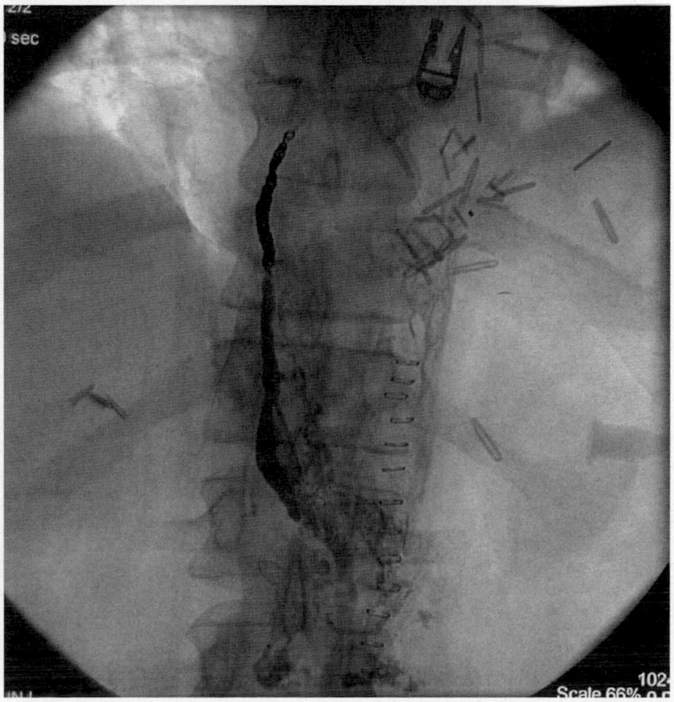

Figure 131-1. An anteroposterior radiograph of the upper abdomen in a patient who has undergone TDE shows coils and radiopaque glue in the thoracic duct.

PREOPERATIVE ASSESSMENT

Preoperative imaging is critical to determining the safest approach because of the close proximity of the cisterna chyli to the right renal artery and aorta. Thin-slice, fat-suppressed, heavily T2-weighted MR imaging of the thoracolumbar region in the coronal and axial planes is used to localize the cisterna chyli and determine its relationship to adjacent structures (Fig. 131-2A). It is also important for the patient to have a normal coagulation profile because the needle will traverse many abdominal and retroperitoneal structures on the way to its periaortic target.

TECHNIQUE

TDE is a 4- to 6-hour event and can be separated into two distinct procedures. A lymphangiogram is performed first to visualize the thoracic duct (see Fig. 131-2B). Once opacified, the thoracic duct is cannulated and embolized. The transit time for oil-based contrast material to travel from the dorsal foot (i.e., lymphangiogram site) to the upper abdomen is extremely variable and is the rate-limiting step for the procedure.

Pedal Lymphangiography

The patient is positioned supine on a fluoroscopy table, and both feet are sterilely prepped. Moderate procedural sedation is employed for patient comfort. Prophylactic intravenous antibiotics are administered.

Because the cisterna chyli is more commonly located in the right upper abdomen, right pedal lymphangiography generally provides for more efficient and definitive opacification of this structure, but either or both feet may be used. Standard pedal lymphangiography is performed by injecting 0.25 to 0.5 mL of methylene blue dye between the web spaces of the toes. The dye is taken up by the lymphatics, which can be visualized as blue streaks under the skin. After 1% lidocaine local anesthesia, a small incision is made on the dorsum of the foot, and a lymphatic vessel is isolated and cannulated with a 30-gauge needle lymphography catheter. The lymphatic is secured to the needle with silk ties, and a gentle test injection is performed with a 3-mL saline syringe to assess for leaks. The lymphography catheter is then connected to an injector, and iodized oil (Lipiodol, Laboratoire André Guerbet, Aulnay-sous-Bois, France) is infused at a rate of 8 to 12 mL per hour to a maximal administered volume of 20 mL. During infusion, serial spot radiographs are obtained of the lower extremity, pelvis, and abdomen to track the cephalad opacification of the lymphatic system (Fig. 131-3). Transit times from the foot to the cisterna chyli are typically 1 to 3 hours. A saline bolus can be administered behind the column of iodized oil, if necessary, to speed its transit through the lymphatics. Once the thoracic duct is visualized, the infusion can be stopped and attention turned to the cisterna chyli and/or dominant lumbar lymphatics for needle cannulation or disruption. The foot incision is

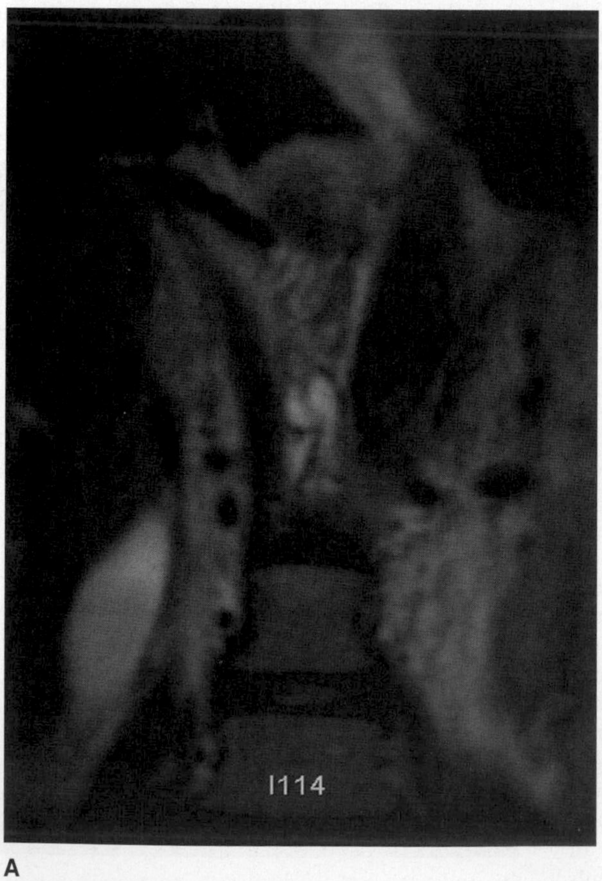

A

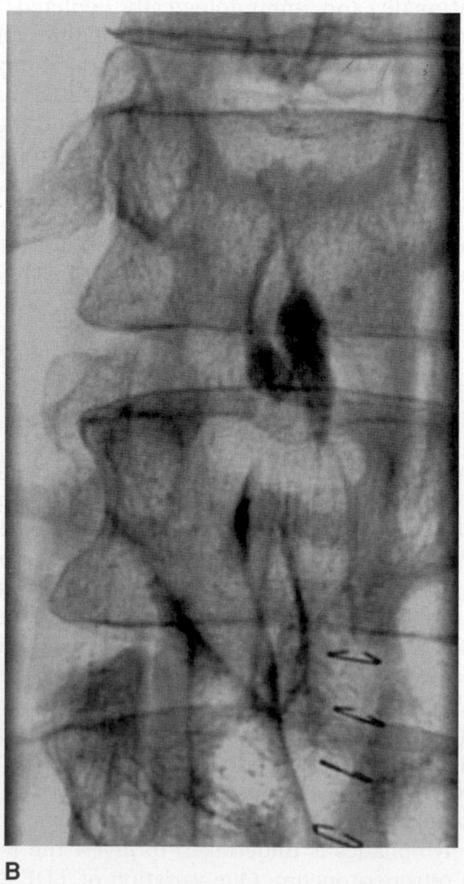

B

Figure 131-2. *A.* A coronal T2-weighted MR image shows the cisterna chyli just anterior to the spine. *B.* Lymphangiography in the same patient shows excellent correlation with the preoperative MRI.

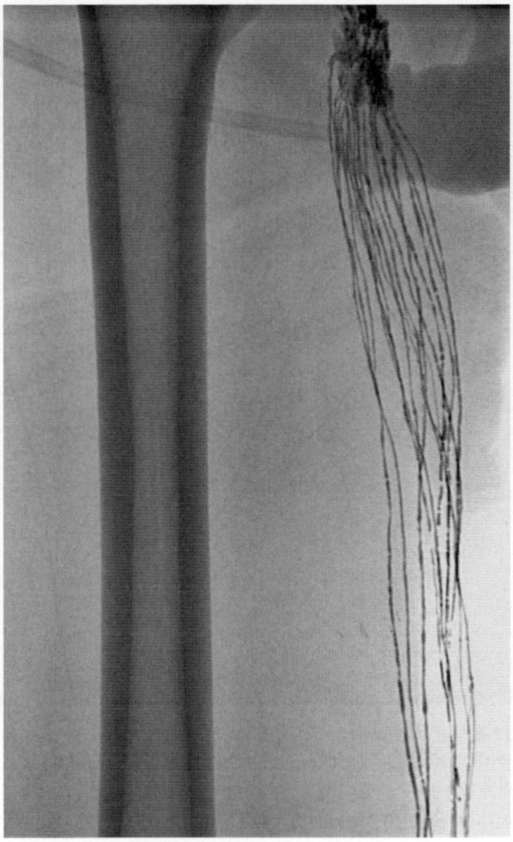

Figure 131-3. An anteroposterior radiograph of the right thigh in a patient undergoing pedal lymphangiography shows multiple lymphatic channels. The transit time from the foot to the abdomen is variable and can be augmented with a saline bolus behind the iodized oil contrast column.

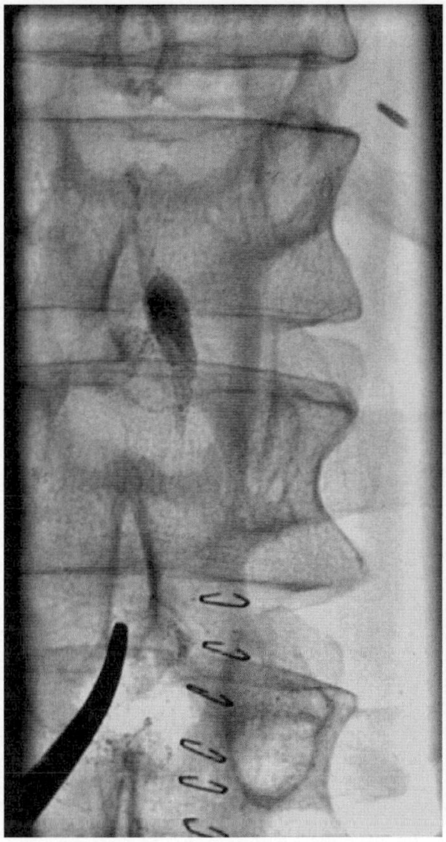

Figure 131-4. An anteroposterior radiograph of the upper abdomen shows the opacified cisterna chyli. A hemostat is placed just right of the midline (at the intended puncture site), and the image intensifier is angled so that it overlies the cisterna. This "gun-site" technique minimizes drifting of the needle as it travels through the abdomen.

closed with 3-0 Prolene vertical mattress sutures and covered with a sterile dressing.

Thoracic Duct Cannulation

Once the cisterna chyli is visualized, the patient's abdomen is prepped from the inferior costal margin to just below the umbilicus. Planning a percutaneous approach requires careful examination of the preoperative MRI. The position of the aorta and right renal artery are referenced to bony landmarks on the scan. A slightly inferior right anterior oblique approach is used most often to avoid these two vascular structures. The approximate starting position is 3 to 5 cm to the right of midline just below the costal margin. After local anesthesia, a small dermatotomy is made, and a 21- or 22-gauge, 15- to 20-cm Chiba needle (Cook Medical, Inc., Bloomington, IN) is directed toward the cisterna chyli using a "gun-site" technique (Fig. 131-4). This technique helps to minimize drifting of the needle as it travels through visceral structures. Just before the needle reaches the cisterna chyli, the C-arm is placed into an anteroposterior position. The needle can be seen "tenting" the lymphatic channels. Entry is made with a brisk and deliberate motion. A 0.018-in, 150-cm stiff guidewire (V-18 Control wire, Boston Scientific, Natick, MA) is advanced into the duct (Fig. 131-5). The needle is exchanged for a microcatheter. Predilation with a 4-French inner dilator and stiffening cannula from a nonvascular access kit (MAK-NV Introducer System, Merit Medical Systems, Inc., South Jordan, UT) is employed if the microcatheter fails to track appropriately. Given the likelihood of transintestinal passage, it is recommended that the access system be kept as small as possible, ideally 3 to 4 French. Direct hand injection of iodinated contrast medium is then performed to locate the site of thoracic duct injury. The point of extravasation should be carefully documented with imaging; in the event TDE is unsuccessful, precise localization of the injury will help guide subsequent surgical en bloc ligation.

Embolization Procedure (a.k.a. Type 1 TDE)

The microcatheter is positioned up to, or ideally across, the site of thoracic duct injury. Embolization is performed by depositing 4- to 6-mm diameter platinum-fibered microcoils (Cook Medical, Inc., Bloomington, IN) along the entire length of the thoracic duct to within a few centimeters of the entry site. As the final step, a 2:1 mixture of ethiodized oil and N-butyl cyanoacrylate with 0.5- to 1-g of tantalum powder (components included in Trufill n-BCA Liquid Embolic System, Codman & Shurtleff, Inc., Raynham, MA) is injected to seal off the lower thoracic duct and lymphatic entry site (Fig. 131-6).

Needle Disruption of Lymphatics (a.k.a. Type 2 TDE)

If cannulation of the thoracic duct is not possible, serial needle passes are made to intentionally disrupt the cisterna chyli and

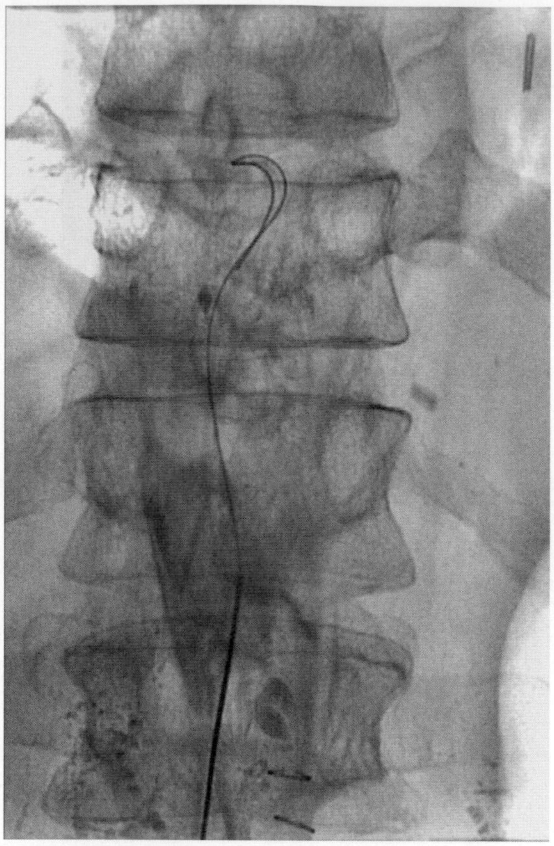

Figure 131-5. A 0.018-in guidewire is advanced through the access needle into the cisterna chyli and the lower thoracic duct. The needle is removed and exchanged for a microcatheter.

adjacent lymphatics. Completion is indicated by the extravasation of contrast in the retroperitoneal space. The needle disruption technique results in the diversion of chyle into the retroperitoneum and decompression of the thoracic duct, allowing the intrathoracic injury to heal.

POSTOPERATIVE CARE

Careful monitoring of the chest tube output is important for determining the success of the procedure. Chest tube output may drop rapidly, but typically, there is a gradual decline of approximately 50% each day. The chest tubes are removed when output is less than 200 mL per day and the patient passes an oral dietary challenge. Routine wound care and dressing changes are required for the pedal cutdown site until the sutures are removed 10 days postprocedure.

PROCEDURE-SPECIFIC COMPLICATIONS

Although solid organs and bowel are traversed with the access system en route to the cisterna chyli and thoracic duct, to date, there have been no reported complications related to this approach. Standard complications of pedal lymphangiography include permanent tattooing of the skin with methylene blue dye, wound infection, and allergic reactions. Iodized oil-related pulmonary complications include hypoxia and chemical

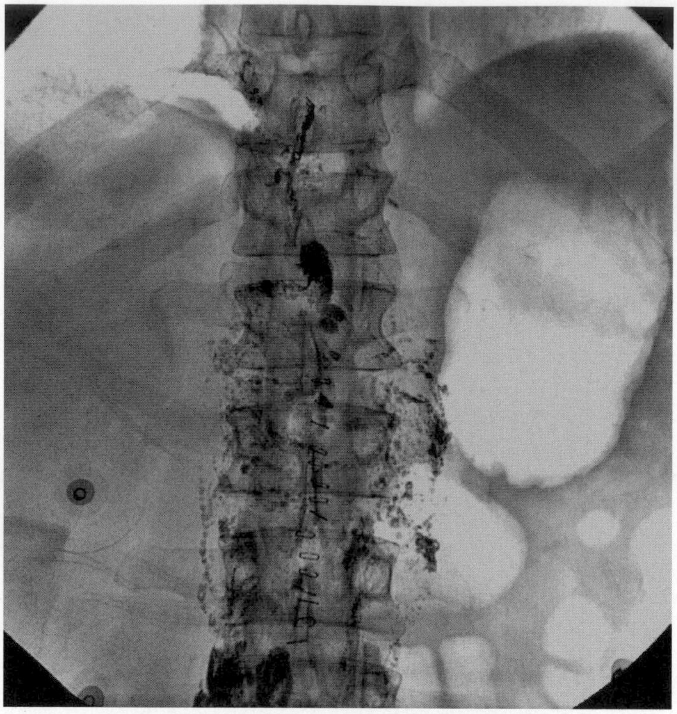

Figure 131-6. An abdominal radiograph after TDE shows coils in the lower portion of the thoracic duct and radiopaque glue throughout the upper abdominal lymphatics.

pneumonitis. Asymptomatic pulmonary embolism from liquid embolic adhesive injected into the thoracic duct has been reported. Overall, early complication rates are very low (3%).[9]

Delayed complications related to TDE are certainly conceivable, given the intentional redistribution of lymphatic flow induced by the procedure. A recent retrospective survey of 169 patients who underwent TDE uncovered several instances of chronic leg swelling, abdominal swelling without evidence of anasarca or ascites, and chronic diarrhea that were classified as "probably related" to the procedure (14.3% overall).[10] This idea is supported by reports of chronic chylous ascites and peripheral lymphedema as possible long-term complications of surgical thoracic duct ligation,[11–13] and protein losing enteropathy after thoracic duct ligation in animal models.[14] A prospective randomized investigation would be required to assess the strength of these apparent relationships.

SUMMARY

Since traumatic chylothorax is a relatively uncommon post-surgical complication, the published data on outcomes after TDE are limited, but highly supportive of the technique. The largest case series to date reviewed the results of 109 patients who underwent TDE and reported an overall clinical success rate of 71%,[9] comparing favorably to the success rate of 73.5% reported in the original case series of 42 patients.[6] Importantly, the success rate for type 1 TDE in the larger series was significantly higher than for type 2 needle disruption (90% vs. 72%), and the use of both coils and liquid embolic adhesive for type 1 TDE was observed to be more effective than the use of coils alone (91% vs. 84%). Overall, TDE is a well-tolerated, minimally

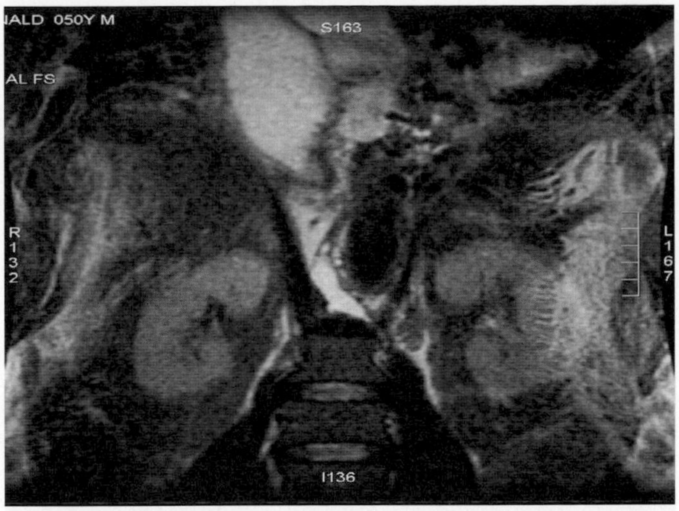

Figure 131-7. The cisterna chyli is demonstrated as a bright white saccular structure on this heavily T2-weighted MR image just anterior to the spine.

invasive, and effective alternative to the reoperation for patients with unremitting traumatic chylothorax.

CASE HISTORY

A 50-year-old man developed a high-output (2 L per day) chyle leak after esophagectomy. The patient did not respond to conservative management and was referred for TDE.

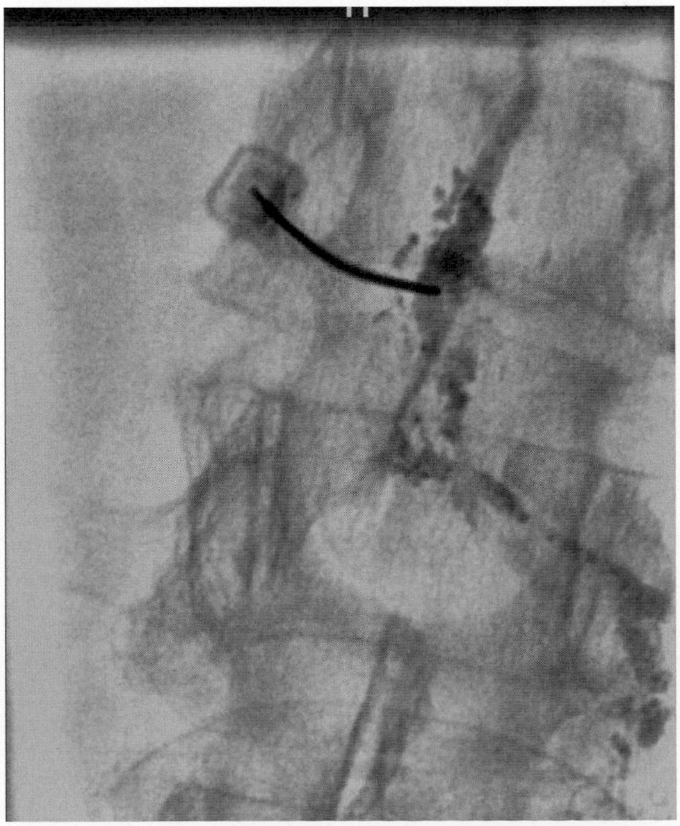

Figure 131-8. A radiograph illustrating the "gun-site" technique. The image intensifier is angled so that the needle overlies the target on fluoroscopy.

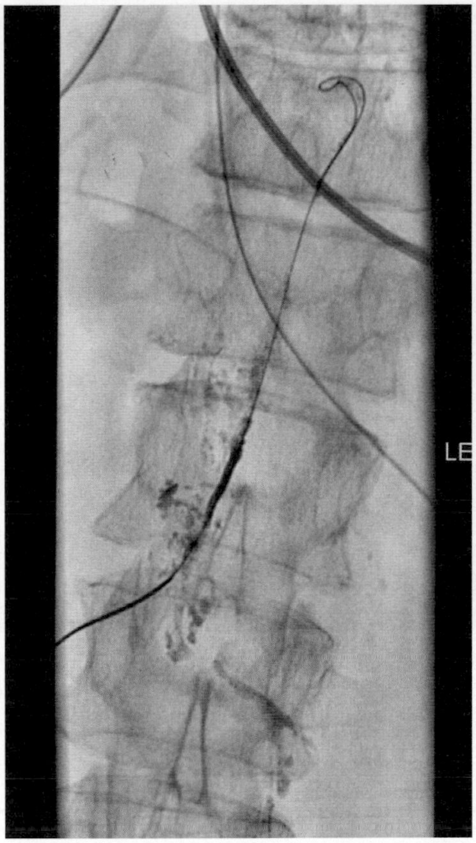

Figure 131-9. A spot radiograph of the upper abdomen shows a 0.018-in guidewire in the lower thoracic duct.

A pre-embolization MRI shows the cisterna chyli (Fig. 131-7). After a right pedal lymphangiogram, the cisterna was opacified with an oil-based contrast agent. The puncture site was located just to the right of midline, and the image intensifier was positioned so that the needle overlay the target lymphatic structure. The "gun-site" technique is illustrated in Figure 131-8. The lymphatic system was cannulated (Fig. 131-9), and iodinated contrast was injected to define the site of thoracic duct injury (Fig. 131-10). The leak then was embolized and sealed using platinum-fibered microcoils and liquid embolic adhesive (Fig. 131-11).

Postoperatively, the effusions decreased by 50% each day, and the chest tubes were removed 3 days later. The patient was discharged home soon thereafter.

EDITOR'S COMMENT

An important principle in management of lymph leaks is the notion of relative resistance. The lymph system is generally a "low-pressure" system that responds to subtle pressure differences. If a lymph drain provides a low-resistance option to lymph flow, the output is likely to continue. Alternatively, graded increases in resistance are likely to encourage lymph flow through alternative pathways. One of the functional consequences of thoracic duct "embolization" may be that it changes the dynamics of lymph flow.

—Steven J. Mentzer

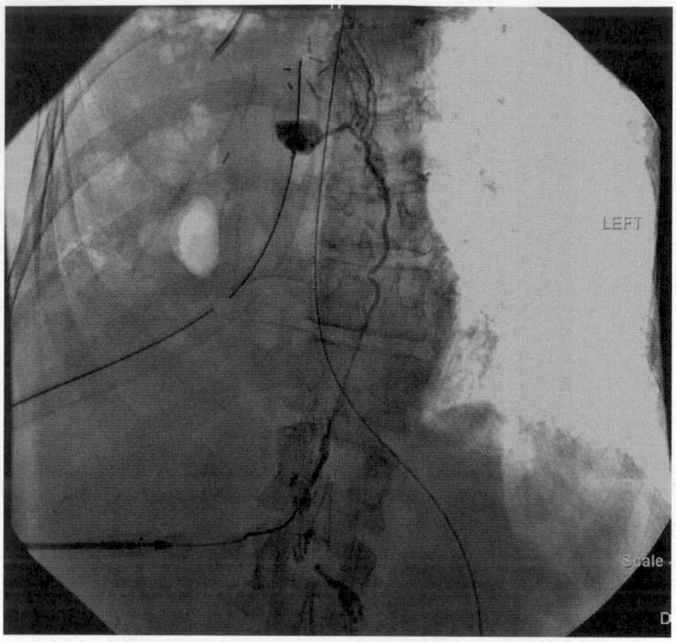

Figure 131-10. Iodinated contrast injection after cannulation of the cisterna chyli shows the site of thoracic duct injury and extravasation of contrast into the right pleural space.

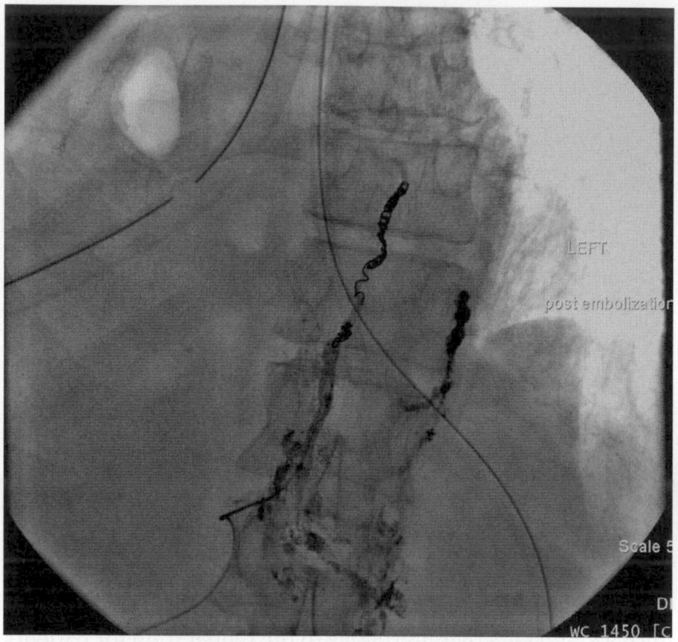

Figure 131-11. Postembolization radiograph demonstrates coils and glue in the lymphatic system. The previously seen leak is now sealed.

References

1. Vallieres E, Karmy-Jones R, Wood DE. Early complications. Chylothorax. *Chest Surg Clin N Am.* 1999;9:609–616.
2. Paes ML, Powell H. Chylothorax: an update. *Br J Hosp Med.* 1994;51(9):482–490.
3. Merigliano S, Molena D, Ruol A, et al. Chylothorax complicating esophagectomy for cancer: a plea for early thoracic duct ligation. *J Thorac Cardiovasc Surg.* 2000;119:453–457.
4. Sieczka EM, Harvey JC. Early thoracic duct ligation for postoperative chylothorax. *J Surg Oncol.* 1996;61:56–60.
5. Cerfolio RJ, Allen MS, Deschamps C, et al. Postoperative chylothorax. *J Thorac Cardiovasc Surg.* 1996;112(5):1361–1365.
6. Cope C, Kaiser LR. Management of unremitting chylothorax by percutaneous embolization and blockage of retroperitoneal lymphatic vessels in 42 patients. *J Vasc Interv Radiol.* 2002;13:1139–1148.
7. Staats BA, Ellefson RD, Budahn LL, et al. The lipoprotein profile of chylous and nonchylous pleural effusions. *Mayo Clin Proc.* 1980;55(11):700–704.
8. Hamm H, Pfalzer B, Fabel H. Lipoprotein analysis in a chyliform pleural effusion: implications for pathogenesis and diagnosis. *Respiration.* 1991;58(5–6):294–300.
9. Itkin M, Kucharczuk JC, Kwak A, et al. Nonoperative thoracic duct embolization for traumatic thoracic duct leak: experience in 109 patients. *J Thorac Cardiovasc Surg.* 2010;139(3):584–589.
10. Laslett D, Trerotola SO, Itkin M. Delayed complications following technically successful thoracic duct embolization. *J Vasc Interv Radiol.* 2012; 23(1):76–79.
11. Christodoulou M, Ris HB, Pezzetta E. Video-assisted right supradiaphragmatic thoracic duct ligation for non-traumatic recurrent chylothorax. *Eur J Cardiothorac Surg.* 2006;29:810–814.
12. Raguse J, Pfitzmann R, Bier J, et al. Lower-extremity lymphedema following neck dissection—an uncommon complication after cervical ligation of the thoracic duct. *Oral Oncol.* 2007;43:835–837.
13. Pimpec-Barthes FL, Pham M, Jouan J, et al. Peritoneoatrial shunting for intractable chylous ascites complicating thoracic duct ligation. *Ann Thorac Surg.* 2011;87:1601–1603.
14. Marshall WH, Neyazaki T, Abrams HL. Abnormal protein loss after thoracic-duct ligation in dogs. *N Engl J Med.* 1965;273:1092–1094.

132 Fibrothorax and Decortication

Thomas J. Birdas and Robert J. Keenan

Keywords: Undrained pleural fluid, trapped or encased lung, organizing empyema, constrictive pleurisy, empyema thoracis, hemothorax, undrained pleural effusion, infections of the pleural space, recurrent effusions after open heart surgery, chronic pneumothorax, tuberculosis, chylothorax, pancreatitis

Fibrothorax is a condition characterized by accumulation of fibrous tissue in the pleural cavity in reaction to undrained pleural fluid. A thick "peel" is formed on both pleural surfaces, eventually preventing complete expansion of the lung. This basic premise explains several other names by which this condition is known: trapped or encased lung, organizing empyema (or hemothorax), and constrictive pleurisy. The process of removing the fibrous peel is called decortication. Delorme used the term for the first time in 1894.[1] The procedure was used primarily in the management of tuberculous pleurisy and later in the management of hemothorax.

PATHOPHYSIOLOGY OF FIBROTHORAX

The main causes of fibrothorax are listed in Table 132-1. The prerequisite for the formation of fibrothorax is the presence of undrained pleural effusion. The ensuing inflammatory response leads to fibrin deposition within the pleural space. This, in turn, is followed by infiltration of macrophages and fibroblasts and eventually formation of a collagen-rich "peel" that covers both the parietal and visceral pleurae and encapsulates the initial fluid collection (Fig. 132-1). At this stage, any attempts at management with thoracentesis are unsuccessful because the fluid quickly reaccumulates in the persistent cavity. Without remedial treatment, the initially thin peel continues to thicken, reaching depths of 2 cm or more.

Undrained pleural effusions also have a significant space-occupying effect and compress the underlying lung parenchyma. With continued organization of the fibrotic peel, the atelectatic portions of the lung become trapped. The same process occurs over the parietal pleura, both on the chest wall and on the diaphragm. The resulting physiologic changes are of the restrictive type. These effects are not always proportional to the thickness of the peel and can occur even with a limited extent of lung entrapment. Hypoxic pulmonary vasoconstriction limits blood flow and results in ventilation/perfusion mismatches. With unilateral disease, hypoxia may be absent at rest. The functional reserve is limited, however, and desaturation is seen with exercise.

Table 132-1

CAUSES OF FIBROTHORAX

Common
Empyema thoracis
Hemothorax
Undrained pleural effusion
Recurrent effusions after open heart surgery
Chronic pneumothorax
Tuberculosis
Uncommon
Chylothorax
Pancreatitis
Unusual infections of the pleural space

CLINICAL PRESENTATION

The most frequent presentation is that of a patient with recurrent or persistent pleural effusion. Careful evaluation is warranted to determine whether fibrothorax is present or likely because this will influence the choice of appropriate management. Prior conditions leading to recurrent effusions and eventually an entrapped lung are often easily identified during history taking. A significant number of patients, however, may lack such a clear correlation. Depending on the underlying etiology and the degree of parenchymal involvement, symptoms may vary. Exertional dyspnea is the most common symptom, usually reported as progressive over a long period of time. Chest discomfort and nonproductive cough are also seen. The most common signs are limited respiratory movement of the affected hemithorax, decreased breath sounds on auscultation, and dullness to percussion.

PREOPERATIVE ASSESSMENT

Imaging techniques are of paramount importance. Standard chest radiographs (Fig. 132-2) demonstrate obliteration of the costophrenic angle and thickened pleural surfaces, initially seen

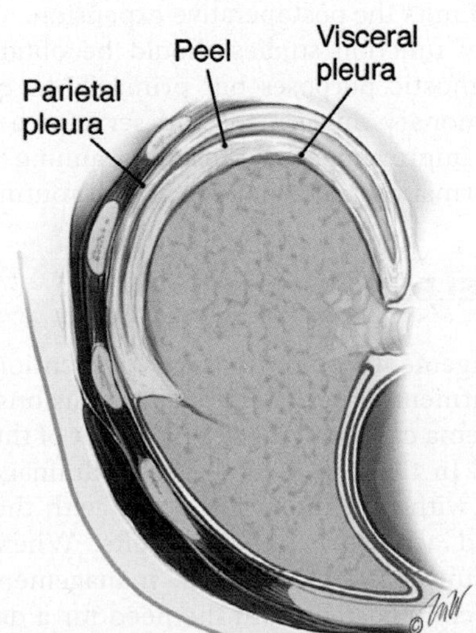

Figure 132-1. Cross section of the lung with fibrous peel encasing the lung.

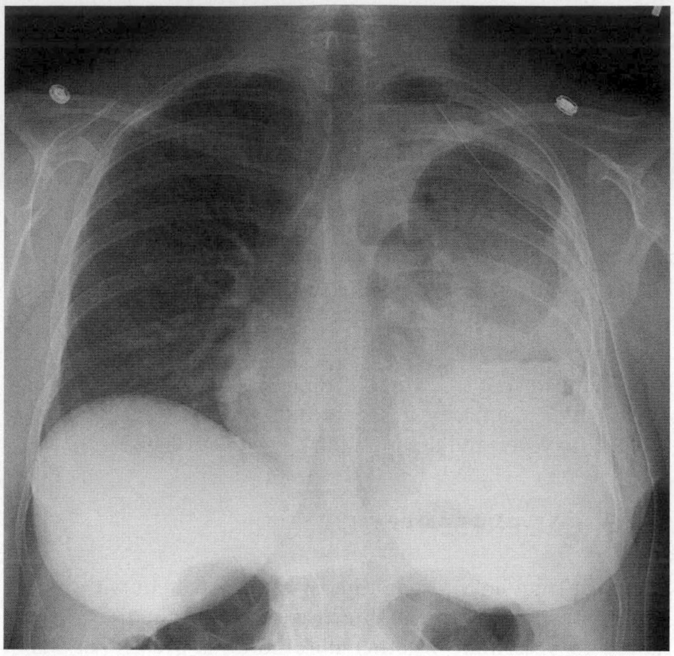

Figure 132-2. Anteroposterior chest x-ray in a young woman with a retained hemothorax.

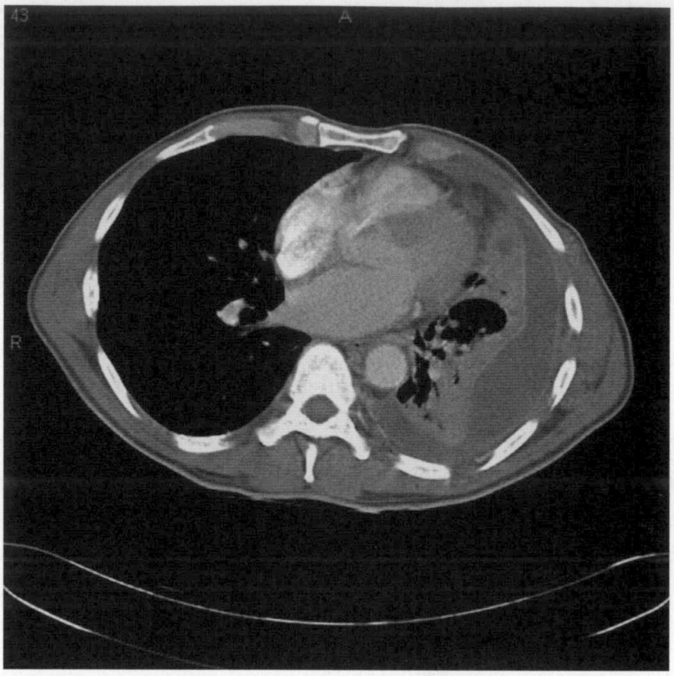

Figure 132-3. Chest CT scan in a patient with fibrothorax secondary to an infected parapneumonic effusion.

over the diaphragmatic surface and the lateral chest wall, progressing superiorly and eventually obliterating the pleural space. The intercostal spaces may be narrowed, and the overall size of the hemithorax may be reduced. Pleural calcifications, when present, can help determine the thickness of the parietal peel.

CT scanning is essential in the evaluation of fibrothorax (Fig. 132-3). In addition to the information regarding the extent of the fibrotic process, the thickness of the peel, the presence of loculations, and potential differentiation from neoplastic pleural disorders (i.e., mesothelioma) are revealed. CT scanning provides useful information about the status of the underlying lung parenchyma. Tuberculous lesions, bronchiectasis, and underlying lung malignancies can be identified. In addition, a reasonable estimation of the effectiveness of the decortication can be made based on the extent of diseased lung parenchyma, which usually limits the postoperative expansion.

Pulmonary function studies should be obtained not so much for diagnostic purposes but primarily to quantify the degree of pulmonary impairment and serve as a measure of postoperative improvement. Perfusion scanning offers little additional information and is not performed routinely.

PATIENT SELECTION

The best management for fibrothorax is prevention. Early and aggressive treatment of persistent pleural effusions, hemothorax, and empyema can avoid the development of the restrictive fibrous peel.[2,3] In the first several weeks, drainage usually is feasible either with tube thoracostomy or with thoracoscopic techniques and achieves excellent results. When treatment is delayed or unsuccessful, however, management decisions become more complicated. Both the need for a decortication and the optimal timing for the operation have to be determined. The decision to proceed with a decortication depends on several factors. The extent of the disease has to be such that it causes significant symptomatology and objective physiologic pulmonary impairment. Patients requiring decortication are those with at least 50% compression of the lung (especially with apical involvement), those with unsuccessful attempts at aspiration, and those with lack of improvement after 6 weeks of conservative management. The nature of the underlying disease is also important. In cases of empyema, failure of initial drainage usually is considered an indication for decortication; the goals of the operation in this setting are not only alleviation of lung constriction but also elimination of the infected pleural space by reexpansion of the lung. In the case of hemothorax, control of coagulation disorders must be addressed before extensive surgery. If the initial intervention has been tube thoracostomy, an early decision, within several days, should be made regarding the necessity of more aggressive surgical evacuation. In patients with tuberculosis, decortication is performed after completion of antituberculous chemotherapy and when there is considerable pleural involvement that does not change despite thoracentesis.

Table 132-2 shows conditions in which decortication is contraindicated. These include patients with significant ipsilateral bronchial obstruction, primary or metastatic pleural malignancy, uncontrolled infection, contralateral disease, and operative risk when it is prohibitively high.

Table 132-2

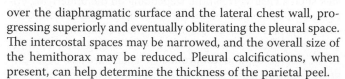

CONTRAINDICATIONS FOR DECORTICATION
Malignant pleural disease
Endobronchial disease preventing lung expansion
Extensive ipsilateral parenchymal disease
Significant operative risk
Chronic debilitation
Fibrothorax with limited subjective or objective impairment

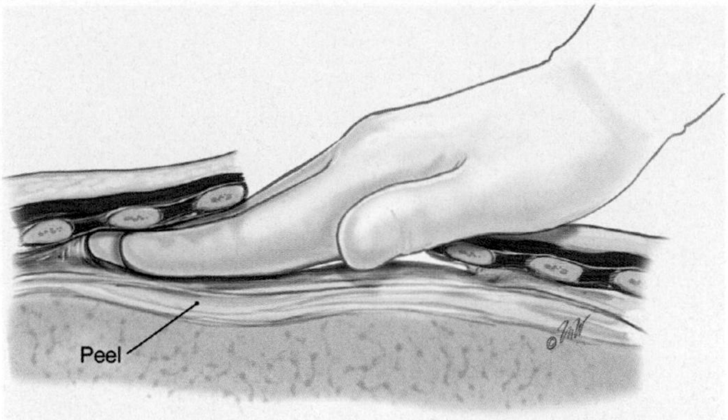

Figure 132-4. Blunt development of the pleural space before inserting the chest retractor.

SURGICAL TECHNIQUE

Conventional Approach

In the majority of patients for whom decortication is performed via a thoracotomy, the classic operative technique suggested by Williams[4] and Samson[5] is still used and will be described briefly in the following text. The basic tenets of the operation include complete pleurolysis, establishment of a decortication plane between the fibrous peel and the visceral pleura, and decortication of all pleural surfaces, including the diaphragm.

After induction of general anesthesia, flexible bronchoscopy is performed to rule out the presence of endobronchial obstruction. The use of a double-lumen endotracheal tube is preferred because frequent ventilatory changes (i.e., intermittent inflation of the affected lung) may be used during the procedure. Although a posterolateral thoracotomy traditionally has been preferred, a muscle-sparing thoracotomy still can be used without impairment in visualization. The chest is entered through the sixth interspace to provide better exposure of the lower lobe and the diaphragm, where the peel is usually thicker and the adhesions denser. Unless the chest is severely contracted and the ribs tightly apposed, rib resection usually is not required. One or two ribs may be shingled posteriorly to facilitate exposure, however.

Before inserting the chest retractor, the pleural space is bluntly developed for a distance of a few centimeters, sometimes in an extrapleural plane as necessary (Fig. 132-4). The need for complete extrapleural dissection is controversial. Most surgeons advocate this maneuver to ensure complete chest wall expansion. The counterargument is that extrapleural dissection may lead to significant bleeding and also can be extremely tedious at the apex of the lung and over the mediastinum. Regardless of whether the parietal pleura is left in place, complete lysis of all pleural adhesions is required. Any loculated spaces are drained and the contents are sent for culture. Concern about contamination of the remainder of the pleural cavity by drainage of such spaces is not justified; the immediate priority in treatment of pleural infections is lung reexpansion and that should be accomplished as completely as possible.

When the visceral peel is encountered, it is incised in layers until the underlying visceral pleura is identified (Fig. 132-5). The most favorable location to initiate the dissection is usually the lateral surface of the lung, away from the diaphragm, where the fibrous peel is usually thicker. The peel then is dissected bluntly off the pleura; we prefer to use a peanut dissector or the tip of a metal sucker for this purpose. The lung usually is kept inflated at this stage to facilitate separation of the peel (Fig. 132-6). As the decortication progresses; however, the inflated lung impairs visualization, and the final stages usually are performed with the lung collapsed. Minor air leaks from the raw surface of the pulmonary parenchyma are unavoidable but heal quickly if the lung is fully reexpanded. Depending on the degree of inflammation and the presence or absence of parenchymal disease, complete decortication may be impossible in certain areas without significant parenchymal injury. In these cases, it is better to leave some layers of the peel behind than to create a severe and difficult-to-manage air leak. In addition, the remaining peel can be incised in several locations, akin to relaxing incisions, thereby allowing some reexpansion of the underlying lung (Fig. 132-7).

After the decortication is complete, hemostasis is obtained, and the pleural cavity is irrigated and drained widely. We prefer to use three chest tubes. Two straight tubes are laid posteriorly in the costovertebral recess and anteriorly to the hilum, respectively, and directed toward the apex. The third (right-angle) tube is placed between the diaphragm and the lung base and directed posteriorly toward the posterior costophrenic recess.

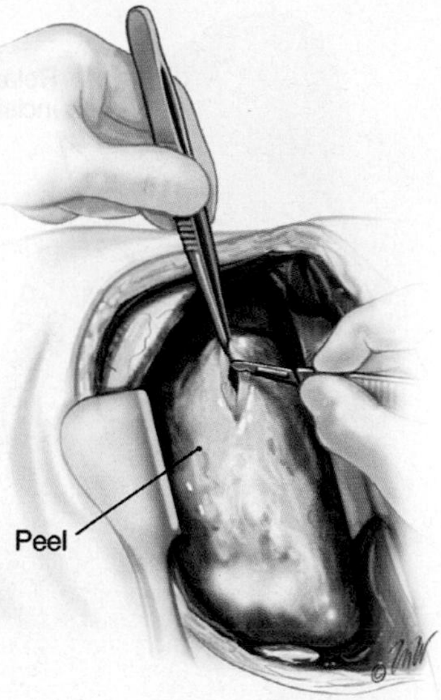

Figure 132-5. The visceral peel is incised in layers until the underlying visceral pleura is identified.

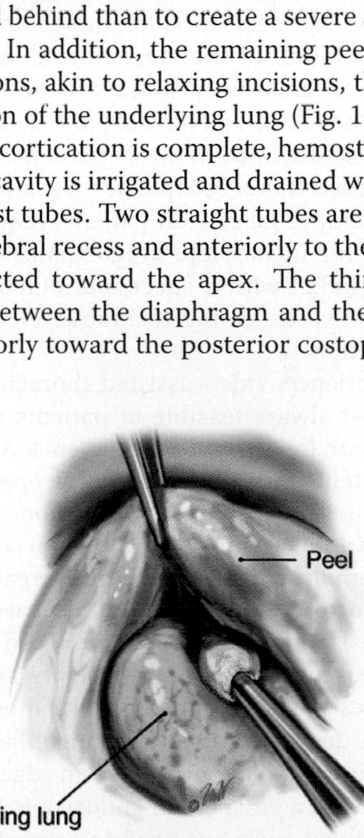

Figure 132-6. The lung is inflated to facilitate separation of the peel.

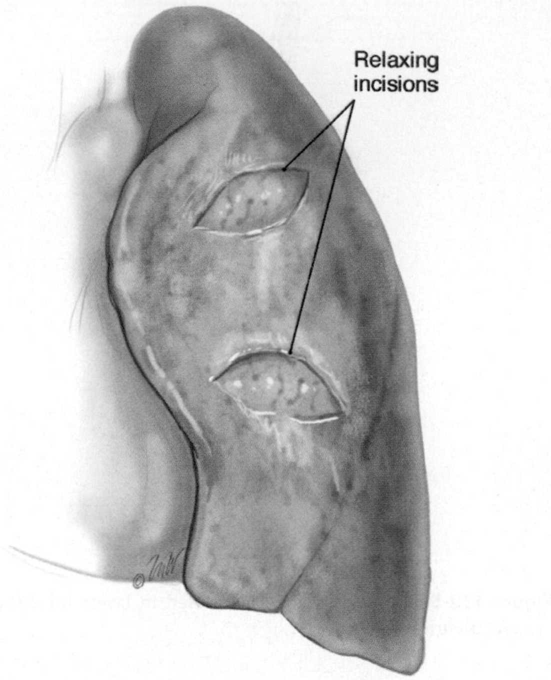

Figure 132-7. When complete decortication is ill-advised, the intact peel is incised in several locations to allow for limited reexpansion of the lung.

THORACOSCOPY

Thoracoscopic (i.e., video-assisted thoracic surgery) drainage of a hemothorax or early-stage empyema has been established as the surgical approach of choice over the last decade.[2,6,7] Its use in cases of organized empyema, as well as other causes of fibrothorax, is not as widely accepted. Cheng et al.[8] reported a small series of decortications for chronic empyema, primarily in patients deemed unfit for thoracotomy. Nine of ten patients had resolution of the empyema. Kim et al.[9] reported on 70 patients who underwent thoracoscopic decortication for empyema with the use of an endoscopic shaver system. Decortication was successful in 65 of the 70 patients. Waller and Rengarajan[10] performed thoracoscopic decortication in 36 patients with organized empyema Fifteen patients required conversion to thoracotomy for incomplete lung expansion, leaving 21 of the 36 patients (58%) with a successful outcome. This report describes in relative detail the technique for formal thoracoscopic decortication.

In our experience, video-assisted thoracic surgical decortication is almost always feasible in patients with fibrothorax not associated with long-standing empyema. A typical example is that of persistent pleural effusion after open heart surgery. These patients present with chronic effusions despite multiple thoracenteses. Another common population consists of trauma patients with hemothorax who have been treated inadequately by tube thoracostomy. Contrary to the cases of organized empyemas, access to the pleural space in these patients is easily obtained thoracoscopically. The lower lobes and varying parts of the upper lobes usually are encased with moderate-thickness fibrous peel and do not expand with lung inflation. The peel is incised with endoscopic scissors. Once an edge is bluntly developed and lifted with a grasper, an endoscopic peanut dissector or the tip of a metal sucker is used to separate the peel from the lung parenchyma (Fig. 132-8). Traction is applied on the peel either directly or, because of limited space, by rolling it on the grasper (Fig. 132-9). Usually it is incised and removed in several pieces, always leaving a small edge so that further dissection is facilitated. The dissection is initiated usually on the convex lateral surface of the lower lobe and extended radially to all directions. Thoracoscopy allows for improved visualization of the lung base and the diaphragm, where the peel is also separated in the same fashion. The pleural space is drained with two chest tubes, usually through the existing ports.

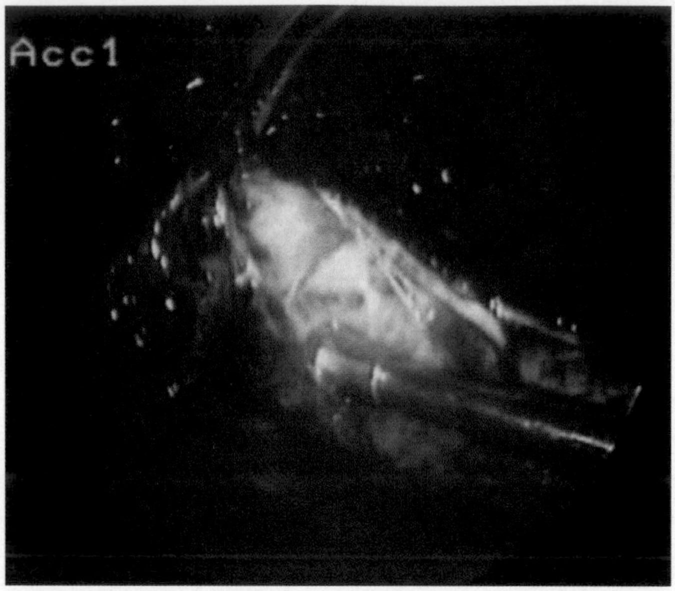

Figure 132-8. Thoracoscopic decortication. The visceral peel is lifted with a grasper and bluntly separated from the parenchyma (in this case with a metal-tip sucker).

POSTOPERATIVE CARE

All tubes are maintained on suction to facilitate drainage of the pleural space and lung expansion. Reexpansion of the lung and obliteration of the pleural space can be enhanced by the use of elective positive-pressure ventilation in the immediate postoperative period. Before the chest tube is removed, or if

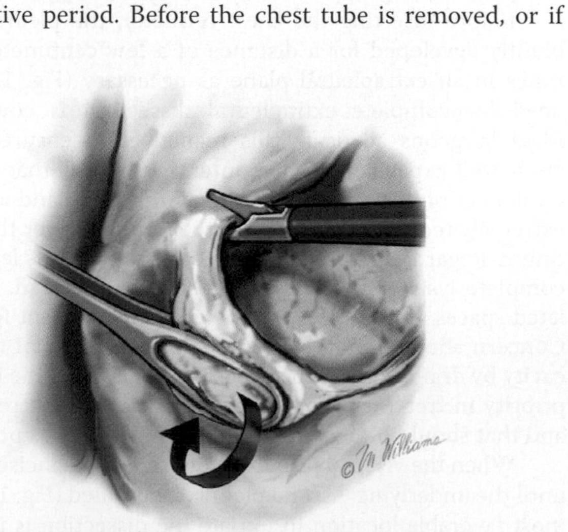

Figure 132-9. Additional traction is applied on the peel by rolling it on the grasper.

the findings on chest x-ray are of concern, a CT scan may be obtained to identify the presence of any undrained collections. If found, a decision regarding chest tube manipulation or additional percutaneous drainage is needed, particularly in cases of empyema. Instillation of fibrinolytic agents may be an additional option, although data for their use in the postoperative setting are lacking. Occasionally, patients may be discharged with one or more chest tubes if there is a persistent air leak or continued drainage.

OUTCOMES

In the recent era, operative mortality for decortication ranges between 0% and 5%, determined primarily by the underlying medical comorbidities. The most common complications are hemorrhage, prolonged air leaks, persistent empyema, and wound infections. Generally, these complications can be minimized with meticulous operative technique, which involves careful dissection and avoidance of parenchymal injuries, and achieves complete lung reexpansion, probably the most important step in controlling the pleural space. In a recent study by Melloni et al,[11] extended duration of symptoms (>60 days) and prolonged conservative management (>30 days) were associated with increased morbidity. The best functional results are achieved in cases where the underlying lung parenchyma is free of any significant disease. In these cases, significant improvements are seen both in vital capacity and in forced expiratory volume in 1 second, as well as in lung perfusion, usually becoming apparent early in the postoperative period and extending up to 3 years after the decortication. The degree of lung reexpansion on chest x-ray correlates well with functional outcomes. Although it is thought that pleural disease of shorter duration usually leads to better results, occasional favorable outcomes have been reported in patients with long-standing tuberculous pleuritic disease.

Failure to achieve a satisfactory outcome is usually due to one of the three factors: underlying parenchymal disease, incomplete operation, or development of postoperative complications. Occasionally, in the presence of a severely affected lung, parenchymal resection may be required because decortication alone will not achieve the desired reexpansion. Concomitant resections not only increase the potential for postoperative complications but also create new space problems, which often require even more extensive surgery (e.g., muscle flaps or thoracoplasty). Careful patient selection and decision making are required in such cases. The attention to meticulous technique that achieves complete lung expansion and avoids significant parenchymal, diaphragmatic, or phrenic nerve injuries cannot be overemphasized.

SUMMARY

The primary cause of fibrothorax is undrained pleural fluid. Exertional dyspnea and chest discomfort are the most common symptoms. Early and aggressive treatment of undrained pleural collections can minimize the risk of developing a restrictive peel. Removal of the peel and complete reexpansion of the lung are keys to the success of decortication.

EDITOR'S COMMENT

A lesson from clinical experience with tuberculous empyema is that the underlying entrapped lung will gradually expand and minimize the residual space; a routine observation in pediatric patients with common bacterial empyemas. This process of gradual adaptation, however, can require months to years. Furthermore, it is unclear if the gradual expansion of the underlying lung is associated with an increase in lung function.

—Steven J. Mentzer

References

1. Deslauriers J, Perrault LP. Fibrothorax and decortication. *Ann Thorac Surg.* 1994;58:267–268.
2. Landreneau RJ, Keenan RJ, Hazelrigg SR, et al. Thoracoscopy for empyema and hemothorax. *Chest.* 1996;109:18–24.
3. Sasse S, Nguyen TK, Mulligan M, et al. The effects of early chest tube placement on empyema resolution. *Chest.* 1997;111:1679–1683.
4. Williams M. The technique of pulmonary decortication and pleurolysis. *J Thorac Surg.* 1950;20:652–654.
5. Samson P. Some surgical considerations in pulmonary decortication. *Am J Surg.* 1955;89:364–371.
6. Grewal H, Jackson RJ, Wagner CW, et al. Early video-assisted thoracic surgery in the management of empyema. *Pediatrics.* 1999;103:e63.
7. Tong B, Hanna J, Toloza E, et al. Outcomes of video-assisted thoracoscopic decortication. *Ann Thorac Surg.* 2010;89:220–225.
8. Cheng YJ, Wu HH, Chou SH, et al. Video-assisted thoracoscopic surgery in the treatment of chronic empyema thoracis. *Surg Today.* 2002;32:19–25.
9. Kim BY, Oh BS, Jang WC, et al. Video-assisted thoracoscopic decortication for management of postpneumonic pleural empyema. *Am J Surg.* 2004;188:321–324.
10. Waller DA, Rengarajan A. Thoracoscopic decortication: a role for video-assisted surgery in chronic postpneumonic pleural empyema. *Ann Thorac Surg.* 2001;71:1813–1816.
11. Melloni G, Carretta A, Ciriaco P, et al. Decortication for chronic parapneumonic empyema: results of a prospective study. *World J Surg.* 2004;28:488–493.

133 Surgical Management of Chylothorax

Christopher T. Ducko and Philip A. Linden

Keywords: Thoracic duct, chyle leak, chylomicrons, congenital chylothorax, lymphovascular malformations, complete thoracic duct atresia, esophagectomy

Chylothorax results from the leakage of chyle from the thoracic duct or one of its lymphatic branches into the pleural space. Common causes include neoplasm and iatrogenic injury. Life-threatening metabolic derangements may occur if chylothorax is not recognized and treated promptly. Numerous maneuvers can be undertaken as part of a conservative approach to treating chylothorax, but surgical intervention is usually the most effective method of achieving definitive results.

ANATOMY AND PHYSIOLOGY

The thoracic duct was first described in humans by Veslingus in 1634. The first successful thoracic duct ligation was performed by Lampson in 1948 for a traumatic chylothorax.[1] Before this time, chylothorax was treated conservatively and associated with a mortality rate of almost 50%. An accurate understanding of the anatomic course of the thoracic duct and common sites of variant anatomy can help to minimize iatrogenic chylothorax and ensure successful surgical intervention through direct repair or mass ligation.

The thoracic duct is a continuation of the cisterna chyli as it passes from the abdomen into the thorax (Fig. 133-1). There are many variations in the course and number of divisions of the thoracic duct. In most individuals, the thoracic duct starts at the cisterna chyli and enters the chest through the aortic hiatus, coursing behind the esophagus between the aorta and azygos vein. The duct runs cephalad in the right hemithorax along the spinal column. At the level of the fifth or sixth thoracic vertebra, the duct crosses to the left hemithorax and continues

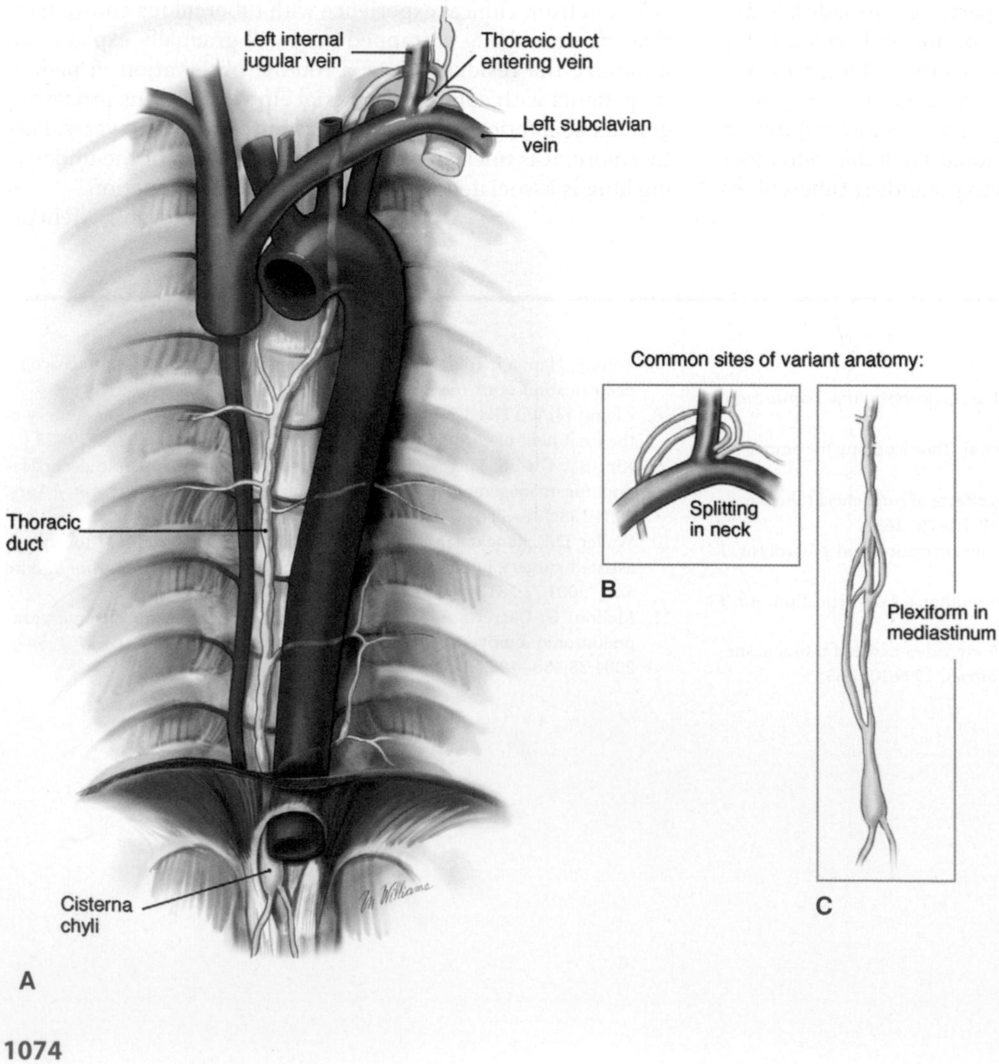

Figure 133-1. The thoracic duct is the primary lymph vessel that carries the lipid products of digestion (fatty chyle) and lymph from the intestines to the left subclavian vein. In the thorax, the duct begins at the level of the cisterna chyli, a lymph sac that lies just below the diaphragm and aortic hiatus, when present. The duct ascends through the right chest, crosses over to the left chest at the fifth or sixth thoracic vertebra, and empties at the angle formed by the left internal jugular and left subclavian veins. This is known as the lymphaticovenous junction *(A)*, and there is a one-way valve at the termination of the thoracic duct. The anatomy may vary. Some common sites of variation are shown in insets *B* and *C*.

cephalad along the left side of the esophagus into the superior mediastinum behind the aortic arch and posterior to the left subclavian artery. The duct terminates at the angle formed by the left internal jugular and left subclavian veins, where it drains into the venous system. Of surgical importance is the consistency in location and paucity of branching of the thoracic duct between the cisterna chyli and the level of the eighth vertebral body in the lower right hemithorax.

Chyle is a milky fluid that consists primarily of proteins, triglycerides, and lymphocytes. Under normal conditions, the thoracic duct transports up to 4 L of chyle per day. Factors that influence flow rate include diet, drug intake, intestinal function, and physical mobility. The flow of chyle is maintained by changes in intraabdominal and intrathoracic pressure along with intrinsic alterations in the muscular tone of the thoracic duct.[2] Valves irregularly spaced throughout the system assist in unidirectional circulation. Although valves may be present throughout the thoracic duct, there is one valve constant in location that lies within 1 cm of the lymphaticovenous junction (see Fig. 133-1, inset A). Drainage of chyle into the rapidly flowing venous system can be explained by the Bernoulli effect, the law governing the behavior of a fluid as it passes from a region of low pressure to a region of high pressure.

Most of the fluid that composes chyle comes from the gastrointestinal tract and liver. It contains high concentrations of digestive products as well as lymphocytes and immunoglobulins.[2] Between 60% and 70% of dietary fat is absorbed via the lymphatic system in the form of chylomicrons. Short and medium-chain fatty acids (i.e., <10 carbon atoms in length) are taken in directly via the portal system. The absorption of dietary fat gives chyle its milky-white color. This explains the high concentration of triglycerides in chyle relative to plasma. Lymphocytes make up 95% of the cellular component of chyle (90% are T-lymphocytes), whereas the concentrations of electrolytes, antibodies, and enzymes approximate those of plasma.[3] Loss of these constituents as a result of injury to the thoracic duct can be quite debilitating from both a nutritional and an immunologic standpoint.

ETIOLOGY OF CHYLOTHORAX

Congenital chylothorax is the most common cause of pleural effusion in the newborn. The condition may result from lymphovascular malformations, complete thoracic duct atresia, or trauma during birth. In the adult, the principal causes of chylothorax are trauma or iatrogenic injury, followed by obstruction or disruption secondary to a neoplastic process. Penetrating injuries to the neck, chest, or abdomen may result in direct ductal damage, whereas blunt trauma may create increased wall tension and distention injury as a result of crushing blows or spinal column hyperextension (Table 133-1).

Iatrogenic injuries occur four times more frequently than blunt or penetrating trauma.[4] These injuries are more common after esophagectomy, but also may be associated with neck dissections, lung resection, aortic surgery, and removal of mediastinal tumors.[5] Postoperative injuries include transection, resection, tangential laceration, and tears of lateral ductal branches. Injury to the thoracic duct also may occur after interventions such as left-sided central line insertion, translumbar angiography, and sclerotherapy for esophageal varices.

Table 133-1

ETIOLOGY OF CHYLOTHORAX
Traumatic
Penetrating
Blunt
Spontaneous
Violent increase in intraabdominal or intrathoracic pressure
Thrombosis of left subclavian vein
Iatrogenic
Postoperative
Esophagectomy
Lung resection
Lymph node dissection
Aortic surgery, near isthmus or descending aorta
Left subclavian surgery
Left-sided central line attempt
Malignancy
Lymphoma
Metastatic disease to mediastinum
Infections
Tuberculosis
Filariasis
Congenital
Birth trauma
Thoracic duct agenesis
Thoracic duct pleural fistula

Malignant ductal obstruction can arise secondary to an intrinsic disease such as intraluminal involvement from neoplastic cells or from extrinsic compression. Seventy percent of malignant duct leaks occur in association with lymphoma.[4]

DIAGNOSIS OF CHYLOTHORAX

Chylothorax is a rare event, with exception of the 5% to 8% incidence of chylothorax associated with esophagectomy. By comparison, the incidence of chylothorax after lung resection is only about 0.5%.[6] The diagnosis of chylothorax is rarely expected or obvious and requires a healthy index of suspicion (Table 133-2). After esophagectomy, chest tube output approaching or exceeding 1 L/day immediately should raise suspicion of a chyle leak, especially if the fluid is milky white. However, high chest tube output simply may be the result of extensive operation, postoperative oozing, or volume overload in the immediate postesophagectomy period. Also, a clear fluid may masquerade as chyle in an unfed patient. For the patient that presents with chylothorax in the nonpostoperative state, shortness of breath or an abnormal chest radiograph will be the presenting symptom or sign, and a number of clinical tests are helpful in making the diagnosis.

Pleural fluid analysis is an aid to diagnosis. A sampling of pleural fluid should be sent for Gram stain, protein and triglyceride determinations, and cell count with differential. Chylothorax is suspected immediately if the fluid is white but neutrophils and bacteria are absent on Gram stain.

The triglyceride level may be even more helpful as a diagnostic aid. A high triglyceride concentration (>110 mg/dL) has a high specificity for chyle leak, whereas concentrations of less than 50 mg/dL are less than 5% likely to be due to a chyle leak. A cholesterol:triglyceride ratio of less than 1 is diagnostic of chyle.[7] Many consider a lymphocyte count of greater than 90% to be equally diagnostic. The presence of chylomicrons in

Table 133-2

ALGORITHM FOR MANAGEMENT OF CHYLOTHORAX

Diagnosis
- Index of suspicion
- New or increasing pleural effusion
  - Thoracentesis
  - Chest tube insertion
- Character of effusion or drainage
  - Triglyceride level >110 mg/dL
  - Lymphocyte count >90%
- Lymphangiography (optional)

Treatment
- Volume of drainage <500 mL/d
- Nonoperative management
  - Nothing by mouth
  - Chest tube drainage for lung expansion
  - Fluid and electrolyte resuscitation
  - Consider total parenteral nutrition
  - Expectant observation for 1–2 wk
    - If drainage remains low, less than 200 mL/d
      - Advance to low-fat diet
      - Remove tube
    - If high-output drainage persists, operative management
- Volume of drainage >500 mL/d
- Operative management
  - Thoracic duct embolization
  - Reexploration with direct repair and/or mass ligation
  - Mass ligation
  - Chemical pleurodesis or pleurectomy
  - Radiation and/or chemotherapy if underlying malignancy is present
  - Pleuroperitoneal shunt

pleural fluid is diagnostic for chyle; however, electrophoresis is necessary to establish their presence. The diagnosis can be confounded if the patient has been fasting or is on an elemental diet. In the proper clinical setting, a fatty-food bolus (e.g., heavy cream) and subsequent increase in chest tube output also can be diagnostic of chylothorax.

Lymphangiography can confirm a chylothorax as well as identify the site of the leak. This type of localization study can prove useful in planning an operative approach for repair, especially when coupled with postlymphangiogram CT imaging.[8] Lymphangiography can demonstrate accessory ducts and the course of the main duct in over 97% of patients.[9]

PREOPERATIVE ASSESSMENT AND DECISION-MAKING

A large, prolonged chyle leak can have several adverse effects. Patients are often already malnourished and/or immunosuppressed as a result of prior surgery or illness. In the presence of a chyle leak, the nutritional and immunologic status of the patient is further compromised. Not only is there a significant loss of fluid and electrolytes (at times, >1.5 L/day), but also a significant number of T-lymphocytes can be lost through the drainage of chyle fluid, resulting in lymphopenia and immunosuppression. Finally, there is depletion of nutritional stores through loss of fats and protein. Accumulation of chyle in the pleural cavity can quickly cause compression of underlying lung, respiratory compromise, and even tension chylothorax. The first priority in managing these patients is adequate drainage of chyle from the thorax, reexpansion of the lung, and assurance of pleural apposition. This is usually best accomplished through placement of a posteriorly directed chest tube. Replacement of IV fluids and electrolytes is initiated. Drainage of chyle should drop significantly with cessation of oral intake; total parenteral nutrition should be instituted immediately if this route is chosen.

Noninterventional Management

We prefer the term noninterventional over conservative because this method of management for large leaks in debilitated patients carries significant risk. Observation is considered optimal management for leaks of low or moderate output (<500 mL/day) in patients who are not severely malnourished. Once the fluid is drained adequately, it is important to have accurate measurements of daily chest tube drainage. Fluids and electrolytes must be checked and replaced. The patient is given nothing by mouth, and total parenteral nutrition is instituted. Alternatively, the patient may be maintained on a very low-fat diet with oral medium-chain triglyceride supplementation. However, any oral intake at all, even without dietary fat, is a stimulus to chyle production. After 1 to 2 weeks, provided the drainage decreases to less than 200 mL/day, an oral low-fat diet may be instituted. If the drainage remains low, the chest tube may be removed. If the drainage persists without feedings or increases with institution of low-fat feedings, intervention is recommended. The use of octreotide, a somatostatin analog, to inhibit chyle production is of theoretical value with equivocal clinical results.[10]

Intervention

Chyle leaks of greater than 500 mL/day are less likely to heal without intervention. (Some surgeons may use a cutoff value of 1 L.). While observation is an option, if the output is not decreased significantly in 7 days, intervention should be considered. In the postesophagectomy patient, however, intervention is mandated as soon as a leak is diagnosed because it is usually high output, the patient is already malnourished and debilitated, and the leak can be fixed readily through intervention.[11] While prophylactic thoracic duct ligation is not undertaken routinely by all surgeons performing esophagectomy, postoperative chylothorax is a serious problem.[12] Routine prophylactic mass ligation of the thoracic duct has been shown to be safe and effective in several studies.[13–15]

With advances in the percutaneous technique and improved results as it has evolved, thoracic duct embolization should be considered first if locally available, especially to avoid reoperation.[6,16] This therapy is becoming more widely available and is effective in the majority of patients with favorable thoracic duct anatomy. A single large duct in the upper abdomen is necessary to perform the procedure, and the anatomy is predetermined by lymphangiogram, CT scan and/or MRI. The cisterna chyli is cannulated percutaneously and the catheter is threaded up the thoracic duct under fluoroscopic guidance. The leak is located and coils and/or glue are injected into the duct. Postembolization injections are performed to verify cessation of the leak.

When the duct was accessed and in the recent study from Kaiser's group, embolization with coils and/or glue was effective in 64 out of 71 patients (90%).[17] Needle interruption of the duct is necessary when the duct cannot be cannulated or embolized, but is less effective at controlling the leak with 13 out of 18 patients (72%) successfully being managed in this fashion. For a detailed description of this technique, see Chapter 131.

If thoracic duct embolization or disruption is not possible or unsuccessful, then surgery is undertaken. The operative approach involves either direct repair of the leak or right-sided mass ligation of the thoracic duct just above the aortic hiatus. We favor mass ligation of the duct over attempt at repair for patients who have had a prior thoracotomy when the leak is difficult to localize, and to avoid potential injury of adjacent structures. More explicitly, this approach avoids the necessity of dissecting around the site of previous aortic surgery or following resection in the neck or chest. In the case of prior neck dissections, potential injury to nearby vital structures such as the phrenic nerve or subclavian vessels is obviated. Right-sided mass ligation of the thoracic duct above the diaphragmatic hiatus can be used to treat a leak in any location.

Alternatively, a direct repair can be attempted with incision made in the right or left chest or neck (if secondary to prior neck surgery or dissection). Usually this repair is performed by using a limited, muscle-sparing thoracotomy because localization of the leak and ligation of the tiny structure with fine sutures are difficult with a purely thoracoscopic approach. Preoperative and/or intraoperative enteral administration of cream via a nasogastric tube or jejunostomy can be very helpful in locating the leak.

Chyle leaks associated with mediastinal lymphoma or neoplasia metastatic to the mediastinum can be difficult to manage. Effective treatment of the underlying malignancy, if possible, with radiation or chemotherapy, often will cause the leak to stop. In instances where the malignancy responds poorly to chemoradiation, numerous interventions have been attempted, including percutaneous embolization of the duct. Ligation or direct repair of the duct may be difficult or impossible owing to the burden of disease. Insertion of a tunneled subcutaneous valved pleuroperitoneal shunt may allow for evacuation of the pleural space and reabsorption in the peritoneum. However, the patient must pump the catheter manually throughout the day. Alternatively, an indwelling pleural catheter can be used for palliative management and is much easier to care for with the help of caregivers or family members.[18] Pleurodesis, either chemical or by complete pleurectomy, is usually the last and least favored option for refractory chylothorax of any etiology, but may stop the leak through obliteration of the pleural space. Chemical pleurodesis can be done using a number of novel substances in addition to standards such as talc or doxycycline, and include elemene, 50% glucose, blood patch, and minocycline irrigation.[19–22]

TECHNIQUE

Thoracic Duct Leak Repair

A direct repair can be considered when the leak has been clearly identified. The site of the leak may be determined preoperatively by placement of right- or left-sided thoracostomy tubes or by the appearance of a milky-white drainage from a neck incision. The traditional approach for a leak in the pleural cavity is a muscle-sparing posterolateral thoracotomy. If the patient has had a recent thoracotomy, the prior incision is reopened either fully or in part with the adjunctive use of thoracoscopy if possible. On the right side, the course of the duct is inspected

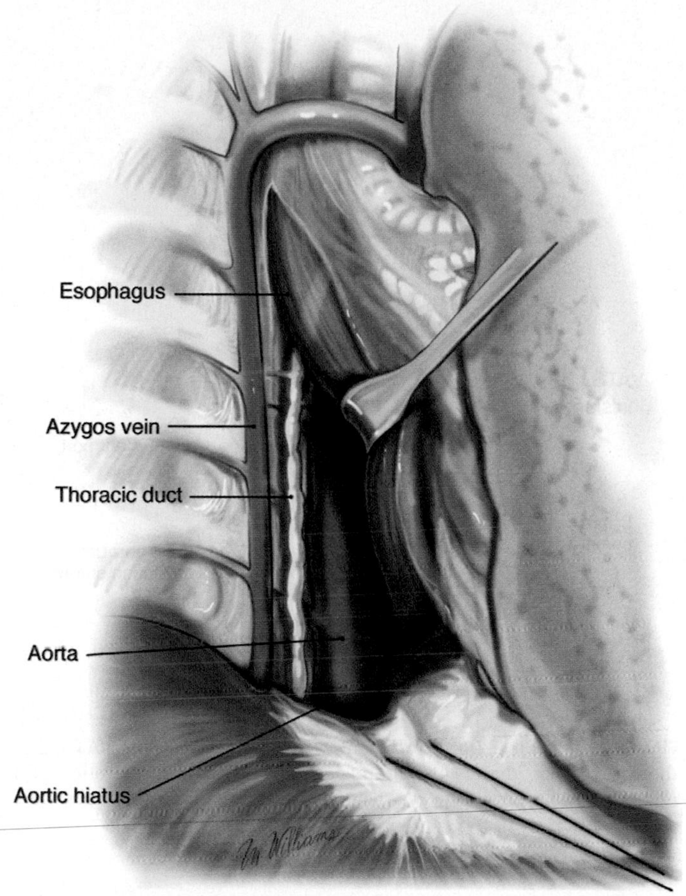

Figure 133-2. Exposure of thoracic duct for direct repair by means of a muscle-sparing posterolateral thoracotomy approach.

between the aorta and azygos vein along the spine (Fig. 133-2). The duct crosses into the left chest at the level of the fifth or sixth vertebral body.

Before incision, up to 1 L or more of heavy cream is administered enterally. A limited posterolateral thoracotomy is performed, sparing the serratus muscle. The chest is entered through the fifth interspace, although for leaks localized to the upper chest a fourth interspace incision can be used. Alternatively, a sixth or seventh interspace incision can be used for leaks localized to the lower chest. Magnifying loops may be helpful in identifying the thoracic duct and the site of leak. A search is conducted along the predicted course of the duct. If the leak is not found, further inspection of all midline operative sites is performed (i.e., sites of mediastinal nodal dissection, aortic surgery, etc.). Near-infrared fluorescence imaging is an up-and-coming modality in visualizing thoracic duct flow and site of leak in a porcine model that should eventually have clinical applications.[23]

The easiest, most secure method of repair is to use a pledgeted fine suture (i.e., 4-0 polypropylene). If a large duct has been interrupted, clips to either side of the duct may be applied, although this method may be less secure than direct suture ligation. The site of repair should be observed before and after repair for several minutes to ensure cessation of the chyle leak. A tissue sealant also can be used in conjunction with repair or ligation, but should not be relied on as the sole treatment.

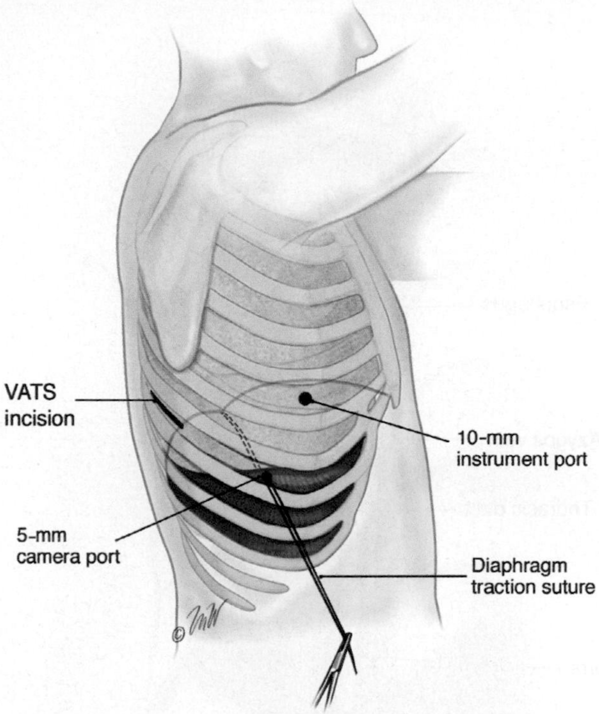

Figure 133-3. Ideal port placement for direct repair with VATS (i.e., thoracoscopy to identify the site of leak and to guide the location of a minithoracotomy utility port). This also may be used for simple mass suture ligation.

Thoracoscopy is sometimes used to identify the site of leak and to guide the location of a minithoracotomy utility port (Fig. 133-3). A 5-mm camera can be inserted in the midaxillary line at approximately the seventh interspace. An additional 10-mm port is placed in the anterior axillary line at approximately the fifth or sixth interspace, and a grasping instrument is used to draw the lung forward. Alternatively, a fan retractor can be used. If the leak is not found, an additional posterior port can be placed behind and inferior to the tip of the scapula and the camera moved to this location. A figure-of-eight heavy silk stitch can be placed in the central tendon near the esophageal hiatus and passed out through the 5-mm port to retract the diaphragm inferiorly and expose the course of the thoracic duct near the diaphragm. Again, direct repair (other than clipping) of a fine thoracic duct can be difficult when following a purely thoracoscopic approach, and a minithoracotomy (i.e., video-assisted thoracic surgery [VATS]) incision placed directly over the leak can simplify the repair.

Mass Ligation of Duct

Mass ligation of the duct can be performed by thoracotomy, VATS, or even entirely by a thoracoscopic approach. In this region, between the diaphragmatic hiatus and the point where the thoracic duct passes over the spine to the left chest, the path of the duct is consistent in nearly all patients, even though the duct itself may have a plexiform configuration (see Fig. 133-1, inset C). A serratus-sparing sixth interspace thoracotomy incision is made, and the lung is retracted forward. The diaphragm is retracted inferiorly. The esophagus, or neoesophagus, is retracted anteriorly. Just above the aortic hiatus, the course of

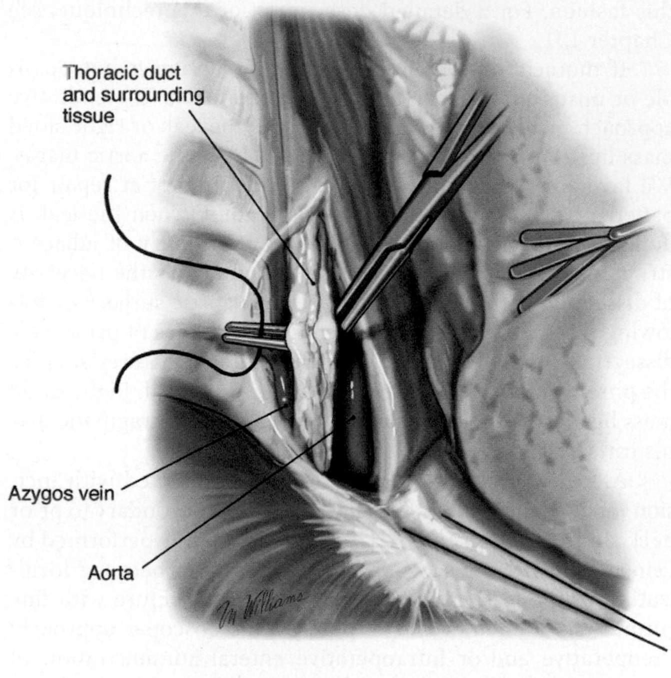

Figure 133-4. Technique for simple mass suture ligation of a thoracic duct leak in the right chest.

the thoracic duct can be visualized between the aorta and azygos vein overlying the spine. The pleura is incised over the edge of the aorta and over the edge of the spine. Several techniques may be used. A large, blunt right-angled clamp is passed under the duct alongside the aorta, onto the surface of the spine, and out again medial to the azygos vein, and a large suture (e.g., 0 silk) is tied around the tissues (Fig. 133-4). Large metal clips can be used instead, and others have even tried a TA stapler or LigaSure (Valley Lab, Denver, CO) device.[24,25]

Alternatively, a size 0 stitch or a smaller, pledgeted stitch could be used to encompass all the tissues between the aorta and azygos vein along the spine. The EndoStitch (Covidien, Mansfield, MA) can also be used. Occasionally, the suture, ligature, or clip may tear or pull through the duct, creating a new leak. Hence the ligation should be inspected carefully for several minutes to verify the integrity of the repair. In addition, the area of original leak should be inspected to ensure that it has fully sealed. One method of knot-tying that is very helpful in avoiding the pulling through of the suture that can be associated with hand-tying in this tight, low space is use of the Ti-Knot (LSI Solutions, Victor, NY) technique. With this device, the suture is placed in similar fashion, either passed under the bundled mass of tissue opened with a clamp or following suture ligature placement, but then the knot is tied down using the device which pulls the sutures through a short metal tie down clip that is crimped tight over the tissue as the surgeon pulls down tension with the instrument.

Thoracoscopic or VATS mass ligation can be performed as described for repair, with the utility incision placed at approximately the eighth interspace, centered over the posterior axillary line. Suture ligation or passage of a large tie around the ductal area can be performed as described earlier, especially with use of the EndoStitch and Ti-Knot. Regardless of surgical access technique, all fibrinous debris should be removed from the chest, and if there is any fibrin peel on the lung, it must be decorticated before closure to ensure complete lung reexpansion. A posteriorly directed drainage tube(s) should be placed.

Postoperative Care

Properly placed thoracostomy drainage tubes are important for continued control of chest drainage and pleural apposition. In theory, fatty foods should not interfere with the patient's recovery once the ductal injury has been controlled, and the diet can be advanced as tolerated. If there is concern regarding the effectiveness of the repair, it may be prudent to keep the patient on a low-fat oral diet and/or with elemental tube feedings. Total parenteral nutrition should be discontinued when the patient is able to achieve full oral intake. The chest tube drainage amount and character should be recorded and monitored closely. The chest tubes can be removed when the drainage is clear and less than 200 mL/day after resumption of a full-fat diet. Chest radiography should be followed to rule out residual effusion not controlled by thoracostomy drainage.

PROCEDURE-SPECIFIC COMPLICATIONS

Failure to Identify or Inadequate Repair of Chyle Leak

Intraoperative administration of enteral cream is an invaluable method of increasing the rate of chyle production, visualizing the leak intraoperatively, and verifying cessation of the leak. Direct closure of the frail-injured duct probably is accomplished most reliably with fine suture (e.g., 4-0 polypropylene) with pledgets. Adjacent tissue is incorporated into the pledgets to compress and seal the duct. Alternatively, if a single, large duct is seen, clips can be used above and below the site of tear. The risk of failure may be somewhat increased with simple clipping because of collaterals with other lymph ducts or the azygos.

Injury to Adjacent Structures

Approaching a duct repair via mass ligation may be useful when one wishes to avoid a duct leak that lies adjacent to a phrenic nerve injury or to a prior surgical site (e.g., aortic repair or replacement).

SUMMARY

A thoracic duct leak can be a life-threatening condition because it often occurs in a malnourished patient recovering from a major illness or surgery. Drainage of the pleural space, reexpansion of the underlying lung, and quantification of the leak are important first steps. Small leaks (typically <500 mL/day) may be given a trial of observation with diet modification or cessation of oral intake and parenteral hyperalimentation. Postesophagectomy leaks and large-volume leaks (>1000 mL/day) almost always require surgical correction. Observation of these leaks for greater than 7 days can have adverse effects on patient outcome. Percutaneous intervention for thoracic duct embolization or disruption of the cisterna chyli is a good strategy to consider before committing to surgical intervention or reoperation.

CASE HISTORIES

Case 1

A 61-year-old man with stage III (T3N1M0) adenocarcinoma of the esophagus underwent esophagectomy after neoadjuvant chemoradiation. A three-incision technique was used for the esophageal resection, including a radical lymphadenectomy and prophylactic thoracic duct ligation. The chest tube drainage persisted after a normal postoperative swallow evaluation and with advancement to a full-liquid diet plus supplemental tube feeds. Despite a dietary restriction of clear liquids and elemental tube feedings, the drainage from the chest tube remained elevated at 800 to 1200 mL/day during the second week of postoperative care. Since the patient was not responding to conservative measures, there was concern that he was in jeopardy of nutritional compromise. Therefore, the patient was evaluated and treated by the interventional radiology team with a percutaneous thoracic duct embolization. A preprocedure MRI revealed suitable anatomy for the percutaneous approach. After a lymphangiogram via a lower extremity cut-down, the cisternal chyli was identified and cannulated. The duct was embolized successfully with coils and embolic agent glue. The chest tube was removed several days later, after the patient was back on a full liquid oral diet plus standard supplemental tube feeds and producing minimal output from the chest tube.

Case 2

A 46-year-old man with tonsillar squamous cell carcinoma underwent resection and left modified radical neck dissection after induction chemotherapy coupled with combined chemoradiation. During dissection in the deep cervical fibrofatty plane, a prominent lymphatic structure representing the thoracic duct was identified and doubly ligated. No active drainage was noted before closure despite provocative Valsalva maneuvers. In the subsequent postoperative period, the neck drainage became milky in color, yielding 900 mL/day. The patient underwent duct ligation by a thoracoscopic approach on the right side. The duct was clearly visible as it coursed through the tissues between the azygos vein and the aorta and crossed over the mediastinum into the left chest at the level of the subcarinal lymph nodes. Clips were used to ligate the duct, which resulted in evidence for proximal dilatation and distal decompression consistent with successful ligation. The chest drain was removed 2 days later with the patient on a full diet.

Case 3

A 59-year-old man with adenocarcinoma of the esophagus underwent esophagectomy after neoadjuvant chemoradiation. The resection was done using a three-incision technique and prophylactic thoracic duct ligation. However, after the operation, chylous drainage was noted with an output of up to 2 L/day. The patient was taken back to the OR for exploration. Two areas were in question for the source of chyle leak, one around the lymph node dissection at the level of the azygocaval junction and the other over the hiatus. The tissue around both areas was ligated with polypropylene sutures and covered with a fibrin sealant (Tisseel, Baxter International, Inc., Biosurgery Division, Deerfield, IL). In addition, a pleurectomy was done to ensure good apposition of the lung to the chest wall for obliteration of the pleural space. The chest tube was removed 3 days later with the patient on a full diet with minimal drainage.

EDITOR'S COMMENT

There is an important practical distinction between surgically induced and tumor-related chylothoraces. Both etiologies can produce identical clinical presentation, fluid chemistries, and cell composition; however, surgical injury to the thoracic duct usually occurs in the setting of an unobstructed lymphatic system. In contrast, tumor-related chylothoraces – typically, a consequence of lymphoma – occur as a result of an obstructed lymphatic system and pose a far more difficult management problem.

—Steven J. Mentzer

References

1. Lampson RS. Traumatic chylothorax; a review of the literature and report of a case treated by mediastinal ligation of the thoracic duct. *J Thorac Surg.* 1948;17:778–791.
2. Paes ML, Powell H. Chylothorax: an update. *Br J Hosp Med.* 1994;51:482–490.
3. Wemyss-Holden SA, Launois B, Maddern GJ. Management of thoracic duct injuries after oesophagectomy. *Br J Surg.* 2001;88:1442–1448.
4. Breaux JR, Marks C. Chylothorax causing reversible T-cell depletion. *J Trauma.* 1988;28:705–707.
5. Merrigan BA, Winter DC, O'Sullivan GC. Chylothorax. *Br J Surg.* 1997;84:15–20.
6. Cerfolio RJ, Allen MS, Deschamps C, et al. Postoperative chylothorax. *J Thorac Cardiovasc Surg.* 1996;112:1361–1365; discussion 5–6.
7. Staats BA, Ellefson RD, Budahn LL, et al. The lipoprotein profile of chylous and nonchylous pleural effusions. *Mayo Clin Proc.* 1980;55:700–704.
8. Deso S, Ludwig B, Kabutey NK, et al. Lymphangiography in the diagnosis and localization of various chyle leaks. *Cardiovasc Intervent Radiol.* 2012;35:117–126.
9. Boffa DJ, Sands MJ, Rice TW, et al. A critical evaluation of a percutaneous diagnostic and treatment strategy for chylothorax after thoracic surgery. *Eur J Cardiothorac Surg.* 2008;33:435–439.
10. Tatar T, Kilic D, Ozkan M, et al. Management of chylothorax with octreotide after congenital heart surgery. *Thorac Cardiovasc Surg.* 2011;59:298–301.
11. Merigliano S, Molena D, Ruol A, et al. Chylothorax complicating esophagectomy for cancer: a plea for early thoracic duct ligation. *J Thorac Cardiovasc Surg.* 2000;119:453–457.
12. Shah RD, Luketich JD, Schuchert MJ, et al. Postesophagectomy chylothorax: incidence, risk factors, and outcomes. *Ann Thorac Surg.* 2012;93:897–903; discussion 903–904.
13. Cagol M, Ruol A, Castoro C, et al. Prophylactic thoracic duct mass ligation prevents chylothorax after transthoracic esophagectomy for cancer. *World J Surg.* 2009;33:1684–1686.
14. Guo W, Zhao YP, Jiang YG, et al. Prevention of postoperative chylothorax with thoracic duct ligation during video-assisted thoracoscopic esophagectomy for cancer. *Surg Endosc.* 2012;26:1332–1336.
15. Lai FC, Chen L, Tu YR, et al. Prevention of chylothorax complicating extensive esophageal resection by mass ligation of thoracic duct: a random control study. *Ann Thorac Surg.* 2011;91:1770–1774.
16. Cope C, Kaiser LR. Management of unremitting chylothorax by percutaneous embolization and blockage of retroperitoneal lymphatic vessels in 42 patients. *J Vasc Interv Radiol.* 2002;13:1139–1148.
17. Itkin M, Kucharczuk JC, Kwak A, et al. Nonoperative thoracic duct embolization for traumatic thoracic duct leak: experience in 109 patients. *J Thorac Cardiovasc Surg.* 2010;139:584–589; discussion 9–90.
18. Jimenez CA, Mhatre AD, Martinez CH, et al. Use of an indwelling pleural catheter for the management of recurrent chylothorax in patients with cancer. *Chest.* 2007;132:1584–1590.
19. Jianjun Q, Song Z, Yin L, et al. Treatment of chylothorax with elemene. *Thorac Cardiovasc Surg.* 2008;56:103–105.
20. Chen Y, Li C, Xu L, et al. Novel treatment for chylothorax after esophagectomy with 50% glucose pleurodesis. *Ann Vasc Surg.* 2010;24:694.e9–e13.
21. Windhaber RA, Holbrook AG, Krysztopik RJ. Blood patch treatment of chylothorax following transthoracic oesophagogastrectomy: a novel technique to aid surgical management. *Ann R Coll Surg Engl.* 2010;92: W10–1.
22. Huang PM, Lee YC. A new technique of continuous pleural irrigation with minocycline administration for refractory chylothorax. *Thorac Cardiovasc Surg.* 2011;59:436–438.
23. Ashitate Y, Tanaka E, Stockdale A, et al. Near-infrared fluorescence imaging of thoracic duct anatomy and function in open surgery and video-assisted thoracic surgery. *J Thorac Cardiovasc Surg.* 2011;142:31–38. e1–e2.
24. Stringel G, Teixeira JA. Thoracoscopic ligation of the thoracic duct. *JSLS* 2000;4:239–242.
25. Khelif K, Maassarani F, Dassonville M, et al. Thoracoscopic thoracic duct sealing with LigaSure in two children with refractory postoperative chylothorax. *J Laparoendosc Adv Surg Tech A.* 2007;17:137–139.

PART 22

CHEST WALL AND STERNAL TUMORS

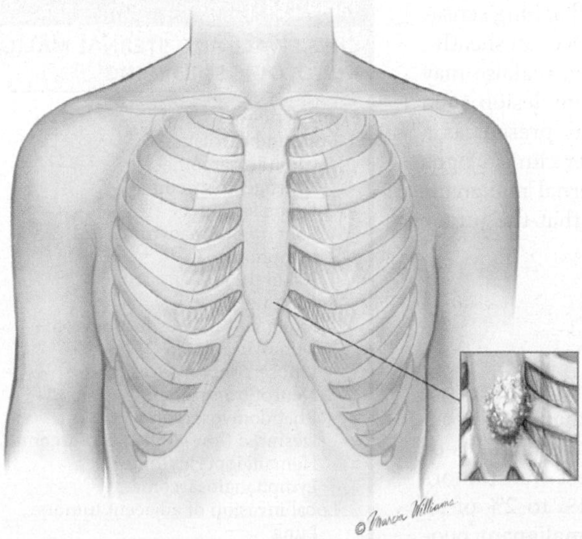

134 Overview of Chest Wall and Sternal Tumors

Yael Refaely

Keywords: Benign and malignant chest wall/sternal tumors, chondroma, chondrosarcoma, osteochondroma, eosinophilic granuloma, Ewing sarcoma, fibrous dysplasia, histiocytoma, lymphoma, osteomyelitis, osteosarcoma, malignant fibrous histiocytoma, radiation-induced sarcoma, rhabdomyosarcoma, solitary plasmacytoma

Chest wall tumors reflect a wide range of the various musculoskeletal diseases. Their infrequency in this unique location generates a diagnostic and therapeutic challenge to the thoracic surgeon. More than half the malignant tumors of the chest wall represent either metastatic lesions from distant organs (i.e., carcinoma or sarcoma) or invasion from contiguous structures such as the breast, lung, pleura, or mediastinum.[1] Primary malignant neoplasms include tumors that arise from soft, cartilaginous, or bony tissues. The most common pathology is sarcoma and, less frequently, solitary plasmacytoma or lymphoma. In many series, the number of patients reported is small because of the rarity of primary chest wall malignant tumors; thus the data on these cases are limited. From these data it can be concluded that approximately 45% of primary malignant chest wall tumors arise from soft tissue sarcomas and 55% appear in cartilaginous or bony tissue.[2]

PRESENTING SIGNS AND SYMPTOMS

The soft tissue chest wall tumor commonly presents as an enlarging mass without pain. Conversely, patients with bone tumors most often have pain as their initial complaint secondary to periosteal damage or expansion. Rapidly expanding lesions more often produce pain and favor a malignant diagnosis. The character of the pain is a persistent, dull aching sensation that is likely related to stretching of the pericostal sheath.

Constitutional complaints such as fever and malaise may accompany Ewing sarcoma. Rarely, a benign bony lesion such as osteomyelitis or eosinophilic granuloma may present as a painful bony mass with fever and malaise. Other clinical signs and symptoms produced by chest wall and sternal malignancies are related to invasion or pressure effects that the tumor exerts on adjacent structures.

DIFFERENTIAL DIAGNOSIS

Chest wall masses can be divided into three main categories: malignant, benign, and nonneoplastic. More than half of all chest wall tumors represent metastases from different sites or local invasion of adjacent tumors. Primary chest wall tumors are relatively uncommon and represent only 1% to 2% of all primary neoplasms. Table 134-1 classifies the malignant neoplasms of the chest wall.

Benign tumors comprise approximately half the primary neoplasms of the chest wall. The most common benign neoplasms in the chest wall are osteochondroma and chondroma. Osteochondroma is the most common benign rib neoplasm and accounts for nearly 50% of this group. It is usually asymptomatic and does not mandate removal. Chondromas usually occur anteriorly at the costochondral junction. The chondroma commonly presents as a slowly enlarging mass that may range from slightly painful to not painful at all. It is impossible to differentiate a chondroma from a chondrosarcoma on clinical and radiographic examination, and microscopic differentiation can be extremely difficult. Therefore, wide surgical excision is recommended for these tumors.

Nonneoplastic conditions include inflammations and cysts. Fibrous dysplasia is a cystic, nonneoplastic lesion characterized by fibrous replacement of the medullary cavity of the rib. It usually manifests as a slowly enlarging, nonpainful mass in the posterolateral rib cage. Excision is not indicated unless it enlarges and becomes painful.

The evaluation of patients with chest wall masses should include a careful history and physical examination, followed by plain film chest x-ray. Particular attention should be paid when there is a history of previous malignancies or if there are recognized risk factors for soft tissue and bone sarcomas. These factors include previous radiation therapy, exposure to chemicals (e.g., vinyl chloride and arsenic), immunodeficiency, prior injury (e.g., scars and burns), chronic tissue irritation (e.g., foreign-body implants), neurofibromatosis, Paget disease, bone

Table 134-1

CHEST WALL AND STERNAL MALIGNANCIES: HISTOLOGIC SUBTYPING

- Primary tumors
  - Bone and cartilage
    - Chondrosarcoma
    - Osteogenic sarcoma
    - Ewing sarcoma
    - Solitary plasmacytoma
    - Lymphoma
    - Askin tumor
  - Soft tissue
    - Malignant fibrous histiocytoma
    - Leiomyosarcoma
    - Liposarcoma
    - Neurofibrosarcoma
    - Rhabdomyosarcoma
    - Desmoid (low-grade fibrosarcoma)
    - Hemangiopericytoma
    - Lymphangiosarcoma
  - Local invasion of adjacent tumors
    - Lung
    - Pleura
    - Breast
    - Mediastinum
    - Skin (melanoma)
  - Metastatic tumors
    - Carcinoma
    - Sarcoma

infarcts, and genetic cancer syndromes (e.g., hereditary retinoblastoma, Li–Fraumeni syndrome, and Gardner syndrome). In most patients, however, no specific etiology can be identified.

DIAGNOSTIC TECHNIQUES

CT Scanning and MRI

CT scanning and MRI play complementary roles in the evaluation of chest wall masses. CT scanning is faster and less expensive and more accurately demonstrates cortical bone distraction from masses arising in the ribs. MRI, on the other hand, is better for depicting infiltration of bone marrow and evaluating the extent of intraspinal and soft tissue involvement. The choice of technique, CT scanning versus MRI, often depends on the clinical question being addressed. CT scanning of the chest is necessary to rule out metastatic disease.

Molecular Imaging

The exact role of ^{18}F-fluorodeoxyglucose PET/CT (18F-FDG PET/CT) scanning in the diagnosis and management of chest wall malignancies has not been fully determined. Substantial evidence supports its use in soft tissue and bone sarcoma. Fuglø et al.[3] retrospectively reviewed FDG PET/CT in 89 patients with high-grade bone and soft tissue sarcoma. They found high sensitivity, specificity, and accuracy, 95%, 96%, and 95%, respectively, for detection of lymph node and distant metastases. They also found that the maximum standardized uptake value (SUV max) of the primary tumor was a strong predictor of survival. A high SUVmax indicated a poor prognosis, a lower value a better prognosis. Nishiyama et al.[4] also found the SUV max value in FDG PET/CT to be an independent predictor of event-free survival and overall survival in 42 patients with chest wall sarcoma. 18F-FDG PET/CT scanning might also be useful in patient management as a tool for biopsy guidance, whole-body staging, therapeutic response assessment, and evaluation of residual mass lesions after treatment. 18F-FDG PET/CT scanning may aid tumor grading but offers inadequate discrimination between low-grade tumors and benign lesions.

Tissue Diagnosis

While obtaining tissue for diagnosis, there are several pitfalls to keep in mind. The skin incision or the Tru-Cut needle tract must not jeopardize subsequent skin flaps. Hematoma must be avoided because it may propel sarcoma cells into and along soft tissue planes. The biopsy must be adequate for pathologic study. Necrotic tissue, hematoma, or inflammatory tissue may be present within the biopsy rather than tumor tissue, and therefore, if there is any question about the adequacy of the tissue specimen, a frozen section to confirm the cancerous tissue should be performed.

Core Needle Biopsy

Percutaneous core needle biopsy was found to be effective and safe for the diagnosis of musculoskeletal masses.[5] It can be performed either by palpation or using image-guided procedures, that is, CT scan, fluoroscopy, or ultrasonography. Welker et al.[5] found that CT-guided biopsy permitted 88% of the patients with suspected sarcomas to undergo a single needle biopsy procedure before the initiation of definitive treatment. Only 7.4% of the masses in their study required open biopsy. Besides being cost-effective, core needle biopsy limits the size of the biopsy tract that must be removed at the time of definitive wide or radical excision. If neoadjuvant therapy is planned, the treatment can be given immediately without waiting for wound healing. It should be emphasized that while evaluating a patient with previous malignancy for suspected chest wall metastasis, fine-needle aspiration should be sufficient for making a diagnosis.

Open Biopsy

Open biopsy should be employed when the needle biopsy is not diagnostic, or for tumors with unusual histologic patterns, when it is important to know whether these patterns are present throughout the whole lesion or confined to small areas of the tumor. In these circumstances, open biopsy will be more informative. Open biopsy also appears to be superior for the diagnosis of cystic bone lesions. These lesions contain substantial amounts of fluid, blood, and necrotic material that are not diagnostic. A biopsy specimen from the wall of the lesion is therefore needed.

Open biopsy can be either excisional or incisional, but any incisional biopsy site must be planned to permit complete excision of its scar with the primary tumor at a subsequent surgical resection. It is accepted that for tumors smaller than 5 cm, *excisional* biopsy should be performed with at least 1-cm margins, while *incisional* biopsy is recommended for tumors greater than 5 cm, taking into consideration future definitive resection. In cases of a primary malignant tumor diagnosed by excisional biopsy, the patient should usually undergo reoperation for radical resection and wider margins.

SPECIFIC TUMORS

Chondrosarcoma

Chondrosarcoma is the most common primary malignant bone tumor of the chest wall. It is more common in males and in the age group of 30 to 60 years. It usually presents on the anterior chest wall, arising from the costochondral arches or sternum. It may occur as the result of malignant degeneration of a benign chondroma. Both chondrosarcomas and benign chondromas present as painful, slow-growing, hard, fixed, and nontender anterior chest wall masses. Radiologic features of both tumors may be indistinguishable; therefore, a histologic diagnosis is required to assess malignancy. Chondrosarcoma has the appearance of a large expanding mass containing chondroid-type calcifications accompanied by a significant soft tissue component that causes distraction of the bone (Fig. 134-1). Current therapy for chondrosarcoma requires adequate surgical excision with a margin of at least 4 cm. Chemotherapy is ineffective, and radiation therapy is used only for patients with tumors that are either not amenable to surgical resection or have positive resection margins. In the Mayo Clinic series,[6] the overall survival rate at 5 years was 92%. The recurrence rate for patients with adequate surgical margins was 10%, compared with 75% in patients with inadequate surgical margins. The 5-year survival rate for patients with adequate surgical margins was 100%, compared with 50% in patients with inadequate surgical margins. Inadequate surgical margins of resection were associated with a significantly decreased overall survival and a higher chance of local recurrence.

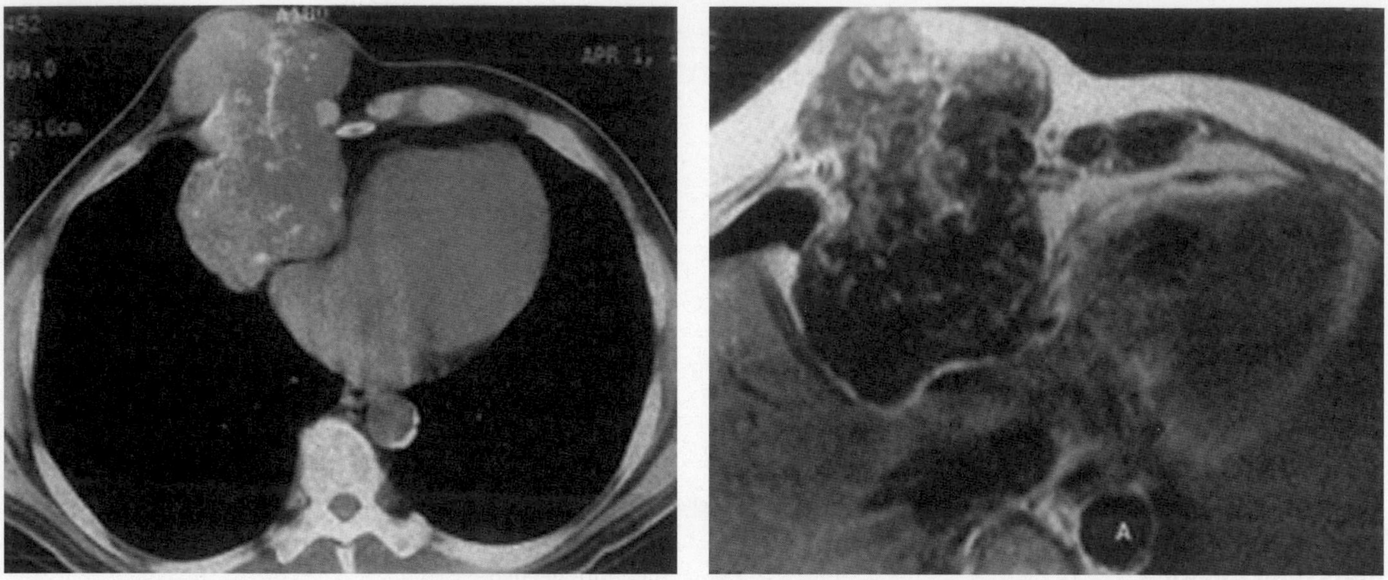

A B

Figure 134-1. Chest wall chondrosarcoma in a 62-year-old man. *A.* Nonenhanced CT scan shows a large mass that arises from the costochondral junction. The mass extends into the subcutaneous tissue and compresses and displaces the heart. *B.* Axial gadolinium-enhanced T_1-weighted MRIs show that the mass is heterogeneous and enhances. (Reproduced with permission from Gladish GW, Slaboff ABM, Munden RF, et al. Primary thoracic sarcomas. *Radiographics.* 2002;22:621–637.)

Osteosarcoma

Osteosarcoma is much less common than chondrosarcoma among primary bony chest wall malignancies. Although osteosarcoma represents the most common primary malignant tumor arising in bone, only 3% arise from the chest wall (Fig. 134-2). Osteosarcomas occur in a bimodal age distribution. Adolescents and young adults are affected most commonly, with a smaller subgroup of patients developing osteosarcoma after age 40. It commonly presents as a rapidly enlarging, painful mass. In older patients, secondary osteosarcoma may develop in preexisting diseases of the bone, such as Paget disease, bone infarction, sites of previous radiation, and so forth. Metastatic disease (lung mostly) is present in one-third of patients at initial presentation, and over two-thirds of patients will develop metastases at some point. For this reason, perioperative chemotherapy is standard treatment, with improved 5-year survival of up to 50% for extremity osteosarcoma. Given that primary osteosarcoma of the chest wall is such a rare tumor, it is permissible to extrapolate the survival benefit of chemotherapy from extremity osteosarcoma, with the exception that tumors

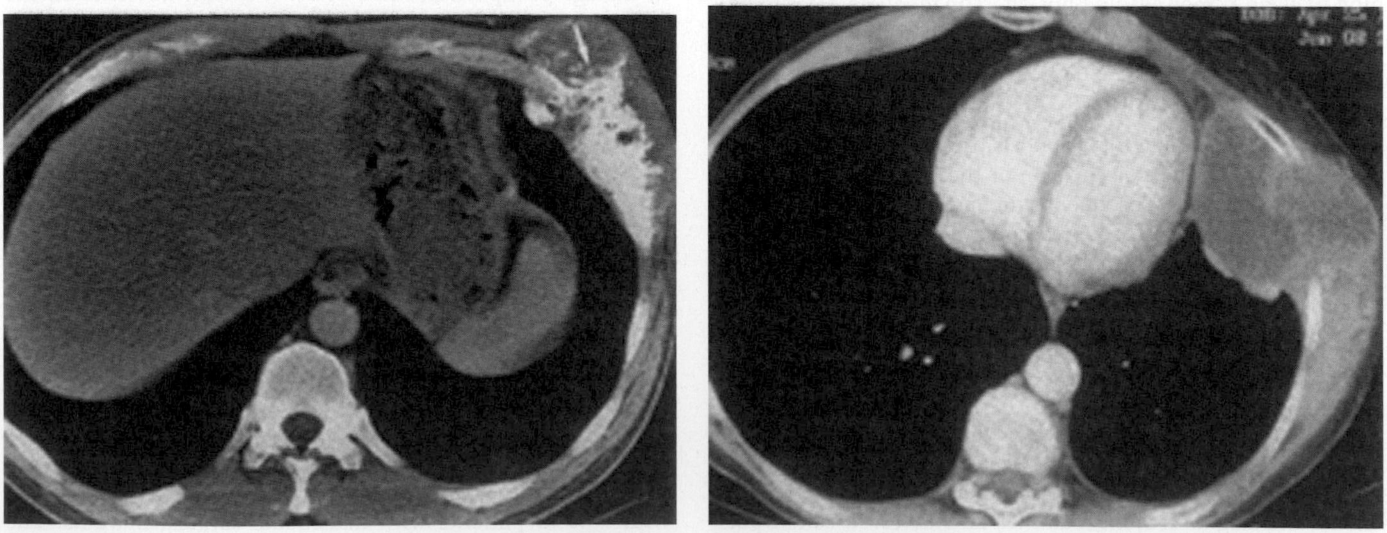

A B

Figure 134-2. *A.* Osteosarcoma in a 43-year-old man. Contrast-enhanced CT scan shows a left-sided chest wall mass with an osteoid matrix (arrow), a finding characteristic of chest wall osteosarcoma. *B.* Osteosarcoma in a 52-year-old woman. Contrast-enhanced CT scan shows a heterogeneous chest wall mass without an ossified matrix. (Reproduced with permission from Gladish GW, Sabloff BAM, Munden RF, et al. Primary thoracic sarcomas. *Radiographics.* 2002;22:621–637.)

presenting in diverse sites may respond differently. Radiotherapy is largely ineffective in treating osteosarcoma.

Solitary Plasmacytoma

Plasmacytoma is a rare tumor that consists of sheets of plasma cells of variable maturity. The histologic features are indistinguishable from those found in multiple myeloma. The presence of multiple myeloma is excluded by the absence of multicentric disease and plasma cell infiltration of the bone marrow. The most common sites are the vertebral column in approximately 50% of the patients, with tumors of the ribs and sternum accounting for 10% to 15% of cases. It is twice as common in men, and it may occur in any age group. The most common mode of presentation in the chest wall is pain without a palpable fixed mass. Radiologic testing usually shows a solitary osteolytic or punched-out bone lesion without evidence of primary tumor. Systemic manifestations such as anemia, hypercalcemia, impaired renal function, immunoglobulinopathy, or elevated Bence–Jones protein are not expected in this disease.

The role of surgery in the management of solitary plasmacytoma of the chest wall is limited to diagnostic biopsy in most settings. Definitive local radiation is the treatment of choice, providing local control in over 90% of patients. Chemotherapy is used if there is evidence of progression to multiple myeloma, such as may occur in 75% of patients.

Ewing Sarcoma

Ewing sarcoma is the most common malignant tumor of the chest wall in children and young adults. It is a small round cell sarcoma that occurs primarily in flat bones and in the midshaft of long bones. Approximately 300 new cases of Ewing sarcoma occur each year worldwide. Only 15% of these cases occur in the chest wall. It arises almost exclusively in white populations. Two-thirds of all cases of Ewing sarcoma are seen in persons younger than 20 years. Over the past two decades, the 5-year survival rate has improved dramatically from 10% to 50% in different series. The improvement in survival is attributed to the availability of newer chemotherapy regimens to treat systemic disease. Most patients will develop metastasis at some point in the course of their disease. Because of the typical systemic nature of this tumor, chemotherapy alone with some form of local therapy is the standard. Shamberger et al.[7] compared the completeness of resection and disease-free survival in patients undergoing initial surgical resection versus those treated with neoadjuvant chemotherapy followed by resection, radiotherapy, or both. Patients with positive resection margins received radiotherapy. They reported 98 patients with Ewing sarcoma of the chest wall. Their 5-year disease-free survival was 56% and did not differ based on timing of surgery or type of local control. However, neoadjuvant chemotherapy decreased the percentage of patients needing radiation therapy. Seventy percent of the patients undergoing initial surgery received radiotherapy compared with 40% of patients who had neoadjuvant therapy and then surgery.

Lymphoma

Among primary chest wall tumors, chest wall lymphoma is uncommon, accounting for fewer than 2% of primary tumors. Few cases of primary malignant lymphoma arising from the pleura, the rib, or the sternum have been reported. Hsu et al.[8] reported their experience in seven patients with non-Hodgkin lymphoma presenting as a solitary chest wall mass. For three patients with chest wall lymphoma as the only site of disease, complete surgical resection followed by chemotherapy was carried out with satisfactory outcome. Most of the patients had B-cell lymphoma. Histologic cell types reported by others include Hodgkin lymphoma and other non-Hodgkin lymphomas.

The primary treatment of choice for lymphoma with or without chest wall involvement is chemotherapy and radiation. It is debatable whether surgical resection followed by adjuvant chemotherapy can provide a survival benefit in some patients in whom the chest wall lymphoma is the only site of disease.

Soft Tissue Sarcoma

Primary soft tissue sarcomas of the chest wall are uncommon. Of the 11,000 new cases of soft tissue sarcoma diagnosed annually in the United States, fewer than 10% arise in the chest wall. A few studies have suggested that soft tissue sarcomas of the chest wall and primary extremity sarcomas have similar prognoses. Both groups have better survival rates than observed in patients with retroperitoneal, head and neck, and visceral soft tissue sarcomas. Gross et al.[9] reviewed 55 surgically treated patients with chest wall soft tissue sarcomas. The median age of their patients was 47.5 years, with a male predominance. Painless mass was the most common initial presentation. The median duration of symptoms was 12 months and is longer than that reported for patients with tumors in other sites. The tumor diameter in most patients was larger than 9 cm. The overall 5-year survival rate was 87.3%. The disease-free survival rates at 5 and 10 years were 75% and 64%, respectively. Tumor size less than 5 cm, low histologic grade, and wide surgical resection were determinants of a better disease-free survival.

Undifferentiated Pleomorphic Sarcoma (Malignant Fibrous Histiocytoma)

Malignant fibrous histiocytoma, now officially referred to as undifferentiated pleomorphic sarcoma, is the most commonly observed soft tissue sarcoma in adults. It generally develops after radiation therapy and may originate in the extremities, retroperitoneum, peritoneal cavity or occasionally the chest wall. It is usually a disease of advanced age and is seen during the sixth and seventh decades of life. It does not have any strong gender preference. In most instances, the patient is asymptomatic, and the appearance is that of a well-defined, lobulated or regular soft tissue mass. On CT scan, histiocytomas enhance heterogeneously with contrast material and rarely contain calcifications (Fig. 134-3). The diagnosis is confirmed by histopathologic and immunohistochemical analysis of tumor tissue. Such sarcomas are highly aggressive and surgery remains the cornerstone of treatment whenever possible. Wide excision with chest wall reconstruction using synthetic mesh or flap reconstruction is advocated for chest wall involvement as these tumors are generally not responsive to chemotherapy or radiation therapy as sole treatment modalities.[10–13]

Rhabdomyosarcoma

Rhabdomyosarcoma is a childhood tumor that has a bimodal age distribution. In adults, it is seen after age 50 and occurs more often in males. It can originate either from chest wall

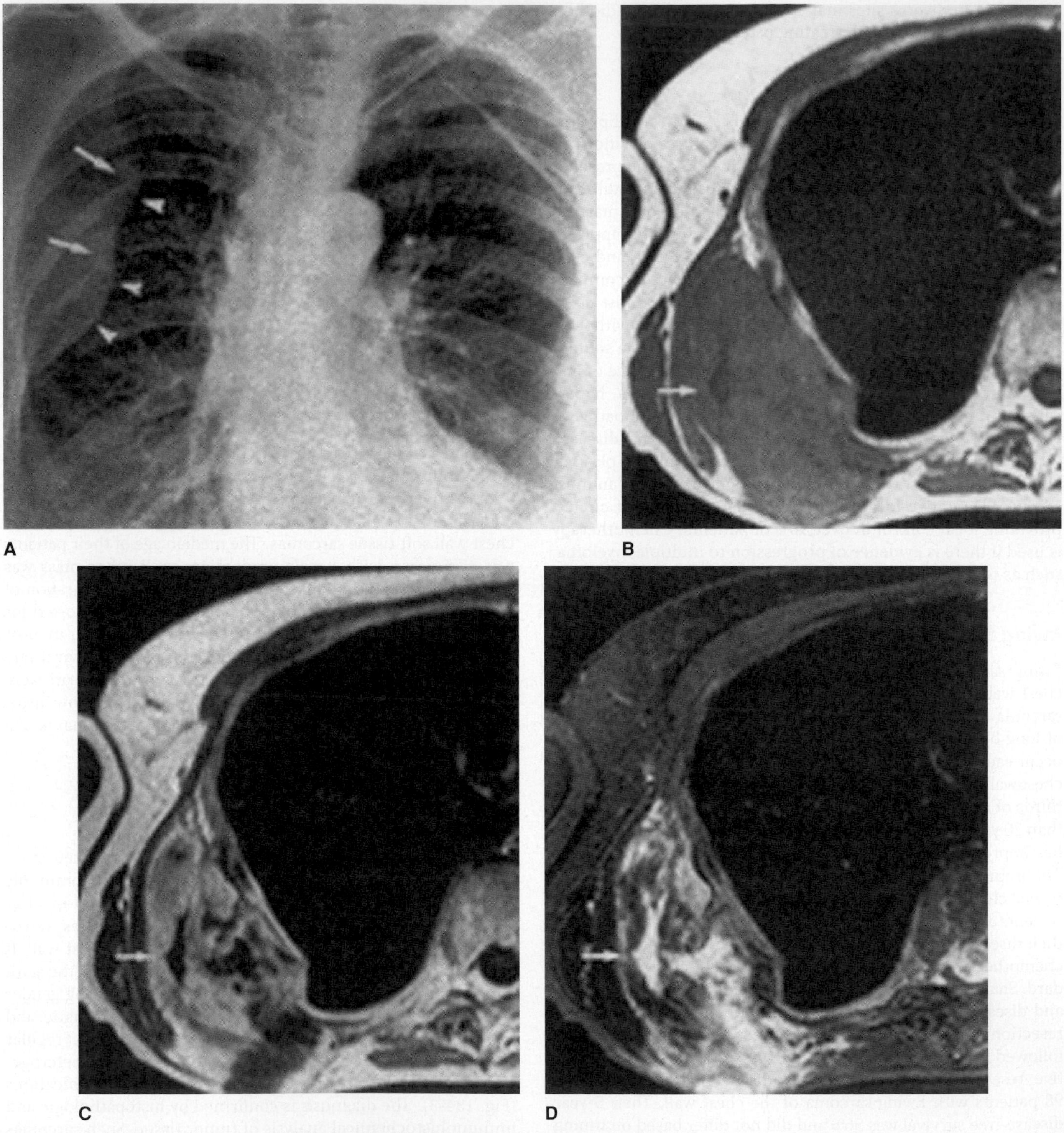

Figure 134-3. Malignant fibrous histiocytoma of the chest wall in a 76-year-old woman. *A.* The chest x-ray shows a large extraparenchymal mass in the right upper hemithorax. MRIs show that the mass has heterogeneous signal intensity and marked enhancement on *B.* Axial T_1-weighted *C.* gadolinium-enhanced T_1-weighted and *D.* fat desaturation T_2-weighted images. (Reproduced with permission from Gladish GW, Sabloff BM, Munden RF, et al. Primary thoracic sarcomas. *Radiographics.* 2002;22:621–637.)

striated muscles or the diaphragm. Prognosis depends on the histopathologic subtype. Alveolar type has a less favorable prognosis than the embryonic and pleomorphic subtypes. Since these tumors can remain clinically silent, they may have already reached large dimensions by the time of diagnosis. There may be necrosis and cystic areas within the mass.

Fibrosarcoma

Fibrosarcoma originates from the connective tissue found in the chest wall. It is the most common cell type among soft tissue sarcomas of the chest wall in children and young adults. It forms a large mass, and on CT scan, foci of calcifications or ossification may be observed.

Desmoid Tumor

Desmoid tumors are slow-growing mesenchymal neoplasms without metastatic potential. They most frequently occur during the second or third decades of life, but can be seen in all age groups. Although the etiology is unknown, genetic predisposition in patients with familial adenomatous polyposis and association with pregnancy have been recognized. Histologically they consist of small numbers of spindle cells with rare mitoses and surrounded by copious stoma. They appear to arise from musculoaponeurotic tissue. Desmoid tumors present high tendency toward local infiltration and invasion. Invasion to surrounding structures results pain, functional limitation, deformity, and even death if vital organs become compromised. Although distant spread has not been documented in long-term follow-up studies, these tumors have a strong propensity to recur locally after resection. In a series of 53 patients who underwent resection for desmoid tumor of the chest wall, Abbas et al.[14] found that the 5-year overall probability of developing a local recurrence was 37.5%.

Surgery remains the gold standard of treatment and achieving microscopic negative margins is the goal of the surgical resection. Nevertheless, it should be noted that while most studies in the past suggested that positive resection margins correlated with high recurrence rate, more recent papers with large number of cases have been questioning this assumption. Moreover, wide negative margins do not further decrease the recurrence rate when compared to microscopically negative margins, whether they frequently compromise functional result. Melis et al. reviewed the current evidences for multimodality management of desmoids and presented the following algorithms: complete surgical excision with negative margins is the goal of treatment but, this should not be achieved at the cost of functional compromise. The most radical example for that might be in a case where upper extremity amputation is needed in order to achieve negative margins. The recommendation in this situation is to reserve amputation only for patients whose limb is already nonfunctional or embrace other tumor related complications. If residual tumor is left behind, treatment options include: reexcision (if this can be safely performed), adjuvant radiation or chemotherapy, or observation. In patients with recurrence, reexcision can be followed by radiation therapy, especially if residual tumor is left behind or if the tumor recurred after complete initial excision.[15]

Patients who have multiple locoregional recurrences despite adequate local therapy are considered for systemic therapy. Additional indications for systemic therapy include unresectable tumors. Options for systemic therapy include anti-inflammatory agents, hormonal agents (e.g., antiestrogens and androgens), systemic chemotherapy, and more recently good tumor response has been observed with kinase directed therapies such as Imatinib and Sorafenib.[16]

Radiation-Induced Sarcomas

Sarcomas are a rare but recognized complication of radiotherapy for chest malignancies and are associated with poor prognosis. In 1948, Cahan et al.[17] established the criteria for the diagnosis of radiation-induced sarcoma (RIS). These criteria are still in use today and include (1) history of radiotherapy, (2) asymptomatic latency period of several years, (3) occurrence of sarcoma within a previously irradiated field, and (4) histologic confirmation of the sarcomatous nature of the post irradiation lesion. The incidence of RIS is considered to be associated with radiotherapy dose. A shorter latency period also was found to be associated with high-dose radiotherapy. Indications for the initial irradiation are most commonly breast carcinoma and lymphoma, but RIS may develop regardless of the initial tumor type. In a review of 351 patients with primary malignant tumors of the chest wall, Schwarz and Burt[18] identified 21 patients with lesions (6%) arising in an irradiated field. A third of the patients in this study with primary osteosarcoma had a tumor arising in the field of prior irradiation (11 of 38 patients). There was no significant difference in survival between malignant chest wall tumors arising in an irradiated field and those arising de novo. The authors concluded that since the outcome after operative therapy appeared to be similar, patients with tumors arising from an irradiated field should be offered identical treatment to those with tumors arising de novo.

In a large-scale series, Kirova et al.[19] reviewed records of 13,472 patients with breast carcinoma who were treated with megavoltage radiotherapy. Of those, 27 patients (0.2%) fulfilled the Cahan criteria. The latency period ranged from 3 to 20 years. Histologic evaluation identified most commonly angiosarcoma (48%), followed by osteosarcoma, undifferentiated sarcoma, histiocytoma, leiomyosarcomas, fibrosarcoma, rhabdomyosarcoma, and myosarcoma. The cumulative RIS incidence was 0.07% at 5 years, 0.27% at 10 years, and 0.48% at 15 years. Standardized incidence ratios were 10.2 for irradiated patients compared with 1.3 for nonirradiated patients. The 5-year actuarial survival rate after diagnosis of RIS was 36%. Since the response to chemotherapy tends to be poor, the treatment for RIS is not different from that for other primary sarcomas and involves a wide resection.

Metastatic Tumors to the Chest Wall

Metastatic disease accounts for 20% to 30% of all chest wall neoplasms. It can occur within the bony thorax or the soft tissues surrounding it. Owing to advances in cancer treatment that prolong survival, there has been a noticeable increase in the prevalence of bone metastasis. Consequently, indications for surgical treatment were expanded mainly for pathologic or high-risk fractures of the limb bones and for compression fractures in the spine. The indication for surgery of a solitary metastasis for which extended survival may be anticipated is controversial. Some thoracic surgeons regard solitary metastasis as a marker for micrometastatic disease and suggest other treatment modalities, whereas others support resection for palliation and possible survival benefit. Manabe and colleagues[20] reviewed their experience with surgical treatment of bone metastasis. They reported long survival for patients with metastases from thyroid, breast and kidney, with median survival of 56, 30, and 30 months, respectively, and short survival for those with metastases from lung and liver carcinoma (median 8 and 13 months, respectively). These findings should be considered when selecting patients for wide resection.

In a review of 703 patients who developed metastatic bone lesions after beginning treatment for breast cancer, Koizumi et al.[21] found that 41% (289) had solitary skeletal metastasis. The sternum was the most common site for solitary skeletal metastasis (98 of 289, or 34%). The patients with solitary skeletal metastasis lived longer than those with multiple metastatic bone lesions (p <0.001). Solitary sternal metastatic lesions remained solitary longer than solitary lesions in anatomic regions other than the sternum ($p < 0.001$) but did not lengthen patient survival times.

Durr et al.[22] retrospectively studied the effect of surgical therapy on a series of 70 patients with breast cancer who were treated surgically for metastasis of the bone. Surgical treatment involved: palliative procedures, radical resections, and biopsies. Of the six patients who were radically resected for solitary bone lesions, five developed systemic progression of the disease. The authors concluded that although patients with solitary bone lesions have a better prognosis, with a 39% chance of living 5 years, radical resection does not significantly improve survival.

Fuchs et al.[23] who retrospectively analyzed the survival rate of 60 patients with solitary bony metastasis from renal cell carcinoma, came to a similar conclusion. Thirteen patients had wide resection, 20 had local stabilization, and 27 patients had no surgical treatment but had adjuvant treatment alone. There was no survival advantage for patients who had a wide resection of the lesion compared with patients who had intralesional resection or intramedullary stabilization alone. These results indicate that wide surgical excision of a solitary bony metastasis from renal cell carcinoma is not mandatory to improve survival. However, wide resection of metastatic lesions may be necessary to prevent local disease progression and complications.

THERAPEUTIC OPTIONS

En bloc surgical resection with negative margins continues to be the most fundamental treatment of most tumors of the chest wall. A minimum 2-cm margin is required for low-grade tumors, and a 4-cm margin with a rib above and below the tumor is required for high-grade sarcoma. Surgical planning requires a team approach that includes a thoracic surgeon and thoracic anesthesiologist and may involve plastic surgeons or spine surgeons for lesions requiring extensive soft tissue resection or vertebral body or dural sac involvement (see Chapter 135). The resection should not be compromised because of concern for closing the defect. It is recommended that a separate plastic surgery team focus on this aspect of patient care. Usually, posterior chest wall defects, protected by either the scapula or the posterior musculature, do not require reconstruction. Lateral and anterior wall defects need to be reconstructed to protect the underlying viscera, improve respiratory function, and for cosmetic reasons. Wide excision with clear margins is the most important prognosticator for long-term survival. An aggressive surgical approach also applies for recurrences because local relapse and pulmonary metastases remain the most common sites of treatment failure (Fig. 134-4).[24]

Adjuvant treatment with chemo- and radiation therapy is used selectively for high-grade sarcomas. It is used routinely for residual disease and positive or equivocal resection margins to gain local control and prevent distant disease. The list of agents with significant activity in soft tissue sarcomas is very short and arguably only includes doxorubicin and ifosfamide. Several other agents such as dacarbazine, cisplatin, and etoposide, to name a few, have marginal activity and are sometimes used in combination. The Sarcoma Meta-analysis Collaboration[25] published an individual patient data meta-analysis of outcomes in 1568 patients from 14 randomized trials of Adriamycin-based adjuvant chemotherapy versus observation control. The median follow-up period was 9.4 years. Soft tissue sarcomas of all sites,

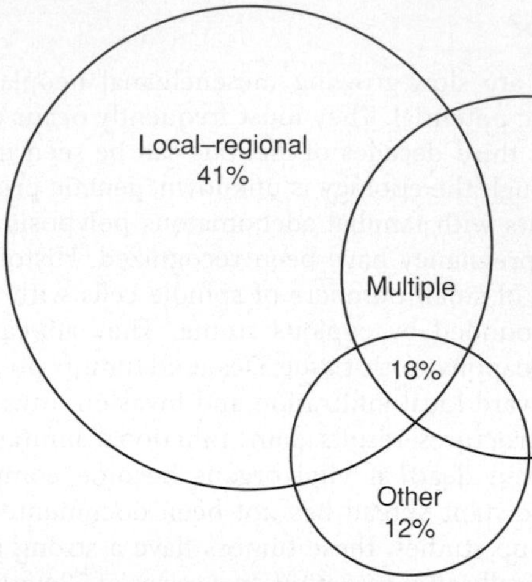

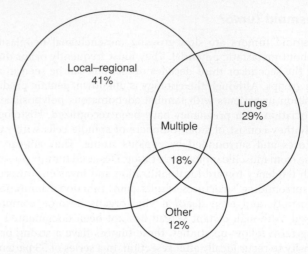

Figure 134-4. Truncal sarcomas: patterns of recurrence. (Used with permission from Sugarbaker P. Management of truncal sarcoma. In: Malawer MM, Sugarbaker P, eds. *Musculoskeletal Cancer Surgery: Treatment of Sarcoma and Allied Diseases.* Boston, MA: Kluwer Academic publishers; 2001:172.)

sizes, grades, and histology were included. This individual patient data meta-analysis showed a significant improvement for adjuvant chemotherapy with respect to time to recurrence (local and distant) and disease-free survival, but only a trend for benefit in overall survival.

Radiotherapy is used mainly for local control, although benefits similar to those seen with extremity sarcoma have not been reported. Because chest wall sarcomas are rare, many of the treatment strategies are extrapolated from treatment strategies for extremity sarcomas. Although similar chemotherapy and radiation sensitivity is frequently noted, this is not always the case. For this reason, neoadjuvant chemotherapy might be considered for patients with large tumors of borderline resectability or with lesions that are known to respond to chemotherapy, such as Ewing sarcoma, osteosarcoma, or malignant fibrous histiocytoma.

The advantages of induction therapy are that it permits the in vivo assessment of chemosensitivity, it theoretically treats occult metastasis, and it may facilitate future surgical dissections and the ability to obtain clean surgical margins if the tumor shrinks with treatment.

PERIOPERATIVE MANAGEMENT AND COMPLICATIONS

The approach to evaluating patients for chest wall resection and reconstruction is basically the same as that used for other major thoracic operations. Careful assessment is crucial to determining the best therapeutic option, as well as minimizing the operative risks. A thorough medical history and physical examination form the basis for any further investigation. Pulmonary function testing must be performed to evaluate patient reserves because a temporary compromise in respiratory function must be expected after the resection. A number of different techniques have been proposed to avoid paradoxical motion of the chest wall and impaired ventilation. Reconstruction with methylmethacrylate has been described in these situations and has gained increasing acceptance because it satisfies the requirements for rigidity, protection, and chest wall remodeling (see Chapters 135, 136). However, it also has been suggested that the rigidity achieved with methylmethacrylate for chest wall reconstruction, highly desired in the early postoperative course, might adversely influence late outcome secondary to stiffness of the chest wall and late pulmonary restriction. Lardinois et al.[26] investigated the impact of methylmethacrylate substitutes on chest wall integrity after extended anterolateral chest wall resection. At 6 months' follow-up they found that there was no significant difference between the preoperative and postoperative forced expiratory volume in 1 second and that concordant chest wall movements during expiration and inspiration were demonstrable by dynamic testing (using cine-MRI) in 92% of patients.

Patients with cardiovascular disease or known risk factors for diabetes, hypertension, or obesity; a history of smoking; or a family history of cardiovascular disease should undergo complete cardiac evaluation accordingly.

Although advanced surgical techniques, use of prosthetic materials for reconstruction, and improvements in anesthesia and postoperative care have reduced the rates of mortality and morbidity, complications occur in approximately 25% of patients. Operative mortality ranges from 0% to 4% in different series. Walsh et al. reported a multidisciplinary approach to primary sarcomas involving the chest wall in 51 patients requiring full-thickness resections. Respiratory complications occurred in 8% of patients, and wound complications occurred in 6% of the patients.[27]

Chapelier et al.[28] reviewed their experience with 38 patients with primary malignant tumors of the sternum who underwent sternal resection and reconstruction. A paradoxical motion occurred in two patients after total sternectomy and rigid replacement of the sternum and in one patient with subtotal sternectomy. These patients required prolonged ventilatory support and needed a tracheostomy. No flap-related complications were observed. Major septic complications occurred in four patients with methylmethacrylate reinforcement, which required removal of the composite prosthesis. Chang et al.[29] from Memorial Sloan–Kettering Cancer Institute reported their experience with reconstruction of complex oncologic chest wall defects in 113 patients. Eighty-four percent of the patients achieved stable chest wall reconstruction with no complications. The most common complications were partial flap loss (necrosis) in 4%, infection in 7%, hematoma in 3%, and delayed wound healing in 2%.

References

1. Pairolero PC, Arnold PG. Chest wall tumors: experience with 100 consecutive patients. *J Thorac Cardiovasc Surg*. 1985;90:367–372.
2. Incarbone M, Pastorino U. Surgical treatment of chest wall tumors. *World J Surg*. 2001;25:218–230.
3. Fuglø HM, Jørgensen SM, Loft A, et al. The diagnostic and prognostic value of (18)F-FDG PET/CT in the initial assessment of high-grade bone and soft tissue sarcoma. A retrospective study of 89 patients. *Eur J Nucl Med Mol Imaging*. 2012;39(9):1416–1424.
4. Nishiyama Y, Tateishi U, Kawai A et al. Prediction of treatment outcomes in patients with chest wall sarcoma: evaluation with PET/CT. *Jpn J Clin Oncol*. 2012;42(10):912–918.
5. Welker JA, Henshaw RM, Jelinek J, et al. The percutaneous needle biopsy is safe and recommended in the diagnosis of musculoskeletal masses. *Cancer* 2000;89:2677–2686.
6. Fong YC, Pairolero PC, Sim FH, et al. Chondrosarcoma of the chest wall: a retrospective clinical analysis. *Clin Orthop*. 2004;427:184–189.
7. Shamberger RC, LaQuaglia MP, Gebhardt MC, et al. Ewing sarcoma/primitive neuroectodermal tumor of the chest wall: impact of initial versus delayed resection on tumor margins, survival, and use of radiation therapy. *Ann Surg*. 2003;238:563–567; discussion 567–568.
8. Hsu PK, Hsu HS, Li AF, et al. Non-Hodgkin's lymphoma presenting as a large chest wall mass. *Ann Thorac Surg*. 2006;81(4):1214–1219.
9. Gross JL, Younes RN, Haddad FJ, et al. Soft-tissue sarcomas of the chest wall: prognostic factors. *Chest*. 2005;127:902–908.
10. Cho KH, Park C, Hwang KE, et al. Primary malignant fibrous histiocytoma of the pleura. *Tuberc Respir Dis (Seoul)*. 2013;74(5):222–225.
11. Yoshida N, Miyanari N, Yamamoto Y, et al. Successful treatment of malignant fibrous histiocytoma originating in the chest wall: report of a case. *Surg Today*. 2006;36(8):714–721.
12. Shikada Y, Yoshino I, Fukuyama S, et al. Completely wide resection of malignant fibrous histiocytoma of the chest wall; expect for long survival. *Ann Thorac Cardiovasc Surg*. 2006;12(2):141–144.
13. Sawai H, Kamiya A, Kurahashi S, et al. Malignant fibrous histiocytoma originating from the chest wall: report of a case and collective review of cases. *Surg Today*. 1998;28(4):459–463.
14. Abbas AE, Deschamps C, Cassivi SD, et al. Chest-wall desmoid tumors: results of surgical intervention. *Ann Thorac Surg*. 2004;78:1219–1223; discussion 1223.
15. Melis M, Zager JS, Sondak VK. Multimodality management of desmoid tumors: how important is a negative surgical margin? *J Surg Oncol*. 2008;98(8):594–602.
16. Gounder MM, Lefkowitz RA, Keohan ML, et al. Activity of Sorafenib against desmoid tumor/deep fibromatosis. *Clin Cancer Res*. 2011;17(12):4082–4090.
17. Cahan W, Woodward H, Higginbotham N. Sarcoma arising in irradiated bone: report of 11 cases. *Cancer*. 1948;1:3–29.
18. Schwarz R, Burt M. Radiation-associated malignant tumors of the chest wall. *Ann Surg Oncol*. 1996;3:387–392.
19. Kirova YM, Vilcoq JR, Asselain B, et al. Radiation-induced sarcomas after radiotherapy for breast carcinoma: a large-scale single-institution review. *Cancer*. 2005;104:856–863.
20. Manabe J, Kawaguchi N, Matsumoto S, et al. Surgical treatment of bone metastasis: indications and outcomes. *Int J Clin Oncol*. 2005;10:103–111.
21. Koizumi M, Yoshimoto M, Kasumi F, et al. Comparison between solitary and multiple skeletal metastatic lesions of breast cancer patients. *Ann Oncol*. 2003;14:1234–1240.
22. Durr HR, Muller PE, Lenz T, et al. Surgical treatment of bone metastases in patients with breast cancer. *Clin Orthop Relat Res*. 2002;396:191–196.
23. Fuchs B, Trousdale RT, Rock MG. Solitary bony metastasis from renal cell carcinoma: significance of surgical treatment. *Clin Orthop Relat Res*. 2005;431:187–192.
24. Sugarbaker P. Management of truncal sarcoma. In: Malawer MM, Sugarbaker P, eds. *Musculoskeletal Cancer Surgery: Treatment of Sarcoma and Allied Diseases*. Boston, MA: Kluwer Academic Publishers; 2001:172.
25. Anonymous. Adjuvant chemotherapy for localised resectable soft tissue sarcoma in adults. Sarcoma Meta-analysis Collaboration (SMAC). *Cochrane Database Syst Rev*. 2000;(2):CD001419.
26. Lardinois D, Muller M, Furrer M, et al. Functional assessment of chest wall integrity after methylmethacrylate reconstruction. *Ann Thorac Surg*. 2000;69:919–923.
27. Walsh GL, Davis BM, Swisher SG, et al. A single-institutional, multidisciplinary approach to primary sarcomas involving the chest wall requiring full-thickness resections. *J Thorac Cardiovasc Surg*. 2001;121:48–60.
28. Chapelier AR, Missana MC, Couturaud B, et al. Sternal resection and reconstruction for primary malignant tumors. *Ann Thorac Surg*. 2004;77:1001–1006; discussion 1006–1007.
29. Chang RR, Mehrara BJ, Hu QY, et al. Reconstruction of complex oncologic chest wall defects: a 10-year experience. *Ann Plast Surg*. 2004;52:471–479; discussion 479.

135 Chest Wall Resection and Reconstruction

David R. Jones

Keywords: Chest wall tumors, skeletal reconstruction, soft tissue reconstruction

Chest wall tumors are uncommon malignancies, whether primary or secondary in nature. Nevertheless, nearly every thoracic surgeon eventually will be asked to evaluate one of these tumors in clinical practice. It is estimated that only 500 index cases of primary malignant chest wall tumors occur in the United States annually,[1] in addition to secondary chest wall tumors, which are, most notably, those related to recurrent breast cancer. Given this relatively low incidence, no one surgeon or surgical group could be expected to have an extensive experience with this tumor type. Having a working knowledge of the surgical principles underlying the management of uncommon chest wall tumors therefore is all the more relevant.

The more common primary chest wall tumors are listed in Table 135-1. Although most of these tumors in the pediatric population are malignant, only approximately half of these tumors are malignant in adults.

TECHNICAL AND ONCOLOGIC PRINCIPLES

The overriding technical principle of chest wall surgery is similar to that of tracheal surgery. Specifically, the procedure consists of two separate but equally important parts – resection and reconstruction – and the technical considerations of each must be assessed independently.

With regard to resection, it is imperative to establish first whether the tumor is primary or metastatic, and if primary, whether it is malignant or benign. This determination may be clear from the patient's history and certain radiographic characteristics of the tumor, but a tissue diagnosis is important for several reasons. If the tumor is benign, an overly aggressive resection and complex reconstruction may not be needed. Alternatively, if the tumor is malignant, one of several different treatment strategies may be required. For example, some of these tumors (e.g., osteosarcoma and plasmacytoma) are best treated nonoperatively initially. Other primary malignant chest wall tumors (e.g., primitive neuroectodermal tumors and some sarcomas) may benefit from induction therapy before a planned surgical resection. Thus, establishing a tissue diagnosis is the first important step in the treatment algorithm for chest wall tumors.

The diagnostic technique selected for biopsy also must adhere to standard oncologic principles. The biopsy site must be placed in a location that can be incorporated into the planned resection specimen. Most chest wall lesions that arise from bone, cartilage, or soft tissues of the chest wall are amenable to diagnosis by core needle biopsy. On the rare occasion that core needle biopsy is not possible or is nondiagnostic, incisional biopsy can be performed, provided that the incision is placed within the margins of the resection specimen, as mentioned earlier. Excisional biopsy also can be used for smaller lesions (<3 cm), and if such lesions are later determined to be malignant, a wider local excision that incorporates the old surgical scar can be performed as a separate procedure.

Resectability represents another important oncologic principle, and it is addressed after the tissue diagnosis has been established. Typically, the determination of resectability involves a radiographic assessment of the involved anatomic structures. If it is determined that resection is possible, the surgeon must decide how the resulting skeletal defect will be handled and whether any additional soft tissue coverage will be required. If it is likely that a muscle flap or omentum or a split-thickness skin graft will be needed, a careful assessment of the suitability of the various tissues and flaps should be made. This assessment is often made with the assistance of a plastic surgeon both familiar and comfortable with soft tissue reconstruction of chest wall defects. The planned resection strategy should ensure a complete R0 resection if at all possible. With advances in chest wall reconstruction (both skeletal and soft tissue) and some intraoperative creativity, nearly any postresection chest wall defect can be managed successfully. Thus the size of a resulting chest wall defect has little, if anything, to do with the resectability of the tumor or extent of the planned resection.

From both a technical and an oncologic perspective, it is important to have an adequate surgical margin around the tumor. This typically requires resection of one uninvolved rib above and below the ribs invaded by the malignant tumor. The medial and lateral margins of resection should be at least 4 to 6 cm. Several reports have documented the importance of a wide

Table 135-1

PRIMARY CHEST WALL TUMORS

Malignant
Chondrosarcoma
Malignant fibrous histiocytoma
Fibrosarcoma
Primitive neuroectodermal tumors (Askin tumor of chest wall, Ewing sarcoma of bone)
Rhabdomyosarcoma
Leiomyosarcoma
Neurofibrosarcoma
Osteosarcoma
Angiosarcoma
Myeloma
Liposarcoma
Desmoid tumor (low-grade fibrosarcoma)
Benign
Chondroma
Lipoma
Osteochondroma
Fibrous dysplasia
Neurilemmoma

local excision (margin of at least 4 cm) resulting in increased disease-free and overall survivals.[2,3] For tumors located in the sternum, the sternum must be removed, although the manubrium may be spared if the tumor affects only the body. The converse is true for isolated manubrial lesions. Additionally, sternal tumors require removal of at least 2 to 3 cm of costal cartilage laterally to ensure R0 resection. If possible, the upper aspect of the manubrium should be preserved because it provides for the majority of anterior chest wall stability.[4] Resection of overlying soft tissue and skin is mandatory if there is any suspicion of tumor involvement.

An essential part of the treatment algorithm is the need for case discussion, including careful review of the pathology in the context of a multidisciplinary tumor conference. Such discussion provides the opportunity for medical and radiation oncologists to examine their potential roles in the treatment plan. This exchange is particularly important if either induction chemotherapy or catheter placement for intraoperative brachytherapy is being considered. In addition, multidisciplinary review of the staging studies and pathology ensures the appropriateness of the treatment plan.

TUMOR-SPECIFIC TREATMENTS

Most benign and malignant chest wall tumors are managed with complete surgical resection. For example, the primary treatment for chondrosarcoma, the most common malignant chest wall tumor, is wide local excision. These lesions are highly chemoresistant and have limited sensitivity to radiation. Selected tumors, however, are better managed with adjuvant therapies.

Induction chemotherapy appears to play a role in the management of some primary chest wall tumors. On the basis of data from extremity sarcoma studies, preoperative Adriamycin-based chemotherapy is used in patients with primitive neuroectodermal tumors and for some soft tissue sarcomas.[5,6] After restaging, wide surgical excision is performed, and many patients complete an additional course of adjuvant chemotherapy secondary to the high rate of systemic failure observed with surgery alone for tumors of this type.[7]

Adjuvant external beam radiation for all primary chest wall tumors typically is reserved for R1 or R2 resections or in cases where the margin, while negative, lies close to the tumor.[8] For instance, the rate of recurrence with an R1 resection of a desmoid tumor of the chest wall is 90%.[9] In contrast, patients with R0 resection for a desmoid tumor have a recurrence rate of 27%, and none of the patients who received adjuvant radiation with an R0 resection developed a recurrence. This suggests that adjuvant radiation may be reasonable in all patients with a desmoid tumor regardless of margin status. The role of adjuvant brachytherapy in the treatment of soft tissue sarcomas of the chest wall is limited by a greater incidence of regional recurrences compared with in-field recurrences. Thus external beam therapy, which covers a larger region of the tumor bed, is preferred.[10] On the other hand, brachytherapy is a useful adjunct to surgical resection for a tumor that has been irradiated previously.

For several tumors, the role of surgery is purely diagnostic. Plasmacytoma is a prime example. These tumors are associated most commonly with multiple myeloma, and even if the patient has no current clinical or laboratory evidence of the disease, he or she frequently develops the disease years later. Therefore, isolated chest wall plasmacytomas typically are treated with external beam radiation alone with very good results. Similar to plasmacytomas, osteosarcomas are often metastatic deposits from long bone (e.g., tibia, femur, or humerus) primaries, although primary chest wall osteosarcomas can arise from the ribs. Regardless of the origin, once the diagnosis is established, both types are treated initially with Adriamycin-based multidrug chemotherapy. Residual primary chest wall osteosarcomas should be resected with wide margins after restaging studies demonstrate the absence of metastatic disease.

PREOPERATIVE ASSESSMENT

After the tissue diagnosis has been established, the patient must be assessed for operability. This process necessitates evaluation of the patient's cardiopulmonary status, age, comorbidities, and performance status.

Once it is clear that the patient is operable, a careful radiographic assessment of the stage and local extent of the tumor is performed. All patients need a CT scan of the chest and upper abdomen, and many will have a PET scan as well. There are few data on the use of PET scans for primary chest wall tumors, particularly those arising from bone or cartilage, but extrapolation from other solid-tumor malignancies suggests that they may be beneficial, particularly with PET-avid tumor types known to metastasize early. Pertinent information supplied from the CT images includes the locoregional extent of the tumor, as well as its proximity to the mediastinum, vertebral bodies, and diaphragm. CT scan also may suggest the presence or absence of metastatic disease in the lung, liver, or adrenals. MRI is reserved for tumors located close to the brachial plexus and subclavian vessels and to resolve any questions about direct involvement of the great vessels or extension into the intervertebral foramina. For soft tissue tumors of the chest wall, it may be difficult to know with certainty if there is bony involvement. No roentgenographic study can definitively include or exclude bone involvement. If the patient has chest wall pain at the tumor site, there is at least an 80% likelihood that bone is involved.

If it appears that the tumor is growing into the underlying lung tissue and that a lung resection may be required, pulmonary function studies also should be performed. If the patient has had a prior surgical procedure, it is imperative to obtain the old operative notes. Likewise, if the patient has received preoperative external beam radiation, the dose and the fields need to be identified before planning the resection and, more particularly, the reconstruction. It is wise to perform a nutritional assessment of the patient and to strongly encourage smoking cessation if applicable. Finally, outpatient consultation with plastic and neurosurgical colleagues can be very helpful, particularly if removal of the tumor requires an extended resection (e.g., vertebral body) or a complex soft tissue reconstruction.

OPERATIVE TECHNIQUE

Anesthesia

General anesthesia usually is provided through a single-lumen endotracheal tube. If there is concern that concomitant pulmonary resection or diaphragm reconstruction may be required, a double-lumen tube should be placed. An epidural catheter is used routinely to help manage postoperative pain.

Patient positioning is critical because there is frequently a need for access to the abdomen, lower back, flank area, and anterior chest wall. Correct patient positioning and incision planning are facilitated in more complex cases by the presence of other members of the multidisciplinary team, who, if needed, can be called on for their input. This is particularly important if plastic surgery assistance is needed for muscle flap harvest and transposition. Concurrent with patient positioning, the patient should receive prophylactic IV antibiotics.

Chest Wall Resection

All previous incisional biopsy sites or old surgical scars need to be incorporated into the planned resection specimen. The overlying skin does not need to be excised if it is viable and free of tumor. If there is a history of significant radiation with obvious skin changes, however, the skin should be excised back to nonradiated, viable skin and underlying soft tissue. The surgical dissection and resection of a chest wall tumor are guided by the principle that a tumor should be palpated but not seen. Thus a wide (4 cm or more) margin of grossly normal soft tissue around the tumor is required as the dissection plane is being developed. This margin may include portions of the overlying chest wall musculature. The extent of chest wall or sternal resection has been discussed previously. It is worth emphasizing the importance of achieving a complete R0 resection and obtaining the necessary surgical margins despite temptations to "limit" the resulting chest wall defect.

The pleural cavity should be entered away from the tumor, and the lung should be inspected and palpated for any nodules suspicious for metastatic disease (Fig. 135-1). This is particularly important with soft tissue sarcomas. It is not uncommon for these tumors to adhere to or directly involve the underlying lung parenchyma. Usually a wide nonanatomic wedge excision

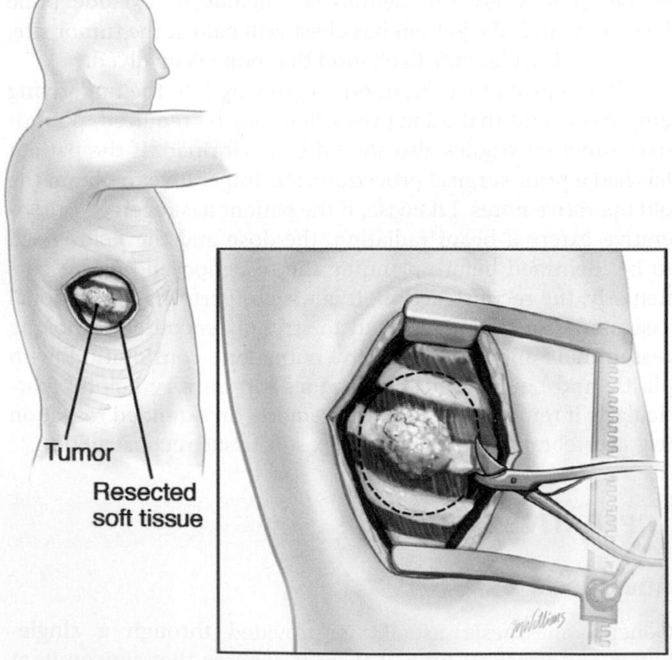

Figure 135-1. After exposing the primary chest wall tumor, rib shears are used to begin the chest wall resection 4 to 5 cm away from the primary malignant tumor.

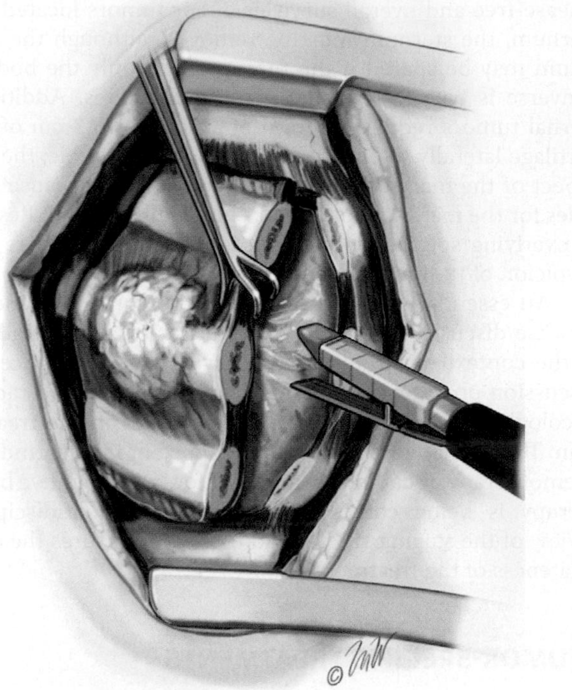

Figure 135-2. The lung parenchyma may be adherent to the primary chest wall tumor. As shown here, this can be taken en bloc with the specimen with the aid of an endo-GIA stapler.

is sufficient to obtain an adequate margin, although occasionally a lobectomy or segmentectomy is required (Fig. 135-2). Alternatively, the tumor may involve the pericardium or more likely the diaphragm. Pericardial reconstruction is necessary for right-sided resections, whereas wide opening of the entire pericardium on the left will suffice. The diaphragm is reconstructed with polytetrafluoroethylene with interrupted 0 Ethibond or Prolene sutures. This reconstruction is commonly performed independent of the chest wall reconstruction, but if the tumor involves portions of the ribs at the insertion site of the diaphragm, that edge of the Gore-Tex (W. L. Gore and Associates, TX, Flagstaff, AZ) will need to be incorporated into the resulting chest wall reconstruction as well.

The extent of chest wall resection typically includes one normal rib above and below the tumor. If an adequate chest wall margin cannot be obtained secondary to proximity to a vital structure, clips should be placed to guide adjuvant radiation therapy. Once the tumor is removed, the specimen should be inspected, and any questionable soft tissue margins should be marked and submitted for frozen-section analysis. A small Blake drain or chest tube should be placed into the pleural cavity through a separate incision.

Skeletal Reconstruction

Attention now turns to the first phase of chest wall reconstruction—the skeletal reconstruction. The choice of prosthetic material should be appropriately rigid, inert, malleable, and if possible, radiolucent to permit follow-up radiographic assessment.[11] Several prosthetic materials are available for reconstruction, including Marlex or Prolene mesh, polytetrafluoroethylene (2-mm thick), and methyl methacrylate placed

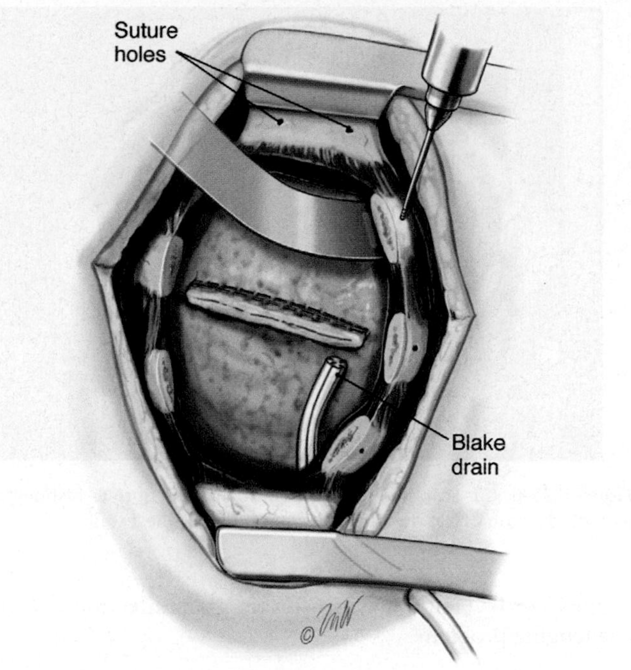

Figure 135-3. A pneumatic drill is used to place holes through the ribs for future placement of sutures, which are required to secure the prosthetic material used for the chest wall reconstruction.

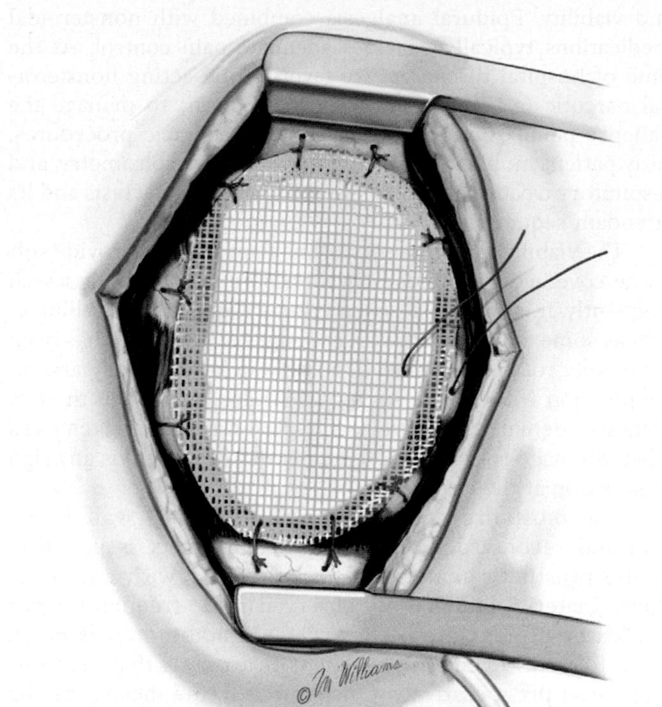

Figure 135-4. The prosthetic chest wall material is secured to the underlying ribs with nonabsorbable suture. A second running layer between the prosthetic material and the intercostal muscles typically is used to help buttress the repair.

between two pieces of Marlex mesh. The choice of material depends on the location of the defect, its size, as well as surgeon preference and experience.[12] We prefer to use the Marlex mesh-methyl methacrylate composite for large defects involving the sternum or anterolateral chest wall, where protection of the underlying cardiovascular structures is most important. The surgeon needs to fashion the methyl methacrylate to fit the defect and the contour of the chest wall and then exhibit all due patience as the substance hardens via an exothermic reaction. For smaller defects, DualMesh polytetrafluoroethylene is quite easy to use and is impervious to fluid and air. Regardless of the prosthetic material chosen, the prosthesis is sewn to the ribs with interrupted nonabsorbable sutures (0 Ethibond or Prolene) placed around the ribs superiorly and inferiorly and through holes drilled into the rib edges laterally and medially. An alternative to placing the sutures around the ribs and their associated neurovascular bundles is to drill holes in the ribs superiorly and inferiorly and place the sutures accordingly (Fig. 135-3). The prosthetic material is then secured in place with a slight amount of tension to confer some rigidity to the chest wall reconstruction (Fig. 135-4).

Occasionally the chest wall defect is very large and the number and length of resected ribs required to remove the tumor and have negative margins are significant. These large defects can be addressed through a combined prosthetic (titanium) rib osteosynthesis and expanded polytetrafluoroethylene (DualMesh).[13] When this approach is used one needs to tailor the DualMesh such that its circumference is approximately 2 cm greater than the defect area. The number of titanium plates that should be used depends on the number of resected ribs, but in general one plate is sufficient for skeletal reconstruction of 2.75 ribs. While uncommon, there can be occasion to need a vertical expandable titanium prosthesis, and these devices are also available. Once the extensive skeletal chest wall defect is reconstructed, one should use a muscle flap to provide additional soft tissue coverage over the combined DualMesh and titanium plate reconstruction.

Chest wall defects that do not require skeletal reconstruction typically are very small (<3 cm) or posterior defects that lie above the fourth rib and are covered by the scapula. One does need to be aware that herniation of the scapular tip into the pleural cavity through an unclosed defect in the fifth or, less commonly, sixth rib can happen and is quite painful. These ultimately will require surgical reintervention.

Soft Tissue Reconstruction

After the skeletal reconstruction is completed, the second phase of chest wall reconstruction begins with mobilization and rotation of the muscle flaps or omentum to provide soft tissue coverage of the defect. This part of the procedure is often performed in conjunction with a plastic surgeon, although for smaller flaps and omentum we have performed the soft tissue coverage ourselves. We typically place Jackson–Pratt drains under the flaps, the harvest sites, or both to help prevent the formation of seromas.

POSTOPERATIVE CARE AND PROCEDURE-RELATED COMPLICATIONS

The postoperative care of the patient who undergoes a chest wall resection and reconstruction centers on adequate pain control, pulmonary hygiene, and assessment of flap integrity and viability. Epidural analgesia combined with nonsteroidal medications typically provides adequate pain control. At the time of hospital discharge, we favor a long-acting nonsteroidal narcotic (e.g., OxyContin or MS Contin) to manage the patient's pain. Common to other major thoracic procedures, early patient mobilization, coughing, incentive spirometry, and respiratory treatments are instituted to avoid atelectasis and its attendant sequelae.

The viability and integrity of the flaps used to provide soft tissue coverage for the chest wall closure need to be assessed frequently. It is typical to observe some slight tissue swelling as well as some faint duskiness at the edges of a flap that has been maximally rotated. This needs to be watched carefully and, in conjunction with plastic surgery, debrided only when there is complete demarcation. Previously placed drains are removed when drainage is less than 30 mL per day or if there is any sign of infection at the drain site.

The most dreaded complication of chest wall resection and reconstruction of the skeletal defect is infection of the prosthetic material. This can occur with any prosthetic material but may be observed more frequently with Marlex or Prolene mesh constructs. In addition, it is much more likely to occur in patients with wounds that are contaminated preoperatively. Once infected, the mesh must be removed to completely eradicate the problem. Deschamps et al.[14] report a 4.6% infection rate in 197 patients undergoing chest wall resection and reconstruction with prosthetic material. Fifty percent of those infected had mesh, and the others had polytetrafluoroethylene. Of note, the mesh was removed in all patients, and the polytetrafluoroethylene was removed in none. Even if the mesh requires removal, the lung commonly adheres to the chest wall, and thus an open pneumothorax is avoided. The wound is managed subsequently with debridement and gauze packing, and healing occurs by secondary intent.

SUMMARY

Resection and reconstruction of the chest wall require a multidisciplinary effort. Optimal results are obtained with aggressive resection of tumor with adequate margins, followed by reconstruction of resulting skeletal and soft tissue defects. Complications are few, although prosthetic graft infection can be a challenging problem.

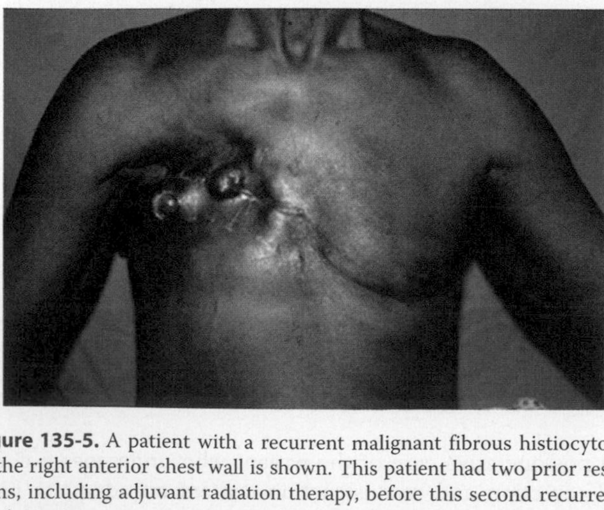

Figure 135-5. A patient with a recurrent malignant fibrous histiocytoma of the right anterior chest wall is shown. This patient had two prior resections, including adjuvant radiation therapy, before this second recurrence of his tumor.

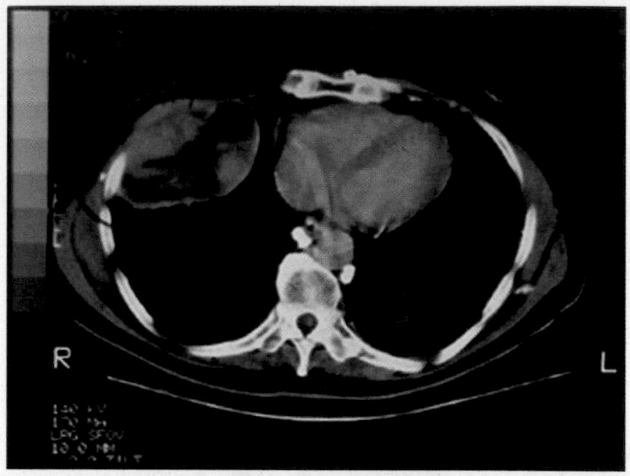

Figure 135-6. CT scan showing a large malignant fibrous histiocytoma with destruction of the ribs along the anterolateral chest wall.

CASE HISTORY

A 62-year-old man had resection of a right anterior chest wall malignant fibrous histiocytoma followed by adjuvant external beam radiation for positive margins. The initial resection included soft tissue only, and no ribs were resected. Two years later he presented with a painful recurrent mass (Fig. 135-5). He had no other complaints, and his performance status was good. CT scan demonstrated a large tumor involving the right anterolateral ribs with possible invasion of the diaphragm and lung (Fig. 135-6). A core needle biopsy of the lesion confirmed recurrent malignant fibrous histiocytoma.

The patient was scheduled for a combined thoracic and plastic surgery chest wall resection and reconstruction. After intubation with a double-lumen endotracheal tube, a wide local chest wall excision of the mass was performed, including all previously irradiated skin and soft tissue. The resection included removal of one noninvolved rib above and below the tumor (Fig. 135-7). The tumor was found at surgery to be invading the lung and diaphragm. A nonanatomic wedge resection of the right lower lobe was performed, and the diaphragm was resected en bloc with the tumor. The diaphragm then was reconstructed with polytetrafluoroethylene. Given the size of the chest wall defect, a methyl methacrylate mesh prosthesis was constructed and used to close the skeletal defect (Fig. 135-8). The resulting soft tissue defect was closed in conjunction with the plastic surgery service using a right transverse myocutaneous rectus abdominis flap. Jackson–Pratt drains were placed at the flap harvest site.

EDITOR'S COMMENT

Although rare, the resection of chest wall tumors and subsequent "pearls" of reconstruction are critically important skills for all thoracic surgeons to master. Failure in either aspect often will significantly impact patient outcome and/or quality of life.

—Yolonda L. Colson

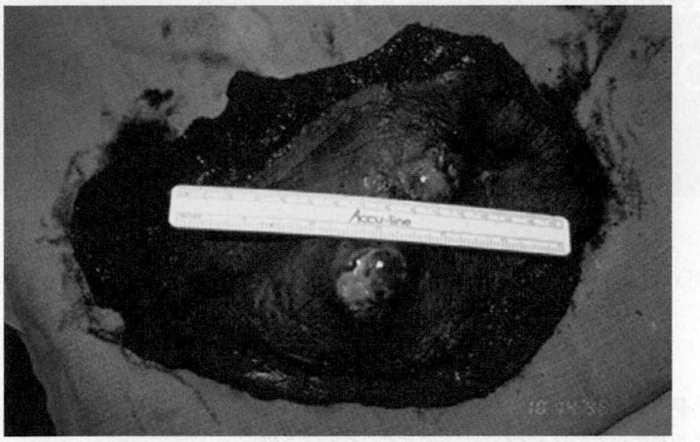

Figure 135-7. The surgical specimen includes overlying skin, soft tissue, and ribs that were involved with tumor. Additional soft tissue margins were necessary to excise all tissue in the prior radiation field.

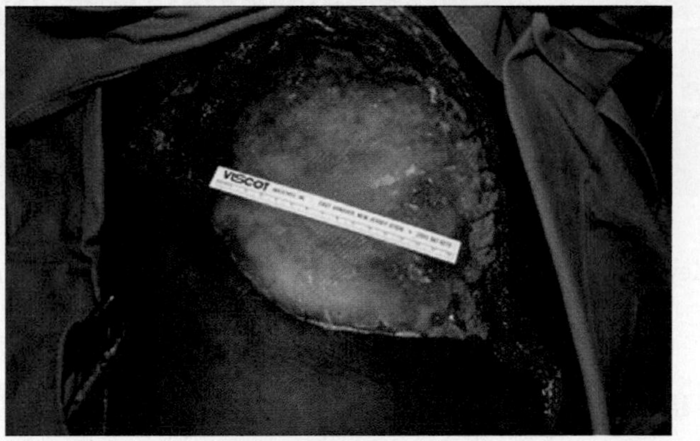

Figure 135-8. After the tumor is resected, the chest wall is reconstructed with methyl methacrylate, as shown here. Note that the chest tubes were surgically placed before chest wall reconstruction. A contralateral rectus abdominis flap was then rotated to provide soft tissue coverage of the defect.

References

1. Graeber G, Jones D, Pairolero P. Primary neoplasms. In: Pearson FG, Cooper JD, Deslauriers J, et al. eds. *Thoracic Surgery*. New York, NY: Churchill Livingstone; 2002:1417–1430.
2. Graeber GM, Snyder RJ, Fleming AW, et al. Initial and long-term results in the management of primary chest wall neoplasms. *Ann Thorac Surg*. 1982;34:664–673.
3. McAfee MK, Pairolero PC, Bergstralh EJ, et al. Chondrosarcoma of the chest wall: factors affecting survival. *Ann Thorac Surg*. 1985;40:535–541.
4. Downey RJ, Huvos AG, Martini N. Primary and secondary malignancies of the sternum. *Semin Thorac Cardiovasc Surg*. 1999;11:293–296.
5. Pisters PW, Ballo MT, Patel SR. Preoperative chemoradiation treatment strategies for localized sarcoma. *Ann Surg Oncol*. 2002;9:535–542.
6. Issels RD, Schlemmer M. Current trials and new aspects in soft tissue sarcoma of adults. *Cancer Chemother Pharmacol*. 2002;49:S4–S8.
7. Gordon MS, Hajdu SI, Bains MS, et al. Soft tissue sarcomas of the chest wall: results of surgical resection. *J Thorac Cardiovasc Surg*. 1991;101:843–854.
8. Alektiar KM, Velasco J, Zelefsky MJ, et al. Adjuvant radiotherapy for margin-positive high-grade soft tissue sarcoma of the extremity. *Int J Radiat Oncol Biol Phys*. 2000;48:1051–1058.
9. Abbas AE, Deschamps C, Cassivi SD, et al. Chest-wall desmoid tumors: results of surgical intervention. *Ann Thorac Surg*. 2004;78:1219–1223; discussion 1223, .
10. Wallner KE, Nori D, Burt M, et al. Adjuvant brachytherapy for treatment of chest wall sarcomas. *J Thorac Cardiovasc Surg*. 1991;101:888–894.
11. LeRoux B, Shama D. Resection of tumors of the chest wall. *Curr Probl Surg*. 1983;20:345–386.
12. Incarbone M, Pastorino U. Surgical treatment of chest wall tumors. *World J Surg*. 2001;25:218–230.
13. Berthet JP, Canaud L, D'Annoville T, et al. Titanium plates and dual mesh: a modern combination for reconstructing very large chest wall defects. *Ann Thorac Surg*. 2011;91:1709–1716.
14. Deschamps C, Tirnaksiz BM, Darbandi R, et al. Early and long-term results of prosthetic chest wall reconstruction. *J Thorac Cardiovasc Surg*. 1999;117:588–591; discussion 591–592.

136 Sternal and Clavicular Chest Wall Resection and Reconstruction

Jeffrey B. Velotta and Jay M. Lee

Keywords: Sternal and clavicular resection and reconstruction, primary or secondary sternal or clavicular malignancy, radiation osteonecrosis

INTRODUCTION

Sternal resection is primarily required for primary or secondary malignancy, infection, or radiation osteonecrosis (radiation osteitis).[1,2] The resulting chest wall defect involving loss of skeleton and often overlying soft tissue depends on tumor extent and type, and severity of infection or radiation necrosis. Full-thickness sternal resections can compromise chest wall stability or have paradoxical respiratory movements, highlighting the importance of proper reconstruction of the thoracic wall and sternum.

Primary tumors of the thoracic skeleton are rare, accounting for 4.5% to 8% of published series of primary bone tumors with 11% in the sternum and 9% in the clavicles.[3] Sternal tumors are classified as primary tumors (i.e., benign or malignant), adjacent tumors with local invasion (i.e., lymphoma or primary neoplasm of lung, breast, pleura, or mediastinum), metastases (i.e., primary neoplasm of breast, lung, or thyroid), and nonneoplastic lesions (i.e., inflammatory masses or bone cysts). The majority of sternal tumors are malignant and frequently represent metastasis or direct invasion by adjacent tumor.[1,4,5] The majority of primary sternal malignancies are bony or cartilaginous in origin.[3–5] The most common primary malignancy of the sternum is chondrosarcoma, and other common primary malignancies include osteosarcoma, solitary plasmacytoma, and Ewing sarcoma.[3–5] Although primary benign tumors of the sternum are rare, the most common benign tumors of the sternum are chondroma and osteochondroma.[6]

Most clavicle tumors are malignant and much more likely to be metastases than primary tumors. Primary neoplasms of the clavicle are rare. The most common primary malignancy of the clavicle is solitary plasmacytoma.[7] Isolated clavicular resection is rare. Indications for resection include (1) exposure of the base of the neck, superior mediastinum, or brachial plexus, (2) tumor, infection, or injury/trauma of the clavicle itself or in association with sternal/chest wall resection, and (3) dysfunction of the sternoclavicular and acromioclavicular joints.[8] Distal clavicle pathology generally entails dysfunction of the acromioclavicular joint which is usually managed by orthopedic surgeons specializing in shoulder reconstruction. The distal end of the clavicle is commonly resected for arthritis and dislocation of the acromioclavicular joint. Partial, medial clavicular resection is required during an anterior approach to superior sulcus tumor resection (Chapter 80).[9] In addition, clavicular resection may be sufficient to provide exposure of the ipsilateral superior mediastinum during head and neck operations obviating the need for a partial or complete median sternotomy.

PATIENT SELECTION AND PREOPERATIVE ASSESSMENT

Careful preoperative evaluation, including assessment of cardiopulmonary reserve, is critical for successful outcome. A detailed history should identify comorbid factors such as advanced age, malnutrition, overall debilitation, and cardiopulmonary disease. Severe respiratory insufficiency is considered a contraindication for extensive sternal resection. There should be a clear understanding of the patient's prior operations with attention to location of previous incisions and radiation treatment history, including location and dosage of exposure. This information is critical in establishing the reconstructive plan, particularly when assessing availability and usability of muscle and omental flaps.

An extent of disease workup to determine appropriateness of resection should be thoroughly investigated. Given the high propensity for metastases to occur in the sternum and clavicle, there should be investigation for a primary tumor elsewhere. Our preference is a whole body PET/CT scan with intravenous contrast to assess for extrathoracic disease. CT scan of the chest with intravenous contrast is the single best radiographic modality to localize and characterize the sternum, clavicle, and chest wall. Thorough knowledge of the extent of involvement by sternal or clavicular pathology (e.g., mediastinal structures, pulmonary parenchyma, ribs, sternum, clavicles, and overlying soft tissues) is readily obtained through CT scanning. Although MRI of the chest is not mandatory in every case, it can be quite helpful in evaluating invasion of the thoracic inlet, brachial plexus, and subclavian vasculature. MRI is also useful in characterizing cartilage and soft tissue, and is more sensitive in evaluating bone marrow edema and replacement than CT. Image guided (CT or ultrasound) core needle biopsy of chest wall and sternal tumors has been shown to be a safe and highly accurate diagnostic modality to determine malignancy, histological subtype, and high-grade differentiation of musculoskeletal tumors.[10] Preoperative tissue diagnosis should be obtained to determine presence and type of malignancy and also to consider neoadjuvant or definitive chemotherapy depending on the tissue diagnosis.[10] On this basis, imaged guided needle biopsy is routinely performed before resection, and incisional biopsy is rarely needed.[10]

Given the rarity of sternal and clavicular mesenchymal tumors, a multidisciplinary team approach to guide management and treatment plans is recommended.[10] Preoperative treatment may be appropriate in some situations (i.e., metastases, high-grade soft tissue sarcoma, osteosarcoma, Ewing sarcoma, and mesenchymal or dedifferentiated chondrosarcoma).

Consultation with a plastic surgeon to devise plans for soft tissue reconstruction may be necessary for complex situations, such as those requiring extensive myocutaneous flaps (Chapter 138).

TECHNIQUE

General Principles

The sternum provides structural support for the thoracic skeletal structures and stabilizes the shoulder girdle through the clavicles. In addition, it provides a protective barrier to the mediastinum, particularly the great vessels and the heart. Surgical principles governing resection of the sternum or clavicle emphasize the importance of a complete resection with clear margins. Repair or reconstruction of these bony defects requires the selection of appropriate prosthetic and/or autologous replacement material. It is important to stabilize the chest wall and sternum to maintain the normal dynamics of respiration and to protect mediastinal structures. Current techniques most often entail the use of rigid prostheses and soft tissue (muscle or omentum) coverage to ensure adequate healing. The use of soft tissue reconstructive techniques is imperative in any irradiated field to prevent incisional dehiscence and wound infection. Local wound complications have attendant risks for prosthetic contamination and may delay initiation of adjuvant therapy depending on the tumor type.

Anesthesia

Preoperative placement of a thoracic epidural is used routinely for postoperative pain management unless contraindications exist, such as coagulopathy, systemic infection, anticipated cardiopulmonary bypass (CPB), or immediate need for postoperative therapeutic anticoagulation. Antibiotic prophylaxis is administered prior to incision. Subcutaneous heparin and pneumatic compression stockings are used for deep vein thrombosis prophylaxis, especially since the majority of patients have an underlying malignancy. General anesthesia is induced with initial single-lumen intubation for bronchoscopic examination followed by exchange to a double-lumen endotracheal tube to facilitate resection in the supine position. Single lung isolation is useful especially if there is involvement of adjacent lung parenchyma, concomitant chest wall or rib resection, or to facilitate resection of the sternochondral junction during sternectomy.

Positioning of the Patient

Sternectomy or claviculectomy generally requires the patient to be in the supine position. The chest and abdomen should be prepped widely to provide adequate access to potential muscle or omental flaps. The thighs should be prepped if skin grafting becomes necessary. Prior to tumor resection, there should be consideration for initial harvest of the pedicled latissimus dorsi muscle flap in the full lateral decubitus position through a vertical incision along the anterior edge of the muscle to the axilla or through a standard posterolateral thoracotomy incision. Sterile prepping of the entire ipsilateral upper extremity can facilitate dissection of the latissimus dorsi muscle but is not mandatory. In this case, all intravenous or arterial catheters should be placed in the contralateral arm. The lateral decubitus position is essential for adequate exposure for optimal latissimus dorsi muscle flap harvest. The dissected muscle flap can be tucked into the axilla and later retrieved during sternal or clavicular resection in the supine position. The latissimus dorsi muscle is our preferred flap for soft tissue coverage following sternectomy or claviculectomy. If the latissimus dorsi muscle is not available or suitable, then the pectoralis major muscle (ipsilateral and/or contralateral), transverse rectus abdominus myocutaneous (TRAM) flap, or omentum are alternatives, and can be harvested in the supine position during or after tumor resection. The pectoralis muscle is ideally suited for upper chest wall/sternal defects. The TRAM and omental flaps can reach essentially any part of the anterior and lateral thorax and sternum. However, the use of a superiorly based pedicled TRAM flap is limited given the need for preservation of ipsilateral internal mammary artery, which is generally resected in total sternectomy.

Supine positioning is the ideal position for sternal or clavicular resection. A transverse shoulder roll can be helpful to allow mild neck extension (Fig. 136-1A). In addition, a slight elevation or lateral decubitus position at 30- to 45-degree rotation ipsilateral to the clavicular resection or concomitant chest wall rib resection will provide a wider field for the tumor resection and ease retrieval of the latissimus dorsi muscle flap from the axilla (Fig. 136-1B). The ipsilateral arm should be tucked to the side. This positioning also facilitates the insertion of a thoracoscope when there is involved lung that requires en bloc resection or to evaluate the entry point into the chest wall lateral to the sternum to ensure that adequate margins are achieved in cases of concomitant sternal and chest wall tumor resection or when there is a significant intrathoracic/mediastinal component compared to the extrathoracic sternal part of the tumor.

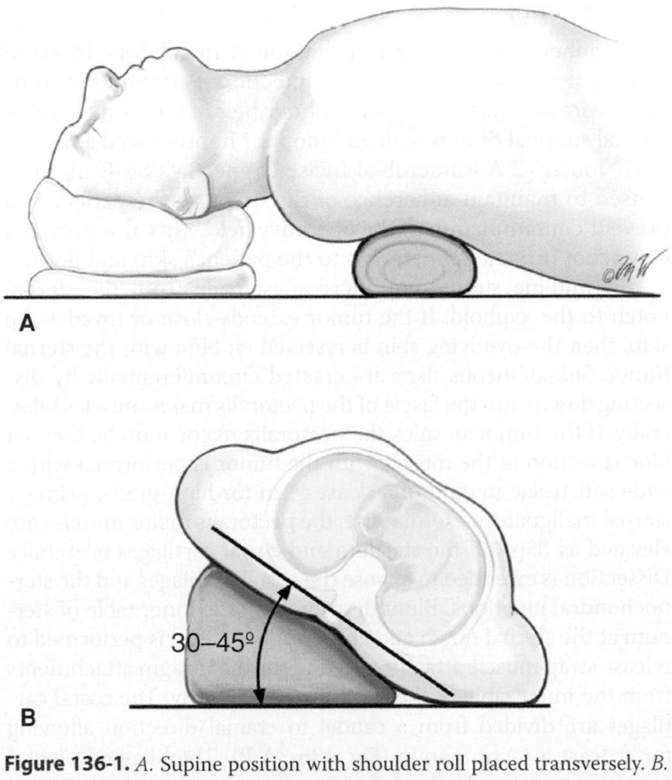

Figure 136-1. *A.* Supine position with shoulder roll placed transversely. *B.* A slight elevation at 30- to 45-degree angle ipsilateral to site of resection.

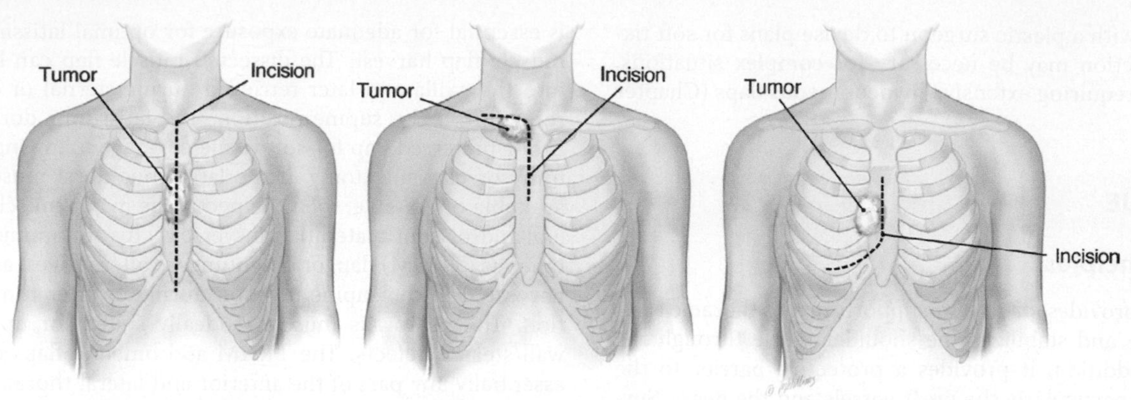

Figure 136-2. Various incisions dependent upon tumor location. *A.* Vertical midline. *B.* Reverse hockey stick. *C.* Hemiclamshell.

Incisions

A variety of incisions can be used depending on the location of the tumor. For a sternal or manubrial tumor, a vertical midline incision is made centered over the portion of the involved manubrium or sternum (Fig. 136-2A). For a clavicular/manubrial tumor, or upper sternal tumor, a reverse hockey stick incision can be made (Fig. 136-2B). For a lower sternal tumor involving the sternochondral junctions or chest wall ribs, a partial hemiclamshell incision (Fig. 136-2C) or lower midline vertical incision can be made. In women, the hemiclamshell incision can be extended from the midline sternum to along the ipsilateral breast crease to permit utilization of the ipsilateral pectoralis muscle and breast tissue for soft tissue coverage during reconstruction. Any previous incisional biopsy scars should be excised in an elliptical manner incorporating the entire open biopsy site.

Total Sternectomy (Resection of Costal Cartilages and Sternum)

Strict adherence to aseptic technique is mandatory to avoid incisional wound and prosthetic infection. Perioperative antibiotics are administered within 1 hour before incision. Antimicrobial surgical drapes with an iodophor impregnated adhesive (3M™ Ioban™ 2 Antimicrobial Incise Drape, 3M, St. Paul, MN) is used to maintain adherence of the drape to the patient and prevent contamination of the operative field. This also prevents contact of prosthetic materials to the patient's skin and flora.

A midline sternotomy incision is made from the sternal notch to the xyphoid. If the tumor extends close or invades the skin, then the overlying skin is resected en bloc with the sternal tumor. Subcutaneous flaps are created circumferentially by dissecting down onto the fascia of the pectoralis major muscles bilaterally. If the tumor invades the pectoralis major muscle, then en bloc resection of the muscle with the tumor is performed with a wide soft tissue margin of at least 4 cm for high-grade, primary sternal malignancies. Otherwise, the pectoralis major muscles are elevated as flaps off the sternum and costal cartilages bilaterally. Dissection is extended to expose the costal cartilages and the sternochondral junctions. Blunt dissection on the inner table of sternum at the sternal notch and at the xyphoid level is performed to release strap muscle attachments and the diaphragm attachments from the inner table of the sternum, respectively. The costal cartilages are divided from a caudal to cranial direction allowing for at least a 4-cm margin (Fig. 136-3A,B). The bilateral pleural cavities are entered. The inferior epigastric arteries are ligated bilaterally. The intercostal neurovascular bundles are ligated and divided. The lower part of the sternum is lifted anteriorly allowing visualization of the sternal undersurface. The anterior mediastinal/pericardial fat, thymus, or pericardium can be resected en bloc if tumor invasion is present. The internal mammary arteries are identified, ligated, and divided bilaterally in the upper sternal area. When the entire sternum is involved by tumor or total sternectomy is required to achieve margin negativity, the sternum is resected in its entirety with the manubrium with or without resecting the clavicular heads. When the manubrium must be resected in its entirety, the sternoclavicular joint can be disarticulated with preservation of the medial clavicular heads bilaterally. In general, the extent of margin clearance is determined primarily by tumor type and grade. For benign and metastatic lesions, negative margins are adequate. For low- and high-grade primary sternal sarcomas, 2- and 4-cm margins are required, respectively. For associated sternal and chest wall tumor resections, one rib above and below the tumor are resected to achieve adequate margins.

Partial Sternectomy

A partial resection of the sternum with or without chest wall and ribs may be sufficient for smaller tumors and is accomplished either by division of the ribs or cartilages bilaterally for centrally located tumors or by division of the ribs or cartilages on the ipsilateral side of an eccentrically located sternal tumor (Fig. 136-4A,B). The tumor is resected with the same principles as described for a complete sternectomy. If complete resectability is not compromised, preservation of at least part of the manubrium or lower part of the sternum can provide chest wall stability and facilitate an easier reconstruction.

Reconstruction Options

Reconstruction after sternal resection is necessary to provide chest wall stability for support of respiration and to protect the underlying organs (e.g., heart and great vessels). Reconstruction is performed at the time of sternal resection unless there is associated infected tissue requiring dressing changes and systemic antibiotics before definitive reconstruction with autologous grafts. Sternal reconstructions entail autologous soft tissue transpositions and prosthetic substitutes.[2,5] Autologous tissue transpositions include omentum and muscle flaps that can be harvested with or without overlying skin (Chapter 138). Prosthetic substitutes include polytetrafluoroethylene (PTFE), methyl methacrylate (MMC), and polypropylene mesh.[2,5]

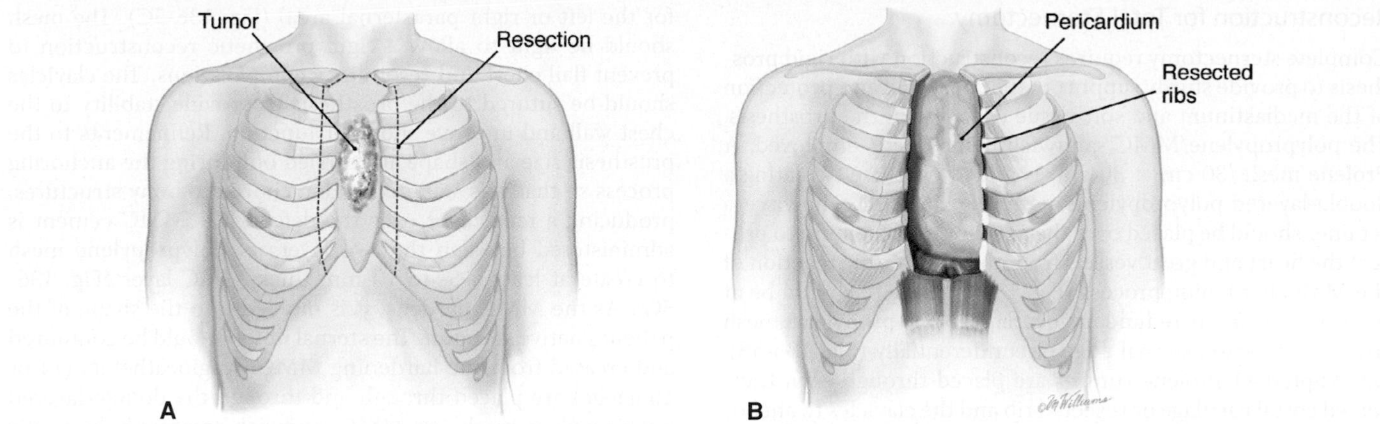

Figure 136-3. Total sternectomy. *A.* Dotted lines represent incision for centrally located sternal tumor allowing for at least 4-cm margins. *B.* Area representing fully resected sternum and associated ribs.

Preferential use of autologous tissue rather than prosthetic substitutes in sternal reconstruction is not clearly established except in cases of infection. Exclusive use of prosthetic materials in cases of active or deep tissue infection is contraindicated for final reconstruction but is appropriate occasionally for interim stabilization during dressing changes. In many instances, definitive reconstruction requires the combined use of prosthetic material and autologous tissue flaps.

PTFE is flexible and durable, and easily conforms to the contour of the chest wall. Although not an essential characteristic, it is impermeable to fluids and gases. It is available in a variety of thicknesses. Gore DualMesh (2-mm thickness) is used most often for chest wall reconstructions and in combined chest wall and partial sternal reconstructions. The radiolucency of this prosthesis permits easier radiographic surveillance for cancer recurrence.

Prolene or Marlex mesh, a double-stitch knit mesh with relative rigidity, is a commonly used polypropylene mesh. It is semipermeable, permitting fibroblast in growth, which is responsible for tenacious incorporation into the surrounding soft tissues.

MMC is a flammable liquid. When activated by an appropriate resin, it develops into a semisolid prosthetic substance that remains malleable for only a brief period (approximately 2 minutes) before it hardens. Since the exothermic reaction can reach temperatures of 50°C, causing necrosis of surrounding tissue, it should be molded to the appropriate contour and allowed to harden without making direct contact with the patient's tissues. Studies have proved that the rigidity and limitation of chest wall movement caused by this prosthetic material do not impair postoperative pulmonary function. MMC is radiolucent. It is commonly used in combination with polypropylene mesh in a sandwich technique discussed in detail below.

Reconstruction for sternal tumors begins with an assessment of size and location of the defect. These factors guide the choice for sternal prosthetic substitutes or autologous tissue transpositions.

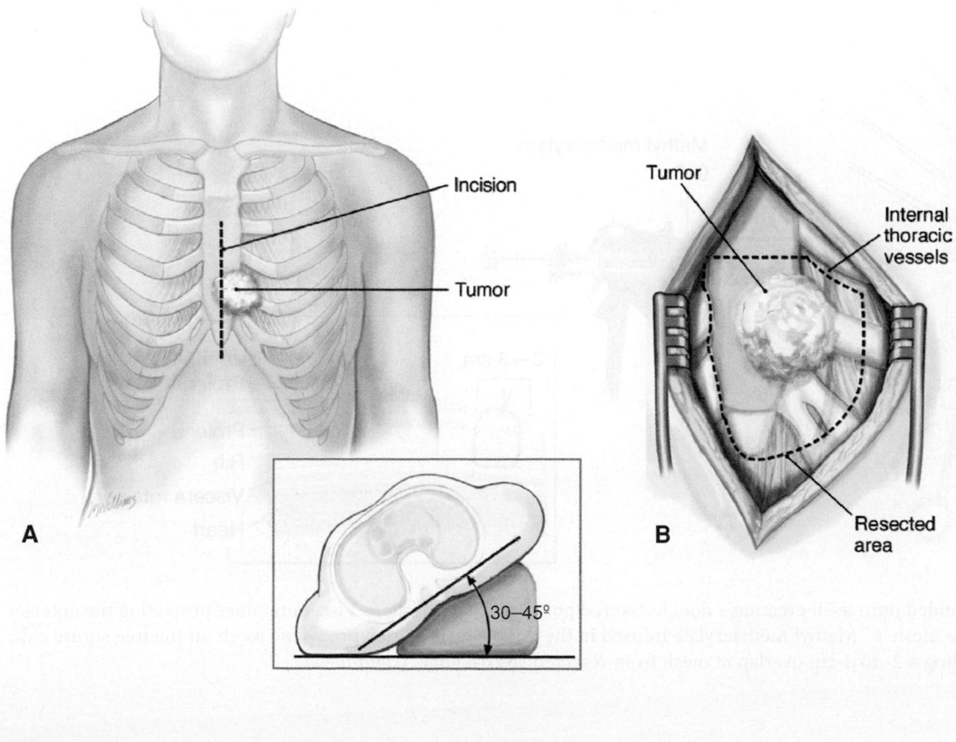

Figure 136-4. Partial sternectomy. *A.* Lower midline vertical incision. *Inset A.* Patient positioned supine with 30- to 45-degree elevation on ipsilateral side of resection. *B.* Resection area for eccentrically located sternal tumor.

Reconstruction for Total Sternectomy

Complete sternectomy requires reconstruction with rigid prosthesis to provide sturdy support to the chest wall and protection of the mediastinum and soft tissue coverage of the prosthesis. The polypropylene/MMC sandwich technique is employed. A Prolene mesh (30 cm × 30 cm) is folded over itself creating a double-layered polypropylene mesh (Fig. 136-5A). The viscera retainer should be placed over the anterior mediastinum to protect the heart and great vessels from the exothermic reaction of the MMC hardening process (Fig. 136-5B). There should be at least a 2- to 3-cm redundant overlap of polypropylene mesh from the resected sternal edge circumferentially (Fig. 136-5B). Interrupted #1 Prolene sutures are placed through each transected costal cartilage or resected rib and the clavicles to anchor the polypropylene mesh to the resected sternal edges. Use of a power drill through the ribs or clavicle may be necessary to allow suture placement through bone. The Prolene sutures are tied down in three of the four sides of the sternal defect (except for the left or right parasternal area) (Fig. 136-5C). The mesh should be tight to allow a rigid prosthetic reconstruction to prevent flail chest and respiratory complications. The clavicles should be sutured to the prosthesis to provide stability to the chest wall and improve shoulder function. Refinements to the prosthesis size and shape are carried out during the anchoring process so that it is sculpted and anchored to bony structures, producing a taut cover over the defect. The MMC cement is administered between the two layers of polypropylene mesh to create at least a 5- to 10-mm thick MMC layer (Fig. 136-5C). As the MMC hardens, it is molded into the shape of the patient's native sternum. The sternal notch should be contoured and created from the hardening MMC. Angiocatheters (14 or 16 gauge) are placed through and through the double-layered polypropylene mesh and MMC sandwich creating holes in the prosthesis to facilitate drainage of any postoperative seroma over the prosthesis into the mediastinum, alleviating the need to place any drains directly over the prosthesis (Fig. 136-5D).

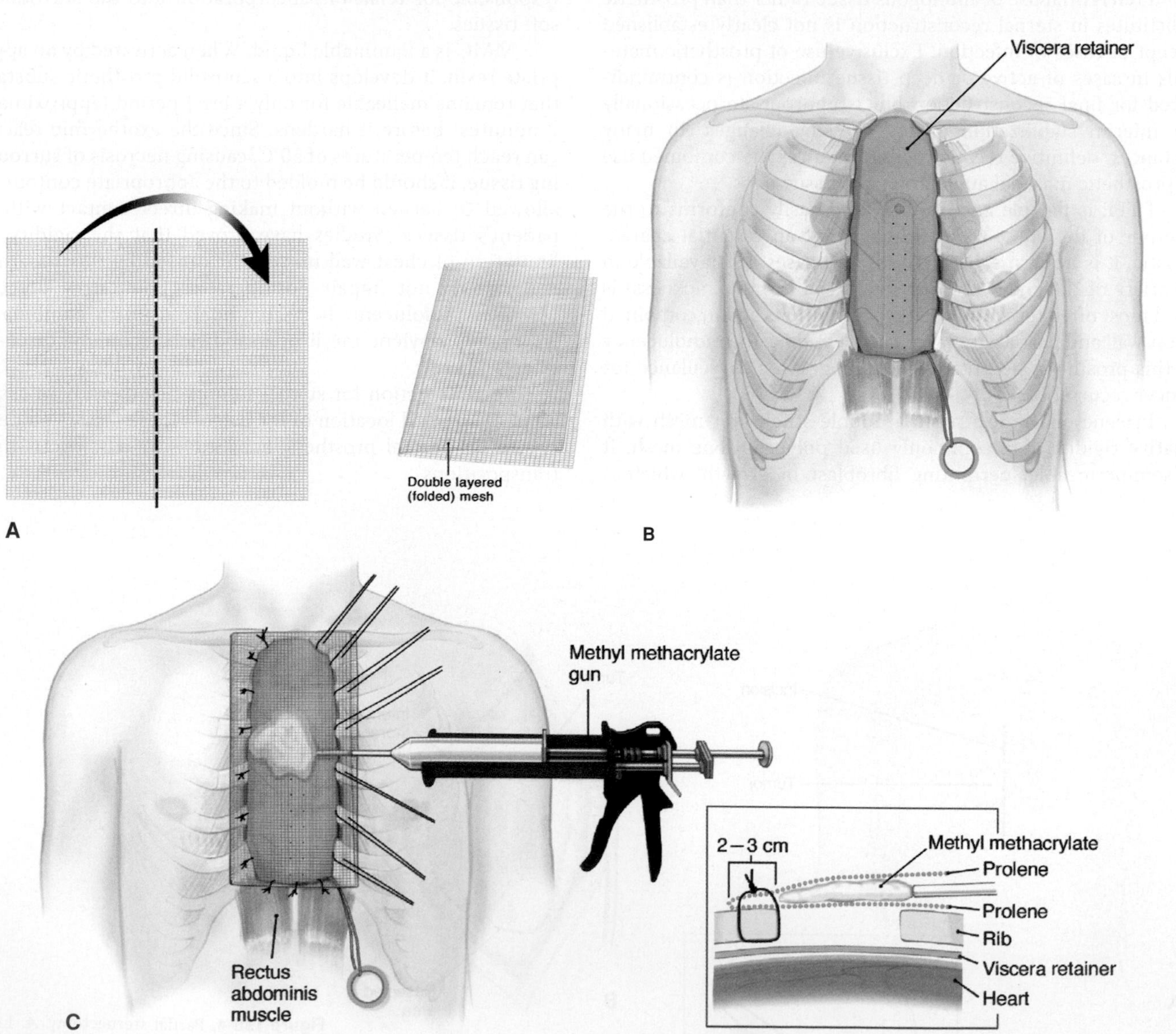

Figure 136-5. *A.* 30 cm × 30 cm prolene mesh folded onto itself creating a double-layered polypropylene mesh. *B.* Viscera retainer protecting the anterior mediastinum with 2-cm overlap of polypropylene mesh. *C.* Methyl methacrylate infused in the double-layered polypropylene mesh on the free suture side. (*Inset C*) Layers from anterior to posterior including a 2- to 3-cm overlap of mesh from resected sternal edge. (*continued*)

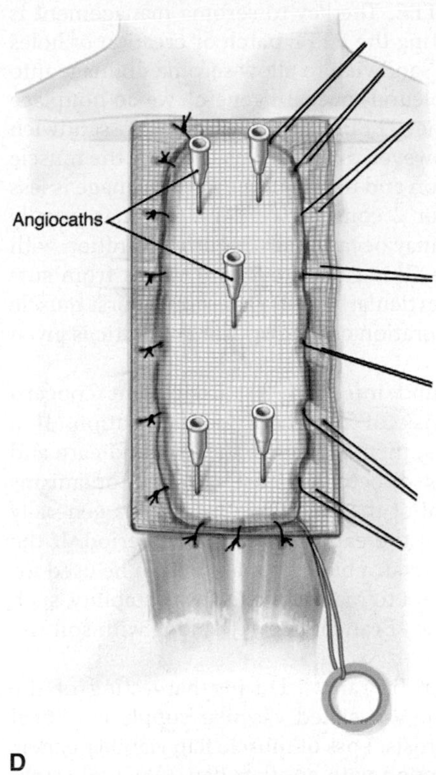

D

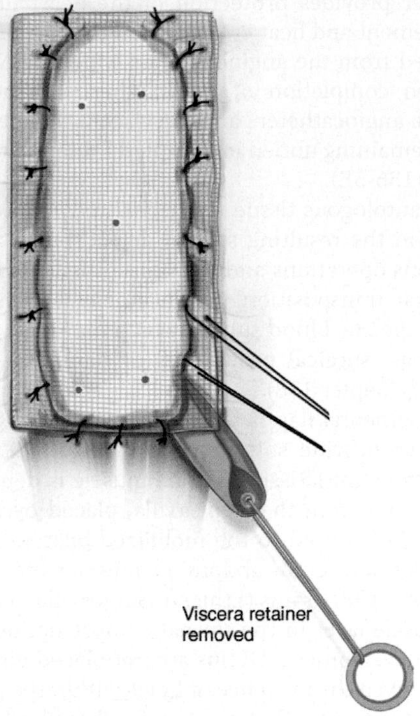

E

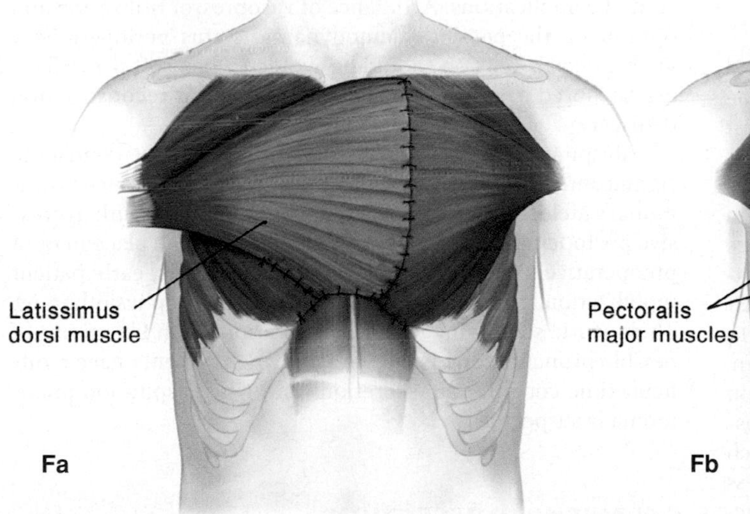

Fa

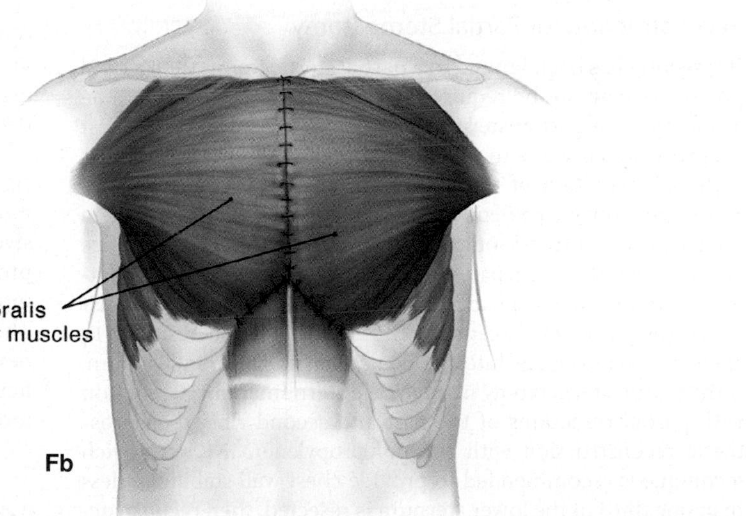

Fb

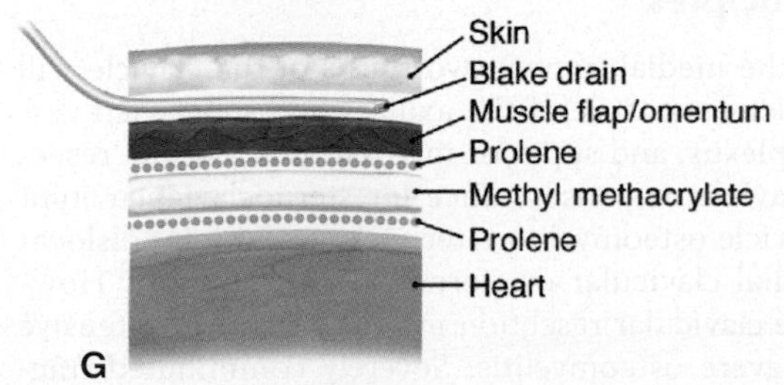

G

Figure 136-5. (*Continued*) *D.* Angiocatheters strategically placed to allow proper drainage of postoperative seroma formation. *E.* Angiocatheters and viscera retainer removed after completion of exothermic reaction. *Fa.* Latissimus dorsi muscle flap sutured to pectoralis major and rectus abdominus muscles. *Fb.* Bilateral pectoralis major muscles sutured together along with rectus abdominus inferiorly. *G.* Layers from anterior to posterior in relation to blake drain and muscle flap placement.

The viscera retainer provides protection of the heart during angiocatheter placement and heat created from the MMC. The needles are removed from the angiocatheters while the MMC is hardening. Upon completion of the exothermic reaction from the MMC, the angiocatheters and the viscera retainer are removed, and the remaining untied interrupted Prolene sutures are tied down (Fig. 136-5E).

The choice of autologous tissue for sternal reconstruction depends not only on the resulting sternal defect, but also on the patient's previous operations and incisions. The viability of muscle and omental transposition, advancement, and island flaps depends on a specific blood supply, which may have been disrupted during past surgical procedures or damaged from radiation exposure (Chapter 138).

The muscle or omental flap is then placed over the sandwiched prosthesis to provide soft tissue coverage. In Figure 136-5F, the use of the right latissimus dorsi muscle is depicted after being brought out from the right axilla, placed over the sternal prosthesis, and sutured to the mobilized bilateral pectoralis major muscles and rectus abdominis muscles inferiorly (Fig. 136-5F,G). Blake (19F) drains (Ethicon, Somerville, NJ) are placed over the muscle layer in the sternal reconstruction site to prevent seroma development. Drains are not placed directly over the prosthesis given the presence of holes within the prosthesis created by the angiocatheters. Drains should also be placed in the muscle harvest sites. The overlying skin is closed over the muscle flap (Fig. 136-5G). Bilateral chest tubes (28F) should be placed for pleural drainage.

Reconstruction for Partial Sternectomy

If resection has been limited to a partial sternectomy, then a rigid prosthesis may not be required depending on the location. The advantage of a partial sternectomy is that it provides the chest wall with stability due to the intact remaining thoracic skeleton. Although resection of the manubrium alone does not require reconstruction, placement of a prosthetic mesh may assist in improving the cosmetic outcome. Our preference in this instance is placement of a PTFE patch and local advancement of the bilateral pectoralis major muscles or use of the latissimus dorsi muscle for soft tissue reinforcement. The PTFE patch is fenestrated to allow seroma drainage into the pleural cavity and mediastinum. If the partial sternectomy involves the sternomanubrial junction with partial resections of the first and second ribs, then prosthetic reconstruction with the polypropylene/MMC sandwich technique is recommended to provide chest wall stability. If less than one third of the lower sternum is resected, then reconstruction is not necessary. However, our preference is placement of a PTFE patch to improve cosmetic outcome. Larger resections of the sternum will expose the heart necessitating reconstruction with the prosthetic sandwich technique. Combined partial sternal and right parasternal chest wall resections can be reconstructed usually with PTFE patch placement. However, combined partial sternal and left parasternal chest wall resections usually require reconstruction with a rigid prosthesis to provide protection of the heart mandating the prosthetic sandwich technique.

Postoperative Care and Complications

The most common complications of sternal resection and reconstruction are seroma formation, wound infection, flap necrosis, reconstruction dehiscence, and respiratory complications (i.e., pneumonia and respiratory failure).[2,5] Seroma development can occur over prosthetic materials, especially after reconstruction with PTFE. The key to seroma management is prevention by fenestrating the PTFE patch or creation of holes through the prosthetic sandwich to allow seroma drainage into the mediastinum and pleural space. In general, we do not place drains directly over the PTFE patch or prosthetic sandwich reconstruction site. However, drains are placed over the muscle flap at the reconstruction and harvest sites until drainage is less than 30 mL per day for 2 consecutive days. Seromas usually resorb over weeks but may occasionally require aspiration with strict sterile technique. This can take 2 to 4 weeks from surgery before removal, particularly at the latissimus dorsi muscle harvest site. A first generation cephalosporin antibiotic is given until drain removal.

Postoperative wound infection is a significant concern given the attendant risk of prosthetic contamination. If a wound infection occurs, then aggressive local wound care and intravenous antibiotics directed against cultured organisms are warranted. Removal of the prosthetic material is generally required, particularly in the early postoperative period. If the prosthesis requires removal, a biologic material can be used for temporary reconstruction to maintain chest wall stability, such as Alloderm (Lifecell Inc., Branchburg, NJ), along with soft tissue flap coverage.

Muscle graft failure is rare.[2,5] During harvesting of the flap, preservation of the associated vascular supply is critical to preventing graft necrosis. Loss of muscle flap viability generally requires reconstruction with another flap. Omental transposition is an excellent alternative in situations of muscle flap related complications. Avoidance of vasopressor utilization and optimizing the patient's hemodynamic status perioperatively are beneficial. Tension should be avoided when soft tissue flaps are anchored to neighboring tissues to prevent reconstruction dehiscence.

Respiratory complications are infrequent but contribute significantly to perioperative mortality.[2,5] The occurrence of pulmonary atelectasis and pneumonia are minimized with aggressive postoperative pain management with routine placement of preoperatively placed thoracic epidural catheters, early patient mobilization, frequent ambulation, and chest physiotherapy. Therapeutic suctioning of airway secretions with liberal use of flexible bronchoscopy is encouraged when patients have a difficult time coughing up secretions and when aspiration pneumonia is suspected.

CLAVICULAR RESECTION

General Principles

Resection of the medial (inner) two thirds of the clavicle will provide sufficient exposure of the axillary and subclavian vessels, brachial plexus, and superior mediastinum. Medial resection of the clavicle may also suffice for sternoclavicular joint infections/clavicle osteomyelitis, sternoclavicular joint dislocation, and medial clavicular or sternoclavicular tumors. However, complete clavicular resection may be needed in extensive tumors and severe osteomyelitis. Severely comminuted fractures, and malunion or nonunion of the clavicle may also warrant complete resection by disarticulating the sternoclavicular and acromioclavicular joints. It has been well documented that the clavicle can be partially or completely resected without resultant disability if performed with proper technique.[8]

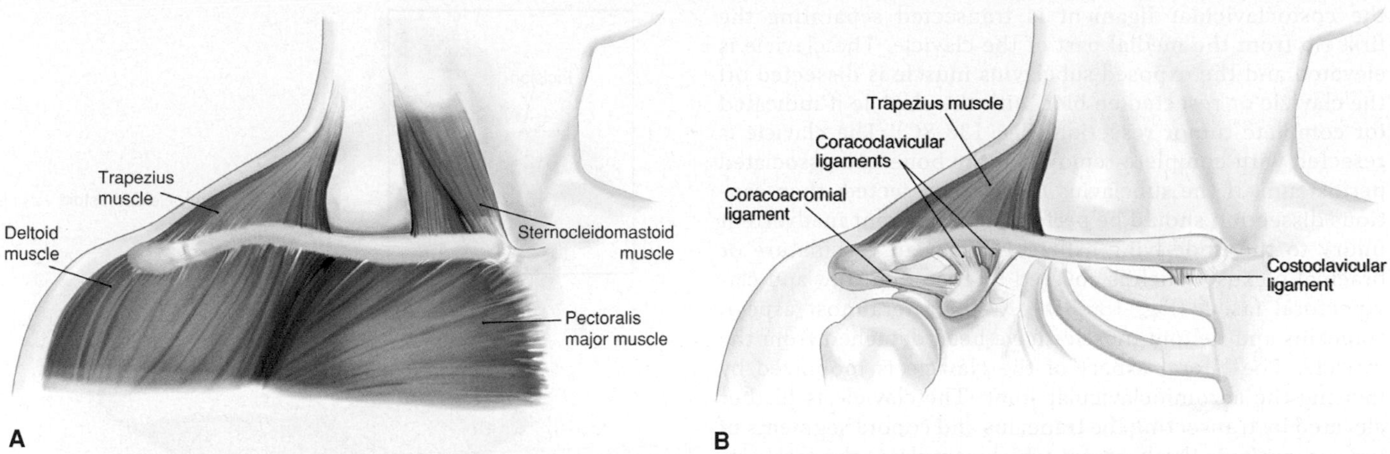

Figure 136-6. *A.* Muscle origin and insertion sites into clavicle. *B.* Pertinent ligament attachment sites in relation to the clavicle.

The sternoclavicular and acromioclavicular joints of the clavicle are stabilized by the ligaments between the clavicle and the first rib (costoclavicular ligament) and the clavicle and the coracoid process (coracoclavicular ligament), respectively (Fig. 136-6A,B). The clavicle has four primary functions: (1) acts as a prop to hold the scapula away from the body during shoulder motion, (2) provides bony framework for muscle origins and insertions (Fig. 136-6A), (3) provides bony protection of the axillary and subclavian vessels and brachial plexus, and (4) transmits the supporting force of the trapezius muscle to the scapula.[8] The sternoclavicular and acromioclavicular joints of the clavicle are stabilized by the ligaments between the clavicle and the first rib (costoclavicular ligament) and the clavicle and the coracoid process (coracoclavicular ligament), respectively (Fig. 136-6B). The costoclavicular ligament prevents lateral displacement of the clavicle by intimately binding the medial part of the clavicle to the first rib. Loss of this ligament results in malfunction and degeneration of the sternoclavicular joint.[8] Based on this anatomic understanding, several sites of resection can be performed with consideration of preserving the shoulder girdle functions balanced by the indication for clavicular resection (Fig. 136-7); the most common resections involving the medial two-thirds of the clavicle (Fig. 136-7B), midclavicle resection with preservation of all ligaments (Fig. 136-7D), and complete clavicular resection (Fig. 136-7E).

In situations where only the medial clavicle is resected, the transection line should extend up to the coracoclavicular ligament. Resection of the costoclavicular ligament will result in anterior displacement of the remaining clavicle with protrusion onto the skin if resection is not performed sufficiently lateral to the coracoclavicular ligament (Fig. 136-7B).

With complete clavicular resection, the functions of acting as a prop to hold the scapula away from the body during shoulder motion and bony protection of the axillary and subclavian vessels and brachial plexus are lost. However, the remaining two functions can be maintained with proper surgical techniques.[8]

Complete Clavicular Resection Technique

The patient is placed in the supine position with a transverse roll between the shoulders. The shoulder ipsilateral to the operative side is gently pulled down with moderate traction. Incision is made along the clavicle from the sternoclavicular to the acromioclavicular joint (Fig. 136-8A). Skin flaps are created superiorly and inferiorly to expose the fascia of the sternocleidomastoid, pectoralis major, deltoid, and trapezius muscles and their attachments to the clavicle. These muscles are detached from the clavicle or resected en bloc with the clavicle (Fig. 136-8B). With mobilization of the sternocleidomastoid and pectoralis major muscles, the medial aspect of the clavicle is dissected and the sternoclavicular joint is disarticulated by incising the capsule, and exposing the articular disc (Fig. 136-8C,D). The disc is severed resulting in disarticulation of the sternoclavicular joint, and

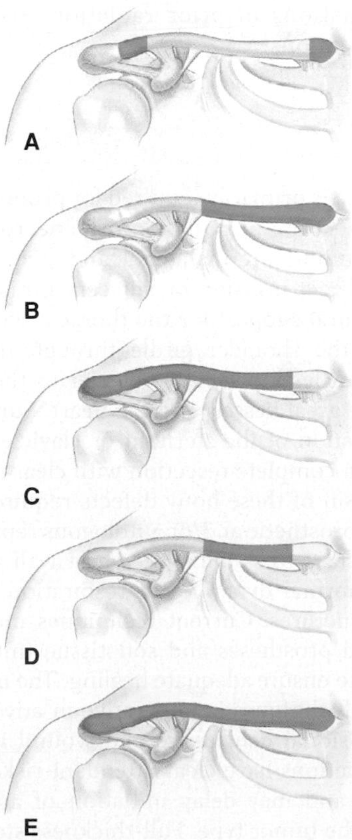

Figure 136-7. Various clavicular resection sites. Shaded areas represent resected portion. *A.* Medial or distal portions of clavicle. *B.* Medial two-thirds of clavicle. *C.* Majority of clavicle except for sternoclavicular joint. *D.* Midclavicle sparing ligaments. *E.* Complete clavicle.

the costoclavicular ligament is transected separating the first rib from the medial part of the clavicle. The clavicle is elevated and the exposed subclavius muscle is dissected off the clavicle or resected en bloc with the clavicle if indicated for complete tumor resection (Fig. 136-8C). The clavicle is resected with complete removal of the bone and associated periosteum. If the subclavius muscle is resected, then cautious dissection should be performed to prevent inadvertent injury to the underlying axillary/subclavian vasculature or brachial plexus, which is covered by the omohyoid and clavipectoral fascia (Fig. 136-8D). At the lateralmost aspect, trapezius and deltoid muscles have been detached from the clavicle. The lateral aspect of the clavicle is mobilized by incising the acromioclavicular joint. The clavicle is further elevated by transecting the trapezius and conoid segments of the coracoclavicular ligament which completes the total clavicular resection (Fig. 136-8E). In order to preserve proper muscle function, the trapezius to deltoid muscles, and the sternocleidomastoid to pectoralis major muscles are sutured together, respectively (Fig. 136-8F).

There is no attempt at reconstructing the resected bony clavicle with prosthesis. However, if there has been extensive resection of the surrounding soft tissue and musculature with resultant defect, then there should be consideration for initial harvesting of the ipsilateral latissimus dorsi muscle prior to clavicle resection as described earlier, or mobilization of the ipsilateral pectoralis major muscle following resection to provide soft tissue coverage of the resection site. The use of muscle flap coverage is encouraged if there is a large soft tissue defect and routinely performed in situations of prior radiation to reduce risk of wound complications.

SUMMARY

Sternal resection is primarily required for primary or secondary malignancy, infection, or radiation osteonecrosis. The majority of sternal tumors are malignant and frequently represent metastasis or direct invasion by adjacent tumor. The sternum provides structural support for the thoracic skeletal structures and stabilizes the shoulder girdle through the clavicles. In addition, it provides a protective barrier to the mediastinum, particularly the great vessels and the heart. Surgical principles governing resection of the sternum or clavicle emphasize the importance of a complete resection with clear margins. Repair or reconstruction of these bony defects requires the selection of appropriate prosthetic and/or autologous replacement material. It is important to stabilize the chest wall and sternum to maintain the normal dynamics of respiration and to protect mediastinal structures. Current techniques most often entail the use of rigid prostheses and soft tissue (muscle or omentum) coverage to ensure adequate healing. The use of soft tissue reconstructive techniques is imperative in any irradiated field to prevent incisional dehiscence and wound infection. Local wound complications have clear attendant risks for prosthetic contamination and may delay initiation of adjuvant therapy depending on the tumor type. Full-thickness sternal resections can be performed with no compromise in chest wall stability or respiratory movements and acceptable morbidity if proper technique in reconstruction of the thoracic wall and sternum are applied.

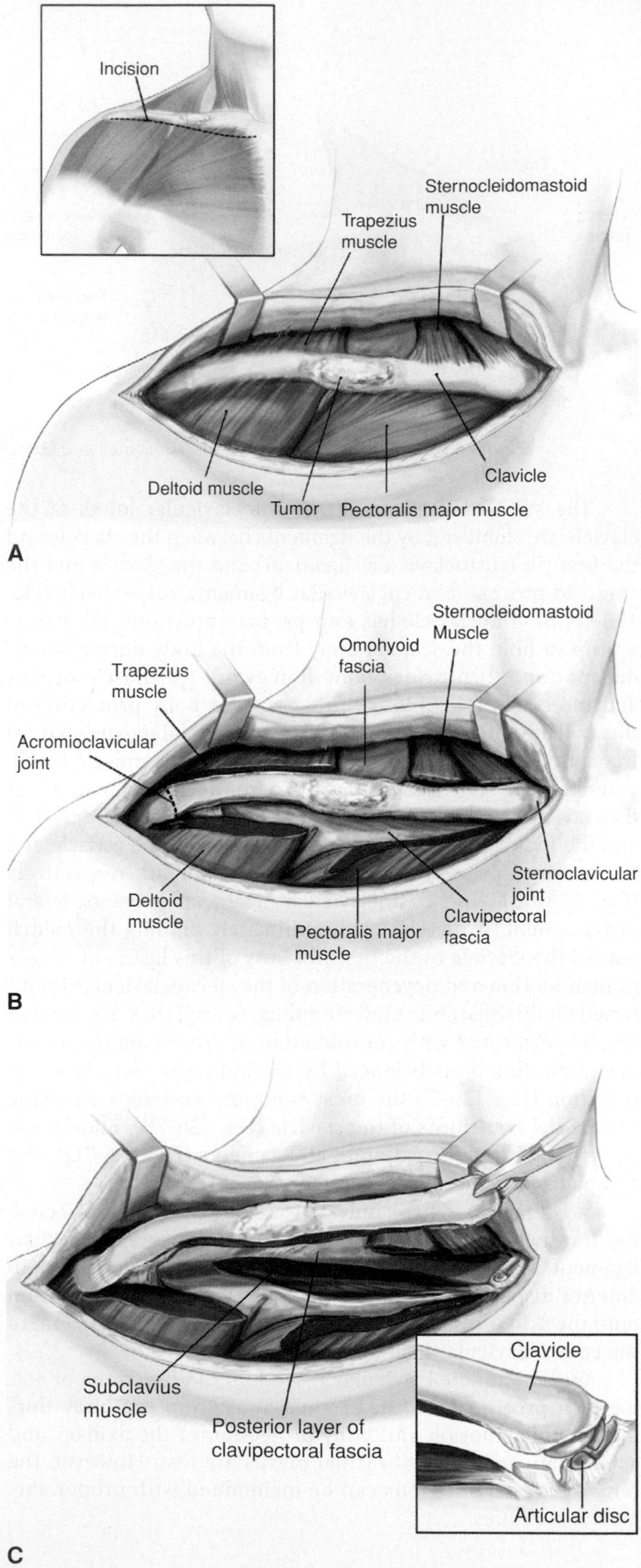

Figure 136-8. *Inset A.* Incision for complete clavicular resection. *A.* Exposure of muscles in relation to clavicle after skin flaps raised. *B.* Muscles resected en bloc or removed from clavicle. *C.* Medial clavicle is dissected after mobilization of sternocleidomastoid and pectoralis major muscles. *Inset C.* Articular disc exposed and incised to allow for disarticulation of sternoclavicular joint. (*continued*)

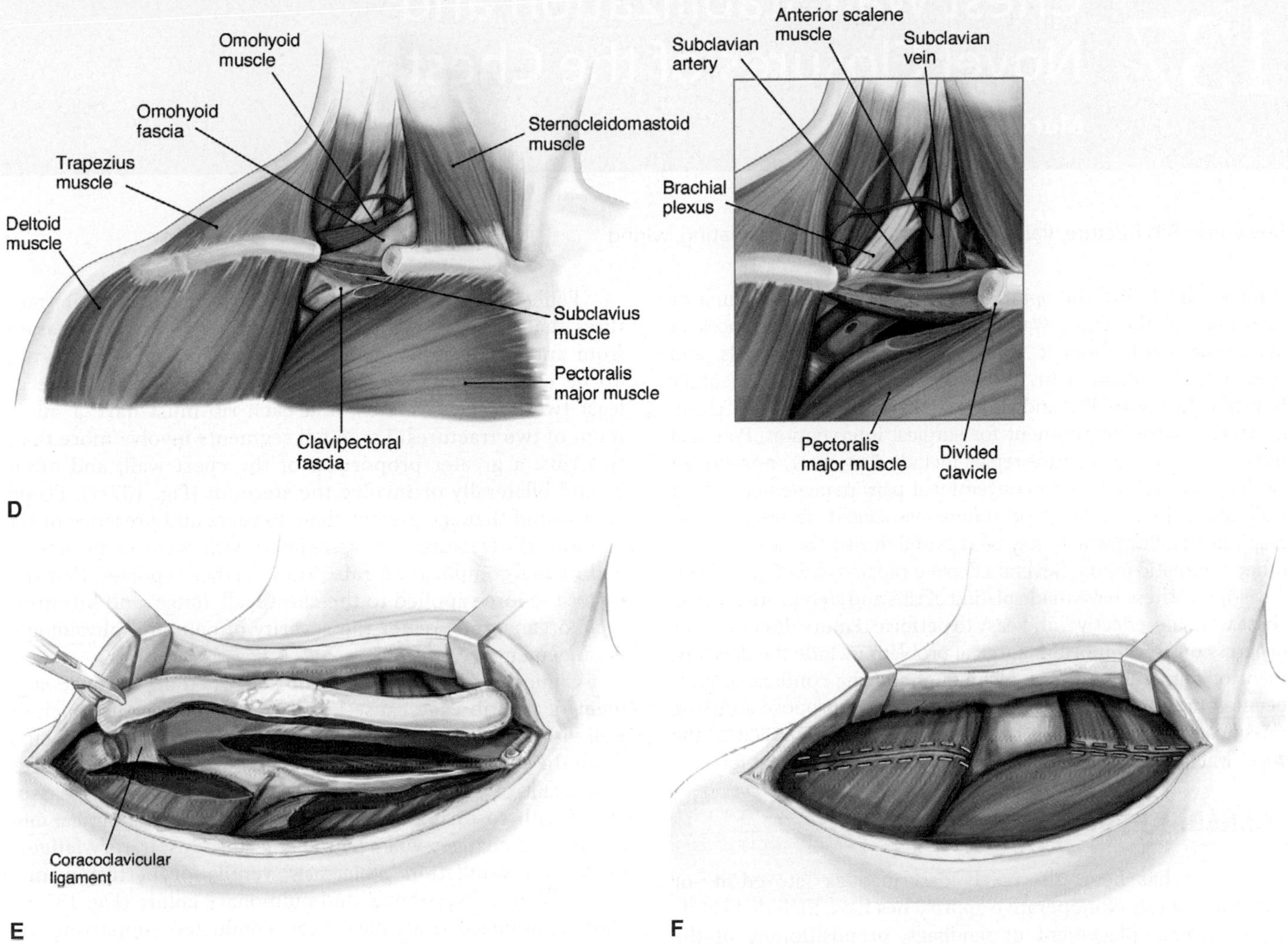

Figure 136-8. (*Continued*) *D and Inset D.* Anatomy of underlying muscle, subclavian vasculature, and brachial plexus (resected clavicle shown to depict anatomy). *E.* Clavicle resection completed with transection of coracoclavicular ligament. *F.* Trapezius to deltoid and sternocleidomastoid to pectoralis major muscles sutured together.

Most clavicle tumors are malignant and much more likely to be metastases than primary tumors. Isolated clavicular resection is rare. Indications for resection include (1) exposure of the base of the neck, superior mediastinum, or brachial plexus, (2) tumor, infection, or injury/trauma of the clavicle itself or in association with sternal/chest wall resection, and (3) dysfunction of the sternoclavicular and acromioclavicular joints. Complete understanding of the clavicular anatomy with associated ligaments and musculature are imperative in surgical planning and preservation of clavicular function.

EDITOR'S COMMENT

The authors have done an excellent job highlighting that the sternum and clavicle are not merely bony structures but rather play important functional roles which must be restored as much as possible through meticulous reconstruction. The detailed anatomical considerations and step-by-step approaches to sternal and clavicular resection and reconstruction demonstrated in this chapter are valuable additions to the repertoire of all thoracic surgeons.

—Yolonda L. Colson

References

1. Pairolero PC, Arnold PG. Chest wall tumors. Experience with 100 consecutive patients. *J Thorac Cardiovasc Surg.* 1985;90:367–372.
2. Arnold PG, Pairolero PC. Chest-wall reconstruction: an account of 500 consecutive patients. *Plast Reconstr Surg.* 1996;98:804–810.
3. Waller DA, Newman RJ. Primary bone tumours of the thoracic skeleton: an audit of the Leeds regional bone tumour registry. *Thorax.* 1990;45:850–855.
4. Martini N, Huvos AG, Burt ME, et al. Predictors of survival in malignant tumors of the sternum. *J Thorac Cardiovasc Surg.* 1996;111:96–105; discussion 105–106.
5. Chapelier AR, Missana MC, Couturaud B, et al. Sternal resection and reconstruction for primary malignant tumors. *Ann Thorac Surg.* 2004;77:1001–1006; discussion 1006–1007.
6. Eng J, Sabanathan S, Pradhan GN. Primary sternal tumours. *Scand J Thorac Cardiovasc Surg.* 1989;23:289–292.
7. Smith J, McLachlan DL, Huvos AG, et al. Primary tumors of the clavicle and scapula. *Am J Roentgenol Radium Ther Nucl Med.* 1975;124:113–123.
8. Abbott LC, Lucas DB. The function of the clavicle; its surgical significance. *Ann Surg.* 1954;140:583–599.
9. Macchiarini P, Dartevelle P, Chapelier A, et al. Technique for resecting primary and metastatic nonbronchogenic tumors of the thoracic outlet. *Ann Thorac Surg.* 1993;55:611–618.
10. Kachroo P, Pak PS, Sandha HS, et al. Chest Wall Sarcomas are accurately diagnosed by image-guided core needle biopsy. *J Thorac Oncol.* 2012;7:151–156.

137 Chest Wall Stabilization and Novel Closures of the Chest

Marcelo C. DaSilva

Keywords: Rib fracture, flail chest, intramedullary rods, plating, wiring

Prior to the 1950s, the approach to treating skeletal trauma or deformity of the chest was largely nonoperative. Advances in anesthesia, cardiothoracic surgery, bioprosthetic materials, and mechanical ventilation in the second half of the 20th century reduced the morbidity and mortality of operating in the chest, creating a safer environment for surgical intervention. Potential indications for rib fracture repair include flail chest, non-united rib fractures refractory to conventional pain management, chest wall deformity or defect, and trauma-associated rib fracture and respiratory failure which may be repaired during thoracotomy for other traumatic injury. Several effective repair systems have been developed. These have made plating of ribs and stabilization of the chest wall safe, effective, and easy to perform. Future directions for progress on this important surgical problem include the development of minimally invasive techniques and the conduct of multicenter, randomized trials. In this chapter, we propose a unique classification for flail chest based on vector force applied to the chest wall and its underlying physiologic response to that force.

GENERAL PRINCIPLES

Flail chest has been alternately described as "stoved-in" or "crushed" chest. Nonoperative approaches have included external strapping, placement of sandbags, or positioning of the patient with the injured side down. These methods have been used with relative success to stabilize unilateral flail chest, but for complex injuries, such as bilateral flail chest, mediastinal flail, and large chest wall soft tissue defects, a different strategy is clearly required. External fixation combined with traction was eventually described and largely used during the initial phase of management of flail chest. The prolonged bed rest necessary for fracture union, however, led surgeons to consider *internal* fixation. Intramedullary "rush nail" fixation was first reported in 1956.[1] Another major factor was the introduction of positive pressure mechanical ventilation. Its adoption and success in preventing respiratory failure in patients with multiple rib fractures and flail chest rendered external fixation/traction obsolete.

By the 1960s and 1970s surgeons recognized that select patients with flail chest might benefit from surgical fixation even after brief periods of mechanical ventilation had failed. Sporadic series attempting rib fracture repair using a number of techniques, including plating, wiring, and intramedullary rods, were reported.[2–9] Brunner was the first to successfully repair a case of sternal flail using a substernal stainless steel prosthesis, the same technique used to reconstruct pectus excavatum.[10]

INDICATIONS

The indications for surgery in flail chest and rib fracture repair are summarized in Table 137-1. Both acute and chronic problems are amenable to surgery.

Flail chest is a complex injury involving multiple rib fractures that cause a segment of the thoracic cage to separate from and move independently of the remaining chest wall. To be classified as flail chest, the segment must involve at least two consecutive ribs, and each rib must have a minimum of two fractures. Large fail segments involve more than two ribs, a greater proportion of the chest wall, and often extend bilaterally or involve the sternum (Fig. 137-1). Flagel et al. found that age greater than 45 years and presence of six or more rib fractures are associated with a worse prognosis and higher complication rate. They further reported that the larger the force applied to the chest wall, lungs, and intrathoracic organs, the greater the severity of pain and physiologic derangement.[11]

Clinically, flail chest is diagnosed when an unstable segment of the rib cage causes paradoxical motion of the chest wall visible on respiration (Fig. 137-2A,B). Sternal flail occurs when the sternum becomes dissociated from the hemithoraces as a result of either unilateral or bilateral rib fractures associated with costochondral dissociation. These anatomical and mechanical changes will eventually lead to respiratory fatigue, inadequate ventilation, atelectasis, ventilation/perfusion mismatch (shunt), hypoxemia, and pulmonary failure (Fig. 137-3). Two randomized trials have been conducted supporting the notion that selected patients with flail chest may experience

Table 137-1

POTENTIAL INDICATIONS FOR REPAIR OF RIB FRACTURE

Flail chest inclusion criteria
• Failure to wean from ventilator
• Paradoxical movement visualized during weaning
• No significant pulmonary contusion
• No significant brain injury
Reduction of pain and disability
• Painful, movable rib fractures
• Failure of narcotics or epidural pain catheter
• Fracture movement exacerbates pain
• Minimal associated injuries (AIS <2)
Chest wall deformity/defect
• Chest wall crush injury with collapse of the structure of the chest wall and loss of thoracic volume
• Severely displaced, multiple rib fractures or tissue defect that may result in permanent deformity or pulmonary hernia
• Severely displaced fractures are significantly impeding lung expansion or rib fractures are impaling the lung
• Patient is expected to survive any other injuries
Symptomatic rib fracture nonunion
• CT scan evidence of fracture nonunion (>2 mos after injury)
• Patient reports persistent, symptomatic fracture movement
• *Thoracotomy for other indications (i.e., "on the way out")*

Adapted from Nirula R, Diaz J Jr, Trunkey DD, et al. *World J Surg.* 2009;33:14–22.

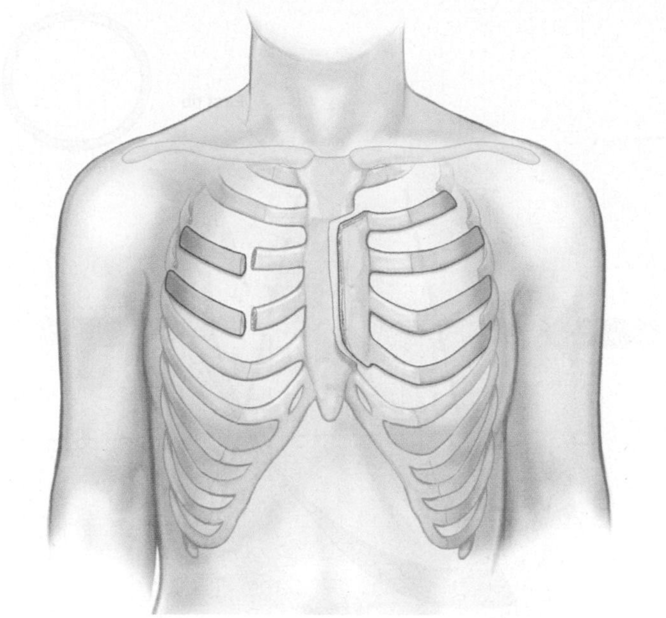

Figure 137-1. Flail chest and flail mediastinum.

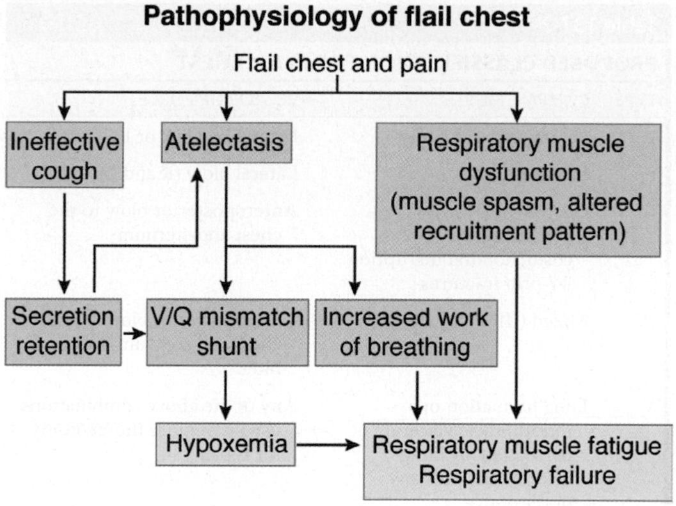

Figure 137-3. The pathophysiology of respiratory failure secondary to flail chest.

short- and long-term benefits from operative repair. The surgically repaired groups in both trials demonstrated significantly fewer days on the ventilator and in the ICU, and had a lower incidence of hospital-acquired pneumonia, better pulmonary function at 1 month follow-up, and a higher rate of return to work at 6 months compared with the nonoperative groups. Visual chest wall deformity or persistent flail chest occurred less frequently in the operative groups, whereas forced vital capacity and total lung capacity were significantly higher in the operative groups at 2 months.[12,13]

Recent, nonrandomized, cohort comparison trials have generally confirmed these findings with the caveat that flail chest repair is usually not advised in patients with significant pulmonary contusions.[14–16] The optimal number of days after injury to perform repair is controversial: one trial randomized patients at 5 days[12] and the other at 36 to 48 hours.[13] In our experience, the repair can be safely performed up to 15 days after injury, before a healing callus begins to form around the fractures, as after this point the callus must be removed to achieve complete alignment of the rib fragments and bony union.

On the basis of our 10-year clinical experience, we developed a new classification for flail chest (Table 137-2), using the vector of the force (blow) applied to the chest (Fig. 137-4) as a guide to determining the optimal approach for treatment of complex chest wall injuries.[17] The chest wall is similar to a ring. When sufficient force is applied to one side of the ring, the energy associated with the force is transmitted to the opposite side. Depending on the magnitude of the force, the structures contained within the chest, such as the lung, heart, and mediastinal structures, may cause the ring to break at *two* points. Most patients presenting with flail chest have unilateral flail segments with minimal respiratory derangement. These injuries are classified as type I. The majority of these patients can be treated with pain management, respiratory therapy, and early ambulation. Patients with type II injuries require repair of at least one side of the chest, since the intrathoracic structures will have absorbed some of the force transmitted to the opposite side.

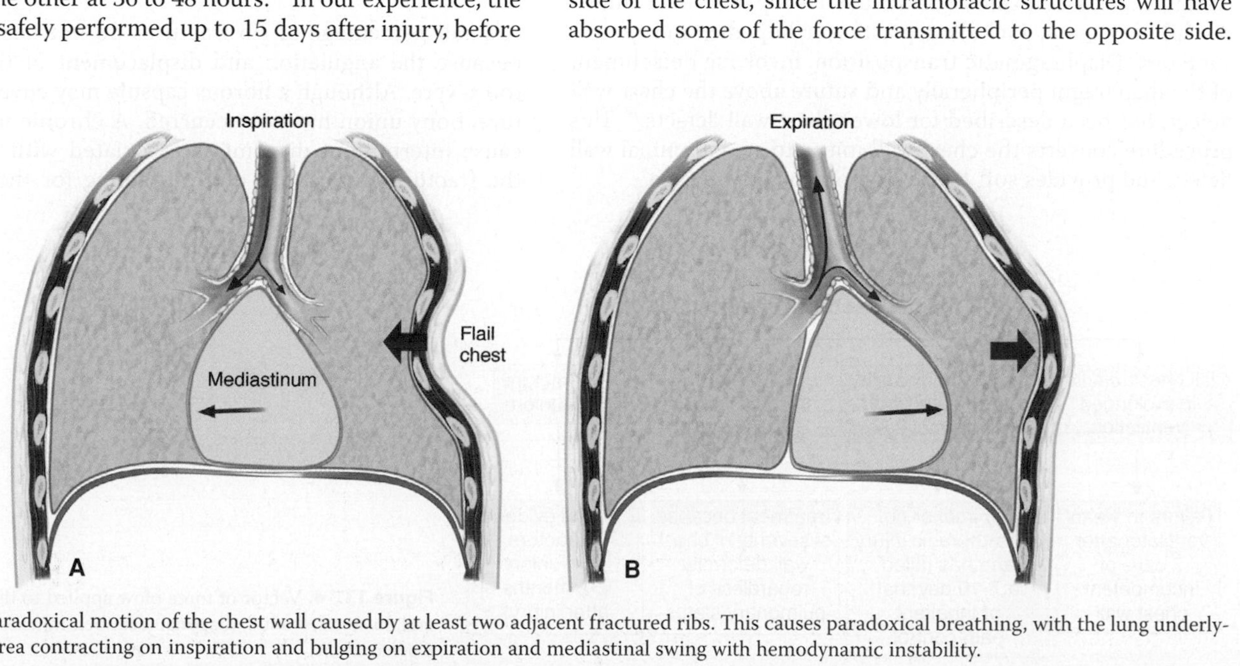

Figure 137-2. Paradoxical motion of the chest wall caused by at least two adjacent fractured ribs. This causes paradoxical breathing, with the lung underlying the injured area contracting on inspiration and bulging on expiration and mediastinal swing with hemodynamic instability.

Table 137-2

PROPOSED CLASSIFICATION FOR FLAIL CHEST

TYPE	COMPARTMENTS	VECTOR OF FORCE
I	Lateral, one side only	Lateral blow (R or L)
II	Bilateral	Lateral blow (R and L)
III	Central Sternal fracture-costochondral disruption +/− rib fractures	Anteroposterior blow to the chest and sternum
IV	Mixed (III + I or II)	Anteroposterior blow to the chest and sternum + lateral blow
V	Lung herniation or intrathoracic visceral herniation, or Lung destruction with any of the above	Any of the above combinations usually require thoracotomy for repair

The exception is the patient who sustains a lateral blow followed by a "counter coup" injury. Patients presenting with type III, IV, and V flail chest have sustained substantial trauma to their chest, and most likely require immediate surgical repair. Figure 137-5 offers a simplified guideline for the management of rib fracture and flail chest.

Chest wall defects/deformities occur in a variety of traumatic circumstances and are characterized by severely displaced rib fractures that visibly deform the chest wall with or without soft tissue loss. Paradoxical motion may not be present in many of these patients, especially in patients with adequate pulmonary reserve. Minimal to moderate-sized tissue defects (<10 × 10 cm) can be caused by penetrating missiles or impalement by surrounding objects during a motor vehicle crash (MVC) or fall. Repair of both rib fractures and soft tissue may be indicated to restore an incompetent or "caved in" segment of the chest wall. Nonoperative management will eventually lead to the development of chest wall herniation. Larger chest wall defects, such as those resulting from close-range shotgun blasts or explosions should be repaired by a multidisciplinary team, including plastic, orthopedic, and neurosurgeons. Diaphragmatic transposition, involving detachment of the diaphragm peripherally and suture above the chest wall defect, has been described for lower chest wall defects.[18] This procedure converts the chest wall injury to an abdominal wall defect and provides soft tissue support for the rib cage.

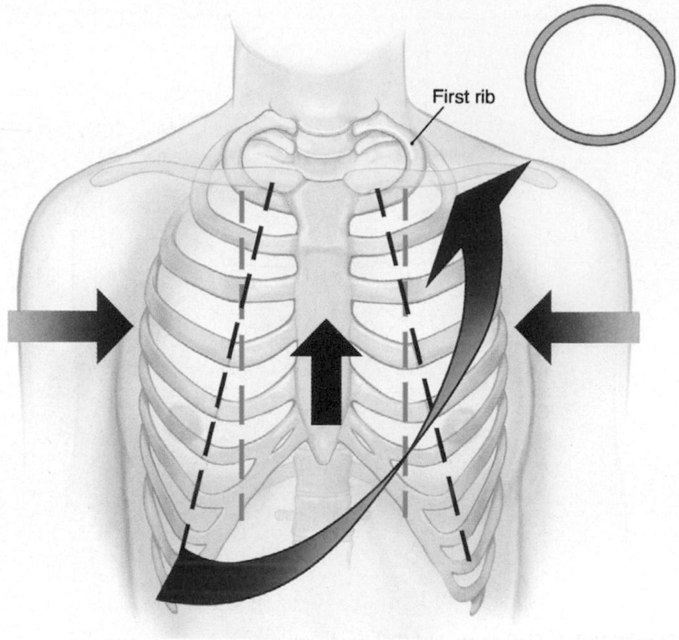
First rib

Figure 137-5. Simplified guideline for repair of rib fractures.

Acute Pain and Disability Reduction

The majority of rib fractures heal without complications and long-term disability. However, patients may present several months after traumatic injury with displaced and movable rib fractures. These patients do not require assisted ventilation, such as BiPAP, but do experience persistent, unrelenting pain with respiration, coughing, or mobilization. Such patients may benefit from having their fractures surgically stabilized. One should exercise clinical judgment, however, and disclose the risks of long-term pain and disability that may persist despite a successful surgical repair.

Nonunion

A small percentage of rib fractures do not heal, presumably because the angulation and displacement of the fracture is too severe. Although a fibrous capsule may envelope the fracture, bony union has not occurred. A chronic nonunion may cause intermittent discomfort associated with movement of the fracture and can be quite disabling for the patient. The

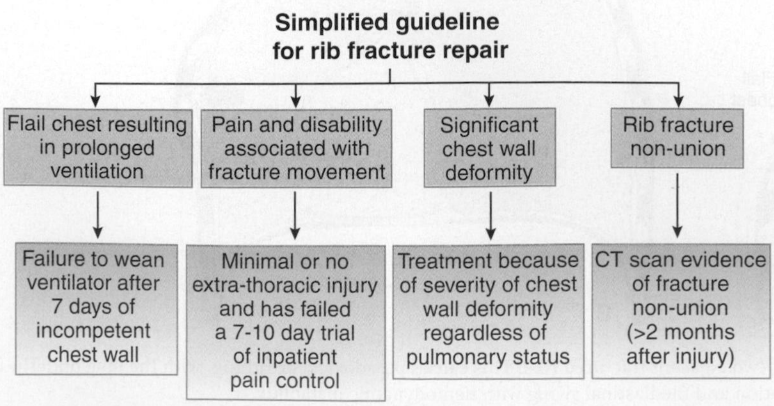
Simplified guideline for rib fracture repair
Flail chest resulting in prolonged ventilation
Pain and disability associated with fracture movement
Significant chest wall deformity
Rib fracture non-union
Failure to wean ventilator after 7 days of incompetent chest wall
Minimal or no extra-thoracic injury and has failed a 7-10 day trial of inpatient pain control
Treatment because of severity of chest wall deformity regardless of pulmonary status
CT scan evidence of fracture non-union (>2 months after injury)

Figure 137-4. Vector of force blow applied to the chest wall, lateral, bilateral, frontal, diagonal (seat belt injuries) and downward displacement.

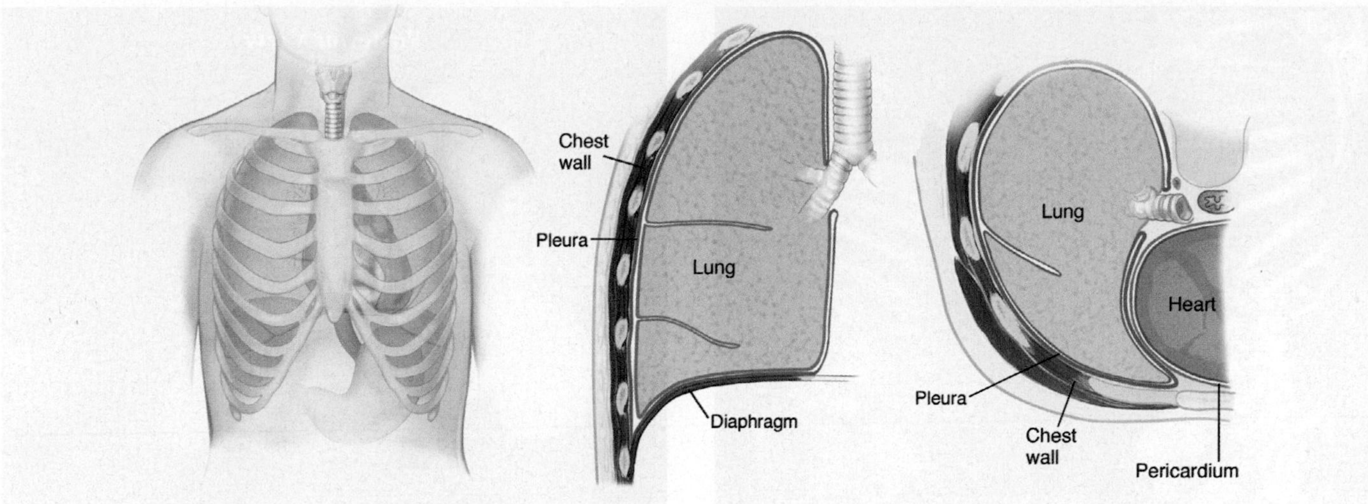

Figure 137-6. Rib cage, lung parenchyma, and mediastinal structures.

rationale for nonunion repair is based on the assumption that without intervention, complete bony healing will not occur. It is of paramount importance that the fibrous callous enveloping the nonunion be resected and a plate placed to fixate the rib ends.

Thoracotomy for Other Indications

A patient with multiple rib fractures or flail chest who needs a thoracotomy for another indication, for example, open pneumothorax, pulmonary laceration, retained hemothorax, or diaphragm laceration, is a candidate for rib fracture repair provided it does not increase the morbidity of the original operation. Otherwise the repair should be delayed and undertaken when the patient is stable. Thoracotomy for nontraumatic indications, for example, tumor resection, also may result in rib fractures that may need to be surgically repaired.

Technical Considerations of Rib Fracture Repair

The goals of rib fracture repair are to target unstable fractures and flail chest segments, improve respiratory function, promote early separation from mechanical ventilator support, ensure early ambulation, decrease the need for prolonged pain medication, decrease recovery time, and accelerate the patient's return to work. The chest anatomy is unique owing to the tight association between the mechanical properties of the chest wall, muscles, and ribs with the underlying lung parenchyma, heart, and mediastinal structures (Fig. 137-6). The human rib thickness ranges from 8 to 12 mm and has a relatively thin (1–2 mm) cortex that surrounds the soft marrow. Individual ribs do not have an abundance of stress tolerance, and the rib with its thin cortex does not hold a cortical screw as well as bone, which has a thicker cortex. Rib fractures may be comminuted, oblique, displaced, or fragmented in several areas along the same rib, further increasing the challenge for a reliable repair. In addition, the intercostal nerve lies along the undersurface of the rib. Intercostal nerve injury during operation or crimping may lead to post-thoracotomy pain syndrome.

TECHNIQUE

Many techniques have been described for repairing rib fractures and flail chest, that is, wire suturing of ribs, intramedullary wires, fixation with various types of plates made of metal or absorbable materials. Anterior plating with bicortical locking screws and intramedullary rods has become the standard of care for these injuries and is a time-tested technique against which innovations should be compared (Fig. 137-7).

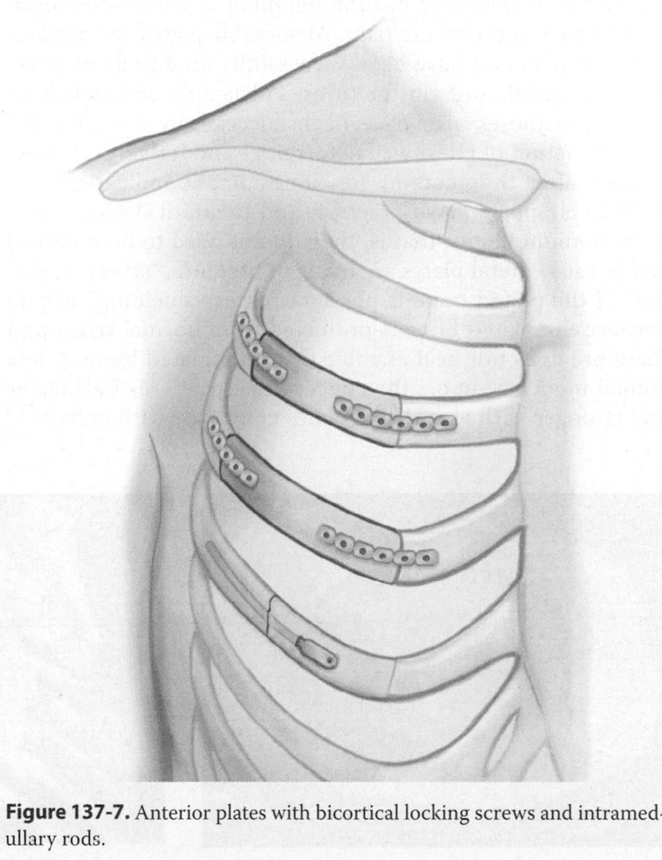

Figure 137-7. Anterior plates with bicortical locking screws and intramedullary rods.

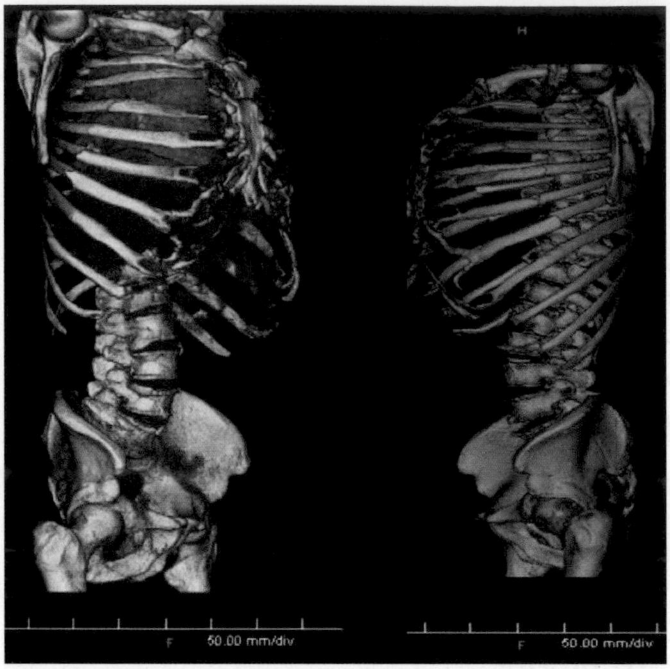

Figure 137-8. Three-dimensional reconstruction of chest CT displaying the type IV flail segment (bilateral chest and sternal fracture with associated central compartment flail).

The Judet strut is a bendable metal plate that grasps the rib with tongs both superiorly and inferiorly without transfixing screws.[4] The fixation of this plate around the inferior margin of the rib usually crimps the intercostal neurovascular bundle. It therefore has the potential to cause intercostal nerve injury and chronic pain. Absorbable plates are polylactide polymers that have been successfully used to fixate maxillofacial, tibial, and rib fractures. Polylactide and polydioxanone prostheses also have been successfully used for the reconstruction of chest wall deformities and for rib reapproximation after thoracotomy for nontraumatic indications.[19,20] Absorbable plates have practical and theoretical advantages over titanium plates, that is, they do not need to be removed and because metal plates are made of titanium, "stress-shielding" of the plated bone is possible. "Stress-shielding" occurs because the plated bone is protected from normal stress and therefore does not heal as robustly as nonplated bone. A few animal models support the concept that fractures heal faster and stronger with absorbable plates compared with metal.[21,22]

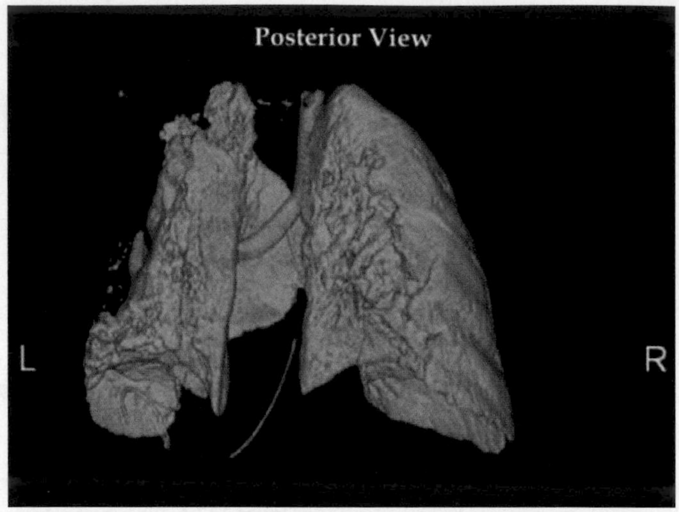

Figure 137-10. Three-dimensional reconstruction of the destroyed lung parenchyma (posterior view).

However, polylactide plates are not bacteriostatic and they may still get infected in vivo.

Preoperative Preparation

The majority of the patients who require surgical repair of rib fractures and flail chest are classified as type III or greater. These patients usually have injuries involving more than one system, such as head trauma, multiple skeletal fractures (spine, pelvis, long bones), abdominal injuries, and lung contusion on positive mechanical ventilation in the ICU. It is important to segregate the degree of respiratory compromise due to flail chest from the degree of compromise caused by the underlying pulmonary contusion and competing injuries. One should be careful not to offer treatment when the degree of physiologic derangement is such that the patient may not be able to tolerate either single lung ventilation or a prolonged surgical procedure. On the other hand, there are a few cases for which performing emergency thoracotomy, lung resection, and rib stabilization is indicated (Figs. 137-8 to 137-11A,B). Three-dimensional CT reconstructions may be useful to completely define all rib fractures and the extent of their displacement and to help plan the surgical approach (Fig. 137-8). A preoperative antibiotic to target gram-positive organisms is given 30 minutes before incision. Video-assisted thoracoscopic surgery (VATS) may be used for pulmonary resections, evacuation of hemothorax,

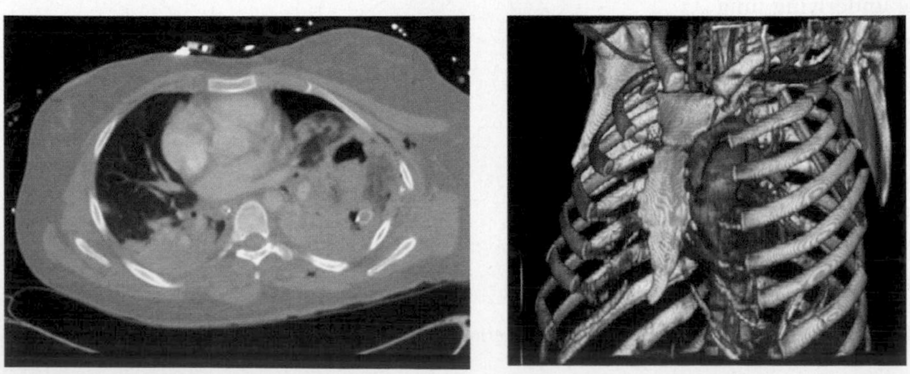

Figure 137-9. CT scan of the chest and three-dimensional reconstruction showing left pneumothorax, hemothorax, traumatic intraparenchymal pneumatocele, left flail chest in a 27-year-old trauma patient.

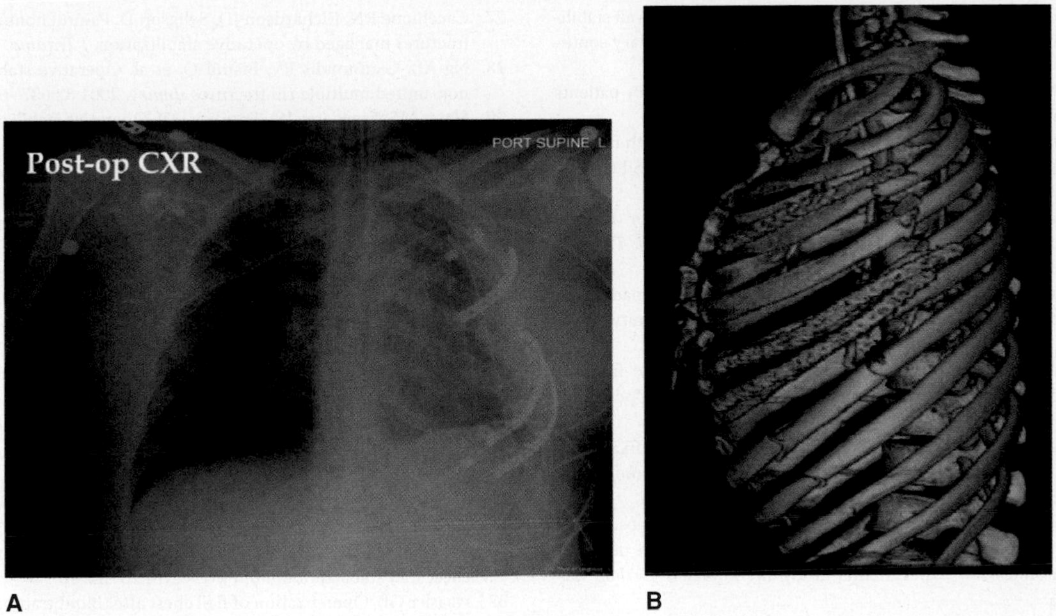

Figure 137-11. *A.* Postoperative chest x-ray, anterior posterior view. *B.* Postoperative three-dimensional reconstruction of chest CT scan. Lateral view.

diaphragmatic repair, and to aid in localizing the flail segment from pushing on the skin surface and observing the exact segment to be repaired. This maneuver can be especially helpful in patients with generous subcutaneous and/or breast tissue.

COMPLICATIONS

Among 650 rib fracture repairs described since 1975, there were eight superficial wound infections (1.2%), four cases of wound drainage without infection (0.6%), two pleural empyemas (0.3%), one wound hematoma, and one persistent pleural effusion.[5–7,11–16,23–41] Fixation failure, including plate loosening or wire migration, occurred in eight patients (1.2%), and postoperative chest wall "stiffness," "rigidity," or "pain" necessitating plate removal was reported in nine patients (1.4%). Rib osteomyelitis was reported in one patient and was ascribed to operative contamination from a preoperative chest tube, which was colonized by *Staphylococcus aureus.*

FUTURE DIRECTIONS

Minimally Invasive Approaches

The advent of three-dimensional reconstruction of chest CT scanning has had a positive impact on the diagnosis and planning of rib fracture repair and flail chest. The addition of intraoperative VATS may improve the surgeon's ability to keep the external exposure to a minimum. Muscle-sparing techniques, along with new instruments and plating systems, permit easy repair. In addition, because we do not recommend plating every segment of the flail chest, since the goal is to promote chest wall stabilization and improve the respiratory mechanics, thoracotomy can sometimes be avoided in favor of minimally invasive approaches. These strategies for minimizing operative dissection should reduce the postoperative morbidity. As well, new technologies and plating systems have been designed exclusively for thoracoscopic repair.

References

1. Crutcher RR, Nolen TM. Multiple rib fracture with instability of chest wall. *J Thorac Surg.* 1956;32:15–21.
2. McDowell AJ, Dykes J, Paulsen G. Early reconstruction of the crushed chest. *Chest.* 1962;41:618–623.
3. Carlisle BB, Sutton JP, Stephenson SE Jr. New technic for stabilization of the flail chest. *Am J Surg.* 1966;112:133–135.
4. Judet R. [Costal osteosynthesis]. *Rev Chir Orthop Reparatrice Appar Mot.* 1973;59:(suppl 1):334–335.
5. Moore BP. Operative stabilization of nonpenetrating chest injuries. *J Thorac Cardiovasc Surg.* 1975;70:619–630.
6. Paris F, Tarazona V, Blasco E, et al. Surgical stabilization of traumatic flail chest. *Thorax.* 1975;30:521–527.
7. Thomas AN, Blaisdell FW, Lewis FR Jr, et al. Operative stabilization for flail chest after blunt trauma. *J Thorac Cardiovasc Surg.* 1978;75:793–801.
8. Albrecht F, Brug E. [Stabilization of the flail chest with tension band wires of ribs and sternum (author's transl)]. *Zentralbl Chir.* 1979;104:770–776.
9. Vecsei V, Frenzel I, Plenk H Jr. [A new rib plate for the stabilization of multiple rib fractures and thoracic wall fracture with paradoxical respiration]. *Hefte Unfallheilkd.* 1979;138:279–282.
10. Brunner L, Hoffmeister HE, Koncz J. [Stabilizing surgical interventions on the thorax in funnel chest corrections and injuries of the bony thorax]. *Med Klin.* 1964;59:515–518.
11. Flagel BT, Luchette FA, Reed RL, et al. Half-a-dozen ribs: the breakpoint for mortality. *Surgery.* 2005;138:717–723; discussion 723–725.
12. Tanaka H, Yukioka T, Yamaguti Y, et al. Surgical stabilization of internal pneumatic stabilization? A prospective randomized study of management of severe flail chest patients. *J Trauma.* 2002;52:727–732; discussion 732.
13. Granetzny A, Abd El-Aal M, Emam E, et al. Surgical versus conservative treatment of flail chest. Evaluation of the pulmonary status. *Interact Cardiovasc Thorac Surg.* 2005;4:583–587.
14. Ahmed Z, Mohyuddin Z. Management of flail chest injury: internal fixation versus endotracheal intubation and ventilation. *J Thorac Cardiovasc Surg.* 1995;110:1676–1680.

15. Voggenreiter G, Neudeck F, Aufmkolk M, et al. Operative chest wall stabilization in flail chest-outcomes of patients with or without pulmonary contusion. *J Am Coll Surg*. 1998;187:130–138.
16. Nirula R, Allen B, Layman R, et al. Rib fracture stabilization in patients sustaining blunt chest injury. *Am Surg*. 2006;72:307–309.
17. DaSilva M, Hamaji M, Jaklitsch M. Management of flail chest with rib plating: a novel surgical approach to the treatment of flail chest. AATS Learning Center Video; 2013.
18. Bender JS, Lucas CE. Management of close-range shotgun injuries to the chest by diaphragmatic transposition: case reports. *J Trauma*. 1990;30:1581–1584.
19. Matsui T, Kitano M, Nakamura T, et al. Bioabsorbable struts made from poly-L-lactide and their application for treatment of chest deformity. *J Thorac Cardiovasc Surg*. 1994;108:162–168.
20. Puma F, Ragusa M, Santoprete S, et al. As originally published in 1992: Chest wall stabilization with synthetic reabsorbable material. Updated in 1999. *Ann Thorac Surg*. 1999;67:1823–1824.
21. Hanafusa S, Matsusue Y, Yasunaga T, et al. Biodegradable plate fixation of rabbit femoral shaft osteotomies. A comparative study. *Clin Orthop Relat Res*. 1995;(315):262–271.
22. Viljanen J, Pihlajamaki H, Kinnunen J, et al. Comparison of absorbable poly-L-lactide and metallic intramedullary rods in the fixation of femoral shaft osteotomies: an experimental study in rabbits. *J Orthop Sci*. 2001;6:160–166.
23. Mouton W, Lardinois D, Furrer M, et al. Long-term follow-up of patients with operative stabilisation of a flail chest. *Thorac Cardiovasc Surg*. 1997;45:242–244.
24. Lardinois D, Krueger T, Dusmet M, et al. Pulmonary function testing after operative stabilisation of the chest wall for flail chest. *Eur J Cardiothorac Surg*. 2001;20:496–501.
25. Kroeker A, Hoke N, Peck E, et al. Long-term morbidity, pain and disability following repair of severe chest wall injury. *J Invest Med*. 2008;56:210.
26. Mayberry JC, Terhes JT, Ellis TJ, et al. Absorbable plates for rib fracture repair: preliminary experience. *J Trauma*. 2003;55:835–839.
27. Cacchione RN, Richardson JD, Seligson D. Painful nonunion of multiple rib fractures managed by operative stabilization. *J Trauma*. 2000;48:319–321.
28. Ng AB, Giannoudis PV, Bismil Q, et al. Operative stabilisation of painful non-united multiple rib fractures. *Injury*. 2001;32:637–639.
29. Slater MS, Mayberry JC, Trunkey DD. Operative stabilization of a flail chest six years after injury. *Ann Thorac Surg*. 2001;72:600–601.
30. Richardson JD, Franklin GA, Heffley S, et al. Operative fixation of chest wall fractures: an underused procedure? *Am Surg*. 2007;73:591–596; discussion 596–597.
31. Menard A, Testart J, Philippe JM, et al. Treatment of flail chest with Judet's struts. *J Thorac Cardiovasc Surg*. 1983;86:300–305.
32. Reber P, Ris HB, Inderbitzi R, et al. Osteosynthesis of the injured chest wall. Use of the AO (Arbeitsgemeinschaft fur Osteosynthese) technique. *Scand J Thorac Cardiovasc Surg*. 1993;27:137–142.
33. Oyarzun JR, Bush AP, McCormick JR, et al. Use of 3.5-mm acetabular reconstruction plates for internal fixation of flail chest injuries. *Ann Thorac Surg*. 1998;65:1471–1474.
34. Engel C, Krieg JC, Madey SM, et al. Operative chest wall fixation with osteosynthesis plates. *J Trauma*. 2005;58:181–186.
35. Hellberg K, de Vivie ER, Fuchs K, et al. Stabilization of flail chest by compression osteosynthesis-experimental and clinical results. *Thorac Cardiovasc Surg*. 1981;29:275–281.
36. Schmit-Neuerburg KP, Weiss H, Labitzke R. Indication for thoracotomy and chest wall stabilization. *Injury*. 1982;14:26–34.
37. Haasler GB. Open fixation of flail chest after blunt trauma. *Ann Thorac Surg*. 1990;49:993–995.
38. Landreneau RJ, Hinson JM, Jr., Hazelrigg SR, et al. Strut fixation of an extensive flail chest. *Ann Thorac Surg*. 1991;51:473–475.
39. Di Fabio D, Benetti D, Benvenuti M, et al. [Surgical stabilization of post-traumatic flail chest. Our experience with 116 cases treated]. *Minerva Chir*. 1995;50:227–233.
40. Balci AE, Eren S, Cakir O, et al. Open fixation in flail chest: review of 64 patients. *Asian Cardiovasc Thorac Ann*. 2004;12:11–15.
41. Beelen R, Rumbaut J, De Geest R. Surgical stabilization of a rib fracture using an angle stable plate. *J Trauma*. 2007;63:1159–1160.

138 Options for Soft Tissue Chest Wall Reconstruction

Dennis P. Orgill, Charles E. Butler, and Neil A. Fine

Keywords: Chest wall reconstruction, latissimus dorsi muscle, pectoralis major muscle, omentum

INTRODUCTION

The bony thorax with its overlying muscles and integument creates a cage that protects the relatively fragile heart, great vessels, lungs, esophagus, and large lymphatics. Disruption of the thorax by trauma, tumor, congenital anomaly, infection, or surgical intervention can have potentially lethal consequences. Advances in cardiac and thoracic surgery have enabled surgeons to operate safely within these cavities. Positive pressure ventilation with the use of selective tubes and bronchial blockers permits surgeons to open the pleural spaces and continue respiration while the pleural cavity is disrupted. Advances in cardiac surgery include cardiopulmonary bypass, intra-aortic balloon pumps, and ventricular assist devices that permit continued or augmented perfusion with oxygenated blood. These advances combined with a better understanding of biomaterials,[1–3] tissue-engineered solutions, and advances in plastic and reconstructive surgery[4–6] have allowed more complex sternal and chest wall defects to be successfully reconstructed. In this chapter we will focus our efforts on the multidisciplinary approach to reconstruction of the chest and highlight the three most common flaps used for large defects: the latissimus dorsi, pectoralis major, and omental flaps.

SURGICAL PRINCIPLES

The chest wall has a robust blood supply provided anteriorly by the internal mammary vessels that arise from the subclavian artery and are connected via intercostals to the aorta. Multiple other arteries including the thoracoacromial trunk, transverse cervical artery, and the thoracodorsal artery provide the blood supply to muscles around the upper chest, back, and shoulders. A thorough understanding of the intricacies of the chest wall vasculature, including angiosomes, will allow the surgeon to design reliable flap coverage for most defects. Occasionally, if regional flaps are insufficient or unavailable, free tissue transfer may be necessary to close selected defects.

Large chest wall defects may benefit from a stable reconstruction of the ribs or rib cartilages to maintain adequate pulmonary function (see also Chapter 137). This is generally performed with a variety of materials including synthetic and biological implants. An understanding of the biomaterial/tissue interface is critical to the proper planning of any reconstructive operation. In addition, the stiffness of the biomaterial should optimally match that of the region being replaced to avoid stress concentrations at the junction between the biomaterial and normal tissue.

Meticulous surgical technique is essential in dissecting flaps and allowing them to survive when transferred. Because of the robust blood supply to the chest skin, many wounds can be closed with moderate tension without breakdown. Many chest wall reconstructive procedures occur before or after radiation therapy. Radiated tissues can be difficult to work with because of increased stiffness and their susceptibility to infection.

Patient Selection

The reconstructive surgeon must carefully match the many possible solutions of a thoracic defect to the needs of the specific patient. Chest wall compliance is a function of age, with older patients developing stiffer costochondral junctions and barrel chests. These patients often can tolerate more options for chest wall reconstruction than a younger patient where movement can result in chest wall instability. Younger patients require careful attention to the donor site and ultimate functional and aesthetic outcome and can tolerate longer, more complicated procedures to achieve these goals. Older, more debilitated patients are better served with a more expeditious and reliable operation that might involve more visible scarring. Chest wall reconstruction is optimally performed in a multidisciplinary setting that often includes reconstructive, thoracic, and cardiac surgery, as well as an experienced anesthesia team. A team that works together often will soon develop a sense for what operations can be safely performed in which patients.

Preoperative Assessment

The reconstructive surgeon needs to evaluate these patients in conjunction with a cardiac or thoracic surgeon to coordinate each portion of the procedure. The nutritional status of the patient as defined by albumin and prealbumin levels can be an important predictor of the ability to heal wounds and achieve a successful closure.[7] A careful history and examination of the patients with regard to previous surgeries is essential to understand which flaps may not be usable based on previous incisions. Flaps ideally should come from areas that have not been heavily irradiated, so an assessment of where radiation therapy has been given is important. Also, many cancer patients may be on chemotherapy, and operative timing should be coordinated so an operation is not required when the patient is neutropenic.

SURGICAL TECHNIQUE

The majority of thoracic reconstructions can be accomplished with one or a combination of the latissimus dorsi, pectoralis major, and omental flaps. Flaps have an independent blood supply and can be transposed into the defect. They fill dead spaces and allow a three-dimensional vascularized surface to deliver antibiotics, heal tissue, and help prevent direct cutaneous exposure of implanted biomaterials in the event of wound separation.

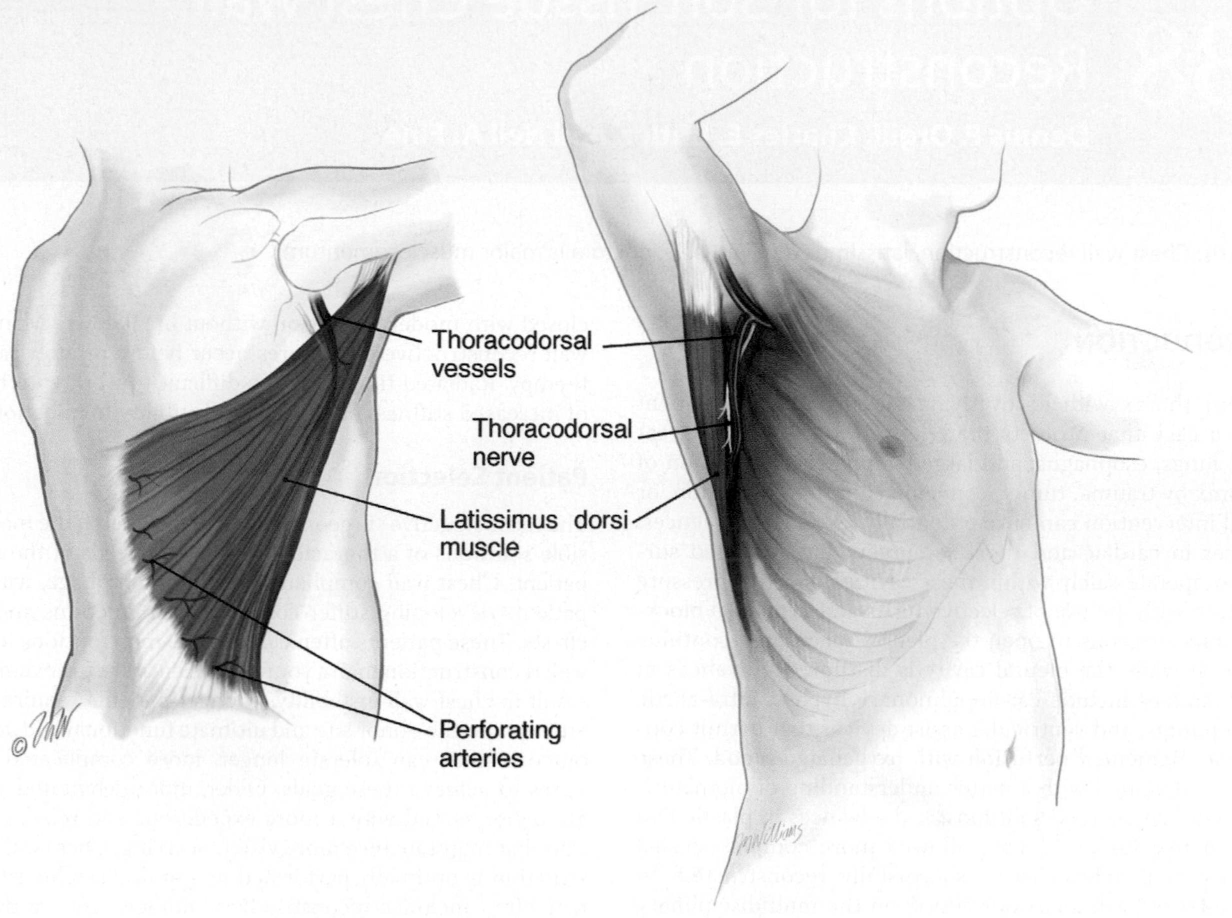

Figure 138-1. Anatomical considerations for the latissimus dorsi muscle.

Latissimus Dorsi Muscle Flap

The latissimus dorsi muscle is the largest muscle in the body. It originates from the thoracic spine and thoracolumbar fascia to the iliac crest and inserts into the humerus (Fig. 138-1). Its major blood supply comes off the thoracodorsal system. The muscle can be accessed through a vertical, horizontal, or oblique incision or endoscopically.[8] The skin and subcutaneous tissues are dissected off the muscle, and the muscle is then dissected off the chest wall. Large perforators off the paraspinous area and thoracolumbar area can be divided with clips or ties. The thoracodorsal pedicle is identified and preserved. The nerve can be left intact, divided, or crushed depending on the desired function of the muscle. For additional pedicle flap reach, the insertion to the humerus can be divided. If the insertion is divided, care must be taken to avoid tension on the pedicle. Suturing the tendinous insertion to the chest wall at a location that provides protection from tension to the pedicle should suffice and also will avoid rotational kinking that can occur if the flap is dissected to the point that it is only attached to the neurovascular bundle. This large muscle reaches nicely into the chest cavity after removing a portion of the second rib and easily covers the hilum. It also can easily reach the anterior mediastinum to cover the heart. With a skin paddle included with the tissue, it can be a useful flap for breast reconstruction or chest wall reconstruction. The distal portion of the flap can sometimes be unreliable because of vascular insufficiency, and caution therefore needs to be taken when the flap is used for defects that are distal to the costal margin. Although loss of latissimus dorsi function results in negligible functional deficit, a split-latissimus dorsi flap can be used to preserve some of its form and function. For many patients who have undergone a standard posterolateral thoracotomy, this muscle is divided and only the superior portion can be used based on the thoracodorsal blood system. The inferior portion can be used for lower thoracic defects based on perforators near the spine. Closure of this defect is generally accomplished with deep dissolvable sutures. Quilting sutures are preferred by many surgeons to reduce the size of the cavity, thus minimizing the risk of postoperative seroma, which has been reported to occur in 20% to 80% of patients.

Pectoralis Major Muscle Flap

The pectoralis major muscle is the largest anterior chest muscle and can be very versatile in treating a variety of chest defects (Fig. 138-2A). Its primary blood supply is from the thoracoacrominal trunk. Access to the muscle can be made through an incision concealed in the inframammary fold. The skin and subcutaneous tissues are dissected off the muscle and the muscle is taken off the chest wall with electrocautery. The perforating vessels off the internal mammary artery are coagulated or ligated and the thoracoacromial trunk is identified and preserved (Fig. 138-2B). For additional length, the medial and lateral pectoral nerves as well

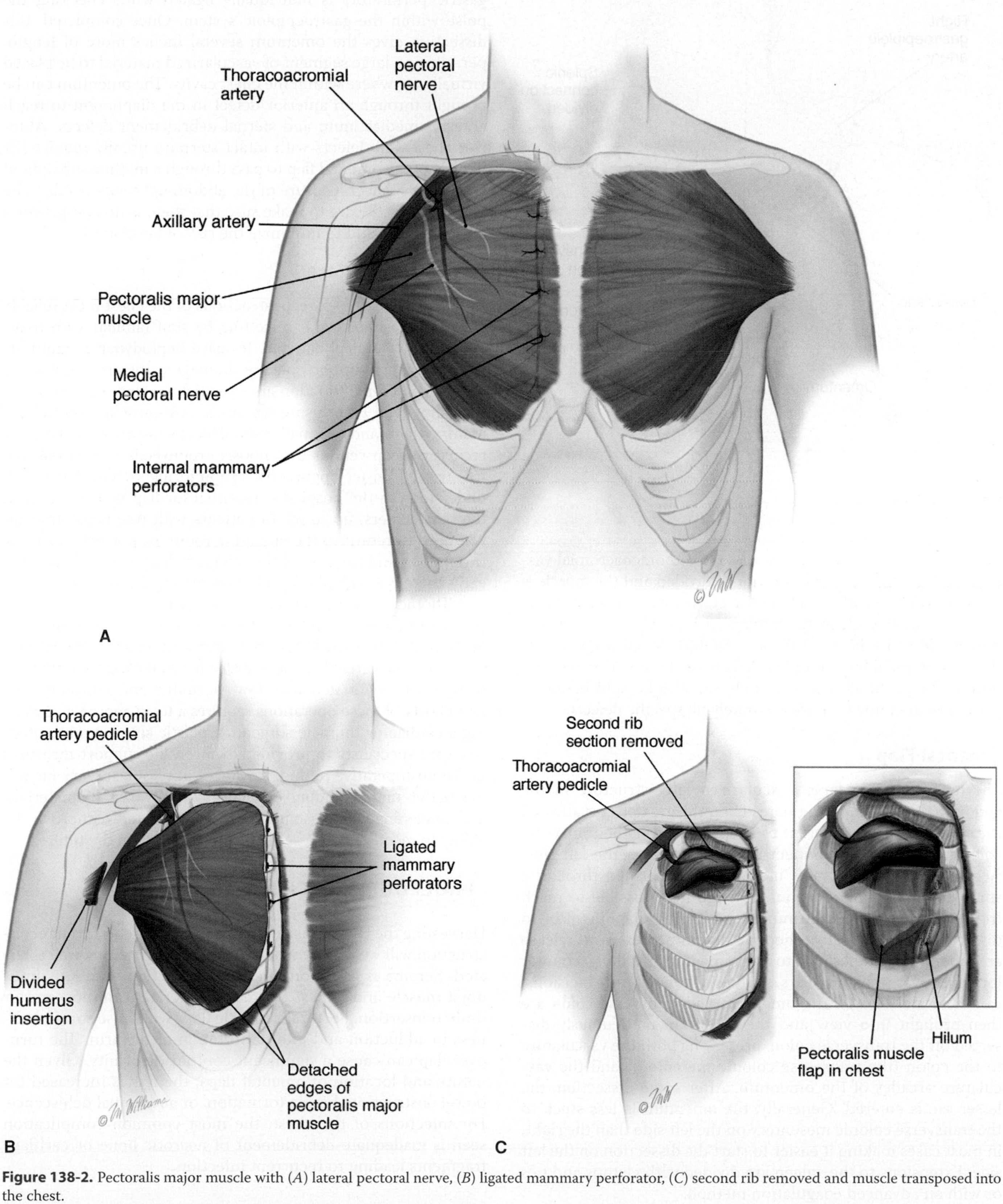

Figure 138-2. Pectoralis major muscle with (*A*) lateral pectoral nerve, (*B*) ligated mammary perforator, (*C*) second rib removed and muscle transposed into the chest.

as the insertion into the humerus can be divided. To cover the hilum, the muscle can be brought through a second rib resection anteriorly (Fig. 138-2C). For cervical esophageal reconstruction, overlying skin can be taken with the flap and fashioned into a tube. For anterior mediastinal reconstructions, the muscle can be transposed over the ribs and easily fills the superior portion of the anterior mediastinum. For lower defects, the muscle is often more efficiently transposed on the perforators from the internal

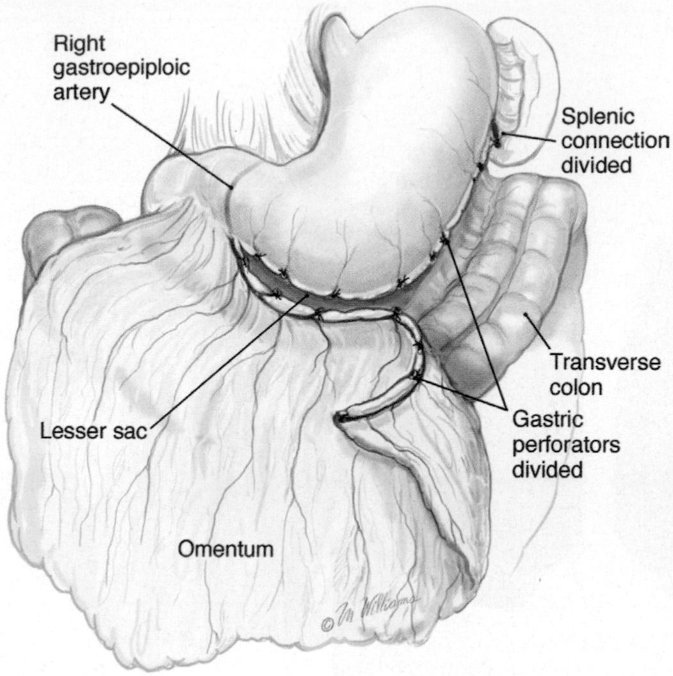

Figure 138-3. Omental flap.

mammary artery system. In this case, the thoracoacromial vascular pedicle and humeral insertion is divided and the muscle is "turned over" medially to fill the defect. As there is usually a perforator between each costal cartilage, it is possible to divide the muscle along its fibers and have multiple small segments of the muscle for filling complex defects of the anterior mediastinum. The pectoralis major muscle can also be split based on perforator anatomy to more accurately fill specific defects.

Omental Flap

The omentum is a large vascularized fatty structure in the abdominal cavity that originates from the greater curvature of the stomach and is adherent to and drapes over the transverse colon (Fig. 138-3). It connects to the spleen on the left side. Access to the omentum is most easily performed through a small upper midline incision, although it is possible to reach from the anterior mediastinum, through the diaphragm or to dissect it endoscopically. The first step in harvest is to release any abdominal adhesions to the omentum. Making counter incisions over previous scars, such as appendectomy incisions, can facilitate release. The omentum and transverse colon are then brought into view and the omentum meticulously dissected off the transverse colon, preserving both the vasculature to the colon (the transverse colonic mesentery) and the vasculature arcades of the omentum. After some dissection, the lesser sac is entered. Generally, the omentum is less stuck to the transverse colonic mesentery on the left side than the right, in most cases making it easier to start the dissection on the left side. Extensions to the spleen are divided with clamps and ties or with an advanced coagulation method.

For anterior mediastinal defects, this amount of dissection may be sufficient. If additional length is needed, it can be acquired from either the right or left gastroepiploic system. Each system should be assessed for patency before dividing any vessels to assure adequate flow to the omental flap. Each of the gastric perforators is individually ligated while checking the pulse within the gastroepiploic system. Once completed, this dissection gives the omentum several inches more of length, permitting a large segment of vascularized material to be placed virtually anywhere within the chest cavity. The omentum can be brought through an anterior defect in the diaphragm to reach anterior mediastinum and sternal debridement defects. Anterior chest wall defects with intact sternum usually require the pedicle of the omental flap to pass through a midline subxiphoid laparotomy defect. Closure of the abdominal cavity needs to be performed with care to make sure that there is no compression on the pedicle and to minimize the risk of herniation.

Postoperative Care

Initial care of complex reconstructions of the chest most reliably occurs in an intensive care setting by staff familiar with treating thoracic surgical patients. Invasive hemodynamic monitoring, ventilatory support, pleural drainage catheters, monitoring of fluids and renal function are essential to avoid morbidity and mortality. Pain relief using narcotics, nonsteroidal anti-inflammatory agents and regional epidural blocks can greatly aid patient recovery. Deep venous thrombosis prophylaxis is essential. For free tissue transfer operations, a monitoring system that is well understood in the hospital is essential for flap success. Even in the best centers, up to 5% of patients with free tissue transfer will need to return to the operating room for potential vascular thrombosis and revision of the microanastomosis. If discovered early, there is a high likelihood of correcting this problem.

Thoracic reconstruction allows treatment of large and complex defects. The combination of new technology such as advanced biomaterials, free tissue transfer, advanced wound care modalities, and vascularized tissue transfer have allowed these defects to routinely be treated with low morbidity and mortality. The complexity of these operations requires a team approach including a cardiac or thoracic surgeon, a plastic surgeon, and intensive care specialists to provide advanced life support measures in the postoperative period. Advances in plastic surgery including better understanding of anatomy, improved biomaterials, and tissue-engineered solutions will undoubtedly improve the ability to reconstruct these challenging defects in the future.

PROCEDURE-SPECIFIC COMPLICATIONS

Harvesting the latissimus dorsi muscle flap for chest wall reconstruction will weaken arm adduction but is generally well tolerated. Seroma is common after reconstruction with latissimus dorsi muscle and is best treated with serial aspiration and/or drain reinsertion. Pectoralis muscle flaps will cause some weakness in adduction and internal rotation of the arm. The turnover flap can cause a significant contour deformity. Given the nature and location of omental flaps, the risk is increased for bowel obstruction, hernia formation, or abdominal dehiscence. For infections of the chest, the most common complication seen is inadequate debridement of necrotic bone or cartilage fragments leading to recurrent infection.

SUMMARY

Chest well reconstruction requires a multidisciplinary approach to patient selection and operative intervention as well as close postoperative monitoring. Advances in plastic surgery have made pedicled flap closure quite reliable. Free tissue transfer is sometimes needed but can generally be avoided by the use of local or regional flaps.

EDITOR'S COMMENT

Given the importance of obtaining negative margins after resection of a chest wall tumor, the ability to resect the necessary chest wall and reconstruct the resultant defect with a variety of tissue flaps is of utmost importance for both the functional and cosmetic benefit of the patient. Early involvement of the plastic surgeon in the planning stages is critical, particularly for planning of the incision to spare as much viable muscle as possible. This chapter highlights the importance of multidisciplinary teamwork for the benefit of the patient.

—Yolonda L. Colson

References

1. McCormack PM. Use of prosthetic materials in chest-wall reconstruction. Assets and liabilities. *Surg Clin North Am*. 1989;69:965–976.
2. Picciocchi A, Granone P, Cardillo G, et al. Prosthetic reconstruction of the chest wall. *Int Surg*. 1993;78:221–224.
3. Hurwitz DJ, Ravitch MM, Wolmark N. Laminated Marlex-methyl methacrylate prosthesis for massive chest wall resection. *Ann Plast Surg*. 1980;5:486–490.
4. Jurkiewicz MJ, Bostwick J 3rd, Hester TR, et al. Infected median sternotomy wound. Successful treatment by muscle flaps. *Ann Surg*. 1980;191:738–744.
5. Colwell AS, Mentzer SJ, Vargas SO, et al. The role of muscle flaps in pulmonary aspergillosis. *Plast Reconstr Surg*. 2003;111:1147–1150.
6. Orgill DP, Austen WG, Butler CE, et al. Guidelines for the treatment of complex chest wounds with negative pressure wound therapy. *Wounds*. 2004;(suppl B):1–23.
7. Michaels BM, Orgill DP, Decamp MM, et al. Flap closure of postpneumonectomy empyema. *Plast Reconstr Surg*. 1997;99:437–442.
8. Fine NA, Orgill DP, Pribaz JJ. Early clinical experience in endoscopic-assisted muscle flap harvest. *Ann Plast Surg*. 1994;33(5):465–469; discussion 469–472.

PART 23

BENIGN CHEST WALL CONDITIONS

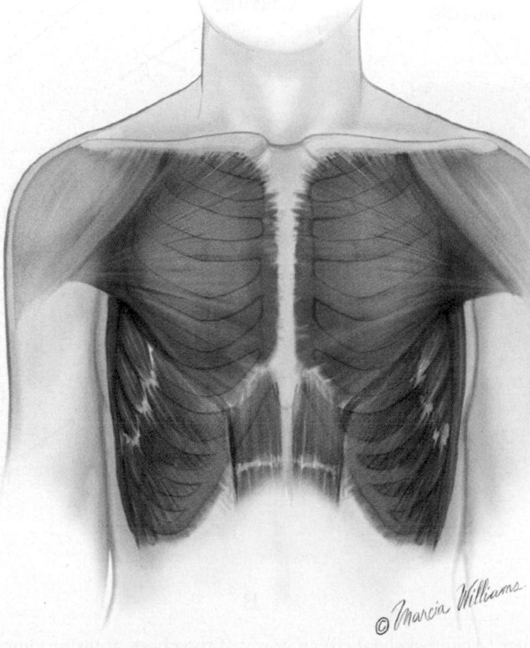

139 Overview: Benign Disorders of Chest Wall

Jacqueline J. Lee and Aneil A. Mujoomdar

Keywords: Pectus excavatum, pectus carinatum, Poland syndrome, chest wall defects, thoracic outlet syndrome, Paget–Schroetter syndrome, hyperhidrosis, chest wall infections

This section on chest wall disorders encompasses benign disorders of the skeletal and muscular chest wall, including congenital deformities of the chest wall, a group of compressive disorders known collectively as *thoracic outlet syndrome*, thoracic sympathectomy for hyperhidrosis, an autonomic disorder involving the sympathetic nerve chain, and management of chest wall infections (Fig. 139-1).

CHEST WALL DEFORMITIES

Congenital chest wall deformities may be categorized as (1) pectus excavatum, (2) pectus carinatum, (3) Poland syndrome, (4) sternal defects, and (5) miscellaneous anterior chest wall defects. While most patients present during childhood, some may present in early adulthood as well.

Pectus Excavatum

Pectus excavatum, or "funnel chest," is a congenital deformity characterized by posterior depression of the middle to inferior portion of the sternum and posterior curvature of the associated costal cartilages (Fig. 139-2). Generally, the manubrium and first and second ribs are normal. The severity of the depression varies and is usually asymmetric with a deviation to the right side. Shamberger and Welch reported that most cases (86%) are diagnosed at or within a few weeks of birth.[1] Although it was once commonly believed that children would "outgrow" this deformity, the severity of the sternal depression may increase during periods of rapid growth.

Pectus excavatum is the most common congenital chest wall deformity in children, with a reported incidence of 1 in 300 to 400 to 1 in 1000 live births. A male predominance is observed, with boys reported to be affected three times more often than girls.[1] The etiology of pectus excavatum is unknown. Theories include intrauterine pressure, rickets, and abnormalities of the diaphragm, including congenital diaphragmatic hernia and diaphragmatic agenesis.[2] Although no clear pattern of inheritance is known, Shamberger and Welch note that 35% of patients report a positive family history for chest wall deformities.[1]

Pectus excavatum may be accompanied by other abnormalities. In a study of 704 children with pectus excavatum, musculoskeletal abnormalities, such as scoliosis or kyphosis, were identified in 19%. Pectus excavatum has been associated with congenital heart defects (1.5%) and connective tissue disorders

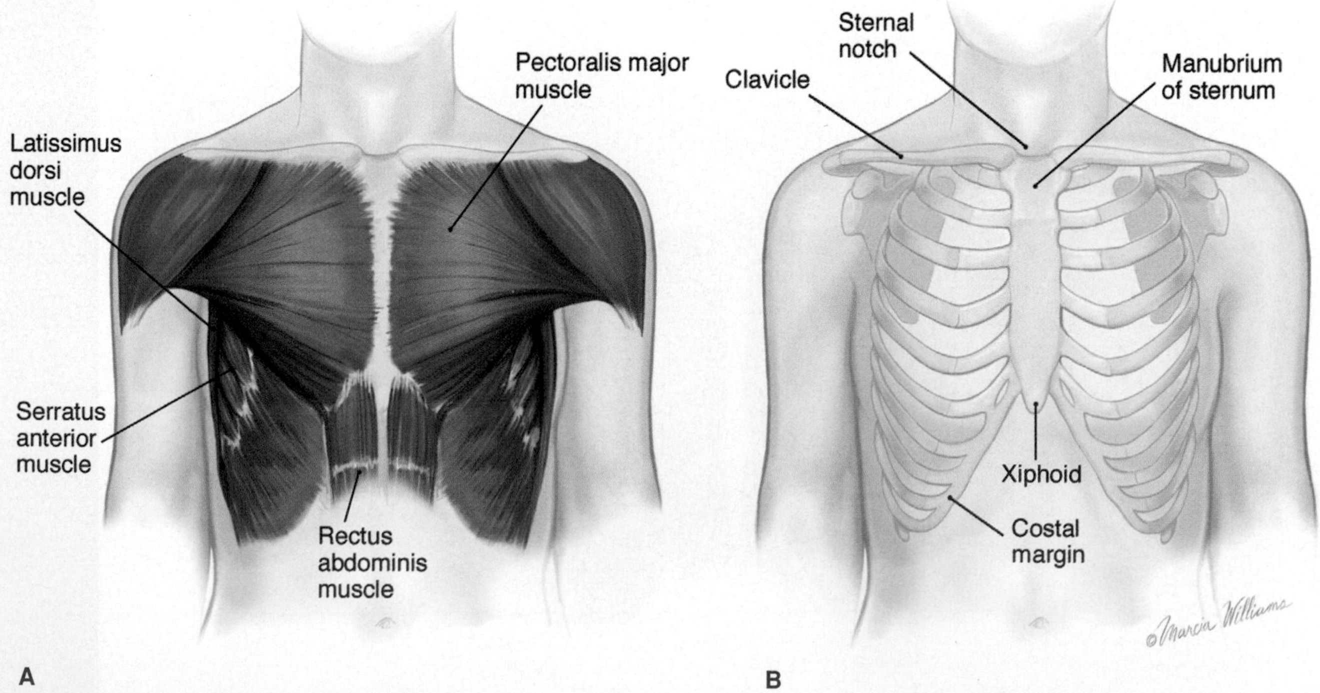

Figure 139-1. Muscular (*A*) and skeletal (*B*) anatomy of the chest, anterior view.

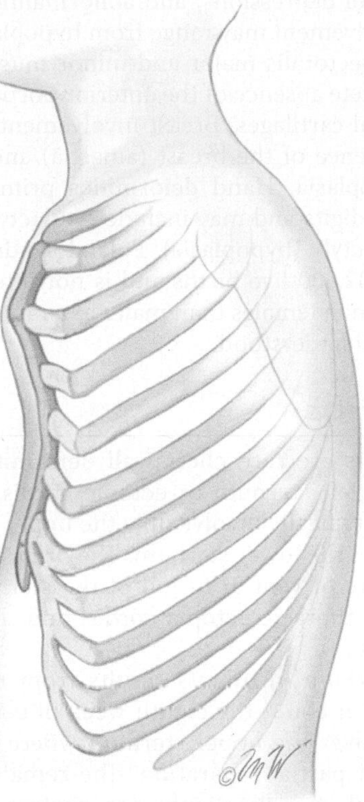

Figure 139-2. Pectus excavatum.

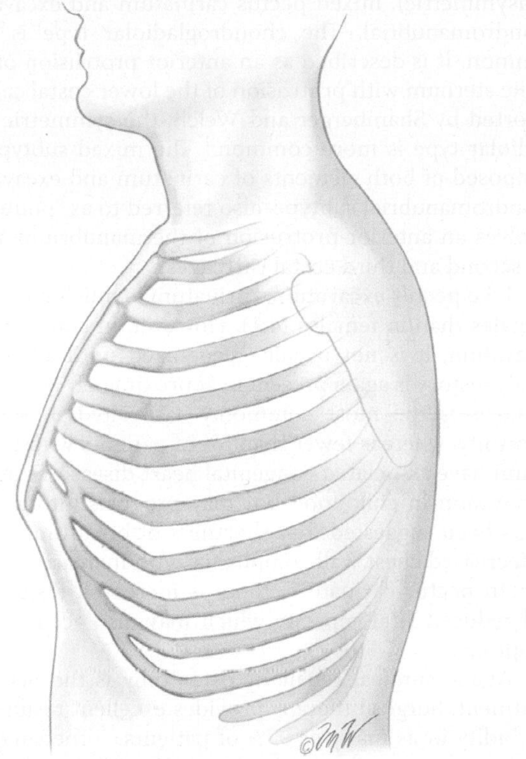

Figure 139-3. Pectus carinatum.

such as Marfan syndrome or Ehlers–Danlos syndrome in up to 6.4%.[3] Although many pediatric patients are asymptomatic, symptoms can worsen with age, with increased physical activity or worsening of deformity during the second growth spurt.[4] A recent multicenter prospective trial demonstrated that approximately two-thirds of patients reported dyspnea or other chest symptoms with limited exercise tolerance (64.5%), shortness of breath at rest (62.1%), and chest pain on exertion (51.1%). Chest pain unrelated to exertion (32%), and palpitations (11%) also were reported. Pain on exertion and at rest was presumably musculoskeletal in origin.[3] In addition, children may experience psychological distress as a consequence of their cosmetic appearance.

Physical examination reveals middle to inferior sternal depression of varying severity. Usually the depression is asymmetric, most commonly with sternal deviation to the right side and subsequent shift of the heart to the left. Many studies have investigated the altered cardiac function by means of electrocardiogram (ECG), echocardiogram, nuclear medicine test, and angiogram. A significant number of patients are found to have right atrial and ventricular compression or mitral valve prolapse. Mitral valve prolapse has been reported in 17% to 65% of patients compared to only 1% in the normal pediatric population. Dysrhythmias have been found in 16% of patients.[5] Most of these studies also have shown decreased exercise tolerance consequent to decreased stroke volume. At rest, the cardiac index is normal, but the response to moderate exertion is below predicted values.

Given the common subjective complaints of shortness of breath, pulmonary function testing has been used in numerous studies to attempt to quantify any abnormality.[6–8] However, the severity of symptoms often does not correlate well with objective findings in pulmonary and cardiac function. In most patients, only a mild-to-moderate (10%–15%) reduction in forced expiratory volume in 1 second (FEV_1) and vital capacity is identified.[3]

There are several methods of "grading" the severity of deformity by radiographic imaging. The pectus (or Haller) index is a ratio between the transverse diameter and anterior–posterior diameter. The transverse diameter is the maximal transverse diameter of the thorax at its widest point. The anterior–posterior diameter indicates the distance between the sternum and the anterior spine at the deepest level of depression.[9] Normal is approximately 2.5, greater than 3.5 is considered abnormal, with greater than 5.0 considered severe. Another method compares the distance from the point closest to the posterior sternum to the anterior spine and the distance between the spine and sternum at the angle of Louis.[1] Unfortunately, neither method consistently correlates the severity of symptoms to an objective index.

Surgery remains the primary form of therapy for these patients. While the cosmetic benefit cannot be debated, the effect on cardiopulmonary function is less clear. A recent meta-analysis of the effect of surgery on long-term follow-up found that most patients experience a decrease in pulmonary function over time, thought to be related to loss of chest wall compliance due to restricted anterior chest wall motion despite symptomatic improvement.[10] From a cardiac standpoint, the data are conflicting. Currently, there is no consensus as to whether surgical repair improves cardiac function.[10–12] The surgical treatment of pectus excavatum is detailed in Chapters 140 and 141.

Pectus Carinatum

Pectus carinatum occurs much less frequently than pectus excavatum, comprising only 10% of chest wall deformities. It is a congenital deformity characterized by outward sternal protrusion with anterior displacement of the middle and lower sternum and associated costal cartilages (Fig. 139-3). Pectus carinatum may be classified as chondrogladiolar (symmetric or asymmetric), mixed pectus carinatum and excavatum, and chondromanubrial. The chondrogladiolar type is the most common. It is described as an anterior protrusion of the body of the sternum with protrusion of the lower costal cartilage. As reported by Shamberger and Welch, the symmetric chondrogladiolar type is more common.[1] The mixed subtype is often composed of both elements of carinatum and excavatum. The chondromanubrial subtype, also referred to as "pouter pigeon," involves an anterior protrusion of the manubrium along with the second and third costal cartilages.

Like pectus excavatum, carinatum is much more common in males than in females (4:1). However, in contrast to pectus excavatum, it is not usually recognized until adolescence. A family history is again present in approximately 30% of patients. Scoliosis is the most commonly associated musculoskeletal deformity, whereas fewer than 5% of patients with pectus carinatum have associated congenital heart disease. Symptoms are uncommon in childhood but may progress into adolescence. It has been suggested that shortness of breath may be related to decreased chest wall compliance with increased chest diameter. In pectus carinatum, there is increased residual volume and reduced vital capacity which may also account for some symptoms.

Again, surgical repair by osteotomy is the main form of treatment. Surgical therapy provides excellent results with low morbidity in as many as 97% of patients.[13] The surgical treatment of pectus carinatum is discussed in Chapter 140.

Poland Syndrome

Poland syndrome is the congenital absence of the pectoralis major and minor muscles associated with syndactyly (fused fingers) (Fig. 139-4). It is also associated with abnormalities of the ribs, chest wall depressions, and abnormalities of the breasts. Thoracic involvement may range from hypoplasia of the sternal head of the pectoralis major and minor muscles with normal ribs, to complete absence of the anterior portions of ribs two to five and costal cartilages. Breast involvement may range from complete absence of the breast (amastia) and nipple (athelia) to mild hypoplasia. Hand deformities primarily involve the central three digits and may include syndactyly (fused fingers) and brachydactyly (hypoplasia). Poland syndrome occurs in 1 in 30,000 to 32,000 live births and is not often familial.[14] It is more common in females than males at a ratio of 3:1. The etiology is not well understood.

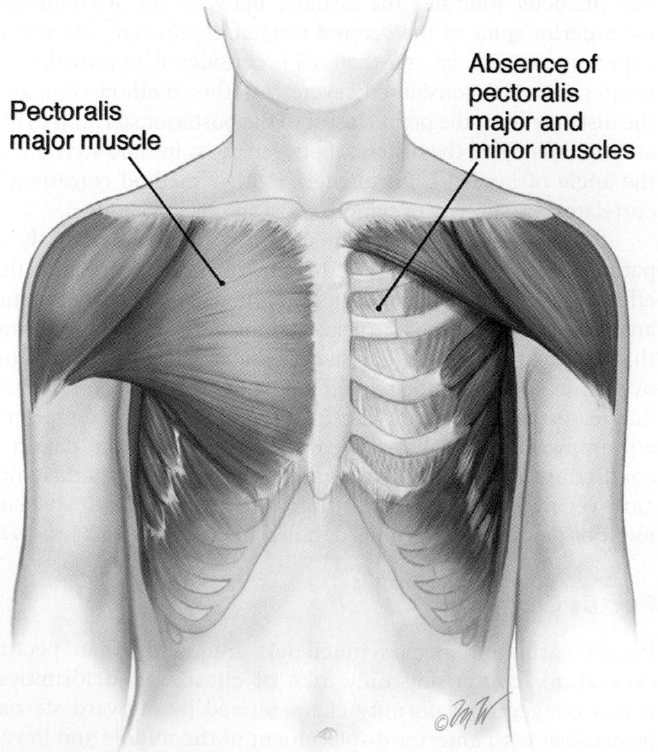

Figure 139-4. Poland syndrome.

Sternal Defects

Sternal defects are rare chest wall deformities that may be classified as cleft sternum or ectopic cordis (Fig. 139-5A,B). Sternal clefts typically involve only the upper sternum; ectopic cordis involves the lower sternum. The presumed embryologic cause is failure of ventral fusion of the sternum, resulting in sternal clefts, thoracic ectopia cordis, and thoracoabdominal ectopia cordis.

Cleft sternum in infants results from nonfusion of the sternal plates at about the eighth week of gestation. The cleft typically involves the upper sternum where the sternum has a complete or partial separation. The remainder of the sternum is normal, as is the diaphragm, pericardium, location of the heart, and overlying skin coverage. Omphaloceles do not occur in these children and it is rarely associated with intrinsic congenital heart disease. In ectopic cordis (thoracic and thoracoabdominal), the sternal cleft involves the inferior portion of the sternum and is associated with an abnormal diaphragm, pericardium, and location of the heart. Intracardiac anomalies are very common. In thoracic ectopic cordis, the lethal factor is the extrathoracic location of the heart without its pericardial coverage. In thoracoabdominal ectopic cordis (the Cantrell Pentology), the associated five features include (1) inferior sternal cleft, (2) anterior diaphragmatic defect, (3) absence of pericardium at the diaphragmatic defect, (4) an omphalocele, and (5) intrinsic cardiac abnormalities.[15] Although surgical repair of isolated cleft sternum is routinely successful, repair of ectopia cordis is associated with a high mortality rate.

THORACIC OUTLET SYNDROME

Thoracic outlet syndrome is a constellation of symptoms that result from compression of elements of the neurovascular bundle (i.e., subclavian artery, subclavian vein, and brachial plexus) as they pass through the thoracic outlet.

The thoracic outlet has three potential spaces for neurovascular compression: the interscalene triangle, the costoclavicular space, and the retropectoralis minor space (Fig. 139-6). The interscalene triangle is bounded anteriorly by the anterior scalene muscle, posteriorly by the middle and posterior scalene muscles, and inferiorly by the first rib. The subclavian artery and the three trunks of the brachial plexus traverse the triangle. The subclavian vein runs beneath the anterior scalene muscle. The costoclavicular space is bounded superiorly by the clavicle, anteriorly by the subclavius muscle, and posteriorly by the first rib and middle scalene muscle.

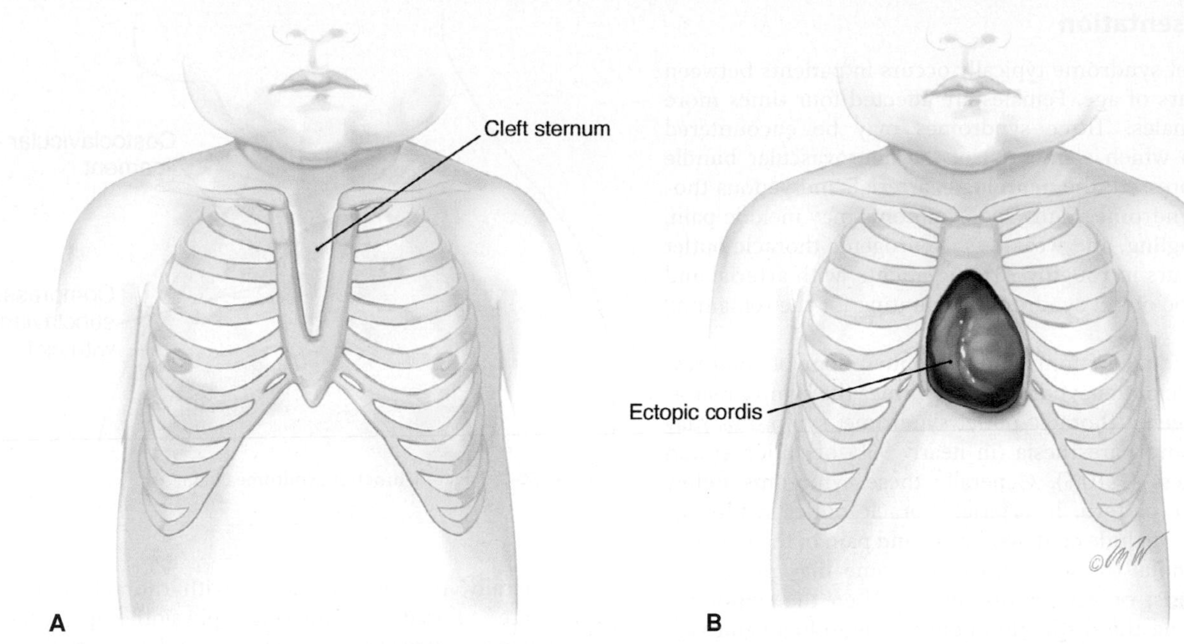

Figure 139-5. Sternal defects: (*A*) cleft sternum, (*B*) ectopic cordis.

The retropectoralis minor space is bounded anteriorly by the pectoralis minor muscle and posteriorly and superiorly by the subscapularis muscle, and posteriorly and inferiorly by the anterior chest wall. Radiographic imaging has shown that in normal subjects, upper extremity elevation does not produce a change in the interscalene triangle but does narrow the costoclavicular and retropectoralis minor spaces.[16] Arterial compression occurs most frequently in the costoclavicular space, followed by the interscalene triangle, whereas neurologic compression occurs equally in the two.

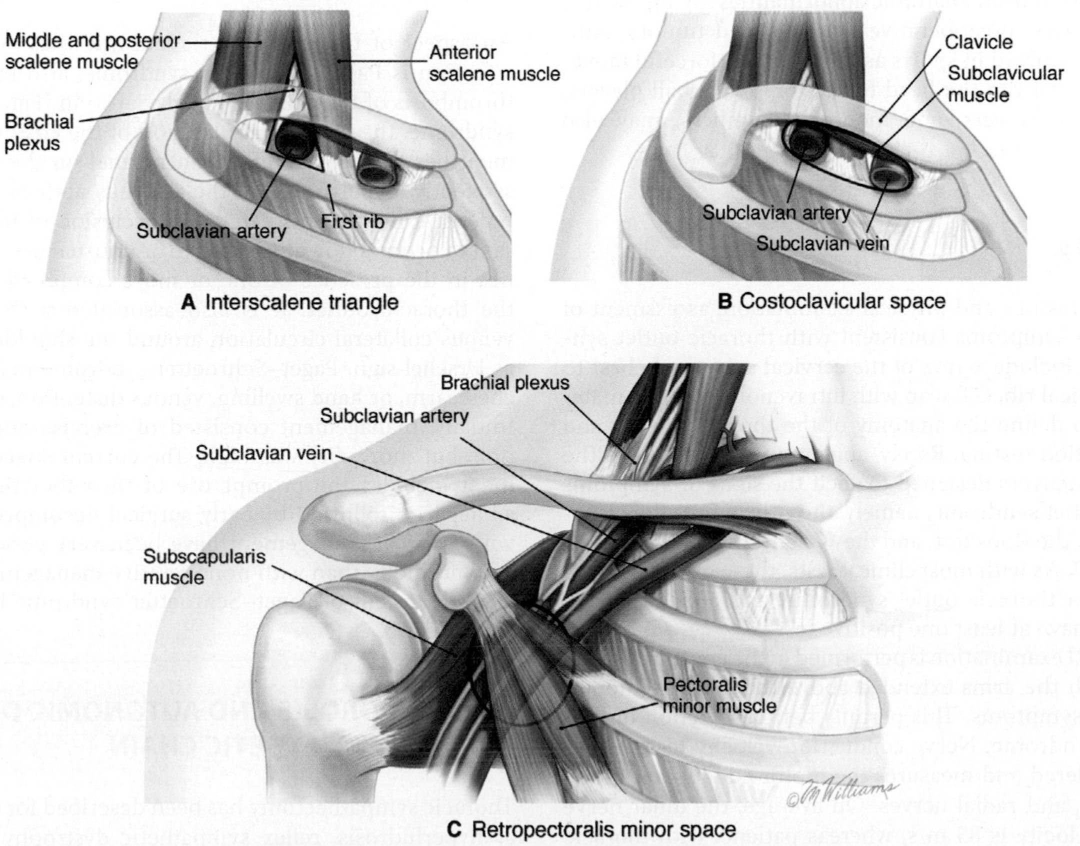

Figure 139-6. Three potential spaces for neurovascular compression.

Clinical Presentation

Thoracic outlet syndrome typically occurs in patients between 20 and 40 years of age. Females are affected four times more often than males. Three syndromes may be encountered depending on which element(s) of the neurovascular bundle is being compressed: the neurologic, arterial, and venous thoracic outlet syndrome. Signs and symptoms may include pain, numbness, tingling, and weakness. Neurogenic thoracic outlet syndrome occurs in roughly 90% of patients, with arterial and venous thoracic outlet syndrome accounting for the remaining 5% to 10%.[17]

The functional anatomy and pathophysiology of compression in thoracic outlet syndrome determines the symptomatology. In neurogenic thoracic outlet syndrome, symptoms may include pain and paresthesia (in nearly 95% of patients) and motor weakness (<10%). Generally these symptoms follow an ulnar nerve pattern. In arterial thoracic outlet syndrome, symptoms may include cold, weakness, and pain in the involved extremity. Venous thoracic outlet syndrome may present as edema, cyanosis, or venous distention. Often the symptoms overlap, blurring the distinction between neurologic and vascular thoracic outlet syndrome.

Thoracic outlet syndrome may be caused by congenital or acquired anatomic abnormalities. Congenital anatomic abnormalities include cervical rib, elongated C7 transverse process, exostosis of the first rib, fibrous band, and supranumerary muscles. A cervical rib is an extra rib originating from the seventh cervical vertebra. In the general population, a cervical rib is present in fewer than 1% and in only 5% to 9% of patients with thoracic outlet syndrome.[18] Fibrous bands arising from the first or cervical rib also may contribute to neurovascular compression. Acquired anatomic abnormalities giving include traumatic injuries, postoperative scarring, and tumors. Athletes who are involved in sports associated with forceful movement of the arm from the head to the torso, like ball players, football players, rowers, and mountain climbers, may also acquire this syndrome.

DIAGNOSIS

Apart from a history and physical examination, assessment of a patient with symptoms consistent with thoracic outlet syndrome should include x-rays of the cervical spine and chest to identify a cervical rib, CT scan with intravenous contrast material or MRI to define the anatomy of the thoracic outlet, and nerve conduction testing. Rarely, angiography is required. The four basic maneuvers designed to elicit the signs or symptoms of thoracic outlet syndrome, namely, the Adson test, the costoclavicular test, the Roos test, and the Wright test, are illustrated in Chapter 143. As with most clinical tests, these maneuvers are not specific for thoracic outlet syndrome, and 56% of normal patients may have at least one positive test.[18]

CT or MRI examination is performed in the neutral position as well as with the arms extended above the head to attempt to reproduce symptoms. This permits better detection of thoracic outlet syndrome. Nerve conduction velocity testing may also be considered and measures the motor conduction of the ulnar, median, and radial nerves. On average, the ulnar nerve conduction velocity is 85 m/s, whereas patients with thoracic outlet syndrome average 53 m/s.[19]

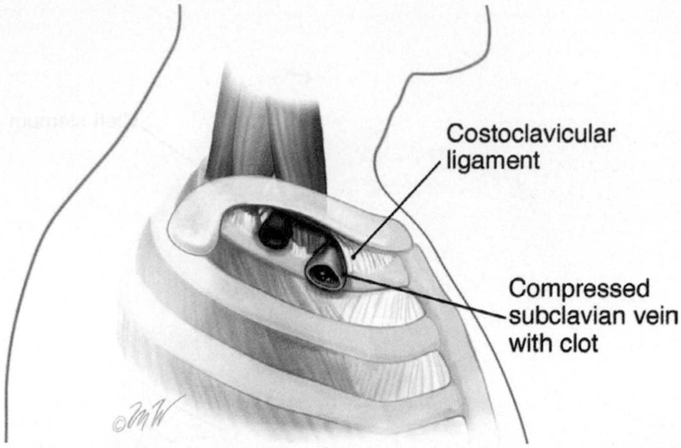

Figure 139-7. Paget–Schroetter syndrome chain.

Generally, patients diagnosed with thoracic outlet syndrome are advised to undertake physiotherapy, including heat massages, active neck massages, scalene anticus muscle stretching, strengthening of the upper trapezius and shoulder girdle, and proper posture instruction. As a rule, patients with an ulnar nerve conduction velocity of greater than 60 m/s do very well with conservative measures, whereas patients with an ulnar nerve conduction velocity of less than 60 m/s do less well and often require surgical intervention. Surgery for thoracic outlet syndrome is discussed in Chapters 142 to 144.

PAGET–SCHROETTER SYNDROME

An aspect of thoracic outlet syndrome that deserves special attention is Paget–Schroetter syndrome, also known as effort thrombosis of the axillary–subclavian vein (Fig. 139-7). In this syndrome, the congenital insertion of the costoclavicular ligament lies further laterally than normal on the first rib. Consequently, hypertrophy of the scalenus anticus muscle due to repetitive movements can cause occlusion of the vein. This is said to occur following excessive or unusual use of the extremities in the presence of one or more compressive elements in the thoracic outlet. It is also associated with subcutaneous venous collateral circulation around the shoulder, also known as Urschel sign. Paget–Schroetter syndrome may present with chest, arm, or hand swelling, venous distention, or aching pain. Initially, management consisted of exercise and anticoagulation, but morbidity was high. The current suggested management includes the prompt use of thrombolytic agents, such as heparin, followed by early surgical decompression. Results with surgical management have been very good, and there is less morbidity than with nonoperative management.[20] The surgical treatment of Paget–Schroetter syndrome is described in Chapter 145.

HYPERHIDROSIS AND AUTONOMIC DISORDERS OF THE SYMPATHETIC CHAIN

Thoracic sympathectomy has been described for disorders such as hyperhidrosis, reflex sympathetic dystrophy (RSD), upper extremity ischemia, Raynaud disease, and splanchnicectomy for pancreatic pain. Hyperhidrosis is a disorder of excessive sweat production. The disorder most commonly affects the axillae, hands, feet, and face. The prevalence of palmar and plantar hyperhidrosis is estimated at 0.6% to 1%, with axillary hyperhidrosis affecting 1.4%. Although diagnostic tests do exist, history provides the diagnosis in most cases. The typical patient is a young adult who is able to give a history of consistent excessive sweating that results in social embarrassment and interference with normal day-to-day activities. A family history may be present in as many as 65% of cases.[21]

The pathophysiology of hyperhidrosis is not well understood. Eccrine glands are distributed around the body, with higher concentrations in areas such as the palms, soles, and forehead. These glands are innervated by the cholinergic fibers of the sympathetic nervous system. Patients with hyperhidrosis do not demonstrate any histopathologic changes in the sweat glands or changes in their numbers. Up to two-thirds of patients report a positive family history. Hyperhidrosis must be differentiated from the secondary effects of neurologic, endocrinologic, metabolic, and other such disorders, as well as febrile illness, malignancy, and drugs.

A wide array of modalities are used in the attempt to treat hyperhidrosis. These include nonsurgical (i.e., topical or systemic) and surgical treatments. Patients with hyperhidrosis generally are initially offered topical agents such as prescription strength antiperspirants that contain 20% aluminum chloride in ethanol (Drysol) or 6.25% aluminum tetrachloride (Xerac). Medications may also have some benefit in selected patients. Anticholingeric agents such as glycopyrrolate (0.5–1 mg) can be used in patients who can tolerate side effects such as dry mouth, urinary retention, or blurred vision. In patients with hyperhidrosis stimulated by emotional events, beta blockers (propranolol 10 mg, two to four times daily) and benzodiazepines may provide some relief of symptoms. However, the duration of these effects may be short. Occasionally, a trial of iontophoresis is offered for palmar or plantar hyperhidrosis. This treatment involves the introduction of ionized substances through the skin by application of direct current. This therapy is appropriate if the patient can tolerate the side effects of tingling, skin irritation, and electric shocks. It has been reported to alleviate symptoms in up to 85% of patients. Botox injections may also be useful in palmar and axillary hyperhidrosis by temporarily reducing sweat production for approximately 3 to 4 months and up to 7 months.[22]

For patients undergoing thoracoscopic sympathectomy, the place where the sympathetic chain is divided also can depend on the primary symptom and underlying disease (Fig. 139-8; see Chapter 146). The recent Society of Thoracic Surgery (STS) expert consensus recommendations for patients with palmar hyperhidrosis are interruption of the sympathetic chain at the top of the third rib (R3) or the top of the fourth rib (R4). An R4 and R5 sympathetic chain interruption is recommended for palmary–axillary, palmar—axillary–plantar, or axillary only hyperhidrosis alone. Patients with craniofacial hyperhidrosis (facial sweating or blushing) generally require division of the chain at R3.[23] Indications for sympathectomy other than hyperhidrosis are not as common and it is less successful. Patients with RSD generally undergo either transthoracic sympathectomy (lower third of the stellate ganglia to R3) or lumbar sympathectomy (L2–L4). Schwartzman et al. reported a high success rate and long-term relief for selected patients with symptom duration less than or equal to 12 months.[24]

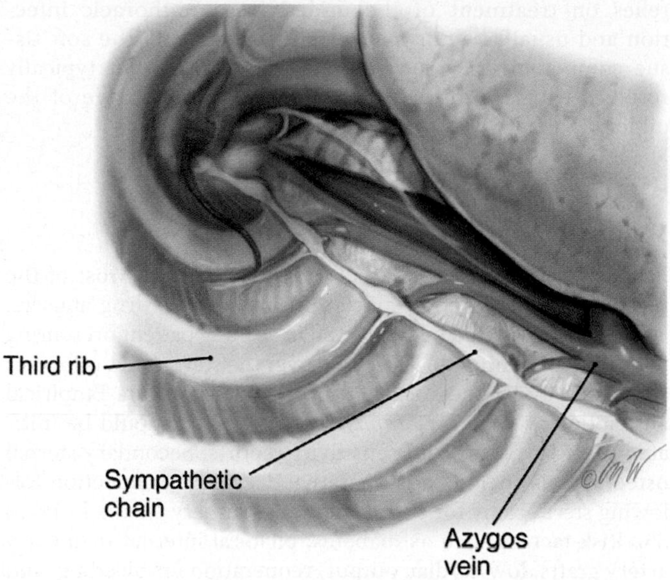

Figure 139-8. Hyperhidrosis, location of sympathetic chain.

Thoracoscopic sympathectomy for Raynaud disease has more variable results. Maga et al. performed thoracoscopic sympathectomy in 25 patients with severe Raynaud disease to assess its effect on microcirculation in the hands of these patients. The basal capillary flow and maximal refilling time were measured and compared with the same measurements obtained in a group of 50 healthy individuals. The basal capillary flow and maximal refilling time improved after the sympathectomy to levels similar to those in the control group. Furthermore, the long-term improvement was maintained during the 5-year follow-up period. The patients' symptom severity scores diminished to zero in the early postoperative period and increased to 28% of their initial value 5 years after the operation.[25]

CHEST WALL INFECTIONS

Infections of the chest wall may be classified as soft tissue infections, infections invading the chest wall, or infections of the cartilage or bony structures.

Soft Tissue Infections

Chest wall soft tissue infections may originate from direct inoculation or hematogenous spread. These infections may be classified as bacterial or nonbacterial, or necrotizing or nonnecrotizing. The clinical presentation varies from only a mildly symptomatic patient to a frankly septic patient. The clinical presentation, as well as treatment, often is dictated by the offending organism. Prompt recognition and intervention is necessary to prevent serious morbidity and potential mortality. Chapter 147 discusses this topic in greater detail.

Empyema Necessitans

Chest wall infections also may originate in the lung parenchyma or pleural space and "invade" the chest wall. Empyema necessitans, or soft tissue infection caused by an undrained pleural or parenchymal infection, is an entity seen more frequently in the days before antimicrobial therapy. Therapy relies on treatment of the underlying intrathoracic infection and usually requires surgical debridement. The soft tissue component may require separate drainage but typically resolves with appropriate debridement and drainage of the underlying empyema.

Cartilage or Bony Infections

Sternal Osteomyelitis

Primary sternal osteomyelitis is a rare condition. Most of the recent cases have been reported in intravenous drug abusers. The diagnosis should be suspected in a young patient presenting with acute inflammatory swelling over the sternum. It is further supported by leukocytosis and positive Gram stain. Empirical antibiotic coverage for *Staphylococcus aureus* should be initiated prior to culture and sensitivity reports. Secondary sternal osteomyelitis such as postoperative deep sternal infection following sternotomy for coronary bypass surgery occurs in 1% to 3%. Risk factors such as diabetes, bilateral internal mammary artery grafts, low cardiac output, reoperation for bleeding, and renal failure have been identified. The first signs of infection may be drainage or discharge from the operative incision or an unstable sternum. Treatment relies on intravenous antibiotics to cover methicillin-resistant *S. aureus* and debridement. Deep sternal infections may require greater debridement and may benefit from soft tissue transposition to aid healing. In chronic sternal osteomyelitis, extensive sternal and chondral debridement with myocutaneous reconstruction provides the most successful results.

Rib Osteomyelitis

Diagnosis of rib osteomyelitis is made based on evidence of local inflammation or clinical symptoms. Imaging studies are performed to confirm the diagnosis and to evaluate for underlying intrathoracic pathology. A review of 106 cases of rib osteomyelitis demonstrated that most cases occurred in children and young adults.[26] Common clinical signs were fever (73%), soft tissue mass (64%), and chest pain (60%). The routes of infection were contiguous spread in 68% and hematogenous spread in 38%. Mycobacterial and bacterial infections accounted for the majority of cases. Therapy entails antimicrobial therapy with or without debridement and resection of all diseased bone.

Sternoclavicular Osteomyelitis

The sternoclavicular joint is an unusual site of septic arthritis. Although spontaneous cases are reported in healthy persons, it is more commonly associated with intravenous drug abuse, indwelling central venous catheters, and immunocompromised patients. Sternoclavicular osteomyelitis usually presents with a slow, progressive onset of chest wall pain that is localized to the sternoclavicular joint or pain referred to the shoulder or neck. Because the sternoclavicular joint capsule is unable to distend, infection spreads rapidly beyond the joint to the nearby mediastinum, pleural space, and brachiocephalic structures. The area is tender to palpation. Fever and leukocytosis are not always present.

In a review of 180 cases of sternoclavicular septic arthritis, the most common risk factor was intravenous drug abuse (21%), followed by infection at a distant site (15%), diabetes mellitus (13%), trauma (12%), and infected central venous access (9%). No underlying medical condition was found in 23% of patients.[27] Median duration of symptoms at presentation was 14 days. *Staphylococcus aureus* was the offending organism in 49% of patients, whereas *Pseudomonas aeruginosa* was found in 10%. Bacteremia was present in 62% of cases and associated osteomyelitis (55%), chest wall abscess or phlegmon (25%), and mediastinitis (13%) were frequently present.

Patients with suspected sternoclavicular joint arthritis should be routinely evaluated by CT scan or MRI. If there is extensive bony destruction with chest wall phlegmon or abscess, retrosternal abscess, mediastinitis, or pleural extension, en bloc sternoclavicular joint resection and possible ipsilateral pectoralis major muscle flap is indicated. Medical management alone, such as intravenous (IV) antibiotics, is associated with a high failure rate. Surgical management starts with a hockey-stick incision made from the medial third of the clavicle down the midline of the manubrium, and en bloc resection of the joint is performed with debridement of bone and soft tissues until they appear healthy. The subclavian vein may be densely adherent to the posterior aspect of the joint capsule. Small wounds can be permitted to heal by secondary intention. Larger wounds may require a soft tissue or muscle flap for coverage. The flap improves wound vascularity and healing, and it protects the great vessels from trauma. Long-term results for both infection control and chest wall function are excellent. Burkhart et al.[28] reported a 7.7% complication rate and 3.8% mortality rate in their series of 26 patients. Specific antibiotic therapy should be based on culture data and continued for 4 weeks in uncomplicated sternoclavicular septic arthritis and for 6 weeks in cases complicated by osteomyelitis or mediastinitis. Functional outcomes generally are excellent, even after sternoclavicular joint resection.[28] Surgical treatment for chest wall infections is discussed in Chapter 147.

BENIGN TUMORS OF THE CHEST WALL

Roughly half of primary chest wall tumors are benign. They may be classified by origin as either soft tissue or bone and cartilage. Benign chest wall tumors typically manifest as slow-growing, palpable masses in asymptomatic patients. The slow growth rate that typifies most benign chest wall tumors is evidenced on radiologic images by well-defined tissue planes, and sometimes by pressure erosions on adjacent bone.[29]

Surgical resection is commonly employed in the treatment of these lesions and the reader is referred to Part 22 (Chapters 134 to 138) for surgical techniques used to resect and reconstruct chest wall tumors.

Benign Soft Tissue Tumors

Primary chest wall soft tissue tumors are not rare. These are typically of mesenchymal origin and can arise from fat, vascular, neural, fibrous, dermal, or muscular tissues. These lesions are comprised of lipomas, fibromas, neurofibromas, lymphangiomas, and hemangiomas. Often these lesions are asymptomatic. Surgical excision is indicated for enlarging masses and for definitive diagnosis to rule out malignancy.

Benign Bone and Cartilage Tumors

Osteochondroma, chondroma, and fibrous dysplasia are the most common forms of benign bone and cartilaginous tumors of the chest wall. Others include eosinophilic granuloma, giant cell tumor, chondroblastoma, and osteoblastoma.

Although relatively rare, osteochondromas are the most common benign rib tumor, encompassing 50% of all nonmalignant rib tumors but only 8% of all rib tumors.[30] They occur commonly in the metaphyseal region of the rib in the bony cortex at the costochondral junction. Tumors characteristically pedunculated with osseous protuberances arising from the surface of the bone. Radiographs may show a cap composed of hyaline cartilage, which may be calcified. Males are affected three times more frequently than females. Surgical resection is indicated for definitive diagnosis since malignant degeneration has been reported.

Chondromas account for approximately 15% of benign rib lesions. These typically arise in the ribs near the costochondral junction anteriorly and may cause pain. These present during the second or third decade of life, equally between men and women. Radiographically, these tumors present as an expansile medullary mass with a thinning cortex. Importantly, they cannot be distinguished from chondrosarcomas, either clinically or radiographically, and thus should be resected for definitive diagnosis and treatment.

Fibrous dysplasia is a benign cystic lesion that presents as a solitary mass. These tumors usually present as a painless asymptomatic mass and account for nearly 30% of all benign chest wall tumors.[30] Fibrous dysplasia is a skeletal developmental anomaly in which mesenchymal osteoblasts fail to undergo normal morphologic differentiation and maturation. The ribs are commonly affected, and the clavicle is occasionally involved. Pain is usually indicative of an underlying pathologic fracture. Radiographs characteristically show unilateral fusiform enlargement and deformity with cortical thickening and increased trabeculation of one or more ribs with amorphous or irregular calcification.[29] Malignant degeneration is rare and resection is indicated for definite treatment.

References

1. Shamberger RC, Welch KJ. Surgical repair of pectus excavatum. *J Pediatr Surg.* 1988;23:615–622.
2. Huddleston CB. Pectus excavatum. *Semin Thorac Cardiovasc Surg.* 2004;16:225–232.
3. Kelly RE Jr, Shamberger RC, Mellins RB, et al. Prospective multicenter study of surgical correction of pectus excavatum: design, perioperative complications, pain, and baseline pulmonary function facilitated by Internet-based data collection. *J Am Coll Surg.* 2007;205:205–216.
4. Neviere R, Montaigne D, Benhamed L, et al. Cardiopulmonary response following surgical repair of pectus excavatum in adult patients. *Eur J Cardiothorac Surg.* 2011;40:e77–e82.
5. Kelly RE Jr. Pectus excavatum: historical background, clinical picture, preoperative evaluation and criteria for operation. *Sem Ped Surg.* 2008;17:181–193.
6. Wynn SR, Driscoll DJ, Ostrom NK, et al. Exercise cardiorespiratory function in adolescents with pectus excavatum: observations before and after operation. *J Thorac Cardiovasc Surg.* 1990;99:41–47.
7. Kaguraoka H, Ohnuki T, Itaoka T, et al. Degree of severity of pectus excavatum and pulmonary function in preoperative and postoperative periods. *J Thorac Cardiovasc Surg.* 1992;104:1483–1488.
8. Lawson ML, Mellins RB, Paulson JF, et al. Increasing severity of pectus excavatum is associated with reduced pulmonary function. *J Pediatr.* 2011;159:256–261.
9. Haller J, Kramer S, Lietman S. Use of CT scans in selection of patients for pectus excavatum surgery: a preliminary report. *J Pediatr Surg.* 1987; 22:905–906.
10. Malek MH, Berger DE, Marelich WD, et al. Pulmonary function following surgical repair of pectus excavatum: a meta-analysis. *Eur J Cardiothorac Surg.* 2006;30:637–643.
11. Guntheroth WG, Spiers PS. Cardiac function before and after surgery for pectus excavatum. *Am J Cardiol.* 2007;99:1762–1764.
12. Malek MH, Berger DE, Housh TJ, et al. Cardiovascular function following surgical repair of pectus excavatum: a meta-analysis. *Chest.* 2006;130:506–516.
13. Fonkalsrud EW, DeUgarte D, Choi E. Repair of pectus excavatum and carinatum deformities in 116 adults. *Ann Surg.* 2002;236:304–312; discussion 312–314, 2002.
14. Shamberger RC, Welch KJ, Upton J 3rd. Surgical treatment of thoracic deformity in Poland's syndrome. *J Pediatr Surg.* 1989;24:760–765.
15. Shamberger R, Welch K. Sternal defects. *Pediatr Surg Int.* 1990;5:156–164.
16. Demondion X, Bacqueville E, Paul C, et al. Thoracic outlet: assessment with MR imaging in asymptomatic and symptomatic populations. *Radiology.* 2003;227:461–468.
17. Urschel HC Jr, Maruf AR. Neurovascular compression in the thoracic outlet: changing management over 50 years. *Ann Surg.* 1998;228:609–617.
18. Atasoy E. Thoracic outlet compression syndrome. *Orthop Clin North Am.* 1996;27:265–303.
19. Urschel HC Jr, Razzuk MA, Wood RE, et al. Objective diagnosis (ulnar nerve conduction velocity) and current therapy of the thoracic outlet syndrome. *Ann Thorac Surg.* 1971;12:608–620.
20. Urschel HC Jr, Patel AN. Surgery remains the most effective treatment for Paget-Schroetter syndrome: 50 years' experience. *Ann Thorac Surgery.* 2008;86:254–260.
21. Ro KM, Cantor RM, Lange KL, et al. Palmar hyperhidrosis: evidence of genetic transmission. *J Vasc Surg.* 2002;35:382–386.
22. Togel B, Greve B, Raulin C, et al. Current therapeutic strategies for hyperhidrosis: a review. *Eur J Dermatol.* 2002;12:219–223.
23. Cerfolio RJ, De Campos JR, Bryant AS, et al. The Society of Thoracic Surgeons expert consensus for the surgical treatment of hyperhidrosis. *Ann Thorac Surg.* 2011;91:1642–1648.
24. Schwartzman RJ, Liu JE, Smullens SN, et al. Long-term outcome following sympathectomy for complex regional pain syndrome type 1 (RSD). *J Neurol Sci.* 1997;150:149–152.
25. Maga P, Kuzdzal J, Nizankowski R, et al. Long-term effects of thoracic sympathectomy on microcirculation in the hands of patients with primary Raynaud disease. *J Thorac Cardiovasc Surg.* 2007;133:1428–1433.
26. Bishara J, Gartman-Israel D, Weinberger M, et al. Osteomyelitis of the ribs in the antibiotic era. *Scand J Infect Dis.* 2000;32:223–227.
27. Ross JJ, Shamsuddin H.Sternoclavicular septic arthritis: review of 180 cases. *Medicine.* 2004;83:139–148.
28. Burkhart HM, Deschamps C, Allen MS, et al. Surgical management of sternoclavicular joint infections. *J Thorac Cardiovasc Surg.* 2003;125:945–949.
29. Tateishi U, Gladish GW, Kusumoto M, et al. Chest wall tumors: radiologic findings and pathologic correlation: 1. Benign tumors. *Radiographics.* 2003;23:1477–1490.
30. Hughes EK, James SLJ, Butt A, et al. Benign primary tumors of the ribs. *Clin Radiol.* 2006;61:314–322.

140 Primary Repair of Pectus Excavatum

Jill M. Zalieckas and Christopher B. Weldon

Keywords: Congenital chest wall defect, open repair, Nuss minimally invasive pectus excavatum repair

Pectus excavatum is the most common congenital anterior chest wall defect, characterized by a posterior depression of the sternum and inferior costal cartilages. The deformity can be present at birth or develop during childhood. The sternal depression may worsen as the child grows, often peaking during pubertal growth. Incidence is reported at 1 per 1000 children. It is more common in males; the male to female ratio is 4:1. The etiology of the defect is unknown, although there is a suggestion of an intrinsic abnormality of costochondral cartilage due to the occurrence of pectus excavatum in patients with connective tissue disorders. Scoliosis is present in up to 20% of patients with pectus excavatum. In addition, a family history of pectus excavatum is present in up to 40% of patients, suggesting a genetic predisposition. Approximately one third of all children with pectus excavatum have a severe deformity that warrants evaluation for surgical repair.[1]

Meyer first attempted surgical repair in 1911 and Sauerbruch in 1913.[1] In 1939, Ochsner and DeBakey reviewed the techniques of repair and reported outcomes with high morbidity and mortality.[1] Ravitch[2] described a technique in 1949 involving division of xiphoid from sternum, excision of deformed costal cartilages, division of intercostal bundles from sternum, transverse sternal osteotomy at junction of manubrium; angling of sternum anteriorly and suturing in position. Welch modified this technique in 1958, emphasizing the preservation of perichondrial sheaths of costal cartilages and preservation of intercostal bundles. This modified Ravitch technique is the basis of current open repair performed 50 years later.[3,4]

In 1998, Nuss reported his 10-year experience with a minimally invasive technique for pectus excavatum repair. This procedure involves placement of an internal stainless steel bar to reshape the chest wall without excision of costal cartilages or sternal osteotomy.[1] The Nuss minimally invasive pectus excavatum repair has become an appealing surgical option to the traditional open repair, with excellent outcomes and a low morbidity.

GENERAL PRINCIPLES

Pectus excavatum includes a spectrum of severity from mild to severe. Mild to moderate deformities can benefit from an exercise and posture program, and yearly follow-up. Those patients with severe deformities should undergo a complete evaluation to define the degree of deformity and physiologic impairments which will aid in determining candidacy for surgical intervention. Approximately two-thirds of patients are treated nonoperatively.[1,4,5]

Although pectus deformities may be present at birth and noticeable in early childhood, it is usually not until older childhood or teenage years that children and their parents seek evaluation and treatment. During puberty, the pectus deformity often deepens and becomes more symptomatic. Patients may describe symptoms of dyspnea on exertion, shortness of breath, exercise intolerance, air hunger, decreased endurance, and pain at the sternal border. Teenagers also present with issues with body image, which can have debilitating and life-altering psychosocial effects.[1,4–6]

The operative technique performed is surgeon dependent. The minimally invasive Nuss procedure has gained widespread acceptance; however, the open technique is still performed and has comparable results. Direct comparisons of outcomes of open and minimally invasive techniques have not been performed in randomized control trials, but there have been several retrospective reviews comparing the two techniques. A meta-analysis by Nasr evaluating the published data comparing the two techniques illustrated that both open and minimally invasive repairs are acceptable techniques, with no significant difference in rate of complication, outcome, postoperative pain management, and hospital length of stay.[7]

Kelly et al. published early results of the Pectus Multicenter Study in 2007, which is a prospective study among 11 centers in the United States, attempting to compare the open and Nuss procedures with respect to complications, effect of repair on cardiopulmonary function, effect on self-image and quality of life, and patient satisfaction with pain management. The study revealed that the majority of centers were performing the Nuss procedure (284 patients) compared to open repair (43 patients). However, early results from this study demonstrated equivalent median hospital length of stay of 4 days, similar complication rates, and successful pain management in both groups.[8]

PATIENT SELECTION/PREOPERATIVE ASSESSMENT

Extensive workup is performed for those patients in whom operative intervention is sought. Patient selection for operative repair is determined by performing a thorough history and physical examination to evaluate the degree of deformity and impairment. Symptoms suggesting cardiorespiratory compromise, pain, or body image issues should be investigated. On physical examination, attention to the depth of depression and associated findings of number of costal cartilages involved, rounded shoulders, protuberant abdomen (due to laxity of rectus abodminis), and presence of scoliosis should be assessed.[1,5]

For those patients who appear to have a moderate-to-severe pectus excavatum deformity, further investigation is warranted. The workup includes CT scan of chest, pulmonary function testing, and echocardiogram. Echocardiogram is used to evaluate right heart function, which may be compromised due to external compression of the sternal deformity. In addition, mitral valve prolapse is associated with up to 35% of patients with pectus excavatum.[3,5] Pulmonary function testing is used to assess baseline function. It may demonstrate decrease in forced vital capacity, forced expiratory volume at

Table 140-1

CRITERIA FOR SURGICAL CORRECTION OF PECTUS EXCAVATUM. TWO OR MORE OF THE FOLLOWING INDICATED FOR SURGICAL REPAIR

1. Progressive or symptomatic pectus deformity
2. Restrictive disease on pulmonary function testing
3. Chest CT with cardiac compression or atelectasis
4. Haller index >3.25
5. Cardiac abnormalities found on echocardiogram (mitral valve prolapse, decreased diastolic filling, bundle branch block)
6. Recurrence

1 second, and decreased oxygen delivery, indicative of restrictive airway disease.[4,5]

Chest CT allows for detailed evaluation of the degree of depression of the sternum, cardiac shift, and compression, as well as providing means to calculate the Haller index. The Haller index is a measure of pectus excavatum severity by measuring the width of the chest between the ribs at the lowest level of the pectus defect in centimeters divided by the height of the chest from the anterior spine to the back of the lowest part of the sternal defect. The quotient of this division is the Haller index. An index greater than 3.25 is considered a severe defect, warranting consideration for repair.[4]

Surgical correction of pectus excavatum is indicated with the presence of two or more of the following criteria: progressive or symptomatic pectus deformity, restrictive disease on pulmonary function testing, chest CT demonstrating cardiac compression or atelectasis, Haller index >3.25, cardiac abnormalities including mitral valve prolapse, decreased diastolic filling due to right heart compression, and recurrence after failed repair (Table 140-1).[4] Although repair of pectus excavatum has been reported from 5 to 29 years of age, the recommended timing of repair is in the middle teenage years. During this time period, the chest wall remains malleable and allows for chest wall maturation while the support bar is still in place. Those patients who have support bars removed before puberty have an increased risk of recurrence.[9,10]

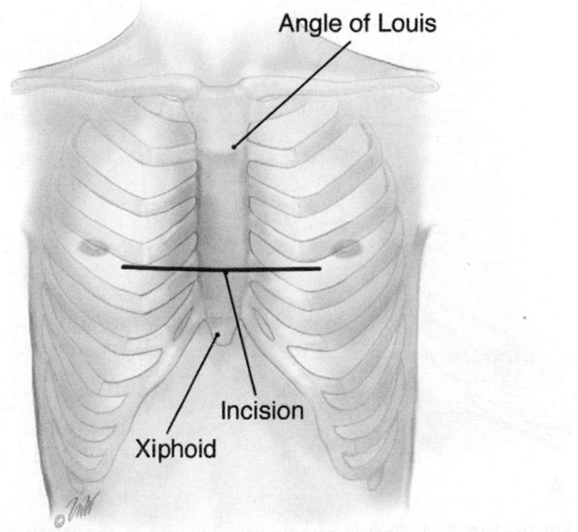

Figure 140-1. A transverse incision is made below and within nipple lines at the level of the inframammary crease.

If a Nuss repair is planned, the preoperative evaluation should also investigate for metal allergy, especially nickel, chromium and copper, or a family history of metal allergy. The standard Lorenz pectus bar is stainless steel, which has been shown to cause allergic reactions in those individuals with metal allergy. Those with a metal allergy and those with history of eczema should have a titanium bar and stabilizer placed instead of the standard stainless steel bar. Titanium bars are shaped by manufacturers in advance of the surgery date.[9]

OPERATIVE TECHNIQUE: OPEN REPAIR

The open technique described by Shamberger and Welch, is depicted in Figures 140-1 to 140-8. Preoperative antibiotics are given and continued for 24 hours postoperatively. A transverse incision is made below and within the nipple lines at the level of the inframammary crease (Fig. 140-1). Skin flaps are elevated and mobilized utilizing electrocautery to the angle of Louis superiorly and xiphoid inferiorly. The pectoral muscle flaps are elevated off the sternum and costal cartilages. This plane is defined by identifying the free area just anterior to the costal cartilages at the junction with the sternum. An empty knife handle is used to develop this plane, and muscle flap is retracted anteriorly with small right angle retractor. The muscle is dissected laterally to the level of the costochondral junctions (Fig. 140-2). The perichondrium is incised anteriorly on the third through fifth ribs, and the pectus elevator is used to preserve the perichondrial sheaths (Fig. 140-3). The cartilage is divided at the sternal junction, held with an Allis clamp, elevated, and excised from the costochondral junction. The costal cartilages of the third through seventh cartilages bilaterally are resected to the costochondral junctions (Fig. 140-4).[3,4]

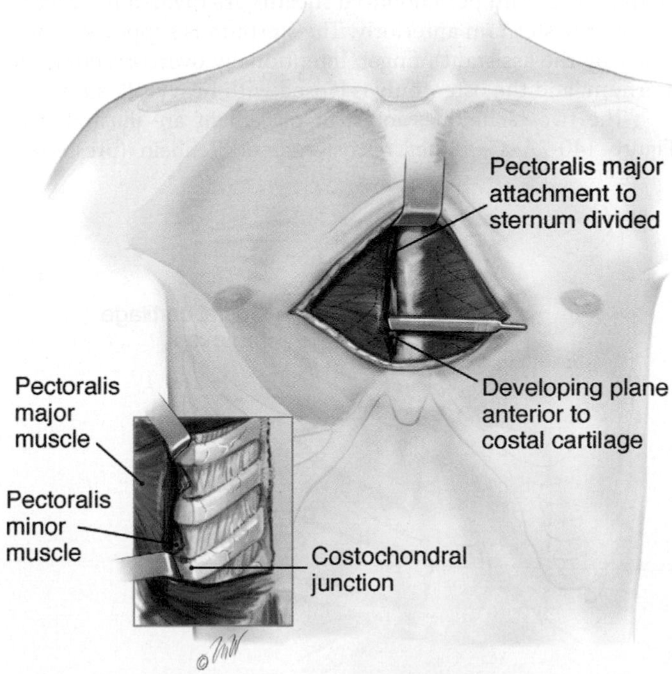

Figure 140-2. Skin flaps are elevated from the angle of Louis to xiphoid. Pectoral muscle flaps are elevated off the sternum and costal cartilages. The pectoral muscles are dissected laterally to the level of the costochondral junctions.

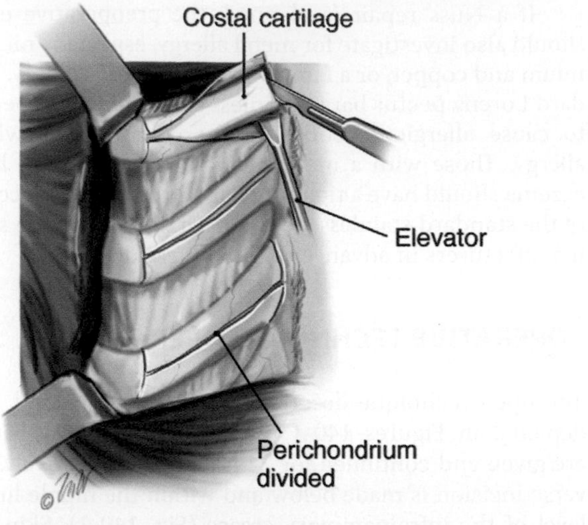

Figure 140-3. Perichondrium is incised anteriorly on third through fifth ribs. An elevator is used to preserve the perichondrial sheaths.

After removing the costal cartilages, a sternal wedge osteotomy is created above the last deformed cartilage at the posterior angulation of the sternum. The wedge osteotomy is accomplished by creating two transverse sternal osteotomies through the anterior cortex with a Hall air drill (Zimmer USA, Inc., Warsaw, IN), approximately 2 to 4 mm apart, and subsequently removing the anterior cortex and cancellous bone (Fig. 140-5).[3,4]

At this point, the procedure diverges depending on whether or not prosthetic struts are used. There is no consensus on the optimal method of reconstruction. The no-strut technique is illustrated in Figure 140-6. The procedure continues by dividing the attachment of the rectus muscle to the sternum with electrocautery and elevating the sternum with towel clips. The xiphoid is divided to allow entry into the retrosternal space. The sixth and seventh perichondrial sheaths are divided in order to elevate the sternum anteriorly. The sternum is supported anteriorly by the assistant's finger, intentionally overcorrecting the sternum, and the osteotomy is closed with heavy silk sutures.[4]

The two techniques for strut placement are illustrated in Figure 140-7A–C. Either retrosternal or Rehbein (presternal) struts may be placed. If a retrosternal strut is used, the perichondrial sheath to the third or fourth rib is divided at the sternal junction. Blunt dissection is performed to develop a retrosternal space for the strut to pass. The strut is secured laterally with two pericostal sutures (Fig. 140-7B). The Rehbein struts are inserted into the marrow of the third or fourth rib and joined to each other medially over the sternum. The sternum is sewn to the arch of the struts to secure the sternum in an anterior position (Fig. 140-7C).[4]

The wound is then irrigated, and a closed suction drain is placed in a right parasternal location at the level of the highest costal cartilage resection and brought through the inferior skin flap to the left of the sternum (Fig. 140-8). The pectoral muscle flaps are sewn to the midline of the sternum. The remaining wound is closed in layers and subcuticular skin closure.[3]

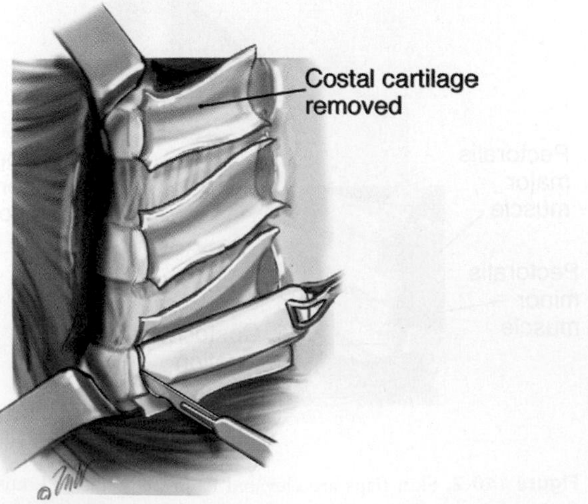

Figure 140-4. Costal cartilages are divided at the sternum, elevated, and resected at the costochondral junction.

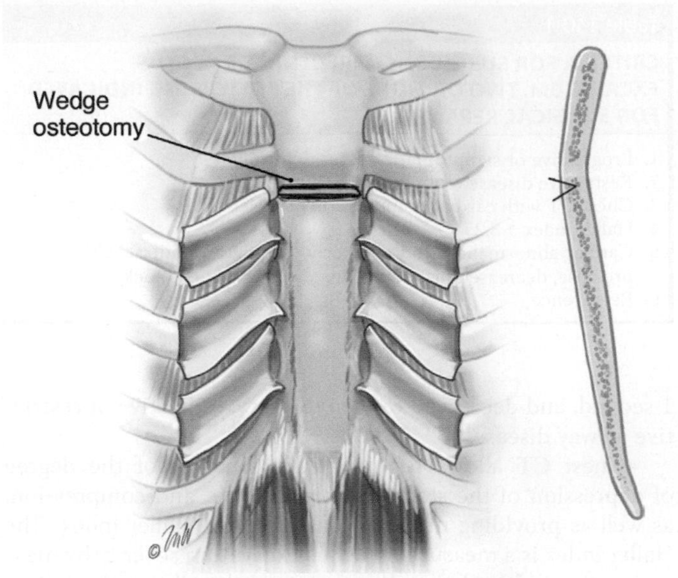

Figure 140-5. Sternal osteotomy is created by making two transverse incisions, approximately 2 to 4 mm apart in the sternum just above the last involved cartilage, which is at the level of the posterior angulation of the sternum. Anterior cortex and cancellous bone are removed.

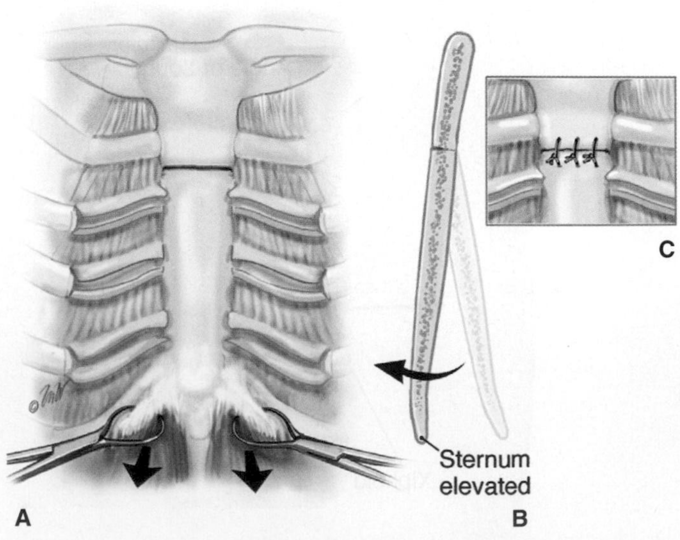

Figure 140-6. *A.* Rectus muscle attachments to the sternum are divided. *B.* This allows elevation of the sternum from the retrosternal space. *C.* The osteotomy is closed with heavy silk suture.

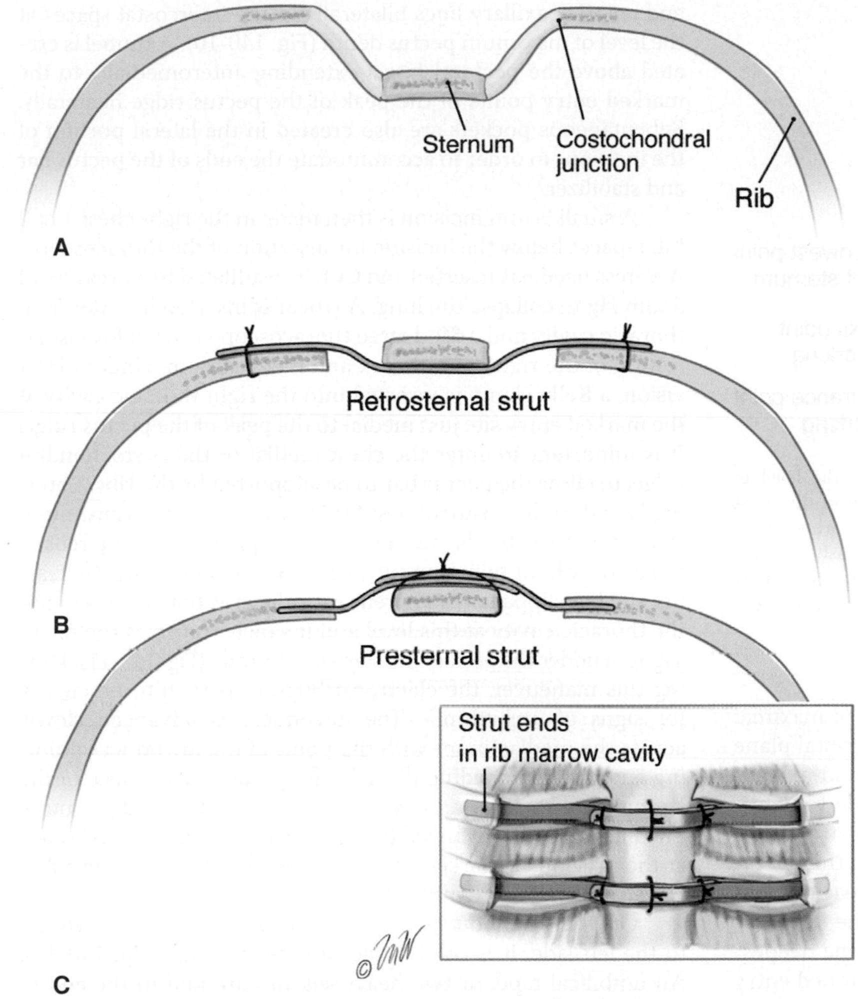

Figure 140-7. *A.* Perichondrial sheath divided at sternal junction. *B.* Retrosternal strut placed and secured with pericostal sutures bilaterally. *C.* Rehbein (presternal) strut placed into marrow and joined medially over sternum. Sternum is sewn to the strut arch, securing it in an anterior position.

OPERATIVE TECHNIQUE: MINIMALLY INVASIVE REPAIR (NUSS)

Nuss first described the minimally invasive pectus excavatum repair in 1998. Modifications of the original repair occurred over the first decade of use, resulting in the technique depicted in Figures 140-9 to 140-14.[9–12]

An epidural catheter is usually placed in the operating room for perioperative pain control. Preoperative antibiotics are given and Foley catheter is placed. The patient is supine on the operating table with arms abducted.

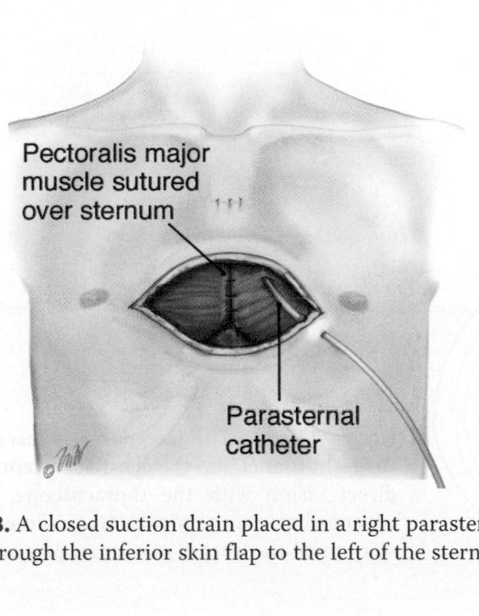

Figure 140-8. A closed suction drain placed in a right parasternal location is brought through the inferior skin flap to the left of the sternum.

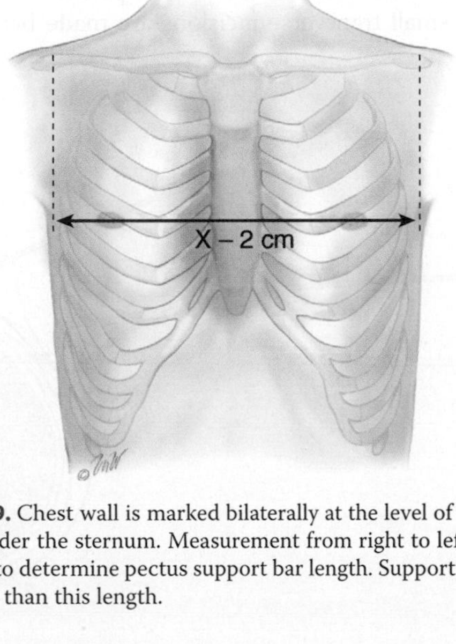

Figure 140-9. Chest wall is marked bilaterally at the level of maximal pectus depth under the sternum. Measurement from right to left mid axillary line is made to determine pectus support bar length. Support bar should be 2 cm shorter than this length.

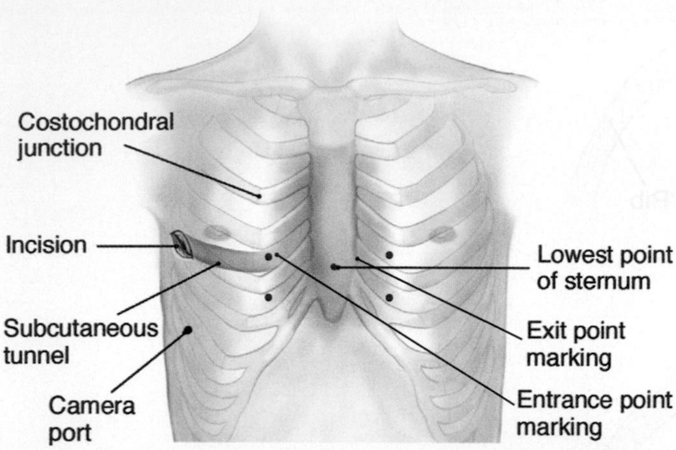

Figure 140-10. The intercostal space that corresponds to the level of maximum pectus depth is marked on the right and left sides of the chest for entry and exit, respectively. Bilateral transverse incisions are made at mid to anterior axillary lines in the intercostal space previously marked. Subcutaneous tunnels are made from each incision to their respective entry and exit points. A 5-mm incision is made 1 to 2 interspaces below the right incision for placement of the thoracoscope.

Each side of the thorax is marked at the level of maximal pectus depth under the sternum, which is the horizontal plane for bar insertion. Measurement from right to left mid-axillary line in the horizontal plane of bar insertion is made to determine the length of the stainless steel Lorenz pectus bar (Walter Lorenz Surgical Inc., Jacksonville, FL) to be used in the operation. The bar should be 2 cm shorter than the measurement from right to left mid-axillary lines (Fig. 140-9). The intercostal spaces that are in the same horizontal plane as the deepest point of the pectus deformity are identified. The planned entry and exit points are marked, which are located on right and left sides of the sternum respectively, medial to the peak of the costochondral ridge. This allows for the pectus bar to be supported by the chest wall while elevating the sternum.[9,12]

After sterile preparation and draping, the bar is bent in a convex shape, leaving a 2 to 4 cm flat middle section to support the sternum. The bar should fit the lateral chest wall on each side without compression or protrusion. If desired, the bar can be preshaped by the manufacturer based on the patient's CT measurements. Two small transverse incisions are made between mid- and anterior axillary lines bilaterally in the intercostal spaces at the level of maximum pectus depth (Fig. 140-10). A tunnel is created above the pectoral fascia extending anteromedially to the marked entry points of the peak of the pectus ridge bilaterally. Subcutaneous pockets are also created in the lateral portion of the incisions in order to accommodate the ends of the pectus bar and stabilizer.[9–11]

A small 5-mm incision is then made in the right chest 1 to 2 interspaces below the incision for insertion of the thoracoscope. A Veress needle is inserted and CO_2 is insufflated to a pressure of 5 mm Hg to collapse the lung. A trocar is inserted into the right thoracic cavity and a 30-degree thoracoscope is used for visualization of the right hemithorax and mediastinum. Under direct vision, a Kelly clamp is inserted into the right thoracic cavity at the marked entry site just medial to the peak of the pectus ridge. It is important to enter the chest medial to the costochondral ridge, to allow the pectus bar to be supported by the ribs. Entering lateral to the costochondral ridge will cause the transmitted force of the bar by the sternum to be applied to the intercostal muscles without bony support, which will result in muscle tearing and bar slippage. The Lorenz introducer is then inserted into the thoracic cavity at this level and it slowly traverses the mediastinum under the peak of the sternal deformity (Fig. 140-11). During this maneuver, the electrocardiogram is monitored closely for signs of arrhythmia. The introducer is advanced slowly across the mediastinum with the point of the introducer pointing anteriorly and riding directly along the undersurface of the sternum, in the plane between the pericardium and sternum. The introducer is advanced to the contralateral intercostal space at the previously marked exit site, medial to the costochondral ridge, and out through the skin.[9,12]

Once the introducer is completely across the mediastinum to the left side, it is used to elevate the sternum (Fig. 140-12). An umbilical tape, or two heavy silk ties are tied to the end of the introducer, which is slowly pulled out, across the mediastinum under direct thoracoscopic guidance (Fig. 140-13A,B). The umbilical tape remains across the substernal tunnel and is tied to the pectus bar, which has been shaped to form the patient's corrected thoracic cavity, and guided through the substernal tunnel under direct vision using the tape for traction (Fig. 140-13C). The pectus bar is inserted with the convexity facing posteriorly. Once the bar is in position across the thorax, it is rotated 180 degrees with the bar flipper (Fig. 140-13D,E). The bar should conform to the shape of the chest wall on each side, without

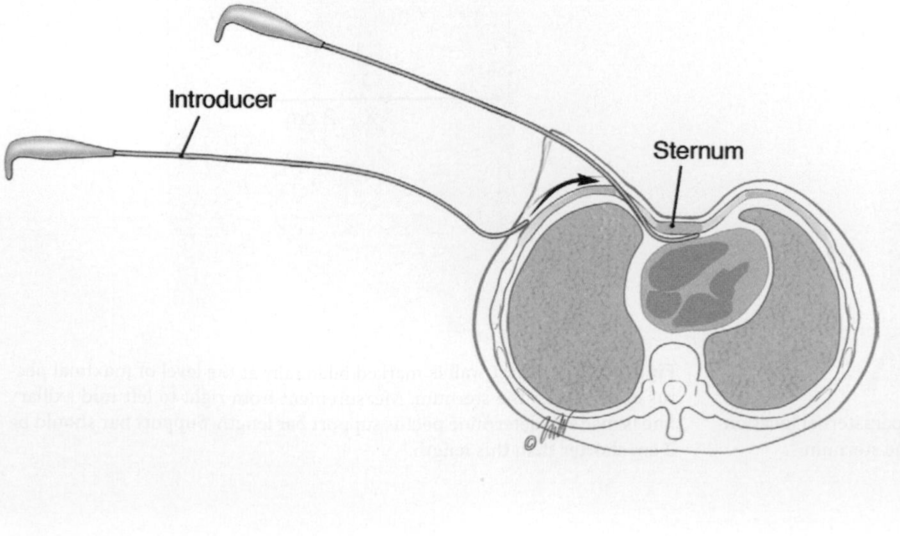

Figure 140-11. The introducer is inserted through the right tunnel into the chest at the entry site under direct vision with the thoracoscope. It is gently advanced across the mediastinum directly under the sternum at the level of maximum pectus depression.

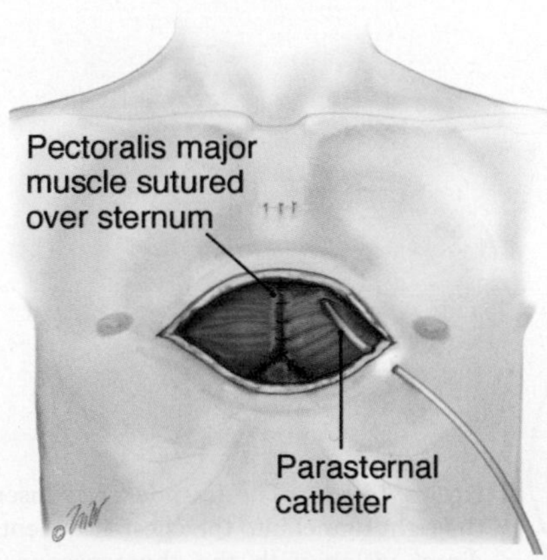

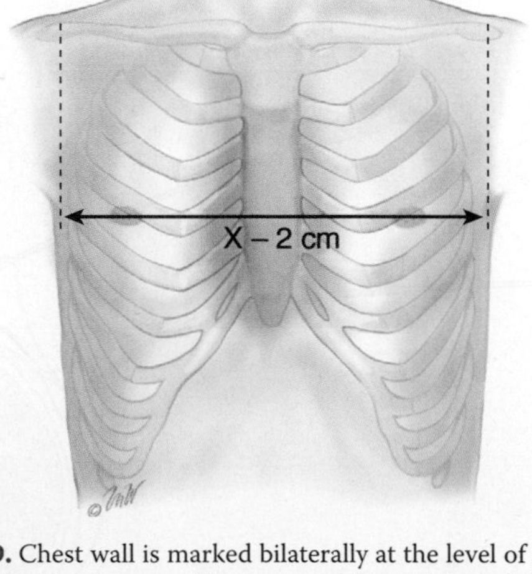

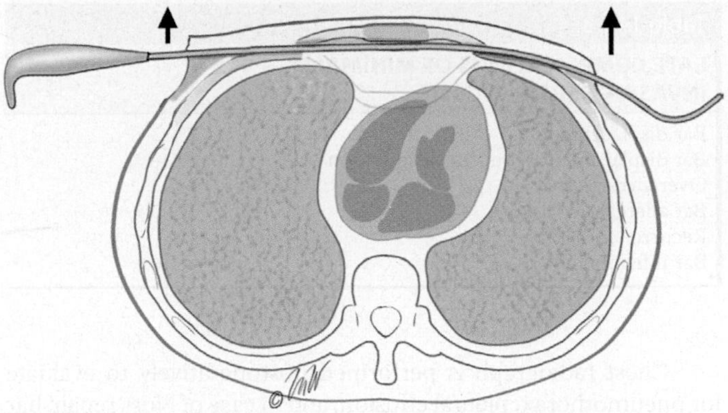

Figure 140-12. The introducer is advanced across the mediastinum and is used to elevate the sternum.

protruding out of the skin or compressing the chest wall (Fig. 140-13F). If further bending of the bar is required, it is flipped and bent using the small Lorenz bar bender. A second bar may be required for adequate correction. This may be inserted one interspace above or below the first bar (Fig. 140-14).[9,13]

After adequate positioning of the bar(s) for correction of the pectus deformity, bar stabilization is performed by placing a stabilizer on the left side and securing into place with number 3 surgical steel in figure-of-eight pattern. Alternatively a heavy nonabsorbable suture such as polypropylene is used with the titanium bar for those with metal allergy (Fig. 140-14, inset). Several heavy 0 or 1 absorbable sutures are used for pericostal suture placement to secure the bar to the underlying rib on the right side. This can be performed under direct vision with the thoracoscope. Additional absorbable 0 sutures are used to secure the fascia of the chest wall to the holes in the bar and stabilizer.[9,12]

Once the bars are secured in place, the incisions are closed in multiple layers. The residual pneumothorax is evacuated after the incisions are closed, by leaving the trocar in the chest, cutting the gas tubing, and placing the tubing in a bowl of saline to create a water seal. The anesthesiologist applies positive pressure ventilation until the CO_2 is evacuated, which is evident by cessation of bubbling in the bowl of saline. The trocar is then removed and site closed in two layers. A chest radiograph is obtained postoperatively to evaluate for residual pneumothorax and baseline bar position.[9–13]

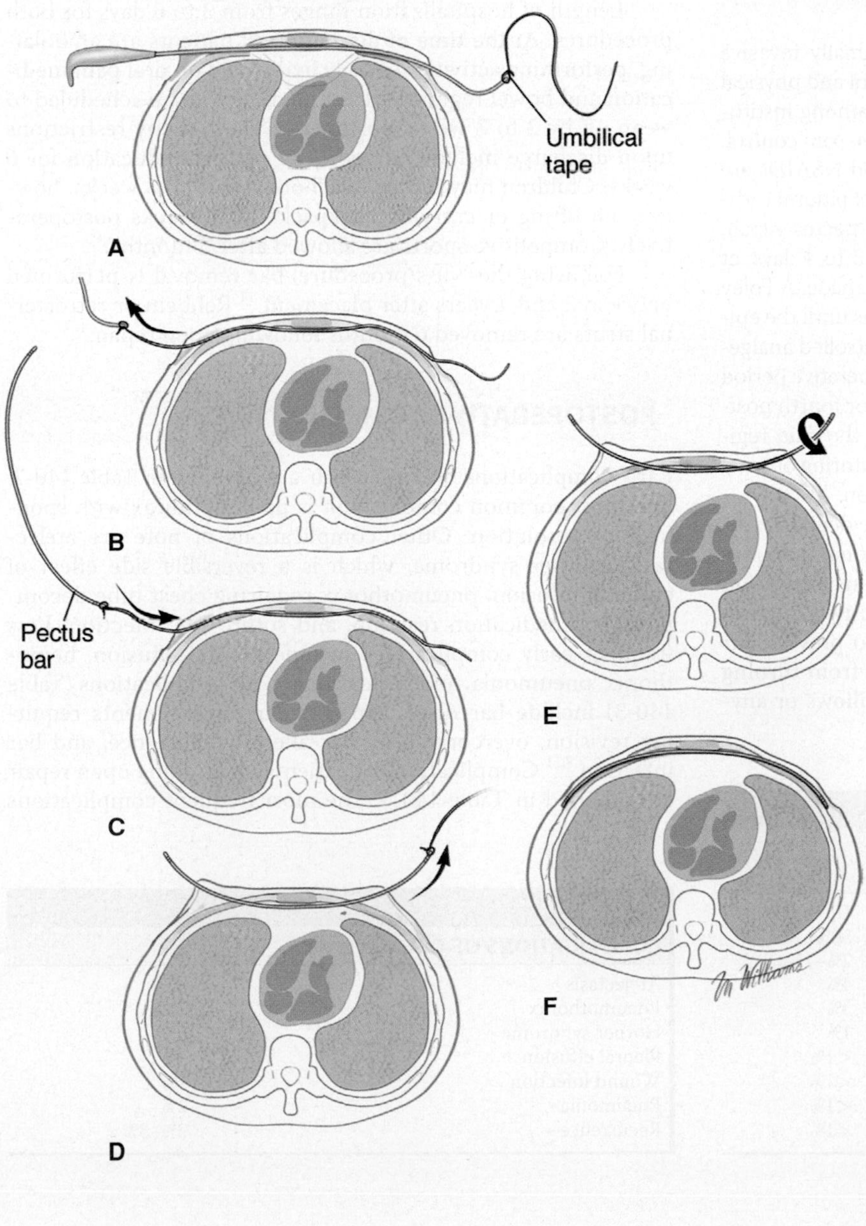

Figure 140-13. *A.* An umbilical tape is tied to the end of the introducer. *B.* The introducer is slowly retracted through the substernal tunnel into the right chest under direct vision, leaving the umbilical tape across the mediastinum. *C.* The umbilical tape is tied to the pectus support bar (shaped to the conformation of the patient's chest wall). *D.* Pectus bar is slowly pulled across the mediastinum into the left chest under direct vision, with the convexity of the bar facing posteriorly. *E.* Bar flipper is used to turn the pectus bar 180 degrees. *F.* The pectus bar should be positioned closely to the chest wall on either side of the thorax.

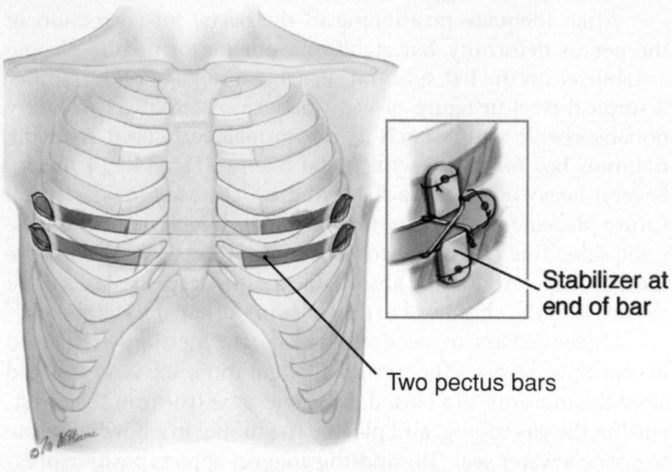

Figure 140-14. A second bar may be required for adequate correction of the pectus deformity. Inset: A stabilizer is placed at the end of the bar on the left side or bilaterally. It is secured with a number 3 surgical steel wire or heavy nonabsorbable suture.

POSTOPERATIVE CARE

Postoperative care following either open or minimally invasive pectus excavatum repair focuses around pain control and physical therapy. Postoperative pain control regimens vary among institutions, but utilize multiple drug regimens for adequate pain control. The combination of narcotics, muscle relaxants and NSAIDs are integral to a successful postoperative pain regimen. Epidural catheters are frequently used for patients undergoing pectus repair. The epidural catheter usually remains in place for 3 to 4 days, at which time the transition to oral pain medication is made. A Foley catheter is placed in the operating room and remains until the epidural is removed. Some institutions use patient-controlled analgesia instead of epidural catheters for the initial postoperative period and transition to oral pain medication on the third or fourth postoperative day. Ketorolac is an effective adjunct to the pain regimen. Attention to adequate IVF hydration and monitoring of renal function is necessary during ketorolac administration.[11,13]

An incentive spirometer is used to encourage deep breathing and prevent atelectasis. Physical and occupational therapies are instituted on the first postoperative day to aid in ambulation and assistance with activities of daily living. Activity restrictions are enforced in the postoperative period to prevent bar slippage. Specific restrictions include restriction from turning on side, twisting, overhead reaching, or use of pillows or anything under shoulders.[7,11]

Table 140-2

EARLY COMPLICATIONS OF MINIMALLY INVASIVE REPAIR (NUSS)

Pneumothorax (with spontaneous resolution)	Up to 60%
Atelectasis	50%
Horner syndrome	7%–15%
Pneumothorax (requiring chest tube decompression)	4%
Medication reaction	3%
Suture site infection	1%
Pneumonia	<1%
Pleural effusion	<1%
Hemothorax	<1%
Pericarditis	<1%

Table 140-3

LATE COMPLICATIONS OF MINIMALLY INVASIVE REPAIR (NUSS)

Bar displacement	5%
Bar displacement requiring reoperation	2%–4%
Overcorrection	3%
Bar allergy	1%–3%
Recurrence	1%
Bar infection	<1%

Chest radiograph is performed postoperatively to evaluate for pneumothorax, pleural effusion, and in case of Nuss repair, bar placement. Perioperative antibiotics continue for 24 hours postoperatively. Clear liquid diet is started on the first operative day and diet is advanced as tolerated on postoperative day one.[4,7,11]

Those undergoing open repair will have a closed suction catheter in the parasternal location in order to prevent fluid accumulation. This is removed when daily output is less than 15 mL over an 8-hour period.[4] Those patients undergoing minimally invasive repair do not require drainage catheters or chest tube placement.[9,11]

Length of hospitalization ranges from 3 to 6 days for both procedures. At the time of discharge, all patients are ambulating, performing activities of daily living, and on oral pain medication and bowel regimens. Pain medications are scheduled to wean off by 2 to 3 weeks postoperatively. Activity restrictions upon discharge include no sports or physical education for 6 weeks. Children may return to school after 2 to 3 weeks, however no lifting or carrying backpacks for 8 weeks postoperatively. Competitive sports are allowed after 3 months.[11]

Following the Nuss procedure, bar removal is performed between 2 and 4 years after placement.[11] Rehbein or retrosternal struts are removed 6 months following open repair.[4]

POSTOPERATIVE COMPLICATIONS

Early complications of Nuss repair are outlined in Table 140-2. The most common complication is pneumothorax with spontaneous resolution. Other complications of note are atelectasis, Horner syndrome, which is a reversible side effect of epidural infusion, pneumothorax requiring chest tube decompression, medication reaction, and suture site infection. Less frequent early complications include pleural effusion, hemothorax, pneumonia, and pericarditis. Late complications (Table 140-3) include bar displacements, bar displacements requiring revision, overcorrection, bar allergy, recurrence, and bar infection.[8,11] Complications of patients undergoing open repair are outlined in Table 140-4. The most frequent complications

Table 140-4

COMPLICATIONS OF OPEN REPAIR

Atelectasis	35%
Pneumothorax	7%
Horner syndrome	5%
Pleural effusion	4%
Wound infection	2%
Pneumonia	2%
Recurrence	2%–3%

include atelectasis, pneumothorax, Horner syndrome, wound infection, pneumonia, pleural effusion, and recurrence.[3,8]

SUMMARY

The repair of pectus excavatum in children is performed safely with no mortality and minimal morbidity with either open repair or the Nuss minimally invasive pectus excavatum repair.[3,7,8] Outcome measures of interest are adequate postoperative pain management and satisfactory surgical result. Although there is no consensus on the optimal pain regimen, multiclass drug regimens for postoperative pain management have been successful in achieving adequate pain control.[11,13] Patients and their parents report significant postoperative change in both physical and psychosocial functioning following pectus excavatum repair.[6] Surgical repair of pectus excavatum can significantly improve body image and limitations on physical activity experienced by patients and should be considered when assessing a patient for surgical repair.[6] Success, as measured by functional improvement, patient satisfaction, and cosmetic results, are generally reported as good to excellent by both patients and providers.[7,11] Review studies evaluating both open and minimally invasive repair demonstrate comparable outcomes with no significant difference in postoperative pain, complications, or duration of hospitalization.[7,8] Therefore, either the open or minimally invasive Nuss pectus excavatum repair can be safely performed with excellent results for those who meet criteria for surgical repair of this congenital chest wall defect.

EDITOR'S COMMENT

This chapter represents a comprehensive review of both open repair and minimally invasive Nuss repair for correction of pectus excavatum. The operative detail given for both approaches is detailed and extremely helpful, given the rarity of these cases in the average thoracic surgery practice and training.

—Yolonda L. Colson

References

1. Kelly RE. Pectus excavatum: historical background, clinical picture, preoperative evaluation and criteria for operation. *Semin Pediatr Surg.* 2008;17:181–193.
2. Ravitch MM. The operative treatment of pectus excavatum. *Ann Surg.* 1949;129(4):429–444.
3. Shamberger RC, Welch KJ. Surgical repair of pectus excavatum. *J Pediatr Surg.* 1988;23(7):615–622.
4. Shamberger RC. Congenital chest wall deformities. In: Grosfeld JL, O'Neill JA, Fonkalsrud EW, et al., eds. *Pediatric Surgery.* 6th ed. Philadelphia, PA: Mosby; 2006:894–921.
5. Colombani PM. Preoperative assessment of chest wall deformities. *Semin Thorac Cardiovasc Surg.* 2009;21:58–63.
6. Kelly RE, Cash TF, Shamberger RC, et al. Surgical repair of pectus excavatum markedly improves body image and perceived ability for physical activity: multicenter study. *Pediatrics.* 2008;122:1218–1222.
7. Nasr A, Fecteau A, Wales PW. Comparison of the Nuss and Ravitch procedure for pectus excavatum repair: a meta-analysis. *J Pediatr Surg.* 2010;45:880–886.
8. Kelly RE, Shamberger RC, Mellins RB, et al. Prospective multicenter study of surgical correction of pectus excavatum: design, perioperative complications, pain and baseline pulmonary function facilitated by internet-based data collection. *J Am Coll Surg.* 2007;205:205–216.
9. Nuss D, Kelly RE. The minimally invasive pectus excavatum repair (Nuss Procedure). In: Holcomb GW, Georgeson KE, Rothenberg SS, eds. *Atlas of Pediatric Laparoscopy and Thoracoscopy.* Philadelphia, PA: Saunders: 2008:305–310.
10. Croitoru DP, Kelly RE, Goretsky MJ, et al. Experience and modification update for the minimally invasive Nuss Technique for pectus excavatum repair in 303 patients. *J Pediatr Surg.* 2002;37(3):437–446.
11. Kelly RE, Goretsky MJ, Obermeyer R, et al. Twenty-one years of experience with minimally invasive repair of pectus excavatum by the Nuss Procedure in 1215 patients. *Ann Surg.* 2010;252(6):1072–1081.
12. Nuss D, Kelly RE. The Nuss procedure for pectus Excavatum. In: Grosfeld JL, O'Neill JA, Fonkalsrud EW, et al., eds. *Pediatric Surgery.* 6th ed. Philadelphia, PA: Mosby; 2006; 921–930.
13. St Peter SD, Weesner KA, Sharp RJ. Is epidural anesthesia truly the best pain management strategy after minimally invasive pectus excavatum repair? *J Pediatr Surg.* 2008;43:79–82.

141 Surgical Repair of Complex (Recurrent) Pectus Excavatum in Adults

Jonathan C. Daniel and Daniel M. Cohen

Keywords: Pectus excavatum, recurrence, modified Ravitch repair, reoperation

Since the first pectus repair was reported by Meyer in 1911, several different techniques have been described.[1,2] The Ravitch procedure, first described in 1949,[3] became the mainstay of repair until Nuss described a minimally invasive repair in the early 1990s.[4] The techniques for primary repair of congenital chest wall deformities, including pectus excavatum, are described in Chapter 140. None of these techniques is perfect, however, and recurrences do occur. Although the incidence of recurrent pectus excavatum in the adult population is most rare, it is usually a consequence of technical failure. The rate of recurrence, although significantly reduced in the hands of a more experienced surgeon, ranges from 2% to 10%.

GENERAL PRINCIPLES

The open repair, described by Ravitch and modified by Haller,[5] involves the excision of all deformed costal cartilages from the sternum to the costochondral junctions. The overlying perichondrium is left intact. This procedure is combined with a transverse sternal osteotomy at the point of maximal declination, elevation of the inferior sternal fragment, and placement of a transverse metal bar or rod to maintain the sternum in this elevated position. The ends of the bar are supported on either side by the bony ribs of the lateral chest wall.[4,6] The bar is left in place until the costal cartridges have regenerated and the chest wall has become firm and rigid. This process usually takes 6 to 9 months in adults.

The rates of recurrence from a series of experienced centers are depicted in Table 141-1. The most common reasons for recurrence may be divided into two categories: technical and disease-related. As with any operation associated with remodeling in which there are several sequential steps to which one needs to adhere, there is a learning curve. Failure to tackle the full extent of the deformity aggressively, inadequate stabilization of the bar resulting in early displacement, premature removal of the bar before adequate healing has taken place, failure to resect the xiphoid process and mobilize the retrosternal space, significant injury to the perichondrial sheaths, and failure to pay sufficient attention to the asymmetry of the defect, all can result in a technical failure of the primary repair.

Patients with connective tissue disorders such as Marfan syndrome are at increased risk for recurrence. In these instances, the repair should be delayed until skeletal maturity has been reached. Also, children who undergo a rapid adolescent growth phase may overcome the benefits of an early repair, resulting in a suboptimal cosmetic outcome. The appropriate timing for surgical correction of a pectus deformity is the subject of controversy and continues to be debated.

Since introduction of the minimally invasive Nuss technique, an increasing number of children are being treated for pectus deformities according to this method. The benefits of the

Table 141-1

RATES OF RECURRENCE FROM VARIOUS SERIES OF INITIAL REPAIR

SOURCE	METHOD OF REPAIR	NUMBER OF PATIENTS	RECURRENCE RATE (%)	REDO OPERATION (%)
Fonkalsrud et al. (2000)[10]	Modified Ravitch with and without bars	375	1.3 (without)	0.8
Gilbert and Zwiren (1989)[11]	Modified Ravitch with and without bars	Without 50 With 32 (14 mesh + bar)	10 (without) 0 (with)	
Haller et al. (1989)[5]	Modified Ravitch, tripod fixation, use of bar in teenagers	460	3	3
Saxena and Willital (2007)[12]	Willital-Hegemann procedure (transsternal and parasternal bars)	1262	1.4 (major) 3.6 (mild)	
Shamberger and Welch (1988)[13]	Modified Ravitch	704	2.7	1.7
Mansour et al. (2003)[14]	Modified Ravitch, no bar	68 (adults only)	1.5	1.5
Jaroszewski and Fonkalsrud (2007)[15]	Modified Ravitch with bar	268 (adults only)	2.2 (mild and moderate)	1.1

Nuss technique include the avoidance of extensive dissection and cartilage resection and smaller incisions. The complications of this procedure include severe postoperative discomfort or pain, longer periods of bar retention before removal, catastrophic injuries to the heart and pulmonary outflow tract, and inadequate cosmetic results with asymmetric defects. Miller and colleagues report a series of children (mean age 11.4 years) who underwent a redo of the minimally invasive repair after a failed initial procedure. The average time to repeat procedure was approximately 9 years.[7] In adults with recurrent pectus deformity, the role of minimally invasive repair is unproved and may not permit a satisfactory or safe repair.

PATIENT SELECTION AND PREOPERATIVE ASSESSMENT

The selection of patients for repair of recurrent pectus deformities should be undertaken very carefully. Unfortunately, not every patient can undergo intervention. In a series of 19 patients who had an original Ravitch procedure and presented with recurrence, three patients had such severe adhesions between the sternum and pericardium that reconstruction was too dangerous to attempt.[8] The most important questions to be answered before undertaking a reoperation include the underlying physiologic status of the patient, the reasons for failure of the primary repair, and the patient's expectations of a satisfactory cosmetic result.

A chest CT scan is a useful tool to assess the degree of deformity and asymmetry, to determine the extent of substernal and pleural adhesions, and to assess the presence of cardiac displacement or compression. This information is helpful in planning and carrying out a successful reoperation. Patients who are considered for reoperation should undergo preoperative physiologic testing, including a battery of pulmonary function tests and an echocardiogram. Should underlying cardiac disease be identified, this needs to be addressed before embarking on an elaborate repair. Patients must be adequately counseled on their reasons for seeking a reoperation and warned of the potential surgical risks, including an unsatisfactory cosmetic result. A multidisciplinary approach with involvement of the plastic surgery service also should be considered.

TECHNIQUE

Anesthesia

The use of an epidural catheter is an important adjunct in patients undergoing reoperation because it will alleviate postoperative pain and reduce morbidity. General anesthesia is necessary because the operation is usually protracted, and there is significant dissection. Hemodynamic monitoring may be necessary depending on the patient's underlying physiologic status. Patients usually are extubated at completion of the repair.

Surgical Management

Reoperative Dissection and Sternal Mobilization

The task of repairing a recurrent pectus deformity may be formidable depending on the nature of the recurrent deformity and the amount of scar tissue encountered. Few centers have had a vast degree of experience with recurrent operations in the adult population.

The incision for the open technique is usually made through the old scar. If the old scar is hypertrophied, it should be excised. The skin and muscle flaps are raised superiorly, inferiorly, and laterally to encompass the full extent of the defect by using the electrocautery unit. Scar tissue may render identification of tissue planes more difficult than in a primary operation, but the dissection needs to be carried down to the chest wall to fully expose the sternum and regenerated cartilaginous matrix.

The subsequent dissection will vary depending on the previous operation. Extensive cartilage resection or injury to the overlying perichondrial sheaths may have resulted in a chaotic array of costosternal connections with no identifiable tissue planes or points of demarcation between one costal cartilage and another. Whereas with a virgin operation, a delicate dissection of the subperichondrial space in a bloodless plane is feasible, in a reoperation, a stone hard outline of the cartilage will be observed, and typically, there is no obvious tissue plane of dissection identified. The goal of the dissection is to excise a sufficient amount of cartilage to achieve adequate anterior mobility of the sternum. (Ideally, a lateral dissection beneath the pectoralis muscles where the territory is less disrupted and the ribs are intact may be pursued.) This frequently also requires detachment of the cartilaginous connections with the sternum and a sternal osteotomy. Both a rongeur and bone cutters can be used to remove the hardened tissue of the fibrocartilaginous plate. Ideally, a layer of scar should be left behind on the chest wall, lateral to the sternum and medial to the osseous portion of the rib, to provide a matrix for hardening and regeneration postoperatively. Careful preservation of the perichondrium is a key maneuver during this stage of the operation.

Osteotomy and Strut Support

As with a primary repair, an osteotomy is performed at the angle of maximal declination. In rare circumstances, creation of a second osteotomy may be required to achieve the best apposition. If the cartilaginous–sternal connections have been severed, they should be reapproximated using an absorbable suture. Then a bar/strut is placed beneath both the sternum and the excised fibrocartilaginous plate to maintain the repair in its desired position (Fig. 141-1). It is critical to choose the correct length, position, and contour of the bar. The bar is passed through the fibrocartilaginous matrix to rest on the bony chest wall above the serratus musculature and should extend from midaxillary line to midaxillary line. To accommodate the desired contour of the chest wall, the bar must be positioned beneath the sternum midway between the point of osteotomy and the sternal tip. The bar should not be bent in too much at its ends because it may erode into the intercostal muscles and penetrate the surface of the lung. Neither should the bar be too straight at its ends such that it rubs on the over-lying skin and is uncomfortable for the patient. The bar is held in position by suturing it to the underlying chest wall and sternum on either side with heavy absorbable sutures. Once the bar is deemed to be in the correct position, a closed drainage system is placed beneath and above the sternum. Secure attachment of the xiphoid to support the rectus muscles and cover the lower chest is critical. The pectoralis major and rectus abdominis muscles are then reapproximated in the midline, and the skin is closed (Fig. 141-2).

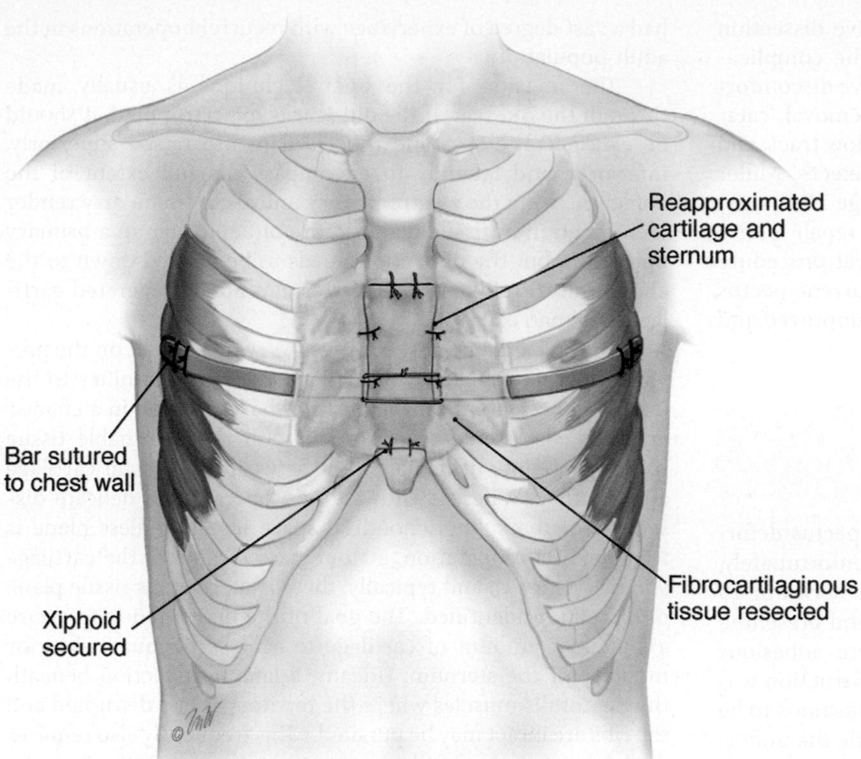

Figure 141-1. A bar or strut is placed beneath the sternum and excised fibrocartilaginous plate to complete the repair. The xiphoid is securely reattached to support the overlying muscles.

Postoperative Management

The patient is extubated at completion of the operation, and postoperative pain is controlled with the use of a continuous thoracic epidural catheter. Early ambulation is encouraged, and a transition toward oral narcotics is made within 48 hours of the operation. The patient can be discharged with the closed drainage system in place 3 to 5 days after operation. The drains are left in place until the drainage is less than 30 mL per day to prevent seroma formation.

The metal bar should be left in place for 6 to 9 months after the operation to prevent recurrence of the deformity.[9] When the time comes to remove the bar, caution is required because scar tissue overgrowth may render removal hazardous. Continuous, slow traction on one end usually results in ready removal of the bar.

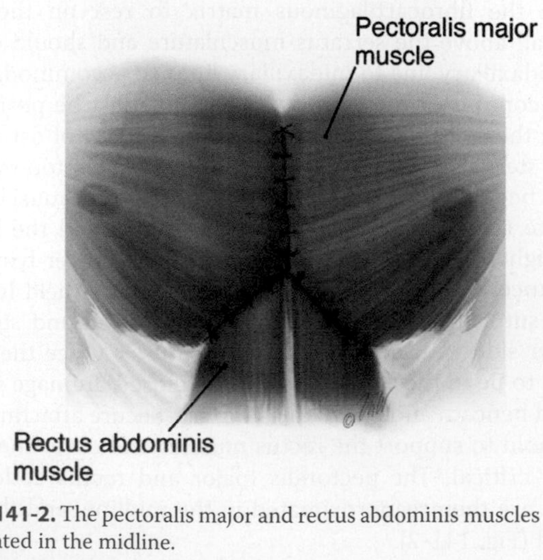

Figure 141-2. The pectoralis major and rectus abdominis muscles are reapproximated in the midline.

COMPLICATIONS

Complications related to recurrent pectus repair are similar to those experienced during routine pectus surgery and include pneumothorax, pneumonia, wound infection, infection of the prosthetic bar, seroma, and bar migration. These have been discussed previously. Recurrence after a redo repair is rare if the preceding principles are maintained.

SUMMARY

For the patient with a pectus excavatum, the condition often represents a significant source of physiologic and psychological stress. Fortunately, this is more widely recognized by all health care practitioners caring for children, and patients are now referred for surgery at an earlier age. As these children progress to adulthood, it can be expected that a small proportion will present with recurrent pectus excavatum deformities that produce symptoms or serious cosmetic concerns. Whether these recurrences are due to imperfect initial operations or other factors, they require operative revision.

The repair of a recurrent pectus excavatum defect can be a complicated ordeal and poses a significant challenge for the surgeon. The decision to undertake a recurrent pectus repair should not be considered lightly and requires a frank discussion with the patient and a realization that the end result may not be cosmetically perfect. The surgical technique used will depend on a number of factors, including the previous operative technique, individual patient factors, and the extent of the underlying fiber-cartilaginous scar tissue. Strict adherence to sound surgical principles, as well as a certain degree of surgical creativity, as our index case illustrates, can lead to a very successful reoperation in most instances.

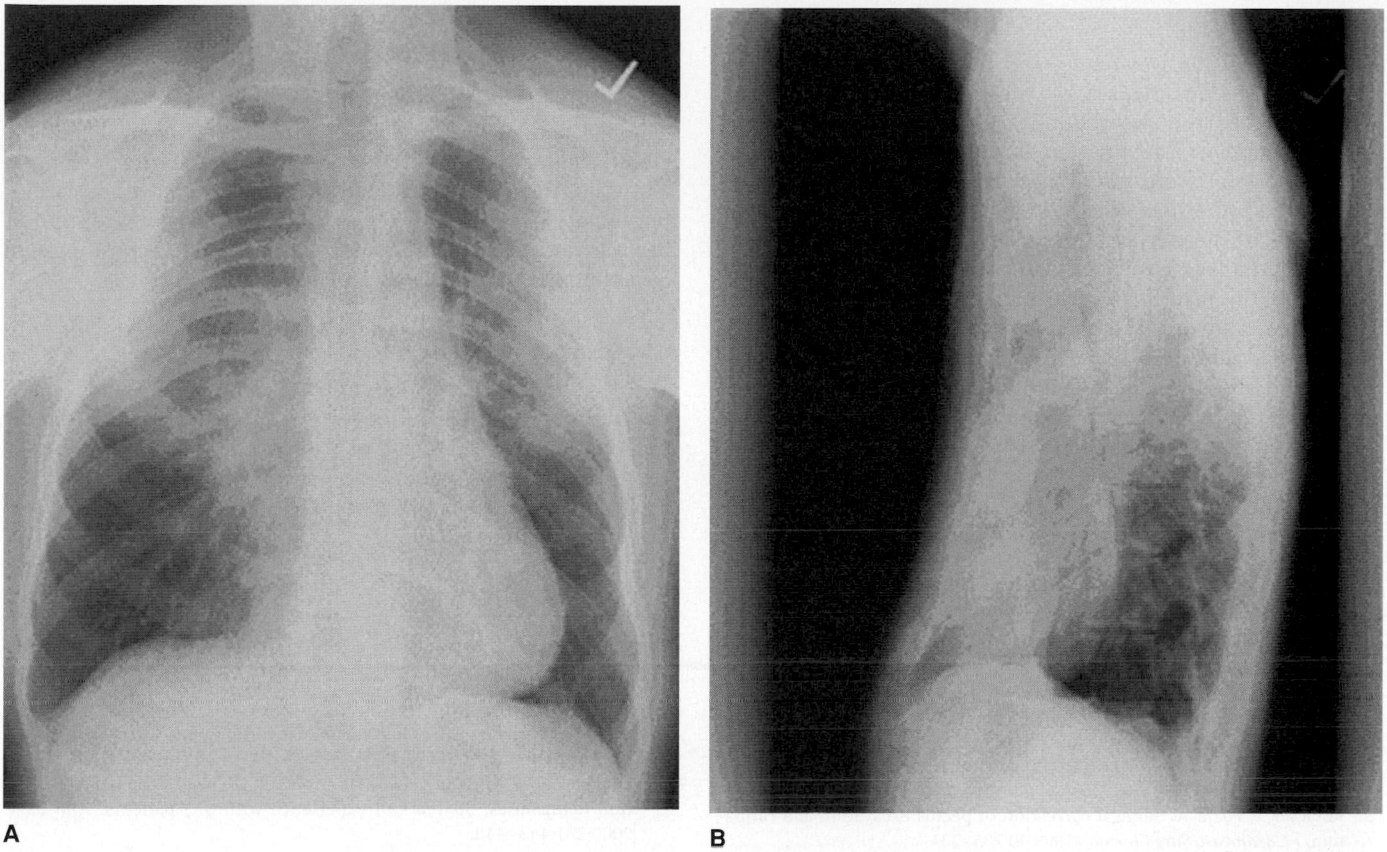

Figure 141-3. Posteroanterior (*A*) and lateral (*B*) chest x-rays for index case.

CASE HISTORY

A 34-year-old man was referred for recurrent pectus excavatum. He had undergone a primary repair of his pectus excavatum deformity as a 3-year-old child. Over the last 10 years, he had been experiencing progressively worsening shortness of breath, resulting in severe limitation of his physical activity. His past medical history was significant for mitral valve prolapse. The patient was otherwise healthy and had no known history of connective tissue disorder or Marfan syndrome.

On physical examination, the patient was tall and slender with a moderate pectus excavatum deformity. The old midline incision was identified over the lower half of the sternum and was well healed. Cardiac examination revealed a middle to late systolic murmur and a midsystolic click consistent with mitral valve prolapse. The lungs were clear to auscultation. Pulmonary function tests demonstrated a forced vital capacity of 3.11 (58%) and a forced expiratory volume in 1 second of 2.82 (63%). A posteroanterior and lateral chest x-ray is shown in Figure 141-3.

A chest CT scan was ordered to better evaluate the extent of the patient's deformity. It is most notable for compression of the right ventricle and displacement of the heart to the left chest, as well as asymmetry of the lung fields (Fig. 141-4).

An echocardiogram was consistent with mild global decreased function, mild mitral regurgitation, and an estimated pulmonary artery systolic pressure of 21 mm Hg plus right atrial pressure. Although the echocardiographic findings were not entirely consistent with his symptoms, the patient was subjectively feeling more tired and had a definite decrease in his exercise tolerance. He wished to have the deformity corrected.

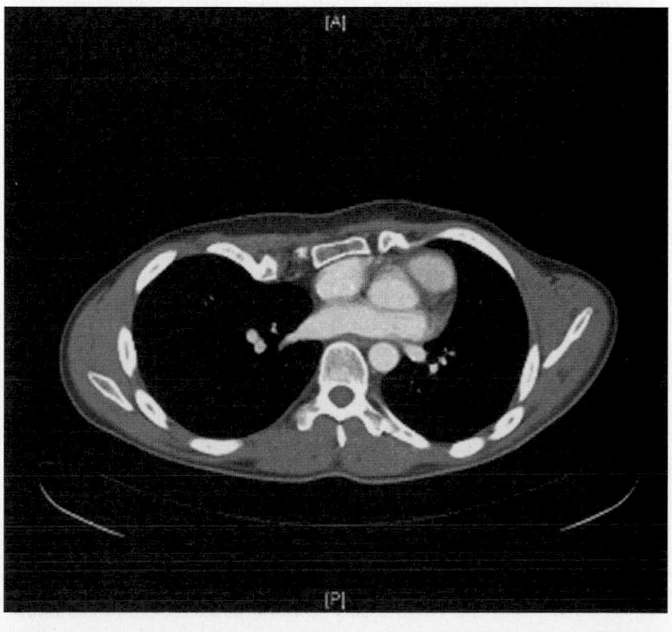

Figure 141-4. Chest CT scan is notable for compression of the right ventricle, leftward displacement of the heart, and asymmetry of the lung fields.

Operation

A midline incision was made, and the old scar was excised. Musculocutaneous flaps were developed bilaterally from the midline to the costochondral junctions and from the point of maximal declination superiorly to the sternoxiphoid junction inferiorly. On inspection, the costal cartilages were noted to be turned inward. The involved cartilages on either side of the sternum were removed, leaving the posterior perichondrium intact. A sternal osteotomy was made just below the manubrium through the anterior and posterior tables, allowing the caudal portion of the sternum to be deflected anteriorly. A second transverse osteotomy was performed about 12 cm inferior to the first to prevent protrusion of the xiphosternal junction. The sternum was then reapproximated using sternal wires, and a bar was used to support the repair.

An omental flap was harvested by extending the incision inferiorly and opening the peritoneal cavity. The omentum was delivered into the wound to fill the large existing space created by correction of the deformity. The pectoral muscles then were reapproximated in the center using absorbable sutures. Closed suction drains were placed, and the remainder of the wound was closed in layers.

The patient was discharged home after 4 days, and the closed suction drains were removed during the first postoperative visit. The patient had marked improvement of his cardiopulmonary function over the ensuing months, and the support bar was removed 1 year later through a small left chest incision as an outpatient procedure.

EDITOR'S COMMENT

The authors have highlighted the key surgical principles important in the surgical repair of a recurrent pectus excavatum, carefully outlining when – and when not – to operate, and reviewing the common technical reasons for recurrence and the pitfalls to avoid.

—Yolonda L. Colson

References

1. Meyer L. Zur chirurgischen behandlung der angeborenen tricterbrust. *Berl Klin Wochens.* 1911;34:1563–1566.
2. Robicsek F, Fokin A. Surgical correction of pectus excavatum and carinatum. *J Cardiovasc Surg (Torino).* 1999;40:725–731.
3. Ravitch MM. The operative treatment of pectus excavatum. *Ann Surg.* 1949;129:429–444.
4. Nuss D, Kelly RE, Jr, Croitoru DP, et al. A 10-year review of a minimally invasive technique for the correction of pectus excavatum. *J Pediatr Surg.* 1998;33:545–552.
5. Haller JA, Jr, Scherer LR, Turner CS, et al. Evolving management of pectus excavatum based on a single institutional experience of 664 patients. *Ann Surg.* 1989;209:578–582; discussion 582–583.
6. Fonkalsrud EW. Current management of pectus excavatum. *World J Surg.* 2003;27:502–508.
7. Miller KA, Ostlie DJ, Wade K, et al. Minimally invasive bar repair for "redo" correction of pectus excavatum. *J Pediatr Surg.* 2002;37:1090–1092.
8. De Ugarte DA, Choi E, Fonkalsrud EW. Repair of recurrent pectus deformities. *Am Surg.* 2002;68:1075–1079.
9. Keshishian JM, Cox PA. Management of recurrent pectus excavatum. *J Thorac Cardiovasc Surg.* 1967;54:740–745.
10. Fonkalsrud EW, Dunn JC, Atkinson JB. Repair of pectus excavatum deformities: 30 years of experience with 375 patients. *Ann Surg.* 2000;231:443–448.
11. Gilbert JC, Zwiren GT. Repair of pectus excavatum using a substernal metal strut within a Marlex envelope. *South Med J.* 1989;82:1240–1244.
12. Saxena AK, Willital GH. Valuable lessons from two decades of pectus repair with the Willital-Hegemann procedure. *J Thorac Cardiovasc Surg.* 2007;134:871–876.
13. Shamberger RC, Welch KJ. Surgical repair of pectus excavatum. *J Pediatr Surg.* 1988;23:615–622.
14. Mansour KA, Thourani VH, Odessey EA, et al. Thirty-year experience with repair of pectus deformities in adults. *Ann Thorac Surg.* 2003;76:391–395; discussion 395.
15. Jaroszewski DE, Fonkalsrud EW. Repair of pectus chest deformities in 320 adult patients: 21-year experience. *Ann Thorac Surg.* 2007;84:429–433.

142 Supraclavicular Approach for Thoracic Outlet Syndrome

Ankit Bharat, Susan E. Mackinnon, and G. Alexander Patterson

Keywords: Neurogenic thoracic outlet syndrome, proximal and distal nerve compression, conservative treatment, first rib resection, scalenectomy

The term *thoracic outlet syndrome* (TOS) describes a condition arising from compression of the subclavian artery, the subclavian vein, and the brachial plexus between the scalene muscles and the first rib (Fig. 142-1). There exists a wide spectrum of patient symptoms, which include vascular and/or neurologic signs. Neurogenic TOS accounts for most cases, whereas venous (2%–3%) and arterial TOS (1%) are relatively rare. Objective vascular studies such as venograms and arteriograms may identify signs of vascular compromise to aid in the diagnosis of arterial or venous TOS, but neurologic findings are more varied, and there is no single specific test to diagnose neurogenic TOS.

The neurologic signs and symptoms of neurogenic TOS can range from mild paresthesias and numbness to intrinsic hand muscle atrophy. There is little controversy in this latter group of patients regarding diagnosis or treatment. However, the diagnosis of TOS is controversial in patients with the neurologic-type complaints of paresthesias, numbness, and pain but with no positive objective test to identify the cause. This chapter focuses on the management and surgical therapy of neurogenic TOS.

GENERAL PRINCIPLES

Many surgeons are highly skeptical of the merits of surgical intervention for patients with TOS because of the high incidence of major complications and the variable reports of successful outcome. Exceptions to this rule include uncommon cases involving vascular compromise and even rarer cases involving severe neurologic muscle atrophy in the hand.[1] Patients with intrinsic hand muscle atrophy that localizes to the level of the brachial plexus with no distal sites of nerve compression are likely to have a cervical rib or anomalous ligamentous band(s) that compresses the lower trunk of the brachial plexus. Compression of the artery may lead to poststenotic dilatation and subsequent thrombosis and embolization. Patients with symptomatic arterial TOS may present with signs and symptoms of microembolization in the digits on the affected side. Venous compression, which usually occurs at the junction of the clavicle and first rib, leads to occlusion and thrombosis. Patients characteristically become symptomatic with evidence of venous congestion after a precipitating physical activity (Paget–Schroetter syndrome).

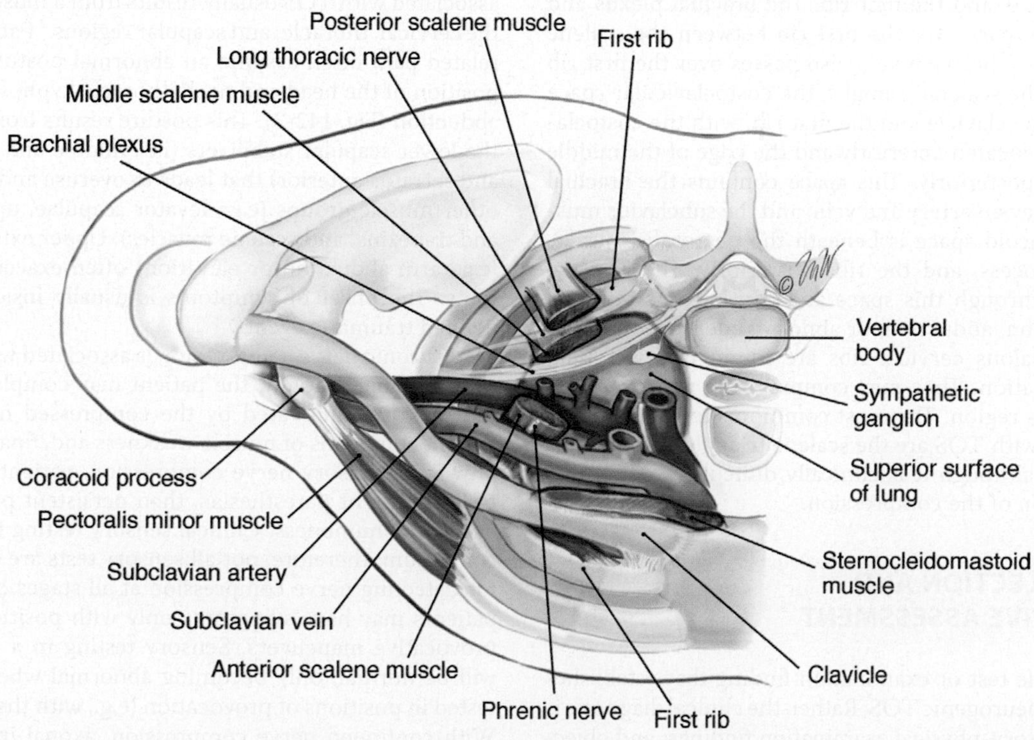

Figure 142-1. Anatomy relevant to thoracic outlet obstruction.

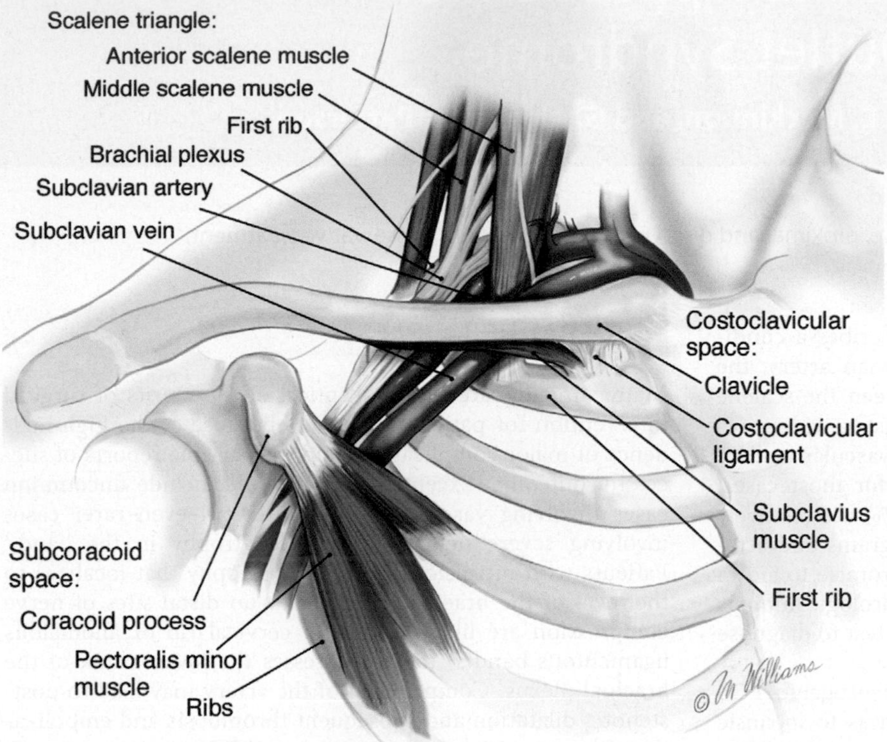

Figure 142-2. The three anatomic spaces that are implicated in brachial plexus compression are the costoclavicular space, the subcoracoid space, and the scalene triangle.

The clinical syndrome (TOS) derives from three anatomic areas in which compression of the neurovascular structures may occur: the scalene triangle, the costoclavicular space, and the subcoracoid space (Fig. 142-2). The scalene triangle is the region bordered by the anterior scalene muscle, the middle scalene muscle, and the first rib. The brachial plexus and subclavian artery pass over the first rib between the scalene muscles, and the subclavian vein also passes over the first rib but external to the scalene triangle. The costoclavicular space is bordered by the clavicle and the first rib, with the costoclavicular ligament located anteriorly and the edge of the middle scalene muscle posteriorly. This space contains the brachial plexus, the subclavian artery and vein, and the subclavius muscle. The subcoracoid space is beneath the pectoralis muscle, the coracoid process, and the ribs posteriorly. The brachial plexus courses through this space and can become tethered with arm elevation, abduction, or abnormal depression of the coracoid. Anomalous cervical ribs are found in fewer than 1% of the population. They may compress the neurovascular structures in this region. The most common sites of compression in patients with TOS are the scalene triangle and the subcoracoid space, although it is clinically difficult to determine the exact location of the compression.

PATIENT SELECTION AND PREOPERATIVE ASSESSMENT

There is no single test or examination finding that establishes the diagnosis of neurogenic TOS. Rather, the clinical diagnosis is based on the history, physical examination findings, and objective tests, such as electrodiagnostic studies of the peripheral nerves, that are used to rule out other more distal compression neuropathies. Chest and neck x-rays are obtained routinely to look for cervical ribs or other bony abnormalities. Paresthesias in the upper extremity may be the result of either compression at the brachial plexus or compression more distally. The pain associated with TOS usually results from a muscle imbalance in the cervical, thoracic, and scapular regions.[2] Patients with TOS-related pain often assume an abnormal posture with forward position of the head and neck, thoracic kyphosis, and scapulae abduction (Fig. 142-3). This posture results from a weakness of the lower scapular stabilizers (i.e., middle and lower trapezius and serratus anterior) that leads to overuse and hypertrophy of other muscle groups (e.g., levator scapulae, upper rhomboids and trapezius, and scalene muscles). Upper extremity activities (e.g., arm abduction or elevation) often exacerbate the symptoms. The onset of symptoms is usually insidious without a defined traumatic event.

Chronic nerve compression is associated with a continuum of symptoms. Initially, the patient may complain of aching in the muscles innervated by the compressed nerve. Later, the patient complains of muscle weakness and, finally, muscle atrophy. With sensory nerve compression, patients complain first of intermittent paresthesias, then persistent paresthesias, and eventually numbness. Clinical sensory testing follows a similar continuum; therefore, not all sensory tests are equally effective for detecting nerve compression at all stages of TOS. Initially, patients may have symptoms only with positional changes or provocative maneuvers. Sensory testing in a resting position will be normal, only becoming abnormal when the patient is tested in positions of provocation (e.g., with the arms elevated). With continued nerve compression, axonal involvement, and wallerian degeneration, the innervation density of the sensory

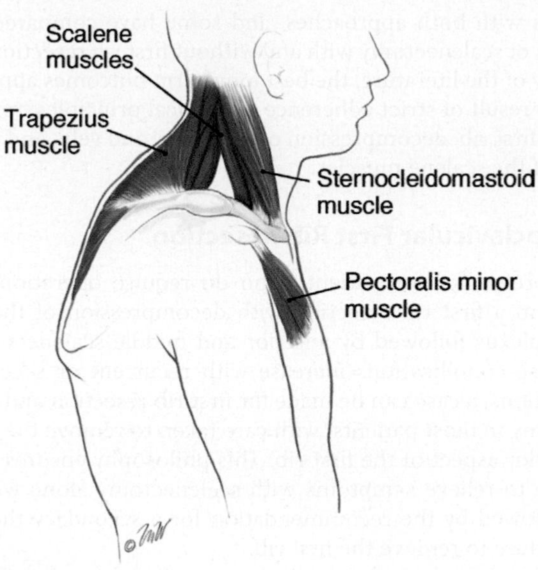

Figure 142-3. Abnormal posterior and muscle imbalance associated with neurogenic TOS results in shortened and hypertrophied scalene, sternocleidomastoid, and pectoralis minor muscles anteriorly. The back muscles (i.e., levator scapulae, upper rhomboid, and trapezius) become overdeveloped to compensate for the weakened serratus anterior and middle and lower trapezius muscles, pulling the head forward.

receptors decreases, and sensory testing with two-point discrimination is abnormal.

It has been hypothesized that proximal compression of a nerve increases its susceptibility to compression injury more distally. Thus, in treating upper extremity neuropathic symptoms, it is important to identify and treat all sites of compression.[3] Distal sites of nerve entrapment, for example, the elbow, forearm, and wrist, should be evaluated carefully and managed conservatively. Clinical evaluation using pressure and positional provocative testing is key to making the diagnosis because electrodiagnostic studies usually do not detect these dynamic sites of nerve compression.[4] Conservative treatment often effectively relieves these distal symptoms, but when surgical intervention is required, surgery at the carpal or cubital tunnel levels is usually more effective than surgical decompression of the thoracic outlet for complete relief of hand paresthesias and numbness. Overlapping symptoms from the cervical disc level or the shoulder are common.

Loss of radial pulse with arm movement on physical examination forms the basis of several clinical tests designed to detect vascular insufficiency, although not effective for the evaluation of neurogenic TOS. In Adson test, the patient is asked to turn his or her head toward the affected side, extend the neck, and inspire deeply. Obliteration of the radial pulse suggests compression. In Roos test, the subject elevates his or her arm to 90 degrees of shoulder abduction and then rotates the arm externally and flexes the elbow for 3 minutes. The patient then is asked to rapidly open and close the hand. A positive test will reproduce the patient's symptoms.

The physical examination of patients with TOS should include documentation of pinch and grip and two-point discrimination, as well as examination of the upper extremity for other compression issues. The cervical spine and rotator cuff are examined as well as the muscles of the parascapular area. Standard tests performed at the wrist are used to assess carpal tunnel syndrome, including Tinel sign, the pressure provocative test, and Phalen test. Care is taken to keep the forearm in a neutral position during testing because extreme supination of the forearm will cause median nerve compression at the pronator teres and lead to a false-positive result. The elbows also must remain extended so as not to provoke signs of cubital tunnel syndrome. One test for median nerve compression in the proximal forearm is to maximally supinate the forearm with pressure applied just proximal to the pronator teres while keeping the wrist in neutral position. If this maneuver produces paresthesias in the distribution of the median nerve, it suggests median nerve compression in the proximal forearm. The radial sensory nerve is provoked by extreme forearm pronation and wrist ulnar deviation. A Tinel sign between the tendons of the extensor carpi radialis longus and the brachioradialis indicates radial sensory nerve compression in the forearm.

The evaluation for cubital tunnel syndrome or ulnar nerve compression at the elbow involves elbow flexion and pressure over the ulnar nerve at the cubital tunnel. The wrist and the forearm are kept in neutral position so as not to provoke median nerve symptoms. Brachial plexus compression in the region of the thoracic outlet is tested by elevating the arms over the head while keeping the wrist neutral, the elbows extended, and the forearms neutral. The examiner evaluates for change in pulse and color while the patient reports any new or increased sensory disturbance in the upper extremity.

Patients with neurogenic TOS typically have an associated muscle imbalance in the cervical scapular area. To evaluate these muscles, the examiner stands behind the patient while the patient slowly elevates the arms above the head. Elbows are kept extended, and the shoulders are forward flexed. The arms then are lowered to the sides from this forward-flexed, elevated position while the examiner observes for winging of the scapula. Winging of the scapula suggests weakness of the serratus anterior muscle. Middle and lower trapezius muscle function is tested by abducting the shoulders with the extremities extended while the arms are elevated above the head from an abducted position. Once again, the arms are lowered slowly to the side. Winging of the scapula suggests a weakness of the middle and lower trapezius muscles. Patients with muscle imbalance in the scapular areas typically have abducted scapulae. Instead of rotating normally with movement of the arms, the scapulae tend to move "up and down" on the back because of overuse of the upper trapezius muscle.

We have described a new test, the *scratch collapse test,* that can be used to identify areas of nerve irritation and/or muscle weakness. To perform this maneuver, the examiner scratches the patient's skin lightly over the area of nerve compression while the patient performs sustained resisted movement of both arms. If the patient has allodynia owing to compression neuropathy, a brief loss of muscle resistance will be elicited. The patient can be scratched lightly at the multiple levels in the neuromuscular pathway to elicit the collapse. When the culprit area is scratched, the muscle collapses. Patients with TOS-related muscle weakness will respond if the examiner just touches along the posteromedial border of the scapula. This test does not rely on patient report and hence is a more objective evaluation method than most clinical tests for nerve compression.[5]

We also rely on a pain questionnaire to assess each patient's symptoms. The questionnaire consists of visual analog scales of pain, questions for patients to describe their pain, and a body diagram for the patient to indicate the location(s) of pain. Responses are considered positive if more than three descriptors are chosen, the body diagram does not follow an anatomic pattern, or if the questionnaire score exceeds 20. Patients who score positive in more than two of these areas are referred for psychological assessment and are not offered immediate surgical intervention. An example of this questionnaire is provided in Table 142-1.[6]

Specific physical therapy protocols that address postural abnormalities, neural mobility, and muscle imbalance relieve the neurologic and muscular symptoms of most neurogenic TOS patients.[3] In our experience, few patients require surgical decompression. When one is evaluating a patient who has "failed" physical therapy, it is important to review the physical therapy regimen. In our experience, a faulty physical therapy program actually can exacerbate the patient's symptoms.

TECHNIQUE

All patients should have an extensive course of appropriate physical therapy before being considered as a surgical candidate. Given the potential for litigation and the controversial nature of the procedure, the patient must be adequately informed of the complexity of the operation and its potential significant surgical complications even with the best surgical technique and care.

The two favored approaches to the treatment of TOS are the transaxillary approach for first rib resection and the supraclavicular approach for anterior and middle scalenectomies with or without first rib resection, the subject of this chapter.[7,8] Reported success rates vary from 75% to 99% when all surgical approaches are considered. In contrast, reoperation on patients in whom the primary operation failed yields improved results in only approximately 15%. There are no randomized clinical trials that compare the transaxillary and supraclavicular approach for TOS decompression. Numerous authors have reported similar results with both approaches, and some have compared outcomes of scalenectomy with and without first rib resection. In a review of the literature, the best long-term outcomes appear to be the result of strict adherence to surgical principles: removal of the first rib, decompression of the artery and vein, and resection of the scalene muscles.

Supraclavicular First Rib Resection

Our preference for patients who do require operation is to perform a first rib resection with decompression of the brachial plexus followed by anterior and middle scalenectomies. Because complications increase with recurrent or secondary operations, a case can be made for first rib resection and scalenectomy in most patients, with care taken to remove the entire posterior aspect of the first rib. This philosophy ensures that a failure to relieve symptoms with scalenectomy alone will not be followed by the recommendation for a secondary thoracic procedure to remove the first rib.

The supraclavicular surgical approach to excise the first rib and release the scalene muscles is our preferred approach. This approach permits direct visualization of the brachial plexus and removal of the cervical rib, if present. Under general anesthesia, the patient is positioned supinely, with a ROHO inflatable sandbag placed between the scapulae and the neck slightly extended toward the nonoperative side. Loupe magnification and microbipolar cautery and a portable nerve stimulator are used. Long-acting paralytic agents are avoided to facilitate intraoperative nerve stimulation. The operative incision is made parallel to and approximately 2 cm above the clavicle in the supraclavicular fossa.

The supraclavicular nerves are identified immediately below the platysma muscle. These nerves are mobilized carefully both proximally and distally, and a vessel loop is placed around them to permit retraction across the operative site throughout the procedure (Fig. 142-4). If these cutaneous nerves are divided inadvertently, the proximal end should be

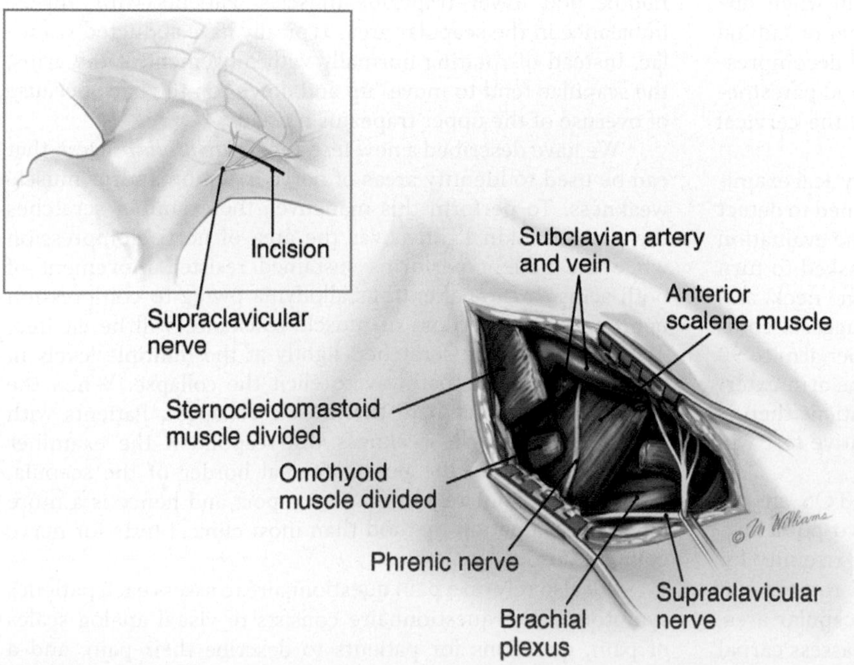

Figure 142-4. For the supraclavicular approach, a 2-cm incision is made above and parallel to the clavicle in the supraclavicular fossa (*inset*). The supraclavicular nerves lie immediately deep to the platysma and should be preserved. The omohyoid muscle is divided after the supraclavicular fat pad has been reflected away. Note the location of the brachial plexus and phrenic nerve in relation to the anterior and middle scalene muscles.

Table 142-1

TOS PATIENT QUESTIONNAIRE

PAIN QUESTIONNAIRE

Name: ______________________________ Date:_____________________________

Age:_______ Sex: Male ____ Female ____ Dominant Hand: Right ____ Left ____ Diagnosis:_________________________

1. Pain is difficult to describe. Circle the words that best describe your symptoms:

Burning	Throbbing	Aching	Stabbing	Tingling	Twisting
Cramping	Cutting	Shooting	Numbing	Vague	Stinging
Indescribable	Pulling	Smarting	Pressure	Coldness	Dull

Other ______________________________

Level of symptoms: place a mark through the line to indicate the level of your pain, if zero is no pain and the end of the line is the most severe pain you can imagine having

2. Mark your average level of pain in the last month:

No Pain ____ Most Severe Pain

3. Mark your worst level of pain in the last week:

Right

No Pain ____ Most Severe Pain

Left

No Pain ____ Most Severe Pain

4. Where is your pain? (Draw on diagram)

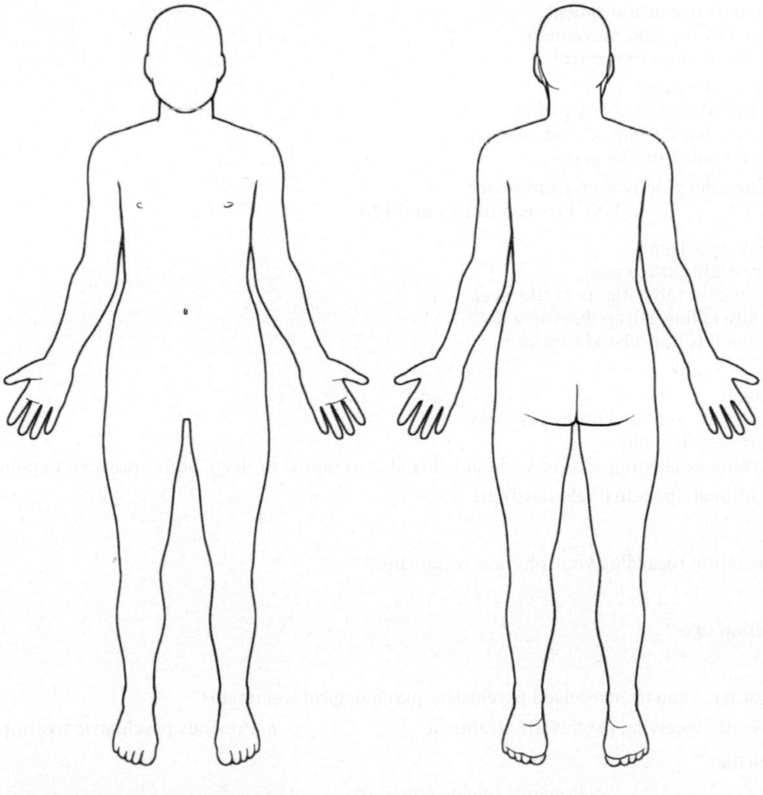

Mark on this scale how your pain has affected your quality of life

0% ____ 100%

Very Little ____ A Large Amount

5. Mark on this scale how depressed you currently feel:

0% ____ 100%

Not at all ____ A Large Amount

(Continued)

Table 142-1 (Continued)

TOS PATIENT QUESTIONNAIRE

PAIN QUESTIONNAIRE

6. Mark your average level of stress 10 the last month:

at home |______________________________|
0

at work |______________________________|
0

7. How well are you able to cope with that stress:

at home |______________________________|
Very Well Not at all

at work |______________________________|
Very Well Not at all

8. How did the pain that you are now experiencing occur?
   a. Sudden onset with accident or definable event
   b. Slow progressive onset
   c. Slow progressive onset with acute exacerbation without an accident or definable event
   d. A sudden onset without an accident or definable event
9. How many surgical procedures have you had in order to try to eliminate the cause of your pain'
   a. None or one
   b. Two surgical procedures
   c. Three or four surgical procedures
   d. Greater than four surgical procedures
10. Does movement have any effect on your pain?
   a. The pain is always worsened by use or movement
   b. The pain is usually worsened by use and movement
   c. The pain is not altered by me use and movement
11. Does weather have any effect on your pain?
   a. The pain is usually worse with dump or cold weather
   b. The pain is occasionally worse with dump or cold weather
   c. Damp or cold weather has no effect on the pain
12. Do you ever have trouble falling asleep or awaken from sleep?
   a. No - Proceed to Question 13 b. Yes - Proceed to 12A and 12B

12A. How often do have trouble falling asleep?
   a. Trouble falling asleep every night due to pain
   b. Trouble falling asleep due to pain most nights of the week
   c. Occasionally having difficulty falling asleep due to pain
   d. No trouble falling asleep which is not related to pain

12B. How often do you awaken from sleep?
   a. Awakened by pain every night
   b. Awakened from sleep by pain more than 3 times per week
   c. Not usually awakened from sleep by pain
   d. Restless sleep or early morning awakening with or without being able to return to sleep, both unrelated to pain

13. Has your pain affected your intimate personal relationships?
   a. No b. Yes
14. Are you involved in any legal action regarding your physical complaint?
   a. No b. Yes
15. Is this a Workers' Compensation case?
   a. No b. Yes
16. Are you presently receiving or have you ever received psychiatric/psychological treatment?
   a. No b. Presently receiving psychiatric treatment c. Previous psychiatric treatment
17. Have you ever thought of suicide?
   a. No b. Yes c. Previous suicide attempts
18. Are you a victim of emotional abuse?
   a. No b. Yes c. No comment
19. Are you a victim of physical abuse?
   a. No b. Yes c. No comment
20. Are you a victim of sexual abuse?
   a. No b. Yes c. No comment
21. Are you presently a victim of abuse?
   a. No b. Yes c. No comment

Table 142-1 (Continued)

TOS PATIENT QUESTIONNAIRE

PAIN QUESTIONNAIRE

22. Are you currently: (Check all that apply)

Employed for wages	____ Yes	____ No
On medical leave	____ Yes	____ No
A homemaker	____ Yes	____ No
Self-employed	____ Yes	____ No
Student	____ Yes	____ No
Retired	____ Yes	____ No
Volunteer	____ Yes	____ No
None of the above	____ Yes	____ No

23. If you are still working, do you?
    a. Work every day at the same pre-pain job
    b. Work every day but the job is not the same as the pre-pain job with reduced responsibility or physical activity
    c. Work occasionally
24. Are you able to do your household chores?
    a. Do same level of household activities without discomfort
    b. Do same level of household chores with discomfort
    c. Do a reduced amount of household chores
    d. Most household chores are now performed by others
25. What medications have you used in the past month?
    a. No medications
    b. List medications: ____

    ____

    ____
26. If you had 3 wishes for anything in the world, what would you wish for?
    1. ____________________
    2. ____________________
    3. ____________________

Modified 1/5/2010.
From: Hendler N, Virnstein M, Gucer P, et al. A preoperative screening test for chronic back pain patients. *Psychosomatics.* 1979;20:801–808.
Mackinnon SE, Dellon AL. Surgery of the Peripheral Nerve. Thieme Medical Publishers; 1988.
Melzack R. The McGill pain questionnaire: major properties and scoring methods. *Pain.* 1975;1:277–299.

cauterized and placed in a deep site, preferably in a muscle bed away from the overlying skin and scar to prevent postoperative neuromatous pain. The omohyoid muscle is identified and divided, and the supraclavicular fat pad is elevated and mobilized proximally. The most lateral portion of the sternocleidomastoid muscle then is divided and, at the conclusion of the procedure, is reapproximated. At this point, the brachial plexus can be palpated between the scalene muscles (Fig. 142-5). The phrenic nerve is identified on the anterior surface of the anterior scalene muscle. There can be an accessory branch of the phrenic nerve that runs within the muscle. The scalene muscle is divided without mobilizing the phrenic nerve to try to avoid excessive manipulation. If the nerve is divided inadvertently, it can be repaired; however, it is unlikely that recovery of diaphragmatic function will be forthcoming because of the long distance to the denervated diaphragm. If the patient experiences respiratory compromise, then consideration can be given for a transfer of a motor intercostal/rectus nerve to the phrenic nerve just above the diaphragm. The long thoracic nerve is located on the posterior aspect or within the middle scalene muscle (Fig. 142-6). A nerve stimulator can be used to identify the nerve, and frequently, two branches of the long thoracic nerve are noted. A vessel loop can be placed around the long thoracic nerve once it is identified (Fig. 142-7). The disposable nerve stimulator is set at its highest stimulation. Even at this setting, if a likely neurologic structure does not respond to direct stimulation, then the tip of the stimulator should be tapped several times on the structure because this maneuver usually will elicit a response. Once the anterior scalene muscle has been divided, the subclavian artery is immediately identified. An umbilical tape is placed around the artery. In patients with TOS, the artery often will be encountered in an elevated position; once it is mobilized and the anterior scalene muscle is divided, it will drop to a more normal location. The middle scalene muscle often will have a fibrous anterior edge. The middle scalene muscle is dissected sharply from the first rib. Care is taken to protect the long thoracic nerve within or behind the middle scalene muscle. The upper, middle, and lower trunks of the brachial plexus can be mobilized as a single unit. Only one branch divides at the trunk level (the suprascapular nerve from the upper trunk). The upper, middle, and lower trunks then are mobilized proximally and distally so that they can be retracted while the first rib is resected. With anterior retraction of the artery and brachial plexus, the first intercostal muscles are sharply dissected, and the midpoint of the first rib is divided. Anterior retraction provides excellent exposure for resection of the posterior first rib back to the spine. Posterior retraction of the plexus and anterior retraction of the artery provide excellent exposure for resection of the anterior portion of the first rib to a point anterior to the subclavian vein. Care is taken to mobilize the C8 and T1 roots because they course above and below the first rib, respectively (Fig. 142-8). Any congenital fibrous bands or thickening of Sibson fascia will be excised.

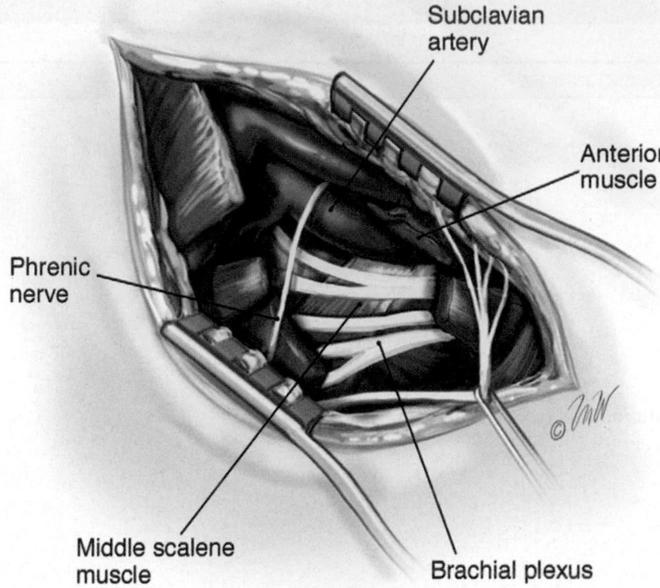

Figure 142-5. Guarding against injury to the phrenic nerve, the surgeon divides the anterior scalene muscle.

A neurolysis of the brachial plexus is needed infrequently, usually only in the cases of a traumatic injury or at the time of recurrent operation. Microinstrumentation and magnification are necessary. Microforceps will hold the epineurium, and straight microspring scissors then will be used to spread and release the epineurium. Care is taken not to damage or breach the perineurium. If the perineurium is violated, then a typical outpouching or herniating of the nerve tissue will be noted.

The first rib is isolated in the midportion of the exposure, where it is visualized most easily, and it is divided under direct vision with the use of a rib cutter. Rongeurs then are used to remove the posterior aspect of the first rib in a piecemeal fashion (see Fig. 142-8). Care is taken to make sure that the most critical portion of the first rib with respect to nerve compression (i.e., the most posterior aspect of the first rib) is totally removed from its spinal attachments. A fine elevator is used to separate the soft-tissue attachments from the first rib. The posterior cut edge of the first rib will be held with a rongeur, and in a twisting, rocking motion, the entire posterior portion of the first rib will be removed so that the cartilaginous components of the first rib articular facets (the costotransverse and costovertebral joints) are identified in the specimen. If periosteum or bony fragments are left at the posterior site, a callus will form subsequently to produce new bone formation, which may result in recurrent compression. If a prolonged transverse process or a cervical rib is present, it is removed with the same technique. The anterior portion of the first rib is removed under direct vision to decompress the neural and vascular elements. An opening of approximately 3 cm then is made in the pleura to facilitate drainage of any postoperative blood away from the

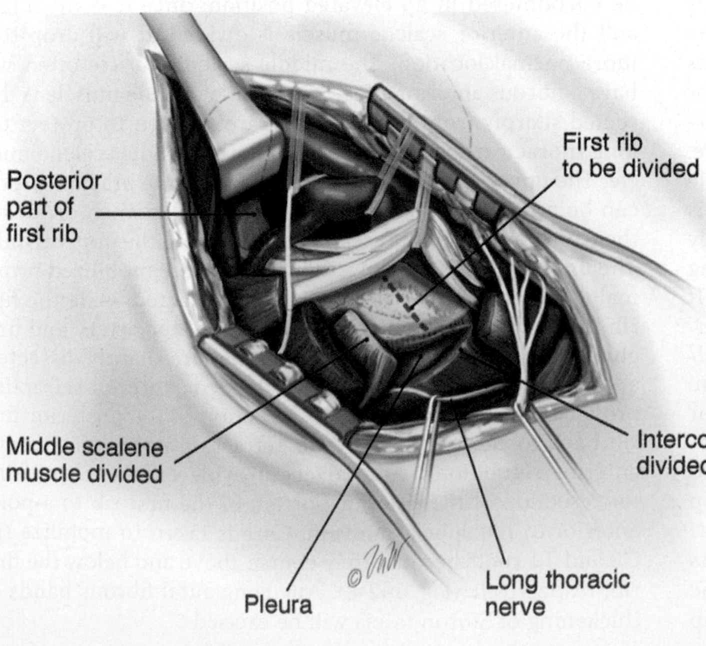

Figure 142-6. Anterior scalene divided, revealing brachial plexus and middle scalene muscle.

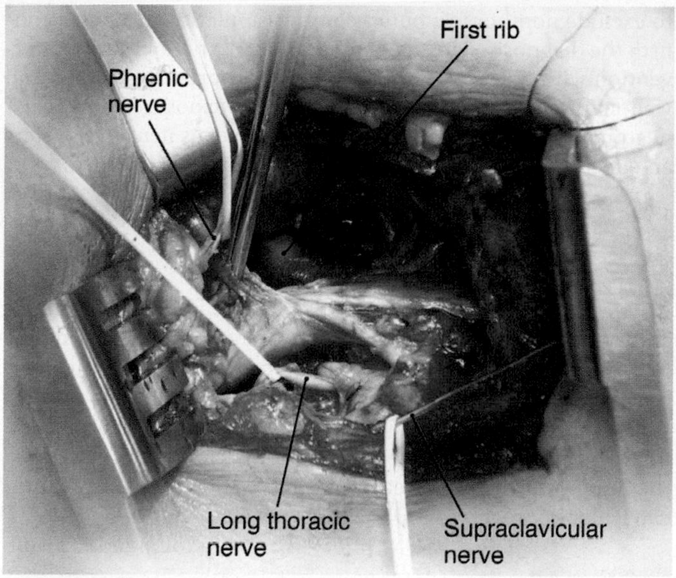

Figure 142-7. Intraoperative view of the phrenic, long thoracic, and supraclavicular nerves in relation to the first rib.

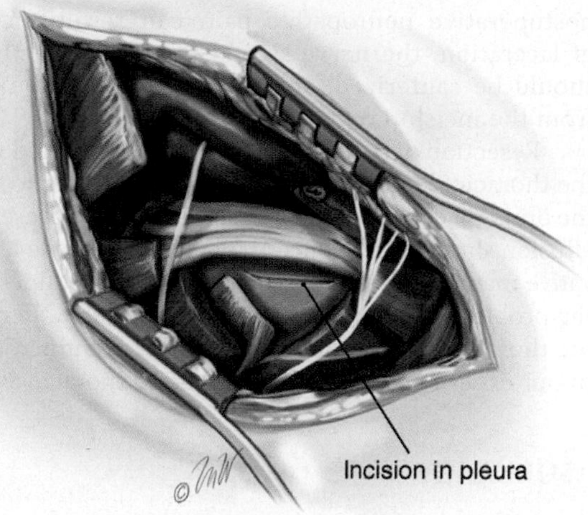

Figure 142-9. A 3-cm incision is made in the pleura for postoperative drainage of blood away from the brachial plexus into the pleural cavity.

brachial plexus into the pleural cavity (Fig. 142-9). Care is taken with this maneuver not to injure the intercostal brachial nerve, which courses across the surface of the dome of the pleura. A Marcaine infusion pump is placed in the incision for postoperative comfort. A simple suction drain in the operative site is used and sealed after wound closure and maximum inflation of the lungs by the anesthesiologist. We have not had to routinely place a chest tube for pneumothorax using this strategy.

POSTOPERATIVE CARE

In the immediate postoperative period, a chest x-ray should be obtained to rule out a pneumothorax. If present, it is typically small and usually does not require a chest tube for drainage. The surgical drain placed during the operation is usually removed on the first postoperative day. The patient should be reexamined to document motor or sensory deficits to the upper extremity. The patient is counseled to resume physical therapy exercises, with emphasis on range of motion. By 6 weeks, the patient should resume a supervised physical therapy program.

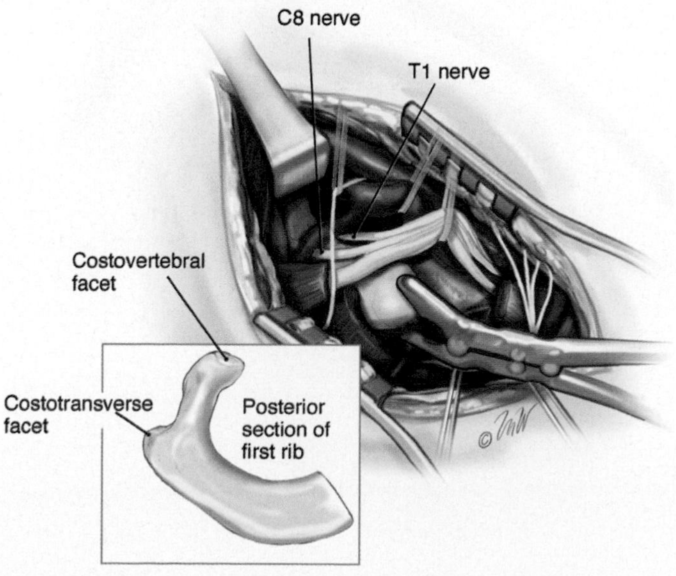

Figure 142-8. The C8 and T1 nerve roots are visualized and protected before rongeurs are used to remove the posterior aspect of the first rib (*inset*). The posterior aspect is the most critical portion of the first rib with respect to nerve compression.

PROCEDURE-SPECIFIC COMPLICATIONS

The most significant complications associated with surgical decompression of the thoracic outlet include injuries to the major neurovascular structures. Injury to the artery and vein are best avoided by careful manipulation and by obtaining proximal control. The surgeon should be prepared to extend the incision or even perform a median sternotomy (e.g., for right-sided innominate artery injury) or thoracotomy (e.g., for left subclavian artery injury) in the event of a difficult-to-control vascular injury.

Injury to nerves may be due to excessive traction or transection. Injury to the phrenic nerve may result in long-term or even permanent paralysis of the diaphragm. Surgical plication of the diaphragm has been used in a patient with respiratory compromise. Injury to the long thoracic nerve may result in a winged scapula. Injury to the sympathetic chain may result in a Horner syndrome. The most devastating injury may be to the lower trunk of the brachial plexus. This may cause constant pain or weakness and significant sensory and motor deficits to the hand. A temporary palsy has been reported to be as high as 10%. We believe that the supraclavicular approach provides for the best visualization of these structures, avoiding unintentional injury.

Even with careful preservation of the supraclavicular nerves (i.e., sensory nerves deep to the platysma), patients routinely will describe diminished sensation in the distribution of the supraclavicular nerves for approximately 6 weeks. To minimize irritation of this area, female patients are discouraged from wearing a bra strap across their surgical site for approximately 1 month after the operation. However, with inadvertent laceration of these small sensory nerves, severe postoperative neuropathic pain can result. In these cases of laceration, the nerve should be mobilized, the distal end should be cauterized, and the nerve should be buried away from the incision region.

Resection of the left first rib can be associated with injury to the thoracic duct. Increased drainage from the wound, or from the drain placed at the time of surgery, or the presence of a large effusion should raise concern for a cervical chyle leak. If conservative management by having the patient fast does not alleviate the problem, the wound should be explored. Often an injury to the thoracic duct or a tributary can be identified and repaired. In our experience, one patient required thoracic duct ligation.

SUMMARY

Neurogenic TOS presents the clinician with a complex array of symptoms and physical signs. Clinical judgment must be used to exclude nonthoracic outlet compression etiology and to confirm the diagnosis. Most patients respond to nonoperative intervention with physical therapy. In the appropriately selected and well-counseled patient, a supraclavicular exposure with scalenectomy, first rib resection, and brachial plexus neurolysis offers an effective and durable treatment for neurogenic TOS.

EDITOR'S COMMENT

TOS, especially Neurogenic TOS, can be difficult to diagnose and treat. Surgical intervention, when appropriate, requires rigorous patient selection, excellent understanding of the anatomy, and adherence to the key surgical principals of first rib removal, neurovascular decompression, and both anterior and middle scalenectomy. The authors have carefully highlighted the important points for each of these critical steps in a supraclavicular approach to TOS within this chapter.

—Yolonda L. Colson

References

1. Mackinnon SE, Novak CB. Clinical commentary: pathogenesis of cumulative trauma disorder. *J Hand Surg.* 1994;19A:873–883.
2. Novak CB, Mackinnon SE. Multilevel nerve compression and muscle imbalance in work-related neuromuscular disorders. *Am J Ind Med.* 2002;41: 343–352.
3. Novak C. Conservative management of thoracic outlet syndrome. *Chest Surg Clin North Am.* 1999;4:747–760.
4. Mackinnon SE, Novak CB. Thoracic outlet syndrome. *Curr Probl Surg.* 2002;39:1070–1145.
5. Cheng CJ, Mackinnon-Patterson B, Beck JL, et al. Scratch collapse test for evaluation of carpal and cubital tunnel syndrome. *J Hand Surg (Am).* 2008;33:1518–1524.
6. Novak C, Mackinnon S. Evaluation of the patient with thoracic outlet syndrome. *Chest Surg Clin North Am.* 1999;4:725–746.
7. Sanders RJ, Hammond SL. Supraclavicular first rib resection and total scalenectomy: technique and results. *Hand Clin.* 2004;20:61–70.
8. Mackinnon S, Patterson G, Colbert S. Supraclavicular approach to first rib resection for thoracic outlet syndrome. In: Andrew W, ed. *Operative Techniques in Thoracic and Cardiovascular Surgery: A Comparative Atlas.* Vol. 10. Philadelphia, PA: WB Saunders; 2005;318–328.

143 Thoracic Outlet Syndromes

Harold C. Urschel, Jr.,* J. Mark Pool, and Amit N. Patel

Keywords: Thoracic outlet syndromes, scalenotomy, nerve compression, vascular compression

INTRODUCTION

Thoracic outlet syndrome (TOS) is a condition that arises from the compression of one or more of the neurovascular structures that traverse the superior aperture of the chest. The name was previously designated according to the etiology of the compression, that is, scalenus anticus, costoclavicular, hyperabduction, cervical rib, or first rib syndrome. Most compressive factors operate against the first rib and produce a variety of symptoms, depending on which neurovascular structures are compressed. These factors, along with common etiologies and symptoms, are illustrated in Figure 143-1. My introduction (H.U.) to TOS came in 1947 at Princeton University, where, as a member of the undefeated freshman football team, my neck was knocked severely to the right, paralyzing my arm for several days. After the season, I was sent by train to Johns Hopkins Hospital to be evaluated by Dr. George Bennett, the eminent orthopedic surgeon who had recently operated on Joe DiMaggio's knee. He made the diagnosis of a cervical rib syndrome on the right and offered me an operation or a brace. Recognizing early that surgery was for others, I tried the brace. A piece of stainless steel covered only with leather was fashioned on my shoulder pad. It extended up past my right ear to prevent my neck from being driven to the right. I used this for the next year. However, in those days, no one wore a facemask, and I was often chagrined to find a piece of nose or face or teeth on the ground after a substantial block from the single-wing formation. For this reason, the NCAA ultimately outlawed the brace. Subsequently, the foam rubber "doughnut" was developed to prevent the neck from being forced to extremes in any direction. It is commonly used today. Conservative treatment, then as now, is usually effective. With no surgery, I contributed significantly to our undefeated team, which produced "Coach of the Year" Charles W. Caldwell, Jr., and the last Heisman Trophy winner in the Ivy League, Richard W. Kazmaier, Jr.

Since my diagnosis in 1947, many changes in the recognition and management of these multiple conditions have evolved. This chapter elucidates the improvements in the diagnosis and management of thoracic outlet neurovascular compression that have transpired over the past 50 years. Recognizing that such procedures as breast implantation and median sternotomy may produce TOS has been revealing. Prompt thrombolysis followed by surgical venous decompression for the Paget–Schroetter

*Deceased.

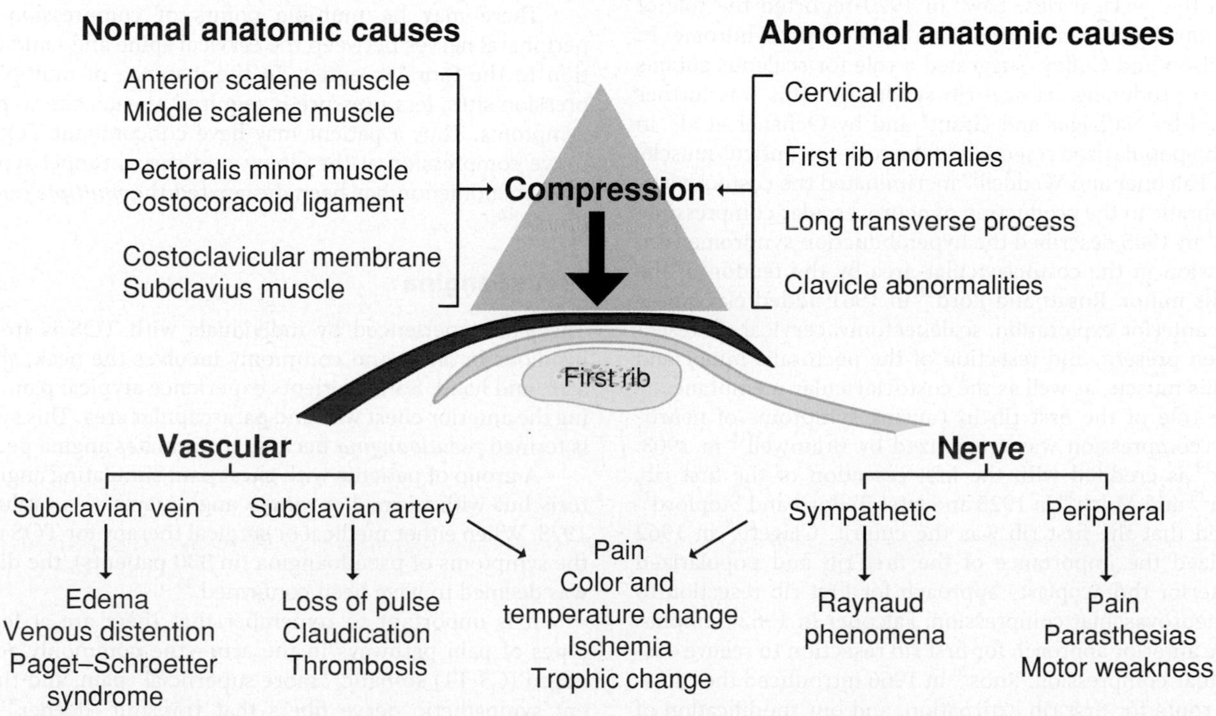

Figure 143-1. Compression factors in the thoracic outlet with the signs and symptoms produced.

syndrome (i.e., effort thrombosis of the axillary–subclavian vein) has improved results in this condition significantly as compared with the conservative anticoagulation approach. Complete first rib extirpation at the initial operation reduces the incidence of recurrent neurologic symptoms or the need for reoperation. Well over 20,000 patients have been evaluated for TOS in my experience; 4914 underwent neurovascular decompression operations, whereas 1721 had reoperations for recurrent symptoms (primarily from other centers). The evaluation of these patients provides the basis for my recommendation for conservative management and the indications for surgical intervention.

The incidence of any type of compression – arterial, venous, or nerve – presenting to the physician varies with the type of referral practice and specialty the particular physician may have. For example, the orthopedist is prone to see a high number of cervical ribs, the neurologist will see nerve compression patients, and a vascular surgeon will see more aneurysms and arterial/venous occlusions. The thoracic surgeon lies somewhere in between. In addition, the kinds of diagnostic techniques that are available may determine which center a patient is attracted to for management of a particular pathology.

HISTORICAL REVIEW

Peet et al. coined the term *thoracic outlet syndrome* to designate compression of the neurovascular bundle at the thoracic outlet.[1] Until 1927, the cervical rib was commonly thought to be the cause of symptoms of this syndrome.[2] Galen and Vesalius were the first to describe the presence of a cervical rib. Hunauld, who published an article in 1742, is credited by Keen[3] as the first observer to describe the importance of a cervical rib in causing symptoms. In 1818, Cooper medically treated symptoms of a cervical rib with some success. In 1861, Coote[4] performed the first operation of cervical rib removal. In 1916, Halsted[5] stimulated interest in dilation of the subclavian artery distal to the cervical ribs. Law[6] in 1920 reported the role of adventitious ligaments in producing cervical rib syndrome. In 1927, Adson and Coffey[7] suggested a role for scalenus anticus muscle in producing cervical rib syndrome. This was further developed by Naffziger and Grant[8] and by Ochsner et al.[9] in 1935, who popularized resection of the scalenus anticus muscle. In 1943, Falconer and Weddell[10] incriminated the costoclavicular membrane in the production of neurovascular compression. Wright[11] in 1945 described the hyperabduction syndrome with compression in the costoclavicular area by the tendon of the pectoralis minor. Rosati and Lord[12] in 1961 added claviculectomy to anterior exploration, scalenectomy, cervical rib resection when present, and resection of the pectoralis minor and subclavius muscle, as well as the costoclavicular membrane.

The role of the first rib in causing symptoms of neurovascular compression was recognized by Bramwell[13] in 1903. Murphy[14] is credited with the first resection of the first rib. Brickner[15] and Milch[16] in 1925 and later Telford and Stopford[17] suggested that the first rib was the culprit. Clagett[18] in 1962 emphasized the importance of the first rib and popularized the posterior thoracoplasty approach for first rib resection to relieve neurovascular compression. Falconer in 1962[19] emphasized the anterior approach for first rib resection to relieve costoclavicular compression. Roos[20] in 1966 introduced the transaxillary route for first rib extirpation, and our modification of his technique is presented in this chapter.

EARLY SCALENOTOMY-NEUROLYSIS SERIES

In the late 1950s and early 1960s, the operation of choice in our practice was the supraclavicular scalenotomy. This procedure involved a partial scalenectomy with neurolysis of the brachial plexus (when indicated) combined with resection of a cervical rib (if present). Early results in 336 patients were extremely good (310 of 336). However, the longer-term follow-up was not as satisfactory. Five-year improvement was present in 150 of 336 patients. However, at 20 years, only 31 of 336 patients were still improved. (We are unable to tell whether this represents 10% or 20% of the total series because 20 patients were lost to follow-up.) For this, and other reasons set forth in the presentation by Dr. O. T. Clagett in 1962,[18] the posterior approach for resection of the first rib, the so-called common denominator for thoracic outlet compression forces, was adopted. Subsequently, the initial operation usually was performed through the transaxillary approach because no muscle division was required, and morbidity for the patient was reduced. The supraclavicular or infraclavicular approach, or a "combined approach," was used for arterial lesions. The posterior approach is now reserved for reoperation in patients with recurrent TOS for removal of rib remnants, regenerated fibrocartilage with neurolysis of C7, C8, and T1 nerve roots, and brachial plexus.

Nerve Compression

The most common symptoms of nerve compression are pain and paresthesias. About 95% of patients exhibit these symptoms; fewer than 10% exhibit motor weakness. Pain and paresthesias are segmental in 75% of cases, and 90% involve the ulnar nerve distribution.[21] TOS can occur in older patients (oldest age 87 years). When nerve compression symptoms occur in patients older than age 60, other causes should be suspected, most frequently degenerative or traumatic cervical spine pathology or cardiac or pulmonary etiologies.

There may be multiple points of compression of the peripheral nerves between the cervical spine and hand in addition to the thoracic outlet. In the instance of multiple compression sites, less pressure is required at each site to produce symptoms. Thus a patient may have concomitant TOS, ulnar nerve compression at the elbow, and carpal tunnel syndrome. This phenomenon has been designated the *multiple crush syndrome*.[22]

Pseudoangina

The pain experienced by individuals with TOS is frequently insidious in onset and commonly involves the neck, shoulder, arm, and hand. Some patients experience atypical pain, involving the anterior chest wall and parascapular area. This symptom is termed *pseudoangina* because it simulates angina pectoris.

A group of patients with chest pain simulating angina pectoris but with normal coronary angiograms was evaluated in 1973. When either medical or surgical therapy for TOS relieved the symptoms of pseudoangina (in 330 patients), the diagnosis was deemed to have been confirmed.[23]

It is important to remember that there are at least two types of pain pathways in the arm—the commonly acknowledged (C5-T1) somatic, "more superficial" pain, and the afferent sympathetic nerve fibers that transmit "deeper" painful stimuli from the heart, esophagus, chest wall, and arm.

The cell bodies of the two types of afferent neurons are situated in the dorsal root ganglia of the corresponding spinal segments. They synapse in the dorsal gray matter of the spinal cord, and the axons of the second-order neurons ascend in the spinal cord up to the brain. Compression of the "superficial" C8-T1 cutaneous afferent fibers elicits stimuli that are transmitted to the brain and recognized as integumentary pain or paresthesias in the ulnar nerve distribution. In contrast, compression of the predominantly "deeper" sensory fibers elicits impulses that are appreciated by the brain as deep pain originating in the arm or the chest wall, even if the source of the impulses is cardiac (referred pain).

The pseudoangina experienced in thoracic outlet compression shares with angina pectoris the same dermatomal distribution. The heart, arm, and chest wall have afferent fibers converging on T2-T5 spinal cord segments, and their cell bodies are located in the corresponding dorsal root ganglia. Referred pain to the chest wall is a component of both pseudoangina and angina pectoris. Because somatic pain is more common than visceral pain, the brain has "learned" from past experience that activity arising in a given pathway is caused by a pain stimulus in a particular somatic area.

DIAGNOSIS AND OBJECTIVE TESTS

A careful history and physical examination are essential for diagnosis. There are four basic maneuvers used to elicit the classical physical signs of thoracic outlet compression.[23,24] These include the Adson test, the costoclavicular test, the Roos test, and the Wright test. The Adson (or scalene) test contracts the anterior and middle scalene muscles, resulting in a decrease in the interscalene triangle and intensifying any preexisting compression of the subclavian artery and brachial plexus. To perform the maneuver, the patient is asked to take and hold a deep breath while extending the neck fully and turning the head toward the involved extremity (Fig. 143-2A). This action should result in a decrease in the radial pulse. The costoclavicular test (military position) narrows the costoclavicular space by narrowing the area between the clavicle and first rib. The maneuver is performed by having the patient hold his shoulders down and backward (Fig. 143-2B). Loss of radial pulse and reproduction of symptoms indicate compression of the neurovascular bundle. The Roos test is performed over 3 minutes by holding both arms at 90 degrees of abduction and external rotation with the shoulders drawn back (Fig. 143-2C). The patient is instructed to open and close the hands slowly for 3 minutes. Numbness or pain will occur in the hands and forearms. The hyperabduction (or Wright) test is performed with the arms hyperabducted to 180 degrees and externally rotated (Fig. 143-2D). Compression is suspected if there is a decrease in radial pulse. As with most clinical tests, these maneuvers are not specific for thoracic outlet syndrome, and 56% of normal patients may have at least one positive test.[23]

The objective test for thoracic outlet peripheral nerve compression in our clinic is the nerve conduction velocity (NCV) test.[25,26] Reduction in NCV below 85 m/s of either the ulnar or median nerves across the thoracic outlet corroborates the clinical diagnosis. More than 8000 NCV studies have been performed annually at Baylor University Medical Center for many years. Approximately 2000 patients per year demonstrate TOS.[27,28]

The electromyogram should be normal and rules out other neuromuscular disorders. With conduction velocities above 60 m/s, the patient is usually improved with appropriate conservative physical therapy.

CONSERVATIVE MANAGEMENT

The principles of conservative management have been outlined by Novak and MacKinnon, as well as by Caldwell and Crane[26,29] Initially, most patients are treated conservatively with physical therapy, except those with vascular problems. The primary goals of physical therapy, for predominately "neurological" patients, are to "open up" the space between the clavicle and first rib, improve posture, strengthen the shoulder girdle, and loosen the neck muscles. This is accomplished by pectoralis stretching, strengthening the muscles between shoulder blades, assumption of good posture, and active neck exercises, including chin tuck, flexion, rotation, lateral bending, and circumduction. It is imperative to rule out other causes of TOS-like symptoms, such as cardiac or pulmonary disease.

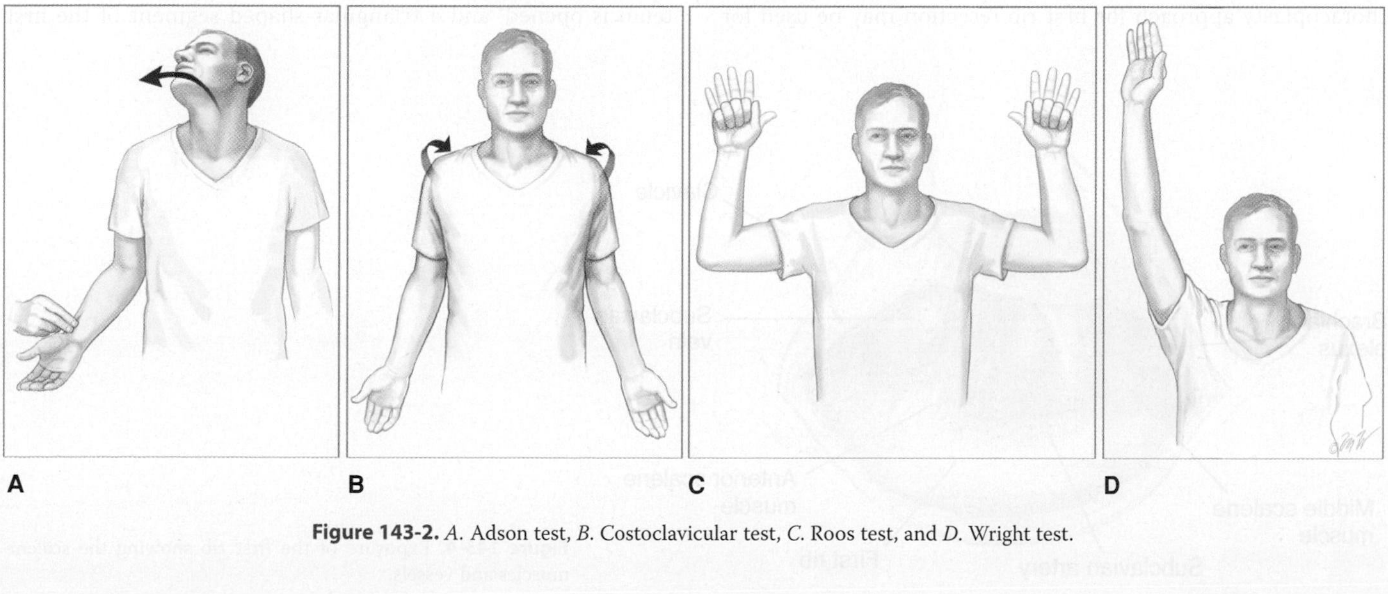

Figure 143-2. *A.* Adson test, *B.* Costoclavicular test, *C.* Roos test, and *D.* Wright test.

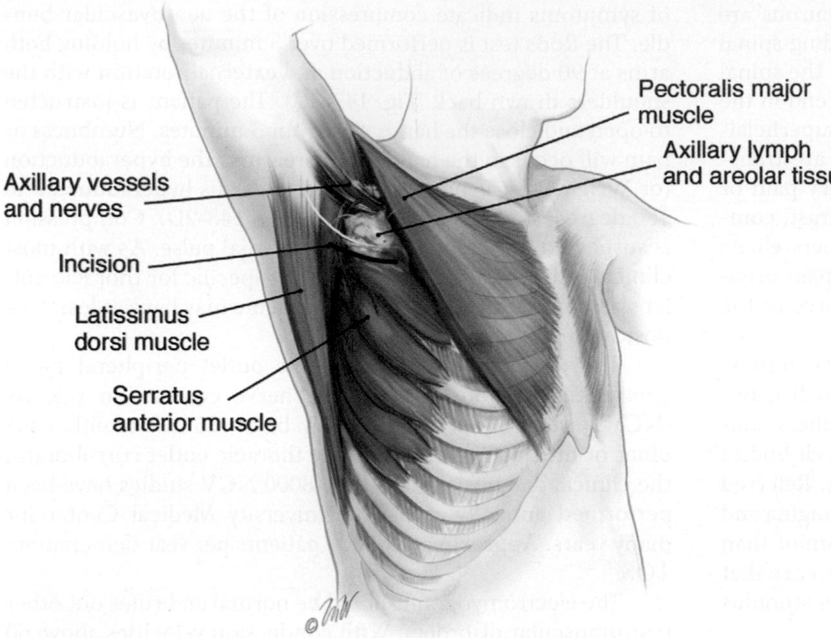

Figure 143-3. A subhairline incision is made for the transaxillary approach to first rib resection.

INDICATIONS FOR SURGERY

Failure of appropriate conservative therapy together with significantly reduced NCVs below 60 m/s (normal 85 m/s) and the elimination of other possible etiologies for the patient's symptoms are the usual indications for surgery of neurological thoracic outlet syndrome.

SURGICAL THERAPY

Initial therapy involves complete first rib resection, anterior scalenectomy, resection of the costoclavicular ligament, and neurolysis of C7, C8, and T1 nerve roots and the brachial plexus through a transaxillary approach (described below).[30] The first rib with the compressive elements also may be removed through the supraclavicular approach.[31] The supraclavicular approach has the disadvantage of working through and retracting the brachial plexus as well as producing a visible scar in women (the preponderant gender with TOS). The posterior thoracoplasty approach for first rib resection may be used for initial therapy, but it is better reserved for reoperation and neurolysis of the brachial plexus (not described).[32,33] Cervical ribs may be removed through any of the approaches described. Dorsal sympathectomy also may be performed with neurovascular decompression through any of the preceding incisions for sympathetic maintained pain syndrome (SMPS), reflex sympathetic dystrophy, causalgia, and Raynaud phenomenon and disease.[33]

TRANSAXILLARY APPROACH TO FIRST RIB RESECTION

The initial surgical therapy involves a complete first rib resection, anterior scalenectomy, resection of the costoclavicular ligament, and neurolysis of the C7, C8, and T1 nerve roots and the brachial plexus through a transaxillary approach. The transaxillary, transthoracic approach is performed through the second interspace with a transverse subhairline incision (Fig. 143-3).

The first rib is exposed, revealing the scalene muscles and vessels (Fig. 143-4). The anterior scalene is divided, the periosteum is opened, and a triangular-shaped segment of the first

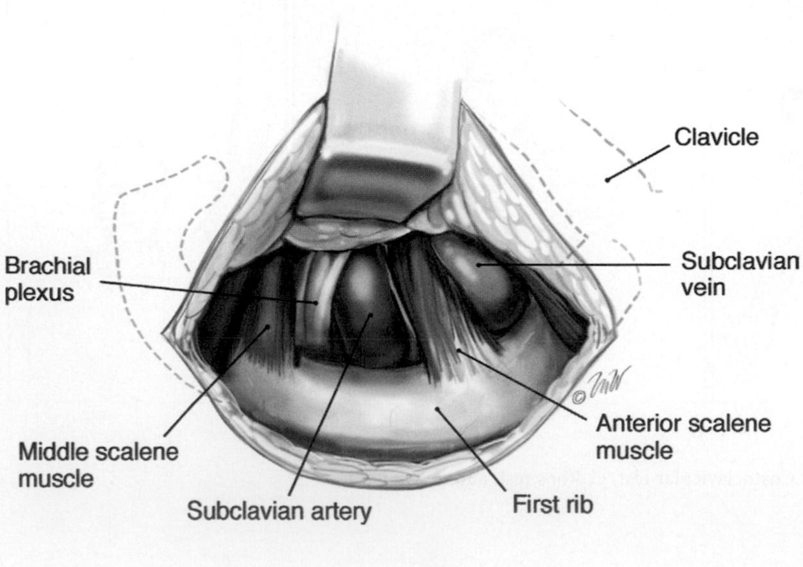

Figure 143-4. Exposure of the first rib showing the scalene muscles and vessels.

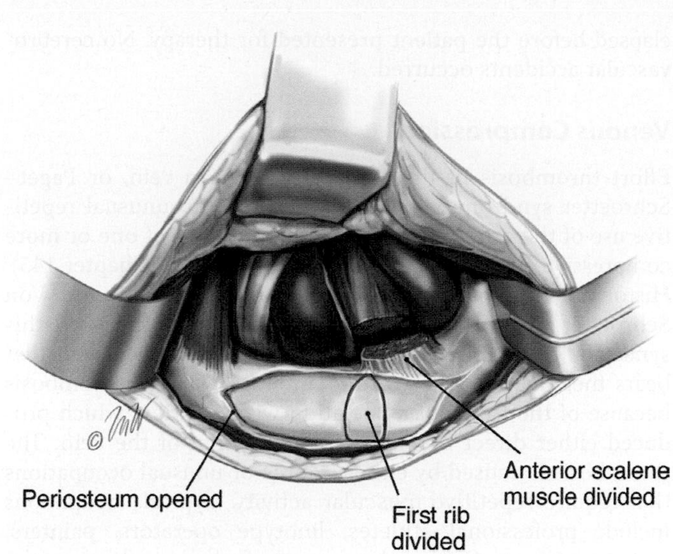

Figure 143-5. A triangular-shaped wedge is excised from the first rib, and the anterior scalene muscle is divided.

rib is excised (Fig. 143-5). The anterior portion of the rib is resected at the cartilage and removed, after which the middle scalene muscle is divided (Fig. 143-6). Next, the posterior section of the rib is resected (Fig. 143-7) with full attention to the T1 and C8 nerve roots to avoid injury. The head and neck of the rib are removed with rongeurs, and the dorsal sympathetic chain is identified and divided through the lower stellate ganglion above the T1 and below the T3 ganglia (Fig. 143-8).

UPPER PLEXUS VERSUS LOWER PLEXUS MANAGEMENT

Most patients with neurologic TOS requiring operation have been managed successfully with transaxillary resection of the first rib. However, for upper plexus (median nerve) compression, Roos and Stoney[34] felt that transaxillary rib resection alone was not enough and that it should be combined with the supraclavicular approach to achieve best results.

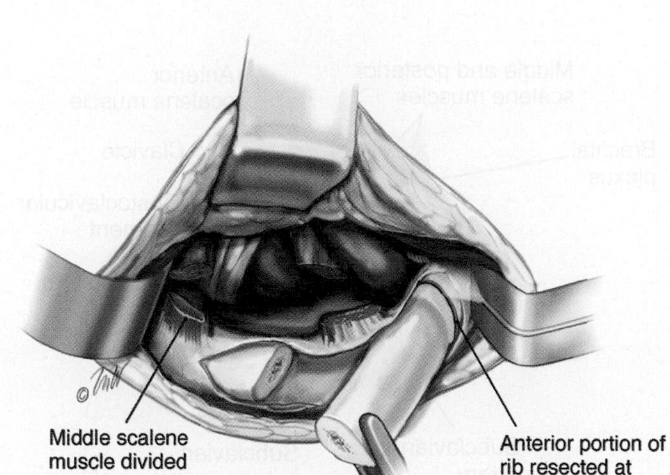

Figure 143-6. The anterior portion of the rib is resected back to the costocartilage. The middle scalene muscle is divided.

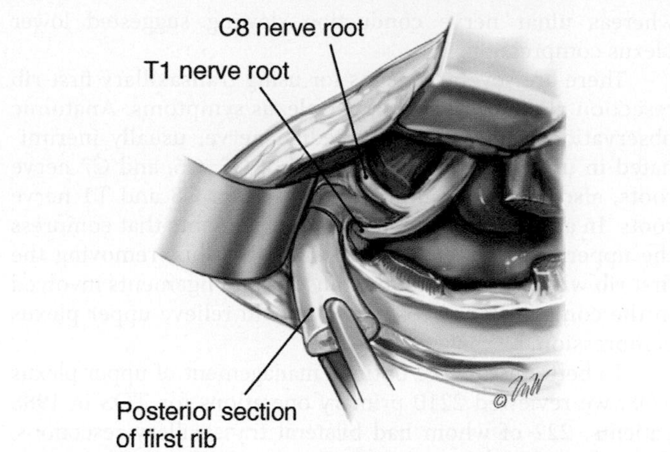

Figure 143-7. The posterior section of the rib is removed, with attention to the T1 and C8 nerve roots.

Upper plexus compression was described initially by Swank and Simeone[31] with symptoms secondary to C5, C6, and C7 nerve root compression. Sensory changes were primarily in the first three fingers and muscle weakness or pain in the anterior part of the chest, triceps, deltoids, and parascapular muscle areas, as well as down the outer arm to the extensor muscles of the forearm. In contrast, lower plexus irritation involves C8 and T1 nerve root compression. It includes sensory changes in the fourth and fifth fingers with muscle weakness or pain from the rhomboid and scapular muscles to the posterior axilla and down the ulnar distribution to the forearm, involving the elbow, flexors of the wrist, and intrinsic muscles of the hand. Roos,[34] Urschel and Razzuk,[35] and Wood and Ellison[36] expanded the upper plexus symptoms to involve pain in the neck, face, mandible, and ear with occipital headaches. Wood and Ellison also noted dizziness, vertigo, and blurred vision in some patients with upper plexus lesions.

In addition to clinical symptoms and signs, median nerve conduction slowing indicated upper plexus compression,

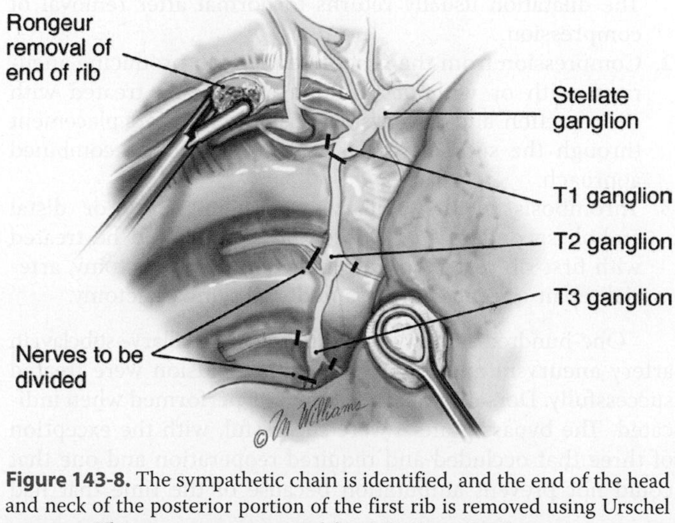

Figure 143-8. The sympathetic chain is identified, and the end of the head and neck of the posterior portion of the first rib is removed using Urschel rongeurs. The nerves are transected from T1 through T3.

whereas ulnar nerve conduction slowing suggested lower plexus compression.

There are several reasons for using transaxillary first rib resection alone to relieve upper plexus symptoms. Anatomic observations show that the median nerve, usually incriminated in upper plexus compression of C5, C6, and C7 nerve roots, also receives significant fibers from C8 and T1 nerve roots. In addition, most muscles and ligaments that compress the upper plexus attach to the first rib. Thus, removing the first rib with release of all the muscles and ligaments involved in the compression theoretically should relieve upper plexus compression.

To better assess the optimal management of upper plexus TOS, we reviewed 2210 primary operations for TOS in 1988 patients, 222 of whom had bilateral transaxillary resections, during a period of 30 years.[35] Two-hundred and fifty operations were for symptoms, signs, and NCVs showing median nerve or upper plexus compression only; 452 were for compression of both the median and ulnar nerves or the combination of upper and lower plexus by symptoms, signs, and NCVs. A total of 1508 operations were carried out for symptoms, signs, and NCVs demonstrating predominantly ulnar nerve or lower plexus compression.

This study of 2210 consecutive operations showed that transaxillary first rib resection with anterior scalenectomy relieves symptoms of the upper plexus (96%) and combined upper and lower plexus (95%) as well as it did for the lower plexus (95%).[35] Wood and Ellison[36] and Sanders[34] independently corroborated these findings. Patients were seen at 3 weeks and 3 months.

VASCULAR COMPRESSION

Arterial Compression

The diagnosis is suspected by history, physical examination, and Doppler studies and confirmed with arteriography.[21] Therapy for arterial compression depends on its degree of involvement.

1. An asymptomatic patient with cervical or first rib arterial compression producing poststenotic dilatation of the axillary–subclavian artery should undergo rib resection, preferably through the transaxillary approach, removing the ribs, both first and cervical, without resecting the artery. The dilatation usually returns to normal after removal of compression.
2. Compression from the first or cervical rib producing aneurysm with or without thrombus should be treated with rib resection and aneurysm excision with graft placement through the supraclavicular and infraclavicular combined approach.
3. Thrombosis of the axillary–subclavian artery or distal emboli secondary to TOS compression should be treated with first rib resection, thrombectomy, embolectomy, arterial repair or replacement, and dorsal sympathectomy.

One-hundred and fifty-one patients with axillary–subclavian artery aneurysm and 62 patients with occlusion were treated successfully. Dorsal sympathectomy was performed when indicated. The bypass grafts[37] were successful, with the exception of three that occluded and required reoperation and one that could not prevent amputation because of the time that had elapsed before the patient presented for therapy. No cerebrovascular accidents occurred.

Venous Compression

Effort thrombosis of the axillary–subclavian vein, or Paget–Schroetter syndrome, is usually secondary to unusual repetitive use of the arm in addition to the presence of one or more compressive elements in the thoracic outlet (see Chapter 145). Historically, Sir James Paget[38] in London in 1875 and Von Schroetter[39] in Vienna in 1884 independently described this syndrome of thrombosis of the axillary–subclavian vein that bears their names. The word *effort* was added to thrombosis because of the frequent association with exertion, which produced either direct or indirect compression of the vein. The thrombosis is caused by either trauma or unusual occupations that require repetitive muscular activity. Typical occupations include professional athletes, linotype operators, painters, and beauticians. Cold and traumatic factors, such as carrying skis over the shoulder, tend to increase the proclivity for thrombosis. Elements of increased thrombogenicity also increase the incidence of this problem and exacerbate its symptoms on a long-term basis.[40] In most patients with thrombosis of the axillary–subclavian vein, the costoclavicular ligament congenitally inserts further laterally than normal.

Pathophysiology

The axillary–subclavian vein traverses the tunnel formed by the clavicle anteriorly, the scalenus anticus muscle laterally, the first rib inferiorly, and the costoclavicular ligament medially (Fig. 143-9).[41]

In patients with thrombosis of the axillary–subclavian vein (Paget–Schroetter syndrome), the costoclavicular ligament congenitally inserts further laterally than normal (Fig. 143-10). When the scalenus anticus muscle, which is lateral to the vein, becomes hypertrophied through activity and exercise, the vein is significantly narrowed. This is not the case when the costoclavicular ligament inserts in a normal place much more medially on the first rib, even when significant scalenus anticus muscle hypertrophy occurs.[42]

The diagnosis is suspected by a careful history and physical examination with Doppler studies and is confirmed by a venogram.

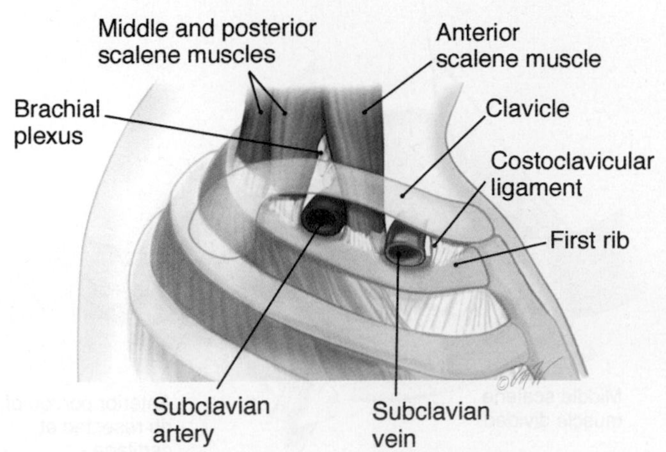

Figure 143-9. Normal anatomy of the thoracic outlet with conventional insertion of the costoclavicular ligament on the first rib.

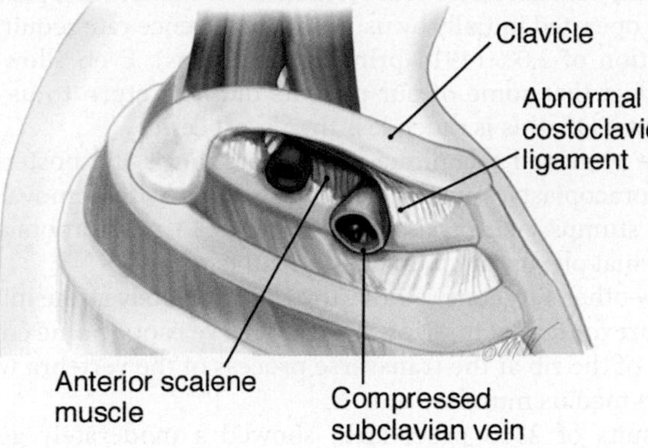

Figure 143-10. Congenital abnormal lateral insertion of the costoclavicular ligament on the first rib with hypertrophy of the scalenus anticus muscle (labeled anterior scalene muscle) lateral to the vein and thrombosis due to compression of the axillary–subclavian vein (Paget–Schroetter syndrome).

Intermittent or partial obstruction should be treated by first rib removal through the transaxillary approach with resection of the costoclavicular ligament medially, first rib inferiorly, and the scalenus anticus muscle laterally. The clavicle is left in place. The vein is decompressed, and all the bands and adhesions are removed.[43,44]

For many years, complete thrombosis Paget–Schroetter syndrome was treated by elevation of the arm and use of anticoagulants, with subsequent return to work. If symptoms recurred, the patient was considered for a first rib resection, with or without thrombectomy, as well as resection of the scalenus anticus muscle and removal of any other compressive element in the thoracic outlet, such as the costoclavicular ligament, cervical rib, or abnormal bands.[21] Thirty-six patients were treated by this approach; only 10 ended with a good to excellent result.

Availability of thrombolytic agents combined with prompt surgical decompression of the neurovascular compressive elements in the thoracic outlet reduced morbidity and the necessity for thrombectomy with substantially improved clinical results, including the ability to return to work.[45,46] This technique involves hospitalizing the patient, and through an antecubital indwelling catheter, a venogram is performed and thrombolytic therapy initiated. After lysis of the clot, prompt first rib resection with removal of compressive elements is performed.[47]

Clinical Observations

Clinical manifestations of "effort" thrombosis of the axillary–subclavian vein in the acute and subacute phases were evaluated in 660 extremities of 638 patients, 22 being bilateral. There were 312 females and 326 males, ranging in age from 16 to 52 years, with a mean of 33 years. Four hundred and sixty-two patients had unusual occupations that involved excessive, repetitive muscular activity of the shoulder, arm, and hand. Potentially aggravating occupations included such sports as golf, tennis, baseball, football, weight lifting, cheerleading, and drill team members, or other pursuits such as painters, beauticians, and linotype operators. The symptoms were usually exacerbated by working overhead, cold temperatures, or having the arm hang down for long periods of time.

Sympathetic Compression

Compression of the sympathetic nerves in the thoracic outlet may occur alone or in combination with peripheral nerve and blood vessels. The sympathetics are intimately attached to the artery as well as the bone. They may be compressed or "irritated" in primary or recurrent TOS situations.

As a cause of atypical chest pain – or pseudoangina – cardiac pain is simulated. Many arterial compressions result in more severe symptoms because of the additive or synergistic sympathetic stimulation. Trauma frequently is associated with the SMPS or reflex sympathetic dystrophy.

For uncomplicated, nontraumatic TOS symptoms, first rib resection alone with neurovascular decompression relieves the sympathetic symptoms without requiring dorsal sympathectomy.

However, if trauma is significant in the etiology, or if causalgia or SMPS is present, concomitant dorsal sympathectomy is routinely required to ameliorate the symptoms. Also, where surgery is required for recurrent TOS symptoms, the relief of accompanying causalgia usually requires dorsal sympathectomy. Initially, dorsal sympathectomies were performed at an interval after traumatic or recurrent TOS operations. However, because of the high necessity index and the inconvenience of a second operation, dorsal sympathectomy is now combined routinely with the initial TOS operative procedure for either trauma or reoperated recurrence patients.[48,49]

Major indications for dorsal sympathectomy include hyperhidrosis, Raynaud phenomenon, Raynaud disease, causalgia, SMPS or reflex sympathetic dystrophy, and vascular insufficiency of the upper extremity (see Chapters 144 and 146). Except for hyperhidrosis, most indications for sympathectomy require the usual diagnostic techniques, including cervical sympathetic block, to assess the relief of symptoms with temporary sympathetic blockade. When Raynaud phenomenon of a minor to moderate degree is associated with TOS, the simple removal of the first rib along with a cervical rib (if present) and stripping of the axillary–subclavian artery (neurectomy) generally relieves most symptoms after the initial operation.[50] It is rarely necessary to perform a sympathectomy unless the Raynaud phenomenon is very severe, in which case a dorsal sympathectomy is carried out with first rib resection (Chapter 144). The only contraindication to dorsal sympathectomy is venous obstruction, that is, Paget–Schroetter syndrome (Chapter 145).

Surgical Approaches for Dorsal Sympathectomy

Historically, the anterior cervical approach to the cervical sympathetic chain has been used.[51] The stellate ganglion lies on the transverse process of C6, and this approach is used by neurosurgeons and vascular surgeons. For hypertension, Urschel and Razzuk[52] popularized the posterior approach with a longitudinal paraspinal incision with the patient in the prone position. Small pieces of the second ribs are removed, and the sympathetic chain is identified in the usual position. This approach has the advantage of allowing bilateral procedures at the same time without changing the patient's surgical position. The most common current approach is the transaxillary, transthoracic approach, which is performed through the second interspace with a transverse subhairline incision.[53] This is more painful than the other approaches, but with video-assisted thoracoscopy, it can be performed with minimal discomfort.[49]

The approach used most frequently for TOS is the transaxillary approach for first rib resection and a dorsal sympathectomy.[48,54] This has the advantage of minimal pain and combines two procedures with low morbidity. Video assistance is also used frequently with this approach.

Dorsal sympathectomy has been performed in 3214 extremities at our institution; 2974 of these were associated with neurologic TOS, causalgia, and SMPS. Two-hundred and forty operations were associated with arterial complications of TOS. In the neurologic TOS patients, 1721 dorsal sympathectomies were related to recurrent disease and reoperation.

On average, symptoms recur in 3 years (range 6 months to 25 years). In 46 patients, symptoms of sympathetic activity were apparent in fewer than 6 months. This is most likely from "sprouting," or failure to strip the artery of its sympathetic nerves. This complication seems to occur less if the bed of the sympathetic chain is cauterized after dorsal sympathectomy. It also can be explained by high circulating concentrations of catecholamines.

The postsympathetic syndrome was observed in 39 patient extremities. This complication involves excessive postoperative pain (lasting as long as 6 months) in several nerve root distributions of the involved extremity and may be the result of injury to the somatic nerve. Unexpected Horner syndrome was noted in 27 patients; in 21 patients, the syndrome was only transient and resolved gradually.

RECURRENT THORACIC OUTLET SYNDROME

Recurrent symptoms, primarily neurogenic, should be documented by objective NCVs. When they are depressed in a symptomatic patient unrelieved by prolonged conservative therapy, he or she should be considered for posterior reoperation. Removal of any rib remnants or regenerated fibrocartilage and neurolysis of the C7, C8, and Tl nerve roots and the brachial plexus are performed.[33] Dorsal sympathectomy is added to minimize the causalgia contribution to symptoms. Depo-Medrol and hyaluronic acid are used to minimize recurrent scars.[55]

We identified two distinct groups of patients who required reoperation: those with pseudorecurrences and those with true recurrences. Pseudorecurrences were observed in 43 patients who were all referred from other surgeons and were never completely relieved of symptoms after the initial operation. They were separated into the following etiologies: mistaken resection of the second rib instead of the first (22 patients), resection of the first rib with a cervical rib left in place (11 patients), resection of a cervical rib with an abnormal first rib remaining (8 patients), and resection of a second rib with a rudimentary first rib left (2 patients).

Two-thousand and five extremities had true recurrences and included patients who were relieved of symptoms after the initial operation but had recurrence of symptoms 4 months to 18 years later. The working and differential diagnoses for recurrence are similar to those for the original operation. Indications for a reoperation are more stringent, in that longer periods of conservative therapy usually are invoked.

In this group, a substantial posterior stump (>1 cm) of the first rib remained in 1560 patients (all referred from outside physicians). Complete resection of the first rib at the initial operation was observed in 161 patients who had recurrent symptoms associated with excessive scar formation on the brachial plexus; 98 were operated initially by us, with a recurrence rate requiring reoperation of 2.0% (4914 primary operations). Even allowing for the fact that some of our patients did not return to us for recurrent TOS, this is much less than most series.

The preferred technique for reoperation is the posterior, high thoracoplasty, muscle-splitting incision with removal of first rib stumps, neurolysis of C7, C8, and T1 nerve roots and the brachial plexus and a dorsal sympathectomy.

Few other surgeons remove the rib completely at the initial procedure for fear of injuring T1 or C8 nerve roots. Some cover the end of the rib at the transverse process of the vertebra with scalenus medius muscle.

Results of 2305 procedures showed a moderately good early effect of a second procedure: 1729 patients had significant improvement (75%), 369 related fair improvement, and only 207 did not feel better. Late results (5-year follow-up) in 528 extremities that underwent a second procedure revealed 396 (75%) with good results and 132 (25%) with fair to poor recovery; 48 patients (3.1%) required a third surgical procedure.

The primary technical factors involved in recurrence seem to be complete extirpation of the rib at the first operation. If a rib remnant is left (as is the case with most surgeons outside our group), osteocytes grow out from the end of the bone and produce fibrocartilage and regenerated bone that compress the nerves. Keloid producers, failure to drain hematomas, and early excessive physical therapy after the first operation also may increase fibrosis. Occasionally, other approaches for reoperation have been used.[56]

Recurrent Arterial Abnormalities

Five patients referred from other physicians (two with false aneurysms, one with a mycotic aneurysm allegedly secondary to trauma at the initial operation, and two with obstructive arterial changes at the thoracic outlet) were reoperated successfully. Vascular reconstructive procedures were performed. In each patient, a saphenous vein bypass graft from the innominate or carotid artery proximally was connected to the brachial artery distally. In the patient with the mycotic aneurysm, the graft was placed first, and the vessels on each side of the aneurysm were ligated. The aneurysm was resected at an interval procedure.

Mortality and Morbidity

There were no deaths in the series of 4914 primary and 1721 reoperative TOS decompressive procedures. The major complication observed was a rib remnant left by the initial surgeon. From this, fibrocartilage and new bone regenerated, producing a high incidence of recurrence. More retractor help (two arm holders) and increased light improved the technique and facilitated the initial operation. This minimized the time of anesthesia, surgery, retractor use, and arm holding.

The pleura is opened at most operations (with the exception of pleurodesis) to provide drainage of blood and fluids, reducing recurrence.

Bleeding requiring reoperation occurred after only 3 of 5008 operations. Significant infection requiring drainage occurred after 9 operations. There were no significant arterial injuries and only one occurrence of postoperative venous bleeding requiring thoracotomy and repair. Venous injuries usually "suck air." Paget–Schroetter syndrome usually is associated with severe inflammation that obliterates the vein and removes its identifying blue color. The axillary structures usually are plastered to the chest wall firmly, making the operation difficult technically.

Significant nerve injuries of the brachial plexus with residual signs occurred in four patients, none of whom could be identified as having had prolonged stretching, inappropriate retraction, or direct surgical injury. Two occurred in diabetic patients and two in older individuals with very prolonged NCVs, suggesting an increased sensitivity to nerve pressure similar to that observed in diabetics.

A review of morbidity from the literature on 881 patients by Dale[57] revealed significant bleeding in 11 (1.4%) and nerve injury of the brachial plexus in 13 (1.5%), of the phrenic nerve in 39 (4.9%), of the long thoracic nerve in 3 (0.1%), and of the recurrent laryngeal nerve in 6 (0.2%). In another 168 patients reported,[58] the phrenic nerve was injured in 6 (4%), the long thoracic and recurrent laryngeal nerves were injured in 1 (0.5%), and Horner syndrome occurred in 9 (6%). Long-term studies,[59,60] as well as other complications, have been reported.[61]

SUMMARY

Over 50 years, many changes have resulted in improved recognition and management of TOS.[62,63] The most remarkable include the use of NCV to obtain a more accurate diagnosis and to follow up with nerve compression patients. Chest pain or pseudoangina can be caused by TOS. Complete rib resection is important at the initial operation to minimize recurrence. Thrombolysis and prompt first rib resection are the optimal treatment for most patients with Paget–Schroetter syndrome. Dorsal sympathectomy is helpful for SMPS, causalgia, and recurrent TOS requiring reoperation. Use of techniques of video-assisted thoracic surgery can reduce the morbidity of the transaxillary approach to first rib resection for TOS.

EDITOR'S COMMENT

We will all miss Dr. Urschel's wit, good humor and stories, and as this chapter clearly demonstrates, thoracic surgery has lost one of the "great ones." Dr. Urschel was a master surgeon with one of the world's largest experiences in TOS and was a true expert in the field. Although he is gone, his contribution to the surgical management of TOS will certainly continue to influence many generations of thoracic surgeons to come.

—Yolonda L. Colson

References

1. Peet RM, Henriksen JD, Anderson TP, et al. Thoracic-outlet syndrome: evaluation of a therapeutic exercise program. *Proc Staff Meet Mayo Clin.* 1956;31:281–287.
2. Borchardt M. Symptomologie und Therapie der Halsripen. *Berl Klin Wochen- schr.* 1901;38:1265.
3. Keen W. The symptomatology, diagnosis and surgical treatment of cervical ribs. *Am J Sci.* 1907;133:173.
4. Coote H. Pressure on the axillary vessels and nerve by an exostosis from a cervical rib; interference with the circulation of the arm; removal of the rib and exostosis; recovery. *Med Times Gas.* 1861;2:108.
5. Halsted W. An experimental study of circumscribed dilation of an artery immediately distal to a partially occluding band, and its bearing on the dilation of the subclavian artery observed in certain cases of cervical rib. *J Exp Med.* 1916;24:271–286.
6. Law A. Adventitious ligaments simulating cervical ribs. *Ann Surg.* 1920;72: 497–499.
7. Adson AW, Coffey JR. Cervical rib: a method of anterior approach for relief of symptoms by division of the scalenus anticus. *Ann Surg.* 1927;85:839–857.
8. Naffziger H, Grant W. Neuritis of the brachial plexus-mechanical in origin: the scalenus syndrome. *Surg Gynecol Obstet.* 1938;67:722–730.
9. Ochsner A, Gage M, DeBakey M. Scalenus anticus (Naffziger). *Am J Surg.* 1935;26:669–695.
10. Falconer M, Weddell G. Costoclavicular compression of the subclavian artery and vein: relation to scalenus syndrome. *Lancet.* 1943;2:539–544.
11. Wright I. The neurovascular syndrome produced by hyperabduction of the arm. *Am Heart J.* 1945;29:1.
12. Rosati L, Lord J. Neurovascular compression syndromes of the shoulder girdle. In: *Modern Surgical Monographs.* New York, NY: Grune & Stratton; 1961.
13. Bramwell E. Lesion of the first dorsal nerve root. *Rev Neurol Psychiatry.* 1903;1:236.
14. Murphy T. Brachial neuritis caused by pressure of first rib. *Aust Med J.* 1910;15:582–586.
15. Brickner W. Brachial plexus pressure by the normal first rib. *Ann Surg.* 1927;85:858–872.
16. Brickner W, Milch H. First dorsal vertebra simulating cervical rib by maldevelopment or by pressure symptoms. *Surg Gynecol Obstet.* 1925;40:30.
17. Telford E, Stopford J. The vascular complications of the cervical rib. *Br J Surg.* 1937;18:559.
18. Clagett OT. Research and prosearch. *Thorac Cardiovasc Surg.* 1962;44: 153–166.
19. Falconer MA, Li FW. Resection of the first rib in costoclavicular compression of the brachial plexus. *Lancet.* 1962;1:59–63.
20. Roos DB. Transaxillary approach for first rib resection to relieve thoracic outlet syndrome. *Ann Surg.* 1966;163:354–358.
21. Urschel HC Jr. Management of the thoracic outlet syndrome. *N Engl J Med.* 1972;286:1140–1143.
22. MacKinnon S, Dellon A. *Surgery of the Peripheral Nerve.* New York, NY: Thieme; 1988.
23. Urschel HC Jr, Razzuk MA, Wood RE, et al. Objective diagnosis (ulnar nerve conduction velocity) and current therapy of the thoracic outlet syndrome. *Ann Thorac Surg.* 1971;12:608–620.
24. Urschel HC Jr, Razzuk M. Thoracic outlet syndrome. In: Sabiston DC, Spencer FC, eds: *Gibbon's Surgery of the Chest.* Philadelphia,PA: Saunders; 1995:536–553.
25. Jebsen RH. Motor conduction velocities in the median and ulnar nerves. *Arch Phys Med Rehabil.* 1967;48:185–194.
26. Caldwell J, Crane C, Krusen E. Nerve conduction studies in the diagnosis of the thoracic outlet syndrome. *South Med J.* 1971;64:210–212.
27. Greep N, Lemmens H, Roos D. *Pain in Shoulder and Arm: An Integrated View.* The Hague: Martinus Nijhoff; 1979.
28. Urschel HC Jr. The John H. Gibbon, Jr., Memorial Lecture: Thoracic outlet syndromes. Annual Meeting of the American College of Surgeons, San Francisco, October 10–15, 1993.
29. Novak C, MacKinnon S. Thoracic outlet syndrome. *Orthop Clin North Am.* 1996;27:747–762.
30. Urschel HC Jr, Paulson D, McNamarra J. Thoracic outlet syndrome. *Ann Thorac Surg.* 1968;6:1–10.
31. Swank R, Simeone F. The scalenus anticus syndrome. *Arch Neurol Psychiatry.* 1944;51:432–445.
32. Urschel HC Jr, Razzuk MA. Thoracic outlet syndrome. In: Glenn WL, Baue AE, Geha AF, eds. *Thoracic and Cardiovascular Surgery.* Norwalk, CT: Appleton-Century-Crofts; 1995.
33. Urschel HC Jr, Cooper J. *Atlas of Thoracic Surgery.* New York, NY: Churchill-Livingstone: 1995.
34. Sanders R. *Thoracic Outlet Syndrome: a Common Sequela of Neck Injuries.* Philadelphia, PA: Lippincott, 1991.
35. Urschel HC Jr, Razzuk MA. Upper plexus thoracic outlet syndrome: optimal therapy. *Ann Thorac Surg.* 1997;63:935–939.

36. Wood VE, Ellison DW. Results of upper plexus thoracic outlet syndrome operation. *Ann Thorac Surg.* 1994;58:458–461.
37. Urschel HC Jr, Razzuk MA. Paget-Schroetter syndrome: what is the best management? *Ann Thorac Surg.* 2000;69:1663–1668.
38. Paget J. *Clinical Lectures and Essays*. London: Longmans Green; 1985.
39. Von Schroetter L. *Erkrankungen der Fegasse*. Vienna: Holder, 1884.
40. Adams JT, DeWeese JA. "Effort" thrombosis of the axillary and subclavian veins. *J Trauma.* 1971;11:923–930.
41. Urschel HC Jr. Anatomy of the thoracic outlet. *Thorac Surg Clin.* 17:4:511–520. Editors: Mark K Ferguson, Jean Deslauriers, FRCS(C). November 2007.
42. Urschel HC Jr. Treatment of deep venous thrombosis in the upper extremity. *Adv Venous Ther.* 2011;188:131–137.
43. Urschel HC Jr, Razzuk MA. Improved management of the Paget-Schroetter syndrome secondary to thoracic outlet compression. *Ann Thor Surg.* 1991;52:1217–1221.
44. Urschel HC Jr, Razzuk MA. Paget-Schroetter syndrome: what is the best management? *Ann Thor Surg.* 2000;69:1663–1669.
45. Urschel HC Jr, Razzuk MA. Improved management of the Paget-Schroetter syndrome secondary to thoracic outlet compression. *Ann Thorac Surg.* 1991;52:1217–1221.
46. Azakie A, McElhinney DB, Thompson RW, et al. Surgical management of subclavian vein effort thrombosis as a result of thoracic outlet compression. *J Vasc Surg.* 1998;28:777–786.
47. Urschel HC Jr, Razzuk MA. Paget-Schroetter syndrome therapy: failure of intravenous stents. *Ann Thor Surg.* 2003;75:1693–1696.
48. Urschel HC Jr. Dorsal sympathectomy and management of thoracic outlet syndrome with VATS. *Ann Thorac Surg.* 1993;56:717–720.
49. Urschel HC Jr. Video-assisted sympathectomy and thoracic outlet syndrome. *Chest Surg Clin North Am.* 1993;3:299–306.
50. Urschel HC Jr, Razzuk M. Thoracic outlet syndrome. In: Shields TW, ed. *General Thoracic Surgery*. Philadelphia, PA: Lea & Febiger; 1994.
51. Hempel GK, Rusher AH Jr, Wheeler CG, et al. Supraclavicular resection of the first rib for thoracic outlet syndrome. *Am J Surg.* 1981;141:213–215.
52. Urschel HC Jr, Razzuk M. Posterior thoracic sympathectomy. In: Malt RA, ed. *Surgical Techniques Illustrated: A Comparative Atlas*. Philadelphia, PA: Saunders; 1958.
53. Atkins HJ. Sympathectomy by the axillary approach. *Lancet.* 1954;266:538–539.
54. Martinez B. Thoracic outlet syndrome. In: Cameron JL, ed. *Current Surgical Therapy*. St Louis: Mosby; 1992:753–757.
55. Urschel HC Jr, Razzuk MA. The failed operation for thoracic outlet syndrome: the difficulty of diagnosis and management. *Ann Thorac Surg.* 1986;42:523–528.
56. Urschel HC Jr, Kourlis H Jr. Thoracic outlet syndrome: a 50-year experience at Baylor University Medical Center. *Proc (Bay Univ Med Cent).* 2007;20:125–135.
57. Dale WA. Thoracic outlet compression syndrome: critique in 1982. *Arch Surg.* 1982;117:1437–1445.
58. Cheng SW, Stoney RJ. Supraclavicular reoperation for neurogenic thoracic outlet syndrome. *J Vasc Surg.* 1994;19:565–572.
59. Lepantalo M, Lindgren KA, Leino E, et al. Long term outcome after resection of the first rib for thoracic outlet syndrome. *Br J Surg.* 1989;76:1255–1256.
60. Goff CD, Parent FN, Sato DT, et al. A comparison of surgery for neurogenic thoracic outlet syndrome between laborers and nonlaborers. *Am J Surg.* 1998;176:215–218.
61. Horowitz SH. Brachial plexus injuries with causalgia resulting from transaxillary rib resection. *Arch Surg.* 1985;120:1189–1191.
62. Urschel HC Jr, Razzuk MA. Neurovascular compression in the thoracic outlet: changing management over 50 years. *Ann of Surg.* 1998;228(4):609–617.
63. Urschel HC Jr, Patel AN. Surgery remains the most effective treatment for Paget-Schroetter syndrome: 50 years' experience. *Ann Thorac Surg.* 2008;86:254–260.

144 Thoracoscopic First Rib Resection with Dorsal Sympathectomy

Miguel Alvelo-Rivera, Amit N. Patel, and Rodney J. Landreneau

Keywords: Thoracic outlet syndromes, hyperhidrosis, Raynaud phenomenon versus Raynaud disease, causalgia, reflex sympathetic dystrophy, vascular insufficiency of the upper extremity, Paget–Schroetter syndrome

Thoracic outlet syndrome (TOS), a term coined by Rob and Standeven,[1] refers to symptomatic compression of the structures of the thoracic outlet (subclavian vessels and brachial plexus) at the superior opening of the chest. It was previously designated as *scalenus anticus, costoclavicular, hyperabduction, cervical rib,* and *first thoracic rib syndromes* according to presumed etiologies. The various syndromes are similar, and the compression mechanism is often difficult to identify. Most compressive factors operate against an osseous structure, most commonly the first rib.[2,3]

SURGICAL ANATOMY

At the superior aspect of the thoracic cage, the subclavian vessels and the brachial plexus traverse the cervicoaxillary canal to reach the upper extremity. The cervicoaxillary canal is divided into two sections by the first rib: the proximal division, composed of the scalene triangle and the costoclavicular space, and the distal division, composed of the axilla (Fig. 144-1). The proximal division is important to achieve acceptable neurovascular decompression. It is bounded superiorly by the clavicle, inferiorly by the first rib, anteromedially by the costoclavicular ligament, and posterolaterally by the scalenus medius (middle scalene) muscle and the long thoracic nerve. The scalenus anticus (anterior scalene) muscle, which inserts on the scalene tubercle of the first rib, divides the costoclavicular space into two compartments: The anteromedial compartment contains the subclavian vein, and the posterolateral compartment contains the subclavian artery and the brachial plexus. The latter compartment, which is bounded by the scalenus anticus (anterior scalene) muscle anteriorly, the scalenus medius (middle scalene) muscle posteriorly, and the first rib inferiorly, is called the *scalene triangle.*

FUNCTIONAL ANATOMY

The cervicoaxillary canal, particularly its proximal division, also termed the *costoclavicular area,* normally has ample space for

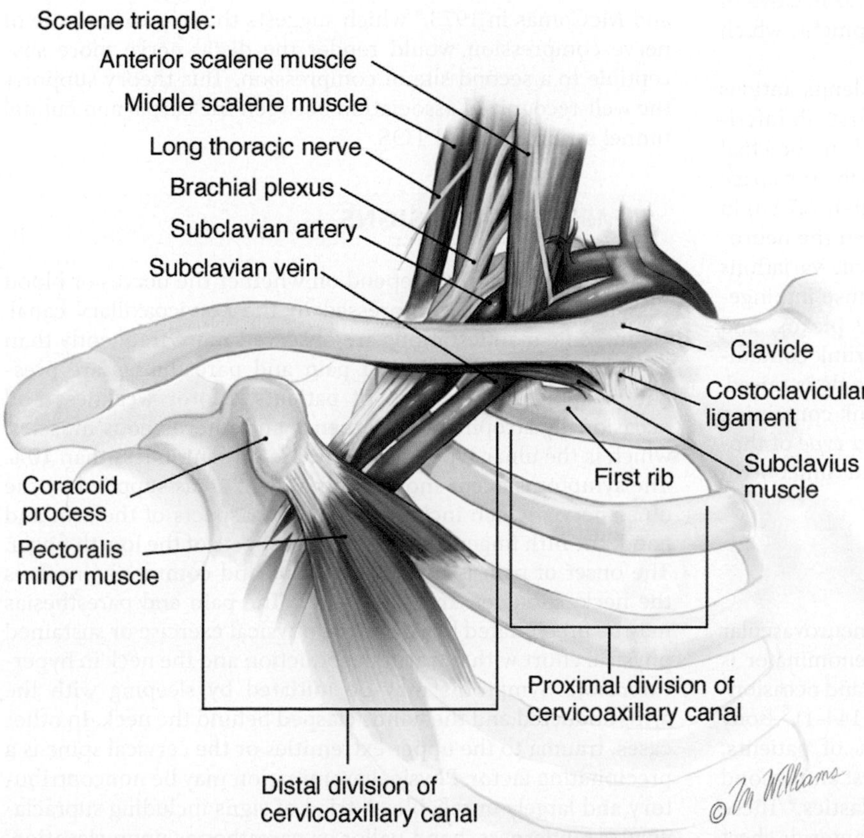

Figure 144-1. The cervicoaxillary canal has a *proximal division* consisting of the scalene triangle and costoclavicular space and a *distal division* composed of the axilla. The proximal division is more susceptible to neurovascular compression.

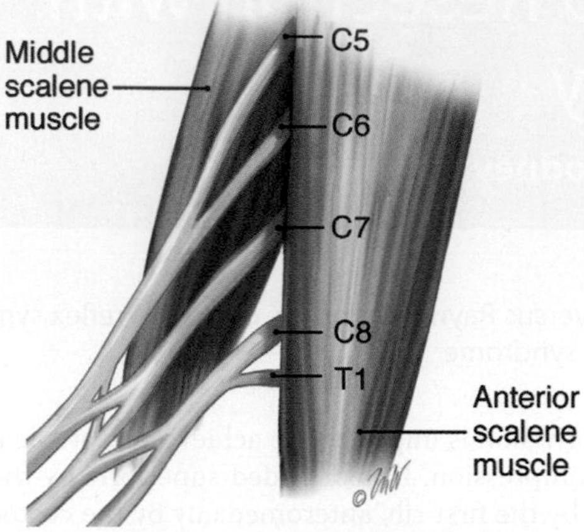

Figure 144-2. Components of the brachial plexus in the scalene triangle.

the passage of the neurovascular bundle without compression. Narrowing of this space occurs during functional motions of the upper extremities. It narrows during abduction of the arm because the clavicle rotates backward toward the first rib and the insertion of the scalenus anticus (anterior scalene) muscle. In hyperabduction, the neurovascular bundle is pulled around the pectoralis minor tendon, the coracoid process, and the head of the humerus. During this maneuver, the coracoid process tilts downward and thus exaggerates the tension on the bundle. The sternoclavicular joint, which ordinarily forms an angle of 15 to 20 degrees, forms a smaller angle when the outer end of the clavicle descends (as in drooping of the shoulders in poor posture), and narrowing of the costoclavicular space may occur. Normally, during inspiration, the scalenus anticus muscle raises the first rib and, thus, narrows the costoclavicular space. This muscle may cause an abnormal lift of the first rib, as in cases of severe emphysema or excessive muscular development, which is seen in young adults.

The scalene triangle, demarcated by the scalenus anticus anteriorly, the scalenus medius posteriorly, and first rib inferiorly, permits passage of the subclavian artery and the brachial plexus, which are in direct contact with the first rib. The space of the triangle is 1.2 cm at its base and approximately 6.7 cm in height. There is a close-fitting relationship between the neurovascular bundle and this triangular space. Anatomic variations may narrow the superior angle of the triangle, cause impingement on the upper components of the brachial plexus, and produce the *upper type* of TOS that involves the trunk containing elements of C5 and C6. If the base of the triangle is raised, compression of the subclavian artery and the trunk containing components of C7, C8, and T1 results in the *lower type* of thoracic outlet syndrome, as described by Swank and Simeone in 1944 (Fig. 144-2).[4]

COMPRESSION FACTORS

Many factors may cause compression of the neurovascular bundle at the thoracic outlet, but the common denominator is deranged anatomy, to which congenital, traumatic, and occasionally, atherosclerotic factors may contribute (Table 144-1).[5] Bony abnormalities are present in approximately 30% of patients, either as cervical rib, bifid first rib and fusion of first and second ribs, clavicular deformities, or previous thoracoplasties.[3] These abnormalities can be visualized on a plain posteroanterior chest film, but special x-ray views of the lower cervical spine may be required in some cases of cervical ribs. A more comprehensive theory of multiple sites of compression was proposed by Upton and McComas in 1973,[6] which suggests that a proximal site of nerve compression would render the distal nerve more susceptible to a second site of compression. This theory supports the well-recognized association between the carpal and cubital tunnel syndromes and TOS.

Table 144-1

ETIOLOGIC FACTORS OF NEUROVASCULAR COMPRESSION SYNDROMES

Anatomic
Potential sites of neurovascular compression
Interscalene triangle
Costoclavicular space
Subcoracoid area
Congenital
Cervical rib and its fascial remnants
Rudimentary first thoracic rib
Scalene muscles
Anterior
Middle
Minimus
Adventitious fibrous bands
Bifid clavicle
Exostosis of first thoracic rib
Enlarged transverse process of C7
Omohyoid muscle
Anomalous course of transverse cervical artery
Brachial plexus postfixed
Flat clavicle
Traumatic
Fracture of clavicle
Dislocation of head of humerus
Crushing injury to upper thorax
Sudden, unaccustomed muscular efforts involving shoulder girdle muscles
Cervical spondylosis and injuries to cervical spine
Atherosclerosis

SYMPTOMS AND SIGNS

The symptoms of TOS depend on whether the nerves or blood vessels or both are compressed in the cervicoaxillary canal. Neurogenic manifestations are observed more frequently than vascular ones. Symptoms of pain and paresthesias are present in approximately 95% of patients. Motor weakness and occasionally atrophy of hypothenar and interosseous muscles, which is the ulnar type of atrophy, are present in less than 10%. The symptoms occur most commonly in areas supplied by the ulnar nerve, which include the medial aspects of the arm and hand, the fifth finger, and the lateral aspects of the fourth finger. The onset of pain is usually insidious and commonly involves the neck, shoulder, arm, and hand. The pain and paresthesias may be precipitated by strenuous physical exercise or sustained physical effort with the arm in abduction and the neck in hyperextension. Symptoms may be initiated by sleeping with the arms abducted and the hands clasped behind the neck. In other cases, trauma to the upper extremities or the cervical spine is a precipitating factor. Physical examination may be noncontributory and largely unreliable. A triad of signs including supraclavicular tenderness, hand pallor or paresthesias upon elevation, and adduction/abduction weakness of digits 4 and 5 (ulnar distribution) has been proposed but is uncommonly obvious and is largely subjective.[7] When present, objective physical findings usually consist of hypesthesia along the medial aspects of the forearm and hand. Atrophy, when evident, is usually described in the hypothenar and interosseous muscles with clawing of the fourth and fifth fingers. In the upper type of TOS, in which components of C5 and C6 are involved in the compression (see Fig. 144-2), pain is usually in the deltoid area and the lateral aspects of the arm. The presence of this pain should raise concern to exclude a herniated cervical disk. Entrapment of C7 and C8 components that contribute to the median nerve produces symptoms in the index and sometimes middle fingers. Compression of components of C5, C6, C7, C8, and T1 can occur at the thoracic outlet by a cervical rib and produce symptoms of various degrees in the distribution of these nerves.

In some patients, the pain is atypical, involving the anterior chest wall or parascapular area, and is termed *pseudoangina* because it simulates angina pectoris. These patients may have normal coronary arteriograms and ulnar nerve conduction velocities decreased to values of 48 m/s and less, which strongly suggests the diagnosis of thoracic outlet syndrome. The shoulder, arm, and hand symptoms that usually provide clues for the diagnosis of TOS may be minimal or absent when compared with the severity of the chest pain, requiring a high index of suspicion. In these patients, the diagnosis of TOS frequently is overlooked, causing significant patient frustration.[8]

Symptoms of arterial compression include temperature changes (usually in the cool range), weakness, easy fatigability of the arm and hand, and pain that is usually diffuse.[3,9] Raynaud phenomenon is noted in approximately 7.5% of patients with TOS.[3] Unlike Raynaud disease, which is usually bilateral, symmetric, and elicited by cold or emotion, Raynaud phenomenon in neurovascular compression usually is unilateral and is more likely to be precipitated by hyperabduction of the involved arm, turning of the head, or carrying heavy objects. Sensitivity to cold also may be present. Symptoms include sudden onset of cold and blanching of one or more fingers, followed slowly by cyanosis and persistent rubor. Vascular symptoms in neurovascular compression may be precursors of permanent arterial thrombosis.[5] When present, arterial occlusion, usually of the subclavian artery, is manifest by persistent coolness, cyanosis, or pallor of the fingers, and in some instances ulceration or gangrene. Palpation in the parascapular area may reveal prominent pulsation, which indicates poststenotic dilatation or aneurysm of the subclavian artery.[10]

Less frequently, the symptoms are those of venous obstruction or occlusion, commonly recognized as effort thrombosis, or Paget–Schroetter syndrome. The condition characteristically results in edema, discoloration of the arm, distention of the superficial veins of the limb and shoulder, and some degree of pain or discomfort. In some patients, the condition is observed on waking; in others, it follows sustained efforts with the arm in abduction. Sudden backward and downward bracing of the shoulders, heavy lifting, or strenuous physical activity involving the arm may constrict the vein and initiate venospasm, with or without subsequent thrombosis. On examination, in patients with definite venous thrombosis, there is usually moderate tenderness over the axillary vein, and a cordlike structure may be felt that corresponds to the course of the vein. The acute symptoms may subside in a few weeks or days as the collateral circulation develops. Recurrence follows with inadequacy of the collateral circulation.

Objective physical findings are more common in patients with primarily vascular as opposed to neural compression. Loss or diminution of radial pulse and reproduction of symptoms can be elicited by the three classic clinical maneuvers (described below)—the Adson or scalene test,[11] the costoclavicular test, and the hyperabduction test.[12]

DIAGNOSIS

The diagnosis of TOS includes history, physical and neurologic examinations, radiographic surveys of the chest and cervical spine, electromyogram, and ulnar nerve conduction velocity (UNCV). In some patients with atypical manifestations, other diagnostic procedures, such as cervical myelography, peripheral or coronary arteriography, and phlebography should be considered. A detailed history and physical examination, together with neurologic examination, often can result in a tentative diagnosis of neurovascular compression. This diagnosis is strengthened when one or more of the classic clinical maneuvers is positive and is confirmed by the finding of decreased UNCV.[9]

Clinical Maneuvers

The clinical evaluation is best based on the physical findings of loss or decrease of radial pulses and reproduction of symptoms that can be elicited by four classic maneuvers (see also Chapter 143).

Adson or Scalene Test

This maneuver tightens the anterior and middle scalene muscles and thus decreases the interspace and magnifies any preexisting compression of the subclavian artery and brachial plexus.[11] The patient is instructed to take and hold a deep breath, extend the neck fully, and turn the head toward the side. Obliteration or decrease of the radial pulse suggests compression.[5,12]

Costoclavicular Test (Military Position, Halstead Maneuver)

This maneuver narrows the costoclavicular space by approximating the clavicle to the first rib and thus tends to compress the neurovascular bundle. Changes in the radial pulse with production of symptoms indicate compression. The shoulders are drawn downward and backward.[5,12]

Roos Test

This maneuver is performed by holding both arms at 90 degrees of abduction and external rotation with the shoulders drawn back. The patient is instructed to open and close the hands slowly for 3 minutes. The test result is positive if the patient experiences numbness or pain in the hands and forearms, or fatigue and heaviness in the shoulders.

Hyperabduction Test (Wright)

When the arm is hyperabducted to 180 degrees, the components of the neurovascular bundle are pulled around the pectoralis minor tendon, the coracoid process, and the head of the humerus. If the radial pulse is decreased, compression should be suspected.[5,12]

Radiographic Findings

Films of the chest and cervical spine are helpful in revealing bone structure-related abnormalities, particularly cervical ribs and bony degenerative changes. If osteophytic changes and intervertebral disk space narrowing are present on plain cervical films, a cervical CT scan or MRI should be performed to rule out bony encroachment and narrowing of the spinal canal and the intervertebral foramina.

Sensory Testing

The range of findings in sensory testing varies according to the severity, chronicity, and degree of functionality required by the patient. Initially, patients may be completely asymptomatic during rest and develop symptoms only during exertion. As the degree of injury increases, these symptoms can become more persistent and severe in nature. Eventually, nerve injury and loss of fibers result in loss of discriminatory function as measured by the two-point discrimination test. The greatest challenge is to be able to diagnose the condition before nerve injury becomes permanent. Provocative testing is used to elicit symptoms in otherwise asymptomatic patients at rest. These include nerve percussion at common entrapment sites (Tinel's test), arm elevation, elbow flexion and wrist flexion (Phalen's sign). Finally, measurements of vibration thresholds, pressure thresholds and innervation density can be used to detect slight degrees of impairment that could be early signs of compression injury. somatosensory evoked potentials (SSEP) have had mixed results in the early diagnosis of TOS and are generally regarded as not useful for early diagnosis.[13,14]

Nerve Conduction Velocity and Electromyography

This test is used widely in the differential diagnosis of the causes of arm pain, tingling, and numbness with or without motor weakness of the hand. Such symptoms may result from compression at various sites: in the spine; at the thoracic outlet; around the elbow, where it causes tardy ulnar nerve palsy; or on the flexor aspects of the wrist, where it produces carpal tunnel syndrome. For diagnosis and localization of the site of compression, cathode-based stimulation is applied at various points along the course of the nerve. Motor conduction velocities of the ulnar, median, radial, and musculocutaneous nerves can be measured reliably. Caldwell et al. [15]have improved the technique of measuring UNCV for evaluation of patients with thoracic outlet compression. Conduction velocities over proximal and distal segments of the ulnar nerve are determined by recording the action potentials generated in the hypothenar or first dorsal interosseous muscles. The points of stimulation are the supraclavicular fossa, middle upper arm, below the elbow, and at the wrist.[9]

Equipment

Electromyographic examination of each upper extremity and determination of the conduction velocities are done with the Meditron 201 AD or 312 or the TECA-3 electromyograph; coaxial cable with three needles or surface electrodes are used to record muscle potentials, which appear as tracings on the fluorescent screen.

Technique

The conduction velocity is determined by the Krusen–Caldwell technique.[16] The patient is placed on the examination table with the arm fully extended at the elbow and in about 20 degrees of abduction at the shoulder to facilitate stimulation over the course of the ulnar nerve. The ulnar nerve is stimulated at the four points by a special stimulation unit that imparts an electrical stimulus with a strength of 350 V with the patient's load, which is approximately equal to 300 V, with a skin resistance of 5000 Ω. Supramaximal stimulation is used at all points to obtain maximal response. The duration of the stimulation is 0.2 ms, except in muscular individuals, for whom it is 0.5 ms. Time of stimulation, conduction delay, and muscle response appear on the screen; time markers occur each millisecond on the sweep. The latency period to stimulation from the four points of stimulation to the recording electrode is obtained from the TECA digital recorder or calculated from the tracing on the screen. Velocities are expressed in meters per second and are calculated according to the following formula:

$$\text{Velocity (m/s)} = \text{distance between points (mm)} \div \text{difference in latency (ms)}$$

Normal UNCVs

The normal values of the UNCVs according to the Krusen–Caldwell technique[15] are $\geq$72 m/s across the outlet, $\geq$55 m/s around the elbow, and $\geq$59 m/s in the forearm. Wrist delay is normally 2.5 to 3.5 ms. Decreased velocity in a segment or increased delay at the wrist indicates either compression, injury, neuropathy, or neurologic disorders. Decreased velocity across the outlet is consistent with TOS. Decreased velocity around the elbow signifies ulnar nerve entrapment or neuropathy. Increased delay at the wrist is encountered in carpal tunnel syndrome.

Grading of Compression

The clinical picture of TOS correlates fairly well with the conduction velocity across the outlet. Any value <70 m/s indicates neurovascular compression. The severity is graded according to the decrease in velocity across the thoracic outlet: Compression is considered slight when the velocity is 66 to 69 m/s, mild when the velocity is 60 to 65 m/s, moderate when the velocity is 55 to 59 m/s, and severe when the velocity is $\leq$54 m/s.

Angiography

Simple clinical observations usually suffice to determine the degree of vascular impairment in the upper extremity. Peripheral angiography[10,17] is indicated in some patients, as in the presence of a periclavicular pulsating mass, the absence of a radial pulse, or the presence of supraclavicular or infraclavicular bruits. Retrograde or antegrade arteriograms of the subclavian and brachial arteries to demonstrate or localize the pathology should be obtained. In cases of venous stenosis or obstruction, as in Paget–Schroetter syndrome, venograms are used to determine the extent of thrombosis and the status of the collateral circulation (Fig. 144-3). In the case of acute venous thrombosis, thrombolysis can be performed immediately after the diagnostic procedure, followed by surgical decompression of the thoracic outlet.

DIFFERENTIAL DIAGNOSIS

TOS should be differentiated from various neurologic, vascular, cardiac, pulmonary, and esophageal conditions (Table 144-2).[5,8,12] Neurologic causes of pain in the shoulder and arm are more difficult to recognize and may arise from involvement of the nervous system in the spine, the brachial plexus, or the peripheral nerves. A common neurologic cause of pain in the upper extremities is a herniated cervical intervertebral

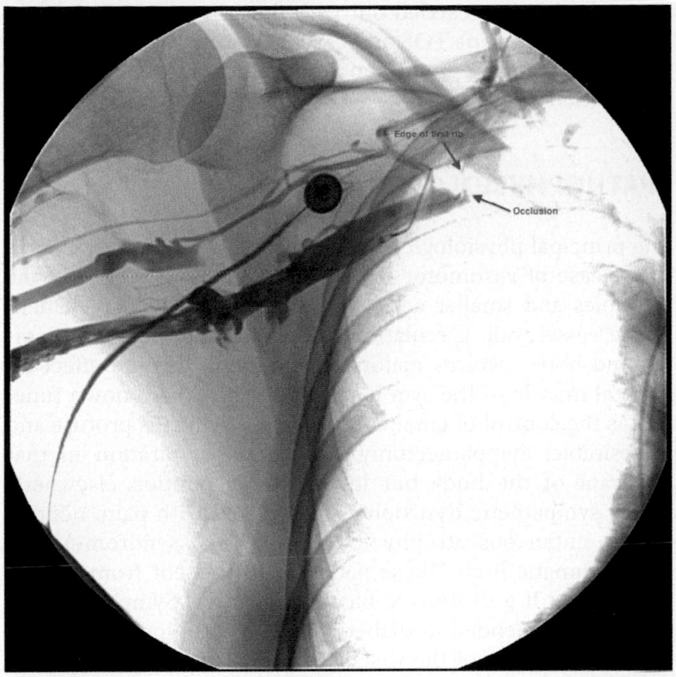

Figure 144-3. Venogram of a patient presenting with acute symptoms of venous occlusion. The patient had pitched a softball game a few hours before she noticed swelling and aching pain on her arm.

disk. The herniation almost invariably occurs at the interspace between the fifth and the sixth or the sixth and the seventh cervical vertebrae and produces characteristic symptoms. Onset of pain and stiffness of the neck is manifested with varying frequency. The pain radiates along the medial border of the scapula into the shoulder, occasionally into the anterior chest wall, and down the lateral aspect of the arm, at times into the fingers. Numbness and paresthesias in the fingers may be present. The segmental distribution of pain is a prominent feature. A herniated disk between the C5 and C6 vertebrae that compresses the C6 nerve root causes pain or numbness primarily in the thumb and to a lesser extent in the index finger. The biceps muscle and the radial wrist extensor are weak, and the reflex of the biceps muscle is reduced or abolished. A herniated disk between the C6 and C7 vertebrae that compresses the C7 nerve root produces pain or numbness in the index finger and weakness of index finger flexion and ulnar wrist extension; the triceps muscle is weak, and its reflex is reduced or abolished. Any of these herniated disks may cause numbness along the ulnar border of the arm and hand owing to spasm of the anterior scalene muscle. Rarely, pain and paresthesias in the ulnar distribution may be related to herniation between the C7 and the Tl vertebrae, which causes compression of the C8 nerve root. Compression of the latter nerve root produces weakness of intrinsic hand muscles.[5,16] Although rupture of the fifth and sixth disks produces hypesthesia in this area, only rupture of the seventh disk produces pain down the medial aspect of the arm.[5] The diagnosis of a ruptured cervical disk is based primarily on the history and physical findings; lateral films of the cervical spine reveal loss or reversal of cervical curvature, with the apex of the reversal of curvature located at the level of the disk involved. Electromyography can localize the site and extent of the nerve root irritation. When a herniated disk is suspected, cervical myelography should be done to confirm the diagnosis.[5,16]

Table 144-2

DIFFERENTIAL DIAGNOSIS OF TOS NERVE COMPRESSION

Cervical spine
Ruptured intervertebral disc
Degenerative disease
Osteoarthritis
Spinal cord tumors
Brachial plexus
Superior sulcus tumors
Trauma-postural palsy
Peripheral nerves
Entrapment neuropathy
Carpal tunnel—median nerve
Ulnar nerve—elbow
Radial nerve
Suprascapular nerve
Medical neuropathies
Trauma
Tumor
Vascular phenomena
Arterial
Arteriosclerosis-aneurysm
Occlusive
Thromboangiitis obliterans
Embolism
Functional
Raynaud disease
Reflex vasomotor dystrophy
Causalgia
Vasculitis, collagen disease, panniculitis
Venous thrombophlebitis
Mediastinal venous obstruction
Malignant
Benign
Other diseases
Angina pectoris
Esophageal
Pulmonary

Another condition that causes upper extremity pain is cervical spondylosis, a degenerative disease of the intervertebral disk and the adjacent vertebral margin that causes spur formation and the production of ridges into the spinal canal or intervertebral foramina. Films and a CT scan of the cervical spine and electromyography help in making the diagnosis of this condition.

Several arterial and venous conditions can be confused with TOS (see Table 144-2); the differentiation often can be made clinically. In atypical patients who present with chest pain alone, it is important to suspect the TOS in addition to angina pectoris. Exercise stress testing and coronary angiography may exclude coronary artery disease when there is a high index of suspicion of angina pectoris.[8,12]

THERAPY

Patients with TOS should be given physiotherapy when the diagnosis is made. Proper physiotherapy includes heat massages, active neck exercises, stretching of the scalenus muscles, strengthening of the upper trapezius muscle, and posture instruction. Because sagging of the shoulder girdle, which is common among the middle-aged, is a major cause in this syndrome, many patients with less severe cases are improved by strengthening the shoulder girdle and by improving posture.[8,12,16]

Most patients with TOS who have UNCVs >60 m/s improve with conservative management. If the conduction velocity is below that level, most patients, despite physiotherapy, may remain symptomatic, and surgical resection of the first rib and correction of other bony abnormalities may be needed to provide relief of symptoms.[3,12]

If symptoms of neurovascular compression continue after physiotherapy, and the conduction velocity shows slight or no improvement or regression, surgical resection of the first rib and cervical rib, when present, should be considered.[3,12] Clagett[2] popularized the high posterior thoracoplasty approach for first rib resection, Falconer and Li[18] emphasized the anterior approach, and Roos and Owens[19] introduced the transaxillary route.

The transaxillary route is an expedient approach for complete removal of the first rib with decompression of the seventh and eighth cervical and first thoracic nerve roots and the lower trunks of the brachial plexus. First rib resection can be performed without the need for major muscle division, as in the posterior approach[2]; without the need for retraction of the brachial plexus, as in the anterior supraclavicular approach[18]; and without the difficulty of removing the posterior segment of the rib, as in the infraclavicular approach. In addition, first rib resection shortens the postoperative disability and provides better cosmetic results than the anterior and posterior approaches, particularly because 80% of patients are female.[3]

INDICATIONS FOR DORSAL SYMPATHECTOMY WITH FIRST RIB RESECTION/MANAGEMENT WITH VIDEO-ASSISTED THORACIC SURGERY

Dorsal sympathectomy and the management of TOS are significantly improved with video assistance through magnification and an improved light system. Video-assisted thoracic surgery (VATS) offers better visualization of anatomic structures in a "deep hole," with an additional bonus of excellent visualization for other members of the team, particularly surgical residents. In addition, for sympathectomy alone, it produces less pain for the patient and a shorter hospitalization.

Video assistance is used in two techniques. One involves sympathectomy through three ports with standard video-assisted thoracic surgery. The second technique involves a transaxillary incision with removal of the first rib using video-assistance magnification and light; the surgeon operates either directly or secondarily while visualizing the image through the television set. This second technique was popularized by Martinez.[20]

Major indications for dorsal sympathectomy include hyperhidrosis, Raynaud phenomenon and Raynaud disease, causalgia, reflex sympathetic dystrophy, and vascular insufficiency of the upper extremity. Except for hyperhidrosis (see Chapter 146), all the other indications require the usual diagnostic techniques, including cervical sympathetic block to assess whether the symptoms are relieved by temporary blockade of the sympathetic ganglia. When Raynaud phenomenon of a minor to moderate degree is associated with TOS, the simple removal of the first rib (and cervical rib, if one is found) and stripping of the axillary–subclavian artery (neurectomy) will relieve most symptoms after the initial operation.[3]

It is rarely necessary to perform a sympathectomy unless the Raynaud's is of a very severe type, in which case a dorsal sympathectomy is carried out with first rib resection. In contrast, with recurrent TOS and causalgia, it has been found that the dorsal sympathectomy should be performed with the initial reoperation procedure.[21,22]

PATHOPHYSIOLOGY

The principal physiologic effect expected of sympathectomy is the release of vasomotor control and hyperactive tone of the arterioles and smaller arteries that have a muscular element in the vessel wall. Circulation to the skin, peripheral extremity, and bone receives major improvement, but the effect on skeletal muscle of the arm is minimal. The other known function is the control of cutaneous sweating, which is profuse and undesirable. Sympathectomy eliminates perspiration in that quadrant of the body but increases perspiration elsewhere. Reflex sympathetic dystrophy is associated with pain, neurasthenia, cutaneous atrophy (Sudeck–Leriche syndrome), and post-traumatic limb. These patients also benefit from a sympathectomy if a diagnostic block is effective. Sympathectomy is not recommended in diabetic neuropathy. Nor should it be performed in any of the vascular vasospastic syndromes until after conservative management, including cessation of tobacco products and institution of beta blockers, peripheral vasodilators, and calcium channel blockers, has been tried.[23]

Preganglionic sympathetic nerves derived from the spinal cord do not follow a corresponding relationship to the accompanying somatic nerves. The cervical ganglia of C1 to C4 are fused into a superior cervical ganglion, C5 and C6 into the middle cervical ganglion, and C7 and C8 into the inferior ganglion, which combines with the ganglion from T1 to the larger stellate ganglion. Cervical ganglionectomy is not used for denervation of the upper extremity because the preganglionic sympathetic outflow from the spinal cord to the arm is usually from T2 to T9, mostly from T2 to T4. In about 10% of cases, T1 preganglionic fibers also supply the upper extremity. To remove the preganglionic fibers to the upper extremity in most patients, removal of paravertebral ganglia T2 and T3 with the interconnecting chain is sufficient. Postganglionic fibers from these two segments often join, and branches then follow the nerves of the brachial plexus. The joined T2 and T3 fibers that bypass the stellate ganglion are known as the *nerve of Kuntz*.[24] To ensure that all the remaining patients who have a T1 connection through the stellate ganglion obtain adequate sympathetic denervation, the lower third of the stellate ganglion also should be removed, as recommended by Palumbo.[25]

Patients with reflex sympathetic dystrophy or sympathetic maintained pain syndrome (SMPS) complain of pain outside a peripheral nerve distribution, and although the injury itself may have been minor, the pain appears out of proportion to the injury. We have seen two types of reflex sympathetic dystrophy or SMPS; one involves the hand or even a majority of the upper extremity, and a second is localized to one or more digits. In no instance can the patient's pain be completely accounted for by an injury to a specific nerve, although injury to a specific nerve may cause the more diffuse symptoms. The patient also demonstrates diminished hand function. Several patients have been referred with a diagnosis of SMPS, and on examination, it is quite apparent that although they may complain of diffuse pain, the hand functions normally with a full range of movement, and motor power is demonstrated. These patients, of course, do not have SMPS. The patient also must demonstrate some joint stiffness. The skin and soft tissue trophic changes demonstrate varying amounts of vasomotor instability, depending on the stage of SMPS.

According to Mackinnon and Dellon,[26] there are early, intermediate, and late stages of SMPS. In the early stages, vasomotor instability is noted, with very dramatic sympathetic overactivity apparent in the hand or digit involved. Instability, with symptoms varying between redness and warmth and cyanosis and sweating, is noted in this early stage. Edema is also a classic finding in the early stage. In the intermediate stage of SMPS, pain is a less dramatic component and is usually elicited by attempts to move the joints. At rest, the patient may be quite comfortable. The edema and vasomotor changes have settled by this time, and the hand has the appearance of a "burned out," dystrophic hand, with marked stiffness and atrophy of the soft tissue noted. The normal wrinkles on the dorsum of the hand are no longer apparent. The fingertips may have a tapered appearance. The nail growth is usually more exaggerated than in the normal hand, and the hand is often cool and pale. The intermediate stage will extend over a number of months. During the late stage, all the superimposed problems of disuse atrophy may take effect. During this stage, problems with the elbow and shoulder are very common, even though the initial SMPS involved only the hand or one or more digits. The degree of pain experienced during the late phase is variable and is often the result of disuse and stiffness. SMPS can affect other areas of the body and has been observed in the foot, face, and penis.

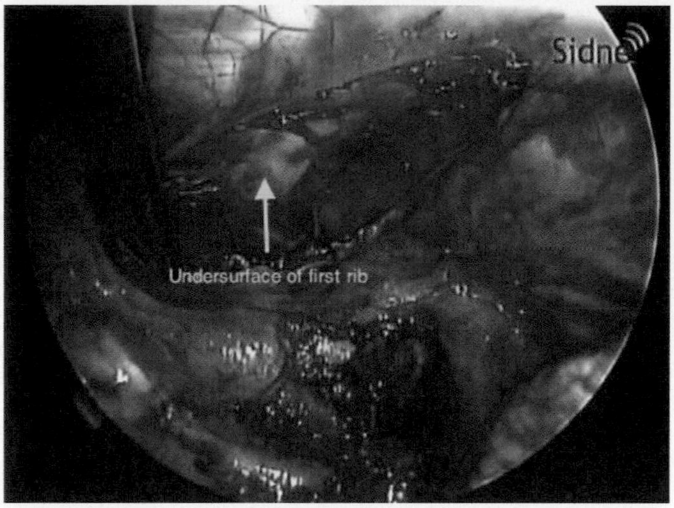

Figure 144-5. Incision of the parietal pleura overlying the first rib.

TECHNIQUE OF TRANSAXILLARY THORACOSCOPIC FIRST RIB RESECTION WITH DORSAL SYMPATHECTOMY

The operated arm is held or suspended over an ether screen. After prepping and draping the axilla, an incision is made below the axillary hairline, between the pectoralis major and latissimus dorsi muscles (Fig. 144-4). The incision is made through the skin and subcutaneous tissue down to the chest wall, and dissection is carried up to the first rib. Care is taken not to injure the intercostal brachial nerve. The videothoracoscope is inserted, and *while watching the screen,* the scalenus anticus muscle is divided at the scalene tubercle.

After collapsing the lung on the operated side, the pleura overlying the underside of the first rib is scored and the rib exposed (Figs. 144-5 and 144-6). A triangular portion of the first rib is removed, with the vertex of the triangle at the scalene tubercle (Figs. 144-7 to 144-9). The costoclavicular ligament is divided medially, and the medial segment of the first rib is removed back to the costal cartilage of the sternum. The posterior segment of the first rib is dissected, with attention to the neurovascular structures, and divided near the transverse process.

The head and neck of the first rib are carefully removed with special, reinforced, Urschel pituitary and Urschel–Leksell rongeurs (Fig. 144-10). Care is taken not to injure the C8

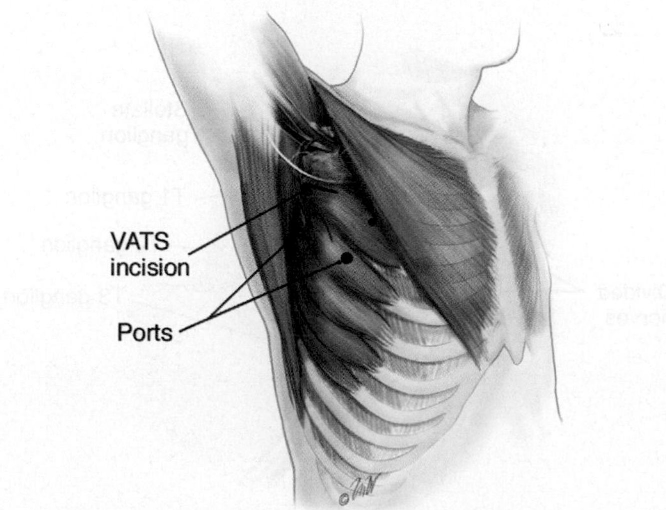

Figure 144-4. Video-assisted thoracic surgery incision and port placement for transaxillary first rib resection with dorsal sympathectomy.

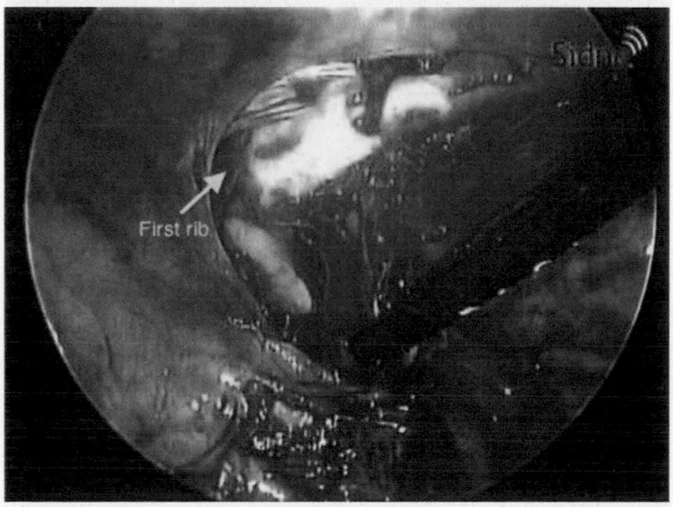

Figure 144-6. Exposure of the underside of the rib.

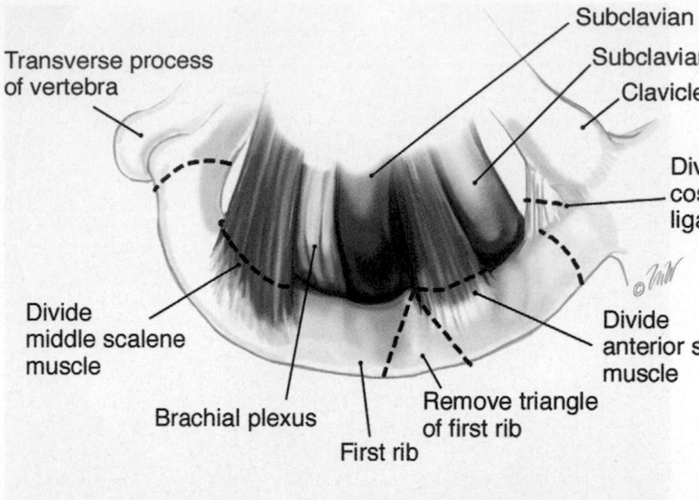

Figure 144-7. A triangular portion of the first rib is removed, with the vertex of the triangle at the scalene tubercle.

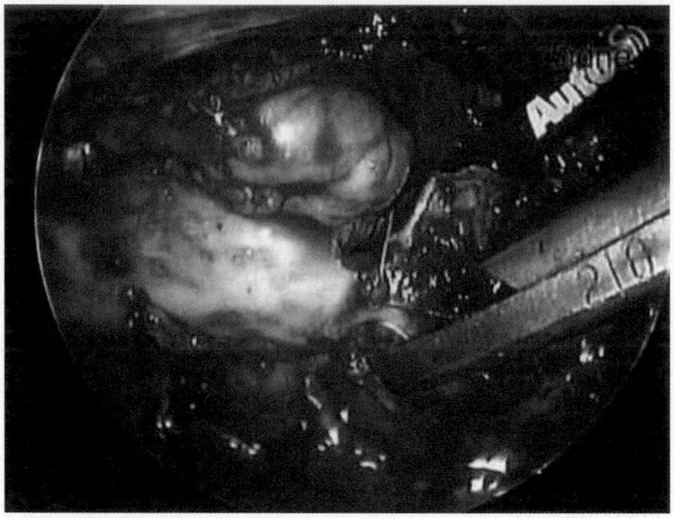

Figure 144-8. Triangular resection of a portion of the rib.

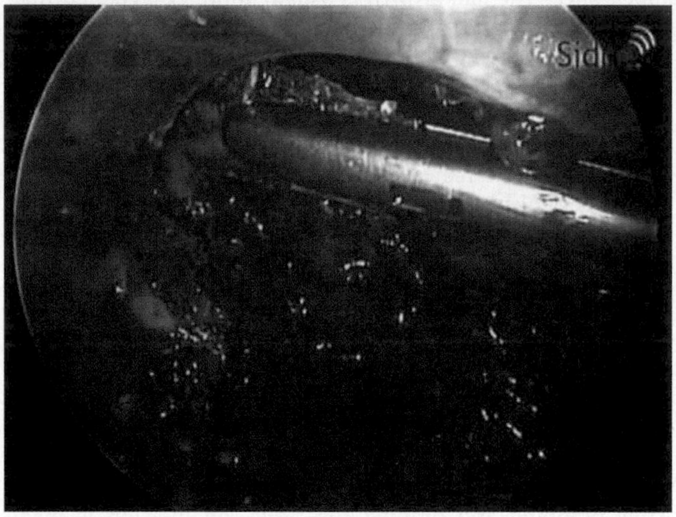

Figure 144-10. Piecemeal resection of the rib with Rongeurs.

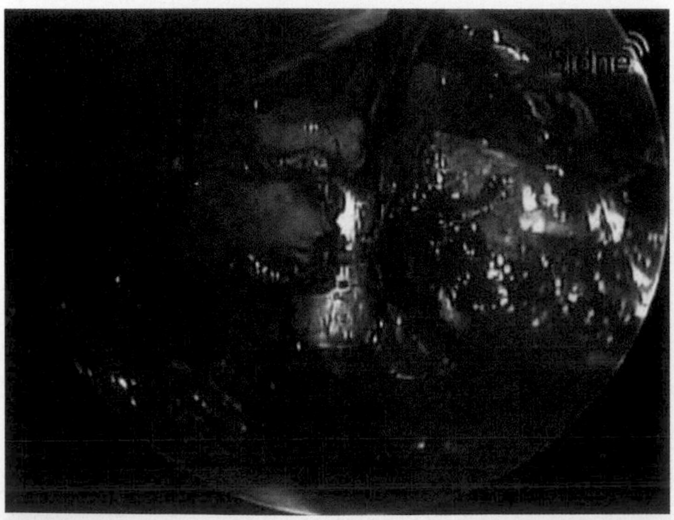

Figure 144-9. Protection of the vascular structures and brachial plexus during rib resection.

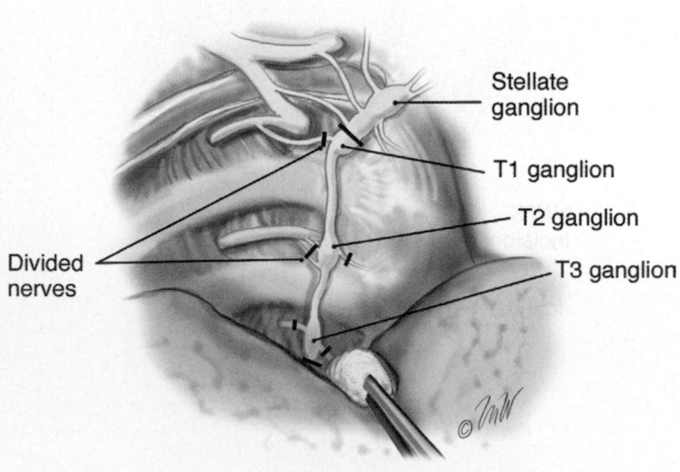

Figure 144-11. T1, T2, and T3 ganglia with the sympathetic chain are removed after clipping the gray and white afferent and efferent rami communicantes.

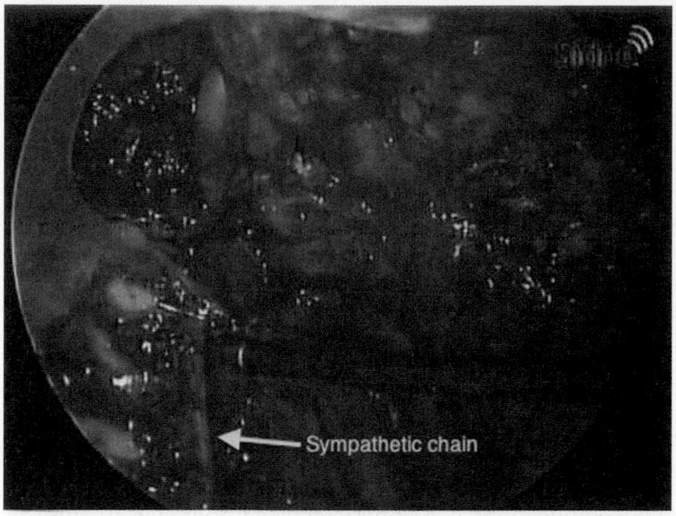

Figure 144-12. Sympathectomy. Notice the wide dissection area around the sympathetic chain to include potential collateral innervation.

and T1 nerve roots. The parietal pleura is dissected inferiorly from the T1 nerve root, and the dorsal sympathectomy chain is exposed (Figs. 144-11 and 144-12). Level T1, T2, and T3 ganglia with the sympathetic chain are removed after clipping the gray and white afferent and efferent rami communicantes (Fig. 144-13). The area is cauterized to minimize sprouting and regeneration. A 20-Fr chest tube is used to expand the lung after closing the incision (Fig. 144-14). A recent report of robotic-assisted first rib resection for Paget Schroetter shows the feasibility of this technique, although further refinement and investigation is needed to determine its role in the management of all the different varieties of TOS.[27]

COMPLICATIONS

Horner Syndrome

If the fibers of C7 and C8 (the upper part of the stellate ganglion) are removed, Horner syndrome results. This involves

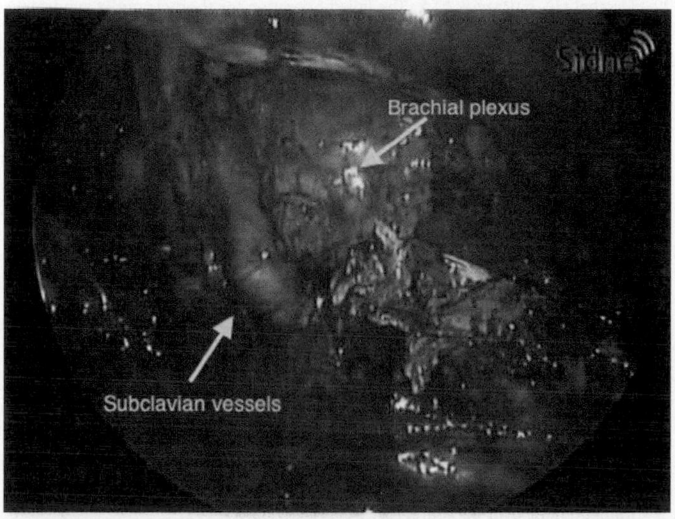

Figure 144-13. Decompressed thoracic outlet structures.

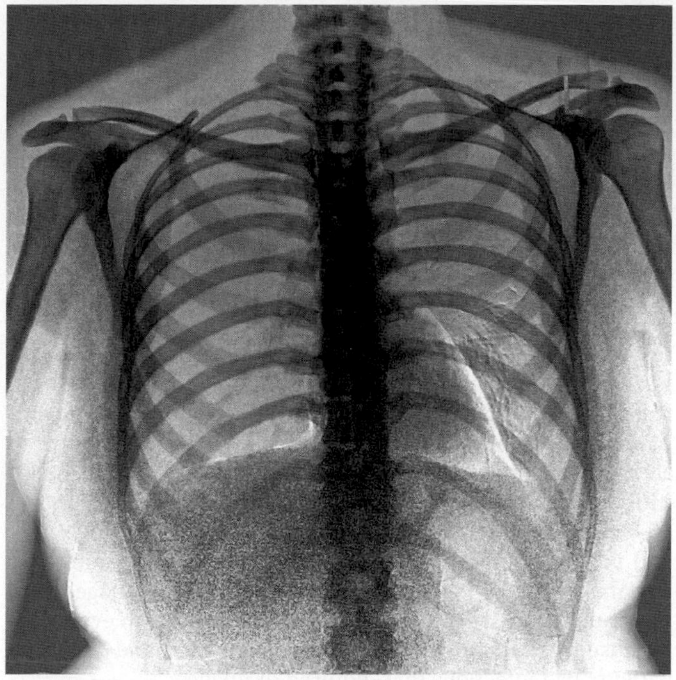

Figure 144-14. Chest radiograph after first rib resection.

miosis, enophthalmos, drooping of the eyelid (ptosis), and flushing of that side of the face with loss of sweating in that area (anhydrosis).[28]

Postsympathetic Neuralgia

The complication of postsympathectomy neuralgia is less common in the upper extremities than in the lower extremities. The pain usually occurs in the shoulder and upper arm on the lateral aspect. Clinical history usually substantiates this diagnosis if the symptoms occur within the first 3 months. The confirmation may be obtained by a test involving skin resistance of pseudomotor activity detection. Tests reveal increased sympathetic activity and suggest a rebound phenomenon from the nonsympathectomized adjacent dermatomes. Rebound may be a regeneration of nerve fibers or an increased response of peripheral nerves to catecholamines. Symptoms usually resolve in 3 to 6 weeks with conservative management. Phenytoin sodium (Dilantin), carbamazepine (Tegretol), and calcium channel blockers all are used in the medical management of these symptoms.[29]

Recurrent Symptoms

Occasionally, following an excellent sympathectomy, with a warm hand and good circulation, recurrent symptoms may recur as early as 3 months. These may be secondary to the regeneration or sprouting and rehooking of nerves or failure to strip the sympathetic nerves from the artery itself and the transfer of sympathetic tone through these nerves. Therefore, it is important to strip the axillary–subclavian artery of its local sympathetic nerves in each case at the initial operation.[30] Also, during the initial procedure, cauterization of the bed of the sympathectomy area produces sympathetic effects that usually last at least 3 years.

RESULTS

In a large series by Urschel,[31] sympathectomy alone or in conjunction with first rib removal for TOS was successful in 926 patients. In only six patients had sympathetic activity recur in less than 6 months. All of these patients were treated conservatively initially. Three required repeat sympathectomy. Postsympathectomy neuralgia occurred in only two of 926 patients. Both these patients were managed successfully in a conservative manner. In the patients in whom Horner syndrome was not created deliberately, four developed the syndrome. All resolved spontaneously in several months. Forty-two cases of Raynaud phenomena were treated successfully with first rib resection alone or with periarterial neurectomy without initial sympathectomy.[31] The results of reoperation are good if an accurate diagnosis is made and the proper procedure is used.[22] More than 1200 patients have been followed up for 6 months to 15 years. All patients improved initially after reoperation, and in 79%, the improvement was maintained for more than 5 years. In 14% of the patients, symptoms were managed with physiotherapy; 7% required a second reoperation, in every case because of rescarring. There were no deaths, and only two patients had infections that required drainage.[31]

SUMMARY

TOS is recognized in approximately 8% of the population. Its manifestations may be neurologic or vascular or both depending on the component of the neurovascular bundle predominantly compressed. The diagnosis is suspected from the clinical picture and usually is substantiated by determination of the UNCV. Treatment is conservative initially, but persistence of significant symptoms is an indication for first rib resection and occurs in approximately 5% of patients with diagnosed TOS. Primary resection is performed preferably through the thoracoscopic transaxillary approach. Symptoms of varying degrees may recur after first rib resection in approximately 10% of patients. Most of the patients improve with physiotherapy, and only 1.6% require reoperation. Reoperation for recurrent symptoms is performed through a high posterior thoracoplasty incision.[21,22,31] Careful patient selection based on clinical data and symptomatology is crucial for good surgical outcomes. Predictors of poor surgical decompressive outcomes include acute ischemia, established sensory or motor deficit, poorly systematized neurologic symptoms on presentation, extended resection of the first rib and severe postoperative complications.[32] A robotic-assisted approach to surgical management has been reported as feasible but remains to be proven safe and effective.

EDITOR'S COMMENT

Again, patient selection, initial conservative management, and surgical resection for specific indications are critically important. Video assistance for the surgical management of TOS, particularly when a dorsal sympathectomy is to be performed, offers better visualization of the anatomic structures important to identify for the safe conduct of this operation.

—Yolonda L. Colson

References

1. Rob CG, Standeven A. Arterial occlusion complicating thoracic outlet compression syndrome. *Br Med J.* 1958;2:709–712.
2. Clagett OT. Research and prosearch. *J Thorac Cardiovasc Surg.* 1962;44:153–166.
3. Urschel HC Jr, Paulson DL, McNamara JJ. Thoracic outlet syndrome. *Ann Thorac Surg.* 1968;6:1–10.
4. Swank W, Simeone F. The scalenus anticus syndrome. *Arch Neurol Psychiatry.* 1944;51:432.
5. Rosati L, Lord J. Neurovascular compression syndromes of the shoulder girdle. In: Rosati L, Lord J, eds. *Modern Surgical Monographs.* New York, NY: Grune & Stratton; 1961.
6. Upton ARM, McComas AJ. The double crush in nerve entrapment syndromes. *Lancet.* 1973;2:359–362.
7. Selmonosky CA, Byrd R, Blood C, et al. Useful triad for diagnosing the cause of chest pain. *South Med J.* 1981;74(8):947–949.
8. Urschel HC Jr, Razzuk MA, Hyland JW, et al. Thoracic outlet syndrome masquerading as coronary artery disease (pseudoangina). *Ann Thorac Surg.* 1973;16:239–248.
9. Urschel HC Jr. Management of the thoracic-outlet syndrome. *N Engl J Med.* 1972;286:1140–1143.
10. Rosenberg JC. Arteriographic demonstration of compression syndromes of the thoracic outlet. *South Med J.* 1966;59:400–403.
11. Adson A. Cervical ribs: symptoms and differential diagnosis for section of the scalenus anticus muscle. *J Int Coll Surg.* 1951;16:546–559.
12. Urschel HC Jr, Razzuk MA. Thoracic outlet syndrome. *Surg Annu.* 1973;5:229–263.
13. Yiannikas C, Walsh JC. Somatosensory evoked responses in the diagnosis of thoracic outlet syndrome. *J Neurol Neurosurg Psychiatry.* 1983;46:234–240.
14. Komanetsky RM, Novak CB, Mackinnon SE, et al. Somatosensory evoked potentials fail to diagnose thoracic outlet syndrome. *J Hand Surg Am.* 1996;21:622–666.
15. Caldwell JW, Crane CR, Krusen EM. Nerve conduction studies: an aid in the diagnosis of the thoracic outlet syndrome. *South Med J.* 1971;64:210–212.
16. Krusen EM. Cervical pain syndromes. *Arch Phys Med Rehabil.* 1968;49:376–382.
17. Lang EK. Roentgenographic diagnosis of the neurovascular compression syndromes. *Radiology.* 1962;79:58–63.
18. Falconer M, Li F. Resection of the first rib in costoclavicular compression of the brachial plexus. *Lancet.* 1962;11:59–63.
19. Roos DB, Owens JC. Thoracic outlet syndrome. *Arch Surg.* 1966;93:71–74.
20. Martinez N. Posterior first rib resection for total thoracic outlet syndrome decompression. *Contemp Surg.* 1979;15:13–21.
21. Urschel HC Jr, Razzuk MA, Albers JE, et al. Reoperation for recurrent thoracic outlet syndrome. *Ann Thorac Surg.* 1976;21:19–25.
22. Urschel HC Jr, Razzuk MA. The failed operation for thoracic outlet syndrome: the difficulty of diagnosis and management. *Ann Thorac Surg.* 1986;42:523–528.
23. Cooley D, Wukasch D. *Techniques in Vascular Surgery.* Philadelphia, PA: Saunders; 1979:211–212.
24. Kuntz A. Distribution of the sympathetic rami to the brachial plexus: its relation to sympathectomy affecting the upper extremity. *Arch Surg.* 1927;15:871–877.
25. Palumbo LT. Upper dorsal sympathectomy without Horner's syndrome. *AMA Arch Surg.* 1955;71:743–751.
26. Mackinnon S, Dellon A. *Surgery of the Peripheral Nerve.* New York, NY: Thieme Medical; 1988:210–214.
27. Gharagozloo F, Margolis M, Meyer M, et al. Robotic Thoracoscopic first rib resection for Paget Schroetter disease. www.ctsnet.org/sections/clinicalresources/thoracic/expert_tech-49.html.
28. Galbraith NF, Urschel HC Jr, Wood RE, et al. Fracture of first rib associated with laceration of subclavian artery: report of a case and review of the literature. *J Thorac Cardiovasc Surg.* 1973;65:649–652.
29. Litwin MS. Postsympathectomy neuralgia. *Arch Surg.* 1962;84:591–595.
30. Urschel HC Jr. Dorsal sympathectomy and management of thoracic outlet syndrome with VATS. *Ann Thorac Surg.* 1993;56:717–720.
31. Urschel HC Jr. Neurovascular compression in the thoracic outlet: changing management over 50 years. *Adv Surg.* 1999;33:95–111.
32. DeGeorges R, Reynaud C, Becquemin JP. Thoracic outlet syndrome surgery: long term functional results. *Ann Vasc Surg.* 2004;18(5):558–565.

145 Thrombosis of the Subclavian Vein: Paget–Schroetter Syndrome

J. Ernesto Molina and Michael T. Jaklitsch

Keywords: Effort thrombosis, venous thoracic outlet syndrome

Paget–Schroetter syndrome is the sudden thrombosis of the subclavian vein in the setting of physical exertion of the arm. This syndrome is also known as effort thrombosis. It is the most extreme presentation of the venous form of thoracic outlet syndrome. It is a rare disease of active young people engaged in physical exertion of the arm (e.g., mechanics, rock climbers, swimmers, and weight lifters). Specifically, it is the forceful movement of pulling the extended arm from over the head down toward the torso that leads to the underlying basis of the disease; hypertrophy of the subclavius and anterior scalene muscles.

The subclavius is a triangular muscle that originates from the groove on the undersurface of the clavicle and inserts by thick tendon into the cartilaginous portion of the first rib. The subclavius muscle depresses the shoulder by drawing the clavicle downward and forward. The anterior scalene muscle arises from the transverse processes of the third to sixth cervical vertebrae and inserts into the scalene tubercle on top of the first rib, separating the subclavian artery and vein. When an arm extended over the head is pulled down vigorously toward the torso, the anterior scalene fixes the first rib into position, anchoring it against the transverse processes of the neck. The subclavius muscle, in turn, anchors on the fixed first rib and pulls the shoulder down by displacing the clavicle.[1]

The sudden and forceful pulling down of the arm toward the torso is accompanied by the powerful contraction of the anterior scalene and subclavius muscles. The hypertrophied subclavius muscle in particular appears to be the cause of the pathologic injury. The sudden and powerful compression of the subclavian vein between these two muscles is sufficient to tear the intima of the vein, and thrombosis occurs (Fig. 145-1). The clot then propagates distally toward the shoulder. Thrombolysis or anticoagulation alone is insufficient to correct the clinical manifestations or to prevent recurrence. First rib resection with division of the two muscles prevents recurrence. The exposure given by an axillary approach to divide these muscles is inadequate and therefore not recommended.[2] A subclavicular approach not only allows division of these muscles but also permits patch angioplasty of the vein.

DIAGNOSIS AND WORKUP

Paget–Schroetter syndrome is a clinical diagnosis confirmed by duplex ultrasound and venogram. The ipsilateral arm frequently is swollen with distended veins up to the shoulder. Range of motion of the arm is impaired as a result of pain. If not treated immediately, the patient may be left with a chronic debilitating condition that limits use of the arm. Lysis of the clot alone or anticoagulation alone is inadequate therapy. The surgeon must be prepared to divide the compressive muscles and to perform a patch angioplasty of the vein to restore its normal caliber. We describe the operative approaches to affect this type of repair.

Paget–Schroetter syndrome is rare, and the average surgeon may see only a few cases across a career. J. Ernesto Molina is a cardiothoracic surgeon at the University of Minnesota who developed an interest in treatment protocols for this disease. He has educated a generation of surgeons from the University of Minnesota program, and this chapter is indebted to his work.[3–6]

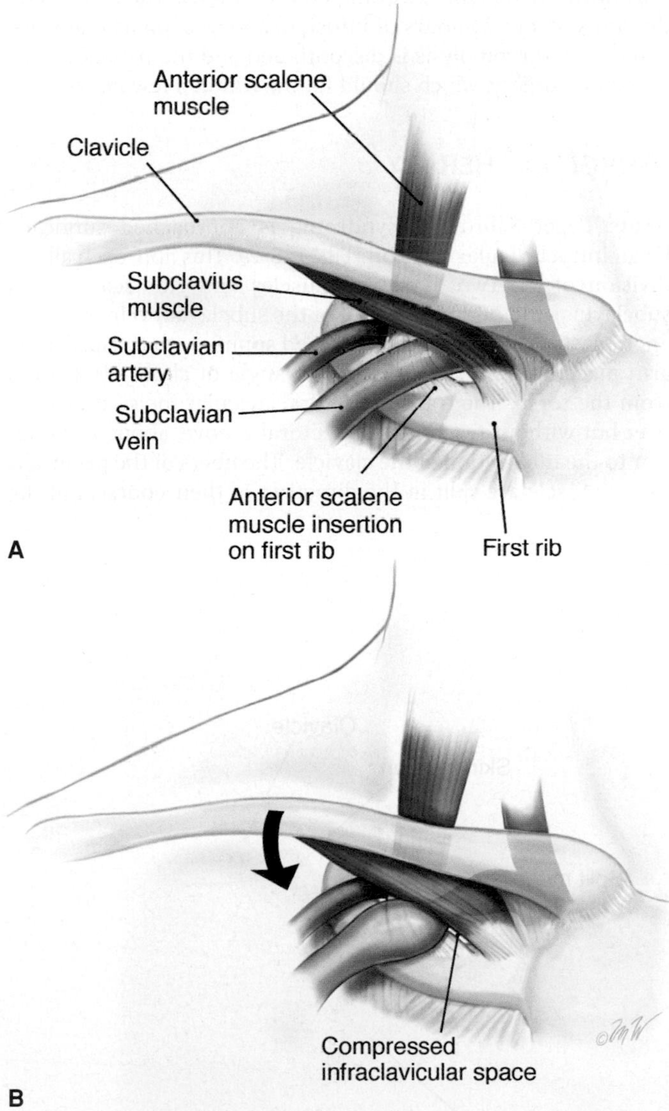

Figure 145-1. *A.* In the relaxed normal position, the subclavian vein runs between the subclavius muscle tendon and the anterior scalene muscle. The floor of the tunnel through which the vein runs is formed by the first rib. *B.* Under tension, the vein is pinched severely between the subclavius tendon and the anterior scalene muscle. The intimal injury evolves into acute thrombosis of the vessel.

The diagnosis of Paget–Schroetter syndrome is based on history, physical examination, and Doppler assessment of the ipsilateral axillary and subclavian veins. The history is one of recent efforts of the ipsilateral arm and sudden pain. The physical examination generally reveals a swollen and functionally impaired forearm and hand. Although distention of arm veins is seen commonly, development of venous collaterals around the shoulder is a late finding and suggestive of a chronic condition. Doppler ultrasound shows venous occlusion with thrombosis of various extent.

At the University of Minnesota since the early 1990s, this diagnosis has been followed by the placement of a venous catheter, which is advanced into the clot. The catheter provides access for a venogram to assess the length of the clot, as well as for local delivery of fibrinolytics. Although urokinase was initially used as our preferred thrombolytic agent in the 1980s, this now has been supplanted by recombinant tissue plasminogen activator (Activase, Alteplase, TNK-TPA). The catheter-directed infusion of thrombolytics at recommended doses is a very safe procedure with no systemic bleeding complications. The clot always dissolves within 24 hours of infusion, and as soon as that stage is reached, thrombolysis is discontinued and the patient is prepared for surgery, which should follow within a few hours.

SURGICAL THERAPY

Acute Paget–Schroetter syndrome is approached surgically by an infraclavicular incision (Fig. 145-2). This approach allows division of the two causative muscles (anterior scalene and subclavius) and permits control of the subclavian vein for patch angioplasty. The patient is positioned supine with the ipsilateral arm placed on an arm board at an angle of about 60 degrees from the torso. The transverse infraclavicular incision extends over but without reaching the pectoral groove, about 1 in inferior to the midsection of the clavicle. The fibers of the pectoralis major muscle are split in the direction of their course, but the muscle is not divided. The first rib is identified as soon as the retromuscular space is reached (Fig. 145-3).

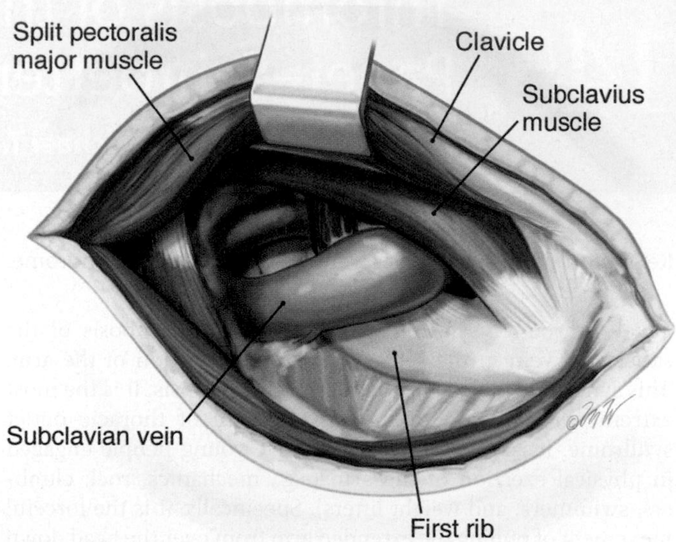

Figure 145-3. The fibers of the pectoralis major muscle are separated, exposing the retromuscular space showing the structures of the thoracic inlet.

The subclavius muscle is identified in the medial aspect of the incision, inserting onto the top surface of the most medial extent of the first rib. The subclavius muscle is divided off its insertion onto the top of the first rib, reflected laterally, and then excised (Fig. 145-4). The subclavian vein is exposed immediately upon removal of the subclavius muscle. The subclavian vein is mobilized and detached from its surrounding tissues. The next *very important step* is to incise the inferior border of the first rib and proceed to detach the inferior periosteum along the entire length of the exposed rib until a space is created behind the rib in the extrapleural plane (Fig. 145-5). This precaution will prevent the occurrence of pneumothorax that sometimes is reported as a complication of this type of surgery. Once the pleura is detached completely from the posterior/inferior

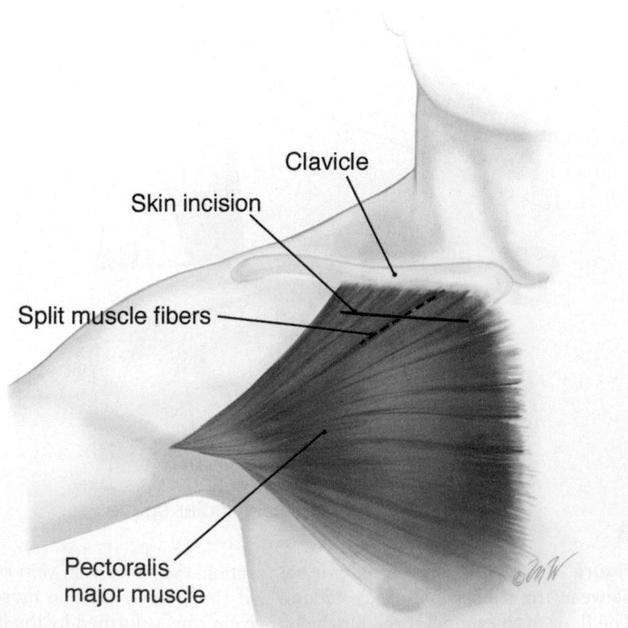

Figure 145-2. Subclavicular incision over the pectoralis major muscle to approach the subclavian vein.

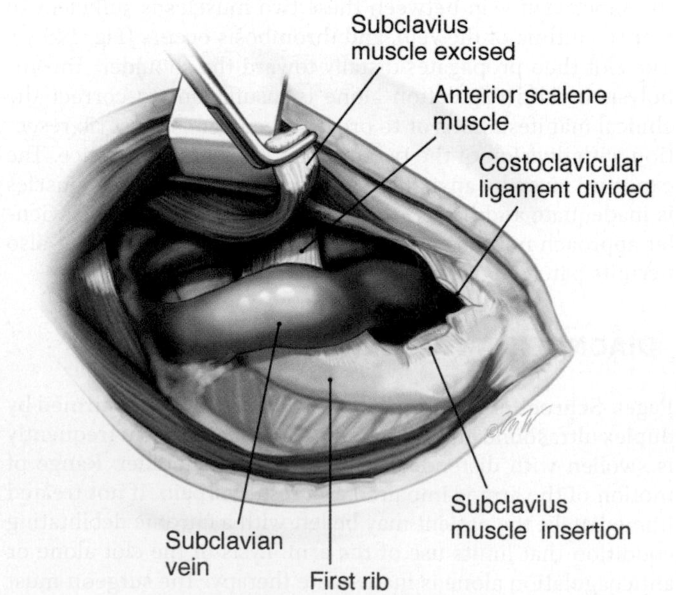

Figure 145-4. The subclavian muscle is identified, divided off its insertion into the top surface of the medial extent of the first rib, and excised. The costoclavicular ligament is divided.

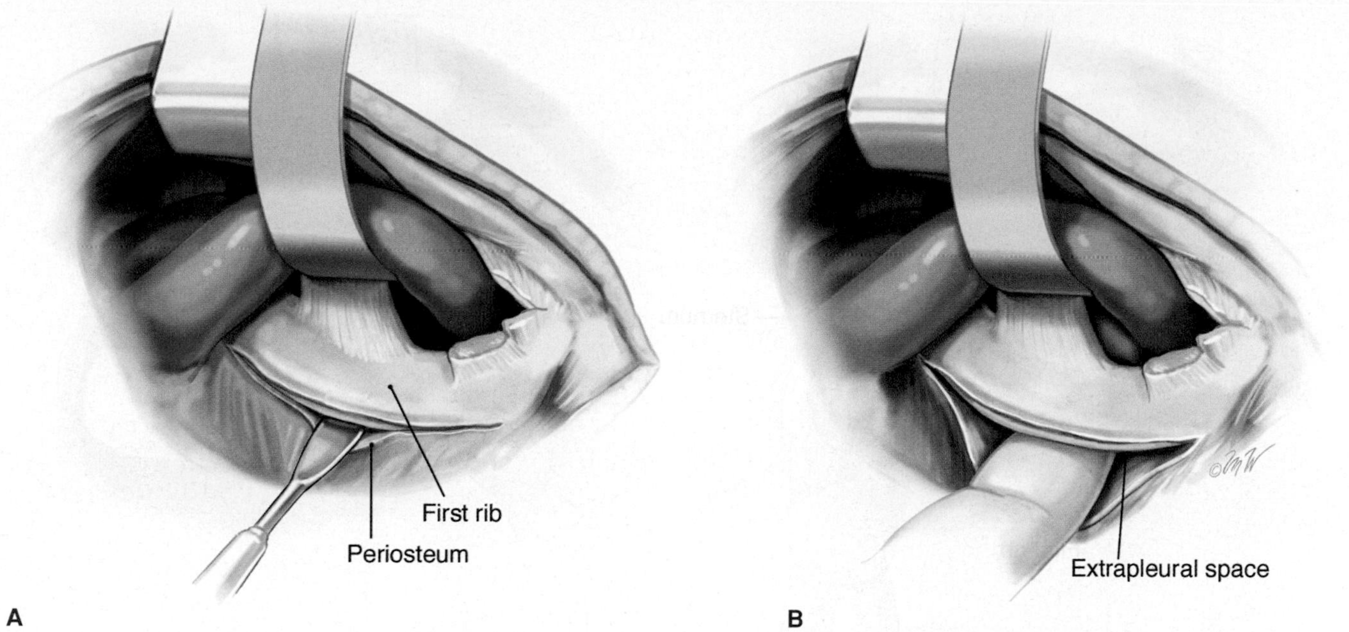

Figure 145-5. *A*. Performing a subperiosteal detachment of the first rib to create an extrapleural space before attempting to divide the anterior scalene muscle is the most important step in this operation to prevent pneumothorax. *B*. The extrapleural space should be large enough to permit digital separation of the pleura from the first rib.

surface of the rib, the pleura is bluntly pushed away from the undersurface of the first rib, and at this point the anterior scalene muscle is safely divided retracting the subclavian vein superiorly (Fig. 145-6). The medial end of the first rib is divided flush to the sternum taking care not to injure the internal mammary vessels.

The first rib is then displaced caudally with downward traction on the broad surface of the rib. If the rib has not yet been divided, this maneuver will stretch the anterior scalene muscle into view posterior to the subclavian vein. This muscle now is divided from its attachment into the scalene tubercle of the midsection of the first rib. The rib is then displaced caudally even more readily. A rib cutter is used to divide the rib posteriorly at the level where the subclavian artery crosses the rib

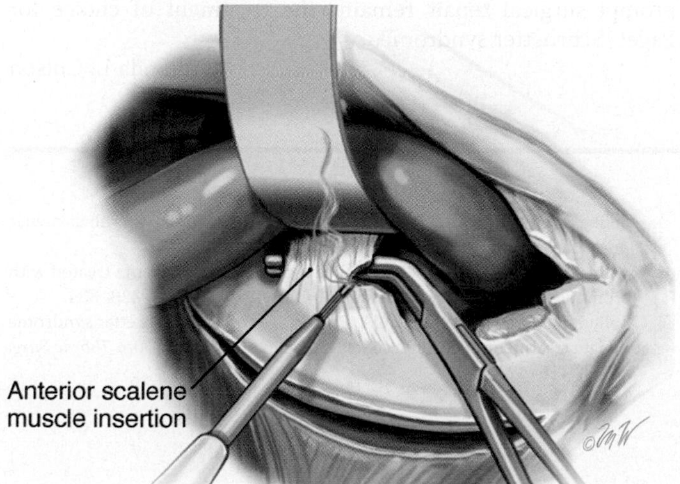

Figure 145-6. The anterior scalene muscle now can be approached safely and divided without injuring the pleura.

(Fig. 145-7). To implant a patch on the vein, vascular clamps are used to obtain both proximal and distal control. To achieve this stage the vein needs to be carefully dissected off the posterior surface of the manubrium of the sternum until the innominate vein can be brought gently into the operative field. The vein is incised longitudinally and a vein patch is used to enlarge the area of stenosis (Fig. 145-8). Saphenous vein harvested from the upper thigh is used for this patch. If a long segment of the vein is stenosed, a long vein patch is constructed using the proximal saphenous vein with its larger diameter.

POSTOPERATIVE CARE

Postoperative anticoagulation is implemented for a total of 8 weeks with warfarin (Coumadin) and clopidogrel (Plavix). Dabigatran may be used instead of the latter drugs, with the advantage that it does not require any periodic blood tests to monitor the level of anticoagulation. Although dextran and low-molecular-weight heparin are used in the early postoperative period, these drugs are discontinued when the international normalization ratio (INR) level reaches the therapeutic range, which is optimally maintained between 2 and 3. To ensure the effectiveness of the operation, a subclavian venogram is obtained the same day of the surgery to assess the status of the vein repair. If significant stenosis persists in any area, placement of an endovascular stent may be necessary. This usually works very well once the extrinsic compression of the vein has been released. For follow-up purposes an ultrasound is obtained the next day after surgery and is repeated at 4 and 8 weeks postoperatively.

SUMMARY

Paget–Schroetter syndrome is an acute thrombosis of the subclavian vein often related to exertional physical activity of

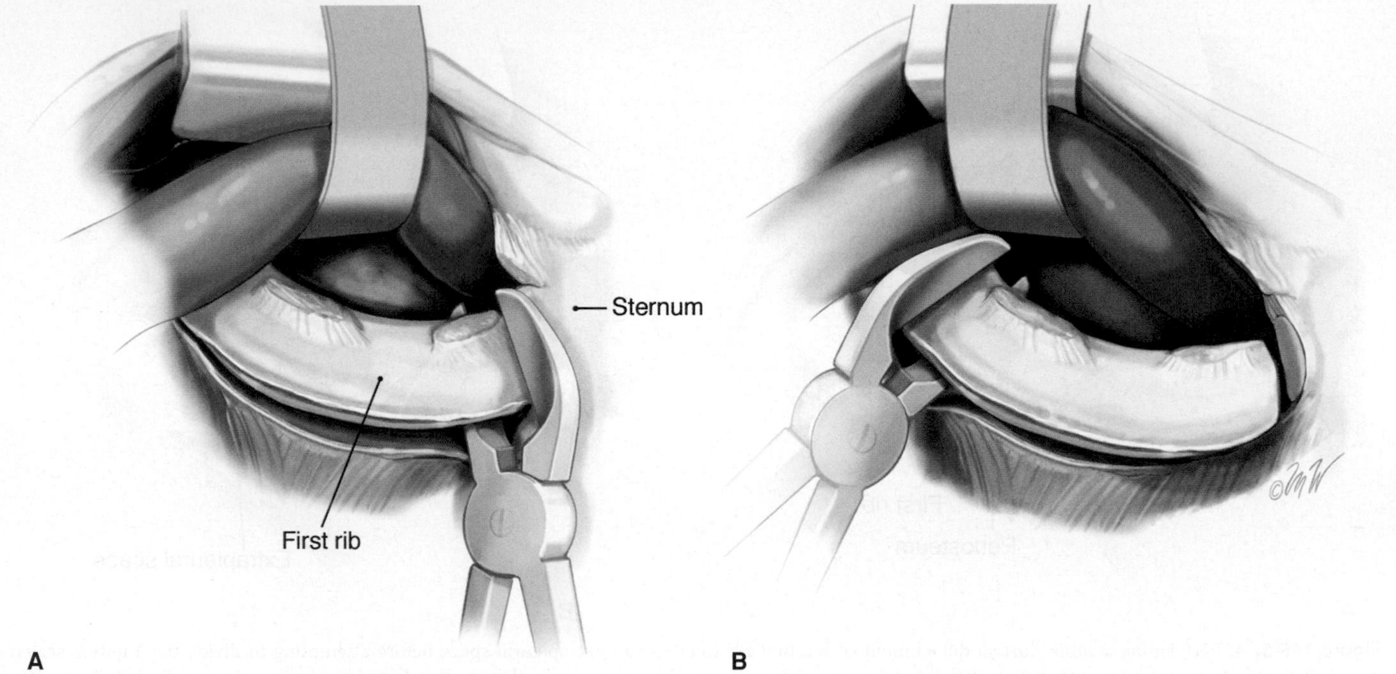

Figure 145-7. *A.* The first rib is divided at its sternal insertion anteriorly and at the level of the subclavian artery posteriorly. *B.* The rib is excised.

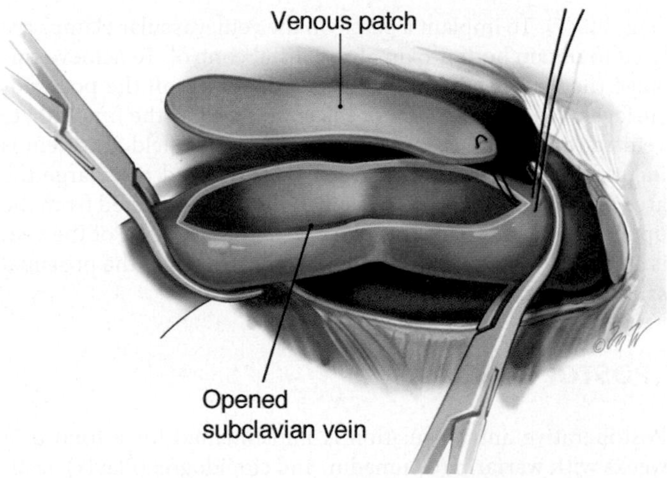

Figure 145-8. Placement of a venous patch over the structure of the subclavian vein.

the arm. It affects mostly young, healthy people and requires emergency care. The standard treatment entails immediate thrombolytic therapy by catheter-directed infusion followed by surgery. The operation involves decompression of the thoracic inlet and reestablishment of the normal caliber and flow of the vein. By following this approach, one can prevent the chronic sequela of total arm vein obstruction and the consequent permanent disability of the patient.

EDITOR'S COMMENT

Despite advancements in the field of interventional radiology and the development of stents, thrombolysis followed by prompt surgical repair remains the treatment of choice for Paget–Schroetter syndrome.

—Yolonda L. Colson

References

1. Gray H. *Anatomy, Descriptive and Surgical.* 15th ed. New York, NY: Bounty Books; 1977.
2. Molina JE. Reoperations after failed transaxillary first rib resections to treat Paget-Schroetter syndrome patients. *Ann Thorac Surg.* 2011;91:1717–1722.
3. Molina JE. Surgery for effort thrombosis of the subclavian vein. *J Thorac Cardiovasc Surg.* 1992;103:341–346.
4. Molina JE: Operative technique of first rib resection via subclavicular approach. *Vasc Surg.* 1993;27:667–672.
5. Molina JE, Hunter DW, Dietz CA. Paget-Schroetter syndrome treated with thrombolytics and immediate surgery. *J Vasc Surg.* 2007;45:328–334.
6. Molina JE, Hunter DW, Dietz CA. Protocols for Paget-Schroetter syndrome and late treatment of chronic subclavian vein obstruction. *Ann Thorac Surg.* 2009;87:416–422.

146 Thoracoscopic Sympathectomy for Hyperhidrosis and Vasomotor Disorders

Amit Bhargava and Steven M. Keller

Keywords: Thermoregulation, sympathetic chain, palmar hyperhidrosis, plantar hyperhidrosis, complex regional pain syndrome

INTRODUCTION

Video-assisted thoracoscopy has largely replaced other approaches to the intrathoracic sympathetic chain. Thoracoscopic sympathectomy is most commonly performed for the treatment of severe palmar hyperhidrosis but can be performed for axillary hyperhidrosis, facial sweating, and facial blushing. In addition, thoracoscopic sympathectomy has been used to treat patients with rare vasomotor disorders and chronic pain syndromes of the upper extremities.

HYPERHIDROSIS

Hyperhidrosis is the pathologic condition of sweating in excess of physiologic requirements for thermoregulation. This excess sweating can be quantified in comparison with the general populace, but patients usually present with a typical history. The typical hyperhidrosis patient is young, between 18 and 25 years old and has had palmar and plantar sweating since early childhood. Parents may recall inordinate wetness of the hands and feet during infancy. Patients may recall grade school classmates refusing to hold their hands because of excessive wetness or teachers scolding them for submitting wet, smudged assignments. Puddles of sweat can accumulate on computer and piano keyboards. Entering adulthood, wet hands adversely affect social interaction and influence career choice.

Sweating is sporadic, occurs during periods of stress or calm, and is usually worse during the summer. Although the degree of hyperhidrosis varies, the sweating is much greater than the dampness associated with stress. Within minutes, a dry hand can become soaked, with sweat dripping to the floor. The volar surface of the fingers, thenar and hypothenar eminences, and palmar skin folds fill with perspiration (Fig. 146-1).

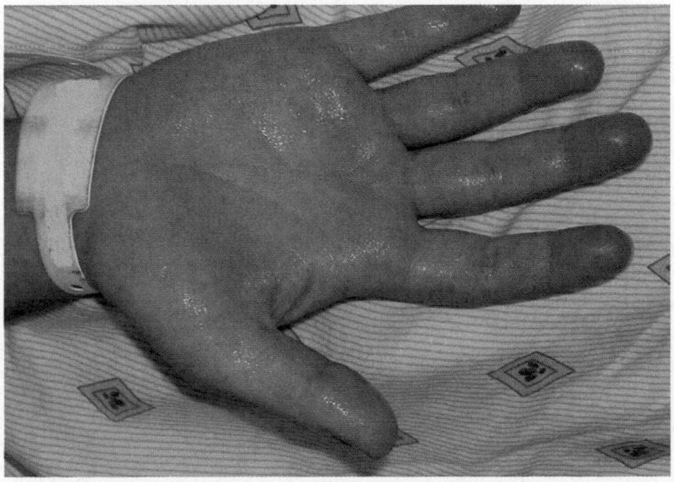

Figure 146-1. Typical appearance of palmar hyperhidrosis. Note wetness on thenar and hypothenar eminences as well as on palmar surface of distal phalanges.

Hyperhidrosis sufferers avoid direct or indirect hand contact and have a handkerchief or tissue always available. Characteristic wiping of the hands on their clothing is noticeable. The damp hands are disguised in social situations by a cold drink held in the right hand. This provides an explanation for the dampness and the need to wipe the hand prior to a handshake.

Concomitant plantar hyperhidrosis occurs in nearly all patients with palmar hyperhidrosis. When walking barefoot, wet footprints are created which are similar to those seen after exiting a shower. Though fungal infections are rare, the constant moistness ruins footwear. Axillary hyperhidrosis with associated garment staining and odor (bromhidrosis) is present in as many as 50% of patients with palmar and plantar hyperhidrosis.[1–4]

Epidemiology

The prevalence of palmar and plantar hyperhidrosis is estimated to be 0.6% to 1% and affects all racial groups.[5] Severe axillary hyperhidrosis affects 1.4% of the United States population.[6] Patients with classic palmar and plantar hyperhidrosis do not have concomitant illnesses. In contrast, generalized hyperhidrosis, which is treated medically, may be associated with thyrotoxicosis, obesity, neurologic diseases, and rare inherited disorders.

Up to 65% of patients who have undergone sympathetic surgery have a familial history of hyperhidrosis.[2,7] In one study, analysis of the kindred data of 49 affected individuals led to the conclusion that the disease allele is present in 5% of the population.[7] One study of 11 families mapped a locus for primary palmar hyperhidrosis to chromosome 14.[8]

Anatomy and Function

Overall, thermoregulation is controlled by the autonomic nervous system with the sympathetic system primarily in control of extremity sweating. Sympathetic fibers originating from spinal levels T1 to T8 ascend in the sympathetic chain and commonly reach the brachial plexus via the stellate ganglia. However, alternate pathways from the T2 and T3 ganglia that bypass the stellate ganglia have been demonstrated.[9] The precise spinal levels responsible for palmar sweating have not been defined. Eccrine sweat glands located in the palm, axilla and face are stimulated by release of acetylcholine from postganglionic neurons.

The sympathetic chain descends vertically within the thorax over the rib heads (Fig. 146-2). Rarely, it is found between the medial border of the rib head and the collus longus muscle.[10] The sympathetic ganglia are located approximately 2 mm cranial to the midportion of the underlying vertebral body.

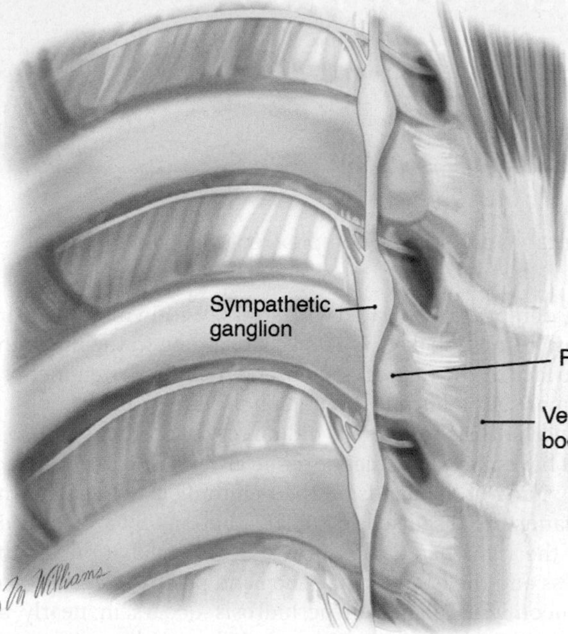

Figure 146-2. The sympathetic chain descends vertically over the rib heads. Descending arterial vessel crosses the right second rib lateral to the sympathetic chain.

Whether hyperhidrosis is emblematic of a global autonomic nervous system dysfunction or it represents a focal abnormality remains unknown. Room temperature resting palmar sweat production is twice normal.[11] The sudomotor skin response is enhanced as a result of shortened nerve recovery time.[12] Palmar sweat production in response to stress is greatly increased (Fig. 146-3). Pulmonary function and resting cardiac function in the supine position are normal when compared with unaffected controls.[13] Plasma catecholamine levels are within normal limits.[14] However, peak exercise heart rate and resting heart rate in the standing position are increased.[13,15] The ultrastructure of hyperhidrotic axillary eccrine glands is normal.[16]

Treatment

Nonoperative

Aluminum chloride hexahydrate, 20% anhydrous ethyl alcohol solution (Drysol™), a highly concentrated liquid preparation of the active underarm antiperspirant ingredient, may be applied daily to the affected area prior to sleep. The effect may be from blockage of the sweat gland ducts or by atrophy of the secretory cells. The hands or feet are covered in plastic wrap to prevent damage to clothing or bedding. Once the desired anhidrosis is obtained, application frequency is decreased but must be continued for lasting effect. Side effects include rash and paradoxical hyperhidrosis. Many patients report therapeutic failure as efficacy in palmar hyperhidrosis has not been assessed in a controlled trial. A randomized trial compared botulinum toxin A to a topical 20% aluminum chloride administration in patients with axillary hyperhidrosis and showed greater effectiveness in the botulinum toxin group, although the study was only 12 weeks in duration.[17]

Botulinum Toxin A (Botox®) stops sweat production by blocking the release of acetylcholine from the postganglionic nerve end. Randomized trials have demonstrated efficacy of this treatment for both palmar and axillary hyperhidrosis.[18,19] Median duration of sweat control varies between 6 and 9 months. Each treatment session involves multiple injections as well. Weakness of the intrinsic muscles of the hand has been reported in 25% to 60% of patients. Botulinum Toxin A injections may represent the treatment of choice for axillary hyperhidrosis.

In one study, iontophoresis was reported to control palmar hyperhidrosis in 82% of 112 patients who underwent daily 15-minute treatment over 8 days.[20] This treatment involves placing the hands or feet in a tap water solution through which electric current flows (Drionic®). Anhidrosis is thought to result from electrically induced precipitation of salts in the sweat ducts. The mean remission was 35 days. Tingling, erythema, and vesicle formation were undesirable side effects.

Oral anticholinergic medications such as glycopyrrolate and oxybutynin have the theoretic ability to block the stimulation of the sweat gland caused by the release of acetylcholine. One hundred and eighty consecutive patients at a single institution were treated with escalating doses of oxybutynin to a maximum of 10 mg per day. Patients were evaluated over a 12-week treatment period, with 80% experiencing improvement in their symptoms and with almost 75% having a quality of life improvement over the 12 weeks. Dry mouth was the most common symptom (70.5%), with 28.7% having severe symptoms. Sixty-eight percent of patients had little to no dry mouth. Very few had other symptoms, including headache (3.6%) and urinary retention (2.8%). One weakness of this study was that 22% of patients were lost to follow-up, leaving open the possibility of a higher failure rate.[21]

Surgery

Interruption of sympathetic innervation may be achieved by transection of the sympathetic chain, crushing the sympathetic chain with clips, or transection of the rami communicante. Resection of ganglia is not necessary, and in fact, it may be difficult to locate the ganglia because of frequent anatomic

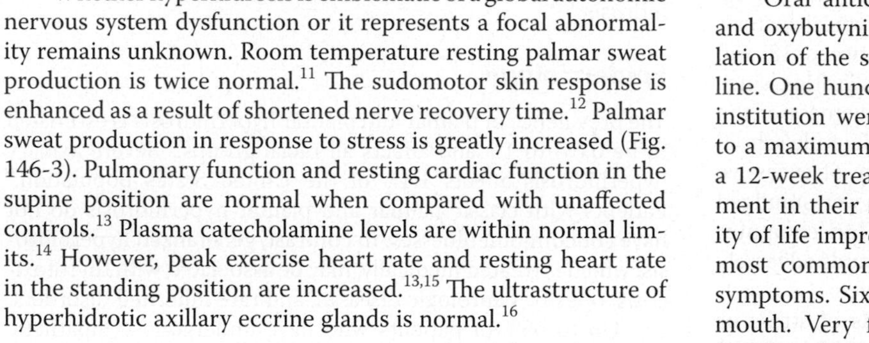

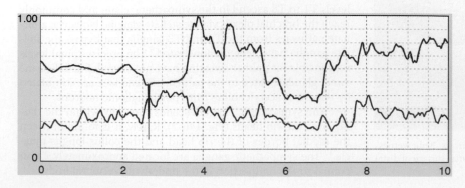

Figure 146-3. Abnormal sweat response. Attachment of the measuring device (Skin Moisture Meter SKD 2000; Skinos Co., LTD, Japan) causes anxiety and the baseline never reaches normal. The response to the stimulus is many times greater than a normal subject. The ordinate is in minutes and the abscissa in cc's moisture. *Upper line*: Thenar eminence. *Lower line*: Forehead (control).

Table 146-1

STS EXPERT CONSENSUS RECOMMENDATIONS[21]

SITE	RECOMMENDED OPERATION[a]
Palmar	R3 or R4
Palmar – Axillary	R4 and R5
Palmar – Axillary – Plantar	
Axillary	R4 and R5 or R5 alone
Craniofacial without blushing	R2 alone or R2 and R3

[a]Cauterizing or clipping to achieve interruption of the sympathetic chain.

variability and the presence of mediastinal fat. Recently, the Society of Thoracic Surgeons (STS) and the International Society on Sympathetic Surgery copublished a consensus opinion regarding hyperhidrosis, recommending a uniform rib-oriented nomenclature for hyperhidrosis surgery (Table 146-1).[22] Cauterization at the third rib would be referred to as "cauterized R3, top."[22] A clipped chain at the fourth rib would be "clipped R4, top."

The thoracic level(s) necessary to achieve the desired anhidrosis while minimizing systemic side effects is not known precisely. Palmar hyperhidrosis has been treated by transecting the sympathetic chain individually over the second (T2), third (T3), or fourth rib (T4) or some combination thereof.[1,2,4,23–30] During the past decade, several randomized controlled trials have evaluated the optimal levels at which to interrupt the sympathetic chain in order to control palmar hyperhidrosis and minimize morbidity.[25–29] The STS expert consensus document reviewed multiple randomized controlled trials, as well as prospective and retrospective studies. For isolated palmar hyperhidrosis, the STS expert consensus group recommends a top of the third rib (R3) or fourth rib (R4) sympathectomy.[8] This recommendation is largely based on two studies: one, a randomized controlled trial of 141 consecutive patients randomized to a cauterized, top R3 or cauterized, top R4 treatment,[29] and the other a larger, retrospective study which compared R4 to R3 and R2 operations.[30] Each study showed very good efficacy in all the groups, but slightly increased wetness in the palms in the R4 groups, although with decreased compensatory hyperhidrosis and decreased incidence of overly dry palms.[29,30] The Expert Consensus Group also makes recommendations regarding other levels of hyperhidrosis. It states that palmar-axillary or axillary sweating can be treated by transecting the sympathetic chain at the R5 level alone or the combined R4 to R5 levels.[22] These recommendations for a uniform nomenclature and levels of interruption were made with the goal of allowing for improved analysis of techniques and outcomes with a view towards the creation of robust evidence-based guidelines.[22] Each specific recommendation for treatment is based on a few small, single-institution studies and should be evaluated by each surgeon in the light of his or her own experience as well. In general, transecting more levels yields more compensatory hyperhidrosis.[31]

Correct identification of the anatomic level is imperative. The second rib is generally the most proximal rib that can be seen within the thorax. It can be reliably identified by a vertical descending arterial branch that originates from the subclavian artery. This vessel forms the second intercostal artery (Fig. 146-4) and crosses the rib 1 cm lateral to the sympathetic chain.[32] The first intercostal space is covered by a fat-pad and the first rib is rarely visible from within the thorax. Additional landmarks are the azygos vein, which lies at the level of the right fifth interspace and the aortic arch, which reaches to the left fourth interspace. The rib number can be determined with certainty by obtaining an intraoperative x-ray after a metallic marker has been introduced into the chest and placed over a rib.

Outpatient bilateral endoscopic thoracic sympathectomy is currently the operation of choice for the surgical treatment of palmar hyperhidrosis. Results are uniformly excellent and virtually all patients will have dry warm hands. Axillary and facial sweating may also be treated in a similar fashion, also with good results. The details of the operation are determined by the level at which the sympathetic chain is clipped or transected.

Technique

General anesthesia is induced with a single lumen endotracheal tube. The patient remains supine and the arms are abducted 90 degrees. The head of the operating table is elevated or the table is flexed into the semi-Fowler position. A 1-cm incision is made over the third interspace in the anterior axillary line lateral to the pectoralis major muscle (Fig. 146-5). CO_2 gas (600–1200 cc) is insufflated via a Veress needle and a 10 mm trochar is introduced under direct vision (VISIPORT*PLUS, Autosuture). The operating thoracoscopic (Karl Storz 26037 AA) is inserted and

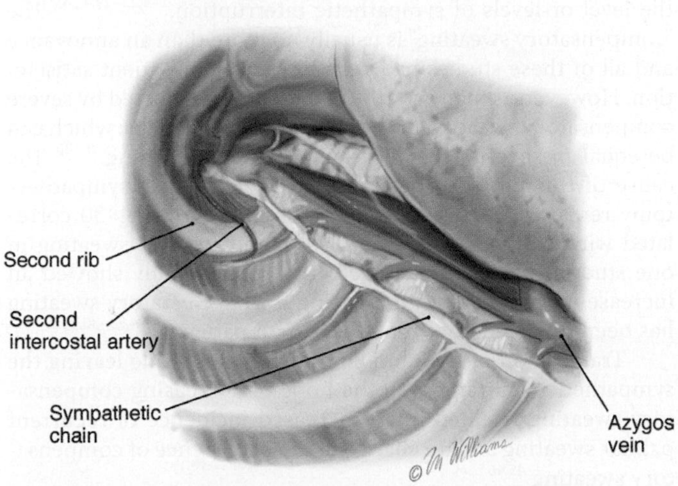

Figure 146-4. The descending arterial vessel crosses the right second rib lateral to the sympathetic chain.

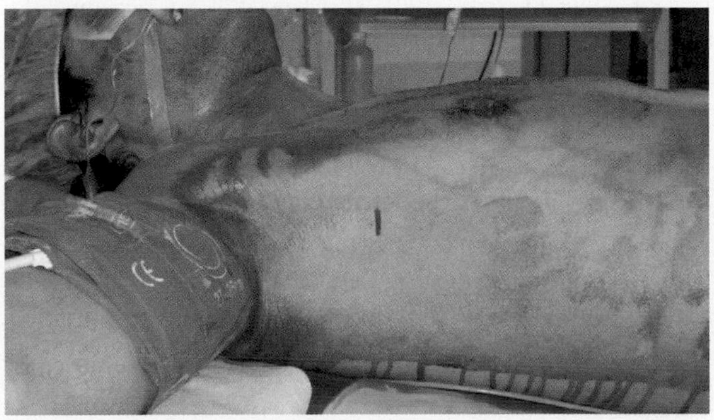

Figure 146-5. The patient is placed in the supine position with both arms perpendicular to the torso. A 1 cm incision is made lateral to the pectoralis major muscle at the level of the axillary hairline.

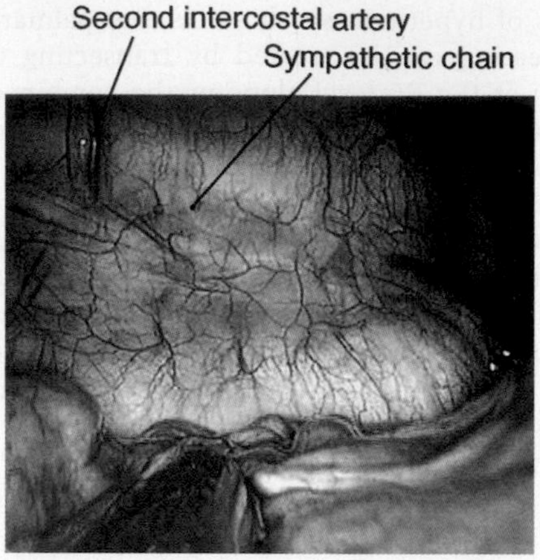

Figure 146-6. Thoracoscopic visualization of sympathetic chain.

the sympathetic chain visualized (Fig. 146-6). A cautery device is introduced via the operating thoracoscope.

Palmar hyperhidrosis is treated by clipping or transection at R3 or R4, whereas palmar hyperhidrosis and concomitant axillary hyperhidrosis can be treated by transecting the sympathetic chain at the R5 level alone or the combined R4 to R5 level. Isolated axillary hyperhidrosis may also be treated by transecting the sympathetic chain at T3 to T4, though subcutaneous axillary Botox® injection is another alternative. Craniofacial hyperhidrosis is treated by transecting the sympathetic chain at the T2 level.[33]

Hemorrhage can occur from venous branches that occasionally cross the sympathetic chain. Rarely, injury to a major arterial or venous vessel is caused by misplacement of the trochar or cautery. In addition, the intercostal vasculature can be injured while placing the trochar. Hemostasis is ascertained and the lung inflated under direct vision as the trochar is withdrawn. The wound is closed and the identical procedure repeated in the contralateral thorax. A postoperative chest x-ray frequently demonstrates small apical pneumothoraces. Chest tubes are not required. When awake and comfortable, the patient is discharged.

Adequate exposure of the sympathetic chain can be achieved with single lung ventilation or intermittent apnea instead of CO_2 gas. The harmonic scalpel may be employed in place of electrocautery. Two 5-mm port sites are required to place crushing clips, the first for the thoracoscope and the second for the automatic clip applier. Smaller incisions have been described by investigators who have access to millimeter diameter scopes and cautery instruments.[34] Intraoperative palmar skin temperature monitoring provides documentation of successful operation[35] and the temperature usually increases by 1.7°C to 2.6°C.[36]

Results of Endoscopic Thoracic Sympathectomy

Palmar hyperhidrosis is cured in virtually all patients who undergo endoscopic thoracic sympathectomy.[1–4,23–29,37] Recurrence during the next few years is reported as 1% to 3%.[1,2,4,24] Quality of life questionnaires consistently demonstrates that >90% of patients are satisfied with the results.[1–4] Compensatory sweating and recurrence are common reasons for dissatisfaction.

Interruption of the upper thoracic ganglia often produces a decrease in plantar sweating. The anatomic basis for this unexpected response is unexplained, but an increase in plantar skin temperature and decrease in the sympathetic skin responses has been documented.[38]

Surgical errors are responsible for early treatment failure. Analysis of 36 patients who underwent reoperation after experiencing resweating within 1 month of operation demonstrated an intact sympathetic chain (11%), incomplete transection (17%), partial regrowth (17%), incorrect ganglia level (11%), slipped clip (30%), and unknown (14%).[38] Some of these failures likely resulted from poor visualization of the sympathetic chain due to pulmonary–chest wall adhesions, overlying vessels, and misidentification of the sympathetic chain.[39,40] The role of the Kuntz nerves is controversial. Late failures are presumably due to nerve regeneration. Endoscopic reoperation is feasible, though the surgeon must be familiar with distorted intrathoracic anatomy and be prepared to perform a thoracotomy.[39,40]

Complications and Sequelae of Surgery

Immediate

Incisional and retrosternal pain exacerbated by cough or deep breathing are the principle postoperative complaints. Narcotic analgesics are generally necessary for the first 48 hours. Patients commonly return to work or school within 3 to 7 days. Anhidrosis of the upper chest and face is expected.

Injury to either intrathoracic or extrathoracic structures can result in delayed postoperative hemorrhage. Significant chest wall bleeding may drain into the pleural space without providing external evidence of hemorrhage. In the presence of unexplained hypotension a repeat chest x-ray and hematocrit are necessary.

Horner syndrome (ptosis, miosis, and anhidrosis) occurs in <1% of patients and results from damage to the sympathetic nerves that pass through the stellate ganglia.[1,2,41] As the optics and collective experience with the procedure has evolved, this has become an exceedingly rare complication. Misidentification of the nerve level or proximal transmission of cautery heat is the presumed mechanism of injury. Ptosis is immediate and frequently permanent.

Chronic

Compensatory Sweating Following proximal thoracic sympathectomy, up to 100% of patients can develop abnormal sweating in previously unaffected regions of the body, depending on the level or levels of sympathetic interruption.[1–4,23–29,42,43] The "compensatory sweating" is usually no more than an annoyance and all of these studies had very high rates of patient satisfaction. However, as many as 10% of patients are affected by severe compensatory sweating of the chest, thighs, and legs, which can be equal in severity to the original palmar sweating.[26–30] The cause of this most serious of sequela of thoracic sympathectomy remains obscure. A body mass index (BMI) >30 correlated with an increased severity of compensatory sweating in one study[44] and another large retrospective study showed an increase in severity with increasing BMI.[30] Gustatory sweating has been reported in as many as 73% of patients.[1–4,23–30,43]

Transection of the rami communicantes while leaving the sympathetic chain intact in the hope of decreasing compensatory sweating resulted in an increased incidence of recurrent palmar sweating and no change in the occurrence of compensatory sweating.[45,46]

Interruption of the T2 ganglia is not necessary to achieve dry palms and indeed, appears to increase compensatory hidrosis.[26,28,30] Two randomized, controlled trials showed interruption of only the T3 ganglia achieved dry hands with improved compensatory sweating compared to either the T2 or T2 to T4 levels.[26,28] Other trials, one a randomized controlled trial and another a large retrospective trial, reported on the interruption of the T4 ganglion. Compensatory sweating was less frequent and more often less severe compared to treatments at the T3 or T2 ganglia.[29,30] These studies and others have led to the STS recommendation for interruption at the R3 or R4 level for palmar hyperhidrosis.

Cardiopulmonary Sympathetic fibers to the heart pass through the upper thoracic ganglia. Following T2 sympathectomy, the resting heart rate at rest and with peak exercise is reduced 13% and 7%, respectively.[43] Exercise capacity and the cardio-respiratory response to exercise remain unchanged.[12]

Prevention and Treatment of Complications

Interruption of the sympathetic chain by application of nerve compressing clips was devised as a potentially reversible procedure in order to ameliorate the symptoms of patients suffering from severe compensatory sweating. Hyperhidrosis is controlled as effectively as with sympathectomy.[7,47] As many as 60% of patients note return of palmar sweating and decrease of compensatory sweating following clip removal.[2,47] Reconstruction of the transected sympathetic chain with a sural nerve graft has been reported.[48] Given the high percentage of patients that will persist with compensatory sweating, the STS Expert Consensus Document suggests that patients be advised to consider a procedure with clips irreversible.[22]

VASOMOTOR DISORDERS AND PAIN SYNDROMES

Arterial Disease

Ablative surgery of the thoracic sympathetic chain has been utilized for many years to treat upper extremity vascular insufficiency due to diseases of the microvasculature. However, there are few reports documenting the efficacy of the thoracoscopic approach. Twenty-eight patients with Raynaud disease, including seven with digital ulceration, underwent thoracoscopic sympathectomy following failure of medical therapy.[49] The sympathetic chain was transected over the T2 to T4 vertebrae using the operative technique previously described for palmar hyperhidrosis. Immediate symptomatic improvement was noted in 93% of patients. All the digital ulcers healed within 1 month of surgery. Eighty-two percent of patients reported recurrence of symptoms within 16 months, though with reduced frequency and severity.

Thoracoscopic sympathetic surgery has also been used to treat ischemia of the upper extremity caused by peripheral arterial obstruction. Fifteen patients with atherosclerosis ($n = 8$), Buerger disease ($n = 4$), and ischemia due to intra-arterial drug injection underwent resection of the sympathetic chain from T2 to T4.[50] Eleven patients had terminal digital necrosis, gangrene, or ulceration. The majority of patients experienced a decrease in pain and five patients had complete healing of the skin ulcers.

Complex Regional Pain Syndromes

The International Association for the Study of Pain created specific definitions for the diagnosis of the complex regional pain syndrome (CRPS).[35] Included within CRPS type I are a group of poorly defined disorders, such as: reflex sympathetic dystrophy, shoulder-hand syndrome, and Sudeck atrophy (Table 146-2). CRPS type II is initiated by a peripheral nerve injury and was commonly known as causalgia. The clinical course of CRPS has been divided into three stages (Table 146-3). Although the pathophysiology of CRPS has not yet been elucidated, a strong relationship to dysfunction of the sympathetic nervous system is well established. Nonoperative treatment of CRPS includes physical therapy, medications, transcutaneous neural stimulation, spinal cord stimulation, and percutaneous sympathetic nerve blocks. There are substantially fewer reports of thoracoscopic sympathetic surgery for this disease than for hyperhidrosis.

Forty-one patients with CRPS type I of the upper extremity were treated with 46 thoracoscopic sympathectomies.[51] The surgical technique was different from that described above for treatment of hyperhidrosis. The sympathetic chain was removed from the inferior aspect of the stellate ganglia to the third or

Table 146-2

COMPLEX REGIONAL PAIN SYNDROMES
Complex Regional Pain Syndrome Type I
Develops after an initiating noxious event. Spontaneous pain or allodynia/hyperalgesia occurs, is not limited to the territory of a single peripheral nerve, and is disproportionate to the inciting event
There is or has been evidence of edema, skin blood flow abnormality, or abnormal sudomotor activity in the region of pain since the inciting event
This diagnosis is excluded by the existence of conditions that would otherwise account for the degree of pain and dysfunction
Complex Regional Pain Syndrome Type II
Develops after a nerve injury. Spontaneous pain or allodynia/hyperalgesia occurs and is not necessarily limited to the territory of the injured nerve
There is or has been evidence of edema, skin blood flow abnormality, or abnormal sudomotor activity in the region of the pain since the inciting event
This diagnosis is excluded by the existence of conditions that would otherwise account for the degree of pain and dysfunction

Table 146-3

STAGES OF COMPLEX REGIONAL PAIN SYNDROME
Stage I
Development of painful limb with or without obvious cause
Burning and sometimes throbbing pain
Diffuse aching
Hypersensitivity to touch or cold
Localized edema
Altered color and temperature
X-ray demonstrates patchy demineralization or appears normal
Stage II (lasts 3–6 mos)
Progression of soft tissue edema
Thickening of skin and articular soft tissues
Muscle wasting
Development of brawny skin
Stage III
Limitation of movement
Contractures of digits
Waxy trophic skin changes
Brittle-ridged nails
Severe demineralization demonstrated on bone x-ray

fourth thoracic ganglia. Prior to transection of the sympathetic chain, a clip was placed across the inferior aspect of the stellate ganglia. All patients had previously undergone successful percutaneous bupivacaine sympathetic blocks to demonstrate the response to interruption of the sympathetic nervous system. Success was defined as greater than a 50% reduction in the patient's basal pain score that persisted for more than 2 days. Postoperative sympathalgia developed in 24% of patients and consisted of new pain over the scapula. In all but one patient, the pain resolved within 90 days. Three months following surgery, 90% of patients reported a >50% reduction in pain and improved limb motion. Although by 1 year post surgery the pain reduction persisted in only 72% of patients, the majority were satisfied with the procedure.

Thoracoscopic sympathectomy of the T2 ganglia was planned in 42 patients with CRPS type II.[52] Prior to surgery, all patients had been treated with a variety of medication. Stellate ganglion blocks (frequently multiple) were performed in all patients, 25 of whom experienced symptomatic improvement. The minimally invasive procedure was successfully completed in 30 patients, but was converted to a supraclavicular approach in 12 patients due to dense adhesions or apical pleural thickening. The intraoperative findings that prevented the thoracoscopic approach were attributed to the multiple stellate ganglion injections. Thirty-two patients reported excellent ($n = 20$) or good results ($n = 12$). Response to sympathectomy did not correlate with the response to stellate ganglion injections. Symptomatic improvement correlated with the thoracoscopic approach and performance of the sympathectomy within 3 months of symptom onset. The beneficial effect persisted throughout the 41-month median follow-up.

SUMMARY

Thoracoscopic sympathectomy is the surgical treatment of choice for patients with severe palmar hyperhidrosis not responsive to medical therapy. Either an R3 or R4 interruption can be made in the thoracic chain, taking care to advise patients about the trade-off between slightly damp hands and the probability of compensatory sweating. Patients must be specifically warned about compensatory sweating which may occasionally be severe. Axillary hyperhidrosis may be treated with an interruption at R5 alone or R4 and R5. Thoracoscopic sympathectomy can also provide relief from symptoms of Raynaud disease and CRPS.

CASE ILLUSTRATION—PALMAR HYPERHIDROSIS

The patient is a 23-year-old male who has had wet hands and feet since early childhood. He reports that sweating occurs intermittently and unpredictably, though it is worsened by stress. The sweat sometimes drips to the floor and is worse during the summer months. Pedal sweating accompanies the palmar hyperhidrosis but he has no history of fungal infections of the feet.

Throughout grammar and high school, teachers wondered why his homework was always wet with smudged ink. During his teenage years he experienced social difficulties due to wet and cold hands. He is now beginning his career in business and is worried that his palmar hyperhidrosis will interfere with his ability to interact with clients. He has tried Drysol™ and Drionic® without success. A younger brother also has palmar hyperhidrosis. The remainder of his medical history is normal.

Physical examination reveals wet hands and feet, with sweat pooling on the volar surface and within the palmar creases. The non-operative and operative treatment of hyperhidrosis, as well as the potential benefits and complications, were discussed in detail. Included in the informed consent is the possibility of a Horner syndrome, a pneumothorax that might require a chest tube, and compensatory sweating, which may be severe. Transection of the sympathetic chain versus application of crushing clips is also discussed. He elects to undergo sympathectomy, which is performed as an outpatient procedure at the R3 and R4 levels. Two weeks following surgery, he reports dry hands and minimal compensatory sweating. He is elated with his new situation and filled with self-confidence.

EDITOR'S COMMENT

Thoracoscopic sympathectomy is performed via single lung ventilation rather than CO_2 insufflation at our institution, with transection versus clipping of the sympathetic chain based on patient factors and surgeon preference.

—Yolonda L. Colson

References

1. Neumayer C, Bischof G, Fugger R, et al. Efficacy and safety of thoracoscopic sympathicotomy for hyperhidrosis of the upper limb. Results of 734 sympathicotomies. *Ann Chir Gynaecol.* 2001;90:195–199.
2. Reisfeld R, Nguyen R, Pnini A. Endoscopic thoracic sympathectomy for hyperhidrosis. *Surg Laparosc Endosc Percutan Tech.* 2002;12:255–267.
3. Neumayer C, Zacherl J, Holak G, et al. Limited endoscopic thoracic sympathetic block for hyperhidrosis of the upper limb. *Surg Endosc.* 2004;18:152–156.
4. Dumont P, Denoyer A, Robin P. Long-term results of thoracoscopic sympathectomy for hyperhidrosis. *Ann Thorac Surg.* 2004;78:1801–1807.
5. Adar R, Kurchin A, Zweig A, et al. Palmar hyperhidrosis and its surgical treatment: a report of 100 cases. *Ann Surg.* 1977;186:34–41.
6. Strutton DR, Kowalski JW, Glaser DA, et al. US prevalence of hyperhidrosis and impact on individuals with axillary hyperhidrosis: results from a national survey. *J Am Acad Dermatol.* 2004;51:241–248.
7. Ro KM, Cantor RM, Lange KL, et al. Palmar hyperhidrosis: evidence of genetic transmission. *J Vasc Surg.* 2002;35:382–386.
8. Higashimoto I, Yoshiura K, Hirakawa N, et al. Primary palmar hyperhidrosis locus maps to 14q11.2-q13. *Am J Med Gen A.* 2006;140:567–572.
9. Cho HM, Lee DY, Sung SW. Anatomical variations of rami communicantes in the upper thoracic sympathetic trunk. *Eur J Cardiothorac Surg.* 2005;27(2):320–324.
10. Wang Y-C, Sun M-H, Lin C-W, et al. Anatomical location of T2–3 sympathetic trunk and Kuntz nerve determined by transthoracic endoscopy. *J Neurosurg (Spine 1).* 2002;96:68–72.
11. Shih CJ, Lin MT. Thermoregulatory sweating in palmar hyperhidrosis before and after upper thoracic sympathectomy. *J Neurosurg.* 1979;50:88–94.
12. Manca D, Valls-Solé J, Callejas MA. Excitability recovery curve of the sympathetic skin response in healthy volunteers and patients with palmar hyperhidrosis. *Clin Neurophysiol.* 2000;111:1767–1770.

13. Noppen M, Herregodts P, Dendale P, et al. Cardiopulmonary exercise testing following bilateral thoracoscopic sympathicolysis in patients with essential hyperhidrosis. *Thorax.* 1995;50:1097–1100.
14. Noppen M, Sevens C, Gerlo E, et al. Plasma catecholamine concentrations in essential hyperhidrosis and effects of thoracoscopic D2-D3 sympathicolysis. *Eur J Clin Invest.* 1997;27:202–205.
15. Noppen M, Dendale P, Hagers Y, et al. Changes in cardiocirculatory autonomic function after thoracoscopic upper dorsal sympathicolysis for essential hyperhidrosis. *J Auton Nerv Syst.* 1996;60:115–120.
16. Bovell DL, Clunes MT, Elder HY, et al. Ultrastructure of the hyperhidrotic eccrine sweat gland. *Br J Dermatol.* 2001;145:298–301.
17. Flanagan KH, King R, Glaseer DA. Botulinum toxin type a versus topical 20% aluminum chloride for the treatment of moderated to severe primary focal axillary hyperhidrosis. *J Drugs Dermatol.* 2008;7:221–227.
18. Karakoç Y, Aydermir EH, Kalkan T, et al. Safe control of palmoplantar hyperhidrosis with direct electric current. *Int J Derm.* 2002;41:602–605.
19. Lowe NJ, Yamuauchi PS, Lask GP, et al. Efficacy and safety of botulinum toxin type a in the treatment of palmar hyperhidrosis: a double-blind, randomized, placebo-controlled study. *Dermatol Surg.* 2002;28:822–827.
20. Naumann M, Lowe NJ, Kumar CR, et al. Botulinum toxin type a is a safe and effective treatment for axillary hyperhidrosis over 16 months. *Arch Dermatol.* 2003;139:731–736.
21. Wolosker N, de Campos JR, Kauffmann P, et al. An alternative to treat palmar hyperhidrosis: use of oxybutinin. *Clin Auton Res.* 2011;21:389–393.
22. Cerfolio RJ, De Campos JR, Bryant AS, et al. The Society of Thoracic Surgeons expert consensus for the surgical treatment of hyperhidrosis. *Ann Thorac Surg.* 2011;91:1642–1648.
23. Drott C. Results of endoscopic thoracic sympathectomy (ETS) on hyperhidrosis, facial blushing, angina pectoris, vascular disorders and pain syndromes of the hand and arm. *Clin Auton Res.* 2003;13(Suppl 1):I26–I30.
24. Lin T S, Kuo S-J, Chou M-C. Uniportal endoscopic thoracic sympathectomy for treatment of palmar and axillary hyperhidrosis: analysis of 2000 cases. *Neurosurgery.* 2002;51(Suppl 2):S84–S88.
25. Katara AN, Domino JP, Cheah W-K, et al. Comparing T2 and T2–3 ablation in thoracoscopic sympathectomy for palmar hyperhidrosis: a randomized control trial. *Surg Endosc.* 2007;21:1768–1771.
26. Li X, Tu Y-R, Lin M, et al. Endoscopic thoracic sympathectomy for palmar hyperhidrosis: a randomized control trial comparing T3 and T2–4 ablation. *Ann Thor Surg.* 2008;85:1747–1751.
27. Munia MAS, Wolosker N, Kaufmann P, et al. Sustained benefit lasting one year from T4 instead of T3-T4 sympathectomy for isolated axillary hyperhidrosis. *Clinics (Sao Paulo).* 2008;63:771–774.
28. Yazbeck G, Wolosker N, Kauffmann P, et al. Twenty months of evolution following sympathectomy on patients with palmar hyperhidrosis: sympathectomy at the T3 level is better than at the T2 level. *Clinics.* 2009;64:743–749.
29. Liu Y, Yang J, Liu J, et al. Surgical treatment of primary palmar hyperhidrosis: a prospective randomized study comparing T3 and T4 sympathicotomy. *Eur J Cardiothorac Surg.* 2009;35:398–402.
30. Chang Y-T, Li H-P, Lee J-Y, et al. Treatment of palmar hyperhidrosis: T4 level compared with T3 and T2. *Ann Surg.* 2007;246:330–336.
31. Weksler B, Blaine G, Souza ZBB, et al. Transection of more than one sympathetic chain ganglion for hyperhidrosis increases the severity of compensatory hyperhidrosis and decreases patient satisfaction. *J Surg Res.* 2009;156:110–115.
32. Chiou TSM, Liao K-K. Orientation landmarks of endoscopic transaxillary T-2 sympathectomy for palmar hyperhidrosis. *J Neurosurg.* 1996;85:310–315.
33. Lin T-S, Fang H-Y. Transthoracic endoscopic sympathectomy for craniofacial hyperhidrosis: analysis of 46 cases. *J Laparoendosc Adv Surg Tech A.* 2000;10:243–247.
34. Lee DY, Yoon YH, Shion HK, et al. Needle thoracic sympathectomy for essential hyperhidrosis: intermediate-term follow-up. *Ann Thorac Surg.* 2000;69:251–253.
35. Stanton-Hicks M, Janig W, Hassenbusch S, et al. Reflex sympathetic dystrophy: changing concepts and taxonomy. *Pain.* 1995;63:127–133.
36. Sáiz-Sapena N, Vanaclocha V, Panta F, et al. Operative monitoring of hand and axillary temperature during endoscopic superior thoracic sympathectomy for the treatment of palmar hyperhidrosis. *Eur J Surg.* 2000;166: 65–69.
37. Wolosker M, De Campos JR, Kauffman P, et al. Evaluation of quality of life over time among 453 patients with hyperhidrosis submitted to endoscopic thoracic sympathectomy. *J Vasc Surg.* 2012;55:154–156.
38. Chen H-J, Liang C-L, Lu K. Associated changes in plantar temperature and sweating after transthoracic endoscopic T2–3 sympathectomy for palmar hyperhidrosis. *J Neurosurg (Spine 1).* 2001;95:58–63.
39. Kim DH, Paik HC, Lee DY. Video assisted thoracoscopic re-sympathectomy surgery in the treatment of re-sweating hyperhidrosis. *Eur J Cardiothorac Surg.* 2005;27:741–744.
40. Lin T-S. Video-assisted thoracoscopic "resympathicotomy" for palmar hyperhidrosis: analysis of 42 cases. *Ann Thorac Surg.* 2001;72:895–898.
41. Gossot D, Kabiri H, Caliandro R, et al. Early complications of thoracic endoscopic sympathectomy: a prospective study of 940 procedures. *Ann Thor Surg.* 2001;71:1116–1119.
42. Lin C-C, Telaranta T. Lin-Telaranta classification: the importance of different procedures for different indications in sympathetic surgery. *Ann Chirurg Gyn.* 2001;90:161–166.
43. Licht PB, Pilegaard HK. Severity of compensatory sweating after thoracoscopic sympathectomy. *Ann Thorac Surg.* 2004;78:427–431.
44. De Campos JRM, Wolosker N, Takeda FR, et al. The body mass index and level of resection. *Clin Auton Res.* 2005;15:116–120.
45. Cho HM, Chung KY, Kim DJ, et al. The comparison of VATS ramicotomy and VATS sympathicotomy for treating essential hyperhidrosis. *Yonsei Med J.* 2003;44:1008–1013.
46. Gossot D, Toledo L, Fritsch S, et al. Thoracoscopic sympathectomy for upper limb hyperhidrosis: looking for the right operation. *Ann Thorac Surg.* 1997;64:975–978.
47. Lin C-C, Mo L-R, Lee L-S, et al. Thoracoscopic T2-sympathetic block by clipping-A better and reversible operation for treatment of hyperhidrosis palmaris: experience with 326 cases. *Eur J Surg Suppl.* 1998;164(Suppl 580): 13–16.
48. van't Riet M, De Smet AAEA, Kuiken H, et al. Prevention of compensatory hyperhidrosis after thoracoscopic sympathectomy for hyperhidrosis. *Surg Endosc.* 2001;15:1159–1162.
49. Matsumoto Y, Ueyama T, Endo M, et al. Endoscopic thoracic sympathicotomy for Raynaud's phenomenon. *J Vasc Surg.* 2002;36:57–61.
50. De Giacomo T, Rendina EA, Venuta F, et al. Thoracoscopic sympathectomy for symptomatic arterial obstruction of the upper extremities. *Ann Thorac Surg.* 2002;74:885–888.
51. Bandyk DF, Johnson BL, Kirkpatrick AF, et al. Surgical sympathectomy for reflex sympathetic dystrophy syndromes. *J Vas Surg.* 2002;35:269–277.
52. Singh B, Moodley J, Shaik AS, et al. Sympathectomy for complex regional pain syndrome. *J Vasc Surg.* 2003;37:508–511.

147 Surgical Treatment of Chest Wall Infections

Sean C. Grondin and Gary A. J. Gelfand

Keywords: Bacterial infections, fungal infections, necrotizing soft tissue infections, osteomyelitis, *Clostridium*, *Aspergillus*, *Actinomycosis*, *Staphylococcus*, *Streptococcus*, *Mycobacterium tuberculosis*, vacuum-assisted closure device

Infections of the chest wall, although uncommon, are important problems for thoracic surgeons. The severity of these infections can range from relatively minor and inconvenient problems to life-threatening situations that require urgent and aggressive care. Since most surgeons will see only a small number of cases in their careers, an organized approach to management is essential. In this chapter, we present our preferred methods of classification, and we review the various aspects of management. Specific topics of significant importance, for example, poststernotomy sternal infections and mediastinitis, are covered in other chapters in this text.

CLASSIFICATION

A review of recent review of the literature suggests that there is no standard or ideal way to categorize chest wall infections. In our experience, classification according to type of organism, anatomic location, and the presence or absence of necrosis is most helpful for organizing the majority of clinical presentations of chest wall infections.

TYPE OF ORGANISM

Bacterial

Bacterial infection is among the most common type of chest wall infection. Although diagnosis may be straightforward on culture, this may not be the case with certain fastidious organisms or if the patient has already received antibiotic therapy. Infections may be mono- or polymicrobial. *Staphylococcus* spp. is a common organism that produces typical features of infection and can vary in appearance from small abscesses to destructive chest wall masses. Although *Staphylococcus* spp. infections may develop without any warning or history, they most commonly arise as a complication of surgical procedures or trauma. *Streptococcal* spp. such as *pneumoniae* and *milleri* are also common culprits and can be related to underlying empyema. Anaerobic organism infections (e.g., *Bacteroides* spp.) can be life-threatening and may arise from the oral cavity as a result of poor dentition with extension into the head and neck, mediastinum, and chest wall. Invasion of the chest wall from an underlying lung infection is not unusual and can be difficult to distinguish from a primary pulmonary malignancy with chest wall invasion. These infections are more common in immunocompromised patients such as diabetics.

Unusual organisms, such as *Actinomyces* spp., can arise in the oropharynx and affect the chest wall and underlying thoracic structures. The most common of these organisms is *Actinomyces israelii*. Aspiration is the most common cause with lower lobes being the predominant area affected. Pulmonary infection from *Actinomyces* spp. may also result in an empyema which in turn may extend into the chest wall.[1] Sulfur granules are pathognomonic of *Actinomyces* infection and are composed of colonies of organisms surrounded by neutrophils.[2]

Fungal

Fungal infections of the chest wall are quite uncommon and typically arise in immunocompromised individuals either as a primary infection or as part of a disseminated infection (see Chapter 103). Occasionally, these types of infection occur after surgical procedures. Fungal organisms that may cause infection include *Aspergillus*, *Candida*, *Rhizopus*, *Mucor*, *Absidia*, and *Phycomyces* spp.[3] Fungal infections can be extremely difficult to eradicate and may require multiple surgical procedures and prolonged antifungal therapy.

Mycobacterial

As with other pathology of the chest, tuberculosis must always be part of the differential diagnosis in chest wall infections. Although the chest wall is not a common initial presentation, cultures to rule out tuberculosis infection should always be sent. Immigration from other parts of the world or a history of immunocompromise should raise the possibility of a tuberculosis infectious etiology.

Parasitic

A high degree of suspicion is necessary to diagnose chest wall parasitic infections. Hydatid disease, leishmaniasis, and cutaneous myiasis are examples of parasitic infections that are difficult to diagnose in patients traveling outside of their endemic regions.

ANATOMIC LOCATION

Bone

Although osteomyelitis can affect any part of the chest skeleton, it more commonly affects the sternum than other parts of the chest wall. Primary infection is rare, with most cases occurring post-sternotomy. Sternal infections after cardiac surgery are well described elsewhere in this text. Primary infections in the absence of surgical intervention are uncommon but can be seen in drug addicts and patients with underlying pulmonary infections with extension into bone. These infections result in destruction of the cancellous bone and impairment of blood supply. Untreated, these infections will result in bone death. Osteomyelitis of the rib is usually localized and associated with procedures, such as chest tube insertion or chest trauma.

Cartilage

Infections of the cartilage arise most commonly after surgical interventions, including cardiac surgery, thoracotomy, and chest tube insertion. Primary infections are extremely uncommon but can be seen, particularly with *Mycobacterium*. Cartilages five through nine are contiguous and therefore an infection arising in any cartilage may spread and be particularly difficult to manage. Common organisms include *Staphylococcus* and *Streptococcus*, but *Escherichia coli* and *Pseudomonas aeruginosa* may also be cultured. The patient presents generally with a draining sinus which is associated with pain and tenderness. Imaging, both computed tomography (CT) of the chest and bone scan, can be helpful. Such infections can be very resistant to therapy and frequently require open debridement and prolonged antibiotic therapy. Large defects can occur if the contiguous cartilages of the costal margin are involved.

One of the more common but nonsurgical entities is painful swelling of the costal cartilages without abnormal histology or suppuration, a condition called Tietze syndrome. Chest pain with swelling of the second costochondral junction is the usual presentation. Pain to deep palpation is common. The differential diagnosis includes underlying neoplasm and infection. CT of the chest may be helpful in ruling out other diagnosis. Symptoms can be severe and long-lived. Conservative management including reassurance, anti-inflammatory medication, and hydrocortisone injections may be helpful. Surgical management in this instance is generally unsuccessful and can easily make matters worse.

Sternoclavicular Joint Infections

Infections of the sternoclavicular joint have been reviewed in a number of journal articles.[4,5] Risk factors include diabetes, immunosuppression, intravenous drug abuse, central venous catheters, and renal failure. Typically, patients may be septic and present with fever, pain, and swelling in the area. Diagnosis is aided by a high degree of suspicion and appropriate imaging such as CT.[6] The most common organism is *Staphylococcus aureus*. Management will depend on several factors including level of acuity, premorbid status, and extent of disease. Although drainage and antibiotics are the mainstays of therapy, more extensive infections can require surgical debridement and, rarely, resection.

NONNECROTIZING SOFT TISSUE INFECTIONS

Infections of the soft tissues covering the thorax can range in severity from common infections, such as furuncles and boils, to superficial cellulitis and abscesses, to more severe, potentially life-threatening necrotizing soft tissue infections (NSTIs).

Superficial Cellulitis

As is the case elsewhere in the body, superficial infections of the thorax often develop from minor injuries such as burns, abrasions, or minor lacerations of the chest. Signs such as swelling and erythema are common. Organisms such as *Staphylococcus aureus* and *Streptococcus epidermidis* are frequently responsible for infections, but other organisms such as *Vibrio* and *Clostridium* spp. have been implicated.[7] Treatment usually involves oral antibiotics for minor infections and intravenous antibiotics for more serious infections.

Abscesses

Chest wall abscesses can develop on any part of the chest wall and usually arise secondary to another infectious site such as an infected thoracotomy wound. Symptoms and signs including localized pain and swelling with fever are usually present along with an elevated white cell count. As with superficial infections, common inciting organisms include *Staphylococcus* and *Streptococcus* species. Unlike plain chest radiographs which are not usually helpful, CT of the chest accurately characterizes and localizes chest wall abscesses. Antibiotic therapy and prompt drainage are the mainstays of treatment and usually result in complete resolution of the problem.[8]

Fungal abscesses of the chest wall may occasionally arise in patients who are immunocompromised due to malnutrition, diabetes, malignancy, or human immunodeficiency virus infection. Imaging by CT is helpful to rule out transmural involvement with associated empyema necessitans. For successful management, surgical debridement along with long-term antibiotic therapy is often necessary.

Treating physicians should always be aware of the possibility of abscess arising from a mycobacterium when a slowly enlarging painful, or sometimes painless, mass is detected on the chest wall. A history of travel to locations with endemic tuberculosis or a patient who is immunocompromised should raise suspicion of mycobacterium infection. Diagnosis can be made on aspiration of abscess fluid using culture. Treatment with antituberculous therapy prior to surgical drainage is preferred with antibiotic therapy lasting 6 to 9 months for eradication.[9]

NECROTIZING SOFT TISSUE INFECTIONS

NSTI of the chest wall are uncommon but are associated with a high morbidity and mortality.[10] Most infections are polymicrobial consisting of various anaerobes and aerobes, including *Streptococcus pyogenes, Peptostreptococcus, Bacteroides, Fusobacterium, and Staphylococcus aureus*. Occasionally, a single organism such as *Clostridium perfringens* may release the toxins that are responsible for rapid soft tissue invasion with subsequent tissue necrosis of the superficial and deep fascia, thrombosis of blood vessels, and ensuing sepsis.

NSTI of the chest wall may develop as a result of other chest infections, such as empyema or infectious due to a contaminated esophageal operation.[11] Postoperative patients demonstrating septic deterioration with evidence of wound infection should have the wound opened and drained. Suspicion of the presence of necrotic tissue mandates urgent wound exploration down to muscle and fascia to rule out NSTI. The absence of gas can mislead the treating physician and result in a diagnostic delay. Delay in management is the leading cause of treatment failure. Wide aggressive surgical debridement of nonviable tissue is mandatory with broad-spectrum antibiotic therapy. Repeat surgical exploration is often necessary to control the infection. These sick patients usually require management in an intensive care unit (ICU) with mechanical ventilation and ionotropic support. The use of hyperbaric oxygen may be beneficial for NSTI of the chest

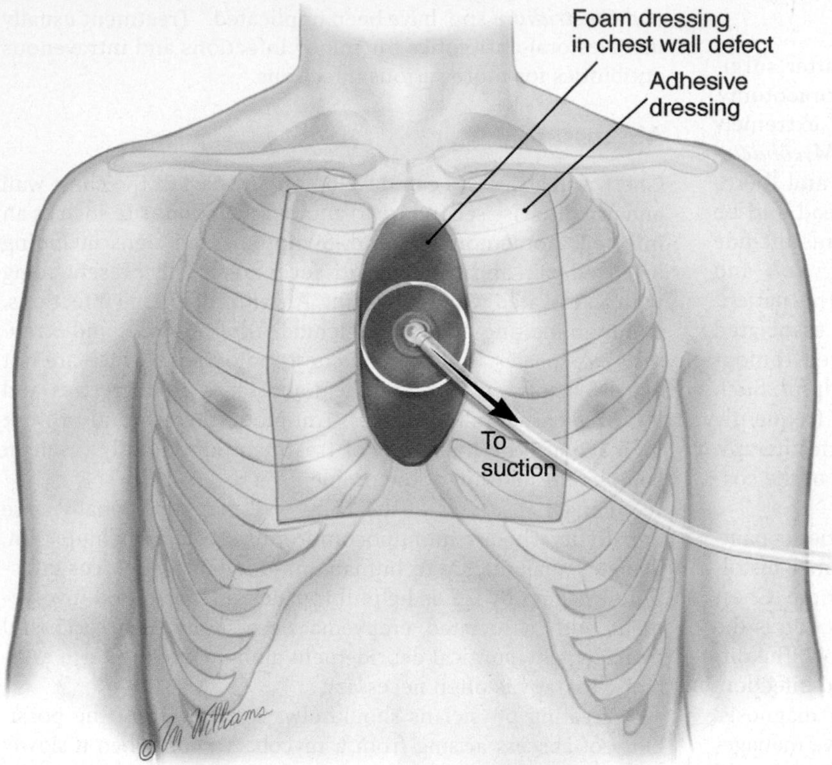

Figure 147-1. Negative-pressure wound therapy with a vacuum-assisted closure device promotes formation of granulation tissue and wound healing.

wall but should not replace wide surgical debridement as the mainstay of treatment.[12]

Despite appropriate care many patients succumb to NSTI. If the patient survives the initial fulminant phase of the infection, the ICU stay often involves a slow healing process associated with challenges of soft tissue wound care and subsequent closure. Obtaining expert advice from reconstructive plastic surgeons is helpful in determining the best approach for closing a chest wall defect created during debridement. Typically, muscle flaps are used for wound closure, although omental flaps may also be necessary (see Chapter 138). In some instances, closure is not possible and healing must occur slowly by secondary intention. Newer techniques for reconstruction that use biologic graft substitutes such as porcine submucosa and treated human cadaver skin are currently being investigated.[13,14]

In recent years, reconstruction after debridement has been facilitated by negative-pressure wound therapy using a vacuum-assisted closure (VAC) device (Fig. 147-1). These devices apply a foam sponge over the wound and allow the removal of wound exudates by regulated suction to encourage granulation tissue formation and wound healing.[15] Over time these devices facilitate dressing changes and contract the wound, thereby minimizing the area requiring future grafting. A detailed description of plastic surgical approaches to chest wall reconstruction is provided in Chapter 138.

SUMMARY

Chest wall infections typically arise in immunocompromised patients and may range in presentation from a discrete lesion to an extensive necrotic life-threatening infection. Inciting organisms can be bacterial, fungal, or parasitic in origin. CT imaging is helpful to determine the extent of disease. Treatment varies depending on the organism and extent of infection. In most cases, debridement and appropriate antibiotic therapy are the mainstays of care. For life-threatening necrotizing infections, early recognition with wide surgical debridement and antibiotic therapy is critical followed by supportive ICU care and careful wound management. Often a multidisciplinary approach is required to plan the extent of debridement and to weigh surgical wound closure options.

EDITOR'S COMMENT

Although these infections are rare, surgeons need to play a central role in the management of chest wall infections as surgical drainage is often a central tenant of treatment. Early, aggressive surgical debridement in patients with NSTIs cannot be stressed enough, as the superficial skin manifestations underestimate the true extent of underlying infection and tissue necrosis.

—Yolonda L. Colson

References

1. Chernihovski A, Loberant N, Cohen I, et al. Chest wall Actinomycosis. *Isr Med Assoc J.* 2007:9(9);686–687.
2. Deshpande M, Kamath A, Allinson K, et al. A 76-year-old lady with chronic cough and a discharging chest wall sinus. *Thorax.* 2011;66(8):733,738–739.
3. Paul S, Zellos L. Surgical treatment of chest wall infections. In: Sugarbaker D, Bueno R, Krasna M, Mentzer S, Zellos L, eds. *Adult Chest Surgery.* 1st ed. New York, NY: McGraw-Hill; 2009:1048–1051.
4. Haddad M, Maziak DE, Shamji FM. Spontaneous sternoclavicular joint infections. *Ann Thorac Surg.* 2002;74(4):1225–1227.

5. Song HK, Guy TS, Kaiser LR, et al. Current presentation and optimal surgical management of sternoclavicular joint infections. *Ann Thor Surg.* 2002;73(2):427–431.
6. Bouaziz MC, Jelassi H, Chaabane S, et al. Imaging of chest wall infections. *Skeletal Radiol.* 2009;38(12):1127–1135.
7. Vinh DC, Embil JM. Rapidly progressive soft tissue infections. *Lancet.* 2005;5(8):501–513.
8. LoCicero J. Infections of the chest wall. In: Shields TW, LoCicero J, Reed CE, Feins RH, eds. *General Thoracic Surgery*. 7th ed. Philadelphia, PA: Lippincott Williams and Wilkins; 2009:633–639.
9. Cho S, Lee EB. Surgical resection of chest wall tuberculosis. *Thorac Cardiovasc Surg.* 2009;57(8):480–483.
10. Urshel JD, Takita H, Antkowiak JG. Necrotizing soft tissue infections of the chest wall. *Ann Thorac Surg.* 1997;64(1):276–279.
11. Blasberg JD, Donington JS. Infections and radiation injuries involving the chest wall. *Thorac Surg Clin.* 2010;20(4);487–494.
12. Jallali N, Withey S, Bulter PE. Hyperbaric oxygen as adjuvant therapy in the management of necrotizing fasciitis. *Am J Surg.* 2005:189(4);462–466.
13. Pu LL. Small intestinal submucosa (Surgisis) as a bioactive prosthetic material for repair of abdominal wall fascial defect. *Plast Reconstr Surg.* 2005;115(7):2127–2131.
14. Abenavoli FM. Usefulness of Alloderm. *Plast Reconstr Surg.* 2005;116(2):677.
15. Venturi ML, Attinger CE, Mesbahi AN, et al. Mechanisms and clinical applications of the vacuum-assisted closure (VAC) device. *Am J Dermatol.* 2005:6(3);185–194.

PART 24

DIAPHRAGM

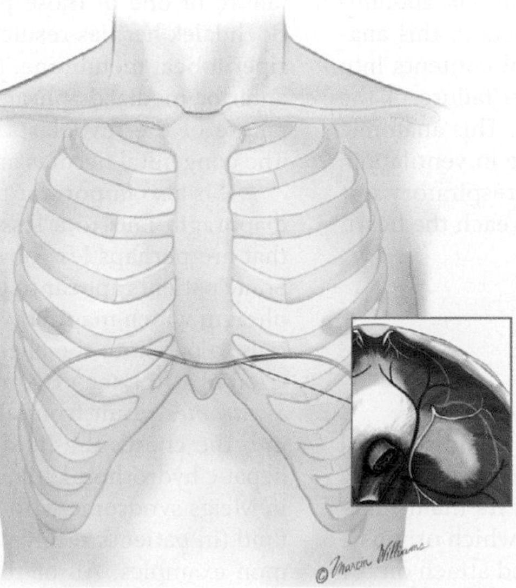

148 Overview of Anatomy, Physiology, and Pathophysiology of the Diaphragm

Joseph B. Shrager

Keywords: Respiration, ventilation, esophageal aperture, aortic aperture, porous diaphragm syndrome

The diaphragm is generally referred to as the main "respiratory muscle"—which is to some extent a misnomer. A better description would be that the diaphragm is the primary muscle of *ventilation.* Its critical physiological role is to serve as the main muscle which moves air into the lungs, where this air, of course, oxygenates the blood. Since delivery of oxygenated blood to all parts of the body is critical to life, and since intact cardiac and respiratory systems are the essential elements to assure that this oxygenated blood is manufactured and delivered, failure of any of the components that makes up either one of these systems results in death or severe disability. *One could thus make a very strong argument that along with the heart and lungs, the diaphragm is one of the three most important organs in the body.*

Just as the heart is the blood pump, the diaphragm is the air pump. Brief consideration will convince the reader that the heart and diaphragm are the only two muscles in the body that are continuously active throughout the life of an individual. If either one of these muscles fails, the individual fails. As the only *skeletal muscle* that is continuously active (the heart is made up of *cardiac* muscle), the diaphragm presents a number of interesting physiological adaptations. Diaphragm muscle fibers demonstrate unique characteristics that permit it to function adequately given this unusual role of constant activity. Further, its special role seems to influence the diaphragm muscle's response to various disease states (e.g., emphysema) and medical interventions (e.g., mechanical ventilation [MV]), such that it often does not respond in the same manner as skeletal muscles in the limbs do under similar circumstances.

Beyond its physiological role, the diaphragm also serves an important anatomic role—separating the mobile abdominal contents from the compressible lung. Defects in this anatomic barrier result in herniation of abdominal contents into the chest, which can lead to both malfunction/failure of the abdominal organs, and dysfunction of the lung. This anatomic role of the diaphragm, like its physiological role in ventilation, serves at bottom to preserve a fully functioning respiratory system such that oxygenated blood can efficiently reach the heart.

ANATOMY

Basic Anatomy and Embryology

The diaphragm is made up of two muscular parts and a central tendon. The muscular portions are the *costal diaphragm and the crural diaphragm.* The costal diaphragm is its main functional component. It is formed by muscle fibers which originate on the lower six ribs and the xiphoid process and attach on the central tendon (Fig. 148-1). The crural diaphragm consists of bundles of muscle fibers that arise from the first three lumbar vertebral bodies and the medial and lateral arcuate ligaments on each side. Although some mistakenly think of the costal diaphragm as being made up of two separate muscles – right and left hemidiaphragms each forming their own separate dome – in fact the diaphragm is a single, continuous organ that spans the midline as one broad dome.

The importance of the diaphragm's role in separating the abdominal from the intrathoracic contents is highlighted by the *apertures in the diaphragm,* through which a number of structures that span each of these cavities must pass. These apertures for the vena cava, the esophagus, and the aorta also allow passage of smaller structures. The vagi and sympathetic trunks pass through the esophageal aperture; the thoracic duct and azygos vein pass through the aortic aperture. Although the apertures are sealed around each of these structures by soft tissue including the mesothelial layer that lines the abdominal surface of the diaphragm and the pleura that lines its thoracic surface, the apertures are nevertheless sites that can allow herniation of visceral contents into the chest. By far the most common *acquired diaphragmatic hernias,* as discussed in Chapter 46, are hiatal hernias through the esophageal aperture.

Congenital diaphragmatic hernias occur at sites that are compromised by failure of the normal embryological development of the diaphragm. In the embryo, the diaphragm is formed by the fusion of the septum transversum, the pleuriperitoneal membrane, the dorsal mesentery, and the lateral body wall mesoderm (Fig. 148-2). There is also a contribution of myoblasts from the third through fifth cervical somites which migrate to contribute to the formation of muscle fibers. The various congenital diaphragmatic defects can be attributed to failure of one of these processes. For example, posterolateral Bochdalek hernias result from failure of the fusion of the pleuriperitoneal membrane. Morgagni hernias, which occur in the anterior, medial diaphragm posterior to the xiphoid, result from failure of the myoblasts from the cervical somites to appear. The congenital hernias are discussed in Chapter 51.

It is also important to note that the barrier function of the diaphragm fails to a lesser extent in other clinical syndromes that are perhaps less obvious than the diaphragmatic hernias. Some patients appear to have "pores" of varying sizes in the diaphragm which may allow intraabdominal fluid and other materials to pass into the chest. These syndromes were first categorized by Kirchner.[1] The most obvious of the *Porous Diaphragm Syndromes* result from abnormal intraabdominal fluid passing into the chest. The fluid may consist of benign ascites (as in hepatic hydrothorax in cirrhotic patients), malignant ascites (as in Meigs syndrome with ovarian cancer), or peritoneal dialysis fluid (in patients receiving PD), as just a few of the more common examples. All of these tend to occur in the right hemithorax, perhaps because peritoneal fluid circulates such that it pools in the right subphrenic space, or because the presence of the liver on the right creates a sumping action upon the right

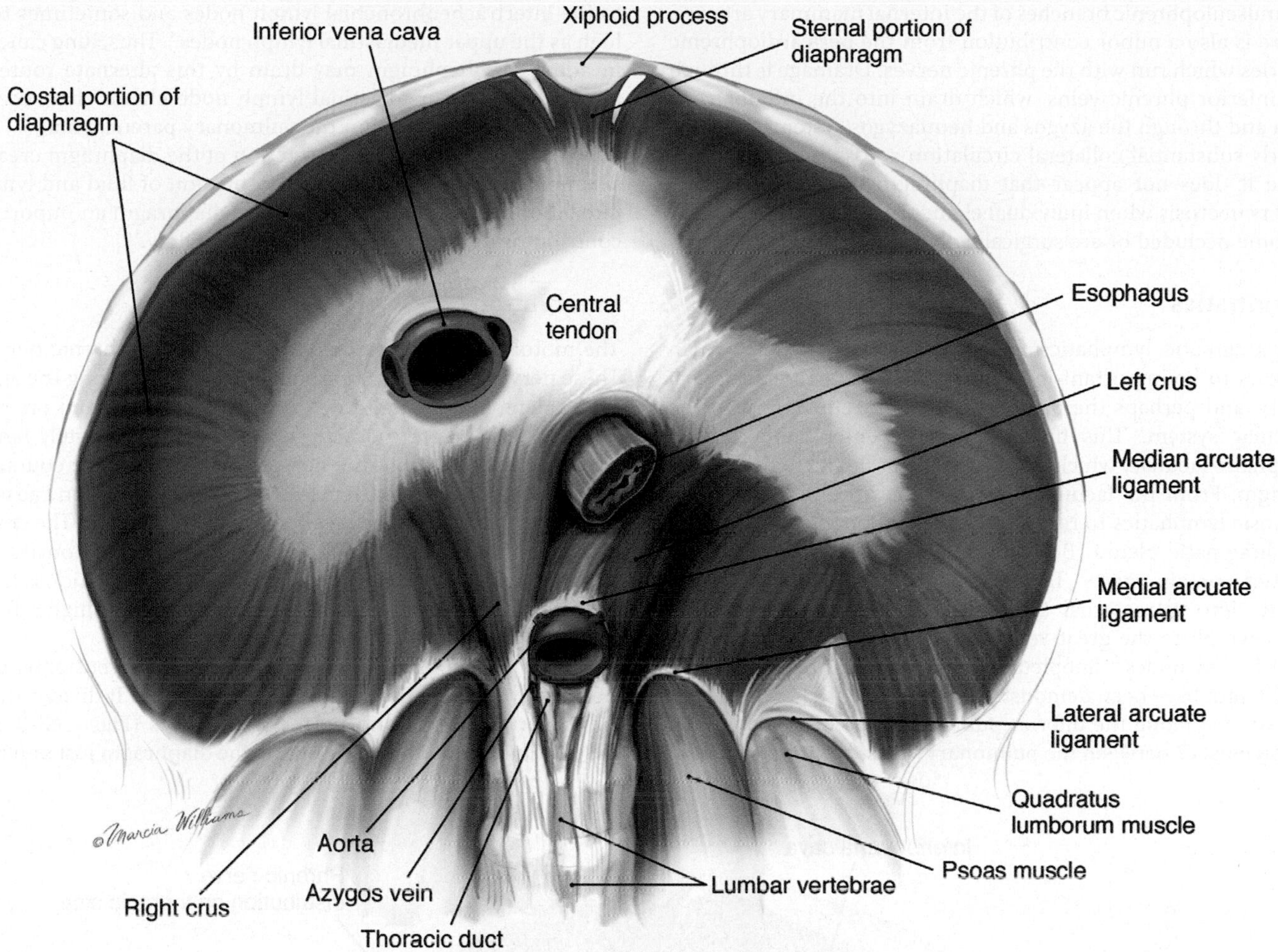

Figure 148-1. The muscle fibers of the diaphragm originate from the posterior lumbar spine (arcuate ligaments) and curve upward to form an aponeurotic sheath known as the central tendon. Several thoracic organs and vessels pass through apertures in the diaphragmatic surface.

hemidiaphragm. These problems can often be solved by: (1) at least temporarily minimizing as much as possible the abdominal fluid component by drainage or medical therapy, and then (2) creating a basilar pleurodesis with talc or mesh that will allow the adherent lung to occlude the pores. Depending upon the chronicity of the pleural effusion, a formal decortication may be required as part of this procedure, and if the pores are large, success may be improved by actual pore suture or stapling rather than relying upon a pleurodesis alone. The thoracic procedure is generally carried out by video-assisted thoracoscopic surgery (VATS). Examples of this type of approach are

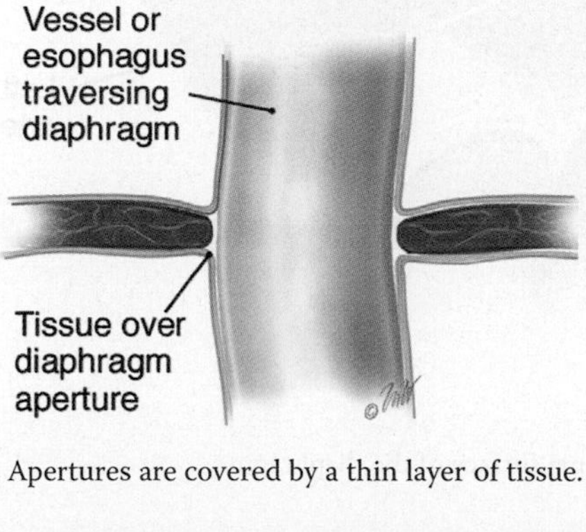

Figure 148-2. Apertures are covered by a thin layer of tissue.

described in publications by Cerfolio and Bryant[2] for hepatic hydrothorax and Mak et al.[3] for effusions related to PD.

Catamenial pneumothorax refers to pneumothorax that occurs cyclically with menses. This is thought to result in some cases from implants of endometriosis on the lung (which may lead to direct leakage of air from the visceral pleural surface during the hemorrhagic phase within the implants), and in other cases from implants on the diaphragm which may in a similar fashion lead to diaphragmatic defects through which air may enter the chest from the peritoneal space. Implants in both of these locations have been identified during thoracoscopic exploration in a high percentage of patients with this syndrome. It is becoming clear that creating a particularly effective pleurodesis at the level of the diaphragm is an important component of successful management of these patients (as with other "porous diaphragm syndromes") in addition to the more standard pleurodesis or pleurectomy covering the remainder of the chest.[4] Resection of any blebs and visceral pleural implants that are seen are of course also performed during these procedures. Hormonal manipulation to prevent menses for several weeks after the time of the surgical procedure has also been suggested.

Blood Supply

The diaphragm's arterial supply derives largely from the right and left inferior phrenic arteries, the intercostal arteries, and the musculophrenic branches of the internal mammary arteries. There is also a minor contribution from the pericardiophrenic arteries which run with the phrenic nerves. Drainage is through the inferior phrenic veins, which drain into the inferior vena cava and through the azygos and hemiazygos systems. There is clearly substantial collateral circulation across the diaphragm, since it does not appear that diaphragm muscle infarcts or suffers necrosis when individual elements of the arterial supply become occluded or are surgically divided.

Lymphatics

Diaphragmatic lymphatics form a specialized system which appears to be important in draining fluid from the peritoneal cavity, and perhaps the pleural cavity, and returning it to the vascular system. This fluid appears to enter subperitoneal lymphatic lacunae, which sit between muscle fibers of the diaphragm. From the lacunae, fluid traverses the diaphragm via intrinsic lymphatics to reach collecting lymphatics beneath the diaphragmatic pleura. Both the intrinsic and collecting lymphatics contain valves. The collecting lymphatics drain principally into retrosternal (parasternal) lymphatic trunks that carry lymph to the great veins after it filters through mediastinal lymph nodes.[5] Subpleural lymphatic channels along the diaphragm have been demonstrated to drain into lymph vessels that ascend along the inferior pulmonary ligaments, along the esophagus, or between the pulmonary veins, before connecting to the intertracheobronchial lymph nodes and sometimes toas high as the upper mediastinal lymph nodes.[6] Thus, lung cancers invading the diaphragm may drain by this alternate route to involve the same mediastinal lymph node chains that receive lymph from tumors within the pulmonary parenchyma.

It is thought that the contraction of the diaphragm creates a sumping action that facilitates absorption of fluid and lymph into all of these channels, making the diaphragm an important contributor to the total volume of lymph flow.

Innervation

The motor supply to the diaphragm is via the phrenic nerves. These nerves run in very reproducible positions along the anterior scalene muscle and down along the mediastinum on each side. It is critical for thoracic surgeons to be intimately familiar with the anatomy of the nerves along their entire course in order to avoid injury to them (likely the most common cause of diaphragm paralysis) during all thoracic procedures. The costal diaphragm's innervation derives from the third and fourth cervical segments, while the crural diaphragm's innervation is from the fifth segment. Thus, spinal cord injury at C4 or higher leads to partial or complete diaphragm paralysis.

The right phrenic nerve passes through the central tendon along the vena cava through the caval aperture. It divides there into anterior, lateral, and posterior branches (Figs. 148-3 and 148-4). On the left, the nerve enters the diaphragm just anterior

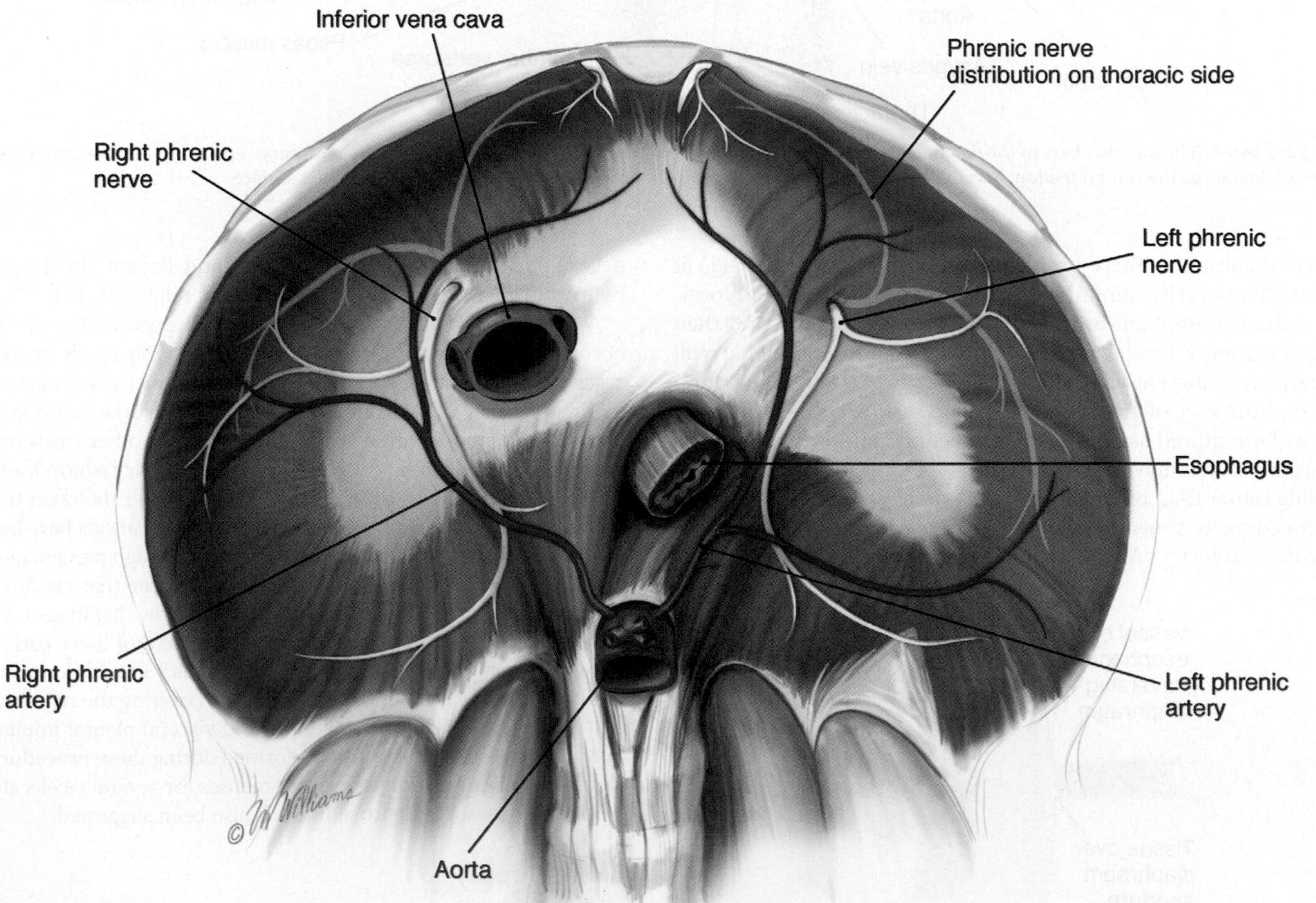

Figure 148-3. Blood supply and innervation from the abdominal surface of the diaphragm.

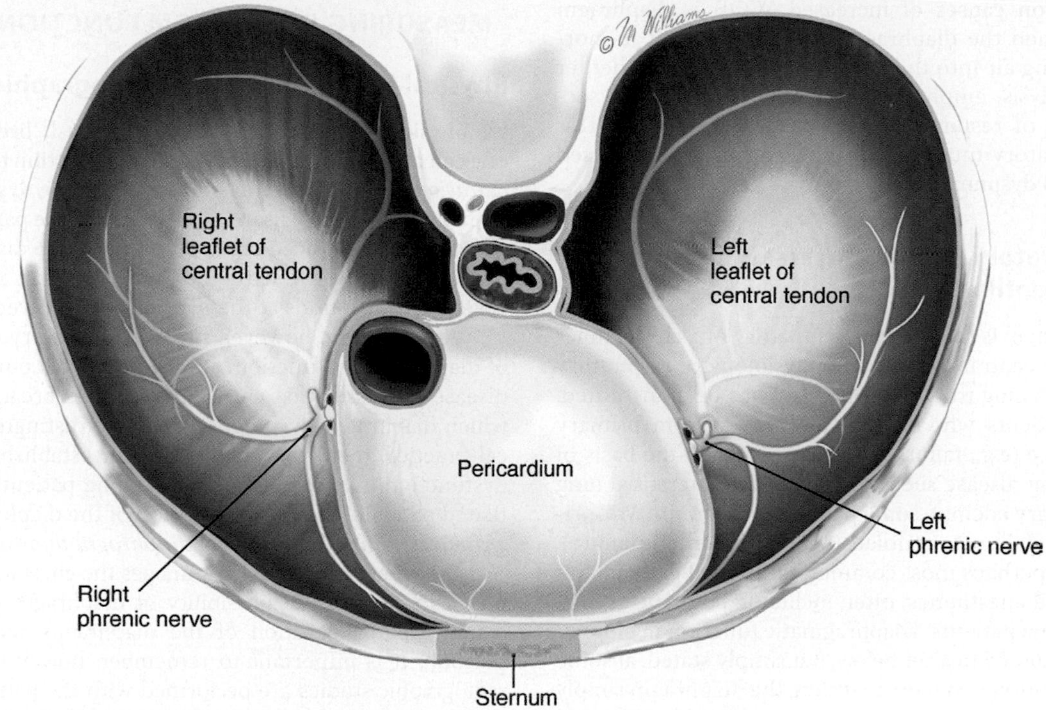

Figure 148-4. Thoracic surface of the diaphragm.

to the central tendon and sends off similar branches. The locations of these branches have implications for the placement of incisions in the diaphragm that will be least disruptive to innervation (see separate chapter on diaphragm incisions).

In normal individuals there is very little or no cross-innervation between the left and right sides of the diaphragm. The right phrenic nerve supplies only the right hemidiaphragm and the left nerve supplies only the left hemidiaphragm. As a result, injury to one nerve only causes major dysfunction to the ipsilateral diaphragm. In experimental animals, there seems to be some ability of the contralateral, healthy phrenic to eventually, partially reinnervate a denervated diaphragm, but it is unclear if this occurs to any clinically significant extent in humans.

PHYSIOLOGY

Role in Ventilation

As a result of its circumferential attachments to the ribs and spine, its attachment to a central tendon, and its sheet-like, domed configuration, when the muscle fibers of the diaphragm contract, the sheet-like muscle descends caudally. Wade measured the displacement of the diaphragm's dome with inspiration at 9.5 cm on average.[7] The diaphragm essentially acts as a piston, descending caudally with contraction. This diaphragmatic descent increases the intrathoracic volume, thereby reducing the intrapleural pressure. A lesser component (approximately 10%) of the reduction in intrapleural pressure with diaphragm contraction results from what is called the "insertional component" – or the diaphragm fibers' insertion on the superior margin of the lower ribs – which during contraction cause the lower ribs to expand outward (the increase in intraabdominal pressure may also contribute to this action). The resulting reduced intrapleural pressure expands the lung, drawing air into the lungs via the airways. As the diaphragm relaxes, it moves passively in a cranial direction, allowing air to passively exit the lung as a result of the intrinsic elastic recoil of the lung tissue and chest wall.

When the diaphragm is dysfunctional or ventilatory requirements are increased by exercise, other inspiratory muscles – which do not contribute much during quiet breathing – may become active. These include mainly the scalene muscles, the parasternal intercostal muscles, the sternocleidomastoid muscles, the transversus abdominis muscle, and possibly the external intercostal muscles.

As in limb muscle, shifts in the distribution of the various muscle fiber types within the diaphragm (e.g., slow or fast fibers) occur in response to certain stressors. These shifts may be adaptive, or in some cases perhaps maladaptive (see below discussion regarding changes in fiber types in emphysema).

Pathophysiology of Dyspnea

The sensation of dyspnea remains poorly understood, but appears to result from a very complicated set of neurophysiological events. Interestingly, it has been clearly shown that dyspnea is far more closely related to respiratory muscle function than it is to FEV_1. To summarize a large body of research in a few sentences, one might say that one of the most important contributor to the sense of dyspnea in many patients is the work of breathing (WOB).

WOB is work performed by the respiratory muscles—chiefly the diaphragm in the absence of expiratory airflow limitation. Its level is determined by the two main types of resistances against which the respiratory muscles must work—the elastic resistance of the lung or chest wall tissues and the frictional resistance of the airways to gas flow (e.g., increased COPD). When WOB is increased, dyspnea results.

One common causes of increased WOB is diaphragm dysfunction. When the diaphragm fails to carry out its normal role of pulling air into the lungs by descending – whether because of paralysis, emphysema, or other causes – the secondary muscles of respiration must become activated. This increased ventilatory muscle activation appears to be sensed by the patient as dyspnea.

Role in Respiratory Failure and Weaning from Mechanical Ventilation

Since the diaphragm is the primary ventilatory muscle, its function is of course central to the pathophysiology of respiratory failure and to weaning from MV once MV has been instituted. While many patients who require MV suffer from primary pulmonary failure (e.g., failure of gas exchange on the basis of parenchymal lung disease such as pneumonia, interstitial lung disease, pulmonary edema), some patients will require MV primarily because of failure to ventilate (i.e., diaphragmatic failure). This situation is perhaps most common in surgical patients following prolonged anesthetics, often including paralytic agents, and in emphysema patients. Diaphragmatic function in emphysema will be discussed further below, but simply stated, at some point in the evolution of hyperexpansion, the diaphragm simply cannot move enough air to maintain an acceptable pCO_2, and at that point the patient will either die or require MV.

Similarly, *weaning* from MV, once pulmonary parenchymal disease has been improved such that oxygenation is adequate, is primarily a function of the adequacy of the diaphragm to move air. The ability to inspire adequately without support would seem to be the *sine qua non* of separation from a ventilator. Thus, it is critical to do everything possible to preserve diaphragm function while a patient is subjected to MV (see below section on *MV-associated diaphragm dysfunction*). And measurements of diaphragm function serve as useful determinants of a patient's readiness for discontinuation of MV (see next section on *measuring diaphragm function*).

MEASURING DIAPHRAGM FUNCTION

Physical Examination and Radiographic Studies

On physical examination in a spontaneously breathing patient, one can often recognize diaphragm dysfunction by reduced *auscultation* of breath sounds on the side of the dysfunction. Even with diaphragm paresis in the absence of true paralysis, one can generally hear reduced breath sounds. When diaphragm elevation is marked in the setting of paralysis, there are often nearly absent breath sounds at the base on the involved side.

Auscultation, however, provides on a very crude estimate of diaphragm dysfunction, and there are of course many other disease processes that can cause reduced breath sounds from which diaphragm dysfunction must be distinguished. In clinical practice, then, the main means of establishing diaphragm dysfunction in spontaneously breathing patients (i.e., nonventilated patients) are (1) the position of the diaphragm on *radiographic examinations* and (2) *diaphragm fluoroscopy*.

Essentially any study that images the chest and upper abdomen can suggest the possibility of diaphragm dysfunction by demonstrating elevation of the diaphragm above its normal position. It is important to remember, however, that different radiographic studies are performed with the patient in different body positions, and that *the dysfunctional diaphragm will move to markedly different apparent degrees of elevation depending upon the body position of the patient.* For example, a patient with diaphragm paralysis will usually demonstrate far less elevation of the involved side of the diaphragm on a PA and lateral chest radiogram (which is obtained with a patient standing upright) than on the scout films from a computed tomogram (CT) of the chest (which is obtained with the patient fully supine) (Fig. 148-5). I suspect that many dyspneic patients have been misdiagnosed to have normal diaphragm function on the basis of PA/lateral chest radiogram showing near-normal diaphragm position.

Diaphragm fluoroscopy (often termed the "sniff test") examines the movement of the diaphragm in real time as the patient

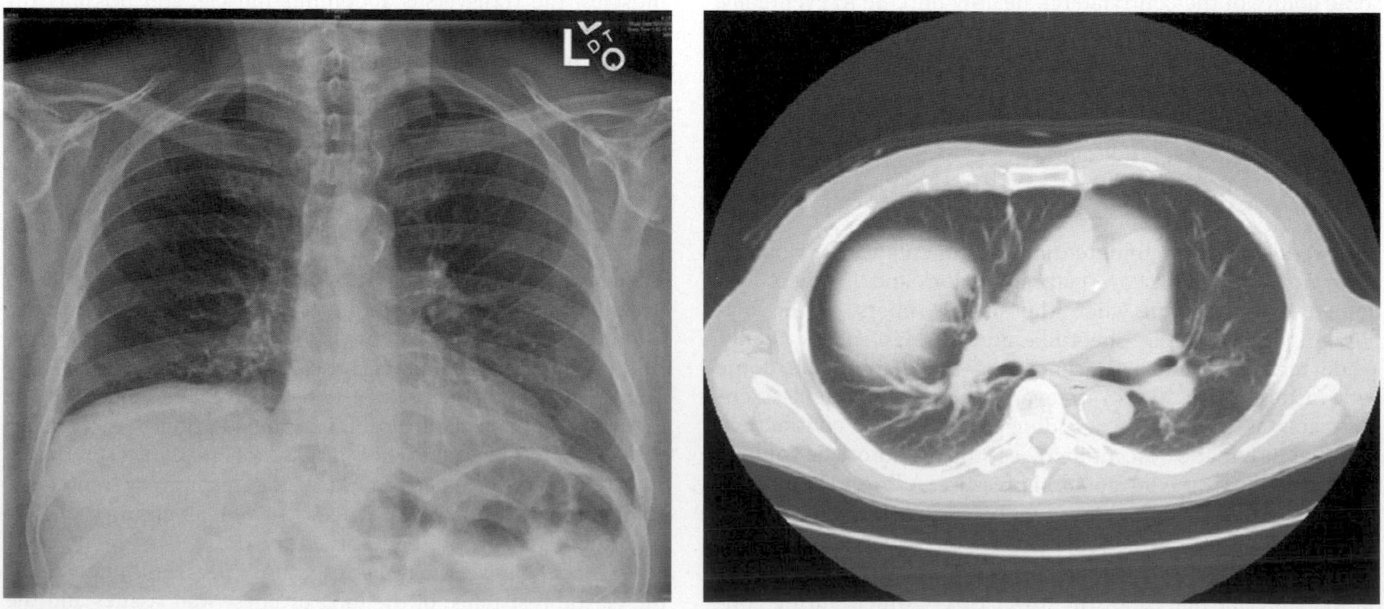

Figure 148-5. PA upright chest radiogram and computed tomogram of the same preoperative patient with a paralyzed right hemidiaphragm. Note that the diaphragm nearly reaches the carina on the CT taken in a supine position, whereas on the upright radiogram the elevation is far less impressive.

is asked to breathe deeply. A diaphragm that is paretic but not paralyzed may show some, but a reduced degree of, descent with deep inspiration, or it may show no motion at all. A fully paralyzed diaphragm will generally show paradoxical elevation during inspiration. This is because the involved side of the diaphragm not only fails to contract and thus fails to descend, but also actually rises in response to the increased negative pressure created in the ipsilateral pleural space as a result of contraction of the uninvolved, fully contractile, contralateral side of the diaphragm. When the intact side of the diaphragm contracts, it conveys a strong negative pressure to its ipsilateral pleural space, which is then conveyed to a lesser degree through the mediastinal structures to the contralateral pleural space, which will therefore result in mild paradoxical elevation of the paralyzed diaphragm.

It is important to remember that there are degrees of diaphragm dysfunction, any of which may cause a patient to be dyspneic, and which may result in less than classic findings on fluoroscopy. In fact, a patient may be dyspneic when the diaphragm is elevated but fully contractile (termed an *eventration*). In this situation, the phrenic nerve may be fully intact, but a structural weakness of the diaphragm muscle leads it to assume a more elevated position. An eventrated diaphragm may descend nearly normally on diaphragm fluoroscopy, but more commonly it appears to descend incompletely, or there may be portions of the diaphragm that descend normally while others do not. Some portions may actually show paradoxical motion. With an eventration, even though the diaphragm may descend, thereby reducing intrapleural pressure and causing inspiration as in normal diaphragm function, if the muscle is significantly elevated it may cause atelectasis of the lung, ventilation/perfusion mismatch, and shunting, which may themselves be causes of dyspnea.

Electromyography

Changes in diaphragmatic electrical activity reflect various aspects of diaphragm contraction. Although perhaps less clinically useful than measurement of maximal inspiratory pressure (MIP) (see below), the "compound motor action potential" (electromyography [EMG] signal) measured at the skin level does correlate with force of contraction. Other information, for example, on whether the diaphragm is fatiguing, can also be learned from more detailed evaluation of the EMG signal characteristics. Phrenic nerve conduction time can be measured with electrodes placed over the rib cage and stimulation of the nerve in the neck. Although not a primary mode of evaluating diaphragm paralysis – a diagnosis which is more easily established by fluoroscopy – nerve conduction time can be useful in the evaluation of phrenic nerve dysfunction when the diagnosis is in doubt.

Maximal Inspiratory Pressure

The most commonly used and clinically useful means of measuring the overall strength of diaphragm contraction are measurements of the maximal amount of negative inspiratory pressure that can be created by a patient at the level of the mouth. Although rarely ordered preoperatively in the evaluation of surgical patients, most pulmonary function laboratories are equipped to measure the MIP. This is done by having the patient inspire maximally from residual volume against an obstructed mouthpiece with only a small leak. It has been suggested that in cardiac surgery, preoperative MIP and MEP are associated with the need for prolonged postoperative ventilation.[8] To my knowledge, a study of whether preoperative MIP is an independent determinant of postoperative pulmonary complications in general thoracic surgical patients has never been carried out.

In the intensive care unit, MIP is commonly used as one of the determinants of whether a ventilated patient is "ready to wean." There are a number of studies that correlate successful weaning with higher levels of inspiratory pressure that are able to be generated. A MIP of less than 30-cm water is generally considered insufficient to support successful weaning. However, more complex formulas combining MIP, respiratory load, and/or minute ventilation have also been proposed to predict successful weaning.[9]

Transdiaphragmatic Pressure

Although used primarily in research applications, the force of diaphragmatic contraction can be more precisely measured by measuring the transdiaphragmatic pressure (Pdi) that is generated and plugging this into a formula that allows calculation of the force of contraction. The Pdi is measured by placing a catheter perorally that has both intraesophageal and intragastric balloons that can measure the intrathoracic and intraabdominal pressures, respectively. The difference between intrathoracic and intraabdominal pressures is the Pdi. Pdimax can be measured while having awake patients inspire maximally against a nearly occluded mouthpiece, or while maximally stimulating the phrenic nerves in the neck in sedated, intubated patients.

Since a variety of factors affect the force of contraction from breath to breath, clearly the more objective measure of diaphragm function is the Pdimax measured during maximal bilateral phrenic nerve stimulation. Since this value is designed to measure the force the diaphragm can create when all of its muscle fibers are maximally recruited, it is a measure that is relatively reproducible and can be used to follow diaphragm function over time far more precisely than with measures such as MIP.

DIAPHRAGM TUMORS

The diaphragm may rarely give rise to primary diaphragmatic tumors. Since the diaphragm is intimately associated with vital organs on both its thoracic and abdominal sides, it is more common for neoplasms of these organs to spread to involve the diaphragm, requiring en bloc resection. We review diaphragm tumors here, since they are not covered elsewhere in this volume.

Primary tumors of the diaphragm are more often benign than malignant, and as one would expect, they arise from muscle or other mesenchymal tissues.[10] The benign tumors most commonly include mesenchymal cysts, lipomas, and fibromas. The malignant tumors are most commonly rhabdomyosarcomas or leiomyosarcomas. These tumors are often asymptomatic at the time of presentation, although pain, cough, or dyspnea is not uncommon.[11]

Secondary tumors that involve the diaphragm most commonly arise from the lungs, the liver, or the gastroesophageal junction. One might also consider tumors of the pleura, such as mesothelioma, that commonly penetrate into the diaphragm to also be secondary tumors of the diaphragm. In each of these cases, diaphragmatic involvement does not preclude cure by diaphragmatic resection along with resection of the primary tumor, but the prognosis is generally worse than without diaphragmatic involvement.[12–14] This may be because of the extensive lymphatic and venous drainage of the diaphragm.

Metastases to the pleural or peritoneal spaces from a variety of tumors may also involve the diaphragm secondarily, but these cases have a very poor prognosis. Cytoreductive peritonectomy[15] and pleurectomy,[16] including diaphragm resection plus adjuvant therapies, have been described for these situations, with some suggestion of benefit. However, there is currently no indication for surgical resection in these cases outside of clinical trials.

It can be quite difficult to determine whether a tumor in the vicinity of the diaphragm is a primary diaphragmatic tumor versus a primary tumor of an adjacent organ secondarily involving the diaphragm. The thin structure of the diaphragm, and its constant movement, render it difficult to accurately image. Fortunately, this determination is often not critical for therapy. It can, however, be helpful for preoperative planning to know if the diaphragm will need to be resected. While CT can suggest loss of normal tissue planes and thus diaphragmatic invasion, its volume averaging effect on curved surfaces can render this less than reliable. Magnetic resonance imaging (MRI) does not have this technical limitation, and a number of studies have suggested that it is more accurate than CT in predicting diaphragmatic involvement.

DIAPHRAGM DYSFUNCTION AND ITS CONSEQUENCES

Paralysis/Paresis

This topic is covered deeply elsewhere in the text. Unilateral diaphragm paralysis is a relatively common condition – whether idiopathic or iatrogenic – and has substantial impact on dyspnea and quality of life. Diaphragm plication is a very effective therapy, substantially improving symptoms and objective measures of pulmonary function. Particularly since it can now reliably be performed by VATS,[17] it should be considered in all patients with paralysis that has persisted for over 6 months. Still, because the diaphragm remains noncontractile after plication, exercise capacity does not generally return to the full preoperative level. Although one might consider direct diaphragm pacing as a more physiological solution, the problem of timing the paced contraction to the normal phrenic nerve impulse and contraction on the contralateral side has limited exploration of this possibility.

Post Thoracotomy Diaphragm Dysfunction

It has been clearly demonstrated in sheep that diaphragm function is less robust following thoracotomy,[18] and that this dysfunction extends at least to 28 days postoperatively. Recovery from this postoperative deficit in diaphragm contractility is somewhat faster following VATS than following thoracotomy.[19] Although one might infer that this compromised diaphragm function following thoracic surgery is a source of pulmonary complications, it would be very difficult to demonstrate this experimentally.

Diaphragm Dysfunction in Emphysema

In emphysema, the progressively increasing volume of the lung gradually pushes the diaphragm caudally until, in severe disease, it has attained a nearly flat, horizontal position quite different from its usual domed, piston-like configuration (Fig. 148-6). In this flatter configuration, the piston-like descent of the diaphragm is obviously severely compromised. Also, the

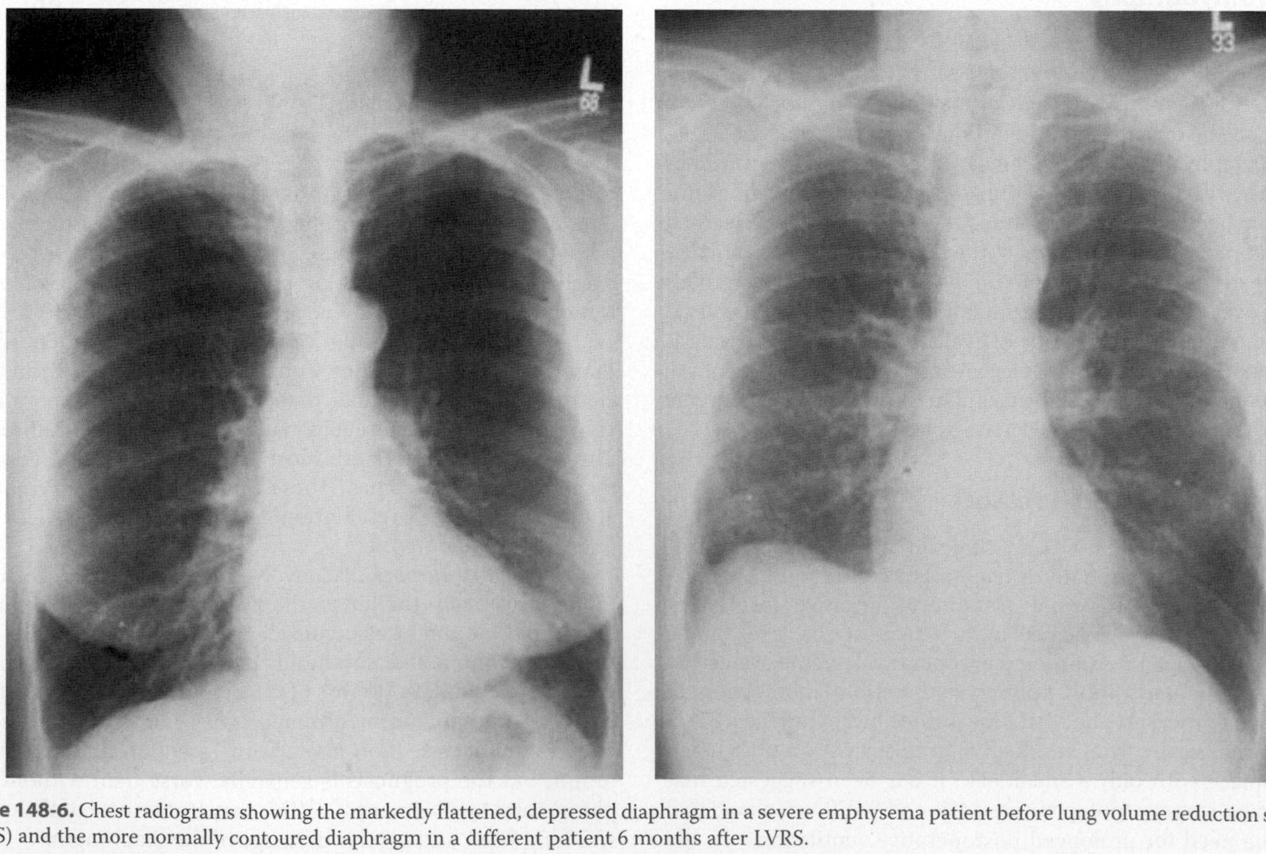

Figure 148-6. Chest radiograms showing the markedly flattened, depressed diaphragm in a severe emphysema patient before lung volume reduction surgery (LVRS) and the more normally contoured diaphragm in a different patient 6 months after LVRS.

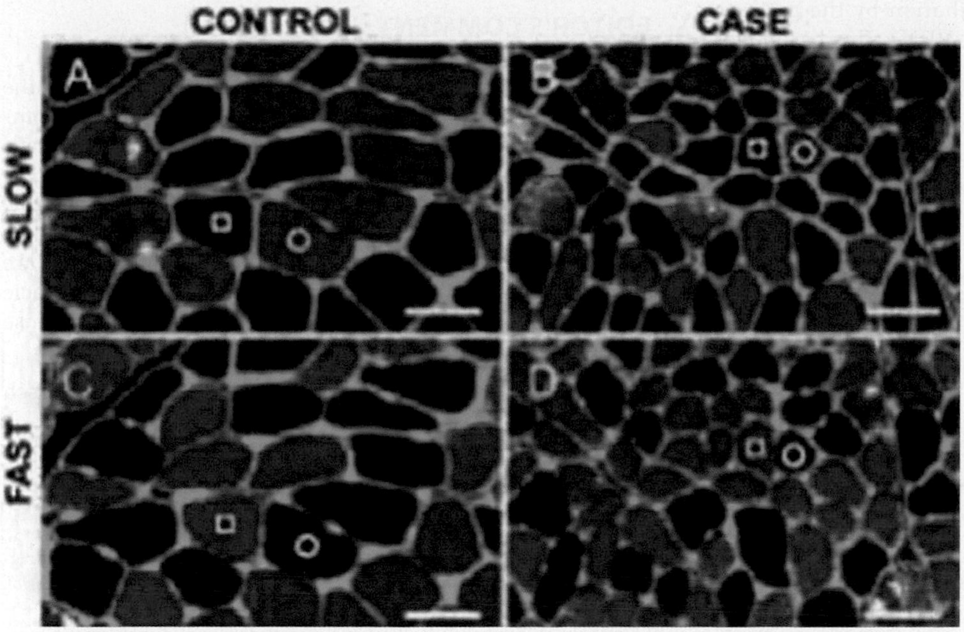

Figure 148-7. Cross sections of immunohistochemically stained human diaphragm muscle biopsies taken after 2 hours of mechanical ventilation (panels *A* and *C*) and after approximately 25 hours of mechanical ventilation (panels *B* and *D*). All panels are taken at the same magnification. Note that both the slow (*A* and *B*) and the fast (*C* and *D*) fibers shrink to approximately 50% of their normal size after even medium-term duration of mechanical ventilation. (Adapted from Levine S, Nguyen T, Taylor N, et al. Rapid disuse atrophy of diaphragm fibers in mechanically ventilated humans. *N Engl J Med.* 2008;358:1327.)

diaphragm's secondary action of expanding the lower rib cage may actually be reversed such that the ribs are drawn inward with contraction, favoring exhalation. The diaphragm is thus an extremely ineffective inspiratory muscle in severe emphysema. This diaphragm dysfunction increases the WOB and forces emphysema patients to recruit their accessory muscles of inspiration to draw air in. This is a major contributor to the severe sensation of dyspnea in these patients.

It is interesting to note that although the contraction of the diaphragm in emphysema is less effective at creating inspiration than in the normal state, it is unlikely that the diaphragm is receiving any less descending neural stimulation. In fact, diaphragm muscle fibers of emphysema patients shift towards a fiber type (slow, oxidative type expressing type I myosin heavy chains [MHCs]) – similar to the adaptations that occur within the leg muscles in a long-distance runner – suggesting that the muscle is in emphysema under greater rather than lesser load.[20] Muscle with more type I fibers may be "adaptive" to the extent that it will be more resistant to fatigue, but on the other hand it cannot generate the same maximal force as a muscle with a greater (normal) proportion of fast myofibers.

After lung volume reduction surgery (LVRS), the diaphragm progressively attains, over a 3- to 6-month period, a more normal, domed configuration and improved function.[21] New sarcomeres are actually laid down within the diaphragm muscle fibers, allowing the now longer fibers to function at their optimal point on their length–tension curve.[22] Along of course with changes within the lung itself, such as improved elastic recoil and V/Q matching, these changes within the diaphragm certainly contribute in a major way to the objective symptomatic improvements obtained by appropriately selected LVRS patients. Remember, dyspnea is more closely related to respiratory muscle function than to FEV_1.

Obesity

As in emphysema, obesity places an increased load on the respiratory muscles including the diaphragm, and they function less effectively. The load in this situation appears to result from reduced chest wall compliance. This results in similar shifts in the diaphragm as seen in emphysema—to a greater proportion of slow fiber types, MHCs, and greater oxidative enzyme capacity (at least in experimental models).[23]

Aging

At age 70 to 80, the maximal contractile force able to be generated by the diaphragm is 20% to 30% lower than at age 20.[24] This seems to result from shifts in the proportions of the various fiber types with age.[25]

Mechanical Ventilation

A very important recent discovery is that even brief periods of full mechanical ventilator support appear to result in rapid and severe (~50%) reduction in diaphragm muscle fiber cross-sectional area in humans (Fig. 148-7).[26] This finding confirmed a substantial amount of data showing this phenomenon in experimental animals.[27] The loss of diaphragm muscle mass with MV is far more rapid than that seen in casted limb muscles, a finding that may be somehow related to the diaphragm's unique, continuous function when compared with limb muscles. The atrophy seems to occur via rapid activation of muscle proteolytic pathways.

Obviously, reduction of muscle fiber size by 50% will translate to a dramatic reduction in the ability of the diaphragm to create inspiratory force. Although it has not been proven with certainty, strong circumstantial evidence exists that this reduction in diaphragm force is a central cause of "failure to wean" and thus the need for prolonged MV in many patients.[28,29] If ventilator-induced diaphragm atrophy (VIDD) could be prevented, it might prevent the major morbidity and mortality rates that are associated with prolonged MV as well as saving millions of health care dollars.

One way to prevent VIDD might be to avoid, where possible, full ventilator support. Using pressure support, or other modes that require an ongoing contribution by the patients diaphragm to inspiration, may prevent VIDD. This has in fact been demonstrated to be effective in rats.[30] However, there are many disease processes and severities in which pressure support modes are impossible to employ. Another approach might be electrical stimulation of the diaphragm when patients require full MV support, although this has not been shown to be effective even in animals as of this writing. Lastly, and perhaps most conveniently, a drug might be developed that would prevent diaphragm atrophy. Such a drug could be administered to all patients at the time they are placed on the ventilator. Work delineating the molecular basis of VIDD is ongoing,[31] and has already yielded drugs showing effectiveness in animal models.[32,33]

EDITOR'S COMMENT

Dr. Shrager presents a clear and concise description of the important anatomy of the diaphragm. I appreciate his comparison of the diaphragm to an "air pump" or "piston." Readers should note the clear explanation of porous diseases of the diaphragm in this chapter. This chapter also addresses the role of the diaphragm in respiratory failure and the feeling of dyspnea. A number of ways of measuring diaphragm function are presented. This is an area of growing understanding in thoracic surgery, and this chapter is a valuable contribution to those wishing to further this field.

—Michael T. Jaklitsch

References

1. Kirschner PA. Porous diaphragm syndromes. *Chest Surg Clin North Am.* 1998;8:449.
2. Cerfolio RJ, Bryant AS. Efficacy of video-assisted thoracoscopic surgery with talc pleurodesis for porous diaphragm syndrome in patients with refractory hepatic hydrothorax. *Ann Thorac Surg.* 2006;82:457.
3. Mak SK, Nyunt K, Wong PN, et al. Long-term follow-up of thoracoscopic pleurodesis for hydrothorax complicating peritoneal dialysis. *Ann Thorac Surg.* 2002;74:218.
4. Marshall MB, Ahmed Z, Kucharczuk JC, et al. Catamenial pneumothorax: optimal hormonal and surgical management. *Eur J Cardiothorac Surg.* 2005;27:662.
5. Abu-Hijleh MF, Habbal OA, Moqattash ST. The role of the diaphragm in lymphatic absorption from the peritoneal cavity. *J Anat.* 1995;186:453.
6. Okiemy G, Foucault C, Avisse C, et al. Lymphatic drainage of the diaphragmatic pleura to the peritracheobronchial lymph nodes. *Surg Radiol Anat.* 2003;25:32.
7. Wade OL. Movements of the thoracic cage and diaphragm in respiration. *J Physiol.* 1954;124:193.
8. Rodrigues AJ, Mendes V, Ferreira PE, et al. Preoperative respiratory muscle dysfunction is a predictor of prolonged invasive mechanical ventilation in cardiorespiratory complications after heart valve surgery. *Eur J Cardiothorac Surg.* 2011;39:662.
9. Jabour ER, Rabil DM, Truwit JD, et al. Evaluation of a new weaning index based on ventilator endurance and the efficiency of gas exchange. *Am Rev Resp Dis.* 1991;144:531.
10. Olafsson G, Rausing A, Holen O. Primary tumors of the diaphragm. *Chest.* 1971;59:568.
11. Limmer KK, Kernstine KH, Grannis FW, et al. Mediastinal diseases, benign or malignant. In: Sugarbaker DJ, ed. *Adult Chest Surgery*. 1st ed. New York, NY: McGraw-Hill; 2009:1053–1067.
12. Riquet M, Porte H, Chapelier A, et al. Resection of lung cancer invading the diaphragm. *J Thorac Cardiovasc Surg.* 2000;120:417.
13. Yokoi K, Tsuchiya R, Mori T, et al. Results of surgical treatment of lung cancer involving the diaphragm. *J Thorac Cardiovasc Surg.* 2000;120:799.
14. Lim MC, Wu CC, Chen JT, et al. Surgical results of hepatic resection for hepatocellular carcinoma with gross diaphragmatic invasion. *Hepatogastroenterology.* 2005;52:1497.
15. Eisenhauer EL, D'Angelica MI, Abu-Rustum NR, et al. Incidence and management of pleural effusions after diaphragm peritonectomy or resection for advanced mullerian cancer. *Gynecol Oncol.* 2006;103:871.
16. Friedberg JS, Mick R, Stevenson JP, et al. Phase II trial of pleural photodynamic therapy and surgery for patients with non-small-cell lung cancer with pleural spread. *J Clin Oncol.* 2004;22:2192.
17. Mouroux J, Venissac N, Leo F, et al. Surgical treatment of diaphragmatic eventration using video-assisted thoracic surgery: a prospective study. *Ann Thorac Surg.* 2005;79:308.
18. Torres A, Kimball WR, Qvist J, et al. Sonomicrometric regional diaphragmatic shortening in awake sheep after thoracic surgery. *J Appl Physiol.* 1989;67:2357.
19. Imanaka H, Kimball WR, Wain JC, et al. Recovery of diaphragmatic function in awake sheep after two approaches to thoracic surgery. *J Appl Physiol.* 1997;83:1733.
20. Levine S, Nguyen T, Kaiser LR, et al. Human diaphragm remodeling associated with COPD: clinical implications. *Am J Respir Crit Care Med.* 2003;168:706.
21. Laghi F, Jubran A, Topeli A, et al. Effect of lung volume reduction surgery on neuromechanical coupling of the diaphragm. *Am J Respir Crit Care Med.* 1998;157:475.
22. Shrager JB, Kim DK, Stedman HH, et al. Sarcomeres are added in series to emphysematous rat diaphragm after lung volume reduction surgery. *Chest.* 2002;121:210.
23. Powers SK, Farkas GA, Demirel H, et al. Effects of aging and obesity on respiratory muscle phenotype in Zucker rats. *J Appl Physiol.* 1996;81:1347.
24. Black LF, Hyatt RE. Maximal respiratory pressures: normal values and relationship to age and sex. *Am Rev Respir Dis.* 1968;99:696.
25. Gosselin LE, Johnson BD, Sieck GC. Age-related changes in diaphragm muscle contractile properties and myosin heavy chain isoforms. *Am J Respir Crit Care Med.* 1994;150:174.
26. Levine S, Nguyen T, Taylor N, et al. Rapid disuse atrophy of diaphragm fibers in mechanically ventilated humans. *N Engl J Med.* 2008;358:1327.
27. Powers SK, Kavazis AN, Levine S. Prolonged mechanical ventilation alters diaphragmatic structure and function. *Crit Care Med.* 2009;37:S347.
28. Jaber S, Petrof BJ, Jung B, et al. Rapidly progressive diaphragmatic weakness and injury during mechanical ventilation in humans. *Am J Respir Crit Care Med.* 2011;183:364.
29. Purro A, Appendini L, De Gaetano A, et al. Physiologic determinants of ventilator dependence in long-term mechanically ventilated patients. *Am J Respir Crit Care Med.* 2000;161:1115.
30. Futier E, Constantin JM, Combaret L, et al. Pressure support ventilation attenuates ventilator-induced protein modifications in the diaphragm. *Crit Care.* 2008;12:116.
31. Tang H, Lee M, Budak MT, et al. Intrinsic apoptosis in mechanically ventilated human diaphragm: linkage to a novel Fos/FoxO1/Stat3-Bim axis. *Faseb J.* 2011;25:2921.
32. Betters JL, Criswell DS, Shanely RA, et al. Trolox attenuates mechanical ventilation-induced diaphragmatic dysfunction and proteolysis. *Am J Respir Crit Care Med.* 2004;170:1179.
33. Powers SK, Hudson MB, Nelson WB, et al. Mitochondria-targeted antioxidants protect against mechanical ventilation-induced diaphragm weakness. *Crit Care Med.* 2011;39:1749.

149 Incision, Resection, and Replacement of the Diaphragm

Daniel C. Wiener and Michael T. Jaklitsch

Keywords: Circumferential incision, central tendon incision, radial incision, patch reconstruction of diaphragm, diaphragm resection

INTRODUCTION

The fan-shaped muscle of the diaphragm arises from the internal circumference of the thorax, with attachments to the sternum, the lower six or seven ribs, and the lumbar vertebral bodies. The muscle fibers also attach posteriorly to the aponeurotic arch of the ligamentum arcuatum externum, which overrides the psoas and quadratus lumborum muscles (Fig. 149-1). Laterally, the fibers of the diaphragm interdigitate with slips from the transversalis muscle of the abdomen to originate from the ribs.[1] The right crus is larger and longer than the left and arises from the bodies of the upper three or four lumbar vertebrae. The left crus arises from the upper two lumbar vertebral bodies.

There are three natural openings within the diaphragm (Fig. 149-2). The aortic opening is the most posterior of the three and is formed from fibers comprising the right and left diaphragmatic crura.[1] This tunnel is actually behind the diaphragm, not within it, and contains the aorta, azygos vein, and thoracic duct. The esophageal hiatus is slightly more ventral in relation to the aortic hiatus and consists of fibers passing between the aorta and the esophagus toward the right crus, as well as fibers converging on the pericardial tendon. The opening of the inferior vena cava lies within the confluence of the tendons of the right hemithorax and the tendon beneath the pericardium.

The muscular diaphragm acts as a boundary between the positive pressure abdominal cavity and the negative pressure

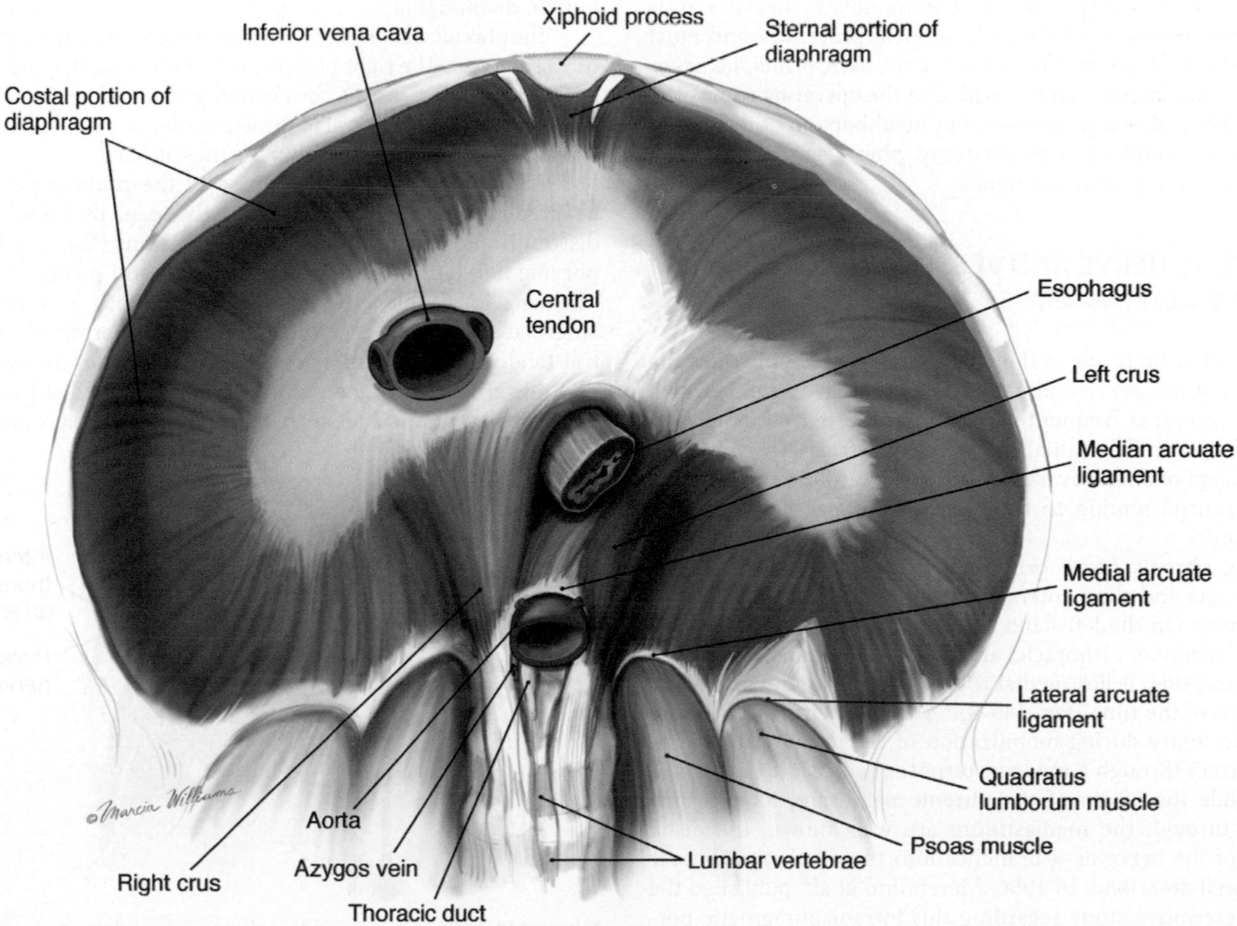

Figure 149-1. The muscle fibers of the diaphragm originate from the posterior lumbar spine (arcuate ligaments) and curve upward to form an aponeurotic sheath known as the central tendon. Several thoracic organs and vessels pass through apertures in the diaphragmatic surface.

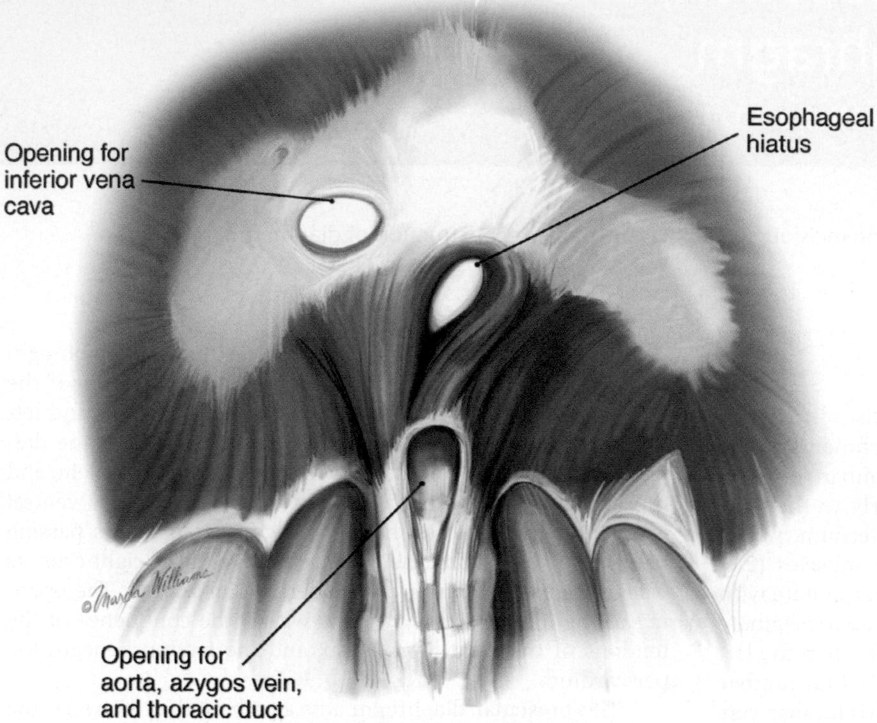

Figure 149-2. Abdominal surface of the diaphragm with three natural openings.

thoracic cavity. Although diaphragmatic disease is infrequent, exposure to the diaphragm is commonplace, because it is visualized during every thoracic surgical procedure and most intraabdominal operations. Therefore the basic principles advocated by this chapter can be verified in the operating room. The diaphragm makes a good fence, but neighbors on both sides of that fence should know its anatomy, physiology, and surgical principles of resection and repair.

PHRENIC NERVE AND VESSEL BRANCHES IN THE DIAPHRAGM

A number of incisions in the diaphragm are possible once the location of the nerve and vessel branches have been learned. These structures frequently lie within the muscle itself and are not seen on the cranial surface of the structure. Therefore, the concept of a neurovascular "manacle" around the junction of the central tendon to the muscle is a very helpful visual mnemonic.

The phrenic nerve originates from the C3, C4, and C5 nerve roots and then enters the chest anterior to the subclavian artery. On the left-hand side, the nerve lies medial to the internal mammary (thoracic) artery 64% of the time, and on the right-hand side, it lies medial to the internal mammary artery only 46% of the time (Fig. 149-3).[2] Thus the left nerve is more prone to injury during mobilization of the left internal mammary artery through a median sternotomy incision.

While the origin of the phrenic nerve and its proximal course through the mediastinum are well known, the distal extent of the nerve as it branches into the diaphragm proper is less well described. In 1956, Merendino et al.[3] published the most descriptive study regarding this intradiaphragmatic portion of the phrenic nerve. Their anatomic findings and drawings are based on electrical stimulation studies and gross dissection in dogs as well as intraoperative dissection of approximately 40 human diaphragms.

The phrenic nerve usually divides at the level of the diaphragm or just above it. The right phrenic nerve enters the diaphragm just lateral to the inferior vena cava within the central tendon. The left phrenic nerve enters lateral to the left border of the heart just anterior to the central tendon within the muscle itself.

The intradiaphragmatic course of the phrenic nerve can be predicted, even when not directly seen, by knowing the distribution of the four main motor divisions (Fig. 149-4). The phrenic nerve first splits into an anterior and posterior trunk. The anterior trunk subsequently divides into a sternal and anterolateral branch near the anteromedial border of the central tendon. The posterior trunk likewise divides into a crural and posterolateral branch along the posteromedial border of the central tendon. The sternal and crural branches are short

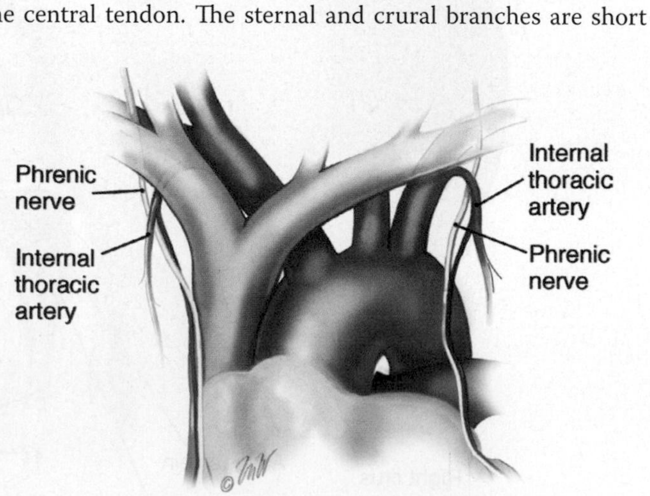

Figure 149-3. Juxtaposition of the phrenic nerve and internal thoracic (mammary) artery on right and left sides creates the potential for phrenic nerve injury, leading to diaphragmatic elevation.

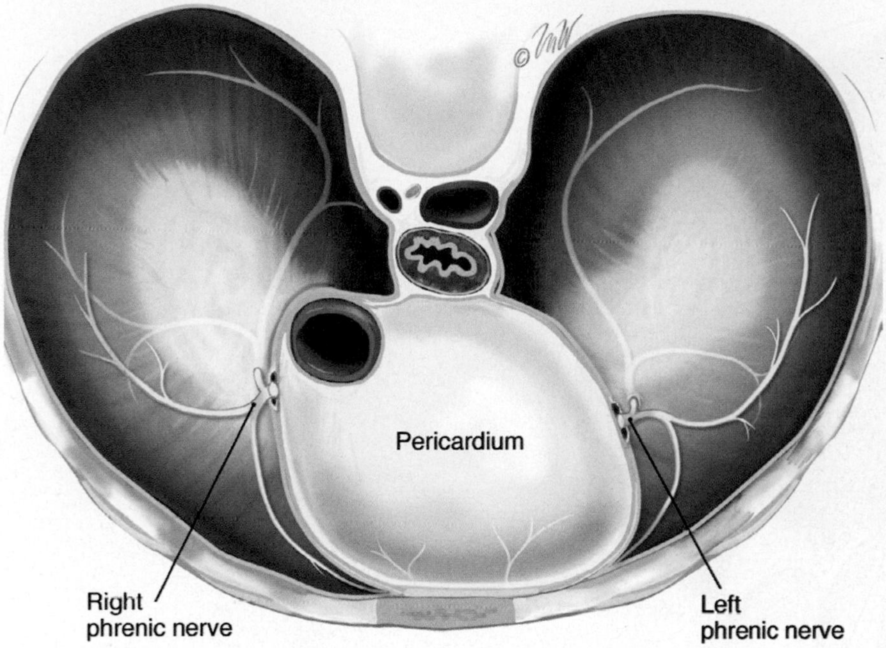

Figure 149-4. The phrenic nerves pierce the diaphragmatic surface and course through musculature invisible to the naked eye.

and continue to run in an anteromedial and posteromedial direction, respectively. The anterolateral and posterolateral branches are much longer and run close to the muscular fiber insertions into the central tendon. These two branches innervate the majority of the diaphragm. Their anatomic relation to one another is often described as a pair of handcuffs or manacles. Often these branches are within the muscle layers and are not readily visible.

The superior phrenic arteries are located on the thoracic surface of the diaphragm (Fig. 149-5). These represent small branches from the lower thoracic aorta and traverse the posterior diaphragm over the top portion of each crus close to the mediastinum.[1] They terminate in small anastomoses with the musculophrenic and pericardiophrenic arteries, which are both branches from the internal mammary artery. These latter two arteries also supply blood to the phrenic nerve and the pericardial fat pad.[4]

The inferior phrenic arteries lie on the undersurface of the crus and the dome of the diaphragm (Fig. 149-6). These are small, paired vessels with frequent anatomic variations. They can originate separately from the aorta above the celiac artery. Alternatively, a common trunk arising from either the aorta or the celiac artery gives rise to these two arteries. Occasionally, one vessel will originate from the aorta, whereas the other emerges from one of the renal arteries. The inferior phrenic arteries then course obliquely superior and lateral along the inferior surface of the diaphragm. The left phrenic artery passes

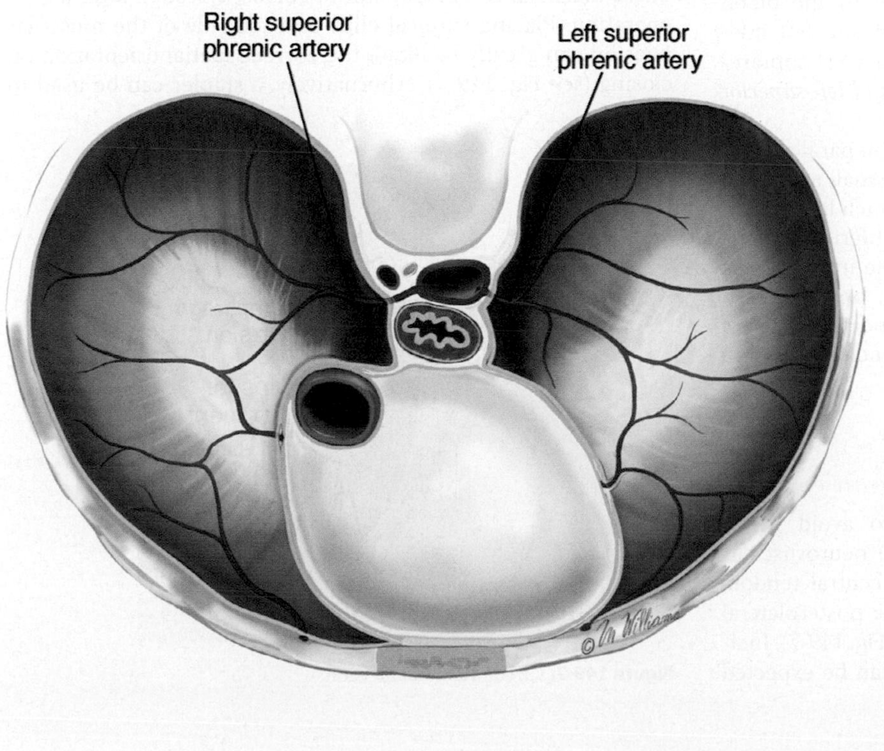

Figure 149-5. Thoracic surface of the diaphragm with phrenic artery anatomy.

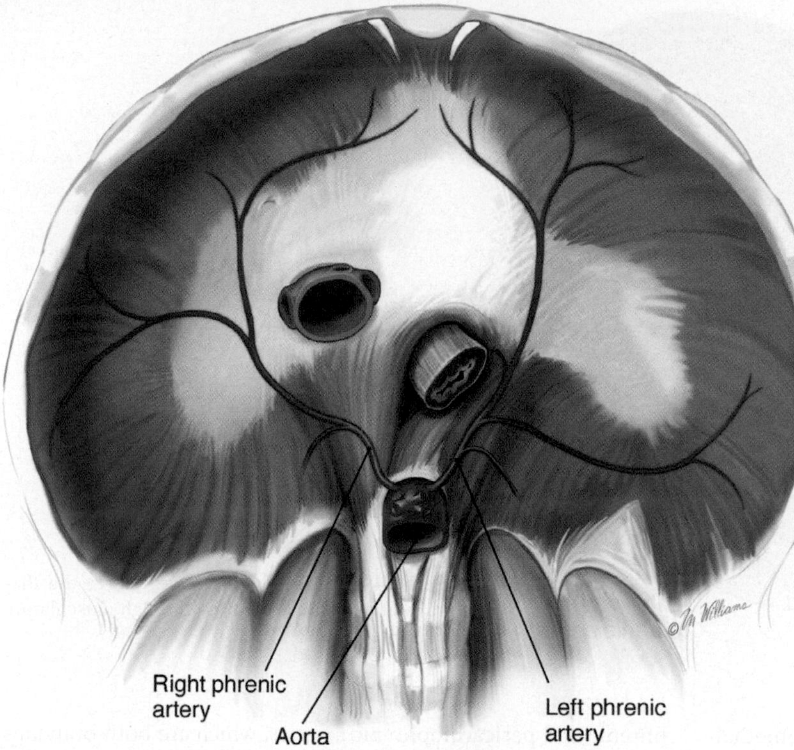

Figure 149-6. Course of the phrenic artery from the abdominal surface of the diaphragm.

posterior to the esophagus and then runs anteriorly along the lateral side of the esophageal hiatus. The right inferior phrenic artery passes behind the inferior vena cava.[1]

Close to the posterior aspect of the central tendon, both the left and right inferior phrenic arteries divide into a medial and lateral branch. The medial branch extends anteriorly, close to the mediastinum. Branches of this vessel traverse the muscular portion of the diaphragm to anastomose with the musculophrenic and pericardiophrenic arteries. The lateral branch of the inferior phrenic artery courses laterally and forms anastomoses with the lower intercostal arteries. The left inferior phrenic artery provides a minor contribution to the blood supply of the lower esophagus. Both the right and left inferior phrenic arteries have branches to the ipsilateral suprarenal gland. These branches are called the *right and left superior suprarenal arteries.*[1]

In general, the venous anatomy in this region parallels that of the arteries. The superior phrenic veins are small and drain anteriorly to the internal mammary vein. The much larger inferior phrenic veins parallel the course of the inferior phrenic arteries. The right vein empties directly into the inferior vena cava. The left vein usually has two branches, one of which drains into the left renal or suprarenal vein and the other of which passes anterior to the esophageal hiatus and empties into the inferior vena cava.[1]

DIAPHRAGMATIC INCISIONS

Diaphragmatic incisions should be placed to avoid major branches of the arteries and nerves. Since the neurovascular bundles are swinging around the edge of the central tendon, incisions should avoid those areas except at the posterolateral edge of the tendon (the open area of the handcuff, Fig. 149-7). Incisions that cross major neurovascular bundles can be expected to result in bleeding, structural weakness, and partial diaphragmatic paresis.

Diaphragmatic incisions can be divided into three groups: circumferential, central tendon, and radial.

Circumferential

Circumferential incisions in the periphery result in little loss of function. These circumferential incisions, however, should lie at least 5-cm lateral to the edge of the central tendon to avoid the posterolateral and anterolateral branches of the phrenic nerve. These incisions can be difficult to correctly realign after a long operation. Placing surgical clips on each side of the muscular incision can greatly facilitate the correct spatial orientation on closing (see Fig. 149-7). Alternatively, a stapler can be used to

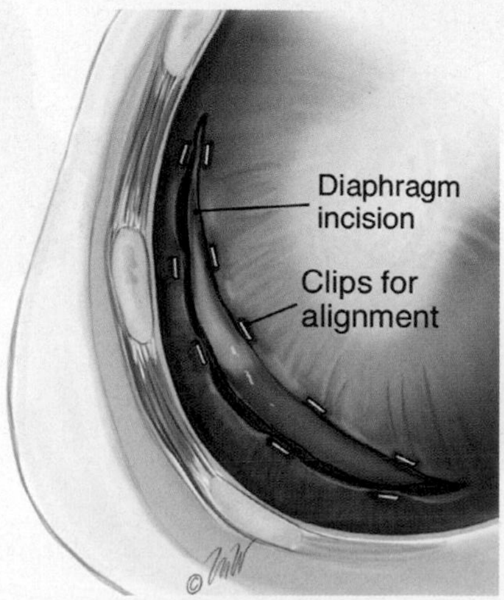

Figure 149-7. Circumferential incision.

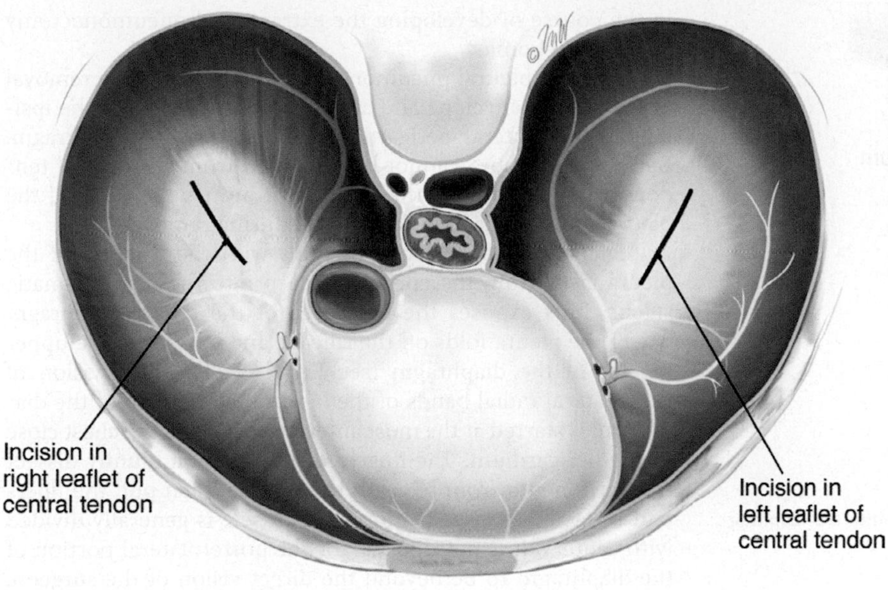

Figure 149-8. Central tendon incision.

divide the muscle, and these staple lines can greatly facilitate reapproximation of the muscle.

Closing suture should be a strong grade to withstand the force of a cough. This can include a monofilament such as 0-Prolene or a braided suture such as 0-Ethibond. Pledgets can help the closure if the muscle is fraying during closure. The incisions can be difficult to close in the face of truncal obesity if the abdominal contents are under pressure. Displacement of the central tendon caudally (toward the feet) in a vigorous manner can produce a nicely approximated edge of muscle that facilitates closure.

Central Tendon

Incisions in the central tendon, as far centrally as within 2 cm of the entrance of the phrenic nerve, do not interrupt any major branch of the nerve itself. This type of incision can provide excellent visualization of the abdomen from the thorax, and vice versa. These incisions are easy to open and close (Fig. 149-8). In general, we recommend that the incision be oriented toward the posterolateral portion of the central tendon if the incision needs to be opened further, as this represents the open area of the manacle, and thus, has the least chance of injuring a neurovascular branch.

Radial

A transverse radial incision made from the posterolateral portion of the tendon and moving centrally is relatively safe because it courses between the distal aspects of the anterolateral and posterolateral branches of the phrenic nerve (i.e., through the opening of the "handcuffs") (Fig. 149-9). The lateral part of this incision roughly correlates to the line of the tip of the scapula along the chest wall.

Radial incisions from the costal margin extending all the way to the esophageal hiatus have previously been advocated for thoracoabdominal incisions and resection of the GE junction. This incision, however, may result in segmental diaphragmatic paralysis if the incision transects the crural or posterolateral branches of the phrenic nerve (see Fig. 149-9).

Pleural and Peritoneal Attachments

The pleurae are tightly adherent to the top surface of the diaphragmatic central tendon and most of the musculature. It is impossible to separate the pleura from the central tendon of each hemidiaphragm. As each pleura curves off the chest wall and folds back on the surface of the diaphragm, there is a circumferential diaphragmatic recess of approximately 1 cm that does not contain pleura (Fig. 149-10).[5]

The peritoneum is less adherent to the undersurface of the diaphragm and can be bluntly mobilized off the diaphragm during extraperitoneal approaches to the abdominal aorta. The plane of dissection lies between the inferior phrenic artery and vein on the muscle side and the peritoneal membrane. The peritoneum separates from the central tendon of the right diaphragm to form the falciform ligament and

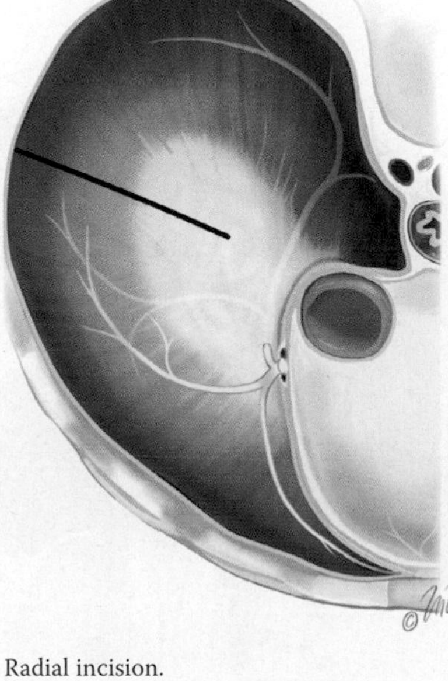

Figure 149-9. Radial incision.

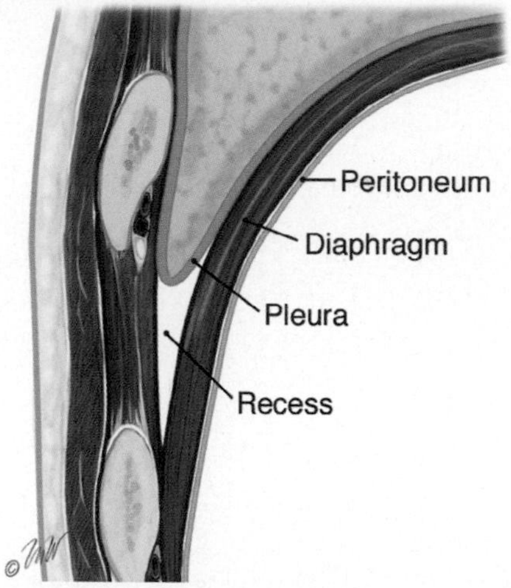

Figure 149-10. The pleurae do not extend all the way into the diaphragmatic recess.

produces an area directly under the central tendon that does not have peritoneal covering. This is known as the *bare area* (Fig. 149-11).

DIAPHRAGMATIC RESECTION AND RECONSTRUCTION WITH PROSTHETIC PATCH

Partial diaphragmatic resections are necessary to remove tumors that have invaded a portion of the diaphragm. The redundancy of the muscle frequently permits primary repair for small to modest resections. Larger defects are easily repaired with the use of a mesh or impermeable graft sutured to the remnant of muscle. We use mesh for patients with lung tissue remaining in the ipsilateral hemithorax, but impermeable grafts for patients who have had a pneumonectomy. The impermeable patches prevent fluid shifts between the thorax and abdomen.

Complete diaphragmatic resection may be required for large tumors invading the diaphragm, such as lung cancer of the lower lobe or sarcomas of the chest. We have gained extensive experience with complete diaphragmatic resection in the course of developing the extrapleural pneumonectomy for mesothelioma.[5]

An extrapleural pneumonectomy is the complete removal of the pleural envelope and all its contents, including the ipsilateral lung, lateral pericardium, and underlying diaphragm. Because the pleura cannot be separated from the central tendon of the diaphragm, the diaphragm must be resected if the pleural envelope is to be kept intact during removal.

Diaphragmatic resection begins with the traction of the pleura away from the chest wall deep into the diaphragmatic sulcus. This exposes the bare area of the lateral diaphragm where the pleura folds off the ribcage and back onto the upper surface of the diaphragm (see Fig. 149-11). The division of these lateral radial bands of the fan-shaped portion of the diaphragm is started at the most anterior portion of the chest close to the pericardium. The fingers of the surgeon bluntly dissect the peritoneum from beneath the muscle, then pull the fibers taut to facilitate visualization. The muscle is generally divided with cautery. It is not unusual for the posterolateral portion of the diaphragm to be beyond the direct vision of the surgeon. Fibers in this area can be bluntly avulsed with minimal risk of bleeding. Once the ligamentum arcuatum externum (external arcuate ligament) is reached in the paravertebral sulcus, the perinephric fat of Gerota fascia, and not the peritoneum, is directly beneath the fan-shaped muscle. This part of the dissection quickly progresses to the lateral margin of the crus. The diaphragm can then be separated from the peritoneum up toward the lateral border of the pericardium. Defects in the peritoneum are closed as they are recognized.

The phrenic nerve is divided. The trileaflet of the diaphragmatic tendon is divided along the line demarcating the central tendon of the ipsilateral muscle from the tendon lying beneath the pericardium. This cut is made medial to the insertion of the phrenic nerve into the anterior muscle. This medial cut is extended along the fused portion of diaphragmatic tendon and pericardium to the inferior vena cava on the right, or the esophageal hiatus on the left.

The only attachment of the diaphragm remaining is the crus. Blunt dissection of the pleura of the deep diaphragmatic sulcus needs to be completed before division of the crus to prevent buttonholing the inferior extent of the posterolateral pleura.

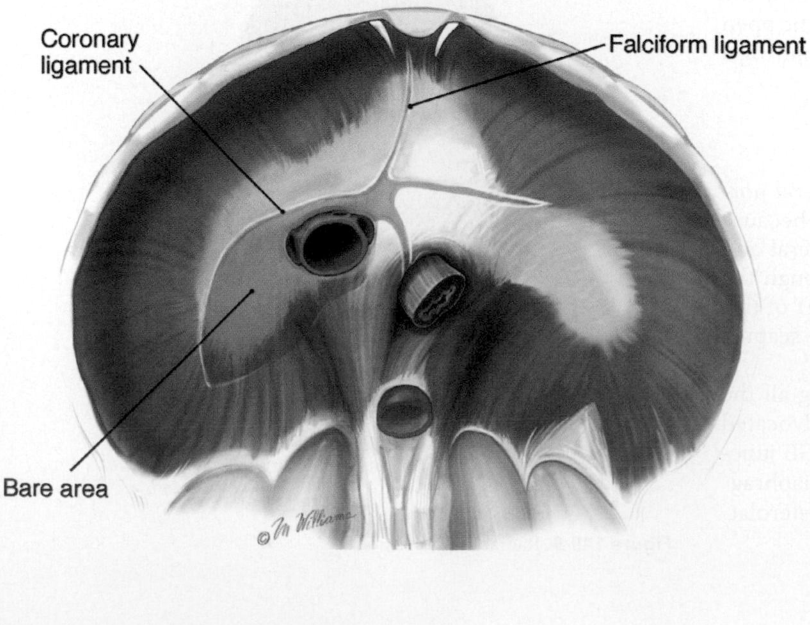

Figure 149-11. The peritoneum does not adhere to the abdominal surface of the right diaphragm where it separates from the central tendon, creating a bare area.

The superior phrenic arteries are surgically inconsequential and rarely identified. The inferior phrenic vessels, however, lie on the deep surface of the crus and are easily seen and ligated. These vessels may bifurcate low over the crus, and a second branch may therefore be found after ligation of a branch thought to be the main trunk. The left inferior phrenic vein usually has two branches, one of which drains into the left renal or suprarenal vein and another that passes anterior to the esophageal hiatus and empties into the inferior vena cava. The right inferior phrenic vein empties directly into the inferior vena cava and therefore requires careful dissection and ligation. Vigorous lateral traction can avulse this vessel from the inferior vena cava, close to the insertion of the hepatic veins. Once these vessels have been divided, the crus is easily divided. This completes the diaphragmatic resection.

The postpneumonectomy space fills with fluid. To prevent fluid shifts between the thorax and abdomen, we use a 2-mm impermeable Gore-Tex prosthetic patch to reconstruct the resected diaphragm. This patch prevents herniation of abdominal contents into the chest, holds the abdominal viscera out of the thoracic radiation field, and also bolsters the contralateral diaphragm by fixing the medial edge of the fan into place. This then facilitates the function of the opposite diaphragm by allowing its central tendon to become the anchor point for the lateral fan fascicles. Without patching the ipsilateral diaphragmatic defect, the contralateral muscle function is compromised.

After the patch has been cut to the shape of the removed diaphragm, the medial edge is sewn to the pericardial tendon with a soft nonabsorbable stitch. We prefer 0-Ethibond for this suture. This suture line runs from the free edge of the divided anterior fan muscles, along the pericardial edge, to either the inferior vena cava or esophageal hiatus. A reliable lateral anchorage system has been devised, requiring a sterilized leatherworking awl. Loops of suture material that have been passed through the lateral edge of the patch are then brought through the chest wall with the awl. The sutures are then passed through a small postage stamp–sized patch of the same material, as well as a sterile plastic button, with the assistance of two angiocaths. The loop of suture is then tied down to itself onto the button, resulting in excellent lateral displacement of the patch.

The posterior mediastinum between the thoracic spine and the inferior vena cava or esophagus is the area where patch ruptures occur, with abdominal contents herniating into the chest. This is due to a lack of strong mediastinal tissue available to anchor the patch. Our group of surgeons have developed the following three potential solutions: (1) a suture anchoring the patch to the anterior spinal ligament, (2) a tongue of extra patch material folded inferiorly along the lumbar spine in simulation of the diaphragmatic crus, and (3) a composite of two patches of 2-mm Gore-Tex stapled together in the middle with a thoracoabdominal (TA) stapler to create a dynamic patch at the center with less tension at the lateral suture lines. The first technique uses the dense spinous ligament to anchor the posterior mediastinal portion of the patch and decreases the free defect between the anterior suture line at the inferior vena cava and the thoracic spine to a few centimeters. The second technique allows the medial portion of the patch to partially displace into the chest, but prevents visceral herniation unless the entire tongue becomes displaced into the chest. The last technique allows the prosthetic patch to "give" without rupture if the patient experiences abdominal distention.

SUMMARY

Diaphragm incisions are straight forward, but require the surgeon to have an understanding of the course of the neurovascular bundles of the phrenic nerve. These branches frequently run on the undersurface of the muscle. Circumferential and central tendon incisions are generally safe. Radial incisions should be oriented to pass between the open arms of the anterior and posterior branches of the phrenic nerve in a posterolateral manner (toward the line of the tip of the scapula).

Diaphragms can be partially or completely resected. Muscle resections require the surgeon to have an understanding of the crural anatomy, the pleural attachments, and the peritoneal attachments. Particular attention should be made to the branches of the phrenic vessels, especially the venous branches draining the hepatic veins. A clever system of attaching the prosthetic patch to the lateral chest wall has been developed by Sugarbaker et al. That technique is described in this chapter.

References

1. Gray H. *Anatomy, Descriptive and Surgical*. Revised American, from the 15th English ed. Pick T, Howden R, eds. New York, NY: Bounty Books; 1977:1257.
2. Owens WA, Gladstone DJ, Heylings DJ. Surgical anatomy of the phrenic nerve and internal mammary artery. *Ann Thorac Surg*. 1994;58:843–844.
3. Merendino KA, Johnson RJ, Skinner HH, et al. The intradiaphragmatic distribution of the phrenic nerve with particular reference to the placement of diaphragmatic incisions and controlled segmental paralysis. *Surgery*. 1956;39:189–198.
4. Garbaccio C, Gyepes MT, Fonkalsrud EW. Malfunction of the intact diaphragm in infants and children. *Arch Surg*. 1972;105:57–61.
5. Sugarbaker DJ, Mentzer SJ, Strauss G. Extrapleural pneumonectomy in the treatment of malignant pleural mesothelioma. *Ann Thorac Surg*. 1992;54:941–946.

150 Plication of the Diaphragm from Above

Michael T. Jaklitsch

Keywords: Diaphragmatic elevation, congenital eventration, phrenic nerve palsy, central tendon plication technique, radial plication technique

The two most common causes of diaphragmatic elevation are congenital eventration of the diaphragm and phrenic nerve palsy.[1,2] Both may require plication of the diaphragm. This chapter specifically focuses on techniques to plicate the diaphragm from above (intrathoracic).

Congenital eventration is the lack of muscle or tendon within the diaphragm. It is a spectrum of disorders that share the underlying cause of impaired fetal myotome migration.[1] Mild cases may only lack the central tendon, while severe cases may lack the central tendon as well as the entire muscular diaphragm. The area of congenitally missing muscle tissue is usually closed with a fused single membrane of pleura and peritoneum. This membrane is generally displaced within the ipsilateral hemithorax owing to the absence of muscle. If only a membrane is present, a patch may be more appropriate than plication.[1] A rim of rudimentary diaphragmatic tissue can generally be found around the lateral contour of the chest with enough substance to hold sutures to anchor the patch. Along the medial side, the patch can be stitched to the pericardium and the anterior thoracic spinal ligaments.

Causes of acquired phrenic nerve paralysis include viral palsy, iatrogenic injury (typically following thoracic surgery or instrumentation around the phrenic nerve above the clavicle), fracture of the first rib and clavicle, or a traction injury to the phrenic nerve. This last mechanism can also be seen in infants following a forceps delivery. The muscle and tendon of the diaphragm are normal, and plication pulls the muscle taut and reduces the compression of the ipsilateral lung.

A flaccid diaphragm compresses the lower lobe of the ipsilateral lung. In addition, if there is a large displacement of abdominal components into the negative pressure thorax, this bulk mechanically shifts the mediastinum with compression of the contralateral lung. Thus, there is atelectasis of the ipsilateral lower lobe, compression of the left atrium, impairment of pulmonary venous blood flow, and contralateral lung compression with additional atelectasis.[2]

Adults with paralyzed diaphragms do not always need plication if they are asymptomatic during normal activity. If they have underlying pulmonary disease, or desire strenuous activity, then plication can offer palliation of dyspnea from a paralyzed diaphragm. If the phrenic nerve is believed to be intact, but injured with the possibility of recovery within 2 years, conservative management will eventually lead to recovery of function. Plication, however, remains a low-risk procedure which continues to be underutilized. The radial plication technique, in particular, is designed to palliate symptoms while providing the maximum probability that the phrenic nerve will recover.

A recent study of patients who underwent unilateral plication via VATS technique documented substantial increases in spirometry readings at 6 months postprocedure.[3] The mechanism for improvement in these patients is the increased tension of the diaphragmatic barrier between the thorax and abdomen. This allows patients to generate a more negative intrapleural pressure than was possible with a floppy, paralytic diaphragm.

CENTRAL IMBRICATION TECHNIQUE

The easiest technique of plication is to place imbricating stitches within the central tendon of the diaphragm.[4,5] These stitches can be readily placed both thoracoscopically and through a minithoracotomy.[6] Sutures that are only placed within the central tendon will not adequately tighten the flaccid diaphragm. If the sutures extend far enough from the edge of the diaphragmatic tendon into the paralyzed muscle, however, they can produce substantial caudal displacement of the tendon towards the abdominal cavity and allow expansion of the ipsilateral lower lobe as well as balancing the mediastinum (Fig. 150-1).[7]

A number of variants of the central tendon repair exist and are performed by thoracoscopic, laparoscopic, or hybrid techniques. With improved videoscopic equipment and experience the trend towards less invasive procedures will continue and may encourage more physicians to refer their patients for surgery.

Mouroux et al.[6] describe a series of 12 patients who underwent thoracoscopic-assisted plication with a utility 5-cm incision. A Duval grasper is used to invaginate the apex of the eventration caudally, creating a fold which is closed in two layers. A VATS reproduction of the traditional pleating or "accordion" repair was performed by Freeman et al.[3] in 22 patients using an Endo Stitch (Ethicon Endo-Surgery, Cincinnati, Ohio) device to create 6 to 8 parallel U stitches for patients with unilateral diaphragm paralysis (Fig. 150-2). Improvement in pulmonary function and quality of life was seen along with a shortened hospital stay compared to patients who underwent thoracotomy. A total thoracoscopic technique with three ports has been described by Kim et al.[8] and uses the additional adjuncts of CO_2 insufflation and steep reverse Trendelenburg position to push the diaphragm down and increase the effective working space. Laparoscopic plication with four working trocars has been performed by Hüttl et al.[9] Retention sutures are placed on the dome of the diaphragm and then used for traction. This allows creation of an intraabdominal fold for plication with 12 to 15 U-type sutures. Finally, to counter the difficulty in placing adequate sutures through minimal access techniques, Moon et al.[10] report grasping and rolling the redundant diaphragm followed by placing noncutting linear endoscopic staplers underneath for creation of folds which are left in situ.

The drawback of all central imbrication techniques is that the majority of the pleats will fold the noncompliant central

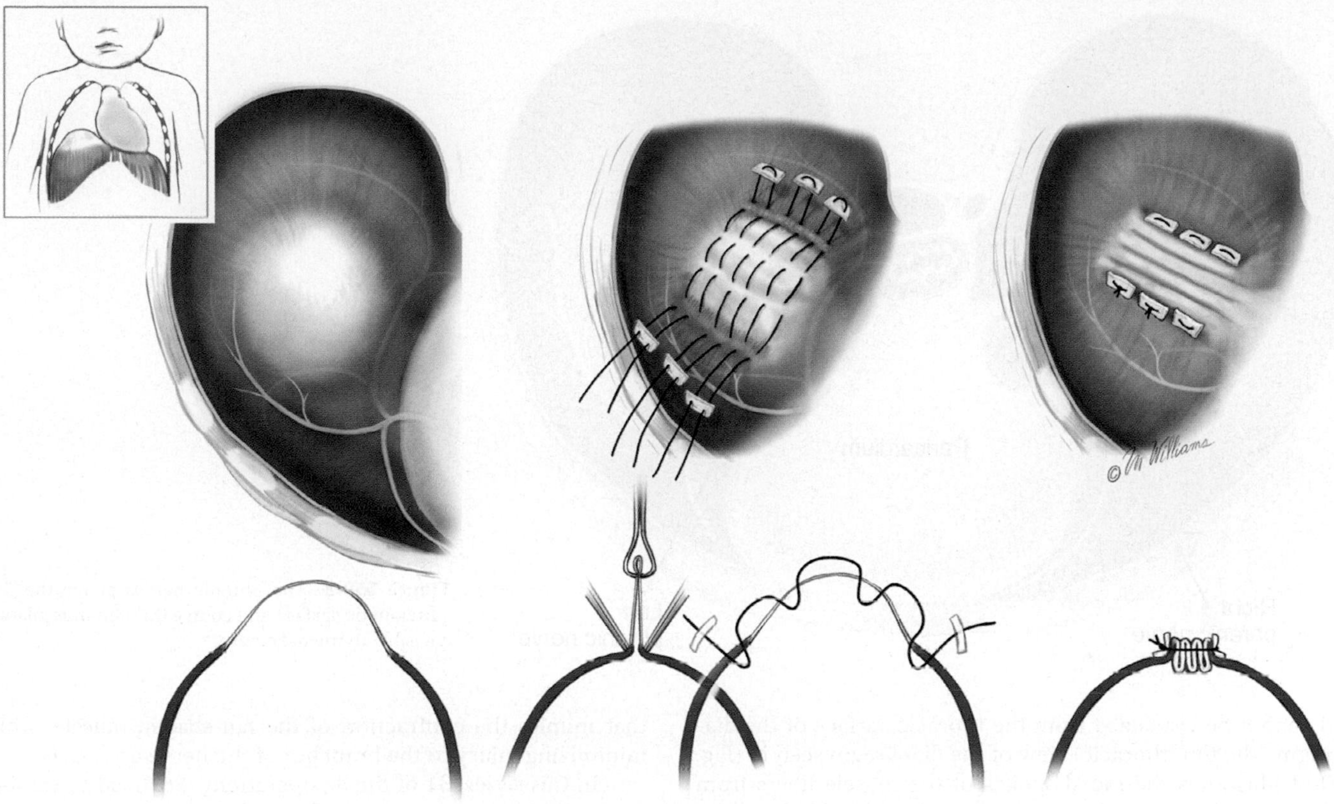

Figure 150-1. The weakened area is identified (*A*), grasped with a Babcock clamp (*B*), and lifted to determine placement and orientation of suture lines. *C.* Linear rows of pledgeted nonabsorbable horizontal mattressed sutures are placed through the weak spot in the diaphragm. *D.* The suture is tightened and the weakened tissues are gathered into pleats, creating a taut diaphragmatic surface.

tendon, and the compliant muscular remnant can be expected to further stretch with time. This will produce a recurrent elevation of the paralyzed diaphragm. It has been my experience that the central tendon pleating technique is associated with reelevation of the diaphragm to the level of the hilum within several years. Long-term follow-up of this technique has included reports of diaphragmatic elevation requiring additional intervention in as many as 19% of treated patients.[11] Furthermore, the phrenic vessels and branches of the nerve travel near the insertion of the muscle into the edge of the tendon

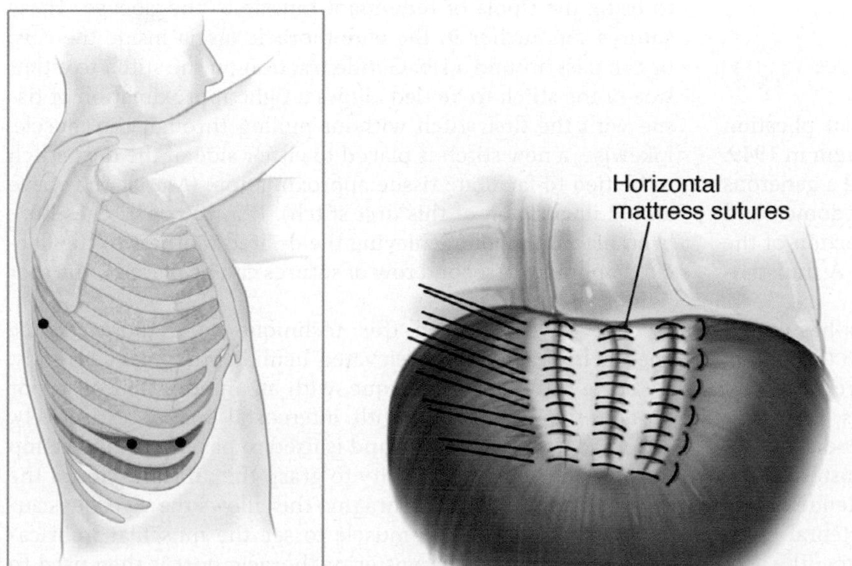

Figure 150-2. *A.* Ideal placement of incisions for thoracoscopic approach using multiple pleat technique. *B.* Similar to the open approach, parallel rows of horizontal mattress sutures are placed and drawn together.

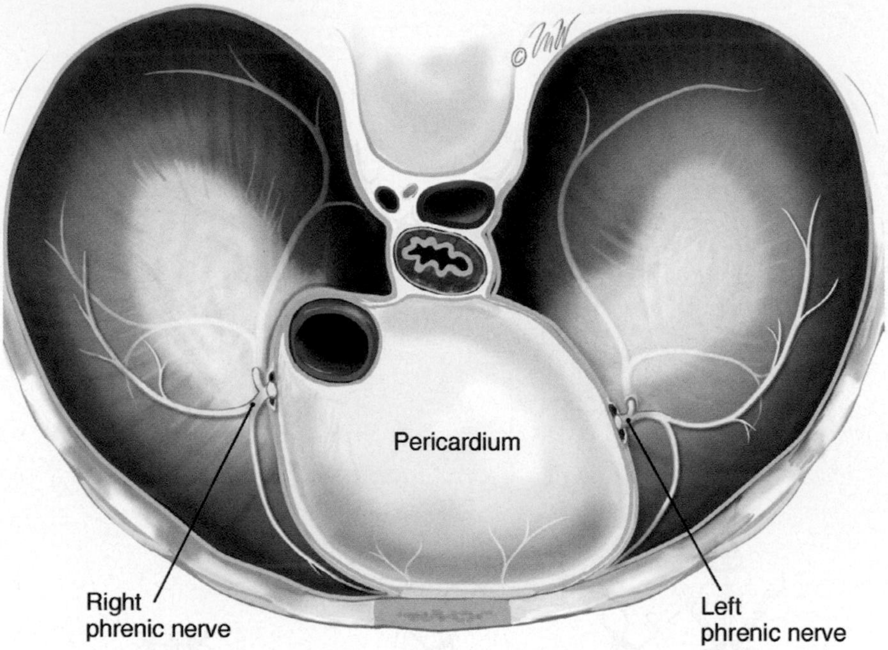

Figure 150-3. The phrenic nerves pierce the diaphragmatic surface and course through musculature invisible to the naked eye.

and cannot be visualized from the thoracic surface of the diaphragm. The top (thoracic) view of the diaphragm seen in (Fig. 150-3) illustrates the radial spokes of the muscle fibers from their origin along the costal margin toward the central tendon. The phrenic nerve can be seen along the mediastinal pleura, but then it pierces the diaphragmatic muscle close to the inferior vena cava on the right and the tip of the acute angle of the heart on the left. The phrenic vessels and phrenic nerve cannot be visualized from the thoracic surface of the diaphragm beyond these areas. Yet, to displace the central tendon adequately, these stitches need to extend into the muscle area, which places the branches of the nerve at risk of injury. The radial plication technique described below allows tightening of the diaphragm with less risk of injury to the hidden branches of the phrenic nerve, allowing reinnervation of a paralyzed nerve with time.

RADIAL PLICATION TECHNIQUE

Dr. David State[12] first described a subcostal radial plication technique for congenital eventration of the diaphragm in 1949. The original description of this technique included a generous incision across the right upper quadrant of the abdomen and placement of radial sutures along the muscular portion of the diaphragm pulling it towards the lateral chest wall. A transthoracic radial plication has also been described.[7,13]

Dr. John Foker at the University of Minnesota has used a transthoracic radial plication technique since 1976 to treat 35 children with elevation of the diaphragm.[14] The repairs were performed with interrupted horizontal mattress pledgeted sutures imbricating the muscular portion of the diaphragm in a radial manner toward the chest wall via a posterolateral thoracotomy (Fig. 150-4). The plication sutures extended in an unbroken band from the xyphoid area to the vertebral body. No sutures were placed along the mediastinal pleura. The goal was to produce a taut diaphragm which appeared as a straight angled line from mediastinum to chest wall on AP view of the chest roentgenogram. We believe that this produces a plication that mimics the contraction of the fan-shaped muscle, while minimizing injury to the branches of the nerve or vessels.

In this series, 31 of the 36 operations (86%) led to extubation within 3 days, even though 15 patients had been ventilator dependent prior to plication.[14] There were no deaths within 30 days, and no morbidity directly attributed to plication. Only 1 (3%) patient suffered a recurrence requiring repeat plication. Twenty-six of these patients survived long-term (median 12 years at time of analysis) and 18 of these patients were reevaluated with diaphragmatic ultrasound in 1996. Some degree of function had returned to 14 (78%) of the diaphragms.

Radial plication depends upon vigorous displacement of the edge of the muscle–tendon interface toward the lateral chest wall. This produces a ripple of muscle folds against the ribcage. Three to four individual pledgeted sutures are placed to bring the ripple of redundant muscle to the ribcage. These sutures can anchor in the endothoracic fascia inside the ribs, or can pass around a rib. Gentle traction on the stitch to either side of the stitch to be tied allows a tight approximation of tissue with the first stitch without pulling through the muscle. Likewise, a new stitch is placed to either side of the next stitch to be tied to facilitate tissue approximation. (Marcia may have an old illustration of this first stitch). If a row of stitches have been placed without achieving the desired tautness to the flaccid diaphragm, a second row of sutures can be placed to further tighten the muscle.

We have extended this technique to a thoracoscopic approach in adults with elevated hemidiaphragms. Currently, we use a three-port technique, with an anterior and posterior port at the sixth and eighth intercostal space, respectively. The third port is subcostal and is used to pass an O-ring clamp through the abdominal cavity to grasp the undersurface of the central tendon of the diaphragm. This allows the vigorous caudal displacement of the muscle to see the muscular imbrications for plication. The posterior thoracic port is then used to plicate the anterior and lateral borders of the muscle, while the anterior thoracic port is used to plicate the lateral and posterior borders.

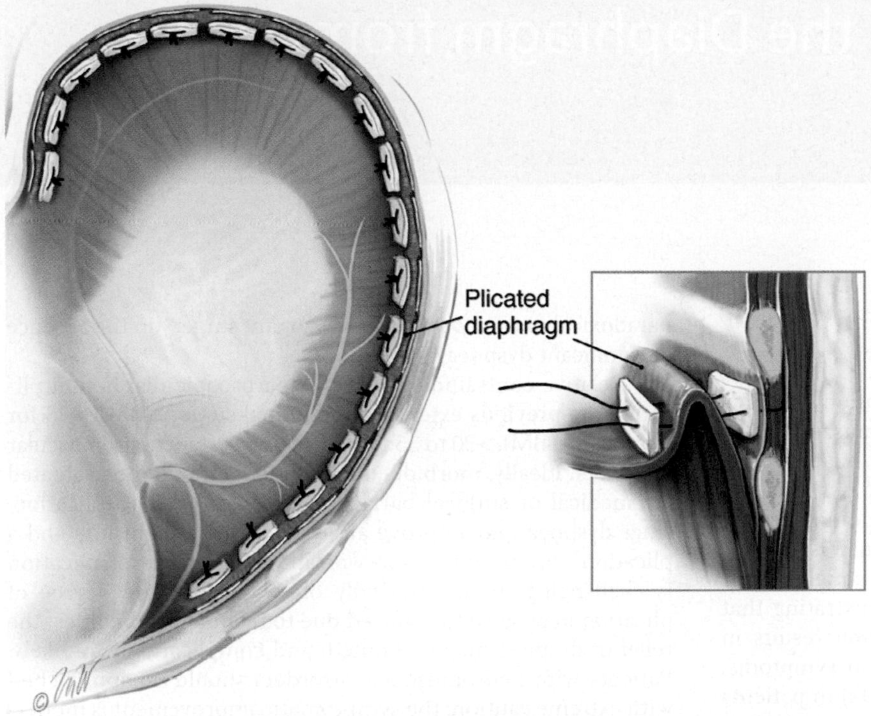

Figure 150-4. Radial plication technique.

SUMMARY

Elevation of an ipsilateral hemidiaphragm can come from a variety of causes. Although rarely a source of significant pulmonary incapacity, it is generally a contributor of dyspnea, that could be relieved with plication.

There are several plication techniques available. Plication from above can be achieved with a central imbrication technique or a radial plication technique. I personally prefer the radial plication technique as taught to me by Dr. John Foker for the reasons stated in this chapter. A randomized study to compare these methods is unlikely because of the rarity of diaphragmatic surgery for ipsilateral paralysis. Most surgeons will continue to practice the procedure with which they are most familiar.

EDITOR'S COMMENT

Most residents are familiar with the central tendon plication technique since it is easy and readily adaptable to a thoracoscopic approach. The radial plication technique is currently more difficult, but could become easier as technology improves. The radial technique has greater promise for being a permanent solution since it prevents the flaccid muscle from stretching with time. Although the radial technique allows a tighter final result, experience is needed to judge a semitaut from a very taut plication. When one considers the role of the diaphragm in dyspnea (Shrager's, Chapter 148), there appears to be a potential future role for diaphragmatic pacing (Ducko's, Chapter 152) or plication techniques (Jaklitsch and Andrade, Chapters 150 and 151) in the treatment of dyspneic syndromes.

—Michael T. Jaklitsch

References

1. Beck W, Motsay D. Eventration of the diaphragm. *Arch Surg.* 1952;65:557–563.
2. Markos J, Grover F, Trinkle J. Paralyzed diaphragm—effect of plication on respiratory mechanics. *J Surg Res.* 1974;16:523–526.
3. Freeman RK, Wozniak TC, Fitzgerald EB. Functional and physiologic results of video-assisted thoracoscopic diaphragm plication in adult patients with unilateral diaphragm paralysis. *Ann Thor Surg.* 2006;81(5):1855–1857.
4. Garbaccio C, Gyepes M, Fonkalsrud E. Malfunction of the intact diaphragm in infants and children. *Arch Surg.* 1972;105:57–61.
5. Schwartz M, Filler R. Plication of the diaphragm for symptomatic phrenic nerve paralysis. *J Pediatr Surg.* 1978;13(3):259–263.
6. Mouroux J, Padovani B, Poirer NC, et al. Technique for the repair of diaphragmatic eventration. *Ann Thorac Surg.* 1996;62;905–907.
7. Shoemaker R, Palmer G, Brown JW, et al. Aggressive treatment of acquired phrenic nerve paralysis in infants and small children. *Ann Thorac surg.* 1981;32(3):251–259.
8. Kim DH, Hwang JJ, Kim KD. Thoracoscopic diaphragmatic plication using three 5 mm ports. *Int J Cardiovasc and Thorac Surg.* 2007;6:280–282.
9. Hüttl TP, Wichmann MW, Reichart B, et al. Laparoscopic diaphragmatic plication. *Surg Endosc.* 2004;18:547–551.
10. Moon SW, Young-Pil W, Yong-Whan K, et al. Thoracoscopic plication of diaphragmatic eventration using endostaplers. *Ann Thorac Surg.* 2000;70:299–300.
11. Smith C, Sade RM, Crawford FA, et al. Diaphragmatic paralysis and eventration in infants. *J Thorac Cardiovasc Surg.* 1986;91:490–497.
12. State D. The surgical correction of congenital eventration of the diaphragm in infancy. *Surgery.* 1949;25:461–468.
13. Sethi G, Reed W. Diaphragmatic malfunction in neonates and infants: diagnosis and treatment. *J Thorac Cardiovasc Surg.* 1971;62(1):138–143.
14. Jaklitsch M. Twenty year experience with peripheral radial plication of the diaphragm. Presented at 33rd Annual Meeting of the Society of Thoracic Surgeons, San Diego, CA: 1997.

151 Plication of the Diaphragm from Below

Rafael Andrade

Keywords: Laparoscopic approach

INTRODUCTION

The abdominal approach for diaphragmatic plication is appropriate in properly selected patients. Open transabdominal plication has been described for unilateral or bilateral diaphragmatic eventration or paralysis in children,[1] but very few data are available on the results of open transabdominal plication in adults. Laparoscopic diaphragm plication was initially described by Hüttl et al. in a report of three patients.[2] We reported our experience with 25 patients demonstrating that the laparoscopic approach to diaphragm plication results in significant short- and mid-term improvements in symptoms, quality of life, and pulmonary function tests (PFTs) in patients with hemidiaphragm paralysis or eventration.[3]

GENERAL PRINCIPLES

The choice of access for diaphragmatic plication is primarily guided by surgeon experience and preference. The minimally invasive approach is preferred over an open approach, since it is associated with less morbidity, although no direct comparisons between open and minimally invasive plication have been reported in the literature. As a general rule, the anterior portion of the hemidiaphragm is easier to access via the abdomen, whereas the posterior portion is more approachable through the chest. Finally, regardless of approach, proper patient selection, safety, and tight imbrication of the entire hemidiaphragm are essential.

The theoretical advantages of a transabdominal approach in comparison with a transthoracic approach are (a) easy intraoperative positioning (supine vs. lateral decubitus), (b) selective ventilation is unnecessary, (c) the abdominal cavity offers ample operating room, (d) there is direct visualization of the intraabdominal organs which reduces the risk of injury during imbrication, and (e) there is less postoperative pain. Disadvantages of transabdominal plication include difficult visualization of the posterior portion of the hemidiaphragm, potential splenic or liver laceration, and technical challenges in centrally obese patients.

PATIENT SELECTION

The potential candidate for diaphragmatic plication must have dyspnea that cannot be solely attributed to another process (e.g., poorly controlled primary lung or heart disease) and must have an elevated hemidiaphragm on a posteroanterior and lateral (PA/LAT chest x-ray. Since the only goal of diaphragm plication is to treat dyspnea; operative intervention is indicated *exclusively* for symptomatic patients. An elevated hemidiaphragm or paradoxical motion *per se* do not warrant surgery in the absence of significant dyspnea.

Relative contraindications to laparoscopic diaphragm plication are previous extensive abdominal surgery, BMI >35 for females and BMI >30 to 35 for males, and certain neuromuscular disorders. Ideally, morbidly obese patients should be evaluated for medical or surgical bariatric treatment prior to plication, since dyspnea may improve after significant weight loss and a plication may no longer be warranted. Any type of plication is challenging in the morbidly obese patient: the degree of plication may be compromised due to technical difficulties, the relief of dyspnea may be limited, and complications are likely. Patients with neuromuscular disorders should be approached with extreme caution; the symptomatic improvement is moderate at best, and complications are common. An individualized multidisciplinary approach is necessary to decide on a plication in patients with morbid obesity or neuromuscular disorders.

PREOPERATIVE ASSESSMENT

Clinical Evaluation

The diagnosis of symptomatic hemidiaphragm paralysis or eventration is primarily clinical, and relies mostly on history, chest x-ray, and the physician's clinical acuity.

The evaluation of a symptomatic patient with diaphragmatic paralysis or eventration should include an objective assessment of dyspnea, physical examination, PFTs, and imaging studies.

Careful history taking about the duration and progression of dyspnea and orthopnea is critical. Any additional causes of dyspnea (e.g., morbid obesity, primary lung disease, heart failure) should be investigated and corrected if possible, since dyspnea secondary to diaphragmatic paralysis or eventration is mainly a diagnosis of exclusion.

All patients with dyspnea secondary to an elevated hemidiaphragm eventration should fill out a standardized respiratory questionnaire to more objectively evaluate the severity of their symptoms and to assess the response to treatment.

Pulmonary Function Tests

PFTs provide certain objectivity to the assessment of dyspneic patients with an elevated hemidiaphragm; however, PFTs are imprecise and do not correlate well with severity of dyspnea or response to plication. Since diaphragm dysfunction reduces the compliance of the chest wall, a restrictive pattern (i.e., low forced vital capacity [FVC] and forced expiratory volume in 1 second [FEV_1]) is often seen.[4]

The diaphragm is a critical mediator of inspiration; therefore, assessing inspiratory PFT parameters (e.g., maximum forced inspiratory flow [FIFmax]) is important.

In addition, FVC should be assessed in the upright and supine position. Supine FVC in healthy individuals can decrease up to 20% from upright values, and supine lung volumes may decrease by 20% to 50% in patients with diaphragmatic eventration or paralysis.

Imaging Studies

Chest x-ray

On a standard full-inspiration PA/LAT chest x-ray, the right hemidiaphragm is normally 1 to 2 cm higher than the left. Hemidiaphragm elevation can be a sign of diaphragmatic paralysis or paralysis; however, this is a nonspecific finding since a variety of pulmonary, pleural, and subdiaphragmatic processes can also cause elevation of the hemidiaphragm. Consequently, further studies may be needed if an elevated hemidiaphragm is noted on a chest x-ray in the presence of dyspnea.

Fluoroscopic Sniff Test

The clinical value of a sniff test is limited in the presence of an elevated diaphragm and dyspnea. The principal role of the sniff test is to help discern the etiology of dyspnea in patients with a less evident primary cause of dyspnea.

During fluoroscopy, patients are instructed to sniff, and diaphragmatic excursion is assessed. Normally, the diaphragm moves caudally. In patients with hemidiaphragmatic paralysis, the diaphragm may (paradoxically) move cranially. Patients with diaphragmatic eventration, however, may also exhibit passive upward movement of the diaphragm when sniffing.

Fluoroscopy findings should be interpreted with caution. First, about 6% of normal individuals exhibit paradoxical motion on fluoroscopy; to increase the specificity of this study, at least 2 cm of paradoxical motion should be noticed. Second, a paralyzed or eventrated hemidiaphragm may move very little or not at all, without paradoxical motion, making the interpretation of the sniff test and the distinction between paralysis and eventration even more challenging.[4]

Computed Tomography

The principal utility of computed tomography (CT) scans is to exclude the presence of a cervical or intrathoracic tumor as the cause of phrenic nerve paralysis or to evaluate the possibility of a subphrenic process as the cause of hemidiaphragm elevation. However, a CT scan is not routinely required if the clinical suspicion of an alternate process is low.

Other Tests

Other diagnostic tests such as ultrasonography, dynamic magnetic resonance imaging, maximal transdiaphragmatic pressure, and phrenic nerve conduction studies are of limited or no value for the clinical evaluation of a dyspneic patient with an elevated hemidiaphragm.[4]

Summary

Potential candidates for laparoscopic diaphragm plication have an elevated hemidiaphragm and dyspnea; the minimal clinical assessment for plication should include history and physical examination, evaluation of the severity of dyspnea with a standardized respiratory quality-of-life questionnaire, a PA/LAT chest x-ray, and PFTs. Fluoroscopic sniff test and CT scan are of value in selected patients.

TECHNIQUE

Anesthesia

The procedure is performed under general anesthesia, with a single-lumen endotracheal tube; selective ventilation is not necessary.

Position

The patient is in the supine position with abducted arms. The abdomen and lower lateral chest wall are prepared and draped to allow access for chest tube placement, a footboard is essential for steep Trendelenburg positioning.

Operative Technique

1. Ports: we use four 12-mm ports; two assistant ports are placed 2 cm parallel to the midline on the opposite site of the elevated hemidiaphragm. The two working ports are placed in the ipsilateral upper quadrant (Fig. 151-1). We insufflate the abdomen with CO_2 at a pressure of 15 mm Hg.
2. Exposure: steep reverse Trendelenburg positioning helps to optimize exposure of the posterior portion of the hemidiaphragm; for a right-sided plication, transection of the falciform ligament is useful for appropriate access to the diaphragm. The thinned-out hemidiaphragm is taut and displaced cranially as a result of the pneumoperitoneum. We make a small perforation at the dome of the diaphragm with electrocautery (Fig. 151-2A). The resultant pneumothorax allows the surgeon to easily pull the hemidiaphragm into the abdominal cavity for suturing (Fig. 151-2B). At this point, we often place a 19 Blake pleural drain through an incision in the anterolateral chest wall to vent the pneumothorax as needed.
3. Stitching: we use pledgeted U-stitches (#2 nonabsorbable, braided suture, 31-mm curved needle). We place the first stitch centrally and as far posteriorly as possible (Fig. 151-3). Traction on the first stitch facilitates exposure for two or three subsequent deeper stitches (Fig. 151-4) to plicate the posterior

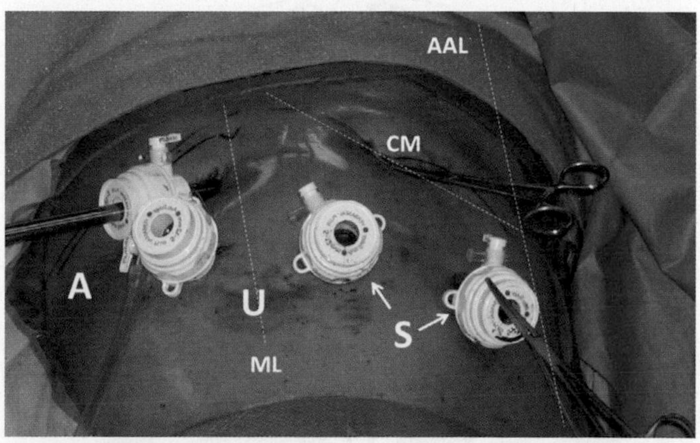

Figure 151-1. Port placement for laparoscopic left hemidiaphragm plication. A, assistant ports (placed about 2 cm parallel to the midline [ML] on the right side); S, surgeon ports (placed about 2 cm above the level of the umbilicus [U] and equidistantly from the midline [ML] and anterior axillary line [AAL]); CM, costal margin.

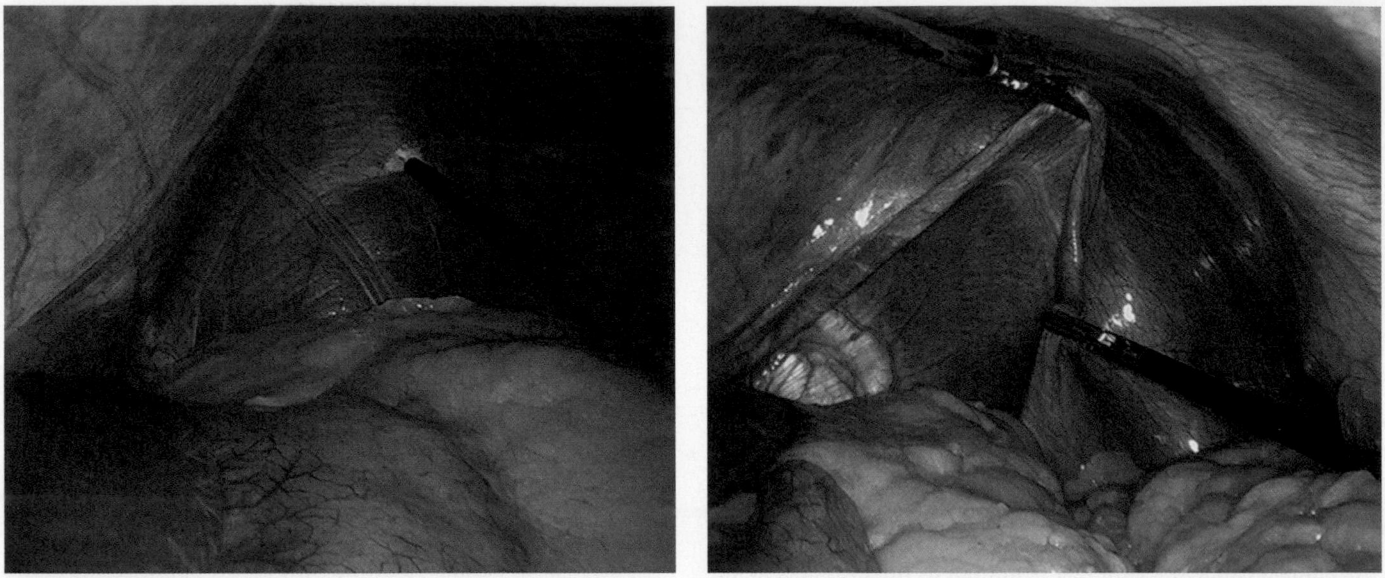

Figure 151-2. Cephalad displacement of the left hemidiaphragm following CO_2 insufflation, the diaphragm is taught and difficult to handle. *A.* A small opening with the electrocautery induces a pneumothorax. *B.* Easy manipulation of the floppy diaphragm.

portion of the hemidiaphragm in an anteroposterior direction (Figs. 151-5 and 151-6). To plicate the anterior portion of the hemidiaphragm we use two or three weaving stitches (Fig. 151-7). The diaphragm must be taught at the end of the procedure (Fig. 151-8). Closure of the initial perforation at the dome occurs with the plication.

4. Tube thoracostomy: we leave the pleural drain in place upon completion of the procedure and verify that it has not been caught in a stitch.
5. Intraoperative management of lower lobe atelectasis: upon completion of the plication, we ask the anesthesia team to ventilate the patient with high tidal volumes and a PEEP of 10 cm H_2O until extubation with the intention to re-expand the lower lobe.

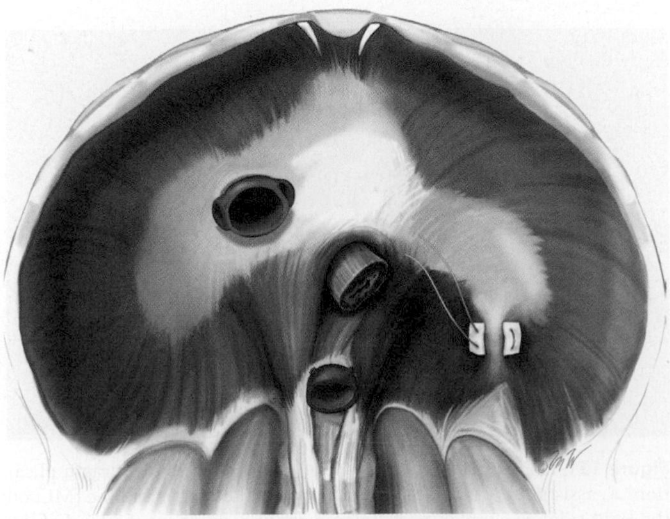

Figure 151-3. Placement of the first stitch in the central portion of the diaphragm.

POSTOPERATIVE MANAGEMENT

Patients should engage in intense pulmonary toilet to re-expand the lower lobe of the ipsilateral lung. The chest tube remains in place until output is less than 200 mL/day; on occasion patients need to be discharged with the chest tube in place. Premature removal of the chest tube can lead to symptomatic pleural effusion. The immediate postoperative chest x-ray should show that the plicated side is lower than the opposite side, with a very acute costophrenic angle (Fig. 151-9). One may also see elevation of the contralateral hemidiaphragm. After 1 month, both hemidiaphragms are about at the same level. We monitor patients with the St. George's Respiratory Questionnaire (SGRQ), PA/LAT chest x-ray, and PFTs at 1 month after discharge and yearly thereafter.

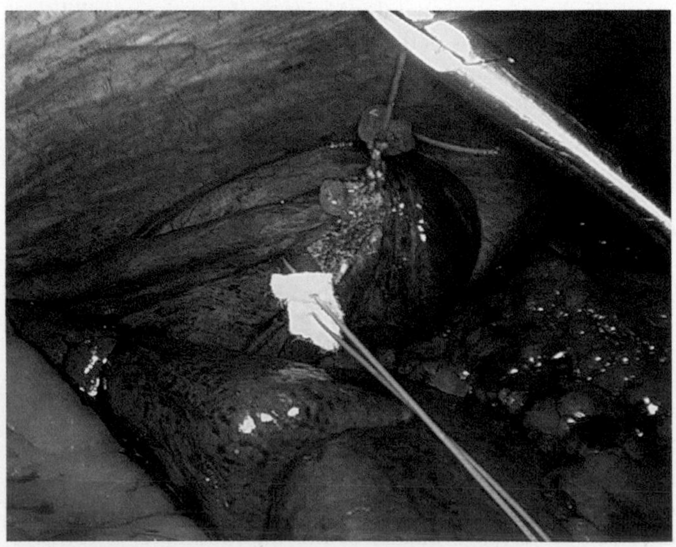

Figure 151-4. Retraction on the first stitch allows exposure for placement of two or three subsequent stitches in anteroposterior direction.

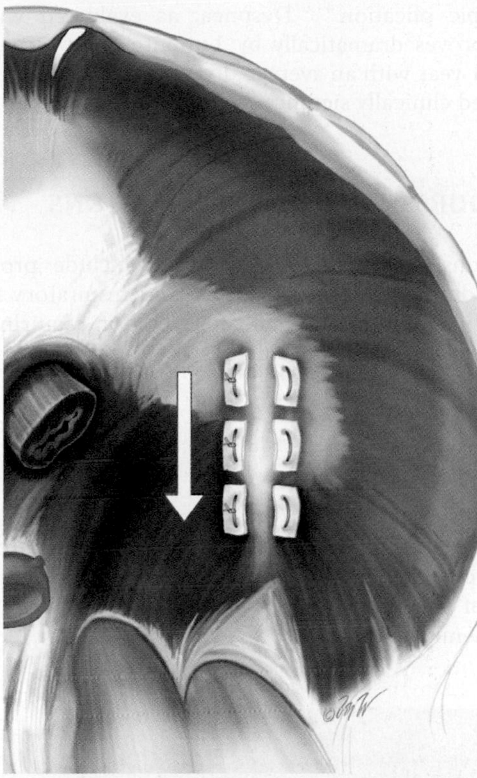

Figure 151-5. Completed posterior plication with three stitches.

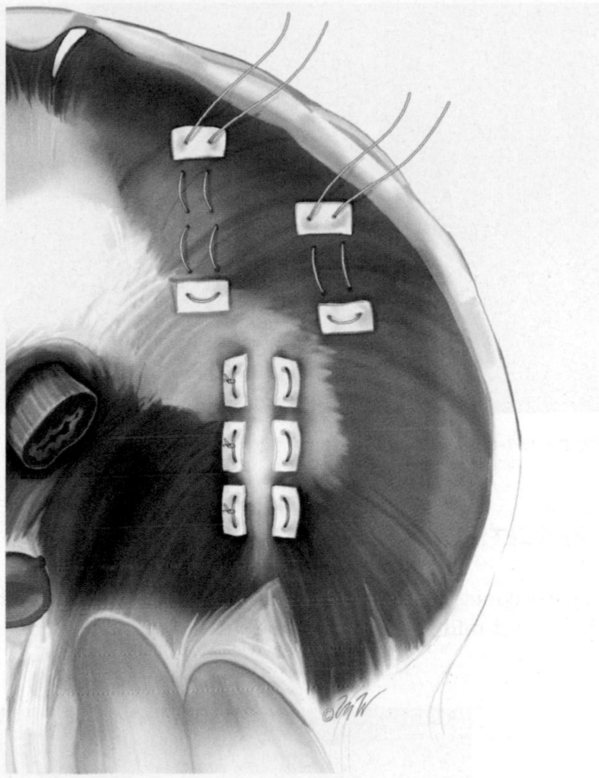

Figure 151-7. Placement of two weaving stitches as outlined in the matching sketch. Tightening of these stitches will complete the anterior plication.

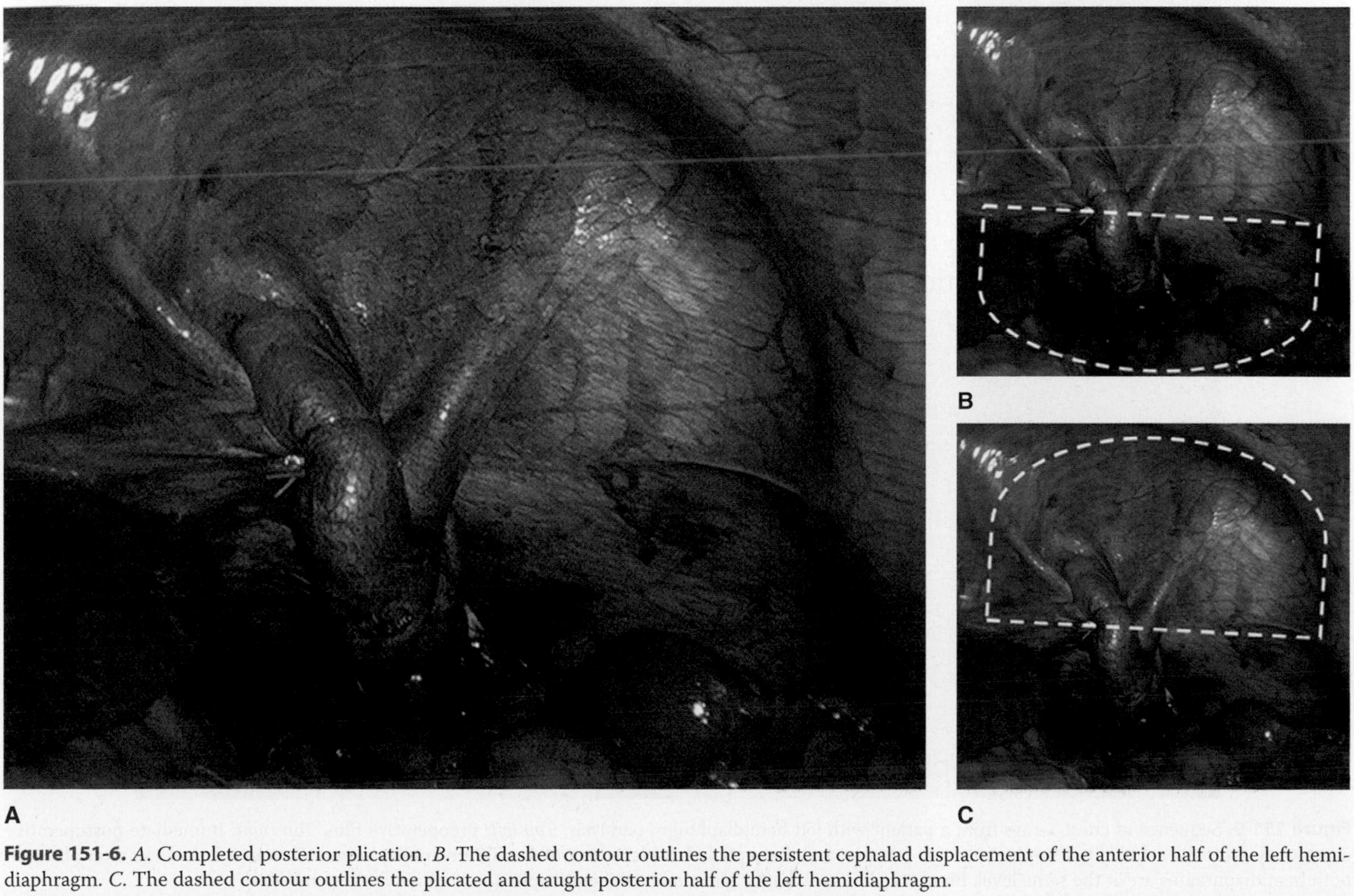

Figure 151-6. *A.* Completed posterior plication. *B.* The dashed contour outlines the persistent cephalad displacement of the anterior half of the left hemidiaphragm. *C.* The dashed contour outlines the plicated and taught posterior half of the left hemidiaphragm.

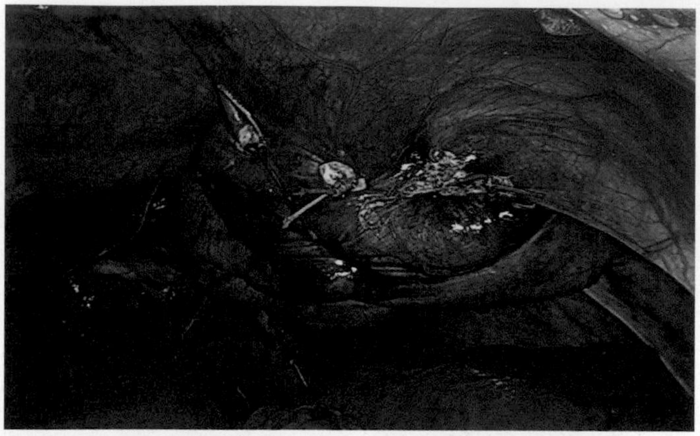

Figure 151-8. Completed plication.

RESULTS

Laparoscopic plication using meticulous technique achieves short- and mid-term results that are comparable to open and thoracoscopic plication.[4–9] Dyspnea, as evaluated with the SGRQ, improves dramatically by 1 month after surgery and persists at 1 year with an average drop of 20 points (>4 points is considered clinically significant).[3]

PROCEDURE-SPECIFIC COMPLICATIONS

Complications of laparoscopic plication include prolonged chest tube drainage (>7 days) in 8%, and respiratory failure, gastrointestinal hemorrhage, splenic laceration requiring splenectomy, stroke and atrial fibrillation in 4% each.

SUMMARY

Properly selected patients with symptomatic diaphragmatic paralysis or eventration benefit significantly from laparoscopic diaphragm plication as long as the surgeon adheres to the basic principles of patient selection, safety, and tight imbrication of the entire hemidiaphragm.

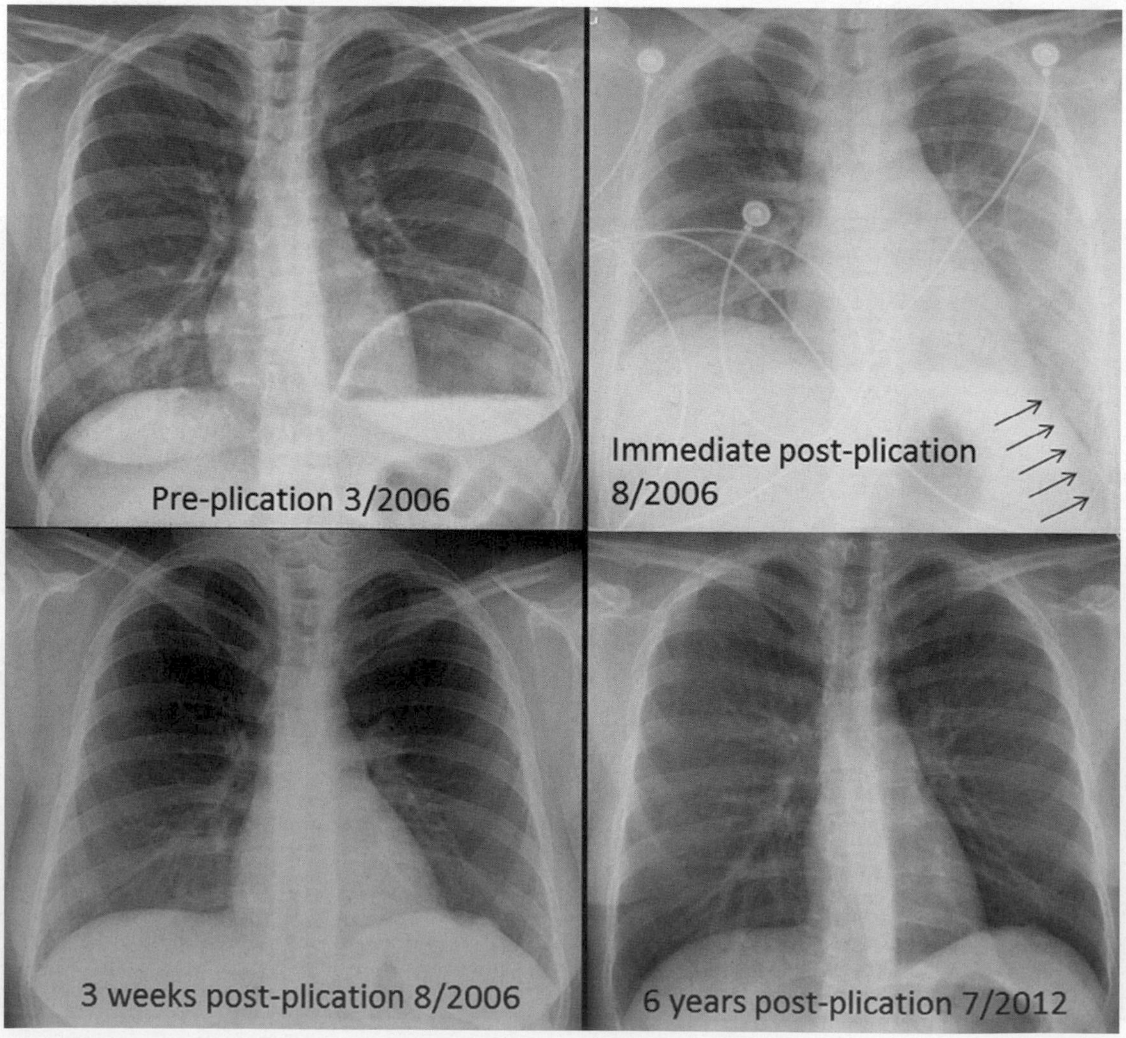

Figure 151-9. Sequence of chest x-rays from a patient with left hemidiaphragm paralysis. *Top left:* preoperative film. *Top right:* immediate postoperative chest x-ray. Note the acute left costophrenic angle (arrows) and the cephalad displacement of the right hemidiaphragm. *Bottom left:* 3 weeks after plication both hemidiaphragms are at the same level. *Bottom right:* 6 years after plication both hemidiaphragms remain at the same level.

ILLUSTRATED CASE HISTORY

A 21-year-old female who underwent chemotherapy and radiation therapy for a non-Hodgkin lymphoma of the mediastinum developed left hemidiaphragm paralysis (Fig. 151-9). She planned to go on vacation prior to scheduled laparoscopic plication, but had to return home early because of dyspnea. She underwent a laparoscopic left hemidiaphragm plication and was discharged on postoperative day 4 after an uneventful recovery. Four months after surgery she was playing ice hockey and keeping pace with her teammates. Six years after surgery, she remains free of dyspnea, and her chest x-ray is almost identical to her chest x-ray from 3 weeks post-plication.

EDITOR'S COMMENT

Laparoscopic diaphragm plication from below is a new technique, and we are pleased to include this description in our book. Dr. Andrade has provided clear instructions in regard to patient selection, positioning, and suture technique. He openly discusses the advantages (easy position, no need for selective ventilation, ample operative space, direct visualization of abdominal organs during suture placement, less pain) and disadvantages (difficulty in visualizing the posterior diaphragm and challenges in central obesity) of this approach. This technique will likely be modified as technology advances, and may prove to be a popular choice for plication.

—Michael T. Jaklitsch

References

1. Kizilcan F, Tanyel FC, Hicsonmez A, et al. The long-term results of diaphragmatic plication. *J Pediatr Surg.* 1993;28:42–44.
2. Hüttl TP, Wichmann MW, Reichart B, et al. Laparoscopic diaphragmatic plication: long-term results of a novel surgical technique for postoperative phrenic nerve palsy. *Surg Endosc.* 2004;18:547–551.
3. Groth SS, Rueth NM, Kast T, et al. Laparoscopic diaphragm plication for diaphragmatic paralysis and eventration: an objective evaluation of short- and mid-term results. *J Thorac Cardiovasc Surg.* 2010;139:1452–1456.
4. Groth SS, Andrade RS. Diaphragm plication for eventration or paralysis: a review of the literature. *Ann Thorac Surg.* 2010;89(6):S2146–S2150.
5. Graham DR, Kaplan D, Evans CC, et al. Diaphragmatic plication for unilateral diaphragmatic paralysis: a 10-year experience. *Ann Thorac Surg.* 1990;49:248–252.
6. Higgs SM, Hussain A, Jackson M, et al. Long term results of diaphragmatic plication for unilateral diaphragm paralysis. *Eur J Cardiothorac Surg.* 2002;21:294–297.
7. Freeman RK, Van Woerkom J, Vyverberg A, et al. Long-term follow-up of the functional and physiologic results of diaphragm plication in adults with unilateral diaphragm paralysis. *Ann Thorac Surg.* 2009;88:1112–1127.
8. Freeman RK, Wozniak TC, Fitzgerald EB. Functional and physiologic results of video-assisted thoracoscopic diaphragm plication in adult patients with unilateral diaphragm paralysis. *Ann Thorac Surg.* 2006;81:1853–1857.
9. Mouroux J, Venissac N, Leo F, et al. Surgical treatment of diaphragmatic eventration using video-assisted thoracic surgery: a prospective study. *Ann Thorac Surg.* 2005;79:308–312.

152 Diaphragm Pacing

Christopher T. Ducko

Keywords: Diaphragm pacing, phrenic nerve, breathing pacemaker, phrenic nerve motor point, respiratory insufficiency

INTRODUCTION

The technique of applying electrical stimulation to the phrenic nerve to induce diaphragm pacing was first described by Cavallo in 1777.[1] Early proponents used this technique for a variety of conditions associated with impaired respiration, including asphyxia (Hufeland, 1783), cholera (Duchenne, 1849), apnea (Israel, 1927), and polio (Sarnoff, 1950).[2] Diaphragm pacing was introduced into contemporary thoracic surgical practice in the 1970s by Glenn, who pioneered its application in patients with central apnea (Glenn, 1966) and quadriplegia (Glenn, 1972).[2–4] With the standard pacing devices, the electrical stimulus is applied at the phrenic nerve, as originally described. However, a newer approach applies the stimulus directly into the muscle at the phrenic nerve motor point for more direct control.[5] The primary conditions amenable to pacing are high cervical spinal cord injuries (i.e., C3–C5) and congenital or acquired central hypoventilation syndrome. Onders et al. have extended pacing via the motor point technique to other populations, including patients with the progressive neuromuscular degenerative disorder, amyotrophic lateral sclerosis (ALS), and other more transient problems, such as intensive care unit patients who demonstrate difficulty weaning from mechanical ventilation.[6,7]

GENERAL PRINCIPLES

The successful application of diaphragm pacing requires a fundamental knowledge of the anatomy and physiology of the respiratory system. A full discussion of the neural control of breathing is beyond the scope of this chapter. Briefly, the major components of the respiratory system include respiratory centers in the brainstem that control voluntary and involuntary breathing through connections to the diaphragm and muscles of respiration via the phrenic and intercostal nerves. Respiratory sensors deliver feedback to the brain via mechanoreceptors and chemoreceptors, which help regulate ventilation based on oxygen and carbon dioxide levels, as well as neural reflexes from smooth muscles in the airways and chest wall. The three respiratory centers in the brainstem include the medullary, which controls rhythmic inspiration and expiration, the apneustic center in the lower pons, which controls the prolongation of inspiration, and the pneumotaxic center in the upper portion of the pons. The latter inhibits inspiration to prevent overexpansion of the lungs.

The diaphragm is innervated by the phrenic nerve bundle, which exits the spinal cord from the upper motor nerve centers in the brainstem at C3 to C5 and passes from the neck between the heart and respective lung to its most distal extent on the hemidiaphragm. The phrenic nerve can be accessed in the cervical region or in the chest. The nerve descends obliquely with the internal jugular vein across the anterior scalene deep to the prevertebral layer of the deep cervical fascia and the transverse cervical and suprascapular arteries. On the left, the phrenic nerve crosses anterior to the first part of the subclavian artery. On the right it lies on the anterior scalene muscle and crosses anterior to the second part of the subclavian artery. On both sides, the phrenic nerve runs posterior to the subclavian vein and anterior to the internal thoracic artery as it enters the thorax.

The right phrenic nerve passes over the innominate artery posterior to the subclavian vein. It then crosses the root of the right lung anteriorly and leaves the thorax by passing through the vena cava hiatus in the diaphragm at the level of T8. The right phrenic nerve passes over the right atrium. The left phrenic nerve passes over the pericardium of the left ventricle and penetrates the diaphragm separately. Within the diaphragm muscle are three branches that split from the main phrenic nerve. These include the anterior or sternal, lateral, and posterior trunks. The location of these branches is relevant to mapping for diaphragm pacer insertion at the motor point. The phrenic nerve must be identified along its course and preserved during thoracic procedures, since severing the nerve will cause paralysis of the corresponding hemidiaphragm. The nerve is easily identified as it passes anterior to the hilum of the corresponding lung.

PATIENT SELECTION

Patients with diaphragmatic paralysis are occasionally referred for thoracic surgical evaluation. Most are found to have unilateral paralysis from idiopathic conditions that can be managed with diaphragmatic plication (see Chapters 150 and 151) if the clinical situation warrants. Select populations, however, may benefit from diaphragm pacing, where the goal is to wean the patient from mechanical ventilation or to avoid it altogether. Patients with partial or total ventilatory insufficiency typically are those with high cervical spinal cord injuries (above C3) and congenital or acquired central hypoventilation syndrome. Select patients with these disorders have an intact phrenic nerve, but the signal required to conduct an impulse from the respiratory centers in the brainstem to the diaphragm is disrupted as a result of injury or underlying disease, that is, axonal degeneration or idiopathic central disconnect, respectively. Diaphragm pacing can provide a significant benefit in this setting. It also may be indicated in other less common conditions including intracranial vascular lesions, tumors, central nervous system infections, syringomyelia, and poliomyelitis. Contrary to initial thoughts on diaphragm pacing, recently it has been shown that pacing may play a valuable role in patients with acute respiratory insufficiency as well as patients with neuromuscular disease, that is, ALS. This paradigm shift may benefit patients by promoting weaning from, or delaying the need for, mechanical ventilation. Careful patient selection is critical to a successful result.

PREOPERATIVE ASSESSMENT

A thorough and careful preoperative evaluation is performed with particular attention to the neurologic and pulmonary systems. Before assessing the status of the patient's phrenic nerve and diaphragm, preexisting conditions must be systematically excluded, particularly any condition that would preclude effective signal conductance or proper oxygenation and ventilation.[8] Patients with advanced neuromuscular disorders, underlying restrictive lung disease, or extensive parenchymal processes, for example, would not be suitable for diaphragm pacing. A detailed survey of the cervical spine, neck, and chest by CT is recommended to rule out underlying mass lesion or organic pathology. Elevated unilateral hemidiaphragm on chest radiography is suggestive of phrenic nerve paralysis, and diaphragm plication should be considered.[9]

The purpose of the preoperative assessment is to verify the integrity of the phrenic nerve, neuromuscular junction, and diaphragm without which diaphragm pacing will not succeed. The current gold standard for phrenic nerve function testing is percutaneous cervical electrical stimulation.[10–12] This study is performed by placing an electrode at the lateral edge of the clavicular head of the sternocleidomastoid muscle. The muscle is retracted medially, and the current is directed posteriorly toward the phrenic nerve. An obvious contraction of the diaphragm should occur after stimulation, if the nerve is intact. Any failure to conduct the nerve evidenced by absence of contraction or prolonged latency of response is a sign of phrenic nerve compromise.

Magnetic stimulation is a noninvasive alternative to percutaneous cervical electrical stimulation, but results of this test must be interpreted with caution, since the body can lateralize function with unilateral nerve injury by activating accessory muscles of respiration and the contralateral diaphragm.[13] An appropriate interval should pass between the time of injury and testing, since the nerves may initially be unresponsive to stimulation. Likewise, patients who fail nerve conduction early after spinal cord injury may show recovery up to 2 years later.[14]

The "sniff test" relies on the fluoroscopic visualization of radioopaque markers that are strategically placed to measure the maximal excursion of the diaphragm on inspiration. The patient in supine position sniffs through his or her nose. This maneuver elicits a brisk downward deflection of the diaphragm if the phrenic nerve is intact. The test is deemed positive when a paradoxical upward shift of the diaphragm is visualized fluoroscopically. Ultrasound and MRI imaging of the diaphragm is an emerging option for visualizing the diaphragm, but is somewhat limited in availability.

For ALS patients, proper patient selection is critical because of the increased risks associated with general anesthesia in patients with neuromuscular degeneration. It is imperative to demonstrate that the diaphragm is capable of stimulation and that the patient has clear evidence of chronic hypoventilation before pacing can be considered. Patients must be 21 years of age or older and cannot have progressed to a forced vital capacity (FVC) of less than 45% predicted. A variety of metrics can be used to document chronic hypoventilation including FVC greater than 50% predicted; maximum inspiratory pressure (MIP) less than 60 cm H_2O; pCO_2 greater than 45 mmHg; and oxygen saturation less than 88% for 5 consecutive minutes during sleep. Phrenic nerve function can be assessed by neurophysiologic testing with EMG, by visualizing diaphragm contraction with full-motion fluoroscopy or by other radiologic techniques including ultrasound or MRI.

DIAPHRAGM PACING DEVICES

The pacing electrode of most phrenic nerve pacemakers is implanted directly on the phrenic nerve either in the chest or in the cervical neck region. In a more recent approach to pacing, the electrode is implanted in the muscle at the phrenic nerve motor point. Most patients with phrenic nerve or diaphragm pacemakers can be successfully weaned from mechanical ventilation for a substantial time each day, if not completely. Even transitory periods of ventilator independence can have a significant impact on the patient's quality of life and significantly reduce overall healthcare costs. The potential exists for expanding this technology to other types of respiratory failure. Application of this technique to ALS or temporary scenarios in difficult-to-wean intensive care unit patients may grow as investigative experience emerges. Although diaphragm pacing is appropriate for only a few select conditions, it is a useful tool and worth mastering. Ample assistance is available online to get started, and the diaphragm pacing manufacturers are knowledgeable and can assist the surgeon through the learning curve. Websites for the two companies available in the United States can be found at www.averybiomedical.com and www.synapsebiomedical.com.

Four pacing systems are available worldwide. These include the Vienna Phrenic Pacemaker (Medimplant, Vienna, Austria), the Atrostim (Atrotech, Ltd., Tampere, Finland), the Avery Mark IV Phrenic Pacemaker (Avery Biomedical, Commack, NY, USA), and the NeuRx Diaphragm Pacing System (DPS; Synapse Biomedical Inc., Oberlin, OH, USA). The first three systems are implanted directly on the phrenic nerve and use an external transmitter with antenna to transmit radiofrequency signals transcutaneously to a receiver implanted subcutaneously.[15–17] The receiver translates the signal into electrical impulses which are delivered to the phrenic nerve electrode to generate contraction of the diaphragm. Diaphragm stimulation and muscle fatigue can be affected by the electrode type which may be unipolar, bipolar, or quadripolar. All three systems seem to rely on the same concept and implantation strategies. Of these three only the Avery device with its monopolar electrode is available in the United States (Fig. 152-1).

The fourth and newest device, the NeuRx DPS, was approved by the Food and Drug Administration under a humanitarian device exemption in 2008. It is available in the United States and many other countries. This technology takes advantage of the phrenic nerve motor point at the level of the diaphragm which is mapped for direct intramuscular electrode implantation. Although it is not fully implantable in its current form, only a few tiny electrode leads exit the skin from a subcutaneous tunnel which serves as a barrier to infection.

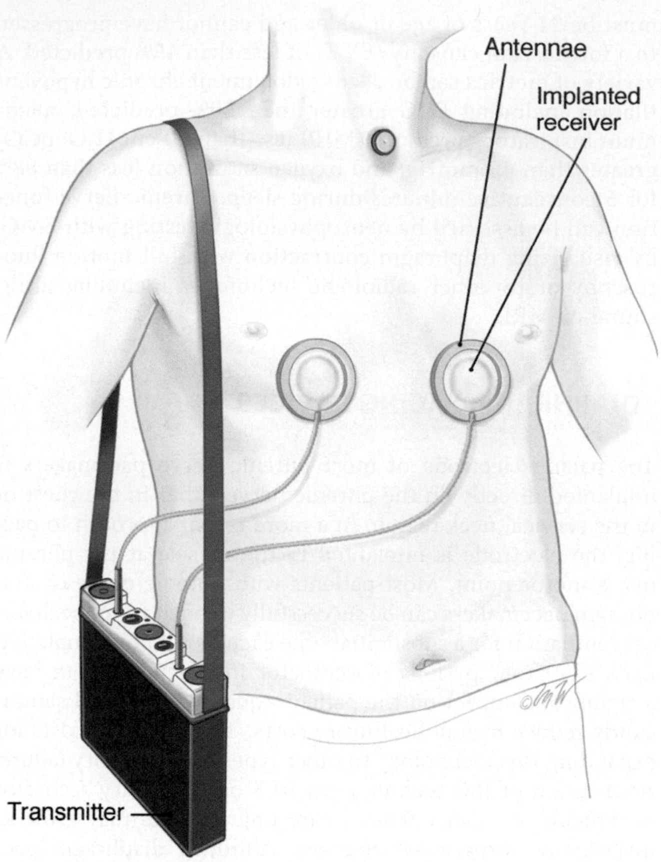

Figure 152-1. Avery Mark IV Phrenic Pacemaker. The portable external transmitter is connected to antennae on the anterior chest wall and used to transmit radiofrequency signals across the skin to the implanted receiver. The receiver stimulates the phrenic nerve via the pacing electrode. Reproduced with permission from Reference 21.

OPERATIVE TECHNIQUES

Implantation and Pacing with the Avery Mark IV Phrenic Pacemaker

Cervical approach: The Avery pacing device can be implanted in the neck via a cervical approach (Fig. 152-2A) or in the chest (Fig. 152-2B) by either open or video-assisted thoracic surgical technique. Technically speaking, cervical implantation fails to capture all of the potential nerve branches, since some accessory phrenic nerve fibers may join the main trunk lower down at the thoracic inlet. This is mainly of theoretical consequence, however, as it does not translate into noticeable differences in pacing abilities between the two levels. The principal advantage of cervical implantation is the possibility of avoiding general anesthesia and double lumen intubation, as the procedure can be performed under conscious sedation or with standard general endotracheal anesthesia. There is a slight increased risk of infection incurred by placing the incision close to a tracheostomy site, which is present in many of these patients.

A 3- to 4-cm transverse incision is made close to the base of the neck with the sternocleidomastoid muscle retracted medially. Dissection is carried down laterally to the phrenic nerve, which can be identified superficial to the anterior scalene muscle. Proper identification is done with a nerve stimulator to visualize ipsilateral diaphragm contraction. The platinum electrode is passed beneath the nerve, and the cuff is anchored with fine polypropylene sutures such that the nerve sits in the cradle with full contact. The lead is then tunneled under the skin above the clavicle and connected to the receiver pocket on the anterior chest wall.

Thoracic approach: A thoracotomy incision can generally be avoided by using minimally invasive access techniques (Fig. 152-2B). The video-assisted thoracic surgical approach can be performed bilaterally in one sitting with double lumen ventilation, but a staged approach is occasionally preferable. A small utility mini-thoracotomy incision is made in the second intercostal space with two thoracoscopic ports inserted in the fifth intercostal space along the midaxillary line and seventh intercostal space along the anterior axillary line. The phrenic nerve is again dissected circumferentially such that the electrode is passed around it and secured to ensure good contact with the nerve. On the right side, the ideal level for insertion is between the azygos junction with the superior vena cava and the cavoatrial junction. On the left side, the preferred site is between the aortic arch and the pulmonary artery.

Regardless of approach, precautions should be taken to prevent devascularization of the phrenic nerve during the dissection. For this reason, one should leave a 2- to 3-mm rim of perineural tissue at the level of the nerve dissection. The wire lead from the thoracic electrode exits via a port incision and then is tunneled to the subcutaneous receiver pocket on the anterior chest wall. A coil of slack lead should be left in the chest to account for lung re-expansion and patient growth, especially in younger children. Diaphragmatic contraction is confirmed and pacing thresholds are determined before closure. In patients with congenital hypoventilation syndrome who are ambulatory, the receiver pocket is often placed overlying the abdominal wall laterally, whereas in tetraplegic patients the chest wall is more commonly used.

NeuRx DPS PACING

With the DPS system, the leads are inserted at the phrenic nerve motor point on the underside of the diaphragm (Fig. 152-3). Inadvertent nerve injury caused by the necessity of implanting the lead directly on the phrenic nerve is thus avoided. The procedure is currently performed laparoscopically. Four ports are used including two 10-mm ports in the supraumbilical and epigastric regions in addition to two lateral 5-mm ports. A portion of the falciform ligament is taken down to improve exposure of both hemidiaphragms. The motor point is then mapped to determine the location of the optimal diaphragm contraction both visually and via pressure measurements using a transducer connected to one of the ports. Once two points of maximal contraction have been mapped on each side for redundancy, a laparoscopic insertion device is used to implant the electrodes (Fig. 152-4A,B).

Each lead is loaded into the shaft of the inserter such that the lead is released into the muscle at the mapped motor point when the device needle tip is pulled back and out. If the needle crosses into the pleural space, it is important to assess for capnothorax. If proper hemodynamics are maintained, treatment may be unnecessary. Otherwise, aspiration and/or temporary chest tube insertion may be required. The leads are each tested with train stimulations to confirm proper capture and then tunneled

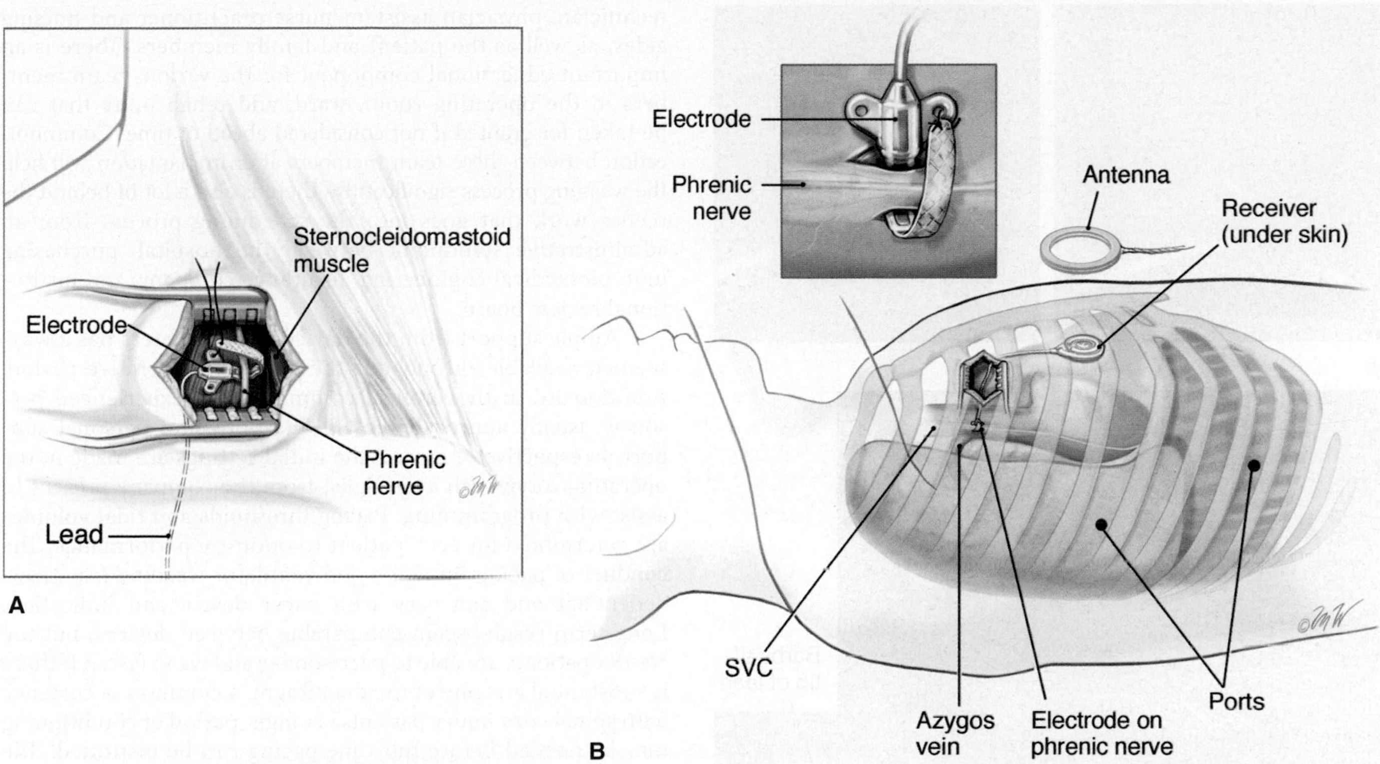

Figure 152-2. Implantation technique for Avery Mark IV Phrenic Pacemaker. *A.* Cervical approach. The sternocleidomastoid muscle is retracted medically and the phrenic nerve is identified superficial to the anterior scalene muscle. The electrode is placed beneath the phrenic nerve and the lead is tunneled under the skin of the anterior chest to the receiver. *B.* Thoracic approach. The receiver translates radiofrequency signals into electrical impulses, which are carried through the implanted electrode to the phrenic nerve that generates contraction of the diaphragm. The electrode is placed under the phrenic nerve (inset) with care not to injure the nerve. Reproduced with permission from Reference 21.

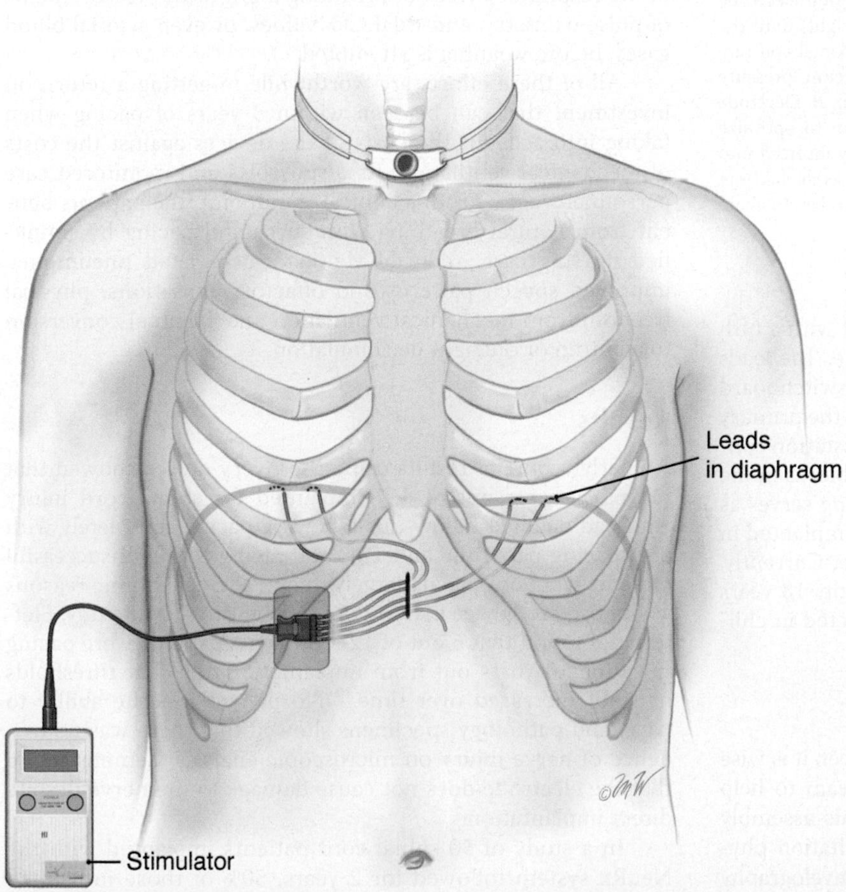

Figure 152-3. NeuRx Diaphragm Pacing System. This device is implanted laparoscopically with two leads inserted into the musculature of each hemidiaphragm. The leads are then tunneled to exit the skin level where they connect with the stimulator. Device settings for each lead are programmed into the stimulator via a clinical work station (not shown).

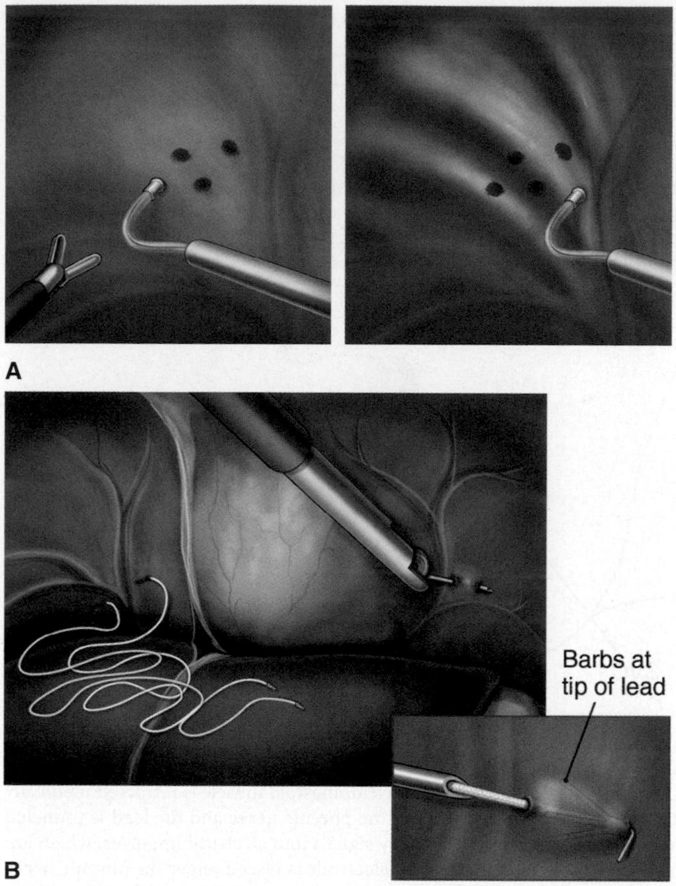

Figure 152-4. *A.* Diaphragm mapping. The laparoscopic view of the right hemidiaphragm during mapping is shown. The mapping electrode is positioned in different areas (left) and then stimulated (right) until the ideal phrenic nerve motor point is found. The point of maximal contraction is determined by measurement of pneumoperitoneum pressure displacement, tidal volumes generated, and visual inspection. *B.* Electrode insertion. Two leads are inserted into each hemidiaphragm to optimize diaphragm contraction. The implantation device is carefully inserted into the muscle at the optimal mapping point and then pulled out as the barbs at the tip of each lead hold the wire electrode in place. Care is taken to avoid inadvertent capnothorax.

out the epigastric port to the right upper quadrant with a fifth subcutaneous lead serving as the ground electrode. The leads are then connected to the stimulator via a small switchboard adapter. Stimulus parameters are programmed into the primary and backup stimulator units using the clinical workstation console. Although the DPS is not completely implantable, as in the case of the phrenic nerve pacemakers, the tunneling serves as a good barrier for infection and the device can be implanted in the outpatient setting with laparoscopic technique. Currently, the NeuRx device is FDA approved only for patients 18 years and older, although clinical trials are being conducted in children aged 5 to 17 years, with encouraging results.

Setup and Perioperative Planning

When embarking on placement of a diaphragm pacer, it is wise for the surgeon to establish a multidisciplinary team to help in the perioperative assessment and planning. This assembly of clinicians can include a pulmonologist, rehabilitation physician, respiratory therapist, neurologist, electromyelography technician, physician assistant/nurse practitioner and nursing aides, as well as the patient and family members. There is an important educational component for the various team members in the operating room, ward, and rehab units that can be taken for granted if not considered ahead of time. Communication between these team members after implantation will help the weaning process significantly. There is also a lot of behind the scenes work that goes into the scheduling process from an administrative standpoint between the hospital, purchasing unit, biomedical engineering, insurance company, and institutional review board.

Ample support from the device manufacturers has always seemed available throughout the entire perioperative period. Additionally, in the surgical community, an experienced person is usually approachable for questions and personal support. Irrespective of device, the initial settings are made in the operating room with a specialist from the company present to assist with programming. Pacing thresholds and tidal volumes are determined for each patient to optimize performance. The conduct of pacing initiation and ventilator weaning is patient-dependent and can vary with pacer device and indication. Long-term results seem comparable between devices, but the NeuRx patients are able to pace sooner and wean faster. If there is substantial atrophy of the diaphragm, a common occurrence with spinal cord injury patients, a longer period of conditioning may be needed before full-time pacing can be instituted. The necessity for conditioning results from the conversion of type I fatigue-resistant slow twitch muscle fibers to the less efficient type II fast twitch fibers during prolonged periods of ventilator dependence. For these patients, progress with conditioning by electrical stimulation is monitored by clinical observation of the respiratory work of breathing along with measurements of pulse oximetry, end-tidal CO_2 values, or even arterial blood gases, before weaning is attempted.

All of these efforts are worthwhile in getting a return on investment that can be seen within 3 years of pacing when taking into account the costs of the devices against the costs of mechanical ventilation, its disposables and monitored care personnel wages. From a clinical standpoint, the patients benefit from natural breathing with successful pacing by simplified nursing care, reduced ventilator-associated pneumonia, improved speech patterns and olfactory sensations, physical freedom from mechanical ventilation and eventual conversion to a button or outright decannulation.

Results

An early report of results using the Avery device showed that in 165 patients out of 477 implanted for spinal cord injury who had detailed follow-up, 47% were pacing completely with 35% pacing part-time and 17% not pacing.[18] The unsuccessful patients were not pacing largely due to socioeconomic reasons as opposed to device malfunction. In a more recent study, Elefteriades found that 6 out of 12 tetraplegic patients were pacing full time 10 years out from implantation and that thresholds had not increased over time.[19] No patient lost the ability to pace, and pathology specimens showed that there was no evidence of nerve injury on microscopic analysis, demonstrating that the electrode does not cause damage to the nerve despite direct implantation.

In a study of 50 spinal cord patients implanted with the NeuRx system followed for 2 years, 50% of those implanted over 6 months were completely off mechanical ventilation while 66% were pacing over 12 hours a day without the need of an attendant.[20] No patient was on the ventilator full time. The longest patient with the device was pacing out a 8 years and another was weaned from mechanical ventilation 28 years after injury. The latter patient took longer to wean from the ventilator, but the case demonstrates that it was still possible effectively pace despite this long period due to the intact phrenic nerves.

In its application to ALS patients, the DPS has been shown by Onders to be an effective means of delaying the inevitable need for mechanical ventilation in this patient population by up to 2 years.[7] In the first 16 ALS patients, the decline in FVC with pacing was 0.9% per month compared to controls of 2.4% per month. Ultrasound studies in several patients showed thickening with improved excursion on fluoroscopy.

Procedure-Specific Complications

By virtue of the differences in implantation schemes, the Avery unit puts the phrenic nerve at greater risk for devascularization or mechanical injury during the dissection and insertion of the electrode. This risk is largely avoided with NeuRx system, which implants at the neuromuscular motor point. While each system is susceptible to device-related infection, the risks are lower with the Avery system, which is completely implantable making percutaneous infection theoretically less likely. Capnothorax is a known complication for the NeuRx system since the electrode is inserted from the underside of the diaphragm and the needle may inadvertently puncture the pleura during insertion. The condition may be symptomatic requiring treatment or occult requiring additional close observation.

Each device is quite durable from a mechanical standpoint, but both may require electrode or electrode component replacement due to wear and tear over time. The Avery electrode on the nerve cannot be removed easily or safely, but the end attached to the receiver can be replaced should the receiver malfunction. The NeuRx electrodes can fray or be damaged outside the body, but are easily spliced back together at the bedside with experience. Additionally, these electrodes implanted in the diaphragm can be simply cut similar to epicardial pacing wires or perhaps carefully pulled out if necessary.

Conclusion

Diaphragm pacing is an uncommon procedure in thoracic surgery. Many patients with unilateral diaphragm paralysis are referred for diagnostic evaluation, but few will be suitable for pacing. Others will have idiopathic, viral, or traumatic etiology that can be managed surgically with diaphragm plication, if clinically warranted. For patients with high cervical spinal cord injury or central hypoventilation (congenital or acquired), the integrity of the phrenic nerve must be carefully evaluated, including full review of the neurologic and pulmonary systems, and careful assessments conducted via diagnostic procedures. During implantation, the ability of the phrenic nerve or motor point to conduct a signal is retested on-the-spot before proceeding to full implantation of the device. All four devices mentioned in this chapter are suitable for pacing. However, the author's experience is limited to the Avery Mark IV and the NeuRx DPS, as these are the only two approved for implantation in the United States. Nevertheless, the surgical access techniques and technical principles are all very similar. Recently, it has been shown that diaphragm pacing may play a valuable role in patients with acute respiratory insufficiency and with the neuromuscular disease, ALS. This expanded indication may benefit patients by promoting weaning long-term result. Future applications of this technique in patients with marginal pulmonary function following high-risk resection, after lung transplantation, or for temporary pacing in the intensive care unit for difficult to wean patients may prove viable but will require further exploration. Thoracic surgeons should keep this enabling technology in their armamentarium.

EDITOR'S COMMENT

Pacing technology has been available for many decades. Unfortunately, only a few thoracic surgeons have developed expertise in this area. A large population of patients can benefit from diaphragmatic pacing. This chapter clearly maps out patient selection, operative technique, and available hardware for use. The specific details provided by Dr. Ducko on available hardware are a particularly valuable resource. The operative intervention is straightforward, and this field can be expected to dramatically expand in the next few years.

—Michael T. Jaklitsch

References

1. Schechter D. Application of electrotherapy to noncardiac thoracic disorders. *Bull N Y Acad Med*. 1970;46:932–951.
2. Glenn WW, Phelps ML. Diaphragm pacing by electrical stimulation of the phrenic nerve. *Neurosurgery*. 1985;17(6):974–984.
3. Glenn WW, Holcomb WG, Gee JB, et al. Central hypoventilation; long-term ventilatory assistance by radiofrequency electrophrenic respiration. *Ann Surg*. 1970;172(4):755–773.
4. Glenn WW, Holcomb WG, McLaughlin AJ, et al. Total ventilatory support in a quadriplegic patient with radiofrequency electrophrenic respiration. *N Engl J Med*. 1972;286(10):513–516.
5. DiMarco AF, Onders RP, Kowalski KE, et al. Phrenic nerve pacing in a tetraplegic patient via intramuscular diaphragm electrodes. *Am J Respir Crit Care Med*. 2002;166(12 Pt 1):1604–1606.
6. Onders RP, Carlin AM, Elmo M, et al. Amyotrophic lateral sclerosis: the Midwestern surgical experience with the diaphragm pacing stimulation system shows that general anesthesia can be safely performed. *Am J Surg*. 2009;197(3):386–390.
7. Onders R. Phrenic nerve and diaphragm motor point pacing. In: Patterson GA, Pearson FG, Cooper JD, et al., *Pearson's Thoracic and Esophageal Surgery*. 3rd ed. Philadelphia, PA: Churchill Livingstone Elsevier; 2008.
8. Qureshi A. Diaphragm paralysis. *Semin Respir Crit Care Med*. 2009;30(3):315–320.
9. Ko MA, Darling GE. Acquired paralysis of the diaphragm. *Thorac Surg Clin*. 2009;19(4):501–510.
10. Chervin RD, Guilleminault C. Diaphragm pacing for respiratory insufficiency. *J Clin Neurophysiol*. 1997;14(5):369–377.
11. Shaw RK, Glenn WW, Hogan JF, et al. Electrophysiological evaluation of phrenic nerve function in candidates for diaphragm pacing. *J Neurosurg*. 1980;53(3):345–354.
12. Alshekhlee A, Onders RP, Syed TU, et al. Phrenic nerve conduction studies in spinal cord injury: applications for diaphragmatic pacing. *Muscle Nerve*. 2008;38(6):1546–1552.

13. Similowski T, Straus C, Attali V, et al. Assessment of the motor pathway to the diaphragm using cortical and cervical magnetic stimulation in the decision-making process of phrenic pacing. *Chest.* 1996;110(6):1551–1557.
14. Lieberman JS, Corkill G, Nayak NN, et al. Serial phrenic nerve conduction studies in candidates for diaphragm pacing. *Arch Phys Med Rehabil.* 1980;61(11):528–531.
15. DiMarco AF, Onders RP, Ignagni A, et al. Inspiratory muscle pacing in spinal cord injury: case report and clinical commentary. *J Spinal Cord Med.* 2006;29(2):95–108.
16. Le Pimpec-Barthes F, Gonzalez-Bermejo J, Hubsch JP, et al. Intrathoracic phrenic pacing: a 10-year experience in France. *J Thorac Cardiovasc Surg.* 2011;142(2):378–383.
17. Mayr W, Bijak M, Girsch W, et al. Multichannel stimulation of phrenic nerves by epineural electrodes. Clinical experience and future developments. *ASAIO J.* 1993;39(3):M729–M735.
18. Glenn WW, Brouillette RT, Dentz B, et al. Fundamental considerations in pacing of the diaphragm for chronic ventilatory insufficiency: a multi-center study. *Pacing Clin Electrophysiol.* 1988;11(11 Pt 2):2121–2127.
19. Elefteriades JA, Quin JA, Hogan JF, et al. Long-term follow-up of pacing of the conditioned diaphragm in quadriplegia. *Pacing Clin Electrophysiol.* 2002;25(6):897–906.
20. Onders RP, DiMarco AF, Ignagni AR, et al. The learning curve for investigational surgery: lessons learned from laparoscopic diaphragm pacing for chronic ventilator dependence. *Surg Endosc.* 2005;19(5):633–637.
21. Kanaan S, Ducko C. Disorders of ventilation: diaphragmatic pacing. In: Fauci AS, ed. *Harrison's Online.* New York, NY: McGraw-Hill Professional; 2010.

153 Long-Term Outcomes After a Congenital Diaphragmatic Hernia Repair: Implications for Adult Thoracic Surgeons

Bradley C. Linden

Keywords: Agenesis of hemidiaphragm, Morgnani hernia

INTRODUCTION

Survival of infants born with congenital diaphragmatic hernias (CDHs), as with many other anomalies in pediatrics, has steadily improved over the last three decades owing to advances in critical care medicine, as well as surgical technique. While early attempts to repair CDH were made in emergent fashion, recognition that the life-threatening issue was not mechanical compression of the lungs or mediastinal structures, but disordered pulmonary vascular reactivity, has been the major advance in improving survival and outcomes. There is wide variation in the technical approach to the repair of these anomalies including variability in pre- and postoperative care, timing of the operation, abdominal or thoracic operative approach, and choice of prosthetic material for closure. The intent of this chapter is to provide the adult thoracic surgeon with a reference for review of the current management of CDH and discuss the impact of having these diaphragmatic defects repaired as an infant or child on general thoracic anomalies/procedures in the adult.

TYPES OF CDH

The most common type of CDH is the Bochdalek hernia (Fig. 153-1). These occur posterolaterally and most commonly on the left. In general, Bochdalek hernias are categorized on the basis of size. Small defects are usually triangular in shape, with the apex medially and the base on the chest wall. Small defects most often are repaired primarily. Medium-sized defects have a larger segment of missing diaphragm, often leading to inability to close by primary repair. These defects may require a prosthetic patch, which usually includes sutures placed around the ribs laterally. The largest defects are commonly referred to as agenesis of the hemidiaphragm, and require nearly complete replacement of the hemidiaphragm with prosthetic patch material. The medium and large defects tend to have vanishingly small amounts of tissue along the esophagus and aorta to which the patch can be sewn. Consequently, gastroesophageal reflux (GERD) is more common in the medium and large defect forms of CDH leading these patients to be more likely to require a fundoplication to control their reflux. Another reason that patients with a patch repair have more reflux is that the patch does not grow as the patient does, and may, therefore, pull on the esophageal hiatus as the patient grows.

Morgagni hernias are located in the midline just posterior to the sternum. These defects can have little to no symptoms. Consequently, Morgagni hernias are most commonly diagnosed with older patients who have chest x-rays for other reasons and a mediastinal mass is seen. These Morgagni defects are commonly closed primarily; however, on rare occasion, a patch may be required. Morgagni defects are also seen in pentalogy of Cantrell, and in that case, are usually bilateral.

Eventration of the diaphragm (Fig. 153-2) occurs in the congenitally thin muscular portion of the hemidiaphragm. It

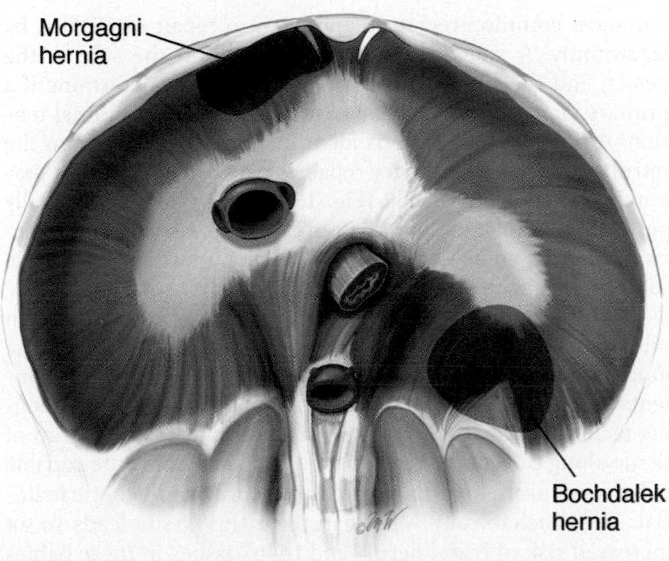

Figure 153-1. Common locations of congenital diaphragmatic hernias.

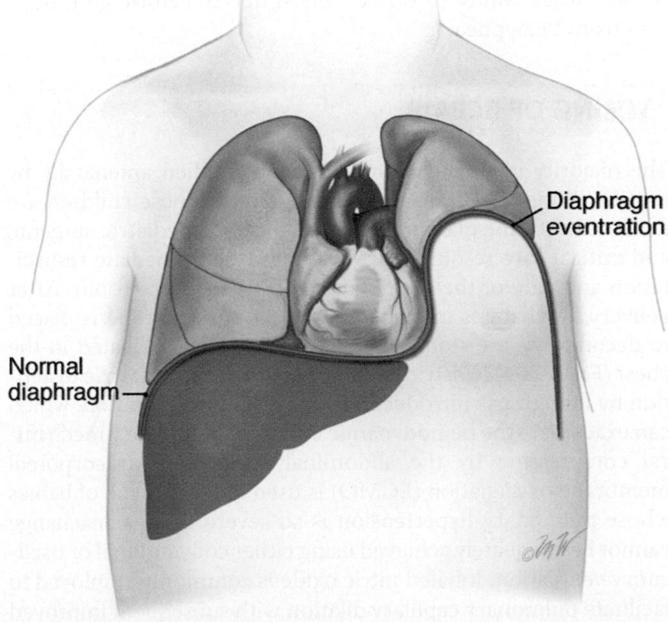

Figure 153-2. Eventration of the diaphragm.

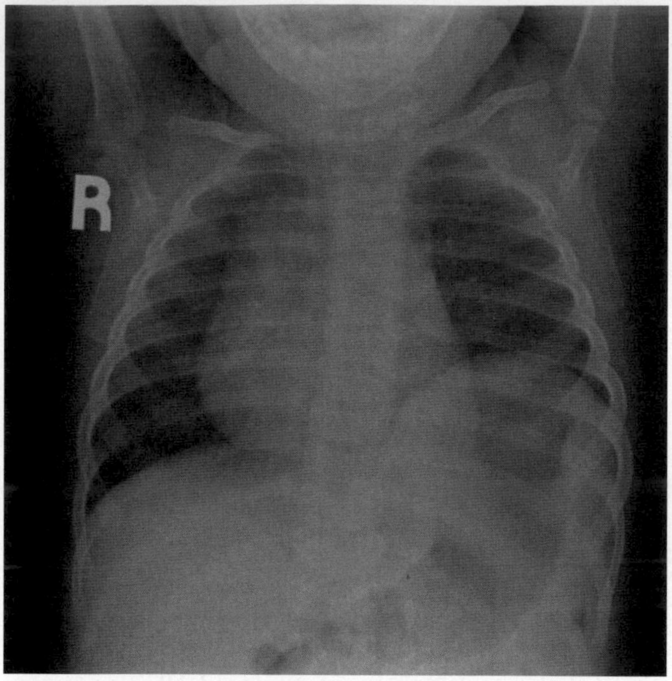

Figure 153-3. Chest x-ray of child with eventration of the left diaphragm.

occurs far more frequently on the right (5:1), as the heart tends to be protective. The eventration occurs anteromedially. It is often mistaken for CDH with an associated membrane sac; however, clinically and anatomically, eventration is a different entity (Fig. 153-3). As depicted in Figure 153-2, anatomically, there is still a small rim of diaphragmatic tissue. Diagnosis of eventration is elucidated either by a fluoroscopic diaphragmatic excursion study or by ultrasound, where paradoxical movement of the diaphragm is seen. Treatment consists of halting this paradoxical movement of the diaphragm though plication of the tissue. Surgical intervention is warranted when there is an inability to wean from a ventilator or when the respiratory status causes failure to thrive—often due to caloric consumption from tachypnea.

TIMING OF REPAIR

The majority of Bochdalek CDHs are identified antenatally by routine ultrasound screening. Consequently, these children are delivered with the planning and presence of a pediatric surgeon, and critical care resources are ready for the immediate resuscitation and care of the baby starting in the delivery room. After delivery, the baby is intubated and a nasogastric tube is placed to decompress the stomach, which is commonly located in the chest (Fig. 153-4). Gastric decompression reduces gastric distention by fluid or gas introduced by the initial resuscitation, which can exacerbate the hemodynamic effects of pulmonary mechanical compression by the abdominal contents. Extracorporeal membrane oxygenation (ECMO) is used for the rescue of babies whose pulmonary hypertension is so severe that gas exchange cannot be adequately achieved using either conventional or oscillatory ventilation. Inhaled nitric oxide is commonly employed to facilitate pulmonary capillary dilation with subsequent improved oxygenation and normalization of serum pH.

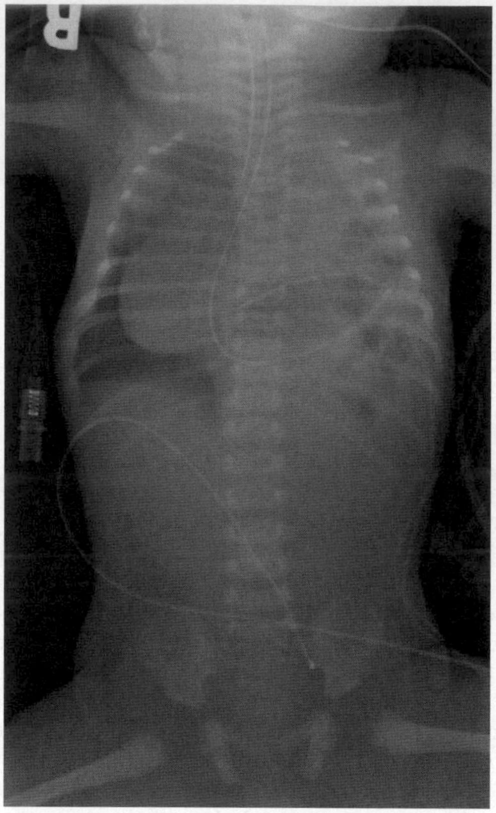

Figure 153-4. Newborn with a left CDH. Note the loops of intestine and nasogastric tube above the diaphragm. Also, there is significant shift of the mediastinal structures to the right.

If conventional ventilation with or without nitric oxide were adequate for the support of the infant, then operation is delayed until hemodynamic stability is achieved. If ECMO is used, then repair can be performed while on ECMO. Morgagni hernias are repaired electively.

METHODS OF REPAIR

The most common technical approach to repair of CDH is by laparotomy. A subcostal incision is made on the side of the defect, and the size of the defect is assessed to determine if a primary closure can be achieved with acceptably minimal tension. A posteromedial rim is identified and dissected from the retroperitoneum. A primary repair is performed when the diaphragmatic defect is small (Fig. 153-5). This repair is usually performed with interrupted sutures of non-absorbable material; however, some surgeons will use long-lasting absorbable sutures such as PDS.

When the diaphragmatic defect is large, a prosthetic patch must be used to close the defect, reduce the compression of the lungs and mediastinal structures, and hold the abdominal contents below the diaphragm. In a patch repair, the most challenging technical task is the creation of a substantial medial rim of tissue along the aorta and esophagus. This rim must be capable of holding suture for either primary closure or prosthetic material. The mechanically weak nature of this tissue leads to an increased risk of hiatal hernia and reflux issues in these babies as they grow. Additionally, sutures may be (unintentionally)

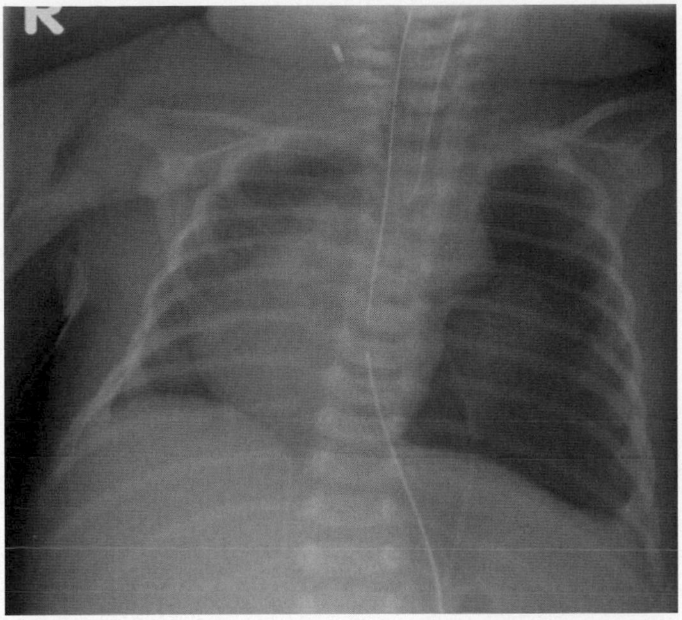

Figure 153-5. CDH after repair. No chest tube was left for this patient. The air reabsorbs with time, and the mediastinum shifts leftward. Note the hypoplastic left lung.

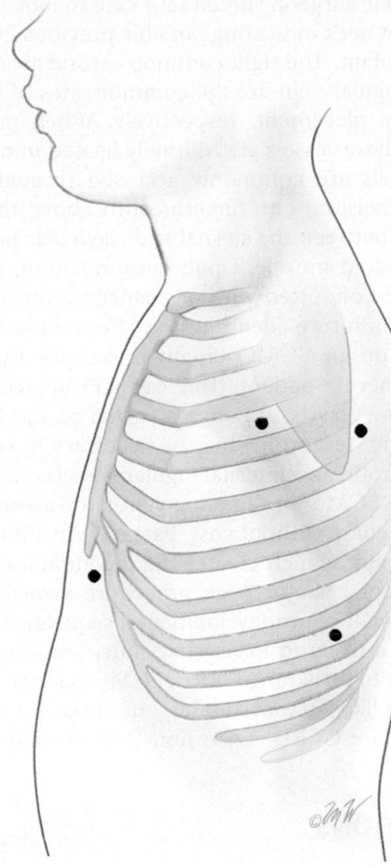

Figure 153-6. Port placement for thoracoscopic repair of congenital diaphragmatic hernia.

placed in the periadventitial tissue on the left lateral edge of the aorta, since in many cases the tissue is essentially nonexistent in this region. The adult general thoracic surgeon should take great care when reoperating in this region, particularly when patch material has been used. Adhesions formed in this area in conjunction with sutures that may have been placed in the adventitia of the aorta, and this leads to substantial risk of aortic injury when reoperations are performed.

Whatever material is used for the repair, the patch is made sufficiently large to avoid tension due to undersizing. With large defects, the patch is secured to the ribs by passing sutures carefully around the rib. As previously discussed, medial sutures may include tissue located close the aorta because of sparse tissue volume in this area. As the child grows, this small patch becomes encapsulated and, if fixed to the ribs, may remain so fixed. Depending on the material used, adhesions will form on both the abdominal and thoracic sides of the diaphragm. While some surgeons use a single patch material such as PTFE, others creates a "sandwich" using one patch material on the thoracic side and a different patch material on the abdominal side in an effort to reduce the chance of recurrence. Consequently, it is certainly beneficial to obtain an operative note that describes the patch construction prior to reoperating. When the defect is too large for primary repair, some surgeons create a split abdominal wall muscle flap by separating the transversalis and internal oblique muscles, and turn the flap upward to patch the diaphragmatic hernia defect.

In the last several years, minimally invasive techniques have been used to repair both Morgagni and Bochdalek hernias. Morgagni hernias usually can be closed primarily often via a laparoscopic approach, although, in rare cases, a patch may be used. Minimally invasive repair of diaphragmatic hernia usually is approached through the chest. Primary repairs are fairly straightforward and have a similar recurrence rate to an open repair. Patch repairs are certainly more technically challenging and these repairs are associated with a modestly higher recurrence rate than when a patch is placed in open fashion.

Recurrence of diaphragmatic hernia can be managed in a minimally invasive fashion (Fig. 153-6). When the recurrence is small, a thoracoscopic approach can allow the placement of interrupted sutures with reduction of the herniated contents. When the recurrence is larger, a full laparotomy may be necessary. Depending on the material used in patch repairs, the spleen, colon, and stomach may be densely adherent to the patch. Dense adhesions also may be present at the gastroesophageal junction making injury to the esophagus or aorta an important concern during operations for recurrent diaphragmatic hernia. Whatever technique is used for CDH repair, surgeons reoperating in the chest or abdomen should be aware that they could encounter recurrence of CDH in the form of breakdown of the primary repair or peri-patch hernia (recurrent hernia).

EXTRACORPOREAL MEMBRANE OXYGENATION

Since its introduction for CDH in 1977, ECMO has become a useful adjunct in the perioperative management of CDH patients. When acidosis and hypoxic respiratory failure persist despite maximal medical therapy, including low-tidal volume ventilation, nitric oxide, inotropes and vasopressors, ECMO is considered.

Once on ECMO, the CDH-associated predicted mortality is 52%. ECMO cannulation can be venovenous or venoarterial.

The adult thoracic surgeon should take care to look for an incision on the right neck indicating possible previous ECMO cannulation as an infant. The right common carotid artery, and the right internal jugular vein are the common sites of inflow and outflow cannula placement, respectively. When patients are decannulated, these vessels are routinely ligated in neonates.

These vessels are commonly accessed through a transverse cervical incision, one fingerbreadth above the clavicle, with dissection between the sternal and clavicular heads of the sternocleidomastoid muscle. Upon decannulation, the vessels are normally tied off, often with permanent sutures to permit the potential for future identification. Recannulation to put a patient back on an ECMO circuit is rare for the repaired diaphragmatic hernia patient. This can still be accomplished through the same vessels, although a partial or, less frequently, complete midline sternotomy may be necessary to recannulate the common carotid and internal jugular vessels.

The role of ECMO in reducing ventilator-associated lung injury does not come without cost. Patients are anticoagulated while on the circuit, which creates the potential for intracerebral/intraventricular hemorrhage, procedure-associated bleeding, and subsequent neurodevelopmental sequelae. Patients on ECMO are more likely to experience nutrition-related issues, including failure to thrive and GERD. ECMO patients are nearly four times more likely to have undergone surgical intervention (fundoplication) for GERD versus non-ECMO counterparts.[1]

COMPLICATIONS

The diagnosis of CDH is associated with a mortality rate of 40% to 50% depending on the population being studied. CDH patients tend to have multisystem disease processes that must be considered when planning an operation later in life. Up to 50% of CDH patients also have associated additional congenital malformations. These early malformations include intestinal atresias, congenital cardiovascular disease, and chromosomal anomalies. High-risk patients who undergo cardiorespiratory failure and are cannulated for ECMO are also at risk for serious neurologic sequelae related to peri-cannulation hypoxemia, thromboembolus, or intraventricular hemorrhage, all of which can have life-long neurologic implications.

Overall, outcomes of patients with CDH are dependent on both the inherent pathophysiological process of the disease as well as the different treatment options used for their treatment. Complications include but are not limited to the following: (1) nerve palsies; (2) recurrence of CHD; (3) chylothorax; (4) small bowel obstructions; and (5) persistent pulmonary hypertension. Long-term sequelae include issues with the thoracic/chest wall and GERD.

Nerve palsies are common following repair of the CDH. The diagnosis can be made in the usual fashion with a follow-up x-ray. This specifically complicates an already dysplastic residual diaphragm. In general, it is important to continue to monitor pulmonary function tests and remaining residual functional capacity; often it is the use of inappropriate high pressure ventilatory strategies in the hypoplastic lung parenchyma that cause long-term sequelae.

Chylothorax can present in as many as 28% of CDH patients following surgical repair. Risk factors include prosthetic patch use, prenatal diagnosis, and ECMO cannulation.[2] Long-term sequelae include and are not limited to nutritional deficiencies, immunologic dysfunction, and the potential for further interventions to correct the persistent loss of proteinaceous and often lymphocyte-rich fluid.

CDH patients are likely to undergo further operations during their lifetime after initial hernia repair. Recurrence is not uncommon following repairs of diaphragmatic hernias. Recurrence may follow both open and thoracoscopic repairs (Fig. 153-7A,B). Recurrence may also follow both primary

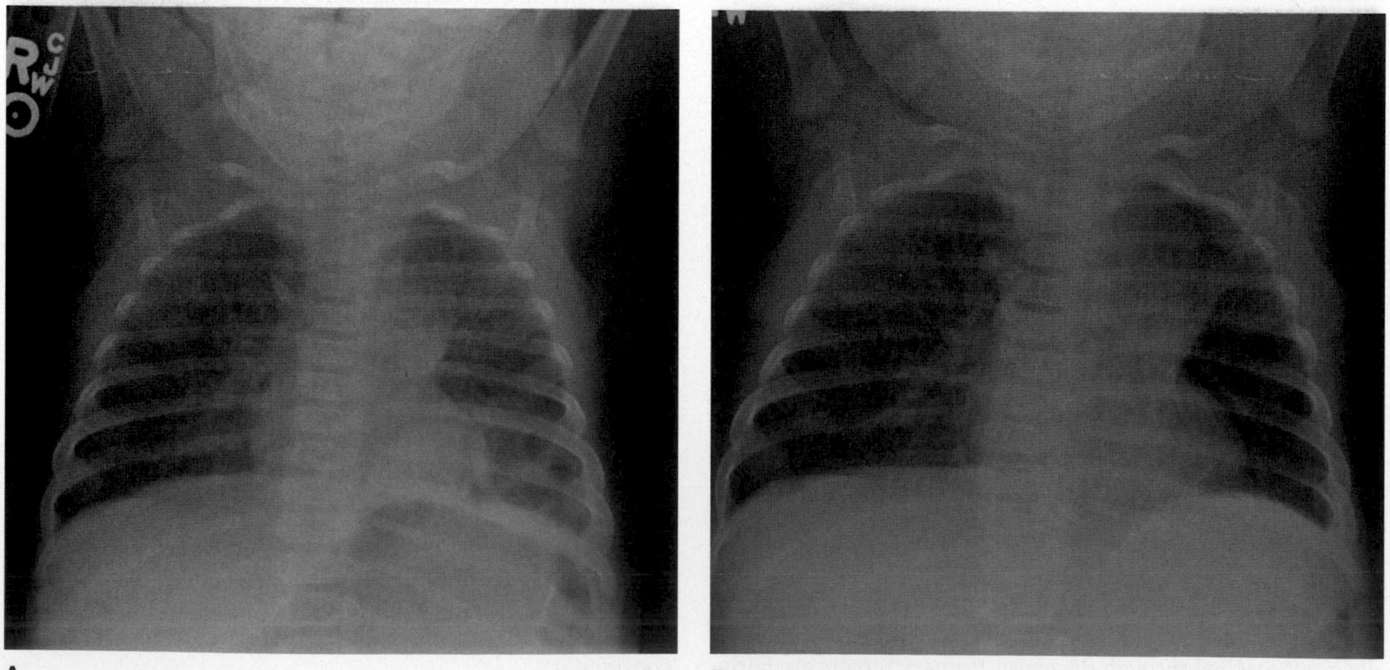

A B

Figure 153-7. *A.* Small late recurrence after thoracoscopic patch CDH repair. *B.* After thoracoscopic repair of recurrence.

and prosthetic patch repairs. According to Guner et al., the incidence of recurrence in all CDH patients ranges from 2% to 45%, where the highest incidence occurs in patients who undergo open repair with patch material.[3] Recurrence likely occurs from the inherent growth of the child, patch stability, and inherent pathophysiology of the diaphragm itself. Up to 50% of patients who receive a patch repair have subsequent recurrence by 3 years of age.[4] ECMO recipients are more likely than their non-ECMO counterparts to undergo subsequent procedures, including antireflux operations, recurrent diaphragmatic hernia repair, Ladd's procedure, tracheostomy, and chest wall reconstruction.[5] Occasionally ECMO patients require an umbilical silo to permit the abdominal space to decompress into the silo, and, therefore, reduce pressure on the repair.[5] These silos can be placed at the time of defect repair, or following closure to relieve abdominal compartment syndrome. Patients with CDH uniformly have intestinal malrotation. Small bowel obstruction occurs in 4% to 20%, attributed to midgut volvulus, incarcerated CDH recurrence, or intestinal adhesions.[4,6] Laparotomy for small bowel obstruction is the second most commonly performed procedure for CDH patients other than repair of hernia recurrence.[5]

Long-term data categorizing outcomes for CDH patients are lacking. CDH patients who require ECMO embody a high-risk patient group. In general, the degree of pulmonary hypoplasia and pulmonary hypertension are the most significant sources of potential morbidity. These patients more commonly have larger defects, which predisposes them to greater risk of recurrence, scoliosis, and chest wall dissymmetry. Up to one-third of CDH patients may exhibit reduced FEV_1 and FVC values compared to otherwise healthy counterparts on pulmonary function testing. CDH patients who are on mechanical ventilation for more than 7 days have significantly lower FEV_1 and VC than patients who were on the ventilator for less time, likely reflecting both their underlying disease severity and effects of ventilator-induced barotrauma.[7] There are few studies documenting the influence of pulmonary hypertension in CDH survivors later in life. While some patients exhibit normal exercise capacity and gas exchange parameters in adulthood,[7] studies have shown approximately one half of children survivors demonstrate evidence of right ventricular hypertension on electrocardiogram.[8]

LONG-TERM ANATOMIC IMPLICATIONS

Chest wall deformities related to abnormal breathing patterns and surgical repair create functional and anatomic barriers for potential thoracic surgery. Apart from intrinsic pulmonary hypoplasia and pulmonary hypertension, chest wall deformities further complicate pulmonary mechanics by adding extraparenchymal lung dysfunction. While scoliosis in young children may be ameliorated by bracing, patients with underlying pulmonary dysfunction often are not suitable candidates for this therapy given the restriction it imposes on chest wall expansion. Studies suggest that lung diffusion capacity, as well as the ability to achieve normal aerobic capacity, is comparable between CDH patients and otherwise healthy controls.[5] The combined obstructive/restrictive disease in adulthood following CDH repair is not well categorized, and warrants careful preoperative attention. Early respiratory insufficiency also predisposes the CDH patient group to tracheostomy. Up to 7% of patients with CDH repair undergo tracheostomy.[5]

Patients may also have scoliosis, as well as chest wall defects, including pectus malformations, and chest dissymmetry. Dissymmetry affects approximately half of CDH patients,[9] with pectus excavatum being the most common type of chest wall deformity,[6] and more common among patients with large defects or patch repairs. Approximately one-fifth of CDH patients undergo pectus excavatum repairs. Patch repair is an independent risk factor for both hernia recurrence and early chest wall deformity. Patients repaired initially with a patch are approximately five times more likely to develop early chest wall deformity or CDH recurrence than primary repair counterparts.[4] Scoliosis is found in up to 13% of CDH survivors. The scoliosis tends to curve toward the side of the hernia (concave), which can make approaches such as thoracoscopy more challenging. There is an association between the size of the patient's hernia defect and the observed degree of scoliosis.[9]

GERD affects up to 80% of CDH survivors.[10] Several theories for the origin of GERD in CDH survivors exist. Abnormal anatomy at the level of the diaphragm (including an absent or attenuated left diaphragmatic crus) as well as medial traction from patch or primary repair can lead to abnormal function of the lower esophageal sphincter. In utero compression of the mediastinal esophagus by herniated viscera is also thought to be a contributor, which has been associated with mega-esophagus in up to 40% of CDH survivors.[8] Long-term follow-up of patients with CDH has found esophagitis in up to 54% of individuals, along with presence of a hiatal hernia in as many as half of CDH survivors.[6]

CONCLUSIONS

Adults who underwent repair of a CDH are coming to the attention of general thoracic surgeons for the treatment of numerous sequelae of their congenital anomalies. This chapter provides a summary of the most common issues to be considered prior to operating on a patient who has survived this previously lethal congenital anomaly. With respect for the multisystem dysfunction, aberrant physiology, and continuity of surgical care of this unique patient group, general thoracic surgeons can be an integral part of the complex care these patients deserve.

References

1. Muratore CS, Utter S, Jaksic T, et al. Nutritional morbidity in survivors of congenital diaphragmatic hernia. *J Pediatr Surg.* 2001;36(8):1171–1176.
2. Guner YS, Chokshi N, Aranda A, et al. Thoracoscopic repair of neonatal diaphragmatic hernia. *J Laparoendosc Adv Surg Tech A.* 2008;18(6):875–880.
3. Zavala A, Campos JM, Riutort C, et al. Chylothorax in congenital diaphragmatic hernia. *Pediatr Surg Int.* 2010;26(9):919–922.
4. Jancelewicz T, Vu LT, Keller RL, et al. Long-term surgical outcomes in congenital diaphragmatic hernia: observations from a single institution. *J Pediatr Surg.* 2010;45(1):155–160; discussion 160.

5. Breckler FD, Molik KA, West KW. Influence of extracorporeal membrane oxygenation on subsequent surgeries after congenital diaphragmatic hernia repair. *J Pediatr Surg*. 2009;44(6):1186–1188.
6. Peetsold MG, Heij HA, Kneepkens CMF, et al. The long-term follow-up of patients with a congenital diaphragmatic hernia: a broad spectrum of morbidity. *Pediatr Surg Int*. 2009;25(1):1–17.
7. Peetsold MG, Vonk-Noordegraaf A, Heij HH, et al. Pulmonary function and exercise testing in adult survivors of congenital diaphragmatic hernia. *Pediatr Pulmonol*. 2007;42(4):325–331.
8. Van Meurs KP, Robbins ST, Reed VL, et al. Congenital diaphragmatic hernia: long-term outcome in neonates treated with extracorporeal membrane oxygenation. *J Pediatr*. 1993;122(6):893–899.
9. Vanamo K, Peltonen J, Rintala R, et al. Chest wall and spinal deformities in adults with congenital diaphragmatic defects. *J Pediatr Surg*. 1996;31(6):851–854.
10. Vanamo K, Rintala RJ, Lindahl H, et al. Long-term gastrointestinal morbidity in patients with congenital diaphragmatic defects. *J Pediatr Surg*. 1996;31(4):551–554.

154 Acute and Chronic Traumatic Rupture of the Diaphragm

Scott C. Bellot and Loring W. Rue, III

Keywords: Diaphragmatic laceration, blunt and penetrating diaphragmatic injuries

The diaphragm, in its role as a musculoaponeurotic structure separating the thoracic and abdominal domains, is subject to injury following blunt or penetrating trauma. Historical accounts documenting diaphragmatic injury date from 1541, when Sennertus described the postmortem finding of delayed herniation of the stomach through a diaphragmatic defect in a patient who had previously suffered a penetrating chest wound. Detailed postmortem findings related to both blunt and penetrating diaphragmatic injuries were reported by Ambroise Pare in the sixteenth century. The first antemortem diagnosis of a traumatic diaphragmatic injury was published by H. I. Bowditch in 1853, who also set forth physical criteria for the diagnosis of traumatic diaphragmatic hernias: (1) prominence and immobility of the left thorax; (2) displacement to the right of the area of cardiac dullness; (3) absent breath sounds over the left thorax; (4) audible bowel sounds in the left chest; and (5) tympany to percussion over the left chest. Riolfi, in 1886, subsequently performed the first successful repair of a diaphragmatic laceration secondary to penetrating trauma. Hedblom, in 1925, reviewed 378 cases of diaphragmatic hernias in the surgical literature, providing a contemporary overview of diagnosis and surgical treatment.

ANATOMY

The diaphragm (dia: across, phragm: fence) is the musculotendinous, dome-shaped structure separating the negative-pressure thoracic cavity and the positive-pressure peritoneal cavity. Embryologically, the diaphragm is derived from the fusion of four distinct structures: the septum transversum, the pleuroperitoneal membranes, the dorsal mesentery of the esophagus, and the body wall musculature. After development is complete, the diaphragm is composed of two distinct muscle groups, costal and crural. The costal muscle group is composed of peripherally located skeletal muscle fibers, whose contraction results in flattening of the diaphragm and lowering of the ribs. The crural muscle group, by contrast, does not contribute significantly to diaphragmatic excursion. The left crus arises from the upper two lumbar vertebrae and the right crus arises from the lateral aspect of the upper three lumbar vertebrae. The interdigitation of the medial tendinous crural fibers anterior to the aortic hiatus forms the median arcuate ligament, and the fibers of the right crus encircle the esophagus. Both costal and crural muscle fibers converge to insert into the aponeurotic central tendon, whose central aspect lies immediately beneath the pericardium (Fig. 154-1). Thoracoabdominal structures traverse the diaphragm through three major openings: the vena cava aperture (T8 vertebral level, containing the vena cava), the esophageal aperture (T10 vertebral level, containing the esophagus and the left and right vagal nerves), and the aortic aperture (T12 vertebral level, containing the aorta, thoracic duct, and the azygos vein (Fig. 154-2).

The diaphragm attaches to the xiphisternum anteriorly, the first three lumbar vertebrae posteriorly, and laterally attaches to the internal surface of the lower ribs, spanning the sixth rib anteriorly to the twelfth rib posteriorly. The phrenic nerves, arising from the anterior rami of the third through fifth cervical nerve roots, supply motor innervation to the diaphragm and sensory innervation to the central tendon and parietal pleura. In addition, the outer portion of the diaphragmatic musculature is innervated by the lower intercostal nerves (T7–T12) secondary to derivation from the somatopleuric mesenchyme during embryologic development. The rich arterial blood supply includes the pericardiophrenic arteries on the superior aspect and branches from the abdominal aorta and intercostal arteries on the inferior surface (Fig. 154-3).

PHYSIOLOGY

As the chief respiratory muscle of the body, the diaphragm is a dynamic structure.

With normal respiration, a 3- to 5-cm diaphragmatic excursion is produced in both directions, providing 75% to 80% of tidal volume. On deep exhalation, the right hemidiaphragm rises anteriorly to the fourth intercostal space, and the left hemidiaphragm to the fifth intercostal space. Both hemidiaphragms ascend to the seventh or eighth intercostal space posteriorly. Clinically useful landmarks for the cephalad extent of diaphragmatic excursion are the nipple line anteriorly and tip of scapula posteriorly.

Diaphragmatic injury may occur secondary to either penetrating or blunt mechanisms. Retrospective reviews have demonstrated the incidence of diaphragmatic injuries to range from 0.8% to 5.8%. Penetrating injuries remain the most common cause of diaphragmatic injuries, outnumbering blunt injury twofold.[1] Penetrating injuries associated with stab wounds, the left hemidiaphragm is more frequently injured due to the preponderance of right-handed assailants. The principal mechanism involved in blunt injury is a sudden and abrupt increase in the pleuroperitoneal pressure gradient, which normally ranges from +7 to +20 cm H_2O. The resulting burst-type diaphragmatic injury results from the transmission of force through the abdominal viscera to the diaphragm.

Injury to the left hemidiaphragm occurs more frequently than that to the right, secondary to the protection afforded the right hemidiaphragm by the liver. Most left-sided diaphragmatic tears are greater than 10 cm long, and rupture typically occurs in the posterolateral aspect due to congenital weakness of the fusion between the costal and lumbar diaphragmatic muscular attachments. Lateral impact motor vehicle collisions are associated with a higher incidence of diaphragmatic ruptures compared to frontal collisions.[2]

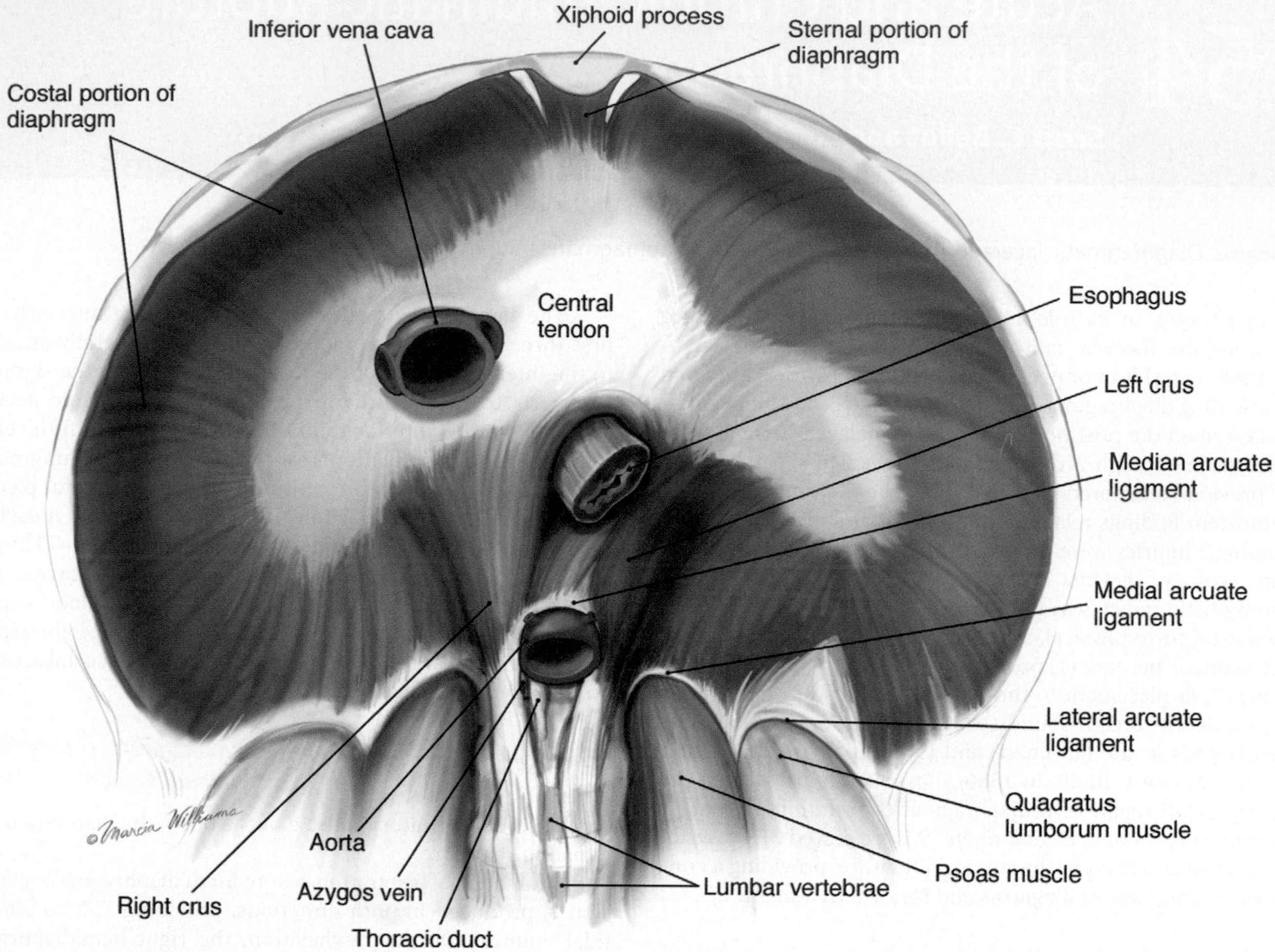

Figure 154-1. The muscle fibers of the diaphragm originate from the posterior lumbar spine (arcuate ligaments) and curve upward to form an aponeurotic sheath known as the central tendon. Several thoracic organs and vessels pass through apertures in the diaphragmatic surface.

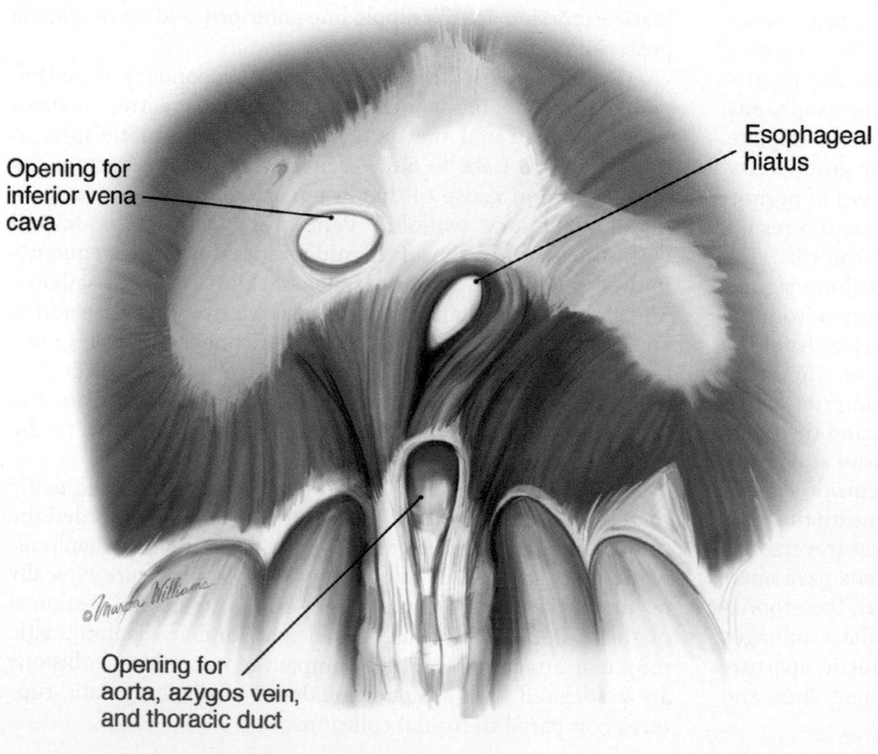

Figure 154-2. Abdominal surface of the diaphragm with three natural openings.

PART 25

MEDIASTINAL DISEASES, BENIGN OR MALIGNANT

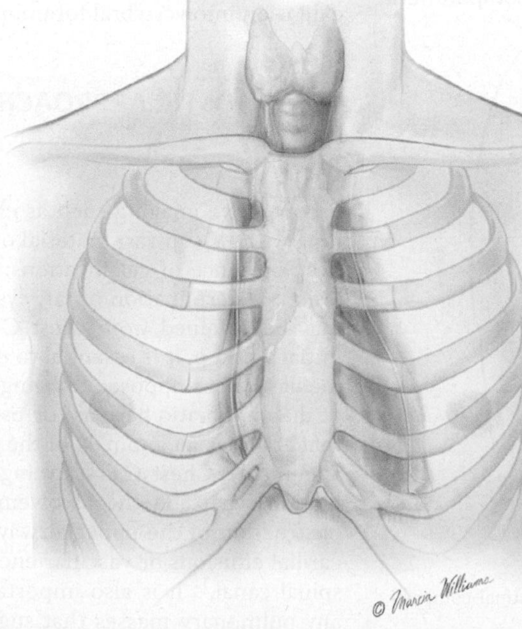

155 Overview of Benign and Malignant Mediastinal Diseases

Stacey Su and Yolonda L. Colson

Keywords: Tumor markers, role of biopsy in diagnosis of mediastinal masses, anterior mediastinal masses, middle mediastinal masses, posterior mediastinal masses, thymoma, lymphoma, thymic cysts, parathyroid adenomas, thyroid goiters, Castleman disease, mesenchymal tumors

The mediastinum is defined as the space between the lungs. It is bordered by the sternum anteriorly, the thoracic inlet superiorly, the diaphragm inferiorly, and the ribs (Fig. 155-1). Mediastinal masses arise from structures that normally reside in the mediastinum, as well as those that migrate through it during development. The mediastinum is compartmentalized into four major spaces based on anatomic landmarks. The superior mediastinum extends from the thoracic inlet to an imaginary line between the angle of Louis and the fourth thoracic vertebral body. The anterior mediastinum spans the back of the sternum to the front of the ascending aorta and pericardium. The posterior mediastinum is located between the posterior pericardium and the spine; this includes the costovertebral sulci. The middle mediastinum lies between the anterior and posterior mediastinal compartments. These divisions are not precise and become less defined as lesions invade or displace adjacent organs, leading to distorted anatomy. Nevertheless, they provide a framework to classify and understand mediastinal diseases. With knowledge of the patient's age, location of the lesion, and presence or absence of sentinel signs and symptoms, a reasonable preoperative diagnosis often can be made.

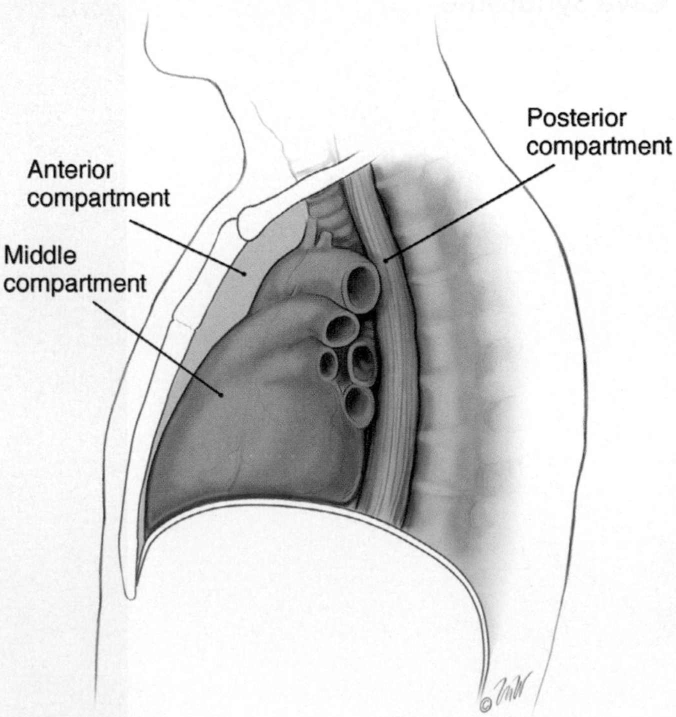

Figure 155-1. The anterior, middle, and posterior mediastinal compartments.

Tumors and cysts occur in the mediastinum across all ages and consist of both benign and malignant entities (see Chapters 161–163). The location of the most frequent mediastinal masses differs by age. In children, the most common lesion is the neurogenic tumor in the posterior mediastinum, which accounts for about half of all mediastinal masses in the pediatric population. By contrast, the most frequent lesion in adults is thymoma in the anterior mediastinum. Posterior mediastinal lesions are less common in adults, whereas thymic lesions are rare in children. The trend is otherwise similar in adults and children, with lymphoma and germ cell tumor as the next most common mediastinal tumors, in order.[1–5]

Most mediastinal masses are asymptomatic, but many can be associated with specific symptoms and signs. Symptoms depend on the size of the lesion, whether it is benign or malignant, and the presence or absence of infection. It is generally agreed that malignant lesions are more likely to be symptomatic than benign lesions.[5,6] Approximately 25% of all mediastinal tumors are malignant in both adults and children. Roughly two-thirds of children are symptomatic at presentation, whereas only one-third of adults have symptoms.[7,8] Most symptoms are related to mediastinal structures that have been either compressed or invaded by tumor. These consist of respiratory symptoms such as cough, stridor, hemoptysis, and dyspnea or pain related to invasion of the chest wall, pleura, or diaphragm.[5,8] Other symptoms and signs may include dysphagia, hoarseness, superior vena cava syndrome (see Chapter 164), pericardial tamponade, Horner syndrome, and reticular pain owing to extension into vertebral foramina.[7]

DIAGNOSTIC APPROACH

Imaging

Preoperative imaging such as chest x-ray and chest CT scanning with IV contrast material offers insight into the size, location, presence of calcifications, and tissue consistency of the lesion. Determination of fat, cystic, or soft tissue components may be obtained from chest CT and/or MRI scan.[9,10] In the initial workup, it is essential to establish that the lesion is truly mediastinal as opposed to being intraabdominal, as in the case of diaphragmatic hernias, or pseudomediastinal, as in a mass that arises as an anomaly of the vascular system (e.g., an aortic aneurysm). Chest CT scanning also provides essential information regarding the involvement of other organs, such as obstruction of the upper airways, presence of pleural or pericardial effusions or vascular encasement, or extension into the spinal canal.[11] It is also important to identify the presence of any pulmonary masses that suggest a primary malignancy or metastatic disease. For the most part, the resolution of helical chest CT scanning makes it unnecessary to pursue further imaging. However, in the case of neurogenic tumors of the posterior mediastinum, MRI can better delineate extension of the mass into the neural foramina and spinal canal. MRI is also used to evaluate processes that involve the great vessels and can obviate the need for IV contrast material administration.[10,11]

In rare instances, radionuclide studies may be useful, as in the case of technetium scans for substernal goiters (see Chapter 157), gallium scans for nonseminomatous germ cell tumors,[12] and [^{131}I]*meta*-iodobenzylguanidine scans for mediastinal neuroendocrine tumors.[13] Angiography and myelography are used infrequently today, given the excellent CT and MRI images that are available, but one possible application of angiography is to show the involvement of the artery of Adamkiewicz by neurogenic tumors.[14] Usually this artery originates from the intercostal arteries at T9 to L2; however, in 15% of individuals, it originates from the T5 to T8 levels and is an important surgical consideration in relation to the risk of postoperative paraplegia.[15]

PET/CT is not routinely utilized except to rule out the presence of extrathoracic or disseminated disease. In select cases, the degree of FDG uptake on PET can suggest the aggressiveness of the tumor.

Laboratory Tests

Useful serum tumor markers in the management of germ cell tumors (GCTs) include beta-human chorionic gonadotropin (β-hCG) and α-fetoprotein (AFP). Eighty percent of patients with nonseminomatous GCTs have elevated AFP, and 30% have elevated β-BCG.[16] Changes in the titer of the markers roughly parallel the increase or decrease of tumor activity.[17] Only 10% of patients with pure seminomas have mildly elevated β-hCG; any elevation in AFP level indicates a mixed germ cell tumor and portends a worse prognosis than for pure seminoma. In addition, elevated AFP levels are nearly diagnostic for nonseminomatous germ cell tumor and obviate the need for tissue biopsy.

Another serum marker useful in the preoperative workup of an anterior mediastinal mass or in patients with a newly diagnosed thymoma is antiacetylcholine receptor antibody because its presence is indicative of myasthenia gravis (MG).[18] However, only one-third of patients with a known thymoma have associated MG; half of all patients with thymoma have no symptoms at all.[19] Occasionally, neuroendocrine tumors of the anterior mediastinum secrete corticotropin-releasing hormone, and very rarely, neurogenic tumors cause hypoglycemia by secreting insulin. Neuroblastomas may be hormonally active and can be detected with measurement of catecholamines or their breakdown products, that is, vanillylmandelic acid and metanephrines, in the urine. Thus, like pheochromocytomas, neuroblastomas may be associated with diarrhea, cramping, and hypertension. Workup of thyroid goiters includes thyroid function tests, and parathyroid tumors in the mediastinum may be associated with an elevated serum level of calcitonin. Elevated serum LDH may be associated with lymphoma and is used as a prognostic marker for progression of this disease.[20]

Biopsy

The surgeon's role in mediastinal disease is to provide histopathologic diagnosis either through surgical excision or through biopsy. Lesions that are small and well circumscribed may be resected without preoperative biopsy, but larger tumors that show evidence of local invasion or that are suspicious for diseases to be treated by nonsurgical means should undergo biopsy.

In the case of lesions that are treated via medical therapy, it is especially important to biopsy adequate tissue not only for diagnosis but also for subclassification, as is the case for non-Hodgkin lymphoma and for malignant germ cell tumors. Subtyping of malignancies involves analysis by immunohistochemistry and flow cytometry. In the initial workup, it is reasonable to consider obtaining a fine-needle aspiration (FNA) by the least-invasive approach: CT-guided transthoracic approach or by endoscopic ultrasound-guided biopsy (either via transbronchial or transesophageal route). However, because of the limited tissue yield, in addition to sampling error and cellular heterogeneity within the lesion, FNA may provide inadequate tissue samples to achieve definitive diagnosis.[21,22] Additional tissue may be obtained by core-needle biopsy or surgical biopsy.

The surgeon has multiple diagnostic techniques that can provide adequate biopsy specimens, including cervical mediastinoscopy, anterior mediastinotomy (Chamberlain procedure), transcervical approach, and video-assisted thoracic surgery (VATS). In many instances, surgical biopsy (e.g., via VATS) has the added benefit of allowing excision of the mass, if so indicated. In the age of minimally invasive techniques, it is rare to perform median sternotomy or thoracotomy for diagnosis alone. With regard to biopsy approaches, biopsy incisions must be planned with consideration for future surgical resection. Similarly, one should be cautious to avoid spilling tumor cells into the pleural spaces because this may prevent subsequent curative resection of the lesion.[21,22]

Anesthetic Considerations

Preoperatively, it is important to discuss anesthetic considerations unique to mediastinal masses, particularly those in anterior and sometimes middle mediastinal locations. In addition to avoiding neuromuscular blocking agents in patients with MG, or hypertension in those with pheochromocytoma, one must realize that patients with large mediastinal masses may have both restrictive and obstructive pulmonary physiology. Large mediastinal masses may displace lung volume and thus result in restrictive impairment. More important, patients with significant extrinsic compression of the airway may have sudden respiratory collapse on induction of general anesthesia. This is attributed to the loss of respiratory drive and the conversion from spontaneous (negative-pressure) to assisted (positive-pressure) ventilation, which maximizes the loss in pressure differential (ΔP) across the point of airway obstruction. In this case, ventilation of the distal airways may not be achieved. Such patients require awake intubation, possibly in the upright position. To avoid general anesthesia, one should consider acquiring tissue diagnosis through less invasive means, if possible (e.g., aspiration of pleural effusion or image-guided percutaneous biopsy), or through an approach under local anesthesia (e.g., suprasternal or anterior mediastinotomy). Although there is no single predictor of anesthetic risk in patients with mediastinal masses, it is advisable to obtain preoperative supine and upright pulmonary function tests and to calculate a tracheal cross-sectional area from a CT scan to delineate patients who are at highest risk for respiratory collapse.[23] Shamberger et al. suggest that those with a peak expiratory flow rate greater than

50% predicted or tracheal area greater than 50% normal can undergo general anesthesia safely.[24,25]

ANTERIOR MEDIASTINAL MASSES

Thymic Tumors

The incidence of thymoma is highest in patients between the ages of 40 and 60 years and is distributed equally between the sexes.[26] In addition to the high association with MG, up to 10% of those with thymoma have other paraneoplastic syndromes, including red blood cell aplasia, hypogammaglobulinemia, inappropriate antidiuretic hormone secretion, systemic lupus erythematosus, or Cushing syndrome.[27] Suggestion of local invasion may be determined by chest CT scan with IV contrast. A well-circumscribed lesion is likely a thymoma, whereas a lesion showing infiltration into surrounding mediastinal structures such as lung or great vessels is likely malignant. Thymomas are classified according to histopathologic (2004 WHO classification) or clinicopathologic criteria (Masaoka staging system).[28,29]

All thymomas are considered to have malignant potential in so far as they may demonstrate local invasiveness and propensity to local recurrence after treatment. Of all thymic tumors, thymic carcinoma and thymic carcinoid have a dismal survival regardless of stage of the disease.[29]

The mainstay of treatment consists of complete surgical resection. Preoperative biopsy of small and well-circumscribed thymic masses is not required, especially if the index of suspicion for lymphoma is low based on the patient's clinical presentation. Biopsy of a large mass with local infiltration should be performed to ascertain diagnosis before resection is pursued, especially if induction chemotherapy and/or radiation is planned.[30] Operative approaches for extended thymectomy generally include median sternotomy (see Chapter 160) with possible extension to thoracosternotomy (hemiclamshell incision) if the pulmonary hilum must be controlled. Maximal exposure of the mediastinum is achieved through a clamshell incision with bilateral thoracosternotomy. According to individual surgeon experience and preference, small thymomas without invasion of surrounding structures may be resected via minimally invasive approach: VATS (see Chapter 159), robotic-assisted, or transcervical approach (see Chapter 158).[31–33]

The goal of surgery is extended thymectomy with resection of thymus and surrounding adipose tissue, extending from the thyroid gland down to the diaphragm. If surrounding structures (such as phrenic nerve, lung, pericardium, great vessels) are involved, they should be resected en bloc with the thymectomy specimen. If there is residual tumor after resection, adjuvant radiation therapy is recommended; cisplatin-based chemotherapy is used in the case of widespread disease. Recurrent local disease after resection may be considered for reoperation. Recent guidelines issued by the International Thymic Malignancy Interest Group (ITMIG) emphasize that the surgeon should specifically orient the resected specimen to delineate margins and discourse with the pathologist, whose report of close or positive margins will determine adjuvant treatment.[34]

While 30% of patients with thymoma have MG, only approximately 10% to 15% of patients with MG have an associated thymoma.[35,36] The indications for thymectomy in MG patients without evidence of thymic masses are controversial, but the American Academy of Neurology recommends that all patients with nonthymomatous MG should be considered for thymectomy to increase the probability of remission or clinical improvement.[37] Thymectomy should not be performed in patients on an emergency basis; symptoms are best managed by plasmapheresis and immunosuppression, followed by thymectomy once the patient is medically optimized. Thymectomy can be performed through a full sternotomy or through less invasive techniques such as the partial upper sternotomy, transcervical approach, VATS, or robotic (see Chapter 159). The VATS technique can be approached from either the left or right side, with each side having its benefits of better exposure of key structures (e.g., aortopulmonary window on left, superior vena cava-innominate vein junction on right).[38] Studies generally have reported the following results from surgical treatment of MG: a remission in 20% to 25% of patients, with 10% to20% being drug-free; improvement in 30% to 50%; no change in 10%; and progression in a few percent.[19]

Complications after thymectomy include the usual post-operative respiratory sequelae, with heightened risk in predisposed MG patients. Thus aggressive pulmonary toilet, early mobilization, adequate pain control, and involvement of the neurologist are of supreme importance to ensure a smooth postoperative recovery. Technical complications include injury to the surrounding structures such as the phrenic nerve, thoracic duct, and innominate vein.

Lymphoma

Hodgkin lymphoma has a peak incidence in the third and fourth decades of life, whereas non-Hodgkin lymphoma is evenly distributed across the first five decades of life. Most patients with lymphoma in the mediastinum usually have systemic disease, but 10% of patients present with primary mediastinal lymphoma.[39] Mediastinal involvement usually manifests as enlarged lymph nodes in the anterior or middle mediastinum; thus patients usually report symptoms related to respiratory compression or pleuropericardial disease. The surgeon's role is limited primarily to obtaining tissue for diagnosis and for subtyping the lymphoma. FNA biopsy is often insufficient for diagnosis, and thus one should proceed to biopsy via the least invasive surgical technique by which adequate tissue can be obtained safely, for example, cervical mediastinoscopy, anterior mediastinotomy, or VATS (see Chapter 159). As in biopsies of all mediastinal masses, frozen sections should be obtained to ensure that the pathologist has sufficient lesional tissue for diagnosis and subsequent studies (e.g., flow cytometry, cytogenetics, molecular analysis).

Germ Cell Tumors

Although extragonadal primary GCTs are uncommon, the mediastinum is the most common location in adults (see Chapter. 163). In the pediatric population, mediastinal GCTs are equally divided between the sexes. In adults, benign GCTs are equal between the sexes, but more than 90% of malignant GCTs occur in males in their third decade of life.[40–42] In males with a potential mediastinal GCT, it is important to exclude a gonadal primary tumor through physical examination and scrotal ultrasound. All patients should have serum levels of β-hCG and AFP measured as part of the initial workup.

Benign teratomas or dermoid cysts are the most common GCT in both children and adults, with a frequency of about two-thirds of all GCT.[43] Fewer than half these lesions are associated with symptoms, and up to 30% have calcifications that are present on chest x-ray. These tumors contain elements derived from all three embryonic germ cell layers and display little tendency toward malignant degeneration. CT scans show well-defined lesions with fatty, cystic, and calcific components. Treatment consists of surgical resection without biopsy.

Among malignant GCT, seminomas comprise more than half the cases. In addition to the routine chest imaging performed for mediastinal lesions, staging abdominal CT scans, scrotal ultrasounds, and PET/CT scans are essential to screen for extrathoracic disease. Serum β-hCG and AFP levels are measured and are low in seminomatous GCTs. Only approximately 10% of patients with GCT have even mildly elevated β-hCG levels, and all patients with pure seminomas have undetectable AFP levels.[41] Because these lesions often infiltrate into surrounding mediastinal structures, open biopsy should be performed to distinguish between seminoma and a mixed tumor. The treatment for pure seminoma is radiation therapy with cisplatin-based chemotherapy. After induction chemotherapy, any residual lesion greater than 3 cm should be resected to ensure the removal of all viable tumor and to determine whether additional adjuvant therapy is necessary.

Mediastinal nonseminomatous GCT portends a worse prognosis, with 80% of patients having at least one site of metastasis at the time of diagnosis. Ninety percent of patients have an elevation in either β-hCG, AFP, or both, and tumor marker levels parallel the clinical activity of the tumor. Despite the presence of elevated tumor markers in the serum, open biopsy must be done to ascertain diagnosis. Treatment consists of cisplatin-based chemotherapy and radiation treatment. Surgical resection is reserved for patients with localized residual tumor after response to chemotherapy or for selected patients with relapse in whom the lesion appears to be a solitary recurrence and is technically resectable.[16]

Thymic Cysts

Thymic cysts are derived from pharyngeal pouches and are universally benign. Usually asymptomatic, they often can grow quite large, compressing nearby structures. Although fluid can be readily visualized by chest CT scan and MRI, cystic components can be present in thymomas and teratomas as well. Excision is curative and excludes other diagnoses.

Parathyroid Adenomas

Approximately 20% of parathyroid glands are ectopic and may be found along the thymic line of descent within the anterior mediastinum. Parathyroid adenomas or hyperplastic glands are hypervascular oval masses seen on chest CT scan with variable contrast enhancement. Ectopic inferior parathyroid glands are the most variable in location and usually are found within the anterior mediastinum; ectopic superior parathyroid glands sometimes may be located in the posterior compartment. Patients in whom preoperative localization is warranted, parathyroid tissue is best localized by ^{99m}Tc sestamibi imaging.[44] Selective parathyroid angiography or venous sampling is done only when results from noninvasive imaging are equivocal.

Thyroid Goiters

Most intrathoracic thyroid goiters are continuous with the cervical gland; only 2% of goiters are primary substernal tumors with vascular supply derived from the chest. On chest CT scan, thyroid goiters have a characteristic multinodular appearance, circumscribed by a smooth surface and containing calcifications and cystic areas.[45,46] Although usually involving the anterior mediastinum, up to 10% of intrathoracic goiters may be located within the posterior mediastinum. Although these usually can be surgically resected via a low cervical collar incision, the incision can be extended to a partial upper sternotomy, if needed (see Chapter 160).

MIDDLE MEDIASTINAL MASSES

The most common masses of the middle mediastinum remain enlarged lymph nodes around the tracheobronchial tree, for which the differential diagnosis includes lymphoma, sarcoidosis, or inflammatory foci resulting from tuberculosis or histoplasmosis. Metastatic disease from lung or esophageal cancer may also manifest as middle mediastinal masses. Surgical biopsy of enlarged lymph nodes is warranted for diagnosis. Nodes located in the aortopulmonary window are accessible for biopsy via an anterior mediastinoscopy, whereas pretracheal, subcarinal, and tracheobronchial nodes can be accessed by endobronchial ultrasound-guided biopsy (EBUS) or cervical mediastinoscopy (see Chapter 156). More distal mediastinal nodes, including perihilar nodes, can be biopsied via EBUS or VATS approach.

Cystic masses comprise approximately 20% of all mediastinal masses. Although cysts can occur at any location within the mediastinum, they are most commonly of foregut origin and thus begin in the middle mediastinum. Bronchogenic and esophageal duplication cysts are malformations that are jointly considered enterogenous cysts. When these lesions have associated vertebral malformations, they are called *neuroenteric cysts.*

Bronchogenic cysts are the most common mediastinal cyst and usually lie in a subcarinal position. Two-thirds of patients present with symptoms related to compression of adjacent structures or obstruction of distal airways with subsequent parenchymal infection.[43] Given their predisposition to infection and potential for malignant degeneration, bronchogenic cysts are best managed with surgical resection via minimally invasive approach or thoracotomy.[47]

Esophageal cysts are lined with either stratified squamous epithelium or gastric mucosa. Sixty percent are found in the lower third of the esophagus and are twice as likely to be located in the right chest rather than the left.[48] They may be found within or adjacent to the esophagus and thus can be found in both the middle and posterior mediastinal compartments. Rarely, they may communicate with the esophageal lumen, and thus a communication or dimpling sometimes can be visualized on esophagoscopy. Like bronchogenic cysts, they have a tendency to become infected; moreover, if they are lined with acid-secreting gastric mucosa, they have the potential to ulcerate and bleed spontaneously. These cysts may be symptomatic by virtue of their enlarging size, causing dysphagia, chest pain, and cardiac arrhythmias. Treatment consists of surgical resection with buttressed closure of any esophageal connection.[49]

Neuroenteric cysts are rare and are always associated with vertebral anomalies, most commonly spina bifida. The vertebral anomalies occur cephalad to the cyst and include fused vertebrae or hemivertebrae. Patients may present with respiratory or neurologic signs and symptoms. If there is any evidence of intraspinal extension, the resection will require a joint effort with a neurosurgeon.

Pericardial cysts are mediastinal masses that are found at the anterior cardiophrenic angle, more commonly on the right than the left side. The cysts are filled with clear serous fluid and may be serially aspirated. If the lesions show radiographic change over time or produce symptoms, resection is indicated.[10] They are otherwise not known to undergo malignant degeneration.

Posterior Mediastinal Masses

Neurogenic tumors comprise 60% of posterior mediastinal tumors and are the most common etiology of masses in this compartment (see Chapter 162).[50,51] They are classified according to the neural cell of origin and may arise from the intercostal nerve sheath, the sympathetic ganglia, or the paraganglionic cells. Neuroblastomas and ganglioneuroblastomas, which arise from sympathetic ganglia, are most common in children and are malignant. Ganglioneuromas, which also arise from the sympathetic ganglia, are most common in young adults and are benign.[6] Tumors of the nerve sheath, schwannomas and neurofibromas, account for 90% of adult neurogenic tumors and are benign; they have a peak incidence in the third and fourth decades.[26,52] Overall, fewer than 5% of neurogenic tumors are malignant. Most are asymptomatic, although malignant forms are associated with symptoms related to compression of surrounding structures, radiculopathy from involvement of nerve roots, and erosion into bone. In addition, neuroblastomas, paragangliomas, and pheochromocytomas can be hormonally active and may be detected by the measurement of serum catecholamines or urine vanillylmandelic acid.

Tumors arising from paraganglionic cells of the sympathetic nervous system include pheochromocytomas and nonchromaffin paragangliomas. Although these tumors can occur within each of the mediastinal compartments, they are commonly thought of as posterior mediastinal tumors. Both types may be functional and secrete hormones. Malignancy is determined by the degree of local invasiveness or the presence of distant metastasis. Paragangliomas, also known as *chemodectomas,* are hypervascular soft tissue masses found in the aortopulmonary window or in the costovertebral sulci. The differential diagnosis for such highly vascularized masses includes Castleman disease and hemangiomas.[43]

Approximately 10% of pheochromocytomas are extraadrenal. As described previously, [^{131}I]*meta*-iodobenzylguanidine scans are used to localize pheochromocytomas to the mediastinum if initial chest CT scan and MRI are unrevealing. It is important to screen patients with pheochromocytomas for the presence of familial syndromes, such as multiple endocrine neoplasia type II, von Hippel–Lindau disease, and neurofibromatosis type I.[53] Careful preoperative blood pressure control using alpha blockade followed by beta blockade is required to prevent hypertensive crises.[54]

Approximately 10% to 20% of posterior mediastinal neurogenic tumors have a spinal canal component.[55] These tumors are called *dumbbell tumors* and consist of a larger posterior mediastinal component with a smaller intraspinal component connected by a narrow foraminal segment. Of patients with dumbbell tumors, 60% to 80% have neurologic symptoms.[51] It is important to have joint preoperative planning for resection by the neurosurgical and thoracic surgical teams. Resection of the intrathoracic component alone can lead to tumor hemorrhage, necrosis of the intraspinal component with subsequent spinal cord compression, or a dural injury with leakage of cerebrospinal fluid and subsequent meningitis.

OTHER MEDIASTINAL MASSES

Castleman Disease

Castleman disease is also known as *angiofollicular lymph node hyperplasia* and represents a heterogeneous array of lymphoproliferative disorders that are associated with HIV and Human Herpes Virus 8. There are three recognized pathologic and clinical variants (hyaline vascular variant, plasma cell variant, and HHV8+ variant) and the disease can be unicentric or multicentric.[56] The unicentric form is characterized by a solitary nodal mass within the mediastinum that significantly enhances on chest CT scan. Castleman disease may occur in any compartment of the mediastinum and may be confused on needle-guided biopsy with other lymphoproliferative disorders such as lymphoma or thymoma. Although usually asymptomatic, it can be associated with cough and dyspnea due to local mass effects. The unicentric form is treated with curative resection.[57] The multicentric form is treated with systemic chemotherapy or immunotherapy.[58]

Mesenchymal Tumors

Mesenchymal tumors include lipomas, hemangiomas, lymphangiomas, fibromas, and their malignant counterparts. Although these may occur in any compartment of the mediastinum, they are found mostly in the anterior mediastinum and should be resected because the presence of malignant degeneration cannot be determined preoperatively.

SUMMARY

Mediastinal masses include a wide variety of diseases and etiologies. A differential diagnosis for a given mediastinal mass is based primarily on patient age, symptoms, and mediastinal location. Most masses require biopsy via anterior/cervical mediastinoscopy or VATS to establish a tissue diagnosis, although lesions classic for thymoma, small localized masses, and posterior mediastinal masses may undergo complete surgical excision for both diagnostic and curative intent. "Secretory" mediastinal masses, such as MG, pheochromocytomas, and thymomas, pose specific perioperative risks and concerns, as do large mediastinal masses that impair the airway. It is critical that the thoracic surgeon be aware of the various mediastinal entities and concerns unique to their treatment.

EDITOR'S COMMENT

Imaging is important for suggesting not only the likely diagnosis, but also the best surgical approach. Mastery of mediastinal imaging is essential for surgeons operating in or around the mediastinum.

—Steven J. Mentzer

References

1. Azarow KS, Pearl RH, Zurcher R, et al. Primary mediastinal masses. A comparison of adult and pediatric populations. *J Thorac Cardiovasc Surg.* 1993;106: 67–72.
2. Davis RD Jr., Oldham HN Jr., Sabiston DC Jr. Primary cysts and neoplasms of the mediastinum: recent changes in clinical presentation, methods of diagnosis, management, and results. *Ann Thorac Surg.* 1987;44: 229–237.
3. Mullen B, Richardson JD. Primary anterior mediastinal tumors in children and adults. *Ann Thorac Surg.* 1986;42:338–345.
4. Takeda S, Miyoshi S, Akashi A, et al. Clinical spectrum of primary mediastinal tumors: a comparison of adult and pediatric populations at a single Japanese institution. *J Surg Oncol.* 2003;83:24–30.
5. Deslauriers J, LeTourneau L, Giubilei F. *Tumors and Masses: Diagnostic Strategies in Mediastinal Tumors and Masses.* New York, NY: Churchill-Livingstone; 2002.
6. Silverman NA, Sabiston DC Jr. Primary tumors and cysts of the mediastinum. *Curr Probl Cancer.* 1977;2:1–55.
7. King RM, Telander RL, Smithson WA, et al. Primary mediastinal tumors in children. *J Pediatr Surg.* 1982;17:512–520.
8. Cohen AJ, Thompson L, Edwards FH, et al. Primary cysts and tumors of the mediastinum. *Ann Thorac Surg.* 1991;51:378–384, discussion 385–386.
9. Graeber GM, Shriver CD, Albus RA, et al. The use of computed tomography in the evaluation of mediastinal masses. *J Thorac Cardiovasc Surg.* 1986;91: 662–666.
10. Brown K, Aberle DR, Batra P, et al. Current use of imaging in the evaluation of primary mediastinal masses. *Chest.* 1990;98:466–473.
11. Moore E. Radiologic evaluation of mediastinal masses. *Chest Surg Clin N Am.* 1992;2:1.
12. Beckerman C, Hoffer PB, Bitran JD. The role of gallium-67 in the clinical evaluation of cancer. *Semin Nucl Med.* 1984;14:296–323.
13. Ilias I, Pacak K. Anatomical and functional imaging of metastatic pheochromocytoma. *Ann N Y Acad Sci.* 2004;1018:495–504.
14. Giudicelli R, Pellet W, Fuentes P, et al. [Danger to spinal cord arterial vascularization during surgery for neurogenic tumors of the posterior mediastinum]. *Ann Chir.* 1991;45:692–694.
15. Doppman J, Dichino G, Omya K. *Selective Arteriography of the Spinal Cord.* St. Louis, MO: WH Green; 1969.
16. Wright CD, Kesler KA, Nichols CR, et al. Primary mediastinal nonseminomatous germ cell tumors. Results of a multimodality approach. *J Thorac Cardiovasc Surg.* 1990;99:210–217.
17. Knapp RH, Hurt RD, Payne WS, et al. Malignant germ cell tumors of the mediastinum. *J Thorac Cardiovasc Surg.* 1985;89:82–89.
18. Kirschner P. Myasthenia gravis and other parathymic syndromes. *Chest Surg Clin N Am.* 1992;2:183.
19. Shamji F, Pearson FG, Todd TR, et al. Results of surgical treatment for thymoma. *J Thorac Cardiovasc Surg.* 1984;87:43–47.
20. Bouafia F, Drai J, Bienvenu J, et al. Profiles and prognostic values of serum LDH isoenzymes in patients with haematopoietic malignancies. *Bull Cancer.* 2004;91:E229–E240.
21. Herman SJ, Holub RV, Weisbrod GL, et al. Anterior mediastinal masses: utility of transthoracic needle biopsy. *Radiology.* 1991;180:167–170.
22. Kern JA, Daniel TM, Tribble CG, et al. Thoracoscopic diagnosis and treatment of mediastinal masses. *Ann Thorac Surg.* 1993;56:92–96.
23. Azizkhan RG, Dudgeon DL, Buck JR, et al. Life-threatening airway obstruction as a complication to the management of mediastinal masses in children. *J Pediatr Surg.* 1985;20:816–822.
24. Shamberger RC. Preanesthetic evaluation of children with anterior mediastinal masses. *Semin Pediatr Surg.* 1999;8:61–68.
25. Shamberger RC, Holzman RS, Griscom NT, et al. Prospective evaluation by computed tomography and pulmonary function tests of children with mediastinal masses. *Surgery.* 1995;118:468–471.
26. Strollo DC, Rosado-de-Christenson ML, Jett JR. Primary mediastinal tumors: part II. Tumors of the middle and posterior mediastinum. *Chest.* 1997;112:1344–1357.
27. Souadjian JV, Enriquez P, Silverstein MN, et al. The spectrum of diseases associated with thymoma. Coincidence or syndrome? *Arch Intern Med.* 1974;134:374–379.
28. Nakagawa K, Asamura H, Matsuno Y, et al. Thymoma: a clinicopathologic study based on the new World Health Organization classification. *J Thorac Cardiovasc Surg.* 2003;126:1134–1140.
29. Detterbeck FC, Nicholson AG, Kondo K, et al. The Masaoka-Koga stage classification for thymic malignancies: clarification and definition of terms. *J Thorac Oncol.* 2011;6:S1710–S1716.
30. Detterbeck FC, Parsons AM. Thymic tumors. *Ann Thorac Surg.* 2004;77: 1860–1869.
31. Sugarbaker DJ. Thoracoscopy in the management of anterior mediastinal masses. *Ann Thorac Surg.* 1993;56:653–656.
32. Lin J, Landreneau R. *Video-Assisted Thoracic Surgery for Mediastinal Tumors and Cysts and Other Diseases within the Mediastinum.* Philadelphia, PA: Lippincott Williams & Wilkins; 2004.
33. Yim AP. Video-assisted thoracoscopic resection of anterior mediastinal masses. *Int Surg.* 1996;81:350–353.
34. Detterbeck FC et al. "Which Way Is Up? Policies and Procedures for Surgeons and Pathologists regarding Specimens of Thymic Malignancy," (*J Thorac Oncol.* 2011;6: S1730–S1738)
35. Osserman KE, Genkins G. Studies in myasthenia gravis: review of a twenty-year experience in over 1200 patients. *Mt Sinai J Med.* 1971;38: 497–537.
36. Lopez-Cano M, Ponseti-Bosch JM, Espin-Basany E, et al. Clinical and pathologic predictors of outcome in thymoma-associated myasthenia gravis. *Ann Thorac Surg.* 2003;76:1643–1649; discussion 1649.
37. Gronseth GS, Barohn RJ. Practice parameter: thymectomy for autoimmune myasthenia gravis (an evidence-based review): report of the Quality Standards Subcommittee of the American Academy of Neurology. *Neurology.* 2000;55:7–15.
38. Yim AP. Thoracoscopic thymectomy: which side to approach? *Ann Thorac Surg.* 1997;64:584–585.
39. Manoharan A, Pitney WR, Schonell ME, et al. Intrathoracic manifestations in non-Hodgkin's lymphoma. *Thorax.* 1979;34:29–32.
40. Sham JS, Fu KH, Choi PH, et al. Primary mediastinal seminoma. *Oncology.* 1990;47:124–127.
41. Nichols CR. Mediastinal germ cell tumors. *Semin Thorac Cardiovasc Surg.* 1992;4:45–50.
42. Nichols CR, Fox EP. Extragonadal and pediatric germ cell tumors. *Hematol Oncol Clin North Am.* 1991;5:1189–1209.
43. Rice TW. Benign neoplasms and cysts of the mediastinum. *Semin Thorac Cardiovasc Surg.* 1992;4:25–33.
44. Krudy AG, Doppman JL, Brennan MF, et al. The detection of mediastinal parathyroid glands by computed tomography, selective arteriography, and venous sampling: an analysis of 17 cases. *Radiology.* 1981;140:739–744.
45. Glazer GM, Axel L, Moss AA. CT diagnosis of mediastinal thyroid. *AJR Am J Roentgenol.* 1982;138:495–498.
46. Chin SC, Rice H, Som PM. Spread of goiters outside the thyroid bed: a review of 190 cases and an analysis of the incidence of the various extensions. *Arch Otolaryngol Head Neck Surg.* 2003;129:1198–1202.
47. Lewis RJ, Caccavale RJ, Sisler GE. Imaged thoracoscopic surgery: a new thoracic technique for resection of mediastinal cysts. *Ann Thorac Surg.* 1992; 53:318–320.

48. Choong CK, Meyers BF. Benign esophageal tumors: introduction, incidence, classification, and clinical features. *Semin Thorac Cardiovasc Surg.* 2003;15:3–8.
49. Cioffi U, Bonavina L, De Simone M, et al. Presentation and surgical management of bronchogenic and esophageal duplication cysts in adults. *Chest.* 1998;113:1492–1496.
50. Ribet ME, Cardot GR. Neurogenic tumors of the thorax. *Ann Thorac Surg.* 1994;58:1091–1095.
51. Yuksel M, Pamir N, Ozer F, et al. The principles of surgical management in dumbbell tumors. *Eur J Cardiothorac Surg.* 1996;10:569–573.
52. Reeder LB. Neurogenic tumors of the mediastinum. *Semin Thorac Cardiovasc Surg.* 2000;12:261–267.
53. Yip L, Lee JE, Shapiro SE, et al. Surgical management of hereditary pheochromocytoma. *J Am Coll Surg.* 2004;198:525–534; discussion 534–535.
54. Keiser H. *Pheochromocytoma and Other Diseases of the Sympathetic Nervous System.* Philadelphia, PA: Lippincott; 1995.
55. Ricci C, Rendina EA, Venuta F, et al. Diagnostic imaging and surgical treatment of dumbbell tumors of the mediastinum. *Ann Thorac Surg.* 1990;50:586–589.
56. Aster J, Brown J, Freedman A. Castleman's disease. *UpToDate.* 2012
57. Rena O, Casadio C, Maggi G. Castleman's disease: unusual intrathoracic localization. *Eur J Cardiothorac Surg.* 2001;19:519–521.
58. Dham A, Peterson BA. Castleman disease. *Curr Opin Hematol.* 2007;14:354–359.

156 Cervical Mediastinoscopy and Anterior Mediastinotomy

Mandeep Singh Saund, Michael Y. Chang, and Steven J. Mentzer

Keywords: Mediastinoscopy, lung cancer, lymphadenopathy

Mediastinoscopy is a surgical technique that permits minimally invasive access to the mediastinum.[1] In most cases, mediastinoscopy is used to biopsy and facilitate the histologic diagnosis of enlarged mediastinal lymph nodes (carcinoma, sarcoidosis, and tuberculosis) and masses (lymphoma, germ cell tumor, and thymoma). Mediastinoscopy currently plays a particularly important role in defining the clinical stage of bronchogenic carcinoma. Staging is the first step toward determining the optimal course of management. Staging directs treatment, implementation of protocols, and permits comparison of treatment between patients.

Cervical mediastinoscopy, first described by Harken,[2] involves a neck incision that facilitates access to the superior mediastinum. Carlens[3] and Pearson[4] popularized a technique using a specially designed mediastinoscope through a suprasternal incision. Cervical mediastinoscopy, however, has limited access to the aorticopulmonary (AP) window. One approach to the AP window is "extended" cervical mediastinoscopy, a rarely used approach in which the mediastinoscope is inserted anterior to the aortic arch between the innominate artery and left carotid artery.[5] A more common approach to the AP window is through an anterior mediastinotomy—so-called anterior mediastinoscopy.[6] Extended and anterior mediastinoscopy are techniques used to sample mediastinal lymph nodes in the AP window. In addition, anterior mediastinoscopy can be used in a variety of parasternal locations to facilitate the biopsy of anterior mediastinal masses to the right or left of midline. Subxiphoid mediastinoscopy is a technique in which the mediastinoscope is used to biopsy anterior masses in the lower mediastinum.

SURGICAL PRINCIPLES

Frequent indications for mediastinoscopy include (1) staging patients with bronchogenic carcinoma,[7] and (2) obtaining tissue diagnoses in patients with unexplained adenopathy.[8] Patients diagnosed with bronchogenic carcinoma are staged using a combination of modalities. Computed tomography (CT) of the chest determines the size and location of the primary tumor in conjunction with any associated lung parenchymal abnormalities (atelectasis, collapse, pneumonia, emphysema, or fibrosis). In addition, the location and size of enlarged mediastinal nodes directs further investigation to stage patients. Mediastinal nodes larger than 1 cm in their short axis are considered suspicious for tumor.

The differential diagnosis of patients with persistent and unexplained adenopathy includes sarcoidosis and lymphoma, but because these diseases may be difficult to distinguish, clinically, histologic confirmation of the diagnosis is usually recommended. Sarcoidosis is characterized by noncaseating granulomas that can readily be distinguished from both Hodgkin and non-Hodgkin lymphomas.

Although cervical mediastinoscopy can be performed with low morbidity and mortality, the potential for catastrophic complications exists. Because of this risk, surgeons must be properly trained in mediastinoscopy. The procedure is usually performed as a day surgery procedure, although it should be performed in a hospital setting because of the potential complications.

The procedure of mediastinoscopy involves a comprehensive exam of the mediastinum informed by CT scan findings. Sampling of the lymph nodes is directed by manual palpation and visual inspection (Fig. 156-1). Cervical mediastinoscopy can sample ipsilateral and contralateral nodes (stations 1, 2, 4, 7) in patients with bronchogenic cancer. The presence of positive contralateral nodes, multistation N2 disease, extracapsular spread, and extension into mediastinal structures (T4) portends a generally poor outcome and usually precludes the patient from surgical therapy. Cervical mediastinoscopy in comparison to CT scans has 90% sensitivity and 100% specificity for determining pathological mediastinal lymph nodes. In lymphomas or inflammatory diseases, lymph node mapping has limited value. The focus of the operation is obtaining an accurate tissue diagnosis.

Anterior mediastinoscopy – performed through an anterior mediastinotomy – is often indicated in patients with a bronchogenic carcinoma of the left upper lobe. The aortopulmonary window contains lymph node stations 5 and 6, which are the first drainage sites of the left upper lobe of the lung. The secondary lymphatic drainage sites of the left upper lobe include lymph node stations 2 L and 4 L, which can be examined by cervical mediastinoscopy.

Ideal Patient Characteristics

Thin patients with no previous surgery in the neck are ideal candidates for mediastinoscopy. Previous cervical mediastinoscopy or mediastinal radiation therapy does not preclude mediastinoscopy, but the procedure has to be performed with caution. The risk of inadvertent injury to an adjacent structure is increased, as is the probability of poor sampling of the various lymph node stations. Large thyroid gland, cervical spine fusion, or cervical spine arthritis make introducing the scope and positioning the patient challenging, but are not absolute contraindications for surgery.[9,10]

Preoperative Assessment

Cervical mediastinoscopy and anterior mediastinotomy are performed under general anesthesia. Candidates for these procedures need to be suitable for general anesthesia. Preoperative assessment includes evaluation of cardiac status, pulmonary

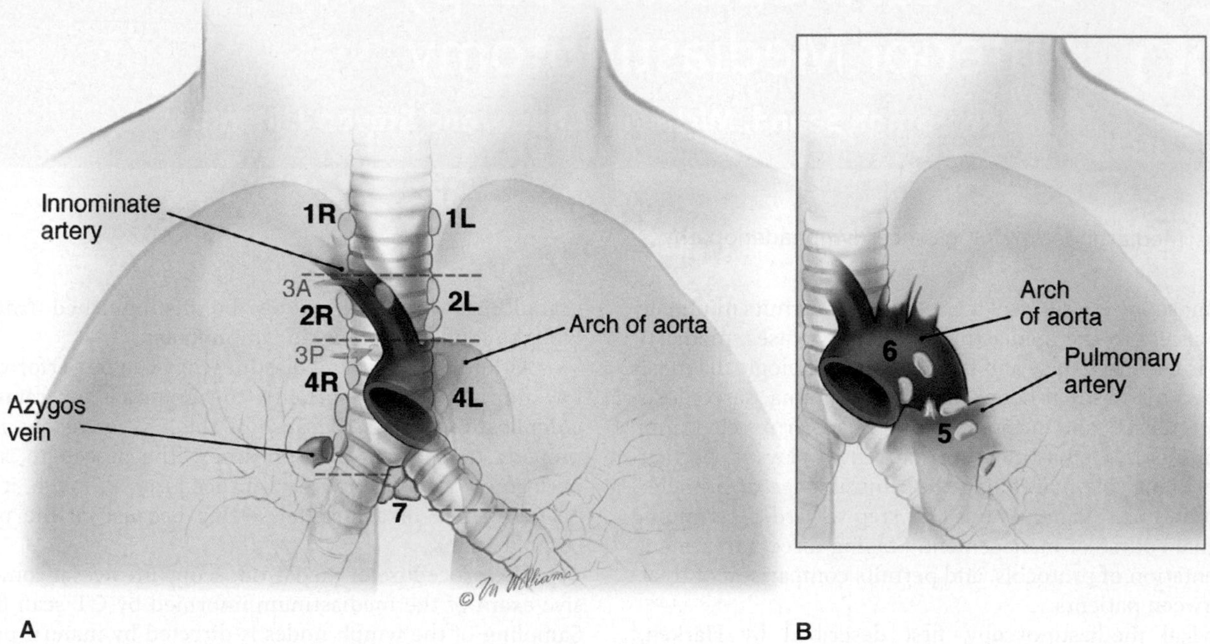

Figure 156-1. (*A*) Cervical mediastinoscopy is ideal for accessing the mediastinal lymph node stations, but has limited value for nodes in the aorticopulmonary window (*B*), which can be accessed via anterior mediastinoscopy.

status, and clinical staging. Clinical stage is determined by history and physical examination, CT scan of the chest including upper abdomen for evaluation of adrenal glands, and PET scan to determine metastasis (locoregional and systemic).

A history of facial swelling and plethora (SVC syndrome), persistent neck or arm pain (Pancoast tumors with brachial plexus involvement), hoarseness (recurrent laryngeal nerve involvement), back pain, and headaches (systemic metastasis) suggests advanced disease that requires evaluation before subjecting patients to cervical mediastinoscopy or anterior mediastinotomy.

Paraneoplastic syndromes (e.g., syndrome of inappropriate antidiuretic hormone secretion [SIADH], Eaton–Lambert Syndrome, dermatomyositis, hypercalcemia) are associated with both small-cell and non–small-cell lung cancers and do not necessarily suggest the patient has metastatic disease. Large scalene or supraclavicular lymph nodes can undergo biopsy at the time of mediastinoscopy. A positive scalene or supraclavicular node renders the patient N3, and not a candidate for surgical resection.

TECHNIQUE

Cervical Mediastinoscopy

Cervical mediastinoscopy is performed under general anesthesia. The patient is positioned with a roll under the shoulders and between the scapulae, which throws back the shoulders and extends the neck to improve tracheal exposure (Fig. 156-2). The head of the operating room table is elevated to 20 to 30 degrees to decrease venous congestion. The neck and entire chest is draped in the event that a median sternotomy is required to manage a major complication.

A 2- to 3-cm incision is made transversely one fingerbreadth (1–2 cm) above the suprasternal notch through skin, subcutaneous tissue, and platysma (Fig. 156-3). The investing layer of deep cervical fascia is identified and the midline divided vertically to separate sternohyoid and sternothyroid muscles, which are retracted laterally. The strap muscles can also be divided, but lateral retraction of these muscles usually provides adequate exposure. Deep to the strap muscles and anterior to the trachea, the pretracheal fascia is identified and divided to enter the pretracheal space.

On the right side of the trachea, the superior vena cava, azygos vein, and tracheobronchial junction form the lateral boundaries of the dissection. On the left, the extent of dissection is limited by the pulmonary artery and arch of the aorta, with the distal extent of dissection to the left tracheobronchial angle.

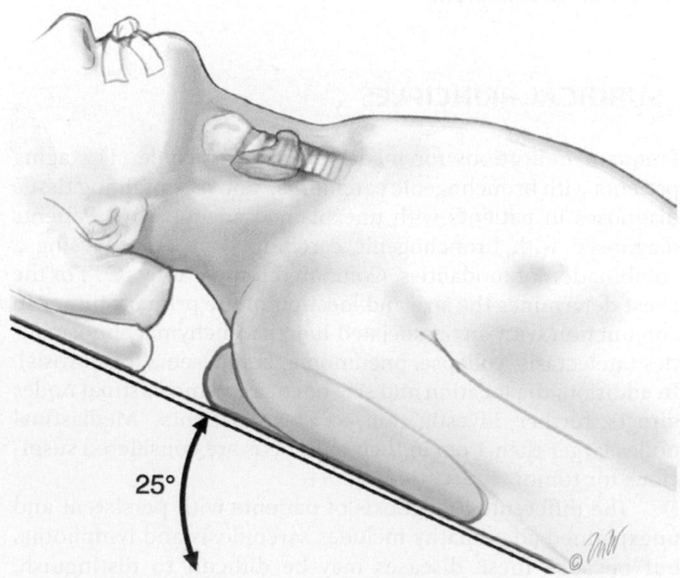

Figure 156-2. A shoulder roll is placed under the shoulders between the scapulae to extend the neck and improve exposure of the trachea.

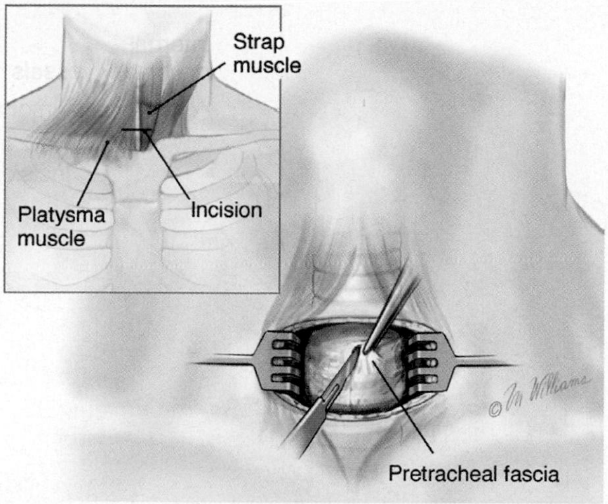

Figure 156-3. A 2- to 3-cm transverse incision is made in the suprasternal notch (*inset*). The pretracheal fascia is identified and the sternohyoid and sternothyroid muscles are divided vertically along the midline.

An index finger is used to break through pretracheal fascia laterally to gain access to pretracheal and paratracheal lymph nodes (stations 2 and 4) (Fig. 156-4). Inability to break through the pretracheal fascia prevents biopsy of lymph nodes that lie anterior and lateral to the pretracheal fascia. The mediastinoscope is inserted along superior surface of the trachea (Fig. 156-5). The subcarinal lymph node (station 7) biopsy is performed by using the tip of the cannula to break through the pretracheal fascia distal to the carina. Gentle blunt dissection of nodes is essential to safely separate the lymph nodes from their surrounding structures.

Normal lymph nodes usually feel rubbery and may have an anthracotic appearance, with gray or bluish-black pigmentation. Close proximity of nodes to vascular structures and inflammatory or malignant adhesions places these structures at risk for inadvertent injury and bleeding. Palpation of pulses or visible pulsations is not a good indicator of vascularity, as the mediastinum is a small confined space and cardiac pulsations

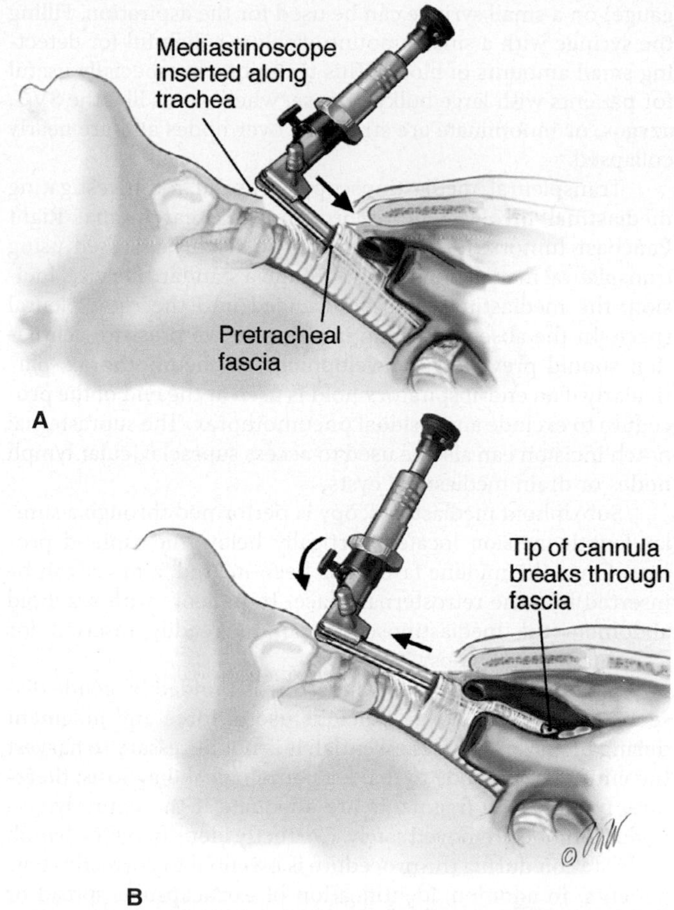

Figure 156-5. *A.* The mediastinoscope is inserted along the trachea. *B.* The tip of the cannula is used to break the fascia distal to the carina to access the subcarinal lymph nodes (station 7).

are transmitted easily to adjoining structures. Careful, gentle, and thorough dissection of the lymph node will usually confirm its identity. However, if there is any doubt as to whether the structure is a lymph node or blood vessel, aspiration of tissues prior to biopsy is recommended. A spinal needle (21–22

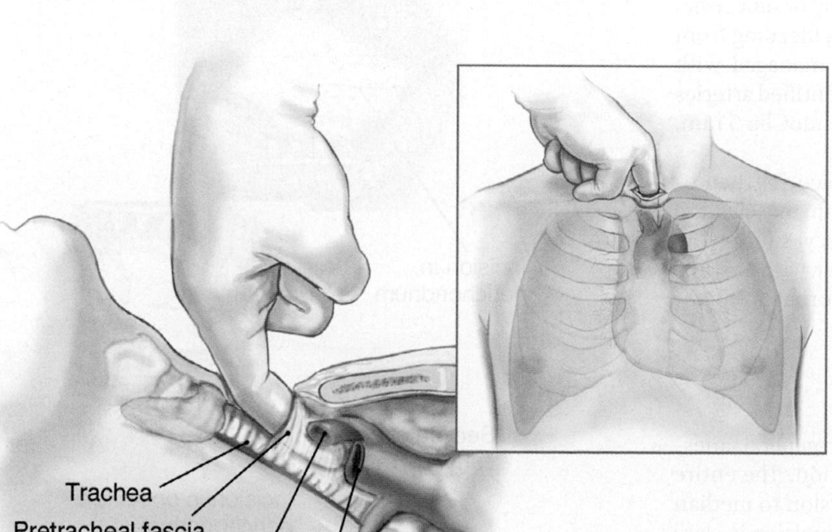

Figure 156-4. An index finger is used to break through the pretracheal fascia laterally to gain access to station 2 and 4 lymph nodes. (*inset*) Blunt finger dissection through the cervical incision.

gauge) on a small syringe can be used for the aspiration. Filling the syringe with a small amount of saline is helpful for detecting small amounts of blood. This technique is especially useful for patients with large bulky disease, where veins like the SVC, azygos, or innominate are stretched over nodes and are nearly collapsed.

Transpleural mediastinoscopy is useful for investigating mediastinal involvement of bronchogenic carcinoma. Right Pancoast tumors, for example, can be readily assessed using transpleural mediastinoscopy. Through a standard cervical incision, the mediastinoscope is advanced into the right pleural space. In the absence of lung injury, positive pressure ventilation should prevent the development of pneumothorax, particularly if an end-inspiratory hold is used at the end of the procedure to exclude any residual pneumothorax. The suprasternal notch incision can also be used to access supraclavicular lymph nodes or drain mediastinal cysts.

Subxiphoid mediastinoscopy is performed through a similar length incision located vertically below the xiphoid process. Once the midline fascia has been incised, a finger can be inserted into the retrosternal space. In patients with scaphoid abdomen, the mediastinoscope can be readily inserted for examination and biopsy.

Bleeding during mediastinoscopy is avoided by gentle dissection of lymph nodes. Judicious use of force and judgment during biopsy of tissue is essential. It is not necessary to harvest the entire lymph node to make a pathological diagnosis; therefore, lymph node fragments are adequate if the entire lymph node cannot be removed safely. Correctly identifying the lymph node station during the procedure is essential to correctly stage patients. In addition, identification of extracapsular spread or involvement of adjoining mediastinal structures is important to correctly stage patients.

Packing of the mediastinal space controls mild bleeding. Removal of the mediastinoscope after packing is helpful in obtaining hemostasis as this allows the tissues to collapse and obliterate the mediastinal space created by the instrument. Lymph node tissue can be cauterized using the metal tip cannula. Thermal energy should be used judiciously because it can spread and cause recurrent laryngeal nerve damage and increase the chances of injury to vascular structures. Biopsy of subcarinal lymph nodes is occasionally associated with brisk bleeding from bronchial arteries. This complication is usually managed with packing as described previously. Occasionally, identified arteries can be clipped with an endoscopic clip applier (EndoClip 5 mm, Autosuture, US Surgical Norwalk, CT, USA).

After completion of the procedure and securing hemostasis, the incision is closed in layers. The strap muscles are approximated in the midline using 3-0 silk or vicryl suture. The platysma can be approximated as a separate layer with absorbable suture. The skin is approximated using absorbable subcuticular suture.

Anterior Mediastinotomy

Anterior mediastinotomy is performed under general anesthesia. The patient is placed in the supine position. The entire chest is draped in the unlikely event that conversion to median sternotomy is required to control bleeding. The incision is classically made in the second intercostal space on the left side (Fig. 156-6). The incision can be as small as 2 cm in length. The incision is made through the skin and subcutaneous fat, and the pectoral muscle fibers are split, to expose underlying intercostal muscles. A small (2 cm) portion of the costal cartilage is excised in the subperichondrial plane. The perichondrium is incised to enter the subperichondrial plane and dissected carefully to avoid injury to the internal mammary vessels and the intercostal vessels and nerve (Fig. 156-7). Alternatively, the intercostal muscles are divided at the superior border of the costal cartilage, the pleura identified, and the mediastinum entered without excision of the cartilage. The internal mammary vessels should be safeguarded and retracted laterally, or identified and ligated.

The mediastinal pleura is swept laterally and the mediastinum is entered. The mediastinoscope can be introduced through this incision into the mediastinum to facilitate dissection and biopsy of lymph nodes or masses. Vagus and phrenic nerves course in cepahlocaudad direction and must not be

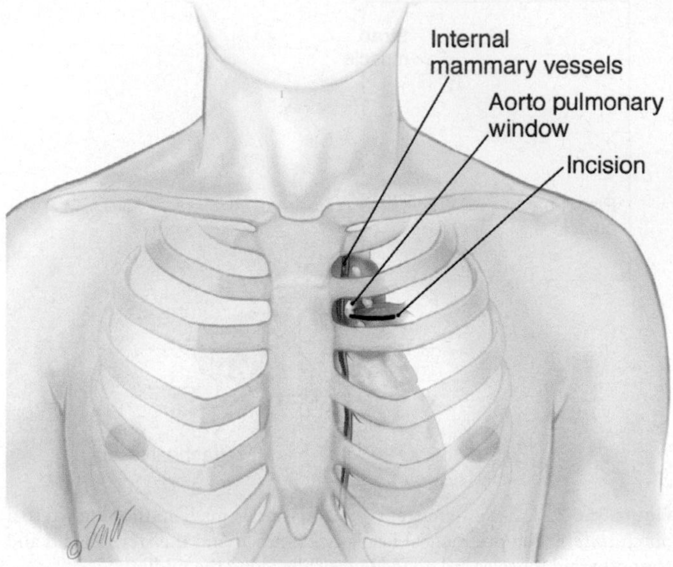

Figure 156-6. A classic 2-cm anterior mediastinotomy incision is made in the second intercostal space on the left side.

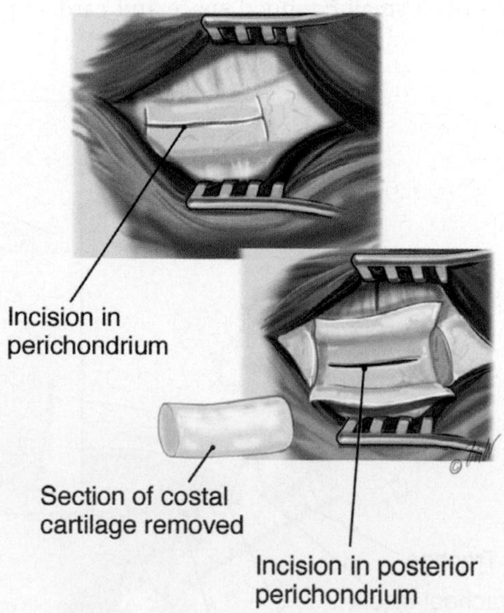

Figure 156-7. A 2-cm portion of the costal cartilage is excised in the subperichondrial plane and the perichondrium is incised to enter the subperichondrial plane.

injured. The level 6 mediastinal lymph nodes are found at the base of the innominate artery near the course of the phrenic and vagus nerves. The level 5 lymph nodes are closer to the proximal pulmonary artery. The entire dissection is typically performed within the mediastinum. The pleura can be opened to examine the hilum of the lung and to perform wedge biopsy of lung tissue. If the pleura is opened or inadvertently injured, placement of a chest tube is not essential as long as there is no injury to the lung. The pleura may be repaired over a red rubber catheter with positive pressures of 30 to 40 cm of H_2O applied to the lung. In the event of lung biopsy or injury to the lung, a chest tube is placed in the pleural space.

After ensuring adequate hemostasis, the incision is closed with reapproximation of the perichondrium with absorbable suture. The pectoral muscle is similarly reapproximated and the skin closed using subcuticular suture. Removal of perichondrium creates a slight, permanent depression on the chest wall after healing. Overall, bleeding from injury to major vascular structures is rare.

Postoperative Care

After cervical or anterior mediastinoscopy, if there is no suspected injury to pleura a chest x-ray is not essential and patients can be discharged home. At most institutions, chest x-rays are still performed to rule out a pneumothorax or new pleural effusion. Diagnosis of a pneumothorax does not mandate tube thoracostomy placement. The size of the pneumothorax, percentage volume loss of lung, and symptoms of the patient dictate placement of a chest tube. After patients are ambulatory, tolerate liquids by mouth, have good pain control, and are able to pass urine, they are discharged to home with oral analgesics, which are typically required for only a few days.

PROCEDURE-SPECIFIC COMPLICATIONS

Cervical Mediastinoscopy

Cervical mediastinoscopy is a safe procedure with mortality rates less than 0.1% and complication rates less than 1%.[9,11] Injudicious use of the biopsy forceps or aggressive attempts to biopsy complete mediastinal lymph nodes may result in hemorrhage. Bleeding is usually minor and can be controlled with packing. Cauterization of bleeding tissue should be performed judiciously. Fortunately, major bleeding from the SVC, azygos vein, brachiocephalic artery or vein, arch of aorta, and pulmonary artery is rare. Major bleeding can occasionally be controlled with packing only and is recommended while arrangements are made to open the chest. Bleeding from major vessels will require a median sternotomy, which provides access to all mediastinal vessels. Alternatively, a thoracotomy may be performed dependent on the location of the suspected injury, resectability of the tumor, and condition of the patient.

Pneumothorax can occasionally develop after mediastinoscopy. Chest x-ray is performed either routinely postoperatively or selectively according to surgeon preference. Pneumothorax is managed nonsurgically, by aspiration or chest tube placement depending on the symptoms and percentage lung volume loss. Injury to pleura can sometimes be recognized by the appearance of a new pleural effusion, caused by mediastinal blood draining into the pleura space. Injury to recurrent laryngeal nerve is more common on the left side because the 2 L and 4 L lymph node stations are located near the nerve in the tracheoesophageal groove. Vocal cord dysfunction is usually transient.

Tracheobronchial injuries can result in subcutaneous emphysema or persistent air leak. The air leak is usually small and needs packing of mediastinum with surgical cellulose. Large injuries require direct or pedicled repair with flaps. Similarly, esophageal injuries are also rare and are usually not recognized immediately. Small, contained esophageal leaks can be managed conservatively by draining the mediastinum via the mediastinoscopy incision. Substantial injuries to the esophagus or a delay in diagnosis may require thoracotomy and repair, or even esophageal exclusion.

Anterior Mediastinotomy

Anterior mediastinotomy is performed less frequently than cervical mediastinoscopy, and there are no large series to determine risk of complications. There is the potential risk of bleeding from the aorta, pulmonary artery and vein, internal mammary vessels, but this is uncommon. Injury to phrenic and vagus nerves is possible, resulting in diaphragmatic paralysis and hoarseness of voice. Removal of costal cartilage is associated with a depression under the skin and occasionally lung herniation.

Caution is to be exercised when performing an anterior mediastinotomy in patients after coronary artery bypass graft (CABG) surgery. The patent internal mammary vessel used to perform bypass must be protected. It runs along the course of the phrenic nerve and lies anterior to the hilum of the lung and mediastinal nodes. It is at risk for injury when gaining access to the mediastinum and during lymph node biopsy. Most surgeons would consider previous CABG surgery with left internal mammary artery as a contraindication to anterior mediastinotomy on the left side.

SUMMARY

Cervical mediastinoscopy is the mainstay for staging of mediastinal lymph nodes in patients with bronchogenic carcinoma. It is also used for biopsy of mediastinal masses. It is an invasive procedure, with extremely low morbidity and mortality. The advent of whole body PET scan and PET-CT scan has improved noninvasive staging of bronchogenic cancer, but has not eliminated the need for mediastinoscopy. Mediastinoscopy continues to play an important role in staging of mediastinal disease. Anterior mediastinoscopy, in contrast, is used to sample lymph nodes in the AP window (stations 5 and 6) in patients with left-sided lung cancer, or to biopsy anterior mediastinal masses.

EDITOR'S COMMENT

Mediastinoscopy is a remarkably simple, yet effective tool for obtaining diagnostic tissue. A skilled mediastinoscopist can obtain tissue from anywhere in the mediastinum with the exception of the posterior inferior mediastinum and the inferior pulmonary ligament. These relative "blind spots" of mediastinoscopy can be effectively explored with thoracoscopy.

—Steven J. Mentzer

References

1. Mentzer S. Mediastinal staging prior to surgical resection. *Op Tech Cardiovasc Thor Surg*. 2005;10:152–162.
2. Harken DE, Black H, Clauss R, et al. A simple cervicomediastinal exploration for tissue diagnosis of intrathoracic disease; with comments on the recognition of inoperable carcinoma of the lung. *N Engl J Med*. 1954;251:1041–1044.
3. Carlens E. Mediastinoscopy: a method for inspection and tissue biopsy in the superior mediastinum. *Dis Chest*. 1959;36:343–352.
4. Pearson FG. Mediastinoscopy: a method of biopsy in the superior mediastinum. *J Thorac Cardiovasc Surg*. 1965;49:11–21.
5. Ginsberg RJ, Rice TW, Goldberg M, et al. Extended cervical mediastinoscopy. A single staging procedure for bronchogenic carcinoma of the left upper lobe. *J Thorac Cardiovasc Surg*. 1987;94:673–678.
6. McNeill TM, Chamberlain JM. Diagnostic anterior mediastinotomy. *Ann Thorac Surg*. 1966;2:532–539.
7. Naruke T, Suemasu K, Ishikawa S. Surgical treatment for lung cancer with metastasis to mediastinal lymph nodes. *J Thorac Cardiovasc Surg*. 1976;71:279–285.
8. Pattison CW, Westaby S, Wetter A, et al. Mediastinoscopy in the investigation of primary mediastinal lymphadenopathy. *Scand J Thorac Cardiovasc Surg*. 1989;23:177–179.
9. Puhakka HJ. Complications of mediastinoscopy. *J Laryngol Otol*. 1989;103: 312–315.
10. Ginsberg RJ. Evaluation of the mediastinum by invasive techniques. *Surg Clin North Am*. 1987;67:1025–1035.
11. Pearson FG, Nelems JM, Henderson RD, et al. The role of mediastinoscopy in the selection of treatment for bronchial carcinoma with involvement of superior mediastinal lymph nodes. *J Thorac Cardiovasc Surg*. 1972;64: 382–390.

157 Resection of Substernal Goiter

Alexander S. Farivar and Eric Vallières

Keywords: **Goiter, substernal thyroid, retrosternal thyroid, multinodular goiter, intrathoracic goiter, total thyroidectomy, collar incision, superior mediastinal mass**

Goiter refers to an enlargement of the thyroid gland. The condition is estimated to affect 5% of the general population. While the definition of substernal goiter varies in the medical literature, goiters usually are considered substernal (also referred to as *mediastinal, intrathoracic*, or *retrosternal*) when more than 50% of the thyroid parenchyma is located below the sternal notch. Such tumors have been a focus of interest for surgeons for over 150 years. Klein is credited with being the first to successfully remove a mediastinal goiter in 1820, although the earliest surgical description of mediastinal thyroid extension dates back to Haller in 1749. Today, substernal goiters are treated by a number of different surgical specialists, including thoracic, general, and head and neck surgeons. Goiters account for as many as 10% to 15% of space-occupying mediastinal lesions and are the most common of the superior mediastinal masses.

Mediastinal goiters are classified as *primary* or *secondary*. Primary mediastinal goiters, also referred to as *ectopic* or *aberrant goiters*, do not possess any direct fibrous or parenchymal connections to the cervical portion of the gland. They are uncommon and represent fewer than 1% of all surgically excised goiters. Ectopic mediastinal thyroid tissue generally lies in proximity to the thymus owing to their shared embryological origins and to an intimate association with the thymothyroid ligament but also has been described in the pericardium and heart. Patients with ectopic thyroid tissue typically are clinically euthyroid, although hyperthyroidism has been described. The blood supply of these goiters originates from a mediastinal source, most commonly a branch from the internal mammary artery, the innominate artery, or the intrathoracic aorta itself. Other criteria used to define a primary mediastinal goiter include a normal or absent cervical thyroid gland, no history of prior thyroid surgery, and a lack of similar pathology in both the cervical and mediastinal portions of the thyroid. Confirmation of an ectopic thyroid gland can occur assuredly only at surgical resection if these criteria are met.[1]

Secondary mediastinal goiters are a much more common clinical entity. As many as 5% to 15% of all goiters demonstrate some extension into the mediastinum. These goiters derive their blood supply from cervical branches of the superior and inferior thyroid arteries and therefore can be resected almost uniformly via a cervical collar incision. One exception to this rule, to be discussed later, is of special importance to the thoracic surgeon.

Substernal goiters are an important clinical entity for a number of reasons. Patients may eventually develop compressive or obstructive symptoms when the goiter, which is confined within the narrow thoracic inlet, begins to exert extrinsic compression on respiratory, esophageal, vascular, and/or neural structures. There is also a risk of malignant degeneration within the substernal goiter, reported to be as high as 15% to 20% in some published series.[2] In most situations, pathologic substernal goiter is an entity that is optimally managed surgically. Medical management in the form of thyroid suppression using exogenous thyroid hormone or radioactive iodine ablation can reduce the size of the gland by up to 20%, but these modalities are only temporizing. Delaying definitive surgical treatment of substernal thyroid goiter may allow for further growth and increase the technical difficulty of the operation and surgical morbidity. Most treating physicians express consensus supporting a surgical approach to the management of *all* substernal goiters.[3]

ANATOMY AND PHYSIOLOGY

The thyroid gland is the first of the endocrine derivatives of the pharynx to develop and originates from the foramen cecum. It descends during the third week to reach its eventual position in the neck. It is postulated that ectopic thyroid tissue in the anterior mediastinum, pericardium, or heart originates from abnormal migration of thyroid tissue rudiments as the heart and great vessels develop in the chest, incorporating thyroid tissue into the mediastinum during embryologic unfolding.

Secondary substernal goiters tend to extend inferiorly from the neck as a result of anatomic factors facilitating downward growth into the mediastinum. The thyroid gland is limited superiorly by both the thyroid and cricoid cartilages, posteriorly by the prevertebral fascia and vertebral bodies, and anteriorly by the strap muscles and cervical fascia. Additional factors promote downward mediastinal growth of the goiter, including the negative intrathoracic pressure generated during respiration, gravity, and the downward traction that occurs during the act of swallowing. As thyroid tissue enlarges over time, it may become entrapped in the thorax and remain undiagnosed until compressive symptoms manifest.

Most substernal goiters extend anteriorly into the mediastinum (>85%), arising from the lower lobes of the thyroid or isthmus. They usually project anterolaterally to the trachea, lie anterior to the recurrent laryngeal nerves (RLNs), and tend to displace the great vessels laterally. Posterior goiters arise from the posterior aspects of the thyroid and descend posterior to the great vessels. Most posterior substernal thyroid goiters (including those arising from the left thyroid lobe) project to the right side of the thorax because the aortic arch and great vessels limit their leftward extension. Complex forms of substernal goiter are associated with more than one extension projecting into both the anterior and posterior mediastinum.

GENERAL PRINCIPLES

Substernal goiters are diagnosed most often in the fifth or sixth decade of life and are more common in women. Published reports describe a myriad of symptoms related to substernal goiters, including dyspnea, stridor, cough, hoarseness, dysphagia, superior vena cava syndrome, Pemberton sign which is evidence of venous engorgement of the face or neck when a patient raises his or her arms above the head, thyrotoxicosis, and Horner syndrome. However, 50% of patients are asymptomatic, with the mass found incidentally on routine physical examination coupled with either a chest x-ray (CXR) or CT scan performed for other indications. The most common symptoms attributable to substernal goiters are respiratory in nature (Table 157-1).[4] Asymptomatic patients may demonstrate abnormal flow–volume loops on spirometry. In advanced cases, patients may have profound respiratory insufficiency. Many patients acknowledge exertional dyspnea on questioning (present in up to 60% of patients), and some have been treated for presumed asthma for years. A choking sensation with or without swallowing is also described commonly. Dysphagia may result from esophageal compression. Compression of neural structures can lead to hoarseness from transient vocal cord paralysis, permanent Horner syndrome when the cervical sympathetic chain is affected, or even less commonly phrenic nerve paralysis. If superior vena cava compression is present, patients can demonstrate Pemberton sign or even signs of superior vena cava syndrome. If Pemberton is suspected, the examiner should hold both the patient's arms above his or her head for 1 minute and watch for distention of neck veins, facial plethora, difficulty swallowing, or worsening of respiratory status, including wheezing and stridor. Patients suffering from superior vena cava syndrome demonstrate these findings without provocative maneuvers. Compression of the carotid artery rarely can result in a transient ischemic attack.

Physical examination often identifies a cervical mass, although the lack of a cervical mass does not exclude the diagnosis of intrathoracic thyroid goiter. In published reports, up to 35% of patients lack a palpable cervical mass on examination. The presence of a substernal component of a cervical goiter is suggested when the caudal margin of the gland is undetectable on examination. Extending the patient's neck may help to define the lower thyroid border. Displacement of the trachea may be evident if the gland is large or asymmetric. Dilated neck veins are an indication of significant blood vessel compression. Dysphonia should be evaluated and is present in up to 30% of patients. Biochemically, the incidence of hyperthyroidism varies widely in the literature from 5% to 50%. Thyrotoxicosis is seen in up to 10% of patients with a substernal goiter.

Table 157-1

SYMPTOMS ATTRIBUTABLE TO SUBSTERNAL GOITERS AT PRESENTATION

Asymptomatic
Abnormal flow–volume loop
Choking sensation, particularly in supine position
Vague chest pain or heaviness
Respiratory
Dyspnea
Orthopnea
Cough
Adult-onset asthma
Respiratory distress/insufficiency
Airway obstruction
Neural
Hoarseness
Horner syndrome
Hemidiaphragm elevation
Esophageal
Dysphagia
Odynophagia
Vascular
Superior vena cava syndrome
Transient ischemic attacks
Pemberton sign
Biochemical
Hyperthyroidism
Thyrotoxicosis
Hypothyroidism

Preoperative Assessment

Radiographic assessment of a substernal goiter includes a CXR, which can demonstrate a mediastinal mass, superior mediastinal widening, tracheal deviation or compression, or all the above (Fig. 157-1). A CXR is negative in up to 30% of patients with a substernal goiter. A substernal thyroid is homogeneous, radiopaque, and smoothly contoured. Focal calcifications may be present. Past chest films may facilitate assessing the rate of growth over time.

Chest CT scans are used to define the full extent and anatomic relationships of the substernal thyroid to surrounding structures and to facilitate preoperative planning. A contrast-enhanced chest CT scan should fully characterize the extent of the thyroid gland, including continuous axial images from the neck into the mediastinum. Thyroid tissue exhibits early and

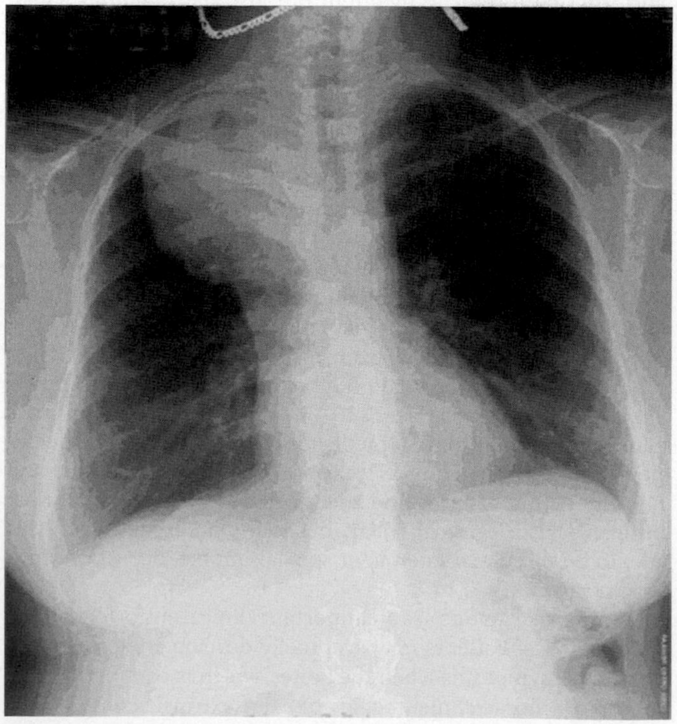

Figure 157-1. Chest x-ray of a patient with a large substernal goiter.

prolonged enhancement after IV contrast administration. IV contrast is also helpful in defining the vascular anatomy and differentiating between blood vessels and lymphadenopathy. Nearly 90% of intrathoracic goiters have borders separated by fat planes from other mediastinal structures. If the CT scan demonstrates a posterior or complex intrathoracic goiter configuration, a careful dissection strategy should be formulated to avoid injury to the RLNs during resection.

While ultrasound is useful for defining anatomy in the neck, it cannot define substernal or posterior thyroid extensions. MRI adds little to preoperative assessment and planning over high-resolution CT scanning. Fine-needle aspiration of thyroid nodules is not necessary for preoperative planning. Malignancy may be missed, and the information does not change the operative approach. The decision to operate is not based on cytopathology.

Evidence of preoperative vocal cord palsy/dysfunction or extracapsular malignancy noted preoperatively in the neck generally mandates preoperative collaboration with a head and neck surgeon. In these situations, it is of utmost importance to preserve the function of the remaining RLNs to avoid the need for tracheostomy postoperatively. Even in patients who present with severe airway compromise and stridor preoperatively, tracheostomy generally is avoided because it does not alleviate the lower tracheal compression that is present, is often technically challenging, and raises the risk of definitive operation. In most of these patients, endotracheal intubation is successful. A preoperative serum thyroid-stimulating hormone measurement should be obtained. If hyperthyroidism is present, medical management with antithyroid medications and beta blockade, as needed, should be undertaken before elective resection.

Pulmonary functioning testing, including spirometry and flow–volume loops, is useful as part of the preoperative evaluation. This testing is not done, however, in patients with severe airway compromise. The presence of abnormalities in flow–volume loops is corroborative evidence of the need for resection in patients with substernal thyroid goiters because abnormalities are indicative of, at least, moderate compromise of airway anatomy by the substernal goiter. Flow–volume loops will demonstrate derangement of the inspiratory phase, suggesting intrathoracic obstruction, or a combined defect, suggesting a fixed obstruction at the thoracic inlet. Postoperative reversal of pulmonary function testing is often not immediate. A prolonged recovery is seen in those with the most severe preoperative airway obstruction.

Surgeons should discuss these patients with the anesthesiologist in advance of surgery, and an adequate anesthetic plan should be formulated before the operation. There is often a significant amount of anxiety and a variable level of comfort of anesthesiologists in regard to airway management of these patients. Close communication between the attending surgeon and the anesthesiologist will lessen the chances for an adverse airway issue to occur on induction of anesthesia.

Indications for Resection

The presence of a substernal goiter (with or without associated symptoms) is an indication for removal. Since mediastinal goiters eventually will cause respiratory problems, resection is indicated if the patient is medically suitable to undergo an operation. These tumors are extremely unlikely to respond to medical therapy and shrink or disappear with thyroid replacement or radioactive iodine suppression, nor can their growth be followed easily over time or translated readily into degrees of anatomic physiologic derangement. Surgery is also indicated in cases of unsuccessful medical therapy (i.e., progressive enlargement of cervical thyroid goiters), thyrotoxicosis in goiters with substernal extension, and to relieve symptoms or effects of extrinsic compression on vital structures, including the trachea, esophagus, nerves, and vessels. Furthermore, surgery will prevent potential airway obstruction and treat overt (abnormal fine-needle aspiration biopsy) or subclinical thyroid malignancy, reported to be as high as 20%.

Substernal thyroid goiters become increasingly difficult to extirpate if resection is delayed until compressive symptoms arise. There is also a small risk of spontaneous or traumatic hemorrhage into a substernal goiter resulting in acute or complete airway compromise, which could be fatal owing to the fixed space of the thoracic inlet and superior mediastinum. Therefore, all patients with a substernal goiter, unless medically unfit for any procedure, should be offered resection and a chance for cure.

SURGICAL TECHNIQUE

The options for surgical approach to a substernal goiter include collar incision, median (partial) sternotomy, thoracotomy, or a combined approach utilizing minimally invasive access (VATS or robot) to mobilize the intrathoracic portion of the gland (Fig. 157-2). Past reviews confirm that most substernal goiters (>90%) can be removed via a collar incision exclusively.[5–8] Exceptions that may best be approached by median sternotomy (partial), thoracotomy (posterolateral or anterior), or minimally invasive techniques (robot) include a primary retrosternal goiter, atypical anatomy, dense adhesions from prior neck or thyroid surgery, inability to deliver the gland into the neck, overt or extracapsular extension of malignancy in the mediastinum, recurrence after previous resection of an intrathoracic goiter, goiters that extend to the tracheal carina or pose significant life-threatening compression of mediastinal structures, and patients who develop significant mediastinal bleeding intraoperatively (Table 157-2).[6] Thoracoscopic approaches (VATS or robotic) to an ectopic thyroid mass may be considered if deemed accessible and safe by the operating surgeon, and the details of VATS approach have been reported previously.[1] We have approached an ectopic thyroid using a robotic approach via the right chest and three arms (Fig. 157-3).

A total or near-total thyroidectomy is performed. Prophylactic antibiotics are administered intravenously. The surgeon should be present in the OR on induction of anesthesia in the event of complete airway obstruction. Patients with significant airway compression or deviation should undergo awake, fiberoptic intubation with variable sedation. Tracheostomy is rarely needed.[9]

The patient is positioned supinely with the arms tucked at the sides. A transverse shoulder roll is positioned behind the upper chest to extend the neck. The anterior neck, chest, and upper abdomen are prepped in their entirety. Access for complete median sternotomy, if necessary, is achieved. The reverse Trendelenburg position is used to diminish venous congestion.

A collar (Kocher) incision approximately 2 cm above the sternal notch is used for initial exploration of thyroid goiter. The platysma is divided using electrocautery, and skin/soft tissue flaps deep to the durable platysma are developed superiorly

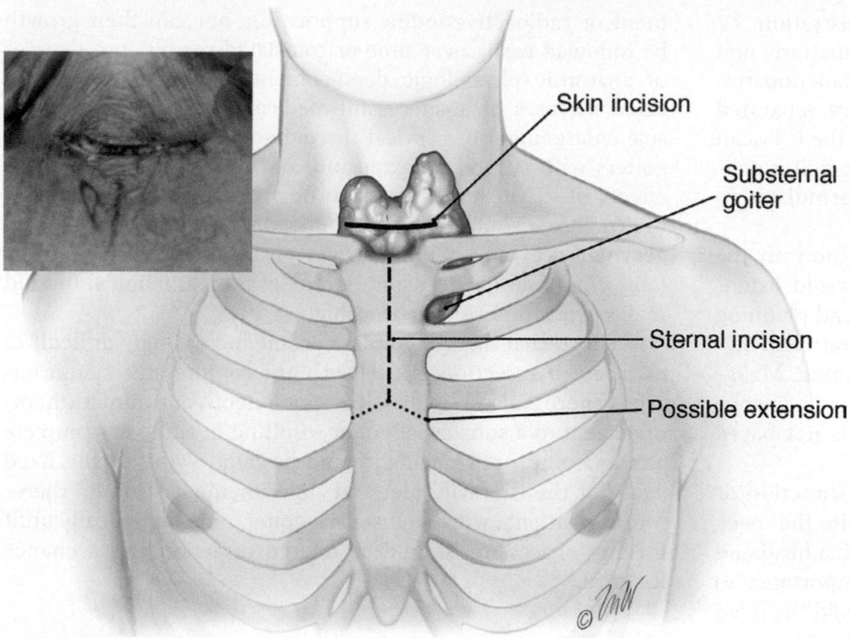

Figure 157-2. Resection of substernal goiter may require a partial sternal incision.

and inferiorly to the level of the hyoid and sternal notch, respectively. Exposure extends to the sternocleidomastoid muscles bilaterally. The strap muscles are exposed for their length and divided in their midline to expose the thyroid capsule. Frequently, the initial position of the neck in extension elevates the substernal goiter from an intrathoracic position to a predominantly extrathoracic position, facilitating complete extirpation of the thyroid gland through the collar incision.

Once access to the thyroid has been completed and exposure optimized, mobilization of the gland is facilitated by elevating the intrathoracic portion of the thyroid and by using blunt finger dissection circumferentially around the gland immediately on the capsule of the thyroid inferior to the middle thyroid vessels. Blunt dissection on the posterior aspect of the manubrium is performed (Fig. 157-4). Some advocate the use of several large sutures (1 or 0 PROLENE noncutting sutures in a figure-of-eight pattern) for traction as the mediastinal portion of the gland is mobilized, whereas others describe the use of a sterile spoon to aid in goiter delivery into the neck (Fig. 157-5). If additional exposure is needed, the strap muscles or medial portions of the sternocleidomastoid muscles can be divided transversely.

Table 157-2

SITUATIONS FOR CONSIDERATION OF AN INTRATHORACIC APPROACH

Primary retrosternal/ectopic goiter
Atypical anatomy
Dense adhesions from prior surgery
Inability to deliver the gland into the neck
Extracapsular extension or known mediastinal malignancy
Recurrent intrathoracic goiter
Prior thyroid surgery, especially for cancer
Goiters that extend to the tracheal carina
Goiters that cause life-threatening compression of mediastinal structures
Significant intraoperative mediastinal bleeding
Adherence to mediastinal pleura

Ligation of the superior and middle thyroid vessels is next accomplished as close to the thyroid capsule as possible. This procedure should be begin on the smaller or most straightforward side of the goiter. Once the superior and middle vessels are ligated, the lateral thyroid is bluntly and sharply medialized by the development of areolar planes along the sides of the goiter. Care should be taken to identify and preserve, if possible, the superior parathyroid glands because the inferior glands may be more difficult to identify. The RLN is identified and preserved. Only careful retraction is used during this portion of the procedure to avoid injury.

The inferior thyroid vessels are ligated close to the thyroid capsule, and the inferior parathyroid glands are identified, if possible. It is not uncommon for parathyroid glands to be removed inadvertently or devascularized during the mobilization of large substernal goiters, especially the bilateral inferior glands. If parathyroid glands are identified and appear to have been injured, incidentally removed, or devascularized, autotransplantation of the minced gland into the sternocleidomastoid mass should be performed. A small frozen section of the presumed parathyroid tissue is obtained before autotransplantation to ensure that parathyroid gland and not lymph node or cancer is being autotransplanted. Once the goiter has been mobilized to the midline, sharp dissection is used to release its attachment to the trachea to avoid inadvertent tracheotomy or airway fire (Fig. 157-6).

There will be times when an intrathoracic extension of a thyroid goiter cannot be delivered safely into the neck via a collar incision. This may not be obvious during preoperative planning or before an attempt at resection is made. An additional approach, including partial (manubrial split) or full sternotomy, thoracotomy, or thoracoscopy (VATS or robot) may be necessary. Incision choice is a clinical decision dictated by the anatomy of the remaining mediastinal component and the comfort level and skill set of the surgeon and should be evident from preoperative scanning coupled with the intraoperative findings and limitations. Primary ectopic thyroid goiters recurring after previous thyroid surgery tend to parasitize mediastinal blood

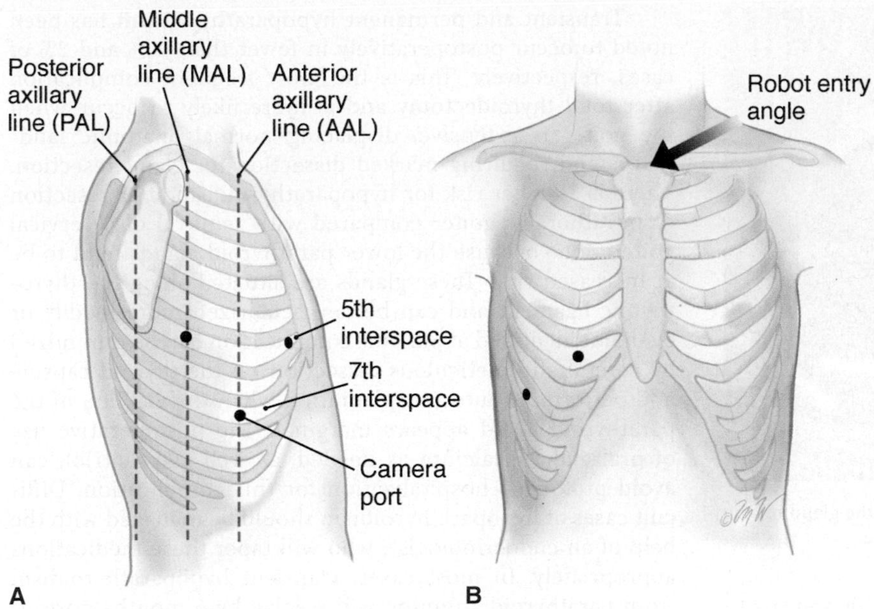

Figure 157-3. *A.* The three ports via the right chest are shown for robotic access for ectopic or substernal components of a thyroid goiter. *B.* Also shown is the angle in which the robot crosses the patient for optimal maneuverability.

vessels, making cervical resection more hazardous. If a thoracoscopic approach is undertaken, resection is accomplished with isolation and ligation of the arterial supply, safe dissection, and identification of the phrenic and/or vagus nerves. The tumor should be removed en bloc and should only be cautiously grasped directly with instruments to ensure complete resection. Thoracoscopic approaches can typically be performed through three ports, with the patients right side bumped and the arm apposed (see Fig. 157-3). A double lumen endotracheal tube is needed and CO_2 insufflation may be utilized. The gland should be positioned directly in a line between the camera and the boom of the docking robot if that approach is undertaken. An intraoperative photograph of an ectopic thyroid removed robotically y is shown in Figure 157-7.

Soft suction drains may be placed at the discretion of the surgeon at the conclusion of the procedure.

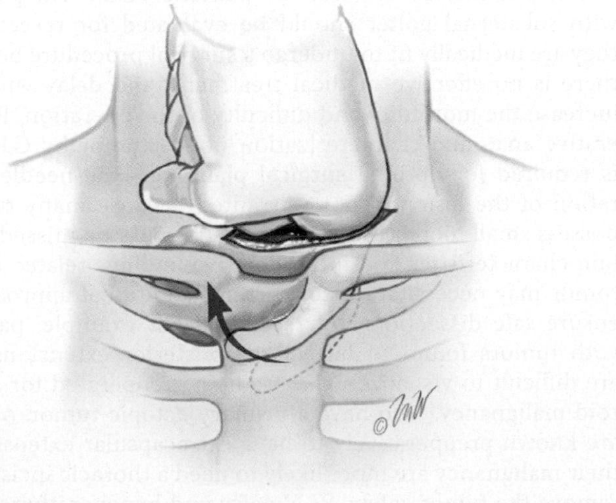

Figure 157-4. Goiters usually can be removed via cervical incision with the use of careful blunt finger dissection to mobilize the gland from its attachment to mediastinal structures. Most large goiters can be removed through a 2-cm collar incision.

Postoperative Complications

Mortality is less than 1% with appropriate preoperative planning, management of the airway, and good surgical technique. Length of stay for an uncomplicated procedure is overnight, and patients can be discharged uneventfully with calcium or calcitriol supplementation as dictated by laboratory values and/or clinical symptoms of hypocalcemia. If a thoracotomy or sternotomy is required, length of stay is increased, although morbidity is not affected.

Occasionally, postoperative hemorrhage has been reported, necessitating a return to the OR for control and hematoma evacuation. The major complications after thyroidectomy for substernal goiter involve injury to the trachea, parathyroid glands, or RLNs. The length of stay for patients with marked intrathoracic extension is increased, as is the need for prolonged intubation. Historically, tracheomalacia was reported as a significant problem in patients with long-standing tracheal

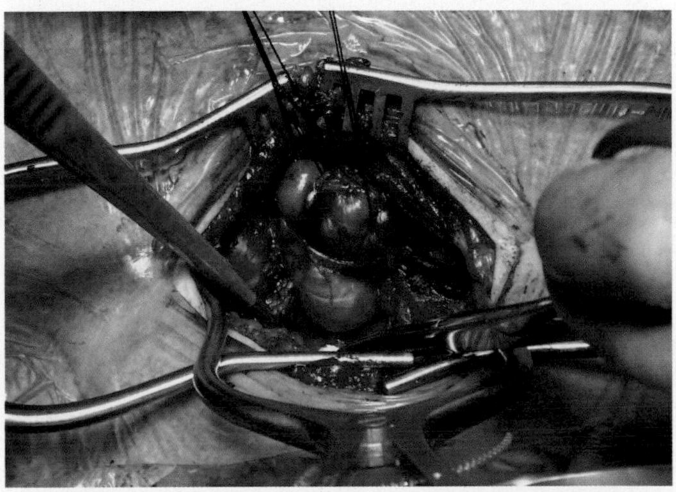

Figure 157-5. Traction stitches (as shown) can be most helpful in delivering a substernal extension of thyroid tissue into the neck incision.

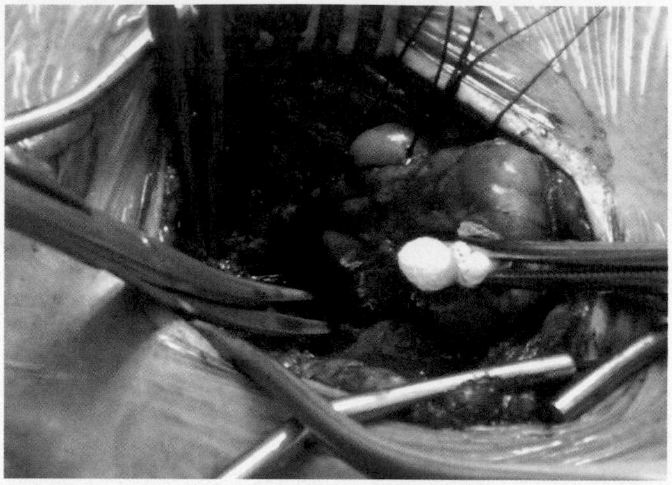

Figure 157-6. Sharp dissection is safest when dissecting the gland off the trachea to avoid inadvertent tracheal injury and airway fire.

compression, although, in more modern series, this appears to be a rare phenomenon (0.001–1.5%). When present, tracheomalacia may result in an extended period of postoperative intubation. One study reported that 10% of patients required extended intubation for airway issues postoperatively, with all patients eventually being extubated by postoperative day 10. However, these patients required multiple attempts at intubation preoperatively, making their need for prolonged postoperative intubation harder to simply attribute to tracheomalacia, as some authors have done. Postoperative airway complications are more likely to occur in older patients with large goiters (>200 g) who demonstrate significant tracheal compression on preoperative imaging. The presence or absence of clinically significant tracheomalacia is best assessed at the time of resection by finger palpation and evaluation of the tracheal walls. The need for tracheostomy at the time of thyroidectomy is rare, and it should be performed only in cases of tracheal infiltration by an undifferentiated cancer or when it can be expected that there is bilateral vocal cord paresis postoperatively. This typically occurs when a patient has a known preoperative unilateral vocal cord palsy from prior thyroid surgery and intraoperative dissection has placed the remaining RLNs at risk.

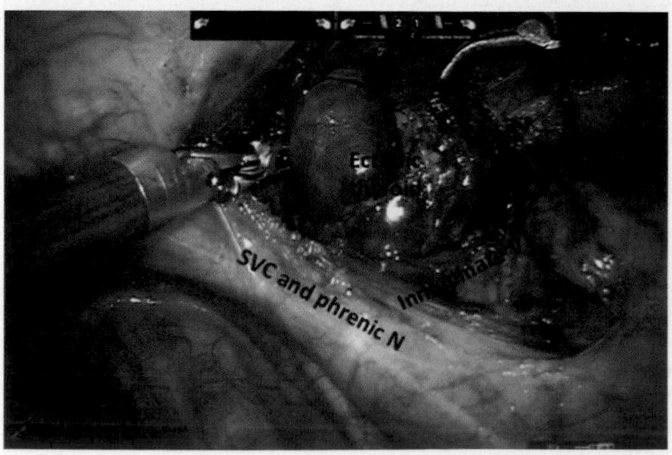

Figure 157-7. An intraoperative photograph of a robotic removal of an ectopic thyroid via the right chest.

Transient and permanent hypoparathyroidism has been noted to occur postoperatively in fewer than 10% and 2% of cases, respectively. This is the most frequent complication after total thyroidectomy and is more likely to occur when the goiter is extensive, displacing normal anatomic landmarks and requiring marked dissection for gland resection. There is a higher risk for hypoparathyroidism after resection of intrathoracic goiter compared with removal of a cervical goiter alone because the lower parathyroid glands tend to be at increased risk. These glands are situated along the thyrothymic ligament and can be devascularized more readily or even not identified at all. This complication can be minimized by careful and meticulous dissection on the thyroid capsule and performing autotransplantation when the viability of the parathyroid gland appears marginal. The postoperative use of oral and IV calcium as needed, as well as calcitriol, can avoid prolonged hospitalization for this complication. Difficult cases of hypoparathyroidism should be managed with the help of an endocrinologist, who will taper these medications appropriately. In most cases, transient hypoparathyroidism from parathyroid stunning will resolve by 6 months postoperatively.

Transient unilateral vocal cord paralysis has been reported to occur after substernal goiter resection in up to 4% of patients and, if suspected postoperatively, warrants consultation with otolaryngology. Permanent RLN paralysis should occur in fewer than 2% of patients with careful surgical technique and dissection. This is more likely to occur in patients with large or extensive intrathoracic goiters or those with extracapsular extension of malignancy.

SUMMARY

Substernal goiters typically are benign neoplasms that can usually be removed via a cervical collar incision. Patients present with a wide variety of symptoms that range in severity from asymptomatic to stridorous requiring emergent intubation. Symptoms experienced by patients are a function of the external compression of vital structures such as the trachea, esophagus, superior vena cava, or nerves such as the RLNs, phrenic, or cervical sympathetic chain. All patients with substernal goiter should be evaluated for resection if they are medically fit to undergo a surgical procedure because there is no effective medical treatment, and delay will only increase the morbidity and difficulty of the operation. Preoperative anatomic characterization of the tumor by CT scan is required for optimal surgical planning. Fine-needle aspiration of the lesion is not warranted because many tumors possess small foci of cancer that likely would be missed. Certain characteristics and intraoperative findings related to the tumor may necessitate a concurrent, additional approach to ensure safe dissection and resection. For example, patients with tumors found to have large posterior extensions that are difficult to visualize, who are being reoperated for a thyroid malignancy, who have a primary ectopic tumor, or who are known preoperatively to have extracapsular extension of their malignancy are more likely to need a thoracic incision to remove the tumor safely. RLN palsy and hypoparathyroidism are complications that may ensue and may warrant close collaboration with otolaryngology or endocrinology to optimize patient care postoperatively.

EDITOR'S COMMENT

Although most large thyroid glands can be removed through a cervical incision, large thyroid glands with their bulk within the thorax will likely require at least partial sternotomy. Also, a feature of thyroid tissue is that it avidly retains intravenous contrast; an imaging characteristic that can be useful for both diagnostic identification and surgical planning.

—Steven J. Mentzer

References

1. Grondin SC, Buenaventura P, Luketich JD. Thoracoscopic resection of an ectopic intrathoracic goiter. *Ann Thorac Surg.* 2001;71:1697–1698.
2. Netterville JL, Coleman SC, Smith JC, et al. Management of substernal goiter. *Laryngoscope.* 1998;108:1611–1617.
3. Erbil Y, Bozbora A, Barbaros U, et al. Surgical management of substernal goiters: clinical experience of 170 cases. *Surg Today.* 2004;34:732–736.
4. Shen WT, Kebebew E, Duh QY, et al. Predictors of airway complications after thyroidectomy for substernal goiter. *Arch Surg.* 2004;139:656–659; discussion 659–660.
5. Arici C, Dertsiz L, Altunbas H, et al. Operative management of substernal goiter: analysis of 52 patients. *Int Surg.* 2001;86:220–224.
6. Sancho JJ, Kraimps JL, Sanchez-Blanco JM, et al. Increased mortality and morbidity associated with thyroidectomy for intrathoracic goiters reaching the carina tracheae. *Arch Surg.* 2006;141:82–85.
7. de Perrot M, Fadel E, Mercier O, et al. Surgical management of mediastinal goiters: when is a sternotomy required? *Thorac Cardiovasc Surg.* 2007; 55:39–43.
8. Torre G, Borgonovo G, Amato A, et al. Surgical management of substernal goiter: analysis of 237 patients. *Am Surg.* 1995;61:826–831.
9. Bennett AM, Hashmi SM, Premachandra DJ, et al. The myth of tracheomalacia and difficult intubation in cases of retrosternal goiter. *J Laryngol Otol.* 2004;118:778–780.

158 Transcervical Thymectomy

Eero Sihvo and Shaf Keshavjee

Keywords: Myasthenia gravis, video-assisted transcervical thymectomy

Myasthenia gravis (MG) is an autoimmune disease mediated by anti-acetylcholine receptor antibodies (AChrab) directed against the acetylcholine receptor region of the post-synaptic membrane. Blocking and accelerated degradation of acetylcholine receptors lead to impaired neuromuscular transmission and muscle weakness.[1] MG has a predilection for the ocular and bulbar muscles, but generalized proximal muscle weakness is also common. Fatigable weakness is the hallmark of MG and the disorder is diagnosed by the clinical presentation, abnormal single-fiber electromyography, repetitive nerve stimulation tests, and elevated ACh and/or anti-MuSK antibodies. Abnormalities of the thymus gland are commonly found in these patients. Of MG patients, 10% to 15% have thymoma. Lymphoid thymic hyperplasia is present in about 70%.[2] Significant data exist to support an immunopathological role of the thymus in the development of autoimmune MG.[3]

ROLE OF SURGICAL THERAPY

The beneficial role of surgery for patients with MG was first described before the middle of the past century.[4] Further clinical reports of the benefits of the thymectomy led to the acceptance of this procedure for patients with generalized MG as a standard of practice. Nonetheless, controversies surrounding the role of thymectomy in the treatment of MG are abound in the literature. The role of thymectomy can be questioned because no randomized, controlled trials comparing the best medical therapy and surgery exist. The changes in intensive care unit (ICU) care, ventilatory support, and the introduction of immunosuppressive therapy also have improved the clinical course of this disease and outcomes. Furthermore, the debate persists because of patient selection and methods of analysis of results vary from center to center. Regardless, surgery is currently considered to increase the likelihood of improvement.[5] Retrospective studies suggest that patients undergoing thymectomy have higher remission rates than those who are treated medically.[6]

In a review, the likelihood of improvement, defined as medication-free remission, asymptomatic on medication, or improved on medication, was two times higher among patients undergoing surgery compared to patients managed medically.[5] The median improvement rates were total remission 25%, asymptomatic with medication 39%, and clinically improved 70%. The benefits of thymectomy are often delayed with 25% achieving remission in the first year, 40% by the end of the second year, and 55% in the third year.[7] These results, however, suggest that other factors in addition to surgery may contribute significantly to the improvement observed after surgery. Currently, an international randomized multicenter study comparing transsternal thymectomy to medical treatment is enrolling patients. It appears that this study has had difficulty enrolling patients, with current evidence favoring thymectomy for generalized, nonthymomatous MG, and also by other less invasive routes.

SURGICAL OPTIONS

The point of debate in the surgical treatment of MG has been the preferred surgical approach. Some centers recommend maximal thymectomy (the Jaretzki approach; transsternal + transcervical) to eliminate the gland and possible extra-anatomical thymic tissue as well,[8] whereas other centers favor a standard transsternal approach, while others have adopted a minimally invasive transcervical thymectomy.[9,10] A more recent surgical innovation is the modification of this procedure with the introduction of video-assisted transcervical thymectomy.[11] During this era of minimally invasive video-assisted surgery, transthoracic thoracoscopic thymectomy has gained popularity, as well. Several variations of this approach exist including unilateral, bilateral, bilateral combined with cervical approach, and robotic. The last surgical innovation for surgical treatment of MG is the infrasternal, either thoracoscopic or mediastinoscopic approach for thymectomy.[12] All procedures allow extracapsular resection of thymus and vary somewhat in the extent of mediastinal fat removal, which may contain foci of thymic tissue. The types of thymectomy have not been compared directly in any randomized study. There is a school of thought which advocated that maximal thymectomy is preferred over more conservative approaches to theoretically achieve a more complete resection of thymic tissue.[13] A combination of transcervical and transsternal approach was recommended to maximize the resection. The outcome data, however, do not support improved results with "maximal thymectomy" over more minimally invasive approaches. Furthermore, approaches that are more patient-friendly are more easily accepted by the patients and their neurologists. To understand the different surgical approaches and categorize the extent of resection of thymus and surrounding tissue, the Myasthenia Gravis Foundation of America (MGFA) has broadly classified varying surgical techniques based on the approach and the extent of surgical resection. The meta-analysis of 21 retrospective studies showing a positive benefit of thymectomy in patients with MG included all types of thymectomy approaches.[5] Furthermore, relatively large case series have shown comparable remission and improvement rates in MG patients with different types of thymectomy.[10,11] Thus, it is not clear at all that more extensive thymectomy procedures are more effective. Statistical reshuffling of crude data from different study reports may show different outcomes for different surgical interventions, but this type of reanalysis in itself may produce flawed results and does not provide definitive evidence of the benefits of one surgical approach over another. Ideally, a randomized trial of the different approaches would need to be done. Currently, no such study is planned and there is no consensus on the optimal surgical approach. Without randomized comparative studies, the decision as to surgical approach must rest on the surgeon's individual experience and facility with each given procedure. The underlying principle for thymectomy for MG remains the same regardless of surgical approach: a safe and complete thymectomy.

All patients should have a CT scan of the thorax before surgery to exclude a thymoma. Although VATS seems to be a safe and feasible approach for early stage thymoma, this approach is controversial and the follow-up times are still short considering that pleural metastases can appear more than 10 years after surgery.[14] Therefore, if a thymoma is present, the preferred surgical approach remains a sternotomy or partial upper sternotomy.

PATIENT SELECTION

Although the current consensus is to use thymectomy for patients with nonthymomatous generalized myasthenia, the role of surgery in other patient groups is much more controversial. In younger patients with ocular MG we recommend surgery, although some clinicians still hesitate to recommend surgery for this group.[15] An important area of debate is the upper age limit for thymectomy. Because older individuals have thymic atrophy rather than hyperplasia, the use of surgery in this group does not appear to have the same theoretical rationale as in younger patients. In addition, one may be concerned that complications of thymectomy are likely to be greater in older patients. This has to be considered, however, in the context of what can be achieved today with improved anesthesia and minimally invasive techniques for thymectomy. There are, in fact, retrospective studies reporting that thymectomy is safe in patients over age 60, and 16% of those patients over age 60 have thymic hyperplasia.[16] Other retrospective series have shown that age does predict outcome in thymectomy for MG with lower response rates in older subjects.[17] Considering the low morbidity of transcervical thymectomy in contrast to the morbidity of chronic immunosuppression in the elderly patient, we currently offer thymectomy to patients over 60 years of age. At the other age spectrum, thymectomy also is not generally recommended in very young children,[18] although it is sometimes necessary in young teenagers with severe MG.

PRE- AND PERIOPERATIVE CARE

The surgical treatment of MG patients should ideally belong to a dedicated team consisting of a thoracic surgeon, anesthesiologist, and neurologist. After the confirmation of the diagnosis of MG, symptoms should be medically stabilized. Cholinesterase inhibitors are used as the first line of therapy. Prednisone and other immunosuppressive agents are available for the persistent symptoms. Steroids are avoided preoperatively, if possible, to avoid the adverse effects on wound healing and infections. Thymectomy is never an emergency, and therefore, the patient's strength and respiratory status should be optimized before the well-planned elective surgery. There is no role for urgent thymectomy in patients with myasthenic crisis, as immediate clinical improvement postoperatively should not be expected. Furthermore, surgery in the setting of myasthenic crisis predisposes the patient to a significantly increased risk of postoperative respiratory failure.[19] The likelihood of prolonged mechanical ventilation is increased in patients with severe generalized weakness and/or with bulbar symptoms, as well. These patients should first be treated with plasmapheresis prior to surgery to optimize their condition. High-dose intravenous immunoglobulin (IVIg) is sometimes used as an alternative to plasmapheresis. Because of the short-lived benefits of these treatments, surgery should be planned in the following 2 to 3 weeks. It should be noted that surgery should not be performed before 5 days after plasmapheresis because of possible coagulation abnormalities related to the treatment. Over the years at the Toronto General Hospital, we have limited the administration of immunosuppressive therapy before surgery, and preoperative stabilization is most often accomplished with pyridostigmine with the addition of plasmapheresis for the higher-grade myasthenic patients only.

Preoperative anesthetic assessment is of importance. The stabilized state of disease can be confirmed just a couple of days before surgery allowing safe same day admission for surgery. Patients should take their morning dose of pyridostigmine as usually scheduled, ideally taken immediately prior to surgery. If surgery is delayed or scheduled for afternoon, another dose of pyridostigmine is given before surgery. No other premedication is administered. Anesthesia can be safely induced with propofol and fentanyl, and maintained with isoflurane and nitrous oxide. Propofol could be used in addition to inhaled anesthetics for maintenance of anesthesia. Muscle relaxation is rarely required. The aim is routine extubation at the end of surgery.

TECHNIQUE OF VIDEO ASSISTED TRANSCERVICAL THYMECTOMY

Transcervical thymectomy was the approach used for the earliest described thymectomies,[20] but was replaced by the transsternal approach by Blalock and his contemporaries midway through the past century.[4] We prefer the video-assisted transcervical thymectomy (VTCT) approach for the treatment of nonthymomatous MG since, despite being a less invasive procedure, it gives excellent bilateral exposure of the thymus, including the lower poles, and permits complete thymectomy. Furthermore, unlike transthoracic video-assisted thymectomies, the transcervical route obviates entry into the pleural spaces, obviates the need for chest tubes, provides enhanced exposure in the neck region, and does not require split lung anesthesia via a double-lumen endotracheal tube.

Relative contraindications to a transcervical approach include prior cervicomediastinal surgery and/or radiation, and cervical spine pathology limiting extension of the neck. Surgery is performed in the supine position with an inflatable bag under the shoulders. The bag is inflated to provide good neck extension. Both arms are tucked in at the sides. The neck and full anterior chest is prepped in case a sternotomy is required. A curvilinear incision is made in the skin at the base of the neck, one finger breadth above the sternal notch, and extended on each side to the medial border of sternocleidomastoid muscle (Fig. 158-1). This incision is extended through the skin and platysma muscle. Flaps are then developed superiorly to the level of the inferior aspect of the thyroid cartilage and inferiorly to

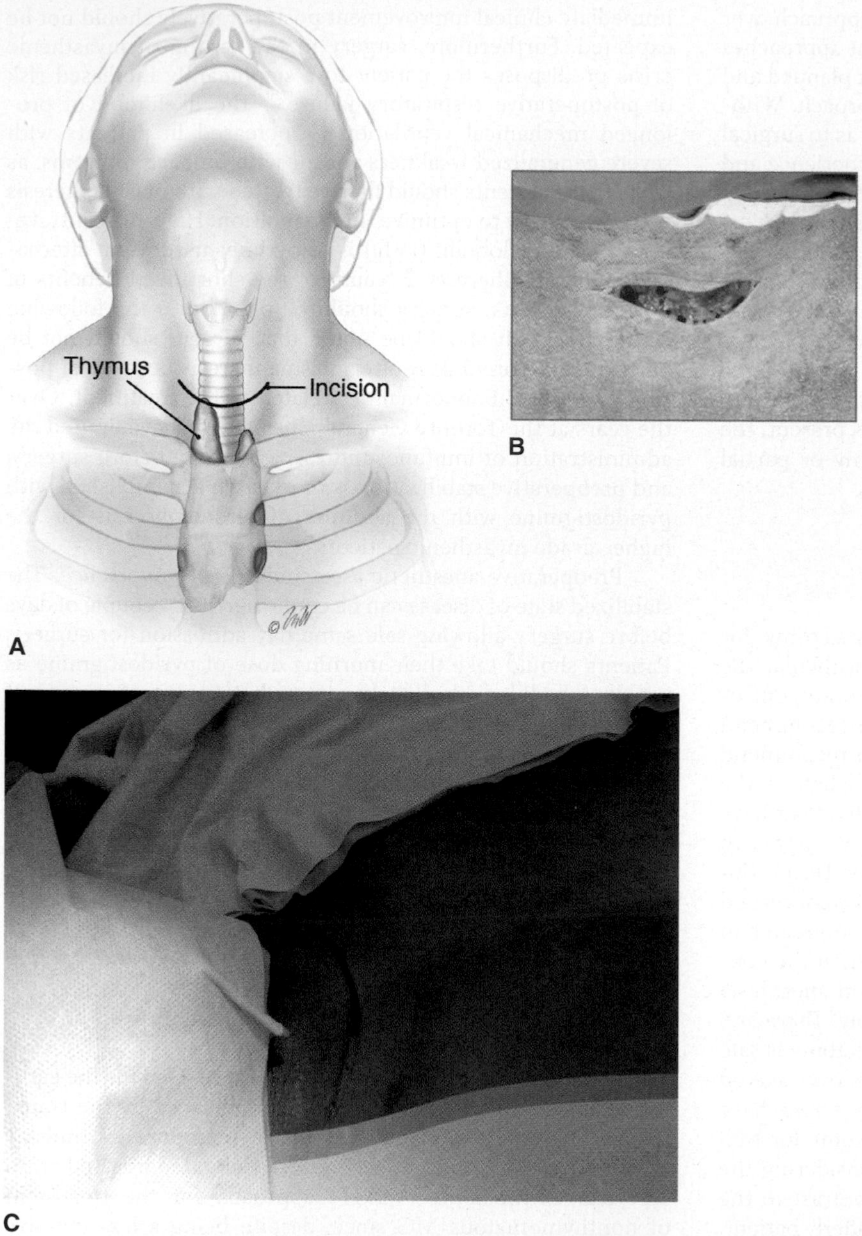

Figure 158-1. An incision is made in the skin at the base of the neck, one finger breadth above the sternal notch, and extended on each side to the medial border of sternocleidomastoid muscle.

the sternal notch. The strap muscles are then split vertically in the midline and elevated bilaterally to expose the superior poles of the thymus gland, which lie opposed to the posterior surface of the sternothyroid muscles. It is imperative that this be done using careful sharp dissection with meticulous attention to control of small blood vessels with electrocautery. A bloodless field makes it significantly easier to delineate thymic tissue from fatty tissue in the neck. Each superior pole of the gland is mobilized near the inferior thyroid vein. The upper pole is divided between ties at the point where the thymic tissue terminates. A heavy silk suture, cut long, is placed on each upper pole and used as a "traction" suture to facilitate orientation and traction of the gland (Fig. 158-2). The superior poles are dissected and pulled up, and the capsule of thymus gland is followed inferiorly to the thoracic inlet.

The retrosternal (retromanubrial) space is cleared to accommodate the placement of the Cooper retractor.[9] The Cooper retractor blade is placed beneath the manubrium to elevate it and open the thoracic inlet (Fig. 158-2). The inflatable pillow that was placed at the start of the procedure is deflated at this point to further improve the thoracic inlet exposure. Care is taken to make sure that the patient's head is not elevated off the operating table by the sternal retractor.

We use a 5-mm 30-degree videothoracoscope at the right lateral aspect of the neck incision to provide light for direct operating and a video magnified view of the operating field on a monitor (Fig. 158-3). The dissection of the gland is carried down into the thorax using primarily blunt dissection. The arterial vessels entering the gland laterally from the internal thoracic artery branches are clipped with stainless steel clips. The thymic veins (there are often several), which drain into the innominate vein, are identified posteriorly and divided between stainless steel clips. The assistance of the videothoracoscope provides good visualization of the lower mediastinum, down

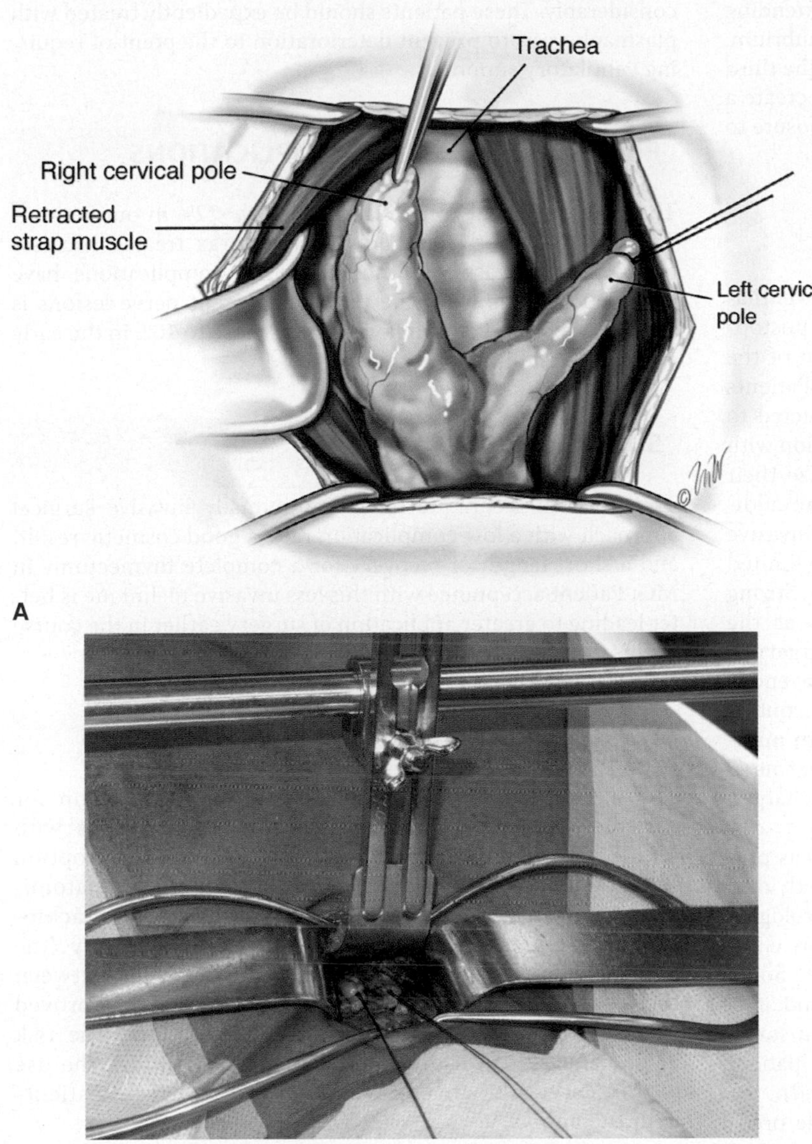

Figure 158-2. Cooper retractor is in place. Sutures are placed on each upper pole and used as a "traction" sutures.

to diaphragm if necessary. The ventilation rate and tidal volume can both be decreased to facilitate exposure in the mediastinum. The dissection of the gland is carried down alternately on both sides until the inferior poles of the gland are clearly identified and a dissecting "peanut" on a long-curved Swedish-Debakey dissector is used to sweep up each inferior pole. The dissector is placed on the pericardium, distal to the inferior pole of the thymus gland, and in a sweeping motion the gland is extracted from the inferior mediastinum. A 7 Jackson-Pratt (JP) drain (Zimmer, Dover, OH) is inserted through a lateral stab wound in the neck, placed down into the mediastinum, and the Cooper retractor is removed. The strap muscles are approximated and the platysma and the skin are closed. Patients are discharged home on the morning after surgery.

In rare instances, if complete thymectomy cannot be performed by removing the thymus and its capsule, the operation is usually converted to a partial upper sternotomy. This is

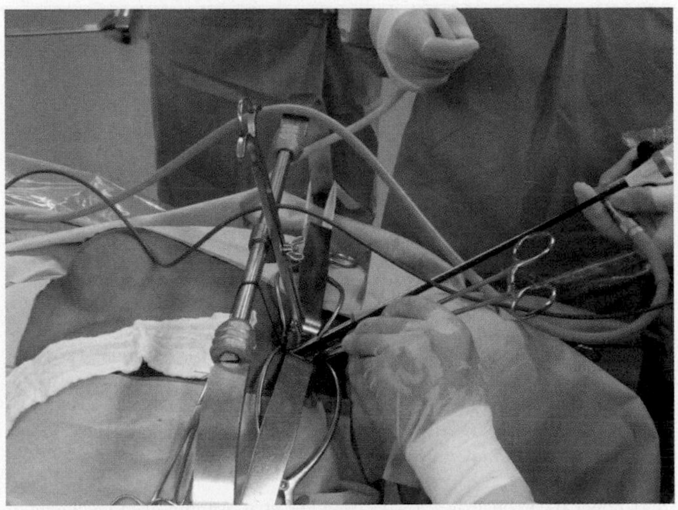

Figure 158-3. Operative view illustrating the position of the telescope and instruments through the cervical incision.

carried out by the addition of a vertical skin incision extending down from the sternal notch to the lower end of manubrium. The sternal bone incision is then extended laterally in the third intercostal space (in a "T") with the oscillating saw to create a partial upper sternotomy, which provides sufficient exposure to easily complete the operation.

POSTOPERATIVE CARE

The patient's respiratory status and requirements for ventilatory support are, by far, the most salient issues in the postoperative period. With careful preoperative preparation of the MG patient, ventilatory issues are rarely a problem. Patients are extubated in the operating room. They are instructed to take their morning dose of anticholinesterase medication with a sip of water immediately preoperatively, to optimize their strength at the time of extubation. They are given an additional dose in the recovery room. With the minimally invasive approach, the need of postoperative analgesia can be limited to acetaminophen with mild narcotics such as codeine. Strong narcotics are rarely required. Oral pyridostigmine at the patient's usual dose is introduced 4 to 6 hours after surgery. If patients are on steroid therapy before surgery, an intravenous stress dose is given on induction and oral steroids are continued at the patient's usual dose the next morning. With minimally invasive approaches today, patients almost never need postoperative care in the ICU and are ready to be discharged early the next day.

Their medications are continued at the same dose as preoperatively. The medications are not altered until 1 month after surgery when they are seen by the surgeon and the neurologist. A period of 3 to 12 months is most often observed before clinical improvement can be seen following thymectomy.[21] Some patients may get transiently worse postoperatively and it is this exacerbation of myasthenic symptoms, rather than surgical considerations, that is the usual reason to keep a patient in the hospital for longer than 1 day. If symptoms worsen, the medication regimen may have to be altered to include prednisone or azathioprine. An occasional patient may deteriorate considerably. These patients should be expediently treated with plasmapheresis to prevent deterioration to the point of requiring ventilatory support.

PROCEDURE-SPECIFIC COMPLICATIONS

The rate of surgical complications is low, <2% in our series.[10] These were hemothorax and pneumothorax treated successfully by conservative methods. Wound complications have been reported, as well. The rate of recurrent nerve lesions is zero. The reported conversion rate was close to 10% in the early experience and is now in the range of 1%.[10,22]

SUMMARY

Transcervical technique offers a minimally invasive surgical approach with a low complication rate, a good cosmetic result, and a short length of recovery for a complete thymectomy in MG. Patient acceptance with this less invasive technique is better leading to greater application of surgery earlier in the course of this disease.

EDITOR'S COMMENT

Transcervical thymectomy is a useful surgical option for patients with thymic hyperplasia; typically, patients with MG. Transcervical thymectomy, however, is not an option for patients with large glands and most thymomas. Anatomically, the transcervical dissection is limited by the brachiocephalic vein posteriorly and the sternum anteriorly (the thymus gland is the only normal anatomic structure between these structures). Although video optics have improved visualization and broadened surgical indications, the risk of inadequate resection or local seeding precludes the use of transcervical thymectomy in the vast majority of patients with thymomas.

—Steven J. Mentzer

References

1. Drachman DB. Myasthenia gravis. *N Engl J Med.* 1994;330:1797–1810.
2. Hohlfeld R, Wekerle H. The role of the thymus in myasthenia gravis. *Adv Neuroimmunol.* 1994;4:373–386.
3. Luo J, Kuryatov A, Lindstrom JM. Specific immunotherapy of experimental myasthenia gravis by a novel mechanism. *Ann Neurol.* 2010;67:441–451.
4. Blalock A. Thymectomy in the treatment of myasthenia gravis. Report of twenty cases. *J Thorac Surg.* 1944;13:316.
5. Gronseth GS, Barohn RJ. Practise parameter: thymectomy for autoimmune myasthenia gravis (an evidence-based review). *Neurology.* 2000 12;55:7–15.
6. Mantegazza R, Baggi F, Antozzi C, et al. Myasthenia gravis (MG): epidemiological data and prognostic factors. *Ann N Y Acad Sci.* 2003;998:413–423.
7. Perlo VP, Arnason B, Poskanzer D, et al. The role of thymectomy in the treatment of myasthenia gravis. *Ann N Y Acad Sci.* 1971 15;183:308–315.
8. Jaretzki A, Wolff M. "Maximal" thymectomy for myasthenia gravis. Surgical anatomy and operative technique. *J Thorac Cardiovasc Surg.* 1988;96: 711–716.
9. Cooper JD, Al-Jilaihawa AN, Pearson FG, et al. An improved technique to facilitate transcervical thymectomy for myasthenia gravis. *Ann Thorac Surg.* 1988;45:242–247.
10. de Perrot M, Bril V, McRae K, et al. Impact of minimally invasive transcervical thymectomy on outcome in patients with myasthenia gravis. *Eur J Cardiothorac Surg.* 2003;24:677–683.
11. Zahid I, Sharif S, Routledge T, et al. Video-assisted thoracoscopic surgery or transsternal thymectomy in the treatment of myasthenia gravis. *Interact Cardiovasc Thorac Surg.* 2011;12:40–46.
12. Murai H, Uchiyama A, Mei FJ, et al. Long-term effects of infrasternal mediastinoscopic thymectomy in myasthenia gravis. *J Neurol Sci.* 2009; 287:185–187.
13. Jaretzki A, Steinglass KM, Molnar J. Thymectomy in the management of myasthenia gravis. *Semin Neurol.* 2004;24:49–62.
14. Pennathur A, Qureshi I, Schuchert MJ, et al. Comparison of surgical techniques for early-stage thymoma: feasibility of minimally invasive thymectomy and comparison with open resection. *J Thorac Cardiovasc Surg.* 2011;141:694–701.
15. Benatar M, Kaminski HJ; Quality Standards Subcommittee of the American Academy of Neurology. Evidence report: the medical treatment of ocular myasthenia (an evidence-based review): report of the Quality Standards Subcommittee of the American Academy of Neurology. *Neurology.* 2007;68: 2144–2149.

16. Tsuchida M, Yamato Y, Souma T, et al. Efficacy and safety of extended thymectomy for elderly patients with myasthenia gravis. *Ann Thorac Surg.* 1999;67:1563–1567.
17. Budde JM, Morris CD, Gal AA, et al. Predictors of outcome in thymectomy for myasthenia gravis. *Ann Thorac Surg.* 2001;72:197–202.
18. Evoli A. Acquired myasthenia gravis in childhood. *Curr Opinion Neurol.* 2010;23:536–540.
19. Gracey DR, Divertie MB, Howard FM Jr, et al. Postoperative respiratory care after transsternal thymectomy in myasthenia gravis. A 3-year experience in 53 patients. *Chest.* 1984;86:67–71.
20. Schumacher, Roth. Thymecktomie bei einem fall von morbus basedowie mit myasthenie. *Mitt Grenzgeb Chir.* 1913;25.
21. Bulkley GB, Bass KN, Stephenson GR, et al. Extended cervicomediastinal thymectomy in the integrated management of myasthenia gravis. *Ann Surg.* 1997;226:324–335.
22. Shrager JB. Extended transcervical thymectomy: the ultimate minimally invasive approach. *Ann Thorac Surg.* 2010;89:S2128–S2134.

159 Thoracoscopic Approach to Thymectomy with Advice on Patients with Myasthenia Gravis

Luis M. Argote-Greene, Michael T. Jaklitsch, and David J. Sugarbaker

Keyword: Thoracoscopic surgical technique

Thoracoscopy is the application of video imaging technology to standard thoracic surgical procedures. The thoracoscopic approach permits indirect visualization of the thoracic cavity without the necessity of performing a full thoracotomy. Before the current era, the standard surgical approach to thymectomy was through a midline sternotomy or a cervical collar incision. In the last two decades, however, thoracoscopic thymectomy has been used increasingly in selected patients as a means of reducing pain and recovery time while maintaining the quality of gland removal, as well as comparable remission and asymptomatic disease rates compared to other minimally invasive and open techniques.[1] Thoracoscopic thymectomy is a good alternative to standard surgical treatment with full sternotomy because it offers excellent visualization (superior to the collar incision) and avoids the morbidity of a sternal division. We enthusiastically advocate a thoracoscopic approach to myasthenia gravis (MG), thymic cysts, thymic masses, and other anterior mediastinal tumors, including small (<2 cm) thymomas.[2,3] Bulky thymomas may be better visualized through a standard sternotomy. In this chapter, we describe our technique for thoracoscopic thymectomy with particular advice on ensuring a complete resection.

For the purposes of this description, we will refer to the superior portions of the H-shaped thymus gland as the *right* or *left cervical horns*, and the inferior portions will be referred as the *right* or *left lobes*.

GENERAL PRINCIPLES

Thoracoscopic thymectomy is well tolerated by patients of any age or gender owing to the minimally invasive nature of this approach. The usual position for a thoracoscopic procedure is the lateral decubitus position. We have lately added slight cervical flexion to permit caudal migration of the cervical horns and easier dissection, which obviates the need for a cervical incision. This position permits adequate instrumentation of the chest and rapid conversion to open thoracotomy in the event of bleeding or extended re-section. The patient must be intubated with a double-lumen endotracheal tube for split-lung anesthesia to permit selective deflation of the right or left lung. A left-sided double-lumen endotracheal tube is preferred because it is safer and easier to intubate the left mainstem bronchus owing to its length. Most thoracoscopic procedures can be performed with three ports: one for the camera and two for instrument access. It is important to place the ports as far apart from each other as possible to provide opposing angles of access to the intrathoracic target. A camera with a 30-degree angled telescope is also recommended for better intrathoracic visualization. Ports that have been placed too close together prevent adequate countertension on the tissues and cause crowding of instruments. A baseball diamond analogy has been used to describe port placement.[4] The camera is at home plate, and the instruments are at first and third base. The target lies between the pitcher's mound and second base. A fourth port can be added later in the procedure to improve exposure and retraction of the specimen. Blake drain is used unless undue air leak or drainage is noted then a single chest tube is preferred.

In the subset of patients with MG, onset of the disease is correlated with gender and age. MG tends to peak in the second and third decades of life for women versus the sixth and seventh decades for men. For women, early resection is associated with a better response. Thus the typical female patient is a young woman between 25 and 30 years of age who has generalized neuromuscular weakness and is seeking to diminish the consequences of lifelong steroid therapy. Since men experience later onset of disease and a greater incidence of thymoma, male patients usually are older than 55 years of age.

PREOPERATIVE ASSESSMENT

Routine preoperative studies include pulmonary function testing, a posteroanterior and lateral chest radiograph, and chest CT scan. The preoperative assessment of patients with MG is performed in collaboration with a team of specialists including the neurologist, anesthesiologist, thoracic surgeon, and pulmonologist. MG is an autoimmune disease resulting from the production of antibodies against the acetylcholine receptors of the neuromuscular synapse. For this reason, patients with severe MG or in crisis may undergo perioperative plasmapheresis or immunoglobulin administration which decreases the level of circulating antibodies.[5] Often on long-term steroid therapy, patients with MG also may receive a steroid stress dose before surgery, with subsequent taper in the first postoperative week.

TECHNIQUE OF THORACOSCOPIC THYMECTOMY

Several approaches to thoracoscopic thymectomy have been described, including right, left, bilateral, and bilateral with cervical incision. In general, we prefer to use the right thoracoscopic approach. It provides better visualization of the junction between the innominate vein and the superior vena cava, the so-called innominate–caval junction (ICJ), and thus a better view of the thymic veins. We have encountered more ease of dissection of the cervical horns by adding neck flexion, which permits caudad migration of the lower anterior neck structures. In addition, since the heart and pericardium are predominantly left-sided structures, there is less room on the left for maneuvering the thoracoscope and other surgical instruments.

Right Thoracoscopic Approach

Position

The patient is anesthetized and intubated with a single-lumen endotracheal tube. A flexible bronchoscope is passed through the lumen and down into the airway to assess for the presence of incidental intraluminal lesions or extrinsic compression. If the airway is clear, a double-lumen endotracheal tube is placed for split-lung ventilation, using the flexible bronchoscope to confirm its position. The mechanics of delivering anesthesia in thoracoscopic procedures are detailed in Chapter 5. It warrants mention, however, that muscle relaxants should be used cautiously in patients with MG, if at all, in view of the goal to withdraw the patient from ventilation as quickly as possible after the operation.

For the right thoracoscopic approach, the patient is placed in the left lateral decubitus position. A roll is placed under the patient's side, elevating the body by approximately 45 to 60 degrees. The easiest way to accomplish this position, we have found, is to place the patient in the full lateral decubitus position and then rotate the patient posteriorly by approximately 30 degrees. The right arm is elevated into a swimmer's position, and slight cervical flexion is achieved. The right chest is prepped and draped in the usual sterile fashion.

Port Placement

Three portals are created in a triangular configuration (Fig. 159-1). The first port (5–20 mm) is placed over the fifth intercostal space (ICS) between the anterior axillary and midaxillary lines. From this location, the chest tube exits the skin anterior to the superior iliac crest of the pelvis, thus preventing chest tube compression or kinking in the postoperative period. This port site is one ICS above the site that we generally use for thoracoscopic procedures of the posterior or midchest (i.e., sixth ICS) and permits use of the curved or straight Foerster (ring-hatched) forceps in the upper anterior mediastinum. The second port (5 mm) is placed in the fifth ICS between the mid- and posterior axillary lines, near the tip of the scapula. The third port (2 cm) is placed at the base of the axilla over the top of the third rib. The size of the ports may vary depending on surgical instrumentation and surgeon preference.

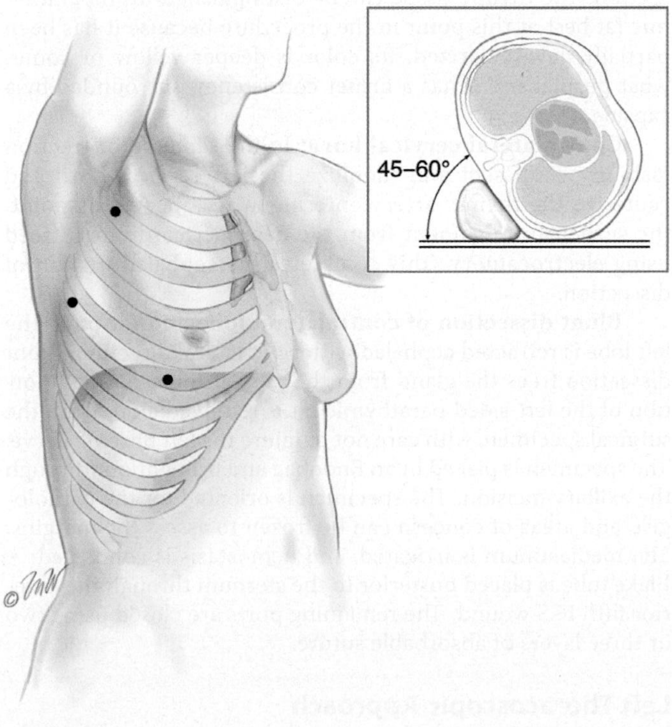

Figure 159-1. For right thoracoscopic thymectomy, the patient is in the left lateral decubitus position and elevated approximately 30 degrees by placing a roll under the patient's side. Three ports are placed in triangular configuration with the patient's arms in swimmer's position.

The camera is placed initially in the anterior fifth ICS port for exploration of the chest. We recommend a 30-degree 5-mm telescopic lens for easy visualization and dissection of the mediastinum. Ventilation is stopped on the right side. The entire thoracic cavity is examined to identify the surgical landmarks, namely, thymus gland, phrenic nerve, superior vena cava, and internal mammary vessels (Fig. 159-2). The posterior diaphragmatic sulcus is examined for "drop metastases."

The camera is moved to the posterior fifth ICS port (5 mm) for the thymic dissection. This produces the classic dissection triangle with the surgeon standing posterior to the patient (Fig. 159-3). The left-hand instruments enter the axillary port, the right-hand instruments enter the anterior fifth ICS port, and the camera eye is between the left and right hands in the posterior fifth ICS port. A fourth port can be created at the surgeon's option and, if so, usually is placed caudally and later in the procedure to aid in dissection of the contralateral side. Placement is based on anatomic considerations, but a fourth port is often located in the seventh ICS in the midaxillary line.

While some surgeons recommend CO_2 insufflation to collapse the lung, we find that it is unnecessary for adequate atelectasis, and its use can compromise the patient physiologically.[6,7] Pneumomediastinum 24 hours in advance of surgery also has been reported as an aid to dissection, but we have no experience with this technique.[8]

For patients with MG, the more complete the anterior mediastinal resection, the better are the chances of improvement. Because of the embryologic origin of the thymus, ectopic thymic cells can be found in the parathymic fat and lower cervical pretracheal area. All anterior mediastinal tissue must be removed, including thymic tissue and pericardial fat pads from phrenic nerve to phrenic nerve (Fig. 159-4).

Mediastinal pleural cuts: The dissection begins from a posteroinferior position, just anterior to the phrenic nerve. We incise using scissors for the mediastinal pleura from the caudal end of the gland to just above the ICJ. A second cut is made in the mediastinal pleura just posterior to the internal mammary artery using cautery. These two pleural incisions come together just cephalad to the ICJ (Fig. 159-5).

Blunt dissection anterior/posterior: Blunt dissection of the mediastinal fat and thymic tissue is performed by developing the avascular plane posterior to the gland and anterior to the pericardium and, likewise, anterior to the gland and posterior to the sternum. This dissection is facilitated by removing the ipsilateral pericardial fat pad. The posterior plane is dissected first because the tissue attachments to the sternum, which suspend the gland anteriorly, assist in visualization of this dissection plane. Once all the parathymic fat has been dissected from the surrounding tissues, the right lobe of the thymus gland is exposed.

Ipsilateral cervical horn: We pull the right cervical horn down from the neck by broadly placing a Foerster forceps

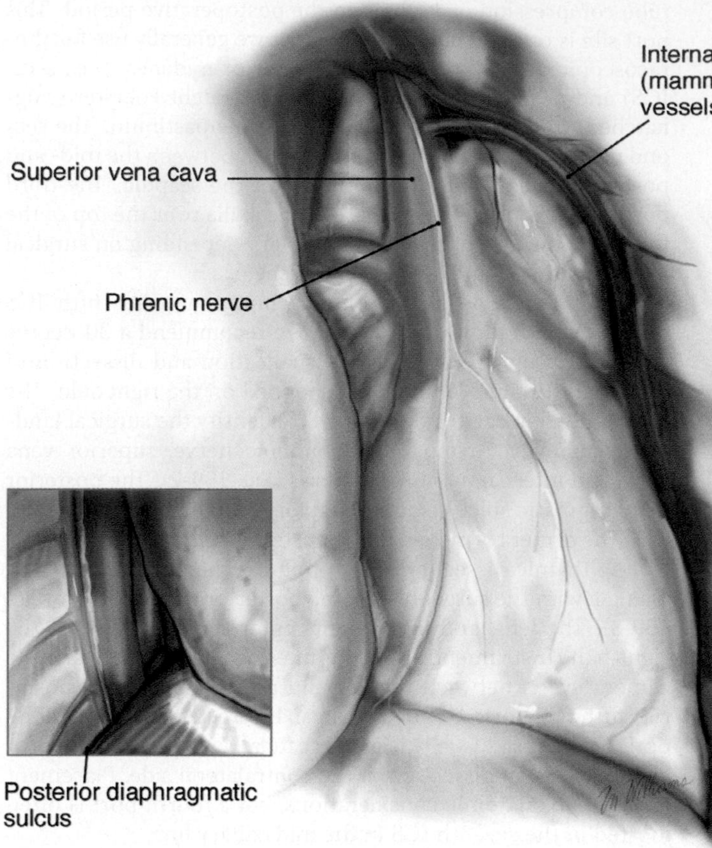

Figure 159-2. Important mediastinal landmarks that are visible with the camera placed in the anterior fifth intercostal port.

across the horn and pulling caudally. A second, ringed Foerster forceps permits a hand-over-hand technique. Electrocautery is used to cauterize the thymic branch from the inferior thyroid artery, which feeds into the thymus at the apex of each of the superior horns of the gland. The cervical horn then is bent back onto itself anteriorly and retracted to the left and caudad, exposing the innominate vein.

Thymic vein: With careful blunt dissection along the innominate vein, it is relatively easy to locate the thymic veins. The thymic veins, usually two or three, can be divided between

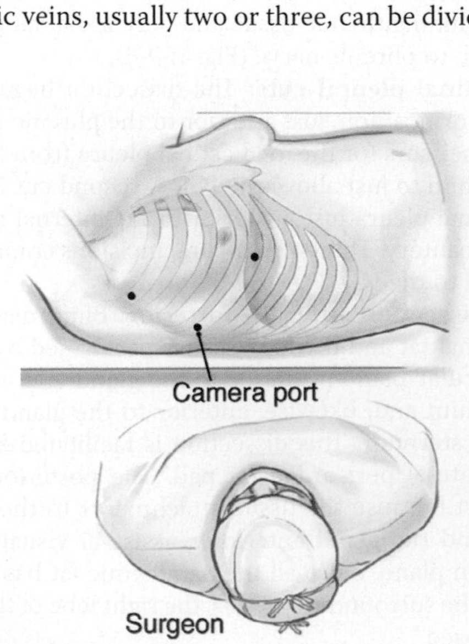

Figure 159-3. For thymic dissection, the camera is moved to the posterior fifth intercostal port.

endoclips. Once these vessels are ligated and divided, the area caudad to the innominate vein opens further with blunt dissection. The thymic tissue can be distinguished from parathymic fat best at this point in the procedure because it has been partially devascularized. Its color is deeper yellow or somewhat purple, and it has a firmer consistency, surrounded by a capsule.

Contralateral cervical horn: In the same blunt traction fashion, we dissect and mobilize the left cervical horn and cauterize the thymic artery entering at its tip. At this point, the suspensory ligament from the deep pericardium is freed using electrocautery. This completes the cephalad margin of dissection.

Blunt dissection of contralateral lobe and fat pad: The left lobe is retracted cephalad with right lateral direction. Blunt dissection frees the gland from the pericardium. A small portion of the left-sided parathymic fat is removed along with the surgical specimen, with care not to injure the left phrenic nerve. The specimen is placed in an Endobag and brought out through the axillary incision. The specimen is oriented for the pathologist, and areas of concern can be frozen to assess the margins. The mediastinum is irrigated, and hemostasis is confirmed. A Blake tube is placed posterior to the sternum through the anterior fifth ICS wound. The remaining ports are closed using two or three layers of absorbable suture.

Left Thoracoscopic Approach

Position

For a left thymectomy, the patient is placed in a 45- to 60-degree right lateral decubitus position with small rolls placed along the

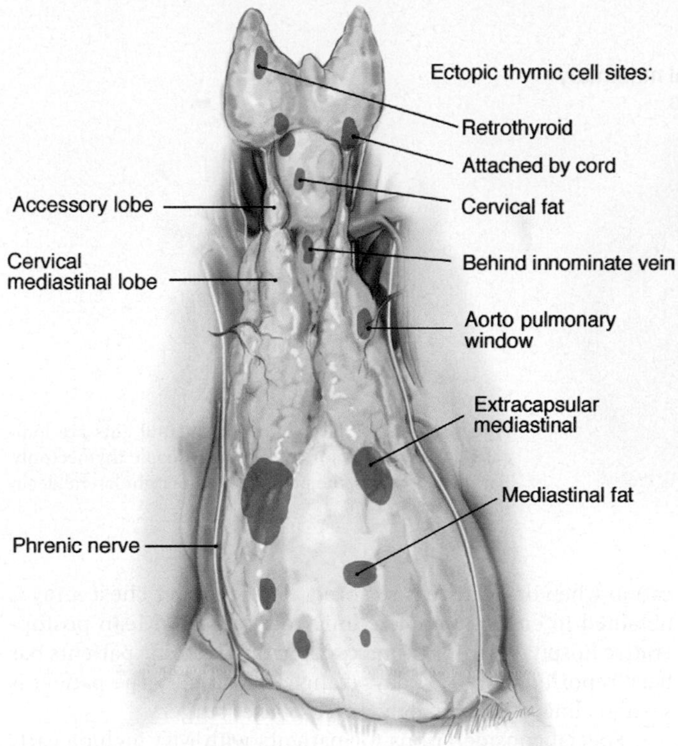

Figure 159-4. Anatomy of the thymus gland with most likely sites of ectopic thymic tissue.

right scapula and behind the patient's hip, and cervical flexion is also warranted.[9]

Ports

The first port is placed in the fifth ICS on the anterior axillary line. The second port is placed between the posterior and midaxillary line in the fifth ICS near the tip of the scapula. The third port is placed at the base of the axillae over the third rib. The best location for the camera is in the posterior port between the left and right instrument ports, with the surgeon standing posteriorly.

Mediastinal pleural cuts: Once the ports have been placed and the mediastinal structures identified, dissection begins with the left thymic lobe. The mediastinal pleura is opened anterior to the phrenic nerve with scissors and posterior to the mammary vessels using cautery (Fig. 159-6).

Blunt dissection anterior/posterior: Blunt dissection is performed posterior and then anterior to the gland.

Ipsilateral cervical horn: Since the left cervical horn is displaced more posteriorly than the right horn because of the contour of the ascending aorta, this may limit the posterior dissection of the upper part of the gland until the left horn has been pulled down from the neck.

Thymic veins: The lateral extent of the innominate vein is usually hidden by mediastinal fat on the left. After the left pole has been dissected, the thymic veins are clipped and divided proximal to the thymus.

Contralateral cervical horn: The right phrenic nerve can be found lateral or just anterior to the superior vena cava. Visualization of this area is not as good from the left approach. This nerve could be injured from blunt traction if the clamps extend beyond the right lateral margin of the gland. Clear visualization and skeletonization of the right cervical horn avoid this injury by displacing the right horn in a posterocaudal manner and pushing the right mediastinal pleura off the right lateral side of the horn and then off the lateral side of the right lobe (Fig. 159-7). The most difficult portion of thymectomy from the left-sided approach is dissection at the ICJ.

The cava and innominate veins form a 120-degree angle at the ICJ, and blunt dissection with an endo-Kitner dissector through the lower anterior port hits this junction at a 45-degree angle (Fig. 159-8). This can lead to injury to one of these structures. Dissection from the upper axillary port tends to avoid this problem.

Blunt dissection of the contralateral lobe and fat pad: The surgeon grasps the right lobe with gentle traction toward the left side, dissecting it bluntly away from the left phrenic nerve.

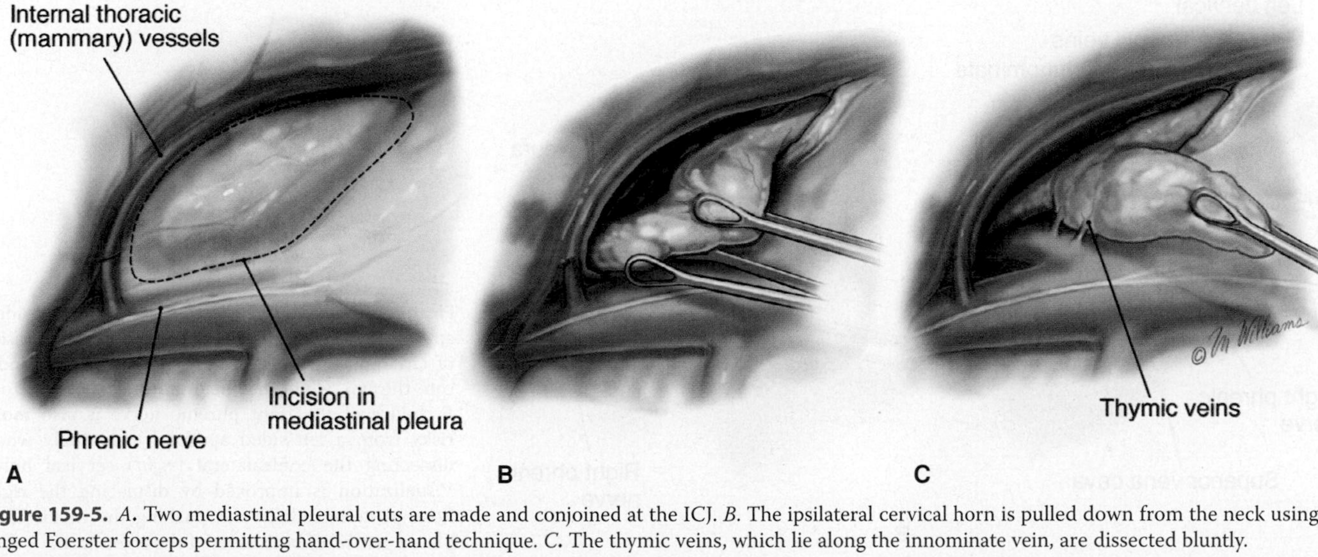

Figure 159-5. *A.* Two mediastinal pleural cuts are made and conjoined at the ICJ. *B.* The ipsilateral cervical horn is pulled down from the neck using two ringed Foerster forceps permitting hand-over-hand technique. *C.* The thymic veins, which lie along the innominate vein, are dissected bluntly.

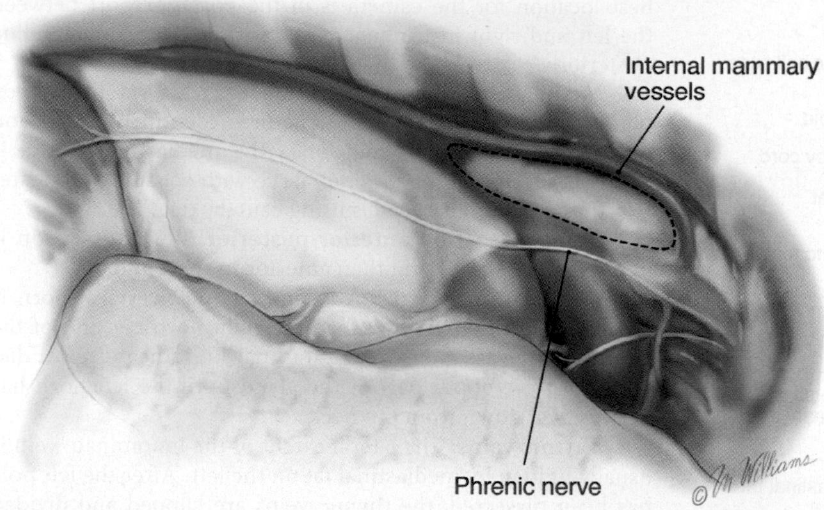

Figure 159-6. Initial mediastinal pleural cuts are indicated (*dashed line*) for a left thoracoscopic thymectomy. For this approach, the patient is in the right lateral decubitus position.

NOTE ON THORACIC CO_2 INSUFLATION

During the last couple of years, we have begun using CO_2 insufflation in the chest. Insufflation is well tolerated to 10–12 cm H_2O. Ports have decreased in size (5 mm) and advanced dissection instrumentation (ultrasonic dissector) is preferred. This has enhanced our ability to extend into the cervical horns of the thymus. Using unilateral or bilateral approaches we have maximized the ectopic thymic tissue extra action with equal results to the open techniques.

Thoracic drainage is done with silastic tubes when needed and most uncomplicated VATS thymectomies are left without a drain nowadays.

POSTOPERATIVE CARE

The Blake drain or chest tube is removed when the effluent is serous and less than 100 mL/d, usually on the first postoperative day. Diet is resumed as tolerated on the first postoperative day. Pain is controlled with IV medications and with oral medication when oral intake is restored. Postoperative chest x-ray is obtained to ensure complete lung reexpansion. Mean postoperative hospital stay for thoracoscopic thymectomy patients has been reported to be 1.64 days (range 0–8 days).[10] The patient is seen in clinic approximately 2 weeks after surgery.

Special considerations for patients with MG include early extubation, preferably before leaving the OR, and careful monitoring of ventilatory function. Before considering tracheal extubation, adequate respiratory function must be ensured. For example, if the patient can lift his or her head for 5 seconds or when the inspiratory force exceeds −25 cm H_2O, the patient can be extubated safely.

PROCEDURE-SPECIFIC COMPLICATIONS

The most serious complications of thoracoscopic thymectomy include iatrogenic injury to the phrenic nerve, which can lead to phrenic nerve palsy and diaphragmatic paralysis. Thorough knowledge of the regional anatomy and meticulous technique, as detailed earlier, including alternating use of scissor (nerve)

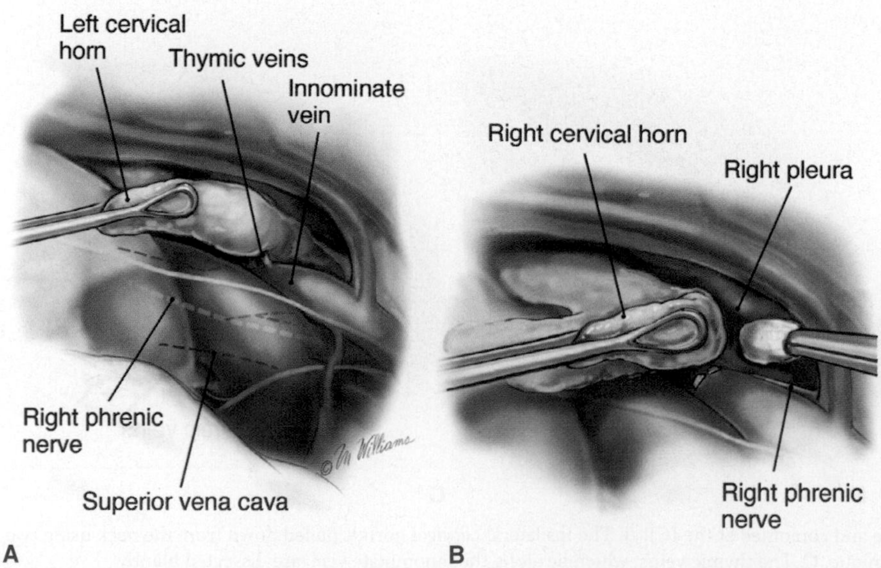

Figure 159-7. Thymic dissection from a left-sided approach is more difficult owing to the necessity of circumnavigating the ICJ. *A. Dashed lines* indicate the ICJ, which lies below the "aortic" horizon. *B.* Injury of the right phrenic nerve is also more risky from a left-sided approach, especially when dissecting the contralateral (*right*) cervical horn. Visualization is improved by displacing the right horn posterocaudally and pushing the mediastinal pleura gently off both sides of the right horn.

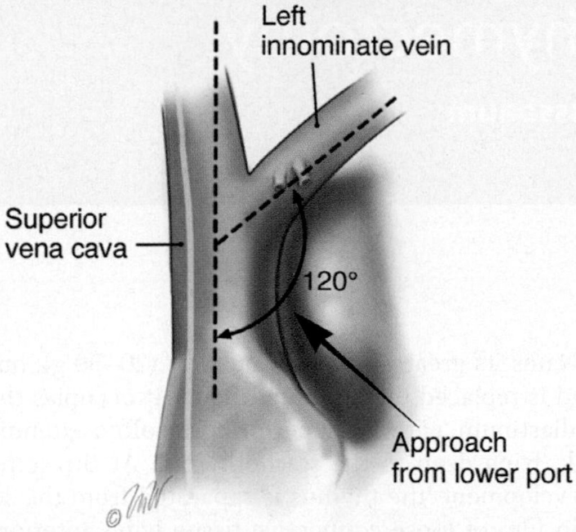

Figure 159-8. The junction between the innominate vein and superior vena cava (ICJ) is encountered when operating from the lower port on the left side. Approaching the dissection through the upper axillary port is recommended to avoid this problem.

versus cautery (vessel) dissection, are the best protection against this sort of injury. Performing the thymectomy from a right approach whenever possible avoids the potential pitfalls of working in the crowded left chest. Other morbidities such as hemorrhage, infection, pneumothorax, pneumonia, failure to wean from the respirator, conversion to thoracotomy, pleural effusion requiring drainage, myocardial infarction, empyema, and pulmonary embolus are managed according to standard practice. In the event of conversion owing to bleeding, we recommend an axillary thoracotomy to control the event and complete the procedure with video-assisted technique.

SUMMARY

Thoracoscopic thymectomy is an excellent alternative to standard surgical treatment with full sternotomy. Its benefits can be enumerated in terms of reduced morbidity and mortality, shorter postoperative recovery, and enhanced cosmesis resulting from avoidance of sternal division.[11] Lately, a retrospective analysis of 57 patients with MG that underwent right three port VATS thymectomy were followed up with strict Myasthenia Gravis Foundation of America (MGFA) Clinical Classification for a minimum of 12 months. The complete stable remission rate was 15% and 28%, for 3 and 5 years, respectively. The asymptomatic disease rate was 59% at 5 years, with a median follow-up of 32 months. This study shows right VATS thymectomy achieves comparable remission and asymptomatic disease rates to other minimally invasive and open techniques.[1] Adequate resection with excellent visualization can be achieved by thoracoscopic technique and meticulous attention to the regional anatomy.

EDITOR'S COMMENT

All surgical approaches to thymectomy have strengths and weaknesses. Transcervical thymectomy allows for excellent visualization of the cephalad horns of the thymus gland, whereas thoracoscopic approaches offer better visualization of the intrathoracic thymic tissue. A potential limitation of all approaches is unrecognized or "ectopic" thymic tissue. Since the thymus gland is derived from the third pharyngeal pouch, just ventral to the inferior parathyroid gland, ectopic thymic tissue can be found anywhere along its descent into the chest.

—Steven J. Mentzer

References

1. Keating CP, Kong YX, Tay V, et al. VATS thymectomy for nonthymomatous myasthenia gravis: standardized outcome assessment using the myasthenia gravis foundation of America clinical classification. *Innovations (Phila).* 2011;6(2):104–109.
2. Pennathur A, Qureshi I, Schuchert MJ, et al. Comparison of surgical techniques for early-stage thymoma: feasibility of minimally invasive thymectomy and comparison with open resection. *J Thorac Cardiovasc Surg.* 2011;141(3):694–701.
3. Davenport E, Malthaner RA. The role of surgery in the management of thymoma: a systematic review. *Ann Thorac Surg.* 2008;86(2):673–684.
4. Jaklitsch M, Harpole D, Roberts J. Video-assisted techniques in thoracic surgery. In: Loughlin K, Brooks D, eds. *Principles of Endosurgery*. Cambridge, MA: Blackwell Scientific Publishers; 1995:230.
5. Gajdos P, Chevret S. Treatment of myasthenia gravis acute exacerbations with intravenous immunoglobulin. *Ann N Y Acad Sci.* 2008;1132:271–275.
6. Mack M. Video-assisted thymectomy. In: Shields T, LoCicero J, Ponn R, eds. *General Thoracic Surgery*. Philadelphia, PA: Lippincott Williams & Wilkins; 2004:2638.
7. Mack MJ. Video-assisted thoracoscopy thymectomy for myasthenia gravis. *Chest Surg Clin N Am.* 2001;11(2):389–405, xi-xii.
8. Mineo TC, Pompeo E, Ambrogi V, et al. Adjuvant pneumomediastinum in thoracoscopic thymectomy for myasthenia gravis. *Ann Thorac Surg.* 1996;62(4):1210–1212.
9. Sugarbaker DJ. Thoracoscopy in the management of anterior mediastinal masses. *Ann Thorac Surg.* 1993;56(3):653–656.
10. Savcenko M, Wendt G, Prince S. Video-assisted thymectomy for myasthenia gravis: an update of a single institution experience. *Eur J Cardiothorac Surg.* 2002;22:978–983.
11. DeCamp MM Jr, Jaklitsch MT, Mentzer SJ, et al. The safety and versatility of video-thoracoscopy: a prospective analysis of 895 consecutive cases. *J Am Coll Surg.* 1995;181(2):113–120.

160 Radical Transsternal Thymectomy

Harry J. D'Agostino, Jr. and Michael S. Nussbaum

Keywords: Surgical technique, myasthenia gravis, thymus, thymoma

The thymus gland is one of the more common structures in the anterior mediastinum that requires surgical extirpation. Most commonly, the indications for thymectomy are either for thymic neoplasm or in the treatment of the autoimmune disorder, myasthenia gravis (MG). Thymus removal should be a safe, straightforward procedure. The key elements in successful and complete thymectomy depend on a comprehensive knowledge of the anatomic and embryologic characteristics of thymic development and the physiology of thymic disease.

The thymus lies in the anterior mediastinum. It is a lymphoepithelial organ that is derived embryologically from the third pharyngeal pouches bilaterally and descends caudally and medially into the mediastinum during gestation, fusing into a bilobed gland. However, fusion and descent are often variable and islands of tissue may be found throughout the neck and mediastinum. In addition to being embedded within the thyroid gland or associated with the parathyroid glands, aberrant thymic rests can occur independently along the entire path of thymic descent (Fig. 160-1).[1] The gland weighs 10 to 35 g at birth, attains its greatest mass in puberty (20–50 g), but involutes and is replaced by fat in adulthood. It occupies the anterior mediastinum, with the superior horns often extending into the neck, lying deep to the sternothyroid. At the completion of its development, the thymus is separated from the sternum by a thin film of loose connective tissue lying anterior to the pericardium and great vessels and is in especially close contact with the left brachiocephalic (innominate) vein. The gland can extend laterally to the phrenic nerves and is partially covered on either side by the pleural reflections. The arterial supply to the thymus is derived principally from the internal thoracic arteries, with contributions from the inferior thyroid, and pericardiophrenic arteries. The veins from both lobes ascend between the lobes posteriorly and usually drain into the left brachiocephalic vein or, rarely, directly into the superior vena cava. The inferior thyroid and thyroid ima veins can receive minor tributaries from the cervical portion of the gland. The phrenic nerves are in immediate proximity to the gland, as are the vagus and recurrent laryngeal nerves. Careful attention to the anatomy is essential for avoiding injury to these vital nerves (Fig. 160-2).

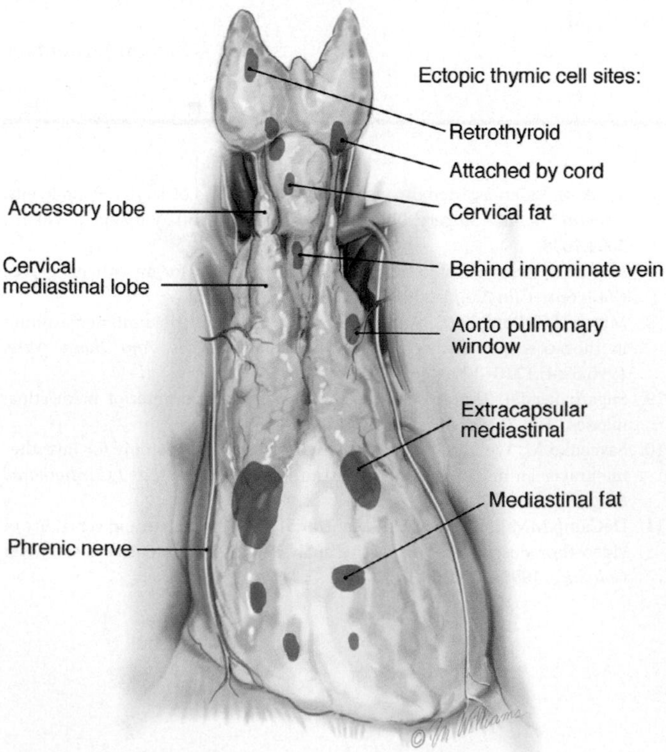

Figure 160-1. The locations of the thymus gland and ectopic extracapsular tissue are shown. There is a high incidence of thymic tissue lateral to the phrenic nerves. Reproduced with permission from Jaretzski A, III. Thymectomy for myasthenia gravis: an analysis of the controversies regarding technique and results. *Neurology*. 1997;48(suppl 5):S52–S63.

The thymus gland is a central lymphoid organ that performs the important immunologic function of transforming null lymphocytes into thymic or T-lymphocytes, which are responsible for cellular immunity. The maturation of T-lymphocytes appears to be promoted by one or more thymic-derived factors, such as the peptide thymosin. The thymus gland is involved in a variety of immunologic, hematologic, endocrine, infectious, and neoplastic diseases. The thymus can display morphologic changes that are associated with abnormal development, immune deficiencies, hyperplasia, and neoplasia. Symptoms may be related to the physical presence of the mass (compression or invasion), associated with a described clinical syndrome (MG, red cell aplasia, or hypogammaglobulinemia), or may be nonspecific (anorexia and fatigue). Failure of the thymus to descend into the anterior mediastinum might account for cervical thymic tissue, which can be mistaken for neoplasm, lymphadenopathy, or an enlarged parathyroid. This aberrant tissue can cause compressive symptoms such as respiratory stridor or dysphagia. In general, symptoms are more common and specific in patients with malignancy, whereas patients with thymic cysts and germ cell tumors have symptoms less frequently.

GENERAL PRINCIPLES

The indications for thymectomy are thymic neoplasm and MG. Thymoma is a neoplastic process of thymic epithelial cells. Often the malignant potential is not determined by the microscopic appearance, but by the behavior in vivo. Even though thymomas may have a benign appearance and a more indolent course, patients with a thymoma should undergo operative

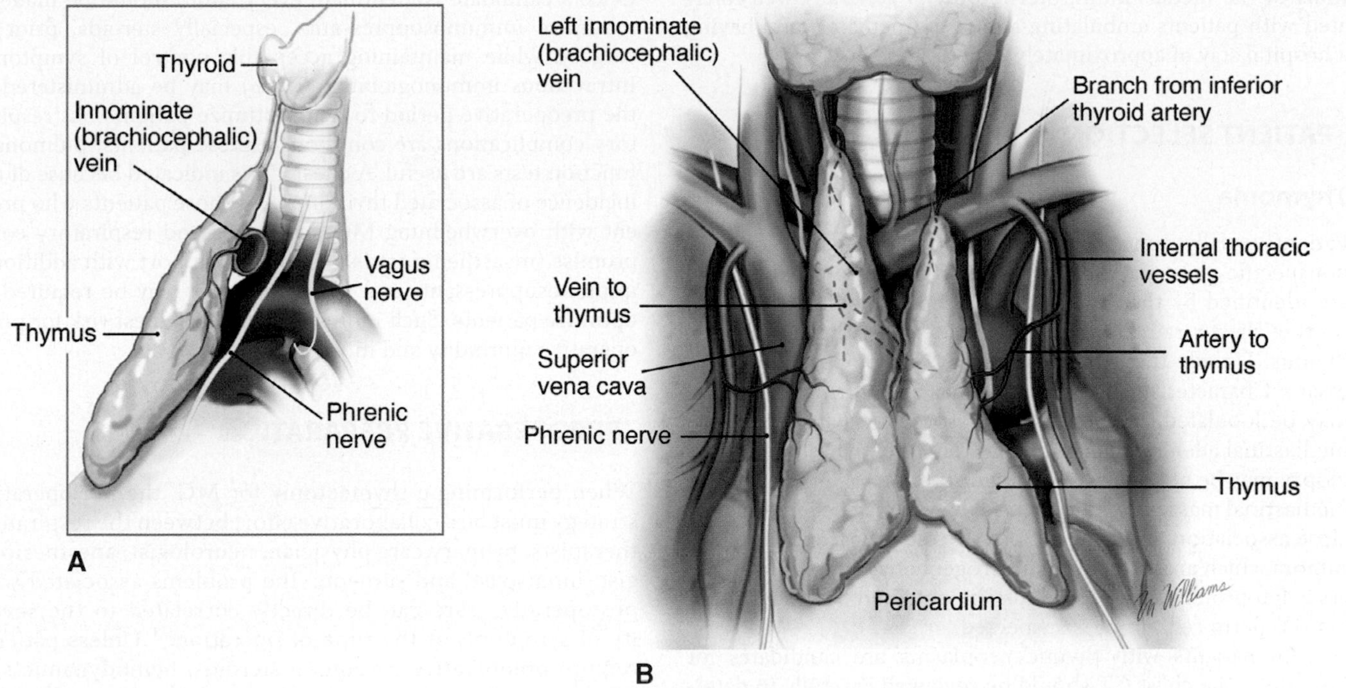

Figure 160-2. The relationships of the thymus gland to critical surrounding structures are shown. The gland and associated tissue may be in close proximity to the phrenic and recurrent laryngeal nerves.

resection due to the potential for invasive spread or morbidity due to local mass effects. For most tumors, a complete resection results in long-term survival. Thus, the majority of thymic abnormalities are treated by surgical extirpation, and it is generally agreed that the excision should be complete. However, the surgical approach to facilitate a complete thymectomy has been a matter of considerable controversy.

MG is a condition characterized by abnormal fatigue of muscles, which worsens as the day progresses, and is relieved by rest. This may be isolated to ocular symptoms, or involve generalized limb weakness. MG is believed to be an autoimmune disease caused by antibodies to acetylcholine receptors at the neuromuscular junction, induced by thymic epitopes. Thymectomy for MG was first described by Blalock, who reported a case of a patient with thymoma who also had MG.[2] Interestingly, he performed this procedure through a partial upper sternotomy, T-ed off at the right third intercostal space. Following resection, the patient noted marked improvement in myasthenic symptoms and was able to discontinue all anticholinergic medications. Since that time, numerous studies have detailed thymic resection for MG, with mostly positive, but variable results. Currently, patients are evaluated according the Osserman classification (Table 160-1).[3] There is consensus that most patients with generalized MG as well as those with debilitating ocular symptoms not controlled by anticholinesterases should undergo thymectomy.[1,4,5] Many authors believe that intervention early in the course of disease (<2 years) also provides a more favorable outcome. However, not all thymic resections are equal in extent, and thus the type of resection performed remains a source of debate.

In most studies, 10% of patients with MG will have an associated thymic neoplasm, which may be identified preoperatively or incidentally in the resected specimen. About 40% of patients with a thymic neoplasm will have MG. Patients without thymoma are more likely to experience an improvement in myasthenic symptoms than those with thymoma.[6]

The presence of ectopic thymic tissue throughout the mediastinum and the problem in differentiating thymus from surrounding fat have led to significant controversy regarding the amount of thymic tissue to be resected and the areas to be explored. Although there is agreement that thymectomy should be complete, the definition is inexact and a multitude of procedures from maximally to minimally invasive have been proposed. Noting the extensive and variable position of extracapsular thymic tissue (see Fig. 160-1), Jaretzski and Wolf[7] described the combined cervical and transsternal approach for maximal removal of all thymic tissue, including potential thymic rests. Cooper et al.[8] described the transcervical thymectomy which removed the bulk of the gland. Other minimally invasive approaches, including video-assisted thoracoscopic surgery (VATS) and robotically assisted surgery, have also been described. The outcomes of these procedures appear to be fairly comparable, although there are no clinical trials directly comparing these procedures and patient selection may bias the results. The transsternal thymectomy is a reasonable approach, providing less morbidity than the combined approach, while offering the exposure necessary to remove almost all thymic tissue, even in the cervical region and in the most inferior por-

Table 160-1

MODIFIED OSSERMAN CLASSIFICATION OF MYASTHENIA GRAVIS[3]

0	Asymptomatic
1	Ocular signs and symptoms
2	Mild generalized weakness
3	Moderate generalized weakness, bulbar dysfunction, or both
4	Severe generalized weakness, respiratory dysfunction, or both

tions of the mediastinum. Sternotomy is generally well tolerated with patients ambulating almost immediately and having a hospital stay of approximately 3 days.

PATIENT SELECTION

Thymoma

Patients usually come to medical attention because of cough or nonspecific chest pain. Many patients are asymptomatic and are identified by the finding of a widened mediastinum on a routine chest x-ray. Chest CT readily identifies the lesion in the thymus. Usually the diagnosis is clear and biopsy is not necessary. Characteristically the lesion has a uniform density and may be lobulated. Masses that are associated with significant mediastinal adenopathy are more likely to be lymphoma and a biopsy may be necessary to distinguish the two. Other anterior mediastinal masses include thyroid, which may be identified by close association with one or both thyroid lobes, and germ cell tumors which are often more heterogeneous. The tumor markers α-fetoprotein and β-HCG may be obtained if a nonseminomatous germ cell tumor is suspected.

All patients with thymic neoplasms are candidates for resection. The chest CT should be reviewed carefully to determine the location and extent of disease. There is sufficient evidence to indicate that completeness of the resection is the most important prognostic factor for most stages of the disease.[9] The staging system most commonly used is the Masaoka–Koga system (Table 160-2) in which staging is determined by the degree of invasion of the capsule and surrounding structures.[10] Stages I and II are treated with operation. For patients with Stage III disease, if a complete resection is anticipated, then surgery is employed.[9] If not, the patients are treated with preoperative chemotherapy followed by surgery.[9] To ensure complete resection, especially in Stage III, the transsternal approach is advocated. Minimally invasive approaches have been proposed, and may be suitable for smaller, lower stage tumors. However, as the overall outcome of thymoma resection is measured by 10-year survival rates, a long period of follow-up will be required to assess the oncologic efficacy of such procedures.

Myasthenia Gravis

Patients with MG are most often under the care of a neurologist and are managed with anticholinergics such as pyridostigmine bromide (Mestinon®), often accompanied by steroids (prednisone). Other immunosuppressants such as azathioprine and mycophenolate mofetil may be used in some patients.

Table 160-2

MASAOKA–KOGA STAGING SYSTEM[10]

STAGE	DEFINITION
I	Grossly and microscopically completely encapsulated tumor
IIa	Microscopic transcapsular invasion
IIb	Macroscopic invasion into thymic or surrounding fatty tissue, or grossly adherent to but not breaking through mediastinal pleura or pericardium
III	Macroscopic invasion into neighboring organs (i.e., pericardium, great vessel, or lung)
IVa	Pleural or pericardial metastases
IVb	Lymphogenous or hematogenous metastases

Once a candidate is identified, every effort should be made to minimize immunosuppressants, especially steroids, prior to surgery, while maintaining acceptable control of symptoms. Intravenous immunoglobulin (IVIG) may be administered in the preoperative period to help optimize patients. As respiratory complications are common in these patients, pulmonary function tests are useful. A chest CT is indicated because of the incidence of associated thymoma. For those patients who present with overwhelming MG symptoms and respiratory compromise (myasthenic crisis), ventilator support with additional immunosuppressants and plasmapheresis may be required to optimize patients. Such individuals are at highest risk for postoperative morbidity and mortality.

PREOPERATIVE PREPARATION

When performing a thymectomy for MG, the perioperative strategy must be a collaborative effort between the respiratory therapists, primary care physician, neurologist, anesthesiologist, intensivist, and surgeon. The problems associated with postoperative care can be directly correlated to the severity of symptoms at the time of operation.[11] Unless patients require preoperative parenteral steroids, hemodynamic stabilization, or plasmapheresis, they can be admitted to the hospital on the day of surgery. In general, anticholinesterase agents (pyridostigmine bromide) should be discontinued 8 hours prior to operation. Discontinuing these medications any earlier, especially in patients with severe myasthenia, can result in a myasthenic crisis, whereas continuing the medications, particularly in patients with mild symptoms, can result in a postoperative cholinergic crisis. In severe cases, an additional intramuscular injection of a small dose of pyridostigmine bromide can be administered just before the operation. Alternatively a continuous infusion of neostigmine may be used in severe cases (total daily dose = total daily dose of pyridostigmine bromide divided by 60).[12] If the patient is on steroids or has received them in the previous few months, perioperative parenteral steroid coverage is provided, beginning with 100 mg of hydrocortisone 1 hour before surgery and continuing every 8 hours for the first 24 hours, then tapered to the preoperative dose. Perioperative antibiotics are administered within 1 hour of the procedure. Usually a first-generation cephalosporin (e.g., cefazolin) suffices. Aminoglycoside antibiotics are contraindicated because they increase the neuromuscular block.

Technique

Anesthesia

A thoracic epidural catheter is often useful for postoperative analgesia. General anesthesia can be performed safely with selective use of agents that do not potentiate the neuromuscular defect. Chemical paralysis is not required for sternotomy. Neuromuscular blocking agents, especially competitive (nondepolarizing) agents should be avoided because of the long-lasting adverse effects on myasthenic patients. Myasthenic patients are very sensitive to the administration of nondepolarizing agents which could result in prolonged postoperative respiratory failure. If needed for intubation, a small dose of a noncompetitive depolarizing agent (succinylcholine) may be used.

Surgical Management

The patient is positioned supine on the operating table and general anesthesia is induced with a single-lumen tube. A double-lumen tube is not necessary. A urinary catheter is placed. An arterial catheter is helpful. A rolled sheet is placed horizontally behind the shoulders. This places the sternum in a horizontal plane. The head and neck may require additional padding to make their position neutral. The arms are padded and tucked at the sides. The neck, chest, and abdomen are prepped and draped. The sternal notch and the xiphoid process are marked. The interspaces are also palpated and a mark placed midway between them. A vertical line connecting these is drawn and the incision is made. The skin incision begins about 2 cm below the sternal notch at approximately the level of the angle of Louis and ends at the inferior border of the xiphoid. Subcutaneous tissue is divided with the knife or electrocautery by palpating the interspaces and spreading the incision while the electrocautery gently "glides" over the tissue, dividing it cleanly and in the midline. This continues until the pectoral fascia is reached. The superior border of the incision is retracted, and the tissue at the sternal notch is divided. There is a large crossing vein in this area which can be avoided by staying close to the manubrium. The interclavicular ligament along the superior border of the manubrium is divided, taking care not to venture too deeply, lest the trachea be encountered. A finger is placed around the notch and a plane of dissection established posterior to the manubrium. The inferior portion of the incision is developed by dividing the linea alba and entering the preperitoneal space. The xiphoid is also divided. Portions of the xiphoid may be calcified and can be divided sharply. A plane is established by blunt finger dissection beneath the inferior border of the sternum. The midline is developed by separating the decussation of the pectoral muscle fibers. This usually (but not always) delineates the midline. The midline can also be determined by palpating the interspaces and marking the midpoint between them. The midline is marked with the electrocautery superficially in the periosteum, especially inferiorly where several small crossing arteries can cause annoying bleeding. The lungs are deflated and the sternum is divided with a saw. This is usually done from superior to inferior, but may be done in the opposite direction depending on the preference of the surgeon. If the xiphoid is calcified or otherwise encumbering, it may be resected at this point. The lungs are reinflated and a laparotomy pad is packed under the sternum. Bleeding points along the edges of the periosteum are cauterized (both anterior and posterior). Hemostasis of the bone marrow is achieved with thrombin Gelfoam® paste or similar material. Bone wax is avoided because it remains in the incision for a long time and can be associated with an increased risk of infection. The sternal halves are elevated and muscular attachments are divided both superiorly (strap muscles) and inferiorly (rectus muscles) to permit better separation of the sternal halves. A sternal retractor is inserted and the sternum is spread.

The standard boundaries for a full thymectomy are the diaphragm inferiorly, the phrenic nerves laterally, and the thyrothymic ligaments superiorly (Fig. 160-3A). Again, the surgeon should be mindful of the areas beyond these boundaries where thymic tissue is often found. Dissection is usually begun on the right. The pleural cavity is opened anteriorly and widely. The lung is packed with a moist warm laparotomy pad. In patients with thymoma, the entire pleural cavity is inspected, including the hemidiaphragm and hilum for any evidence of tumor spread. The mediastinal pleura is incised 1 cm anterior to the phrenic nerve (Fig. 160-3B). Extreme caution is advised because the nerve courses medially in the superior portion of the field. The lateral edge of the incised pleura is elevated and any fatty tissue deep to the phrenic nerve is carefully swept anteromedially. Occasionally small branches of the pericardiophrenic vessels can cause bleeding. These may be packed, clipped, or controlled with the ultrasonic shears but electrocautery should be strictly avoided. All fatty tissue is swept anteriorly and superiorly. Sharp dissection is used to separate the gland from the pericardium. If the pericardium is densely adherent (such as in a thymoma), it is resected with the thymus.

The left side of the gland is addressed in similar fashion with some minor differences. Inferiorly, the phrenic nerve is more posterior and may be more difficult to see, especially if the ventricle is prominent (Fig. 160-3C). Rotating the operating table to the right and placing gentle traction on the pericardium may improve exposure. More superiorly the nerve again is medial and can be injured.

The gland and mediastinal fat are separated from the pericardium by sharp dissection and swept superiorly (Fig. 160-3D). The branches from the internal mammary artery are usually small and can be ligated or sealed with the ultrasonic shears, again taking care to avoid the phrenic nerve. Division of the arterial branches allows the en bloc specimen to be rotated upward, exposing the undersurface of the gland and the draining veins (Fig. 160-3E). In the sulcus between the superior vena cava and the aorta, fatty tissue may be found, and this is dissected en bloc with the specimen. Tissue may also be found deep to the left brachiocephalic vein and this is removed also. In the region of aortopulmonary window there is often additional thymic tissue. Great care is taken in dissecting this area to avoid phrenic nerve injury. Furthermore, the recurrent laryngeal nerve is also in this area and may be injured. The venous tributaries of the thymus are ligated and divided.

The superior horns are now dissected. In this region, the lateral boundaries between thymic tissue and other mediastinal fat are often indistinct. The thymus is retracted inferiorly and blunt dissection is performed in a superior direction, deep to the sternothyroid muscles, with a Küttner dissector (Fig. 160-3F). This reveals the thyrothymic ligaments. They contain small branches of the inferior thyroid vessels, which are ligated and divided.

The resected specimen should include all fatty thymic tissue, thyrothymic ligaments, and mediastinal pleural sheets. The wide mediastinal exposure obtained by opening both pleural spaces not only ensures complete thymus removal but also helps safeguard the phrenic and vagus nerves.

In patients with thymic neoplasms, gross evidence of invasiveness is the most important prognostic sign of malignancy. Malignant thymic tumors are notorious for local extension and lack of distant metastases as well as a deceptively benign appearance on microscopic examination. When a thymoma is present, the same extensive removal of thymic tissue is performed *en bloc* with the thymoma. If the pericardium, lungs, brachiocephalic vein, or sternal periosteum are adherent to the tumor, they are removed en bloc, because tumor invasion can be present.

In patients with thymoma, invasion of a phrenic nerve may be encountered and a decision will be required as to whether to sacrifice the nerve. Preoperative assessment, including analysis

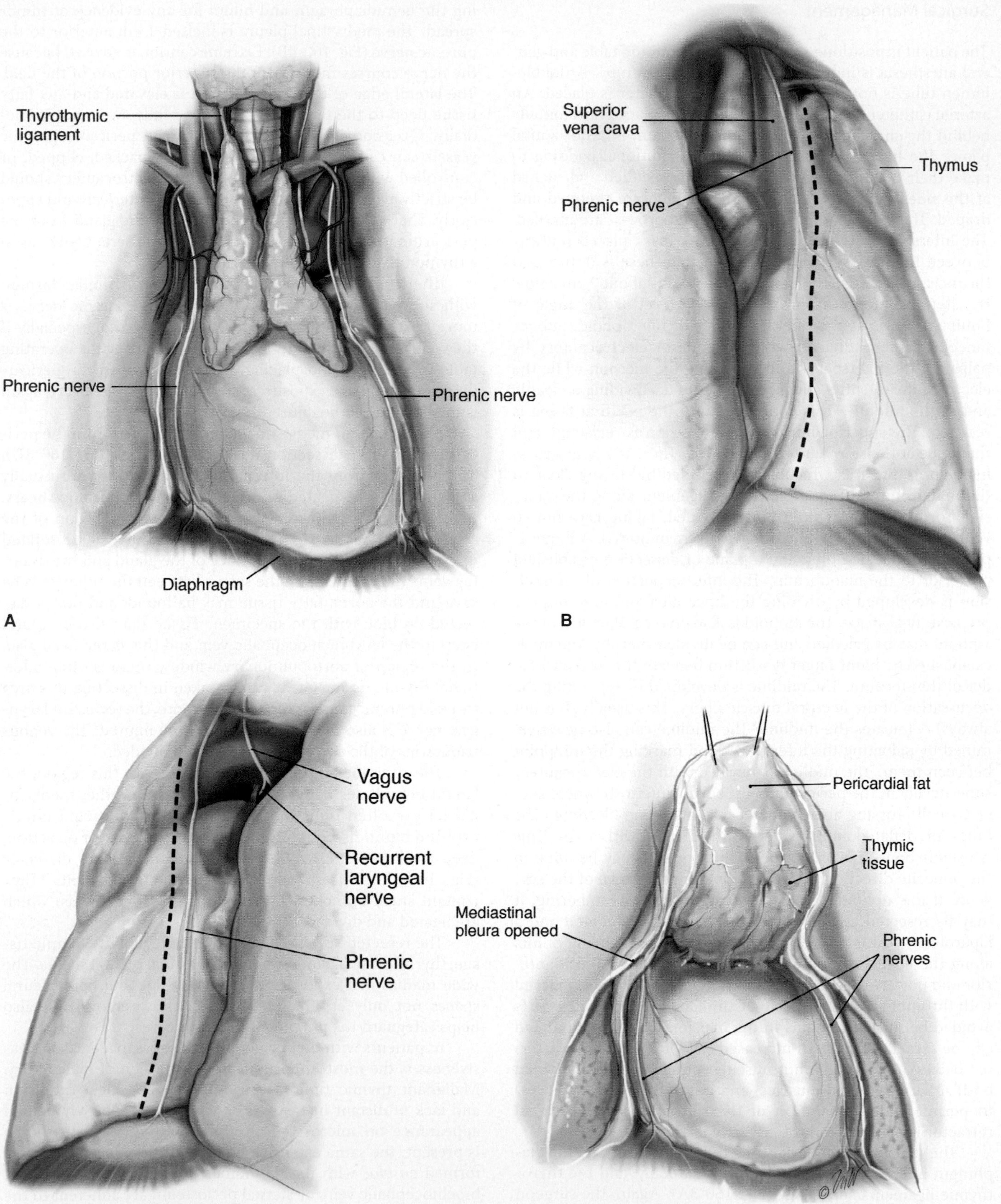

Figure 160-3. *A.* Median sternotomy gives excellent exposure of the thymus. The boundaries of resection are the diaphragm inferiorly, phrenic nerves laterally, and the thyrothymic ligaments superiorly. *B.* The dissection is begun on the right side. An incision is made 1 cm anterior to the phrenic nerve. All tissue is swept toward the midline. *C.* On the left, the phrenic nerve may be more readily exposed with table positioning and traction on the pericardium. Note the position of the vagus and recurrent laryngeal nerves. *D.* The thymus, along with the adherent mediastinal pleura, is elevated from the pericardium and separated from the phrenic nerves bilaterally. (*continued*)

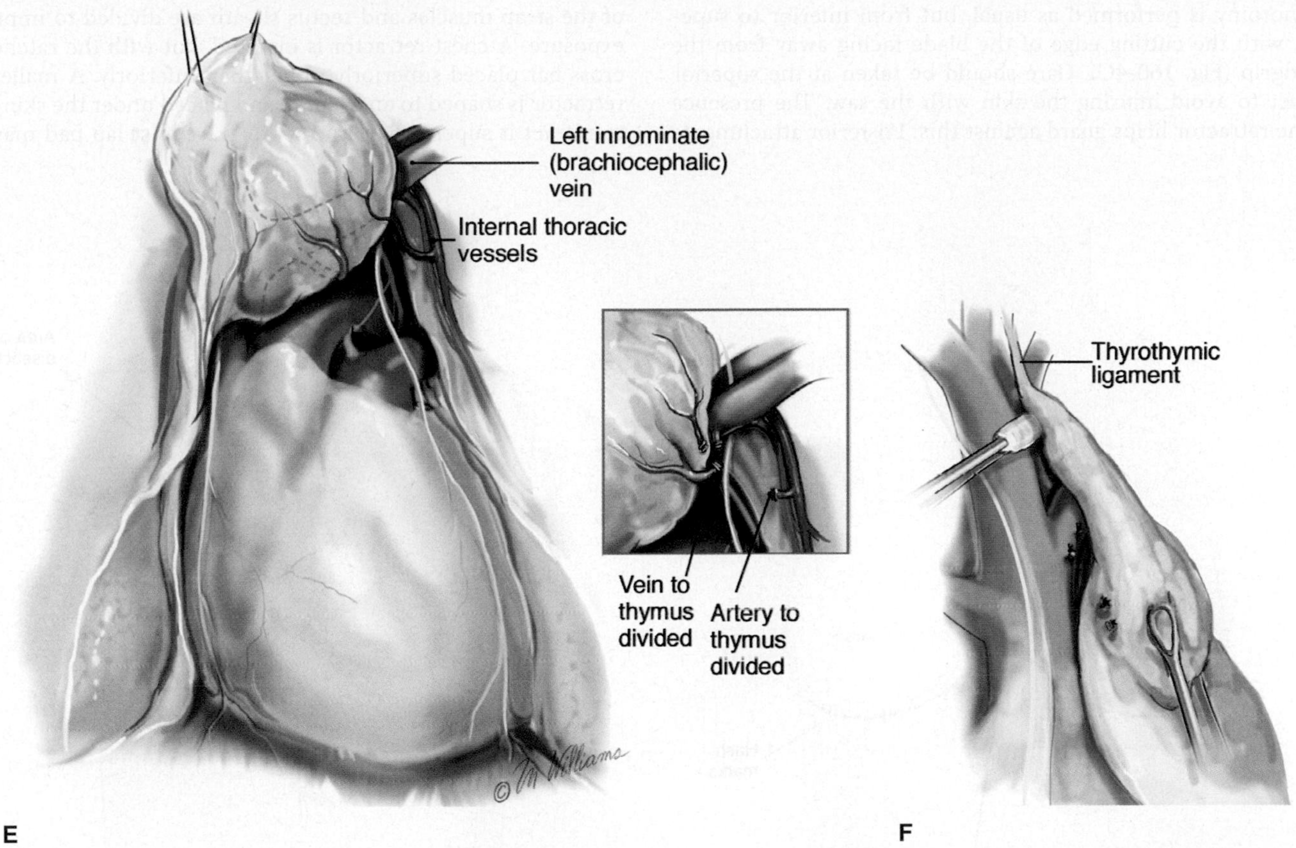

Figure 160-3. (*Continued*) *E.* Division of the branches from the internal thoracic arteries allows the en bloc specimen to be rotated upward, exposing the undersurface of the gland and the draining veins. (*Inset*) The left brachiocephalic vein is exposed and the thymic veins isolated and divided between ligatures or clips. *F.* Gentle inferior traction on the thymus facilitates dissection of the superior horns. The thyrothymic ligaments are dissected with a Küttner dissector, then ligated and divided.

of pulmonary function tests, will help guide the decision-making. A nonfunctional nerve may be resected. Likewise, a patient with good pulmonary function can tolerate a unilateral nerve resection. Otherwise, postoperative radiation can be used to control residual unresected tumor.

After resection of the gland, the area is surveyed for potential additional thymic tissue. Any bleeding points are secured. Drainage tubes are placed in both pleural spaces. These may be conventional chest tubes or large round multichannel silastic drains (e.g., #19 or #24). They are exited inferolaterally. The sternum is closed with heavy steel wire, such as #6 or #7. The wires are twisted and buried in the tissue. The remainder of the incision is closed in layers. Careful attention to sternal closure is important, especially for patients who are receiving steroids.

Cosmetic Technique

In young women with cosmetic concerns, a radical transsternal thymectomy is still possible using the bilateral submammary skin incision popularized by Laks and Hammond.[13] The authors have used this approach for the last two decades and have found it to give excellent exposure of the mediastinum and thymus, including the thyrothymic ligaments. The technique is as follows.

The mammary crease is marked with the patient standing. Once anesthesia is induced, a pad is placed beneath the back to elevate the chest. Arms are tucked and padded appropriately, ensuring adequate access to the anterior axillary lines. The incision is marked and is actually placed about 5 mm below the mammary crease to avoid breast tissue (Fig. 160-4A). The apex of the incision should be at the level of the xiphisternal junction. A gentle curve is placed there rather than a pointed incision in order to preserve blood supply. The marking line is carried out to the anterior axillary line on each side, although this length of incision is usually not necessary. Several marks (hash marks) are placed at various intervals along the incision line and perpendicular to it in order to align the tissue properly for reapproximation at the close of the procedure.

The neck, chest, and abdomen are prepped and draped. The incision is carried out symmetrically to about the midclavicular line bilaterally. Additional length can be added, again symmetrically, if necessary. The incision is carried through subcutaneous tissue to the pectoral fascia. A plane of dissection is created superficial to the fascia on each side. This is first carried inferiorly for 1 to 2 cm for reapproximation later. The linea alba and xiphoid are divided at this point. The dissection is carried superiorly superficial to the pectoral fascia, progressively elevating the skin and subcutaneous tissue. Care is taken not to undermine the nipple–areolar complex which may cause sensory deficits in this area. The flap of skin and subcutaneous tissue raised resembles a bell-shaped curve, with its apex at the sternal notch (Fig. 160-4B). Dissection is continued until the sternal notch is reached. Dissection in the area of the notch may be facilitated with a right-angled clamp. The flap is retracted superiorly and midline is marked. The median sternotomy is performed as usual, but from inferior to superior, with the cutting edge of the blade facing away from the handgrip (Fig. 160-4C). Care should be taken at the superior aspect to avoid injuring the skin with the saw. The presence of the retractor helps guard against this. Posterior attachments of the strap muscles and rectus sheath are divided to improve exposure. A chest retractor is inserted, but with the ratcheted cross bar placed superiorly rather than inferiorly. A malleable retractor is shaped to an S-curve and placed under the skin flap to retract it superiorly (Fig. 160-4D). A moist lap pad may be

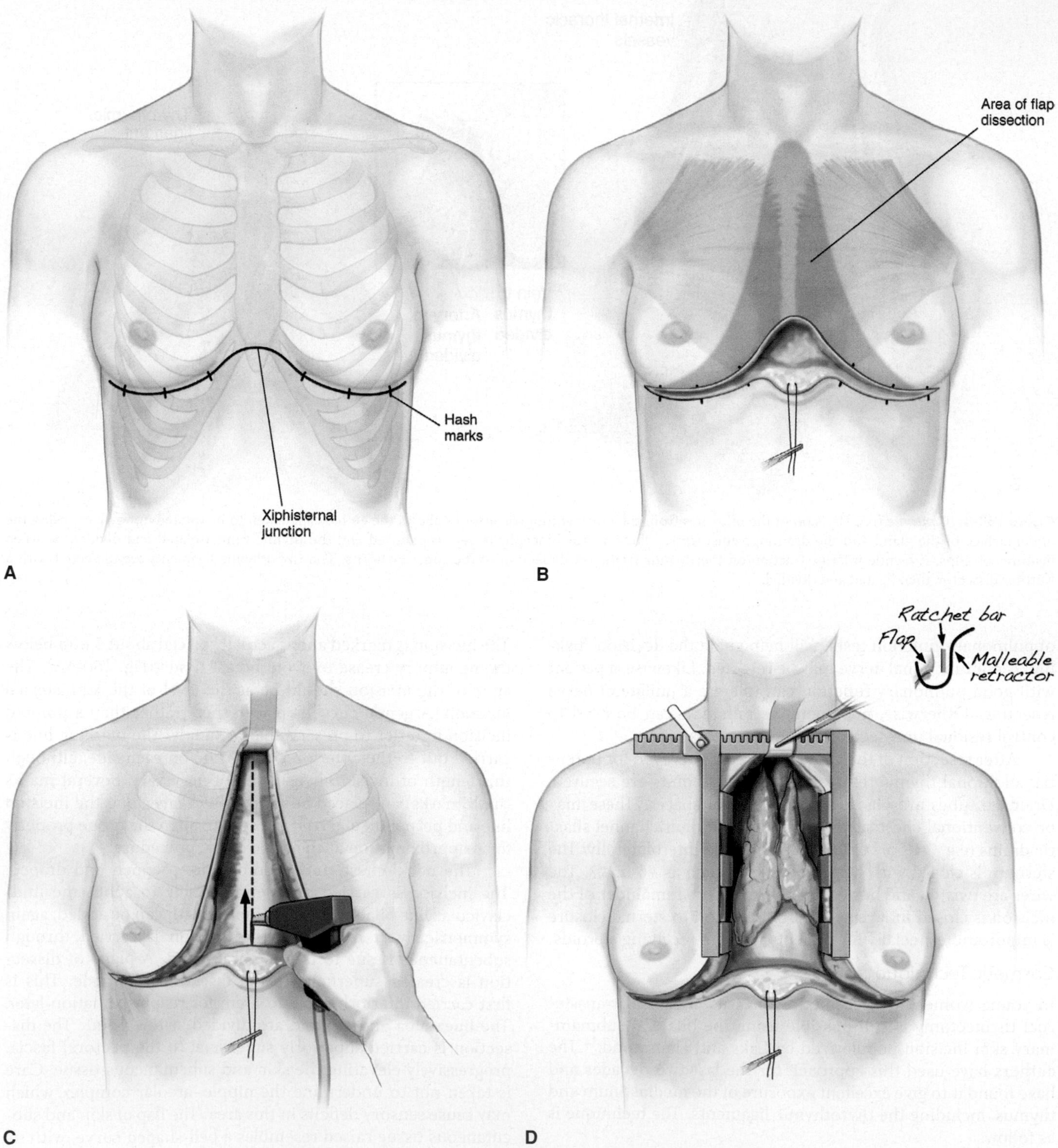

Figure 160-4. *A*. For the submammary technique, the mammary crease is identified with the patient standing. The incision is marked 5 mm below the crease. The apex of the incision is at the xiphisternal junction. Hash marks are placed at intervals to aid in reapproximating the tissue at closure. *B*. The flap is developed superficial to the pectoralis fascia, and carried superiorly in a "bell-shaped" curve, avoiding the undermining of the nipple–areolar complex. (*continued*)

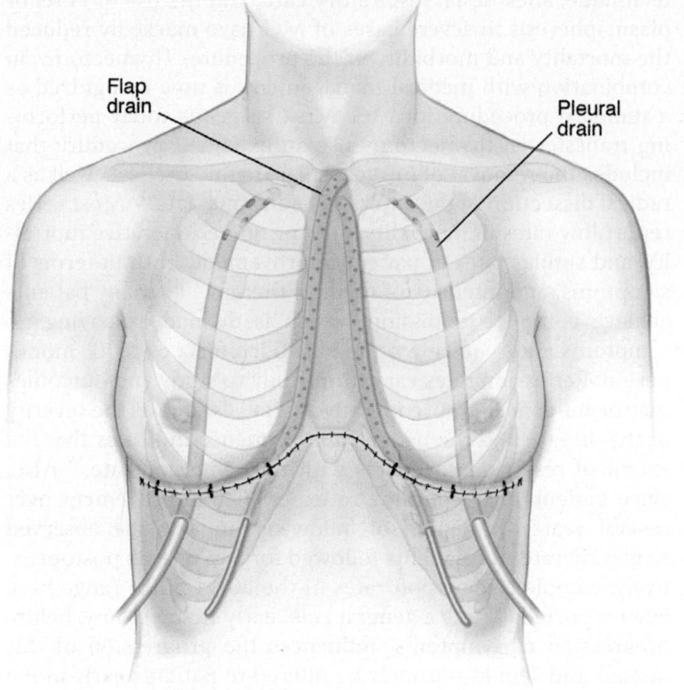

E

Figure 160-4. (*Continued*) *C.* The flap is retracted superiorly and the sternum is divided from inferior to superior. The cutting blade of the saw faces away from the handgrip. Care is taken to avoid injury to the skin with blade. *D.* The retractor is placed with the ratchet bar at the superior end of the incision. A malleable retractor is bent in an S-shape and retracts the superior border of the flap. A moist laparotomy pad may be used to cushion the flap. The retractor is secured to the ratchet bar with a Kocher clamp. Excellent exposure of the thymus is achieved. *E.* The completed procedure. Placement of pleural and flap drains is shown. Sternal wires are not shown.

placed to cushion the flap. The malleable is held in place against the cross bar using a Kocher clamp. This provides exposure to the most superior portion of the field. The thymectomy is performed as previously described. The surgeon will find that the thyrothymic ligaments are easily dissected and divided.

Closure is accomplished in the following manner. The pleural cavities are drained with large round Blake drains which are exited below the submammary incision on each side. The chest is closed with heavy steel wire. The wire ends are curved and twisted into the tissue on each side and pressed flat, typically with the flat end of the wire cutter. Musculofascial tissue may be approximated to cover the wires, although this tissue may be thin superiorly. The linea alba is reapproximated with absorbable suture.

The subcutaneous flap is drained with two #10 flat silastic drains, again exited below the incision line. The subcutaneous tissue is reapproximated with interrupted absorbable sutures using the "hash marks" to ensure proper alignment. Then, the subcutaneous tissue is run with absorbable suture. One or two layers may be used. The skin is closed with an absorbable subcuticular suture (Fig. 160-4E). Steri-strips® may be applied. A gauze dressing is applied, but need only be secured with tape inferiorly, thus keeping adhesive off the breast skin. The pleural drains may be placed to bulb suction or to a water seal drainage system using straight or Y-shaped connectors. The #10 flat drains are placed to bulb suction.

Postoperative care is as described below. The pleural drains may be removed within the first day or two. The flap drains are left in place until drainage is no more than 10 mL per day. The patient may be discharged with the drains in place and instructed to measure the drainage each day. The drains may be removed at a postoperative visit. Any seromas that form can be needle aspirated. Patients are counseled about paresthesias of the anterior chest, which usually resolve within a few weeks.

POSTOPERATIVE CARE

Patients are usually extubated in the operating room at the conclusion of the procedure. Fluids are administered moderately as there is little "third-spacing." An infusion rate of 3/4 to full calculated maintenance is sufficient. Urine output is monitored but is usually adequate. Nausea is uncommon, and patients can resume oral intake in the evening or the following day. Intravenous fluids are discontinued at that time. Perioperative antibiotics are discontinued within 24 hours. It is not necessary to continue these until the chest drains are removed, and there are no data to support this practice. Anticholinergic agents are resumed immediately after surgery. If the patient received a "stress dose" of steroid preoperatively, this is rapidly tapered down to the patient's preoperative dose. Pleural tubes are removed when the drainage has decreased to less than 200 to 300 mL per day. Assuming the lungs were handled with the usual gentleness, air leaks are rarely a problem.

Pain control in thymectomy patients is usually straightforward. Sternotomy incisions are associated with less pain than most other chest incisions. Epidural catheters, when present, are usually removed on the second postoperative day as oral analgesia is introduced. For those patients without epidural catheters, patient-controlled analgesia (PCA) pumps are effective and can be supplemented with parenteral ketorolac.

Tapering of medications in patients with MG begins at various times after operation, depending on the judgment of the neurologist caring for the patient. In most patients, tapering can be started in the early postoperative period. However, some patients require more gradual attempts at weaning. This situation is particularly true for patients on large preoperative doses of steroids and patients who had long-standing symptoms before the operation. Such individuals can require anywhere from weeks to months after the operation to begin a substantial tapering in dosage.

PROCEDURE-SPECIFIC COMPLICATIONS

For patients with pulmonary compromise preoperatively, especially patients with MG, postoperative pulmonary insufficiency is very common, with attendant ventilator dependence and possible pneumonia. Strict attention to pulmonary physiotherapy, including aerosol treatments, suctioning, postural drainage, percussion, and periodic bronchoscopy, is important. Measurement of forced vital capacity is the most useful tool to monitor pulmonary function perioperatively. Optimization of MG continues, including steroids and even plasmapheresis if needed. A postoperative myasthenic crisis is rare, but when it occurs, the patient is unable to maintain an open airway, clear secretions, or provide adequate ventilatory exchange because of failing muscle function. If the patient develops respiratory difficulties or signs of an exacerbation of myasthenic symptoms, a trial dose of edrophonium chloride should be given. If this medication results in prompt improvement in the patient's strength, small doses of a long-acting anticholinesterase drug such as pyridostigmine bromide (approximately one-thirtieth of the oral dose) should be cautiously administered by intramuscular or very slow intravenous injection until a salutary effect is achieved. The patient should be monitored for signs of overmedication. These include diaphoresis, muscle fasciculation, excessive salivation, myosis, and wheezing.[11] Stress doses of steroids should be used concomitantly. If rapid improvement does not ensue, plasmapheresis should be started and continued for 3 days and then every other day until symptoms can be controlled by oral medications.

Fortunately, the incidence of postoperative myasthenic crisis is rare today, likely reflecting sound preoperative management, and the mortality rate has declined markedly over time.[14] In the 1950s, the mortality rate of a patient with a myasthenic crisis was approximately 80%. It decreased to 6% in the 1970s, and 4% in 1994. This overall decrease in the mortality can be directly attributed to advances in the management of the critically ill patient.[14]

Another concerning postoperative complication is phrenic nerve injury. This can be devastating in a patient with MG. However, since the nerves are easily visualized, this complication should be avoidable in essentially all cases. Techniques to avoid nerve injury include (1) maintaining a 1-cm margin anterior to the nerves when incising the mediastinal pleura, especially superiorly; (2) avoiding traction on the nerve or pedicle when dissecting thymic tissue; (3) leaving small remnants of fatty (potentially thymic) tissue when found adherent to the phrenic pedicles; and (4) avoiding cautery of small bleeding points along the incised margin. A patient with a thymic neoplasm who has had a phrenic nerve resected may be observed postoperatively. If pulmonary compromise becomes apparent, a minimally invasive diaphragmatic plication may be performed.

One rare complication is that of recurrent laryngeal nerve injury. This can occur while dissecting thymic tissue in the aortopulmonary window. Here the phrenic and recurrent nerves are often close together and injury to either structure can occur. Extreme caution is observed while dissecting in this area.

RESULTS

Previously, the mortality and considerable morbidity associated with transsternal thymectomy in MG were primarily caused by respiratory complications. Improvements in the surgical technique, anesthesia, respiratory care, and the use of IVIG or plasmapheresis in severe cases of MG have markedly reduced the mortality and morbidity of the procedure. Thymectomy, in combination with medical management, is now recognized as a standard procedure for MG. Most surgeons today performing transsternal thymectomy use an extended procedure that includes the removal of intracapsular thymic tissue as well as a radical dissection of the anterior mediastinal fat.[5,15] Most series report low rates of morbidity, little or no perioperative mortality, and similar rates of patient improvement, both in terms of symptoms, and intensity of medical therapy.[15,16] Many patients achieve complete remission, which is defined as having no symptoms and requiring no medications for a 6- to 12-month period. Remission rates vary from study to study and outcomes may be influenced by preoperative variables such as the severity of the disease and the patient mix. Evidence indicates that the extent of resection correlates with the remission rate.[16] Also, since patients may continue to experience improvement over several years, the length of follow-up impacts the observed remission rate. For patients followed for 5 to 6 years postoperatively, complete remission rates in the 30% to 50% range have been reported.[15,16] As a general rule, early thymectomy, before progression of symptoms, influences the progression of this disease and should routinely be offered to patients early in the course of their disease.

Long-term outlook for patients with thymoma is very good following resection. Overall, the 10-year survival rate for Stages I and II is approximately 75% to 80% and for Stage III, 45%.[17] Long-term follow-up in these patients is important for optimal outcome.

SUMMARY

Radical transsternal thymectomy for both thymoma and MG can be accomplished with minimal morbidity and mortality. The overwhelming evidence that thymic tissue normally resides outside of the intracapsular thymus supports the use of an extended procedure that includes removal of the intracapsular thymic tissue as well as radical dissection of the anterior mediastinal fat. Open and cosmetic techniques are viable options. Minimally invasive approaches, such as transcervical, video thoracoscopic, and robotically assisted means have been developed and may demonstrate equivalent results when larger studies and longer follow-up are available.

ILLUSTRATED CASE HISTORY

A 61-year-old man noted ptosis as well as diplopia and his primary care physician referred him to an ophthalmologist who made a preliminary diagnosis of ocular MG. Subsequent neurologic evaluation revealed physical signs of generalized MG. The patient also noted some difficulty with chewing, excessive drooling, and a change in his speech to a more nasal tone. Laboratory testing showed a markedly elevated serum acetylcholine receptor antibody. He was treated with pyridostigmine bromide 60 mg four times daily, and noted some improvement, but was not at his baseline. The neurologist recommended a surgical evaluation for thymectomy. During the encounter, he became progressively weaker, had more difficulty keeping his head up, and phonation became more nasal. He denied any

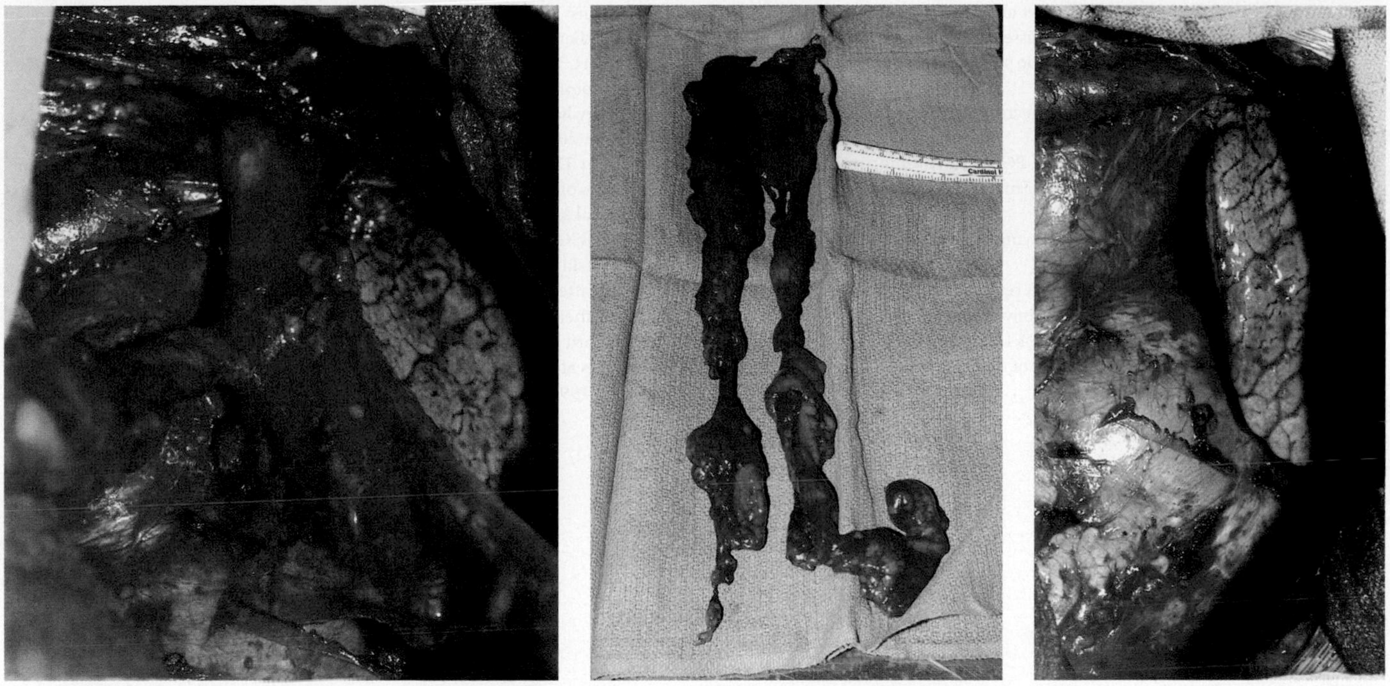

A B C

Figure 160-5. *A*. Dissection of thymus off of the brachiocephalic vein including the left pleura. *B*. Radical thymectomy specimen. *C*. Operative bed post-thymectomy.

other significant medical problems. A CT scan of the chest revealed no evidence of thymoma. Elective transsternal thymectomy was recommended.

In preparation for surgery the patient received an echocardiogram and pulmonary function testing which were normal. Electrolytes and a complete blood count were within normal limits. He was started on a beta blocker, atenolol 25 mg a day, beginning 1 week before surgery. An epidural catheter was placed perioperatively for pain management. He underwent an uncomplicated transsternal thymectomy that removed a 430 g thymus (Fig. 160-5A–C). He was extubated in the operating room and admitted to the intensive care unit on 2 L nasal cannula O_2. FVC was noted to be 800 mL. On the night of surgery, the patient was given an intravenous dose of pyridostigmine bromide which improved his respiratory effort. On the morning of the first postoperative day, he was started on clear liquids and restarted on his oral medications. A repeat FVC was noted to be 1.2 L. Later that day he was transferred to a surgical floor and advanced to a regular diet. On postoperative day 2, the patient sat in a chair without difficulty. His lungs were fully expanded on his postoperative chest x-ray. Output from the chest tubes was less than 150 mL per shift without an air leak, and they were removed. This was followed by removal of the epidural and urinary catheters. The patient ambulated without difficulty and tolerated a regular diet. He was discharged to home on the third postoperative day on oral narcotic analgesics as well as his preoperative pyridostigmine and atenolol. Final histology on the thymectomy specimen revealed thymic hyperplasia with germinal centers.

Over the course of the next 6 months, the patient noted moderate subjective improvement in his muscle strength. The ptosis and diplopia resolved. His neurologist successfully tapered the pyridostigmine bromide down to 30 mg QID with plans to continue a gradual taper as long as the patient continued to improve.

EDITOR'S COMMENT

The traditional argument for radical thymectomy is the infrequent, but real, incidence of ectopic or discontinuous thymic tissue. In addition, visual inspection is frequently inaccurate; that is, the thymus gland may resemble the surrounding fat tissue and microscopic thymic tissue cannot be grossly identified. The argument against radical thymectomy is that most patients do not need a radical dissection; certainly, the relative benefit of the operation for most patients is unclear. Furthermore, some of the potential sites of ectopic thymic tissue (roughly paralleling the potential sites of ectopic parathyroid tissue) are not addressed even with radical thymectomy. Perhaps reflecting an acknowledgment of both arguments, most surgeons are selective in their use of radical thymectomy.

—Steven J. Mentzer

References

1. Jaretzki A III. Thymectomy for myasthenia gravis: an analysis of the controversies regarding technique and results. *Neurology.* 1997;48(suppl 5):S52–S63.
2. Blalock A, Mason MF, Morgan HJ, et al. Myasthenia gravis and tumors of the thymic region. *Ann Surg.* 1939;110(4):544–561.
3. Calhoun RF, Ritter JH, Guthrie TJ, et al. Results of transcervical thymectomy for myasthenia gravis in 100 consecutive patients. *Ann Surg.* 1999;230(4):555–559.
4. Jaretzki A, Steinglass KM, Sonett JR. Thymectomy in the management of myasthenia gravis. *Semin Neurol.* 2004;24(1):49–62.

5. Stern LE, Nussbaum MS, Quinlan JG, et al. Long-term evaluation of extended thymectomy with anterior mediastinal dissection. *Surgery.* 2001;130(4):774–778.
6. Zielinski M. Management of myasthenic patients with thymoma. *Thorac Surg Clin.* 2011;21(1):47–57.
7. Jaretzki A III, Wolf M. "Maximal" thymectomy for myasthenia gravis. *J Thorac Cardiovasc Surg.* 1988;96(5):711–716.
8. Cooper JD, Al-Jilaihawa AN, Pearson FG, et al. An improved technique to facilitate transcervical thymectomy for myasthenia gravis. *Ann Thorac Surg.* 1988;45(3):242–247.
9. Venuta F, Anile M, Disco D, et al. Thymoma and thymic carcinoma. *Eur J Cardiothorac Surg.* 2010;37(1):13–25.
10. Koga K, Matsuno Y, Noguchi M, et al. A review of 79 thymomas: modification of staging system and reappraisal of conventional division into invasive and non-invasive thymoma. *Pathol Int.* 1994;445(5):359–367.
11. Kernstine K. Preoperative preparation of the patient with myasthenia gravis. *Thorac Surg Clin.* 2005;15(2):287–295.
12. Wilkins KB, Bulkley GB. Thymectomy in the integrated management of myasthenia gravis. *Adv Surg.* 1999;32:105–133.
13. Laks H, Hammond GL. A cosmetically acceptable incision for the median sternotomy. *J Thorac Cardiovasc Surg.* 1980;79(1):146–149.
14. Keesey JC. Clinical evaluation and management of myasthenia gravis. *Muscle Nerve.* 2004;29(4):484–505.
15. Meyer DM, Herbert MA, Sobhani NC, et al. Comparative clinical outcomes of thymectomy for myasthenia gravis performed by extended transsternal and minimally invasive approaches. *Ann Thorac Surg.* 2009;87(2):385–390.
16. Zielinski M, Hauer L, Hauer J, et al. Comparison of complete remission rates after 5 year follow-up of three different techniques of thymectomy for myasthenia gravis. *Eur J Cardiothorac Surg.* 2010;37(5):1137–1143.
17. Regnard J-F, Magdeleinat P, Dromer C, et al. Prognostic factors and long-term results after thymoma resection: a series of 307 patients. *J Thorac Cardiovasc Surg.* 1996;112(2):376–384.

161 Resection of Benign Anterior and Middle Mediastinal Cysts and Tumors

Ciaran J. McNamee

Keywords: Endocrine tumors, benign thymic tumors, teratoma, mediastinal cysts (i.e., bronchogenic, pericardial, foregut, and thymic cysts), benign mediastinal mesenchymal tumors, Castleman disease

Primary benign anterior and middle mediastinal tumors arise from mediastinal structures either as benign neoplastic processes or as a result of inflammation. They may also occur as a result of local extension of adjacent compartment organ growth into the neighboring space or as a result of the arrest of embryonic cells traversing this compartment with later tumor growth. Uncommon primary mediastinal tumors usually are of mesenchymal origin. These tumors represent fewer than 10% of primary mediastinal tumors and have a higher prevalence and malignant potential in children.[1]

Primary mediastinal tumors are divided for the convenience of diagnosis and surgical approach into three compartments: anterior, middle, and posterior. Each compartment is defined by theoretic anatomic borders (Fig. 161-1) and each is specific for certain tumors. These compartments are described as follows.

Anterior mediastinum: This compartment is bounded anteriorly by the sternum and posteriorly by the pericardium, the aorta, and the brachiocephalic vessels. The thoracic inlet comprises the superior border, and the inferior border is demarcated by the diaphragm. Tumors in the superior aspect of this compartment largely derive from tissues native to or passing through this compartment or extending down from the neck. Tumors in the inferior aspect consist primarily of hernias that extend superiorly from the abdomen or pericardial fat pad extensions or pericardial or mesothelial cysts.

Middle mediastinum: This compartment is bounded by the anterior and posterior reflections of the pericardium, and it stretches from the thoracic inlet to the diaphragm. It is probably best described as the space that lies between the anterior and posterior mediastinum.

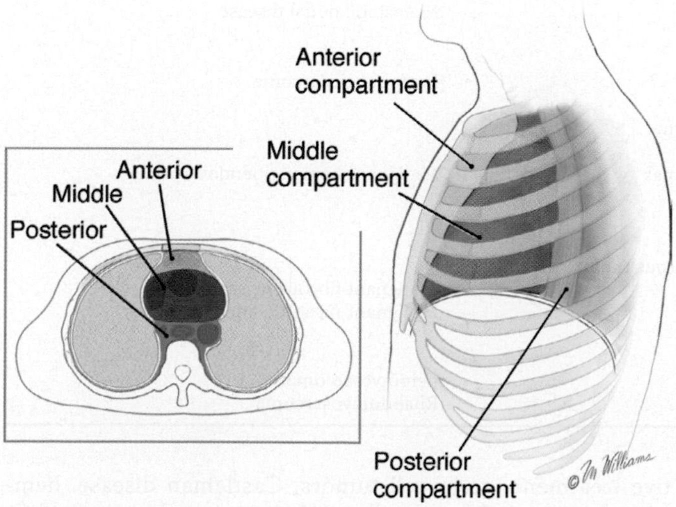

Figure 161-1. Mediastinal tumors are divided for the convenience of diagnosis and surgical approach into three compartments: anterior, middle, and posterior.

Posterior mediastinum: This compartment is defined anteriorly by the posterior trachea and the pericardium and it extends to the vertebral column including the paraspinal areas with vertical dimensions from the apex of the thoracic cavity to the diaphragm.

This chapter focuses on benign anterior and middle mediastinal tumors and the common surgical methods used to deal with these tumors. It should be noted that histologic overlap may occur between benign and malignant tumors arising from similar tissues in the same compartment as noted in Table 161-1. In addition, it may be clinically and pathologically difficult to distinguish a benign from a malignant mediastinal mass (even if cystic) until the specimen has been removed and fully examined pathologically.

The differentiation on clinical grounds between benign and malignant mediastinal tumors is dependent on three major factors: mediastinal location, patient age, and the presence or absence of symptoms.[2,3] Younger patients are more likely to suffer from neurogenic tumors (the majority are benign), lymphomas, or germ cell tumors (the majority are benign teratomas) compared with older patients, who tend to have anterior mediastinal tumors, which are more often malignant.[4–8] Benign tumors are commonly asymptomatic; thus they often are discovered as incidental findings accompanying parallel investigations for other health problems. Malignant tumors are commonly symptomatic,[3,5] possibly related to tumor size, complications of local compression, or systemic symptoms. Malignant mediastinal tumor product expression (e.g., adrenocorticotropic hormone, β-human chorionic gonadotropin, α-fetoprotein, calcium, parathyroid hormone, and acetylcholine receptor antibody levels) or the systemic consequences of these tumors (e.g., myasthenia gravis, pure red blood cell anemia, and agammaglobulinemia), may be indicative of the malignant potential in a mediastinal mass.

The pragmatic value of preoperative confirmation of benign from malignant mediastinal disease impacts not only survival and tumor recurrence but also allows for greater freedom with respect to surgical approaches. Surgical standards mandate the use of larger incisions for malignant mediastinal tumors to allow for tumor removal without local dissemination and to account for factors of size, diffuse adherence, hypervascularity, and local invasion to adjacent structures.[9] However, this is not the case for benign tumors, where with respect to surgical approach the only constraints are complete tumor removal, patient safety, and procedural morbidity.

Radiographic presentations of these tumors are often nonspecific and may be difficult to distinguish from malig-

Table 161-1

BENIGN AND MALIGNANT TUMORS OF THE ANTERIOR AND MIDDLE MEDIASTINUM

BENIGN TUMORS	BENIGN WITH POSSIBLE MALIGNANT ASSOCIATION	MALIGNANT TUMORS
Thymic origin		
Thymic hyperplasia		
Lymphoid (follicular)		
True hyperplasia		
Idiopathic		
Rebound		
Thymic cysts	Thymic cyst associated with thymoma	Thymoma
		Thymic carcinoma
Thymolipoma	Thymic neuroendocrine tumor	
Germ cell origin		
Teratoma	Cystic teratoma with malignant elements	Malignant germ cell tumor
Immature teratoma (<15 yrs)		Seminoma
Mature teratoma with <50% immature elements		Nonseminomatous germ cell tumor
		Teratoma with malignant transformation
Mesothelial cysts		
Bronchogenic cysts		Malignant bronchogenic cysts
Esophageal duplication cysts		Malignant esophageal duplication cysts
Pericardial cysts		
Hydatid cysts		
Endocrine cell origin		
Ectopic thyroid		
Mediastinal thyroid goiter		Mediastinal thyroid cancer
Parathyroid adenoma		Mediastinal parathyroid cancer
Parathyroid hyperplasia		
Parathyroid mediastinal cyst		
Paragangliomas		
	Chemodectoma (nonsecreting)	Malignant paraganglioma
	Paraganglioma (functioning)	
Neurogenic origin		
Benign nerve sheath tumors		Malignant nerve sheath tumors
Schwannoma (Neurilemmoma)		Malignant schwannomas
Neurofibroma		Malignant Neurofibromas
		Neurogenic fibrosarcomas
Sympathetic nerve origin		
Ganglioneuroma	Neuroblastoma	
	Ganglioneuroblastoma	
Mesenchymal tumors		
Adipose tissue		
Lipoma		
Lipoblastoma		Liposarcoma
Hibernoma		
Vascular/congenital tissue		
Congenital vascular anomalies		
Nodal enlargement		
Inflammatory causes		
Lymphoma		Metastatic nodal disease
Granulomatous causes		
Castleman disease		
Lymphangioma (cystic hygroma in children)		Lymphangiosarcoma
Lymphangiomatosis		
Hemangioma	Hemangioendothelioma	
Hemangiopericytoma	Angiosarcoma	
Epithelioid	Hemangioendotheliomas	Malignant hemangioendothelioma
Lymphangiohemangioma		
Fibrous tissue		
Fibromatosis	Fibrosarcoma	
Solitary fibrous tumor	Malignant solitary fibrous tumor	
		Malignant fibrous histiocytoma
		Malignant mesothelioma
Muscle tissue		
Angiomyolipoma		
Leiomyoma		Leiomyosarcoma
Rhabdomyoma		Rhabdomyosarcoma

nant tumors as outlined in Table 161-2.[10] However, serum tumor markers, contrast enhancement, and ultrasound or CT-guided mediastinal biopsy may help to distinguish malignant from benign tumors.[11] This is particularly important for mediastinal tumors which may benefit from preoperative treatment (germ cell tumors, Castleman disease, hemangiomas, and thymomas) and for tumors that are generally treated nonsurgically (lymphomas and multicentric Castleman disease). MRI is often used to determine the presence of vascular anatomy or tumor invasion and PET scan

Table 161-2

RADIOGRAPHIC CHARACTERISTICS OF CYSTIC ANTERIOR AND MIDDLE MEDIASTINAL MASSES

CYSTIC	FAT DENSITY	CYSTIC WITH SOLID COMPONENT	SOLID
Teratoma	Teratoma	Teratoma	Germ cell tumor
Thymic cyst	Thymoma lipoma	Thymoma with cyst	Thymoma or cancer
Foregut cyst	Morgagni hernia	Thyroid	Thyroid goiter
Pericardial cyst	Lymphoma		
Parathyroid adenoma	Inflammatory disease with abscess		
CONTRAST DELINEATION FOR DETERMINATION OF ANTERIOR AND MIDDLE MEDIASTINAL MASSES			
Contrast enhancement	HIDA scan	PET scan	Octreotide scan
Vascular abnormalities			
Parathyroid adenomas	Parathyroid adenoma		
Castleman disease			
Mesenchymal vascular tumors			

may be helpful to distinguish benign from malignant thymic conditions.[12,13]

BENIGN ANTERIOR MEDIASTINAL TUMORS

Benign anterior mediastinal tumors commonly comprise benign thymic masses, endocrine tumors, teratomas (benign), lymphoid hyperplasia or uncommon mesenchymal tumors.

Thymic Tumors

Benign thymic tumors consist of thymic hyperplasia, thymic cysts, thymolipomas, and lymphoepithelial thymomas. The management of diffuse thymic enlargement, if not associated with systemic autoimmune disease or parathymic symptoms, may depend on the presence or absence of symptoms which may denote true thymic pathology warranting thymic biopsy or thymectomy. In a review of asymptomatic, diffusely enlarged thymus glands, symptomatic patients were found in 22% of cases to have underlying malignancy, whereas no malignancy was found in asymptomatic patients.[14]

a. True thymic hyperplasia which is present when there is an increase in the normal components of the thymus gland and the normal organoid framework of the thymus gland is maintained. This type of hyperplasia may occur as a result of rebound thymic reconstitution following thymic depletion associated with antiretroviral therapy, following chemotherapy or stress, as an idiopathic condition, or in association with autoimmune diseases such as hyperthyroidism.[15]
b. Lymphofollicular thymic hyperplasia occurs in conjunction with increased lymphocytic B cell follicular production within germinal centers. It is associated with expanded B and T cell populations that lie outside the normal epithelial framework of the gland and is typically associated with systemic autoimmune disease such as myasthenia gravis.[16]

The separation of true thymic hyperplasia from lymphofollicular thymic hyperplasia is important therapeutically, since surgical resection of the thymus gland is beneficial only for hyperplasia associated with myasthenia gravis or other parathymic syndromes.[17] It is recommended that surgery for thymic hyperplasia (described in Chapters 137–139) should be performed only after resolution of the hypothyroid state unless signs of malignancy are present (invasion, calcifications, cysts, or septations).[18] Thymic cysts may be congenital or acquired.[19,20] The congenital form is usually unilocular, whereas the acquired form is generally multilocular and accompanied by inflammation. Malignancy is uncommonly associated with thymic cysts.[21,22] Thymic cysts present a clinical dilemma in distinguishing between benign thymic cysts and tumors with cystic degeneration occurring with invasive thymoma. The treatment of thymic cysts is controversial, as to whether they should be followed, aspirated, or removed. Excision is suggested if a thymic tumor cannot be excluded.

Thymolipoma is an uncommon benign hamartomatous tumor of the thymus composed of mature adipose cells and lymphoepithelial cells in various proportions. It may be associated with autoimmune-induced systemic diseases such as Graves disease, pure red blood cell neoplasia, aplastic anemia, hypogammaglobulinemia, myasthenia gravis, and Hodgkin disease. The etiology of this tumor is unknown; calcifications and cystic degeneration may occur, in the lymphoepithelial component, which may lead to the diagnosis of a mediastinal lipoma. Surgical resection is the treatment of choice which may also resolve accompanying systemic autoimmune symptoms.[23,24]

Endocrine Tumors

Substernal or intrathoracic goiter may account for anywhere between 3% and 6% of mediastinal masses. These goiters rarely receive their blood supply from mediastinal vessels.[25] Surgery for mediastinal goiter is described in Chapter 136. Ectopic thyroid glands can also present in the mediastinum with compressive symptomatology.[26]

Parathyroid adenomas can occur in the mediastinum; 20% of patients with parathyroid adenomas have tumors that extend into the mediastinum, but most can be extracted by a neck incision. Parathyroid cysts are rare (106 cases reported worldwide)[27] and usually associated with the inferior parathyroid glands; the majority occupy the middle mediastinum and the rest lay in the anterior mediastinum. These cysts are classified as functioning or nonfunctioning on the basis of elevated serum parathyroid hormone levels.[27] Mediastinal and neck exploration is necessary for functioning ectopic mediastinal parathyroid adenomas or cysts, which occur in 2% of patients; such glands may be reached by thoracoscopic exploration.[28] Nonfunctioning parathyroid cysts can be either removed, aspirated, or sclerosed[1,27]; removal is recommended for all functioning cysts and those that are large enough to cause compressive symptoms or recur after aspiration. Accurate preoperative localization of these glands can be obtained with selective venous sampling for parathyroid hormone levels, technetium sestamibi scans, CT scans of the chest and neck, or combined sestamibi CT scans which, if positive, also can aid with intraoperative localization by gamma probe thoracoscopic identification of the tumor. Confirmation of tumor removal may be achieved by intraoperative parathormone assay.[29,30]

Paragangliomas are sympathetic and parasympathetic chromaffin cells are derived from their associated paraganglioma. Between 10% and 50% are hereditary and may be associated with neurofibromatosis type I, von Hippel–Lindau syndrome, Carnery syndrome, and rarely multiple endocrine neoplasia type II. Germline mutations in three genes encoding subunits of succinate dehydrogenase (SDH) or mitochondrial complex II are associated with the familial form of this disease. In particular, one subunit (SDH B) is associated with a malignant form of this disease,[31] although malignancy can occur in the absence of this gene mutation.[32] This tumor can present in a cystic form[33] either with or without hypertension from catecholamine release, and it is highly vascularized and predominantly occurs in the anterior and middle mediastinum.[33,34] Surgical resection may be extensive and may require both α blockade and cardiopulmonary bypass.[34,35]

TERATOMAS

Teratomas account for 5% to 10% of all mediastinal tumors, with 95% occurring in the anterior mediastinum (primarily found in the thymus)[16,36] and 3% to 5% in the posterior mediastinum.[37,38] In the pediatric population, 7% of germ cell tumors are found in the mediastinum while it is the most common site for extragonadal germ cell tumor in adults There is no sex predilection, and most patients present without symptoms with large tumors[16] Benign teratomas include mature teratomas (45%–75% of patients), mature teratomas with immature elements comprising less than 50% of the volume, and immature teratomas, which occur almost exclusively in patients younger than age 15.[5,39] Symptoms related to these tumors usually include pain and occasionally cough, with the possible expectoration of hemoptysis, hair, or sebum.[37] Complete excision of mediastinal teratomas is strongly desired to prevent malignant somatic transformation of teratomatous elements[40] or the complications of compressive conditions or chronic fistula formation with infection.[41] Resection of these tumors may be difficult to do by a VATS approach because of dense adhesions to neighboring structures and the need for adequate incisions for large tumor delivery.[37] The prognosis for cystic teratoma containing immature or malignant elements is age-dependent; in the pediatric population these tumors behave in a benign fashion; however, they can be very aggressive in adults.[16,36]

CASTLEMAN DISEASE

Castleman disease is a benign form of marked lymph node hyperplasia caused by human rhadinovirus infection of the B-cell population, usually occurring in the mediastinum (70% of patients); it commonly occurs in the anterior compartment, but it can occur in any lymphatic area or rarely in nonnodal areas.[42,43] Histologically, it is divided into the hyaline-vascular form (91% of patients, commonly in a solitary location) and the plasma cell form (9% of patients, likely found in multicentric locations). These tumors are unusual and may portend other malignancies such as Kaposi sarcoma and lymphoma, which are strongly associated with HIV positive patients.[44] The unicenter hyaline-vascular form usually is benign, and recurrence occurs only rarely after complete surgical removal, although vascular neoplasms and occasionally lymphomas may occur in long-term follow-up.[42,43,45] The plasma cell variant is often multicentric and aggressive, particularly if associated with HIV positive patients.[44] Its proliferative potential may be attributed to high levels of the cytokine interleukin 6, which may induce Kaposi-like endothelial vascular neoplasms and lymphomas. The solitary and multicentric plasma cell forms of Castleman disease are strongly associated with infection by human herpesvirus 8, which may induce interleukin 6 production by virally encoded particles into native strands of DNA.[45,46]

Surgical resection, is the primary treatment of the localized forms of both types of Castleman disease. Preoperative angiography and embolization may be helpful to reduce the increased vascularity of these tumors.[42,43] Surgery for the multicentric form of this disease is limited to biopsy provision for pathologic determination or possibly debulking for early-stage disease combined with rituximab and chemotherapy.[44] Anti-human monoclonal antibodies against interleukin 6 and anti-CD20 monoclonal antibodies against CD20+ B-lymphocytes are potential treatment strategies for the multicentric variant of Castleman disease, once the diagnosis is confirmed histologically.[42,47] Other potential molecular targets for this disease are human herpesvirus 8 and angiogenesis factors.[47]Both variants of the disease require long-term surveillance for vascular tumors or lymphomas.

BENIGN MIDDLE MEDIASTINAL TUMORS

Cystic Mediastinal Abnormalities

The classification of mediastinal cysts is based on the tissue of origin and encompasses bronchogenic cysts and esophageal duplication cysts of foregut origin (50%–60% of mediastinal cysts) thymic cysts (15% of mediastinal cysts), mesothelial-derived pericardial/pleural cysts, and other miscellaneous cysts.[48] Foregut cysts are believed to result from abnormal budding or division of the primitive foregut[49,50] and share a similar embryogenesis to congenital cystic lesions of the lung parenchyma.[50,51] In a broad sense, these disease entities are categorized into bronchopulmonary foregut malformations, such as pulmonary sequestration, congenital cystic adenomatoid malformation, congenital lobar emphysema, and bronchogenic pulmonary cysts. Mediastinal cystic disease can be broadly divided into unilocular and multilocular forms with varying solid components as shown in Table 161-2.[52] It is important to remember that although unusual, mediastinal cysts (other than pericardial cysts) can contain malignant elements.[21,48,53,54]

BRONCHOGENIC AND PERICARDIAL CYSTS

Mediastinal cysts may arise from numerous sources and include lymphangiomas (i.e., cystic hygromas), meningoceles, thymic cysts, parathyroid cysts, pericardial cysts, pancreatic

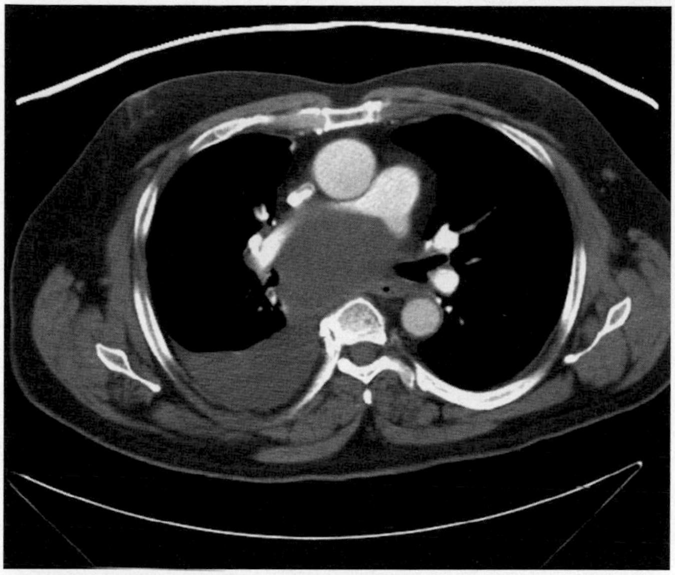

Figure 161-2. Bronchogenic cyst compressing pulmonary artery.

cysts, thoracic duct cysts, teratomatous cysts, and foregut cysts (e.g., bronchogenic, esophageal, and neurenteric). Mediastinal cysts are reported to represent 18% to 25% of all primary mediastinal mass lesions. Bronchogenic cysts and pericardial cysts are the most common mediastinal cysts.[48,55,56] Bronchogenic cysts are found most commonly in the middle mediastinum (Fig. 161-2), but they also may occur uncommonly in the anterior and posterior mediastinal compartments, as described by Ribet et al. and Cioffi et al.[57,58] Bronchogenic cysts often present with or develop symptoms of pain, dyspnea, dysphagia, or infection. In contrast, pericardial cysts in adults typically are asymptomatic and present as an incidental finding on routine chest roentgenograms.[48] Diagnosis usually is confirmed by chest CT scan demonstrating a simple cyst with low attenuation. All foregut cysts (bronchogenic and esophageal duplication cysts) should be excised if possible owing to the high likelihood of compressive or infective symptom development.[48,59,60] Endoesophageal aspiration of foregut duplication cysts is not recommended because there is a high likelihood of infection associated with this approach. The difficulty with managing foregut duplication cysts by endoscopic ultrasound evaluation is that they may appear to be noncystic because of mucinous involvement of the cyst contents. Mediastinal benign cysts often represent ideal lesions for resection by minimally invasive techniques.[58,61] Surgical excision offers the advantages of complete and definitive treatment, elimination of the mediastinal mass and prevention of any potential complications, relief of symptoms when present, and histologic evaluation. It is important to emphasize that these cysts can be very adherent and difficult to excise from adjacent vital structures. Incomplete resection may result in recurrence or continued fluid production by the residual cyst wall; when the cyst cannot be removed completely, partial excision with cautery destruction of the epithelial mucosal lining is an acceptable alternative, as described by Ferguson.[62]

Pericardial cysts result from failure of one or more fetal lacunae to coalesce into the pericardium. They commonly appear as unilocular cysts and contain clear, water-like fluid. Most pericardial cysts are found in the right costophrenic angle, and as many as a third of patients may have associated symptoms. Unlike bronchogenic cysts, which carry a risk of infection, pericardial cysts usually follow a benign course and infrequently need intervention. Resection with excision by either a thoracoscopic or open technique is recommended for symptomatic lesions and when the diagnosis is uncertain.[63,64]

BENIGN MEDIASTINAL MESENCHYMAL TUMORS

Mesenchymal tumors of the mediastinum are rare, constituting fewer than 5% to 10% of all primary mediastinal tumors. However, vigilance is required as 55% of these tumors are malignant, and they may occupy any compartment (see Table 161-1).[1,5] These tumors derive from elements of tissues native to the area; although combinations of tissue types occur, including tissue composites of adipose, vascular, and lymphatic tissue.

Adipose Tissue

Excess accumulation of adipose tissue can occur as a spectrum of disease in the mediastinum, and different forms of lipomatous mediastinal infiltration not associated with other mediastinal tumors can be described as follows.

Exaggerated Response to Systemic Disease

Mediastinal lipomatosis is seen with excess steroid production, hypercortisolism (i.e., Cushing syndrome), or with excess ACTH production.

Localized accumulations of fat may occur, such as increased pericardial fat pads or Morgagni hernia with omental fat. These are seen in the right anterior lower mediastinal compartment.

Localized Benign Conditions

Lipomas or hibernomas (brown fat tumor) are benign accumulations of adipose tissue. Either tumor may occur in any compartment, although the anterior compartment is often favored.[1,65]

Lipoblastoma represents a benign localized form of cells with a range of adipocyte maturation with myxoid changes and a vascular network that can be differentiated from liposarcoma by cytogenetics. The diffuse infiltrative form of this benign tumor has been termed lipoblastomatosis. Surgical resection is the treatment of choice but carries a recurrence rate of 9% to 22%.[66]

Vascular tumors

Benign vascular and lymphatic anomalies are best classified by division into the following categories: malformations, neoplasms, reactive proliferations, and ectasias. Malformations are congenital and may grow proportionally with age and do not involute, whereas neoplasms due to endothelial proliferation appear after birth and may spontaneously regress. Reactive vascular proliferations are associated with trauma or infection, and ectasias present with dilations of preexisting vessels without an increase in their number.[67]

These vascular malformations are divided into high-flow and low-flow categories. The high-flow arteriovenous malformations include angiomatosis which may involve multiple planes of tissues and intramuscular hemangiomas. Low-flow malformations include the following.

Hemangiomas

Hemangiomas are the most common benign vascular mediastinal tumor included in this category. These are usually well-encapsulated but may also present as infiltrative lesions or with a solid/cystic appearance. These vascular abnormalities have a low-flow state which predisposes to the formation of phleboliths and thromboses possibly leading to pulmonary emboli. They may be associated with the Maffucci, Klippel–Trénaunay, or blue bleb nevus syndrome. There are three histological variants, cavernous (most common), capillary, and venous. Surgical excision is recommended for all variants and the surgical dissection may be aided by interferon-2α if they are considered unresectable because of tissue infiltration.

Benign Vascular Neoplastic Disease

Angiomyolipomas include varying amounts of fat with abnormal blood vessels and smooth muscle cells and may be associated with tuberous sclerosis complex or lymphangioleiomyomatosis.[68]

Epithelioid hemangioendothelioma is a low-grade malignancy of epithelial cells with histologic features intermediate between hemangioma and angiosarcoma. The tumor is present with a benign histology; however, there is a 20% metastatic rate at 5 years. Treatment is by resection with radical lymphadenectomy; recurrence and metastases may benefit from radiation and chemotherapy.[1]

Hemangiopericytoma: These are benign-appearing tumors occurring in adults and sometimes are associated with hypoglycemia which although histologically bland may often metastasize. Surgical resection is the treatment of choice as radiation therapy and chemotherapy have not been shown to be effective.[1,69]

Benign Lymphatic Abnormalities

Lymphangiomas/cystic hygromas are benign multicystic or cavernous proliferations of lymphatic endothelium which may occur in children as an extension into the mediastinum from cervical lymphangioma. In adults, they may arise in the anterior mediastinum without a cervical component. These tumors are associated with several syndromes (e.g., Gorham disease which represents a dysplastic disorder of the bones and nonskeletal soft tissue of the mediastinum, Klippel–Trénaunay syndrome, a triad of soft and bony hypertrophy of the extremities), hemangiomas or lymphangiomas, Servelle–Noques disease (congenital or acquired malformation of the lymphatics and absence of the cisterna chyli), and lymphangiomatosis (diffuse and infiltrative form of lymphangioma which dissects through collagen and tissue planes to involve other visceral organs). These tumors unlike congenital hemangiomas do not spontaneously regress and are best treated by surgical resection which may be difficult because of their infiltrative nature. They are often associated with intractable chylous pleural or pericardial effusions or they may cause severe intractable chylous effusions.

Benign Mediastinal Nerve Tumors

Mediastinal benign nerve tumors include nerve sheath tumors (schwannomas or neurilemmoma), ganglion tumors, and paraganglion tumors (described under mediastinal endocrine tumors). Schwannomas are the most common neurogenic tumor of the thorax and may involve any thoracic nerve although they commonly occur in the posterior mediastinum.

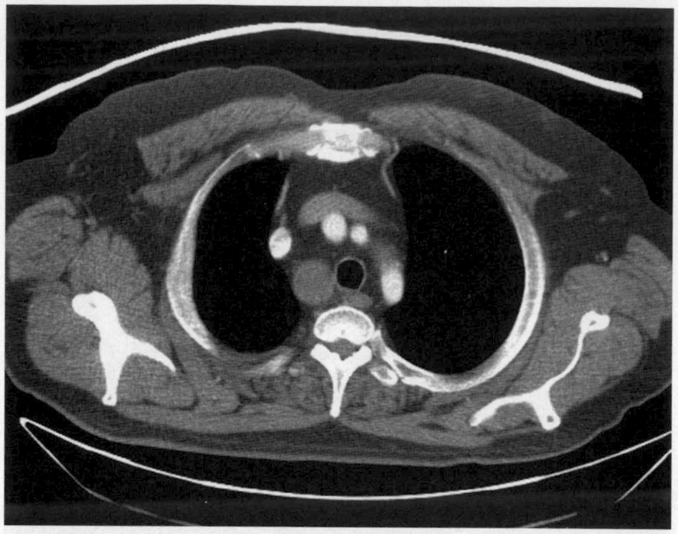

Figure 161-3. Schwannoma of the vagus nerve.

Usually they are benign and present as a solitary mass from the vagus nerve in the middle mediastinum (Fig. 161-3)[70] or from nerves associated with the esophagus.[71] Surgical excision is recommended because of compressive symptomatology and to exclude the potential for malignancy.

Benign Mediastinal Fibrous Abnormalities

Mediastinal fibrous lesions include multiple forms of fibromatosis (idiopathic mediastinal fibrosis, and fibrosis following histoplasmosis infection or after radiation) and solitary fibrous tumor of the mediastinum.

Idiopathic mediastinal fibrosis can rarely occur (93.3%) in association with retroperitoneal fibrosis and is best treated with steroid therapy which is approximately 80% effective.[72] The mediastinal fibrosis that occurs following histoplasma infection can lead to fibrosis and calcification within the mediastinum, which can cause occlusion of major vessels and airways.[73] Mediastinal fibrosis with chylous effusions also may occur following mediastinal radiation.[74] Scattered case reports of solitary fibrous tumors of the mediastinum are found in the literature; this tumor arises from stromal fibroblastic cells that are positive for CD34. Symptoms may arise from compression or invasion of mediastinal structures which may require extensive surgery including cardiopulmonary bypass for removal.

Benign Mediastinal Muscle Tumor

Approximately two thirds of benign esophageal tumors are leiomyomas; the remaining benign esophageal tumors are mostly polyps and cysts. Benign esophageal tumors are described in Chapter 28. Angiomyolipomas are tumors of fat, smooth muscle cell, and tortuous blood vessels, but involvement of the mediastinum rarely occurs (6 cases reported in 2004) primarily involving the middle or posterior mediastinum.[75] Surgical resection is the treatment of choice with attention to their extensive vascular supply.

Surgical Resection of Benign Anterior and Middle Mediastinal Masses

Surgery for mediastinal masses in adults requires an assessment of anesthetic risk for perioperative cardiorespiratory

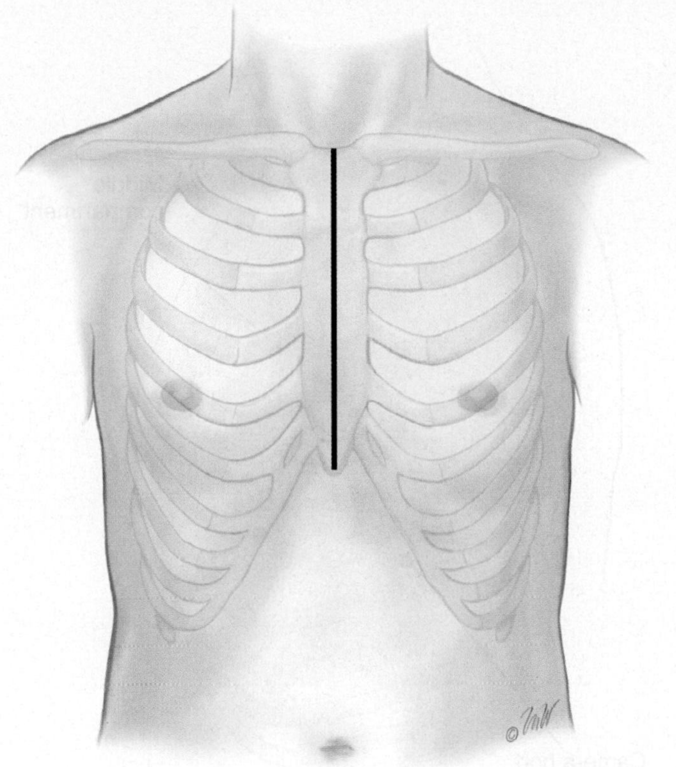

Figure 161-4. Partial or complete sternotomy with anterior thoracotomy.

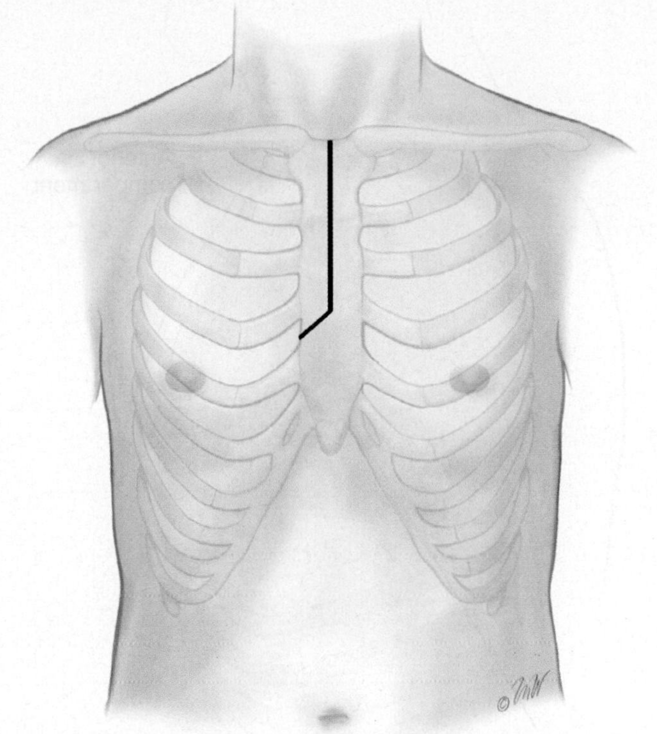

Figure 161-5. Partial or vertical sternotomy.

complications from airway or cardiovascular compression as well as the operative approach. In general, the pediatric population is more susceptible to cardiorespiratory complications than adults because of the smaller more compressible airways in the pediatric population.[76] Predictors for high-risk adult patients for these complications include the following: severe postural symptoms, stridor, cyanosis, tracheal compression >50%, tracheal compression with associated bronchial compression, pericardial effusion or SVC syndrome.[76,77] The operative approaches for benign mediastinal abnormalities range from open procedures involving a sternotomy (vertical sternotomy, partial sternotomy, clamshell procedure, or extended sternotomy) (see Figs. 161-4 to 161-6) to creative solutions involving minimal-access sternal-sparing approaches to avoid the morbidity of a sternotomy.

Minimal-Access Surgery for Anterior or Middle Mediastinal Tumors

The selection of minimal-access surgical approach for mediastinal tumors will depend on the size and location of the tumor (anterior/superior, anterior/inferior, or middle mediastinum) as well as the invasion or involvement of neighboring structures. The thoracic surgeon contemplating a VATS approach for mediastinal surgery should be prepared to convert to either a thoracotomy or a sternotomy as appropriate for unexpected mediastinal findings. Access to the anterior mediastinum by minimal-access approaches, which may be facilitated by the use of a robot, can be performed with single- or two-lung ventilation. Bilateral lung ventilation with small tidal volumes for anterior tumors may be as effective as single-lung ventilation if the patient is positioned appropriately such that low lung ventilation does not obscure the area of interest in the mediastinum. The patient may be placed supine or with the chest elevated 30 degrees, which permits anterior visualization with two-lung ventilation. Middle or posterior mediastinal VATS surgery or the full lateral position will require absence of ventilation to the ipsilateral lung.

In general, benign anterior mediastinal tumors are accessed primarily from the chest that the abnormality points to with camera ports placed in the fifth or sixth intercostal

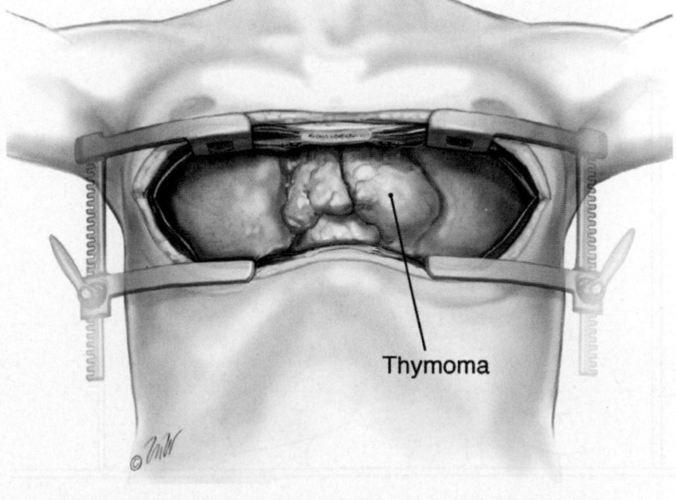

Figure 161-6. Surgical procedures that permit wide margins to prevent local recurrence are considered standard therapy for thymoma. Shown here is a bilateral clamshell incision.

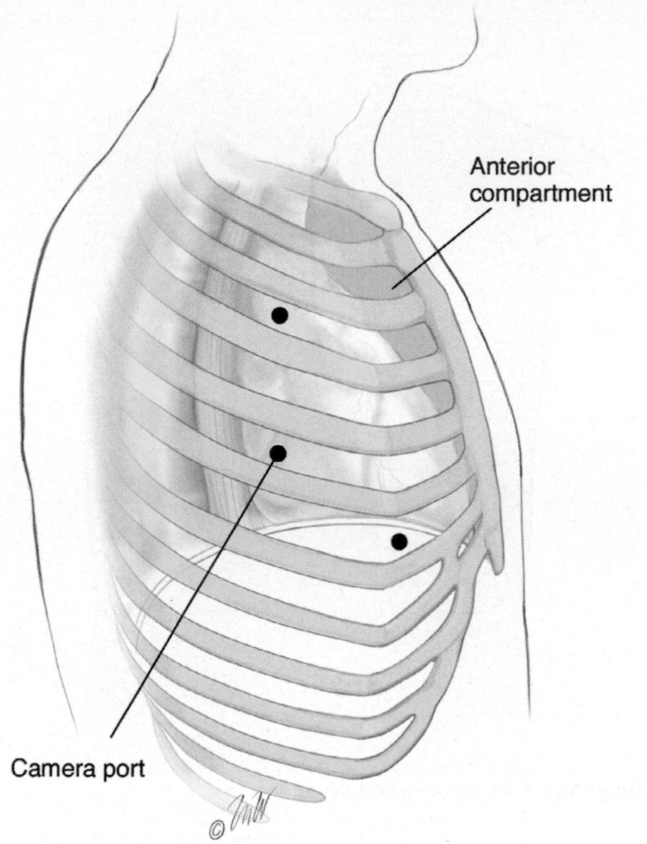

Figure 161-7. Port placement for a VATS approach to benign anterior mediastinal tumors via the right chest.

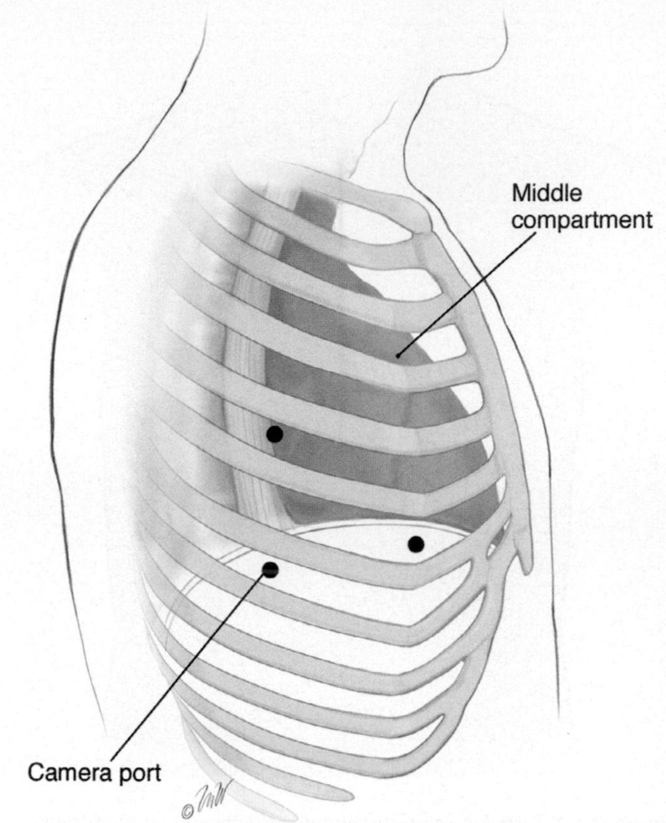

Figure 161-9. Port placement for a VATS approach to benign middle mediastinal tumors from the right chest.

space in the midaxillary line (Fig. 161-7). Other accessory ports for manipulation and removal of the tumor are placed in the second to fourth intercostal spaces as needed. The contralateral chest also can be accessed for dissection of the abnormality from the contralateral side as well as direct observation of both the phrenic nerves. Unique techniques to improve visualization of the operative field in the anterior mediastinum are a sternal lift procedure (Fig. 161-8)[78] and a video-assisted subxiphoid approach, as described by Hsu et al.[79] Cystic lesions of the mediastinum may be dissected or marsupialized more easily if they are decompressed by intraoperative needle aspiration; the caveat is the concern for malignant cystic elements and the potential for intraoperative spillage. Bipolar or unipolar cautery or a Harmonic scalpel will help dissect these tumors from surrounding structures while minimizing bleeding from small vessels. Middle mediastinal benign tumors are also accessed principally from the right chest with the camera port placed in the fourth or fifth intercostal space in the midaxillary line (Fig. 161-9).

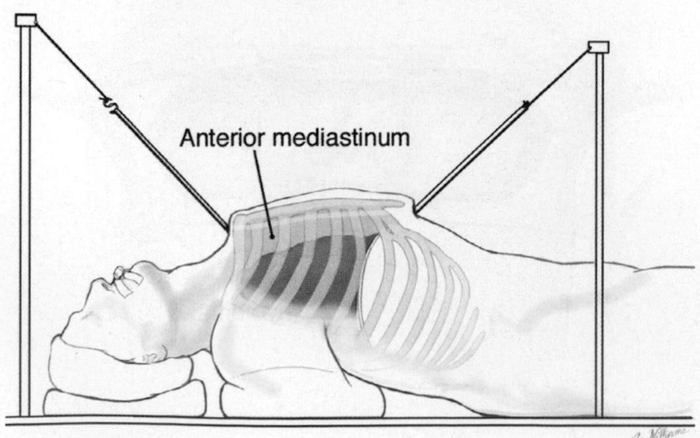

Figure 161-8. A sternal lift procedure can improve visualization of the anterior mediastinal operative field.

SUMMARY

It is important to separate benign anterior and middle mediastinal lesions from their malignant counterparts. This often can be done on the basis of location, age, symptoms, and biochemical markers. The differentiation of benign from malignant tumors on the basis of radiographic criteria may be difficult even when aided by CT or ultrasound-guided biopsy. Surgical resection for benign mediastinal abnormalities is often performed for symptoms of compression of contiguous structures, the risk of future infection, for control of systemic endocrine abnormalities or to exclude malignancy. Minimally invasive techniques have been introduced that permit sternal-sparing surgery for the removal of benign mediastinal tumors. Sternotomy approaches may be still required, however, for benign large tumors, hypervascular tumors, or those with significant adhesions to surrounding mediastinal structures.

EDITOR'S COMMENT

Historically, mediastinal cysts and benign conditions were surgical conditions because preoperative imaging was limited or misleading. In contrast, modern imaging techniques not only clarify the likely diagnosis, but also estimate the likelihood of secondary complications (local compression, infection, etc.). With advances in imaging technology, an increasing percentage of these patients will not require surgery.

—Steven J. Mentzer

References

1. Macchiarini P, Ostertag H. Uncommon primary mediastinal tumours. *Lancet Oncol.* 2004;5:107–118.
2. Wychulis AR, Payne WS, Clagett OT, et al. Surgical treatment of mediastinal tumors: a 40 year experience. *J Thorac Cardiovasc Surg.* 1971;62:379–392.
3. Duwe BV, Sterman DH, Musani AI. Tumors of the mediastinum. *Chest.* 2005;128:2893–2909.
4. Davis RD Jr, Oldham HN Jr, Sabiston DC Jr. Primary cysts and neoplasms of the mediastinum: recent changes in clinical presentation, methods of diagnosis, management, and results. *Ann Thorac Surg.* 1987;44:229–237.
5. Priola AM, Priola SM, Cardinale L, et al. The anterior mediastinum: diseases. *Radiol Med.* 2006;111:312–342.
6. Grosfeld JL. Primary tumors of the chest wall and mediastinum in children. *Semin Thorac Cardiovasc Surg.* 1994;6:235–239.
7. Saenz NC, Schnitzer JJ, Eraklis AE, et al. Posterior mediastinal masses. *J Pediatr Surg.* 1993;28:172–176.
8. Simpson I, Campbell PE. Mediastinal masses in childhood: a review from a paediatric pathologist's point of view. *Prog Pediatr Surg.* 1991;27:92–126.
9. Roviaro G, Varoli F, Nucca O, et al. Videothoracoscopic approach to primary mediastinal pathology. *Chest.* 2000;117:1179–1183.
10. Quint L. Imaging of anterior mediastinal masses. *Cancer Imaging (Special Issue).* 2007;7:S56–S62.
11. Date H. Diagnostic strategies for mediastinal tumors and cysts. *Thorac Surg Clin.* 2009;19:29–35, vi.
12. Kumar J, Seith A, Kumar A, et al. Chest wall and mediastinal nodal aspergillosis in an immunocompetent host. *Diagn Interv Radiol.* 2009;15:176–178.
13. Ustaalloglu BB, Seker M, Bilici A, et al. The role of PET-CT in the differential diagnosis of thymic mass after treatment of patients with lymphoma. *Med Oncol.* 2011;28:258–264.
14. Singla S, Litzky LA, Kaiser LR, et al. Should asymptomatic enlarged thymus glands be resected? *J Thorac Cardiovasc Surg.* 2010;140:977–983.
15. Desforges-Bullet V, Petit-Aubert G, Collet-Gaudillat C, et al. [Thymic hyperplasia and Graves' disease: a non-fortuitous association. case report and review of literature]. *Ann Endocrinol (Paris).* 2011;72:304–309.
16. den Bakker MA, Oosterhuis JW. Tumours and tumour-like conditions of the thymus other than thymoma; a practical approach. *Histopathology.* 2009;54:69–89.
17. Suto Y, Araga S, Sakuma K, et al. Myasthenia gravis with thymus hyperplasia and pure red cell aplasia. *J Neurol Sci.* 2004;224:93–95.
18. Boyd JD, Juskevicius R. Mediastinal neoplasms in patients with Graves disease: a possible link between sustained hyperthyroidism and thymic neoplasia? *Thyroid Res.* 2012;5:5.
19. Petroze R, McGahren ED. Pediatric chest II: Benign tumors and cysts. *Surg Clin North Am.* 2012;92:645–658, ix.
20. Wick MR. Cystic lesions of the mediastinum. *Semin Diagn Pathol.* 2005;22:241–253.
21. Zaitlin N, Rozenman J, Yellin A. Papillary adenocarcinoma in a thymic cyst: a pitfall of thoracoscopic excision. *Ann Thorac Surg.* 2003;76:1279–1281.
22. Honda S, Morikawa T, Sasaki F, et al. Cystic thymoma in a child: a rare case and review of the literature. *Pediatr Surg Int.* 2007;23:1015–1017.
23. Damadoglu E, Salturk C, Takir HB, et al. Mediastinal thymolipoma: an analysis of 10 cases. *Respirology.* 2007;12:924–927.
24. Moran CA, Rosado-de-Christenson M, Suster S. Thymolipoma: clinicopathologic review of 33 cases. *Mod Pathol.* 1995;8:741–744.
25. Kanzaki R, Higashiyama M, Oda K, et al. Surgical management of primary intrathoracic goiters. *Gen Thorac Cardiovasc Surg.* 2012;60:171–174.
26. Guimaraes MJ, Valente CM, Santos L, et al. Ectopic thyroid in the anterior mediastinum. *J Bras Pneumol.* 2009;35:383–387.
27. McKay GD, Ng TH, Morgan GJ, et al. Giant functioning parathyroid cyst presenting as a retrosternal goitre. *ANZ J Surg.* 2007;77:297–304.
28. Kumar A, Kumar S, Aggarwal S, et al. Thoracoscopy: the preferred method for excision of mediastinal parathyroids. *Surg Laparosc Endosc Percutan Tech.* 2002;12:295–300.
29. Wei B, Inabnet W, Lee JA, et al. Optimizing the minimally invasive approach to mediastinal parathyroid adenomas. *Ann Thorac Surg.* 2011;92:1012–1017.
30. Weigel TL, Murphy J, Kabbani L, et al. Radioguided thoracoscopic mediastinal parathyroidectomy with intraoperative parathyroid hormone testing. *Ann Thorac Surg.* 2005;80:1262–1265.
31. Young WF Jr. Paragangliomas: clinical overview. *Ann N Y Acad Sci.* 2006;1073:21–29.
32. Ayala-Ramirez M, Feng L, Johnson MM, et al. Clinical risk factors for malignancy and overall survival in patients with pheochromocytomas and sympathetic paragangliomas: primary tumor size and primary tumor location as prognostic indicators. *J Clin Endocrinol Metab.* 2011;96:717–725.
33. Ortega PF, Sosa LA, Patel M, et al. Cystic paraganglioma of the anterior mediastinum. *Ann Diagn Pathol.* 2010;14:341–346.
34. Brown ML, Zayas GE, Abel MD, et al. Mediastinal paragangliomas: the mayo clinic experience. *Ann Thorac Surg.* 2008;86:946–951.
35. Wald O, Shapira OM, Murar A, et al. Paraganglioma of the mediastinum: challenges in diagnosis and surgical management. *J Cardiothorac Surg.* 2010;5:19.
36. McKenney JK, Heerema-McKenney A, Rouse RV. Extragonadal germ cell tumors: a review with emphasis on pathologic features, clinical prognostic variables, and differential diagnostic considerations. *Adv Anat Pathol.* 2007;14:69–92.
37. Allen MS. Presentation and management of benign mediastinal teratomas. *Chest Surg Clin N Am.* 2002;12:659–664, vi.
38. Wood DE. Mediastinal germ cell tumors. *Semin Thorac Cardiovasc Surg.* 2000;12:278–289.
39. Dulmet EM, Macchiarini P, Suc B, et al. Germ cell tumors of the mediastinum. A 30-year experience. *Cancer.* 1993;72:1894–1901.
40. Muramatsu T, Nishii T, Ohmori K, et al. Mature cystic teratoma with malignant transformation to adenocarcinoma. *Ann Thorac Surg.* 2011;91:1971–1973.
41. Wagner RB. The history of mediastinal teratoma. *Chest Surg Clin N Am.* 2000;10:213–222, xi.
42. Shahidi H, Myers JL, Kvale PA. Castleman's disease. *Mayo Clin Proc.* 1995;70:969–977.
43. Seirafi PA, Ferguson E, Edwards FH. Thoracoscopic resection of Castleman disease: case report and review. *Chest.* 2003;123:280–282.
44. Talat N, Schulte KM. Castleman's disease: systematic analysis of 416 patients from the literature. *Oncologist.* 2011;16:1316–1324.
45. Pauwels P, Dal Cin P, Vlasveld LT, et al. A chromosomal abnormality in hyaline vascular Castleman's disease: evidence for clonal proliferation of dysplastic stromal cells. *Am J Surg Pathol.* 2000;24:882–888.
46. El-Osta HE, Kurzrock R. Castleman's disease: from basic mechanisms to molecular therapeutics. *Oncologist.* 2011;16:497–511.
47. Dham A, Peterson BA. Castleman disease. *Curr Opin Hematol.* 2007;14:354–359.
48. Le Pimpec-Barthes F, Cazes A, Bagan P, et al. [Mediastinal cysts: clinical approach and treatment]. *Rev Pneumol Clin.* 2010;66:52–62.
49. Sirivella S, Ford WB, Zikria EA, et al. Foregut cysts of the mediastinum. Results in 20 consecutive surgically treated cases. *J Thorac Cardiovasc Surg.* 1985;90:776–782.
50. Takeda S, Miyoshi S, Inoue M, et al. Clinical spectrum of congenital cystic disease of the lung in children. *Eur J Cardiothorac Surg.* 1999;15:11–17.
51. St-Georges R, Deslauriers J, Duranceau A, et al. Clinical spectrum of bronchogenic cysts of the mediastinum and lung in the adult. *Ann Thorac Surg.* 1991;52:6–13.
52. Kim JH, Goo JM, Lee HJ, et al. Cystic tumors in the anterior mediastinum. Radiologic-pathological correlation. *J Comput Assist Tomogr.* 2003;27:714–723.

53. Tsai JH, Lee JM, Lin MC, et al. Carcinoid tumor arising in a thymic bronchogenic cyst associated with thymic follicular hyperplasia. *Pathol Int.* 2012;62:49–54.
54. Olsen JB, Clemmensen O, Andersen K. Adenocarcinoma arising in a foregut cyst of the mediastinum. *Ann Thorac Surg.* 1991;51:497–499.
55. Takeda S, Miyoshi S, Minami M, et al. Clinical spectrum of mediastinal cysts. *Chest.* 2003;124:125–132.
56. Magee M, Hazelrigg S, Boley T. *Mediastinal Cysts.* Philadelphia, PA: Saunders; 2000.
57. Ribet ME, Copin MC, Gosselin B. Bronchogenic cysts of the mediastinum. *J Thorac Cardiovasc Surg.* 1995;109:1003–1010.
58. Cioffi U, Bonavina L, De Simone M, et al. Presentation and surgical management of bronchogenic and esophageal duplication cysts in adults. *Chest.* 1998;113:1492–1496.
59. Turkyilmaz A, Eroglu A, Subasi M, et al. Intramural esophageal bronchogenic cysts: a review of the literature. *Dis Esophagus.* 2007;20:461–465.
60. Kirmani B, Sogliani F. Should asymptomatic bronchogenic cysts in adults be treated conservatively or with surgery? *Interact Cardiovasc Thorac Surg.* 2010;11:649–659.
61. Weber T, Roth TC, Beshay M, et al. Video-assisted thoracoscopic surgery of mediastinal bronchogenic cysts in adults: a single-center experience. *Ann Thorac Surg.* 2004;78:987–991.
62. Ferguson MK. Thoracoscopic management of pericardial disease. *Semin Thorac Cardiovasc Surg.* 1993;5:310–315.
63. Najib MQ, Chaliki HP, Raizada A, et al. Symptomatic pericardial cyst: a case series. *Eur J Echocardiogr.* 2011;12:E43.
64. Song J, Costic JT, Seinfeld FI, et al. Thoracoscopic resection of unusual symptomatic pericardial cysts. *J Laparoendosc Adv Surg Tech A.* 2002;12:135–137.
65. Baldi A, Santini M, Mellone P, et al. Mediastinal hibernoma: a case report. *J Clin Pathol.* 2004;57:993–994.
66. Amra NK, Amr SS. Mediastinal lipoblastomatosis: report of a case with complex karyotype and review of the literature. *Pediatr Dev Pathol.* 2009;12:469–474.
67. Sheth S, Lai CK, Dry S, et al. Benign vascular tumors and tumor-like proliferations. *Semin Diagn Pathol.* 2008;25:1–16.
68. Morita K, Shida Y, Shinozaki K, et al. Angiomyolipomas of the mediastinum and the lung. *J Thorac Imaging.* 2012;27:W21–W23.
69. Lee KH, Song KS, Kwon Y, et al. Mesenchymal tumours of the thorax: CT findings and pathological features. *Clin Radiol.* 2003;58:934–944.
70. Huang TW, Yang MH, Cheng YL, et al. Vagus nerve schwannoma in the middle mediastinum. *Thorac Cardiovasc Surg.* 2010;58:312–314.
71. Kassis ES, Bansal S, Perrino C, et al. Giant asymptomatic primary esophageal schwannoma. *Ann Thorac Surg.* 2012;93:e81–e83.
72. Bahler C, Hammoud Z, Sundaram C. Mediastinal fibrosis in a patient with idiopathic retroperitoneal fibrosis. *Interact Cardiovasc Thorac Surg.* 2008;7:336–338.
73. Davis AM, Pierson RN, Loyd JE. Mediastinal fibrosis. *Semin Respir Infect.* 2001;16:119–130.
74. Lee SC, Kueh YK, Lehnert M, et al. Characteristics and prognosis of KI-1 positive anaplastic large cell lymphoma in Asians. *Aust N Z J Med.* 1998;28:790–794.
75. Amir AM, Zeebregts CJ, Mulder HJ. Anterior mediastinal presentation of a giant angiomyolipoma. *Ann Thorac Surg.* 2004;78:2161–2163.
76. Bechard P, Letourneau L, Lacasse Y, et al. Perioperative cardiorespiratory complications in adults with mediastinal mass: incidence and risk factors. *Anesthesiology.* 2004;100:826–834; discussion 5A.
77. Blank RS, de Souza DG. Anesthetic management of patients with an anterior mediastinal mass: continuing professional development. *Can J Anaesth.* 2011;58:853–859, 60–67.
78. Takeo S, Sakada T, Yano T. Video-assisted extended thymectomy in patients with thymoma by lifting the sternum. *Ann Thorac Surg.* 2001;71:1721–1723.
79. Hsu CP, Chuang CY, Hsu NY, et al. Comparison between the right side and subxiphoid bilateral approaches in performing video-assisted thoracoscopic extended thymectomy for myasthenia gravis. *Surg Endosc.* 2004;18:821–824.

162 Neurogenic Tumors of the Posterior Mediastinum

Sidhu P. Gangadharan

Keywords: Nerve sheath tumors, neurofibroma, neurilemmoma, von Recklinghausen disease, ganglion cell tumors, ganglioneuroma, neuroblastoma, paraganglion cell tumors, granular cell tumors

Neurogenic tumors arise in tissues derived from the embryonic neural crest. Further classification is based on whether the tumor cell originates from nerve sheath, nerve cells (ganglia), paraganglia, or peripheral nerve (Table 162-1). In the thorax, the latter nerve is represented by the intercostal nerve. The chief impediment to understanding thoracic neurogenic tumors is the lack of uniformity in the nomenclature used in the published literature, and thus multiple descriptors exist at each taxonomic level (Table 162-2). This chapter relies on the nomenclature endorsed by the most recent revision of the World Health Organization classification of tumors derived from neural tissue.[1]

Neural crest-derived tissues can be found throughout the body. In the thorax, neurogenic tumors are found most commonly in the posterior mediastinum (63%–96%).[1–6] In fact, neurogenic tumors account for 75% of all posterior mediastinal neoplasms.[3] The epidemiology of neurogenic tumors depends primarily on whether the patient is an adult or a child. Although one-third of mediastinal tumors diagnosed and treated in children are neurogenic, the incidence is only 12% to 14% in adults.[7,8] Adults also have a lower rate of malignancy (5%–10% in adults compared with 40%–60% in children) (Fig. 162-1).[1,7] The most common neurogenic tumors in adults arise from the nerve sheath (e.g., neurilemmoma and neurofibroma), whereas in pediatric populations the cells of origin are the ganglia (e.g., ganglioneuroma and neuroblastoma) (Table 162-3).[1,9,10]

NEUROGENIC TUMORS

The mainstay of treatment for neurogenic tumors, benign or malignant, is complete surgical extirpation. Since most neurogenic tumors are benign, the rationale for resection is to prevent symptoms related to local growth, confirm the diagnosis (i.e., exclude malignancy and determine other options for treatment), and avoid the remote possibility of malignant degeneration.[3] The exceptions to this strategy involve cases of advanced neuroblastoma and ganglioneuroblastoma. Although these tumors are encountered more commonly in pediatric practice, we address them in this chapter to give a comprehensive understanding of mediastinal tumor biology. Specific treatments are presented by tumor type.

Nerve Sheath Tumors

Benign nerve sheath tumors have an excellent prognosis, with negligible rates of local recurrence after complete resection.[2,11,12] One should not expect, even after subtotal resection, that recurrence (or continued growth) of a benign nerve sheath tumor will adversely affect long-term survival.[1,5] Surgical resection of benign tumors is indicated to ascertain diagnosis, prevent or alleviate effects from local invasion, and avoid the rare malignant transformation of a benign lesion.

Approximately 30% to 45% of patients with neurofibromas also carry a diagnosis of neurofibromatosis, and the presence of multiple neurofibromas or a single plexiform tumor is highly suggestive of this link.[13] von Recklinghausen disease also may be associated with ganglion cells tumors, neurilemmoma, and malignant peripheral nerve sheath tumors, with the incidence of malignancy severalfold higher than that of the general population.[2,5,11] In cases of malignant peripheral nerve sheath tumors, von Recklinghausen disease confers a worse prognosis.[5,13] Postoperative radiation has been used to obtain local control of malignant peripheral nerve sheath tumors, but the efficacy of this strategy remains unproved.[1,2,12] There is no effective adjunctive cytotoxic chemotherapy.[1,2,5,12] Recent advances in targeted therapies have yielded promising results using bevacizumab and erlotinib for vestibular schwannoma in the setting of neurofibromatosis type 2.[14–17] Whether this may translate to the adjuvant or palliative setting

Table 162-1

CLASSIFICATION OF NEUROGENIC TUMORS

ORIGIN	TUMOR		BENIGN	MALIGNANT	ASSOCIATED BIOLOGICAL ACTIVITY
Nerve sheath	Neurilemmoma		X		
	Neurofibroma		X		
	Granular cell tumor		X	X	
	Malignant peripheral nerve sheath tumor			X	Insulin-releasing substance
Ganglion cell	Ganglioneuroma		X		Catecholamines, vasoactive intestinal polypeptide (VIP)
	Ganglioneuroblastoma			X	
	Neuroblastoma			X	
Paraganglion cell	Paraganglioma	Functioning	X	X	Catecholamines
		Nonfunctioning	X	X	
Intercostal nerve	Primitive neuroectodermal tumor			X	

Table 162-2

NEUROGENIC TUMOR NOMENCLATURE

TUMOR	ALSO KNOWN AS
Neurilemmoma	Schwannoma, neurilemmoma, neurinoma
Granular cell tumor	Myoblastoma
Malignant peripheral nerve sheath tumor (MPNST)	Malignant schwannoma, neurosarcoma, neurofibrosarcoma, malignant fibroma, malignant tumor of nerve sheath origin (MTNSO)
Paraganglioma (functioning)	Pheochromocytoma
Paraganglioma (nonfunctioning)	Chemodectoma, paraganglionoma
Primitive neuroectodermal tumor (PNET)	Peripheral neuroectodermal tumor, peripheral neuroepithelial tumor, Askin tumor

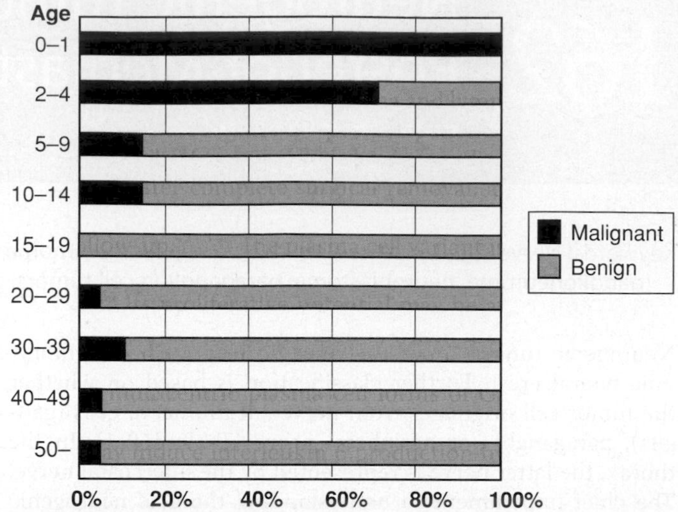

Figure 162-1. Malignancy rate according to the patient's age. (Reproduced with permission from Takeda S, Miyoshi S, Minami M, et al. Intrathoracic neurogenic tumors: 50 years' experience in a Japanese institution. *Eur J Cardiothorac Surg.* 2004;26:807–812.)

for mediastinal peripheral nerve sheath tumors remains to be seen however.

Granular cell tumors are found rarely in the posterior mediastinum.[18] Such tumors are thought to arise from the Schwann cell and can be found throughout the body.[19] Few granular cell tumors are malignant (2%–3%).[20] Complete surgical resection is the treatment of choice. Absent a total resection, the local recurrence rate may be as high as 20%.[18]

Ganglion Cell Tumors

Neuroblastoma is a tumor that is seen rarely in adults. Most cases are diagnosed in children under 5 years of age.[4] The International Neuroblastoma Staging System has established disease stages that span from local tumor growth to lymph node involvement and distant metastasis.[21] Patients with early-stage disease are treated by surgical resection. Intermediate-risk patients are treated with a combined chemotherapeutic regimen (e.g., cyclophosphamide/doxorubicin), potentially with the addition of etoposide, surgical resection, and adjuvant radiation. Advanced-stage disease with evidence of dissemination of tumor to distant sites is treated aggressively with chemotherapy, sometimes in conjunction with bone marrow transplantation.[9,22] A report on incompletely resected posterior mediastinal neuroblastomas in a pediatric population noted that thoracic neuroblastoma tends to demonstrate better 5-year survival rates than extrathoracic tumors. Moreover, the presence of positive margins on the resected specimen did not alter the excellent prognosis.[23] The adult literature is far less developed than that of children, but surgical resection with chemotherapy and possible adjuvant radiation has been reported to be effective for long-term survival and freedom from recurrence.[24]

Ganglioneuroma represents the benign end of the spectrum of ganglion cell tumors and is diagnosed at a median age of 6.5 years, in contrast to the 22-month age observed with neuroblastoma.[22,25] A recent report on children with thoracic ganglion cell tumors noted that with an age <1 year, nearly all (92%) had neuroblastomas, whereas with age ≥ 1 year, ganglioneuroblastomas and neuroblastomas were found in near-equal distribution (39% and 37%), with a significant number of ganglioneuroma as well (24%).[26] The histology of ganglioneuroma reveals mature ganglion cells, whereas neuroblastoma contains neuroblasts. Ganglioneuroblastoma has a mixture of these immature and mature cell types. It is the presence of immature tumor cells that confers the risk of malignancy to neuroblastomas and ganglioneuroblastomas,

Table 162-3

COMPARISON OF CHILDREN AND ADULTS FOR HISTOLOGIC TYPE OF NEUROGENIC TUMOR

HISTOLOGIC CLASS	ADULTS, 86 CASES	CHILDREN, 60 CASES	*p* VALUE
Gender	M/F: 48/38	M/F: 27/33	0.20
Malignancy (%)	Benign/Malignant, 81/5 (5.8%)	Benign/Malignant, 35/25 (41.7%)	<0.001
Ganglioneuroma	18 (M/F: 8/10)	33 (M/F: 17/16)	<0.001
Schwannoma	37 (M/F: 21/16)	0	<0.001
Neurofibroma	28 (M/F: 16/12)	2 (M/F: 0/2)	<0.001
Neuroblastoma	0	18 (M/F: 8/10)	<0.001
Ganglioblastoma	0	5 (M/F: 1/4)	0.023
PNET	0	2 (M/F: 1/1)	0.081
Neurofibrosarcoma	2 (M/F: 2/0)	0	0.23
Pheochromocytoma	1 (M/F: 1/0)	0	0.40
Others	2 (M/F: 0/2)	0	0.23

M/F, male/female; PNET, primitive neuroectodermal tumor.

Used with permission from Takeda S, Miyoshi S, Minami M, et al. Intrathoracic neurogenic tumors-50 years' experience in a Japanese institution. *Eur J Cardiothorac Surg.* 2004;26(4):807–812.

and these tumors generally are grouped together for purposes of assigning treatment and analyzing outcomes.[22] The 5-year survival of posterior mediastinal ganglioneuroblastoma has been reported to be as high as 88%, which exceeds survival with neuroblastoma.[27] Surgical resection of ganglioneuroma should be curative for this benign tumor.

Paraganglion Cell Tumors

Paraganglion cell tumors can be functioning or nonfunctioning, and either type has the possibility of being malignant or benign.[28–31] Local invasion, as evidenced by vertebral collapse, spinal cord compression, or contiguous neural, pleural, or lung involvement, is a hallmark of malignant paragangliomas that is seen much less frequently with benign cases.[30] Surgical resection is the standard treatment, with en bloc resection of involved structures, if possible.

PREOPERATIVE ASSESSMENT

Neurogenic tumors exhibit bioactivity. This feature, along with immunohistochemistry, can be harnessed for diagnostic purposes (see Table 162-1). For example, paragangliomas produce catecholamines, which may account for the characteristic symptoms of hypertension, headache, diaphoresis, and palpitations associated with adrenal pheochromocytomas. Similarly, immunostaining may detect chromogranin and S-100 protein.[28] Adults with neurogenic tumors, however, generally are asymptomatic. As few as 16% to 37% of patients exhibit symptoms or signs related to the tumor.[1,5] In children, when considering all mediastinal tumors, most specifically neurogenic tumors, the absence of symptoms tends to favor a malignant diagnosis.[4,5] In adults, perhaps as a result of the very low incidence of malignancy, the presence or absence of symptoms does not accurately predict malignancy.[5] The most common symptom reported by adults is pain, whereas in children respiratory symptoms, such as cough or dyspnea, predominate.[1,5]

The workup of a patient with a posterior mediastinal mass must begin with a thorough physical examination and accurate history. A review of symptoms may detect evidence of local growth or invasion (e.g., pain, dyspnea, stridor, cough, dysphagia, neuropathy, or Horner syndrome), bioactivity (e.g., catecholamine, vasoactive intestinal peptide, or insulin-releasing substance production), or associated syndromes (e.g., von Recklinghausen and neurofibromas). Rarely, evidence of cord compression from tumor extension within the spinal canal may be detected by history and physical examination.[32]

Imaging with CT scanning is ordered to define the morphology and location of the tumor, as well as some features of local invasion, such as bony or airway involvement (Fig. 162-2).[33] Features such as enhancement and homogeneity of density on CT scan can help differentiate different types of neurogenic tumors.[34–36] A tumor size greater than 10 cm has been correlated with malignancy, as well as the findings of pleural effusion and significant mediastinal displacement.[5] When the neural foramen is effaced by tumor on CT scan and intraspinal extension is suspected (known as a dumbbell tumor), MRI should be acquired to further define the anatomy.[33] In practice, unless the mass is fully circumscribed by pleura on CT scan or small enough that involvement of the foramen obviously is excluded by anatomy alone, an MRI should be ordered to clarify the relationship of the tumor to the neural foramen and spinal canal. The intraoperative dissection of the tumor (described later) may be markedly altered by extension through the neural foramen. Similar to CT scanning but perhaps more specific, MRI also can be used to narrow the differential diagnosis of a posterior mediastinal mass because several common neurogenic tumors have characteristic appearances on MRI.[37] Magnetic resonance or conventional arteriography also can be used to identify the artery of Adamkiewicz for dumbbell tumors located in the lower posterior mediastinum (T8–L1) (Fig. 162-3). This practice has been advocated as part of the preoperative workup to minimize spinal cord ischemia during resection.[38] Finally, the tumor bioactivity may be targeted with radiologic modalities such as $[^{123}\text{I}]$meta-iodobenzylguanidine (MIBG) scanning, which detects neuroblastomas or functioning paragangliomas.[39] MIBG scanning may detect occult multifocal disease or metastatic deposits and is used to monitor for recurrence after therapy. More recently, PET scanning has been examined as an alternative to MIBG scanning.[40] Recent studies involving PET scans have used $[^{18}\text{F}]$fluorodopamine, $[^{18}\text{F}]$fluorohydroxyphenylalanine, $[^{11}\text{C}]$epinephrine, or $[^{11}\text{C}]$hydroxyephedrine to detect paragangliomas, neuroblastomas, and ganglioneuromas by targeting characteristic metabolic pathways.[41] In the case of the more common neurilemmomas and neurofibromas, however, standard PET scanning has not been found to very specific or sensitive and thus would not be recommended for a standard workup.[42–44]

Laboratory testing includes 24-hour urinary homovanillic acid, vanillylmandelic acid, and metanephrine, as well as serum- and urine-free catecholamine levels in cases of suspected functioning paragangliomas or some tumors of ganglion cell origin that produce catecholamines. In cases where catecholamine excess was found, preoperative preparation was broadened to include the initiation of the α-blocking agent, phenoxybenzamine, 2 weeks before the planned tumor resection to minimize the likelihood of hypertensive crises. Occasionally, β-blockade may be instituted (after the α-blockade is established) for heart rate or arrhythmia control.

Insulin and glucose levels are checked when a malignant peripheral nerve sheath tumor is suspected of secreting an insulin-releasing substance that could lead to hypoglycemia. Electrolytes and serum vasoactive intestinal protein levels are monitored in patients who report persistent diarrhea because this raises the suspicion of a ganglion cell tumor that is producing excess vasoactive intestinal protein.[45] Adjunctive preoperative workup, such as pulmonary function testing or cardiac risk stratification, is pursued on a case-by-case basis. For example, a cardiopulmonary workup might be warranted if there is tumor-related airway obstruction or lung parenchymal collapse or with excess catecholamine production that has led to hypertension and other cardiovascular sequelae.

A final preoperative consideration is whether one should obtain a biopsy to confirm the diagnosis prior to definitive resection. The differential diagnosis of a posterior mediastinal mass includes bronchogenic or esophageal duplication cysts,[46] metastatic disease to the pleura, soft tissue tumors,[47] infectious/inflammatory diseases such as tuberculosis and sarcoidosis,[48] pleural-based neoplasms such as solitary fibrous tumor,[49] lymphoma,[50] Castleman disease,[51] pulmonary sequestration,[52] and lateral thoracic meningocele.[53] In Figure 162-4 is an unusual presentation of an intercostal artery aneurysm which was initially suspected to be a posterior neurogenic

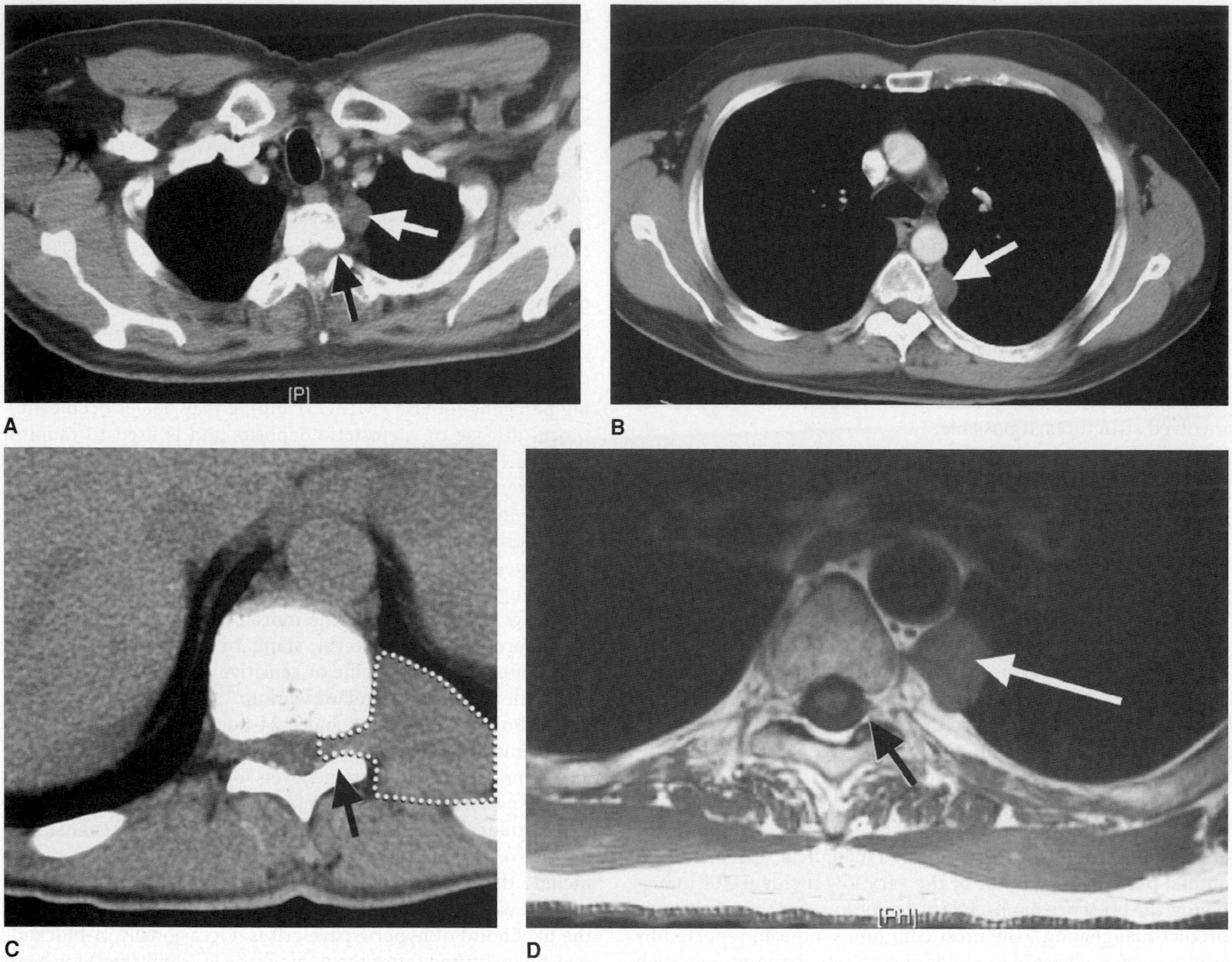

Figure 162-2. CT and MRI appearance of neurogenic tumors. *A*. Neurilemmoma (*white arrow*) clearly not invading the neural foramen (*black arrow*) on CT scan. *B*. Neurilemmoma (*white arrow*) in closer proximity to neural foramen on CT scan. *C*. Neurilemmoma (*dotted white outline*) invading neural foramen (*black arrow*) on CT scan. *D*. Neurilemmoma (*white arrow*) in proximity to neural foramen (*black arrow*) but not extending into it on T1-weighted MRI.

tumor. More unusual posterior mediastinal masses that have been mistaken for possible neurogenic tumors have included pancreatic pseudocysts, extramedullary hematopoiesis, achalasia, pulmonary sequestration, thoracic splenosis, variant azygos lobe, and teratoma.[52,54–59] Fine-needle aspiration may provide a diagnosis for neurogenic tumors, but cytology alone potentially may be misleading.[60–62] Because the treatment of most neurogenic tumors in the posterior mediastinum involves complete surgical resection, in most cases a preoperative biopsy will not alter the surgical plan.

TECHNIQUE

The classic approach for most posterior mediastinal masses is a lateral or posterolateral thoracotomy.[3] A double-lumen endotracheal tube is used to obtain lung isolation for exposure. Preoperative bronchoscopy or esophagoscopy is considered when the tumor may involve aerodigestive structures, although, in practice, this is a rare necessity. Because of the predominance of benign neurogenic tumors in the adult population, en bloc resection of major adjacent structures (e.g., vertebral body or chest wall) is not usually required. Rather, the mass is enucleated from its subpleural origin. The site of the thoracotomy is determined by the level of the tumor. In cases of neurilemmomas, the nerve root may be preserved with careful dissection of the tumor after incising the epineurium, but this is often not possible. Neurofibromas are intercalated with the nerve fibers, and thus the nerve root is taken en bloc with the tumor.[63]

Dumbbell tumors pose a special challenge for complete resection because of extension into the neural foramen and spinal canal. Approximately 10% of benign nerve sheath tumors have this type of anatomy.[13] Complications such as hemorrhage within the spinal canal leading to neurologic deficits or dural leak can arise with improperly approached dumbbell tumors secondary to excessive traction on the nerve root or improper control of vascular structures (see Fig. 162-3).[2,64,65] In addition, thoracotomy alone may provide only enough exposure for an incomplete resection, leaving tumor in the foramen and spinal canal, with the consequences of continued tumor progression and eventual spinal cord compression.[3] Various approaches have been described for resection. The degree of foraminal

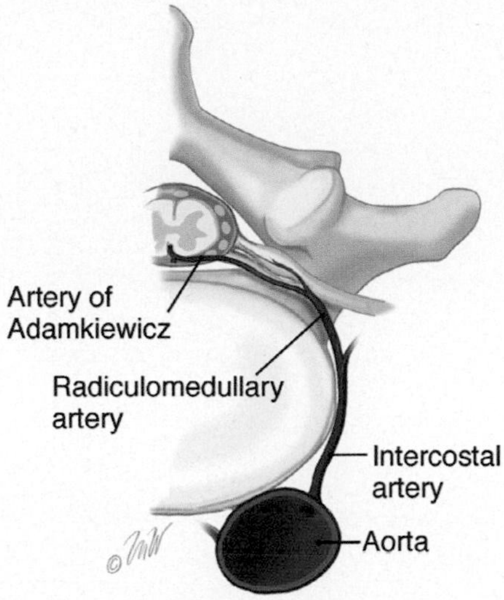

Figure 162-3. Artery of Adamkiewicz. Inadequate control of vascular structures can lead to dural leak.

involvement dictates the need for a spinal approach in addition to the transthoracic resection. In some cases, the tumor simply may extend to the distal aspects of the neural foramen, where it widens the foramen but does not truly extend into the spinal canal. Such tumors still may be resected solely via a thoracic approach, taking care not to avulse the nerve root and injure the spinal cord by using meticulous dissection and control of any incised dura to prevent cerebrospinal fluid leak.[66] For true dumbbell tumors with intraspinal extension, some have advocated removal of the intraspinal portion via laminectomy for immediate decompression of the spinal cord and relief of symptoms, followed by resection of the intrathoracic portion as a second procedure.[67,68] Grillo et al.[69] removed dumbbell tumors via a single posterolateral thoracotomy with a "hockey-stick" extension that extended vertically over the middle of the spinous processes. The vertical aspect of the skin incision traversed 5 cm superior and inferior to the level of the involved foramen, and thus a skin flap was created to access the desired site of thoracotomy superior to the level of the horizontal skin incision. An update on this technique reported minimal morbidity, and it was noted that the order of the thoracotomy and intrathoracic tumor mobilization and laminectomy or hemilaminectomy for the intraspinal resection was not fixed. Rather, it depended on surgeon preference.[38] In general, a full laminectomy is not necessary to mobilize a unilaterally oriented tumor (Fig. 162-5).[70] Whether a single incision or combined chest and back approach is used, the goal of obtaining a complete resection with minimal risk of bleeding and cerebrospinal fluid leak is paramount.

In the last 20 years, video-assisted thoracic surgery (VATS) has been used to resect posterior mediastinal neurogenic tumors.[66,71–73] Conversion rates of thoracoscopy to open thoracotomy for resection of neurogenic tumors had been reported to be as high as 17% in early series, but the more modern series note rates around 2% to 4%.[71–76] Although the operative time is longer, the advantages of the thoracoscopic approach include quicker recovery, as evidenced by a shorter length of stay and quicker return to work.[77] A prospective trial comparing the two techniques has not been done. Long-term freedom from recurrence has been reported with the thoracoscopic technique.[76]

The camera and port sites are similar to those used for standard thoracoscopic lung resection (Fig. 162-6). The videoscope generally is introduced into the chest in the seventh interspace in the middle to posterior axillary line. A port is placed anteriorly to retract the lung away from the paravertebral space. One or two additional ports then are placed for dissection, with the locations determined by the level of the tumor. The resected tumor is removed in a specimen bag to avoid contamination of the port site. This technique has been used for resection of dumbbell tumors as well, in conjunction with a spinal approach either before or after the thoracic dissection.[78,79]

The advent of robotic-assisted thoracoscopic surgery has seen several reports that have described successful robotic thoracoscopic resection of neurogenic tumors.[80–83] The ports may

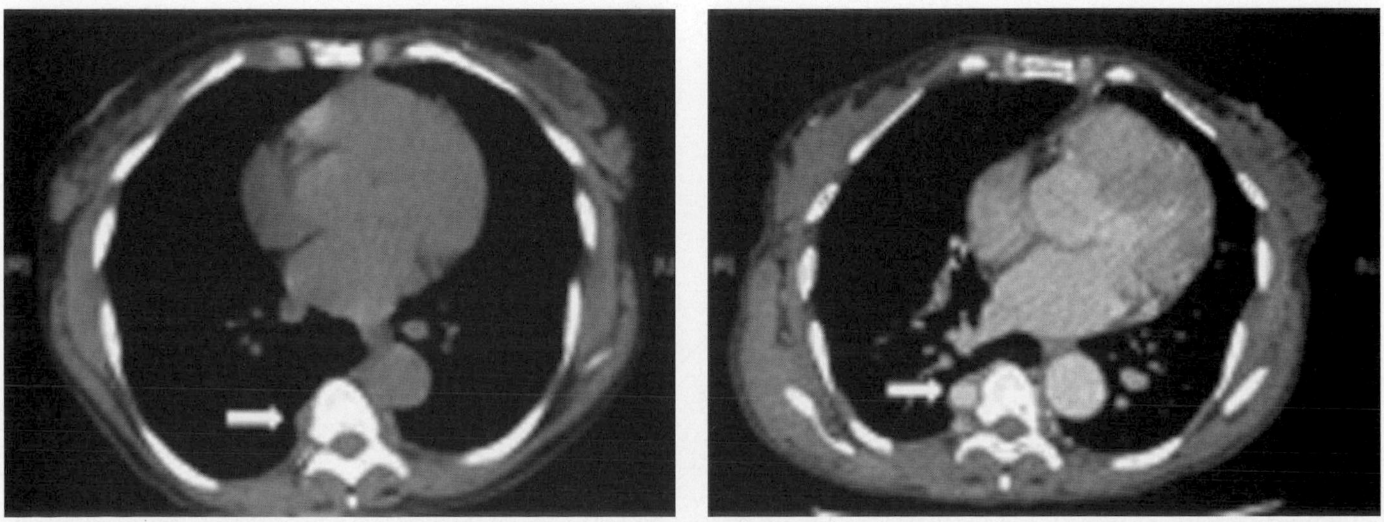

A B

Figure 162-4. Posterior mediastinal mass mimicking a neurogenic tumor: intercostal artery aneursym. *A.* Non-contrast chest CT scan shows paraspinal mass (*white arrow*). *B.* Two years later the paraspinal mass (*white arrow*) has enlarged considerably and is defined as a vascular structure with the administration of intravenous contrast.

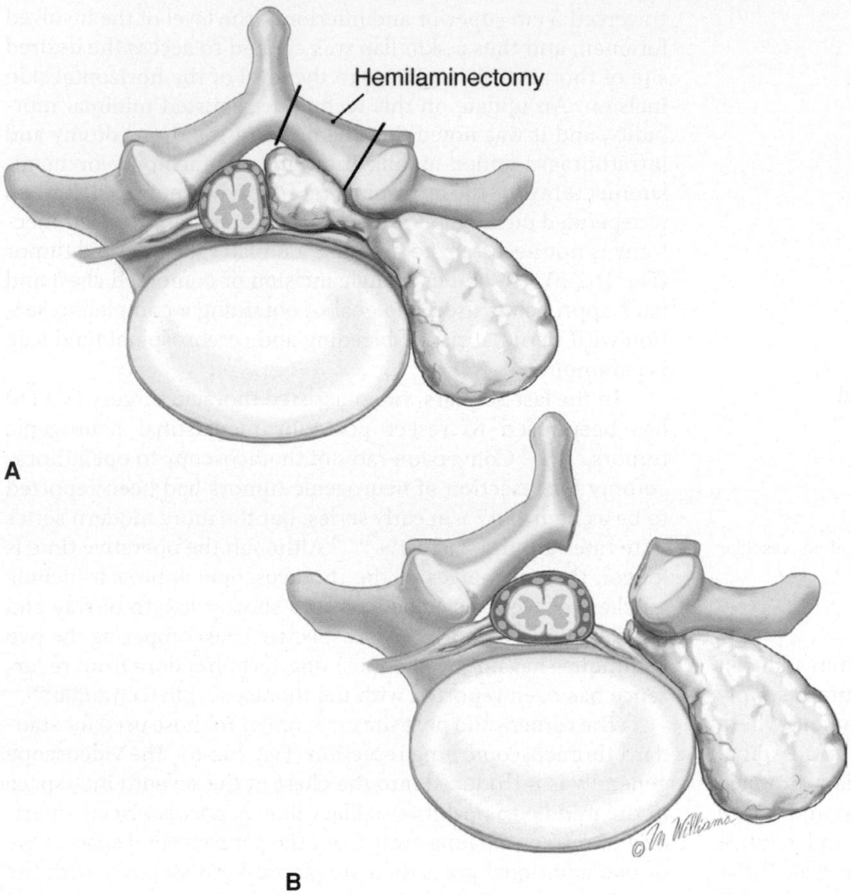

Figure 162-5. Approach for dumbbell tumors. *A.* Hemilaminectomy (*black arrow*). *B.* Resection of intraspinal component of tumor prior to thoracic approach.

be placed in a similar fashion to those used for robotic-assisted thoracoscopic lobectomy,[84] or may be triangulated using the camera port at the inferior apex.[85] In either case, inferior and superior posterior mediastinal tumors require different robot docking angles to maximize robot-arm mobility. The largest series of robotic posterior mediastinal neurogenic tumor resections (41 cases) was included in a recent report on robotic use for posterior mediastinal pathology. There were no conversions to thoracotomy, significant bleeding, or other operative morbidity noted.[84]

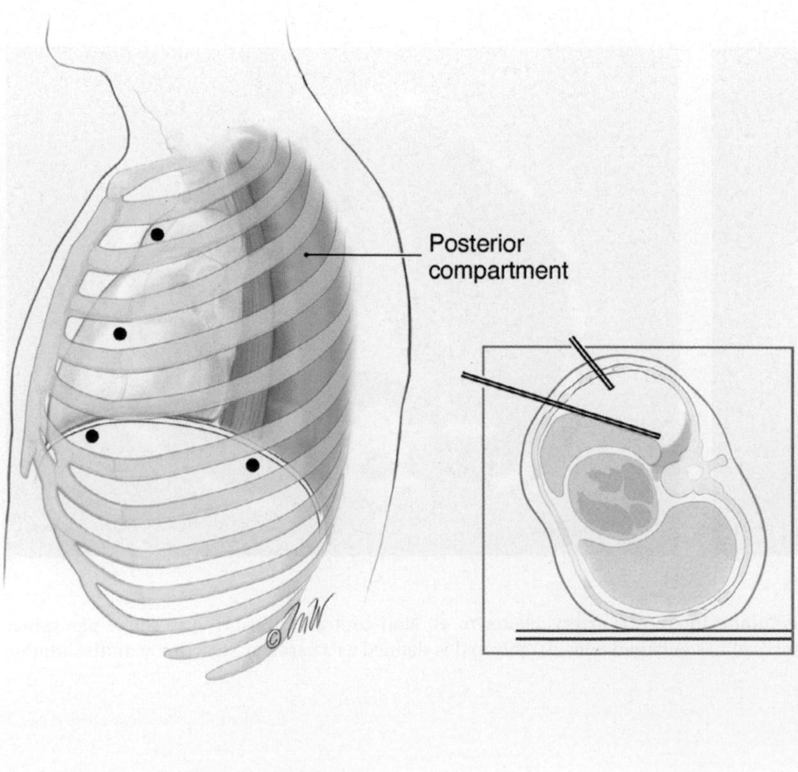

Figure 162-6. Ideal port placement for access to posterior mediastinal compartment.

Postoperative Management

Patients undergoing neurogenic tumor resection are managed similarly to any patient who has undergone thoracotomy or thoracoscopy. Chest drains are removed early (i.e., on the day of surgery or postoperative day 1) based on output and re-expansion of the lung. Patients are extubated in the OR, and early mobilization is advocated. The performance of a hemilaminectomy in patients with dumbbell tumors should not dissuade this practice. Diet may be resumed in short order as tolerated. Analgesia is delivered via patient-controlled analgesia devices or orally in VATS patients. Discharge on the day of the surgery or postoperative day 1 is anticipated.

The management of patients with paragangliomas warrants special attention to heart rate and blood pressure because doses of pharmacologic agents may be reduced or withdrawn preoperatively. For example, because of its prolonged half-life, the dose of the α-blocker phenoxybenzamine usually is reduced immediately prior to surgery to prevent postoperative hypotension. Although β-blockers may be continued through the perioperative period for cardioprotective effects, the dose likewise may be reduced.

Complications

Hemorrhage requiring spinal cord decompression has been described.[2,64] Postoperative assessment after resection of a neurogenic tumor should include a detailed neurologic examination, even with a purely thoracic (i.e., nondumbbell) tumor resection. Of note, the preoperative physical assessment also should document the neurologic examination in detail to distinguish preoperative deficits from the untoward sequelae of resection.

Management of the dura when tumor invades the neural foramen requires meticulous dissection and attention to the possibility of a dural leak. A cerebrospinal fluid leak into the chest, necessitating a pleural drain, can add to the already negative intrathoracic pressures of inspiration and may be difficult to manage conservatively. Thus, the sleeve on the nerve root should be controlled with a hemoclip or suture before the proximal margin of resection is divided. Intraoperatively, if any cerebrospinal fluid is detected, further application of suture, clips, fibrin glue, or a fascial patch may be used to control the leak.[66] In the immediate postoperative interval, chest drains are placed on water seal as opposed to suction. In some patients, a lumbar drain can be used to reduce the potential flow gradient of cerebrospinal fluid into the pleural space.[66] If the dural leak is noted postoperatively, reoperation and laminectomy will be required occasionally to close the dural defect.[5]

Other complications are related to the extent of resection, and these possibilities should be conveyed when obtaining the preoperative informed consent. Depending on the scope of the intended resection, these may include recurrent nerve palsy (vagus), Horner syndrome (sympathetic chain), neuralgia/paresthesia/hypesthesia/neuropraxia (nerve root, brachial plexus), and dyspnea (lung, phrenic nerve).[1–3,5] Other complications, such as wound infection, atelectasis, post-thoracotomy or post-thoracoscopic port neuralgia, and chylothorax, are managed with standard measures.

SUMMARY

Most thoracic neurogenic tumors are found in the posterior mediastinum, and most posterior mediastinal neoplasms are neurogenic in origin. Adequate preoperative workup includes elucidation of any functional symptoms or symptoms of local invasion. The radiologic workup must definitively assess for neural foraminal and spinal canal involvement by tumor, which could change the approach from solely thoracic to a combined spinal and thoracic procedure with involvement of a neurosurgical team. Most adult neurogenic tumors are benign, and surgical resection affords excellent survival and freedom from recurrence in most cases.

EDITOR'S COMMENT

The management of presumed neurogenic tumors requires an appreciation of the clinical context. In the elderly patient with comorbidities, the statistical likelihood of benignity is a prudent rationale for surveillance. Alternatively, an otherwise healthy patient may warrant surgical intervention, given the nonzero frequency of events such as malignant neurogenic tumors and unexpected malignant diagnoses (e.g., mesothelioma, thymic implant, etc.).

—Steven J. Mentzer

References

1. Takeda S, Miyoshi S, Minami M, et al. Intrathoracic neurogenic tumors-50 years' experience in a Japanese institution. *Eur J Cardiothorac Surg.* 2004;26(4):807–812.
2. Ardissone F, Andrion A, D'Alessandro L, et al. Neurogenic intrathoracic tumors. A clinicopathological review of 92 cases. *Thorac Cardiovasc Surg.* 1986;34(4):260–264.
3. Davidson KG, Walbaum PR, McCormack RJ. Intrathoracic neural tumours. *Thorax.* 1978;33(3):359–367.
4. Davis RD Jr, Oldham HN Jr, Sabiston DC Jr. Primary cysts and neoplasms of the mediastinum: recent changes in clinical presentation, methods of diagnosis, management, and results. *Ann Thorac Surg.* 1987;44(3):229–237.
5. Ribet ME, Cardot GR. Neurogenic tumors of the thorax. *Ann Thorac Surg.* 1994;58(4):1091–1095.
6. Yamaguchi M, Yoshino I, Fukuyama S, et al. Surgical treatment of neurogenic tumors of the chest. *Ann Thorac Cardiovasc Surg.* 2004;10(3):148–151.
7. Azarow KS, Pearl RH, Zurcher R, et al. Primary mediastinal masses. A comparison of adult and pediatric populations. *J Thorac Cardiovasc Surg.* 1993;106(1):67–72.
8. Blegvad S, Lippert H, Simper LB, et al. Mediastinal tumours. A report of 129 cases. *Scand J Thorac Cardiovasc Surg.* 1990;24(1):39–42.
9. Reeder LB. Neurogenic tumors of the mediastinum. *Semin Thorac Cardiovasc Surg.* 2000;12(4):261–267.
10. Reed JC, Hallet KK, Feigin DS. Neural tumors of the thorax: subject review from the AFIP. *Radiology.* 1978;126(1):9–17.
11. Gale AW, Jelihovsky T, Grant AF, et al. Neurogenic tumors of the mediastinum. *Ann Thorac Surg.* 1974;17(5):434–443.
12. Shields TW, Reynolds M. Neurogenic tumors of the thorax. *Surg Clin North Am.* 1988;68(3):645–668.
13. Strollo DC, Rosado-de-Christenson ML, Jett JR. Primary mediastinal tumors: part II. Tumors of the middle and posterior mediastinum. *Chest.* 1997;112(5):1344–1357.
14. Plotkin SR, Halpin C, McKenna MJ, et al., Erlotinib for progressive vestibular schwannoma in neurofibromatosis 2 patients. *Otol Neurotol.* 2010;31(7):1135–1143.
15. Plotkin SR, Singh MA, O'Donnell CC, et al. Audiologic and radiographic response of NF2-related vestibular schwannoma to erlotinib therapy. *Nat Clin Pract Oncol.* 2008;5(8):487–491.

16. Plotkin SR, Singh MA, O'Donnell CC, et al. Hearing improvement after bevacizumab in patients with neurofibromatosis type 2. *N Engl J Med.* 2009;361(4):358–367.
17. Mautner VF, Nguyen R, Kutta H, et al. Bevacizumab induces regression of vestibular schwannomas in patients with neurofibromatosis type 2. *Neuro Oncol.* 2010;12(1):14–18.
18. Machida E., Haniuda M, Eguchi T, et al. Granular cell tumor of the mediastinum. *Intern Med.* 2003;42(2):178–181.
19. Ordonez NG, Mackay B. Granular cell tumor: a review of the pathology and histogenesis. *Ultrastruct Pathol.* 1999;23(4):207–222.
20. Angeles RM, Papari M, Malecki Z. Pathologic quiz case: a 43-year-old woman with an incidentally detected posterior mediastinal mass. Granular cell tumor of the posterior mediastinum. *Arch Pathol Lab Med.* 2005;129(1):e27–e28.
21. Brodeur GM, Pritchard J, Berthold F, et al. Revisions of the international criteria for neuroblastoma diagnosis, staging, and response to treatment. *J Clin Oncol.* 1993;11(8):1466–1477.
22. Lonergan GJ, Schwab CM, Suarez ES, et al. Neuroblastoma, ganglioneuroblastoma, and ganglioneuroma: radiologic-pathologic correlation. *Radiographics.* 2002;22(4):911–934.
23. Horiuchi A, Muraji T, Tsugawa C, et al. Thoracic neuroblastoma: outcome of incomplete resection. *Pediatr Surg Int.* 2004;20(9):714–718.
24. Shimizu M, Shimizu T, Adachi T, et al. Long-term survival in adult mediastinal neuroblastoma. *Jpn J Thorac Cardiovasc Surg.* 2003;51(7):326–329.
25. Geoerger B, Hero B, Harms D, et al. Metabolic activity and clinical features of primary ganglioneuromas. *Cancer.* 2001;91(10):1905–1913.
26. Demir HA, Yalçin B, Büyükpamukçu N, et al. Thoracic neuroblastic tumors in childhood. *Pediatr Blood Cancer.* 2010;54(7):885–889.
27. Adam A, Hochholzer L. Ganglioneuroblastoma of the posterior mediastinum: a clinicopathologic review of 80 cases. *Cancer.* 1981;47(2):373–381.
28. Moran CA, Suster S, Fishback N, et al. Mediastinal paragangliomas. A clinicopathologic and immunohistochemical study of 16 cases. *Cancer.* 1993;72(8):2358–2364.
29. Noorda RJ, Wuisman PI, Kummer AJ, et al. Nonfunctioning malignant paraganglioma of the posterior mediastinum with spinal cord compression. A case report. *Spine.* 1996;21(14):1703–1709.
30. Odze R, Begin LR. Malignant paraganglioma of the posterior mediastinum. A case report and review of the literature. *Cancer.* 1990;65(3):564–569.
31. Victor S, Anand V, Andappan P, et al. Malignant mediastinal chemodectoma. *Chest.* 1975;68(4):583–584.
32. Rosenfeld JV, Kevau I, Jacob O, et al. Dumbbell schwannoma causing acute spinal cord compression: case report. *P N G Med J.* 1994;37(1):40–44.
33. Kuhlman JE, Bouchardy L, Fishman EK, et al. CT and MR imaging evaluation of chest wall disorders. *Radiographics.* 1994;14(3):571–595.
34. Kumar AJ, Kuhajda FP, Martinez CR, et al. Computed tomography of extracranial nerve sheath tumors with pathological correlation. *J Comput Assist Tomogr.* 1983;7(5):857–865.
35. Ikezoe J, Sone S, Higashihara T, et al. CT of intrathoracic neurogenic tumours. *Eur J Radiol.* 1986;6(4):266–269.
36. Lee JY, Lee KS, Han J, et al. Spectrum of neurogenic tumors in the thorax: CT and pathologic findings. *J Comput Assist Tomogr.* 1999;23(3):399–406.
37. Sakai F, Sone S, Kiyono K, et al. Intrathoracic neurogenic tumors: MR-pathologic correlation. *AJR Am J Roentgenol.* 1992;159(2):279–283.
38. Shadmehr MB, Gaissert HA, Wain JC, et al. The surgical approach to "dumbbell tumors" of the mediastinum. *Ann Thorac Surg.* 2003;76(5):1650–1654.
39. Ilias I, Pacak K. Diagnosis and management of tumors of the adrenal medulla. *Horm Metab Res.* 2005;37(12):717–721.
40. Shulkin BL, Hutchinson RJ, Castle VP, et al. Neuroblastoma: positron emission tomography with 2-[fluorine-18]-fluoro-2-deoxy-D-glucose compared with metaiodobenzylguanidine scintigraphy. *Radiology.* 1996;199(3):743–750.
41. Ilias I, Shulkin B, Pacak K. New functional imaging modalities for chromaffin tumors, neuroblastomas and ganglioneuromas. *Trends Endocrinol Metab.* 2005;16(2):66–72.
42. Roger PA, Berna P, Merlusca G, et al. [Schwannoma of the vagus nerve: diagnostic strategy and therapeutic approach]. *Rev Mal Respir.* 2012;29(1):70–73.
43. Sadok Boudaya M, Dechaud C, Gossot D, et al. [Benign schwannoma with high uptake of 18 fluorodeoxglucose (PET-Scan)]. *Rev Mal Respir.* 2009;26(1):63–65.
44. Hsu CH, Lee CM, Wang FC, et al. Neurofibroma with increased uptake of [F-18]-fluoro-2 deoxy-D-glucose interpreted as a metastatic lesion. *Ann Nucl Med.* 2003;17(7):609–611.
45. Auringer ST, Cox D. Thoracic ganglioneuroma presenting with the watery diarrhea, hypokalemia, achlorhydria (WHDA) syndrome. *Applied Radiology Online.* 2000;29(3).
46. Divisi D, Battaglia C, Crisci R, et al. Diagnostic and therapeutic approaches for masses in the posterior mediastinum. *Acta Biomed Ateneo Parmense.* 1998;69(5-6):123–128.
47. Gladish GW, Sabloff BM, Munden RF, et al. Primary thoracic sarcomas. *Radiographics.* 2002;22(3):621–637.
48. Rockoff SD, Rohatgi PK. Unusual manifestations of thoracic sarcoidosis. *AJR Am J Roentgenol.* 1985;144(3):513–528.
49. Sung SH, Chang JW, Kim J, et al. Solitary fibrous tumors of the pleura: surgical outcome and clinical course. *Ann Thorac Surg.* 2005;79(1):303–307.
50. Filly R, Bland N, Castellino RA. Radiographic distribution of intrathoracic disease in previously untreated patients with Hodgkin's disease and non-Hodgkin's lymphoma. *Radiology.* 1976;120(2):277–281.
51. Erdogan A, Eser I, Ozbilim G. Posterior mediastinal localization of Castleman's disease: report of a case. *Surg Today.* 2004;34(9):772–773.
52. Lupinski RW, Agasthian T, Lim CH, et al. Extralobar pulmonary sequestration simulates posterior neurogenic tumor. *Ann Thorac Surg.* 2004;77(6):2203–2204.
53. Heselson NG, Goldberg S. Intrathoracic meningocele: a report of two cases. *S Afr Med J.* 1976;50(53):2108–2110.
54. Bizekis CS, Pua B, Glassman LR. Thoracic splenosis: mimicry of a neurogenic tumor. *J Thorac Cardiovasc Surg.* 2003;125(5):1155–1156.
55. Falk RH. A posterior mediastinal mass diagnosed by echocardiogram. *Chest.* 1995;108(5):1447–1448.
56. Gentry SE, Harris MA. Posterior mediastinal mass in a patient with chest pain. *Chest.* 1995;107(6):1757–1759.
57. Kline RM, Reyna PA, Reyna TM. Azygous lobe presenting as a posterior mediastinal mass in a 2-year-old boy. *J Pediatr Surg.* 1998;33(12):1829–1830.
58. Kurosaki Y, Tanaka YO, Itai Y. Mature teratoma of the posterior mediastinum. *Eur Radiol.* 1998;8(1):100–102.
59. Moran CA, Suster S, Fishback N, et al. Extramedullary hematopoiesis presenting as posterior mediastinal mass: a study of four cases. *Mod Pathol.* 1995;8(3):249–251.
60. Bressler EL, Kirkham JA. Mediastinal masses: alternative approaches to CT-guided needle biopsy. *Radiology.* 1994;191(2):391–396.
61. Gupta RK, Dowle CS. A case of neurilemoma (schwannoma) that mimicked a pleomorphic adenoma (an example of potential pitfall in aspiration cytodiagnosis). *Diagn Cytopathol.* 1991;7(6):622–624.
62. Kara M., Ozkan M, Sak SD, et al. Giant ancient schwannoma of the posterior mediastinum cytologically misdiagnosed as a malignant tumour. A case report. *Acta Chir Belg.* 2002;102(6):464–466.
63. Murphey MD, Smith WS, Smith SE, et al. From the archives of the AFIP. Imaging of musculoskeletal neurogenic tumors: radiologic-pathologic correlation. *Radiographics.* 1999;19(5):1253–1280.
64. Akwari OE, Payne WS, Onofrio BM, et al. Dumbbell neurogenic tumors of the mediastinum. Diagnosis and management. *Mayo Clin Proc.* 1978;53(6):353–358.
65. Shamji FM, Todd TR, Vallières E, et al. Central neurogenic tumours of the thoracic region. *Can J Surg.* 1992;35(5):497–501.
66. Han PP, Dickman CA. Thoracoscopic resection of thoracic neurogenic tumors. *J Neurosurg.* 2002;96(Suppl 3):304–308.
67. Castelein RM, MacEwen GD. A dumbbell (hourglass) neurofibroma of the spine in a patient with von Recklinghausen's disease. A case report with twelve-year follow-up. *Arch Orthop Trauma Surg.* 1984;102(4):216–220.
68. King D, Goodman J, Hawk T, et al. Dumbbell neuroblastomas in children. *Arch Surg.* 1975;110(8):888–891.
69. Grillo HC, Ojemann RG, Scannell JG, et al. Combined approach to "dumbbell" intrathoracic and intraspinal neurogenic tumors. *Ann Thorac Surg.* 1983;36(4):402–407.
70. Pompili A., Caroli F, Cattani F, et al. Unilateral limited laminectomy as the approach of choice for the removal of thoracolumbar neurofibromas. *Spine.* 2004;29(15):1698–1702.
71. Hazelrigg SR, Boley TM, Krasna MJ, et al. Thoracoscopic resection of posterior neurogenic tumors. *Am Surg.* 1999;65(12):1129–1133.

72. Liu HP, Yim AP, Wan J, et al. Thoracoscopic removal of intrathoracic neurogenic tumors: a combined Chinese experience. *Ann Surg*. 2000;232(2):187–190.
73. Riquet M, Mouroux J, Pons F, et al. Videothoracoscopic excision of thoracic neurogenic tumors. *Ann Thorac Surg*. 1995;60(4):943–946.
74. Lacreuse I, Valla JS, de Lagausie P, et al. Thoracoscopic resection of neurogenic tumors in children. *J Pediatr Surg*. 2007;42(10):1725–1728.
75. Barrenechea IJ, Fukumoto R, Lesser JB, et al. Endoscopic resection of thoracic paravertebral and dumbbell tumors. *Neurosurgery*. 2006;59(6):1195–1201; discussion 1201–1202.
76. Ponce FA, Killory BD, Wait SD, et al. Endoscopic resection of intrathoracic tumors: experience with and long-term results for 26 patients. *J Neurosurg Spine*. 2011;14(3):377–381.
77. Bousamra M 2nd, Haasler GB, Patterson GA, et al. A comparative study of thoracoscopic vs open removal of benign neurogenic mediastinal tumors. *Chest*. 1996;109(6):1461–1465.
78. Heltzer JM, Krasna MJ, Aldrich F, et al. Thoracoscopic excision of a posterior mediastinal "dumbbell" tumor using a combined approach. *Ann Thorac Surg*. 1995;60(2):431–433.
79. Konno S, Yabuki S, Kinoshita T, et al. Combined laminectomy and thoracoscopic resection of dumbbell-type thoracic cord tumor. *Spine*. 2001;26(6):E130–E134.
80. Ruurda JP, Hanlo PW, Hennipman A, et al. Robot-assisted thoracoscopic resection of a benign mediastinal neurogenic tumor: technical note. *Neurosurgery*. 2003;52(2):462–464; discussion 464.
81. Yoshino I, Hashizume M, Shimada M, et al. Video-assisted thoracoscopic extirpation of a posterior mediastinal mass using the da Vinci computer enhanced surgical system. *Ann Thorac Surg*. 2002;74(4):1235–1237.
82. Morgan JA, Ginsburg ME, Sonett JR, et al. Advanced thoracoscopic procedures are facilitated by computer-aided robotic technology. *Eur J Cardiothorac Surg*. 2003;23(6):883–887; discussion 887.
83. Weissenbacher A, Bodner J. Robotic surgery of the mediastinum. *Thorac Surg Clin*. 2010;20(2):331–339.
84. Cerfolio RJ, Bryant AS, Minnich DJ. Operative techniques in robotic thoracic surgery for inferior or posterior mediastinal pathology. *J Thorac Cardiovasc Surg*. 2012;143(5):1138–1143.
85. Kajiwara N, Kakihana M, Usuda J, et al. Extended indications for robotic surgery for posterior mediastinal tumors. *Asian Cardiovasc Thorac Ann*. 2012;20(3):308–313.

163 Malignant Primary Anterior Mediastinal Tumors

Prashant C. Shah and Ciaran J. McNamee

Keywords: Thymoma, thymic carcinoma, seminoma, nonseminomatous germ cell tumor, teratoma, mediastinal lymphoma, Hodgkin lymphoma, non-Hodgkin lymphoma

Among the three mediastinal compartments, the anterior compartment has the greatest potential for developing a primary mediastinal malignancy. Malignant tumors often are symptomatic and have considerable bulk compared with their benign counterparts. The most common primary malignant tumors of the anterior mediastinum include invasive thymomas, seminomas, nonseminomatous germ cell tumors (GCTs), malignant teratomas, and lymphomas. Commonly, at presentation, these masses manifest clinical symptoms as a result of either extrinsic compression of neighboring mediastinal structures or due to paraneoplastic syndromes. It is important to identify the specific pathology of these tumors, as each of these clinical entities requires a unique treatment strategy with different clinical outcome and prognosis.

ANATOMY AND PATHOLOGY

The anatomy of the three mediastinal compartments is outlined and reviewed in Chapters 155 and 161. The anterior compartment differs from the middle and posterior compartments in that it has a higher rate of malignant tumors. In a study of over 400 patients with primary mediastinal tumors, malignancy was identified in 59% of anterior compartment tumors as compared with only 29% for middle compartment and 16% for posterior compartment tumors in adults.[1,2] Malignancy is also dependent on age and the presence of symptoms. Children are more likely to develop lymphoma or malignant neurogenic tumors.[3] The presence of symptoms foretells malignant disease in 85% of patients, while only 46% of patients with symptoms have benign disease.[1,4] Posterior compartment mediastinal tumors are described in Chapter 162 and the middle mediastinal compartment is described in Chapter 161.

The three primary malignant mediastinal tumors that commonly occur in the anterior compartment are thymic tumors, GCTs, and lymphomas (Fig. 163-1). Each of these tumors can be further divided into subtypes, each possessing a unique tumor biology which influences treatment and outcomes. Mesenchymal tumors are uncommon, comprising less than 10% of anterior mediastinal tumors, and can be divided into tumors of vascular origin, lymphatic origin, or tumors of connective tissue origin.[5]

Thymoma and Thymic Tumors

Thymic tumors are the most frequently identified primary mediastinal tumor in adults and although they originate in

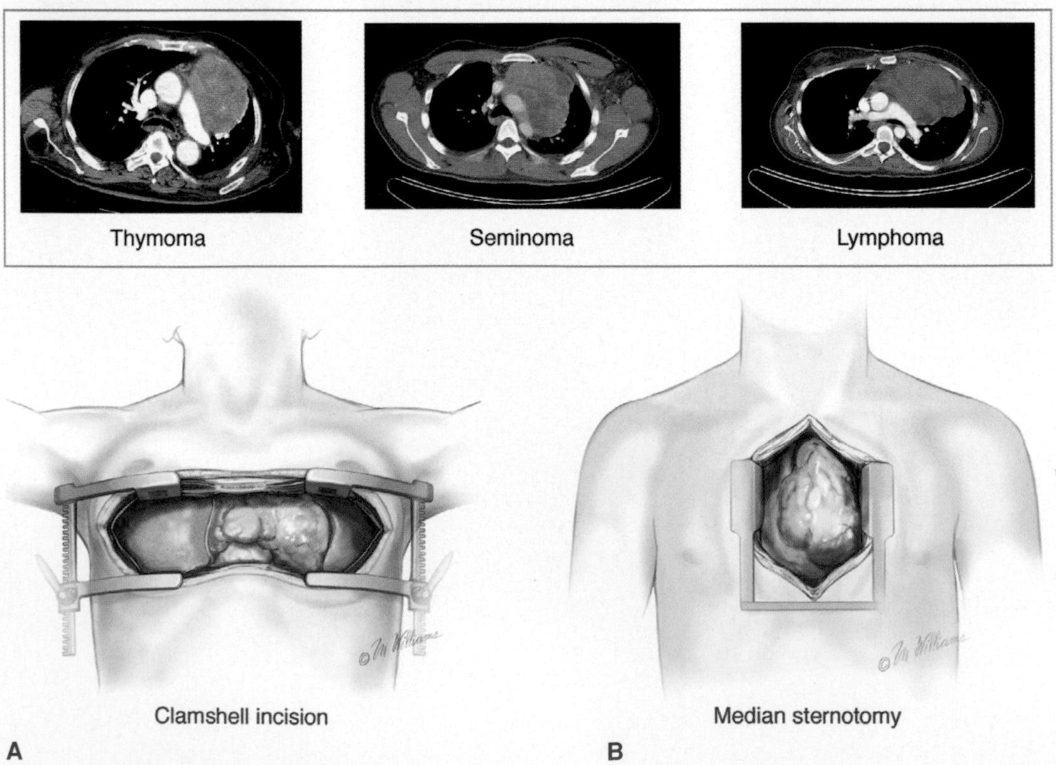

Figure 163-1. The three primary malignant tumors that occur in the anterior compartment are thymoma, seminoma, and lymphoma. Clamshell incisions (*A*) and median sternotomy (*B*) provide access for wide surgical margins.

the anterior mediastinum they may invade other neighboring structures or cavities. Thymic tumors are pathologically subclassified as noninvasive (encapsulated) thymomas, invasive thymomas, thymic carcinomas, and neuroendocrine thymic tumors. Of these thymic tumors, noninvasive thymomas are defined by encapsulation, without involvement of other surrounding structures. Invasive thymomas may ostensibly possess benign appearing features on histologic examination but they may also demonstrate malignant properties with invasion past the capsule into contiguous structures.[6] This extracapsular invasion can occur irrespective of size, such that at least 30% of thymomas may demonstrate invasion of surrounding mediastinal fat.[6,7] It has likewise been recognized that "noninvasive" thymoma pathology does not necessarily predict a "benign" clinical outcome. Stage I thymomas (i.e., well-encapsulated tumors without invasion) have been found to recur and metastasize, although these recurrences are usually indolent.[8] Thymic cancers do not possess the bland histologic features of thymoma; they demonstrate cellular atypia, mitoses, and necrosis and lack the organoid features of a normal thymus gland.[9–11] Neuroendocrine tumors of the thymus are rare; the most common histologic type is carcinoid tumors (typical and atypical). These thymic neuroendocrine tumors carry a worse prognosis as compared to carcinoid tumors of the lung.[12]

Thymoma

Clinically, thymomas may be associated with paraneoplastic syndromes. Myasthenia gravis is the most common parathymic syndrome, occurring in 45% of thymoma patients (range 10%–67%), followed by pure red blood cell aplasia (2%–5%) and hypogammaglobulinemia (2%–5%).[13] These tumors are also known to be associated with other neuromuscular syndromes, hematologic syndromes, autoimmune disorders, endocrine disorders, as well as immunodeficiency syndromes.[7] While prognosis is variable for the majority of these parathymic syndromes, symptoms of myasthenia gravis may improve postthymectomy for thymoma. However the neuromuscular improvement is not to the same extent that is observed in patients with thymic hyperplasia suggesting the possibility of a different pathway for antibody production with thymoma as compared to hyperplasia.[14]

The classification of thymomas is geared to prognosis and is based on extent of tumor invasiveness and tumor histology. Two different staging schemes have been proposed to accommodate both of these systems. I. Currently, the Masaoka staging system is used most widely for clinical staging (Table 163-1). This staging classification emphasizes a correlation between the extent of tumor involvement/invasion and prognosis. However, it is primarily based on local or distant extracapsular invasion and does not include the complex

Table 163-1

MASAOKA THYMOMA STAGING SYSTEM

Stage I	Encapsulated tumor without gross or microscopic capsular invasion
Stage IIA	Macroscopic invasion into surrounding mediastinal fat or pleura
Stage IIB	Microscopic capsular involvement
Stage III	Gross invasion of neighboring organs
Stage IVA	Pleural or pericardial spread
Stage IVB	Lymphatic or hematogenous metastases

Table 163-2

WORLD HEALTH ORGANIZATION CLASSIFICATION OF THYMOMA

A (medullary)	Thymoma with spindle or oval epithelial cells with little nuclear atypia and few lymphocytes.
AB (mixed)	Thymoma with features of A mixed with lymphocytes.
B1 (organoid)	Thymoma that resembles the normal functioning thymus with cortical and medullary areas.
B2 (cortical)	Thymoma with plump epithelial cells among a large population of lymphocytes.
B3 (epithelial)	Thymoma with epithelial cells with a round or polygonal shape with mild atypia in a sheetlike growth. They are admixed with a minor component of lymphocytes.
C (carcinoma)	Thymic tumor with obvious atypia and features that do not resemble thymus tissues. These tumors lack immature lymphocytes; if any are present, they are mature and mixed with plasma cells.

histology of thymic tumors, which many believe is relevant for determining overall clinical prognosis. To this end, a World Health Organization (WHO) classification (Table 163-2) was created.[15–18] This classification includes all thymic tumors, and differentiates thymomas according to separate morphology.[19] Each subsequent subtype in this classification (ranging from A to B3) demonstrates increasing abnormal histology of epithelial cells in proportion to lymphocytes with preserved organoid features, which is correlated with survival. Type C thymic tumors (thymic carcinoma) in comparison to thymomas demonstrate cytologic features of malignancy, a lack of encapsulation, and adherence to, or invasion of, mediastinal structures. These tumors fail to recapitulate the normal thymus tissue and may resemble malignant neoplasms from other organs.[20]

The prognosis for these tumors depends on three interrelated parameters: histologic features (i.e., WHO classification), staging (i.e., Masaoka classification), and the completeness of resection.[18] These three factors determine the invasiveness and metastatic potential of these tumors. Lymphatic or hematogenous involvement of these tumors is uncommon; however, local recurrence can occur, even for encapsulated tumors without capsular invasion after resection.[13] Long-term survival for thymoma has been directly related to stage, extent of resection, and histology.[21]

As part of the initial evaluation, thymic tumors require a complete chest and upper abdomen computed tomography (CT) scan to delineate the full extent of disease. The CT attenuation (fat attenuation vs. water attenuation) as well as the calcification and contrast pattern may be helpful to discriminate between the different anterior mediastinal tumors.[22] Positron emission tomography (PET) is not an obligatory investigation for this malignancy but may serve in difficult situations to discriminate thymic hyperplasia from thymic tumors and may also help to confirm metastatic disease.[23,24] Magnetic resonance imaging (MRI) is primarily useful with large tumors to identify the anatomy and possible invasion of vascular structures which may be distorted by tumor bulk. Preoperative biopsy has long been debated regarding its usefulness in the assessment of thymic tumors. Biopsy is considered unnecessary, particularly when there is substantial evidence of a parathymic syndrome, if the tumor is considered small (and possibly well encapsulated), and there is little likelihood of a competing diagnosis (e.g., germ cell tumor, lymphoma). In all other instances, a preoperative biopsy is helpful to determine appropriate therapy for the mediastinal tumor. Preoperative pathology has been found to be most useful in the differentiation between thymic tumors and lymphoma particularly because the latter is usually treated non-surgically.[13] Practical experience has demonstrated that biopsy tract seeding following thymic biopsy is a rather rare phenomenon. However, this does not address the practical concern of conversion of a Masaoka stage I thymoma to a Masaoka stage II thymoma by extrinsic capsular needle invasion.

In the preoperative investigation of an anterior mediastinal mass, patients with clinically suspected thymic tumors should be assessed for myasthenic signs and symptoms. If myasthenia gravis is suspected, an assay for antiacetylcholine receptor antibody titer will be diagnostic and will help to obviate the need for a preoperative biopsy. If the diagnosis is still unclear, all male patients should undergo a testicular examination, as well as serology for alpha-fetoprotein (AFP) and beta-human chorionic gonadotropin (beta-HCG), to help exclude the possibility of a malignant germ cell tumor. If the diagnosis is still elusive, biopsy is mandatory.

With respect to surgical resection, the surgical literature is divided between those who recommend traditional sternotomy with removal of both the tumor and its surrounding tissue to prevent local recurrence from microscopic invasion, and those who advocate a sternal-sparing procedure (i.e., thoracoscopic approach).[8,25] The perioperative considerations and surgical techniques for these different approaches are discussed in Chapters 159 and 160. Transcervical thymectomy is not an option for patients with thymomas or thymic tumors (Chapter 158); it is reserved specifically for patients with thymic hyperplasia or nonthymomatous thymic conditions.[26] Thoracoscopic approaches may be used for small (<4 cm), well-encapsulated thymomas and thymic cysts, but are not recommended for bulky or invasive thymomas or thymic tumors.[8,27] Large (>4 cm) or invasive thymomas (i.e., stage II or higher) may require a transsternal approach to help facilitate exposure and completeness of resection. In the preoperative setting, it may often be difficult to determine whether a small thymoma has an invasive component. Invasiveness may be predicted clinically or radiographically, based on the association of myasthenia gravis (primarily associated with B1, B2, and B3 thymomas), presence of calcifications, or a flat or irregular surface, as compared with a round or oval shape (as seen with encapsulated thymomas).[19] If invasion of surrounding structures is suspected, a transsternal radical thymectomy is recommended to decrease the local recurrence rate as well as to avoid future concerns as to the value of a re-do procedure for microscopic disease.

Complete thymus resection is the procedure of choice for thymomas with Masaoka stages I and II, as well as limited stage III cases. It is recommended that patients with more extensive thymomas (e.g., stages III and IVa) with obvious invasion or intrathoracic spread should undergo neoadjuvant chemotherapy, followed by complete surgical resection. Thymomas are chemosensitive, with objective response rates of 67% to 100%, and complete response rates of 33% (range 7%–57%). Complete surgical resection following induction chemotherapy yields response rates of 69% to 92%, although results likely depend on surgical expertise.[28] Some centers advocate induction chemotherapy protocols for thymomas >5 cm, and as treatment for locally recurrent thymomas prior to reoperation.[29]

Thymomas are also largely radiosensitive, and postoperative radiation therapy is increasingly utilized, particularly for locally advanced thymic tumors (e.g., stages II and III). Postoperative radiation was historically reserved for incomplete resections, but is now recommended by most large centers, particularly for stages II and III thymomas, even when resection is deemed complete.[30] The present available data, however, does not support improvement in survival or overall recurrence, but does suggest that mediastinal recurrence may be reduced.[31] Thus, radiation therapy immediately following resection for these tumors is reasonable, as is treatment for recurrences not amenable to reresection. Long-term surveillance is mandatory given the indolent biology of these tumors.

Chemotherapy is the primary modality for treatment of stage IV thymomas. Select patients with stage IVa thymomas, however, should be treated with neoadjuvant chemotherapy, followed by complete resection of all clinically evident disease. This has resulted in significantly improved 5-year and 10-year survivals (78% and 65%, respectively) for stage IVa patients.[32] However, for resection to be "complete," all pericardial and pleural implants should be widely excised, sometimes requiring pleurectomy, as well as lung resection (extrapleural pneumonectomy), in addition to thymectomy. Patients with evidence of extrathoracic disease (e.g., stage IVb) are not considered surgical candidates and are best treated with maintenance chemotherapy protocols. There is no established role for radiation therapy for stage IV disease.

Thymic Carcinomas

Thymic carcinomas (WHO type C) are not associated with parathymic syndromes, but instead cause symptoms of local compression or invasion. These tumors are markedly aggressive and invasive. Most are either squamous cell carcinomas or are lymphoepithelioma-like carcinomas. Roughly, about two-thirds of thymic carcinomas are high grade, and one-third are low grade. The low-grade thymic carcinomas are usually well localized, whereas the high-grade types are usually found to have extensive spread, at presentation.[9] While there is no established protocol for treatment of thymic carcinomas, most authors advocate a trimodality approach, including neoadjuvant chemoradiation followed by complete surgical resection.[33] Complete surgical resection can only be performed in one-third of patients, and survival is markedly better for low-grade thymic carcinomas.[5,13] Prognosis is poor for patients with nodal involvement, with a distant metastasis, with high-grade histology, or those with an incomplete resection.[34]

Other Thymic Tumors

Thymic neuroendocrine tumors are rare, accounting for fewer than 5% of anterior mediastinal tumors. They can be further subdivided into typical thymic carcinoids (low-grade), atypical thymic carcinoids (intermediate-grade), and thymic small-cell carcinomas (high-grade).[35] Collectively, they are all aggressive tumors compared with neuroendocrine tumors in other locations. Fifty percent of patients with a thymic carcinoid have an endocrine abnormality (e.g., Cushing syndrome or multiple endocrine neoplasia [MEN] syndrome). Expression of the carcinoid syndrome is, however, very rare.[35] Complete surgical resection, if possible, is the desired approach, because thymic carcinoids respond poorly to adjuvant therapy. Surgical debulking for extensive thymic carcinoids is warranted in selected cases, as this may help to palliate symptoms and prolong survival.[36] Octreotide therapy has also been shown to help palliate symptoms, particularly if the thymic carcinoid is associated with an endocrine syndrome. Thymic small-cell carcinomas are exceedingly rare, but likewise are aggressive, and are usually found to have extensive metastases on presentation. Surgery should only be offered for those with limited disease, or those who demonstrate a significant clinical response after induction therapy. Overall prognosis and survival is poor.[35]

PRIMARY MEDIASTINAL GERM CELL TUMORS

Mediastinal GCTs are thought to arise from an embryogenic error during the migration of germ cells to the gonads. They account for 50% to 75% of extragonadal GCTs and for 10% to 15% of primary mediastinal masses in adults.[7] They are predominantly located in the anterior mediastinal compartment, and are divided into four types.

1. Benign teratomas. These tumors may present as immature or mature lesions. A tumor is defined as mature if it has fewer than 50% immature elements. Mature benign teratomas can present in both prepubescent and postpubescent patients. Immature benign teratomas have more than 50% immature elements and are found primarily in prepubescent patients.[7,37] These tumors are discussed in Chapter 161.
2. Malignant teratomas. Malignant teratomas are the most common malignant GCT; they are defined as having more than 50% immature elements. These teratomas typically have a malignant component, associated with a GCT, epithelial malignancy (e.g., squamous cell carcinoma or adenocarcinoma), sarcoma, or a mixed malignancy. They present primarily in postpubescent patients.
3. Seminomas. These tumors are the second most frequent primary malignant GCTs, second only to teratomas. They occur almost exclusively in postpubescent male patients <45 years of age.
4. Nonseminomatous germ cell tumors (NSGCTs). These tumors are further subdivided into yolk sac tumors (endodermal sinus tumors), embryonal carcinomas, and choriocarcinomas. As with seminomas, these tumors are found almost exclusively in postpubescent male patients <40 years of age.[5,38]

As part of the initial investigation, tumor marker serology (AFP and beta-HCG) may often be helpful for the diagnosis of these tumors as well as for treatment protocols. These tumor markers should be obtained in all adult male patients at the first clinical encounter. A positive result implies a malignant NSGCT; a negative result, however, does not exclude a GCT malignancy, as pure teratomas and seminomas do not elaborate these tumor markers (Table 163-3).[39] Because testicular GCTs have a metastatic affinity for the anterior mediastinum, all adult male patients should undergo a testicular examination and a testicular ultrasound study as well. The evaluating clinician should have a low threshold for obtaining a transthoracic needle biopsy, particularly when the tumor marker serology and testicular examination are both negative, and the diagnosis is still elusive.[28] A chest and abdomen CT scan study is mandatory in all patients, as it will help to elaborate all sites of

Table 163-3

TUMOR MARKER SEROLOGY FOR GERM CELL TUMOR DIFFERENTIATION

GERM CELL TUMOR SUBTYPE	AFP	BETA-HCG
Embryonal carcinoma	+	–
Choriocarcinoma	–	+
Yolk sac tumor	+	+
Seminoma	–	–
Teratoma	–	–
Teratoma with embryonal carcinoma	+	–
Teratoma with choriocarcinoma	–	+

metastatic disease. PET scan has great potential for the evaluation of persistent or recurrent disease particularly when salvage surgery is considered.[40,41]

MALIGNANT TERATOMAS

Malignant teratomas are generally found only in the postpubescent population and represent teratomas that have undergone malignant transformation or have another associated GCT malignancy contained within. Most often, these teratomas are found to have a germinal layer that has transformed into frank malignancy, such as sarcoma, adenocarcinoma, or squamous cell carcinoma.[38] Unlike their benign counterparts, malignant teratomas in the adult patient are more often symptomatic with increased size on presentation, and compress adjacent mediastinal structures. As a result, adult patients with a malignant teratoma generally have symptoms of fatigue, weight loss, cough, dyspnea, and chest pain. On histology, they are typically solid and have a high composition of poorly differentiated tissue.

Preoperatively, if serum tumor markers (AFP and beta-HCG) are elevated, one should suspect the presence of NSGCT elements within the teratoma.[39] These patients should undergo surgical resection after an induction course of intensive chemotherapy targeted against the nonseminomatous elements. Conversely, if tumor marker serology and preoperative biopsy is negative for GCT involvement, surgery should be undertaken as first-line therapy. Teratomas associated with epithelial carcinoma or sarcoma are notoriously resistant to induction chemotherapy regimens.[38] Use of induction therapy should be avoided preoperatively in these cases. The presence of GCT elements in a teratoma is associated with a recurrence rate of 25%. However, if the malignant element is a sarcoma (commonly rhabdosarcoma or angiosarcoma), the prognosis is grave, and recurrence is common. Adjuvant treatment should be considered after resection in cases of malignant sarcomatous transformation to help prevent recurrence.[37,38] When teratoma recurrences and metastases are identified, they should be treated aggressively with surgery, provided all sites of disease can be reasonably resected.

Seminomas

Mediastinal seminomas are the second most frequent primary malignant mediastinal GCTs, accounting for about 37% of all mediastinal GCTs.[42] These tumors occur almost exclusively in adult males between ages 15 and 45 years, predominantly in Caucasian males. Although they are considered slow-growing, indolent tumors, mediastinal seminomas often are found to be rather large (>5 cm) at initial presentation.[43] Most patients have vague symptoms at presentation, while a minority has symptoms that are due to extrinsic compression of adjacent structures. Seminomas typically are also found to have early metastatic potential, with about 60% to 70% of patients identified to have metastases to bone, brain, lung, liver, or locoregional lymph nodes. CT imaging often demonstrates these masses as compressing other nearby structures, but rarely with an invasive component; they typically have a homogeneous appearance on CT scan.

All male patients should undergo serum tumor marker testing (AFP and beta-HCG) to exclude the possibility of NSGCT elements. While AFP and beta-HCG are very specific for NSGCTs and mixed GCTs (Table 163-3), pure seminomas have been demonstrated to have mildly elevated levels of beta-HCG (<100 mIU/mL) but are not known to elaborate AFP.[39] If any AFP is present, or if beta-HCG is moderately elevated (>500 mIU/mL), then the mediastinal mass is regarded as having nonseminomatous elements or mixed GCT components; these patients are then treated with a NSGCT regimen. If AFP and beta-HCG are both negative, then a CT-guided needle biopsy should be done to provide a tissue diagnosis.[44] All male patients must undergo a bimanual testicular examination, testicular ultrasound, and a chest/abdomen CT scan study to help identify all sites of potential GCT disease.

Despite having a high metastatic affinity, mediastinal seminomas are very chemosensitive and radiosensitive, and thus, have a very favorable prognosis (88% 5-year survival), akin to gonadal seminomas.[5,7] Primary first-line therapy with the use of platinum-based chemotherapy has resulted in remission rates >95%.[45] The multiagent regimen found to be most efficacious for treating seminomas includes cisplatin, bleomycin, etoposide, and vinblastine. When persistent or residual disease is identified radiographically after a course of intense chemotherapy, adjuvant radiation therapy is recommended. If persistent or new metastatic disease is identified after initial chemotherapy, then measures such as dose escalation or change in chemotherapy agents should be undertaken first.

Because of the excellent results obtained with chemotherapy and radiation, surgery does not have a primary role in the treatment of mediastinal seminomas. Previously, surgery had been advocated in the adjuvant setting after a course of chemotherapy to help query the presence of persistent, viable tumor.[46] While surgery can still be helpful in this regard, most have now advocated additional chemotherapy or radiation therapy when there is persistent radiographic evidence of disease.[47] There are nonetheless several reports of previously treated "pure seminomas" whereby surgery after chemotherapy did identify teratomatous elements that had not been previously recognized. In these rare instances, surgery may have an adjunctive role, but should not be incorporated into a routine treatment regimen for mediastinal seminomas.

Nonseminomatous Germ Cell Tumors

Like mediastinal seminomas, mediastinal NSGCTs occur almost exclusively in adult male patients <40 years of age. There are several different histologic subtypes in this group, all of which have similar tumor biology but behave differently than pure seminomas. For this reason, they are grouped together as NSGCTs. About 45% to 50% of mediastinal GCTs are found to have NSGCT histology. While teratocarcinomas and yolk sac tumors (endodermal sinus tumors) are more commonly encountered and collectively account for more than 75% of all mediastinal NSGCTs, the other histologies (mixed GCT, choriocarcinoma, and embryonal carcinoma) are not rare and do account for the other 25% of mediastinal NSGCTs.[42]

On initial presentation, mediastinal NSGCTs are identified as large, infiltrating masses that frequently invade and compress adjacent mediastinal structures. These tumors are typically known for their rapid growth and early metastatic potential. Over 85% of patients are found to have metastatic disease at presentation, usually involving lung, pleura, liver, or locoregional or distant lymph nodes.[48] Upon imaging of these tumors, CT scan often demonstrates an obvious local compressive and invasive component, as well as an inhomogeneous appearance, due to multiple areas of hemorrhage and necrosis within the mass.[49]

All adult male patients suspected of having a mediastinal GCT should undergo serum tumor marker testing (AFP and beta-HCG), a bimanual testicular exam, a testicular ultrasound, and a chest/abdomen CT scan, during the initial evaluation. When tested together, AFP and beta-HCG have a high specificity for NSGCT, whereby about 90% of patients with an NSGCT will have either an elevated AFP or beta-HCG.[39] A positive result is regarded as diagnostic for NSGCT and will help to obviate the need for a diagnostic biopsy. A CT-guided needle biopsy should only be reserved for those with negative AFP and beta-HCG results, where the diagnosis is still in question.[44]

Because each of the mediastinal NSGCT subtypes is known to have aggressive tumor biology with early invasion and metastases, local forms of therapy (e.g., surgery or radiation) are contraindicated as a first-line measure. Instead, it is now standard practice to begin initial treatment for a mediastinal NSGCT with four cycles of intensive cisplatin-based combination chemotherapy. Although still dismal, this treatment strategy has resulted in a 42% 5-year survival.[50] The most common agents used alongside cisplatin are etoposide, bleomycin, and vinblastine.

After chemotherapy, patients should undergo reimaging scans and repeat serology (AFP and beta-HCG) testing to help determine therapeutic response. When both the CT scan and serology are normal (no evidence of residual disease), no further therapy is required beyond close surveillance. If CT imaging does identify a residual abnormality, or if surveillance imaging identifies relapse, then surgery should be considered when complete resection is possible. In this setting, elevated tumor markers (AFP and beta-HCG) are not a contraindication for resection, since further chemotherapy has proven to be ineffective. Expectations of postchemotherapy pathology for mediastinal NSGCTs include teratoma (34%), residual NSGCT (31.4%), and necrosis/fibrosis (25.5%).[50] The remaining patients have demonstrated non-GCT histology (e.g., epithelial carcinoma or sarcoma). In these instances, surgical resection has proved to be diagnostic and curative. When residual viable GCT is identified in the final pathology, adjuvant chemotherapy should be given to help prevent recurrence. If the initial postchemotherapy CT scan demonstrates unresectable persistent disease, a multi-disciplinary approach including surgery is the only reasonable option for these patients who may demonstrate induction chemotherapy resistance.[45,51]

Overall poor prognostic factors for mediastinal NSGCT patients include persistently elevated tumor markers postchemotherapy, persistent unresectable disease postchemotherapy, and presence of viable tumor after resection.[50,52]

MEDIASTINAL LYMPHOMA

Mediastinal lymphoma commonly occurs as a manifestation of systemic disease; however, in 5% of cases, the mediastinum is the only site of disease occurrence. Primary mediastinal lymphoma is derived from thymic lymphocytes. Commonly, if the thymic lymphocytes develop into lymphoma, they devolve into Hodgkin lymphoma (HL); however, they also may degenerate into non-Hodgkin B-cell lymphoma (NHL) or lymphoblastic lymphoma (LL).[5,7] Mediastinal lymphoma accounts for 20% of mediastinal tumors in adults and 50% of mediastinal tumors in children. These tumors may occur in any compartment, but typically, HL has a predilection for the anterior mediastinum. The diagnosis is often achieved by CT-guided core needle biopsy. Surgery is required only for diagnostic purposes, such as for CT-guided biopsy failures or to diagnose residual masses after chemotherapy.

Hodgkin Lymphoma

Although HL only represents 25% of all lymphomas, it is the most common subtype of the primary mediastinal lymphomas, representing about 70% of mediastinal cases. Typically, it has a bimodal distribution, most commonly affecting young adults (ages 15–35 years) and older adults (age >55 years).[53] Although there is a near equal gender distribution, males with HL have higher mortality than their female counterparts.

There are four specific histologic HL subtypes: nodular sclerosis, lymphocyte-predominant, mixed cellularity, and lymphocyte-depleted. The nodular sclerosis subtype is the most common, but the lymphocyte-predominant subtype has the best prognosis. The classic Reed–Sternberg cell is not only highly characteristic, but also pathognomonic for HL.

The clinical presentation of mediastinal HL is varied, ranging from those who are completely asymptomatic to those with persistent "B-type" symptoms (e.g., fevers, chills, night sweats, and weight loss). The majority of patients will have palpable cervical or supraclavicular disease on initial presentation, either as evident lymphadenopathy or a bulky mediastinal mass.[54]

In the diagnostic evaluation of a mediastinal mass, it is important to obtain chest/abdomen/pelvis CT imaging as well as PET imaging, particularly when lymphoma is suspected and is high in the differential.[55] Prebiopsy imaging will help guide and determine the least invasive means to obtain diagnostic tissue most accessibly. While CT-guided fine-needle aspiration (FNA) often does not confer sufficient tissue for diagnosis of lymphoma, a core-needle biopsy may be more helpful. In other cases, particularly when the disease is centrally located and inaccessible, surgical measures are required for biopsy, such as cervical mediastinoscopy, anterior mediastinotomy (Chamberlain procedure), thoracoscopy, or, rarely, thoracotomy. Once a tissue diagnosis is obtained, staging is completed with serology and a bone-marrow biopsy.

The primary treatment modality for HL is chemoradiation therapy for early-stage disease, and combination chemotherapy with adriamycin (doxorubicin), bleomycin, vinblastine, and dacarbazine (ABVD), for more advanced stages. With this treatment standard, very high complete-remission rates (90% for early-stage HL, and 82% for advanced-stage HL) have been achieved.[56,57] HL patients with relapsing disease are candidates for high-dose chemotherapy, followed by autologous stem-cell transplant. Prognosis is still favorable in this group, as demonstrated by a 76% 5-year survival after treatment.[58]

Non-Hodgkin Lymphoma

Patients with NHL often present with diffuse disease, with 85% of patients presenting with systemic symptoms. About 5% of NHL patients have a primary mediastinal component, and are termed as having primary mediastinal B-cell lymphoma (PMBL). PMBL most commonly affects young adults (ages 20–40 years) and has a slightly greater predilection for females.[59] On presentation, these patients are commonly identified to have symptoms related to compression of adjacent mediastinal structures. One-third of these PMBL patients will present with superior vena cava syndrome, while many others will present with dysphagia, hoarseness of voice, phrenic nerve palsy, productive cough, or chest pain. PMBL often can be infiltrative, and can invade lung, pleura, chest wall, diaphragm, pericardium, and supraclavicular fossae. However, unlike the other subtypes of NHL, PMBL rarely has extrathoracic disease or spread.[59]

The diagnostic and staging workup for NHL is similar to that used for HL patients. Adequate tissue sampling is necessary to differentiate the different subtypes of mediastinal lymphoma. On histology, PMBL is manifest as numerous medium-sized or large-sized B cells with abundant cytoplasm. In ambiguous cases, flow cytometry and immunophenotyping can distinguish PMBL from the other subtypes of NHL.[59] Treatment for PMBL consists of multidrug chemotherapy with the addition of rituximab.[60] Those with acute compressive symptoms (e.g., superior vena cava syndrome) usually achieve relief with this standard regimen, without the need for adjunctive radiation. Postchemotherapy residual masses can either be treated with radiation therapy or consolidation with autologous stem-cell transplant. When treatment failures occur in PMBL patients, they usually are identified in the first 6 to 12 months. Recurrences after 2 years are rare for PMBL patients, unlike HL patients. Recurrences are best treated with high-dose chemotherapy and autologous stem-cell transplant.[61]

Lymphoblastic Lymphoma

Although LL is a rare subtype of NHL, it is regarded as a highly aggressive tumor of T-cell phenotype. It is the most common mediastinal lymphoma in children, but can also affect young adults (ages 15–30 years) and older adults (age >50 years). However, patients with LL are typically male adolescents.[62] On presentation, these patients are found to have diffuse disease, with mediastinal involvement, with bone marrow involvement, and with about 10% having central nervous system involvement.[62] When LL is suspected, the diagnostic and staging workup should be done expeditiously to allow for prompt initiation of treatment.

Treatment for LL consists of high-dose intensive multidrug chemotherapy. These multiagent regimens have resulted in a complete-remission rate of 80%, and a 5-year survival of 45%. Low-dose maintenance chemotherapy is typically instituted for about 2 years after initial treatment. Radiation therapy is generally reserved for large residual masses postchemotherapy. Recurrences and refractory disease is best treated with high-dose chemotherapy and autologous stem-cell transplant.[62]

Malignant Anterior Mesenchymal Tumors

These include tumors of adipose tissue (liposarcoma), vascular tissue (hemangioendothelioma, hemangiopericytoma and angiosarcoma), lymphatic tissue (lymphangiosarcoma and lymphangiopericytoma), connective tissue (fibrosarcoma, malignant fibrous histiocytoma, inflammatory fibrosarcoma), skeletal tissue (osteosarcoma, chondrosarcoma), and muscular origin (leiomyosarcoma, rhabdomyosarcoma).[5,7] These tumors are fortunately rare as they are often very aggressive and may require combination therapy including chemotherapy and radiation therapy with surgical therapy if possible.

SUMMARY

Primary malignant anterior mediastinal masses include a variety of tumor subtypes, each with unique tumor biology and patient presentation. The clinical presentation and radiographic appearance may help to distinguish the possible underlying pathology. Minimally invasive tissue sampling techniques may be needed to corroborate the diagnosis. Tumor marker serology (e.g., AFP and beta-HCG) should be routinely obtained in young adult male patients with an anterior mediastinal mass, as often this serology can be diagnostic for a malignant GCT. Staging generally requires both CT scanning and may include PET imaging.

Definitive treatment options and the order of treatment sequences are dependent on tumor type and stage. While surgery plays a primary role for treatment of early-stage thymomas, advanced thymic tumors, and certain GCTs may be best dealt with by a multimodality approach. Surgery may be helpful in a diagnostic role for seminomas and lymphomas; however, with advanced anterior mediastinal malignancies, surgery may be an adjunct to oncologists for the resection of residual malignant anterior mediastinal masses after chemotherapy. The prognosis is variable for each of the different tumor subtypes, but does largely depend on treatment response.

EDITOR'S COMMENT

Almost all patients with large mediastinal tumors, in the >8 cm range, will benefit from a multimodality approach. A critical surgical task is to help establish an accurate histologic diagnosis and facilitate treatment planning, a task complicated by cell type heterogeneity within many mediastinal tumors. Ample biopsies and a preliminary identification of "lesional tissue" by pathologists during the operation are essential for an accurate diagnosis.

—Steven J. Mentzer

References

1. Davis RD Jr, Oldham HN Jr, Sabiston DC Jr. Primary cysts and neoplasms of the mediastinum: recent changes in clinical presentation, methods of diagnosis, management, and results. *Ann Thorac Surg.* 1987;44(3):229–237.
2. Garey CL, Laituri CA, Valusek PA, et al. Management of anterior mediastinal masses in children. *Eur J Pediatr Surg.* 2011;21(5):310–313.
3. King RM, Telander RL, Smithson WA, et al. Primary mediastinal tumors in children. *J Pediatr Surg.* 1982;17(5):512–520.
4. Azarow KS, Pearl RH, Zurcher R, et al. Primary mediastinal masses. A comparison of adult and pediatric populations. *J Thorac Cardiovasc Surg.* 1993;106(1):67–72.
5. Macchiarini P, Ostertag H. Uncommon primary mediastinal tumours. *Lancet Oncol.* 20045(2):107–118.
6. Lewis JE, Wick MR, Scheithauer BW, et al. Thymoma. A clinicopathologic review. *Cancer.* 1987;60(11):2727–2743.
7. Priola AM, Priola SM, Cardinale L, et al. The anterior mediastinum: diseases. *Radiol Med.* 2006;111(3):312–342.
8. Roviaro G, Varoli F, Nucca O, et al. Videothoracoscopic approach to primary mediastinal pathology. *Chest.* 2000;117(4):1179–1183.
9. Suster S, Rosai J. Thymic carcinoma. A clinicopathologic study of 60 cases. *Cancer.* 1991;67(4):1025–1032.
10. Blumberg D, Burt ME, Bains MS, et al. Thymic carcinoma: current staging does not predict prognosis. *J Thorac Cardiovasc Surg.* 1998;115(2):303–308; discussion 308–309.
11. Suster S, Moran CA. Thymic carcinoma: spectrum of differentiation and histologic types. *Pathology.* 1998;30(2):111–122.
12. Chaer R, Massad MG, Evans A, et al. Primary neuroendocrine tumors of the thymus. *Ann Thorac Surg.* 2002;74(5):1733–1740.
13. Detterbeck FC, Parsons AM. Thymic tumors. *Ann Thorac Surg.* 2004;77(5):1860–1869.
14. Okumura M, Inoue M, Kadota Y, et al. Biological implications of thymectomy for myasthenia gravis. *Surg Today.* 2010;40(2):102–107.
15. Detterbeck FC. Clinical value of the WHO classification system of thymoma. *Ann Thorac Surg.* 2006;81(6):2328–2334.
16. Kondo K, Yoshizawa K, Tsuyuguchi M, et al. WHO histologic classification is a prognostic indicator in thymoma. *Ann Thorac Surg.* 2004;77(4):1183–1188.
17. Suster S. Diagnosis of thymoma. *J Clin Pathol.* 2006;59(12):1238–1244.
18. Suster S, Moran CA. Thymoma classification: current status and future trends. *Am J Clin Pathol.* 2006;125(4):542–554.
19. Okumura M, Shiono H, Minami M, et al. Clinical and pathological aspects of thymic epithelial tumors. *Gen Thorac Cardiovasc Surg.* 2008;56(1):10–16.
20. Hasserjian RP, Strobel P, Marx A. Pathology of thymic tumors. *Semin Thorac Cardiovasc Surg.* 2005;17(1):2–11.
21. Okumura M, Fujii Y, Shiono H, et al. Immunological function of thymoma and pathogenesis of paraneoplastic myasthenia gravis. *Gen Thorac Cardiovasc Surg.* 2008;56(4):143–150.
22. Quint L. Imaging of anterior mediastinal masses. *Cancer Imaging (Special Issue).* 2007;7:S56-S62.
23. Sung YM, Lee KS, Kim BT, et al. 18 F-FDG PET/CT of thymic epithelial tumors: usefulness for distinguishing and staging tumor subgroups. *J Nucl Med.* 2006;47(10):1628–1634.
24. Ustaalioglu BB, Seker M, Bilici A, et al. The role of PET-CT in the differential diagnosis of thymic mass after treatment of patients with lymphoma. *Med Oncol.* 2011;28(1):258–264.
25. Cheng YJ, Kao EL, Chou SH. Videothoracoscopic resection of stage II thymoma: prospective comparison of the results between thoracoscopy and open methods. *Chest.* 2005;128(4):3010–3012.
26. Deeb ME, Brinster CJ, Kucharzuk J, et al. Expanded indications for transcervical thymectomy in the management of anterior mediastinal masses. *Ann Thorac Surg.* 2001;72(1):208–211.
27. Pennathur A, Qureshi I, Schuchert MJ, et al. Comparison of surgical techniques for early-stage thymoma: feasibility of minimally invasive thymectomy and comparison with open resection. *J Thorac Cardiovasc Surg.* 2011;141(3):694–701.
28. Evans TL, Lynch TJ. Role of chemotherapy in the management of advanced thymic tumors. *Semin Thorac Cardiovasc Surg.* 2005;17(1):41–50.
29. Port JL, Ginsberg RJ. Surgery for thymoma. *Chest Surg Clin N Am.* 2001; 11(2):421–437.
30. Uematsu M., Yoshida H, Kondo M, et al. Entire hemithorax irradiation following complete resection in patients with stage II-III invasive thymoma. *Int J Radiat Oncol Biol Phys.* 1996;35(2):357–360.
31. Ogawa K, Uno T, Toita T, et al. Postoperative radiotherapy for patients with completely resected thymoma: a multi-institutional, retrospective review of 103 patients. *Cancer.* 2002;94(5):1405–1413.
32. Huang J, Rizk NP, Travis WD, et al. Feasibility of multimodality therapy including extended resections in stage IVA thymoma. *J Thorac Cardiovasc Surg.* 2007;134(6):1477–1483; discussion 1483–1484.
33. Greene MA, Malias MA. Aggressive multimodality treatment of invasive thymic carcinoma. *J Thorac Cardiovasc Surg.* 2003;125(2):434–436.
34. Kondo K, Monden Y. Lymphogenous and hematogenous metastasis of thymic epithelial tumors. *Ann Thorac Surg.* 2003;76(6):1859–1864; discussion 1864–1865.

35. Moran CA, Suster S. Neuroendocrine carcinomas (carcinoid tumor) of the thymus. A clinicopathologic analysis of 80 cases. *Am J Clin Pathol.* 2000;114(1):100–110.
36. Best LA, Westbrook BM, Trastek VF, et al. Surgery in the management of mediastinal carcinoid. *J Cardiovasc Surg (Torino).* 1994;35(6 Suppl 1):133–135.
37. Dulmet EM, Macchiarini P, Suc B, et al. Germ cell tumors of the mediastinum. A 30-year experience. *Cancer.* 1993;72(6):1894–1901.
38. Dominguez Malagon H, Perez Montiel D. Mediastinal germ cell tumors. *Semin Diagn Pathol.* 2005;22(3):230–240.
39. Nichols CR. Mediastinal germ cell tumors. Clinical features and biologic correlates. *Chest.* 1991;99(2):472–479.
40. De Giorgi U, Pupi A, Fiorentini G, et al. FDG-PET in the management of germ cell tumor. *Ann Oncol.* 2005;16(Suppl 4):iv90–94.
41. Buchler T, Dusek P, Brisuda A, et al. Positron emission tomography and clinical predictors of survival in primary extragonadal germ cell tumors. *Klin Onkol.* 2012;25(3):178–183.
42. Moran CA, Suster S. Primary germ cell tumors of the mediastinum: I. Analysis of 322 cases with special emphasis on teratomatous lesions and a proposal for histopathologic classification and clinical staging. *Cancer.* 1997;80(4):681–690.
43. Martini N, Golbey RB, Hajdu SI, et al. Primary mediastinal germ cell tumors. *Cancer.* 1974;33(3):763–769.
44. Chhieng DC, Lin O, Moran CA, et al. Fine-needle aspiration biopsy of nonteratomatous germ cell tumors of the mediastinum. *Am J Clin Pathol.* 2002;118(3):418–424.
45. Bokemeyer C, Nichols CR, Droz JP, et al. Extragonadal germ cell tumors of the mediastinum and retroperitoneum: results from an international analysis. *J Clin Oncol.* 2002;20(7):1864–1873.
46. Kolodziejski L, Duda K, Niezabitowski A, et al. Occurrence of malignant non-germ cell components in primary mediastinal germ cell tumours. *Eur J Surg Oncol.* 1999;25(1):54–60.
47. Motzer R, Bosl G, Heelan R, et al. Residual mass: an indication for further therapy in patients with advanced seminoma following systemic chemotherapy. *J Clin Oncol.* 1987;5(7):1064–1070.
48. Israel A, Bosl GJ, Golbey RB, et al. The results of chemotherapy for extragonadal germ-cell tumors in the cisplatin era: the Memorial Sloan-Kettering Cancer Center experience (1975 to 1982). *J Clin Oncol.* 1985;3(8):1073–1078.
49. Levitt RG, Husband JE, Glazer HS. CT of primary germ-cell tumors of the mediastinum. *AJR Am J Roentgenol.* 1984;142(1):73–78.
50. Kesler KA, Rieger KM, Hammoud ZT, et al. A 25-year single institution experience with surgery for primary mediastinal nonseminomatous germ cell tumors. *Ann Thorac Surg.* 2008;85(2):371–378.
51. Hartmann JT, Einhorn L, Nichols CR, et al. Second-line chemotherapy in patients with relapsed extragonadal nonseminomatous germ cell tumors: results of an international multicenter analysis. *J Clin Oncol.* 2001; 19(6):1641–1648.
52. Sakurai H, Asamura H, Suzuki K, et al. Management of primary malignant germ cell tumor of the mediastinum. *Jpn J Clin Oncol.* 2004;34(7):386–392.
53. Medeiros LJ, Greiner TC. Hodgkin's disease. *Cancer.* 1995;75(Suppl 1):357–369.
54. Mauch PM, Kalish LA, Kadin M, et al. Patterns of presentation of Hodgkin disease. Implications for etiology and pathogenesis. *Cancer.* 1993; 71(6):2062–2071.
55. Seam P, Juweid ME, Cheson BD. The role of FDG-PET scans in patients with lymphoma. *Blood.* 2007;110(10):3507–3516.
56. Ferme C, Eghbali H, Meerwaldt JH, et al. Chemotherapy plus involved-field radiation in early-stage Hodgkin's disease. *N Engl J Med.* 2007;357(19):1916–1927.
57. Canellos GP, Anderson JR, Propert KJ, et al. Chemotherapy of advanced Hodgkin's disease with MOPP, ABVD, or MOPP alternating with ABVD. *N Engl J Med.* 1992;327(21):1478–1484.
58. Ferme C, Mounier N, Diviné M, et al. Intensive salvage therapy with high-dose chemotherapy for patients with advanced Hodgkin's disease in relapse or failure after initial chemotherapy: results of the Groupe d'Etudes des Lymphomes de l'Adulte H89 Trial. *J Clin Oncol.* 2002;20(2):467–475.
59. van Besien K, Kelta M, Bahaguna P. Primary mediastinal B-cell lymphoma: a review of pathology and management. *J Clin Oncol.* 2001;19(6):1855–1864.
60. Coiffier B, Lepage E, Briere J, et al. CHOP chemotherapy plus rituximab compared with CHOP alone in elderly patients with diffuse large-B-cell lymphoma. *N Engl J Med.* 2002;346(4):235–242.
61. Popat U, Przepiork D, Champlin R, et al. High-dose chemotherapy for relapsed and refractory diffuse large B-cell lymphoma: mediastinal localization predicts for a favorable outcome. *J Clin Oncol.* 1998;16(1):63–69.
62. Thomas DA, Kantarjian HM. Lymphoblastic lymphoma. *Hematol Oncol Clin North Am.* 2001;15(1):51–95; vi.

164 Resection of Patients with Superior Vena Cava Syndrome

Gary W. Chmielewski and Michael J. Liptay

Keyword: Superior vena cava obstruction

Thoracic surgeons are routinely involved with patients with superior vena cava obstruction (SVCO) and on occasion are called upon to resect the superior vena cava (SVC) in the course of treatment. This chapter will summarize overall management principles, indications for SVC resection, the proper patient evaluation with coordination of care, intraoperative considerations, and postoperative care principles to ensure a successful outcome.

GENERAL PRINCIPLES AND GUIDELINES

General thoracic surgeons serve the patient with SVCO in three ways. First and most commonly they are involved in the workup and diagnosis of the patient who presents with the spectrum of SVCO symptoms and a chest mass on radiographic studies. Second, a patient with severe symptoms from SVCO will need expedient management of life-threatening symptoms. Similar to approaching the patient with esophageal cancer a "Captain of the Ship" is needed in both above situations which often will require the coordination of care of a multidisciplinary team (oncology, radiation oncology, interventional radiology, pathology) and nonoperative means of treatment will often be utilized (radiation, chemotherapy, stenting, thrombolytic therapy). Last, the thoracic surgeon may be called upon to resect the SVC for benign or malignant disease.

When called upon to evaluate the patient with SVCO the thoracic surgeon should classify the patient by severity of the SVCO symptoms, achieve an expedient tissue diagnosis, coordinate the care of the multidisciplinary team of physicians, and evaluate if there is any role for therapeutic surgical intervention especially if the patient has a diagnosis of non–small-cell lung cancer (NSCLC), thyroid/thymic cancer, or germ cell neoplasm.

Approximately 35% of SVCO patients will be asymptomatic or have only mild symptoms of head and neck edema and cyanosis. Moderate-to-severe symptoms will be seen in 60% of patients manifested by increasing degrees of cerebral edema resulting in visual disturbances, headache, laryngeal edema, and diminished cardiac reserve. Patients will present with life-threatening symptoms 5% of the time.[1]

See proposed grading system for superior vena cava syndrome (Table 164-1).

As proposed by Detterbeck, patients with grade 4 symptoms require a venogram, urgent stenting, and possible thrombolytics. Patients with grade 1, 2, and 3 symptoms require tissue diagnosis and multidisciplinary discussion to decide on treatment modality based on particular tumor response to a specific modality. Surgery is usually considered for NSCLC, thymoma, thymic carcinoma, or a residual germ cell mass. Chemoradiotherapy is the mainstay of treatment for patients with small-cell lung cancer, lymphoma, or germ cell tumor. Supportive care only may be indicated for patients with treatment refractory tumors or poor performance status.

See treatment algorithm of superior vena cava syndrome (Table 164-2).

Indications: Malignancy is the most common (90%) cause of SVCO usually due to bronchogenic carcinoma (>50% cases) with mediastinal lymphomas or germ cell neoplasms accounting for the rest.[2] Occasionally, patients with SVCO of a benign etiology (sarcoidosis, histoplasmosis, fibrosing mediastinitis, iatrogenic thrombosis) may benefit from venous reconstruction to establish flow from the superior venous system to the right atrium.[3,4]

Table 164-1

GRADING SYSTEM FOR SVCO

GRADE	CATEGORY	ESTIMATED INCIDENCE (%)	DEFINITION[a]
0	Asymptomatic	10	Radiographic superior vena cava obstruction in the absence of symptoms
1	Mild	25	Edema in head or neck (vascular distention), cyanosis, plethora
2	Moderate	50	Edema in head or neck with functional impairment (mild dysphagia, cough, mild or moderate impairment of head, jaw or eyelid movements, visual disturbances caused by ocular edema)
3	Severe	10	Mild or moderate cerebral edema (headache, dizziness) or mild/moderate laryngeal edema or diminished cardiac reserve (syncope after bending)
4	Life threatening	5	Significant cerebral edema (confusion, obtundation) or significant laryngeal edema (stridor) or significant hemodynamic compromise (syncope without precipitating factors, hypotension, renal insufficiency)
5	Fatal	<1	Death

[a]Each sign or symptom must be thought to be due to superior vena cava obstruction and the effects of cerebral or laryngeal edema or effects on cardiac function. Symptoms caused by other factors (e.g., vocal cord paralysis, compromise of the tracheobronchial tree, or heart as a result of mass effect) should not be considered as they are due to mass effect on other organs and not superior vena cava obstruction.

Source: Reproduced with permission from Yu, JB, Wilson, LD, Detterbeck, FC. Superior vena cava syndrome-a proposed classification system and algorithm for management. *J Thorac Oncol. 2008;3:811.* Copyright ©2008 Lippincott Williams & Wilkins.

Table 164-2

TREATMENT ALGORITHM OF SUPERIOR VENA CAVA SYNDROME

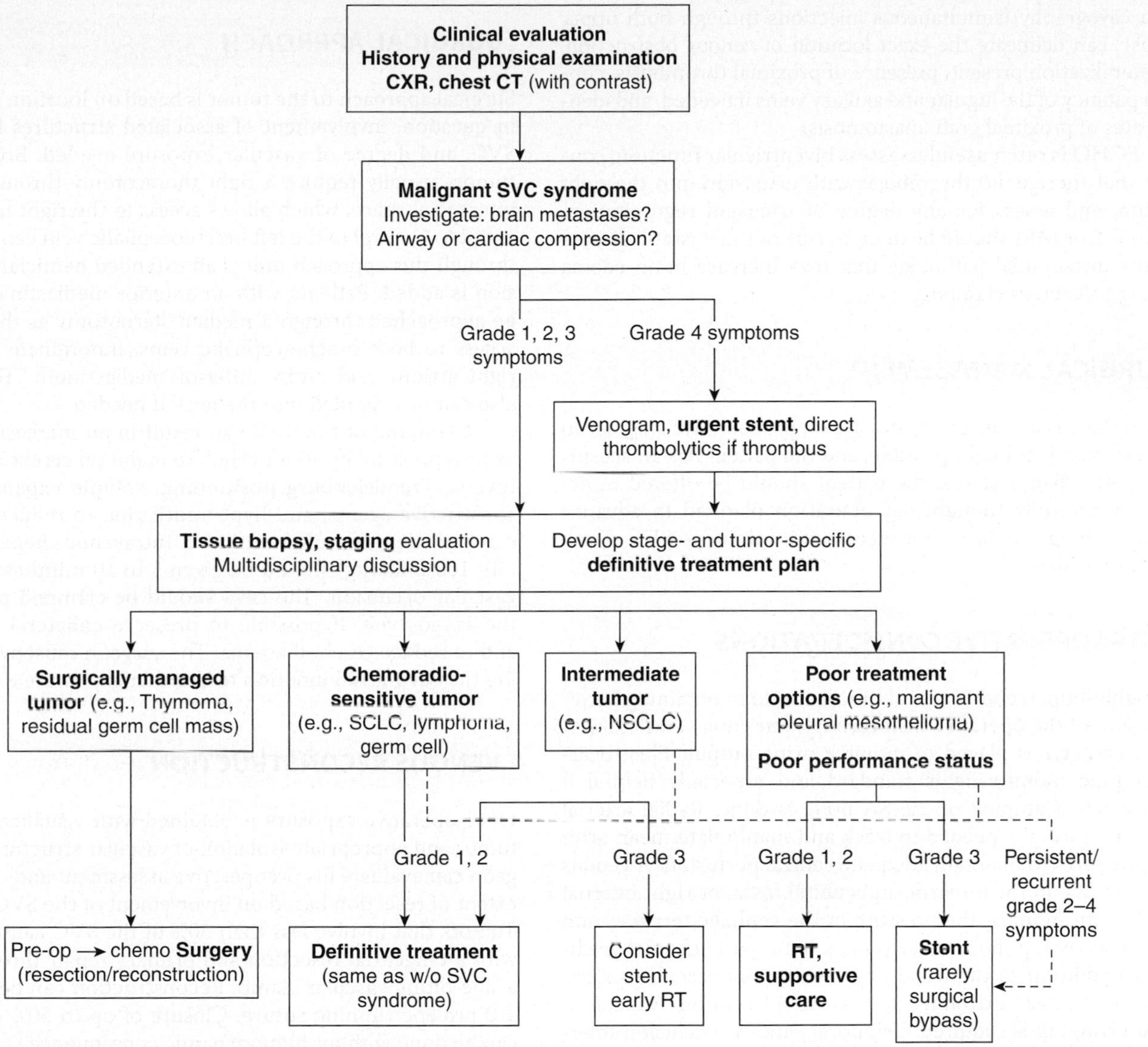

NSCLC, non–small-cell lung cancer; SCLC, small-cell lung cancer.

Reproduced with permission from: Yu, JB, Wilson, LD, Detterbeck, FC. Superior vena cava syndrome-a proposed classification system and algorithm for management. J Thorac Oncol. 2008;3:811. Copyright ©2008 Lippincott Williams & Wilkins.

PATIENT SELECTION

When approaching the patient with a malignant tumor involving the SVC, complete resection of all diseases should be the goal. Overall, patients should have acceptable ECOG performance status of 0 to 1 because of the potential moderate morbidity associated with surgery. For patients with a diagnosis of lung cancer, acceptable pulmonary functions on the higher end of normal are required because of the extent of resections and possible need for sacrifice of the phrenic nerve.[5] Right-sided lung cancers with SVC involvement require a lobectomy at the minimum, and sleeve resection or pneumonectomy is often required.

Preoperative Evaluation and Imaging

Goals are to obtain a tissue diagnosis, establish the proper stage of disease, facilitate planning of the vascular reconstruction if needed, and predict the ability to achieve a complete (R0) resection.

Core-needle biopsy (CT or US guided), mediastinoscopy,[6,7] mediastinotomy bronchoscopy, EBUS, EUS, and VATS biopsies can all be utilized to confirm the diagnosis and lymph node or other sites of potential metastatic involvement. Fusion PET-CT can focus on areas of potential metastatic sites.

The surgeon must have complete understanding of the venous anatomy involved, in particular the site and extension of venous obstruction, the presence of proximal thrombosis, the degree of venous collateralization (complete or incomplete), and the site where the proximal graft anastomosis can be made. Besides initial workup with plain chest roentography a chest CT scan with contrast, magnetic resonance venography,[8] or superior vena cavography (simultaneous injections through both upper limbs)[2] can delineate the exact location of venous obstruction, collateralization present, presence of proximal thrombosis, confirm patency of the jugular and axillary veins if needed, and identify sites of proximal graft anastomosis.

ECHO is often useful to assess biventricular function, confirm that there is no thrombosis with extension into the right atrium, and assess for any degree of tricuspid regurgitation. Brain CT or MRI should be done to rule out metastatic disease or any intracranial pathology that may increase brain edema during SVC cross clamping.

SURGICAL MANAGEMENT

When there is no metastatic disease on preoperative staging, an R0 resection is thought possible, and the patient has an acceptable performance status, the patient should be offered resection. A carefully thought-out operation planned in advance will go a long way to insure success and minimize SVC clamp times if needed.

INTRAOPERATIVE CONSIDERATIONS

A double-lumen endotracheal tube is useful in obtaining better exposure of the operative field through one-lung ventilation. A Foley catheter is placed to monitor urine output. Electrocardiographic monitoring is standard and especially helpful if inadvertent clamping of the SA node is done. Radial arterial line monitoring is needed to track and manipulate mean arterial pressures to maintain adequate central perfusion. A venous pressure line in the forearm, antecubital fossa, or right internal jugular can monitor the pressure in the cephalic territory and help in assessing the arterial-venous brain parenchymal gradient. In addition to the usual upper extremity vascular access, large bore lower extremity access should also be available if caval clamping is required. Temporary inflow occlusion tolerance will be facilitated by intravascular fluid expansion. Vasoactive agents can also be used once volume status is optimized.

See intraoperative checklist (Table 164-3).

Table 164-3

CHECKLIST OF INTRAOPERATIVE CONSIDERATIONS

- Double-lumen endotracheal tube
- Arterial line for mean arterial perfusion pressure monitoring
- Lower extremity venous access
- Intravascular fluid expansion
- Cephalic territory venous pressure monitoring
- Reverse Trendelenburg position if SVC clamping required
- Vasoactive agents to elevate cerebral profusion pressure
- Intravenous heparin sodium (50–100 units/kg) 5–10 min before vascular occlusion
- Clamp SVC proximal to azygos vein to preserve collateral circulation and reduce cerebral edema if possible
- Absolutely avoid clamping at cavo-atrial junction to avoid injury to the SA node
- Hyperventilation to reduce vasogenic cerebral edema
- Safety briefing with operative team at the beginning and throughout the case concerning procedure steps, equipment and materials needed, cerebral protection issues, and plans to address hemodynamic instability

SURGICAL APPROACH

Surgical approach to the tumor is based on location of the mass in question, involvement of associated structures besides the SVC, and degree of vascular exposure needed. Bronchogenic tumors usually require a right thoracotomy through the fifth intercostal space, which allows access to the right hilum, SVC, and RA. Control of the left brachiocephalic vein can be difficult through this approach unless an extended hemiclamshell incision is added. Patients with an anterior mediastinal mass will be approached through a median sternotomy as this provides access to both brachiocephalic veins, innominate vein, SVC, right atrium, and entire anterior mediastinum. The incision also can be extended into the neck if needed.

Clamping of the SVC can result in an increase of cranial venous pressure by 40 mm Hg.[9] To maintain cerebral perfusion reverse Trendelenburg positioning, volume expansion, vasoconstrictive agents, and hyperventilation to reduce vasogenic cerebral edema should be utilized. Intravenous heparin sodium (50–100 units/kg) should be given 5 to 10 minutes before any vascular occlusion. The cava should be clamped proximal to the azygos vein if possible to preserve collateral circulation and to reduce cerebral edema. The surgeon must avoid clamping the cavo-atrial junction to avoid injury to the SA node.

VENOUS RECONSTRUCTION

Once operative exposure is obtained with visualization of the tumor and appropriate isolation of vascular structures, the surgeon can evaluate his preoperative assessment and confirm the extent of resection based on involvement of the SVC by tumor. Tumors that involve less than 30% of the SVC can be handled with a tangential resection and primary repair through use of a side-biting vascular clamp. Reconstruction can be done with 4-0 prolene running suture. Closure of up to 50% of the cava can be done without hemodynamic consequence.

Tumors with 30% to 50% involvement of the SVC may best be served by resection of the SVC and patch repair Figure 164-1. Bovine pericardium or autologous pericardium has been used with success.[10–13]

Tumors with greater than 50% involvement of circumference of the SVC will require complete resection and reconstruction (Figure 164-2A–E). PTFE-ringed Gore-Tex (W.L. Gore and Associates, Flagstaff, Arizona) is the most commonly used material for reconstruction today, mainly because of its ease of use and ability to avoid compression. Cryopreserved arterial allograft, spiral saphenous vein, and pericardial tubes have all been reported as possible conduits.[9,10,14,15]

Dartevelle proposes that SVC revascularization can be classified into four options: truncal, solitary to the left brachiocephalic vein, solitary to the right brachiocephalic vein, or rarely to both brachiocephalic veins. The proximal conduit anastomosis in SVC revascularization should be performed to the side that is technically easiest and has the most viable blood flow with ligation of the contralateral side in almost all cases. Endovascular staplers facilitate division of the cava and major venous branches.

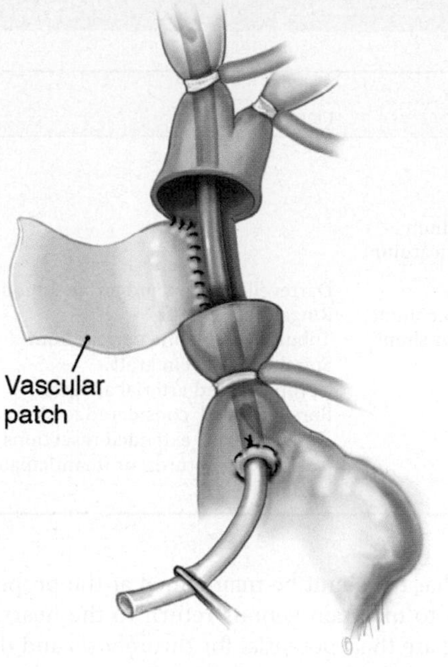

Figure 164-1. For 30% to 50% tumors, resection and patch repair of the SVC with bovine or autologous pericardium has been used with success.

Truncal: Truncal replacement requires a tumor-free zone on both brachiocephalic veins. Once proximal (brachiocephalic vein confluence) and distal (cavo-atrial) control is obtained, the involved segment is removed. A straight (not ringed) PTFE graft (#14 –20) is used for reconstruction. Sizing of the conduit is variable and can be done visually at the time of resection. A 5-0 prolene is used to perform the proximal (SVC to graft) anastomosis, and then the distal (graft to atrial) anastomosis. Before tightening down the distal anastomotic sutures the proximal clamp is released, the graft is flushed with heparinized saline, and deaeration is done.

Left brachiocephalic vein: A ringed PTFE graft (#12 –14) is used to prevent kinking. Minimal dissection should be done on the left brachiocephalic vein trunk to prevent rotation. This usually requires a long portion of graft that should be tailored in a gentle curve to prevent kinking after the sternotomy is closed. Sequence of anastomosis and deairing is as previous. The distal anastomosis can be done to the distal caval stump, atrial appendage (clear any muscle chords), or atrium proper.

Right brachiocephalic veins: Once again a ringed PTFE graft (#12 or #14) is used. The direction of the graft is vertical, so kinking risks are minimal. The proximal anastomosis can be difficult because the resulting right brachiocephalic stump can be very short.

Both brachiocephalic veins: This is the rarest of reconstruction situations. It is technically more demanding and because of the competing blood flows it has the highest chance of graft thrombosis. It is reserved for the patient who has already had resection of either the right or left internal jugular vein from thyroid cancer surgery. Y-grafts should be avoided because of the increased thrombogenicity of Gore-Tex to Gor-Tex surfaces. The right limb should be anastomosed to the SVC stump and the left limb to the right atrium.

See summary of SVC reconstruction options (Table 164-4) and diagram (Fig. 164-1).

HEMODYNAMIC INSTABILITY CONSIDERATIONS

The surgeon must be prepared along with his team for dealing with hemodynamic compromise when clamping the SVC and its major tributaries. The steps in dealing with this would be well discussed during the surgical "time out" as a safety briefing at the beginning of the case. The degree of obstruction of the SVC predicts the potential deleterious cascade of events that can ensue if clamping of the SVC is required. Patients with complete SVCO may have little hemodynamic compromise once the SVC is clamped because of the extensive collateral circulation that will maintain blood flow back to the heart. In this situation the "clamp and go" technique will usually suffice. With adequate intravascular volume and pressor agents inflow occlusion for over 30 minutes should be well tolerated without

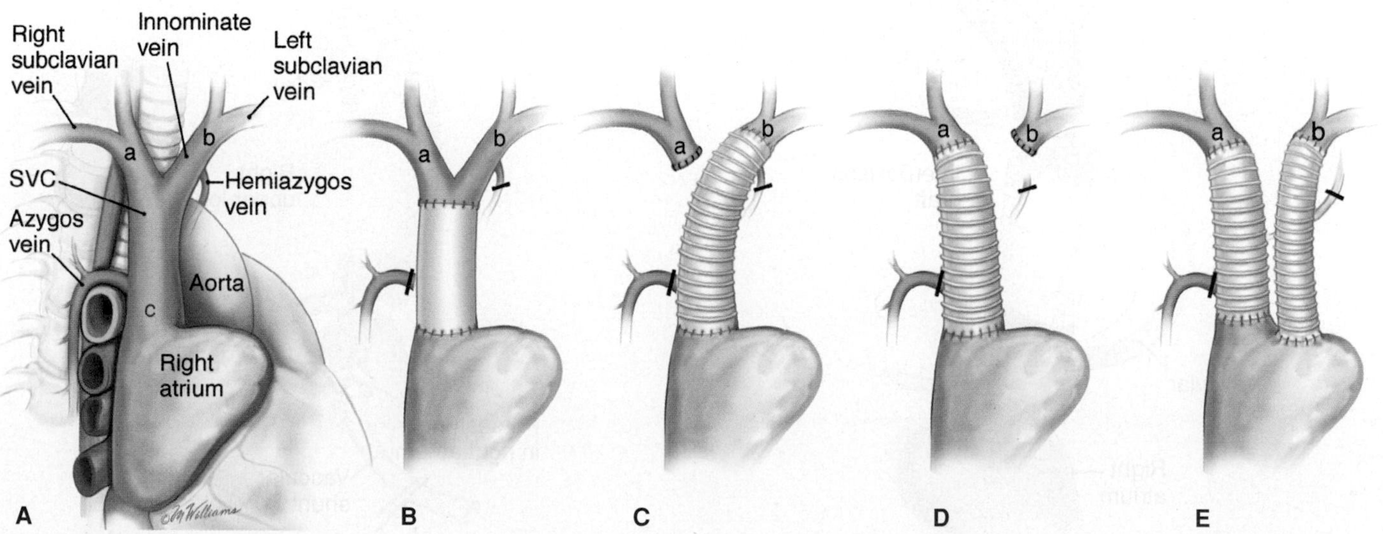

Figure 164-2. *(A)* SVC revascularization can be classified into four options: *(B)* truncal, *(C)* solitary to the left brachiocephalic vein, *(D)* solitary to the right brachiocephalic vein, or rarely *(E)* to both brachiocephalic veins.

Table 164-4

SVC RESECTION TECHNIQUE OPTIONS SUMMARY

PERCENT CIRCUMFERENTIAL INVOLVEMENT OF SVC	TECHNIQUE	ADJUNCT	COMMENTS
<30%	Tangential SVC resection and primary repair		
30%–50%	Resection and patch repair	Bovine pericardium Autologous pericardium	
>50%	Resection and vascular reconstruction	No shunt External vascular shunt Internal vascular shunt	Dartevelle "clamp and go" technique Ringed PTFE graft Tubularized bovine pericardium Spiral venous vein graft Cryopreserved arterial allograft
		CPB	Rarely needed; considered for intraoperative hemorrhage, extended resections involving cardiac structures, or unanticipated resection issues

hemodynamic compromise or sequelae of cerebral edema. Conversely, clamping the SVC in patients with partial SVCO may result in decreased cardiac inflow and outflow, increased venous pressure in the cephalic territory, and changes in the cerebral arterial-venous gradient leading to brain ischemia and intracranial bleeding. When SVC clamping results in unstable hemodynamics, clamp times over 60 minutes are anticipated, or the SVC needs to be clamped below the azygos vein shunting (external vascular shunting or internal vascular shunting) should be considered.[5] Warren et al., have advocated either an external or internal shunt for such occurrences.[10] An external vascular shunt can be inserted through proximal and distal SVC 4-0 prolene purse-string sutures (Fig. 164-3). A partial or complete resection of the SVC can be accomplished without interrupting venous return to the heart using these techniques. An internal shunt can be placed through a right atrial 4-0 prolene purse-string suture (Fig. 164-4). The shunt is maneuvered to the level of the innominate veins. Venous tapes can be secured to establish SVC isolation while shunting the venous return into the right atrium. It is critical that the shunt be maintained at the proper depth and orientation to maintain venous return to the heart. Drawbacks of shunting are their potential for thrombosis and the cluttering of the operative field making the distal anastomosis difficult. The use of cardiopulmonary bypass has been described in the literature but appears to be rarely needed. Indications may be when an extremely prolonged clamp time is anticipated, massive bleeding is encountered during the course of resection, extended resection of cardiac structures are planned, or unanticipated need for SVC resection discovered at the time of operation. This last instance is a situation that should be avoided at all costs as "being prepared" is an absolute for these cases.

To complete an R0 resection often times other structures besides the cava are involved necessitating resection. If a mediastinal tumor involves both sides of the chest, the surgeon should work from left to right to gain exposure for caval resection and reconstruction. The remaining right-sided portion of the tumor resection can then be completed. For right-sided bronchogenic tumors (especially those involving the carina or main PA) caval

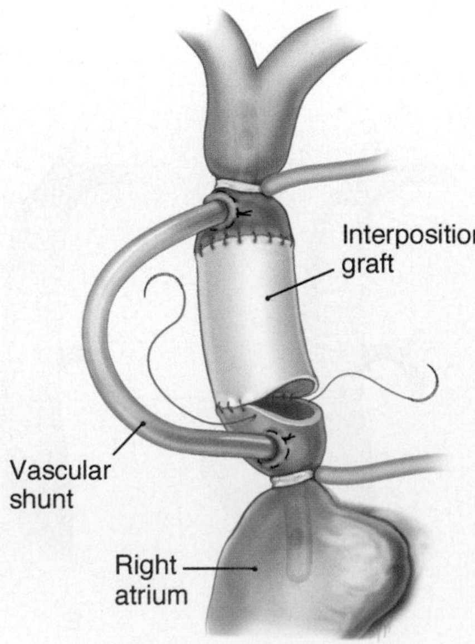

Figure 164-3. An external vascular shunt can be inserted through proximal and distal SVC 4-0 prolene purse-string sutures.

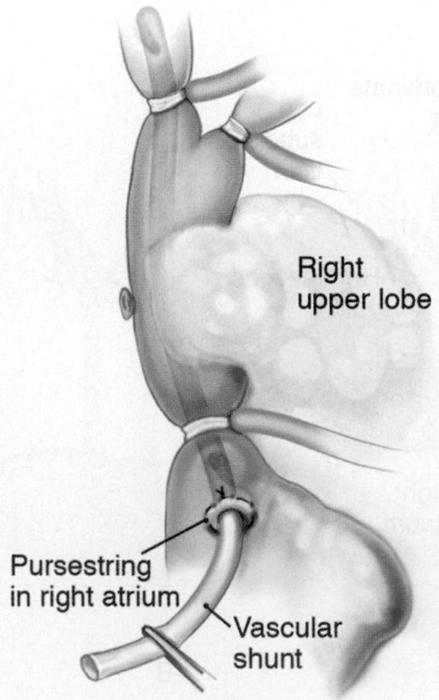

Figure 164-4. View of the internal vascular shunt placed through a right atrial 4-0 prolene purse-string suture.

Table 164-5

SUMMARY OF RESULTS OF SVC RESECTION

AUTHOR	YEAR	NUMBER	LUNG CA	N2 (%)	MORTALITY (%)	5-YEAR SURVIVAL(%)
Lanuti	2009	19	9	3 (33)	5	43
Spaggiari	2007	70	52	21 (40)	7.7	31
Suzuki	2004	40	40	15 (38)	10	24
Shargall	2004	23	15	7 (47)	14	37
Spaggiari	2004	109	109	55 (50)	12	21
Warren	1998	11	9	NR	9	36
Dartevelle	1997	22	6	2 (33)	7	31
Thomas	1994	15	15	6 (40)	7	24
Summary					**9%**	**31%**

resection and reconstruction is usually done first followed by the pulmonary resection. Care must be taken to avoid bacterial seeding of any graft material during pulmonary resection.

Standard drains should be placed to promote lung expansion and a dry postoperative field with one caveat; any drains should not be in contact with the graft material to avoid seeding of bacteria on the conduit. A combination of a chest tube and Blake or Jackson-Pratt drain can be efficacious in this situation.

POSTOPERATIVE CARE

Anticoagulation started in the OR usually is not actively reversed with protamine. Heparin sodium is maintained in the postoperative period at 1 to 2 mg/kg. Once the chest drains are removed, the patient can be converted to oral agents (Coumadin). The more collateral venous circulation that has developed may induce a higher likelihood of graft thrombosis because of competitive flow. If graft thrombosis is suspected ultrasound or venography should be carried out to confirm and delineate any graft kinking or other technical error that would require a reoperation. More likely is a spontaneous thrombosis that can be treated by interventional radiology through catheter techniques, thrombolytics, and further anticoagulation.

The patient should be maintained in a 30 to 45 degree upright position. If a unilateral reconstruction was done to only one of the brachiocephalic veins, the contralateral arm should be elevated above the heart on pillows or a padded bedside table to decrease limb swelling.

Manipulation of the sinus node can result in postoperative sick sinus syndrome. Placement of a temporary or permanent pacemaker may be indicated.

Standard early ambulation and encouragement of pulmonary hygiene should be done as in any thoracic procedure along with DVT prophylaxis.

OUTCOMES OF RESECTION FOR MALIGNANT DISEASE

Review of the literature of resection for patients with SVCO of a malignant etiology shows a 5-year survival of 31% against a 9% operative mortality. The presence of metastatic N2 nodes has less favorable outcomes. Patients with malignant mediastinal tumors that cause SVCO historically do better than those with bronchogenic carcinoma that involves the cava.[11,16] See summary of results of SVC resection (Table 164-5).

SUMMARY

Patients with SVCO can be best treated with a multidisciplinary approach to their evaluation led by a thoracic surgeon. Surgery with resection of tumor, SVC, and reconstruction is often indicated for malignant etiologies (NSCLC, thymoma, residual germ cell tumor). Optimal results are achieved in patients who can undergo an R0 resection of all known diseases. Superior vena caval resection and reconstruction techniques can help achieve this goal.

CASE HISTORY

A 41-year-old male presented to the thoracic surgical services with grade 1 symptoms of SVCO (head and neck edema, mild cyanosis, plethora). An 8- × 14-cm mass was demonstrated on CT scan of the chest (Fig. 164-5). Core-needle biopsy was

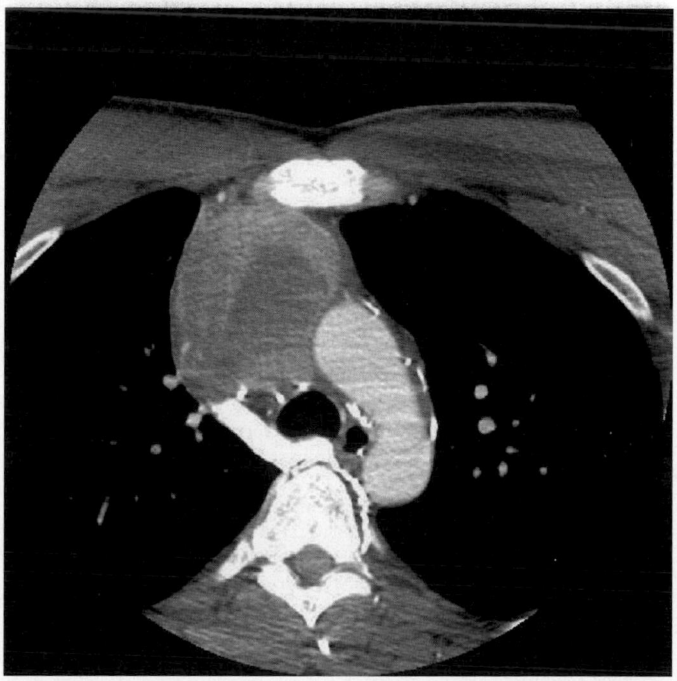

Figure 164-5. Chest CT revealing 8-cm × 14-cm mass on the superior vena cava.

interpreted as a thymic carcinoid tumor. Because of concern with resectability and the acute nature of the SVCO he received cisplatinum-based chemotherapy for three cycles and mediastinal radiation to 4800 cGy.

The patient was then restaged after treatment with fusion PET/CT. No metastatic disease was found and surgical resection was planned. The patient had a median sternotomy done with isolation of the right and left brachiocephalic veins, innominate veins, and significant venous tributaries. The pericardium was widely opened exposing the SVC-RA junction. After dissection of the mass a caval resection would be required as planned preoperatively. A clamp and go technique was utilized without need for pressors after adequate volume expansion. After clamping the SVC and right and left brachiocephalic veins, the venous structures were divided with endovascular staplers. Brisk bleeding was found and controlled with oversewing after localizing to the azygos system which was adherent in the tumor mass. The right atrium was opened and cleared of chordae tendineae and a 14-mm ringed Gore-Tex graft was fashioned with a bevel and anastomosed with 4-0 prolene to the right atrial appendage. After checking this anastomosis for hemostasis the graft was fashioned in a gentle curve back to the left brachiocephalic vein and another 4-0 prolene anastomosis was completed, the graft deaired, and the clamps released (Fig. 164-6). No reversal agents were given. Heparin was maintained in the postoperative period and held prior to chest tube removal. The patient was converted to oral anticoagulation in the postoperative period after the chest tubes were removed on postoperative day 2. He was discharged home and had no evidence of disease until 14 months later when he presented with a symptomatic pericardial effusion and lung metastasis. He succumbed to metastatic disease in spite of salvage chemotherapy 18 months after resection.

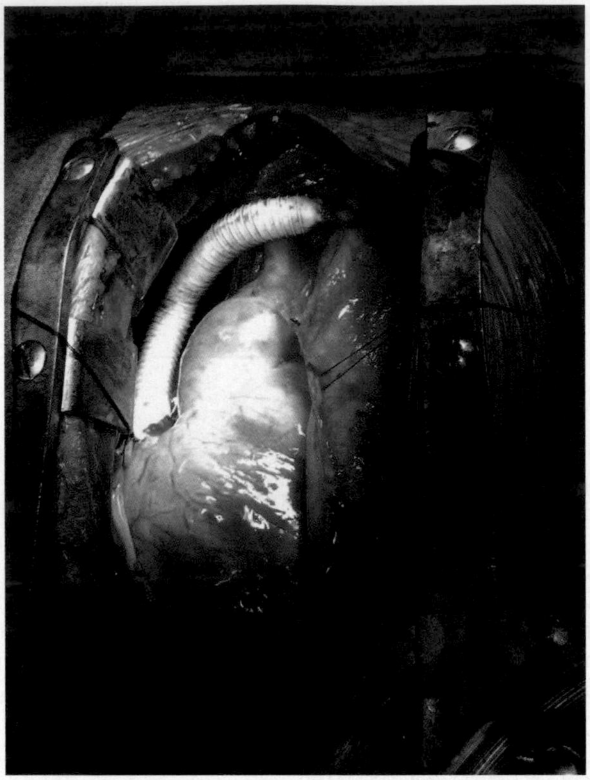

Figure 164-6. Intraoperative appearance of the completed repair, with graft fashioned in a gentle curve back to the left brachiocephalic vein.

EDITOR'S COMMENT

The evolution of superior vena caval reconstruction techniques provides a valuable example of why thoracic surgeons need to constantly reevaluate our assumptions about locally advanced cancer. Evolving surgical techniques may offer options for patients whose disease was previously considered "inoperable." Importantly, this reassessment must be made in the context of the individual patient's disease process and physiologic reserve.

—Steven J. Mentzer

References

1. Yu JB, Wilson LD, Detterbeck FC, Superior vena cava syndrome–a proposed classification system and algorithm for management. *J Thorac Oncol.* 2008;3(8):811–814.
2. Wudel LJ Jr, Nesbitt JC. Superior vena cava syndrome. *Curr Treat Options Oncol.* 2001;2(1):77–91.
3. Narayan D, Brown L, Thayer JO. Surgical management of superior vena caval syndrome in sarcoidosis. *Ann Thorac Surg.* 1998:66(3):946–948.
4. Kalra M, Gloviczki P, Andrews JC, et al. Open surgical and endovascular treatment of superior vena cava syndrome caused by nonmalignant disease. *J Vasc Surg.* 2003;38(2):215–223.
5. Garcia A, Flores RM. Surgical management of tumors invading the superior vena cava. *Ann Thorac Surg.* 2008;85(6):2144–2146.
6. Pop D, Venissac N, Nadeemy AS, et al. Video-Assisted Mediastinoscopy in Superior Vena Cava Obstruction: To Fear or not to Fear? *J Thorac Oncol.* 2011;7:386–389.
7. Dosios T, Theakos N, Chatziantoniou C. Cervical mediastinoscopy and anterior mediastinotomy in superior vena cava obstruction. *Chest.* 2005;128(3):1551–1556.
8. Lin J, Zhou KR, Chen ZW, et al. Vena cava 3D contrast-enhanced MR venography: a pictorial review. *Cardiovasc Intervent Radiol.* 2005;28(6):795–805.
9. Nesbitt JC, Gary WG. *Thoracic Surgical Oncology: Exposures & Techniques.* Philadelphia, PA: Lippincott Williams & Wilkens; 2003.
10. Warren WH, Piccione WJ Jr, Faber LP. As originally published in 1990: superior vena caval reconstruction using autologous pericardium. Updated in 1998. *Ann Thorac Surg.* 1998. 66(1):291–292; discussion 292–293.
11. Spaggiari L, Leo F, Veronesi G, et al. Superior vena cava resection for lung and mediastinal malignancies: a single-center experience with 70 cases. *Ann Thorac Surg.* 2007;83(1):223–229; discussion 229–230.
12. Inoue H, Shohtsu A, Koide S, et al. Resection of the superior vena cava for primary lung cancer: 5 years' survival. *Ann Thorac Surg.* 1990;50(4):661–662.
13. Grunenwald DH, Resection of lung carcinomas invading the mediastinum, including the superior vena cava. *Thorac Surg Clin.* 2004;14(2):255–263; vii.
14. Spaggiari L, Veronesi G, D'Aiuto M, et al. Superior vena cava reconstruction using heterologous pericardial tube after extended resection for lung cancer. *Eur J Cardiothorac Surg.* 2004;26(3):649–651.
15. Gomez-Caro A, Martinez E, Rodríguez A, et al. Cryopreserved arterial allograft reconstruction after excision of thoracic malignancies. *Ann Thorac Surg.* 2008;86(6):1753–1761; discussion 1761.
16. Lanuti M, De Delva PE, Gaissert HA, et al. Review of superior vena cava resection in the management of benign disease and pulmonary or mediastinal malignancies. *Ann Thorac Surg.* 2009;88(2):392–397.

PART 26

NEW HORIZONS

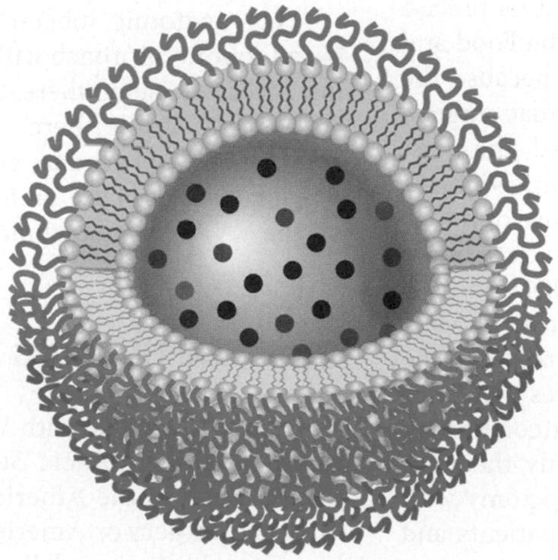

165 Robotics: Lobectomy

Bernard J. Park

Keywords: Robotic lobectomy, da Vinci Surgical System, mediastinal and hilar lymph node dissection

INTRODUCTION

Lobectomy via minimally invasive video-assisted thoracic surgery (VATS) has proved to be a feasible and oncologically acceptable approach for non–small-cell lung cancer (NSCLC) and other isolated tumors and conditions. However, despite multiple studies showing clear benefits over a traditional thoracotomy approach, such as decreased length of stay, decreased short-term postoperative pain, and fewer complications,[1–3] VATS is still not accepted as the standard approach for anatomic resection, and is only slowly being implemented more widely. The explanation is likely multifactorial including (1) technical issues, such as two-dimensional imaging and limited maneuverability of instrumentation; (2) lack of adequate training; and (3) concerns about the consequences of major vascular injury with a closed chest approach.

To address the perceived technical limitations of conventional minimally invasive platforms, a master–slave robotic surgical system was developed (da Vinci Surgical System, Intuitive Surgical, Sunnyvale, California). The major advances were the three-dimensional visual system that reestablished binocular vision and wristed instrumentation capable of seven degrees of freedom enabling more natural bimanual movement for precise dissection. Initially, the system was approved by the Food and Drug Administration for cardiothoracic surgery because the original intent was to achieve true closed chest cardiac surgery. This, however, has not been fully realized. Instead, the most common applications that evolved were for pelvic procedures—prostatectomy and hysterectomy. Similarly, while use of robotics for general thoracic surgical procedures dates back to initial case reports in the early 2000s, it was not until 2004 and 2006 that actual series of robotic lobectomies were reported by Melfi et al. and Park et al., respectively.[4,5] These centers reported the initial technique and early perioperative experiences that demonstrated feasibility, safety, and concordance of outcomes with the largest series of VATS lobectomies. Subsequently, there has been a steadily increasing interest in robotic lobectomy with additional publications with greater numbers of patients and various modifications of the technique.[6–8]

This chapter will focus on review of the general principles and clinical aspects of robotic lobectomy with an emphasis on patient selection, preoperative preparation, technical aspects, and perioperative outcomes.

GENERAL PRINCIPLES

The guiding principle that must be remembered when one is considering utilizing robotic surgical systems for any procedure is that the robot is a tool like any other in the art of surgery. It is up to the surgeon to use his or her best judgment as to whether its use is appropriate and in the best interest of the patient. Robotic procedures are simply minimally invasive procedures, that are performed with a different, perhaps more advanced technology that has unique advantages and disadvantages. In the case of pulmonary lobectomy the robotic approaches that have been described all conform to the consensus criteria of a standard VATS lobectomy put forth in the Cancer and Leukemia Group B (CALGB) prospective, multi-institutional registry study (CALGB 39802).[9] For early stage NSCLC (node-negative, peripheral tumors ≤3 cm) this definition includes: absence of rib-spreading, minimal incision size (no greater than a 4–8 cm access incision with 0.5-cm port incisions), videoscopic guidance at all times, and traditional hilar dissection with individual ligation and division of lobar structures. Adhering to these principles the authors were able to demonstrate that VATS lobectomy is associated with acceptable morbidity and mortality. Similarly, multiple independent centers have demonstrated the feasibility and safety of robotic lobectomy[4–8] while adhering to these same universal aspects of minimally invasive thoracic surgery established for VATS lobectomy. Moreover, a recent multicenter study by Park et al.[10] also demonstrated excellent long-term oncologic results of robotic lobectomy in the treatment of early NSCLC.

For anatomic lobectomy the author practices a VATS-based robotic approach with a small (3–4 cm), non–rib-spreading access incision whereas others advocate a complete portal approach.[7,8] While there are minor technical differences, the conduct of the procedure and utilization of the robotic technology for dissection are uniform. Major emphasis will be placed on the VATS-based technique.

ROBOTIC TRAINING AND ACCREDITATION

Currently, much like with VATS lobectomy neither the American Board of Thoracic Surgery nor any governing surgical society, such as the American College of Surgeons, Society of Thoracic Surgery or American Association of Thoracic Surgery has any published guidelines for the training and accreditation of surgeons and operating room teams for the performance of robotic thoracic procedures. As a result, each hospital typically has developed its own policies. Hospitals uniformly mandate that surgeons attend an intensive, 2-day training course given by Intuitive Surgical® that is comprised of didactic instruction regarding the system components followed by simulation training for basic skills and cadaver-based training for specific procedures. It is critical for specialty-specific personnel – operating room nurses, surgical technicians, and bedside assistants – to be formally trained on the basics of system functioning, instrument changes, and position of the surgical cart. This is typically done by the robotic company representative. It is common, but not required for the prospective robotic surgeon to observe an established practitioner to become familiar with specific index procedures. This author cannot stress enough how critically important case observation is during the training and prior to implementation of robotics into treatment of patients.

Once the entire surgical team has received the appropriate training, institutions usually will allow implementation of the robotic system into procedures under the supervision and guidance of a case proctor, defined as a surgeon with documented clinical experience independently performing robotic procedures. The console surgeon is typically required to perform between three and as many as ten proctored cases before being granted independent robotic procedure privileges. Some hospitals require that eligible proctors themselves have performed a minimum number of cases, while the majority has no such requirement. In fact, most institutions do not mandate that the proctor be specialty-specific—thus, a robotic urologist may proctor a thoracic surgeon. While this may be in compliance with a specific institutional requirement, this type of implementation is ill advised. The ideal situation is for the training surgeon to observe an experienced robotic surgeon in their respective field and then enlist that individual, if possible, to serve as the case proctor. This maximizes the continuity of training and, consequently, patient safety during clinical implementation.

PATIENT SELECTION AND PREOPERATIVE ASSESSMENT

The theoretical benefit of utilizing robotic technology is to replicate what can be done through VATS or almost entirely what can be done through a thoracotomy. Patients eligible for robotic lobectomy include those with suspicious or biopsy-proven NSCLC or other pathologic tumors or disease processes confined to the lung and ipsilateral hemithorax. This should be verified through computed tomography (CT) of the chest and whole body positron emission tomography (PET/CT). For NSCLC, suspicious mediastinal nodal or extrathoracic disease warrants further invasive staging to identify patients with advanced disease requiring multimodality or systemic therapy only. Patients should have adequate cardiopulmonary status and performance status to tolerate lobectomy. Specifically, cardiac disease should be asymptomatic and stable on medication and preoperative pulmonary function tests should demonstrate a postoperative predicted forced expiratory volume in 1 second (FEV_1) and diffusion capacity (D_{LCO}) above 40% of predicted. Borderline postoperative predicted lung function should be further investigated by quantitative lung scanning and/or exercise testing. Smoking cessation for active smokers should be aggressively advocated.

As with any new surgical technique or approach, careful selection of initial cases is critical to success and progression. While scenarios such as large tumors (>5 cm), extensive hilar or mediastinal disease, postinduction therapy, chest wall invasion, extensive adhesions, and need for bronchial or vascular sleeve resection do not absolutely preclude a robotic approach, it is wise to avoid these conditions until a sufficient experience with most straightforward cases has been developed. Informed consent for the use of robotic assistance should be obtained as a distinct portion of the procedure.

OPERATIVE TECHNIQUE

Preparation of the Robot

The operating room technical staff sets up the robotic surgical system (surgical cart, surgeon's console, vision system) in the room (Fig. 165-1). In the beginning of the case the nursing staff power up the system, run the appropriate diagnostics, and drape the robotic arms and camera. This requires two individuals and typically takes 5 to 10 minutes for staff who are trained and are familiar with the process and occurs prior to or while the patient is undergoing induction of anesthesia and positioning.

Anesthesia Considerations

Standard methods of general anesthesia and single-lung ventilation are employed via either double-lumen endotracheal tube placement or bronchial blocker. The patient is placed in a maximally flexed, lateral decubitus position, and single-lung ventilation is initiated. Depending on the size of the operating room, it will often be necessary to move the table away from the anesthesia machine and angle the foot of the table away from the surgical cart (Fig. 165-2). This establishes enough space to dock the robot. Care must be taken to insure that sufficient length of the circuit tubing is available during this positioning, and the anesthesia team must be comfortable that there is adequate access to the patient's airway once docking of the robotic system has taken place.

Initial Exploration and Docking of the Robot

Initial thoracic exploration is conducted with the robotic thoracoscope through a 12-mm trocar in the eighth intercostal space

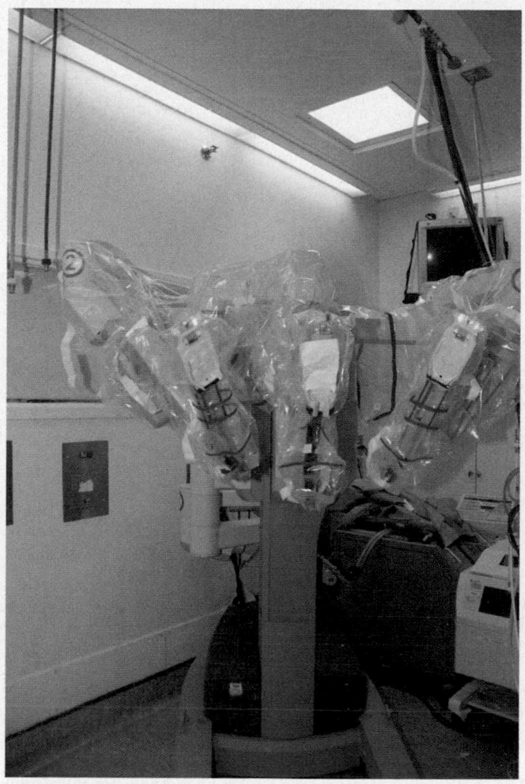

Figure 165-1. Robotic surgical cart draped and prepared for docking.

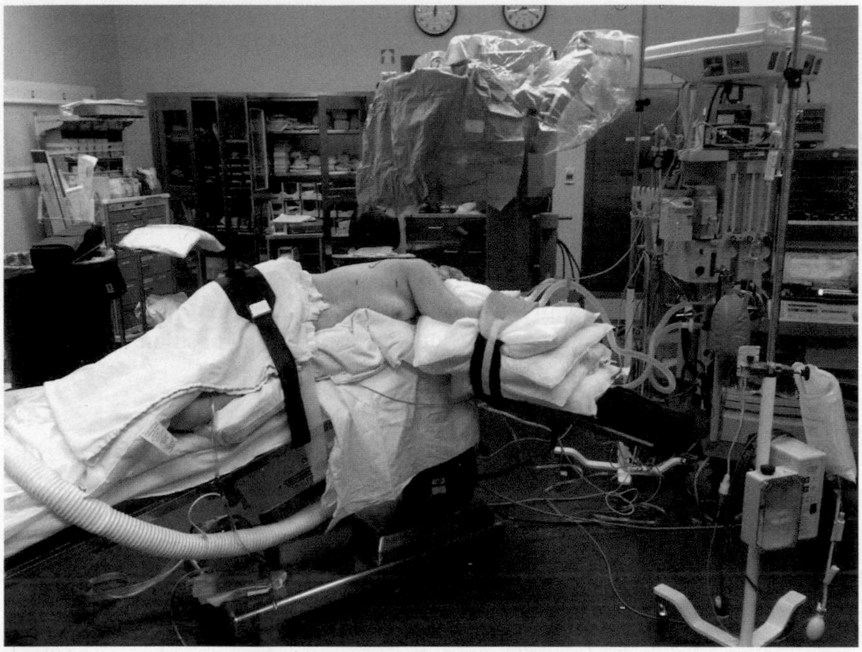

Figure 165-2. Table positioning prior to docking.

(ICS) just posterior to the anterior axillary line (Fig. 165-3) to verify tumor location, establish a tissue diagnosis if necessary, assess resectability and appropriateness of the robotic approach, and to place the additional incisions prior to docking. A 1-mm incision is placed posterior to the tip of the scapula in the ninth ICS just above the diaphragm. The 3- to 4-cm access incision is placed in the fourth or fifth ICS in the midaxillary line. A fourth incision may be employed posteriorly in the fifth or sixth ICS in line with the ninth ICS incision if so desired. Once the skin incisions have been made, the surgical cart is brought into position from the posterior aspect of the patient with the center column and camera arm angled over the scapula at an approximately 45-degree angle with respect to the longitudinal axis of the patient (Fig. 165-4). This allows for the field of dissection to include the hilar structures and the majority of the chest. When docking the surgical cart, it is important to avoid positioning the surgical cart too close to the patient and maintain adequate spacing between ports (handbreadth). This will eliminate instrument arm conflicts and maximize range of motion of the instruments.

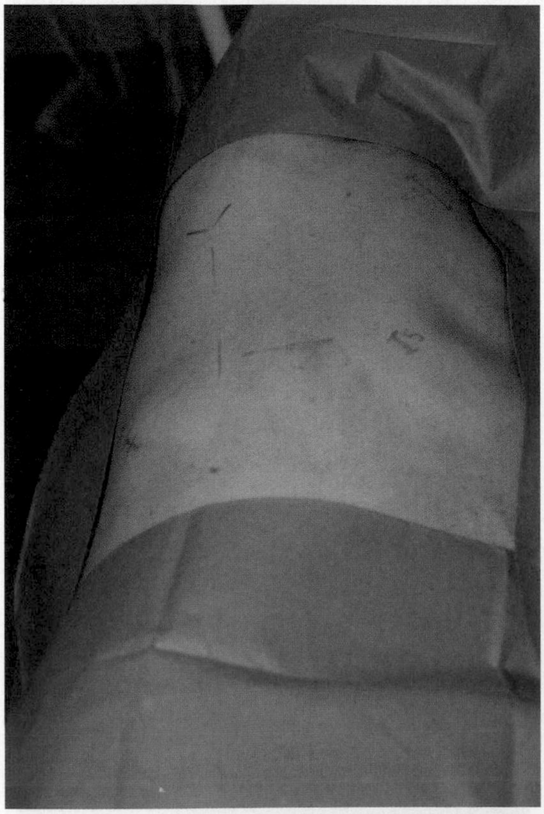

Figure 165-3. Incision strategy for VATS-based robotic pulmonary resection.

Once the surgical cart is in position the camera arm is attached first to the trocar, and the robotic thoracoscope is introduced and secured to the camera arm. The 8-mm metallic robotic trocars are introduced through each of the other incisions and attached to their respective arms. This is accomplished under direct vision both from outside the patient and

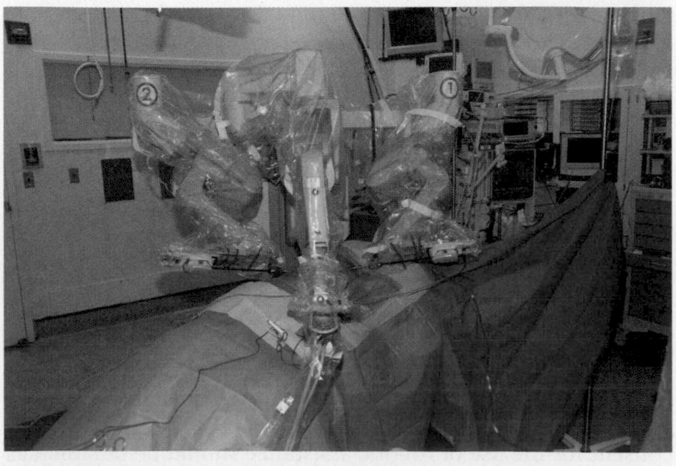

Figure 165-4. Docking of the surgical card for lobectomy.

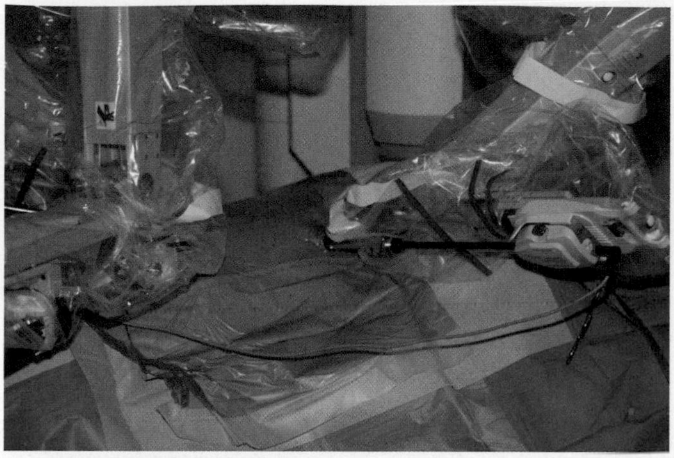

Figure 165-5. Positioning of the instrument arm through the access incision.

from within the patient's thorax. In the case of the access incision the trocar is placed in the midpoint of the incision with room above and below to introduce additional instruments (lung retractor, suction). Care must be taken to ensure that each instrument arm has full range of motion and does not collide with one another or with the patient (Fig. 165-5).

Once the trocars are in place and attached to the robotic arms, the surgical instruments are introduced under direct thoracoscopic vision. A Cadiere forceps is most commonly controlled by one hand for grasping tissue, and a cutting instrument (monopolar spatula, Maryland bipolar, monopolar hook) is used in the other hand. If the fourth arm is employed, it is typically used for a lung grasper or suction irrigator. After the instruments have been introduced the operating surgeon moves to the surgeon's console. The bedside assistant stands at the anterior aspect of the patient and provides additional exposure through the access incision.

Completely Portal Robotic Lobectomy (CPRL-4)

Cerfolio et al.[8] have developed a robotic incision strategy that avoids an access incision under the premise that no exposure of the intrathoracic cavity to air may have additional benefits over and above lack of rib spreading. There are four robotic arm incisions, all placed in the sixth ICS spaced 9 to 10 cm apart beginning from the midaxillary line to the paraspinal area (Fig. 165-6). In addition, there is a fifth, nonrobotic 15-mm assistant access port through which the endovascular staplers are passed. The surgical cart is then brought in over the head of the patient, with the camera view replicating the traditional thoracotomy view.

Mediastinal and Hilar Lymph Node Dissection

Dissection is performed with the Cadiere forceps and the monopolar cautery spatula. Wherever possible, the entire nodal packet is removed without fracturing the nodes into fragments (Fig. 165-7). Large bronchial or lymphatic vessels can be clipped, and when indicated suspicious lymph nodes are sent for frozen section analysis to identify occult N2 disease. For a right upper lobectomy it is easier to perform the paratracheal node dissection after the specimen has been removed. Similarly, it is often advantageous to perform the subcarinal lymphadenectomy by retracting the stump of the lower lobe to elevate the mediastinum.

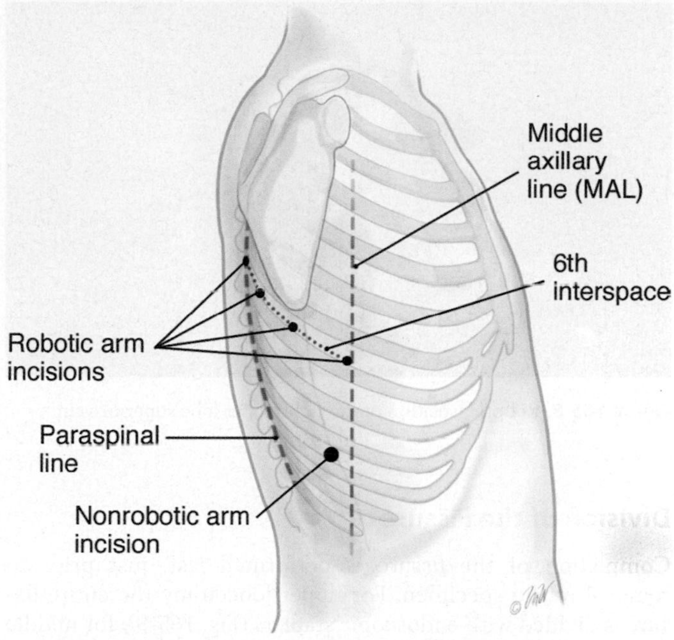

Figure 165-6. Incision strategy for a CRPL-4 approach.

Hilar Dissection

If there are no contraindications to lobectomy, individual isolation of the hilar structures proceeds with dissection around the hilar vessels and bronchi performed through a combination of cautery, sharp, and blunt dissection. Complete removal and labeling, rather than sweeping of all regional nodal tissue is performed both for adequate staging and to facilitate isolation of the hilar structures. When either a vessel or the bronchus is mobilized sufficiently, the Cadiere forceps are used to isolate the structure, using the seven degrees of freedom to articulate the instruments at near right angles to do so (Fig. 165-8). Ligation and division of the named vessels and bronchus are performed with endovascular staplers introduced either through the posterior inferior or access incision. This requires temporary removal of one of the robotic trocars followed by replacement of the arm after stapler firing.

The precise order in which the structures are divided depends on the particular lobectomy being performed and the approach (anterior vs. posterior/fissural). Therefore, the specific steps for each lobectomy will not be reviewed in detail.

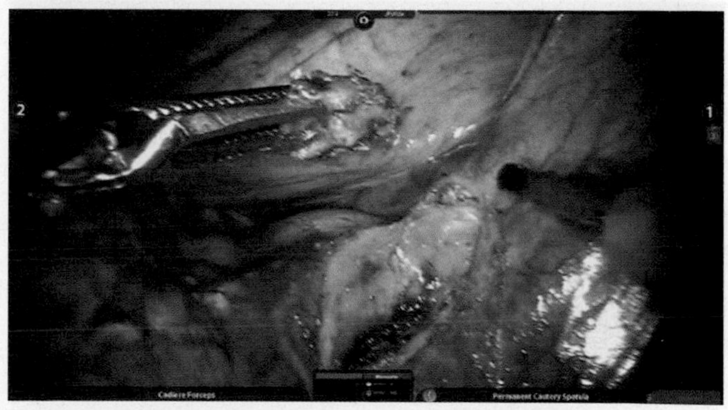

Figure 165-7. Right-sided interlobar hilar lymph node dissection.

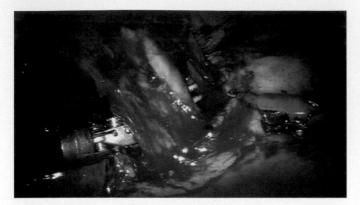

Figure 165-8. Robotic isolation of the right upper lobe superior vein.

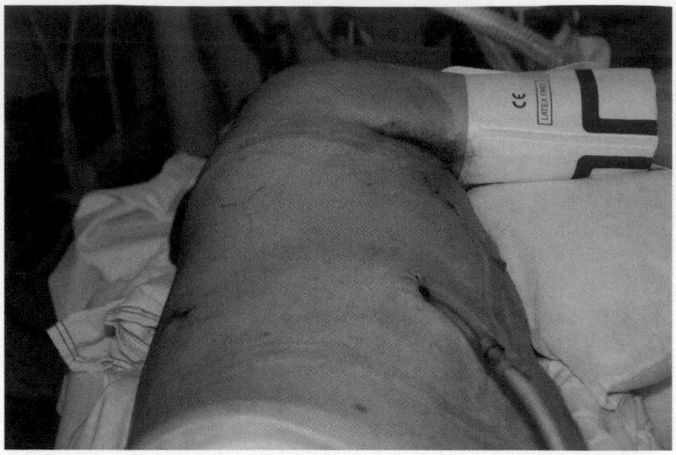

Figure 165-10. Incision closure following right robotic lobectomy.

Division of the Fissure

Completion of the fissure is performed last, just prior to removal of the specimen. For upper lobectomy the entire fissure is divided with endoscopic staplers (Fig. 165-9); for middle and lower lobectomies the anterior portion of the fissure is often divided with electrocautery in the course of dissection of the hilar structures. The remaining posterior portion of the fissure is then completed using the endoscopic staplers.

Specimen Removal

The completed lobectomy specimen should be placed in a durable laparotomy sac and removed through the access incision in the case of a VATS-based incision strategy or by enlarging one of the port incisions in a completely portal approach. In the event that the primary tumor is large the access incision may have to be enlarged to remove the specimen without inadvertently fracturing the ribs.

Termination of the Procedure

Once the specimen has been removed and the systematic lymphadenectomy or sampling has been completed the surgical arms can be undocked from the trocars, and the cart can be moved away from the patient. The trocars should be removed, and a single drainage chest tube placed through the anterior inferior camera incision and positioned with the tip at the apex of the chest posteriorly. The lung should be reinflated under direct thoracoscopic vision with the robotic scope placed in the access incision. The remaining wounds are closed in a standard fashion (Fig. 165-10).

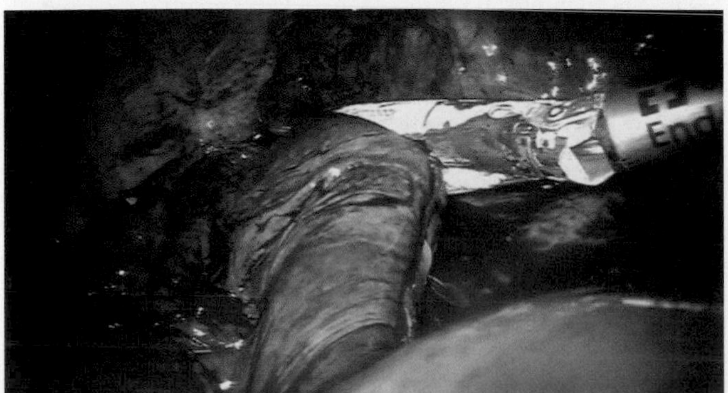

Figure 165-9. Division of the horizontal fissure during robotic lobectomy.

POSTOPERATIVE CARE

Standard postoperative lobectomy management should be undertaken. In virtually all cases, patients should be extubated in the operating room and brought initially to the postanesthesia care unit. Chest tubes may be left to water seal unless the immediate postoperative radiograph demonstrates a large air space. Patient-controlled analgesia should be initiated through the use of an epidural or a peripheral narcotic combined with either intraoperative intercostal blocks or continuous subpleural local anesthetic infusion. Patients may be transferred to a surgical floor with telemetry. Early ambulation and chest physiotherapy is critical to prevent hypoventilatory atelectasis and pneumonitis. Removal of the chest tube should be performed once there is no evidence of air leak and fluid drainage is sufficiently diminished. Commonly, patients can be discharged once the chest tube is discontinued provided there are no other concomitant complications and pain control on oral medication is sufficient.

PROCEDURE-SPECIFIC CONSIDERATIONS

Potential intraoperative and postoperative complications are no different with a robotic approach to lobectomy than VATS lobectomy. Major perioperative morbidity and mortality are consistent with the largest and best series of VATS lobectomies.[10] However, there are unique aspects to robotic thoracic procedures and lobectomy that need to be considered.

1. *Lack of tactile feedback.* The robotic arms do not impart haptic feedback to the console (operating) surgeon. Therefore, both the console surgeon and the bedside assistant must be constantly vigilant about inadvertent injury to either the external patient or surrounding internal structures by the instrument arms or the instruments themselves. Externally, care must be taken to insure that the arms do not compress any part of the patient with undue force for a prolonged

period of time. Internally, the surgeon must pay close attention to the visual feedback to prevent direct traction injury and compression injury by the shaft or heel of the instruments to adjacent structures.

2. *Visual magnification.* The robotic thoracoscope by design has greater magnification compared with the optics of the conventional camera. This is quite beneficial when working in a narrow, confined space, but results in decreased overall perspective view. This can be a disadvantage in the chest when one is attempting to delineate anatomic boundaries, such as lobar versus segmental structures or location of the minor fissure. It is critical to zoom out to the farthest extent possible when a greater overall view is required.
3. *Hemorrhage.* While the threat of catastrophic hemorrhage during major pulmonary resection is not unique to robotic procedures, absence of the operating surgeon at the bedside for immediate intervention is a necessary condition of the current master–slave robotic system. There are several strategies to maximize safety and minimize patient morbidity in the event of significant vascular injury. First, anticipation of a potential injury and maintaining a low threshold for conversion is key. Second, there must be a sponge stick ready and available for the bedside assistant to use for temporary tamponade of a bleeding vessel. Third, the bedside staff must be poised for rapid instrument removal and undocking of the surgical cart in preparation for conversion. With proper training this can be executed in less than 1 minute, and use of robotic technology should never impede timely management of potentially catastrophic bleeding.

SUMMARY

Robotic lobectomy is a feasible, safe, and oncologically sound surgical treatment for early-stage lung cancer. The technique is reproducible across multiple centers and yields results consistent with the best seen with conventional VATS. It should not be considered experimental, but an accepted minimally invasive thoracic surgical technique. Successful and safe implementation into clinical practice requires preparation and commitment on an institutional and multidisciplinary team level. The future directions for study of this technology include further refinement of the technique, validation of the adequacy of the oncologic results, and determining methods to compare it with conventional VATS and thoracotomy techniques.

EDITOR'S COMMENT

The overall setup for robotic lobectomy and the unique considerations through the eye of an experienced "insider" make this chapter particularly valuable to surgeons interested in robotic thoracic surgery.

—Yolonda L. Colson

References

1. McKenna RJ Jr, Houck W, Fuller CB. Video-assisted thoracic surgery lobectomy: experience with 1,100 cases. *Ann Thorac Surg.* 2006;81:421–426.
2. Onaitis MW, Petersen RP, Balderson SS, et al. Thoracoscopic lobectomy is a safe and versatile procedure. *Ann Surg.* 2006;244:420–425.
3. Flores RM, Park BJ, Dycoco J, et al. Lobectomy by video-assisted thoracic surgery (VATS) versus thoracotomy for lung cancer. *J Thorac Cardiovasc Surg.* 2009;138:11–18.
4. Melfi FMA, Ambrogi MC, Lucchi M, et al. Video robotic lobectomy. *MMCTS.* 2005;(628):000448. Available at http://mmcts.ctsnetjounals.org/cgi/content/full/2005/0628/mmcts.
5. Park BJ, Flores RM, Rusch VW. Robotic assistance for video-assisted thoracic surgical lobectomy: technique and initial results. *J Thorac Cardiovasc Surg.* 2006;131:54–59.
6. Veronesi G, Galetta D, Maisonneuve P, et al. Four-arm robotic lobectomy for the treatment of early-stage lung cancer. *J Thorac Cardiovasc Surg.* 2010;140:19–25.
7. Ninan M, Dylewski MR. Total port-access robot-assisted pulmonary lobectomy without utility thoracotomy. *Eur J Cardiothorac Surg.* 2010;38:231–232.
8. Cerfolio RJ, Bryant AS, Skylizard L, et al. Initial consecutive experience of completely portal robotic pulmonary resection with 4 arms. *J Thorac Cardiovasc Surg.* 2011;142:740–746.
9. Swanson SJ, Herndon JE, D'Amico TA, et al. Video-assisted thoracic surgery lobectomy: report of CALGB 39802-a prospective, multi-institutional feasibility trial. *J Clin Oncol.* 2007;25:4993–4997.
10. Park BJ, Melfi F, Mussi A, et al. Robotic lobectomy for non-small cell lung cancer (NSCLC): long-term oncologic results. *J Thorac Cardiovasc Surg.* 2012;143:383–389.

166 Robotics: Esophagectomy

David B. Graham and Kemp H. Kernstine

Keywords: Robotic esophagectomy, robot-assisted transhiatal esophagectomy, robot-assisted extended lymphadenoesophagectomy

INTRODUCTION

The first report of minimally invasive esophagectomy (MIE) appeared in the early 1990s. Whether thoracoscopic, laparoscopic, transhiatal, or combined, MIE evolved as a result of several goals: to reduce thoracotomy-related chest wall discomfort and postoperative debility; to achieve a more frequent R0 rate and better lymphadenectomy; and to achieve superior local control compared with the MIE transhiatal esophagectomy.[1,2] Robotic-assisted esophageal resection emerged onto the surgical literary scene in 2003 and 2004 with the transhiatal esophagectomy and 3-field esophagolymphadenectomy, respectively. The advantages of robotic technology that are brought to this procedure include multi-articulated instruments with 7 degrees of rotational freedom, referred to as the EndoWrist®, simulating normal wrist movements thus differentiating the robotic system from standard videoscopic techniques; and the three-dimensional (3D) imaging provided by the double optic system allowing depth perception that improves surgical precision. Subsequent case series over the last decade have accomplished many of these goals while conferring clinical advantages of minimally invasive surgery (MIS), thus paving a road for the different methods of the robotic-assisted esophagectomy.

GENERAL PRINCIPLES

Robotic esophagectomy has been performed for high-grade dysplasia, invasive carcinoma, and severe surgically failed esophageal dysfunction. Esophageal cancer is the most common indication, although not readily accepted by the esophageal surgical community. The nihilists believe the sole benefits of MIE are a new conduit for swallowing and some staging information, and that radiation and chemotherapy are critical for long-term survival. Others believe that resection not only provides palliation, but also reduces the likelihood of local–regional recurrence and, if performed correctly, will improve survival. Collaborative efforts have found that depth of esophageal wall penetration and location of tumor are important for determining the extent of lymphadenectomy. Key factors for surgical and clinical success must follow a few general rules: (1) achieve an R0 resection; (2) provide adequate staging by performing an extensive lymphadenectomy assisted by knowledge of the tumor location, cell type, as well as information from high-resolution computed tomogram (CT), FDG-positron emission tomography, and endoscopic ultrasound; and (3) minimize local–regional recurrence, postoperative pain, and procedural-related morbidity and mortality.

An open technique using wide resection can be compromised because of the lack of visibility inherent in a thoracotomy exposure and articulations necessary to perform a thorough lymphadenectomy. In addition, the significant torque on the chest wall required to obtain the best visibility increases the likelihood for postoperative discomfort. Aforementioned robotic advantages, we feel, solve limitations of prior approaches thus extending clinical benefits to the patient.

PATIENT SELECTION

The preoperative evaluation is no different for robotic surgery than for the conventional open surgical procedure. The history and physical examination are integral components in the initial phases of surgical decision making. Further workup may include CXR, CT chest/abdomen, FDG-positron emission tomography, barium swallow, upper endoscopy, bronchoscopy, endoscopic ultrasound, pulmonary function testing, and cardiopulmonary exercise testing. We do not exclude patients based on BMI, ASA status, or age. Higher values on each of these measures actually may benefit from a minimally invasive approach rather than a thoracotomy. On the other hand, those patients with marginal pulmonary or cardiac reserve may have difficulty with single-lung ventilation and carbon dioxide insufflation, which are typically employed in robotic techniques. We place all of our patients in a preoperative physiotherapy program for conditioning.

PREPROCEDURE TECHNICAL CONSIDERATIONS

There is little guidance in the literature regarding the planning and preparation necessary for an efficient thoracic robotic procedure. Robotic work, in the chest, even more than in the abdomen, requires additional planning, skills, and knowledge of the anatomy and an understanding of the limitations of the technology. Creation and maintenance of a skilled operating room robotically oriented team is absolutely imperative to facilitate communication and to minimize operating room time. The bedside surgical assistant provides key exposure, mobilization, and suctioning. An operating nurse and support nursing staff, as well as an experienced anesthesiologist, who can perform single-lung ventilation and hemodynamically support the patient, are critical to maintaining the flow of the procedure.

Patient Positioning

The rigidity of the chest wall and the movement of the heart, lungs, and mediastinum present technical challenges and specific techniques are used to optimize exposure. In general, for the chest portion, if that is the first portion of the procedure and if we are not planning an in-the-chest anastomosis, we place the patient in the prone and a slightly reverse Trendelenburg position. The weight of the mediastinal and lung structures fall toward gravity, exposing the normally less visible areas thus providing more room for dissection and countertraction.

We also introduce CO_2 insufflation to distend the mediastinum creating more space for dissection. It also compresses the ipsilateral lung and diaphragm, helps to evacuate any smoke from the cautery or harmonic dissection device, and helps to keep the lens clean. We typically use a pressure of 5 to 15 mm Hg at a maximal flow rate, although we often start with low pressures and slowly advance the pressure after the patient has hemodynamically adjusted. For the chest, we most often use the 0-degree scope as it provides a better peripheral view, often a limitation in the chest, and we rarely need the angled vision afforded by the 30-degree scope.

Lower esophageal, periesophageal, and diaphragmatic procedures may be best performed transabdominally in a supine position. Robotic arm ports placed at varying distances beneath each costal margin and a periumbilically placed videoscope optimize the robotic transhiatal thoracic access. Through this approach, most procedures in the lower mediastinum can be performed; however, limitations of the current robotic arms and instruments prevent accessibility beyond the level of the mid-mediastinum. Therefore, for example, a transhiatal robotic esophagectomy with extensive lymphadenectomy would be very difficult to perform in most patients. These aspects will need to be addressed in the future to improve utility.

Port Placement

Like patient positioning, proper port placement is critical. The intended operative area should be drawn on the chest using the CT scan and surface landmarks as a guide. In the case of esophagectomy, the scope of visibility for the chest exposure is quite large, encompassing the entire cranial–caudal length of the thorax.

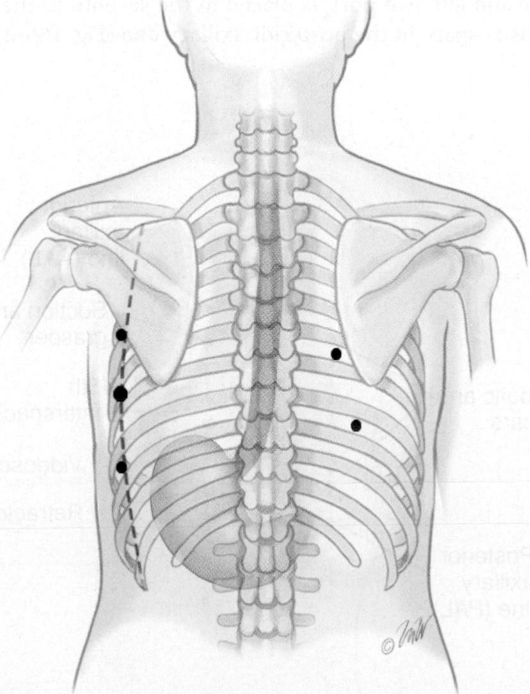

Figure 166-1. Port placement for prone portion of the procedure.

For the prone portion of the procedure, we place five ports in the chest, each about 10 to 15 cm apart, three of them in a line along the area of the esophagus toward the posterior axillary line with the central port view at the center of the esophagus (or the most critical part of the dissection), (Fig. 166-1). As a rule, the robotic chassis or bedside cart is brought in exactly opposite the viewing scope, keeping the pathology to be dissected or removed between the camera port and the base of the bedside robotic cart.

Additional ports are placed, as necessary, for a fourth robotic arm or accessory instruments to be used by the surgical assistant for retraction or dissection assistance. Occasionally, the robotic arms and instruments do not sufficiently reach the target and specific maneuvers may be necessary: inserting the trocars further into the chest; moving the trocar into a different intercostal space through the same skin incision; adding positive end-expiratory pressure to the opposing lung thereby pushing the mediastinum closer to the reach of the robotic instruments; and/or removing some of the CO_2 pressure used during the procedure. For better exposure, the partially open fan retractor (US Surgical, Norwalk, CT) or the paddle retractor (US Surgical) are safe, and may provide sufficient retraction of the lung, the heart, and great vessels.

OPERATIVE TECHNIQUES

The first case reports of robotic esophagectomy were published in 2003[3] and 2004.[4] Since that time there have been four different reports in the literature: (1) the chest only approach; (2) the robotically assisted transhiatal esophagectomy, initially coined the robot-assisted transhiatal esophagectomy (RATE) procedure; (3) the robotically assisted esophagolymphadenectomy, a modification of the three-hole or McKeown approach, termed the robot-assisted extended lymphadenoesophagectomy (RALE) procedure; and (4) the robotically assisted Ivor Lewis approach with an intrathoracic esophagogastrostomy, termed the robot-assisted Ivor Lewis esophagectomy (RILE) procedure. As with the MIE and the open thoracotomy approaches, there are many different steps and many different techniques used to perform each of those steps. Thus, the merits of the overall approach and the successes or failures should not be attributed to the robot or the general approach. Robotic surgery is still in its infancy and even more so with its use in esophagectomy and alimentary tract reconstruction.

Literature Review

The conventional open approach and the thoracoscopic MIS approach have shortcomings. The conventional open esophagectomy has a reported morbidity of 40% to 80%.[5] The published institutions have an in-hospital mortality of approximately 5%.[5] In the largest published VATS esophagectomy series, the major and minor morbidity was 32% and 55%, respectively, with 1.4% mortality.[6] A recent comparative review article from the Netherlands demonstrated nicely the benefits of MIE versus open techniques. Calculated means showed a significant decrease in estimated blood loss (EBL), hospital and ICU stays, number of harvested lymph nodes, lower morbidity (especially pulmonary complications), and mortality (1.9% vs. 4.5%).[7] A recent review compared nine robotic case series to the study by Verhage. This found even further improvement in the robotic group with respect to operating times (−6%), EBL (−22%), ICU stay (−42%), major complications (−45%), and lymph node retrieval (+27%).[8] They also found comparative rates for robotic versus laparoscopic approaches in the length-of-hospital stay and mortality rates (15.6 vs. 15.9 days, 2.4% vs. 1.3%, respectively).

Critically important, the robotic approach has been shown to be oncologically sound and similar to that found in the open non-MIS esophagectomy cases. In a recent review article appraising the literature on robotic esophagectomy, R0 resections were noted in 76% to 100% of patients, the median lymph node retrieval was 14 to 38, and disease-specific recurrence rate was 14%.[8] There is insufficient information to provide long-term survival in robotic esophagectomy patients; however, a few studies have reported >50% survival at >15 months.[9–12] Currently, there is insufficient data to make any conclusions, but as a tool, robotics can potentially offer as rigorously sound a cancer operation as the more standard open procedures.

Tables 166-1 and 166-2 highlight the relevant case reports and series in tabular format.[6–19] It summarizes each according to the technique type and various metrics related to their preoperative, intraoperative data, and surgical outcomes. As was shown in multiple series, the Dutch group, for example, noted that their complication rate was initially high, approximately 60%, which subsequently improved after they gained experience. As with the open technique, the most common complication was pulmonary-related albeit abated. The location and histology type of the primary lesion was most commonly in the lower third of the esophagus and adenocarcinoma, respectively. Neoadjuvant therapy was given at variable rates, according to institutional protocol. Conversion rates were low (mean 4%, range 0%–15%) and were mainly related to difficulties with adhesions or bleeding. The median operating room time varied relating to surgeon experience and technique: chest only averaged 6½ hours, RATE averaged 4¾ hours, RALE averaged 11 hours, and RILE averaged 9 hours, but this represents a very early experience and most surgeons are reporting shorter times with greater experience. The higher later two times attributed to the inherently more complex total robotic esophagectomy approach. The median intraoperative blood loss also varied relating to technique: chest only averaged 380 mL, RATE averaged 75 mL, RALE averaged 588 mL, and RILE averaged 400 mL. Obviously, these are very rough estimates as data variability within the case series limit true averages. The R0 rate for the series was >76% and often as high as 100% in many series. The average number of lymph nodes retrieved and/or examined was 21 among the studies. The anastomosis was mostly performed in the neck (only a few RILE patients) and the leak rate was reportedly as high as 33% and as low as 0% with an average of 17%. Regarding the anastomosis, it was quite surgeon or institution specific; most performed either a side-to-side linear stapling technique[20] or a circular stapling technique. Still, advocates of a hand-sewn technique report lower leak rates than the average.[19] For the group overall, the average length-of-hospital stay and perioperative 30-day mortality was 11.75 days and 1.3%, respectively.

The abdominal portion of the procedure varied among the different reports. A gastric tube, created using a stapling technique, was used in all of the cases. The width and length of the gastric tube varied; however, most proposed a narrow tube around 3 to 4 cm. The use of pyloroplasty varied. Most did not perform any intervention on the pylorus; however, Weksler routinely performed a standard pyloroplasty and Cerfolio preferred botulinum injections.

Chest Only

To date, this technique is the most commonly reported in the literature. Advantages of the robotic technique, namely, improved 3D visualization and instrument maneuverability, are quite evident during the thoracic dissection. Resections of the pericardium, portions of the diaphragm, and other adjacent structures are afforded by this technology. Rather than placing a retractor or an encircling loop such as a Penrose drain around the esophagus to pull it up out of its bed, this technology allows the surgeon to dive into the periesophageal areas and into the opposite chest tube for a more complete lymphadenectomy. Furthermore, it allows dissection down to the hiatus and up into the superior sulcus, areas that were previously difficult to reach with either the MIE or open thoracotomy techniques. The abdominal portion of the procedure is either performed by open laparotomy or by laparoscopy, rather than robotically. As a result of this greater detailed resection, the robotic procedure operative times should be expected to be somewhat longer than the MIE technique.

After double-lumen endotracheal intubation and placement of a measured length of nasogastric tube, the patients are positioned in the lateral decubitus to slightly prone and strapped securely to the operating table. It is important to note that the distance of the insertion of the NG tube is important later in the procedure so the tube can be pulled back out of the stomach before creation of the gastric conduit. The right arm is well padded and positioned over the ear with the elbow below the horizontal plane of the right shoulder. The operating table is tilted as far anteriorly as possible so that the patient is 30 to 45 degrees from prone.

Five puncture wounds are made in the right midanterolateral chest. A 12-mm trocar is placed in the fifth to the sixth intercostal space in the anterior axillary line. A second port, an 8-mm robotic and right arm port, is placed in the posterior axillary line just anterior to the border of the scapula in the third to the fourth intercostal space. A third port, the second 8-mm robotic and left arm port, is placed in the seventh to the eighth intercostal space in the posterior axillary line (Fig. 166-2).

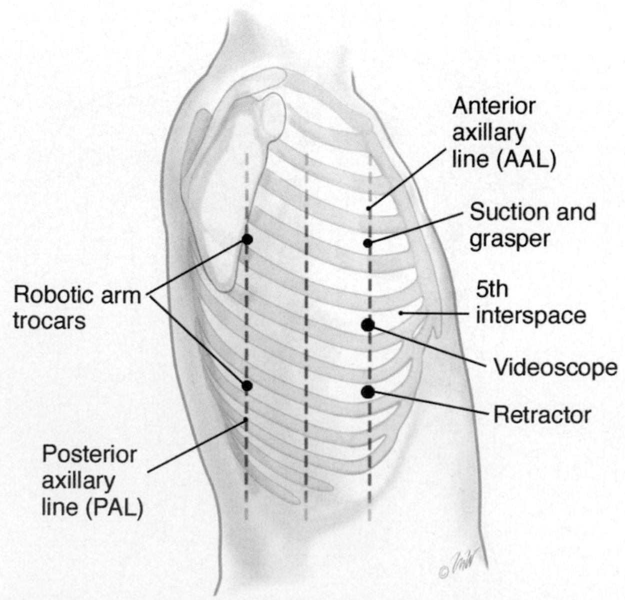

Figure 166-2. Chest only port placement.

Table 166-1

LITERATURE REVIEW OF ROBOTIC ESOPHAGECTOMY—PREOPERATIVE AND INTRAOPERATIVE FINDINGS

AUTHOR	YEAR	TECHNIQUE	*n*	ADENO (%)	DISTAL OR GEI (%)	NEOADJ (%)	STAGE	ABD LN DISSECTION	THORACIC LN DISSECTION	PYLORUS INTERVENTION	LOCATION OF ANASTOMOSIS	SPECIMEN EXTRACTION	ANASTOMOSIS METHOD	
Horgan *USA*	2003	RATE	1	100	100	0	1	D1	Sampling	None	Cervical	Neck	2-layer	
Kernstine *USA*	2004	RALE	1	100	100	100	2b	D2	MLND	None	Cervical	Neck	Linear stapler	
Bodner *Austria*	2005	Chest only	4	25	75	NR	1b–3a	NR	NR	NR	Cervical	Neck	NR	
Van Hillegersberg *The Netherlands*	2006	Chest only	21	48	62	14	1–4 a	D1 Left gastric	MLND	NR	Cervical	Abdomen	1-layer	
Anderson *USA*	2007	Chest only (*n* = 22) RATE (*n* = 1) Abd Only (*n* = 2)	25	NR	100	68	NR	D2	MLND	None	Neck Neck Chest	Neck Neck Chest	Linear stapler	
Kernstine *USA*	2007	Chest only (*n* = 6) RALE (*n* = 8)	14	57	71	64	2b–4	D2	MLND	None	Chest	Neck	Linear stapler	
Kernstine [a] *USA*	2008	RILE	39	NR	NR	NR	NR	D1	MLND	Botulinum?	Cervical selective chest	Neck	Linear stapler	
Galvani *USA*	2008	RATE	18	100	NR	NR	0–2 a	D1	Sampling	None	Cervical	Neck	Linear stapler, 2-layer	
Boone *The Netherlands*	2009	Chest only	47	61	74	6	1–4b	D1 Left gastric	MLND	NR	Cervical	Abdomen	1-layer	
Sutherland *USA*	2010	RATE	36	88	NR	38	NR	NR	Sampling	NR	Cervical	Neck	Circular stapler	
Kim *South Korea*	2010	Chest only RALE (*n* = 4)	21	5	52	14	1–4	D1	MLND	None	Cervical	Neck	Stapled: 19 linear, 2 circular	
Clark (meta-analysis) *England*	2010	Chest only RATE	130	NR	70	NR	1–4	NR	NR	NR	Both	Neck	Both	
Weksler *USA*	2012	Chest only	11	90	NR	37	0–3	D1	MLND	Pyloroplasty	Cervical	Abdomen	Stapled	
Cenfolio *USA*	2012	Chest only	22	82	NR	91	1–3 c	D1	Left gastric	MLND	Botulinum	Chest	Chest	2-layer (73%) Stapled (27%)
Dunn *USA*	2012	RATE	40	90	92.5	42	1–4	D1	Left gastric	MLND	Pyloroplasty	Cervical	Neck	Circular stapler

[a]Denotes unreported surgeon case series.

Table 166-2

LITERATURE REVIEW OF ROBOTIC ESOPHAGECTOMY—SURGICAL OUTCOMES

AUTHOR	YEAR	TECHNIQUE	*n*	RO (%)	CONVERSION (%)	OR Time (min)	EBL (mL)	Lymph nodes	LOS (days)	Complications	Survival and Mortality
Horgan *USA*	2003	RATE	1	100	0	246	50	NR	8	leak: 100%	NR
Kernstine *USA*	2004	RALE	1	100	0	660	900	NR	8	None	100% DFS 6 mo
Bodner *Austria*	2005	Chest only	4	100	0	173 (160–190)	NR	12 (8–19)	14 (10–42)	leak: 0% chyle leak: 17%	50% DFS 5 mo mortality: 0%
Van Hillegersberg *The Netherlands*	2006	Chest only	21	76	14	450 (370–550)	950 (250–5300)	20 (9–30)	18 (11–182)	leak: 14%	NR mortality: 5%
Anderson *USA*	2007	Chest only ($n = 22$) RATE ($n = 1$) Abd only ($n = 2$)	25	100	0	482 (391–646)	350 (100–1600)	22 (10–49)	11 (5–64)	leak: 16% chyle leak: 8%	100% DFS 6 mo mortality: 0%
Kernstine *USA*	2007	Chest only ($n = 6$) RALE ($n = 8$)	14	100	7	672 (570–780)[a]	275 (50–950)[a]	18 (10–32)	NR	leak: 14%	87% DFS 17 mo mortality: 0%
Kernstine[a] *USA*	2008	RILE	39	NR		544 (427–782)	400 (25–1700)	NR	10 (5–66)	NR	NR
Galvani *USA*	2008	RATE	18	76	0	267 (180–365)	54 (10–450)	14 (7–27)	10 (4–38)	leak: 33% chyle leak: 5.5%	61% DFS 22 mo mortality: 0%
Boone *The Netherlands*	2009	Chest only	47	95	15	450 (360–550)	625 (150–5300)	29 (8–68)	18 (10–182)	leak: 21% pulm: 44%	50% DFS 15 mo mortality: 6%
Sutherland *USA*	2010	RATE	36	NR	0	312 (226–491)	97 (25–300)	NR	NR	leak: NR incarc HH: 19.4%	NR NR
Kim *South Korea*	2010	Chest only RALE ($n = 4$)	21	95	0	410 (310–510)	150 (50–2300)	38 (24–52)	21 (11–45)	leak: 19%	NR mortality: 0%
Clark (metaanalysis) *England*	2010	Chest only RATE	130	90	7	377	226	21	16	leak: 18% pulmonary: 25% major compl:31%	NR mortality: 2.4%
Weksler *USA*	2012	Chest only	11	100	NR	445 (306–536)	150 (50–600)	19 (10–47)	7 (5–16)	leak: 9.1%	NR mortality: 0%
Cerfolio *USA*	2012	Chest only	22	100	0	367 (290–453)	60 (30–120) 75 (40–800)	18 (15–28) 17 (15–26)	7 (6–10) 7 (6–32)	leak: 9% chyle leak: 4.5%	100% DFS 5 mo mortality: 0%
Dunn *USA*	2012	RATE	40	95	12.5	311 (226–491)	100 (25–300)	20 (3–38)	9 (6–36)	leak: 25%	50% DFS 20 mo mortality: 2.5%

[a]Denotes unreported surgeon case series.

The robot is then brought into position from the posterior direction or back of the patient. The robotic arms are placed through the 8-mm trocars, and the 0-degree videoscope is placed through the 12-mm trocar. Two accessory trocars are placed, both at the level of the anterior axillary line. The first, a 5-mm trocar, is placed at the level of the third intercostal space, and the second, a 12-mm trocar, is placed at the level of the sixth to the seventh intercostal space. The upper trocar is used for suctioning and grasping instruments, whereas the lower trocar is used for access to place a fan retractor for the lung, the suctioning and grasping instruments, and the sutures used for ligation of the thoracic duct. CO_2 is insufflated to 10 mm Hg of pressure to evacuate cautery smoke and to compress the lung away from the surgical site.

Initially, the hook cautery and Caudiere grasper (Intuitive Surgical) are used to dissect along the anterior aspect of the esophagus just at the pericardial bulge cephalad to the inferior pulmonary vein. The dissection is continued inferiorly to the esophageal hiatus, with the inferior pulmonary ligament and adherent lung taken down as necessary for access to the periesophageal nodes, completely cleaning the pericardium, hiatus, and left pleura. Both hila are cleared of nodal tissue and taken contiguously with the specimen. The periaortic–spinal–azygos nodes are removed. The dissection is continued along the azygos vein, which is preserved when the vein is uninvolved, as determined by CT scan, endoscopic ultrasound, and direct visual assessment. Small lymphatic tributaries seen under high robotic magnification are endoclipped through the accessory port or even robotically.

The supra-azygos esophagus and periesophageal tissue are resected into the thoracic apex, well into the neck. First, over the intended resection area, the pleura is scored with the hook cautery. Then the associated peritracheal nodes and the right vagus nerve are transected with the ultrasonic shears, reducing the potential of electrical transmission to the recurrent laryngeal nerve. The posterior and rightward aspect of the trachea and the thoracic peritracheal and cervical spaces are completely cleaned of periesophageal tissue, and the dissection is continued into the thoracic inlet.

At the level of the diaphragm, the thoracic duct is triply ligated, encompassing all the tissue beneath the remaining intact pleura between the azygos vein and the aorta with 2-0 Ethibond on an SH needle. At the conclusion of the chest phase, two drains are placed: a 19-Fr round fluted drain through the lower accessory trocar along the diaphragm and an additional 19-Fr drain to the superior aspect of the thoracic cavity, through the upper accessory trocar. A thorough multilevel intrathoracic intercostal nerve block is then performed using dilute 0.25% Marcaine mixture (1:1 with injectable saline). The robotic arms are removed and the robotic bedside cart is moved away from the patient.

Robot-Assisted Transhiatal Esophagectomy

This procedure is likely best for patients who have or are suspicious for early-stage disease. Procedure allows for extensive celiac axis lymph node resection and fairly aggressive lower mediastinal lymph node removal, but the mid- and upper esophagus is minimally addressed, if at all. The anastomosis is performed in the neck through a variety of techniques.

After single endotracheal intubation and placement of a measured length of nasogastric tube (the distance of the insertion is important later in the procedure so the tube can be pulled back out of the stomach before creation of the gastric conduit), the patients are positioned supine and reverse Trendelenburg.

The head is turned upward and to the patient's right, exposing the left neck. The upper extremities are placed by the side, and the legs are placed together. After skin preparation and the placement of drapes, a 5-cm transverse incision is made in the left neck 3 cm above the medial left clavicle. The dissection is continued deeply and medially toward the spine, transecting the omohyoid muscle for exposure. The previously mobilized and dissected esophagus is encircled with a Penrose drain, and the incision packed with an antibiotic-soaked surgical sponge to prevent the later escape of CO_2 from the peritoneal cavity.

The abdominal phase is performed next. Six puncture wounds in the abdomen are performed, for two 8-mm robotic arm trocars and the 12-mm robotic viewing trocar placed supraumbilically via a Veress needle. (Fig. 166-2) A distance of 10 to 12 cm is maintained from either of the robotic arms and also placed 10 to 12 cm superior to the transverse plane of the supraumbilically placed videoscope site. Two 5-mm trocars are placed beneath each costal margin in the anterior axillary line and a 12-mm trocar is placed in the left midclavicular line at the umbilicus level. The abdomen is inflated to 15 mm Hg of CO_2 pressure.

The robot is then brought into position from the cephalad direction. After these trocars have been positioned and before the gastric dissection, a percutaneous small bowel feeding tube (Ross Flexiflow Lap J, 10-Fr; Ross Products Division, Abbott Laboratories, Columbus, OH, USA) is placed 20 cm from the ligament of Treitz with "T-fasteners." A diamond-flexed table-mounted self-retaining liver retractor exposing the esophageal hiatus is placed through the right 5-mm accessory port. The robot then is brought into position from the head of the operating table, and the three robotic arms are placed through the 8-mm trocars located 8 cm subcostally in the right and left midclavicular lines. The 30-degree down videoscope is placed through the supraumbilical 12-mm trocar.

A ProGrasp is placed in the left robotic arm (patient's right side) and a harmonic scalpel is placed in the right. Using the harmonic scalpel, the lesser omentum is transected from the base of the liver up to the esophageal hiatus approximately 2 cm away from the right gastroepiploic arcade. The short gastric arteries are taken, with preservation of the right gastroepiploic arcade along its entirety, to the right gastroepiploic vein at the transverse mesentery. The pyloric attachments are transected to free the pylorus, allowing mobilization sufficient to reach toward the esophageal hiatus. No Kocher maneuver is performed. To relax the pylorus to prevent gastric outlet obstruction due to vagal denervation, we then inject 100 U of Botulinum toxin A into four quadrants of the pylorus, raising a definite wheal in each location. Additional nodes are resected from the splenic hilum along the splenic artery to the origin of the left gastric artery and along the celiac axis and common hepatic artery. We ligate the left gastric artery with either an endostapler or a robotic Hem-o-lok clip. We perform a retrogastric dissection along the antrum to the gastroduodenal artery.

The lesser omentum is divided widely to expose the right crus. All of the diaphragmatic attachments around the circumference of dislocation are taken, exposing the right and left crus. We make a small anterior incision in the hiatus. A 1-in Penrose drain is placed around the distal aspect of the esophagus/gastroesophageal junction. This allows for download retraction on the esophagus. We then begin the mediastinal dissection widely immediately adjacent to the diaphragm and the mediastinal pleura, leaving the mediastinal pleura intact. We continue the dissection cephalad avoiding injury to the aorta, mediastinal pleura, and airways. To assist in the mediastinal dissection, we decrease the peritoneal pressure approximately 5 mm Hg and use a 0-degree scope. We continue dissection within the mediastinum as cephalad as possible.

Next, the gastric conduit is created. Approximately 4 to 5 cm cephalad from the origin of the right gastric artery along the lesser gastric curve, the gastric wall is cleared of perigastric tissue. A 4-cm-wide (from the greater curvature) gastric tube is created with a linear endostapler requiring approximately 8 to 10 firings. The most cephalad aspect of the gastric tube is then sutured to the most distal aspect of the specimen with two widely spaced figure-of-eight 0-Ethibond sutures (Ethicon, Inc., Cincinnati, OH, USA) to avoid later twisting of the conduit when it is pulled up in the posterior mediastinum.

Because we are often unable to reach the cervical incision site, we will undock robotic arms and move the bedside cart away and then use a cervical mediastinal scope to perform the remainder of the upper periesophageal dissection through the left neck wound. Once this is achieved, we then replace the videoscope into the abdomen and watch the conduit as it is passed through the esophageal hiatus up into the patient's cervical incision for extraction. The previously placed nasogastric tube is pulled back far enough to divide the esophagus at an appropriate location and the cephalad aspect of the gastric tube is transected using the thick tissue stapler. The end is imbricated with interrupted 3-0 Ethibond sutures. Through an incision on the mesenteric side of the gastric tube, a side-to-side functional end-to-end stapled anastomosis is performed as described by Orringer. After the nasogastric tube is positioned in the conduit at the lower aspect of the mediastinum level, the remaining portion of the anastomosis is closed with interrupted Ethibond. Air is instilled via the nasogastric tube to check for any leak and reinforce the anastomosis as necessary. We also imbricate the upper third of the conduit with interrupted 3-0 Ethibond in order to secure the staple line and to avoid the staple line injury to the adjacent trachea and bronchi. Before neck fascia and skin closure, a small soft flat multiholed drain is placed in the neck beneath the platysma, avoiding the perimeter of the anastomosis, and brought out from an inferior and separate stab wound. After the wound is irrigated, it is closed in layers with Vicryl suture.

We redock the robotic bedside cart and loosely reapproximate the hiatus. The anterior gastric conduit serosa is sutured to each esophageal hiatus crus with two figure-of-eight 3-0 Ethibond sutures to reduce the risk of later periconduit herniation. Care is taken to avoid injury to the gastroepiploic blood supply. Any adjacent omentum is positioned around the lower aspect of the dissection and occasionally sutured into place. The 12-mm port sites are closed with 0-Vicryl to prevent port site herniation.

Robot-Assisted Extended Lymphadenoesophagectomy

This procedure is like the modified McKeown technique. The mediastinal dissection is performed through a transthoracic route first and, in the second stage, the abdominal dissection and the creation of the gastric conduit are performed with the anastomosis performed through a cervical incision in the neck. Extensive lymphadenectomy is performed in the abdomen and the mediastinum with only the deep cervical lymph nodes resected.

After double-lumen endotracheal intubation and placement of a measured length of nasogastric tube (the distance of the insertion is important later in the procedure so the tube can be pulled back out of the stomach before creation of the gastric conduit), the patients are positioned in the lateral decubitus to slightly prone and strapped securely to the operating table. The right arm is well padded and positioned over the ear with the elbow below the horizontal plane of the right shoulder. The operating table is tilted as far anteriorly as possible so that the patient is 30 to 45 degrees from prone.

The thoracic portion of the procedure follows the Chest Only technique (please refer to operative details in the Chest Only section). Following the chest dissection, the patient next is positioned supinely and reintubated with a single-lumen endotracheal tube. The head is turned upward and to the patient's right, exposing the left neck. The upper extremities are placed by the side, and the legs are placed together. After skin preparation and the placement of drapes, a 5-cm transverse incision is made in the left neck 3 cm above the medial left clavicle. The dissection is continued deeply and medially toward the spine, transecting the omohyoid muscle for exposure. The previously mobilized and dissected esophagus is encircled with a Penrose drain, and the incision packed with an antibiotic-soaked surgical sponge to prevent the later escape of CO_2 from the peritoneal cavity.

The abdominal phase is performed next. Six puncture wounds in the abdomen are performed, for two 8-mm robotic arm trocars and the 12-mm robotic viewing trocar placed supraumbilically via a Veress needle. A distance of 10 to 12 cm is maintained from either of the robotic arms. Two 5-mm trocars are placed beneath each costal margin in the anterior axillary line and a 12-mm trocar is placed in the left midclavicular line at the umbilicus level. The abdomen is inflated to 15 mm Hg of CO_2 pressure.

After these trocars have been positioned and before the gastric dissection, a percutaneous small bowel feeding tube (Ross Flexiflow Lap J, 10-Fr; Ross Products Division, Abbott Laboratories, Columbus, OH, USA) is placed 20 cm from the ligament of Treitz with "T-fasteners." A diamond-flexed table-mounted self-retaining liver retractor exposing the esophageal hiatus is placed through the right 5-mm accessory port. The robot is then brought into position from the head of the operating table, and the two robotic arms are placed through the 8-mm trocars located 8 cm subcostally in the right and left midclavicular lines. The 0-degree videoscope is placed through the supraumbilical 12-mm trocar.

A ProGrasp is placed in the left robotic arm (patient's right side) and a harmonic scalpel is placed in the right. Using the harmonic scalpel, the lesser omentum is transected from the base of the liver up to the esophageal hiatus approximately 2 cm away from the right gastroepiploic arcade. The short gastric arteries are taken, with preservation of the right gastroepiploic arcade along its entirety, to the right gastroepiploic vein at the transverse mesentery. The pyloric attachments are transected to free the pylorus, allowing mobilization sufficient to reach toward the esophageal hiatus. No Kocher maneuver is performed. To relax the pylorus to prevent gastric outlet obstruction due to vagal denervation, we then inject 100 U of

Botulinum toxin A into four quadrants of the pylorus, raising a definite wheal in each location. Additional nodes are resected from the splenic hilum along the splenic artery to the origin of the left gastric artery and along the celiac axis and common hepatic artery. We ligate the left gastric artery with either an endostapler or a robotic Hem-o-lok clip. We perform a retrogastric dissection along the antrum to the gastroduodenal artery.

Next, the gastric conduit is created. Approximately 4 to 5 cm cephalad from the origin of the right gastric artery along the lesser gastric curve, the gastric wall is cleared of perigastric tissue. A 4-cm wide (from the greater curvature) gastric tube is created with a linear endostapler requiring approximately 8 to 10 firings. The most cephalad aspect of the gastric tube is then sutured to the most distal aspect of the specimen with two widely spaced figure-of-eight 3-0 Ethibond sutures to avoid later twisting of the conduit when it is pulled up in the posterior mediastinum. The ventilator and the suction on the chest drains are briefly discontinued, and the Penrose drain is used as a handle to pull the specimen carefully up through the neck incision, with the conduit watched closely as it is pulled to the neck.

Once the conduit has been pulled to reach the neck, at the esophageal hiatus level, the anterior gastric conduit serosa is sutured to each esophageal hiatus crus with two figure-of-eight 3-0 Ethibond sutures to reduce the risk of later periconduit herniation. Care is taken to avoid injury to the gastroepiploic blood supply. The abdominal phase is now complete, and the robot is moved away from the patient to allow access to the left neck incision site. The abdominal trocar sites are closed.

The previously placed nasogastric tube is pulled back far enough to divide the esophagus at an appropriate location and the cephalad aspect of the gastric tube is transected using the thick tissue stapler. The end is imbricated with interrupted 3-0 Ethibond sutures. Through an incision on the mesenteric side of the gastric tube, a side-to-side functional end-to-end stapled anastomosis is performed (45- × 4.1-mm linear endostapler and a 60- × 4.1-mm transverse stapler). After the nasogastric tube is positioned in the conduit at the lower aspect of the mediastinum level, the remaining portion of the anastomosis is closed with interrupted Ethibond. Air is instilled via the nasogastric tube to check for any leak and reinforce the anastomosis as necessary. We also imbricate the upper third of the conduit with interrupted 3-0 Ethibond in order to secure the staple line and to avoid the staple line injury to the adjacent trachea and bronchi. Before neck fascia and skin closure, a small soft flat multiholed drain is placed in the neck beneath the platysma, avoiding the perimeter of the anastomosis, and brought out from an inferior and separate stab wound. After the wound is irrigated, it is closed in layers with Vicryl suture.

Robot-assisted Ivor Lewis Esophagectomy

This two-step procedure is likely best for patients with gastroesophageal junction and lower third lesions. As with the RATE, it allows for a wide lymph node dissection in the abdomen, but provides better access of the mediastinum compared to the open transthoracic route. The anastomosis is performed above the level of the azygos vein; usually at the level of the superior sulcus.

After double-lumen endotracheal intubation (for later single-lung ventilation) and placement of a measured length of nasogastric tube (the distance of the insertion is important later in the procedure so the tube can be pulled back out of the stomach before creation of the gastric conduit), the patients are positioned supine and reverse Trendelenburg in order to begin the abdominal portion of the procedure (see operative details highlighted in the RALE section) with the upper extent of the periesophageal mediastinal dissection in the lower fifth of the esophagus. No neck incision is required as the anastomosis will be performed in the chest.

Once the abdominal portion is completed, the bedside cart is undocked and moved away from the patient. The patient is positioned in the left lateral decubitus and slightly prone. The right arm is well padded and positioned over the ear with the elbow below the horizontal plane of the right shoulder.

Five port sites are marked on the patient's right chest. At the level of the seventh rib posteriorly, a 4- to 5-cm incision is made along the rib. We remove a 6-cm segment of rib and make a wide parietal pleural incision. Through this wound, an Alexis laparoscopic wound protector is placed including the Gelport accessory. All thoracoports are positioned as in the RALE section. The patient is positioned approximately 15 to 30 degrees anterior and in reverse Trendelenburg.

The bedside robotic cart is brought in from the patient's head and the arms docked. A robotic ProGrasp instrument is used in the left arm and a robotic Harmonic scalpel in placed in the right arm. The dissection is started at the lower portion of the esophagus and continued cephalad (see operative details highlighted in the RALE section). We attempt to preserve the mediastinal pleura above the azygos vein while performing the periesophageal dissection at that location.

A portion of the esophagus at the desired proximal resection line is cleared and divided with a thick tissue endostapler inserted from the Gelport. With an additional ProGrasp in the right arm we carefully pull the specimen and conduit into the chest avoiding any twisting or deserosalization of the conduit. An EEA stapler is then passed through the Gelport and subsequently through a gastrotomy located on the mesenteric side of the gastric conduit. Anesthesia then passes a 25-mm OrVil (Covidien, Mansfield, MA) anvil into the upper esophageal remnant. The receptacle on the OrVil docks with the EEA spike creating a side-to-end anastomosis. A thick tissue endostapler transects the remaining portion of the specimen and closes the final gastrotomy. The specimen is removed through the posterior incision and through the Gelport wound protector. The nasogastric tube is repositioned and an air leak test is performed after instilling the chest with saline. Two robotic needle holders are used to imbricate the anastomosis and any suspicious areas along the conduit with interrupted 0 Ethibond. A remnant of omentum is wrapped around the anastomosis. The previously intact upper mediastinal pleura is secured over the perianastomotic tissue, holding it into place with interrupted 0 Ethibonds. Two #19 Blake drains are strategically placed both anterior and posterior to the conduit and brought out through the port sites and loosely secured in place with chromic suture to prevent intrathoracic migration. Intrathoracic intercostal nerve blocks are performed as aforementioned and port sites closed using Vicryl suture.

POSTPROCEDURE CARE

Patients are extubated in the operating room and sent to the Thoracic Intensive Care Unit for overnight recovery. A barium swallowing study is performed on the fifth postoperative day, first through the nasogastric tube at various levels and under slight pressure and then via a standard swallowing study, assessing for gastric conduit emptying as well as for any evidence of anastomotic conduit leak. For the patients without a suspicious defect or leak, the diet is advanced to five small liquid feedings per day. If there is any concern, the tube is left in place, and the study repeated in 3 to 5 days. D10W is started at 10 mL through the feeding tube in the recovery room and not advanced to tube feeding until the patient has flatus, bowel sounds, and on examination a nondistended abdomen. Patients are typically discharged on the sixth to seventh postoperative day. During follow-up, the chest drains are left until certain criteria have been met: acceptable interpretation of chest x-ray (no effusions), low output (<100 mL/day), no concern for chyle leak (negative milk/cream test, normal consistency of drain effluent, <110 mg/dL triglycerides in drain effluent), nor concern for esophageal leak (normal esophagram, minimal output, low amylase count in drain effluent). Oral liquids are initiated at approximately 2 to 3 weeks and slowly advanced. The patients are encouraged to use nonnarcotic pain alternatives rather than narcotics by postoperative day 2.

PROCEDURE-SPECIFIC COMPLICATIONS

Complications encountered in robotic thoracic surgery are similar to those with standard videoscopic techniques. Theoretical limitations, including the loss of haptic feedback and having the surgical console away from the sterile operating field, pose unique risks due to the inherent nature of "telesurgery"; however, this has not been an imposing factor in clinical use. Other risks include trocar site complications (bleeding, infection), injury to the surrounding organs (lung, heart, vasculature, nerves, diaphragm, bowel, etc.), and anesthetic risks (heart attack, stroke), infection, pneumonia, hemorrhage, and death.

SUMMARY

We are witnessing the birth of the robotics era. Advances and refinements in robotic-assisted techniques and equipment continue to push the limits of exploration in the surgical care of patients. There are physiologic, immunologic, and clinical reasons for exploring robotic surgery. Published data support a favorable trend for MIS, especially in terms of lowering mortality, morbidity, length of stay, recovery, and pain control, and should be offered for those who are acceptable operative candidates. During cancer resection, robotic methods tend to minimize lung manipulation, reduce surgical seeding, improve visibility, and extend lymph node dissection, which may ultimately improve survival. We have described robotic advantages over standard videoscopic surgery as well as numerous robotic techniques for esophageal resection (chest only, RATE, RILE, RALE) which can be chosen based on location of pathology and surgeon experience.

EDITOR'S COMMENT

An excellent review of the literature and step-by-step guide of the important factors for a successful robotic esophagectomy via several different techniques.

—Yolonda L. Colson

References

1. Kent MS, Schuchert M, Fernando H, et al. Minimally invasive esophagectomy: state of the art. *Dis Esophagus.* 2006;19(3):137–145.
2. Dantoc M, Cox MR, Eslick GD. Evidence to support the use of minimally invasive esophagectomy for esophageal cancer: a meta-analysis. *Arch Surg.* 2012;147(8):768–776.
3. Horgan S, Berger RA, Elli EF, et al. Robotic-assisted minimally invasive transhiatal esophagectomy. *Am Surg.* 2003;69(7):624–626.
4. Kernstine KH, DeArmond DT, Karimi M, et al. The robotic, 2-stage, 3-field esophagolymphadenectomy. *J Thorac Cardiovasc Surg.* 2004;127(6):1847–1849.
5. Hulscher JB, Tijssen JG, Obertop H, et al. Transthoracic versus transhiatal resection for carcinoma of the esophagus: a meta-analysis. *Ann Thorac Surg.* 2001;72(1):306–313.
6. Luketich JD, Alvelo-Rivera M, Buenaventura PO, et al. Minimally invasive esophagectomy: outcomes in 222 patients. *Ann Surg.* 2003;238(4):486–494; discussion 94–95.
7. Verhage R J, Hazebroek E J, Boone J, et al. Minimally invasive surgery compared to open procedures in esophagectomy for cancer: a systematic review of the literature. *Minerva Chir.* 2009;64:135–146.
8. Clark J, Sodergren MH, Purkayastha S, et al. The role of robotic assisted laparoscopy for oesophagogastric oncological resection; an appraisal of the literature. *Dis Esophagus.* 2011;24(4):240–250.
9. Kernstine KH, DeArmond DT, Shamoun DM, et al. The first series of completely robotic esophagectomies with three-field lymphadenectomy: initial experience. *Surg Endosc.* 2007;21(12):2285–2292.
10. Boone J, Schipper M E, Moojen W A, et al. Robot-assisted thoracoscopic oesophagectomy for cancer. *Br J Surg.* 2009;96:878–886.
11. Galvani CA, Gorodner MV, Moser F, et al. Robotically assisted laparoscopic transhiatal esophagectomy. *Surg Endosc.* 2008;22(1):188–195.
12. Dunn DH, Johnson EM, Morphew JA, et al. Robot-assisted transhiatal esophagectomy: a 3-year single-center experience. *Dis Esophagus.* 2012;26(2):159–166.
13. Bodner JC, Zitt M, Ott H, et al. Robotic-assisted thoracoscopic surgery (RATS) for benign and malignant esophageal tumors. *Ann Thorac Surg.* 2005;80(4):1202–1206.
14. van Hillegersberg R, Boone J, Draaisma WA, et al. First experience with robot-assisted thoracoscopic esophagolymphadenectomy for esophageal cancer. *Surg Endosc.* 2006;20(9):1435–1439.
15. Anderson C, Hellan M, Kernstine K, et al. Robotic surgery for gastrointestinal malignancies. *Int J Med Robot.* 2007;3:297–300.
16. Sutherland J, Banerji N, Morphew J, et al. Postoperative incidence of incarcerated hiatal hernia and its prevention after robotic transhiatal esophagectomy. *Surg Endosc.* 2011;25:1526–1530.
17. Kim DJ, Hyung WJ, Lee CY, et al. Thoracoscopic esophagectomy for esophageal cancer: feasibility and safety of robotic assistance in the prone position. *J Thorac Cardiovasc Surg.* 2010;139(1):53–59.
18. Weksler B, Sharma P, Moudgill N, et al. Robot-assisted minimally invasive esophagectomy is equivalent to thoracoscopic minimally invasive esophagectomy. *Dis Esophagus.* 2012;25(5):403–409.
19. Cerfolio RJ, Bryant AS, Hawn MT. Technical aspects and early results of robotic esophagectomy with chest anastomosis. *J Thorac Cardiovasc Surg.* 2013;145(1):90–96.
20. Orringer MB, Marshall B, Iannettoni MD. Eliminating the cervical esophagogastric anastomotic leak with a side-to-side stapled anastomosis. *J Thorac Cardiovasc Surg.* 2000;119:277–288.

167 Robotics: Thymectomy

Bernard J. Park

Keywords: Myasthenia gravis, robotic thymectomy, thymic carcinoid, thymoma, thymic cysts, thymic hyperplasia

INTRODUCTION

The standard treatment of isolated disorders of or related to the thymus is typically thymectomy. Indications include known or suspected thymoma, thymic carcinoid tumor, myasthenia gravis (MG) with or without concomitant thymoma, and benign thymic lesions, such as cysts or discrete hyperplasia. Regardless of the indication, complete thymectomy is the ultimate goal in order to avoid retention of ectopic thymic tissue. This is felt to be particularly important in the surgical management of MG.[1] The most common surgical approach to thymectomy is the classic transsternal approach (Chapter 160), which has proved effective and safe, both in the setting of thymic neoplasms and MG.[2]

In the case of MG, however, many patients and neurologists are hesitant to undergo transsternal thymectomy despite evidence demonstrating clinical improvement because of concerns about perioperative morbidity, pain, and cosmesis. As a result, alternative surgical approaches were developed, including the transcervical method, the video-assisted thoracic surgery (VATS) thymectomy, and most recently robotic thymectomy. VATS thymectomy attempted to replicate complete thymectomy performed under direct, intrathoracic vision but eliminating the morbidity associated with dividing and spreading the sternum.[3] Meyer et al.[4] showed in a single-institution cohort study of VATS versus transsternal thymectomy for MG that there were equivalent clinical outcomes and improved perioperative results (need for postoperative ventilation and length of stay). Despite this, minimally invasive VATS thymectomy never became a widely accepted technique, and significant controversy still exists regarding the optimal surgical approach to thymectomy.

The reason for this controversy is unclear, but similar to VATS lobectomy, it is likely due to a combination of factors, including the technical limitations of an unstable two-dimensional camera platform and limited maneuverability of instrumentation. These issues are especially enhanced in the limited confines of the anterior mediastinum. It was precisely for this application that the master–slave robotic surgical system was developed (da Vinci Surgical System; Intuitive Surgical, Sunnyvale, CA). The three-dimensional (3D) visual system and wristed instrumentation was specifically designed for closed chest cardiothoracic surgery in the anterior and middle mediastinum. However, while this original indication has never been widely realized, other indications evolved, including thymectomy. The earliest case reports consist of only patients with nonthymomatous MG,[5,6] but subsequent series have included those with encapsulated thymic lesions as well.[7–10]

This chapter reviews the general principles and clinical aspects of robotic thymectomy with an emphasis on patient selection, preoperative preparation, technical aspects, and perioperative outcomes.

GENERAL PRINCIPLES

The guiding principle that must be remembered when one is considering utilizing robotic surgical systems for thymectomy is that the ultimate goal is to perform complete resection without violating the capsule of the thymus or any associated lesion. It is up to the surgeon to decide whether this can be safely and appropriately achieved though a minimally invasive robotic approach. The incision strategy, conduct of the procedure, and postoperative management between VATS and robotic thymectomy are similar. Ruckert et al.[11] were among the first to standardize the steps of minimally invasive thymectomy into a 10-step procedure. In their single-institution retrospective study, they compared outcomes of using this standard approach by VATS or robotics in a cohort of matched patients with MG and showed that while immediate perioperative outcomes were indistinguishable, on the basis of long-term follow-up (42 months) those treated by robotics had a higher cumulative complete remission rate (39.25% vs. 20.3%, $p = 0.01$).

In the case of thymic neoplasms, the size, location (right- or left-side predominant) and extent of lesion, influence the choice of operative approach, yet these are not the most compelling factors in deciding whether robotic assistance is feasible. Rather, how these factors determine the likelihood of achieving complete macroscopic and microscopic resection without violating oncologic principles is paramount. Marulli et al. [12] recently described a multicenter European experience of patients undergoing robotic thymectomy for early-stage thymoma. All patients had Masaoka stage I or II tumors and, despite a range of diameters from 1 to 12 cm, demonstrated a 5-year survival rate of 90%.

ROBOTIC TRAINING AND ACCREDITATION

Currently, much like with VATS thymectomy, there are no established guidelines for the training and accreditation of surgeons and operating room teams for performance of robotic thoracic procedures. As a result, each hospital center has developed its own policies regarding the credentialing of individual practitioners. Most uniformly mandate that surgeons attend an intensive, 2-day training course given by Intuitive Surgical® that is comprised of didactic instruction regarding the system components followed by simulation training for basic skills and cadaver-based training for specific procedures. It is critical for specialty-specific personnel, including operating room nurses, surgical technicians and bedside assistants, to be formally trained on the basics of system functioning, instrument changes, and position of the surgical cart. This is typically done by the robotic company representative. It is common, but not required for the prospective robotic surgeon to observe an established practitioner in order to become familiar with specific index procedures. This author cannot stress enough how critically important case observation is during training and prior to implementing robotics into the treatment of patients.

Once the entire surgical team has received the appropriate training, institutions usually will allow implementation of the robotic system into procedures under the supervision and guidance of a case proctor, defined as a surgeon with documented clinical experience independently performing robotic procedures. The console surgeon is typically required to perform 3 to 10 proctored cases before being granted independent robotic procedure privileges. Some hospitals require that eligible proctors themselves have performed a minimum number of cases, while the majority has no such requirement. In fact, most institutions do not mandate that the proctor be specialty-specific. Thus, a robotic urologist may proctor a thoracic surgeon. While this may be in compliance with a specific institutional requirement, this type of implementation is ill-advised. The ideal situation is for the training surgeon to observe an experienced robotic surgeon in their respective field and then enlist that individual, if possible, to serve as the case proctor. This maximizes the continuity of training and, consequently, patient safety during clinical implementation.

PATIENT SELECTION AND PREOPERATIVE ASSESSMENT

MG with or Without Thymoma

It is well accepted that thymectomy is most effective in younger patients with generalized MG with the goal of symptom improvement, decreased medication requirement, and for some, complete remission. Its role in patients with pure ocular MG or late onset of disease is less clear as ocular MG typically has a better overall prognosis and is less likely to resolve following thymectomy. However, up to 70% of patients who present with ocular symptoms only eventually progress to more generalized disease. Thus, in this patient population, the emphasis must be placed on prevention of disease progression. Patients with generalized disease diagnosed at an older age should be counseled about the realistic chances of benefit from thymectomy because even minimally invasive approaches can have long-term adverse effects.

The extent and severity of muscle weakness should be carefully elicited and documented. Patients should see their neurologist preoperatively for optimization of their medical treatment. In patients with severe weakness, preoperative treatment with either plasmapheresis or intravenous immunoglobulin therapy may be required. Patients should be prepared for the possibility of postoperative mechanical ventilation and myasthenic crisis. It is critical for the neurologist, anesthesiologist, and surgical team to work closely to achieve the best results. Recent imaging of the chest is advised preoperatively as 25% of patients with MG will have a concomitant thymoma. Although a computed tomography (CT) of the chest with intravenous contrast is preferred, magnetic resonance imaging (MRI) with and without contrast is also suitable.

Thymoma

Patients with known or suspected thymoma should undergo a recent CT chest with intravenous contrast to ascertain the size and extent of the lesion (Fig. 167-1). Particular attention should be paid to the possibility of invasion of surrounding structures, such as the lung, pericardium, and phrenic nerves. In addition, it is important to note if the tumor is located predominantly on one side or centrally as this may determine from which side the procedure will be approached. Careful assessment in the history and physical examination should be directed at eliciting any suspicion of undetected MG, as one-quarter of patients with newly diagnosed thymoma will have concomitant MG. As with any new surgical technique or approach, careful selection of initial cases is critical to success and progression. While scenarios such as large (>5 cm) tumors and/or those with suspected gross invasion of the thymic capsule into surrounding structures or prior sternotomy do not absolutely preclude a robotic approach, it is wise to avoid these conditions until a sufficient experience has been developed with the most straightforward cases. Informed consent for the use of robotic assistance should be obtained as a distinct portion of the procedure.

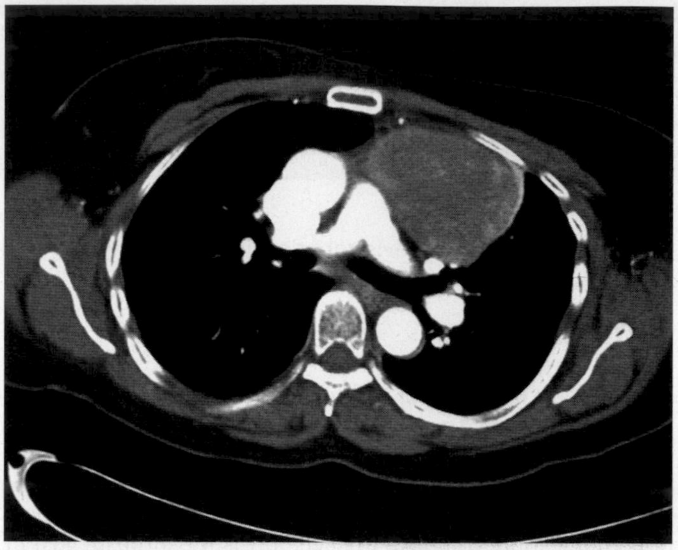

Figure 167-1. Preoperative CT chest in a patient with a thymoma.

All patients considered for thymectomy should have adequate cardiopulmonary and performance status to tolerate single-lung ventilation and possible intrathoracic CO_2 insufflation. Patients with significant smoking history, diminished exercise tolerance or a history of chronic obstructive pulmonary disease should probably undergo preoperative pulmonary function testing. Smoking cessation for active smokers should be aggressively advocated.

OPERATIVE TECHNIQUE

Preparation of the Robot

The operating room technical staff sets up the robotic surgical system (surgical cart, surgeon's console, vision system) in the room (Fig. 167-2). In the beginning of the case, the nursing staff power up the system, run the appropriate diagnostics, and drape the robotic arms and camera. This requires two individuals and typically takes 5 to 10 minutes for staff who are trained and familiar with the process and occurs prior to or while the patient is undergoing induction of anesthesia and positioning.

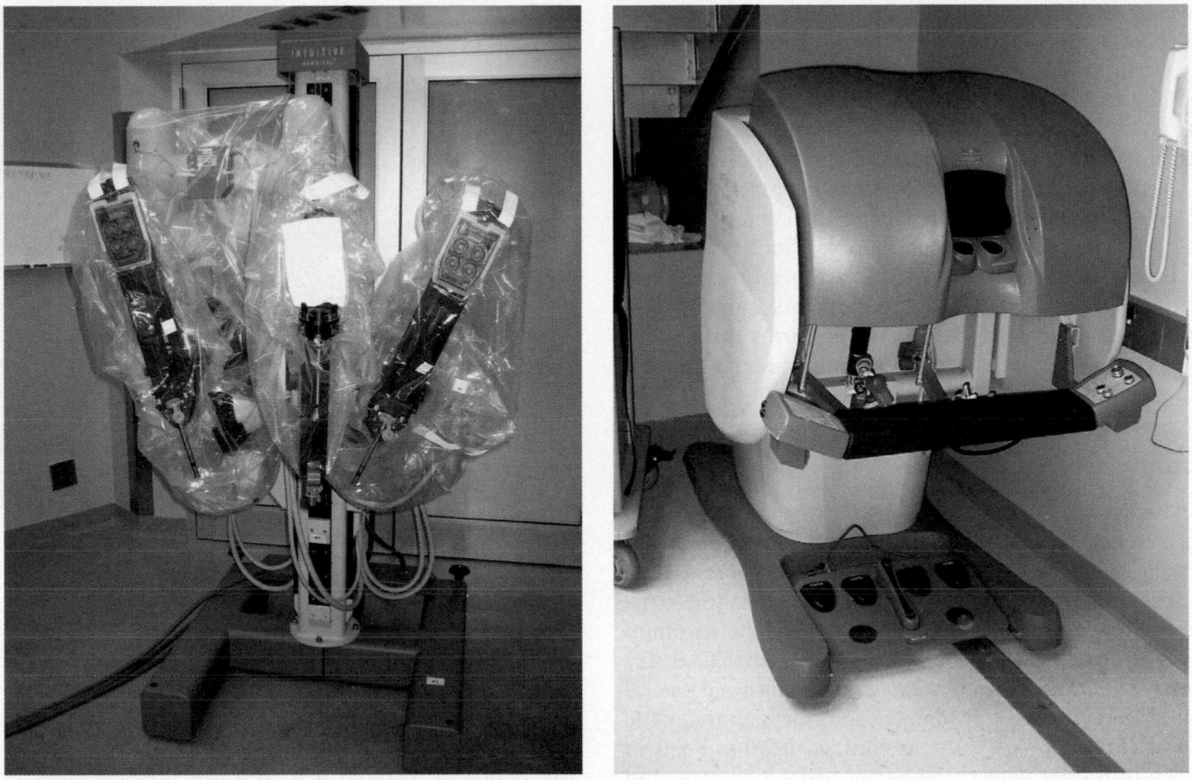

A B

Figure 167-2. Robotic surgical system. *A.* Surgical Cart. *B.* Surgeon console.

Anesthesia Considerations and Patient Positioning

Standard methods of induction of general anesthesia and endotracheal intubation are used. Single-lung ventilation via either double-lumen endotracheal tube placement or bronchial blocker, while not mandatory, greatly facilitates the procedure and can be initiated early once correct tube position has been verified bronchoscopically or clinically. Patients with MG are exquisitely sensitive to nondepolarizing muscle relaxants, and their use should be avoided as much as possible. Anesthesia can be maintained with volatile, inhalational agents. If muscle relaxation is necessary, a reduced dose of intermediate-acting nondepolarizing agents can be employed at the beginning of the procedure.

The patient is placed in a supine position with the ipsilateral side elevated 30 degrees with a gel roll or padding placed longitudinally below the tip of the scapula. The contralateral arm is padded and tucked. The ipsilateral arm should be slightly abducted, padded and placed on an armboard that is fully adducted in line with the operating room table so that the arm and shoulder are below the anterior chest. The operating table is moved away from the anesthesia machine and angled with the foot of the table away from the surgical cart. This establishes enough space to dock the robot which will be positioned at the contralateral side. Thus, with a left-sided robotic approach, the left side of the patient is elevated with the robotic cart docked from the right side of the table. Care must be taken to insure that sufficient length of the circuit tubing is available during this positioning, and the anesthesia team must be comfortable that there is adequate access to the patient's airway once docking of the robotic system has taken place. The entire neck and chest below the xiphoid process should be prepped and draped in the event that a transsternal or contralateral incision is needed.

Initial Exploration and Docking of the Robot

Robotic thymectomy is a three-incision, three-arm procedure. Initial thoracic exploration is conducted with the robotic thoracoscope through a 12-mm port in the fifth or sixth intercostal space (ICS) in the anterior axillary line. Use of CO_2 insufflation to 8 to 10 mm Hg is generally well tolerated and enhances the visualization and working space by increasing the anteroposterior diameter of the chest. The anesthesia team should be alerted to the initiation of insufflations so that they may monitor the patient's airway and blood pressure. When operating on the left side, care must be taken in making this initial incision as it will be quite close to the pericardium. The camera port should be placed without the use of a sharp trocar and CO_2 insufflation should be initiated prior to placing the subsequent ports.

The remaining ports are 8 mm reusable metal robotic ports placed under robotic thoracoscopic visualization. Because the working space is limited, it is critical to space the ports at least one handbreadth apart to avoid arm collisions that will limit full range of motion of the instruments in the chest. The second port is placed in the sixth or seventh ICS in the inframammary crease in the midclavicular line. The last port is placed in the third or fourth ICS anterior to the anterior axillary line. Once all three ports have been placed, the surgical cart is brought into position from the contralateral side with the center column and camera arm in a line between the camera port and the contralateral shoulder. It is important to position the arms within the working range and avoid having them too close to the ports and the patient as this will limit the working range of the instruments.

Once the surgical cart is in position, the camera arm is attached first to the 12-mm port. The camera arm and port are used to elevate the anterior chest wall for increased visualization. The robotic thoracoscope is introduced and secured to the camera arm. A 0-degree scope is preferred for the initial dissection and avoids excessive torque in the interspace. The remaining ports are attached to the robotic arms, and the surgical instruments are introduced under direct thoracoscopic vision. A Cadiere forceps is most commonly controlled by one hand for grasping tissue, and a cutting instrument (monopolar spatula, Maryland bipolar, monopolar hook) is used in the other hand. After the instruments have been introduced, the operating surgeon moves to the surgeon's console. The first assistant remains at the table and performs instrument exchanges as needed. A separate, nonrobotic assistant port is typically not required.

Thymectomy

Dissection is initiated by incising the mediastinal pleural medial to the phrenic nerve. It is easiest to begin in the midpoint of the pericardium where fat content is lowest. The perithymic and pericardial fat is mobilized along the entire length of the phrenic nerve from cephalad to caudad off of the pericardium as far toward the contralateral chest as is convenient. CO_2 insufflation greatly facilitates dissection once the mediastinal pleural is divided. Dissection at the ipsilateral anterior diaphragmatic recess can be limited by instrument conflict. It often helps in this situation to retract with the superior instrument arm and divide the tissue with the inferior arm.

Next, the mediastinal pleural just posterior to the posterior table of the sternum is incised from the thoracic inlet to the diaphragm and from the ipsilateral to the contralateral pleural space. The contralateral pleura is divided completely, allowing dissection up to the contralateral phrenic and for greater manipulation of the specimen as the mobilization proceeds. The dissection continues cephalad and toward the contralateral pleural space by dividing en bloc all attachments of the specimen to the pericardium. Visualization of tissue at the limits of the contralateral pleural space is improved through the use of the 30-degree robotic thoracoscope.

Once the majority of the specimen has been mobilized off the pericardium toward the neck, the ipsilateral portion of the innominate vein is identified. The superior horns are bluntly separated from the innominate vein. The thymic veins are isolated and divided either by serial clips or through the use of the robotic harmonic scalpel. Similarly, the superior horns are freed from the surrounding attachments, pulled inferior out of the neck and either clipped and divided or resected by harmonic scalpel. It is useful to place a clip of one of the horns for proper orientation of the specimen once ex vivo. Visualization can be improved by allowing the already mobilized portion to fall into the contralateral pleural space. After all of the tissue from the thoracic inlet has been freed, the remaining attachments to the anterior surface of the pericardium medial to the contralateral phrenic should be divided. At this point, if not done so previously, a change to the 30-degree thoracoscope in a downward orientation will facilitate identification and avoidance of the phrenic nerve.

Specimen Removal

Once the entire gland and surrounding tissue have been completely mobilized, the inferior port may be removed. Removing the specimen from this incision is preferable because the rib space is widest in the anterior position. When the thymoma or other thymic mass is larger than the initial incision, the incision should be enlarged with an Anchor™ tissue retrieval bag (Anchor Products Company, Addison, Illinois) or other suitable bag is placed through it to retrieve the specimen. A durable nylon bag is preferred to plastic to minimize the chance of rupture and spillage. A conventional thoracoscopic grasper can be introduced in the superior port manually and used to grasp the specimen. The sac should be positioned such that the full extent of the bag may be opened toward the contralateral chest. Once the specimen is placed into the bag, it is removed (Fig. 167-3).

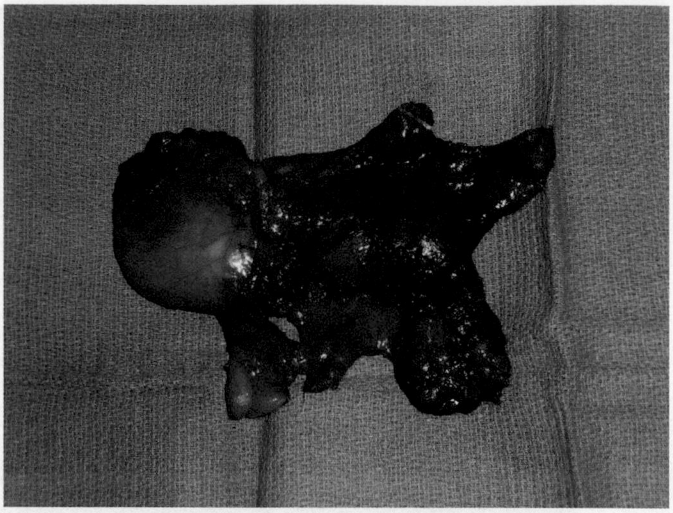

Figure 167-3. Robotic thymectomy specimen.

Termination of the Procedure

After the specimen has been removed, the operative bed should be inspected for any signs of active or potential bleeding. Any blood or clots should be irrigated and removed. The ports are then removed, and a single chest tube is placed through the camera incision and positioned with the tip at the apex of the ipsilateral chest or in the anterior mediastinum. The lung should be reinflated under direct thoracoscopic vision with the robotic scope placed in the inferior incision. The remaining wounds are closed in a standard fashion.

POSTOPERATIVE CARE

Standard postoperative management should be undertaken. In virtually all cases, patients can be extubated in the operating room and brought initially to the postanesthesia care unit. The chest tube may be left to water seal. Patient-controlled analgesia should be initiated through the use of a preoperatively placed epidural or a peripheral narcotic combined with intraoperative intercostals blocks. Patients may be transferred to a surgical floor with telemetry. If the immediate postoperative chest radiograph shows no evidence of pneumothorax or effusion, and there is no air leak, the chest tube may be removed immediately. Chest physiotherapy and early ambulation should be provided and encouraged. In patients with MG, their preoperative medications should be resumed and regular checks of oxygen saturation and incentive spirometry should be performed for early detection of respiratory muscle weakness. Commonly, patients can be discharged the following day provided there are no other concomitant complications; and pain control on oral medication is sufficient.

PROCEDURE-SPECIFIC CONSIDERATIONS

Potential intraoperative and postoperative complications are no different with a robotic approach to thymectomy than VATS or transsternal thymectomy. However, there are unique aspects to robotic thoracic procedures and thymectomy that need to be considered.

1. Lack of tactile feedback: The robotic arms do not impart haptic feedback to the console (operating) surgeon. Therefore, both the console surgeon and the bedside assistant must be constantly vigilant about inadvertent injury to either the external patient or surrounding internal structures by the instrument arms or the instruments themselves. Externally, care must be taken to insure that the arms do not compress any part of the patient with undue force or for a prolonged period of time. Internally, the surgeon must pay close attention to the visual feedback to prevent direct traction injury and compression injury by the shaft or heel of the instruments to adjacent structures.
2. Visual magnification: The robotic thoracoscope by design has greater magnification compared with the optics of the conventional camera. This is quite beneficial when working in a narrow, confined space, but results in decreased overall perspective view. This can be a disadvantage in the chest when one is attempting to delineate anatomic boundaries. It is critical to zoom out to the farthest extent possible when a greater overall view is required.
3. Hemorrhage: While the threat of hemorrhage during thymectomy is not unique to robotic procedures, absence of the operating surgeon at the bedside for immediate intervention is a necessary condition of the current master–slave robotic system. There are several strategies to maximize safety and minimize patient morbidity in the event of significant vascular injury. First, anticipation of a potential injury and maintaining a low threshold for conversion is key. Second, there must be a sponge stick ready and available for the bedside assistant to use for temporary tamponade of a bleeding vessel. Third, the bedside staff must be poised for rapid instrument removal and undocking of the surgical cart in preparation for conversion. With proper training, this can be executed in less than 1 minute, and use of robotic technology should never impede timely management of potentially catastrophic bleeding.
4. Right or left-sided approach: Robotic thymectomy is typically performed from a unilateral approach, and there is much debate regarding the optimal side from which robotic thymectomy should be approached. Advocates of a right-sided approach feel that there is initially more room to safely place the ports and initiate dissection. In addition, identification of the innominate vein from the right is technically easier than from the left. The main weakness of a right-sided approach is that the left phrenic nerve is more difficult to visualize, particularly near the thoracic inlet. Proponents of a left-sided approach feel that identification of the right phrenic is easier, as is dissection high into the neck. The innominate vein, however, is more difficult to identify from the left, and the pericardium is very close to the chest wall during initial exploration and docking. Most agree, however, that in the case of a mass that is predominantly located on one side, the thymectomy should be approach from the same side as the mass.
5. No touch technique: Robotic thymectomy, particularly in the setting of a known or suspected thymoma, should be conducted with a no-touch technique with respect to both the thymic tissue and the lesion, if present, to avoid seeding of the anterior mediastinum and pleural spaces with either tumor or retained thymic tissue. This is particularly important with respect to robotic technology where there is no haptic feedback. Thus, during active retraction, it is critical to grab only perithymic tissue. As the specimen becomes more mobilized and especially when a mass is involved, a better strategy is to use the closed instrument to push rather than grab the specimen. If adequate retraction and exposure cannot be accomplished without increased risk of tearing and spillage, conversion to a transsternal approach should be considered.

SUMMARY

Robotic thymectomy is a safe and feasible method of accomplishing complete thymectomy for surgical treatment of MG and thymic neoplasms. The 3D high-definition visual system and wristed instrumentation are ideal for the anterior mediastinum. The procedure can be performed with minimal morbidity and an expected hospital stay of just 1 to 2 days. As with any procedure, patient selection, preoperative preparation, and multidisciplinary care are critical for success.

EDITOR'S COMMENT

The risks and benefits of robotic thymectomy are outlined. The "insider's" tips as to how to do this better are important for anyone new to robotic surgery.

—Yolonda L. Colson

References

1. Jaretzki A, Penn AS, Younger DS, et al. Maximal thymectomy for myasthenia gravis. Results. *J Thorac Cardiovasc Surg*. 1988;95:747–757.
2. Masaoka A, Yamakawa Y, Niwa H, et al. Extended thymectomy for myasthenia gravis patients: a 20-year review. *Ann Thorac Surg*. 1996;62:853–859.
3. Mack MJ, Landreneau RJ, Yim AP, et al. Results of video-assisted thymectomy in patients with myasthenia gravis. *J Thorac Cardiovasc Surg*. 1996;112:1352–1360.
4. Meyer DM, Herbert MA, Sobhani NC, et al. Comparative clinical outcomes of thymectomy for myasthenia gravis performed by extended transsternal and minimally invasive approaches. *Ann Thorac Surg*. 2009;87:385–391.

5. Rea F, Bortolotti L, Girardi R, et al. Thoracoscopic thymectomy with the 'da Vinci' surgical system in patient with myasthenia gravis. *Interact Cardiovasc Thorac Surg.* 2003;2:70–72.
6. Ashton RC, Jr, McGinnis KM, Connery CP, et al. Totally endoscopic robotic thymectomy for myasthenia gravis. *Ann Thorac Surg.* 2003;75:569–571.
7. Bodner J, Wykypiel H, Greiner A, et al. Early experience with robot-assisted surgery for mediastinal masses. *Ann Thorac Surg.* 2004;78:259–266.
8. Ruckert JC, Ismail M, Swierzy M, et al. Thoracoscopic thymectomy with the da Vinci robotic system for myasthenia gravis. *Ann N Y Acad Sci.* 2008; 1132:329–335.
9. Augustin F, Schmid T, Sieb M, et al. Video-assisted thoracoscopic surgery versus robotic-assisted thoracoscopic surgery thymectomy. *Ann Thorac Surg.* 2008;85:S768–S771.
10. Freeman RK, Ascioti AJ, Van Woerkom JM, et al. Long-term follow-up after robotic thymectomy for nonthymomatous myasthenia gravis. *Ann Thorac Surg.* 2011;92:1018–1023.
11. Ruckert JC, Swierzy M, Ismail M. Comparison of robotic and nonrobotic thoracoscopic thymectomy: a cohort study. *J Thorac Cardiovasc Surg.* 2011;141:673–677.
12. Marulli G, Rea F, Melfi F, et al. Robot-aided thoracoscopic thymectomy for early-stage thymoma: a multicenter European study. *J Thorac Cardiovasc Surg.* 2012;144:1125–1132.

168 Sentinel Node Mapping in Lung Cancer

Yolonda L. Colson, Michael J. Liptay, and Denis Gilmore

Keywords: Sentinel lymph nodes, lymphatic mapping, metastatic nodal disease

RATIONALE OF SENTINEL LYMPH NODE MAPPING AND BIOPSY

Early in the nineteenth century, Virchow implicated lymph nodes in the process of the local spread of solid tumors to a more widespread systemic disease. The node identified by Virchow is specifically located in the left supraclavicular region. In the modern vernacular, the term sentinel lymph node (SLN) describes the first lymph node to receive drainage from any solid tumor in any anatomic region. It was not until 1989 that the concept of SLN biopsy, as it is currently known, was first made popular based on studies by Morton et al.[1] A feasibility study using blue dye was translated into a successful clinical trial in patients with melanoma. Their results indicated that biopsy and analysis of SLNs accurately reflected the tumor status of the lymph node basin. SLN biopsy was introduced in breast cancer patients shortly thereafter.[2] Further studies supported SLN biopsy as a way to identify patients at highest risk for locoregional recurrence and metastatic spread, and, therefore, most likely to benefit from adjuvant therapy. SLN mapping aids in the identification of lymph nodes at highest risk of metastasis and allows for more detailed analysis to detect early metastatic disease thus identifying patients who may benefit from adjuvant therapy. While SLN biopsy is standard in both breast cancer and melanoma patients, a number of factors have led to slower adoption in patients with non-small cell lung cancer (NSCLC).

NODAL DISEASE IN LUNG CANCER

Lung cancer is the leading cause of cancer deaths among both men and women in the US, with an estimated 170,000 new cases and 160,000 deaths reported each year.[3] Even in patients with stage I disease thought to have undergone curative resection, recurrence rates remain high at nearly 40%.[4] This high incidence of recurrent disease in stage I lung cancer patients suggests that these patients are currently understaged and undertreated. In fact, retrospective analysis has demonstrated that nearly 15% to 20% of N0 patients harbor "occult" metastatic disease when nodes are histologically scrutinized in the manner done for breast cancer and melanoma.[5] Not surprisingly, patients with occult nodal disease exhibit poorer survival and increased rates of recurrence. Despite all the recent clinical advances in lung cancer therapy, the best predictor of patient outcome following surgical resection remains the presence or absence of metastatic disease to lymph nodes. To improve survival of patients with surgically resectable lung cancer, detailed intraoperative lymph node evaluation is needed to more accurately stage patients and identify candidates for early adjuvant therapy.

SLN mapping seeks to identify the first lymph node to harbor metastatic disease from a nearby tumor and has become an integral part of patient selection for adjuvant treatment in solid malignancies such as breast cancer and melanoma. The two primary benefits of SLN mapping in breast cancer and melanoma have been (1) limiting the extent of lymph node dissection in the axilla or groin and (2) focused pathologic assessment of specific "at risk" nodes. In lung cancer surgery, the morbidity of mediastinal node dissection or sampling is low; however, lymph node drainage patterns are complex and variable, and thus the primary utility of SLN mapping is to identify those nodes at highest risk for metastatic disease and to facilitate the focused assessment of such nodes. The ability to conduct more detailed histologic and molecular analysis on the identified SLN would allow for better patient selection for subsequent adjuvant therapy in hopes of improving survival and decreasing locoregional recurrence. Although the goal of detecting micrometastatic disease prospectively via SLN mapping in lung cancer is sound, conventional SLN mapping techniques using radioisotopes or blue dye have not been successfully translated to the thorax, and currently this important therapeutic intervention is not clinically available for the care of lung cancer patients.

Several factors unique to the lung, including the presence of intrapulmonary and anthracotic (black) lymph nodes, have made identification of SLN with blue dye more difficult in lung cancer patients. Furthermore, "shine through" of radioactivity from the tumor injection site to nearby nodes in the mediastinum and hilum has hampered reliable SLN identification using radioisotopes in the thorax. In this chapter, we review prior attempts at SLN identification in non-small cell lung cancer and discuss recent research findings using indocyanine green (ICG) dye and near-infrared (NIR) fluorescence imaging to improve SLN mapping in patients with early-stage lung cancer.

SLN MAPPING IN NONSMALL CELL LUNG CANCER

SLN biopsy is currently the standard of care in both melanoma and breast cancer patients, but these methods have not been successfully translated to NSCLC. Unfortunately, only approximately 45% of surgeons completely remove lymph nodes from the hilum and mediastinum at the time of surgical resection.[6] In addition, lymphatic drainage patterns are highly variable in the lung, making it difficult to predict the draining lymph node basin that should be sampled, and it is unknown whether the specific SLN for a patient is even included in the conventional surgical lymphadenectomy specimens. Furthermore, skip metastases to the N2 nodal station have been shown to bypass the nearby N1 stations and are present in an estimated 20% of cases.[7] By removing only the nodes included with the resection specimen and failing to sample hilar and mediastinal nodes, surgeons are missing these skip metastases.

In addition to potentially missing nodal disease during surgical resection, current conventional histologic analysis may also miss micrometastatic disease in removed nodes. This prospect is particularly worrisome as nearly 16% of patients with histologically node-negative lung cancer and up to 27.5% of patients with subcentimeter adenocarcinomas are found to harbor evidence of occult micrometastatic disease or disseminated tumor cells within sampled nodes when these nodes are analyzed retrospectively with more time-intensive "SLN" histologic analysis techniques. Furthermore, Liptay et al. recently demonstrated in an analysis of 104 patients with lung cancer, and Takizawa in a series of 157 lobectomies, that the SLN was the only positive node present in 36% to 37% of node-positive patients.[7,8] This is important information, since failure to remove this node or to identify metastatic disease histologically leaves the patient with untreated occult micrometastatic disease which has been shown to correlate with a threefold increase in recurrence and a significant decrease in patient survival.[8] To impose more focused histologic analysis on all lymph nodes removed during a lung resection is impractical. However, if SLN mapping could identify a small subset of nodes for the pathologists to scrutinize, focused histological and molecular examination could be performed on these nodes to better identify micrometastasis.

EARLY CLINICAL TRIALS

Conventional means of SLN mapping using blue dye and radioactive have been attempted in NSCLC but have remained unreliable secondary to physical properties of both the tracer and the lung. The initial attempt at SLN biopsy in lung cancer was performed in 1999 by Little et al.[9] Thirty-six patients underwent intraoperative injection of blue dye with a SLN identified in only 47% of patients. Low success rates were attributed to the learning curve associated with the injection technique in presence of anthracotic nodes. The authors acknowledged an unacceptably low rate of SLN identification, but advocated for the addition of radiolabeled tracers to improve sensitivity and specificity. Unfortunately, however, this combination proved unsuccessful.

Intraoperative radioactive tracers were first used for SLN mapping in lung cancer by Liptay et al. in 2000.[10] Intraoperative injection of technetium 99 resulted in successful radioisotope migration in 81% of patients and SLN identification in almost 87%. Roughly a quarter of the SLNs identified were located in the mediastinum representing skip metastasis. Furthermore, SLN analysis on previously deemed negative nodes detected occult micrometastatic disease in 24% of these patients. The SLN was the only metastatic node in just over a third of patients. As a result of this initial Phase I study, a multicenter Phase II trial under the direction of Cancer and Leukemia Group B (CALGB) research cooperative focused on intraoperative injection of technetium 99 in patients with suspected stage I NSCLC. Unfortunately, accrual was less than 50% and of those enrolled, only 51% of patients had an SLN identified. Poor accrual and the low success rate was attributed to logistical issues of organizing nuclear medicine, surgery, and pathology for intraoperative injection and analysis, and cumbersome regulations for radioactivity handling in addition to a difficult learning curve of the injection technique.[11] Less than optimal results obtained with either blue dye or radioisotopes led to different variations of the technique in an effort to increase the sensitivity and specificity of SLN identification in lung cancer. Owing to the fact that lymphatic vessels may be disrupted during intraoperative incision and dissection, Nomori et al. hypothesized that preoperative CT-guided injection and intraoperative injection via a transbronchial approach may improve results, but findings were similar to the initial studies by Liptay et al.[12] with successful SLN identification reported in only 81% of patients. Shine-through effect, residual radioactivity, and possible decreased lymphatic density or impaired lymphatic flow in COPD patients were also thought to contribute to these less than optimal results. Even more worrisome, however, was the increased morbidity noted with this technique. The preoperative injection was associated with complications of bleeding, pneumothorax, and potential tumor seeding along the injection track. These studies demonstrate that SLN mapping with single-agent blue dye or radioisotope is not optimal, but that a combined approach may be warranted.

Two separate groups attempted combining both blue dye and radioisotopes to aid in the detection of SLN in patients with lung cancer. Schmidt et al. used intraoperative injection of both blue dye and Tm-99, achieving a SLN identification rate of 81%.[13] Tiffet et al. was the second group to evaluate intraoperative injection of both markers, but again demonstrated suboptimal results, identifying the SLN in only 13 of 24 patients (54%).[14] The technical difficulties associated with each of these approaches included visualization of blue dye within anthracotic nodes, intrathoracic use of the Geiger counter to identify radioisotopes, and anatomical differences in patients, all of which were thought to contribute to the low accuracy in SLN identification. In addition to these technical issues, potential risks of radioactivity to the surgeon, operating room personnel, patient, and pathologist raise legitimate concerns that hampered adoption of this technique.

The search for a better technique has led surgical groups to innovate by exploring nonradioactive agents that not only promise more reliable and accurate SLN identification but also the potential for therapeutic intraoperative targeting of nodal metastases (Table 168-1).

Table 168-1

EARLY RESULTS OF SENTINEL NODE MAPPING IN LUNG CANCER

GROUP	YEAR	TECHNIQUE	SUCCESS RATE (%)
Little et al.[9]	1999	Blue dye	47
Liptay et al.[10]	2000	Radioisotope	81
Liptay et al.[11]	2009	Multicenter radioisotope trial	51
Nomori et al.[12]	2007	Preoperative radioisotope	81
Schmidt et al.[13]	2002	Intraoperative blue dye/radioisotope	81
Tiffet et al.[14]	2005	Intraoperative blue dye/radioisotope	54

NEAR-INFRARED IMAGING FOR SLN MAPPING IN LUNG CANCER

Recent large animal and Phase I/II clinical trials have investigated the use of Near-Infrared (NIR) imaging for the identification of SLNs in breast, skin (melanoma), stomach, colon, and lung.[15,16] These studies have used optimized NIR lymphatic tracers, the most common of which is ICG dye, since it is FDA-approved for intravenous use in the calculation of cardiac outputs and ophthalmologic angiography. The success rates for SLN identification in these studies have approached 100% with doses of peritumoral ICG ranging from 0.1% to 5% of the conventional dose used intravenously. Peritumoral injection of ICG can quickly and reliably migrate in real time to draining lymph node basins permitting rapid and accurate SLN identification in an operative setting. Invisible NIR light penetrates deep into tissue allowing detection of fluorescent signal at a depth of 1 cm in solid tissue. Unique NIR cameras are now commercially available with the spectral sensitivity to provide safe NIR excitation with simultaneous intraoperative imaging of visible reflected light and the NIR fluorescence emitted from the ICG fluorophore. Separation of the visible and NIR fluorescent light allows simultaneous acquisition of color and NIR fluorescence images with high signal to background ratios with subsequent overlay of the two images (Fig. 168-1). This approach results in a single, intraoperative procedure whereby SLNs can be visualized but the surgical field remains unaltered by radioactivity or discoloration. This approach is particularly attractive because it allows direct videoscopic images of the necessary anatomic landmarks within the surgical field and extremely low background signal from biologic tissues thus permitting accurate surgical dissection. In large animal studies, NIR–SLN mapping has demonstrated a high success rate in identification of a single SLN station (>90%) with only occasional identification of a split lymphatic channel to two separate SLNs (<10%). Furthermore, this approach is nontoxic, without exposure risk to the patient or hospital personnel or the need for special biologic or disposal precautions.

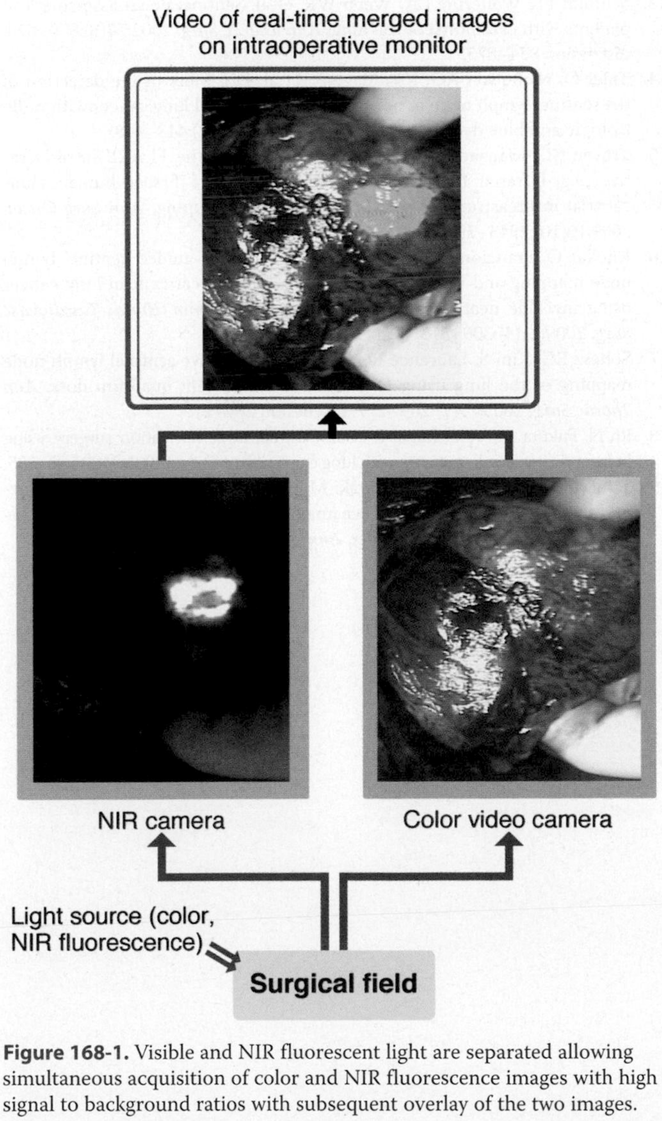

Figure 168-1. Visible and NIR fluorescent light are separated allowing simultaneous acquisition of color and NIR fluorescence images with high signal to background ratios with subsequent overlay of the two images.

One of the first studies to look at the use of NIR-imaging for SLN mapping in the lung was performed by Soltesz et al. in a swine model using NIR-fluorescent quantum dots.[17] Quantum dots are semiconductor nanocrystals that contain an inorganic core of cadmium telluride, an inorganic shell of cadmium selenide, and an outer organic coating of solubilizing oligomeric phosphines. The intraparenchymal injection of quantum dots did result in SLN identification in all animals tested regardless of the lobe of the lung evaluated, and confirmed that SLN identification was also possible for the lung. Unfortunately, although quantum dots offer excellent lymphatic mapping and SLN identification, they have not been aggressively pursued for clinical use because of concerns over the possibility of heavy metal toxicity in patients. Therefore, additional preclinical studies were performed to establish the feasibility of SLN mapping in lung tissue using the organic FDA-approved fluorophore ICG. These large animal pulmonary studies demonstrated evidence of an NIR fluorescent signal within the SLN within 10 minutes of intraparenchymal ICG injection, establishing the potential of NIR imaging as a rapid, safe, and accurate means of SLN mapping for the lung.

Based on these successful preclinical studies in swine, we and others have assessed the safety and feasibility of NIR imaging using ICG for SLN identification in patients with early-stage non-small cell lung cancer. In a study by Ito et al., whereby ICG was used at high concentrations to visibly see migration with the naked eye, an SLN was identified in only 7 of 38 patients with lung cancer (<20%) as detection was limited to evidence of stained lymph nodes.[18] However, Yamashita et al. demonstrated that when ICG detection utilized intraoperative fluorescent imaging, SLNs were identified in 80.3% of the lung cancer patients studied using 10 mg of ICG.[19] Our current Phase I clinical trial has utilized both an open platform (FLARE) and thoracoscopic (Novadaq SpyScope) NIR system to conduct a dose escalation study to optimize intraoperative mapping of SLN in lung cancer. The current technique consists of intraparenchymal, peritumoral injection in each of four quadrants around the tumor, followed by a short period of ventilation to improve lymphatic flow of ICG (Fig. 168-1). To date, successful SLN identification in 80% of patients undergoing lung resection has been obtained with the injection of only 1 mg ICG in an ICG–albumin mixture. Future goals of this study are to optimize the ICG dose and determine whether the SLN identified using NIR imaging would have been missed during a conventional lymphadenectomy, and if focused analysis of the identified SLN will identify occult metastatic disease in patients currently classified as "node negative" by non-SLN techniques.

CONCLUSION

The best predictor of survival for patients with surgically resectable disease is the presence or absence of metastatic disease in regional lymph nodes. However, even in the setting of complete surgical resection, 30% to 50% of patients with early-stage lung cancer will develop recurrent disease, proving that current approaches are inadequate to accurately stage nodal disease in patients with lung cancer. SLN identification with concomitant focused histologic analysis for micrometastatic disease could identify patients that may benefit from adjuvant therapy and thus improve patient survival. Despite limited success with standard approaches for SLN identification, recent investigations suggest that SLN mapping using NIR imaging may prove to be a safe, rapid, and feasible approach to improve staging in lung cancer patients. Future studies are required to further optimize the ICG dose and technique, and to assess the efficacy and clinical impact of SLN analysis on the use of adjuvant therapy and subsequent patient outcomes.

EDITOR'S COMMENT

The future of SLN mapping in lung cancer is on the horizon and will become feasible for all with future advances in technology. The hope is that through better staging and treatment planning, SLN mapping will improve outcomes for patients with lung cancer.

—Yolonda L. Colson

References

1. Morton DL, Wen DR, Wong JH, et al. Technical details of intraoperative lymphatic mapping for early stage melanoma. *Arch Surg.* 1992;127(4):392–399.
2. Giuliano AE, Kirgan DM, Guenther JM, et al. Lymphatic mapping and sentinel lymphadenectomy for breast cancer. *Ann Surg.* 1994;220(3):391–398; discussion 398–401.
3. Howlader N NA, Krapcho M, Neyman N, et al. SEER Cancer Statistics Review, 1975–2008, National Cancer Institute.
4. Mountain CF. Revisions in the International System for Staging Lung Cancer. *Chest.* 1997;111(6):1710–1717.
5. Kubuschok B, Passlick B, Izbicki JR, et al. Disseminated tumor cells in lymph nodes as a determinant for survival in surgically resected non-small-cell lung cancer. *J Clin Oncol.* 1999;17(1):19–24.
6. Tsang GM, Watson DC. The practice of cardiothoracic surgeons in the perioperative staging of nonsmall cell lung cancer. *Thorax.* 1992;47(1):3–5.
7. Takizawa T, Terashima M, Koike T, et al. Lymph node metastasis in small peripheral adenocarcinoma of the lung. *J Thorac Cardiovasc Surg.* 1998;116(2):276–280.
8. Liptay MJ. Sentinel node mapping in lung cancer. *Ann Surg Oncol.* 2004;11(3 Suppl):271S–274S.
9. Little AG, DeHoyos A, Kirgan DM, et al. Intraoperative lymphatic mapping for non-small cell lung cancer: the sentinel node technique. *J Thorac Cardiovasc Surg.* 1999;117(2):220–224.
10. Liptay MJ, Masters GA, Winchester DJ, et al. Intraoperative radioisotope sentinel lymph node mapping in non-small cell lung cancer. *Ann Thorac Surg.* 2000;70(2):384–389; discussion 389–390.
11. Liptay MJ, D'Amico T A, Nwogu C, et al. Intraoperative sentinel node mapping with technitium-99 in lung cancer: results of CALGB 140203 multicenter phase II trial. *J Thorac Oncol.* 2009;4(2):198–202.
12. Nomori H. Sentinel node mapping in lung cancer: the Japanese experience. *Semin Thorac Cardiovasc Surg.* 2009;21(4):316–322.
13. Schmidt FE, Woltering EA, Webb WR, et al. Sentinel nodal assessment in patients with carcinoma of the lung. *Ann Thorac Surg.* 2002;74(3):870–874; discussion 874–875.
14. Tiffet O, Nicholson AG, Khaddage A, et al. Feasibility of the detection of the sentinel lymph node in peripheral non-small cell lung cancer with radio isotopic and blue dye techniques. *Chest.* 2005;127(2):443–448.
15. Troyan SL, Kianzad V, Gibbs-Strauss SL, et al. The FLARE intraoperative near-infrared fluorescence imaging system: a first-in-human clinical trial in breast cancer sentinel lymph node mapping. *Ann Surg Oncol.* 2009;16(10):2943–2952.
16. Khullar O, Frangioni JV, Grinstaff M, et al. Image-guided sentinel lymph node mapping and nanotechnology-based nodal treatment in lung cancer using invisible near-infrared fluorescent light. *Semin Thorac Cardiovasc Surg.* 2009;21(4):309–315.
17. Soltesz EG, Kim S, Laurence RG, et al. Intraoperative sentinel lymph node mapping of the lung using near-infrared fluorescent quantum dots. *Ann Thorac Surg.* 2005;79(1):269–277. discussion 269–277.
18. Ito N, Fukuta M, Tokushima T, et al. Sentinel node navigation surgery using indocyanine green in patients with lung cancer. *Surg Today.* 2004;34(7):581–585.
19. Yamashita S, Tokuishi K, Miyawaki M, et al. Sentinel node navigation surgery by thoracoscopic fluorescence imaging system and molecular examination in non-small cell lung cancer. *Ann Surg Oncol.* 19(3):728–733.

169 Genomics, Molecular Markers, and Targeted Therapies in Non Small-Cell Lung Cancer

Daniel Morgensztern and Roy S. Herbst

Keywords: Cancer genomics, epidermal growth factor receptor inhibitors, EML4-ALK fusion genes

INTRODUCTION

Lung cancer is the most frequent invasive malignancy and the common cause of cancer death worldwide with an estimated 1.60 million new cases and 1.37 million deaths in 2008.[1] Non small-cell lung cancer (NSCLC), the broad category that accounts for approximately 87% of all patients with lung cancer, usually presents at an advanced stage, where the treatment is essentially palliative. The survival improvement for unselected patients with metastatic NSCLC has been modest, with a large surveillance, epidemiology, and end results (SEER) study, from the periods 1990–1993 to 2002–2005, showing increased survivals at 1 and 2 years of 13.2% to 19.4% and 4.5% to 7.8%, respectively.[2] More recently, however, there has been a significant improvement in the understanding of the biology of lung cancer, with the discovery of new targets and development of several drugs with novel mechanisms of action. This chapter reviews the current knowledge of cancer genomics, the use of molecular markers, and results from clinical trials that are changing the therapeutic landscape of NSCLC.

CANCER GENOMICS

Genomics is defined as the study of the entire set of genetic information of a person, encoded in the structure of deoxyribonucleic acid (DNA). *Cancer genomics* is the study of DNA-associated abnormalities associated with the development of cancer. The DNA in normal cells is constantly damaged by environmental and normal cellular processes. Although the majority of the damage is repaired, a small fraction is converted into fixed mutations. Mutations may be broadly subdivided into germline and somatic. Whereas germline mutations are present in the fertilized egg, inherited from the parents and therefore present in all somatic cells, the somatic mutations are acquired after conception. Although somatic mutations are distributed throughout the genome, a subset of them occurs in key genes. These "driver mutations" are implicated in oncogenesis by allowing the malignant clone to expand more than the normal cells. In contrast, the "passenger mutations" are carried along during clonal expansion, do not contribute to cancer development, and are not associated with growth advantage.[3,4]

The majority of malignancies is sporadic and occurs as a consequence of the accumulation of genomic alterations that lead to dysregulation of protein-encoding genes. As normal cells evolve to a neoplastic state, they acquire several essential complementary capabilities including sustained proliferative signaling, resistance to apoptosis, evasion of growth suppressors, and induction of angiogenesis, invasion, and metastasis.[5] Cancer cells, however, often are physiologically dependent or "addicted to" to the continued activity of specific oncogenes, and this dependency has been explored for drug discovery.[6] The pivotal study of chronic myeloid leukemia that showed excellent response rates (RRs) and good tolerability for imatinib in patients who progressed after interferon therapy, validated the concept of targeting driver mutations and essentially started the era of targeted therapy in cancer treatment.[7]

Recent advances in DNA sequencing have permitted significant advances in cancer genomics. The major breakthrough came with the development of next-generation sequencing, also known as second-generation sequencing, which increased the efficiency for detecting the main types of somatic cancer genome alterations including nucleotide substitutions, small insertions and deletions (indels), copy number gains or losses, chromosomal rearrangements, and microbe infections.[8] Platforms for massive parallel DNA sequence reads, such as the 454 Genome Sequencer FLX, Illumina Genome Analyzer and Applied Biosystems SOLiD, combined with powerful computational methods derived from significant progress in bioinformatics, made possible the sequencing of exome, transcriptosome, and epigenome.[9]

MOLECULAR MARKERS

Molecular markers, also known as biomarkers, are defined as a characteristic that can be objectively measured and evaluated as an indicator of normal biologic processes, pathogenic processes, or pharmacologic responses to a therapeutic intervention.[10] *Prognostic markers* provide information about the natural history of the disease by describing outcomes independently of therapeutic intervention. Their main applications are to evaluate which patients should be treated. This information is particularly useful in the adjuvant setting.[11,12] *Predictive markers* in contrast, provide information on the probability of benefit or toxicity from a specific therapy, and therefore guide the choice of therapy. Since cancer therapy typically benefits only a small fraction of patients, the identification of those most likely to respond to each specific treatment is one of the top priorities in new drug development.

TARGETED THERAPY IN NON–SMALL-CELL LUNG CANCER

NSCLC is broadly subdivided into three main histologies, namely, adenocarcinomas, squamous cell carcinomas, and large cell carcinomas. Traditionally, patients with advanced stage NSCLC, good performance status, and no specific contraindications have been treated as a single entity with platinum-based doublets. With this empirical approach, modern third-generation regimens have shown an RR of 19%, median time to progression (TTP) 3.6 months, median overall survival

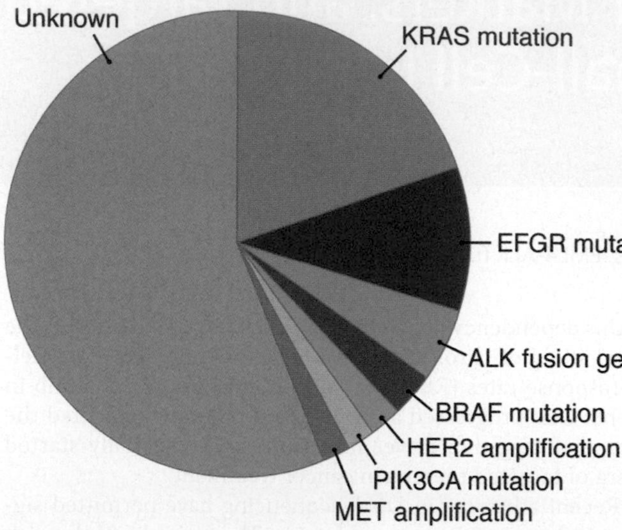

Figure 169-1. Common driver mutations in lung adenocarcinomas with approximate frequency in unselected patients.

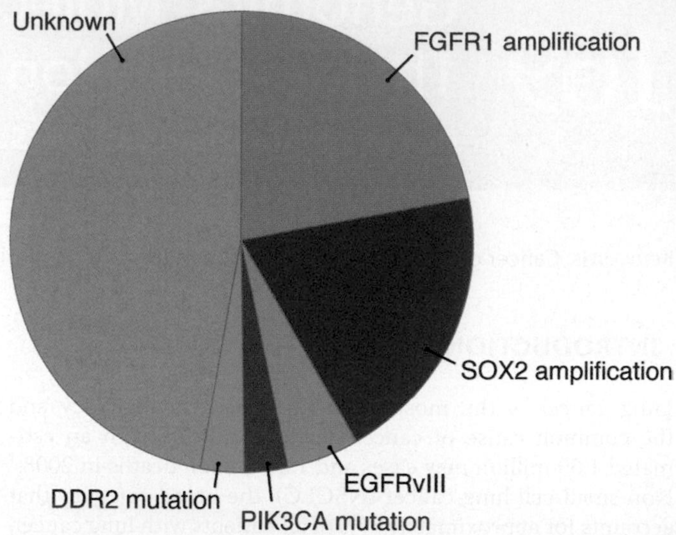

Figure 169-2. Common mutations in squamous cell lung carcinomas with approximate frequency.

(OS) 7.9 months, and 1-year OS of 33%.[13] These regimens are associated with significant toxicity and reached a plateau in efficacy. Therefore, treatment has been chosen based on personal preferences and toxicity profile.

The advances in DNA sequencing made a significant impact on the understanding and treatment of NSCLC through the identification of multiple driver mutations. These driver mutations occur mostly in the genes encoding signaling proteins, particularly the tyrosine receptor kinases (TKIs).[14] It soon became clear that a substantial percentage of lung cancer patients harbor mutant signaling proteins, encoded by "driver mutations," which could be used as targets for drug therapy. Most of the initial mutations were described predominantly or exclusively in patients with adenocarcinoma histology, including those in the epidermal growth factor receptor (*EGFR*), *KRAS, BRAF, PIK3CA*, and other genes, as well as the anaplastic kinase lymphoma (*ALK*) fusion gene (Fig. 169-1). The most common abnormalities in patients with squamous cell carcinomas are amplifications of fibroblast growth factor receptor 1 (*FGFR1*) and *SOX2* and mutations of *DDR2* and *PIK3CA*, with the amplifications each occurring in 20% of cases in an almost mutually exclusive pattern, and the mutations occurring in less than 5% of patients (Fig. 169-2).[15–17]

EPIDERMAL GROWTH FACTOR RECEPTOR INHIBITORS

The EGFR is a transmembrane receptor tyrosine kinase that belongs to a family of four related proteins, also including ERBB2 (HER2), ERBB3 (HER3), and ERBB4 (HER4). Each receptor consists of three domains including extracellular ligand-binding, transmembrane domain, and intracellular. Upon binding to one of the ligands, the inactive EGFR monomers undergo conformal changes that lead to homodimerization or heterodimerization with the other members of the family, most commonly HER2, which lacks a specific ligand, followed by autophosphorylation of tyrosine residues within the cytoplasmic tail, which work as docking sites for several proteins leading to activation of downstream intracellular signaling pathways.[18] EGFR may be targeted by two broad mechanisms, monoclonal antibodies, and small-molecule tyrosine kinase inhibitors (TKIs). The promising results from randomized phase II studies comparing chemotherapy alone or in combination with the anti-EGFR monoclonal antibody cetuximab in previously untreated patients[19] led to the two large randomized phase III trials evaluating the role of cetuximab in this setting. The first study, the FLEX trial,[20] randomized 1125 chemotherapy-naïve patients with EGFR-expressing tumors to cisplatin plus vinorelbine alone or in combination with cetuximab. The cetuximab arm was associated with increased RRs (36% vs. 29%, $p = 0.01$), identical progression-free survival (PFS) of 4.8 months, and a modest improvement in median OS (11.3 vs. 10.1 months, $p = 0.04$). In the BMS099 trial,[21] 676 patients were randomized to carboplatin, a taxane (either paclitaxel or docetaxel) with or without cetuximab. Compared to chemotherapy alone, the cetuximab arm improved the RRs (25.7% vs. 17.2%, $p = 0.007$) but did not lead to a significant improvement in PFS (4.4 vs. 4.2 months, $p = 0.23$) or median OS (9.6 vs. 8.3 months, $p = 0.16$). In the correlative study evaluating *KRAS* mutations, *EGFR* mutations, *EGFR* protein expression, and *EGFR* copy number, there were no predictive markers for response to cetuximab.[22] In contrast to monoclonal antibodies, the discovery of predictive molecular markers for response to EGFR TKIs in NSCLC resulted in a marked improvement in the outcomes from the initial studies in unselected populations to the most recent trials restricted to patients harboring the specific driver mutation.

The initial experience with EGFR TKIs showed good tolerance to gefitinib, with the most common side effects including rash, diarrhea, nausea, and anorexia.[23–26] Among the combined 100 heavily pretreated patients with NSCLC enrolled into the phase I studies, 10 had partial response and an additional 24 achieved stable disease, increasing interest for gefitinib in this setting and leading to the development of phase II studies. The Iressa Drug Evaluation in Advanced Lung Cancer (IDEAL) I and II studies were conducted simultaneously worldwide and in the United States, respectively.[27,28] Both studies enrolled previously treated patients and had two arms consisting of gefitinib at doses of 250 or 500 mg daily. RRs were observed in approximately 10% of Caucasian patients and 18% of Japanese patients with no significant differences according to the treatment doses. The treatment was overall well tolerated, with predicted toxicities similar to the phase I trials. Attempts to increase the RR by combining either gefitinib[29,30] or erlotinib[31] to chemotherapy did not improve outcomes compared to chemotherapy alone. RRs to erlotinib or gefitinib compared to placebo in two randomized clinical trials enrolling previously treated patients with NSCLC were 8.9% and 8%, respectively, reflecting a modest efficacy for EGFR TKIs in unselected populations.[32,33] Nevertheless, subset analyses from multiple studies identified subgroups of patients most likely to respond to EGFR TKIs based on clinical characteristics including good performance status, women, never smokers, adenocarcinoma histology, and Asians.[27,32,33] The first breakthrough toward personalized medicine in patients with NSCLC occurred in 2004, when two independent groups described the association between activating *EGFR* tyrosine kinase mutations and response to EGFR TKIs.[34,35] The majority of *EGFR*-activating mutations are a point deletion in exon 21 with the substitution of arginine for leucine (L858R) and a small in-frame deletion of four amino acids around the LREA motif centered at codons 746 to 750 in exon 19. These mutations were present more commonly in patients with the same previously described clinical characteristics that predicted response to EGFR TKIs, explained the earlier observations, and provided the first genotype-driven therapy in NSCLC. In a pooled analysis of 268 *EGFR*-mutant patients treated with TKIs, 210 patients (78%) responded, compared to 68 out of 659 (10%) patients with wild-type *EGFR*.[36] Several prospective phase II studies evaluated the use of EGFR TKIs in patients with activating mutations, with RRs ranging from 55% to 84%, PFS from 8.9 to 12.9 months, and 1-year survival from 73% to 83%.[37–42] Since the RRs and PFS for TKIs in patients with activating *EGFR* mutations were clearly superior to historical studies using chemotherapy, the next step was to perform a direct comparison in the first-line setting.

Five randomized clinical trials compared TKIs to standard chemotherapy with platinum doublets as the first-line therapy in advanced NSCLC (Table 169-1). The Iressa Pan-Asia Study (IPASS) compared gefitinib to chemotherapy with carboplatin and paclitaxel as first-line therapy in patients with advanced lung adenocarcinoma that were either nonsmokers or former light smokers, the former defined as smoking less than 100 cigarettes in their lifetime and the latter as a total of 10 packs or less having quit at least 15 years prior to enrollment.[43] The study randomized 1217 patients from 87 centers in a 1:1 ratio. *EGFR* mutation was present in 261 (59.7%) of the 437 patients with available data. In the overall population, PFS was longer in those treated with gefitinib compared to chemotherapy (HR 0.74, 95% CI 0.65–0.85; p <0.001). RRs for gefitinib in mutated and wild-type tumors were 71.2% and 1%, respectively, whereas responses to chemotherapy were 47.3% in mutated tumors and 23.5% in wild-type. Gefitinib was associated with a significant improvement in the PFS among patients with *EGFR* mutation (HR 0.48, 95% CI 0.36–0.64; p <0.001) but shorter PFS among those with wild-type tumors (HR 2.85, 95% CI 2.05–3.98; p <0.001). Median OS, however, was not statistically significant, reaching 18.6 and 17.3 months in those treated with gefitinib and chemotherapy, respectively. In the subsequent biomarker analysis study of the IPASS, *EGFR* mutation, as expected, was the strongest predictive biomarker for PFS and tumor response to gefitinib compared to chemotherapy.[44] Maemondo and colleagues[45] randomized 230 *EGFR* mutant patients from 43 institutions in Japan to gefitinib or carboplatin plus paclitaxel. Similar to IPASS, both RR (73.7% vs. 30.7%, p <0.001) and median PFS (10.8 vs. 5.4 months, p <0.001) favored the gefitinib arm. Although the gefitinib arm was numerically superior, neither median survival (30.5 vs. 23.6 months) nor 2-year survival (61.4% vs. 46.7%) reached statistical significance (p = 0.31), perhaps caused by the high crossover rate, where 94.6% of patients progressing on chemotherapy received second-line gefitinib with a RR of 58.5%. The West Japan Oncology Group (WJTOG) 3405[46] randomized 172 *EGFR* mutant patients to gefitinib or chemotherapy with cisplatin and docetaxel. Both RRs (62.1% vs. 32.2%, p <0.001) and median PFS (9.2 vs. 6.3 months, p <0.001) were significantly better in the gefitinib arm. The OPTIMAL trial[47] was the first randomized study comparing erlotinib to chemotherapy in the first-line setting. In this study, 165 *EGFR* mutant patients from 22 centers in China, were randomized to erlotinib or carboplatin plus gemcitabine. Similar to the gefitinib trials, the RR (83% vs. 36%, p <0.001) and median PFS (13.1 vs. 4.6 months, p <0.001) were significantly higher in the targeted therapy arm. The EURTAC trial,[48] conducted in a Caucasian population, randomized 153 patients to erlotinib or platinum-based chemotherapy. The preliminary results, reported in an abstract

Table 169-1

RANDOMIZED CLINICAL TRIALS COMPARING TYROSINE KINASE INHIBITORS AND CHEMOTHERAPY AS FIRST-LINE THERAPY

STUDY	ARMS	PATIENTS	RESPONSE RATE (%)	MEDIAN PFS	MEDIAN OS
IPASS	Gefitinib	261[a]	71.2	9.5 m	18.6 m
	Carbo-Pac		47.3	6.3 m	17.3 m
Maemondo	Gefitinib	230	73.7	10.8 m	30.5 m
	Carbo-Pac		30.7	5.4 m	23.6 m
WJTOG 3405	Gefitinib	172	62.1	9.2 m	30.9 m
	Cisp-Doc		32.2	6.3 m	Not reached
OPTIMAL	Erlotinib	165	83	13.1 m	NR
	Carbo-Gem		36	4.6 m	NR
EURTAC	Erlotinib	153	54.5	9.4 m	22.9 m
	Chemotherapy		10.5	5.2 m	18.8 m

Carbo, Carboplatin; Pac, Paclitaxel; Cisp, Cisplatin; Doc, Docetaxel; NR, Not reported.
[a]*EGFR* mutant subset.

presented at the American Society of Clinical Oncology meeting, showed a significant improvement in RR (54.5% vs. 10.5%, $p < 0.001$) and PFS (9.4 vs. 5.2 months, $p < 0.001$), whereas the median OS improvement did not reach statistical significance (22.9 vs. 18.8 months, $p = 0.42$). Taken collectively, these five randomized clinical trials showed a consistent improvement in RRs and PFS for TKIs in patients with activating *EGFR* mutations. Although numerically superior, the increased median OS in the targeted therapy arms was not statistically significant, most likely caused by the crossover occurring in patients progressing on chemotherapy. As the result of these randomized clinical trials, the American Society of Clinical Oncology recommended that patients with NSCLC should have their tumors tested for *EGFR* mutation to determine whether the first-line chemotherapy should be an EGFR TKI or chemotherapy.

EML4-ALK FUSION GENES

The EML4-ALK fusion oncogene results from the fusion of the N-terminal portion of the protein encoded by the echinoderm microtubule-associated protein-like 4 (*EML4*) gene with the intracellular signaling portion of the ALK receptor tyrosine kinase on the short arm of chromosome 2.[49] ALK-positive patients are usually younger than the wild-type counterparts, never or light smokers, and have histology characterized by more than 10% signet ring cells.[50] Kwak and colleagues[51] evaluated the role of the ALK inhibitor crizotinib in 82 patients with advanced NSCLC and ALK rearrangement by fluorescence in situ hybridization (FISH), which was defined as positive if more than 15% of scored tumors had split *ALK*5' and 3' probe signals or isolated 3' signals. Among the enrolled patients, 62 (76%) were never smokers and only 5 (5%) were chemotherapy-naïve. The treatment was well tolerated with mild nausea and diarrhea as the most common toxicities. RRs were observed in 47 (53%) patients, whereas 27 (33%) had stable disease, and 6 (7%) had progressive disease. The estimated probability of PFS at 6 months was 72% with median PFS not reached. Based on these results, crizotinib received accelerated FDA approval for patients with advanced NSCLC and *ALK*-positive tumors. The PROFILE 1014 (NCT01154140) is a phase III trial comparing crizotinib to platinum plus pemetrexed as first-line therapy in patients with translocation or inversion involving the *ALK* gene locus.

OTHER MUTATIONS

Unlike *EGFR* mutations and *ALK* gene rearrangements, *KRAS* mutations are more commonly observed in smokers. The presence of *KRAS* mutations has been associated with primary resistance to EGFR TKIs. However, RRs to gefitinib or erlotinib are uncommon in patients without activating *EGFR* mutations, regardless of *KRAS* mutation status. Since the mutations are mutually exclusive, the lack of responses may be mostly because of the absence of *EGFR* mutants in comparison to unselected populations from earlier studies. Furthermore, the effects of *KRAS* mutations in the PFS or OS remain undetermined. Therefore, it remains unclear whether the KRAS mutation status should be used to select patients for treatment with EGFR TKIs.[52] There are currently no specific drugs for KRAS mutations. BRAF mutations are present in approximately 3% to 4% of patients with lung adenocarcinoma, occurring mostly in current or former smokers.[53,54] The V600E mutations account for approximately half of BRAF mutations in NSCLC and may potentially be targeted by vemurafenib (PLX4032), a drug that has been recently approved by the FDA for patients with B600E BRAF mutated melanomas because of the significant RRs in this population compared to the control arm of dacarbazine.[55] *MET* amplifications occur more commonly in patients developing secondary resistance to EGFR TKIs, although it may also be present in a small percentage of previously untreated NSCLC patients.[56] *PIK3CA* and *FGFR1* mutations occur more commonly in patients with squamous cell carcinomas and there are several specific inhibitors currently being developed for each of them. *DDR2* mutations, also more common in squamous cell carcinomas, were found to confer sensitivity to dasatinib and nilotinib in preclinical studies.[57]

In summary, advances in DNA sequencing have permitted significant improvements in the understanding of cancer genomics, with the discovery of new driver mutations that have been used as therapeutic targets for drug development. In NSCLC, the use of EGFR TKIs resulted in significant RRs and survival among patients with *EGFR*-activating mutations, with improved PFS compared to standard chemotherapy in this population. Similarly, remarkable results were observed in the initial studies with crizotinib, which is currently being compared to chemotherapy in patients with ALK rearrangement. It has become clear that NSCLC represents a very heterogenic disease with multiple molecularly defined subsets. Although the development of therapies tailored according to the cancer genome of each patient has showed promising results only in the small fraction of patients studied thus far, it has already changed the therapeutic paradigms in several malignancies and has the potential for significant improvements in outcomes for a larger population of NSCLC patients in the near future through the conduct of new trials based on predictive molecular markers, which are becoming an integral part of treatment decisions.

EDITOR'S COMMENT

The recent advances in cancer genomics have revolutionized the approach to treatment of NSCLC patients, with thoracic surgeons playing important roles in both surgical resection of the primary tumor or biopsy of advanced disease to provide sufficient tumor for sequencing.

—Yolonda L. Colson

References

1. Jemal A, Bray F, Center MM, et al. Global cancer statistics. *CA Cancer J Clin.* 2011;61:69–90.
2. Morgensztern D, Waqar S, Subramanian J, et al. Improving survival for stage IV non-small cell lung cancer: a surveillance, epidemiology, and end results survey from 1990 to 2005. *J Thorac Oncol.* 2009;4:1524–1529.
3. Stratton MR, Campbell PJ, Futreal PA. The cancer genome. *Nature.* 2009;458:719–724.
4. Stratton MR. Exploring the genomes of cancer cells: progress and promise. *Science.* 2011;331:1553–1558.
5. Hanahan D, Weinberg RA. Hallmarks of cancer: the next generation. *Cell.* 2011;144:646–674.

6. Weinstein IB. Addiction to oncogenes – the Achilles heel of cancer. *Science.* 2002;297:63–64.
7. Druker BJ, Talpaz M, Resta DJ, et al. Efficacy and safety of a specific inhibitor of the BCR-ABL tyrosine kinase in chronic myeloid leukemia. *N Engl J Med.* 2001;344:1031–1037.
8. Meyerson M, Gabriel S, Getz G. Advances in understanding cancer genomes through second-generation sequencing. *Nat Rev Genet.* 2010;11:685–696.
9. Wong KM, Hudson TJ, McPherson JD. Unraveling the genetics of cancer: genome sequencing and beyond. *Annu Rev Genomics Hum Genet.* 2011;12:407–430.
10. Biomarkers Definitions Working Group. Biomarkers and surrogate endpoints: preferred definitions and conceptual framework. *Clin Pharmacol Ther.* 2001;69:89–95.
11. Dancey JE, Dobbin KK, Groshen S, et al. Guidelines for the development and incorporation of biomarker studies in early clinical trials of novel agents. *Clin Cancer Res.* 2010;16:1745–1755.
12. Sawyers CL. The cancer biomarker problem. *Nature.* 2008;452:548–552.
13. Schiller JH, Harrington D, Belani CP, et al. Comparison of 4 chemotherapy regimens for advanced non-small-cell lung cancer. *N Engl J Med.* 2002;**346**:92–98.
14. Pao W, Iafrate AJ, Su Z. Genetically informed lung cancer medicine. *J Pathol.* 2011;223:230–240.
15. Ohashi K, Pao W. A new target for therapy in squamous cell carcinoma of the lung. *Cancer Discov.* 2011;1:23–24.
16. Weiss J, Sos ML, Seidel D, et al. Frequent and focal FGFR1 amplification associates with therapeutically tractable FGFR1 dependency in squamous cell lung cancer. *Sci Transl Med.* 2010;2:62–93.
17. Turner NC, Seckl MJ. A therapeutic target for smoking-associated lung cancer. *Sci Transl Med.* 2010;2:62ps56.
18. Hynes NE, Lane HA. ERBB receptors and cancer: the complexity of targeted inhibitors. *Nat Rev Cancer.* 2005;5:341–354.
19. Butts CA, Bodkin D, Middelman EL, et al. A randomized phase II study of gemcitabine/platinum with or without cetuximab as first-line therapy for patients with advanced/metastatic non–small-cell lung cancer (NSCLC). *J Clin Oncol.* 2007;25:5777–5784.
20. Pirker R, Pereira JR, Szczesna A, et al. Cetuximab plus chemotherapy in patient with advanced non-small-cell lung cancer (FLEX): an open-label randomized phase III trial. *Lancet.* 2009;373:1525–1531.
21. Lynch TJ, Patel T, Dresibach L, et al. Cetuximab and first-line taxane/carboplatin chemotherapy in advanced non-small-cell lung cancer: results of the randomized multicenter phase III trial BMS099. *J Clin Oncol.* 2010;28:911–917.
22. Khamb ata-Ford S, Harbison CT, Lowell L, et al. K-Ras mutation status, EGFR mutation status and increased EGFR gene copy number do not predict for cetuximab benefit in BMS099, a phase III study of cetuximab and first-line taxane/carboplatin in advanced non-small cell lung cancer. *J Clin Oncol.* 2010;28:918–927.
23. Ranson M, Hammond LA, Ferry D, et al. ZD1839, a selective oral epidermal growth factor receptor-tyrosine kinase inhibitor, is well tolerated and active in patients with solid, malignant tumors: results of a phase I trial. *J Clin Oncol.* 2002;**20**:2240–2250.
24. Herbst RS, Maddox AM, Rothenberg ML, et al. Selective oral epidermal growth factor receptor tyrosine kinase inhibitor ZD1839 is generally well-tolerated and has activity in non-small-cell lung cancer and other solid tumors: results of a phase I trial. *J Clin Oncol.* 2002;20:3815–3825.
25. Baselga J, Rischin D, Ranson M, et al. Phase I safety, pharmacokinetic, and pharmacodynamic trial of ZD1839, a selective oral epidermal growth factor receptor tyrosine kinase inhibitor, in patients with five selected solid tumor types. *J Clin Oncol.* 2002;**20**:4292–4302.
26. Nakagawa K, Tamura T, Negoro S, et al. Phase I pharmacokinetic trial of the selective oral epidermal growth factor receptor tyrosine kinase inhibitor gefitinib ('Iressa', ZD1839) in Japanese patients with solid malignant tumors. *Ann Oncol.* 2003;**14**:922–930.
27. Fukuoka M, Yano S, Giaccone G, et al. Multi-institutional randomized phase II trial of gefitinib for previously treated patients with advanced non-small-cell lung cancer (The IDEAL 1 Trial). *J Clin Oncol.* 2003;21: 2237–2246.
28. Kris MG, Natale RB, Herbst RS, et al. Efficacy of gefitinib, an inhibitor of the epidermal growth factor receptor tyrosine kinase, in symptomatic patients with nonsmall cell lung cancer: a randomized trial. *JAMA.* 2003;**290**:2149–2158.
29. Herbst RS, Giaccone G, Schiller JH, et al. Gefitinib in combination with paclitaxel and carboplatin in advanced non-small-cell lung cancer: a Phase III trial —INTACT 2. *J Clin Oncol.* 2004;**22:**785–794.
30. Giaccone G, Herbst RS, Manegold C, et al. Gefitinib in combination with gemcitabine and cisplatin in advanced non-small-cell lung cancer: a Phase III trial — INTACT *1. J Clin Oncol.* 2004;**22**:777–784.
31. Herbst RS, Prager D, Hermann R, et al. TRIBUTE: a Phase III trial of erlotinib hydrochloride (OSI-774) combined with carboplatin and paclitaxel chemotherapy in advanced non-small-cell lung *cancer. J Clin Oncol.* 2005;**23:**5892–5899.
32. Thatcher N, Chang A, Parikh P, et al. Gefitinib plus best supportive care in previously treated patients with refractory advanced non-small-cell lung cancer: results from a randomised, placebo-controlled, multicentre study (Iressa Survival Evaluation in Lung Cancer). *Lancet.* 2005;**366**:1527–1537.
33. Shepherd FA, Rodrigues Pereira J, Ciuleanu T, et al. National Cancer Institute of Canada Clinical Trials Group. Erlotinib in previously treated non-small-cell lung cancer. *N Engl J Med. 2005;353:*123–132.
34. Lynch TJ, Bell DW, Sordella R, et al. Activating mutations in the epidermal growth factor receptor underlying responsiveness of non small-cell lung cancer to gefitinib. *N Engl J Med. 2004;350:*2129–2139.
35. Paez JG, Janne PA, Lee JC, et al. EGFR mutations in lung cancer: correlation with clinical response to gefitinib therapy. *Science.* 2005;304:1497–1500.
36. Sequist LV, Bell DW, Lynch TJ, et al. Molecular predictors of response to epidermal growth factor receptor antagonists in non-small cell lung cancer. *J Clin Oncol.* 2007;25:587–595.
37. Asahina H, Yamazaki K, Kinoshita I, et al. A phase II trial of gefitinib as first-line therapy for advanced nonsmall cell lung cancer with epidermal growth factor receptor mutations. *Br J Cancer. 2006;95:*998–1004.
38. Sunaga N, Tomizawa Y, Yanagitani N, et al. Phase II prospective study of the efficacy of gefitinib for the treatment of stage III/IV non-small cell lung cancer with EGFR mutations, irrespective of previous chemotherapy. *Lung Cancer.* 2007;56:383–389.
39. Inoue A, Suzuki T, Fukuhara T, et al. Prospective phase II study of gefitinib for chemotherapy-naive patients with advanced non-small-cell lung cancer with epidermal growth factor receptor gene mutations. *J Clin Oncol.* 2006;24:3340–3346.
40. Sutani A, Nagai Y, Udagawa K, et al. Gefitinib for non-small-cell lung cancer patients with epidermal growth factor receptor gene mutations screened by peptide nucleic acid-locked nucleic acid PCR clamp. *Br J Cancer.* 2006;95:1483–1489.
41. Tamura K, Okamoto I, Kashii T, et al. West Japan Thoracic Oncology Group. Multicentre prospective phase II trial of gefitinib for advanced non-small cell lung cancer with epidermal growth factor receptor mutations: results of the West Japan Thoracic Oncology Group trial (WJTOG0403). *Br J Cancer.* 2008;98:907–914.
42. Sequist LV, Martins RG, Spigel D, et al. First-line gefitinib in patients with advanced non-small-cell lung cancer harboring somatic EGFR mutations. *J Clin Oncol.* 2008;26:2442–2449.
43. Mok TS, Wu YL, Thongprasert S, et al. Gefitinib or carboplatin-paclitaxel in pulmonary adenocarcinoma. *N Engl J Med.* 2009;362:947–957.
44. Fukuoka M, Wu YL, Thongprasert S, et al. Biomarker analyses and final overall survival results from a phase III, randomized, open-label, first-line study of gefitinib versus carboplatin/paclitaxel in clinically selected patients with advanced non-small-cell lung cancer in Asia (IPASS). *J Clin Oncol.* 2011;29:2866–2874.
45. Maemondo M, Inoue A, Kobayashi K, et al. Gefitinib or chemotherapy for non-small-cell lung cancer with mutated EGFR. *N Engl J Med.* 2010;362:2380–2386.
46. Mitsudomi T, Morita S, Yatabe Y, et al. Gefitinib *versus* cisplatin plus docetaxel in patients with non-small-cell lung cancer harbouring mutations of the epidermal growth factor receptor (WJTOG3405): an open label, randomised phase 3 trial. *Lancet Oncol.* 2010;11:121–128.
47. Zhou C, Wu YL, Chen G, et al. Erlotinib versus chemotherapy as first-line treatment for patients with advanced EGFR mutation-positive non-small-cell lung cancer (OPTIMAL, CTONG-0802): a multicentre, open-label, randomised, phase 3 study. *Lancet Oncol.* 2011;12:735–742.
48. Rosell R, Gervais R, Vergnenegre A, et al. Erlotinib versus chemotherapy (CT) in advanced non-small cell lung cancer (NSCLC) patients (p) with epidermal growth factor receptor (EGFR) mutations: interim results of the European Erlotinib Versus Chemotherapy (EURTAC) phase III randomized trial. *J Clin Oncol.* 2011;29:Abstract 7503.

49. Soda M, Choi YL, Enomoto M, et al. Identification of the transforming *EML4–ALK* fusion gene in non-small-cell lung cancer. *Nature.* 2007;448:561–566.
50. Shaw AT, Yeap BY, Mino-Kenudson M, et al. Clinical features and outcome of patients with non-small-cell lung cancer who harbor *EML4–ALK*. *J Clin Oncol.* 2009;27:947–957.
51. Kwak EL, Bang Y-J, Camidge R, et al. Anaplastic lymphoma kinase inhibition in non-small-cell lung cancer. *N Engl J Med.* 2010;363: 1693–1703.
52. Roberts PJ, Stinchcombe TE, Der CJ, et al. Personalized medicine in non-small-cell lung cancer: is KRAS a useful marker in selecting patients for epidermal growth factor receptor-targeted therapy? *J Clin Oncol.* 2010;28:4769–4788.
53. Paik PK, Arcila ME, Fara M, et al. Clinical characteristics of patients with lung adenocarcinomas harboring *BRAF* mutations. *J Clin Oncol.* 2011;29:2046–2051.
54. Marchetti A, Felicioni L, Malatesta A, et al. Clinical features and outcome of patients with non-small-cell lung cancer harboring *BRAF* mutations. *J Clin Oncol.* 2011;29:3574–3579.
55. Chapman PB, Hauschild A, Robert C, et al. Improved survival with vemurafenib in melanoma with BRAF V600E mutation. *N Engl J Med.* 2011;363:2507–2516.
56. Pao W, Girard N. New driver mutations in non-small-cell lung cancer. *Lancet Oncol.* 2011;12:175–180.
57. Hammerman PS, Sos ML, Ramos AH, et al. Mutations in the *DDR2* kinase gene identify a novel therapeutic target in squamous cell lung cancer. *Cancer Discov.* 2011;1:OF76–OF87.

170 Genomics, Molecular Markers, and Targeted Therapies in Esophageal Cancer

Jules Lin and Andrew C. Chang

Keywords: Esophageal neoplasms, gastric cardia, gastric neoplasms, genetics, review

INTRODUCTION

Esophageal carcinomas remain a leading cause of cancer-related death worldwide, and the prognosis remains poor with 5-year overall survival of only 17%.[1] In the mid-1990s, esophageal adenocarcinoma (EAC) overtook squamous cell carcinoma (ESCC) as the most common esophageal cancer in the United States.[2,3] Risk factors include smoking, obesity, and Barrett metaplasia secondary to gastroesophageal reflux, whereas infection with *Helicobacter pylori* appears to be protective.[4]

The development of EAC is a multistep process involving numerous genetic changes. According to Hanahan and Weinberg, tumorigenesis involves six hallmark characteristics including self-sufficient growth, insensitivity to antigrowth signals, evasion of apoptosis, sustained angiogenesis, a limitless replicative potential, and tissue invasion and metastasis.[5] The genetic changes involved in the metaplasia–dysplasia–adenocarcinoma sequence of EAC will be presented in this review. Whether further characterization of the molecular events leading to EAC will provide new targets for diagnosis, prevention, or treatment remains to be established.

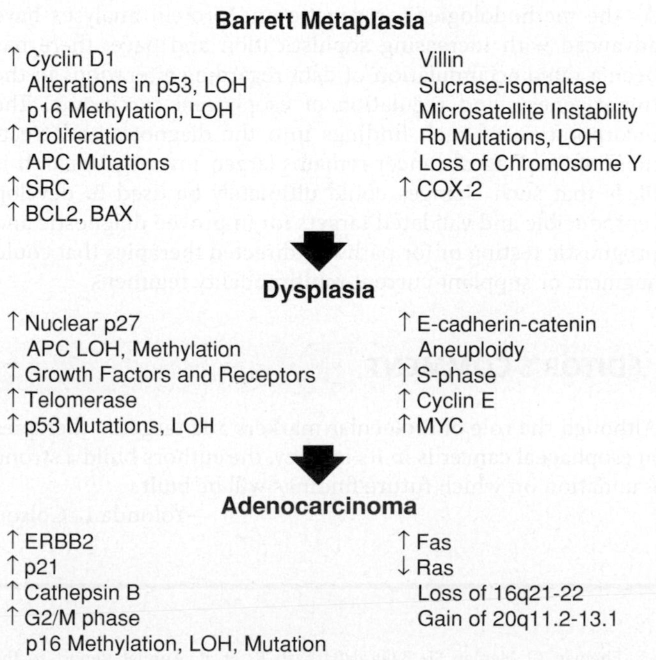

Figure 170-1. Genetic changes involved in the progression from Barrett metaplasia to esophageal adenocarcinoma. Many of the early changes persist as the lesions progress to dysplasia and adenocarcinoma. With permission from Lin J, Beer DG. Molecular biology of upper gastrointestinal malignancies. *Semin Oncol.* 2004;31(6):476–486.

MOLECULAR EVENTS AND THE PROGRESSION TO ESOPHAGEAL CARCINOMA

During the progression from dysplastic Barrett esophagus to EAC a number of molecular events have been identified (Fig. 170-1),[6] including altered expression of tumor suppressor genes such as *p53* and *p16*, cyclin-dependent kinase inhibitor 2 A (CDKN2 A), and involvement of oncogenes including *myc*, *EGFR*, *HER2/neu*, and *c-Met*.[7–10] Cell cycle markers including polyploidy and aneuploidy also have been identified early in the dysplasia–adenocarcinoma sequence.[11–13]

With the development of high-throughput microarray technologies and concomitant analytic methodologies,[14] investigators have sought to identify genes,[15,16] proteins, or important regulatory elements such as microRNAs[17] or protein kinases[18] among which patterns of expression either might distinguish between esophageal dysplasia and carcinoma, or might identify tumors with more likelihood to respond to specific treatment regimens. At the chromosomal level, alterations of gene copy number, such as by gene amplification or deletion, are being characterized in ever-increasing number and detail.[19] Such copy-number alterations may be associated with EAC progression and advancing stage.[20] Investigators also have catalogued copy-neutral changes, particularly loss of heterozygosity, associated with EAC, using single nuclear polymorphism (SNP) microarrays.[21–23] Genome sequencing techniques likely will provide further detailed characterization of gene rearrangements that are important in the pathophysiology of esophageal cancers, as has been demonstrated in a number of solid-tumor malignancies.[24]

As more studies are published that identify associations between genetic changes and the progression to EAC, it is readily apparent that there is wide variability among such alterations between one individual and another. Such variability may limit the diagnostic and prognostic utility for any one putative marker to only a small percentage of tumors. It also appears that there can be considerable genetic heterogeneity even within a tumor, reflecting the evolutionary nature of neoplastic progression. Measurement of such clonal diversity appears to be a strong predictor of the progression from Barrett esophagus to EAC, independent of the actual genetic events, such as loss of heterozygosity, frameshift or deletion mutations, or abnormal changes in promoter methylation status, that comprise this heterogeneity.[25,26]

BIOMARKER STUDIES

Clinical trials evaluating the efficacy of preoperative chemotherapy with concurrent radiation therapy consistently have demonstrated pathologic complete response (ypT0N0 Mx) of approximately 20% to 30% among patients who undergo subsequent esophageal resection.[27–30] Pathologic complete response has been associated as a significant determinant for long-term disease-free and overall survival.[31] Conversely for patients who have either partial or no tumor response to preoperative chemoradiation, there does not appear to be a survival benefit but rather an overall detriment. Thus identification of predictive markers for response to preoperative therapy potentially can direct nonresponders to alternative treatment regimens while limiting the toxicity of first-line chemoradiation strategies and subsequent esophageal resection.

Molecular markers may be developed for a number of clinical applications, and can be categorized broadly as diagnostic, prognostic, and predictive.[32] For patients with esophageal carcinomas, most putative biomarkers remain unproven for broad application in terms of analytic validity (accuracy and reliability of the measured analyte), clinical validity (accuracy and reliability of detecting or predicting a clinically defined disorder) and clinical utility (i.e., providing added value for patient management decision making).[33] Several small cohort studies have identified possible markers for response to preoperative chemotherapy with or without radiation therapy, although large-scale validation studies remain to be completed. [34] Such markers include genes associated with chemotherapy metabolism such as thymidylate synthase (TYMS), thymidine phosphorylase (TP), dihydropyrimidine dehydrogenase (DPD), and methylenetetrahydrofolate reductase (MTHFR), all of which participate in the metabolism of 5-fluorouracil,[35,36] or glutathione S-transferase π (GSTP) and the excision cross-complementing gene 1 (ERCC1), both of which have been associated with response to platinum-based chemotherapy.[37,38]

TARGETED THERAPY

Molecular analysis has identified a number of potential mechanisms and genes of interest, for which targeted therapy may be feasible. Amplification of one such therapeutic target, *ERBB2*, appears to be a frequent event in EAC,[8,10] and such amplification also has been associated with worse overall prognosis.[39] The *HER2* gene encodes a receptor tyrosine kinase transmembrane receptor, $p185^{HER2}$, that is targeted by the humanized anti-$p185^{HER2}$monoclonal antibody, trastuzumab (Herceptin, Genentech, South San Francisco, CA).

Although a panoply of genetic changes in genes such as *cyclin D1, p16INK4 A, p27KIP1, p53, EGFR,* and *c-ErbB2 (HER2/neu)* have been associated with the development of esophageal carcinoma, measurement of altered expression in such genes of interest or their protein products does not appear to provide any prognostic advantage over standard measures such as tumor stage or regional lymph node involvement.[40] Such potential markers still can be utilized in directing targeted therapy as such pharmacologic agents become available, as demonstrated by an ongoing cooperative group study of patients diagnosed with *HER2/neu*-overexpressing esophageal carcinomas. For this phase III study, patients with documented *HER2/neu* overexpression will receive the receptor tyrosine kinase inhibitor, trastuzumab (Genentech, San Francisco, CA) in addition to preoperative chemotherapy (cisplatin, 25 mg/m^2 and paclitaxel, 50 mg/m^2 weekly for 6 weeks) with thoracic radiation (50.4 Gy), followed by esophageal resection. In the phase I/II study preceding this phase III trial, 14 of 19 patients (74%) had either 3+ HER2 expression by immunohistochemistry, or an increase in *HER2* gene copy number (*HER2* gene amplification or high polysomy) by fluorescence in situ hybridization. Enrolled patients had T3N0 or T3N1 (AJCC, 6th edition) esophageal cancers. Of the fourteen patients with HER2 overexpression, eight were found to have a complete clinical response, defined as no evidence of tumor at posttreatment esophagoscopy with biopsies. Of the five patients who had HER2 expression less than 3+ by immunohistochemistry and no evidence of gene copy number increase, one patient was found to have a complete clinical response. The median survival of all patients was 24 months and the 2-year survival was 50%.[41]

Among patients with unresectable gastric cancer, including subjects with esophagogastric junction (cardia) carcinomas, whose tumors had overexpression of *HER2/neu*, an open label, randomized phase III trial demonstrated that the addition of trastuzumab to standard regimens of cisplatin and 5-fluorouracil or capecitabine improved overall survival without any observed difference in the number of grade 3 or 4 adverse events.[42]

SUMMARY

Esophageal cancer, particularly EAC, is a heterogeneous solid organ malignancy that is diagnosed at more advanced stages in more than 60% of patients and as such remains highly lethal.[1] As the methodologies for genetic and protein analyses have advanced with increasing sophistication and pace, there has been a rapid accumulation of data regarding alterations in the tumorigenesis and regulation of esophageal carcinoma. The incorporation of such findings into the diagnosis and treatment of esophageal cancer remains largely investigational. It is likely that such changes could ultimately be used to develop reproducible and validated targets for improved diagnostic and prognostic testing or for pathway-directed therapies that could augment or supplant current multimodality regimens.

EDITOR'S COMMENT

Although the role of molecular markers and targeted therapies in esophageal cancer is in its infancy, the authors build a strong foundation on which future findings will be built.

—Yolonda L. Colson

References

1. Siegel R, Naishadham D, Jemal A. Cancer statistics, 2012. *CA A Cancer J Clin.* 2012;62:10–29.
2. Pohl H, Welch HG. The role of overdiagnosis and reclassification in the marked increase of esophageal adenocarcinoma incidence. *J Natl Cancer Inst.* 2005;97:142–146.
3. Eheman C, Henley SJ, Ballard-Barbash R, et al. Annual Report to the Nation on the status of cancer, 1975–2008, featuring cancers associated with excess weight and lack of sufficient physical activity. *Cancer.* 2012;118:2338–2366.
4. Holmes RS, Vaughan TL. Epidemiology and pathogenesis of esophageal cancer. *Semin Radiat Oncol.* 2007;17:2–9.

5. Hanahan D, Weinberg RA. Hallmarks of cancer: the next generation. *Cell.* 2011;144:646–674.
6. Lin J, Beer DG. Molecular biology of upper gastrointestinal malignancies. *Semin Oncol.* 2004;31:476–486.
7. Miller CT, Lin L, Casper AM, et al. Genomic amplification of MET with boundaries within fragile site FRA7G and upregulation of MET pathways in esophageal adenocarcinoma. *Oncogene.* 2006;25:409–418.
8. Miller CT, Moy JR, Lin L, et al. Gene amplification in esophageal adenocarcinomas and Barrett's with high-grade dysplasia. *Clin Cancer Res.* 2003;9:4819–4825.
9. Chiang PW, Beer DG, Wei WL, et al. Detection of erbB-2 amplifications in tumors and sera from esophageal carcinoma patients. *Clin Cancer Res.* 1999;5:1381–1386.
10. al-Kasspooles M, Moore JH, Orringer MB, et al. Amplification and overexpression of the EGFR and erbB-2 genes in human esophageal adenocarcinomas. *Int J Cancer.* 1993;54:213–219.
11. Chao DL, Sanchez CA, Galipeau PC, et al. Cell proliferation, cell cycle abnormalities, and cancer outcome in patients with Barrett's esophagus: a long-term prospective study. *Clin Cancer Res.* 2008;14:6988–6995.
12. Lin L, Wang Z, Prescott MS, et al. Multiple forms of genetic instability within a 2-Mb chromosomal segment of 3q26.3-q27 are associated with development of esophageal adenocarcinoma. *Genes Chromosomes Cancer.* 2006;45:319–331.
13. Reid BJ, Levine DS, Longton G, et al. Predictors of progression to cancer in Barrett's esophagus: baseline histology and flow cytometry identify low- and high-risk patient subsets. *Am J Gastroenterol.* 2000;95:1669–1676.
14. Eisen MB, Spellman PT, Brown PO, et al. Cluster analysis and display of genome-wide expression patterns. *Proc Natl Acad Sci USA.* 1998;95:14863–14868.
15. Selaru FM, Zou T, Xu Y, et al. Global gene expression profiling in Barrett's esophagus and esophageal cancer: a comparative analysis using cDNA microarrays. *Oncogene.* 2002;21:475–478.
16. Kimchi ET, Posner MC, Park JO, et al. Progression of Barrett's metaplasia to adenocarcinoma is associated with the suppression of the transcriptional programs of epidermal differentiation. *Cancer Res.* 2005;65:3146–3154.
17. Hu Y, Correa AM, Hoque A, et al. Prognostic significance of differentially expressed miRNAs in esophageal cancer. *Int J Cancer.* 2010;128(1):132–143.
18. Lin L, Bass AJ, Lockwood WW, et al. Activation of GATA binding protein 6 (GATA6) sustains oncogenic lineage-survival in esophageal adenocarcinoma. *Proc Natl Acad Sci USA.* 2012;109:4251–4256.
19. Beroukhim R, Mermel CH, Porter D, et al. The landscape of somatic copy-number alteration across human cancers. *Nature.* 2010;463:899–905.
20. Paulson TG, Maley CC, Li X, et al. Chromosomal instability and copy number alterations in Barrett's esophagus and esophageal adenocarcinoma. *Clin Cancer Res.* 2009;15:3305–3314.
21. Nancarrow DJ, Handoko HY, Smithers BM, et al. Genome-wide copy number analysis in esophageal adenocarcinoma using high-density single-nucleotide polymorphism arrays. *Cancer Res.* 2008;68:4163–4172.
22. Wiech T, Nikolopoulos E, Weis R, et al. Genome-wide analysis of genetic alterations in Barrett's adenocarcinoma using single nucleotide polymorphism arrays. *Lab Invest.* 2009;89:385–397.
23. Gu J, Ajani JA, Hawk ET, et al. Genome-wide catalogue of chromosomal aberrations in barrett's esophagus and esophageal adenocarcinoma: a high-density single nucleotide polymorphism array analysis. *Cancer Prev Res (Phila).* 2010;3:1176–1186.
24. Maher CA, Kumar-Sinha C, Cao X, et al. Transcriptome sequencing to detect gene fusions in cancer. *Nature.* 2009;458:97–101.
25. Maley CC, Galipeau PC, Finley JC, et al. Genetic clonal diversity predicts progression to esophageal adenocarcinoma. *Nat Genet.* 2006;38:468–473.
26. Merlo LM, Shah NA, Li X, et al. A comprehensive survey of clonal diversity measures in Barrett's esophagus as biomarkers of progression to esophageal adenocarcinoma. *Cancer Prev Res (Phila).* 2010;3:1388–1397.
27. Walsh TN, Noonan N, Hollywood D, et al. A comparison of multimodal therapy and surgery for esophageal adenocarcinoma. *N Engl J Med.* 1996; 335:462–467.
28. Urba SG, Orringer MB, Turrisi A, et al. Randomized trial of preoperative chemoradiation versus surgery alone in patients with locoregional esophageal carcinoma. *J Clin Oncol.* 2001;19:305–313.
29. Vallbohmer D, Holscher AH, DeMeester S, et al. A multicenter study of survival after neoadjuvant radiotherapy/chemotherapy and esophagectomy for ypT0N0M0R0 esophageal cancer. *Ann Surg.* 2010;252:744–749.
30. van Hagen P, Hulshof MCCM, van Lanschot JJB, et al. Preoperative chemoradiotherapy for esophageal or junctional cancer. *N Engl J Med.* 2012;366:2074–2084.
31. Chirieac LR, Swisher SG, Ajani JA, et al. Posttherapy pathologic stage predicts survival in patients with esophageal carcinoma receiving preoperative chemoradiation. *Cancer.* 2005;103:1347–1355.
32. Febbo PG, Ladanyi M, Aldape KD, et al. NCCN Task Force Report: evaluating the clinical utility of tumor markers in oncology. *J Natl Compr Canc Netw.* 2011;9:S1–S32.
33. Teutsch SM, Bradley LA, Palomaki GE, et al. The Evaluation of Genomic Applications in Practice and Prevention (EGAPP) Initiative: methods of the EGAPP Working Group. *Genet Med.* 2009;11:3–14.
34. Maher SG, Gillham CM, Duggan SP, et al. Gene expression analysis of diagnostic biopsies predicts pathological response to neoadjuvant chemoradiotherapy of esophageal cancer. *Ann Surg.* 2009;250:729–737.
35. Langer R, Specht K, Becker K, et al. Association of pretherapeutic expression of chemotherapy-related genes with response to neoadjuvant chemotherapy in Barrett carcinoma. *Clin Cancer Res.* 2005;11:7462–7469.
36. Langer R, Specht K, Becker K, et al. Comparison of pretherapeutic and posttherapeutic expression levels of chemotherapy-associated genes in adenocarcinomas of the esophagus treated by 5-fluorouracil– and cisplatin-based neoadjuvant chemotherapy. *Am J Clin Pathol.* 2007;128:191–197.
37. Moore-Joshi M-B, Shirota Y, Danenberg KD, et al. High gene expression of *TS1*, *GSTP1*, and *ERCC1* are risk factors for survival in patients treated with trimodality therapy for esophageal cancer. *Clin Cancer Res.* 2005;11:2215–2221.
38. Schneider S, Uchida K, Brabender J, et al. Downregulation of TS, DPD, ERCC1, GST-Pi, EGFR, and HER2 gene expression after neoadjuvant three-modality treatment in patients with esophageal cancer. *J Am Coll Surg.* 2005;200:336–344.
39. Brien TP, Odze RD, Sheehan CE, et al. HER-2/neu gene amplification by FISH predicts poor survival in Barrett's esophagus-associated adenocarcinoma. *Hum Pathol.* 2000;31:35–39.
40. Langer R, Von Rahden BHA, Nahrig J, et al. Prognostic significance of expression patterns of c-erbB-2, p53, p16INK4 A, p27KIP1, cyclin D1 and epidermal growth factor receptor in oesophageal adenocarcinoma: a tissue microarray study. *J Clin Pathol.* 2006;59:631–634.
41. Safran H, DiPetrillo T, Akerman P, et al. Phase I/II study of trastuzumab, paclitaxel, cisplatin and radiation for locally advanced, HER2 overexpressing, esophageal adenocarcinoma. *Int J Radiat Oncol Biol Phys.* 2007;67:405–409.
42. Bang YJ, Van Cutsem E, Feyereislova A, et al. Trastuzumab in combination with chemotherapy versus chemotherapy alone for treatment of HER2-positive advanced gastric or gastro-oesophageal junction cancer (ToGA): a phase 3, open-label, randomised controlled trial. *Lancet.* 2010;376:687–697.

171 Nanoparticle Therapy in Lung Cancer

Kimberly A. Zubris, Mark W. Grinstaff, and Yolonda L. Colson

Keywords: Drug delivery, nanometer scale, pharmacokinetics

INTRODUCTION

Nanoparticles (NPs) are colloidal particles ranging in size from approximately 10 to 1000 nm in diameter and can be synthesized from a variety of materials (e.g., lipids, polymers, metals, and ceramics). Due to their unique properties, NPs have found increasing applications in medicine from drug delivery to imaging.

In the drug delivery arena, NPs are able to address many of the difficulties encountered during the administration of therapeutic compounds. The encapsulation of drugs within NPs can increase the solubility of insoluble drugs, improve pharmacokinetics through sustained release, alter biodistribution, protect sensitive drugs from low pH environments or enzymatic alteration, and, in some cases, provide targeting of the drug to the desired tissues.[1] Modern drug discovery and developmental technologies have yielded a wide array of small molecule and biologic drugs for the treatment of many diseases; however the requirements for these compounds to be successfully commercialized and translated into the clinic are challenging.

CANCER TREATMENT WITH NANOPARTICLES

Oncology is one field of medicine where NP-mediated drug delivery systems can potentially have a significant impact since issues with solubility and pharmacokinetics have limited the clinical application of many new, potentially effective anticancer drug candidates. There are several classes of promising NP drug delivery systems, including drug nanocrystals, liposomes, micelles, dendrimers, and polymeric NPs (Fig. 171-1).[2] Drug nanocrystals are simply pure drugs that have been processed down to nanometer sizes.[3] The extremely small particle size increases the surface area of the drug, thereby increasing solubility. In contrast, liposomes are spherical lipid bilayers measuring a few nanometers in diameter.[4] When used as a drug delivery vehicle, insoluble drugs can be transported within the hydrophobic environment of the lipid bilayer, whereas soluble drugs are contained within the internal aqueous compartment inside the liposome, thereby altering the pharmacokinetics and biodistribution of the native drug. Like liposomes, micelles are also composed of phospholipids. In aqueous solution, a micelle is formed by spontaneous self-assembly resulting in the exposure of the hydrophilic head regions to the surrounding solvent and aggregation of the hydrophobic tails at the micelle center. The core of the micelle can thereby contain small hydrophobic molecules such as therapeutic drugs, while remaining stable in aqueous solution. Dendrimers are highly branched molecules that can be used to deliver drugs via two different methods. Drugs can either be attached to the outer functional groups of the dendrimer branches, or encapsulated within the dendrimers to form a drug-dendrimer supermolecular assembly. Finally, polymeric NPs, which encapsulate drug within various polymers, tend to be more stable than liposomes and can increase the effective solubility of hydrophobic drugs. In addition, unlike liposomes, several polymeric systems appear to allow programmable, or at least controlled, drug release through the manipulation of the structure and composition of the polymer used to prepare the particles.[1,5,6]

NANOPARTICLES FOR THE TREATMENT OF LUNG CANCER

Despite the potential survival advantage seen with adjuvant chemotherapy in patients with later stage lung cancer, the overall benefits of systemic treatment in lung cancer patients with early stage disease are often outweighed by the incidence of common systemic side effects. Two of the most common drugs used in

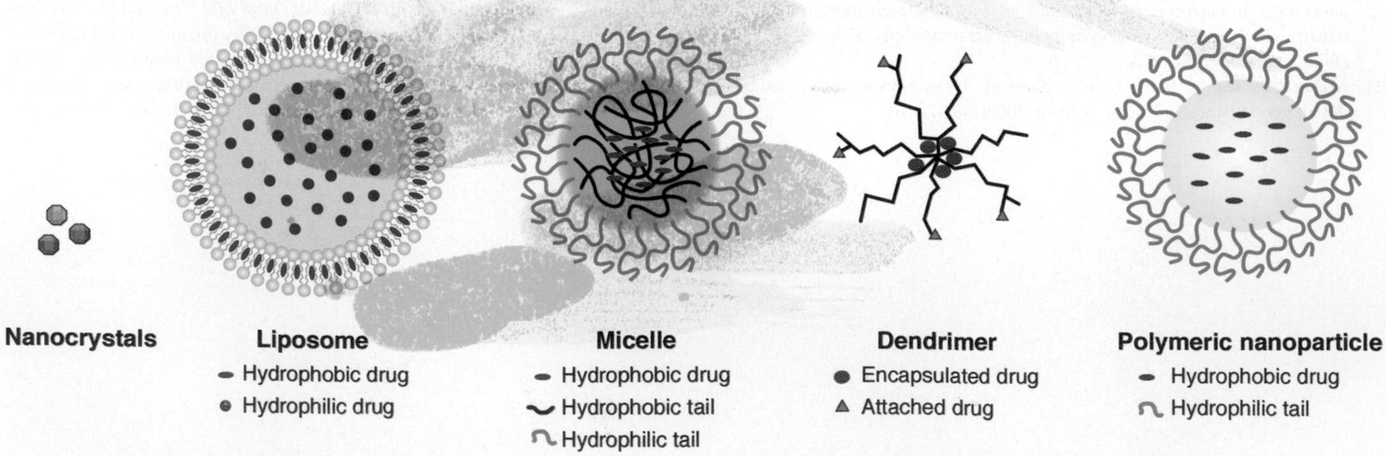

Figure 171-1. Schematic diagram of different types of nanoparticles used for drug delivery.

lung cancer treatment are paclitaxel and docetaxel, which are both extremely hydrophobic and are difficult to deliver due to poor solubility. In its current clinical formulation, paclitaxel is delivered in a Cremophor EL (polyethoxylated castor oil) and ethanol mixture, which is thought to be responsible for many of the toxic side effects associated with paclitaxel treatment. Furthermore, drug distribution within the lung parenchyma is suboptimal since systemically administered chemotherapeutics may be rapidly excreted, leaving only a small percentage of the total dose locally available to prevent growth of recurrent lung tumors. For example, when paclitaxel is given as a single intravenous (IV) bolus dose, maximum drug levels are reached within 0.5 hours and only 0.5% of the total dose is delivered to the lung tissue.[9] In contrast, drug-loaded NPs can potentially be targeted to the lungs or specific tissues following IV injection, oral delivery, or inhalation.[10] Therefore, in an effort to improve tissue delivery, decrease side effects, and prevent drug resistance secondary to enhanced cellular efflux, several NP formulations have been proposed for use in the treatment of patients with non–small-cell lung cancer (NSCLC). The current chapter will discuss several promising experimental approaches, including micelles, liposomes, covalently modified paclitaxel conjugates, and polymeric NPs.

Micelles

Zhang et al.[11] have described ~20 nm paclitaxel-loaded Pluronic P123/F127 mixed micelles (PF-PTX), prepared by thin-film hydration. PF-PTX were developed to both deliver drug and to overcome multidrug resistance by inducing apoptosis through loss of mitochondrial membrane potential and subsequent ATP depletion. PF-PTX micelles contain paclitaxel within the hydrophobic core of the particle and demonstrate a nearly 70% decrease in tumor volume compared with standard paclitaxel in a human A549 lung tumor xenograft model in mice.[11]

Liposomes

Liposomes provide a hydrophobic environment within the lipid bilayer and a hydrophilic internal compartment to allow delivery of different payloads. Paclitaxel liposomes have been evaluated in a Phase I study to treat patients with malignant pleural effusions secondary to NSCLC. However, the most successful application of liposomal delivery relevant to lung cancer has been with anthracycline chemotherapeutic agents. As opposed to the hydrophobic taxanes, use of anthracyclines such as doxorubicin is not limited by solubility issues, but rather by cardiac toxicity which occurs with cumulative exposure of these agents to healthy tissues. Therefore liposomes are an appropriate candidate for anthracycline delivery since agents like doxorubicin can be readily loaded into the hydrophilic core of the liposome. The most common formulations include liposomal doxorubicin and polyethylene glycol (PEG)-ylated liposomal doxorubicin (PLD).

Liposomal doxorubicin and PLD delivery systems consist of a liposomal bilayer surrounding an aqueous core containing the drug doxorubicin HCl, with and without a PEG coating, respectively (Fig. 171-2). The hydrophilic PEG coating, serves to decrease systemic clearance of the liposome by the reticuloendothelial system, thereby delivering more drug to the desired tissues. Although efficacy did not differ significantly between liposomal and conventional formulations of doxorubicin in clinical trials of breast cancer patients, liposomal or PLD did significantly reduce the number of patients developing cardiac toxicity. Liposomal doxorubicin has also shown efficacy in

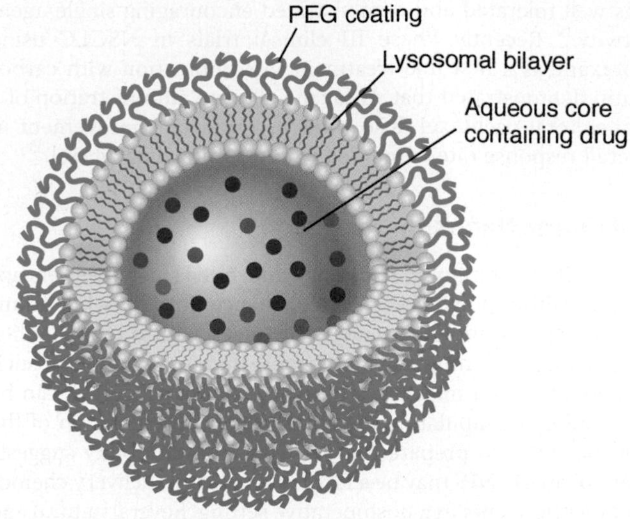

Figure 171-2. Schematic diagram of PEG-ylated liposomal doxorubicin. Doxorubicin HCl is encapsulated within the aqueous core.

patients with locally advanced or metastatic NSCLC that failed platinum-based first-line chemotherapy.[16,17] The use of doxorubicin loaded liposomes is therefore a key example of how nanocarriers can improve delivery of effective chemotherapeutic agents by simply minimizing their toxicity on healthy tissues.

Besides enabling the improved delivery of established chemotherapeutics such as paclitaxel, doxorubicin, and camptothecin (CPT), NP drug delivery is also being explored for use in delivering newly developed drugs that are limited by solubility. For example, Agashe et al.[18] recently reported a novel curcuminoid, CLEFMA, as a potent antiproliferation agent that induces autophagic cell death in lung cancer cells. CLEFMA is a highly hydrophobic compound, and therefore a drug-in-cyclodextrin-in-liposome formulation was developed. This formulation demonstrated more potent antiproliferative activity in vitro in lung adenocarcinoma H441 cells than naturally occurring curcumin, while having no effect on the proliferation of healthy lung fibroblasts. Additionally, tumor volume in nude rats bearing xenograft H441 tumors was significantly reduced following treatment with CLEFMA liposomes as compared to liposome-only controls.[18]

Nanoparticle Bound Conjugates

As an alternative to physical encapsulation of paclitaxel within a particle, the drug may also be formulated with a protein for protein-stabilized NP delivery. The most successful example of this approach is NP albumin bound (*nab*)-paclitaxel, also known as Abraxane®. This is the most recent NP drug delivery system to be approved for clinical use by the FDA. Abraxane is a protein-stabilized paclitaxel suspension created by subjecting paclitaxel to high-pressure homogenization in the presence of human serum albumin, resulting in a colloidal suspension of paclitaxel NPs. This formulation provides the ability to administer paclitaxel without the use of Cremophor EL, allowing quicker administration and higher maximum tolerated doses while reducing adverse events. Preclinical studies with Abraxane have shown improved tumor penetration, higher plasma clearance, and a larger volume of distribution compared to conventional paclitaxel. In addition, results from NSCLC Phase I/II trials with weekly IV Abraxane therapy have indicated that *nab*-paclitaxel was well tolerated and demonstrated encouraging single-agent activity.[19] Recently Phase III clinical trials in NSCLC using Abraxane as a first-line treatment in combination with carboplatin demonstrated that Abraxane allowed administration of a higher total paclitaxel dose with a significant improvement in overall response rate compared to conventional paclitaxel.[20]

Polymeric Nanospheres

Due to its hydrophobic nature, paclitaxel has also been encapsulated within polymeric NPs to enhance delivery while minimizing complications secondary to issues with drug solubility. Polymeric NPs tend to be more stable than other carriers, such as liposomes and micelles, and their delivery properties can be adjusted by manipulating the structure and composition of the polymer used to prepare the particles. This flexibility suggests that polymeric NPs may be a favorable means to delivery chemotherapeutic agents in a postoperative setting. Several natural and synthetic polymers have been investigated for the preparation of polymeric NPs, including chitosan, methacrylic acid copolymers, and polycaprolactone, but poly(lactic acid) (PLA) and poly(lactic-co-glycolic acid) (PLGA) are the most widely studied due to availability, biocompatibility, and FDA-approved status.

PLGA systems are simple to synthesize, can be functionalized for tumor targeting, and have been explored for the delivery of many agents, including anticancer drugs. Despite promising in vivo results in small animal models and the appeal of PLGA as a biocompatible FDA-approved polymer, PLGA NPs have at least one significant limitation—particles afford rapid "burst" release of the encapsulated drug (>50% release in 10–48 hours) regardless of NP location. Drug release before NPs reach the tumor may therefore reduce the benefit of using a localized drug delivery system.[24] Furthermore, a recent study suggests that PLGA NPs are not readily taken up by cells and thus deliver their payload by extracellular drug release and/or direct drug transfer to contacting cells.[24]

To improve the relatively low tumor-targeting efficiency of bare PLGA NPs, several studies have focused on modifying the surface of these NPs. For example, surfaces of paclitaxel-loaded PLGA NPs surface modified with covalently bound wheat germ agglutinin (WGA) were found to have superior antiproliferation activity against A549 human NSCLC cells in vitro compared with conventional formulations of paclitaxel. The increased efficacy was attributed to a more efficient intracellular accumulation of paclitaxel via WGA-receptor mediated uptake. A single intratumoral injection of these NPs was also shown to inhibit growth of A549 tumor nodules in mice over a period of 25 days and tumor volume shrank to baseline within 2 days.[25] Similarly, other investigators have utilized chitosan modification to enhance lung specificity or tumor targeting.

Another chemotherapeutic agent commonly used in the treatment of lung cancer is CPT, a natural plant alkaloid, which has shown a broad spectrum of antitumor activity against a range of solid tumors. The effective delivery of CPT to tumor targets presents a challenge however, due to the drug's insolubility in water, structural instability, and high toxicity to healthy tissue cells. Because of these toxic side effects, CPT needs to be administered frequently in limited doses to achieve the desired drug efficacy. NPs have therefore been explored as a means to provide sustained release of controlled amounts of CPT over a prolonged period. One example of a CPT-loaded polymer formulation is 100 to 300 nm particles synthesized from highly hydrophobic, biodegradable poly(ω-pentadecalactone-co-butylene-co-succinate) (PPBS) copolyesters.[26] In vivo studies using a 7-day established subcutaneous LLC tumor model demonstrated that PPBS NPs loaded with 12% to 22% CPT showed increased cellular uptake, higher cytotoxicity against murine Lewis lung carcinoma cells in vitro and better antitumor efficacy in vivo.[26]

A new area of investigation is the use of NP drug delivery for the prevention of lung cancer recurrence. Local recurrence of lung cancer following lobectomy for Stage I patients occurs in 7% to 9% of patients.[27] However, many patients with lung cancer have poor pulmonary function due to age and/or the effects of smoking, therefore surgical removal of a significant amount of lung tissue is not a clinically viable option for these patients. Consequently, these patients often undergo a more limited wedge resection with the trade-off being higher locoregional tumor recurrence. The recurrence rate for such patients is nearly three times higher than in patients undergoing lobectomy.[27] Therefore, a drug delivery system capable of preventing recurrence at the tumor–tissue interface would potentially extend the benefit of surgical therapy with improved clinical outcomes to patients previously deemed unacceptable candidates for lobectomy.

Recently, pH-responsive paclitaxel-loaded NPs, prepared using methacrylate-based polymers, have been developed for local application at the surgical resection margin to reduce the rate of cancer recurrence.[28] These NPs are designed to focus chemotherapy delivery within tumor cells through a unique mechanism. Upon endocytosis by the tumor cell, exposure of the NP to the acidic pH of the endosome results in cleavage of a pH-responsive "protecting group" which triggers NP expansion and subsequent intracellular drug release (Fig. 171-3). These paclitaxel-loaded expansile nanoparticles (Pax-eNP) have been shown to prevent the initial in vivo tumor growth of Lewis lung carcinoma in mice, whereas more conventional paclitaxel-loaded nonexpansile NPs, empty expansile NPs, or even a 10-fold higher dose of paclitaxel alone did not.[28] Subsequent studies with a more robust and clinically relevant model of tumor recurrence after surgical resection, have shown that local delivery of Pax-eNP immediately after

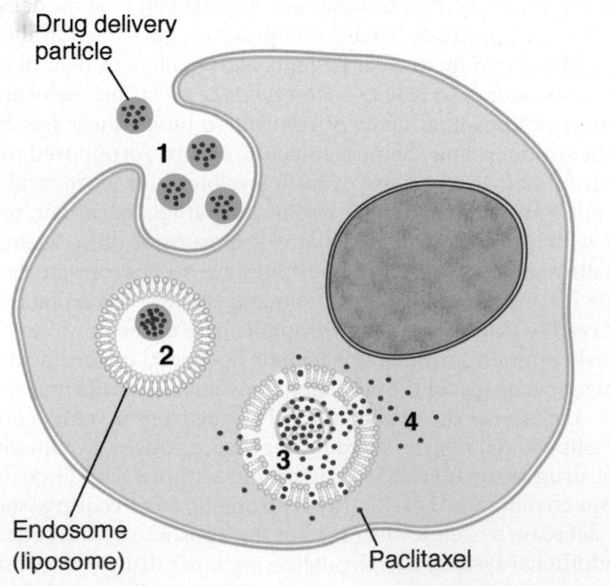

Figure 171-3. Diagram of intracellular paclitaxel delivery via expansile nanoparticles. Pax-eNP enter the cell via endocytosis (1) whereby the nanoparticle becomes entrapped within the endosome (2). The acidic environment of the endosome (pH 5–6) results in expansion of eNP with subsequent release of the encapsulated chemotherapeutic agent, paclitaxel (3).

resection of established tumors prevented local recurrence.[29] In these studies, subcutaneous Lewis lung carcinoma implants were excised when tumor volume reached 300 mm, and animals were treated with a 300 μg dose of either IV paclitaxel or as a local injection of pax-eNP. A single dose of pax-eNP placed within the tumor bed at the time of surgical resection delayed tumor recurrence and modestly prolonged survival compared to the current clinical formulation of the paclitaxel in Cremophor EL/ethanol.[29]

CONCLUSIONS

Due to their unique properties, NPs have the potential for application in a wide range of fields, and are being increasingly used as a means of drug delivery. Specifically, NPs are being developed to address many of the difficulties encountered when administering therapeutic compounds. Their use for anticancer drug delivery is especially of interest as NPs can improve delivery of the chemotherapeutic agents to cancer cells while minimizing toxicity to healthy tissues.

Current research on NP therapy in cancer encompasses a variety of approaches differing in NP material composition, method of delivery, type of therapeutic drug delivered, and the specific disease target. Many of the NP formulations being studied today show improved efficacy over conventional treatments or equivalent efficacy with reduced incidence of side effects. However, continued development of NP systems for the delivery of chemotherapeutics will provide ways of maximizing the benefits derived from current and future therapeutic compounds, with the ultimate goal of advancing adjuvant cancer therapy, decreasing tumor recurrence and improving the lives of lung cancer patients.

EDITOR'S COMMENT

New improved methods of delivering effective drugs to the site of the tumor are critical to future advances in lung cancer care. This chapter reviews the promise of a wide variety of NP drug delivery systems.

—Yolonda L. Colson

References

1. Sahoo SK, Labhasetwar V. Nanotech approaches to drug delivery and imaging. *Drug Discov Today*. 2003;8(24):1112–1120.
2. Ganta S, Devalapally H, Shahiwala A, et al. A review of stimuli-responsive nanocarriers for drug and gene delivery. *J Control Release*. 2008;126(3):187–204.
3. Date AA, Patravale VB. Current strategies for engineering drug nanoparticles. *Curr Opin Colloid Interface Sci*. 2004;9(3–4):222–235.
4. Barratt GM. Therapeutic applications of colloidal drug carriers. *Pharm Sci Technolo Today*. 2000;3(5):163–171.
5. Mitra S, Gaur U, Ghosh PC, et al. Tumour targeted delivery of encapsulated dextran-doxorubicin conjugate using chitosan nanoparticles as carrier. *J Control Release*. 2001;74(1–3):317–323.
6. Shah LK, Amiji MM. Intracellular delivery of saquinavir in biodegradable polymeric nanoparticles for HIV/AIDS. *Pharm Res*. 2006;23(11):2638–2645.
7. Arriagada R, Bergman B, Dunant A, et al. Cisplatin-based adjuvant chemotherapy in patients with completely resected non-small-cell lung cancer. *N Eng J Med*. 2004;350(4):351–360.
8. Strauss GM, Herndon JE, Maddaus MA, et al. Adjuvant paclitaxel plus carboplatin compared with observation in stage IB non-small-cell lung cancer: CALGB 9633 with the Cancer and Leukemia Group B, Radiation Therapy Oncology Group, and North Central Cancer Treatment Group Study Groups. *J Clin Oncol*. 2008;26(31):5043–5051.
9. Sparreboom A, Van Tellingen O, Nooijen WJ, et al. Tissue distribution, metabolism and excretion of paclitaxel in mice. *Anticancer Drugs*. 1996;7(1):78–86.
10. Azarmi S, Roa WH, Löbenberg R. Targeted delivery of nanoparticles for the treatment of lung diseases. *Adv Drug Deliv Rev*. 2008;60(8):863–875.
11. Zhang W, Shi Y, Chen Y, et al. Enhanced antitumor efficacy by paclitaxel-loaded Pluronic P123/F127 mixed micelles against non-small cell lung cancer based on passive tumor targeting and modulation of drug resistance. *Eur J Pharm Biopharm*. 2010;75(3):341–353.
12. Wang X, Zhou J, Wang Y, et al. A phase I clinical and pharmacokinetic study of paclitaxel liposome infused in non-small cell lung cancer patients with malignant pleural effusions. *Eur J Cancer*. 2010;46(8):1474–1480.
13. Zhao P, Wang H, Yu M, et al. Paclitaxel-loaded, folic-acid-targeted and TAT-peptide-conjugated polymeric liposomes: in vitro and in vivo evaluation. *Pharm Res*. 2010;27(9):1914–1926.
14. Liu KK, Zheng WW, Wang CC, et al. Covalent linkage of nanodiamond-paclitaxel for drug delivery and cancer therapy. *Nanotechnology*. 2010;21(31):315106.
15. Yang R, Yang SG, Shim WS, et al. Lung-specific delivery of paclitaxel by chitosan-modified PLGA nanoparticles via transient formation of microaggregates. *J Pharm Sci*. 2009;98(3):970–984.
16. Numico G, Castiglione F, Granetto C, et al. Single-agent pegylated liposomal doxorubicin (Caelix®) in chemotherapy pretreated non-small cell lung cancer patients: a pilot trial. *Lung Cancer*. 2002;35(1):59–64.
17. Koukourakis MI, Koukouraki S, Giatromanolaki A, et al. Liposomal doxorubicin and conventionally fractionated radiotherapy in the treatment of locally advanced non–small-cell lung cancer and head and neck cancer. *J Clin Oncol*. 1999;17(11):3512–3521.
18. Agashe H, Sahoo K, Lagisetty P, et al. Cyclodextrin-mediated entrapment of curcuminoid 4-[3,5-bis(2-chlorobenzylidene-4-oxo-piperidine-1-yl)-4-oxo-2-butenoic acid] or CLEFMA in liposomes for treatment of xenograft lung tumor in rats. *Colloids Surf B Biointerfaces*. 2011;84(2):329–337.
19. Rizvi NA, Riely GJ, Azzoli CG, et al. Phase I/II trial of weekly intravenous 130-nm albumin-bound paclitaxel as initial chemotherapy in patients with stage iv non-small-cell lung cancer. *J Clin Oncol*. 2008;26(4):639–643.
20. Socinski MA, Bondarenko IN, Karaseva NA, et al. Results of a randomized, phase III trial of nab-paclitaxel (nab-P) and carboplatin (C) compared with cremophor-based paclitaxel (P) and carboplatin as first-line therapy in advanced non-small cell lung cancer (NSCLC) (Abstract LBA7511). *J Clin Oncol*. 2010;28(20 Suppl):2055–2062.
21. Feng Z, Zhao G, Yu L, et al. Preclinical efficacy studies of a novel nanoparticle-based formulation of paclitaxel that out-performs Abraxane. *Cancer Chemother Pharmacol*. 2010;65(5):923–930.
22. Chung Y-I, Kim JC, Kim YH, et al. The effect of surface functionalization of PLGA nanoparticles by heparin- or chitosan-conjugated Pluronic on tumor targeting. *J Control Release*. 2010;143(3):374–382.
23. Chakravarthi SS, Robinson DH. Enhanced cellular association of paclitaxel delivered in chitosan-PLGA particles. *Int J Pharm*. 2011;409(1–2): 111–120.
24. Xu P, Gullotti E, Tong L, et al. Intracellular drug delivery by poly (lactic-co-glycolic acid) nanoparticles, revisited. *Mol Pharm*. 2008;6(1):190–201.
25. Mo Y, Lim L-Y. Paclitaxel-loaded PLGA nanoparticles: potentiation of anticancer activity by surface conjugation with wheat germ agglutinin. *J Control Release*. 2005;108(2–3):244–262.
26. Liu J, Jiang Z, Zhang S, et al. Poly([omega]-pentadecalactone-co-butylene-co-succinate) nanoparticles as biodegradable carriers for camptothecin delivery. *Biomaterials*. 2009;30(29):5707–5719.
27. Landreneau RJ, Sugarbaker DJ, Mack MJ, et al. Wedge resection versus lobectomy for stage I (T1 N0 M0) non-small-cell lung cancer. *J Thorac Cardiovasc Surg*. 1997;*113*(4):691–698; discussion 698–700.
28. Griset AP, Walpole J, Liu R, et al. Expansile nanoparticles: synthesis, characterization, and in vivo efficacy of an acid-responsive polymeric drug delivery system. *J Am Chem Soc*. 2009;131(7):2469–2471.
29. Liu R, Khullar OV, Griset AP, et al. Paclitaxel-loaded expansile nanoparticles delay local recurrence in a heterotopic murine non-small cell lung cancer model. *Ann Thorac Surg*. 2011;91:1077–1084.

172 Ex Vivo Lung Perfusion

Marcelo Cypel and Shaf Keshavjee

Keywords: Lung transplantation, lung donor shortage, Toronto technique for ex vivo lung perfusion

INTRODUCTION

Lung transplantation is a life-saving therapy for patients suffering from end-stage lung diseases. The number of patients waiting for lung transplantation, however, greatly exceeds the number of donor lungs available. Moreover, only about 15% of lungs from multiorgan donors are deemed usable for transplantation.[1] Most potential lungs are considered unsuitable as the result of injury that occurs with brain death and ICU-related complications (i.e., barotrauma or lung edema associated with fluid resuscitation). Since primary graft dysfunction leads to severe early and long-term consequences for lung transplant recipients, transplant teams tend to be very conservative in their selection of donor lungs. As a result, fewer organs are selected and the wait list mortality may climb as high as 30% to 40%.[2,3] While the current cornerstone of clinical lung preservation is to limit the metabolic rate of the donor lung by hypothermia, this strategy best serves lungs meeting ideal acceptance criteria. The current donor organ shortage has prompted most donor programs to use increasing numbers of extended criteria organs, where lung function is not as assured as with an ideal lung. The ex vivo phase of organ preservation, prior transplantation into the recipient, provides a window of opportunity for further evaluation and even resuscitation of these compromised lungs. To take advantage of this opportunity, however, it is necessary to preserve the donor organs under normothermic or near-normothermic conditions. One strategy, termed ex vivo lung perfusion (EVLP), attempts to simulate in vivo conditions through ventilation and perfusion of the donor lung graft. One important advantage of normothermic perfusion is that it maintains the active metabolic functions of the lung, providing an opportunity for continued assessment of the organ during the ex vivo phase of organ preservation, active treatments, and restoration of normal function. This chapter focuses on the resurgence of EVLP, important technical aspects, clinical outcomes, and future perspectives.

Normothermic EVLP—Historical Perspectives

Originally proposed in 1938 by Carrel for organs in general and then in 1970 by Jirsch et al. for the evaluation and preservation of lungs in cases of distant procurement, attempts at EVLP in those eras failed because of an inability to maintain the air/fluid barrier integrity within the lung, which led to the development of edema and increased pulmonary vascular resistance in the donor lung.[4,5] For most of the past century, EVLP systems were used in small animal studies of lung physiology. More recently, normothermic perfusion became a research focus as a preservation alternative in experimental models of lung, liver, and kidney transplantation.[6–11]

Experimental Work

The resurgence of EVLP as a potential tool in lung transplantation started with the work of Steen et al.[12] This group described EVLP as a method to reassess lungs after uncontrolled donation from cardiac death donors (DCD),[13] since these organs cannot *be evaluated* in vivo. A lung perfusion specific solution (Steen® solution) with optimal osmolarity and high dextran content was developed by this group.[12,14] After Steen's publications, other groups demonstrated the feasibility of blood-based short-term EVLP (30–90 minutes) to evaluate lung function in animal models of donation after cardiac death and experimentally using injured human lungs deemed unsuitable for transplantation.[15–21] However, even in this most current era of EVLP, attempts to perfuse ex vivo lungs for greater than 2 hours have largely failed, as extended perfusion times lead to the development of pulmonary edema and an increase in the pulmonary vascular resistance meaning that the system, itself, inflicts some degree of injury.[22]

With the vision that ex vivo treatment and repair of injured organs would, in general, require an ex vivo period lasting longer than 2 hours, we developed a protective EVLP system and strategy with the goal of maintaining lungs in the EVLP system for at least 12 hours without causing additional injury to the lungs (currently known as the Toronto technique of EVLP, see details below). Several important modifications were made to achieve 12 hours of perfusion stability. These included (1) an *acellular* perfusate, (2) a closed circuit with protective low perfusion pressure (pulmonary artery pressure [PAP] 10–13 mm Hg) and stable positive left atrial (LA) pressure (5 mm Hg), and (3) a protective mode of mechanical ventilation (tidal volume of 7 mL/kg, rate of 7 breaths per minute [bpm], with a positive end-expiratory airway pressure [PEEP] of 5 cmH_2O). In our early work with normal pig lungs, lung function was stable during 12 hours of normothermic EVLP.[23] This stability during prolonged EVLP translated into excellent posttransplant lung function, absence of edema formation, and preserved lung histology after transplantation. The acellular perfusion assessment of lung function accurately correlated with posttransplant graft function, and the addition of red blood cells did not provide additional functional information compared to acellular perfusate alone.[23] This study provided the proof of concept that EVLP is able to maintain *normal* donor lungs for a prolonged period of time without damaging the organ. Further examination was then performed to determine the impact of prolonged EVLP using *injured* ischemic donor lungs.[24] Pig donor lungs were cold preserved for 12 hours and subsequently divided into two groups: cold static preservation (CSP) or normothermic EVLP for a further 12 hours (total 24 hours of preservation). EVLP preservation resulted in significantly better lung oxygenation and lower edema formation rates after transplantation

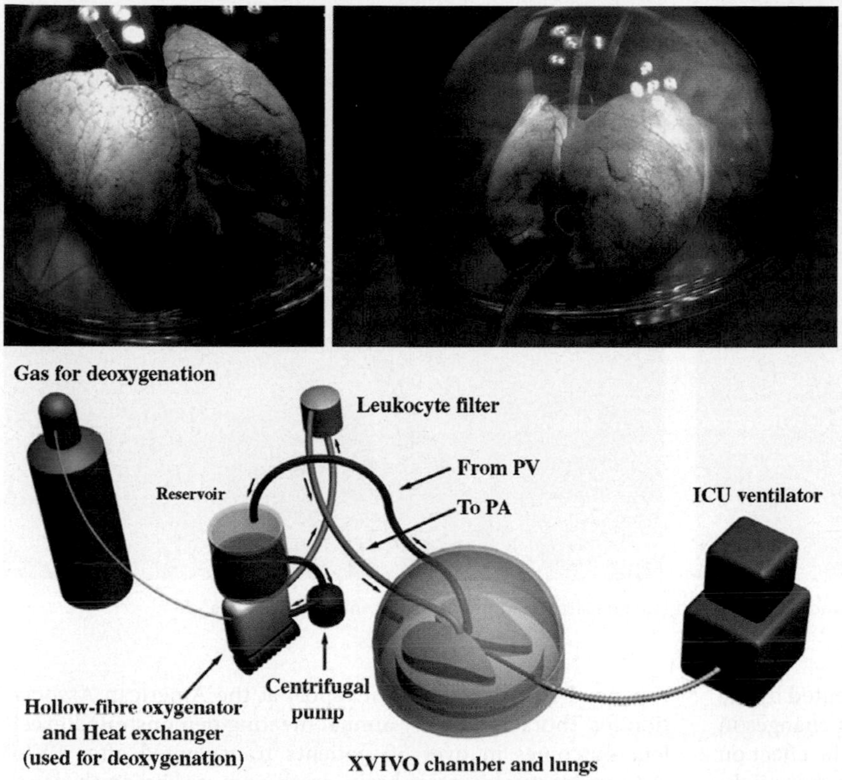

Figure 172-1. Components of ex vivo lung perfusion circuit. The perfusate is circulated by a centrifugal pump passing through a membrane gas exchanger and a leukocyte-depletion filter before entering the lung block through the pulmonary artery. A filtered gas line for the gas-exchange membrane is connected to an H-size tank with a specialty gas mixture of oxygen (6%), carbon dioxide (8%), and nitrogen (86%). A heat exchanger is connected to the membrane gas exchanger to maintain the perfusate at temperature. Pulmonary artery flow is controlled by the centrifugal pump and measured using an electromagnetic flow meter. The outflow oxygenated perfusate returns through the left atrial cannula to a hard-shell reservoir. Lungs are ventilated with a standard ICU-type ventilator. The lungs are contained in a specifically designed lung enclosure (XVIVO, Vitrolife).

when compared to CSP. Alveolar epithelial cell tight junction integrity, evaluated by zona occludens-1 protein staining, was disrupted in the cell membranes after prolonged CSP but not after EVLP.

TORONTO TECHNIQUE FOR EVLP

The components and set up of the circuit are demonstrated in Fig. 172-1. The EVLP perfusion and ventilation strategy is shown in Table 172-1. The preparation of the donor lungs occurs on the back table with the lungs immersed in a CSP solution. Specifically designed funnel-shaped cannulas with built in pressure sensors (XVIVO cannulas, Vitrolife) are attached to the LA and pulmonary artery (PA). The lungs are then transferred from the back table to the XVIVO chamber.

Table 172-1

VENTILATION AND PERFUSION STRATEGY DURING EVLP

Ventilation	
Tidal volume	7 mL/kg
PEEP	5 cm H_2O
Frequency	7 breaths per minute
I/E ratio	1/2
Recruitment	1 every hour to PawP 20 cm H_2O
Perfusion	
Pump flow	40% estimated donor CO
Pulmonary artery pressure	7–13 mm Hg
Left atrial pressure	3–5 mm Hg
Perfusate exchange	250 cc every hour
Perfusate composition	Steen solution, heparin, antibiotics, solumedrol
Perfusate pH	6.8–7.4
Perfusate pCO_2	35–45 mm Hg

The PA cannula is connected to the circuit and anterograde flow (PA–LA) is initiated at 150 mL/min with the perfusate at room temperature. The temperature of the perfusate is then gradually increased to 37°C over the next 30 minutes. Before increasing flow beyond this level, a careful check of the system is made. The PA and LA pressure readings are double-checked. When a temperature of 32 to 34°C is reached (usually over 20 minutes), ventilation is started and the perfusate flow rate is gradually increased to the target flow (40% of estimated donor cardiac output) within 60 minutes. Once ventilation is started, the flow of gas (86%N_2, 6%O_2, 8%CO_2, Praxair) that will deoxygenate and provide carbon dioxide to the inflow perfusate via the gas exchange membrane is initiated (started at 1 L/min) and titrated to maintain inflow perfusate pCO_2 between 35 and 45 mm Hg. Steroids, antibiotics, and heparin are added to the perfusate prior to EVLP initiation. Recruitment lung maneuvers are performed every hour to an airway peak pressure of 25 cmH_2O. Ex vivo bronchoscopic examination and x-rays of the lungs are performed every 2 hours. Every 2 hours, 250 cc of perfusion solution is exchanged for a fresh perfusate.

Assessment of Lungs During EVLP

Current donor lung evaluation is a clinical process greatly dependent on the judgment of the surgeon. While some evaluation does occur prior to retrieval, that is., chest x-rays and ICU bronchoscopy, the majority of the evaluation leading to the decision of utilization occurs at a single time point—the time of organ retrieval. EVLP allows the decision of lung utilization to be made at a later time point in the transplantation process (which is very useful in the case of donors after cardiac death) and allows for the use of more objective parameters. During EVLP, lung functional parameters can be monitored carefully and trends in compliance and airway pressure can be

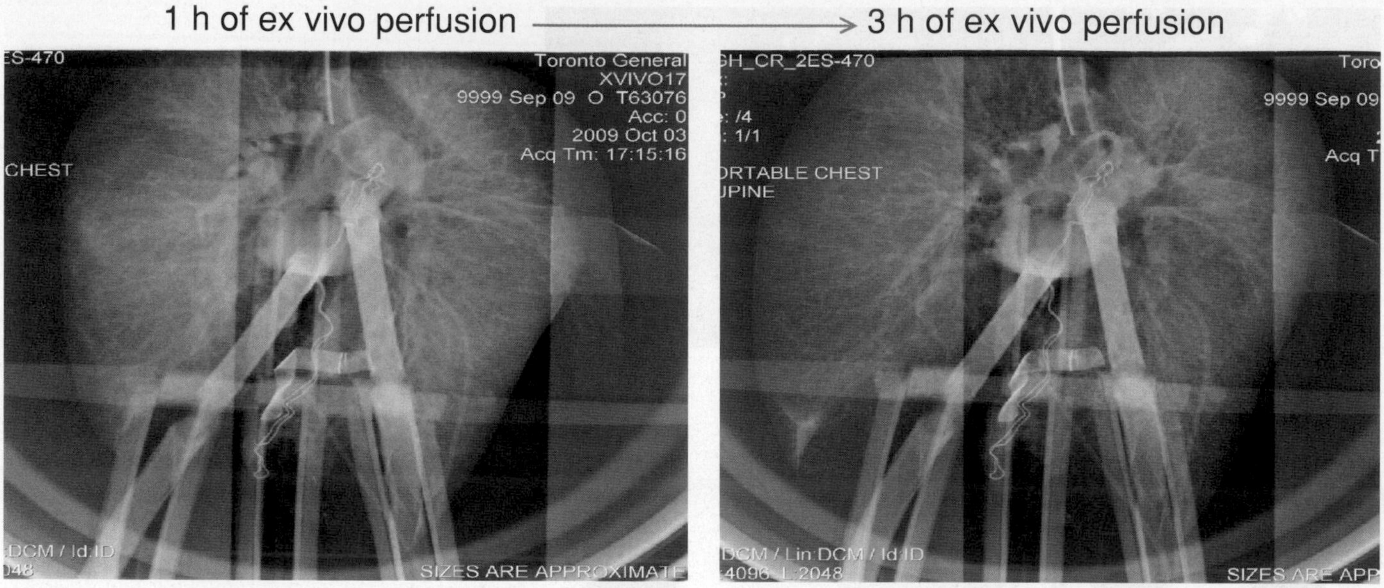

Figure 172-2. Ex vivo x-ray at 1 hour and 3 hours of EVLP demonstrating improvement in interstitial edema.

detected over at least a few hours. Injury, as represented by the development of edema during EVLP, is reflected in changes in compliance and airway pressure and this precedes the effect on perfusate pO_2.[25] To reduce the effect of atelectasis that might occur during donor lung transport, the baseline time point should be 1 hour after warming the perfusate and after careful recruitment of the lung. All subsequent physiological measurements (compliance, airway pressures, PVR, and perfusate pO_2) can be compared to this time point. A cut-off, or normal value, is often sought for lung evaluation, but compliance and resultant airway pressure is based in part on lung volume and thus can fall within a large range of values. With this strategy, the trend of values becomes more important than the absolute values themselves. In general a P/F >400 mm Hg and stability or improvements of other functional parameters and ex vivo lung x-ray are required to accept the lungs for transplantation (Fig. 172-2). Perfusate biomarkers have now been extensively studied and will certainly assist in the overall organ assessment in the near future.

Clinical Outcomes with EVLP

The first clinical use of an EVLP system was described by Steen et al.[14] in 2001 to briefly assess lung function from a donor after cardiac death. The same group reported their experience with 60 to 90 minutes of blood-based perfusion to assess six high-risk donor lungs prior to transplantation. These case reports showed acceptable outcomes; however, the mean time in the intensive care unit was longer in recipients of perfused lungs compared to conventional transplantation (13 vs. 7 days).[26,27]

The first prospective clinical trial using EVLP was recently completed at the University of Toronto and the results were recently published.[28] In this study, 20 EVLP lung transplants were performed after 4 hours of EVLP using the acellular protective ventilation/perfusion strategy.[23,24] This trial demonstrated that extended acellular normothermic EVLP is safe for the assessment of high-risk donor lungs, and similar early outcomes were obtained compared to conventionally selected and transplanted donor lungs. This experience has been rapidly expanded and a more recent report at the American Association for Thoracic Surgery annual meeting demonstrated excellent outcomes in over 50 patients transplanted after EVLP assessment/treatment of brain death and cardiac death donor lungs. In this study, incidence of PGD 3 at 72 hours was 2% in EVLP and 8.5% in controls. Thirty-day mortality (4% in EVLP; 3.5% controls, $p = 1.00$) and 1-year survival (87% in EVLP; 86% controls, $p = 1.00$) were similar in both groups. Other groups have equally reported their promising experience with the technique, mostly in a form of published abstracts. The Vienna group recently reported very good outcomes after EVLP lung transplantation using initially unsuitable lungs.[29]

Potentials of EVLP in Lung Transplantation

Normothermic preservation demonstrates great promise for resuscitating injured donor lungs. Given that the majority of potential donor lungs are injured by a variety of mechanisms including brain death, contusion, aspiration, infection, edema, and atelectasis, one can imagine that targeted therapies for each of these injuries could be delivered ex vivo for repair and greatly increase the donor lung pool. The requirements for perfusion for repair compared to perfusion solely for evaluation differs by the time requirements. While the majority of lungs can be evaluated within 2 to 4 hours of perfusion, repair will require longer noninjurious stable perfusion while potential treatments are administered.

Early studies in the use of EVLP for lung repair have been reported, many still only in abstract form. Each of these studies have been targeted at a different form of donor lung injury and it is this breadth of exploration that will ultimately result in an arsenal of ex vivo lung therapy techniques applicable to each uniquely injured donor lung. Pulmonary edema is a common injury in donor lungs due to brain death physiology and/or ICU fluid management prior to retrieval. Unlike the in vivo situation, use of terbutiline was found to accelerate the clearance of alveolar fluid during perfusion.[30] Another common mechanism of injury is aspiration. Inci et al.[31] have attempted to improve porcine lungs injured by acid aspiration.

By lavaging the donor lung with surfactant during EVLP, they were able to achieve improved graft function when compared with controls. A significant number of lungs are rejected for suspicion of infection or pneumonia, making the delivery of high doses of antibiotics during EVLP an attractive therapy. Both the Newcastle and Toronto groups have early data showing potential reduction in the burden of infection following EVLP antimicrobial therapy.[32,33]

EVLP-based gene and cellular therapy have also been explored. We have shown that ex vivo gene therapy with an adenoviral vector is effective and additionally attractive because of the reduced vector-associated inflammation. Furthermore, this strategy can easily fit into the logistical flow of clinical lung transplantation, simplifying adoption.[34] We have demonstrated that EVLP-based IL-10 gene therapy of rejected human donor lungs resulted in improved function and reduced biomarkers of inflammation suggesting that IL-10 gene therapy could possibly increase the resilience of all donor lungs to reperfusion injury.[35] Lee et al.[36] have shown that the delivery of mesenchymal stem cells to EVLP lungs can restore endothelial barrier permeability and alveolar fluid balance after endotoxin-induced lung injury.

Finally, EVLP may be a strategy to minimize cold ischemia if the lungs are inserted in the circuit immediately after organ retrieval and transported on mobile EVLP systems. A clinical trial is currently under way in the international INSPIRE trial using the Organ Care Systems machine.[37,38] Compelling experimental and clinical data demonstrate that continuous mobile normothermic perfusion is superior to a combination of short intervals of cold ischemic preservation (currently used for transportation of the lungs to the EVLP site), but additional normothermic evaluation and treatment will be needed to justify the conversion to this strategy considering the logistical challenges and the added economic expenses needed for mobile normothermic perfusion of lungs.

CONCLUSION

Ever since the development of clinical lung transplantation, transplant clinicians and scientists have sought to reduce injury and maximize safe preservation time during the storage and transport of donor lungs. Key advancements in lung preservation in the form of hypothermia, inflated storage, and Perfadex flush have culminated in the maturation of lung transplantation into a standard of care for end-stage lung disease. Currently, the emphasis of lung preservation is shifting from slowing down organ death to that of facilitating organ recovery and regeneration prior to implantation. This has led to the emergence of normothermic EVLP as a strategy for lung preservation. Though EVLP is effective for lung preservation alone, its true potential lies in facilitating lung assessment, recovery, and repair. Development of an ex vivo treatment arsenal ranging in complexity from pharmacologic to gene and cellular therapies may one day allow for a personalized medicine approach to the donor organ. The personalized or targeted repair of donor lung injuries specific to each individual lung may finally allow clinicians to realize the full potential of the donor organ pool.

EDITOR'S COMMENT

This chapter provides both historical and practical knowledge about this new technology with enormous potential to profoundly change the practice of clinical lung transplantation in the immediate future.

—Yolonda L. Colson

References

1. Punch JD, Hayes DH, LaPorte FB, et al. Organ donation and utilization in the United States, 1996–2005. *Am J Transplant.* 2007;7:1327–1338.
2. De Meester J, Smits J, Persijn G, et al. Listing for lung transplantation: life expectancy and transplant effect, stratified by type of end-stage lung disease, the Eurotransplant experience. *J Heart Lung Transplant.* 2001;20:518–524.
3. Lederer DJ, Arcasoy SM, Wilt JS, et al. Six-minute-walk distance predicts waiting list survival in idiopathic pulmonary fibrosis. *Am J Respir Crit Care Med.* 2006;174;659–664.
4. Carrel A, Lindbergh CA. The culture of whole organs. *Science.* 1935;81:621–623.
5. Jirsch DW, Fisk RL, Couves CM. Ex vivo evaluation of stored lungs. *Ann Thorac Surg.* 1970;10:163–168.
6. Brasile L, Stubenitsky BM, Booster MH, et al. Solving the organ shortage: potential strategies and the likelihood of success. *ASAIO J.* 2002;48:211–215.
7. Brasile L, Stubenitsky BM, Booster MH, et al. Overcoming severe renal ischemia: the role of ex vivo warm perfusion. *Transplantation.* 2002;73:897–901.
8. Brasile L, Buelow R, Stubenitsky BM, et al. Induction of heme oxygenase-1 in kidneys during ex vivo warm perfusion. *Transplantation.* 2003;76:1145–1149.
9. Brasile L, Stubenitsky BM, Booster MH, et al. NOS: the underlying mechanism preserving vascular integrity and during ex vivo warm kidney perfusion. *Am J Transplant.* 2003;3:674–679.
10. Brasile L, Stubenitsky BM, Haisch CE, et al. Repair of damaged organs in vitro. *Am J Transplant.* 2005;5:300–306.
11. Imber CJ, St Peter SD, Lopez de Cenarruzabeitia I, et al. Advantages of normothermic perfusion over cold storage in liver preservation. *Transplantation.* 2002;73:701–709.
12. Steen S, Liao Q, Wierup PN, et al. Transplantation of lungs from non-heart-beating donors after functional assessment ex vivo. *Ann Thorac Surg.* 2003;76:244–252.
13. Daemen JW, Kootstra G, Wijnen RM, et al. Nonheart-beating donors: the Maastricht experience. *Clin Transpl.* 1994;303–316.
14. Steen S, Sjöberg T, Pierre L, et al. Transplantation of lungs from a non-heart-beating donor. *Lancet.* 2001;357:825–829.
15. Aitchinson JD, Orr HE, Flecknell PA, et al. Functional assessment of non-heart-beating donor lungs: prediction of post-transplant function. *Eur J Cardiothorac Surg.* 2001;20:187–194.
16. Rega FR. Vanaudenaerde BM, Wuyts WA, et al.. IL-1beta in bronchial lavage fluid is a non-invasive marker that predicts the viability of the pulmonary graft from the non-heart-beating donor. *J Heart Lung Transplant.* 2003;24:20.
17. Rega FR, Jannis NC, Verleden GM, et al. Long-term preservation with interim evaluation of lungs from a non-heart-beating donor after a warm ischemic interval of 90 minutes. *Ann Surg.* 2003;238:782–792.
18. Neyrinck AP, Van De Wauwer C, Geudens N, et al. Comparative study of donor lung injury in heart-beating versus non-heart-beating donors. *Eur J Cardiothorac Surg.* 2006;30:628–636.
19. Egan TM, Haithcock JA, Nicotra WA, et al. Ex vivo evaluation of human lungs for transplant suitability. *Ann Thorac Surg.* 2006;81:1205–1213.
20. Snell GI, Oto T, Levvey B, et al. Evaluation of techniques for lung transplantation following donation after cardiac death. *Ann Thorac Surg.* 2006;81:2014–2019.

21. Wierup P, Haraldsson A, Nilsson F, et al. Ex vivo evaluation of nonacceptable donor lungs. *Ann Thorac Surg.* 2006;81:460–466.
22. Erasmus ME, Fernhout MH, Elstrodt JM, et al. Normothermic ex vivo lung perfusion of non-heart-beating donor lungs in pigs: from pretransplant function analysis towards a 6-h machine preservation. *Transplant Int.* 2006;19:589–593.
23. Cypel M, Yeung JC, Hirayama S, et al. Technique for prolonged normothermic ex vivo lung perfusion. *J Heart Lung Transplant.* 2008;27:1319–1325.
24. Cypel M, Rubacha M, Yeung J, et al. Normothermic ex vivo perfusion prevents lung injury compared to extended cold preservation for transplantation. *Am J Transplant.* 2009;9:2262–2269.
25. Koike T, Yeung JC, Cypel M, et al. Kinetics of lactate metabolism during acellular normothermic ex vivo lung perfusion. *J Heart Lung Transplant.* 2011;30:1312–1319.
26. Ingemansson R, Eyjolfsson A, Mared L, et al. Clinical transplantation of initially rejected donor lungs after reconditioning ex vivo. *Ann Thorac Surg.* 2009;87:255–260.
27. Haraldsen P, Lindstedt S, Metzsch C, et al. A porcine model for acute ischaemic right ventricular dysfunction. *Interact Cardiovasc Thorac Surg.* 2014; 18: 43–48.
28. Cypel M, Yeung JC, Liu M, et al. Normothermic ex vivo lung perfusion in clinical lung transplantation. *N Engl J Med.* 2011;364:1431–1440.
29. Aigner C, Slama A, Hötzenecker K, et al. Clinical ex vivo lung perfusion–pushing the limits. *Am J Transplant.* 2012;12:1839–1847.
30. Frank JA, Briot R, Lee JW, et al. Physiological and biochemical markers of alveolar epithelial barrier dysfunction in perfused human lungs. *Am J Physiol Lung Cell Mol Physiol.* 2007;293:L52–L59.
31. Inci I, Ampollini L, Arni S, et al. Ex vivo reconditioning of marginal donor lungs injured by acid aspiration. *J Heart Lung Transplant.* 2008;27:1229–1236.
32. Andreasson A, Karamanou DM, Perry JD, et al. The effect of ex vivo lung perfusion on microbial load in human donor lungs. *J Heart Lung Transplant.* 2014;29:S94.
33. Yeung JC, Cypel M, Machuca TN, et al. Physiologic assessment of the ex vivo donor lung for transplantation. *J Heart Lung Transplant.* 2012;31:1120–1126.
34. Yeung JC, Wagnetz D, Cypel M, et al. Ex vivo adenoviral vector gene delivery results in decreased vector-associated inflammation pre- and post-lung transplantation in the pig. *Mol Ther.* 2012;20:1204–1211.
35. Cypel M, Liu M, Rubacha M, et al. Functional repair of human donor lungs by IL-10 gene therapy. *Sci Transl Med.* 2009;1:4–9.
36. Lee JW, Fang X, Gupta N, et al. Allogeneic human mesenchymal stem cells for treatment of E. coli endotoxin-induced acute lung injury in the ex vivo perfused human lung. *Proc Natl Acad Sci U S A.* 2009;106:16357–16362.
37. Warnecke G, Moradiellos J, Tudorache I, et al. *J Heart Lung Transplant.* 2012;31:S115.
38. Souilamas R, Souilamas JI Jr, Saueressig M, et al. Advanced normothermic ex vivo lung maintenance using the mobile Organ Care System. *J Heart Lung Transplant.* 2011;30:847–848.

173

Keywords: Endoscopic submucosal resection, esophageal cancer, mucosal cancer, ligation technique, transparent cap technique

Endoscopic resection (ER) of early neoplastic lesions in the gastrointestinal tract has become increasingly important in recent years, both as a diagnostic tool and as a method of performing definitive treatment when the cancer meets certain criteria in which the risk of lymph node metastasis is negligible.[1]

INDICATIONS FOR ENDOSCOPIC RESECTION OF EARLY ESOPHAGEAL CARCINOMA

Adenocarcinoma in Barrett Esophagus

The indications for ER in esophageal adenocarcinoma are high-grade intraepithelial neoplasia (HGIN) and mucosal cancer. Risk stratification should be carried out in accordance with known risk factors such as grade of differentiation, lymphatic or venous infiltration, and the infiltration depth of the carcinoma. The limitations of ER in early Barrett cancers should be submucosal infiltration or infiltration of the lamina muscularis mucosa in combination with another risk factor, such as poor tumor differentiation or lymphatic and venous infiltration. The largest series ever published on endoscopic treatment of early Barrett neoplasia showed a long-term complete response in 94.5% of patients. Long-term survival of patients treated for Barrett neoplasia in this series did not significantly differ from that of the normal German population with the same age and gender distribution.[2]

Squamous Cell Carcinoma of the Esophagus

In esophageal squamous cell neoplasia (SCN), ER should only be carried out if the carcinoma is limited to the mucosal layer as has been shown in several publications.[3,4]

PREPROCEDURE ASSESSMENT

Accurate staging is mandatory before endoscopic treatment of early esophageal cancer. The most important part of the staging procedure entails careful evaluation of the neoplasia and the borders of the lesion using a high-resolution endoscope, and a thorough search for multifocal neoplasia. In addition, the macroscopic type of the lesion should be determined, as it has been shown to have significant correlation with infiltration depth.[5,6] Conventional endoscopic ultrasound (EUS) and EUS with miniprobes (20 or 30 MHz) can be carried out to evaluate the depth of infiltration and the lymph node status of the tumor. However, the accuracy of T staging is limited, particularly for distinguishing between the important stages of T1 m and T1 sm. The diagnostic accuracy of submucosal cancer ranges from 33% to 85%.[7–11] Underdiagnosis by EUS has been shown in 12.5% to 67% of cases.[7,8] In contrast, EUS is highly accurate in differentiating T1 and T2 tumors.[9]

ENDOSCOPIC RESECTION TECHNIQUES

"ER" is the general term for the different resection techniques used to treat neoplastic and uncertain lesions in the gastrointestinal tract. The term "endoscopic mucosal resection" is widely used; however, it is misleading because significant proportions of the submucosal layer are also resected, which is important in the case of submucosal infiltration of the tumor.

Endoscopic Resection with a Ligation Device

A common method is ER with a ligation device, also used for ligation of esophageal varices. With this method, the target lesion (Fig. 173-1A) is sucked into the cylinder of the ligation device (Fig. 173-1B) and a rubber band is then released to create a pseudopolyp that has the rubber band at its base (Fig. 173-1C). After this, the pseudopolyp is resected with a reusable snare underneath the rubber band to achieve larger resection specimens (Fig. 173-1D).

Several ligation devices are available: single-use devices, multiple usable ligators or ligation devices with multiple rubber bands. Another useful development is a ligation cylinder that has six rubber bands and a facility for advancing a snare through the working channel of a regular endoscope. This enables the endoscopist to perform up to six resections without the necessity of withdrawing and reintroducing the endoscope. This device is widely used for piecemeal resection of larger neoplastic lesions.

Endoscopic Resection with a Transparent Cap

The cap technique was introduced by Inoue and Endo[12] almost 20 years ago. When ER is performed with the cap technique, a specially developed transparent plastic cap is attached to the end of the endoscope. After submucosal injection under the target lesion, usually with a saline-epinephrine solution, the lesion is sucked into the cap and resected with a diathermy snare that has previously been loaded onto a specially designed groove on the lower edge of the cap. Marking the borders of the lesion either with electrocautery using the tip of the snare or an APC probe is recommended before performing the resection, because injecting underneath a discrete neoplastic lesion often makes it difficult to identify the borders of the target lesion afterward.

Ulcerated lesions often have fibrosis, which attaches the submucosa to the lamina muscularis propria, resulting in failure of the lesion to lift as is frequently found in tumors with

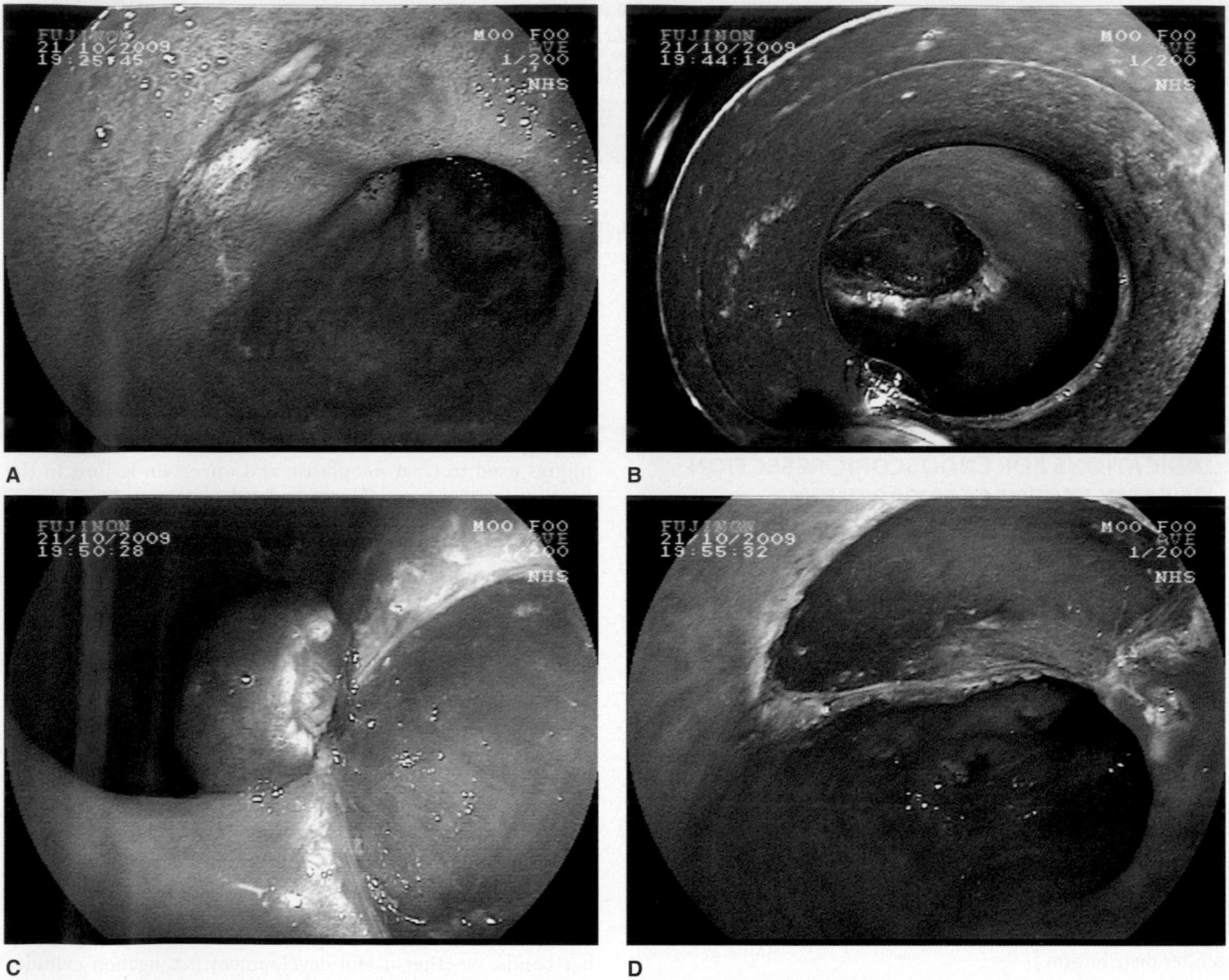

Figure 173-1. Endoscopic resection with a ligation device.

submucosal infiltration. In these cases, ER is not advisable, or should only be performed with caution. Larger lesions can usually be resected completely with the piecemeal technique, but this method seems to be associated with a higher recurrence rate.

Endoscopic Submucosal Dissection

The endoscopic submucosal dissection (ESD) procedure in the treatment of early gastric cancer was first described by Hosokawa and Yoshida[13] and Ono et al.[14] They used an insulated-tip knife to obtain a large resection specimen with the neoplasm resected en bloc (Fig. 173-2E). Once the borders of the neoplastic lesion have been adequately visualized, the borders are marked with electrocautery at a distance of 5 to 10 mm from the margin of the carcinoma (Fig. 173-2A). Then submucosal injection of fluid is performed to elevate the lesion from the muscular layer, and the mucosa surrounding the lesion is circumferentially cut outside the markings. Finally, the submucosal connective tissue is dissected with a dedicated knife (Fig. 173-2B). Visible vessels can be coagulated with the top of the knife or a coagulation forceps to prevent bleeding (Fig. 173-2C and D). The fluid used for submucosal injection could be isotonic saline solution or a solution of hyaluronic acid with additives including a dye, such as indigocarmine; a composition defined by the individual endoscopist. A wide variety of different knives are used for ESD, including the insulated-tip knife, Hook knife, flex knife, needle knife, triangle-tip knife, flush knife, and hybrid knife. With the flush and hybrid knife, submucosal injection and dissection can be performed at the same time without changing the instruments. The size of the resected specimen obtained with ESD can extend up to more than 10 cm in diameter. Because of the high complication rate in inexperienced endoscopists, practice with ESD models is highly recommended to become familiar with this technique. Afterward, ESD procedures should be carried out in the stomach, then in the rectum, before this method is used for esophageal lesions. ESD is a demanding, time-consuming technique with a flat learning curve.

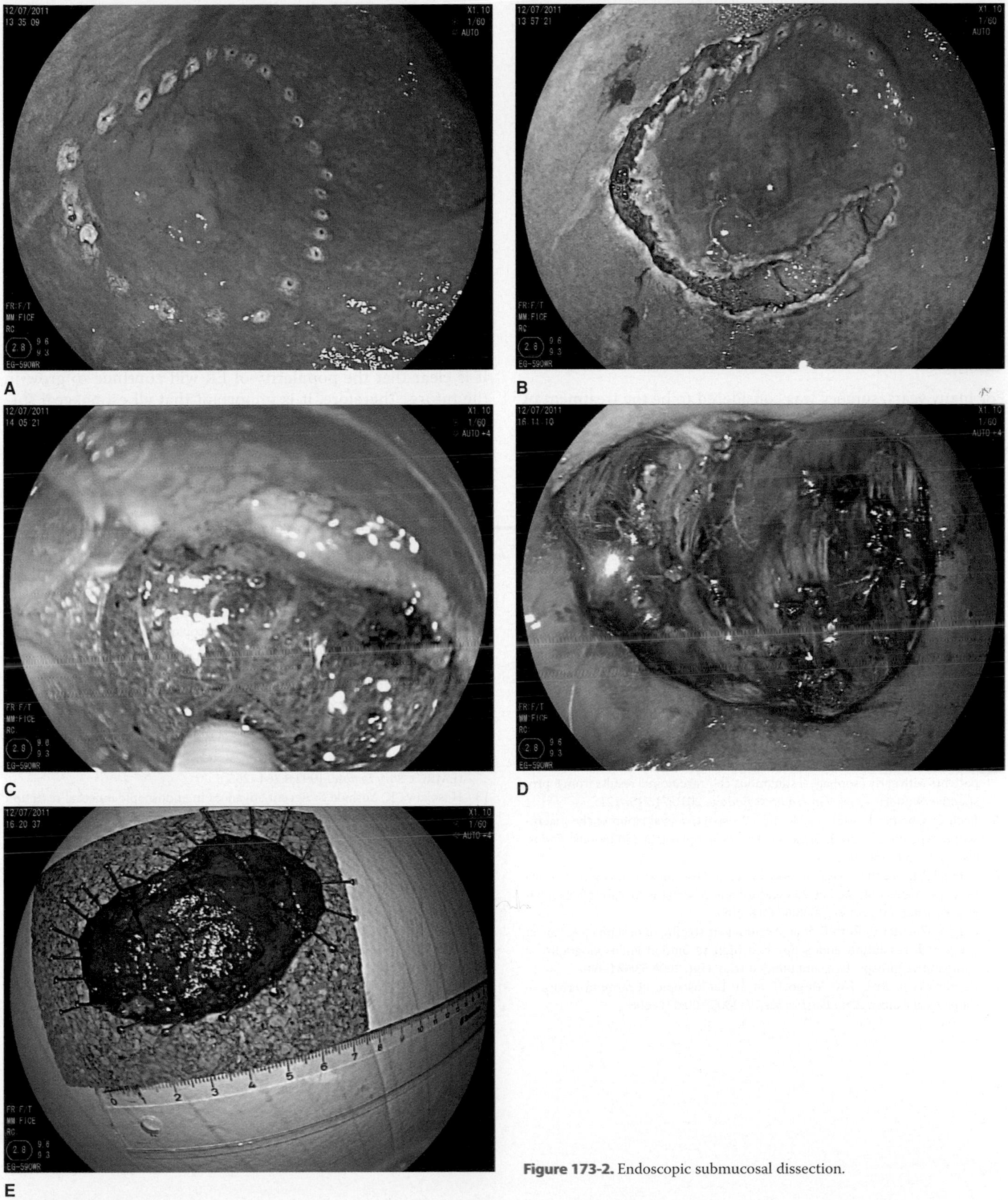

Figure 173-2. Endoscopic submucosal dissection.

PROCEDURE-SPECIFIC COMPLICATIONS

A prospective randomized trial with 100 consecutive ERs in 70 patients comparing ER performed with a ligation device versus ER with a cap was able to demonstrate that there is no difference in the complication rate.[15] One minor bleeding incident occurred in each group, but no severe complications were seen.

Another randomized study from the Amsterdam group, performing esophageal piecemeal resection in 84 patients, showed a comparable complication rate between ER with a multiband ligator and cap resection, with four perforations.[16] A recently published European multicenter study has shown that ESD is associated with a substantial complication rate, including perforations that require surgery and bleeding.

SUMMARY

For many years, surgery was considered to be the treatment of choice for early neoplastic lesions of the esophagus. Surgery, however, is associated with a 30-day mortality of 1% to 5% and significant morbidity in 30% to 50% of cases, even in high-volume centers.

Because of these data, local treatment methods have been introduced and investigated in several studies. ER with a ligation device or using the cap technique has been proved to be safe. However, ESD should be strictly limited to experienced endoscopists who are familiar with this method. In contrast to ablative treatment methods, such as photodynamic therapy, argon plasma coagulation, cryotherapy, and radiofrequency ablation, ER, regardless of the resection technique used, allows histologic assessment of the resected specimen to assess the depth of infiltration of the tumor and determine whether lymphatic infiltration (L-status) or blood vessel involvement (V-status) is present. These significant advantages of ER are the main reason why ER, regardless of type, should be preferred over all ablative treatment methods.

EDITOR'S COMMENT

It is clear that the popularity of ER will continue to grow in the future. Therefore, it is important that all esophageal surgeons read this practical discussion of the several approaches to ER, so as to understand both the risks and benefits of this technology.

—Yolonda L. Colson

References

1. Pech O, May A, Rabestein T, et al. Endoscopic resection of early oesophageal cancer. *Gut*. 2007;56:1625–1634.
2. Pech O, Behrens A, May A, et al. Long-term results and risk factor analysis for recurrence after curative endoscopic therapy in 349 patients with high-grade intraepithelial neoplasia and mucosal adenocarcinoma in Barrett's oesophagus. *Gut*. 2008;57:1200–1206.
3. Pech O, Gossner L, May A, et al. Endoscopic resection of superficial esophageal squamous-cell carcinomas: western experience. *Am J Gastroenterol*. 2004;99:1226–1232.
4. Repici A, Hassan C, Carlino A, et al. Endoscopic submucosal dissection in patients with early esophageal squamous cell carcinoma: results from a prospective Western series. *Gastrointest Endosc*. 2010;71:715–721.
5. Pech O, Gossner L, Manner H, et al. Prospective evaluation of the macroscopic types and location of early Barrett's neoplasia in 380 lesions. *Endoscopy*. 2007;39:588–593.
6. Peters FP, Brakenhoff KP, Curvers WL, et al. Histologic evaluation of resection specimens obtained at 293 endoscopic resections in Barrett's esophagus. *Gastrointest Endosc*. 2008;67:604–609.
7. May A, Guenter E, Roth F, et al. Accuracy of staging in oesophageal cancer using high resolution endoscopy and high resolution endosonography: a comparative, prospective, and blinded trial. *Gut*. 2004;53:634–640.
8. Zuccaro G Jr, Rice TW, Vargo JJ, et al. Endoscopic ultrasound errors in esophageal cancer. *Am J Gastroenterol*. 2005;100:601–606.
9. Pech O, May A, Günter E, et al. The impact of endoscopic ultrasound and computed tomography on the TNM staging of early cancer in Barrett's esophagus. *Am J Gastroenterol*. 2006;101:2223–2229.
10. Rampado S, Bocus P, Battaglia G, et al. Endoscopic ultrasound: accuracy in staging superficial carcinomas of the esophagus. *Ann Thorac Surg*. 2008;85:251–256.
11. Chemaly M, Scalone O, Durivage G, et al. Miniprobe EUS in the pretherapeutic assessment of early esophageal neoplasia. *Endoscopy*. 2008;40:2–6.
12. Inoue H, Endo M, Takeshita K, et al. A new simplified technique of endoscopic esophageal mucosal resection using a cap-fitted panendoscope (EMRC). *Surg Endosc*. 1992;6:264–265.
13. Hosokawa K, Yoshida S. Recent advances in endoscopic mucosal resection for early gastric cancer. *Gan To Kagaku Ryoho*. 1998;25(4):476–478.
14. Ono H, Kondo H, Gotoda T, et al. Endoscopic mucosal resection for treatment of early gastric cancer. *Gut*. 2001;48:225–229.
15. May A, Gossner L, Behrens A, et al. A prospective randomized trial of two different endoscopic resection techniques for early stage cancer of the esophagus. *Gastrointest Endosc*. 2003;58:167–175.
16. Pouw RE, van Vilsteren FG, Peters FP, et al. Randomized trial on endoscopic resection-cap versus multiband mucosectomy for piecemeal endoscopic resection of early Barrett's neoplasia. *Gastrointest Endosc*. 2011;74:35–43.Keywords: Surgical technique, myasthenia gravis, thymus, thymoma

Index

C

F

G

H

I

Q

R

S

T

U

V